CURRENT SURGICAL THERAPY

CURRENT SURGICAL THERAPY

10th edition

JOHN L. CAMERON, MD
FACS, FRCS(Eng)(hon), FRCS(Ed)(hon), FRCSI(hon)
The Alfred Blalock Distinguished Service Professor
Department of Surgery
The Johns Hopkins Medical Institutions
Baltimore, Maryland

ANDREW M. CAMERON, MD, PhD
FACS
Assistant Professor of Surgery
Department of Surgery
The Johns Hopkins Medical Institutions
Baltimore, Maryland

ELSEVIER
SAUNDERS

1600 John F. Kennedy Blvd.
Ste 1800
Philadelphia, PA 19103-2899

CURRENT SURGICAL THERAPY   ISBN: 978-1-4377-0823-3
Copyright © 2011, 2008, 2004, 2001, 1998, 1995, 1992, 1989, 1986, 1984 by Mosby, Inc., an affiliate of Elsevier Inc.

Notice

Knowledge and best practice in this field are constantly changing. As new research and experience broaden our understanding, changes in research methods, professional practices, or medical treatment may become necessary.

Practitioners and researchers must always rely on their own experience and knowledge in evaluating and using any information, methods, compounds, or experiments described herein. In using such information or methods they should be mindful of their own safety and the safety of others, including parties for whom they have a professional responsibility.

With respect to any drug or pharmaceutical products identified, readers are advised to check the most current information provided (i) on procedures featured or (ii) by the manufacturer of each product to be administered, to verify the recommended dose or formula, the method and duration of administration, and contraindications. It is the responsibility of practitioners, relying on their own experience and knowledge of their patients, to make diagnoses, to determine dosages and the best treatment for each individual patient, and to take all appropriate safety precautions.

To the fullest extent of the law, neither the Publisher nor the authors, contributors, or editors, assume any liability for any injury and/or damage to persons or property as a matter of products liability, negligence or otherwise, or from any use or operation of any methods, products, instructions, or ideas contained in the material herein.

Library of Congress International Standard Serial Number   ISSN 0835-3689

Acquisitions Editor: Judith Fletcher
Developmental Editor: Roxanne Halpine Ward
Publishing Services Manager: Patricia Tannian
Project Manager: Carrie Stetz
Project Manager: Jayavel Radhakrishnan
Design Direction: Louis Forgione

Printed in the United States of America
Last digit is the print number: 9 8 7 6 5 4 3 2 1

CONTRIBUTORS

Herand Abcarian, MD
Chairman
Division of Colon and Rectal Surgery
John H. Stroger Hospital of Cook County;
Professor of Surgery
University of Illinois at Chicago
Chicago, Illinois

MANAGEMENT OF RECTOVAGINAL FISTULA

Fizan Abdullah, MD, PhD
Associate Professor
Division of Pediatric Surgery
Assistant Program Director
Residency in General Surgery
Johns Hopkins University School of
Medicine
Baltimore, Maryland

*EXTRACORPOREAL LIFE SUPPORT FOR
RESPIRATORY FAILURE*

Michael A. Abramson, MD
Resident in Radiology
Georgetown University Hospital
Washington, DC

PRIMARY SCLEROSING CHOLANGITIS

Christopher J. Abularrage, MD
Division of Vascular Surgery and
Endovascular Therapy
The Johns Hopkins Hospital;
Assistant Professor of Surgery
Johns Hopkins University School of Medicine
Baltimore, Maryland

AORTOILIAC OCCLUSIVE DISEASE

Reid B. Adams, MD
Claude A. Jessup Professor of Surgery
Chief, Division of Surgical Oncology
Chief, Hepatobiliary and Pancreatic
Surgery
Director, Gastrointestinal Oncology
Program
University of Virginia Health System
Charlottesville, Virginia

BILE DUCT CANCER

John H. Adamski II, MD, MPH
Assistant Professor of Surgery
R. Adams Cowley Shock Trauma Center
University of Maryland School of Medicine
Baltimore, Maryland

ENDOCRINE CHANGES IN CRITICAL ILLNESS

Steven A. Ahrendt, MD
Associate Professor
Department of Surgery
University of Pittsburgh
Pittsburgh, Pennsylvania

CYSTIC DISORDERS OF THE BILE DUCTS

Nita Ahuja, MD
Assistant Professor
Department of Surgery
Johns Hopkins Hospital
Baltimore, Maryland

*USE OF [¹⁸F]-2-FLUORO-2-DEOXY-
D-GLUCOSE POSITRON EMISSION
TOMOGRAPHY IN THE MANAGEMENT OF
COLORECTAL CANCER*

Hasan B. Alam, MD
Associate Professor of Surgery
Harvard Medical School;
Director of Research
Division of Trauma, Emergency Surgery,
and Surgical Critical Care
Director of Surgical Critical Care/Acute
Care Surgery Fellowship Program
Massachusetts General Hospital
Boston, Massachusetts

DAMAGE CONTROL OPERATION

John C. Alverdy, MD, FACS
Sarah and Harold Lincoln Thompson
Professor
Executive Vice Chair
Department of Surgery
Director Minimally Invasive Surgery
University of Chicago Pritzker School of
Medicine
Chicago, Illinois

ACUTE PANCREATITIS

**David N. Armstrong, MD, FRCS, FACS,
FASCRS**
Georgia Colon and Rectal Surgical Clinic
Atlanta, Georgia

ANORECTAL ABSCESS AND FISTULA

George J. Arnaoutakis, MD
Surgical Resident
Johns Hopkins Hospital
Baltimore, Maryland

SMALL BOWEL OBSTRUCTION

Alejandro Arnold, MD
General Surgery
Shawnee Mission Medical Center
Shawnee Mission, Kansas

*LAPAROSCOPIC MANAGEMENT OF
COMMON BILE DUCT STONES*

Zachary M. Arthurs, MD
Department of Vascular Surgery
Cleveland Clinic Foundation
Cleveland, Ohio

*MANAGEMENT OF PERIPHERAL ARTERIAL
EMBOLI*

Horacio J. Asbun, MD, FACS
Professor of Surgery
Director of Hepatobiliary and Pancreas
Surgery
Mayo Clinic Florida
Jacksonville, Florida

*LAPAROSCOPIC REPAIR OF
PARAESOPHAGEAL HERNIAS*

Nancy L. Ascher, MD, PhD
Professor and Chair
Department of Surgery
University of California at San Francisco
San Francisco, California

*THE ROLE OF LIVER TRANSPLANTATION IN
PORTAL HYPERTENSION*

Theodor Asgeirsson, MD
Assistant Director of Outcomes Research
Spectrum Health
Department of Colorectal Surgery
Michigan State University College of
Human Medicine
Grand Rapids, Michigan

COLON CANCER

Stanley W. Ashley, MD
Frank Sawyer Professor and Vice
Chairman
Program Director, General Surgery
Residency
Department of Surgery
Brigham and Women's Hospital
Harvard Medical School
Boston, Massachusetts

*MANAGEMENT OF PANCREATIC
PSEUDOCYST*

Gildy V. Babiera, MD
Associate Professor
Department of Surgical Oncology
University of Texas MD Anderson Cancer
Center
Houston, Texas

*MANAGEMENT OF RECURRENT AND
METASTATIC BREAST CANCER*

James H. Balcom IV, MD
Vascular and Endovascular Surgery
North Shore Medical Center
Salem, Massachusetts;
MGH/North Shore Center for Outpatient
Care
Danvers, Massachusetts

ACUTE MESENTERIC ISCHEMIA

Zsolt J. Balogh, MD, PhD, FRACS, FACS
Professor and Director of Traumatology
Department of Traumatology
John Hunter Hospital
University of Newcastle
Newcastle, Australia

*ABDOMINAL COMPARTMENT SYNDROME
AND MANAGEMENT OF THE OPEN
ABDOMEN*

Farzaneh Banki, MD
Assistant Professor
Department of Cardiothoracic and Vascular
Surgery
University of Texas
Houston, Texas

PARAESOPHAGEAL HIATAL HERNIA

Adrian Barbul, MD, FACS
Surgeon-in-Chief
Sinai Hospital;
Professor of Surgery
Johns Hopkins Medical Institutions
Baltimore, Maryland

INTRAABDOMINAL INFECTIONS

**Philip S. Barie, MD, MBA, FIDSA,
FACS, FCCM**
Professor of Surgery and Public Health
Weill Cornell Medical College
New York, New York

ACUTE KIDNEY INJURY

Todd W. Bauer, MD
Assistant Professor of Surgery
Department of Surgery
University of Virginia
Charlottesville, Virginia

BILE DUCT CANCER

David E. Beck, MD
Chairman
Department of Colon and Rectal Surgery
Ochsner Clinic Foundation
New Orleans, Louisiana

*USE OF STENTS FOR COLONIC
OBSTRUCTION*

Mazen I. Bedri, MD
Johns Hopkins University School of
Medicine
Baltimore, Maryland

LYMPHEDEMA

Manijeh Berenji, MD
Fellow, Surgical Research Laboratory
New York Medical College
Valhalla, New York

CUTANEOUS MELANOMA

David L. Berger, MD
Director of the Colo-Rectal Surgery
Program
Massachusetts General Hospital;
Associate Professor of Surgery
Harvard Medical School
Boston, Massachusetts

GALLSTONE ILEUS

Thomas A. Bergman, MD
Assistant Chief of Neurosurgery
Hennepin County Medical Center;
Associate Professor of Neurosurgery
University of Minnesota
Minneapolis, Minnesota

SPINE AND SPINAL CORD INJURIES

Stepheny D. Berry, MD
Co-director, Medical/Surgical ICU
Department of Surgery
Carilion Clinic
Roanoke, Virginia

INJURY TO THE SPLEEN

Richard P. Billingham, MD
Clinical Professor
Department of Surgery
University of Washington;
Swedish Colon and Rectal Clinic
Seattle, Washington

*PREOPERATIVE BOWEL PREPARATION: IS IT
NECESSARY? _*

Elisa H. Birnbaum, MD
Professor of Surgery
Washington University School of Medicine
St. Louis, Missouri

*RADIATION INJURY TO THE LARGE AND
SMALL BOWEL*

James H. Black III, MD, FACS
The Bertram M. Bernheim, MD, Associate
Professor of Surgery
Division of Vascular and Endovascular
Surgery
Johns Hopkins Hospital
Baltimore, Maryland

BUERGER DISEASE

Kirby I. Bland, MD
Fay Fletcher Kerner Professor and
Chairman
Department of Surgery
Senior Advisor to the Executive Director
Comprehensive Cancer Center
University of Alabama at Birmingham
Birmingham, Alabama

*DUCTAL AND LOBULAR CARCINOMA IN SITU
OF THE BREAST*

Grant V. Bochicchio, MD, MPH, FACS
Professor of Surgery
University of Maryland School of Medicine;
Director of Clinical and Outcomes Research
R Adams Cowley Shock Trauma Center;
Deputy Chief of Surgery and
Chief of Surgical Critical Care
BVAMC
Baltimore, Maryland

ENDOCRINE CHANGES IN CRITICAL ILLNESS

Philippe Bouchard, MD, FRCSC
Colon & Rectal Surgery Specialist
Division of Colorectal Surgery
Mayo Clinic Arizona
Scottsdale, Arizona

PILONIDAL DISEASE

Judy C. Boughey, MD
Assistant Professor of Surgery
Department of Surgery
Mayo Clinic
Rochester, Minnesota

SCREENING FOR BREAST CANCER

Steven P. Bowers, MD, FACS
Assistant Professor of Surgery
Mayo Clinic Florida
Jacksonville, Florida

*LAPAROSCOPIC REPAIR OF
PARAESOPHAGEAL HERNIAS*

Colin M. Brady, MD
Division of Vascular Surgery
Emory University
Atlanta, Georgia

*MANAGEMENT OF INFECTED VASCULAR
GRAFTS*

Steven B. Brandes, MD, FACS
Professor of Surgery
Division of Urologic Surgery
Washington University School of Medicine
St. Louis, Missouri

*RETROPERITONEAL INJURIES: KIDNEY AND
URETER*

Peter Brant-Zawadzki, MD
Vascular Surgery Fellow
Department of Surgery
Division of Vascular Surgery
University of Wisconsin
Madison, Wisconsin

FEMOROPOPLITEAL OCCLUSIVE DISEASE

Kenneth L. Brayman, MD, PhD, FACS
Professor of Surgery and Medicine
Nabi Professor of Transplantation
Division Chief, Transplant Surgery
Director, Renal, Pancreas & Islet Transplant
Programs
Director, Center for Cellular
Transplantation and Therapeutics
Director, Transplantation Services,
University of Virginia Health System
University of Virginia
Charlottesville, Virginia
TRANSPLANTATION OF THE PANCREAS

Stacy A. Brethauer, MD
Assistant Professor of Surgery
Cleveland Clinic Lerner College of Medicine
Cleveland Clinic
Cleveland, Ohio
*LAPAROSCOPIC SURGERY FOR SEVERE
OBESITY*

Malcolm V. Brock, MD
Associate Professor of Surgery
Associate Professor of Oncology
Johns Hopkins Hospital
Baltimore, Maryland
VIDEO-ASSISTED THORACIC SURGERY

Benjamin S. Brooke, MD, PhD
Chief Resident
Department of Surgery
Johns Hopkins University
Baltimore, Maryland
*MANAGEMENT OF RECURRENT CAROTID
ARTERY STENOSIS*

James T. Broome, MD
Assistant Professor of Surgery
Division of Surgical Oncology and
Endocrine Surgery
Vanderbilt University Medical Center
Nashville, Tennessee
*SMALL BOWEL CARCINOID/
NEUROENDOCRINE TUMORS*

Carl J. Brown, MD, MSc, FRCSC
Head
Division of General Surgery
St. Paul's Hospital;
Clinical Assistant Professor of Surgery
University of British Columbia
Vancouver, Canada
COLORECTAL POLYPS

F. Charles Brunicardi, MD
Professor and Chairman
Michael E. DeBakey Department of Surgery
Baylor College of Medicine
Houston, Texas
MALLORY-WEISS SYNDROME

Thomas M. Brushart, MD
Brushart Professor of Hand Surgery
Johns Hopkins Orthopaedics
Baltimore, Maryland
HAND INFECTIONS

Timothy G. Buchman, PhD, MD
Professor of Surgery and of Anesthesiology
Director
Center for Critical Care
Emory University School of Medicine
Atlanta, Georgia
*MULTIPLE ORGAN DYSFUNCTION AND
FAILURE*

Eileen M. Bulger, MD
Professor of Surgery
University of Washington
Harborview Medical Center
Seattle, Washington
*NECROTIZING SKIN AND SOFT TISSUE
INFECTION*

J. Bracken Burns, DO
Assistant Professor
Department of Surgery
University of Florida College of Medicine;
Medical Director
Trauma One Flight Services
Shands Jacksonville Medical Center
Jacksonville, Florida
*MANAGEMENT OF EXTREMITY
COMPARTMENT SYNDROME*

Ronald W. Busuttil, MD, PhD
Distinguished Professor and Executive
Chairman
David Geffen School of Medicine at UCLA
Department of Surgery;
Chief
Division of Liver and Pancreas
Transplantation
Director
The Pfleger Liver Institute
Los Angeles, California
CAVERNOUS LIVER HEMANGIOMA

John Byrne, MCh, FRCSI (Gen)
Attending Vascular Surgeon
Albany Medical College
The Institute for Vascular Health and
Disease
Albany, New York
ATHEROSCLEROTIC RENOVASCULAR DISEASE

Glenda G. Callender, MD
Assistant Professor of Surgery
Division of Surgical Oncology
Department of Surgery
University of Louisville
Louisville, Kentucky
MANAGEMENT OF ESOPHAGEAL TUMORS

Mark P. Callery, MD
Division of General Surgery
Beth Israel Deaconess Medical Center
Harvard Medical School
Boston, Massachusetts
UNUSUAL PANCREATIC TUMORS

Richard P. Cambria, MD
Division of Vascular and Endovascular
Surgery
Massachusetts General Hospital
Harvard Medical School
Boston, Massachusetts
*OPEN REPAIR OF ABDOMINAL AORTIC
ANEURYSMS*

Andrew M. Cameron, MD, PhD, FACS
Assistant Professor of Surgery
Department of Surgery
Johns Hopkins Medical Institutions
Baltimore, Maryland
CLOSTRIDIUM DIFFICILE COLITIS
*EXPOSURE TO BLOOD-BORNE PATHOGENS
IN THE OPERATING ROOM*

**John L. Cameron, MD, FACS,
FRCS(Eng)(hon); FRCS(Ed)(hon);
FRCSI(hon)**
The Alfred Blalock Distinguished Service
Professor
Department of Surgery
Johns Hopkins Medical Institutions
Baltimore, Maryland
CLOSTRIDIUM DIFFICILE COLITIS

Jeffrey Campsen, MD
Transplant Surgeon
Baylor Regional Transplant Institute
Dallas, Texas
*MANAGEMENT OF BUDD-CHIARI
SYNDROME*

Joseph A. Caprini, MD, FACS, RVT
Louis W. Biegler Chair of Surgery
Division of Vascular Surgery
NorthShore University HealthSystem
Evanston, Illinois;
Clinical Professor of Surgery
University of Chicago Pritzker School of
Medicine
Chicago, Illinois
*THROMBOSIS PROPHYLAXIS IN GENERAL
SURGERY*

Jonathan Carter, MD
Assistant Professor of Surgery
University of California, San Francisco
San Francisco, California
*LAPAROSCOPIC REPAIR OF RECURRENT
INGUINAL HERNIAS*

Abigail S. Caudle, MD
Assistant Professor
Department of Surgical Oncology
University of Texas MD Anderson Cancer
Center
Houston, Texas
*MANAGEMENT OF RECURRENT AND
METASTATIC BREAST CANCER*

Eugene P. Ceppa, MD
Minimally Invasive Surgery Fellow
Department of General Surgery
Duke University Medical Center
Durham, North Carolina
BENIGN BILIARY STRICTURES

Marisa Cevasco, MD, MPH
Resident in Surgery
Brigham and Women's Hospital
Harvard Medical School
Boston, Massachusetts
*MANAGEMENT OF PANCREATIC
PSEUDOCYST*

Elliot L. Chaikof, MD, PhD
Chairman
Department of Surgery
Surgeon-in-Chief
Beth Israel Deaconess Medical Center
Harvard Medical School
Boston, Massachusetts
*MANAGEMENT OF INFECTED VASCULAR
GRAFTS*

Sricharan Chalikonda, MD
Director
General Surgery Robotics Program
Department of Hepatopancreaticobiliary
Surgery
Digestive Disease Institute
Cleveland Clinic
Cleveland, Ohio
*LAPAROSCOPIC BYPASS FOR PANCREATIC
CANCER*

Vinay Chandrasekhara, MD
Senior Clinical Fellow
Department of Gastroenterology
Johns Hopkins Hospital
Baltimore, Maryland
ESOPHAGEAL FUNCTION TESTS

**Vivek Chaudhry, MBBS, FACS,
FASCRS**
Section Head Surgical Endoscopy
Director Research Division of Colon and
Rectal Surgery
John H. Stroger Jr Hospital of Cook County;
Assistant Professor
University of Illinois at Chicago;
Instructor
Rush University Medical School;
Lecturer
Chicago Medical School
Chicago, Illinois
CONDYLOMA ACUMINATA

Haiquan Chen, MD
Department of Cardiothoracic Surgery
The Cancer Hospital of Fudan University
Shanghai, China
*LAPAROSCOPIC TREATMENT OF
ESOPHAGEAL MOTILITY DISORDERS*

Herbert Chen, MD, FACS
Vice-Chair
Department of Surgery
Professor of Surgery and Biomedical
Engineering;
Chief
Endocrine Surgery
University of Wisconsin
Leader
Endocrine Cancer Disease Group
University of Wisconsin Carbone Cancer
Center
Madison, Wisconsin
PRIMARY HYPERPARATHYROIDISM

Aaron M. Cheng, MD
Assistant Professor
Division of Cardiothoracic Surgery
University of Washington
Seattle, Washington
MEDIASTINAL MASSES

Michael A. Choti, MD, MBA, FACS
Jacob C. Handelsman Professor of Surgery
Professor of Surgery and Oncology
Vice Chair
Department of Surgery
Johns Hopkins Hospital
Baltimore, Maryland
*RADIOFREQUENCY ABLATION OF
COLORECTAL LIVER METASTASES*

Kathleen K. Christians, MD
Associate Professor
Department of Surgery
The Medical College of Wisconsin
Milwaukee, Wisconsin
*VASCULAR RECONSTRUCTION DURING THE
WHIPPLE OPERATION*

A. Britton Christmas, MD, FACS
Trauma, Surgical Critical Care, and Acute
Care Surgery
Department of Surgery
Carolinas Medical Center
Charlotte, North Carolina
VENA CAVA FILTERS

Heidi Chua, MD
Assistant Professor of Surgery
College of Medicine
Mayo Clinic
Rochester, Minnesota
SURGICAL MANAGEMENT OF CONSTIPATION

Albert K. Chun, MD
Instructor of Radiology
Brigham and Women's Hospital
Harvard Medical School
Boston, Massachusetts
*TRANSHEPATIC INTERVENTIONS FOR
OBSTRUCTIVE JAUNDICE*

Alice Chung, MD
Department of Breast & Endocrine
John Wayne Cancer Institute
Saint John's Health Center
Santa Monica, California
*LYMPHATIC MAPPING AND SENTINEL
LYMPHADENECTOMY*

Orlo H. Clark, MD
Professor of Surgery
University of California, San Francisco
Mt. Zion Medical Center
San Francisco, California
MANAGEMENT OF THYROID NODULES

**Sean P. Cleary, MD, MSC, MPH,
FRCSC**
Pancreatic and Hepatobiliary Surgery
Toronto General Hospital;
Assistant Professor
University of Toronto
Toronto, Ontario, Canada
*MANAGEMENT OF CYSTIC DISEASE OF THE
LIVER*

**Christine S. Cocanour, MD, FACS,
FCCM**
Professor of Surgery
Division of Trauma and Emergency Surgery
University of California Davis Medical
Center
Sacramento, California
COLONIC VOLVULUS

Panna A. Codner, MD, FACS
Assistant Professor of Surgery
Division of Trauma/Critical Care
Department of Surgery
Medical College of Wisconsin
Milwaukee, Wisconsin
INJURIES TO THE SMALL AND LARGE BOWEL

Thomas H. Cogbill, MD
Program Director Emeritus
General Surgery Residency
Department of General & Vascular Surgery
Gundersen Lutheran Medical Center
La Crosse, Wisconsin
*ABNORMAL OPERATIVE AND
POSTOPERATIVE BLEEDING*

Patrick S. Collier, BS
The DeWitt Daughtry Family Department
of Surgery
University of Miami Miller School of
Medicine
Miami, Florida

*VASCULAR ACCESS SURGERY: AN EMERGING
SPECIALTY*

Mark F. Conrad, MD, MMSc
Division of Vascular and Endovascular
Surgery
Massachusetts General Hospital;
Assistant Professor in Surgery
Harvard Medical School
Boston, Massachusetts

AORTOILIAC OCCLUSIVE DISEASE

Joel D. Cooper, MD
Professor of Surgery
Chief
Division of Thoracic Surgery
University of Pennsylvania Health System
Philadelphia, Pennsylvania

MANAGEMENT OF TRACHEAL STENOSIS

Cybil Corning, MD
Assistant Professor of Surgery
Division of Colon and Rectal Surgery
University of Illinois at Chicago
Chicago, Illinois

ANAL FISSURE

Vicente Cortes, MD, FACS
Attending Trauma Surgeon and Director
Trauma Intensive Care Unit
Allegheny General Hospital Shock Trauma
Center
Pittsburgh, Pennsylvania

MANAGEMENT OF RECTAL INJURIES

Joseph S. Coselli, MD
Professor of Surgery and Cullen Foundation
Endowed Chair
Division of Cardiothoracic Surgery
Michael E. DeBakey Department of Surgery
Baylor College of Medicine
Texas Heart Institute at St. Luke's Episcopal
Hospital
Houston, Texas

*MANAGEMENT OF DESCENDING THORACIC
AND THORACOABDOMINAL AORTIC
ANEURYSMS*

Randall O. Craft, MD
Chief Resident Associate
Department of General Surgery
Mayo Clinic Arizona
Scottsdale, Arizona

*LAPAROSCOPIC PARASTOMAL HERNIA
REPAIR*

Martin A. Croce, MD, FACS
Professor of Surgery
Chief, Trauma and Surgical Critical Care
University of Tennessee Health Science
Center
Memphis, Tennessee

INJURY TO THE SPLEEN

Jessica Crow, PharmD
Clinical Pharmacy Specialist
Johns Hopkins Hospital
Baltimore, Maryland

CARDIOVASCULAR PHARMACOLOGY

Robert F. Cuff, MD, FACS
Division of Vascular and Endovascular
Specialists
Spectrum Health Medical Group
Assistant Clinical Professor of Surgery
Michigan State University
College of Human Medicine
Grand Rapids, Michigan

*COAGULOPATHY IN THE CRITICALLY ILL
PATIENT*

Joseph J. Cullen, MD
Professor of Surgery
University of Iowa Carver College of
Medicine;
Chief of Surgical Services
Veterans Affairs Medical Center
Iowa City, Iowa

MANAGEMENT OF SMALL BOWEL TUMORS

Steven C. Cunningham, MD
Department of Surgery
The Johns Hopkins University School of
Medicine
Baltimore, Maryland;
Department of Surgery
Saint Agnes Hospital
Baltimore, Maryland

*MANAGEMENT OF PRIMARY MALIGNANT
LIVER TUMORS*

Myriam J. Curet, MD, FACS
Professor
Department of Surgery
Stanford University
Stanford, California

*MANAGEMENT OF COMMON BILE DUCT
STONES*

Alan P.B. Dackiw, MD, PhD
Department of Surgery
Division of Endocrine and Oncologic
Surgery
Johns Hopkins Hospital
Johns Hopkins University School of
Medicine
Baltimore, Maryland

LAPAROSCOPIC ADRENALECTOMY

Nabil N. Dagher, MD
Assistant Professor of Surgery
Division of Transplantation
Department of Surgery
Johns Hopkins Hospital
Baltimore, Maryland

*EXPOSURE TO BLOOD-BORNE PATHOGENS
IN THE OPERATING ROOM*

R. Clement Darling III, MD
Professor of Surgery
Albany Medical College;
Chief
Division of Vascular Surgery
Albany Medical Center Hospital;
The Institute for Vascular Health and
Disease
Albany, New York

ATHEROSCLEROTIC RENOVASCULAR DISEASE

Nancy E. Davidson, MD
Director
University of Pittsburgh Cancer Institute
and UPMC Cancer Centers
Professor of Medicine and Pharmacology
and Chemical Biology
University of Pittsburgh School of Medicine
Pittsburgh, Pennsylvania

*ADVANCES IN ADJUVANT AND
NEOADJUVANT THERAPY FOR BREAST
CANCER*

John J. Degliuomini, MD, FACS
Assistant Professor of Surgery
New York Medical College
Valhalla, New York

CUTANEOUS MELANOMA

Amy C. Degnim, MD
Associate Professor of Surgery
Department of Surgery
Mayo Clinic
Rochester, Minnesota

SCREENING FOR BREAST CANCER

Conor P. Delaney, MD, MCh, PhD
Chief
Division of Colorectal Surgery
Vice-Chair
Department of Surgery
University Hospitals Case Medical Center;
The Jeffrey L. Ponsky Professor of Surgery
Case Western Reserve University
Cleveland, Ohio

CROHN'S COLITIS

Ronald P. DeMatteo, MD, FACS
Vice Chair
Department of Surgery
Chief
Division of General Surgery Oncology
Leslie H. Blumgart Chair in Surgery
Memorial Sloan-Kettering Cancer Center
New York, New York

GASTROINTESTINAL STROMAL TUMORS

Steven R. DeMeester, MD
Department of Surgery
University of Southern California
Keck School of Medicine
Los Angeles, California

*MANAGEMENT OF PHARYNGEAL
ESOPHAGEAL (ZENKER) DIVERTICULA*

Tom R. DeMeester, MD
Professor and Chairman Emeritus
Department of Surgery
University of Southern California
Keck School of Medicine
Los Angeles, California

PARAESOPHAGEAL HIATAL HERNIA

Daniel T. Dempsey, MD
Professor and Chairman of Surgery
Temple University
Philadelphia, Pennsylvania

MANAGEMENT OF DUODENAL ULCER

**Ashwin L. deSouza, MS, MRCSEd,
DNB, FCPS, MNAMS**
Fellow
Minimally Invasive and Laparoscopic Colon
and Rectal Surgery
University of Illinois at Chicago
Chicago, Illinois

MANAGEMENT OF RECTOVAGINAL FISTULA

E. Gene Deune, MD, MBA
Associate Professor
Johns Hopkins Department of Orthopedic
Surgery
Co-Director Hand Surgery Division
Johns Hopkins Plastic Surgery
Director Hand Surgery Section,
Microsurgery
Johns Hopkins Hospital
Baltimore, Maryland

ELECTRICAL AND LIGHTNING INJURIES

Wayne C. DeVos, MD, PhD
Berks Colorectal Surgical Associates
West Reading, Pennsylvania

*COLONIC PSEUDOOBSTRUCTION (OGILVIE
SYNDROME)*

Justin B. Dimick, MD, MPH
Assistant Professor of Surgery
Research Scientist
Center for Healthcare Outcomes & Policy
University of Michigan
Ann Arbor, Michigan

MEASURING OUTCOMES IN SURGERY

Timothy R. Donahue, MD
Assistant Professor
Departments of Surgery and Molecular and
Medical Pharmacology
David Geffen School of Medicine at UCLA
Los Angeles, California

GALLSTONE PANCREATITIS

FLUID AND ELECTROLYTE THERAPY

Jonathan M. Dort, MD, FACS
Associate Professor of Surgery
Virginia Tech Carilion School of Medicine;
Clinical Associate Professor of Surgery
University of Virginia
Charlottesville, Virginia

*CHEST WALL TRAUMA, HEMOTHORAX, AND
PNEUMOTHORAX*

Eric J. Dozois, MD
Associate Professor of Surgery
Division of Colon and Rectal Surgery
Mayo Clinic
Rochester, Minnesota

*MANAGEMENT OF SOLITARY RECTAL ULCER
SYNDROME*

Elizabeth Dreesen, MD
Assistant Professor of Surgery
Trauma Medical Director
University of North Carolina School of
Medicine
Chapel Hill, North Carolina

ACID-BASE DISORDERS

Quan-Yang Duh, MD, FACS
Professor and Chief
Section of Endocrine Surgery
Department of Surgery
University of California, San Francisco
San Francisco, California

*LAPAROSCOPIC REPAIR OF RECURRENT
INGUINAL HERNIAS*

**Scott A. Dulchavsky, MD, PhD, FACS,
FCCM**
Roy D. McClure Chair of Surgery
Henry Ford Hospital;
Professor of Surgery, Molecular Biology,
and Genetics
Wayne State University School of Medicine
Detroit, Michigan

*THE SURGEON'S USE OF ULTRASOUND IN
THORACOABDOMINAL TRAUMA*

Mark D. Duncan, MD, FACS
Associate Professor of Surgery and
Oncology
Johns Hopkins University School
of Medicine;
Chief of Surgical Oncology
Johns Hopkins Bayview Medical Center
Baltimore, Maryland

ACUTE APPENDICITIS

ACUTE CHOLECYSTITIS

Umamaheshwar Duvvuri, MD, PhD
Assistant Professor
Department of Otolaryngology
University of Pittsburgh School of Medicine
Pittsburgh, Pennsylvania

*MANAGEMENT OF THE ISOLATED NECK
MASS*

**Soumitra R. Eachempati, MD, FACS,
FCCM**
Professor of Surgery and Public Health
Weill Cornell Medical College;
Director
Surgical Intensive Care Unit
Chief
Trauma Services
New York Weill Cornell Center
New York, New York

ACUTE KIDNEY INJURY

Jeffrey Eakin, MD
Chief Resident
Department of Surgery
The Ohio State University Medical Center
Columbus, Ohio

ACHALASIA

Frederic E. Eckhauser, MD
Professor of Surgery
Johns Hopkins Hospital
Baltimore, Maryland

SMALL BOWEL OBSTRUCTION

Barish H. Edil, MD
Assistant Professor of Surgery and Oncology
Johns Hopkins University
Baltimore, Maryland

HEPATIC ABSCESS

LAPAROSCOPIC APPENDECTOMY

Eric D. Edwards, MD, FACS
Attending Surgeon
St. Mary Medical Center
Langhorne, Pennsylvania

LAPAROSCOPIC INGUINAL HERNIORRAPHY

Meghan Edwards, MD
Surgical Resident
University of Utah
Salt Lake City, Utah

RECURRENT INGUINAL HERNIAS

David T. Efron, MD, FACS
Associate Professor of Surgery, Anesthesia
and Critical Care Medicine
The Johns Hopkins School of Medicine;
Chief, Division of Acute Care Surgery
Director of Adult Trauma
Johns Hopkins Hospital
Baltimore, Maryland

*SPLENIC SALVAGE PROCEDURES:
THERAPEUTIC OPTIONS*

LIVER INJURY

Jonathan E. Efron, MD, FACS, FASCRS
Associate Professor
The Mark M Ravitch, MD, Endowed
Professorship in Surgery
Chief of the Ravitch Division
Johns Hopkins University
Baltimore, Maryland

PILONIDAL DISEASE

Philip A. Efron, MD
Assistant Professor of Surgery and
Anesthesiology
Co-Director, Laboratory of Inflammation
Biology and Surgical Science
Associate Medical Director, Trauma ICU;
Surgical Critical Care Fellowship Director
Division of Acute Care Surgery and Surgical
Critical Care
University of Florida, Health Science Center
Gainesville, Florida
SPLENIC SALVAGE PROCEDURES:
THERAPEUTIC OPTIONS

E. Christopher Ellison, MD
Associate Vice President of Health Sciences
and Vice-Dean for Clinical Affairs
The Robert M. Zollinger Professor and
Chair
Department of Surgery
Ohio State University College of Medicine
Columbus, Ohio
ZOLLINGER-ELLISON SYNDROME

Trevor A. Ellison, MD
Resident in General Surgery
Johns Hopkins University
Baltimore, Maryland
LAPAROSCOPIC APPENDECTOMY

Amgad El Sherif, MD
Department of Surgery
The Heart, Lung, and Esophageal Surgery
Institute
University of Pittsburgh Medical Center
Pittsburgh, Pennsylvania
VIDEO-ASSISTED THORACIC SURGERY

Guillermo A. Escobar, MD
Assistant Professor of Surgery
Section of Vascular Surgery
University of Michigan Health System
Ann Arbor, Michigan
MANAGEMENT OF RUPTURED ABDOMINAL
AORTIC ANEURYSMS

Domenic P. Esposito, MD, FACS
Professor of Neurosurgery
Director of Neurotrauma
University of Mississippi Medical Center
Department of Neurosurgery
Jackson, Mississippi
TRAUMATIC BRAIN INJURY

Douglas B. Evans, MD
Donald C. Ausman Family Foundation
Professor of Surgery
Chairman
Department of Surgery
Medical College of Wisconsin
Milwaukee, Wisconsin
VASCULAR RECONSTRUCTION DURING THE
WHIPPLE OPERATION

Heather L. Evans, MD
Assistant Professor of Surgery
Department of Surgery
Harborview Medical Center
University of Washington
Seattle, Washington
ELECTROLYTE DISORDERS

Peter J. Fabri, MD, PhD
Professor of Surgery
Professor of Industrial Engineering
University of South Florida
Tampa, Florida
MANAGEMENT OF DIVERTICULOSIS OF THE
SMALL BOWEL

Ronald M. Fairman, MD
The Clyde F. Barker–William Maul Measey
Professor of Surgery
Chief, Division of Vascular Surgery and
Endovascular Therapy
Vice-Chairman for Clinical Affairs,
Department of Surgery
Hospital of the University of Pennsylvania
Philadelphia, Pennsylvania
ENDOVASCULAR TREATMENT
OF ABDOMINAL AORTIC ANEURYSMS

Houssam Farres, MD
Surgical Critical Care Fellow
Johns Hopkins University School of
Medicine
Baltimore, Maryland
CLOSTRIDIUM DIFFICILE COLITIS

Richard H. Feins, MD
Professor of Surgery
Division of Cardiothoracic Surgery
University of North Carolina at Chapel Hill
Chapel Hill, North Carolina
ESOPHAGEAL STENTS

David V. Feliciano, MD
Professor of Surgery
Emory University School of Medicine;
Surgeon-in-Chief
Grady Memorial Hospital
Atlanta, Georgia
PANCREATIC AND DUODENAL INJURIES

Charles M. Ferguson, MD
Associate Professor of Surgery
Division of General Surgery
Massachusetts General Hospital
Boston, Massachusetts
SPIGELIAN, LUMBAR, AND OBTURATOR
HERNIAS

Mark K. Ferguson, MD
Professor of Surgery
Section of Cardiac and Thoracic Surgery
Department of Surgery
The University of Chicago
Chicago, Illinois
MANAGEMENT OF ESOPHAGEAL TUMORS

Cristina R. Ferrone, MD
Assistant Professor of Surgery
General Surgery
Harvard University
Massachusetts General Hospital
Boston, Massachusetts
BENIGN LIVER TUMORS

George S. Ferzli, MD, FACS
Professor of Surgery
SUNY Health Science Center at Brooklyn;
Chairman
Department of Surgery
Lutheran Medical Center
Brooklyn, New York
LAPAROSCOPIC INGUINAL HERNIORRHAPHY

Alessandro Fichera, MD, FACS,
FASCRS
Associate Professor
Program Director
Colon and Rectal Surgery Training Program
University of Chicago
Chicago, Illinois
LAPAROSCOPIC MANAGEMENT OF CROHN'S
DISEASE

Aaron S. Fink, MD
Professor of Surgery
Emory University School of Medicine;
Chief Surgical Consultant
VA Southeast Network 7;
Attending Surgeon
Veterans Affairs Medical Center Atlanta
Atlanta, Georgia
LARGE BOWEL OBSTRUCTION

David Fink, MD
Research Fellow
Bioengineering Institute of Advanced
Surgery and Endoscopy
University of Chicago;
General Surgery Resident
Massachusetts General Hospital
Boston, Massachusetts
ACUTE PANCREATITIS

Rhonda Fishel, MD, MBA, FACS
Associate Chief of Surgery
Sinai Hospital
Baltimore, Maryland
POSTOPERATIVE RESPIRATORY FAILURE

Kerry Fisher, MD, FACS
General Surgeon
Intermountain Medical Center
Salt Lake City, Utah
RECURRENT INGUINAL HERNIAS

William E. Fisher, MD
Professor
Michael E. DeBakey Department of Surgery
Director
Elkins Pancreas Center
Baylor College of Medicine
Houston, Texas
MALLORY-WEISS SYNDROME

Timothy C. Fitzgibbons, MD, FACS
Assistant Clinical Professor
Orthopaedic Surgery
Creighton University;
Clinical Associate Professor
Department of Orthopaedics
University of Nebraska Medical Center
Omaha, Nebraska
DIABETIC FOOT

James W. Fleshman, MD
Professor of Surgery
Chief
Section of Colon and Rectal Surgery
Washington University School of Medicine
St. Louis, Missouri
MANAGEMENT OF TOXIC MEGACOLON

Lewis M. Flint, MD, FACS
Editor-in-Chief
Selected Readings in General Surgery
Division of Education
American College of Surgeons
Chicago, Illinois
PELVIC FRACTURES

Tanya R. Flohr, MD
General Surgery Resident
University of Virginia Health System
Department of Surgery
University of Virginia
Charlottesville, Virginia
HEMORRHOIDS

Jaime I. Flores, MD
Plastic Surgeon
University of Miami
Miami, Florida
LYMPHEDEMA

Sara P. Fogarty, DO
General Surgery Resident
Sinai Hospital
Baltimore, Maryland
POSTOPERATIVE RESPIRATORY FAILURE

Paul J. Foley, MD
Fellow
Division of Vascular Surgery and
Endovascular Therapy
Department of Surgery
Hospital of the University of Pennsylvania
Philadelphia, Pennsylvania
*ENDOVASCULAR TREATMENT OF
ABDOMINAL AORTIC ANEURYSMS*

Yuman Fong, MD
Murray F. Brennan Chair in Surgery
Department of Surgery
Memorial Sloan-Kettering Cancer Center;
Professor of Surgery
Weill Cornell Medical College
New York, New York
MANAGEMENT OF GALLBLADDER CANCER

Charles M. Friel, MD
Associate Professor of Surgery
Section of Colon and Rectal Surgery
University of Virginia
Charlottesville, Virginia
HEMORRHOIDS

Eric R. Frykberg, MD
Professor
Department of Surgery
University of Florida College of Medicine;
Chief
Division of General Surgery
Shands Jacksonville Medical Center
Jacksonville, Florida
*MANAGEMENT OF EXTREMITY
COMPARTMENT SYNDROME*

Joseph C. Fuller, BS
The DeWitt Daughtry Family Department
of Surgery
University of Miami Miller School of
Medicine
Miami, Florida
*VASCULAR ACCESS SURGERY: AN EMERGING
SPECIALTY*

Michele A. Gadd, MD
Assistant Professor
Harvard Medical School
Department of Surgery
Massachusetts General Hospital
Boston, Massachusetts
*MANAGEMENT OF BENIGN BREAST
DISEASE*

Philippe Gailloud, MD
Division of Interventional Neuroradiology
Department of Radiology and Radiological
Science
Johns Hopkins University Hospital and
School of Medicine
Baltimore, Maryland
*ENDOVASCULAR TREATMENT OF CAROTID
ARTERY OCCLUSIVE DISEASE*

Charles Galanis, MD
General Surgery
Johns Hopkins Medical Center
Baltimore, Maryland
ACUTE PULMONARY EMBOLISM

James J. Gallagher, MD
Assistant Professor of Surgery
Weill Cornell Medical College;
Assistant Attending Surgeon
New York-Presbyterian Hospital
Weill Cornell Medical Center
New York, New York
BURN WOUND MANAGEMENT

Scott F. Gallagher, MD, FACS
Associate Professor
Department of Surgery
University of South Florida College of
Medicine (USF Health);
Vice Chief
Department of Surgery
Tampa General Hospital
Tampa, Florida
*MANAGEMENT OF DIVERTICULOSIS OF THE
SMALL BOWEL*

Bryan A. Gaspard, MD
Resident in Neurosurgery
University of Mississippi Medical Center
Jackson, Mississippi
TRAUMATIC BRAIN INJURY

Colleen B. Gaughan, MD
Assistant Professor of Surgery
Temple University
Philadelphia, Pennsylvania
MANAGEMENT OF DUODENAL ULCER

Susan L. Gearhart, MD
Department of Surgery
Johns Hopkins Hospital
Baltimore, Maryland
DIVERTICULAR DISEASE OF THE COLON

David A. Geller, MD
Richard L. Simmons Professor of Surgery
Director
UPMC Liver Cancer Center
Thomas E. Starzl Transplantation Institute
Department of Surgery
University of Pittsburgh Medical Center
Pittsburgh, Pennsylvania
LAPAROSCOPIC LIVER RESECTION

Christos S. Georgiades, MD, PhD, FSIR
Associate Professor of Radiology & Surgery
Vascular & Interventional Radiology
Johns Hopkins University
Baltimore, Maryland
*TRANSJUGULAR INTRAHEPATIC
PORTOSYSTEMIC SHUNT*

Jean-Francois H. Geschwind, MD
Professor of Radiology, Surgery & Oncology
Director, Interventional Radiology Center
Johns Hopkins University School of
Medicine
Baltimore, Maryland
*TRANSJUGULAR INTRAHEPATIC
PORTOSYSTEMIC SHUNT*

Bashar Ghosheh, MD
General Surgery Resident
University of Mississippi Medical Center
Jackson, Mississippi

*MANAGEMENT OF ANEURYSMS OF THE
EXTRACRANIAL CAROTID AND VERTEBRAL
ARTERIES*

Samuel A. Giday, MD
The Robert E. Meyerhoff Professor of
Medicine
Division of Gastroenterology and
Hepatology
Johns Hopkins Hospital
Baltimore, Maryland

ASYMPTOMATIC (SILENT) GALLSTONES

**Armando E. Giuliano, MD, FACS,
FRCSEd**
Chief of Science and Medicine
John Wayne Cancer Institute
Saint John's Health Center
Santa Monica, California;
Clinical Professor of Surgery
University of California, Los Angeles
Los Angeles, California

*LYMPHATIC MAPPING AND SENTINEL
LYMPHADENECTOMY*

Natalia Glebova, MD, PhD
Resident in Halsted General Surgery
Training Program
Johns Hopkins University School of
Medicine
Baltimore, Maryland

BUERGER DISEASE

Nelson H. Goldberg, MD, FACS
Professor of Surgery
Division of Plastic Surgery
University of Maryland School of Medicine
Baltimore, Maryland

*MANAGEMENT OF ABDOMINAL WALL
DEFECTS*

Jerry Goldstone, MD, FACS, FRCSE
Professor of Surgery
Case Western Reserve University School
of Medicine;
Chief Emeritus
Division of Vascular Surgery and
Endovascular Therapy
University Hospitals Case Medical Center
Cleveland, Ohio

BRACHIOCEPHALIC RECONSTRUCTION

Suman Golla, MD, FACS
Associate Professor
Department of Otolaryngology
University of Pittsburgh School of Medicine
Pittsburgh, Pennsylvania

*MANAGEMENT OF THE ISOLATED NECK
MASS*

Jessica E. Gosnell, MD
Assistant Professor of Surgery
University of California San Francisco
Mt. Zion Medical Center
San Francisco, California

MANAGEMENT OF THYROID NODULES

Jeffrey R. Gourley, MD
Department of Radiology
Virginia Hospital Center
Arlington, Virginia

*TRANSHEPATIC INTERVENTIONS FOR
OBSTRUCTIVE JAUNDICE*

Jay A. Graham, MD
Department of Surgery
Massachusetts General Hospital
Boston, Massachusetts

*HEPATIC MALIGNANCY: RESECTION VERSUS
LIVER TRANSPLANTATION*

Jayleen Grams, MD, PhD
Assistant Professor
Department of Surgery
University of Alabama at Birmingham
Birmingham, Alabama

LAPAROSCOPIC GASTRIC SURGERY

Michael P. Grant, MD, PhD, FACS
Division Head
Oculoplastic Surgery
Director
Ocular and Orbital Trauma Center
Wilmer Eye Institute at Johns Hopkins
Baltimore, Maryland

*EVALUATION AND MANAGEMENT OF
FACIAL INJURIES*

Ana M. Grau, MD, FACS
Associate Professor of Surgery
Division of Surgical Oncology and
Endocrine Surgery
Vanderbilt University
Nashville, Tennessee

*SMALL BOWEL CARCINOID/
NEUROENDOCRINE TUMORS*

Axel Grothey, MD
Professor of Oncology
Mayo Clinic Rochester
Rochester, Minnesota

*NEOADJUVANT AND ADJUVANT TREATMENT
FOR COLORECTAL CANCER*

Marlon A. Guerrero, MD
Assistant Professor of Surgery
University of Arizona
Tucson, Arizona

*SECONDARY AND TERTIARY
HYPERPARATHYROIDISM*

Jose G. Guillem, MD, MPH
Professor of Surgery
Department of Surgery
Memorial Sloan-Kettering Cancer Center
New York, New York

RECTAL CANCER

Adil H. Haider, MD, MPH, FACS
Assistant Professor of Surgery,
Anesthesiology and Critical Care Medicine
Division of Acute Care Surgery: Trauma,
Emergency Surgery and Critical Care;
Co-Director
Center for Surgery Trials and Outcomes
Research
Johns Hopkins University School
of Medicine;
Assistant Professor of Health Policy and
Management
Johns Hopkins Bloomberg School of Public
Health
Baltimore, Maryland

THE ABDOMEN THAT WILL NOT CLOSE

Bruce Lee Hall, MD, PhD, MBA
Professor of Surgery
School of Medicine
Professor of Healthcare Management
Olin Business School
Barnes Jewish Hospital
Washington University in Saint Louis;
Associate Chief of Surgery
St. Louis Veterans' Affairs Medical Center
St. Louis, Missouri

HYPERTHYROIDISM

David C. Han, MD
Associate Professor of Surgery and
Radiology
Vice Chair for Education
Department of Surgery
Penn State Hershey Medical Center
Hershey, Pennsylvania

*POPLITEAL AND FEMORAL ARTERY
ANEURYSMS*

John W. Harmon, MD
Professor of Surgery
Hendrix Burn/Wound Laboratory
Johns Hopkins University School of
Medicine
Baltimore, Maryland

ACUTE APPENDICITIS

Kristi L. Harold, MD
Associate Professor of Surgery
Chair
Division of General Surgery
Director of Minimally Invasive Surgery
Mayo Clinic Arizona
Phoenix, Arizona

*LAPAROSCOPIC PARASTOMAL HERNIA
REPAIR*

Amy P. Harper, MSN, ACNP-BC
Division of Interventional Radiology
George Washington University Hospital
Washington, DC

*TRANSHEPATIC INTERVENTIONS FOR
OBSTRUCTIVE JAUNDICE*

Hobart W. Harris, MD, MPH
J. Englebert Dunphy Professor of Surgery
Chief, Division of General Surgery
Department of Surgery
University of California, San Francisco
San Francisco, California

*MANAGEMENT OF ENTEROCUTANEOUS
FISTULAS*

Samad Hashimi, MD
Fellow
Cardiothoracic Surgery
University of Iowa Hospitals and Clinics
Iowa City, Iowa

ESOPHAGEAL PERFORATION

Heitham T. Hassoun, MD
Associate Professor of Cardiovascular
Surgery
The Methodist Hospital Physician
Organization
DeBakey Heart & Vascular Center
Houston, Texas

GANGRENE OF THE FOOT

Elliott R. Haut, MD, FACS
Associate Professor of Surgery and
Anesthesiology and Critical Care Medicine
Division of Acute Care Surgery
Department of Surgery
Johns Hopkins University School of
Medicine;
Director
Trauma/Acute Care Surgery Fellowship
Johns Hopkins Hospital
Baltimore, Maryland

*AIRWAY MANAGEMENT IN THE TRAUMA
PATIENT*

*COAGULATION OF TRAUMA: PATHOGENESIS,
DIAGNOSIS, AND TREATMENT*

Marie-Noëlle Hébert-Blouin, MD
Peripheral Nerve Fellow
Department of Neurologic Surgery
Mayo Clinic
Rochester, Minnesota

NERVE INJURY AND REPAIR

Richard F. Heitmiller, MD
JMT Finney Chairman of Surgery
Union Memorial Hospital
Baltimore, Maryland

GASTROESOPHAGEAL REFLUX DISEASE

J. Michael Henderson, MB, ChB
Department of Hepato-pancreato-biliary
and Transplant Surgery
Digestive Disease Institute
Cleveland Clinic
Cleveland, Ohio

THE ROLE OF SHUNTING PROCEDURES

B. Todd Heniford, MD, FACS
Chief
Division of Gastrointestinal and Minimally
Invasive Surgery
Chief of Surgery
Carolinas Medical Center
Charlotte, North Carolina

*STAGING LAPAROSCOPY FOR
GASTROINTESTINAL CANCER*

Peter K. Henke, MD
Professor of Surgery
Section of Vascular Surgery
University of Michigan
Ann Arbor, Michigan

*VENOUS THROMBOEMBOLISM: DIAGNOSIS,
PREVENTION, AND TREATMENT*

H. Franklin Herlong, MD
Associate Professor of Medicine
Johns Hopkins School of Medicine
Baltimore, Maryland

HEPATIC ENCEPHALOPATHY

Jonathan M. Hernandez, MD
Surgery Resident
Department of Surgery
University of South Florida
Tampa, Florida

REFRACTORY ASCITES

Philip J. Hess Jr, MD
Associate Professor
Thoracic and Cardiovascular Surgery
University of Florida
Gainesville, Florida

ACUTE AORTIC DISSECTIONS

Jonathan R. Hiatt, MD
Professor and Chief
Division of General Surgery
Vice Chair for Education
Department of Surgery
David Geffen School of Medicine at UCLA
Los Angeles, California

FLUID AND ELECTROLYTE THERAPY

O. Joe Hines, MD
Department of Surgery
David Geffen School of Medicine at UCLA
Los Angeles, California

*PALLIATIVE THERAPY FOR PANCREATIC
CANCER*

Richard A. Hodin, MD
Professor of Surgery
Harvard Medical School;
Surgical Director
MGH Crohn's and Colitis Center
Department of Surgery
Massachusetts General Hospital
Boston, Massachusetts

*APPROACH TO LOWER GASTROINTESTINAL
BLEEDING*

John P. Hoffman, MD, FACS
Professor of Surgery
Fox Chase Cancer Center
Temple University School of Medicine
Philadelphia, Pennsylvania

*ADJUVANT AND NEOADJUVANT THERAPY
FOR PANCREATIC CANCER*

Johnny C. Hong, MD, FACS
Assistant Professor of Surgery
Surgical Director, Living Donor Liver
Transplant Program
Medical Director, Liver Transplant Service
Liver Transplantation and Hepatobiliary
Surgery
Division of Liver and Pancreas
Transplantation
Department of Surgery
David Geffen School of Medicine at UCLA
Los Angeles, California

ECHINOCOCCAL DISEASE OF THE LIVER

Toshitaka Hoppo, MD, PhD
Research Assistant Professor
Division of Thoracic and Foregut Surgery
Department of Cardiothoracic Surgery
University of Pittsburgh Medical Center
Pittsburgh, Pennsylvania

MINIMALLY INVASIVE ESOPHAGECTOMY

Jan K. Horn, MD, FACS
Professor of Clinical Surgery
University of California, San Francisco
San Francisco, California

GAS GANGRENE

Francis J. Hornicek, MD, PhD
Associate Professor of Orthopedic Surgery
Harvard Medical School
Boston, Massachusetts

MANAGEMENT OF SOFT TISSUE SARCOMAS

Rydhwana Hossain, MSIV
George Washington University Medical
Center
Washington, DC

*TRANSHEPATIC INTERVENTIONS FOR
OBSTRUCTIVE JAUNDICE*

Thomas J. Howard, MD
Willis D. Gatch Professor of Surgery
Indiana University School of Medicine
Indianapolis, Indiana

PANCREAS DIVISUM AND OTHER VARIANTS OF DOMINANT DORSAL DUCT ANATOMY

David B. Hoyt, MD, FACS
Executive Director
American College of Surgeons
Chicago, Illinois

PENETRATING ABDOMINAL TRAUMA

Jennifer E. Hrabe, MD
Surgery Resident
Department of Surgery
University of Iowa Carver College of Medicine
Iowa City, Iowa

MANAGEMENT OF SMALL BOWEL TUMORS

Tjasa Hranjec, MD
Surgery Resident
Department of Surgery
University of Virginia
Charlottesville, Virginia

MANAGEMENT OF PANCREATIC ABSCESS

Tracy L. Hull, MD
Professor of Surgery
Department of Colon and Rectal Surgery
Cleveland Clinic College of Medicine
Case Western Reserve University
Cleveland Clinic Foundation
Cleveland, Ohio

MANAGEMENT OF FECAL INCONTINENCE

Mark D. Iannettoni, MD, MBA
Johann L. Ehrenhaft Professor of Cardiothoracic Surgery
Director, Cardiothoracic Surgery
Physician Executive Director, UI Heart and Vascular Center
University of Iowa Hospitals & Clinics
Iowa City, Iowa

ESOPHAGEAL PERFORATION

David A. Iannitti, MD
Clinical Associate Professor of Surgery
University of North Carolina
Chapel Hill, North Carolina;
Chief, HPB Surgery
Carolinas Medical Center
Charlotte, North Carolina

LAPAROSCOPIC PANCREATIC RESECTION

Kamran Idrees, MD
Surgical Oncology Fellow
Department of Surgery
University of Pittsburgh
Pittsburgh, Pennsylvania

CYSTIC DISORDERS OF THE BILE DUCTS

Elizabeth A. Ignacio, MD
Assistant Professor of Radiology
George Washington University School of Medicine
Washington, DC

TRANSHEPATIC INTERVENTIONS FOR OBSTRUCTIVE JAUNDICE

Tim A. Iseli, MBBS
Staff Surgeon
Department of Otolaryngology, Head & Neck Surgery
Royal Melbourne Hospital
Melbourne, Victoria, Australia

SKIN LESIONS: EVALUATION, DIAGNOSIS, AND MANAGEMENT

Hiromichi Ito, MD
Research Fellow
Department of Surgery
Brigham and Women's Hospital
Boston, Massachusetts

PRIMARY SCLEROSING CHOLANGITIS

Heather Jacene, MD
Assistant Professor of Radiology
Johns Hopkins Hospital
Baltimore, Maryland

USE OF [^{18}F]-2-FLUORO-2-DEOXY-D-GLUCOSE POSITRON EMISSION TOMOGRAPHY IN THE MANAGEMENT OF COLORECTAL CANCER

Lana L. Jackson, MD
Department of Otolaryngology
Medical College of Georgia
Augusta, Georgia

TRACHEOSTOMY

Lenworth M. Jacobs, MD, MPH
Professor of Surgery and Chairman
Department of Traumatology and Emergency Medicine
University of Connecticut School of Medicine
Hartford Hospital
Hartford, Connecticut

USE OF ANTIBIOTICS IN SURGICAL PATIENTS

Lisa K. Jacobs, MD
Associate Professor of Surgery
Johns Hopkins University
Baltimore, Maryland

MANAGEMENT OF MALE BREAST CANCER

Sanjay Jagannath, MD, AGAF, FASGE
The Melissa I. Posner Institute for Digestive Health and Liver Disease;
Director
Center for Comprehensive Pancreatic Care;
Mercy Medical Center
Baltimore, Maryland

ESOPHAGEAL FUNCTION TESTS

Nicholas Jaszczak, MD
Fellow
Acute Care Surgery
Johns Hopkins Hospital
Baltimore, Maryland

LIVER INJURY

Vijay Jayaraman, MD
Trauma Fellow
Department of Traumatology and Emergency Medicine
Hartford Hospital
Hartford, Connecticut

USE OF ANTIBIOTICS IN SURGICAL PATIENTS

Juan Carlos Jimenez, MD, FACS
Assistant Professor
Division of Vascular Surgery
UCLA School of Medicine
Attending Surgeon
Ronald Reagan-UCLA Medical Center
UCLA Olive View Medical Center
UCLA Santa Monica Hospital
Santa Monica, California

UPPER EXTREMITY ARTERIAL OCCLUSIVE DISEASE

Judy Jin, MD
Resident
Department of Surgery
MetroHealth Medical Center
Case Western Reserve University
Cleveland, Ohio

MANAGEMENT OF THYROID CANCER

Blair A. Jobe, MD, FACS
Professor of Surgery
Department of Cardiothoracic Surgery
University of Pittsburgh Medical Center
Pittsburgh, Pennsylvania

MINIMALLY INVASIVE ESOPHAGECTOMY

Jennifer E. Joh, MD
Breast Surgical Oncology Fellow
H. Lee Moffitt Cancer Center & Research Institute
Tampa, Florida

CUTANEOUS MELANOMA

Eric K. Johnson, MD, FACS, FASCRS
Assistant Professor of Surgery
Uniformed Services University of the Health Sciences
Chief, Colorectal Surgery and Surgical Endoscopy
Eisenhower Army Medical Center
Fort Gordon, Georgia

ANORECTAL ABSCESS AND FISTULA

Jonas T. Johnson, MD
The Dr. Eugene N. Myers Professor and
Chairman of Otolaryngology
Department of Otolaryngology
University of Pittsburgh School of Medicine
Pittsburgh, Pennsylvania

*MANAGEMENT OF THE ISOLATED NECK
MASS*

Lynt B. Johnson, MD, MBA
Robert J. Coffey Professor
Chairman, Department of Surgery
Georgetown University Hospital
Washington, DC

*HEPATIC MALIGNANCY: RESECTION VERSUS
LIVER TRANSPLANTATION*

Michael Johnson, MD
Department of Hepato-pancreato-biliary
and Transplant Surgery
Digestive Disease Institute
Cleveland Clinic
Cleveland, Ohio

THE ROLE OF SHUNTING PROCEDURES

Sreenivasa Jonnalagadda, MD
Professor of Medicine
Director of Pancreatic and Biliary
Endoscopy
Division of Gastroenterology
Washington University in St. Louis
St. Louis, Missouri

ACUTE CHOLANGITIS

Gregory J. Jurkovich, MD
Professor of Surgery
University of Washington
Chief of Trauma
Harborview Medical Center
Seattle, Washington

DIAPHRAGMATIC INJURIES

Stefan S. Kachala, MD
Resident
Department of Surgery
New York Presbyterian
Weill Cornell Medical Center
New York, New York

*ABLATIVE THERAPIES IN BENIGN AND
MALIGNANT BREAST DISEASE*

Anthony N. Kalloo, MD
The Moses and Helen Golden Paulson
Professor of Gastroenterology
Chief
Division of Gastroenterology and
Hepatology
Johns Hopkins Hospital
Baltimore, Maryland

*OBSTRUCTIVE JAUNDICE: ENDOSCOPIC
THERAPY*

Giorgos C. Karakousis, MD
Fellow in Surgical Oncology
Memorial Sloan-Kettering Cancer Center
New York, New York

GASTROINTESTINAL STROMAL TUMORS

Ryan D. Katz, MD
Attending Hand Surgeon
Division of Hand Surgery
The Curtis National Hand Center
Union Memorial Hospital
Baltimore, Maryland

ELECTRICAL AND LIGHTNING INJURIES

Thomas Keane, MD
Clinical Assistant Professor
Department of Radiology
Johns Hopkins Medical Institutions
Baltimore, Maryland

*ACUTE PERIPHERAL ARTERIAL AND BYPASS
GRAFT OCCLUSION: THROMBOLYTIC
THERAPY*

Electron Kebebew, MD, FACS
Senior Investigator
Head of Endocrine Oncology Section
National Cancer Institute
Bethesda, Maryland

*SECONDARY AND TERTIARY
HYPERPARATHYROIDISM*

K. Craig Kent, MD
A.R. Curreri Professor of Surgery
Chairman
Department of Surgery
University of Wisconsin School of Medicine
and Public Health
Madison, Wisconsin

FEMOROPOPLITEAL OCCLUSIVE DISEASE

Tara S. Kent, MD
Division of General Surgery
Beth Israel Deaconess Medical Center
Harvard Medical School
Boston, Massachusetts

UNUSUAL PANCREATIC TUMORS

Mouen Khashab, MD
Department of Medicine and Division of
Gastroenterology and Hepatology
Johns Hopkins Medical Institute
Baltimore, Maryland

ASYMPTOMATIC (SILENT) GALLSTONES

Arman Kilic, MD
Resident
Department of Surgery
Johns Hopkins Hospital
Baltimore, Maryland

*LAPAROSCOPIC TREATMENT OF
ESOPHAGEAL MOTILITY DISORDERS*

Elizabeth Min Hui Kim, MD
Massachusetts General Hospital
Boston, Massachusetts

*MANAGEMENT OF THE AXILLA IN BREAST
CANCER*

Yongsik Kim, MD, PhD
Assistant Professor
Department of Internal Medicine
Korea University College of Medicine
Seoul, Korea

*OBSTRUCTIVE JAUNDICE: ENDOSCOPIC
THERAPY*

Jonathan C. King, MD
Resident
Department of Surgery
University of California Los Angeles
Los Angeles, California

*PALLIATIVE THERAPY FOR PANCREATIC
CANCER*

Tari A. King, MD, FACS
Associate Attending Surgeon, Breast Service
Jeanne A. Petrek Junior Faculty Chair
Memorial Sloan-Kettering Cancer Center
Associate Professor of Surgery
Weill Medical College of Cornell
New York, New York

*CELLULAR, BIOCHEMICAL, AND MOLECULAR
TARGETS IN BREAST CANCER*

**Andrew W. Kirkpatrick, MD, FRCSC,
FACS**
Regional Director of Trauma
Professor of Critical Care Medicine and
Surgery
Departments of Critical Care Medicine
and Surgery
Foothills Medical Centre
University of Calgary
Calgary, Alberta, Canada

*THE SURGEON'S USE OF ULTRASOUND IN
THORACOABDOMINAL TRAUMA*

Allen Kong, MD
Assistant Clinical Professor
Department of Surgery
University of California, Irvine
Orange, California

PENETRATING ABDOMINAL TRAUMA

Richard A. Kozarek, MD
Director, Digestive Disease Institute
Department of Gastroenterology
Virginia Mason Medical Center
Seattle, Washington

MANAGEMENT OF CHRONIC PANCREATITIS

Mark J. Krasna, MD
Medical Director
The Cancer Institute
St. Joseph Medical Center
Program in Health Policy
University of Maryland at Baltimore
Towson, Maryland

*NEOADJUVANT AND ADJUVANT THERAPY
FOR ESOPHAGEAL CARCINOMA*

Helen Krontiras, MD
Associate Professor
Department of Surgery
University of Alabama at Birmingham
Birmingham, Alabama

INFLAMMATORY BREAST CANCER

David Kuwayama, MD
Department of Surgery
Division of Vascular Surgery
Johns Hopkins University
School of Medicine
Baltimore, Maryland

*ABDOMINAL AORTIC ANEURYSM AND
UNEXPECTED ABDOMINAL PATHOLOGY*

**Edward C.S. Lai, MD, FRCS(Ed),
FRACS, FCSHK, FHKAM, FACS**
Department of Surgery
Pedder Clinic
Hong Kong SAR, China

*LAPAROSCOPIC MANAGEMENT OF
PANCREATIC PSEUDOCYST*

Alysandra Lal, MD, MPH
Assistant Professor of Surgery
Medical College of Wisconsin
Milwaukee, Wisconsin

*VASCULAR RECONSTRUCTION DURING THE
WHIPPLE OPERATION*

Glenn M. LaMuraglia, MD
Division of Vascular and Endovascular
Surgery
Department of Surgery
Massachusetts General Hospital
Harvard Medical School
Boston, Massachusetts

*FALSE ANEURYSMS AND ARTERIOVENOUS
FISTULAS*

Kwan N. Lau, MD
Section of Hepato-Pancreatico-Biliary
Surgery
Division of GI and Minimally Invasive
Surgery
Department of Surgery
Carolinas Medical Center
Charlotte, North Carolina

LAPAROSCOPIC PANCREATIC RESECTION

Harish Lavu, MD
Assistant Professor of Surgery
Jefferson Medical College
Jefferson Pancreas, Biliary and Related
Cancer Center
Thomas Jefferson University
Philadelphia, Pennsylvania

PERIAMPULLARY CANCER

Peter F. Lawrence, MD
Vascular Surgery
UCI College of Medicine
Los Angeles, California

*UPPER EXTREMITY ARTERIAL OCCLUSIVE
DISEASE*

Karl A. LeBlanc, MD, MBA, FACS
Surgeons Group of Baton Rouge/Our Lady
of the Lake Physician Group
Director and Fellowship Program Chairman
Minimally Invasive Surgery Institute;
Adjunct Professor
Pennington Biomedical Research Center
Baton Rouge, Louisiana;
Clinical Professor
Department of Surgery
Louisiana State University School of
Medicine
New Orleans, Louisiana

*INCISIONAL, EPIGASTRIC, AND UMBILICAL
HERNIAS*

Anna M. Ledgerwood, MD
Professor
School of Medicine
Department of Surgery
Detroit Receiving Hospital
Detroit, Michigan

PENETRATING NECK TRAUMA

Scott A. LeMaire, MD
Professor of Surgery, Molecular Physiology
and Biophysics
Director of Research, Division of
Cardiothoracic Surgery
Michael E. DeBakey Department of Surgery
Baylor College of Medicine
Texas Heart Institute at St. Luke's Episcopal
Hospital
Houston, Texas

*MANAGEMENT OF DESCENDING THORACIC
AND THORACOABDOMINAL AORTIC
ANEURYSMS*

Barry C. Lembersky, MD
Clinical Associate Professor of Medicine
University of Pittsburgh Cancer Institute
Pittsburgh, Pennsylvania

*ADVANCES IN ADJUVANT AND
NEOADJUVANT THERAPY FOR BREAST
CANCER*

William H. Leukhardt, MD
Department of Surgery
MetroHealth Medical Center Campus
Case Western Reserve University School of
Medicine
Cleveland, Ohio

*ANTIFUNGAL THERAPY IN THE SURGICAL
PATIENT*

Ryan Li, MD
Resident Physician
Department of Otolaryngology-Head and
Neck Surgery
Johns Hopkins Hospital and Health System
Baltimore, Maryland

ACUTE APPENDICITIS

Keith D. Lillemoe, MD, FACS
Jay L. Grosfeld Professor and Chairman
Department of Surgery
Indiana University School of Medicine
Indianapolis, Indiana

*INTRADUCTAL PAPILLARY MUCINOUS
NEOPLASMS OF THE PANCREAS*

**Pamela A. Lipsett, MD, MHPE, FACS,
FCCM**
Professor of Surgery, Anesthesiology,
Critical Care Medicine, and Nursing
Program Director, General Surgery and
Surgical Critical Care
Department of Surgery
Johns Hopkins University Schools of
Medicine and Nursing
Baltimore, Maryland

CLOSTRIDIUM DIFFICILE COLITIS

Evan C. Lipsitz, MD
Associate Professor of Surgery
Chief
Division of Vascular and Endovascular
Surgery
Montefiore Medical Center and the Albert
Einstein College of Medicine
Bronx, New York

PROFUNDA FEMORIS RECONSTRUCTION

Alex G. Little, MD
Chair and Professor
Department of Surgery
Wright State University
Dayton, Ohio

DISORDERS OF ESOPHAGEAL MOTILITY

Charles E. Lucas, MD
Professor of Surgery
Wayne State University
School of Medicine
Detroit, Michigan

PENETRATING NECK TRAUMA

James D. Luketich, MD
Henry T. Bahnson Professor of Surgery
Chairman
Department of Cardiothoracic Surgery
Director
The Heart, Lung, and Esophageal Surgery
Institute
University of Pittsburgh Medical Center
Pittsburgh, Pennsylvania
*LAPAROSCOPIC TREATMENT OF
ESOPHAGEAL MOTILITY DISORDERS*

Ying Wei Lum, MD
Vascular Surgery Fellow
Division of Vascular and Endovascular
Surgery
Department of Surgery
Johns Hopkins Hospital
Baltimore, Maryland
RAYNAUD SYNDROME

Sean P. Lyden, MD
Associate Professor of Surgery
Department of Vascular Surgery
Cleveland Clinic Foundation
Cleveland, Ohio
*MANAGEMENT OF PERIPHERAL ARTERIAL
EMBOLI*

Bruce V. MacFadyen, MD, FACS
Moretz/Mansberger Distinguished Professor
Chairman
Department of Surgery
Medical College of Georgia
Augusta, Georgia
LAPAROSCOPIC CHOLECYSTECTOMY

Maria Lucia L. Madariaga, MD
Resident
Department of Surgery
Massachusetts General Hospital
Boston, Massachusetts
*MOTILITY DISORDERS OF THE STOMACH
AND SMALL BOWEL*

Thomas H. Magnuson, MD
Associate Professor of Surgery
Johns Hopkins University School of
Medicine
Baltimore, Maryland
MORBID OBESITY

Ronald V. Maier, MD
Jane and Donald D. Trunkey Professor and
Vice Chair of Surgery
Department of Surgery
Harborview Medical Center
University of Washington
Seattle, Washington
ELECTROLYTE DISORDERS

Martin A. Makary, MD, MPH
Associate Professor of Surgery
Johns Hopkins University School of
Medicine;
Associate Professor of Health Policy &
Management
Johns Hopkins University School of Public
Health
Baltimore, Maryland
BENIGN GASTRIC ULCER

Rohit Makhija, MD
Division of Colorectal Surgery
University Hospitals Case Medical Center
Cleveland, Ohio
CROHN'S COLITIS

Mark A. Malangoni, MD, FACS
Professor of Surgery
Case Western Reserve University School of
Medicine
MetroHealth Medical Center Campus
Cleveland, Ohio
*ANTIFUNGAL THERAPY IN THE SURGICAL
PATIENT*

Mahmoud B. Malas, MD, MHS, FACS
Department of Surgery
Division of Vascular Surgery
Johns Hopkins University School of
Medicine
Baltimore, Maryland
*ABDOMINAL AORTIC ANEURYSM AND
UNEXPECTED ABDOMINAL PATHOLOGY*

*MANAGEMENT OF RECURRENT CAROTID
ARTERY STENOSIS*

Paul N. Manson, MD, FACS
Professor and Head
Division of Plastic and Reconstructive
Surgery
Johns Hopkins Hospital
Baltimore, Maryland
*EVALUATION AND MANAGEMENT OF
FACIAL INJURIES*

FROSTBITE AND COLD INJURIES

Peter W. Marcello, MD, FACS, FASCRS
Vice Chairman
Department of Colon & Rectal Surgery
Lahey Clinic
Burlington, Massachusetts
LAPAROSCOPIC COLORECTAL SURGERY

Jeffrey M. Marks, MD, FACS
Associate Professor
Department of Surgery
University Hospitals Case Medical Center
Cleveland, Ohio
NOTES: WHAT THE FUTURE HOLDS

Michael R. Marohn, DO, FACS
Associate Professor of Surgery
Johns Hopkins University School of
Medicine
Baltimore, Maryland
*CYSTS, TUMORS, AND ABSCESSES OF THE
SPLEEN*

Terri R. Martin, MD
Department of Surgery
Carolinas Medical Center
Charlotte, North Carolina
*STAGING LAPAROSCOPY FOR
GASTROINTESTINAL CANCER*

Tomas D. Martin, MD
Professor
Thoracic and Cardiovascular Surgery
University of Florida
Gainesville, Florida
ACUTE AORTIC DISSECTIONS

Douglas J. Mathisen, MD
Chief, Cardiothoracic Surgery
Massachusetts General Hospital;
Hermes C. Grillo Professor of Thoracic
Surgery
Harvard Medical School
Boston, Massachusetts
*MANAGEMENT OF ACQUIRED ESOPHAGEAL
RESPIRATORY TRACT FISTULA*

Brent D. Matthews, MD
Department of Surgery
Section of Hepatobiliary/Pancreatic Surgery
Washington University School of Medicine
St. Louis, Missouri
LAPAROSCOPIC SPLENECTOMY

Peter J. Mazzaglia, MD
General Surgeon
The Warren Alpert Medical School of
Brown University
Providence, Rhode Island
ADRENAL INCIDENTALOMA

John E. McDermott, MD
Department of Surgery
Swedish-Providence Medical Center
Seattle, Washington
DIABETIC FOOT

David W. McFadden, MD, MBA
Stanley S. Fieber Professor and Chairman
Fletcher Allen Healthcare
University of Vermont College of Medicine
Burlington, Vermont
GASTRIC ADENOCARCINOMA

Christopher R. McHenry, MD, FACS, FACE
Vice Chairman Department of Surgery
MetroHealth Medical Center;
Professor of Surgery
Case Western Reserve University
Cleveland, Ohio
MANAGEMENT OF THYROID CANCER

Robert C. McIntyre Jr, MD
Professor of Surgery
University of Colorado Denver School of
Medicine
Denver, Colorado
BLOOD TRANSFUSION THERAPY

Elisabeth C. McLemore, MD
Assistant Professor
University of California, San Diego
San Diego, California
*USE OF STRICTUREPLASTY IN CROHN'S
DISEASE*

Robin S. McLeod, MD
Angelo and Alfredo De Gasperis Families
Chair in Colorectal Cancer and IBD
Research
Zane Cohen Clinical Research Unit
Samuel Lunenfeld Research Institute
Mount Sinai Hospital;
Professor of Surgery and Health Policy,
Management and Evaluation
University of Toronto
Toronto, Canada
COLORECTAL POLYPS

John D. Mellinger, MD, FACS
Professor and Chair of General Surgery
Residency Program Director
Southern Illinois University School of
Medicine
Springfield, Illinois
LAPAROSCOPIC CHOLECYSTECTOMY

Nicholas Melo, MD
Chief Resident
Department of Surgery
Massachusetts General Hospital
Boston, Massachusetts
ACUTE MESENTERIC ISCHEMIA

Genevieve B. Melton, MD
Assistant Professor
Department of Surgery
Faculty Fellow
Institute for Health Informatics
University of Minnesota
Minneapolis, Minnesota
*MANAGEMENT OF CHRONIC ULCERATIVE
COLITIS*
ACUTE APPENDICITIS

Andrew J. Meltzer, MD
Fellow in Vascular Surgery
New York-Presbyterian Hospital
New York, New York
*SPIGELIAN, LUMBAR, AND OBTURATOR
HERNIAS*
ACUTE MESENTERIC ISCHEMIA

W. Scott Melvin, MD
Professor of Surgery
Chief
Division of General and Gastrointestinal
Surgery
Director
Center for Minimally Invasive Surgery
The Ohio State University
Arthur G. James Cancer Hospital and
Research Institute
Columbus, Ohio
ACHALASIA

Maria Clara Mendoza, MD
Post Doctoral Research Associate
Fogarty International Center Research
Fellow
Department of Surgery
University of Pittsburgh
Pittsburgh, Pennsylvania
*NUTRITIONAL SUPPORT IN THE CRITICALLY
ILL*

Ryan Messiner, DO
Fellow in Vascular Surgery
Penn State Hershey Medical Center
Hershey, Pennsylvania
*POPLITEAL AND FEMORAL ARTERY
ANEURYSMS*

Anthony A. Meyer, MD, PhD
Colin G, Thomas Jr, MD, Distinguished
Professor and Chair
Department of Surgery
University of North Carolina
at Chapel Hill
Chapel Hill, North Carolina
ACID-BASE DISORDERS

William C. Meyers, MD, MBA
Senior Associate Dean
Chairman of Surgery
Director of Core Performance Center
Drexel University College of Medicine
Philadelphia, Pennsylvania
ATHLETIC PUBALGIA: "THE SPORTS HERNIA"

Fabrizio Michelassi, MD
Lewis Atterbury Stimson Professor
Chairman
Department of Surgery
Weill Cornell Medical College;
Surgeon-in-Chief
New York-Presbyterian Hospital at Weill
Cornell
New York, New York
CROHN'S DISEASE OF THE SMALL BOWEL

Keith W. Millikan, MD, FACS
Professor of Surgery
Rush University
Chicago, Illinois
INGUINAL HERNIA

Thomas J. Miner, MD, FACS
Assistant Professor of Surgery
Director
Department of Surgical Oncology
Associate Residency Program Director
The Warren Alpert Medical School of
Brown University
Rhode Island Hospital
Providence, Rhode Island
ADRENAL INCIDENTALOMA

Jeffrey F. Moley, MD
Chief of Endocrine and Oncologic Surgery
Professor of Surgery
School of Medicine
Barnes Jewish Hospital
Washington University in St. Louis;
Staff Surgeon
St. Louis Veterans' Affairs Medical Center
St. Louis, Missouri
HYPERTHYROIDISM

Frederick A. Moore, MD, FACS, FCCM
Head
Division of Acute Care Surgery
Department of Surgery
The Methodist Hospital;
Professor of Surgery
Weill Cornell Medical College
Houston, Texas
*ABDOMINAL COMPARTMENT SYNDROME
AND MANAGEMENT OF THE OPEN
ABDOMEN*
BLOOD TRANSFUSION THERAPY

Ellen H. Morrow, MD
Resident
Department of Surgery
Stanford University School of Medicine
Stanford, California
*MANAGEMENT OF PANCREATIC ISLET CELL
TUMORS EXCLUDING GASTRINOMA*

Monica Morrow, MD, FACS
Chief, Breast Service
Department of Surgery
Anne Burnett Windfohr Chair of Clinical
Oncology
Professor of Surgery
Weill Cornell Medical College
Memorial Sloan-Kettering Cancer Center
New York, New York
*CELLULAR, BIOCHEMICAL, AND MOLECULAR
TARGETS IN BREAST CANCER*

Angela K. Moss, MD
Resident
Department of Surgery
Massachusetts General Hospital
Harvard Medical School
Boston, Massachusetts

*APPROACH TO LOWER GASTROINTESTINAL
BLEEDING*

Fady Moustarah, MD, MPH, FRCSC
General Surgery
Advanced Laparoscopic and Bariatric
Surgery Fellow
Endocrinology and Metabolism Institute
Cleveland Clinic Foundation
Cleveland, Ohio

*LAPAROSCOPIC SURGERY FOR SEVERE
OBESITY*

Sami Mufeed, MD, FACS
Assistant Professor of Surgery
Cairo University School of Medicine
Cairo, Egypt

BENIGN GASTRIC ULCER

Roberta L. Muldoon, MD, FACS
Assistant Professor of Surgery
Colon and Rectal Surgery
Vanderbilt University
Nashville, Tennessee

*RECTAL PROLAPSE AND OBSTRUCTIVE
DEFECATION*

Ashok Muniappan, MD
Instructor in Surgery
Division of Thoracic Surgery
Department of Surgery
Massachusetts General Hospital
Harvard Medical School
Boston, Massachusetts

*MANAGEMENT OF ACQUIRED ESOPHAGEAL
RESPIRATORY TRACT FISTULA*

Erin H. Murphy, MD
Vascular Research Fellow
Department of Vascular Surgery
Stanford University Medical Center
Stanford, California

*MANAGEMENT OF TIBIOPERONEAL
OCCLUSIVE DISEASE*

Peter Muscarella II, MD, FACS
Associate Professor
Department of Surgery
Gastrointestinal Surgery
Ohio State University Medical Center
Columbus, Ohio

*SPLENECTOMY FOR HEMATOLOGIC
DISORDERS*

Maurice Y. Nahabedian, MD
Associate Professor of Plastic Surgery
Georgetown University Hospital
Washington, DC

*BREAST RECONSTRUCTION AFTER
MASTECTOMY: INDICATIONS, TECHNIQUES,
AND RESULTS*

**Lena M. Napolitano, MD, FACS, FCCP,
FCCM**
Professor of Surgery
Division Chief, Acute Care Surgery
Associate Chair, Department of Surgery
Director, Trauma and Surgical Critical Care
University of Michigan School of Medicine
Ann Arbor, Michigan

SURGICAL SITE INFECTIONS

William H. Nealon, MD
Professor of Surgery and Vice Chairman for
Clinical Affairs
Department of Surgery
Vanderbilt University School of Medicine;
Associate Surgeon-in-Chief
Vanderbilt University Hospital
Nashville, Tennessee

*PANCREATIC DUCTAL DISRUPTIONS
LEADING TO PANCREATIC FISTULA,
PANCREATIC ASCITES, OR PLEURAL
EFFUSIONS*

Todd Neideen, MD
Assistant Professor
Division of Trauma/Critical Care
Department of Surgery
Medical College of Wisconsin
Milwaukee, Wisconsin

INJURIES TO THE SMALL AND LARGE BOWEL

Leigh A. Neumayer, MD, FACS
Professor of Surgery
University of Utah School of Medicine;
Co-Director
Integrated Breast Program
Huntsman Cancer Hospital
Salt Lake City, Utah

RECURRENT INGUINAL HERNIAS

Naeem A. Newman, MD
Fellow, Center for Surgical Outcomes
Research
Department of Surgery
Johns Hopkins University School of
Medicine
Baltimore, Maryland

BENIGN GASTRIC ULCER

Hien T. Nguyen, MD
Minimally Invasive Surgery Fellow
Johns Hopkins University School of
Medicine
Baltimore, Maryland

*CYSTS, TUMORS, AND ABSCESSES OF THE
SPLEEN*

Kevin Tri Nguyen, MD, PhD
Clinical Instructor
HPB Surgery
Department of Surgery
University of Pittsburgh Medical Center
Pittsburgh, Pennsylvania

LAPAROSCOPIC LIVER RESECTION

Mehrdad Nikfarjam, MD, PhD, FRACS
Lecturer, University of Melbourne
Department of Surgery
Austin Health
Melbourne, Australia

*ENDOLUMINAL APPROACHES TO
GASTROESOPHAGEAL REFLUX DISEASE*

NOTES: WHAT THE FUTURE HOLDS

Jeffrey A. Norton, MD
Robert L. and Mary Ellenburg Professor of
Surgery
Chief
Division of General Surgery
Stanford University School of Medicine
Stanford, California

*MANAGEMENT OF PANCREATIC ISLET CELL
TUMORS EXCLUDING GASTRINOMA*

Charles S. O'Mara, MD
Clinical Professor of Surgery
University of Mississippi Medical Center
Jackson, Mississippi

*MANAGEMENT OF ANEURYSMS OF THE
EXTRACRANIAL CAROTID AND VERTEBRAL
ARTERIES*

Raymond P. Onders, MD
Margaret and Walter Remen Chair in
Surgical Innovation
Director of Minimally Invasive Surgery
University Hospitals Case Medical Center
Case Western Reserve University School of
Medicine
Cleveland, Ohio

NOTES IN THE INTENSIVE CARE UNIT

H. Leon Pachter, MD
The George David Stewart Professor and
Chair
Department of Surgery
New York University School of Medicine
New York, New York

*MANAGEMENT OF ADRENAL CORTICAL
TUMORS*

Theodore N. Pappas, MD
Chief, Gastrointestinal Surgery
Duke University Medical Center
Durham, North Carolina

BENIGN BILIARY STRICTURES

Manish Parikh, MD
Assistant Professor of Surgery
Director of Bariatric and Minimally Invasive Surgery
Bellevue Hospital
Department of Surgery
New York University School of Medicine
New York, New York
MANAGEMENT OF ADRENAL CORTICAL TUMORS

Jason Park, MD, MEd
Department of Surgery
University of Manitoba
Winnipeg, Manitoba, Canada
RECTAL CANCER

Jose L. Pascual, MD, PhD, FRCS(C), FRCP(C)
Assistant Professor of Surgery
Division of Traumatology, Critical Care and Emergency Surgery
Department of Surgery
University of Pennsylvania School of Medicine
Philadelphia, Pennsylvania
THE SEPTIC RESPONSE

Virendra I. Patel, MD
Instructor in Surgery
Massachusetts General Hospital
Harvard Medical School
Boston, Massachusetts
OPEN REPAIR OF ABDOMINAL AORTIC ANEURYSMS

Russell K. Pearl, MD, FACS, FASCRS
Associate Professor of Surgery and Biomedical Visualization
University of Illinois at Chicago
Chicago, Illinois
CONDYLOMA ACUMINATA

Andrew B. Peitzman, MD
Mark M. Ravitch Professor of Surgery
Department of Surgery
University of Pittsburgh
Pittsburgh, Pennsylvania
BLUNT ABDOMINAL TRAUMA

John H. Pemberton, MD
Professor of Surgery
College of Medicine
Mayo Clinic
Rochester, Minnesota
SURGICAL MANAGEMENT OF CONSTIPATION

Bruce A. Perler, MD, MBA
Julius H. Jacobson II Professor of Surgery
Chief
Division of Vascular Surgery and Endovascular Therapy
Director of the Vascular Noninvasive Laboratory
Johns Hopkins University School of Medicine and the Johns Hopkins Hospital
Baltimore, Maryland
CAROTID ENDARTERECTOMY

Nancy D. Perrier, MD, FACS
Professor of Surgery
Department of Surgical Oncology
Chief, Section of Surgical Endocrinology
MD Anderson Cancer Center
Houston, Texas
MANAGEMENT OF PHEOCHROMOCYTOMAS

Catherine E. Pesce, MD
General Surgery Resident
Johns Hopkins Hospital
Baltimore, Maryland
MANAGEMENT OF MALE BREAST CANCER
MANAGEMENT OF THYROIDITIS

Joseph B. Petelin, MD, FACS
Clinical Associate Professor
Department of Surgery
University of Kansas School of Medicine;
Director
Surgix Minimally Invasive Surgery Institute & Fellowship
Kansas City, Kansas
LAPAROSCOPIC MANAGEMENT OF COMMON BILE DUCT STONES

Jeffrey H. Peters, MD
Professor and Chairman
Department of Surgery
University of Rochester School of Medicine & Dentistry
Rochester, New York
MANAGEMENT OF BARRETT ESOPHAGUS

Henrik Petrowsky, MD
Department of Surgery
The Dumont-UCLA Transplant Center
David Geffen School of Medicine at UCLA
Ronald Reagan-UCLA Medical Center
Los Angeles, California
CAVERNOUS LIVER HEMANGIOMA

Jason M. Pfluke, MD
Assistant Professor of Surgery
Wilford Hall Medical Center
Lackland Air Force Base
San Antonio, Texas
ENDOSCOPIC TREATMENT OF BARRETT ESOPHAGUS

Scott R. Philipp, MD
Assistant Professor
Department of Surgery
Associate Program Director
General Surgery Residency
University of Missouri, Columbia
Columbia, Missouri
LAPAROSCOPIC VENTRAL AND INCISIONAL HERNIA REPAIR

Bradley J. Phillips, MD
Burn Director
Surgical ICU Director
Swedish Medical Center
Englewood, Colorado
BURNS: FLUID, NUTRITION, AND METABOLICS

Greta L. Piper, MD
Fellow
Trauma and Acute Care Surgery
Department of Surgery
University of Pittsburgh
Pittsburgh, Pennsylvania
BLUNT ABDOMINAL TRAUMA

Henry A. Pitt, MD
Professor and Vice Chair
Department of Surgery
Indiana University School of Medicine
Indianapolis, Indiana
HEPATIC ABSCESS

Louis R. Pizano, MD, MBA, FACS
Associate Professor of Surgery
Chief
Division of Burns
Associate Director
Trauma and Surgical Critical Care Fellowship Program
DeWitt Daughtry Family Department of Surgery
University of Miami, Miller School of Medicine
Miami, Florida
BLUNT CARDIAC INJURY

Jeffrey L. Ponsky, MD, FACS
Oliver H. Payne Professor and Chairman
Department of Surgery
Case Western Reserve University;
Surgeon-in-Chief
University Hospitals Case Medical Center
Cleveland, Ohio
ENDOLUMINAL APPROACHES TO GASTROESOPHAGEAL REFLUX DISEASE

Jason D. Prescott, MD, PhD
Department of Surgery
Yale University School of Medicine
New Haven, Connecticut
PERSISTENT OR RECURRENT HYPERPARATHYROIDISM

Peter J. Pronovost, MD, PhD
Professor
Department of Anesthesia and Critical Care
Medicine
Johns Hopkins University School of
Medicine;
Director, Quality and Safety Research
Group
Director, Adult Critical Care Medicine
Medical Director, Innovation in Quality
Patient Care
Baltimore, Maryland

*CENTRAL LINE–ASSOCIATED BLOODSTREAM
INFECTIONS: A NOVEL APPROACH TO
PREVENTION*

Gerd D. Pust, MD
Fellow, Trauma and Surgical Critical Care
Jackson Memorial Hospital
DeWitt Daughtry Family Department of
Surgery
University of Miami, Miller School of
Medicine
Miami, Florida

BLUNT CARDIAC INJURY

Aliaksei Pustavoitau, MD
Assistant Professor
Department of Anesthesia and Critical Care
Medicine
Johns Hopkins University School of
Medicine
Baltimore, Maryland

CARDIOVASCULAR PHARMACOLOGY

Juan Carlos Puyana, MD
Associate Professor of Surgery and Critical
Care
Secretary Treasurer, Pan-American Trauma
Society
University of Pittsburgh
Pittsburgh, Pennsylvania

*NUTRITIONAL SUPPORT IN THE CRITICALLY
ILL*

Umair Qazi, MD, MPH
Department of Surgery
Division of Vascular Surgery
Johns Hopkins University School of
Medicine
Baltimore, Maryland

*ABDOMINAL AORTIC ANEURYSM AND
UNEXPECTED ABDOMINAL PATHOLOGY*

Robert R. Quickel, MD, FACS
Director of Surgical Critical Care
Department of Surgery
Hennepin County Medical Center;
Assistant Professor of Surgery
University of Minnesota Medical School
Minneapolis, Minnesota

SPINE AND SPINAL CORD INJURIES

Jin H. Ra, MD
Fellow in Surgical Critical Care
Department of Surgery
Division of Trauma
Hospital of the University of Pennsylvania
Philadelphia, Pennsylvania

THE SEPTIC RESPONSE

Ariel N. Rad, MD, PhD
Assistant Professor of Surgery
Division of Plastic & Reconstructive Surgery
Johns Hopkins Hospital
Baltimore, Maryland

LYMPHEDEMA

Martin G. Radvany, MD
Division of Interventional Neuroradiology
Department of Radiology and Radiological
Science
Johns Hopkins University School of
Medicine and Johns Hopkins Hospital
Baltimore, Maryland

*ENDOVASCULAR TREATMENT OF CAROTID
ARTERY OCCLUSIVE DISEASE*

Janice F. Rafferty, MD
Chief
Division of Colon and Rectal Surgery
Clinical Professor of Surgery
University of Cincinnati College of
Medicine
Cincinnati, Ohio

MANAGEMENT OF PRURITUS ANI

Reza Rahbari, MD
Clinical Fellow
Surgical Oncology
Surgery Branch
National Cancer Institute
National Institutes of Health
Bethesda, Maryland

*SECONDARY AND TERTIARY
HYPERPARATHYROIDISM*

Margarita Ramos, MD, MPH
Resident
Brigham and Women's Hospital
Boston, Massachusetts

*GLUCOSE CONTROL IN THE POSTOPERATIVE
PATIENT*

Bruce J. Ramshaw, MD, FACS
Chairman
Department of General Surgery
Halifax Health
Daytona Beach, Florida

*LAPAROSCOPIC VENTRAL AND INCISIONAL
HERNIA REPAIR*

Arthur Rawlings, MD, MDiv
Minimally Invasive Fellow
Washington University
St. Louis, Missouri

LAPAROSCOPIC SPLENECTOMY

Patrick R. Reardon, MD, FACS
Chief
Section of Foregut Surgery
Director
Methodist Hospital Minimally Invasive
Surgery Training Program;
Surgical Director
Methodist Hospital Reflux Center;
Medical Director
Methodist Hospital Bariatric Surgery
Program
Houston, Texas

*LAPAROSCOPIC 360-DEGREE
FUNDOPLICATION*

Howard A. Reber, MD
Professor and Chief
Division of Gastrointestinal Surgery
Director
UCLA Center for Pancreatic Diseases
Department of Surgery
David Geffen School of Medicine at UCLA
Los Angeles, California

GALLSTONE PANCREATITIS

Jennifer G. Reeder, MD
University of Pittsburgh Cancer Institute
UPMC Cancer Pavilion
Pittsburgh, Pennsylvania

*ADVANCES IN ADJUVANT AND
NEOADJUVANT THERAPY FOR BREAST
CANCER*

Tobi Reidy, DO
Fellow
Indiana University School of Medicine
Colon and Rectal Surgery Residency
Kendrick Regional Center
Mooresville, Indiana

MANAGEMENT OF PRURITUS ANI

Andrew Reifsnyder, MD
Department of Radiology
University Medical Center
Brackenridge Hospital
Austin, Texas

MANAGEMENT OF PRURITUS ANI
ACUTE PULMONARY EMBOLISM

Thomas F. Reifsnyder, MD
Assistant Professor of Surgery
Division of Vascular Surgery
Johns Hopkins Hospital
Baltimore, Maryland

ACUTE PULMONARY EMBOLISM

Andrew S. Resnick, MD, MBA
Executive Director
Penn Medicine Clinical Simulation Center;
Assistant Professor of Surgery
Division of Gastrointestinal Surgery
Department of Surgery
University of Pennsylvania
Philadelphia, Pennsylvania

*MANAGEMENT OF CHRONIC MESENTERIC
ISCHEMIA*

William O. Richards, MD
Director of Laparoendoscopic Surgery
Vanderbilt University School of Medicine
Nashville, Tennessee

CURRENT TREATMENT OF ACHALASIA

Erwin Rieder, MD
Legacy Health System
Portland, Oregon

NOTES: WHAT IS CURRENTLY POSSIBLE?

John P. Roberts, MD
Professor
Department of Surgery
Chief of the UCSF Transplant Service
University of California, San Francisco
San Francisco, California

*THE ROLE OF LIVER TRANSPLANTATION IN
PORTAL HYPERTENSION*

Raymond E. Robinson, BS
Department of Anesthesia and Critical Care
Medicine
Johns Hopkins University School of
Medicine
Baltimore, Maryland

*CENTRAL LINE–ASSOCIATED BLOODSTREAM
INFECTIONS: A NOVEL APPROACH TO
PREVENTION*

Thomas N. Robinson, MD
Associate Professor
Department of Surgery
University of Colorado School of Medicine
Aurora, Colorado

*PREOPERATIVE ASSESSMENT OF THE
ELDERLY PATIENT: FRAILTY*

Aurelio Rodriguez, MD, FACS
Associate Director of Trauma Surgery
Sinai Hospital
Baltimore, Maryland

MANAGEMENT OF RECTAL INJURIES

Jose M. Rodriguez-Paz, MD
Department of Anesthesiology and Critical
Care Medicine
Johns Hopkins University School of
Medicine
Baltimore, Maryland

*CENTRAL LINE–ASSOCIATED BLOODSTREAM
INFECTIONS: A NOVEL APPROACH TO
PREVENTION*

Selwyn O. Rogers, Jr, MD, MPH
Associate Professor of Surgery
Harvard Medical School
Division of Trauma, Burn, and Surgical
Critical Care
Brigham and Women's Hospital
Boston, Massachusetts

*GLUCOSE CONTROL IN THE POSTOPERATIVE
PATIENT*

Mark Romig, MD
Assistant Professor
Department of Anesthesia and Critical Care
Medicine
Johns Hopkins University School of
Medicine
Baltimore, Maryland

CARDIOVASCULAR PHARMACOLOGY

Glen S. Roseborough, MD
Adjunct Assistant Professor of Surgery
Johns Hopkins University
Salem CardioVascular Associates
Salem, Oregon

RAYNAUD SYNDROME

Alexander S. Rosemurgy, MD
Surgical Director
Digestive Disorders
Tampa General Hospital;
Medical Director
Center for Advanced Medical Learning and
Simulation
University of South Florida
Tampa, Florida

REFRACTORY ASCITES

Eben L. Rosenthal, MD
Julius Hicks Professor of Surgery
Division of Otolaryngology–Head
and Neck Surgery
University of Alabama at Birmingham
Birmingham, Alabama

*SKIN LESIONS: EVALUATION, DIAGNOSIS, AND
MANAGEMENT*

Daniel C. Rossi, DO
Associate, Colorectal Surgery
Geisinger Health System
Wilkes-Barre, Pennsylvania

*PREOPERATIVE BOWEL PREPARATION: IS IT
NECESSARY?*

Gedge D. Rosson, MD
Assistant Professor
Director of Breast Reconstruction
Division of Plastic, Reconstructive and
Maxillofacial Surgery
Department of Surgery
Johns Hopkins University School of
Medicine
Baltimore, Maryland

LYMPHEDEMA

Bashar Safar, MD
Assistant Professor
Division of General Surgery
Colon and Rectal Surgery Section
Washington University School of Medicine
St. Louis, Missouri

MANAGEMENT OF TOXIC MEGACOLON

Barry A. Salky, MD
Professor of Surgery
Chief (Emeritus)
Division of Laparoscopic Surgery
Mount Sinai Hospital
New York, New York

LAPAROSCOPIC GASTRIC SURGERY

Rachel J. Santora, MD
Resident
Department of Surgery
Methodist Hospital
Houston, Texas

GANGRENE OF THE FOOT

Shawn N. Sarin, MD
Assistant Professor of Radiology
and Surgery
George Washington University Hospital
Washington, DC

*TRANSHEPATIC INTERVENTIONS FOR
OBSTRUCTIVE JAUNDICE*

Robert G. Sawyer, MD, FACS
Professor of Surgery and Public Health
Sciences
Chief
Division of Acute Care Surgery and
Outcomes Research
University of Virginia School of Medicine
Charlottesville, Virginia

MANAGEMENT OF PANCREATIC ABSCESS

VENTILATOR-ASSOCIATED PNEUMONIA

Harry C. Sax, MD
Professor of Surgery
Department of Surgery
Brown University
Miriam Hospital
Providence, Rhode Island

*MANAGEMENT OF SHORT BOWEL
SYNDROME*

Thomas M. Scalea, MD
Physician in Chief
R. Adams Cowley Shock Trauma Center;
Francis X. Kelly Professor of Trauma
Director, Program in Trauma
University of Maryland School of Medicine
Baltimore, Maryland

ENDOCRINE CHANGES IN CRITICAL ILLNESS

Philip R. Schauer, MD
Professor of Surgery
Cleveland Clinic Lerner College of Medicine
Cleveland, Ohio

*LAPAROSCOPIC SURGERY FOR SEVERE
OBESITY*

A. Frederick Schild, MD, FACS
Professor and Clerkship Director
Florida International University
Herbert Wertheim College of Medicine
Miami, Florida

*VASCULAR ACCESS SURGERY: AN EMERGING
SPECIALTY*

C. Max Schmidt, MD, PhD, MBA, FACS
Department of Surgery
Indiana University School of Medicine
Indianapolis, Indiana

*INTRADUCTAL PAPILLARY MUCINOUS
NEOPLASMS OF THE PANCREAS*

John G. Schneider, MD
Resident, General Surgery
University of Vermont
Burlington, Vermont

GASTRIC ADENOCARCINOMA

Martin A. Schreiber, MD, FACS
Professor and Chief
Division of Trauma, Critical Care, and
Acute Care Surgery
Oregon Health & Science University
Portland, Oregon

*INITIAL EVALUATION AND RESUSCITATION
OF THE TRAUMA PATIENT*

**Douglas J.E. Schuerer, MD, FACS,
FCCM**
Associate Professor of Surgery
Washington University in St. Louis
Section of Acute and Critical Care Surgery
St. Louis, Missouri

*RETROPERITONEAL INJURIES: KIDNEY AND
URETER*

Richard D. Schulick, MD, FACS
Professor of Surgery and Oncology
John L. Cameron Professor of Alimentary
Tract Surgery
Chief
Division of Surgical Oncology
Director
Hepatopancreatobiliary Fellowship
Johns Hopkins University School of
Medicine
Baltimore, Maryland

*MANAGEMENT OF PRIMARY MALIGNANT
LIVER TUMORS*

C. William Schwab, MD, FACS
Professor of Surgery
University of Pennsylvania School of
Medicine;
Chief
Division of Traumatology, Surgical Critical
Care & Emergency Surgery
Hospital of the University of Pennsylvania
Philadelphia, Pennsylvania

THE SEPTIC RESPONSE

Michael A. Schweitzer, MD
Associate Professor of Surgery
Johns Hopkins University School of
Medicine
Baltimore, Maryland

MORBID OBESITY

Christopher Scortino, MD
Surgical Chief Resident
Johns Hopkins University School of
Medicine
Baltimore, Maryland

MORBID OBESITY

Anthony J. Senagore, MD, MBA
VP Research and Education
Spectrum Health;
Professor of Surgery
Michigan State University/CHM
Grand Rapids, Michigan

COLON CANCER

Stephen M. Sentovich, MD
Chief
Section of Colon and Rectal Surgery
Associate Professor of Surgery
Boston University School of Medicine
Boston, Massachusetts

MANAGEMENT OF ANORECTAL STRICTURE

Boris Sepesi, MD
General Surgery Resident
University of Rochester Medical Center
Rochester, New York

MANAGEMENT OF BARRETT ESOPHAGUS

Melanie W. Seybt, MD
Assistant Professor
Department of Otolaryngology
Associate Surgical Director of Thyroid
Center
University of Georgia Medical Center
Augusta, Georgia

TRACHEOSTOMY

Amit Shah, MD
Fellow in Vascular Surgery
Montefiore Medical Center and the Albert
Einstein College of Medicine
Bronx, New York

PROFUNDA FEMORIS RECONSTRUCTION

Paul C. Shellito, MD
Associate Visiting Surgeon
Massachusetts General Hospital;
Assistant Professor of Surgery
Harvard Medical School
Boston, Massachusetts

TUMORS OF THE ANAL REGION

Alexander D. Shepard, MD
Head, Division of Vascular Surgery
Henry Ford Hospital;
Professor of Surgery
Wayne State University School of Medicine
Detroit, Michigan

AXILLOFEMORAL BYPASS

Kirti Shetty, MD
Medical Director of Liver Transplantation
Georgetown University
Washington, DC

*HEPATIC MALIGNANCY: RESECTION VERSUS
LIVER TRANSPLANTATION*

Jason K. Sicklick, MD
Assistant Professor of Surgery
Division of Surgical Oncology
Moores UCSD Cancer Center
University of California, San Diego
San Diego, California

MANAGEMENT OF GALLBLADDER CANCER

Eric J. Silberfein, MD
Division of Vascular Surgery and
Endovascular Therapy
Michael E. DeBakey Department of Surgery
Baylor College of Medicine
Houston, Texas

MANAGEMENT OF PHEOCHROMOCYTOMAS

Ronald P. Silverman, MD, FACS
Associate Professor of Surgery
University of Maryland School of Medicine;
Adjunct Associate Professor of Plastic
Surgery
Johns Hopkins School of Medicine
Baltimore, Maryland;
Senior Vice President and Chief Medical
Officer
KCI Corporation
San Antonio, Texas

*MANAGEMENT OF ABDOMINAL WALL
DEFECTS*

Rache M. Simmons, MD
Professor of Surgery
Anne K. and Edwin C. Weiskopf Professor
of Surgical Oncology
Joan and Sanford Weill Medical College of
Cornell University
New York Presbyterian Hospital
New York, New York

*ABLATIVE THERAPIES IN BENIGN AND
MALIGNANT BREAST DISEASE*

Ronald F. Sing, DO, FACS, FCCM
Associate Professor of Surgery
School of Medicine, University of North
Carolina at Chapel Hill;
Faculty
Department of Surgery
Carolinas Medical Center
Charlotte, North Carolina

VENA CAVA FILTERS

Barbara L. Smith, MD, PhD
Associate Professor of Surgery
Harvard Medical School;
Director, Breast Program
Massachusetts General Hospital
Boston, Massachusetts

MANAGEMENT OF THE AXILLA IN BREAST CANCER

C. Daniel Smith, MD, FACS
Professor and Chair
Department of Surgery
Surgeon-in-Chief
Mayo Clinic Florida
Jacksonville, Florida

ENDOSCOPIC TREATMENT OF BARRETT ESOPHAGUS

Maurice A. Smith, MD
Department of Surgery
Division of Thoracic Surgery
Appalachian Regional Hospital
Beckley, West Virginia

PRIMARY TUMORS OF THE CHEST WALL

R. Stephen Smith, MD, RDMS, FACS
Vice Chair
Professor of Surgery
Director of Surgical Education
Virginia Tech Carilion School of Medicine;
Clinical Professor of Surgery
University of Virginia
Charlottesville, Virginia

PRIMARY TUMORS OF THE CHEST WALL

CHEST WALL TRAUMA, HEMOTHORAX, AND PNEUMOTHORAX

Michael J. Snyder, MD, FACS
Program Director, Colon and Rectal Surgery
Clinical Associate Professor
University of Texas Medical School
Houston, Texas

IS A NASOGASTRIC TUBE NECESSARY FOLLOWING ALIMENTARY TRACT SURGERY?

Helen Sohn, MD
Department of Surgery
University of Southern California
Keck School of Medicine
Los Angeles, California

MANAGEMENT OF PHARYNGEAL ESOPHAGEAL (ZENKER) DIVERTICULA

David I. Soybel, MD
Professor of Surgery
Harvard Medical School
Senior Staff Surgeon
Brigham and Women's Hospital
Boston, Massachusetts

MOTILITY DISORDERS OF THE STOMACH AND SMALL BOWEL

Michael P. Spencer, MD
Associate Professor
Department of Surgery
University of Minnesota
St. Paul, Minnesota

MANAGEMENT OF CHRONIC ULCERATIVE COLITIS

Robert J. Spinner, MD
Professor
Departments of Neurologic
Surgery, Orthopedics and Anatomy
Mayo Clinic
Rochester, Minnesota

NERVE INJURY AND REPAIR

Nicholas J. Spoerke, MD
General Surgery Resident
Oregon Health & Science University
Portland, Oregon

EMERGENCY DEPARTMENT THORACOTOMY

Scott R. Steele, MD
Chief, Colon & Rectal Surgery
Madigan Army Medical Center
Fort Lewis, Washington

ANORECTAL ABSCESS AND FISTULA

Sharon L. Stein, MD
Assistant Professor of Surgery
Case Western Reserve University;
Division of Colorectal Surgery
University Hospitals
Case Medical Center
Cleveland, Ohio

CROHN'S DISEASE OF THE SMALL BOWEL

Kent A. Stevens, MD, MPH
Assistant Professor of Surgery
Division of Acute Care Surgery
Johns Hopkins Hospital
Baltimore, Maryland

AIRWAY MANAGEMENT IN THE TRAUMA PATIENT

Robert P. Sticca, MD, FACS
Chairman and Professor
Department of Surgery
University of North Dakota School of
Medicine and Health Sciences
Grand Forks, North Dakota

MANAGEMENT OF PERITONEAL SURFACE MALIGNANCY

Gregory V. Stiegmann, MD
Professor of Surgery
Head
Division of Gastrointestinal, Tumor and
Endocrine Surgery
University of Colorado Denver School
of Medicine
Denver, Colorado

ENDOSCOPIC THERAPY FOR ESOPHAGEAL VARICEAL HEMORRHAGE

Jerry Stonemetz, MD
Clinical Associate
Department of Anesthesia
Johns Hopkins University
Baltimore, Maryland

PREOPERATIVE PREPARATION OF THE SURGICAL PATIENT

Steven M. Strasberg, MD
Pruett Professor of Surgery
Department of Surgery Section
of Hepatobiliary-Pancreatic and
Gastrointestinal Surgery
Washington University School of Medicine
St. Louis, Missouri

ACUTE CHOLANGITIS

Michael B. Streiff, MD
Associate Professor of Medicine and
Pathology
Division of Hematology
Medical Director
Anticoagulation Management Service and
Outpatient Clinics;
Medical Director
Special Coagulation Laboratory
Johns Hopkins Medical Institutions
Baltimore, Maryland

COAGULOPATHY OF TRAUMA: PATHOGENESIS, DIAGNOSIS, AND TREATMENT

Stacey Su, MD
Division of Thoracic Surgery
University of Pennsylvania Health Systems
Philadelphia, Pennsylvania

MANAGEMENT OF TRACHEAL STENOSIS

Joseph F. Sucher, MD, FACS
Assistant Professor of Surgery
Weill Cornell Medical College/
The Methodist Hospital
Houston, Texas

ABDOMINAL COMPARTMENT SYNDROME AND MANAGEMENT OF THE OPEN ABDOMEN

Marc Sussman, MD
Assistant Professor of Surgery
Johns Hopkins University School
of Medicine
Baltimore, Maryland

PRIMARY TUMORS OF THE THYMUS

David E.R. Sutherland, MD, PhD
Professor
Division of Transplantation
Director
Schulze Diabetes Institute
Department of Surgery
University of Minnesota
Minneapolis, Minnesota

TRANSPLANTATION OF THE PANCREAS

Lee L. Swanstrom, MD
Clinical Professor of Surgery
Oregon Health Sciences University;
Director
MIS and GI Surgery Division
Legacy Health System
Portland, Oregon
NOTES: WHAT IS CURRENTLY POSSIBLE?

Maakan Taghizadeh, MD
Clinical Instructor
House Staff
Department of Surgery
Ohio State Medical Center
Columbus, Ohio
*SPLENECTOMY FOR HEMATOLOGIC
DISORDERS*

Mark A. Talamini, MD
M.J. Orloff Family Professor and Chairman
Department of Surgery
University of California, San Diego
San Diego, California
*USE OF STRICTUREPLASTY IN CROHN'S
DISEASE*

John L. Tarpley, MD
Professor of Surgery and Anesthesiology
Program Director, General Surgery
Vanderbilt University;
Chief
General Surgery
VATVHS
Nashville, Tennessee
*SMALL BOWEL CARCINOID/
NEUROENDOCRINE TUMORS*

Servet Tatli, MD
Assistant Professor of Radiology
Department of Radiology
Brigham and Women's Hospital
Harvard Medical School
Boston, Massachusetts
*MANAGEMENT OF PANCREATIC
PSEUDOCYST*

Spence M. Taylor, MD
Senior Assistant Dean for Academic Affairs
Greenville Hospital System University
Medical Center;
Chairman and Clinical Professor
Department of Surgery
University of South Carolina School of
Medicine
Greenville, South Carolina
*TREATMENT OF VASCULOGENIC
CLAUDICATION*

David J. Terris, MD, FACS
Porubsky Professor and Chairman,
Department of Otolaryngology
Surgical Director of Thyroid Center
University of Georgia Medical Center
Augusta, Georgia
TRACHEOSTOMY

Geoffrey B. Thompson, MD
Professor of Surgery
College of Medicine
Chief
Endocrine Surgery
Department of Surgery
Mayo Clinic
Rochester, Minnesota
NONTOXIC GOITER

L. William Traverso, MD
Clinical Professor of Surgery
University of Washington
Seattle, Washington;
Director, Center for Pancreatic Disease
St Luke's Hospital System
Boise, Idaho
MANAGEMENT OF CHRONIC PANCREATITIS

Donald D. Trunkey, MD, FACS
Professor Emeritus
Department of Surgery
Oregon Health & Science University
Portland, Oregon
EMERGENCY DEPARTMENT THORACOTOMY

Peter I. Tsai, MD
Assistant Professor of Surgery
Division of Cardiothoracic Surgery
Michael E. DeBakey Department of Surgery
Ben Taub General Hospital
Baylor College of Medicine
Houston, Texas
*MANAGEMENT OF DESCENDING THORACIC
AND THORACOABDOMINAL AORTIC
ANEURYSMS*

Susan Tsai, MD
Assistant Professor
Surgical Oncology
Johns Hopkins Hospital
Baltimore, Maryland
*USE OF [¹⁸F]-2-FLUORO-2-DEOXY-
D-GLUCOSE POSITRON EMISSION
TOMOGRAPHY IN THE MANAGEMENT OF
COLORECTAL CANCER*

Theodore N. Tsangaris, MD, FACS
Associate Professor of Surgery
Chief of Breast Surgery
Division of Oncology
Director
Johns Hopkins Avon Foundation Breast
Center
Sidney Kimmel Comprehensive Cancer
Center at Johns Hopkins
Baltimore, Maryland
BREAST CANCER: SURGICAL THERAPY

Robert Udelsman, MD, MBA
Carmalt Professor of Surgery and Oncology
Department of Surgery
Yale University School of Medicine
New Haven, Connecticut
*PERSISTENT OR RECURRENT
HYPERPARATHYROIDISM*

Konstantin Umanskiy, MD
Assistant Professor
Department of Surgery
University of Chicago
Chicago, Illinois
*LAPAROSCOPIC MANAGEMENT OF CROHN'S
DISEASE*

Gilbert R. Upchurch, Jr, MD
Professor and Chief
Division of Vascular and Endovascular
Surgery
University of Virginia
Charlottesville, Virginia
*MANAGEMENT OF RUPTURED ABDOMINAL
AORTIC ANEURYSMS*

Marshall M. Urist, MD
Champ Lyons Professor and Vice Chair
Department of Surgery
University of Alabama at Birmingham
Birmingham, Alabama
INFLAMMATORY BREAST CANCER

Harold C. Urschel, Jr, MD
Chair of Cardiovascular & Thoracic Surgical
Research, Education & Clinical Excellence
Baylor University Medical Center;
Professor of Cardiovascular & Thoracic
Surgery
University of Texas
Southwestern Medical School
Dallas, Texas
THORACIC OUTLET SYNDROMES

Parsia A. Vagefi, MD
Department of Surgery
Massachusetts General Hospital
Harvard Medical School
Boston, Massachusetts
GALLSTONE ILEUS

Philbert Y. Van, MD
General Surgery Resident
Oregon Health & Science University
Portland, Oregon
*INITIAL EVALUATION AND RESUSCITATION
OF THE TRAUMA PATIENT*

Kyle J. Van Arendonk, MD
Resident in Surgery
Johns Hopkins University School of
Medicine
Baltimore, Maryland
ACUTE CHOLECYSTITIS

Jean-Nicolas Vauthey, MD, FACS
Professor of Surgery
Chief, Liver Service
MD Anderson Cancer Center
Houston, Texas
*MANAGEMENT OF CYSTIC DISEASE
OF THE LIVER*

Nirmal K. Veeramachaneni, MD
Assistant Professor of Surgery
Thoracic Surgery
University of North Carolina at Chapel Hill
Chapel Hill, North Carolina
ESOPHAGEAL STENTS

George C. Velmahos, MD, PhD, MSEd
John F. Burke Professor of Surgery
Harvard Medical School;
Chief
Division of Trauma, Emergency Surgery,
and Surgical Critical Care
Massachusetts General Hospital
Boston, Massachusetts
DAMAGE CONTROL OPERATION

Anthony C. Venbrux, MD
Professor of Radiology and Surgery
Director
Cardiovascular and Interventional
Radiology
George Washington University Medical
Center
Washington, DC
*TRANSHEPATIC INTERVENTIONS FOR
OBSTRUCTIVE JAUNDICE*

Charles M. Vollmer, Jr, MD
Attending Surgeon
Beth Israel Deaconess Medical Center
Assistant Professor of Surgery
Harvard Medical School
Boston, Massachusetts
UNUSUAL PANCREATIC TUMORS

Frank K. Wacker, MD
Professor of Radiology
Chairman
Department of Radiology
Hannover Medical School
Hannover, Germany
*ACUTE PERIPHERAL ARTERIAL AND BYPASS
GRAFT OCCLUSION: THROMBOLYTIC
THERAPY*

Marc K. Wallack, MD, FACS
Chief of Surgery
Metropolitan Hospital Center
New York, New York;
Professor of Surgery
Vice Chairman
Department of Surgery
New York Medical College
Valhalla, New York
CUTANEOUS MELANOMA

R. Matthew Walsh, MD
Professor of Surgery and Vice-Chair
Rich Family Distinguished Chair of
Digestive Diseases
Digestive Diseases Institute
Cleveland Clinic
Cleveland, Ohio
*LAPAROSCOPIC BYPASS FOR PANCREATIC
CANCER*

Grace J. Wang, MD
Assistant Professor of Surgery
Division of Vascular Surgery and
Endovascular Therapy
Department of Surgery
Hospital of the University of Pennsylvania
Philadelphia, Pennsylvania
*MANAGEMENT OF CHRONIC MESENTERIC
ISCHEMIA*

Jennifer Y. Wang, MD
Division of Colon and Rectal Surgery
Mayo Clinic
Rochester, Minnesota
*MANAGEMENT OF SOLITARY RECTAL ULCER
SYNDROME*

Thomas N. Wang, MD, PhD
Associate Professor of Surgery
Section of Surgical Oncology
University of Alabama at Birmingham
Birmingham, Alabama
*DUCTAL AND LOBULAR CARCINOMA IN SITU
OF THE BREAST*

Joshua A. Waters, MD
Department of Surgery
Indiana University School of Medicine
Indianapolis, Indiana
*INTRADUCTAL PAPILLARY MUCINOUS
NEOPLASMS OF THE PANCREAS*

Michael T. Watkins, MD, FACS, FAHA
Associate Professor of Surgery
Division of Vascular and Endovascular
Surgery
Department of Surgery
Massachusetts General Hospital
Harvard Medical School
Boston, Massachusetts
*FALSE ANEURYSMS AND ARTERIOVENOUS
FISTULAS*

Christopher M. Watson, MD
Clinical Assistant Professor of Surgery
University of South Carolina
Department of Trauma, Acute Care Surgery,
and Surgical Critical Care
Palmetto Health
Columbia, South Carolina
VENTILATOR-ASSOCIATED PNEUMONIA

Alexandra L.B. Webb, MD, FACS
Assistant Professor
Division of GI and General Surgery
Emory University School of Medicine
Atlanta VA Medical Center
Decatur, Georgia
LARGE BOWEL OBSTRUCTION

John A. Weigelt, DVM, MD
Associate Dean of Clinical Quality
Milt and Lidy Lunda/Charles Aprahamian
Professor of Surgery
Chief Division of Trauma/Critical Care
Medical College of Wisconsin
Milwaukee, Wisconsin
INJURIES TO THE SMALL AND LARGE BOWEL

Eric G. Weiss, MD
Vice Chairman
Department of Colorectal Surgery
Clinical Professor of Surgery
Florida International University School of
Medicine
Cleveland Clinic Florida
Weston, Florida
ANAL FISSURE

Edward E. Whang, MD
Associate Professor of Surgery
Department of Surgery
Brigham and Women's Hospital
Harvard Medical School
Boston, Massachusetts
PRIMARY SCLEROSING CHOLANGITIS

Eric B. Whitacre, MD, FACS
Director
Breast Center of Southern Arizona
Tucson, Arizona
*ROLE OF STEREOTACTIC BREAST BIOPSY IN
THE MANAGEMENT OF BREAST DISEASE*

D. Brandon Williams, MD
Assistant Professor of Surgery
Division of General Surgery
Vanderbilt University
Nashville, Tennessee
CURRENT TREATMENT OF ACHALASIA

Bruce G. Wolff, MD
Chair
Division of Colon and Rectal Surgery
Professor of Surgery
College of Medicine
Mayo Clinic
Rochester, Minnesota
SURGERY FOR POLYPOSIS SYNDROMES

Christopher Wolfgang, MD, PhD
Assistant Professor of Surgery and Oncology
Cameron Division of Surgical Oncology
Johns Hopkins University School of
Medicine and Johns Hopkins Hospital
Baltimore, Maryland
ISCHEMIC COLITIS

Patricia Wong, MD
Assistant Professor of Medicine
Division of Gastroenterology
Johns Hopkins School of Medicine
Baltimore, Maryland
HEPATIC ENCEPHALOPATHY

Douglas E. Wood, MD
Professor and Chief
Division of Cardiothoracic Surgery
Endowed Chair in Lung Cancer Research
University of Washington
Seattle, Washington
MEDIASTINAL MASSES

Bhupender Yadav, MD
Vascular & Interventional Radiology
Pediatric Radiology
Washington, DC
TRANSHEPATIC INTERVENTIONS FOR OBSTRUCTIVE JAUNDICE

Stephen C. Yang, MD
The Arthur B. and Patricia B. Modell
Professor in Thoracic Surgery
Chief of Thoracic Surgery
Surgical Curriculum and Clerkship Director
Director, Thoracic Oncology Program
Department of Surgery
Johns Hopkins Hospital
Baltimore, Maryland
PRIMARY TUMORS OF THE CHEST WALL

Charles J. Yeo, MD
Samuel D. Gross Professor and Chairman
Department of Surgery
Co-Director
Jefferson Pancreas, Biliary and Related
Cancer Center
Jefferson Medical College
Philadelphia, Pennsylvania
PERIAMPULLARY CANCER

Sam S. Yoon, MD
Division of Endocrine and Oncology
Surgery
Department of Surgery
Hospital of the University of Pennsylvania;
Department of Cancer Biology
University of Pennsylvania School of
Medicine
Philadelphia, Pennsylvania
MANAGEMENT OF SOFT TISSUE SARCOMAS

Christopher J. You, MD
Attending Surgeon
Assistant Program Director
Union Memorial Hospital
Baltimore, Maryland
GASTROESOPHAGEAL REFLUX DISEASE

Y. Nancy You, MD, MHSc
Assistant Professor
Department of Surgical Oncology
University of Texas MD Anderson Cancer
Center
Houston, Texas
SURGERY FOR POLYPOSIS SYNDROMES

Yassar Youssef, MD
Chief Resident Surgery
Department of Surgery
Sinai Hospital
Baltimore, Maryland
INTRAABDOMINAL INFECTIONS

Stéphane Zalinski, MD
Service de Chirurgie Digestive et Viscérale
Hôpital Saint-Antoine, Assistance Publique
Hôpitaux de Paris
Université Pierre et Marie Curie
Paris, France
MANAGEMENT OF CYSTIC DISEASE OF THE LIVER

Gideon A. Zamir, MD
Department of Surgery
Hadassah Medical Center
Jerusalem, Israel
TRANSPLANTATION OF THE PANCREAS

Christopher K. Zarins, MD
Chidester Professor of Surgery
Stanford University Medical Center
Stanford, California
MANAGEMENT OF TIBIOPERONEAL OCCLUSIVE DISEASE

Martha A. Zeiger, MD, FACS, FACE
Professor of Surgery, Oncology, Cellular and
Molecular Medicine
Chief, Endocrine Surgery
Co-Director of Basic and Translational
Research, Department of Surgery
Johns Hopkins University School of
Medicine
Baltimore, Maryland
MANAGEMENT OF THYROIDITIS

Michael E. Zenilman, MD
Clarence and Mary Dennis Professor
Department of Surgery
SUNY Downstate Medical Center
Brooklyn, New York
PREOPERATIVE ASSESSMENT OF THE ELDERLY PATIENT: FRAILTY

Michael A. Zimmerman, MD
Associate Professor of Surgery
University of Colorado, Denver
Aurora, Colorado
MANAGEMENT OF BUDD-CHIARI SYNDROME

PREFACE

The first edition of *Current Surgical Therapy* was published in 1984. The text has thus been in existence for 26 years. Each edition has included new features, and this one is no exception. The first and most obvious is that there are now two editors. My son, Andrew, has joined the effort. He is a general/transplant surgeon and brings a new perspective to *Current Surgical Therapy*. First and foremost, he is familiar with a new generation of younger surgeons, who have much to contribute to this book. The two of us now span several decades of surgeons who are potential contributors to this publication. When I finally step down as editor of *Current Surgical Therapy*, Andrew will be more than capable of carrying on the effort. The text continues to be perhaps the most popular surgical book in this country, and as long as it fulfills a need, we plan to continue its publication. In addition, it is a special privilege and honor for the two editors to be able to review contributions from surgeons around the country, and indeed from around the world, on what they believe is current surgical therapy for virtually all general surgical topics. It is an enjoyable task and keeps these two surgeons, who care for surgical patients and operate daily, current on all general surgical topics.

The tenth edition contains more than 270 chapters. This is twice the number of chapters in the first edition of *Current Surgical Therapy*. The length, however, has been held constant through the last few editions in an effort to keep the text at a manageable size. As with prior editions, nearly every chapter is written by a new author. All authors have contributed their specific thoughts on the current surgical therapy of the disease about which they are experts. Thus, to obtain a broader view of the topic, the reader should review the contributions of other experts in the last two or three editions of *Current Surgical Therapy*.

As with past editions, disease presentation, pathophysiology, and diagnosis are discussed only briefly, with the emphasis being on current surgical therapy. When an operative procedure is discussed, an effort has been made to contain brief and concise descriptions, with figures and diagrams when possible. *Current Surgical Therapy* is written for surgical residents, fellows, and fully trained surgeons in private practice or an academic setting. Many have told us that it is an excellent text to review prior to taking the general surgical boards or recertifying. In addition, medical students have given us feedback that they believe the text is of value to them. However, *Current Surgical Therapy* is not written principally for medical students. We believe a more classic surgical textbook with substantial sections on disease presentation, diagnosis, and pathophysiology is more appropriate for medical students.

We remain grateful to the many surgeons throughout the country, as well as the international surgeons, who participated in creating this textbook. Most of the potential authors that we solicit respond enthusiastically to the opportunity to present their expert views. Their efforts obviously are what make this textbook a success. In addition, Andrew and I could not have compiled this textbook without the herculean efforts of Ms. Irma Silkworth, who has been involved with virtually all of these editions, and Ms. Bonnie Bowling, my administrative assistant.

Both editors continue to enjoy and thrive in our chosen profession of general surgery. In recruiting medical students into our specialty over the last 40 years, I have used the statement, "If you pick a profession you love, you never have to work the rest of your life." In our view, that profession is general surgery.

Finally, we would like to dedicate this edition, as with others, to the surgical house staff at The Johns Hopkins Hospital, who are the "best of the best."

JOHN L. CAMERON, MD
ANDREW M. CAMERON, MD

CONTENTS

Trauma And Emergency Care

NATURAL ORIFICE TRANSLUMINAL ENDOSCOPIC SURGERY

THE ESOPHAGUS

ESOPHAGEAL FUNCTION TESTS

Vinay Chandrasekhara, MD, and Sanjay Jagannath, MD

MOTILITY DISORDERS

Esophageal motility disorders often present with patients reporting dysphagia, or difficulty swallowing. The act of swallowing is complex and depends on neural innervation, both motor and sensory, and coordinated muscular activity. Dysphagia often results when there is an interruption in this complex neuromuscular process.

Swallowing disorders are broadly classified into *oropharyngeal* or *esophageal,* depending on their anatomic site of origin. Obtaining a detailed dysphagia history is often helpful in determining whether the disorder is oropharyngeal or esophageal. However, differentiation and diagnosis of an esophageal dysmotility condition require further diagnostic testing.

The focus of this chapter is to review diagnostic testing modalities for esophageal motility diseases and provide a brief overview of commonly encountered motility disorders.

DIAGNOSTIC TESTS FOR ESOPHAGEAL DISEASES

Radiographic Imaging

Radiographic tests of the esophagus include conventional fluoroscopic studies or cross-sectional imaging. An esophagram, or barium swallow, is often performed as a biphasic examination in which double-contrast and single-contrast techniques are used. Because the act of swallowing is a dynamic process, a complete examination of the esophagus should include video, or a cine, recording to better assess oropharyngeal function and esophageal motility. Indications for a videoesophagram are listed in Table 1.

A properly conducted videoesophagram allows the physician to comment on oropharyngeal function, morphology of the esophagus, esophageal motility, the appearance of the mucosal surface, evaluation of the gastroesophageal junction and the presence or absence of spontaneous gastroesophageal reflux, and the efficiency of secondary wave clearance. A videoesophagram is sensitive for detecting certain motility disorders, such as achalasia (94%) and scleroderma (100%); however, it is relatively insensitive for detecting most other motility disorders.

At times, it can be difficult to decide whether to obtain a radiographic imaging test prior to endoscopy or to proceed directly to esophagogastroduodenoscopy. A videoesophagram is recommended as the initial diagnostic test in conditions such as suspected cricopharyngeal bar, esophageal web, small diverticula, subtle Schatzki ring, early achalasia, and complex esophageal stricture, where the esophagram will provide a "road map" to guide the endoscopist.

Cross-sectional imaging with computed tomography is helpful for evaluating extraluminal esophageal disease, including the staging of esophageal carcinoma and evaluation for esophageal trauma. CT will identify esophageal changes, such as thickening of the esophagus, but it is not recommended as the primary imaging modality for evaluation of mucosal disease or motility disorders. Magnetic resonance imaging has the capability to produce high-quality multiplanar images without using ionizing radiation, but it has limited usefulness for evaluating esophageal diseases because of motion artifact and long imaging times.

Endoscopy

Endoscopic evaluation is necessary to confirm or establish a diagnosis for most esophageal disorders, particularly when surgery is being considered. A list of indications for standard upper endoscopy has been recommended by the American Society for Gastrointestinal Endoscopy. A modified list of these indications that applies to surgical practice is listed in Table 2.

Esophageal Anatomy

Endoscopic evaluation for esophageal disorders begins with a good view of the vocal cords and aryepiglottic folds, which can appear inflamed in patients with chronic gastroesophageal reflux. The upper esophageal sphincter (UES) consists of the cricopharyngeus muscle and is best seen on final withdrawal of the endoscope. Upon entering the esophagus, the mucosa can be carefully inspected for signs of mucosal inflammation or luminal irregularities such as esophageal webs, rings, or strictures. It is also important to assess whether the esophagus appears distended or atonic, which is suggestive of a motility disorder.

At the level of the aortic arch, the striated muscle of the upper esophagus transitions to smooth muscle in the distal half of the esophagus. Patients with dysphagia should have random biopsies sampled from the distal and proximal esophagus to evaluate for eosinophilic esophagitis, particularly if the endoscopic examination demonstrates a corrugated "feline" esophagus, with multiple concentric rings and/or linear furrows (Figure 1). In patients with long-standing gastroesophageal reflux disorder (GERD), the squamocolumnar junction proximal to the lower esophageal sphincter (LES) should be carefully inspected for signs of Barrett esophagus (Figure 2), which appears as a salmon-colored discoloration in the distal esophagus. If this is

TABLE 1: General indications for videoesophagram

Globus sensation

Dysphagia

Nasal regurgitation

Noncardiac chest pain

Suspected postoperative complications

TABLE 2: Indications for upper endoscopy

A. Upper abdominal symptoms that persist despite an appropriate trial of medical therapy
B. Upper abdominal symptoms associated with other alarm signs or symptoms suggesting worrisome organic disease (e.g., anorexia, weight loss, gastrointestinal bleeding) or in patients older than 45 years
C. Patients older than 45 years with new onset of abdominal symptoms (regardless of alarm features)
D. Dysphagia or odynophagia
E. Persistent or recurrent esophageal reflux symptoms despite appropriate therapy (includes typical symptoms of GERD and/ or extraesophageal symptoms of GERD, such as aspiration, unexplained laryngeal symptoms, unexplained chronic cough or asthma, and recurrent sinusitis)
F. Other conditions in which the presence of upper GI pathology might modify other planned management
G. For confirmation and/or histologic confirmation of radio-graphic lesions (e.g., ulcers, strictures, masses)
H. Upper gastrointestinal bleeding
I. To assess acute injury after caustic ingestion
J. Removal of foreign body
K. Removal of selected polypoid lesions
L. Placement of feeding or drainage tubes (e.g., oral, percutane-ous endoscopic gastrostomy, and nasojejunal feeding tubes)
M. Dilatation of stenotic lesions
N. Palliative management of malignant dysphagia (e.g., stent placement)
O. Management of achalasia (e.g., botulinum toxin injection, pneumatic balloon dilatation)

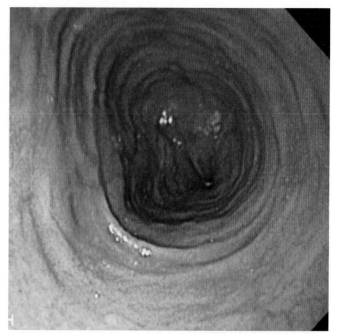

FIGURE 1   Eosinophilic esophagitis. Mucosal rings consistent with "trachealization" of the esophagus.

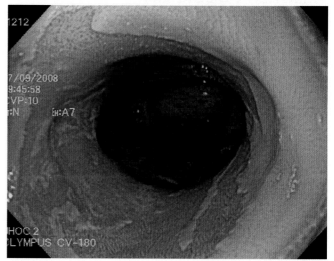

FIGURE 2   Salmon-colored mucosal changes of the esophagus seen in BE.

detected on endoscopy, the extent of the lesion should be noted to classify the disorder as *short segment* (<3 cm) or *long segment* (>3 cm), with multiple four-quadrant biopsies obtained to assess for dysplasia.

The LES consists of a ring of thickened smooth muscle at the gastroesophageal junction. Once the endoscope has entered the stomach, the endoscopist will note if the gastric wall is poorly distensible and typically performs endoscopic retroflexion to assess the cardia and gastroesophageal junction. This allows for identification of a hiatal hernia, assessment of the competency of the LES, and evaluation for an esophageal malignancy infiltrating into the cardia, which is not always seen in forward view (Figure 3).

Endoscopic Therapy

Several endoscopic therapies can be used at the time of endoscopy. Dilatation with transendoscopic balloons, or with serial dilators over an endoscopically placed guidewire, can be used to dilate obstructing lesions such as benign or malignant strictures, Schatzki ring, or esophageal web. Botulinum toxin (Botox) can be injected into the LES if achalasia, or incomplete relaxation of the LES, is suspected. In cases where superficial esophageal abnormalities are identified (e.g., dysplastic tissue), ablative techniques such as radiofrequency ablation, cryotherapy, and endoscopic mucosal resection may be useful. Such ablative modalities should be conducted only in well-defined clinical scenarios.

Endoscopic Ultrasonography

Endoscopic ultrasonography (EUS) is an imaging modality that combines endoscopy and 5 to 12 MHz ultrasonography. It is routinely used for a transmural evaluation of the esophagus. EUS is the most sensitive imaging modality for evaluating the different layers of the esophageal wall, particularly for infiltrative or malignant disease. EUS is routinely combined with fine needle aspiration to sample irregularities that are seen deeper than the mucosal layer, and it can be used for sampling adjacent structures, including lymph nodes.

The most common scenario in which EUS is useful is in the evaluation of patients with malignant dysphagia. The accuracy of EUS for T and N staging of esophageal cancer is between 80% and 85%, and it remains the standard of care of locoregional staging (Figure 4).

Substaging of T1 tumors (e.g., in Barrett esophagus) is possible with EUS, which may have clinical significance regarding therapeutic options. Abnormal motility occurs in several gastrointestinal diseases, and EUS can be used in biomechanical and motility studies. Three-dimensional EUS, elastography, and strain-rate imaging are new techniques that may be promising in imaging the gastrointestinal tract and in the examination of gut motility. However, it should be emphasized that, at this time, EUS plays a limited role, if any, in the management of nonobstructive causes of esophageal dysmotility.

Esophageal Manometry

Once structural causes of dysphagia have been ruled out, the evaluation should focus on motility abnormalities. Esophageal manometry is considered the gold standard for assessing esophageal motor function. It is the only modality that can define the pressure profile of peristalsis and allow measurement of LES pressure.

Conventional manometry uses three to eight sensors, positioned at various points throughout the esophagus, to measure pressure

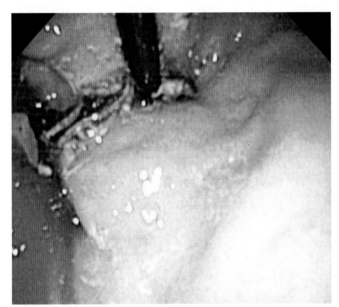

FIGURE 3 Retroflexed view of gastric cardia showing submucosal tumor infiltration from esophageal cancer.

changes that help assess the contractile pattern of the esophagus. Recent advances in transducer technology allow for a larger number of sensors to be placed closely together, thereby capturing pressure measurements as a continuum throughout the esophagus. This ability to measure pressure changes throughout the esophagus, along with improvements in software capturing and graphic data presentation with topographical display methodology, have led to the exciting development of high-resolution manometry. This new technology offers the ability to simplify the procedural setup, eliminate motion artifact, simplify the ability to interpret data, and allow for a more sophisticated interpretation of esophageal motility. Indications for esophageal manometry are summarized in Table 3.

Technical Considerations

For conventional manometry, a solid-state or water-perfused catheter system is used. The manometry catheter is swallowed until all the sensor sites are in the stomach, and the catheter is then pulled back in increments of 0.5 cm to 1 cm to measure the resting pressure of the LES, esophageal body, and upper esophageal sphincter (Figure 5). Once the resting pressures have been calibrated, the catheter is positioned across the entire esophagus to record pressure changes during swallowing. The contraction and relaxation of the UES, the body of the esophagus, and the LES are recorded with 10 consecutive swallows of a 5 mL bolus of water (Figures 6 to 9), and those values are compared to standardized normal values (Tables 4 to 6). Plotting the pressure values with the passage of the water bolus allows for detection of abnormal peristalsis and sphincter dysfunction. These patterns form the basis of esophageal dysmotility conditions.

Recent advances in manometry technology have led to the development of high-resolution manometry, which uses a catheter-based system with multiple sensors, typically 1 cm or less apart, at the level of the UES and LES. Ideally, the sensors should span from the pharynx to the stomach, thereby eliminating the need to pull back the catheter to measure resting pressures, such as with conventional manometry. Again, pressure measurements are recorded both in the resting phase and during 10 consecutive swallows. The information is then presented as a topographic display (Figure 10).

DIAGNOSTIC TESTS FOR GASTROESOPHAGEAL REFLUX

Acid exposure in the esophagus is measured by using an intraluminal pH probe with one of two methods: either an intraluminal tube with a nasopharyngeal catheter or a wireless Bravo pH probe (Medtronic, Minneapolis, MN). Both methods provide the physician with similar data, particularly relating to the amount of time the esophagus is exposed to acid reflux. When this information is correlated with a symptom log, it is possible to determine whether the patient's symptoms are related to acid exposure within the esophagus. This

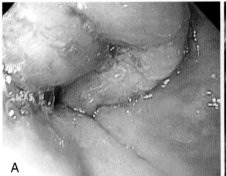
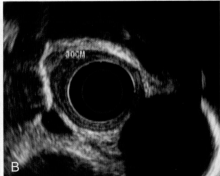
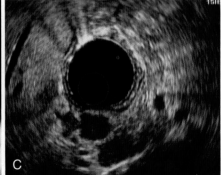

FIGURE 4 **A,** Endoscopic picture of malignant esophageal stricture. **B,** EUS image showing T3 lesion. **C,** Malignant celiac lymphadenopathy.

information is commonly expressed by using six standard parameters (Table 7) to calculate a DeMeester score, also referred to as a *composite pH score*. A score below 14.72 (95th percentile of normal patients) is considered physiologic, whereas a score greater than 14.72 is considered abnormal. Acid exposure in the esophagus may be physiologic, and it is recorded according to the position of the patient (supine or erect) and the relation of acid exposure to meals, particularly postprandial reflux (Figure 11); however, pH monitoring can also be used while a patient is on therapy to determine if there is adequate acid suppression with proton-pump inhibitor (PPI) treatment. The data collected from each individual's test are compared to normal values derived from data from healthy volunteers. The Bravo probe is often the patient-preferred method for pH monitoring because it is placed

at the time of upper endoscopy and does not require an extended time with a nasopharyngeal catheter. The Bravo probe is placed 5 cm above the LES and wirelessly transmits data to a recorder worn by the patient.

Esophageal Impedance

Impedance monitoring is a method used to measure bolus transport by measuring the resistance to electrical conductivity of the esophagus and its contents. Impedance measurement works by using low AC voltage to apply an electrical potential between two electrodes on a catheter separated by an isolator. The circuit can be closed by the surrounding material spanning these electrodes. Because air, liquid, and esophageal mucosa have unique impedance characteristics, it is easy to identify the material that is bridging the electrodes. Air is resistant to current flow and thus has a high impedance value, and liquid has a low impedance value (Figure 12). Esophageal tissue has an indeterminate impedance range and is used as a baseline during monitoring. By having multiple electrodes along a catheter system, identifying changes in impedance makes it possible to determine the direction of bolus transport within the esophagus, and it allows detection of a bolus that has cleared the esophagus (Figures 13 and 14).

Multichannel intraluminal impedance (MII) is a new technology that incorporates impedance, transducers for pressure measurement for manometric readings, and a pH probe into one catheter. As a result, MII is utilized for the same indications as esophageal manometry as well as for detection and measurement of acid and nonacid gastroesophageal reflux.

TABLE 3: Indications for esophageal manometry

1. Dysphagia—for the assessment of functional disorders after structural causes have been ruled out
2. Noncardiac chest pain—to assess for esophageal dysmotility as a cause of symptoms
3. Diagnosis or confirmation of a suspected motility disorder
4. Preoperative assessment of esophageal motility prior to planned surgery
5. Postoperative assessment—to detect response to surgery or confirmation of response to treatment, or to assess the cause of persistent symptoms after surgery

---

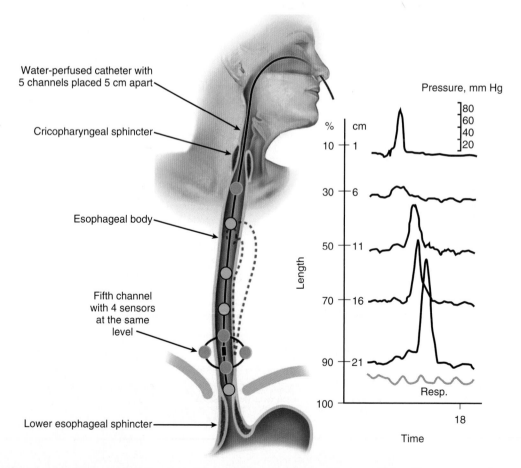

FIGURE 5 Esophageal manometry: a water-perfused or solid-state catheter is positioned in the esophagus. The sensors are 5 cm apart and, in this catheter, there are four radially placed sensors at the same level to measure the LES.

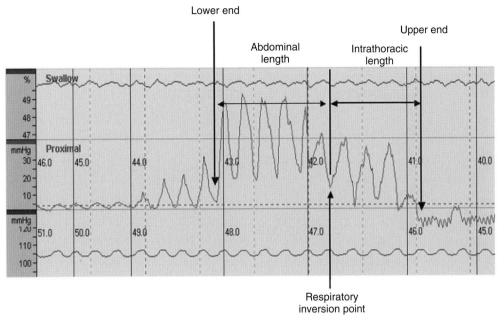

FIGURE 6 A normal LES. The total length is divided into a thoracic and abdominal segment at the respiratory inversion point. Baseline pressures in the stomach are measured at the end-expiratory phase of respiration. Note that the pressure in the thoracic esophagus is negative.

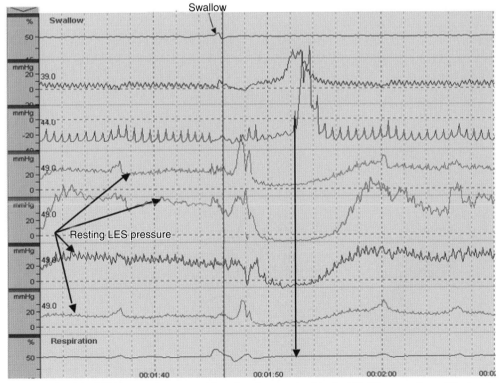

FIGURE 7 A relaxation study of the LES. Four probes are positioned at the same level in the LES. After a swallow of 5 mL water, the sphincter pressure drops to baseline, demonstrating complete relaxation. The uppermost probe, 5 cm above the LES, shows a contraction response to a swallow.

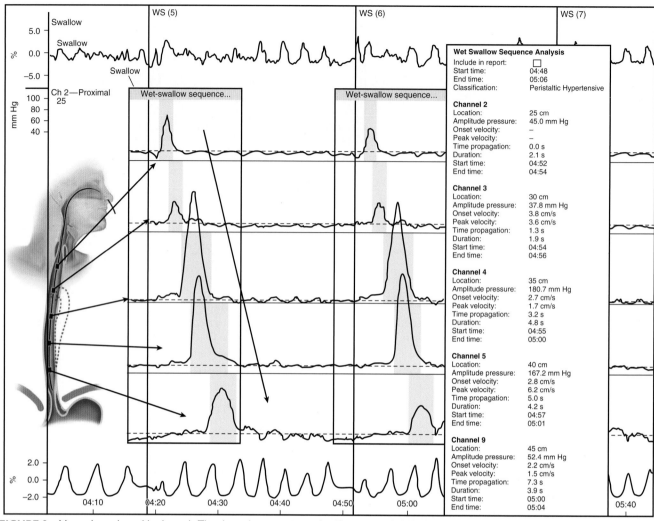

Wet Swallow Sequence Analysis
Include in report: ☐
Start time: 04:48
End time: 05:06
Classification: Peristaltic Hypertensive

Channel 2
Location: 25 cm
Amplitude pressure: 45.0 mm Hg
Onset velocity: –
Peak velocity: –
Time propagation: 0.0 s
Duration: 2.1 s
Start time: 04:52
End time: 04:54

Channel 3
Location: 30 cm
Amplitude pressure: 37.8 mm Hg
Onset velocity: 3.8 cm/s
Peak velocity: 3.6 cm/s
Time propagation: 1.3 s
Duration: 1.9 s
Start time: 04:54
End time: 04:56

Channel 4
Location: 35 cm
Amplitude pressure: 180.7 mm Hg
Onset velocity: 2.7 cm/s
Peak velocity: 1.7 cm/s
Time propagation: 3.2 s
Duration: 4.8 s
Start time: 04:55
End time: 05:00

Channel 5
Location: 40 cm
Amplitude pressure: 167.2 mm Hg
Onset velocity: 2.8 cm/s
Peak velocity: 6.2 cm/s
Time propagation: 5.0 s
Duration: 4.2 s
Start time: 04:57
End time: 05:01

Channel 9
Location: 45 cm
Amplitude pressure: 52.4 mm Hg
Onset velocity: 2.2 cm/s
Peak velocity: 1.5 cm/s
Time propagation: 7.3 s
Duration: 3.9 s
Start time: 05:00
End time: 05:04

FIGURE 8   Normal esophageal body study. The channels are positioned at 5 cm intervals. With each wet swallow of 5 mL water, there is a peristaltic pressure response. A software program calculates the height, duration, and propagation of each swallow response.

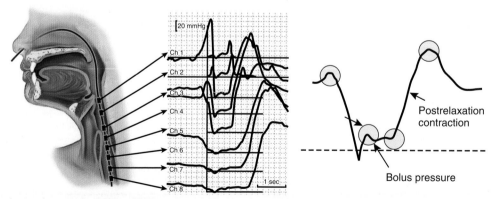

FIGURE 9   Normal cricopharyngeal sphincter (CPS) swallow study using an eight-channel catheter. The channels are 1 cm apart. In the diagram on the left, two channels are in the pharynx, three are in the CPS, and three are in the esophagus. On swallowing, the resting CPS pressure falls precipitously (diagram on the right). This pressure drop is followed by a brief bolus pressure rise before a postrelaxation contraction. Channel 5 demonstrates that the relaxation of the lower part of the sphincter occurs before the relaxation of the upper part.

TABLE 4: Normal LES parameters in 50 healthy volunteers (after Zaninotto and DeMeester, 1988)

LES Measurements	Mean	SD	Median	Maximum	Minimum	PERCENTILE 2.5	5
Pressure (mm Hg)	14.87	5.14	13.8	25.6	5.2	6.1	8
Abdominal length (cm)	2.18	0.72	2.2	5	0.8	0.89	1.1
Overall length (cm)	3.65	0.68	3.5	5.5	2.4	2.4	2.6

TABLE 5: Normal values for swallow responses in the esophageal body

Medians (5th and 95th percentiles)

	Wet Swallows	Dry Swallows
Amplitude (mm Hg)		
Level I	88 (40–177)	74 (26–154)
Level II	40 (14–94)	28 (14–74)
Level III	76 (30–164)	52 (26–142)
Level IV	93 (38–180)	61 (20–148)
Level V	93 (36–190)	78 (22–172)
Duration (sec)		
Level I	2.3 (1.5–4.3)	2.3 (1.4–3.9)
Level II	3.1 (1.8–4.8)	2.8 (1.0–4.5)
Level III	3.3 (2.4–5.2)	3.1 (1.8–4.6)
Level IV	3.6 (2.6–5.7)	3.4 (2.0–5.6)
Level V	3.7 (2.4–7.0)	3.6 (2.4–6.4)
Slope (mm Hg/sec)		
Level I	99 (22–222)	72 (25–153)
Level II	30 (9–61)	22 (6–61)
Level III	52 (20–117)	40 (14–96)
Level IV	66 (25–120)	45 (14–102)
Level V	62 (23–120)	47 (16–104)
Propagation speed (cm/sec)		
Level I	2.4 (1.5–4.6)	2.8 (1.6–6.2)
Level II–III	2.8 (1.9–6.2)	3.1 (1.9–8.3)
Level III–IV	3.8 (1.9–8.3)	4.5 (1.8–8.3)
Level IV–V	2.6 (1.3–8.3)	3.5 (1.7–12)
Level I–IV	2.9 (2.2–3.7)	3.3 (2.3–4.4)
Level I–V	2.9 (2.1–4)	3.4 (2.2–5)

From Costantini M, Bremner RM, Hoeft SF, et al: Normal esophageal motor function: a manometric study of 134 healthy subjects, *Gastroenterology* 104:A1407, 1993.

TABLE 6: Normal swallow responses for the cricopharyngeal sphincter

	Median	5th Percentile	95th Percentile
Length of UES (cm)	5.0	4.1	5.1
Resting pressure (mm Hg)	61.0	40.0	87.0
Bolus pressure (mm Hg)	13.3	11.2	15.7
Pharyngeal pressure (mm Hg)	52.0	46.4	56.5
Minimal residual pressure (mm Hg)	0.5	−2.3	3.2
Maximal residual pressure (mm Hg)	11.3	8.9	14.5
Relaxation time (sec)	0.58	0.546	0.60
Time of initiation of relaxation (sec)			
Upper UES	−0.10	0.19	−0.43
Lower UES	−0.28	−0.401	−0.19

DISORDERS OF ESOPHAGEAL MOTILITY

Achalasia

Achalasia, the most common motility disorder, is defined as failure or incomplete relaxation of the LES accompanied by an absence of peristalsis in the esophageal body. The LES is hypertensive in approximately 50% of patients with achalasia. The cause of achalasia remains unknown, but the hallmark pathologic feature is a decreased number of inhibitory ganglion cells. An esophagram is a good screening test, and the classic findings are a dilated esophagus and tapering at the gastroesophageal junction that creates a "bird's beak" appearance (Figure 15). However, a diagnosis of achalasia cannot be made without first ruling out pseudoachalasia—any condition that masquerades as achalasia, such as malignancy—with upper endoscopy and careful evaluation of the gastroesophageal junction. Manometry, which is used to confirm the diagnosis, classically demonstrates aperistalsis with an incomplete or failed relaxation of the LES after a swallow (Figure 16). Medical options for treatment of achalasia include calcium channel blockers, nitrates, or sildenafil. Endoscopic options include botulinum toxin injections into the LES and pneumatic dilatation, and surgical options include a surgical myotomy.

Hypertensive Lower Esophageal Sphincter

A patient with an LES pressure above the 95th percentile of normal and symptoms of dysphagia or noncardiac chest pain is deemed to have a hypertensive LES. The exact value will differ according to the method used for measurement, but this condition can only be diagnosed with manometry. The distinguishing features between hypertensive LES and achalasia are listed in Table 8.

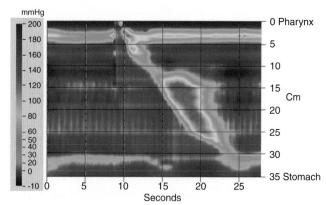

FIGURE 10   High-resolution manometry demonstrating a normal swallow. *(Courtesy John O. Clarke III, MD.)*

TABLE 7: Measured parameters during 24-hour esophageal pH monitoring

1. Percent total time pH <4
2. Percent upright time pH <4
3. Percent supine time pH <4
4. Number of reflux episodes
5. Number of reflux episodes ≥5 minutes
6. Longest reflux episode (in minutes)

Mechanically Defective Lower Esophageal Sphincter

An LES is considered to be mechanically defective when one or more of the components is abnormal (pressure <6 mm Hg, total length <2 cm, abdominal length <1 cm). The chance of gastroesophageal reflux is 74% when one component is defective, 75% with two defective components, and 92% with three defective components.

Diffuse Esophageal Spasm

Diffuse esophageal spasm (DES) is an uncommon condition that accounts for 3% to 10% of all motility abnormalities. DES is characterized by uncoordinated contractions of the esophagus that typically result in symptoms of chest pain, dysphagia, or both. The esophagram may be abnormal, but manometry is usually required to make the diagnosis (Figure 17); however, the manometric findings often do not correlate with symptoms. This disorder is typically characterized by disordered rather than high-pressure esophageal contractions.

Medical treatment options include nitrates and sildenafil, and reports in the medical literature show that tricyclic antidepressants may be useful for the treatment of noncardiac chest pain. Using PPIs to treat concomitant gastroesophageal reflux may be helpful. A long myotomy for refractory diffuse esophageal spasm can be effective in up to 70% of patients.

Hypercontractile "Nutcracker" Esophagus

Hypercontractile, or "nutcracker," esophagus is a manometric diagnosis defined by one of the following characteristics: 1) high-pressure contractions (>180 mm Hg) or 2) the duration of swallow responses exceeding 7 seconds in patients who have either chest pain or dysphagia (Figure 18). The peristaltic contractions propagate normally in the esophagus, and the LES relaxes appropriately. Diltiazem has been shown to lower the mean distal peristaltic pressures and has a tendency to reduce chest pain; however, these results are not reliably reproducible. As in DES, nitrates, sildenafil, PPIs, and tricyclic antidepressants may be useful for the treatment of noncardiac chest pain.

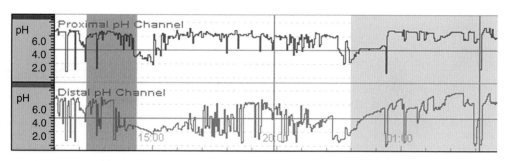

FIGURE 11   Esophageal pH measurement. Dual pH probes (placed 15 cm apart) have recorded the 24-hour acid exposure to the esophagus. Acid exposure is abnormal at both sites. The software program has reported six parameters of measurement and has calculated a mathematical (DeMeester) score from the components, which is abnormal for the upper probe recording (lower probe results not included here). Post *Pr*, postprandial; *HH:MM*, hours and minutes.

Reflux Table - Proximal

	Total	Meal	Supine	Upright	PostPr	Other
Duration of period (HH:MM)	21:11	00:30	06:59	14:11	03:59	02:00
Number of refluxes	40	1	6	35	11	9
Number of long refluxes (>5 [min])	3	0	1	3	0	0
Duration of longest reflux (min)	30	0	8	30	1	1
Time pH <4 ([min])	74	0	14	60	5	4
Fraction time pH <4 ([%])	5.9	0.2	3.4	7.1	2.1	4.1

DeMeester score, proximal
Total score = 21.3, DeMeester normals less than 14.72 (95th percentile)

Ineffective Esophageal Motility

Ineffective esophageal motility is characterized by either decreased distal esophageal peristaltic wave pressures, with amplitudes greater than 30 mm Hg, or an absence of esophageal contractions in greater than 30% of wet swallows (Figure 19). A distinguishing feature between ineffective esophageal motility and achalasia is that the resting LES pressure is typically decreased or absent in ineffective

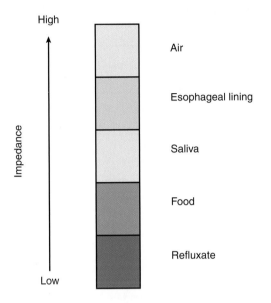

FIGURE 12   Diagram illustrating the range of impedance measurements with different refluxates.

esophageal motility. Systemic conditions, such as scleroderma, can be associated with ineffective esophageal motility. Unfortunately, in esophageal scleroderma, there are no standard treatment options besides PPIs and lifestyle modifications. Patients are advised to eat small meals, remain standing or upright after eating, chew food well, and take acid-reducing medications.

Nonspecific Esophageal Motor Disorder

Nonspecific esophageal motor disorder refers to an esophageal motility disorder that does not have features of a named motility disorder. These abnormalities are often not associated with dysphagia and are not specific. Examples of frequently encountered nonesophageal motor disorders are triple-peaked and retrograde contractions. Systemic diseases such as diabetes mellitus, hypothyroidism, and amyloidosis can be associated with nonspecific esophageal motor abnormalities.

Hiatal Hernia

Although technically a structural disorder, manometric features of a hiatal hernia are well described. The LES is displaced proximally from the diaphragm so that two pressure profiles, also known as a "double hump," with an intervening plateau can be seen (Figure 20).

SUMMARY

The diagnosis of a surgically amenable esophageal disorder can be made from a careful history along with diagnostic testing. Often several diagnostic tests need to be performed to accurately determine whether a patient is a good surgical candidate and to preoperatively evaluate the type and extent of disease to determine the type of surgery required. The management of complex esophageal disorders requires the multidisciplinary effort of a gastroenterologist, a radiologist, and a surgeon.

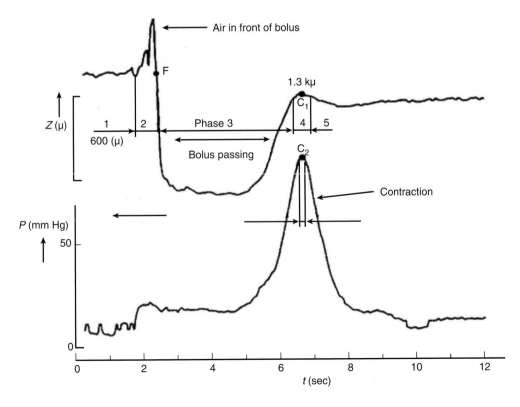

FIGURE 13   The upper diagram illustrates the pattern of impedance when a bolus is swallowed. An initial impedance rise signifies the swallowing of air prior to the bolus passage. The duration of the bolus in the esophagus is demonstrated. The lower diagram is a manometry recording taken simultaneously and demonstrates the esophageal contraction.

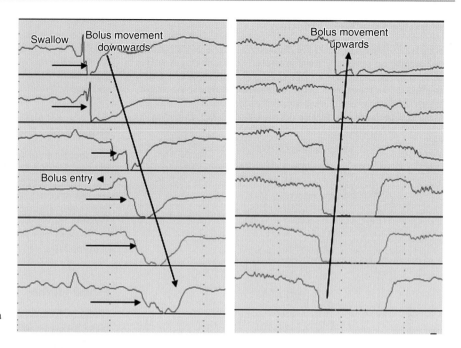

FIGURE 14   Impedance study showing anterograde and retrograde movements of a swallowed bolus.

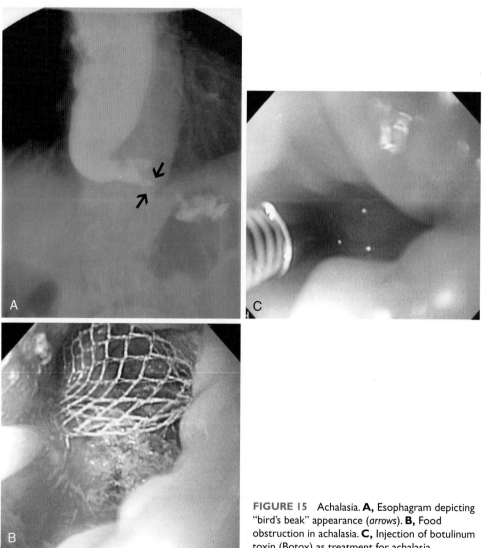

FIGURE 15   Achalasia. **A,** Esophagram depicting "bird's beak" appearance (*arrows*). **B,** Food obstruction in achalasia. **C,** Injection of botulinum toxin (Botox) as treatment for achalasia.

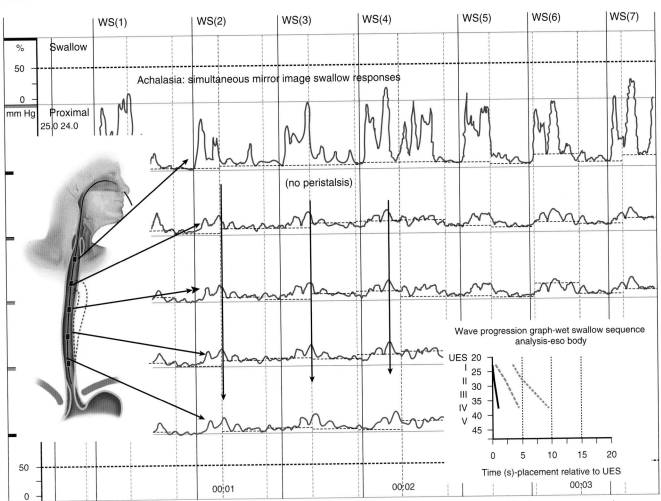

FIGURE 16   Achalasia. A swallow study in the esophageal body demonstrates mirror-image swallow responses (simultaneous responses). *eso,* esophageal; *s,* seconds.

TABLE 8: Distinguishing features between a hypertensive LES and achalasia

	Hypertensive LES	Achalasia
Relaxation of LES	Usual	Fails or incomplete
Negative intrathoracic pressure	+	Usually positive
Peristaltic swallow responses	+	Never

LES, lower esophageal sphincter

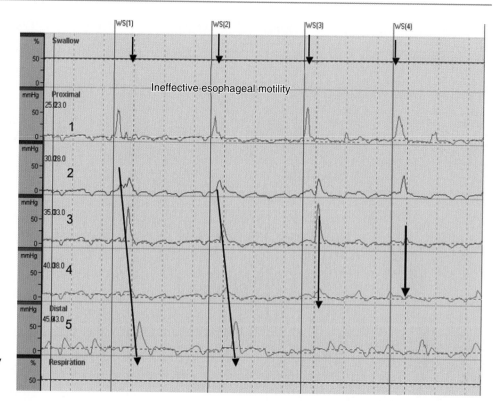

FIGURE 17 Diffuse esophageal spasm. More than 30% of the swallow responses are simultaneous, and the remaining responses are peristaltic.

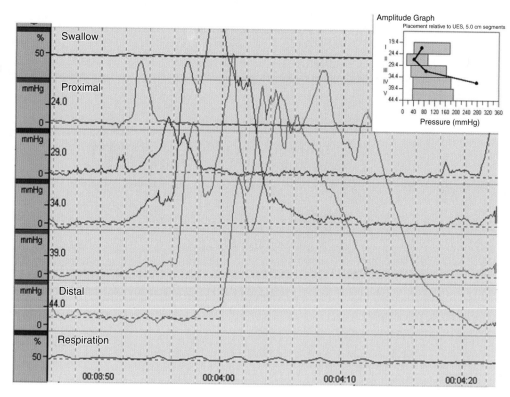

FIGURE 18 A hypercontracting esophageal body is designated a "nutcracker" esophagus if the pressures are >180 mm Hg and if the patient complains of chest pain or dysphagia.

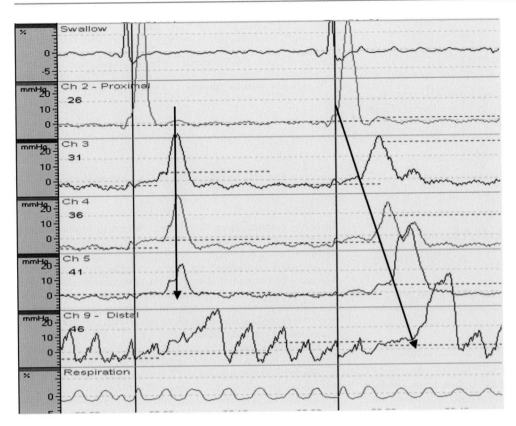

FIGURE 19 Ineffective esophageal motility. Thirty percent or more of the contractions are less than 30 mm Hg, and/or 30% of the contractions are nonpropulsive.

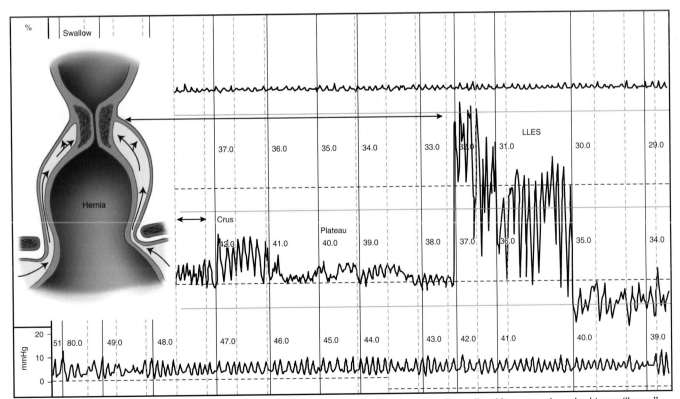

FIGURE 20 Manometric features of a hiatal hernia. There is a "double hump," a hiatal pressure "hump," and lower esophageal sphincter "hump," with an intervening plateau of pressure. The diagram on the left demonstrates the origin of the two humps from the crura and the intrinsic lower esophageal sphincter.

SUGGESTED READINGS

Bremner CG, DeMeester TR, Bremner RM, et al: *Esophageal motility testing made easy*, St Louis, 2001, Quality Medical Publishing.

Bremner CG, DeMeester TR, Huprich J, et al: *Esophageal disease and testing*, London, 2005, Taylor and Francis.

Gockel I, Lord RVN, Bremner GC, et al: The hypertensive lower esophageal sphincter: a motility disorder with manometric features of outflow obstruction, *J Gastrointest Surg* 7:692, 2003.

Schuster MM, Crowell MD, Koch KL: *Schuster atlas of gastrointestinal motility in health and disease, part II: motility tests for the gastrointestinal tract*, ed 2, London, 2002, BC Decker.

Tutuian R, Castell DO: Clarification of the esophageal function defect in patients with manometric ineffective esophageal motility: studies using combined impedance-manometry, *Clin Gastroenterol Hepatol* 2:230, 2004.

GASTROESOPHAGEAL REFLUX DISEASE

Richard F. Heitmiller, MD, and Christopher J. You, MD

HISTORY

Over the last 60 years, huge strides in the understanding and treatment of gastroesophageal reflux disease (GERD) have been made. These include discovering the association of hiatal hernia with reflux symptoms, defining the pathogenesis of reflux symptoms, considering esophagitis with reflux, developing new and more effective medical treatments, defining the safety and effectiveness of open surgical antireflux procedures, and introducing laparoscopic surgical methods. Now, gastroesophageal reflux is referred to even in the lay public realm as GERD, and at least one antireflux medication is in the list of the top 10 prescribed medications worldwide.

Despite the progress made in the understanding and treatment of GERD, controversy regarding *surgical* treatments remains. Bias against surgical treatments persists with many referring physicians. Unacceptable variations are often seen in outcome, depending on the operating surgeon, and there is a lack of agreement on whom should be considered for surgery, what approach to use, and when to proceed.

PREOPERATIVE EVALUATION

The objectives of the preoperative evaluation shown in Table 1 are to 1) confirm the presence of reflux, 2) define esophagogastric anatomy, and 3) rule out any motility disorders of *both* the esophagus and stomach. The complete list of options to fulfill all the preoperative objectives listed above is long and rigorous. It is up to the individual surgeon to decide how detailed the workup needs to be; however, the surgeon must be certain of the preoperative findings or else risk an adverse outcome and an unhappy patient. As a rule, patients who are referred for potential reoperative surgery need a comprehensive evaluation beforehand.

Confirm the Presence of Gastroesophageal Reflux Disease

Symptoms are the most common tip-off that a patient has GERD. This is especially true when a patient has the classic symptoms of heartburn (pyrosis): regurgitation, a salty salivary hypersecretion known as *waterbrash,* and dysphagia. Symptoms of chest pains, vague indigestion, or tiredness from esophagitis-induced anemia are much less specific for GERD. Patients may have respiratory symptoms, including dyspnea on exertion, cough, wheezing, hoarseness, and asthma. Respiratory symptoms can occur with gastrointestinal (GI) symptoms or on their own.

Antireflux medications are now so effective that many internists use a medication trial as a means of confirming GERD after symptoms suggest the diagnosis. Medications sometimes become less effective with time, however; and beware the patient who never responds to medical therapy at all, as this is often indicative that the symptoms are not from GERD.

Radiographic studies that use contrast esophagography are readily available and are an excellent screening test for GERD because such studies define esophagogastric (EG) anatomy and can identify reflux with moderate accuracy. An experienced radiologist who knows specifically that GERD is the suspected diagnosis can increase the accuracy of this test. Acidification of the swallowed contrast (Bernstein test) is also reported to increase the radiographic diagnosis of reflux. Upper GI endoscopy with esophageal mucosal biopsies that demonstrate esophagitis supports the clinical diagnosis of GERD. The gold standard for identifying, quantifying, and correlating reflux events with clinical symptoms is the pH probe study. This test is not always available nor is it tolerated in all patients, but it is helpful information to have if you can get it.

Define Esophagogastric Anatomy

Important anatomic features that should be screened for are the presence or absence of hiatal hernia; type of hiatal hernia; length of esophagus, if there are concerns of "short esophagus"; and mucosal pathology to determine whether Barrett mucosa, dysplasia, or cancer is present. Contrast swallowing studies and endoscopy generally will provide these anatomic data. Computed tomography of the chest and upper abdomen can give more specific information if there is a

TABLE 1: Preoperative evaluations

1. Confirm the presence and severity of reflux
   a. Reflux symptoms
   b. Clinical response to medications
   c. Contrast esophagography
   d. Esophagoscopy
   e. pH probe studies
2. Define esophagogastric anatomy
   a. Contrast esophagography
   b. Esophagoscopy with biopsy
   c. Chest CT
3. Rule out esophagogastric motility disorders
   a. Manometry
   b. Video contrast swallowing studies
   c. Nuclear medicine esophageal and gastric emptying studies

TABLE 2: Surgical indications and contraindications

1. Indications
   a. Patient wishes to control symptoms without medication
   b. Medical therapy is no longer effective
   c. GERD with prominent regurgitation component
   d. Paraesophageal hiatal hernia
   e. Complications of reflux
      i. Esophagitis
      ii. Bleeding
      iii. Stricture
      iv. Mucosal ulceration
2. Contraindications
   a. Elevated body mass index
   b. Barrett mucosa with HGD or adenocarcinoma
   c. Comorbidities with high surgical risk
   d. Portal hypertension

complex hiatal hernia, a concern about diaphragmatic anatomy, or suspicion of a mass.

Rule Out Motility Disorders

An occult motility disorder of the esophagus or stomach can result in a potentially disastrous outcome after antireflux surgery, especially if a complete fundoplication has been used. Esophageal motility problems may result in heightened or continued pain and dysphagia after fundoplication. Occult poor gastric emptying leads to gas bloat syndrome after antireflux surgery. Esophageal manometry accurately defines esophageal and lower esophageal sphincter (LES) function; however, this test is not universally available and is often not tolerated by patients. Radionuclide gastric emptying studies accurately document and measure the degree of gastric dysmotility. In our experience, a video contrast swallowing study, specifically one used to look at EG motility, has proved to be a well-tolerated and accurate screening test for occult motility disorders.

INDICATIONS

Selection of patients for antireflux surgery has become much easier with the dramatic improvement in medical management. There are two reasons for this. The first is the general rule that if medical antireflux therapy does not produce at least short-term improvement in patient symptoms, there is little hope of success with surgery. The second reason is that more aggressive and effective medical treatments have significantly reduced the prevalence of reflux-induced esophageal damage. Indications for surgery are listed in Table 2. These include patients who, although successfully treated medically, wish to have surgery to stop antireflux medications; patients whose symptoms have recurred despite medications; and patients with a severe component of regurgitation symptoms, complications of reflux (persistent esophagitis, bleeding, ulceration, stricture), and a paraesophageal component to the hiatal hernia.

Patients with Barrett esophagus (BE) are discussed in this section but could be included under contraindications as well. Those who advocated early and aggressive surgical treatment of antireflux patients with BE did so because it was hypothesized that medical management did not prevent, and could possibly even promote, the progression of BE to high-grade dysplasia (HGD) and adenocarcinoma. Although results with surgery have demonstrated success in treating symptoms and decreasing the length of BE in some patients,

it has not been proven that surgery is superior to medical management to prevent the development of dysplasia and cancer.

CONTRAINDICATIONS

The list of contraindications is less well defined. Patients with a markedly elevated body mass index probably would do better with weight-loss measures instead of antireflux surgery. High-risk surgery patients and those with elevated portal venous pressure should stay on medical management.

For young adult patients who want to end successful medical management, we encourage them to consider waiting on surgery. Antireflux surgery, although very effective, does not necessarily last indefinitely; the complexity of later surgery increases, and its effectiveness decreases with multiple attempts.

Patients with HGD should not be treated with antireflux surgery because of its imminent invasive malignant potential. Instead, patients should be considered for close follow-up, mucosal ablation, or esophagectomy.

SURGICAL TREATMENT OPTIONS

GERD results from incompetent function of the LES. It is remarkable that medical therapy works as well as it does given that it does nothing to address LES function. The objective of surgery, on the other hand, is to re-create a competent LES and thereby stop GERD. This is accomplished by *fundoplication*. Historically, the type of fundoplication has been associated with the name of the surgeon responsible for its development, use, and promotion. Examples are Nissen (complete, 360 degree wrap), Belsey (partial, 270 degree wrap), Hill (fundoplication and posterior gastropexy), and Toupet (anterior partial wrap). Not to diminish the huge impact of these antireflux surgery pioneers, we feel that it is clearer to describe antireflux surgery by incision approach and whether a complete or partial fundoplication is used. Regardless of whether a chest, abdominal, or laparoscopic approach is used, all share the same objectives. These are to reduce the hiatal hernia (if present) and thereby return the EG junction back into the abdomen, tighten the hiatus, protect the vagus nerve, and create a competent LES by means of fundoplication.

Chest Approach

Advantages of a chest (thoracic) approach include the following:

1. Patient weight is not a significant issue. Heavier patients do not pose as much of a technical challenge as they would using a laparotomy.
2. When operating on the EG junction region, it is technically easier to extend the surgery through the diaphragm into the abdomen than it is to be in the abdomen and work up into the chest.
3. A patient with a short esophagus can be managed with a Collis lengthening procedure to restore the EG junction into the abdomen.
4. The chest provides an adhesion-free approach in patients with previous open upper abdominal surgery.

Technique

A left thoracotomy through the seventh interspace usually works well. Always look at a patient's chest film to assess the level of the left hemidiaphragm to ensure that the incision does not need to be higher or lower: if it is too low, the left hemidiaphragm is in the way; too high, and it is hard to work in the region of the hiatus. Encircle the esophagus approximately midway between the inferior pulmonary vein and the hiatus. This point could be higher if there is a large hiatal hernia.

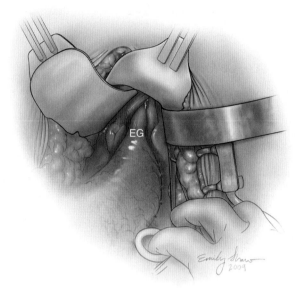

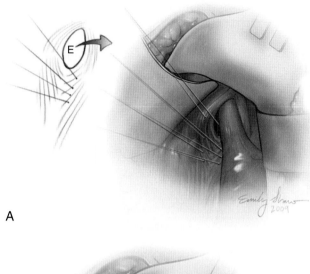

A

FIGURE 1 The exposure of the esophageal hiatus is demonstrated after mobilizing the liver and retracting it laterally. The hiatus is exposed and the esophagogastric junction is reduced into the abdomen. The distal 5 cm of esophagus and proximal stomach are circumferentially mobilized. *(Courtesy Emily Shaw.)*

Protect the vagus, and stay out of the right side pleura—it is closer than you think. Mobilize the distal esophagus, and enter the peritoneum at the hiatus anteriorly. If there is a hiatal hernia, open the sac and debride the thoracic component. Mobilize the proximal stomach along both the lesser and greater curvature, resect the EG junction fat pad, and place the sutures to tighten the crus, but do not tie them (sutures are posterior to the esophagus). Add a fundoplication, tie the crural sutures, and close over a chest tube. The classic transthoracic fundoplication is the partial, 270 degree wrap as described and promoted by Belsey.

Abdominal Approach

Advantages of an open abdominal approach include the following:

1. Laparotomy is a less painful incision than thoracotomy.
2. Abdominal exploration is possible. Patients with GI symptoms may have associated pathology that can be assessed at surgery.
3. Complete fundoplication is easily performed.
4. Associated procedures may be added, such as highly selective vagotomy or pyloric drainage.

Technique

An upper midline abdominal incision is used, and a nasogastric (NG) tube is placed. we prefer to use the upper hand retractor; one blade attachment lifts the left costal margin, and the other holds the mobilized left tip of the liver up toward the right shoulder to expose the hiatus. It is possible to work around the unmobilized liver, but we believe that the exposure described removes a great deal of variability from the surgical equation and optimizes exposure (Figure 1).

The proximal 5 cm of stomach is circumferentially mobilized by dividing short gastric and lesser curvature vessels. Dissection is kept close to the stomach wall on the lesser curvature to protect the vagus nerve. The lower 4 to 5 cm of esophagus is circumferentially mobilized, and the EG junction fat pad is removed. The left and right crus of the hiatus are identified (Figure 2), the EG junction is reduced into the abdomen, and the hiatus is narrowed with interrupted sutures placed posterior to the esophagus. These are tied.

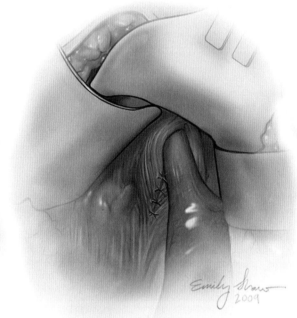

B

FIGURE 2 **A,** Esophageal crural sutures are placed to narrow the hiatus. Sutures are placed posterior to the esophagus and progressively angled to displace the esophagus (*E*) anteriorly and slightly to the left. **B,** The completed crural repair shows a snug hiatus with the esophagogastric junction in the abdomen without tension. *(Courtesy Emily Shaw.)*

With a Maloney bougie in place, a 360 degree fundoplication is constructed (Figure 3). We have found that larger bougies, 50 to 56 Fr, work best. The fundoplication must be over the lower esophagus, not the stomach, and is designed to be 2.5 to 3.0 cm in length. Each fundoplication stitch incorporates the esophageal muscular wall to minimize the chance for wrap migration. The bougie is removed, the NG tube is left behind, and the laparotomy is closed.

Laparoscopic Approach

Advantages of the minimally invasive approach include the following:

1. The patient experiences less discomfort than with open incisions.
2. There is no need to leave in an NG tube postoperatively.
3. A shorter hospital stay and faster return to full activity can be expected.

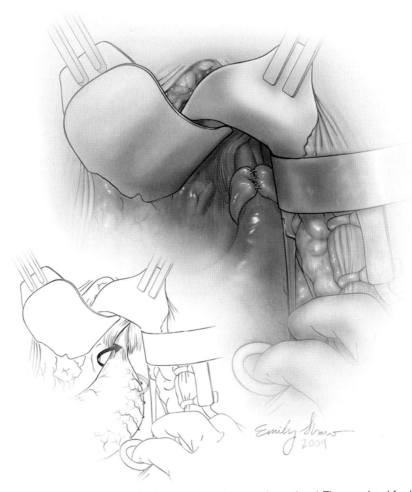

FIGURE 3   Fundoplication is performed by passing the fundus posterior to the esophagus *(inset)*. The completed fundoplication should measure 2.5 to 3.0 cm in length. Note the position of the fundal wrap over the distal esophagus, proximal to the esophagogastric junction. *(Courtesy Emily Shaw.)*

4. The approach provides access to explore the abdomen.
5. Associated procedures can be performed.
6. Complete or partial fundoplication is possible.

Technique

Patient positioning and port placement are key factors to consider for the operation. Patients are positioned in the lithotomy position so that the surgeon can stand in the midline at the foot of the bed. Both arms are tucked at the patient's sides. The assistant stands at the patient's left, and standard laparoscopic monitoring is used, with two screens placed on either side of the patient's shoulders.

Issues to consider regarding port placement are maintaining normal hand-eye axis, length of the instruments and camera, camera size, and suture method. We use a 10 mm port for the camera in a midline supraumbilical position and a 10 mm port for the surgeon's right hand at the left subcostal margin, midclavicular line. A 5 mm port for the surgeon's left hand is placed along the right subcostal margin, just medial to the mid-clavicular line. A 5 mm trocar for the assistant is then inserted at the left subcostal margin, anterior axillary line. Finally, another port is placed near the xiphoid and removed to allow for placement of a liver retractor. After port placement, the patient is placed at a 30 to 45 degree reverse Trendelenberg position.

Laparoscopic surgical objectives are the same as with the open abdominal methods: the hiatus is dissected out, the EG junction is reduced into the abdomen, and the lower esophagus and proximal stomach are circumferentially mobilized in preparation for fundoplication. Dissection is started at the angle of His. With care, this can often be done bluntly and only occasionally requires the use of an energy device.

Once the left crus is identified, attention is then turned to just below the spleen, where division of the gastrosplenic ligament is begun. It is imperative that the surgeon, whose left hand is retracting the stomach medially, and the assistant, whose instrument is retracting the gastrosplenic ligament laterally, work together to provide gentle tension. The lesser sac is entered by blunt dissection, and the short gastric vessels are divided by using the ultrasonic dissector to the angle of His.

Care must be taken that the active blade of the ultrasonic dissector comes fully across the vessel, that the tip of the blade is not touching another vessel, and that undue tension is not placed on the tissues. Instead of lifting up on the tissues with the ultrasonic dissector, a slight torquing motion of the ultrasonic dissector tends to give the right amount of additional tension and facilitates a clean, bloodless dissection. Remember to stay approximately 1 cm off the greater curvature of the stomach.

Attention is turned to the medial aspect of the stomach, where the pars flaccida is opened. The gastrohepatic ligament is then divided up to the right crus. Remember that a replaced left hepatic artery should be identified and preserved. The phrenoesophageal membrane is divided using careful application of the ultrasonic dissector, and the plane between the medial border of the right crus and esophagus is then developed. Finally, remaining attachments of the gastrophrenic ligament are divided.

The left and right crus are identified. Approximately 4 cm of esophagus are circumferentially mobilized, and clear visualization of the retroesophageal window is established. Posterior closure of the crura is performed using nonabsorbable suture. Typically, three to four sutures are required. For widely dilated hiatal openings, some have suggested placing anterior crural sutures, and others have used a bioprosthetic mesh. Key considerations here are that 1) the bioprosthetic mesh is not used to bridge the left and right crus but rather to reinforce the approximated crura, and 2) the mesh should span three sides of the hiatus, and never circumferentially.

After ensuring sufficient gastric mobility, the stomach fundus is then passed behind the esophagus. The fundus is elevated on either side of the esophagus in a back-and-forth motion to allow for a floppy closure that is clearly above the GE junction and over the esophagus. A 50 to 56 Fr bougie is inserted, and three nonabsorbable sutures, each incorporating the esophageal muscular wall, are placed to complete the fundoplication. The bougie and liver retractor are removed, the pneumoperitoneum is reversed, ports are removed, and all skin incisions are closed.

POSTOPERATIVE MANAGEMENT

Open Surgical Cases

After surgery, patients are kept NPO, on intravenous fluids, with NG drainage. Intravenous GI prophylaxis is used. The addition of metachlopramide (10 mg every 6 hours), started immediately after surgery, hastens return of GI function and thereby shortens length of stay by several days. The NG tube is removed on postoperative day 1 or 2. Patients are kept NPO until there is evidence of return of GI function, which is usually postoperative day 3 to 5. The diet is then advanced within 1 day to soft solids, and patients are discharged home. Projected discharge day is postoperative day 4 to 5. On discharge, patients are kept on oral GI prophylaxis and metachlopramide (10 mg orally twice per day). Both medications are to be stopped approximately 3 to 4 weeks after discharge.

Laparoscopic Surgical Cases

Patients are admitted to the floor, and medications for pain and nausea are administered as appropriate. Patients are not continued on proton-pump inhibitor therapy. Clear liquids are given the day of surgery, and the patient is advanced to a soft diet just before discharge, typically on postoperative day 1.

Redo Antireflux Surgery

Patients with recurrent symptoms after prior antireflux surgery represent a challenging problem. The preoperative evaluation must be complete and must clearly demonstrate the anatomic (i.e., paraesophageal hernia) or physiologic (i.e., recurrent reflux) process; it must adequately correlate the abnormality with the presenting symptoms and identify an abnormality that can be corrected with redo surgery. There is a limitation to the number of times that redo antireflux surgery can be safely attempted, so reoperative procedures must be carefully considered. Do not blindly explore a patient if you cannot identify the source of the patient's symptoms or correlate them with your findings. When offering redo surgery to patients, they must understand the risks and reduced expectations (compared with first-time surgery) for a favorable outcome. Consider all of the incisional options to reduce the impact of previous adhesions.

At the time of surgery, the plan should be to take down and redo the antireflux surgery to ensure everything is again set in place for a favorable outcome. Despite the technical challenges of redo surgery, the postoperative management is much the same as for first-time surgery.

Outcome

Mortality rates less than 1% are reported for antireflux surgery, regardless of approach. Redo antireflux surgery, even though potentially much more complicated, also has a similarly low mortality rate. Operative complications include splenic injury with bleeding; esophageal, gastric, or other visceral injury with leak; and pneumothorax (with laparoscopic approach). These complications are reported in up to 2% of patients. Many patients experience early postoperative satiety and some dysphagia to solid foods. These generally resolve within 6 weeks. Relief of symptoms occurs in 90% of patients following surgery, but success rates for redo surgery decrease by 10% or more with each surgery. Symptoms of reflux should be better immediately upon resumption of oral intake. Patients do not need to "heal" for the fundoplication to work, and failure rates of complete fundoplication of 1% per year are quoted.

Length of hospital stay is 4 to 7 days for open surgery, and recovery is approximately 4 weeks. Laparoscopic surgery results in length of stay and recovery times approximately half that of open cases.

SUGGESTED READINGS

DeMeester TR, Bonavina L, Albertucci M: Nissen fundoplication for gastroesophageal reflux disease: evaluation of primary repair in 100 consecutive patients, *Ann Surg* 204:9–20, 1986.

Hill LD: An effective operation for hiatal hernia: an eight-year appraisal, *Ann Surg* 166:681–692, 1967.

Hunter JG, Smith CD, Branum GD, et al: Laparoscopic fundoplication failures: patterns of failure and response to fundoplication revision, *Ann Surg* 230:595–604, 1999.

Jobe BA, Wallace J, Hansen PD, et al: Evaluation of laparoscopic Toupet fundoplication as a primary repair for all patients with medically resistant gastroesophageal reflux, *Surg Endosc* 11:1080–1083, 1997.

Skinner DB, Belsey RHR: Surgical management of esophageal reflux and hiatal hernia: long-term results with 1,030 cases, *J Thorac Cardiovasc Surg* 53:33–54, 1967.

Watson DI, Jamieson GG: Antireflux surgery in the laparoscopic era, *Br J Surg* 85:1173–1184, 1998.

Endoluminal Approaches to Gastroesophageal Reflux Disease

Mehrdad Nikfarjam, MD, PhD, and Jeffrey L. Ponsky, MD

THERAPY OVERVIEW

Laparoscopic fundoplication is currently the most effective therapy for long-term management of gastroesophageal reflux disease (GERD). There is, however, increasing interest in the role of endoluminal therapies for treatment of patients with GERD who wish to minimize proton pump inhibitor (PPI) use without undergoing a major operative intervention.

Various endolumninal therapies have previously been described. All aim to prevent or reduce gastroesophageal reflux by one or more of the following: 1) reduction of transient lower esophageal sphincter (LES) relaxation, 2) increase in baseline lower esophageal length, 3) decrease in distal esophageal luminal diameter, 4) re-creation of the angle of His, 5) formation of a gastroesophageal valve, or 6) reduction of compliance of the gastric cardia and fundus.

Indications and Contraindications

It is estimated that 30% to 40% of patients with GERD do not respond to standard doses of a PPI. In a high percentage of cases, symptoms recur shortly after the cessation of therapy. Patients with documented GERD confirmed by 24-hour pH monitoring and manometry are potential candidates for endoluminal therapy, which appears particularly suited to those for whom the morbidity and mortality associated with antireflux surgery appear overly prohibitive. It may also be especially appropriate when surgical intervention is likely to be extremely difficult due to previous abdominal operations or following failed antireflux surgery.

All patients require a diagnostic endoscopy to assess for complications of gastroesophageal reflux and exclude other diagnoses. Currently, most endoluminal techniques are limited to patients with GERD symptoms without significant esophagitis (grade 2 or higher), esophageal stricture, esophageal motility disorders, biopsy-proven Barrett esophagus, or a hiatal hernia greater than 3 cm. In some studies, obesity (based on a body mass index >35 kg/m^2) has been used as an exclusion criterion for an endoluminal approach, but this does not appear to be a true contraindication.

Technique

Several endoluminal therapies have been previously described. Some techniques have been abandoned due to adverse effects or clear lack of efficacy. Currently approved endoluminal therapies for GERD involve either mechanical suturing in the region of the gastroesophageal (GE) junction or application of radiofrequency (RF) energy to this area. Although conscious sedation is adequate in some cases, these therapies tend to be performed with the patient under general anesthesia because treatment times can be prolonged and it minimizes risks of aspiration. In the case of full-thickness suturing techniques, prophylactic antibiotics are recommended to reduce the incidence of postprocedure leukocytosis and fever.

Endoluminal Gastroplication

Several endoluminal suturing techniques for plication at the level of the GE junction have been trialed with variable success. This includes Esophyx (EndoGastric Solutions, Redmond, Wash.), the Bard EndoCinch procedure (Bard Endoscopic Technologies, Billerica, Mass.), and the NDO Full-Thickness Plicator (NDO Medical, Mansfield, Mass.). Each technique is described here; however, Esophyx is the main plication device currently available for the treatment of GERD.

Esophyx

Esophyx is an instrument used for transoral incisionless fundoplication (TIF). The procedure is performed under general anesthesia with the patient in the left lateral decubitus position.

The system consists of a disposable device that rides axillary over a standard endoscope. The procedure is usually performed by two physicians; one operates the endoscope, and the other operates the device. The endoscope is threaded through the device, and both are passed into the stomach. Using a built-in vacuum invaginator, the device is able to partly engage the distal esophagus at the squamocolumnar junction (SCJ) and reduce a small hiatal hernia when present. This also allows the distal esophagus to be partly invaginated into the stomach. Gastric tissue is drawn downward between the esophagus and the body of the instrument with a helix retractor portion of the device engaging the fundus and used to mold a valve (Figure 1).

Polypropylene H-fasteners are then passed full thickness across the tissue to create a 2 to 5 cm long serosa-serosa flap. This process is performed posteriorly and continues anteriorly to create an omega-shaped valve of approximately 200 to 300 degrees circumference, attaching the gastric fundus to the anterior and left lateral wall of the esophagus slightly below the esophagogastric (EG) junction. The device is then withdrawn, and the newly created valve is examined.

The procedure generally takes 60 to 90 minutes to complete. TIF was initially designed to construct an anterior 270 degree partial fundoplication; studies in progress are assessing the efficacy of 360 degree full-thickness plication.

EnodoCinch Suturing System

The EndoCinch system consists of a suturing capsule, a knot pusher, and a suture cutter attached to a standard endoscope. The procedure is performed with the patient in a left lateral decubitus position.

An overtube is initially inserted into the esophagus using a standard endoscope; the device is attached to the endoscope and inserted though the overtube with the capsule at the tip positioned 1 to 2 cm below the SCJ. Suction is applied to capture a fold of tissue, a needle is deployed through it, and a suture is passed through the needle with a T-tag to allow commencement of plication. Afterward, the suction is turned off and the device is withdrawn.

The suture tag is reloaded into the needle, and the device is reinserted and rotated to take a second bite of tissue 1 to 2 cm away from the first bite. The device is then withdrawn, an extracorporeal knot is formed, and the scope, with its knot pusher and cutter attachment, is inserted. Sutures are secured together using a ceramic plug, and the suture is cut (Figure 2).

Generally, four separate plications between 0.5 and 2.5 cm below the SCJ are performed with the scope inserted and removed for each complete plication; these sutures are not generally full thickness. This procedure requires 60 minutes or more to complete.

The NDO Full-Thickness Plicator

The NDO Full-Thickness Plicator is a suturing device used to restore the valvular mechanism of the LES, altering the angle of His and

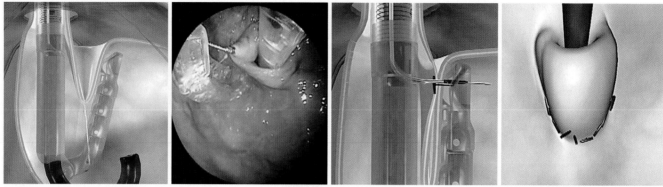

FIGURE 1   Esophyx system (EndoGastric Solutions) demonstrating sequence of fundoplication. Gastric tissue is drawn downward between the esophagus and the body of the instrument with a helix retractor. Fastners are then passed across the tissue, and the process is repeated several times (completed plication shown).

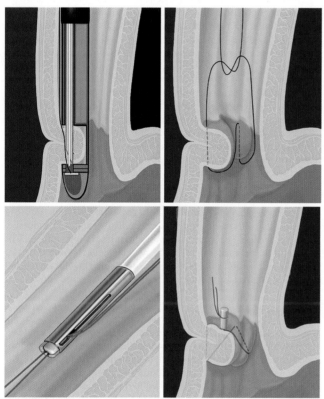

FIGURE 2   EndoCinch (Bard Endoscopic Solutions) suturing system. Two separate endoscopic "bites" of tissue are taken and secured with the device, creating an endoluminal plication.

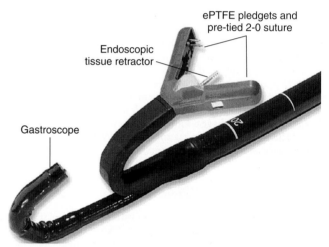

FIGURE 3   Full-thickness plicator. Note helical endoscopic tissue retractor and pre-tied sutures and pledgets.

reducing compliance of the cardia and fundus. The procedure is generally performed under conscious sedation.

The plicator consists of a reusable instrument, a single-use helical tissue retractor, and a suture-based implant. The device has a 6 mm channel through which a gastroscope is inserted. An initial endoscopy is performed and a Savary guidewire is passed, over which a 54 Fr dilator and 60 Fr overtube are passed into the esophagus; the dilator and guidewire are then removed, and the plicating device is inserted (Figure 3).

The tissue retracting component of the device engages the gastric mucosa 1 cm distal to the SCJ and is advanced up to the serosal layer, under endoscopic visualization, in the retroflexed position. The arms of the device are then closed, and an implant that consists of a 2-0 polypropylene suture between two polytetrafluoroethylene bolsters and two titanium retention bridges is deployed, creating

a full-thickness plication. The device is disengaged and removed, which creates a plication in the gastric cardia.

Generally, a single plication is performed, but some have advocated placement of two transmural sutures in the anterior gastric cardia for possible greater efficacy. The procedure generally takes less than 20 minutes to complete.

Radiofrequency Energy

The Stretta system (Mederi Therapeutics, Greenwich, Conn.) gained FDA approval for use in 2000. The procedure is often performed with the patient under conscious sedation in the left lateral decubitus position. The therapy uses RF energy to induce thermal injury to the LES, resulting in scarring and collagen deposition at the GE junction. This reduces the compliance of the LES and decreases the frequency of transient LES relaxations, possibly by interruption of vagal afferent signals to the brainstem.

The Stretta system consists of a catheter connected to a four-channel RF generator (Figure 4). A 30 Fr bougie tip, a balloon surrounded by four radially oriented nickel-titanium 22-gauge needle electrodes, and delivery sheath forms the catheter system. The device also has one channel for suction and one for irrigation.

A standard endoscopy is performed to measure the the SCJ. A guidewire is inserted though the working channel, and the endoscope is then removed. Under fluoroscopic guidance, the surgeon passes the catheter system over the guidewire into the stomach, and the device is withdrawn and positioned approximately 2 cm above the SCJ. The balloon is inflated to a pressure of 2.5 psi, and the needle electrodes are deployed into the mucosa, submucosa, and muscularis, where RF energy is delivered to the tissues for 90 seconds via the generator. A feedback thermostat maintains a temperature of 85° C within the esophageal musculature, and continuous delivery of chilled water through the catheter systems maintains a mucosal temperature below 50° C.

Next, the needle electrodes are withdrawn, the balloon is deflated, the catheter is rotated 45 degrees, and the process is repeated with a total of eight lesions created in a radial manner. The catheter is advanced at 0.5 cm increments, and the procedure is repeated at various levels, extending from 2 cm below to 1.5 cm above the SCJ, with a total of six sets of treatments (Figure 5).

At the end of the procedure, the treated region is inspected with repeat passage of the endoscope to confirm the correct treatment site. The entire procedure takes approximately 40 minutes to complete.

Other Methods

Bulking methods, or injection of synthetic substances or devices into the GE junction, have been trialed but abandoned because of significant complications or clear lack of efficacy. These include Enteryx (Boston Scientific, Natick, Mass.), Gatekeeper Reflux Repair (Medtronic, Minneapolis, Minn.), and Plexiglas systems.

Outcomes

The outcomes of endoluminal therapies for GERD vary according to the type of procedure, but no technique to date has the same proven long-term effectiveness as antireflux surgery. There are no

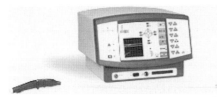

FIGURE 4 Stretta RF generator and catheter system (Mederi Therapeutics).

well-designed randomized controlled trials that have compared the effectiveness of these therapies with antireflux surgery.

The Esophyx system is emerging as an effective endoluminal therapy with lasting results. A multicenter European trial consisting of 86 patients treated by Esophyx has been reported. Two patients sustained upper esophageal perforations at the time of device insertion, and the procedure was abandoned. Another patient had intraluminal bleeding that was treated successfully by endoscopic clipping. Otherwise, adverse events were mild and included abdominal pain (15%), sore throat (8%), and nausea (8%). At 12 months, 73% of patients in this series had clinically significant improvement in GERD-related quality-of-life scores, and 81% had complete cessation of PPI use. Overall, 56% were cured based on symptom reduction and discontinuation of PPI use. The esophageal acid exposure time was significantly reduced or normalized in 61% of patients, with significant increases in resting LES pressures. Two-year follow-up was provided for 14 patients in the series at one of the centers, and none in this group had any adverse effects. Heartburn was eliminated in 93%, daily PPIs were eliminated in 71%, and 79% of patients overall achieved complete cure or remission. Intact reconstructed valves were noted in all cases on endoscopy. In 10 patients with a small hiatal hernia, the herniation was eliminated in six (60%). North American study of the Esophyx system is limited to a report of eight patients, and moderate effectiveness was shown.

The safety and effectiveness of the EndoCinch device has been assessed in a number of studies, and it appears to be effective in reducing GERD symptoms at short-term follow-up. There are a few reports of significant postprocedural bleeding, but overall the procedure appears to be associated with minimal side effects. One small, randomized, sham versus EndoCinch study reported in abstract form showed fewer episodes of heartburn and reduced esophageal acid exposure compared with the sham-treated patients. Promising results were also reported in a prospective case series of 85 patients, with resolution of heartburn (52%) and regurgitation (77%) assessed 2 years after intervention. Only one patient (1.1%) experienced significant dysphagia, managed by suture removal. Reports from other centers have not been so promising due to suture loss in the majority of patients. In a single-center study involving 70 patients, 80% continued to have symptoms or required significant PPI use after 18 months

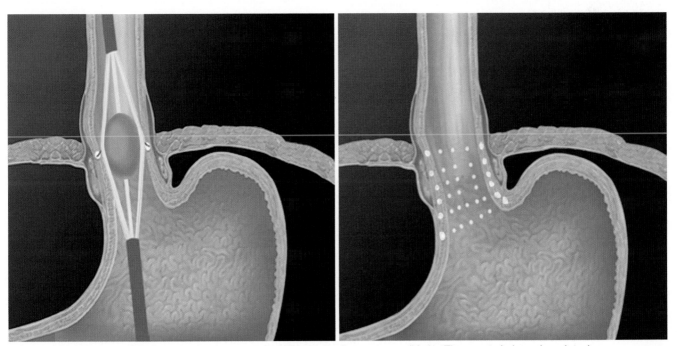

FIGURE 5 RF energy delivery systems to the LES using the Stretta system (Mederi Therapeutics); the end result is shown.

of follow-up evaluation. No residual sutures were visible on endoscopy in 26% of these cases.

Favorable short-term results have been obtained with the NDO Full-Thickness Plicator. The procedure is generally safe. However, FDA reports of adverse effects include pneumoperitoneum, pneumothorax, airway compromise, and distal esophageal perforation. The most common complications are mild pharyngitis and epigastric pain that almost always resolves spontaneously within a week of the procedure. In a sham-controlled, randomized trial, 78 patients received plication and 81 patients underwent sham procedure. At 12 months, 65% of intervention patients showed greater than 50% improvement in GERD health-related quality-of-life scores compared with 20% in the sham group. However, only 57% percent of patients achieved complete PPI cessation compared with 25% of sham patients. In addition, median time of esophageal acid exposure was significantly reduced in the plication group. There is also some evidence from both 3-year and 5-year follow-up studies that report maintenance of GERD symptom improvement and reduction in PPI use after full-thickness plication. Recent studies suggest that two plications, rather than one, may increase the efficacy of this procedure.

The Stretta procedure has been well studied, with evidence demonstrating effective symptom control at short- and mid-term follow-up. The procedure is generally safe. In an open-label trial, there was a 9% complication rate, but all were self-limited. These included fever (without leukocytosis), transient chest pain or dysphagia, sedation-induced hypotension, allergy to topical anesthesia, and superficial mucosal injury from catheter insertion. In FDA reports of postmarketing events, an esophageal perforation after forceful postprocedure emesis and a death related to cardiac arrhythmia and aspiration pneumonia were reported. In a controlled trial of 64 patients from eight centers, randomized into a sham group (n = 29) and active treatment (n = 35), significant improvements in symptom control were noted in the Stretta group at 6 months. There was no difference, however, in median esophageal acid exposure. Favorable mid-term results after the Stretta procedure have been observed in a study of 77 patients at 2 years postintervention. Sixty percent of patients either no longer required PPI therapy or had their dose reduced by at least 50%. In a nonrandomized study comparing the Stretta procedure with laparoscopic fundoplication, no differences were observed between the procedures with regard to reflux and dyspepsia symptoms. However, PPI use was eliminated in 97% of patients following laparoscopic surgery compared with 58%

after the Stretta procedure. More recent 3-year follow-up studies confirm that the Stretta procedure is not very effective in providing long-term symptom control.

SUMMARY

The minimally invasive management of GERD continues to evolve with the advent of endoluminal therapies. This is particularly important given the high number of patients who depend on PPI therapy but are either reluctant or unable to undergo antireflux surgery. Both endoscopic plication techniques and RF treatments appear to offer good short- and mid-term symptom relief. Endoluminal full-thickness plication techniques at present appear to be most effective based on both symptom control and esophageal pH studies. The Esophyx system attempts to endoscopically replicate surgical fundoplication and appears to be particularly promising.

With all these techniques, long-term outcome reports are limited, and the need to compare endoluminal techniques in randomized trials to laparoscopic fundoplication remains. Additional studies examining the utility of such procedures in patients with recurrent symptoms after antireflux surgery should also be considered. These studies should help clarify which patients will benefit the most from an endoluminal approach.

Suggested Readings

Cadière GB, Buset M, Muls V, et al: Antireflux transoral incisionless fundoplication using Esophyx: 12-month results of a prospective multicenter study, *World J Surg* 32(8):1676–1688, 2008.

Chen D, Barber C, McLoughlin P, et al: Systematic review of endoscopic treatments for gastro-oesophageal reflux disease, *Br J Surg* 96(2):128–136, 2009.

Dundon JM, Davis SS, Hazey JW, et al: Radiofrequency energy delivery to the lower esophageal sphincter (Stretta procedure) does not provide long-term symptom control, *Surg Innov* 15(4):297–301, 2008.

Jeansonne LO 4th, White BC, Nguyen V, et al: Endoluminal full-thickness plication and radiofrequency treatments for GERD: an outcomes comparison, *Arch Surg* 144(1):19–24, 2009.

Pearl JP, Marks JM: Endolumenal therapies for gastroesophageal reflux disease: are they dead? *Endosc* 21(1):1–4, 2007.

Rothstein R, Filipi C, Caca K, et al: Endoscopic full-thickness plication for the treatment of gastroesophageal reflux disease: a randomized, sham-controlled trial, *Gastroenterology* 131(3):704–712, 2006.

Management of Barrett Esophagus

Boris Sepesi, MD, and Jeffrey H. Peters, MD

CLINICAL FEATURES

Barrett esophagus (BE) is a pathologic change of the esophageal mucosa from its normal squamous lining to columnar epithelium. Barrett epithelium is associated with a marked increase (40 to 50 times) in the risk of esophageal adenocarcinoma. It is an acquired abnormality caused by chronic gastroesophageal reflux disease

(GERD) and occurs in at least 10% to 15% of patients with GERD. It is typically diagnosed in white men older than 50 years who are overweight or obese with a prolonged history of gastroesophageal reflux. First reported in 1950, and still a rare finding in the 1960s, its prevalence has markedly increased over the past 50 years. BE was reported in 1 per 1000 endoscopies in the early 1980s; by the late 1990s, it was reported in up to 60 per 1000 endoscopies.

The clinical management of patients with BE has historically been focused on the treatment of the underlying GERD rather than on specific interventions aimed at the Barrett epithelium. This paradigm is changing, however, as new technologies offer effective endoscopic ablation; combined with effective reflux control, complete squamous reepithelialization has become widespread. Endoscopic ablation is now widely used for dysplastic BE and is under investigation as a treatment paradigm for nondysplastic epithelium.

Studies comparing GERD patients with and without intestinal metaplasia (IM) have identified multiple factors associated with BE:

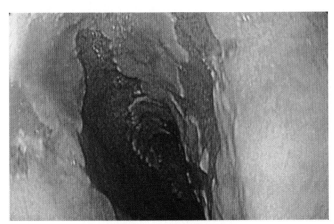

FIGURE 1   Long-segment BE.

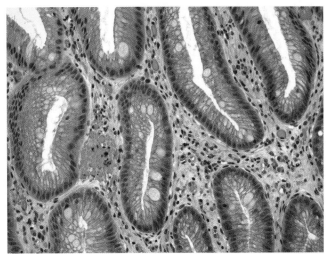

FIGURE 2   BE/IM with goblet cells.

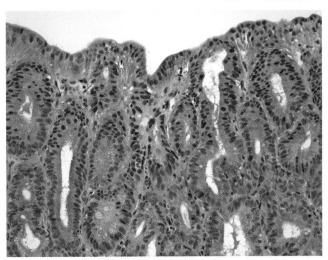

FIGURE 3   BE/IM with HGD.

an earlier age of onset and greater severity of reflux symptoms; high prevalence of an incompetent gastroesophageal barrier and hiatal hernia, often with poor esophageal motility; increased frequency of erosive esophagitis, ulceration, or stricture; and markedly high esophageal acid exposure. Recent evidence also suggests a direct link between increasing body mass index, visceral fat, metabolic syndrome, and BE. The severity of symptoms and abnormal diagnostic studies tend to increase as the degree of esophageal mucosal injury progresses, from erosive esophagitis to short-segment (<3 cm) BE to long-segment (>3 cm) BE (Figure 1). Thus irrespective of any concern for the development of dysplasia or adenocarcinoma, the presence of BE is a sign of severe GERD and, as such, it is an indication for aggressive antireflux therapy.

The definition of BE has evolved considerably over the past 10 to 20 years and continues to be debated. Classically, it was defined by two key criteria: 1) the presence of endoscopically evident columnar mucosa extending more than 3 cm into the esophagus and 2) the presence of IM (goblet cells) on histology. The concept of short-segment BE—less than 3 cm of endoscopically visible tissue confirmed histologically as IM—emerged in the late 1990s, and this type is now found almost twice as often as the long-segment variety.

Identification of short-segment BE requires that 1) the endoscopist recognize what may be quite small areas of columnar-lined esophagus (CLE) and 2) that the endoscopist biopsy the area; both of these are a source of error and debate. Finally, recent studies identifying areas of adenocarcinoma in the absence of IM, coupled with molecular studies showing similar genetic defects in intestinalized (IM goblet cells) and nonintestinalized columnar epithelium, have raised doubt as to the importance of requiring the presence of goblet cells for the diagnosis. Current guidelines in the United Kingdom, for example, do not require IM for the diagnosis. Thus whether the finding of columnar lining without histologic IM and histologic IM without the endoscopist recognizing columnar lining should be called BE is currently debated. If so, the potential pool of patients with the diagnosis would increase considerably.

Histologically, BE is classified as either nondysplastic IM (Figure 2), low-grade dysplasia (LGD), high-grade dysplasia (HGD; Figure 3), or indefinite for dysplasia. The finding "indefinite for dysplasia" often occurs in the presence of inflammation; in this situation, patients should be placed on high-dose (40 mg twice daily) proton pump inhibitor (PPI) therapy and should undergo repeat biopsies 4 to 6 weeks later. Variability studies have shown that the agreement among pathologists on the degree of dysplasia is often moderate to poor ($\varkappa$ = 0.2 to 0.6); therefore presence of HGD should be confirmed by two independent expert gastrointestinal pathologists, preferably those who have validated their findings in esophagectomy specimens.

The diagnosis of BE has significant implications for a patient, ranging from an increase in life insurance premiums to the heightened risk of developing esophageal adenocarcinoma. Although possibly cost effective in the high-risk population (white men older than 50 years with 5 or more years of GERD symptoms), no current recommendations exist for screening the general population for BE. However, once diagnosed, patients should undergo periodic endoscopic surveillance, including four-quadrant biopsies every 2 cm, aimed at identification of any progression of the epithelial change into dysplasia or adenocarcinoma.

The interval for surveillance has been a point of debate and likely should be individualized based upon patient characteristics, such as the type of BE and the patient's age, race, sex, body mass index, and other known risk factors. Current guidelines for nondysplastic BE recommend 3- to 5-year surveillance intervals, potentially too long a wait for some patients. Patients with LGD should be rebiopsied in 3 months and at least every 6 to 12 months unless ablation is undertaken. Those with HGD should undergo four-quadrant mapping biopsies every 1 cm of the CLE every 3 months, with endoscopic mucosal resection of visible mucosal irregularities and or ablation/resection. Considering the controversy, the ideal is likely an individual approach that takes into account local experience and expertise and availability of new therapies for BE.

TREATMENT OF NONDYSPLASTIC BARRETT ESOPHAGUS

Medical Therapy and Chemoprophylaxis

The main therapeutic goal for patients with IM is effective and durable GERD symptom control. Additional important consideration is given to complete eradication of metaplastic epithelium at risk for cancer and the prevention of its reoccurrence. Medical therapy typically uses PPIs to achieve symptom control, coupled with endoscopic surveillance, the rationale for which is the identification of dysplasia.

The impact of medical therapy on cancer prevention is not proven. A prospective trial of PPIs versus a placebo would be unethical due to the withholding of acid-reducing medications for patients with reflux symptoms. The large randomized AspECT trial underway in the United Kingdom is designed to randomize 5000 patients with BE to low- and high-dose PPI therapy (initial interim analysis of the trial is expected in 2011). Along with long-term acid suppressive therapy, initial evidence shows that inhibition of cyclooxygenase-2 (COX-2) with aspirin or selective nonsteroidal antiinflammatory drugs (rofecoxib) may be useful in prevention of esophageal adenocarcinoma. It remains to be seen whether the combination of PPIs and COX-2 inhibitors will have the desired chemopreventive effect.

Antireflux Surgery

Antireflux surgery continues to be an excellent treatment option in most patients with BE, as it reestablishes the barrier at the gastroesophageal junction. It is important to keep in mind that the presence of BE is generally a sign of the severe GERD commonly associated with a large hiatal hernia, stricture, poor motility, or shortened esophagus; these anatomic and physiologic features make successful antireflux surgery a challenge in this population.

Preoperatively, identification of esophageal shortening, compromised esophageal body motility, and the extent of dysplasia have significant bearing on surgical treatment decision and selection of the appropriate antireflux procedure. Failure to recognize anatomic shortening of the esophagus compromises a tension-free repair, potentially leading to increased failure rates of laparoscopic fundoplication in patients with BE. Careful analysis of endoscopic findings and a video barium esophagogram focusing on stricture and hiatal hernia less than 5 cm, which are associated with a short esophagus, should help circumvent this problem.

The presence of poor esophageal body motility is characterized by contraction amplitudes less than 30 mm Hg in the distal esophageal segment or greater than 40% of simultaneous waves on manometry. When faced with such a scenario, a partial fundoplication has been advocated based on a fear that a complete 360 degree Nissen fundoplication will result in an unacceptably high rate of dysphagia. Partial fundoplication is, however, not as effective in preventing reflux, which challenges the clinician to make a choice between the risks of recurrent reflux versus postoperative dysphagia.

Preliminary outcomes have been reported from a large, multicenter trial underway in the United Kingdom (the LOTUS trial) comparing the medical and surgical management of patients with BE. Laparoscopic antireflux surgery was compared with dose-adjusted esomeprazole (20 to 40 mg daily). Operative complications, pH testing 6 months after treatment, Gastrointestinal Symptom Rating Scale, and Quality of Life in Reflux and Dyspepsia (QOLRAD) scores were assessed at 3 years. Sixty patients with BE were randomized to either esomeprazole (n = 28) or laparoscopic antireflux surgery (n = 32). As objectively documented by esophageal pH studies, GERD was significantly better controlled in the surgery group (P = .002). Mean GSRS and QOLRAD scores were similar between the two therapies, and no differences in postoperative complications were seen among patients with and without BE. The authors of that study concluded that in a well-controlled surgical environment, laparoscopic antireflux surgery is as good or better than optimized medical therapy.

Progression and Regression

Studies focusing on progression of Barrett epithelium or regression of dysplasia compared the effects of medical and surgical antireflux therapy. The aim of a prospective randomized trial by Parrilla and colleagues (2003) was to study the long-term results of medical and surgical antireflux therapy on progression of metaplasia to dysplasia and adenocarcinoma.

In the trial, 101 patients were randomly assigned to either a medical group (n = 43), who received either an H2 antagonist or omeprazole and a surgical group (n = 58), who underwent Nissen fundoplication. A 5-year median follow-up was achieved in the medical group, and a 6-year median follow-up was achieved in the surgical group, which showed significantly less (P < .05) esophagitis and stricture after treatment. Although complete disappearance of IM was not observed in either group, 20% of patients in the medical group developed dysplasia, and 25% of these developed HGD. Newly diagnosed dysplasia occurred in 6% (n = 3) of surgical patients; two had evidence of HGD.

In a subgroup analysis, patients with successful Nissen fundoplication had a significantly decreased risk (P < .05) of progression to dysplasia and adenocarcinoma. Authors of that study concluded that the risk of progression to dysplasia is similar in both groups, and that they cannot recommend Nissen fundoplication as the treatment of choice in all patients with BE. At the same time, they pointed out that when the operation successfully prevents reflux, progression to dysplasia and adenocarcinoma is significantly lowered compared with medical therapy.

The efficacy of Nissen fundoplication versus medical therapy in the regression of LGD in patients with BE was studied by Rossi and colleagues (2006), who used screening endoscopy of 6592 patients to identify 327 patients with IM. The final analysis involved 35 patients self-selected into medical and surgical treatments. The aim of the study was to evaluate the difference between 20 mg omeprazole twice daily (n = 19) and standardized laparoscopic Nissen fundoplication (n = 16) on the natural course of LGD.

In the group getting medical treatment, a regression of LGD to IM was observed in 63% of patients on endoscopic biopsy 12 months after initiation of treatment; this regression was confirmed in all patients at 18 months. In the surgical group, the observed regression 12 months after Nissen fundoplication occurred in 94%, and at 18 months, 100% of patients had no evidence of LGD on biopsy. Multivariate logistic regression identified only laparoscopic Nissen fundoplication to be significantly associated with the probability of regression of LGD (odds ratio = 15.53, P = .0033).

TREATMENT OF DYSPLASTIC BARRETT ESOPHAGUS

Progression of nondysplastic Barrett epithelium to either LGD or HGD represents significant neoplastic advancement and should trigger a more intensive biopsy and treatment protocol. Dysplasia develops in 3% to 5% of BE patients per year and is the single most important risk factor for further deterioration to cancer.

A large, retrospective population-based analysis of endoscopy and pathology reports from 1976 to 2001 was conducted by Alcedo from Spain (2009). The aim was to asses changes in incidence and prevalence of BE. After dividing the study period into four quartiles, researchers observed an increase in incidence of BE diagnosis, from 0.73 to 9.73 cases per 100,000 persons, with adjusted increase in prevalence from 6.5 to 76 cases per 100,000. The incidence of dysplasia was 2.13% per year—1.78% for LGD and 0.36% for HGD—giving a

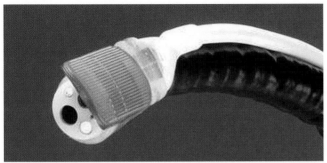

FIGURE 4   HALO⁹⁰ device. *(Courtesy BÂRRX Medical.)*

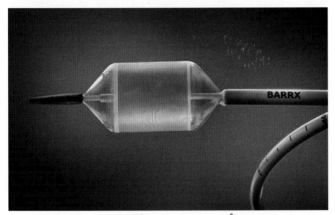

FIGURE 5   HALO³⁶⁰ device. *(Courtesy BÂRRX Medical.)*

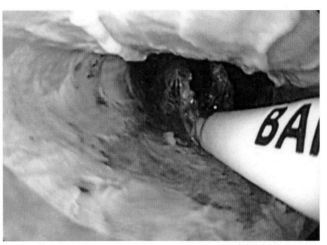

FIGURE 6   Metaplastic esophageal mucosa treated with a radiofrequency ablation HALO³⁶⁰ device. *(Courtesy BÂRRX Medical.)*

total incidence of dysplasia of 1 per 47 patient-years. The incidence of adenocarcinoma during follow-up was 0.5% per year for an incidence of 1 per 210 patient-years. Several prospective cohort studies have suggested that 4% to 5% of BE patients per year will develop dysplasia.

Although the significance and natural course of dysplasia continue to be debated, two large, prospectively followed cohorts of patients with HGD and one retrospectively reviewed experience showed that cancer will be identified in approximately 25% of patients with HGD at 1.5 years, 50% at 3 years, and up to 80% at 8 years. The potential 20% error rate in the pathologic diagnosis of HGD notwithstanding, the majority of patients with HGD will have an invasive adenocarcinoma identified during the 5- to 10-year surveillance, although a minority may not. Therefore the motivation to eradicate precancerous dysplastic epithelium by any means is high.

Ablation

Currently used methods for eradication of dysplastic Barrett epithelium include photodynamic therapy, cryoablation, radiofrequency ablation (RFA), and endoscopic resection. An arguably exciting advance in the management of dysplastic BE has been the development of the HALO³⁶⁰ & ⁹⁰ System (BÂRRX Medical, Sunnyvale, Calif; Figures 4 and 5), which uses a balloon-based endoscopically guided technique for elimination of both nondysplastic and dysplastic Barrett epithelium (Figure 6).

The device consists of a heat-generating balloon with tightly spaced coils on its surface that conduct high-frequency radiowaves. The ablation procedure begins with a sizing balloon that estimates the diameter of the metaplastic esophagus. The appropriate size RFA catheter is then positioned in apposition to the metaplastic tissue, and the balloon is inflated to a standardized pressure (0.5 atm), effectively flattening the esophageal folds to allow a homogeneous ablation. This is followed by a high-power, ultrashort (~300 msec) burst

of energy that results in a uniform ablation (~1000 μm) of the muscularis mucosa. The depth of injury has been calibrated in dosimetry studies to the depth of the epithelium, thus avoiding deep circumferential damage that may result in scarring and strictures.

Initial studies of appropriate energy dose, safety, and efficacy of this device were performed in animals and in resected surgical specimens. In both the porcine model and in human esophagectomy patients, ablation depth was directly related to energy density delivered, with 8 to 12 J/cm² resulting in complete removal of the epithelium. Within this intensity range, there was no submucosal injury or stricture observed, whereas an intensity greater than 20 J/cm² produced deeper submucosal injury.

Studies of the efficacy of RFA have evolved rapidly. In the first clinical report, Sharma et al (2007) reported on the use of this device in a multicenter dosimetry trial in patients (n = 32) with nondysplastic IM (AIM-I). The procedure was performed on an outpatient basis, using conscious sedation, with a median procedure time of 24 minutes. Single applications of 8, 10, and 12 J/cm² energy densities were evaluated. The procedure was well tolerated, and there were no strictures or buried glands. Pathology was performed by a centralized pathology service. After one treatment, most patients treated at 8 J/cm² had residual IM, whereas 10 and 12 J/cm² resulted in a 40% and 36% complete response (CR) rate, respectively (CR considered to be no histologic evidence of IM on four-quadrant biopsies). Given the equivalence of 10 and 12 J/cm², all patients were treated a second time with 10 J/cm², resulting in a CR of 67% at 1 year.

Fleischer and colleagues (2008) performed a larger follow-on study to AIM-I, called *AIM-II*, which included longer segment (2 to 6 cm), nondysplastic IM. Median procedure time was 26 minutes. A single energy-density setting was evaluated, 10 J/cm² (2X). The procedure was well tolerated, and there were no strictures or buried glands. At 12 months, CR was 52%. Those patients with persistent IM at 1 year typically exhibited focal disease only, in the form of small islands (average clearance in the group with residual disease was 90%).

A uniform and reproducible depth of ablation can be achieved following these key recommendations: 1) very high power (300 W), 2) ultrashort energy-delivery time (<300 msec), 3) tightly spaced bipolar electrode array (<250 μm between electrodes), 4) standardized wall tension with balloon dilation, 5) standardized energy density (Joules of energy delivered to each cm² of epithelium [J/cm²]), and 6) a large surface area on the electrodes (>30 cm²).

Outcomes of Radiofrequency Ablation

Unlike previous ablative therapies, RFA achieves successful reversion to squamous epithelium in up to 97% of patients with nondysplastic BE when a balloon-based device (HALO³⁶⁰) is used for the initial ablation, followed by "touch-up" ablations of focal areas of metaplasia with a smaller, flat device (HALO[90]). In contrast with a 20% stricture rate associated with previous ablative techniques, the RFA stricture rate in published studies is low (0% to 1%). The absence of buried Barrett epithelium following RFA suggests high efficacy of this technique in ablating metaplastic mucosa. The high rate of CR, safety, and cost effectiveness make RFA therapy ideal for patients with nondysplastic Barrett epithelium and LGD. Sharma and colleagues (2008) evaluated this device in patients with LGD using an energy of 12 J/cm² applied two consecutive times. They reported a CR rate of 100% for LGD and 60% for IM at 1 year, with no strictures or buried glands.

Despite the success and safety profile of RFA, recommendations on the routine use of endoscopic ablation of nondysplastic BE in clinical practice remain controversial. All clinical trials have so far been conducted in specialized centers with expert endoscopists and pathologists, with close patient follow-up. The challenge for routine clinical practice remains personnel training, uniform patient follow-up, and the ability to use advanced techniques to critically assess for more advanced disease, such as early carcinoma. These challenges may prove to be daunting, and the procedure may turn out to be ineffective in routine clinical practice and potentially lead to undesirable outcomes.

The use of RFA for BE with dysplasia was studied by Bergman and colleagues (2008) from The Netherlands, who reported on 44 patients with HGD and/or early neoplasia treated with RFA following initial endoscopic resection (ER) of the visible lesions. Careful patient selection was paramount in this trial, which excluded all patients with submucosal cancer. Of 75% of patients who underwent ER prior to ablation, 16 had intramucosal carcinoma, 12 had HGD, and 3 had LGD. Successful eradication of dysplasia occurred in 43 of the 44 patients.

In a large multicenter sham-controlled U.S. trial (2009), 127 patients with dysplastic BE were randomly assigned in a 2:1 ratio to receive ablation or a sham procedure. The primary study outcome was complete eradication of dysplasia and IM at 12 months. In patients with LGD, complete eradication of dysplasia occurred in 90.5% after ablation compared with 22.7% of sham controls ($P < .001$). Similarly, ablation eradicated HGD in 81% compared with 19% of those in the control group ($P < .001$). Patients randomized into an ablation group had complete eradication of IM in 77.4%; they also had less disease progression ($P = .03$) and fewer cancers (1.2% vs. 9.3%, $P = .045$) than controls. The stricture rate in this trial was 6%, and only one patient had gastrointestinal hemorrhage.

As demonstrated in the data above, RFA technology challenges the treatment paradigm of dysplastic BE and early cancer. With longer patient follow-up and continued technologic evolution, the role of RFA in the treatment algorithm of dysplastic and nondysplastic BE will likely become certain.

Endoscopic Resection

ER is another important technique necessary in the armamentarium of a surgeon treating patients with BE. Patients with BE and HGD or early intramucosal carcinoma have been recommended for esophagectomy as a curative procedure, providing they are suitable candidates for surgical intervention. While the curability rate of esophagectomy in this setting is high, the role of esophagectomy has been challenged due to the perception of excessive operative morbidity and mortality rates, particularly in low-volume centers.

ER was initially introduced into clinical practice as an additional method to standard imaging techniques for diagnoses and staging of visible mucosal abnormalities suspicious for dysplasia or early esophageal carcinoma. With increasing experience, ER is now offered as a potentially curative treatment, either alone or in conjunction with RFA, for patients with dysplastic BE or early esophageal neoplasia. Considering traditional teaching of surgical oncologic principles, such as adequate tumor resection margin and lymphadenectomy, it

is not surprising that considerable controversy now exists regarding optimal treatment strategy for patients with HGD and early carcinoma.

First done in Japan, ER was found to be a safe and potentially curative technique for squamous cell carcinomas with low risk of intramural spread as defined by the criteria: 1) tumor size no greater than 2 cm, 2) infiltration to lamina propria, 3) no greater than half the esophageal circumference, and 4) an absence of lymphatic or vascular invasion. Following Japanese experience, ER was adopted in the United States and Europe as an excisional biopsy of visible mucosal irregularities in two applications: 1) as a large biopsy guiding further tailored therapy or 2) as a curative procedure for tumors with low risk of nodal spread. A clear advantage of ER over ablative therapies for treatment of dysplasia or early neoplasia is the preservation of specimens for histopathologic examination and staging; ER also allows for the assessment of the completeness of resection.

The rationale of ER as a curative therapy is predicated upon a thorough understanding of the histology of the esophageal wall. LGD and HGD represent a neoplastic process limited to the epithelial layer. Penetration of the basement membrane to the bottom edge of the muscularis mucosa is classified as *intramucosal carcinoma;* invasion beyond muscularis mucosa is classified as *submucosal carcinoma.* The potential for nodal metastasis for HGD is likely zero; for intramucosal cancer, it is approximately 2%. However, submucosal penetration is associated with a 20% to 30% prevalence of nodal metastasis. Although some authors have suggested that superficial submucosal invasion carries the same risk of nodal spread as intramucosal carcinoma, the curative potential of ER for these tumors is not uniformly accepted. Therefore ER is appropriate as a curative therapy for tumors limited only to mucosa.

Evaluation and Technique of Endoscopic Resection

A thorough and careful endoscopic assessment of the entire esophageal mucosa is mandatory prior to any consideration of ER for a discrete nodule (Figure 7) because multiple subtle mucosal abnormalities may exist and be missed by a hurried or inexperienced examiner. A variety of technologies and techniques are available for improved visualization of mucosal abnormalities, including high-resolution endoscopy, virtual chromoendoscopy, narrow-band imaging (Figure 8), or staining with a number of dyes such as acetic acid, methylene blue, or indigo carmine.

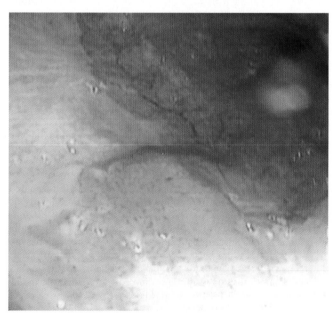

FIGURE 7   Visible lesion on endoscopy.

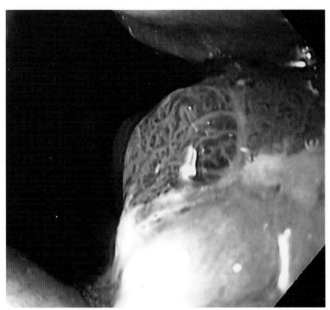

FIGURE 8   Visible lesion on endoscopy (view augmented with narrow-band imaging).

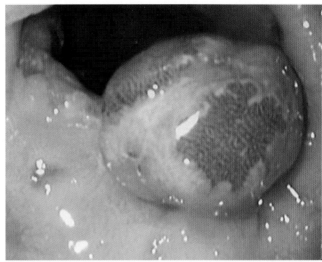

FIGURE 9   Pseudopolyp of visible lesion created with suction cap and rubber band.

Once a localized tumor is detected, endoscopic ultrasound may be used to determine the depth of esophageal wall invasion. Although endoscopic ultrasound has been shown to be beneficial in differentiating T1, T2, and T3 esophageal tumors, its accuracy in differentiating the fine, often microscopic difference between intramucosal (T1A) and submucosal (T1B) tumors is limited. ER should be used in any visible nodules because it provides a specimen for histopathologic examination and confirmation of both tumor depth and differentiation; this information is invaluable for definitive therapy planning. The benefit of ER in patients with BE has been seen in corrections of the grading of dysplasia or neoplasia in 40% of patients.

Current eligibility criteria for the use of ER as a definitive therapy include 1) focal HGD or a T1A intramucosal tumor on the basis of histopathologic examination without evidence of lymph node involvement or systemic disease on staging evaluation, 2) a lesion less than 2 cm in diameter, 3) polypoid or flat without ulceration, 4) well or moderately differentiated, and 5) without evidence of lymphovascular invasion. It is also important to stress that all patients undergoing treatment for focal HGD or a tumor must be informed about the option of ER, which has been the standard of care. An absolute contraindication for ER is tumors invading muscularis propria or beyond (T2 or T3).

There are several techniques described for ER, and all share the same principle: isolation of the target lesion with subsequent resection using a snare cautery device. Initial isolation can be accomplished with submucosal injection of saline, with or without dilute epinephrine, or with a cap-and-suction technique with or without band ligation. Some polypoid lesions maybe excised with a simple snare.

The injection technique commonly uses 10 to 20 mL of saline with 1:100,000 epinephrine injected into the submucosal layer, which effectively separates the mucosal layer. An alternative method is to create a pseudopolyp (Figure 9) by raising and isolating the target lesion with specially designed cap (Olympus EMR-001, Olympus America, Center Valley, Penn.) and applying a rubber band using a variceal banding device (Duette Multiband Mucosectomy System; Cook Medical, Bloomington, Ind., or Bard Six-Shooter; Bard Interventional Products, Billerica, Mass.) to the base of the elevated mucosa. The pseudopolyp is then excised, either above or below the rubber band (Figure 10), using snare electrocautery. The excised specimen (Figure 11) is retrieved

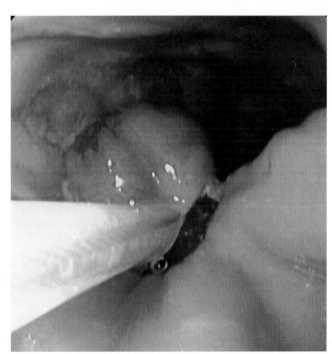

FIGURE 10   Snaring of the pseudopolyp.

with a net or polypectomy grasper, and the specimen is tacked to a small piece of corkboard, preserving the margins and allowing the measurement of its diameter.

The importance of an experienced pathologist examining and reporting on the specimen cannot be overemphasized. A complete report should include comments on lateral and deep margins, depths of tumor invasion, presence or absence of lymphatic or vascular invasion, and degree of tumor differentiation. Unavailability of a pathologist experienced with such an assessment should prompt sending the specimen to a center of excellence, as subtleties in histopathologic evolution affect subsequent treatment decisions.

Potential risks of ER include bleeding, perforation, stricture, or inadequate treatment that leaves positive margins or associated nodal disease untreated. Bleeding is commonly self-limited;

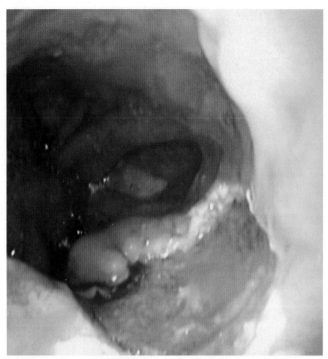

FIGURE 11   Excised lesion.

more brisk bleeding can be treated with dilute epinephrine injection, electrocautery, or endoscopic clip application. The most dreaded complication, perforation, requires significant judgment and skill to avoid further morbidity. Strictures are treated with serial dilations. Although positive lateral margins maybe treated with another ER, some providers may opt to refer the patient for esophagectomy.

It is important to emphasize that a patient undergoing ER agrees to not only the actual ER procedure but also to an intensive endoscopic surveillance initially every 1 to 3 months and lasting years, perhaps a lifetime, with a possibility of further ER or esophagectomy.

Outcomes After Endoscopic Resection

The most quoted data regarding outcomes of ER come from Ell and colleagues, from Wiesbaden, Germany. They first reported on ER for treatment of HGD and early esophageal adenocarcinoma in 2000, in 64 patients treated with ER alone. Complete remission was observed in 82.5% of patients after a mean of 1.3 ± 0.6 treatment sessions at 8 to 12 months of follow-up. Fourteen percent of patients developed recurrent or metachronous tumors, and all were retreated with ER.

More recently and so far the largest series on ER in early esophageal adenocarcinoma was published by the same group (Ell et al, 2007). The cohort of 100 patients was selected from 667 patients referred for evaluation of intraepithelial neoplasia. During a mean of 1.47 resections per patient, there were no major complications. Argon plasma coagulation and photodynamic therapy were added to ER treatment of short- and long-segment BE. Complete R0 local remission was achieved in 99 of 100 patients after a mean of 1.9 months and a maximum of three resections. Metachronous or recurrent lesions occurred in 11% of cases, and all were successfully treated with another ER.

There were two non–cancer-related deaths in the group, and overall 5-year survival was estimated at 98%. Surveillance protocol in this study included follow-up endoscopies at 1, 2, 3, 6, 9, and 12 months and then every 6 months until 5 years. Every other visit included endoscopic ultrasound, computed tomography, and abdominal ultrasound.

Available data advocate for the feasibility of ER in a highly select group of patients with HGD or early intramucosal carcinoma treated at a specialty center under intensive surveillance. Whether similar results could be achieved in general nonspecialty community centers remains unknown. For now, we recommend that these patients be referred to specialty centers with availability of multispecialty teams composed of esophageal surgeons, gastroenterologists, and pathologists with specific interest and experience in this disease process.

Esophageal Resection (Esophagectomy)

Historically, the standard therapy, esophagectomy, has been challenged as the most appropriate therapy for HGD. Criticism of this approach emphasizes the magnitude of the procedure, the potential for postoperative morbidity and mortality, and the negative impact on quality of life that foregut reconstruction can impose. Other treatment strategies, especially a variety of endoscopic mucosal therapies, are becoming more commonly used as alternatives to esophagectomy, particularly in high-risk patients. However, each less invasive alternative has its own potential risks and limitations that must be weighed against perceived advantages.

To make informed comparisons among each of the treatment alternatives for HGD, understanding data regarding the outcomes of both endoscopic therapy and esophagectomy for HGD is essential. In a review of 22 published reports between 1987 and 2007 on outcomes of esophagectomy, Williams and colleagues (2007) indentified 530 patients who underwent esophagectomy for HGD. The perioperative mortality rate, one of the most scrutinized outcomes, was found to be 0.94%; in 17 reports, it was 0%.

It should be emphasized that mortality rates of esophagectomy are reported for all stages and types of esophageal cancer, and despite much progress and a decrease in mortality rate for this procedure below 4% in high-volume centers, the tendency to report historically high mortality values of 8% to 10% erroneously persists. Lack of dysphagia and weight loss with resultant malnutrition, no need for preoperative neoadjuvant therapy, and perhaps a better immunologic milieu of patients with HGD, compared with cancer patients, are some of the plausible explanations of lower mortality rates of esophagectomy for HGD. Moreover, the physiologic outcome and quality of life following esophagectomy for HGD remains good. In the same study, it was found that patients consumed a median of three meals per day, and two thirds of patients considered their eating pattern to be normal or only mildly affected; most (76%) were able to eat an unrestricted diet.

The main advantage of esophagectomy over any endoscopic therapy is an absolute eradication of an organ with impending transformation into carcinoma. For a patient more interested in peace of mind than in intensive endoscopic follow-up, esophagectomy may be a better solution. When considering treatment alternatives for dysplastic BE, a patient should be presented with all treatment options, and therapy should be individualized.

SUMMARY

The rising prevalence of BE parallels the rising incidence of esophageal adenocarcinoma in the Western world. Current management strategy of this disease requires thorough knowledge of histologic epithelial types at the esophagogastric junction, excellent endoscopic skills, application of new technologies, and critical thinking and good judgment in patient selection for potential surgical antireflux therapy or esophagectomy. Although recent technologic advancements have broadened the therapeutic armamentarium, much remains to be learned about the prevention and management of BE.

SELECTED READINGS

Atwood SE, Lundell L, Hatlback JG, et al: Medical or surgical management of GERD patients with Barrett's esophagus the LOTUS trial 3-year experience, *J Gastrointest Surg* 12(10):1646–1654, 2008.

Chandrasoma PT, DeMeester TR: *GERD: reflux to esophageal adenocarcinoma*, Burlington, Mass, 2006, Elsevier.

Pech O, May A, Rabenstein T, et al: Endoscopic resection of early oesophageal cancer, *Gut* 56(11):1625–1634, 2007.

Pech O, Behrens A, May A, et al: Long-term results and risk analysis for recurrence after curative endoscopic therapy in 349 patients with high-grade intraepithelial neoplasia and mucosal adenocarcinoma in Barrett's oesophagus, *Gut* 57(9):1200–1206, 2008.

Pouw RE, Gondrie JJ, Sondermeijer CM, et al: Eradication of Barrett esophagus with early neoplasia by radiofrequency ablation, with or without endoscopic resection, *J Gastrointest Surg* 12(10):1627–1636, 2008.

Shaheen N, Sharma P, Overholt BF, et al: Radiofrequency ablation in Barrett's esophagus with dysplasia, *N Engl J Med* 360(22):2353–2355, 2009.

ENDOSCOPIC TREATMENT OF BARRETT ESOPHAGUS

Jason M. Pfluke, MD, and C. Daniel Smith, MD

HISTORY

In 1950, Norman Ruppert Barrett, a British physician, published a description of an ulcer in the distal esophagus associated with esophagitis and columnar epithelium. At that time, the association with chronic inflammation and adenocarcinoma was not known. Today, Barrett esophagus (BE) describes the replacement of the normal squamous epithelial lining of the esophagus by intestinalized columnar epithelia, also known as *intestinal metaplasia* (IM), most commonly in association with chronic gastroesophageal reflux disease (GERD). Conservative estimates suggest that 3% to 12% of patients with GERD will have BE, and this prevalence increases with age, with up to 25% of people older than 50 years with some degree of BE. This means from 2 to 20 million Americans may have BE—clearly a significant public health issue.

The importance of BE lies not only in its association with GERD but in its association with esophageal adenocarcinoma, especially the progression of nondysplastic BE to dysplasia and eventual adenocarcinoma if GERD is left untreated or undertreated. BE can be clinically silent, and up to 10% of patients with BE will already have dysplasia at the time of initial diagnosis; nearly 7% will have frank adenocarcinoma at first presentation. Left unmanaged, 24% of patients with nondysplastic BE will progress to dysplasia or adenocarcinoma over the first 4 years after initial diagnosis. Overall, those with BE are 30 to 125 times more likely to develop esophageal adenocarcinoma than those without BE. The risk of progression to high-grade dysplasia (HGD) is 0.9% per year, and progression to adenocarcinoma 0.5% per year.

With the natural history of BE being one of progression over time, early detection and management before the development of dysplasia is ideal. Endoscopic management of BE starts with screening strategies that include an esophagogastroduodenoscopy (EGD), for any patient with persistent GERD symptoms despite adequate medical therapy, and a baseline EGD at or around age 50 years. If nondysplastic BE is found, surveillance endoscopy every 1 to 3 years is recommended, until there is no evidence of progression. If low-grade dysplasia (LGD) is found, endoscopy with extensive biopsies should be performed every 6 to 12 months. If HGD is found, treatment must be considered, because in this setting, 10% to 30% of patients will already have progressed to adenocarcinoma, and 15% to 60% will progress to esophageal cancer within 5 years.

When considering the management of BE, a strategy for lasting treatment of GERD must be decided to manage the diseased epithelium, and available options must be weighed when the risk of esophageal cancer is high enough to consider esophagectomy. To affect one condition without the other commits the patient to the ongoing risk of the diseased epithelium and its progression, and esophagectomy is a fairly morbid procedure with significant, long-lasting lifestyle consequences.

TREATMENT OF GASTROESOPHAGEAL REFLUX DISEASE

Treatment with acid-suppressing medication alone does not result in regression of BE, likely due to the continued exposure of the distal esophagus to refluxed gastric content. Antireflux surgery, and in particular, a well-done 360 degree fundoplication, provides durable control of all gastric reflux, including nonacid refluxate, and leads to regression of BE in up to 30% of patients. Any patient with BE who is a reasonable surgical candidate should at least be made aware of this option and be given an opportunity to talk to a skilled and knowledgeable esophageal surgeon. Currently, the presence of BE is a contraindication for endoscopic management of GERD.

Management of Diseased Epithelium

Until more recently, management of the diseased epithelium involved only surveillance endoscopy and esophagectomy if HGD or adenocarcinoma developed. Endoscopic ablation techniques have been developed over the years, reserved largely for advanced disease in patients who were poor surgical candidates. In those with HGD or cancer who could tolerate esophagectomy, it has been the gold standard of care; but although esophagectomy offers the most definitive treatment of HGD or adenocarcinoma, even when performed using minimally invasive techniques, it is a morbid procedure that leaves the patient with less than optimal upper gut function.

In an effort to eliminate dysplastic BE before malignant transformation, recent advances in endoscopic therapies can achieve resection and/or ablation of HGD or early adenocarcinoma, effecting an esophageal-sparing cure in these more advanced states.

Principles of Endoscopic Treatment

It is known that ablation of Barrett epithelium leads to removal of the IM and repopulation with normal squamous cells. Several different techniques have applied this principle to the treatment of BE with varying success and complication rates. Appropriate and adequate depth of ablation is a key factor in determining effectiveness, durability, and side effects. The optimal depth of ablation should extend down to include the muscularis mucosa, allowing for complete ablation of metaplastic cells without the risk of developing subsquamous islands of BE during the healing stage (Figure 1). Ablating deeper into the submucosa results in high rates of stricture and other complications.

Human Esophagus

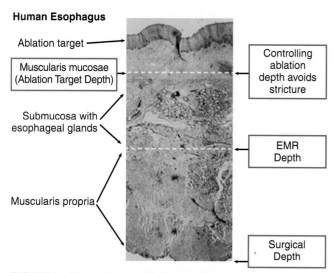

FIGURE 1   Histopathology slide showing the layers of the esophagus, indicating the depth of resection with endoscopic treatments of BE.

Mucosal Ablation Techniques

Laser ablation, argon plasma coagulation, multipolar electrocoagulation, and cryotherapy techniques are all examples of techniques that have been described and applied but are declining in use. This is largely because each has been plagued by complications, primarily due to the lack of reliable uniform ablation of Barrett segments, poorly controlled depth of ablation, and the requirement of multiple repeat treatments to achieve adequate ablation. Published reports initially demonstrated encouraging results with each of these approaches, but long-term follow-up showing high recurrence rates, development of subsquamous metaplasia, and stricture has limited the clinical use of these techniques.

Photodynamic therapy (PDT) and radiofrequency ablation (RFA) have emerged as the two most applied and successful endoscopic treatments of the diseased esophageal epithelium. PDT involves use of an intravenously administered photosensitizing drug that is selectively taken up and concentrated in neoplastic Barrett cells. Nonthermal light in the 630 to 635 nm wavelength is delivered at the time of endoscopy, and a photochemical reaction occurs, resulting in mucosal destruction and ablation of BE.

Overholt and colleagues (2006) reported the results of a prospective, randomized, controlled trial comparing PDT with porfimer sodium and omeprazole versus omeprazole alone in the treatment of BE with HGD in 208 patients. After randomization, patients in the treatment arm underwent one to three PDT sessions. Patients in both groups underwent surveillance endoscopy, with biopsy every 3 months until four consecutive quarterly biopsies were negative for HGD, then every 6 months thereafter. Complete ablation of HGD at 24 months was observed in 77% of patients who underwent PDT, compared with 39% in the control group, and 13% of patients in the PDT group progressed to adenocarcinoma compared with 28% in the control group.

Side effects were significant in the treatment group. Photosensitivity reactions (69%), esophageal strictures (36%), vomiting (32%), and chest pain (20%) were reported in the patients undergoing PDT. The stricture rate was higher in those undergoing repeat treatments, but stricture occurred even in patients with a single treatment. Although not explicitly reported in this study, recurrence of subsquamous intestinal metaplasia is also a concern following PDT, with most studies reporting a rate of 30% on follow-up.

This and other studies have confirmed that PDT is effective in the treatment of BE, with most studies reporting a 77% to 88% success rate in the ablation of HGD. The high incidence of esophageal strictures, photosensitivity reactions, and subsquamous metaplasia are drawbacks of this approach. To address these concerns, investigations

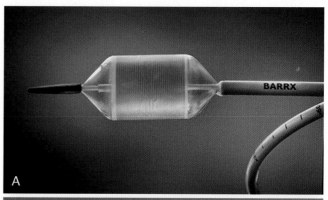

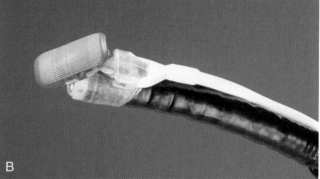

FIGURE 2   **A,** RF catheter used for circumferential ablation of BE. **B,** RF catheter used for focal ablation of small patches of BE or residual disease.

are ongoing to identify the optimal dosimetry in PDT and to develop novel photosensitizing agents.

RFA involves the delivery of bipolar energy through a tightly coiled wire array at a very controlled and precise duration and intensity. This wire array is wrapped around a balloon (Figure 2, *A*) such that when the balloon is positioned over the IM and inflated, the esophageal mucosa effaces the wire array in a precise and reproducible manner, thereby ablating the mucosa to a controlled and predictable depth. With this predictable and controlled depth of ablation, deep injury to the esophagus is avoided, thereby decreasing esophageal stricture and other complications. Initial treatment is performed using this circumferential ablation technique, whereas subsequent treatments employ a focal ablation probe for residual disease (Figure 2, *B*). Seventy percent of those so treated have complete ablation of all diseased mucosa in one treatment, and the remainder achieve complete ablation in one or two subsequent sessions. Encouraging results with this technique have been reported by Roorda and colleagues (2007) in the treatment of nondysplastic and dysplastic BE.

In a multicenter, uncontrolled Ablation of Intestinal Metaplasia (AIM) trial, 70 patients with nondysplastic BE segments 2 to 6 cm in length were treated with circumferential RFA. Patients underwent one or two ablation sessions. At 12-month follow-up, biopsy revealed complete eradication of intestinal metaplasia in 70% of patients. In an extension of this trial, 62 of 70 patients consented to additional evaluation and treatment. Patients underwent an average of 1.9 additional sessions with focal ablation for residual disease. Biopsies at 30-month follow-up demonstrated complete elimination of intestinal metaplasia in 98% of patients, with no evidence of buried glandular mucosa. Side effects were minor, consisting primarily of self-limited chest pain, nausea, or fever, all of which resolved without treatment. There were no strictures identified in this study group.

Smith and colleagues reported the use of RFA in the treatment of eight patients with BE undergoing esophagectomy for HGD with or without adenocarcinoma. BE segments ranged from 4 to 10 cm. Immediately preceding esophagectomy, patients were treated with circumferential RFA. Ten ablation zones were created in the eight patients and, after esophagectomy, multiple sections from the ablation zones were analyzed histologically. Nine of 10 ablation zones demonstrated complete removal of all intestinal metaplasia and HGD. In the one treatment failure, there remained a single focus of HGD attributed to inadequate overlap of the treatment zones.

In a recent multicenter, prospective, sham-controlled trial, 127 patients with dysplastic BE were randomized to receive RFA or a sham upper endoscopy with biopsy only. Both groups were given proton-pump inhibitors (PPIs). Subjects with HGD underwent endoscopic ultrasound (EUS) demonstrating the absence of lymphadenopathy or esophageal wall abnormalities. Patients in the ablation group received up to four ablation sessions, performed at baseline, 2, 4, and 9 months. Patients with LGD underwent surveillance biopsies at 6 and 12 months, and patients with HGD underwent surveillance biopsy at 3, 6, 9, and 12 months. Ninety-two percent of patients completed the study and, at 12-month follow-up, 90.5% of LGD patients in the RFA group achieved complete eradication of dysplasia compared with only 22.7% in the control group. Among patients with HGD, 81% in the RFA group achieved complete eradication of dysplasia compared with only 19% of the control group. Eradication of all IM occurred in 77.4% of patients in the RFA group, regardless of dysplasia type, compared with 2.3% in the control group. Among patients with HGD, 2.4% in the RFA group progressed to adenocarcinoma compared with 19% in the control group. Subsquamous IM was identified in 5.1% of the RFA patients compared with 40% of the control group.

In this trial, the complication rate was low. One patient experienced upper GI bleeding, which was treated endoscopically. No perforations or procedure-related deaths occurred. Five patients developed esophageal strictures (6%), all of which were treated successfully with endoscopic dilatation. Chest discomfort occurred more frequently in the ablation group, but it had resolved in most patients 8 days after the procedure.

Many other trials have reported similarly encouraging results using RFA in the endoscopic treatment of BE. Favorable complication and side-effect profiles and uniform ablation confined to the muscularis mucosa are key benefits of this approach. Longer follow-up data and additional randomized, controlled trials will further establish the scope of use of this technique and, in particular, will explore its use in nondysplastic BE to further establish indications for this technique.

TREATMENT OF ADVANCED BARRETT ESOPHAGUS

In patients who are good surgical candidates who have HGD or early esophageal cancer, minimally invasive esophagectomy (MIE) remains the most conservative treatment to eliminate risk or cure early esophageal cancer, but it is also the most invasive, and traditional esophagectomy has a mortality rate of up to 10% and morbidity in as many as 50% of patients. Because of this, less invasive approaches to esophagectomy, and even esophageal-sparing treatments, have been developed. These include MIE and endoscopic mucosal resection (EMR) alone or in combination with mucosal ablation (described earlier in this chapter).

MIE is covered elsewhere in this text, but suffice it to say for this discussion that although it has significantly decreased the morbidity and mortality over traditional esophagectomy, MIE remains a complex procedure, with a 1% mortality rate and up to 20% perioperative morbidity rate, particularly with pulmonary complications that accompany the commonly needed single-lung ventilation and thoracic dissection. Also, although lifesaving in the case of esophageal cancer, functional outcomes related to upper gut function remain less than ideal, thus making esophageal-sparing approaches conceptually appealing for those with HGD or T1 esophageal malignancies.

When combined with EUS, EMR is a promising technique that allows the identification and resection of focal areas of concern within a bed of IM while preserving the esophagus and its function. With this, EMR promises potential cure of early esophageal cancer through endoscopic complete resection of suspicious lesions otherwise identifiable and managed only through esophagectomy. EMR also offers more precise staging of these areas through an assessment of depth of invasion of focal lesions before committing to esophagectomy.

After EUS staging to include an assessment or periesophageal lymph nodes and areas suspicious for advanced cancer (focal nodularity or potential deep invasion), EMR consists of submucosal injection of fluid to elevate the lesion and excision using a suction cap and snare device. The resected specimen includes mucosal and submucosal layers, thereby providing pathologic information about depth of invasion, and potentially providing a curative resection. Using this approach, EMR has been applied in the treatment of dysplastic BE, nondysplastic BE, and early adenocarcinoma.

Ell and colleagues reported results of localized EMR in the treatment of 100 patients with low-risk adenocarcinoma arising in BE. All patients underwent preenrollment EUS to assess depth of invasion and lymph node status. Patients with a more advanced tumor stage (greater than T1), lymph node involvement, or metastasis were excluded, as were patients who did not meet low-risk criteria as outlined by the Japanese Society for Endoscopy for low risk in early gastric cancer.

Ninety-nine percent of patients experienced a complete local eradication (R0 resection), and all patients underwent rigorous surveillance endoscopic examinations. At a median follow-up of 33 months, 11 metachronous lesions (11%) were identified and treated successfully with repeat EMR, and 11 episodes of minor bleeding (11%) occurred. No strictures were reported during this follow-up period. Forty-nine percent of the patients underwent some type of ablative therapy following R0 resection of the cancer, and all patients were continued on acid-suppressive therapy.

In the largest published series to date, Pech and colleagues (2008) reported long-term results of endoscopic treatment of BE in 349 patients, 61 with HGD and 288 with intramucosal adenocarcinoma. All patients underwent EUS prior to enrollment. EMR alone was performed in 279, with a median of 2.1 resections each. Fifty-five patients were treated with PDT using 5-aminolevulinic acid, 13 patients with residual HGD after EMR were subsequently treated with PDT, and 2 patients were treated with argon plasma coagulation.

Among all treatment groups, complete response of neoplastic changes was observed in 96.6%. At a median follow-up of 63 months, metachronous lesions were identified in 21.5%. These patients all underwent endoscopic retreatment, and 95.7% achieved a long-term complete response. The complication rate was low in this series of patients, with a stenosis rate of 5.1% in patients undergoing EMR (15 of 292).

A recent review of published literature on total endoscopic resection of BE with HGD or early intramucosal cancer was reported by Seewald. Reported success rates ranged from 70% to 100%, with stricture rates ranging from 0% to 70%. The trials reviewed were nonrandomized, noncontrolled trials of relatively small sample sizes.

Large, randomized, controlled trials of EMR with long-term follow-up are underway to further assess the precise role of EMR in the treatment of BE. Most published series include multiple different nonrandomized treatment arms combined with various ablative therapies. In many reports, the challenge to EMR has been the high stricture rate due to extensive resection of the submucosa. On the other hand, localized and more limited EMR is associated with short-term recurrence rates of 11% to 30%. This raises the prospect of a role for combination therapy for advanced disease, where EMR is followed by ablation of the remaining IM and even HGD.

With combination therapy, EMR is used to resect suspicious areas. Based on pathology results from resected areas, a decision can be made as to whether to proceed to esophagectomy (T2 lesion or positive radial margin of resection) or to use ablation to manage

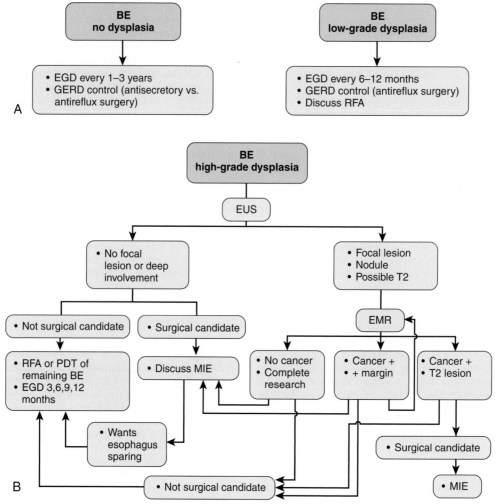

FIGURE 3   A, Treatment algorithm for nondysplastic and LGD in BE. **B,** Treatment algorithm for BE with HGD.

the remaining mucosa, followed by surveillance and definitive anti-reflux treatment. An algorithm for comprehensive management of BE, including the use of multimodal therapy, is presented in Figure 3. Clearly, EMR has been shown to be effective in the treatment of dysplastic BE and early adenocarcinoma, and it will continue to play a significant role in the endoscopic treatment of BE, likely in combination with ablative therapies.

Finally, new imaging technologies are allowing earlier detection of BE and better endoscopic staging. One such technology is confocal endoscopy, which promises to allow image-based pathologic diagnosis, and when combined with EUS, diagnosis and staging in a single endoscopic session. Ultimately this would result in diagnosis and treatment in the same session, thereby decreasing the risk and cost of multiple procedures and finding BE at an earlier stage, one more amenable to esophageal-sparing management strategies.

SUMMARY

Endoscopic therapies for BE are progressing quickly and promise to offer esophageal-sparing approaches to what have traditionally been considered conditions only treatable with esophagectomy, namely BE

with LGD or HGD and early esophageal cancer. RFA alone or in combination with EMR achieves complete eradication of dysplastic BE in a significant number of patients. Management of patients with BE requires a comprehensive treatment strategy providing consideration of both esophageal-sparing strategies using endoscopic techniques and esophagectomy.

SUGGESTED READINGS

Fleischer DE, Overholt BF, Sharma VK, et al: Endoscopic ablation of Barrett's esophagus: a multicenter study with 2.5 year follow-up, *Gastrointest Endosc* 68:867, 2008.

Shaheen NJ, Sharma P, Overholt BF, et al: Radiofrequency ablation in Barrett's esophagus with dysplasia, *N Engl J Med* 360:2277, 2009.

Sharma VK, Wang KK, Overholt BF, et al: Balloon-based, circumferential, endoscopic radiofrequency ablation of Barrett's esophagus: 1-year follow-up of 100 patients (with video), *Gastrointest Endosc* 65:185, 2007.

Smith CD, Bejarano PA, Melvin WS, et al: Endoscopic ablation of intestinal metaplasia containing high-grade dysplasia in esophagectomy patients using a balloon-based ablation system, *Surg Endosc* 21:560, 2006.

Pouw RE, Sharma VK, Bergman JJ, Fleischer DE: Radiofrequency ablation for total Barrett's eradication: a description of the endoscopic technique, its clinical results and future prospects, *Endoscopy* 40:1033, 2008.

Paraesophageal Hiatal Hernia

Farzaneh Banki, MD, and Tom R. DeMeester, MD

DEFINITION

An abdominal hernia is a protrusion of the abdominal cavity beyond its walls through a fascial or muscular opening or defect. Hiatal hernias are a protrusion through a muscular opening in the diaphragm, usually the diaphragmatic esophageal hiatus, and are classified based on their radiographic or endoscope appearance. The most common is type I, also called a *sliding hernia,* which represents approximately 95% of all hiatal hernias. The phrenoesophageal ligament is attenuated and stretched out, and this laxity allows the migration of the gastroesophageal junction (GEJ) into the thoracic cavity.

Type II is a paraesophageal hiatal hernia (PEH), characterized by the herniation of the gastric fundus through the diaphragmatic hiatus anterior and alongside the lower thoracic esophagus. The posterolateral attachments of the phrenoesophageal ligaments remain intact and maintain the GEJ below the diaphragmatic hiatus. An anterior weakness in the phrenoesophageal ligament and the enlarged diaphragmatic esophageal hiatus allows the formation of an intrathoracic sac, which lets the fundus and body of the stomach rotate anteriorly and cephalad into the thorax. The cause for the enlarged diaphragmatic esophageal hiatus is unknown but is hypothesized to be a developmental abnormality of the diaphragm as it forms from the costal margin and moves toward the center. A "pure" type II PEH seldom occurs.

The majority of cases are type III, a combination of type I and II, in which the GEJ is herniated above the diaphragm, and the fundus is herniated alongside the esophagus above the GEJ (Figure 1). When more than 30% of the stomach is herniated into the chest, the term *giant paraesophageal hernia* is used to describe the condition. When nearly all of the stomach is within the chest, the term *intrathoracic stomach* is used to describe the condition (Figure 2). When other organs such as the colon, small intestine, or spleen are present in the sac in addition to the stomach, the hernia is classified as a type IV. PEH must be differentiated from *parahiatal hernia,* a very rare condition in which the stomach herniates through a defect in the diaphragm adjacent to the esophageal hiatus (Figure 3).

CLINICAL MANIFESTATION

Patients with PEH vary from having no symptoms at the time of an incidental finding of the hernia to reporting symptoms of chest and epigastric pain, dysphagia, nausea, vomiting, palpitations, postprandial shortness of breath, and aspiration manifested by chronic cough, choking, dyspnea, and wheezing. Chest pain, the most common complaint, is usually substernal, postprandial, and often thought to be cardiac in origin. The complaint of heartburn may or may not be present.

Most symptoms of PEH are due to the volvulization of the stomach: attached at the GEJ and pylorus, the stomach rotates to an upside-down position as it ascends into the hernia sac. The dependent portion of the GEJ prevents the evacuation of swallowed air that collects in the volvulized body of the stomach. The distended stomach can compress the distal esophagus and cause dysphagia, or

it can compress the lung and cause shortness of breath. The most common laboratory finding is chronic blood loss anemia from erosions of the engorged gastric mucosa secondary to the gastric distension and compression of the gastric veins at the hiatus. PEHs can be life threatening in that the volvulized distended stomach can lead to a cascade of catastrophic events, such as excessive bleeding or acute gastric obstruction with incarceration, strangulation, and perforation.

PATHOPHYSIOLOGY

Hiatal hernias are caused by a combination of factors: 1) enlargement of the esophageal hiatus due to developmental defects, 2) an increased abdominal thoracic pressure gradient, 3) altered collagen metabolism, and 4) depletion of elastic fibers in the phrenoesophageal membrane with aging. The hiatal enlargement and attenuated phrenoesophageal ligament allows the formation of a hernia sac anterior to the esophagus. The abdominal thoracic pressure gradient encourages the migration of the gastric fundus and body into the hernia sac and sets the stage for volvulization of the stomach.

PEH is the most common cause of gastric volvulus in both adults and children. Less frequent causes are eventration of the diaphragm, diaphragmatic defects caused by trauma, or congenital defects such as a Bochdalek hernia, commonly seen in children. Eventration of the left diaphragm can allow the stomach to volvulize within the abdomen. This is called a *primary gastric volvulus* and is often associated with symptoms similar to those of a gastric volvulus that occurs with a PEH.

There are two ways the stomach can rotate when a volvulus occurs. The most common form is *organoaxial rotation,* when the greater curvature of the stomach rotates horizontally on its longitudinal axis between the pylorus and the GEJ. Rarely, the stomach rotates vertically on a line parallel to the gastrohepatic ligament, a condition known as *mesenteroaxial rotation* (Figure 4).

Diagnosis and Assessment

The diagnosis of PEH is based on radiographic and endoscopic findings; physical examination frequently provides little information.

Chest Film

A retrocardiac air-fluid level on a routine chest film is suggestive of gastric volvulus and is a common mode of discovery of PEH.

Videoesophagram

Videoesophagram is especially helpful in the assessment of patients suspected of having PEH. The study illustrates the anatomy, including the organoaxial volvulus of the stomach (Figure 5), and the presence of other intraabdominal organs in the chest. The videoesophagram also evaluates the esophageal transport of barium into the stomach to assess esophageal motility. If there is poor esophageal transport or clearance of barium, motility of the esophageal body should be assessed prior to surgical therapy.

Upper Endoscopy

The upper endoscopy should be performed by the operating surgeon to assess the amount of herniated stomach, the degree of gastric volvulus, the extent of venous engorgement and ulceration of the gastric mucosa, and the presence of esophagitis and ulceration in the distal esophagus.

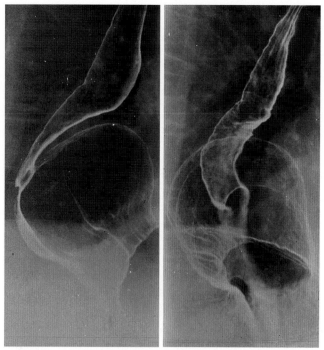

FIGURE 1 An air contrast/barium radiogram showing a type III hiatal hernia composed of a type I and a type II hernia. The GEJ has slid above the diaphragm, as in a type I hernia, and the fundus of the stomach is herniated along side the esophagus above the GEJ, as in a type II hernia.

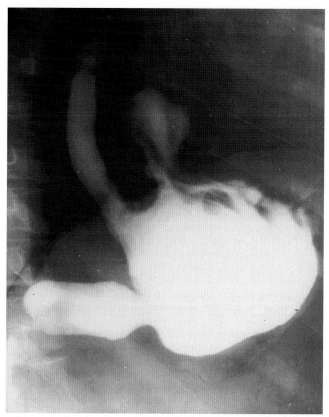

FIGURE 3 A radiogram obtained from an upper gastrointestinal barium study showing a rare parahiatal hernia, in which the stomach herniates through a defect in the diaphragm adjacent to the esophageal hiatus.

Esophageal Motility Study

It is particularly important to assess the motility of the esophageal body prior to surgery in patients whose esophageal clearance of barium on the videoesophagram is abnormal. The passing of a motility catheter can be challenging, and at times impossible, due to the altered anatomy. In this situation the motility catheter should be placed into the stomach at the time of endoscopy. It is not unusual for the lower esophageal sphincter (LES) pressure to be increased in patients with PEH because the herniated stomach exerts pressure on the LES, causing a false elevation. Measuring the location of the LES also helps in positioning the pH probe or capsule to determine the degree of esophageal acid exposure.

24- to 48-Hour Esophageal pH Monitoring

We do not routinely obtain esophageal pH monitoring in patients with PEH because the results usually do not change the management of the condition. Some surgeons advocate repairing only the hernia in patients who have normal esophageal acid exposure. There is limited support for this approach in the literature, and usually the degree of dissection necessary to remove the hernia sac makes performing an antireflux procedure a necessity.

THERAPY

Most physicians agree that patients with a symptomatic PEH need to be surgically treated. In contrast, controversy exists over the management of patients who are asymptomatic or have only mild symptoms. The concept of "watchful waiting" for patients with an asymptomatic PEH has been advanced by some surgeons because episodes of gastric

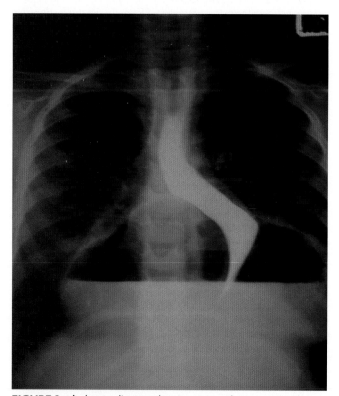

FIGURE 2 A chest radiogram showing an intrathoracic stomach. The esophagus and stomach are filled with contrast, which illustrates the size of the distended stomach and the dependent position of the GEJ.

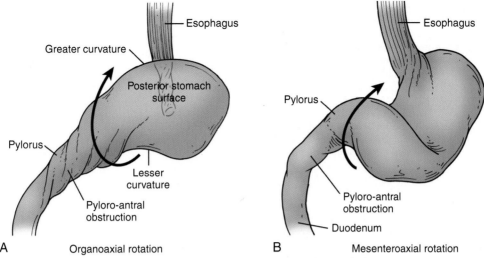

A   Organoaxial rotation   B   Mesenteroaxial rotation

FIGURE 4   The two ways the stomach can rotate when a volvulus occurs.

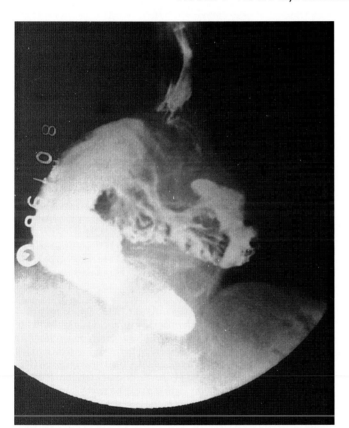

FIGURE 5   A radiogram obtained from a videoesophagram, showing an organoaxial volvulus of the stomach. Notice the stomach is upside down, and the GEJ is in a dependent position below the volvulized gastric body.

incarceration and strangulation are rare after the age of 60 years; even if an emergency operation is required, the difficulty of the procedure is not as challenging as was thought in the past. Other physicians observe a lower threshold for surgical treatment, sighting the low but existing risk for future complications and the improved success of the minimally invasive approach as the reason. In our experience, it is uncommon to see patients with a PEH who are asymptomatic; consequently, most hernias are repaired. The occasional asymptomatic patient is educated about the progressive nature of this disease and the future risks, although low, of aspiration, gastric incarceration,

obstruction, bleeding, strangulation, perforation, and death. Most asymptomatic patients, especially those who wish to travel, elect to have the hernia repaired, particularly if it can be done laparoscopically.

Surgical Approach

Traditionally, a PEH was repaired through a thoracotomy or laparotomy incision with a morbidity rate of 20%, a mortality rate of 2%, and a median length of stay of 7 days. The development of laparoscopic surgery has allowed the repair of these complicated hernias by a minimally invasive approach, with reported mortality rates of 0.5% and a median length of stay of 3 days. During 40 years of experience, our surgical approach has evolved from an open transthoracic approach to an open transabdominal approach and eventually to a laparoscopic approach.

Surgical Challenges in the Repair of Paraesophageal Hiatal Hernia

Laparoscopic repair of PEH is challenging and should be performed by expert laparoscopic surgeons who are familiar with the anatomy of the cardia and the principles of antireflux surgery. The operation needs to be done systematically and meticulously. The risk of gastric perforation is higher compared with the repair of type I hernias due to the large hernia sac that extends high in the mediastinum and the altered anatomy of the posterior hiatus and gastrohepatic ligament. The posterior vagal nerve is usually separated from the esophagus and can be easily injured. The important steps of the operation are covered here.

Excision of the Hernia Sac

PEH is often seen with a large hernia sac that extends high in the mediastinum and commonly adheres to the right and left crus, pleura, pericardium and, at times, the inferior pulmonary veins. The gastrohepatic ligament can be displaced high in the mediastinum, making the anatomy confusing for an inexperienced surgeon.

The first step in correcting this is to reduce the herniated organs into the abdomen as much as possible. An extra retraction port may be necessary to keep them reduced. An avascular plane is developed at the lip of the diaphragmatic esophageal hiatus, and the sac is bluntly dissected off intrathoracic structures. If moderate bleeding ensues, it is likely that the proper plane has not been correctly identified; dissection of the sac can generally be done with minimal bleeding in an avascular plane.

When completely mobilized, the sac is reduced into the abdomen and excised by dividing the sac down to the anterior wall of the esophagus and around the GEJ. Complete dissection and excision of the hernia sac are crucial for a successful repair, and care should be taken not to injure the vagal nerves during excision of the sac.

Isolation of the Posterior Vagal Nerve

We routinely dissect and isolate the posterior vagal nerve during the dissection of the right posterior wall of the sac. The nerve commonly lies to the right of the esophagus and aorta, close to the posterior chest wall.

Management of Short Esophagus

The diagnosis of a short esophagus should be suspected if the patient has a stricture, a long-segment Barrett esophagus on endoscopy, or a short esophageal length on manometry. These clinical markers are only suggestive of a short esophagus. Shortening of esophageal length occurs with progressive mucosal disease, but the individual variation is considerable. Consequently, there is no definitive threshold at which a short esophagus can be readily identified.

The only absolute way to identify a clinically significant shortened esophagus is by an inability to surgically mobilize 3 cm of the distal esophagus into the abdomen. If 2 to 3 cm of true esophagus lie below the posterior border of the diaphragmatic esophageal hiatus without applying tension, the esophagus is not shortened. Less than 2 cm of abdominal esophagus can place sufficient tension on a repair to cause it to herniate or disrupt over time. It is important to realize that the diaphragm contracts 30,000 times per day to carry out the work of respiration, and the esophagus contracts 1000 times a day swallowing. Consequently, unless the repair is free of tension, breakdown can be expected.

The best management of a short esophagus is to perform a lengthening procedure, originally described by Dr. Lee Collis and called a *gastroplasty*. Initially the procedure was done through a transthoracic approach. Later, a technique for performing a Collis gastroplasty via a transabdominal approach was described. The technique consists of passing a 48 Fr bougie down the esophagus and making a circular opening in the stomach with an end-to-end anastomosis stapler 4 cm from the GEJ and closely adjacent to the indwelling bougie. A gastrointestinal anastomosis (GIA) stapler is used to divide the stomach parallel and snugly against the bougie, between the circular opening and the GEJ. This provides 4 to 5 cm of additional esophageal length (Figure 6).

A Nissen fundoplication is constructed around the neoesophagus. The procedure allows for a tension-free fundoplication and results in an effective antireflux mechanism. It is possible for the procedure to leave a small segment of acid-secreting gastric mucosa proximal to the intact fundoplication. Although not desirable, it is accepted over the risk of having an almost certain reherniation of the antireflux repair. Complications of the procedure are persistent dysphagia from a gastroplasty tube that is too small and ischemia of the gastroplasty tube that leads to ulceration, bleeding, necrosis, and stricture. To avoid the latter, every effort should be made not to devascularize the lesser curvature.

Today, advances in technology have made it possible for a Collis gastroplasty to be performed laparoscopically by excising a wedge of fundus along the greater curvature, as shown in Figure 7. An endo-GIA stapler is used first to divide the stomach from the greater curvature down to an indwelling 48 Fr bougie and then parallel to and snugly along the bougie to the GEJ. The angles to perform these maneuvers can be difficult but are made simpler by adding a retraction port in the right flank, at the level of the umbilicus, and inserting the endo-GIA stapler for the second step through the retraction port in the left flank.

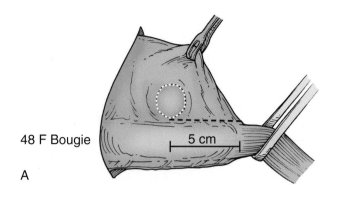

48 F Bougie

A

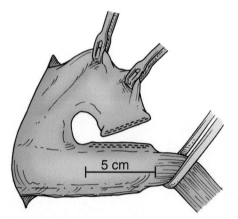

B

FIGURE 6   An open transabdominal Collis gastroplasty. **A,** An EEA stapler is passed through the stomach along the lesser curvature adjacent to a bougie and 5 cm from the GEJ. **B,** The stomach is divided along the bougie for a distance of 5 cm with a GIA stapler. This creates an extra 5 cm of esophageal length. The portion of fundus superior to the EEA excised circle is amputated, and the remaining fundus and body of the stomach are advanced cephalad to form the fundoplication around the newly constructed gastroplasty tube.

Management of a Wide Crura

The wide crural openings in patients with PEH require particular attention because obtaining a permanent crural closure is the Achilles heel of the repair. In patients with PEH, it is common for the crura to fail to develop properly, so the opening between the right and left crus is greater than 4 cm and more circular than oval in shape (Figure 8). This is too wide to close effectively without tension. Furthermore, in patients with PEH, the right crus can be atretic and may hold sutures poorly, resulting in tearing of the crural muscle, separation of the crural closure, and reherniation of the repair.

To prevent reherniation, pledgets of Surgisis (Cook Biotech, West Lafayette, Ind.) are used to reinforce the closure. Three centimeter pledgets of Surgisis with 0-0 Ethibond suture (Ethicon, Somerville, NJ) are used to approximate the crural closure. A second row of double-0 Ethibond figure-eight stitches are used to secure the closure; stitches should incorporate large bites of crural muscle. The last figure-eight stitch should be placed after the bougie used to size the Collis gastroplasty and the fundoplication have been removed. The crura are approximated snugly around the esophagus, and crural sutures are tied using the Ti-Knot device (LSi Solutions, Victor, NY), to approximate the crura without tension or strangulation of the muscle. A 4 × 5 cm piece of absorbable Vicryl mesh (Dermabond; Ethicon, Somerville, NJ) is laid over the crural closure and anchored with BioGlue (CryoLife, Kennesaw, Ga.). The Vicryl mesh and BioGlue, while absorbed, induce the infiltration of permanent fibrous tissue.

Division of Short Gastric Vessels

Division of short gastric vessels allows a complete mobilization of the stomach for construction of a fundoplication, rather than performing a fundic wrap with only the anterior fundic wall. The stubs of the short gastric vessel provide a landmark for keeping the fundoplication in the proper plane. At the completion of the fundoplication, the greater curvature, identified by the location of the stubs of the short gastric vessels, should remain on the left side of the abdomen in the exact location as before construction of the fundoplication. This prevents twisting the fundoplication and narrowing the fundoplication.

Reconstruction of Nissen Fundoplication

Following the division of short gastric vessels, a draw stitch is placed on the posterior fundic wall of the stomach 6 cm down from the GEJ along the greater curvature at mid width on the posterior fundic wall. With gentle dissection the posterior vagus nerve is isolated from the esophagus, and the tail of the draw stitch is used to pull the posterior fundic lip of the fundoplication through the window between the posterior vagus nerve and the esophagus. The anterior fundic lip is formed by pulling the anterior fundic wall over the anterior wall of the esophagus.

The anterior and posterior fundic lips are approximated using 2-0 pledgetted Proline sutures (Ethicon) over the 48 Fr bougie used to size the gastroplasty tube, incorporating the right lateral esophageal wall between the lips. If a gastroplasty was not done, a 60 Fr bougie

is used. The nylon suture pulls through tissue smoothly and avoids hematoma formation.

The approximated lips of the fundoplication are placed in the right anterolateral position to keep the stomach in its normal plane (Figure 9). Pledgetted stitches are used to avoid early disruption of the repair from unexpected gastric distension or patient retching during recovery from anesthesia. One well-oiled 2-0 silk stitch is added cranial and caudal to the fundoplication to give it a length of 1.5 to 2 cm. The bougie is removed, the fundoplication is retracted to the left, and the closure of the hiatus is finished with additional figure-eight sutures.

Recurrence After Repair of PEH

One of the most concerning complications following the repair of paraesophageal hernias has been the lack of long-term durability and recurrent herniation. The rate of recurrent hernias has been

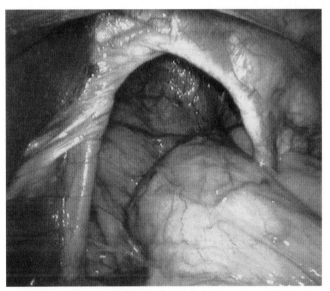

FIGURE 8   A laparoscopic view of an enlarged esophageal hiatus. Note that the right and left crura are separated by more than 4 cm and will require a reinforced closure.

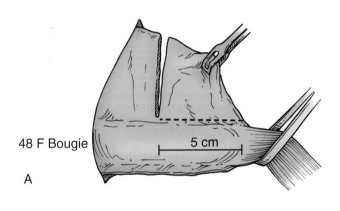

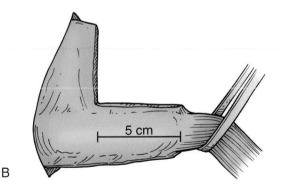

FIGURE 7   A laparoscopic Collis gastroplasty. **A,** The stomach is divided with an endo-GIA from the greater curvature down to a 48 Fr bougie placed along the lesser curvature and 5 cm from the GEJ. **B,** A wedge of stomach is removed by dividing the stomach with an endo-GIA along the bougie up to the GEJ. This usually requires that the endo-GIA is placed through the left lateral flank port. The remaining fundus and body of the stomach are advanced cephalad to form the fundoplication around the newly constructed gastroplasty tube.

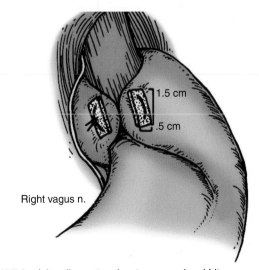

FIGURE 9   A line illustration showing a completed Nissen fundoplication with the posterior fundic lip brought through the window between the posterior vagal nerve and the posterior esophageal wall and securing the fundoplication in the right anterolateral position. The technique for closing the esophageal hiatus is not shown.

TABLE 1: Summary of operative tips to construct a durable fundoplication

1. Excision of the hernia sac
   a. Develop an avascular plane between the hernia sac and the surrounding structures.
   b. Reduce and completely excise the hernia sac.
   c. Identify and protect the vagal nerves.
2. Esophaeal mobilization
   a. Mobilize the distal half of the esophagus.
   b. Ensure an intraabdominal length of 2 to 3 cm.
3. Assessment of esophageal length
   a. Assess the tension-free abdominal esophageal length; if unable to obtain 2 to 3 cm of tension-free esophageal abdominal length, perform a Collis gastroplasty.
4. Construction of a posterior window for the posterior fundic lip of the fundoplication
   a. Separate the posterior vagus nerve with gentle dissection.
   b. Make a window by dividing its mesentery longitudinally.
5. Construction of the fundoplication
   a. Take down the short gastric vessels over the upper third of the greater curvature.
   b. Draw the posterior fundic lip of the fundoplication between the esophagus and the posterior vagus nerve.
   c. Construct the fundoplication over a 60 Fr bougie.
   d. Place the fundoplication in the right anterolateral position.
   e. Use 2-0 pledgetted Proline sutures with generous bites to approximate the anterior and posterior fundic lip to form the fundoplication.
   f. Use 2-0 silk stitches caudal and cranial to the pledgets to give a fundoplication of 1.5 to 2 cm.
6. Closure of the enlarged crura
   a. Reduce the crural opening with two to three U stitches of double-0 Ethibond over Surgisis pledgets.
   b. Approximate the crural edge with large, figure-eight double-0 Ethibond sutures.
   c. Cover the crural closure below the esophagus with a patch of Vicryl mesh anchored with the application of BioGlue.

reported to be 10% after a transthoracic approach, 15% after an open transabdominal approach, and from 2.5% to 42% after a laparoscopic approach. After 40 years of experience with the procedure, we have concluded that the most common cause of recurrence is a short esophagus or an enlarged crural opening. Operative tips to prevent recurrence of a PEH repair are shown in Table 1.

SUMMARY

PEHs make up less than 5% of all hiatal hernias but account for most of the hiatal hernia complications. They are unique in that the normal posterior phrenoesophageal ligament anchors the GEJ within the abdomen, and the body and fundus of the stomach herniate through a large esophageal hiatus and into a large anterior, peritoneal-lined sac.

Chest pain and dysphagia are the most common symptoms. The most common complication of a paraesophageal hiatal hernia is an intermittent esophageal obstruction from compression of the distal esophagus by the distended, herniated stomach. The most common laboratory finding is chronic blood loss and anemia from erosions in the engorged gastric mucosa secondary to compression of the gastric veins at the hiatus. Videoesophagram and upper endoscopy are essential for diagnosis.

Traditionally, PEHs were repaired through a thoracotomy or laparotomy incision, but the development in laparoscopic surgery has allowed repair of these hernias by a minimally invasive approach. The key steps of the operation are 1) excision of the hernia sac, 2) isolation of the posterior vagus nerve, 3) complete esophageal mobilization, 4) freeing the fundus by taking down the short gastric vessels, 5) performing a Collis gastroplasty if a short esophagus is encountered, 6) reinforcing the crural closure with absorbable pledgets and mesh, and 7) reconstructing a durable Nissen fundoplication.

It is important to recognize that an antireflux operation is different than the surgical removal of a diseased organ. In the former, the anatomy of an organ is rearranged to improve its function. In this situation, surgical technique is paramount to a good outcome. Over time the procedure has been improved by surgeons who follow their patients' recovery and adjust their technique based on analysis of patient outcome. The laparoscopic repair of a PEH is challenging and needs to be performed in a systematic and meticulous manner by experienced laparoscopic surgeons who have a good grasp of esophageal physiology and the principles of antireflux surgery.

SUGGESTED READINGS

Gastal OL, Hagen JA, Peters JH, et al: Short esophagus: analysis of predictors and clinical implications, *Arch Surg* 134:633–636, 1999.

Hashemi M, Peters JH, DeMeester TR, et al: Laparoscopic repair of large paraesophageal hernia: objective follow-up reveals high recurrence rate, *J Am Coll Surg* 190(5):553–560, 2000.

Oelschlager BK, Pellegrini CA, Hunter J, et al: Biologic prosthesis reduces recurrence after laparoscopic paraesophageal hernia repair: a multicenter, prospective, randomized trial, *Ann Surg* 244(4):481–490, 2006.

Pierre AF, Luketich JD, Fernando HC, et al: Results of laparoscopic repair of giant paraesophageal hernias: 200 consecutive patients, *Ann Thorac Surg* 74:1909–1916, 2002.

Patel HJ, Tan BB, Yee J: A 25-year experience with open primary transthoracic repair of paraesophageal hiatal hernia, *J Thorac Cardiovasc Surg* 127:843–849, 2003.

Skinner DB, Belsey RH: Surgical management of esophageal reflux and hiatus hernia: long-term results with 1030 patients, *J Thorac Cardiovasc Surg* 53(1):33–54, 1967.

Zehetner J, Lipham JC, Ayazi S, et al: A simplified technique for intrathoracic stomach repair: laparoscopic fundoplication with Vicryl mesh and BioGlue crural reinforcement, *Surg Endosc* 24:675–679, 2009.

Management of Pharyngeal Esophageal (Zenker) Diverticula

Helen Sohn, MD, and Steven R. DeMeester, MD

DIVERTICULA

Esophageal diverticula are unusual but interesting abnormalities that can develop in any part of the esophagus. Most commonly they are found in the cervical esophagus; in this location, they are known as *Zenker diverticula.* There are two etiologies for esophageal diverticula: *pulsion* and *traction,* with pulsion representing the most common form in the United States. A pulsion diverticulum develops as a consequence of a motility abnormality in the esophagus distal to the site of the diverticulum.

A Zenker diverticulum is a pulsion diverticulum that occurs secondary to repetitive pharyngeal pressure on a food bolus that is delayed by a dysfunctional cricopharyngeus muscle. Over time this pressure causes a herniation of the esophageal mucosa through a weak point called a *Killian dehiscence,* located superior to the cricopharyngeus muscle at its junction with the inferior constrictor muscle. Pulsion diverticula are not composed of the entire wall of the esophagus and are therefore considered false diverticula. Radiographically, they typically have a wide neck, rounded contour, and retain contrast on a barium swallow.

Symptoms associated with pulsion diverticula are often initially related to the underlying motility abnormality, but as the size of the diverticulum increases, some symptoms may develop secondary to the pouch itself. Although dysphagia is often the primary symptom, as the pouch enlarges, regurgitation becomes a more prominent symptom and may prompt a diagnosis of gastroesophageal reflux disease (GERD) unless a careful history is obtained. Careful questioning in these patients will elicit the important information that the regurgitated material tastes bland, not bitter, and often includes pills or small food particles, suggesting that the regurgitated material is food and fluid that never made it to the stomach. Other symptoms attributable to a Zenker diverticulum are halitosis, cough, and aspiration of debris retained within the pouch. The larger the pouch, the more troublesome these symptoms may be for the patient.

Surgery is the only effective therapy for esophageal diverticula. Dilatation of the cricopharyngeus muscle and its temporary paralysis with Botox injections have been attempted with limited success, and even if dysphagia is improved, these therapies do not address the pouch. Given the absence of effective nonsurgical therapy and the relative safety of most of these procedures, symptomatic patients with an esophageal diverticulum should be considered for surgical therapy regardless of age.

The surgical plan for patients with a Zenker diverticulum includes myotomy of the dysfunctional cricopharyngeus muscle and either excision or suspension of the diverticulum based on its size and location. Alternatively, some Zenker diverticula are amenable to a transoral endoscopic approach. Regardless of the approach, failure to divide the dysfunctional cricopharyngeus muscle leads to a high rate of recurrence and increases the risk of a leak from the suture or staple line if the diverticulum has been excised.

PREOPERATIVE ASSESSMENT

The physical examination of patients with an esophageal diverticulum is generally unrevealing, even when a large Zenker diverticulum is present. However, if a transoral approach for correction of the condition is being considered, it is important to assess the patient's ability to adequately open the mouth and extend the neck.

The best way to visualize an esophageal diverticulum is with a barium swallow, although our preference is a video swallow esophagogram; in addition to showing the size and location of the diverticulum, it provides information about the efficacy of bolus transport by the esophageal body. The barium study should also be used to assess for hiatal hernia or other potential abnormalities associated with the presence of GERD. Upper endoscopy is useful both to measure the size of the diverticulum and to evaluate the esophageal mucosa for any abnormalities, particularly in elderly patients, for whom it is essential to rule out malignancy.

Esophageal manometry, although important in patients with a mid or distal esophageal diverticulum to evaluate for an underlying motility abnormality, is unnecessary in patients with a Zenker diverticulum because the cause is always dysfunction of the cricopharyngeus muscle. Underlying conditions that explain the dysfunction include scarring or fibrosis from injury, cervical spine procedures or radiation therapy, and neurologic abnormalities such as can occur with a stroke. In younger patients with a Zenker diverticulum, often no clear reason for the dysfunction is apparent and GERD is often present; it is reasonable to wonder about the potential association of proximal reflux in the development of Zenker diverticula.

Even though the cause of a Zenker diverticulum is cricopharyngeus muscle dysfunction, results from a motility test are often normal. In this area of the esophagus, the muscle is skeletal rather than smooth, and events happen quickly and are hard to capture on standard motility testing. If an esophageal motility study is planned, it is usually necessary to pass the motility catheter using endoscopic guidance because the catheter may otherwise coil in the diverticulum. Motility abnormalities that may be recognized with a Zenker diverticulum include evidence of outflow obstruction, such as increased bolus pressure in the pharyngeal contraction wave, and incomplete or discoordinated relaxation of the cricopharyngeus with a swallow.

OPERATIVE TECHNIQUE

Transcervical Cricopharyngeal Myotomy and Diverticulectomy or Suspension

The traditional approach for repair of a Zenker diverticulum is transcervical, with the patient positioned supine and the neck extended. An incision is made in the left neck along the anterior border of the sternocleidomastoid muscle. The muscle and carotid sheath are retracted laterally. The omohyoid, sternothyroid, and sternohyoid muscles are divided to facilitate exposure of the entire cervical esophagus.

The Zenker diverticulum will be located posterior to the cricoid cartilage, sheathed in multiple layers of fibrous tissue that must be teased apart to permit exposure of the base of the diverticulum. Once exposed, a longitudinal myotomy on the posterolateral aspect of the cervical esophagus is started just inferior to the base of the diverticulum. It should extend inferiorly to the thoracic inlet, where it is carried superiorly through the muscular ring of the cricopharyngeus at the base of the diverticulum.

Typically, the muscle in the area of the base of the diverticulum is quite thick and fibrotic. Once released, the diverticulum should be clearly visualized. To ensure that all of the dysfunctional fibers are divided, we also incise the lower fibers of the inferior pharyngeal constrictor superiorly from the base of the diverticulum proximally for 1 to 2 cm. In addition, the edges of the divided muscle should be bluntly dissected to widely splay open the mucosa and permit identification and division of any residual circular muscle fibers.

Next, the diverticulum is either suspended or excised. Diverticula 2 cm or less in size are easily suspended by tacking the tip of the diverticulum with 3-0 Prolene to the precervical fascia as high up in the neck as necessary to fully upend the pouch. Larger pouches are difficult to fully upend and are best excised using a thoracoabdominal (TA) stapler with a 52 Fr bougie in the esophagus to prevent narrowing of the esophageal lumen. The staple line and/or myotomy can be checked for leaks by passing a nasogastric tube into the area and insufflating air to distend the mucosa while the neck incision is filled with saline. This also provides an opportunity to ensure sufficient mucosal distension with no residual bands throughout the area of the myotomy.

Before neck closure, it is critical to ensure perfect hemostasis because a hematoma requiring reexploration can develop from even small vessels secondary to coughing or straining as the patient awakens from anesthesia. We leave a small, closed suction drain in place and approximate the platysma and skin to complete the operation.

Transoral Endoscopic Stapled Diverticulotomy

A transoral endoscopic approach is another option for treating a Zenker diverticulum. This approach is attractive largely because it eliminates the neck incision, but it is limited; the pouch must be at least 3 cm in length, and the patient must be able to extend the neck and open the mouth widely. Inability to adequately extend the neck and open the mouth widely makes placement of the rigid Weerda diverticuloscope (Karl Storz, Tuttingen, Germany) diverticuloscope difficult to impossible. If the diverticulum is less than 3 cm in length, it will not permit adequate division of the dysfunctional cricopharyngeus muscle, leading to persistent or recurrent symptoms.

Patients with evidence of malignancy inside the pouch are also not candidates for a transoral stapling technique and instead require excision of the pouch. Although the procedure is quick and well tolerated—and in suitable patients, it produces excellent relief of dysphagia and regurgitation symptoms—patients must be warned of the possibility of chipped teeth secondary to insertion of the rigid scope. In addition, most patients have tongue swelling for a day or two after the procedure.

Before the procedure commences, a 30 mm gastrointestinal anastomosis (GIA) laparoscopic stapler is modified by cutting off the tip of the stapler with an orthopedic circular saw, such that the knife blade and the staple line reach the end of the modified tip. The tip should be smoothed with a rasp or file. The patient is placed under general anesthesia and positioned supine with the neck extended, and the Weerda diverticuloscope is inserted carefully under direct visualization and advanced into the esophagus. It is helpful to have a pediatric flexible esophagoscope to facilitate placement of the rigid scope. The goal is to advance the longer anterior blade into the true lumen of the esophagus while the shorter posterior blade is advanced into the diverticulum.

Once positioned, the blades of the scope are separated to permit clear visualization of the cricopharyngeus muscle band (Figure 1). Using a laparoscopic needle holder, 3-0 Prolene traction sutures are placed on each side of the cricopharyngeus muscle (Figure 2). With gentle traction on these stitches, the bar is held in position as the modified GIA stapler is inserted and fired (Figure 3). Several applications of the stapler are typically necessary to divide the muscle bridge all the way to the tip of the diverticulum (Figure 4). In this fashion, the cricopharyngeus muscle is divided, and the pouch is incorporated into the esophagus to create a single common cavity. If the diverticulum is less than 3 cm in length, the cricopharyngeus muscle will not be adequately divided, leading to a high rate of symptomatic failure and a significant risk for the development of a recurrent diverticulum. It is important to modify the stapler to minimize the amount of residual pouch with the transoral approach, since even a 1 cm remnant can lead to persistent symptoms of regurgitation. While it is nearly impossible to completely eliminate the pouch, it has been our experience that patients with less than 4 to 5 mm of residual pouch remain asymptomatic.

POSTOPERATIVE CARE

Patients are kept NPO after the procedure until the following day, or 24 to 48 hours longer when the diverticulum has been excised. We typically obtain a Gastrografin esophagogram before starting oral feeds, both to document the integrity of the myotomy, with or without a staple line, and to verify that the patient is able to swallow without aspiration.

COMPLICATIONS AND RESULTS

Major morbidity is uncommon, but potential complications include a leak from the myotomy or suture line if the diverticulum was excised, mediastinitis, fistula formation, hoarseness from vocal cord paralysis, incomplete myotomy, luminal stenosis, and wound infection. Long-term complications include recurrence. The likelihood of a recurrent diverticulum is reduced when a myotomy is performed compared with diverticulectomy alone. A good or excellent outcome is reported by the majority of patients.

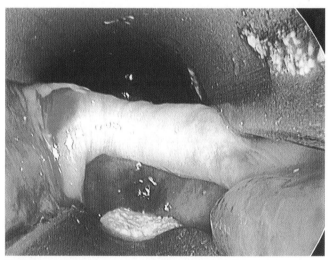

FIGURE 1   Diverticuloscope positioned with the longer, upper blade in the true lumen of the esophagus and the shorter blade in the diverticulum (*lower left*). The cricopharyngeus muscle band is clearly seen between the blades.

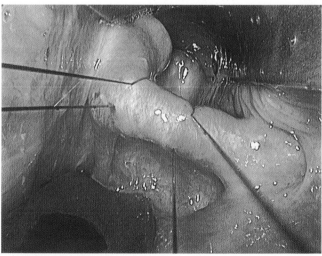

FIGURE 2   Traction sutures in place in preparation for the stapling.

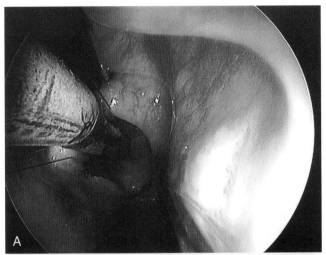

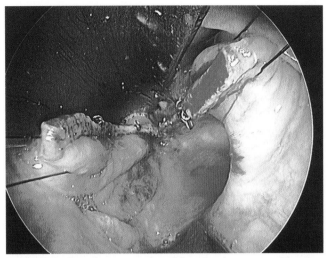

FIGURE 4   Complete transection of the cricopharyngeus achieved with multiple loads of a 30 mm GIA stapler. A common chamber has now been created between the true esophageal lumen and the diverticulum, and the dysfunctional cricopharyngeus muscle has been completely divided.

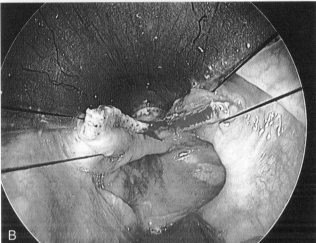

FIGURE 3   **A,** Modified 30-mm GIA stapler inserted and ready. **B,** Partial transection of the cricopharyngeus after use of a single 30 mm GIA stapler. Note the residual pouch.

SUMMARY

Zenker diverticula are an uncommon but interesting esophageal abnormality. They develop as a consequence of an underlying esophageal motility disorder in the cricopharyngeus muscle. All symptomatic patients should be considered surgical candidates because there is no effective medical therapy. Surgical treatment for a pulsion diverticulum, such as a Zenker diverticulum, requires alleviating the outflow obstruction with an esophageal myotomy coupled with diverticulectomy or diverticulopexy. These objectives can be accomplished with transoral stapling of the cricopharyngeus muscle and creation of a common cavity between the esophageal lumen and the pouch in selected patients with a pouch at least 3 cm in depth. Careful patient evaluation and technical precision during the procedure will ensure excellent results.

SUGGESTED READING

Aly A, Devitt PG, Jamieson GG: Evolution of surgical treatment for pharyngeal pouch, *Br J Surg* 91:657–664, 2004.

Bremner CG, DeMeester TR: Endoscopic treatment of Zenker's diverticulum, *Gastrointest Endosc* 49:126–128, 1999.

Nehra D, Lord RV, DeMeester TR, et al: Physiologic basis for the treatment of epiphrenic diverticulum, *Ann Surg* 235:346–354, 2002.

Salerno CT, Mitchell JD, Whyte RI: Congenital and acquired esophageal diverticula. In Yang SC, Cameron DE (eds): *Current therapy in thoracic and cardiovascular surgery*, St Louis, 2004, Mosby Elsevier, pp 432–435.

CURRENT TREATMENT OF ACHALASIA

William O. Richards, MD, and D. Brandon Williams, MD

HISTORY

In 1672, Sir Thomas Willis first described the symptoms of achalasia in a patient who was unable to swallow liquids. The initial treatment was esophageal dilatation using a carved whalebone with a sponge attached to its tip. In North America, esophageal achalasia is a rare idiopathic motility disorder that affects 1 in 100,000 individuals, yet it is the most commonly diagnosed primary esophageal motility disorder, second only to gastroesophageal reflux disease (GERD) as the most common functional esophageal disorder requiring surgical intervention.

Achalasia is a benign, idiopathic disorder caused by progressive neuronal degeneration in the mesenteric plexus of Auerbach, which results in a nonrelaxing, hypertensive lower esophageal sphincter (LES) and aperistalsis of the body of the esophagus. Peak incidence is between 20 and 50 years of age, and the most common clinical features are progressive dysphagia, to both solids and liquids, and regurgitation. Achalasia is also a risk factor for the development of esophageal cancer, presumably as a consequence of chronic esophagitis due to stasis. One recent study reported an increased risk of cancer 140-fold over that of the general population.

DIAGNOSIS

Typically, patients note progressive dysphagia to both solids and liquids. Symptoms of chest pain, regurgitation of undigested food, and failure to clear acid from the esophagus are frequently misdiagnosed as GERD, based on clinical history alone, in early achalasia. Weight loss is generally modest in nature, and many patients maintain their weight despite progressive symptoms.

Achalasia is a motor disorder of the esophagus composed of two distinct abnormalities that must be satisfied for diagnosis: 1) aperistalsis of the body of the esophagus in the distal smooth muscle segment of the esophageal body and 2) incomplete or absent relaxation of the LES with deglutition. Additional manometric findings that are characteristic but not necessary for the diagnosis of achalasia include elevated LES pressure and elevated intraesophageal body pressure compared to the pressure found within the stomach.

A complete and absolute manometric diagnosis of achalasia should be obtained prior to therapeutic intervention. In classic achalasia, low-amplitude aperistaltic contractions occur within the body of the esophagus. A variant of achalasia called *vigorous achalasia* is characterized by aperistalsis but with pressures less than 60 mm Hg produced in the body of the esophagus. Patients with vigorous achalasia have more chest pain associated with their disease and have less esophageal dilation than patients with classic end-stage achalasia.

A barium swallow will show repetitive nonperistaltic contractions and incomplete relaxation of the LES that is not coordinated with wet swallows. A telltale "bird's beak" deformity of the distal esophagus and LES is seen with failure of the barium to pass (Figure 1). In later stages the esophagus can be dramatically dilated to the point that the esophagus takes on the appearance of the sigmoid colon.

Endoscopy should be performed in all patients suspected of having achalasia to ensure that there is not a proximal gastric cancer infiltrating the LES causing pseudoachalasia.

TREATMENT MODALITIES

There are basically four modalities that can be used for the treatment of achalasia: 1) medical treatment, 2) endoscopic Botox injection, 3) pneumatic dilatation, and 4) surgical myotomy.

Medical Treatment

Many drugs have been tried for treatment of achalasia, but they are generally considered only in patients who are not candidates for surgery or other treatment modalities. Isosorbide dinitrate has been shown to reduce LES pressure transiently after sublingual administration. Calcium channel blockers act to block calcium uptake in the smooth muscle cells and reduce LES pressure. In one study, nifedipine was able to reduce LES pressure 30% to 40% after sublingual administration of 20 mg. However, subsequent placebo-controlled crossover trials have found only minimal clinical improvement with nifedipine.

Multiple prospective studies have demonstrated the effectiveness of botulinum toxin A injection (Botox) for relief of symptoms that typically lasts 3 to 12 months in 50% to 60% of patients. A randomized trial of 80 patients compared Botox injection, two treatments spaced 1 month apart, with surgical myotomy with fundoplication.

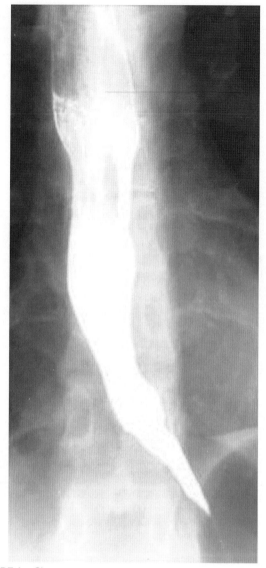

FIGURE 1   Characteristic upper gastrointestinal radiography in achalasia, with a distal tapered narrowing, the so-called "bird's beak" deformity.

Only 6 months after treatment, 45% of the Botox group experienced a recurrence of symptoms. In a 2-year follow-up, the probability of being symptom free was much higher in the myotomy group: 87.5% versus 34%. Another drawback to the use of Botox is that repeated injections sclerose the gastroesophageal junction (GEJ), making surgical myotomy more difficult and more prone to result in mucosal injury.

Endoscopic pneumatic dilatation of the LES may be the most effective nonsurgical treatment for achalasia. A recent review article by Campos (2009) showed an initial improvement of symptoms in 84.8% of patients after dilatation. However, with longer follow-up, the success rate steadily declined to 58.4% by 36 months. The other major problem with dilatation is the risk of perforation. The same article reported an average perforation rate of 1.6%.

Csendes and colleagues (1989) performed a randomized trial comparing pneumatic dilatation in 39 patients to myotomy with anterior fundoplication in 42 patients. Two patients in the dilatation group (5%) incurred a perforation that required immediate surgery. After 5-year median follow-up, 98% of the surgery group had absent or mild dysphagia compared with only 73% undergoing dilatation.

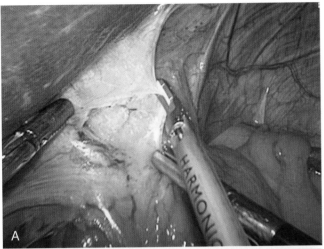

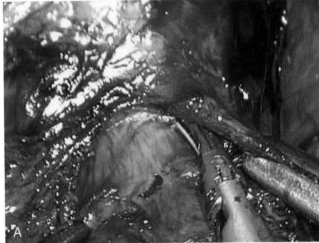

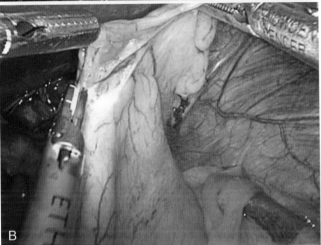

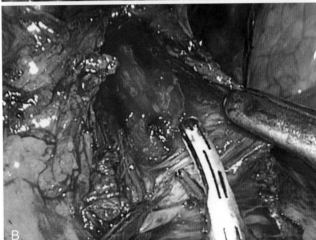

FIGURE 2 **A,** Opening the phrenoesophageal membrane. **B,** Excising the gastroesophageal fat pad.

FIGURE 3 Performing the esophageal myotomy. **A,** Separating the superficial linear muscle fibers. **B,** Dividing the deeper circular muscle layer.

Surgical Treatment

The first approach to surgical esophagomyotomy was described in 1913 by Ernest Heller using an abdominal approach with an anterior and posterior myotomy of the LES. The current operative technique is performed laparoscopically and involves an anterior longitudinal myotomy and usually some variant of partial fundoplication to prevent free reflux of gastric acid into the esophagus.

Surgical Technique

Preoperatively, patients should be kept on a liquid diet for 3 days to reduce the amount of solid undigested food in the esophagus. They need to be intubated in such a fashion as to reduce the risk of aspiration. The patient is then positioned and secured to allow a steep reverse Trendelenburg position. A 10 mm trocar is placed 15 cm below the xiphoid process to the left of midline via an open Hasson technique or with an optical trocar, and a pneumoperitoneum is established. A table-mounted liver retractor is placed through a stab incision in the subxiphoid area, and the left lobe of the liver is lifted to expose the hiatus. A 5 mm trocar and a 10 mm trocar are placed in the right upper quadrant as the two working ports. A final 5 mm port for the assistant is placed in the left upper quadrant adjacent to the costal margin.

The phrenoesophageal membrane is opened and the gastroesophageal fat pad is excised, exposing the GEJ (Figure 2). The anterior vagal trunk is then identified and preserved. Only the anterior

portion of the esophagus is dissected in order to preserve the posterior attachments of the phrenoesophageal ligament and the esophageal hiatus. The myotomy is performed by splitting the longitudinal esophageal muscular fibers and dividing the circular muscle fibers with the scissors or the harmonic scalpel (Figure 3). Electrocautery is used sparingly to avoid inadvertent mucosal perforation, and a gauze sponge can be helpful in maintaining exposure. Once the submucosal plane has been entered, the myotomy is carried proximally 5 to 6 cm from the GEJ and distally 2 to 3 cm onto the anterior gastric wall.

Once the myotomy is complete, the muscle edges are separated from the underlying mucosa on both sides for approximately 50% of the esophageal circumference. This should lead to a distinctive view of a bulging, unobstructed mucosa of the lower esophagus (Figure 4). Endoscopy is performed to ensure no residual obstruction at the GEJ and to rule out perforation. If perforation occurs, it is repaired laparoscopically with interrupted 5-0 monofilament absorbable sutures and a gentle intracorporeal knot-tying technique.

We routinely perform a Dor fundoplication to reduce gastroesophageal reflux (GER) and to buttress a mucosal repair. After mobilizing the upper third of the fundus by dividing the short gastric vessels, the top part of the cardia is sutured to the left crural pillar and to the left side of the myotomy, at the most superior aspect, with a nonabsorbable suture. Next, the anterior surface of the gastric cardia and fundus are folded upward and toward the patient's right side, placing the anterior gastric wall over the myotomy. Two additional sutures are then placed. The uppermost suture anchors the fundic

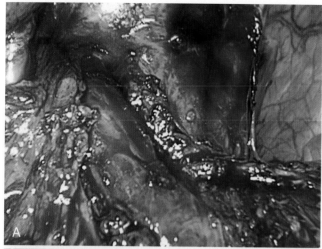

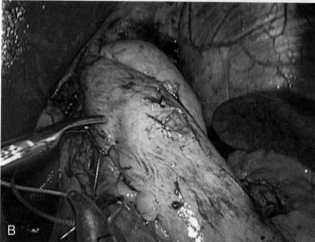

FIGURE 4 Completed myotomy. **A,** Exposed mucosa. **B,** Dor fundoplication.

flap to the right side of the myotomy to incorporate the right crural pillar. With the last suture, the fundus is joined with the inferior aspect of the right side of the myotomy (see Figure 4).

Controversies

Length of Myotomy

Wright and colleagues (2007) retrospectively reviewed the results from 52 patients treated with a 1 to 2 cm myotomy and Dor fundoplication compared with 63 patients given at least a 3 cm myotomy and Toupet fundoplication. With a median follow-up of almost 4 years, the dysphagia severity score was significantly less in the extended myotomy group (3.1 vs. 4.8). Also, significantly fewer patients in that group required reintervention for dysphagia (5% vs. 10%), and no significant difference was observed in heartburn, esophageal acid exposure, or LES pressure between the groups.

Heller Myotomy plus Dor Fundoplication

Studying 50 patients treated with Heller myotomy alone, Burpee and colleagues reported that 30% complained of significant heartburn. Of the 30 patients postoperatively tested with 24-hour pH probe surveillance or endoscopy, 60% had objective evidence of reflux. Even more concerning, 23% had objective reflux without subjective heartburn. Although these findings suggest the need to perform an antireflux

operation at the time of myotomy, the concern is that doing so will impair the degree of dysphagia relief from the myotomy.

To address this controversial question, we performed a double-blind, parallel-group randomized trial to test the effect of adding a Dor fundoplication to the Heller myotomy. The study randomized 21 patients to Heller alone and 22 to Heller plus Dor fundoplication. Both groups had a similar postoperative LES pressure (13.7 mm Hg in the Heller group and 13.9 mm Hg in the Heller-plus-Dor group), and an equal improvement in the dysphagia was reported by each group. However, adding the Dor fundoplication significantly reduced pathologic GER, defined as distal esophageal acid exposure greater than 4.2% of the time on a 24-hour pH probe study. The incidence of pathologic GER was 47.6% in the Heller group and 9.1% in the Heller-plus-Dor group. The Heller-only group also had a significantly higher median acid exposure to the distal esophagus (4.9% vs. 0.4%).

In another study, Rice and colleagues (2005) retrospectively reviewed the results of 149 patients treated with a Heller myotomy, 88 of which also received a Dor fundoplication. They found a higher resting postoperative LES pressure in the Heller-plus-Dor group (18 vs. 13 mm Hg). The percentage of time with a pH less than 4 in the distal esophagus was significantly less in the Heller-plus-Dor group, especially when the subject was supine (upright, 0.4% vs. 2.9%; supine, 0% vs. 5.8%). Importantly, there was no difference in barium height and width on an esophageal emptying study.

Heller Myotomy plus Toupet Fundoplication

Many surgeons have been reluctant to use what they consider to be an inadequate antireflux procedure, such as the Dor, and have performed a 270 degree Toupet fundoplication. Several studies have reported excellent results with a Heller myotomy plus a Toupet fundoplication, with relief of dysphagia and low rates of postoperative reflux. Arain and colleagues (2004) retrospectively compared 41 Heller-plus-Dor patients with 23 Heller-plus-Toupet patients and found no significant difference in dysphagia resolution or in the use of proton pump inhibitors. Nevertheless, no randomized trials to date have compared the Dor and the Toupet fundoplication in conjunction with a Heller myotomy.

Heller Myotomy plus Nissen Fundoplication

Arguments for a 360-degree fundoplication center on the inadequacy of partial fundoplications to control pathologic GER. Recent studies, however, indicate that a Nissen fundoplication is not an appropriate procedure after Heller myotomy because of the impaired esophageal clearance with the complete wrap. Rebecchi and colleagues (2008) performed a randomized controlled trial of Heller plus Dor versus Heller plus Nissen in 144 patients. With a mean follow-up of more than 10 years, a minimum follow-up of 5 years, and 138 patients available for testing, no significant difference was found in GER symptoms between the groups, but dysphagia was significantly more common in the Heller-plus-Nissen group (15% vs. 2.8%).

Sigmoid Esophagus

Some surgeons believe that a markedly dilated esophagus with a tortuous, angulated shape indicates a severity of dysfunction that necessitates esophagectomy or certainly avoidance of a fundoplication. However, Mineo and Pompeo (2004) showed excellent results with Heller myotomy plus Dor fundoplication in 14 patients with a sigmoid esophagus due to achalasia. After 24 months of follow-up, they showed a mean decrease in esophageal diameter of 10 mm and an improvement in dysphagia, regurgitation, and quality of life similar to that achieved by patients with an earlier stage of achalasia.

Patti and colleagues (1999) divided their series into four groups, depending on the severity of esophageal dilation and the presence of a sigmoid shape, and found that neither size nor shape of the

TABLE 1: Outcomes after laparoscopic Heller myotomy

Author	Year	Patients	Follow-up (Median Months/Range)	Relief of Dysphagia (%)	Length of Stay (Median Days/Range)	Perforations (%)	Reflux (%)
Zaninotto	2008	407	30 (N/A)	90.4	5 (N/A)	3.9	6*
Torquati	2006	200	42.1 (N/A)	85	1 (1–3)	6	N/A
Smith	2006	209	20 (1–108)	82.8	N/A	N/A	2
Portale	2005	248	43 (1–131)	88	5 (3–11)	4	7*
Bonatti	2005	75	64 (10–131)	84	2 (1–6)	4	11
Khaianchee	2005	121	9 (6–48)	91	1.7 (N/A)	6.6	13*
Arain	2004	78	24 (6–100)	77	N/A	0	17
Perrone	2004	100	26 (6–72)	96	1.2 (1–4)	3	N/A
Oelschlager	2003	110	26 (1–85)	90	N/A	N/A	23

*Based on postoperative 24-hour pH recording.
N/A, not applicable

esophagus affected the relief of dysphagia following Heller myotomy plus Dor fundoplication. Ultimately, none of those patients required esophagectomy.

OUTCOMES

Medium- to long-term results of laparoscopic Heller myotomy have been reported worldwide (Table 1). Most studies indicate 85% or more patients report dysphagia and regurgitation improvement or resolution. Complications are rare and usually minor. In a recent large meta-analysis, Campos and colleagues (2009) reported a 6.3% complication rate and a 0.1% mortality rate after laparoscopic Heller myotomy.

Predictors of Outcome

Younger age (<40 years), male sex, absence of esophageal dilation, and lower basal LES pressure are predictors of a worse response to pneumatic dilatation. Arain and colleagues performed a multivariate analysis of preoperative variables and found that only a high resting LES predicted resolution of dysphagia after Heller myotomy. A study from our institution (Torquati, 2006) found patients with a preoperative LES pressure less than 35 mm Hg were 21.3 times more likely to have dysphagia relief from myotomy.

It is generally agreed that prior endoscopic therapy makes a Heller myotomy more difficult to perform. Smith and colleagues (2006) showed that previous pneumatic dilatation or Botox injection nearly tripled the risk of operative complications (9.7% vs. 3.6%). Furthermore, the rate of operative failure, defined as persistent or recurrent symptoms or need for further treatment, nearly doubled (19.5% vs. 10%). These findings suggest endoscopic therapy should be reserved for poor surgical candidates.

SUMMARY

Treatment of achalasia has evolved over the past decade, and there are sufficient data to recommend laparoscopic Heller myotomy with a Dor or Toupet fundoplication as the current best therapy for most patients with achalasia. Patients who are too physically unfit to safely undergo a surgical procedure and those with a life expectancy of less than 2 years would benefit from endoscopic injection of Botox and may see improvement with use of oral nifedipine. There is good level I data to suggest that long-term relief of dysphagia after pneumatic dilatation is significantly less than that achieved by surgical myotomy, and there is a significant perforation rate after pneumatic dilatation. Laparoscopic Heller myotomy with partial fundoplication provides the most durable and effective treatment of dysphagia and also provides effective prevention of pathologic acid exposure in the distal esophagus.

SELECTED READINGS

Csendes A, Velasco N, Graghetto I, Henriquez A: A prospective randomized study comparing forceful dilatation and esophagomyotomy in patients with achalasia of the esophagus, *Gastroenterology* 80:789–795, 1981.

Katsinelos P, Kountouras J, Paroutoglou G, et al: Long-term results of pneumatic dilation for achalasia: a 15 years' experience, *World J Gastroenterol* 11(36):5701–5705, 2005.

Richards WO, Torquati A, Holzman MD, et al: Heller myotomy versus Heller myotomy with Dor fundoplication for achalasia: a prospective randomized double-blind clinical trial, *Ann Surg* 240(3):405–415, 2004.

Wright AS, Williams CW, Pellegrini CA, et al: Long-term outcomes confirm the superior efficacy of extended Heller myotomy with Toupet fundoplication for achalasia, *Surg Endo* 21:713–718, 2007.

Zaninotto G, Annese V, Costantini M, et al: Randomized controlled trial of botulinum toxin versus laparoscopic Heller myotomy for esophageal achalasia, *Ann Surg* 239:364, 2004.

DISORDERS OF ESOPHAGEAL MOTILITY

Alex G. Little, MD

MOTILITY DISORDERS

Achalasia, the most common disorder of esophageal motility, was previously discussed in this section. In addition, disorders of esophageal motility associated with the development of pulsion diverticula of the esophagus are likewise considered elsewhere. This chapter focuses on the remaining disorders of esophageal motility as identified in Table 1.

Diffuse Esophageal Spasm

Diffuse esophageal spasm (DES) is a disorder characterized clinically by chest pain, dysphagia, or both. The chest pain varies in severity and frequency but is typically substernal and more likely to suggest angina than heartburn. The pathophysiology is defined by esophageal motility studies, which show that more than 20% of esophageal contractions are simultaneous rather than peristaltic. However, if 100% of the contractions are simultaneous, the diagnosis is achalasia. Confusion can be created by older publications, which describe DES as a disorder of high-amplitude contractions. This is inaccurate. DES is a disorder of the swallow-induced pattern of contractions rather than a pressure abnormality. The lower esophageal sphincter (LES) characteristics are typically normal—another distinction from achalasia.

The medical literature suggests that the first phase of treatment, once the diagnosis has been secured, is reassurance to the patient that this is not a life-threatening situation. Usually, these patients will have undergone cardiac evaluation, so reassurance that their heart is not the source of the pain and that this is a benign esophageal disorder will satisfy many patients. However, when symptoms persist and the patient remains troubled despite reassurance, the next step is to evaluate the patient for the possibility of gastroesophageal reflux disease (GERD) with 24-hour pH monitoring of the esophagus. Although the exact correlation and prevalence are not known, at least some patients have GERD as the underlying inciting event; when it is appropriately treated, their symptoms will subside. Accordingly, if GERD is identified, appropriate and aggressive medical management should be started. Consideration of a surgical antireflux operation should be based on the standard criteria including, most importantly, the failure of medical management to control the symptoms.

When reassurance is ineffective, symptoms persist, and the patient is not found to have GERD, surgical myotomy can be considered. Unfortunately, the results of myotomy are not consistently predictable; consequently, it is reserved for a small number of patients and should only be performed when all other conservative measures have failed and the patient has been made aware of the unpredictability of the outcome.

Since the simultaneous contractions are typically more prevalent in the distal rather than the proximal esophagus, my preference is to begin with a laparoscopic approach rather than a minimally invasive or open thoracic approach. Port placement for the procedure is shown in Figure 1, A.

After mobilizing the gastroesophageal junction (GEJ) laterally and anteriorly, leaving the posterior attachments undisturbed, the fat pad at the GEJ is mobilized using ultrasonic shears, moving from the patient's left to the patient's right. This clearly exposes the operative area and elevates and moves the left anterior vagus nerve toward the patient's right. A temporary holding stitch between the fat pad and the right side of the hiatus keeps the fat and the vagus out of the field.

I perform a myotomy starting on the distal esophagus, and I recommend going as far proximal as the surgeon feels is safe and prudent, so that the entire region of abnormal motility is addressed (this is not necessary for achalasia). I carry the myotomy distally across the GEJ and on to the stomach. The muscle edges must be vigorously spread from each other to prevent them healing together.

It is true that the LES is normal in most patients, but I fear that poor esophageal emptying may be the consequence of a myotomy with an intact LES. I perform a Dor fundoplication to reduce the incidence and/or severity of postoperative GERD.

A video-assisted thoracic approach can be used if preferred by the surgeon; however, it is a necessity if a myotomy of the mid to upper esophagus is required to address all areas of abnormal motility. Figure 1, B, illustrates the port locations for this procedure.

Hypercontracting Esophagus

The diagnosis of hypercontracting esophagus, sometimes more imaginatively termed the *nutcracker esophagus*, is present in patients with high-pressure esophageal contractions, usually in excess of 180 mm Hg. Symptomatically, these patients do not differ from patients with DES and may have chest pain, dysphagia, or both. The pain is nonspecific in character, usually is substernal, and is distinguishable by the patient from heartburn.

Again, treatment begins by reassuring the patient that the cause of the pain is the esophagus and not the heart. Second, a search for GERD is appropriate. As with DES, at least some patients will have acid reflux as a precipitating event causing pain. Management of the reflux will result in a diminishing, if not a complete disappearance, of the symptoms.

Surgical myotomy is reserved for the very few. In fact, results of myotomy for hypercontracting esophagus are even less satisfactory than for DES. It is very tempting for the surgeon to see these high-pressure contractions and assume that reduction in pressure will result in relief, but in fact this is quite frequently not the case; myotomy should be performed rarely, if at all, in these patients. The poor results from myotomy correlate with the observation that the patient's pain is not perceived simultaneously with the high-pressure contractions.

CONNECTIVE TISSUE DISORDERS

Connective tissue disorders frequently affect the smooth muscle of the gastrointestinal tract and may involve the distal esophagus. The most frequent culprits are scleroderma and systemic lupus erythematosus, which weaken the distal smooth muscle of the esophagus

TABLE 1: Disorders of esophageal motility

Disorder	Symptoms	Motility Findings
DES	Chest pain, dysphagia	>20% simultaneous contractions Normal LES
Hypercontracting esophagus	Chest pain, dysphagia	Esophageal contractions >180 mm Hg Normal or high-pressure LES
Connective tissue disorders	GERD symptoms	Weak or absent LES Weak or absent distal contractions

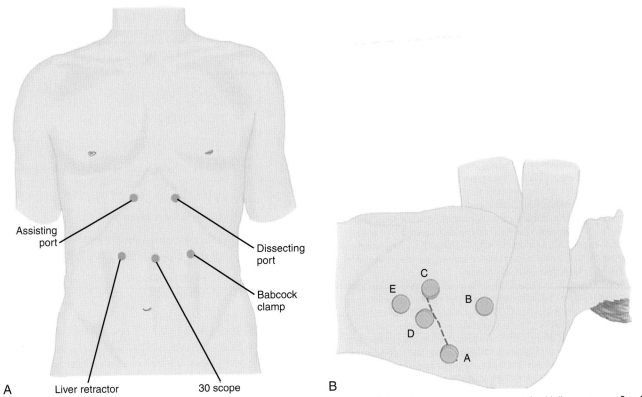

FIGURE I **A,** Laparoscopic port placement for Heller myotomy. **B,** Video-assisted thoracic surgery port placement for Heller myotomy. *Port A, cautery; port B, retraction; port C, grasper; port D, optional utility; port E, camera. (From Patti M, Fisichella P. In Wilmore D, Cheung L, Harken A, et al (eds): ACS surgery, New York, 2003, WebMD.)*

to the extent that no LES can be detected, and the distal esophagus does not contract.

The result of this esophageal involvement is florid reflux through the essentially nonexistent LES into a flaccid distal esophagus that is unable to clear itself. These patients, then, have severe GERD and are at risk for stricture development. Management of the reflux should be aggressive to prevent stricture formation, and antireflux surgery must be considered if the patient remains symptomatic despite medical therapy, has regurgitation, or persistent esophagitis is detected. The antireflux operation of choice is a partial fundoplication, such as a Toupet procedure, rather than a complete Nissen wrap. The incomplete wrap is less likely to combine with the weak esophageal contractions to cause dysphagia than the complete and more obstructive wrap of the Nissen fundoplication.

SUGGESTED READINGS

Richter JE: Oesophageal motility disorders, *Lancet* 358(9284):823–828, 2001.
Smout AJ: Advances in esophageal motor disorders, *Curr Opin Gastroenterol* 24(4):485–489, 2008.
Herbella FA, Raz DJ, Nipomnick I, et al: Primary versus secondary esophageal motility disorders: diagnosis and implications for treatment, *J Laparoendosc Adv Surg Tech* 19(2):195–198, 2009.
Patti MG, Gorodner MV, Galvani C, et al: Spectrum of esophageal motility disorders: implications for diagnosis and treatment, *Arch Surg* 140(5):442–448, 2005.
Ferguson MK, Little AG: Angina-like chest pain associated with high-amplitude peristaltic contractions of the esophagus, *Surgery* 104:713–719, 1988.

MANAGEMENT OF ESOPHAGEAL TUMORS

Glenda G. Callender, MD, and Mark K. Ferguson, MD

ESOPHAGEAL CANCER

Esophageal cancer is the sixth leading cause of death from cancer worldwide. In the United States, approximately 13,000 men and 3500 women were diagnosed with esophageal cancer in 2009; approximately 11,500 men and 3000 women will die from the disease. Risk factors for esophageal cancer are listed in Table 1. More than 90% of esophageal and gastroesophageal junction cancers are squamous cell carcinomas or adenocarcinomas. Other histologies, such as gastrointestinal stromal tumor, primary small cell carcinoma, leiomyosarcoma, melanoma, lymphoma, and carcinoid, are rare. Over the past quarter of a century, the incidence of esophageal adenocarcinoma in the United States and Western Europe has risen sixfold, a change that is largely related to growing problems with gastroesophageal reflux disease, obesity, and resultant Barrett esophagus.

Most patients with esophageal cancer present with dysphagia (50% to 75%) and/or weight loss (50% to 60%). Approximately 25% are diagnosed on endoscopy performed for reflux or for Barrett esophagus surveillance. Odynophagia may occur in 20% of patients. Symptoms such as dyspnea, cough, hoarseness, and retrosternal pain or back pain are rare but are usually suggestive of extensive, locally advanced disease. Physical examination is often unremarkable. Early signs of cachexia may be appreciated, and obvious signs of metastatic disease—such as a pleural effusion, hepatomegaly, or a palpable left supraclavicular (Virchow's) node—may be encountered.

Although barium swallow is sometimes the first test performed for the workup of dysphagia, the diagnosis is best established with esophagogastroduodenoscopy (EGD) and biopsy. Once the diagnosis of cancer is confirmed, routine staging studies include endoscopic ultrasound; computed tomography of the chest, abdomen, and pelvis; and ^{18}F-fluorodeoxyglucose positron emission tomography (^{18}F-FDG-PET).

Endoscopic ultrasound, especially when accompanied by fine needle aspiration biopsy, is the most sensitive tool for evaluating the depth of invasion of the primary tumor as well as involvement of regional lymph nodes. Endoscopic mucosal resection (EMR) can provide even greater accuracy of tumor depth staging than endoscopic ultrasound in patients with early-stage cancers. Histologic analysis of the specimen can definitively distinguish high-grade dysplasia or carcinoma in situ from invasive cancer. It is most useful in areas of Barrett esophagus and early lesions.

Esophageal cancer is staged according to the American Joint Committee on Cancer (AJCC) tumor node metastasis (TNM) staging system. Table 2 defines the AJCC 2009 variables of TNM, histologic grade, and cancer location for esophageal cancer. Table 3 provides the AJCC 2009 stage groups for esophageal adenocarcinoma and squamous cell carcinoma. Figures 1 and 2 illustrate the risk-adjusted survival curves for esophageal adenocarcinoma and squamous cell carcinoma according to the AJCC 2009 stage groups.

TABLE 1: Risk factors for esophageal cancer according to histologic type

Squamous Cell Carcinoma
Tobacco
Alcohol
Caustic injury
Achalasia
Low socioeconomic status
Prior head and neck cancer
Prior thoracic irradiation
Plummer-Vinson syndrome
Tylosis A
Frequent consumption of hot beverages
Frequent consumption of smoked meats
Adenocarcinoma
Barrett esophagus
Gastroesophageal reflux disease
Obesity
Tobacco
Prior thoracic irradiation
Medications that reduce lower esophageal sphincter tone

TABLE 2: AJCC definitions of TNM, histologic grade, and cancer location for esophageal cancer

Definition of TNM	
Primary tumor (T)	
TX	Primary tumor cannot be assessed
T0	No evidence of primary tumor
Tis	High-grade dysplasia
T1	Tumor invades lamina propria or submucosa
T2	Tumor invades muscularis propria
T3	Tumor invades adventitia
T4a	Resectable tumor invades adjacent structures such as pleura, pericardium, and diaphragm
T4b	Unresectable tumor invades adjacent structures such as aorta, vertebral body, and trachea
Regional lymph nodes (N)	
Regional lymph node is defined as any periesophageal lymph node from cervical periesophageal lymph nodes to celiac lymph nodes	
N0	No regional lymph node metastases
N1	1 to 2 positive regional lymph nodes
N2	3 to 6 positive regional lymph nodes
N3	7 or more positive regional lymph nodes
Distant metastases (M)	
M0	No distant metastases
M1	Distant metastases
Definition of Histologic Grade	
G1	Well differentiated
G2	Moderately differentiated
G3	Poorly differentiated
G4	Undifferentiated
Definition of Cancer Location	
Upper thoracic	Proximal tumor margin is 20 to 25 cm from incisors
Middle thoracic	Proximal tumor margin is >25 to 30 cm from incisors
Lower thoracic	Proximal tumor margin is >30 to 40 cm from incisors
Gastroesophageal junction	Includes tumors whose epicenter is in the distal thoracic esophagus, gastroesophageal junction, or within the proximal 5 cm of the stomach that extend into the gastroesophageal junction or esophagus

From *AJCC Cancer Staging Manual,* ed 7, American Joint Committee on Cancer, New York, 2010, Springer.

TABLE 3: AJCC stage groups for esophageal adenocarcinoma and squamous cell carcinoma

HISTOLOGY	ADENOCARCINOMA		SQUAMOUS CELL CARCINOMA		
Stage	TNM	Grade	TNM	Grade	Location
0	TisN0M0	G1	TisN0M0	G1	Any
IA	T1N0M0	G1-2	T1N0M0	G1	Any
IB	T1N0M0	G3	T1N0M0	G2-3	Any
	T2N0M0	G1-2	T2-3N0M0	G1	Lower
IIA	T2N0M0	G3	T2-3N0M0	G1	Upper, middle
			T2-3N0M0	G2-3	Lower
IIB	T3N0M0	Any	T2-3N0M0	G2-3	Upper, middle
	T1-2N1M0	Any	T1-2N1M0	Any	Any
IIIA	T1-2N2M0	Any	T1-2N2M0	Any	Any
	T3N1M0	Any	T3N1M0	Any	Any
	T4aN0M0	Any	T4aN0M0	Any	Any
IIIB	T3N2M0	Any	T3N2M0	Any	Any
IIIC	T4aN1-2M0	Any	T4aN1-2M0	Any	Any
	T4bNAnyM0	Any	T4bNAnyM0	Any	Any
	TAnyN3M0	Any	TAnyN3M0	Any	Any
IV	TAnyNAnyM1	Any	TAnyNAnyM1	Any	Any

From *AJCC Cancer Staging Manual*, ed 7, American Joint Committee on Cancer, New York, 2010, Springer.

Management of Early Disease

Screening programs are not practical or cost effective in the United States or in Western Europe, where the overall incidence of esophageal cancer is very low; as a consequence, most patients present with regionally advanced or metastatic disease. However, in patients who undergo endoscopy for gastroesophageal reflux disease or for surveillance of Barrett esophagus, high-grade dysplasia (HGD) or early-stage esophageal cancer is often diagnosed.

The management of HGD in the setting of Barrett esophagus is controversial. Older literature has consistently reported that coexisting invasive cancer is found in 40% of patients with Barrett HGD, which supports traditional recommendations for early esophagectomy in these patients. However, more recent reports suggest that patients with Barrett HGD are more likely to have carcinoma in situ or intramucosal carcinoma rather than early invasive cancer. The incidence of invasive cancer in the resected esophageal specimen in these patients is as low as 12%. Therefore, because of the morbidity and mortality associated with esophagectomy, some centers are now advocating more conservative approaches for these patients: intensive surveillance for HGD (EGD every 3 months, with four-quadrant biopsies every 1 cm along the length of the Barrett segment); focal EMR for localized areas of HGD; or complete eradication of the Barrett segment, with EMR for high-risk areas and mucosal ablation for the remaining columnar epithelium.

Conventional esophagectomy is indicated for the management of most early invasive cancer (T1N0M0) because this approach removes the tumor and any occult lymph node metastases. The risk of lymph node metastasis in the setting of clinical T1N0 disease *limited to the lamina propria* (previously T1a) is less than 5%. Therefore less invasive therapies such as EMR, endoscopic ablation (e.g., photodynamic or laser), or vagal-sparing esophagectomy can be considered in this setting. Vagal-sparing esophagectomy does not include a complete lymphadenectomy but preserves the vagus nerves and maintains better blood supply to the gastric conduit than conventional esophagectomy. Postoperative physiology is therefore better preserved than after conventional esophagectomy, and patients experience less dumping and better gastric emptying. The risk of lymph node metastasis in T1N0 esophageal cancer *with tumor penetration into the submucosa* (previously T1b) is greater than 30%; thus conventional esophagectomy is warranted. Approaches for conventional esophagectomy are described in the next section.

Management of Regionally Advanced Disease

Multimodal Therapy

The optimal management of regionally advanced, nonmetastatic esophageal cancer (T2-4aN0-3) is controversial. Surgery has historically been the mainstay of therapy for this patient population. However, dismal outcomes after surgery alone have generated interest in multimodal therapy. A combination of surgery, radiation, and chemotherapy represents the current practice in the management of resectable esophageal cancer in the United States, although there is little evidence supporting such combined therapy over surgery alone. In fact, in most other Western countries, esophagectomy is the standard of care for most resectable esophageal cancers.

Preoperative radiation therapy followed by surgery has been compared to surgery alone in at least half a dozen randomized, controlled trials and two large meta-analyses. No statistically significant difference in outcome was observed in any of those studies. This is not a

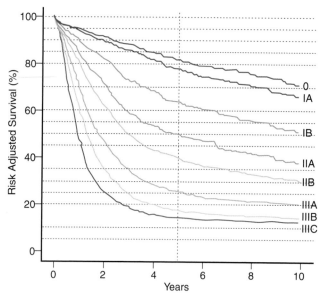

FIGURE 1 Risk-adjusted survival for esophageal adenocarcinoma according to AJCC (ed 7, 2009) stage groups. *(Data from AJCC Cancer Staging Manual, ed 7, American Joint Committee on Cancer. New York, 2010, Springer.)*

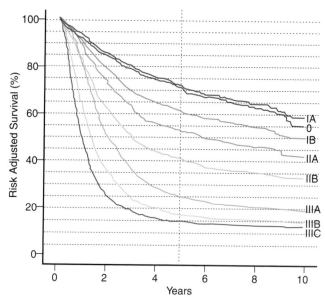

FIGURE 2 Risk-adjusted survival for esophageal squamous cell carcinoma according to the AJCC (2009) stage groups. *(Data from AJCC Cancer Staging Manual, ed 7, American Joint Committee on Cancer. New York, 2010, Springer.)*

surprising result; radiation and surgery both represent locoregional therapy.

Preoperative chemotherapy followed by surgery has been compared to surgery alone in at least six randomized, controlled trials and four meta-analyses. One randomized, controlled trial of 802 patients demonstrated a modest survival benefit in the arm that received induction fluorouracil and cisplatin compared with the arm that received surgery alone (median survival of 16.8 months compared with 13.3 months). One meta-analysis of 2051 patients also demonstrated a modest survival benefit at 5 years for the induction chemotherapy arm compared with the surgery alone arm. However, none of the many remaining studies demonstrated any benefit to preoperative chemotherapy.

At least a dozen randomized controlled trials and meta-analyses have evaluated preoperative chemoradiation followed by surgery (trimodal therapy) compared with surgery alone. Only one randomized, controlled trial demonstrated a survival benefit for the arm that received trimodal therapy (fluorouracil, cisplatin, 40 Gy) compared with the arm that received surgery alone. The remaining studies have not demonstrated a benefit to preoperative chemoradiation. Three meta-analyses have demonstrated a statistically significant but modest survival benefit for patients receiving trimodal therapy compared with surgery alone.

As has been the case in certain other malignancies, response to neoadjuvant chemoradiation has been shown to predict outcome. Approximately 20% to 25% of patients who undergo neoadjuvant chemoradiation followed by surgery are found to have a pathologic complete response. This patient cohort demonstrates considerably longer 5-year survival (>50%) than patients without a pathologic complete response.

It is generally accepted that patients with regionally advanced disease (T3-T4a or any regional nodal involvement) who undergo surgery without preoperative therapy should undergo adjuvant therapy. This is an approach that has largely been unsubstantiated by the literature. The lack of clear benefit of any single combination of therapies has led some to question whether surgery is even a necessary part of the treatment paradigm of esophageal cancer. Currently there is insufficient evidence to support this point of view.

Patients with T4b tumors are generally considered unresectable, and treatment with radiotherapy and chemotherapy is most appropriate. Controversy exists regarding indications for resection in patients with an advanced T stage (T3, T4a) in the presence of multiple involved lymph nodes (more than six); the poor long-term survival in such patients suggests that bimodal treatment with chemotherapy and radiation therapy is most appropriate for this small subgroup.

Surgical Considerations

The objectives of surgical therapy for esophageal cancer are to remove the tumor and associated lymph nodes with clear margins to achieve the goals of local control of disease, improved long-term survival, and resumption of a normal diet. However, the optimal surgical approach is controversial with regards to incisions, the appropriate extent of lymph node dissection, and the extent of soft tissue resection.

Incisions

Options for a surgical approach include transthoracic esophagectomy (TTE), transhiatal esophagectomy (THE), and a variety of approaches to minimally invasive esophagectomy (MIE). TTE uses right thoracotomy and laparotomy incisions, and the anastomosis to the conduit may be created either high in the chest (traditional Ivor Lewis, or "two-hole" approach) or in the neck (McKeown modification of the Ivor Lewis operation, or "three-hole" approach). For a distal esophageal tumor, an exclusive left thoracotomy can be used with the abdominal portion of the operation performed through the chest by taking the diaphragm down peripherally. THE does not use a thoracotomy and instead is performed through a laparotomy and a left cervical incision with blunt dissection of the intrathoracic esophagus and a cervical anastomosis. MIE involves right thoracoscopic mobilization of the esophagus and lymph node–bearing tissue, laparoscopic mobilization of the stomach, and a high intrathoracic or cervical anastomosis. Regardless of the surgical approach, a gastric conduit is the preferred option for reconstruction. Therefore the right gastroepiploic artery must be preserved during gastric mobilization; colon or jejunal interpositions are alternatives if the stomach is unusable.

Theoretical advantages of direct-vision approaches (TTE, MIE) include the ability to control bleeding vessels, a more complete lateral soft tissue resection, and a more complete lymph node dissection. However, TTE is also associated with higher morbidity related to respiratory complications; if an intrathoracic anastomosis is performed, an anastomotic leak can lead to mediastinitis with devastating consequences. On the other hand, THE avoids the morbidity of a thoracotomy, and a cervical anastomotic leak can be managed by merely opening the wound at the bedside. However, THE does not allow for equivalent lymphadenectomy, as the intrathoracic esophagus is bluntly dissected with little visualization, which can lead to understaging. There also exists an increased risk of injury to intrathoracic structures such as the azygos vein, which can be difficult to control without direct vision. Four randomized, prospective trials have evaluated outcomes following TTE versus THE and have demonstrated no important differences in morbidity between approaches other than an increased incidence of pulmonary complications after TTE and an increased incidence of anastomotic leak after THE. The trials also failed to demonstrate any statistically significant difference in survival between the two groups.

MIE is a relatively new approach to esophagectomy for cancer. Versions of MIE include laparoscopic THE, hybrid MIE with either the thoracic or abdominal portions done through an open incision, and totally minimally invasive MIE with either a high intrathoracic or a cervical anastomosis. A growing body of literature has addressed the effectiveness of MIE compared with TTE and/or THE. There is clearly a significant learning curve associated with MIE, with an increase in the incidence of complications evident during the first 30 to 50 procedures. Nonetheless, in high-volume centers, this technique has been demonstrated to be safe and appears to have equivalent outcomes compared with open approaches in terms of lymph node retrieval and survival.

Nodal Dissection

The extent of lymphadenectomy that should be performed during esophageal cancer resection is another area of considerable controversy. Lymphadenectomy achieves two goals: staging and local control. The number of lymph nodes required for accurate staging is not agreed upon, but the suggested range in the literature ranges from 15 to 30.

The submucosal lymphatic drainage system of the esophagus is extensive and complex (Figure 3). Labeling studies indicate no single

or simple pattern of spread to lymph nodes regardless of the location of the primary tumor; thus the use of sentinel node mapping for esophageal cancer has not been shown to have much benefit. This varied pattern of spread indicates the need to perform an extensive nodal dissection if a complete lymphadenectomy for esophageal cancer is the surgeon's goal.

Approximately 80% of patients with T2 or deeper tumors will have positive lymph nodes, indicating that nodal dissection is appropriate for most patients undergoing esophagectomy for cancer. Proponents of aggressive lymph node dissection believe that extended lymphadenectomy improves survival by achieving optimal local control. THE can include a formal abdominal lymphadenectomy, but the intrathoracic lymph nodes are dissected bluntly, if at all. TTE and MIE can include a formal two-field (thoracic and abdominal) or three-field (thoracic, abdominal, and cervical) lymph node dissection. The literature has consistently reported that 20% to 40% of patients with mid-or distal esophageal tumors, including squamous cell carcinomas and adenocarcinomas, have involved cervical lymph nodes. This suggests that a more extensive nodal dissection may improve long-term survival. However, although several retrospective and cohort studies have demonstrated improved 5-year survival rates for patients who underwent three-field versus two-field lymphadenectomy, a randomized controlled trial did not demonstrate any statistically significant difference in survival. One of the major criticisms of any study that demonstrates increased survival after extended lymphadenectomy is that sampling more lymph nodes allows for more accurate staging; therefore differences in outcome may be explained by stage migration alone. At this time, there is insufficient evidence to support an extended lymphadenectomy during esophagectomy for esophageal cancer.

Extent of Soft Tissue Resection

The "en bloc" esophagectomy was popularized in the 1980s to include a buffer zone of soft tissue, resected in continuity with the esophagus, to avoid violating tissue planes and thus reduce local recurrence of cancer.

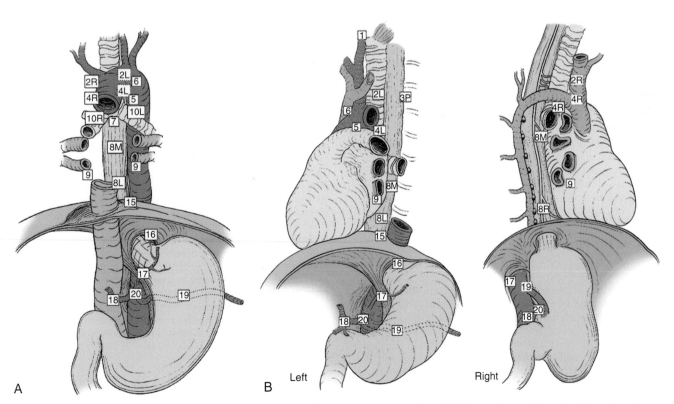

FIGURE 3   Esophageal lymph node map. **A,** Anterior perspective. **B,** Lateral perspectives. *(From AJCC Cancer Staging Manual, ed 7, American Joint Committee on Cancer. New York, 2010, Springer.)*

The extent of soft-tissue dissection originally included the azygos vein, thoracic duct, contralateral pleura, posterior pericardium, and a rim of diaphragm for tumors of the gastroesophageal junction. Currently the extent of dissection for en bloc esophagectomy includes the azygos vein, thoracic duct, and a rim of diaphragm for tumors of the distal esophagus. No randomized studies have been performed to compare local recurrence rates or long-term survival between standard resection and en bloc resection. At present there is no conclusive information suggesting a benefit to the more extensive en bloc resection.

Other Controversies

Other controversies in the surgical technique of esophagectomy include whether to perform a gastric emptying procedure (pyloroplasty or pyloromyotomy) after esophagectomy, and whether a feeding jejunostomy should routinely be placed. In general, the literature supports routinely performing a gastric emptying procedure because it improves gastric emptying, avoids pyloric obstruction, and does not lead to significantly more dumping or bile reflux. The literature does not support the routine placement of a feeding jejunostomy tube unless the patient has experienced severe preoperative weight loss; perioperative nutritional support can be accomplished by nasojejunal feeding or total parenteral nutrition, if necessary. However, placement of a feeding jejunostomy at the time of esophagectomy provides an optimal means of nutritional support for patients who have postoperative complications, permits early introduction of enteral nutrition to help prevent bacterial overgrowth and translocation, and permits nutritional supplementation in an outpatient setting for patients who are unable to resume satisfactory oral intake prior to hospital discharge. Many of these latter factors have not been considered in studies evaluating the routine use of jejunostomy feeding tubes after esophagectomy.

Postoperative Management

After surgery, patients should remain in a monitored setting overnight. A restrictive approach to intravenous fluids is usually appropriate, especially in patients who have had a thoracotomy, to help prevent pulmonary complications. Chest tube management is routine. If a feeding jejunostomy has been placed, tube feedings are initiated at a low rate on postoperative day one and advanced slowly to goal on subsequent days. A nasogastric tube that traverses the anastomosis is kept in place until there is evidence of return of bowel function, usually 3 to 5 days. There is no evidence that routine evaluation of the anastomosis with barium swallow is necessary; after the nasogastric tube has been discontinued, the patient's diet may be advanced slowly as tolerated. Workup for an anastomotic leak (chest radiograph, barium swallow, or chest computed tomography) is initiated only if clinically indicated by fever or leukocytosis on or after postoperative day 3; new onset of supraventricular tachycardia; or other unexplained signs of sepsis such as confusion, hypotension, arterial desaturation, or sinus tachycardia.

Follow-up and Surveillance

Recurrence after surgical treatment for esophageal cancer usually occurs in the first 2 years, and the median time to recurrence is about 8.5 months; approximately 75% of patients who recur do not survive beyond 2 to 3 years. Therefore a strategy of intensive follow-up in the early postoperative years is reasonable. Patients who undergo EMR or other local therapy for Tis or T1 disease are followed with EGD every 3 months for the first year and then annually. Patients who undergo esophagectomy are followed with history and physical exam every 3 months for the first 2 years and then annually. There are no clear guidelines regarding when to obtain imaging and routine bloodwork (blood count, chemistries, liver function tests). A reasonable strategy is to obtain a computed tomographic image of the chest and abdomen every 6 months for 2 years and then annually until 5 years. There is no known advantage to obtaining routine bloodwork. EGD should be performed for patients who report dysphagia to differentiate between benign stricture formation and recurrent cancer. Surveillance EGD is performed every 2 years. beginning at 2 years postoperatively, to screen for the development of Barrett esophagus in the esophageal remnant and to evaluate for recurrent or new cancers.

Management of Metastatic Disease

Approximately 50% of patients who develop esophageal cancer in the United States have metastatic disease at the time of diagnosis. Chemotherapy and radiation are options for patients with metastatic disease, although survival is dismal. Response to therapy (tumor shrinkage of at least 50%) may occur in 15% to 50% of patients, depending upon which regimen of chemotherapy is used, and this is often sufficient to palliate symptoms. However, survival in patients whose symptoms are palliated is still usually less than a year.

Palliative esophagectomy in the setting of metastatic disease is seldom necessary because endoscopic dilatation and/or esophageal stent placement is usually effective. Indications for surgical resection include bleeding, perforation, and the rare situation in which dysphagia or an esophageal airway fistula cannot be palliated with an endoluminal stent.

Other Tumors

Esophageal gastrointestinal stromal tumors account for 1% to 5% of all esophageal malignancies. Treatment is surgical resection with wide local excision of the tumor and adherent tissues. An extensive lymphadenectomy is not necessary. Enucleation or local resection is possible for some small tumors (<2 cm). For larger lesions, neoadjuvant imatinib may provide some shrinkage, but subsequent esophagectomy is usually necessary.

Primary small cell carcinoma of the esophagus accounts for approximately 1% of all esophageal malignancies and carries a poor prognosis. Early dissemination of tumor cells is characteristic, and most patients have metastases to liver and lungs at the time of presentation. Management is similar to that for small cell carcinoma of the lung: chemotherapy and radiation therapy are the best options with little role for surgery.

Other forms of cancer such as esophageal melanoma, lymphoma, leiomyosarcoma, and carcinoid tumors are extremely rare. Esophageal melanoma is typically extremely aggressive and is usually metastatic at the time of diagnosis. For locoregional melanoma without metastasis, esophagectomy with lymph node dissection is indicated. However, survival is usually about half that of an equal-stage cutaneous melanoma. The treatment of esophageal lymphoma is similar to the treatment of lymphoma elsewhere in the body: chemotherapy and radiation. Surgery is reserved for diagnosis and the treatment of complications. Overall prognosis is good, with 5-year survival approaching 75%. The treatment for esophageal leiomyosarcoma is usually esophagectomy, although there are some reports of long-term cure with local resection only. Esophageal carcinoid usually does not present with carcinoid syndrome and can be locally aggressive, although there are too few cases reported in the literature to draw any firm conclusions regarding prognosis. Treatment is esophagectomy with lymphadenectomy.

Benign submucosal tumors, such as leiomyoma and schwannoma, are enucleated, usually via a thoracoscopic approach. Lymphadenectomy is not necessary, and the risk of local recurrence is minimal.

SUMMARY

Although it is relatively uncommon, esophageal cancer remains a challenging disease process. The incidence of adenocarcinoma is rising rapidly in the United States, and survival remains poor, even for patients who have surgically resectable disease at the time of diagnosis. Multimodal therapy has provided some promise of better outcomes, but earlier detection, additional therapies, and identification of subpopulations that respond well to specific therapies are clearly necessary.

SUGGESTED READINGS

Altorki N, Kent M, Ferrara C, et al: Three-field lymph node dissection for squamous cell and adenocarcinoma of the esophagus, *Ann Surg* 236:177, 2002.

Hammoud ZT, Kesler KA, Ferguson MK, et al: Survival outcomes of resected patients who demonstrate a pathologic complete response after neoadjuvant chemoradiation therapy for locally advanced esophageal cancer, *Dis Esoph* 19:69, 2006.

Konda VJA, Ross AS, Ferguson MK, et al: Is the risk of concomitant invasive esophageal cancer in high-grade dysplasia in Barrett esophagus overestimated? *Clin Gastroenterol Hepatol* 6:159, 2008.

McKian KP, Miller RC, Cassivi SD, et al: Curing patients with locally advanced esophageal cancer: an update on multimodality therapy, *Dis Esoph* 19:448, 2006.

Omloo JMT, Lagarde SM, Hulscher JBF, et al: Extended transthoracic resection compared with limited transhiatal resection for adenocarcinoma of the mid/distal esophagus: five-year survival of a randomized clinical trial, *Ann Surg* 246:992, 2007.

Peyre CG, DeMeester SR, Rizetto C, et al: Vagal-sparing esophagectomy: the ideal operation for intramucosal adenocarcinoma and Barrett with high-grade dysplasia, *Ann Surg* 246:665, 2007.

Rice TW, Zuccaro G Jr, Adelstein DJ, et al: Esophageal carcinoma: depth of tumor invasion is predictive of regional lymph node status, *Ann Thorac Surg* 65:787, 1998.

NEOADJUVANT AND ADJUVANT THERAPY FOR ESOPHAGEAL CARCINOMA

Mark J. Krasna, MD

INDICATIONS

Esophageal cancer incidence is rising faster than any other malignancy in Western countries. In Asia, it still represents the most common malignancy, with areas that approach epidemiologic proportions. The etiologies of the two main cancer types, adenocarcinoma and squamous cell carcinoma, are different, which gives rise to differences in pathogenesis, location, and clinical presentation.

In brief, squamous cell carcinoma remains a disease of the upper to mid-esophagus, most commonly associated with alcohol and tobacco consumption. There is a marked disparity in the development of these malignancies among minority populations, particularly African Americans, and in the Far East. Squamous cell lesions tend to invade locally and involve the airway and other adjacent structures. They are usually diagnosed at an advanced stage, after causing severe dysphagia with obstruction of greater than 50% to 75% of the esophageal lumen. Lymph node (LN) spread for these lesions is typically in the regional mediastinal nodes and in the cervical LN chain, as described by Akiyama and colleagues in 1981.

Adenocarcinoma of the esophagus typically occurs in the distal esophagus and gastroesophageal junction (GEJ). The majority of these cases are related to reflux esophagitis with metaplasia of the distal squamous mucosa to columnar epithelium. Unfortunately, as is the case for squamous cell carcinoma, over two thirds of these lesions present with locoregional spread to LNs in the lower mediastinum and upper abdomen, including the celiac LNs.

Staging is crucial; newer algorithms for the approach to these lesions show a benefit with a stage-specific approach, as has been shown in patients with lung cancer. Endoscopy is now often the first diagnostic test, although most patients will undergo a barium swallow at some point. Following the establishment of a tissue diagnosis, computerized tomography scanning of the chest and upper abdomen is recommended to identify any evidence of metastatic disease, particularly to the liver and lungs, and to rule out regional LN spread.

Our current approach uses routine fluorodeoxyglucose positron emission tomography as the next step to confirm or rule out further evidence of unresectability based on metastatic spread. If necessary, minimally invasive testing can be used to confirm suspicious lesions by needle biopsy (fine needle aspiration [FNA]). If no evidence of metastatic disease is present, these patients next undergo esophageal ultrasound (EUS) (Figure 1). This relatively new technology has revolutionized the approach to staging these patients by ensuring a greater than 80% T-staging and 75% LN-staging accuracy pretreatment.

In those rare cases where suspicious lesions remain that have not been confirmed by EUS-guided FNA, a staging thoracoscopy and laparoscopy is done. This ensures greater than 94% accuracy in pretreatment staging. Once the final clinical stage is determined, a multidisciplinary team approach is used to determine the best way to treat patients in a stage-specific fashion.

TECHNIQUE

There are many challenges to performing combination therapy in patients with esophageal cancer. Delivery of therapeutic doses of chemotherapy and radiation can lead to increased perioperative morbidity and mortality even in the best centers. This is balanced with the fact that performing surgical resection followed by adjuvant chemotherapy or chemoradiation rarely allows a full dose of therapy to

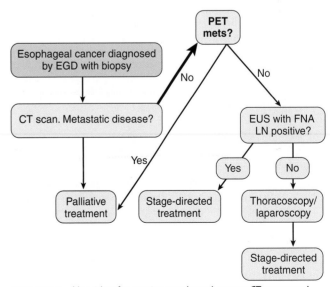

FIGURE 1 Algorithm for staging esophageal cancer. *CT*, computed tomography; *EGD*, esophagogastroduodenoscopy; *mets*, metastases; *PET*, positron emission tomography.

be administered. Our preferred approach for the last 2 decades has therefore been neoadjuvant chemotherapy with concurrent radiation therapy at full curative doses followed by surgical resection.

The challenge of operating on the patient after induction therapy can be overcome by meticulous preoperative patient selection, careful use of energy in the operative field, judicious allowance of perioperative fluids, and an experienced team of nurses and intensivists in the postoperative period. In my opinion, the single most important factor, however, remains careful intraoperative technique with meticulous preparation of the gastric conduit, thorough LN dissection, and attention to detail while performing the anastamosis.

Surgical Technique

Although speed is not essential, a stepwise, standardized approach can facilitate this very complex surgery and still allow it to be completed safely in less than 4 hours. We generally use an Ivor Lewis laparotomy with right thoracotomy technique for adequate exposure of the esophageal bed and maximum LN dissection. Alternatively, for patients with proximal extension above the carina (24 cm or above when measuring from the incisors), we prefer a modified McKeown or so-called *three-hole approach,* where the right thoracotomy is done first, with complete esophageal mobilization proximally to the plane around the cervical prevertebral fascia, and distally to include a cuff of diaphragm at the hiatus. Following this, the patient is placed supine, and a combined, simultaneous laparotomy with a left-neck approach is used, usually with two surgeons, to facilitate a rapid dissection.

After dissection of the GEJ, the crurae are exposed by careful sharp dissection of the peritoneum just below the inferior pericardiophrenic vein. The surgeon's right index finger is placed around the esophagus, and a Penrose drain is wrapped around the GEJ for retraction. While preserving the right gastroepiploic artery, all branches inferiorly are divided using the harmonic scalpel with great care to avoid thermal injury to the pedicle by staying 2 cm from the vessel (alternatively, these branches are divided between ties).

This dissection continues laterally to the left; at the point of the short gastric vessels, the dissection comes closer to the gastric serosa, dividing the short gastrics again with the harmonic scalpel, occasionally reinforcing them with hemoclips. The left gastric artery and vein are indentified, and lymph nodes in this region are dissected; we then divide the vessels with a single firing of an endoscopic linear vascular stapler (Figure 2).

Now, a point along the lesser curvature is chosen, generally between the fourth and fifth branches of the gastric arcade; after dividing the gastrohepatic omentum, multiple firings of the stapler are used to create a gastric conduit. By using multiple short firings

parallel to the greater curvature, a long conduit can be prepared that can easily reach the neck if needed (Figure 3) The proximal tube continues toward the apex of the fundus, allowing a 5 cm margin distal to the actual GEJ. It is our practice that after induction chemoradiation, we leave an additional wide margin of 5 cm above and below the edge of the radiation field, not just above the tumor. This will ensure the best possible tissue for anastamosis (Figure 4).

After placement of a feeding jejunostomy, the abdomen is closed with interrupted sutures to avoid dehiscence and postoperative hernias, and the patient is turned to the lateral decubitus position and prepared for a right thoracotomy through the fifth intercostal space using selective lung ventilation.

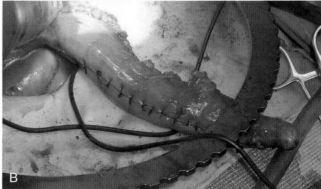

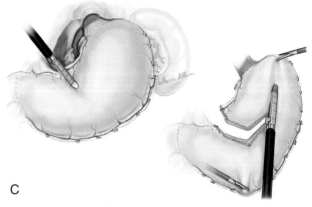

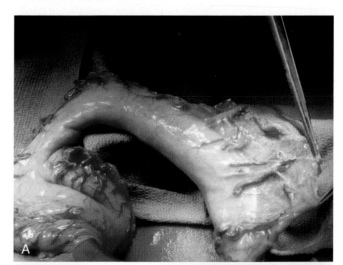

FIGURE 2   Division of left gastric artery and vein using the endostapler.

FIGURE 3   A and **B,** Formation of gastric conduit after multiple firings of the endostapler. **C** Drawing of gastric conduit formation. *(Reprinted with permission from Sugarbaker D, Bueno R, Krasna M, et al: Adult chest surgery, New York, 2009, McGraw Hill.)*

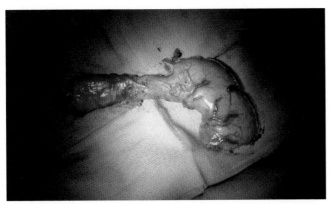

FIGURE 4   Esophagogastrectomy specimen of the resection.

The pleura is incised anterior to the esophagus, along the posterior edge of the pericardium, up to the azygos arch, and down to the hiatus posteriorly along the edge of the aorta. The surgeon's finger is now placed around the esophagus, and a Penrose drain is inserted as a retractor. With careful retraction, alternating posteriorly and then anteriorly, each of the bronchial arteries and direct aortic branches can be individually ligated as the esophagus specimen bloc is separated from the mediastinum.

After opening the peritoneum previously dissected from below, including a cuff of diaphragm with the specimen, the surgeon retrieves the stomach conduit from below with gentle traction and delivers it into the chest. This avoids tension or torsion of the conduit. We now take care not to deliver excessive length of the conduit to avoid an S-shaped loop postoperatively, which can cause dysphagia and postoperative pain. The anastamosis is then created using a hand-sewn, two-layer technique with silk mattress seromuscular sutures and interrupted 3-0 polydioxanone (PDS) sutures for the mucosa (Figure 5).

Recently, an endoscopic linear stapler forming a side-to-side stapled anastamosis has been used, with the anterior wall closed with hand sutures. Alternatively, a third technique involves the use of a circular stapler, either passed transorally or by making a gastrotomy in the specimen side. In an attempt to minimize leaks postoperatively, we have been using an intercostal muscle flap routinely as a way of reinforcing the staple line/anastamosis when patients have received preoperative chemoradiation (Figure 6).

Results

Surgery, chemoradiotherapy, or a combination of these techniques is the accepted treatment for the management of locally advanced esophageal cancer. The overall 5-year survival with multimodal treatment for esophageal cancer is about 40%, but despite many clinical trials and retrospective reviews, no treatment modality has proven superior.

NEOADJUVANT THERAPY

Preoperative radiation therapy is designed to reduce tumor size and risk of tumor spread during surgical manipulation. With one exception, none of the preoperative radiation trials demonstrated survival benefit. A meta-analysis concluded that survival was not improved with neoadjuvant radiotherapy, and it should not be recommended for patients for whom surgical resection was indicated.

The purported benefit of preoperative chemotherapy is the elimination of micrometastases, downstaging of the tumor, reduction of tumor recurrences, and improved surgical resectability. In patients with localized, resectable tumors, chemotherapy-related toxicity can occasionally result in prolonged delay or even cancellation of planned

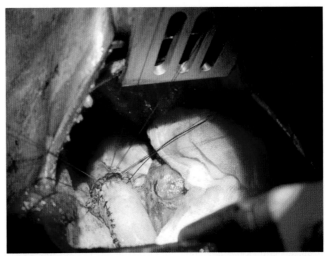

FIGURE 5   Esophagogastrotomy anastomosis in the right chest.

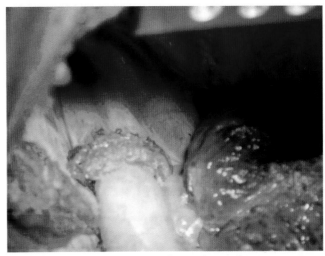

FIGURE 6   Intercostal muscle flap reinforcing the anastomosis.

surgical resection. Several randomized prospective trials comparing neoadjuvant chemotherapy plus surgery with surgical resection alone have been published with mixed results. The North America Intergroup Trial (INT 0113) randomized 467 patients with resectable esophageal adenocarcinoma (54%) and squamous cell carcinoma (46%). Two-year survival rates were 35% and 37%, respectively (not significant). The U.K. Medical Research Council Group (MRC OE02) randomized 802 patients with resectable esophageal adenocarcinoma (67%) and squamous cell carcinoma (33%). Patients who received preoperative chemotherapy had a significant improvement in median (17.2 months vs. 13.3 months) and 2-year (43% vs. 34%) survival rate. Patients did not generally undergo all their postoperative chemotherapy treatments in these studies.

The addition of radiation to a chemotherapeutic regimen before esophagectomy downstages the primary tumor, increases resectability rate, eliminates micrometastases, and improves overall survival. The study by Walsh and colleagues (1996) randomized 113 patients with adenocarcinoma to receive preoperative cisplatin and 5-fluorouracil with radiotherapy (58 patients) or surgery alone (55 patients). Patients who received preoperative chemoradiotherapy had a median survival of 16 months, versus 11 months for the group treated with surgery alone, and a 3-year survival rate of 32% versus 6%, respectively ($P = .01$).

Tepper and colleagues (2008) have demonstrated survival benefit from neoadjuvant chemoradiotherapy compared with surgery alone in the Cancer and Leukemia Group B 9781 study (CALGB). In that study, patients were randomized to receive surgery alone or two cycles of cisplatin and 5-fluorouracil with concurrent radiotherapy followed by surgery. Although the trial was closed prematurely after 2 years due to lack of accrual, a total of 56 patients were treated. Results were recently published that showed a median survival of 4.5 years versus 1.8 years in favor of trimodal therapy, with a 5-year survival of 39% versus 16% ($P = .020$).

ADJUVANT THERAPY

Radiotherapy following esophagectomy has been suggested to sterilize occult micrometastases and therefore increase cure rate and prolong survival. The data from studies randomizing to surgery versus adjuvant external beam radiotherapy indicated that postoperative radiation following curative esophagectomy provided no overall survival benefit but might be harmful from the significant side effects from the radiation. One study published by Xiao et al (2003) randomized 495 patients with esophageal cancer into surgery plus adjuvant radiotherapy (n = 220) and surgery alone (n = 275). The study showed that the overall 5-year survival rate for the surgery plus radiotherapy versus surgery alone was 41.3% versus 31.7%. There were concerns about the results because of lack of consent of the patients, and the large number of, and the rationale for, withdrawals from the study.

There has been only one published, prospective randomized trial comparing adjuvant chemotherapy with surgery alone in resectable esophageal cancer, by Ando and colleagues in 1997. Using cisplatin and vindesine as the postoperative regimen, 100 patients were randomized. There was no significant difference in the median and 5-year survival.

A prospective randomized trial comparing adjuvant chemoradiotherapy with surgery alone in locoregionally advanced esophageal cancer was published by Rice et al (2003), in which 83 patients were randomized (31 received adjuvant therapy and 52 received surgery alone). The median and 4-year survival were 28 versus 14 months and 44% versus 17% respectively, which suggests that adjuvant chemoradiotherapy provides an overall survival benefit for patients with locoregionally advanced esophageal cancer. Other data from gastric cancer trials support a similar conclusion.

SUMMARY

Neoadjuvant chemoradiotherapy for locally advanced esophageal carcinoma provides a survival advantage, particularly in patients downstaged to pathologic complete response status, although the results of randomized controlled trials are conflicting. Current standard of care is surgery for stage I and II disease, with a 5-year survival of 25% to 60%, respectively. The role of adjuvant chemo/radiotherapy is currently unclear except as the standard of care for nonsurgical patients with advanced esophageal carcinoma.

SUGGESTED READING

Akiyama H, Tsurumaru M, Kawamura T, et al: Principles for surgical treatment for carcinoma of the esophagus: analysis of lymph node involvement. *Ann Surg* 194:438, 1981.

Kelsen DP, Ginsberg R, Pajak TF, et al: Chemotherapy followed by surgery compared with surgery alone for localized esophageal cancer, *N Engl J Med* 339:1979–1984, 1998.

Krasna MJ, Jiao X, Mao Y, et al: Thoracoscopy/laparoscopy in the staging of esophageal cancer: the Maryland experience, *Surg Laparosc Endosc* 12(4):213–218, 2002.

Medical Research Council Oesophageal Cancer Working Group: Surgical resection with or without preoperative chemotherapy in oesophageal cancer: a randomized controlled trial, *Lancet* 359:1727–1733, 2002.

Rice TW, Mason DP, Murphy SC, et al: T2N0M0 esophageal cancer. *J Thorac Cardiovasc Surg* 133:317–324, 2007.

Tepper JE, Krasna MJ, Niedzwiecki D, et al: Phase III trial of trimodality therapy with cisplatin, fluorouracil, radiotherapy and surgery compared with surgery alone for esophageal cancer: CALGB 9781, *J Clin Oncol* 26:1086–1092, 2008.

Walsh TN, Noonan N, Hollywood D, et al: A comparison of multimodality therapy and surgery for esophageal adenocarcinoma, *N Engl J Med* 335:462–467, 1996.

Xiao ZF, Yang Z, Liang J, et al: Value of radiotherapy after radical surgery for esophageal carcinoma: a report of 495 patients. *Ann Thorac Surg* 75:331–336, 2003.

ESOPHAGEAL STENTS

Nirmal K. Veeramachaneni, MD, and Richard H. Feins, MD

HISTORY

Esophageal cancer is the seventh leading cause of cancer death in men and the eighth most common cause of cancer worldwide. Although complete surgical resection remains the mainstay of therapy, most patients are not candidates for surgical resection. Palliative treatment to relieve progressive dysphagia includes chemoradiation, brachytherapy, photodynamic therapy, and endoscopic strategies, including tumor ablation with laser or mechanical dilatation and stent placement.

It is beyond the scope of this chapter to discuss all of these palliative strategies. We focus the discussion on mechanical palliative strategies (stents) to treat the complications of obstruction and the utility of stents in the management of esophageal fistula.

The first clinically used stents date back to the 1950s. These early stents were essentially tubes made of silicon or plastic with a fixed diameter. They were placed by retrograde traction via open gastrostomy and often required dilatation of the malignant stricture. A pilot bougie would need to be placed orally and retrieved via the gastrostomy for the stent to be pulled into place. Endoscopic strategies evolved, eliminating the need for gastrostomy, but this strategy resulted in the placement of stents with limited internal diameter. Although these stents were useful in permitting the swallowing of oral secretions, most patients were unable to resume a normal diet. The use of these types of fixed-diameter, rigid stents is now largely of historical interest. The limited diameter of the stents and their rigid profiles meant that they could not conform to an angulated or tortuous esophagus. These factors, and the need to dilatate malignant strictures, resulted in an unacceptable perforation rate.

The advent of a self-expanding metal (SEM) stent has paved the way for modern treatment strategies. A number of manufacturers offer SEM stents with slight differences in material and delivery systems. Given the rapid changes in technology, it is beyond the scope of this chapter to review the technical details of each product. We can, however, offer general principles applied in the design of these products and offer comparisons between the different types. Unlike conventional stents, SEM stents are offered in a low-profile delivery system that may be deployed using conventional fiberoptic endoscopic techniques that employ fluoroscopy with the patient under conscious sedation or general anesthetic.

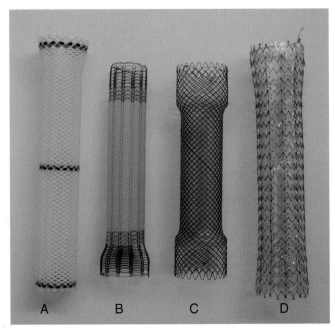

FIGURE 1 The surgeon should note the wide array of stent designs available for use in the esophagus. Covered stents are more prone to migration due to less tissue ingrowth, whereas uncovered stents are more prone to restenosis because they permit ingrowth. Some stents are designed to permit repositioning, which is often facilitated by incorporation of a "lasso" at the end of the stent. This lasso can be grasped with endoscopic forceps to permit repositioning into the appropriate position. Pictured are four commonly used stents in the United States. **A,** Polyflex, Boston Scientific. Polyester stent lined with silicone. **B,** Ultraflex, Boston Scientific. Partially covered nitinol stent. Notice that the ends are not covered. **C,** Evolution, Cook (Bloomington, Ind.). Partially covered nitinol stent. Notice that the ends are not covered. **D,** Alimaxx-E, Merit Medical Systems. Completely covered nitinol stent.

Stents are available uncovered, partially covered, and completely covered (Figure 1). SEM stents are composed of either stainless steel or nitinol, a nickel-titanium alloy that is tightly wound as wire coils or mesh around a small delivery device. A completely plastic expandable stent is also available (Polyflex, Boston Scientific, Natick, Mass.). Although the metals in stents are made to be inert, resistant to corrosion, and nonallergenic even in patients who are allergic to nickel, when the stent coils embed into the esophageal mucosa or submucosa, they do trigger a mild inflammatory response with fibrosis that reduces the risk of stent migration.

Nitinol stents are made from a single wire and can be easily removed if completely covered. The advantage of nitinol is that this alloy has thermal shape memory characteristics that enable it to expand at body temperature to fit the shape of a particular lesion. Covered designs are available for most SEM stents, with a covering of polyurethane or silicone. Most covered stents have "flared" proximal and distal ends that remain bare and uncovered to provide additional luminal anchorage. Covered stents are believed to have less tumor ingrowth but can potentially be more susceptible to stent migration, especially in high-risk areas such as the distal esophagus. Additional security of placement is provided by the radial expansive force of the stent after deployment, which allows it to expand to its final shape and diameter.

Today, most stents have a covered design, but stents are available in a wide variety of diameters and lengths to fit various strictures. The most commonly used stent is probably the 10 cm long, 17 to 23 mm diameter covered SEM stent. The increased internal diameter of the fully deployed stent lets the patient return to a more normal diet.

The design of the stent must be carefully considered prior to insertion. Early stents consisted of uncovered bare metal. Although initially effective, the rapid ingrowth of tissue and the inflammatory response of the mucosa to the metal made these stents problematic in the long term. Partially covered stents minimize this problem, but even the small, exposed areas at the ends of the stents may result in obstruction. Their putative advantage is to minimize migration, but this is countered by the problems of stent ingrowth. In our clinical practice, considering the palliative indication for stent placement, we have used fully covered stents (Polyflex or Alveolus [Merit Medical Systems, Inc., South Jordan, Utah]) almost exclusively and have accepted the increased risk of stent migration. The self-expanding plastic stents have a migration rate of up to 25%.

STENT PLACEMENT TECHNIQUE

In the United States, esophageal stents are available in a variety of lengths, from 60 to 150 mm, with internal diameters of 17 to 23 mm. Stents are available in a low-profile delivery system, and various manufacturers differ in the type of deployment mechanism. It is important that the surgeon become familiar with the deployment mechanism to avoid stent misplacement or migration.

The basic tools required to place a stent include fluoroscopic capabilities, radiopaque markers (paper clips usually suffice), esophageal dilators, a guidewire, and a flexible endoscope. The procedure may be performed with the patient under either conscious sedation or general anesthetic; we tend to favor the latter.

Before placing the stent, the physician identifies the proximal and distal extent of the stricture. Radiopaque markers are placed on the patient's skin to mark the extent of the stricture, and a guidewire is placed to traverse the stricture. If the endoscope cannot traverse the stricture, gentle dilatation may be required. Unlike older plastic stents, minimal dilatation is required, although it may be necessary to place a small-diameter stent initially, with a need for further dilatation and a larger stent at a later time. Under fluoroscopic guidance, the delivery system is placed over the guidewire, aligned with the skin markers, and deployed. Positioning is then confirmed both fluoroscopically and endoscopically. Endoscopic grasping forceps can be used to reposition the stent if required. Gentle balloon dilatation inside the stent may be required if the stent appears to be buckled or improperly seated. The expansile process of the stent continues, especially with nitinol stents, and can be augmented when the patient drinks warm liquids.

Special Considerations

Tumor location must be carefully considered prior to stent placement. Tumors located at the gastroesophageal junction (GEJ) pose the problem of an incompetent antireflux mechanism after stent placement. Patients may benefit from proton pump inhibitors to mitigate the symptoms of gastroesophageal reflux, but SEM stents with a windsock-type antireflux valve have been developed to minimize reflux. In small studies, the incidence of reflux was minimized with no compromise in dysphagia improvement. We have been able to manage patients with high-dose proton pump inhibitors after placement of stents near the GEJ.

Seating the stent at the GEJ may also pose a problem. A large portion of the distal stent may be in the lumen of the stomach, with no anchoring. Repositioning of the stent may be required. In this instance, a partially covered stent or uncovered stent may be the better option, or using a stent with the wire on the outside of the covering to promote tissue anchoring without tissue ingrowth.

Additional problems are posed by the natural angulation of the GEJ. A larger stent may be required to overcome these barriers, but this may result in increased pressure-related complications such as ulceration. The stomach may also be the site of injury due to the protrusion of the stent into the stomach. We favor frequent radiographs in the early postprocedure period to monitor for stent migration.

Stents placed in the cervical esophagus also pose a special challenge for the surgeon. They are generally less well tolerated by the patient due to increased risks of aspiration and proximal migration, and globus sensation may limit their use. Prior to deployment of a stent in the proximal esophagus, the airway must be inspected to ensure no compromise. We typically place a small savory dilator, similar in diameter to the stent we intend to place into the esophagus, and perform bronchoscopy to ensure no airway problems.

Esophageal stents have also been used in selective cases of esophageal perforation, fistula, and anastamotic disruption. This is typically done when open surgical intervention is not possible and the patient is not in a severe septic state, although some investigators (Freeman et al, 2009) have extended their criteria. A covered stent is placed to exclude the site of perforation or fistula, but only after the sinus tract or cavity arising from the site of perforation has been well drained. The goal of this intervention is to limit ongoing contamination. Once the abscess cavity has been drained; the fistulous tract is allowed to scar in.

After a number of weeks, the patient undergoes a repeat barium swallow study and a computed tomographic scan of the chest to ensure no ongoing leak and complete obliteration of the abscess cavity. Only after both of these goals have been reached is the stent removed. Once the stent has been removed, we repeat the swallow study to ensure lack of an ongoing leak prior to resuming oral intake. Careful attention must be given to ensure that the patient does not develop an abscess or suffer from sepsis caused by ongoing contamination.

A similar strategy has been employed in patients requiring palliation of a tracheoesophageal fistula caused by malignancy. The esophageal stent prevents ongoing contamination of the lung. A tracheal stent may need to be placed in addition to the esophageal stent to ensure adequate palliation.

POSTOPERATIVE CARE

Most patients tolerate the placement of an esophageal stent with few severe problems. The development of pain and chest discomfort is expected from the radial force of esophageal dilation and stent placement and may be avoided by not oversizing the stent. However, persistent and severe pain is unusual, and the physician must be suspicious

of the possibility of a perforation. There should be a low threshold to obtain a contrast swallow study, and some physicians routinely obtain a swallow study after the placement of an esophageal stent.

It is our routine practice to observe the patient for 24 hours after the placement of an esophageal stent. If the patient has no symptoms of severe pain, we begin a liquid diet. If the stent was placed near the GEJ, or traversed the GEJ, the patient is started on a proton pump inhibitor and advised to sleep with the head of the bed elevated. Prior to discharge, chest and abdominal radiographs are obtained to document the location of the stent.

SUMMARY

The goal of this review was to provide a framework to guide the choice of stent. It is impossible to review all of the manufactured stents available today; with improvements in technology, new designs are actively being marketed. There is no compelling evidence to favor one stent over another, but it is critical to understand the properties of the stent the surgeon is going to deploy and to understand the pitfalls of the various designs. Most of the available literature is marked by small studies with few patients randomized between the various manufactured stents. The lack of large randomized trials has resulted in no single SEM stent being declared superior to another.

The advent of SEM stents has supplanted the use of fixed-diameter plastic stents. As a class, SEM stents are easier to deploy and have lower stent-related mortality compared with their plastic counterparts, decreased risk of esophageal perforation, and less stent migration. The choice of covered versus uncovered SEM stent influences the risk of migration at tumor ingrowth.

REFERENCES

1. Yakoub D, Fahmy R, Athanasiou T, et al: Evidence-based choice of esophageal stent for the palliative management of malignant dysphagia, *World J Surg* 32(9):1996–2009, 2008.
2. Knyrim K, Wagner HJ, Bethge N, et al: A controlled trial of an expansile metal stent for palliation of esophageal obstruction due to inoperable cancer, *N Engl J Med* 28; 329(18):1302–1307, 1993.
3. Freeman RK, Van Woerkom JM, Vyverberg A, et al: Esophageal stent placement for the treatment of spontaneous esophageal perforations, *Ann Thorac Surg* 88(1):194–198, 2009.

ESOPHAGEAL PERFORATION

Mark D. Iannettoni, MD, MBA, and Samad Hashimi, MD

MORBIDITY AND MORTALITY

Esophageal perforation is generally considered a life-threatening condition. Despite advances in surgery and intensive care medicine, mortality rates ranging from 10% to 40% have been reported in the literature. Delay in diagnosis has catastrophic implications, leading to sepsis and death. Early aggressive surgical intervention is preferred to avoid increased mortality and reduce long-term morbidity. The incidence of esophageal perforation will most likely continue to increase as the number and complexity of endoscopic procedures performed increase. Factors that influence mortality are 1) age, 2) general medical condition of the patient, 3) the location of the perforation, 4) the cause, and 5) the presence or absence of intrinsic esophageal disease.

Conservative management has been used with some success, but patients have to be carefully selected and monitored closely when attempting nonoperative therapy, and strict adherence to established tenets must be observed. In general, however, we favor early aggressive surgical management.

PATHOPHYSIOLOGY

Early diagnosis and intervention can help avoid the lethal complications of sepsis and death. The negative intrathoracic pressure increases the leakage of esophageal and gastric contents into the mediastinum, which can induce a chemical injury resulting in a necrotizing infection. The direction and descent of mediastinal infection depends on the site of perforation. An inferior and posterior perforation can allow descent into the posterior mediastinum as well as up into the neck, and a cervical or pharyngeal perforation can result in extension into the anterior or posterior mediastinum. This occurs through the fascial planes demonstrated in the diagram in Figure 1.

Structural abnormalities or anatomic weakness in the muscle wall can account for an increase in localized perforations, such as

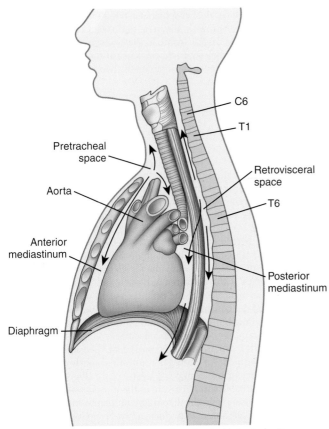

FIGURE 1   Direction of descent of mediastinal infections. *(From Patterson A, Cooper JD, Deslauriers J, et al: Pearson's thoracic and esophageal surgery, ed 3, Philadelphia, 2008, Churchill Livingstone.)*

at the level of the cricopharyngeus. At this level there are not only changes in the anatomic structure of the esophagus but also an anatomic weakness in the cervical esophagus with posterior displacement. In the case of Boerhaave syndrome, there is a rapid rise in the intraluminal esophageal pressure through a patent lower esophageal sphincter (LES) during vomiting. This increase, combined with lack of relaxation of cricopharyngeal muscle, can lead to transmural rupture of the esophageal wall. Usually the rupture is located on the left posterolateral wall of the lower third of the esophagus 2 to 3 cm proximal to gastroesophageal junction (GEJ). This area is structurally and inherently weakened as the longitudinal muscle fibers taper out before passing into the stomach wall.

CLINICAL FEATURES

The etiology of the esophageal perforation is important and requires an astute clinician. The location of the injury is an important part of the information because it determines the surgical approach for its treatment. Although time elapsed between the injury and intervention is important, it has less to do with the type of repair than it does with aiding in outlining the postoperative course and the morbidity associated with the injury. Table 1 shows a few causes of esophageal perforation.

Most patients with cervical perforation will complain of neck pain that is worse with swallowing or neck flexion, and cervical crepitus may be evident. Thoracic esophageal perforation can manifest with epigastric or substernal pain. Most patients will soon become febrile and develop leukocytosis. Depending on the timing of plain radiographs (chest or lateral cervical radiographs), these may be completely normal or may show evidence of pleural effusion, which

TABLE 1: Causes of esophageal perforation

Instrumentation	Esophagoscopy, transesophageal echocardiography, pneumatic dilatation, placement of intraesophageal tubes, traumatic endotracheal intubation
Postsurgical	Mediastinoscopy, thyroid surgery, anterior spinal surgery, vagotomy, antireflux surgery, thoracic aneurysm resection
Trauma	Penetrating, foreign body, caustic ingestion
Barotrauma	Vomiting, blunt chest trauma
Tumor	Esophageal, lung, mediastinal
Infection	Tuberculosis, histoplasmosis, AIDS

develops within 24 hours, anterior displacement of trachea and esophagus, or a widening of the retrovisceral space. Classically, dissection of air along the subcutaneous planes or into the mediastinum has been considered a hallmark of esophageal perforation.

DIAGNOSIS

Once the diagnosis is suspected, most authorities favor obtaining an esophagogram (Figure 2). Esophagograms are usually performed with water-soluble contrast material to help confirm the location of the perforation. The study should be followed with thin barium if no leak is seen, but there is a high clinical suspicion of a leak. Our preference is to start directly with thin barium to determine if a leak is present, because if a large leak is detected, intervention is almost always required. And because barium is inert, the risk of aspiration-induced chemical pneumonitis that occurs with water-soluble contrast agents is eliminated.

Although computed tomography (CT) technology has improved tremendously over the last decade, barium swallow still remains the gold standard for diagnosing esophageal perforation. Although false-negative rates as high as 10% have been reported, it still remains the study of choice for the detection of esophageal injury. If clinical suspicion remains high despite a negative study, the study can be repeated after several hours. A CT can be used as an adjunct in the setting of high clinical suspicion to help identify mediastinal inflammation, abscess, and emphysema. An upper endoscopy in the setting of thoracic perforation following a contrast esophagogram is essential to evaluate the associated pathology that either accompanies the perforation or that caused it. Upper endoscopy and contrast esophagogram are of great value in visualizing small mucosal tears. Although extreme care and caution must be exercised in performing the endoscopy, the fears of worsening the injury are outweighed by the information that is obtained by this procedure.

THERAPY

Regardless of the location of injury, prompt resuscitation with intravenous fluids and administration of broad-spectrum antibiotics to cover upper digestive tract organisms is a must. We favor antibiotics to cover anaerobes, fungi, and both gram-positive and gram-negative organisms. Nasogastric decompression is also important, and the nasogastric tube can be inserted during the esophagram to avoid inadvertent worsening of the injury; a chest tube should be inserted to drain the pleural effusion. The surgical management of the perforation, however, will depend on the location of injury.

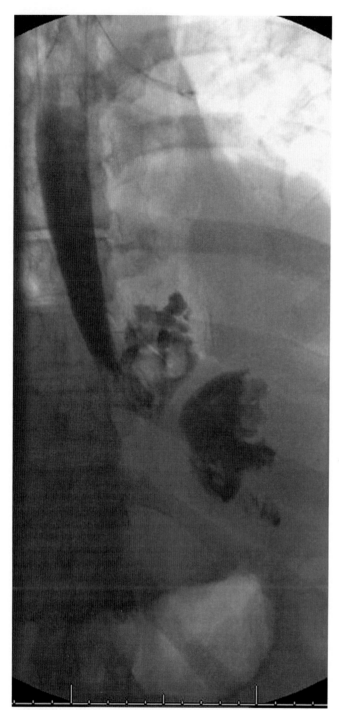

FIGURE 2   Barium swallow demonstrating a lower esophageal perforation.

Cervical Perforation

Prompt surgical management not only reduces morbidity and mortality, but also the length of hospital stay. We prefer a left-sided neck incision over the anterior border of the sternocleidomastoid muscle (Figure 3). Retract the carotid sheath and internal jugular vein laterally, and the trachea and esophagus medially, then bluntly enter the retroesophageal space along the prevertebral fascia, taking care to avoid injury to the recurrent laryngeal nerve. Finger dissection should be carried out down to the posterior mediastinum to drain all collections, both in a proximal and distal direction. Once the perforation is identified, close the defect with absorbable sutures.

An injury to the cervical esophagus is frequently not identifiable in this region. However, with adequate drainage a cervical perforation will heal without direct closure in the absence of distal obstruction from intrinsic pathology. In the presence of concomitant tracheal injury, a pedicled muscle flap to separate the two repairs is essential.

Thoracic Perforation

There must be no delay in bringing the patient to the operating room once the diagnosis of a perforation has been established. For the upper two thirds of the thoracic esophagus, the injury is approached from a right thoracotomy through the fourth or fifth intercostal space. For injuries in the lower third of the esophagus, the approach is through a left-sided thoracotomy through the sixth or seventh intercostal space. Depending on the etiology of perforation, one can attempt primary repair, diversion, or esophagectomy. It is of utmost importance to know whether there is evidence of intrinsic esophageal disease and the underlying pathology, as this will guide the operative intervention and determine the functional outcome for these patients.

Primary repair is the preferred approach and should be considered in all cases regardless of the time course; however, underlying pathology must be considered and will determine the short- and long-term outcomes both from a functional and a success standpoint. Primary repair requires opening the muscular layers above and below the injury to better visualize the mucosal defect, then a two-layer closure can be performed. An endo-gastrointestinal anastomotic stapler can be used to perform the mucosal layer closure (Figures 4 and 5), followed by absorbable suture closure of the muscle layer. The stomach, pleura, or muscle from the diaphragm or intercostals can be used to buttress the repair; failure to perform a two-layer closure can result in an inadequate repair subject to recurrent leaks and possible fistula formation. Finally, the pleural cavity is irrigated and drained via chest tubes.

In cases where the injury occurred proximal to a long stricture, or where there is evidence of esophageal carcinoma, our preferred treatment is esophagectomy with immediate reconstruction. It is also of paramount importance that distal obstruction to the site of primary repair be eliminated. If there are multiple sites of obstruction not amenable to correction, an esophagectomy is warranted.

Intraabdominal Perforation

The steps taken to repair an intraabdominal perforation are similar to those needed for a thoracic perforation: debridement, drainage, two-layer closure, and buttressing of the repair. The injury can be approached via laparotomy or laparoscopy, and perforations are best treated by closure and fundoplication. If the injury and perforation are secondary to a procedure for a motor disorder, this disorder must be addressed prior to repair. For example, if a perforation occurs with a known diagnosis of achalasia, then a contralateral myotomy and partial fundoplication should be performed, and a decompressive gastrostomy is highly recommended.

Nonoperative Management

Nonoperative management can be considered for patients whose injury suggests a contained mucosal defect with leakage of contrast back into the esophagus. We would perform an upper endoscopy to evaluate the extent of injury. The patient would need to be kept NPO and on IV fluids and antibiotics for at least 3 days, then the diet can be slowly advanced. If at any time the patient develops signs of sepsis, emergent operative intervention must be undertaken.

Patient selection is of utmost importance. Appropriate patients include those with 1) intraluminal dissection, 2) transmural perforation that drains back into the esophagus, 3) no associated distal

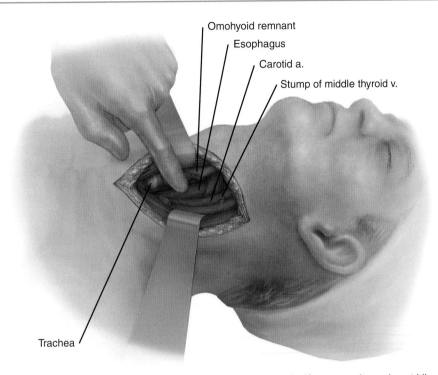

Omohyoid remnant
Esophagus
Carotid a.
Stump of middle thyroid v.
Trachea

FIGURE 3 Make an incision over the anterior border of the sternocleidomastoid muscle. If necessary, ligate the middle thyroid vein and inferior thyroid artery. Retract the trachea and thyroid gland medially to help expose the esophagus. *(From Cooke DT, Lau CL: Primary repair of esophageal perforation. Op Tech Thor Cardiovasc Surg 13(2):126-137, 2008.)*

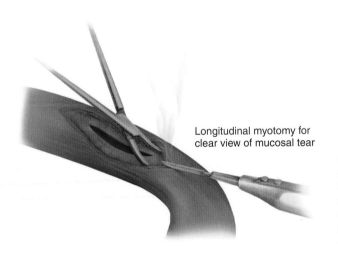

Longitudinal myotomy for clear view of mucosal tear

FIGURE 4 Mucosal injury is usually more extensive than the apparent muscular defect. A longitudinal myotomy is performed until the full extent of the mucosal tear is apparent. The mucosa is debrided as necessary to freshen edges. *(From Cooke DT, Lau CL: Primary repair of esophageal perforation. Op Tech Thor Cardiovasc Surg 13(2):126–137, 2008.)*

obstruction, 4) a perforation that is not in the abdominal cavity, 5) no evidence of systemic sepsis, and 6) no evidence of esophageal carcinoma. Despite strict adherence to these criteria, up to 20% of patients managed nonoperatively develop complications within 24 hours that require surgical intervention.

Minimally Invasive Techniques

Minimally invasive surgery (MIS) offers a magnified view of the entire operative field but has many limitations. Over the next decade, the use of MIS will undoubtedly increase as surgeons become more proficient at thoracoscopy and laparoscopy. Combining endoscopy and thoracoscopy allows the surgeon to submerge the suspected area under irrigation and insufflate the esophagus

to precisely localize the area of injury and identify the area of perforation. If the area is smaller than 1 cm, a primary repair can be performed thoracoscopically or laparoscopically, depending on the proficiency of the operating surgeon. In cases of larger perforation and extensive inflammation, we would recommend an open repair. MIS is still associated with longer operation times and limited operative options.

Endoscopic Stenting and Clipping

The use of endoluminal stenting, which was previously used in cases of inoperable neoplasm, has increased over the last few years. Successful management of early esophageal perforation with stenting has been described in the setting of perforation secondary to endoscopic instrumentation, foreign body ingestion, and even Boerhaave syndrome. Stents have been successful when used in the setting of minimal mediastinal contamination. The use of stents needs to be individualized through a multidisciplinary team approach involving the endoscopist and surgeon.

REFERENCES

Patterson A, Cooper JD, Deslauriers J, et al: *Pearson's thoracic and esophageal surgery*, ed 3, Philadelphia, 2008, Churchill Livingstone.

Greenfield LJ, Mulholland MW, Oldham KT, et al: *Surgery: scientific principles and practice*, ed 3, Philadelphia, 2001, Lippincott Williams & Wilkins.

Bresadola V, Terrosu G, Favero A, et al: Treatment of perforation in healthy esophagus: analysis of 12 cases, *Langenbeck's Arch Surg* 393:135–140, 2008.

Rubesin S, Levine MS: Radiologic diagnosis of esophageal perforation, *Radiol Clin North Am* 41:1095–1115, 2003.

Fadoo F, Ruiz DE, Dawn SK, et al: Helical CT esophagography for evaluation of suspected esophageal perforation or rupture, *AJR* 182:1177–1179, 2004.

Vogel SB, Rout WR, Marin TD, Abbitt PL: Esophageal perforation in adults: aggressive conservative treatment lowers morbidity and mortality, *Ann Surg* 241(6):1016–1023, 2005.

Freeman RK, Van Woerkom JM, Ascioti AJ: Esophageal stent placement for treatment of iatrogenic intrathoracic esophageal perforation, *Ann Thorac Surg* 83:2003–2008, 2007.

Wu JT, Mattox KL, Wall MJ Jr: Esophageal perforation: new perspectives and treatment paradigms, *J Trauma* 63:1173–1184, 2007.

Port JL, Kent MS, Korst RJ, et al: Thoracic esophageal perforations: a decade of experience, *Ann Thorac Surg* 75:1071–1074, 2003.

Brinster CJ, Singhal S, Lee L, et al: Evolving options in management of esophageal perforation, *Ann Thorac Surg* 77:1475–1483, 2004.

Cooke DT, Lau CL: Primary repair of esophageal perforation, *Op Tech Thor Cardiovasc Surg* 13:126–137, 2008.

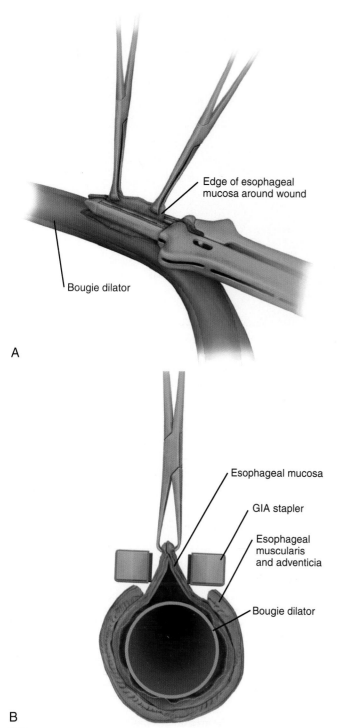

FIGURE 5   A 40 Fr or 46 Fr Maloney bougie is inserted into the lumen, the esophageal mucosal edges are grasped and approximated with Allis clamps or interrupted sutures, and the mucosa is closed with a 3.5 mm load. GIA, gastrointestinal anastomosis. *(From Cooke DT, Lau CL: Primary repair of esophageal perforation. Op Tech Thor Cardiovasc Surg 13(2):126–137, 2008.)*

BENIGN GASTRIC ULCER

Naeem A. Newman, MD, Sami Mufeed, MD, and
Martin A. Makary, MD, MPH

SYMPTOMS

Despite the increased use of proton-pump inhibitors (PPIs), earlier treatment of *Helicobacter pylori,* and decreased long-term use of non-steroidal antiinflammatory drugs (NSAIDs), gastric ulcers remain a common and important diagnosis among patients with epigastric pain or a perforated viscus. A gastric ulcer can present in many ways, ranging from subtle findings in the outpatient setting to late-stage sepsis in the emergency department. It is also important to remember that most benign gastric ulcers never present to a medical professional, and many more never present to a surgeon, as most ulcers heal on their own given the rich blood supply of the stomach (Figure 1). However, proper diagnosis and treatment of gastric ulcer remains a classic problem for the astute surgeon in both the inpatient and outpatient settings.

INCIDENCE

Despite its declining incidence, benign gastric ulcer still represents one of the most common upper gastrointestinal (GI) problems. It is most common in older men, with a peak incidence between 55 and 65 years of age. The three main risk factors for gastric ulcer are NSAIDs, cigarette smoking, and *H. pylori* infection.

Most gastric ulcers are subclinical, and many do not require surgery. It is estimated that 10% to 35% of patients diagnosed with gastric ulcer will develop a serious complication such as a perforation or stricture. Most importantly, because a gastric malignancy will commonly ulcerate through the stomach mucosa, it is critical to consider a potential malignancy when treating a new gastric ulcer because 10% of all gastric ulcers are malignant. For this reason, a biopsy of the ulcer is recommended to rule out malignancy. Ulceration from malignancy is less likely in younger patients and in those with a history of NSAID use or of gastric ulcers. Conversely, a new ulcer in an older patient without a plausible explanation for having an ulcer is more worrisome for malignancy.

Recognizing the consideration of risk factors for malignant ulcers, this chapter will focus on the clinical diversity, manifestations, and surgical treatment of benign ulcers of the stomach.

ETIOLOGY

In the absence of chronic use of NSAIDs or Zollinger-Ellison syndrome, *H. pylori* infection is considered the main cause of gastric peptic ulcer. In fact, 85% to 90% of patients with gastric ulcer are colonized with *H. pylori,* and without treating the *H. pylori* infection 80% of gastric ulcers recur within 1 year of treatment. Following the eradication of the *H. pylori* infection, recurrence of the ulcer is rare.

NSAIDs are known to break the gastric mucosal barrier, most notably with chronic use. Patients with abdominal pain and arthritis, back pain, or another condition requiring chronic use of NSAIDs should be suspected of having a benign gastric ulcer. The most classic presentation is that of an older patient in the emergency department with epigastric pain and a history of arthritis. Sometimes the addition of referred left shoulder pain from a perforation is present.

Another common presentation of benign gastric ulcer is the transplant or lymphoma patient who takes steroids. Prolonged use of corticosteroids not only causes gastric ulcers, it also blurs the clinical presentation because steroids can mask abdominal pain. Any patient who takes steroids long term and develops sudden and worsening abdominal pain should be considered for a gastric ulcer. Gastric ulcers are also common in patients who abuse alcohol, which is often coupled with cigarette smoking, both of which decrease the gastric mucosal defense barrier.

Finally, gastric ulcers can occur in postoperative patients. Studies show that patients with stress ulcers have a mortality rate up to four times higher than patients who do not have stress ulceration and bleeding. The literature has demonstrated that in critically ill surgical patients, the only risk factors associated with clinically significant bleeding from stress ulcers were mechanical ventilation for more than 48 hours and coagulopathy. The practice of stress ulcer prophylaxis in non–critically ill patients is generally not recommended. Prophylactic agents include antacids, H2-receptor blockers, sucralfate, proton pump inhibitors (PPIs) prostaglandin analogs, and nutrition.

CLINICAL PRESENTATION

Patients with uncomplicated gastric ulcers report bouts of epigastric pain following meals. The pain is sometimes referred to the back. About 20% to 40% of patients describe bloating, belching, or symptoms suggestive of gastroesophageal reflux; another 30% to 40% of patients with gastric ulcers experience nightly pain. This pattern is believed to be the result of increased gastric acid secretion, which occurs after meals and during the late night and early morning hours, when circadian stimulation of gastric acid secretion is the highest. Although gastric ulcers can cause generalized visceral pain, the pain can be more focal within the epigastrium. Palpation often does not reveal tenderness over the epigastrium.

Gastric ulcer complications present with a more profound clinical picture. Recurrent ulcers at the pylorus can result in stricture formation and cause a gastric outlet obstruction. Gastric ulcers can bleed, especially when a blood vessel is visible in the base of the ulcer on endoscopy. While many of these ulcers can be injected and cauterized endoscopically, some require surgical resection. Before the bleeding lesion is identified endoscopically, patients often present with hematemesis or melena. Perforation will present with acute epigastric pain and tenderness with guarding and rigidity of abdominal muscles. Obstruction will present with persistent nausea and vomiting.

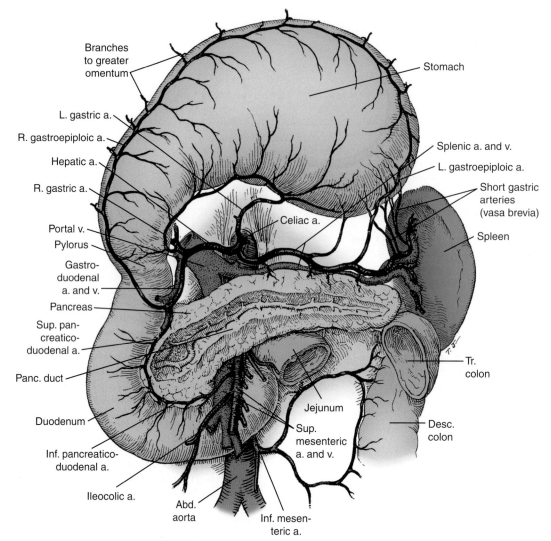

FIGURE 1 Blood supply to the stomach. *L,* Left; *a.,* artery; *R,* right; *v.,* vein; *Sup.,* superior; *Panc.,* pancreatic; *Inf.,* inferior; *Abd.,* Abdominal; *Tr.,* transverse; *Desc.,* descending. *(From Yeo NN: Shackelford's surgery of the alimentary tract, ed 6, Philadelphia, 2007, Saunders, p 719.)*

UBT - urea labeled isotope, isotope labelled urea CO₂ indicates

DIAGNOSIS

Patients seen in the outpatient setting can be evaluated for *H. pylori* by antibody detection tests and urea breath tests (UBTs). Antibody detection by serologic or whole-blood testing is safe, easy to perform in the outpatient setting, and inexpensive. Serologic testing should be considered for patients with no symptoms of complicated gastric ulcer who have a history of documented ulcers but have not received treatment for *H. pylori*. The nonradioactive and radioactive UBTs are more sensitive, specific, and expensive than serologic and whole-blood antibody detection tests and are better suited for follow-up testing to verify eradication. False-negative results with UBTs are infrequent but can occur for patients currently or recently taking an antisecretory drug, bismuth subsalicylate, or an antimicrobial agent.

Another noninvasive test was recently developed that detects antigen in the stool of patients with active *H. pylori* infection. Although only a few studies have been performed thus far, stool antigen testing has sensitivity and specificity similar to those of serologic testing and seems to be as effective as UBTs in screening for *H. pylori*.

For inpatients with a suspected gastric ulcer without perforation, an upper endoscopy is recommended to biopsy the ulcer and test for *H. pylori* so that the appropriate treatment can be started. When endoscopy is indicated, the test of first choice for *H. pylori* is a urease test of an antral specimen. This test can only be used in patients not taking bismuth-containing medications, PPIs, or antimicrobials within the previous 4 weeks, because these medications decrease the test's sensitivity.

Since blood in the gastric lumen may also compromise a urease test of an antral specimen, alternative testing may include histological examination of a specimen taken a distance from the ulcer crater and serologic testing. Upper endoscopy is routinely performed with a minimum of 10 biopsies from the ulcer to exclude malignancy and evaluate for *H. pylori*. A rapid urease test or a histologic visualization can demonstrate the bacteria in a mucosal specimen. In the absence of a gastric mucosal sample, *H. pylori* can be diagnosed initially by serology, and follow-up is done with a urea breath test 4 weeks after the end of treatment.

Because testing is expensive, confirmation of *H. pylori* eradication is not necessary in all treated patients. Patients with documented peptic ulcers or with complicated or refractory ulcers should have eradication verified after therapy. This can be done by repeat endoscopy or UBT. Antibody detection by serologic or whole-blood testing is not reliable for confirming eradication and therefore should not be used. The results of studies examining the role of the stool antigen test for determining posttreatment eradication have been inconsistent; therefore this test is not currently recommended. Eradication cannot be verified until at least 4 weeks after the last dose of an antimicrobial and at least 7 days after the last dose of a PPI. All patients should be followed up clinically to assess symptom response and recurrence. Absence of symptoms upon the completion of antimicrobial therapy in patients who were previously symptomatic has been shown to be a sensitive and specific indicator of eradication of *H. pylori*.

Management of *H. Pylori*

The advent of effective antacid medications in the 1970s dramatically reduced the number and type of operations that were required to address complications of gastric ulcers. Because 85% to 90% of patients with gastric ulcer are colonized with *H. pylori* bacteria, the treatment of uncomplicated gastric ulcer is medical and aimed at alleviating the symptoms, achieving ulcer healing, and preventing its recurrence.

For all patients with gastric ulcers, regardless of the presenting complication, some universal principles should be followed. Indications for steroids should be evaluated so they can be discontinued if feasible, and NSAIDs should be discontinued if possible. In addition, PPIs should be prescribed to promote ulcer healing. If *H. pylori* is demonstrated, triple therapy should be initiated with metronidazole and clarithromycin or amoxicillin for 10 to 14 days along with PPIs. This therapy achieves eradication in 90% of cases. Endoscopy is typically repeated 6 weeks later to ensure healing of the gastric ulcer.

Ulcer Location

To help guide treatment, gastric ulcers are classified into five types based on their location and acid-secretory status. Type I gastric ulcers are the most common (60%) and occur along the lesser curvature just proximal to the incisura at the histologic transition between the fundus and the antrum. In type II gastric ulcers (15%), there are two simultaneous ulcers: one in the body of the stomach, usually around the incisura, and another in the duodenum. The ulcer in the duodenum can be active or healed. A type III gastric ulcer is prepyloric (20%). Type III ulcers are typically found within 2 to 3 cm from the pylorus and can be multiple. Only type II and III gastric ulcers are associated with acid hypersecretion and require an acid-reducing operation. A type IV gastric ulcer (<10%) occurs high on the lesser curve, near the gastroesophageal junction (GEJ). A type V gastric ulcer may occur anywhere in the stomach; it is caused by medications such as NSAIDs, and it heals once these drugs are stopped (Figure 2).

ELECTIVE SURGICAL MANAGEMENT

The indication for elective surgical therapy in patients with gastric ulcer is failure of an ulcer to completely heal after an adequate trial of medical therapy. Traditionally, 12 weeks of antisecretory therapy has been considered an adequate trial; however, most patients are currently given an additional 12-week trial. Failure to respond to adequate and correct medical therapy should significantly raise the suspicion of malignancy. Other possible causes for intractable ulcers include Zollinger-Ellison syndrome, persistent or resistant *H. pylori* infection, a noncompliant patient, occult use of NSAIDs, and motility disorders.

High-quality preoperative endoscopy is essential to direct surgical therapy. Endoscopic injection of dye (tattooing) at the ulcer site can guide the surgeon during the operation. Tattooing is especially useful when the ulcer operation of choice is performed laparoscopically.

Type I

Type I gastric ulcer is not associated with hyperacidity, and the elective operation of choice is a distal gastrectomy, which includes the ulcer in the resected specimen. A gastroduodenal (Billroth I) reconstruction is preferred, although gastrojejunostomy (Billroth II) is an acceptable alternative when a tension-free anastomosis is possible (Figure 3).

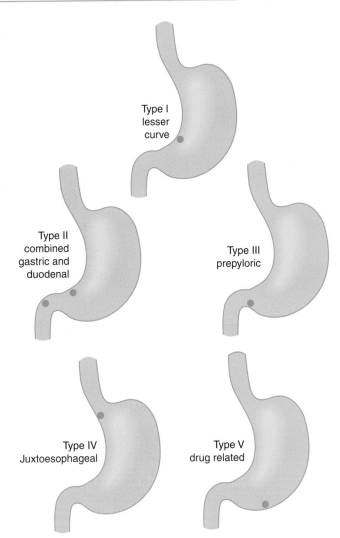

FIGURE 2 Types of gastric ulcers. *(From Matthews JB, Silen W: Operations for peptic ulcer disease and early operative complications. In Sleisenger MH, Fordtran JS [eds]: Gastrointestinal disease, Philadelphia, 1993, Saunders.)*

Type II and Type III

The elective operation of choice for patients with type II or III gastric ulcers, who are acid hypersecretors, is an antrectomy that includes the gastric ulcer. Since acid secretion has been recognized to be associated with these types of ulcers, adding a truncal vagotomy has traditionally been recommended. However, given the potential morbidity of a vagotomy—diarrhea, delayed gastric emptying, dysphagia, dumping, regurgitation—postoperative treatment with PPIs is preferred. We reserve vagotomy for rare cases in which the patient is particularly noncompliant and has a history of complicated and recurrent ulcer disease.

Type IV

A type IV gastric ulcer is challenging to the surgeon because it is located close to the GEJ. Different techniques are used depending on the size of the ulcer and its proximity to the GEJ. The Pauchet procedure is performed on ulcers that are 2 to 5 cm away from the GEJ, if the stomach can be securely closed without narrowing the gastric inlet. This entails distal gastrectomy along the lesser curvature, with vertical extension to include the ulcer, followed by Billroth I or II

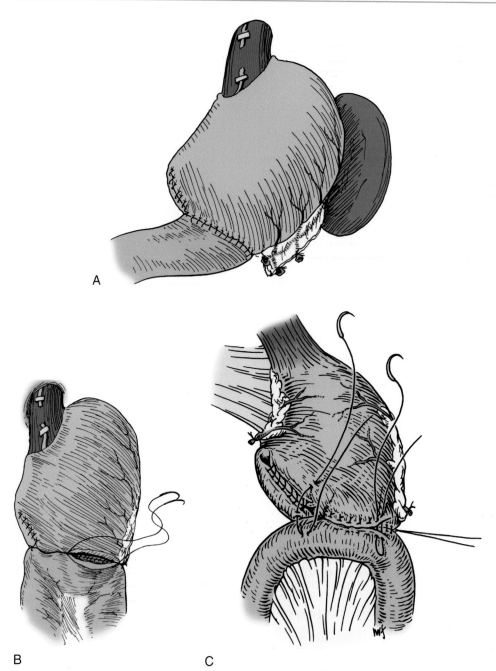

FIGURE 3 **A,** Bilroth I ulcer. **B** and **C,** Bilroth II ulcers. (**A** and **B** from Soybel DI, Zinner MJ: Stomach and duodenum: operative procedures. In Zinner MJ, Schwartz SI, Ellis H [eds]: Maingot's abdominal operations. Stamford, CT, 1997, Appleton & Lange, pp 1105, 1112. **C** from Mulholland MW: Atlas of gastric surgery. In Bell RH Jr, Rikkers LF, Mulholland MW [eds]: Digestive tract surgery, Philadelphia, 1996, Lippincott-Raven, p 352.)

anastomosis. The Csendes procedure is an option for ulcers 2 cm or less from the GEJ, where most of the stomach is resected up to the GEJ, including the ulcer followed by a Roux-en-Y gastrojejunostomy. Proximal ulcers near the GEJ can also be managed with excision and coverage of the hole with an anastomosis to a Roux limb of the jejunum, if it cannot be closed primarily due to narrowing (Figure 4).

Giant Gastric Ulcers

A giant gastric ulcer is an ulcer with a diameter of 3 cm or greater. Most giant gastric ulcers are located along the lesser curvature. The incidence of an underlying malignancy for these large ulcers ranges up to 30%. With this higher incidence of malignancy and the increased risk of complications, early surgical treatment is warranted,

following a thorough workup for cancer. A computed tomographic (CT) scan and colonoscopy are important prior to exploration of such giant ulcers. For ulcers that have either penetrated or cannot be dissected free of adjacent organs, an en bloc resection may be warranted if an occult or obvious malignancy is present.

MANAGEMENT OF GASTRIC ULCER PERFORATION

Nonoperative Management

For select, nonseptic patients, nonoperative management of a perforated benign gastric ulcer can be considered. Nonsurgical treatment can occasionally be successful in a stable patient without peritonitis

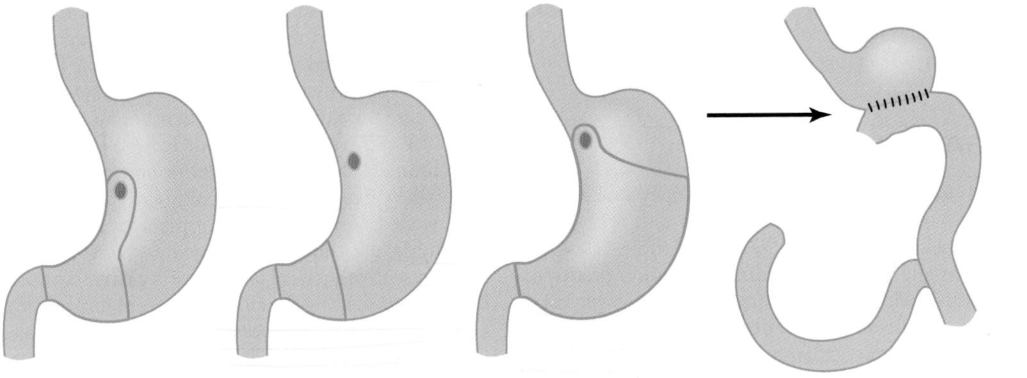

| Pauchet's procedure | Kelling-Madlener procedure | Csendes procedure (esophagogastrojejunostomy) |

FIGURE 4 Operations for ulcers near the gastroesophageal junction (type IV). *(Modified from Seymour NE: Operations for peptic ulcer and their complications. In Feldman M, Scharschmidt BF, Sleisenger MH [eds]: Gastrointestinal disease, Philadelphia, 1998, WB Saunders.)*

in whom a water-soluble contrast upper GI series documents a sealed perforation. Both the ulcer and the effects of peritoneal soilage are managed with antibiotic therapy, nasogastric suction, and suppression of gastric acid secretion.

A critical aspect of this method of nonoperative management is the necessity for reassessment of the patient every few hours by physical examination. If evidence of peritonitis progresses, or if evidence of regression is not observed within 12 hours, surgery is indicated to rule out another cause of peritonitis or releaking from the ulcer. In this case of nonsurgical management of a sealed perforation, a follow-up endoscopy should be done after 6 weeks to confirm healing and obtain tissue biopsy.

Surgical Management

Perforated gastric ulcers are commonly associated with NSAID use. Plain radiology of the chest with the patient in the erect position reveals the characteristic free air under the diaphragm. In a stable patient with perforated gastric ulcer, the preferred surgical procedure is distal gastrectomy, including the ulcer, followed by Billroth I anastomosis. Vagotomy is rarely indicated and is reserved for noncompliant patients with recurrent type II and type III ulcers with no other reason in their history to have an ulcer. The effectiveness of PPIs and the recognized morbidity of vagotomy have essentially eliminated the indication for vagotomy today.

In an unstable patient or a patient with multiple comorbidities, simple patching of the perforation with omentum can be life saving. Whenever excision of a perforated gastric ulcer is not performed, an intraoperative or comparable future endoscopic biopsy is useful to exclude malignancy in patients without a known etiology for their ulcer. Testing and treating *H. pylori* should not be forgotten in emergency admissions.

Management of Gastric Ulcer Bleeding

Although it is self-limited in the majority of cases (80%), a bleeding gastric ulcer still has an appreciable mortality rate. The first step in managing a bleeding gastric ulcer is to resuscitate and achieve hemodynamic stability. Endoscopy with the use of heater probe coagulation, injection therapy, or both can usually stop the active bleeding and allow stabilization of the patient. Endoscopic control of the bleeding is often successful in averting the need for emergent surgery. At minimum, endoscopy allows for appropriate localization and a semielective procedure.

In addition to enabling a biopsy for malignancy and *H. pylori*, endoscopy assesses the likelihood of recurrent bleeding. The two

characteristics at endoscopy that predict a high rebleeding risk (50% to 80%) are *active pulsatile bleeding* or a *visible vessel*. Conversely, nonpulsatile bleeding or an adherent clot seen at endoscopy are associated with a low risk of rebleeding. Occasionally, a nuclear medicine bleeding scan can suggest the possibility of a bleeding gastric ulcer, and an angiogram can definitively locate the site of a bleeding ulcer. However, endoscopy is the gold standard method to diagnose and treat the vast majority of bleeding gastric ulcers.

The surgery of choice depends on the type of ulcer, and the operation chosen needs to accomplish the same goals for elective ulcer surgery described above. When endoscopy is not available or successful, usually due to inadequate local resources or a large burden of clot in the stomach, and the patient has a rapid rate of bleeding, an emergency operation may be indicated. Such an emergency exploration for bleeding may also be indicated when an unstable bleeding patient cannot be supported with blood products until a high-quality endoscopic intervention is available. In suboptimal situations of emergency bleeding without preoperative localization, the stomach is opened through an anterior gastrotomy and examined for a bleeding source. In rare situations, ligation of the blood supply to the stomach or even near-total gastrectomy are indicated, although this situation is extremely rare. In such a case, the blood supply to the stomach is ligated (gastric devascularization) without ligating the short gastric arcade. However, the lack of preoperative localization can make such a "blind" surgical approach risky; thus it should be avoided when possible.

Management of Gastric Ulcer Obstruction

Gastric outlet obstruction is usually a complication of a scarred duodenal ulcer, rather than a gastric ulcer, but occasionally strictures can form from recurrent gastric ulcers. Initially, for acute obstruction, a nasogastric tube is inserted for gastric decompression for a few days; this should be performed first, together with correction of fluid and electrolyte imbalance and treatment with antisecretory drugs, and endoscopy should be done for evaluation of the obstruction, type of ulcer, tissue biopsy, and occasionally for therapeutic balloon dilatation, especially in the acute type of obstruction. Endoscopic dilatation or stenting of strictures can provide temporary relief of symptoms but should not replace definitive surgical management, unless palliation at the end of life is the goal.

For chronic obstruction, antrectomy is the procedure of choice. In this setting, it is important for the surgeon to assess the duodenal stump before transection of the duodenum. Scarring often precludes a Billroth I reconstruction and may also make a Billroth II reconstruction dangerous because of the risk of a duodenal stump leak. If there is concern about safe closure of the duodenal stump, an alternative is to perform a diverting gastrojejunostomy.

STRESS GASTRITIS

Acute stress gastritis is characterized by multiple superficial erosions that begin in the proximal region of the stomach and occasionally progress distally. Stress gastritis usually develops within 2 days of a major traumatic event and is usually minimal. Common predisposing clinical conditions include multiple traumas, often with hypotension and massive transfusion; sepsis, often with acute respiratory distress syndrome or systemic inflammatory response syndrome; multiple organ failure; burns (Curling's ulcer); central nervous system injury (Cushing's ulcer); and steroid use. Prophylaxis remains the ideal way to deal with the risk of stress gastritis. This is achieved through proper management of the stress-causing events and antisecretory agents or sucralfate.

Diagnosis and Therapy

Endoscopy is the best means to diagnose stress ulcers. Treatment starts with resuscitation through blood transfusion and correction of any coagulopathy. A nasogastric tube has to be inserted for performing saline lavage and gastric decompression. In the majority of cases, such measures are sufficient to achieve cessation of bleeding. Antisecretory agents are given to minimize the damage caused by gastric acidity. After lavage of the stomach, endoscopic measures confirm the

diagnosis and establish the extent of disease; and with heater probe coagulation and injection, the bleeding can be stopped. If bleeding persists, angiographic embolization of the left gastric artery or infusion of vasopressin is typically the next step and has been reported to decrease transfusion requirements but not mortality.

If bleeding still persists or recurs, surgery is the last resort. One technique is to make an anterior gastrotomy and secure the bleeding points by deep figure-eight sutures. Occasionally, partial gastrectomy is needed. Rarely, in cases of persistent bleeding, near-total gastrectomy is the only remaining life-saving procedure. An additional, nonresective surgical procedure is gastric devascularization, in which all vessels feeding the stomach, except for the short gastric arcade, are ligated. Gastric devascularization is worth considering in a patient who is unstable or who has severe underlying medical problems because this procedure can be performed more rapidly than near-total gastrectomy.

SUGGESTED READINGS

Lau JY, Sung JJ, Lam YH, et al: Endoscopic retreatment compared with surgery in patients with recurrent bleeding after initial endoscopic control of bleeding ulcers, *N Engl J Med* 340(10):751–756, 1999.
Bertleff MJ, Halm JA, Bemelman WA, et al: Randomized clinical trial of laparoscopic versus open repair of the perforated peptic ulcer: the LAMA trial, *World J Surg* 33(7):1368–1373, 2009.
Poultsides GA, Kim CJ, Vignati PV, et al: Angiographic embolization for gastroduodenal hemorrhage: safety, efficacy, and predictors of outcome, *Arch Surg* 143(5):457–461, 2008.
Marshall C, Ramaswamy P, Leaper DJ, et al: Evaluation of a protocol for the non-operative management of perforated peptic ulcer, *Br J Surg* 86:131–134, 1999.

MANAGEMENT OF DUODENAL ULCER

Colleen B. Gaughan, MD, and Daniel T. Dempsey, MD

HISTORY

Duodenal ulcer remains a common malady today. But elective operation for intractability has virtually disappeared because of a better understanding of the pathophysiology of the disease and more effective medical treatment with powerful antisecretory agents, such as proton pump inhibitors (PPIs) and H2 receptor antagonists, and *Helicobacter pylori* eradication (Table 1). Duodenal ulcer remains a surgical disease, however, because operation is often required for ulcer complications that include bleeding, perforation, and obstruction.

In 2006, there were about 60,000 hospitalizations for duodenal ulcer in the United States, and 3.7% of those patients died in the hospital. Interestingly the hospital mortality rate for gastric ulcer in about 86,000 admissions was significantly lower (2.1%). Ten percent of hospitalized patients with peptic ulcer required surgery that year, and the operative mortality rate was 11%.

Most patients (90%) with duodenal ulcer have *H. pylori* infection and/or recent use of nonsteroidal antiinflammatory drugs (NSAIDs) or aspirin. Zollinger-Ellison syndrome (gastrinoma) remains an important part of the differential diagnosis, particularly if the ulcer

diathesis is hard to treat or if the ulcer is distal to the first portion of the duodenum, where 90% of duodenal ulcers are located. Gastrinoma is rare, however, and only 1% to 2% of patients with newly diagnosed duodenal ulcer will turn out to have Zollinger-Ellison syndrome. Other important pathophysiologic factors in duodenal ulcer are smoking, psychological stress, steroid or cocaine use, and probably gastroduodenal dysmotility.

TABLE 1: Some treatment regimens for *Helicobacter pylori**

Regimen 1
PPI†
Clarithromycin 500 mg bid (10–14 days)
Amoxicillin 1 g BID or metronidazole 500 mg BID (10–14 days)
Regimen 2
PPI†
Bismuth subsalicylate 2 tablets daily (14 days)
Metronidazole 250 mg four times daily (14 days)
Tetracycline 500 mg four times daily (14 days)

*Eradication rates with either regimen of 85% to 90%.
†PPIs have in vitro activity against *H. pylori*.

MEDICAL MANAGEMENT OF DUODENAL ULCER

The majority of patients with duodenal ulcer are treated medically with acid suppression, eradication of *H. pylori,* and abstention from NSAIDs or aspirin. *Helicobacter* infection is usually diagnosed by serology, antral biopsy (histology and/or urease test), and/or C-labeled urea breath test. The latter is most useful in documenting clearance of the infection after the completion of anti-*Helicobacter* therapy. If *H. pylori* infection is eliminated and NSAIDs and aspirin are avoided, acid suppression medication may be stopped in about 2 months with a low likelihood of recurrent ulcer. Patients at risk for ulcer recurrence and those with ulcer complications should continue PPIs indefinitely, particularly those who require NSAIDs, aspirin, steroids, or anticoagulants (Figure 1). It would not seem unreasonable to suggest that all patients admitted to a hospital with duodenal ulcer complications should remain on acid-suppressing medication indefinitely.

Surgical Management

The main indications for operation in duodenal ulcer disease are bleeding, perforation, obstruction and, rarely, intractability. The surgical options to manage duodenal ulcer disease include simple closure or oversewing, highly selective vagotomy (HSV), vagotomy and drainage (pyloroplasty or gastrojejunostomy), and vagotomy and antrectomy (Table 2).

As already stated, the number of elective operations for duodenal ulcer has decreased dramatically over the last 40 years. There has also been a more modest but significant decrease in the number of urgent operations for peptic ulcer disease over the last 15 to 20 years, probably because of better medical management and the increased use and effectiveness of endoscopic hemostatic therapy (Figure 2). There is clearly a trend away from the use of truncal vagotomy and gastric resection in the surgical treatment of peptic ulcer, and some cases of perforation or obstruction can be handled laparoscopically. Cheap,

safe, and readily available PPIs and H2 receptor antagonists make the small risk (about 10%) with truncal vagotomy—dumping, diarrhea, and gastroparesis—increasingly difficult to justify in many surgical patients, particularly in patients who can be relied upon to comply with postoperative medical management.

The routine use of definitive ulcer operations—especially truncal vagotomy, pyloroplasty, and/or antrectomy—to prevent recurrent ulcer in all surgical patients with duodenal ulcer complications becomes illogical when we know that maintenance PPIs and the avoidance of NSAIDs and aspirin, together with *Helicobacter* eradication, will minimize the risk of ulcer recurrence. However, PPIs should NOT be relied upon to compensate for an ill-conceived or poorly executed operation, particularly in patients requiring surgery in the setting of failed medical management for duodenal ulcer.

The number of elective operations done for duodenal ulcer disease has declined dramatically since the introduction of H2 blockers and, subsequently, PPIs. The discovery that the eradication of *H. pylori* and the avoidance of NSAIDs and aspirin could prevent the recurrence of peptic ulcer disease has had an additional impact on elective duodenal ulcer surgery and has made intractability an uncommon indication for operation. Indeed today's surgeon should not be anxious to operate for intractable duodenal ulcer, particularly in the asthenic or medically high-risk patient because the likelihood of a suboptimal clinical result is high. Remember that the majority of surgical publications dealing with outcomes following elective operation for duodenal ulcer are from the premodern era, before

TABLE 2: Operations commonly (++++) and uncommonly (+) performed for duodenal ulcer

Indication	Patch or Oversew	HSV	V + D or HSV + GJ	V + A
Perforation	++++	+++	++	+
Bleeding	++++	+	+++	++
Obstruction	0	0	+++	++++
Intractable	0	+++	++	+

V+D, Vagotomy plus drainage; *GJ,* gastrojejunoscopy; *V+A,* vagotomy and antrectomy.

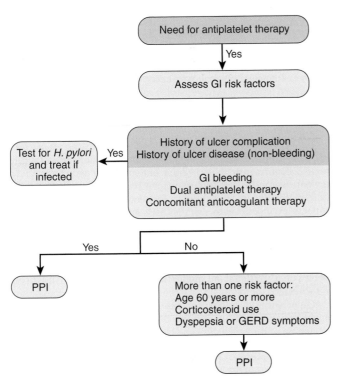

FIGURE 1 Antiplatelet therapy in patients at risk for ulcer complications.

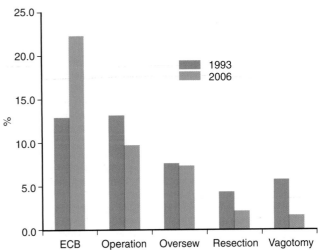

FIGURE 2 Percentage of patients hospitalized in the United States during 1993 and 2006 with peptic ulcer treated with endoscopic control of bleeding *(ECB),* surgery, oversew/patch, resection, and vagotomy.

the development of PPIs and the discovery of *H. pylori*. The patient referred to the surgeon today for intractability is very different from the majority of the subjects in those studies, most of whom would be cured by medical therapy today. Not surprisingly, most of these patients did well with elective ulcer surgery in the previous era.

Perforated Duodenal Ulcer

Although bleeding is more common than perforation, perforation is more likely to be fatal (Table 3). In 2006, hospitalized patients with perforated peptic ulcer had a mortality rate of 10.6% compared with a mortality rate of 2.5% in hospitalized patients with bleeding peptic ulcer. Over 90% of patients with perforated duodenal ulcer show symptoms of acute abdomen, peritonitis, and/or pneumoperitoneum on plain radiograph or computed tomography (CT) scan. After a brief period of fluid resuscitation and intravenous antibiotics, these patients should be taken to the operating room for open or laparoscopic repair and peritoneal washout. The very occasional stable patient with a radiologically documented sealed perforation may be cautiously managed nonoperatively.

Usually the perforation is on the anterior surface of the postpyloric duodenum and is less than 5 mm in diameter. Simple omental patch closure and peritoneal irrigation (5 to 10 L warm saline) is satisfactory treatment for most patients. Attempts to close the perforation primarily typically result in a bigger hole, as the sutures pull through the inflamed tissue. Instead, the perforation is plugged with viable tension-free omentum held in place by absorbable sutures placed through healthy seromuscular tissue adjacent to the opening. We usually irrigate the peritoneal cavity until clear before we repair the perforation, and if there is extensive peritoneal exudate, we remove only what can be debrided quickly and atraumatically. After the perforation is sealed, the integrity of the repair is tested by insufflating air under gentle pressure via the nasogastric (NG) tube. A closed-suction drain is placed in Morrison's pouch, and the NG tube is secured in position.

Although prevention of relapse is an important consideration in patients with perforated duodenal ulcer, the effectiveness and side effects of definitive ulcer operations in this setting must be considered within the context of the patient's risk for ulcer recurrence and expected compliance with prescribed medical treatment. The definitive ulcer surgery for perforated duodenal ulcer, highly selective vagotomy (HSV) or truncal vagotomy and drainage, is probably unnecessary in many cases but should be considered in patients who have clearly failed medical management or who have a documented history of significant chronic duodenal ulcer disease. An example of the former would be a patient who develops a perforated duodenal ulcer despite optimal medical management; an example of the latter would be a patient with a previous hospitalization for an endoscopically visualized bleeding duodenal ulcer. Patients with obvious risk factors for ulcer recurrence who cannot afford, tolerate, or comply with long-term acid-suppression medication should be considered for HSV. Definitive surgery should be avoided in patients with shock, multiple medical problems, or perforation older than 24 hours.

Laparoscopic repair of perforated duodenal ulcers and juxtapyloric ulcers is safe and effective for selected patients in experienced hands; however, it should be avoided in patients with hemodynamic instability, multiple medical problems, and long-standing peritonitis. The addition of laparoscopic HSV or the Taylor procedure (posterior truncal vagotomy and anterior seromyotomy or anterior parietal cell vagotomy) is a reasonable consideration in the stable low-risk patient in need of a definitive operation. Large or complex duodenal perforations are best treated with an open technique.

Typically, we begin a liquid diet on the second or third postoperative day, after an upper GI study—first with water-soluble contrast, then barium—confirms both no leakage and adequate gastric emptying. Antibiotics are discontinued after 24 hours unless established purulent peritonitis or abscess was found, in which case antibiotics are continued until the patient is afebrile with normal white blood count. PPIs are given intravenously then orally, and treatment for

TABLE 3: Determinants of in-hospital death for peptic ulcer disease

	Year: 1993 (n = 40,792)	Year: 2006 (n = 31,676)
Age (yr)	1.05 (1.05, 1.05)*	1.04 (1.04, 1.05)*
Sex (female)	0.84 (0.75, 0.93)†	0.87 (0.75, 1.00)
Peptic ulcer site		
Duodenum (vs. stomach)	1.14 (1.02, 1.27)‡	1.48 (1.28, 1.72)*
Unspecified (vs. stomach)	1.26 (1.02, 1.56)‡	1.28 (0.91, 1.81)
Complication		
Hemorrhage	2.24 (1.93, 2.59)*	2.19 (1.78, 2.71)*
Perforation	11.10 (9.64, 12.79)*	12.06 (9.79, 14.85)*
Obstruction	1.35 (1.08, 1.69)†	1.09 (0.72, 1.66)
Comorbidity score		
1 (vs. 0)	1.98 (1.77, 2.22)*	1.79 (1.54, 2.09)*
≥2 (vs. 0)	2.01 (1.60, 2.53)*	2.43 (1.96, 3.03)*
Teaching hospital	1.23 (1.09, 1.39)*	1.13 (0.97, 1.31)
Urban hospital	1.33 (1.14, 1.55)*	1.35 (1.07, 1.71)‡
Hospital region		
Midwest (vs. Northeast)	0.77 (0.65, 0.90)†	0.64 (0.52, 0.79)*
South (vs. Northeast)	0.90 (0.77, 1.04)	0.78 (0.64, 0.94)†
West (vs. Northeast)	0.75 (0.63, 0.89)*	0.69 (0.55, 0.86)*

Data are odds ratios (95% confidence interval) from the logistic regression model. Both regressions were weighted to reflect national estimates.
*$P < .001$
†$P < .01$
‡$P < .05$

H. pylori is prescribed if serology is positive. If postoperative leakage occurs, confirmed by bilious drain output and/or radiologic study, the patient can be managed nonoperatively if doing well, but clinical deterioration is an indication for reoperation. Upon discharge, patients are instructed to avoid NSAIDs and aspirin and to continue oral PPI therapy for 2 months. Perhaps all patients without an acid-reducing procedure should remain on PPIs or H2 receptor antagonists indefinitely. Whether all such patients would be better off with HSV is unknown. Patients treated for *H. pylori* are scheduled for a carbon-labeled urea breath test in 1 month to confirm eradication. All patients are scheduled for follow-up with the surgeon and gastroenterologist.

Other surgical options to treat perforated duodenal ulcer that might be useful for a large and/or inconveniently located hole include intubation of the perforation and serosal jejunal patching. An omental patch or plug may still be useful even for large perforations. We add *triple intubation*—gastrostomy, feeding jejunostomy, and retrograde jejunostomy for duodenal decompression—to the repair of the unusually difficult duodenal perforation. Gastrectomy is rarely, if ever, indicated in the repair of perforated duodenal ulcer. It is too radical

How much inflammation?

for the routine case, and it makes the repair of the difficult duodenal perforation more complex by creating a difficult duodenal stump.

Bleeding Duodenal Ulcer

The incidence of bleeding secondary to peptic ulcer disease has not significantly changed since the advent of H2 blockers, PPIs, and *Helicobacter* therapy. This may be partially explained by the increased use of NSAIDs and aspirin, together with the increased age and medical comorbidities of hospitalized ulcer patients. Recent analysis suggests that in 2006, 73% of peptic ulcer hospitalizations in the United States were for bleeding, and 2.5% of these patients died. The number of operations for bleeding peptic ulcer has probably decreased somewhat because of advances in pharmacotherapy and endoscopic treatment. In 1993, 13.1% of patients admitted to hospital for peptic ulcer, 72% of whom were admitted for bleeding, required surgery compared with 9.7% in 2006, of whom 73% were admitted for bleeding. Interestingly, over that period, endoscopic treatment of bleeding ulcer increased from 12.9% in 1993 to 22.2% in 2006 (see Figure 2). Increasing age and hemorrhage remain significant independent predictors of death in hospitalized patients with peptic ulcer, and the operative mortality rate in bleeding ulcer is 10% to15% (see Table 3).

All hospitalized patients with significant duodenal ulcer bleeding should be on a continuous infusion of PPIs. Patients with hypotension, transfusion requirement, or posterior duodenal ulcer should have surgical consultation. Attempted endoscopic control—with cautery, epinephrine injection, and sometimes clips—is the first line of invasive therapy for bleeding duodenal ulcer disease. This treatment decreases the need for emergent operation. If bleeding recurs, the surgeon should be involved in the decision to repeat endoscopic therapy or proceed with surgical intervention. Factors predicting the likelihood of failure of endoscopic therapy (e.g., hemodynamic instability, visible vessel, ulcer greater than 2 cm, deep posterior duodenal ulcer, transfusion requirement of more than four units in 24 hours) should be considered in this decision. Though repeat endoscopic treatment may be effective, surgery is necessary in patients with refractory or continued bleeding.

Most of the bleeding duodenal ulcers requiring operation are posterior lesions in the proximal duodenum. There are three surgical options: simple oversewing, oversewing with vagotomy and drainage, and oversewing with vagotomy and antrectomy. In hemodynamically unstable patients and in those with multiple comorbidities, control of bleeding by simple oversewing of the ulcer is the procedure of choice. An anterolateral duodenotomy allows access to the posterior ulcer. If bleeding is vigorous, a Kocher maneuver permits compression of the ulcer between the thumb anteriorly and the fingers posteriorly. Heavy permanent suture material on a stout needle is used to oversew the bleeding vessel in the base of the ulcer with an over-and-over stitch, or U stitch. Multiple sutures may be necessary, and once initial hemostasis has been achieved, the area should be gently abraded with the suction tip to determine hemostasis with certainty. When the bleeding ulcer is postbulbar, care should be taken to avoid injury to the common bile duct. The duodenotomy is then closed in two layers. Vagotomy is *not* performed, and postoperative intravenous infusion of PPIs is continued.

In hemodynamically stable, low-risk patients, definitive ulcer surgery can be considered. The duodenotomy may be extended by choice or of necessity, proximally through the pylorus, and closed as either a Heineke-Mikulicz or Finney pyloroplasty. Truncal vagotomy or HSV is added. In sturdy, hemodynamically stable patients with a chronic history of ulcer problems, truncal vagotomy and antrectomy with Billroth II reconstruction (or Roux reconstruction if 50% distal resection is performed) is a reasonable operation for bleeding duodenal ulcer. However, before committing to this operation, the surgeon must consider the duodenal stump because the ulcer should be oversewn whether or not it is excluded from the food stream. Will the duodenum be transected and closed distal to the ulcer, and the ulcer bed oversewn? Or will the duodenum be transected proximal to the ulcer, and the ulcer oversewn through the open end of the duodenum,

which is then closed? The latter is the more likely scenario; regardless, the surgeon should think twice about gastric resection if a difficult duodenal closure seems likely.

Reconstruction via gastrojejunostomy diverts the acid and food away from the ulcer bed. Although the operative risk of gastric resection for bleeding ulcer is higher than the operative risk of vagotomy and drainage, the rebleeding rate is higher with vagotomy and drainage, and the in-hospital mortality rate is probably comparable between the two procedures. If patients rebleed following vagotomy and drainage, antrectomy is indicated. Angiographic embolization can be useful in the occasional problematic patient with bleeding duodenal ulcer. *Helicobacter* status is determined postoperatively, if not preoperatively, and continuous intravenous PPIs are continued.

Obstructing Duodenal Ulcer

Some duodenal ulcer patients come in with edematous functional obstruction of the gastric outlet. These patients usually have pain, nausea, and vomiting of fairly short duration (days). Typically these patients improve with NG suction and intravenous PPIs and they do not require operation; esophagogastroduodenoscopy reveals edema and active ulceration.

Patients with obstructing duodenal ulcer that requires operation often have chronic symptoms (weeks or months) and typically have weight loss, nausea, and vomiting. A succussion splash and/or distended epigastrium may be evident on physical examination, and most of the time the endoscopist cannot get the endoscope through the pylorus or duodenal bulb because of cicatrix. An upper GI study shows a distended stomach and a very narrow gastric outlet. Durable relief of symptoms does not result from gastric decompression with NG suction and PPI infusion, and some invasive treatment is usually necessary.

Practically speaking, three treatment options for chronic gastric outlet obstruction from duodenal ulcer disease are available: (1) endoscopic balloon dilatation, (2) laparoscopic or open HSV and gastrojejunostomy (HSV/GJ), and (3) vagotomy and antrectomy. Balloon dilatation may work in about half of the patients for up to 2 years, but multiple dilatations are often necessary. HSV/GJ has been shown in a randomized clinical trial to be comparably effective to vagotomy and antrectomy for obstructing duodenal ulcer disease. Understandably, HSV/GJ is an attractive option for the laparoscopic surgeon. But the reader is reminded that by far the most common cause of gastric outlet obstruction in the modern era is cancer—gastric, pancreatic, and duodenal—and this lesion may be difficult to detect laparoscopically in the patient presumed, often erroneously, to have obstructing ulcer disease. False-negative preoperative endoscopic biopsies and radiologic studies can be misleading. We have operated on two patients for obstructing duodenal ulcer in the last 5 years, both of whom were found to have duodenal cancer requiring a Whipple operation. One disadvantage of both balloon dilatation and laparoscopic HSV/GJ for obstructing duodenal ulcer is that unsuspected cancer is more likely to be missed than with open vagotomy and antrectomy.

The standard surgical treatment for obstructing duodenal ulcer is vagotomy and antrectomy with Billroth II reconstruction, but the surgeon should consider whether this choice will create a difficult duodenal stump. Following Billroth II reconstruction, we position the NG tube in the afferent limb, with side holes proximal and distal to the anastomosis, for postoperative duodenal and gastric decompression. Gastrostomy and/or jejunostomy are useful adjunct procedures in patients operated on for obstructing ulcer because return of gastric motor function may be slow. This can limit early full oral alimentation, necessitating prolonged postoperative nutritional support and gastric decompression.

Intractable Duodenal Ulcer

Patients with intractable duodenal ulcer fall into a small but difficult group in whom some as yet unrecognized pathophysiologic factor or factors may be present. Alternatively, compliance with medical

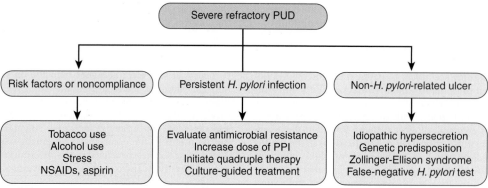

FIGURE 3   Possible causes of intractable duodenal ulcer. *PUD*, Peptic ulcer disease.

management may be suboptimal, and typical causes may go undiagnosed (Figure 3). Regardless, many of these patients will do poorly after major ulcer operation. Truncal vagotomy and gastric resection should be eschewed in this group, particularly in thin female patients.

If surgery for intractable duodenal ulcer is necessary, HSV is the safest operation, though it may be no more effective that indefinite PPI treatment. HSV/GJ is a reasonable option, if the patient can be relied upon to continue PPIs to minimize the occurrence of marginal ulceration. The advantage of GJ over pyloroplasty as a drainage procedure is that if intolerable dumping develops, the former is reversible, but the latter is not. Prior to definitive operation for intractability, patients should be treated empirically for *H. pylori*, no matter the result. NSAIDs and aspirin should be stopped and compliance assessed with salicylate level and bleeding time. Smoking should be stopped and compliance assessed with urine nicotine level, and gastrinoma should also be ruled out.

Giant Duodenal Ulcer

Giant duodenal ulcer (>2 cm) can be a manifestation of an aggressive ulcer diathesis or unusually weak mucosal defenses. Giant duodenal ulcers more often present the surgeon with intraoperative challenges, such as large and inconveniently located perforations or exsanguinating hemorrhage. A more aggressive ulcer operation may be warranted in the low-risk patient with giant duodenal ulcer. Patients with perforated giant duodenal ulcer should be considered for definitive ulcer operation in addition to repair of the perforation. Patients with bleeding giant duodenal ulcer should be considered for vagotomy and antrectomy.

Difficult Duodenal Stump

The routine closure of the proximal duodenum during distal gastrectomy is most easily accomplished with a gastrointestinal anastomosis or thoracoabdominal stapler (blue cartridge). A two-layer suture closure is also straightforward in the routine case. But occasionally ulcer location or size, or the extensiveness of the inflammation and/or scar, may render secure duodenal closure very difficult. Though best avoided, this situation can test the mettle of the experienced surgeon, who knows that operative mortality skyrockets with postoperative duodenal leakage.

If the ulcer has destroyed the posterior duodenal wall, the anterior edge of the open duodenum is sewn to the proximal or distal lip of the ulcer with interrupted suture. Secure hemostasis in the ulcer bed must be accomplished. The integrity of the closure is tested by placing the tip of the NG tube at the ligament of Treitz, through the GJ, and distending the duodenum with air. Additional sutures may be necessary to render the duodenal closure airtight, and the healthy omentum is sewn over the closure.

Postoperative duodenal decompression may be accomplished via duodenostomy placed retrograde through the proximal jejunum (our preference) or placed in the lateral duodenum (*lateral duodenostomy*). Only as a last resort should the duodenal stump be closed around a tube (*end duodenostomy*) because leakage is the rule. Jejunal serosal patch is typically not helpful in closing the difficult duodenum, but a Roux limb anastomosed to the end of the open duodenum can occasionally be useful. Gastrostomy and feeding jejunostomy should be considered in patients with difficult duodenal closure. Although the aforementioned NG tube, strategically positioned with the tip in the afferent limb near the distal duodenum, can be relied upon for postoperative decompression of the *routine* duodenal closure, it should not be relied upon as the sole means of duodenal decompression for the unusually difficult duodenal stump.

Marginal Ulcer/Recurrent Ulcer

An ulcer that occurs following GJ is typically in the perianastomotic region, most commonly distal to the anastomosis (on the jejunal side). This is referred to as a *marginal ulcer*, and the most common associated operation nowadays is probably Roux-en-Y gastric bypass for morbid obesity. In that setting the differential diagnosis includes large gastric pouch, ischemia, NSAID or aspirin use, chronic perforation, smoking, gastrinoma, and excluded antrum following revisional gastric bypass surgery. When a recurrent or marginal ulcer develops following vagotomy and drainage or vagotomy and antrectomy for duodenal ulcer, the differential diagnosis includes, in addition to those above, inadequate vagotomy, retained antrum (after Billroth II or Roux-en-Y), long afferent limb (after Billroth II), and recurrent or persistent *Helicobacter* infection. The best test for completeness of truncal vagotomy is the serum pancreatic polypeptide response, or gastric acid output, during sham feeding. These responses are mediated through intact vagal trunks, and they should both be significantly blunted following a complete truncal vagotomy.

Retained or excluded antrum results when the acid-secreting proximal stomach is disconnected from the intact antrum. Since antral acidification, the physiologic brake on antral gastrin secretion, now does not occur, hypergastrinemia results. This causes acid hypersecretion in the proximal gastric pouch, which may lead to marginal ulceration. The hypergastrinemia of retained antrum syndrome is distinguished from that of gastrinoma by secretin infusion, which substantially increases gastrin levels in gastrinoma but not in retained antrum syndrome.

Aggressive acid suppression, *Helicobacter* treatment if appropriate, and abstinence from NSAIDs, aspirin, and tobacco may result in satisfactory long-term healing of recurrent and marginal ulcers. Reoperation should be considered when a surgically remediable situation is identified, and marginal ulcer persists or recurs. Thoracoscopic truncal vagotomy is a straightforward option for incomplete vagotomy. If laparotomy is performed, distal resection of the gastric remnant, including the gastrojejunostomy, with reanastomosis removes the recurrent or marginal ulcer. Truncal vagotomy should be considered unless hazardous. Retained or excluded antrum should be resected, and a large proximal gastric remnant should be partially resected, and a long afferent limb should be shortened. The reoperating surgeon must realize that conversion of a Billroth I gastroduodenostomy or a Billroth II GJ to a Roux-en-Y GJ in the setting of recurrent peptic ulcer is destined to fail (i.e., result in another marginal ulcer), unless the long-term acid-secretory capacity of the gastric remnant is substantially reduced and local mucosal defenses maximized (no NSAIDs, no smoking). Roux-en-Y reconstruction in this setting is ill advised if the proximal gastric remnant exceeds 30% normal gastric size.

REFERENCES

Harbison SP, Dempsey DT: Peptic ulcer disease [review], *Curr Probl Surg* 42(6):346–454, 2005.

Wang YR, Richter JE, Dempsey DT: Trends and outcomes of hospitalizations for peptic ulcer disease in the United States, 1993 to 2006, *Ann Surg* 251:51–58, 2010.

Dempsey DT: The stomach. In Brunicardi F, Andersen D, Billiar T, et al: *Schwartz principles of surgery*, New York, 2009, McGraw Hill.

ACG/AHA 2008 expert consensus document on reducing the gastrointestinal risks of antiplatelet therapy and NSAID use: a report of the American College of Cardiology Foundation Task Force on Clinical Expert Consensus Documents, *Circulation* 118:1894–1909, 2008.

Bhatt DL, Scheiman J, Abraham NS, et al: American College of Cardiology Foundation Task Force on Clinical Expert Consensus Documents, *Circulation* 118:1899–1904, 2008.

Guzzo JL, Duncan M, Bass BL, et al: Severe and refractory peptic ulcer disease: the diagnostic dilemma—case report and comprehensive review, *Dig Dis Sci* 50(11):1999–2008, 2005.

Csendes A, Burgos AM, Smok G, et al: Latest results (12-21 years) of a prospective randomized study comparing Billroth II and Roux-en-Y anastomosis after a partial gastrectomy plus vagotomy in patients with duodenal ulcers, *Ann Surg* 249(2):189–194, 2009.

Wu X, Zen D, Xu S, et al: A modified surgical technique for the emergent treatment of giant ulcers concomitant with hemorrhage in the posterior wall of the duodenal bulb, *Am J Surg* 184(1):41–44, 2002.

Behrman SW: Management of complicated peptic ulcer disease, *Arch Surg* 140:201–208, 2005.

Schwesinger WH, Page CP, Sirinek KR, et al: Operations for peptic ulcer disease: paradigm lost, *J Gastrointest Surg* 5(4):438–443, 2001.

Katkhouda N, Mavor E, Mason RJ, et al: Laparoscopic repair of perforated duodenal ulcers: outcome and efficacy in 30 consecutive patients, *Arch Surg* 134:845–850, 1999.

ZOLLINGER-ELLISON SYNDROME

E. Christopher Ellison, MD

HISTORY

Since the initial presentation of the two index cases in 1955, there have been over 1000 patients reported, and in excess of 3300 published articles, on the Zollinger-Ellison Syndrome (ZES). Although a rare cause of ulcer disease, ZES has not only affected our understanding and treatment of gastric hypersecretion and neuroendocrine tumors, it has also ushered in the field of gastrointestinal endocrinology.

It is known that ZES is caused by the secretion of gastrin by neuroendocrine tumors located in the duodenum, pancreas, and at ectopic sites. All of these tumors should be considered potentially malignant. Gastrin induces profound acid secretion that leads to ulcer disease and, in some cases, diarrhea. Historically, total gastrectomy was required to treat gastric acid hypersecretion, but this is rarely if ever necessary today. Current treatment of the ulcer disease is with proton pump inhibitors (PPIs), and surgery is directed at cancer control.

This chapter provides a review of gastrinoma that includes 1) gastrin physiology, 2) molecular pathogenesis, 3) clinical presentation, 4) diagnosis, 5) treatment of sporadic and familial gastrinoma, 6) management of metastatic disease, and 7) staging and prognosis.

GASTRIN PHYSIOLOGY

Gastrin is synthesized in the G cells, open-ended endocrine cells found predominantly in the gastric antrum. G cells are present in smaller numbers in the duodenal mucosa, and gastrin release is controlled by chemical, neural, and mechanical stimuli. It is stimulated by digestive proteins, notably phenylalanine and tryptophan, and by calcium, epinephrine, achlorhydria, and gastric distention. Gastrin release is inhibited by beta blockade.

Vagal parasympathetic control is complex because it has both stimulatory and inhibitory actions. Activation of vagal cholinergic reflexes by hypoglycemia or sham feeding stimulates gastrin release, and atropine blocks gastrin stimulation. Truncal vagotomy causes an increase in basal and food-stimulated gastrin release, and hypergastrinemia occurs.

Studies suggest that vagotomy interrupts cholinergic inhibitory pathways. In addition, a variety of peptides have been shown to affect gastrin release. In normal physiology, gastrin release is stimulated by bombesin, or gastrin releasing peptide (GRP), and is inhibited by somatostatin, secretin, glucagon, gastric inhibitory peptide (GIP), and vasoactive intestinal peptide (VIP).

PATHOGENESIS OF GASTRINOMA

Although some advances have occurred in our understanding of the molecular pathogenesis of gastrinoma and other endocrine tumors, many details in tumorogenesis are still unknown. The molecular pathogenesis of gastrinoma may involve oncogenes, specifically c-myc and HER-2/neu, and tumor-suppressor gene mutations, MEN-1 gene, DPC4/Smad, and p16INK4a. Markers for aggressive biologic behavior of neuroendocrine tumors, such as gastrinomas, include oncogenes, RET-protooncogene, overexpression of endothelial growth factor receptors (EGF-R and IGFIr), chromosomal abnormalities, chromosome 1q, chromosome 22q, and the X chromosome. The involvement of the tumor-suppressor gene for multiple endocrine neoplasia type I (MEN-1) on chromosome 11q13 has been most studied.

MEN-1 Gene

The MEN-1 gene encodes menin, which is principally a nuclear protein that alters tumor growth factor beta signaling, regulates nuclear factor kappa-beta (NFKB) transcription, and may function in DNA repair and synthesis. MEN-1 gene alterations have been studied in familial and sporadic gastrinoma. MEN-1–associated endocrine tumors demonstrate loss of loss of heterozygosity (LOH) in 11q13, the chromosomal location of the *MEN-1* gene in approximately 50% of cases. LOH in the *MEN-1* gene is reported in 0% to 40% of patients with sporadic gastrinomas.

The importance of the *MEN-1* gene is due to the possibility of a hyperplasia-to-neoplasia transition during tumorogenesis. The *MEN-1* gene alterations seem to be of fundamental importance in the pathogenesis of familial and sporadic gastrinomas but may not be a determinant of aggressive tumor growth or metastases.

CLINICAL PRESENTATION

ZES is usually diagnosed in the fifth decade of life, and although it may occur in children, adolescents, and the elderly, it is diagnosed between the ages of 20 and 60 about 90% of the time. Patients with *MEN-1* have onset of the disease at a younger age (33 years vs. 44 years for sporadic cases). The correct diagnosis is rarely made at initial presentation: sporadic gastrinoma patients are correctly diagnosed only 2% of the time initially, compared with 5% with *MEN-1*. The most frequent initial diagnosis is idiopathic peptic ulcer disease, noted in 75%, or diarrheal conditions, noted in 20%. The average duration of symptoms prior to diagnosis is 5 to 6 years.

Despite numerous publications and widespread awareness of ZES, delay in diagnosis persists. Analysis of reported series indicates several features that should lead the physician to suspect ZES and to perform the recommended testing and thereby shorten the delay in diagnosis. These telltale features include 1) the combination of abdominal pain, diarrhea, and weight loss; 2) recurrent or refractory ulcers; 3) prominent gastric rugal folds, secondary to the trophic effect of gastrin, seen on endoscopy; and 4) GI symptoms with or without ulcers occurring in a *MEN-1* patient.

DIAGNOSIS

Fasting Serum Gastrin

The measurement of fasting serum gastrin, taken once a patient has been off PPIs for 72 hours, is the initial diagnostic test performed in a patient suspected of having ZES. Gastrin is determined by radioimmunoassay; however, fasting hypergastrinemia alone is insufficient to establish the diagnosis. A number of medical conditions associated with achlorhydria may cause hypergastrinemia, including pernicious anemia, atrophic gastritis, and pharmacologic acid suppression. Several conditions that cause fasting hypergastrinemia are associated with acid hypersecretion, including *Helicobacter pylori* infection, gastric outlet obstruction associated with peptic ulceration, antral G-cell hyperplasia, retained antrum, short bowel syndrome, and renal failure. Collectively, these other conditions are far more common than ZES.

The absolute level of gastrin is not diagnostic of ZES. Only 30% of those afflicted have gastrin levels over 1000 pg/mL, and only 60% have levels over 500 pg/mL. In addition, many patients with nongastrinoma hypergastrinemia also exhibit gastrin levels in this range. All patients require a secretin-stimulation test to confirm the diagnosis. In addition, patients with a normal fasting gastrin level in the presence of symptoms of ZES should have a gastrin-stimulation test. Finally, the absolute level of fasting gastrin is associated with the degree of acid secretion, a pancreatic primary location, tumor size, and extent of disease, but it is not predictive of gastrinoma associated with MEN-1 and is unrelated to prognosis.

Secretin Provocative Test

Secretin is known to cause stimulation of gastrin in ZES. The effect is mediated through secretin receptors on gastrinoma cells. It is not necessary to discontinue PPIs for this test. It is recommended that secretin 0.4 mg/kg body weight be administered by intravenous push

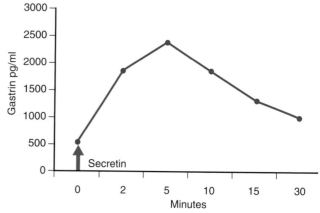

FIGURE 1   Secretin-provocative test in gastrinoma.

with determinations of gastrin at 0, 2, 5, 10, 15, and 30 minutes. Gastrin levels may increase with other conditions as well, but usually not to the same magnitude.

What constitutes a positive test? The most widely used criterion since 1980 is an increase in postsecretin gastrin of 200 pg/mL. To limit false-negative tests, the National Institutes of Health (NIH) recommends use of more than 120 pg/mL. However, most authorities use an increment greater than 110 pg/mL to define a positive secretin test (Figure 1). In modern experience, false-negative secretin test results have been reported in ZES in up to 1.5% of patients. The false-positive rate is reported as zero in nonachlorhydric patients. In achlorhydric patients, false-positive secretin tests are more common.

Evaluation for *MEN-1*

It is well established that 25% of patients with gastrinoma may have *MEN-1*. Many of these patients may have no family history. Twenty-five percent of both the NIH and the literature patients lacked a family history of *MEN-1*, and ZES was the initial clinical manifestation of *MEN-1* in 45% of patients.

The diagnosis of MEN-1 may be separated from the initial diagnosis of ZES by many years. Of patients with *MEN-1*, about 30% to 45% may present with ZES initially and then subsequently develop hyperparathyroidism. Hence, it is recommended that all patients with gastrinoma be screened for *MEN-1* with serum measurement of calcium, phosphorus, parathyroid hormone, and prolactin at initial presentation and periodically during postdiagnosis evaluation and follow-up.

Imaging for Tumor Localization

Imaging tests recommended include ultrasound (US), computed tomography (CT), magnetic resonance imaging (MRI), angiography, somatostatin scintigraphy (SS) using [^{111}In-DTPA-DPhe1] octreotide, and endoscopic ultrasound (EUS). In addition, selective arterial secretin or calcium stimulation with sampling from the hepatic veins has proven helpful in localization of gastrinomas. Based on current information, the overall success of preoperative localization approaches 60% to 80% (Table 1).

Although SS had greater sensitivity than all other conventional studies combined, it was unable to detect about one third of all lesions found at surgery. The results seem to be correlated with tumor size and location because SS can detect 30% of gastrinomas less than 1.1 cm, 64% of those 1.1 to 2 cm, and 96% of those greater than 2 cm, but it misses small duodenal tumors (Figure 2). Test results are more often positive in *MEN-1*. Imaging is negative in 3% of *MEN-1* and 34% of sporadic cases and may miss up to 40% of lesions found at surgery.

EUS has a high sensitivity for detection of pancreatic gastrinoma, which ranges from 75% to 100% (mean, 85%); however, the sensitivity

TABLE I: Sensitivity (percent positive) of various imaging test for gastrinoma

Test	Primary Tumor	Liver Metastases
US	9	46
CT	31	42
MRI	30	71
Angiography	28	62
SS	58	92

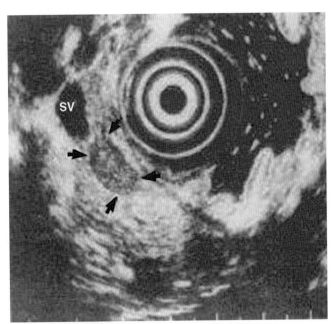

FIGURE 3   EUS showing a primary gastrinoma in the uncinate process.

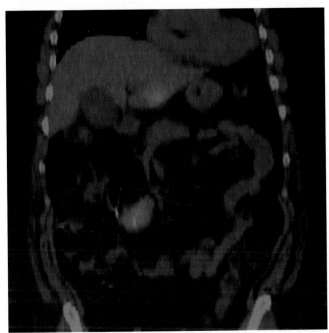

FIGURE 2   SS showing a liver metastasis and retroperitoneal tumor.

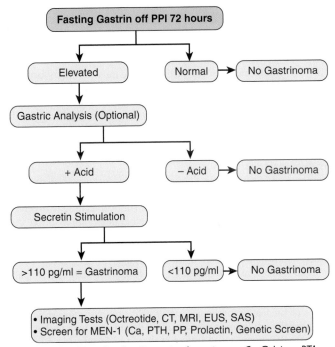

FIGURE 4   Algorithm for diagnosis of gastrinoma. *Ca,* Calcium; *PTA,* parathyroid hormone.

for detection of duodenal gastrinomas is 25% to 63% (mean, 43%; Figure 3). The procedure allows for cytologic evaluation of primary tumors as well as lymph nodes, and endoscopy will detect about 11% of duodenal gastrinomas.

Fluorine-18 (F-18) fluorodeoxyglucose positron emission tomography (FDG-PET) is an imaging modality with a high sensitivity for malignant tumors. Recent studies have indicated the limited value of FDG-PET in identifying pancreatic endocrine tumors. In one study the sensitivity was 53%. At present FDG-PET does not have a routine role in the localization of gastrinoma. The recommended diagnostic algorithm is shown in Figure 4.

TREATMENT OF ZOLLINGER-ELLISON

Medical Treatment of Gastric Acid Hypersecretion

The treatment of gastric acid hypersecretion is of primary importance in gastrinoma. It is accomplished with PPIs and includes omeprazole, lansoprazole, rabeprazole, pantoprazole, and esomeprazole. PPI dosing should be titrated based on symptoms and documented ulcer healing. PPI doses greater than those commonly recommended for typical ulcer disease are usually required. Most studies indicate that lifelong treatment with PPIs is relatively risk free in ZES. With prolonged PPI treatment, periodic assessment of vitamin B12 levels may be warranted.

Surgical Treatment of Gastrinoma

Sporadic Gastrinoma

Imaging of primary gastrinoma will be possible in 60% to 80% of sporadic ZES patients. These patients should be offered surgical exploration. Patients with negative localization tests may be recommended to have exploration as well, but there is a possibility that no tumor may be identified in as many as 15% of image-negative patients. The majority of primary gastrinomas are in the gastrinoma triangle (Figure 5). The principles of exploration include 1) a wide Kocher maneuver to permit careful examination of the head of the pancreas and uncinate process, 2) mobilization of the body and tail

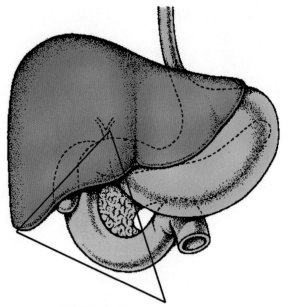

FIGURE 5 The gastrinoma triangle.

of the pancreas to permit bimanual palpation, 3) intraoperative ultrasound, 4) duodenotomy for exploration of the duodenal mucosa, and 5) sampling of lymph nodes in the gastrinoma triangle.

Duodenal Gastrinoma

The duodenum has been reported to be the most common location for gastrinomas. The increased frequency was seen following the incorporation of routine duodenotomy in ZES patients undergoing abdominal exploration to improve detection of gastrinoma in this location. Duodenal gastrinomas may be found in over 60% of patients having direct duodenal exploration compared with less than 20% in whom other techniques were used, such as external palpation or duodenal transillumination.

In sporadic gastrinoma, duodenal primaries are usually in the first and second portion of the duodenum, but in some cases they may be in the third and fourth portion. The surgical technique involves making a lateral duodenotomy in the longitudinal direction at the junction of the first and second portion. Initially, this is about 3 cm in length, but it may be extended either proximally or distally to allow better exposure for removal of the gastrinoma.

The mucosa of the duodenum is inspected visually and by palpation, because gastrinoma in this location is submucosal in nature and often small (<2 mm), typically less than 1 cm. Brunner gland hyperplasia that accompanies gastric acid hypersecretion may produce small nodules in the proximal duodenum that may mislead the surgeon. If a nodule is identified, it should be locally excised and a frozen section obtained. The surgeon should continue to inspect the duodenum for other nodules, as multiple primaries may coexist.

The porta hepatis in the area of the gastrinoma triangle should be explored and lymph nodes excised. The pancreas should be assessed by palpation and intraoperative ultrasound (IOUS), as some patients with sporadic gastrinoma may have duodenal and pancreatic primary tumors.

Lymph Node Primary Tumors

Current experience indicates that 1) primary lymph node (LN) gastrinomas may occur in approximately 10% of sporadic cases; 2) they do not occur in MEN-1 patients; 3) the designation as a lymph node primary should be tentative until 10 years after surgery because a true primary may be detected with subsequent follow-up; 4) patients require yearly assessment with fasting and secretin-stimulated serum gastrin levels; and 5) long-term disease-free and disease-specific survival is possible in this group of patients.

Pancreatic Primary Tumors

Approximately 50% of gastrinomas occur in the pancreas. Identification requires exposure of the pancreas as previously described. IOUS may be helpful. The finding of a pancreatic tumor does not negate the possibility of a duodenal primary tumor; duodenotomy is required. In general, tumors smaller than 2 cm in the uncinate process or head of the pancreas may be enucleated, unless they involve the pancreatic duct. Involvement in the pancreatic duct may be determined by IOUS.

Lesions larger than 2 cm, or those involving the pancreatic duct, generally require pancreaticoduodenectomy. Lesions in the body and tail of the pancreas often are near the pancreatic duct, and unless they clearly protrude from the surface of the gland, they require distal pancreatectomy and splenectomy.

The role of pancreaticoduodenectomy in gastrinoma is controversial. Most centers with considerable experience in treating ZES do not recommend routine Whipple procedures, particularly for patients with sporadic disease. The decision to perform pancreaticoduodenectomy should be based on individual patient considerations, the patient's general medical condition and tumor size. Further discussion of this topic is included in the section on surgical treatment of gastrinoma in MEN-1.

Results of Surgery in Sporadic Zollinger-Ellison Syndrome

The definition of a biochemical cure following surgery for ZES is a normal fasting and secretin-stimulated gastrin level. Initial cure rates range from 35% to 60%, but with long-term follow-up, recurrent hypergastrinemia may occur in nearly 40%. Surgical resection increases disease-specific survival in sporadic gastrinoma—98% for operated and 74% for nonoperated patients at 15 years and 60% versus 20% at 20 years.

Gastrinoma in MEN-1

There is no disagreement that the hyperparathyroidism in MEN-1 requires surgical treatment. If the patient has synchronous ZES, the parathyroid disease should be managed initially in the majority of cases because this reduces serum gastrin levels by removing the constant stimulation from hypercalcemia. The procedure is either subtotal parathyroidectomy (3.5 gland) or total parathyroidectomy and autotransplantation of parathyroid tissue.

In contrast, there is controversy regarding the role of surgery for gastrinoma in MEN-1. Most studies report that biochemical cure of ZES in MEN-1 rarely occurs; however, we reviewed 56 patients who underwent surgical resection of gastrinoma in MEN-1, and seven patients were cured (11.3%).

The role of surgery for the patient with ZES and MEN-1 is determined by imaging: *image-negative* patients should be observed and should not undergo exploration, given the low cure rates with surgery; *image-positive* patients with no distant metastases to liver or bone should undergo exploration for surgical resection because resection has been shown to improve survival independent of a biochemical cure. The NIH group recommends surgery in patients with index lesions greater than 2 to 2.5 cm.

The results of targeted resection continue to show low cure rates but prolonged survival. The NIH group found that although cure was infrequent, patients with advanced tumors who underwent surgical resection had the same survival as patients with limited disease and those without identifiable tumor, which suggests that surgical resection of locally advanced neuroendocrine tumors offers a survival benefit in MEN-1.

TABLE 2: Elements of staging of gastrinoma

Stage	Tumor	Lymph Node	Distant Metastases
0	T0	N0	M0
1	T1	Any N	M0
2	T2–3	Any N	M0
3	T 4	Any N	M1

T0, no primary tumor; *T1*, primary tumor ≤1 cm; *T2*, primary tumor 1.2 to 2.0 cm; *T3*, primary tumor 2.1 to 2.9 cm; *T4*, primary tumor ≥3 cm

From Ellison EC, Sparks J, Verduci JS, et al: 50-year appraisal of gastrinoma: recommendations for staging and treatment, *J Am Coll Surg* 202:897–905, 2006.

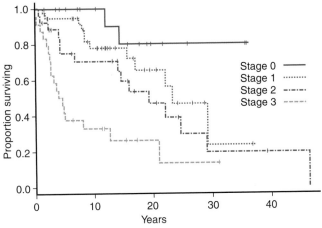

FIGURE 6 Gastrinoma survival by stage.

The Ohio State University Group (2006) group reported 26 patients with MEN-1, and those with complete gross resection had a 10- and 20-year disease-specific survival of 100% and 80%, respectively, compared with 40% at both intervals for the incomplete resection. However, eugastrinemia was only achieved in one patient (6%).

Groups using surgical procedures that included aggressive, targeted tumor excision with distal pancreatectomy, pancreaticoduodenectomy, or total pancreatectomy focused on the field defect in MEN-1 and report variable rates of biochemical cure and prolonged survival. There are frequent late recurrences in the pancreatic remnant, but the results of resection are superior for insulinoma compared with gastrinoma.

Many patients with MEN-1 live many years after the diagnosis without radical surgery and have a relatively indolent course. Hence, many surgeons are reluctant to perform radical surgery, particularly total pancreatectomy. Considering the rarity of cure and the indolent natural course of the disease, the targeted approaches combined with distal pancreatectomy that preserve the head of the pancreas and duodenum seem more prudent. Such an approach avoids the short- and long-term risk of radical surgery and increases survival if complete gross resections are accomplished even without normalization of the postoperative gastrin. Debulking of gastrinoma does not increase survival; hence patients with extensive metastatic disease or locoregional spread that precludes complete resection receive little benefit from surgical resection.

TREATMENT OF METASTATIC DISEASE

The treatment options for hepatic metastases are surgical resection, radiofrequency ablation, hepatic artery embolization, hepatic artery chemoembolization, liver transplantation, chemotherapy, biotherapy, and radiolabeled therapy using somatostatin.

It is difficult to consider the results for surgical resection of gastrinoma in isolation; most series include a combination of pancreatic neuroendocrine tumors and carcinoids. The general consensus is that surgical resection improves survival in patients with neuroendocrine tumors metastatic to the liver, with a 5-year survival that ranges from 70% to 100%. Poor prognostic factors are age greater than 50 years, bilobar disease, and extensive tumor burden.

Considering published studies and data presented to date, there exists low-level evidence supporting liver transplantation in this setting, but its application should be restricted to selected patients who have had the primary tumor removed previously and who have not responded to conventional treatment of liver metastases that included a trial of somatostatin therapy, and who are younger than 50 years and perhaps demonstrate low Ki67 and regular E-cadherin staining.

If the patient is not a surgical candidate, the surgeon is advised to refer the patient to a medical oncologist with experience in neuroendocrine tumors. The monograph referred to in the Suggested Readings has reviewed other modalities of treatment on this topic.

Staging and Survival

Table 2 shows the elements of a staging system for gastrinoma. Survival by stage is shown in Figure 6. This is accurate for sporadic and MEN-1–related ZES.

SUGGESTED READINGS

Zollinger RM, Ellison EH: Primary peptic ulcerations of the jejunum associated with islet cell tumors of the pancreas, *Ann Surg* 142:709–728, 1955.

Stabile BE, Morrow DJ, Passaro E Jr: The gastrinoma triangle: operative implications, *Am J Surg* 147(1):25–31, 1984.

Melvin WS, Johnson JA, Sparks J, et al: Long-term prognosis of Zollinger-Ellison syndrome in multiple endocrine neoplasia, *Surgery* 114:1183–1188, 1993.

Corleto VD, Delle Fave G, Jensen RT: Molecular insights into gastrointestinal neuroendocrine tumours: importance and recent advances, *Dig Liver Dis* 34:668–680, 2002.

Norton JA, Alexander HR, Fraker DL, et al: Comparison of surgical results in patients with advanced and limited disease with multiple endocrine neoplasia type 1 and Zollinger-Ellison syndrome, *Ann Surg* 234(4):495–505, 2001.

Norton JA, Warren RS, Kelly MG, et al: Aggressive surgery for metastatic liver neuroendocrine tumors, *Surgery* 134(6):1057–1063, 2003.

Norton JA, Jensen RT: Resolved and unresolved controversies in the surgical management of patients with Zollinger-Ellison syndrome, *Ann Surg* 240:757–773, 2004.

Ellison EC, Sparks J, Verducci JS, et al: Fifty-year appraisal of gastrinoma: recommendations for staging and treatment, *J Am Coll Surg* 202:897–905, 2006.

Tonelli F, Fratini G, Nesi G, et al: Pancreatectomy in multiple endocrine neoplasia type 1–related gastrinomas and pancreatic endocrine neoplasias, *Ann Surg* 244(1):61–70, 2006.

Ellison EC, Johnson JA: The Zollinger–Ellison Syndrome: a comprehensive review of historical, scientific and clinical considerations, *Curr Probl Surg* 46:1–108, 2009.

MALLORY-WEISS SYNDROME

William E. Fisher, MD, and F. Charles Brunicardi, MD

HISTORY

Although George Kenneth Mallory and Soma Weiss are most famous for the syndrome that bears their names, both focused their careers and made contributions in other areas. Weiss was a Hungarian physiologist and biochemist who immigrated to the United States after World War I. He qualified in medicine in 1923 and initially worked at Cornell University before moving to Harvard Medical School, where he became physician-in-chief at the Peter Bent Brigham Hospital in 1939. Most of his contributions were in the field of cardiovascular disease and pharmacology. Mallory was an American pathologist who spent his entire career in Boston, where he was born. He received his medical degree from Harvard Medical School in 1926 and subsequently worked at Boston City Hospital and the Mallory Institute of Pathology, founded by and named after Mallory's father, Frank B. Mallory. The younger Mallory's main interests were in diseases of the liver and kidneys.

In 1929, Mallory and Weiss described 15 cases of severe, painless, massive, upper gastrointestinal (GI) hemorrhage caused by a tear in the mucosa of the distal esophagus. They described six additional cases in 1932. In subsequent decades, reports of the syndrome were sporadic because a specific diagnosis of this type of upper GI hemorrhage was difficult, and the syndrome was thought to be rare. However, in the 1970s, the diagnosis was facilitated by widespread use of flexible upper endoscopy. A greater incidence of these lesions was subsequently appreciated, as well as a large number of causal factors in addition to alcohol abuse. Mallory-Weiss syndrome is now understood to include all causes of linear mucosal lacerations of the gastroesophageal junction (GEJ) that lead to upper GI hemorrhage.

DEFINITION, PRESENTATION, AND ASSOCIATED CONDITIONS

A Mallory-Weiss tear is a disruption of the mucosa of the distal esophagus, usually caused by anything that produces prolonged violent retching or vomiting. Mallory-Weiss syndrome is not to be confused with Boerhaave syndrome, a rare condition in which the distal esophagus is perforated due to vomiting. Mallory-Weiss syndrome is now thought to be the cause of about 5% to 15% of all cases of upper GI bleeding.

In the 15 cases originally described by Mallory and Weiss, the mucosal tear was described as caused by vomiting due to excessive alcohol ingestion; however, other causes of these linear tears in the distal esophageal mucosa are now appreciated. For example, the tear can sometimes be caused by violent coughing or a seizure. There also is an association of this tear with eating disorders such as bulimia, and it can sometimes occur during pregnancy (hyperemesis gravidarum of childbirth) and has been described in chemotherapy-associated emesis. Blunt abdominal trauma and cardiopulmonary resuscitation also have been associated with the syndrome.

No matter what the etiology, violent retching seems to be the common denominator. Apparently, the pylorus closes while the stomach and abdominal wall contract violently, creating a large pressure gradient between the proximal stomach and distal esophagus. Elevation of the GEJ into the low-pressure thoracic cavity causes a rapid pressure increase inside the distal esophagus, which stretches and tears the mucosa.

Although not present in every case, the classic history is violent emesis or retching followed by hematemesis. As many as half of the patients affected do not give this history. Most patients do have hematemesis, emesis of bright red blood; however, if bleeding is brisk, they may present with hematochezia, bright red blood in the stool, and syncope due to hemorrhagic shock. Abdominal pain is an uncommon complaint. A minority (about 10%) will present with melena, dark stool due to digested blood from a slower upper GI hemorrhage. As with all cases of GI hemorrhage, a history of the use of aspirin, nonsteroidal antiinflammatories, or anticoagulant medications should be sought.

DIAGNOSIS AND CURRENT THERAPY

As with all GI bleeding, the first priority of management is an assessment of the severity of bleeding and hemodynamic stability. Large-bore intravenous access is rapidly established, and blood samples are immediately sent for analysis of hemoglobin, hematocrit, platelets, coagulation parameters, type, and crossmatch. Serial assessments of hemoglobin, blood pressure, pulse, and urine output are monitored. Resuscitation with crystalloid or blood products is given as necessary.

The next step in the diagnosis and management is flexible upper endoscopy. Frequent lavage is often required to achieve an adequate view. All potential sources of upper GI hemorrhage need to be considered. Therefore evaluation of the entire mucosal surface of the esophagus, stomach, and duodenum is necessary, including a retroflexed view of the GEJ.

Most Mallory-Weiss tears will be found just below the GEJ on the lesser curve side. The second most common site is on the greater curve side, followed by posterior and then anterior sites. Most cases (75% to 90%) involve a single tear, but multiple tears are possible. Thorough examination is important because as many as one third or more patients will have additional coexisting potential sources of upper GI bleeding.

Bleeding is self-limited in 80% to 90% of patients with Mallory-Weiss syndrome and thus is of little interest to the surgeon. In fact, due to normal repair mechanisms of the esophageal mucosa, the tear has been documented to heal in as little as 2 or 3 days. Therefore, if there is no active bleeding at the time of endoscopy, which is witnessed in the majority of cases, antacids and observation as an outpatient is the recommended treatment (Figure 1).

A variety of endoscopic methods that include injection, coagulation, band ligation and, most recently, hemoclips are available for those patients found to have active bleeding. Sometimes a combination of methods is used. Some data exist from case series and randomized, prospective trials comparing outcomes using these techniques. Injection of alcohol (sclerotherapy) or epinephrine has been reported to be highly successful in stopping bleeding and preventing recurrent bleeding, and multipolar electrocoagulation also is reported to be highly successful in achieving hemostasis. Esophageal perforation has been reported as a rare complication of these techniques.

Endoscopic banding has been successful for the control of variceal hemorrhage and has more recently been applied to Mallory-Weiss tears with active bleeding. Patients with cirrhosis and a Mallory-Weiss tear warrant special consideration. Due to the presence of portal hypertension with vascular congestion or even esophageal varices and liver dysfunction, a Mallory-Weiss tear in these patients is more likely to result in massive hemorrhage. Such patients also are more likely to bleed again and warrant close observation. Endoscopic banding might be particularly attractive in patients who also have esophageal varices.

Hemoclips offer the potential advantage of less tissue injury. Two recent randomized, prospective trials of endoscopic hemoclip placement for bleeding Mallory-Weiss tears reported 100% success in

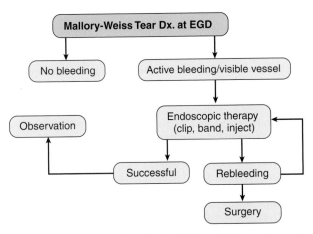

FIGURE I   Treatment algorithm for Mallory-Weiss syndrome. *Dx,* Diagnosis.

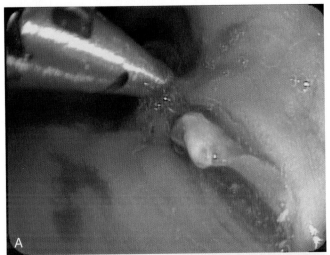

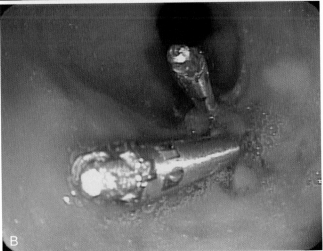

FIGURE 2   Endoscopic views of Mallory-Weiss tear being treated with hemoclips. *(Courtesy Isaac Raijman, MD, associate professor, Department of Gastroenterology, Baylor College of Medicine.)*

achieving hemostasis and a negligible incidence of recurrent hemorrhage (Figure 2). In randomized trials, results with hemoclips have been equal to injection of epinephrine and endoscopic banding. In practice, the choice of technique currently depends on the available local endoscopic expertise.

Currently, a need for surgical treatment is extremely rare in patients who present with upper GI hemorrhage due to a Mallory-Weiss tear. However, hemodynamic instability and hemorrhagic shock can occur. Initial treatment of severe hemorrhage usually is transfusion and endoscopic therapy with one of the above techniques. It is uncommon for patients to rebleed, but when this occurs, the problem usually is approached with repeat endoscopy. Patients with shock at initial presentation and active bleeding at initial endoscopy are at increased risk of recurrent bleeding. Surgery is reserved for patients who fail to stop bleeding with endoscopy. It is critically important to localize the site of bleeding and potential sites of coexistent bleeding prior to laparotomy if at all possible.

For a bleeding Mallory-Weiss tear, the surgical approach is usually through a midline laparotomy and longitudinal gastrotomy near, but not through, the GEJ. Once visualized, the tear is directly sutured with absorbable suture. The gastrotomy can be closed in two layers with a running absorbable suture reinforced with silk Lembert sutures. A postoperative nasogastric tube is not necessary.

Carefully selected patients might be approached with a combined endoscopic and laparoscopic technique. The advantage of such a technique is to avoid a gastrotomy. Laparoscopic exposure can be obtained using five ports; one port is placed above the umbilicus for the camera, and two working ports are placed along each costal margin. The distal esophagus and GEJ are exposed, and the bleeding site is localized with intraoperative upper endoscopy. Care must be taken to avoid unnecessary insufflation of air and distension of the stomach and small intestine. Full-thickness absorbable sutures are placed using intracorporeal laparoscopic techniques.

It must be stressed that patients requiring surgery for a bleeding Mallory-Weiss tear are often unstable and have multiple comorbid conditions responsible for their failure to stop bleeding with endoscopy. Laparotomy may be the best and most rapid way to provide the needed hemostasis.

■ SUMMARY

Mallory-Weiss syndrome is a linear tear in the distal esophageal mucosa, usually on the lesser curve side, caused by any condition associated with forceful vomiting and retching. The condition is usually of little interest to the surgeon because bleeding is self-limited in 90% of patients, and the tear quickly heals spontaneously. When intervention is required, endoscopic methods are highly successful, and surgery is required in less than 1% of patients.

S U G G E S T E D   R E A D I N G S

Cho YS, Chai HS, Kim HK, et al: Endoscopic band ligation and endoscopic hemoclip placement for patients with Mallory-Weiss Syndrome and active bleeding, *W J Gastroentrol* 14(13):2080–2084, 2008.

Higuchi N, Akahoshi K, Sumida Y, et al: Endoscopic band ligation therapy for upper gastrointestinal bleeding related to Mallory-Weiss syndrome, *Surg Endosc* 20(9):1431–1434, 2006.

Park CH, Min SW, Sohn YH, et al: A prospective randomized trial of endoscopic band ligation vs. epinephrine injection for actively bleeding Mallory-Weiss syndrome, *Gastrointest Endosc* 60(1):22–27, 2004.

Morales P, Baum AE: Therapeutic alternatives for the Mallory-Weiss tear, *Curr Treat Options Gastroenterol* 6:75, 2003.

Weiss S, Mallory GK: Lesions of the cardiac orifice of the stomach produced by vomiting, *JAMA* 98:1353, 1932.

Mallory GK, Weiss S: Hemorrhages from lacerations of the cardiac orifice of the stomach due to vomiting, *Am J Med Sci* 178:506, 1929.

GASTRIC ADENOCARCINOMA

David W. McFadden, MD, MBA, and John G. Schneider, MD

HISTORY

Epidemiology and Pathogenesis

The incidence of gastric cancer in the United States has fallen considerably since the 1930s, when it was the leading cause of cancer mortality in the United States and Europe. In 2008, over 21,000 new cases were diagnosed, and 13,000 deaths were attributed to gastric cancer, according to estimates by the American Cancer Society.

Internationally, gastric cancer is the fourth most common malignancy and second leading cause of cancer-related death. There is considerable geographic variation in the incidence of gastric adenocarcinoma. Japan, Korea, and areas of South America have the highest incidences, and North America, Australia, and portions of Northern Africa have the lowest. The incidence of distal gastric cancer is decreasing, but that of proximal tumors is increasing, suggesting the etiology of gastric cancer may differ based on tumor location.

Known risk factors include *Helicobacter pylori* infection, gastric polyps, exposure to nitrosamines, tobacco use, previous gastric surgery, pernicious anemia, and family history. Although few gastric cancers result from genetic predisposition, it is important to be aware of specific mutations, such as E-cadherin, so appropriate genetic counseling and screening can be offered to patients and their families.

Pathology

Over 90% of malignant gastric tumors are classified as adenocarcinomas. There are two distinct subtypes: *intestinal* (well differentiated) and *diffuse* (poorly differentiated). The intestinal type is more common in high-risk populations and older patients and tends to form glands because it is derived from the gastric mucosa and is more frequently associated with blood-borne metastases. The diffuse type is more common in women and younger patients. It is thought to arise from the lamina propria and spreads via submucosal infiltration. Lymphatic metastases are common, and the prognosis is less favorable with the diffuse type. In recent years, proximally located and diffuse-type tumors have been increasing in incidence in Western cultures. However, distal lesions continue to predominate in Japan and other parts of the world. The etiology for this trend is unknown and likely multifactorial.

Diagnosis and Staging

Unfortunately, symptoms of gastric cancer, such as nausea and epigastric pain, are vague and mimic those of benign gastrointestinal disorders. Thus the majority of tumors are diagnosed at advanced stages. Physical examination is often unremarkable; however, late findings such as a palpable abdominal mass, the classically described "Sister Mary Joseph" (periumbilical) and Virchow (left supraclavicular) nodes, and Blumer's shelf (prerectal metastases palpated during rectal exam) are infrequently observed.

Endoscopy is the diagnostic examination of choice. Frequently, endoscopic ultrasound (EUS) is used as an adjunctive test to determine the depth of the tumor or lymph node involvement with accuracy up to 80% and 50%, respectively. Computed tomography is used primarily for detection of metastatic disease, and diagnostic laparoscopy can aid in the detection of unresectable disease because it identifies metastatic disease in up to 30% of patients with negative cross-sectional imaging.

Peritoneal washings should be collected during these procedures because they offer further prognostic information. A recent investigation of patients who underwent R0 resection after laparoscopic confirmation of no visible metastases showed that the mean survival for individuals with negative peritoneal cytology was 98.5 months compared with 14.8 months for patients with positive cytology.

The American Joint Committee on Cancer and International Union against Cancer (AJCC/UICC) system is the most commonly used pathologic staging criteria (Table 1). Tumor (T) stage is defined by the depth of gastric wall invasion. T1 lesions invade into the lamina propria or submucosa. T2a tumors penetrate into the muscularis propria, and T2b cancers invade the subserosa. T3 lesions invade the serosa without extension into adjacent structures. Finally, T4 is characterized by involvement of adjacent organs. Nodal (N) status is determined by the number of lymph nodes involved. N1 involves metastases in 1 to 6 regional nodes, N2 from 7 to 15 regional nodes, and N3 more than 15 nodes. To obtain accurate staging, the surgical specimen should contain at lease 15 lymph nodes for examination.

SURGERY

Primary Resection

Surgical excision remains the cornerstone of curative therapy for gastric cancer. The objective is to perform a complete resection with negative margins (R0 resection). This can be accomplished via subtotal or total gastrectomy; randomized controlled trials have shown no difference in survival when comparing these operations. Due to the propensity of gastric cancer to spread in the submucosa, gross margins of at least 5 cm are preferable. The management of microscopically positive margins (R1 resection) is a contentious issue. Recent Italian studies have shown that resection line involvement may not affect prognosis in early (T1) gastric cancers. However, reexcision for advanced tumors does improve survival independently of lymph node status. Thus the decision to reoperate should be considered carefully based on the patient's overall condition and treatment goals.

Lymphadenectomy

The extent of lymphadenectomy continues to be controversial. Historically, nodal resection has been defined by the proximity to the stomach. A D0 dissection is when no effort is made to resect nodes, typically during palliative resection. D1 lymphadenectomy refers to excision of perigastric nodes, and D2 dissection includes nodes located along the main trunks of the celiac axis.

The Japanese Society for Research in Gastric Cancer (JSRGC) standardized the extent of resection and lymphadenectomy in the early 1980s. Since that time, several retrospective studies from Japan have demonstrated significant survival advantage with extended D2 resection. However, several prospective, randomized trials done in Western countries have not reproduced these findings. Notably, the Dutch Gastric Cancer Group trial comparing D1 and D2 lymphadenectomy, as defined by the JSRGC and performed under the tutelage of an experienced Japanese surgeon, did not show improvement in survival with higher postoperative morbidity. Similarly, the British Medical Research Council investigation of D1 and D2 lymphadenectomy showed a significant increase in postoperative morbidity without improvement in either overall or recurrence-free survival. In these trials, distal pancreatectomy and splenectomy were included in D2 resection, and subgroup analyses suggested that these procedures

TABLE 1: AJCC/UICC gastric cancer staging system

Tumor:	Tx	Primary tumor cannot be assessed		
	T0	No evidence of primary tumor		
	Tis	Carcinoma in situ: intraepithelial tumor without invasion of lamina propria		
	T1	Tumor invades lamina propria or submucosa		
	T2	Tumor invades muscularis propria or subserosa		
	T2a	Tumor invades muscularis propria		
	T2b	Tumor invades subserosa		
	T3	Tumor invades serosa (visceral peritoneum) without invasion of adjacent structures		
	T4	Tumor invades adjacent structures		
Nodes:	Nx	Regional lymph nodes cannot be assessed		
	N0	No regional lymph node metastases		
	N1	Metastases in 1 to 6 regional lymph nodes		
	N2	Metastases in 7 to 15 regional lymph nodes		
	N3	Metastases in more than 15 regional lymph nodes		
Metastases:	Mx	Distant metastases cannot be assessed		
	M0	No distant metastases		
	M1	Distant metastases		
Stages:	0	Tis	N0	M0
	IA	T1	N0	M0
	IB	T1	N1	M0
		T2a/b	N0	M0
	II	T1	N2	M0
		T2a/b	N1	M0
		T3	N0	M0
	IIIA	T2a/b	N2	M0
		T3	N1	M0
		T4	N0	M0
	IIIB	T3	N2	M0
	IV	T4	N1–3	M0
		T1–3	N3	M0
		any T	any N	M1

contributed to the morbidity of patients undergoing extended lymph node dissection. D1 and D2 resections without pancreatosplenectomy have subsequently been compared in nonrandomized, single-center trials that demonstrated comparable morbidity and improved survival after D2 resection.

Aggressive lymphadenectomy is also beneficial because it allows for accurate staging. Review of patients undergoing R0 resection at Memorial Sloan-Kettering Cancer Center demonstrated that the number of positive nodes, rather than their location, was a key determinant of prognosis. Examination of at least 15 nodes increases prognostic accuracy and results in improved survival at all stages. This observation is likely due to a reduction in understaging or stage migration when more lymph nodes are examined.

Operative Technique

Prior to commencing with resection and lymphadenectomy, the peritoneal cavity is examined for undiagnosed metastases. If a neoadjuvant protocol is considered, diagnostic laparoscopy should be performed. After the confirmation of resectability, the avascular plane between the transverse colon and greater omentum is divided sharply, and the greater omentum is dissected off the colon (Figure 1, A). The anterior sheath of the transverse mesocolon is separated along an avascular plane down to the pancreas (Figure 1, B). The pancreatic capsule should be taken selectively because there is limited evidence regarding oncologic benefit. Next, the short gastric vessels and lateral omental attachments are taken down (Figure 1, C). We prefer to use ultrasonic coagulating devices for our dissection.

The type of resection that is planned determines the extent of dissection along the greater curvature. The duodenum is then isolated and transected using a gastrointestinal anastomosis (GIA) stapler 2 to 3 cm distal to the pylorus, with close attention to avoiding a retained antral remnant (Figure 1, D). Dissection continues along the porta hepatis toward the celiac vessels to include all nodal tissue anterior to the portal vein (Figure 1, E). Lymph nodes between the common hepatic artery and superior portion of the pancreas are reflected toward the celiac axis. The left gastric artery is identified and divided at its base, and nodal tissue is swept off the right crus of the diaphragm (Figure 1, F). The splenic artery is dissected along the superior portion of the pancreas, and the lymph node dissection continues toward the splenic hilum. Here, the proximal portion of the specimen is divided, either sharply for a total gastrectomy or with a GIA stapler for a subtotal gastrectomy. Proximal margins are routinely sent for frozen section to confirm microscopic tumor clearance. The gastrointestinal tract can be reconstructed with Roux-en-Y esophagojejunostomy following total gastrectomy and either Billroth II or Roux-en-Y gastrojejunostomy after subtotal gastrostomy. We favor the Roux-en-Y for its lack of bile reflux into the gastric remnant.

COMBINED MODALITY THERAPY

Adjuvant Therapy

Unfortunately, many patients who undergo curative R0 resection will have recurrent disease within 2 years of surgery. Locoregional and distant recurrences happen with comparable frequency; thus significant attention has been given to combined modality therapies following resection of gastric cancer.

Numerous trials have investigated postoperative chemotherapy with or without radiation and have failed to demonstrate survival benefits. Recently, the Intergroup 0116 prospective randomized controlled trial that compared 5-fluorouracil (5-FU) and leucovorin plus external beam radiation to observation demonstrated improvement in both overall and relapse-free survival in the treatment group (Figure 2). Based on this investigation, this regimen has become the standard of care in the United States. However, this study has been

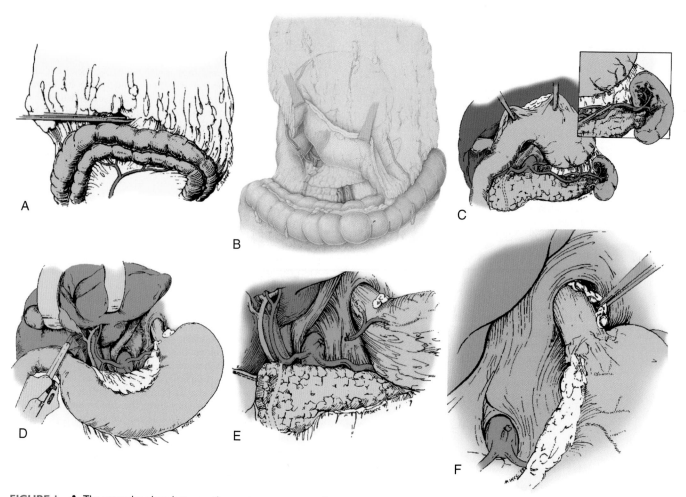

FIGURE 1   A, The avascular plane between the greater omentum and transverse mesocolon is incised. **B,** The greater omentum is dissected off of the colon along the avascular plane between the anterior and posterior sheaths of the transverse mesocolon. Dissection is carried down to the level of the pancreas. **C,** The lateral attachments of the stomach and short gastric vessels are divided. **Inset:** The splenic artery is dissected along the superior border of the pancreas. Nodal tissue is dissected down to the level of the splenic hilus. **D,** The duodenum is identified and divided with the GIA linear stapler. **E,** Nodal dissection proceeds from the porta hepatis toward the celiac axis along the superior border of the pancreas. The left gastric artery is divided at its origin. **F,** Nodal dissection continues along the right diaphragmatic crus and esophageal hiatus. The left paracardial nodes are taken during total gastrectomy.

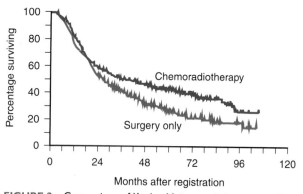

FIGURE 2   Comparison of Kaplan-Meier survival curves analyzing the influence of adjuvant chemoradiation and extent of nodal dissection. Overall survival of patients randomized to surgery alone (median survival = 27 months, n = 275) and surgery and chemoradiation (median survival = 36 months, n = 281; P = .005). *(From MacDonald JS, Smalley SR, Stenning SP, et al: Chemotherapy after surgery compared with surgery alone for adenocarcinoma of the gastroesophageal junction, N Engl J Med 345:725; 2001.)*

criticized for poor standardization of surgical therapy. Complete resection with D2 lymphadenectomy was recommended in the study, but only 10% of patients actually underwent this procedure. The majority of patients (54%) underwent a D0 resection.

The survival benefit from adjuvant chemoradiation is not expected to surpass that of surgery alone when tumors are accurately staged with standardized lymph node resection. Recent studies from Japan have investigated an alternative chemotherapeutic agent, S-1. This drug is a combination of tegafur (prodrug of 5-FU), 5-chloro-2, 4-dihydroxypyridine, and oxonic acid. The Adjuvant Chemotherapy Trial of TS-1 for Gastric Cancer (ACTS-GC) trial, a large randomized phase III study, demonstrated a survival benefit in patients with stage II or III disease who received this treatment following D2 resection. Importantly, these results assume that D2 resection is the standard resection and therefore have limited application in the treatment of Western patients.

Neoadjuvant Therapy

In addition to the criticisms of surgical therapy in the Intergroup 0116 trial, only 64% of patients were able to complete the regimen of postoperative chemoradiation. Likely benefits of preoperative

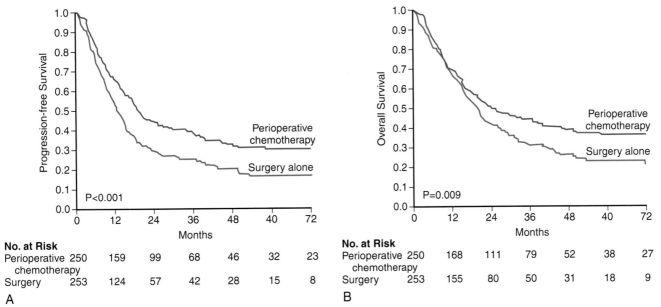

FIGURE 3 Kaplan-Meier survival curves comparing surgery alone with surgery plus perioperative epirubicin, cisplatin, and fluorouracil chemotherapy. Both progression-free survival (**A**) and overall survival (**B**) were lengthened with the addition of chemotherapy. *(From Cunningham D, Allum WH, Stenning SP, et al: Perioperative chemotherapy versus surgery alone for resectable gastroesophageal cancer, N Engl J Med 355:17, 2006.)*

administration that include improved patient tolerance, ability to assess disease response in vivo, and tumor downstaging have sparked significant interest in neoadjuvant therapy. The British Medical Research Council's Adjuvant Gastric Infusional Chemotherapy (MAGIC) trial comparing perioperative epirubicin, cisplatin, and 5-FU to surgery alone demonstrated improved overall and progression-free survival in addition to improved resectability (Figure 3). Presently, neoadjuvant therapy is recommended for patients with T2 or higher tumors.

PROGNOSIS

Traditionally, outcomes have been predicted based on the AJCC staging system. However, there is significant variability within stage groups, making prognostication for individual patients quite difficult. Surgeons from Memorial Sloan-Kettering have developed a postoperative nomogram for predicting survival that is more accurate than AJCC staging alone (Figure 4). This was accomplished by including age, sex, number of positive and negative lymph nodes, depth of invasion, and histotype. Subsequent analyses at large-volume centers in both the United States and Europe have validated this model, and using it may allow for more careful stratification of treatment groups in future clinical trials. Discovery and implementation of additional prognostic markers, such as E-cadherin levels, could improve the accuracy of the nomogram.

PALLIATION

Due to the grim prognosis of advanced gastric cancer and the inability to complete curative resection in about half of the patients who have it, understanding palliation is imperative when treating patients. The utility of surgical therapy in palliation is controversial. Palliative gastrectomy is associated with significant morbidity (>50%) and mortality rates. While this is presumably due to the deconditioned state of patients with advanced gastric cancers, this procedure cannot be universally justified for relief of symptoms. Follow-up studies of patients in whom elective gastrectomy was aborted due to detection of metastases at the time of operation found that only half required intervention for symptoms of advanced tumors, and just over 10% needed operative interventions.

SUMMARY

Even though the incidence of gastric adenocarcinoma has declined significantly in the United States over the last century, there is a trend toward more proximal and biologically aggressive tumors. Surgical excision continues to be the foundation of curative therapy for patients with operable disease. R0 resection optimizes outcomes, and extended lymphadenectomy enhances staging accuracy and may provide marginal survival benefit. At present, the optimal timing and form of adjuvant treatment remains unknown. Additional research is needed to define the role chemoradiation will play in treatment of advanced disease.

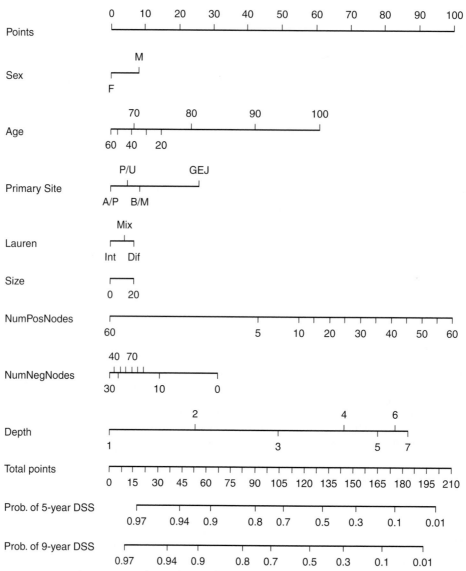

FIGURE 4 Gastric cancer postoperative nomogram for prediction of disease-specific survival after curative R0 resection. *(From Kattan MW, Karpeh MS, Mazumdar M, Brennan MF, et al: Postoperative nomogram for disease-specific survival after an R0 resection for gastric carcinoma, J Clin Oncol 21:3647; 2003.)*

SUGGESTED READINGS

Cunningham D, Allum WH, Stenning SP, et al: Perioperative chemotherapy versus surgery alone for resectable gastroesophageal cancer, *N Engl J Med* 355:11–20, 2006.

Hartgrink HH, Van De Velde CJH, Putter H, et al: Extended lymph node dissection for gastric cancer: who may benefit from final results of the randomized Dutch Gastric Cancer Group Trial, *J Clin Oncol* 22:2069–2077, 2004.

Macdonald JS, Smalley SR, Benedetti J, et al: Chemoradiotherapy after surgery compared with surgery alone for adenocarcinoma of the stomach or gastroesophageal junction, *N Engl J Med* 345:725–730, 2001.

Novotny AR, Schumacher C, Busch R, et al: Predicting individual survival after gastric cancer resection: validation of a U.S.-derived nomogram at a single high-volume center in Europe, *Ann Surg* 243:74–81, 2006.

GASTROINTESTINAL STROMAL TUMORS

Giorgos C. Karakousis, MD, and Ronald P. DeMatteo, MD

HISTORY

Gastrointestinal stromal tumor (GIST) is the most common mesenchymal-derived tumor of the intestinal tract, but it is rare overall and accounts for just over 1% of all gastrointestinal neoplasms. Its incidence is estimated to be approximately 5000 cases per year in the United States. Its incidence has increased in the past decade in part from the use of immunohistochemistry that has allowed for the reclassification of some tumors formerly considered to be leiomyomas or leiomyosarcomas.

Thought to originate from the interstitial cell of Cajal, an intestinal pacemaker cell, treatment of GIST has become a paradigm for effective molecularly targeted therapy of solid tumors. In 1998, Hirota and colleagues initially described a gain of function mutation in the *KIT (CD117)* protooncogene in the majority of GISTs. Just 3 years later, Joensuu and colleagues described the dramatic response of a patient with advanced GIST to imatinib mesylate (Gleevec, STI571; Novartis Pharmaceuticals, Basel, Switzerland), an inhibitor of the tyrosine kinases ABL, BCR-ABL, KIT, and platelet-derived growth factor receptor (PDGFR).

With approximately 80% of GIST patients demonstrating response or stability to imatinib therapy compared with the approximately 5% response with prior conventional chemotherapy, the median survival in patients with metastatic disease has shifted from 15 months prior to tyrosine kinase inhibitors to nearly 5 years. Targeted therapy has revolutionized the treatment of patients with metastatic GIST and those undergoing resection of primary localized GIST.

CLINICAL PRESENTATION

The mean age of presentation for GIST patients is approximately 60 years of age, with a slight male predominance. Most GIST tumors are thought to be sporadic, with only a few familial cases reported in the literature, harboring either a germline mutation in the *KIT* protooncogene or the PDGFRα receptor. Small (<2 cm) GISTs are often discovered incidentally in the workup of other conditions.

Many patients with larger tumors will present with vague abdominal discomfort or an abdominal mass. About a quarter of patients will present with GI bleeding due to erosion of the overlying mucosa. Intestinal obstruction from GIST tumors is uncommon, since GISTs, like other sarcomas, will typically displace rather than invade adjacent structures; occasionally, however, they may serve as a lead point for intussusception. Dysphagia and jaundice are rare presenting symptoms in patients with GISTs of the esophagus and duodenum, respectively.

Most GISTs (60%) are located in the stomach, while 25% to 30% are in the small intestine; approximately 10% originate in the esophagus or rectum. Rarely, GISTs will arise from the colon or mesentery. The liver and peritoneum are the most frequent sites of initial metastasis, and lymph node metastases are rare, except in pediatric patients. The biology of GIST in children is further distinguished by multifocal disease, a female predominance, and absence of a KIT or PDGFRα mutation.

DIAGNOSIS AND PROGNOSTIC FACTORS

Because of their relative rarity, GISTs can often pose a diagnostic challenge to clinicians. Cross-sectional imaging with computed tomography or magnetic resonance imaging of the abdomen and pelvis may show a hypervascular mass that appears intimately associated with the GI tract. GISTs of the stomach, particularly when large, may be misconstrued as primary liver tumors such as hemangiomas. The degree of involvement of adjacent structures by these tumors is often difficult to interpret from preoperative imaging and may often be overestimated (Figure 1). Upper endoscopy or colonoscopy may reveal a submucosal mass and, less commonly, an ulcerated lesion if the mucosa has been disrupted. Often, however, endoscopic evaluation will be unrevealing. Frequently, these tumors will display avidity by fluorodeoxyglucose positron emission tomography (FDG-PET). Although its role in establishing a diagnosis is limited, PET may play a role in assessing the extent of disease in patients with suspected metastases and in assessing early biologic response to imatinib or other agents in tumors resistant to imatinib.

Recent reports have suggested the sensitivity for diagnosing GIST of the stomach using fine needle aspiration (FNA) may be as high as 70% to 80%. If endoscopic biopsy is not feasible or inconclusive, percutaneous biopsy may not be necessary if the diagnosis is suggested by radiologic imaging. In contrast, biopsy is frequently performed in metastatic disease prior to the initiation of tyrosine kinase inhibitor therapy.

Careful pathologic evaluation of tissue by conventional hematoxylin and eosin staining and immunohistochemistry usually establishes the diagnosis of GIST, which frequently expresses both smooth muscle and neural elements. But the single most important immunohistochemical marker for characterization of these tumors is the product of the *KIT* protooncogene, or *CD117,* which is found in approximately 95% of cases. The *KIT* protooncogene found on chromosome 4q11-q12 codes for a transmembrane tyrosine kinase receptor, whose activation initiates an intracellular signaling cascade that influences a variety of cellular functions that include proliferation, differentiation, and adhesion. GISTs harbor gain-of-function mutations in the *KIT* protooncogene, leading to constitutive activation of the receptor. These mutations occur most frequently in exon 11 (70%); mutations at other sites, such as exon 9 (10%) or exon 13 or 17 (1% to 2%), occur less commonly. Recent data demonstrate an association between the specific exon mutation type and imatinib responsiveness and clinical outcome (exon 9 mutations demonstrating a worse clinical behavior than exon 11 mutations). A small percentage of GISTs (5%) instead harbor mutations in PDGFRα.

The three most important clinical and histopathologic factors found to be independently predictive of recurrence of localized GIST following resection are mitotic rate, tumor size, and tumor location. We recently created and validated a nomogram based on these three factors to predict the likelihood of tumor recurrence following removal of primary GIST (Figure 2).

TREATMENT

Primary GIST

Preoperative assessment and staging of a primary GIST can typically be accomplished with a CT scan of the abdomen and pelvis and chest radiograph. At exploration, careful examination of the abdomen for peritoneal metastases or liver metastases should be undertaken. In assessing resectability, great care should be given to avoid excessive tumor manipulation, which may lead to disruption of the often friable tumor with subsequent bleeding or intraperitoneal dissemination of the tumor.

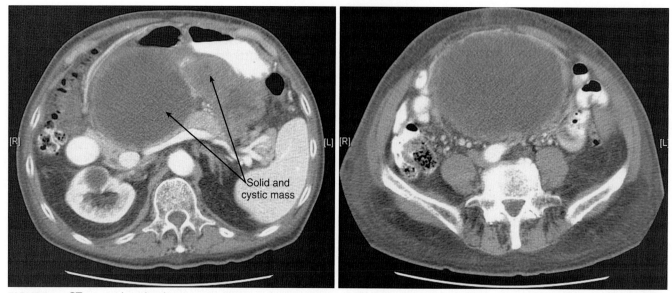

FIGURE 1   CT scan with oral and intravenous contrast of a patient with a large GIST with solid and cystic components extending from the upper abdomen to the pelvis. Upon laparotomy, the patient was noted to have a 15 cm cystic component connected to a 7 cm solid GIST, originating from the stomach, which did not invade the liver or other organs. The entire mass was completely removed with only a limited (wedge) resection of normal stomach.

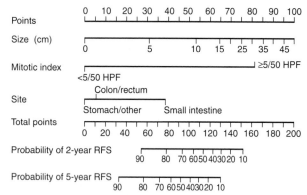

FIGURE 2   A nomogram predicting likelihood of 2-year and 5-year recurrence-free survival (*RFS*) after primary GIST resection based on size, mitotic index, and site of tumor. Points are assigned for each prognostic factor by drawing a line vertically to the "Points" line. The sum of the point contributions from the three factors is used to determine the 2-year and 5-year RFS by drawing a vertical line to the respective "Probability" lines. *HPF*, High-power field. *(From Gold JS, Gönem M, Guttierez J, et al: Development and validation of a prognostic nomogram for recurrence-free survival after complete surgical resection of localised primary gastrointestinal stromal tumour: a retrospective analysis, Lancet Oncol 10:1045-1052, 2009.)*

Primary GISTs will typically displace and not infiltrate adjacent structures, and limited resection of the organ of origin is often sufficient. However, for tumors in inopportune locations—such as near the gastroesophageal junction (GEJ), duodenum, or distal rectum—more extensive en bloc resections may be necessary.

Because of the exceedingly low incidence of nodal metastases with GIST, routine regional lymph node dissections or proximal mesenteric transection is usually not required. Generally, a 1 to 2 cm margin is recommended when resecting GIST tumors, and wedge resection of the involved organ is therefore usually adequate. In the case of microscopically positive margins following resection, the decision to remove additional tissue should be tempered by the difficulty in accurately identifying the area of potential residual disease on reexploration and the lack of evidence supporting a clear

association of microscopically positive margins with poorer survival outcomes. Large tumors likely have the capacity to shed cells intraperitoneally, and achieving negative microscopic margins for these tumors may not be indicative of true microscopic clearance of disease. Laparoscopic resection of primary GISTs can be undertaken by surgeons experienced in this approach, although the same general principles of minimal tumor manipulation and complete gross resection apply.

Recent results from a large double-blind, randomized, controlled trial (American College of Surgeons Oncology Group Z9001) of over 700 patients support the use of imatinib mesylate in the adjuvant setting after resection of primary GIST tumors 3 cm or larger (Figure 3). Patients receiving imatinib at 400 mg daily displayed a 1-year recurrence-free survival of 98% compared with 83% for those receiving placebo. In the subset analysis for patients with tumors 10 cm or larger, there was an approximately 40% difference in recurrence-free survival at 1 year favoring the imatinib group. The trial results led to FDA approval of adjuvant imatinib in 2008. The drug is fairly well tolerated with few side effects reported, most notably diarrhea, abdominal discomfort, dermatitis, and periorbital or peripheral edema. The optimal duration of adjuvant therapy with imatinib has not been clearly defined and is the subject of current clinical investigation. A trial is underway investigating the impact and toxicity of prolonged (5 years) adjuvant therapy with imatinib in patients at moderate or high risk for tumor recurrence.

Neoadjuvant therapy with imatinib for patients with resectable primary GIST has been reported to be safe. It appears to be particularly helpful in patients with large GISTs with extensive organ involvement, duodenal GISTs, low rectal GISTs, or those near the GEJ, where downsizing the viable tumor may alter the nature of the operation and decrease the need for more extensive resections. Early detection of a tumor response with imatinib therapy can be discerned by a decrease in tumor density on contrast-enhanced CT. Changes in tumor size typically occur later.

The 2009 National Comprehensive Cancer Network (NCCN) guidelines recommend follow-up computed tomographic scans of the abdomen and pelvis after complete resection of primary tumor every 3 to 6 months for the first 5 years and annually thereafter. Less frequent and shorter duration follow-up can probably be safely achieved in patients with low-risk tumors (<2 cm), although the natural history of small GISTs is not well defined.

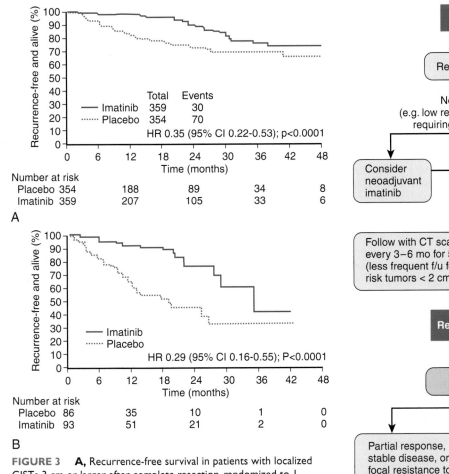

A

B

FIGURE 3   A, Recurrence-free survival in patients with localized GISTs 3 cm or larger after complete resection, randomized to 1 year adjuvant imatinib therapy versus placebo. **B,** Subset analysis of randomized patients with tumor size 10 cm or greater. *HR,* Hazard ratio; *CI,* confidence interval. *(Data from the American College of Surgeons Oncology Group (ACOSOG) Z9001 trial: DeMatteo RP, Ballman KV, Antonescu CR, et al: Adjuvant imatinib mesylate after resection of localised, primary gastrointestinal stromal tumor: a randomised, double-blind, placebo-controlled trial, Lancet 373:1097, 2009.)*

Recurrent and Metastatic Gastrointestinal Stromal Tumor

The most frequent sites of recurrence for GIST are intraabdominal, such as on the surfaces of the peritoneum, or metastases to the liver. Rarely, tumors will recur in bone or in the lung. The median time to recurrence is 18 to 24 months. For patients with recurrent disease who are not currently on imatinib therapy, the initial approach is to begin therapy with imatinib and assess tumor response. A similar approach should be used for patients who present initially with metastatic disease, except in those instances where the patient is symptomatic or there is minimal metastatic disease, in which case surgical intervention can be considered. Approximately 80% of patients with metastatic disease will demonstrate either a partial response (50% to 60%) or stable disease with imatinib therapy. The 2-year survival of patients with metastatic disease treated with imatinib is as high as 70% to 80% compared with approximately 40% in the pre-imatinib era, and the median survival in this group is now 5 years.

Unfortunately, seldom will therapy with imatinib result in the complete regression of tumors, and the majority of patients will eventually develop progressive disease or resistance to therapy, with a median time to progression of about 18 months. This resistance frequently reflects additional mutations in the *KIT* protooncogene, typically

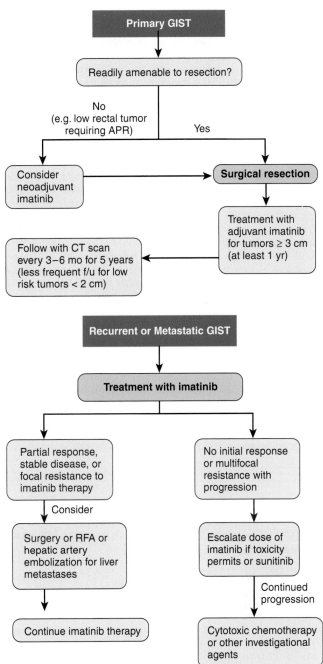

FIGURE 4   Schematic approach to patients with GIST. Approaches to treat liver metastases from GIST include surgical resection, radiofrequency ablation *(RFA),* and hepatic artery embolization. *APR,* Abdominoperineal resection; *F/u,* follow-up. *(Adapted From Gold JS, DeMatteo RP: Combined surgical and molecular therapy: the gastrointestinal stromal tumor model, Ann Surg 244:176, 2006.)*

in exons 13, 14, or 17. Because the maximum response to imatinib therapy is usually achieved by 2 to 6 months, we advocate careful consideration of patients with recurrent or metastatic disease for other interventions, including surgical options, if possible after this time.

In a study of 40 patients with metastatic GIST from our institution who were treated initially with imatinib therapy, those patients demonstrating stable or partial response to imatinib therapy that were taken for surgical resection had a 61% 2-year progression-free survival and 100% overall survival. By comparison, those with unifocal resistance (one tumor increasing in size) who were on imatinib therapy had a

2-year overall survival of 36% after surgery, and those with multifocal resistance (more than one tumor increasing in size) had a median progression-free survival of 3 months and a 1-year overall survival of 36%.

Based on these results and those from other investigators, we do not recommend surgery for patients with multifocal resistance. Other approaches that have been used successfully in the treatment of liver metastases include radiofrequency ablation and hepatic artery embolization.

For patients on imatinib therapy with multifocal resistance or with metastatic disease initially unresponsive to therapy, increasing the dose of imatinib or changing the targeted agent to sunitinib malate (Sutent, SU11248; Pfizer Pharmaceuticals, New York) may yield a clinical response. Sunitinib, which is used also in the treatment of renal cancer, is another selective inhibitor of *KIT* and PDGFRα receptor but also has activity against the vascular endothelial growth factor receptor and other tyrosine kinase receptors (flt-3, RET, CSF1R). Response to sunitinib in patients resistant to imatinib therapy can be as high as 40%, and sunitinib may have particular clinical applications in patients without *KIT* mutation or with a *KIT* exon 9 mutation compared with imatinib. Patients continuing to progress on sunitinib should be considered for other tyrosine kinase inhibitors. A schematic approach to patients with primary, recurrent, and metastatic GISTs is shown in Figure 4.

SUMMARY

With the advent of tyrosine kinase inhibitors, the treatment of GIST has served as a paradigm for effective molecularly targeted therapy; it requires a multidisciplinary approach by general and specialty surgeons, medical oncologists, gastroenterologists, and interventional radiologists. Although the past decade has witnessed dramatic results from imatinib therapy in the metastatic and adjuvant settings, the emergence of resistance to prolonged targeted therapy has presented new challenges and questions to clinicians.

Defining the optimal duration of targeted treatment in the adjuvant setting, the role of neoadjuvant therapy, and the optimal time for other interventions (surgical or interventional radiology) are just a few of the questions currently under investigation. Further understanding of the aberrations at the genetic level will undoubtedly lead to new drug developments and perhaps multiagent approaches to overcome drug resistance. The management of recurrent and metastatic GIST will continue to provide valuable lessons for the treatment of other solid malignancies as effective therapies for them become available.

SUGGESTED READING

DeMatteo RP, Ballman KV, Antonescu CR, et al with American College of Surgeons Oncology Group (ACOSOG) Intergroup Adjuvant GIST Study Team: Adjuvant imatinib mesylate after resection of localised, primary gastrointestinal stromal tumor: a randomised, double-blind, placebo-controlled, *Lancet* 373:1097–1104, 2009.

DeMatteo RP, Gold JS, Saran L, et al: Tumor mitotic rate, size, and location independently predict recurrence after resection of primary gastrointestinal stromal tumor (GIST), *Cancer* 112:608–615, 2008.

DeMatteo RP, Maki RG, Singer S, et al: Results of tyrosine kinase inhibitor therapy followed by surgical resection for metastatic gastrointestinal stromal tumor, *Ann Surg* 245:347–352, 2007.

Demetri GD, von Mehren M, Blanke CD, et al: Efficacy and safety of imatinib mesylate in advanced gastrointestinal stromal tumors, *N Engl J Med* 347:472–480, 2002.

Gold JS, Gonen M, Gutierrez A, et al: Development and validation of a prognostic nomogram for recurrence-free survival after complete surgical resection of localised primary gastrointestinal stromal tumour: a retrospective analysis, *Lancet Oncol* 10:1045–1052, 2009.

MORBID OBESITY

Christopher Scortino, MD, Michael A. Schweitzer, MD, and Thomas H. Magnuson, MD

OVERVIEW

The prevalence of morbid obesity continues to increase throughout industrialized nations. In the United States, nearly 6% of adults are classified as severely obese, with a body mass index (BMI) greater than 40. Medical therapies for weight reduction are, on the whole, unsuccessful at achieving and maintaining significant weight loss in the severely obese population. Bariatric surgery continues to be the only durable method to achieve sustained weight loss for most patients. As a result, over 200,000 bariatric procedures are performed in the United States annually. The four most common operations are Roux-en-Y gastric bypass, laparoscopic adjustable gastric band, duodenal switch with biliopancreatic diversion, and vertical sleeve gastrectomy. These operations achieve weight loss either by restriction of calorie intake (gastric band and sleeve gastrectomy), intestinal malabsorption of calories (duodenal switch), or a combination of restriction and malabsorption (gastric bypass).

PATIENT SELECTION

The National Institutes of Health issued a consensus statement in 1991 regarding the effectiveness of bariatric surgery, outlining patient selection criteria that are still in place today (Table 1). Patients are considered candidates for bariatric surgery if they have a BMI of 40 kg/m^2 or greater, or a BMI between 35 and 40 kg/m^2 if an obesity-related comorbidity, such as diabetes or hypertension, is present. In general, appropriate candidates for surgery should demonstrate prior unsuccessful attempts at medically supervised weight-reduction programs and have realistic expectations regarding the long-term outcomes achieved with surgery. Relative contraindications include inability to comply with postoperative requirements and follow-up, active alcohol or substance abuse, and uncontrolled psychiatric disease.

The evaluation of potential patients for bariatric surgery should involve a multidisciplinary team approach. This team should include a dietician and a mental health professional familiar with bariatric surgery. Their purpose is to obtain a complete past dietary and behavioral eating history, educate the patient on postoperative dietary expectations, examine the social support structure, and ensure that any psychiatric or behavioral disorders are optimally controlled. At the Johns Hopkins Center for Bariatric Surgery, all patients are required to attend a multidisciplinary preoperative education seminar. Postoperative participation in support groups is also encouraged.

TABLE 1: Indications for bariatric surgery for morbid obesity

1. BMI of 40 kg/m^2 or greater
2. BMI 35 to 40 kg/m^2 with significant obesity-related comorbidities (hypertension, diabetes)
3. Unsuccessful attempt at weight loss by nonoperative means
4. Clearance by dietician and mental health professional
5. No medical contraindications to surgery

The age limits for surgery have expanded considerably over the last decade. Select centers now offer surgery to adolescent patients 16 to 17 years old and to patients over the age of 70 years, with overall good results.

OPERATIVE PROCEDURES

Most bariatric surgical procedures are now performed laparoscopically, with a hospital stay of 2 days or less. Open surgery may be required in patients undergoing revisional surgery, those with prior extensive abdominal operations and adhesions, or patients with extreme obesity (BMI >70). On the morning of surgery, all patients should receive appropriate antibiotics and subcutaneous unfractionated or low molecular weight heparin to help minimize the risk of venous thromboembolism.

Laparoscopic surgery involves the use of steep reverse Trendelenburg position, and the patient must be appropriately placed on the operating room table, with a footboard and with arms and legs secured. We have found that the safest way to enter the abdomen in morbidly obese patients is in the left upper quadrant under direct vision, using a device that allows visualization of the abdominal wall layers during entry with a zero-degree laparoscope (12 mm Visiport; Autosuture, Norwalk, Conn.).

Laparoscopic Roux-en-Y Gastric Bypass

Gastric bypass (Figure 1) is the most common bariatric procedure performed in the United States (60% to 70% overall). It has been demonstrated in numerous reports to achieve durable long-term weight loss and remission of metabolic disease with a reasonably low complication rate.

We perform the procedure using five laparoscopic trocars—three 12 mm and two 5 mm—and a subxiphoid puncture for placement of a Nathanson liver retractor. The jejunum is initially divided approximately 40 cm distal to the ligament of Treitz with a 60 mm white stapler cartridge (Endo-GIA Universal XL; Autosuture, Norwalk, Conn.). The mesentery is divided with a gray stapler cartridge and ultrasonic shears (AutoSonix XL; U.S. Surgical, Norwalk, Conn.). The proximal biliopancreatic limb of jejunum is then anastomosed to the distal segment of jejunum 75 to 100 cm distal to the point of division. We perform this anastomosis in a side-to-side fashion using a white Endo-GIA stapler cartridge. The mesenteric defect is closed with a running suture to help minimize the risk of internal hernia.

Next, the patient is placed in steep reverse Trendelenburg position. Dissection is performed at the angle of His, to expose the left crus, and at the gastrohepatic ligament, to gain access to the lesser sac. Division of the neurovascular bundle on the lesser curve side of the stomach, just distal to the left gastric vein, is accomplished using a gray vascular cartridge. Multiple 60 mm blue staple cartridges are then used to transect the stomach up to the angle of His, creating a vertically oriented, 20 mL proximal gastric pouch. Any bleeding at the staple lines is easily controlled with clips or suture ligation.

We routinely bring the Roux limb of jejunum up to the gastric pouch in an antecolic-antegastric orientation. This seems to reduce the incidence of internal hernia and is simpler to perform than the retrocolic-retrogastric approach. The gastrojejunostomy is performed by first suturing the side of the Roux limb to the gastric pouch staple line. A small enterotomy is made just proximal to the end of the Roux limb, and a similarly sized gastrotomy is made in the pouch for the placement of the Endo-GIA stapler. The stapler is loaded with a 45 mm blue cartridge to create the gastrojejunostomy, using only the first 30 mm of the staple cartridge.

After the stapler is fired, a stay suture is placed on the lesser curve (right) side of the opening, and the suture is used to retract the anastomosis to the left and anterior side, thereby exposing the posterior side. A running 2-0 suture is placed posterior on the left side and

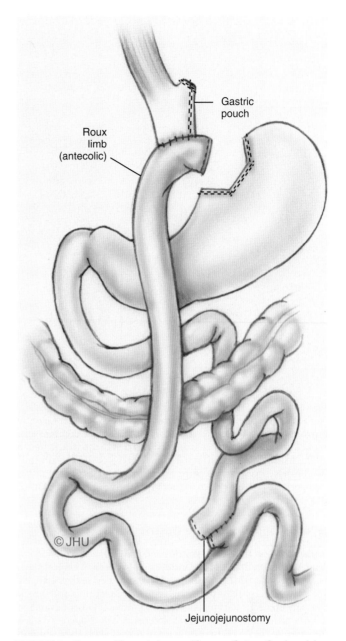

FIGURE I   Roux-en-Y gastric bypass. *(Courtesy Corinne Sandone, Johns Hopkins University.)*

continuously run to the stay suture on the right side to which it is tied.

A blunt 32 Fr round-end bougie is then passed from the mouth through the gastrojejunal anastomosis and into the Roux limb. The bougie can be seen through the opening formed after the stapler is removed. A stay suture is placed at the halfway point of the opening between the end stay sutures. This stay suture and the stay suture on the left (angle of His) side are used to elevate the tissue so that the 60 mm blue cartridge can be used to close the openings. The stapler is brought down on top of the bougie, while the tissue to be transected is retracted. This firing will close most of the opening, and the small remaining defect on the right side is readily closed with a 2-0 suture.

The gastrojejunostomy is completed by running a 2-0 suture to cover the entire anterior portion in a second layer. The resultant anastomosis is approximately 12 mm in diameter. A leak test can be performed by clamping the Roux limb just distal to the anastomosis and insufflating air, via an endoscope or orogastric tube, while the gastric pouch and anastomosis are submerged in saline.

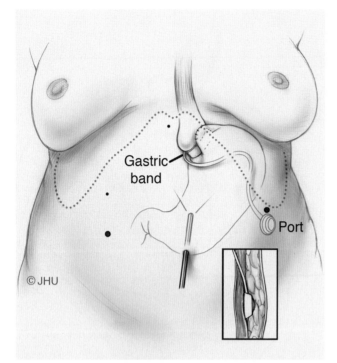

FIGURE 2   Laparoscopic adjustable gastric band. *(Courtesy Corinne Sandone, Johns Hopkins University.)*

The mesenteric defect between the Roux limb mesentery and the transverse mesocolon is then closed up to the level of the transverse colon. If desired, a drain can be placed adjacent to the gastric pouch, but it is usually removed prior to hospital discharge. If clinically indicated in select patients, we perform a gastrografin swallow study on postoperative day one or two to check for leakage or obstruction.

Laparoscopic Adjustable Gastric Band

The laparoscopic adjustable gastric band (LAGB) received Food and Drug Administration approval in 2002 and has been in clinical use in the United States since that time. It is the only device that is adjustable after surgery, allowing for tightening or loosening of the band via a subcutaneous port placed for fluid injection. Other advantages of the band include relative ease of placement, lack of operative staple lines or need for bowel transection, and reversibility. The band does require, however, an average of five to six adjustments in the first year after surgery, and its success depends in part on patient compliance and close follow-up.

The LAGB procedure (Figure 2) is routinely performed using two 12 mm trocars, one 5 mm trocar, and a 15 mm trocar for band placement. The liver is retracted, similar to the gastric bypass, with a Nathanson retractor. Dissection is first performed bluntly at the angle of His, freeing up attachments for later insertion of the band. The gastrohepatic ligament adjacent to the lesser curve of the stomach is then divided with electrocautery. The right crus is identified, its inferior anterior surface is scored using electrocautery, and the anterior peritoneal tissue is divided. Two graspers are used to carefully dissect in this plane of tissue posterior to the gastroesophageal junction.

An articulating dissector is then placed from the right crus side up toward the angle of His; it is then flexed to a right angle and locked in place. The adjustable band is placed in the abdomen through the 15 mm trocar in the left upper quadrant. The band is then secured to the articulating dissector and brought around the stomach, as the dissector is withdrawn; the band is locked into place with a slightly diagonal orientation up toward the angle of His. Two sutures are then placed from the fundus to the proximal stomach around the band, securing

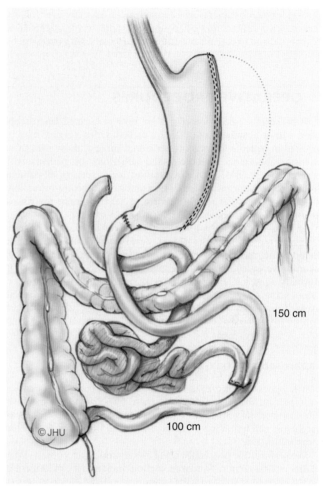

FIGURE 3   Duodenal switch with biliopancreatic diversion. *(Courtesy Corinne Sandone, Johns Hopkins University.)*

the band in place and minimizing the possibility of band migration or herniation. The band tubing is brought out through the left upper quadrant trocar site, where it is secured to the subcutaneous injection port. Fascia is cleared in this area, and the port is secured to the fascia with care so as not to entrap or kink the band tubing.

Laparoscopic Duodenal Switch with Biliopancreatic Diversion

The laparoscopic duodenal switch with biliopancreatic diversion (DS-BPD) is primarily a malabsorptive operation that involves preservation of the gastric pylorus and creation of a short, 100 cm ileal "common channel," where food and biliopancreatic enzymes are allowed to mix. Because of the potential for malabsorption-related nutritional deficiencies and the complexity of the operation, DS-BPD is the least common bariatric operation performed (5% to 10% overall).

The first step in the DS-BPD (Figure 3) involves dividing the small bowel 250 cm from the ileocecal valve. The proximal end of bowel is then anastomosed to the distal ileum 100 cm from its juncture with the cecum. The patient is then placed in steep reverse Trendelenburg position, and a liver retractor is placed to retract the left lateral segment of the liver. A vertical sleeve gastrectomy is then performed over a 48 Fr bougie to reduce the size of the stomach while leaving the pylorus intact. The duodenum is divided approximately 3 to 4 cm distal to the pylorus with a blue staple cartridge.

The Roux limb is then brought antecolic up to the end of the proximal duodenum, and a side-to-side anastomosis performed. With the

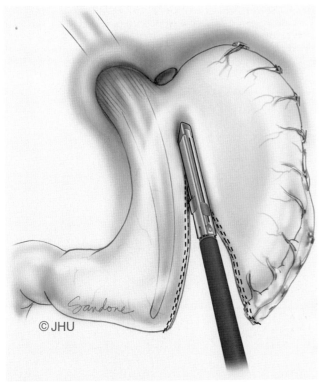

FIGURE 4 Laparoscopic vertical sleeve gastrectomy. *(Courtesy Corinne Sandone, Johns Hopkins University.)*

Roux limb clamped, an air-leak or liquid dye test can be performed via an orogastric tube to check for possible leaks at the stomach staple line or ileoduodenal anastomosis. The mesenteric defect is then closed between the Roux limb mesentery and the transverse mesocolon, and a closed suction drain is left near the stomach and the ileoduodenal anastomosis.

Laparoscopic Vertical Sleeve Gastrectomy

Of the commonly performed bariatric procedures, the laparoscopic vertical sleeve gastrectomy (LVSG) is the most recent to be introduced, and only limited outcomes data (5 years) are available. Because it is primarily restrictive, long-term outcomes will likely parallel those of the adjustable band. Unlike the band, however, the LVSG does not involve an implanted foreign body that can potentially erode or migrate, and it does not require frequent adjustments. The sleeve resection may also achieve weight loss by impacting satiety. Serum levels of ghrelin, a proappetite hormone produced in the fundus, are reduced after the LVSG because that area of the stomach has been resected. In addition, the sleeve procedure is not reversible because a partial gastrectomy is performed; but it can be converted to a gastric bypass or duodenal switch later if greater weight loss is desired.

The LVSG (Figure 4) is performed using one 5 mm and three 12 mm trocars. With the liver retracted, the short gastric vessels along the greater curve of the stomach are divided, beginning near the antrum and extending to the angle of His. A 40 Fr bougie is placed in the stomach and directed along the lesser curve. The stomach is then divided with the stapler (blue or green cartridge) using the bougie as a guide, beginning 6 cm from the pylorus on the greater curve side and continuing up to the angle of His. The staple line can be oversewn with a running absorbable suture. Alternatively, an absorbable staple buttress material may also be used to help prevent bleeding. Air or liquid dye can be infused via an orogastric tube into the newly created "sleeve" to rule out a leak. The lateral stomach specimen is then removed from one of the trocar sites, and we routinely place a drain in the left upper quadrant.

OUTCOMES AND COMPLICATIONS

After any procedure, patients are seen in follow-up at 2 weeks after surgery and then at 3, 6, 12, 18, and 24 months and yearly thereafter. Patients are maintained on a pureed, high-protein diet for the first month after surgery and are gradually advanced to solid food. LAGB patients receive their first band fill, the injection of fluid into the subcutaneous port to tighten the band, at 6 weeks and then every 2 months as needed, depending on restriction and weight loss. All patients receive multivitamin, calcium, and vitamin B_{12} supplements. This is especially important for gastric bypass and DS-BPD patients, who are at higher at risk for malabsorption and possible malnutrition. Supplemental iron should also be considered for menstruating women.

Weight loss after gastric bypass and DS-BPD occurs primarily in the first 12 to 18 months after surgery and averages approximately 70% and 80% excess weight loss (EWL), respectively. Expected EWL after the LAGB and the sleeve gastrectomy is somewhat less (40% to 50%) and occurs over a longer time (2 to 3 years). Perhaps the most important outcome measure after bariatric surgery, however, is remission of obesity-related metabolic diseases, such as type 2 diabetes. Over 70% to 80% of patients with diabetes will experience complete remission after gastric bypass or DS-BPD. The more restrictive operations, LAGB and LVSG, usually result in remission rates of 50% to 60%. Similar remission rates are seen for other metabolic diseases such as hypertension, sleep apnea, hyperlipidemia, and fatty liver disease.

The main complications of bariatric surgery are seen primarily in the early perioperative period. Mortality is usually less than 1% and is primarily attributable to pulmonary emboli or sepsis secondary to anastomotic or staple-line leakage. Persistent and unexplained tachycardia (>120 beats/min) postoperatively should raise suspicion for leakage and prompt an appropriate workup. Patients with a history of pulmonary emboli or an inherited coagulopathy should be considered for additional prophylaxis, such as vena caval filter insertion or extended anticoagulation with low molecular weight heparin after hospital discharge. The incidence of pulmonary emboli or leakage in most reported series is usually less than 1%.

Vitamin B_{12}, calcium, iron, vitamin D, and protein deficiencies can all occur in the first year after surgery and require nutritional monitoring. Vitamin B_1 deficiency can occur in patients with protracted vomiting after surgery and may present with extremity parasthesias and confusion. Lower extremity weakness and parasthesias can also be seen with vitamin B_{12} deficiency. Anastomotic stenosis and obstruction at the gastrojejunostomy in the first few months after surgery occur in less than 5% of patients after gastric bypass and can usually be managed with endoscopic dilatation. Late symptoms of bowel obstruction after gastric bypass should raise the suspicion for a possible internal hernia, which may require operative repair. Overall complication rates after bariatric surgery in most reports are less than 15%.

In general, the results of weight-loss surgery are excellent, with the majority of patients losing more than 50% of their excess weight. Approximately 10% to 15% of patients either will not achieve significant weight loss or will partially regain their weight after 2 to 3 years. These patients usually respond to dietary counseling, although some may require operative revision or conversion to a more malabsorptive procedure.

Unfortunately, there is currently a lack of evidence-based data to help health care providers decide which primary operation will result in the best outcome for an individual patient. It is important for patients and providers to understand that weight-loss surgery is not designed to achieve a cosmetic result but rather to reverse obesity-related disease and improve overall health and quality of life. Patients need to be aware that although most operations are reversible, weight-loss surgery should be viewed as a lifelong commitment to behavioral and dietary modification and medical supervision.

Suggested Readings

Adams TD, Gress RE, Smith SC, et al: Long-term mortality after gastric bypass surgery, *N Engl J Med* 357:753, 2007.

Buchwald H, Avidor Y, Braunwald E, et al: Bariatric surgery: a systemic review and meta-analysis, *JAMA* 292:1724, 2004.

Melton G, Steele K, Schweitzer MA, et al: Suboptimal weight loss after gastric bypass surgery: correlation of demographics, comorbidities, and insurance status with outcomes, *J Gastrointest Surg* 12:250, 2008.

Schweitzer MA, Lidor A, Magnuson TH: 251 consecutive laparoscopic gastric bypass operations using a 2-layer gastrojejunostomy technique with a zero leak rate, *J Laparoendosc Adv Surg Tech* 16:83, 2006.

SMALL BOWEL OBSTRUCTION

George J. Arnaoutakis, MD, and Frederic E. Eckhauser, MD

OVERVIEW

Although surgical techniques and innovations continue to evolve, obstruction of the small bowel remains a common and vexing clinical problem. In the early 1900s, hernias represented the most common cause of small bowel obstruction (SBO). However, that pattern has shifted; today, postoperative adhesions are the most common cause, accounting for nearly 75% of all SBOs.

With the advent of laparoscopic surgery, the incidence of SBO has not changed. One third of all obstructions due to adhesive disease will manifest within 1 year following initial laparotomy, with two thirds of these events occurring in the initial postoperative period. Hernia is the second most common cause of SBO; tumors, typically arising from metastatic colorectal cancer, are the third leading cause. Intussusception (Figures 1 and 2), bezoar, gallstone ileus, Crohn's disease, and volvulus are all interesting medical conditions that infrequently result in SBO.

Approximately one fourth of all patients with SBO will need an operation during the index admission, and patients who undergo initial operative management have fewer recurrent obstructive episodes (Foster, 2007). Landercasper and colleagues (1993) documented a 42% risk of subsequent obstruction in the 10 years following initial SBO. The rate of recurrence was 29% in patients treated surgically and 53% for patients managed nonoperatively.

As with etiology, prior surgical history, partial versus complete obstruction, first occurrence versus numerous recurrences, comorbidities, patient condition, and imaging results all contribute to the surgeon's judgment in pursuing nonoperative management. However, where appropriate, the timely decision to operate may avoid the untoward effects of inappropriate delay, including bowel incarceration and strangulation. In the setting of full-thickness necrosis and perforation, septic shock may ensue with devastating consequences, and many series report mortality rates greater than 33% in the setting of bowel ischemia.

INITIAL EVALUATION

During the initial evaluation of patients with suspected SBO, the primary objectives are to gauge the degree of metabolic derangement and volume depletion and to assess the need for and expediency of surgery. As with many surgical conditions, determining the correct diagnosis and management strategy hinges on a focused yet thorough history and physical examination.

Usual complaints with SBO include nausea, vomiting, distension, crampy abdominal pain that is periumbilical, and decreased flatus and bowel movements; episodic diarrhea can also be consistent with partial obstruction. The constellation of symptoms will vary based on three factors: (1) the *anatomic site* of the obstruction (proximal versus distal), (2) the *elapsed time* between onset and presentation, and (3) the *severity* of the obstruction (complete vs. partial).

Physical assessment should evaluate signs of systemic shock and also concentrate on the abdominal examination. A chemistry profile will detect metabolic derangements, and a finding of leukocytosis or lactic acidemia supports the presence of bowel ischemia. Novel biomarkers suggestive of mucosal ischemia, such as intestinal fatty-acid binding protein, hold promise for diagnosing enterocyte necrosis but are not yet widely used in clinical practice.

Initial radiographic evaluation begins with plain x-ray films of the abdomen (supine and erect) and an upright chest radiograph. An upright chest radiograph is of paramount importance to inspect for pneumoperitoneum and also for evidence of aspiration in a patient with a history of vomiting. A simple SBO is associated with air-fluid levels, dilated loops of intestine, and absence of colonic gas on plain film radiographs.

In the past, a small bowel series was the next imaging study used, but it has been replaced by computed tomography (CT) scan, which has the resolution to assess the degree of obstruction and can also elucidate the cause, such as the presence of a mass (Figure 3) or a hernia with subsequent obstruction (Figure 4). In addition, CT has high sensitivity for detecting strangulation and pneumoperitoneum indicative of a perforation, and is particularly useful in the early postoperative setting to rule out ischemia, intraabdominal abscess, or morbidity as the underlying cause. It is also useful in patients with a history of malignancy to differentiate potentially recurrent disease from adhesions (Figure 5). In patients with many comorbidities in

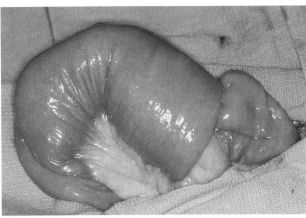

FIGURE I   Small bowel intussusception.

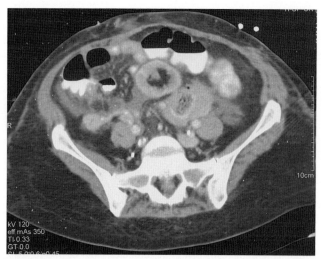

FIGURE 2   CT scan of small bowel intussusception with typical target sign.

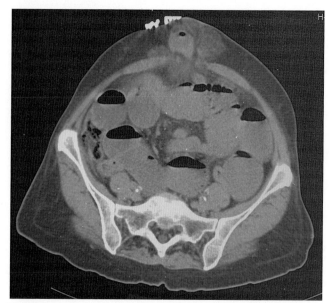

FIGURE 4   CT scan of complete small bowel obstruction due to incisional hernia.

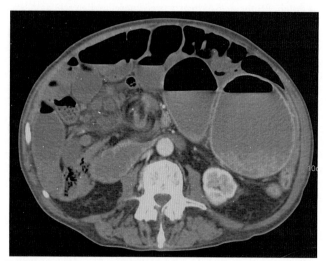

FIGURE 3   CT scan of small bowel volvulus with notable mesenteric torsion.

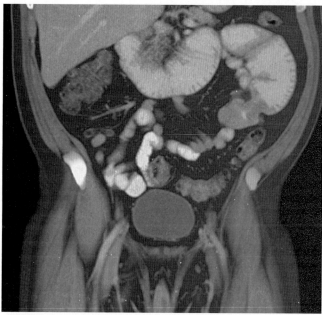

FIGURE 5   Coronal image of CT scan showing mass in proximal small bowel with decompressed loops of small bowel distal to obstruction.

whom nonoperative management is preferred, CT scan is the preferred serial imaging study because of the ability to detect subtle signs of bowel ischemia, such as wall thickening, free peritoneal fluid, or pneumatosis intestinalis.

A newer application of CT technology is CT enterography, in which intraluminal distension is achieved with administration of large volumes of oral contrast such as water-methylcellulose solution. This modality is most often used to diagnose patients with Crohn's disease–related strictures, and its benefit is high-resolution imaging of the bowel wall; however, it is impractical in the patient with gastrointestinal (GI) distress who is nauseated and vomiting.

A small bowel series is useful in patients undergoing nonoperative management who do not exhibit signs of strangulation yet fail to resolve the obstruction. Enteroclysis, in which the proximal small bowel is accessed by fluoroscopic guidance and then instilled with air and contrast for delineating the bowel wall, has an even more limited application; however, both modalities of contrast study are highly predictive of eventual spontaneous resolution if contrast reaches the cecum within 24 hours. A recent Cochrane review found that water-soluble contrast administration does not improve resolution of SBO, but it may shorten hospital stay in patients managed nonoperatively (Abbas, 2007). Barium impaction occurs very infrequently following a small bowel series, typically in patients with severe dehydration. However,

the surgeon should be vigilant for this clinical scenario, which will worsen the severity of the SBO.

Ultrasound remains an important modality in the evaluation of patients with suspected SBO, and some authors have shown ultrasound to be more sensitive and specific than plain radiographs alone. This test is especially useful in pregnant patients or as a bedside test in the critically ill.

A distinction should be made between SBO and nonobstructive motility disorders such as paralytic ileus or pseudoobstruction. Some extent of paralytic ileus occurs following the majority of open abdominal operations, and motility disorders can occur as a result of recent major surgery, abdominal trauma, mesenteric ischemia, electrolyte disturbances, or peritonitis. Many of the symptoms of motility disorders overlap those of SBO, but an accurate diagnosis can be made with a careful history and appropriate radiographic examination.

NONOPERATIVE MANAGEMENT

Vigorous fluid resuscitation and correction of electrolyte disorders underpin the initial therapeutic goals of both nonoperative and pre-operative management strategies. Patients with protracted vomiting prior to presentation will exhibit a hypochloremic, hypokalemic metabolic alkalosis with concomitant paradoxic aciduria. Placing a Foley catheter to measure urinary output, establishing adequate intravenous access, and reassessing hemodynamic and electrolyte status are all essential in the initial management.

Because unabated intraluminal distension leads to mucosal ischemia, GI decompression is paramount in the treatment of SBO. Historically, the tube used for decompression had been a matter of debate, but it has become less so in recent years. A standard nasogastric (NG) tube provides symptomatic relief, prevents added gas and fluid accumulation proximally, and enables the serial assessment of antegrade fluid movement. Care should be taken to ensure that nasoenteric tubes are properly functioning because they render the lower and upper esophageal sphincters incompetent and pose a theoretical risk of aspiration. Although long intestinal tubes are more cumbersome to place, they may increase resolution of SBO, making them an especially useful adjunct in patients who are poor operative candidates.

In patients undergoing serial abdominal examination and attempted nonoperative management, the use of narcotics has been debated. Many studies have shown that experienced clinicians are wrong over 50% of the time in predicting the presence of necrotic bowel, and abdominal pain is an unreliable predictor of strangulation. Moreover, there are several patient populations in whom narcotic medications should not be withheld: a postoperative patient, chronic pain patients, trauma patients, and those patients with known intraabdominal cancer. A patient with an escalating need for narcotic medication who does not fit into one of these groups likely warrants operative exploration.

It is important to identify those patients most likely to succeed with a nonoperative approach. Patients with low-grade partial SBOs are prone to spontaneous resolution with conservative interventions such as bowel rest, NG decompression, and appropriate fluid resuscitation. These patients demonstrate improving pain, decreased distension, and improving imaging studies. Their diet can be slowly advanced as they continue to show clinical improvement. Occasionally, a small bowel series or enteroclysis can be useful in those patients who do not achieve complete resolution of the obstruction.

In the absence of systemic signs, patients presenting with an early postoperative obstruction following abdominal surgery also deserve an attempt at nonoperative management. Some series report the rate of spontaneous resolution to exceed 90%. When pursuing a nonoperative approach, these patients and those with incomplete low-grade bowel obstruction benefit from a period of total parenteral nutrition (TPN) to prevent the sequelae of negative nitrogen balance.

Patients with multiple prior episodes of bowel obstruction, especially those with a history of spontaneous improvement, warrant an attempt at conservative management. In addition, patients who have undergone numerous abdominal operations should be treated nonoperatively if possible. As long as the patient remains clinically stable and shows signs of improvement, the prudent surgeon will avoid reentering a hostile abdomen.

Crohn's disease typically will cause incomplete obstruction. If the obstructive episode represents an initial symptomatic event for a specific site of obstruction or stricture, then initially these patients should be managed conservatively. Patients with Crohn's disease will also benefit from steroids or other immunosuppressive therapy, and these measures are not reported to increase infection risk in the perioperative period.

Blunt abdominal trauma may also result in SBO; this most commonly occurs in children but may affect adults as well. The obstruction typically arises due to intramural hematoma and most frequently involves the duodenum. In patients who do not have peritonitis, nonoperative management is appropriate and will likely include the use of TPN because these episodes occasionally take weeks to resolve. Imaging studies can be useful in guiding the timing of gradually reintroducing food.

In very rare situations, early evacuation of intramural hematoma may be necessary. This intervention is infrequently needed; obstruction typically resolves between 2 and 4 weeks. If symptoms of obstruction persist beyond 4 weeks, it is important to consider possible progression to fibrosis. Surgery should be reserved for patients who develop fibrosis, which will require either a gastrojejunostomy or duodenojejunostomy to bypass the area of fibrotic narrowing.

OPERATIVE MANAGEMENT

More than 25% of inpatients admitted because of SBO will require an operation. Patients with complete or high-grade partial SBO are most likely to need surgery, with less than 20% successfully managed nonoperatively. Significant abdominal pain consistent with peritonitis, high fever, tachycardia, and leukocytosis are all worrisome situations that warrant expeditious surgical intervention. Surgery should also be strongly considered for patients who are clinically stable but who do not demonstrate any improvement within 24 hours of nonoperative treatment.

SBO is unlikely due to adhesions without a prior history of abdominal surgery; therefore this group of patients warrants operative management. Incarcerated hernia, tumor, or the initial presentation of Crohn's disease should be considered. The objectives of surgery are to relieve the obstruction and also address the underlying etiology with appropriate operative treatment, including tumor resection or hernia repair.

Patients with a history of intraabdominal malignancy can be difficult to manage. When patients have known recurrent disease, many surgeons pursue nonoperative therapy. However, studies have shown that two thirds of these patients have a lesion amenable to surgical correction, such as an adhesive band or a resectable area of malignant disease. The remaining third likely harbor carcinomatosis. This diagnosis can be extremely difficult to ascertain with preoperative imaging, with studies noting significant interobserver variability. Unless the surgeon is certain of the presence of carcinomatosis, patients with a known history of intraabdominal malignancy should undergo operative management. Obstructions occurring soon after the initial cancer operation are more likely due to recurrent malignancy, whereas adhesions become the more probable cause when obstructions develop at a later time.

Intussusception is a more common clinical entity in the pediatric population than in adults, and one must worry about a pathologic lead point, such as a tumor, when an adult presents with this condition. In children the risk of malignancy is very low, and intussusception can usually be treated with radiographic decompression. In contrast, 50% of adult patients will harbor a malignancy, and operative management is usually required.

A history of numerous SBOs usually represents a challenging problem in that a majority of these patients have undergone multiple abdominal operations, making the technical difficulty much greater. If a patient with recurrent obstructions does not respond to a prolonged course of nonoperative management, including use of TPN, surgery is warranted.

In the setting of a repeat laparotomy, most surgeons prefer a long midline incision and enter the peritoneal space through a previously unopened portion if possible. Many times there will not be a clearly defined site of obstruction. These patients require careful adhesiolysis to free the small intestine. In selected situations, especially in the setting of numerous prior SBOs, placement of a long intestinal tube may be considered. Such tubes should be left in place for approximately 2 to 3 weeks.

Other rare sources of intraluminal obstruction include bezoar, gallstone ileus, and possibly barium from previous radiographic studies. These conditions generally cause complete obstruction that warrants surgery. Patients with gallstone ileus usually have radiographically apparent stones within the intestinal lumen, usually in the distal ileum; pneumobilia from a biliary-enteric fistula; and SBO. Appropriate management begins with milking the stone retrograde and performing an enterotomy in a region of proximally dilated small bowel to extract the stone. Partial bowel resection for severely impacted stones is occasionally necessary. The entire small intestine should be examined for remaining stones. Additionally, cholecystectomy and repair of the biliary-enteric fistula should be performed. If the fistula occurs between the distal common bile duct and the duodenum, the definitive repair necessitates closure of the fistula and biliary reconstruction with a Roux-en-Y choledochojejunostomy.

Patients who experience early postoperative SBO are more likely to respond to nonoperative management. However, in patients who do not respond, the timing of reexploration is critical. If based on the clinical situation that the patient has not required reoperation within the first 7 to 10 days, then the most prudent course is to delay until 4 weeks postoperatively, as the clinical picture permits. During the 10- to 30-day postoperative window, as part of the healing process, adhesions are vascular, cohesive, and thickened.

Special Technical Considerations

Once the obstruction has been resolved at the time of surgery, the surgeon must perform a diligent and complete determination of bowel viability. The bowel often will clearly be pink and unequivocally viable, and this assessment can be rendered with subjective criteria. Occasionally this decision is more difficult, and some subjective signs, such as motility, may be misleading. When this situation arises, the surgeon should exercise patience. Irrigating the peritoneal cavity with warm saline and ensuring the prior placement of external forced-air warming blankets will help maintain normothermia. The wound should be covered to minimize further heat and fluid loss, and 10 minutes should elapse.

If upon reinspection viability remains questionable, two maneuvers can be used: Doppler and fluorescein. Bulkley et al (1981) reported a series showing that intravenous fluorescein (1000 mg) and Woods lamp illumination more accurately assess bowel viability than standard Doppler or subjective assessment. Laser Doppler velocimetry holds more promise than standard Doppler but is not as widely available and is less practical than fluorescein administration. If a large segment of bowel appears threatened, and after these maneuvers viability is not clearly established, many surgeons advocate returning to the operating room in 24 hours for a repeat assessment. If the segment in question is very limited, much of the effort exerted to determine viability is better spent performing a resection at the initial operation.

Some surgeons recommend luminal decompression as an important maneuver to promote blood flow to the distended, edematous, and previously obstructed bowel segment. There is also the belief that this technique enables easier closure of the abdomen. The surgeon can manually milk enteric contents in the retrograde direction to reach the NG tube. This must be conducted in close communication with the anesthesiology team to ensure a properly functioning NG tube to prevent possible aspiration; and great care must be taken handling the bowel, as extensive manipulation of the bowel wall may result in traumatic injury. If a bowel resection is necessary, decompression can be accomplished by briefly inserting a soft drainage catheter into the proximal bowel lumen prior to completing the planned bowel anastomosis.

Laparoscopy

With newer technological innovations, the role of laparoscopy in the management of patients with SBO continues to evolve. Although there are no clear contraindications, patients with massive bowel distension, multiple prior laparotomies, or early postoperative obstruction, or who exhibit obvious peritonitis are not good candidates for the laparoscopic approach.

Initial trocar placement within the abdominal cavity should be performed using the open technique to avoid underlying bowel injury. Additional ports can then be inserted with the advantage of direct vision. Atraumatic grasping instruments, strategic operating table positioning, and examining the entire course of the bowel, starting at the ileocecal valve, all improve success rates with the laparoscopic approach. Some series cite 80% success rates at resolving bowel obstruction laparoscopically, and retrospective data suggest this approach may result in earlier return of bowel function and shorter hospital stays (Szomstein, 2006).

Adhesion Prevention

Much of the focus in preventing SBO revolves around managing adhesion formation. Early procedures, such as the Noble plication, described suturing the bowel during abdominal surgery into anatomic patterns that would seem to prevent obstruction formation. This technique is advocated by some surgeons but is not widely practiced.

There are many chemical agents that have been studied to prevent postoperative adhesions. Nonsteroidal antiinflammatory drugs, steroid solutions, lubricants, chemotherapeutic agents, fibrinolytic compounds, and dextran have all been used. None of these chemicals produces a significant decrease in the development of bowel obstruction, and some have resulted in increased postoperative infection complications.

Currently, bioresorbable membrane technology harbors the most promise in adhesion prevention. Several currently available are Intercede (oxygenated regenerated cellulose; Ethicon, Somerville, NJ) and Seprafilm (sodium hyaluronate–based carboxymethylcellulose; Genzyme, Cambridge, Mass.). These materials usually consist of a thin transparent film and can be difficult to handle. A newer material, SurgiWrap (polylactide; MAST Biosurgery, San Diego, Calif.), is a bioresorbable sheet that is easier to handle; it reinforces fascial strength and minimizes formation of intraabdominal adhesions.

Studies have shown that these adhesion barriers are effective at preventing adhesions to intraabdominal surfaces on which they are placed. A recent Cochrane review concluded that these materials decrease adhesion severity; however, there is no effect on the rate of SBO or the need for reoperations (Kumar, 2009). One could argue that their main benefit, as of now, remains easier reentry into a patient who has undergone prior abdominal operations.

SUGGESTED READINGS

Abbas S, Bissett IP, Parry BR: Oral water-soluble contrast for the management of adhesive small bowel obstruction, *Cochrane Database Syst Rev*, 2007:CD004651.
Bulkley GB, Zuidema GD, Hamilton SR, et al: Intraoperative determination of small intestinal viability following ischemic injury: a prospective, controlled trial of two adjuvant methods (Doppler and fluorescein) compared with standard clinical judgment, *Ann Surg* 193:628, 1981.
Foster NM, McGory ML, Zingmond DS, et al: Small bowel obstruction: a population-based appraisal, *J Am Coll Surg* 203:170, 2006.
Kumar S, Wong PF, Leaper DJ: Intra-peritoneal prophylactic agents for preventing adhesions and adhesive intestinal obstruction after non-gynaecological abdominal surgery, *Cochrane Database Syst Rev* CD005080, 2009.
Szomstein S, Lo Menzo E, Simpfendorfer C, et al: Laparoscopic lysis of adhesions, *World J Surg* 30:535, 2006.

CROHN'S DISEASE OF THE SMALL BOWEL

Sharon L. Stein, MD, and Fabrizio Michelassi, MD

OVERVIEW

Crohn's disease is a transmural inflammatory process that affects the gastrointestinal (GI) tract from mouth to anus and may cause septic, obstructive, neoplastic, or hemorrhagic complications. The etiology of Crohn's disease is unknown, but it appears to be autoimmune in origin and is associated with Northern European descent and increased socioeconomic status.

There is currently no cure for Crohn's disease; pharmacologic and surgical interventions are aimed at the control of symptoms and prevention of long-term complications, which include disease recurrence and malabsorptive syndromes from loss of functional intestinal length. Approximately 70% of patients with Crohn's disease will require surgery for their disease, and in 50% disease will recur and require a second operation. Treatment of Crohn's disease is best performed in collaboration with experts that include a gastroenterologist, surgeons, radiologists, pathologists, nutritionists and, when needed, enterostomal therapists and psychologists.

Patients with Crohn's disease often present with nonspecific symptoms such as abdominal pain, bloating, diarrhea, and anorexia. Pain may be diffuse or localized. Patients may experience chronic intermittent GI distress that helps differentiate Crohn's disease from acute processes such as appendicitis. Approximately 40% of patients will have involvement of the terminal ileum; the colon is involved in approximately 20% of patients, 10% of patients have isolated disease in the jejunum and ileum, and 10% have isolated involvement of the anus. The remaining patients have disease in multiple locations throughout the GI tract.

Diagnosis of Crohn's disease is based on an accurate history and physical exam, including anal examination, and on a combination of several of the following studies: (1) upper endoscopy to evaluate gastroesophageal and duodenal disease, (2) colonoscopy to characterize colonic or ileal disease, (3) traditional small bowel contrast studies or advanced computed tomographic (CT) enterography to reveal intraluminal manifestions that include fistulas, and (4) traditional CT with oral contrast to evaluate extraluminal complications such as intraabdominal abscesses or inflammatory masses.

MEDICAL MANAGEMENT

Crohn's disease is unusual in its diversity of presentation and disease phenotype. The Vienna Classification divided Crohn's disease into three major phenotypes: *stricturing, fistulizing, and inflammatory* disease. When recurring, disease tends to reappear in the same anatomic location: small bowel disease tends to present in a similar distribution, ileocolic disease most frequently recurs at the site of prior anastomosis, and colonic disease tends to reappear in the colon. Similarly, disease behavior frequently follows familiar patterns: stricturing disease recurs with strictures, fistulizing disease with fistulas, and inflammatory disease with phlegmonous masses.

Inflammatory disease is often the most responsive to medical therapy. Inflammation is typically treated with a number of medications including aminosalicylate (5-ASA) derivatives, steroids, antibiotics, immunomodulators, or biologics. When successful, partial obstructions, intermittent abdominal pain, diarrhea, and anorexia may resolve. In general, stricturing disease is less responsive to medical

management. Occasionally, strictures can be dilatated with endoscopic balloon interventions; but in general, endoscopic treatment is limited by inaccessibility, fixed strictures, and disease recurrence. Ultimately, most strictures require definitive surgical treatment. Extensive or disabling perineal fistulizing disease can be treated with biologic therapy, shown to reduce both the incidence and symptoms of fistulization.

Initial management of Crohn's disease is medical unless a complication has evolved, such as abscess; cutaneous, vaginal, or urinary fistulas; perforation; obstruction; GI hemorrhage; or malignancy. Medical management is typically pharmacologic in nature and focuses on reduction of inflammation and autoimmune reaction in the short term and maintenance of remission in the long term. For this reason, immunologic medications such as steroids, antimetabolites, and anti–tumor necrosis factor-alpha (TNF-α) medications are frequently used.

Therapies used in the treatment of Crohn's disease are listed in Figure 1 and can be used in either a bottom-up or top-down approach. In a bottom-up approach, milder medications with lesser side-effect profiles are prescribed initially, with increasing strength of medications if milder medications fail. The premise in a top-down approach is that naïve disease responds more favorably to "big guns" and surgery; biologics and immunologics are used more liberally early in the disease course.

Derivatives of 5-ASA, including sulfasalazine and mesalamine, are antiinflammatory derivatives used orally or transrectally to treat mild to moderate Crohn's disease and maintain remission. These 5-ASA agents are formulated to allow targeted distribution of medication to a specific intestinal target with 70% response rates. Although 5-ASA derivatives decrease inflammation through the arachidonic acid pathway, use of nonsteroidal antiinflammatory drugs (NSAIDs) such as ibuprofen and ketorolac are associated with worsening disease flares and should not be given to patients with Crohn's disease. Derivatives of 5-ASA are not associated with increased perioperative complications and can be maintained until the operation and resumed immediately after surgery.

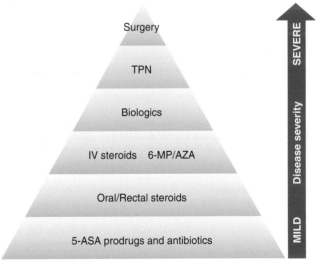

FIGURE 1 Medications and interventions used in the treatment of Crohn's disease. Treatment is initiated with medications at the bottom of the pyramid for mild disease. If disease progresses, treatment progresses up the pyramid in the typical "bottom-up" approach. Recently, a "top-down" approach has been utilized; patients with severe disease are initially treated with stronger medications, such as biologics, and early utilization of surgery to quickly quell active disease and prevent further progression. *TPN,* total parenteral nutrition; *IV,* intravenous; *6-MP,* 6-mercaptopurine; *AZA,* azathioprine; *5-ASA,* aminosalicylates. *(From Scherl E, Weitzman G, Feuerstadt P: Crohn's and colitis crossroads update 2006: part 2, Gastroenterology & Endoscopy News, 2006; 4:31-36.)*

Steroids are used orally, intravenously, or rectally for the acute treatment of moderate to severe disease. In the short term, steroids decrease inflammation in 60% to 80% of patients and allow for improved intestinal function, but long-term steroid dependence is associated with significant side effects that include growth retardation, osteopenia, cushingoid features, systemic hypertension, glomerular nephritis, cataracts, necrosis of the head of the femur, and adrenal suppression. Patients on long-term steroids are at risk of perioperative adrenal crisis that can result in hemodynamic instability, unless stress doses of steroids are administered perioperatively. In addition, long-term use of steroids can result in poor wound healing, increased risk of infection, or other perioperative problems. Long-term use of steroids may complicate diagnosis by masking signs and symptoms of disease, including early findings of peritonitis.

Antibiotics are often used in conjunction with other medications for the treatment of acute inflammation and perianal disease. Fluoroquinolones, metronidazole, and rifaximin are commonly used. Antibiotics have not been shown to be detrimental when used in the perioperative setting, but recent reports show an increase in the prevalence of *Clostridium difficile* in patients with inflammatory bowel disease, which may be associated with antibiotic usage.

Immunologics such as azathioprine and 6-mercaptopurine are useful for the maintenance of remission for 40% to 60% of patients, but the slow onset of action limits their efficacy in acute disease flares. Immunologics are antimetabolites that inhibit ribonucleic acid synthesis, much like chemotherapeutic agents. Side effects include pancreatitis, bone marrow suppression, and flulike symptoms. Immunologics have not been shown to complicate postoperative course when urgent surgery is needed.

Biologics are the most recent addition to the Crohn's disease pharmacologic armamentarium, with response rates up to 70%, including patients with fistulizing disease. Biologics such as TNF-α antagonists (infliximab, adalimumab) reduce T-cell proliferation, decreasing inflammation in patients with Crohn's disease. Medications are delivered intravenously or subcutaneously, and side-effects of the medications include infusion reactions, increased risk of infection, and lymphoma.

Some evidence suggests that use of these agents in the perioperative period may increase the risk or severity of perioperative infection. Unfortunately, studies are retrospective, heterogeneous, and poorly powered, limiting their clinical validity; further data are necessary to fully elucidate the associated risks. Our practice is to avoid operating on patients with therapeutic levels of biologics, if possible, for up to 12 weeks; unfortunately, this is rarely possible. Patients on biologics are frequently referred to the surgeon when failure of medical treatment occurs.

Patients with Crohn's disease may require nutritional supplementation secondary to intestinal dysfunction. Absorption may be decreased secondary to inflammation or stricture. Bacterial overgrowth in prestenotic dilated intestinal loops may contribute to malabsorption. Fat-soluble vitamins such as vitamins A, D, E, and K may be reduced secondary to ileal disease or prior resections.

Chronic disease may cause anemia, and patients with profuse diarrhea may have protein wasting or hypovolemia. Treatment of Crohn inflammation may reverse some of these findings, but supplementation with fluids, iron, blood products, and parenteral vitamins may also be required. Parenteral nutrition may be required in extreme cases of malabsorption.

INDICATIONS FOR SURGICAL MANAGEMENT

Indications for surgical intervention are multiple. Although inflammatory disease will often respond to pharmaceutical treatment, stricturing disease is often refractory to medical treatment and requires surgical resection. Progression of disease that includes complete obstruction, fistulization, abscess, presence of neoplasia, or

TABLE 1: Indications for surgical intervention in Crohn's disease

Acute	Subacute	Elective
Perforation	Neoplasia	Recurrent/medically
Sepsis	Abscess	refractory disease
Hemorrhage	Obstruction	Failure to wean/steroid
Toxic megacolon	Symptomatic fistula	dependence
	Refractory diarrhea	Growth retardation
	Malnutrition	(pediatric)

In almost all scenarios, except in an unstable patient or one with a perforation, an attempt at medical treatment may be appropriate. Patients with Crohn's disease often respond to medical interventions that include steroids, antibiotics, and bowel rest. Patients should be monitored closely by a surgical team. Failure to improve is an indication for immediate surgical intervention.

occurrence of GI hemorrhage are indications for surgical intervention, as indicated in Table 1.

The most common indication for surgical intervention is medically refractory Crohn's disease. Disease symptoms continue or worsen with therapy, or patients are unable to tolerate pharmacologic treatment. Patients may continue to lose weight; they have substantial diarrhea, or recurrent abdominal pain despite best medical therapy, and they may choose to undergo surgery.

Failure to wean from steroids is a frequent indication for surgical intervention. Other patients may choose not to undergo treatment with medical therapies known for substantial side effects, such as risk of infection, hepatic dysfunction, and bone marrow suppression. Growth retardation secondary to chronic disease and use of medications, including steroids, are an indication for surgery in up to 50% of children with Crohn's disease.

Obstructive disease occurs as a result of inflammation or stricturing disease. If obstructive symptoms remit with medical treatment, patients may choose to continue with medical management. Progressive disease is a common feature; therapy often fails to relieve symptoms, and surgery may be required. Patients may come in with a partial or complete obstruction; in patients with a history of previous surgery, bowel obstruction secondary to adhesions should be included in the surgeons' differential diagnosis.

Internal fistulas may be asymptomatic and do not necessarily require resection. A large fistula from proximal to distal intestine may cause a functional bypass of absorptive intestinal surface and consequent diarrhea or malabsorption, requiring surgical intervention. In addition, enterocutaneous or colocutaneous fistulas, fistulas to the vagina following hysterectomy, or fistulas to the bladder are often symptomatic and require surgical resection.

Inflammatory masses and abscesses typically cause abdominal pain and obstruction; in severe cases, they progress to fistula or become the source of systemic sepsis. They may be palpated on exam or noted on computed tomography (CT). When patients are stable, initial treatment consists of draining the liquid component with ultrasound or CT guidance. Antibiotics are prescribed until the surrounding inflammation has resolved. In most cases surgical intervention will ultimately be necessary, but a period of initial bowel rest aids in decreasing inflammation and facilitates operation. If necessary, parenteral nutrition can be used for nutritional supplementation while the abscess resolves and inflammation subsides.

Patients with Crohn's disease are at increased risk of neoplasia. In patients without inflammatory bowel disease, the incidence of small bowel cancer tends to decrease from proximal to distal small bowel; in Crohn's disease the incidence increases along the length of the small bowel and mimics disease distribution. Sporadic small bowel cancers form a mass or growth; in Crohn's disease, patients' cancers are often found without an associated mass lesion, which complicates diagnosis and screening.

Bleeding and toxic megacolon are both common indications for surgery in ulcerative colitis, but these are rare in the treatment of Crohn's disease. GI hemorrhage can originate from the small bowel or colon. Localization techniques, including endoscopy and angiogram, can be helpful in treatment or at least preoperative planning. Tagged red blood cell scans may help to discern small bowel from large bowel hemorrhage, but these rarely have the degree of precision in localizing the source of bleeding, which is required for targeted surgical therapy; intraoperative enteroscopy can help identify the source of bleeding. Toxic megacolon occurs in the setting of Crohn's colitis, and significant dilation of the colon with signs of leukocytosis, fever, or sepsis are indications for immediate surgical intervention.

Technical Considerations of Surgical Intervention

Thorough preoperative evaluation is paramount to successful operative outcomes in patients with Crohn's disease. Such patients may be dehydrated from chronic diarrhea and may have electrolyte imbalances that should be addressed prior to surgery. Malnutrition, anemia, and vitamin deficiencies are common and may require preoperative repletion.

Knowledge of preoperative medications is necessary. Chronic use of steroids demands perioperative administration of stress doses of steroids (usually intravenous hydrocortisone 100 mg before surgery, and then every 8 hours in the first 24 hours, followed by a rapid taper is sufficient to avoid the consequences of adrenal insufficiency). Recent use of biologics may increase postoperative risk of septic complications and anastomotic dehiscences.

Preoperative mapping of the extent of disease aids in operative planning and appropriate informed consent. Colonoscopy helps to evaluate the extent of colonic disease; CT scan, enteroscopy, and small bowel follow-through studies evaluate small bowel disease and the presence of abscesses or fistulas. Upper endoscopy elucidates the extent of gastroesophageal and duodenal disease.

Understanding of past surgical interventions is vital to prevent inadvertent injury to a matted segment of intestine that may be a prior strictureplasty and to ensure that remaining intestinal segments are adequately vascularized for anastomosis after resection of diseased areas. Length and extent of prior resections will help determine how essential it is to spare bowel and therefore how desirable it is to select strictureplasty over resection.

In patients with complicated, recurrent disease, it is not uncommon to discover unexpected intraoperative disease; up to 50% of fistulas are not diagnosed preoperatively, and diseased segments distal to an obstruction often lack radiographic findings of active disease. Informed consent should include discussion of possible additional surgical treatments, including resection or ostomy.

Any operation on a patient with Crohn's disease should commence with a thorough evaluation of the entire abdomen (see Figure 2). The small bowel should be inspected from the ligament of Treitz to the ileocecal valve, with measurements recording the total length of the small intestine and the extent and location of diseased segments; the intraperitoneal portion of the colon should also be examined and evaluated.

In Crohn's disease, only symptomatic and severely diseased segments should be resected. Findings of mild disease, including creeping fat and corkscrew vessels, are not indications for resection. Resection to microscopically negative margins has not decreased disease recurrence, and it causes unnecessary resection of additional bowel length. When operating on a patient with small intestinal obstructing disease, particular attention should be given to the bowel distal to the disease segment. When an upstream segment is obstructed or narrowed, downstream disease may be asymptomatic until after the resection, when narrowing and stricturing may cause an early postoperative "recurrence."

A Foley catheter may be used to grossly evaluate narrowed disease segments for consideration of resection or strictureplasty. After gentle insertion of the catheter in the intestinal loop, through an enterotomy

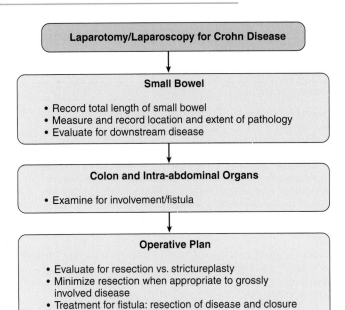

FIGURE 2   Operative plan for Crohn's disease. Whether performed laparoscopically or using open technique, appropriate abdominal exploration is critical to a successful operation. The small bowel should be run from the ligament of Treitz to the ileocecal valve and the location and extent of disease should be recorded. Small intestine distal to any obstruction should be examined for stricture or disease. The colon, vagina, and bladder should be evaluated for disease involvement or fistula when clinically indicated. After full exploration, an operative plan should be created that includes consideration of strictureplasty when appropriate.

at the anticipated site of resection or strictureplasty, the Foley balloon is inflated to 2 cm and gently pulled through the segments of the intestine that appear grossly narrowed. Any site where the inflated Foley balloon does not pass easily should be carefully examined and considered for additional resection or strictureplasty.

Most commonly, diseased segments of small intestine are resected with a primary anastomosis. A functional-end anastomosis, stapled side-to-side, allows for the most ample intestinal lumen at the site of the anastomosis. The proximal and distal intestinal ends are placed parallel to each other and stapled longitudinally with a linear gastrointestinal anastomosis stapler on the antimesenteric side of the bowel. The intestinal crotch is buttressed with a 3-0 Vicryl or silk suture. The staple line is examined, submucosal bleeding is controlled with electrocautery, and the common enterotomy is then stapled closed with a single thoracoabdominal linear stapler.

Hand-sewn anastomoses are most commonly used when there are disparities in the thickness of the two bowel loops to be anastomosed. We start with an interrupted layer of 3-0 silk Lembert (seromuscular) sutures on the back wall. A running layer of 3-0 Vicryl is used to approximate all layers of the bowel, typically run from the middle of the back wall of the anastomosis in each direction. After closing the enterotomy, a front wall of Lembert sutures is completed.

Malabsorption following small bowel resection is a direct correlate with the quantity of small bowel resected. Loss of the terminal ileum, which plays a specialized role in the absorption of fat, fat-soluble vitamins, and bile, may lead to vitamin deficiencies and increased diarrhea. When less than 100 cm of small bowel remains, severe malnutrition and diarrhea may occur. Any resection in a patient with Crohn's disease should consider the risk of future short gut syndrome and malabsorption.

To avoid the risk of short gut syndrome, bowel-sparing techniques or strictureplasties have become preferred alternatives, when technically

TABLE 2: Relative and absolute contraindications to strictureplasty*

Absolute	Relative
Perforation neoplasia	Abscess
Fistula	Long, severely narrowed segments†
Severe malnutrition	

*As techniques improve, fewer contraindications exist to strictureplasty.
†In the presence of a long, severely narrowed segment of small bowel preceded and followed by a loop with sequential strictures, the middle segment can be resected; the proximal and distal diseased loop may be preserved as part of a side-to-side isoperistaltic strictureplasty.

feasible, to bowel resection in Crohn patients. Strictureplasty provides an alternative to intestinal resection. By preserving bowel length and alleviating a narrow bowel lumen, strictureplasty reestablishes adequate intestinal patency while preserving bowel length.

Contraindications to strictureplasty, relative and absolute, are listed in Table 2. For short, isolated segments, a Heineke-Mikulicz strictureplasty can be used. A Finney strictureplasty is useful for longer segments but has the unwanted side effect of a capacious intestinal side diverticulum. The Michelassi strictureplasty offers an option for more extensive small bowel disease. Lengths of up to 150 cm have been successfully maintained using this technique.

Strictureplasty provides a favorable risk/benefit ratio: longer operative time and slightly increased incidence of postoperative bleeding are exchanged for decreased recurrence rate, preservation of bowel length, and possible restoration of bowel function. Endoscopic and radiographic evidence exists that demonstrates restitution of normal appearance after strictureplasty; histopathologic evidence indicates quiescence of disease in the strictureplastied segment with the possibility of restitution of absorptive function to previously diseased bowel. Details of techniques of strictureplasty are presented elsewhere in this text.

Fistulas are treated with resection of the primary diseased segment and closure of the opening on the target organ, if necessary. In the majority of cases, fistulas originate from a diseased segment of intestines and drain into an innocent bystander loop of bowel. This commonly occurs between two loops of small bowel or between the diseased terminal ileum and the sigmoid colon. Recurrent disease of the neoterminal ileum may fistulize to the duodenal sweep, or primary disease from the transverse colon may fistulize to the stomach or fourth portion of the duodenum.

After resection of the primary diseased segment, the bystander segment should be closed primarily. Care should be taken to avoid narrowing the unaffected segment of bowel by closing in a transverse direction; if the fistulous opening on the target loop is large, very edematous, or situated on the mesenteric side, a segmental resection with primary anastomosis may be necessary. Fistulas to the bladder can be oversewn in one or two layers, and vaginal and uterine fistulas often heal spontaneously after resection of the primary diseased intestine. Overlaying the repair with epiploic appendices or omentum can aid in the success rate of the repair and prevent recurrence of the fistula. Enterocutaneous or colocutaneous fistulas need debridement of the fistulous tract through the aponeurotic and cutaneous planes of the abdominal wall, with complete drainage of intervening abscesses.

Surgery for Crohn's disease can be performed laparoscopically. Challenges facing the laparoscopic approach include matted loops of bowel, adhesions, fistulas, thickened Crohn mesentery, and prior surgical interventions. There are currently no strict contraindications to laparoscopic surgery in a patient with Crohn's disease; in experienced hands, it can be treated using minimally invasive techniques with outcomes comparable to open techniques.

Several studies, including two randomized control trials and a meta-analysis, demonstrate that although laparoscopic surgery results in longer operative times, length of stay is decreased, functional recovery is enhanced, and postoperative complications and recurrence rates are comparable. Even patients with prior open surgery may have success rates approaching 80% for treatment of recurrence laparoscopically.

When performing laparoscopic surgery, access to the abdominal cavity is typically obtained through a periumbilical incision; but in the case of prior abdominal surgery, fistulizing disease, or large abscess, the site of entry should be away from the diseased segment or scarring to minimize risk of injury to intestines attached to the anterior abdominal wall. Either a Veress needle or open Hassan technique can be used. Two 5 mm trocars are generally placed to triangulate with the camera port. Ideally, the camera is located in line between the surgeon and the area of disease and in between the two operating trocars.

Using intestinal graspers, the bowel is inspected in an orderly fashion, from the ligament of Treitz to the ileocecal valve or to a previous ileocolic anastomosis. In the case of extensive adhesions, the surgeon should recognize a personal comfort level and ability to continue laparoscopically. Large complicated phlegmons may be better approached using open technique to prevent additional injury. Dissection of the mesentery should be done with care; Crohn mesentery is significantly thickened, and 5 mm energy devices may be inadequate to fully control bleeding with a single firing. We prefer a midline incision for specimen removal, protected with a flexible wound retractor; this incision can be utilized again should the patient require additional subsequent surgery.

RECURRENCE OF DISEASE

Recurrence is a significant concern in patients with Crohn's disease. Almost 50% of patients have signs of endoscopic recurrence by 1 year after surgery, and up to 50% will require a second surgery, often with disease in the same location as the prior intervention. Use of nicotine has been correlated with increased recurrence rates in multiple studies, and patients should be strongly counseled to stop smoking after surgery. Cessation of smoking reduces the chances of long-term disease recurrence by 50%. Other less well-elucidated factors also play a role in disease recurrence; disease phenotype, granulomas, and prior recurrence are risk factors for future surgical interventions.

Immunoprophylaxis with early postoperative medical therapy has been advocated because of the high risk of recurrence, particularly in patients with severe disease or multiple prior surgeries. Patients may be prescribed antibiotics, 5-ASA agents, immunomodulators, or biologics within 10 days of surgical intervention. Metronidazole has been shown to decrease the rate of endoscopic recurrence when used for 3 months postoperatively, and 5-ASA agents have been shown to reduce recurrence rates in postoperative patients by up to 30%, particularly in patients with terminal ileal disease and long disease duration. Results with use of azathioprine and 6-mercaptopurine show a decrease in recurrence rates up to 50%. Preliminary data on the postoperative use of biologics suggest that this category of drugs may also play a substantial role in recurrence prevention.

SUGGESTED READINGS

Fichera A, Lovadina S, Rubin M, et al: Patterns and operative treatment of recurrent Crohn's disease: a prospective longitudinal study, *Surgery* 140(4):649–654, 2006.

Michelassi F, Taschieri A, Tonelli F, et al: An international, multicenter, prospective, observational study of the side-to-side isoperistaltic strictureplasty in Crohn's disease, *Dis Colon Rectum* 50(3):277–284, 2007.

Milsom JW, Hammerhofer KA, Bohm B, et al: Prospective, randomized trial comparing laparoscopic vs. conventional surgery for refractory ileocolic Crohn's disease, *Dis Colon Rectum* 44:1–9, 2001.

Yamamoto T: Factors affecting recurrence after surgery for Crohn's disease, *World J Gastroenterol* 11(26):3971–3979, 2005.

USE OF STRICTUREPLASTY IN CROHN'S DISEASE

Mark A. Talamini, MD, and Elisabeth C. McLemore, MD

OVERVIEW

Crohn's disease is a chronic and frequently unremitting inflammatory disorder that affects the gastrointestinal (GI) system. Transmural inflammation can occur anywhere in the GI tract, from the oral cavity to the anus, but Crohn's disease predominantly affects the small bowel, colon, rectum, and perianal region.

The etiology of Crohn's disease is still not fully determined. Current treatment is based on a variety of systemic and local immunomodulators, antiinflammatory agents, and more recent biologics, such as tumor necrosis factor-alpha antagonists. Unlike ulcerative colitis, in which the intestinal manifestations of the disease are cured with removal of the colon and rectum, surgery is directed at treating the complications of Crohn's disease and should not be considered curative, but rather an adjunct to careful and effective medical therapy. Surgery should be considered only after careful consultation with the patient and with a gastroenterologist experienced in the medical management of Crohn's disease.

The transmural inflammation of the bowel wall in Crohn's disease can lead to abscess formation, enteroenteral fistula, enterocutaneous fistula, perforation, and stricture. Stricture formation most commonly becomes symptomatic when it occurs in the small bowel. The primary surgical treatment of symptomatic Crohn's disease is resection of the involved bowel with either restoration of intestinal continuity or a stoma. Unfortunately, a high percentage of patients develop recurrence despite maximal medical management and previous surgery. In patients with recurrent complications, repeated bowel resection may lead to short bowel syndrome with vitamin and nutrient malabsorption and volume depletion. Strictureplasty is a useful surgical technique that relieves the obstructive symptoms caused by small bowel strictures, while preserving intestinal length. Overall surgical objectives for complications of Crohn's disease are listed in Table 1.

INDICATIONS AND PREOPERATIVE PREPARATION

The etiology of bowel stricture formation is most likely related to repeated episodes of inflammation, resolution, and remodeling of the bowel wall, leading to replacement of the normally pliable tissue with a thickened, nonpliable bowel wall segment that eventually narrows the lumen, which will ultimately lead to obstructive symptoms. The time course of this process will vary from patient to patient and may be modified by medications such as steroids, immunomodulators, or biologic TNF-α antagonists. Over time, the involved segment of bowel may become less responsive to increasingly aggressive medical management, and surgical intervention will become necessary for obstructive symptoms.

Strictureplasty may be performed in ileal, jejunal, duodenal, and ileocolic anastamotic strictures. Strictureplasty for colonic strictures has been performed with less frequency, as the incidence and concern for neoplasm is increased in colonic strictures, making resection the standard treatment. The nature of the stricture and the amount of the remaining bowel are key factors in determining whether a strictureplasty is appropriate. Strictureplasty is not an option in the setting of bowel perforation or extensive inflammatory phlegmon in the involved segment of bowel. Distant sites of abscess or phlegmon are not a contraindication for strictureplasty, but the procedure has less of a role in severely thickened bowel or in an extremely long, strictured segment. The indications and contraindications for strictureplasty are listed in Table 2 and Table 3, respectively.

The preoperative evaluation and preparation in patients with obstructive Crohn's disease is extensive. Patients should have received optimal medical therapy for their disease, and any septic focus should be controlled with antibiotics, percutaneous drainage, or both. Nutritional status should be evaluated, and patients who are nutritionally compromised should undergo nutritional repletion, either by a liquid enteral diet or parenteral nutrition, to reverse their catabolic state before surgery to reduce postoperative complications.

The key for optimal surgical outcome is clearly defining the scope and nature of the patient's past and current disease activity. Obtaining a thorough history of prior operations and operative reports is helpful to determine the patient's anatomy. Colonoscopy should be performed to determine whether any colonic disease might require surgical treatment. Any colonic stricture must undergo biopsies to rule out the possibility of malignancy. Although colonic strictureplasty may be considered if there is a real need to preserve colonic length, the risk of an occult malignancy in a colonic stricture is relatively high, and resection should be the standard treatment.

The extent of small bowel disease should be defined preoperatively. Traditionally, a small bowel series is used to map the distribution of disease activity. This study provides information on the number and length of strictures, the presence of any unsuspected enteroenteral fistulae, the presence of any contained perforations, and an estimate of small bowel length. Newer techniques, such as computed tomographic and magnetic resonance enterography, provide images that offer additional information that a small bowel study may not reveal, such as an occult abscess or phlegmon or evidence of disease distal to a high-grade obstruction.

A final important preoperative planning step is to discuss the possible need for a temporary or permanent stoma. Stoma sites should be marked on the patient's abdomen preoperatively, even if there is only a small chance that a stoma will be needed; this is because unexpected intraoperative findings may change the scope of the operation and necessitate a stoma, and proper preoperative stoma marking is important for successful long-term stoma function and care.

TABLE 1: Surgical objectives for complications of Crohn's disease

Preoperative Objectives

- Maximize or exhaust nonsurgical treatment options prior to surgery
- Surgical intervention should be limited to the treatment of symptomatic complications of Crohn's disease
- Evaluate nutritional status prior to surgery
- Consider supplemental nutrition to improve nutritional parameters prior to surgery when nutritional status is poor

Intraoperative Objectives

- Spare bowel length
- Utilize alternative strategies to resection when appropriate to preserve sufficient length of the remaining bowel and minimize the propensity for short bowel syndrome
- Spare the ileocecal valve when possible
- Biopsy any suspicious ulcers or mucosa for malignancy

TABLE 2: Indications for strictureplasty

- Diffuse involvement of the small bowel with strictures
- Prior small bowel resection greater than 100 cm
- Rapid recurrence of Crohn's disease with obstruction
- An obstructing, fibrotic small bowel stricture without associated sepsis

TABLE 3: Contraindications to strictureplasty

- Albumin level >2 g/dL
- Free or contained perforation of the bowel associated with the stricture
- Phlegmonous inflammation, internal fistula, external fistula involving affected site
- Stricture close in proximity to a resection site
- Multiple strictures within a short segment in a patient who has not had prior small bowel resections or in a patient with sufficient small bowel length
- Any stricture with pathologic evidence of dysplasia or malignancy

TABLE 4: Stricture length and recommended strictureplasty technique

Stricture	Recommended Technique
Short (<10 cm)	Heineke-Mikulicz
Medium (10 to 20 cm)	Finney
Long (>20 cm)	Side-to-side isoperistaltic

Surgical Strategy

Strictureplasty should be considered an option in any patient with Crohn's disease who presents with obstructive symptoms. The goal is to prevent significant bowel loss related to resection. In patients requiring multiple operations, the surgeon must be concerned about loss of bowel length, which may result in short bowel syndrome. The length of bowel necessary for support by oral nutrition varies from patient to patient, but in general at least 100 to 125 cm of small bowel is considered necessary to avoid supplemental intravenous alimentation or hydration. Some patients who have lived with chronically obstructed bowel may be able to tolerate shorter lengths of remaining bowel because of physiologic adaptation.

Another important consideration when evaluating a patient with obstructive Crohn's disease is the possibility of an occult malignancy. It is recommended that any stricture being prepared for strictureplasty have a specimen taken during the operation for frozen-section analysis to rule out dysplasia or malignancy. This is particularly important in patients in whom a previous bypass procedure has been performed.

Operative Techniques

On initial exploration of the abdomen, all evidence of disease should be carefully noted, and obvious strictures should be marked. Each area of involved bowel should be examined for any other pathology that might preclude a strictureplasty, such as a fistula or localized abscess.

The length of bowel remaining in situ must be determined. If the patient has adequate bowel length, and the strictures are close to each other, a single resection and anastomosis, rather than multiple strictureplasties, may be performed. However, if residual bowel length is a concern, strictureplasties are indicated. It is also important at the end of the operation to document the remaining length of small bowel by actual intraoperative measurement.

Visual and tactile external evaluation of the bowel may not identify all small bowel strictures. A number of techniques have been described to evaluate the internal diameter of the small bowel lumen intraoperatively. These techniques all rely on the introduction into the bowel of a device, most commonly a balloon-tipped catheter, that can be passed along its length to assess any obstructions to easy passage. The best technique for introducing the balloon is through the enterotomy made for the first strictureplasty. A long jejunal Baker tube with an inflatable balloon at the distal end is utilized at many institutions. The tube is passed to the end of the small bowel manually, and then the balloon is inflated with 12 to 15 mL of saline to approximately 1.5 cm in diameter. Points along the length of the small bowel where easy passage of the balloon is hindered are marked for potential strictureplasty with easily identifiable suture material, as clips may be dislodged inadvertently with manipulation.

Although there is no defined upper limit to the number of strictureplasties that can be safely performed, each strictureplasty site represents a potential site for a leak. A postoperative leak can be a catastrophic complication in a patient with Crohn's disease. Therefore the decision to perform multiple strictureplasties, instead of a single resection, must be weighed carefully.

The technique used to perform a strictureplasty depends on the length of the stricture (see Table 4). Strictures less than 10 cm are best dealt with using a strictureplasty technique derived from the Heineke-Mikulicz pyloroplasty performed for pyloric stenosis. A Heineke-Mikulicz strictureplasty (Figure 1) is performed by first placing two 3-0 sutures, either nonabsorbable or absorbable, on the side of the bowel at the middle of the stricture to act as stay sutures, after the bowel is opened along the antimesenteric edge. The surgeon evaluates the bowel by making an antimesenteric longitudinal incision with electrocautery. This incision divides the stricture and should be carried out at an equal distance of 1 to 2 cm proximally and distally into normal, thin-walled, nondiseased bowel. For ease of closure, it is essential that the longitudinal incision stay truly on the antimesenteric border.

It is important to obtain excellent hemostasis, because bleeding from a strictureplasty site is one of the most common and troubling postoperative complications. Labeling the mesentery at each strictureplasty site with radiopaque metal clips may assist with discrimination between multiple sites in the event of postoperative hemorrhage. Selective mesenteric angiography with intraarterial vasopressin infusion will control most episodes of bleeding. If bleeding continues despite conservative medical therapy, the metallic clips may help localize the bleeding strictureplasty site and prevent the need to open all of the strictureplasty sites to localize the bleeding at the time of surgery. Alternatively, India ink blue dye can be injected at the time of selective mesenteric angiography for intraoperative localization.

Mucosal biopsies of the stricture for frozen-section analysis are obtained to rule out the presence of dysplasia or malignancy. This is especially important if an ulcer is noted. The stay sutures are pulled perpendicular to the long axis of the bowel (see Figure 1), and the enterotomy is closed in one or two layers. This transverse-closure strictureplasty technique is ideal for short strictures but not for longer ones.

There are general surgical principles that should be followed irrespective of the strictureplasty technique being performed (Table 5). The bowel wall should be incised along the antimesenteric margin. The antimesenteric incision should extend 1 to 2 cm beyond the diseased segment. A biopsy should be performed and should include tissue from any suspicious ulcers and mucosa to exclude malignancy.

Prior to closure of the enteroenterostomy, meticulous attention should be paid to obtaining excellent hemostasis to prevent postoperative bleeding. Closure of the strictureplasty can be performed with an absorbable or nonabsorbable suture in a one- or two-layer fashion. Consider labeling the mesentery at the strictureplasty site with a

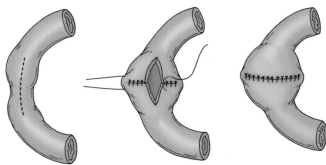

FIGURE 1 A Heineke-Mikulicz strictureplasty on an isolated stricture. In this drawing, a single-layer everting technique is performed to close the longitudinal enterotomy transversely, reconstructing an unobstructed lumen.

TABLE 5: Strictureplasty strategy for all techniques

- Incise bowel wall along the antimesenteric margin
- Extend incision 1 to 2 cm beyond the diseased segment
- Biopsy any suspicious ulcers and mucosa to exclude carcinoma
- Obtain excellent hemostasis
- Closure with an absorbable or nonabsorbable suture in a one- or two-layer fashion
- Label mesentery at strictureplasty site with metallic clip

radiopaque metallic clip to serve as a future reference for localization of bleeding postoperatively in the setting of multiple strictureplasties.

Lastly, the steps and intraoperative evaluation of the open technique should be followed if a robotic or laparoscopic-assisted strictureplasty is performed. These principles should not be compromised for the sake of smaller incisions.

Other configurations for strictureplasty may be useful and are designed for the treatment of longer strictures or for multiple strictures in a short segment of bowel. The Finney strictureplasty, named after the Finney pyloroplasty, resembles a side-to-side anastomosis (Figure 2). This strictureplasty may be useful in a patient with a medium-length stricture (10 to 20 cm) or for a segment with multiple short strictures closely grouped together with intervening dilated, short segments of bowel.

In the Finney technique, the bowel is folded at the stricture, and the normal proximal and distal bowel are brought alongside one another. If a hand-sewn technique is used, there are two options. First, if the strictured area is mildly stenotic and the bowel is of reasonable quality, the entire stricture may be opened along the antimesenteric border, and a hand-sewn, essentially side-to-side anastomosis may be performed along the length of the enterotomy (Finney strictureplasty, Figure 2). Second, if the stricture is too tight or the bowel is not suitable for suturing, then a true side-to-side anastomosis between the proximal and distal normal bowel can be performed, leaving the strictured segment in place as a short bypassed segment (Jaboulay strictureplasty, Figure 3). Similarly, if a stapling device is used, a side-to-side anastomosis can be fashioned between the normal proximal and distal bowel, leaving the strictured segment in continuity. There is some concern with the Jaboulay strictureplasty technique in that it merely results in a bypassed segment. Although the segment is short, there are potential long-term ramifications, including bacterial overgrowth and malignant degeneration.

In patients with two strictures in close proximity, a modification of the Heineke-Mikulicz strictureplasty technique has been created. The bowel is entered on the antimesenteric border, and both strictures are divided, as is the normal intervening segment. The resulting long enterotomy is closed transversely (Figure 4).

When the bowel is markedly dilated proximal to a short stricture, the size discrepancy between the proximal and distal normal

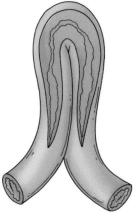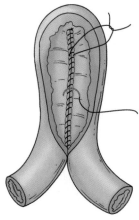

FIGURE 2 A Finney strictureplasty can be used for the treatment of a long stricture. The enteroenterostomy is performed after the stricture is divided along the antimesenteric border, and the involved bowel is folded onto itself in a U shape. The cut edges of the bowel on the interior of the U are sutured together as the back wall of the anastomosis and the outer edges are sutured together as the front wall.

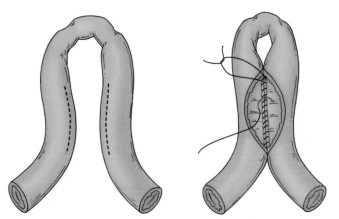

FIGURE 3 A Jaboulay strictureplasty can be used to bypass a stricture that is too narrow or a stricture in which the bowel is not suitable for suturing.

bowel often precludes a Heineke-Mikulicz strictureplasty. In these cases, a Moskel-Walske-Neumayer strictureplasty can be performed (Figure 5). This strictureplasty technique is essentially a Y-to-V advancement flap closure of the stricture. The stricture is opened along the antimesenteric border as a Y-shaped enterotomy, with the Y portion in the dilated bowel just proximal to the stricture. The strictured segment is then pulled apart, and the antimesenteric segment of the proximal dilated bowel is advanced into the strictured area and closed in a transverse fashion; one side of the closure is normal bowel along the entire length, and the other comprises the two strictured bowel edges.

Long strictures (>20 cm) or a series of strictures in close proximity are less common and more difficult to treat. In these patients, a long segment of bowel that would result in a prohibitively extensive resection can be retained as a side-to-side isoperistaltic strictureplasty, described by Tichansky in 1992 (Figure 6). In this technique, the bowel is completely divided transversely at the middle of the strictured segment. Unlike other strictureplasties, the mesentery is divided perpendicular to the long axis of the bowel to permit the two segments of bowel to be overlapped and positioned side to side along the entire length of the divided segments. Both strictured segments are opened along the antimesenteric border, and the antimesenteric faces of bowel are sewn to one another in an isoperistaltic fashion. This technique results in no bypassed segments of bowel.

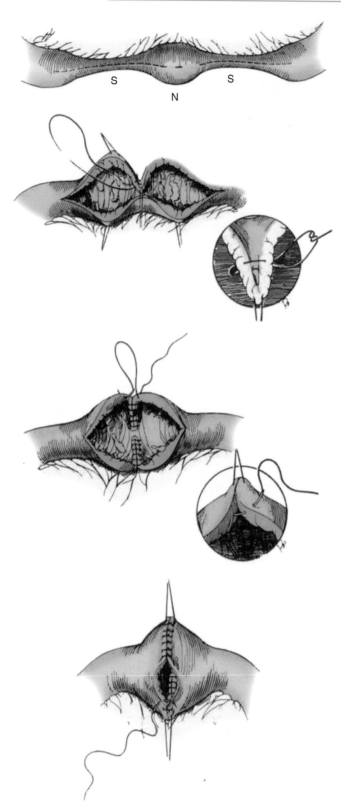

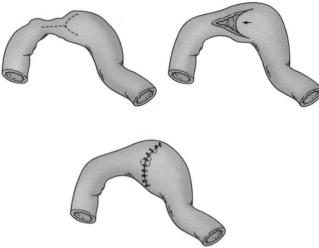

FIGURE 5   The Moskel-Walske-Neumayer strictureplasty is used when there is a significant size difference between the proximal and distal bowel segments adjacent to a short stricture. Instead of a longitudinal incision, a Y-shaped enterotomy is performed and then closed in a transverse fashion. *(From Tichansky D, Cagir B, Yoo E, et al: Dis Colon Rectum 43:911–919, 2000.)*

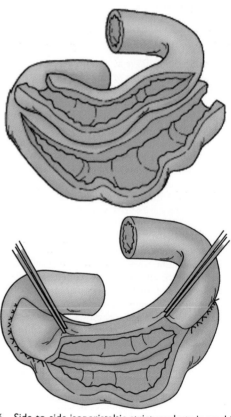

FIGURE 6   Side-to-side isoperistaltic strictureplasty is used for a long segment of involved bowel that would require resection because of multiple consecutive strictures. The involved bowel is divided in the middle of the segment, and in a minimal portion of mesentery, to allow the two segments to be slid over one another and laid side to side in an isoperistaltic fashion. An enteroenterostomy is performed, with the two cut edges closest to one another closed as a back wall and the others closed as the front wall. *(From Tichansky D, Cagir B, Yoo E, et al: Dis Colon Rectum 43:911–919, 2000.)*

FIGURE 4   A modified Heineke-Mikulicz strictureplasty can be used for two short-segment strictures that are close to one another with a normal or dilated segment of bowel between them.

Recurrent terminal ileal stricture formation at a prior ileocolic resection and anastamosis can be managed with a Finney strictureplasty. A long ileocolostomy is constructed to relieve the obstruction in the diseased bowel segment. This technique can also be performed in select patients undergoing a first operation for obstructive terminal ileal Crohn's disease. This technique should be limited to use in patients with obstruction due to fibrosis of the bowel wall with luminal narrowing; it should not be used in the treatment of fistulizing, phlegmonous terminal ileal disease with obstruction.

Colonic strictureplasty has limited appeal because the colon is not essential for nutrient absorption, and an isolated colonic stricture has a 7% incidence of harboring an occult malignancy. However, there may be patients in whom preservation of colonic mucosal surface area in the setting of an existing short bowel is important for fluid and electrolyte homeostasis. In this rare circumstance, an isolated colonic strictureplasty may be performed after the stricture has been extensively biopsied to ensure that there is no evidence of dysplasia or malignancy.

RESULTS

Overall, the literature supports the safety and efficacy of strictureplasty in the treatment of obstructing small bowel Crohn's disease. The majority of studies report acceptable operative morbidity and recurrence rates comparable to traditional surgical resection. A few small series of laparoscopic-assisted strictureplasties have also been reported with similar results.

Strictureplasty has been shown to relieve obstructive symptoms in patients with Crohn's disease; patients demonstrate weight gain, improved food tolerance, and reduction or discontinuation of steroid usage. In addition, patients who undergo strictureplasty alone appear to have an equal likelihood of requiring reoperation when compared with patients who undergo strictureplasty combined with bowel resection.

In 2009, Greenstein and colleagues reported that the number of strictures and the number of strictureplasties performed have been shown to be associated with an increased recurrence rate. The reoperative rate at 5 years for patients with fewer than four strictureplasties is 14%, versus 33% for patients with more than four. This is likely a reflection of disease severity and may be useful as a prognostic indicator for future recurrence.

Endoscopic and imaging evaluation after strictureplasty have revealed complete morphologic disease regression in a variety of case series reports. The mechanism of inflammation regression remains unknown. One theory postulates that the relief of obstruction diminishes the degree of focal bacteria and food allergens driven into the ulcerations and fissures in narrow, higher-pressure diseased segments, thereby decreasing the local inflammatory response.

One of the largest systematic reviews and meta-analyses of the safety and efficacy of strictureplasty for Crohn's disease was published by Fazio, Yakayki, and Tekkis in 2007 (Tables 6 and 7). A total of 3259 strictureplasties were performed in 1112 patients with Crohn's disease, with a mean of three at one operation (range, 1 to 21). A bowel resection for long strictures, perforation, fistula, or abscess was performed in 61% of these patients (660 of 1086). The overall complication rate was 13% (142 of 1057) for jejunum and/or ileum strictureplasty. The most common complications were septic complications in 4% (leak, fistula, or abscess in 39 of 1057 patients), of which 44% required reoperation for sepsis. Other complications included hemorrhage 3% (35 of 1057), ileus 2% (24 of 1057), wound infection 2% (19 of 1057), and bowel obstruction 1% (11 of 1057).

Risk factors for complications included hypoalbuminemia, preoperative weight loss, emergency operations, and presence of an intraabdominal abscess with peritoneal contamination, anemia, and older age. Risk factors for recurrence included younger age, short duration of disease, and short interval since previous resection. The recurrence rate for jejunum and/or ileum strictureplasty was 39%, and recurrence requiring reoperation occurred in 30% of patients (312 of 1038), with a median follow-up duration of 107 months.

TABLE 6: Technique used in 3081 strictureplasties in 1112 patients

Type of Strictureplasty	%	N
Heineke-Mikulicz	81%	2,499
Finney	10%	321
Side-to-side isoperistaltic	5%	148
Not specified	4%	113

TABLE 7: Stricture location in 3081 strictureplasties in 1112 patients

Location	%	N
Jejunum and/or ileum	94%	2242
Anastamotic strictureplasty	4%	99
Duodenal	1%	35
Colonic	1%	27
Not specified	22%	678

An international multicenter prospective observational study of side-to-side isoperistaltic strictureplasty in 184 patients with obstructive Crohn's disease was published in 2009 by Michelassi and colleagues. The length of diseased bowel ranged from 21 to 64 cm. The overall complication rate ranged from 6% to 21% at the various centers. The most common complications were hemorrhage (2%), anastamotic leak (1%), and bowel obstruction (1%). Symptomatic recurrence requiring reoperation occurred in 22% (41 of 184 patients), and the average interval to recurrence was 35 months.

SUMMARY

Strictureplasty is an integral part of the surgical management of patients with obstructive jejunoiloeal Crohn's disease and ileocolonic recurrence. The primary role of strictureplasty is to preserve small bowel length in a patient population prone to recurrence and multiple surgical interventions over a lifetime. The most commonly performed strictureplasty is the Heineke-Mikulicz technique; the length of the stricture dictates the technique of strictureplasty to be used. Patients with complications of Crohn's disease that require surgery should have a thorough preoperative evaluation and consultation with a gastroenterologist experienced in inflammatory bowel disease.

Suggested Readings

Greenstein AJ, Zhang LP, Miller AT, et al: Relationship of the number of Crohn's strictures and strictureplasties to postoperative recurrence, *J Am Coll Surg* 208(6):1065–1070, 2009.

Schmidt CM, Talamini MA, Kaufman HS, et al: Laparoscopic surgery for Crohn's disease: reasons for conversion, *Ann Surg* 233:733–739, 2001 [erratum in *Ann Surg* 234, 2001].

Spencer MP, Nelson H, Wolff BG, et al: Strictureplasty for obstructive Crohn's disease: the Mayo experience, *Mayo Clin Proc* 69:33–36, 1994.

Takayuki Y, Fazio VW, Tekkis PP: Safety and efficacy of strictureplasty for Crohn's disease: a systematic review and meta-analysis, *Dis Colon Rectum* 50:1968–1986, 2007.

Tjandra JJ, Fazio VW: Techniques of strictureplasty, *Perspect Colon Rectal Surg* 5:189–198, 1992.

MANAGEMENT OF SMALL BOWEL TUMORS

Jennifer E. Hrabe, MD, and Joseph J. Cullen, MD

OVERVIEW

Small bowel mucosa comprises approximately 75% of the length and 90% of the absorptive surface area of the digestive system, yet only 2% of new digestive system cancers each year occur in the small intestine. Men and patients in their sixth through eighth decades of life are most likely to be affected. While the incidence of primary small intestine cancers is on the rise, the numbers are still quite low. The American Cancer Society estimates that each year, more than 6000 new small bowel malignancies are found, and more than 1000 people die from the disease.

Several reasons for the low incidence of small bowel tumors have been proposed, including the rapid transit of contents through the small bowel, lower bacterial load, a high amount of lymphoid tissue, rapid turnover of epithelial cells, and decreased inflammation owing to the liquidity and alkaline nature of small bowel contents.

Signs and symptoms of these tumors are usually nonspecific and include abdominal pain, distension, nausea, vomiting, obstruction, and occult bleeding. Vague symptoms, limited findings on examination, and failure to obtain or correctly interpret diagnostic tests have all been implicated as delaying the diagnosis of small intestine cancers. Because of this, more than 50% of patients have nodal or distant metastases at presentation.

Diagnosing small bowel tumors has historically been made difficult due to limited means of gaining access to distal portions of the small bowel. Commonly noted studies have included small bowel follow-through, enteroclysis, computed tomography (CT) scans, ultrasound, magnetic resonance imaging (MRI), upper endoscopy, and push enteroscopy. Wireless capsule endoscopy (Figure 1) and double-balloon endoscopy have become increasingly more common.

Capsule endoscopy offers the advantage of being less invasive while providing visualization of the entire small intestine. Its disadvantage is that it cannot distinguish benign lesions from malignant ones, nor can it be used to determine mural involvement from biopsy tissues. Double-balloon endoscopy also offers the potential to inspect the entire small intestine, although complete enteroscopy is not always possible; the procedure is more invasive, but it allows biopsies and resection of polyps.

The treatment of small bowel neoplasms has not changed significantly over the past two decades, and surgery continues to be the primary therapy for most types. Thus it is not entirely surprising that long-term survival for small bowel cancers has remained relatively unchanged for the last 20 years.

CARCINOID/NEUROENDOCRINE TUMORS

Tumor Characteristics

Gastrointestinal carcinoid tumors, more recently referred to as *neuroendocrine tumors,* are a diverse range of slow-growing neoplasms arising from enterochromaffin cells found throughout the crypts of Lieberkühn. Although neuroendocrine tumors can secrete a variety of biologically active amines and hormones, serotonin is the most commonly secreted. Carcinoids can occur anywhere along the gastrointestinal (GI) tract, though approximately 45% occur in the small intestine, most commonly in the ileum. The average tumor size at presentation is less than 2 cm.

Up to one third of cases of carcinoid tumors of small intestine are multifocal, and more than 50% of patients have nonlocalized disease at the time of diagnosis. Mesenteric lymph node metastases are common, and an estimated 40% to 80% of GI carcinoids spread to the mesentery. Though a rare tumor, the incidence of carcinoid tumors increased 340% from 1973 to 2004. In fact, carcinoids are now the most common small bowel tumor reported to the National Cancer Database, with adenocarcinoma close behind.

Clinical Presentation

Patients with carcinoid tumors may present with abdominal pain and obstructive symptoms. Obstruction is often due to fibrosis around the tumor, which can cause adhesions of intestinal loops and stricturing of the bowel. Fibrosis around mesenteric metastases can cause contraction of the mesentery or fixation of the mesentery to the retroperitoneum, which can lead to kinking and obstruction via fibrous bands. Encasement of mesenteric vessels by tumor and fibrosis can lead to venous stasis and even ischemia in portions of the small bowel. An estimated 10% of patients will present with carcinoid syndrome, with typical manifestations including cutaneous flushing, excessive diarrhea, and bronchoconstriction. Right-sided heart disease, due to endocardial fibrotic plaques and valvular dysfunction, is estimated to occur in less than half of those patients exhibiting carcinoid syndrome.

Diagnosis

While duodenal carcinoids are often identified on endoscopy, jejunal and ileal carcinoids are frequently diagnosed late, when patients undergo surgical exploration for bowel obstruction and GI bleeding. Biochemical diagnosis of carcinoids may be done by measurement of 5-hydroxyindolacetic acid in a 24-hour urine sample, or by serum analysis of chromogranin A, which is believed to be a superior screening test. Common imaging studies for localizing carcinoid tumors include abdominal CT, MRI, and somatostatin receptor scintigraphy (octreotide scan). Octreotide scanning is a useful initial imaging method, with a diagnostic sensitivity estimated to be 80% to 90%. Additionally, it can help predict tumor response to treatment with somatostatin receptor analogs.

Treatment

Surgery is usually the most effective treatment for averting both local tumor effects, such as obstruction and bleeding, and symptoms caused by the secreted bioactive agents. Because metastatic spread to regional lymph nodes is common, small intestine carcinoids warrant an en bloc resection with extensive lymphadenectomy and wide resection of the mesentery. The abdomen should be carefully inspected for multicentric lesions and liver metastases. If liver metastases are identified, the primary tumor should still be resected to diminish later complications such as obstruction, perforation, and bleeding.

In the case of duodenal tumors, small lesions may be resected endoscopically. However, if the tumor is in proximity to the ampulla, a pancreaticoduodenectomy may be necessary to obtain complete resection. The role of surgery in metastatic disease is not well defined, but resection of bowel, mesenteric tumors, lymph node and hepatic metastases, and fibrotic areas may improve symptoms and quality of life. Extensive resections in metastatic disease may even prolong survival, though it is estimated that 90% of the disease needs to be resected to achieve

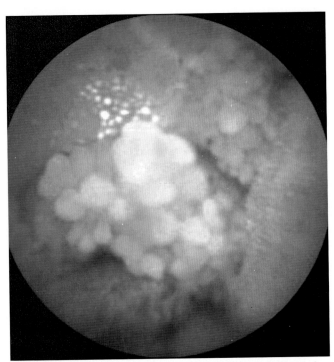

FIGURE 1 Wireless capsule endoscopic findings of an endoluminal mass in the proximal jejunum. Patient had anemia, and upper GI endoscopy and colonoscopy did not reveal a source of the chronic bleeding. Exploratory laparotomy and small bowel resection revealed adenocarcinoma.

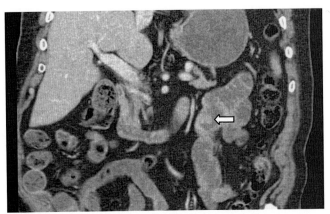

FIGURE 2 Coronal sections of a CT scan demonstrating a protruding mass (arrow) in the patient who had the wireless capsule endoscopy in Figure 1.

palliation. Tumor debulking may also improve the efficacy of pharmacologic therapy by reducing the bioactive substances secreted.

Long-acting somatostatin analogs have been shown to be highly effective in controlling carcinoid syndrome symptoms. Routine preoperative administration can prevent carcinoid crisis, which is characterized by excessive cutaneous flushing, hyperthermia, shock, arrhythmias, and bronchial obstruction. Somatostatin analogs, interferons, and single-agent chemotherapy result in marginal tumor responses. The overall 5-year survival for carcinoid tumors is 60% to 65%, ranging from 96% for stage I to 43% for stage IV disease. Age greater than 55 years, male sex, primary tumor size greater than 1 cm, and distant metastases negatively affect outcome. Approximately 85% of patients with carcinoid tumors can be expected to have liver metastases; therefore life-long surveillance is critical.

ADENOCARCINOMA

Tumor Characteristics

Adenocarcinoma is the second most common malignancy of the small intestine, comprising approximately 33% of small bowel cancers. It most commonly occurs in the duodenum, though in patients younger than 50 years, jejunal adenocarcinoma is more prevalent. It is associated with a variety of other diseases and syndromes, including Crohn disease (ileal adenocarcinoma), celiac disease (jejunal adenocarcinoma), familial adenomatous polyposis (duodenal adenocarcinoma), hereditary nonpolyposis colorectal cancer, and Peutz-Jeghers syndrome.

Clinical Presentation

More than 50% of patients are found to have advanced disease at presentation; 24% have distant metastases, and less than one third have nodal involvement. Clinical presentation depends on the extent and location of disease and can include abdominal pain, obstructive symptoms, and biliary obstruction caused by periampullary masses.

Diagnosis

Periampullary lesions can be diagnosed by upper endoscopy, endoscopic ultrasound, and magnetic resonance cholangiopancreatography. Cancers distal to the ligament of Treitz are more amenable to video capsule endoscopy and double-balloon endoscopy. Advanced adenocarcinomas may appear on barium contrast studies as "apple core" lesions: short, annular, narrowed portions that show evidence of mucosal ulceration and appear rigid and unchanging with compression. On CT (Figure 2), adenocarcinomas often appear as a protruding polyp or as a constricting circumferential mass that demonstrates moderate enhancement following intravenous contrast administration.

Treatment

The primary treatment and only potential for cure of small bowel adenocarcinoma continues to be surgical resection. For periampullary and proximal duodenal lesions, pancreaticoduodenectomy is usually required. Distal duodenal cancers are treated with segmental resection and lymphadenectomy. Jejunal and ileal tumors require segmental bowel resection with a wide resection of the lymph node–bearing mesentery, and terminal ileal tumors are treated with ileocolectomy.

Patients with intraabdominal metastases at the time of their initial surgery should be palliated to relieve obstruction or control hemorrhage. In advanced disease, proximal GI obstruction can be treated with endoscopic stents or by placement of gastric or gastrojejunostomy tubes, which decompress and also provide nutritional support. The 5-year observed survival is approximately 30%, with a median survival of 20 months. Factors negatively affecting survival include male sex, age greater than 55 years, tumor location in the duodenum or ileum, and the presence of distant metastases.

GASTROINTESTINAL STROMAL TUMORS

Tumor Characteristics

Gastrointestinal stromal tumors (GISTs) are most frequently found in the stomach (50%) and the small bowel (25%); within the small bowel, they are more likely to be in the jejunum. Duodenal GISTs are more commonly located in the second portion of the duodenum.

Most GISTs arise from the bowel wall, and they can grow into the mucosa and cause ulceration, or they can protrude toward the serosal side; 75% are diagnosed in patients older than 50 years. Aggressive GISTs have a defined pattern of metastasis to the liver and throughout the abdomen, usually as innumerable serosal-based nodules. Importantly, these tumors rarely metastasize to lymph nodes, and extraabdominal spread is unusual except in advanced disease.

Clinical Presentation

Presenting complaints include obstructive symptoms, abdominal discomfort, early satiety, and abdominal distension due to the space-occupying nature of these masses. Blood loss can occur when GISTs erode through the bowel wall or lead to intraperitoneal rupture.

Diagnosis

Performing preoperative biopsy for tissue diagnosis is generally discouraged, especially if the tumor is easily resectable. GISTs are soft, fragile masses, and biopsies increase the risk of tumor hemorrhage and dissemination. Biopsy may be appropriate when planning neoadjuvant therapy with imatinib, whether for localized, potentially resectable lesions whose surgical morbidity would be improved by tumor size reduction or for unresectable or metastatic lesions.

Radiographic evaluation often includes CT of the abdomen and pelvis with contrast. Attention should be given to the liver and peritoneum, the most common sites of metastases. Chest CT can be performed to assess for rare lung metastases. Staging and determination of surgical resection is generally based on CT findings, and the characteristic finding is of a smooth and well-circumscribed mass in the bowel wall that demonstrates exophytic growth, and larger GISTs may demonstrate central necrosis or hemorrhage.

Treatment

Treatment depends on the extent of disease. For localized disease, resection is the primary therapy. The abdomen must be thoroughly explored for peritoneal and liver metastases. The goal is complete gross resection with an intact pseudocapsule. Careful handling of these tumors is critical to avoid rupture and tumor dissemination. Some evidence has suggested that patients whose complete resection is complicated by tumor rupture have a shortened survival compared with those who do not have tumor rupture.

Surgery should consist of a segmental resection of the affected bowel, though periampullary tumors may require a pancreaticoduodenectomy. An en bloc resection is performed for adjacent organs adherent to the mass, again with the goal of maintaining an intact capsule. Because GISTs rarely metastasize to lymph nodes, routine lymphadenectomy is not recommended. The role of laparoscopy in managing GISTs is evolving. Laparoscopic resection of gastric GISTs has been successful and is acceptable for tumors less than 5 cm; however, the data describing outcomes for resection of small intestine GISTs are limited.

Preoperative administration of imatinib should be considered for marginally resectable GISTs in patients whose surgical morbidity would be improved by reducing the size of the tumor preoperatively and for unresectable or metastatic GISTs. Those patients needing preoperative imatinib must be monitored closely because their disease can progress rapidly and render their tumors unresectable. A baseline CT followed by subsequent CT, with or without positron emission tomography scans, can be used to monitor therapeutic effect. The timing of follow-up imaging varies with the extent of disease. Current recommendations include follow-up imaging 2 to 4 weeks after initiating therapy for less extensive GISTs and 3 months for unresectable or metastatic GISTs.

Up to 50% of patients develop tumor recurrence within 5 years and eventually succumb to the disease. Postoperative administration of imatinib has been shown to prolong recurrence-free survival and thus is recommended as an alternative to observation. The duration of treatment is still to be determined, but it is recommended that patients with intermediate to high-risk GISTs be treated for a minimum of 12 months. Imatinib should also be given postoperatively to patients with incomplete resection, recurrent disease, and metastatic disease.

The decision to reoperate for grossly positive margins should be tailored to each patient. In patients with new or progressing lesions despite medical therapy, surgery should be considered, especially for those lesions that appear potentially easy to resect. The 5-year overall observed survival for patients with a GIST is 40%. Factors that negatively affect prognosis include tumor size, mitotic index per high-powered field, male gender, age greater than 55 years, metastases, poorly differentiated tumors, and involved margins. Small bowel tumors carry a higher risk of progression than gastric tumors.

NON-HODGKIN LYMPHOMA

Tumor Characteristics

GI lymphomas are the most frequently occurring extranodal lymphomas. Primary lymphomas of the small intestine consist of a variety of non-Hodgkin lymphoma subtypes, which vary significantly in tumor behavior, response to chemotherapy, and prognosis. These subtypes include diffuse, large B-cell lymphoma, the most frequently encountered GI lymphoma; mucosa-associated lymphoid tissue (MALT) lymphoma; and immunoproliferative small intestinal disease. MALT tumors are associated with chronic antigenic stimulation, such as with *Helicobacter pylori* infection and autoimmune diseases, which leads to the proliferation of lymphoid tissue. The small intestine is the second most common location of GI lymphomas after the stomach, though the incidence in the small intestine is increasing. Within the small intestine, these lymphomas are more prevalent in the ileum.

Lymphoma is the most common malignancy affecting bowel mesentery. Primary GI lymphomas often involve only one site, whereas secondary lymphomas usually have multiple sites of involvement. In addition, primary lymphomas can spread such that they are difficult to distinguish from secondary tumors. Patients with celiac disease have up to a twentyfold relative risk for GI lymphoma, most commonly non-Hodgkin T-cell lymphoma. Patients with HIV and low CD4 count are at risk for developing B-cell GI lymphomas, which often have a high grade of malignancy and a poor prognosis.

Clinical Presentation

Patients report nonspecific symptoms, such as intermittent abdominal pain, fatigue, diarrhea, weight loss, and occasionally fever. GI bleeding, obstruction, and perforation are less common manifestations.

Diagnosis

Radiographic evaluation includes a CT scan, which characteristically demonstrates a large, homogenous mass. These tumors often show less contrast enhancement compared with other malignancies. Variable mural thickening is seen, from marked thickening with B-cell lymphoma to more moderate thickening with T-cell lymphoma. Diagnosis of lymphoma requires a tissue biopsy so that studies including immunohistochemistry, flow cytometry, and cytogenetic and molecular genetic evaluation can be performed. These allow classification of the lymphoma and ultimately determine optimal treatment and prognosis.

Treatment

Optimal treatment of GI lymphoma remains poorly defined. Chemotherapy has variable cure rates. Certain tumors, such as diffuse large cell lymphomas, respond to chemotherapy; others, such as anaplastic lymphomas, demonstrate resistance to chemotherapeutic agents. For localized, early-stage lymphomas, surgical resection of all gross disease plays a critical role in preventing complications, such as perforation and obstruction, and improving prognosis.

For advanced, disseminated tumors involving multiple organs, surgical treatment is limited to obtaining tissue for diagnosis and palliating any complications caused by the malignancy. The prognosis for GI lymphoma varies with the tumor subtype. The 5-year observed survival across subtypes is approximately 50%. Factors that negatively affect patient survival include male sex and age greater than 75 years.

METASTASES

The majority of GI tumors are metastases, most often from melanoma, lung cancer, and breast cancer. Metastases to the small bowel can occur via direct invasion, hematogenous spread, lymphatic spread, and intraperitoneal seeding. The most common presentation of metastasis is small bowel obstruction, though ascites, mesenteric ischemia, perforation, and bleeding can also be seen. Unfortunately, small bowel metastases indicate an advanced stage of the primary neoplasm, so treatment usually is focused on alleviating symptoms. Small bowel obstructions are treated in the standard fashion: with nasogastric decompression, bowel rest, and intravenous hydration. Failure of conservative treatment necessitates surgical intervention, typically resection of obstructed or intussuscepted bowel with primary anastomosis.

Patients with diffuse carcinomatosis are high-risk operative candidates who must be medically optimized prior to undergoing surgery. In those patients whose tumors are so advanced that definitive treatment cannot be performed, placement of a gastrostomy tube or an ostomy for decompression may be considered. Before any surgery, however, it is useful to repeat tumor staging to define the patient's prognosis.

BENIGN TUMORS

Not unlike their malignant counterparts, benign small intestine tumors often go undetected. Approximately 50% are asymptomatic, and those patients who are symptomatic most commonly present with abdominal pain and bleeding. Despite their benign nature, endoscopic or surgical resection is usually indicated to obtain adequate tissue for diagnosis and to reduce the risk of subsequent complications, such as bleeding and obstruction.

Adenomas

Adenomas can develop throughout the small intestine but are most common in the duodenum. Similar to colonic adenomas, small intestinal adenomas are classified histologically as *tubular, tubulovillous,* and *villous,* and they are precursors of adenocarcinoma. Risks of malignant transformation include size greater than 1 cm, a high grade of dysplasia, and villous subtype. Nearly one third of excised villous duodenal tumors are malignant. Patients with familial adenomatous polyposis have a significantly higher prevalence of duodenal adenomas as well as a much greater risk of duodenal adenocarcinoma. In fact, periampullary carcinoma is now the leading cause of death in these patients.

Although endoscopic evaluation is a common and useful means of evaluating these tumors, endoscopic biopsies have been shown to miss malignancies. Treatment of small intestinal adenoma varies by the pathology. Local excision may be appropriate for small tumors.

For villous tumors of the duodenum, treatment recommendations vary from local excision to pancreas-sparing duodenectomy to pancreaticoduodenectomy. Patients whose tumor has no features that raise concerns for malignancy—such as ulceration, severe dysplasia on preoperative biopsy, or dilation of pancreatic and common bile ducts—may be treated with local excision; if any of the aforementioned worrisome traits are present, pancreaticoduodenectomy should be considered.

Because of the high rate of tumor recurrence with local excision (up to 30% at 5 years) and the potential for recurrence as invasive cancer, regular endoscopic surveillance postoperatively is required. Villous tumors of the duodenum that recur after local excision call for pancreaticoduodenectomy. Patients with familial adenomatous polyposis and duodenal tumors showing high-grade dysplasia should undergo either pancreas-sparing duodenectomy or pancreaticoduodenectomy.

Lipomas

Small intestine lipomas have little or no malignant potential and are unlikely to cause symptoms. Symptoms, when they do occur, are usually related to obstruction, bleeding, and intussusception. Lipomas will show up on CT as a homogenous mass with the density of fat. On barium studies they appear as smooth, radiolucent, well-circumscribed intramural masses whose size and form change with peristalsis and pressure. Small, asymptomatic lipomas can be treated conservatively, whereas symptomatic lipomas or those greater than 2 cm should be resected.

Hamartomas

Hamartomatous polyps consist of a smooth muscle core arising from the muscularis mucosa and extending into the polyp. They usually occur in multiples and in varying sizes and shapes. These hamartomas are characteristic of Peutz-Jeghers syndrome, an autosomal dominant condition. They occur throughout the bowel and in varying number, from solitary polyps to hundreds coating the intestine. The polyps can cause abdominal pain, intussusception, obstruction, and GI bleeding. Though rare, Peutz-Jeghers hamartomas are associated with an increased risk of adenocarcinoma. Invasive treatment of these polyps, either endoscopic or surgical, should be limited to removing symptomatic polyps or polyps that are rapidly enlarging.

Hemangiomas

Hemangiomas of the small intestine are rare masses consisting of capillaries or blood-filled endothelial-lined spaces. Hemangiomas often become symptomatic, with either acute or chronic bleeding and rarely with obstruction, intussusception, or perforation. Treatment of symptomatic hemangiomas includes local excision or segmental resection. For appropriately sized and located lesions, endoscopic sclerotherapy and angiographic embolization may be used.

SUGGESTED READINGS

Bilimoria KY, Bentrem DJ, Wayne JD, et al: Small bowel cancer in the United States: changes in epidemiology, treatment, and survival over the last 20 years, *Ann Surg* 249(1):63–71, 2009.

Hatzaras I, Palesty JA, Abir F, et al: Small-bowel tumors: epidemiologic and clinical characteristics of 1260 cases from the Connecticut tumor registry, *Arch Surg* 142(3):229–235, 2007.

Kingham TP, DeMatteo RP: Multidisciplinary treatment of gastrointestinal stromal tumors, *Surg Clin North Am* 89(1):217–233, 2009.

Schnirer II, Yao JC, Ajani JA: Carcinoid—a comprehensive review, *Acta Oncol* 42:672–692, 2003.

SMALL BOWEL CARCINOID/ NEUROENDOCRINE TUMORS

Ana M. Grau, MD, James T. Broome, MD, and
John L. Tarpley, MD

OVERVIEW

Carcinoids are neuroendocrine neoplasms that most frequently occur in the gastrointestinal (GI) tract, where they originate from endocrine cells that populate the submucosa. These tumors were originally described by Langhans in 1867 and Lubarsch in 1888. Later, in 1907, Oberndorfer referred to them as *karzinoide*, or "carcinoma-like," because of their relative indolent nature compared with carcinomas. Gosset and Masson described silver salt–reducing granules in these tumors and originated the concept that carcinoid tumors are composed of argentaffin cells derived from Kulchitsky or enterochromaffin (EC) cells of the small intestine.

Carcinoids are histologically and biochemically diverse tumors. Perhaps the most widely used classification of carcinoids is based on anatomical location, with serotonin-containing EC cell carcinoids being more commonly located in the ileum. More recently, the World Health Organization (WHO) classification published in 2000 uses the general terms *neuroendocrine tumor* and *neuroendocrine carcinoma* instead of *carcinoid*.

Data from both the National Cancer Database (NCDB) and the Surveillance Epidemiology and End Results (SEER) databases were analyzed for small bowel malignancies and demonstrated that of 67,843 patients with small bowel malignancies, 37.4% had carcinoid tumors and 36.9% had adenocarcinomas; the remaining patients had stromal tumors or lymphomas. Interestingly, the incidence of small bowel carcinoids has increased fourfold from 1985 to 2005, surpassing adenocarcinomas as the most common small bowel tumor sometime in the mid 1990s.

The median age of presentation for small bowel carcinoid is 66 years, and 52.4% of patients are male. Carcinoids were located in the ileum in 45%, followed by the duodenum in 18%, jejunum in 6%; diffuse or undetermined carcinoids were located in the remaining patients. Small bowel carcinoids can be multicentric in up to 30% of patients, and noncarcinoid neoplasms are associated with small bowel carcinoids in up to 29% of patients. Although the incidence of duodenal carcinoids is also increasing, tumors located in the duodenum and jejunum currently are more often adenocarcinomas, and tumors found in the ileum are more likely to be carcinoids.

Carcinoids are white, yellow, or gray firm submucosal nodules in the wall of the intestine (Figure 1). They may protrude into the lumen as polyps, and the overlying mucosa may be intact or ulcerated. The primary lesions are usually small; however, metastatic deposits of carcinoids in the lymph nodes, mesentery, and liver may be quite large. Involvement of the subserosa and adjacent mesentery stimulates an intense desmoplastic reaction (Figure 2, *B*) that may lead to mesenteric fibrosis, intestinal kinking, retraction, and partial or intermittent bowel obstruction. The infiltrative growth and the local release of serotonin and other substances results in the formation of dense fibrosis, which may affect mesenteric vessels and cause ischemia and venous congestion. Microscopically, the tumors are composed of sheets of small, round, well-differentiated neuroendocrine cells that can be identified by silver impregnation staining or by immunohistochemical staining for neuroendocrine markers, such as chromogranins.

CLINICAL PRESENTATION

Small bowel carcinoid tumors are often asymptomatic because they grow slowly in the intestinal wall. Initially, symptoms are vague with a long history of episodic abdominal pain that progresses to cramping, abdominal distension, nausea and vomiting, diarrhea, and weight loss. Ultimately, the primary tumor and mesenteric involvement may result in small bowel obstruction, ischemia, or bleeding. In about 30% to 45% of patients, the diagnosis is made at the time of exploration for small bowel obstruction or ischemia, which is most often secondary to venous thrombosis due to the intense mesenteric desmoplastic reaction. In another subset of patients, the diagnosis is made by detection of liver metastasis identified on imaging studies or celiotomy. These patients may or may not have associated carcinoid syndrome. Large tumor burden in the liver can result in hepatomegaly. Other sites of dissemination are the skeleton, lungs, central nervous system, mediastinal and peripheral lymph nodes, ovaries, breast, and skin.

As many as 20% to 30% of patients with a small bowel carcinoid develop signs of carcinoid syndrome, such as flushing, secretory diarrhea, palpitations, intolerance to some foods or alcohol, right-sided valvular heart disease, and bronchoconstriction. These manifestations are associated with the release of various substances from the tumor, which may include serotonin, histamine, dopamine, vasoactive intestinal peptide, 5-hydroxytryptophan (HTP), and prostaglandins.

The liver can detoxify substances released by the primary and mesenteric tumors, as these are carried through the portal circulation to the liver. Carcinoid syndrome develops when vasoactive substances produced by the tumor enter the systemic circulation without undergoing metabolic degradation by the liver. Therefore the syndrome most commonly occurs when there is metastatic involvement of the liver, or when there is a large burden of retroperitoneal tumor involvement that drains into the systemic circulation, bypassing the liver.

Carcinoid heart disease, or *neoplastic infiltrative cardiomyopathy*, develops in as many as two thirds of patients with carcinoid syndrome and is caused by the effects of circulating serotonin. It is characterized by unique fibrous plaques that preferentially involve the right side of the heart. Those with left-sided disease are likely to have right-to-left cardiac shunts. Carcinoid heart disease may require heart surgery or valve replacement, and it is responsible for about 50% of deaths in these patients.

DIAGNOSIS

From 30% to 50% of patients with a small bowel carcinoid are diagnosed at the time of operation for bowel obstruction, ischemia, or bleeding. For patients suspected of having a small bowel carcinoid who come in with GI symptoms, carcinoid syndrome, or incidental imaging findings, additional studies are available.

Biochemical Studies

Carcinoid tumors of the small bowel can be diagnosed by the demonstration of elevated levels of the serotonin metabolite 5-hydroxyindolacetic acid (5-HIAA) in 24-hour urinary samples collected under strict dietary restrictions. It has been shown that 5-HIAA has a sensitivity of 73% for localized disease and 100% for metastatic disease, and it has a specificity of 100% in predicting the presence of midgut carcinoid.

Chromogranin A is a glycoprotein released by tumor cells, and it can be measured in plasma. The levels of chromogranin A are increased in more than 80% of patients with carcinoid tumors, but its specificity is low for small bowel carcinoids. False-positive chromogranin A tests can be caused by atrophic gastritis, renal impairment,

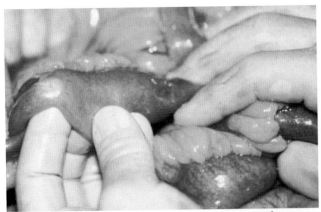

FIGURE I   Midgut carcinoid in the terminal ileum. *(From Åkerström G, Hellman P, Hessman O, et al: Midgut carcinoid tumors: surgical treatment and prognosis, Best Pract Res Clin Gastroenterol 19(5):717, 2005.)*

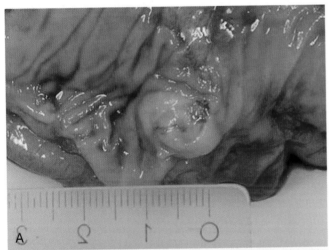

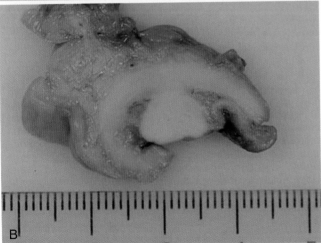

FIGURE 2   **A,** Macroscopic image of a 1.5 cm tumor of the terminal ileum. **B,** Cross-section of the surgical preparation. *(From Bellutti M, Fry LC, Schmitt J, et al: Detection of neuroendocrine tumors of the small bowel by double balloon enteroscopy, Dig Dis Sci 54:1050, 2009.)*

inflammatory bowel disease, or use of proton pump inhibitors. There is a correlation between chromogranin A levels, tumor load, and prognosis, and chromogranin A measurement is currently being used as a tumor marker for monitoring of disease progress and surveillance of recurrence.

Imaging and Endoscopic Studies

Because primary small bowel carcinoid tumors are often small in size, they are not typically seen on computed tomography (CT) scan. Lesions are more often identified on contrast CT scan once involvement of the mesentery or liver is evident. A mesenteric tumor with radiating densities is highly suggestive of mesenteric metastasis of a small bowel carcinoid, with calcifications present in more than 50% of those lesions (Figure 3).

Contrast enhancement aids in the evaluation of involvement of the major mesenteric vessels by assessing tumor mass and resectability and defining the extent of liver involvement. Liver metastases are generally hypervascular, and tumor necrosis may produce central, heterogeneous nonenhancing regions within the metastases, giving lesions a rim-like pattern of enhancement (Figure 4).

Magnetic resonance tomography can sometimes better demonstrate the extent of liver metastasis. A significant percentage of small bowel carcinoids overexpress somatostatin receptors, which have high affinity for the somatostatin analogue octreotide. Octreoscan and somatostatin receptor scintigraphy (SRS) with labeled octreotide is routinely used to determine metastatic spread and has more than 90% sensitivity (Figure 5).

Standard positron emission tomography (PET) scan is used less in the setting of well-differentiated tumors; however, the use of PET with specific tracers for neuroendocrine tumors, such as labeled HTP or dihydroxyphenylalanine, may allow for better sensitivity in the detection of small primary tumors and lymph node metastases.

Duodenal carcinoids are endoscopically accessible lesions that may be further characterized by endoscopic ultrasound (EUS) to determine the extent of disease. Echocardiogram should be performed on patients with carcinoid syndrome to evaluate for valvular disease and congestive heart disease, which can be detected in up to 70% of patients.

Localization of the Primary Tumor

A primary small bowel carcinoid may not be seen on imaging, and thus a patient with chronic abdominal pain may be labeled as having irritable bowel syndrome. Ileocolonoscopy should be performed to rule out synchronous neoplastic disease and may identify carcinoid tumors in the terminal ileum/ileocecal valve. Capsule endoscopy can be useful after small bowel enteroclysis studies have failed to detect the primary tumor, and it can be used to screen the small bowel in patients with a suspected small bowel carcinoid.

Double-balloon enteroscopy (DBE) can be performed through the oral or the anal route. The combined approach allows for complete small bowel examination in 86% of patients. DBE allows for direct access to the lesion for histologic diagnosis and for India ink marking for intraoperative localization.

TREATMENT

Although treatment of a small bowel carcinoid should be a multidisciplinary effort, surgery is the primary treatment for most patients. Specific issues in the preoperative assessment of patients with small bowel carcinoids include 1) determination of the extent of local and distant disease, 2) identification of synchronous carcinoid and noncarcinoid tumors, 3) fluid and electrolyte repletion, 4) pharmacologic treatment of carcinoid syndrome, and 5) detection of cardiac abnormalities.

Preoperative management of patients with carcinoid tumors should include prophylactic measures against potential carcinoid crisis precipitated by anesthesia and operative stress. Although the risk of carcinoid crisis is higher for patients with carcinoid syndrome, all patients with carcinoid tumors are at risk. Prophylactic measures include perioperative administration of the somatostatin analog octreotide (100 µg subcutaneously three times daily). Carcinoid crisis

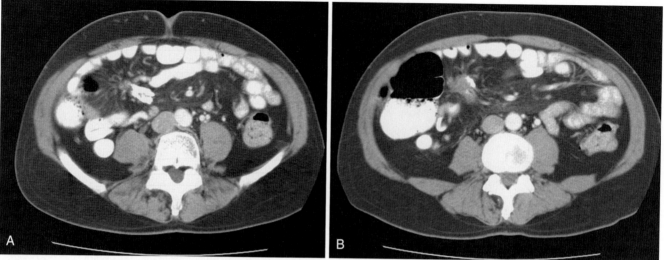

FIGURE 3   Abdominal CT scan illustrating a mesenteric tumor with radiating densities and calcifications.

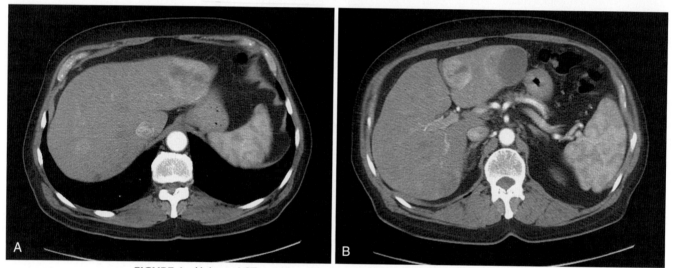

FIGURE 4   Abdominal CT scan illustrating liver metastases from a small bowel carcinoid.

may be treated with bolus intravenous octreotide (100 μg IV push) followed by an octreotide infusion, antihistamines, hydrocortisone, and albuterol as needed.

Duodenal Carcinoids

Duodenal carcinoids should be removed unless there is widely metastatic disease, markedly limited life expectancy, or increased surgical risk. Even in the face of metastatic disease, these lesions may be removed if they occur with complications, such as uncontrollable bleeding, or if the metastases are in the liver only and they are potentially resectable.

Different options for resection are available, and there is still considerable controversy on the selection of treatment modalities for these lesions. Lesions smaller than 1 cm may be locally treated by endoscopic resection, provided there is no evidence of lymph node involvement by imaging, SRS and, ideally, EUS. Lesions between 1 and 2 cm and periampullar lesions may be amenable to transduodenal excision; the concern again is for retained lymph node metastases. Large (>2 cm) duodenal carcinoids and lesions with associated lymph node involvement should be treated by duodenal resection, which most often requires pancreaticoduodenectomy.

Jejunum/Ileum

Most patients with small bowel carcinoids will initially be seen for intestinal obstruction. The diagnosis in these patients may be suspected and is typically made after celiotomy and resection. Findings at celiotomy may include a relatively small ileal mass and large mesenteric metastases with surrounding mesenteric fibrosis. The entire bowel should be inspected for additional synchronous lesions (seen in approximately 30% of patients). If feasible, the primary tumor and mesenteric metastases should be removed by wedge resection of the mesentery and limited intestinal resection.

Lymph node metastases should be cleared by high dissection around the mesenteric artery and its branches. If this cannot be accomplished at the time of emergency operation, there is a role for reoperation, after the patient has been evaluated for synchronous carcinoid and noncarcinoid tumors and for extent of disease and resectability. In cases of severe desmoplastic reaction around the superior mesenteric vessels, radical resection may not be possible. Wedge resection in the fibrotic and contracted mesentery may compromise the superior mesenteric vessels and devascularize a large extent of small bowel, leading to short bowel syndrome.

Careful preoperative mapping with CT scan or MRI is indicated to assess resectability. Because most small bowel carcinoids will

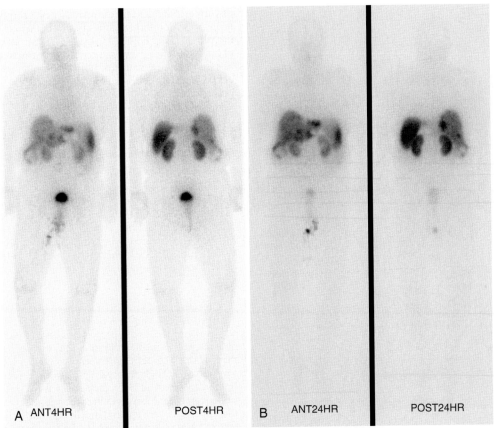

A ANT4HR   POST4HR   B ANT24HR   POST24HR

FIGURE 5   Octreoscan in the same patient as Figure 4, illustrating uptake pattern in liver metastases from a small bowel carcinoid.

originate in the terminal ileum, the mesenteric tumor mass may be mostly situated to the right of the superior mesenteric artery. This may allow for resection and preservation of vascular supply to the remaining small bowel. In these cases, mobilization of the right colon and small bowel mesentery to the level of the lower pancreatic border may help identify the extent of disease. The superior mesenteric vessels should be identified and followed dorsally in the elevated mesenteric root. Arteries and veins can then be dissected free from surrounding tumor. Vascular collaterals and arcades should be preserved, and intestinal resection should be reserved until dissection of the mesenteric tumor is complete, in an effort to determine bowel viability (Figure 6).

Tumor multicentricity should be carefully assessed and should not be a contraindication for resection. In asymptomatic patients, prophylactic resection of mesenteric tumor is recommended because it may later become more difficult to manage. Cholecystectomy should be considered during abdominal operation because many patients on long-term somatostatin analogs will develop gallstones.

Metastatic Disease

Over 60% of patients will have nonlocalized disease at diagnosis, and approximately 50% of patients will be seen initially with liver metastases. Surgical resection remains the gold standard in the treatment of liver metastases. Patients resected for cure have a survival rate of 60% to 80% at 5 years. According to the European Neuroendocrine Tumor Society (ENETS) consensus meeting, the minimal requirements for resection with curative intent are (1) resectable well-differentiated liver disease with acceptable morbidity (~30%) rate and a less than 5% mortality rate, (2) absence of right heart insufficiency, and (3) absence of extraabdominal metastases or diffuse peritoneal carcinomatosis.

Care should be taken to ensure adequate and functional residual liver parenchyma postoperatively. If the primary tumor is still present, it should be removed at that time. One- or two-step procedures may be undertaken, depending upon the complexity of the resection. If heart surgery is also required, it should be undertaken about 3 months prior to liver surgery.

Besides resection, other options for management of liver metastases include ablative procedures, embolization, transplantation, and molecular targeted radionuclide therapy, alone or in combination with medical treatment. Liver metastases causing functional symptoms that do not respond to medical treatment can be treated with palliative debulking procedures with a high probability of symptom control.

In patients with diffuse unresectable liver metastases, or in those who have life-threatening hormonal disturbances refractory to medical therapy, liver transplantation may be an option in well-selected candidates. Long-term cure is still exceptional for these patients. The most frequently used ablative technique is radiofrequency ablation (RFA), although other techniques described include cryotherapy and laser-induced thermotherapy. These techniques can be used effectively as antitumor treatment and to relieve symptoms in patients with liver metastases, either as sole therapy or in combination with resection. RFA has the potential to be delivered percutaneously under image guidance, which may be useful for nonoperative candidates. The use of RFA is not recommended for patients with tumors over 5 cm or those near vital structures, large vessels, and central bile ducts.

Because the blood supply of liver metastases is predominantly arterial, transcatheter arterial embolization or chemoembolization (TACE) may be used in patients with unresectable liver disease, although there is no proof that TACE is superior to embolization alone in these patients. Objective tumor responses and effective control of symptoms can be seen in over 50% of patients. Transarterial

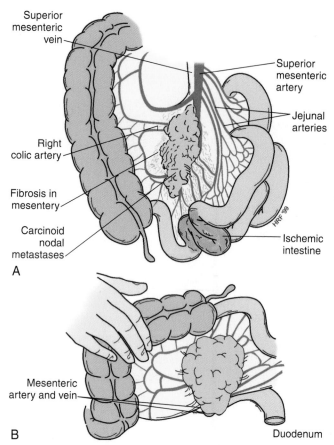

FIGURE 6 Resection of midgut carcinoid primary tumor and mesenteric metastasis. **A,** Mesenteric tumor may extensively involve the mesenteric root. **B,** Mobilization of cecum, terminal ileum, and mesenteric root allows the tumor to be lifted, approached also from a posterior angle, and separated from duodenum, pancreas, and main mesenteric vessels with preservation of intestinal vascular supply and intestinal length. *(From Åkerström G, Hellman P, Hessman O, et al: Midgut carcinoid tumors: surgical treatment and prognosis, Best Pract Res Clin Gastroenterol 19(5):717, 2005.)*

embolization should be performed only in centers staffed with experienced surgeons, and it is contraindicated in patients with portal vein thrombosis and hepatic insufficiency. Figure 7 summarizes the treatment approach to liver metastases without extrapancreatic spread.

Biotherapy

Long-Acting Somatostatin Analogs

Somatostatin analogs are effective in reducing hypersecretion-related symptoms in patients with carcinoid syndrome. A reduction of biochemical markers can be seen in 40% to 60% of patients, and symptomatic improvement is seen in 40% to 80% of patients. The duration of the effects varies, and the antiproliferative effect of somatostatin analogs is limited. Partial or complete responses are seen in less than 10% of patients; however, stabilization of progression of disease occurs in 24% to 57% of patients with documented tumor growth before initiation of treatment.

Therapy is initiated with short-acting analogs, followed by depot formulations that can be given every 4 weeks; these should be titrated individually. Side effects may include abdominal discomfort, flatulence, steatorrhea, malabsorption, and gallstone formation. Monitoring of the efficacy of therapy is done by observing patient symptoms and urinary 5-HIAA, plasma serotonin, and plasma substance P levels. Interferon-α treatment is recommended as second-line treatment of functioning tumors with a low proliferation rate. Its effect is not as rapid, and its toxicities are more pronounced than those of somatostatin analogs. Biochemical and symptoms control can be seen in up to 50% of patients, with partial tumor size responses of 10% to 15%.

Peptide-Receptor Radionuclide Therapy

Targeting of somatostatin receptors with radiolabeled somatostatin analogs is a promising option for the treatment of somatostatin-receptor–positive endocrine tumors, and it may soon become the therapy of choice for patients with metastatic or inoperable disease. Treatment with somatostatin analogs labeled with ^{111}In, ^{90}Y, or ^{177}Lu can result in symptomatic improvement, although tumor remission is seldom achieved with ^{111}In-labeled analogs. An objective response was achieved in 9% to 33% of patients treated with ^{90}Y-DOTATOC, with a median duration of response of 30 months.

Objective and minor responses to ^{177}Lu-octreotate were achieved in 29% and 16% of patients, respectively; stable disease was present in 35%, and progressive disease was present in 20% of patients, with a median duration of response of 40 months. Treatment with ^{177}Lu-octreotate seems to confer a survival benefit of several years. High tumoral uptake of radioactivity on SRS and limited numbers of liver metastases were predictive factors for tumor remission. Adverse effects of peptide receptor radionuclide therapy (PRRT) are few and mostly mild with the use of renal protective agents. Serious, delayed adverse effects, such as myelodysplastic syndrome or renal failure, are rare. In summary, the data on PRRT compare favorably with those on the few alternative treatment approaches, such as chemotherapy.

Chemotherapy

Chemotherapy for neuroendocrine tumors includes treatment with combinations of streptozotocin, doxorubicin and 5-fluorouracil, cisplatin and etoposide, and dacarbazine. The benefits of chemotherapy for small bowel carcinoids are very limited.

FOLLOW-UP AND PROGNOSIS

From the study of large numbers of patients from the NCDB and SEER trials, some prognostic factors have been identified: patients older than 55 years, male, of black race/ethnicity, and with tumors larger than 1 cm, distant metastasis, and involved margins have been associated with a less favorable prognosis. The 5-year observed survival rate was 65% for small bowel carcinoids, and it appears to be improving with active and combined medical and surgical treatment.

Although a formal staging system is lacking, tumors are often grouped by the extent of spread at diagnosis. *Localized* refers to a tumor confined to the organ in which the tumor originated. *Regional* refers to involvement of surrounding structures, including lymph nodes and contiguous organs. *Distant* refers to spread beyond the nearby structures to other organs.

Presence of liver metastases and carcinoid heart disease have been the most significant adverse prognostic factors. Patients with inoperable liver metastases had a 5-year survival of approximately 50%, and survival was 40% with inoperable liver and mesenteric metastases. Recommended follow-up depends on the extent of disease and includes history and physical examination, chromogranin A and 5-HIAA, abdomen and pelvis CT scan or MRI, and other imaging studies, such as octreoscan, as clinically indicated.

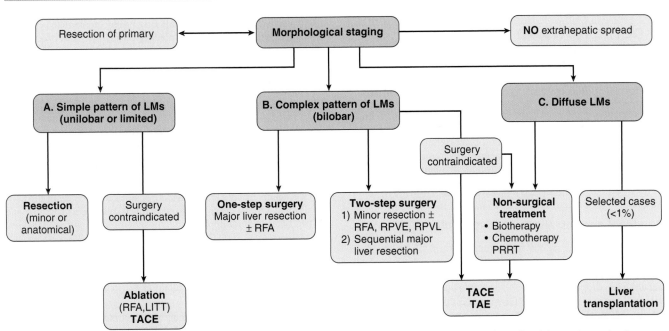

FIGURE 7 Treatment approach to liver metastases without extrahepatic spread. The first line of therapy in limited unilobar and complex liver disease without extrahepatic spread is surgical resection with or without local ablative techniques. Patients with diffuse liver disease, and those who are poor surgical candidates, may be treated with biotherapy, chemotherapy, TACE, or TAE. In specially selected candidates with diffuse metastases, liver transplantation may be an option. *LM*, Liver metastasis; *PRRT*, peptide receptor radiotherapy; *RFA*, radiofrequency ablation; *RPVE*, right portal vein embolization; *RPVL*, right portal vein ligation; *LITT*, laser-induced thermotherapy; *TACE*, transcatheter arterial chemoembolization; *TAE*, transcatheter arterial embolization. *(From Steinmüller T, Kianmanesh R, Falconi M, et al: Consensus guidelines for the management of patients with liver metastases from digestive (neuro)endocrine tumors: foregut, midgut, hindgut, and unknown primary, Neuroendocrinology 87:47, 2008.)*

SELECTED READINGS

Åkerström G, Hellman P, Hessman O, et al: Management of midgut carcinoids, *J Surg Oncol* 89:161, 2005.
Bilimoria KY, Bentrem DJ, Wayne JD, et al: Small bowel cancer in the United States, *Ann Surg* 249:63, 2009.
Eriksson B, Klöppel G, Krenning E, et al: Consensus guidelines for the management of patients with digestive neuroendocrine tumors: well-differentiated jejuna-ileal tumor/carcinoma, *Neuroendocrinology* 87:8, 2008.

Levy AD, Sobin LH: Gastrointestinal carcinoids: imaging features with clinicopathologic comparison, *RadioGraphics* 27:237, 2007.
Steinmüller T, Kianmanesh R, Falconi M, et al: Consensus guidelines for the management of patients with liver metastases from digestive neuroendocrine tumors: foregut, midgut, hindgut, and unknown primary, *Neuroendocrinology* 87:47, 2008.
van Essen M, Krenning EP, Kam BLR, et al: Peptide-receptor radionuclide therapy for endocrine tumors, *Nat Rev Endocrinol* 5:382, 2009.

MANAGEMENT OF DIVERTICULOSIS OF THE SMALL BOWEL

Scott F. Gallagher, MD, and
Peter J. Fabri, MD, PhD

OVERVIEW

Although diverticulosis of the small bowel remains relatively uncommon, appropriate management is clinically important. The reported prevalence from multiple autopsy series ranges from 0.3% up to 5%. Diverticulosis of the small bowel has been observed in approximately 1% of small bowel contrast studies done for any reason; however, the radiology literature reports diverticulosis in up to 6% of small bowel contrast studies for symptoms. Most small bowel diverticula are asymptomatic, with estimates that fewer than 4% cause symptoms.

Small bowel diverticula can be congenital or acquired and can be classified as *true diverticula,* which contain all layers of the intestinal wall, or *false diverticula,* which contain only mucosa, submucosa, and serosa. Diverticula can occur in the duodenum, jejunum, and ileum. Most asymptomatic small bowel diverticula are identified incidentally at celiotomy or on radiographic study and usually are managed nonoperatively; advances in endoscopy have also increased the recognition and diagnosis. Resection of jejunoileal diverticula has been advocated because they are the most likely to become symptomatic or develop complications.

A fair amount of literature exists addressing the management of complications from diverticulosis of the small bowel. There have been hundreds of publications; most are case reports that include reviews of the literature. Some larger series have attempted to extrapolate the findings to the general population, but the utility of doing so may be limited.

DETECTION AND MANAGEMENT OF ASYMPTOMATIC SMALL BOWEL DIVERTICULOSIS

Incidentally Discovered Small Bowel Diverticulosis

In the current era of radiologic imaging combined with advances in endoscopy, diverticulosis of the small bowel is increasingly being diagnosed. Despite the seeming increase in detection, there has not been a notable increase in those diverticula that become symptomatic. Most are truly discovered incidentally while still asymptomatic.

Duodenal and Intraluminal Diverticula

Duodenal diverticula are the most common form of diverticulosis of the small bowel, accounting for approximately 45% of all diverticula. Duodenal diverticula are usually solitary and asymptomatic, and although they are found in 1% to 6% of all upper gastrointestinal (GI) radiologic series, they are discovered even more commonly at autopsy. Fortunately, less than 1% become symptomatic because surgical intervention carries significant morbidity and mortality.

Duodenal diverticula can develop congenitally or they can be acquired. In addition to those classically described, pseudodiverticula, or windsock diverticula, can also occur congenitally in the duodenum as prolapses of mucosa or an incompletely divided congenital septum. They typically arise from the second portion of the duodenum and can extend as far as the fourth portion. Frequently, pseudodiverticula are associated with other congenital anomalies: malrotation, omphalocele, annular pancreas, congenital biliary cysts, and various cardiac and urinary congenital abnormalities. Symptoms vary depending on the size and location, especially with regard to proximity to the ampulla of Vater.

Asymptomatic diverticula, by definition, are incidentally discovered upon radiographic or endoscopic examination and at celiotomy for some other complaint. Because most are asymptomatic and remain so, it has become the standard recommendation to not operate or resect any asymptomatic small bowel diverticula.

Interestingly, there is statistical justification for operating only on symptomatic diverticula of the small bowel, which is infrequent; only 1% are symptomatic, and even fewer than that ever come to operation. Conversely, there is also statistical justification for not operating on asymptomatic diverticula. It has been calculated by Zani and colleagues that 758 patients with incidental Meckel diverticulum would need to undergo intestinal resection to prevent one death.

Jejunoileal Diverticula

Diverticula arising in the jejunum and ileum account for 25% of all small bowel diverticulosis; however, they are the most likely to become symptomatic, but only about 10% will. They are commonly multiple: 80% occur in the jejunum, 15% occur in the ileum, and 5% occur in both.

These jejunoileal (false) diverticula are thought to develop as a result of myoneural abnormalities and dysmotility in the migrating motor complexes, which leads to spastic contractions that result in prolonged, increased intraluminal pressures. This is thought to lead to the formation of false diverticula over many years. Enteroclysis is the best radiographic study to evaluate jejunoileal diverticula and confirm the diagnosis; however, the use of capsule endoscopy is gaining an increased role in the diagnosis and evaluation of jejunoileal diverticula, especially when diverticula are symptomatic but not infected.

As with most other diverticulosis of the small bowel, surgical excision is not warranted in an asymptomatic patient with jejunoileal diverticula or with any diverticula discovered incidentally; in addition, there has been no proven role for prophylactic resection.

Meckel Diverticula

Meckel diverticula are the most common congenital small bowel abnormality and account for the remaining 25% of small bowel diverticulosis. A Meckel diverticulum is the remnant, from failure of obliteration, of a persistent portion of the proximal vitelline (omphalomesenteric) duct, which connects the embryonic midgut to the yolk sac. It only occurs on the antimesenteric border of ileum as a true diverticulum, which contains all layers of the intestinal wall.

Meckel diverticula are located approximately 2 feet from the ileocecal valve. One of every two Meckel diverticula (50%) contains one of two types of heterotopic tissue, most commonly *gastric* (75%) but also *pancreatic* (15%). The "rule of two" states that Meckel diverticula occur twice as commonly in males in 2% of the population and become symptomatic in 2% of cases usually within the first 2 years of life; they can extend over 2 inches in length and predominantly cause two types of symptoms, *bleeding* and *obstruction*.

The lifetime risk of an asymptomatic Meckel diverticulum is very low. Most Meckel diverticula will become symptomatic within the first 2 years of life and certainly by the age of 18 years. Based on 19 autopsy studies, of which seven were reported postnatal autopsies, Meckel diverticulum had a prevalence of 1.23%. Mortality from Meckel diverticulum is low (<0.001%) and is most common in the pediatric population. Incidentally discovered Meckel diverticula should be left in situ because the risk of postoperative complications from resection outweighs the risk of late complications.

A comprehensive, systematic review done by Zani and colleagues (2008) found no compelling evidence in the literature to support prophylactic resection of incidentally discovered Meckel diverticulum at operation for an unrelated condition, even in young children. Per the previous edition of this text, "[Upon] review of the literature, most surgeons do not recommend resection for an incidental Meckel diverticulum in a patient 18 years or older." Nonetheless, palpable evidence of ectopic tissue; prior diverticulitis, hemorrhage, or intussusception; or the presence of a mesodiverticular band serve as relative indications. It is widely agreed that symptomatic or incidentally discovered Meckel diverticula in a young child should be resected.

MANAGEMENT OF SYMPTOMATIC SMALL BOWEL DIVERTICULA

Duodenal Diverticula

The investigational modalities of choice for duodenal diverticula includes esophagogastroduodenoscopy and endoscopic retrograde cholangiopancreatography. These two modalities have become the cornerstone of visualizing duodenal diverticula, especially to clarify the relationship with and proximity to the ampulla of Vater and any contiguous biliary or pancreatic ductal structures. Increasingly, computed tomography (CT), especially with multiplanar reconstructions, and magnetic resonance cholangiopancreatography are being utilized for imaging, often to better characterize findings on standard contrast radiography.

Symptomatic duodenal diverticula are often the most difficult to manage because they usually include or are adjacent to the ampulla of Vater and biliary and pancreatic ductal structures. Operative management is reserved for when the patient cannot undergo endoscopic therapy or after failure of endoscopic therapy, which usually includes sphincterotomy as well as temporary stent placement.

Operative treatment of duodenal diverticula can be difficult, and it is associated with significant morbidity and mortality, especially in inexperienced hands. Keys to a successful operative approach include several important factors: (1) a wide Kocher maneuver,

(2) clarification of the anatomic relationship of the diverticulum to biliary and pancreatic ductal structures, (3) identification of *all* biliary and pancreatic ductal structures, (4) liberal use of intraoperative ductal stents, and (5) transverse or oblique closure of the duodenum and sometimes a Thal patch, including cholecystectomy, with any operation for duodenal diverticula. A thorough description of treatment options appears in the previous (ninth) edition of this text.

Jejunoileal Diverticula

Symptomatic jejunoileal diverticulitis is most often diagnosed using contrast-enhanced CT. After enteroclysis, uninfected symptomatic jejunoileal diverticula are increasingly being evaluated by push enteroscopy, double-balloon endoscopy, and capsule endoscopy with an expanding role in the diagnosis and evaluation. Jejunoileal diverticulitis can be managed nonoperatively; however, symptomatic diverticula may warrant more aggressive treatment. Jejunoileal diverticula can present as diverticulitis, refractory inflammation, obstruction, perforation, and hemorrhage.

Most recommendations support segmental resection of jejunoileal diverticula when necessary, especially to prevent narrowing of the small bowel. The real possibility of postoperative complications, a reason to not operate when asymptomatic, is the reason for at least considering incidental appendectomy at the same time.

Meckel Diverticula

Meckel diverticula can become symptomatic in many ways. Most commonly, acid produced by ectopic gastric mucosa causes ulceration along the mesenteric border of the ileum; of those with hemorrhage, 95% show evidence of ectopic gastric mucosa. Meckel diverticula is also a common cause of chronic and acute GI hemorrhage in young patients, and it is an important cause of hemorrhage in the entire pediatric population, although it also occurs in adults.

Diagnostic modalities usually include some form of angiography or nuclear scintigraphy. Angiography can be useful during active hemorrhage because it can show bleeding into the diverticulum or distal small bowel. Angiography is even more useful when it demonstrates a persistent right vitelline artery arising from the superior mesenteric artery, or an enlarged, long, nonbranching, embryonic ileal artery leading to the diverticulum.

The most useful arteriographic finding is a nonbranching end artery in the right lower abdomen containing a cluster of small, irregular arteries at its distal distribution. These often contain irregular arteries in the wall of the diverticulum and vitelline artery remnants as well as increased parenchymal blush from the ectopic gastric mucosa lining the diverticulum.

Meckel scintigraphy uses technetium-99m pertechnetate, which is concentrated then excreted by mucus-producing cells (gastric mucosa). It is important to remember that a Meckel scan identifies ectopic gastric mucosa, not the hemorrhage. To obtain a quality study, it is often necessary to obtain oblique, lateral, or postvoid films to distinguish a diverticulum; the activity in a Meckel diverticulum should occur at about the same time as activity in the stomach. Depending on the facility and the skill of the radiologist, the sensitivity of a Meckel scan is reportedly 75% to 85% and supposedly can be increased by pretreatment with pentagastrin or glucagon.

In adults, Meckel diverticula commonly show up as small bowel obstruction (45%). Once adequately resuscitated, obstruction is managed as quickly as possible, usually by wedge excision and primary closure or amputation with a surgical stapler.

Diverticulitis (25%) within a Meckel diverticulum is often indistinguishable from acute appendicitis and is managed by segmental resection and primary ileoileostomy. Hemorrhage (20%) and ulcer are also managed by segmental resection and primary ileoileostomy. At operation for hemorrhage, segmental resection is necessary because the ulcer is typically on the mesenteric border of the ileum, opposite the Meckel diverticulum on the antimesenteric border and occasionally distal to it. Despite improved diagnostic modalities, enteroclysis, angiography, and scintigraphy, most bleeding Meckel diverticula are diagnosed at celiotomy.

Appendectomy should be contemplated, and often undertaken, at any operation for a symptomatic Meckel diverticulum, to prevent any future diagnostic dilemmas.

Suggested Readings

Akhrass R, Yaffe MB, Fischer C, et al: Small-bowel diverticulosis: perceptions and reality, *J Am Coll Surg* 184(4):383–388, 1997.
Chiu EJ, Shyr YM, Su CH, et al: Diverticular disease of the small bowel, *Hepatogastroenterology* 47(31):181–184, 2000.
Kouraklis G, Glinavou A, Mantas D, et al: Clinical implications of small bowel diverticula, *Imaj* 4(6):431–433, 2002.
Thompson JN, Salem RR, Hemingway AP, et al: Specialist investigation of obscure gastrointestinal bleeding, *Gut* 28(1):47–51, 1987.
Zani A, Eaton S, Rees CM, et al: Incidentally detected Meckel diverticulum: to resect or not to resect?, *Ann Surg* 247:276–281, 2008.

Motility Disorders of the Stomach and Small Bowel

Maria Lucia L. Madariaga, MD, and David I. Soybel, MD

patients undergoing manipulation of the abdominal viscera during laparotomy and especially during colectomy; in a subset of these patients (10% to 20%), ileus is prolonged. In addition, there are medical illnesses in which motility of the stomach and/or small intestine requires the surgeon's evaluation because the condition is in the differential diagnosis of a surgical condition, or it requires surgical intervention for relief of symptoms. A guiding principle in most cases is that surgical intervention generally should be considered for patients with disabling symptoms, after reasonable efforts at medical management have failed.

OVERVIEW

The surgeon encounters motility disturbances of the stomach and small intestine in patients who have undergone vagotomy and in those who require reconstruction following partial or total gastric resection. Paralysis of the small intestine is routinely observed in

GASTROPARESIS

Gastroparesis is the syndrome associated with delayed gastric emptying in the absence of mechanical obstruction. Emptying of solids is more often compromised than that of liquids; indeed, poor tolerance of a liquid diet is predictive of poor outcome.

Idiopathic gastroparesis has been reported in an estimated 4% of the adult population, with an overwhelming female majority and a mean age of onset of 34 years. It is present in up to 50% of patients with type 1 diabetes and 30% of those with type 2 diabetes. Symptoms of delayed gastric emptying, requiring gastroenterostomy for drainage, were reported in 15% to 20% of the first groups of patients who underwent truncal vagotomy for treatment of peptic ulcer. Similar rates have been reported in patients undergoing fundoplication for gastroesophageal reflux, gastric bypass surgery, pylorus-preserving Whipple procedure, esophagectomy, and heart/lung transplant.

Gastroparesis is also reported as a side effect of certain medications—including opiates, anticholinergics, and calcium channel blockers—and as a complication of viral infection, connective tissue disease, thyroid dysfunction, metabolic abnormalities (hyperglycemia, hypokalemia, hypomagnesemia), and neuromuscular disorders.

The predominant symptoms are nausea, vomiting, early satiety, and bloating in the upper abdomen; these form the basis of the gastroparesis cardinal symptom index, which is used to assess and standardize the severity of disease, although it may not always reliably predict delayed gastric emptying in symptomatic patients. Other symptoms may include postprandial fullness, abdominal pain, and weight change.

A classification scheme of gastroparesis severity has been proposed, delineating three categories: *mild, compensated,* and *severe* gastroparesis. In mild (grade 1) gastroparesis, symptoms are easily controlled, and nutrition is maintained on a regular diet or with minor dietary modifications. In compensated (grade 2) gastroparesis, symptoms are partially controlled by pharmacotherapy, nutrition is maintained with dietary modifications, and hospital admissions are rare. In severe (grade 3) gastroparesis, symptoms are refractory to medical therapy, nutrition via oral route is compromised, and hospital admissions are frequent.

Initial evaluation includes a computed tomographic (CT) scan and upper endoscopy to exclude mechanical obstruction due to peptic ulcer disease or malignancy; serologic and hematologic studies should be undertaken to evaluate nutritional and metabolic abnormalities. The gold standard for diagnosis is gastric emptying scintigraphy of a technetium 99m sulfur-colloid–labeled low-fat, egg-white meal, with scintigraphy at 1, 2, and 4 hours after meal ingestion in the upright position. Medications that affect gastric emptying should be discontinued 48 to 72 hours in advance, and blood glucose level in diabetics should be below 275 mg/dL on the day of testing. More than 10% retention of the solid meal after 4 hours is abnormal, with 62% specificity and 93% sensitivity. Intravenous (IV) prokinetics may be given after 4 hours to determine whether the patient is a "responder" or "nonresponder."

Other radiographic techniques that may be less desirable due to lack of standardization, reliance on operator technique, radiation exposure, or relative unavailability include ingestion of radiopaque markers, which show an abnormal response if they remain in the stomach 6 hours after ingestion. Serial transabdominal ultrasound, which measures when antral area/volume returns to fasting baseline, is only reliable for liquid emptying, which is rarely impaired in patients with severe gastroparesis. Magnetic resonance imaging (MRI) with gadolinium measures semisolid gastric emptying and shows reduced velocity of antral propagation waves, and CT with 99-Tc pertechnetate that accumulates within the gastric wall provides real-time measurements of wall motion.

Other tests that may assist in diagnosis include stable isotope breath tests, swallowed capsule telemetry, and manometry. In the breath test (80% specificity, 86% sensitivity), a solid meal is labeled with ^{13}C-octanoate, which is rapidly absorbed by the small intestine, metabolized by the liver, and expelled by the lungs as $^{13}CO_2$ during expiration. A gastric emptying curve can be calculated by measuring the concentration of $^{13}CO_2$ over time. Normal half times of solid emptying (<109 minutes) and liquid emptying (<75 minutes) correlate well with scintigraphy.

A swallowed capsule (83% specificity, 82% sensitivity) can continuously measure changes in pH, pressure, and temperature to determine gastric transit time. Antroduodenal manometry measures gastroduodenal contractility and evaluates responses to prokinetic agents, but its use is limited due to its invasive nature and the need for gastrointestinal (GI) motility expertise to perform the test and analyze results. None of these objective measures of gastric function clearly correlates with symptoms; thus they cannot be used to select patients for intervention or to predict the ensuing response.

Management of gastroparesis is centered on nutritional and metabolic support, reducing symptoms, and addressing the underlying cause (Figure 1). The first approach should be dietary modification. The patient should be advised to partake of multiple small meals and avoid fibers and fats, which tend to slow gastric emptying. Since liquid emptying is often preserved in gastroparesis, noncarbonated fluids can be taken throughout the meal, and appropriate liquid caloric supplementation can be used if solids are not tolerated. Diabetic patients should maintain optimal glycemic control. For enteral access, jejunostomy tubes are preferred over nasogastric (NG) and gastrostomy tubes; low-osmolarity tube feeds are used, and parenteral nutrition should be considered when the patient is severely malnourished (>10% unintentional weight loss in 6 months) or is unable to maintain weight by oral intake alone.

The next line of therapy uses medication. It is common for patients to be on a combination of prokinetic and antiemetic agents, selected by trial and error, to control nausea, vomiting, and bloating. Commonly these medications have no effect on abdominal pain or early satiety, but prokinetic agents enhance GI tract contractility.

Currently, only two prokinetic medications are available for use in the United States for the indication of gastroparesis. Erythromycin (50 to 250 mg three times daily, 30 minutes before meals), a macrolide antibiotic that also acts as a motilin receptor agonist, is the most potent stimulant of solid and liquid gastric emptying in its IV form. A meta-analysis of 36 clinical trials found that erythromycin was the most potent stimulant of gastric emptying, and that erythromycin and domperidone are most effective in reducing gastroparesis symptoms. Metoclopramide (10 mg orally 30 minutes before meals and at bedtime)—acting as a serotonin 5-HT4 receptor agonist, dopamine D2 receptor antagonist, and direct stimulator of smooth muscle contraction—is effective for short-term symptomatic relief for up to several weeks, but it has not been definitively shown to improve gastric emptying. Metoclopramide is inferior to erythromycin in terms of symptomatic relief. Domperidone (10 to 20 mg three to four times daily, 30 minutes before meals), a peripheral dopamine D2 receptor antagonist, improves gastroparesis symptoms and reduces hospital admissions, but studies have not uniformly observed accelerated gastric emptying. Domperidone also has potent central antiemetic action. Although used in several other countries, including Canada, for diabetic gastroparesis and for its antiemetic actions in other settings, it is only available in the United States through a Food and Drug Administration investigational new drug application via local institutional review boards.

Other options for off-label use include Bethanechol, a smooth-muscle muscarinic agonist that increases contraction in the gastric fundus and antrum, but it has significant adverse effects and should only be used if standard prokinetic and antiemetic therapy fails. New agents under clinical investigation include motilin receptor agonists (azithromycin, mitemcinal, atilmotin, ghrelin), dopamine antagonists/serotonin agonists (itopride, sulpiride, mosapride, renzapride), and others (pyridostigmine, nizatidine, cholecystokinin receptor antagonists, sildenafil).

Antiemetics are used to alleviate some of the most disabling symptoms of gastroparesis. Several classes of agents may be helpful, including phenothiazines (prochlorperazine and thiethylperazine), serotonin 5-HT4 receptor antagonists (ondansetron, granisetron, and dolasetron) and antihistamines (diphendyramine, dimenhydrinate, and meclizine). Retrospective studies of diabetic gastroparesis patients suggest that tricyclic antidepressants at low doses may ameliorate nausea and vomiting.

Pylorospasm can contribute to delayed gastric emptying in some patients. Endoscopic injection of botulinum toxin A in the pylorus is an off-label indication that may provide relief of functional gastric

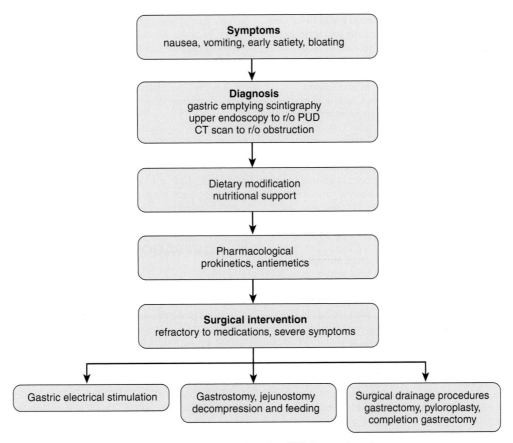

FIGURE 1   Gastroparesis algorithm, *PUD*, Peptic ulcer disease.

outlet obstruction by inhibiting acetylcholine release. Symptoms are reduced with respect to placebo only in highly selected patients (female, age <50 years, nondiabetic, non-postsurgical etiology); even so, symptoms return by 6 months after injection.

For medically refractory or severe gastroparesis, surgical intervention may be required. The most common procedure is gastric electrical stimulation (GES), which is covered in this chapter; it has an incompletely understood mechanism of action but has proven to be the most promising therapy. Supportive measures are also beneficial; gastrostomy and jejunostomy tubes can be used for decompression and feeding, respectively. Gastrectomy, pyloroplasty, and surgical drainage procedures may be offered as a last resort, though data demonstrating efficacy are limited. Conversion from a Billroth I to a Billroth II, although tempting, is rarely an effective intervention. Completion gastrectomy with preservation of a small cuff of gastric tissue may have some long-term benefits, but up to 25% of patients still require some form of parenteral support.

GES is approved as a humanitarian device for drug-refractory gastroparesis and can be currently obtained only at centers that obtain 1-year approval from an FDA-designated institutional review board. Electrodes are placed laparoscopically within the seromuscular layer of the stomach, over the pacemaker area, about 10 cm proximal to the pylorus on the greater curvature of the gastric antrum. Intraoperative endoscopy should be performed to confirm that the electrodes have not perforated the mucosa of the gastric lumen. Leads from the electrodes connect to a pulse generator implanted in the subcutaneous layer of the anterior abdominal wall (the battery life of the Enterra gastric electrical stimulation system [Medtronic, Minneapolis, Minn.] is 6 to 8 years). The low-energy, high-frequency (12 cycles/min) settings currently used have significant antiemetic effect and improve overall quality of life, even though contractility and gastric emptying remain unaffected. Other stimulus parameters may entrain intrinsic gastric electrical activity, elicit propagating contractions,

foster better glycemic control, and, in the morbidly obese population, induce weight loss by reducing appetite.

Clinical trials of stimulation indicated that patients experience 75% to 80% reduction in symptoms, primarily nausea and vomiting, usually within 6 weeks; long-term benefits last 3 to 4 years. Factors associated with a favorable clinical response include primary symptoms of nausea and/or vomiting, independence from narcotic analgesics, and diabetic rather than idiopathic gastroparesis. The strongest adverse effect is infection, which requires device removal (10%).

Newer methods are being developed to achieve temporary endoscopic or percutaneous placement of electrodes. In addition, endoscopically placed mucosal GES may help determine who may be a nonresponder (estimated up to 30% of patients, depending on the cause) before deciding upon this course of therapy. The clinical research consortium on gastroparesis has up-to-date information about current clinical trials (http://www.jhucct.com/gpcrc).

ROUX STASIS SYNDROME

Roux stasis syndrome is encountered following Roux-en-Y gastrojejunostomy. It encompasses symptoms of nausea, vomiting, early satiety, and abdominal pain that arise from Roux limb stasis, delayed gastric emptying, or both. About 25% to 30% of patients who undergo Roux-en-Y gastrojejunostomy subsequently develop Roux stasis syndrome. It occurs predominantly in women and more frequently in cases where the Roux-en-Y limb is greater than 40 cm in length. Dysfunction of both the gastric remnant and the Roux limb results in a continuum of symptoms that may be indistinguishable from those of gastroparesis; however, pure Roux limb dysfunction is generally a late complication, with an onset on the order of months to years.

The diagnosis of Roux stasis syndrome is based on clinical criteria that include epigastric fullness, postprandial pain, nausea, and vomiting. The relative importance of gastric remnant versus Roux limb dysfunction in the manifestation of disease is difficult to discern in the individual patient, particularly because measuring Roux limb transit is not straightforward. Delayed gastrojejunal transit can be demonstrated by scintigraphy; however, interpretation may be difficult due to the reconstructed anatomy, and normal values vary by institution.

Another way to measure motility in the Roux limb is by manometry, though this practice is not widespread. Vagal function can be assessed by measuring the pancreatic polypeptide response to insulin-induced hypoglycemia (PP test). Upper GI series or endoscopy are used to exclude mechanical obstruction.

Medical treatment for Roux stasis syndrome with prokinetics, antiemetics, and minimal use of narcotics has been studied in small patient populations, with demonstrated efficacy in only about 50% of cases. Cisapride provided long-lasting symptomatic relief from pain, fullness, nausea, and vomiting, and it improved transit in about 40% of patients. IV erythromycin significantly reduced gastric emptying time. Bethanechol has also been shown to give short-term symptomatic improvement and decreased gastric retention, but 50% of patients subsequently required total or near-total gastrectomy for recurrent symptoms. Electrical pacing of the Roux limb is currently an experimental treatment in animals only.

Remedial surgical intervention should be pursued when medical therapy fails. Completion gastrectomy is successful in improving symptoms in about 43% of patients, with nausea, need for TPN, and retained food at endoscopy as negative prognostic indicators. The "uncut" Roux procedure may be performed to prevent dysfunction of the intestinal limb (Figure 2). In brief, after vagotomy and antrectomy, Billroth II reconstruction is performed, the afferent limb is stapled closed, and a side-to-side anastomosis between the afferent limb and efferent limb is made 40 cm distal to the gastrojejunostomy. By avoiding jejunal transection, this procedure maintains neuromuscular continuity between the Roux limb and its natural pacemaker. Patients experience about 20% improvement in symptoms relative to the conventional procedure, most likely due to aboral propagation of contractions, because gastric emptying is not affected. However, the risk of staple dehiscence is high, resulting in postoperative alkaline reflux gastritis and esophagitis.

Initial reports demonstrated that rho-shaped Roux-en-Y reconstruction (similar to that described by N.C. Tanner in the 1940s) was effective in reducing Roux stasis syndrome (Figure 3). In this procedure, after transection of the jejunum, 30 cm of distal jejunum is fashioned into a rho shape (jejunojejunostomy), the gastric remnant is anastomosed to the top of the rho (gastrojejunostomy), and the proximal jejunum is anastomosed to the mid jejunum 20 cm distal to the gastrojejunostomy (jejunojejunostomy). The anticipated locus of ectopic pacing is located at the top of the rho-shaped intestine, and the outlet from the stomach flows in two directions. However, the most recent prospective randomized, controlled trial compared conventional versus rho Roux-en-Y procedures and found no significant difference in delayed gastric emptying or any other secondary endpoints.

Another reconstruction option after subtotal gastrectomy is Noh's operation, which combines the concepts of uncut Roux-en-Y and jejunal interposition and aims to preserve physiologic passage through the duodenum (Figure 4). After subtotal gastrectomy, the reconstruction consists of a purse-string jejunal occlusion, end-to-side gastrojejunostomy, side-to-end jejunoduodenostomy, and a side-to-side jejunojejunostomy. Patients who underwent Noh's operation had about a 10% to 20% lower rate of Roux stasis syndrome over time than patients who underwent conventional Roux-en-Y gastrojejunostomy.

POSTVAGOTOMY DIARRHEA

Diarrhea occurs in about 20% of patients after truncal vagotomy; it is severe and debilitating in 2% to 4%. The prevalence of postvagotomy diarrhea (PVD) is much lower, almost nonexistent, after proximal selective vagotomy, especially when celiac and hepatic branches of the vagus are preserved. In a 24-hour period, a patient typically experiences up 20 watery bowel movements that bear no relationship to meals and occur even while asleep. Diarrhea may be explosive, which can lead to malnutrition, weight loss, and orthostatic symptoms from hypovolemia.

The pathophysiology of PVD is to date unclear, but a combination of impaired gastric relaxation and bile acid malabsorption have been suggested. Complete vagotomy alters intraluminal acidity and gastric motility, facilitating bacterial overgrowth that in turn causes diarrhea. Hepatic and celiac denervation impairs the amplitude and coordination of gallbladder contractility with gastric contractility such that the gallbladder distends, a large bile load is delivered into the small intestine, and the capacity of the enterohepatic circulation is overwhelmed. Direct action of bile acids in the colon and delivery of high solute load results in secretory and osmotic diarrhea enriched with bile salts. Interestingly, PVD is more likely to be found after vagotomy in patients who have had prior cholecystectomy, further implicating the pathogenetic role of bile salts.

The difficulty in diagnosing PVD is that diarrhea itself is common after any abdominal operation. Increased levels of bile salts in

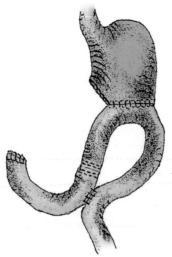

FIGURE 2 The "uncut" Roux procedure.

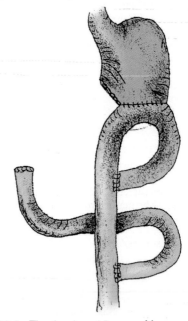

FIGURE 3 The rho-shaped Roux-en-Y reconstruction.

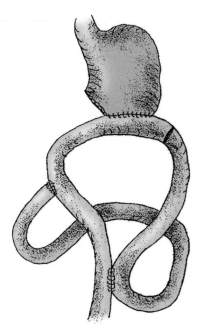

FIGURE 4 Noh's operation.

the feces are consistent with a diagnosis of PVD but do not exclude other primary conditions. Entities such as bacterial overgrowth, malabsorption, infection (particularly *Clostridium difficile*), obstruction, and inflammatory bowel disease should be ruled out. Medications may cause diarrhea by altering intestinal transit time, luminal osmolality, or ion transport; they may also result in nutrient maldigestion or malabsorption or changes in intestinal flora.

Most cases of PVD are self-limited and resolve over time. The first approach should be dietary modification: small, frequent low-fat meals with limited fluids and bulking agents (psyllium, pectin, fiber) to prolong transit time are ideal. Codeine phosphate (60 mg) and loperamide (12 to 24 mg) inhibit GI transit time and have proven efficacy in the short-term management of PVD symptoms. Cholestyramine binds excessive diarrheogenic bile salts and significantly reduces stool volume but it is poorly tolerated and has unconfirmed long-term benefit. One case series documents relief of refractory PVD after initiation of verapamil for cardiac indications, but the mechanism is not clear. Octreotide is not effective for this indication and may exacerbate symptoms by inhibiting pancreatic exocrine function.

The conservative approach, if effective, should resolve symptoms by 18 months after vagotomy. If patients continue to have incapacitating symptoms refractory to medication, the entire GI tract should be assessed by endoscopy before remedial surgery. Correcting rapid gastric emptying may be effective for vasomotor dumping symptoms that are at times associated with cases of PVD, but it does not influence diarrhea. The more successful approach aims to slow small bowel transit. Previously, a 10 cm antiperistaltic jejunal interposition segment about 70 to 100 cm from the ligament of Treitz was used to slow small bowel transit with mixed results—and added risk of episodic partial obstruction. A more successful and better tolerated procedure creates a passive, nonpropulsive segment using a 10 to 12 cm onlay reversed ileal graft about 30 cm from the ileocecal junction. Use of any of these procedures is a last resort for patients with disabling symptoms.

POSTGASTRECTOMY DUMPING

The term *dumping* was first used in 1922 to describe radiographic observations of rapid gastric emptying in patients with vasomotor and GI complaints after gastrectomy. About 25% to 50% of patients who undergo gastrectomy, gastroenterostomy, vagotomy, or Rouxen-Y gastric bypass experience some form of the dumping syndrome, but less than 5% of these patients have severe, disabling symptoms that require medical or surgical management.

Premature rapid emptying occurs because loss of reservoir function and pyloric sphincter mechanisms conspire with vagal denervation to decrease the stomach's ability to relax and accommodate, increasing intragastric pressure and forcing rapid passage of contents, especially liquids, to the duodenum. Additionally, after gastrojejunostomy, duodenal feedback inhibition of gastric emptying is lost. Rapid gastric emptying is accompanied by gut hormone release, such as glucagon-like peptide (GLP-1), which elicits sympathetic activation, and enteroglucagon, which inhibits absorption of sodium and water from the small intestine, resulting in explosive diarrhea. The incidence and severity of dumping is proportional to the rate of gastric emptying.

The dumping syndrome can be further characterized into early versus late dumping, but in practice, it may be difficult to distinguish between the two. Most patients suffer from early dumping or a combination of both early and late dumping. Early dumping symptoms occur within 60 minutes after a meal and involve GI and vasomotor complaints. Rapid emptying of hyperosmolar food boluses into the small bowel induces osmotic fluid shifts into the gut lumen, causing distension and increases in both the amplitude and frequency of bowel contraction. A variety of vasoactive and prosecretory neurotransmitters are then released, causing splanchnic as well as systemic vasodilation and resulting in relative hypovolemia. As a result, in addition to crampy abdominal pain, nausea, vomiting, bloating, and diarrhea, patients also experience palpitations, diaphoresis, weakness, flushing, and an intense urge to lie down.

Late dumping symptoms occur about 1 to 3 hours after a meal and are secondary to reactive hypoglycemia. The entry of carbohydrates into the small bowel and the absorption of glucose causes GLP-1 release and an exaggerated insulin response. Patients then become hypoglycemic, with a concurrent surge of catecholamines, resulting in symptoms of lightheadedness, palpitations, diaphoresis, tremulousness, and confusion. Rapid weight loss and malnutrition may ensue from fear of eating. Other causes of postprandial hypoglycemia, such as insulinoma and noninsulinoma pancreatogenous hypoglycemic syndrome, should be considered in the appropriate clinical context.

The diagnosis of dumping syndrome can be confirmed by provocation testing. Plasma glucose, hematocrit, and heart rate are measured after ingestion of a 50 g oral glucose load at 30 minute intervals over 3 hours. The test is positive if hypoglycemia (<50 mg/dL), rise in hematocrit (>3%), or rise in heart rate (> 10 beats/min) is seen, along with reproduction of the patient's symptoms. Rapid gastric emptying can be assessed by solid-meal scintigraphy, according to the 2008 consensus statement by the American Neurogastroenterology and Motility Society and the Society of Nuclear Medicine, which recommended imaging at 0, 1, 2, and 4 hours after ingestion of a low-fat egg-white meal. The ^{13}C-acetic acid and hydrogen breath tests use bacterial fermentation of glucose as a surrogate for gastric emptying.

Dumping symptoms usually improve over time with dietary modifications. Patients should be advised to eat small meals, avoid fluid intake while eating solids and for the first 2 hours postprandially, and minimize ingestion of simple carbohydrates. The addition of nonabsorbable polysaccharides such as pectin, guar gum, and glucomannan can modify glucose absorption and alleviate severe dumping symptoms resulting from reactive hypoglycemia.

If dumping persists, pharmacologic interventions should be considered. Alpha-glucosidase inhibitor acarbose attenuates the postprandial increase of plasma glucose by preventing digestion of complex polysaccharides and sucrose at the intestinal brush border. Acarbose has demonstrated long-term efficacy in limiting dumping symptoms, but fermentation of the unabsorbed carbohydrates causes the undesirable side effects of diarrhea and flatulence. A second option is somatostatin analog octreotide (tid about 30 minutes prior to each meal). Octreotide (50 to 100 µg IV every 8 hours; increase by 100 µg/dose at 48-hour intervals to a maximum dose of 500 µg every 8 hours) effectively controls the symptoms of dumping syndrome by slowing gastric emptying, inhibiting secretion of insulin and enteric peptides, and mitigating postprandial hemodynamic changes via hormonal release and splanchnic vasoconstriction.

Treatment reduces dumping symptoms by 50% in the short term; by comparison, long-term use has no well-demonstrated efficacy and is associated with side effects, particularly steatorrhea and cholelithiasis. Different formulations, such as the depot long-acting octreotide (Sandostatin-LAR), are as effective as subcutaneous octreotide and get a better quality-of-life rating by patients.

Remedial surgery is not always effective, so it is reserved for patients who have symptoms that do not improve over time and are refractory to medications. The surgical approach aims to recreate gastric reservoir function and to prevent rapid and uncontrolled delivery of food into the proximal intestine. Multiple options exist, but a formal comparison of their relative efficacies has not been done. Of all the reported options, antiperistaltic jejunal interposition loops and conversion Roux-en-Y gastrojejunostomy are generally thought to provide the most satisfactory results.

Patients who experience dumping after pyloroplasty should undergo pyloric reconstruction. Patients with prior Billroth II or Billroth I gastrectomy should undergo conversion to Roux-en-Y gastrojejunostomy, which slows motility by interrupting the migrating motor complexes and introducing retrograde jejunal contractions. Another option is conversion from Billroth II to Billroth I, which restores physiologic delivery of the meal to the duodenum, but it is ineffective in 25% of patients.

Finally, jejunal interposition can be used both as a meter and as a reservoir depending on the segment's orientation: a 10 cm antiperistaltic jejunal interposition segment can serve as a pylorus to delay transit, and a 10 to 20 cm isoperistaltic loop would dilate over time and serve as a reservoir. The antiperistaltic segment can also be interposed in the efferent limb of a Billroth II gastrojejunostomy or in a Coux-en-Y limb in an effort to slow motility.

ILEUS OF THE SMALL INTESTINE

Ileus and pseudoobstruction both refer to impaired forward peristalsis in the absence of a mechanical obstruction. The term *pseudo-obstruction* mainly pertains to the colon and is not discussed in this chapter. It is important to distinguish between a normal *postoperative ileus* and a *paralytic ileus*. The distinction is predominantly one of time since operation, and it is based on circumstance. Normal postoperative ileus (POI) is less severe and lasts no more than 5 days; a prolonged POI (PPOI) occurs with protracted signs or symptoms of abdominal distension, bloating, diffuse and persistent abdominal pain, nausea, vomiting, inability to pass flatus, and inability to tolerate an oral diet.

It is sometimes difficult to distinguish between prolonged paralytic ileus and early postoperative mechanical bowel obstruction (usually due to hernia, thick adhesions, or misplaced sutures). Clinically, the presence of intense colicky pain, feculent emesis, or rapidly progressing pain or distension is more suggestive of small bowel obstruction than PPOI. Localized tenderness, fever, tachycardia, and peritoneal signs suggest bowel ischemia or perforation necessitating emergent surgical intervention.

Risk factors for protracted ileus include overuse of narcotics, spinal cord injury, severe pelvic fractures, peritoneal or retroperitoneal inflammation, and sepsis. Other medications such as anticholinergics, phenothiazines, calcium channel blockers, and tricyclic antidepressants may also impair motility. Metabolic disturbances such as ketoacidosis, hypomagnesemia or hypermagnesemia, hypercalcemia, hyponatremia, and hypokalemia may prolong ileus.

When the patient's postoperative ileus has extended beyond the expected period, plain films of the abdomen reveal gas in segments of both the small and large bowel. To differentiate early postoperative obstruction from ileus, contrast studies or CT scans are helpful but should be used sparingly. In the absence of acute symptoms, CT is useful if other abdominal pathology, such as an abscess, could be contributing to the clinical picture. CT with oral contrast has a sensitivity and specificity of 90% to 100% in distinguishing ileus from a complete postoperative small bowel obstruction. However, CT is less reliable in distinguishing ileus from partial obstruction of the small intestine (Figure 5).

A number of interventions have been described as adjuncts for reducing the duration of a normal postlaparotomy ileus. The goals in management of postoperative ileus are to prevent uncomfortable distension, vomiting, and aspiration. For many years, the mainstay of therapy was the use of NG suction to prevent accumulation of swallowed air and secreted fluids in an alimentary tract not yet coordinating flow distally. Subsequent studies have demonstrated that the putative benefit does not compensate for risks of aspiration and the discomfort of the tube.

In elective abdominal cases such as colectomy, NG tubes are used selectively in patients who are felt to be at risk for complications of ileus, based on the surgeon's judgements about intraoperative findings or manipulations such as prolonged handling and packing of the bowel, anticipation of intensive use of narcotics or other antikinetic agents, presence of sepsis or peritonitis, or extensive blood loss. In patients not selected for NG suction, nothing is allowed by mouth, or only sips are allowed, until evidence is found that ileus is likely resolving by listening for bowel sounds or for the patient's report of "rumbles." IV fluids are necessary until the patient can be advanced to full intake of requirements, usually after flatus is passed.

Adjuncts to minimizing the normal interval of postoperative ileus include use of thoracic/high abdominal epidural catheters for management of pain and correction of disturbances in serum electrolytes, minerals, and endocrine function (hypothyroidism, adrenal insufficiency). Fluid imbalances in the body also may influence return of bowel function following laparotomy.

In one study, patients undergoing colectomy received a restricted perioperative fluid-resuscitation regimen or a standard, more liberal fluid resuscitation. The restricted group had a quicker passage of flatus and moved their bowels earlier, leading in part to shorter hospital stays. Subsequent studies have not uniformly suggested that recovery from ileus is faster with temperance in fluid resuscitation. However, this benefit, as well as others, may be more clearly observed when fluid therapy is directed by physiologic assessments of volume status.

Gum chewing has attracted attention as a simple and inexpensive means of accelerating return of bowel function. A number of prospective randomized trials have been conducted to test the hypothesis that gum chewing results in earlier passage of flatus and bowel movement in patients undergoing laparoscopic colectomy. No conclusive evidence has been obtained to demonstrate a clear benefit of gum chewing for all patients undergoing laparotomy or even colectomy, although subgroup analysis suggests some patients may benefit.

Prokinetic agents such as metoclopramide, cisapride (currently not approved by the FDA), and erythromycin have been evaluated for their efficacy in shortening the duration of POI. For ileus following upper GI procedures (e.g., pancreaticoduodenectomy), such medications may be effective in promoting gastric emptying but have not proved efficacious in management of ileus after general abdominal or pelvic procedures. Opioid antagonists such as alvimopan and methylnaltrexone are peripherally acting opioid antagonists and do not cross the blood-brain barrier. In a number of studies, alvimopan has been shown to hasten postoperative GI recovery following bowel surgery and abdominal hysterectomy. In one study where an overall benefit was not observed, subgroup analysis showed a benefit to patients who received patient-controlled, intravenously administered opiate analgesia, suggesting that prolonged ileus may be shortened if opiates are being used regularly to control pain. However, cardiovascular and neoplastic risks with the use of alvimopan have precluded its widespread use. Currently FDA approval for alvimopan is limited to perioperative care after partial large or small bowel resections with primary anastomosis and does not extend to protracted ileus.

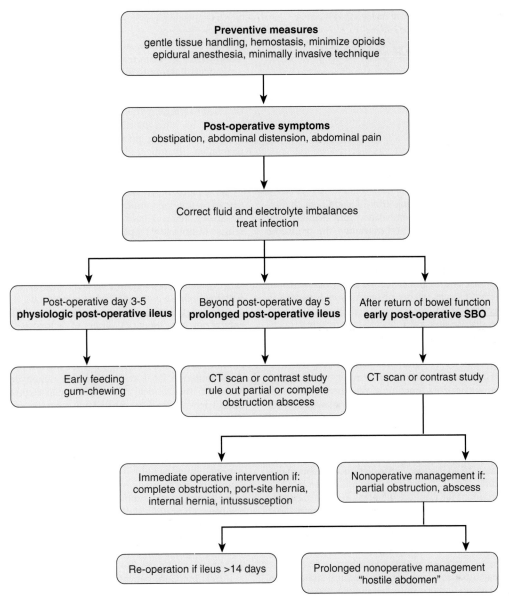

FIGURE 5   Ileus algorithm. *SBO,* Small bowel obstruction.

Along with pharmacologic measures, it should be emphasized that, in otherwise routine laparotomy or laparoscopy, gentle handling of tissues, meticulous attention to hemostasis, and application of sound principles of wound management are likely to have the greatest impact on optimizing recovery from ileus and minimizing the incidence of prolonged ileus. Efforts to reduce incision size and time spent handling the intestines through the use of laparoscopic approaches clearly improves recovery from ileus in some if not all patients undergoing standardized intraabdominal procedures such as colectomy.

Suggested Readings

Abell TL, Camilleri M, Donohoe K, et al: Consensus recommendations for gastric emptying scintigraphy: a joint report of the American Neurogastroenterology and Motility Society and the Society of Nuclear Medicine, *Am J Gastroenterol* 103(3):753–763, 2008.

Becker G, Blum HE: Novel opioid antagonists for opioid-induced bowel dysfunction and postoperative ileus, *Lancet* 373 (9670):1198–206, 2009.

Didden P, Penning C, Masclee AA: Octreotide therapy in dumping syndrome: analysis of long-term results, *Aliment Pharmacol Ther* 24(9):1367–1375, 2006.

Hasler WL: Gastroparesis: symptoms, evaluation, and treatment, *Gastroenterol Clin North Am* 36(3):619–647, 2007.

van der Mijle HC, Beekhuis H, Bleichrodt RP, et al: Transit disorders of the gastric remnant and Roux limb after Roux-en-Y gastrojejunostomy: relation to symptomatology and vagotomy, *Br J Surg* 80(1):60–64, 1993.

MANAGEMENT OF SHORT BOWEL SYNDROME

Harry C. Sax, MD

OVERVIEW

Short bowel syndrome is a devastating clinical condition characterized by malabsorption, electrolyte imbalance, and malnutrition, often leading to significant morbidity and mortality. The syndrome is not uniformly tied to a specific length of bowel. Patients with normal small bowel who require resection due to embolus, trauma, or internal hernia can survive and adapt with as little as 75 cm of small bowel, assuming an intact pylorus and ileocecal valve. Once the colon is no longer in the circuit, up to 150 cm of small bowel is necessary for eventual independence from parenteral nutrition. Patients with inherent small bowel disease such as Crohn's disease require proportionately more bowel, and the severity of their syndrome is often variable and is affected by underlying disease activity.

Although modern critical care techniques often save patients who have undergone massive resection, their long-term survival and quality of life depend on maximizing function of the remaining bowel. If that is not possible, reduction of complications associated with parenteral nutrition and efforts to augment enteral absorption are paramount.

After massive enterectomy, the remaining bowel undergoes both morphologic and physiologic change. Initially, villous hypertrophy and hyperplasia occur with an increase in the surface area. This manifests clinically as a reduction in the massive fluid and electrolyte loss seen early after resection. However, the adaptive increase in nutrient transport efficiency lags and is influenced by multiple factors that include the location of remaining bowel, the ability to feed enterally, and patient's own degree of volitional intake.

This chapter focuses on the management of the patient with short bowel syndrome, stressing nutritional support, pharmacologic options that may increase adaptation, and surgical strategies to maximize remaining bowel function or to determine when definitive therapy with transplantation is appropriate (Table 1).

NUTRITION AND INITIAL PHARMACOLOGIC THERAPY

Optimizing and maintaining nutritional status is important for adaptation subsequent to surgery, and it is central to long-term survival. Although most patients in the early postoperative period require total parenteral nutrition (TPN), even small amounts of enteral nutrition are key to accelerating adaptation and reducing septic complications. Enteral access should be achieved by gastrostomy at the initial surgery or subsequent second look. Placement of a permanent tunneled catheter at the time of the initial or early subsequent bowel resection is not recommended due to the high rate of bacteremia and sepsis during the initial recovery. A percutaneous subclavian line used solely for TPN is appropriate and preferable to internal jugular lines due to difficulty in maintaining a dressing as well as proximity to tracheostomy sites.

Initial TPN management focuses on meeting baseline requirements with a moderate stress factor. A solution that provides 1.5 g protein/kg/day with a total caloric load of 30 kcal/kg/day is adequate. Many patients are hyperglycemic due to sepsis or surgical stress, and a mixed fuel substrate with reduced dextrose (15%) and 25% of calories as fat provides adequate nonprotein calorie/nitrogen ratios; insulin drips are often required.

Patients have quite high fluid and electrolyte losses from stomas and third spacing. Direct measurement of ostomy or fistula electrolytes will guide replacement with supplemental parenteral fluids as opposed to frequent altering of the TPN. Enteral nutrition is trialed at 10 mL/hr. With gastric feeds, this can be intact protein with the goal of maintaining gut immune integrity and stimulating further adaptation. The tube feedings are increased slowly at a rate of 5 to 10 mL/hr/day, closely monitoring ostomy output and the development of metabolic acidosis.

Most patients benefit from agents that slow motility, such as tincture of opium, loperamide, or phenoxylate. Octreotide, a somatostatin analog, reduces fluid and electrolyte losses, but it also inhibits release of normally tropic hormones, slows subsequent adaptation, and is associated with hyperglycemia. Nonetheless, control of large fluid and electrolyte losses, especially in patients with ill-fitting stoma devices or fistulae, aids management during the early phase. The short-term analog is utilized initially, moving to the once-monthly, sustained-release compound when appropriate.

After surviving the surgery, patients are encouraged to increase enteral nutrition intake. A variety of factors specify the appropriate diet. The presence of a colon aids in fluid and electrolyte absorption, and soluble fiber supplementation creates short-chain fatty acids and provides additional calories. Diets are high in protein (30% of calories), limited in fat, and 40% complex carbohydrates. Patients who have had massive ileal resections should receive fats as medium-chain triglycerides. Oral rehydration solutions are higher in electrolytes than conventional sports drinks and are encouraged to maintain euvolemia.

The role of glutamine in the maintenance of gut health as well as adaptation continues to emerge. Glutamine is a conditionally essential amino acid; it is the primary fuel for the enterocyte, and it supports gut immune function. Conventional TPN does not contain glutamine, and supplementation either intravenously or orally has been advocated. Multiple studies that combine oral glutamine, parenteral growth hormone, and a specialized diet have shown transient improvement in nutrient uptake and a reduction in TPN dependence. It appears that dietary education is key to long-term success. Glutamine, if supplemented orally, is dosed at 0.5 gm/kg/day.

After resection, patients become hypersecretory with high levels of serum gastrin. Reduction of gastrointestinal (GI) secretion is appropriate with either H2 antagonists or proton pump inhibitors. A secondary advantage is permissive serum hypergastrinemia, a further tropic signal for the gut. Patients with multiple resections, especially those who may have strictures or defunctionalized segments, develop bacterial overgrowth leading to diarrhea and further fluid and electrolyte losses. Rotating treatment with nonabsorbable antibiotics, such as tetracycline or polymyxin, aids in controlling these losses but has not been shown to have a direct effect on nutrient absorption.

Hormonal Augmentation of Small Bowel Adaptation

Small bowel adaptation involves both an increase in the surface area as well as an increase in the efficiency of nutrient absorption through increased numbers and increased density of amino acid and glucose transporters. Early studies recognized this was mediated through gut hormonal signaling, and numerous putative trophic factors have been studied to accelerate small bowel adaptation after resection. The three that appear to have the greatest potential are growth hormone, epidermal growth factor, and glucagon-like peptide 2.

Human growth hormone (HGH) is a 191–amino acid anabolic protein that initiates cell division and regulates nutrient metabolism with the stimulation of protein synthesis and gluconeogenesis. HGH is released from the anterior pituitary gland and appears to mediate

TABLE 1: Management stategies for short bowel syndrome

Management Strategies
1. Acute phase
a. Treat postoperative complications
b. Maintain full support via the parenteral route
c. Initiate low-rate trophic enteral feeds
d. Document amount and site of remaining bowel and underlying disease
2. Early adaptation (up to 1 year postsurgery)
a. Increase enteral nutrition to tolerance; supplement with glutamine
b. Achieve permanent parenteral access, if indicated
c. Maximize antiperistaltic agents
d. Octreotide for high output ostomy or fistula
e. Dietary counseling
f. Clinical trials of trophic growth factors
3. Long-term adaptation (>1 year postsurgery)
a. Recruit bypassed bowel
b. Bowel-lengthening procedure (Bianchi or STEP)
c. Monitor for development of TPN-associated complications, and refer for transplant prior to recurrent sepsis, thrombosis, or end-stage liver disease

its effect through insulin-like growth factor 1. Because of its anabolic effects, HGH was purported to accelerate adaptation after massive resection. However, the effects were transient, and most of the significant results were seen in animals, with initiation soon after the surgery. The dosage of growth hormone of 0.10 mg/kg/day is associated with fluid retention, joint pain, and hyperglycemia, especially in older adults. Although HGH has been approved by the Food and Drug Administration for use in patients with short bowel syndrome, it appears that maximal effects occur when it is used as part of an overall program of intestinal rehabilitation, including clear dietary manipulation and optimal TPN management.

Epidermal growth factor (EGF) is a 53–amino acid peptide from saliva and pancreaticobiliary secretions that bathe the GI tract. EGF receptors are distributed throughout the gut and, in an animal model, overexpression of EGF leads to massive villous hypertrophy and hyperplasia. Removing the source of EGF by sialectomy inhibits adaptation after resection. Exogenous EGF supplementation may also play a role in maintaining gut health and reducing the incidence of necrotizing enterocolitis in neonates. In animals, EGF alone and in combination with HGH increases nutrient transport during the early phase of small bowel adaptation. This effect has been seen for both amino acid and glucose transporters. Unfortunately, EGF is not available commercially, although an investigational new drug application has been approved. Because EGF is primarily produced in the GI tract, and feedings further stimulate secretion, the optimal route to increase EGF exposure at the enterocyte level is through enteral feedings.

Perhaps the most promising trophic hormone is glucagon-like peptide 2 (GLP-2). Released from the L cells in the ileum and colon, it is encoded by the proglucagon gene. GLP-2 has a wide series of actions that include not only structural adaptation of the small bowel but also upregulation of jejunal nutrient transport. It has effects on motility and slows gastric emptying, which meters nutrients to the remaining bowel. GLP-2 itself has a very short half-life. Initial studies with infusions showed significant improvements in intestinal absorption of energy, wet weight, and nitrogen.

The development of a long-acting GLP-2 agonist (teduglutide) offers significant potential benefit for the patient with short gut. In

multiple human trials, doses are in the range of 0.10 mg/kg/day, and the major side effect is abdominal pain and obstructive symptoms due to significant gut hypertrophy. As phase III trials are completed, it is likely that GLP-2 will be a significant adjunct to the improvement of residual bowel function, however the optimal timing and duration of its use not yet clear.

SURGICAL CONSIDERATIONS IN SHORT BOWEL SYNDROME

From a surgical point of view, the focus is on recruiting the maximum amount of absorptive capacity, slowing motility, and recognizing early that the patient will not adapt and should be referred for intestinal transplantation prior to the development of parental nutrition–associated liver failure.

At initial surgery, it is optimal to obtain enteral access via gastrostomy. Prophylactic cholecystectomy is appropriate, and a liver biopsy will provide a baseline to define any abnormalities prior to the development of TPN-associated liver disease. Residual bowel length and location should be included in the operative report.

The recruitment of bypassed intestine carries with it both advantages and disadvantages. Reintroducing colon back into the digestive circuit leads to improvement in fluid, electrolyte, and eventually nutrient absorption. However, in patients with significant ileal resections, bile acid diarrhea may increase output to the point that the patients develop perianal excoriation and begin to restrict their volitional intake. The author has found it useful in this situation to accept the loss of a small portion of the absorptive capacity of the rectum by creating an end-sigmoid colostomy at the time of ileostomy or jejunostomy take down. Patients at this point are already quite accepting of their ostomy, and the ability to reduce fluid losses and increase absorption is often beneficial.

There have been multiple scattered reports regarding the use of reversed segments, nipple-valve constructions, and colonic interpositions. The theoretical advantage of slowing intestinal motility is outweighed by frequent obstructions and the lack of a suitable volume of patients at a single center to report consistent positive results. These procedures are not recommended.

As the bowel adapts, it also dilates. This dilation does not necessarily lead to improvement of overall absorption, but it can be used to the patient's advantage to create a longer alimentary segment. In the 1980s, Bianchi recognized that the mesentery has two leaves, and by dividing between these leaves, a dilated segment of bowel can be split longitudinally and reanastomosed to create double the length (Figure 1). Results have been reported in multiple series, the larger series reporting 20 to 25 patients. Bowel length was increased between 25% and 60%, and metabolic studies showed an increase in absorption of fat and a slowing of transit. Initial follow-up, in some cases of up to 6 years, reported that about 80% of patients were able to come off of TPN or have significant reductions. However, the Bianchi procedure is technically demanding, and misadventures in splitting the small bowel mesentery can lead to loss of what was previously viable bowel.

Recognizing these risks, an alternate bowel-lengthening procedure, the serial transverse enteroplasty, or STEP procedure, was created (Figure 2). The mesentery remains intact, but the bowel is plicated using a stapler, alternatively from the mesentery and antimesenteric edges. Since the normal diameter of the small bowel is 2 cm, the staple lines are controlled to reproduce this diameter in what would otherwise be a dilated bowel. The STEP procedure increases bowel length up to 50%. Follow-up at up to 2 years has shown a 60% TPN wean rate. As the total number of patients reported with the STEP grew, a registry was created that is now available for following these patients long term (http://www.childrenshospital.org/cfapps/step/index.cfm). As of March 2009, 44 hospitals have submitted at least one patient to the registry.

Intestinal transplantation has evolved to yield excellent outcomes despite the overall critically ill nature of the patients. The 1-year

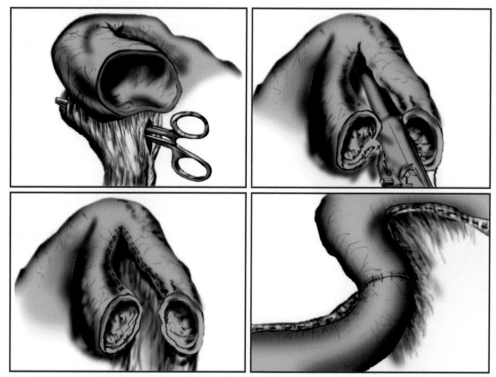

FIGURE 1   Bianchi procedure. *(Courtesy Jon S. Thompson, University of Nebraska Medical Center.)*

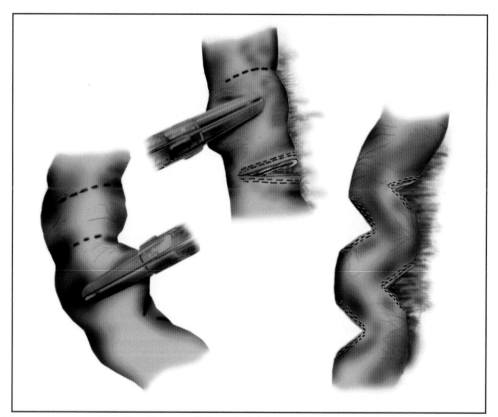

FIGURE 2   Serial transverse enteroplasty. *(From Thompson JS: Surgical rehabilitation of the intestine in short bowel syndrome, Surgery 135:465, 2004.)*

patient survival from high-volume centers is 80%, and 3-year survival is 50%. Combined multivisceral transplant, including liver and small bowel, offers hope to patients who have a significantly shortened life expectancy due to short bowel syndrome combined with progressive liver disease or multiple areas of vascular thrombosis. The greater challenge is the early recognition of the patient for whom adaptation will not take place and in whom TPN-associated liver disease is likely. Many of these patients have an ultra-short gut (<60 cm in adults and <30 cm in children) as well as the inability to tolerate even small amounts of enteral nutrition. Recurrent bouts of line sepsis and fungemia are other significant factors predicting that long-term TPN will not be an option. In these patients, early referral for transplantation is appropriate.

There is a small but increasing number of patients who receive isolated small bowel segments from living, related donors. Because the ischemia time is short, and human leukocyte antigen matching is optimal, results are quite promising. There is increased technical difficulty in the recipient operation, however, because the vessels are distal arcades of the superior mesenteric artery, which are smaller.

SUMMARY

Short bowel syndrome is extremely challenging and requires the experience of a multidisciplinary team. Initial therapy should concentrate on preserving length, maintaining nutritional status, and optimizing enteral nutrient absorption. The early utilization of trophic factors, especially GLP-2, appears to offer promise to those patients with marginal bowel length for whom acceleration of adaptation may allow weaning or a reduction in TPN. In patients with dilated bowel, the Bianchi or STEP procedures both increase bowel

length and transit time, although the patient should be referred to a center with adequate experience in both of these highly technical procedures. Finally, the continued improvement in outcome of small bowel transplantation makes it a suitable alternative to patients who do not have recoverable small bowel function or who have developed intractable complications related to TPN-induced liver disease, recurrent infections, or vascular thrombosis.

SUGGESTED READINGS

Langnas AN, Goulet AN, Quigley O, et al. editors: *Intestinal failure: diagnosis management and transplantation*, Oxford UK, 2008, Blackwell Publishing.
Modi BP, Javid DJ, Jaksic T, et al: First report of the international serial transverse enteroplasty data registry: indications, efficacy, and complications, *J Am Coll Surg* 204:365–371, 2007.
Ray EC, Anissar NE, Sax HC: Growth factor regulation of enterocyte nutrient transport during intestinal adaptation, *Am J Surg* 183:361–371, 2002.
Seydel AS, Miller JH, Sarac TP, et al: Octreotide diminishes luminal nutrient transport activity, which is reversed by epidermal growth factor, *Am J Surg* 171:267–271, 1996.

MANAGEMENT OF ENTEROCUTANEOUS FISTULAS

Hobart W. Harris, MD, MPH

OVERVIEW

Enterocutaneous fistulas are a common and frequently vexing clinical problem for general surgeons. The 15% to 25% mortality rate associated with these fistulas is most commonly due to sepsis and multisystem organ failure. Over the past two decades, the clinical spectrum of enterocutaneous fistulas has shifted with the emergence of the enteroatmospheric (or exposed) fistula. In these fistulas, the fistulous opening is located within an open wound or abdomen and is frequently surrounded by a bed of granulation tissue, making them especially challenging to manage. Regardless of the variant, no patient benefits more from a multidisciplinary care team approach than those with enterocutaneous fistulas. The team should include general surgeons, nurses, enterostomal therapists, social workers, and nutritionists who are familiar with the complex and varied problems these patients often have.

DEFINITIONS, CLASSIFICATION, AND PROGRESSION

A *fistula* is an abnormal communication between two epithelialized surfaces, in contrast to a *sinus*, which is an abnormal communication between an epithelialized surface and a source of infection. An *enterocutaneous* fistula is an abnormal communication between the intestinal lumen and the skin. Enterocutaneous fistulas are classically associated with a triad of sepsis, fluid and electrolyte abnormalities, and malnutrition, and they can be classified by anatomy, etiology, or physiology.

Anatomically, an enterocutaneous fistula is identified by the segment of the intestinal tract from which it originates (e.g., *colo*cutaneous, *gastro*cutaneous). The etiologic classification is based on the underlying disease process responsible for the fistula. For example, up to 20% of all enterocutaneous fistulas are due to Crohn's disease. The physiologic classification of enterocutaneous fistulas is dependent on the daily output, segregating them into low- (<200 mL/day), moderate- (200 to 500 mL/day), and high-output (>500 mL/day) fistulas.

Enteroatmospheric fistulas are also classified based on the nature of the surrounding wound. A *deep* enteroatmospheric fistula is one in which the effluent drains freely into the abdominal cavity, resulting in diffuse peritonitis and abdominal sepsis. In contrast, a *superficial* enteroatmospheric fistula is one in which the effluent drains onto a granulating abdominal wound. Under these circumstances, the peritoneal space is excluded from the intestinal contents, greatly reducing the risks of sepsis. A deep enteroatmospheric fistula is an uncontrolled infection that renders the patient hypercatabolic, whereas a superficial enteroatmospheric fistula is largely a wound management problem.

The natural progression of enterocutaneous fistulas is that approximately one third will close spontaneously, provided the patient receives adequate fluid resuscitation, sepsis is eliminated, and nutritional support is optimized. However, several factors inhibit spontaneous fistula closure (Table 1), including infection, malnutrition, steroids, prior radiation, a foreign body (including hernia mesh), high fistula output, a short fistula tract, distal intestinal obstruction, malignancy, or chronicity with epithelialization of the fistula tract.

MANAGEMENT

The basic management principles for enterocutaneous fistulas have been derived and refined over the past 60 years and include fluid resuscitation, control of the fistula output, drainage of infection, nutritional support, skin and wound care, and closure of the fistula.

Resuscitation of the Patient

The first goal in managing a patient with an enterocutaneous fistula is fluid resuscitation and correction of associated electrolyte and acid–base imbalances. Hypokalemia is the most common electrolyte

TABLE 1: Factors that inhibit spontaneous fistula closure

Foreign body, which includes hernia mesh
Radiation
Infection or inflammatory bowel disease (e.g., Crohn's disease)
Epithelialization or a fistula tract less than 2 cm
Neoplasia
Distal obstruction

abnormality and must be aggressively corrected. Losses from high-output fistulas should be assessed and replaced several times a day. Fistula output from the upper gastrointestinal (GI) tract is best replaced with normal saline solution supplemented with potassium. Duodenal fistulas are often associated with the loss of pancreatic secretions and bile, producing a metabolic acidosis that requires replacement of sodium bicarbonate. Since it is impossible to predict the exact electrolyte losses, the higher the volume of the fistula output, the lower the threshold should be for directly measuring the composition of the effluent to guide targeted fluid and electrolyte therapy.

Control of the Fistula

Controlling an enterocutaneous fistula entails the complete evacuation and collection of the intestinal effluent. This can be as simple a matter as placing a stoma appliance over a small fistulous opening in the skin or as complex as the highly customized wound dressing needed to control enteroatmospheric fistulas. Vacuum-assisted wound devices are a recent and powerful addition to the armamentarium of fistula care. When successful, these devices simplify wound care, reduce the frequency of dressing changes, and may even accelerate fistula closure by promoting wound healing. Adequately controlling the fistula output not only helps achieve and maintain fluid and electrolyte homeostasis, it is essential to protecting the surrounding skin and soft tissue. Intestinal contents can be extremely caustic and irritating, resulting in significant pain and tenderness for the patient and a potentially serious threat to successful fistula treatment.

Another critical aspect of controlling the fistula involves an aggressive search for undrained intraabdominal or subcutaneous abscesses. Controlling any associated infection helps stabilize the patient, and it reduces the risk of systemic sepsis and reduces overall caloric needs. Whereas most experts recommend defining the fistula anatomy as a mandatory component of fistula care, I do so on a selective basis, obtaining fistulograms in approximately 10% of patients, only when such anatomic definition is likely to affect my overall operative strategy.

Nutritional Support

Optimal nutritional support is the next priority. Baseline nutritional requirements are 20 kcal/kg/day of carbohydrate and fat and 0.8 g/kg/day of protein but can increase to 30 kcal/kg/day and 1.5 to 2.5 g/kg/day, respectively, in patients with high-output fistulas. The relative merit of enteral versus parenteral nutrition in patients with enterocutaneous fistulas is a subject of ongoing research and debate. In my practice, approximately two thirds of patients will require long-term total parenteral nutrition (TPN). However, I consider enteral feeding preferable whenever feasible. Feeding via the gut preserves the intestinal mucosal barrier as well as the immunologic and hormonal function of the intestinal tract. In addition, enteral nutrition is easy to implement, relatively inexpensive, and is associated with a lower

overall complication rate than TPN, especially in the outpatient setting.

When managing a patient with an enterocutaneous fistula, it is often worth trying to convert from intravenous to enteral feedings, with a close eye kept on the patient's clinical symptoms and fistula output. Should enteral feedings result in nausea, vomiting, abdominal distension, or abdominal pain, or should the fistula output increase dramatically, the enteral feeding trial should be discontinued. Instituting an enteral diet should not result in converting a low-output fistula to a high-output fistula. And although octreotide, a long-acting somatostatin analog, has been used in the management of enterocutaneous fistulas, it has not been proven to promote fistula closure or improve overall outcome. Frequently, simply adding bulk-forming agents to the diet can convert a difficult-to-manage fistula into one that is more readily controlled with simple stomal appliances.

Regardless of route, nutritional support must be initiated with care and caution in severely malnourished patients due to the risk of the refeeding syndrome, which usually occurs within a few days of starting nutritional support. Affected patients develop fluid and electrolyte disorders, especially hypophosphatemia, along with neurologic, pulmonary, cardiac, neuromuscular, and hematologic complications. Most of the physiologic effects result from a sudden shift from fat to carbohydrate metabolism and a sudden increase in insulin levels after refeeding, which leads to increased cellular uptake of phosphate. The risk of inducing refeeding syndrome can be reduced by correcting fluid, electrolyte, and vitamin abnormalities before starting modest levels of nutritional support, and by gradually advancing to the feeding rate goal over several days, thereby giving the patient time to adjust to the new feeding regimen.

Skin and Wound Care

Care of the surrounding skin and associated open wounds is a very important component of successfully managing enterocutaneous fistulas, and it is something that I am concerned about from the time of the initial diagnosis. Proper skin and wound care can frequently be the major determinant both of patient comfort and the ability to manage these complex wounds on an outpatient basis. In addition, the quality of the surrounding skin has significant implications for the definitive management of enterocutaneous fistulas.

Certain special cases pose unique wound care challenges, including situations where the wound has such irregular topography that a standard stoma appliance cannot be used. In such cases, an enterostomal therapist can prove invaluable in designing a custom dressing, often with associated suction catheters and other materials used to control the effluent, thereby creating a stable, manageable wound. Another special case is that of the enteroatmospheric fistula that is surrounded or contained within a bed of granulation tissue, as is frequently seen in patients recovering with an open abdomen. I have successfully managed these fistulas by using a fistula vac technique, wherein a split-thickness skin graft is placed to provide skin coverage to surround the fistula site (Figure 1). This technique utilizes a modified vacuum-assisted wound closure device that effectively excludes the intestinal effluent from the skin graft, thus allowing the graft to heal. Once the graft is healed, a standard stoma appliance can be used to control the fistula output.

Ultimately, maintaining the health of the skin and soft tissue surrounding the fistula is as important as each of the preceding therapeutic goals. Whereas healthy and supple soft tissue will facilitate fistula closure—whether that closure is spontaneous or surgical—inflamed, ulcerated, or infected skin will impede wound healing.

Definitive Repair

The definitive repair of an enterocutaneous fistula falls into one of two broad categories: either the fistula will spontaneously close, or it will require a surgical procedure. In either case, if nutrition and oxygen

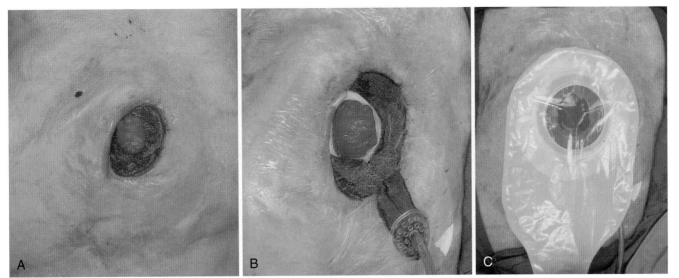

FIGURE 1 Wound management using the fistula vacuum-assisted closure technique.

delivery to the wound are optimized, one third of fistulas can be expected to close within 4 to 6 weeks. If a fistula fails to close within that time frame, then it is unlikely to do so with further waiting. It is important to search for and remedy any and all complicating factors to provide the patient with the best chances of spontaneous fistula closure. However, most often, enterocutaneous fistulas require definitive surgical repair.

The first issue to consider in cases that require surgery is the timing of the operation. I generally wait a minimum of 12 to 16 weeks before definitive repair, temporizing this decision by the patient's overall clinical status. Ideally, the patient should have a serum albumin level above 3.0 g/dL, and if a skin graft had to be placed to facilitate wound management, the graft must pass the "pinch test" before reoperation; the pinch test entails simply pinching the split-thickness skin graft that has been placed around the enteroatmospheric fistula. If the skin graft is seen and felt to separate readily from the underlying soft tissue when pinched, a less technically challenging subsequent operation can be assured.

Several basic strategies and tips are important in the surgical management of enterocutaneous fistulas. The first stage of the operation is an exploratory laparotomy with lysis of adhesions sufficient to allow for the complete definition of the patient's intestinal anatomy. This is critically important, because the segments of the intestine that are involved with the fistula or fistulas must be clearly identified, as must the approximate length of the small intestine, and how any planned bowel resection might affect the patient's overall intestinal physiology. Clear definition of the intestinal anatomy is also important to exclude intestinal stenoses and bowel obstructions.

The second stage of the operation is the decision to either resect or repair the injured intestines. The decision to resect rather than repair the bowel requires the surgeon to balance the risk of a recurrent enterocutaneous fistula versus that of the patient developing short gut syndrome due to excessive intestinal resection. The third and final stage of the operation is closure of the abdomen, which is often complicated by the need to repair an associated ventral hernia.

When attempting to achieve the first two stages of surgical repair, the responsible surgeon must allow adequate time for the operation. Ideally, these procedures should be the first operation of the day, and everything possible should be done to reduce any associated time pressures, thus creating a relaxed, low-stress operating room environment that will facilitate a meticulous lysis of adhesions. Antibiotic prophylaxis should include coverage of gram-negative enteric organisms, as would be done for a colon resection, because it is impossible to anticipate the number and location of potential enterotomies.

The operation generally begins by using prior surgical incisions and, when possible, extending these incisions into virgin territory. Since entering the peritoneal cavity is a critical early technical milestone, I prefer sharp dissection over electrocautery for both entering the abdomen and lysing intraabdominal adhesions. Although advantageous in terms of hemostasis, electrocautery does not provide the same level of fine control for dissecting tissues in a layer-by-layer fashion. Furthermore, sharp dissection affords tactile feedback that can help the surgeon distinguish between scar tissue and underlying viscera and thus avoid enterotomies.

The importance of a thorough lysis of adhesions that allows inspection of the bowel from the ligament of Treitz to the rectum cannot be overestimated. However, if the patient has a "frozen" abdomen, in which there is such extensive scar tissue that separating individual loops of intestine is dangerous, the surgical procedure may need to be aborted. Creating multiple enterotomies can convert a manageable situation into a lethal disaster. Still, thorough lysis of adhesions and running the bowel ultimately helps the surgeon plan the extent of bowel resection necessary to safely reestablish intestinal continuity.

While lysing adhesions, the surgeon should identify all areas where there is concern about a possible bowel injury, including partial-thickness serosal injuries. I tag areas of concern with loosely tied, 4-0 silk suture tags. Thus at the stage at which I am determining the extent of any bowel resection, I can easily identify all potential injuries as part of that assessment. The surgeon should resist any temptation to primarily repair a fistula, as this is associated with a 40% to 50% fistula recurrence rate. Ultimately, my goal is to minimize the number of anastomoses needed at the conclusion of the procedure. For example, two or three bowel injuries or a couple of fistulous openings that can be removed by resecting a modest length of small bowel is preferable to several bowel resections in series that result in multiple, adjacent anastomoses. I prefer hand-sewn, two-layer bowel anastomoses with an inner layer of a monofilament absorbable suture and an outer layer of silk sutures. These anastomoses are frequently constructed in a side-to-side but functional end-to-end, two-layer manner; they are safe and are associated with a lower risk of fistula recurrence than the more rapid, stapled anastomoses.

Once the abdomen has been entered, the adhesions lysed, the fistulous segments of intestine resected, and intestinal continuity reestablished, the last challenge is to close the abdominal wall. Since fistulas are frequently associated with fascial dehiscences, it is best to repair these ventral hernias with prosthetic material rather than closing the wound primarily. As these cases are at the very least clean contaminated, the general recommendation is to use either an absorbable mesh or a biological prosthetic to repair the hernia. Absorbable meshes, such as Vicryl or Dexon, dissolve within 60 to 90 days; therefore, choosing to use an absorbable mesh requires the patient to subsequently undergo a definitive ventral hernia repair using permanent mesh. Alternatively, the use of a biologic prosthetic, of which there are several choices—including products derived from human or porcine dermis, bovine pericardium, or porcine intestinal submucosa—may preclude the need for a second procedure. Although it is impossible to determine which of the various biologic prosthetics is the most effective based on the currently available data, I have had good overall success using a porcine dermal product containing cross-linked collagen.

SUMMARY

In conclusion, enterocutaneous fistulas are a common and challenging clinical problem, with a mortality rate of 15% to 25%. The enteroatmospheric fistula is an increasingly frequent and especially challenging type of fistula that requires unique strategies for successful management. The basic principles of management include fluid resuscitation and correction of associated electrolyte and acid-base imbalances, controlling the fistula output, robust nutritional support, diligent skin and wound care, and definitive surgical repair in those patients whose fistulas do not spontaneously close. A multidisciplinary team approach to the care and management of enterocutaneous fistulas affords the patient the best chance for a successful and durable outcome.

SUGGESTED READINGS

Everson AR, Fischer JE: Current management of enterocutaneous fistulas, *J Gastrointest Surg* 10:455, 2006.

Goverman J, Yelon JA, Platz JJ, et al: The fistula VAC, a technique for management of enterocutaneous fistulae arising within the open abdomen: report of 5 cases, *J Trauma* 60:428, 2006.

Schecter WP, Hirshberg A, Chang DS, et al: Enteric fistulae: principles of management, *J Am Coll Surg* 209:484-491, 2009.

PREOPERATIVE BOWEL PREPARATION: IS IT NECESSARY?

Richard P. Billingham, MD, and Daniel C. Rossi, DO

HISTORY

Mechanical bowel preparation (MBP) for elective colorectal operations was first introduced in the nineteenth century. Prior to this, fecal diversion and wound healing by secondary intention were routinely used. Infectious complication rates for elective colorectal operations continued at the rate of 30% to 50% up until the 1970s, when research determined that anaerobic flora were the predominant causative agents of infection. These data heralded the use of mechanical and antibiotic preoperative bowel preparation, which have been a mainstay of practice for the past 30 years.

Over the last decade, however, an increasing body of evidence has challenged the necessity of preoperative bowel preparation. The purpose of this chapter is to review the traditional practice of mechanical and antibiotic bowel preparations, but more importantly, to challenge the dogma that preoperative bowel preparation is a necessity for all elective colorectal operations.

MECHANICAL BOWEL PREPARATION

Mechanical preparation of the bowel has traditionally consisted of ingestion of oral osmotics and a clear liquid diet the day before surgery to reduce the colonic fecal mass. Mechanical preparation itself, however, has no effect on the species or concentration of organisms in residual fluid within the colon at the time of operation.

Oral cathartics traditionally utilized are isosmotic polyethylene glycol (PEG) solution or insoluble hyperosmolar salts containing phosphate or magnesium. A colonoscopy study by Ker found no difference in the efficacy of preparations using either 90 mL of sodium phosphate, 2 L PEG solution with 20 mg of oral bisacodyl, or 4 L PEG administered the day before surgery; no significant differences were seen for cleanliness, time to complete colonoscopy, or polyp detection. Patients did, however, experience less emesis, nausea, abdominal bloating, and cramping with the low-volume sodium phosphate preparation, compared with the 2 L or 4 L preparations.

Mechanical preparation can be advantageous for colon surgery because it facilitates passage of intraluminal staplers and heightens tactile sensation of tumor by having reduced the colonic stool volume.

It is also of benefit should intraoperative colonoscopy become necessary. The use of mechanical preparations, however, is not without risk. Higher rates of mucosal barrier loss and increased inflammation with lymphocyte and polymorphonucleocyte infiltration of the bowel wall have been associated with mechanical preparations. Documented patient side effects include emesis, nausea, abdominal pain, dehydration, and electrolyte derangement.

The use of sodium phosphate preparations garnered the attention of the Food and Drug Administration in 2006, when it mandated a Boxed Warning for their prescription, citing concerns about the risk for acute phosphate nephropathy; the product has since been unavailable. The introduction of 2 L PEG preparations has allowed patients to drink less volume to achieve equally efficacious bowel cleansing compared with traditional 4 L PEG preparations.

Is Mechanical Bowel Preparation Still Warranted?

Contrary to traditional mandates for elective colorectal surgery, several published studies over the past decade have advocated the omission of preoperative bowel preparation; however, none of them have been U.S. studies. As previously mentioned, mechanical preparation has been shown to cause dehydration, electrolyte disturbances, and patient discomfort. Jung found that only 30% of patients said they would undergo MBP again, and that 52% of patients required assistance from either a relative or hospital staff for completing the preparation. Jung also found no significant difference for postoperative pain, nausea, or time to initiation of diet; he did, however, find a significantly longer time to return of bowel function with the use of MBP. Incomplete colonic cleansing with mechanical preparations has also been associated with increased intraoperative contamination and surgical site infections from spillage of liquid stool.

Studies by both Zmora and Bretagnol found no significant difference in postoperative anastomotic leak rates among individuals who underwent elective colorectal anastomosis with or without mechanical preparation. A significantly longer hospital stay was, however, witnessed for the MBP group. The study by Bretagnol found significantly higher extraabdominal infectious complications for the MBP group. Zmora also documented that the omission of MBP in elective laparoscopic colectomy showed no significant differences compared with MBP for anastomotic leak or complication rates; a trend toward increased conversion to laparotomy was seen, yet this remained insignificant.

The 2009 Cochrane Review meta-analysis of 13 randomized controlled trials encompassing 4777 patients found no statistical evidence that MBP is of benefit in elective colorectal surgery. In a similar meta-analysis of 14 randomized controlled trials, Slim found no statistical significance for anastomotic leakage, abdominal or pelvic abscesses, or wound sepsis. In fact, when considering all surgical site infections, the group that did not have MBP was significantly favored. In a randomized prospective multicenter study of 1354 patients, Contant (2007) similarly found a 5% anastomotic leak rate regardless of whether mechanical bowel preparation was utilized. Subgroup analysis showed no difference in anastomotic leak rates or septic complications for anastomoses occurring below the peritoneal reflection. Although a slightly higher rate of abscess formation occurred in the non-MBP group, the abscesses were of little clinical significance, as the number of reinterventions, length of stay, and mortality rate were not affected. Rates of septic complications, fascial dehiscence, death, hospital duration, and days until resumption of diet were similar between both groups.

ANTIBIOTIC BOWEL PREPARATION

Oral antibiotic preoperative bowel preparation has historically been advocated to decrease the bacterial count of the colon at the time of surgery. Research by Nichols and Condon (1972) championed the use of preoperative oral antibiotics in addition to the mechanical preparation, documenting a decrease in surgical site infections from 43% to 9%. The Nichols-Condon antibiotic preparation originally consisted of 1 g of neomycin and 1 g of erythromycin base administered 19, 18, and 9 hours before the surgery start time.

Poor patient compliance and colitis associated with oral antibiotic ingestion are areas for concern. Wren and colleagues found a significant increase in *Clostridium difficile* colitis when using cathartics with intravenous and oral antibiotics versus using cathartics and intravenous antibiotics alone.

Given the risks associated with preoperative oral antibiotics, compliance issues on the part of the patient, and data supporting the use of parenteral antibiotics alone, the national Surgical Care Improvement Project (SCIP) guidelines require only parenteral antibiotics, administered within 60 minutes prior to the surgical incision.

SUMMARY

Despite the historical perspectives advocating the use of preoperative bowel preparation, the current literature reveals that its elimination for colorectal operations has no deleterious effects on anastomotic leak or surgical site infection. Although there are often some advantages to the omission of MBP for the patient, we believe that it can be advantageous for left-sided colorectal surgeries by facilitating passage of intraluminal staplers and heightening tactile sensation of tumor by having reduced the colonic stool volume. It is also beneficial if the need for intraoperative colonoscopy becomes necessary, and for ease of manipulation of the colon during laparoscopic colectomy. Oral antibiotics have been abandoned for a single-dose, broad-spectrum, parenteral antibiotic administered in compliance with SCIP guidelines.

SUGGESTED READINGS

Bretagnol F, Alves A, Ricci A, et al: Rectal cancer surgery without mechanical bowel preparation, *Br J Surg* 94(10):1266–1271, 2007.

Contant CM, Hop WG, van't Sant HP, et al: Mechanical bowel preparation for elective colorectal surgery: a multicentre randomised trial, *Lancet* 370(9605):2112–2117, 2007.

Guenaga KK, Matos D, Wille-Jorgensen P: Mechanical bowel preparation for elective colorectal surgery, *Cochrane Database Syst Rev* 2009(1): CD001544.

Hayashi MS, Wilson SE: Is there a current role for preoperative non-absorbable oral antimicrobial agents for prophylaxis of infection after colorectal surgery? *Surg Infect (Larchmt)* 10(3):285–288, 2009.

Jung B, Lannerstad O, Pohlman L, et al: Preoperative mechanical preparation of the colon: the patient's experience, *BMC Surg* 7:5, 2007.

Ker TS: Prospective comparison of three bowel preparation regimens: Fleet phosphosoda, two-liter and four-liter electrolyte lavage solutions, *Am Surg* 74(10):1030–1032, 2008.

Slim K, Vicant E, Launay-Savari MV, et al: Updated systematic review and meta-analysis of randomized clinical trials on the role of mechanical bowel preparation before colorectal surgery, *Ann Surg* 249(2):203–209, 2009.

Wren SM, Ahmed N, Jamal A, et al: Preoperative oral antibiotics in colorectal surgery increase the rate of *Clostridium difficile* colitis, *Arch Surg* 140(8):752–756, 2005.

Zmora O, Mahajna A, Bar Zakai B, et al: Is mechanical bowel preparation mandatory for left-sided colonic anastomosis? Results of a prospective randomized trial, *Tech Coloproctol* 10(2):131–135, 2006.

Zmora O, Lebedyev A, Hoffman A, et al: Laparoscopic colectomy without mechanical bowel preparation, *Int J Colorectal Dis* 21(7):683–687, 2006.

DIVERTICULAR DISEASE OF THE COLON

Susan L. Gearhart, MD

OVERVIEW

Diverticular disease is a term that refers to a variety of clinical presentations associated with the presence of diverticulae, or "outpouchings," of the wall of the colon. The incidence of the disease is highest among Westernized populations and is estimated to affect 30% of individuals by the age of 60 years and 60% of individuals over the age of 80 years. In the United States, diverticular disease results in over 200,000 hospitalizations annually, making it the fifth most costly gastrointestinal (GI) disorder.

The vast majority of patients with colonic diverticulosis are asymptomatic; only 20% develop the disease, and only about 1% require surgical intervention. Acute uncomplicated diverticulitis characteristically presents with left lower quadrant abdominal pain and fever. In less than 25% of patients, signs of generalized peritonitis indicate the presence of colonic perforation. Diverticular perforation with peritonitis or abscess formation, fistulization to the bladder or vagina, or colonic stricturing define complicated diverticular disease (Table 1). Finally, hemorrhage from a colonic diverticulum is the most common cause of hematochezia in patients over the age of 60 years. This chapter discusses the surgical indications and management of this disease.

CONTROVERSIES IN THE SURGICAL MANAGEMENT OF DIVERTICULAR DISEASE

Historically, controversy existed over whether or not a colostomy should be placed at the initial operation for complicated diverticular disease, which led to the Hinchey classification system for the management of complicated diverticular disease (Figure 1). In the late 1980s, the development of image-guided percutaneous drainage techniques revolutionized the management of several diseases, including diverticular disease, and it allowed for interval colonic resection once the acute process had improved. We now recognize that primary resection with anastomosis is usually safe and feasible

TABLE 1: Presentation and incidence of findings in acute diverticular disease

Uncomplicated Disease: 75% to 80%
• Abdominal pain • Fever • Leukocytosis • Anorexia/obstipation
Complicated Disease: 20% to 25%
• Abscess: 16% • Perforation: 10% • Stricture: 5% • Fistula: 2%

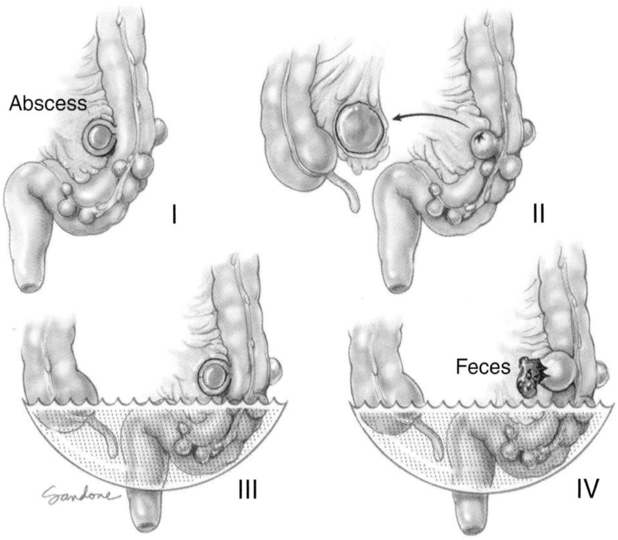

FIGURE 1 Schematic of the Hinchey classification of complicated diverticular disease. *(Courtesy Corinne Sandone.)*

with laparoscopic or open techniques in most cases. However, more recent controversies revolve around the need for surgery in uncomplicated and complicated diverticular disease with abscess formation. These controversial issues are addressed throughout the text.

UNCOMPLICATED DIVERTICULAR DISEASE

Evaluation

The diagnosis of uncomplicated diverticular disease is best made based on computed tomography (CT) with findings of sigmoid diverticula, thickened colonic wall (>4 mm), and inflammation within the pericolonic fat (Figure 2). In 16% of patients, an abdominal abscess may be present (management of this is discussed below, in the section on complicated diverticular disease). Suspected acute diverticulitis that does not meet CT criteria or is not associated with a fever of leukocytosis is not diverticular disease. Other conditions that can mimic diverticular disease include irritable bowel syndrome, ovarian cyst, endometriosis, acute appendicitis, and pelvic inflammatory disease.

Colonoscopy or barium enema should not be performed in the acute setting because of the higher risk of colonic perforation associated with insufflation or insertion of barium-based contrast material under pressure. However, a sigmoid malignancy can masquerade as diverticular disease, and therefore a colonoscopy should be performed 4 to 6 weeks following an attack.

MANAGEMENT

Asymptomatic diverticular disease discovered on imaging studies or at the time of colonoscopy is best managed with dietary alterations. Studies have suggested that a fiber-enriched diet decreases colonic transit time and prevents hypertonicity within the sigmoid colon, which is a part of the pathophysiology of this disease. Patients should be instructed to eat 30 g of soluble fiber and to consume 64 oz of caffeine- and alcohol-free beverages a day. Historically, patients were instructed to avoid nut consumption, since this was thought to encourage an attack by poorly digested nut particles lodging in diverticula. However, Strate and colleagues (2008) demonstrated in a large cohort study no increased incidence of diverticular disease among men who consumed nuts regularly.

The mainstay of treatment for acute uncomplicated diverticular disease is bowel rest and antibiotics. Patients with mild diverticular symptoms can be managed by their primary care physician as an outpatient. Nearly 75% of patients hospitalized for their disease will respond to nonoperative management with a suitable antimicrobial regimen. A limited diet is recommended until abdominal pain resolves. The most frequent bacteria involved in diverticulitis are *Escherichia coli, Proteus, Klebsiella, Enteroccocus,* and *Bacteroides fragilis.* The current recommended antimicrobial coverage is trimethoprim–sulfamethoxazole or ciprofloxacin and metronidazole. Unfortunately, this does always cover enterococci, and the addition of ampicillin to this regimen for nonresponders is recommended. The usual course of antibiotics is 7 to 10 days. In addition, newer studies have indicated that the addition of rifaximin, a poorly absorbed broad-spectrum antibiotic, in combination with soluble fiber significantly improves patients' GI symptoms.

In low-risk patients, surgical therapy can be considered after at least two documented attacks of diverticulitis requiring hospitalization or in those patients who do not improve on medical therapy. Preoperative risk factors influencing postoperative mortality include higher American Society of Anesthesia (ASA) class and preexisting organ failure. Recently, several studies have indicated that medical therapy can be continued beyond two attacks without an increase risk of perforation or need for colostomy. A large retrospective cohort study showed that only 13% of over 2000 patients managed nonoperatively at the time of their initial presentation had recurrent symptoms, and all were managed well nonoperatively. Furthermore, reserving colectomy for patients with several episodes of diverticulitis may provide a more optimal risk-to-benefit ratio for patients with diverticulitis. Salem and colleagues published a decision analysis showing that performing colectomy after the fourth rather than the second episode of diverticulitis resulted in fewer deaths, fewer colostomies, and significant cost savings (hospitalizations).

Finally, counseling patients that a preemptive elective colectomy is necessary to avoid the possibility of an emergent colectomy and stoma in the future may not be accurate; the majority of emergent colostomies were performed on patients who had not had antecedent diverticular events.

The exact indications for surgery in uncomplicated diverticular disease remain under discussion, but the trend does favor nonoperative therapy and individualizing surgery for a particular indication. The indications that have been addressed are age, health, and quality of life. The relationship of age to the management of uncomplicated diverticular disease has always been debated. Recent data suggest that although younger patients (<50 years) may have a higher likelihood to develop recurrent episodes and complicated disease that eventually will require surgery, they should follow the guidelines recommended for all ages. Furthermore, patients who are immunocompromised are at higher risk for perforation, and surgery should be contemplated

TABLE 2: Principles of elective resection for diverticular disease

- The procedure can be performed with either open or laparoscopic techniques.
- Ureteric stents are placed to aid in identifying the ureters, especially in severe disease.
- Moblization of the splenic flexure due to a foreshortened mesocolon is often required.
- Primary resection is from the proximal rectum, where tenia coli coalesce, to the normal caliber proximal colon with minimal diverticula.
- Oncological operation is performed with en bloc resection, and higher vascular ligation in malignancy cannot be ruled out.
- During a reversal of a Hartmann procedure, if a complete sigmoid resection was not performed at the initial operation, remove the residual rectosigmoid colon to minimize the chance for recurrence.

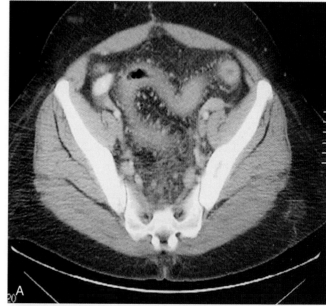

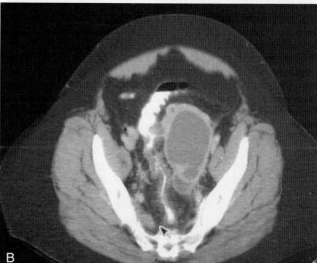

FIGURE 2   CT demonstrating the characteristic findings seen on CT scan of a patient with acute uncomplicated (**A**) and complicated (**B**) diverticular disease.

earlier rather than waiting for further episodes of diverticular disease to occur. Recurrent attacks of diverticular disease can cause significant alterations in quality of life with regard to bowel function; these should also be taken into consideration with regard to the specific management plan.

The steps in the elective management of acute diverticulitis are outlined in Table 2. This procedure can be performed using open or laparoscopic techniques. It should be emphasized that the dissection should be carried down to the rectum, and a colorectal anastomosis should be performed. Recurrent disease following resection is a known phenomenon related to retained distal sigmoid colon. Mobilization of the splenic flexure is required in the majority of cases to facilitate an anastomosis to healthy proximal colon. The benefits of a laparoscopic resection over an open resection include earlier return of bowel function, less narcotic use, decreased length of stay, and earlier return to work.

Complicated Diverticular Disease

As previously stated, *complicated diverticular disease* is defined as diverticulitis associated with abscess formation (Hinchey I and II) or perforation (Hinchey III and IV), fistula formation, and colonic stricture. There remains some controversy regarding surgical versus nonsurgical management for complicated diverticular disease, however, nonoperative management is less common, and frequently less acceptable to the patient, than uncomplicated diverticular disease. The goals of surgical management of complicated diverticular disease include controlling sepsis, eliminating fistula or intestinal obstruction, removing diseased colon, and restoring intestinal continuity. These goals should be achieved while minimizing morbidity, length of hospitalization, and cost and maximizing survival and quality of life. Figure 3 demonstrates the operative procedures performed for complicated disease. Table 3 lists the operations most commonly performed based upon Hinchey classification and the predicted morbidity and mortality.

Conventional management of Hinchey stages I and II is percutaneous drainage of accessible intraabdominal abscesses 5 cm or larger. Resolution of the abscess will occur in 75% of patients. If the abscess persists, the percutaneous drain is reassessed by CT scan and may need to be adjusted or upsized. In rare cases, operative intervention may be necessary. Paracolic abscesses smaller than 5 cm may resolve with antibiotic therapy alone. Following drainage, a colonoscopy is recommended, and surgical resection should be offered to the patient as an option. In selected cases, nonoperative therapy may be

considered. Recent studies have demonstrated lower than expected recurrence rates following nonoperative management. This is especially true for paracolic abscess formation than for distant abscesses (Hinchey I vs. Hinchey II), where the recurrence rate has been reported to be higher.

Contraindications to percutaneous drainage include poor percutaneous route of access, pneumoperitoneum, and fecal peritonitis (Hinchey stage IV). Urgent operative management is the treatment of choice for peritonitis and perforated diverticular disease. Prior to surgery, these patients may be hemodynamically unstable, and resuscitation with fluids and broad-spectrum antibiotics should be initiated. The safest option when treating patients with severe sepsis and generalized peritonitis is limited resection with colostomy (Hartmann procedure, Figure 3). If the dissection is not taken down to the rectum, it is important to resect the distal sigmoid at the time of reversal of the Hartmann procedure. If the patient is too unstable, an abdominal washout, omental pedicle graft, and proximal diversion can be performed.

Drains should be left in the paracolic gutters to assist in preventing abscess formation. It is best to avoid too much mobilization of

TABLE 3: Outcomes associated with the Hinchey classification and the operative procedures recommended for each stage

Hinchey Stage	Characteristics	Operative Procedure	Anastomotic Leak Rate	Overall Morbidity
Stage I	Pericolic or intramesenteric abscess	Resection with primary anastomosis without diverting stoma	3.8%	22%
Stage II	Pelvic abscess	Resection with primary anastomosis ± diversion	3.8%	30%
Stage III	Generalized purulent peritonitis without intestinal communication	Hartmann procedure vs. diverting colostomy and omental pedal graft	—	0% vs. 6% mortality
Stage IV	Fecal peritonitis with intestinal communication	Hartmann procedure vs. diverting colostomy and omental pedicle graft	—	6% vs. 2% mortality

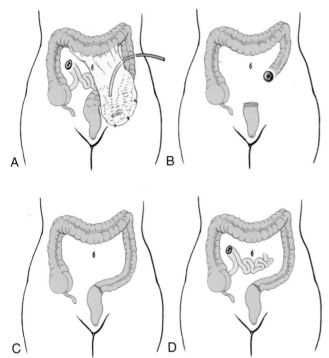

FIGURE 3 Operative procedure performed for complicated diverticular disease. **A,** Proximal diversion with drainage and omental patch. **B,** Hartmann procedure. **C,** Resection with primary anastomosis. **D,** Resection with primary anastomosis and diversion.

the colon if the contamination is extensive, as this may lead to contamination and abscess formation as well as loss of otherwise helpful resection planes. If the contamination is limited, a resection with an anastomosis can be performed. If preferred, the fecal stream can be diverted proximal to the anastomosis until complete healing is assured.

Colonic fistulae as a result of diverticular disease are commonly found to attach to the bladder or vaginal cuff in patients who have had a hysterectomy. Patients show evidence of pneumaturia, fecaluria, recurrent urinary tract or vaginal infections, and passage of flatus or stool through the vagina. The recurrent infections can be disabling to the patient, and quality of life is poor. Endoscopic evaluation is a necessity to rule out malignancy. Surgical resection either through an open or laparoscopic technique is the treatment of choice, however, conversion rates to an open procedure are reportedly higher than uncomplicated diverticular disease with the laparoscopic approach.

Once the disease is resected, closure of the bladder or vaginal defect is not required. If present, omentum can be secured to the site of fistula formation. Foley catheter drainage should be maintained for 5 days following surgery, and a cystogram is performed prior to the catheter's removal to assess for complete bladder healing.

Repeated episodes of diverticulitis can result in the development of a colonic stricture. Often patients are seen following routine colonoscopy, in which the stricture prohibits the procedure from being performed. In an asymptomatic patient without any proximal lesion, surgery is not mandated. Alternatively, a barium enema or virtual colonoscopy can be performed to ensure that the lumen is patent and no other colonic lesions are present. In the event of an acute large bowel obstruction secondary to stricture, surgery is indicated. Bridge intraluminal stenting of benign strictures has been less successful than reported for the management of an obstructing cancer, and it is not recommended. On-table colonic lavage can be useful; however, frequently the proximal colon is dilated and is not suitable for an anastomosis. If this is the case, a colostomy is required.

Diverticular Hemorrhage

Approximately 50% of patients presenting with lower GI hemorrhage will be bleeding from a colonic diverticulum. However, diverticular disease is often to blame when no source is identified. Patients at increased risk for bleeding tend to be hypertensive, have atherosclerotic disease, and regularly use nonsteroidal antiinflammatory drugs. Most bleeds are self-limited and stop spontaneously with bowel rest. However, in 10% to 20% of patients, a surgical intervention will be required to stop the bleeding. The lifetime risk of rebleeding from diverticular disease is 25%; however, as patients continue to have ongoing bleeding episodes, the risk of rebleeding is doubled.

Although, it is more common for diverticular bleeding to originate in the right colon, attempts should be made to localize the source of bleeding prior to resection. Methods for localization of diverticular bleeding include colonoscopy, nuclear scintigraphy, and angiography. For the diagnostic and therapeutic management of mild, self-limited diverticular bleeding, colonoscopy is most beneficial. The success rate for identification of the source of bleeding is 72% to 86%. However, if massive bleeding occurs, prompt attention should be given to resuscitation and stabilization before any intervention. Large-bore vascular access should be obtained, and intravenous fluid and blood administered. A properly placed nasogastric tube can be used to identify an upper GI cause of bleeding in 18% of patients. If the patient is stable, acute bleeding is best managed by angiography or surgery. Unfortunately, nuclear scintigraphy has not always been precise at localization of the bleeding site, and the accuracy of the procedure is time and reader dependent. The two most common techniques include sulfur colloid scan and tagged red blood cell scan. The rate of hemorrhage must be at least 0.1 mL/min to be detectable, and the suggested accuracy from this test ranges from 24% to 91%.

Mesenteric angiography can localize the bleeding site in patients who have ongoing bleeding of 1 mL/min and can occlude it successfully with a coil in 80% of cases. The patient can then be followed closely with or without repetitive endoscopy to look for evidence of colonic ischemia. With newer techniques of highly selective coil embolization, the rate of colonic ischemia is less than 10%, and the risk of acute rebleeding is less than 25%. Alternatively, a selective, progressive infusion of vasopressin can be given to stop the hemorrhage. However, this has been associated with significant complications, including myocardial infarction and intestinal ischemia, which may limit maximizing the dose. Furthermore, rebleeding occurs in 50% of patients once the infusion is stopped.

Surgical therapy for massive lower intestinal bleeding is rare and is associated with significant rates of morbidity and mortality. It has been reported that the incidence of postoperative morbidity and mortality increases after a transfusion of more than 10 units of packed red blood cells in 24 hours. Therefore current recommendations are for unstable patients, or for any patient who has had a 6-unit bleed within 24 hours, surgery should be performed. Patients with presumed bleeding from diverticular disease requiring emergent surgery without localization should undergo an exploratory laparotomy to identify any other possible source within the colon or small bowel. On-table enteroscopy can be performed. If no source is identified, and it appears that the colon may have been the cause, a total abdominal colectomy should be performed. The rate of recurrent bleeding is higher if the surgeon elects to do a more limited resection without precise localization of the bleeding site. In patients without severe comorbidities who are stable, surgical resection with a primary anastomosis can be performed.

Right-Sided (Cecal) Diverticular Disease

Diverticulitis of the cecum is rare in Western countries; however, this presentation is much more common than left-sided disease in the Asian population. Patients tend to be younger, and symptoms are right lower quadrant pain, fever, and leukocytosis. Frequently, this disease is confused with acute appendicitis, Crohn's disease, or carcinoma, and the diagnosis of acute diverticulitis of the cecum is made intraoperatively. The most common procedure performed is a right hemicolectomy or ileocecectomy. This can be performed with an open or laparoscopic technique. In Asian countries, where this presentation is more common, patients have been successfully treated nonoperatively with antibiotics.

Recurrent Disease

Recurrent abdominal symptoms following surgical resection for diverticular disease are estimated to occur in 10% of patients. The cause of recurrent symptoms results from either inadequate resection of the primary diseased colon or misdiagnosis. If there is a retained segment of diseased rectosigmoid colon following the initial resection, the risk of recurrent disease can be up to 20%. The most common scenario in which this happens is during a reversal of a Hartmann procedure, and the surgeon fails to identify retained rectosigmoid colon. Other reasons for the relapse of symptoms include irritable bowel syndrome and inflammatory bowel disease. Patients undergoing surgical resection for presumed diverticulitis and symptoms of abdominal cramping and irregular, loose bowel movements consistent with irritable bowel syndrome have functionally poorer outcomes.

Suggested Readings

Collins D, Winter D: Elective resection for diverticular disease: an evidence-based review, *World J Surg* 32:2429–2433, 2008.

Rocco R, Baxter N, Read T, et al: Is the decline in the surgical treatment for diverticulitis associated with an increase in complicated diverticulitis? *Dis Colon Rectum* 52:1558–1563, 2009.

Rocco A, Compare D, Caruso F, Nardone G: Treatment options for uncomplicated diverticular disease of the colon, *J Clin Gastroenterol* 43:803–808, 2009.

Strate L, Liu Y, Syngal S, et al: Nut, corn, and popcorn consumption and the incidence of diverticular disease, *JAMA* 300(8):907–914, 2008.

Management of Chronic Ulcerative Colitis

Michael P. Spencer, MD, and Genevieve B. Melton, MD

ULCERATIVE COLITIS

Ulcerative colitis (UC) is an idiopathic disorder characterized by mucosal and submucosal inflammation of the colon and rectum. The clinical course remains variable with associated diarrhea, bloody stools, and tenesmus that ranges from mild to severe. Toxic megacolon and perforation should be uncommon occurrences in a patient jointly managed by a gastroenterologist and a surgeon. Unfortunately, there is still a lack of consensus on the optimal medical management and timing of surgical intervention for the steroid refractory patient. What is becoming increasingly clear is that emergent colectomy limits surgical options, it is associated with higher perioperative morbidity rates, and it can compromise long-term function. While the majority of patients with UC respond to medical therapy alone, approximately 25% to 30% eventually require surgical intervention for intractable disease, malignant transformation, fulminate colitis, or side effects of medical management.

Epidemiology and Clinical Presentation

UC and Crohn's disease (CD) were initially thought to be different forms of the same disease. Most commonly, the onset of UC occurs in the teens or twenties; a second peak occurs in patients aged 40 to 60 years. Although familial clustering of inflammatory bowel disease (IBD) often occurs, genetics appears to be but one of several implicating factors. Concordance is seen in 10% of identical twins with UC compared with 3% of fraternal twins, and a positive family history of either UC or CD is seen in less than 10% of UC patients.

The diagnosis of UC is typically made using a combination of clinical factors, endoscopic and radiographic studies, histopathology, and serologic markers. Disease distribution is almost diagnostic with UC patients, who typically have rectal involvement and contiguous extension of the proximal colon but no small bowel disease other than occasional backwash ileitis.

When seen initially, most patients have predominantly distal disease (80%), although a minority will have pancolitis (20%). Approximately 10% of UC patients will show evidence of fulminant colitis, which can progress to toxic megacolon; these patients have a dilated and thickened colon, a septic clinical picture, and a high risk of colonic perforation. Acute infectious colitis must be ruled out first, and stool should be sent for fecal leukocytes and colonic pathogens. When clinically appropriate, stool should also be sent to culture for *Clostridium difficile*, *Cytomegalovirus*, *Cryptosporidium*, and *Giardia*.

Patients should undergo endoscopic examination, ideally with full colonoscopy, including ileal intubation with biopsies; notes should also be made on the disease distribution. Many clinicians also routinely obtain a radiographic study to evaluate the small bowel, such as a small bowel series, computed tomographic enterography, magnetic resonance enterography, or capsule endoscopy. Serology testing can be helpful in disease diagnosis. Perinuclear antineutrophil cytoplasmic antibodies (p-ANCA) are associated with UC, whereas anti-*Saccharomyces cerevisiae* antibodies (ASCA) are expressed in patients with CD; unfortunately, neither p-ANCA nor ASCA are highly sensitive.

A firm diagnosis of UC or CD may not be possible in approximately 10% of patients. These patients with *indeterminate* colitis are usually treated the same as those with UC, and nearly half will eventually manifest CD. The natural history of UC typically involves disease flares followed by periods of relative remission. A small minority of patients with left-sided disease (10%) will progress to disease extension proximal to the splenic flexure. In patients initially seen with pancolitis, over half will progress to surgery within 10 years.

Operative Indications

Improved medical treatment for moderate to severe UC, particularly the use of biologic agents like infliximab, have reduced the frequency of toxic colitis. Thus the most common indication for surgical treatment is intractability of disease; dysplasia, cancer, anemia, and side effects from medical therapy are less frequent considerations for surgical intervention (Table 1). The most common indication for acute colectomy with UC is fulminant colitis with or without perforation. Signs and symptoms consistent with severe colitis include more than eight bloody bowel movements daily, tachycardia, anemia, and a fever as evidenced by a temperature higher than 37.5° C. Patients with severe colitis who fail to respond to intravenous steroids within 48 to 72 hours, and/or a trial of cyclosporine or infliximab, should be considered for surgical intervention. In its most severe form, fulminant colitis can progress to toxic megacolon, with increased systemic disease that includes fever, abdominal tenderness, hypoalbuminemia, leukocytosis, tachycardia, and a dilated colon. Perforation occurs in approximately a fourth of these patients. Dermatologic and ocular manifestations of UC often improve in response to colectomy; however, other manifestations, such as primary sclerosing cholangitis and ankylosing spondylitis, appear to act independently of intestinal disease.

Because primary sclerosing cholangitis is associated with a higher incidence of dysplasia and carcinoma, this is a relative indication for surgery when UC has been present for an extended period. The development of cancer in the setting of UC is related to the severity and length of disease. After the first 8 to 10 years, during which the risk of cancer is low, the incidence increases approximately 1% to 2% annually thereafter. Furthermore, cancer can develop in the setting of colitis in flat-appearing mucosa and is thought to occur etiologically along a separate pathway. For these reasons, surveillance colonoscopy is recommended annually, starting at 8 to 10 years of disease with UC. Dysplasia is considered to be an indication for proctocolectomy. The presence of low-grade dysplasia is associated with cancer in 20% of patients, as opposed to high-grade dysplasia, which is associated with cancer in 50%.

Acute Surgery

When surgery is performed in the acute or emergent setting, the procedure of choice remains an open total abdominal colectomy with end ileostomy. Even with the hand port, laparoscopic techniques often require excessive manipulation of the already friable colon, increasing the risk of perforation and postoperative morbidity. Management of the rectal stump is an important consideration, as the rectum can be inflamed and edematous in this setting. Options include stapled transection at the rectosigmoid junction or preserving a long, distal rectosigmoid segment with exteriorization of the proximal stump in the subcutaneous tissue. Both options should preserve the superior rectal vessels and preserve the pelvic peritoneum. The mucus fistula can be matured or left closed and fixed to the anterior fascia and exteriorized simply by opening the skin at a later date if needed. We generally utilize a rectal tube as well, to keep the rectum decompressed and allow dependent drainage. Exteriorization reduces the risk of a pelvic abscess, prevents injury to pelvic structures, and facilitates future pelvic dissection. The optimal timing of proctectomy, with or without a restorative procedure, is variable and depends on the patient's clinical improvement, which usually takes several months or more.

Elective Surgery

Procedure selection depends on a variety of factors, including patient age, functional status, operative indication (such as low rectal cancer), baseline defecatory function, and patient preferences. Procedures are aimed at removal of diseased tissue, restoration of intestinal continuity, or construction of an end or continent ileostomy. With elective intervention, traditional open approaches and, more recently, minimally invasive approaches are acceptable, provided standard principals of resection are maintained (Table 2).

Total Proctocolectomy with End Ileostomy

The classic operative procedure for UC is total proctocolectomy with end ileostomy, which is curative, as it removes all colorectal disease. The main disadvantage of this procedure is the need to have a permanent end ileostomy. Because in most cases, the procedure is not done for a malignancy with UC, an intersphincteric dissection is often possible for the perineal proctectomy, which facilitates a layered closure of the perineum and lowers the risk of perineal wound problems.

TABLE 1: Indications for operation

Emergent	Urgent	Elective
Colonic perforation	Fulminant colitis >72 hr	Intractable disease
Acute hemorrhage	Anemia	Dysplasia/cancer
Toxic megacolon		Side effects of medication

TABLE 2: Surgical options for ulcerative colitis

Emergent/Urgent	Elective
• Subcolectomy and ileostomy • ± Distal mucus fistula	• Proctocolectomy and permanent ileostomy • Proctocolectomy and IPAA ± diverting ileostomy • Colectomy and ileal rectal anastomosis • Proctocolectomy and continent ileostomy

Total Abdominal Colectomy with Ileorectal Anastomosis

Patients with minimal rectal disease who understand the risks of rectal malignancy, are willing to undergo frequent ongoing surveillance, and wish to have a sphincter-preserving procedure may be candidates for total abdominal colectomy with ileorectal anastomosis. Important long-term considerations with this procedure include the increased risk of cancer in the rectal stump (approximately 10% at 20 years), a 10% incidence of fecal incontinence and a 10% risk of ongoing proctitis necessitating protectomy.

Intraoperatively, the abdominal colon is removed, and an ileorectal anastomosis is formed, typically at the level of the sacral promontory. The anastomosis can be hand-sewn or stapled in a variety of configurations; the end-to-side (Baker) anastomosis can mitigate the size discrepancy between ileum and rectum. The risk of anastomotic leak is low (~3%), and problems with sexual and urinary function are largely avoided. Patients can expect to have multiple daily bowel movements, which are often managed with antidiarrheal agents and/or fiber.

Continent Ileostomy

The continent ileostomy, or Kock pouch, is formed using ileum to create a nipple valve and pouch reservoir. The valve prevents emptying of the pouch spontaneously; patients intermittently insert a catheter to empty the pouch. The pouch reservoir is created in an S or W configuration, and the valve is formed by intussusception of the efferent limb of the pouch. Problems with the continent ileostomy include fistula, valve incompetence, pouchitis, and difficulties with valve intubation. Although utilized more often in several Northern European centers, continent ileostomies are only rarely created in the United States because of high revision rates (approximately 50%) and the increased use of restorative proctocolectomy.

Restorative Proctocolectomy

The technique of restorative proctocolectomy, first reported by Parks, has become the operative procedure of choice in patients with UC. Several terms are used for the procedure, including *ileal pouch–anal anastomosis* (IPAA), *restorative proctocolectomy,* or *pelvic pouch.* IPAA should not be performed in the setting of fulminant colitis, baseline incontinence, high operative risk, a low rectal cancer, or in most cases of Crohn's colitis. Patients with fulminant colitis should be managed first with total abdominal colectomy followed by clinical recovery and possible future pouch creation.

There are several possible approaches for creation of a pelvic pouch. Although a two-stage procedure is most often performed (proctocolectomy with IPAA and diverting loop ileostomy, followed by ileostomy takedown), a three-stage procedure (total abdominal colectomy with end ileostomy, completion proctectomy with IPAA and diverting loop ileostomy, and ileostomy takedown) is most appropriate for patients with fulminant colitis or malnutrition or for those receiving high doses of steroids or anti–tumor necrosis factor-α agents or for other clinical issues where sepsis risk is increased and can be modified following recovery from surgery.

Although some centers routinely use a single-stage procedure without any proximal diversion, this approach has been associated with a higher incidence of septic complications. An alternative, modified two-stage approach is to perform a total abdominal colectomy with end ileostomy followed by a proctectomy and IPAA without a protective proximal stoma. This approach has been gaining favor, given the decreased potential for pelvic sepsis in healthy patients who are no longer on medical therapy.

To begin, the patient should be positioned in a modified lithotomy position, which allows both abdominal and perineal fields to be accessed. Following abdominal colectomy with preservation of the ileocolic trunk by staying near the cecum for division of the right colonic mesentery, the ileal attachments are mobilized. The most

dependent arcade of ileum, just proximal to the distal small bowel staple line, can be brought inferiorly to assess length. In general, the pouch should reach several centimeters beyond the pubic symphysis to assure adequate length. Technically, creation of IPAA is often more difficult in taller and/or obese (particularly male) patients in whom the length of the small bowel mesentery can limit the reach of the pouch into the pelvis.

Several maneuvers have been described to improve the reach of the pelvic pouch. First, the small bowel mesentery should be fully mobilized, including division of the attachments at the level of the third portion of the duodenum. Second, the peritoneum over the distal small bowel mesentery can be scored on the anterior and posterior surface, generally gaining an additional 1 to 2 cm. In addition, a full-thickness defect or window can be created in the small bowel mesentery, or the surgeon may selectively ligate small vessels in the mesenteric arcade to increase length even more. Some recommend using Doppler to confirm adequate perfusion prior to dividing vessels, which can be most helpful if the mesentery is inflamed or scarred. Finally, the ileocolic vessel can also be ligated near its origin.

Pouch configuration is also an important consideration when reach is an issue. While the J-pouch is performed most often, the S-pouch generally provides superior length and is a better fit than the W-pouch in the tight male pelvis, which is the most common scenario when length is an issue. Care must be taken to minimize the length of the efferent limb of the S-pouch to 2 cm or less to avoid the risk of obstructive defecation.

In some cases, reach remains inadequate following all of these maneuvers. Options then include aborting the procedure for a permanent ileostomy, deferring IPAA formation and sewing the pouch into the pelvis to allow for the mesentery to possibly lengthen, or performing an abdominal colectomy at the first procedure and deferring IPAA to a later date.

The J-pouch is most commonly utilized due to the relative ease of construction and reliable function. The pouch length is generally 15 to 20 cm and is most frequently constructed with several firings of the gastrointestinal anastomosis stapler, introduced through an enterotomy at the apex of the pouch. The anal anastomosis is performed using either a double-staple or hand-sewn technique with mucosectomy. The major advantage of the double-stapled technique is overall improved fecal continence with maintenance of the anal transition zone and better sensation. However, mucosectomy can minimize issues with cuffitis and possibly neoplasia. When looking at all patients with IPAA, including patients with familial adenomatous polyposis, the results with respect to the oncologic benefit of mucosectomy are debatable. Most surgeons would, however, recommend a mucosectomy in any patient with a known cancer or dysplasia in the rectum.

With the double-stapled technique, a stapler is placed across the rectal stump just above the level of the levators, taking care not to incorporate the levator muscles, prostate, or vagina. This is done most often with a TA-30 (Covidien, Dublin, Ireland) or a Contour (Ethicon, Somerville, NJ) stapler. The specimen is removed, and an EEA stapler is used with the anvil secured into the apex of the pouch using a purse-string suture.

Mucosectomy is performed with the perineal operator dividing the mucosa at the level of the dentate line and dissecting proximally several centimeters through the anal canal and just above the levator muscles. This dissection can be facilitated by locally injecting submucosal epinephrine to raise the mucosa and maintain hemostasis and by using the Lone Star retractor (Lone Star Medical Products, Stafford, Tex.) to improve visualization. Once the specimen is removed, the pouch is hand-sewn to the anus using approximately eight absorbable sutures.

Although originally described as an open abdominal procedure, IPAA can also be performed using a laparoscopic approach. Several laparoscopic techniques have been described, including pure laparoscopic procedures, hand-assisted laparoscopic surgery, and laparoscopic-assisted procedures in which the abdominal colon is removed laparoscopically, and the proctectomy and pouch are performed with an open approach.

Outcomes following laparoscopic surgery for IPAA have not been widely reported, and no long-term advantages or disadvantages have been demonstrated to either approach. In general, surgeons should use an approach in which they have sufficient experience; however, although laparoscopic mobilization of the rectum is equivalent to open approaches, distal rectal transaction and stapling are difficult with current stapling devices.

Results and Complications. IPAA has several immediate postoperative complications and long-term issues that must be considered. Small bowel obstruction is commonly seen in up to 25% of patients following IPAA. The most common causes of obstruction are loop ileostomy–related complications such as internal hernia, stenosis, adhesions, and volvulus involving the ileostomy. Sepsis is the next most common complication, and it can have long-term implications for pouch function. Formation of pelvic abscess immediately following IPAA often occurs as a result of a leak, which may be less morbid in the setting of diversion with a loop ileostomy. In more severe cases, the leak can manifest itself as a fistula intraabdominally or to the perineum or vagina.

Patients at greatest risk for leaks and abscess formation are those on high-dose steroids; some reports have implicated anti–tumor necrosis factor-α agents as well. Anastomotic leaks can lead to long-term functional impairment and higher pouch excision rates. Although fistula during the immediate postoperative period or following takedown of a loop ileostomy is most likely technical in etiology, spontaneous fistula that occurs in a delayed fashion may occur as a result of CD. Management strategies have poor overall success and include seton placement, fibrin glue or plug, ileoanal flap, or vaginal flap. Diversion with a proximal stoma, except in the immediate postoperative period, is rarely an adequate approach to healing a fistula, but it can benefit those patients undergoing an anal repair.

Urinary and sexual dysfunction, as well as fertility problems, can occur following restorative proctocolectomy. Most of the morbidity appears to occur as a result of injury to the parasympathetic trunks; this can result in urinary retention, which is most often transient. Around 5% of men can have impotence and retrograde ejaculation, and women can suffer from dyspareunia (~5%), difficulty having an orgasm, or leaking during intercourse (2%). Fertility is also decreased following IPAA, most likely from adhesion formation; some surgeons advocate the use of placing Seprafilm around the ovaries with the intention of decreasing scar formation.

Expected bowel function following IPAA includes increased bowel movements (average five to eight daily) and some stool seepage. In several large studies, patients were satisfied with these outcomes 95% of the time. Pouchitis, which results in inflammation of the pouch with increased frequency and urgency of defecation, occurs in up to 50% of UC patients with IPAA at some point. After a single episode, only 15% have chronic symptoms, but over half will have an additional episode within 2 years. Diagnosis is made with pouchoscopy and histology. The pouch appears inflamed, and the mucosa is friable with occasional ulceration. Biopsies should be taken to confirm the clinical diagnosis. The etiology of pouchitis remains unknown, but treatment with antimicrobial agents, typically metronidazole and/or ciprofloxacin, is highly effective. Probiotics may also be helpful in prevention of pouchitis. A small subset of patients will have recurrent or chronic pouchitis, which may lead to pouch excision or additional medical treatment.

IPAA stricture or narrowing is typically not serious and can most often be managed with finger dilation in the office. Occasionally, the narrowing can be the result of a more serious problem such as ischemia, tension, cuffitis, a healed leak, or fistula. IPAA stricture should be managed closely, as a chronic stricture can lead to pouch dilation, which can alter function. Cuffitis is seen uncommonly following IPAA with a stapled technique, where the anal transition remains. Symptoms are similar to pouchitis but also often include bloody bowel movements and pain in the perianal region. The most common treatment is 5-acetylsalicylic acid suppositories.

Although cancer following IPAA for ulcerative colitis is rare, both the cuff of the rectum and the pouch are at risk. Mucosectomy is designed to decrease the risk of cancer; however, malignancy has been reported in patients following mucosectomy. Patients at greatest risk appear to be those with previous dysplasia or cancer and those with primary sclerosing cholangitis. Pouch failure with the need for permanent stoma and/or end ileostomy occurs in 5% to 10% of patients at large volume centers. Sepsis and Crohn's disease are two of the greatest risk factors for this. Other risk factors appear to be hand-sewn anastomosis, fistula formation, and tension on the pouch.

SUGGESTED READINGS

Bernstein CN, Shanahan F, Weinstein WM: Are we telling patients the truth about surveillance colonoscopy in ulcerative colitis? *Lancet* 343(8889): 71–74, 1994.

Chey WY, Hussain A, Ryan C, et al: Infliximab for refractory ulcerative colitis, *Am J Gastroenterol* 96(8):2373–2381, 2001.

Collins RH Jr, Feldman M, Fordtran JS: Colon cancer, dysplasia, and surveillance in patients with ulcerative colitis: a critical review, *N Engl J Med* 316(26):1654–1658, 1987.

Ekbom A: The epidemiology of IBD: a lot of data but little knowledge. How shall we proceed? *Inflamm Bowel Dis* 10(suppl 1):S32–S34, 2004.

Gan SI, Beck PL: A new look at toxic megacolon: an update and review of incidence, etiology, pathogenesis, and management, *Am J Gastroenterol* 98(11):2363–2371, 2003.

Gemlo BT, Wong WD, Rothenberg DA, et al: Ileal pouch–anal anastomosis: patterns of failure, *Arch Surg* 127(7):784–786, 1992.

Gorgun E, Remzi FH, Goldberg JM, et al: Fertility is reduced after restorative proctocolectomy with ileal pouch–anal anastomosis: a study of 300 patients, *Surgery* 136(4):795–803, 2004.

Kock NG: Intra-abdominal "reservoir" in patients with permanent ileostomy: preliminary observations on a procedure resulting in fecal "continence" in five ileostomy patients, *Arch Surg* 99(2):223–231, 1969.

Loftus CG, Egan LJ, Sandborn WJ: Cyclosporine, tacrolimus, and mycophenolate mofetil in the treatment of inflammatory bowel disease, *Gastroenterol Clin North Am* 33(2):141–169, 2004.

MacRae HM, McLeod RS, Cohen Z, et al: Risk factors for pelvic pouch failure, *Dis Colon Rectum* 40(3):257–262, 1997.

Oakley JR, Jagelman DG, Fazio VW, et al: Complications and quality of life after ileorectal anastomosis for ulcerative colitis, *Am J Surg* 149(1):23–30, 1985.

Parks AG, Nicholls RJ, Belliveau P: Proctocolectomy with ileal reservoir and anal anastomosis, *Br J Surg* 67(8):533–538, 1980.

Sagar PM, Lewis WJ, Holdsworth PJ, et al: One-stage restorative proctocolectomy without temporary defunctioning ileostomy, *Dis Colon Rectum* 35(6):582–588, 1992.

MANAGEMENT OF TOXIC MEGACOLON

Bashar Safar, MD, and James W. Fleshman, MD

OVERVIEW

Toxic megacolon (TM) is a serious, life-threatening condition that can result as a complication of ulcerative colitis, Crohn's colitis, and infectious colitides such as pseudomembranous colitis. TM was first described in 1950 by Marschak and colleagues as a complication of colitis, and it is defined as segmental or total colonic distension of 6 cm in the presence of acute colitis and signs of systemic toxicity.

Rapid dilation of the proximal colon produces the radiographic picture. The thickened, severely inflamed distal colon is, however, the segment of colon in which perforation is imminent; moreover, pneumatosis can be seen radiographically. The dilated proximal colon will only perforate if the inflammatory process has weakened the wall of the cecum. Most commonly the point of perforation is the splenic flexure, where a walled-off perforation is found in a phlegmon involving the colon, spleen, and omentum.

Systemic manifestations of toxicity distinguish patients with megacolon from those with colonic dilation due to other causes, such as colonic pseudoobstruction or Hirschsprung disease. Aggressive conservative management is increasingly advocated and may spare some patients an operation. However, prompt recognition of disease severity and surgical intervention may be life saving.

INCIDENCE AND ETIOLOGY

TM can result from any disease that results in inflammation of the colon. Although it is most readily recognized as a complication of inflammatory bowel disease (IBD), other causes include pseudomembranous colitis, *Salmonella*, *Shigella*, *Campylobacter*, *Entamoeba*, and ischemic colitis (Table 1).

The incidence of the syndrome varies based on the etiology and the study population. The incidence of TM in IBD has been the most extensively reported and has been estimated to range between 1% and 5% of patients with IBD. However, the incidence is believed to be decreasing due to improved medical management of patients with severe colitis. Conversely, pseudomembranous colitis, which occurs in up to 1% of hospitalized patients, is responsible for an increasing number of patients with TM.

In recent years *Clostridium difficile* infections were observed to be more frequent, more severe, more refractory to standard therapy, and more likely to relapse than previously described. These observations have occurred throughout North America and Europe and have been attributed to a new strain (BI/NAP1/027) of *C. difficile*. In a recent report of *C. difficile* toxicolitis, only 10% of cases required admission to intensive care, and 2.5% required an emergency colectomy. Other causes of TM are exceedingly rare.

The mechanisms responsible for the toxic dilatation of the colon are not fully understood and likely involve a combination of factors, including severe inflammation and local mediator release. Inflammatory damage to colonic mucosa due to severe colitis seems to extend into the smooth muscle layer in TM, resulting in damage and paralysis. Bacterial translocation occurs and results in bacteremia and the toxic/septic response.

Nitric oxide generated by severely inflamed smooth muscle cells in the colonic wall may play an important role in dysmotility and

atony, resulting in dilation of the colon proximal to the severely inflamed segment, which in turn leads to the development of TM. In fact, *toxic megacolon* may be a misnomer, because the dilated segment is not the toxic segment, nor is it the cause of the syndrome. In the majority of patients experiencing toxicity from colitis, there is minimal dilation. Thus the terms *severe toxic colitis* or *fulminant colitis* are more accurate.

A number of factors can lead to the induction or exacerbation of colonic dysmotility and dilation. These include hypokalemia, antimotility agents, opiates, anticholinergics, antidepressants, barium enema, and colonoscopy. These, combined with an inflammatory process, can be deadly.

DIAGNOSIS

Patients with IBD are at highest risk of developing TM early on in the disease course. Up to one third of patients with IBD develop colonic dilation within 3 months of their diagnosis, and another two thirds do so within the first 3 years. The mean duration of disease before developing TM has been reported to be between 3 and 5 years.

Toxic megacolon must be suspected in all patients who come in with abdominal distension, diarrhea, and systemic toxicity. In patients with IBD, dilation of the proximal, less inflamed colon frequently complicates severe distal colitis. In such cases the diagnosis is often preceded or accompanied by severe bloody diarrhea, fever, chills, and abdominal pain. Patients are thought to develop TM when massive colonic distension and functional obstruction ensues and results in worsening signs of systemic disease, including tachycardia and hypotension. The physical exam is often remarkable for significant abdominal tenderness, localized or generalized.

The diagnosis of toxic megacolon should be suspected based on physical and radiographic findings, so a thorough history and physical are crucial. History of previous bouts of IBD (extent of colonic involvement, previous therapy, extracolonic manifestations), recent use of certain medications (broad-spectrum antibiotics, steroids, antimotility agents, chemotherapy), foreign travel, HIV status, and recent barium enema must be carefully elicited.

Jalan and colleagues described the best accepted clinical criteria for diagnosis as any three of the following: fever of 101.5° F (38.6° C) or higher, heart rate 120 beats/min or higher, white blood cell count greater than 10.5×10^6/L, or anemia. Patients should also have one of the following: dehydration, mental changes, electrolyte disturbances, or hypotension.

A plain abdominal radiograph can aid in making the diagnosis and is crucial in following the disease course. Dilation of the ascending or transverse colon is typical and can vary from 6 cm, which is suggestive of the diagnosis, to as much as 15 cm. The absolute width of the colon is not as important as the rate of expansion along with the overall clinical condition. Small bowel as well as gastric distension may also be present and may be a significant predictor of TM and multiorgan dysfunction in severe ulcerative colitis. Thickening and edema of the wall of the transverse and left colon, with a thin trail of luminal air or none at all, is the typical finding on the left side.

An initial CT scan of the abdomen and pelvis can confirm the diagnosis and exclude pneumatosis or colonic perforation. In addition, CT scan may be useful to determine the etiology of the colonic dilation and exclude other causes of colonic distension, such as obstructing colon cancer or a diverticular stricture. Pronounced thickening of the colonic wall is more suggestive of *C. difficile* and IBD as the causative factor.

Laboratory tests should be obtained to both confirm the diagnosis and identify any correctable abnormality. Anemia and leukocytosis are frequently present. Electrolyte abnormalities are common, due to the severe inflammation, and they lead to increased fluid loss from the colon; salt and water losses can lead to severe dehydration and hypokalemia. Hypoalbuminemia may herald a poor prognosis. Stool

TABLE 1: Causes of toxic megacolon

Inflammatory

Ulcerative colitis

Crohn's disease

Infectious

Bacterial
- *Clostridium difficile* pseudomembranous colitis
- *Salmonella* (typhoid and nontyphoid)
- *Shigella*
- *Campylobacter*
- *Yersinia*

Parasitic
- *Entamoeba histolytica*
- *Cryptosporidium*

Viral
- Cytomegalovirus colitis

Other

Ischemia

Kaposi sarcoma

samples should be sent for culture, sensitivity, and *C. difficile* toxin assay. Blood cultures should be considered, as bacteremia occurs in up to 25% of patients with TM.

Limited endoscopy may be useful, but mistreatment can result in significant harm to the patient. Endoscopy is especially useful in patients with no previous diagnosis of IBD. Complete colonoscopy should be avoided due to the high risk of perforation, however, biopsies can identify inclusion bodies in the case of cytomegalovirus colitis; pseudomembranes in the rectum and sigmoid colon suggest *C. difficile* colitis.

THERAPY

Management of patients with TM and severe acute fulminant colitis necessitates a multidisciplinary approach with early surgical consultation. Communication between the admitting team and the surgical team is crucial. Clear management goals should be defined at the time of diagnosis, and criteria for continuing medical management versus surgical intervention should be set out at the outset and communicated to the patient and the patient's family. An aggressive attempt at medical management is warranted; however, in the absence of measurable improvement or any deterioration, surgical intervention should be instituted early to avoid the high rate of morbidity and mortality associated with colonic perforation.

Medical Therapy

All patients with TM should be admitted to the intensive care unit. Bowel rest and decompression with nasogastric tube is recommended, along with frequent clinical assessment by the nursing and medical staff. Complete blood counts, electrolytes, and serial abdominal plain films are reviewed every 12 hours initially and then daily as the patient improves. Anemia, dehydration, and electrolyte deficits, particularly hypokalemia, may aggravate colonic dysmotility and should be treated aggressively. All antimotility agents, opiates, and anticholinergics should be discontinued. Patients should be given prophylaxis for both gastric stress ulcerations and deep venous thrombosis. Broad-spectrum antibiotics are recommended to reduce septic complications. Significant improvement in the intensive care management of these patients has led to a significant decrease in morbidity and mortality in recent years.

Management of Patients with Inflammatory Bowel Disease

Patients known to suffer from IBD who show signs and symptoms of TM should be managed as mentioned above with the addition of high-dose intravenous steroids. A typical dose is hydrocortisone 100 mg every 8 hours or an equivalent dose of other intravenous steroids. High-dose steroids have not been shown to result in higher risk of colonic perforation.

Aminosalicylic acid products have no role in the management of TM. They are used in patients with mild to moderate disease, and their clinical efficacy is not proven in severe disease. Other immunosuppressive medication, such as cyclosporin and anti–tumor necrosis factor-alpha (TNF-α) agents, have been successfully used in the management of severe steroid-refractory colitis, however their use in patients with TM has not been substantiated beyond anecdotal case reports. Their use is not recommended for the management of TM.

Frequent patient repositioning resulting in redistribution of air in the lumen of the colon has been reported to be successful in decompressing colonic distension in patients with TM. The true value of this technique has not been confirmed by randomized trial, however, the intervention is fairly simple and should be attempted. Medical therapy is reported to be successful in 50% to 75% of patients with TM.

Management of Patients Without Irritable Bowel Disease

Management of patients with other diseases follows the same medical principle of aggressive supportive therapy and bowel rest. In addition, depending on the cause, other interventions may also be appropriate.

Clostridium Difficile *Colitis*

Withdrawal of the offending antibiotics and initiation of oral vancomycin 500 mg four times daily taken with intravenous metronidazole 500 mg three times daily are effective in the majority of patients. Patients with severe ileus may have the vancomycin delivered through an enema preparation or by colonoscopic spraying of the mucosa. A recent review suggested that earlier surgical intervention may be lifesaving. Patients who survived had lower white blood cell count, less preoperative multisystem organ failure, were less likely to be on pressors preoperatively, and were more likely to be operated on sooner than patients who did not survive.

In another study, leukocytosis greater than $50,000/mm^3$ and lactate at concentrations greater than 5 mmol/L were found to predict mortality. Both of these reports suggest that earlier intervention saves lives. Most patients warrant an aggressive medical management trial with close observation; however, in the presence of any deterioration, delaying surgical intervention may result in higher rates of morbidity and mortality.

The surgical management of patients with TM secondary to *C. difficile* colitis is similar to that in patients with IBD.

Surgical Therapy

Free perforation, massive hemorrhage, and progression of colonic dilatation are absolute indications for surgery. Failure to improve within 48 hours is a relative indication. Some authorities suggest continuing medical therapy for up to 7 days in the absence of any signs of deterioration, but proponents of early surgical intervention highlight the high mortality rate once colonic perforation occurs (40% vs. 9%). Goligher's popular dictum to "save the patient, not the colon" was based on a study that reduced the rate of perforation from 32.5% to 11.6%, and mortality rate from 20% to 7%, by means of early surgery. The investigators concluded that surgery should be performed shortly after diagnosis. D'Amico and colleagues confirmed this finding; they suggested that lower mortality (13%) can be achieved by surgical intervention at the time of diagnosis with no trial of medical therapy. However, as mentioned above, medical management can be effective in 50% to 75% of patients and should be instituted without delay. Patients should be observed closely for signs of deterioration, but the length of medical management should be limited to 7 days, provided the patient is stable clinically or improving.

Subtotal colectomy and end ileostomy is the treatment of choice, once surgery is deemed necessary. Due to the amount of dilatation in the colon, laparoscopy should be avoided in patients with TM.

Upon admitting a patient with TM, the enterostomal therapist should be consulted as soon as possible for marking the site of an end ileostomy; a generous midline incision is used to gain access to the abdominal cavity. Mechanical bowel preparation should be avoided.

Once the abdomen is entered, the bowel should be handled with care; the bowel is fragile, and the likelihood of intraoperative perforation is high. The hepatic flexure and splenic flexure should be mobilized and the colonic mesentery divided close to the bowel wall to avoid damage to retroperitoneal structures, including the ureters and nerves. The colon mesentery can be divided with Kelly clamps and ties; alternatively, a hemostatic coagulation device can be employed. The rectum should be divided as low as possible to avoid a rectal stump blowout, and the staple line should be marked with long, permanent sutures for future identification. A large mushroom catheter is left in the rectum, taped to the inside of the thigh to prevent dislodgment, for continued drainage of the rectal stump.

The patient is transported postoperatively back to the intensive care unit, where fluid resuscitation and further support are provided (e.g., ventilatory support, antibiotics, pressure support as needed). The nasogastric tube may be removed and enteric feeds initiated upon resumption of gastric motility. The rectal tube should remain in place for a minimum of 5 days, or until the patient is ready to be discharged; perioperative antibiotics should be discontinued within 24 hours, unless a perforation is encountered. Intravenous steroids should be weaned rapidly to the patient's preoperative dose over the course of a few days.

Outcomes

Mortality as a consequence of TM has improved markedly within the last 30 years. Jalan and colleagues reported an overall mortality rate of 45% in 1969, but studies with no deaths were being published by the end of the 1970s.

Teeuwen and colleagues reviewed the literature for colectomy in 1257 colitis patients who were operated on in an acute setting (urgent or emergency colectomy). Over the past 3 decades, three has been a shift in incidence: TM has become less common (71.1% from 1975 through 1984 to 21.6% from 1995 through 2005) than severe acute colitis not responding to conservative treatment (16.5% from 1975 through 1984 to 58.1% from 1995 through 2007). Mortality rate

decreased from 10.0% to 1.8%, and the review suggests that improvement in medical management of IBD may be responsible for the decrease in incidence of TM and overall mortality.

SUMMARY

TM is a severe, life-threatening emergency that can result from a variety of conditions, but it is most commonly associated with severe ulcerative colitis. Improved medical management has resulted in a decrease in its incidence due to IBD; however, increasing use of broad-spectrum antibiotics has lead to a sharp increase secondary to *C. difficile* colitis. Early recognition and multidisciplinary management are crucial if significant morbidity and mortality are to be avoided.

SUGGESTED READINGS

Ali SO, Welch JP, Dring RJ: Early surgical intervention for fulminant pseudomembranous colitis, *Am Surg* 74:20, 2008.

Ausch C, Madoff RD, Gnant M, et al: Aetiology and surgical management of toxic megacolon, *Colorectal Dis* 8:195, 2006.

D'Amico C, Vitale A, Angriman I, et al: Early surgery for the treatment of toxic megacolon, *Digestion* 72:146–149, 2005.

Gan SI, Beck PL: A new look at toxic megacolon: an update and review of incidence, etiology, pathogenesis, and management, *Am J Gastroenterol* 98:2363, 2003.

Goligher JC, Hoffman DC, DeDombal FT, et al: Surgical treatment of severe attacks of ulcerative colitis, with special reference to the advantages of early operation, *Br Med J* 4:703–706, 1970.

Grieco MB, Bordan DL, Geiss AC, et al: Toxic megacolon complicating Crohn's colitis, *Ann Surg* 191:75–80, 1980.

Jalan K, Sircus W, Card WI, et al: An experience of ulcerative colitis, I. Toxic dilation in 55 cases, *Gastroenterology* 57:68–82, 1969.

Latella G, Vernia P, Viscido A, et al: GI distension in severe ulcerative colitis, *Am J Gastroenterology* 97:1169–1175, 2002.

Pepin J, Valiquette L, Cossette B: Mortality attributable to nosocomial *Clostridium difficile*–associated disease during an epidemic caused by a hypervirulent strain in Quebec, *CMAJ* 173(9):1037–1042, 2005.

Pepin J, Vo TT, Boutros M, et al: Risk factors for mortality following emergency colectomy for fulminant *Clostridium difficile* infection, *Dis Colon Rectum* 52:400–405, 2009.

Sheth SG, LaMont JT: Toxic megacolon, *Lancet* 351:509, 1998.

Strauss RJ, Flint GW, Platt N, et al: The surgical management of toxic dilatation of the colon: a report of 28 cases and a review of the literature, *Ann Surg* 184:682, 1976.

Teeuwen PH, Stommel MW, Bremers AJ, et al: Colectomy in patients with acute colitis: a systematic review, *J Gastrointest Surg* 13:676–686, 2009.

CROHN'S COLITIS

Rohit Makhija, MD, and
Conor P. Delaney, MD, MCh, PhD

CROHN'S DISEASE

Crohn's disease (CD) was first described by Crohn, Ginsberg, and Oppenheimer in 1932, when it was called *regional ileitis*. The annual incidence of CD is 3 per 100,000, and the prevalence is 10 to 15 per 100,000. The highest incidence is in Scandinavian countries and Scotland, followed by the United Kingdom and the United States; however, the incidence is rising in the United States.

Two age groups show an increased incidence of CD, with prevalence in the second and third decades and in the sixth and seventh decades of life. However, 10% of patients are younger than 18 years. Females are affected more than males, and it is more common in Jewish patients and whites compared with nonwhites. Smoking confers another major risk factor, particularly for recurrence after treatment.

ETIOLOGY

The etiology of CD is unclear, but several theories have been proposed, including that it is an immune-mediated response to an unknown infectious agent or the result of a defective mucosal barrier or genetic defect. The NOD2/CARD15 gene has been associated with CD, and abnormal T cell responses are seen frequently. CD involves only the small intestine in a third of patients, small intestine

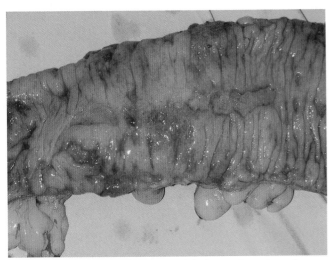

FIGURE 1 Colon showing transmural thickening, linear bear claw ulceration, and mucosal inflammation.

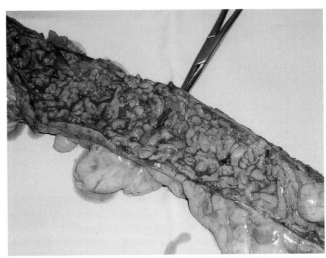

FIGURE 2 Section of colon showing ulceration, wall thickening, and a fistula tract.

and colon in a third, and colon alone in a third; but it may affect any part of the gastrointestinal (GI) tract, from the mouth to the anus. Extraintestinal manifestations are common, such as uveitis and primary sclerosing cholangitis, however, these are less common than in ulcerative colitis (UC).

Macroscopically, there are areas of disease interspersed with normal bowel. Involved segments are rubbery, thickened, and edematous with creeping mesenteric fat that wraps around the bowel surface. Three main disease patterns are seen: *inflammatory* (edematous), *stricturing* (fibrotic), and *penetrating* (fistulizing). Reactive lymphadenopathy of mesenteric nodes is common; the lumen is narrowed and may be strictured in a segmental fashion. The mucosa shows inflammation and serpentine ulceration with a cobblestone appearance (Figure 1).

Fissures develop that can erode through the bowel wall to involve surrounding structures such as the vagina, bladder, and other parts of the bowel (Figure 2). Sometimes fissures can result in perforated bowel or intraabdominal abcesses that may track to the cutaneous surface, becoming enterocutaneous or colocutaneous fistulas. Characteristic histologic features include transmural inflammation, neutrophilic infiltration, blunting of villi, lymphoid aggregates, crypt abscesses, and ulceration. Noncaseating granulomas are seen in 35% of patients. Muscular hypertrophy and submucosal fibrosis lead to thickening of the bowel wall with subsequent stricture formation.

Accurate pathologic diagnosis of Crohn's colitis is essential, as it influences the medical management of the disease as well the surgical management. However, in 10% of patients, differentiation from UC may not be possible, resulting in the pathologic diagnosis of indeterminate colitis. A significant number of these patients go on to develop features of CD. Crohn's colitis affects the rectum in 50% patients, unlike UC, in which it inevitably does.

Colonic involvement may be segmental, or patients can show signs of pancolitis. Perianal CD is associated with colitis more than half the time and with proctitis in more than 90% of patients, unlike UC. The distribution within the colon is segmental in 40%, total in 31%, and left sided in 29%.

CLINICAL FEATURES

The clinical features of Crohn's colitis are variable and range from relatively minor symptoms to peritonitis. The usual pattern is of episodic, crampy abdominal pain, diarrhea, and weight loss. This may be associated with lethargy, anorexia, and pyrexia. Some patients show features of complicated disease, such as massive bleeding, fulminant colitis, intestinal obstruction, or intraabdominal sepsis. It has

been proposed that Crohn strictures progress from inflammatory lesions to more fibrotic ones. It would appear that the inflammatory strictures are more amenable to medical management, whereas the fibrotic lesions are unresponsive and thus require surgery.

The major differential diagnosis is UC, and it is important to try and obtain pathologic clarity of diagnosis. Stool should be checked to exclude infectious causes of colitis; samples should be sent to look for ova and parasites, especially for newly diagnosed patients and those with severe acute flares of their disease. Barium enema may be helpful, but it is a relatively insensitive test and has been largely replaced by computed tomography (CT).

Direct visualization with colonoscopy (with ileal intubation) and biopsy is the best method for diagnosis. Colonoscopy is important for diagnosis, as well as to delineate the extent of disease. Segmental disease is common; however, some patients may have pancolitis, either macroscopically or microscopically. Further, patients with established Crohn's colitis should have a small bowel series to look for segmental lesions in the small bowel.

CT is a good tool for visualizing colonic thickening, mesenteric fat stranding, and abscesses. Radiolabeled white cell scanning can be used to outline areas of active inflammation, but it is rarely required.

MEDICAL MANAGEMENT

Medical management includes a combination of 5-aminosalicylic acid (5-ASA) products, corticosteroids, and immunomodulatory agents. A number of 5-ASA products are available such as oral preparations, enemas, suppositories, and retention enemas. Topical preparations have minimal side effects and are useful for left-sided colonic disease as well as for proctitis. Oral prednisolone 40 to 60 mg daily can also be used, ideally on a short-term basis with a rapid taper once symptoms have resolved. Budesonide (less first-pass mechanism) 9 mg is as effective as prednisone with less adrenal suppression. Metronidazole and ciprofloxacin have a role in the management of mild colonic Crohn's colitis, however the efficacy is less than steroids, and there may be long-term side effects, such as peripheral neuropathy.

Azathioprine and 6-mercaptopurine are useful agents both for maintaining remission and for their steroid-sparing effect; however, patients must be assessed for thiopurine methyltransferase deficiency before starting therapy to avoid the risk of adverse effects. Intravenous infliximab infusion (monoclonal anti–tumor necrosis factor-alpha [TNF–α] antibody) has a role in patients unresponsive to steroids, antibiotics, and immunomodulators. It also plays a role in the treatment of fistulating CD. Cessation of smoking is vital, particularly in reducing the incidence of recurrences.

SURGERY

CD differs from UC in that surgery is not curative but simply has the goal of dealing with the symptomatic area of the intestine, to return the patient to a good quality of life for as long as possible. About 80% of Crohn's patients will need surgery at some point, and many of these will need reoperation. Of patients with Crohn's colitis, 50% will need surgery within the first 10 years; 25% will need a permanent ileostomy. Surgery should therefore be used cautiously and conservatively, for clear-cut indications.

The patients are complex, the disease is recurrent, and reoperative surgery in this setting can be a challenging undertaking. Because of this, patients should be thoroughly assessed and fully counseled. Psychological support may help, as most patients have overlying psychiatric issues as a result of long-standing illness. Malnutrition should be corrected, and some patients may need a period of parenteral nutrition. All patients with CD must be urged to stop smoking, as this increases the recurrence risk after surgery. If the bowel is not obstructed, patients should undergo mechanical bowel preparation, as this facilitates the operation.

Indications for Surgery

Failure of Medical Management

Failure of medical management remains the commonest indication for surgery (Table 1). Patients may have progressive symptomatic disease despite best medical management, or they may be intolerant to the side effects of medical therapy. Despite advances in immunomodulatory therapy, the incidence of patients coming to surgery has not decreased in the last two decades.

Stricture and Obstruction

Crohn's colitis may result in obstruction from inflammatory strictures, fibrosing disease, or an inflammatory mass. Adhesions from previous surgery are unlikely to be responsible for colonic obstruction. Initial management is conservative, consisting of nasogastric tube decompression, fluid and electrolyte balance correction, and nutritional support. Steroids may have an effect, if the process is inflammatory rather than fibrotic. Endoscopic dilation of strictures is an option in experienced hands, but there is a risk of perforation during the procedure. Long-term results of dilation are unknown, but it may help avoid emergency surgery.

All strictures should be biopsied at endoscopy to detect malignancy, and all strictures should essentially be regarded as malignant until proven otherwise, usually by examination of a resection specimen. Recurrent strictures after surgical resection are usually not at anastomotic sites.

Perforation and Intraabdominal Abscess

Abscesses result from perforation and are best detected by CT scan. The initial management of intraabdominal abscess is conservative and consists of antibiotics, bowel rest, and radiological drainage, where amenable. Surgical treatment is warranted if the abscess cannot be drained radiologically or in the presence of signs of peritonitis or progressive sepsis. Surgery involves laparatomy/laparoscopy with drainage of abscess and resection of the involved portion of colon. Patients treated with immunosuppression who have an abscess frequently require creation of a diverting stoma, at least temporarily. Interval surgery is indicated when symptoms persist despite radiologic drainage.

TABLE 1: Indications for surgery

Failure of Medical Management
Stricture/obstruction
Perforation/Intraabdominal Abscess
Acute severe colitis, fulminant colitis, toxic megacolon Dysplasia/neoplasia Major lower gastrointestinal bleeding
Fistula Formation
Extracolonic manifestations Growth retardation in children

Acute Severe Colitis/Fulminant Colitis/Toxic Megacolon

Patients with Crohn's colitis may have symptoms similar to UC with abdominal distension, systemic inflammatory response syndrome, and a distended abdomen with megacolon on plain abdominal radiographs (>6 cm transverse colon). Conservative management consists of bowel rest; intravenous fluids; assignment to a specialized unit, possibly the intensive care unit; steroids (except for infectious colitis); and frequent clinical and radiologic reassessment.

Crohn's colitis can be insidious, and the physiologic response and immunosuppression sometimes hides the severity of colonic inflammation. Timing of surgery is crucial; time to respond must be balanced against the mounting systemic inflammatory response and the possibility of perforation. In the setting of perforation, mortality rates have historically been as high as 20% to 30%.

Dysplasia/Neoplasia

As with UC, colorectal cancer risk is elevated in patients with Crohn's colitis and can be three times that seen in the normal population. The guidelines for colonoscopic surveillance are similar in both Crohn's colitis and UC. Indications for surgery would be overt neoplasia, high-grade dysplasia, or the presence of a dysplasia-associated lesion/mass. Controversy exists regarding the management of low-grade dysplasia.

Major Lower Gastrointestinal Bleeding

An occasional patient will need surgery for persistent bleeding. Colonoscopy should be done to find the source of bleeding, to exclude other causes, and with a therapeutic intent. Mesenteric angiography is unlikely to help in this situation, and surgery is indicated. This may change the operation required, as the standard subtotal colectomy and end ileostomy may still leave a bleeding source in the rectum.

Fistula Formation

Fistulae may develop between almost any adjacent organ in CD. The usual sites are small bowel (particularly terminal ileum to adjacent sigmoid colon), bladder, colon, stomach, and vagina. Fistulae are suggested by urinary tract infections, pneumaturia, particulate matter in urine, hematuria, passage of fecal matter or air per vagina, feculent vomiting without evidence of distal bowel obstruction, and abdominal pain. A variety of investigations can be used to discern the location, such as contrast studies, cystoscopy, and GI endoscopy.

If the symptoms are minimal or manageable, surgery may be deferred until symptoms worsen or the patient becomes dependent on antibiotics to maintain quality of life. There are reports of successful management of fistulizing abdominal CD with infliximab, but in the majority of patients, treatment requires segmental resection of the colon with en bloc resection of the fistula. In ileosigmoid fistula, the inflammation is often only in the ileal side, and formal sigmoid resection may be avoided by excising the involved area and primarily closing the defect in the sigmoid colon.

Extracolonic Manifestations

Progressive extraintestinal manifestations of CD may resolve with surgery, with the exception of primary sclerosing cholangitis and ankylosing spondylitis.

Growth Retardation in Children

Childhood CD is treated more aggressively than CD in adults. A combination of malnutrition and the effects of medical therapy render children with CD prone to growth failure. Growth hormone can help mitigate the effects of medical therapy, in early cases; recognition of growth failure is an important indication for surgery before termination of long bone growth and epiphyseal closure.

Operations

Mechanical bowel preparation is generally used for elective cases along with antibiotic prophylaxis and deep vein thrombosis prophylaxis.

Emergency Surgery

Emergency surgery is indicated for toxic megacolon, major lower GI bleed, perforation, abscess with peritonitis, and severe acute colitis that does not respond to medical management. The usual management is total or subtotal abdominal colectomy with terminal ileostomy. The rectum is left intact, as emergency proctectomy is a major undertaking with high morbidity, difficult access to friable edematous tissues, and major blood loss. Emergency rectal resection should be reserved for unremitting bleeding from the rectum after all endoscopic measures have failed or in the event of rectal perforation.

The incision should be midline, as there is a likelihood that access to the abdominal cavity will be needed again, and this keeps ostomy sites available. After assessing the peritoneal cavity and the abdominal organs, the small and large bowel should be fully assessed for disease. If the colon alone is involved, proceed with total abdominal colectomy. The surgeon must be particularly cautious about dealing with the raw mesenteric edges and the vessels; the thickened tissues are prone to bleeding if care is not taken. In the usual fashion, care should be taken to avoid injury to the ureters, duodenum, stomach, and other abdominal organs.

The rectal stump is left long enough so it may reach the lower end of the midline wound. The rectum may be closed if it is minimally inflamed. However, the surgeon may have to make a mucous fistula if the rectum is grossly inflamed with friable tissues; the mucous fistula is brought out in the lower end of the wound. If the rectum is closed, there is a concern it may open up intraabdominally and cause sepsis. The closed rectal stump is therefore buried within the lower end of the midline wound as a potential mucus fistula. Additionally, the rectum may be drained by a large Foley catheter or daily digitation, although the use of drains is avoided unless there is a specific reason, such as indurated abscess cavity walls. The splenic flexure is generally difficult in these patients and should be left until last, after mobilization of the transverse and descending colon, to permit maximum control in case of spillage of stool, and to avoid tearing frail, damaged tissues.

Proctectomy

After emergency colectomy, more than half the patients will require completion proctectomy for continuing perianal CD or for proctitis. If the rectum is involved in the inflammation, the risk of neoplasia warrants either close surveillance or proctectomy. For inflammatory disease, the perineal dissection should be in the intersphincteric plane. Proctectomy and end colostomy is rarely used for isolated proctitis, as the disease usually progresses proximally; therefore a proctocolectomy and end ileostomy is usually the preferred option.

Segmental Colectomy

With colocolic or ileosigmoid anastomosis, following the vascular supply is an option in a small number of patients with segmental colonic disease such as a stricture or fistula. If an inflammatory phlegmon involves an adjacent organ, a fistula should be suspected, and intraopearive measures taken to confirm this. If the small bowel is involved, the affected segment should be resected.

Often the sigmoid colon overlies the bladder, and it is unclear whether there is a definite fistula. In such a situation, one can fill the bladder with methylene blue to localize a leak. A urinary cather should be left for 2 days postoperatively, and a cystogram should be obtained prior to removing the catheter. Patients who have undergone extensive small bowel resection are candidates to have as much colon preserved as possible, especially the ileocecal valve. Segmental colectomy does not prevent recurrence, and the rates are similar to those seen elsewhere in the GI tract, as opposed to panproctocolectomy, in which the recurrence rates are lower (~25%).

The goals of surgery are resection of palpably abnormal colon and anastomosis to visibly healthy bowel. Microscopic disease at resection margins is not predictive of a higher recurrence rate, therefore resection to visibly and palpably healthy bowel is sufficient. In the presence of gross sepsis, fecal diversion is indicated in this population of chronically unwell patients.

Surgery for CD can be a challenging exercise, and great care is required to avoid anastomotic leak in this population. The basic principles of colonic surgery should be carefully followed with careful attention paid to the vascularity of the ends being joined together. It is our practice to visually assess flow in the marginal artery by checking for pulsatile bleeding from the cut edge. The anastomosis should be carefully constructed without tension.

Total Abdominal Colectomy with Ileorectal Anastomosis

In about a quarter of patients who need total abdominal colectomy, the rectum is spared; in such a situation, ileorectal anastomosis is a viable option. Quality of life and satisfaction is better in patients who can avoid an ileostomy, making this a popular option in suitable candidates. Ileorectal anastomosis may be offered to patients with mild proctitis or anorectal disease, as long as the sphincters are functional and rectal compliance is good. A comprehensive discussion is advisable, as there is a risk of recurrence and disease progression in the retained rectum; about one half of such patients will need to have a proctectomy with end ileostomy in 10 years. Rectal compliance is assessed by insufflation on rigid sigmoidoscopy as well as anophysiology studies. The sphincter function is assessed by digital rectal examination to assess basal tone and squeeze. Anophysiology may help in cases of doubtful sphincter function. In the presence of a narrow rigid rectal tube, functional results are likely to be poor, and there is a risk of anastomotic leak.

In selected patients with proximal rectal disease, a short rectal stump may be left in place, and a 10 cm ileal pouch may be fashioned and anastomosed to the rectal stump. This provides adequate function and reduces the usual irritation seen with a smaller rectal reservoir.

Panproctocolectomy with Terminal Ileostomy

Panproctocolectomy with terminal ileostomy is the treatment option for colorectal CD with the lowest recurrence rate, although at the price of a permanent ileostomy. It is indicated in patients with multiple or large segments of colonic involvement, along with rectal disease, or in patients with perianal as well as colonic CD. Recurrent disease elsewhere in the GI tract occurs in about 20% at 10 years, and some patients will require ileostomy revision for stoma problems or CD in the ileal segment.

Rectal dissection can be challenging, and proponents of close perimuscular dissection within the mesorectal plane state a proposed advantage of reduced incidence of damage to the pelvic autonomic nerves and less resultant sexual dysfunction. The disadvantage is excessive blood loss from dissecting within the mesorectum. However, the majority of surgeons favor a mesorectal plane of dissection for a number of reasons, such as familiarity with the procedure, low rates of pelvic nerve damage in experienced hands, and a relatively bloodless field.

The perineal dissection is carried out in the intersphincteric plane, allowing a smaller perineal wound with better healing. In extensive perineal dissection, the excision field should be widened to include the diseased perineal tissues. Rarely, for extensive perineal disease, plastic flap reconstruction may be necessary. Delayed healing of the perineal wound can be a problem in many patients, and it may take several months of wound care to induce healing. Occasionally, wound sinuses may develop that need probing and excision. Sometimes, contrast studies may be required to exclude perineal enterocutaneous fistula.

Ileoanal Pouch Reconstruction

Ileoanal pouch reconstruction is the gold standard of treatment for UC; however, CD has generally been considered a contraindication to pouch surgery because of the risk of recurrent disease. Of patients who undergo emergency total abdominal colectomy, 10% to 15%

have indeterminate colitis, and some of these have undergone ileal pouch–anal anastomosis after a full discussion. Subsequently 40% to 55% developed CD with pouch failure or fistula to the bladder, vagina, or perianal skin, however, many patients manage to retain their pouch for many years.

Laparoscopic Surgery

In recent years, a laparoscopic approach to surgery for CD has been shown to offer faster recovery, reduced costs, and lower morbidity. The majority of colonic operations—such as segmental colectomy, total proctocolectomy, or a diverting loop ileostomy—can be performed laparoscopically with all the related benefits. Complicated reoperative colonic laparoscopic surgery and rectal surgery has been performed with good results in experienced hands.

SUGGESTED READINGS

Casillas S, Delaney CP: Laparoscopic surgery for inflammatory bowel disease, *Dig Surg* 22(3):135–142, 2005.

Duepree HJ, Senagore AJ, Delaney CP, et al: Advantages of laparoscopic resection for ileocecal Crohn's disease, *Dis Colon Rectum* 45(5):605–610, 2002.

Strong SA, Koltun WA, Hyman NH, et al: Practice parameters for the surgical management of Crohn's disease, *Dis Colon Rectum* 50(11):1735–1746, 2007.

Wolf JM, Achkar JP, Lashner BA, et al: Afferent limb ulcers predict Crohn's disease in patients with ileal pouch–anal anastomosis, *Gastroenterology* 126(7):1686–1691, 2004.

ISCHEMIC COLITIS

Christopher Wolfgang, MD, PhD

OVERVIEW

Ischemic colitis is a condition that mainly affects the elderly, but in rare instances, it can occur in younger individuals. Ischemic colitis occurs when the metabolic demand of the colon exceeds oxygen and nutrient delivery. This may be the result of a complete disruption of blood flow to the colon but is more commonly due to a low-flow state in which susceptible regions of the colon become transiently ischemic.

Ischemic colitis exists as a spectrum of conditions, ranging from transient self-limiting ischemia that results in abdominal pain and diarrhea to severe, permanent disruption of blood flow that results in necrosis, peritonitis, and sepsis. The latter condition carries a high risk of mortality. The true incidence of ischemic colitis is unknown, because a large number of indolent cases resolve spontaneously and are never brought to medical attention.

Many of the risk factors of ischemic colitis parallel those of other vascular diseases, such as coronary artery and peripheral vascular disease; these include advancing age, hypertension, smoking, and diabetes. Additional risk factors include operations often performed on patients with these risk factors, such as cardiopulmonary bypass and aortic repair. A recent study has estimated that the incidence of ischemic colitis ranges from 4.5 to 44 cases per 100,000 person-years. In addition, it has been reported that 1 in every 1000 hospital admissions is due to ischemic colitis. It is likely that the incidence will

continue to increase with the increase in the proportion of elderly individuals in Western societies.

Ischemic colitis was first described by Boley and colleagues (1963) as a sequela of aortic surgery. Currently, ischemic colitis is a well-recognized condition that results from various underlying etiologies that go beyond this original description. This chapter reviews current understanding of ischemic colitis with an emphasis on diagnosis and management. Guidelines for the diagnosis and management of ischemic colitis have recently been developed by the American Gastroenterological Association, and more information is available on this topic online at http://www.gastro.org.

THE ETIOLOGY OF COLONIC ISCHEMIA

Blood Supply to the Colon

The colon is supplied by branches of the superior mesenteric artery (SMA), inferior mesenteric artery (IMA), and internal iliacs (Figure 1). The SMA gives rise to the *middle colic artery*, which supplies the transverse colon, approximately from the hepatic flexure to the splenic flexure; the *right colic artery*, which supplies the ascending colon and proximal hepatic flexure; and the *ileocolic artery*, which supplies the terminal ileum, cecum, and proximal ascending colon. The IMA gives rise to the *left colic artery*, which supplies the descending colon and distal splenic flexure, and the *sigmoid* and *superior hemorrhoidal arteries*, which supply the sigmoid and proximal rectum, respectively. The proximal rectum is additionally supplied by the *middle hemorrhoidal arteries*, which arise from the internal iliac arteries bilaterally.

A rich network of anastomotic connections exists among the various arterial pedicles. Although these connections are clearly present based on physiology, the nomenclature of these structures

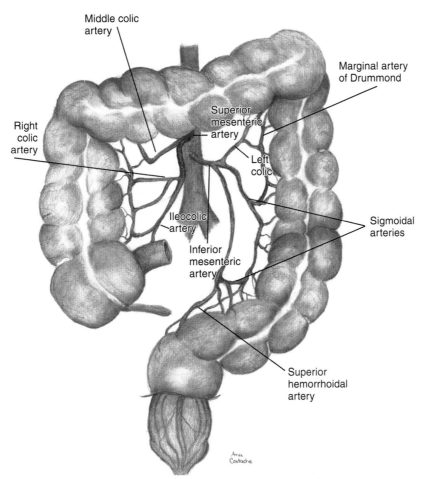

FIGURE 1   Blood supply to the colon. *(Courtesy Ana Costache.)*

is variable (Lange et al, 2007). In the majority of individuals, a marginal artery, *arcus paracolicus,* courses from the cecum to the rectum. Eponyms for this structure and confusion with other arterial arcades have resulted in inconsistent usage of terms to describe the arterial anatomy supplying the colon. In the most generally promulgated version, this vessel is called the *marginal artery of Drummond,* in the area of the splenic flexure; it is absent in approximately 5% of the population. Additionally, the entire marginal artery has often been referred to as the *arch of Riolan,* in honor of the seventeenth-century anatomist who described visceral blood supply in a an early anatomic text entitled *Opera Anatomica.*

It has been argued by some that the arch of Riolan is actually an arterial arcade distinct from the marginal artery that connects the SMA and IMA in a minority of individuals. The evaluation of Riolan's original writings does not clarify which structure represents the arch of Riolan. In any case, a network of collateralization of blood flow exists within the colonic mesentery and likely varies significantly within individuals. Disruption of this network through vascular disease, colonic resection, or ligation of the IMA may predispose individuals to the development of ischemic colitis; but due to individual variability in anatomy, this effect is not uniform throughout the population.

In addition to the macroscopic interconnections of the SMA, IMA, and iliac arteries, a microscopic network of collateralization exists within the bowel wall. The intramural vascular network is not as robust in the colon compared with the small bowel; thus disruption of terminal braches supplying a segment of colon is less well tolerated than in the small bowel, and it more commonly results in ischemia in the colon.

Certain segments of colon called *watershed areas* are more susceptible to ischemia than others. These include the right colon, splenic flexure, and the sigmoid colon. The rectum is seldom affected by ischemia due to its dual blood supply. The distribution of the right colon is susceptible to low-flow states, such as heart failure, sepsis, and causes of sudden hypotension, such as hemorrhage. A reduction of visceral blood pressure below 40 mm Hg is sufficient to predispose this region to ischemia (Chang, 2007). The vasa recti in this region traverse a relatively long distance and are prone to spasm in response to transient reductions in blood flow. Ischemia in this location is seldom associated with an identifiable vascular lesion on arteriogram, and pulses are maintained in the main vascular pedicles.

A second ischemic insult that affects the proximal right colon and cecum is embolic events. The ileocolic branch that supplies this region is a terminal branch of the SMA and is a straight shot for emboli entering this vessel. When compared with sigmoid ischemia, ischemic insult of the right colon, regardless of etiology, more often takes a more fulminant course that requires an operation. The splenic flexure is susceptible to ischemia due to its relatively remote location from the middle colic and left colic arteries, which both supply this region. Moreover this area is even more sensitive to ischemia in the minority of individuals who lack a marginal artery of Drummond as described above. Finally, the sigmoid colon normally receives its blood supply from the IMA. This vessel is often chronically occluded in the aged population due to vascular plaque. Moreover, the IMA is sometimes sacrificed in both traditional and endovascular repair of aortic aneurysms. Under these circumstances, the blood supply to the sigmoid colon is derived from collateral flow originating from the middle colic (SMA) superiorly and the middle rectal (iliac) inferiorly.

In addition to the common causes of ischemic colitis that result from disruption of blood flow in individuals with diseased vessels, a wide range of conditions may result in colonic ischemia. These conditions also affect younger individuals (age 18 to 50 years), who have no apparent vascular risk factors, and they follow the demographics of the underlying disease; for example, the distension caused by colonoscopy has been reported to result in intestinal ischemia in rare cases.

There also is a strong association between chronic constipation and intestinal ischemia. A detailed list of etiologies of ischemic colitis is shown in Table 1. Notable conditions associated with ischemic colitis include hypercoagulable states, cocaine use, and extreme physical activity. It has been reported that 28% of patients with ischemic colitis have some type of hypercoagulable state compared with less than 10% of the general population. Very rarely, extreme exercise such as marathon running has been found to result in transient mild ischemic colitis that is often self-limited and corrected with rehydration. The etiology behind this is thought to be a combination of shunting blood from viscera to muscles and dehydration.

Pathophysiology

In the initial phase of compromised blood flow to the colon, the first histologic changes that become apparent are mucosal edema and hemorrhage within the mucosa and submucosa. If blood flow is restored during this phase, little damage is incurred by the colon. In cases where the disruption of blood supply is more prolonged, these changes are followed by sloughing and ulceration of the mucosa. Healing of these ulcers occurs through fibrosis and granulation tissue infiltrated by iron-rich macrophages. In profound defects of perfusion, mucosal ulceration proceeds to transmural necrosis and colonic perforation. This process is irreversible and results in peritonitis, sepsis, and death in patients who do not undergo aggressive treatment.

Classification

The natural history of ischemic colitis generally follows two patterns: *transient nongangrenous ischemia* or *fulminant gangrenous ischemia*. It is important to make a clinical distinction between the two, because it will dictate management and predict outcome. Approximately 85% of cases of ischemic colitis are of the nongangrenous type and, of these, half will resolve spontaneously. In some patients, a chronic form of nongangrenous ischemic colitis is manifested by colonic strictures or segmental colitis. In patients with gangrenous ischemic colitis, emergent surgical intervention is required to resect necrotic colon and control peritonitis. Not surprisingly this form of ischemic colitis results from a more profound disruption of blood flow and is associated with a higher mortality.

Clinical Presentation and Diagnosis

Ischemic colitis is generally a disease of the elderly. Signs and symptoms are nonspecific and are also found in a large number of other abdominal conditions. Individuals with nongangrenous ischemic colitis often experience vague, poorly localized abdominal pain followed by diarrhea and passage of blood per rectum. Most often the melena or hematochezia associated with these cases is minor and does not require a blood transfusion. Significant hematochezia with severe anemia should suggest an alternative diagnosis. In patients with more severe forms of nongangrenous ischemic colitis, pain may be localized and is often associated with systemic signs of infection, such as a low-grade fever or leukocytosis. Abdominal exams in these patients will often elicit peritoneal signs. Patients with gangrenous ischemic colitis will appear septic

TABLE 1: Etiology of ischemic colitis

Relatively Common
Low-flow states/hypotension
Shock (septic, hemorrhagic, hypovolemic, cardiogenic)
Arterial emboli (usually SMA)
Cholesterol
Thrombus
Arterial thrombosis (usually IMA)
Colonic obstruction
Constipation
Volvulus
Neoplasm
Adhesion
Hernia
Surgical/iatrogenic
Cardiopulmonary bypass
Aortic surgery or stent graft placement
Colectomy with disruption of marginal artery
Medications
Vasopressin
Cocaine
Digoxin
Estrogens
Pseudoephedrine
Phenylephrine

Relatively Uncommon
Hypercoagulable states
Protein S or C deficiency
Antithrombin III deficiency
Anticardiolipin antibodies
Paroxysmal nocturnal hemoglobinuria
Vasculitis
Systemic lupus erythematosus
Polyarteritis nodosa
Rheumatoid arthritis
Thromboangitis obliterans
Sickle cell disease
Long-distance running, extreme physical exertion

with fever, tachycardia, hypotension, and peritonitis. Patients who do not undergo aggressive management of this condition will rapidly deteriorate.

Since the signs and symptoms of ischemic colitis are nonspecific, the key to making this diagnosis is a high index of suspicion. Factors such as patient age, history of vascular disease, risk of embolic and thrombotic events, and recent operations should be considered. The known risk factors for ischemic colitis are listed in Table 2. The workup of a patient with colonic ischemia is often in a debilitated patient with abdominal pain, and commonly a computerized tomography (CT) scan is obtained prior to endoscopy. In ischemic colitis without perforation, segmental thickening of the colonic wall is the most common finding. This discovery is nonspecific and can be seen in other conditions such as infectious colitis. In addition, plain films are often obtained, which may demonstrate thumb-printing indicative of submucosal edema. Colonic distension and pneumoperitoneum are later signs, found in perforated gangrenous ischemic colitis.

Once the diagnosis of ischemic colitis is entertained, the gold standard confirmatory test includes colonoscopy or sigmoidoscopy. Endoscopy is often performed without a bowel preparation and under low insufflation to avoid exacerbation of existing ischemia. Findings of ischemia include pale or cyanotic appearing mucosa, mucosal edema with petechial bleeding, hemorrhagic nodules, and ulcerations. The involvement is often segmental with an abrupt transition to normal mucosa within the well-perfused areas of colon. The hallmark finding is a linear ulcer running longitudinally, typically along the antimesenteric border of the mucosa, called the *single-stripe sign*. However, the absence of this finding does not preclude colonic ischemia.

Historically, a barium enema was used in the workup of a patient showing symptoms of ischemic colitis. However, its use has been supplanted by the use of endoscopy and CT, which are more specific. Angiography is rarely performed in the workup for ischemic colitis, unless other conditions coexist, such as more diffuse visceral ischemia. Since colonic ischemia is most often due to diminished perfusion at the arteriolar level, and large vessel flow is maintained, arteriography is seldom useful. Moreover, in the majority of cases, flow is spontaneously restored to the colon by the time arteriography is obtained.

The differential diagnosis of ischemic colitis should include infectious causes of colitis such as *Salmonella, Shigella, Campylobacter, Yersinia,* toxogenic *E. coli,* and ova and parasites. Stool samples should be sent to evaluate for pathogens, particularly in those patients who have been hospitalized within the past 72 hours. In addition, *Clostridium difficile* should be considered in any patient who has been treated with antibiotics.

TREATMENT

The treatment of ischemic colitis depends on the clinical circumstances. In general, nongangrenous ischemic colitis resolves spontaneously or with supportive care, while gangrenous colitis requires emergent operation. Figure 2 shows a flow diagram that guides the decision making in the management of a patient with ischemic colitis.

Surgical intervention is usually not required in the acute setting for patients with nongangrenous ischemic colitis. Patients with mild ischemic colitis can be treated with clear liquids and broad-spectrum antibiotics as an outpatient. Close follow-up is required for those patients treated outside of the hospital, because worsening colitis can occur in a minority of patients. More severe cases require hospitalization, and their initial treatment begins with bowel rest, aggressive intravenous fluid resuscitation, and broad-spectrum antibiotics. These treatments reduce the metabolic demand of the mucosa and ensure adequate vascular volume; the antibiotics serve the purpose of reducing the risk of peritonitis or sepsis caused by bacterial translocation across compromised colon. Although this practice has essentially no level I evidence in humans, animal studies strongly suggest infectious complications and survival are improved when antibiotics are administered in the setting of ischemic colon.

Cardiac function should be optimized through medical management, and a Swan-Ganz catheter may be necessary to guide these measures in patients with known cardiac dysfunction. The addition of supplemental oxygen may maximize oxygen delivery in relatively hypoperfused colon. All medications known to promote colonic ischemia (see Table 1) should be discontinued or avoided. In addition to the above measures, patients with an associated ileus should have a nasogastric tube placed. When significant distal colonic distension is present, the careful placement of a rectal tube may result in symptomatic relief and might even improved microvascular perfusion of the decompressed colon. Oral cathartics and bowel preparations should be avoided, because they may exacerbate the ischemia or increase the risk of perforation.

Patients should be monitored closely with frequent vital signs taken and serial abdominal exams at the very least. Patients with numerous comorbidites or more severe colitis may be best served in an intensive care unit with continuous monitoring. Once a diagnosis of ischemic colitis is made, serial abdominal radiographs (flat plate, upright, and chest) may be useful in following the degree of ileus, colonic distension, or the development of pneumoperitoneum.

Despite these measures, approximately 20% of patients will go on to develop refractory or worsening symptoms and will require an operation. Indications that a patient is failing expectant management include continuing or worsening fever, tachycardia, oliguria, acidosis, or development of peritonitis. Patients undergoing operation during the acute phase of ischemic colitis, either initially or following non-operative management, have a risk of mortality in the range of 50% to 80%.

Urgent operations for ischemic colitis should include resection of all compromised colon, a thorough washout and exploration of the abdomen, and almost invariably the creation of a stoma. For patients with right-sided colonic ischemia, a right hemicolectomy with an end ileostomy and a long Hartmann pouch or mucus fistula should be performed. In cases of ischemia to the splenic flexure, a left hemicolectomy should be performed that includes the transverse colon, just distal to the left branch of the middle colic artery, and ends at the proximal rectum. For left-sided lesions, an

TABLE 2: Risk factors for ischemic colitis

Vascular disease
Coronary artery disease
Peripheral vascular disease
Small vessel disease (diabetes)
Recent hypotension
Hemorrhage
Sepsis
Heart failure
Recent surgery
Aortic surgery
Cardiopulmonary bypass
History of colonic surgery

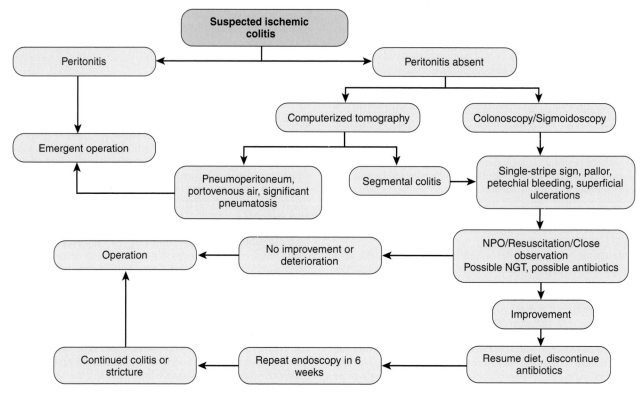

FIGURE 2   Proposed treatment algorithm for a patient with ischemic colitis.

end colostomy and Hartmann pouch should be created. Care must be taken to ensure the colon is resected to the level of healthy margins. The serosal appearance may be deceptive because of potentially unrecognized mucosal or submucosal ischemia. This can be avoided by the intraoperative evaluation of the margins of resection by a pathologist using a frozen-section preparation and light microscopy to ensure viability. In most cases, however, examination of the opened colon by the surgeon will address this potential pitfall.

At operation, if the small bowel appears to also be potentially ischemic, a second-look laparotomy, following 24 to 48 hours of aggressive resuscitation, may be helpful. In addition, if areas of colon or small bowel are not clearly ischemic on visual routine inspection, the administration of fluorescein dye (100 mg/5 mL IV) followed by a Wood's lamp evaluation may be useful. Doppler signals and palpable pulses within the colonic mesentery do not rule out ischemia, because it is mainly a disease of small vessels. For this same reason embolectomy, vascular bypass, and endarterectomy rarely play a role in the care of these patients.

In patients who go on to develop chronic sequelae of ischemia following initial nonoperative management, such as strictures that lead to obstruction, may need to undergo a segmental colectomy under routine conditions. These operations are tailored to resect the diseased areas and may allow for more limited resections and primary colonic anastomosis. As with colonic resection in the acute setting, painstaking care must be taken to ensure the margins of resection are well perfused in patients who have already proven to have marginal colonic perfusion. In this regard, strong consideration to the creation of a stoma should be given, even in the elective setting. Stomas created in both emergent and elective operations should not be reversed for at least 3 months, and certainly not until the patient has nutritionally and physiologically recovered from the ischemic event. Many patients who undergo emergent colectomy with the creation of a stoma for ischemic colitis will never have their stoma reversed due to the significant associated comorbidites in this population.

SUMMARY

Ischemic colitis is a condition that mainly affects the elderly but in rare instances can occur in younger individuals. Ischemic colitis occurs when the metabolic demand of the colon outstrips oxygen and nutrient delivery. This may be the result of a complete disruption of blood flow to the colon but is more often due to a low-flow state in which susceptible regions of the colon become transiently ischemic. Ischemic colitis exists as a spectrum of conditions, ranging from transient self-limiting ischemia to severe permanent disruption of blood flow and necrosis.

The natural course of ischemic colitis generally follows two patterns: transient nongangrenous ischemia and fulminant gangrenous ischemia. This is an important clinical distinction to make, because it dictates subsequent management and predicts outcome. Since the signs and symptoms of ischemic colitis are nonspecific, the key to making this diagnosis is a high index of suspicion. Factors such as patient age, history of vascular disease, risk of embolic and thrombotic events, and recent operations should be considered. The treatment of ischemic colitis depends on the clinical circumstances. In general, nongangrenous ischemic colitis resolves either spontaneously or with supportive care once the insult is removed. Patients with gangrenous ischemic colitis require emergent operation for a colonic resection and abdominal washout.

Suggested Readings

Green B, Tendler D: Ischemic colitis: a clinical review, *South Med J* 98:217–222, 2005.

Koutroubakis I: Ischemic colitis: clinical practice in diagnosis and treatment, *World J Gastroenterol* 14(48):7302–7308, 2008.

Lange J, Komen N, Akkerman G, et al: Riolan's arch: confusing, misnomer, and obsolete: a literature survey of the connection(s) between the superior and inferior mesenteric arteries, *Am J Surg* 193:742–748, 2007.

Sreenarasimhaiah J: Diagnosis and management of ischemic colitis, *Curr Gastroenterol Rep* 7:421–426, 2005.

CLOSTRIDIUM DIFFICILE COLITIS

John L. Cameron, MD, Andrew Cameron, MD, PhD, Houssam Farres, MD, and Pamela A. Lipsett, MD

OVERVIEW

Although rare in the preantibiotic era, pseudomembranous colitis was first recognized by J.M. Finney and William Osler in 1893 and was primarily associated with gastric, colonic, or pelvic surgery. In the early 1970s, the disease became known as *clindamycin colitis* because of strong links to that particular antibiotic; *Clostridium difficile* was thereafter proved to be the cause.

Since 2002, renewed interest in *C. difficile* has been stimulated by epidemic outbreaks in hospitals in Canada, the United States, United Kingdom, and The Netherlands secondary to a hypervirulent strain of *C. difficile*, with high recurrence and increased severity. *C. difficile*–associated diarrhea (CDAD) is a major cause of nosocomial and antibiotic-associated diarrhea (10% to 30%), and it is the commonest recognized cause of pseudomembranous colitis (96% to 100%).

EPIDEMIOLOGY

The overall attack rate of antibiotic-associated diarrhea in hospitals is 3.2% to 29%. More than 300,000 cases of CDAD occur annually in the United States alone, with an incidence among hospitalized and long-term care patients of 25 to 60 cases per 100,000 bed-days. The risk of acquiring *C. difficile* while hospitalized directly relates to length of hospital stay, with 13% colonization after 2 weeks and 50% at greater than 4 weeks of hospitalization. Overall, approximately 20% of hospitalized patients become colonized, whereas 8% develop diarrhea.

Several studies have reported recent increases in both incidence and severity of CDAD worldwide. This pattern is now attributed to a new strain of *C. difficile*, alternatively designated as BI, NAP1, or ribotype 027 toxinotype III. Although this strain had been isolated as far back as 1984, it has recently emerged as a public concern with the development of fluoroquinolone resistance. In Oregon, a 1994 to 2000 cohort of patients with CDAD had a 15.3% mortality rate compared with 3.5% mortality rate during the previous 10 years.

On average, each case of CDAD adds $2000 to $5000 to the yearly cost of health care. The mean lifetime cost for recurrent CDAD has been estimated at nearly $11,000 per patient, and overall, *C. difficile* adds an estimated $1 billion in health care costs in the United States annually.

C. difficile is a highly resistant spore that has been isolated and cultured from soil; swimming pools; and salt, fresh, and tap water. In the hospital setting, it has been cultured from telephones, call buttons, shoes of health care workers, fingernails, and numerous other objects. *C. difficile* is transmitted via the fecal-oral route, either directly (hand carriage by health care workers and patient-to-patient contact) or indirectly (from contaminated environments). *C. difficile* has been found in infected patients' rooms up to 40 days after discharge.

Because most cases of disease appear to be caused by acquisition of the organism from an exogenous source, rather than from endogenous colonization, the cornerstones of prevention of CDAD are handwashing and avoiding inappropriate use of antibiotics; hands must be cleansed with soap and water, rather than alcohol rubs, to kill spores on the hands. In epidemic situations, the restriction of antibiotic formularies to prevent the indiscriminate use of fluoroquinolones in addition to infection control, disposable gloves, single-use disposable thermometers, and hand washing with soap and water is credited for decreasing the rates of CDAD.

RISK FACTORS

Antibiotic use is clearly the major risk factor for CDAD. Normal intestinal flora exert a protective effect, known as *colonization resistance*, against *C. difficile* by depleting carbon sources required for *C. difficile* growth, preventing access to adherence sites, and producing inhibitory substances. Antibiotics alter this normal gut flora, allowing overgrowth of *C. difficile*. Although longer duration of antibiotic use confers greater risk of CDAD, cases following a single dose, such as for perioperative prophylaxis, have been reported.

Although initially attributed to clindamycin use, CDAD can be caused by any antimicrobial; clindamycin, penicillins, cephalosporins, and fluoroquinolones are most commonly associated with CDAD. Cephalosporins and fluoroquinolones have higher attributable risk for CDAD given their higher usage rates compared with clindamycin.

Host factors play an essential role in determining outcome after exposure to antibiotics and to *C. difficile* (Table 1). Host immune response plays a particularly vital role in determining whether patients become colonized or develop clinical disease. Serum immunoglobulin (Ig) G and IgA and mucosal IgA all appear to be involved in protection.

Despite adequate therapy, *C. difficile* infection recurs in 20% of patients. Risk factors for relapse are prolonged antibiotic usage, prolonged hospitalization, age over 65 years, diverticulosis, and any other comorbid conditions.

PATHOPHYSIOLOGY

The primary initiating event in CDAD is disruption of the normal protection barrier provided by the intestinal flora during treatment with antibiotics or antineoplastic agents. Ingestion of toxigenic strains of *C. difficile* by fecal-oral transmission allows for colonization and multiplication of the vegetative form throughout the colon,

TABLE 1: Identified intrinsic and extrinsic risk factors associated with *Clostridium difficile* infection

Intrinsic Patient Risk Factors	
Age	Severity of illness
Ongoing infection	Renal failure
Hematologic malignancy	Transplant patient
Debilitated/bedridden	Burns
Bowel obstruction/ileus	Hypoalbuminemia
Extrinsic Patient Risk Factors	
Antibiotics	
Agents that alter gastrointestinal motility	Gastrointestinal surgery
Laxatives and narcotics	Proton pump inhibitor use
Enteral tube feeding	

facilitated by a reduced microbial ecosystem. Although the vegetative form is normally destroyed by gastric acid, the spores are acid resistant and vegetate in the small bowel.

The pathogenicity locus that includes the genes for toxins A and B are always present in toxigenic isolates and absent from nontoxigenic isolates. Toxin A is considered primarily an enterotoxin that has some cytotoxic properties. Toxin B is a cytotoxin that induces cytopathogenic effects in numerous tissue-culture cell lines. Both toxins interfere with the actin cytoskeletons of intestinal epithelial cells, rendering the cells nonfunctional. Disassembly of the actin cytoskeleton can then lead to disruption of the intestinal epithelium and excessive fluid leakage. Both toxins A and B are potent stimulators of the inflammatory cascade and the proinflammatory cytokines—such as tumor necrosis factor-α, interleukin (IL)-1, IL-6, and IL8—and the prostaglandin pathway, as evidenced by massive infiltration of neutrophils, macrophages, and lymphocytes in the intestinal (colonic) mucosa. This is why patients with *C. difficile* can require massive amounts of fluids for resuscitation.

PRESENTATION

The spectrum of disease produced by toxigenic strains of *C. difficile* is quite variable, from asymptomatic infection or mild diarrhea to severe disease that results in toxic megacolon, multisystem failure, and death. Symptoms can begin within the first day of antibiotic use or up to 6 weeks after completion of the antibiotic course. Most commonly, symptoms develop within 4 to 9 days after exposure to an antibiotic. Mild disease is defined as diarrhea without any systemic symptoms, such as fever or hemodynamic changes. Moderate disease may result in profuse diarrhea, abdominal distension or pain, fever, tachycardia, and oliguria, but it responds readily to volume resuscitation. It is not generally appreciated or recognized by clinicians that *C. difficile* colitis can present without diarrhea, usually with distended abdomen and severe leukocytosis.

Severe or fulminant disease may result in occult bleeding, severe oliguria, or hemodynamic instability that requires vasopressor support and/or mechanical ventilation. Fulminant colitis develops in 1% to 3% of cases and can lead to ileus, toxic megacolon, intestinal perforation, and death. The first warning sign may be diminishing diarrhea due to decreased colonic muscle tone. Other clues to the diagnosis include fever without obvious cause, unexplained leukocytosis, distended abdomen with or without generalized tenderness, recent or present antibiotics, and obtundation in the critical care unit. The clinician must have a high degree of suspicion about this diagnosis in an at-risk patient population. Patients who have mild disease should not be treated with the same aggressiveness as those with fulminant disease.

DIAGNOSIS AND MANAGEMENT

The most sensitive diagnostic laboratory test for detecting *C. difficile* is the toxin B–detecting tissue-culture method. Unfortunately, the test can take 24 to 48 hours, diminishing its usefulness in establishing a definitive diagnosis before treatment. Stool culture also has high sensitivity and specificity but is labor intensive. Because of the increased turnaround time associated with stool cultures (72 to 96 hours), and the fact that asymptomatic carriers also test positive, few laboratories perform stool cultures.

Rapid enzyme immunoassay is a methodology used to quickly detect toxin A or B. Although turnaround time is significantly shorter than with other methodologies (a few hours) and specificity is high (95% to 100%), 100 to 1000 pg of toxin A or B must be present to yield a positive result, and assay sensitivity ranges from 65% to 85%. Enzyme-linked immunosorbent assays differ in their abilities to detect toxin subtypes. Two reagent categories exist: one can detect toxin A or B, and one detects only toxin A. Reagents that detect only

toxin A can be problematic, because 1% to 2% of all *C. difficile* strains produce toxin B exclusively and would not be detected using the toxin A–specific reagents.

Also available for *C. difficile* detection is the latex agglutination assay, which detects glutamate dehydrogenase, a constitutively expressed enzyme in *C. difficile* strains. While this assay offers rapid turnaround time, sensitivity drops to 58% to 68%, and specificity is 90% to 96%. Because sensitivities, specificities, cost, and turnaround times differ for each methodology, individual laboratories have developed real-time polymerase chain reaction diagnostics for *C. difficile* detection that targets tcdB (sensitivity, 93%; specificity, 97%; positive predictive value, 76%; negative predictive value, 99%). To best utilize the information obtained from these possible tests, clinicians should identify which test is used at their hospital.

The diagnosis may also be made endoscopically by detection of ulcers, plaques, and pseudomembranes (in 90% of fulminant colitis cases, vs. 23% in mild cases). The pathognomonic lesion is characteristically raised, yellowish, and usually 2 to 10 mm in diameter with "skipped" areas of normal mucosa; but in severe disease, lesions may coalesce to form plaques. There is a risk of perforation with any colonoscopy or sigmoidoscopy in the setting of frail and/or fulminant colitis.

Radiographs of the abdomen may be normal, or they may show adynamic ileus, colonic dilation, thumb printing, or haustral thickening. These nonspecific findings are not helpful in the most serious cases. CT, however, may be quite helpful in suggesting this diagnosis (Figure 1) because the scan may show an edematous and thick-walled colon with thumbprinting in the case of fulminant colitis. Other findings include the presence of pericolic stranding, ascites, pancolitis, and megacolon.

To reduce vancomycin resistance, current guidelines still recommend the first-line use of metronidazole over vancomycin, except in patients with severe disease or as noted (Table 2). Best responses to metronidazole are usually seen within 7 days of therapy. Longer therapeutic courses of metronidazole may be associated with refractory strains and increased disease severity that merits more aggressive therapy.

Although apparently susceptible to metronidazole, the new strain of *C. difficile* may not respond as well to treatment with metronidazole. Recent studies reveal a high rate of failure of metronidazole. Accordingly, it seems prudent to use vancomycin as the initial therapy when facing a virulent organism or if risk factors for severe disease or fulminant colitis are present. Intracolonic vancomycin preparations have been suggested as an alternative treatment for refractory and

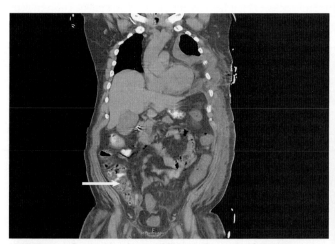

FIGURE I   Coronal cut from a CT scan of a patient following thoracoabdominal surgery with fever and elevated white blood cell count. Note the thickened right colon with thumbprinting and poor contrast filling (*arrow*). This patient recovered after treatment with vancomycin and metronidazole.

persistent CDAD. Intracolonic vancomycin is often combined with oral or IV metronidazole or oral vancomycin. The use of various dosage regimens of intracolonic vancomycin has been reported, and the use of intracolonic vancomycin is based only on anecdotal evidence.

Cholestyramine and colestipol, anion-exchange resins, are thought to bind toxin B and are adjunctive treatment options for patients with CDAD. However, significant drug interactions can occur with their use, including the binding and possible inactivation of vancomycin.

As previously noted, only a small number of patients with diarrhea will have *C. difficile* as an identified cause of their diarrhea. For the patient who is otherwise well, treatment should follow the identification of *C. difficile* toxin as the pathogen, risk factors should be modified, and specific therapy, as noted in Table 2, should be undertaken.

C. difficile should be suspected in any patient with severe diarrhea who has had recent antibiotic exposure and any combination of fever, tachycardia, oliguria, or marked leuckocytosis. These patients should have aggressive resuscitation, and empiric treatment should begin, often with intravenous metronidazole because of intolerance to oral intake. A stool specimen should be sent for testing, but treatment should not be delayed when serious illness is present. Computed tomography (CT) may suggest the diagnosis by the presence of *C. difficile* findings, as previously described. Because the most severe cases of *C. difficile* may present without diarrhea, this diagnosis must be suspected in any patient who is severely ill without an identified cause, especially in the presence of abdominal distension and severe leuckocytosis. A CT scan should be considered in this patient population, and if consistent with the diagnosis, treatment should be initiated with intravenous metronidazole.

The decision to operate on a patient with *C. difficile* colitis requires substantial mature judgment and balance between the probable benefits of removing a source of ongoing toxicity and the possibility of removing a colon that would have responded to therapy with additional time. Thus the clinician must carefully monitor the response to therapy, which should occur within hours of aggressive treatment. Ongoing signs of organ failure, shock, and requirement for vasopressors should prompt serious consideration of colectomy for therapy. Obvious indications for surgical intervention are colonic perforation and toxic megacolon.

In published retrospective series, delayed intervention was found to be the one factor most associated with death. Because the decision to proceed with colectomy is not rigorously formulaic, the surgeon must consider the underlying diseases of the patient, the trajectory and rate of response to therapy, the probability that the toxicity and severity of illness is solely attributable to *C. difficile*, and of course the preferences of the patient. Reported rates of surgery necessitated by *C. difficile* infection range from 0.39% of 3300 toxin-positive assays in a 6-year survey (before 1994) to 7.5% in a more recent series. In the setting of CDAD due to the hypervirulent strain (NAP1/027), some patients progressed from severe disease to death in less than 48 hours.

Once a decision has been made to operate for *C. difficile* colitis, a total abdominal colectomy should be performed. The surgeon should not be dissuaded by the external appearance of the colon, which may be surprisingly benign appearing. Almost universally, the colon will be extremely edematous and boggy, often containing liters of fluid. Pericolic inflammation and serous sterile ascites are commonly seen. Occasionally, especially if surgery is delayed, a necrotic wall with or without colon perforation may be seen.

Although no prospective randomized trials evaluating the surgical treatment for fulminant colitis have been performed, subtotal abdominal colectomy with end ileostomy remains the procedure of choice for fulminant colitis. The surgeon should not consider segmental resection because they believe the disease is confined to one area of the colon. Given the severity of the patient's illness, the operation should be performed in the most expeditious manner. Thus the operation should performed open, typically ligating the mesenteric vessels before they branch, to facilitate the most expedient resection. The intraperitoneal portion of the colon should be removed and the rectum divided at or near the peritoneal reflection with a 4.5 mm stapling device. This allows removal of the greatest amount of tissue, and it offers the potential for a functional reconstruction after recovery.

PROGNOSIS

The outcome of patients with fulminant colitis due to *C. difficile* will of course depend on the selection of patients for surgical intervention and the timing of that intervention. A very liberal and aggressive approach toward treating with colectomy will have an excellent clinical result when mortality is considered the end point, but patients may have had an unnecessary colectomy. A recent publication suggested that patients who are older than 70 years, with marked leuckocytosis (>30,000 mm^3) and either intubation or vasopressors, may have a mortality rate higher than 50%; but without these signs, all survived. Treatment with colectomy improved outcome.

A recent report of long-term outcome after surgery for fulminant *C. difficile* infection demonstrated an overall 5-year survival of 16%, but only 20% of these patients had their gastrointestinal continuity

---

TABLE 2: Adjunctive and drug interventions for the treatment of *Clostridium difficile* colitis

- Discontinue offending antibiotics or narrow the spectrum of agents.
- Replace fluid and electrolyte losses.
- Avoid antiperistaltic agents.
- Do not treat asymptomatic colonization.
- Re-treat first-time recurrences with the same regimen used to treat the initial episode.
- When possible, antibiotics should be avoided for 2 months after infection resolution.

Disease Severity	Available Route	Recommended Antibiotic
Asymptomatic	Not recommended	Not recommended
Mild/moderate disease	Oral/NGT route is tolerable Oral/NGT route is NOT tolerable	PO metronidazole 250-500 mg qid IV metronidazole 500 mg q6h or vancomycin retention enemas if no improvement
Critically ill patient, severe or fulminant disease	Oral/NGT route is tolerable Oral/NGT route is NOT tolerable	PO vancomycin 125-500 mg qid with or without IV metronidazole 500 mg q6h Vancomycin retention enemas with or without IV metronidazole 500 mg q6h

NGT, Nasogastric tube

restored. These data suggest that we have not perfected the decision making about the timing of this therapy, nor have we decided who should undergo aggressive surgical therapy and who should not.

SUGGESTED READINGS

Bartlett JG: Narrative review: the new epidemic of *Clostridium difficile*-associated enteric disease, *Ann Intern Med* 145:758–764, 2006.

Dallal RM, Harbrecht BG, Boujoukas AJ, et al: Fulminant *Clostridium difficile*: an underappreciated and increasing cause of death and complications, *Ann Surg* 235(3):363–372, 2002.

Hermsen JL, Dobrescu C, Kudsk KA: *Clostridium difficile*: a surgical disease in evolution, *J Gastrointest Surg* 12(9):1512–1517, 2008.

Lamontagne F, Labbe A-C, Haeck O, et al: Impact of emergency colectomy on survival of patients with fulminant *Clostridium difficile* colitis during an epidemic caused by a hypervirulent strain, *Ann Surg* 245:267–272, 2007.

Lipsett PA, Samantaray DK, Tam ML, et al: Pseudomembranous colitis: a surgical disease? *Surgery* 116:491–496, 1994.

Miller AT, Tabrizian P, Greenstein AJ, et al: Long-term follow-up of patients with fulminant *Clostridium difficile* colitis.

Morris AM, Jobe BA, Stoney M, et al: *Clostridium difficile* colitis: an increasingly aggressive iatrogenic disease? *Arch Surg* 137:1096–1100, 2002.

Sailhamer EA, Carson K, Chang Y, et al: Fulminant *Clostridium difficile* colitis: patterns of care and predictors of mortality, *Arch Surg* 144(5):433–439, 2009.

Zerey M, Paton BL, Lincourt AE, et al: The burden of *Clostridium difficile* in surgical patients in the United States, *Surg Infect (Larchmt)* 8(6):557–566, 2007.

LARGE BOWEL OBSTRUCTION

Alexandra L.B. Webb, MD, and Aaron S. Fink, MD

ETIOLOGY

Large bowel obstruction is a serious and rapidly progressive disease process that frequently requires urgent surgical intervention. Large bowel obstruction may result from either dynamic (mechanical) or adynamic causes. The most common etiologies for mechanical large bowel obstruction in adults are colorectal carcinoma (90%), volvulus (5%), and diverticulitis (3%). Additional causes of mechanical large bowel obstruction are listed in Table 1. Colonic pseudoobstruction (Ogilvie syndrome) is the most common cause of adynamic obstruction.

The onset and pattern of symptoms may provide clues to the etiology of the obstruction. Acute or relapsing symptoms are common with volvulus. Subacute presentation, with a gradual progression of symptoms, is more consistent with malignancy or inflammatory bowel disease. Given the smaller lumen on the left side of the colon, as well as the solid consistency of the stool in this location, malignant obstruction is more common on the left side of the colon than on the right.

The age of the patient can also provide clues; in children, Hirschsprung disease and imperforate anus (neonates) are common causes of large bowel obstruction; in the elderly, malignancy and diverticulitis are the leading causes. Past surgical history may offer further insight into the etiology of colon obstruction. For example, patients with prior colectomy may develop anastomotic recurrence or stricture. Patients with a history of aortic surgery may have an ischemic stricture.

CLINICAL PRESENTATION

History

Abdominal distension is the most frequent initial symptom of large bowel obstruction. Nausea, vomiting, and obstipation are also common. Emesis of brownish, foul-smelling (feculent) material typically signifies high-grade or complete obstruction. Patients with partial obstruction are usually able to pass some flatus or stool, but those with complete obstruction are unable to pass either.

The history may again provide useful clues to the etiology of obstruction. The time course of the patient's symptom evolution may suggest a potential etiology. Chronic weight loss and passage of melanotic bloody stools suggest malignancy; acute onset of nausea, vomiting, and abdominal distension is consistent with volvulus. Recurrent episodes of left lower quadrant abdominal pain suggests diverticulitis as a cause, but the symptoms of large bowel obstruction may be indistinguishable from those of small bowel obstruction.

Abdominal Examination

Patients with large bowel obstruction are usually noted to have abdominal distension and tympany. Bowel sounds may be high-pitched in early stages of obstruction, but as the disease progresses, bowel sounds may become diminished or absent. Abdominal distension without tenderness or bowel sounds may also suggest pseudoobstruction. Fever, focal tenderness, or signs of peritonitis should raise concerns for diverticulitis or complications of large bowel obstruction, such as bowel ischemia or perforation.

Examination of Inguinal and Femoral Regions

It is essential to perform a thorough examination of the inguinal and femoral regions in patients with suspected small or large bowel obstruction. An incarcerated left inguinal hernia may contain the sigmoid colon; this situation can lead to sigmoid obstruction as well as ischemia.

Digital Rectal Examination

The examination focuses on identifying rectal pathology that may be causing the obstruction. In addition, the contents of the rectal vault can be determined. An empty rectal vault is suggestive of obstruction proximal to the level reached by the examining finger. If stool

TABLE 1: Causes of adult large bowel obstruction

Neoplasm (benign or malignant)
Volvulus (sigmoid, cecal, or transverse colon)
Diverticulitis
Ischemic colitis
Inflammatory bowel disease
Incarcerated hernia
Intussusception
Colonic pseudoobstruction
Fecal impaction

is present, fecal occult blood testing should be performed; a positive result reflects mucosal injury, which suggests the possibility of malignancy, inflammation, or ischemia.

DIAGNOSIS

Laboratory Studies

Initial laboratory studies should include a complete blood count and electrolytes. In addition, coagulation studies (type and screen) and a lactate level are frequently indicated.

Abdominal Radiographs

A flat and upright abdominal series can be diagnostic of colonic obstruction. These images can often differentiate between small bowel and colonic obstruction and can frequently identify the etiology of the obstruction. If the films demonstrate free intraperitoneal air, emergent surgical exploration is indicated. Other notable findings include presence of air in the colon (to differentiate from small bowel obstruction), presence of air in the rectum (to determine partial vs. complete obstruction), and presence of pathognomonic findings of colonic volvulus. The classic radiographic appearance of sigmoid volvulus has been described as that of a bent inner tube, coffee bean, or omega loop. The loop consists of two markedly distended limbs of colon, extending from the left lower quadrant, with the loop pointing toward the right upper quadrant. Although less common, cecal volvulus may have the appearance of a comma; a dilated loop of colon is apparent in the mid-abdomen, often with loops of small bowel seen to the right of the colon (Figure 1).

Regardless of the etiology of obstruction, a cecal diameter greater than 10 to 12 cm should raise concern for impending perforation. The cecum is the portion of the colon with the thinnest wall and the largest diameter, rendering it most susceptible to perforation. Emergent decompression should be considered in these patients, either via endoscopy or by laparoscopic or open surgical intervention.

Enema

Water-soluble contrast enema can confirm the presence of mechanical obstruction of the colon. In addition, it can localize the site of obstruction and facilitate surgical planning. In cases of functional obstruction or fecal impaction, contrast enema may be therapeutic as well as diagnostic (Figure 2).

If high-grade partial or complete large bowel obstruction is suspected, barium should be avoided; barium retained above the site of obstruction can rapidly inspissate and adhere to the proximal colon, making subsequent surgical intervention difficult. Additionally, if perforation is present, barium can produce extensive peritoneal reaction.

If intussusception is detected in an adult, reduction should not be attempted via contrast enema. In contrast to the pediatric population, the lead point in adults frequently contains a pathologic portion that should be resected.

Computed Tomographic Scan

CT scan is not the optimal study to evaluate for large bowel obstruction. It is difficult to identify intraluminal mass lesions with this modality, even when rectal contrast is given. CT scan may be useful, however, in patients known to have malignant obstruction, as it can delineate the presence and extent of metastatic disease and aid in surgical planning.

TREATMENT

Patient Preparation

Intravenous resuscitation with crystalloid and electrolyte correction should be ensured in all patients. A nasogastric tube should be inserted, and urine output should be closely monitored as a measure of adequate resuscitation; insertion of a Foley catheter is required.

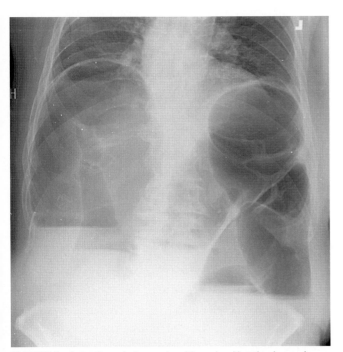

FIGURE 1   Large bowel obstruction. Note the dilated colon and air-fluid levels; the haustra can also be seen, distinguishing large bowel obstruction from small bowel obstruction.

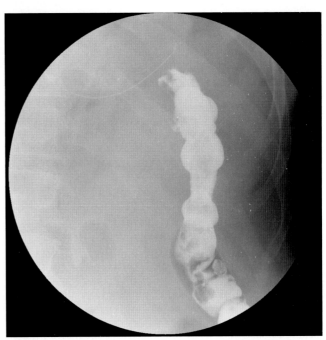

FIGURE 2   Gastrografin enema demonstrates obstruction at the splenic flexure. Note the blunt termination of the column of contrast.

Partial Obstruction

If a patient is able to pass some stool and flatus, preoperative bowel preparation may be possible. If successfully accomplished, the potential need for ostomy creation and two-stage surgery is greatly reduced. A "slow prep," consisting of magnesium citrate, 5 to 10 oz per day, given over 3 to 4 days may be attempted if the patient cannot tolerate a standard Go-Lytely preparation. Oral antibiotics are given the day before the planned procedure. Resection of the affected area with primary anastomosis is typically the procedure of choice in patients who have successfully completed a bowel preparation.

Complete Obstruction

In the case of total obstruction, therapy depends on the etiology of the obstruction. If complete obstruction is due to malignancy, urgent surgical intervention is indicated. Surgical options include a diverting loop ostomy or resection of the lesion with end stoma.

Treatment of Etiologies

Malignancy

The segment of colon or rectum containing the mass should be resected with 5 cm proximal and distal margins (2 cm for distal rectal margin). Wide excision of the mesentery should be performed. In the case of left-sided malignancy with a right-sided perforation, subtotal colectomy should be performed.

Volvulus

In patients with sigmoid volvulus without signs of peritonitis or perforation, colonoscopy with reduction of the volvulus and placement of a rectal tube may be attempted. If reduction is successful, bowel preparation and single-stage surgery should be performed. If unsuccessful, resection with colostomy may be necessary. On-table colonic lavage with primary anastomosis has also been described for patients with sigmoid volvulus.

Do not attempt colonoscopic decompression in patients with cecal volvulus. Surgical resection can often be accomplished as a single-stage procedure that includes primary anastomosis. Cecopexy may also be performed if there is no sign of vascular compromise in the right colon.

Diverticular Disease

Typically, sigmoid colectomy with a Hartmann pouch is performed in patients with obstruction due to diverticulitis. However, on rare occasions, the inflammation may be so severe that resection is not safe. In these circumstances, a diverting loop colostomy should be created, leaving the diseased segment in situ. Because it is never possible to completely exclude malignancy in this situation, interval colonoscopy and subsequent resection should be planned.

Hernia

If a hernia is the cause of colon obstruction, careful attention should be paid to the condition of the bowel. Exploration through a groin incision is appropriate if bowel compromise is not suspected; however, if there is a high suspicion for compromise, exploration should be carried out via a midline laparotomy incision to fully inspect and possibly resect the involved segment of colon. If colon resection is necessary, mesh repair should be avoided; a tissue repair of the hernia should be performed instead.

Intussusception

In contrast to the pediatric population, intussusception in adults is typically caused by a mass lesion, which may be a benign polyp, malignancy, or hyperplastic submucosal lymphoid tissue. Therefore radiographic decompression should be avoided as primary therapy. Surgical exploration with resection is indicated in most cases to ensure the identification and removal of any malignant or premalignant mass lesion. In the case of benign lesions, surgical resection significantly reduces the likelihood of recurrence.

Stenting

The first colonic stents were placed in the early 1990s, and treatment involved the use of stents designed for other locations in the gastrointestinal (GI) tract. Stents may be placed exclusively with fluoroscopic guidance in the radiology suite or with combined endoscopic and fluoroscopic guidance, typically in the GI suite or in the operating room. Either endoscopy or water-soluble contrast-enhanced fluoroscopy is used to identify the lumen and the stricture. The obstructed segment is then traversed with a guidewire, which is subsequently used to guide stent deployment, either through the endoscope or over the wire. Complications include bleeding, perforation, recurrent obstruction, and stent migration.

Colorectal cancer is the most frequent indication for stenting. Stents can be placed on a temporary basis and used as a bridge to definitive resection, allowing for bowel preparation and one-stage surgery with primary anastomosis. Stents can also be used as primary therapy for palliation to avoid a stoma, either in patients with end-stage malignancy or in those for whom operative risk is prohibitive.

Stents are most effective in lesions of the left colon that are more than 5 cm from the anus; stents have been used in the distal rectum and right colon as well with acceptable results. Clinical success is defined as successful one-stage resection of the malignant lesion, avoiding colostomy creation. When performed for malignancy, 80% to 90% clinical success rates have been reported.

Colonic stents may be used for benign disease as well as malignancy, but there are less data available regarding their use in such indications. As experience with colonic stent placement grows, and as technology continues to improve, the indications will certainly expand (Figure 3).

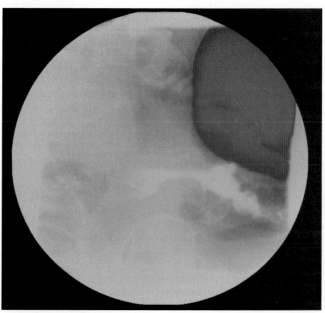

FIGURE 3   Colonic stent placement. *(Courtesy Dr. Mohammad Wehbi.)*

Pseudoobstruction

Although acute colonic pseudoobstruction, or Ogilvie syndrome, is described elsewhere, a brief description is included here because psuedoobstruction must be part of the differential diagnosis in patients with signs of large bowel obstruction. Typically, patients are elderly, bedridden, and frequently are nursing home residents. There is usually a history of chronic constipation. The hallmark of this syndrome is massive abdominal distension with air present through the colon. An aggressive bowel regimen that includes oral laxatives and enemas usually produces resolution. Pharmacologic treatment may also succeed in colonic decompression. Neostigmine, guanethidine, and erythromycin have all been used successfully for this indication; however, colonoscopic decompression is sometimes required.

Fecal Impaction

Fecal impaction may cause large bowel obstruction. It is most common in elderly patients, patients with chronic constipation, and patients taking narcotic pain medications. If fecal impaction is noted on digital rectal examination, digital disimpaction should be performed to the degree possible. This can be followed by warm tap water or soapsuds enemas to further evacuate obstructing stool. Daily radiographs of the kidneys, ureters, and bladder should document improvement.

SUMMARY

Large bowel obstruction can be caused by a number of disease processes, and at some point, most cases of mechanical large bowel obstruction require surgical intervention. Whenever possible, preoperative bowel preparation and single-stage surgery with primary anastomosis is preferred. If complete obstruction is present, two-stage surgery is usually necessary, with resection (if possible) and diversion initially, followed by a second procedure to close the stoma. The use of colonic stents may allow for patients who otherwise would be treated with resection and colostomy to undergo bowel preparation, allowing single-stage surgery.

SUGGESTED READINGS

Campbell S, Verma R, MacFie J, et al: The management of malignant large bowel obstruction: ACPGBI position statement, *Colorectal Dis* 9(suppl 4):1–17, 2007.

De Giorgio R, Knowles CH: Acute colonic pseudo-obstruction, *Br J Surg* 96(3):229–239, 2009.

Dionigi G, Villa F, Rovera F, et al: Colonic stenting for malignant disease: review of literature, *Surg Oncol* 1(16 Suppl):S153–S155, 2007.

Kam MH, Tang CL, Chan E, et al: Systematic review of intraoperative colonic irrigation vs. manual decompression in obstructed left-sided colorectal emergencies, *Int J Colorectal Dis* 24(9):1031–1037, 2009.

Trompetas V: Emergency management of malignant acute left-sided colonic obstruction, *Ann R Coll Surg Engl* 90(3):181–186, 2008.

USE OF STENTS FOR COLONIC OBSTRUCTION

David E. Beck, MD

OVERVIEW

Colonic obstruction is a common clinical problem in the United States. The majority of obstructions are due to malignant processes. Approximately 8% to 29% of patients with colorectal cancer initially show symptoms of partial or complete bowel obstruction, most of which are left sided and either stage III or IV. There are several options for managing patients with large bowel obstruction. Usually, patients are resuscitated with intravenous fluid, evaluated with a contrast study—such as water-soluble enema (Figure 1), computed tomographic scan, or colonoscopy—and then taken to surgery.

Surgical options for right-sided lesions usually involve a segmental resection and an ileocolic anastomosis or ileostomy, depending on the status of the bowel, status of the patient, and the experience of the surgeon. Management of left-sided lesions may comprise a segmental resection and colostomy, a subtotal colectomy and ileorectal anastomosis, or ileostomy. These emergency procedures have an associated mortality rate of 10% to 30% and a morbidity rate of 10% to 36%.

Due to age and comorbidities, many patients who receive ostomies do not have their stomas closed, and the time spent recovering from therapy or morbidity or complications from surgery often delays or prevents chemotherapy and radiotherapy. Quality of life and the cost of ostomy supplies have also been issues. These limitations have encouraged development of other options, most notably self-expanding intraluminal stenting, which can be used for palliation or as a bridge to surgery (i.e., converting an emergency procedure to an elective one). The use of stents for nonmalignant obstruction has been limited and not especially optimistic.

INDICATIONS

Since their introduction in 1991, colonic stents have become an important method of palliation for obstruction in colorectal cancer patients, especially those with unresectable metastatic disease. These self-expanding metallic stents can potentially dilate the lumen to a near-normal diameter, providing quick relief of symptoms and, in some cases, allowing endoscopic or radiologic assessment of the proximal colon.

Stents can be placed in patients using minimal sedation, without need of prior endoscopic dilatation, and with a low risk of complications such as perforation or tumor fracture. Moreover, these stents can be placed across relatively long lesions by overlapping stents in a "stent within a stent" fashion. Most patients with benign strictures are better managed with traditional operative techniques because the morbidity associated with stents in this patient group has been prohibitive.

TECHNIQUE

A number of intralumenal stents are currently available (Table 1). There are coated and uncoated stents that range in predeployment diameter from 10 to 30 Fr and postdeployment diameter of 20 to 35 mm and from 40 to 120 mm in length. They can be deployed through the scope (TTS), with or without guidewires, or passed under fluoroscopic control over an endoscopically or fluoroscopically placed guide wire. My preference is an Enteral Wallflex (Boston Scientific, Mason, Ohio) 120 mm in length. TTS stents are easier to place through proximal or angulated lesions.

In the technique I use, patients are taken to the endoscopy unit and placed on a fluoroscopically capable table. After monitors and nasal oxygen are placed, the patient is put in a left lateral position and sedated. A colonoscope is inserted and advanced to the obstructing lesion (Figure 2). Fluoroscopy is used to observe the lesion location, and the patient's position is altered to obtain the best fluoroscopic view. If the lumen appears tight, a flexible guidewire in inserted through the working port of the colonoscope; under direct vision, it is gently passed across the obstruction (Figure 3). If the lumen is not too tight, the stent may be passed across the lesion.

Fluoroscopy confirms that the wire or catheter has passed through the lesion. If a guidewire was used, a TTS stent is then passed through the scope over the guidewire and passed across the lesion. Radiopaque markers help position the stent across the obstructing lesion. Under fluoroscopic visualization, the stent is slowly deployed

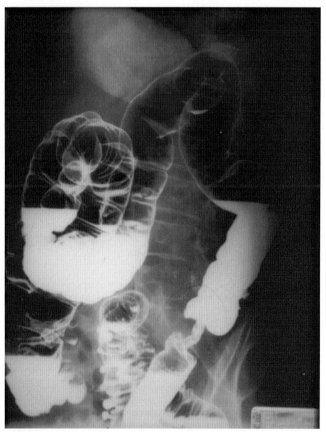

FIGURE 1   Contrast enema demonstrating an obstructive colonic lesion.

(Figure 4). Some repositioning is possible prior to complete stent deployment; optimally, the configuration of the deployed stent will have a flare proximal and distal to the stricture with a narrowed neck at the stricture. Successful deployment is often associated with a rush of gas or colonic contents through the deployed stent. Following successful deployment, a contract study or plain film will confirm appropriate deployment (Figure 5).

If the stricture is long, or the stent does not have adequate extension across the stenosis, a second stent can be placed overlapping a portion of the initial stent. Attempting to pass the colonoscope through the stent after deployment should be avoided; the metal edges of the stent can damage the colonoscope (Figure 6).

RESULTS

Stenting has been more successful in shorter, distal lesions and with colonic primaries. Technical failure is usually due to inability to pass a guidewire or stent catheter across the obstruction, usually because of the angulation of the tumor. Clinical failure is usually defined as failure to relieve the obstruction or the occurrence of a major complication.

Three reviews have evaluated the safety and efficacy of stents in dealing with colorectal malignant obstruction. The first examined 29 publications composed 598 patients. Technical success was achieved in 92% and clinical success in 88%. A successful bridge to surgery was accomplished in 85% of 162 stent insertions, and the mean time to surgery was 8.9 days (range, 1 to 115 days).

A second review of 54 case series (1198 patients) by Sebastian and colleagues found that stenting was technically successful as a bridge to surgery in 92% of 407 cases and clinically successful in 72%. In 791 patients who received palliative therapy, the technical success was 93% and clinical success was 91%. Complications included perforation in 3.8%, stent migration in 11.8%, and reobstruction in 7.3%.

The third review included 88 articles, 15 of which were comparative. The median rates of technical and clinical success were 96.2% and 92%, respectively. The median time between stenting and elective surgery was 5.8 days (range, 2 to 16 days). The review concluded that stenting followed by elective surgery appeared to be safer and more effective than emergency surgery, with higher rates of primary anastomosis, lower rates of colostomy, shorter hospital stays, and lower overall complication rates.

In a retrospective series of 80 patients who underwent colonic stent placement for malignant large bowel obstruction, stents were successfully placed in 70 patients (87.5% overall technical success rate). Satisfactory symptomatic relief and clinical decompression was achieved in 67 patients (83.7% overall clinical success rate). Two perforations occurred in this series, one of which resulted in death. Other complications included stent migration resulting in expulsion, reobstruction, and intractable tenesmus. Stenting of cancers in the mid and low rectum may result in debilitating urgency and incontinence.

Law and colleagues studied 52 patients with malignant obstruction secondary to either primary or recurrent disease, who underwent

TABLE 1: Available stents

Stent	Manufacturer	Composition	Deployment	Size (Diameter/Length)
WallFlex	Boston Scientific	Elgiloy	TTS	27–30 mm/60–120 mm
WALLSTENT	Boston Scientific	Stainless steel	TTS	
Z-Stent	Cook Medical Inc.	Stainless steel	OTW	25–40 mm/120 mm
Ultraflex Precision	Boston Scientific	Nitinol	OTW	25–30 mm/57–117 mm

OCW, Over the wire

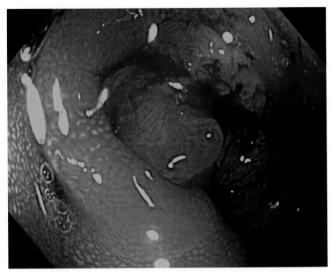

FIGURE 2   Colonoscopic view of obstructing lesion.

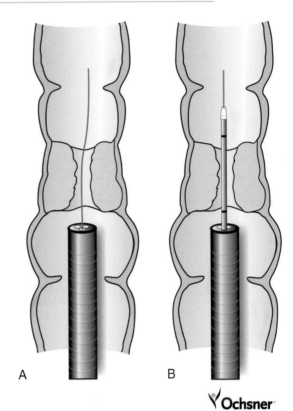

A   B

 Ochsner

FIGURE 4   Undeployed stent is passed through stricture. *(Courtesy Ochsner Clinic Foundation.)*

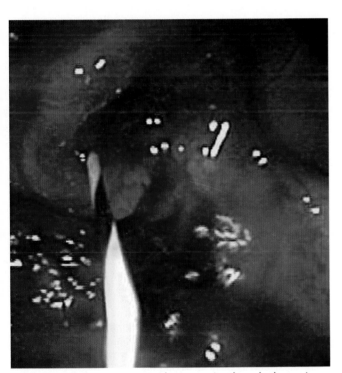

FIGURE 3   Endoscopic view, guidewire passing through obstructing lesion.

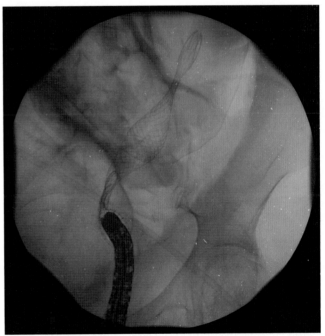

FIGURE 5   Radiograph of stent in place.

stent placement by colorectal surgeons and reported that 50 out of 52 were successfully palliated. One patient had a perforation, and in another patient obstruction was not relieved because of multiple sites of obstruction. The complication rate in this series was 25%; migration was the most common complication (15.4%), followed by reobstruction secondary to tumor ingrowth (3.8%), perforation, colovesical fistula, and severe tenesmus (2% each). Surgery was required in 17.3%, mostly due to complications or recurrent obstruction. Complications reported in the literature on colonic stents include stent malpositioning, migration, tumor ingrowth (through the stent interstices), tumor overgrowth (beyond the ends of a stent), perforation, stool impaction, bleeding, tenesmus, and postprocedure pain. The insertion technique and type of stent remain under discussion.

SUMMARY

The published data suggest that in experienced hands, an initial attempt at stent placement by a highly skilled multidisciplinary team is the preferred option. Endoscopic procedures can serve as a bridge to surgery in potentially curable, fit patients and can provide effective and durable palliation for selected patients with malignant obstruction.

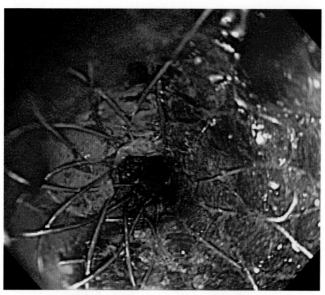

FIGURE 6   Endoscopic view of deployed stent.

Gandrup P, Lund L, Balslev I: Surgical treatment of acute malignant large bowel obstruction, *Eur J Surg* 158(8):427–430, 1992.

Govindarajan A, Naimark D, Coburn NG, et al: Use of colonic stents in emergent malignant left colonic obstruction: a Markov chain Monte Carlo decision analysis, *Dis Colon Rectum* 50:1811–1824, 2007.

Khot UP, Lang AW, Murali K, et al: Systemic review of the efficacy and safety of colorectal stents, *Br J Surg* 89:1096–1102, 2002.

Kim JS, Hur H, Min BS, et al: Oncologic outcomes of self-expanding metallic stent insertion as a bridge to surgery in the management of left-sided colon cancer obstruction: comparison with nonobstructing elective surgery, *W J Surg* 33:1281–1286, 2009.

Law WL, Choi HK, Lee YM, Chu KW: Palliation for advanced malignant colorectal obstruction by self-expanding metallic stents: prospective evaluation of outcomes, *Dis Colon Rectum* 47(1):39–43, 2004.

Repici A, Adler DG, Gibbs CM, et al: Stenting of the proximal colon in patients with malignant large bowel obstruction: techniques and outcomes, *Gastrointest Endosc* 66(5):940–964, 2007.

Sebastian S, Johnston S, Geoghegan T, et al: Pooled analysis of the efficacy and safety of self-expanding metal stenting in malignant colorectal obstruction, *Am J Gastroenterol* 99:2051–2057, 2004.

Watt AM, Faragher IG, Griffin TT, et al: Self-expanding metallic stents for relieving malignant colorectal obstruction: a systemic review, *Ann Surg* 246:24–30, 2007.

SELECTED READINGS

Camunez F, Echenagusia A, Simo G, et al: Malignant colorectal obstruction treated by means of self-expanding metallic stents: effectiveness before surgery and in palliation, *Radiology* 216(2):492–497, 2000.

Deans GT, Krukowski ZH, Irwin ST: Malignant obstruction of the left colon, *Br J Surg* 81(9):1270–1276, 1994.

COLONIC PSEUDOOBSTRUCTION (OGILVIE SYNDROME)

Wayne De Vos, MD, PhD

OVERVIEW

Acute colonic pseudoobstruction is characterized by the development of significant colonic distension in the absence of any detectable organic cause. Sir William Heneage Ogilvie first described the condition in his 1948 publication of two patients found on exploration for obstruction to have no evidence of mechanical blockage but to have tumor invading the retroperitoneal sympathetic nerve bed at the celiac plexus. He suggested that the pathologic process involved a derangement of the autonomic nervous system, though he incorrectly hypothesized that a loss of sympathetic input and subsequent unopposed parasympathetic input caused relaxation and consequent distension of the colon.

For reasons not fully understood, an imbalance in the autonomic input to the colon does develop, as suggested by Ogilvie; however, rather than a relative increase in parasympathetic tone, current evidence favors a relatively increased sympathetic tone and/or decreased parasympathetic tone, the combination of which yields an adynamic—and, consequently, functionally obstructing—distal colon and a relaxed proximal colon. The term *pseudoobstruction* was coined by Dudley in 1958; *acute* differentiates the disease from chronic processes, such as chronic idiopathic intestinal pseudoobstruction.

PRESENTATION

Colonic pseudoobstruction occurs more commonly in the elderly age group, favors men slightly, and generally presents with the relatively rapid development of abdominal distension, tympany, and anorexia. Nausea and vomiting and constipation or diarrhea may also be present but are not predictive of bowel viability; bowels sounds are variable and of no great assistance. Pain and tenderness may also be present at presentation, and although worrisome, they are not diagnostic for ischemia. Elevated white blood cell count and fever, however, support ischemia or impending perforation. Electrolyte derangement (e.g., hypokalemia) is common and should be addressed promptly.

In a review by Vanek and colleagues, common clinical settings that contribute to the development of pseudoobstruction include trauma or orthopedic procedures (18.6%); obstetric, gynecologic, or pelvic operations (19.1%); infection (10%); cardiac event (10%); and neurologic event (9.3%). Less commonly, pulmonary events, electrolyte imbalance, or pharmaceutical causes (e.g., narcotics, antidepressants, or anticholinergics) may be involved. Pseudoobstruction has also been described following renal transplant, stroke, and in patients with connective tissue disorders. Rarely, pseudoobstruction may develop spontaneously.

DIFFERENTIAL DIAGNOSIS

Distal colonic obstruction and infectious or inflammatory etiologies *must* be ruled out prior to initiation of treatment. Plain films of the abdomen are a useful and inexpensive method to rule out perforation, generalized ileus, or suggestion of a distal colonic obstruction, and it also assists in serial measurement of colonic dilation. Advances in computerized tomography (CT) have greatly increased its utility, and CT can assist in differentiation of distal obstruction, ischemia, perforation, or toxic megacolon from infection or inflammatory bowel disease. Water-soluble enema also remains a very sensitive, specific, and occasionally therapeutic method of diagnosis and differentiation from mechanical obstruction.

TREATMENT

In the patient in whom ischemia and perforation are not suspected, treatment begins with observation, fasting, electrolyte correction, cessation of narcotics and anticholinergics, and serial exams. Nasogastric tube decompression is rarely necessary, and rectal tube placement, although useful in the presence of persistent diarrhea, has not been found to be therapeutic for pseudoobstruction. Plain films and laboratory studies should be repeated at least daily. Pharmacologic treatment is reasonable for up to 72 hours and has been shown to result in resolution of pseudoobstruction in the majority of patients. Invasive measures can be considered early in the patient's disease course, if pharmacologic treatment is contraindicated or after 2 to 3 days have elapsed without signs of resolution. If at any time increasing abdominal pain or clinical and laboratory signs of sepsis are observed, operative intervention must be considered.

Based on the premise that antagonism of increased sympathetic input will have a therapeutic effect, cholinergic agonists have been studied and found to be an effective method of resolving colonic pseudoobstruction. A 1 to 2 mg intravenous dose of the cholinesterase inhibitor neostigmine has been found to significantly reduce colonic distension in the majority of patients within 30 minutes, though in up to 40% of cases, a second dose may be required secondary to recurrent colonic dilation; it can be administered as soon as 2 to 3 hours after the initial dose. Neostigmine administration requires cardiac monitoring for at least 30 minutes, given its systemic cholinergic effect, and it should be administered with the patient in supine position. Atropine (1 mg) should be readily available in the event of symptomatic bradycardia. Other side effects of neostigmine include bronchospasm, abdominal cramping, nausea, and increased salivation. Neostigmine should not be given if ischemia or perforation are suspected, the patient's baseline heart rate is less than 60 beats/min, systolic blood pressure is less than 90 mm Hg, or in the presence of second- or third-degree heart block without a pacer, in a patient with bronchospasm requiring ongoing treatment, in pregnancy, or in the context of renal failure with a baseline creatinine greater than 3 mg/dL.

With failure of pharmacologic and noninvasive treatment, colonoscopy is an effective though tedious and difficult tool for decompression of the colon; it has been found to be successful in 40% to 80% of patients, although a second intervention may be required 24 to 48 hours later in 20% of patients. The exam should be performed by an experienced endoscopist using a large-bore colonoscope with frequent irrigation and suctioning. Colonoscopy has been found to be most effective when the cecum is reached, and it should be done without preparation and with minimal further insufflation; series have reported a 2% risk of perforation. Consideration can be given to the placement of a colonic tube, spanning the length of the colon, to assist in continued decompression. The actual benefit of this is unclear given the high success rate of colonoscopy alone.

A recent small, prospective, randomized trial studying the effect of oral administration of polyethelyne glycol (PEG) after successful pharmacologic or endoscopic decompression of the colon showed that administration of 29.5 g of PEG daily resulted in no recurrence of cecal dilation in the treatment group versus 33% in the nontreatment group.

The cecum carries the highest risk of perforation, according to the law of LaPlace, which describes the direct relationship between tube diameter and wall tension. A cecal diameter greater than 12 cm is accepted as a threshold over which more invasive intervention should be considered. In patients who are considered at prohibitive surgical risk, the placement of a cecostomy—either percutaneous or guided by CT, endoscopy, or laparoscopy—is a reasonable option for urgent cecal decompression, given its minimally invasive approach. Risks include peritonitis, failure to effectively treat the entire colon, and abdominal wall cellulitis. No controlled trials comparing cecostomy with more invasive intervention have been published, and enthusiasm for this technique is overshadowed by its potential morbidity.

When nonoperative intervention or minimally invasive techniques have been unsuccessful, and the patient has not shown signs of recovery within 5 to 6 days, operative intervention with laparotomy must be considered. In the patient who shows signs of ischemia, necrosis, or perforation, exploration should be completed promptly. No data exist to compare the benefit of a venting colostomy to resection and end ostomy, and choice of operative therapy will depend on patient stability and intraoperative findings.

Consideration of segmental or total abdominal colectomy depends on the extent of the disease, and given the common finding of significant comorbidities in these patients, the operation is most commonly completed with a colostomy or ileostomy with or without a colonic mucous fistula. A 30% to 50% mortality rate following resection has been reported in the literature, though this number is most certainly reflective of patient condition at the time of operation.

PROGNOSIS

Ogilvie syndrome most often presents in the hospital setting, and the patient's comorbidities are an important predictor of survival. With conservative nonoperative treatment, successful resolution and survival is observed in 80% of patients; but with progression to ischemia and necrosis or perforation, a mortality rate of up to 60% is observed. Generally, persistent megacolon after 5 to 6 days is a negative prognostic indicator for successful nonoperative treatment, and the operation performed will depend on intraoperative findings and the stability of the patient. With vigilance, proper monitoring and resuscitation, and timely operative intervention in the event of progression to ischemia or necrosis, colonic perforation can be avoided and mortality rates are kept low. In spite of appropriately rendered care, however, mortality rates of 15% to 30% are to be expected, reflecting the burden of significant comorbidities commonly observed in patients who develop acute colonic pseudoobstruction.

SUGGESTED READINGS

Batke M, Cappell MS: Adynamic ileus and acute colonic pseudo-obstruction, *Med Clin N Am* 92:649–670, 2008.

Choi JS, Lim JS, Kim H, et al: Colonic pseudo-obstruction: CT findings, *Am J Roentgen* 190:1521–1526, 2008.

Di Giorgio R, Knowles CH: Acute colonic pseudo-obstruction, *Br J Surg* 96:229–239, 2009.

Ponec RJ, Saunders MD, Kimmey MB: Neostigmine for the treatment of the acute colonic pseudo-obstruction, *N Engl J Med* 341:137–141, 1999.

Sgouros SN, Vlachogiannakos J, Vassiliadis K, et al: Effect of polyethelene glycol electrolyte-balanced solution on patients with acute colonic pseudoobstruction after resolution of colonic dilation: a prospective, randomized placebo-controlled trial, *Gut* 55:638–642, 2006.

Vanek VW, Al-Santi M: Acute pseudo-obstruction of the colon (Ogilvie's syndrome): an anaylsis of 400 cases, *Dis Colon Rectum* 29:203–210, 1986.

COLONIC VOLVULUS

Christine S. Cocanour, MD

OVERVIEW

The term *volvulus* is derived from the Latin *volvere*, which means to twist or turn about. When applied to the colon, it refers to the rotation of the gut on its own mesenteric attachment. This twisting can produce either a partial or complete obstruction. Although the rotation of the gut on its mesentery rarely compromises the arterial supply to the gut, it does cause venous congestion, which if left untreated leads to infarction.

The epidemiology of colonic volvulus varies with geographic location. In Westernized nations, 2% to 4% of all intestinal obstructions are attributed to volvulus. If obstruction is limited to the colon, volvulus causes 10% to 15% of colonic obstruction. In non-Westernized nations, volvulus causes 20% to 50% of all intestinal obstructions. The difference in incidence is due to the difference in occurrence of predisposing factors.

The risk of colonic volvulus occurs anytime there is an excessively mobile colon. Anything that causes chronic stretching of the colon is a predisposing factor. This can be congenital but is most often the result of external forces, such as chronic constipation or a high-fiber diet. Nursing home patients are at risk for developing volvulus due to their relatively low-fiber diet, chronic constipation, and lack of exercise. Megacolon, whether from hypothyroidism, Parkinson, Hirschsprung, or Chagas disease predisposes to colonic volvulus. Ogilvie syndrome, with its chronically dilated colon, can also lead to the development of volvulus. Interestingly, pregnancy can cause stretching of the colon that can lead to volvulus.

The incidence of volvulus is greatest in the sigmoid colon (65% to 80%). The age of patients who develop sigmoid volvulus has increased over the years; it is currently seen in patients with a mean age of 70 years. The cecum is the second most common location of volvulus, with an incidence of 15% to 30%. Its mean age of presentation is 50 years. Volvulus involving the transverse colon or splenic flexure is much less common, with an incidence of 2% to 5% involving the transverse colon and only 1% involving the splenic flexure.

SIGMOID VOLVULUS

In the United States, sigmoid volvulus is most likely to occur in the elderly, in patients with psychiatric or neurologic disease, or in institutionalized patients. All are patients likely to have chronic constipation. Pediatric patients are the next largest population that develops sigmoid volvulus, but the majority of these patients are found in less industrialized nations. Roundworm infestation, or Chagas disease, caused by the parasite *Trypanosoma cruzi*, is the most common cause in pediatric patients. Chagas disease is appearing in United States–Mexican border towns and in poverty-stricken areas of the United States with a high proportion of South American immigrants. Hirschsprung disease is also a potential predisposing factor in the pediatric population.

Volvulus of the sigmoid colon occurs when the sigmoid is anatomically disproportionately long compared with its mesenteric base. The degree of torsion can vary from 180 degrees (found in 35% of patients with sigmoid volvulus) to 540 degrees (found in 10% of patients with sigmoid volvulus). About 50% of patients with sigmoid volvulus will have a 360-degree twist. Although torsion can be found in either a clockwise or counterclockwise direction, it is usually counterclockwise and is usually situated 15 to 25 cm from the anus.

Sigmoid volvulus may present insidiously with intermittent cramping, a vague feeling of lower abdominal discomfort, and progressive abdominal distension. There may have been similar episodes in the past that resolved spontaneously after passage of large amounts of flatus and stool. Nausea, vomiting, dehydration, and obstipation are all late symptoms. Sigmoid volvulus also occurs as an abdominal emergency with acute distension, colicky pain in the left lower quadrant, and no flatus or stool. Vomiting occurs late, and distension may progress to the point of compromising respiratory and cardiac function.

On physical exam, the patient has a distended, tympanitic abdomen with diffuse abdominal tenderness. There may or may not be an abdominal mass that is palpable. The rectal exam will reveal an empty ampulla.

Patients characteristically are seen late in their course. The presence of peritoneal signs and fever indicate possible strangulation. Perforation of the sigmoid is unusual because the sigmoid colon in older patients is usually thickened.

The diagnosis of sigmoid volvulus can be made 80% of the time with a plain abdominal radiograph. The air-distended bowel has the appearance of a bent inner tube. In the past, a barium enema was often used for diagnosis, and the appearance of a "bird's beak" or "ace of spades" at the point of obstruction was diagnostic. Five percent of the time, a barium enema was also successful in reducing the volvulus. Barium enema is contraindicated if strangulation is suspected, as it is likely to cause perforation. If strangulation with gangrene is suspected, CT of the abdomen may be helpful, especially if a "whirl sign" is present (see Figure 3).

Since 1947, nonoperative reduction of the volvulus has been the initial treatment of choice for patients who show no signs of intestinal ischemia. Decompression can be done with either a rigid or flexible endoscope. Success rates of 70% to 90% are reported with only a 2% mortality rate in those without gangrene; another 2% will spontaneously reduce, and perforation will occur 1% to 3% of the time; decompression alone has a 40% to 90% recurrence rate.

The site of torsion is often at 15 cm. If the torsion occurs higher, flexible endoscopy is more often successful because it allows aspiration of colon contents above the site of the obstruction, which can relieve the massive distension. Once the colon is decompressed, a rectal tube, which must pass the point of torsion, is then left in place for 48 to 72 hours. Surgery can then be scheduled as an elective procedure, preferably at the same admission.

If the colon fails to decompress or strangulation is suspected, surgery is required. Emergency resection has a mortality rate of 31% versus 8% for elective resection. Gangrenous colon occurs in less than 10% of patients in industrialized countries but may be as high as 25% in patients in developing countries. If gangrenous bowel is identified, the involved area must be excised *without* untwisting the volvulus. If untorsed, the unblocked vessels and lymphatics can unleash a flood of mediators and bacteria that can result in hypotension, acute organ failure, and death. Mortality rates following emergency resection with gangrenous bowel range from 18% to 75%; death in patients with viable bowel is reported in 0% to 10% of patients.

Reconstruction following bowel resection is controversial and ranges from colostomy with mucous fistula to Hartmann procedure or primary anastomosis. Although primary anastomosis in unprepared left colon was previously discouraged, over the past two decades, trauma surgeons have had acceptable results for both primary repair and anastomosis in unprepared bowel. A number of series have also shown primary anastomosis to have a decreased mortality rate of 0% to 33% with a mean of 13.8%, versus a mortality of 0% to 50% with a mean of 26% in patients given a colostomy. Whether this is due to the decision to place colostomies in unstable patients or due to the mortality associated with additional surgery is unclear.

In my practice, I favor primary anastomosis unless the patient is hemodynamically unstable, cold, acidotic, or if the bowel has questionable viability. In those instances, I will leave the patient in discontinuity until the metabolic and hemodynamic instability is corrected, and then I bring the patient back for a second look. At this second operation, the bowel may be more amenable to a primary anastomosis.

When the bowel is viable, sigmoid resection versus nonresection is controversial. Resection has been considered the procedure of choice because its recurrence rate of 1.2% is significantly lower than for nonresection procedures. If megacolon is present, a total or subtotal resection is advised. If dysmotility is documented in the entire colon preoperatively, a subtotal resection is recommended.

Improvements in laparoscopy have increased options for those patients considered at high risk for resectional surgery. Colopexy can be done either laparoscopically or as an open procedure; it has a mortality rate of 11% with a recurrence rate of 22%. Mesosigmoidoplasty has been reported with a mortality rate of 0%, and a recurrence rate from 1.6% to 29% is reported. Extraperitonealization of the sigmoid colon and mesenteropexy are also described. Percutaneous endoscopic colopexy has also been reported. Figure 1 provides an algorithm for the management of sigmoid volvulus.

CECAL VOLVULUS

Cecal volvulus accounts for 1% of all causes of intestinal obstruction and approximately 18% to 44% of colonic volvulus. It occurs from 2.8 to 7.1 per million people per year and is generally seen in those aged 30 to 60 years. Interestingly the age and sex distribution has shifted toward the older female patient, with the typical presentation in a 53-year-old woman; the female/male ratio is 1.4:1.

Around 11% to 25% of the population have a cecum that is sufficiently mobile to allow torsion; in autopsy studies, it is 400 times as common as actual clinical incidence of torsion. The two anatomic requirements for volvulus are 1) an improper developmental fusion of the cecal and ascending colon mesentery with the posterior parietal peritoneum and 2) restriction of the bowel at a fixed point, whether from an adhesion, abdominal mass, or scarring from a calcified lymph node. In 90% these are 180 to 360 degree axial twists around the mesenteric pedicle of the ileocecal artery.

Cecal volvulus is often associated with vascular compromise and increased mortality. *Cecal bascule* is a variant of cecal volvulus in which the cecum folds anteromedial to the ascending colon, causing a flap-valve occlusion at the site of flexion.

Cecal volvulus can be triggered by multiple causes; among these are adhesions from previous surgery, congenital bands, pregnancy, malrotation, obstructing lesions of the left colon, colonoscopy, travel in a nonpressurized plane, and colonic atony/ileus. Interestingly, marathon runners are at risk if they have congenital hypofixation coupled with a thin and flexible mesentery.

Diagnosis is notoriously difficult; the presentation of cecal volvulus is often atypical, and radiologic signs may be absent. Its clinical presentation is usually generalized abdominal pain with mild intermittent cramping, often of sudden onset. It can be accompanied by nausea, vomiting, constipation—all the signs and symptoms of bowel obstruction.

The diagnosis can sometimes be made from a a plain abdominal film in which there is a rounded focal collection of air in distended bowel with haustral creases in the left upper quadrant, resembling either a coffee or kidney bean, as seen in Figure 2. The bowel gas pattern may not be characteristic because the right colon and/or the cecum can be displaced to any portion of the abdominal cavity, making cecal volvulus mimic sigmoid volvulus. A single air-fluid level in the dilated cecum may be seen anywhere in the abdomen. A CT of the abdomen is diagnostically superior to plain films. However, its use remains controversial, and it is advocated only when the plain film and clinical exam are inconclusive. It is also helpful when a patient is seen in the late stages of cecal volvulus because it may help identify ischemia and perforation. The use of 3-D reconstruction may further improve its diagnostic capabilities. A whirl sign is characteristic of a volvulus on CT (Figure 3). Three-dimensional reconstruction may show a coffee bean sign similar to a plain radiograph (see Figure 2) and occasionally a bird's beak sign at the point of obstruction.

Although nonoperative decompression by colonoscopy or barium enema has been reported, because of the high risk for bowel ischemia, operative management is usually required. Gangrenous cecum is reported 23% to 100% of the time. If the bowel is nonviable, then right hemicolectomy is the treatment of choice; just as in sigmoid volvulus, the volvulus should not be reduced; this may result in irreversible shock. If the bowel's viability is unclear, plan a second look. When the bowel is viable, detorsion alone is not recommended because the recurrence rate ranges from 20% to 75%. A right hemicolectomy has a reported mortality rate of 0% for those with viable colon and a mortality rate of 9% to 17% in patients with nonviable colon. Since the offending portion of the colon is removed, its recurrence is zero. For patients too fragile to undergo

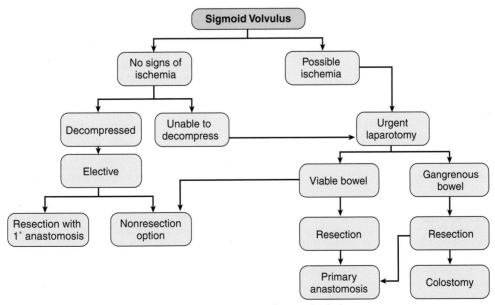

FIGURE 1 Management of sigmoid volvulus.

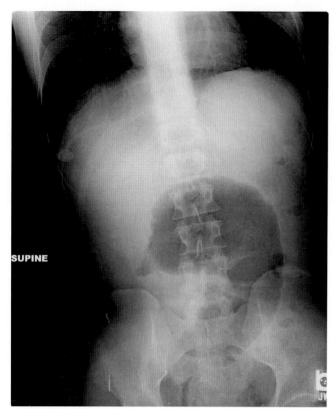

SUPINE

FIGURE 2 A plain abdominal film showing a focal collection of air resembling a coffee or kidney bean, which is typical for cecal volvulus.

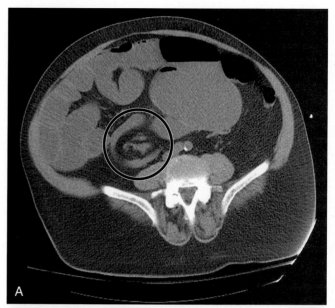

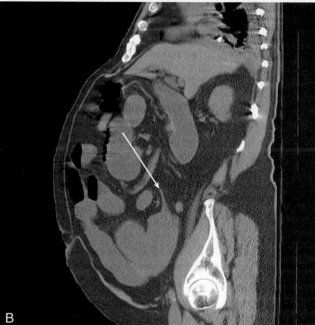

FIGURE 3 **A,** The black circle outlines a "whirl sign" that is sometimes seen with both cecal and sigmoid volvulus. **B,** This sagittal reconstruction of an abdominal CT of a patient with cecal vovlulus has a "bird's beak" appearance at the point of obstruction as indicated by the *white arrow*.

resection, cecopexy where the right colon is anchored to the parietal peritoneum (including laparascopic cecopexy) is described; recurrence with cecopexy is reported from 0% to 40%, with an average of 16% recurrence of volvulus after cecopexy, and mortality rates are relatively low (0% to 18%).

Cecostomy has been advocated in the past. Placement of a tube through the cecal wall that exits through the abdominal wall does allow decompression of the distended segment; however, attendant complications of gangrene, cecal necrosis, intraperitoneal leakage, fistula, and a recurrence rate of 2% to 14%, with a mortality rate of 0% to 40%, make it somewhat less desirable. Both cecostomy and cecopexy are best used only if the cecal wall is healthy and of normal thickness. A small case study of combined cecopexy and cecostomy reported no recurrence and no mortality.

TRANSVERSE COLON VOLVULUS

Volvulus of the transverse colon accounts for only 2% to 5% of all colonic volvulus. It most commonly presents in middle age with a 2:1 female predominance, and symptoms are typical of a large bowel obstruction. Preoperative diagnosis is difficult; principles of treatment are the same as for cecal volvulus; however, mortality rates are high after detorsion alone.

SPLENIC FLEXURE VOLVULUS

The splenic flexure is the least common site of colonic volvulus and accounts for 1% of all colonic volvulus. Its etiology is either from a congenital absence of the gastrocolic, phrenocolic, and splenocolic ligaments or from operative injury to those ligaments. Its management requires either fixation or resection. Splenic flexure colostomy has been reported.

SUMMARY

Colonic volvulus is a rare cause of intestinal obstruction. Sigmoid volvulus, the most common type, can often be identified early from plain films alone. If successfully detorsed, additional options for treatment become available, including sigmoidoplasty or mesenteroplexy; however, resection with primary anastomosis is considered the procedure of choice in hemodynamically stable patients because of its low recurrence rate. Compromised bowel requires emergent resection and either primary anastomosis or a Hartmann procedure, depending upon the status of both patient and bowel. Cecal volvulus is often more difficult to diagnose and nearly always requires resection and anastomosis.

SUGGESTED READINGS

Jones IT, Fazio VW: Colonic volvulus: etiology and management, *Dig Dis Sci* 7:203–209, 1989.

Madiba TE, Thomson SR: The management of sigmoid volvulus, *J R Coll Surg Edinb* 45:74–80, 2000.

Madiba TE, Thomson SR: The management of cecal volvulus, *Dis Colon Rectum* 45:264–267, 2002.

Mehendale VG, Chaudhari NC, Mulchandani MH: Laparoscopic sigmoido-pexy by extraperitonealization of sigmoid colon for sigmoid volvulus, *Surg Laparosc Endosc Percutan Tech* 13:283–285, 2003.

Moore CJ, Corl FM, Fishman EK: CT of cecal volvulus: unraveling the image, *AJR Am J Roentgenol* 177:95–98, 2001.

Oren D, Atamanalp SS, Aydinli B, et al: An algorithm for the management of sigmoid colon volvulus and the safety of primary resection: experience with 827 cases, *Dis Colon Rectum* 50:489–497, 2007.

Utpal D, Ghosh S: Single-state primary anastomosis without colonic lavage for left-sided colonic obstruction due to acute sigmoid volvulus: a prospective study of 197 cases, *ANZ J Surg* 73:390–392, 2003.

RECTAL PROLAPSE AND OBSTRUCTIVE DEFECATION

Roberta L. Muldoon, MD

OVERVIEW

Rectal prolapse, or procidentia, is a full-thickness prolapse of the rectum beyond the anus. Internal intussusception, on the other hand, is an internal prolapse that does not pass beyond the anus; mucosal prolapse is not full thickness. It is important to distinguish these different types of prolapse, because the management is different for each.

Obstructive defecation is the inability to successfully pass a bowel movement secondary to abnormalities of the pelvic floor, which are either structural or functional. Structural abnormalities might include stricture, rectocele, or enterocele. Functional abnormalities include paradoxic contraction of the puborectalis muscle. Again, it is important to correctly diagnose the abnormality, because the treatment is different for each.

ETIOLOGY AND PRESENTATION

Rectal Prolapse

The exact etiology of rectal prolapse is still unknown; however, it is thought to be related to chronic constipation and straining. It has been found that some common anatomic findings are associated with rectal prolapse. These include a deep cul-de-sac (pouch of Douglas), a redundant sigmoid colon, pelvic floor muscle weakening, internal and external anal sphincter weakening, pudendal neuropathy, and lack of normal fixation to the rectum. It is difficult to know whether these findings precede or are a result of the constipation and straining.

Patients are usually seen initially with complaints of tissue prolapsing from the rectum. They will often state that the rectum will only prolapse with Valsalva, however more severe cases can progress to the point that the prolapse will occur with minimal to no straining. Some prolapses will reduce spontaneously, and other patients will report needing to manually reduce the prolapsed rectum. Occasionally, the rectal prolapse is associated with rectal bleeding. The majority of patients are women (6:1 ratio), and it is usually seen after the fifth decade. Up to 70% of patients will have some degree of fecal incontinence associated with rectal prolapse, and symptoms of constipation are seen in 15% to 65% of patients.

Obstructive Defecation

Patients with obstructive defecation will often report sensations of incomplete evacuation, excessive straining, and the need for assistance to pass stool, including the use of laxatives, enemas, or digital manipulation. The etiology is not clearly understood, and again it is difficult to determine whether the anatomic findings are actually the cause or the result of the chronic constipation.

A rectocele is the bulging of the rectum into the vagina through a weakened rectovaginal septum. It is thought that the rectovaginal septum weakens with age and parturition, allowing the rectocele to develop. Rectoceles less than 2 cm are typically asymptomatic and are accepted as a normal finding. Rectoceles may coexist with other pelvic floor prolapses including sigmoidocele, enterocele, intussusceptions, or perineal descent.

One of the functional etiologies of obstructive defecation is a nonrelaxing puborectalis muscle. This is often referred to as *nonrelaxing puborectalis syndrome* or *paradoxic contraction* of the puborectalis muscle, which acts as a sling around the rectum. It is normally in a contracted state, which causes angulation of the rectum and assists with continence. When the action to defecate is initiated, the muscle relaxes. This allows straightening of the rectum and eases evacuation of the stool through the rectum and out the anus. In a patient with paradoxic muscle contraction, upon initiation of a bowel movement the muscle contracts further, thus increasing the acute angle of the rectum and preventing passage of stool. The more the patient strains, the less successful the evacuation.

EVALUATION

The evaluation of rectal prolapse and obstructive defecation begins with a complete history and physical examination. It is important to have a full understanding of the patient's symptoms so that associated problems can also be addressed. The physician must inquire about the duration of symptoms, whether the patient is constipated, and, if so, the frequency of bowel movements must be determined, along with what specifically needs to be done to successfully pass a stool. If laxatives alone are needed, this may suggest colonic inertia. If manual digitation is necessary, this may suggest the presence of a rectocele. If the patient reports prolapse, it is important to know how much tissue prolapses, what triggers the prolapse, and what must be done to reduce the tissue once it has prolapsed. It is also important to get a good understanding of associated symptoms, such as incontinence, leakage, or straining during defecation.

The initial examination can be done with the patient in either the lateral decubitus position or the prone jackknife position. External examination may reveal a patulous anus, frequently seen with full-thickness rectal prolapse. Digital rectal examination is then performed. The sphincter muscle should be assessed for resting tone, squeeze, and the possibility of sphincter defects. The puborectalis muscle should also be assessed by asking the patient to contract the pelvic floor muscles and then to Valsalva; the examiner should feel relaxation of the muscle when the patient is bearing down. If the muscle does not relax, this may signify paradoxic motion of the puborectalis muscle. Anoscopy should be performed to look for mucosal abnormalities such as hemorrhoids, strictures, or ulcerations. The patient should be asked to perform the Valsalva maneuver to reproduce the presence of a prolapse, and the prolapse should be assessed for length as well as whether it is mucosal, hemorrhoidal, or full thickness. If the prolapse is not reproducible in this position, the patient should be examined while seated on the commode.

Colonoscopy should be performed in these patients to rule out polyps or cancerous lesions. Other tests may be necessary to fully evaluate these patients and their defecatory problems. Manometry is used to assess the sphincter complex, and electromyography is useful for assessing the presence of paradoxic puborectalis muscle contraction. Defecography or dynamic magnetic resonance imaging is useful in assessing the coexistence of other pelvic floor disorders such as rectoceles, enteroceles, cystoceles, pelvic floor descent, or internal intussusception. Defecography can also help diagnose paradoxic puborectalis muscle contraction.

It is important to note that rectoceles and intussusceptions are common findings on defecography. In one study of asymptomatic women, rectoceles were found in 81% and intussusceptions were found in 35%. The mere presence of these is not an indication for surgical repair. Transrectal ultrasound is useful in assessing for possible sphincter defects, and colonic transit studies are important for the diagnosis of colonic inertia. With these studies, the subjects ingest markers, and follow-up abdominal films are taken on days 3, 5, and 7 to follow the transit of the markers through the gastrointestinal tract. All markers should be passed by day 5 in a normal study, and abnormal studies suggest either colonic inertia or obstructive defecation based on the distribution of the markers. If colonic inertia is found and not addressed and corrected, the patient will likely continue to have straining and constipation and will be prone to experience failure of any procedure performed to correct the rectal prolapse or obstructive defecation.

RECTAL PROLAPSE TREATMENT OPTIONS

Conservative treatment is limited with full-thickness rectal prolapse, and it includes the use of fiber and laxatives to minimize straining and prevent constipation. Biofeedback and pelvic floor exercises can also be used. These methods of treatment are more successful in treating internal intussusception and mucosal prolapse but will rarely be successful in the treatment of full-thickness rectal prolapse.

A large number of procedures, and variations on those procedures, have been proposed over the years for the treatment of rectal prolapse in an attempt to find the best treatment option. Many of the earlier procedures have been abandoned because of high recurrence and complication rates. The procedures performed to correct rectal prolapse can be divided into two categories: those performed from the *abdominal approach* and those performed from the *perineal approach*. Preoperative mechanical bowel preparation is recommended for all patients undergoing rectal prolapse repair, and appropriate preoperative antibiotics should also be administered.

Abdominal Approach

Rectopexy

For rectopexy, the patient is placed in the lithotomy position, and a lower midline or Pfannenstiel incision is made. The peritoneum along the rectum is incised to allow access to the presacral avascular plane, which is then developed sharply down to the pelvic floor. The lateral dissection is taken down to the middle hemorrhoidal vessel only, thus preserving the pelvic nerves. The anterior peritoneum is incised to

further free the rectum if necessary, and the rectum is then pulled up and out of the pelvis and secured to the sacrum by placing four to six sutures to attach it to the presacral fascia. The majority of studies in the literature show a 0% mortality rate and a recurrence rate typically less than 3%. Continence has been shown to improve with this procedure; however, the effect on constipation symptoms has not been consistent.

Rectopexy with Mesh

This procedure also involves full mobilization of the rectum as described above; however, the fixation is performed using a type of prosthesis or mesh. The material used has varied greatly over the years and has included nylon, polypropylene (Prolene, Marlex), polyglactin (Vicryl), and polyglycolic acid (Dexon). The mesh can be placed either in the anterior position (Ripstein procedure) or the posterior position. Ripstein recommended placing the mesh in front of the rectum and then wrapping it around to secure it to the sacrum, which restores the rectum to its natural anatomic position. Review of the literature for this procedure reveals a mortality rate of 0% to 2.8% and a recurrence rate of 0% to 13%. Although incontinence does seem to improve after the procedure, similar to suture rectopexy, improvement in constipation has not been consistent. One possible complication of this procedure is obstructive defecation. For this reason, a modification was made that included having a split in the anterior mesh.

In the posterior repair, the mesh is secured to the lateral and posterior aspects of the rectum, leaving the anterior portion free to expand as necessary. The mesh is then secured to the presacral fascia. Early studies used the polyvinyl alcohol sponge (Ivalon) for fixation. Though the mortality rate was low (0% to 3%), and the recurrence rate was also low (3%), the Ivalon sponge was abandoned due to the increased risk of infection associated with its use. Both absorbable and nonabsorbable materials have been used for fixation, and studies have shown similar outcomes for each. Use of mesh does carry a risk of infection, and this risk is increased if the mesh rectopexy is combined with resection. When comparing suture rectopexy and mesh repairs, there is no clear advantage of the use of mesh over suture repair.

Resection Rectopexy

Resection rectopexy includes complete mobilization of the rectum along with resection of the redundant portion of sigmoid colon. The left colon is mobilized in preparation for resection. The splenic flexure should not be mobilized, because the splenocolic ligament will help to reduce recurrence. The redundant sigmoid colon is resected, and a tension-free anastomosis is performed. Once this is completed, a suture rectopexy can be performed. The advantage of this procedure is that redundant tissue is removed, the rectum is returned to its normal location with fixation, and associated symptoms of constipation are also addressed.

Resection alone is not an acceptable treatment for rectal prolapse. These procedures should be combined with suture rectopexy and not mesh placement because of the increased risk of infection with mesh placed during a colon resection. Resection rectopexy has a mortality rate less than 7% and a recurrence rate of 0% to 5%, and constipation was found to improve with this procedure (Table 1).

Division or Preservation of the Lateral Attachments

Division of the lateral attachments may result in denervation of the rectum secondary to injury of the parasympathetic nerves. Review of the literature reveals that with division of the lateral attachments, a worsening of constipation was seen in 14% to 48% of patients, and improvement with continence was seen in 13% to 64%. With preservation of the lateral attachments, improvement in constipation was seen in 17% to 83% of patients, and improvement in continence was seen in 11% to 75% of patients. There is a potential for increased recurrence with preservation of the lateral attachments, presumably from incomplete mobilization of the rectum; however, the benefit of improvement of constipation does outweigh the risk of increased recurrence.

Laparoscopic Versus Open Procedures

The benefits of laparoscopic surgery have been seen with many procedures. There were concerns that prolapse procedures performed laparoscopically might result in a higher recurrence rate because the beneficial scarring would presumably be lessened. Studies performed comparing laparoscopic repairs to open repairs revealed no difference with regard to morbidity, mortality, constipation, incontinence, or recurrence rates. As seen with other procedures performed laparoscopically, patients did have a shorter length of stay and better cosmesis (Table 2).

TABLE 1: Open abdominal procedures

Procedure	Mortality Rates	Morbidity Rates	Recurrence Rates
Suture rectopexy	0%	9.3%–20%	0%–9%
Ripstein procedure	0%–2.8%	3.7%–33%	0%–12%
Posterior mesh repair	0%–1%	15%–28%	0%–6%
Resection rectopexy	0%–6.7%	7.1%–17.2%	0%–5%

TABLE 2: Laparoscopic abdominal procedures

Procedure	Mortality Rates	Morbidity Rates	Recurrence Rates
Suture rectopexy	0%	9%–19%	0%–7%
Posterior mesh repair	0%	8%–14%	0%–4%
Resection rectopexy	0%	8%–13%	0%

Perineal Approach

Delorme Procedure

Mucosal stripping of the rectum for correction of rectal prolapse was described by Delorme in 1899. The procedure can be performed with general, regional, or local anesthesia, and it can be performed with the patient in either the lithotomy or prone jackknife position. First, the prolapse is everted, and local anesthetic with epinephrine is injected circumferentially just proximal to the dentate line. A circumferential mucosal incision approximately 1 to 1.5 cm proximal to the dentate line is made. Next, the mucosa is dissected free from the muscle circumferentially to the apex of the prolapse. The circular muscle is then plicated, the redundant mucosa is excised, and the mucosal anastomosis is performed.

Although this procedure has a low mortality rate, the morbidity rate ranges from 0% to 50%, and the recurrence rate is 5% to 30%. It has been suggested that a lead point of prolapse higher than what can be reached with a mucosal dissection or major perineal descent (>9 cm on straining) might lead to failure of this procedure (Figure 1).

Perineal Proctosigmoidectomy (Altemeier)

The perineal proctosigmoidectomy was first described by Auffret in 1882. The procedure was further advocated by Miles in 1933; however, it was popularized in the United States in 1971 by Altemeier.

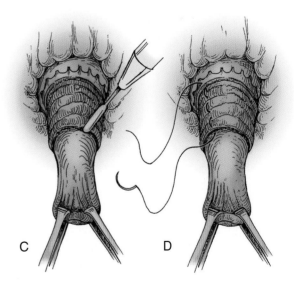

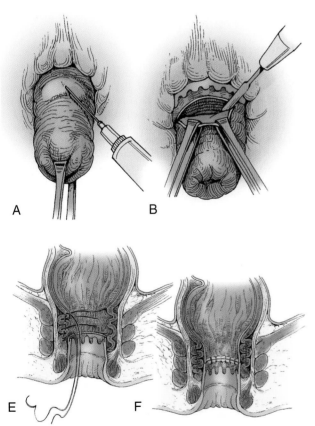

FIGURE 1   Mucosal proctectomy (Delorme). **A,** Submucosal infiltration with epinephrine solution. **B,** Circumferential mucosal incision. **C,** Dissection of mucosa away from muscular layer. **D** and **E,** Plicating stitch including cut edge of mucosa and muscular wall. **F,** Completed anastomosis. *(From Whitlow CB: Rectal prolapse and intussusceptions. In Beck DE [ed]: Handbook of colorectal surgery, St Louis, 1997, Quality Medical Publishing, pp 274–298.)*

This procedure also can be performed with general, regional, or local anesthesia. The patient is positioned in either the prone jackknife or lithotomy position, and the rectal prolapse is everted. Local anesthetic with epinephrine is injected circumferentially just proximal to the dentate line, and a circumferential incision is made approximately 1 cm proximal to the dentate line and then deepened, so full-thickness dissection is performed. The abdominal cavity is entered, allowing division of the mesentery and its vessels, thus freeing up the redundant sigmoid colon.

It is possible at this point to palpate the abdominal cavity to make sure the redundant colon has been fully mobilized. A levatorplasty can also be performed, either anteriorly of posteriorly. The colon is then divided, and the anastomosis is performed using interrupted absorbable sutures. Overall, the mortality rate from this procedure is very low; morbidity is 0% to 25%, and the recurrence rate ranges from 0% to 18% (Figure 2; Table 3).

RECTAL PROLAPSE: CHOOSING THE RIGHT OPERATION

Abdominal procedures should be performed in healthy patients who can tolerate an operation because of the lower recurrence rates seen with these types of procedures. In addition, many different materials can be used to fix the rectum to the sacrum, but there is no clear

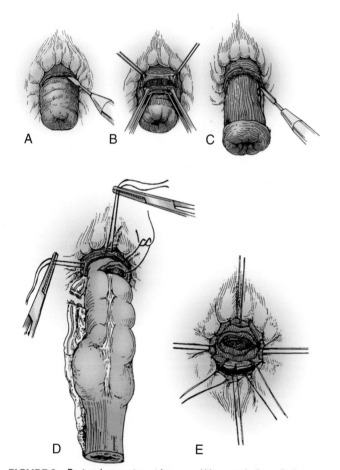

FIGURE 2   Perineal rectosigmoidectomy (Altemeier). **A** to **C,** Full-thickness excision of the outer cylinder of the prolapse. **D,** Mesenteric vessels ligated; stay sutures placed in distal edge of inner cylinder. **E,** Anastomosis of the distal aspect of the remaining colon to the rectal stump. *(From Whitlow CB: Rectal prolapse and intussusception. In Beck DE [ed]: Handbook of colorectal surgery, St Louis, 1997, Quality Medical Publishing, pp 274–298.)*

benefit of the type of mesh used versus suture with regard to recurrence rate. Infection rates, however, are higher when prosthetic material is used. It is recommended that patients with rectal prolapse without constipation undergo an abdominal rectopexy with preservation of the lateral attachments.

Laparoscopic expertise has been shown to decrease length of stay and has improved cosmesis with no difference in morbidity or recurrence rates. Patients with rectal prolapse and constipation without evidence of colonic inertia benefit from resection rectopexy with preservation of the lateral attachments.

Perineal procedures are typically reserved for those with comorbidities that would preclude an abdominal operation or for those who cannot tolerate general anesthesia. Perineal procedures avoid the complications seen with abdominal surgeries, and they can be performed with either regional or local anesthesia. The perineal procedures, however, have a higher recurrence rate compared with the abdominal procedures. The perineal proctosigmoidectomy is favored for full-thickness rectal prolapse in the frail patient. This procedure has been shown in the literature to have lower mortality and morbidity rates as well as a lower recurrence rate compared with the Delorme procedure.

In certain situations the perineal proctectomy may be the preferred choice of operation even in younger, healthier patients, such as those with incarcerated or gangrenous prolapse and in younger men and women who wish to avoid possible sexual dysfunction complications. Recently, the trend has been to perform the perineal procedures on younger patients because of the shorter recovery time, reduced pain, and reduced disruption to the patient's normal activities. These benefits must be carefully weighed against the increased risk of recurrence.

OBSTRUCTIVE DEFECATION TREATMENT OPTIONS

Nonoperative Treatment

All patients should first be treated with conservative medical management. This includes a high-fiber diet with the goal to ingest 25 to 35 g of fiber per day. Increased fluid intake is also encouraged, and laxatives and enemas may also be helpful.

For patients with paradoxic puborectalis syndrome, the treatment options include conservative measures as mentioned above, along with the use of biofeedback. Biofeedback is a conditioning treatment in which information about a physiologic process is converted to a simple visual or auditory signal to enable the patient to learn to control a particular function. For treatment of paradoxic puborectalis syndrome, an anal plug electrode is placed into the anus and connected to the biofeedback device. The patient is then asked to contract the external sphincters and note the response. The patient is then asked to bear down as if passine a stool and to note the response. With instruction, the straining attempts can be altered to become successful and purposeful, but the success of this procedure is highly dependent on the involvement and determination of the patient. The initial success rate of biofeedback ranges from 31% to 89% with no risk to the patient. These results are not necessarily sustained, and in one study, the success rate dropped over time to 25%.

TABLE 3: Perineal procedure outcomes

Procedure	Mortality Rates	Morbidity Rates	Recurrence Rates
Delorme	0%–7%	2%–50%	5%–30%
Perineal proctosigmoidectomy (Altemeier)	0%	0%–25%	0%–12.5%

A second nonoperative treatment that has been proposed is Botox injections; botulinum toxin is a potent neurotoxin that causes paralysis of the muscles by presynaptic inhibition of acetylcholine release. Botox is injected into the puborectalis muscle in an attempt to decrease the contraction of the muscle, but there has been no consensus as to the amount of Botox to inject. Early studies suggest an initial success rate of up to 70%; however, that number dropped to 33% over time. The effect persists for about 3 months, so repeat injection may be necessary to maintain a beneficial outcome. Most studies also reported minimal complications. When compared with biofeedback, it was found that though the initial success was higher for those treated with Botox, the results dropped off and were comparable with the passage of time.

Operative Treatment

There is no role for surgery for the treatment of paradoxic puborectalis syndrome and only a very limited role for surgery in the treatment of internal intussusception. The STARR procedure (stapled transanal rectal resection) was proposed for the treatment of symptomatic rectoceles and intussusception. This procedure is performed with the patient in the lithotomy position under regional or local anesthesia. Using a circular stapler, a portion of the anterior wall of the rectum is removed, and a second firing is used to remove a portion of the posterior wall of the rectum.

The rationale is to restore the normal anatomy and function by excising the redundant tissue. The overall success of the procedure was 60% to 65%; however, with stricter adherence to exclusion criteria, the success rate in one study increased to 89.4%. Selection in this later study was very strict and only included those subjects with symptomatic rectocele or intussusception; those with colonic inertia, anismus, other pelvic floor dysfunction, anal incontinence, tenesmus, or pelvic floor descent were all excluded. Postoperative complications included persistent anal pain, rectal bleeding, anal incontinence, and recurrence of symptoms. If the surgeon performing the operation is an expert in the evaluation and treatment of pelvic floor abnormalities and disorders, and in the use of the PPH stapler, and if the surgeon adheres to strict patient selection, success should be achievable.

SUMMARY

Defecatory problems such as rectal prolapse and obstructive defecation can be difficult to treat. Proper evaluation and diagnosis is important so that proper treatment selection can be made. With special consideration to preoperative symptoms and good technique, rectal prolapse can be successfully treated with good outcomes. Surgery has a limited role in the treatment of obstructive defecation, however, but it can be beneficial when patients are appropriately selected for treatment.

Suggested Readings

Glasgow SC, Birnbaum EH, Kodner IJ, et al: Recurrence and quality of life following perineal proctectomy for rectal prolapse, *J Gastrointest Surg* 12:1446–1450, 2008.

Jayne DG, Schwandner O, Studo A: Stapled transanal rectal resection for obstructed defecation syndrome: one-year results of the European STARR Registry, *Dis Colon Rectum* 52:1205–1212, 2009.

Madiba TE, Baig MK, Wexner SD: Surgical management of rectal prolaspe, *Arch Surg* 140:63–73, 2005.

Purkayastha S, Tekkis P, Athanasiou T, et al: A comparsion of open vs. laparoscopic abdominal rectopexy for full-thickness rectal prolapse: a meta-analysis, *Dis Colon Rectum* 48:1930–1940, 2005.

Raftopoulos Y, Senagore AJ, Di Giuro G, et al: Recurrence rates after abdominal surgery for completed rectal prolapse: a multicenter pooled analysis of 643 individual patient data, *Dis Colon Rectum* 48:1200–1206, 2005.

Tou S, Brown SR, Malik AI, et al: Surgery for complete rectal prolapse in adults, *Cochrane Database Syst Rev* 4: CD001758, 2008.

Management of Solitary Rectal Ulcer Syndrome

Jennifer Y. Wang, MD, and Eric J. Dozois, MD

OVERVIEW

Solitary rectal ulcer syndrome (SRUS) describes a condition characterized by difficult evacuation, rectal bleeding, pain, and mucus discharge. It is occasionally associated with partial or full-thickness rectal prolapse. Patients describe prolonged time on the toilet, incomplete evacuation, excessive straining, and digitations to help evacuate stool.

Despite the name of the syndrome, an ulcer is not always seen on endoscopic or proctoscopic exam. Furthermore, when ulcerations are present, they may be multiple, and they may be associated with a polypoid mass. The lesions are typically on the anterior rectal wall, although they can be found on any aspect and may even be circumferential. Lesions are usually found 5 to 10 cm from the anus. Because the macroscopic appearance can be that of an ulcer or of a polypoid or flat lesion, it is important to perform a biopsy to rule out cancer or colitis. Solitary rectal ulcers have a distinct histologic finding of fibromuscular obliteration of the lamina propria, which differentiates it from other conditions, such as malignancy.

Traditionally it was thought that difficult evacuation led to excessive straining and possibly self-instrumentation to stimulate defecation, which led to rectal trauma, bleeding, and formation of the rectal ulcer. While the etiology of SRUS is still not entirely clear, an important component of the syndrome appears to be rectal intussusception and outlet obstruction. While defecography is not required for diagnosis, it demonstrates intussusception in 38% to 100% of cases. Rectocele is frequently seen in women, and delayed evacuation is seen in most of the imaging studies. Anorectal testing is not required for diagnosis, but findings may suggest those who will respond better to certain therapies.

In one series, pelvic dyssynergia was seen in 82% of subjects; in comparison with healthy controls, those with SRUS exhibited less anal relaxation and lower thresholds for first sensation, desire to defecate, and urge to defecate. Balloon expulsion times were also somewhat prolonged. These patients may benefit from biofeedback therapy. A recent study using dynamic pelvic MRI identified the absence of normal mesorectosacral fixation, resulting in anorectal redundancy and pelvic floor descent. These anatomic abnormalities seen in patients with SRUS are important when considering treatment because the underlying problem, not just the ulcer, must be treated.

INDICATIONS FOR TREATMENT

Many patients suffer from symptoms long before they seek treatment; management can also be delayed because of frequent misdiagnoses, such as hemorrhoids or inflammatory bowel disease. Once the proper diagnosis is made, treatment options should begin with conservative measures. Treatment goals are to heal the ulcer; manage bleeding, particularly if severe; and relieve the painful defecation. For those refractory to conservative treatment, surgery can be considered.

NONSURGICAL TREATMENT

Dietary Modification

Since part of the pathophysiology of SRUS relates to disordered defecation, dietary modification to improve bowel habits can be beneficial in some patients. Increased dietary fiber, or fiber supplementation and fluid intake with or without stool softeners, results in improvement of symptoms in 19% to 70% of patients with SRUS.

Topical

Topical therapies to promote ulcer healing—such as enemas of steroids, sulfasalazine, and sucralfate—are not useful for long-term treatment because they do not address the underlying problem that resulted in the ulceration. However, topical therapies have been shown to provide symptomatic relief, particularly sucralfate enemas, and they can be used in conjunction with other nonsurgical treatments.

Biofeedback

Biofeedback addresses the underlying defecation disorder. Short-term results are good, although with long-term follow-up the benefits appear to diminish. Biofeedback sessions are typically conducted with a therapist every 1 to 2 weeks for a total of four or five sessions. The sessions involve practice expelling a balloon from the rectum with electromyographic feedback for pelvic floor training; in addition, the patient is advised about normal bowel habits and diet, and patients are encouraged to continue practicing the exercises after their therapy sessions have ended.

In a series of 11 patients with SRUS, at 1 week after completion of biofeedback therapy, one third of patients had complete endoscopic resolution of the rectal ulcer, and another one third had more than 50% healing of the ulcer. The study also reported significant improvement in a validated bowel symptom score. However, in another series of 13 patients with a longer follow-up (36 months), only 33% felt they had ongoing benefit from the biofeedback. It is difficult to assess the role of patient compliance and underlying psychological factors in failure of a sustained improvement from biofeedback. However, this is a noninvasive treatment with little risk for complication; therefore it should be one of the first measures implemented.

SURGICAL TREATMENT

Surgery is typically reserved for patients with more severe or refractory symptoms, such as full-thickness rectal prolapse or bleeding that requires blood transfusion. Behavioral therapy and biofeedback may serve as important adjuncts to surgery because there is a risk for recurrence if habits of excessive straining and prolonged time on the toilet are not addressed. Local excision of the ulcer has been described and may be useful if a pathologic diagnosis has not been confirmed, and transanal endoscopic microsurgery for performing such excision has also been described. However, poor healing of the wound is a concern, especially when these ulcers are caused by a component of ischemia and repeated trauma to the area.

To address the anatomic issue of rectoanal or internal rectal intussusception, a combination of rectal tissue resection and rectopexy should be considered. Rectopexy can be performed laparoscopically or as an open procedure. When rectopexy is performed alone, improvement in the solitary rectal ulcer can be seen. However, postoperative constipation or difficulty evacuating the rectum occurs in about 50% of patients, and this could potentially result in recurrence of the rectal ulcer.

In a series of surgical procedures for SRUS at St. Mark's Hospital in London, 49 of 81 patients had rectopexy performed, with 22 failures at a median of 90 months' follow-up; 19 underwent further procedures, and 14 ultimately ended with a colostomy. In that same series, nine patients had a Delorme procedure with four failures, and three of those underwent further surgery.

Alternative primary surgical options include low anterior resection, which has higher morbidity than the other procedures and should be reserved as a last alternative; colostomy is another option that many patients would prefer to avoid.

When rectopexy is combined with sigmoid resection, long-term results may be improved and more sustained when compared with rectopexy or resection alone. In a series of 27 women with rectoanal intussusception, seven of whom had solitary rectal ulcers, by 6 months postoperatively, 80% were satisfied with the functional results of their surgery, and all rectal ulcers had healed.

More recently, stapled transanal rectal resection (STARR) has been described for management of SRUS. It has been successfully used for management of internal rectal prolapse and hemorrhoids, and its application to SRUS makes sense, because it removes the redundant rectal tissue that is believed to be resulting in ulcer formation. A prospective evaluation of 10 patients undergoing STARR with the procedure for prolapse and hemorrhoids device showed zero ulcer recurrences with a mean follow-up of 27 months; after 12 months, 80% reported good to excellent satisfaction.

SUMMARY

An awareness of SRUS is important for its timely diagnosis. Therapy must be directed not to the ulcer itself but to the underlying cause, which is likely a combination of rectoanal intussusception and pelvic floor dyssynergia with outlet obstruction. Dietary modification is a simple first step, with varying degrees of effectiveness. Biofeedback appears to only be effective in about one third of patients, and the majority of patients do not have long-term sustained improvement. Surgical candidates must be carefully selected, but when they are, resection rectopexy or STARR procedures can have good results in terms of healing the rectal ulcer, with at least 80% patient satisfaction. However, patients may benefit most from a combination of surgery and behavioral therapy.

SURGICAL MANAGEMENT OF CONSTIPATION

Heidi Chua, MD, and John H. Pemberton, MD

OVERVIEW

Constipation is one of the most common gastrointestinal complaints, resulting in over 2 million physician visits per year and accounting for more than $1 billion in sales of over-the-counter laxatives. Self-reported constipation is more common in women, and it increases with age. Constipation is defined by these parameters:

- Straining during a bowel movement more than 25% of the time
- Hard stools more than 25% of the time
- Incomplete evacuation more than 25% of the time
- Two or fewer bowel movements in a week
- Having to use manual maneuvers (digital evacuation, support of the pelvic floor) more than 25% of the time

There are several causes of constipation; these are outlined in Table 1, along with the common medications associated with constipation. Care should be taken to elucidate this information to appropriately counsel and manage patients.

EVALUATION

History

Evaluation for constipation starts with a history and physical exam. Frequency of bowel movements is as important as symptoms experienced between bowel movements, such as bloating and pain. If symptoms of bloating and pain are predominant, a diagnosis of irritable bowel syndrome may be more likely. A detailed dietary history with regard to fiber intake, medications, and activity level may reveal the reason for constipation.

Physical Exam and Endoscopy

On physical exam, the abdomen, perineum, and rectum must be examined in the supine and sitting (straining) positions. Colonoscopy, barium enema, and endoscopy—such as anoscopy, rigid proctoscopy, or flexible sigmoidoscopy—are an important part of the evaluation of patients with constipation.

Testing

Physiologic function of the pelvic floor is assessed by anal manometry with balloon expulsion. Manometry measures resting and squeeze pressure of the sphincter muscles. It also measures intraanal and intrarectal pressures with a transanally inserted catheter, which is then withdrawn slowly. With this device, presence of the rectoanal inhibitory reflex is confirmed. The absence of this reflex raises the possibility that the patient has Hirschsprung disease, but it may be noted in Chagas disease or after an ileoanal or coloanal anastomosis. Balloon expulsion is performed using a small balloon filled with 50 mL of fluid, which is placed in the rectum; the patient is asked to expel the balloon. Balloon expulsion may be done sitting on the commode or, as in our institution, in the left lateral decubitus position.

Although controversial, pudendal nerve terminal motor latency (PNTML) and electromyogram (EMG) testing assess the status of the striated muscle of the sphincter complex. PNTML uses an electrode mounted to the examiner's finger, which is introduced into the rectum. The electrode is positioned in close proximity to the ischial spine, and the time between the electrical stimulus and the external sphincter contraction is the PNTML value. EMG is the recording of the electrical activity of the external sphincter muscle.

Care must be taken when interpreting test results because many patients may have pelvic floor injuries from chronic straining; likewise, normal subjects may have abnormal physiologic testing and still have normal defecation. Colonic transit scintigraphy or Sitz marker study may be used to quantify colon motility. Anatomic imaging of the pelvic floor with defecating proctogram or dynamic pelvic magnetic resonance imaging allows images to be recorded in real time with simultaneous assessment of gynecologic abnormalities that may affect defecation. The algorithms outlined in Figures 1 through 3 provide a summary guide to evaluating these patients.

DIAGNOSIS

By using the tests outlined above, patients with chronic constipation can be categorized in the following diagnostic groups:

1. Colonic inertia/slow-transit constipation
2. Pelvic floor dysfunction (obstructive defecation syndrome, nonrelaxing or paradoxic puborectalis, descending perineum syndrome)
3. Slow transit constipation with pelvic floor dysfunction
4. Congenital (Hirschsprung disease)
5. Idiopathic (irritable bowel syndrome)
6. Rectocele, enterocele, and sigmoidocele

Colonic Inertia (Slow-Transit Constipation)

Colonic inertia, or slow-transit constipation (STC), is caused by a dysmotility disorder of the colon, the cause of which is unknown. Findings on evaluation include a normal colonoscopic exam or the presence of melanosis coli in the setting of chronic laxative use. A tortuous and redundant colon is sometimes a part of this disease, but not its cause, and is visualized by barium exam. Results of anal manometry with balloon expulsion are normal, but if patients are unable to expel the balloon, a diagnosis of pelvic floor dysfunction in addition to STC must be considered.

Pelvic floor imaging with defecating proctogram or dynamic MRI reveals normal defecatory function with relaxation of the puborectalis muscle, widening of the anorectal angle, and the absence of extraanatomic abnormalities. The diagnostic modality of choice for functional assessment is the colon transit study (colonic scintigraphy) or Sitz marker study. With the colon transit study, patients ingest a meal of radiolabeled isotope, and multiple abdominal images are obtained. In addition to colonic transit time, gastric and small bowel transits are calculated with the scintigraphy tests, and images are obtained up to 48 hours after ingestion of the isotope. Colon transit will be prolonged with normal stomach and small bowel motility in patients with colonic inertia. A simpler Sitz marker study is performed by ingesting capsules filled with radiopaque rings. Radiographic images are taken on days 3 and 5. Patients with normal colonic motility should expel 40% and 80% of the markers on days 3 and 5 respectively. The pattern of leftover rings also supports a diagnosis of colonic inertia when they are scattered throughout the entire colon; rings clustered in the rectosigmoid area may be more indicative of pelvic floor dysfunction.

TABLE 1: Common medical conditions and medications associated with constipation

Conditions	Medications	Other
Cancer	Opiates	Depression
Extrinsic compression	Anticholinergic agents	Cognitive impairment
Strictures	Tricyclic antidepressants	Cardiac disease
Rectocele	Calcium channel blockers	Immobility
Postsurgical status	Antiparkinson drugs	Autonomic neuropathy
Megacolon	Sympathomimetics	Degenerative joint disease
Anal fissure	Antipsychotics	
Metabolic	Diuretics	
Diabetes	Antihistamines	
Hypothyroidism	Antacids, especially those with calcium	
Hypercalcemia		
Hypokalemia	Calcium supplements	
Hypomagnesemia	Iron supplements	
Uremia	Antidiarrheal agents	
Heavy metal poisoning	Nonsteroidal antiinflammatory drugs	
Myopathies		
Amyloid		
Scleroderma		
Neuropathies		
Parkinson's disease		
Spinal cord injury or tumor		
Multiple sclerosis		
Cerebrovascular disease		

(From Locke GR 3d, Pemberton JH, Phillips SF: AGA technical review on constipation, *Gastroenterology* 119:1766–1778, 2000.)

Pelvic Floor Dysfunction

Obstructive Defecation Syndrome

Obstructive defecation may be mistaken by some patients for chronic constipation. Symptoms include frequent trips to the bathroom to complete evacuation, the need to digitally evacuate, and the constant feeling of fullness. The pathophysiology and cause are poorly understood.

Nonrelaxing Puborectalis or Paradoxic Puborectalis Contraction

Severe chronic constipation with difficulty evacuating may be due to a nonrelaxing puborectalis muscle. The puborectalis is a striated muscle that arises from the symphysis pubis and loops around the rectoanal flexure, pulling it forward. On radiographic images, the muscle makes an indentation on the lower rectum. At rest, the muscle is contracted, accentuating the anorectal angle. When defecating, the puborectalis relaxes, opening the anorectal angle; in the act of defecation, the anal canal opens and shortens. In patients with nonrelaxing puborectalis, the muscle paradoxically tightens, the anorectal angle becomes more acute, and defecation is not achieved. EMG studies show the paradoxic increase in the recruitment of external sphincter and puborectalis muscle fibers during defecation. Abnormal EMG results can also be seen in normal subjects; therefore a single abnormal EMG in the absence of other symptoms does not support the diagnosis of pelvic floor dysfunction.

Descending Perineum Syndrome

Constipation also occurs in patients whose perineum bulges down on defecation, and it is best demonstrated while patients are on the commode. The etiology of this condition has been attributed to nerve injury during childbirth or chronic excessive straining.

Slow-Transit Constipation with Pelvic Floor Dysfunction

Some patients have both STC and pelvic floor dysfunction. Colonoscopy or barium enema findings are similar to findings in patients with STC, but physiologic testing will be abnormal as outlined above.

Hirschsprung Disease

A congenital disease usually diagnosed in the pediatric population, Hirschsprung disease may present in adults as chronic constipation. Diagnosis may be difficult, but the absence of the rectal inhibitory reflex on anal manometry is suggestive. The *rectal inhibitory reflex* refers to the relaxation of the internal sphincter muscle that occurs when the rectum is distended, and its spontaneous recovery. However, the diagnosis of Hirschsprung disease is not made on the absence of this reflex alone but is usually diagnosed definitively on rectal biopsy as an absence of ganglion cells in the mesenteric and submucosal plexuses with the presence of hypertrophied nerve trunks.

Rectocele, Enterocele, and Sigmoidocele

Although not the cause of chronic constipation—but rather the sequelae—rectocele, enterocele, and sigmoidocele mimic the symptoms of difficult defecation by causing obstruction to the fecal stream. Colonoscopic evaluation will reveal a normal colon and rectum. Physiologic testing may not reveal any abnormalities, and colonic transit should be normal.

Rectocele is a protrusion of the rectal wall into the vagina. It can be of various sizes and may be asymptomatic. The mere presence of a rectocele does not warrant its repair. Patients have to be counseled that rectoceles are a result of constant straining and thus are the result, and not the cause, of their constipation.

An enterocele is a peritoneum-lined sac that herniates through the pelvic floor between the vagina and the rectum. There are four types of enteroceles: *congenital, traction, pulsion,* and *iatrogenic.* Congenital enteroceles are rare and may result from a connective tissue disorder. Traction enteroceles are secondary to uterine and vaginal prolapse, and cystocele and rectocele occur commonly with traction enteroceles. Pulsion enteroceles occur secondary to prolonged increases in abdominal pressure or massive prolapse. Iatrogenic enteroceles occur postoperatively, but the pathophysiology of enteroceles is unknown. Symptoms are complex because these occur concomitantly with other vaginal support defects. Symptoms include pelvic pressure, vaginal protrusion, or pelvic prolapse. Physical exam is in the lithotomy position; patients are asked to cough or strain, and the enterocele can be seen as a bulge at the apex of the vagina.

The more elusive sigmoidocele, perhaps better termed a *pouch of Douglas protrusion,* requires careful history and physical examination with radiographic imaging support to detect. It occurs when a redundant cul-de-sac of Douglas protrudes through the anterior wall of the rectum to form a mass that sometimes protrudes through the anus or impinges on the rectum at the level of the anorectal ring. Symptoms mimic obstructive defecation by compressing the rectum, which can be visualized on defecography or magnetic resonance imaging.

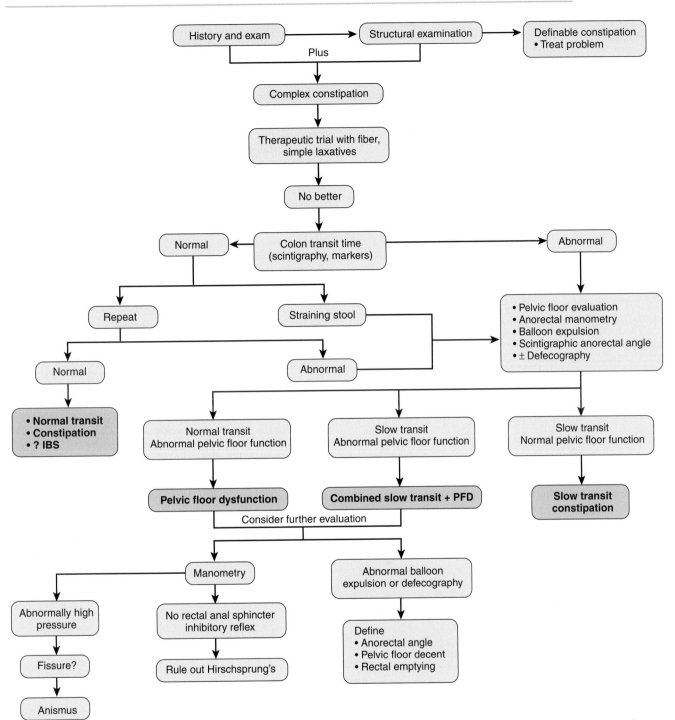

FIGURE 1 Evaluation of constipation. *PFD,* Pelvic floor dysfunction. *(From Pemberton JH, Swash M, Henry MM: The pelvic floor: its functions and disorders, Philadelphia, 2001, Saunders Elsevier.)*

TREATMENT

Colonic Inertia or Slow-Transit Constipation

Surgical treatment of STC is abdominal colectomy with ileorectal anastomosis (IRA), preferably performed laparoscopically. With the use of the hand port for hand-assisted laparoscopic surgery, the procedure is performed quite efficiently. The operation starts with mobilization of the entire colon to the rectosigmoid junction. The anastomosis is created between the terminal ileum and the top of the rectum at the sacral promontory. The ileorectal anastomosis is fashioned either end to end or side to end. As the presacral space is entered, care must be taken to preserve the sympathetic nerves. In the appropriate patient, the results improve quality of life dramatically, but patients must be cautioned that they will have frequent loose stools.

A study of the long-term results of IRA in patients with STC from our institution showed that IRA provided long-term durable symptomatic relief with improvement in patients' quality of life. With a median follow up of 5.7 years, the average number of bowel movements was four per day, and improvement of constipation and satisfaction with bowel function was 98% and 85%, respectively.

Pelvic Floor Dysfunction

Obstructive Defecation Syndrome

The mainstay of therapy for obstructive defecation syndrome (ODS) attributed to pelvic floor dysfunction is nonsurgical: pelvic floor retraining. A more recent surgical treatment is the stapled transanal rectal resection (STARR), which involves resection of circumferential full-thickness rectal wall in two firings of a stapler (Figures 4 and 5). The stapling device is the same for treating prolapsing hemorrhoids.

The procedure starts with the patient in the lithotomy position. The anoscope is inserted into the anal canal and secured to the skin with silk sutures. Several rows of half-circumferential purse-string sutures with 2-0 Prolene are placed, starting a few centimeters above the dentate line; sutures placed too close to the top of the hemorrhoidal plexus will result in bleeding. The purse-string sutures include the mucosa, submucosa, and the muscular layer of the rectal wall; they are placed sequentially, until the proximal extent of the rectocele is reached.

The number of rows of plicating sutures will differ for each patient based on the size of the rectocele. Prior to firing the stapler, the posterior rectal wall is protected by a narrow, malleable retractor. Care is taken to inspect the posterior vaginal wall to prevent its incorporation into the staple line; failure to do so may result in a rectovaginal fistula. The stapler is inserted into the rectum and fired, and bleeding is controlled with suture ligation with 2-0 Vicryl. The posterior rectal wall is managed in the same fashion.

Patients report minimal pain and are discharged in 2 to 3 days. Contraindications for this procedure include a prior history of left or distal colorectal resection, history of hemorrhoid surgery, fecal incontinence, concomitant urogenital prolapse, and inflammatory bowel disease.

Long-term outcomes with this operation are unknown. The largest series to date is a multicenter trial from Spain, in which 104 patients diagnosed with ODS were treated with STARR. They were followed at 1, 3, and 6 months and then annually. At 1 year, a decrease in the Wexner constipation score was observed, from 13.5 to 5.1. Fecal incontinence and urgency were present in a small group of patients, but most resolved over time. Morbidity was minimal, with bleeding in three patients that required surgery. There were no reports of rectovaginal fistula, pelvic sepsis, or anastomotic leak. A recent report (Harris et al, 2009) compared STARR with standard

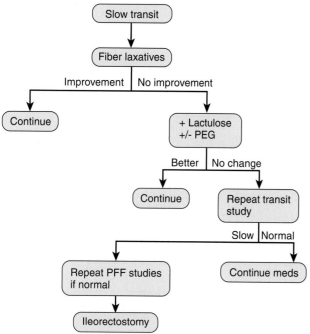

FIGURE 2 Management of STC. *PEG*, polyethylene glycol; *PPF*, pelvic floor function. *(From Pemberton JH, Swash M, Henry MM: The pelvic floor: its functions and disorders, Philadelphia, 2001, Saunders Elsevier.)*

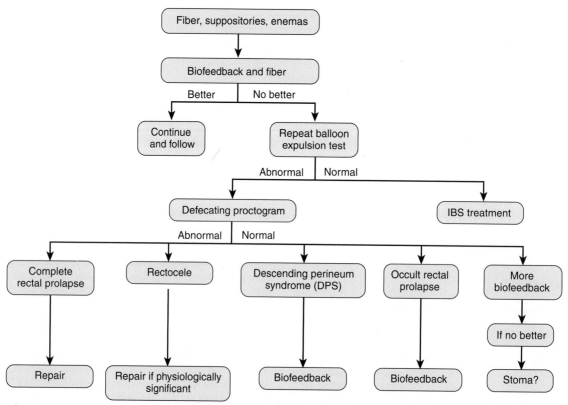

FIGURE 3 Posterior pelvic floor dysfunction. *(From Pemberton JH, Swash M, Henry MM: The pelvic floor: its functions and disorders, Philadelphia, 2001, Saunders Elsevier.).*

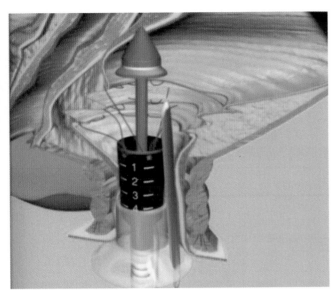

FIGURE 4 STARR procedure: Insertion of the stapler after placement of purse-string sutures in the anterior rectal wall. (Courtesy Medtronic.)

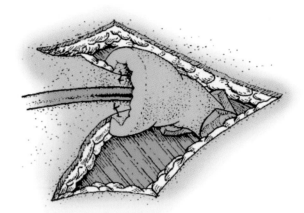

FIGURE 6 Creation of the Malone antegrade continence enema (MACE) with the appendix open and a flap of skin fishtailed into the appendix. (From Griffiths DM, Malone PS: The Malone antegrade continence enema, J Pediatr Surg 30(1):68-71, 1995.)

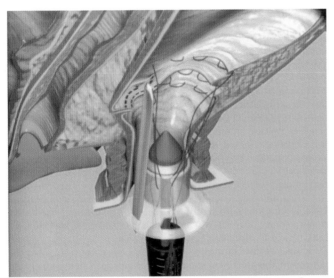

FIGURE 5 STARR procedure. Insertion of the stapler after placement of purse-string sutures in the posterior rectal wall. (Courtesy Medtronic.)

transvaginal repair of rectoceles. The study reported shorter operating times and less blood loss but at the expense of higher complication rates.

In an effort to further evaluate the efficacy of this new modality, the European Stapled Transanal Rectal Registry was initiated in 2006, and outcomes after 1 year in 2224 patients were recently reported. This registry is a nonrandomized, multicenter audit established to assess the short-term outcome of STARR with data from the United Kingdom, Italy, and Germany. A total of 1588 complications were reported in 1011 patients (morbidity of 36%), with urgency as the most common complaint (20%), followed by persistent pain (7.1%) and urinary retention (6.9%). Bleeding was reported in 5%, and fecal incontinence was reported in 1.8%; however, two serious complications were reported—rectal necrosis that required diversion and rectovaginal fistula—but no deaths occurred. Other studies have shown

multiple problems in these patients after STARR, and the procedure is currently performed *very* infrequently in the United States.

Nonrelaxing Puborectalis or Paradoxic Puborectalis Contraction

Treatment for patients with nonrelaxing puborectalis or paradoxic puborectalis contraction is biofeedback and pelvic floor retraining geared toward relaxation of the puborectalis muscle. Repetitive physical therapy may be required to achieve the desired results of muscle relaxation. In our institution, a 2-week intensive pelvic floor retraining program is the treatment of choice.

If physical therapy fails, *Clostridium botulinum* toxin injection has been described in some small studies. The toxin is injected directly into the muscle, usually under ultrasound or EMG guidance. Initial results were promising, but symptoms recurred after a few months, requiring reinjection. Another treatment option involves sacral nerve stimulation, but this option is currently not available in the United States. There are currently no surgical treatment options for nonrelaxing puborectalis.

Descending Perineum Syndrome

There is no surgical treatment for this condition. Even with aggressive pelvic floor retraining, the success rates are dismal.

Slow-Transit Constipation with Pelvic Floor Dysfunction

It is critical that patients with STC and pelvic floor dysfunction be identified prior to any surgical management because their treatment regimen should start with aggressive pelvic floor retraining and reassessment of colonic transit. Patients who do not respond to surgical management of colonic inertia with abdominal colectomy and IRA may, on further evaluation, have undiagnosed pelvic floor dysfunction.

Hirschsprung Disease

Treatment for Hirschsprung disease depends on the length of the aganglionic segment. Patients with a short segment of diseased bowel may do well on medical management alone. Longer segments may require coloanal anastomosis or a permanent stoma. In a small minority of patients, ileal pouch–anal anastomosis has been performed.

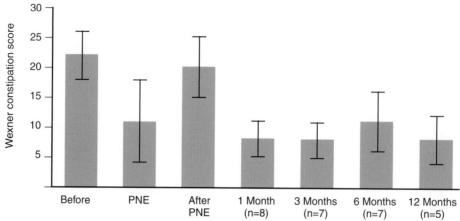

FIGURE 7 Wexner constipation score with sacral nerve stimulation for treatment of constipation. *(From Holzer B, Rosen HR, Novi G, et al: Sacral nerve stimulation in patients with severe constipation, Dis Colon Rectum 51:524–530, 2008.)*

TABLE 2: Quality of Life SF-36 results with sacral nerve stimulation for treatment of constipation

	Prestimulation (n = 19)	6-Month Follow-up (n = 7)	P value
Physical functioning	52.82 (±21.43)	70.29 (±25.01)	<.001
Role, physical	46.57 (±29.54)	61.15 (±27.73)	<.001
Bodily pain	49.44 (±21.19)	61.02 (±23.93)	<.001
General health	53.34 (±19.52)	56.37 (±21.27)	<.033
Vitality	45.23 (±27.28)	64.82 (±29.37)	<.001
Social functioning	53.43 (±26.57)	71.06 (±25.37)	<.001
Role, emotional	65.99 (±45.2)	74.09 (±37.87)	<.001
Mental health	57.81 (±20.63)	68.39 (±22.0)	<.001

From Holzer B, Rosen HR, Novi G, Ausch C: Sacral nerve stimulation in patients with severe constipation, *Dis Colon Rectum* 51:524–530, 2008.

Rectocele, Enterocele, and Sigmoidocele

Repair of rectoceles is accomplished transvaginally or transrectally, depending on the surgeon's preference. Primary repair of the attenuated rectovaginal septum or use of mesh has been described, along with the STARR procedure discussed earlier. Treatment of the enterocele can be accomplished vaginally, abdominally, or laparoscopically and will involve the urogynecologist. Treatment of the sigmoidocele in women involves uterosacral plication, and a gynecologic surgeon is often consulted.

Other Treatment Options for Constipation

Antegrade enemas have been suggested for patients with idiopathic chronic constipation. The concept was derived from the pediatric population, which has been shown to gain benefit from the Malone antegrade continence enema procedure. Done open or laparoscopically, the procedure is simple if the appendix is still present: The right colon is mobilized to allow the appendix to be exteriorized to the level of the skin, and the tip of the appendix is opened and fishtailed with a flap of skin inset and sutured for ease of entubation

and to decrease risk of stenosis (Figure 6). Patients initiate irrigation when bowel function returns, and the patient determines frequency of intubation and irrigation, but it is recommended that the stoma be intubated daily or twice daily for patency. In the absence of the appendix, a tubularized transverse cecal flap can be fashioned. Irrigants via the tube can be normal saline, phosphate enema, or both.

Sacral Nerve Stimulation

Sacral nerve stimulation is also a consideration for patients with chronic constipation, although it is not as well studied in this setting as it is in patients with urinary and fecal incontinence. A recently published prospective nonrandomized study included patients with STC, defined as less than two bowel movements per week despite aggressive medical management, and patients with rectal outlet obstruction, defined as incomplete rectal emptying or defecation that requires digital manipulation.

All patients were extensively evaluated. After implantation of the device, patients were followed at 1, 3, 6, and 12 months. The Wexner constipation score, Quality of Life SF-36 questionnaire, and the bowel diary were completed during this period. Initially, 19 patients were identified, and 8 patients (42%) underwent permanent implantation. No complications were identified in the short follow-up period of 11 months (range, 2 to 20). Wexner score and Quality of Life SF-36 were both improved with SNS (Figure 7 and Table 2).

Results of this study and others are clearly encouraging, but the efficacy of this treatment modality is unknown. Large multicenter, prospective, randomized trials are needed to further investigate the role of SNS in patients with chronic constipation; sacral nerve stimulation is not yet an FDA-approved procedure in the United States.

Stomas

Stomas are good options for patients with chronic constipation, whether with an ileostomy or colostomy. Colostomy is indicated in patients with STC. In the setting of a colostomy, patients may opt to irrigate the stoma.

SUMMARY

Chronic constipation is a vexing problem for both patient and physician. A multidisciplinary team comprising a gastroenterologist, colorectal surgeon, and urogynecologist, along with physical therapy, are essential in management of this condition. The key to successful management of this heterogenous patient population is systemic evaluation to categorize physiologic and anatomic abnormalities accurately; only then will treatment be successful.

SUGGESTED READINGS

Arroyo A, Gonzalez-Argente FX, Garcia-Domingo M, et al: Prospective multicentre clinical trial of stapled transanal rectal resection for obstructive defaecation syndrome, *Br J Surg* 95:1521–1527, 2008.

Camilleri M, Thompson WG, Fleshman JW, et al: Clinical management of intractable constipation, *Ann Int Med* 121(7):520–528, 1994:1.

Griffiths DM, Malone PS: The Malone antegrade continence enema,, *J Pediatr Surg* 30(1):68–71, 1995.

Harris MA, Ferrara A, Gallagher J, et al: Stapled transanal rectal resection vs. transvaginal rectocele repair for treatment of obstructive defecation syndrome, *Dis Colon Rectum* 52(4):592–597, 2009.

Hassan I, Pemberton JH, Young-Fadok TM, et al: Ileorectal anastomosis for slow-transit constipation: long-term functional and quality of life results, *J Gastrointest Surg* 10:1330–1337, 2006.

Holzer B, Rosen HR, Novi G, Ausch C: Sacral nerve stimulation in patients with severe constipation, *Dis Colon Rectum* 51:524–530, 2008.

Jayne DG, Schwander O, Stuto A: Stapled transanal rectal resection for obstructed defecation syndrome: one-year results of the European STARR Registry, *Dis Colon Rectum* 52:1205–1214, 2009.

Locke GR 3d, Pemberton JH, Phillips SF: AGA technical review on constipation, *Gastroenterology* 119:1766–1778, 2000.

RADIATION INJURY TO THE LARGE AND SMALL BOWEL

Elisa H. Birnbaum, MD

OVERVIEW

The treatment of gynecologic, urologic, and rectal malignancies has evolved over the years, and a multimodal treatment approach has significantly affected the management of these malignancies. Radiation therapy plays an ever-increasing role in the treatment of pelvic tumors. Improved resectability, decreased recurrence, and improved mortality rates are a few of the benefits seen with the addition of radiation. However, as the use of radiation for pelvic malignancies has expanded, subsequent complications from the effects of ionizing radiation on the gastrointestinal tract have also developed. Many of these complications do not develop until years after treatment, making cause and effect associations more difficult. The understanding of the short- and long-term effects of radiation has advanced, and efforts are ongoing to avoid injury caused by radiation. Although some of the complications are unavoidable, some basic principles help both minimize the occurrence of and treatment for the complications.

Radiation injury is biphasic. Acute injury occurs during administration of radiation therapy because of the disruption of rapidly dividing cells at the base of the crypts. Flattening of the villi leads to subsequent alteration in the absorptive and resorptive functions of the intestine, which causes diarrhea, cramping, anismus, and occasional bleeding. These early effects are encountered almost immediately upon administration of treatment; however, changes in protocol, altering the method of delivery, and the withholding of chemotherapy can alter the early acute effects of radiation.

Chronic injury is characterized by progressive obliterative endarteritis, which in turn leads to submucosal and transmural fibrosis and ischemia. Unfortunately, the chronic long-term effects can occur years after treatment and are often affected by factors not within the treating physician's control. These chronic pathologic changes lead to noncompliance of the bowel wall, fibrosis, strictures, fistulization, and hemorrhage. Understanding the risk factors that lead to chronic injury is valuable in minimizing these long-term, life-altering problems.

RISK FACTORS

Risk factors for both acute and chronic radiation injury have been defined. The strongest correlation with injury is the dose of radiation delivered (Table 1). Total radiation dose and the rate of administration are key factors in the incidence of bowel complications. Approximately 1% to 5% of patients receiving 4500 cGY can be expected to experience radiation-induced complications. If 6500 cGY is administered, 50% of patients experience complications at 5 years. Small bowel is more radiosensitive than the colon or rectum; the rectum can tolerate approximately 5500 cGY, but at doses greater than 7500 cGY, 25% to 50% of patients experience chronic rectal complications.

Risk factors that compound the effects of radiation or increase the likelihood that higher doses will be delivered to a segment of bowel have been identified. High doses given over a short time interval increase the acute effects of radiation. Concomitant administration of chemotherapy increases the tumorcidal effect of radiation but also increases tissue susceptibility to ionizing radiation.

Acute-phase toxicities are more likely to occur in patients receiving chemotherapy in conjunction with radiation than in those receiving radiation alone. Other factors that impair tissue oxygenation increase the probability that tissue injury will occur even with standard doses of radiation. Diabetes, atherosclerosis, vasculitis, and a history of smoking increase injury to small vessels and compound the effect of the progressive vasculitis seen with radiation injury. Patients who require extended fields to treat their tumor burden are more prone to enteric damage because a larger volume of small bowel is included within the radiation field. Previous abdominal and pelvic surgery increases the likelihood that loops of small bowel will be adherent in the pelvis and receive higher doses than bowel that is not fixed. The terminal ileum is frequently injured by pelvic irradiation because of fixation within the pelvis secondary to adhesions. Although the rectum can tolerate higher doses of radiation than the small bowel, it is more commonly affected by radiation due to its fixed location within the pelvis.

TREATMENT OF COMPLICATIONS

Treatments for complications are directed toward symptom relief. Antimotility agents and occasionally antiinflammatory agents are used to treat the acute effects of radiation such as diarrhea, cramping, anismus, and mucositis. Mesalamine and steroid enemas have been reported to be effective, although no single treatment has been shown to be more effective than another in the acute setting. Low-residue or elemental diets may help improve absorption, and intravenous hydration and total parenteral nutrition are occasionally needed for seriously debilitated patients. Fractionating the radiation dose or delaying the treatment allows most patients to resolve the acute toxicity.

Chronic effects occur months to years after radiation has been completed, and management should be tailored to the severity of clinical complaints. Diarrhea and fecal incontinence can occur if the small bowel, colon, or rectum become noncompliant. Fibrosis of the small bowel can lead to malabsorption and malnutrition. Strictures can occur within the small bowel or rectum because of progressive

TABLE 1: Common radiation doses

Site	Dose (cGY)	
Rectal	5000	Preoperative or postoperative ± chemotherapy
Anal	5000	+ Chemotherapy
Uterine	5000	Postoperative
Prostate	7500–8000	
Cervical	5000 8000	Postoperative Definitive therapy

ischemic vasculitis and can result in episodic, progressively worsening obstructive symptoms. Fistulae can occur between loops of bowel, bladder, or vagina, often at prior surgical sites. When surgery is unavoidable for a patient with chronic radiation injury, complications that can occur include inadvertent enterotomies, serosal injuries, or anastomoses that do not heal, leading to intraabdominal abscesses and fistulae.

A thorough workup should be performed prior to surgical intervention for radiation injury. The prognosis of the original carcinoma should be considered, and a workup for metastatic disease should be performed. Computed tomography (CT), magnetic resonance imaging, or positron emission tomography scanning can be used to distinguish between radiation fibrosis and recurrent tumor. Biopsies of rectal fistulae should be done to rule out recurrent carcinoma, and further evaluation of the colon and small bowel with contrast studies (either thin barium or water-soluble contrast) may help determine the number and extent of fistulae and strictures. Fistulography may be helpful to assess enterocutaneous or enterovaginal fistulae, and colonoscopy may help determine the extent and severity of colonic involvement. Capsule endoscopy should not be performed because of the risk of impaction of the foreign body in a tight radiation stricture.

Radiation Proctitis

Bleeding is usually secondary to acute or chronic radiation proctitis. In the acute setting, the rectum appears edematous and erythematous with evidence of mucosal sloughing. These symptoms and findings usually resolve at the completion of treatment. Deep biopsies and excision of hemorrhoids during this phase should be avoided because of the potential for the development of nonhealing wounds. In the chronic phase, the rectal mucosa is paler with visible telangiectasias. Radiation proctitis associated with treatment of urologic malignancies is often seen on the anterior wall of the rectum, where the greatest dose has been delivered.

Treatment for radiation proctitis is directed toward symptom relief. For mild symptoms, enemas of sucralfate, steroids, and short-chain fatty acids have been used; but their effectiveness is questionable and there is little evidence to support their routine use. Hyperbaric oxygen has also been used to treat radiation proctitis, although most series include a small number of patients with variable success rates. Proximity to a hyperbaric oxygen chamber and the need for multiple treatments limit the accessibility of this treatment for most patients.

Treatment of the telangiectatic vessels can be managed using ablative techniques delivered via the endoscope. Nd:YAG lasers and argon-beam coagulation produce a superficial burn over the affected mucosa. The equipment for argon-beam coagulation is more readily available and is used more frequently by experienced endoscopists. Repeat treatments may be required to control the hemorrhage, and the durability of response has not been completely evaluated. Ulceration and perforation at the treatment site are an uncommon but real concern and have been reported to occur.

Topical formalin, either as a 4% rectal instillation or a 10% topical application, has been advocated for the treatment of mucosal bleeding secondary to radiation proctitis. Early results show this treatment to be effective. Topical formalin causes a chemical cauterization of the friable mucosal vessels. The technique is simple to perform, either in the office or in an outpatient setting. After protecting the perianal skin with Vaseline gauze and packing the rectum above the area to be treated, 4% formalin solution is instilled into the rectum via a proctoscope. The formalin is left in contact with the rectal mucosa for approximately 2 to 3 minutes and is then suction evacuated. A slight blanching of the mucosa is typically seen. Alternatively, 10% formalin can be used as a topical application, using long, cotton-tipped applicators directly on the site. Repeat applications can be done every 2 to 4 weeks until bleeding has stopped.

Several small studies have shown a 60% to 90% success rate with 4% irrigation with minimal relapse. Similarly, in a recent small study utilizing 10% topical application, 90% of patients stopped bleeding after three to four treatments. Patients who re-bled were retreated successfully. No prospective studies of topical formalin are available, and no long-term results have been published in the literature. Perianal pain is commonly reported, although other serious complications are rare. Ulcerations and worsening of rectal strictures can also occur, so follow-up is necessary.

Radiation Enteritis

Radiation enteritis can lead to malabsorptive symptoms when long segments of small bowel have been affected. Resection of the involved small bowel will not restore function, because the remaining bowel may not be able to maintain adequate nutrition and hydration. If the terminal ileum is involved, chronic diarrhea and electrolyte imbalance may occur because of the bowel's inability to reabsorb bile salts. Symptomatic treatment with cholestyramine and antimotility agents may minimize symptoms of diarrhea.

When the fibrotic damage progresses, the resultant chronic stricturing causes obstructive symptoms. Patients typically experience multiple episodic small bowel obstructions that can grow progressively worse over time. In addition, multiple strictures may occur, which makes determining the exact site of obstruction difficult.

Initial management of patients with symptomatic radiation enteritis is with low-residue or elemental diets and occasionally total parenteral nutrition. Surgery is reserved for patients with severe symptoms and complications due to tight strictures. The surgical options are resection of the affected segments with reanastomosis versus bypass of the obstructive segments.

In the past, bypass was widely practiced because it was felt to be a simpler and lower risk operation; however, this technique does not eliminate the narrowed segments, and it can lead to bacterial overgrowth, abscess formation, risk of further disease progression, and perforation. In a study by Regimbeau (2001), patients who had undergone bypass surgery were compared with patients who had resections for radiation enteritis. Postoperative morbidity was approximately 30% for each group, and the leak rate was similar among bypass and resected patients. Reoperations were more common in the patients treated with bypass (50%) compared with 34% of those patients who were resected. The 5-year survival, however, was better with patients who had undergone resection (71% vs. 51%).

Bypass can be useful in patients with dense pelvic adhesions; however, even with meticulous dissection, the risk to the patient is great. It is imperative that an afferent and efferent limb be identified. The bypass anastomosis should be done between two loops of healthy, nonirradiated bowel if possible to minimize complications of leaks and future strictures (Figure 1).

Generally, resection with anastomosis is the preferred approach to chronic small bowel strictures that result from radiation. The use of nonirradiated intestine for at least one component of the anastomosis is advocated. If the terminal ileum is involved, it may be necessary to

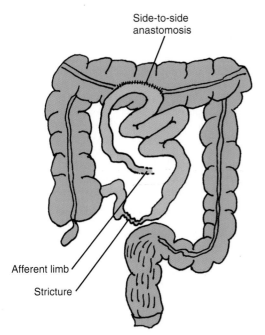

Side-to-side anastomosis

Afferent limb

Stricture

FIGURE I   Side-to-side small bowel–transverse colon anastomosis bypassing a strictured segment of terminal ileum.

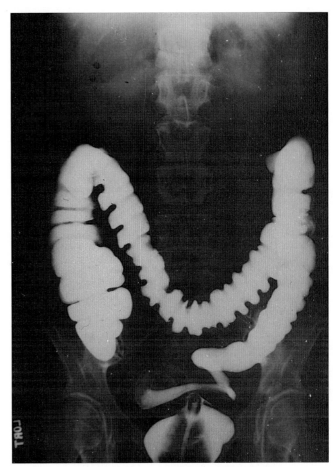

FIGURE 2   Chronic radiation of the rectum.

perform the anastomosis to the transverse colon, which is frequently out of the pelvis and undamaged by radiation. Careful dissection and minimal manipulation of small bowel can minimize damage to uninvolved loops of bowel. Repair of all enterotomies and all areas of serosal injury may minimize postoperative fistulization.

Stricturoplasty for short-segment strictures has been described as an alternative to resection. This technique has been described and used for multiple strictures, usually related to Crohn's disease. Studies using similar techniques for radiation strictures are limited, and this technique should only be used in patients with diffuse short-segment disease who have few other options available.

If the area of stricture is in the rectum or sigmoid colon (Figure 2), resection with anastomosis is possible. A proximal, nonirradiated segment of colon should be mobilized in an effort to maximize anastamotic healing. Air testing the anastomosis may help to identify areas of concern, and proximal diversion with a loop ileostomy should be done if there is any question about the security of the repair, or if the repair is done in the lower rectum. If the lower rectum is noncompliant or anastomosis is deemed risky, a permanent diverting colostomy is recommended.

Fistulizing complications should be managed as conservatively as possible. The type of surgery depends on how proximal within the gastrointestinal tract the fistula occurs and the organ to which the fistula connects. A fistula from the proximal small bowel typically has prohibitively high outputs, affecting nutrition and hydration. Pouching an enterocutaneous fistula is difficult due to the high outputs and the typically flat fistulae often found within healing wounds. Resection with anastomosis is preferable to diversion or bypass for proximal fistulae.

Enteric fistulae involving the genitourinary tract or vagina can be handled in a similar manner, with resection and anastomosis preferred over bypass. In some situations this cannot be accomplished safely; alternatively, the fistula can be left intact but excluded. The segment of bowel containing the fistula can be divided proximal and distal to the fistula, leaving a short segment of well-vascularized bowel containing the actual fistula attached to the bladder or vagina. The patient may have persistent mucus discharge because the bypassed or excluded segment of bowel remains attached to the bladder or vagina.

Patients who develop enterocutaneous fistulae pose numerous challenges. While it is tempting to try to reoperate and close the fistula, it is better to hydrate, improve nutritional support, drain any sepsis, and allow the fistula to mature. Reoperation can be done 3 to 6 months later, when the acute inflammatory process has abated.

Radiation-induced rectovaginal and rectourethral fistulae may represent technical mistakes or recurrent carcinoma and can occur years after treatment. Technical mistakes resulting from the incorporation of the vaginal cuff in a staple line during a low anterior resection may result in symptomatic fistulae that occur shortly after surgery. Diagnosis is made by patient symptoms, vaginal examination, cystoscopy, and proctoscopy.

Contrast studies can identify where the fistula is, within the rectum or sigmoid, if the site is not evident on proctoscopic examination. CT scans are highly sensitive in the identification of air within a noninstrumented bladder, indicating a colovesical fistula. Recurrent malignancy must be ruled out, and biopsies of the fistula tract need to be done. Radiation-induced fistulae will not heal by primary intention or bowel rest. Total parenteral nutrition may decrease symptoms and improve nutrition, but spontaneous closure of radiation-induced fistulae is rare.

Resection is the preferred approach for upper rectal fistulae. Healthy, nonirradiated proximal colon can be sutured to the low rectum or anal canal. Abdominal approaches include resection of the involved rectum with creation of a neorectum, utilizing a colonic J-pouch or straight coloanal anastomosis (Figure 3). Occasionally, omentum or rectus flaps can be used to interpose healthy tissue between the colonic anastomosis and the affected organ. Temporary fecal and urinary diversion should be performed to allow healing of the new anastomosis. Permanent diversion with a proximal diverting colostomy can be used as definitive therapy for patients with comorbidities.

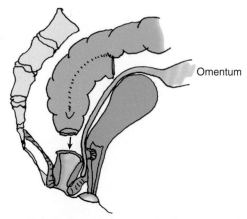

Omentum

FIGURE 3 Abdominal approach to a midlevel rectovaginal fistula, demonstrating the use of a colon J-pouch. The coloanal anastomosis is below the level of the posterior vaginal defect, which is left open to granulate closed. This may also be done with a straight anastomosis. The omental flap is an important additional buttress between the vagina and colon, serving to separate the strictures and reduce the probability of recurrent fistulization.

The goal of surgical management of mid to low rectal fistulae is to close the fistula and preserve anal sphincter function. Avoidance of pelvic dissection and use of a perineal approach may be preferable for low rectovaginal or rectourethral fistulae. Gracilis, martius, and buccal flaps have been described for reconstructing large defects. Temporarily diverting the stream of stool and urine is advisable in all reconstructive cases; if possible, an omental interposition flap should be used to bring healthy tissue between the anastomosis and the fistula.

Strategies for Prevention of Radiation Enteritis

Improvements in radiation technology have resulted in more specific and more localized radiation delivery. Over the years, radiation oncologists have altered their technique to minimize the acute effects of radiation and to minimize tissue exposed. Multiplanar delivery systems have been developed to administer radiation therapy in an effort to decrease delivery to the small bowel while increasing the dose to the targeted organ. Three-dimensional conformal radiation therapy and intensity modulation help reduce radiation morbidity, and patient positioning and blocking helps shield other organs during the delivery of radiation. Filling the bladder prior to treatment helps to displace small bowel from the pelvis. Excluding small bowel from the pelvis in cases where postoperative radiation is necessary will help minimize the amount of exposure while the small bowel recedes. Using the retroverted uterus, closing retroperitoneal tissues of the pelvic inlet, and packing the pelvis with omentum have been described. Absorbable mesh slings and adhesive barriers such as Seprafilm attempt to minimize the number of pelvic adhesions

and thus minimize the amount of bowel exposed to postoperative radiation.

There is much discussion in the literature regarding the use of preoperative versus postoperative radiation for the treatment of rectal carcinomas. Administering radiation prior to surgical intervention has been advocated by many to avoid toxicity related to bowel fixed in the pelvis. In addition, the majority of the irradiated tissue (rectum) is removed at the time of surgery, allowing an anastomosis to be created with one nonirradiated limb of bowel. Even so, there are real concerns regarding anastomotic healing with preoperative radiotherapy, particularly when adjuvant chemotherapy has been used. The use of a temporary diverting ileostomy is recommended when performing a low anastomosis after chemoradiation.

Surgical Strategies for Treatment of Radiation Enteritis

The natural history of radiation enteritis is progressive. The majority of clinical presentations of radiation injury are nonemergent, and careful clinical assessment of the patient helps to identify other comorbid conditions. Nutrition and hydration should be aggressively managed, and sepsis resulting from undrained collections should be identified and corrected. Evaluation for metastatic disease and radiologic and endoscopic assessment should help localize the affected organs. Management should be tailored to the severity of the complaint, and therapeutic interventions should begin with the least invasive intervention.

Chronic radiation injury cannot be reversed; therefore the goals of treatment should be to optimize quality of life while minimizing the morbidity and mortality of therapeutic intervention. Surgical exploration, when undertaken, should be meticulous, and operative time should be allotted accordingly. Adhesiolysis should be limited, and all serosal injuries should be repaired. Resection and anastomosis with nonirradiated bowel should be performed if possible, and bypass surgery should be used only if there is no other approach.

It is not uncommon for patients who have had surgery to have further complications, which occur in approximately 50% of those who survive the initial surgery. Many of these require further treatment and/or surgical intervention.

SUGGESTED READINGS

Haas EM, Bailey HR, Farragher I, et al: Application of 10 percent formalin for the treatment of radiation-induced hemorrhagic proctitis, *Dis Colon Rectum* 50:213–217, 2007.

Marshall GT, Thirlby RC, Bredfeldt JE, et al: Treatment of gastrointestinal radiation injury with hyperbaric oxygen, *Undersea Hyperb Med* 34:35–42, 2001.

Onodera H, Nagayama S, Mori A, et al: Reappraisal of surgical treatment for radiation enteritis, *World J Surg* 29:459–463, 2005.

Regimbeau JM, Panis Y, Gouzi JL, et al: Operative and long-term results after surgery for chronic radiation enteritis, *Am J Surg* 182:237–242, 2001.

Turina M, Mulhall AM, Mahid SS, et al: Frequency and surgical management of chronic complications related to pelvic radiation, *Arch Surg* 143:46–52, 2008.

SURGERY FOR POLYPOSIS SYNDROMES

Y. Nancy You, MD, MHSc, and Bruce G. Wolff, MD

OVERVIEW

Polyposis syndromes can be classified by polyp histology into two categories: *adenomatous polyposis syndromes,* which include familial adenomatous polyposis (FAP) and *mutY* human homologue–associated polyposis (MAP), and *hamartomatous polyposis syndromes,* which include Peutz-Jegher syndrome, juvenile polyposis, and the *PTEN* hamartomatous polyposis syndromes. Rare diseases such as hyperplastic or serrated polyposis, Cronkhite-Canada syndrome, and others are not discussed here.

Surgery in polyposis syndromes often involves complex decision making. Because the genetic basis of disease cannot be eliminated, the goal of surgery is to minimize the malignant threat while preserving function and quality of life (QOL). The surgeon should also recognize the need for multidisciplinary care and should consider referring the patient to a polyposis registry.

Familial Adenomatous Polyposis

Patients with more than 100 adenomas, or with fewer adenomas but a positive family history, meet the clinical criteria for FAP. In its classic form, patients develop at least 100 polyps starting in the teenage years, and they develop colorectal cancer (CRC) by a median age of 39 years. Patients with attenuated FAP are diagnosed 10 to 15 years later, have fewer polyps (median, 25 polyps), and have a lower lifetime risk for CRC. Extracolonic manifestations of FAP include desmoid tumors, congenital hypertrophy of the retinal pigment epithelium, osteomas, and cutaneous lesions, most commonly epidermoid cysts and fibromas. Variants of classic FAP are Gardner syndrome—colonic polyposis with osteomas, soft tissue desmoids, or cutaneous lesions—and Turcot syndrome, colonic polyposis with central nervous system tumors. Patients with FAP face a near-certain risk of CRC and elevated risks for soft tissue (desmoids), periampullary, pancreatic, papillary thyroid, central nervous system, hepatobiliary, and other cancers.

A germline mutation in the *APC* gene is identified in more than 90% of patients with FAP, using whole-gene sequencing and gene duplication/deletion analyses. Most mutations lead to a truncated APC protein, which normally functions as a tumor suppressor in the *wnt*-signaling pathway and in intercellular adhesions. Several clinically relevant genotype-phenotype correlations have been observed (Table 1).

COLORECTAL DISEASE

Indications

Surgical consultation may be sought for either symptomatic or asymptomatic patients. The most common presenting symptoms are bleeding and diarrhea. Up to 25% of FAP patients may present de novo; cancer must be suspected in these patients until proven otherwise because the reported incidence of CRC in this group may be as high as 60%. Asymptomatic patients under a surveillance program typically seek help when 1) polyps develop advanced histology, such as high-grade dysplasia or invasive carcinoma; 2) endoscopic

management is no longer adequate or feasible; or 3) the patient desires prophylactic surgery. When suspicious or large (>1.0 cm) adenomas appear, or when cancer cannot be ruled out, the patient should be managed according to oncologic principles.

Operative Choices

Common operative procedures performed in FAP patients include total proctocolectomy with end ileostomy (TPC), total abdominal colectomy with ileorectostomy (IRA), and total proctocolectomy with ileal–anal pouch anastomosis (IPAA). Construction of a continent Koch pouch is only performed in select centers today. Laparoscopic and other minimally invasive techniques have been shown to be safe and feasible for each of these procedures and should be strongly considered when expertise is available.

Decision-Making Factors

Choosing the optimal procedure for an individual patient requires close collaboration among the surgeon, gastroenterologist, geneticist, and patient. Several factors may need to be considered.

Disease Phenotype, Risk of Future Malignancy, and Surveillance

The choice between IRA and IPAA requires a careful assessment of the number, size, and histology of the rectal polyps and the difficulty of endoscopic surveillance and interventions. The patient's genotype, family history, and extracolonic disease phenotype should also be known.

An IRA leaves rectal mucosa at risk for malignant transformation. The reported risk of metachronous rectal cancer is 13% to 25% after 15 to 25 years, and it may be as high as 30% by age 60 years. Risk factors include a phenotype of multiple rectal adenomas, increasing age, and genotype. In a recent study, Nieuwenhuis and colleagues (2009) stratified 475 FAP patients by their genotype and predicted their polyp burden. In patients with attenuated, intermediate, or severe polyp burdens, the 20-year cumulative risk of rectal cancer after IRA was 3.7%, 9.3%, and 8.3%, respectively. The associated 20-year risk of secondary proctectomy was 10%, 39%, and 61%. Therefore current consensus favors IRA for patients with a personal and family history of low rectal polyp burden (<20 polyps) and an attenuated phenotype.

Relative contraindications for IRA include a rectal lesion greater than 3 cm, severe dysplasia, and any colorectal malignancy. Patients who choose IRA should commit to close postoperative surveillance and should be informed of the risks of rectal cancer and secondary proctectomy. There is evidence, however, that because IRA has been reserved only for properly selected patients, the rate of metachronous rectal cancer is not as high as previously reported. A four-nation long-term follow-up study by Bulow and colleagues (2009) demonstrated a decrease from 10% to 2% in the recent decade.

On the other hand, an IPAA accomplishes near-complete removal of rectal mucosa and eliminates the risk of rectal cancer. However, patients should still be surveyed endoscopically after an IPAA because adenoma can develop in the ileal pouch at estimated rates of 7%, 35%, and 75% with 5, 10, and 15 years of follow-up, respectively. Although malignant transformation is rare, it has been reported in the literature. In addition to rectal disease, IPAA may be favored in patients predisposed to duodenal or desmoid diseases. IPAA is thought to alter bile salt absorption via the enterohepatic circulation, leading to decreased secondary bile acid production and lessened duodenal exposure to intestinal carcinogens. Biasco and colleagues (2006) reported a lower incidence of advanced duodenal adenoma

TABLE 1: Select phenotype-genotype correlations reported in FAP

Mutation Location	Phenotypic Findings
Codon 1309	Most frequent mutation in FAP; high number of polyps; polyps found at early age (20s)
5' end (codons 1–177) 3' end (codons 1580 and higher)	Attenuated polyposis; <100 polyps; found in the fourth or fifth decades
Codons 168–1580 (except 1309)	Intermediate polyposis; >100 polyps; found in the second or third decades
Codon 1250–1464	Severe/profuse polyposis; >1000 polyps; found in the first or second decades
Codons 976 and 1067	Duodenal adenoma
Codons 1220–1440	Gardner syndrome; desmoid tumors, osteomas, and epidermoid cysts
Codons 1444–1580	Desmoids
Codons 311–1444 or whole gene deletion	Congenital hypertrophy of retinal pigmented epithelium
5' to codon 1220	Thyroid cancer

after IPAA than after IRA (8% vs. 50%) and advocated IPAA for patients with duodenal disease. Additionally, because intraabdominal desmoids may prevent construction of a secondary IPAA after initial IRA, some favor IPAA as the initial procedure in such patients.

Oncologic Requirement

The procedure of choice in patients with dysplasia or invasive cancer is TPC to remove all at-risk mucosa. Whether reconstruction via an IPAA is feasible depends on several factors. First, proximal ligation of the ileocolic vascular bundle during an oncologic resection may limit the mesenteric reach and/or jeopardize the vascular supply to the terminal ileum, making ileal pouch construction not feasible. Second, patients with advanced rectal cancer may require pelvic radiation. Although little literature exists on the subject, surgeons are generally reluctant to construct an IPAA in an irradiated field for concerns of anastomotic complications and fistula formation in the short term and pouch dysfunction and sphincter damage in the long term. Third, the presence of intraabdominal desmoids or upper gastrointestinal (GI) malignancy may preclude IPAA. Desmoid tumors may present as flat plaques that pucker or contract bowel mesentery and limit its reach into the deep pelvis. Extensive resection or reconstruction of the upper GI tract for periampullary tumors may also make construction of IPAA impractical. Thus indications for TPC with an end ileostomy include locally advanced rectal cancer, poor sphincter function, or preclusion of IPAA.

Morbidity, Functional Outcomes, and Quality of Life

Abdominal colectomy with IRA is a relatively simple procedure that does not involve pelvic dissection or a temporary ileostomy. Postoperative ileus may occur in 26% of the patients, but the anastomotic leak rate is low. On the other hand, IPAA is technically demanding; it involves pelvic dissection and often a diverting ileostomy. The overall morbidity rate is high, perhaps over 30%, with a 5% to 10% risk

for intraabdominal abscess and anastomotic leak. Finally, TPC with end ileostomy eliminates anastomotic complications but does involve pelvic dissection.

Functional outcomes of IRA and IPAA have been compared extensively. Hassan and colleagues (2005) found no difference in incontinence or urgency. The median number of daytime stools was six after IPAA and five after IRA, and the number of nighttime stools was two and one, respectively. A meta-analysis by Aziz and colleagues (2006) summarizing 12 observational studies found that IRA patients had decreases in bowel frequency, nighttime defecation, and incontinence pad use compared with IPAA patients.

Although this meta-analysis did not report differences in sexual function, a recent Scandinavian study showed that female fecundity may be reduced to only 54% of normal levels after IPAA, whereas it was unchanged after IRA. A survey of 109 patients after IPAA at our institution by Larson and colleagues (2006) found worsened sexual function among female patients when compared with population norms. Despite these functional deficits, however, most longitudinal studies of QOL find that patients adapt over time; the reported postoperative QOL at 1 year appears to be similar to that of the general population.

Taken together, these findings highlight the importance of assessing a patient's medical comorbidities, ability to withstand potential complications, and baseline bowel and sexual function during preoperative consultation. The surgeon should also aim to understand the patient's priorities and preferences.

Timing of Surgery

For patients with dysplasia or malignancy, surgery should take place as soon as it is convenient, but the optimal time for prophylactic surgery is elusive. Factors to consider may include disruption of life events, plans for reproduction, and the risk of desmoid formation. In young patients, it may be preferable to delay surgery until a growth spurt is finished, emotional maturity is reached, and disturbance of social life and schooling can be minimized. In addition, surgical intervention can trigger desmoid formation. Data from the Familial Gastrointestinal Cancer Registry of 887 patients followed over 25 years showed that girls who underwent colectomy before age 18 years were 1.8 times more likely to develop desmoid tumors when compared with women who underwent colectomy after age 18 years. No difference was observed among male patients.

Because genotype and family history also influence the risk of desmoids, a selective approach postponing colectomy in high-risk young female patients may be prudent. Sexual dysfunction and reproductive complications are risks of pelvic dissection. In a survey of 160 patients who underwent IPAA in Finland, the probability of pregnancy after 2 years of trying was significantly reduced when compared with the control group (56% vs. 91%); at our institution, a higher rate of cesarian section was found among 43 women who had a successful pregnancy after IPAA.

These concerns have led some to advocate a staged approach in which IRA is performed first and IPAA is performed after childbearing is complete. St Mark's Hospital in London recently reported that such an approach with secondary IPAA was not feasible in 8% of the attempted patients; the main reason was intraabdominal desmoid disease. When it was technically feasible, however, no difference was found in rates of morbidity and functional outcomes, except for a higher rate of wound infection in the secondary IPAA group (9% vs. 1%).

Technical Considerations

During an IRA, colonic resection is typically uncomplicated. In malignant cases, oncologic principles of en bloc resection, high vascular ligation, and adequate nodal harvest must be respected. The anastomosis should be placed within the rectum, identified either by taenia coli convergence or by the transition from rectal to colonic mucosa via intraoperative endoscopy. A rectal stump shorter than 10 to 15 cm may be associated with poor reservoir compliance and function and should be avoided. If a staged IPAA is planned in the future, it is advisable to not enter the presacral plane during the primary IRA to facilitate future pelvic dissection. Finally, several anastomotic configurations are possible. An end-to-side anastomosis may be favored for better anastomotic blood supply and less ischemia, and an end-to-end anastomosis avoids blind ends and may facilitate postoperative endoscopic surveillance.

Most commonly, IPAA is formed with a J-pouch configuration. Mesenteric reach may be difficult in obese patients or in tall, slender young men. The ease of a tension-free reach should be assured and can be increased by transversely scoring the peritoneum over the superior mesenteric artery and completely mobilizing the mesentery near the pancreatic head and duodenum. Absence of twisting in the mesentery, proper orientation of the pouch, and no small bowel loops sneaking behind the pouch are ensured prior to making the anastomosis.

The specific technique of anastomosis has been debated. Compared with a stapled IPAA, hand-sewn IPAA with mucosectomy is technically demanding. A meta-analysis of 21 comparative studies found worsened nighttime continence and manometric measurements after mucosectomy. However, with more complete removal of rectal mucosa, a trend toward lower rates of dysplasia in the anal transition zone (ATZ) was observed (7.2% vs. 18.5%). Therefore, in general, if adenomas are present within the ATZ, hand-sewn IPAA with mucosectomy should be performed. When a stapled IPAA is chosen, the transverse staple line should be placed within 1 to 2 cm of the dentate line, such that when the circular stapler is fired, the last 1 cm of rectal mucosa is removed in the distal donut. For adenomas that develop after an IPAA, treatment is controversial. Reported options have included medical treatment with cyclooxygenase (COX)-2 inhibitors, endoscopic removal of adenomas that developed, transanal excision, pouch readvancement, and complete pouch excision.

Redo pelvic procedures in patients with FAP, including pouch excision, are technically difficult. Since tissue planes have been obliterated, careful dissection is needed to avoid injury to surrounding structures; this may be aided by placement of ureteral stents. Consideration should be given to referring the patient to clinicians experienced with these procedures.

Desmoid Tumors

Desmoid tumors consist of differentiated fibroblasts and myofibroblasts within a collagenous stroma; they affect 10% to 20% of FAP patients and represent the major cause for morbidity and mortality after colorectal disease is addressed. Risk factors for desmoid development include prior surgical trauma, family history, hormonal factors (estrogen exposure), and location of the *APC* mutation beyond codon 1400. Over 80% of the desmoids in FAP are intraabdominal; the rest involve the abdominal wall, trunk, or limbs. Intraabdominal desmoids can vary from sheet-like plaques that infiltrate along the small bowel mesentery to large masses that cause obstruction or fistula. Currently, two staging systems exist for desmoid tumors, and one is dedicated to intraabdominal desmoids (Tables 2 and 3).

Surgical treatment of intraabdominal desmoid tumors has been marked by technical difficulty, serious perioperative morbidity (up to 36%), and high recurrence rate (up to 88%). The general reluctance to operate on these patients has led to a stage-specific tiered approach. With increasing stage of disease, treatment may escalate from observation only to COX-2 inhibitors for stage I disease, hormonal therapy (tamoxifen or raloxifene) for stage II disease, and cytotoxic agents (vinblastine, methotrexate, adriamycin) and newer targeted agents (imatinib) for stage III and IV disease. Operative indications may include pain, fistula, obstruction, perforation, and failed medical treatment. The operative goal must be clearly defined preoperatively; tumor resectability is assessed early, and intestinal bypass or proximal diversion should be utilized to effectively palliate symptoms. Unplanned mesenteric devascularization or serosal injuries leading to massive bowel resection should be avoided.

TABLE 2: Staging systems for desmoid tumors: the DES system*

	D (cm)	Rate of Doubling Size (mo)	Location
0	Minimal lesion (desmoplastic reaction)	Unknown at diagnosis	Unknown
1	<5	>24	Extraabdominal
2	5–10	12–24	Abdominal wall
3	10–20	6–12	Mesentery without obstruction
4	>20	1–6	Mesentery with obstruction

*Diameter, expansion, and site.
Modified from Peterschulte G, Lickfeld T, Moeslein G: The desmoid problem, *Chirurg* 71:894–900, 2000.

TABLE 3: Staging system for intraabdominal desmoid tumors

Grade	Description
I	Asymptomatic, <10 cm maximum diameter, and not growing
II	Mildly symptomatic, <10 cm maximum diameter, and not growing
III	Moderately symptomatic (bowel/ureteric obstruction), 10–20 cm, or slowly growing
IV	Severely symptomatic, >20 cm, or rapidly growing

Modified from Church J, Berk T, Bomann BM, et al: Staging intraabdominal desmoid tumors in familial adenomatous polyposis: a search for a uniform approach to a troubling disease, *Dis Colon Rectum* 48:1528–1534, 2005.

Surgical treatment of abdominal wall desmoids, on the other hand, may be undertaken with more enthusiasm. If a large abdominal wall defect is anticipated, preoperative consultation with reconstructive surgical colleagues may be beneficial. Adjunctive treatments, such as preoperative radiation and postoperative sulindac, have been used to help decrease local recurrence rates.

Ampullary and Periampullary Disease

Duodenal adenomas develop in nearly all patients with FAP, but the lifetime risk of duodenal carcinoma is only 5% to 10% by age 60 years; therefore prophylactic surgery for duodenal disease is not recommended, and endoscopic surveillance is emphasized. The most widely used risk stratification is the Spigelman staging system, which predicts the risk of malignancy based on polyp number, size, and histology (Table 4). Low-risk patients are scoped every 1 to 3 years and undergo observation and medical or endoscopic treatments. On the other hand, high-risk patients are surveyed every 6 to 12 months.

Medical therapy with COX-2 inhibitors and endoscopic options including snare polypectomy, endoscopic mucosal resection, and argon-beam plasma coagulation; photodynamic therapy may be utilized to control duodenal disease. Operative intervention, however, is indicated for stage IV disease, failed local or endoscopic therapy, or true carcinoma. For duodenal lesions larger than 1 cm, or with severe

TABLE 4: Spigelman staging system for duodenal familial polyposis and risk of invasive malignancy

	SCORE		
	1	**2**	**3**
Number of lesions	1–4	5–20	>20
Maximum size (mm)	1–4	5–10	>10
Histology	Tubular	Tubovillous	Villous
Dysplasia	Mild	Moderate	Severe

Spigelman Stage	Scores	Risk Stratification Category	Risk of Invasive Cancer (10-Year Follow-up)*
0	0	Low	0%
I	1–4	Low	0%
II	5–6	Low	2%
III	7–8	High	2%
IV	9–12	High	36%

*Data from Groves CJ, Saunders B, Spigelman A, et al: Duodenal cancer in patients with familial adenomatous polyposis: results of a 10 year prospective study, *Gut* 50:636, 2002.

dysplasia, endoscopic ultrasound and abdominal imaging should be done to complete staging. Operative choices include standard or pylorus-sparing pancreaticoduodenectomy (PD) or pancreas-sparing duodenectomy (PSD).

In a literature review, de Castro and colleagues (2009) found comparably significant perioperative mortality (1% vs. 3%) and morbidity (51% vs. 46%) rates after PSD versus PD, although PSD is technically demanding; a small cuff of at-risk duodenal mucosa may be left around the ampulla, but postoperative anatomy allows easier endoscopic surveillance. The major drawbacks of PD are the 2 cm of duodenum preserved beyond the pylorus and the altered anatomy, making endoscopic surveillance difficult. In practice, the choice between PD and PSD will likely depend on local expertise and the surgeon's experience.

MYH-*Associated Polyposis*

Clinical identification of patients with *MYH*-associated polyposis (MAP) is difficult because there is no distinctive phenotype. Most patients exhibit phenotypic overlap with attenuated FAP, with fewer than 10 adenomas usually found in the fourth decade of life and few extracolonic manifestations. However, MAP is an autosomal recessive disease characterized by biallelic germline mutations in *MYH;* its protein product functions in the base excision repair pathway to correct base-pair mismatches that result from oxidative damage. Biallelic carriers have an 80% cumulative lifetime risk of colorectal cancer by age 70 years.

Testing for *MYH* mutation should be pursued in patients with 15 or more adenomas, recessive inheritance, and no germline *APC* mutation. The reported biallelic *MYH* mutation rate in such patients ranges from 7.5% to 69%, depending on colonic polyp severity. In young patients with phenotypic overlap with hereditary nonpolyposis colorectal cancer who test negative for mismatch repair gene defects, the biallelic *MYH* mutation rate has been reported to be 2%.

Patients with MAP should undergo annual or biannual endoscopic surveillance, starting between the ages of 25 and 30 years. The surgical management of MAP is similar to that for FAP, but because of the wide variation in the disease phenotype, decision making is individualized.

Peutz-Jegher Syndrome

Peutz-Jegher syndrome (PJS) is characterized by gastrointestinal hamartomas, mucocutaneous melanotic macules, and significantly elevated risks for cancer in multiple organs. Patients without a known family history are typically diagnosed between the ages of 10 and 30 years, after being seen for bowel obstruction or intussusception, bleeding, or melanotic macules. In up to 70% of PJS patients, mutation in the *STK11/LKB1* gene can be identified. These mutations result in abnormal cell cycle metabolism and cell polarity.

Patients with PJS need a multiorgan surveillance program; in addition to the GI tract, other at-risk organs include the pancreas, lung, breast, cervix (*adenoma malignum*), and ovaries (sex cord tumor with annular tubules) in women and in the testes (Sertoli cell) in men. In this population, the estimated cumulative lifetime risk of developing any cancer is 85% by age 70 years, and malignancies account for the main cause of death.

Indications for operative intervention are 1) symptomatic disease, 2) an asymptomatic polyp larger than 1.5 cm and not amendable to endoscopic management, or 3) malignancy. Intraoperatively, the extent and distribution of all polyps needing intervention should be mapped by palpation, transillumination, and intraoperative endoscopy. For those not amenable to removal via endoscope, enterotomy and polyp excision and/or bowel resection may be needed.

Sites of enterotomy or resection are strategically planned to minimize both the number of suture lines and the length of resected bowel. In addition, some advocate a policy of "clean sweep" surgery to remove all visible polyps in the hopes of decreasing the need for subsequent reexploration. Finally, *pseudoinvasion,* in which normal epithelial cells are seen in the submucosa or muscularis, is a well-described phenomenon in PJS, and distinguishing it from true malignancy may be difficult. When doubt exists, however, it is better to intraoperatively err on the side of performing a wide oncologic resection rather than leaving the patient with an inadequately treated malignancy.

Juvenile Polyposis

Juvenile polyposis (JP) is a hamartomatous polyposis syndrome defined by three criteria: 1) more than five juvenile polyps in the colorectum, 2) multiple juvenile polyps in the upper and lower GI tract, or 3) any number of juvenile polyps with known family history of JP. Germline mutations in either *SMAD4* or *BMPR1A* genes are found in 40% of the patients, while *ENG* may account for additional cases. Both *BMPR1A*, a cell-surface receptor, and *SMAD4*, a cytoplasmic protein mediatior, are critical in the tumor growth factor-β cell–signaling pathway.

Patients with JP vary in disease onset, polyp burden, and polyp distribution, but they most commonly present with anemia, bleeding, polyp prolapse, protein-losing enteropathy, and intussusception. Such patients face elevated risks for colorectal, gastric, small bowel, and pancreatic cancers. Howe and colleagues (1998) described a 38% risk for colorectal cancer and a 21% risk for upper GI cancer, and they recommend upper and lower endoscopies starting at age 15 years or when patients become symptomatic. Colectomy should be reserved for those patients with a high polyp burden, suspected cancer, or severe symptoms such as anemia, obstruction, and protein-losing enteropathy. Postoperative surveillance should be continued because of high rates of polyp recurrence. Finally, when bleeding, obstruction, or malignant gastric disease warrants operative intervention, subtotal or total gastrectomy may be required.

JP should be distinguished from other autosomal-dominant *PTEN* hamartomatous polyposis syndromes. Patients with Bannayan-Riley-Ruvalcaba syndrome exhibit a characteristic phenotype of macrocephaly, lipomas, and pigmented macules of the body and penis. Those with Cowden syndrome exhibit macrocephaly, trichilemmomas, and gingival papillomatous papules; these patients should also be evaluated for thyroid, breast, and endometrial cancers.

Selected Readings

Aziz O, Athanasiou T, Fazio VW, et al: Meta-analysis of observational studies of ileorectal versus ileal pouch–anal anastomosis for familial adenomatous polyposis, *Br J Surg* 93(4):407–417, 2006.

Church J, Simmang C: Practice parameters for the treatment of patients with dominantly inherited colorectal cancer (familial adenomatous polyposis and hereditary nonpolyposis colorectal cancer), *Dis Colon Rectum* 46(8):1001–1012, 2003.

da Luz Moreira A, Church JM, Burke CA: The evolution of prophylactic colorectal surgery for familial adenomatous polyposis,, *Dis Colon Rectum* 52(8):1481–1486, 2009.

Howe JR, Mitros FA, Summers RW: The risk of gastrointestinal carcinoma in familial juvenile polyposis,, *Ann Surg Oncol* 5(8):751–756, 1998.

Nieuwenhuis MH, Bulow S, Bjork J, et al: Genotype predicting phenotype in familial adenomatous polyposis: a practical application to the choice of surgery, *Dis Colon Rectum* 52(7):1259–1263, 2009.

Sieber OM, Lipton L, Crabtree M, et al: Multiple colorectal adenomas, classic adenomatous polyposis, and germline mutations in, *MYH, N Engl J Med* 348(9):791–799, 2003.

Sturt NJ, Clark SK: Current ideas in desmoid tumours, *Fam Cancer* 5(3):275–285, 2006.

COLON CANCER

Theodor Asgeirsson, MD, and Anthony J. Senagore, MD, MBA

OVERVIEW

Colon and rectal malignancies continue to be the second most common cause of cancer death, after lung cancer, with over 50,000 deaths per year in the United States. *Colon cancer* is defined as a lesion within the large bowel above the rectosigmoid junction at the reconstitution of the circumferential longitudinal muscle layer from the taenia coli. Adenocarcinoma of the colon accounts for over two thirds of colorectal malignancies, and despite aggressive screening guidelines, it shows up initially as advanced disease more than 60% of the time. Survival is clearly superior in earlier stage disease; therefore early detection, better implementation and compliance with screening modalities, and prompt surgical intervention are the mainstays for better patient survival in colon cancer. Despite moderate 5-year survival benefits after reresection of recurrent disease, only 10% of recurrences are resectable, with curative intent limiting salvage of treatment failures.

SCREENING AND PRESENTATION

In the United States, reduction in the incidence of distal colorectal malignancies and, to a lesser extent, cancer-specific mortality have contributed to policies for broader implementation of screening colonoscopy; in Europe, the same trends have not been as clear. Colonoscopy is the screening tool of choice in the United States, and epidemiologic trends in colon cancers point to the emphasis of adequate prep quality, cecal intubation, and removal of clinically significant adenomatous lesions.

Revised colorectal cancer screening guidelines from the American Cancer Society have been endorsed by The American Society of Colon and Rectal Surgeons. These guidelines divide the population into three categories based on risk of colorectal cancer: *average* (65% to 75% of population), *moderate* (20% to 30%), and *high* (6% to 8%). Screening for average-risk individuals should begin at age 50 years and includes annual digital rectal exam and either fecal occult blood testing yearly and flexible sigmoidoscopy every 5 years or total colon exam every 5 to 10 years (colonoscopy or double-contrast barium enema and proctosigmoidoscopy). *Moderate risk* is defined as one or

more first-degree relatives with colorectal cancer or a personal history of colorectal neoplasia. In this population, screening includes colonoscopy every 5 years, either beginning at age 40 years or at an age 10 years younger than the youngest affected relative. If the patient has a personal history of a significant adenomatous polyp (>1 cm), the patient should undergo colonoscopy annually until colonoscopy results are negative for significant polyps, and then move to less frequent colonoscopic follow-up every 5 years. *High-risk* individuals are those with a hereditary or genetic predisposition, such as familial adenomatous polyposis, hereditary nonpolyposis colorectal cancer, or inflammatory bowel disease lasting longer than 10 years. These patients should be screened annually once the diagnosis is confirmed, and family members should receive genetic counseling and testing. Prophylactic or therapeutic abdominal colectomy with ileorectal anastomosis or total proctocolectomy are the appropriate interventions if premalignant or malignant lesions are found during screening.

The majority of colon cancers are sporadic neoplasms found during routine physical exam or screening colonoscopy in asymptomatic patients. When symptomatic, the location of the tumor dictates the symptomatology. Right-sided lesions present with anemia, vague abdominal pain, weight loss, and changes in bowel habits. Left-sided lesions are more likely to present with changes in bowel habits, rectal bleeding, and abdominal pain. Left-sided colon cancers are more likely to present with obstruction compared with the right side, which may likely be explained by differences in bowel diameter and stool consistency.

DIAGNOSIS

After identification of colon cancer, a thorough evaluation is required to rule out synchronous cancers (6%) and significant polyps. If colonoscopy cannot be performed, an air contrast barium enema or computed tomography (CT) colonography are acceptable alternatives for full colonic evaluation. Surgery remains the mainstay of therapy after complete endoscopic evaluation of the colon for other lesions. A detailed family history of colon cancer should be determined because, as previously mentioned, 6% to 8% of colon cancers are hereditary. The patient should then be assessed for surgical risk, including comorbidities and a physical exam focusing on cardiopulmonary assessment and hepatosplenomegaly, abdominal masses, or ascites indicative of advanced disease. Of note, 10% of colorectal cancers present with liver metastasis.

Advanced disease is seen most commonly with local invasion to adjacent structures (e.g., duodenum, pancreas, kidney) and/or metastasis to the liver via portal venous drainage or to the lungs via hematogenous spread. CT of the abdomen remains the most cost-effective tool for preoperative assessment of extent of disease. A chest radiograph should also be performed, and any suspicious lesions should be evaluated with CT of the chest. The value of obtaining these studies as part of the preoperative evaluation not only minimizes the risk of any intraoperative surprises but also may alter the approach to initial care. Positron emission tomography (PET) scans offer little value in the assessment of primary lesions but may be advantageous in recurrent or metastatic disease treatment schema.

Laboratory work should be based on comorbid conditions and clinical presentation. Anemia should be assessed and managed preoperatively. Preoperative carcinoembryonic antigen (CEA) is routinely used for advanced and metastatic disease and may be a predictor of poor outcome based on clearance of elevated levels prior to resection.

Choice of surgical resection is based upon accurate localization of the primary lesion, exclusion of family cancer syndromes, extent of disease, and operative risk assessment. In addition, tattooing of polyps or cancer sites should be performed in lesions that may be nonpalpable or when laparoscopic resection is considered.

Staging

The TNM staging system is currently the accepted universal staging system for colorectal cancer. This system was developed by the American Joint Committee on Cancer (AJCC) in cooperation with the TNM Committee of the International Union Against Cancer. Revisions have been made in current editions of stage II and stage III, with subgroupings based on survival and relapse data (Table 1).

TABLE 1: TNM classification for colorectal cancer staging

Stage 0	Tis, N0, M0
Stage I	T1, N0, M0
	T2, N0, M0
Stage IIA	T3, N0, M0
Stage IIB	T4, N0, M0
Stage IIIA	T1, N1, M0
	T2, N1, M0
Stage IIIB	T3, N1, M0
	T4, N1, M0
Stage IIIC	Any T, N2, M0
Stage IV	Any T, any N, M1
5-Year Survival	
Stage I	70%–95%
Stage II	54%–65%
Stage III	39%–60%
Stage IV	0%–16%

Primary tumor (**T**): *Tis*, carcinoma in situ: intraepithelial or invasion of the lamina propria; *T0*, no evidence of primary tumor; *T1*, tumor invades submucosa; *T2*, tumor invades muscularis propria; *T3*, tumor invades through the muscularis propria into the subserosa or into nonperitonealized pericolic or perirectal tissues; *T4*, tumor directly invades other organs or structures and/or perforates visceral peritoneum.
Regional lymph nodes (**N**): *N0*, no regional lymph node metastasis; *N1*, metastasis in one to three regional lymph nodes; *N2*, metastases in four or more regional lymph nodes.
Distant metastasis (**M**): *M0*, no distant metastasis; *M1*: distant metastasis.
(From the American Joint Committee on Cancers: *AJCC cancer staging manual*, ed 7, New York, 2010, Springer.)

▮ SURGICAL MANAGEMENT

Resection for colon cancer is the mainstay of curative treatment and requires advanced anatomic knowledge of the intraperitoneal and retroperitoneal components of the large bowel. In addition, anatomic distribution of feeding vessels, watershed areas, and lymphatic drainage dictates the limits of resections. The goal of surgical therapy is complete resection of the primary lesion, primary feeding vessel, adjacent organs if local invasion is present, and the regional lymph nodes to yield an R0 resection. Resection margins should be 2 to 5 cm.

Intraoperative evaluation of metastatic disease cannot be underestimated. Liver, peritoneal surfaces (ovaries, diaphragm), omentum, and paraaortic lymph nodes should be assessed for metastatic disease.

The basic tenets of an oncologically appropriate colon cancer resection require ligation of the appropriate arterial and venous blood supply to provide adequate lymph node clearance and resection of sufficient bowel length to provide clear proximal, distal, and radial margins and appropriately vascularized segments for a tension-free anastomosis. The cecum, ascending colon, and hepatic flexure are fed by the ileocolic, right colic, and branches of the middle colic artery, which requires a formal right or extended right colectomy (the middle colic artery needs to be taken), depending on the anatomic location of the lesion.

The transverse colon is fed mainly by the middle colic artery. Transverse colectomies can be complicated by difficulty in creating a safe, well-vascularized, and tension-free anastomosis, so an extended left or right colectomy may be a safer option. The sigmoid, descending, and splenic flexure are fed by the inferior mesenteric, left, and branches of the middle colic artery, respectively. In a fashion similar to the right side, it may require segmental or extended resection involving the middle colic artery. If a synchronous lesion is found in a different anatomic segment of the colon during or prior to resection, a subtotal colectomy should be considered.

Laparoscopic Colectomy

Prospective randomized trials have shown that oncology outcomes for laparoscopic colon resection are equivalent to open colon resection. With increasing adoption of this technique, the postoperative benefits are becoming clearer, with decreased length of stay and reduced incidence of postoperative ileus compared with open resections. In the past, concerns with this technique in regard to maintaining oncologic principles, port site metastasis, technical feasibility, and length of operative time limited the generalized use of laparoscopy for colon cancer resection. In experienced hands, however, all oncologic priniciples can be maintained. Operative time is comparable to open resection, and with meticulous specimen handling and extraction techniques, port site metastases are no more common than incisional metastases in open colon cancer resections. Prior limitations of technical feasibility will be reduced, as will the learning curve, as more general surgeons and colorectal surgeons are trained in advanced laparoscopy. The emphasis of training in laparoscopic colectomy for colon cancer should be on safe bowel handling, medial to lateral dissection, and acknowledgement that early conversion to open colectomy if required is in the patient's best interest.

Importance of Adequate Lymph Node Assessment

Prognosis after colon cancer resection is dependent on multiple factors. Tumor invasion (T stage) and lymph node involvement (N stage) most strongly correlate with 5-year survival in curative colon cancer resection, and current guidelines for postoperative adjuvant chemotherapy are based on lymph node involvement. T1 lesions have a 9% to 10% risk of lymph node involvement, T2 lesions have a 25%

risk, and T3 lesions have a 45% risk. The National Comprehensive Cancer Network (NCCN) recommends that no fewer than 12 nodes be microscopically examined to determine the nodal status accurately. Although controversial as a quality measure, this assessment is thought to avoid understaging patients with presumed stage II disease and therefore offers the possible benefit of adjuvant chemotherapy.

The key components of successful lymph node evaluation are a complete anatomic lymphadenectomy and an understanding between surgeon and pathologist of the importance of histologic evaluation of resected nodes. Variations in immunologic responses to lesions may explain differences in lymph node retrieval among patients in some cases. Additional pathological techniques, such as fat clearing, may be required to increase lymph node retrieval from resected specimen. Sentinel lymph node mapping is experimental, and its value as part of staging, particularly as an indicator of effective adjuvant chemotherapy, has not been defined.

Special Circumstances

Obstructing cancers require careful preoperative physiologic evaluation and resuscitation of the patient prior to surgical intervention, because operative mortality is increased significantly in these situations. The presence of impending perforation often precludes preoperative evaluation for synchronous colonic neoplasia and metastatic disease; therefore intraoperative evaluation of the local extent of disease and of the liver will be relied upon to guide the procedure.

The presence of significant colonic distension and fecal loading impacts the ability to safely perform a segmental colectomy with primary anastomosis. Surgical options include subtotal colectomy for left-sided obstruction; on-table colonic lavage with segmental colectomy, with or without diverting loop ileostomy; or Hartmann resection. The latter option is typically reserved for extreme situations or for patients in whom the colostomy is likely to be permanent because of the higher complexity of the Hartmann closure. Right-sided obstructing lesions are most typically managed by right hemicolectomy and primary anastomosis.

Colonic stenting has been advocated as a bridging step to relieve colonic obstruction, particularly left-sided colonic obstruction. Small series have demonstrated safety and efficacy in converting the procedure to a one-stage segmental resection. However, the limited data make assessment of comparative effectiveness difficult with respect to risk of perforation or migration of the stent. Cost of the stents is also significant, therefore more evaluation is required to define the true place of stenting in the algorithm of obstructive colon cancer.

In a similar fashion, a perforated colon requires careful but prompt surgical evaluation. For patients with perforation and peritonitis, abdominal washout and resection of perforated bowel with fecal diversion is a way to minimize the risk of overwhelming sepsis. If not involved in the perforation, removing tumor is based on hemodynamic stability of the patient during intervention. Locally contained perforations with abscess may be drained percutaneously, and further evaluation is performed before formal resection. If resection and anastomosis are performed, it would be unwise not to protect the anastomosis with a diverting ostomy to minimize the risk of septic complications from anastomotic disruption.

Multiple modalities are available for treatment of liver metastases, including palliative chemotherapy, surgical resection, and radiofrequency ablation. Thorough evaluation of the liver is required to make the best estimate of the anatomic location of such lesions, taking into account proximity to major vascular and biliary structures. Surgical resection must spare 15% of the liver parenchyma to allow adequate function. CT, PET, magnetic resonance imaging, and intraoperative ultrasound may be used for such evaluation, and accurate staging and precise surgical technique may result in 25% to 30% 5-year survival in such situations.

The approach to a patient with a primary colon cancer and resectable liver cancer has become more complex based upon several possible approaches: 1) resection of the colonic segment, followed by chemotherapy and delayed liver resection; 2) resection of the liver disease, followed by delayed colonic resection; or 3) simultaneous liver and colonic resection. In experienced hands, the last option can be performed safely, but the operative risk is clearly higher than with the other two approaches. A nonbleeding, nonobstructing colonic lesion offers the potential for a liver-first approach. A colon-first approach offers the potential to avoid risk related to hepatectomy in patients who will demonstrate early development of multilobar disease. Future investigation of these approaches is required to define the optimal strategy.

Prophylactic oophorectomy should not be performed routinely, although it may decrease the risk of ovarian cancer in postmenopausal patients or in those with family cancer syndromes. Surgeons need to be aware that up to 30% of advanced colon and rectal cancers may have metastases to the ovaries, however, this pattern of involvement may actually be hematogenous spread rather than local extension from the colon. Identification of an ovarian mass in the setting of advanced colorectal cancer should be considered metastatic, and bilateral oophorectomy is the appropriate approach.

En bloc resection refers to resection of tumors and adjacent structures in locally advanced colon and rectal cancer. It is important to recognize that survival for patients with direct extension of colon cancer is related to nodal status, assuming an R0 resection is performed on the primary disease. As always, oncologic principles should be followed and free tumor margins achieved, which may require duodenectomy, pancreatectomy, total abdominal hysterectomy/bilateral salpingo-oophorectomy, or partial or total nephrectomy in addition to colonic resection.

Adjuvant Therapy

About 30% to 70% of all node-positive (stage III) patients develop recurrence of their disease, and adjuvant chemotherapy has been shown to increase 5-year survival 10% to 15% in this patient population. Current recommendations are that all medically appropriate node-positive patients receive adjuvant chemotherapy for 6 months after colon cancer resection. Newer publications have shown response in high-risk stage II (T4, poor histologic grade, peritumoral lymphovascular involvement, obstruction, T3 with local perforation, and close or positive margins), and there has been a shift toward treating these individuals with adjuvant chemotherapy.

Despite some variation in regimens of adjuvant chemotherapy, all chemotherapeutic regimens are 5-fluorouracil based, although the most typical regimen includes leucovorin and oxaliplatin. Increasing knowledge of processes at the molecular level is showing promise in detecting optimal responders to adjuvant chemotherapy and chemoresistance, as has been suggested in microsatellite instability tumors, the association with wild type K-RAS, and sensitivity to antiepidermal growth factor agents. Radiation therapy has no defined role in current guidelines for treatment of colon cancer.

Follow-up

Follow-up strategies after colon cancer resection are implemented in the hopes of early identification of recurrent disease at a point where curative intervention is possible. The recommended strategies have ranged from intensive imaging and biochemical evaluation to much less aggressive symptom-based assessment. Despite multiple strategies, only 10% of recurrences are resectable with curative intent, albeit with the potential for 25% to 30% 5-year survival after treatment. A reasonable approach to surveillance after curative resection includes quarterly office history and physical examination with CEA assay and annual CT scan of the abdomen, chest radiograph, and colonoscopy (primarily for metachronous polyps or cancers). Because 60% to 80% of recurrences occur within 2 years of colon cancer resection, and 90% occur within 5 years, this strategy (office visit and CEA) can be applied for the first 2 years and then every 6 months for 2 years. After a normal colonoscopy at the first anniversary, colonoscopy can be deferred to every 3 years. The risk of metachronous polyps is 30% to 56%, and the risk of a metachronous cancer is 2% to 8%. After 5 years, surveillance is likely of limited value.

Suggested Readings

Benson AB 3d, Schrag D, Sommerfield MR, et al: American Society of Clinical Oncology recommendations on adjuvant chemotherapy for stage II colon cancer, *J Clin Oncol* 22:3408–3419, 2004.

Byers T, Levin B, Rothenberger D, et al: American Cancer Society guidelines for screening and surveillance for early detection of colorectal polyps and cancer: update 1997, American Cancer Society Detection and Treatment Advisory Group on Colorectal Cancer, *CA Cancer J Clin* 47:154–160, 1997.

The COLOR: Study Group: Impact of hospital case volume on short-term outcome after laparoscopic operation for colonic cancer, *Surg Endosc* 19:687–692, 2005.

Fleshman J, Sargent DF, Green E, et al: Laparoscopic colectomy for cancer is not inferior to open surgery based on 5-year data from the COST study group trial, *Ann Surg* 246(4):655–664, 2007.

Horner MJ, Ries LAG, Krapcho M et al, editors: *SEER Cancer Statistics Review, 1975–2006*, Bethesda, MD, November 2008, National Cancer Institute, http://seer.cancer.gov/csr/1975_2006, based on SEER data submission.

Otchy D, Hyman NH, Simmang C, et al: Practice parameters for colon cancer, *Dis Colon Rectum* 47(8):1269–1284, 2004.

Rectal Cancer

Jason Park, MD, MEd, and Jose G. Guillem, MD, MPH

OVERVIEW

An estimated 148,810 new cases of colorectal cancer were diagnosed in the United States in 2008, about 28% of which occurred in the rectum. Despite the development of screening guidelines and significant advances in combined therapeutic modalities, colorectal cancer remains the second leading cause of cancer-related deaths in the United States, after lung cancer, with an estimated 49,960 cancer deaths from colon or rectal cancer in 2008.

The medical literature contains various and sometimes discrepant definitions for the junction of the colon and rectum, and these discrepancies can lead to uncertainty when assigning patients to colon or rectal cancer treatment protocols. Anatomically, the rectum extends from the rectosigmoid junction to the anal canal (Figure 1). However, from an oncologic standpoint, it is the distal 10 to 12 cm (withstanding individual variation) in the extraperitoneal pelvis that constitutes the rectum. Cancers that occur proximal to this level, in the intraperitoneal rectum, behave more like colon cancers with regard to recurrence patterns and prognosis.

This chapter reviews the preoperative evaluation and clinical staging of patients with rectal cancer and management options based on stage of disease, highlighting in particular the role of sequenced multimodal therapy (surgery, radiation therapy, and chemotherapy). Important practical considerations regarding surgery and other technical approaches for patients with rectal cancer are also discussed.

PREOPERATIVE EVALUATION

History and Physical Examination

A complete history and physical examination by the surgeon are essential components of the initial evaluation of rectal cancer patients. The history should include a detailed family history to assess for the possibility of a hereditary or familial syndrome. In addition, when an ostomy is a consideration, preoperative counseling with an enterostomal therapist should be offered when available.

A complete physical examination of patients with rectal cancer includes a digital rectal examination (DRE) and rigid sigmoidoscopy. The DRE enables assessment of size, degree of fixation, and location of disease relative to the upper part of the anorectal ring. Rigid sigmoidoscopy is usually performed in conjunction with the DRE. It allows delineation of tumor orientation (anterior, lateral, or posterior) and circumferential involvement, evaluated as a percentage of the entire bowel wall circumference, and it allows the most precise measurement of tumor distance from the anal verge. This information is useful in preoperative planning to help determine the need for neoadjuvant treatment and the likelihood of preserving anorectal function. A full colonoscopy should also be performed, because at least 5% of patients with rectal cancer will have synchronous lesions that may alter treatment plans. In addition to basic laboratory blood tests, a baseline carcinoembryonic antigen (CEA) level is also recommended, mainly for postoperative surveillance purposes.

Preoperative Imaging Studies

Accurate pretreatment imaging is needed to 1) delineate the depth of tumor penetration through the rectal wall, 2) assess whether locoregional lymph nodes (LN) are involved, and 3) determine the absence or presence of metastatic disease. The most common imaging studies currently used to acquire this information for rectal cancer are endorectal ultrasound (ERUS), magnetic resonance imaging (MRI), computed tomography (CT), and positron emission tomography (PET) scans.

Both ERUS and pelvic MRI can provide important preoperative locoregional staging information for rectal cancer. The choice between these two studies depends in part on local expertise, institutional resources, and accessibility. ERUS is an office-based procedure that can be used to clinically assess the depth of bowel wall penetration (T stage) and LN involvement (N stage). Figure 2 shows a schematic view of the layers of the rectum as seen on ERUS, and it gives an example of the normal layers of the rectal wall.

In the literature, the accuracy of staging by ERUS is variable and ranges from 63% to 96% for T stage and 63% to 86% for N stage. However, a recent review suggests that the accuracy for locoregional staging by ERUS may be overestimated in the literature, with a decline in accuracy noted over time and the lowest accuracy being reported in the more recent literature. Accurate staging by ERUS is highly operator dependent, and a steep learning curve applies for learning to perform and interpret ERUS.

Phased-array MRI is a relatively new modality that offers improved soft tissue resolution, which makes it useful to assess for breaches of the mesorectal fascia and potential tumor involvement with surrounding pelvic structures. In determining bowel wall penetration, MRI and ERUS have comparable overall accuracy rates, but MRI appears to be more accurate for T3/T4 lesions. Nodal staging is comparable between MRI and ERUS. Although MRI is less operator dependent than ERUS, its use may be limited by cost and accessibility.

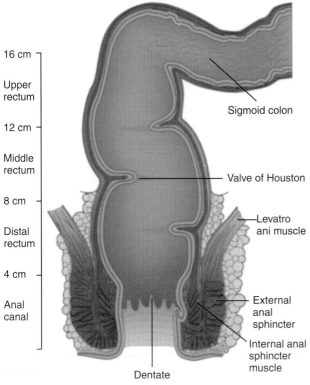

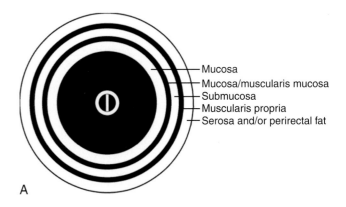

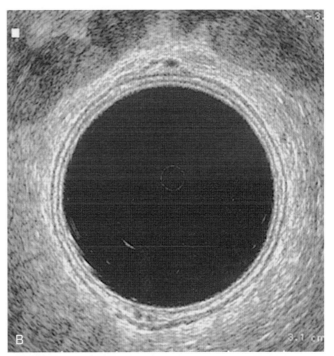

FIGURE 1   Anatomy of the rectum.

FIGURE 2   Layers of the rectal wall. **A,** Schematic drawing of the layers of the rectal wall seen on ERUS. **B,** Example of an ERUS image of the normal layers of the rectal wall in a male patient. (**B** *from Kim HJ, Wong WD: Role of endorectal ultrasound in the conservative evaluation of rectal cancer, Semin Surg Oncol 19:360, 2000.*)

CT of the abdomen and pelvis are mainly used in primary rectal cancer to assess for intraabdominal metastasis. CT may also provide some information regarding adjacent organ involvement in advanced cases, but it is less accurate than both ERUS and MRI for T- and N-staging purposes, which limits its role in locoregional staging.

PET is being used with increased frequency to stage various cancers, but data are limited for examining its role in primary rectal cancer. PET has not been shown to offer an advantage over ERUS or MRI with regard to locoregional staging, and PET is not routinely indicated as an initial imaging study for evaluating patients with primary disease. However, PET and especially PET-CT can detect distant metastasis and may help to differentiate lesions that are indeterminate, particularly nonregional LNs and liver and lung lesions, on other conventional diagnostic imaging modalities.

The ultimate goal of the preoperative workup is to accurately stage the patient's disease in a timely and cost-effective manner. Given the multitude of imaging modalities from which to choose, it is important to understand the type of information that each provides and to have specific reasons for ordering each test. During the initial workup of primary disease, our practice is to include ERUS for locoregional staging and intravenous contrast-enhanced CT of the chest, abdomen, and pelvis to assess for intraabdominal and lung metastasis. Patients in whom locally advanced T4 rectal cancer is suspected undergo a phased-array pelvic MRI to obtain more detail regarding possible involvement of pelvic structures and to assess resectability. We selectively obtain PET-CT scans when it is necessary to further characterize indeterminate distant lesions found on abdominopelvic and chest CT.

Staging

Following the diagnosis of rectal cancer, the patient is clinically staged by integrating the history and physical examination with the results of preoperative imaging studies. The clinical stage is then used to select the most appropriate treatment strategies for individual patients. Although the imaging studies described above form the current standard of care, there are clear limitations to these studies, and the implications of either clinically understaging or overstaging disease must be recognized. Implicit to this discussion is the continued need to develop techniques to improve the clinical staging of rectal cancer.

Definite pathologic staging is carried out after surgical resection. Currently, the International Union Against Cancer (UICC) TNM classification is the preferred system to stage rectal cancer. The most recent version of the TNM staging system (seventh edition, 2010) further subdivides stage II, III, and IV disease to better reflect prognosis within these groups (Table 1). The American Joint Commission on Cancer (AJCC) recommends the histologic examination of a minimum of 12 LNs to adequately assess nodal status and accurately stage patients.

Management Based on Clinical Stage

Deciding on the optimal treatment plan for patients with rectal cancer can be a complex and highly individualized process. Multimodal therapy that combines radiation therapy (RT), chemotherapy, and surgery

TABLE 1: AJCC TNM staging system for colon and rectal cancers

Primary Tumor (T)

TX	Primary tumor cannot be assessed
T0	No evidence of primary tumor
Tis	Carcinoma in situ: intraepithelial or invasion of lamina propria*
T1	Tumor invades submucosa
T2	Tumor invades muscularis propria
T3	Tumor invades through the muscularis propria into pericolorectal tissues
T4a	Tumor penetrates to the surface of the visceral peritoneum
T4b	Tumor directly invades or is adherent to other organs or structures

Regional Lymph Nodes (N)

NX	Regional lymph nodes cannot be assessed
N0	No regional lymph node metastasis
N1	Metastasis in one to three regional lymph nodes
N1a	Metastasis in one regional lymph node
N1b	Metastasis in two to three regional lymph nodes
N1c	Tumor deposits in the subserosa, mesentery, or nonperitonealized pericolic or perirectal tissues without regional nodal metastasis
N2	Metastasis in four or more regional lymph nodes
N2a	Metastasis in four to six regional lymph nodes
N2b	Metastasis in seven or more regional lymph nodes

Distant Metastasis (M)

M0	No distant metastasis
M1	Distant metastasis
M1a	Metastasis confined to one organ or site (e.g., liver, lung, ovary, nonregional node)
M1b	Metastases in more than one organ or site or the peritoneum

ANATOMIC STAGE/PROGNOSTIC GROUPS

Stage	T	N	M	Dukes*	MAC*
0	Tis	N0	M0	–	–
I	T1	N0	M0	A	A
	T2	N0	M0	A	B1
IIA	T3	N0	M0	B	B2
IIB	T4a	N0	M0	B	B2
IIC	T4b	N0	M0	B	B3
IIIA	T1-T2	N1/N1c	M0	C	C1
	T1	N2a	M0	C	C1
IIIB	T3-T4a	N1/N1c	M0	C	C2

Continued

TABLE 1: AJCC TNM staging system for colon and rectal cancers—cont'd

		ANATOMIC STAGE/PROGNOSTIC GROUPS			
Stage	T	N	M	Dukes*	MAC*
	T2-T3	N2a	M0	C	C1/C2
	T1-T2	N2b	M0	C	C1
IIIC	T4a	N2a	M0	C	C2
	T3-T4a	N2b	M0	C	C2
	T4b	N1-N2	M0	C	C3
IVA	Any T	Any N	M1a	–	–
IVB	Any T	Any N	M1b	–	–

*Dukes B is a composite of better (T3/N0/M0) and worse (T4/N0/M0) prognostic groups, as is Dukes C (any T/N1/M0 and any T/N2/M0). MAC is the modified Astler-Coller classification.
(From the *AJCC cancer staging manual*, ed 7, New York, 2010, Springer–Verlag.)

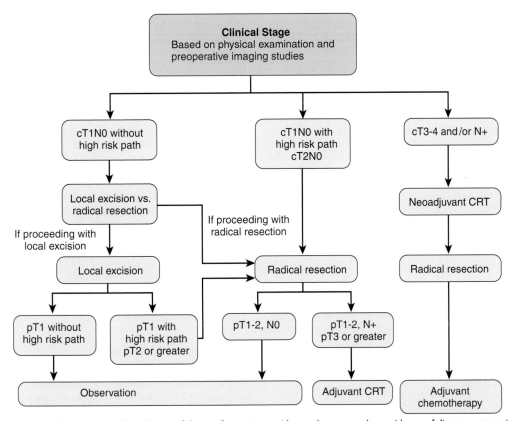

FIGURE 3 Treatment algorithm based on clinical stage of disease for patients with rectal cancer and no evidence of distant metastasis. *C,* clinical stage; *P,* pathologic stage. *High-risk path* refers to 1) poor differentiation, 2) the presence of lymphovascular or perineural invasion, or 3) deep submucosal invasion (sm2 or sm3). NOTE: Local excision can be considered in patients who have a significant medical contraindication to major abdominal surgery or who make the informed decision to avoid the short-term morbidity, functional consequences, and possible stoma associated with radical surgery with full knowledge that local excision is associated with a significantly higher recurrence rate and may compromise their chances of cure.

is accepted as the standard of care for patients with rectal cancers, although the precise type and sequence of modalities depends on the stage at presentation. Particularly complex cases should be reviewed in the setting of a multidisciplinary tumor board. A proposed algorithm for the treatment of patients with rectal cancer is presented in Figure 3.

Even with the advances made in combined modality therapy, surgery remains the cornerstone of curative treatment for rectal cancer.

Early rectal cancers (stage I) can be definitively treated by surgery alone; however, patients with more advanced (stage II and III) rectal cancers are treated with neoadjuvant therapy prior to surgery to decrease the risk of recurrence and optimize oncologic outcomes.

The surgical options for individual patients depend largely on the location and extent of disease, although patient factors, such as comorbid medical conditions and baseline anorectal function, are also considered. The main surgical approaches for rectal cancer include local excision procedures such as polypectomy, transanal excision, or transanal endoscopic microsurgery and radical procedures that involve a transabdominal low anterior resection (LAR) or abdominoperineal resection (APR). The goals of surgical resection with curative intent are complete resection of the primary tumor with adequate margins, an anatomically complete lymphadenectomy of draining LNs, and en bloc resection of contiguously involved structures.

Carcinoma In Situ and T1N0 Rectal Cancer

Local excision is commonly used as a treatment strategy for carcinoma in situ (CIS) and small adenocarcinomas limited to the rectal mucosa. Local excision aims to fully excise the rectal lesion with negative margins, but regional LNs are generally not removed. These procedures are appealing because they are associated with lower operative morbidity and better preservation of long-term anorectal function compared with more radical resection. Treatment by local excision may also allow some patients to avoid a permanent colostomy.

Many authors have attempted to develop and validate criteria that are purportedly associated with low-risk T1 cancers to identify those patients who might be suitable for treatment by excision as definitive therapy without compromising oncologic outcomes. Some of these criteria are listed in Table 2. However, even when strict selection criteria for local excision are applied, local recurrence is common, with documented local recurrence rates in the range of 11% to 29% in most series with long-term follow-up. A large, retrospective review of patients who underwent surgery for T1 rectal cancers at Memorial Sloan-Kettering Cancer Center found an estimated 5-year local recurrence rate of 15% for patients treated with local excision compared with 3% for patients selected for treatment with radical resection. Long-term follow-up suggests that local excision may also be associated with decreased disease-specific survival and overall survival.

From an oncologic standpoint, the main problems with local excision are the risk of unresected regional LN disease and incomplete pathologic staging because regional nodes are not pathologically assessed. Retrospective data on patients who underwent radical resection for T1 rectal cancer suggest the prevalence of LN metastasis may be as high as 18%. Patients who undergo local excision may have LN metastases that are not identified and are therefore not treated surgically or with adjuvant therapy, which likely accounts for the higher local recurrence rates seen with excision alone. In patients who develop a pelvic recurrence of rectal cancer after local excision,

salvage surgery is possible in selected cases, but the outcomes are rather poor when the early stage of the initial disease is considered. Data from a single institution series showed a postsalvage actuarial 5-year DSS of just over 50% in these highly selected patients.

Given the high local recurrence rate, these data would argue against local excision as definitive treatment for T1 rectal cancers, even for those with favorable histologic features. Local excision should be limited to cases of cancer in which a significant medical contraindication to major abdominal surgery exists—or the patient has low-risk disease and makes the informed decision to avoid the short-term morbidity, functional consequences, and possible permanent colostomy related to radical surgery, with full knowledge that local excision is associated with a significantly higher recurrence rate and may compromise chances of cure.

Complete local excision is acceptable as definitive treatment for small CIS of the rectum, although patients who undergo local excision for a lesion that is thought to be CIS on biopsy but is later found to be invasive cancer after excision should be considered for radical resection, again depending on the above factors. Radical resection is associated with low recurrence rates and offers the more definitive surgical treatment for T1 rectal cancers.

T2N0 Rectal Cancer

For tumors that appear to invade the musclaris propria without LN involvement (T2N0) on preoperative evaluation, the standard treatment is radical resection in patients who are acceptable operative candidates. If LNs are found to be involved on subsequent pathologic examination of the resected specimens, postoperative adjuvant chemoradiation (CRT) is recommended.

In very select clinical T2N0 rectal cancers, preoperative external-beam RT can be considered when a bulky tumor in close proximity to the upper part of the anorectal sphincter precludes sphincter preservation. A good response to RT may sufficiently reduce tumor bulk to allow the surgeon to perform an LAR, which might not have been possible otherwise. One small, retrospective series reported on 27 patients with T2N0 distal rectal cancers on preoperative staging who refused APR despite the consulting surgeon's judgment that it was required. These selected patients were treated with a long course of pelvic RT, without concurrent chemotherapy, followed by resection 4 to 7 weeks later. Of these, 78% percent were subsequently able to undergo resection with a sphincter-preserving procedure, and these patients had an actuarial 5-year disease-free survival of 77% with a median follow-up of 55 months. Although these results show promise, it should be recognized that if the tumor directly invades the anorectal sphincter, a restorative procedure is unlikely, even when a complete response to RT is achieved.

Locally Advanced Rectal Cancer

In patients with transmural and/or node-positive (T3/T4 and/or N+) disease without evidence of distant metastases, the sequence of neoadjuvant CRT followed by radical resection results in superior local control compared with initial surgery followed by CRT. Long-term follow-up data suggest that this treatment approach affords durable oncologic outcomes in properly selected patients. Guillem and colleagues (2005) reported on 247 consecutive patients who were treated with standardized CRT regimens followed by resection with total mesorectal excision (TME). With a median follow-up of 44 months, the recurrence rate in this study population was found to be 23% (2% local recurrence only, 19% distant recurrence, and 2% local and distant recurrence), with an estimated 10-year recurrence-free survival of 62% and a 10-year overall survival of 58%.

There is, however, some debate as to whether all patients with locally advanced rectal cancer require preoperative CRT. Several retrospective analyses suggest that a subset of patients with low-risk disease (T3N0M0 lesions with negative margins and favorable histologic features) may not derive a significant benefit from RT. Unfortunately,

---

TABLE 2: Criteria for local excision of rectal cancers

Tumor Location and Size

Location within 8 cm of anal verge

Size <3 cm and involving less than one third of the circumference of the rectum

Clinical features

Mobile, nonfixed

T1/N0 on pretreatment imaging

Histologic Features

Well to moderately differentiated

No lymphovascular or perineural invasion

T1 lesion on final histologic examination

Modified from the National Comprehensive Cancer Network: *Practice guidelines in oncology rectal cancer,* v.3 2010. Available at www.nccn.org.

limitations with current imaging modalities make it impossible to pre-operatively select with certainty those patients with low-risk T3N0 disease. A large multiinstitutional review found that 22% of patients who received preoperative CRT for clinically staged T3N0 rectal cancer by ERUS or MRI actually had node-positive disease on pathologic review of resected specimens. Because preoperative CRT may reduce the total number of LNs and may also sterilize mesorectal LNs, the true rate of patients clinically staged as having T3N0 who actually have node-positive disease may be even higher, perhaps as high as 40%. Although the risks of overstaging T3 rectal cancer have been recognized (18% of patients with clinically staged T3N0 disease actually had T2N0 disease, according to data from the German Rectal Cancer Group), it is possible that twice as many are understaged based on the above findings. These data would support preoperative CRT for patients with clinical T3N0 rectal cancers staged by ERUS or MRI because understaged patients would otherwise require postoperative CRT, which is associated with inferior local control, higher toxicity, and poor functional outcomes. Moreover, these data highlight some of the limitations of clinical staging by ERUS and MRI and clearly underscore the ongoing need to improve the pretherapy staging of rectal cancer.

Distant Metastatic (M1) Disease

Patients with distant metastasis represent a heterogenous population for whom it is difficult to define an all-encompassing strategy. These complex and challenging cases should be discussed within the context of a multidisciplinary team. Treatment strategies are mainly based on factors related to 1) the primary lesion (related symptoms, resectability), 2) the extent of metastases (sites, resectability), and 3) the patient (age, comorbidities, ability to withstand major surgery, wishes regarding quality of life).

A strategy directed at curative intent can be adopted in patients with a resectable primary tumor and limited, resectable metastatic disease. In these cases, systemic chemotherapy is commonly used as the initial treatment modality. After restaging, resection of the primary and metastatic disease can be considered as either combined or staged operations. Alternatively, up-front surgical resection, as either combined or staged procedures, can be considered in patients with limited metastatic disease.

In selected patients with stage IV disease, systemic chemotherapy may provide effective palliation that obviates the need for surgery. Some patients with a symptomatic primary tumor may, however, require a diverting colostomy or endoscopic rectal stent as a bridge to definitive treatment or for palliation in incurable cases.

NEOADJUVANT AND ADJUVANT THERAPIES

The reader should be aware of the some of the landmark trials that have contributed to the understanding of rectal cancer and how combined modality therapy is optimally applied to treat patients with this disease.

The 1990 National Institute of Health Consensus Conference recommended postoperative CRT for patients with stage II or III rectal cancers, but these recommendations were based on trials that were conducted prior to the widespread implementation of TME-based surgery. More recent, well-designed, and adequately powered randomized trials on combined therapeutic modalities that incorporate TME have caused us to reexamine the treatment paradigm for rectal cancer. Some of these trials are discussed here.

The Dutch Colorectal Cancer Group assessed whether adding preoperative RT (5 x 5 Gy) to TME surgery improved oncologic outcomes in patients with locally advanced rectal cancers. On long-term follow-up, RT was found to improve 5-year local recurrence rates (5.6% for the RT plus TME group vs. 10.9% for the TME-alone group), without affecting OS. This study established a benefit with preoperative RT, even when optimal surgical resection with TME is performed.

The German Rectal Cancer Group compared preoperative to postoperative CRT (long-course RT with concurrent chemotherapy) for patients with stage II or III disease. Preoperative CRT was found to be associated with fewer acute and chronic toxicities and an improved 5-year local recurrence rate (6% vs. 13% for the postoperative group).

Together, these data support neoadjuvant therapy followed by TME-based surgical resection as standard care for patients with stage II or III rectal cancer. Most centers in North America prefer preoperative long-course CRT, whereas short-course RT is still commonly used in Europe. Surgical resection is usually performed 6 to 8 weeks after completing long-course neoadjuvant therapy. This interval allows for maximal tumor response to the CRT, while also giving patients time to recuperate from the toxicities sometimes associated with CRT. Some authors have suggested that patients who have a significant or complete response to neoadjuvant therapy can be treated with transanal incision or even observation alone. However, at this time, most surgeons in North America would not consider this the standard of care for locally advanced rectal cancer. The American College of Surgeons Oncology Group (ACOSOG) has initiated a phase II trial with aggressive neoadjuvant CRT followed by local excision for clinically staged T2N0 rectal cancers, which may expand the indications for nonradical resection. At present, however, patients should undergo definitive radical resection after neoadjuvant therapy unless they are part of a clinical trial.

After surgical resection, the current National Comprehensive Cancer Network (NCCN) guidelines recommend further adjuvant chemotherapy for all patients who received neoadjuvant CRT. The results of the recent multicenter Quick and Simple and Reliable (QUASAR) trial, which found a small reduction in the relative risk of recurrence and death with adjuvant chemotherapy over observation alone, would appear to support the NCCN recommendations. However, an overall survival benefit for adjuvant chemotherapy has not been a consistent finding in most modern randomized trials on locally advanced rectal cancers where neoadjuvant CRT is given.

SURGICAL CONSIDERATIONS

Transanal Excision

Lesions considered amenable to a transanal excision must be accessible from the anal canal and located below the peritoneal reflection. The proximal limit of the resection is usually 6 to 8 cm from the anal verge. The goal of local excision is full-thickness excision of the rectal lesion with negative margins. We use electrocautery to mark a 1 cm margin circumferentially around the tumor, and then we incise the rectal wall full thickness down to the perirectal fat. The specimen is removed in one piece, oriented and pinned on a board prior to fixation, and brought to the pathologist by the surgeon. We prefer to close the defect in the rectum with absorbable suture, and we are careful to ensure that the rectal lumen is not significantly narrowed. Postoperative complications are usually minor and may include bleeding, local infection, and urinary retention.

Transanal Endoscopic Microsurgery

Transanal endoscopic microsurgery (TEM) can be used to excise mid and upper rectal lesions that might otherwise be inaccessible with a standard transanal approach. TEM requires a specialized 40 mm diameter endoscope and long endoscopic operating equipment. Carbon dioxide insufflation facilitates exposure, while a binocular microscope on the TEM endoscope provides a constant, sixfold-magnified three-dimensional view of the operative field. The technical principles that apply to transanal local excision, with respect to full-thickness excision and negative circumferential margins, also apply to TEM excision. Tumors as high as 10 cm anteriorly, 15 cm laterally, and 18 cm posteriorly can be excised with the TEM approach. However, very distal rectal lesions are often not amenable to TEM because of difficulty maintaining an adequate seal around the scope.

Radical Resection

Radical resection for rectal cancer involves resection of the tumor and rectum en bloc with its blood and lymphatic supply (i.e., the mesorectum). A sphincter-preserving low anterior resection (LAR) is the preferred approach to radical resection, as long as it is technically feasible and oncologically appropriate. With proper training and experience, it can usually be safely performed when cancers are located more than 1 cm from the upper portion of the anorectal ring, as long as the patient has a favorable body habitus and pelvic anatomy. Generally, slender patients with wide pelvises provide more favorable conditions for sphincter-preserving surgery, and obese patients and those with long, narrow pelvises pose a technical challenge that can preclude a restorative procedure.

Contraindications to LAR include tumor invasion into the anal sphincter or levator muscles. Significantly impaired preoperative anorectal function is a relative contraindication because it often leads to poor postoperative bowel function. An abdominoperineal resection is preferred in situations where a margin-negative resection would result in loss of anal sphincter function leading to fecal incontinence.

During the planning and conduct of radical surgery for rectal cancer, the following must be considered: 1) TME, 2) autonomic nerve preservation, 3) negative circumferential and distal margins, and 4) sphincter preservation and restoration of bowel continuity and function, when possible. The following sections discuss each of these principles.

Total Mesorectal Excision

In 1979, Heald and colleagues described and popularized the TME technique for rectal cancer, which has since gained widespread acceptance. Even though it has never been assessed in a large, prospective, randomized trial, the TME technique has consistently been associated with significantly lower locoregional failure rates, ranging from 3% to 7%, compared with historic and contemporary controls. The markedly low local recurrence rates associated with TME have made it the standard of care in the surgical management of rectal cancer.

Total mesorectal excision is defined as the complete excision of the visceral mesorectum with pelvic nerve preservation; the *mesorectum* refers to the fatty tissue that encompasses the rectum. It contains lymphatic elements from the rectum and is encased by visceral fascia. TME entails sharp dissection in the areolar plane between the visceral fascia that envelops the rectum and mesorectum and the parietal fascia overlying the sacrum and pelvic sidewall structures (Figure 4). When properly performed, TME results in en bloc removal of the primary rectal cancer and mesorectum as an intact "package." The TME sharp dissection technique facilitates the identification and preservation of the pelvic autonomic nerves and is also associated with high negative circumferential resection margin (CRM) rates. For most middle and low rectal cancers, the entire mesorectum is mobilized and resected. Cancers in the upper rectum, usually located above 10 cm from the anal verge, can be treated with a tumor-specific excision in which the mesorectum is divided at a right angle to the bowel 5 cm distal to the mucosal edge of the tumor.

Autonomic Nerve Preservation

Autonomic nerve preservation, as promoted by Enker and colleagues (1995), requires an understanding of the anatomy of the pelvic nerves (Figure 5). The sympathetic nerves of the pelvis originate from the T12 to L3 ventral nerve roots, which form the superior hypogastric plexus. Distal to the aortic bifurcation, the superior hypogastric plexus gives rise to the hypogastric nerves, and these may be intimately associated with the visceral fascia of the mesorectum. The parasympathetic nerves of the pelvis, *nervi erigentes,* arise from the S2 to S4 ventral nerve roots. These join the sympathetic hypogastric nerves on the pelvic sidewall to form the inferior hypogastric plexus.

Injury to the pelvic autonomic nerves can be associated with significant genitourinary dysfunction and morbidity. Damage to the

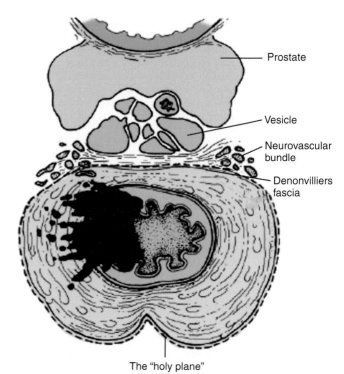

The "holy plane"

FIGURE 4   Schematic representation of the relationship of the mesorectum to the anterior anatomic structures in a male patient. The neurovascular bundle contains the nerves responsible for erection, ejaculation, and aspects of bladder function. *(From Heald RJ, Moran BJ: Embryology and anatomy of the rectum, Sem Surg Oncol 15:70,1998.)*

sympathetic hypogastric nerves can result in increased bladder tone and reduced bladder capacity, as well as with impaired ejaculation in men. Damage to the parasympathetic system can result in voiding difficulties from increased tone in the bladder neck, as well as with erectile dysfunction in men and impaired vaginal lubrication in women.

Circumferential Resection Margin

The CRM *status* refers to the adequacy of the surgical resection margin relative to the 360 degree radial extension of the primary tumor, which may include extension into the mesorectum and adjacent extrarectal soft tissue. The prognostic significance of a negative CRM in the presence of an intact mesorectum has been well established. A review of patients enrolled in the Dutch TME study found that CRMs less than 2 mm were associated with an increased local recurrence rate (16% vs. 6% for margins ≥2 mm). Moreover, CRMs 1 mm or less were associated with a significantly higher risk of distant metastasis (78% vs. 13% for margins >1 mm) and shorter survival.

Distal Resection Margin

Distal resection margins (DRMs) of 2 to 5 cm have been the traditional standard in rectal cancer surgery. However, multiple recent studies have narrowed these limits by showing that occult disease extending beneath the mucosal edge of the tumor is uncommon, especially after CRT. Recent whole-mount pathologic analyses on specimens from selected patients who underwent CRT followed by resection found intramural extension beyond the gross mucosal edge of residual tumor in only 2 (1.8%) of 109 patients. Moreover, when extension was present, it was limited to a distance 0.95 mm or less in both cases. These results compare very favorably to data in the literature documenting distal spread beyond the mucosal edge of tumor in only 10% of patients, all of which occurred in poorly differentiated, node-positive lesions.

Retrospective data suggest that margins as small as 1 cm may not compromise oncologic outcomes. A review from our institution found

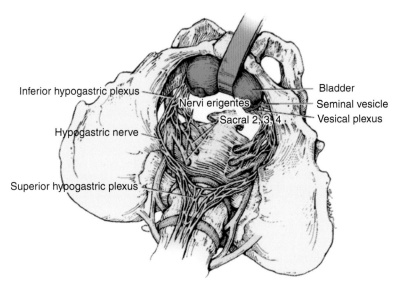

Inferior hypogastric plexus

Nervi erigentes

Hypogastric nerve

Sacral 2, 3, 4

Superior hypogastric plexus

Bladder

Seminal vesicle

Vesical plexus

FIGURE 5   Diagram of pelvic nerve anatomy. *(From Guillem JG: Ultra-low anterior resection and coloanal pouch reconstruction for carcinoma of the distal rectum, World J Surg 21:722, 1997.)*

that local control and RFS with 3 years of follow-up after neoadjuvant CRT and TME-based resection were not significantly different when patients with DRMs less than or equal to 1 cm were compared with those with DRMs greater than 1 cm. We advocate striving for a DRM of at least 2 cm for most rectal cancers, even after preoperative CRT. However, a histologically negative DRM less than 1 cm is acceptable in carefully selected patients in the absence of adverse histologic features, particularly in situations where an APR may be required for a wider margin. In cases where the DRM status is uncertain, we suggest obtaining an intraoperative frozen section of the distal margin.

Reconstruction Options Following Low Anterior Resection

Various reconstructive techniques, including colonic J-pouches (CJPs) and transverse coloplasty pouches (TCPs), have been developed in an attempt to improve functional outcomes over a straight anastomosis (SA) after a very low anterior resection.

Multiple randomized studies have compared CJPs to SA, and the majority of these show better short-term functional outcomes with CJPs (Figure 6); however, it has been difficult to demonstrate a measurable difference in quality of life between these two techniques. Five randomized trials have compared CJPs to TCPs. In two of these trials, better functional outcomes were seen with CJPs; the other three trials showed comparable outcomes. In addition, comparisons of TCPs to SA have not found consistent differences in functional outcomes, although these analyses have been underpowered.

Taken together, these data support a functional benefit to reconstruction with a CJP over SA, but the benefit of a TCP over SA is uncertain. We prefer a CJP reconstruction after a very low anterior resection. However, when a CJP is not technically feasible, usually because of a disproportionately bulky colonic mesentery and narrowed pelvis, we favor performing an SA.

Temporary Diversion Following Low Anterior Resection

Data from randomized studies demonstrate a reduction in the incidence of anastomotic leaks when diverting stomas are performed after an LAR. A large, randomized trial from Sweden found that diverting stomas decreased the symptomatic leak rate (10.3% in the diverted group compared with 28% in the nondiverted control group) after restorative LAR for rectal cancer. Another interesting finding from this study was the low likelihood of stoma reversal in patients who were not initially diverted but who later developed anastomotic leaks. A large population-based study suggested that factors associated with anastomotic leakage after anterior resection included male gender, a low anastomosis (≤6 cm from the anal verge), preoperative RT, and

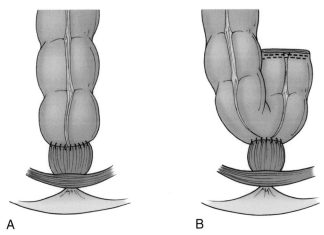

A   B

FIGURE 6   Illustrated comparison of a straight coloanal anastomosis *(left)* and a coloanal anastomosis with a colonic J-pouch *(right)*. *(Adapted from Sailer M, Fuchs KH, Fein M, Thiede A: Randomized clinical trial comparing quality of life after straight and pouch coloanal reconstruction, Br J Surg 89:1109, 2002.)*

the presence of adverse intraoperative events. Although exceptions do exist, we tend to perform a diverting loop ileostomy on most patients with a coloanal anastomosis and on those who have received preoperative external-beam RT. The ileostomy reversal is usually scheduled 6 to 8 weeks following surgery. However, when postoperative chemotherapy is required, reversal is postponed for several weeks beyond completion of chemotherapy. In these cases, an interim office visit and DRE are recommended to ensure that the anastomosis remains patent because diversion may result in narrowing.

Abdominoperineal Resection

Abdominoperineal resection (APR) refers to a combined abdominal and perineal approach to resect the rectum and mesorectum en bloc, along with the anus, surrounding perineal soft tissue, and pelvic floor musculature. An end colostomy is then created. APR is associated with higher morbidity when compared with LAR, mainly from complications of the perineal wound, as well as lower scores in most, but not all, studies that examine patients' self-reported quality of life after rectal cancer surgery.

APR is usually performed with the patient in the supine lithotomy position. However, several European centers have reported on extended perineal dissections with patients in a prone position. The prone technique involves a wide perineal dissection to a point laterally where the levator musculature originates on the pelvic sidewall. Because of the wide dissection, tissue-flap reconstruction of the pelvic floor is required. Authors who endorse this approach contend it results in a more cylindrical specimen compared with the standard APR specimens, which may narrow where the mesorectum disappears at the level of the sphincters. Nonrandomized data suggest that the cylindrical APR approach is associated with the ability to obtain a greater amount of tissue around the tumor specimen and lower rates of CRM involvement compared with standard APR specimens. However, these studies need to be interpreted with caution, as they are small in size and retrospectively review highly selected patients. Extended resections may be useful when tumor infiltrates the pelvic floor. However, the clinical indications for the cylindrical APR approach require further clarification before this technique can be recommended on a routine basis.

Minimally Invasive Approaches to Radical Resection

The application of minimally invasive techniques to rectal cancer surgery represents a significant advancement in the surgical management of rectal cancer. The Conventional versus Laparoscopic-Assisted Surgery in Colorectal Cancer (CLASICC) trial from the UK Medical Research Council randomized 794 patients with colorectal cancer, of whom 381 (48%) had rectal primaries, to laparoscopic-assisted or open resection. In the subgroup of rectal cancer patients who underwent LAR, a trend was seen toward a higher rate of involved CRMs in the laparoscopic-assisted group compared to the open-resection group, but this did not translate into any significant differences between groups with regard to local control, 3-year DFS, or OS. There was, however, a trend toward worsened sexual function for men in the laparoscopic-assisted group.

Although the results of the CLASICC and smaller emerging trials show that minimally invasive surgery for rectal cancer is feasible, further data on the long-term oncologic outcomes are needed before laparoscopic techniques can be recommended for mid to low rectal cancers, particularly with regard to the TME portion of the procedure. Currently, the multicenter Colorectal Cancer Laparoscopic or Open Resection (COLOR) II and the National Cancer Institute–sponsored ACOSOG Z6051 trials are accruing patients to further address these issues.

SUGGESTED READINGS

Bentrem DJ, Okabe S, Wong WD, et al: T1 adenocarcinoma of the rectum: transanal excision or radical surgery? *Ann Surg* 242:472–477, 2005.

Guillem JG, Chessin DB, Cohen AM, et al: Long-term oncologic outcome following preoperative combined modality therapy and total mesorectal excision of locally advanced rectal cancer, *Ann Surg* 241:829–836, 2005.

Guillem JG, Chessin DB, Shia J, et al: A prospective pathologic analysis using whole-mount sections of rectal cancer following preoperative combined modality therapy: implications for sphincter preservation, *Ann Surg* 245:88–93, 2007.

Guillem JG, Diaz-Gonzalez JA, Minsky BD, et al: cT3N0 rectal cancer: potential overtreatment with preoperative chemoradiotherapy is warranted, *J Clin Oncol* 26:368–373, 2008.

Heald RJ, Moran BJ, Ryall RD, et al: Rectal cancer: the Basingstoke experience of total mesoretal excision, 1978-1997, *Arch Surg* 133:894–899, 1998.

Jayne DG, Guillou PJ, Thorpe H, et al: Randomized trial of laparoscopic-assisted resection of colorectal carcinoma: 3-year results of the UK MRC CLASICC Trial Group, *J Clin Oncol* 25:3061–3068, 2007.

Minsky BD, Guillem JG: Multidisciplinary management of resectable rectal cancer. New developments and controversies, *Oncology (Williston Park)* 22:1430–1437, 2008.

Nash GM, Weiser MR, Guillem JG, et al: Long-term survival after transanal excision of T1 rectal cancer, *Dis Colon Rectum* 52:577–582, 2009.

Park J, Neuman HB, Weiser MR, et al: Randomized clincial trials in rectal and anal cancers, *Surg Oncol Clin North Am* 19:205–223, 2010.

Peeters KC, Marijnen CA, Nagtegaal ID, et al: The TME trial after a median follow-up of 6 years: increased local control but no survival benefit in irradiated patients with resectable rectal carcinoma, *Ann Surg* 246:693–701, 2007.

Sauer R, Becker H, Hohenberger W, et al: Preoperative versus postoperative chemoradiotheraphy for rectal cancer, *N Engl J Med* 351:1731–1740, 2004.

Skandarajah AR, Tjandra JJ: Preoperative loco-regional imaging in rectal cancer, *ANZ J Surg* 76:497–504, 2006.

TUMORS OF THE ANAL REGION

Paul C. Shellito, MD

FIRST CONSIDERATIONS

An understanding of anorectal anatomy is important for the evaluation and treatment of anal tumors (Figure 1). The anal canal is the most distal portion of the gastrointestinal (GI) tract, and it is surrounded by sphincter musculature; it extends from the anorectal ring proximally to the anal verge distally. The anal canal is 4 to 5 cm long (slightly longer in males than in females). The anorectal ring corresponds to the upper border of the sphincter muscles at the puborectalis. The anal verge corresponds to the lower border of the sphincters and is the point at which anoderm meets the hair-bearing perianal skin. The dentate line bisects the anal canal and is the demarcation between glandular or transitional mucosa proximally and squamous mucosa distally. Transitional epithelium extends for about 1 cm proximal to the dentate line, and it has has rectal, urothelial, and squamous features. Above the transitional epithelium is glandular mucosa, the same as in the rectum. Anoderm is the modified squamous epithelium that lies between the dentate line and the anal verge.

It is similar to skin, except that it is thin, and hair follicles and sweat glands are absent. Also, a rich supply of nerves makes it particularly sensitive. Perianal skin is the epithelium caudal to the anal verge, and it is the same as skin elsewhere in the body. The term *anal margin*, an unfortunate and inexact term, is sometimes used to refer to the perianal skin that extends 5 cm from the anal verge circumferentially. The lymphatic drainage proximal to the dentate line is primarily along the superior rectal artery, within the mesorectum to the inferior mesenteric lymph nodes, and occasionally laterally to the internal iliac lymph nodes. The lymphatic drainage below the dentate line (anoderm and perianal skin) is primarily to the inguinal and femoral nodes but occasionally to the superior rectal/mesorectal lymphatics.

The symptoms of anal tumors are nonspecific. Bleeding, pain, and the sensation of a mass are common, but there may be only itching, burning, or discharge. Frequently, anal tumors are completely asymptomatic and are discovered only incidentally. The physical appearance of an anal tumor may be nonspecific also. The lesion may be flat or raised, and the surface may be verrucous, erythematous, or scaly. An ulcer may be present, especially if there is malignancy. Other anorectal lesions—such as hemorrhoids, fistulas, or fissures—may coexist with anal tumors to confuse the picture.

For the initial evaluation of any patient with an anorectal lesion, it is best to carry out a four-part examination in everyone in addition to a general history and physical exam that includes examination of the inguinal nodes. The four parts include the following:

- Careful anal inspection, with good exposure and good light
- Digital exam

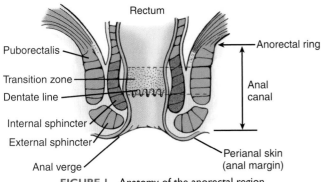

Rectum

Puborectalis

Anorectal ring

Transition zone

Anal canal

Dentate line

Internal sphincter

External sphincter

Perianal skin (anal margin)

Anal verge

FIGURE 1   Anatomy of the anorectal region.

- Anoscopy
- Sigmoidoscopy, preferably flexible sigmoidoscopy

Colonoscopy may be added if necessary. Any suspicious or persistent anal lesion should be biopsied because malignancy may have an unexpected appearance. If an examination or biopsy is difficult to do in an office, evaluation under anesthesia is appropriate.

NONINVASIVE LESIONS

Noninvasive anal lesions include condyloma acuminatum, anal intraepithelial neoplasia (AIN) and, rarely, Paget's disease.

Condylomata Acuminatum

Condylomata acuminatum, or anal warts, are caused by human papilloma virus (HPV). HPV infects the skin and mucous membranes of the anogenital area. The infection may be asymptomatic and without visible lesions, or it may cause warts—the most common clinical manifestation of HPV. Anogenital HPV is also strongly associated with AIN and squamous cell carcinoma (SCC), which may coexist with condyloma acuminatum. There are numerous subtypes of HPV: subtypes 6 and 11 most frequently cause benign anogenital warts. Transmission is usually by genital contact with infected individuals (who may have an asymptomatic infection). Digital contact or fomites might also spread HPV. Condyloma acuminatum is the most common sexually transmitted disease (STD), and its incidence is increasing. Anal warts can occur without anoreceptive intercourse, however. The risk factors for anal warts include a higher number of sexual partners, the presence of other STDs, human immunodeficiency virus (HIV) infection, and immunosuppression.

Condylomata acuminatum are fleshy exophytic or sessile verrucous growths of variable size. They may be gray, pink, or skin colored, less than 1 mm in diameter or several centimeters in size, and may be nearly flat or quite exophytic. Only a few may be present, or they may be innumerable. They may be found on the perianal skin; in the anal canal (but only at or below the level of the dentate line); and on the penis, vulva, vagina, cervix and, occasionally, the groin. Most cause no symptoms other than bothersome growths, although they may cause much psychological distress. Anoscopy is particularly important in patients with anal condylomata because intraanal lesions often coexist with perianal lesions, and the former may be missed without a directed examination. Although anal warts usually have a typical appearance, biopsy and/or excision should always be done to confirm the diagnosis and rule out invasive cancer.

The options for treatment of condylomata acuminatum include excision/cauterization in the operating room (probably the most effective treatment), topical office treatments, and topical treatments applied by the patient at home. The goal is destruction and removal of all gross warts. Nevertheless, the virus can never be eradicated, so recurrence of condylomata acuminatum can be a stubborn problem,

especially in immunosuppressed or HIV-positive patients. It is difficult to generalize about recurrence rates or cure rates, because it depends on how extensive the warts are, how aggressive the physician is with treatment, and how careful the follow-up is. Probably over 50% of immunocompetent patients can be cured, but immunodeficient patients rarely so.

Excision/cauterization is best done under anesthesia, unless there are only a few warts present. A careful examination under anesthesia is important, so that intraanal lesions are not missed. After a meticulous search, all lesions should be excised or thoroughly cauterized, with an effort to minimize damage to normal surrounding epithelium. If cauterization is done, at least some representative lesions should be excised for biopsy to confirm the diagnosis. Laser has no advantage over excision or electrocauterization. Anal stenosis is a risk if large areas are excised or cauterized. Repeated operations are often required to eradicate warts.

Office treatments include podophyllin, cryotherapy, and trichloroacetic acid (TCA). All usually require repeated applications to eradicate condylomata. Podophyllin is an antimitotic plant resin (active agent: podophyllotoxin). It is teratogenic in animals, so it is not approved for use in pregnancy. Also, any necessary biopsies should be done *before* starting podophyllin, since the agent can produce dysplastic histologic changes. The minimum amount of podophyllin necessary to cover the lesions should be applied and allowed to dry, avoiding contact to the normal surrounding epithelium. It cannot be used in the anal canal.

Cryotherapy can be carried out with liquid nitrogen and a cotton-tipped applicator. It can be used in the anal canal through an anoscope. TCA (80%) is probably the easiest topical agent to use. The end of a toothpick-sized wooden applicator is dipped in the acid and dabbed onto the warts for chemical cauterization. The acid turns the tissue white, so it is easy to gauge the therapeutic effect. TCA can also be used in the anal canal.

Patient-applied home treatments include podofilox, 5-fluorouracil (5-FU) cream, and imiquimod. A side effect for all of them is perianal skin inflammation, which at least to some extent may be necessary for the agent to work. Gloves should be used to apply these treatments, after washing and drying the anal area. The relative efficacy of these agents is unknown.

Podofilox (Condylox) is 5% podophyllotoxin and is available as a solution or gel. It is applied twice daily for 3 days and then stopped for 4 days, and the cycle can be repeated for up to 4 weeks. Its restrictions are the same as for podophyllin. The antimetabolite 5-FU is sold as a 5% cream (Efudex). It is often used for condylomata acuminatum or AIN, although it is not Food and Drug Administration (FDA) approved for this. It is applied once a day, or two to three times a week, for up to 10 weeks. Imiquimod (Aldara) is a 5% cream that is FDA approved. It enhances the local immune response, although its exact mechanism of action is unknown. Most patients and physicians find it the easiest to use; it is applied three times a week for up to 16 weeks (apply at bedtime, and wash off in the morning). It is not for use within the anal canal. The accompanying skin inflammation may be more acceptable to patients if it is explained to them that this is part of the mechanism of action.

Recommendation

All patients with newly diagnosed or suspected condylomata acuminatum should be taken to the operating room for a careful examination under anesthesia, including anoscopy to find intraanal lesions, which may be subtle. Excision/cauterization with extensive biopsies can then be done to confirm the diagnosis and rule out AIN and cancer. On follow-up office exam, small recurrences can be treated in the office with TCA. If recurrent warts are frequent or persistent, imiquimod can be added. Probably all immunosuppressed or HIV patients should be offered imiquimod after initial excision/cauterization. Some physicians routinely use imiquimod as adjuvant treatment for 6 weeks after excision/cauterization in all patients.

Giant condyloma acuminatum (Buschke-Loewenstein tumor) is a rare form of this condition. This large, exophytic tumor is marked by local invasion into surrounding tissues. Although the rate of local recurrence is high, distant metastases are unlikely. About half contain foci of invasive SCC, but this does not seem to correlate with recurrence or prognosis. Local invasion and recurrence are the major sources of morbidity. The treatment is complete excision if possible, but sometimes abdominoperineal resection (APR) is required if there is deep tissue involvement. The role of chemoradiation in the treatment of giant condyloma acuminatum is unclear. It has been used for unresectable or recurrent tumors, as well as for neoadjuvant treatment of extensive disease, but the response is unpredictable.

Anal Intraepithelial Neoplasia

AIN is probably the precursor to invasive SCC. Numerous other terms—*carcinoma in situ* (CIS), *anal dysplasia, anal squamous intraepithelial lesion* (SIL), and *Bowen's disease*—have been used to refer to this lesion, which can be a source of confusion. AIN is subdivided into grades I, II, and III for low-, moderate-, and high-grade dysplasia. SIL often refers to cytologic changes seen on Pap smear and is subdivided into low-grade (LSIL), high-grade (HSIL), and invasive cancer. Traditionally, the term *Bowen's disease* most often referred to a discrete macroscopic area of red, thickened, or eczematous epithelium of squamous cell CIS on the perianal skin, probably corresponding to AIN grade III. The term has no certain definition, however, and is therefore best avoided. These terms all refer to dysplasia in the squamous epithelium, which has a spectrum of severity leading to invasive cancer.

HPV infection strongly correlates with AIN and is suspected to be the causative agent. HPV subtypes 16 and 18 are associated with the greatest risk of AIN and cancer. AIN can affect the perianal skin and anal canal, including the anal transition zone. It may cause macroscopic lesions such as warts, tumors, ulcers, or eczematous plaques. Alternatively, microscopic changes may occur in grossly appearing normal epithelium, and the patient may be asymptomatic, so the diagnosis can be difficult. AIN tends to be multifocal. Probably most cases of SCC are preceded by AIN, but only a small minority of patients with AIN progress to cancer. The risk factors for AIN and anal SCC include HPV infection, anal warts, multiple sexual partners, men who have sex with men (MSM), anoreceptive intercourse, other sexually transmitted diseases, cervical dysplasia or cancer, smoking, immunosuppression (such as in transplant patients), and HIV infection. It is unclear whether the increased risk of AIN in this last category is a direct effect of HIV or is due to the associated immune deficiency. Highly active antiretroviral therapy (HAART) has had no apparent effect upon HPV infection, AIN, or SCC.

There is no consensus about the best management of AIN because of difficulties with detection and treatment and uncertainty about its malignant potential. It would seem logical that eradication of AIN would prevent later progression to cancer, as is the case with cervical dysplasia. Nevertheless, AIN is difficult and cumbersome to detect, and there is no clearly effective treatment for it. Furthermore, excision or ablation of AIN can cause appreciable morbidity, including pain, stricture, incontinence, and prolonged healing time. The morbidity is especially pronounced in HIV-positive individuals and in patients who are otherwise immunosuppressed. AIN is a virally induced, frequently multifocal "field defect" that can affect any part of the anogenital area, and the virus and AIN can exist in normal-appearing epithelium. Thus it is not surprising that surgical treatments often fail to eradicate it. Positive resection margins are common, even after careful mapping of the lesion; recurrences are frequent, even with negative margins.

Furthermore, the natural history and malignant potential of AIN is unclear. It is not known how likely it is that AIN will progress to

cancer, but it is probably a low risk; AIN seems to be much less dangerous than cervical dysplasia. For high-grade AIN, the risk of invasive carcinoma is probably on the order of 5% to 10% in immunocompetent patients. On the other hand, the course of AIN in HIV-positive and immunosuppressed individuals is a greater concern; up to 50% will progress to invasive cancer. The prevalence of HPV and AIN is unknown, but because these lesions are often subclinical, the figure is probably much higher than would be suggested just by the number of individuals who come to medical attention. It is also uncertain whether the detection and eradication of AIN decreases the risk of subsequent cancer or improves survival. It is worth remembering that even when SCC appears, chemoradiation is often curative, with avoidance of a colostomy.

The options for managing AIN range from aggressive intervention to watchful waiting. Anal Pap smears can be done to screen for SIL, although anal cytology correlates poorly with the histology of confirmed lesions. There is no proof of benefit for anal Pap smears, but it is nevertheless probably worthwhile in high-risk individuals. If the Pap smear is positive, the patient should undergo careful physical exam, including anoscopy. For established AIN, mapping by frozen-section biopsies and wide local excision of macroscopically and microscopically abnormal areas is the most aggressive treatment. However, this can lead to large, open wounds, skin grafts, or flap closures, with the associated morbidity alluded to above, so it is best avoided. Another treatment option is high-resolution anoscopy (HRA), which is done either in an office or in the operating room. The anus and perineum are swabbed with 3% to 5% acetic acid, and the area is examined with 10-power magnification, such as with a colposcope. The abnormal areas turn "aceto white," which is suggestive but not diagnostic of AIN. In addition, Lugol iodine can be applied; mature squamous epithelium, which contains glycogen, stains a deep brown, whereas only light yellow staining in an aceto-white area is suggestive of high-grade AIN. Suspicious lesions can then be biopsied, excised, or destroyed by cautery, infrared coagulation, cryotherapy, or TCA; such targeted therapy minimizes damage to surrounding normal tissue. Retrospective studies have suggested that this approach may reduce the likelihood of progression to cancer compared with expectant management. On the other hand, periodic HRA is inconvenient and time consuming for both the patient and the physician, and it is painful for the patient. Furthermore, there is no evidence that eradicating AIN affects survival. Periodic treatment courses with imiquimod or 5-FU cream have been used with some success. The most conservative option is close clinical follow-up alone, with periodic physical exams and anoscopy, and biopsy or excision of suspicious lesions as they appear (warts, tumors, or ulcers).

Recommendation

Be attentive but conservative with AIN. If only reasonably small and isolated macroscopic lesions are present, locally excise them, but avoid large or wide excisions and ablations. Biopsies or resection margins that are positive for AIN can be accepted, as long as the epithelium looks grossly normal; just continue to closely follow the patient, and biopsy suspicious macroscopic lesions if they appear. If there are wide areas of irregular or thickened epithelium that are difficult to assess, prescribe a course of imiquimod for some weeks and then reevaluate the patient. Imiquimod may be worth using, even in relatively normal appearing epithelium, if microscopic AIN is present. Be especially attentive to immunodeficient patients and MSM. If invasive SCC is discovered, treat it as described below.

Paget Disease

Paget disease of the anus (extramammary Paget disease) is a very uncommon lesion. The origin of this intraepithelial adenocarcinoma is unclear, but it probably arises from apocrine glands.

A characteristic Paget's cell is present on histologic examination which is a large and vacuolated cell with clear, pale cytoplasm and a large hyperchromatic nucleus. Paget's disease typically presents as an erythematous or eczematous area of epithelium. About half of Paget's disease cases are associated with a synchronous internal malignancy, often a colorectal adenocarcinoma, which may or may not be contiguous. Therefore colonoscopy is indicated. Sometimes an invasive carcinoma is within the anal Paget's lesion itself. If no invasive cancer is present, the treatment is wide local excision. Preoperative biopsies for mapping are important, or at least intraoperative frozen-section pathologic analysis of margins, because the Paget's cells may extend beyond the gross margin of the lesion. After excision, primary closure may be done for a small lesion, but skin grafting or flap closure may be required for larger resections. Paget's disease may be multifocal, and local recurrences occur in about 20% of patients, even with negative resection margins, so follow-up is important. If the Paget's lesion contains invasive cancer, the treatment is the same as for rectal adenocarcinoma.

INVASIVE LESIONS

Invasive lesions of the anus include SCC, adenocarcinoma, and melanoma. Rarely, lymphoma, sarcoma, neuroendocrine tumor (carcinoid), and GI stromal tumor may occur.

Squamous Cell Carcinoma

For SCC of the anus, it is important to determine whether the lesion is located within the anal canal or on the perianal skin, because this greatly affects the treatment and prognosis. Carcinomas of the perianal skin are much less common and less aggressive than anal canal cancers. The behavior of SCC of the perianal skin is similar to skin cancers elsewhere in the body, and the treatment is the same: wide local excision, and the prognosis is very good. Nevertheless, when cancers lie at or near the anal verge, or if they extend into the anal canal at all, they are best classified as anal canal lesions and treated as such.

The evaluation of SCC of the anal canal begins with a physical exam that includes careful attention to the inguinal lymph nodes, anoscopy, and biopsy of the primary tumor. Anal cancers occasionally present with prominent adenopathy within the mesorectum, which may overshadow the primary tumor. Flexible sigmoidoscopy or colonoscopy is usually wise, to rule out other colorectal lesions. The tumor should be biopsied, but it need not be excised. Except for a rare, tiny SCC of the anal canal, local excision alone is inadequate primary treatment. Furthermore, removing the tumor does not improve results with chemoradiation; it also risks sphincter damage and delays the initiation of chemoradiation. In addition, chest and abdominal CT scans should be done, and perhaps PET scanning. Prognosis in SCC largely correlates with the size of the primary tumor and the presence or absence of lymph node metastases. Staging has little impact upon treatment decisions, however, because at least initially, virtually all tumors are best treated with chemoradiation regardless of stage.

Numerous histologic subtypes of anal canal SCC/epidermoid carcinoma exist: transitional cell carcinoma, basaloid carcinoma, cloacogenic carcinoma, large-cell keratinizing carcinoma, and large-cell nonkeratinizing carcinoma. But these distinctions have little clinical relevance; the treatment and prognosis are the same for all of them.

Chemoradiation has replaced abdominoperineal resection (APR) as the preferred primary treatment for SCC of the anal canal. Medical treatment avoids a colostomy and is associated with a better survival than radical resection. 5-FU and mitomycin-c are standard for chemotherapy. Concomitant radiation is delivered to the primary tumor and the regional lymph nodes, usually including those in the groin. If the groin nodes are clinically involved—as suggested by examination, position emission tomography (PET) scan, or needle biopsy—a boost dose of radiation is delivered there. Inguinal lymph node dissection usually should be avoided, because chemoradiation is most often sufficient to control groin metastases. Furthermore, groin dissections often lead to wound-healing problems and chronic lower extremity edema. Chemoradiation is generally effective for this cancer, with a 70% to 90% 5-year survival. Nevertheless, the regimen can be difficult because of hematologic toxicity, perineal desquamation, diarrhea or tenesmus, and anal pain. Treatment-related toxicity is worse in HIV-positive patients, although the treatment response seems to be as good as in other patients.

A difficult management decision arises when a small or microscopic SCC is found incidentally, after excision of a presumed benign lesion, such as a hemorrhoid. The choice is either to accept the local excision that has been done as adequate treatment (or perhaps to reexcise the area) or to give chemoradiation. Unfortunately, the specimen is often difficult to orient, and the resection margins may be uncertain or inadequate. And because the location and extent of possible residual cancer is usually uncertain, reexcision may not be practical. Therefore standard chemoradiation is usually best.

After chemoradiation of SCC of the anal canal, the patient should be followed up with periodic physical exams with anoscopy. The tumor may take a long time to regress; 12 weeks should be allowed to elapse before reassessing the patient. Random biopsies of apparently normal epithelium are not helpful. If residual or recurrent cancer is discovered after 12 weeks, patients without metastases are candidates for APR. Perhaps 40% to 50% can be salvaged by this, but there is appreciable morbidity associated with radical resection in this situation, especially with perineal wound healing problems. Therefore it is usually best to carry out a simultaneous flap closure of the perineum (gracilis flap, rectus abdominus flap) with APR. Rarely, if a groin node recurrence appears after chemoradiation without disease elsewhere, the patient is a candidate for inguinal node dissection, but at the cost of a high complication rate. Sometimes only AIN is found after chemoradiation. Although in this circumstance, there is a good chance that invasive cancer will appear later; it is appropriate simply to observe these patients, and APR can be at least postponed, if not avoided altogether.

Adenocarcinoma

Adenocarcinoma of the anal canal should be treated in the same way as rectal adenocarcinoma: APR with or without neoadjuvant chemoradiation and postoperative adjuvant chemotherapy. Occasionally, local excision is appropriate for a small and very early stage tumor.

Melanoma

Anal melanoma often has an unusual appearance. Frequently it is not pigmented, and it may not resemble a malignancy. Surgery is indicated, since anal melanoma does not respond to radiation or chemotherapy. Unfortunately, however, the prognosis is poor, and this is equally true regardless of whether radical resection or local excision are done. Therefore if it is possible to carry out wide local excision with negative margins, this is the preferable treatment. Similarly, if distant metastases are present, local excision may be best—or no surgery, depending on the patient's overall condition. If the melanoma is too large for local excision, and there are no distant metastases, APR is appropriate. There is about a 30% 5-year disease-free survival for patients who undergo curative resection, both for APR and local excision. The benefit of adjuvant radiation, chemotherapy, and interferon is uncertain.

Other Tumors

Anorectal lymphoma is usually treated with chemoradiation. Sarcomas can occasionally be treated with local excision, but they are usually so large at presentation that radical resection is required. Adjuvant radiation treatment is frequently helpful before resection for sarcomas. Neuroendocrine tumors (carcinoids) can be treated by local excision if they are small, and by radical resection if they not. Similarly, GI stromal tumors are treated by local or radical resection, depending on tumor size.

SELECTED READINGS

Abbasakoor F, Boulos PB: Anal intraepithelial neoplasia, *Br J Surg* 92:277–290, 2005.

Chin-Hong PV, Palefsky JM: Human papillomavirus anogenital disease in HIV-infected individuals, *Dermatol Ther* 18:67–76, 2005.

Cummings BJ: Current management of anal canal cancer, *Semin Oncol* 32(suppl 9):S123–S128, 2005.

Fleshner PR, Chalasani S, Chang GJ, et al: Practice parameters for anal squamous neoplasms, *Dis Colon Rectum* 51:2–9, 2008.

Moore HG, Guillem JG: Anal neoplasms, *Surg Clin North Am* 82:1233–1251, 2002.

Ryan DP, Compton CC, Mayer RJ: Carcinoma of the anal canal, *N Engl J Med* 342:792–800, 2000.

Vukasin P: Anal condyloma and HIV-associated anal disease, *Surg Clin North Am* 82:1199–1211, 2002.

Yeh JJ, Shia J, Hwu WJ, et al: The role of abdominoperineal resection as surgical therapy for anorectal melanoma, *Ann Surg* 244:1012–1017, 2006.

USE OF [¹⁸F]-2-FLUORO-2-DEOXY-D-GLUCOSE POSITRON EMISSION TOMOGRAPHY IN THE MANAGEMENT OF COLORECTAL CANCER

Susan Tsai, MD, Heather Jacene, MD, and Nita Ahuja, MD

OVERVIEW

The imaging technique of [¹⁸F]-2-fluoro-2-deoxy-D-glucose positron emission tomography (¹⁸F-FDG PET) has become a useful tool in assessing patients with a broad variety of malignancies. In comparison with cross-sectional imaging modalities that identify anatomic changes, ¹⁸F-FDG PET allows for the detection of alterations in metabolic activity, helping to differentiate benign from malignant processes. ¹⁸F-FDG PET has been utilized in a variety of clinical scenarios, from initial staging to assessment of treatment response to the management of recurrent disease. Although ¹⁸F-FDG PET is widely used in the management of several malignancies, including lung and esophageal cancer and melanoma, the indications for its use in colorectal cancer are more selective but are rapidly evolving. This chapter will discuss potential applications for ¹⁸F-FDG PET in the management of colorectal cancer.

PET SCANS

First developed in the early 1970s, ¹⁸F-FDG PET is a nuclear medicine technology whose theoretical principles are based upon observations made by Warburg: that cancer cells exhibit enhanced glycolysis and often have increased expression of epithelial glucose transporter proteins, as well as key enzymes, such as hexokinase and pyruvate dehydrogenase, that lead to enhanced glucose metabolism.

¹⁸F-FDG PET utilizes a radionuclide, fluorine-18 (¹⁸F), attached to a glucose analog. Administration of ¹⁸F-FDG promotes competition at the binding sites of the glucose transporter. Once internalized within the cell, unlike glucose, ¹⁸F-FDG cannot be metabolized and accumulates within the cell. The resultant intensity of the FDG signal is proportional to the amount of accumulated ¹⁸F-FDG in the cell. PET scanners indirectly detect the positron emission that is a result of ¹⁸F-FDG decay and generates the pattern of distribution, which can be reconstructed in sagittal, coronal, or axial planes.

With increasing frequency, PET scans are often fused with CT or MRI images to allow correlation of anatomic detail with biologic activity. A number of studies have demonstrated improved accuracy of integrated ¹⁸F-FDG PET/CT compared with ¹⁸F-FDG PET alone. The sensitivity, specificity, and positive and negative predictive values of ¹⁸F-FDG PET/CT in detecting pelvic recurrences in colorectal patients (98%, 96%, 90%, and 97%, respectively) is superior to ¹⁸F-FDG PET alone (82%, 65%, 73%, and 75%, respectively). Furthermore, several studies comparing ¹⁸F-FDG PET/CT with or without intravenous contrast have found that the addition of IV contrast further increases the sensitivity and accuracy of the exam.

In a recent study of 187 patients with colorectal metastases undergoing ¹⁸F-FDG PET/CT with and without intravenous contrast, the sensitivity, specificity, and accuracy of PET/contrast-enhanced CT were 93.2%, 95.8%, and 94.7%, respectively, whereas those of PET/non–contrast-enhanced CT were 89.2%, 94.8%, and 92.4%, respectively; those of enhanced CT were 79.7%, 93.8%, and 87.6%, respectively. Increasingly, ¹⁸F-FDG PET/CT with intravenous contrast is evolving as the preferred form of ¹⁸F-FDG PET imaging.

¹⁸F-FDG PET scans require cautious interpretation based on the clinical scenario. Normal tissues that have high glucose metabolism, such as brain and myocardium, as well as organs through which ¹⁸F-FDG is excreted (kidney and bladder) will exhibit ¹⁸F-FDG uptake. Small bowel and colon also exhibit physiologic uptake, which may sometimes be confused with malignancy. In addition, the sensitivity of ¹⁸F-FDG PET is dependent on the difference in ¹⁸F-FDG uptake between normal and abnormal tissues. Because of competition between glucose and ¹⁸F-FDG for uptake into abnormal cells, patients are required to fast 4 to 6 hours before the study. In many cases, the exam will not be performed in patients with elevated serum glucose levels because of higher false-negative rates.

The sensitivity and specificity of PET scans are dependent on a variety of factors, including size and tumor biology. Because of limitations in spatial resolution, the sensitivity of PET for tumors less than 1 cm is unreliable. Tumor biology also dictates relative ¹⁸F-FDG PET avidity. In particular, ¹⁸F-FDG PET is less sensitive in detecting mucinous colorectal cancer than nonmucinous (58% vs. 92%). The degree of histologic dysplasia also affects FDG avidity. In a study of colorectal polyps, low-grade dysplasia, high-grade dysplasia, and early carcinoma were visualized in 13%, 67%, and 75% of patients, respectively.

Although PET scans are commonly used in the detection of malignancy, it is important to note that benign conditions that have an increased utilization of glucose may also exhibit high ^{18}F-FDG uptake, including inflammatory processes such as infection, scarring, or inflammatory bowel disease. In general, the level of FDG uptake is highest in malignancies; however, there may be areas of overlap that may lead to equivocal interpretation. Finally, the timing of PET scanning in relation to treatment is also important, as FDG avidity can be increased after radiotherapy and reduced after chemotherapy. In particular, chemotherapy has been associated with a 40% decrease in tumor cell hexokinase activity, which is the rate-liming glycolytic enzyme. Accordingly, ^{18}F-FDG PET performed within 4 weeks of chemotherapy may be associated with higher false-negative rates.

Screening

The utility of ^{18}F-FDG PET in the routine screening of colorectal cancer is unproven, and no prospective trials have incorporated ^{18}F-FDG PET as a screening modality. Current recommendations for screening recommend fecal occult blood tests, endoscopy, or barium enema. Colonoscopy and barium enemas are able to detect over 90% of colorectal cancers. Approximately 30% of screening colonoscopies detect a new colorectal cancer in average-risk patients.

Colonoscopies serve both diagnostic and therapeutic purposes; they are performed ubiquitously and are relatively inexpensive. In contrast, the availability ^{18}F-FDG PET is more limited and is associated with a significant cost, ranging from $3000 to $6000. In addition, any suspicious finding on ^{18}F-FDG PET would likely require a colonoscopy for pathologic diagnosis. Given the current cost limitations and the need for additional procedures, ^{18}F-FDG PET is unlikely to play a pivotal role in the screening of primary colorectal cancer.

Staging

Preoperative staging serves a different purpose in patients with colon cancer compared with those with rectal cancer. In colon cancer patients, the aim of preoperative staging is to identify patients with metastatic disease. Asymptomatic patients with metastatic disease may receive systemic therapy rather than an initial resection of the primary tumor. In those patients who have metastatic disease confined to the liver or lung, several recent series have reported 5-year survival rates of up to 60% after metastasectomy. Prolonged survival rates are in part due to improved surgical techniques and chemotherapy, but they are also the result of careful patient selection. Currently, one of the most compelling indications for ^{18}F-FDG PET is in the evaluation of patients undergoing metastasectomy. CT scans have a reported sensitivity of 61% to 64% and a specificity of 91% to 94% in detecting extrahepatic metastatic disease, and MRI yields similar results.

Several studies have demonstrated ^{18}F-FDG PET to be superior to all other conventional imaging modalities in detecting metastatic disease, with sensitivity of 79% to 100% and specificity of 73% to 100%. In patients being considered for resection who have high-risk clinical features, initial staging ^{18}F-FDG PET identified unresectable disease in 23% of patients. Furthermore, based on the ^{18}F-FDG PET findings, clinical management was changed in 40% of patients. In the setting of colon cancer staging, ^{18}F-FDG PET (PET/CT) should be considered in patients with high clinical suspicion of metastatic disease, or in those patients being considered for metastasectomy to rule out other occult metastatic disease (see Table 1 for a summary of indications for PET scans in colorectal cancer).

In contrast, for patients with rectal cancer, staging is important not only to identify the presence of metastatic disease, but also to identify patients with advanced locoregional disease who will benefit from neoadjuvant therapies. Increasingly, ^{18}F-FDG PET/CT has been utilized to characterize both locoregional and metastatic disease in patients with rectal cancer (Figures 1 and 2).

Traditionally, rectal cancer staging has involved delineating T (primary tumor) and N (regional lymph nodes) involvement with endorectal ultrasound (ERUS) or magnetic resonance imaging (MRI). The additional benefit of ^{18}F-FDG PET to ERUS or MRI staging has been limited, since the resolution of ^{18}F-FDG PET does not allow for

TABLE 1: Summary of evidence to support use of ^{18}F-FDG PET in colorectal cancer

Indication	Summary of Evidence	Recommendations
Primary diagnosis and staging	Two studies in primary rectal cancer staging find ^{18}F-FDG PET to affect management in 14% to 27% of cases. No studies support ^{18}F-FDG PET in routine staging of colon cancer.	^{18}F-FDG PET should be used selectively in patients with primary colon cancer screening in the setting of high clinical suspicion of metastatic disease. ^{18}F-FDG PET may be considered in the staging of primary rectal cancer.
Treatment response	Several studies have suggested that change in observed SUV after neoadjuvant chemoradiation predicts long-term outcomes. Single study has not correlated ΔSUV after neoadjuvant chemoradiation to histopathologic response.	Changes in ^{18}F-FDG PET response may be related to treatment efficacy, but further investigation is required to confirm this relation.
Evaluation of recurrence	^{18}F-FDG PET and ^{18}F-FDG PET/CT are more sensitive than CT or MRI in the detection of recurrent disease. ^{18}F-FDG PET is accurate in distinguishing between scar and tumor recurrence. The addition of ^{18}F-FDG PET to restaging affects further clinical management in up to 40% of cases.	^{18}F-FDG PET should be considered in the restaging of patients with suspected colorectal recurrence.
Preoperative staging before metastasectomy	^{18}F-FDG PET is more sensitive than CT in detecting extrahepatic recurrences. ^{18}F-FDG PET is superior to other conventional imaging in identifying unresectable metastatic disease.	^{18}F-FDG PET should be considered in the restaging of patients with suspected colorectal recurrence.

Δ SUV, Change in standardized uptake value

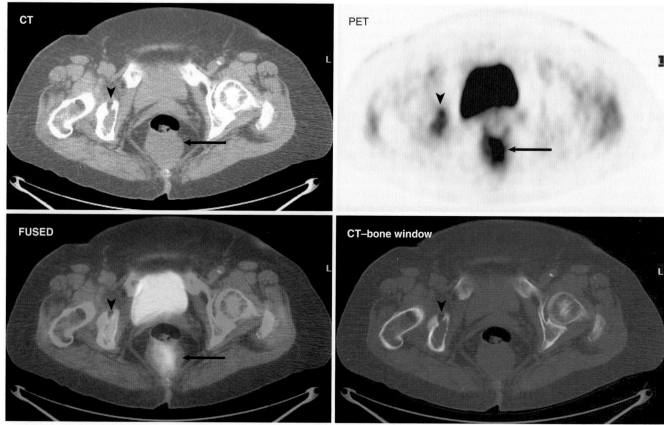

FIGURE 1 Patient with rectal cancer who has synchronous bony metastasis to the pelvis. The *arrow* shows the FDG-avid primary rectal cancer; the *arrowhead* shows the bony metastases. Normal bladder activity is seen anterior to the primary rectal tumor.

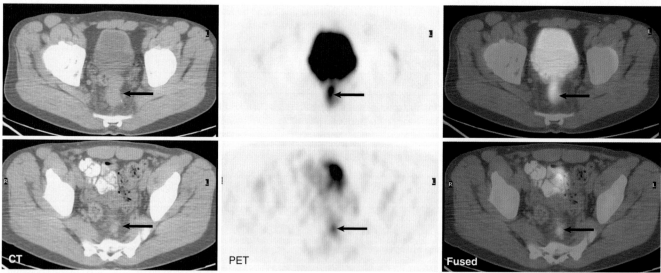

FIGURE 2 Patient preoperatively staged with T3N0 rectal cancer by endorectal ultrasound 10 cm from anal verge. Preoperative ¹⁸F-FDG PET-CT demonstrated intense FDG uptake in the primary tumor (*upper panel, arrow*). A focus of uptake fusing to a soft-tissue nodule superior to the primary tumor was highly suspicious for nodal metastasis (*lower panel, arrow*). Patient received neoadjuvant chemoradiotherapy followed by surgery. Final pathology demonstrated 13 positive lymph nodes.

differentiation between T stages, and signal overlap from the primary tumor complicates the detection of nodal metastasis (sensitivity 22% to 29%). More recently, however, two studies have examined staging patients with rectal cancer using combined ¹⁸F-FDG PET/CT imaging. In two small, single-institution series, the addition of PET/CT to conventional CT, MRI, and/or ERUS resulted in a change from the initial staging in 31% to 38% of patients. One study found that patients with low rectal cancers in particular were more often restaged based on additional PET/CT findings. In both studies, patients were most often restaged due to identification of occult regional (iliac or inguinal) lymph node metastases. Patients were both upstaged and downstaged, resulting in a significant change in management in 14% to 27% of patients.

Although PET/CT is not routinely used in the staging of rectal cancer, it has the potential to alter treatment strategies. Further studies are needed to identify which patients may benefit from preoperative PET/CT staging. However, for the purpose of preoperative staging, ^{18}F-FDG PET/CT is clearly superior to ^{18}F-FDG PET in characterizing locoregional disease.

Assessment of Treatment Response

Because ^{18}F-FDG PET has the ability to provide functional information about a tumor's metabolic activity, it has been evaluated as a means to predict response to chemotherapy or radiotherapy. In several tumor types, it has been shown that changes in tumor metabolic activity on ^{18}F-FDG PET precede radiographic evidence of response, allowing for earlier detection of treatment efficacy. For colorectal cancer, one series has reported the sensitivity and specificity of ^{18}F-FDG PET in identifying response to neoadjuvant chemoradiation to be 100% (CT, 54%; MRI, 71%) and 60% (CT, 80%; MRI, 67%), respectively. Furthermore, ^{18}F-FDG PET response to neoadjuvant therapy has been correlated with survival outcomes. In a small, single-institution series, the change in ^{18}F-FDG PET standardized uptake value (ΔSUV) greater than 62.5% after neoadjuvant chemoradiation in rectal cancer patients correlated with improved disease-specific and recurrence-free survival.

Other studies have corroborated the finding that changes in ^{18}F-FDG PET signal following neoadjuvant therapy is predictive of disease-free and overall survival. Interestingly, only one study has been performed examining the relationship of ^{18}F-FDG PET to histopathologic response. In this study of 30 patients, 40% of patients had a false-negative ^{18}F-FDG PET/CT, with positive and negative predictive values of 83% and 33%, respectively. Several explanations have been offered to correlate the disparate results of this study with previous published reports on outcome.

Further investigation is necessary to determine whether any relationship exists between ^{18}F-FDG PET response and histopathologic response. If a significant metabolic response can be correlated to histopathologic response, patients may be selected for more aggressive surgical procedures or for close observation in the setting of a complete response. Conversely, lack of ^{18}F-FDG PET response may identify patients with biologically aggressive disease who are unlikely to benefit from surgery.

^{18}F-FDG PET may be useful in the assessment of response after radiofrequency ablation (RFA) for the treatment of metastatic colorectal cancer lesions. In this setting, conventional radiographic response criteria for cross-sectional images such as CT and MRI may be unreliable due to the inability to distinguish between treatment artifact, such as hemorrhage, and residual tumor. Alteration in anatomy after RFA may also complicate the identification of local recurrences. ^{18}F-FDG PET may improve post-RFA evaluation by utilizing the presence of metabolic activity. Successful ablation is typically represented as an area of photopenia on ^{18}F-FDG PET/CT and can be used to correlate the observed structural changes seen with conventional imaging to assess completeness of ablation.

Initial concerns that RFA may create an inflammatory response that may confound ^{18}F-FDG PET interpretation remain unclear. In a study of ^{18}F-FDG PET after RFA, seven of eight patients had no inflammatory uptake on ^{18}F-FDG PET performed within 2 days of treatment. The timing of the PET scan after RFA seems to be an important consideration. These preliminary findings need to be validated in larger prospective trials. However, ^{18}F-FDG PET may serve as a tool to assess RFA completeness and monitor for recurrence after therapy.

Management of Colorectal Recurrence

After surgery for colorectal cancer, up to 50% of patients will develop recurrent disease. Of these patients, 10% to 15% may be offered surgical resection. Recurrences may be identified clinically, biochemically (with rising CEA), or by changes seen on conventional imaging modalities. The sensitivity and specificity of serum CEA measurements are 59% and 84%, respectively. The sensitivity of conventional diagnostic imaging in detecting colorectal recurrences ranges from 52% to 78%. In contrast, ^{18}F-FDG PET has been reported to have the greatest sensitivity and specificity in the detection of both local recurrences and metastatic disease. A recent meta-analysis of 11 studies found ^{18}F-FDG PET to have an overall sensitivity and specificity rate of 97% and 76%, respectively.

Although no evidence is available to support the use of ^{18}F-FDG PET in routine surveillance following curative resection, both ^{18}F-FDG PET and ^{18}F-FDG PET/CT have an established role in the care of patients with suspected recurrent disease. In particular, ^{18}F-FDG PET is useful in three clinical scenarios: 1) in patients with rising CEA but radiographically occult disease, 2) in the evaluation of indeterminate or equivocal lesions seen on standard imaging modalities, and 3) for the exclusion of other sites of metastatic disease in patients being considered for curative metastasectomy. Up to 70% of patients with asymptomatic recurrent colorectal disease will present with elevated serum CEA levels, often without any accompanying radiographic findings to suggest recurrence. In this setting, up to 90% of recurrences are intraabdominal, but only a small percentage will be amenable to curative resection. The inability to identify the site of disease radiographically limits any subsequent treatment strategies to either observation or to empiric second-look laparotomy.

Alternatively, ^{18}F-FDG PET imaging may be used to detect previously radiographically occult metastases (Figure 3). In a study of 22 patients with colorectal cancer who developed a rising CEA level but had a normal CT scan, ^{18}F-FDG PET had a positive predictive value of 89% and a negative predictive value of 100%. In another prospective study of patients with elevated serum CEA levels, patients underwent extensive preoperative staging with CT, MRI, bone scan, colonoscopy, and ^{18}F-FDG PET and CEA scan. Patients were then taken to the operating room for a second-look laparotomy; the patients were explored twice, once by a surgeon blinded to the ^{18}F-FDG PET scan results and once by an unblinded surgeon, to identify metastatic disease. In this study, ^{18}F-FDG PET was superior to all imaging studies in identifying sites of recurrence and was accurate in predicting unresectable disease in 90% of patients. These studies suggest that ^{18}F-FDG PET may be useful in identifying sites of recurrence in patients with a rising CEA without a radiographic correlate.

It is often difficult to distinguish posttherapy changes from local recurrence. In particular, after surgical resection and radiation therapy, scarring and fibrosis may be difficult to distinguish from local recurrence based on conventional imaging modalities. Although CT and MRI are both accurate at detecting pelvic masses after colorectal surgery, they are unreliable in distinguishing between scarring and tumor recurrence. These lesions may be observed over a period of time for growth to determine malignant potential, however, this also risks losing a window of resectability.

Increasingly, ^{18}F-FDG PET has been studied as a means to differentiate between scarring and tumor recurrence. Multiple studies have demonstrated ^{18}F-FDG PET to be superior to CT in this differentiation. More recently, ^{18}F-FDG PET/CT has been shown to improve the ability of ^{18}F-FDG PET to distinguish between benign and malignant disease. In the largest series, 62 patients who had previously undergone low anterior resection or abdominoperineal resection were evaluated with ^{18}F-FDG PET or ^{18}F-FDG PET/CT for locoregional recurrence. ^{18}F-FDG PET/CT was superior in distinguishing between scar and tumor, with sensitivity and specificity of 98% and 96% and positive and negative predictive values of 90% and 97%.

Finally, ^{18}F-FDG PET has increasingly been utilized in the staging of patients with recurrent colorectal cancer prior to metastasectomy. Over 60% of patients with colorectal cancer develop metastases, with the liver being the most common site of disease. It is well established that resection of colorectal liver metastases can result in a survival advantage for selected patients, however, a rigorous search for occult

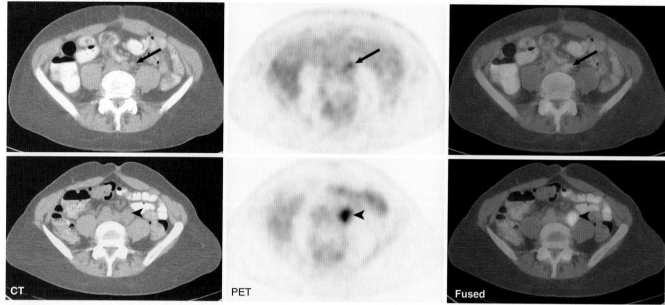

FIGURE 3   Patient with a history of stage II colon cancer and normal CEA. ^{18}F-FDG PET-CT scan demonstrated a normal-sized node, with moderate uptake, suspicious for recurrence (*upper panel, arrow*). Repeat ^{18}F-FDG PET-CT several months later (*lower panel*) confirmed progressive disease (*arrowhead*). At surgery, patient was found to have recurrent cancer.

metastases should be performed prior to any attempts at curative metastasectomy.

Despite improvement in CT and MRI technology, several studies have reported nontherapeutic laparotomy rates from 9% to 50%. At our institution, with preoperative CT or MRI, the nontherapeutic laparotomy rates approached 10%. The addition of ^{18}F-FDG PET has reduced the rate of nontherapeutic laparotomy (5.6% vs. 12.4%, $P = .09$, odds ratio of 0.42). In a double-blind prospective comparative study, the sensitivity of ^{18}F-FDG PET in detecting hepatic metastasis was comparable to CT; however, ^{18}F-FDG PET was more sensitive at detecting extrahepatic disease. CT scan fails to identify extrahepatic disease in up to one third of patients. In another series of high-risk patients being considered for liver resection, the addition of ^{18}F-FDG PET changed clinical management in 40% of patients, of which 23% avoided surgery because of unresectable disease. In the setting of metastatic disease, ^{18}F-FDG PET may yield important additional information and should be considered in the workup prior to curative metastasectomy.

SUMMARY

^{18}F-FDG PET is a sensitive and specific test for the evaluation of primary and recurrent colorectal cancer. In addition, most centers now utilize the combination of ^{18}F-FDG PET/CT for its superior sensitivity and specificity. The use of ^{18}F-FDG PET scans in colorectal cancer is becoming more ubiquitous, however, its application should be individualized. Although it is routinely used in the staging of several malignancies, including lung and esophageal cancer, the benefit of ^{18}F-FDG PET as a staging tool in all colorectal cancers is unproven; however, an increasing body of literature supports its use in the staging of primary rectal cancer.

The most well-established use of ^{18}F-FDG PET for colorectal cancer is in the management of recurrent disease. In this setting, ^{18}F-FDG PET may facilitate the detection of occult or ambiguous disease and may significantly impact clinical management. The use

of ^{18}F-FDG PET to evaluate treatment response is evolving, and the routine use of ^{18}F-FDG PET for surveillance is yet to be defined. The major limitations of its widespread application are related to the cost of the procedure as well as its availability. Currently, Medicare reimburses ^{18}F-FDG PET imaging for the initial treatment strategy (previously called *diagnosis and initial staging*) and the subsequent treatment strategy of colorectal cancer, which includes treatment monitoring, restaging, and detection of recurrent disease.

A small number of European studies have found the application of ^{18}F-FDG PET in colorectal cancer management to be cost effective, with an incremental cost savings of over $3000 per patient because of the elimination of contraindicated surgical procedure and therapies, but this finding remains to be reproduced in the United States.

SUGGESTED READINGS

Davey K, Heriot AG, Mackay J, et al: The impact of 18-fluorodeoxyglucose positron emission tomography–computed tomography on the staging and management of primary rectal cancer, *Dis Colon Rectum* 51(7):997–1003, 2008.

Even-Sapir E, Parag Y, Lerman H, et al: Detection of recurrence in patients with rectal cancer: PET/CT after abdominoperineal or anterior resection, *Radiology* 232(3):815–822, 2004.

Fong Y, Saldinger PF, Akherst T, et al: Utility of 18F-FDG positron emission tomography scanning on selection of patients for resection of hepatic colorectal metastases, *Am J Surg* 178(4):282–287, 1999.

Gearhart SL, Frassica D, Rosen R, et al: Improved staging with pretreatment positron emission tomography/computed tomography in low rectal cancer, *Ann Surg Oncol* 13(3):397–404, 2006.

Guillem JG, Moore HG, Akhurst T, et al: Sequential preoperative fluorodeoxyglucose-positron emission tomography assessment of response to preoperative chemoradiation: a means for determining long-term outcomes of rectal cancer, *J Am Coll Surg* 199(1):1–7, 2004.

Libutti SK, Alexander HR Jr, Choyke P, et al: A prospective study of 2-[18F] fluoro-2-deoxy-D-glucose/positron emission tomography scan, 99mTc-labeled arcitumomab (CEA scan), and blind second-look laparotomy for detecting colon cancer recurrence in patients with increasing carcinoembryonic antigen levels, *Ann Surg Oncol* 8(10):779–786, 2001.

Neoadjuvant and Adjuvant Treatment for Colorectal Cancer

Axel Grothey, MD

OVERVIEW

Colorectal cancer (CRC) is the second leading cause of cancer mortality in the United States. In 2009, an estimated 146,970 new cases of cancer of the colon and rectum were diagnosed in the United States, and 49,920 deaths were associated with this disease. Almost 40% of patients with newly diagnosed colorectal carcinoma have locoregional spread of the disease at diagnosis, and 20% have distant metastasis.

Surgical resection is the foundation of a curative approach in both colon and rectal cancer. The emergence of distant metastasis after potentially curative resection, the most common form of tumor recurrence, is due to the presence of micrometastatic spread that occurred before or during the actual surgery. The goal of postoperative adjuvant chemotherapy is to eradicate these micrometastases and thereby increase the chance for long-term cure.

In rectal cancer, because of the special anatomic challenges for locally curative resection, chemotherapy is routinely and preferably complemented by preoperative neoadjuvant radiation therapy to reduce the risk of local recurrence. It is important to note that the majority of patients will not actually benefit from adjuvant or neoadjuvant therapy because they are either cured by surgery alone or experience a recurrence in spite of therapy. Unfortunately, our understanding is rudimentary when it comes to selecting groups of patients that might benefit from adjuvant therapy, and the decision to use such treatment is mainly based on an assessment of the risk of recurrence in view of the anatomical tumor stage. Molecular markers and signatures that will help refine the assessment of prognosis of patients are in development, and perhaps eventually these will also serve as predictive tools to identify patients who will benefit from specific adjuvant therapies.

STAGING

Formal CRC staging is essential to establish the risk of recurrence and to ensure that the goals of care are curative rather than palliative. The National Comprehensive Cancer Network (NCCN) recommends that the preoperative workup for colon and rectal cancers include a colonoscopy, complete blood counts, comprehensive electrolyte panel, carcinoembryonic antigen (CEA) serum level, computed tomography (CT) scan of abdomen, pelvis, and chest, and a pathologic review. In general, the preoperative workup in rectal cancer is similar to that of colon cancer, with the optional addition of pelvic magnetic resonance imaging (MRI) or endoscopic ultrasound (EUS) to help better define the depth of invasion and lymph node spread. Accurate preoperative staging is critical, because rectal cancer therapy often includes a neoadjuvant radiation or radiochemotherapy component, which can lead to downstaging of the primary tumor and lymph node metastases. Positron emission tomography (PET) is not routinely indicated but is often used if there are suspicious findings on the CT scan that suggest disease outside the colon and rectum. It should also be considered mandatory before surgical resection of limited metastatic, stage IV disease (e.g., liver metastasis).

The true pathologic stage is defined after the appropriate surgical procedure. Upon its introduction in 1987 by the American Joint Committee on Cancer (AJCC), the TNM (*T*, primary tumor; *N*, regional lymph nodes; *M*, distant metastasis) staging system has largely replaced the Dukes and other older staging systems for CRC. The most recent revision of the AJCC staging system (seventh edition) came into effect in January 2010 (Table 1). As demonstrated in Table 2, the 5-year survival rates for both colon and rectal cancer are stage dependent. For patients with stage I disease, surgery alone is the treatment of choice, because the 5-year survival is greater than 90%. As discussed in this chapter, the more extensive the disease and the more aggressive the tumor biology, the greater the benefit of the adjuvant therapy.

ADJUVANT CHEMOTHERAPY FOR COLON CANCER

Stage III Colon Cancer

The initial trial presented in the early 1990s that established adjuvant chemotherapy as the standard of care in stage III colon cancer used a combination of 5-fluorouracil (5-FU) and levamisole administered for 12 months. A 10% to 20% improvement in 5-year survival was documented for patients receiving postoperative adjuvant fluorouracil-based chemotherapy. Evidence from newer trials demonstrated that 5-FU combined with leucovorin (5-FU/LV) provides a superior outcome, with 6 months of therapy being adequate to achieve this survival benefit. For more than a decade, the standard in adjuvant therapy remained unchanged because of the lack of novel agents with relevant activity in CRC. This changed when oxaliplatin, irinotecan, and the oral 5-FU prodrug capecitabine were utilized for the treatment of advanced CRC, with combination regimens of infusional 5-FU plus either irinotecan or oxaliplatin demonstrating high antitumor efficacy.

Worldwide, seven phase III trials were conducted to evaluate the value of the novel chemotherapeutic agents irinotecan, oxaliplatin, and capecitabine in the adjuvant setting. To set the stage for the conduct and interpretation of these trials and their results, a large retrospective meta-analysis confirmed that for adjuvant colon cancer, 3-year disease-free survival (DFS) can serve as an definitive surrogate marker for 5-year overall survival (OS). This finding had a major effect on clinical trial design and end-point definition in subsequent studies of adjuvant therapy for colon cancer. Based on these findings, the FDA recognized 3-year DFS as an appropriate end point for full approval of a regimen for colon cancer. Subsequently, a series of phase III adjuvant trials was presented and published that has shaped the current standard of adjuvant therapy (Table 3).

One trial established 6 months of oral capecitabine as a safe and at least equally effective alternative to conventional intravenous bolus 5-FU/LV (Mayo Clinic regimen) for stage III colon cancer. Three trials confirmed the value of oxaliplatin as a component of adjuvant chemotherapy for stage II and III colon cancer. The results of the pivotal Multicenter International Study of Oxaliplatin/5-FU/LV in the Adjuvant Treatment of Colon Cancer trial clearly demonstrated that oxaliplatin plus infusional 5-FU/LV (FOLFOX) is superior to 5-FU/LV in terms of 3-year DFS. In a subgroup analysis, only the rise in DFS for patients with stage III disease was statistically significant, providing an absolute benefit in approximately 8% to 10% (hazard ratio, 0.76; 95% confidence interval, 0.62 to 0.92). Consequently, oxaliplatin was approved as part of adjuvant treatment for stage III colon cancer in November 2004.

In unselected patients with stage II disease, the DFS with FOLFOX compared with 5-FU/LV alone was approximately 3.5%, but it exceeded 5% for patients with stage II tumors with clinical

TABLE 1: American Joint Committee on Cancer (AJCC) TNM classification of colon cancer

Primary Tumor (T)	
Tis	Carcinoma in situ
T1	Tumor invades submucosa
T2	Tumor invades muscularis propria
T3	Tumor invades through muscularis propria or subserosa
T4	Tumor directly invades other organs or structures
T4a	Perforation of visceral peritoneum
T4b	Invasion of adjacent organs
Regional Lymph Nodes (N)	
N0	No regional lymph node (LN) metastases
N1	Metastases in one to three regional LNs
N1a	One LN positive
N1b	Two to three LNs positive
N2	Metastases in four or more regional LNs
N2a	Four to six LNs positive
N2b	More than six LNs positive
Distant Metastases (M)	
M0	No distant metastases
M1	Distant metastases

From *The AJCC cancer staging manual*, ed 7, Philadelphia, 2010, Springer.

TABLE 2: TNM classification, staging, and survival

TNM Category	% of Patients	TNM Stage	5-Year Survival (%)
T1 N0	9.9	I	97.4
T2 N0	11.8	I	96.8
T3 N0	36.7	IIA	87.5
T4a N0	4.6	IIB	79.6
T4b N0	2.8	IIC	58.4
T1-2 N1a	1.7	IIIA	90.7
T1-2 N1b	1.1	IIIA	83.0
T1 N2a	0.3	IIIA	79.0
T2 N2a		IIIB	
T1-2 N2b	0.1	IIIB	74.2
T3 N1a	8.0	IIIB	74.2
T3 N1b	8.3	IIIB	65.3
T3 N2a	4.8	IIIB	53.4
T3 N2b	2.9	IIIC	37.3
T4a N1a	1.2	IIIB	67.6
T4b N1a	0.8	IIIC	38.5
T4a N1b	1.3	IIIB	54.0
T4b N1b	0.8	IIIC	31.2
T4a N2a	0.9	IIIC	40.9
T4b N2a	0.7	IIIC	23.3
T4a N2b	0.6	IIIC	21.8
T4b N2b	0.6	IIIC	15.7

Data from *The AJCC cancer staging manual*, ed 7, Philadelphia, 2010, Springer.

high-risk features (undifferentiated tumors, T4, perforation, obstruction, fewer than 10 lymph nodes identified, angiolymphatic invasion). A recent update demonstrated a significant improvement in 6-year (not 5-year) OS for patients with stage III colon cancer, but not for unselected patients with stage II colon cancer, when an oxaliplatin-based regimen was used as adjuvant therapy. Results of the National Surgical Adjuvant Breast and Bowel Project (NSABP) C-07 trial further strengthened the role of oxaliplatin-based regimens in the adjuvant treatment of colon cancer.

Most recently, data from the phase III XELOXA trial randomized 1886 patients with stage III colon cancer to either bolus 5-FU/LV (Mayo Clinic or Roswell Park regimen) or a combination of capecitabine and oxaliplatin (XELOX). The use of XELOX was associated with an incremental increase in DFS at 3 years of 4% (71% vs. 67%), which is similar to the results obtained in the other two adjuvant oxaliplatin-based trials.

Although regimens based on irinotecan and oxaliplatin are thought to be equally effective as palliative therapy for advanced colorectal cancer, none of the three phase III trials using combination regimens of irinotecan with 5-FU/LV demonstrated significantly superior efficacy regarding 3-year DFS compared with 5-FU/LV alone. Similar to irinotecan, both monoclonal antibodies with clear activity in metastatic colorectal cancer, bevacizumab and cetuximab, failed to provide clinical benefit as measured by 3-year DFS when added to FOLFOX as adjuvant therapy for colon cancer.

Based on these results, the standard adjuvant chemotherapy for stage III colon cancer is an oxaliplatin-containing regimen (FOLFOX or bolus 5-FU/LV plus oxaliplatin [FLOX] or XELOX) administered for 6 months. Capecitabine and 5-FU/LV should be reserved for patients who are not considered optimal candidates for oxaliplatin. Initial analysis suggested that the efficacy and tolerability of FOLFOX is largely identical for patients younger and older than age 70 years. However, updated results of the MOSAIC trial and a meta-analysis of the MOSAIC and NSABP C-07 trials demonstrated that patients older than 70 years do not derive any benefit with regard to DFS and OS from the use of oxaliplatin, not even in a stage III setting. Thus the use of FOLFOX as adjuvant therapy should be limited to the fit and biologically young–appearing older patient population.

Stage II Colon Cancer

For patients with stage II disease, the role of adjuvant chemotherapy remains controversial; the results from a series of clinical trials demonstrated a trend toward improved recurrence-free survival and overall survival (hazard ratio, 0.80; 95% confidence interval, 0.56 to 1.15). Findings from two pooled retrospective analyses showed

TABLE 3: Results of selected recent phase III adjuvant trials in colon cancer

Trial	Stage (% of Patients)	Regimen	3-Year DFS (%)	P Value HR (95% CI)	6-Year OS (%)	P Value HR (95% CI)
X-ACT N = 1987	III	Mayo Cape	61.0 64.6	P = .0525 0.87 (0.75–1.0)	NA	
Oxaliplatin Regimens						
MOSAIC N = 2246	II/III (40/60)	LV5FU2		P < .001 0.77 (0.65–0.90)	76.0	P = .046 0.84 (0.71–1.00)
		FOLFOX			78.5	
	II	LV5FU2		0.82 (0.60–1.13)	86.8	P = .986 1.00 (0.70–1.41)
		FOLFOX			86.9	
	III	LV5FU2		0.75 (0.62–0.89)	68.7	P = .023 0.80 (0.65–0.97)
		FOLFOX			72.9	
NSABP C-07 N = 2407	II/III (29/71)	RP	71.6	P < .004 0.79 (0.67–0.93)	73.5	P = .06 0.85 (0.72–1.01)
		FLOX	76.5		78.3	
XELOXA	III	RP/Mayo	67.0	P = .0045 0.80 (0.69–0.93)	NA	
N = 1886		XELOX	71.0			

HR, Hazard ratio; *CI,* confidence intervals; *Cape,* capecitabine; *Mayo,* Mayo Clinic bolus 5-FU/LV regimen; *RP,* Roswell Park bolus 5-FU/LV regimen; *LV5FU2,* bolus/infusional 5-FU/LV regimen; *FOLFOX,* bolus/infusional 5-FU/LV plus oxaliplatin; *FLOX,* bolus 5-FU/LV plus oxaliplatin; *XELOX,* capecitabine plus oxaliplatin; *NA,* not available.

conflicting results. One analysis suggested a 30% risk reduction, translating into an approximate 8% absolute reduction in mortality, whereas a similar pooled data set showed no benefit from adjuvant chemotherapy. An analysis of Medicare data revealed that more than 50% of patients in the United States with stage II colon cancer receive postoperative adjuvant chemotherapy. In view of these data, and the UK QUASAR (QUick And Simple And Reliable) trial, it appears that unselected patients with stage II colon cancer (i.e., not distinguished between high-risk and low-risk stage II) will have a 3% benefit in 3-year DFS and OS with bolus 5-FU/LV as adjuvant chemotherapy.

Current American College of Clinical Oncology (ASCO) recommendations suggest that not all patients with stage II tumors should receive adjuvant chemotherapy, but that a discussion should be had with patients about their individual benefit/risk ratio when utilizing adjuvant chemotherapy in stage II colon cancer. Efforts have been made to individualize the baseline prognosis and to predict the benefits of chemotherapy for patients with resected colon cancer. As a result, two Web-based tools are available to provide data of this type (an adjuvant therapy calculator developed by the Mayo Clinic and Adjuvant! online). Although neither of these tools is infallible, but they can provide helpful information. Over the last few years, our understanding of stage II colon cancer has made significant advances, leading to a refinement in the identification of the patient population and in the treatment options considered appropriate as adjuvant therapy in this setting.

First of all, it has been shown that the addition of oxaliplatin to 5-FU does not improve OS in unselected stage II colon cancer, and that even in patients with so-called high-risk stage II colon cancers, the use of oxaliplatin might improve DFS but not OS. With regard to

staging, T4N0 tumors (stage IIB according to the AJCC sixth edition, or stage IIB/IIC per the seventh edition) have clearly been associated with poor prognosis, worse than for T3N1 colon cancers.

In addition, the number of lymph nodes identified in the surgical specimen has routinely been correlated with clinical outcomes. This finding appears to go beyond the fact that the number of analyzed lymph nodes will enhance accurate staging; unknown biological factors potentially reflecting the immunocompetence of the patient have been discussed to explain this phenomenon. Other clinical parameters such as obstruction/perforation at presentation, undifferentiated histology, perineural infiltration, and lymphovascular invasion might be helpful to further characterize the prognosis of patients with stage II colon cancer, although not all of these parameters have been validated in multivariate analyses.

More recently, novel approaches to identify single molecular factors or molecular signatures as prognostic markers in colon cancer have shown promising results. In fact, various studies have confirmed that those 10% to 20% of stage II tumors that exhibit a defective mismatch repair (MMR-D) or microsatellite unstable (MSI-H) phenotype have an excellent prognosis but are potentially 5-FU resistant, and such patients should thus not receive adjuvant 5-FU. Unfortunately, with the exception of MSI-H/MMR-D tumors, no further predictive markers for chemosensitivity in adjuvant colon cancer have been identified.

Molecular techniques might also be helpful to enhance the correct classification of stage II cancers as truly lymph-node negative. For instance, the detection of guanylyl cyclase 2C (GCC), an enzyme exclusively expressed in luminal cells of the intestinal tract, in lymph nodes of cancers characterized as stage II by conventional means has been associated with poor prognosis.

NEOADJUVANT AND ADJUVANT THERAPY FOR RECTAL CANCER

Cancers arising in the rectum are associated with a higher overall risk of recurrence than with similar stages of colon cancer. In particular, locoregional failures can occur in 25% to 50% of patients who undergo potentially curative surgery without further perioperative therapy, most likely because of close surgical margins. The reason for local recurrence in rectal cancer is believed to be the anatomic location of the rectum and the challenge this presents to the surgeon, particularly surgeons practicing in low-volume hospitals. Increasing evidence suggests that local excision should be restricted to patients with T1 rectal cancer without high-risk factors. For all other stages, total mesorectal excision (TME) has emerged as the preferred surgical technique. This technique honors natural tissue planes and decreases the chance for local seeding and subsequent recurrence. In combination with preoperative or postoperative chemoradiation, local recurrence rates of less than 10% at 5 years can be achieved.

Recognition of the significant morbidity and potential mortality associated with local relapse has led to the use of both preoperative and postoperative radiation therapy as additional regional treatment options designed to reduce local recurrence. Two different approaches have been used in this regard: short-term, high-dose radiation, commonly delivered as daily 5 Gy for 5 days (5 x 5) immediately before surgery, or prolonged combined-modality therapy with radiosensitizing chemotherapy administered parallel to radiation to a total dose of 50.4 Gy (45 + 5.4 Gy local boost) over 5 to 6 weeks, followed by a 3- to 4-week interval before curative surgery.

It is important to note that only the longer chemoradiation approach is able to downstage tumors and cause tumor shrinkage that might allow sphincter-preserving surgery. Both treatment approaches, however, have been associated with a decrease in locoregional failure, but prevention of local recurrence has not uniformly been associated with improved overall survival. However, the results of one Swedish trial in which 1168 patients were randomly assigned to either 5 days of high-dose radiation therapy (to 25 Gy) in the week just before surgery or to surgery alone demonstrated a reduction in local recurrences (11% vs. 27%, $P < .001$) and a survival advantage at 5 years (58% vs. 48%, $P = .004$) for preoperative radiation therapy. A subsequent Dutch trial using the same radiation technique in combination with quality-controlled TME surgery confirmed a low rate of local recurrence (at 2 years, 2.4% vs. 8.4%, $P < .001$) but failed to demonstrate a survival benefit. It is of note, however, that the local recurrence rate of tumors more than 10 cm from the anal verge was not significantly affected.

Although the shorter, high-dose preoperative radiation strategy is most commonly used in Scandinavia and in European countries, U.S. oncologists have historically preferred combined-modality therapy with preoperative and postoperative chemoradiation. Findings from two studies of postoperative adjuvant chemoradiation demonstrated that 5-FU–based chemotherapy plus radiation was more effective than radiation or surgery alone in preventing both local and distant recurrence. Results from another trial showed that prolonged infusion of fluorouracil was superior to bolus administration during radiation therapy, providing a 3-year DFS advantage. This finding confirms that protracted delivery of chemosensitizing agents concomitant with radiation is the best way to deliver combined-modality therapy. In clinical practice, capecitabine administered twice daily parallel to radiation has become a widely used substitute for continuous infusion of 5-FU, although definitive results of trials comparing capecitabine with 5-FU as radiosensitizers are not available yet.

The long-standing question about whether preoperative or postoperative chemoradiation delivers improved outcome was definitively answered by the results of a large German randomized trial that compared standard, continuously infused 5-FU plus radiation either before or after quality-controlled TME. Patients undergoing preoperative combined-modality therapy had a lower rate of local recurrence (at 5 years, 6% vs. 13%), a lower rate of acute and chronic toxicities,

and a significantly higher rate of sphincter preservation compared with postoperative chemoradiation ($P = .006$). This trial established preoperative neoadjuvant radiochemotherapy with 5-FU as a radiosensitizer as new standard of care for stage II and III rectal cancers.

Subsequent studies are trying to further improve the local control rate by incorporating additional radiosensitizing agents, such as oxaliplatin, and biologic agents into the preoperative treatment phase. Current studies also are seeking to enhance the activity of the postoperative adjuvant therapy by using regimens effective against colon cancer, such as FOLFOX with or without the addition of novel biologic agents.

POSTTREATMENT SURVEILLANCE

The majority of patients with colorectal cancer can undergo surgery with curative intent following diagnosis. Unfortunately, depending on the stage, 30% to 50% of these patients will relapse with distant metastasis. Unlike most other solid tumors, salvage resection of solitary metastases or oligometastases to the liver and lungs may result in either long-term DFS or possible cure.

The best approach to surveillance remains controversial. The NCCN recommendations are similar to American Society of Clinical Oncology guidelines (see Table 4): history and physical every 3 months for 2 years, and then every 6 months for years 3 to 5; CEA every 3 months for 2 years, and then every 6 months for years 3 to 5; and a colonoscopy within 1 year following resection (within 3 to 6 months if the patient presented with obstruction, and a complete preoperative colonoscopy could not be performed), and then every 1 to 3 years on the basis of the findings. Chest, abdominal, and pelvic CT scans may be considered annually for patients at high risk for recurrence, including those with poorly differentiated histologic grade and perineural or venous invasion. If the patient is postmetastasectomy for synchronous liver disease, the recommendation for CT scans may be increased to every 3 to 6 months. PET scans are not recommended during regular surveillance, however, some evidence supports their use in the situation of a rising CEA without CT evidence of disease.

CURRENT RECOMMENDATIONS

The magnitude of benefit from adjuvant therapy appears to be proportional to the risk of relapse on the basis of pathologic stage (Figure 1). For stage III (node-positive) patients, the evidence supports the use of adjuvant chemotherapy for 6 months following resection. FOLFOX and XELOX are considered the standard of care, at least for patients younger than 70 years. Capecitabine and intravenous

---

TABLE 4: Guidelines of the National Comprehensive Cancer Network (NCCN) for colorectal cancer surveillance after curative surgery

- History and physical exam every 3 to 6 months for 2 years, then every 6 months for a total of 5 years
- CEA every 3 to 6 months for 2 years, then every 6 months for a total of 5 years for T2 or greater lesions
- Chest/abdomen/pelvis CT annually for 3 years for patients at high risk for recurrence
- Colonoscopy at 1 year, unless no preoperative colonoscopy due to obstructing lesion, then colonoscopy in 3 to 6 months
  - If advanced adenoma found, repeat in 1 year
  - If no advanced adenoma found, repeat in 3 years, then every 5 years

From National Comprehensive Cancer Network: *The NCCN practice guidelines for colon and rectal cancer,* ed 2. Available at http://www.nccn.org. Accessed April 12, 2010.

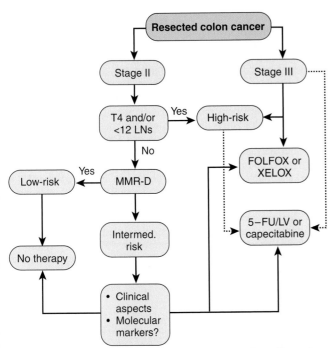

FIGURE 1   Algorithm for use of adjuvant treatment for colorectal cancer.

5-FU/LV are reasonable alternatives if patients are not candidates for oxaliplatin. Irinotecan-based regimens cannot be recommended in the adjuvant setting. Likewise, the anti–vascular endothelial growth factor monoclonal antibody bevacizumab and the epidermal growth factor receptor antibodies cetuximab and panitumumab play no role in the adjuvant therapy of colorectal cancer.

For unselected stage II (node-negative) patients, the absolute benefit of adjuvant therapy appears to be real but much smaller. In stage II colon cancer, patients with T4 tumors should receive treatment according to guidelines established for stage III disease, in light of their poor prognosis. This would lead to the recommendation of an oxaliplatin-based adjuvant therapy (FOLFOX or XELOX) for most of these patients. A similar approach can be considered for patients in whom less than 12 lymph nodes have been identified in the surgical specimen—after the case has been discussed with the pathologist.

If neither of these two high-risk features is present, an MMR-D or MSI-H phenotype should be excluded from adjuvant therapy, because these cancers have an excellent prognosis (3-year DFS of 90% to 95%) and very likely will not benefit from adjuvant therapy. For the remaining group of intermediate-risk patients, clinical factors—age, comorbidities, tumor differentiation, bowel obstruction/perforation, lymphovascular invasion, perineural invasion—and potential future molecular signatures could provide further data on prognosis; it is hoped that such predictive information will lead to further refinement of our adjuvant approach to patients with stage II colon cancer.

In rectal cancer, preoperative chemoradiotherapy is the preferred treatment for patients with locally advanced rectal cancer, given that it is associated with a superior overall compliance rate, an improved rate of local control, reduced short- and long-term toxicity, and an increased rate of sphincter preservation in patients with low-lying tumors. As an alternative, the less commonly used short-course radiation therapy may also be beneficial.

Suggested Readings

Andre T, Boni C, Mounedji-Boudiaf L, et al: Oxaliplatin, fluorouracil, and leucovorin as adjuvant treatments for colon cancer, *N Engl J Med* 350:2343–2351, 2004.

Andre T, Boni C, Navarro M, et al: Improved overall survival with oxaliplatin, fluorouracil, and leucovorin as adjuvant treatment in stage II or III colon cancer in the MOSAIC trial, *J Clin Oncol* 27:3109–3116, 2009.

Benson AB 3d, Schrag D, Somerfield MR, et al: American Society of Clinical Oncology recommendations on adjuvant chemotherapy for stage II colon cancer, *J Clin Oncol* 22:3408–3419, 2004.

Chang GJ, Rodriguez-Bigas MA, Skibber JM, et al: Lymph node evaluation and survival after curative resection of colon cancer: systematic review, *J Natl Cancer Inst* 99:433–441, 2007.

Desch CE, Benson AB 3d, Somerfield MR, et al: Colorectal cancer surveillance: 2005 update of an American Society of Clinical Oncology practice guideline, *J Clin Oncol* 23:8512–8519, 2005.

Gill S, Loprinzi CL, Sargent DJ, et al: Pooled analysis of fluorouracil-based adjuvant therapy for stage II and III colon cancer: who benefits and by how much? *J Clin Oncol* 22:1797–1806, 2004.

Gray R, Barnwell J, McConkey C, and the QUASAR Collaborative Group: Adjuvant chemotherapy versus observation in patients with colorectal cancer: a randomised study, *Lancet* 370:2020–2029, 2007.

Gunderson LL, Jessup JM, Sargent DJ, et al: Revised TN categorization for colon cancer based on national survival outcomes data, *J Clin Oncol* 28:264–271, 2010.

Heald RJ, Ryall RD: Recurrence and survival after total mesorectal excision for rectal cancer, *Lancet* 1:1479–1482, 1986.

International Multicentre Pooled Analysis of B2 Colon Cancer Trials (IMPACT B2) Investigators: Efficacy of adjuvant fluorouracil and folinic acid in B2 colon cancer, *J Clin Oncol* 17:1356–1363, 1999.

Kapiteijn E, Marijnen CA, Nagtegaal ID, et al: Preoperative radiotherapy combined with total mesorectal excision for resectable rectal cancer, *N Engl J Med* 345:638–646, 2001.

Mamounas E, Wieand S, Wolmark N, et al: Comparative efficacy of adjuvant chemotherapy in patients with Dukes' B versus Dukes' C colon cancer: results from four National Surgical Adjuvant Breast and Bowel Project adjuvant studies (C-01, C-02, C-03, and C-04), *J Clin Oncol* 17:1349–1355, 1999.

NCCN: *Practice guidelines for colon and rectal cancer*, ed 2, 2010. Available at http://www.nccn.org Accessed April 12, 2010.

Ribic CM, Sargent DJ, Moore MJ, et al: Tumor microsatellite-instability status as a predictor of benefit from fluorouracil-based adjuvant chemotherapy for colon cancer, *N Engl J Med* 349:247–257, 2003.

Sargent DJ, Wieand HS, Haller DG, et al: Disease-free survival versus overall survival as a primary end point for adjuvant colon cancer studies: individual patient data from 20,898 patients in 18 randomized trials, *J Clin Oncol* 23:8664–8670, 2005.

Sauer R, Becker H, Hohenberger W, et al: Preoperative versus postoperative chemoradiotherapy for rectal cancer, *N Engl J Med* 351:1731–1740, 2004.

Tsai HL, Chu KS, Huang YH, et al: Predictive factors of early relapse in UICC stage I-III colorectal cancer patients after curative resection, *J Surg Oncol* 100:736–743, 2009.

COLORECTAL POLYPS

Carl J. Brown, MD, and Robin S. McLeod, MD

OVERVIEW

A colorectal polyp is an intraluminal mass lesion arising from the mucosa of the colon and rectum. A number of other lesions can present as luminal masses, such as lipomas, carcinoid tumors, and leiomyomas, but they are covered by normal mucosa. Thus they should not be referred to as *polyps*.

The molecular alterations that lead to the development of colorectal polyps have become increasingly understood. This improved knowledge of the correlation between histology and genotype has provided a change in recommendations related to treatment and risk reduction of cancer. Colonic polyps may also be a component of a variety of acquired or familial syndromes, many of which are potentially malignant conditions. These polyposis syndromes are described in more detail in this section of text but are reviewed briefly here.

The importance of colorectal polyps is related primarily to the risk of malignancy, which has led to a significant increase in the use of screening colonoscopy. Larger polyps may also prompt treatment as a result of hemorrhage, obstruction, or intussusception. Endoscopic evaluation of polyps frequently allows complete excision of the lesion, but at the least, it allows for histological confirmation of the polyp type. Flexible endoscopy has proven to be a safe and highly effective means of treating colorectal polyps.

HISTOPATHOLOGY OF POLYPS

Hyperplastic Polyps

The relationship between hyperplastic polyps and colon cancer is controversial. However, the risk appears to be only slightly increased. Hyperplastic polyps contain an increased number of glandular cells with decreased cytoplasmic mucus, but they lack nuclear hyperchromatism and stratification. These types of polyps are not considered neoplastic and generally do not confer a higher risk of colorectal cancer, especially small polyps located in the rectum.

Factors associated with an increased risk for malignancy with hyperplastic polyps include large polyp size (>1 cm diameter); right colon lesions; a mixed adenoma/hyperplastic histology; more than 20 hyperplastic colonic polyps; familial hyperplastic polyposis; and a family history of colorectal cancer. Serrated adenomas represent a type of polyp previously classified as hyperplastic; however, these lesions appear to carry an increased risk of colon cancer, as do typical adenomas. These serrated polyps tend to be larger, rightsided, and associated with *BRAF* genetic mutations and DNA metrication.

Hamartomas

A second histologic category of colorectal polyps is hamartomas, which occur most commonly in association with one of three autosomal-dominant familial syndromes: *Peutz-Jeghers syndrome, juvenile polyposis,* and *Cowden syndrome*. Historically, these syndromes have been considered benign; however, it is now clear that these lesions have malignant potential, and patients with these syndromes should undergo regular colonoscopic surveillance.

Peutz-Jeghers syndrome results from a mutation of the *STK11* gene and is associated with a typical phenotype that includes perioral pigmented spots and multiple hamartomatous small bowel polyps. The polyps in this syndrome may be complicated by intussusception, bleeding, and obstruction early in life. After the third decade of life, there is a 2% to 13% risk for gastrointestinal (GI) cancer for this population.

Juvenile polyposis is diagnosed when a young patient has 10 or more hamartomatous GI polyps. Lesions frequently occur in the colon but may develop anywhere within the G1 tract. The initial symptom is often bleeding resulting from autoamputation of the polyp. The mutations in this syndrome occur in the *SMAD4/DPC4* and PTEN genes. Colon cancer affects up to 50% of those with juvenile polyposis and may occur in the fourth decade of life.

A final syndrome of juvenile and other hamartomatous polyps within the colon and throughout the gastrointestinal tract is Cowden syndrome. It results from a mutation of the *PTEN* gene. Colorectal cancer is not an established major risk in this syndrome, and no specific surveillance is recommended.

Adenoma

Approximately 10% to 25% of average-risk asymptomatic patients older than 50 years have an adenomatous polyp. These lesions are characterized by histologic architecture that may be tubular (65% to 85%), tubulovillous (10% to 25%), or villous (5% to 10%). Advanced lesions are defined by size greater than 1 cm and the presence of villous architecture, severe dysplasia, or carcinoma. Identification of a distal adenoma on flexible sigmoidoscopy should prompt a complete colonoscopy because of the approximately 20% to 40% risk of proximal neoplastic lesions. Conversely, a small hyperplastic polyp in itself is not an indication for colonoscopy.

The causal relationship between adenomas and colorectal cancer has been called the *adenoma–carcinoma sequence*. This relation is supported by the following data: 1) almost all colon cancer arises within an adenoma, as evidenced by residual polyps in many colon cancers; 2) an approximately 30% incidence of synchronous adenomas is seen in colon cancer resection specimens; 3) risk of colon cancer increases with larger and increasing numbers of adenomatous polyps; 4) the incidence of colorectal cancer is high in patients with familial adenomatous polyposis; and 5) the risk is 4% after 5 years and 14% after 10 years in unresected polyps.

The development of colorectal polyps and subsequent cancer is believed to be the result of a cascade of sequentially accumulated genetic mutations. These mutations are a combination of loss-of-function and gain-of-function defects. Mismatch repair genes are directly tied to hereditary nonpolyposis cancer syndrome. They are also identified in 15% of sporadic colon cancers. Similarly, the adenomatous polyposis coli (APC) mutation is the causal mutation in familial adenomatous polyposis, but the mutation is also seen in more than 80% of sporadic colon cancers and appears to be an early mutation leading to sporadic adenomatous polyps. Although 50% to 80% of benign polyps harbor the APC mutation, the transition to malignancy requires additional mutations. The loss of the gene *Deleted in Colon Cancer* (*DCC*) appears to play a key role in the transition to a more advanced adenoma because of dysfunction of a neural cell adhesion molecule receptor and alterations in apoptosis.

Another commonly altered gene is *p53*, which normally allows for arrest of the cell cycle to provide sufficient time for either DNA repair or apoptosis if the damage is too severe. A mutation of *p53* appears to be a key component in the transition from advanced adenoma to carcinoma. In addition, the *K-ras* gene is involved in signal transduction from the cell membrane to the nucleus and gain-of-function mutation leads to increased replication and development of exophytic growth of adenomas. This mutation can be found in more than 50% of colon cancers.

COLONOSCOPIC POLYPECTOMY

Polypectomy has proven to be an effective means of colorectal cancer prevention, because it allows for identification of the mucosal lesions and their removal. Most endoscopists recommend removal of lesions greater than 5 mm using biopsy polypectomy and a snare for larger lesions. Snare excision provides a larger specimen, and the stalk (or base) can be evaluated histopathologically to allow better definition of the level of superficial malignancy. Large lesions may be removed using a piecemeal excisional technique, which will allow for sequential excision of the entire lesion. In some cases, these larger sessile lesions may be better treated with injection of saline in the submucosal plane to separate the lesion from the muscularis propria and to allow safer removal of the lesion with electrocautery. When larger polyps are removed, it is important to tattoo the area with India ink, in case there are cancerous changes in the polyp necessitating further evaluation, or possible resection, of that segment of the colon.

Endoscopic mucosal resection (EMR) is a technique that incorporates saline injection and a suction cautery attachment on a conventional colonoscope. This approach is useful in flat lesions that are difficult to ensnare with standard loops. Narrow-band imaging (NBI) colonoscopy, which uses only blue (415 nm) and green (540 nm) wavelengths, with the intent of making blood vessels and neoplasia stand out, can be helpful in ensuring that the entire polyp has been removed. Relative contraindications to colonoscopic polypectomy include anticoagulation, bleeding diathesis, acute colitis, or signs of invasive malignancy (central ulceration, hard or fixed lesion, necrosis, inability to "raise" the lesion with submucosal injection).

With modern techniques, complications with colonoscopic polypectomy are uncommon and usually mild. The risk of death is approximately 1 in 14,000. The most common serious complications of colonoscopy are bleeding and perforation. Postpolypectomy bleeding occurs in 4.8 per 1000 patients after colonoscopic polypectomy and may occur immediately or days later, after clot dissolution. Most postpolypectomy bleeds stop spontaneously, and persistent bleeds can usually be controlled with repeat endoscopy and cauterization or clipping. Rarely, interventional angiography or colectomy are necessary. Bleeding risk should be minimized by ensuring that warfarin and aspirin are discontinued 5 days prior to polypectomy, and clopidogrel should be withheld for 7 days.

Colonic perforation occurs in up to 0.1% of patients undergoing polypectomy. The majority of patients who present with free air identified after polypectomy may be observed and treated with intravenous antibiotics. However, patients should be carefully followed as inpatients for any signs of clinical deterioration, worsening physical examination findings, or signs of infection, which would indicate laparotomy. An alternative approach is early laparoscopic primary repair of the defect, unless there is significant fecal soiling, peritonitis, or identification of an obvious malignancy requiring resection. Identification of the perforation is usually straightforward. However, occasionally it can be difficult to find the hole; positioning the patient in lithotomy to facilitate intraoperative colonoscopy for identification of the site of perforation is advised.

Postpolypectomy syndrome—manifested by abdominal pain, fever, and leukocytosis—can occur in up to 0.3% of patients after polypectomy. The pathophysiology is likely a microperforation and bacterial translocation related to cautery injury. Patients can be treated with fasting, intravenous antibiotics, and close observation until symptoms resolve.

In 2008, the American Cancer Society, in collaboration with the U.S. Multisociety Task Force on Colorectal Cancer and the American College of Radiology, updated their guidelines for screening and surveillance for colorectal cancer and adenomatous polyps (Table 1). Current recommendations for surveillance after polypectomy are based on the risk of recurrent neoplasia after the index colonoscopic polypectomy.

TABLE 1: Current guidelines for colorectal cancer screening after polypectomy

Risk Category	Recommended	Interval
Previous History of Polyp		
One to two small tubular adenomas	Colonoscopy	5 to 10 years
1. Three to ten small adenomas *or* 2. One adenoma >1 cm *or* 3. A polyp with villous or high-grade dysplasia	Colonoscopy	3 years
>10 adenomas	Colonoscopy	<3 years
Sessile adenomas removed piecemeal	Colonoscopy	3 to 6 months

Increased risk is defined as 1) three or more adenomas removed, 2) high-grade dysplasia, 3) villous features, 4) an adenoma greater than or equal to 1 cm in size, or 5) a large adenoma removed piecemeal. Lower risk is defined by one or two small (<1 cm) tubular adenomas with no high-grade dysplasia. High-risk patients should have a repeat colonoscopy at 3 years, and low-risk patients may safely defer colonoscopy for 5 to 10 years. Patients with hyperplastic polyps may defer for the same 10-year follow-up recommended for those at average risk (Figure 1).

Although colonoscopy is the best method for detecting polyps, two studies of patients undergoing back-to-back colonoscopies suggest that polyps bigger than 1 cm may be missed in as many as 6% to 14% of patients. However, the miss rate of invasive cancer is considered to be lower than 5%. There is evidence to suggest that prolonging the withdrawal time to at least 6 minutes during colonoscopy can improve neoplasia detection rates. Thus patients should be warned that relevant symptoms, such as rectal bleeding or change in bowel habits, should be investigated.

APPROACH TO THE MALIGNANT POLYP

Most premalignant adenomatous polyps are amenable to endoscopic removal for definitive treatment. Colonoscopic removal of these polyps has been shown to reduce the risk of colon cancer. However, up to 5% of polyps that appear grossly benign will contain invasive cancer. The risk of cancer correlates to the size of the polyp, and polyps larger than 2 cm may contain invasive cancer in 30% of cases. It is for this reason that even if cancer is not suspected, the area should be tattooed. If not, it may be difficult to identify the site of the polypectomy at a later date, if there is malignancy, and further evaluation and treatment is required.

Pathologically, a malignant polyp is defined by adenocarcinoma that invades into (but no deeper than) the submucosal layer of the bowel wall. By definition, a malignant polyp is a T1 colon cancer. It is important to distinguish a malignant polyp from a polyp with carcinoma in situ or high-grade dysplasia, in which changes are confined to the mucosa and lamina propria. These entities have no metastatic potential and are cured by polypectomy, if the pathologic assessment is adequate, and the specimen has been completely removed (Table 2).

In a malignant polyp that has been removed with negative margins, the main reason to proceed with a formal segmental resection is to harvest the associated lymph nodes in the mesentery. The risk of lymph node metastasis in malignant polyps is 8% to 15%. This is a relatively low risk, and in some patients, this risk approaches the mortality associated with colon resection.

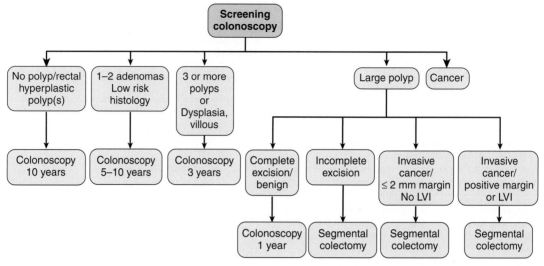

FIGURE I Algorithm for outcomes with screening colonscopy. *LVI,* Lymphovascular invasion.

TABLE 2: Pathologic features of malignant polyps

Haggitt level:	Submucosal invasion in polyp head (1), neck (2), stalk (3), and base (4) and/or submucosal invasion in a sessile polyp (4)
Submucosal invasion:	Invasion in upper third of submucosa (sm1), middle third (sm2), or deep third (sm3)
Tumor grade:	Well, moderately, or poorly differentiated
Tumor budding:	Absence or presence of clusters of malignant cells in the submucosa remote from the main site of submucosal invasion

Listed in order of escalating risk of lymph node metastasis.

In 1985, Haggitt proposed a classification of malignant polyps designed to predict lymph node metastasis. In 64 patients who had a malignant polyp excised, Haggitt demonstrated that polyps with invasive cancer at the base of a pedunculated polyp or any sessile polyp had a 25% risk of lymph node involvement, but all other polyps had less than a 5% risk of lymphatic spread.

Although Haggitt's classification is still important in assessing the risk of lymph node involvement, other pathologic features also help advise clinicians about the risk of lymph node metastasis. In retrospective studies, the features most predictive of adverse outcomes such as lymph node metastasis or recurrence with clinical follow-up are tumor grade, tumor budding, and lymphovascular invasion. In the absence of any of these features, the risk of adverse outcome is less than 1%. However, if a malignant polyp has any one of these features, the risk of adverse outcome is 20%. If a polyp has two or more of these features, the risk of adverse outcome increases to 36%. Further evaluation of these features may better define patients who can be spared major surgery.

The American College of Gastroenterology guidelines state that malignant polyps may be treated with endoscopic removal and close surveillance when:

- The polyp is completely excised.
- The polyp can be accurately assessed with respect to the depth of invasion, grade of differentiation, and completeness of the excision of the carcinoma.
- The cancer is not poorly differentiated.

- There is no vascular or lymphatic involvement.
- The margin of excision is not involved.

All other malignant polyps should be considered for surgical resection. However, even with some high-risk features, patients with malignant polyps and serious medical comorbidities are best managed with close surveillance and nonsurgical treatment.

SUGGESTED READINGS

Bond JH: Polyp guidelines: diagnosis, treatment, and surveillance for patients with colorectal polyps. Practice Parameters Committee of the American College of Gastroenterology, *Am J Gastroenterol* 95(11):3053–3063, 2000.

Damore LJ 2d, Rantis PC, Vernava AM 3d, Longo WE: Colonoscopic perforations: etiology, diagnosis, and management, *Dis Colon Rectum* 39(11):1308–1314, 1996 [review].

Heresbach D, Barrioz T, Lapalus MG, et al: Miss rate for colorectal neoplastic polyps: a prospective multicenter study of back-to-back video colonoscopies, *Endoscopy* 40(4):284–290, 2008.

Huh KC, Rex DK: Advances in colonoscope technique and technology, *Rev Gastroenterol Disord* 8(4):223–232, 2008 [review].

Kaltenbach T, Friedland S, Soetikno R: A randomised tandem colonoscopy trial of narrow-band imaging versus white light examination to compare neoplasia miss rates, *Gut* 57(10):1406–1412, 2008 [Epub Jun 3, 2008].

Levin B, Lieberman DA, McFarland B, et al. for the American Cancer Society Colorectal Cancer Advisory Group, U.S. Multisociety Task Force, American College of Radiology Colon Cancer Committee: Screening and surveillance for the early detection of colorectal cancer and adenomatous polyps, 2008: a joint guideline from the American Cancer Society, the U.S. Multisociety Task Force on Colorectal Cancer, and the American College of Radiology, *CA Cancer J Clin* 58(3):130–160, 2008 [Epub Mar 5, 2008].

Rapuri S, Spencer J, Eckels D: Importance of postpolypectomy surveillance and postpolypectomy compliance to follow-up screening: review of literature, *Int J Colorectal Dis* 23(5):453–459, 2008 [Epub Jan 9, 2008].

Rex DK, Cutler CS, Lemmel GT, et al: Colonoscopic miss rates of adenomas determined by back-to-back colonoscopies, *Gastroenterology* 112(1):24–28, 1997.

Timothy SK, Hicks TC, Opelka FG, et al: Colonoscopy in the patient requiring anticoagulation, *Dis Colon Rectum* 44(12):1845–1848, 2001.

Ueno H, Mochizuki H, Hashiguchi Y, et al: Risk factors for an adverse outcome in early invasive colorectal carcinoma, *Gastroenterology* 127(2):385–394, 2004.

Winawer SJ, Zauber AG, Fletcher RH, et al: Guidelines for colonoscopy surveillance after polypectomy: a consensus update by the U.S. Multisociety Task Force on Colorectal Cancer and the American Cancer Society, *CA Cancer J Clin* 56(3):143–159, 2006.

Management of Peritoneal Surface Malignancy

Robert P. Sticca, MD

OVERVIEW

The management of peritoneal carcinomatosis has changed dramatically over the past three decades. Historically, peritoneal involvement in most malignancies has been considered an incurable, fatal event. In most cases, attempts at surgical removal of peritoneal malignancies were fraught with incomplete resections or the failure to recognize microscopic residual disease, which resulted in early recurrence and death. Consistently poor outcomes caused the surgical community to avoid operative intervention in patients with malignant peritoneal involvement. Systemic chemotherapy was largely ineffective due to poor penetration into the peritoneal cavity and limited activity of chemotherapeutic agents against the primary tumor. Current treatment methods for peritoneal malignances were developed in the 1970s and 1980s; these have been used increasingly in the treatment of peritoneal surface tumors, both primary and metastatic, with a resultant improvement in disease-free and overall survival and the potential for cure in some situations.

The involvement of the peritoneal surface in malignancies is a common problem, and prognosis varies with the type of malignancy (Table 1). Although peritoneal involvement can occur in extraabdominal malignancies, it is most common with cancers of the gastrointestinal (GI), reproductive, and genitourinary tracts. The primary peritoneal malignancies, primary peritoneal carcinoma and malignant peritoneal mesothelioma, are uncommon malignancies that are treatable with current management techniques. By far, the greatest impact of current treatment methods is on other intraabdominal malignancies, which often involve the peritoneum with metastatic disease (appendiceal, colorectal, gastric, pancreatic, and ovarian), whose incidence far exceeds that for primary peritoneal malignancies.

RATIONALE FOR CURRENT TREATMENT

The principles of treatment of peritoneal surface malignancies are similar to those for management of most other solid tumors but with a few notable exceptions. As with most solid tumors, the obtainable degree of surgical removal is one of the most important prognostic factors in the ultimate outcome of peritoneal malignancy. Optimal treatment of a malignancy involving the peritoneum requires cytoreductive surgery (CRS), or debulking of the tumor, with the goal of complete removal of all *visible* disease. Depending on the amount of disease present, the surgical procedure can be long and tedious, but the goal remains the same: removal and/or ablation of all visible disease. As opposed to other solid tumors, removal of the tumor with a margin of normal tissue does *not* result in elimination of the disease; in the treatment of peritoneal malignancies, it is recognized and accepted that there will be residual microscopic cancer cells remaining in the peritoneal cavity after the surgical procedure.

Upon completion of CRS, it is virtually impossible to ensure that all microscopic disease has been removed from the abdominal cavity; by the very nature of the peritoneal involvement, there are almost always residual malignant cells remaining in the peritoneal cavity.

In fact, historical evidence indicates that in most cases, there remain residual malignant cells after attempted CRS, as demonstrated by the quick intraperitoneal recurrence and eventual demise of most patients with malignant peritoneal involvement.

This phenomenon has led to the development of additional techniques for treatment of the residual disease after surgical debulking, namely hyperthermic intraoperative intraperitoneal chemotherapy (HIPEC). The advantages of HIPEC in the treatment of peritoneal malignancies are numerous. These include:

1) The residual malignant cells are directly exposed to higher doses of chemotherapy than would be possible with systemic chemotherapy.
2) The addition of heat, which potentiates the chemotherapy, also increases its penetration into malignant cells. Heat itself is preferentially cytotoxic to malignant cells.
3) Toxicity of the chemotherapy agents is not an issue for the patient, as these are delivered while the patient is under general anesthesia.

Perhaps nowhere else in oncology is the effect of tumor biology on the outcome of therapy as evident as it is with peritoneal surface malignancies. There is a direct relationship between the type and grade of the tumor and the recurrence rate and outcome of the treatment. One of the key biologic characteristics of treatable peritoneal surface malignancies is the ability to spread through the peritoneal cavity by direct attachment and proliferation, while lacking the ability to spread by hematogenous or lymphatic routes. This is common with the low-grade mucinous peritoneal surface malignancies, such as *pseudomyxoma peritonei* and appendiceal cancers. This characteristic makes low-grade peritoneal surface malignancies ideal candidates for locoregional therapy, which successfully eradicates the malignant cells within the peritoneum. Many reports in the literature document the significantly better recurrence rates and survival in low-grade peritoneal surface malignancies with CRS and HIPEC.

Conversely, higher grade tumors often encountered with colorectal, pancreatic, and gastric cancer have a higher propensity to metastasize by hematogenous or lymphatic routes, and they are often associated with recurrence outside the peritoneal cavity despite the best attempts to control disease within the peritoneum. In fact, the long-term outcome in the treatment of peritoneal surface malignancies is inversely proportional to the tumor's grade and ability to metastasize by extraperitoneal routes; thus the biologic capabilities of a malignancy involving the peritoneal surface should be considered when planning for a major intervention such as CRS and HIPEC. It is not practical to remove large amounts of disease in a highly aggressive tumor, as there is high likelihood of intraperitoneal recurrence and distant metastases within months. Optimal situations for CRS and HIPEC include tumors that 1) are low grade, 2) lack the ability to metastasize hematogenously or lymphatically, and 3) are surgically resectable with the techniques currently in use for CRS.

SURGICAL MANAGEMENT

Cytoreductive Surgery

The goal of CRS is the complete elimination of all detectable malignant involvement of the peritoneal surfaces. It is only necessary to remove areas of visible disease and the attached peritoneum, as one of the characteristics of many peritoneal surface malignancies is their propensity to involve the peritoneal surfaces without invading deeper into the underlying tissues of the abdominal wall or organs on which they are found. The debulking procedure begins with a generous midline incision and evaluation of all areas where malignant nodules are noted. The surgeon can then plan the steps for the cytoreductive procedure in a systematic fashion, removing tumor deposits from any or all of the six major areas of the abdominal cavity when they are involved (Table 2).

TABLE 1: Estimated incidence of peritoneal carcinomatosis by primary disease site

Type of Malignancy	Estimated Annual Incidence in U.S.	Estimated Annual Incidence of Peritoneal Involvement
Primary peritoneal cancer	1000	1000
Malignant peritoneal mesothelioma	400	400
Appendiceal cancer	1500	1350
Colorectal cancer	146,970	31,000
Gastric cancer	21,130	10,000
Ovarian cancer	21,550	18,000
Pancreatic cancer	42,470	2500
Endometrial cancer	42,160	1500
Sarcoma	10,660	500

TABLE 2: Major areas of disease involvement of peritoneal carcinomatosis

Right upper quadrant and porta hepatis
Omentum, spleen, and lesser sac
Left upper quadrant and stomach
Colon and colic gutters
Small bowel and mesentery
Pelvic peritoneum and pelvic organs

The decision to pursue a complete cytoreduction (curative procedure) versus a palliative debulking procedure can sometimes be difficult and depends on several factors: 1) the surgeon's experience, 2) the availability of HIPEC treatment, 3) the type and grade of malignancy, 4) the condition of the patient, and 5) the degree of peritoneal involvement. When it is determined that a complete cytoreduction is indicated, the procedure ensues with removal of all visible tumor deposits by organ resection and peritoneal stripping procedures in the major areas of involvement.

The techniques of peritoneal stripping for all major areas of the abdominal cavity have been well described in the literature by Sugarbaker. By using traction and electrocautery on a high setting, the peritoneum strips away easily, as it is thickened by the peritoneal surface malignancy. Electrocautery is mandatory for the numerous small blood vessels between the underlying tissue and the peritoneum will bleed extensively. These vessels may be enlarged due to the vascular growth factors generated by the malignancy.

When the disease is confluent in any of the major areas, complete peritonectomy of that area is necessary. Because of the many areas of potential sequestering of the malignancy throughout the recesses within the peritoneal cavity, the debulking procedure requires a meticulous and diligent approach to remove all disease. Every attempt should be made to obtain a completeness of cytoreduction (CC) score of 0 (Figure 1); this will enable the HIPEC to eliminate any residual malignant cells after the debulking procedure.

Experimental evidence has demonstrated that the chemotherapy agents used in the HIPEC portion of the procedure will penetrate up to 2.5 mm; therefore the potential for curative resection is dependent

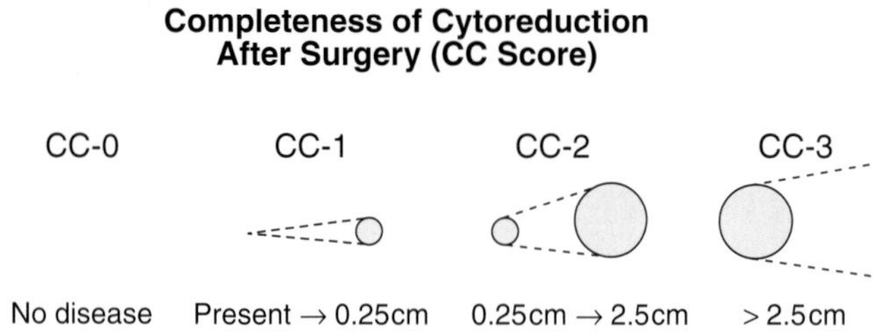

Completeness of Cytoreduction After Surgery (CC Score)

CC-0   CC-1   CC-2   CC-3

No disease   Present → 0.25cm   0.25cm → 2.5cm   > 2.5cm

FIGURE 1   Completeness of cytoreduction. *Circles* represent largest visible malignant nodule after the completion of the cytoreductive surgery. CC-0 or CC-1 score is necessary for a curative procedure.

on a cytoreductive procedure that removes all disease greater than 2.5 mm (CC score of 0 or 1).

When the disease extensively involves an organ, and removal of the peritoneal surface malignancy is impractical, that organ should be removed. Organs commonly removed in CRS include the gallbladder, spleen, sigmoid colon, upper rectum, uterus, ovaries, and portions of the small bowel and colon. Ideally all visible tumor deposits will be removed, but in some cases, this is not feasible.

In situations where there are small deposits of tumor on many surfaces of the small bowel and mesentery, it is appropriate to ablate those deposits larger than 2 mm that cannot be resected. Ablation of small tumor deposits is performed with electrocautery on a high setting, resulting in vaporization of the smaller tumor nodules. As opposed to other forms of oncologic surgery, the surgeon should remember that CRS is not designed to be curative in itself, as the presence of residual microscopic and small macroscopic disease is accepted. The subsequent HIPEC is a necessary part of any curative procedure and will eliminate any residual microscopic disease less than 2.5 mm in depth.

After all disease is removed, the HIPEC treatment is performed. Upon completion of HIPEC, gastric and bowel anastomoses are performed if necessary. In addition, all bowel surface serosal defects are repaired. It is important to delay bowel anastomosis and serosal repairs until after the HIPEC to allow all surfaces to come in contact with the chemotherapy, which will eradicate any residual tumor cells in those areas. In cases where prior surgery has left areas of fibrosis and scarring, it is necessary to lyse all adhesions, as well as to resect the thicker areas of adhesions, to expose all of the fibrotic tissue to the heated chemotherapy. Experimental evidence has shown that tumor cell surface molecules preferentially adhere to adhesions, which can serve as a focus for later tumor cell growth and recurrence of the malignancy.

Each area of CRS has unique technical characteristics that the operating surgeon must be cognizant of when performing an optimal surgical debulking. The sequence of the cytoreductive procedures often depends upon the amount of disease and the location of involvement. When disease involves most of the six areas, the debulking procedure often begins in the right upper quadrant, proceeding around the abdomen in a clockwise fashion.

TECHNICAL CONSIDERATIONS FOR PERITONECTOMY BY SITE

Right Upper Quadrant Peritonectomy

The right upper quadrant is commonly involved in peritoneal surface malignancies because of the normal flow pattern of ascitic fluid within the abdomen. When this fluid contains malignant cells, they often seed the peritoneal surfaces along the right colic gutter, extending to the right hemidiaphragm, and also involve the recesses posterior to the liver. When involvement of these surfaces is widespread, a peritoneal stripping is required. This is begun on the right mid abdominal wall, stripping the anterior abdominal wall peritoneum cranially and laterally removing all peritoneum along the abdominal wall, extending this dissection to the diaphragmatic peritoneum.

The dissection on the muscular portion of the diaphragm generally proceeds without difficulty, but the surgeon must exercise caution medially, where the tendinous portion of the diaphragm is encountered. In this area the diaphragm is only a few millimeters thick and is easily penetrated, exposing the pleural cavity to the tumor cells, which should be avoided if possible. If the peritoneal surface malignancy is invasive of the diaphragm so as to necessitate resection, or if the diaphragm is entered inadvertently, immediate repair of the diaphragm should be performed to prevent dissemination of the malignant cells into the pleural cavity.

The most posterior recesses adjacent to the inferior vena cava, extending cranially to the suprahepatic vena cava, must be carefully stripped, using care not to disrupt the accessory hepatic veins and the veins to the caudate lobe. These areas are commonly involved with disease on the diaphragmatic peritoneum.

Inferiorly the dissection merges into the dissection of the gallbladder and porta hepatis. If involvement of the gallbladder and porta hepatis are found, the gallbladder should be removed, and the peritoneum should be stripped from the porta hepatis full circumferentially, dissecting out and preserving the major structures in the porta. It is important to remove all disease posterior to the porta hepatis, extending into the lesser sac and around the caudate lobe medially.

Omentectomy, Splenectomy, and Lesser Sac

This portion of the CRS may be performed first, if a large volume of disease on the omentum precludes access to the upper abdomen. The omentum is removed from the colon along the avascular plane. The greater omentum is removed from the stomach at the greater curvature, ligating all of the short gastrics. The spleen is mobilized and removed with the omentum; when there is disease on the splenic surface, it is not practical to attempt removal, as the exposed splenic parenchyma will bleed continuously. The distal tail of the pancreas may be transected with a stapling device and removed with the spleen, especially when disease in the area of the splenic hilum or the tail of the pancreas is in close association with the splenic hilar vessels. After the omentum and spleen are removed, the lesser sac is exposed by retracting the stomach anteriorly. In general, involvement of the lesser sac is not significant, as it is protected by the stomach, omentum, and transverse colon.

In some cases, tumor cells gain access to the lesser sac through the foramen of Winslow. When extensive involvement in the lesser sac is seen, the peritoneum should be stripped; in patients with a few scattered nodules, the nodules can be resected individually or ablated. When completed, this dissection leads to the left upper quadrant dissection, which is now better exposed due to the removal of the spleen and mobilization of the stomach.

Left Upper Quadrant and Stomach

The left diaphragm and left upper quadrant are less often involved with significant peritoneal carcinomatosis, partially because the splenocolic ligament and omentum form barriers to ascitic fluid flow to the left upper quadrant. When the peritoneum on the left diaphragm is involved, the stripping procedure is very similar to that for the right diaphragm. Again, care is taken to avoid entry into the pleural cavity, especially at the tendinous portion of the diaphragm medially. The peritoneum covering the intraabdominal portion of the esophagus can be stripped in continuity with the diaphragmatic dissection.

The lesser omentum and recesses adjacent to and posterior to the caudate lobe of the liver should be carefully evaluated and resected if disease is present. Care should be exercised at the superior aspect of this dissection, posterior to the left lobe of the liver, as there may be a small, extrahepatic portion of the left hepatic vein that can be entered inadvertently and cause excessive bleeding. When involved, the lesser omentum is removed, carefully dissecting out the structures of the celiac axis, including the left gastric artery; however, every attempt should be made to preserve the left gastric artery; it is the only remaining blood supply to the stomach. Ligation of the left gastric artery will generally result in gastric ischemia, resulting in partial or total gastrectomy. In my experience, even when involved with malignancy, the celiac arterial structures usually can be dissected out, stripped of disease, and preserved to maintain blood supply to the stomach.

The postoperative nutritional consequences of total gastrectomy in this procedure are significant. In addition, the quality of life after total gastrectomy can be poor. Extensive disease on the stomach may require distal gastrectomy, but disease on the proximal stomach is often limited and can be treated with ablation techniques. This allows preservation of the proximal stomach, provided the left gastric artery blood supply is intact.

Colon and Colic Gutters

The left and right colic gutters are commonly involved with peritoneal carcinomatosis when the disease is widespread. The peritoneum can be stripped from the anterior abdominal wall posteriorly to remove all peritoneum in the colic gutters, extending this dissection to the colonic mesentery. When significant disease is seen on the colon, colectomy should be considered. Small deposits on the colonic surfaces can be electrevaporated, but for large deposits or confluent disease, segmental colectomy should be considered. It is helpful to preserve as much colon as possible, as this may enable the patient to return to a more normal pattern of bowel function after all treatments are completed. Because of the extensive dissection and removal of tissue, it is usually possible to anastomose any portion of residual colon to the rectal stump after the pelvic resections are complete.

When disease volume makes it impossible to salvage any significant portion of the colon, subtotal colectomy may be necessary. Subtotal colectomy with subsequent ileorectal anastomosis is well tolerated, especially in younger patients. After the HIPEC is completed, the remaining colon can be anastomosed to the rectal stump using an end-to-end anastomosis stapler.

Small Bowel and Mesentery

The small bowel and small bowel mesentery can be involved to varying degrees, especially with higher grade malignancies. Areas of heavy involvement should be resected keeping in mind the necessary amount of small bowel needed for adequate nutrient absorption (at least 150 cm). Malignant nodules on the small bowel mesenteric peritoneal surfaces can often be removed primarily without taking the underlying blood supply to the small bowel. Larger tumor nodules on the small bowel peritoneal surfaces can be removed with the outer layers of the muscularis propria, as long as the serosal defects are repaired after the HIPEC is completed.

Smaller tumor nodules on the small bowel surfaces can be electroevaporated with the cautery on a high setting; the HIPEC will penetrate into the residual coagulated tissue, provided it is less than 2 mm thick, and eradicate any residual cancer cells. An area where tumor nodules have a propensity to grow is at the border of the mesentery and the small bowel surface. When these nodules are larger or are from higher grade, invasive malignancies, resection is often required. In some cases resection of the nodules at the border of the mesentery, with preservation of the collateral blood supply to the small bowel, can be accomplished.

The terminal ileum is often involved with bulky disease and can be resected en bloc with the right colon if necessary. After the HIPEC treatment is completed, small bowel anastomoses and serosal tears are repaired. Small bowel anastomoses can be performed with gastrointestinal anastomosis staplers, but it is advisable to oversew the staple lines with Lembert sutures, as leaks and fistulas are common postoperative complications of CRS. Small bowel serosal defects should be repaired transversely with invaginating Lembert sutures to prevent subsequent stenosis of the small bowel.

Pelvic Peritoneum and Pelvic Organs

As the most dependent portion of the abdominal cavity, the pelvis is commonly involved with peritoneal carcinomatosis, and it is often the site of the greatest disease volume. With bulky disease in the pelvis and cul de sac, it is usually necessary to remove the sigmoid colon and rectum down to the level of the nonperitonealized portion of the rectum below the peritoneal reflection.

After the sigmoid colon is transected at the appropriate level, the peritoneum can be stripped from the level of the pelvic inlet caudally and full circumferentially, allowing an en bloc resection of the pelvic peritoneum and pelvic organs. Anteriorly the peritoneum is stripped from the anterior abdominal wall and bladder; it is stripped laterally from the pelvic sidewalls posteriorly, taking care to identify and preserve the ureters.

In females the uterus and ovaries are taken en bloc with the rectum and pelvic peritoneum by ligating and transecting the blood supply to these organs. The vagina is transected below the cervix, leaving the rectum as the final attachment of the pelvic peritonectomy specimen. The deep pelvic peritoneum is dissected below the level of the peritoneal reflection, and the rectum is transected below the peritoneal reflection to remove all disease. This usually leaves a rectal stump of 8 to 10 cm, which facilitates a subsequent colorectal or ileorectal anastomosis.

After the HIPEC an anastomosis can be constructed to the rectal stump, or the rectal stump can be left closed for subsequent anastomosis at a later date. If the anastomosis is performed at the time of the CRS and HIPEC, it is necessary to create a diverting ileostomy, as the danger of a leak at the rectal anastomosis is significant, and the consequences can be disastrous.

MEDICAL TREATMENT

Hyperthermic Intraoperative Intraperitoneal Chemotherapy

HIPEC is an essential part of the successful management of peritoneal surface malignancy. After optimal CRS, this treatment is necessary to eradicate the residual macroscopic or microscopic malignant cells within the peritoneal cavity. Although several techniques have been described for HIPEC treatment in peritoneal surface malignancies, the basic principles of all techniques are the same. These include 1) the delivery of a high dose of a chemotherapeutic agent to all peritoneal surfaces at risk for malignancy, 2) exposure of the peritoneal surface to a solution heated 5° to 7° C higher than normal body temperature, and 3) circulation of the heated chemotherapy solution to maintain a constant temperature and exposure of peritoneal surfaces to the HIPEC solution.

Several devices used to heat and circulate the chemotherapy solution have been developed and approved for use in both the United States and Europe. These consist of a pump with an associated heat exchanger to circulate and heat the HIPEC solution. A diagram of one setup is shown in Figure 2.

HIPEC Technique

After the CRS is completed, the inflow and outflow catheters are placed, and the abdominal wall skin is temporarily closed with a running monofilament suture. Temperature probes are placed on the inflow and outflow catheters to monitor the temperature of the solution at these points in the circuit. The carrier solution, 1.5% peritoneal

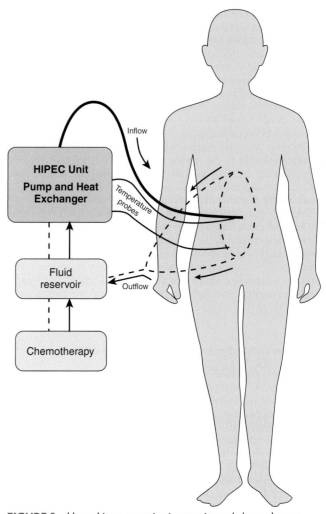

FIGURE 2 Heated intraoperative intraperitoneal chemotherapy diagram. After cytoreductive surgery (CRS), the heated chemotherapy solution is circulated for 90 minutes at inflow temperatures of 44° to 46° C.

dialysate solution, is then circulated through the circuit until an outflow temperature of approximately 40° to 42° C is reached.

The chemotherapy agent is then added to the dialysate solution and circulated for 90 minutes. During this time the abdomen is constantly agitated, and the operating table position is shifted to maximize perfusion to the different areas of the abdomen: Trendelenburg position, upper abdomen; left side down position, left abdomen and colic gutter; right side down position, right abdomen and colic gutter; reverse Trendelenburg position, lower abdomen and pelvis. In addition with the four-catheter drainage technique, preferential perfusion of the various areas of the abdomen can be accomplished by clamping the outflow catheters on the side of the abdomen opposite the side where maximal perfusion is desired.

Several safeguards are instituted to protect the patient from the toxic effects of the heat and chemotherapy. Preoperatively, the patient is placed on a cooling blanket that is used during the HIPEC to keep the core temperature within a range of 36° to 39° C. During the perfusion the ambient temperature in the operating room is turned down to 60° F, while the patient's core temperature is monitored with an esophageal and bladder temperature probe.

To minimize chemotherapy-induced renal toxicity from absorbed chemotherapy during the procedure, which is more of a problem when extensive peritoneal stripping is performed, the patient's urine output is maintained at 400 mL/hr during the HIPEC treatment using generous amounts of intravenous crystalloid solutions and diuretics if necessary.

Type of Chemotherapy

The chemotherapy agent used for HIPEC is dependent on the type and grade of the primary malignancy. Currently there is not universal agreement on the chemotherapy agents or doses used, as there have not been clinical trials performed that compare the various agents for specific peritoneal surface malignancies. In general, the low-grade, noninvasive peritoneal surface malignancies are treated with intraperitoneal mitomycin C, and the higher grade malignancies are treated with mitomycin C plus an additional agent, such as doxorubicin, cisplatin, or oxaliplatin. The concentration ratio for exposure of tumor cells to chemotherapy by intraperitoneal compared to systemic routes ranges from 16 times greater (oxaliplatin) to 500 times greater (doxorubicin).

PATIENT SELECTION

Appropriate patient selection is crucial in the decision to perform CRS and HIPEC for peritoneal surface malignancies. Many factors enter into this decision, including patient age, comorbidities, tumor type and grade, extent of disease, and biologic behavior of the malignancy. CRS and HIPEC place a large physiologic stress on patients, therefore those with significant physiologic deficits resulting from age and comorbidities should not be considered candidates for this treatment.

The magnitude of the stress often is dependent on the amount of surgical debulking necessary, which should be taken into account when evaluating or referring a patient for CRS and HIPEC. The HIPEC alone is often well tolerated when extensive dissection and debulking are not necessary, as is the case with low-volume disease. Age alone should not be considered exclusionary for CRS and HIPEC; as with many other major surgical procedures, the physiologic status of the patient is much more predictive of a successful outcome than age alone. The biologic behavior of the malignancy should also be considered; patients with high-grade, rapidly progressive malignancies fare worse than those with low-grade indolent malignancies, so those with high-grade disease may not be appropriate candidates for a procedure of this magnitude.

Current indications for CRS and HIPEC include those listed in Table 3. As shown in the table, some indications are accepted as the standard of care by many who manage peritoneal malignancies. These indications are supported by multiple studies in the literature showing improved outcomes with CRS and HIPEC. Other indications should be considered investigative at this time, although reports

in the literature that do support the use of CRS and HIPEC or HIPEC alone in these situations.

Although most low-grade, noninvasive peritoneal surface tumors are candidates for CRS and HIPEC regardless of tumor volume, the higher grade, invasive malignancies should only be considered for CRS and HIPEC when low-volume disease is present. The criteria for low-volume disease are not well defined, but they generally refer to patients with disease limited to one or two areas of the abdomen or scattered tumor nodules in several areas without bulky or confluent disease.

With the advent of improved chemotherapy agents for gastrointestinal cancers in the past decade, selected patients with high-volume, aggressive, high-grade peritoneal surface malignancies can be treated with neoadjuvant chemotherapy. If response to the neoadjuvant therapy is good, with documented tumor reduction, the patient can then be considered for CRS and HIPEC. It is unusual to find a complete pathologic response with neoadjuvant therapy alone. Even in the best responders, there often is residual disease, albeit small, after treatment with systemic chemotherapy.

INDICATIONS FOR, AND OUTCOMES OF, TREATMENT BY SITE OF ORIGIN

Primary Peritoneal Malignancies

Patients diagnosed with both malignant peritoneal mesothelioma and primary peritoneal cancer are generally considered candidates for CRS and HIPEC, regardless of tumor volume, because of the propensity of these malignancies to spread via intraperitoneal routes. Primary peritoneal cancer is often treated like ovarian cancer, but many feel that peritoneal cancer is a distinct clinical and pathologic entity and should be treated accordingly. Current long-term survival rates for all stages of disease approach 50% for malignant peritoneal mesothelioma, but in the primary peritoneal cancers, long-term survival is lower (15% to 25%). Most published series on primary peritoneal cancer report treatment with CRS and systemic therapy rather than with HIPEC.

Intra-abdominal Malignancies

Pseudomyxoma Peritonei

All patients diagnosed with pseudomyxoma peritonei from mucinous cystadenomas of the appendix should be treated with CRS and HIPEC. These patients are ideal candidates for this treatment

TABLE 3: Current indications for CRS and HIPEC

Disease or Condition	Example	Accepted	Under Investigation
Noninvasive peritoneal carcinomatosis, any volume	Pseudomyxoma peritonei	X	
Malignant peritoneal mesothelioma (MPM), any volume	MPM	X	
Invasive cancer, low volume	Colorectal cancer	X	
Gastrointestinal cancer with positive cytology or perforation	Gastric cancer		X
Recurrent ovarian cancer unresponsive to systemic chemotherapy	Recurrent ovarian cancer		X
Gastrointestinal cancer with invasion of adjacent organs or positive margins	Colorectal cancer		X
Ovarian cancer, initial diagnosis of stage IIIB or IIIC	Ovarian cancer		X
Malignant ascites (for palliation)	Pancreatic cancer	X	
Noninvasive sarcomatosis, any volume	Recurrent retroperitoneal fibrosarcoma	X	

because of the low grade of the malignancy, which is very sensitive to the locoregional therapy of CRS and HIPEC. The pseudomyxoma peritonei syndrome (i.e., the presence of large amounts of mucinous ascites) can be present in other, more invasive intraabdominal cancers; but when the histology reveals a low-grade lesion with a ruptured mucinous cystadenoma of the appendix, aggressive therapy with CRS and HIPEC should be undertaken. Long-term survival as high as 90% has been reported in this situation.

Appendiceal Cancer

Cancers of the appendix are the paradigm for the use of CRS and HIPEC. Almost all appendiceal cancers with peritoneal involvement should be considered for CRS and HIPEC because there is often diffuse intraperitoneal dissemination prior to any extraabdominal metastases. The rate of success and long-term survival of CRS and HIPEC therapy is dependent on the grade and invasiveness of the tumor. After CRS and HIPEC, reported 5-year survivals for low-grade appendiceal malignancies is in the range of 70% to 80%, but in the higher grade appendical cancers, the 3-year survival is 45% to 55%. Recent reports in the literature indicate that the long-term survival for high-grade appendiceal cancers is more closely related to the ability to obtain a complete cytoreduction than to the grade of the tumor.

Colorectal Cancer

Colorectal cancers with low-volume peritoneal involvement should be considered for CRS and HIPEC. A recent consensus statement from peritoneal carcinomatosis experts recommended this treatment for all patients with intraperitoneal metastases from colorectal cancer who do not have distant disease, when complete cytoreduction is possible. High-volume intraperitoneal disease or extraabdominal metastases are generally considered contraindications to CRS and HIPEC in colorectal cancer. Currently, peritoneal involvement from colorectal cancer is probably the most common indication for CRS and HIPEC because of the higher incidence of this disease compared with other peritoneal surface malignancies.

It is estimated that involvement of the peritoneum occurs in up to 60% of cases of recurrent colorectal cancer. Reported 3-year survival rates for colorectal cancer patients who have undergone CRS and HIPEC range from 25% to 65%. Additionally, in the only prospective randomized trial comparing CRS and HIPEC with conventional therapy, the median disease-specific survival was significantly prolonged (12.6 vs. 22.2 months, $P = .028$) in patients with peritoneal carcinomatosis of colorectal origin who were treated with CRS and HIPEC.

Gastric Cancer

Gastric cancer commonly involves the peritoneal cavity, with up to a third of early gastric cancer patients demonstrating positive cytology, when techniques such as polymerase chain reaction are used to detect malignant cells. Later stages of gastric cancer have higher rates of peritoneal involvement. CRS and HIPEC have been used in stage II and III gastric cancer patients, but it has been difficult to show a survival advantage because of the aggressive behavior of gastric adenocarcinoma and the propensity it has for developing distant metastases. After complete cytoreduction (CC score 0), the reported 5-year survival rates using CRS and HIPEC range from 21% to 32%. Locally advanced gastric cancers, as well as peritoneal-only recurrences of gastric cancer, should be considered for CRS and HIPEC.

Ovarian Cancer

The biologic properties of ovarian malignancies would seem to make them ideal candidates for the use of CRS and HIPEC. Ovarian malignancies predominantly spread intraperitoneally, often until late in the course of the disease. The value of debulking surgery followed by subsequent systemic chemotherapy in stage II and III ovarian cancer is well documented in the gynecologic oncology literature.

Recently, the value of postoperative intraperitoneal chemotherapy has also been shown to confer a survival benefit for stage III ovarian cancer. The use of CRS and HIPEC as the initial treatment in stage III ovarian cancer has not been adequately evaluated, even though there is room for improvement in the outcomes using current treatment regimens; stage III survival rates are 15% to 40%. A prospective randomized trial comparing current treatment (CRS plus postoperative intraperitoneal and systemic chemotherapy versus CRS with HIPEC plus systemic chemotherapy) as initial treatment for stage III ovarian cancer would answer this question. The use of CRS and HIPEC has been studied in patients with recurrent ovarian cancer with peritoneal involvement. In this situation, median survival ranged from 22 to 54 months in reported series. Improved overall 5-year survival of 57% after CRS and HIPEC compared with 17% without HIPEC has also been reported in small series.

Other Cancers

The use of CRS and HIPEC in various malignancies with peritoneal metastases has been reported. The numbers of patients in these reports are low, making it difficult to determine the absolute value of this therapy in these tumors. Current philosophy toward the use of CRS and HIPEC in unusual tumors with peritoneal involvement would indicate that almost any patient in this type of clinical situation could be considered for this treatment, provided the appropriate patient selection criteria are used. Patients with adequate physiologic reserve with tumors that have demonstrated the appropriate biologic characteristics and lack of distant metastases would fit these criteria.

MORBIDITY AND MORTALITY OF CRS AND HIPEC

Multiple series in the literature have reported mortality rates of 0% to 5% and morbidity rates of 27% to 52% for CRS and HIPEC. The major morbidities associated with these procedures include small bowel fistulas, intraabdominal abscesses, hematologic complications, anastomotic leaks, pancreatitis, and postoperative bleeding. The mortality and major morbidity rates are proportional to the magnitude of surgical resection necessary to achieve an adequate cytoreduction. Extensive CRS coupled with the HIPEC predisposes patients to postoperative complications. With increasing experience and judicious patient selection, major morbidity and mortality rates have decreased. Many centers are now reporting mortality rates of 0% for large series of patients treated with CRS and HIPEC.

PERITONEAL CARCINOMATOSIS PROGRAMS

Beginning a program to manage peritoneal surface malignancies requires a major commitment from the physicians involved and from the sponsoring institution. Necessary resources from the institution include the HIPEC equipment; availability of operative time and staff for extended cases, critical care, and surgical and oncologic nursing support; pharmacy support; and availability of appropriate rehabilitation, social, and outpatient services. Education regarding the use and handling of chemotherapy-contaminated solutions and waste is necessary for operating room, recovery room, critical care unit, and surgical floor staff. Surgical staff must be prepared for the long operative times, prolonged postoperative inpatient stays, and outpatient recovery.

Active programs in the management of peritoneal carcinomatosis should manage at least 5 to 10 cases per year to maintain surgeon and staff familiarity and experience with the procedure and postoperative care. Despite the challenges in developing and maintaining a peritoneal carcinomatosis program, the results achieved more than justify the time and expense of the program. These programs offer peritoneal carcinomatosis patients the potential for extended survival and cure for a disease that was once considered hopeless.

SUGGESTED READINGS

Esquivel J, Sticca R, Sugarbaker P, et al: Cytoreductive surgery and hyperthermic intraperitoneal chemotherapy in the management of peritoneal surface malignancies of colonic origin: a consensus statement, *Ann Surg Oncol* 14:128, 2007.

Foltz P, Wavrin C, Sticca R: Heated intraoperative intraperitoneal chemotherapy: the challenges of bringing chemotherapy into surgery, *AORN J* 80:1055, 2004.
Reuter NP, Macgregor JM, Woodall CE, et al: Preoperative performance status predicts outcome following heated intraperitoneal chemotherapy, *Am J Surg* 196:909, 2008.
Sticca RP, Dach BW: Rationale for hyperthermia with intraoperative intraperitoneal chemotherapy agents, *Surg Oncol Clin North Am* 12:689, 2003.
Sugarbaker PH: Peritonectomy procedures, *Surg Onc Clin North Am* 12:703, 2003.
Verwaal VJ, van Ruth S, Witkamp A, et al: Long-term survival of peritoneal carcinomatosis of colorectal origin, *Ann Surg Oncol* 12:65, 2005.

ACUTE APPENDICITIS

**Genevieve B. Melton, MD, Ryan Li, MD,
Mark D. Duncan, MD, and John W. Harmon, MD**

OVERVIEW

Historically, it is believed that British surgeon Claudius Amyand performed the first appendectomy during the repair of an inguinal hernia in 1735. However, inflammation of the appendix, including subsequent clinical sequelae of abscess and perforation, was first described in 1886 by Reginald Fitz.

Today, acute appendicitis is the most common surgical emergency of the abdomen, with more than 250,000 appendectomies performed annually in the United States. Although the diagnosis of appendicitis in a young man with acute abdominal pain localized to the right lower quadrant can be clear-cut, the clinical diagnosis may be less straightforward in women of childbearing age and in those at the extremes of age. In these patients, appendicitis can still be a challenging clinical entity to diagnose in a timely, accurate, and cost-effective manner.

Important considerations for surgeons and areas of debate include investigative radiology tests, such as computed tomography (CT) and ultrasonography, and the use of laparoscopy as a diagnostic and therapeutic approach. As with other etiologies of the acute abdomen, early and accurate recognition of patients requiring urgent operative repair should be the overriding principle in the workup and treatment of patients with suspected appendicitis. Delayed diagnosis in the treatment of acute appendicitis is associated with higher rates of perforation with resultant increased morbidity and mortality.

PRESENTATION OF ILLNESS

Appendicitis is most frequently a disease of young and healthy individuals. The location, timing, and character of pain and associated symptoms are key factors to elicit in understanding the presentation of the disease. The classic symptoms are cramping and intermittent abdominal pain that usually begins in the periumbilical or epigastric region with subsequent migration to the right lower quadrant. As the course of appendicitis progresses, pain progresses from intermittent and cramping to constant and sharp in nature. If the appendix does not lie in an anterior or pelvic position, the diagnosis of appendicitis may be more difficult, leading to potential delay. In particular, a retrocecal appendix may not cause local signs of peritonitis.

The timing of nausea can also help to distinguish appendicitis, in which nausea follows the pain, from gastroenteritis, in which nausea typically precedes pain. In addition, most patients with gastroenteritis show evidence of anorexia. A low-grade fever is often present in uncomplicated appendicitis; high fevers are atypical for simple appendicitis and may be a sign of perforation, appendiceal abscess, or another disease process. Other clinical entities to be considered in the differential diagnosis include urinary tract infection, renal calculi, gastroenteritis, gynecologic diagnoses such as ruptured ovarian cyst or pelvic inflammatory disease, cholecystitis, diverticulitis, or small bowel obstruction.

PATHOPHYSIOLOGY

The exact pathophysiology of acute appendicitis is not entirely clear, but the prevailing theory is that appendiceal luminal obstruction is the key mechanism. In children, lymphoid hyperplasia, often in the setting of infection or dehydration, is thought to be the most common etiology of obstruction.

In the adult population, fecaliths are the main causes of obstruction leading to acute appendicitis; other causes are scarring, which is rare, or tumor. Obstruction causes distension of the lumen of the appendix, yielding increased intramural and intraluminal pressures. This leads to lymphatic and vascular compromise with ischemia and then necrosis of the appendix with associated bacterial overgrowth. In the first 24 hours, the great majority of patients have inflammation and possibly necrosis, with perforation uncommon. Approximately two thirds of patients with perforated appendicitis have had symptoms for more than 48 hours. Early in appendicitis, the most common bacteria are aerobic organisms. In contrast, late appendicitis is associated with mixed infections. Common organisms associated with late appendicitis are *Escherichia coli*, *Streptococcus* spp., *Proteus* spp., *Bacteroides fragilis*, and *Pseudomonas* spp.

DIAGNOSIS

History and Physical Examination

Initial features in the history are typically nonspecific, including indigestion, change in bowel habits, and malaise. Following this, patients most typically experience visceral-type pain in the periumbilical or sometimes epigastric region that is characteristically intermittent, poorly localized, and often not terribly severe. Nausea and vomiting, which can occur, usually follow the onset of pain. Similarly, fever may be present and usually occurs following the onset of pain. The presence of high fever (>39.4° C) may be a sign of a perforated appendix.

Early stages of appendicitis may not elicit tenderness on physical examination, but signs of localized inflammation or peritonitis occur as the disease progresses. Patients with an appendix in the anterior position typically have tenderness in the right lower quadrant near McBurney's point, two thirds of the distance from the umbilicus to the anterior superior iliac spine, often associated with peritoneal signs. In contrast, patients with a retrocecal appendix often have less impressive tenderness. Tenderness in patients with a pelvic appendix is often below McBurney's point. These patients often have symptoms of dysuria, urinary frequency, diarrhea, or tenesmus. Several classical maneuvers on physical examination that aid in the diagnosis of appendicitis are described (Table 1).

Laboratory Examination

Laboratory tests are not a primary diagnostic modality in appendicitis, although they are helpful in ruling out other conditions and in assessing metabolic derangements from dehydration and other electrolyte abnormalities. The white blood cell count in patients with simple appendicitis is typically mildly elevated, but it may be normal in 30% of cases. More than 95% of patients, however, have a left shift in their differential.

Urinalysis is useful for ruling out a urinary tract infection or a stone in the urinary tract. Sterile pyuria or hematuria is observed in approximately a third of patients with appendicitis because of secondary inflammation of the bladder and ureter. In sexually active or menstruating women, a urinary β-human chorionic gonadotropin is mandatory to rule out pregnancy, including possible ectopic pregnancy. Cervical cultures may also need to be obtained if pelvic inflammatory disease is suspected.

Imaging Studies

In general, a patient with a history and physical examination strongly suggestive of appendicitis should undergo prompt appendectomy without further imaging studies. When the presentation of appendicitis is not typical and the diagnosis is unclear, radiographic studies are key clinical tools. Abdominal x-rays in patients with appendicitis may demonstrate a fecalith, loss of the psoas shadow, deformity of the outline of the cecum, or a "sentinel loop" of small bowel in the right lower quadrant. However, plain films need not be routinely performed in patients with appendicitis because these findings are often subtle and not sensitive or specific for appendicitis.

The two most widely used radiologic modalities for the diagnosis of appendicitis are ultrasonography and CT. The strengths and weaknesses of each modality were analyzed in a systematic review by Terasawa and colleagues (2004). The authors demonstrated that CT had an overall sensitivity of 0.94 (confidence interval [CI], 0.91 to 0.95) and specificity of 0.95 (CI, 0.93 to 0.96), whereas ultrasonography had an overall sensitivity of 0.86 (CI, 0.83 to 0.88) and a specificity of 0.81 (CI, 0.78 to 0.84) with a positive likelihood ratio of 5.8 (CI, 3.5 to 9.5).

Findings strongly suggestive of acute appendicitis on standard abdominal CT scan include 1) a thick wall (>2 mm), often with "targeting" that may be concentrically thickened, indicating inflammation of the appendix; 2) increased diameter of the appendix (>7 mm); 3) an appendicolith (seen in 25% of cases); 4) a phlegmon or abscess; or 5) free fluid. Stranding of the adjacent fatty tissues in the right lower quadrant is usually also seen (Figure 1).

Air in the appendix or a contrast-filled appendiceal lumen without other abnormalities on CT virtually eliminate appendicitis as a diagnosis. However, appendicitis is not excluded if the appendix is not visualized on CT scan. If patients come in early in their course, only minimal inflammatory changes may be seen. CT is also useful in diagnosing an appendiceal abscess (Figure 2) and can guide percutaneous drainage of the abscess.

Some have advocated the use of CT with rectal contrast alone and the use of thin cuts through the right iliac fossa, a so-called *appendiceal CT*. In contrast to complete abdominal CT, which takes up to 2 hours to perform with standard oral preparation, appendiceal CT can be performed in 15 minutes. The main disadvantage of this technique is that it may not reveal pathology in other portions of the abdomen; therefore workup of patients must

TABLE 1: Maneuvers on physical examination in patients with suspected appendicitis

Maneuver	Description
Rovsing sign	Palpation of the left lower quadrant that elicits pain in the right lower quadrant
Obturator sign	Pain with internal rotation of the hip (pelvic appendix)
Iliopsoas sign	Extension of the right hip that elicits pain in the right hip (retrocecal appendix)

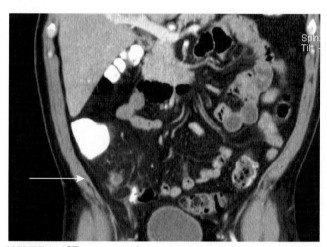

FIGURE 1   CT scan, coronal view, demonstrating acute appendicitis with increased diameter of the appendix and right lower quadrant stranding.

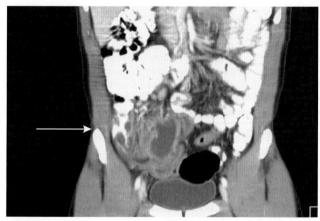

FIGURE 2   CT scan, coronal view, demonstrating periappendiceal abscess.

continue if the study is negative. The question of which study is superior remains an area of debate. Practically, the type of CT performed can often depend on institutional preference and clinician experience.

Ultrasonography can be particularly useful for examining pelvic pathology in women, especially with the technique of endovaginal ultrasound. Findings on ultrasonography suggestive of appendicitis include a thickened wall (>2 mm), increased appendiceal diameter (>6 mm), or free fluid. Whereas CT is performed with a low-variability protocol and can often be interpreted by the surgeon, ultrasound is highly operator dependent and may require a radiologist to interpret. Ultrasound can also be difficult to perform well in obese patients and in patients with a large amount of bowel gas overlying the appendix.

MANAGEMENT OF APPENDICITIS

General Management Issues

In all cases of suspected appendicitis, patients should have fluid and electrolyte abnormalities corrected, and appropriate antibiotics should be administered. Andersen and colleagues (2005) examined antibiotic use for suspected appendicitis with a systematic review. The authors included 45 studies with 9576 patients and compared antibiotic treatment versus placebo in patients with suspected appendicitis, both uncomplicated and perforated, undergoing appendectomy. Use of antibiotics was found to be superior to placebo with respect to wound infection, intraabdominal abscess, and length of stay, with no apparent difference according to the method (open or laparoscopic) of appendectomy.

If nonperforated appendicitis is suspected, surgery is indicated using either a traditional open or laparoscopic approach. Because of the acute nature of the condition, patients with acute appendicitis are frequently cared for by the on-call surgeon. The choice of procedure is dictated primarily by the experience of the treating surgeon, which may vary significantly, even within an institution.

Laparoscopic appendectomy is rapidly becoming the more common approach. Following surgery for nonperforated appendicitis, most patients are discharged within 24 to 48 hours. General requirements for discharge include being afebrile for 12 to 24 hours and tolerance of a diet. Patients are started on clear liquids following surgery and advanced as tolerated to an unrestricted diet. It is our practice to continue antibiotics for up to 24 hours after surgery in patients with nonperforated appendicitis; there is only evidence that perioperative antibiotics are beneficial, and no firm guidelines are available for exact antibiotic timing with current clinical evidence.

Perforation or rupture of the appendix may be suspected preoperatively or may not be confirmed until the time of surgery. In either case, prompt appendectomy is suitable. In most cases, appendectomy can be performed in standard laparoscopic or open fashion. Rarely, if necrosis is extensive and tissue quality is poor, an ileocecectomy may be required. Antibiotic coverage in patients following appendectomy for perforated appendicitis should involve 5 to 10 days of broad-spectrum antibiotics. Typical regimens include single therapy with piperacillin/tazobactam or triple therapy with ampicillin, gentamicin, and metronidazole.

Patients may also have a postoperative ileus, and their diet should be advanced only as bowel function clinically returns. These patients are at risk for postoperative abscess, and a high clinical suspicion for abscess is warranted in those with fevers or ileus persisting beyond 3 to 5 days following appendectomy for perforated appendicitis.

In the case of periappendiceal abscess, the management algorithm is less straightforward and should be tailored to the individual patient. Treatment options include immediate appendectomy or percutaneous drainage, typically with interval appendectomy. Patients who have a well-delineated appendiceal abscess respond best to initial percutaneous drainage with CT guidance. The goal of percutaneous drainage is to allow inflammation to subside. This may alleviate the potential need for extended bowel resection and can help to stabilize an otherwise ill patient. These patients require an extended course of broad-spectrum antibiotics.

In patients undergoing initial percutaneous drain placement, it is our practice to follow this in 6 to 8 weeks with an interval appendectomy, with the rationale that these patients are at risk for recurrent inflammation. Recent studies have challenged this notion, citing low rates of subsequent appendectomy in patients followed nonoperatively after CT-guided drainage of appendiceal abscess. Further evaluation of this strategy is required before it can be clearly advocated.

Older patients should be considered for a colonoscopy or barium enema after resolution of the acute abscess to rule out colonic pathology (e.g., diverticular disease or malignancy) as the etiology for periappendiceal abscess before surgical intervention, particularly if no surgery is planned.

Laparoscopic versus Open Approach

Surgical options include both open and laparoscopic approaches. Although laparoscopic appendectomy may require longer operative time and greater hospital costs, it has also been associated with less postoperative pain and possibly a shorter hospital stay.

Laparoscopic surgery may be especially helpful in the treatment of patients whose diagnosis is less certain. A systematic Cochrane review examined the diagnostic and therapeutic differences between the two approaches. The review included 54 studies, of which 45 compared laparoscopic appendectomy to open appendectomy in adults. Most consistently, laparoscopic appendectomy was associated with a decreased wound infection rate (approximately half the risk) and increased intraabdominal abscess rate (approximately twice the risk). The review also suggested a reduction in hospital stay by 1.1 days using the laparoscopic approach; with laparoscopic appendectomy, the return to normal activity and work was 6 and 3 days earlier, surgery was 12 minutes longer, pain decreased an average of 9 points of 100 on a visual analog scale, and hospital costs were increased.

The benefit of diagnostic laparoscopy was most evident in fertile women, in whom the rate of negative appendectomy with no final diagnosis was decreased. From these reports, most advocate laparoscopy if the clinician's index of suspicion is moderate to high, but several other items remain in the differential diagnosis. In particular, women may benefit from a laparoscopic approach, which may reveal other pelvic pathology, which has traditionally resulted in higher rates of negative appendectomies in this population. The laparoscopic approach can also be helpful in obese patients in whom exposure with the standard open approach may require a larger incision.

Open Surgical Approach

The traditional open surgical approach involves an incision approximately 4 cm long centered over McBurney's point, lateral to the rectus sheath. It cannot be overemphasized that by staying lateral to the rectus sheath, anatomic clarity is easily achieved. This incision can be oblique along skin folds or transverse, which is more easily extended for increased exposure. We also find that the transverse incision provides a better cosmetic result during the healing process.

The dissection is carried through the subcutaneous tissues to the external oblique fascia, which is then sharply incised. The muscle-splitting technique is then used to bluntly separate the external oblique fibers, followed by the internal oblique and transversus abdominis muscle fibers. The peritoneum is carefully entered. This layer-by-layer anatomic exercise is one of the joys of general surgery.

On entry to the peritoneal cavity, turbid or murky fluid may be encountered; we do not advocate culture of peritoneal fluid because the results so rarely affect clinical management. Cultures typically reveal multiple organisms that require broad-spectrum antibiotic coverage.

To locate the appendix, a finger is swept lateral to medial in the right paracolic gutter. If the appendix is not found with this maneuver, the taenia coli can be followed to the base of the cecum, where the appendix originates. After the appendix is located, adhesions can be freed from the appendix and any surrounding structures, and the appendix can be delivered through the incision with care to avoid tearing and possible spilling of enteric contents.

The mesoappendix is divided between Rienhoff clamps and tied off using 3-0 absorbable suture. The appendix is then gently clamped at its base, where it is tied with 2-0 absorbable suture. Any fecalith is manually dislodged, and the appendix is sharply excised. The appendiceal stump is cauterized to prevent mucocele formation. If the appendiceal stump appears weak or necrotic, this base may be inverted into the cecum using a purse-string suture or Z-stitch. The surgical bed should then be thoroughly irrigated with an antibiotic solution.

Closure of the incision is performed in layers with absorbable suture; peritoneum is closed with a running 2-0 suture, and the internal oblique fascia is closed with an interrupted 0-0 suture. Irrigation is performed between each layer, and the external oblique fascia is closed with an interrupted 0-0 suture and may be infused with local anesthetic to improve analgesia. The skin is closed with 4-0 absorbable suture or surgical staples.

Primary closure is the general rule for nonperforated appendicitis because wound infection is less likely. In the case of perforated appendicitis, skin closure options include primary closure as described earlier, loose partial closure, delayed primary closure, or secondary closure. If heavy fecal contamination is present, secondary closure is our general practice; loose partial closure with gauze packing between sutures is suitable for most other cases of perforated appendicitis.

Laparoscopic Surgical Approach

The laparoscopic approach for appendectomy can be performed using a variety of port placement configurations and techniques. Once adequate general anesthesia has been administered, decompression of the stomach and bladder is performed using a nasogastric or orogastric tube and a Foley catheter. Port placement has been described with a variety approaches, but the general principle is port triangulation to allow adequate visualization and exposure. We use a Hassan technique to directly place an umbilical 10 mm port for the camera.

Following general inspection of the abdomen with a 45 degree, 10 mm camera to confirm the pathology, two trocars are placed under direct visualization: A single 12 mm port is placed in the left abdomen, inferior to the umbilical port, and a single 5 mm port placed in the suprapubic region along the midline. At the start of the procedure, two atraumatic graspers are placed into the left lower quadrant and suprapubic ports.

The appendix is identified, grasped at its tip with an alligator grasper, and retracted anteriorly and superiorly. This maneuver exposes the mesoappendix, which can then be divided using ligaclips, endostapler with vascular cartridge, LigaSure (Valleylab, Boulder, Colo.), or harmonic scalpel. The appendix is further cleared of any adhesions, and attention is then focused on division of the appendix from the cecum.

We routinely have used the 30 mm reticulating laparoscopic gastrointestinal anastomosis stapler with 3.5 mm blue cartridge for division of the appendix. Care must be taken to fire the device across healthy, unaffected tissue, which may include a portion of the cecum. The divided appendix is delivered through the 12 mm port site using an EndoCatch bag (U.S. Surgical, Norwalk, Conn.) to avoid wound contamination. One liter of antibiotic-containing saline irrigation is routinely employed with the suction irrigator. If an obvious abscess cavity is seen, the abscess should be evacuated thoroughly and a drain placed. This is uncommon, because even ruptured appendicitis rarely requires a drain.

Negative Appendectomy

Historically, up to 20% of patients with suspected appendicitis were found intraoperatively to have a normal appendix. This number may differ in the era of routine CT imaging. If a normal appendix is encountered intraoperatively, it is important to address other possible etiologies and to remove the normal appendix to avoid possible confusion about future abdominal pain. Removal of the appendix is especially important if the procedure is performed using a standard, open, right lower quadrant incision. Other causes to look for

explicitly in the operating room include terminal ileitis, Meckel diverticulitis, mesenteric adenitis, cholecystitis, colonic diverticulitis, and pathology of the uterus, ovary, or fallopian tubes.

Crohn's disease adds complexity to the management of appendiceal disease. For patients with Crohn's disease in the ileocecal distribution, rates of fistulization are significant (15% to 20%) after appendectomy. If surgical exploration is pursued, and the appendix is found to be uninvolved, appendectomy should be performed. If the appendix is included in a generalized ileeocecal inflammatory process, the appendix should not be removed but rather treated as part of the larger mass. Resection should be reserved for patients with stricture (obstructive symptoms), fistula, or failure of medical management.

There may be rare patients with a low suspicion for acute appendicitis for whom it is important to rule appendicitis out definitively. In such patients, if the appendix is normal, diagnostic laparoscopy without appendectomy may be an appropriate choice. But our routine is to remove the appendix even if it is normal, to prevent confusion in the future should symptoms recur.

SPECIAL CONSIDERATIONS

Children

Age is one of the predominant factors in the consideration of acute appendicitis. Children with acute appendicitis often have associated diarrhea and may not have symptoms of anorexia. Despite reluctance on the part of some practitioners to expose children to radiation, CT has been demonstrated to be highly accurate in the diagnosis of appendicitis and can be helpful in those with an atypical presentation. In neonates and infants, the differential diagnoses include mid gut volvulus, pyloric stenosis, Meckel diverticulitis, and intussusception.

Elderly

Although diverticulitis and colonic neoplasms are more common in the elderly and can have symptoms similar to appendicitis, appendicitis in the elderly is not uncommon; the estimated incidence in patients older than 65 years is approximately 1 in 2000. Elderly patients often may not be able to give a detailed history, and the acute abdomen may come with few or minimal subtle signs. CT is particularly helpful in this setting. Again, if a normal appendix is found intraoperatively, other causes of symptoms, including perforated colon cancer or diverticulitis of the cecum or sigmoid colon, should be sought.

Pregnancy

The most common general surgery emergency in pregnancy is acute appendicitis. The incidence of acute appendicitis is estimated at 0.1% of all deliveries, and it occurs with equal frequency during all three trimesters.

The pregnant patient with suspected appendicitis can be difficult to diagnose. As the uterus enlarges, the appendix is pushed more cephalad, making the location of tenderness typically in the right upper quadrant or right flank. Ultrasound may be helpful in making the diagnosis and is preferred in early pregnancy to avoid the possible teratogenic effects of ionizing radiation. Late in pregnancy, when the effects of ionizing radiation are fewer, CT can be particularly helpful.

The diagnosis and treatment of appendicitis in a timely manner is especially important in pregnancy because of the potential devastating effects on the fetus. Whereas nonperforated appendicitis carries a fetal mortality rate of less than 5%, perforated appendicitis is associated with a fetal mortality rate of more than 20%. Although appendicitis occurs equally during all trimesters of pregnancy, perforated appendicitis occurs most frequently in the third trimester, when diagnosis can be particularly challenging, again underscoring the importance of early recognition and management.

Immunocompromised Patients

Immunocompromised states include organ transplantation, immunosuppressive therapy for autoimmune or neoplastic pathology, and AIDS. These patients may show only mild tenderness on examination, but they have other issues that should be considered in their differential diagnosis, including mycobacterial infection, cytomegalovirus, and fungal infections. In addition, enterocolitis is an important cause of abdominal pain and fever in patients with neutropenia, which can occur secondary to chemotherapy.

CT is an important tool for the diagnostic workup of these patients, which can be particularly challenging. Although it is important to be clinically cautious in immunocompromised patients, it is also essential not to delay operative treatment in patients in whom there is a strong suspicion of appendicitis.

SUGGESTED READINGS

Andersen BR, Kallehave FL, Andersen HK: Antibiotics versus placebo for prevention of postoperative infection after appendicectomy, *Cochrane Database Syst Rev* (3):CD001439, 2005.

Harrell AG, Lincourt AE, Novitsky YW, et al: Advantages of laparoscopic appendectomy in the elderly, *Am Surg* 72(6):474, 2006.

Morris KT, Kavanagh M, Hansen P, et al: The rational use of computed tomography scans in the diagnosis of appendicitis, *Am J Surg* 183(5):547, 2002.

Rao PM, Rhea JT, Novelline RA, et al: Effect of computed tomography of the appendix on treatment of patients and use of hospital resources, *N Engl J Med* 338(3):141, 1998.

Roberts KE: True single-port appendectomy: first experience with the "puppeteer technique", *Surg Endosc* 23(8):1825, 2009.

Sauerland S, Lefering R, Neugebauer EA: Laparoscopic versus open surgery for suspected appendicitis, *Cochrane Database Syst Rev* (4):CD001546, 2004.

Sporn E, Petroski GF, Mancini GJ, et al: Laparoscopic appendectomy: is it worth the cost? Trend analysis in the U.S. from 2000 to 2005, *J Am Coll Surg* 208(2):179, 2009.

Terasawa T, Blackmore CC, Bent S, et al: Systematic review: computed tomography and ultrasonography to detect acute appendicitis in adults and adolescents, *Ann Intern Med* 141(7):537, 2004.

Wei HB, Huang JL, Zheng ZH, et al: Laparoscopic versus open appendectomy: a prospective randomized comparison, *Surg Endosc*, Jun 11, 2009.

HEMORRHOIDS

Tanya R. Flohr, MD, and Charles M. Friel, MD

ANATOMY

The normal anal canal encloses three regions of fibrovascular cushions beneath the epithelium; these contain submucosa, blood vessels, smooth muscle, and connective tissue. These cushions are located in the left lateral, right posterior, and right anterior regions of the canal. Normally, the fibrovascular cushions contribute 15% to 20% of the resting anal pressure. They work in conjunction by congesting and filling with blood to prevent fecal incontinence during times of increased abdominal pressure and decreased anal tone. The term *hemorrhoid* is reserved for when one of these cushions becomes abnormally large and produces symptoms.

Hemorrhoids are subcategorized based on their location relative to the dentate line. Those occurring below the dentate line are *external hemorrhoids,* which are covered with anoderm and have sensory innervation. *Internal hemorrhoids,* those found above the dentate line, are covered with thin, often friable mucosa; they have no sensory innervation. Internal hemorrhoids are further classified based on their degree of prolapse (Table 1).

ETIOLOGY

The etiology of hemorrhoids remains uncertain. The pathophysiology of hemorrhoid development may occur secondarily to elevated anal sphincter pressures, abnormal dilation of the internal hemorrhoidal venous plexus, distension of the arteriovenous anastomosis, prolapse of the cushions and surrounding adjacent tissue, or any combination of the aforementioned factors. These changes might also be the consequences of hemorrhoidal disease.

While their direct cause remains unknown, it is likely that hemorrhoids occur secondarily to constant straining with defecation. Most commonly, patients affected have histories of constipation, diarrhea, or prolonged efforts at defecation. Normally, during the process of evacuation, the voluntary sphincter contracts to return any residual fecal matter to the rectum. In an attempt to completely evacuate the anal canal, extended straining compounded by inadequate fiber intake, long periods on the commode, or conditions with elevated intraabdominal pressure—such as pregnancy, ascites, or other similar states—can contribute to the development of the disease.

INCIDENCE

The exact incidence of hemorrhoids is unknown because people who suffer from hemorrhoids are often reluctant to seek medical attention. Therefore the reported cases likely underrepresent the prevalence. In the United States, the reported prevalence is 4.4%, with approximately 10 million people affected. There is a peak incidence for both genders between 45 and 60 years of age, and occurrence before the age of 20 years is rare; whites are more likely to be affected than are African Americans.

TABLE 1: Classification of internal hemorrhoids

Grade I	No prolapse but bleeding
Grade II	Prolapse with spontaneous reduction
Grade III	Prolapse requiring manual reduction
Grade IV	Prolapse that is not amenable to reduction secondary to thrombosis/incarceration

Although no direct evidence of hereditary predisposition has been found, family history might contribute to the incidence, especially because diet and bowel habits are interrelated with routine and environment. Women during pregnancy are at increased risk of developing hemorrhoids because of a gestational increase in circulating blood volume and a compressing gravid uterus, leading to venous engorgement and stasis. Elderly patients are also at greater risk of developing hemorrhoids because of digestive disturbances and weakened structures supporting the anal canal.

SYMPTOMS

Generally, the symptoms caused by hemorrhoids include bleeding, swelling, prolapse, pruritus, hygiene problems, and pain. Painless bleeding is the most frequent complaint. The bleeding associated with hemorrhoids is often bright red due to its arterial source. Patients will report blood with wiping after a bowel movement or blood seen dripping or squirting into the toilet. Bleeding not associated with a bowel movement is uncommon. Atypical symptoms of bleeding include bleeding that is not bright red or blood that is mixed with stool; often this suggests a more proximal source of bleeding, which requires further evaluation.

Prolapse of internal hemorrhoids below the dentate line can occur with straining. The prolapse and the associated swelling of the involved tissue can cause fecal leakage and poor hygiene. Additionally, the frequent soiling of the surrounding perianal skin can cause pruritus. Although patients may experience leakage associated with large prolapsing hemorrhoids, frank incontinence is unusual and should prompt the physician to look for sphincter defects with anal ultrasound and anal manometry. Because one of the major complications associated with any anorectal surgery is incontinence, it is important to clearly document preoperative bowel function and identify any anatomic abnormalities before proceeding with surgical intervention.

External hemorrhoids, because of their location and innervation with somatic fibers, can cause discomfort and pain. Pain associated with external hemorrhoids occurs most often with thrombosis (Figure 1). This pain generally subsides after 48 to 72 hours. Acute pain associated with internal hemorrhoids occurs with incarceration and strangulation after prolapse, leading to thrombosis and eventual necrosis (Figure 2). The pain associated with these hemorrhoids can require exam under anesthesia. Infrequently, emergent intervention is needed. If no thrombosis is readily obvious on exam, the source of pain is likely due to another cause, such as abscess, fissure, or trauma to the area.

DIFFERENTIAL DIAGNOSIS

Any symptom in the anal region is commonly attributed to "hemorrhoids." However, several other conditions cause anorectal symptoms; these include anal fissures, abscesses, fistulas, perianal Crohn's disease, skin tags, condyloma acuminata, hypertrophied anal papillas, melanoma, rectal prolapse, rectal or colon polyps, and carcinoma. Fortunately, most of these diagnoses are readily apparent on thorough examination. Evaluation should include a digital rectal exam and anoscopy. Bleeding and discomfort associated with a perianal mass may represent an anal cancer or a low rectal cancer. Too frequently these cancers are often misdiagnosed, being dismissed as "hemorrhoids" by both patients and physicians. Therefore, even in the presence of obvious hemorrhoids, the astute physician must consider more ominous reasons for bleeding and consider full endoscopic evaluation.

Hemorrhoids and *rectal varices* are not synonymous. The collateral circulation that develops in the setting of portal hypertension causes blood from the portal system to divert into the systemic circulation via the middle and inferior hemorrhoidal veins. The resulting rectal varicosities are located more proximally in the anal canal and rectum and are best treated with procedures that reduce portal hypertension.

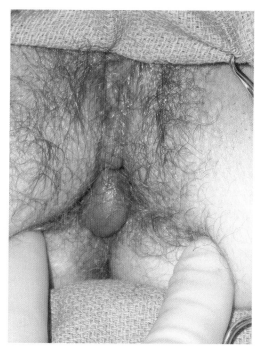

FIGURE 1   Thrombosed external hemorrhoid.

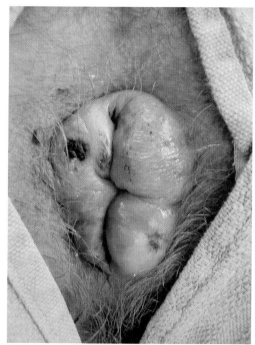

FIGURE 2   Prolapsed and thrombosed internal hemorrhoids.

Moreover, multiple studies have been unsuccessful in demonstrating any increased incidence of hemorrhoids in patients with portal hypertension.

TREATMENT

Medical Management

Lifestyle modifications to treat hemorrhoids should be suggested for all patients with hemorrhoids, regardless of grade. Grade I, II, and often grade III internal hemorrhoids will respond to these changes.

The mainstay of these modifications includes dietary changes, specifically increased fluid and fiber intake. Patients should drink approximately 6 to 8 (12 oz) glasses of fluid daily. Fiber intake should be increased to 25 to 30 grams per day. Dietary supplements such as psyllium or hydrophilic colloid are often required in addition to changing food preferences. The increased dietary fiber works by adding bulk to stools, which are more formed and occur at decreased frequency. In a meta-analysis reviewing 378 participants randomized to either fiber or a nonfiber laxative, fiber laxatives were associated with a 53% reduction in hemorrhoid symptoms, including 50% less bleeding.

Patients should also be encouraged to improve anal hygiene. Excessive scrubbing of the perianal area should be avoided; wiping gently with moist facial or baby wipes and frequent sitz baths can be useful in relieving discomfort and promoting cleanliness. Avoiding foods that can cause diarrhea should also be suggested; similarly, constipating foods and medications should be avoided. Regular toilet regimens must be promoted, and patients should be told not to sit on the commode for prolonged periods of time, not to read on the toilet, and not to defer the urge to defecate. When bleeding is a major component, medications that exaggerate bleeding, such as nonsteroidal antiinflammatory drugs (NSAIDs), should be stopped when possible.

There are multiple over-the-counter topical treatments containing various agents, including local anesthetics, corticosteroids, vasoconstrictors, antiseptics, protectants, and astringents. These mostly help with improving hygiene and alleviating associated pruritus and discomfort; however, no clinical trials have proven efficacy for preventing prolapse or bleeding. Care should be taken with topical corticosteroids; their extended use can thin perianal skin. Purified flavonoids derived from citrus fruit have been shown to stop the bleeding from grade I and II hemorrhoids, but their long-term treatment benefits are not known.

Rubber Band Ligation

Rubber band ligation is a simple and effective procedure for the treatment of hemorrhoids that can be done easily in the office setting. Although rubber band ligation can successfully treat grades I, II, and III internal hemorrhoids, it is best suited for grade I hemorrhoids that are bleeding but with minimal prolapse. External hemorrhoids should not be treated with rubber band ligation because of their somatic innervation.

The procedure is relatively easy to perform (Figure 3). For anxious patients, sedation and anesthesia can improve the exam and results, but it is generally not necessary. For a "one-handed" band delivery, some instruments use suction to pull the hemorrhoidal column into the banding device. If such an instrument is not available, two operators are required: one to maintain the anoscope, the other to hold the grasping and banding device. One or two bands should be delivered around the base just proximal to the internal anal cushion to constrict the blood supply, creating a zone of necrosis. Placing the band promotes an inflammatory response that leads to ulcer formation, tissue scarring, and fixation to the rectal wall. The band is retained for 2 to 10 days.

The procedure is generally well tolerated. Patients will feel a lump with band application, which may cause some discomfort. The amount of discomfort associated increases with the number of hemorrhoids treated per visit. Although multiple hemorrhoids can be treated safely at one time with rubber band ligation, most surgeons will elect to treat one hemorrhoid at a time. If repeat banding is required, it is best performed after 4 weeks, when the inflammation has resolved. Severe pain can result from placing the band too close to the dentate line; these bands should be removed. Usually, moderate discomfort can be relieved with sitz baths, mild analgesics, and avoidance of constipation.

Rubber band ligation has a reported overall complication rate of 0.5% to 8%. Significant complications are rare. The most common immediate problem can be a vasovagal reaction following the procedure. Therefore patients should rise slowly after the procedure and should be monitored with blood pressure checks. For patients who do feel faint, simply having them lie down for a short time will resolve these symptoms.

Although minor bleeding is common after a rubber band ligation, severe bleeding can also happen when the necrotic tissue sloughs off the anal wall. This significant bleeding may even occur 1 to 2 weeks after the procedure. To prevent bleeding complications, aspirin, NSAIDs, and other blood thinners should be adjusted or avoided periprocedure. Patients requiring chronic anticoagulation may be best treated with an alternative approach, such as sclerotherapy. If bleeding does take place, it can be stopped with local epinephrine injection or suture placement. Uncommonly, critical bleeding needs to be tamponaded by placing a large caliber urinary catheter in the rectum and inflating the balloon so that it is tight against the anal ring until definitive operative treatment can be done.

Pelvic sepsis after rubber band ligation has been reported. A total of five deaths, two life-threatening cases of sepsis, and three cases of severe pelvic cellulitis requiring debridement have been recorded. Symptoms from this rare condition include pelvic pain, perineal cellulitis, fever, and urinary retention. Patients with these symptoms need prompt evaluation to diagnose this rare but life-threatening complication.

Rubber band ligation is very effective for treating patients with grade I and II hemorrhoids, with a success rate exceeding 75%. Although other authors have reported success using rubber band ligation for patients with grade III hemorrhoids, in our experience these patients are best treated with operative intervention. Additionally, rubber band ligation is more successful than sclerotherapy for the treatment of hemorrhoids. The complication rate of rubber band ligation is less than hemorrhoidectomy and equivalent to sclerotherapy, making it a well-tolerated procedure. For these reasons, rubber band ligation is our office procedure of choice.

Sclerotherapy

Sclerotherapy is an alternative procedure that can be performed in the office setting. The therapy has been used for centuries and is currently recommended for the treatment of grade I and II internal hemorrhoids. The technique involves the injection of an irritant at the base of the hemorrhoid, eliciting an inflammatory reaction, edema, and intravascular thrombosis, causing eventual scarring. To perform sclerotherapy, an anoscope is passed into the anal canal and distal rectum. The anoscope is subsequently withdrawn until the hemorrhoid and surrounding mucosa prolapse over the opening of the scope. Either of two types of irritants can then be injected: Approximately 1 to 2 mL of an oil-based irritant, either arachis or cottonseed oil containing 5% phenol, is injected with an 18 gauge spinal needle into the hemorrhoid base. Alternatively, 1 to 2 mL of an aqueous irritant, such as ethanolamine oleate (Ethamolin; QOL Medical, Kirkland, Wash.) can be injected with a 25 gauge spinal needle directly into the hemorrhoid. Direct pressure is applied over the site of injection to ensure bleeding cessation.

There are multiple benefits of sclerotherapy. The treatment is easy to perform, inexpensive, and requires little time. Injections can be performed without anesthetic. One to two hemorrhoids can be injected per visit, and patients experience little discomfort associated with the procedure.

Serious complications associated with the procedure are rare (0.02%). A burning, dull pain lasting for up to 48 hours after treatment can occur, especially with repeated injections. During the procedure, the clinician should avoid directly injecting the irritant into the hemorrhoidal vessels, as it has been known to precipitate precordial and upper abdominal pain. If periprostatic parasympathetic nerves are directly injected, the patient can have erectile dysfunction.

Local infections and abscesses rarely occur. A more severe complication, pelvic sepsis, can occur up to 5 days after injection, with

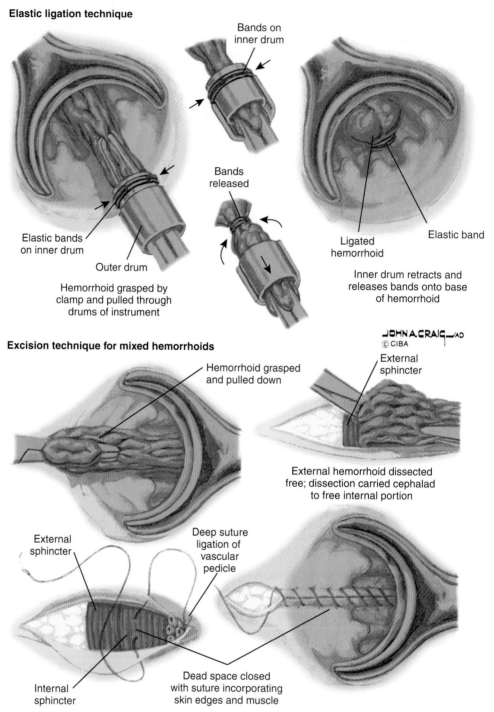

Elastic ligation technique

Bands on inner drum

Elastic bands on inner drum

Outer drum

Hemorrhoid grasped by clamp and pulled through drums of instrument

Bands released

Ligated hemorrhoid

Elastic band

Inner drum retracts and releases bands onto base of hemorrhoid

Excision technique for mixed hemorrhoids

Hemorrhoid grasped and pulled down

External sphincter

External hemorrhoid dissected free; dissection carried cephalad to free internal portion

External sphincter

Deep suture ligation of vascular pedicle

Internal sphincter

Dead space closed with suture incorporating skin edges and muscle

JOHN A. CRAIG _AD
© CIBA

FIGURE 3   Rubber band ligation and closed hemorrhoidectomy.

symptoms of fever; perianal pain, sometimes radiating down the leg; watery discharge; urinary retention; and other signs of sepsis. Although the incidence of pelvic sepsis is rare, its diagnosis requires immediate surgical intervention and broad-spectrum antibiotics. Treated patients should be instructed to contact their treating physician immediately if they experience these symptoms.

Sclerotherapy is also recommended for the treatment of hemorrhoids in immunocompromised patients. Successful treatment of more complicated grade III internal hemorrhoids in AIDS patients has also been reported. Treatment with sclerotherapy avoids potential surgical complications in patients with poor overall general health.

As with other hemorrhoid treatments, patients should be given the appropriate dietary education and instructed to take bulking

agents and sitz baths and to use mild analgesics for relief of procedure-associated discomfort. For grade II hemorrhoids, sclerotherapy improves symptoms for approximately 75% of patients. Generally, hemorrhoid symptoms can be initially controlled with sclerotherapy; however, the treatment is the least durable treatment performed in the office setting.

Other Procedures

Coagulation of hemorrhoidal tissue can be accomplished by applying energy in various forms directly to the effected tissue. The coagulation causes local injury, resulting in the hemorrhoid sloughing off and promoting scarring at the hemorrhoidal base. All of these procedures are performed using a slotted anoscope. Infrared coagulation, the most popular of these techniques, can be used to treat grade I, II, and III internal hemorrhoids. The procedure is fast, can be performed easily, and has few complications.

In coagulation therapy, an infrared light beam produced by a tungsten–halogen lamp is focused on the hemorrhoidal apex at two to four separate sites for 1.5 second pulses. The infrared energy penetrates the hemorrhoidal tissue, causing the temperature to rise to about 100° C, effectively resulting in the boiling of intracellular fluids and tissue destruction. The beam coagulates to a depth of 1 to 3 mm, and destruction of the tissue is highly focal. The procedure feels like a sharp pinprick. Most physicians recommend two to three repeat treatments at 2-week intervals.

Infrared coagulation has a success rate of 67% to 96%, which is similar to rubber band ligation or sclerotherapy for the treatment of grade I and II internal hemorrhoids. Infrared coagulation does not, however, treat substantial prolapsing tissue. Because of decreased pain associated postoperatively with the procedure, some surgeons favor infrared coagulation over rubber band ligation. However, rubber band ligation seems to have better long-term efficacy compared with infrared coagulation.

Bipolar coagulation and direct current electrotherapy are two other procedures that involve energy application directly to the hemorrhoidal tissue. Both procedures are excellent for controlling bleeding but do not treat significant prolapse. Both procedures are well tolerated with the most common postoperative complications being bleeding and pain.

External Hemorrhoid Treatment

External hemorrhoid treatment involves dietary management, avoidance of constipation, and proper anal hygiene with delicate washing, similar to the conservative management of internal hemorrhoids. Resection of exclusively external hemorrhoids is rarely indicated. The treatment of thrombosed external hemorrhoids depends on the associated symptoms. Pain with acute thrombosis worsens within 24 hours and subsides in a few days; it often can be temporarily relieved with sitz baths and mild analgesics. If a patient complains of intolerable pain associated with external hemorrhoid thrombosis, the underlying clot can be removed under local anesthesia, leaving the skin edges to heal by secondary intention.

To prevent recurrence, excision should include the overlying skin and not just incision with enucleation of the clot. Surgical management, if indicated for pain, should occur within the first 24 hours of thrombosis. Otherwise, the cumulative pain associated with external hemorrhoid thrombosis and subsequent surgery is worse than the initial pain. Topical application of 0.3% nifedipine cream can also treat the pain associated with external hemorrhoids through antiinflammatory and smooth muscle–relaxing properties.

Surgical Management

For patients with large grade III or IV internal hemorrhoids, mixed (internal and external) hemorrhoids, large external hemorrhoids, and patients who have failed or could not tolerate office procedures, surgical management is offered.

Preoperative preparation includes stopping anticoagulants prior to the procedure. If patients have any symptoms of incontinence, they should be evaluated using anal manometry and ultrasound to look for sphincter defects. Patients should be prepped with an enema on the morning of operation. Generally, prophylactic antibiotics are not necessary except for those patients considered high risk for bacterial endocarditis by the American Heart Association.

These procedures can be done under general anesthesia, spinal anesthesia, or with local anesthetics and sedation. Patients are placed in either the lithotomy or prone jackknife position. For our practice, prone positioning allows for better visualization and more working area, enabling an assisting surgeon room to participate. The buttocks are taped apart for adequate exposure. If incarcerated prolapsed hemorrhoids are obstructing visualization, attempts should be made for manual reduction. A perianal block with local anesthetic and epinephrine is performed by injecting the four quadrants around the anus, making sure to infiltrate both the superficial submucosa and deep intersphincteric space. A total of 30 mL of 0.25% bupivicaine with epinephrine is recommended for the perianal block.

Surgical Hemorrhoidectomy

Ferguson first developed the closed hemorrhoidectomy in 1952. The procedure can be done as an outpatient and can be used to excise one to three hemorrhoids. The anal canal is exposed with an anal retractor, and the hemorrhoid is grasped and retracted using a hemostat. Care should be taken not to excessively retract the anal canal, which may cause more pain and also risks injury to the anal sphincter.

An elliptical incision using electrocautery or sharp dissection is made around the hemorrhoidal complex (see Figure 3). Excision can also be performed using the LigaSure (Valleylab, Boulder, Colo.) or harmonic scalpel (Johnson and Johnson Gateway, Piscataway, NJ). A hemostat or 3-0 Vicryl suture can be placed at the pedicle site to control potential bleeding from the contained vascular complex.

For surgical hemorrhoidectomies, adequate bridges of normal anoderm should be left for healing. If not, wound healing can lead to stricture formation and anal stenosis. The hemorrhoid is then dissected off the underlying internal sphincter muscles, which should be visualized. To prevent sphincter injury and incontinence, the surgeon needs to correctly identify the proper dissection planes. The wound is finally closed with a 3-0 chromic running suture extending out to the anoderm.

Most commonly the incisions are closed. However, if gangrenous hemorrhoids are being excised, or if other signs of infection are present, the incision can be left open. This open hemorrhoidectomy is also known as the *Milligan-Morgan procedure*. However, closing the wounds is more hemostatic and is our preferred technique. Hemostasis can also be achieved with electrocautery and suture ligation.

Postoperatively, minor bleeding, drainage, and pain are to be expected. However, serious complications for both closed and open hemorrhoidectomies are rare. The most serious complications are anal incontinence, anal stenosis, and significant bleeding. These complications are best avoided by careful technique and attention to dissection planes. To avoid stenosis, always begin with the largest hemorrhoid, and be careful to leave at least 1 cm of normal anoderm between suture lines. If there is a concern about causing an anal stenosis, it is better to leave residual hemorrhoidal tissue than to risk this dreaded complication. Passing clots is a sign of significant hemorrhage and requires prompt evaluation. The bleeding occurs at the wound edges or at the remaining vascular pedicle and frequently occurs late, up to 1 to 2 weeks after the procedure. Anal examination with anesthesia might be needed for adequate visualization and treatment. The reported rate of serious hemorrhage in one study of patients undergoing surgical hemorrhoidectomy was 0.9%.

The most common minor complication is urinary retention. To minimize this risk, intravenous fluids should be limited during these short procedures. Patients should be instructed to void before discharge. If patients do have difficulty voiding, they can be instructed to soak in a warm bath, which may relieve some of the discomfort and promote voiding. However, for persistent urinary retention, a urinary catheter should be placed. These symptoms nearly always resolve once the postoperative swelling subsides.

Postoperative care should include analgesics and sitz baths for 20 minutes or more, several times per day. Nonsteroidal medications can be very helpful. Constipation must be avoided in this postoperative period, and normal bowel habits should be encouraged. If patients fail to move their bowels within the first 48 hours, a gentle laxative may be used to help prevent fecal impaction, which is very painful.

Patients should also be told to expect sutures to loosen with the first bowel movement.

Procedure for Prolapsing Hemorrhoids

The procedure for prolapsing hemorrhoids (PPH) was first described by Longo in 1998, proposed as an alternative to conventional surgical hemorrhoidectomy. Although this procedure is also known as the *stapled hemorrhoidectomy,* the name is actually a misnomer because the hemorrhoidal tissue is not removed. *Hemorrhoidopexy* is a more accurate name for this procedure. The PPH can be done quickly in the outpatient setting with any range of anesthesia. Another benefit is that the procedure allows for the single treatment of multiple large internal hemorrhoids. Since no hemorrhoidal tissue is resected, this procedure is best suited for patients with large internal hemorrhoids with a minimal external component. The procedure requires an extensive knowledge of the anatomy and experience with a specialized stapler. Therefore an international task force has established guidelines for surgeons to practice the PPH, and only those who have undergone formal training should attempt the procedure.

The PPH utilizes a special 33 mm circular stapler to resect a ring of distal rectal mucosa and submucosa proximal to the hemorrhoid. By resecting this tissue, the redundant tissue of the hemorrhoid is pulled proximally and subsequently fixed to the rectal wall. The resection also interrupts the blood supply feeding the hemorrhoid, decreasing hemorrhoidal engorgement.

To start, the patient is placed prone in jackknife position. An operating anoscope is inserted into the rectum for visualization (Figure 4). A circumferential purse-string suture is placed in the mucosa and submucosa approximately 2 to 4 cm proximal to the dentate line, above the apex of the hemorrhoid. Great care should be taken placing this suture, as it determines the procedure outcome. The great distance above the dentate line prevents any involvement of areas with somatic innervation. Each bite of the purse-string suture should be placed at the same circumferential level, without large gaps in between.

The stapler is introduced transanally, and the purse-string suture is tied around the shaft, drawing the redundant tissue into the jaws of the stapler. In female patients, prior to firing the stapler, the surgeon should ensure no purse-string suture involvement of the vaginal septum by palpating the common wall between the rectum and the vagina. The stapler is then fired, and the circumferential band of rectal mucosa proximal to the hemorrhoid is removed, pulling the hemorrhoids upward. The surgeon should pay meticulous attention to the staple line to ensure hemostasis, because bleeding at the staple line is not uncommon. Bleeding vessels should be oversewn. The result of PPH is shown in (Figure 5).

As with other hemorrhoidal procedures, minor complications including discharge, minimal bleeding, discomfort, and urinary retention. In a retrospective review of 3711 patients who underwent the PPH, 12.3% experienced these minor complications. Pain in particular can occur if the staple line is placed too far distally. Thrombosis of residual hemorrhoidal tissue can also lead to pain.

If the purse-string suture is too deep, the PPH can inadvertently remove some smooth muscle with the mucosa. Therefore to prevent sphincter injury, great care must be taken to ensure that the staple line is within the distal rectum and not in the anal canal. When this is done, the procedure rarely causes incontinence. Nonetheless, patients with known sphincter dysfunction should not be treated with this procedure. Other serious complications include secondary hemorrhage, rectal perforation, retropneumoperitoneum, rectovaginal fistula, anastomotic dehiscence, and retroperitoneal and pelvic sepsis. Fortunately, in the hands of trained surgeons, these complications are rare; however, although rare, these serious complications are probably more common with the PPH than with surgical hemorrhoidectomy.

The PPH does provide a treatment option for hemorrhoids that has less severe postoperative pain and shorter recovery time as compared with surgical hemorrhoidectomy. In a meta-analysis of 10 randomized controlled studies comparing the PPH to conventional surgical hemorrhoidectomy for the treatment of grade III and IV internal hemorrhoids, patients undergoing the PPH had significantly shorter hospital stays, less pain, and a decreased need for postoperative analgesia. However, a Cochrane review of seven trials and 537 patients showed that the PPH is associated with a higher rate of hemorrhoid recurrence compared with conventional surgery (odds ratio, 3.85; confidence interval, 1.47 to 10.07; $P = .006$). Therefore, although excellent outcomes with minimal postoperative pain can be achieved with the PPH, the traditional surgical hemorrhoidectomy remains the gold standard with regard to preventing hemorrhoid recurrence.

New Techniques

Hemorrhoidal artery ligation (HAL) is a new technique that entails ligation of the terminal branches of the superior rectal artery. By ligating these feeding vessels, hemorrhoidal engorgement is diminished, reducing the symptoms of the hemorrhoids. This new technique utilizes a special proctoscope with a Doppler transducer to indentify and ligate feeding arteries.

For the procedure, patients are placed in lithotomy or prone position and are either given spinal or local anesthesia with sedation.

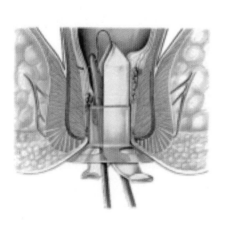
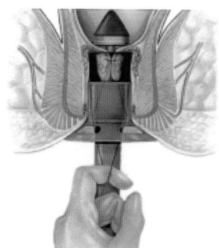
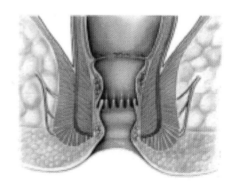

FIGURE 4   Procedure for prolapsing hemorrhoids (PPH).

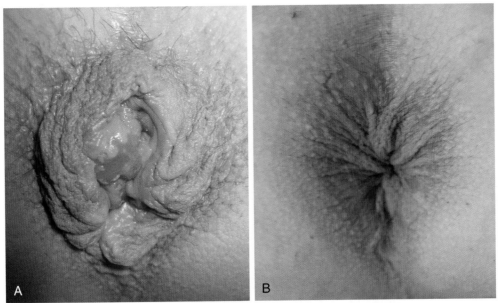

FIGURE 5   **A,** Prolapsing internal hemorrhoids. **B,** Appearance following PPH.

A perineal block is performed. The special proctoscope is introduced transanally, and intraluminal arteries are located approximately 2 cm proximal to the dentate line. An average of six arteries can be located and ligated using the lateral ligation window of the proctoscope. Ligation of the arteries is performed using a 2-0 synthetic braided suture. Topical anesthesia with a xylocaine gel–covered sponge placed in the anal canal can minimize postoperative discomfort. The complications experienced are minimal and are similar to the PPH. In addition, HAL can be used in combination with rectoanal repair (RAR), which is a transanal rectomucopexy performed to lift and secure the prolapsed hemorrhoid back into a normal anatomic position. The combination of the two procedures in a small prospective single-center study showed a 12 month prolapse recurrence rate of 11%.

SUMMARY

Hemorrhoids are a common anorectal condition in aging adults. The most common complaint is bleeding. Despite the finding of hemorrhoids on exam, patients with bleeding who are at risk for carcinoma and lack colorectal screening require a more extensive workup to rule out a more concerning pathology.

Conservative management with dietary changes and adjustments in bowel regimen usually can improve symptoms associated with small, less severe hemorrhoids. Several procedures exist that do not require surgery and can be performed in the office setting for treating hemorrhoids that do not respond to conservative measures. These procedures have similar complications and outcomes. For these reasons many surgeons will adopt one preferred procedure to be used in their office.

Additionally, many strategies for the surgical treatment of severe hemorrhoids have been developed. The treatment plan should be tailored to the severity and grade of the hemorrhoids and to the patient's wishes. Our practice generally incorporates a combination of conservative treatment, rubber band ligation for less severe hemorrhoids, and either closed hemorrhoidectomy or the PPH for those hemorrhoids requiring surgical management. We discuss with our patients undergoing surgery the tradeoff between less pain but more recurrence with the PPH when compared with a closed hemorrhoidectomy, and then we tailor the treatment to patient concerns.

SUGGESTED READINGS

Alonso-Coello P, Guyatt GH, Heels-Ansdell D, et al: Laxatives for the treatment of hemorrhoids, *Cochrane Rev* (4):CD004649, 2005.

Jayaraman S, Colquhoun PH, Malthaner R: Stapled versus conventional surgery for hemorrhoids, *Cochrane Rev* (4):CD005393, 2006.

Kaidar-Person O: Hemorrhoidal disease: a comprehensive review, *J Am Coll Surg* 204(1):102–117, 2007.

Nienhuijs SW, de Hingh IHJT: Conventional versus LigaSure hemorrhoidectomy for patients with symptomatic hemorrhoids, *Cochrane Rev* (1):CD006761, 2009.

Scheyer M, Antonietti E, Rollinger G, et al: Doppler-guided hemorrhoidal artery ligation, *Am J Surg* 191(1):89-93, 2006.

Anal Fissure

Cybil Corning, MD, and Eric G. Weiss, MD

DEFINITION

An *anal fissure* is a painful linear tear in the skin or anoderm overlying the internal anal sphincter distal to the dentate line. Fissures may be classified as *acute* or *chronic* depending on their time course and associated findings. Although the distinction is not always entirely clear based on the physical exam, determining the chronicity of the fissure may guide your treatment algorithm.

Acute anal fissures, as the name implies, are typically present for less than 6 to 8 weeks. In addition, they do not have the associated findings of an external skin tag, or "sentinel pile," or a hypertrophied anal papilla. More than 90% of fissures are found in the posterior midline, although they can be found in conjunction with anterior midline fissure or solely in the anterior midline in a small percentage of patients (10%). Anterior anal fissures are seen in women more frequently than in men, but in general, anal fissures affect males and females with equal distribution. Typically, this is a condition of young adults, but it may be found in patients of all ages. Fissures identified in positions other than the anterior or posterior midline should arouse suspicions of other underlying conditions, including Crohn's disease, ulcerative colitis, syphilis, tuberculosis, leukemia, cancer, and HIV infection.

ETIOLOGY

There are many theories as to the etiology of anal fissure. Although passage of a hard stool that causes trauma and disruption of the anoderm is believed to be the most common initiating event, constipation is not present in all patients. Diarrhea with associated multiple bowel movements can also cause trauma to the anal canal, leading to a fissure. Occasionally, other forms of trauma from digital rectal examination, endoscopy, or anoreceptive intercourse can be the inciting event.

The most widely agreed upon factor contributing to anal fissure and persistence of anal fissure is increased resting anal pressure and the sequelae of this state. Many physiologic studies have confirmed the presence of resting hypertonia in the internal anal sphincter in the great majority of patients with anal fissure. Treatment of this condition is frequently targeted at decreasing this elevated resting pressure, also known as *mean anal resting pressure* (MARP). Abcarian and colleagues (1982), based on the work of Nothmann and Schuster, found that 90% of patients with anal fissure had findings of high MARP and an overshoot phenomenon, demonstrated on anal manometry with a lower threshold for stimulation of overshoot in these patients. They suggest that this overshoot phenomenon, or spasm of the sphincter mechanism, is responsible for the difficulty in healing anal fissures. Furthermore, sphincterotomy contributes to fissure healing, because it widens the anal canal, resulting in decreased stretching of the anoderm, subsequently triggering the overshoot; this is in addition to decreasing resting pressure, which is further described later.

Other studies have investigated anodermal blood flow in animal and cadaveric experiments. Klosterhalfen (1988), demonstrated the vascular anatomy of the rectum and anus with angiography. There is consistently a vessel-deficient area in the posterior midline. This work has given credence to the theory that anal fissures have poor healing in part related to decreased blood flow in this area. Consequently, improvement in blood flow has been demonstrated in patients with documented decreases in the resting hypertonia, which

has been ultimately associated with healing of the fissure. Other theories explore the anatomy of the anal canal; some attribute decreased support or adherence of the anal mucosa to the underlying structure of the external anal sphincter, predisposing it to shear injury and contributing to difficult healing.

Dietary factors also play a role in fissure-in-ano. The risk for development of anal fissure is decreased in patients who consume a high-fiber diet with a large amount of raw fruits, vegetables, and whole grains. This is an important modifiable factor in conservative treatment of this disease and is combined with all forms of intervention. According to some sources, patients are at higher risk if they consume white bread, roux sauces, bacon, and sausage. Notably, consumption of coffee, tea, and alcohol has not been associated with increased risk despite the common assumption that these exacerbate anal fissure.

SYMPTOMS

Characteristically, patients will report a very sharp pain provoked with defecation that frequently lasts for minutes to hours after defecation. This is the most common symptom identified. In addition, rectal bleeding associated with defecation is seen in many of these patients. Patients will note bright red blood, most often on the toilet tissue, but it can also be seen in the toilet bowl. It is not, however, uniformly present.

The anxiety about the pain caused by the passage of stool can lead to constipation and fecal impaction. Pain with defecation may lead to spasm of the sphincter mechanism, contributing to the hypertonicity of the anal canal and exacerbating the symptoms in a vicious cycle.

Other symptoms may occur with fissure-in-ano, including mucous anal discharge, urinary retention, and dyspareunia. These are less frequent than the cardinal symptoms of pain and bleeding.

PHYSICAL EXAM

The diagnosis of an acute anal fissure can almost entirely be made based on the patient's history. The story is often so characteristic that our clinic nurses have diagnosed these patients before finishing their intake and abbreviated history. All that is often required on the physical exam is gentle retraction of the buttocks with or without retracting the anal skin to see a linear tear in the anoderm. It is unnecessary, rarely tolerated, and very painful to continue with the exam if the diagnosis is confirmed on inspection.

Care must be taken, however, if no fissure is actually identified to ensure that the patient does not have perianal sepsis. It is possible in patients without an external or overt manifestation of an abscess, such as an intersphincteric postanal space or submucosal abscess, to have a similar presentation. In these situations an examination under anesthesia or anal ultrasound, which may be tolerated, is mandatory to rule out these abscesses.

In a chronic anal fissure, two other physical findings may be identified. Proximally in the anal canal, a hypertrophied anal papilla can be seen; distally, on the perianal skin, patients will frequently have an associated sentinel pile or tag. This is an area of heaped-up anoderm. Additionally, in a chronic fissure, anoscopic exam is usually better tolerated. In this scenario, fibers of the sphincter muscle may be clearly identified at the base of the ulcer.

TREATMENT

The treatment of anal fissure can be either medical or surgical in nature. Depending on the chronicity of the fissure and etiology, some measures may be more efficacious than others.

Nonsurgical treatment of anal fissures initially may consist of conservative measures, including stool softeners, bulking agents, sitz baths, and local anesthetic ointment with or without a topical steroid, based on preference. This is termed "best supportive care" in studies, when compared with other medical and surgical therapies, and would include dietary manipulations to decrease anorectal trauma with passage of a hard stool. Fiber agents titrated to desired consistency of soft but formed with at least one bowel movement daily can be recommended. There is not one "gold standard" recipe, but Jensen (1987) demonstrated fewer recurrences of anal fissure with patients receiving 5 g of unprocessed bran three times daily when compared to placebo or 2.5 g of bran three times daily. Stool softeners such as docusate, MiraLax, or other nonstimulants may also achieve this goal with few long-term side effects. Sitz baths should be taken in a tub of warm water twice daily. This is most effective if performed once after defecation and once before bedtime. These maneuvers can be tried for up to 4 weeks, reasonably, followed by repeat examination. This approach will be most effective in a patient with a very new fissure; if symptoms do not resolve fairly expediently, it may be necessary to escalate treatment.

Although many pharmacologic treatments have been tried with varying degrees of success, a Cochrane analysis of nonsurgical treatment published in 2009, in addition to several other meta-analyses, have fairly consistently found that certain medical therapies can be applied with a high chance of cure. The actual efficacy varies, however, and only nitroglycerin ointment, calcium channel blockers, and botulinum toxin were significantly better than placebo in a comparison of multiple randomized controlled trials. Although each of these agents works somewhat differently, the effect of the chemical sphincterotomy is essentially the same, with relaxation of the internal anal sphincter (IAS) the goal. Detailed discussion of medical management of fissure-in-ano in this chapter is limited to these agents; however, other medications found in the literature include L-arginine, alpha-blockers, phosphodiesterase inhibitors, potassium channel openers, oral or transdermal nitroglycerin, and oral calcium channel blockers.

Nitroglycerin ointment, or glyceryl trinitrate (GTN), has been studied extensively in the treatment of anal fissure. The organic nitrate compound has been demonstrated to be the main chemical neurotransmitter in the neurons mediating relaxation of the IAS. When applied to the anal mucosa, GTN works by diffusion across the mucosa, binding to cellular receptors and releasing nitric oxide. This, in turn, allows relaxation of the IAS and thus improves anodermal blood flow via vasodilation, with reduction in mean resting anal pressure. When compared with placebo, efficacy was significantly better (48.6% vs. 37%), but almost 50% percent of those initially cured had recurrence. The most common side effect is headache, which does limit its use. The best results with fewest side effects were found with 0.2% to 0.4% ointment applied to the anal skin three times daily. One study found that the presence of a sentinel pile, an indicator of chronic anal fissure, predicted failure of treatment with GTN.

Patients should begin to notice an improvement in symptoms in several days to a week. Full results may not be achieved for 4 to 6 weeks. In those patients with resolution of pain but persistent fissure on exam, it is appropriate to continue topical GTN for an additional 4 to 6 weeks followed by reexamination. Most of these patients will see resolution of the fissure by the next exam. Calcium channel blockers, such as nifedipine and diltiazem, offer an alternative in topical treatment of anal fissure. They have been shown to cause a decrease in maximum anal resting pressure by antagonizing smooth muscle contraction of the IAS. Calcium channel blockers were found to be equivalent in efficacy to GTN in the same Cochrane review, with fewer associated side effects, particularly a lack of headaches. One noted side effect was anal itching; for this we prescribe diltiazem 2% ointment applied three times daily. Because of the relatively mild side-effect profile and our institution's success with this treatment, this is typically our first-line therapy in addition to the nonpharmacologic adjuncts.

It is important to note that both topical calcium channel blockers and nitroglycerin require a compounding pharmacy. Diltiazem powder can be combined with either a petroleum base to make an ointment or a cream base. Nitroglycerin powder is only compounded with a petroleum base. Patients will need to be educated in regard to where they can purchase the ointment, and the physician should also be wary of inadvertently applying nitroglycerin at a higher percentage (e.g., 2%), which will significantly increase side effects without increasing the likelihood of desired effect.

Botulinum toxin A (Botox) is an additional method of chemical sphincterotomy. Also fairly well studied, Botox has been found to be equivalent to the pharmacologic agents previously mentioned, approaching 50% initial healing rates. It is an appealing method of chemical sphincterotomy for several reasons: Once injected, the effects of the botox injection on the IAS may last up to 3 months. This requires minimal additional effort by patients. Botox may be a good option in patients for whom continence is a particular concern. Although incontinence is a potential side effect, this complication is self-limited, and patients will return to their prior level of continence once the effect of the toxin resolves. Overall, patients report fewer side effects than with GTN ointment. A 100 unit vial of toxin is diluted with 2 mL of normal saline. Then, 20 to 40 units of toxin are injected into the IAS on either side of the fissure (Figure 1).

Surgical Treatment

Anal fissure has been recognized and treated by surgical means for many years. Sphincter stretching was initially reported as a method of treatment, and many variations of the technique have been described, including the use of digital traction, anal dilators, and balloon dilators. Each of these methods works by disrupting the sphincter mechanism to some degree. Proponents of sphincter stretching believe that if it is done in a cautious and controlled manner, incontinence is rare, there are no incisions, and patients have quick relief from complaints and rapidly return to routine activities. Critics of this form of treatment cite reports about uncontrolled trauma to both the inter-

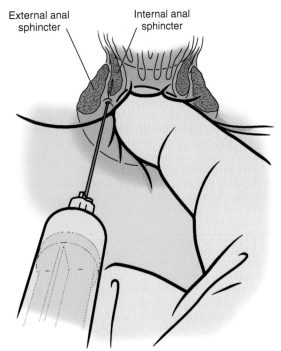

FIGURE 1   The internal anal sphincter is palpated and identified with the nondominant hand, facilitating Botox injection directly into the muscle.

nal and external anal sphincters, as seen on ultrasonography, and a historically high rate of incontinence.

Pneumatic balloon dilation (PBD) has gained renewed interest recently. Studies by Renzi and colleagues in Italy have shown good results. A lubricated 40 mm or 60 mm long anal balloon is inserted into the anal canal and positioned with 10 mm protruding from the anus. The balloon is then rapidly inflated to 20 psi, maintained for 6 minutes, then deflated and removed. When compared to lateral internal sphincterotomy (LIS, discussed below) healing rates were 92% versus 83%. Only one patient in that population of 65 had recurrence, and it was in the LIS group. Incontinence was reported in 0% in the PBD group and in 16% in the LIS group. Other researchers have also demonstrated a relatively low rate of incontinence, about 4% to 24%.

Sphincter stretching as a surgical technique has been largely supplanted by LIS; with healing rates reported as high as 95% for chronic anal fissures, none of the aforementioned treatments is as effective as LIS. There are several techniques for dividing the lateral internal sphincter, but it is recognized that lateral sphincterotomy is associated with the fewest incidences of incontinence, flatus, or seepage when compared with posterior sphincterotomy with associated keyhole deformity. Recurrence rates are also comparatively low, at 5% or less. Incontinence is considered the major risk, and the rates in the literature vary from less than 1% to 30% or higher, but quality and technique vary widely in these studies.

Technique

LIS can be performed under general, regional, or local anesthesia. The patient is positioned according to the surgeon's preference, in prone jackknife, lithotomy, or lateral decubitus position. Using a Pratt bivalve retractor, the IAS is stretched. Using either an open technique or a closed technique, the IAS is divided proximally to the level of the dentate line. In the open technique, a radial incision is made at the intersphincteric groove to the dentate line to expose the fibers of the IAS, which are then divided with Metzenbaum scissors under direct visualization (Figure 2).

The incision may be closed or left open, but the closed technique also requires placing the IAS on stretch and inserting a number 11 scalpel in the intersphincteric groove, parallel to the muscle, to the level of the dentate, and then turning the blade into the lumen, thus dividing the sphincter (Figure 3). Alternatively, a small incision may be made in the mucosa, and the straight-bladed scalpel is placed in the submucosal plane; the blade is then away from the lumen, toward the external anal sphincter, and the IAS is divided that way.

The surgeon must be careful to avoid injury to the external sphincter. Numerous reports of postoperative incontinence have been associated with inadvertent division of the external anal sphincter. Hemostasis is achieved with pressure, and the minimal incision is left open to allow drainage. Postoperatively the patient continues the fiber supplementation with daily intake of 15 to 25 g of fiber, divided twice or three times daily, and takes sitz baths with warm water for 10 minutes after defecation and before bedtime. At the time of operation, it is safe to surgically address a large sentinel pile or hemorrhoids, if necessary. Division of the sphincter on the left or right side is essentially a matter of surgeon preference.

Historically, sphincterotomies were performed in the posterior midline to avoid an additional break in the anal mucosa. These patients frequently developed what is known as a *keyhole deformity*. Because the divided sphincter in this location leaves the patient with a persistent deep groove, this interferes with complete closure of the sphincter at rest, and patients may have associated seepage or soiling. In 1967, Dr. Parks suggested lateral placement of the sphincterotomy, and this became popularized in 1989 by Notars and has since been adopted by most colorectal surgeons. Sphincterotomy may be performed on the right or left side, however, the right side is preferred, to perform the sphincterotomy between the two

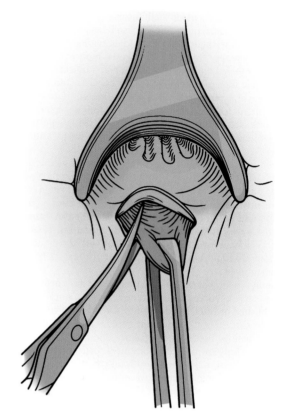

FIGURE 2 The internal sphincter is grasped with an Allis clamp, pulled partially through the wound, and transected for 4 to 5 mm.

hemorrhoidal columns on the right rather than at the base of the left lateral hemorrhoid.

Other surgical procedures for chronic anal fissure include fissurectomy with various advancement flaps. These procedures are ideal for patients without demonstrated hypertonia in the IAS (maximum resting pressure <85) on manometry. The concomitant finding of a subcutaneous fistula tract in some patients with anal fissure can interfere with surgical healing. For these patients, too, fissurectomy and flap may be of benefit.

Fissurectomy requires a U-shaped midline incision at the site of the fissure and dissection of the IAS to free it from the skin and mucosa. The fissure and associated pile or papilla, if present, is excised, and a superficial midline sphincterotomy is then performed to the dentate line. The mucosa is then reapproximated with absorbable suture if easily performed; or, if required, local or rotational flaps are raised in the anal skin, and then the fissurectomy site is closed.

Long-Term Results

Although the rate of incontinence varies widely in the literature, it is likely that true permanent incontinence occurs in 1% or fewer patients; depending on the definition of incontinence used and the depth of questioning, this rate may vary. Most commonly, incontinence is transient and occurs as gas incontinence alone. When meticulous technique is employed in identification of the internal sphincter, this complication is minimized. Julio Garcia-Aguilar and colleagues (1996) have demonstrated a correlation between length of sphincterotomy and incontinence. To some extent, they recognized that the method of sphincterotomy also contributed to development of incontinence and found that open techniques had more extensive sphincterotomies with higher resultant rates of incontinence.

Recurrence can occur in the long or short term. If a repeat trial of the conservative measures noted above fail and surgical intervention is entertained, the surgeon must consider the previous operations

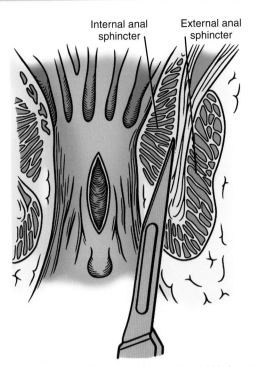

Internal anal sphincter   External anal sphincter

FIGURE 3 For closed sphincterotomy, a number 11 blade is inserted into the intersphincteric groove, and the distal 4 to 5 mm of the internal sphincter are transected. A finger within the anal canal is used to judge the extent of the transection and to avoid mucosal injury.

and history of obstetric trauma and revisit the patient's medical history. Investigation for Crohn's disease and anal ultrasound to evaluate the sphincter structure should be performed. On endoanal ultrasound (EAUS), initial sphincterotomy is identified to be inadequate, either because it only involved the superficial IAS, or it did not extend

proximally to the dentate or beyond the area of hypertonia. In these situations, a repeat LIS should carry little additional risk of incontinence than the original procedure. However, in cases where the IAS has clearly been divided as demonstrated either on EAUS or on manometry, repeat procedures to the IAS carry a much higher risk of incontinence and should be avoided.

Follow-up

It is important to reevaluate patients after resolution of symptoms, especially those with acute anal fissure. Physical examination is initially limited by patient discomfort; however, on follow-up it is necessary to properly evaluate the patient for other abnormalities. For example, a patient with initial complaints of bleeding and pain may have resolution of pain after treatment of anal fissure, but colonoscopy should be considered to rule out other sources of bleeding, particularly in older patients and in those with family history of colorectal pathology. Anoscopy and proctoscopy should be performed in patients with atypical fissures when Crohn's disease or other infectious etiologies are entertained. Additional follow-up testing should be based on risk factors.

SELECTED READINGS

Gordon PH, Nivatvongs S: *Principles and practice of surgery for the colon, rectum, and anus*, ed 3, London, 2007, Informa Healthcare.
Nelson RL: Nonsurgical therapy for anal fissure, *Cochrane Rev* (4):CD003431, 2006.
Nelson RL: Operative procedures for fissure in ano, *Cochrane Rev* (1):CD002199, 2010.
Wolff BG, Fleshman JW, Beck DE, et al: *The ASCRS textbook of colon and rectal surgery*, Philadelphia, 2006, Springer.

ANORECTAL ABSCESS AND FISTULA

Scott R. Steele, MD, Eric K. Johnson, MD, and David N. Armstrong, MD

INTRODUCTION

Anorectal abscess is a debilitating condition originating from a cryptoglandular infection in the anal canal in about 90% of patients, and it remains one of the more common anorectal conditions encountered in general surgical practice. In approximately 50% of patients, a fistula-in-ano subsequently develops, which usually requires surgical correction to prevent recurrent abscess and address symptoms. Without definitive closure of the fistula tract, patients experience persistent purulent drainage, intermittent perianal swelling and tenderness, followed by spontaneous discharge. In 1976, Parks and colleagues categorized fistulas based on their anatomical course relative to the sphincter complex (Figure 1): *intersphincteric, transsphincteric, suprasphincteric,* and *extrasphincteric.*

Fistulas may also be classified as *simple* or *complex*. Simple fistulas include intersphincteric and low transsphincteric tracts. Complex fistulas encompass high transsphincteric fistulas, suprasphincteric and extrasphincteric fistulas, multitract fistulas, fistulas with blind extensions, horseshoe fistulas, and fistulas associated with inflammatory bowel disease, radiation, or malignancy. Given the attenuated nature of the anterior sphincter complex in women, fistulas in this location may also be considered complex.

Several new surgical modalities have been introduced in recent years for the treatment of complex anorectal fistula: the anal fistula plug (AFP); the button plug, or Rectovaginal Plug (RVP; Cook Surgical, Bloomington, Ind.), and the ligation of the intersphincteric fistula tract (LIFT) procedure. This new generation of procedures emphasizes an important principle of sphincter-sparing techniques in anorectal fistula surgery and seeks to minimize injury to the anal sphincter mechanism. The principles of each of these new surgical modalities recognizes that fistula-in-ano is a simple hydrostatic system, wherein the primary opening is the high-pressure source of fluid passing through a conduit, the fistula, to the low-pressure opening, the secondary opening in the perianal skin. When these simple and logical engineering principles are applied to fistula surgery, new surgical modalities and devices evolve to treat fistula-in-ano without the disfiguring, painful, and morbid surgeries of the past. These new modalities are addressed in this chapter.

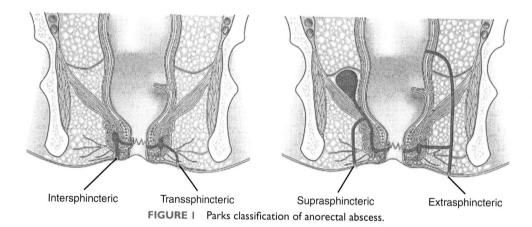

Intersphincteric   Transsphincteric   Suprasphincteric   Extrasphincteric

FIGURE 1   Parks classification of anorectal abscess.

ANORECTAL ABSCESS

The vast majority of anorectal abscess are cryptoglandular in origin; however, they may also result from Crohn's disease, trauma, or iatrogenic causes (e.g., proctectomy, ileal pouch). Regardless of the source, these abscesses are classified based on location into *perianal, ischiorectal, intersphincteric,* and *supralevator* (see Figure 1). In addition, abscesses originating in the deep postanal space may extend to the ischiorectal fossa unilaterally (hemihorseshoe) or bilaterally (horseshoe abscess). Depending on the location and size of the abscess, patients may complain of a variety of symptoms, ranging from local pain, tenderness, and a fluctuant mass (perianal and ischiorectal abscess) to normal external findings with deep-seated rectal pain (intersphincteric abscess) or even abdominal pain (supralevator abscess).

INITIAL EVALUATION

The diagnosis of anorectal abscess is most often made based on the patient's history and physical examination. However, it is important to distinguish anorectal abscess from other perianal suppurative processes such as *hidradenitis suppurativa,* low pilonidal abscess, or infected sebaceous cyst. In addition, the presence of large "elephant ear" skin tags or multiple fistulas suggesting Crohn's disease should be noted because this may require a more detailed workup and conservative surgical approach.

Perianal and ischiorectal abscesses almost always present as a characteristic tender, fluctuant mass; patients with intersphincteric or supralevator abscesses may have a paucity of external findings, with only pelvic or rectal tenderness or fluctuance on digital rectal examination. Careful inspection may reveal other clues: a prior surgical drainage site or an old fistulotomy scar. Palpation of the perianal area and gentle digital rectal examination may reveal the subtle "fullness" of an intersphincteric abscess or the distinctive "boggy" feel of a supralevator abscess.

In the setting of an acute abscess, anoscopy and sigmoidoscopy should be deferred. Presence of cellulitis or fasciitis should be noted and should trigger a more aggressive surgical approach combined with antibiotic therapy. In general, laboratory evaluation adds little useful information but may be useful in patients with complex comorbidities such as diabetes, HIV, or other immunosuppressive diseases, where it can be used to monitor resolution of sepsis and confirm adequate systemic response to surgical drainage.

IMAGING STUDIES

Although anorectal abscesses are most commonly diagnosed based on clinical findings, adjunctive radiologic studies can occasionally provide valuable information in certain situations. Pelvic computed tomography (CT) scan or magnetic resonance imaging can be helpful in identifying occult abscesses such as supralevator, deep postanal

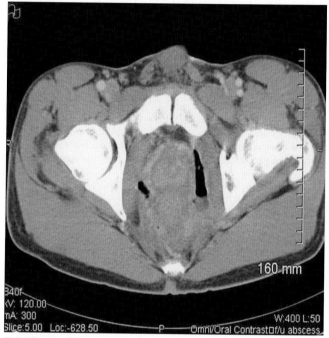

FIGURE 2   CT demonstrating deep postanal space infection with horseshoe extension.

space, and deep ischiorectal or intersphincteric abscess. Another useful role for pelvic CT is in the morbidly obese; identifying deep anorectal abscess may be extremely difficult in this population, and pelvic CT can prove to be an invaluable aid to directing surgical drainage (Figure 2).

TREATMENT

Operative Management

As with any abscess, the mainstay of treatment of anorectal abscesses is adequate surgical drainage. In general, most perianal abscesses can be safely drained in the outpatient setting under local anesthesia (0.25% Marcaine with 1:200,000 epinephrine). Care should be taken to make the incision with the goal of ensuring adequate drainage; we use a cruciate incision of generous proportions over the point of maximum fluctuance. If tolerated, gentle exploration of the cavity breaks up loculi of pus and ensures adequate dimensions of the opening. Packing is an individual decision: Our preference is surgical drainage, followed by several days of frequent soaks or sitz baths to irrigate the cavity and prevent premature closing. With adequate initial drainage, surgical packing is usually not required, but it can be useful to assist in hemostasis or to prevent premature closing in a deep abscess cavity.

If the abscess is deep seated or difficult to locate, or if the patient is anxious or obese, incision and drainage are best performed under anesthesia; this provides more adequate drainage of the abscess cavity and permits insertion of a draining seton if the primary opening can be identified.

The majority of intersphincteric abscesses may be safely drained into the rectum by performing an internal sphincterotomy over the cavity itself. Supralevator abscesses generally arise from an intrabdominal source such as perforated diverticulitis, and CT drainage by interventional radiology is the preferred technique. Concomitant treatment of the source (usually diverticulitis) is obviously also important.

Horseshoe Abscess

Deep postanal space and horseshoe or hemihorseshoe abscesses require special attention. In this case, the crypt of origin is located in the posterior midline, and the resulting abscess is located in the deep postanal space and may extend laterally into one or both ischiorectal fossae. Due to the complex anatomy of the deep postanal space and horseshoe abscess, a surgically conservative approach is best. These patients have frequently had multiple prior surgeries, and there is significant potential for anorectal incontinence.

The initial drainage procedure involves drainage of the deep postanal space abscess. This is best performed by making a small incision between the tip of the coccyx and the anal verge and gently separating the fibers of the external sphincter using a pair of hemostats, working progressively toward the deep postanal space. Having found the abscess, the hemostats are gently passed through the posterior midline (12 o'clock position) primary opening, and a draining seton (vessel-loop) is tied loosely around the posterior sphincter mechanism. Lateral counterdrains are inserted into each lateral ischiorectal extension and tied loosely. By performing this procedure, the source of the abscess (primary opening), the deep postanal space, and the lateral extensions are drained without compromising the sphincter mechanism. After 6 to 8 weeks of drainage, the horseshoe fistula is then addressed with a modified Hanley procedure, AFP, or alternative technique.

Antibiotics

The first principle in treating anorectal sepsis is drainage of the underlying abscess. Antibiotics may be useful in some scenarios, such as with cellulites or fasciitis and in patients with complex comorbidities, underlying immunosuppression, systemic symptoms, or failure to improve after drainage. Antibiotics are the primary treatment modality in patients with profound immunosuppression (neutrophil counts <500 to 1000/mm³) and a lack of fluctuance on examination. Finally, guidelines from the American Heart Association (AHA) recommend preoperative antibiotics before incision and drainage of infected tissue in patients with prosthetic valves, previous bacterial endocarditis, congenital heart disease, and in heart transplant recipients with valve pathology. Unlike prior AHA recommendations, antibiotic prophylaxis is no longer recommended in patients with routine mitral valve prolapse.

FISTULA-IN-ANO

There are two basic, important principles to be followed when treating patients with anal fistulas: First, it is important to accurately establish the relation of the fistula tract to the internal and external sphincter as defined in the Parks classification (see Figure 1). Second, it is important to accurately identify the location of the causative primary opening.

Physical examination under adequate anesthesia in the operating room is the best method for determining the course of a fistula. In addition to careful use of a fistula probe, injecting hydrogen peroxide into the external opening will help identify the internal opening in more than 80% of patients; Goodsall's rule helps predict the location of the internal opening by dividing the anal canal into anterior and posterior segments via an imaginary transverse line through the anal verge (Figure 3). Fistulous tracts with external openings posterior to this line tend to generally follow a course to the posterior midline (12 o'clock position) crypt, such as horseshoe (Figure 4) or hemihorseshoe fistulas (Figure 5). Anterior fistulas tend to track in a radial fashion internally to the dentate line. The most common exception to Goodsall's rule is the horseshoe fistula (with primary opening at posterior midline) and long tracts that extend into the anterior quadrants of the anal canal. Other exceptions are iatrogenic fistula, Crohn's disease, and in women with anterior openings, in whom a higher percentage will track to the anterior midline.

Imaging Studies

Fistulography, in which contrast is injected into the external opening under fluoroscopic imaging, has reported accuracy rates of 16% and has been replaced by more accurate modalities such as ultrasound, CT, and MRI.

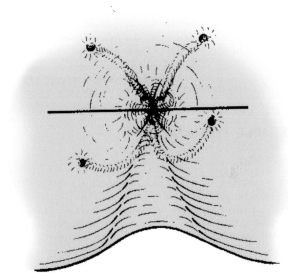

FIGURE 3 Goodsall's rule. (From Keighley MRB, Fazio VW, Pemberton JH, et al: *Atlas of colorectal surgery*, New York, 1996, Churchill Livingstone.)

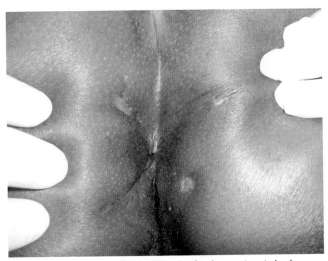

FIGURE 4 Horseshoe fistula. Note the fistula openings in both ischiorectal fossae.

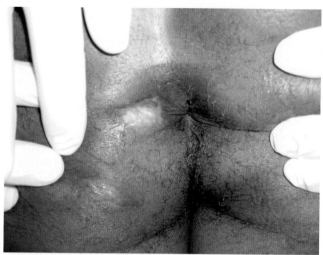

FIGURE 5   Hemihorseshoe fistula. Note the fistula openings in the left ischiorectal fossa.

Ultrasound is a useful tool to identify fistula tracts and secondary extensions. Combining 3-D ultrasound with hydrogen peroxide injection through the external opening has demonstrated comparable accuracy rates to MRI, with concordance rates of up to 90%. Pelvic CT has much more limited use in fistula disease, as soft tissue differentiation with CT lacks sensitivity and specificity. MRI with or without endoanal coils has accuracy rates greater than 90% for mapping fistula tracts and identifying the internal opening.

SIMPLE FISTULA

Fistulotomy

Although a number of advances have been made in recent years in the management of complex anorectal fistula (AFP, RVP, and LIFT procedure), it is important not to underestimate the role of fistulotomy, which remains the preferred technique for intersphincteric and low transsphincteric fistula repair (Figure 6, *A*). If necessary, hydrogen peroxide may be injected into the external opening to locate the internal (primary) opening (Figure 6, *B*). After dividing the skin and anoderm overlying the tract, the fibers of the internal sphincter (Figure 6, *C* and *D*) are then divided to the intersphincteric plane (Figure 6, *E*).

As a practical rule of thumb, two landmarks are helpful. First, the junction between the proximal and middle third of the external sphincter, the distal margin of the levator ani muscle, is located at the level of the dentate line. Second, the distal third of the external sphincter (low transsphincteric fistula) can usually be divided without significant anorectal incontinence. As the proportion of the external sphincter divided increases to half of the external sphincter (mid-transshpincteric fistula) to two thirds of the external sphincter (deep-transsphincteric fistula), the incidence of postfistulotomy incontinence increases.

Ideally, the fistulotomy incision should be marsupialized, in which the edges of the tract are sutured to its base, minimizing the amount of exposed open wound and thereby minimizing healing time (Figure 6, *F*). With proper patient selection, fistulotomy is associated with success rates of 92% to 97%, and recurrence rates approach zero. As with any other fistula surgery, failure to accurately identify the internal opening leads to recurrent fistula formation; and the importance of this critical step, even with simple fistulotomy, cannot be overemphasized.

Although it is generally safe to divide the distal third of the external sphincter, these broad generalizations must take other factors into consideration, such as preoperative continence status, anterior fistula in a female, complex fistulas, and prior fistula surgery. Under these

circumstances, newer modalities of sphincter-sparing surgery (AFP, LIFT) should be considered.

COMPLEX FISTULA

Fibrin Glue

After tract debridement, the combination of thrombin and fibrinogen injection obliterates the tract (Figure 7). The glue is reconstituted and injected into the external opening. The internal opening may be sutured to retain the glue; however, there is no evidence that this increases success rates. Although success rates with fibrin glue are low, the procedure has no significant complications and can be repeated if the fistula persists. Fibrin glue use in conjunction with the AFP has also been described.

Anal Fistula Plug

The AFP is a bioprosthetic plug used to close the primary (internal) fistula opening, and it serves as a matrix for the obliteration of the fistula tract. In this technique, the plug is initially rehydrated for 1 to 2 minutes prior to insertion into the primary opening. The plug is then pulled through the tract until light resistance is met before being sutured securely in the internal opening using a 2-0 vicryl or similar absorbable suture (Figure 8, *A* and *B*). The excess plug is trimmed from the external opening at the skin level while ensuring that this secondary opening is open to allow for drainage.

Prior to inserting the AFP, setons are useful; they drain any residual sepsis, mature the tract, and facilitate surgical insertion of the plug. Patients must be instructed to avoid heavy lifting or straining for at least 2 weeks after surgery to avoid extruding the plug. Patient selection and avoiding excessive postoperative activity are the keys to successful outcomes with the AFP. The best outcomes are achieved in deep-transsphincteric (or deeper) fistulas, fistulas with long tracts, and narrow-gauge fistulas. To avoid extrusion of the AFP, the plug must be firmly anchored to the primary opening. Various techniques have been described to anchor the plug, but the key is to firmly secure it to the internal opening. With appropriate patient selection, proper technique, and careful postoperative management, most series report success rates of 40% to 60%.

Button Plug or Rectovaginal Plug

Excessive patient activity after the AFP procedure has led to a number of plug extrusions, which led to a second generation "button" plug, or RVP (Figure 9, *A* and *B*). The RVP incorporates a conventional AFP attached to a nonabsorbable button using absorbable suture material. The RVP has the advantage that it is simpler to suture and is difficult to extrude. The button is sutured to the anoderm at the primary opening using 2-0 Vicryl and a UR6 needle (Figure 9, *C* and *D*). As with the AFP, the tip is amputated at skin level. These sutures dissolve 2 to 3 weeks postoperatively, and the button is passed per rectum, leaving the plug securely lodged in the fistula tract. The button plug affords a simpler means of closing the primary opening of complex fistula tracts and follows the same sphincter-preserving principles as the AFP.

Setons

Setons have been used for thousands of years in the treatment of fistula-in-ano, from descriptions by Hippocrates (circa 460–370 BCE) and even earlier by the Indian surgeon Sushruta (circa 800 BCE) with the use of Kshara sutra chemical setons. In this method, the seton (i.e., the suture or silastic vessel loop) is passed through the fistula tract to

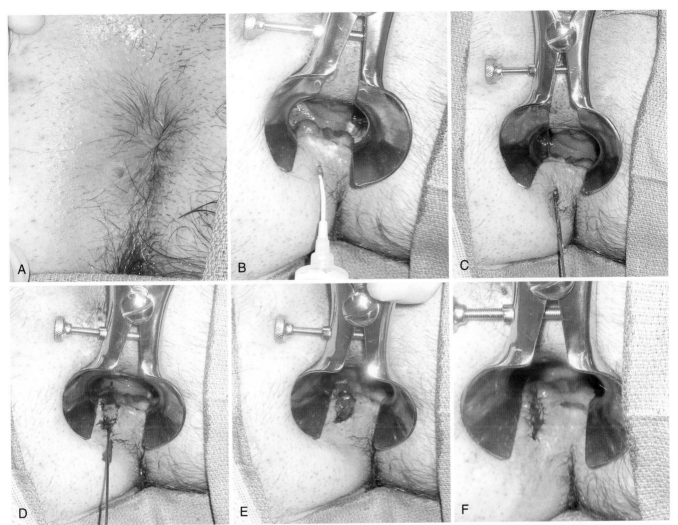

FIGURE 6 **A,** Intersphincteric fistula (secondary opening). **B,** Peroxide is used to locate the internal (primary) opening. **C,** A fistula probe is inserted from the secondary to primary opening. **D,** Skin and anoderm are divided to expose the fibers of the internal sphincter. **E,** The internal sphincter is divided to complete the sphincterotomy. **F,** Fistuloplasty is performed to decrease exposed tissue.

drain the inflammatory process and/or cause fibrosis. Setons may be used in the form of either "draining" or "cutting" setons. Draining, or loose, setons are placed to drain anorectal sepsis or inflammation. Depending on the underlying disease process, these may be left in place for a short time (for sepsis resolution, planned AFP, or LIFT) or long term (Crohn patients). Our preference for seton material is a vessel loop: It has a sufficiently narrow diameter to be nonirritating for the patient; it is elastic, so it can be tightened easily; and it can be kept reasonably clean.

Cutting setons are used to divide sphincter muscle slowly to produce a gradual fistulotomy with scarring of the tract over the course of several weeks or months. The skin and anoderm overlying the fistula are divided prior to tightening the seton around the sphincter muscle. Cutting setons are progressively tightened to maintain the necessary erosive forces; this can be performed in the office setting without additional anesthesia. Wide variations are reported, from 4 to more than 60 weeks, for the seton to completely erode through the muscle.

Cutting setons are a useful compromise option for fistula tracts that are too deep for safe fistulotomy but too superficial for a successful AFP procedure. In spite of this, cutting setons have a surprisingly high rate of incontinence, probably due to overly aggressive tightening of the seton, which causes it to "cut" through the sphincter too quickly.

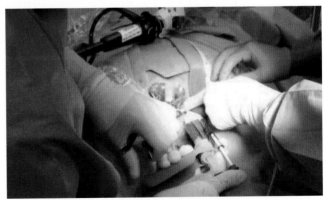

FIGURE 7 Fibrin glue injected into the secondary fistula opening.

In the setting of complex anal fistulas, setons are more commonly used as a staged procedure, with initial seton placement to control active perianal sepsis (Figure 10, *A*), followed by a secondary procedure (endoanal advancement flap, fibrin glue, AFP, or LIFT) 6 to 8 weeks later (Figure 10, *B*). As history attests, loose draining setons are a safe and simple surgical option when the best course of action is not clear.

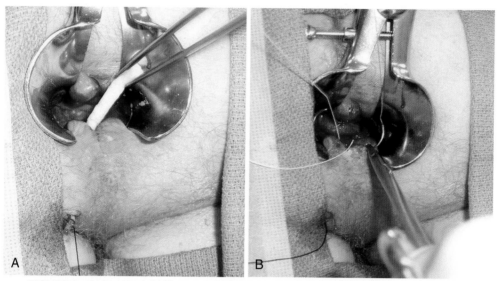

FIGURE 8   **A,** Insertion of AFP into primary opening. **B,** AFP is anchored at the primary opening.

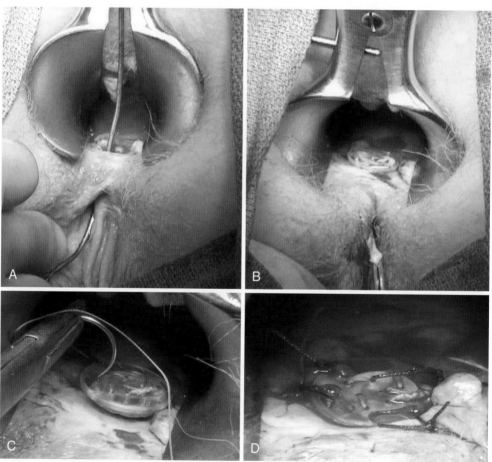

FIGURE 9   **A,** Complex rectoperineal fistula. **B,** Insertion of "button" plug. **C,** Button is sutured to the anorectal mucosa. **D,** Button prevents extrusion. The plug is passed after 2 weeks.

Endoanal Advancement Flap

Endoanal advancement flap is another sphincter-sparing technique that avoids dividing a significant amount of the sphincter. This procedure consists of curettage of the tract and mobilization of a segment of proximal, well-vascularized anorectal mucosa, submucosa, and underlying muscle to cover the site of the sutured internal opening.

The flap should be a minimum of 1 to 2 inches long; the base should be wider than the apex and should overlay the fistula tract without tension. The fistula-bearing apex of the flap is excised and secured using 2-0 Vicryl or chromic catgut. The lateral margins are closed using a running-locking suture, and finally the apex is closed with interrupted sutures.

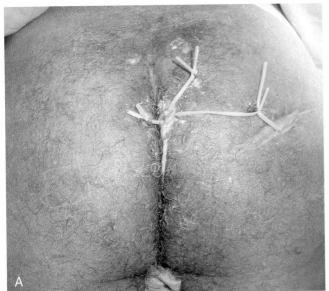

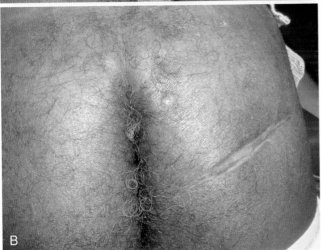

FIGURE 10 A, Setons in complex fistula-in-ano. **B,** Appearance 6 weeks after closure of the primary opening using an AFP.

In general, initial healing rates are 77% to 100%, but long-term success rates range from 13% to 56%. The most common reasons for failure are flaps made too small and excessive tension on the flap. While the sphincter is not "divided" with this repair, mild or moderate incontinence is still reported in up to 38% of patients.

LIFT Procedure

The ligation of the intersphincteric fistula tract (LIFT) procedure is a relatively new sphincter-sparing technique first described in 2007 by Rojanasakul and colleagues. In this procedure, a curvilinear incision is made over the intersphincteric groove, and the fistula tract is identified and surgically isolated in the intersphincteric plane (Figure 10, A and B). The fistula tract is then ligated and divided, and the incision is closed (Figure 10, C and D). As there is no division of the sphincter muscle, impaired continence is usually minimal. This technique has been described on low and high transsphincteric fistulas. Early success rates vary from 58% to 94% of patients. In general, complications are few and minor, with anal pain and postoperative fissure reported. Higher rates of success have been demonstrated after seton drainage for 6 to 8 weeks.

HORSESHOE FISTULA

As described under horseshoe abscess, horseshoe fistula is one of the most complex and potentially morbid conditions faced in modern anorectal surgery. Hanley (1965) reported his original procedure for horseshoe fistula, which involved complete division of the posterior 12 o'clock sphincter mechanism down to the deep postanal space. Counterdrains were placed though each lateral extensions and were removed several weeks afterwards. Not surprisingly, this aggressive procedure obliterated the source of the fistula, but at the inevitable price of a high incidence of anorectal incontinence. This was followed by the modified Hanley procedure (1990), in which the posterior sphincter was divided gradually by using a cutting seton placed around the 12 o'clock sphincter mechanism. As with any cutting seton, this was serially tightened until the posterior sphincter was divided, and it was tethered by resulting scar tissue. This was a longer process (average of 8 months); success rates were lower, but incontinence rates were also lowered.

The recent introduction of the AFP, RVP, and other minimally invasive procedures provide an alternative to these traditional surgeries. Insertion of an AFP into the primary opening of the horseshoe complex is designed to close the primary opening of the entire fistula complex without dividing any sphincter muscle.

CROHN'S DISEASE

Patients with Crohn's disease pose a particular challenge in the treatment of perianal fistula disease, with perianal pathology present in up to 40% to 80% of Crohn patients (Figure 11). Unlike standard fistula disease, advances in medical treatment have been extremely helpful in addressing perianal Crohn's disease. Topical 10% metronidazole (SLA Pharma, Leavesden, UK) is a simple, inexpensive, and effective means of controlling pain and discharge from anorectal Crohn disease before, after, or as an alternative to surgery. Tumor necrosis factor alpha (TNF-α) antibodies have been shown to decrease drainage from Crohn fistulas in spite of the persistence of tracts demonstrated on ultrasound.

The use of surgery in anorectal Crohn's disease should be very conservative, because the postoperative inflammatory response is often florid and incapacitating. Fistulas in Crohn's disease characteristically ignore the anatomic rules of cryptoglandular tracts and are frequently termed *nonanatomic*. Crohn fistulas are often multiple, complex, and have extensive sphincter involvement (Figures 12 and 13). Yet, patients with Crohn's disease may also have low-lying simple fistulas, where fistulotomy is safe and effective. Given the chronicity of the disease and high frequency of disease relapse, maximum preservation of sphincter function is essential. With proper patient selection, healing rates following fistulotomy are reported in over 50% of patients, and anorectal incontinence rates may be as low as 10%.

For complex fistulas associated with Crohn's disease, long-term placement of loose setons combined with TNF-α therapy results in satisfactory symptom control and avoids the pitfalls of surgery in this condition. For more difficult Crohn fistulas, such as rectovaginal fistula, the principles of sphincter-sparing surgery are paramount. AFP and RVP are most successful in longer, narrower tracts, and advancement flaps may be considered in selected patients with no active proctitis. A subset of patients have such extensive and aggressive disease that even maximum TNF-α therapy and seton placement are unsuccessful, requiring proctocolectomy and end ileostomy.

SUMMARY

Significant advances have been made in recent years in the treatment of anorectal fistula, and new devices and techniques have become available for sphincter-sparing surgery. In spite of this, traditional

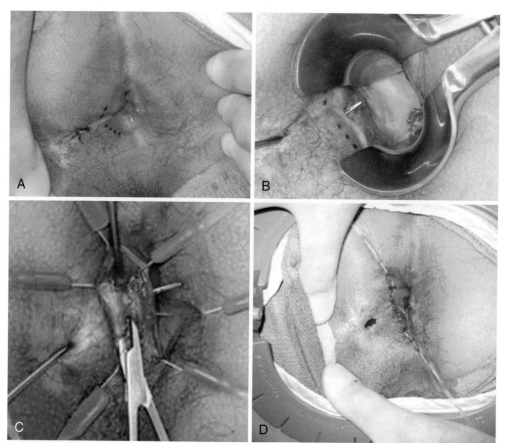

FIGURE 11 LIFT procedure. **A,** Draining seton is inserted to "mature" the tract. **B,** Curvilinear incision made over the intersphincteric groove. **C,** Fistula tract is isolated in the intersphincteric plane, ligated, and divided. **D,** The incision is closed.

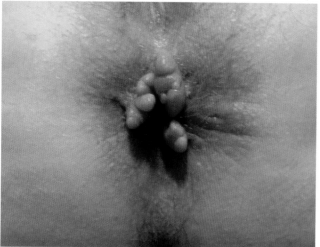

FIGURE 12 Perianal Crohn's disease with classical "elephant ear" skin tags.

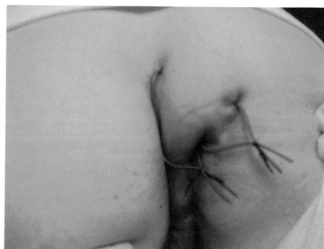

FIGURE 13 Multiple complex Crohn extrasphincteric fistulas with draining setons.

surgeries such as fistulotomy and traditional devices such as setons remain the workhorses in the treatment of this disease. As the role of biologic devices such as the AFP and procedures such as the LIFT repair evolve, we will hopefully witness continued evolution in technique and improved outcomes. Until then, the goals of surgery for anorectal abscess and fistula remain to drain all perineal sepsis, provide the highest closure rate for fistula disease, and maximize sphincter preservation.

SUGGESTED READINGS

Armstrong DN: Anal fistula, *Semin Colon Rectal Surg* 20:1–62, 2009.
Parks AG, Gordon PH, Hardcastle JD: A classification of fistula-in-ano, *Br J Surg* 63:1–12, 1976.

MANAGEMENT OF ANORECTAL STRICTURE

Stephen M. Sentovich, MD

EVALUATION

An anorectal stricture is a nonspecific narrowing that occurs anywhere along the anal canal from the pelvic floor proximally to the anal verge distally. The vast majority of anorectal strictures are iatrogenic and related to previous anorectal surgery. When too much anoderm is excised, most commonly during hemorrhoidectomy, an anorectal stricture can result. Thus most anorectal strictures are associated with a deficiency of anoderm due to previous surgery. All of the potential causes of anorectal stricture are shown in Table 1.

Patients with anorectal strictures complain of constipation, a decrease in stool caliber, and difficult or incomplete evacuation. Often they will report using laxatives, enemas, and suppositories to assist with evacuation. Some patients will also have associated fecal incontinence, which may alter therapy, so it is important to document every patient's continence status. Physical examination will confirm the diagnosis and classify the degree of stricture. A *mild anorectal stricture* is tight but still allows digital examination. A *moderate anorectal stricture* requires a forceful digital examination that usually can be performed only under anesthesia. A *severe anorectal stricture* does not allow digital examination. For patients with moderate to severe anorectal strictures, an exam under anesthesia is often necessary to fully evaluate the severity and extent of the stricture and biopsy it to rule out malignancy.

INDICATIONS AND TREATMENT

Treatment should be offered to all patients with symptomatic anorectal strictures. The overall goal of treatment is to correct the anorectal stricture and preserve continence. Patients should be warned prior to treatment about the risk of incontinence following treatment. Patients with mild anorectal strictures should be treated medically with stool-bulking agents and possibly anal dilatation. Patients with moderate to severe anorectal strictures usually require surgical intervention. Patients with anorectal strictures immediately following anorectal surgery should be treated with bulking agents and stool softeners; often these early postoperative strictures will resolve after 3 to 6 months of medical therapy.

In patients with inflammatory bowel disease (IBD) or a history of pelvic radiation therapy, surgical options are limited by the potential for nonhealing wounds after surgery. For these patients, bulking agents, anal dilatation, and stricturotomy are the mainstays of treatment. If more extensive surgery (advancement flap) is undertaken in these patients, and nonhealing develops, a permanent colostomy may become necessary. Any patient with IBD or any previously irradiated patient with an anorectal stricture should understand this risk prior to any surgical intervention.

Treatment should also be offered to patients with asymptomatic anorectal strictures if their underlying disease is neoplastic, infectious, or inflammatory (i.e., IBD). After identification of these patients with anoscopy and biopsy/culture, diagnosis-specific treatment should be initiated.

MEDICAL TREATMENT

Medical treatment of anorectal strictures uses bulking agents (fiber) and stool softeners to allow for the passage of soft, naturally dilating bowel movements; this can be effective treatment for patients with mild anorectal strictures. In addition, anal dilators can be used, but they are limited in their effectiveness because trauma from repeated dilatation can result in additional scarring and stricture. Thus anal dilatation is most useful on a limited basis, in patients who are not good operative candidates or in those who have IBD or a history of pelvic radiation.

SURGICAL TREATMENT

Stricturotomy and Stricturoplasty

For mild to moderate short anorectal strictures, stricturotomy and stricturoplasty can be effective treatments. Patients with anorectal strictures after low coloanal anastomosis, ileal pouch–anal anastomosis, or stapled hemorrhoidectomy are ideal candidates for this technique. In the operating room, a small anoscope is used to visualize the stricture, which is divided longitudinally in three or four quadrants. The resulting wounds can be left open (my preference) or closed transversely with an absorbable 3-0 suture. For short, mild anorectal strictures, I have found stricturotomy highly successful. If this technique should fail, an advancement flap should be offered.

Advancement Flaps

The most effective treatment for a moderate to severe anorectal stricture is an advancement flap. Although several flap types have been described, all are based on the technique of scar excision followed by the advancement of normal local tissue into the resulting defect. Thus advancement flaps directly correct the deficiency in anoderm associated with anorectal strictures. All flaps require an adequate blood supply and sufficient mobilization to eliminate any tension. A variety of anoscopes and the Lone Star retractor (Lone Star Medical Products, Stafford, Tex.) assist in the exposure.

For severe anorectal strictures, nasal speculums can be particularly useful to obtain adequate visualization. Preoperatively, patients undergo full mechanical bowel preparation and are administered parenteral antibiotics. In the operating room, patients are placed in the prone jackknife position for the best exposure.

Y-V and V-Y Flaps

The Y-V and V-Y flaps are simple advancement flaps (Figures 1 and 2). The Y-V flap has a narrow tip that is subject to ischemia; it transfers minimal tissue into the anal canal. Consequently, when there is a significant deficiency of anoderm, the Y-V flap is not the best option. The V-Y flap, however, has a broader tip that is more suitable to correct larger deficiencies of anoderm proximally, but distally the flap narrows, making it less effective for longer anorectal strictures. Given the limitations of the Y-V and V-Y flaps, my preference for a local advancement flap is the house flap.

House Flap

The house flap is the local advancement flap that has sufficient width and mobility to correct anorectal strictures involving the entire length of the anal canal (Figure 3). After excising the scar to release the anorectal stricture, the house-shaped flap is mobilized with a larger underlying subcutaneous fat pad by dissecting on an angle away from

TABLE 1: Etiology of anorectal stricture

Previous Surgery

Hemorrhoids

Fistula

Fissure

Congenital malformation repair

Coloanal/ileal pouch–anal anastomosis

Neoplasia-Related

Bowen disease and Paget disease

Giant condyloma acuminatum

Squamous cell cancer of anus

Verrucous carcinoma

Rectal adenocarcinoma

Post radiation

Miscellaneous

Inflammatory bowel disease

Sphincter hypertrophy

Laxative abuse

Trauma

Tuberculosis

Sexually transmitted diseases

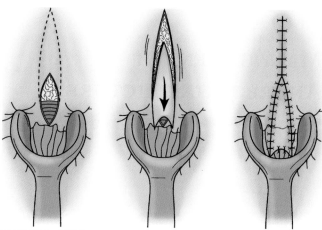

FIGURE 2 V-Y flap. After a longitudinal incision is made over the strictured area, a V-shaped incision is made in the perianal skin, with the wide area of the V oriented proximally into the anal canal. The resultant island of tissue is advanced into the anal canal and sutured in place. The donor site is then closed, leaving the inverted Y configuration of final suture lines. *(From Liberman H, Thorson AG: How I do it: anal stenosis, Am J Surg 179:325; 2000.)*

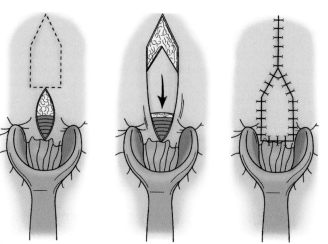

FIGURE 3 House flap. After an incision is made overlying the strictured area, a transverse incision is made at each end of the initial incision, and the edges are undermined, allowing the wound to assume a rectangular shape. The flap is then configured in perianal skin in the shape of a house. The base is oriented proximally and the roof distally. "Walls" of the house are of the same length as the initial incision made in the anal canal. The width of the flap is designed to accommodate the width of the rectangular wound. The island of tissue is mobilized into a defect in the anal canal and sutured in place with 2-0 absorbable sutures. The "roof" of the house allows the donor site to be primarily closed with 3-0 absorbable sutures. *(From Liberman H, Thorson AG: How I do it: anal stenosis, Am J Surg 179:325; 2000.)*

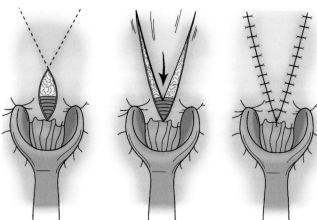

FIGURE 1 Y-V flap. An initial relaxing incision is made overlying the area of the stricture. This corresponds to the vertical limb of the Y. Distally, diagonal limbs of the Y are created in the perianal area, and the resultant flap, in the shape of a V, is sutured to the apex of the relaxed wound. *(From Liberman H, Thorson AG: How I do it: anal stenosis, Am J Surg 179:325; 2000.)*

the flap, which is sufficiently mobilized circumferentially so it can be advanced into the anal canal without tension. The "floor" of the house flap is then secured proximally using deep, muscle-anchoring bites with 2-0 absorbable suture. The "walls" of the house flap are then closed with 3-0 absorbable suture. Finally, the donor site is closed

with 3-0 absorbable suture. The apex of the "roof" of the house flap is often left open to allow for drainage. If stricture is still present after a single flap, a second house flap can be performed in another quadrant. To resurface the entire anal canal, four separate house flaps, one in each quadrant, can be performed.

S Flap

For the rare patient with extensive or recurrent anorectal stricture, the best option is either multiple house flaps or the S (rotational) flap. With the S flap, large areas are mobilized bilaterally and then rotated and advanced into the anal canal (Figure 4).

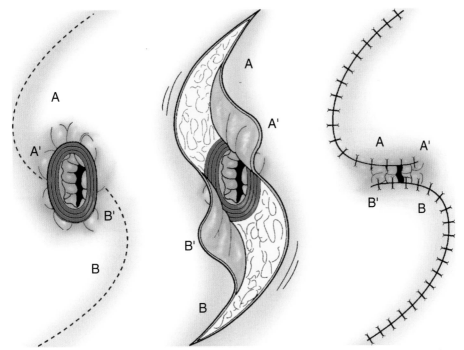

FIGURE 4   S flap. Areas of scar tissue within the anal canal are excised. A full-thickness flap in the shape of an S is configured in the perianal area. After adequate mobilization is achieved, the flap is rotated to cover the resulting defect in the anal canal. *(From Liberman H, Thorson AG: How I do it: anal stenosis, Am J Surg 179:325; 2000.)*

Results

Simple stricturotomy/stricturoplasty and single-quadrant house flaps can be performed as outpatient procedures. Multiple house flaps or rotational flaps usually require a 1 to 2 day hospital stay. Pain control is achieved using nonnarcotic medications for many patients, but narcotic medications are necessary for patients with multiple, extensive flaps. Topical anesthetic ointments may also be beneficial. A high-fiber diet, mild laxatives, and sitz baths are also recommended. Patients commonly have drainage and occasional bleeding until all of their wounds have healed.

Results with the house flap have found 89% of patients clinically improved with an 82% satisfaction rate. Recurrence rates are unknown but are presumably very low. With respect to continence, I avoid sphincterotomy at the time of advancement flap, unless the sphincter muscle is deemed to contribute to the stricture. Thus I rarely divide the sphincter muscle and have successfully preserved continence. Despite this precaution, long-term fecal incontinence can occur, and patients should be warned prior to surgery. Conservative treatment of incontinence with bulking agents and antidiarrheal medications usually resolves these patients' symptoms.

SUGGESTED READINGS

Christensen MA, Pitsch RM Jr, Cali RL, et al: "House" advancement pedicle flap for anal stenosis, *Dis Colon Rectum* 35:201–203, 1992.

Liberman H, Thorson AG: How I do it: anal stenosis, *Am J Surg* 179(4): 325–329, 2000.

Sentovich SM, Falk PM, Christensen MA, et al: Operative results of house advancement anoplasty, *Br J Surg* 83:1242, 1996.

MANAGEMENT OF PRURITUS ANI

Janice F. Rafferty, MD, and Tobi Reidy, DO

OVERVIEW

Pruritus ani is a broad term describing any sensation in the perianal region that induces the urge to scratch. It can be either a symptom or a diagnosis. Primary (idiopathic) pruritis accounts for 50% to 90% of cases. In general, pruritis ani affects 1% to 5% of the population, with males more commonly affected than females. Most patients are between 40 and 70 years of age, and there is a tendency for symptoms to be worse at night and in warm, moist climates.

Pruritus ani is characterized by an intense sensation of itch. This is mediated by nociceptive C-fibers existing in high density at the dermal–epidermal junction of the perianal skin. Although these fibers are distinctively known as *pain fibers,* in the presence of local innocuous irritants such as histamine, kallikrein, bradykinin, papain, trypsin, serotonin, prostaglandins, opioids, or neuropeptides, these nerve endings are stimulated with varying results. The nerve impulse is carried via the spinothalamic tract, ultimately to the thalamus, where itching is perceived rather than pain.

When scratching the itch becomes uncontrollable, mechanical skin breakdown occurs, with further exposure to irritants and worsening of the impulse to scratch. Patients with pruritis ani often suffer social embarrassment and depression and often resort to extensive self-treatments, frequently worsening the condition or leading to chronic changes before consultation is sought.

ETIOLOGY

Idiopathic pruritus ani (IPA) is a diagnosis of exclusion; all secondary causes must be ruled out to treat it effectively. Although this is a simple statement, there are so many secondary causes that even the astute surgeon may struggle and thereby extend morbidity and possibly mortality. A directed history and full physical examination is of paramount importance.

Anatomic and Physiologic Precursors

In most instances, an anatomic or physiologic derangement results in fecal leakage or contamination. Stool containing exotoxins, intestinal lysosymes, endopeptidases, trypsin, and kinase cause chemical skin irritation and breakdown. Neural stimulation ensues, itch is perceived, and ultimately scratching begins (Table 1).

Dermatologic, Allergic, and Infectious Precursors

Virtually any disease that affects the skin, locally or diffusely, can affect the perianal skin (Table 2).

Dietary and Drug Precursors

Specific foods and drugs have been studied to delineate their effects on the gastrointestinal tract. Certain foods cause changes in both the anal sphincter pressure and intestinal transit time. Increased exposure of perianal skin to undigested food and drugs leads to irritation and sensitization and exaggerated anal reflexes (Table 3). Coffee in particular, both decaffeinated and regular, is noted to decrease resting internal anal sphincter pressures.

Systemic Disease Precursors

Many systemic diseases, most likely already diagnosed in a patient with pruritis, are associated with perianal disease. If no preexisting diagnosis is known, signs and symptoms obtained through detailed history and physical can reveal causes such as diabetes mellitus, end-stage renal disease, hepatic diseases associated with hyperbilirubinemia, thyroid disorders, and blood dyscrasias. Each of these can cause perianal skin irritation and pruritis.

Autoimmune Precursors

It has been proposed by Shafik that epithelial remnants of the anorectal sinuses, a structure that normally regresses by birth, can persist into adulthood. These remnants are buried in the anal submucosa and become pruritogenic when they release submucosal irritants and secondary metabolic byproducts. Because they are self-derived, a so-called *autoimmune inflammatory reaction* can cause pruritis.

Idiopathic Precursors

As previously stated, IPA is a diagnosis of exclusion. It is unclear, despite numerous studies, whether it should be classified as a functional disease. Physiologic studies clearly demonstrate that in those with idiopathic pruritus ani, the anal sphincter relaxes in response to rectal distension more readily than controls. This leads to abnormal rectoanal inhibitory reflex (RAIR) and therefore lowers the threshold for internal anal sphincter relaxation. This has been confirmed by saline retention testing, which shows those with IPA can only hold 600 mL compared with 1300 mL in controls.

TABLE 1: Anatomic and physiologic precursors of pruritis ani

Chronic diarrhea	Chronic constipation
Anal creases	Anal fissure
Colorectal or anal cancer	Adenomatous polyps
Hemorrhoids	Rectal prolapse
Anal dyskinesia	Sphincter weakness
Skin tags	Fistula-in-ano

TABLE 2: Dermatologic, allergic, and infectious precursors of pruritis ani

Dermatologic precursors:	Psoriasis, seborrheic keratosis, intertrigo, lichen planus, lichen atrophicus, atopic dermatitis, benign familial pemphigus, acanthosis nigricans, vitiligo, Bowen disease, Paget disease, erythrasma
Allergic precursors:	Soaps, perfumes, detergents, dyes, wipes, toilet paper, clothing
Infectious precursors:	*Staphylococcus* spp., *Streptococcus* spp. (β-hemolytic, groups A, B, and G), sexually transmitted diseases (syphilis, gonorrhea, herpes, papilloma virus), *Herpes zoster,* dermatophytoses, scabies, pediculosis, parasites, folliculitis, furuncles, abscess

TABLE 3: Dietary and drug precursors of pruritis ani

Food precursors:	Coffee, tea, soda, beer, chocolate, dairy, citrus, tomatoes
Drug precursors:	Colchicines, quinidine

DIAGNOSIS

A detailed history and physical examination are critical to establishing the potential causes of pruritis ani. Specific and detailed questions about toileting habits, bowel regimens, perianal hygiene, previous perianal operations, use of over-the-counter medications, and dietary intake must be answered. In addition, it is important to know the number of trips to the toilet each day, time spent sitting on the commode, consistency of the stool that is passed, cleansing regimen, and whether the patient wears a pad in the undergarments. Many patients are hesitant to describe such personal information in detail, so a comfortable, supportive office visit is encouraged.

Optimal exposure through appropriate patient positioning and bright lighting are important to a good exam of the perineum. Placing the patient in the prone, jackknife position is a good way to optimally expose the entire perineum. The availability of an anoscope and proctoscope will facilitate a thorough exam of the anal canal and distal rectum, where often the source of pruritis can be found. Asking the patient to sit on a commode and strain can also be very revealing, as it can demonstrate hemorrhoidal prolapse, mucosal prolapse, or complete rectal prolapse, all of which can be secondary causes of perianal irritation. Inspect lymph node basins of the groins bilaterally, as well as other areas of skin, for evidence of chronic irritation or other primary skin diseases. Be prepared to obtain scrapings, do biopsies, and take cultures to facilitate diagnosis.

TREATMENT

Because of the myriad things that cause IPA, treatment can be complex and requires patience on the part of both physician and patient. Starting with simple remedies, such as mild topical drying agents or antiinflammatory agents, and advancing to more aggressive interventions if needed is recommended. Remind the patient that being too fastidious with perineal hygiene and overuse of topical over-the-counter agents can actually cause worsening of the symptoms rather than improvement. Historically, there are very few studies defining a mandatory treatment algorithm, but most sources agree on one basic tenet: interruption of the vicious cycle. Obviously, if a secondary cause is evident, treatment with surgical excision, antibiotic, or antifungal therapy should be given.

Reassurance

Reassurance is a mainstay of therapy. After ruling out malignancy, reiteration that time and patience will likely result in relief will greatly alleviate the anxiety that invariably plagues patients with IPA.

Elimination

First, counsel the patient to remove all possible irritants. This includes all soaps and harsh toilet paper. Discourage wearing any synthetic or dyed materials as undergarments, and suggest a change to undyed cotton. Remove all foods known to cause perianal irritation, and counsel on tobacco cessation.

Education

It is critical to explain the importance of healthy toileting habits and appropriate levels of attention to hygiene. Also, dietary counseling will allow the patient to take control of the problems that can arise from certain foods, especially those high in acidity, and caffeine. After the patient eliminates all potential dietary causes of pruritis, consider allowing the reintroduction of foods, one by one, at 2-week intervals; this may help pinpoint the offending dietary product.

Instruct the patient to gently cleanse the perianal area twice daily and after any bowel movement with plain warm water (sitz baths) or a nonalkalotic soap. Warm tap water enemas after bowel movements may clear the anal canal and distal rectum of residual irritants and may be soothing as well. The patient should follow by obtaining a dry perianal field—pat the area dry and, if possible, use a blow dryer. Antifungal powder may be applied regardless of fungal infection presence to effect dryness. Consider avoiding cornstarch, which may act as a medium for bacterial growth and can exacerbate symptoms. Finally, tell the patient to tuck a dry cotton ball at the anal margin to absorb seepage and moisture.

Control

The primary reason patients come in for evaluation is to cure the itch. Prior to leaving the office, specific therapy should be offered. To interrupt the cycle of pruritus ani, start by controlling seepage and leakage. This, in part, can be achieved by starting the patient on a bulking agent and high-fiber diet. In addition, antimotility agents can be given to decrease transit time, thereby decreasing water content of the stool and possibly minimizing seepage.

Supply the patient with topical therapy as well. Topical anesthetics offer quick, albeit temporary, relief. Unfortunately, many of these agents are short lived and are often abused. If utilized under supervision and strict instruction, agents such as menthol, phenol, camphor, or a combination of these can be a soothing addition and can extend the period of relief between episodes. Risk of maceration is lower with topical treatment prescribed as creams instead of ointments, especially if used sparingly. Topical mineral oil, lanolin, witch hazel, glycerin, pramoxine, and oatmeal combinations are all available options that can provide comfort if used sparingly.

Reassessment

If these therapies do not lead to relief, more intense intervention may be warranted. Reevaluation should be done periodically until symptoms are manageable.

Invasive Topical Therapy

A few novel options are have been described and can be considered when intense IPA cannot be cured with the usual remedies described above. Topical capsaicin has been shown by Lysy to decrease itch via desensitization; it binds to the capsaicin receptor, which results in a depressant effect on the synthesis, storage, and release of substance P, a nucleopeptide known to be a mediator of pain and itch. Capsaicin is prescribed as topical cream in varying strengths, ranging from 0.006% to 0.075%, and it can be applied up to three times daily. Duration of therapy is based on tolerance and outcome.

Another controversial treatment is the application of topical steroids. Great debate surrounds the use of topical steroids because of the potential for adverse effects. Most notably, continuous use of mid- and high-dose topical steroids can lead to atrophy of the perianal skin in a short amount of time (2 to 4 weeks). This can result in further skin breakdown, interfering with healing and worsening the original complaint. Keeping this in mind, there may still be a place for supervised, time-limited use of these agents. Successful outcomes have been documented, especially when used as "induction" of treatment. In this situation, a 1% steroid cream is applied up to three times daily and is tapered down over 1 to 2 weeks. During this time, a barrier cream is also introduced, such as zinc oxide or other commercially available barriers, to offset the risk of skin breakdown from mechanical irritation. Once the patient has been weaned off steriods, conservative measures and treatments can then be introduced to decrease the chance of recurrence.

The application of Berwick's dye has been described, and it may have some last-ditch utility for the refractory IPA patient. Berwick's dye is a combination of gentian violet, brilliant green, and alcohol. It is applied to the affected perianal skin and then covered with tincture of benzoin. This application forms an impervious layer that will last for approximately 3 days if washed with only warm water. Its success is caused by creation of a stinging sensation with eventual desensitization of the perianal skin. Itch is ultimately reduced or subsides, allowing reepithelialization.

Oral Therapy

The primary goal of any treatment in pruritus ani is to quell the itch and promote reepithelialization of the skin. The use of antihistamines has been investigated, but the results of studies with nonselective antihistamines have shown no benefit. Doxepin, a psychotherapeutic tricyclic compound, has been noted to be 1000 times as potent as Benadryl in relieving itch. It, too, comes with numerous side effects and is not always a viable long-term option, although it may provide relief for intense, acute-phase IPA.

Injections and Anal Tattoo

Other unconventional therapies have been described. These treatments have been studied in small series with varying results. Nonetheless, some report excellent outcomes, and in refractory cases, they may be the only remaining option.

Methylene blue injection and tattooing of the perianal region have been studied. A solution of 5 mL to 30 mL of 0.5% to 1% methylene blue and normal saline (with or without lidocaine or bupivicaine) is introduced into the intradermal, intracutaneous, and subcutaneous perianal tissue, inducing hypoesthesia. Again, as with almost all treatments discussed, this is thought to chemically de-innervate the area. In small series, this treatment has been reported to eliminate 80% of all pruritus after the first treatment and up to 90% after a second treatment.

Other attempted treatments include alcohol injection therapy, phototherapy, cryotherapy, radiation, and surgery. All purport to desensitize, but none have been studied microscopically. No widespread acceptance exists based upon side effects and poor outcomes.

SUMMARY

Pruritus ani is intrinsically complex in its origin and ultimate treatment. It demands a trusting relationship between physician and patient and patience in the pursuit of adequate treatment. No delineated treatment algorithm exists, but with clinical awareness and exclusion of secondary causes, a basic progression of conservative to aggressive and even unconventional therapy has been suggested.

SELECTED READINGS

Gordon P, Nivatvongs S: *Principles and practice of surgery for the colon, rectum, and anus,* ed 3, New York, 2007, Informa Healthcare, pp 247–257.
Lysy J: Topical capsaicin: a novel and effective treatment for idiopathic intractable pruritus ani, *Gut* 52(9):1323–1326, 2003.
Mentes BB: Intradermal methylene blue injection for the treatment of intractable idiopathic pruritus ani, *Tech Coloproctol* 8:11–14, 2004.
Siddiqi S: Pruritis ani, *Ann R Coll Surg Engl* 90:457–463, 2008.

MANAGEMENT OF FECAL INCONTINENCE

Tracy L. Hull, MD

INTRODUCTION

Uncontrollable loss of flatus or stool, while not life threatening, can be humiliating for patients. Heightened awareness over the last two decades has provided a platform for patients to discuss this issue with health care providers. The first step when interviewing a patient who has concerns with inability to control stool is a comprehensive history. This starts with questions to delineate the exact nature of the material that cannot be controlled (gas, mucus, or liquid or solid stool), the frequency of stool loss, and if the patient wears a pad. Further inquiry into stool habits include using the Bristol stool scale (Figure 1) to characterize the stool because some patients will report diarrhea as fecal incontinence; questions about fecal urgency, which may be related to problems with rectal storage and sensation, are also helpful.

Medications can exacerbate problems with stool control, especially if the medication leads to looser stools. Detective work—asking about prescription, over-the-counter, and herbal medications—is needed to rule these out as a potential contributor to the problem. Additionally, past medical and surgical treatment can affect bowels; cholecystectomy, bowel resection, anal surgery, abdominal or pelvic radiation, back injury, and obstetrical history need to be investigated. Many times this type of comprehensive history takes considerable time.

The physical exam should focus on the perineal region. The anus should be examined, looking to see if it is closed at rest. Scars or deformities, anal tags, hemorrhoids, and the status of the perineal body are noted. Asking the patient to squeeze provides the opportunity to see if the muscle moves uniformly, or if an area seems to be devoid of muscle. Examination while straining may show vaginal prolapse or anal mucosal prolapse.

Next, a digital exam is performed, and the patient is again asked to squeeze and strain to determine movement of the sphincter complex and lower rectum. It is important to differentiate anal sphincter movement versus puborectalis muscle movement, which could give the impression of sphincter squeezing. Evaluation of the anal sensation can be performed by stroking the anal skin with a Q-tip and looking for contraction of the anal muscle (anal wink). This may guide treatment recommendation, but it is not uniformly done by caregivers who treat incontinence.

All patients older than 50 years should have a standard screening colonoscopy. Those with no risk factors who are younger should have a tailored evaluation of their colon and/or rectum. Other testing, such as anal physiology and anal ultrasound, is individually ordered when needed to guide treatment. For instance, a patient with an obvious anterior sphincter defect would not need anal ultrasound prior to repair. Patients with pudendal nerve prolongation and anterior sphincter defects may still be offered a sphincter repair but should be counseled preoperatively regarding possible suboptimal results.

After a comprehensive history and tailored physical exam, the exact perceived scope of the problem is discussed with the patient. It is important to outline realistic treatment goals because it is nearly impossible to produce perfect bowel habits. Treatment options usually consist of a combination of several therapies individualized to each person's problem.

One other point is that assessing success of treatments in the published literature is extremely difficult. Many fecal incontinence severity scores have been devised, and no single score is the gold standard. This is due to the incredible complexity of describing fecal incontinence; it covers an extensive range, from incontinence of gas, mucus, liquid stool, or solid stool, and encompasses fecal urgency and the patient's perception of ideal bowel habits. Quality of life as it pertains to fecal control is somewhat easier to measure and report, but again, no gold standard exists.

MEDICAL TREATMENT

Control Diarrhea

The first consideration is to control diarrhea. Simply starting medications to slow the bowel down can give significant improvement for many patients. Agents such as loperamide or diphenoxylate are the most commonly used. The amount must be individualized and may start with one pill each morning, increased to a maximum of eight daily. If one pill each morning is too much, the liquid form with a decrease in the dose can be tried. Use of these medications with psyllium daily may also change the consistency of the stool and may

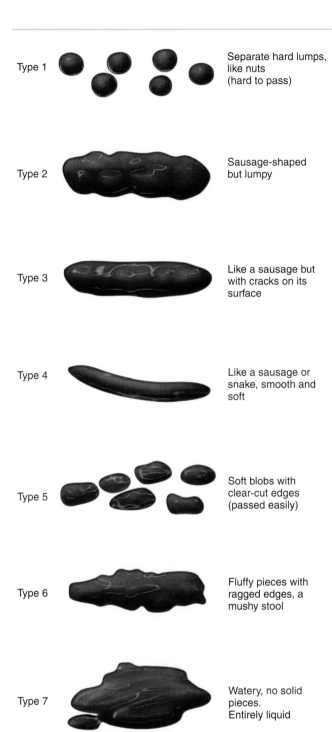

Type 1 — Separate hard lumps, like nuts (hard to pass)

Type 2 — Sausage-shaped but lumpy

Type 3 — Like a sausage but with cracks on its surface

Type 4 — Like a sausage or snake, smooth and soft

Type 5 — Soft blobs with clear-cut edges (passed easily)

Type 6 — Fluffy pieces with ragged edges, a mushy stool

Type 7 — Watery, no solid pieces. Entirely liquid

FIGURE I   The Bristol stool scale is extremely helpful when taking a history, to document exact stool habits and the form of the stool. It allows the health care provider and the patient to communicate on the same level and narrow down the type of stool. This will guide treatment recommendations. For instance, a patient may describe multiple episodes of type 2 stool as "diarrhea," when the health care provider would not consider this type of formed stool diarrhea. *(From Lewis SJ, Heaton KW: Stool form scale as a useful guide to intestinal transit time, Scand J Gastroenterol 32(9):920-924; 1997.)*

provide a better substrate for rectal detection. Pectin found in the grocery store is another agent that will thicken stool. Cholestyramine, 4 to 16 gm daily in divided doses, may be considered for diarrhea after cholecystectomy or right hemicolectomy. Small doses with slow increases help avoid bloating and gas pain.

Diet

Some foods can lead to problems, particularly with significant fecal urgency. One common culprit that can be detected upon close questioning of patients is the dinner salad, especially one eaten at a restaurant. A food diary may uncover other offenders, such as fresh fruits or milk products. Sorbitol ingestion is another forgotten agent that can lead to loose stools and may also cause incontinence. Eliminating any suspected offenders and noting improvement strengthens this point.

Enema Treatment

Some forms of fecal leakage are amendable to rectal washout or enema treatments. There are various methods to provide a washout. Using an asepto-type syringe and instilling tap water after a stool is one method used for patients who leak small amounts after defecation has been completed; this allows the rectum to be cleansed of residual debris. Another technique is to administer a Fleet enema and then rinse out the container. It can be used 4 to 5 more times and filled with tap water until the plastic cracks and does not hold fluid.

A variation of this approach is the surgical creation of access to the proximal colon to instill an antegrade enema. Using the appendiceal orifice or terminal ileum, the goal is to create a small stoma that can be cannulated so water can be instilled daily to every other day. This provides an antegrade enema that flushes out stool and cleans the colon. The premise is that a colon devoid of stool cannot have leakage. This is not a new surgical procedure, but it is gaining new acceptance worldwide in large centers that specialize in advanced treatment of fecal incontinence. Technical problems with the ostomy and leakage continue to make it a challenging surgical procedure.

Biofeedback

Formal behavior modification training in the form of biofeedback has been shown to significantly improve fecal continence. Comparing studies is difficult because there is no standardized treatment regiment. It is important to have a therapist providing treatment who is tolerant, experienced, and enthusiastic. During treatment sessions, multiple areas are addressed, which include pelvic floor strength training, improved coordination between the rectum and anal area, and improved sensation of the rectum to note smaller volumes of stool. Results have varied considerably, most likely because there is no standardized technique, and the reporting of results varies tremendously. It does appear that if improvement is realized, these positive results are sustained long term.

■ SURGICAL TREATMENT

Sphincter Repair

For women who have sustained an obstetrical injury with a resultant anterior anal sphincter defect, a sphincter repair is considered. Overlap of the two ends of the muscle is the preferred method, although end-to-end approximation has been positively reported. Interestingly, in centers outside the United States, sphincter repair has been questioned as a preferred treatment. Centers outside the United States have approval to use sacral neuromodulation (discussed later), which influences their algorithm.

The long-term results of sphincter repair have also been disappointing, with few to no women totally continent at a 10-year follow-up; however, its low cost and simplicity allow it to remain a viable choice. Repair does improve symptoms for some women, and further improvement may be realized by combining repair with other nonsurgical treatments. Timing of repair after an obstetrical

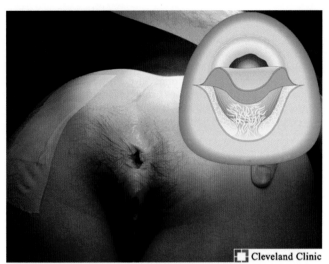

FIGURE 2   For an overlapping sphincter repair, the patient is placed in the prone position and pressure points are padded. A Foley catheter is placed, and the buttocks are taped apart. An incision is usually made in a curvilinear fashion over the perineal body distal enough from the anal verge to avoid ischemic compromise of the skin flap. *(Courtesy the Cleveland Clinic Foundation, Cleveland, Ohio.)*

injury is an important consideration. Surgery must be delayed until all perineal tissue is healed and soft. This may take 3 to 6 months after the birth trauma. Emotional support for the new mother is also needed because dealing with a new baby and fecal incontinence can be overwhelming. However, the surgeon must be firm and avoid repair until the tissue is pliable to provide the best chance of success.

Physiologic age should not be a deterrent. Women in their 90s have gained improved quality of life after sphincter repair. Figures 2 through 5 outline surgical technique for overlapping sphincter repair.

For patients with leakage due to a defined anal trauma, such as fistulotomy where the ends can be delineated, reapproximation, or overlap, if it can be performed, can improve symptoms. Specific planning with anal endosonography can guide important decisions, such as incision placement.

Postanal Repair

Posterior plication of the anal sphincter was envisioned for patients with an intact sphincter to elongate the cylinder of muscle and accentuate the normal anorectal angle at rest. When introduced in 1970s, initial results led to enthusiasm for this procedure, but long-term good results are unclear and have been reported in a range from 30% to 65% of patients. Nonetheless, posterior repair is still considered in patients with an intact sphincter and fecal leakage, where the only other option would be a colostomy.

Artificial Bowel Sphincter

The artificial bowel sphincter (ABS) was patterned after the artificial urinary sphincter. It consists of three implanted elements connected by tubing. A cuff encircles the anus; this is connected to a pump, which is located in the labia in women and the scrotum in men. The pump is then connected to a storage balloon placed in the space of Retzius. At baseline, there is fluid in the cuff. When defecation is desired, the pump is compressed five to eight times. This transports fluid from the cuff to the balloon. An automatic valve then allows the fluid to slowly trickle back into the cuff over the next 8 minutes.

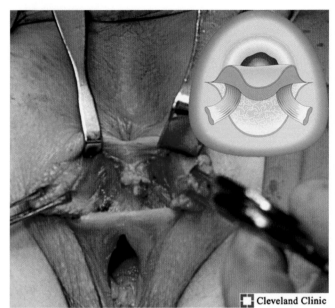

FIGURE 3   Dissection is carried out laterally, and the ischiorectal fossa is identified. With scarring it may be difficult, but usually there is a change in the globular nature of the fat when the fossa is entered. The medial border of the ischiorectal fossa is the external anal sphincter muscle. Remembering this landmark allows easy identification of the muscle, which can then be traced to the severed end. The scar tissue is not dissected from the muscle end, as this provides more substance and it is hoped will also help prevent sutures from pulling through native muscle. The same process is carried out on the other side. It is usually not feasible to separate the internal and external sphincter, and they will be overlapped as one entity. *(Courtesy the Cleveland Clinic Foundation, Cleveland, Ohio.)*

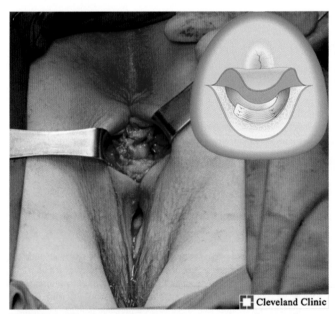

FIGURE 4   The two muscle ends are freed enough to allow overlap, preferably without undue tension. Experimenting with overlapping one side over the other and vice versa will allow the surgeon to view which side overlaps the best (usually one side will lay over the other with less tension). Sutures are placed to allow the overlap in a vest-over-pants fashion. I prefer three or four 2-0 delayed absorbable sutures. Some surgeons always perform a levatorplasty, but I prefer to individualize adding these additional sutures, as the chance of causing dyspareunia increases with levatorplasty. *(Courtesy the Cleveland Clinic Foundation, Cleveland, Ohio.)*

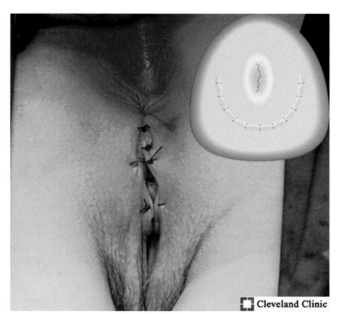

Cleveland Clinic

FIGURE 5 The skin can be closed in many ways. The illustration shows laying the skin flap down and reapproximating it. However, usually the perineal body is lengthened, and the transverse type incision must be closed longitudinally, as shown in the photo. The suture is usually 3-0 absorbable, placed in a simple or mattress fashion. The mid portion can be left open for drainage, or a wick-type drain can be left in the mid portion and positioned in the "dead space," usually on the vaginal side, for several days. The object is to prevent any serous fluid or minor blood ooze from accumulating and becoming infected. The Foley is usually removed on the first day, and I prefer to keep the patient in the hospital at least overnight for pain control and for IV antibiotics. I then discharge them with an additional 5 days of oral antibiotics. *(Courtesy the Cleveland Clinic Foundation, Cleveland, Ohio.)*

Considerable issues with infection and technical malfunction are associated with this device, even after the operator has mastered the learning curve. Problems can be seen in up to 35% or more of patients that lead to explant. However, for those who have an absent or completely defective sphincter mechanism, and a colostomy is their only option, ABS should be considered.

SECCA

There has been renewed interest in the SECCA procedure. Done as an outpatient technique, radiofrequency energy via short needles is delivered in up to 32 targeted areas in the anal sphincter complex to deliver a calculated heat injury. This is believed to produce collagen contraction and deposition that remodels the anal muscle and improves function. The company that initially manufactured the equipment has stopped production. Mederi Therapeutics, Inc. (Greenwich, Conn.) has gained the rights and technology and restarted equipment production, and the treatment will soon be available again. SECCA is targeted to patients with an intact sphincter and minor leakage of fecal material.

Colostomy

While having a colostomy is never an ideal solution, it is recommended when other options fail or are not practical. Having a colostomy allows some who are chained to their toilets the opportunity

to leave their home and function in society. It is important to have potential stoma placement locations marked prior to surgery to avoid poor positioning. Placing the stoma in a crease that precludes a reliable appliance seal will not improve the quality of life for a patient. Some patients may elect to irrigate their colostomy, which allows them to place a small pouch or bandage over the stoma between irrigations. A specialist such as an enterostomal therapy nurse can provide crucial assistance in education, selection of the most optimal pouching equipment, emotional support, and advice in marking the patient before surgery.

INVESTIGATIONAL TREATMENTS IN THE UNITED STATES

Stimulated Graciloplasty

Detaching the gracilis muscle from its distal insertion and wrapping it around the anus, while preserving the proximal nerve and blood supply, is an accepted treatment for fecal incontinence. Addition of a stimulator converts the muscle from type II (short-acting, fast-twitch) to type I (long-acting, slow-twitch) voluntary fibers. Sustained fiber contraction is needed to provide optimum improvement. The stimulator is no longer available in the United States, but it is available in other countries. Like the ABS, there is a high rate of technical complications with this treatment, which has led to reduced enthusiasm to perform it.

Sacral Neuromodulation

Sacral neuromodulation (SNM) has been used for treatment of fecal incontinence outside the United States since the mid-1990s. It is approved in the United States for urinary incontinence, and a large multiinstitutional trial in the United States has been completed in an effort to attain Food and Drug Administration (FDA) approval for bowel issues. This therapy is performed in two stages, which provide the unique ability to gauge therapeutic success prior to implantation. In the first stage, a lead is implanted in the S3 or S4 foramen, and the lead is connected to a temporary external pacemaker. If improvement is seen, a permanent pacemaker is implanted 2 to 3 weeks later beneath the fat pad of the upper buttock. The permanent pacemaker is the same size and shape of most conventional heart pacemakers. This treatment is used extensively outside the United States for patients with an intact but suboptimal functioning sphincter muscle and for muscles with defects. Published studies have shown significant improvement in incontinence scores and quality of life measurements for this therapy.

Injectables

Injection of agents, such as a patented form of silicone injected into the anal canal, has been reported to help some patients with minor fecal incontinence. It is not clear if injection in the submucosa or intersphincteric groove is the ideal location. No injectable agent is FDA approved in the United States, but various studies are underway to obtain results in an effort to obtain FDA approval.

SUMMARY

Management of fecal incontinence is complex, as many factors influence fecal control. There are numerous nonsurgical and surgical options, therefore a detailed history is essential to plan the best combination of treatment for each patient. For a health care provider not associated with a specialized center, nonsurgical and basic surgical treatment can be offered. For patients who do not experience

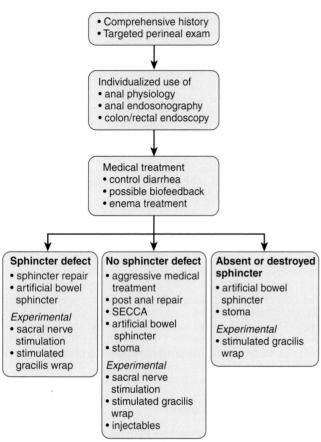

satisfactory improvement in their quality of life after basic treatment, referral to a specialized center should be considered. These patients may qualify for advanced surgical treatment usually performed at these specialized centers. Figure 6 is a general algorithm for treatment considerations.

Selected Readings

Baeten CG, Kuijpers HC: Incontinence. In Wolff BG, Fleshman JW, Beck DE, et al (eds): *The ASCRS textbook of colon and rectal surgery*, New York, 2007, Springer Science and Business Media, pp 653–664.

Hanaway CD, Hull TL: Fecal incontinence, *Obstet Gynecol Clin North Am* 35(2):249–269, 2008.

Hull TL, Zutshi M: Fecal incontinence. In Walters M, Karram M, (eds): *Urogynecology and reconstructive surgery*, Philadelphia, ed 3, 2007, Mosby, pp 309–319.

Lewis SJ, Heaton KW: Stool form scale as a useful guide to intestinal transit time, *Scand J Gastroenterol* 9:920–924, 1997.

Zutshi M, Hull T, Bast J, et al: Ten year outcome after anal sphincter repair for fecal incontinence, *Dis Colon Rectum* 52:1089–1094, 2009.

FIGURE 6   Algorithm outlining various points to be considered when formulating a treatment plan to manage fecal incontinence.

Management of Rectovaginal Fistula

Ashwin L. deSouza, MS, MRCSEd, DNB, and Herand Abcarian, MD

INTRODUCTION

Rectovaginal fistulae constitute one of the most frustrating conditions to treat. Although not life threatening, they are associated with significant morbidity that greatly influence social well-being, sexual activity, and overall quality of life. With a limited number of surgeons conversant in its management, patients with rectovaginal fistulae often present to tertiary referral centers after multiple failed procedures.

Almost all reported literature on the management of rectovaginal fistula is made up of individual case series, each with a small number of patients. It is therefore difficult to objectively compare the results of the different treatment options available. The diverse etiology, numerous treatment options, and lack of randomized trials make it difficult to formulate evidence-based guidelines to optimally manage this condition.

This chapter emphasizes the surgical management of rectovaginal fistula and presents broad treatment guidelines based on current reported literature.

ETIOLOGY

Obstetric injury is the most common cause of rectovaginal fistula. Approximately 2% of all vaginal deliveries are associated with third- and fourth-degree perineal tears, and 3% of these patients will subsequently develop a rectovaginal fistula. Fistulae arising from obstetric injury are often associated with anterior defects in the anal sphincter, leading to some degree of fecal incontinence.

Crohn's disease follows closely as the second most common cause, with 20% to 40% of patients developing either an anorectal or rectovaginal fistula. Rectovaginal fistulae are more likely associated with large bowel compared with small bowel involvement, and it can occur in up to 10% of women with Crohn's disease. Rectovaginal fistulae of Crohn etiology have a high recurrence rate and often require multiple procedures before healing can be achieved.

Surgical trauma, anorectal infection, vaginal or anal neoplasm, and radiation therapy for malignancy constitute the other less common causes (Table 1).

CLINICAL MANIFESTATION

Patients usually present with symptoms of passage of gas or feces through the vagina, although this is often misinterpreted as anal incontinence. Sometimes the clinical presentation may be less obvious, with complaints of a persistent vaginal discharge, dyspareunia, or repeated urinary tract infections.

Because the majority of rectovaginal fistulae are low, digital examination can often locate the indurated fistulous tract. Meticulous

TABLE 1: Rectovaginal fistula etiology

Obstetric injury	Forceps delivery, episiotomy (posterior midline), prolonged labor, third- and fourth-degree perineal lacerations
Inflammatory bowel disease	Crohn's disease
Postsurgical	Anorectal surgery (fistulotomy) Vaginal surgery (hysterectomy, rectocele repair) Abdominal surgery (hysterectomy, low anterior resection, pouch procedure)
Infectious	Cryptoglandular abscess, diverticulitis, tuberculosis
Neoplastic	Anal canal, rectum, vagina, cervix
Radiation induced	External beam radiotherapy, brachytherapy

TABLE 2: Surgical options

Surgical Approach	Procedures
Transanal	Fistulotomy Endorectal advancement flap Rectal sleeve advancement Fibrin glue Bioprosthetics
Transvaginal	Vaginal advancement flap
Transperineal	Episioproctotomy plus layered closure Overlapping sphincteroplasty Interposition flaps
Transabdominal	Primary repair plus omental flap Rectal resection plus coloanal anastomosis and omental flap

examination with an anoscope or speculum usually reveals the granulation tissue around the opening of the fistula, which can be gently probed to delineate the tract. However, not all rectovaginal fistulae are evident on an initial clinical examination. If a high degree of clinical suspicion exists, a thorough examination under anesthesia is justified, especially in patients with Crohn's disease, in whom the activity of disease in the rectum can also be evaluated. On occasion, injection of dilute methylene blue in hydrogen peroxide into the primary opening of a fistula may aid in defining the secondary opening.

The goals of preoperative evaluation are to identify the fistula, determine the etiology, and evaluate the extent of the causative pathology and surrounding injuries. Endoanal ultrasound (EAUS) is an important diagnostic tool to determine defects in the anal sphincter complex, and it can also serve to delineate additional occult collections in complex fistula tracts. Hydrogen peroxide–enhanced transanal ultrasound has also been advocated to map complex fistulae. Pelvic and endorectal MRI are useful diagnostic modalities that are especially popular in European countries.

Tests to determine the functional status of the pelvic floor and anal sphincter are indicated if there is a history of sphincter injury or any degree of incontinence. Anorectal manometry to determine sphincter dysfunction and pudendal nerve terminal motor latency to detect nerve damage are two useful tests to evaluate the function of the pelvic floor. Undiagnosed sphincter injury or pudendal nerve damage could compromise an otherwise successful repair.

After complete workup of the perineum, an evaluation of the entire colon in cases of rectal malignancy, and the small bowel in cases of Crohn's disease, is mandatory. Thus additional workup could include a small bowel series, colonoscopy, barium enema, and a computed tomography scan.

CLASSIFICATION OF RECTOVAGINAL FISTULAE

Rectovaginal fistulae may be classified according their relation to the sphincter complex as *high* (above the sphincter complex) or *low* (at or below the level of the sphincters, also known as *anovaginal*). The low fistula is almost always caused by obstetric trauma and is often associated with sphincter disruption.

Rectovaginal fistulae have also been classified as *simple* or *complex*. Simple fistulae are located in the middle or lower portion of the rectovaginal septum, are less than 2.5 cm in diameter, and are caused by local trauma or sepsis. A complex fistula, on the other hand, is usually greater that 2.5 cm, is located in the upper portion of the rectovaginal septum, and is secondary to causes other than trauma and infection, such as neoplasia, diverticulitis, or inflammatory bowel disease.

PREOPERATIVE PREPARATION

The type of preoperative preparation is largely subjective but usually varies with the type of procedure planned for the repair. For simple advancement flaps, a phosphate enema on the morning of the procedure is usually adequate. For more extensive repairs, such as an overlapping sphincteroplasty or an interposition flap, a full mechanical bowel prep is preferred. Perioperative antibiotics and deep venous thrombosis prophylaxis can be administered as per institutional protocol.

SURGICAL MANAGEMENT

Fistulae due to obstetric injury, which occur in the immediate postpartum period, require at least 3 months for the acute inflammation to subside and for fibrosis to develop. In the interim, symptoms can be improved with stool-bulking agents or with induced mild constipation using loperamide or other antidiarrheals. Once inflammation subsides, a thorough evaluation of the sphincter mechanism should be undertaken to delineate the extent of sphincter disruption.

The presence of sepsis is an absolute contraindication for any attempt at surgical repair, making drainage of abscesses and collections the first step in management. A loose noncutting seton is usually placed through the fistula tract and kept in place until the infection subsides; this may take as long as 3 months, even longer in patients with Crohn's disease.

There are four surgical approaches to repair a rectovaginal fistula: *transanal, transabdominal, transvaginal,* and *transperineal.* Table 2 lists the various surgical options of each approach.

Transanal Approach

Fistulotomy

A fistulotomy involves laying open the fistula tract, which may or may not be excised. This is often performed as a two-stage procedure, in which a noncutting seton is first placed through the fistula to allow for drainage and fibrosis. In the second stage, the seton is removed by dividing the remaining tissue to lay open the tract.

Although a fistulotomy results in successful healing, it involves division of varying thicknesses of the external sphincter muscles. This causes a keyhole deformity, which almost always results in some degree of incontinence, often permanent. Hence a fistulotomy, although only indicated for superficial fistulae, is rarely used.

Endorectal Advancement Flap

Endorectal advancement flap forms the mainstay of treatment for low rectovaginal fistulae and is best suited for patients who do not have disruption of the sphincter muscles. The procedure is usually performed in the outpatient setting and with the patient in prone position, which offers excellent exposure to the anterior rectal wall. Both the anus and vagina are prepped, and a probe is inserted through the fistula from the vagina into the rectum. A trapezoid flap is then outlined with the base cephalad and twice the width of the apex. The flap consists of the rectal mucosa, submucosa, and a portion of the underlying internal sphincter, including the fistula opening at the apex; this is raised in cephalad manner using needle-tip electrocautery. A sufficient length of flap should be mobilized 3 to 4 cm proximal to the fistula opening to ensure a tension-free closure after excision of the fistula. Injection of a dilute epinephrine solution facilitates dissection and minimizes blood loss.

After the flap is elevated, the fistula tract is curetted to remove all granulation tissue, and the defect in the remaining muscle layer (internal sphincter) is closed with a few interrupted absorbable sutures. The tip of the flap is then excised to remove the fistula opening, and the flap is advanced caudad and sutured in place with 3-0 interrupted absorbable sutures to close the wound. The vaginal opening is left open to facilitate drainage. Postoperative care includes a high-fiber diet, sitz baths, and stool softeners to avoid fecal impaction.

The endorectal advancement flap offers the advantages of performing the repair from the high-pressure side of the fistula and of preserving sphincter integrity. Short-term success rates for rectal advancement flaps alone vary from 42% to 68%, although higher success rates have been reported by adding a sphincteroplasty, if a sphincter defect exists.

Rectal Sleeve Advancement

In the presence of limited circumferential or stricturing disease in the distal rectum (e.g., Crohn's disease), a rectal sleeve advancement can be attempted. The procedure involves mobilization of the proximal rectum, resection of the involved distal portion, and restoration of continuity with an anorectal anastomosis.

Kraske Approach

The patient is placed in a semiprone jackknife position, and an incision is made just to the left of the midline, extending from the sacrococcygeal joint to the external anal sphincter. The incision is deepened, and the distal portion of the coccyx is excised. The pelvic floor muscles are then divided in the midline down to the rectum, which is circumferentially mobilized superiorly as far as possible and distally up to the anal canal. The rectum is then transected at the level of the pelvic floor. A circumferential mucosectomy is then performed from the level of the dentate line up to the level of rectal transection. The fistulous tract is completely excised, and the defect in the rectovaginal septum is closed with a few interrupted absorbable sutures. The vaginal defect may be left open for drainage. The mobilized rectum is then advanced to the dentate line and sutured in a single layer with interrupted sutures.

Transabdominal Approach

The patient is placed in the lithotomy position, and the rectum is mobilized anteriorly and posteriorly in standard fashion, right down to the pelvic floor, keeping the lateral vascular supply intact. The rectum is then transected at the pelvic floor, completing the abdominal part of the procedure. The transanal exposure and anastomosis is as described in the Kraske approach.

A rectal sleeve advancement can only be offered if the proximal rectum is normal and is most appropriate in patients with limited, circumferential disease in the distal rectum. Closure rates of 54% to 87% have been described for a rectal sleeve advancement flap in studies with a follow-up greater than 2 years.

Fibrin Glue

Fibrin glue attempts to seal the fistula tract with a fibrin plug, which allows for ingrowth of fibrous tissue that permanently closes the fistula with minimal dissection and no sphincter disruption. However, experience with fibrin glue in rectovaginal fistulae has been very limited because of disappointing results. Extrusion of the fibrin plug due to the short length of the fistula tract is the predominant cause of failure.

Bioprosthetics

Two bioprosthetics have been used for rectovaginal fistulae, the bioprosthetic mesh (Surgisis ES; Cook Surgical, Bloomington, Ind.) and the Rectovaginal Fistula Plug (RVP; Cook Surgical, Bloomington, Ind.). Both products are made from lyophilized porcine intestinal submucosa, which provides a matrix for ingrowth of host connective tissue.

The bioprosthetic mesh is used as an interposition graft. The rectovaginal septum is dissected through a perineal incision, and the fistula is excised. After closure of the rectal and vaginal openings, the rehydrated mesh is placed between the rectum and vagina with an adequate overlap over the rectal and vaginal closures; it is sutured in position with a few interrupted absorbable sutures, keeping the mesh as taut as possible.

The bioprosthetic rectovaginal fistula plug is tapered at one end to facilitate insertion. A fistula probe is introduced from the vaginal to the rectal opening, and the tapered end of the plug is tied to the probe using a suture. The probe is then withdrawn, pulling the plug with it and lodging the button at the broader end at the rectal opening. The excess plug at the rectal end is then excised, and the plug is sutured in position using absorbable sutures, closing the rectal mucosa over the plug. The vaginal opening is left open, and the excess plug is trimmed at this level. The short length of the fistula tract poses the same problem with the plug as with fibrin glue, making the plug only suitable for rectovaginal fistulae that are well over 1 cm in length.

The experience with bioprosthetics as a whole in rectovaginal fistulae is very small. Success rates of fistula closure using interposition techniques have been reported from 66% to 86%

Transvaginal Approach

Vaginal Advancement Flap

Using a technique similar to the rectal advancement flap, a flap of vaginal mucosa is raised, and the fistula tract is excised. The rectal mucosa is closed separately, over which the defect in the rectovaginal septum is approximated with interrupted absorbable sutures. The apex of the flap is then trimmed to excise the fistula opening and is sutured into position to close the wound.

The primary advantage of a vaginal flap is the use of healthy, pliable, and well-vascularized vaginal tissue, even though the repair is on the low-pressure side of the fistula. A vaginal flap is easier to mobilize than a rectal flap, especially in the presence of anorectal stenosis. In a recent comparative analysis of 11 studies, no difference was found in the closure rates between a rectal and vaginal advancement flap in rectovaginal fistulae due to Crohn's disease.

Transperineal Approach

Episioproctotomy and Layered Closure

This repair converts the fistula into a fourth-degree perineal tear by dividing all the tissue between the rectum and vagina through the perineal body. A layered closure is then performed to close the rectal mucosa, the rectal and vaginal muscular walls, and finally the vaginal mucosa. The greatest disadvantage of this procedure is the creation of a full-thickness defect in the anal sphincter. If the repair should fail, the patient will be fully incontinent. For this reason, this procedure should only be attempted in patients with documented existing sphincter disruption and incontinence.

Overlapping Sphincteroplasty

This technique is ideal for patients with concomitant sphincter injury. The detailed technique of an overlapping sphincteroplasty is described elsewhere in this text but essentially involves dissection and mobilization of the external sphincter through a transperineal approach. Very often the sphincter is so attenuated at the site of injury that the healthy ends of the sphincter can be overlapped and sutured into position without dividing or excising any tissue. This technique has the advantage of not worsening the degree of incontinence should the repair fail, while still achieving the same end result. In the presence of sphincter injury, the addition of an overlapping sphincteroplasty to a rectal advancement flap has been reported to greatly increase the success rates

Interposition Flaps

Patients with multiple failed attempts at repair usually have relative ischemia in the surrounding tissues. The interposition of healthy, vascularized tissue in the rectovaginal septum can theoretically increase the chance of successful closure but with a potential risk of de novo dyspareunia. The gracilis and bulbocavernosus flaps are the two most described pedicled flaps for rectovaginal fistula. Although not mandatory, fecal diversion is usually recommended, either before or at the time of the flap procedure.

The approach is usually via a perineal incision between the posterior fourchette of the vagina and the anal verge. The incision is deepened to expose the rectovaginal septum, which is then dissected proximal to the level of the fistula by about 2 cm. The fistula is then completely excised, and the rectal and vaginal defects are closed primarily.

The gracilis muscle has only vestigial function, and a reliable vascular pedicle enters the muscle laterally in its upper third. The muscle of either leg can be used and is harvested through an incision in the medial aspect of the thigh. The harvested muscle is then tunneled through the subcutaneous tissue at the groin and brought out at the perineal incision. This is then placed between the rectum and vagina and held in position using a few interrupted absorbable sutures. The success rate of the gracilis muscle flap has been reported to be as high as 75%.

A Martius flap, using the bulbocavernosus muscle with the overlying fat in the labia majora, is based on the perineal branch of the pudendal artery and is placed in the rectovaginal septum in similar fashion. As with all interposition flaps, this repair has the potential risk for increased postoperative dyspareunia, but there are usually no complaints related to labial function or cosmesis. The success rate with this procedure has been reported to vary from 50% to 93.8%.

Transabdominal Approach

An abdominal approach is best suited to repair high rectovaginal fistulae, which are usually a complication of anterior resection, hysterectomy, or diverticulitis. The rectum is dissected down to the level of the fistula, which is then divided to expose the rectal and vaginal openings. If the rectal wall is healthy and pliable, the fistula opening can be debrided and closed primarily. However, if the surrounding rectum is unhealthy, a resection with primary coloanal anastomosis may be considered. The vaginal opening is then closed, and a pedicled omental flap is placed between the two closures and held in position with a few interrupted sutures.

Sometimes, a low rectovaginal fistula may require an abdominal approach. After the failure of multiple local procedures, further attempts at repair with manipulation of local tissues have a very slim chance of success. A transabdominal approach in this setting has the advantage of resecting all ischemic tissue and bringing down well-vascularized tissues to the anal canal.

The procedure entails mobilization of the rectum and separation of the rectovaginal septum down to the pelvic floor. The fistula openings in the rectum and vagina are then debrided and closed perineally with interrupted absorbable sutures. An omental flap, based on either the left or right gastroepiploic artery, is prepared and placed in the pelvis. Working from the perineum, the lower rectovaginal septum is dissected free. The omental flap is then brought down into the rectovaginal septum and sutured to the subcutaneous tissue of the perineum. Additional sutures are placed to anchor the omentum to the levator ani along the lateral pelvic walls for tension-free interposition (Figure 1). Although this is a major surgical procedure, it brings vascularized omentum into the rectovaginal septum between the rectal and vaginal closures and may be the only option for successful closure in patients with multiple failed procedures.

TREATMENT GUIDELINES

Fecal Diversion

There is no consensus on the indications of proximal fecal diversion in rectovaginal fistulae, as it has been shown that a stoma does not necessarily ensure the success of a repair. However, after two failed attempts, surgeons are more inclined to place a diverting stoma prior to or at the time the third procedure is attempted. Repairs using interposition pedicle flaps are also more likely to be protected with a proximal stoma.

Choice of Repair

Considering the diverse etiology, the large number of surgical options, and the lack of randomized evidence, deciding on a line of treatment is often a daunting task. The choice of procedure is largely governed by the type of fistula (low or high, simple or complex), the etiology, the status of the sphincter mechanism, the number of prior failed attempts, and the functional status of the patient.

The results reported for each procedure vary greatly, and no procedure yields consistent results. It should be appreciated that almost any procedure for rectovaginal fistula is going to fail in a significant number of patients. This is why irreversible steps, like full-thickness sphincter division, which might make the patient worse should the repair fail, are best avoided.

Probably the first point to consider when deciding on a line of treatment is the status of the sphincter mechanism. Documented defects in the anal sphincter with associated incontinence require an overlapping sphincteroplasty. This procedure is often combined with a rectal advancement flap and is the most commonly used first-line option in low fistulae resulting from obstetric trauma.

In the absence of sphincter injury, either a rectal or vaginal advancement flap can be considered as first-line options. Although the results for both procedures are more or less similar, a rectal advancement flap puts the repair on the high-pressure (rectal) side of the fistula and is often preferred over the vaginal flap. However, a rectal flap necessitates the presence of a healthy rectum and is best

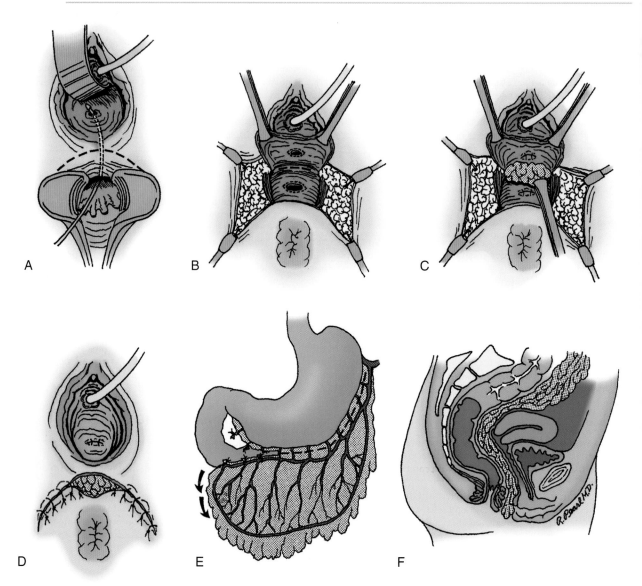

FIGURE 1   A, Probe delineating fistula. *Dashed line* indicates incision site. **B,** Posterior wall of vagina dissected from anterior rectal wall. Fistula sites debrided. Peritoneal cavity entered at apex of plane between vagina and rectum (*dashed line*). **C,** Fistula openings closed with interrupted polyglactin sutures. Mobilized omentum pulled down between vaginal and rectal repairs. **D,** Omentum sutured to subcutaneous tissue of perineum. Center of incision left open for drainage. **E,** Technique of omental mobilization based on left gastroepiploic artery as major blood supply. **F,** Lateral view showing completed interposition. *(Courtesy Russell Pearl, MD.)*

avoided in the presence of poorly controlled Crohn's proctitis or in the presence of stricturing rectal disease.

If a rectal flap fails as the first procedure, it would probably be better to try the vaginal flap at the second attempt rather than to repeat the rectal flap. After failure of both a rectal and vaginal flap, the surgeon has the option of repeating a flap procedure or of considering an interposition pedicle flap. If the local tissues are still healthy and pliable, a repeat flap can be attempted. However, it should be appreciated that at every subsequent procedure, the success rate decreases further. Multiple failed attempts (more than three) render the rectovaginal septum and surrounding tissue ischemic, and further attempts at local repair are less likely to succeed. Interposition flaps should then be considered with appropriate counseling in view of the potential for de novo dyspareunia. Either a gracilis or Martius flap are acceptable alternatives.

Because experience with bioprosthetics is limited, definitive recommendation on their use is impossible. However, because bioprosthetics rely on tissue ingrowth from surrounding tissue, an ischemic rectovaginal septum would probably not be the best environment for

a bioprosthetic mesh. If the proximal rectum is healthy, a distal proctectomy with a coloanal anastomosis will resect the diseased distal rectum, bring healthy proximal rectum to the anal canal, and also provide the opportunity to place a pedicled omental flap in the ischemic rectovaginal septum.

SPECIAL CONSIDERATIONS

Radiation-Induced Fistulae

With the increased use of both brachytherapy and external-beam radiation in the treatment of pelvic malignancies, radiation-induced complications are likely to increase. The first step in management of radiation-induced rectovaginal fistulae is to rule out the presence of residual or recurrent malignancy. This requires detailed imaging and an examination under anesthesia with multiple biopsies of areas of irregularity or random biopsies if no irregularity exists. Once the presence of malignancy has been ruled out, the condition of the rectum, vagina, and surrounding perineal tissues needs to be evaluated.

It is mandatory to wait at least 6 months after the completion of radiation before any repair is attempted. This allows for the full effect of radiation to be realized and for the surrounding tissue to recover. If the local tissues are healthy, a rectal or vaginal advancement flap can be attempted. However, it should be appreciated that because the repair is being performed with radiated tissue, it is less likely to succeed. If one attempt at local repair fails, subsequent attempts will most likely be futile. Interposition flaps using nonradiated tissue (e.g., gracilis flap) or a resection of the involved rectum with a coloanal anastomosis and omental interposition then remain the best available options and are preferable to the classic Bricker procedure.

Crohn's Disease

Almost every patient with Crohn's proctitis and a rectovaginal fistula will require an examination under anesthesia and drainage with a noncutting seton until the infection and inflammation subsides. This is also essential to optimize medical therapy. After quiescence of the acute episode, definitive therapy for the rectovaginal fistula can be pursued.

Local repair is the initial choice in most cases of Crohn-associated rectovaginal fistulae. If the rectum is relatively free from disease, and the rectal wall is pliable, a rectal advancement flap can be attempted. However, in the presence of rectal scarring, this procedure is best avoided. The alternatives include an anocutaneous flap, rectal sleeve advancement, or vaginal flap. An anocutaneous flap can only be done if the anal skin is soft and supple, which is often not the case in patients with Crohn's disease, although a success rate of 70% has been reported for this procedure. The vaginal advancement flap is another alternative for which good healing rates have been reported, especially when a portion of the levator ani muscle is interposed between the rectal and vaginal walls below the flap of vaginal mucosa. Closure rates using this technique have been reported to be as high as 92.3%; however, a 40% to 60% success rate is probably more realistic in Crohn's disease.

Crohn-associated rectovaginal fistulae have an overall poor prognosis with a recurrence rate that varies from 25% to 50%. It is therefore very important to elaborately counsel patients and set realistic treatment goals. In patients with poorly controlled proctitis, surgical options are very limited. Quite often patients are symptomatic from the abscesses associated with the repeated flare-ups of Crohn's proctitis. Prolonged seton drainage for 12 to 18 months epithelializes the fistula tract and limits further episodes of abscess. Very often, patients with multiple failed procedures prefer prolonged seton drainage to a total proctocolectomy and permanent ileostomy, which is the procedure of last resort.

Malignancy

The only definitive treatment of malignant rectovaginal fistulae is an en block surgical extirpation of the fistulous tract with the mass and any contiguous organs involved in the malignant process. This often requires a posterior or total pelvic exenteration. A diverting stoma is often placed to decrease symptoms, while the patient receives neoadjuvant therapy. The patient should then be reevaluated following adjuvant treatment to determine the extent of response and fitness for a major surgical procedure. In patients of good performance status with a satisfactory response to adjuvant therapy, a pelvic exenteration may be considered. However, very few patients fall into this group, and treatment remains palliative in most cases.

ACKNOWLEDGEMENTS

The authors wish to thank Russell Pearl, MD for his contribution of the artwork for this chapter.

SELECTED READINGS

Ellis CN: Outcomes after repair of rectovaginal fistulas using bioprosthetics, *Dis Colon Rectum* 51(7):1084–1088, 2008.

Lefèvre JH, Bretagnol F, Maggioro L, et al: Operative results and quality of life after gracilis muscle transposition for recurrent rectovaginal fistula, *Dis Colon Rectum* 52:1290–1295, 2009.

Ruffolo C, Scarpa M, Bassi N, Angriman I: A systemic review on advancement flaps for rectovaginal fistula in Crohn's disease: transrectal versus transvaginal approach, *Colorectal Dis*, Aug 5, 2009. [epub ahead of print].

Schouten WR, Oom DM: Rectal sleeve advancement for the treatment of persistent rectovaginal fistulas, *Tech Coloproctol*, 13:289–294, 2009.

Venkatesh KS, Ramanujam P: Surgical treatment of traumatic cloaca, *Dis Colon Rectum* 39(7):811–816, 1996.

CONDYLOMA ACUMINATA

Vivek Chaudhry, MBBS, and Russell K. Pearl, MD

OVERVIEW

Condyloma acuminata, or genital warts, is a symptom of infection caused by the human papilloma virus (HPV). This double-stranded DNA virus is one of the most common sexually transmitted diseases. Of the more than 100 HPV genotypes, type 6 and 11 are low-risk types associated with genital warts; high-risk HPV types 16, 18, 31, 33, 45, and 59 are associated with anogenital squamous cell cancers. Genital warts are present in approximately 1% of the general population.

Although sexual transmission is common, fomite transmission in bathrooms and swimming pools, autoinoculation, and puerperial transmission causing respiratory papillomatosis are known to occur.

Direct contact with virus-laden secretions through abrasions of the anogenital macerated skin allows the virus to infect the basal keratinocytes, and proliferation of the keratinocytes causes the genital wart.

Initial infection during teenage years soon after the onset of sexual activity is often cleared within a year. The virus often lies dormant in the basal squamous cells, and many late recurrences of condyloma are due to reactivation of the latent virus. Conversely, small warts may resolve spontaneously. Currently there is no cure for this disease.

Genital warts affect the squamous epithelium and transition zone of the anal canal, perianal skin, scrotum, penis, meatus, groins, vulva, vagina, and cervix. Bleeding, itching, presence of a mass, and difficulty with hygiene are the usual presenting complaints. Rapid growth, ulceration, pain, fixity, and blue-black discoloration should alert the clinician to consider neoplasia. The diagnosis is readily apparent on a careful genital examination, digital rectal examination, and anoscopy with the patient in prone jackknife (Figure 1) or Sims position. Strong focused lighting is essential, and a proctoscopy table is an added advantage. The pelvic and oral cavity should also be examined.

The warts can appear as flat, dome-shaped, keratotic, or cauliflower types. The cauliflower type is most common and appears on non–hair-bearing, partially keratinized squamous epithelium, typically on the anoderm. The lesions may be single, clusters, plaques, or pedunculated. Symmetrical lesions from autoinoculation can occur. Warts may vary in size from microscopic lesions visible on high-resolution colposcopy or anoscopy to giant condylomas greater than 10 centimeters (Figure 2, *A* and *B*).

Differential diagnosis includes molluscum contagiosum, seborrheic keratosis, condyloma lata, squamous or basal cell carcinoma, squamous carcinoma in situ, melanoma, and dysplastic nevus. Large, persistent, symptomatic lesions and lesions in immunosuppressed patients are indications for treatment, even though therapy does not eliminate the risk of transmission or recurrence. The treatment goal is to eradicate all visible warts with preservation of normal intervening anoderm.

Topical therapy is indicated for small, scattered condylomas or as an adjunct to surgical therapy to prevent recurrence. The most common topical agents are listed in Table 1.

TOPICAL THERAPY

Physician-Applied Podophyllin Resin

Podophyllin resin (Podocon-25) is a nonstandardized extract from plant families *Coniferae* and *Berberidaceae* containing podofilox (podophyllotoxin), 4-dimethylpodophyllotoxin, α-peltatum, and β-peltatum. It binds to tubulin to prevent the formation of microtubules, which results in mitotic arrest and tissue necrosis. Podocon-25 is a 25% solution in tincture of benzoin and is approved for physician-directed therapy for moist warts with up to a 10 cm^2 surface area. It is ineffective in dry areas, such as the scrotum, penile shaft, and labia majora. Podophyllin resin is contraindicated in pregnancy and is not appropriate for intranal or mucous membrane disease.

A cotton-tipped applicator is used to apply a thin layer directly to the wart, which is then allowed to air dry. Use 1 drop at a time and

allow drying between drops until the area is covered. Total volume should be limited to less than 0.5 mL per treatment session. Cotton gauze may be left on for a few minutes to prevent inadvertent application to uninvolved skin. Patients are advised to wash the area 2 to 4 hours later and avoid sexual contact for 24 hours. Local side effects include erythema, pain, and irritation. Systemic side effects are nausea, vomiting, diarrhea, paresthesia, polyneuritis, paralytic ileus, pyrexia, leukopenia, thrombocytopenia, and coma caused by increased toxic absorption and are associated with large treatment areas (>10 cm^2) or allowing the resin to absorb for an extended time.

Podofilox (Condylox)

Podofilox (Condylox) is formulated as a standardized preparation. The 0.5% gel is used for perianal disease and is approved for patient-directed therapy. Use the minimum amount to cover the lesion and apply twice daily (morning and evening) with applicator tip or finger for 3 consecutive days, then withhold use for 4 consecutive days. This 1-week cycle may be repeated up to four times or until there is no visible wart tissue. Daily dose should be less than 0.5 g, and treatment area should be limited to 10 cm^2 or less of wart tissue. Additional applications increase the rate of local adverse reactions and systemic absorption. If there is incomplete response after four treatment cycles, discontinue treatment and consider an alternative treatment.

Trichloroacetic Acid

Trichloroacetic acid (Tri-Chlor; TCA) is a topical cauterizing agent. TCA rapidly penetrates and cauterizes skin, keratin, and other tissue. Care should be taken to prevent overapplication because the solution is thin and extremely caustic. It can be applied to intra-anal disease and during pregnancy. Side effects include burning, pruritus, and tenderness.

Imiquimod

The exact mechanism of action of imiquimod (Aldara) is unknown. It is an immunomodulator and induces mRNA encoding cytokines, including interferon-α at the treatment site. Apply a thin layer to the affected areas once daily three times per week on nonconsecutive nights just prior to sleep. The cream should be left on the skin for 6 to 10 hours and then washed off with mild soap and water.

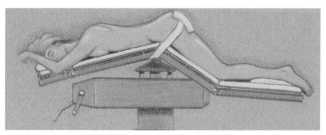

FIGURE 1   Prone jackknife position.

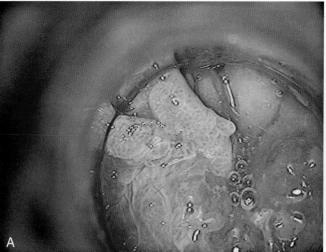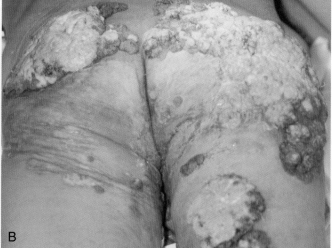

FIGURE 2   **A,** High-resolution anoscopy image showing small condyloma at the dentate line. The anal pap smear showed low-grade squamous intraepithelial lesion. **B,** Extensive giant condyloma.

TABLE 1: Most common topical agents for treatment of condyloma acuminata

Treatment	Mechanism of Action	Dose	Note	Success %	Recurrence (%)
Provider Applied					
Podophyllin resin (25%), 25% suspension in tincture of benzoin	Induces tissue necrosis by disruption of the mitotic spindle	Apply as a thin layer with cotton-tipped applicator, allow to air-dry, weekly for three applications. Avoid sexual contact, bathing, and contact with uninvolved skin.	Contains mutagenic flavonoids—avoid during pregnancy. Limit to <10 cm² to avoid systemic toxicity (nausea, vomiting, abdominal pain, bone marrow, liver, neurologic side effects). Not indicated for intra-anal disease.	45–88	4–38
BCA/TCA 30% to 70%	Acid is corrosive, denatures proteins Minimal absorption	Apply weekly, sparingly with cotton-tipped applicator, allow to air dry	Thin liquid, tendency to spread if over-applied. Local pain, ulceration may follow. Can be used intraanally and during pregnancy.	63–70	
Cryotherapy, liquid nitrogen	Induces cold necrosis	Freeze with cryoprobe 1 to 2 mm beyond visible wart. Local anesthesia and two freeze–thaw cycles may be used for larger lesions.	Requires training and experience; it is difficult to assess depth of destruction. Blistering and wound pain result if overtreated or with larger lesions.	27–40	38–73
Patient Applied					
Imiquimod 5%	Immunomodulator induces macrophages to produce cytokines IL-2, IFN-α	Apply cream to effected area at night three times a week; wash in morning for up to 16 weeks Adjunctive use after other therapies may reduce recurrence.	Mild to severe erythema and burning may result; severe inflammation results if applied to nonintact skin. Most appropriate for small, scattered lesions. Not useful for intraanal disease. Safety during pregnancy is unknown, and contraception is advised.	27–54	13–19
Podofilox (Condylox) 0.5% gel, solution, or cream	Tissue necrosis by disrupting mitotic spindle	Twice daily for 3 consecutive days/week for 2 to 4 weeks.	Local irritation results. Limit use to <10 cm². Devoid of mutagenic flavonoids. Safety during pregnancy is unknown, and contraception is advised.	37	4–38

BCA, Bichloroacetic acid; IFN-α, interferon-α; IL-2, interleukin-2; TCA, trichloroacetic acid.

Percutaneous absorption is minimal. Continue therapy until there is a total clearance of warts or for a maximum of 16 weeks (median time to complete wart clearance is about 10 weeks). In a double-blind placebo-controlled trial, eradication of baseline warts was observed in 50% of patients treated with 5% imiquimod cream and in 11% of patients who received vehicle cream. Clinically, the onset of effect is gradual, with most patients (83%) showing some response to treatment in 4 weeks. Median time to complete clearance was 8 weeks for females and 12 weeks for males; however, wart clearing may take up to 16 weeks. The response rate may be lower in immunosuppressed patients (an 11% response rate was reported in one study of HIV-infected patients).

Systemic, topical, or intralesional interferon has been evaluated and cannot be recommended in the routine treatment of warts due to inconsistent results, side effects, and cost. Topical 5-fluorouracil (5-FU) cream has been used in small case series and in patients with extensive anal intraepethelial neoplasia (AIN). It is a mutagen and teratogen, so it is contraindicated in pregnancy and is not recommended for routine use for the treatment of warts. Cidofovir is a nucleoside analog that inhibits viral polymerases. It has been used systemically to treat cytomegalovirus (CMV) and herpes. Topical application for warts requires further studies to establish its efficacy.

In our practice small, scattered condylomas on the perianal skin are treated with patient-applied imiquimod or podofilox, and patients are reexamined after 8 to 12 weeks. Physician-applied 25% podophyllin resin is an alternative; it is applied in the office once a week for three to four applications, though a recent randomized trial showed patient-applied Condylox was superior to physician-applied podophyllin. Surgical excision and fulguration is indicated for atypical presentation, larger warts, and recalcitrant disease.

SURGICAL TREATMENT

Surgical treatment of condyloma is usually administered under monitored anesthesia care, spinal anesthesia, or general anesthesia with the patient in a prone jackknife or lithotomy position. Gluteal folds are retracted with 3 inch tape applied parallel to the gluteal crease and pulled forward and laterally; the greater trochanter is positioned at the table break, and a pubic gel pad is positioned over the table break. Proper positioning ensures that the anal canal axis is at right angles to the floor with protection of the external genitalia (see Figure 1).

Prophylactic antibiotics and bowel prep are unnecessary. Application of 3% to 4% acetic acid (small gauze wrapped around a cotton-tipped application, applied through an anoscope) for 1 to 2 minutes enhances visualization of the lesions. Discrete lesions are sharply excised with scissors, and the base is fulgurated with electrocautery. Smaller lesions are fulgurated directly, the eschar is wiped away

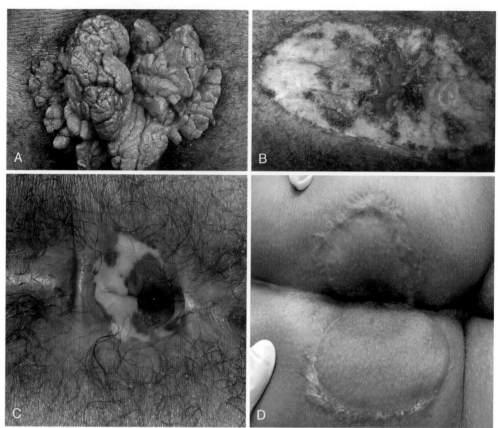

FIGURE 3   **A,** Confluent condyloma of the anal margin. **B,** Intraoperative image after resection. **C,** Postoperative image at 2 months demonstrating healing with anal stenosis. **D,** Postoperative image demonstrating healed result after bilateral dermal advancement flap.

gently, and the base is electrocoagulaed to ensure destruction of tissue to the upper dermis. Intranal lesions are excised and fulgurated.

Care is taken to avoid nuisance bleeding from too deep a fulguration over the hemorrhoidal plexus. Large, firm, and discrete lesions should be sent for histopathologic examination, and the site of excision must be documented accurately. Anatomical terms *left, right anterior,* and *posterior* are preferred over terminology based on clock positions because the patient position is variable.

Postoperative management consists of tepid water baths or showers three times a day and after every bowel movement (sitz baths), pain medications, stool softeners, and dry gauze dressings to the perianal area. The patient is seen within 2 weeks and every 4 weeks until wounds heal completely. Patients are followed for 3 months for the first year, for 6 months for the second year, and annually after that. Early recurrent lesions are treated with topical agents. In patients prone to early recurrence, prophylactic use of topical agents may be useful but are limited by severe irritation if applied to healing wounds. Postoperative bleeding and infection are infrequent. Caution should be taken to prevent large open wounds in patients with AIDS with low CD4 counts (<200), high viral loads, and wasting. The mere presence of HIV is not a contraindication to surgical therapy.

Anal stenosis can occur if circumferential lesions are treated or care is not taken to preserve normal anoderm. Staged excisions have been proposed but have no proven benefit. Mild anal stenosis can be treated with a high-fiber diet and anal dilatation. More severe stenosis can be treated with unilateral or bilateral dermal advancement flap anoplasty (Figure 3, *A* to *D*). Anoplasty at initial excision is unnecessary in most cases and carries the risk of recurrent condyloma growing under the flap.

Laser therapy for anogenital warts is used infrequently. It is expensive and requires special equipment and training with no particular advantage. Any given treatment carries a 40% to 75% chance of clearing and a 25% to 50% chance of recurrence. Recurrence is responsible for a prolonged course for the patient. Treatment failure is commonly caused by improper selection or use of a therapeutic modality. At the present time, all treatments are comparable in effectiveness.

It is important to educate patients to tell sexual partners that they have this infection. Condoms may decrease but do not completely prevent transmission. Treatment of genital lesions may not eliminate infectivity. Women with external genital warts or whose male partners have lesions should have a Pap smear, and investigations for other STDs should be done if suspected.

GIANT CONDYLOMA

Giant condyloma, or Buscke-Loewenstein tumor, has local malignant potential frequently presenting with fistulae and invasion into deeper structures. The definition of *giant* is unclear, and lesions more than 5 to 10 cm, especially with locally invasive pathology with increased mitosis, marked papillomatosis, and thickened, discrete ridges qualify. Invasive squamous cell carcinoma (SCC) can develop or be present in up to one half of the patients and needs to be ruled out by generous biopsies. This is in comparison with 1.8% incidence of SCC in 330 patients with condyloma reported by Abcarian and Prasad (1976).

Wide local excision is the treatment of choice. Oral retinoids and imiquimod have been tried as adjunctive therapies for smaller lesions. Reconstruction with skin grafts, flaps, or abdominoperineal resection may be necessary for larger lesions. Reports that include a patient in our experience have shown a lesion that responded completely to chemoradiation therapy (5-FU, mitomycin C, and 5040 cGy radiation). However, recurrence rates as high as 66% have been reported. Radical resection after failure of local surgery and chemoradiation often require reconstruction with rectus abdominus or other myocutaneous flaps to ensure healing of the large perineal wound (Figure 4, *A* to *F*).

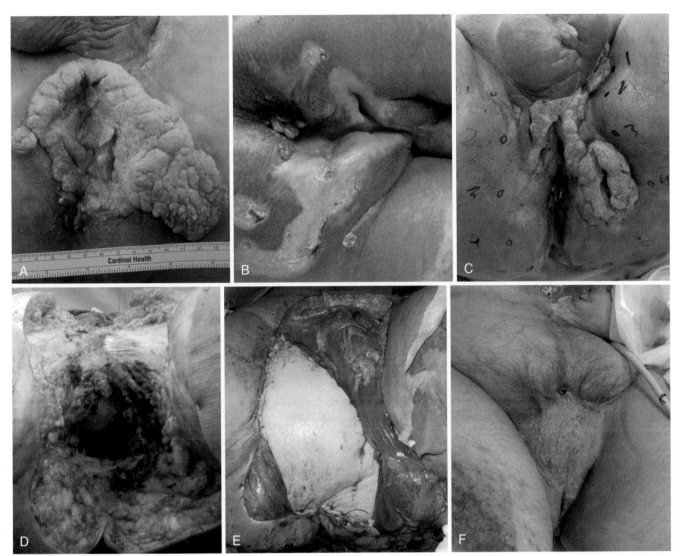

FIGURE 4   **A,** Giant condyloma extending to base of scrotum with focus of microinvasive carcinoma. **B,** Complete clinical regression after treatment with 5-FU, mitomycin C, and 5400 cGy radiation. **C,** Recurrence of disease, now involving scrotum, urethra, and bone. **D,** Recurrence of treated abdominoperineal resection with en bloc resection of genitalia, pubic bone, and perineum. **E,** Reconstruction with bilateral vertical rectus abdominus musculocutaneous flaps and skin graft. **F,** Postoperative image demonstrating complete healing of the perineum.

CONDYLOMA IN FISTULA-IN-ANO

Patients with condylomas in a fistula-in-ano should be tested for HIV and biopsied in the operating room to rule out invasive carcinoma. Fistulotomy with fulguration of condylomas is appropriate if the fistula is superficial and there is no concern of incontinence. Frequently, however, the fistulas are transphincteric in partially continent patients with advanced HIV disease and medication-induced diarrhea. Long-term draining setons with frequent destruction of lesions is the most appropriate therapy for now.

CONDYLOMA WITH DYSPLASIA

Anal Pap and High-Resolution Anoscopy

Anal cancer and dysplasia incidence is increasing, especially in homosexual men with HIV. Additional risk factors for dysplasia and cancer are HIV infection, transplantation, cervical or vulvar neoplasia, smoking, condyloma, and anal intercourse; highly active antiretroviral therapy has not decreased the incidence of disease.

Anal cytology has equivalent sensitivity and specificity to cervical cytology in detecting anal cancer precursors. Terminology used in describing cytological findings is similar to cervical Pap: atypical squamous cells of undetermined significance (ASC-US) and low-grade (LSIL) or high-grade squamous intraepithelial neoplasia (HSIL).

Abnormal cytology should trigger colposcopic examination of the anal canal with biopsy and destruction of suspicious lesions. Colposcopic abnormalities of coarse and fine punctation, mosaicism, abnormal vessels, and raised aceto-white lesions are looked for, recorded, biopsied, and photographed. The lesions are classified as low-grade (LGAIN, AIN grade 1, and condyloma) or high-grade anal intraepithelial neoplasia (HGAIN, AIN grades 2 and 3). LGAIN can be watched or treated, and HGAIN is treated with TCA, infrared coagulation, or electrocautery with topical anesthesia. Patients with larger or more extensive lesions require colposcopic-directed destruction with electrocautery in the operating room.

Hybrid capture-II HPV DNA detection test can identify any of a group of 13 high-risk type HPVs and in some studies has been shown to have a high sensitivity and acceptable specificity in detecting HSIL.

There is limited information about the natural course of HGAIN. Concern about the efficacy and side effects of treatment has limited

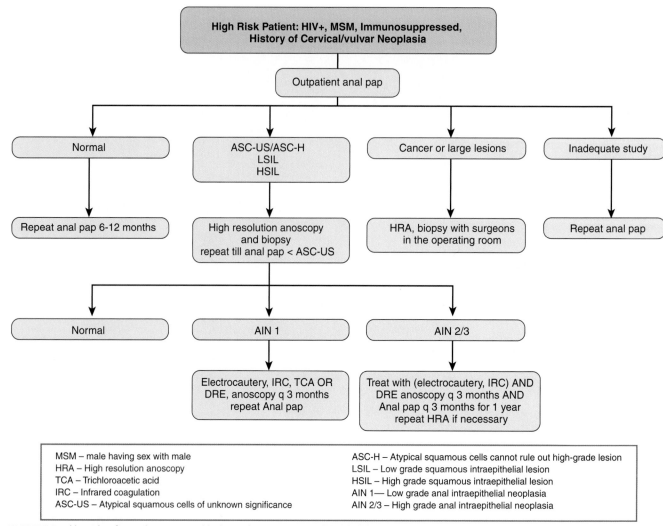

FIGURE 5   Algorithm for anal pap test and high-resolution anoscopy. *(Modified from Palefsky JM, Rubin M: The epidemiology of anal human papillomavirus and related neoplasia, Obstet Gynecol Clin North Am 36[1]:187-200, 2009.)*

the acceptability of anal cytology/high-resolution anoscopy to a few centers. A recent report of 246 patients over 10 years with high-grade lesions showed that though recurrence was common (57), only a quarter of these required surgery; most were treated with office-based HRA procedures for an overall success rate of 78%.

Efficacy improves with experience. Until data and expertise with this technique become more widespread, clinicians should be vigilant for anal cancer; at the minimum, clinicians should perform routine visual inspection and digital rectal examination. Figure 5 demonstrates the protocol used at our institution.

HUMAN PAPILLOMA VIRUS VACCINE

Early attempts at an autologous vaccine from wart extracts injected subcutaneously showed excellent response in 84% with only 5% patients not responding. Modern vaccines are prepared with recombinant genetic engineering techniques.

Prophylactic Vaccine

The current FDA-approved prophylactic HPV (*VLP*, viruslike particle capsid protein) quadrivalent vaccines protect against 70% of HPV 16– and HPV 18–associated anogenital cancers, and

90% of anogenital warts are caused by two strains of HPV (6 and 11). HPV vaccination (Gardasil) has been approved for girls and young women from 9 to 26 years of age, and the FDA has recently approved Gardasil for use in adolescent boys to prevent warts. Many experts feel that boys and young men would benefit from a vaccine that protects against HPV infection, especially anogenital warts, as well as penile and anal carcinomas. Studies are underway to increase the cross-genotype neutralizing capacity of VLP-based vaccines with the incorporation of the L2 (minor capsid protein) vaccines.

Therapeutic Vaccine

Host cell transformation results when HPV viral protein E6 binds to p53, and E7 deactivates pRb and certain cyclin-dependent kinase inhibitors. Therapeutic vaccines against the HPV E6 and E7 viral proteins are being tested, especially in the HIV population. They have been shown to be safe and well tolerated in small studies. Most report moderate reversible injection-site reactions and up to a fourfold increase in anti–HPV 16 antibody and a threefold increase in interferon-γ levels compared with prevaccination levels. The therapeutic efficacy is unknown, though case reports showing tumor response in metastatic cervical cancer from anti–HPV 18 are encouraging. The results of future studies are eagerly anticipated. It is possible that in the near future, anogenital warts and cancers will be prevented and treated with a vaccine.

SUMMARY

Condyloma acuminata is a sexually transmitted disease caused by nononcogenic HPV, usually types 6 and 11. Visual anogenital examination, digital rectal examination, and anoscopy with good exposure and lighting is crucial for accurate diagnosis of anogenital disease. Surgical excision and fulguration with or without adjunctive topical therapy is the primary therapy for larger, atypical, or recalcitrant disease. Preservation of normal skin and anoderm is critical because recurrences are common, and all therapies have similar efficacy. Patients and partners should be counseled and tested for other sexually transmitted diseases if indicated. Screening and treatment of high-grade AIN with high-resolution anoscopy is available and is practiced in a few specialized centers, but it has unproven efficacy in preventing anal cancer. At minimum, clinicians are advised to perform frequent anoscopy and digital rectal examination, especially in the immunosuppressed population. HPV vaccines may play an important role in prevention and treatment of anogenital warts and cancers.

SUGGESTED READINGS

Abcarian H, Sharon N: Immunotherapy in treatment of anal condyloma acuminatum, *Surg Forum* 27(62):127–129, 1976.
Anderson JS, Hoy J, Hillman R, et al: A randomized, placebo-controlled, dose-escalation study to determine the safety, tolerability, and immunogenicity of an HPV-16 therapeutic vaccine in HIV-positive participants with oncogenic HPV infection of the anus, *J Acquir Immune Defic Syndr* 52(3):371–381, 2009.

Edwards L, Ferenczy A, Eron L, et al: Self-administered topical 5% imiquimod cream for external anogenital warts, *Arch Dermatol* 134:25–30, 1998.
Goldstone SE, Hundert JS, Huyett JW: Infrared coagulator ablation of high-grade anal squamous intraepithelial lesions in HIV-negative males who have sex with males, *Dis Colon Rectum* 50(5):565–575, 2007.
Hellberg D, Svarrer T, Nilsson S, et al: Self-treatment of female external genital warts with 0.5% podophyllotoxin cream (Condyline) vs. weekly applications of 20% podophyllin solution, *Int J STD AIDS* 6(4):257–261, 1995.
Hoyme UB, Hagedorn M, Schindler AE, et al: Effect of adjuvant imiquimod 5% cream on sustained clearance of anogenital warts following laser treatment, *Infect Dis Obstet Gynecol* 10(2):79–88, 2002.
Koutsky LA, Ault KA, Wheeler CM, et al: A controlled trial of a human papillomavirus type 16 vaccine, *N Engl J Med* 347(21):1645–1651, 2002.
Palefsky JM, Berry JM, Jay N, et al: The epidemiology of anal human papillomavirus and related neoplasia, *Obstet Gynecol Clin North Am* 36:187–200, 2009.
Pineda CE, Rubin M, High-resolution anoscopy targeted surgical destruction of anal high-grade squamous intraepithelial lesions: a ten-year experience, *Dis Colon Rectum* 51(6):829–835, 2009.
Wiley DJ, Douglas J, Beutner K, et al: External genital warts: diagnosis, treatment, and prevention, *Clin Infect Dis* 35(suppl 2):S210–S224, 2002.
Wolf BG, Fleshman JW, et al: *The ASCRS textbook of colon and rectal surgery*, ed 1, New York, 2007, Springer.

PILONIDAL DISEASE

Philippe Bouchard, MD, and Jonathan E. Efron, MD

ETIOLOGY

Originally thought to be secondary to remnants of a congenital appendage in the gluteal cleft, pilonidal disease is now postulated to originate from a penetration of hairs in the subcutaneous tissue of the intergluteal cleft, causing foreign body reaction, inflammation, and potential abscess formation. High recurrence rates despite adequate excision, occurrence of pilonidal sinuses at nongluteal locations, and a propensity for the disease in hirsute individuals all support the acquired, as opposed to congenital, theory of etiology.

Called "Jeep driver's disease" during World War II, pilonidal disease is more commonly seen in individuals with sedentary occupations or in those whose occupation results in repeated mild trauma to the perineum, such as truck drivers. Pilonidal disease is three to four times more common in men, with an incidence of 26 per 100,000. The average age of diagnosis is between 20 and 35 years.

DIAGNOSIS

The spectrum of clinical symptoms ranges from acute abscess formation to chronic draining sinus tracts. An acute pilonidal abscess is the usual first manifestation of the disease, which occurs with swelling, redness, pain in the midline gluteal cleft area, and sometimes spontaneous drainage. Sinus tract formation in the midgluteal area, with or without cyclical drainage and pain, represents the more chronic

form of the disease. The identification of midline pits during physical exam confirms the diagnosis (Figure 1); these are referred to as the *primary opening.*

Multiple pits may be identified along the gluteal cleft. Sinus tracts extend cephalad in the majority of the cases. Tezel has described a classification scheme for pilonidal disease. Type I is asymptomatic disease, identified by the presence of gluteal cleft pits; type II refers to an acute pilonidal abcess; type III represents symptomatic disease limited to the navicular area, which is defined as the borders of the intergluteal sulcus (natal cleft); type IV is extensive disease that extends outside the natal cleft; and type V refers to recurrent disease (Table 1).

Differential Diagnosis

The differential diagnosis of pilonidal disease includes perianal abscess or fistula, hidradentis suppurativa, or granulomatous diseases such as syphilis or tuberculosis. When the suspected pilonidal tract extends caudally close to the anus, it is imperative to rule out perianal fistula as a cause for the tract. Osteomyelitis with draining sinus and actinomycosis of the sacral area are rare diagnoses that may mimic pilonidal sinus tracts; these should be ruled out in recurrent disease.

PILONIDAL ABSCESS

Primary treatment of a pilonidal abscess is incision and drainage. Oral or intravenous antibiotic therapy without concomitant drainage is inadequate. Drainage can usually be performed without a general anesthetic; the incision should be made parallel and at least 1 cm lateral to the midline, thereby allowing for adequate healing.

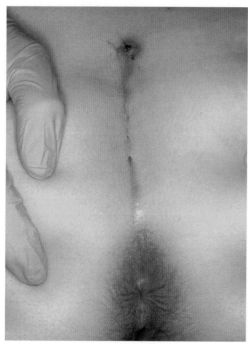

FIGURE 1   Midline pits in the gluteal cleft represent a classic finding of pilonidal disease.

TABLE 1: Clinical classifications of sacrococcygeal pilonidal disease according to the navicular area concept

Type	Definition
I	Asymptomatic
II	Acute pilonidal abscess
III	Symptomatic disease limited to navicular area
IV	Extensive disease that extends outside the navicular area
V	Recurrent disease after any kind of definitive pilonidal surgery

From Tezel E: A new classification according to navicular area concept for sacrococcygeal pilonidal disease, *Colorectal Dis* 9(6):575-576, 2007.

A cruciform or elliptic incision is performed with removal of the skin to avoid early skin closure and recurrence of abscess formation.

Antibiotic coverage is usually not necessary but may be required in immunocompromised patients and in those with significant cellulitis or diabetes. Antibiotic coverage should be broad in nature, with both aerobic and anaerobic coverage. With adequate drainage, packing is not necessary; when used, it is often associated with increased pain. Patients are instructed to use a sitz bath or handheld shower two to three times a day to keep the area clean and to apply dry dressings after cleaning. The skin surrounding the wound should be shaved weekly, either at home or in the surgeon's office, until complete healing has occurred. Many patients (approximately 60%) will have resolution of their pilonidal disease with this conservative approach.

It is crucial to not perform a definitive excision of the pilonidal disease and pits in the face of acute infection. This leads to more extensive surgery with significantly larger wounds, increased risk of wound complications, and increased chances of recurrence.

TABLE 2: Surgical options for the treatment of pilonidal sinus

Midline Approach
Sinus excision: open vs. marsupialization vs. closure
Unroofing and Curettage
Asymetric or oblique excision
Karydakis procedure
Bascom: open vs. closure
Cleft
Flaps
Rhomboid
V-Y advancement
Z-plasty
Gluteal myocutaneous
Others
Phenolization
Vacuum-assisted closure

PILONIDAL SINUS

As with all surgical patients, prior to intervention the surgeon must determine the extent of disease, symptoms, and prior interventions. Patients' expectations and occupations may also influence the treatment, and patients should be informed about healing time of the proposed procedure and the risk of recurrence. The final aesthetic result is important for many individuals, and they should be informed that if a flap procedure is utilized, it will change the appearance and orientation of the gluteal cleft, leaving a more apparent scar.

Indications for surgical intervention include chronic pain, recurrent abscesses, or chronic drainage; asymptomatic pilonidal pits do not require excision. Multiple treatments are available for the management of pilonidal disease, including various surgical approaches (Table 2). The treatment chosen is based on the extensiveness of the disease and whether the disease is primary or recurrent, and it is hoped that the chosen procedure will be less morbid than the disease.

NONSURGICAL APPROACH

For asymptomatic or only mildly symptomatic patients with draining pilonidal sinuses, a conservative approach may be reasonable. Some authors have reported resolution of small sinuses by treating the patient with only repeated shavings. The patient is instructed to shave a 5 cm strip circumferentially around the gluteal cleft weekly until complete healing occurs. No data are available on whether persistent shaving is required after healing. Laser hair removal has been described as an alternative to shaving with good results.

Injection of phenol into the sinus tracts has also been described. Between 1 and 2 mL of 80% phenol is injected into the tracts to induce inflammation and scarring. This procedure is quite painful and is often performed under anesthesia, which requires hospitalization for pain control after treatment. Great care must be taken to avoid phenol contact with the surrounding skin, and shaving the area and maintaining the area free of hair during healing is essential.

SURGICAL TECHNIQUES

Preoperative Care and Positioning

Perioperative antiobiotic use has not been proven to improve wound complication rates, recurrence rate, or healing times; therefore only standard preoperative antibiotics are recommended. A perioperative antibiotic may be considered when a more extensive surgery is performed, such as a rotational flap with drains left in place. The surgery may be performed under a local anesthetic with sedation or under a regional anesthesia, but it is often performed under general anesthesia to ensure airway control. All patients are positioned in the prone position, with or without a jackknife, and the buttocks are often taped apart to allow for visualization of the gluteal cleft.

Midline Approaches

Unroofing

Prior to prepping the patient, hair surrounding the guteal cleft is shaved. After prepping and draping, the pilonidal pits are probed utilizing a fistulotomy probe, and the tract is opened along its entire length (Figure 2). The fibrous tract is curetted and cauterized to remove debris and remaining hair; it can be left open and packed, or the dermis can be marsupialized to the baseline fistula tract using an absorbable suture. The surgeon must be sure that all sinus tracts are unroofed; leaving unopened tracts correlates with an increased recurrence rate.

Postoperatively, patients are seen on a weekly basis, and the surrounding skin is shaved to prevent hair growth into the wound. Complete healing is usually accomplished at 6 weeks (Table 3), but patients often will have only minimal discomfort after 2 weeks and can return to their normal activities. Healing time depends on the size of the wound and on the patient's body habitus. Unroofing reduces the size of the wound by approximately 50% compared with complete sinus excision. A success rate of 90% is possible with diligent postoperative care that ensures no hair regrowth.

Sinus Excision

Midline excision consists of complete removal of the pits and sinus tracts originating from the pilonidal disease. A margin of a few millimeters of normal skin is adequate for excision, and although it is not required to excise the tissue down to the presacral fascia, it may be required, depending on the depth of the sinus tracts. This technique is associated with a long healing time, up to 2 months, and it provides no advantage over unroofing and marsupialization. Prior to excision, it is often beneficial to probe the sinus with a lacrimal cannula or a fistulotomy probe to define the extent of the sinus tracts. Another technique utilizes the injection of methylene blue into the pits or sinus tract openings to fully define the extent of the tracts.

Four options are available for dealing with the open wound. It may be left opened, the dermis may be marsupialized, an attempt at primary closure may be undertaken, or vacuum suction may be applied to attempt to accelerate wound closure. Patients who have open wounds take longer to heal and have greater wound care requirements than those who are primarily closed, but recurrence rates are up to 40% higher in patients with primary closure, so it is generally not recommended. Within the first 2 weeks, most wounds primarily closed in the midline will dehisce secondary to lateral pressure created by sitting, requiring extensive wound care.

Marsupialization is felt to provide some benefit over the open-wound procedure by decreasing the wound size, which decreases the healing time and also prevents premature closure of the wound. This benefit, however, has been difficult to clearly define. Marsupialization

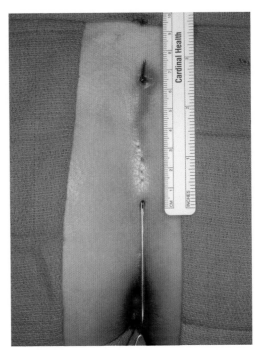

FIGURE 2 Probing the fistula tract. The first step prior to unroofing the pilonidal sinus.

is performed with resorbable suture by tacking the dermal edge of the skin to the base of the wound (Figure 3).

As with unroofing, the average healing time of marsupialization is 6 weeks, with a recurrence rate of approximately 4% to 8%. Follow-up care is similar to unroofing. Finally, placing a vacuum dressing after excision or unroofing has been reported and may be useful when a large defect is created to help facilitate dressings and wound closure. Limited data are available on this technique, and recurrence rates are not known.

Asymmetric or Oblique Techniques

Bascom Procedure

This technique involves a lateral approach off the natal cleft without flap formation. Initially the midline pits are removed through a 2 to 4 mm elliptical incision or using a punch biopsy. An incision is then made 2 cm lateral and parallel to the natal cleft, and dissection is continued medially until the pilonidal sinus tracts are accessed (Figure 4). Curettage of the cavity is performed to remove all debris and granulation tissue. Initially the technique was described leaving the lateral defect open with packing to close by secondary intention. Some surgeons now opt for closing the lateral defect. This technique is relatively simple, with an average healing time of 3 weeks. Long-term results are similar to those of the midline approach (see Table 3).

Cleft Bascom Procedure

This technique was developed for the treatment of recurrent pilonidal disease with the goal to lateralize the natural cleft with a skin flap. The first step is to remove an asymmetric ellipse of skin off the midline that includes the midline pits (Figure 5). The fat is not excised. The midline cavity is cleaned, and debris is removed with curettage. A skin flap is raised from the opposite side and sutured to cover the defect to create a shallow sulcus. Wound breakdown and infection are the main complications of that technique (see Table 3).

TABLE 3: Surgical results and recurrence rates

Procedure	IP or OP	Dressing Changes Required	Time to Healing (Average)	Infection (%)	Wound Breakdown (%)	Recurrence (%)
Sinus excision with an open wound	OP	Yes	6–13 weeks	<5	NA	2–10
Unroofing and curettage with or without marsupiliazation	OP	Yes	6–8 weeks	0–2	NA	4–8
Midline excision and closure	OP	No	2–3 weeks	0–35	1, 5–7	1–21
Karydakis	IP	No	2 weeks	1.8	1.8–8.5	0.9–4.4
Bascom	OP	Depends	3 weeks	4–8	0–7	8–10
Cleft	OP	No	3–11 days	1–22	8–16	1–3
Rhomboid	IP	No	4–6 weeks	1–6	1–3	2–5
V-Y advancement	IP	No	4–6 weeks	0–4	0–8	0–10
Z-plasty	IP	No	4–6 weeks	1–6	1–8	2–8
Gluteal myocutaneous	IP	No	NS	NS	NS	NS

IP, Inpatient procedure; *OP,* outpatient procedure; *n/a,* not applicable; *n/s,* not specified

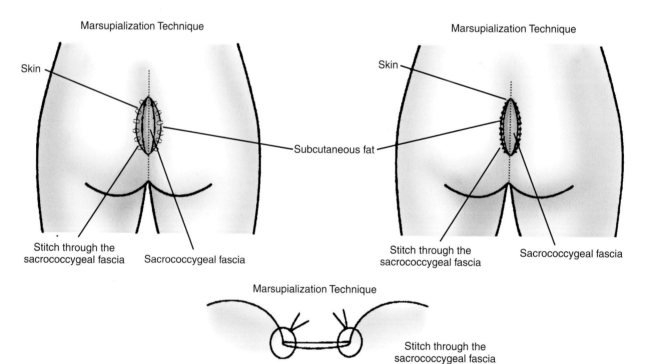

FIGURE 3   Marsupialization technique. *(From Lee PJ, Raniga S, Biyani DK, et al: Sacrococcygeal pilonidal disease, Colorectal Dis 10:639–652, 2008.)*

Karydakis Procedure

Karydakis was the first to propose excision and wound closure away from the midline. Because of poor midline healing of the midgluteal area, the lateralization or abolition of the natal cleft was theorized to increase wound healing. This technique is an asymmetrical excision of the midline until the sacral fascia is reached. A lateral advancement flap with subcuateous tissue is raised to close the defect away from the natal cleft (Figure 6). This technique can be used for recurrent midline pilonidal sinus disease. Reported results from multiple series are good, with low documented recurrence rates (see Table 3).

Flaps

Flap closures can be used for either large primary defects or to treat recurrent disease. Some authors have advocated using a flap closure for type III midline disease. Our preference is to utilize rotational

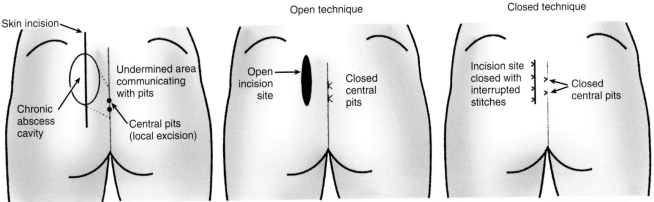

FIGURE 4 Bascom technique. *(From Lee PJ, Raniga S, Biyani DK, et al: Sacrococcygeal pilonidal disease, Colorectal Dis 10:639–652, 2008.)*

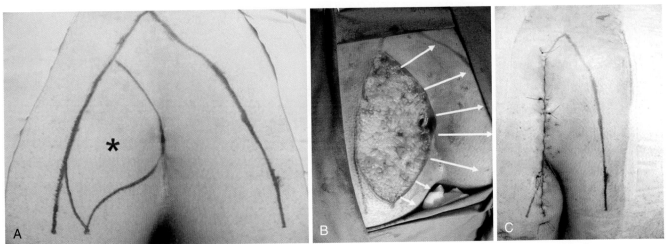

FIGURE 5 Cleft technique. *(From Tezel E, Bostanci H, Anadol AZ, et al: Cleft lift procedure for sacrococcygeal pilonidal disease, Dis Colon Rectum 52[1]:135–139, 2009.)*

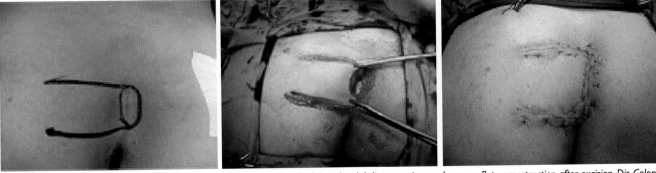

FIGURE 6 Karydakis procedure. *(From Mahdy T: Surgical treatment of the pilonidal disease: primary closure or flap reconstruction after excision, Dis Colon Rectum 51:1816–1822, 2008.)*

flaps primarily for recurrent disease or for extensive disease outside of the natal cleft. Closure of a pilonidal excision site with a rotational flap is a more extensive intervention compared with the other procedures previously described, and it usually necessitates hospitalization for a period of 2 to 5 days with bed rest. Some studies have documented earlier return to work and normal activity with a rotational flap; however, this point is still debated. As with all rotational flaps, failure or significant infection of the flap can lead to a more complex and difficult wound to manage.

The principles behind flap closure include flattening of the natal cleft with an orientation change of the midline fold. This causes

significant scarring and cosmetic changes. Patients should be informed prior to surgery of this potential change in appearance of the buttocks, with loss of the natal cleft, especially when using a rotational flap for simple pilonidal disease.

Rhomboid (Limberg) Flap

Initially, the diseased area is resected to the presacral fascia utilizing a diamond-shaped incision. A rhomboid-shaped flap is mobilized full thickness down to the gluteal fascia, and the flap is rotated to cover the defect (Figure 7). Drawing the flap contour before starting the

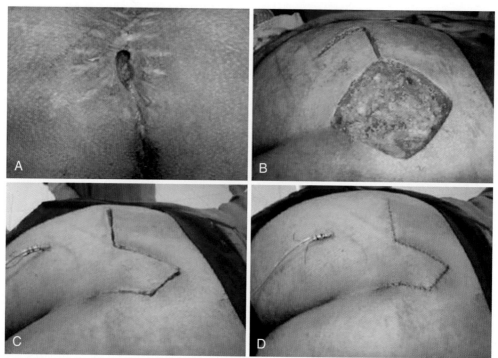

FIGURE 7   Rhomboid (Limberg) flap. **A,** Preoperative recurrent sinus. **B,** Excision of the sinus after design of flap. **C,** Raising of the flap. **D,** Closure of the wound with suction drain. *(From el-Khadrawy O, Hashish M, Ismail K, et al: Outcome of the rhomboid flap for recurrent pilonidal disease, World J Surg 33:1064–1068, 2009.)*

surgery helps to clearly define the excision site and the size of the flap. Lateralization of the distal part of the midline suture line to create an asymmetric flap has been shown to decrease wound infection and separation. This flap is utilized often because its broad pedicle is well vascularized, which decreases the risk of necrosis and avoids a midline suture line.

V-Y Advancement Flap

Depending on the size of the defect created, these flaps can be either unilateral or bilateral. The pilonidal disease is excised in its entirety using a triangular or oval incision. A triangular or V incision is then made with the apex laterally, and the pedicle is mobilized past the gluteal fascia. The flap is rotated medially, and the lateral aspect is closed in a straight line to create the Y-shaped incision. Medial closure is either directly to the retained skin on the opposing side of the buttock or on the vertical edge of a second flap on the opposing side (Figure 8). This flap is often used bilaterally for recurrent disease with large defects. The midline incision may have breakdown, which increases the risk of recurrence.

Z-Plasty

In Z-plasty, the pilonidal disease is resected in an oval fashion. Superior and inferior flaps of skin and subcutaneous tissue are then raised above the gluteal fascia from incisions made 30 degrees from the excision site (Figure 9). Once the flaps have been raised, they are rotated; the superior incision is placed inferiorly, and the inferior flap is placed superiorly. This flap avoids the midline suture line and flattens the gluteal cleft.

Gluteus Musculocutaneous Flap

This flap is often used for larger defects, where muscle and subcutaneous tissue are deemed necessary to fill the defect created after the excision. A semilunar flap of skin, subcutaneous tissue, and gluteus muscle is raised and rotated into the defect (Figure 10). This flap also

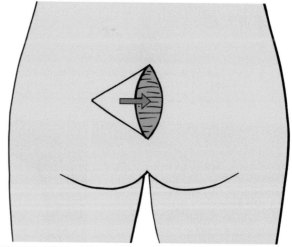

FIGURE 8   V-Y flap. *(Adapted from Nursal TZ, Ezer A, Caliṣkan K, et al: Prospective randomized controlled trial comparing V-Y advancement flap with primary suture methods in pilonidal disease, Am J Surg 199:170–177, 2009.)*

flattens and eliminates the gluteal cleft and avoids a midline suture line. Because the flap includes muscle tissue, it is associated with a longer recovery and is often reserved for filling defects created from a prior flap failure.

Surgical Results of Flaps

The various flap procedures described generally carry the same morbidity and complication rate (2% to 8%) with the exception of the gluteus flap, which has increased morbidity. They usually require 3 to 5 days of hospitalization after the procedure to allow for pain control. Common complications include bleeding and infection and flap separation. Randomized trials have generally shown the rhomboid or Limberg flap to have better results than the others, with lower

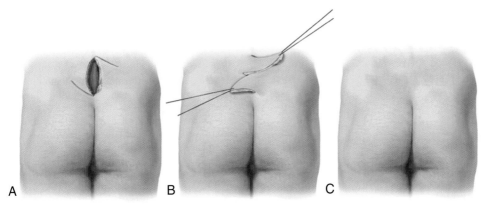

FIGURE 9   Z-plasty closure after midline excision. **A,** After sinus excision, limbs of the Z are marked at an angle 30 degrees to the long axis of the wound. **B,** Full-thickness flaps are raised and transposed. **C,** The wound is closed. *(Adapted from Nivatvongs S: Pilonidal disease. In Gordon P, Nivatvongs S, (eds): Principles and practice of surgery for the colon, rectum, and anus, St Louis, 1992, Quality Medical.)*

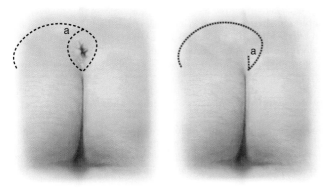

FIGURE 10   Gluteus maximus rotational flap. After sinus excision, the flap is rotated into place as shown.

complication rates; but the choice of flap is based on the anatomy of the pilonidal disease to be excised and the size of the defect created. Recurrence rates range from 4% to 8% (see Table 3).

CANCER AND PILONIDAL DISEASE

Squamous cell carcinoma is the most common neoplasm to arise in chronic pilonidal sinuses, but the presence of cancer in a sinus is rare. Concerning findings such as rapidly expanding ulcers, friable lesions with elevated edges, or a fungating mass should alert the surgeon to the possibility of a neoplasm, and a prompt biopsy of the lesion's edges should be performed. If a cancer is confirmed, primary therapy is wide local excision that includes the presacral fascia with flap closure.

SUMMARY

A pilonidal sinus is a common disorder with multiple therapeutic options. Surgical intervention can be quite invasive and disabling; when formatting a treatment plan, initial interventions should be as simple as possible. Acutely inflamed or infected pilonidal abscesses should be drained but not resected. A recurrence rate of 40% after incision and drainage requires resection after infection.

Primary excision or unroofing, with or without marsupialization, seems to be a simple, reproducible technique for midline sinus, and it has a better initial outcome with respect to recovery and complications compared with rotational flaps. The key to ensuring that disease does not recur is to keep the wound clean and free of surrounding hair until completely healed. The Bascom approach is an attractive alternative for navicular pilonidal disease, and it offers the advantage of a faster healing time.

In the event of a recurrence, resection with flap closure is recommended. The specific flap used for defect closure is chosen according to surgeon comfort and the size and location of the defect. Those flaps that offset the midline suture and eliminate the gluteal cleft tend to have better results with lower recurrence rates. Finally, newer techniques of wound management, such as vacuum dressing, may assist in healing larger defects and in avoiding rotational flaps in the future. Further experience with this technique is required prior to widespread recommendation.

SUGGESTED READINGS

Al-Khamis A, McCallum I, King PM, et al: Healing by primary versus secondary intention after surgical treatment for pilonidal sinus [review]. The Cochran Collaboration, 2009, John Wiley & Sons.

el-Khadrawy O, Hashish M, Ismail K, Shalaby H: Outcome of the rhomboid flap for recurrent pilonidal disease, *World J Surg* 33:1064–1068, 2009.

Karakayali F, Karagulle E, Karabulut Z, et al: Unroofing and marsupialization vs. rhomboid excision and Limberg flap in pilonidal disease: a prospective, randomized, clinical trial, *Dis Colon Rectum* 52:496–502, 2009.

Lee PJ, Raniga S, Biyani DK, et al: Sacrococcygeal pilonidal disease, *Colorectal Dis* 10:639–652, 2008.

Mahdy T: Surgical treatment of the pilonidal disease: primary closure or flap reconstruction after excision, *Dis Colon Rectum* 51:1816–1822, 2008.

APPROACH TO LOWER GASTROINTESTINAL BLEEDING

Angela K. Moss, MD, and Richard A. Hodin, MD

DEFINITION

Lower gastrointestinal bleeding (LGIB) is defined as bleeding that originates distal to the ligament of Treitz. Responsible for 20% of all GI bleeds, its initial symptoms are hematochezia and the passage of maroon or bright red blood or blood clots per rectum. Nevertheless, the most common cause of hematochezia is *upper GI bleeding* (UGIB). Because classic signs of UGIB, such as hematemesis and melena, may be absent, the initial evaluation of hematochezia should include nasogastric aspiration. If copious nonbloody bile returns, UGIB can be largely ruled out and evaluation for LGIB can proceed. Otherwise, further workup for UGIB, such as with esophagogastroduodenoscopy (EGD), should be prioritized.

The severity of LGIB can be classified as *minor, major,* or *massive*. Patients with minor LGIB are hemodynamically stable and are generally evaluated as outpatients. The most common causes of minor LGIB are anorectal disorders such as hemorrhoids and fissures, although inflammatory bowel disease (IBD), infectious colitis, arteriovenous malformations, polyps, and colon cancer should be considered as potential sources. Major LGIB is associated with hemodynamic instability, altered mental status, and the need for 2 units or more of blood. Once a patient requires more than 10 units of blood, he or she is categorized as having massive LGIB. This overview focuses on the etiology, diagnosis, and treatment of major and massive LGIB.

ETIOLOGY OF MAJOR AND MASSIVE LOWER GASTROINTESTINAL BLEEDING

The most common cause of major and massive LGIB in adults is colonic diverticulosis (Table 1). These small outpouchings form in relatively weak areas of the colon wall, where the vasa recta penetrate the muscularis layer to reach the submucosa and mucosa. Risk factors for bleeding include advanced age, anticoagulation medications, diabetes mellitus, and ischemic heart disease. Even though most diverticula are found in the left colon, diverticular bleeding often originates from the right colon. Presentation is usually abrupt, heralded by painless hematochezia. Although 70% to 90% of diverticular bleeds resolve spontaneously, rebleeding occurs in 20% to 40% of patients. Inflammatory changes are classically absent in diverticular bleeding, and diverticulitis does not increase the risk.

Bleeding from a colonic neoplasm is believed to result from erosions or ulcerations on the luminal surface of tumors, and it tends to be low grade and recurrent. Endoscopic therapy is generally limited to biopsy of suspicious masses and evaluation for synchronous lesions.

Hemorrhagic colitis may reflect underlying infectious, ischemic, inflammatory, radiation-induced, or vasculitis-associated disease. Endoscopically the colon may appear friable, edematous, erythematous, or ulcerated. Infectious colitis typically presents abruptly with crampy abdominal pain and bloody diarrhea. The most common pathogens are enterohemorrhagic *Escherichia coli, Shigella* spp., *Campylobacter jejuni,* and *Entamoeba histolytica.*

Ischemic colitis also generally presents with the acute onset of crampy abdominal pain. In some patients the pain is more severe than the degree of tenderness on examination, but in others the degree of pain is minimal. The splenic flexure and sigmoid colon, having the poorest collateral blood flow, are most frequently involved. The diagnosis of ischemic colitis is based on clinical suspicion, though biopsy is useful in distinguishing it from other causes of colitis. Bleeding is frequently self-limited in ischemic colitis, and the prognosis depends on correcting the underlying hypoperfusion. Exacerbations of inflammatory bowel disease may present with bloody diarrhea, though life-threatening hemorrhage only rarely occurs.

Angiodysplasias are small vascular malformations thought to arise from intermittent low-grade obstruction of submucosal veins. Though unusual in the general population (noted on less than 1% of screening colonoscopies), their prevalence increases with age, accounting for 20% to 30% of cases of hematochezia in patients older than 65 years. Angiodysplasias may occur throughout the colon, but the most common site of bleeding is the cecum. Endoscopically, they appear as flat, bright red lesions. Presentation is similar to diverticular bleeding in that it tends to be painless, self-limiting, and episodic; but because the origin is venous rather than arterial, bleeding is generally less brisk and more often occult.

Postpolypectomy hemorrhage is the most common postpolypectomy complication, and it can occur immediately or up to several weeks after the procedure. Early bleeding arises from inadequate cauterization of the polypectomy site, and delayed bleeding is thought to be due to sloughing of the eschar that covered a blood vessel. Risk factors include removal of large, sessile, right-sided polyps and resumption of anticoagulation after the procedure. Though bleeding is usually self-limited, patients with active, severe bleeding should undergo immediate colonoscopy after stabilization.

Surgical causes of bleeding include aortoenteric fistulae and anastomotic bleeding. Aortocolonic fistula formation with severe hemorrhage has been reported from several weeks to years after aortic graft surgery. Fistulization to small bowel—generally the duodenum where it crosses anterior to the aorta—is somewhat more frequent. Staple-line hemorrhage from colonic anastomoses is rare and usually self-limited but occasionally may be severe enough to require procedural intervention. Endoscopic evaluation allows for treatment options, including epinephrine injection, coagulation, or clipping, and it may obviate the need for operative revision.

Severe hematochezia is unusual in children and merits special consideration. Serious causes in neonates include necrotizing enterocolitis and malrotation complicated by midgut volvulus. Sources of hemorrhage relatively unique to children include intussusception, bleeding from a Meckel diverticulum, and juvenile polyps.

General risk factors for LGIB include advanced age and the use of anticoagulants or platelet aggregation inhibitors. Though underappreciated, nonsteroidal antiinflammatory drug use can damage the colon and small bowel in addition to the upper GI tract. Risk factors for death in patients with LGIB include severity of bleeding, advanced age, intestinal ischemia, and comorbid illness.

DIAGNOSTIC ASSESSMENT AND THERAPY

Resuscitation and Stabilization

Initial management of all patients with evidence of severe bleeding must include large-bore intravenous access and volume resuscitation. Blood products should be transfused as needed to correct anemia, coagulopathy, and thrombocytopenia. The ideal transfusion trigger depends on the individual patient's age and comorbidities.

TABLE 1: Etiology of acute LGIB

Source of Bleeding	(%)
Diverticulosis	33
Cancer/polyp	19
Colitis /ulcer (inflammatory bowel disease, infectious colitis, ischemic colitis, radiation colitis, vasculitis, and inflammation of unknown origin)	18
Angiodysplasia	8
Anorectal (hemorrhoids, anal fissures, and idiopathic rectal ulcers)	4
Other (postpolypectomy bleeding, aortocolonic fistula, trauma from fecal impaction, and anastomotic bleeding)	8
Unknown	16

Sources of LGIB determined from review of seven series including 1333 patients with acute LGIB (Zuckerman GR, Prakash C: Acute lower intestinal bleeding. Part II: etiology, therapy, and outcomes, *Gastrointest Endosc* 49: 228–238, 1999).

Colonoscopy

Colonoscopy is the initial examination of choice for both diagnosis and treatment of LGIB, though severe bleeding can rarely preclude colonoscopy. Advantages of colonoscopy are the capability for precise localization (53% to 97% accuracy) and treatment of lesions, as well as the ability to obtain tissue for biopsy. Disadvantages include risk of perforation, need for sedation or general anesthesia, and need for bowel preparation. Although some experts advocate unprepped colonoscopy, generally a rapid preparation is given so that initial colonoscopy is performed within the first 24 hours of admission (purge colonoscopy). Endoscopic treatment options are multiple and include polypectomy, epinephrine injection, direct-contact thermal coagulation, argon plasma coagulation, application of metal clips to lesions, and band ligation of internal hemorrhoids or rectal varices.

Angiography

Angiography is an important diagnostic tool for patients with hematochezia when endoscopy cannot localize the bleeding site. It provides imaging of the entire mesenteric system with high specificity but low sensitivity, requiring a bleeding rate of at least 1 mL/min. It allows for therapeutic transcatheter techniques including infusion of vasopressin (requires prolonged catheterization times) and superselective transcatheter embolization, which is the preferred treatment. Vessel occlusion is performed using microcoils or sponge particles made of polyvinyl alcohol or gelatin. In appropriate cases, when angiography fails to localize bleeding, anticoagulants or thrombolytics may be applied in attempts to provoke bleeding.

Drawbacks to angiography include the risk of access-site thrombosis or hemorrhage, dissection or distal embolization in target vessels, contrast nephropathy, allergic reactions, and also bowel ischemia, which has become infrequent with the development of superselective techniques.

Nuclear Studies

In a tagged red blood cell scan, technetium-labeled red blood cells are infused intravenously, and scanning is performed at several intervals to identify potential bleeding sites. Serial scans may allow for source identification in patients with intermittent bleeding. Compared with angiography, they are more sensitive, allowing for identification of bleeding as slight as 0.1 mL/min, but serial scans can be difficult to interpret and are therefore much less specific for the precise localization of the bleeding site.

Some have used the nuclear test as an initial screen prior to proceeding with the more invasive angiographic approach. Meckel scans are useful in children who present with severe hematochezia. Intravenous 99m-Tc pertechnetate is taken up and secreted by mucoid cells of the gastric mucosa. Because ectopic gastric mucosa is the source of bleeding from a Meckel diverticulum, the test is both sensitive and specific.

Helical Computed Tomographic Scan

The use of arterial phase multidetector-row computed tomographic (CT) scan has been described to identify extravasated contrast in the bowel lumen, but its utility for localization of LGIB has yet to be established. Although it is noninvasive and relatively easy to obtain, limitations include risks of intravenous contrast, potential for image artifacts that obscure contrast extravasation, and the need for active bleeding at a rate of approximately 0.4 mL/min.

Small Bowel Evaluation

Despite evaluation with the above modalities, bleeding sources may still not be evident, and further evaluation of the small bowel may be warranted. Push enteroscopy allows visualization and limited therapeutic interventions of the first 50 to 80 cm of the jejunum. For capsule endoscopy, the patient swallows a pill-sized wireless imaging system that traverses the small bowel and takes serial pictures over several hours. It has become the diagnostic procedure of choice in patients with obscure GI bleeding; it is very well tolerated and has a higher diagnostic yield than all other diagnostic modalities. Drawbacks include the lack of therapeutic potential, the length of the study, and occasional retention of the capsule by a partial small bowel stenosis, which may require surgical intervention.

Double-balloon enteroscopy is a relatively new technique that allows visualization of the entire small bowel through alternating advancement of the enteroscope and an overtube, both of which have a balloon on the end that provides friction against the intestinal wall. Biopsies may be taken, and therapies such as electrocoagulation and epinephrine injection may be used. Disadvantages include the need for sedation or general anesthesia and the requirement for a highly specialized gastroenterologist. Double-balloon enteroscopy may be useful for patients with a capsule endoscopy study showing a lesion that requires biopsy or is amenable to therapeutic intervention, or for those patients in whom suspicion of small bowel pathology is high despite a negative capsule endoscopy.

Barium studies have no role in the acute evaluation of LGIB, as they will almost never identify a bleeding source, and the presence of barium in the bowel can be problematic for subsequent endoscopy or surgery.

OPERATIVE MANAGEMENT

Surgical intervention should be considered a last resort in patients with LGIB. It is reserved for patients with persistent hemodynamic instability despite aggressive resuscitation, the need for four or more blood transfusions in 24 hours or 10 units overall, or in the setting of recurrent severe bleeding. Operative intervention during the same hospitalization in these situations is associated with a better long-term outcome. Surgical evaluation may entail exploratory laparotomy alone or combined with intraoperative enteroscopy to evaluate the small bowel, isolating a short segment at a time.

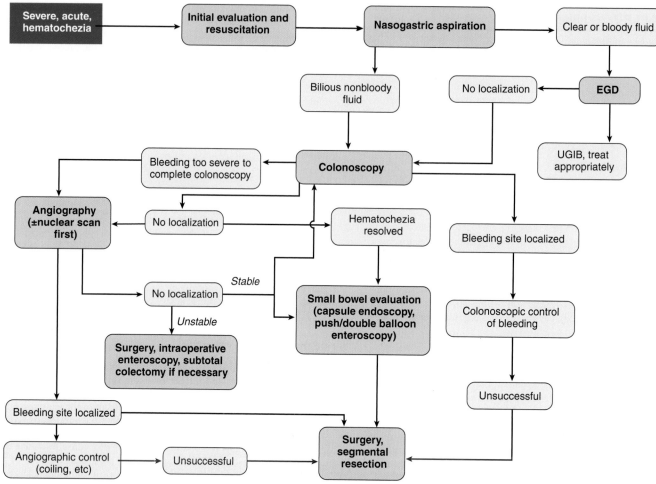

FIGURE 1   Management algorithm for hematochezia. *EGD,* Esophagogastroduodenoscopy.

Operative management of LGIB has long been a controversial subject. What is clear is that blind segmental resection based on clinical suspicion alone has an unacceptably high rate of rebleeding and should not be performed. There is an emerging consensus that with successful preoperative localization of bleeding, segmental intestinal resection may be considered with the understanding that it bears a higher risk of rebleeding (0% to 14%) than subtotal colectomy (0% to 4%). Subtotal colectomy, however, carries a higher risk of intractable diarrhea.

Because morbidity and mortality increase if rebleeding necessitates relaparotomy, some surgeons advocate subtotal colectomy, even if the bleeding source is identified. Nevertheless, several studies have shown comparable mortality rates for subtotal colectomy and segmental resection. Because subtotal colectomy so adversely affects quality of life, the common management is to perform subtotal colectomies only for unstable patients with unidentifiable bleeding sites or for bleeding from ulcerative colitis. Primary anastomosis may be considered only if the patient is hemodynamically stable.

When blood is seen in the small intestine during emergency exploratory laparotomy, a source can sometimes be identified by palpation of a mass, visualization of abnormal vessels on the mesenteric border, or identification of small bowel diverticula. When multiple small bowel diverticula are present, surgical devascularization of the diverticula on the mesenteric border followed by inversion with seromuscular sutures may be successful, but this can only be done if the bleeding site is identified and/or if the diverticula are localized to a short segment of the bowel.

While LGIB resolves on its own in 80% of cases, it recurs in 25% of cases. After a patient's second major bleeding episode, prophylactic resection is usually recommended (assuming the site has been localized), because the risk of rebleeding increases and exceeds 50% after the second episode. Risk factors for rebleeding include severity of the first bleed, major medical comorbidities, and the need for anticoagulation.

SUMMARY

Management of LGIB requires initial examination and resuscitation of the patient followed by early diagnostic localization and treatment of the bleeding source (Figure 1). Bleeding often stops on its own or is controllable with colonoscopy and angiography. Surgical intervention should be reserved for cases of refractory and/or recurrent bleeding and should be pursued only when the precise source of the bleeding has been identified.

SUGGESTED READINGS

Czymek R, Kempf A, Roblick UJ, et al: Surgical treatment concepts for acute lower gastrointestinal bleeding, *J Gastrointest Surg* 12:2212–2220, 2008.

Farner R, Lichliter W, Kuhn J: Total colectomy versus limited colonic resection for acute lower gastrointestinal bleeding, *Am J Surg* 178:587–590, 1999.

Lewis M: Bleeding colonic diverticula, *J Clin Gastroenterol* 42:1156–1158, 2008.

Miller M, Smith TP: Angiographic diagnosis and endovascular management of nonvariceal gastrointestinal hemorrhage, *Gastroenterol Clin N Am* 34:735–752, 2005.

Song LMWK, Baron TH: Endoscopic management of acute lower gastrointestinal bleeding, *Am J Gastroenterol* 103:1881–1887, 2008.

Management of Cystic Disease of the Liver

Sean P. Cleary, MD, Stéphane Zalinski, MD, and Jean-Nicolas Vauthey, MD

OVERVIEW

Nonparasitic cystic lesions of the liver are a common finding. In previous decades these were frequently identified as incidental findings at laparotomy. With the increasing utilization of imaging modalities, particularly ultrasound (US) and computed tomography (CT), cystic lesions of the liver are now frequently identified incidentally on radiologic examinations performed for a diverse set of indications.

The prevalence of liver cysts is thought to be in the range of 5% and thus represents a common condition surgeons encounter. Although the majority of these lesions are benign and asymptomatic, the evaluation of hepatic cysts should include a careful assessment of potential associated symptoms and the differentiation of benign versus neoplastic lesions. Decisions on which cysts warrant intervention and the various treatment options available further add to the clinical dilemma that surgeons face in managing these lesions.

Several classification schemes have been suggested for cystic lesions of the liver (Table 1). Cysts can be considered true or false cysts depending on the presence or absence of an epithelial lining. Alternatively, they may be classified as congenital versus acquired or benign versus malignant. Infectious cysts (e.g., hepatic abscess) or parasitic cysts (hydatid cysts) are discussed elsewhere in this book.

CLINICAL PRESENTATION

The initial signs and symptoms in patients with hepatic cysts are highly variable and depend on the type of cyst, its size and location in relation to intrahepatic structures, and the presence of possible complications. The majority of liver cysts are asymptomatic and are identified as incidental findings on abdominal imaging performed for other indications or at surgery. Symptoms are more common in neoplastic and traumatic cysts than in congenital cysts, and cysts are more frequently seen in women.

Although cysts can be identified at any age, symptoms most often appear in the fourth and fifth decades of life. Vague abdominal pain or discomfort are the most common first symptoms, followed by a sensation of fullness or of a mass. The mass effect of very large cysts or multiple cysts can result in early satiety or gastric or intestinal obstruction that results in nausea and vomiting, or even extrinsic compression of bile ducts that can cause jaundice, depending on the level of obstruction. Acute abdominal pain can occur with intracystic hemorrhage, causing sudden cyst enlargement and distension of the Glisson capsule. Rare complications of cysts that can result in symptoms include cyst torsion, rupture, or secondary bacterial infection.

DIAGNOSTIC EVALUATION

The purpose of the diagnostic evaluation of liver cysts is to determine the presence or absence of premalignant or malignant features (Table 2); identify signs of complications, such as infection, rupture, or hemorrhage; and localize, measure, and account for potential multiple lesions within the liver. In virtually every patient, these goals can be accomplished by using modern noninvasive imaging modalities.

Because the majority of incidentally discovered cystic lesions are simple cysts, the objective of imaging studies is to confirm the diagnosis by ruling out the presence of neoplastic features such as multilocular lesions, septae, papillary projections, and thickening or enhancement of the cyst wall. The presence of mural calcifications and daughter cysts are features of parasitic or hydatid cysts, which are reviewed in a separate chapter. The presence of debris within a cyst may be indicative of intracystic hemorrhage, parasitic cysts, or malignant features and should warrant further investigation. A central hypodensity associated with mural enhancement, perilesional edema, and associated venous thrombosis may be indicative of a pyogenic hepatic abscess.

The evaluation of simple hepatic cysts should be limited and straightforward, but the assessment of cysts with more complex features may require a coordinated, systematic, multimodal approach. The workup of small lesions (<1 cm) may be particularly difficult because the miniscule size may challenge the resolution capabilities of imaging techniques; therefore workup requires a multimodal approach, possibly with serial imaging over time. Whenever possible, imaging studies should be performed at a single institution to allow for evaluation of previous studies, assess for changes in size and character in longitudinal follow-up, and allow a comparison of cyst features using different imaging techniques.

Ultrasound

US is the primary imaging modality for cystic lesions of the liver. It is readily available, inexpensive, and noninvasive, and it can provide significant and highly reliable information about cyst size and characteristics. The sensitivity and specificity of US in the evaluation of hepatic cysts is greater than 90%. Of primary importance, US can

TABLE 1: Classification of cysts

1. True cysts
   A. Congenital
      i) Simple cysts
      ii) Adult polycystic liver disease
         - Associated with autosomal-dominant polycystic kidney disease
         - Autosomal-dominant polycystic liver disease without renal cysts
      iii) Bile duct related
         - Caroli disease, bile duct duplication, peribiliary cysts
   B. Acquired
      i) Primary neoplastic
         - Biliary cystadenoma
         - Biliary cystadenocarcinoma
         - Other: Cystic sarcoma, squamous cell carcinoma
      ii) Secondary neoplastic
         - Metastatic mucinous neoplasms from pancreas, ovary
         - Cystic degeneration of metastases: Colon, pancreas, kidney, neuroendocrine tumor

2. False cysts
   i) Hepatic abscess
   ii) Posttraumatic hematoma or biloma

TABLE 2: Characteristics of simple and neoplastic liver cysts

Simple Cyst	Neoplastic Cyst
Thin, imperceptible homogenous wall	Thick, enhancing irregular wall
Unilocular	Papillary projections, mural nodules
Low-density fluid (<10 HU)	Multilocular, multiple enhancing septae
Normal CEA CA 19-9 in fluid	Higher density (>10 HU), mucinous fluid
May contain blood or bile	Elevated CEA and/or CA 19-9

reliably differentiate between solid and cystic lesions, and it can guide the overall management of hepatic lesions.

On US, simple hepatic cysts appear as homogenous anechoic lesions with smooth contours without a perceptible wall or septations. Acoustic enhancement of the back wall of the cyst can be seen due to the lack of absorption and reflection of US waves by the cyst fluid and wall compared with the hepatic parenchyma. The presence of heterogenous material within the cyst should raise suspicion of neoplasia, but it may also be related to hemorrhage in the cyst. Blood within a simple cyst appears echogenic on US, but it should be mobile, and it should move with changes in patient position.

The role of contrast-enhanced US appears to be limited to the characterization of cystic lesions, which appear as enhancement defects on all phases of contrast US and can be mistaken for hypovascular metastases if not assessed properly on gray-scale US. The use of contrast may help delineate enhancement of the cyst wall or septae in cases of biliary cystadenoma, cystadenocarcinoma, or pyogenic

abscess. Finally, US may be useful in delineating complications associated with mass effect caused by cysts, including intrahepatic biliary dilation or vascular compression and impingement.

Computed Tomography

CT is extremely useful in characterizing lesions within the liver relative to their size, location, and relationship to intrahepatic biliary and vascular structures. CT can also be helpful in defining the relationship between liver cysts and surrounding viscera and in differentiating between intrahepatic lesions and extrahepatic lesions with compression or invasion of the liver.

The ideal assessment of liver cysts would include the use of intravenous contrast and complete visualization of the liver in the arterial portal venous, hepatic venous, or delayed venous phases. Hepatic cysts should appear as nonenhancing on CT scan. Similar to ultrasound, it should show well-defined borders and no identifiable wall or cyst content.

Simple cysts contain low-density fluid (i.e., <10 Hounsfield units [HU]) that is homogenous. Occasionally it can be difficult to differentiate between cysts and solid, low-attenuating lesions on CT, and US may be important in clarifying the nature of these lesions. As with other imaging modalities, the presence of a thickened, irregular wall; papillary projections; septations; or high-density (>10 HU) inhomogenous fluid should be regarded as suspicious and prompt further investigation.

Magnetic Resonance Imaging

Although magnetic resonance imaging (MRI) should rarely be considered the first imaging modality in the assessment of hepatic cysts, it can be very useful in the evaluation of complex lesions. Simple cysts appear as hypointense lesions in T1-weighted images and hyperintense lesions on T2-weighted images. Hemorrhage into a cyst can increase the signal on T1-weighted images, as can the presence of the mucinous material that can be found in cystadenomas and cystadenocarcinomas. Many of the previously mentioned suspicious features seen on other imaging modalities can be seen on MRI, although the spatial resolution of MR technology may lag behind that of CT and US for small lesions. MR cholangiopancreatography (MRCP) can be useful in delineating the anatomy and relationship with the biliary system in cases of Caroli disease or intrahepatic cysts with bile duct communication.

Other Investigations

Plain radiographs have a limited role in the evaluation of cysts. Routine chest or abdominal x-rays can rarely reveal calcifications in the cyst wall or demonstrate displacement of abdominal viscera or the diaphragm. Routine laboratory tests are usually normal, but they may detect biliary obstruction in large cysts or, rarely, hepatic synthetic dysfunction with advanced polycystic disease.

Ecchinococcal serology should be performed in patients with complex cysts to rule out hydatid disease. Biochemical and cytologic analysis of cyst fluid has a limited role in the evaluation and management of uncomplicated simple cysts, but it may be helpful in discriminating between simple and neoplastic cysts in difficult cases. The fluid contained within uncomplicated simple cysts should be thin, acellular, and straw colored. Dark fluid within cysts may be the result of intracystic hemorrhage. The presence of elevated levels of bilirubin in the cyst fluid indicates a communication between the cyst and biliary tree and should influence management. The presence of mucin, atypical cells, or elevated CA 19-9 or CEA levels in fluid should be indicators of a neoplastic process, but it cannot reliably discriminate between benign and malignant lesions.

COMMON CYSTIC LESIONS OF THE LIVER AND THEIR MANAGEMENT

Simple Cysts

Simple hepatic cysts are congenital and are the most common cystic lesion, found in up to 5% of the population. Multiple theories have been suggested regarding the pathogenesis of these cysts, including failure of the intralobular bile ducts to fuse with the interlobular bile ducts, obstruction of aberrant bile ducts, and malformation of foregut epithelial cells. Cysts are lined by a simple epithelium that secretes water and electrolytes in a composition similar to serum. About 50% of patients have a single cyst; although multiple cysts are common, rare cases of patients with innumerable cysts may be difficult to distinguish from inherited forms of polycystic liver disease.

The evaluation of patients with simple cysts should begin with a careful, focused history and physical examination. During this evaluation, it is important to remember that 80% to 95% are asymptomatic and do not require further evaluation or treatment. Symptoms may include pain, abdominal fullness or discomfort, increasing abdominal girth, and early satiety, which are due in large part to mass effect and compression of adjacent structures and are therefore more common in larger cysts (>8 cm). Hemorrhage into a cyst can cause pain as well as an increase in cyst diameter on serial imaging. Pedunculated cysts are reported to be prone to torsion or potential rupture and can be considered for treatment.

Since most cysts are asymptomatic and have no malignant potential, the indications for the treatment of simple cysts are limited to symptomatic cysts and situations where diagnostic uncertainty exists. Asymptomatic cysts discovered incidentally or at laparotomy do not require treatment; symptomatic or complex cysts require further evaluation.

Percutaneous aspiration of cyst fluid, often under ultrasound guidance, can provide immediate decompression, but it is associated with a 100% recurrence rate. Although simple aspiration is not an effective treatment strategy, it can be of benefit in two ways: it provides a fluid sample for biochemical and cytologic analysis in difficult or complex cases, and by providing immediate decompression, aspiration can be used as a therapeutic test to determine whether abdominal symptoms are related to mass effect caused by a cyst. Prior to any invasive procedure for a liver cyst, it is mandatory to rule out any other etiology, such as infectious conditions (hydatidosis) or cystic neoplasm.

The recurrence of cysts after simple aspiration is due to the occlusion of the needle defect in the cyst wall and persistent fluid secretion from the epithelial lining. As a result, aspiration has been combined with injection of a sclerosing solution that damages the epithelial cells, which impairs their ability to secrete fluid and leads to fibrotic obliteration of the cyst. Several sclerosing solutions have been used, including 95% to 99% ethanol, iophendylate, tetracycline, doxycycline, minocycline, and hypertonic saline, all with relatively comparable results.

The procedure begins with aspiration and inspection of cyst fluid. The presence of bile in the cyst fluid or the confirmation of biliary communication on contrast injection or with endoscopic retrograde cholangiopancreatography (ERCP) is a contraindication to sclerosis. Once the cyst is emptied, an equivalent of 25% of the cyst volume, or a maximum of 100 mL of the sclerosing solution, is injected into the cyst. The patient is then asked to periodically change positions to ensure contact of the entire cyst wall with the sclerosing agent.

After approximately 10 minutes, the sclerosing agent is drained, and the catheter is removed. Large cysts may require repeated injections of the sclerosing agent to maximize the chance of effective treatment. Postprocedural complications are usually minor and include pain, transient fever, nausea, and vomiting. Pain can be minimized with the addition of local anesthetic to the sclerosing solution, and prompt removal of the catheter can reduce the risk of leakage of sclerosing solution. The rate of symptomatic recurrence of cysts treated with aspiration and sclerosis is 5% to 10%.

Surgical treatment of hepatic cysts is highly effective and should be considered only in patients with symptoms or complex cysts (Figure 1). The terms *fenestration, marsupialization,* and *deroofing* all refer to the same technique, which involves the resection of a large portion of the cyst wall to allow the fluid produced by the epithelium to drain into the peritoneal cavity to be reabsorbed by the peritoneum.

More than 80% of symptomatic cysts are amenable to surgical treatment, which is ideally suited for large, superficial, or anterior lesions that can be fenestrated with minimal resection of liver parenchyma. In most centers, this procedure is done laparoscopically with reduced postoperative pain and a shortened hospital stay compared with open procedures. Optimal results are obtained when the cyst is opened widely, with as much of the cyst wall resected, or using thermal ablation with electrocautery; however, care must be taken during ablation not to damage underlying critical vascular or biliary structures.

A laparoscopic approach allows excellent visualization of the cyst interior lining and allows inspection for potential neoplastic lesions not seen on imaging; it also facilitates identification of bile leaks, which can be suture ligated intraoperatively. If a bile leak cannot be excluded, a drain can be left in the cyst cavity to allow for inspection of the fluid postoperatively. Persistent postoperative bile leaks can be managed successfully endoscopically with ERCP and sphincterotomy.

Alternate surgical approaches to simple hepatic cysts have been described, including enucleation and formal hepatic resection. Although these techniques have the advantage of a negligible recurrence rate, such procedures are associated with significantly higher morbidity than either laparoscopic fenestration or aspiration and sclerosis.

Once it has been determined that intervention is required, the choice of treatment technique can be difficult. In medically fit patients with superficial, large, symptomatic cysts, we advocate a laparoscopic cyst fenestration as the first-line treatment. Primary treatment with aspiration and sclerosis is reserved for medically unfit patients or for cysts not easily accessible with a laparoscopic approach. Laparoscopic fenestration for recurrence after aspiration and sclerosis is often a difficult procedure associated with a higher complication rate; therefore we prefer a surgical approach as first-line therapy.

Polycystic Liver Disease

Polycystic liver disease (PCLD) is a rare condition characterized by the presence of multiple diffuse cystic lesions (Figure 2). However, unlike polycystic kidney disease, no widely accepted definition of

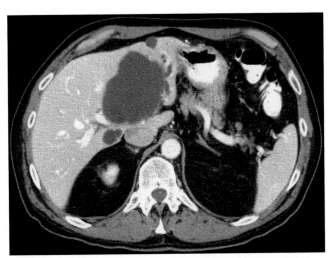

FIGURE I   Enhanced CT revealing a large, low-attenuation cystic lesion within segment IV with proximal bile duct obstruction. Although this cyst presented features of a simple cyst on imaging, it was an indication for resection due to biliary obstruction.

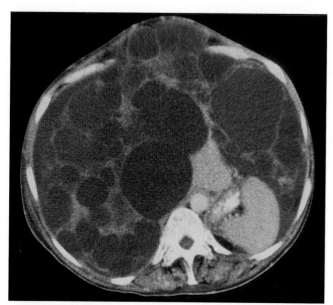

FIGURE 2   Enhanced CT revealing a multicystic liver with loss of the segmental liver anatomy and almost complete disappearance of the normal parenchyma due to an aggregate of cysts with radiologic features of simple cysts.

PCLD differentiates it from cases of multiple simple cysts. Cases of PCLD generally have more diffuse hepatic involvement, a familial pattern, and involvement of other organs, although some authors have suggested five or six cysts as the cutoff between PCLD and multiple simple cysts. The genetic basis for PCLD has been recognized in two autosomal-dominant disorders: PCLD associated with autosomal-dominant polycystic kidney disease (ADPKD) and autosomal-dominant polycystic liver disease without renal involvement (ADPLD).

Polycystic liver disease associated with ADPKD was first described by Bristow in 1856 with a prevalence estimated between 0.01% and 0.13% of the population. Cysts are thought to arise from bile duct overgrowth and failure of intralobar ducts to involute or connect with extralobular bile ducts. This failure of duct development results in the formation of biliary microhamartomas known as *von Meyenburg complexes*; cell proliferation and fluid secretion lead to cyst formation, predominantly in the peripheral regions of the liver. Centrally located cysts may arise from dilated peribiliary glands. The genetic basis of ADPKD has been defined, involving mutations in either chromosome 16 or chromosome 4, affecting the genes encoding the proteins polycystin-1 and -2, respectively.

The frequency of hepatic involvement in ADPKD has been increasing, from 40% to 50% in early series to 75% to 90% more recently as a result of improved survival from the associated kidney disease due to dialysis and renal transplantation. Liver involvement in ADPKD increases with age, female gender, and the severity of the renal disease. A distinct form of autosomal-dominant PCLD without kidney involvement (ADPLD) was recognized in the 1980s. It is less common than ADPKD, with a prevalence of 0.01%, and it is associated with a mutation in the hepatocystin gene located on chromosome 19.

Whether associated with ADPKD or ADPLD, polycystic liver disease is asymptomatic in the majority of cases. The intervening displaced liver parenchyma usually retains its function, and cases of hepatic failure are extremely rare. Symptoms, if present, are most often related to hepatomegaly with resulting mass effect and can be associated with abdominal fullness, pain, early satiety, shortness of breath, and nausea or vomiting. Obstruction of the inferior vena cava by the enlarged liver can result in lower limb edema or Budd-Chiari syndrome and may be more common after nephrectomy in cases

of ADPKD. Compression of the portal vein can lead to ascites and portal hypertension, and jaundice from compression of the biliary system has also been reported. Cyst infection is an uncommon but potentially fatal complication that may occur with right upper quadrant pain, fever, and leukocytosis. Infections are usually caused by Gram-negative bacteria, and blood cultures are positive in over half of infected patients.

US and CT may be helpful in identifying which cyst is infected, although this is often difficult. Such patients are best managed with drainage of the infected cyst, if it can be localized, and intravenous antibiotics. Extrahepatic manifestations of PCLD include not only renal disease but also intracranial aneurysms associated with both ADPKD and ADPLD.

Patients with PCLD are classified based on CT findings according to the number, size, and distribution of cysts and the amount of liver parenchyma between cysts. This classification scheme, proposed by Gigot (Table 3), provides a basis for comparing patients and serves as a guide for formulating treatment plans in symptomatic patients. Although most patients with PCLD are asymptomatic, treatment is indicated in those who develop significant symptoms.

Many centers have traditionally advocated a conservative approach to PCLD, with intervention reserved for patients with end-stage disease characterized by severe disability, weakness, and profound malnutrition. Understandably, treatment in these end-stage patients was associated with high morbidity and mortality rates and has led many to advocate a more aggressive approach to treat PCLD patients earlier in their disease course.

Secretion of electrolytes and fluid by the cyst epithelium has been shown to be stimulated by secretin. Drugs that reduce secretin release, namely cimetidine and somatostatin, have been suggested to decrease the rate of cyst growth and fluid reaccumulation after treatment, but their use has only been reported anecdotally. Treatment for patients with PCLD should be directed at reducing the size of cysts and the liver without compromising hepatic function.

Radiologic workup should involve the careful evaluation of cyst size, number, and location as well the anatomy of residual liver tissue. Treatment techniques utilized in simple cysts may be useful in treating adult PCLD patients with a limited number of large cysts (type 1). The use of aspiration and sclerosis of cysts in PCLD is associated with a much higher recurrence rate (25% to 50%) than in simple cystic disease because of the more rigid nature of the liver, which limits the ability of cysts to properly collapse. As a result, aspiration and sclerosis should be used only in patients who are not candidates for other treatment modalities. Fenestration may be used in patients with type 1 and 2 PCLD with superficial anterior cysts; recurrence rates after laparoscopic and open procedures appear similar (10% to 15%), with lower morbidity in laparoscopic cases. The most common postoperative morbidity in these cases appears to be ascites, and recurrence is highest in large cysts because of failure of the stiff PCLD liver to collapse and wall off the residual cyst.

For patients with more complex type 2 and 3 disease, a combination of fenestration and resection allows a more thorough debulking and removal of affected segments. Despite a higher morbidity rate than fenestration alone, fenestration and resection are associated with both a lower recurrence rate and more durable relief of symptoms.

Liver transplantation is gaining acceptance as a viable treatment option for patients with type 2 and 3 disease characterized by diffuse small cysts with little intervening normal parenchyma. Early experience with transplantation was limited to patients with PCLD and "lethal exhaustion" characterized by intractable pain, cachexia, and fatigue. High complication rates in transplanting these severely debilitated patients have led some centers to become reluctant to transplant polycystic patients, but others have advocated earlier intervention. In these patients the benefits of treatment must be weighed against the long-term effects of immunosuppression and risks of surgery. In cases of ADPKD, combined liver and renal transplantation may be particularly effective.

TABLE 3: Gigot classification of polycystic liver disease

Category	Description
Type 1	Limited number (<10) of large cysts (>10 cm) with large areas of normal parenchyma
Type 2	Diffuse involvement of the parenchyma by medium-sized cysts with large areas of uninvolved liver tissue
Type 3	Massive and diffuse involvement of the liver by small and medium-sized cysts with very little spared parenchyma

Cystadenoma

Cystadenomas are uncommon and account for less than 5% of all liver cysts. They are predominantly asymptomatic lesions that are more common in women and are detected frequently as incidental lesions in the fourth and fifth decade of life. The radiologic appearance on US, CT, and MRI can help distinguish cystadenomas from simple cysts (see Table 2); they often appear as complex lesions, with enhancing wall with mural nodularity or papillary projections, that contain higher density mucinous fluid and may be multilocular(Figure 3). In cases of diagnostic uncertainty, cyst fluid aspiration may be helpful in revealing the presence of mucin, atypical cells, or elevated CEA/CA 19-9, which are all suggestive of a neoplastic cyst. Histologic examination of the cyst wall reveals a cuboidal or low columnar cell lining.

Cystadenomas can be classified into two categories based on the presence of a deeper layer of dense mesenchymal stroma composed of well-vascularized atypical spindle cells lying below the cuboidal cell layer. The mesenchymal stromal type of cystadenoma is found almost exclusively in women and is associated with risk of malignant progression to cystadenocarcinoma.

Cystadenomas are premalignant lesions seen in both sexes; the presence of intestinal metaplasia in the cyst wall may be an early hallmark of malignant progression. The presence of invasion of the liver or adjacent structures is indicative of malignancy, but differentiating cystadenomas and cystadenocarcinomas can be difficult. Cyst fluid aspiration and biopsy are not helpful in differentiating benign and malignant lesions.

Because of the risk of malignancy, the use of cyst aspiration and sclerosis, fenestration, or cyst jejunostomy is not indicated in the treatment of cystadenomas. Rather, surgical treatment with either enucleation or resection should be considered in patients diagnosed with this lesion. Enucleation can be used in cases of superficial lesions with no evidence of malignancy. The technique involves complete resection of the cyst wall by developing the avascular plane between the wall and the liver parenchyma produced by a pseudocapsule in some cysts. Enucleation allows the preservation of the hepatic parenchyma and vascular and biliary structures.

Careful pathologic evaluation of the cyst wall should include a careful examination for intestinal metaplasia and invasive cancer. Formal hepatic resection is indicated in cases where malignancy is suspected, and it may be more appropriate for benign lesions deep within the parenchyma or for those who have a biliary communication.

Traumatic Cysts

Intrahepatic hematomas and bilomas may be seen after blunt trauma, and they can be diagnosed anywhere from a few days to years after an injury. Because the majority of blunt hepatic injuries are managed conservatively, the majority of these patients do not require operative

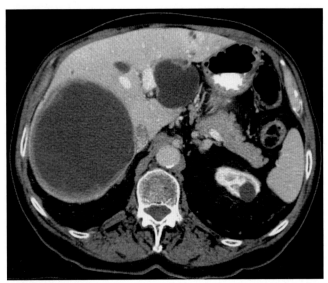

FIGURE 3 Enhanced CT revealing two complex cystic lesions with septations and enhancement of cyst wall consistent with the diagnosis of cystadenoma.

management. If an injury is associated with a persistent bile leak, progressive enlargement of a traumatic cyst can lead to pain and compressive symptoms. Decompression of the biliary system by ERCP and sphincterotomy may relieve the pressure caused by bile leak. Rare cases of enlarging symptomatic cysts can be treated by surgical drainage and ligation of the biliary communication. Otherwise, all asymptomatic traumatic cysts should be managed conservatively.

Ciliated Hepatic Foregut Cyst

Ciliated hepatic foregut cysts are rare lesions: less than 100 are reported in the literature. Most lesions are asymptomatic, and they are equally common in males and females. As with most cystic lesions, symptoms arise from mass effect and can be associated with pain progressing to jaundice or portal hypertension in severe cases.

These lesions are thought to arise from detachment and migration of respiratory epithelium from the tracheobronchial diverticulum during embryogenesis. They are most commonly located in segment IV and appear as unilocular hypoechoic lesions on US, which can make them difficult to differentiate from a simple cyst. Some cysts will have heterogeneous dense fluid that can appear as hyperintense areas on T1-weighted MRI images.

Histologically, cysts are lined by a ciliated, pseudostratified columnar epithelium, followed by a loose subepithelial connective tissue, a smooth muscle layer, and an outer layer of tough fibrous tissue. Cysts contain viscous or mucinous green or brown aspirate, and this fluid may reveal atypical ciliated columnar cells in many cases. Cases detected in children may have a biliary communication. Most lesions are benign but several cases of cysts containing squamous cell carcinoma via a metaplasia–carcinoma progression have been observed. The presence of malignancy risk indicates that resection should be advocated in these cases.

SUGGESTED READINGS

Abdalla EK, Forsmark CE, Lauwers GY, et al: Monolobar Caroli's disease and cholangiocarcinoma, *HPB Surg* 11(4):271–276, 1999.

Cowles RA, Mulholland MW: Solitary hepatic cysts, *J Am Coll Surg* 191:311–321, 2000.

Dixon E, Sutherland FR, Mitchell P, et al: Cystadenomas of the liver: a spectrum of disease, *Can J Surg* 44:371–376, 2001.

Que F, Nagorney DM, Gross JB Jr, Torres VE: Liver resection and cyst fenestration in the treatment of severe polycystic liver disease, *Gastroenterology* 108(2):487–494, 1995.

Russell RT, Pinson CW: Surgical management of polycystic disease, *World J Gastroenterol* 13:5052–5059, 2007.

Taylor BR, Langer B: Current surgical management of hepatic cyst disease, *Adv Surg* 31:127–149, 1998.

Vauthey JN, Maddern GJ, Blumgart LH: Adult polycystic disease of the liver, *Br J Surg* 78:524–527, 1991.

Vauthey JN, Maddern GJ, Kolbinger P, et al: Clinical experience with adult polycystic liver disease, *Br J Surg* 79(6):562–565, 1992.

ECHINOCOCCAL DISEASE OF THE LIVER

Johnny C. Hong, MD

OVERVIEW

Echinococcosis, which is often referred to as *cystic hydatid disease* or *echinococcal disease,* is the result of an infection with adult and larval stages of the tapeworm *Echinococcus,* which affects both humans and other mammals. The adult form of the parasite is present in canids (wolves, foxes, jackals, coyote, dogs); the larval form is found in wild cervids (deer, elk), livestock, and humans. Among the four known species, *Echinococcus granulosus* and *Echinococcus multilocularis* are most commonly associated with hydatid disease in humans. Although *Echinococcus* infection is endemic in Central Asia, South America, and the Mediterranean basin, echinococcal disease occurs worldwide as a result of travel and immigration.

The life cycle of *Echinococcus* requires a definitive host, which is often a dog, and intermediate hosts, such as sheep, goats, or other herbivores. Humans are an accidental intermediate host in the evolution of this parasite. Human infection occurs with ingestion of *E. granulosus* eggs by the host from contaminated vegetables or through contact with infected animals or soil. After ingestion, the embryos penetrate the intestinal wall and travel through circulation and result in hydatid disease anywhere in the body, with the liver being the most frequently involved organ (55% to 80%) followed by the lung (10% to 40%). Echinococcosis in humans may result in asymptomatic infection or severe, potentially fatal disease. Although surgery remains the primary treatment modality for hydatid liver disease, chemotherapy and nonoperative approaches are important adjuncts to surgery and are viable therapeutic options for a select group of patients. This chapter focuses on the current management of echinococcal disease of the liver.

PATHOLOGY

An understanding of the pathologic changes in hepatic hydatid disease is essential for selecting the appropriate diagnostic studies and treatment. The wall of the active cyst in the intermediate host consists of two layers. The inner germinal layer is where the actual echinococcal scolices and daughter cysts develop and then float in the cystic fluid. A cyst contains hundreds to thousands of protoscolices. The outer, acellular layer is usually 2 to 5 mm thick and is composed of a reactive fibrous layer of host tissue called *pericyst,* which contains calcification in approximately 50% of cases.

Expansion of the main cyst may erode into branches of the bile duct and cause infection of the hydatid cyst and/or rupture into body cavities of the chest and abdomen. However, approximately one third of large, long-standing hydatid cysts have communications between the cyst cavity and some part of the biliary system. many mature cysts may become calcified and inactive, containing no live elements. Patients with inactive, mature cysts often are asymptomatic and have false-negative serologic test results.

DIAGNOSIS

Diagnosis of *Echinococcus* can be extremely challenging because the initial signs and symptoms are nonspecific and may not differ much from other forms of liver disease. The most useful means of diagnosis must include a clinical evaluation with a high index of suspicion in regard to epidemiologic data, serologic tests, and noninvasive imaging studies.

CLINICAL MANIFESTATIONS

Hepatic hydatid cysts tend to grow slowly, displacing normal hepatic parenchyma and adjacent organs rather than infiltrating them. Because of this, patients can remain asymptomatic for a long time. With increasing use of noninvasive imaging studies, hydatid cysts of the liver are often discovered before symptoms occur. Typical signs and symptoms are usually nonspecific and may include abdominal mass, abdominal pain from expansion of the cyst, symptoms of infection, or obstructive jaundice related to rupture into the biliary tract. Patients with exceptionally large cysts may also present with signs of vena cava compression or portal hypertension. Although uncommon, hydatid cyst may rupture into the peritoneal cavity, resulting in a more dramatic clinical presentation characterized by acute abdominal pain, anaphylaxis, and shock.

LABORATORY TESTS

The liver function test, particularly transaminase levels, may remain normal, even in extremely large cysts. Cholestatic enzymes, alkaline phosphatase, and γ-glutamyl transferase (GGT) can be mildly elevated in approximately one third of patients, especially in those with biliary involvement. White blood cell counts are elevated only if the cyst has become secondarily infected. Although eosinophilia is present in 20% to 25% of infected patients, it is a nonspecific finding.

Special diagnostic techniques, such as specific enzyme-linked immunosorbent assay (ELISA), yield sensitivity rates from 64% to 100% independent of disease stage and site of the cyst. Other tests include immunoelectrophoresis, which has a diagnostic value of 91% to 94% for hepatic cysts and approximately 70% for pulmonary cysts; hydatid antigen blotting has a sensitivity of 95% and specificity of 100%.

IMAGING

Ultrasonography (US) and computed tomography (CT) are the most widely used noninvasive studies. US is the preferred first-line imaging method for hydatid cyst, with specificity in the range of 90%. To facilitate selection of treatment modalities, the World

TABLE 1: WHO-IWGE classification of hepatic echinococcal cysts

Type of Cyst	Status	Ultrasound Features	Remarks
CL	Active	Signs not pathognomonic, unilocular, no cyst wall	Usually early stage, not fertile; differential diagnosis necessary
CE 1	Active	Cyst wall, hydatid sand	Usually fertile
CE 2	Active	Multivesicular, cyst wall, rosette-like	Usually fertile
CE 3	Transitional	Detached laminated membrane, "water lily" sign, less round, decreased intracystic pressure	Starting to degenerate, may produce daughter cyst
CE 4	Inactive	Heterogenous hypoechogenic or hyperechogenic degenerative contents; no daughter cyst	Usually no living protoscolices; differential diagnosis necessary
CE 5	Inactive	Thick, calcified wall, calcification partial to complete; not pathognomonic, but highly suggestive of diagnosis	Usually no living protoscolices

Health Organization Informal Working Group on Echinococcosis (WHO-IWGE) has proposed a standardized ultrasonographic classification of hydatid disease based on the functional state of the parasite (Table 1).

Cross-sectional imaging with CT and magnetic resonance imaging (MRI) complements information obtained on US. CT and MRI provide additional structural details and show more precisely the location and depth of the cyst within the liver, data essential for planning surgical treatment. The two most important lesions to distinguish from hydatid cyst are a congenital simple cyst and a biliary cystadenoma (Figure 1, Table 2). Characteristic features on imaging include a unilocular or complex cyst with a thick wall, often with calcification, and the presence of daughter cysts (Figure 1, A1).

Communication of the hydatid cyst with the biliary tract may occur in up to 25 % of patients. Endoscopic retrograde cholangiopancreatography (ERCP) provides valuable information in defining the bile duct anatomy and visualizing connections between the cyst and the biliary system before surgery. Although ERCP is mandatory when the patient has complications such as cholangitis or jaundice, it should be performed selectively in patients who are asymptomatic with uncomplicated hydatid liver disease.

TREATMENT

Once hydatid disease is diagnosed, treatment should be initiated so that secondary complications can be prevented. Hydatid disease treatment should center on complete elimination of the parasite and prevention of disease recurrence with minimum morbidity and mortality. There are three therapeutic modalities for hepatic hydatid cysts: *systemic chemotherapy, surgery,* and a treatment known as *puncture, aspiration, injection, reaspiration* (PAIR). Surgery is still the mainstay treatment modality for hepatic hydatid cyst. However, chemotherapy and PAIR are recommended as alternatives to surgery, especially for patients who cannot tolerate surgery or who refuse it. Selection of the most appropriate treatment for hepatic hydatid cysts depends on the health of the patient, characteristics of the cysts (number, size, location), and presence of associated complications.

FIGURE 1 A comparison of computed tomography scans. **A,** Hepatic echinococcal cysts. **B,** Congenital cyst. **C,** Cystadenoma. For echinococcal cyst, **A1** demonstrates a single cyst with calcification and daughter cyst caused by *E. granulosa.* **A2** shows multiple small cysts characteristic of *E. multilocularis* infection. *(Courtesy Barbara M. Kadell, MD, Professor of Radiology, David Geffen School of Medicine at University of California, Los Angeles.)*

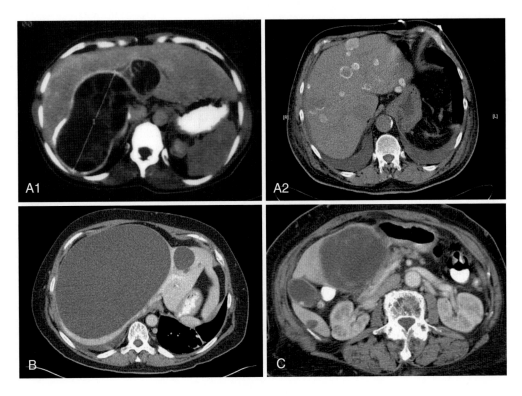

TABLE 2: Hepatic cyst disease: Differential features on imaging studies

Characteristics	Hydatid Cyst	Congenital Cyst	Cystadenoma
Configuration	Cyst within cyst	Single or multiple ± septations	Single ± septations
Wall character	Thick, uniform ± calcification	Thin, uniform	Mural nodules
Cyst contents	Daughter cysts Hydatid sand	Low density	Low density

Medical Therapy

Benzimidazole compounds, such as mebendazole and albendazole, are the agents of choice for medical treatment of echinococcal disease. Albendazole has replaced mebendazole as the most effective first-line drug therapy for hydatid cyst because of its better intestinal absorption and tissue distribution, resulting in a higher cystic fluid concentration. The indicated dosage of albendazole is 10 to 15 mg/kg per day postprandially in two divided doses. More recently, praziquantel, a synthetic isoquinoline–pyrazine derivative, has been used in combination with albendazole. This combination may be more effective than albendazole monotherapy.

When used as the primary treatment modality, chemotherapy has been associated with treatment failure in up to 70% of patients. Medical treatment therefore should be used in conjunction with percutaneous drainage or surgery. According to the WHO guidelines, preoperative administration of albendazole should begin between 1 and 4 days before surgery; if mebendazole is used, it must begin 3 months before surgery. Postoperative medical treatment remains controversial but is generally not indicated when there is no cyst spillage and the cyst has been completely removed.

Percutaneous Aspiration, Injection, and Reaspiration

PAIR is a minimally invasive technique consisting of percutaneous aspiration of the hydatid cyst under ultrasonic guidance, followed by the injection of a protoscolicide into the cyst cavity and, finally, reaspiration of the cyst contents. By reducing the size and volume of the cyst, the cyst wall thickens, the cavity decreases, and the cyst solidifies.

Patients undergoing PAIR typically receive oral benzimidazole therapy for 1 week before and 28 days after the procedure. Different scolicidal agents (20% sodium chloride solution or 95% ethanol) can be used during PAIR; however, 20% sodium chloride is most commonly used. Hypertonic saline has a high density and high attenuation on CT imaging, which allows for evaluation of proper contact of the scolicidal agent with the cyst wall. In general, 95% ethanol is avoided, particularly if a communication between the cyst and the biliary system is suspected. Studies have shown that there is immediate detachment of the inner germinal layer from the pericyst after injection of the scolicidal agent.

Following PAIR, the cyst fluid can be assessed to confirm the success of the procedure and the viability of any remaining protoscolices. PAIR is usually well tolerated. Possible complications include infection and leakage during the drainage, which can result in fever or anaphylaxis. Cyst decompression can also result in cyst-biliary fistula, which requires management with ERCP.

The indications for PAIR are WHO-IWGE ultrasonographic classification CE1, CE2, and CE3 cysts; infected cysts; multiple cysts, if accessible to puncture; absolute contraindication for surgery; refusal of surgery; pregnancy; and relapse after surgery. However, PAIR is contraindicated in patients younger than 3 years; in patients who are uncooperative; and for complicated cysts, cysts that are not accessible to puncture, or cysts in unfavorable or risky locations.

The most recent large multicenter report by the WHO-IWGE demonstrated that PAIR is a safe and effective therapeutic tool. In 765 patients with abdominal cysts treated with PAIR as a primary procedure, the overall complication rate was 14.7%, the recurrence rate was 1.57%, and one patient (0.13%) died of anaphylactic shock. Only 2 (0.26%) of the 765 patients required surgery after treatment failure with PAIR. The follow-up was more than 5 years in 75 patients and less than 5 years in the remaining 690 cases. Further studies are needed to determine the long-term outcomes of PAIR before it can be accepted as a first-line therapy of hydatid cyst. However, PAIR is a viable alternative to surgery in select cases, when carefully planned and executed by a multidisciplinary team that includes the surgeon, interventional radiologist, and chemotherapist.

Surgery

Surgery remains the treatment of choice in hepatic hydatid disease in patients who are good surgical candidates. The principles of the surgery are to inactivate the scolices, prevent spillage of the cyst contents, completely eliminate the viable cyst contents, manage the residual cyst cavity, and correct any cyst-related complications. Surgical options for hepatic hydatid disease range from conservative procedures—such as simple cyst drainage and partial cystectomy, with or without omentoplasty—to radical procedures such as pericystectomy, liver resection and, rarely, liver transplantation. The conservative techniques focus on sparing hepatic tissue and removing the parasite and leaving part or most of the pericyst in situ. In contrast, more radical procedures remove the entire pericyst, with or without entering the cyst itself. Whether the surgeon should routinely use a conservative versus radical approach to hepatic hydatid disease remains controversial. Nevertheless, the type of surgical approach should be based on the size, site, and type of the cyst as well as the surgeon's expertise.

Conservative Surgery

Simple drainage and partial cystectomy is best suited for cysts on the periphery of the liver. Before entering the cyst, packing of the operative field with scolicide-soaked gauzes is necessary to minimize the risk of peritoneal soilage and contamination. The cyst contents are then inactivated by aspirating the cyst with a closed system and infusing the scolicidal agent in the empty cavity (Figure 2, A). If the cyst fluid is bile stained, or if connection with bile ducts has previously been identified on ERCP, intracavitary scolicidal agents should be avoided.

After evacuating the cyst contents and the scolicidal agent, the cyst should be unroofed, and part of the cyst wall should be removed so that the cavity can be fully explored. Any remaining debris should be cleared (Figure 2, B). The cyst cavity should then be filled with an omental pedicle (Figure 2, C).

Radical Surgery

Radical surgery for hydatid cyst ideally includes complete removal of the cyst along with the pericyst, including any exocyst and adjacent liver parenchyma. This approach is the best treatment for all forms of hydatid cysts, particulary those with large biliary-cyst fistulae.

Pericystectomy

Total pericystectomy can be performed with either an open or a closed technique. In the open technique, the cyst content is removed and scolicdal agents are infused before excision of the pericyst wall. The surgeon must be certain not to spill the cyst contents when opening the cyst cavity. The pericyst wall is removed using electrocautery or a dissector (Figure 3). Open pericystectomy is recommended for

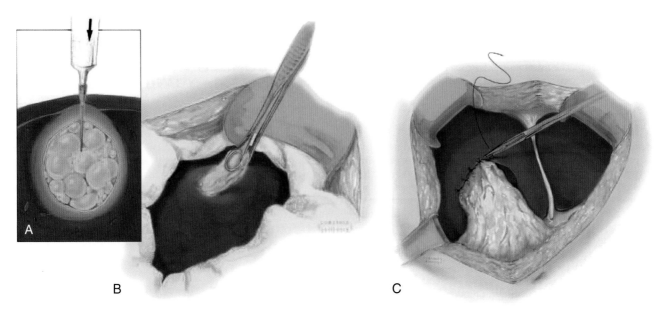

FIGURE 2 Open cyst drainage and evacuation. **A,** The cyst contents are inactivated by aspirating the cyst using a closed system, followed by infusion of the scolicidal agent into the empty cavity. **B,** The cyst is then unroofed and part of the cyst wall removed so that debris can be cleared. **C,** Finally, the cyst cavity is filled with an omental pedicle. *(From Cameron JL, Sandone C: Atlas of surgery: gallbladder and biliary tract, the liver, portosystemic shunts, the pancreas, Hamilton, ON, Canada, 1990, BC Decker.)*

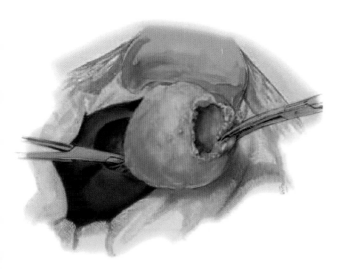

FIGURE 3 Pericystectomy can be performed with removal of the calcified pericyst either using electrocautery or a dissector. *(From Cameron JL, Sandone C: Atlas of surgery: gallbladder and biliary tract, the liver, portasystemic shunts, the pancreas, Hamilton, ON, Canada, 1990, BC Decker.)*

large cysts and when the cyst wall is thin and the risk of cyst rupture during manipulation is high.

For moderately large cysts that are located peripherally with a thick cyst wall and do not involve the major central vascular and biliary structures, the closed technique is preferred. With the closed technique, the whole cyst is removed en bloc, including the adventitia, without resection of healthy liver tissue. A plane is identified outside the pericyst, and pericystectomy is performed without manipulating the contents of the cyst. During the removal of the pericyst, blood vessels and biliary structures are controlled with clips or sutures. Interoperative ultrasonography may be useful to determine the relationship of the cyst to vascular and biliary structures within the liver parenchyma. The advantages of closed pericystectomy include leaving no adventitia and eliminating scolicidal agents. However, the closed method is more technically demanding because hepatic parenchymal transection is required.

Liver Resection

Nonanatomic wedge resection is preferred over pericystectomy if the cut surface of the liver after removal of the cyst is anticipated to be smaller with wedge resection. Compared with pericystectomy, wedge resection does not result in ischemic pedunculated peripheral hepatic tissue. Formal anatomic liver resection is indicated in cases of large multilocular cysts localized in either the right or left hemiliver, for large hydatid cysts that have destroyed one or more liver segments, or if the cyst is near major vascular or biliary structures.

When the development of the cyst distorts adjacent vessels and bile ducts and becomes densely adherent to major vessels, radial excision that leaves behind a small portion of the pericyst attached to the major vascular structures should be considered. This remnant portion of the pericyst should not contain a biliary fistula or an exocyst. Hepatic resection should also be considered in complicated cysts with large biliary fistulae; this method allows closure of the bile duct away from the area of biliary-cyst fistulae.

In general, liver resection in indicated when other, more conservative surgical therapies have failed or are contraindicated (e.g., with deep-seated, centrally located cysts) and should only be performed after an accurate assessment of the hepatic anatomy and when there is adequate hepatic parenchymal volume in the future liver remnant.

Liver Transplantation

In unusual circumstances, when the hydatid disease is not amendable to any standard treatment or when the disease has produced serious local complications and remains confined to the liver, liver transplantation may be the only potential curative therapy. Compared with *E.*

granulosa, which frequently occurs as a single cyst, *E. multilocularis* can result in a more complicated disease process known as *alveolar echinococcosis.* In this variation of the disease, multiple cysts can form throughout the liver, leading to fulminant liver failure from biliary sclerosis, Budd-Chiari syndrome, or sclerosing cholangitis. Although this clinical scenario is rare, orthotopic liver transplantation is a viable treatment option and a life-saving modality.

Intraoperative Management of Biliary-Cyst Communication

The presence of a biliary-cyst communication should be investigated in all patients, regardless of the type of surgical procedure performed. Although preoperative ERCP can be helpful in identifying biliary-cyst communications, a history of cholangitis or the presence of large cysts involving numerous hepatic segments should especially be suspected of harboring a biliary-cyst communication. An intraoperative finding of bile-stained cyst fluid warrants further investigation. After opening the pericyst, leave a dry pad on the inner surface of the cyst while applying gentle pressure on the gallbladder. Staining of bile on the pad is highly suggestive of the presence of a biliary-cyst fistula. In such cases, an intraoperative transcystic cholangiography is performed to identify the site of communication.

Communications smaller than 5 mm are closed with sutures. After excision of the cyst, a methylene blue test through a transcystic duct tube is helpful in identifying overlooked small biliary fistulae. For biliary communications larger than 5 mm, the surgical management may be more challenging. If simple drainage or partial cystectomy are planned, common duct exploration with choledochoscopy is warranted. After closing a large duct, a T-tube is used to decompress the biliary tree. In cases in which the large bile duct has been disrupted, surgical options include an internal drainage with Roux-en-Y intracystic hepaticojejunostomy or conversion to formal hepatic resections, thereby eliminating the need for bile duct exploration, repair, and T-tube drainage.

Laparoscopic Surgical Approaches

When a laparoscopic approach has been chosen to manage hydatid disease of the liver, the same principles of open surgery must be adhered to. The laparoscopic approach can involve simple drainage, partial cystectomy, or even total pericystectomy. Although the laparoscopic approach may allow a more detailed examinatin of the cyst, this approach has not gained wide acceptance. The major disadvantages of laparoscopy are the limited area of manipulation, difficulty in controlling spillage of cyst content into the peritoneal cavity during puncture of hydatid cyst under high pneumoperitoneum intrabdominal pressure, and difficulty in aspirating the thick cyst contents. Various techniques have been suggested to minimize cyst content spillage, including fixing the cyst to the abdominal wall with a customized, umbrella-shaped trocar and suction device, peritoneal lavage using protoscolicidal solutions, and creation of a perihepatic protoscolicidal pool by maintaining the patient in the Trendelenburg position during laparoscopic hydatid surgery. At present, there is no prospective randomized clinical trial comparing the laparoscopic approach with conventional open treatment.

OUTCOME FOLLOWING TREATMENT OF HEPATIC HYDATID DISEASE

With advances in perioperative care and intraoperative techniques, the morbidity and mortality associated with the surgical treatment of hepatic hydatid disease have decreased dramatically. Shock secondary to protoscolice spillage should be a rare occurrence when the appropriate preoperative chemotherapy and intraoperative techniques have been used. For uncomplicated hydatid disease, morbidity and mortality have been reported to be in the range of 20% and 1%, respectively; in contrast, patients with complicated disease have a higher reported morbidity and mortality, in the range of 30% to 50% and 5%, respectively.

SUMMARY

In general, the therapeutic approach to patients with hepatic hydatid disease should center on complete elimination of the parasite and prevention of disease recurrence with minimum morbidity and mortality. Surgery is still the main therapeutic option for patients who are good surgical candidates, particularly for type CE2, CE4, and CE5 cysts. PAIR offers excellent outcomes and should be considered in patients who are poor surgical candidates or who refuse surgery. Patients with WHO-IWGE classification CL, CE1, CE2, and CE3 cysts can often be treated with a combination of chemotherapy and PAIR. Although PAIR may be possible for treatment of CE2 cysts when the number of daughter cysts is low, surgery is often necessary when there are numerous daughter cysts. The standard of care for hepatic echinococcal cyst is still evolving, and further prospective randomized studies are needed to establish the ideal treatment.

SUGGESTED READINGS

Balik AA, Basoglu M, Celebi F, et al: Surgical treatment of hydatid cyst of the liver: review of 304 cases, *Arch Surg* 134:166–169, 1999.

Filice C, Brunetti E, Bruno R, Crippa FG: Percutaneous drainage of echinococcal cysts (PAIR—puncture, aspiration, injection, reaspiration): results of a worldwide survey for assessment of its safety and efficacy, WHO-Informal Working Group on Echinococcosis—PAIR Network, *Gut* 47:156–157, 2000.

Khuroo MS, Wani NA, Javid G, et al: Percutaneous drainage compared with surgery for hepatic hydatid cysts, *N Engl J Med* 337:881–887, 1997.

WHO Informal Working Group: International classification of ultrasound images in cystic *Echinococcus* for application in clinical and field epidemiological settings, *Acta Tropica* 85:253–261, 2003.

Yagci G, Ustonsoz B, Kaymakcioglu N, et al: Results of surgical, laparoscopic, and percutaneous treatment for hydatid disease of the liver: 10 years experience with 355 patients, *World J Surg* 29:1670–1679, 2005.

CAVERNOUS LIVER HEMANGIOMA

Henrik Petrowsky, MD, and Ronald W. Busuttil, MD, PhD

OVERVIEW

Hepatic cavernous hemangiomas are the most common benign liver tumors, with an incidence in autopsy series of up to 7%. Hepatic hemangiomas have a female predominance, with a female/male ratio of 5:1, and are most frequently detected in middle-aged women. Hemangiomas arise from endothelial cells that differ from normal sinusoidal lining cells in terms of phenotype and function. These endothelial cells build multiple vascular channels, which are the basic elements of hemangiomas. Hepatic hemangiomas obtain their blood supply mainly from the hepatic artery.

PATHOGENESIS AND PATHOLOGY

Hemangiomas appear as dark, reddish purple, soft, hypervascular lesions. They are usually well circumscribed and demarcated by a pseudocapsule that facilitates enucleation as a definitive surgical treatment. Most clinical series show that hemangiomas are more frequently located in the right lobe, which may simply reflect the significantly larger volume of the right lobe.

Cavernous hemangiomas mostly present as an intraparenchymal lesion but are sometimes pedunculated (Figure 1). The vasculature of these lesions, which is composed of endothelial cells and collagen, may be asanguinous or blood filled. The lumens are often occluded by thrombi because of the prothrombotic conditions and abnormal blood flow in these irregularly shaped vascular channels. As expected, the immunohistochemical phenotype is characterized by the endothelial markers CD31, CD34, and factor VIII–related antigen. The growth pattern of hepatic hemangiomas is related to vascular ectasia rather than hyperplasia or hypertrophy.

Because of the female predominance in middle-aged women and the observation of accelerated growth at puberty, during pregnancy, or with oral contraceptive use, estrogen was implicated as playing an important role in the pathogenesis of cavernous hemangiomas. Although estrogen receptors were found in some hemangioma specimens, the estrogen-driven theory has never been proved.

CLINICAL PRESENTATION

The majority of hemangiomas are asymptomatic and are often discovered incidentally by imaging for some other reason or during autopsy. Large hemangiomas might present as a right upper quadrant mass, hepatomegaly, or abdominal distension during physical examination. Depending on size and anatomic localization, hepatic hemangiomas can cause a variety of nonspecific symptoms, such as abdominal pain, discomfort, nausea, vomiting, early satiety resulting in weight loss, dysphagia, and dyspepsia. Abdominal pain and vague discomfort are the most frequent presentations in symptomatic patients.

The pathogenesis of pain is related to the stretching of the Glisson capsule or by the development of thrombosis within hepatic hemangiomas. Capsule stretching stimulates nociceptive afferent nerve fibers, resulting in visceral pain that is often difficult to describe. In many cases, patients describe discomfort that is dull in nature and nonspecifically localized in the right upper abdominal quadrant. Capsule stretching by hemangioma can also result in referred visceral pain, where pain is usually perceived at the cutaneous level. This type of referred pain is generally more localized than the nonreferred visceral pain and frequently affects the right shoulder region, particularly on deep inspiration.

Large hemangiomas can also result in a mass effect or compression or displacement of gastrointestinal (GI) organs or the biliary tract (Figure 2). Especially large hemangiomas in the left lobe may compress the stomach, resulting in early satiety and weight loss in severe cases. Also, large hemangiomas involving segments IVb, V, and/or VI can cause compression of the duodenum, which can result in gastric outlet obstruction with nausea and vomiting or biliary tract obstruction with jaundice.

Although it is conceivable that a hemangioma could rupture and cause intraperitoneal hemorrhage, this is an extremely rare event. A recently published systematic review of 10 surgical series on hemangiomas showed that spontaneous rupture occurred in less than 0.2% of all patients. Those with hemangioma rupture and intraperitoneal hemorrhage may report sudden abdominal pain and display severe hypertension. Another unusual but serious complication of hepatic hemangiomas is the development of Kasabach-Merritt syndrome, which is characterized by severe thrombocytopenia secondary to platelet trapping by the abnormal endothelium within hemangiomas. This condition can become life threatening with the development of secondary consumptive coagulopathy. Although this syndrome has its highest incidence in early infancy and is mostly related to subcutaneous hemangiomas, several cases have been reported in adult patients with giant hepatic hemangiomas.

Diagnostic Imaging

The majority of hemangiomas are discovered incidentally with abdominal imaging performed for an unrelated condition. Hemangiomas have characteristic imaging features that make their diagnosis relatively straightforward and preclude extensive blood testing or biopsy. The majority of hemangiomas are detected by abdominal ultrasound because this technique is the most frequently used abdominal imaging modality. On ultrasound, hemangiomas typically appear as well-circumscribed lesions, usually with a homogeneous hyperechoic signal. If hemangiomas contain more dense material, such as fibrosis or calcification, the ultrasound image also may have some hypoechoic portions.

Magnetic resonance imaging (MRI) is the best imaging technique for hemangioma, but it is also the most expensive. On MRI, hemangiomas have a bright signal intensity on T2-weighted images (Figure 3), and they show the typical peripheral enhancement after administration of contrast media. This imaging technique has the highest sensitivity (85%) and specificity (95%) among all imaging modalities and is therefore the preferred first-line diagnostic tool in establishing and differentiating the diagnosis.

CT scan is another frequently used alternative imaging tool in diagnosing hemangiomas, especially for patients with claustrophobia or implanted metal devices. Although hemangiomas are frequently missed on native CT scans because of their isodense appearance, contrast-enhanced CT scans also show the typical findings of peripheral enhancement during the arterial phase (Figure 4) and washout during the venous phase with peripheral retention of contrast.

Another complementary diagnostic modality with similar sensitivity and specificity is single photon emission CT with technetium-labeled red blood cells. However, this technique has its limitations when the lesion is smaller than 3 cm and deeply located.

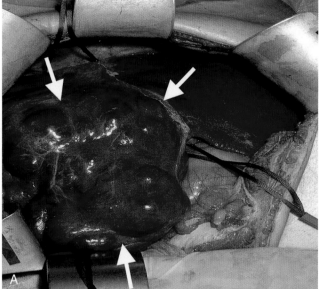

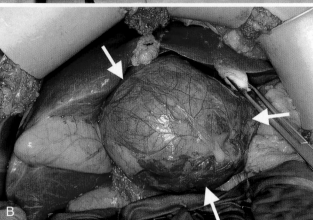

FIGURE 1   A, Intraoperative picture of an intraparenchymal giant hemangioma (*arrows*) occupying segments IVb, V, and VI. **B,** A pedunculated giant hemangioma (*arrows*) arising from the left lobe.

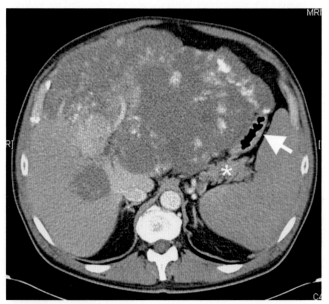

FIGURE 2   Contrast-enhanced CT scan of a giant hemangioma showing a mass effect with compression of stomach (*arrow*) and left laterally displaced pancreas (*asterisk*).

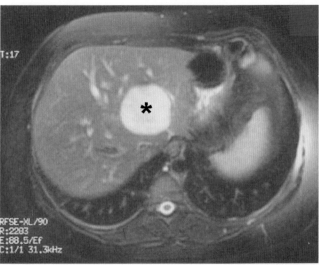

FIGURE 3   MRI shows hepatic hemangioma (*asterisk*) with high signal intensity on T2-weighting.

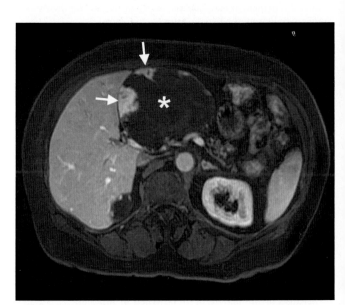

FIGURE 4   Contrast-enhanced CT scan of a giant hemangioma (*asterisk*) with the typical peripheral nodular enhancement (*arrows*) during the early arterial phase.

OPERATIVE TREATMENT

Indications

The vast majority of patients with hemangiomas have no symptoms and do not require surgical treatment. Indications for operative treatment are summarized in Figure 5. The most frequent indications for surgical removal are significant symptoms such as severe pain or mass-effect symptoms on GI organs or the biliary tree as previously described (see Figure 2). These symptoms are more likely to occur with increasing size of the hemangioma. However, anatomic localization, with close proximity to other anatomic structures (biliary tree) or organs (stomach, intestine), determines the severity of symptoms and must be considered when evaluating surgical treatment.

Because many hemangioma-associated symptoms are nonspecific, the physician and surgeon must rule out that these symptoms are not caused by other pathologic conditions involving intraabdominal organs (esophagus, stomach, duodenum and intestine, gallbladder,

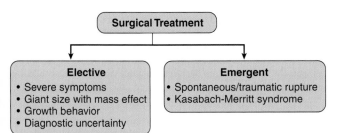

Surgical Treatment

Elective	Emergent
• Severe symptoms • Giant size with mass effect • Growth behavior • Diagnostic uncertainty	• Spontaneous/traumatic rupture • Kasabach-Merritt syndrome

FIGURE 5   Surgical treatment algorithm for elective and emergent indications for surgical resection of hepatic hemangiomas.

pancreas, and kidney) or extraabdominal organs (heart, lungs, musculoskeletal structures) before proceeding with a surgical treatment. Once other potential conditions are excluded, surgical treatment is determined by the severity of symptoms.

Another important indication for surgical resection is if the malignancy cannot be excluded. Although hemangiomas show many characteristic radiologic features, certain lesions may show atypical imaging, which results in diagnostic uncertainty. In these cases, a surgical approach to the suspected liver lesion is justified. On the other hand, if hepatic lesions show the characteristic imaging features of hemangioma but reveal clear growth behavior during follow-up, surgical removal may be justified before the lesions become so large as to cause severe symptoms. As mentioned, in the vast majority of patients hemangiomas can be clearly distinguished from malignant hepatic tumors.

Although spontaneous or traumatic rupture of a hemangioma occurs very rarely, this event can cause life-threatening intraperitoneal bleeding, which requires emergent treatment. The most suitable strategy in these patients is resuscitation, arterial embolization of the bleeding liver lesion, followed by surgical resection. In those cases where interventional embolization is unsuccessful, emergent surgery is indicated. Another condition that requires emergent treatment is the development of Kasabach-Merritt syndrome with severe coagulopathy. Although many other nonoperative strategies have been used to control this syndrome, the gold standard treatment is the removal of the underlying hemangioma, which might be hazardous in the presence of severe coagulopathy but will correct consumptive coagulopathy.

Technical Aspects

Depending on the size and the location, liver hemangiomas can be removed either by laparoscopy or laparotomy. The decision for a laparoscopic or open approach follows the same principles applied to other benign liver tumors. The ideal lesion for a laparoscopic approach is a small, superficial, localized lesion or a lesion localized within the left lateral liver segments (segments II and III).

Giant hemangiomas and lesions that are deeply located within the right lobe or at the dome of the right liver might be better approached through an open operation. A recent Cochrane Library review demonstrated that elective surgery for hemangiomas is safe, as reflected by a low mortality rate of 0.4%. Although there are no guidelines, many liver surgeons prefer enucleation of hemangiomas along the pseudocapsule whenever feasible. This procedure offers the advantage of maximal preservation of functional liver tissue, less blood loss, and probably fewer complications. If the dissection plane strictly follows the pseudocapsule, the likelihood for bile duct leaks is lower compared with parenchymal dissection. However, giant hemangiomas that occupy the entire right lobe or are deeply located within the right lobe might be difficult to enucleate and are better managed through anatomic resection. Enucleation and resection of hemangiomas follow the same rules as for all other liver tumors (Figure 6).

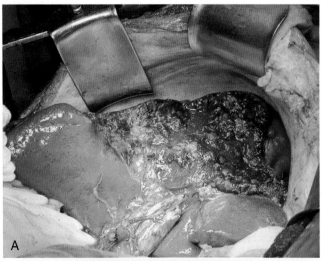

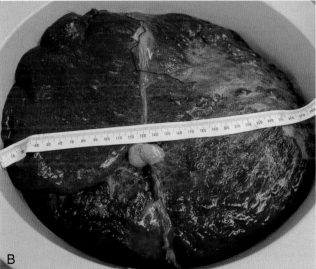

FIGURE 6   **A,** Intraoperative sites after enucleation of a giant hemangioma in the left lobe. View of enucleation surface. (The preoperative image of this case is shown in Figure 2.) **B,** Enucleated hemangioma specimen measuring 27 inches.

Although use of the Pringle maneuver in liver resection is debatable, inflow occlusion may be beneficial in assisting enucleation of large hemangiomas for several reasons. First, since hemangiomas are highly vascularized tumors, inflow occlusion minimizes the blood loss during enucleation. Second, inflow occlusion offers the advantage of decreasing blood flow to the hemangioma, which makes it compressible; this is of particular advantage when shrinking facilitates the dissection. Inflow occlusion of less than 30 minutes is usually well tolerated without significant ischemia-reperfusion injury. If the enucleation or resection takes significantly longer than 30 minutes, intermittent clamping can be applied. With this technique, the inflow occlusion is released for 5 minutes to allow reperfusion of the liver followed by another cycle of inflow occlusion. It is important that gentle pressure be applied to the hemangioma during reperfusion to avoid refilling and reexpansion of the tumor.

Orthotopic liver transplantation has been used in extraordinarily rare cases, when symptomatic giant hemangioma cannot be technically removed, or the remnant liver mass is too small for sufficient function. Also, liver transplantations are performed using donor organs with cavernous hemangiomas. Small hemangiomas can be left in situ, whereas giant hemangiomas can be enucleated or resected ex situ or in situ.

NONOPERATIVE TREATMENT

Nonoperative treatment modalities are reserved for patients with symptomatic hemangiomas who refuse surgery or would not tolerate a major surgical procedure because of severe comorbidities. In these cases, transarterial chemoembolization, percutaneous radiofrequency ablation, and radiation therapy are possible alternatives for nonoperative treatment, although success rates are not well documented, and these modalities cannot be recommended as first-line treatment.

SUMMARY

Cavernous hemangiomas are the most common benign liver tumors. The majority of hemangiomas are discovered incidentally and do not require any treatment. The typical finding of hemangiomas on contrast-enhanced CT and MRI is a peripheral nodular enhancement.

Severe symptoms and diagnostic uncertainty are the most common indications for surgical treatment. It is important before surgery to rule out other extrahepatic pathology that could mimic the symptoms. The surgical removal of hemangiomas has been proven a safe and effective treatment. Whenever feasible, enucleation should be preferred over anatomic resection due to maximal preservation of remnant liver tissue and minimal blood loss.

SUGGESTED READINGS

Baer HU, Dennison AR, Mouton W, et al: Enucleation of giant hemangiomas of the liver: technical and pathologic aspects of a neglected procedure, *Ann Surg* 216:673, 1992.
Colli A, Fraquelli M, Massironi S, et al: Elective surgery for benign liver tumours, *Cochrane Database Syst Rev* 1, CD005164, 2007.
Lerner SM, Hiatt JR, Salamandra J, et al: Giant cavernous liver hemangiomas: effect of operative approach on outcome, *Arch Surg* 139:818, 2004.
Yoon SS, Charny CK, Fong Y, et al: Diagnosis, management, and outcomes of 115 patients with hepatic hemangioma, *J Am Coll Surg* 197:392, 2003.

BENIGN LIVER TUMORS

Cristina R. Ferrone, MD

OVERVIEW

With widespread use of radiographic imaging studies, benign liver tumors are being identified with increasing frequency. These lesions are often identified incidentally in the presence or absence of liver disease. They are usually asymptomatic, with a benign natural history, and therefore are simply observed. Surgical resection is indicated if the patient is symptomatic, if malignancy cannot be ruled out, or if the lesion has the potential for malignant transformation or clinical complications. Patients with lesions that require life-long surveillance because of the potential for malignant transformation or clinical complications may be better served with surgical resection, provided they are good surgical candidates.

Making a definitive diagnosis is the most crucial aspect in the clinical management of patients with liver lesions. Some lesions can be accurately diagnosed based on their imaging studies, but others will require a biopsy. Once the diagnosis is made, the natural history and clinical picture of the patient will guide the management of disease.

CAVERNOUS HEMANGIOMA

Presentation

Hepatic hemangiomas are the most common benign liver tumor, and they can occur at any age. Hemangiomas occur in about 1% to 20% of the general population; they have a female predilection, with a 5:1 female/male ratio. The mean age of the hemangioma patient is 45 years. Hemangiomas occur equally in the left and right sides of the liver and are usually less than 5 cm in size, but they can be as large as 32 cm. Patients are usually asymptomatic; however, large lesions can become symptomatic. As the lesions increase in size, they can cause compression of adjacent organs and hemorrhage; they can also alter coagulation or cause inflammation, which can present with low-grade fever, weight loss, abdominal pain, anemia, thrombocytosis, and an increased fibrinogen level.

A rare complication is Kasabach-Merritt syndrome, which manifests as a coagulopathy resulting from intravascular coagulation, clotting, and fibrinolysis within the hemangioma. The localized coagulopathy can result in death in 20% to 30% of patients due to systemic fibrinolysis and thrombocytopenia. Another very rare complication is intratumoral hemorrhage, which can occur spontaneously or after anticoagulation therapy.

Hepatic hemangiomas in infants and children can often be accompanied by multiple cutaneous hemangiomas. Unlike in adults, large hemangiomas can be dangerous in children because they can cause significant shunting that can lead to hepatomegaly and congestive heart failure. These children are often managed medically with diuretics and inotropes. For patients refractory to medical management, hepatic arterial embolization can be considered as a temporizing measure. Luckily, most pediatric hemangiomas regress after the first year of life and do not require any intervention.

Pathogenesis

Hemangiomas arise from the endothelial lining of blood vessels. The pathogenesis is poorly understood, but there may be a hormonal link. Some lesions have estrogen receptors and show evidence of growth during high-estrogen states such as puberty and pregnancy. This correlation with estrogen may account for the higher prevalence of hemangiomas in women. Macroscopically the lesions are flat with a red-blue color, and may develop fibrosis, calcifications, and thrombosis as they get larger. Microscopically the lesions are composed of cavernous vascular spaces with fibrous septa lined by flattened endothelium.

Radiographic Appearance

Hemangiomas can frequently be diagnosed by imaging. Contrast computed tomography (CT) demonstrates peripheral followed by centripetal enhancement of the lesion. This pattern is pathognomonic for hemangiomas. On delayed scans, the entire lesion enhances. Magnetic resonance imaging (MRI) with gadolinium is also helpful in making the diagnosis because the lesions are hypointense on T1-weighted sequences and strongly hyperintense on T2-weighted images (Figure 1). Biopsy of the lesion should be restricted to atypical cases in which imaging cannot make the diagnosis because there is a small risk of bleeding with needle biopsy.

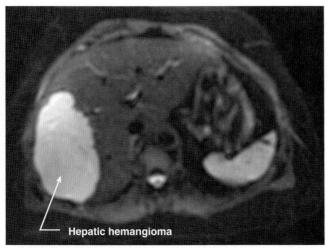

FIGURE 1 Hepatic hemangioma. MRI with T2-weighted image of a 13 cm hepatic hemangioma. The lesion is hyperintense.

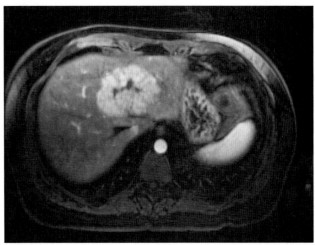

FIGURE 2 Arterial phase gadolinium-enhanced MRI demonstrates hypervascular appearance of FNH with characteristic central scar.

Management

No treatment is necessary for asymptomatic hemangiomas. Surgical resection should only be considered if patients develop symptoms or complications, or if malignancy cannot be excluded. Surgical options include open or laparoscopic enucleation or hepatic resection. Enucleation may have less morbidity than hepatic resection, specifically a lower biliary fistula rate. Symptomatic patients may be considered for liver transplantation if the lesions are unresectable. If patients require an intervention but are not surgical candidates, radiation or hepatic artery embolization can be considered.

Technical Tip

The main blood supply is from the arterial system, so extrahepatic ligation of the right or left hepatic artery can provide vascular control. The dissection should be carried out in the avascular plane, between the hemangioma and the normal hepatic parenchyma. An ultrasonic dissection device can be helpful. The large, raw surface can be treated with the argon beam, and the cavity can be filled with omentum.

FOCAL NODULAR HYPERPLASIA

Presentation

Focal nodular hyperplasia (FNH) is the second most common benign hepatic lesion, and similar to hemangiomas, it has a predilection for females. It is most commonly diagnosed in women between 30 and 50 years of age. These lesions are not stimulated by oral contraceptives. Most lesions are asymptomatic, but larger lesions may be symptomatic because of pressure on adjacent organs. Pedunculated lesions can torse on their pedicle, resulting in acute episodes of pain. The majority of lesions are solitary, but multiple lesions are observed in 20% to 30% of patients. Liver function tests are usually normal, but elevation of alkaline phosphatase and γ-glutamyl transferase may be observed.

Pathogenesis

FNH is considered to be a hyperplastic reaction to an arterial malformation that results in hyperperfusion of the liver parenchyma leading to hepatocellular hyperplasia. This hypothesis is supported by molecular data demonstrating that FNH is a polyclonal regenerative process. Macroscopically FNH is a well-circumscribed, unencapsulated lesion characterized by a central fibrous scar. Microscopically

FNH is composed of benign-appearing hepatocytes arranged in nodules delineated by fibrous septa that originate from the central scar. The large septa are composed of dystrophic vessels, ductal proliferation, and inflammatory cells. Malignant transformation has not been reported.

Radiographic Appearance

The diagnosis of FNH can often be made with imaging. A central scar is the most characteristic imaging feature, however, a central scar can also be seen with fibrolamellar hepatocellular carcinoma, hepatic adenomas, and metastatic lesions.

FNH is hypodense or isodense on the precontrast CT scan, but it enhances rapidly during the arterial phase of the scan. During this phase, the lesion contour is well demarcated, and the central scar is hypodense. The lesion's enhancement decreases during the portal phase, and it becomes isodense to the liver on the delayed images, on which the central scar and septa can demonstrate increased uptake of contrast because of the slow uptake of contrast in these fibrotic elements. FNH is isointense or hypointense on T1-weighted MRI images, and it is isointense or slightly hyperintense on T2-weighted images. The minimal difference between the FNH and the normal liver is due to the normal hepatocytes in FNH; this is important in making the diagnosis. The central scar is hypointense on T1-weighted images and strongly hyperintense on T2-weighted images. Gadolinium administration results in hyperintensity of the lesion during the arterial phase, followed by isointensity during the portal venous phase. The central scar becomes hyperintense on delayed imaging.

Imaging is usually diagnostic, with most studies demonstrating a higher sensitivity and specificity for MRI rather than CT or ultrasound. If neither CT nor MRI can make the diagnosis of FNH, a sulfur colloid scan can be performed. FNHs contain Kupffer cells, which take up sulfur colloid, whereas hepatic adenomas do not. Lastly, biopsy should be considered if imaging cannot firmly establish the diagnosis.

Management

When asymptomatic, there is no treatment for FNH, as long as the diagnosis has been confirmed with certainty. FNH has no risk of malignant potential or complications in men or in women. There is no evidence to support avoiding pregnancy or discontinuing oral contraceptives. Follow-up of these lesions is not necessary, unless they become symptomatic. Surgical resection is only indicated in symptomatic patients or in cases of diagnostic uncertainty. If liver resection is indicated, a margin of normal hepatic parenchyma is safer than enucleation because of large veins that frequently surround these lesions.

HEPATOCELLULAR ADENOMA

Presentation

Adenomas are benign liver neoplasms that are strongly associated with oral contraceptive and androgen use. The incidence is estimated to be 0.1 per year per 100,000 in non–oral contraceptive users and 3 to 4 per 100,000 in long-term oral contraceptive users. The duration of oral contraceptive use and the dose of estrogen increase the risk of developing a hepatic adenoma. Androgen and anabolic steroid use can also increase the risk for developing adenomas, which can also occur spontaneously, or they may be associated with underlying metabolic diseases such as iron overload due to β-thalassemia, type I or III glycogen storage disease, and diabetes mellitus.

Small adenomas are usually found incidentally, but large lesions can cause abnormal liver function tests, pain, or a sensation of upper abdominal fullness. Larger lesions can cause elevations in γ-glutamyl transferase and alkaline phosphatase. As these lesions increase in size, especially over 5 cm, the risk of hemorrhage and infarction increases. The risk of spontaneous bleeding can be as high as 20% to 40%. These patients can experience severe abdominal pain, hemoperitoneum, and hypovolemic shock. Hemodynamic instability is rare unless patients are anticoagulated. The risk of malignant transformation is approximately 10%, with the risk being higher for men than for women.

Most lesions are solitary, but in 10% to 30% of patients, multiple adenomas are identified. Hepatic adenomatosis is defined as more than 10 adenomas. Patients are more likely to have pain, hepatomegaly, and impaired liver function. There is also a higher risk of rupture. These lesions tend to be diffuse, making complete surgical resection difficult. Hepatic artery embolization and radiofrequency ablation can be used in conjunction with resection, and liver transplantation can be considered.

Pathogenesis

Macroscopically these lesions contain subcapsular vessels that can be as large as 30 cm. The lesions can be pedunculated, resulting in torsion and a significant amount of pain. Microscopically these lesions consist of benign hepatocytes arranged in a trabecular pattern with thin vessels throughout. Malignant transformation can occur, but it is rare.

Radiographic Appearance

MRI is the most helpful imaging modality for adenomas, because the lesions are hyperintense or isointense on T1-weighted images and mildly hyperintense on T2-weighted images. The presence of a fatty component can be assessed by fat-suppressed imaging. Signal heterogeneity is considered one of the most constant features of adenomas. Contrast-enhanced CT scans demonstrate hypervascular lesions on the arterial phase, which become isodense or hypodense on the portal phase due to arteriovenous shunting (Figure 3). Distinctive radiologic findings that can help distinguish adenomas from FNH include the smooth surface, presence of a capsule, and presence of necrosis or hemorrhage. Imaging can often reliably differentiate FNH from an adenoma. Unfortunately, imaging is frequently unable to differentiate between an adenoma and a hepatocellular carcinoma.

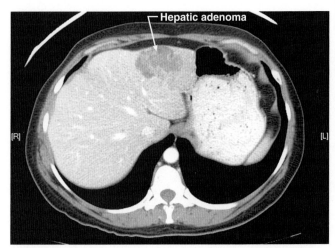

FIGURE 3 Hepatic adenoma. Abdominal CT scan demonstrating a 5 cm hepatic adenoma in the left lobe of the liver.

Management

Surgical resection of these lesions should be performed to relieve symptoms, prevent bleeding, or to prevent malignant transformation. Lesions smaller than 3 cm should be observed with serial imaging and α-fetoprotein levels. Patients should be encouraged to discontinue oral contraceptives. In patients with adenomas greater than 4 cm, surgical resection should be strongly considered. Anatomic or segmental resections, either open or laparoscopic, are the best option. A wide margin is not necessary, because the majority of these lesions are benign. A ruptured adenoma has a mortality of 8%; however, by delaying surgery, the operative risks can be reduced. Patients should be stabilized and should undergo selective hepatic arterial embolization followed by elective resection.

Similar to those with solitary adenomas, patients with multiple adenomas tend to be women on oral contraceptives or women with type I glycogen storage disease. Patients with adenomas greater than 4 cm have a risk of bleeding, and the risk of malignant transformation is approximately 10%. Surgical resection should be performed for all adenomas greater than 5 cm, which may require a staged resection if the patient has bilobar disease.

CYSTIC TUMORS

Simple Cysts

Simple cysts are almost always asymptomatic, and they are usually discovered incidentally. Approximately 50% of patients have solitary cysts with sizes ranging from 5 to 20 cm. Right upper quadrant pain, early satiety, and upper abdominal fullness usually do not occur until the cyst is greater than 8 cm. These lesions are thought to be due to abnormal embryonal development of intrahepatic biliary ducts, which lack a connection to their extrahepatic counterparts. Histologically the cysts consist of a single layer of columnar or cuboidal epithelium with minimal surrounding fibrous stroma. The cyst usually contains a straw-colored serous fluid without bile.

Radiographic Appearance

Ultrasound is usually sufficient to diagnose a simple cyst. These cysts have thin walls that do not enhance on CT or MRI. No internal septations or masses should be visualized.

Management

No intervention is required for asymptomatic cysts. Cysts causing symptoms in patients who are poor operative candidates can be managed with aspiration and injection of a sclerosing agent. In operative candidates, patients with symptomatic cysts larger than 5 cm should be taken to the operating room for a laparoscopic or open cyst unroofing. The cyst wall should be examined closely for any mural nodules or irregularities to rule out malignancy. If the cyst fluid is bilious rather than straw colored, a communication with the biliary system needs to be identified and ligated.

Technical Tips

When unroofing a cyst, the opening should be made as large as possible, avoiding areas with overlying hepatic parenchyma. This will allow the cyst fluid to drain into the peritoneal cavity and minimize the risk of cyst recurrence due to cyst closure.

Complex Cysts

Multiple Cysts

Polycystic liver disease is an inherited autosomal-dominant condition often seen in conjunction with polycystic renal cysts. Polycystic liver disease, unlike polycystic kidney disease, rarely leads to hepatic insufficiency. Most patients are asymptomatic, until they develop advanced disease, at which time they often develop abdominal pain and fullness in the right upper quadrant. To relieve symptoms, a limited hepatic resection in conjunction with aggressive cyst fenestration can be performed. Unfortunately, relief is only temporary, as the disease progresses and cysts recur. Hepatic transplantation is rarely considered unless the patient develops portal hypertension and hepatic failure.

Cystadenomas

Cystadenomas are benign cysts with malignant potential. Surgical resection should be considered whenever a cystadenoma is diagnosed. These cysts are slow growing, multilocular, and lined with a single layer of cuboidal or columnar epithelium surrounded by thickened stroma. Mesenchymal tissue is required to make the diagnosis.

Presentation

Cystadenomas can grow as large as 20 cm, resulting in abdominal fullness, loss of appetite, and pain. Jaundice can occur if the cyst compresses the biliary tree or fistualization allows for the cyst contents to obstruct the biliary tree.

Contrast enhanced CT and MRI scans demonstrate multiple internal septations, irregular borders, calcifications, and a thick stromal layer. Mural nodules can also be seen, which should heighten the clinician's concern for a cystadenocarcinoma.

Technical Tips

Cystadenomas need to be removed in their entirety, because the cyst wall carries the potential for malignant transformation. An enucleation can be performed for cystadenomas, but if there is a suspicion

for malignancy, a formal hepatic resection should be considered. Unroofing of the cyst should not be performed.

Echinococcal Cysts

Pathogenesis

Echinococcal or hydatid cysts should be considered in the differential diagnosis for patients who have traveled to or from endemic areas, such as the southwestern United States, Scotland, Greece, or other parts of Europe. The tapeworm *Echinococcus* infects dogs, but humans, sheep, cattle, and pigs are intermediary hosts. The intermediary hosts are infected by ingestion of parasite eggs via direct contact with an infected animal or by ingestion of contaminated food or water. Cysts can be found in the liver, lung, brain, and kidney.

Presentation

Most patients are asymptomatic, but a few will complain of fever and abdominal pain. Rarely, the cysts will rupture, and the patient will suffer anaphylactic shock. CT and MRI scans will demonstrate thick-walled cysts with calcifications containing debris. Septations and daughter cysts may also be identified within the cysts. Routine blood work can demonstrate eosinophilia; however, the diagnosis is confirmed with serologic tests.

Management

Prior to surgical manipulation of these cysts, patients should be treated with albendazole or mebendazole. The surgeon should plan to perform a complete enucleation of all of the cysts. Cyst drainage or fenestration is not recommended because of the risk of anaphylaxis with spillage of cyst contents and the risk of recurrence.

Technical Tips

The area around the cyst should be carefully packed with a layer of laparotomy pads with a protoscolicidal agent such as 20% hypertonic saline, 0.5% centrimide/0.05% chlorhexadine, or 10% povidone-iodine on top of saline-soaked gauze. Great care should be taken to minimize cyst manipulation to avoid rupture, and complete cyst removal should be performed, including removal of any daughter cysts.

SUGGESTED READINGS

Charny CK, Jarnagin WR, Schwartz LH, et al: Management of 155 patients with benign liver tumours, *Br J Surg* 88(6):808–813, 2001.

Deneve JL, Pawlik TM, Cunningham S, et al: Liver cell adenoma: a multicenter analysis of risk factors for rupture and malignancy, *Ann Surg Oncol* 16(3):640–648, 2009.

Yoon SS, Charney CK, Fong Y, et al: Diagnosis, management, and outcomes of 115 patients with hepatic hemangioma, *J Am Coll Surg* 197(3):392–402, 2003.

MANAGEMENT OF PRIMARY MALIGNANT LIVER TUMORS

Steven C. Cunningham, MD, and
Richard D. Schulick, MD

OVERVIEW

The majority of malignant liver tumors treated by surgeons are either hepatocellular carcinoma (HCC), intrahepatic cholangiocarcinoma (ICC), or metastatic colorectal cancer (mCRC). Because mCRC is covered elsewhere in this book, this chapter focuses on HCC and ICC. The best chance for a cure of either of these two diseases is surgical extirpation, either via resection, typically for ICC, or transplantation or resection for HCC. Unfortunately, many patients are initially seen with advanced disease that is not amenable to resection or transplantation; however, these patients are candidates for other therapies, including liver-directed therapies and palliative care.

GENERAL PREOPERATIVE PREPARATION

Although major hepatic resection has become increasingly safe in recent decades, the potential exists for serious morbidity; therefore all patients being considered for resection should undergo preoperative optimization and risk stratification regarding medical comorbidities. Nutritional status and treatable cardiac, pulmonary, and renal disease warrant special attention.

The functional liver remnant (FLR) is the volume of liver parenchyma that will remain to support the patient following resection. When a large amount of liver is expected to be resected, volumetrics for the FLR may be formally assessed using computer algorithms. The minimum acceptable volume of the FLR depends on the health of the liver parenchyma: 20% to 30% for normal liver, 30% to 40% for liver with steatohepatitis, and 40% to 50% or more for cirrhosis. If less than the minimum is estimated to remain after a proposed resection, the patient is not a candidate for a single-stage resection. Although two-stage resection may be performed to allow an inadequate FLR to hypertrophy to sufficient size, this strategy is more frequently applied in patients with bilateral mCRC. For patients with HCC or ICC, preoperative portal vein embolization to induce hypertrophy to attain a sufficient FLR is an option.

In addition to the volume of the FLR, the patient's hepatic function should also be assessed. The simplest evaluation of liver function begins with serum liver panel: prothrombin time and albumin provide a measure of protein synthesis; alkaline phosphatase and γ-glutamyl transferase (GGT) provide a measure of cholestasis; and bilirubin provides a measure of the uptake, conjugation, and excretion of bile. Transaminases provide a measure of hepatocyte necrosis. More sophisticated tests of liver function exist, many of which measure the clearance of substances such as antipyrine, caffeine, lidocaine, or indocyanine green, although these tests are not commonly performed in the United States.

More commonly, the Child-Turcotte-Pugh (CTP) scoring system is used to risk stratify patients with underlying cirrhosis. Classically, patients with CTP class A liver disease may be expected to have a baseline perioperative mortality of 10%, which nearly triples for patients with class B (~30%) and class C (>80%) liver disease. Similarly, the presence of portal hypertension is a reliable surrogate for increased risk of perioperative complications. The presence of an enlarged spleen, low platelet count, or varices may suggest the presence of portal hypertension.

Since 2002, the United Network for Organ Sharing has used the Model for End-Stage Liver Disease (MELD) score to prioritize patients in need of a liver transplantation. The score is calculated from the serum bilirubin, INR (prothrombin time), and the creatinine values, and ranges from 6 to 40; it provides a measure of prognosis related to liver disease.

SPECIFIC CONSIDERATIONS

Hepatocellular Carcinoma

HCC is the most common primary malignant liver tumor worldwide. Although the incidence is highest in Asia and sub-Saharan Africa, the incidence in the United States has been increasing in recent years. Risk factors include hepatitis B and C and cirrhosis of any etiology. Most patients with HCC in fact have cirrhosis, those with the fibrolamellar variant being a notable exception.

The presence of cirrhosis often makes radiologic diagnosis more difficult because regenerative nodules, dysplastic nodules, and HCC all may have a similar appearance. Nevertheless, computed tomography (CT) and magnetic resonance imaging (MRI) are often able to distinguish HCC. Most small HCC nodules, for example, enhance homogenously on arterial phase CT imaging, but the contrast tends to wash out during the portal venous phase. Regenerative nodules, however, enhance most during the portal venous phase, and dysplastic nodules tend not to display a washout of contrast material. MRI is even more effective than CT at diagnosing HCC because areas of carcinoma demonstrate signal intensity changes distinct from cirrhotic liver parenchyma. T1-weighted images of HCC are generally hypointense, and T2-weighted images are generally hyperintense.

Underlying cirrhosis presents not only a diagnostic difficulty but a therapeutic one, especially for patients with early HCC on well-compensated cirrhosis. The question for these patients is whether resection or transplantation is a most appropriate first therapeutic step. Transplantation is ideal for patients with technically resectable HCC with severe cirrhosis because both the HCC and the underlying liver disease are treated simultaneously. There is controversy, however, regarding those patients with early cirrhosis and a small, solitary HCC that is amenable to either resection or transplantation.

Intrahepatic Cholangiocarcinoma

ICC is the second most common primary malignant liver tumor. Its incidence has also increased markedly over recent decades for reasons that are unclear. Risk factors for the development of cholangiocarcinoma include sclerosing cholangitis (8% to 20% lifetime risk) and choledochal cysts (3% to 28% lifetime risk). Risk is doubled for patients of Asian descent, and it increases 1.5-fold for males. Of the three gross subtypes of ICC—mass forming, periductal infiltrating, and intraductal—the periductal infiltrating type is associated with the worst prognosis.

Contrast-enhanced CT may demonstrate a rim of peripheral enhancement with upstream biliary dilatation. On both CT and MRI, the contrast enhancement often persists in delayed phases. T2-weighted MRI images show ICC to be a high-intensity lesion that tends not to have a visible capsule on MRI, which may help to distinguish it from HCC or other lesions.

Cholangiocarcinoma is an uncommon indication for liver transplantation. Although initial results were disappointing, recent studies evaluating pretransplant adjuvant therapy have shown more promise for perihilar cholangiocarcinomas, but transplantation for ICC continues to return disappointing results and should be considered inappropriate outside of clinical trials.

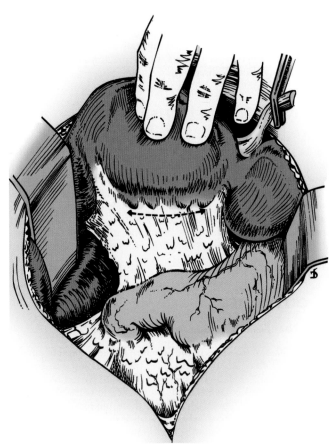

FIGURE 1   Lowering the hilar plate. To lower the hilar plate, the initial incision is made where the Glisson capsule reflects to the lesser omentum. *(From Blumgart LH, editor: Surgery of the liver, biliary tract, and pancreas, ed 4, Philadelphia, 2007, Saunders, p 462.)*

RESECTION WITH CURATIVE INTENT

HCC and ICC are both resected using standard hepatectomy techniques. In accordance with standard principles of hepatic resection, these masses are considered resectable if there is no extrahepatic disease, if the resection is anticipated to be margin negative, and if sufficient FLR can be maintained with adequate hepatic portal and arterial inflow, hepatic venous outflow, and biliary drainage. For patients in whom insufficient FLR is a likely possibility, preoperative ipsilateral portal vein embolization is an option to cause hypertrophy of the FLR.

Resections may be broadly categorized into anatomic and nonanatomic techniques. Small, peripheral lesions are optimally positioned for nonanatomic, or wedge, resection. Larger or more central lesions typically require formal anatomic resection such as segmentectomy, sectionectomy, hemihepatectomy, or extended hepatectomy. In open surgery, these operations are best approached through a right subcostal incision with an upper midline component, extended as necessary. Laparoscopic techniques continue to be developed and are an option in carefully selected patients.

Following access to the abdominal cavity, the operation commences with a search for metastatic disease. For major anatomic resections, the appropriate portion of the liver should be mobilized by dividing the round, falciform, and ipsilateral triangular ligaments. Once the liver is mobilized, intraoperative ultrasound is used to evaluate the intrahepatic anatomy and the extent of intrahepatic disease and to plan the operation.

The hepatic artery and portal vein inflow vessels may be controlled in the hilum of the liver. Alternatively, these inflow pedicles may be approached intraparenchymally after initiating parenchymal transection, or by performing small hepatotomies to gain access. Exposure of the proximal hepatic ducts, especially the left hepatic duct, may be facilitated by initially lowering the hilar plate (Figure 1). Once inflow has been controlled, control of the appropriate hepatic venous outflow is performed. If the right hepatic vein is to be exposed, the inferior vena cava ligament (Makuuchi's ligament) should be divided with scissors or with an endostapler (Figure 2). The hepatic veins may be suture ligated or stapled (Figure 3). Alternatively, the hepatic veins may be divided later, from within the parenchyma.

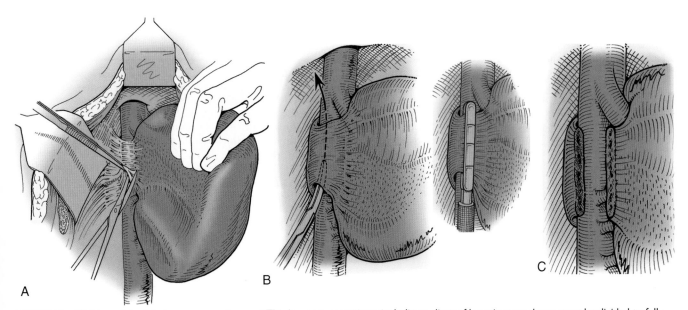

A   B   C

FIGURE 2   Division of the inferior vena cava ligament. This ligament, sometimes including a sliver of hepatic parenchyma, must be divided to fully expose the IVC, the entire extrahepatic right hepatic vein, and the posterior right liver. *(From Blumgart LH, editor: Surgery of the liver, biliary tract, and pancreas, ed 4, Philadelphia, 2007, Saunders, p 1354.)*

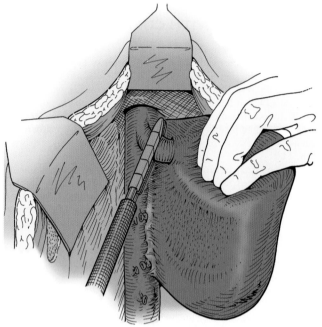

FIGURE 3   Division of the right hepatic vein. With the liver retracted to the left, the right hepatic vein may be rapidly and safely divided using an Endo GIA stapler with a vascular load. *(From Blumgart LH, editor: Surgery of the liver, biliary tract, and pancreas, ed 4, Philadelphia, 2007, Saunders, p 1364.)*

The method of transecting the parenchyma is largely a matter of surgeon preference, and a variety of techniques are available, including simple finger-clamp and Kelly-clamp fracture; ultrasonic, tissue-sealing, and water-jet dissection; and stapling. In all cases, small vessels and ducts may be clipped, but larger ones require ligature or stapling. An intermittent Pringle maneuver may further decrease bleeding but should be used sparingly. Maintaining the central venous pressure at or below 5 mm Hg has been shown to be associated with decreased blood loss and improved outcomes.

PALLIATION

Because many patients are seen initially with unresectable HCC and ICC, palliative management warrants special mention, and purely symptomatic treatment is indeed is the best option for many patients. The goal of palliative management is to provide long-term symptomatic relief, typically with biliary drainage. Although endoscopically placed biliary stents have a high rate of initial success in relieving biliary obstruction, their utility is often limited by frequent obstruction and need for replacement. Self-expanding metallic stents provide greater patency than plastic stents but can be difficult or impossible to change when they do obstruct. Percutaneous stents have several advantages, including access to multiple, isolated areas of the intrahepatic biliary tree, ease of revision, and the possibility to transition to internalized drainage. Operative biliary-enteric bypass provides reliable and durable relief of obstructive jaundice and may be performed

on any patient found at initial exploration to be unresectable. However, owing to the greater incidence of mortality and morbidity compared with the above interventions, operative biliary-enteric bypass is not the best option for patients whose imaging strongly suggests advanced, unresectable disease.

LIVER-DIRECTED THERAPY

The decision regarding treatment of patients with HCC and ICC need not be strictly binary (i.e., curative-intent resection vs. pure palliation). Nonresectional liver-directed therapy is a valuable option for patients who have unresectable disease at initial diagnosis. The most common modalities currently in use are thermal ablation (microwave or radiofrequency), embolization (chemoembolization or bland embolization), percutaneous ethanol injection, and directed radiotherapy. While initial results are promising, more randomized controlled trials are required to better define the role and benefit of these modalities.

OUTCOMES

Hepatocellular Carcinoma

Since 2000, in most series in the literature on the surgical treatment of HCC within the Milan criteria, liver transplantation is associated with improved overall 5-year survival (50% to 81%) and recurrence rates (2% to 18%) compared with liver resection (31% to 78% and 65%, respectively; Table 1). However, these improved rates often come at the cost of increased perioperative morbidity and mortality, an inability to use pathologic information to guide the decision of salvage transplantation, and limited organ availability resulting in waiting list drop-offs due to tumor progression.

A recent international, multiinstitutional series of early stage HCC found that although resection patients did have shorter 5-year overall and disease-free survival, they had tumors with more advanced pathologic features. This study also found that the survival advantage associated with liver transplantation was attenuated for patients whose MELD score was 8 or lower. Factors associated with worse survival following surgical treatment of HCC include large tumor size, positive margin status, major and microscopic vascular invasion, and increasing degrees of liver fibrosis.

Intrahepatic Cholangiocarcinoma

In one of the largest series on cholangiocarcinoma, resectability rates were reported to range from 30% to 50%. In that series of 564 operations, 44 (8%) were ICC, and 66% of those were resectable. While complication rates following resection of cholangiocarcinoma range widely, from 10% to 60%, resection of intrahepatic tumors is associated with a lower complication rate compared with perihilar and distal resections.

Following resection of ICC, 5-year survival ranges from 44% to 63% (Table 2) and is worse in patients with positive margin status, positive lymph node status, larger tumor size, and less differentiation. Palliated patients tend to survive less than 12 months.

TABLE 1: Review of series comparing resection and liver transplant for HCC or cirrhosis

Author (Year)	N RSX	N LT	Overall 5YS RSX	Overall 5YS LT	Mb (%) RSX	Mb (%) LT	Mt (%) RSX	Mt (%) LT	Rec (%) RSX	Rec (%) LT
Figueras (2000)	35	85	51%	60%	NR	6.7	NR	NR	65	7
De Carlis (2001)	131	91	38%	65%	NR	NR	4	18	62	7
Shabahang (2002)	44	65	57% 3YS	66% 3YS	NR	NR	7	7	NR	NR
Bigourdan (2003)	20	17	36%	71%	30	47	5	0	30	18
Margarit (2005)	37	36	78%	50%	NR	NR	2.7	5.6	59	11
Poon (2007)	204	43	68%	81%	35	44	3.4	0	NR	NR
Cillo (2007)	131	40	31%	63%	NR	NR	5.3	7.5	53	2
Del Gaudio (2008)	80	293	66	58	NR	79	0	5	49	9
Bellavance (2008)	245	134	46%	66%	49	65	1.6	1.5	50	14

Modified from Cunningham SC, Tsai S, Marques HP, et al: Management of early hepatocellular carcinoma in patients with well-compensated cirrhosis, *Ann Surg Oncol* 16:1820, 2009.

RSX, Resection; *LT,* liver transplantation; *5YS,* 5-year survival; *3YS,* 3-year survival; *Mb,* morbidity; *Mt,* mortality; *NR,* not reported; *Rec,* recurrence.

TABLE 2: Review of series: ICC treated by resection

Author, Location (Year)	Resected (N)	5-Year Survival, R0	5-Year Survival, All	Mortality (%)
Pichlmayr, Germany (1995)	32	NR	17%	6
Jan, Taiwan (1996)	41	44%	27%	0
Casavilla, Pittsburgh (1997)	34	NR	31%	7
Lieser, Rochester (1998)	32	45%	NR	NR
Madariaga, Pittsburgh (1998)	34	51%	35%	6
Valverde, France (1999)	30	NR	22%	3
Inoue, Japan (2000)	52	55%	36%	2
Weber, New York (2001)	33	NR	31%	3
DeOliveira, Baltimore (2006)	34	63%	40%	2

Modified from DeOliveira ML, Cunningham SC, Cameron JL, et al: Cholangiocarcinoma: 31-year experience with 564 patients at a single institution, *Ann Surg* 245:755, 2007.

NR, not reported.

SUGGESTED READINGS

Bellavance EC, Lumpkins KM, Mentha G, et al: Surgical management of early-stage hepatocellular carcinoma: resection or transplantation? *J Gastrointest Surg* 12:1699, 2008.

Cunningham SC, Choti MA, Bellavance EC, et al: Palliation of hepatic tumors, *Surg Oncol* 16:277, 2007.

Cunningham SC, Tsai S, Marques HP, et al: Management of early hepatocellular carcinoma in patients with well-compensated cirrhosis, *Ann Surg Oncol* 16:1820, 2009.

DeOliveira ML, Cunningham SC, Cameron JL, et al: Cholangiocarcinoma: 31-year experience with 564 patients at a single institution, *Ann Surg* 245:755, 2007.

HEPATIC MALIGNANCY: RESECTION VERSUS LIVER TRANSPLANTATION

Jay A. Graham, MD, Kirti Shetty, MD, and Lynt B. Johnson, MD, MBA

OVERVIEW

Primary hepatic malignancies include several different groups of neoplastic lesions that originate in the liver. The most common neoplastic conditions are predominantly associated with hepatocellular carcinoma (HCC) and cholangiocarcinoma. Although each of these diseases has differing etiologies and tumorogenesis patterns, surgical therapy is the only *true* opportunity for a curative outcome for both cancers. Although success has been reported with transplantation for selected extrahepatic cholangiocarcinoma patients, resection has remained the only reasonable choice for intrahepatic cholangiocarcinoma. The management of HCC, however, has evolved to include several different options; these include surgical resection, liver transplantation (LT), transarterial chemoembolization (TACE), percutaneous ethanol injection (PEI), radiofrequency ablation (RFA), systemic chemotherapy, and localized intratumoral radiation.

Most patients with HCC are diagnosed at advanced stages. In the setting of advanced disease, survival is dismal; untreated patients only live 3 to 6 months. In patients with limited tumor burden, an evaluation for possible surgical treatment is of paramount importance. This appraisal begins with the question of whether resection or liver transplantation would be of best benefit to the patient. At present this question has sparked a great debate within the transplant and oncology communities.

The Milan criteria published in 1996 showed excellent 5-year survival rates following LT in those with cirrhosis and stage I or II HCC. However, applicability of this finding has been tempered by access to LT and the availability of donor organs. Long waiting list times can often lead to progression of the disease. Although the United Network for Organ Sharing (UNOS) adoption of the Model for End-Stage Liver Disease (MELD) exemption status for HCC helped decrease the time to LT for patients with HCC, the core problem of organ shortage still exists. Consequently, partial liver resection remains a viable option for suitable patients, with the intention of curative hepatectomy.

Liver resection is associated with a significant risk of HCC recurrence over time and the development of de novo HCC within the cirrhotic liver remnant. In patients with cirrhosis and portal hypertension, hepatic decompensation may occur due to inadequate regeneration of the remnant liver. Therefore hepatic resection may best be limited to patients whose hepatic synthetic function is excellent, who lack portal hypertension, and who otherwise may not be optimal LT candidates.

Another approach is to offer hepatic resection as an initial therapy, followed by LT if and when there is either recurrence or development of de novo malignancy. However, this concept of liver resection as a bridge to "salvage" liver transplantation is controversial for several reasons: First, LT may be complicated by past hepatic surgery. Second, the pattern of recurrence may be too aggressive to allow for LT. Ultimately, the physician team must lay the framework for treatment in the context of tumor staging, presence of portal hypertension, extent of resection required, age of the patient, presence of comorbidities, and the impact of organ usage and availability.

EPIDEMIOLOGY

Responsible for up to 1 million deaths, HCC is the most common primary neoplasm of the liver and the fifth most common cancer worldwide. Chronic hepatitis B virus infection is the predominant risk factor for HCC in Asia and Africa. In the Western world and Japan, chronic hepatitis C virus infection accounts for the majority (over 60%) of HCC.

In the United States, population studies have demonstrated a dramatic increase in the incidence of HCC from 1.4 per 100,000 between 1975 and 1977 to 6.4 between 2001 and 2005. This increased incidence has been accompanied by a shift to a younger population (those between the ages of 45 and 60 years). HCC is now associated with the fastest growing death rate among cancers in the United States. These trends are believed to be a result of the maturation of the population infected by hepatitis C during the 1960s and 1970s. Ultimately, the incidence of HCC in the United States is expected to further increase over the next 2 to 3 decades, which will contribute to the significant health care burden associated with this disease.

SURVEILLANCE FOR HEPATOCELLULAR CARCINOMA

The overall 5-year survival rate for untreated symptomatic HCC is less than 5%. By contrast, survival rates associated with surgical therapy for early stage HCC approach 75% to 80% at 5 years. Clearly, early diagnosis and appropriate management of HCC is of paramount importance to promote favorable outcomes. In theory, surveillance strategies for HCC should significantly affect patient survival. However, this is an area fraught with controversy and plagued by the lack of controlled data.

Definition of at-Risk Populations

The decision to enter a patient into a surveillance program depends on the risk of HCC, that is, the incidence of HCC within the population. Decision analysis has been utilized to provide guidelines for surveillance. In general, an intervention is considered effective if it increases longevity by about 3 months and can be achieved at a cost less than $50,000 per year of life gained. It has been suggested that patients with liver disease be offered surveillance when the risk of HCC is 1.5% per year or greater. Hepatitis B carriers represent a uniquely high-risk population, and cost efficacy analysis in this population suggests that surveillance becomes cost effective once HCC incidence exceeds 0.2% per year. The American Association for the Study of Liver Diseases (AASLD) recommends surveillance only in specific groups of patients (Table 1).

Surveillance Tests

Serologic

The performance characteristics of α-fetoprotein (AFP) has been best studied. A value of 20 ng/mL is believed to provide the optimal balance between sensitivity and specificity; however, its sensitivity at this level is only 60%, and specificity is about 75%. This makes AFP an inadequate screening test for HCC. Other serologic tests such as des-γ-carboxy prothrombin (DGCP), also known as *prothrombin induced by vitamin K absence* (PIVKA II), have not been shown to be useful as a screening test.

Radiologic

The test most commonly used is ultrasonography (US), with a sensitivity of 65% to 80% and a specificity over 90%. However, US is operator dependent and may be unreliable in obese subjects. The use of CT

TABLE 1: Groups in which HCC surveillance is recommended

Liver Disease	Annual HCC Incidence
Hepatitis B Carriers*	
Documented cirrhosis	2.5% to 5%
Asian males ≥0 yr	0.4%
Asian females ≥50 yr	0.2%
Africans >20 yr	0.3%
Family history of HCC	0.2%
Hepatitis C	
Cirrhosis	2% to 8%
Bridging fibrosis	Increased
Other Etiologies of Cirrhosis	
Alcohol-induced	0.5% to 1%
Hemochromatosis	3% to 4%
NASH	Increased
Other	Unclear

*For carriers not listed, risk of HCC varies, and surveillance should be invidualized.
NASH, Nonalcoholic steatohepatitis

scan and MRI as a screening test cannot be recommended given their expense and lack of availability in many areas of the world.

Surveillance Interval

An interval between 6 and 12 months has been proposed based on tumor doubling times. Therefore current guidelines advocate the use of US at 6- to 12-month frequency to screen for HCC in high-risk patients. The use of AFP alone is strongly discouraged; thus it is best used in conjunction with imaging studies.

Efficacy of Surveillance Programs

There is only one randomized controlled trial of surveillance versus no surveillance that has demonstrated a survival benefit. This large Chinese study recruited 18,816 patients who had markers of current or prior hepatitis B infection. Adherence to surveillance was under 60%, but HCC-specific mortality was reduced by 37% in the surveillance arm. Several retrospective and clinic based studies have concluded that surveillance in a high-risk population has a beneficial effect in early detection of HCC, leading to improved access to liver transplantation and enhanced survival.

DIAGNOSIS OF HEPATOCELLULAR CARCINOMA

The detection of a suspicious lesion on a surveillance scan should prompt further investigation. Dynamic imaging is always necessary to confirm the diagnosis of HCC. The primary modality utilized depends on the institution and local expertise. The options are a triple-phase CT scan, gadolinium-enhanced MRI, or contrast US, which is not readily available in the United States. Characteristic imaging features of HCC include

arterial vascularization with "washout" in the early or delayed venous phase. Such examinations should be conducted in specialized centers and must be read by radiologists with experience in liver imaging.

Utility of Tissue Biopsy in Hepatocellular Carcinoma: Should All Liver Masses Be Biopsied?

The discussion regarding biopsy of a suspicious liver mass takes on its greatest weight in the context of LT, which has become an increasingly important therapeutic option for patients with early HCC. Accurate diagnosis before transplantation is essential for the appropriate allocation of donor livers. Analysis of explant livers from 606 patients who underwent LT under the exceptional case policy for patients with HCC revealed that at least 31% of patients receiving transplants for early HCC (tumor size <2 cm) were misdiagnosed on the basis of imaging examinations performed before transplantation, and these lacked explant evidence of a malignancy. A dilemma thus emerges regarding potential LT patients; accurate diagnosis is of paramount importance, but seeding poses a greater threat because it converts such individuals from potential transplant candidates to those with metastatic disease.

This has generated a great deal of heated debate in terms of the best approach to these patients. Both the AASLD and the European Association for the Study of the Liver (EASL) have issued guidelines for clinical practice that are remarkably similar. They take into account the size of the mass, AFP level, and imaging characteristics.

A Brief Overview of Current AASLD Guidelines (Updated July 2010)

The utility of AFP in the diagnosis of HCC has been questioned in view of recent data suggesting suboptimal sensitivity and specificity. Current guidelines suggest that the diagnosis of HCC must rely on radiologic and histologic characteristics.

Lesion Diameter Greater than 1 cm

If characteristic imaging features (previously described) are noted on a four-phase multidetector CT scan (MDCT) or contrast-enhanced MRI, this is considered diagnostic of HCC. If one imaging study is inconclusive, a second study should be performed. If both are inconclusive, mass biopsy may be considered.

Lesion Diameter Under 1 cm

These lesions are most likely to represent cirrhotic nodules, not HCC. Close follow-up at 3-month intervals is recommended with the imaging modality used to document the lesion.

Biopsy of a liver lesion suspicious for HCC may be undertaken in the following circumstances:

To establish a diagnosis of HCC: Best used in lesions that lack diagnostic imaging characteristics and that are eligible for either resection or LT.

To optimize the use of LT: If the patient does not otherwise require or qualify for LT, the threshold for HCC diagnosis should be higher and biopsy should be used.

The main drawback to biopsy is the risk of tumor seeding along the needle tract, estimated to be in the range of 0 to 5.1%, with a median of 2.67%. The consequences of seeding can be devastating because it would essentially exclude curative surgery as a treatment option.

MANAGEMENT OF HEPATOCELLULAR CARCINOMA

The optimal management of HCC should include a multidisciplinary approach that incorporates surgeons, hepatologists, diagnostic and interventional radiologists, pathologists, and oncologists. Management options vary depending on hepatic function, stage of HCC, the patient's performance status, and local expertise.

One of the most important determinants of management is the stage of HCC, and at least seven different staging systems have been proposed. Of these, the Barcelona Clinic Liver Cancer (BCLC) system appears to have several advantages over other staging systems. First, it incorporates tumor stage, hepatic function impairment, patient performance status, and clinical symptoms. Second, it is linked to a proposed treatment algorithm that ties outcomes to stage of disease based on currently published response rates to various systems (Figure 1).

The Modified BCLC Staging System

Very Early Stage Hepatocellular Carcinoma (Stage 0)

Patients at stage 0 are very difficult to identify based on current imaging modalities. Such individuals have a single lesion less than 2 cm in size, with preserved liver function, normal portal pressure and bilirubin, and they meet other criteria for Child-Turcotte-Pugh (CTP) classification A (Table 2). Theoretically, if such patients are treated with surgical or ablative therapies, the expected survival is excellent. In practice, a nodular liver lesion less than 2 cm is often difficult to definitively diagnose as HCC on imaging studies, and biopsy is often technically challenging. Even if a definite diagnosis is made, these patients would not be eligible for MELD exception points and thus would not likely be allocated a deceased donor organ for transplantation. Hepatic resection is therefore the treatment of choice in such patients.

Early Stage Hepatocellular Carcinoma (Stage A)

Patients at stage A have preserved liver function (CTP class A or B) and either a single tumor smaller than 5 cm or up to three nodules, each 3 cm or smaller. Resection can be considered when there is a single tumor, normal bilirubin, and no portal hypertension. LT is best offered with a single tumor smaller than 5 cm associated with hepatic synthetic impairment or up to three nodules, each less than 3 cm.

Adjuvant ablative techniques can be considered in these patients when the waiting times for deceased organs is long. Alternatively, living donor liver transplantation can be offered if there is a suitable live donor volunteer.

Intermediate Stage Hepatocellular Carcinoma (Stage B)

Patients at stage B have preserved liver function (CTP class A or B) but have large or multifocal disease without evidence of macrovascular invasion, extrahepatic spread, or cancer-related symptoms. They are usually candidates for transarterial chemoembolization (TACE). HCC is notoriously resistant to standard chemotherapy, and molecular targeted therapies have emerged as attractive new options for treatment. Sorafenib tosylate (Nexavar; Bayer Healthcare, Wayne, NJ) is an oral multitargeted tyrosine kinase inhibitor that blocks tumor cell proliferation by inhibition of Raf kinase, (mitogen activated protein kinase and extracellular regulated kinase pathways). In a large, phase III randomized controlled multicenter trial involving 602 patients who were randomized to oral sorafenib versus placebo, sorafenib resulted in an improvement in median survival (10.7 vs. 7.9 months) and a delay in time to progression (5.5 vs. 2.8 months).

Advanced Stage Hepatocellular Carcinoma (Stage C)

Patients at stage C have cancer-related symptoms, macrovascular invasion, or distant metastases. Their survival at 1 year is estimated at approximately 50%. If no evidence of portal vein invasion or distant metastases is found, then TACE can still be considered in addition to sorafenib. If macrovascular invasion or distant metastases are found, systemic treatments such as sorafenib or other anticancer therapeutics, especially in the setting of clinical trials, is preferred.

Terminal Stage Hepatocellular Carcinoma (Stage D)

Patients at stage D have deterioration of their physical capacity, advanced tumor burden, and major impairment of liver function (CTP class C). Such patients have limited therapeutic options, and their median survival is less than 3 months. These patients are best suited for palliative care.

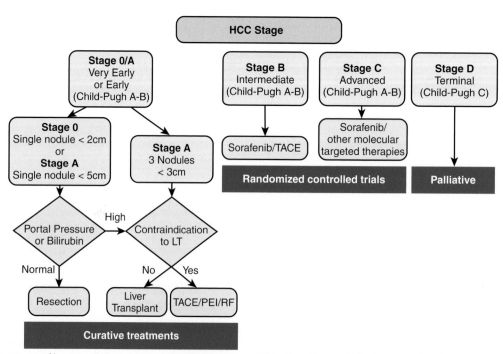

FIGURE 1   Management of hepatocellular carcinoma. Modified Barcelona Clinic Liver Cancer (BCLC) staging classification and treatment schedule.

TABLE 2: CTP classification

Variable	Points
Encephalopahy	
None	1
1-2	2
3-4	3
Ascites	
Absent	1
Slight	2
Moderate	3
Serum Bilirubin (mg/dL)	
1.0-2.0	1
2.1-3.0	2
>3.0	3
Serum Albumin (g/dL)	
>3.5	1
2.8-3.5	2
<2.8	3
Prolongation of Prothrombin Time (sec)	
1-3	1
4-10	2
>10	3

CTP class A (a total of 5 to 6 points) indicates good hepatic function, class B (7 to 9 points) indicates intermediate function, and class C (>10 points) indicates poor function.

Surgical Options for Hepatocellular Carcinoma: Hepatic Resection Versus Liver Transplantation

The end result of a successful surveillance program is to identify patients at an early stage of disease, such that they are candidates for potentially curative surgical therapies, such as tumor resection or liver replacement. Surgical therapies are feasible for patients who have very early or early stage HCC by the BCLC staging system. It should be noted that the level of evidence for these therapeutic options is limited to cohort investigations. There are no randomized controlled trials that compare resection with LT or treatment with no treatment. Therefore therapeutic plans should be based on a careful evaluation that incorporates the principles of tumor morphology, liver anatomy, hepatic synthetic reserve, patient performance status, portal hypertension, and treatment efficacy. Resource availability and local expertise should also be taken into account. Although LT is a well developed and accessible resource in the Western world, it has limited application in developing countries.

Surgical Resection

Hepatic resection can be an effective treatment for very early or early stage HCC in well-selected candidates. Long-term 5-year survival of 50% to 70% can be expected. However, only 20% of patients are amendable to surgery, given that HCC is often multicentric at initial presentation. For patients with very early or early stage HCC, the decision to perform resection or liver transplantation can be difficult and is often influenced by local expertise. Simply put, no straightforward algorithm exists that is accepted by all liver centers.

One advantage of hepatic resection is the expediency of the treatment. In most situations when a living donor is not readily available, tumor progression can occur while awaiting a deceased donor organ due to the long waiting list times. Even with the HCC MELD exception, the average time from listing to transplantation is 6.9 months. Given the likelihood of HCC growth during this time, and a very real possibility of upstaging beyond the limits set forth by the Milan criteria, there has been extensive support for primary resection. In transplant centers with long waiting times, ablative therapy, most often RFA and/or TACE, is employed to minimize the risks of waitlist drop-off due to tumor progression. Some transplant centers have also treated patients with sorafenib to delay tumor progression in those awaiting LT.

Recently, Kamiyama published data on 501 patients who underwent primary curative resection of HCC, half of whom were selected solely on the basis of the Milan criteria. Interestingly, this study was similar to the Milan analysis, except that HCC was treated initially with resection and not LT. In this study no recurrence occurred in 45% of the patients satisfying Milan criteria. However these results should be interpreted cautiously, as the rate of recurrence is much higher than the published recurrence rate of similar patients transplanted.

The Milan study sheds light on the impact of disease-free survival by tumor size, and more importantly presupposes the drastic consequence of interval unmitigated tumor growth on the LT wait lists. Although patients were transplanted along the strict criteria for limited disease, pathologic analysis of explanted liver tissue showed that 13 patients had tumor growth that would have eliminated them from the study. These patients had an overall actuarial survival of only 50% and recurrence-free survival of 59% at 5 years; those within Milan criteria had rates of 85% overall survival and 92% disease-free survival.

Implicit in these findings is that earlier intervention can limit tumor growth and offer better outcomes. This interpretation has shaped the view that initial hepatectomy with curative intent can be considered a reasonable first-line treatment for prevention of HCC progression in patients with preserved liver function. Moreover, assessing the role of hepatectomy in the context of bridge therapy has in many ways made this procedure seem even more appropriate as a first-line treatment. Recently, Belghiti showed that salvage transplantation after hepatectomy had equivalent 5-year survival rates compared to primary LT. However, there are some dissenting voices, most notably Bismuth's, whose recent study was critical of salvage transplantation; he noted that hepatic resection impairs later transplantability and affects overall survival.

A practical approach is to evaluate patients not only on the basis of their tumor stage but also in the context of the clinical stage of the underlying cirrhosis and the age of the patient. Resection of the tumor is the preferred treatment for those who have no evidence of cirrhosis. However, noncirrhotic patients account for 40% of those affected by HCC in Asia but only 5% in the United States.

Preserved hepatic function is best demonstrated by normal portal pressure as evidenced by hepatic vein wedge pressure, normal platelet count, absence of varices or splenomegaly, and normal bilirubin levels. In some countries, indocyanine green clearance is used to ascertain hepatic function, but this test is rarely used in the United States.

In a young patient with limited HCC and cirrhosis, the long-term outcome likely still favors transplantation, as the risk of HCC recurrence after hepatic resection is generally 10% to 15% per year on a cumulative basis. Thus patients generally have approximately a 40% to 50% recurrence rate at 5 years following resection. Patients with an otherwise long life expectancy are likely to have recurrence in their lifetime. Salvage transplantation may not be feasible if the recurrence pattern is aggressive and multifocal.

Underlying cirrhosis is problematic from the standpoint of hepatic resection not only because of compromised synthetic reserve but also because cirrhosis significantly impairs the liver's ability to regenerate following surgery. For now, the prevailing sentiment is that patients with a single tumor and preserved hepatic function without evidence of portal hypertension can be treated by limited partial hepatectomy.

Summary of Appropriate Resection Candidates

Adequate Hepatic Reserve

Classically, the CTP classification (see Table 2) had been used to select patients for resection. However, this is known to have inconsistent predictive value when used alone.

Absence of Portal Hypertension

Most studies conclude that the presence of portal hypertension is a useful predictor of poor outcomes. Clinical evidence of esophageal varices or ascites is a clear indicator of portal hypertension, and such patients do not require further evaluation. Less obvious indicators are splenomegaly and/or a platelet count over 100,000/mm³. If doubt still exists, hepatic vein catheterization with measurement of the portosystemic pressure gradient (<10 mm Hg is acceptable) may be performed.

Several studies have demonstrated that a normal bilirubin concentration and the absence of measurable portal hypertension are the best predictors of excellent outcomes after surgery. Those with portal hypertension will develop postoperative complications, mainly ascites, with a 5-year survival of under 50%. The worst outcomes are noted in those with an elevated bilirubin and portal hypertension, with 30% 5-year survivals.

Tumor Characteristics

Most groups restrict surgery to patients with solitary tumors in a favorable location for resection. The remaining residual remnant should be at least 50% or more of total liver volume. Size of the tumor is not a clear contraindication, although it is a surrogate marker for vascular invasion.

Outcomes of Resection

Several variables affect the risk of recurrence following resection: these include tumor size, number of tumors, vascular invasion, and the width of the resection margin. The recommended upper limit of tumor size for consideration of resection has been argued, noting a significantly higher 5-year recurrence rate in patients with tumors larger than 5 cm than in those whose tumors are smaller than 5 cm (43% vs. 32%, respectively). Similarly, multinodular tumors have been determined to have an increased tendency to recur. A large study of 1000 HCC patients reported a 5-year survival after resection of single tumors of 57%; for patients with three or more nodules, it was 26%. Overall survival after surgical resection in carefully selected patients ranges between 60% and 70% at 5 years. However, tumor recurrence rate exceeds 50% at 5 years because of recurrence and de novo tumor formation.

LIVER TRANSPLANTATION

In the early 1990s, transplantation for HCC was associated with dismal outcomes because it was considered a last-ditch effort in those with advanced HCC. A dramatic change in the approach to HCC management may be attributed to the study published in 1996 by Mazzaferro and colleagues. This provided the first substantial

---

TABLE 3: Milan criteria of eligibility for LT

Presence of a tumor ≤5 cm in diameter in patients with single hepatocellular carcinomas

or

≤3 tumor nodules, each 3 cm or less in diameter, in patients with multiple tumors

---

prospective results demonstrating excellent survival with LT for early HCC. Termed the *Milan criteria,* this landmark study showed a 5-year disease-free survival rate of 83% when LT was performed in patients who satisfied distinct criteria. These critieria required the presence of a single tumor lesion less than 5 cm or no more than three lesions, each no more than 3 cm in diameter, without evidence of vascular invasion or distant metastases (Table 3). These remarkable findings have ignited the debate on which curative treatment is best for the patient with early stage HCC. Some surgeons believe that the Milan criteria should be strictly adhered to for many reasons, least of which is the superiority of LT as treatment of HCC. However, others feel that resection is a viable first step in the management of very early or early stage HCC.

Prior to the Milan group's published experience in the *New England Journal of Medicine* in 1996, a preceding series had reported a dismal success rate, with 5-year survival ranging from 15% to 48%. In fact, in 1989 the U.S. Department of Heath and Human Services declared that HCC was a contraindication for LT. The reasons for the lack of success was that "optimal" patients for LT were those deemed unresectable because of large multinodular tumors. In 1993, Bismuth and colleagues first showed the converse to be true. Later, the historically significant Milan criteria further changed this perception, demonstrating that the restriction of LT to those with limited disease yielded superior survival.

Currently, LT is considered the standard of care for HCC treatment in the setting of advanced cirrhosis and early tumors. Providing the widest margins possible, LT for limited disease and no extrahepatic spread or vascular invasion gives the patient unparalleled disease-free survival. Interestingly, the Milan criteria study showed that LT was performed across all CTP classes without any discernible differences in outcome. At present most transplant centers in the United States adhere to these selection criteria, although the number of exceptional points awarded and the minimum size for a unifocal tumor have been modified to ensure fairness for patients requiring LT for other indications. Therefore LT, in theory, is the optimal therapeutic option for HCC; it simultaneously removes the tumor and underlying cirrhosis, thus minimizing the risk of HCC recurrence. As stated previously, earlier selection criteria for LT were broad, leading to poor results with recurrence rates of approximately 50% and 5-year survival rates less than 40%. The currently recommended UNOS criteria (one lesion ≤5 cm or a maximum of three lesions <3 cm in diameter) have shown tremendous promise, with reported 5-year survival rates over 70% and recurrence rates nearing 15%.

The tumor-burden criteria for transplantation for HCC as established by the Milan group are largely accepted. Expanded selection criteria (a single lesion of ≤6.5 cm or up to three lesions, none of which are larger than 4.5 cm, with a maximum combined tumor bulk of ≤8.0 cm) have been proposed by Yao and colleagues at the University of California in San Francisco. LT in such candidates is controversial, with short-term outcomes similar to those who are within the Milan criteria, but recent long-term data have shown a divergence of outcomes with longer term follow-up. Still, survival is better than without liver transplantation. Given the large number of HCC patients considered for LT, the struggle is to keep a balance between HCC and non-HCC recipients.

Based on the radiologic diagnosis of the number and size of lesions, MELD exception points are awarded for HCC with the expectation that liver transplantation is accomplished in a reasonable period of time. The exception points for HCC are based on 3-month pretransplantation risk of progression. Patients with solitary lesions 2 cm and larger but less than 5 cm or up to three lesions, each smaller than 3 cm, currently receive a MELD score of 22. For each 3-month interval that they remain on the wait list, a greater number of exception points are awarded, based on an expected increase of 10% in the 3-month mortality rate. However, some reasonable dissent has been expressed regarding this distribution scheme, which ignores underlying liver dysfunction as an additional measure for listing priority.

The role of downstaging of tumors that are outside of conventional UNOS criteria for LT has been explored. Downstaging is HCC-directed therapy that aims at reducing the size and/or number of HCC lesions. Studies have shown that successful tumor downstaging can be achieved in up to 70% of the patients treated in a protocol with one or more therapeutic modalities, including TACE, RFA, or PEI. Subsequently, successful LT was accomplished in nearly half of these patients. Although encouraging, longer follow-up is needed to assess further the risk of HCC recurrence after LT before downstaging can be recommended and adopted. The role of salvage LT after initial resection of HCC is less clear. Overall, suboptimal outcomes have been observed with this strategy compared with primary LT for HCC.

Given the shortage of donors, and in attempts to shorten the waiting time for deceased donor liver transplantation, living donor liver transplantation (LDLT) has been shown to be an alternative to deceased donor liver transplantation, with approximately 4000 cases done worldwide for all indications. LDLT is a complex procedure that is associated with a donor morbidity of 20% to 40% and a donor mortality of 0.3% to 0.5%. With that, consideration of ethical, societal, and legal issues are vital to successful implementation of LDLT for HCC treatment. A recent retrospective analysis of the U.S. experience noted that the disease-free survival following LDLT was lower than that of deceased donor LT. LDLT recipients had a higher rate of HCC recurrence within 3 years than deceased donor LT. Some of the difference may be explained by the fact that with short waiting times for LDLT, patients who may have demonstrated progression and subsequently dropped off the deceased donor list were able to undergo LDLT, thus skewing the results. In LDLT the need to preserve the recipient vena cava may also result in compromise of tumor margin. Thus the role of LDLT, particularly for those outside of ideal criteria, needs further evaluation. Cost analyses have shown that LDLT is cost effective if waiting times exceed 7 months.

SUMMARY

Appropriate management of HCC depends largely on tumor stage and the stage of the underlying cirrhosis. Hepatic resection remains a reasonable choice in patients with preserved liver function and early stage HCC. Despite the fact that recurrence rates may be high relative to LT, primary attempts at curative resection in patients with limited progression is beneficial for three reasons. First, resection alleviates the concern of unmitigated tumor growth beyond the Milan criteria, while patients linger on transplant wait lists. Second, salvage transplantation after resection has been shown to be somewhat effective and therefore makes the case for hepatectomy as a first-line treatment. Thirdly, resection with potential cure eliminates the burdens of life-long immunosuppression. Moreover, LT may offer the best hope for a cure in patients with cirrhosis and HCC, as transplantation not only removes the tumor but also the remaining at-risk hepatic parenchyma.

Less controversy surrounds patients with moderate to severe cirrhosis and early stage HCC. Here the right procedure is to perform LT because the gross margins give excellent disease-free survival rates, and engraftment of the new organ corrects the underlying cirrhosis. For patients with advanced multifocal disease, TACE, RFA, and intratumoral radiation have shown some promise for limited survival advantage.

Recent trials comparing sorafenib to placebo confirmed the first efficacious systemic chemotherapy for unresectable HCC. In unresectable HCC, sorafenib increased survival by 44% when compared with placebo-treated patients, and it increased the time to radiologic evidence of tumor progression. In patients with multifocal disease and advanced decompensated cirrhosis, supportive palliative care provides the most reasonable treatment option.

In coming years, the liver surgeon will be increasingly confronted with the question of the most appropriate treatment for HCC given the rise in HCV. This complex problem must be understood within the context of numerous factors that include the clinical stage of the underlying liver parenchyma and the morphologic stage of tumor burden. Priority for liver transplantation will likely be weighted more for patients with underlying hepatic dysfunction. This also may result in a greater role of resection in early stage HCC in patients with preserved hepatic function. Ultimately, the surgical community must subscribe to a multifaceted approach that increases early diagnosis and rates of efficacious surgical therapy.

SUGGESTED READINGS

Adam R, Azoulay D, Castaing D, et al: Liver resection as a bridge to transplantation for hepatocellular carcinoma on cirrhosis: A reasonable strategy? *Ann Surg* 238:508–518, discussion 518-509, 2003.

Belghiti J: Resection and liver transplantation for HCC, *J Gastroenterol* 44(suppl) 19:132–135, 2009.

Bruix J, Sherman M: Management of hepatocellular carcinoma, *Hepatology* (Baltimore, Md) 42:1208–1236, 2005.

Choi D, Kim SH, Lim JH, et al: Detection of hepatocellular carcinoma: combined T2-weighted and dynamic gadolinium-enhanced MRI versus combined CT during arterial portography and CT hepatic arteriography, *J Comput Assist Tomogr* 25:777–785, 2001.

Freeman RB, Mithoefer A, Ruthazer R, et al: Optimizing staging for hepatocellular carcinoma before liver transplantation: a retrospective analysis of the UNOS/OPTN database, *Liver Transpl* 12:1504–1511, 2006.

Kamiyama T, Nakanishi K, Yokoo H, et al: Recurrence patterns after hepatectomy of hepatocellular carcinoma: implication of Milan criteria utilization, *Ann Surg Oncol* 16(6):1560–1571, 2009.

Krinsky GA, Lee VS, Theise ND, et al: Hepatocellular carcinoma and dysplastic nodules in patients with cirrhosis: prospective diagnosis with MR imaging and explantation correlation, *Radiology* 219:445–454, 2001.

Llovet JM, Fuster J, Bruix J: The Barcelona approach: diagnosis, staging, and treatment of hepatocellular carcinoma, *Liver Transpl* 10:S115–S120, 2004.

Llovet JM, Bruix J: Novel advancements in the management of hepatocellular carcinoma in 2008, *J Hepatol* 48(suppl 1):S20–S37, 2008.

Llovet JM, Ricci S, Mazzaferro V, et al: SHARP investigators study group: 2008, *New Engl J Med* (359):378–390, 2008.

Mazzaferro V, Regalia E, Doci R, et al: Liver transplantation for the treatment of small hepatocellular carcinomas in patients with cirrhosis, *N Engl J Med* 334:693–699, 1996.

Yao FY, Kerlan RK Jr, Hirose R, et al: Excellent outcome following downstaging of hepatocellular carcinoma prior to liver transplantation: an intention-to-treat analysis, *Hepatology* 48:819–827, 2008.

Zhang BH, Yang BH, Tang ZY: Randomized controlled trial of screening for hepatocellular carcinoma, *J Cancer Res Clin Oncol* 130:417–422, 2004.

RADIOFREQUENCY ABLATION OF COLORECTAL LIVER METASTASES

Michael A. Choti, MD, MBA

OVERVIEW

Liver metastases from colorectal cancer are the most frequent hepatic malignancies in the United States. Although surgical resection remains the only established potentially curative option for patients with isolated hepatic metastases, many patients are not candidates for resection. Moreover, many patients have disease recurrence within the liver following resection, and few are candidates for re-resection. For these reasons, increasing interest has been focused on ablative approaches for the treatment of unresectable metastases. Radiofrequency ablation (RFA) has become the most commonly used, and perhaps the most promising, modality for tumor ablation.

RFA is a nonextirpative technique of local therapy that uses a form of alternating electrical current to achieve thermal destruction. The radiofrequency energy is supplied by a generator attached to a needle electrode and dispersive grounding electrodes. The generator applies a high-frequency alternating electrical current, causing ionic agitation that heats the volume of tissue in the area of the electrode tip. Cell death is due to irreversible coagulation of proteins and DNA. By targeting the device within the targeted tumor, the tumor and surrounding adjacent liver are thermally destroyed.

RADIOFREQUENCY ABLATION DURING LAPAROTOMY AND LAPAROSCOPY

One advantage of RFA over other ablative approaches, such as cryotherapy, is that it can be performed with percutaneous, open, or laparoscopic approaches. In all cases, the tumor must be clearly seen during treatment with contrast-enhanced computer tomography (CT), magnetic resonance imaging (MRI), or ultrasound (US). Although any of these imaging modalities may be used during percutaneous RFA, intraoperative ultrasound (IOUS) is used for laparoscopic or open procedures.

To prepare the patient, grounding electrodes are placed on the back or legs; care must be taken to ensure adequate skin contact to avoid cutaneous burns. Four grounding pads placed on the thighs provide sufficient surface area to avoid burn injuries at the grounding pad sites when using up to 2000 mA of current.

When performing RFA during open laparotomy, careful exploration of the abdominal cavity should first be performed to exclude the presence of extrahepatic malignancy; this should include assessment of peritoneal surfaces and periportal nodal regions. The liver is then carefully inspected by both palpation and IOUS. When previous biopsy has not been obtained, core biopsy under IOUS guidance should be considered.

Careful planning of the zone of ablation is necessary to achieve complete necrosis of the target lesion. In some cases, using an expandable multielectrode needle of sufficient size, complete ablation can be achieved with a single application, deploying the electrode from the center of the tumor. For example, a 3 cm spherical tumor and 1 cm margin can be treated with a device deployed to produce a 5 cm (diameter) volume of necrosis. Newer electrode technology using higher energy and low-volume hypertonic saline infusion can produce zones of coagulation necrosis as large as 7 cm in diameter.

Tumor size and location can preclude effective RFA with curative intent. Tumor sizes larger than 4 to 5 cm are associated with an increased incidence of local recurrence. The location of a tumor near the main portal pedicles is considered a relative contraindication to RFA. In addition to the inability to achieve an effective ablation due to the high blood flow, ablation near the porta hepatis can result in injury and stricture of a central bile duct.

Once the target tumor is identified with the IOUS transducer, the RFA electrode needle is inserted under US guidance (Figure 1). Optimally, the electrode is advanced parallel to and within the plane of the transducer, so the entire path of the needle can be visualized. When using a multielectrode needle, the array is deployed within the tumor, and the position is confirmed with US in two planes. With some RFA devices, central ablation can first be performed by partially deploying the array and sequentially advancing the electrodes to the desired volume.

Monitoring during thermal ablation can be performed using a variety of methods. Some RFA devices have the capacity to measure tissue temperatures with thermisters located at the tips of the electrodes. Alternatively, tissue impedance and current can be monitored during treatment. With some devices, the power output is adjusted automatically to control impedance and maintain tissue temperature between 70 and 105° C. The ablation zone is visualized by US during treatment. Typically, local miniscule gas bubble formation results in hyperechogenicity within the treated tissue (Figure 2).

Laparoscopic RFA offers the advantage of a minimally invasive procedure with the ability to visualize the abdominal cavity and perform the therapy using IOUS. With this approach, patients are treated under general endotracheal anesthesia, typically in the supine position. In most cases, the procedure can be done with two or three ports. The liver is typically partially mobilized, and viscera within 2 cm of the intended ablation zone are moved away. Laparoscopic cholecystectomy can be performed when a target lesion is in close proximity to the gallbladder. The RFA electrode is placed into the abdominal cavity through a percutaneous approach and does not require the placement of an additional port. The needle is placed within the tumor under US guidance, and ablation is performed and monitored as it is with the open technique (Figure 3).

IMAGING FOLLOWING RADIOFREQUENCY ABLATION

The optimal method for evaluating the efficacy of RFA treatment using imaging modalities is not well defined. The presence of residual viable tumor tissue after RFA can be detected using contrast-enhanced CT or MRI, using criteria similar to those following percutaneous ethanol injection therapy. However, unlike hepatocellular carcinoma, colorectal carcinoma liver metastases are often hypovascular, and determination of postprocedure necrosis and tumor viability is difficult. Perhaps more useful in assessing the success of ablation is the size, shape, and location of the necrosis zone on a postprocedural scan relative to the preprocedure images (Figure 4).

A contrast-enhanced CT or MRI should be performed within 30 days following RFA treatment. Serial follow-up imaging of the liver is then recommended. However, as with other ablative approaches, interpretation of these images can be difficult at times, as a hypoattenuating lesion may persist for months to years despite complete tumor destruction. In most cases, a local recurrence is characterized by an increase in the lesion size on serial scans or evidence of new areas of contrast enhancement. ^{18}F-fluorodeoxyglucose position emission tomography (FDG-PET) may be useful in assessing recurrent disease provided it is acquired after the postablation inflammation has subsided, typically after 3 months.

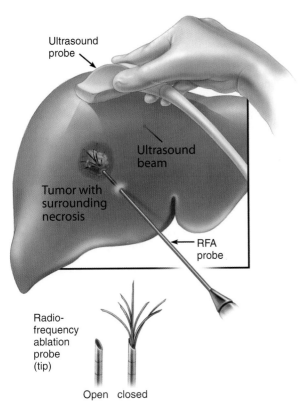

FIGURE 1   Radiofrequency ablation during open laparotomy using IOUS guidance. *(From Johns Hopkins Gastroenterology and Hepatology: Hepatocellular carcinoma (liver cancer): Therapy. Available at http://www.hopkins-gi.org. Accessed June 15, 2010.)*

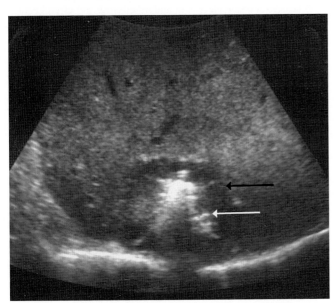

FIGURE 2   IOUS image during RFA. Hyperechoic microbubble formation along multitine RFA electrode *(white arrow)* within hypoechoic liver metastasis *(black arrow)*.

OPERATIVE APPROACHES VERSUS PERCUTANEOUS RADIOFREQUENCY ABLATION

Many of the published reports evaluating RFA of liver metastases have relied on percutaneous electrode insertion under imaging guidance. The principal advantage of the percutaneous approach compared

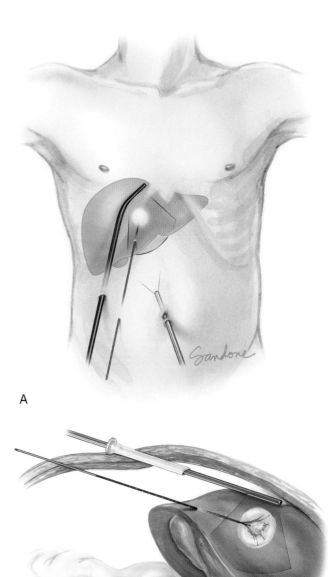

FIGURE 3   Laparoscopic approach when performing operative RFA using IOUS guidance. **A,** Placement of ports. **B,** Position of IOUS and RFA probes. *(From Cameron JL, Sandone C: Atlas of gastrointestinal surgery vol 1, ed 2, 2008, BC Decker, p 182.)*

with operative approaches is the lower associated morbidity and cost. However, performance of ablation during laparotomy or laparoscopy offers several advantages. One benefit is that of enhanced staging, as laparotomy and laparoscopy afford the opportunity to identify both hepatic and extrahepatic metastases not visualized on preoperative imaging. About 10% to 20% of patients who undergo exploration with the intent to resect colorectal liver metastases are found at laparotomy to have additional metastases that either preclude or significantly alter the planned resection. Many of these operative findings can be detected via laparoscopy as well. In addition, intraoperative US can frequently detect lesions that are not visible with transabdominal US, CT, or MRI.

In addition, laparotomy affords the opportunity to combine ablation with surgical resection. It is important to point out that following ablation of tumors larger than 5 cm, the local recurrence rate is

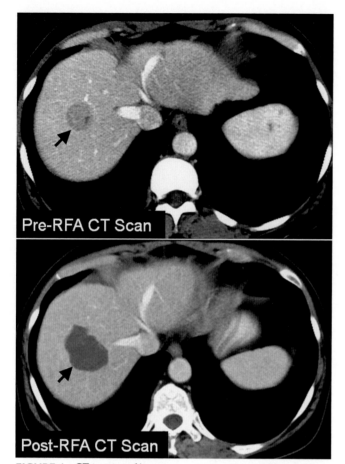

Pre-RFA CT Scan

Post-RFA CT Scan

FIGURE 4 CT imaging of hepatic metastasis prior to RFA and 4 days following ablation.

reported 5-year survival rates in the range of 30% or more. In addition, several studies have attempted to compare outcomes of resection versus outcome of ablation, and most demonstrated RFA to be associated with a worse disease-free and overall survival compared with resection.

In considering these results, it must be realized that important prognostic and treatment-related variables differ between the two cohorts when compared retrospectively. In a methodologic analysis, Tsai and colleagues found that standard statistical techniques may be insufficient to adjust for the confounding differing variables in these uncontrolled comparative studies.

Comparisons of resection versus RFA can also be problematic, as the adequacy of RFA at the time of the procedure is often poorly documented. Whereas resection has an element of quality control (e.g., R status), RFA currently has no such quality control regarding completeness of therapy. In a recent Clinical Evidence Review by the American Society of Clinical Oncology on RFA of hepatic metastases from colorectal cancer, the authors acknowledged a paucity of quality evidence and emphasized a compelling need for more clinical trials to determine the efficacy and utility of RFA for patients with hepatic colorectal metastases.

SUMMARY

Although surgical resection remains the treatment of choice as potentially curative therapy for colorectal carcinoma liver metastases, advances in RFA technology have provided patients and physicians with new treatment options for those with localized unresectable disease. RFA can play a role as an adjunct to resection, used in combination or as an alternative to hepatectomy, when tumor distribution, location, or patient comorbid disease precludes safe extirpative surgery. As with resection, the goal should be complete, margin-negative tumor destruction when possible. Sound surgical judgment with fastidious probe placement and monitoring and careful patient selection will optimize utilization of RFA and best serve patients with advanced colorectal cancer.

SUGGESTED READINGS

Crocetti L, de Baere T, Lencioni R: Quality improvement guidelines for radiofrequency ablation of liver tumours, *Cardiovasc Intervent Radiol* 33(1): 11–17, 2010.

Gleisner AL, Choti MA, Assumpcao L, et al: Colorectal liver metastases: recurrence and survival following hepatic resection, radiofrequency ablation, and combined resection–radiofrequency ablation, *Arch Surg* 143(12):1204–1212, 2008.

Mulier S, Ruers T, Jamart J, et al: Radiofrequency ablation versus resection for resectable colorectal liver metastases: time for a randomized trial? An update, *Dig Surg* 25(6):445–460, 2008.

Tsai S, Pawlik TM: Outcomes of ablation versus resection for colorectal liver metastases: Are we comparing apples with oranges? *Ann Surg Oncol* 16(9):2422–2428 2009.

Wong SL, Mangu PB, Choti MA, et al: American Society of Clinical Oncology 2009 clinical evidence review on radiofrequency ablation of hepatic metastases from colorectal cancer, *J Clin Oncol* 20, 28(3):493–508, 2010.

unacceptably high. Accordingly, a significant fraction of patients with "unresectable" liver tumors can be fully treated only by the combination of resection of larger lesions and ablation of smaller lesions.

OUTCOMES FOLLOWING RADIOFREQUENCY ABLATION

Unlike hepatic resection, in which long-term efficacy is relatively established, evidence of the benefit of RFA for treatment of hepatic colorectal metastases has been limited and inconsistent. There are no published randomized controlled trials examining its use in this disease, so the data are largely based on single-arm, retrospective, and prospective studies.

In the published literature, local recurrence rates range from less than 10% to as high as 50%. Data on the survival benefit of RFA have been similarly contradictory. Some studies have reported 5-year survival of less than 20% following RFA, whereas other studies have

HEPATIC ABSCESS

Barish H. Edil, MD, and Henry A. Pitt, MD

OVERVIEW

Hepatic abscesses are uncommon, accounting for only 1 of every 4500 to 7000 hospital admissions. Liver abscesses require early diagnosis and treatment because they are a source of significant morbidity and mortality.

Hepatic abscesses can be divided into three major categories: *pyogenic, amoebic,* and *fungal.* Pyogenic abscesses represent the majority of liver abscesses in developed countries and tend to contain polymicrobial aerobic and anaerobic bacteria. Amebic abscesses are due to *Entamoeba histolytica,* which has a high endemic prevalence in Mexico, the Indian subcontinent, Indonesia, and tropical Africa. The majority of patients with amebic liver abscesses in the United States will have a history of recent travel to an endemic area. Fungal abscesses are less common and are typically caused by *Candida* species. However, fungal liver abscesses are on the rise with the increase in immunocompromised patients. Another category of liver abscess being seen more frequently are those that occur after direct or hepatic artery ablative procedures for liver tumors.

Over the last several decades, significant changes have occurred in the etiology, presentation, and treatment of liver abscesses. Both interventional radiologists and biliary endoscopists may play a major role in the management of these patients. However, hepatopancreatobiliary surgeons also need to be knowledgeable and must play an active role in diagnosis and management of patients with liver abscesses.

PYOGENIC HEPATIC ABSCESS

Pyogenic hepatic abscesses are uncommon, but without proper diagnosis and timely management, they can develop into a potentially lethal condition. Liver abscesses were first described by Hippocrates around the year 400 BCE. In the early twentieth century, pyogenic liver abscess was a young man's disease, most commonly resulting from appendicitis, as described by Oschner's landmark paper in 1934.

In the second half of the twentieth century, pyogenic liver abscesses shifted from younger patients with relatively benign etiologies to older, more debilitated patients who were developing infections from a biliary source, frequently with an underlying malignancy. In the twenty-first century, a more aggressive approach to the management of hepatic tumors has resulted in another, more subtle shift from biliary to hepatic malignancies as the underlying etiology.

Pathophysiology

Pyogenic abscesses can develop from multiple potential sources: 1) the biliary ductal system in the form of ascending cholangitis, typically from malignant obstruction; 2) the portal blood flow, from pylephlebitis originating from appendicitis or diverticulitis; 3) direct extension from adjacent disease, such as severe cholecystitis; 4) trauma from injury or liver-directed therapy; 5) the hepatic artery, from septicemia originating from a distant source; and 6) a cryptogenic process. In one of the largest Western series at Johns Hopkins Hospital, 40% of pyogenic liver abscesses were biliary in origin, and an underlying malignancy was the cause in the majority of these patients.

The types of bacteria isolated from the blood and the bile in patients with pyogenic hepatic abscesses vary with the underlying pathologic process (Table 1). For example, if choledocholithiasis is the underlying etiology, *Escherichia coli, Klebsiella* spp., and *Enterococcus* will be isolated most commonly. However, if the patient has an unresectable biliary malignancy and has received multiple courses of antibiotics, *Pseudomonas* spp., other multiple resistant gram-negative aerobes, vancomycin-resistant *Enterococcus* (VRE), and yeast will be more likely pathogens. On the other hand, if either diverticulitis or appendicitis is the cause, gram-negative aerobes and *Bacteroides fragilis* will be isolated most frequently. Patients with severe forms of cholecystitis are likely to harbor anaerobes such as *Clostridium perfringens* and *Bacteroides* spp. in addition to typical biliary bacteria. When a subcutaneous abscess is the cause, *Staphylococcus* spp. will be the most common pathogen, and methicillin-resistant *Staphylococcus aureus* (MRSA) is becoming more common. In addition, if endocarditis is the etiology, enterococcal and staphylococcal pathogens are most likely. Finally, anaerobes are somewhat more common in cryptogenic abscesses.

Diagnosis

The classic initial symptom of pyogenic hepatic abscess is fever, which occurs in more than 90% of patients. Approximately one half of those with abscess will have abdominal or right upper quadrant pain. On physical examination the liver may be tender and enlarged, or the patient may appear jaundiced. Other frequent complaints include malaise, anorexia, and nausea. Occasionally, the diaphragm is involved, resulting in pleuritic chest pain, cough, or dyspnea. Pyogenic liver abscesses rarely rupture, so frank peritonitis is unusual; however, severe sepsis may occur in patients with an underlying biliary malignancy and following liver-directed therapy; or transplantation may be the mode of presentation, without significant pain or physical findings.

Over the past 40 years, advances in imaging have dramatically improved the diagnosis of patients with pyogenic hepatic abscesses. Plain films may show an abnormality 50% of the time, including an elevated right hemidiaphragm, right pleural effusion, right lower lobe atelectasis, abnormal extraluminal gas in the right upper quadrant, or portal venous gas if pylephlebitis is the source. Ultrasound (US) may be useful for initial screening for hepatic abscess; it has a sensitivity of 80% to 95% and is excellent in evaluating the gallbladder and intrahepatic bile ducts. However, US may be of limited utility in obese patients and for lesions located in the right lobe under the diaphragm.

In comparison, computed tomography (CT) is more sensitive (95% to 100%) in the detection of abscesses. With CT the abscess can have variable images, but the presence of gas and rim enhancement with intravenous contrast is very suggestive of a hepatic abscess (Figure 1). CT also allows for a more thorough evaluation of the abdomen to detect the underlying cause. Magnetic resonance imaging (MRI) of the liver is an equally sensitive technique, but it may be more costly and is not available for guiding percutaneous drainage.

Treatment

If not diagnosed and treated appropriately, pyogenic hepatic abscess is associated with a significant mortality rate. Management must include treatment of both the liver abscess and the underlying source. Therapy has changed significantly from the days when operative drainage was the definitive treatment to the present day, when surgery is rarely required.

The majority of pyogenic hepatic abscesses are managed by antibiotic administration, radiologic confirmation, and drainage. When pyogenic abscess is confirmed by CT scan, and no intraabdominal

TABLE 1: Underlying etiology and bacteriology

Etiology	Bacteriology
Biliary, benign	*Escherichia coli* *Klebsiella* spp. *Enterococcus*
Biliary, malignant	*Pseudomonas* spp, Multiply resistant GN aerobes VRE Yeast
Diverticulitis/appendicitis	GN aerobes *Bacteroides fragilis*
Severe cholecystitis	See Biliary, benign *Clostridium perfringens* *Bacteroides* spp.
Subcutaneous abscess	*Staphylococcus* spp. MRSA
Endocarditis	*Enterococcus* spp. *Staphyloccus* spp.
Cryptogenic	Anaerobes

GN, Gram negative

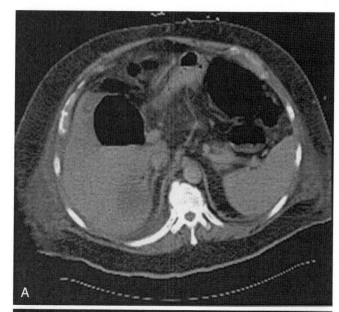

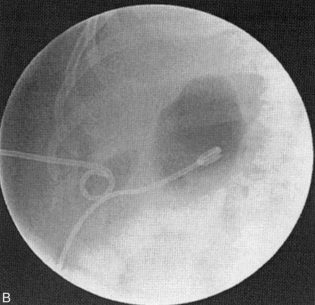

FIGURE 1 **A,** CT scan demonstrating a large pyogenic liver abscess with an air-fluid level in segment VI of the liver. **B,** Radiograph demonstrating percutaneous drainage.

source requires operative intervention, initial management should include systemic antibiotics and percutaneous drainage. In patients with small hepatic abscesses and no biliary obstruction, prolonged intravenous antibiotics may be employed without drainage. When an intraabdominal source for the infection requires an operation, the liver abscess can be drained surgically in concert with management of the primary problem (Figure 2).

Antibiotics

When a pyogenic hepatic abscess is suspected, blood cultures are drawn and empiric, broad-spectrum intravenous antimicrobial therapy is started, until therapy can be focused by the culture results. If drainage is not undertaken, aspiration may be performed to determine the bacteriology. As outlined above, the bacteria found usually correspond to the source (Table 1).

Because the bacterial source of a hepatic abscess can be variable, broad-spectrum antibiotics are used initially, but the choice of empiric antibiotics may vary with the presumed source. For example, for a presumed biliary source, gram-negative aerobe and enterococcal coverage might include broad-spectrum single agents such as piperacillin-tazobactam, ticarcillin-clavulanate, or meropenem. However, if the patient has had multiple episodes of cholangitis and has indwelling stents, double coverage for pseudomonal species, and an agent such as linezolid for VRE, might be an appropriate start. For a presumed colonic source, the combination of a fluoroquinolone or a third-generation cephalosporin with metronidazole would provide appropriate coverage. For severe cholecystitis, a broad-spectrum penicillin should be included to cover *Clostridia,* and the addition of metronidazole for *Bacteroides* would be a reasonable starting combination. If subcutaneous abscess or endocarditis is the presumed source, inclusion of vancomycin for MRSA would be appropriate.

Once the actual bacteria are isolated and sensitivities are determined, the antibiotic regimen should be adjusted if possible to more specific, less broad, and less costly agents. Parenteral administration of antibiotics should be continued for 10 to 14 days. Classically, antibiotic treatment has been recommended for 4 to 6 weeks; however,

shorter antibiotic duration may be appropriate if adequate drainage has been achieved. Even when prolonged antibiotics are indicated for multiple small abscesses with no abdominal source, oral antibiotics may be substituted for home IV antibiotics.

Drainage

Intravenous antibiotics have decreased the mortality rate of patients with pyogenic hepatic abscesses; however, most patients also will require abscess drainage, either by percutaneous catheter placement, closed aspiration, or surgery. As imaging and interventional techniques have evolved, the standard of care for drainage has moved away from surgical to percutaneous procedures. At Johns Hopkins from 1973 to 1993, 45% of patients were treated with a percutaneous drain; many of these, especially later in the series, involved multiloculated abscesses.

Rajak and colleagues in 1998 compared catheter placement with percutaneous aspiration and found that the success rate was superior with catheter placement (60% vs. 100%). Percutaneous catheter placement involves the insertion of an 8 to 14 Fr pigtail catheter over a guidewire under imaging guidance. The abscess cavity is then studied by the injection of contrast through the catheter. Finally, the catheter is left to gravity or suction, until complete resolution of the drainage and collapse of the abscess cavity has occurred (Figure 1 *B*). Percutaneous drainage is not appropriate for patients with multiple large abscesses, a known intraabdominal source that will require surgery, ascites, or if transpleural drainage is required.

Percutaneous needle aspiration involves imaging-guided drainage of the abscess without placement of the catheter. The benefits of needle aspiration are decreased cost, less invasiveness, and avoidance of drain discomfort. In 2004, Yu and colleagues performed a prospective randomized trial of 64 carefully selected patients to compare aspiration with drainage and concluded that they were equivalent. In this study, aspiration resulted in less liver trauma, was more comfortable for the patient, and was less expensive. On the other hand, aspiration may need to be repeated because recurrence of the abscess is higher with this approach. Thus controversy persists regarding the relative value of percutaneous needle aspiration and catheter drainage of pyogenic abscess.

Patients will usually require surgical drainage if percutaneous drainage has failed, if the underlying source requires surgery, or if a bleeding diathesis, ascites, or multiple abscesses are present. Even though the need for surgical therapy has changed with the improvement of percutaneous drainage, surgery continues to play a complementary role in the care of patients with hepatic abscesses.

Prior to the availability of systemic antibiotics, great effort was taken to avoid contamination of the peritoneum, which involved surgical drainage by an extraperitoneal approach. However, with modern antibiotics, the transperitoneal approach is favored when the underlying pathology is located in the abdomen or pelvis, multiple abscesses require drainage, or a bile duct exploration is indicated.

Current technique involves access through a transperitoneal exploration by a midline or subcostal incision. After the underlying pathology in the abdomen is addressed, the liver is evaluated by palpation; intraoperative US is helpful in locating abscesses. The area to be drained is then isolated from the rest of the abdomen with towels, and aspiration of the abscess is performed to obtain fluid for culture (Figure 3). A tract is then created through the hepatic parenchyma toward the cavity, ideally to drain in a dependent fashion. Next, the cavity is irrigated and suctioned to remove purulence and minimize contamination. The tract should then be enlarged and the abscess debrided to break up any loculated pockets of purulence. A large caliber drain is placed in the abscess cavity, and the perihepatic area

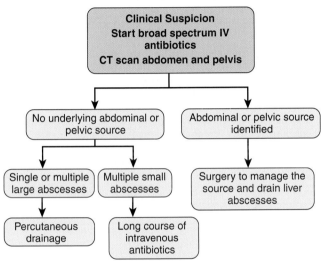

FIGURE 2   Algorithm for managing pyogenic hepatic abscesses.

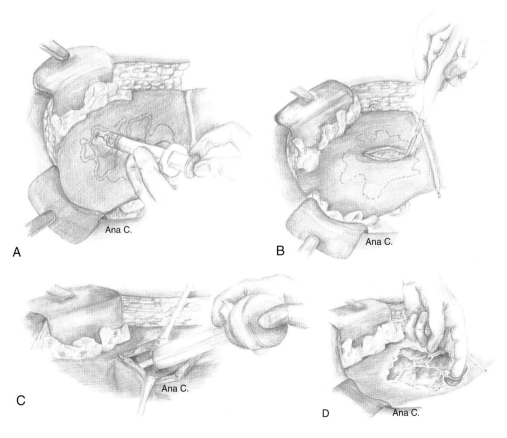

A   B

C   D

FIGURE 3   **A,** Abscess aspiration for aerobic and anaerobic culture. **B,** Incision of the liver capsule to drain the abscess. **C,** Irrigation of abscess cavity. **D,** Manual disruption of loculations. *(Illustrations by Ana Costache.)*

around the abscess may also be drained; however, these drains are brought out through separate incisions. All hepatic abscesses should be biopsied to rule out tumor as well as to evaluate for trophozoites of *E. histolytica*.

Occasionally, an inflammatory mass that is resistant to these treatments develops in patients who have had multiple percutaneous drainage procedures and several rounds of antibiotics. In addition, patients who have chronic biliary obstruction and have undergone multiple biliary drainage procedures may present with an abscess isolated to one lobe. In these unusual circumstances, hepatic-sparing liver resection may be considered to remove the diseased portion of liver; however, these patients are prone to profound sepsis with liver manipulation, therefore hepatectomy should be undertaken cautiously (Table 2).

AMEBIC HEPATIC ABSCESS

Amebiasis is a relatively common global parasitic infection caused by the protozoan *E. histolytica*, with the highest incidence in tropical and subtropical climates. Amebiasis typically affects men between the ages of 20 and 40 years. In the United States amebic abscess is uncommon. However, with the increase in travel, the presence of human immunodeficiency virus, and the large immigrant population from endemic areas in the world, physicians need to be familiar with this possible diagnosis.

Amebic liver abscess is the most common extraintestinal location of amebiasis, but amebic liver abscess occurs in only 1% of patients with amebiasis. After fecal-oral contamination, the cyst passes through the stomach to the intestine, where pancreatic enzymes start to digest the outer cyst wall, releasing the trophozite into the intestine where it multiples. Typically, the patient develops amebic dysentery alone. However, in rare patients, the parasite invades through the intestinal mucosa into the mesenteric lymphatics and veins and enters the liver, where it forms into an abscess. The most common complication of amebic abscesses is rupture into the surrounding organs, such as direct extension into the pleuropulmonary space or rupture into the pericardium or peritoneum. The diagnosis and management of pyogenic and amebic abscesses differs, and these differences are reviewed.

Diagnosis

The presentation of amebic abscesses may be acute with fever and right upper quadrant pain or less specific with weight loss, fever, and abdominal pain. Amebic liver abscess usually does not present at the same time as colitis but within a year after the initial infection. Unlike pyogenic abscess, the patient will not be jaundiced or have underlying biliary disease. Also, a majority of patients are younger than 50 years and have a history of travel to an endemic location. The definitive diagnosis of amebic liver abscess is by identification of *E. histolytica* trophozites in the pus or by serum antibodies to the ameba. The majority (75% to 80%) of amebic liver abscesses show up as a single focus in the right lobe.

Treatment

With the introduction of metronidazole decades ago, surgical drainage of amebic abscess has become virtually obsolete. Drainage procedures (surgical or percutaneous) are only required now in circumstances in which a questionable diagnosis, bacterial coinfection, or complications from the amebic abscess exist.

Antibiotics

The mainstay for treatment of invasive amebiasis is metronidazole. Tinidazole and ornidazole are other nitroimidazole derivatives that are effective treatments; however, they are not currently available in the United States. Metronidazole is able to reach high concentrations in the

TABLE 2: Pearls for pyogenic hepatic abscesses

- The most common organisms isolated from pyogenic liver abscess are gram negative; however, due to increased use of indwelling biliary stents, infection with other organisms—such as *Pseudomonas*, *Streptococcus*, and fungal species—has increased.
- Bacteriology and initial antibiotics should be tailored to the presumed underlying source.
- Aspiration of liver abscess should be undertaken in most patients, unless the abscess is small, because it provides rapid relief of symptoms and renders samples for culture.
- Percutaneous drainage is usually required, and open surgery should be reserved for selected patients.

liver. Current recommendations for metronidazole are 750 mg three times a day for 5 to 10 days. Caution should be taken in pregnant and breastfeeding mothers because metronidazole does cross the placenta and is secreted in breast milk. Ninety-five percent of patients respond after 10 days of therapy; however, 5% to 15% are resistant to metronidazole. Luminal antimicrobials, such as paromomycin and iodoquinol, should also be used to eradicate intestinal colonization because 10% of patients will relapse without luminal amebicidal agents.

A second-line luminal agent, diloxanide furoate, is available from the U.S. Centers for Disease Control for patients who clinically do not respond to paromomycin or iodoquinol. Follow-up stool examination is recommended after completion of therapy to ensure eradication of the infection.

Drainage

Blessmann and colleagues (2003) performed a prospective randomized trial to determine whether any significant benefit was obtained by adding aspiration to antibiotics for the treatment of amebic abscesses. In this study aspiration did not improve the outcomes. Therefore image-guided percutaneous treatment is used only in the following circumstances: 1) if no clinical response is seen after 5 to 7 days of antibiotics, and 2) if an abscess is at high risk for rupture, especially a large abscess in the left lobe. If the complication of rupture or extension does occur, percutaneous drainage is useful in treating pulmonary, peritoneal, or cardiac complications. Percutaneous drainage is rarely required for this disease, and the need for surgical intervention is even less common. However, the unusual situations in which surgery is required include hemorrhage, erosion into surrounding organs, or sepsis due to a secondarily infected amebic abscess that has failed percutaneous treatment.

Results

The vast majority of patients with amebic abscesses will defervesce and start showing improvement after 3 days of therapy. However, if not treated in a timely fashion, this condition can be fatal, with mortality rates ranging as high as 15% to 20%. Several patient factors that are independent predictors of mortality include 1) a bilirubin greater than 3.5 mg/dL, 2) encephalopathy, 3) an abscess volume greater than 500 mL, 4) an albumin less than 2 g/dL, and 5) multiple abscesses. In addition, patients with complications of the abscess, rupture, or direct extension as previously described will have a worse outcome.

In conclusion, amebic abscesses have an excellent outcome with medical management, and drainage procedures are reserved for patients who do not respond to medical therapy. Patients will have clinical improvement with amebicidal therapy more rapidly than radiologic resolution will be observed. Complete radiologic resolution may take up to 9 months, and follow-up imaging is advised (Table 3).

TABLE 3: Pearls for amebic liver abscesses

- Only 10% to 20% of patients with amebic liver abscess have a history of diarrhea.
- Treat the intestinal infection to prevent relapse of amebic liver abscess. Failure to use luminal amebicidal agents after metronidazole in cases of amebic abscess results in a 10% relapse rate.
- Failure to show response to antiamebic medication requires evaluation for polymicrobial infection with bacteria.
- Amebic abscess usually responds clinically to antimicrobial therapy in 3 to 7 days, although imaging takes several months to show resolution.
- Percutaneous drainage is rarely required.

FUNGAL HEPATIC ABSCESS

Bacteria and parasites constitute the majority of hepatic abscesses, but the incidence of fungal liver abscesses has been increasing. The majority of monomicrobial fungal abscesses are seen in immunocompromised patients, such as patients receiving chemotherapy for leukemia or those with HIV infection. Mixed bacterial and fungal abscesses typically occur in patients with biliary malignancies who have had long-term indwelling stents and have been frequently treated with antibiotics.

Treatment

Treatment of fungal abscesses follows the same principles as treatment for pyogenic hepatic abscesses, focusing on antimicrobial agents and drainage. Drainage is again by simple aspiration, percutaneous drainage, or surgical drainage. About 80% of fungal abscesses contain *Candida* spp.; the next most common fungal organisms are *Aspergillus* and *Cryptococcus*. Historically, amphotericin B was the first-line therapy, but micafungin and caspofungin are currently the agents of choice. It is imperative that an adequate course be employed; an earlier analysis suggested that inadequate treatment with amphotericin B was associated with a high mortality rate. Oral fluconazole may be employed after initial intravenous therapy if *Candida albicans* is the cause. Patients with mixed fungal and bacterial abscesses also should receive appropriate antibiotics for the isolated bacteria.

Results

Fungal abscesses of the liver are a significant source of mortality. The series from Johns Hopkins that analyzed fungal infections from 1973 to 1993 reported that all four patients with monomicrobic fungal abscesses with fungemia died. However, those patients who received a complete course of amphotericin B and did not have fungemia survived. In mixed fungal and bacterial abscesses, the overall mortality rate was 50%; however, adequate amophotericin B treatment resulted in a lower mortality rate (20% vs. 62%). In conclusion, even though fungal hepatic abscesses carry a high mortality rate, early administration of modern antifungal agents for the prevention of fungemia should improve survival.

SUGGESTED READINGS

Blessmann J, Binh HD, Hung DM, et al: Treatment of amebic liver abscess with metronidazole alone or in combination with ultrasound-guided needle aspiration: a comparative, prospective and randomized study, *Trop Med Int Health* 8:1030–1034, 2003.

Huang CJ, Pitt HA, Lipsett PA, et al: Pyogenic liver abscess: changing trends over 42 years, *Ann Surg* 223:600–609, 1996.

Lipsett PA, Huang CJ, Lillemoe KD, et al: Fungal hepatic abscess: characterization and management, *J Gastrointest Surg* 1:78–84, 1997.

Rajak C, Gupta S, Jain S, et al: Percutaneous treatment of liver abscess: needle aspiration versus catheter drainage, *Am J Roentgenol* 170:1035–1039, 1998.

Yu SC, Ho SS, Law WY, et al: Treatment of pyogenic liver abscess: prospective randomized comparison of catheter drainage and needle operation, *Hepatology* 39:932–938, 2004.

PORTAL HYPERTENSION

THE ROLE OF SHUNTING PROCEDURES

J. Michael Henderson, MB, ChB, and Michael Johnson, MD

OVERVIEW

Surgical shunting procedures for decompression of varices are no longer a significant part of the management repertoire in managing patients with portal hypertension. Over the last half century, shunts have contributed to both managing patients and understanding portal hypertension, but this has changed dramatically in the last 20 years, such that patients are now better managed with pharmacologic therapy, endoscopic management of varices, radiologic decompression of portal hypertension when indicated, and liver transplantation. The significant advances in patient care using these modalities have largely been supported by randomized trials; many have been led by surgeons, and all have clearly been of benefit to patients.

This chapter takes a high-level look at the current status of the management of portal hypertension and puts in context the few residual indications for shunt procedures. The key steps in this evolution of the management of patients with portal hypertension have been team management and standardization of best practices.

The complex team required to manage patients with portal hypertension is composed of hepatologists, surgeons, endoscopists, radiologists, pathologists, and intensivists. This team needs to be aware of the current evidence and the broad range of options available to optimize management of patients with portal hypertension and its complications.

Standardization of best practices requires 1) protocols for the evaluation of patients with portal hypertension; 2) protocols for managing patients with varices that have not bled, managing acute variceal bleeding, and preventing variceal rebleeding; and 3) protocols for management of other complications of portal hypertension.

Finally, experts on the team should have complete knowledge of the capabilities of pharmacologic therapy for portal hypertension, and they should be fully abreast of the technologic components of endoscopic therapy and have a standardized approach to radiologic decompression with transjugular intrahepatic portosystemic shunts (TIPS). In addition, the effort should include a fully trained transplant team capable of creating surgical decompressive shunts when indicated.

This chapter briefly examines the best approaches for patient evaluation and current treatments and looks in more detail at the surgical options when indicated.

PATIENT EVALUATION

Patients with portal hypertension require an evaluation that includes 1) assessment of their underlying liver disease, 2) imaging studies, and 3) endoscopy. Liver disease is evaluated from a complete history and clinical findings, such as jaundice, ascites, and muscle wasting. In addition, appropriate lab tests and, when necessary, liver biopsy and specialized tests may be helpful. The combination of these allows for further grading of the severity of the liver disease, such as with a Child-Turcotte-Pugh or Model for End-Stage Liver Disease score that will further guide treatment decisions (Tables 1 and 2).

Imaging studies focus on liver morphology and vasculature. Liver ultrasound, possibly augmented by computed tomographic scan or magnetic resonance imaging, provides most of the imaging needed. Morphology focuses on the size of the liver and any focal lesions suspicious for hepatocellular carcinoma. The other component of imaging assesses the venous and arterial anatomy of the liver, particularly for patency of the portal vein and its main tributaries.

Endoscopic evaluation is focused on varices and portal hypertensive gastropathy. The size, extent, and risk factor of varices are considered when making treatment decisions, and evaluation should include an accepted grading system.

MEDICAL MANAGEMENT

Time Points of Therapy for Varices

Table 3 summarizes the different time points of therapy and the main treatment options. The team needs to develop and implement protocols to manage patients for prophylaxis, acute variceal bleeding, and prevention of recurrent variceal bleeding. Therapies that may be used at these points are pharmacologic management, endoscopic treatment, TIPS, surgical shunt, and liver transplant. This table ranks an approach to the use of these treatments at each of these points.

Prophylaxis

Pharmacologic therapy with a β-blocker is the mainstay for preventing an initial bleed. Occasionally, endoscopic banding may be indicated for large varices or for patients intolerant to β-blockers. There is no indication for TIPS or surgical shunting in prophylaxis, and the only time liver transplant may be used is with advanced end-stage liver disease as the indication for transplant rather than just varices.

Acute Variceal Bleeding

Primary management is with pharmacologic therapy and endoscopic banding. For the 10% of patients in whom acute bleeding recurs or is not controlled with these steps, TIPS may be indicated. There are no

TABLE 1: Child-Turcotte-Pugh classification

Parameter	1 Point	2 Points	3 Points
Serum bilirubin (mg/dL)	<2	2–3	<3
Albumin (g/dL)	>3.5	2.8–3.5	<2.8
Prothrombin time (↑ sec)	1–3	4–6	>6
Ascites	None	Slight	Moderate
Encephalopathy	None	1–2	3–4

TABLE 2: Model for End-Stage Liver Disease score for liver disease severity

$$\text{Score} = 0.957 \times \log_e \text{creatinine (mg/dL)} + 0.378 \\ \times \log_e \text{bilirubin (mg/dL)} + 1.120 \log_e \text{INR}$$

INR, International normalized ratio

TABLE 3: Role of therapy options and different time points in managing variceal bleeding

	Pharmacotherapy	Endoscopic Therapy	TIPS	Surgical Shunt	Liver Transplant
Prophylaxis	+++	+	–	–	+
Acute variceal bleed	+++	+++	++	–	–
Prevention of recurrent bleed	+++	+++	++	+	++

+++, primary therapy; ++, secondary; +, occasional; –, not indicated

roles for surgical shunting or liver transplant to manage acute variceal bleeding.

PREVENTION OF RECURRENT BLEEDING

Pharmacologic therapy with β-blockers and a course of endoscopic banding to obliterate varices are the primary management of patients to prevent recurrent bleeding after they are stabilized from an acute bleed. These will control variceal bleeding in 80% of patients. In patients who either re-bleed through this primary treatment or have recurrent high-risk varices, other treatments may be indicated. In patients with well-preserved liver function and recurrent bleeding, TIPS is the next treatment option. Surgical decompression with selective shunt has been shown to be as effective as TIPS but is not as widely available and therefore remains an option rather than recommended treatment. In patients with progressive liver disease and recurrent bleeding, liver transplant becomes the treatment of choice.

The above recommendations are for patients with cirrhosis as the cause of their portal hypertension. In reviewing the current role for surgical shunts, other populations of patients need to be considered, as do geographic differences in diseases and available treatments. For example, patients with portal hypertension secondary to extrahepatic causes, such as portal vein thrombosis, have well-preserved liver function; if they show recurrent variceal bleeding through pharmacologic and endoscopic therapy, they may be ideal candidates for a

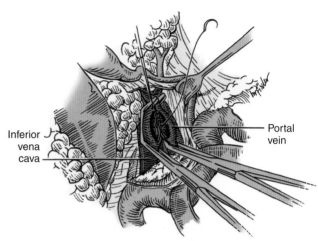

FIGURE 1 Side-to-side portacaval shunt. The hepatic flexure of the colon and duodenum have been mobilized inferiorly and the bile duct retracted medially. The portal vein and IVC have been fully mobilized to permit side-to-side anastomosis. *(From Bell RH Jr, Rikkers LF, Mulholland MW [eds]: Digestive tract surgery: a text and atlas, Philadelphia, 1996, Lippincott-Raven.)*

surgical shunt if their splenic vein is open. Similarly, patients in India with noncirrhotic portal fibrosis and well-preserved liver function may not have good access for treatment that requires repeated visits for endoscopic therapy or TIPS follow-up, so they also may be good candidates for a selective shunt. Other populations that may benefit from surgical shunts are patients in remote locations, who only get one chance at control of variceal bleeding; patients with schistosomiasis; and patients with acute Budd-Chiari syndrome. In this latter population, the need is for sinusoidal decompression, which can be achieved with a side-to-side portacaval shunt.

Although all of these patients can have decompression achieved with TIPS, the long-term durability is less sure, and management may be better served with a vein-to-vein surgical shunt. At the present time, it is incumbent upon the team managing such patients to have full working knowledge of these options and to have a defined management algorithm for patients with portal hypertension of all etiologies.

SURGICAL SHUNT PROCEDURES

Surgical shunts fall into the broad categories of *total decompressive shunts, partial decompressive shunts,* and *selective shunts.* These shunts are illustrated in the figures that follow.

The difference among these three options lies in the degree of maintenance of portal perfusion. All three provide decompression of gastroesophageal varices with greater than 90% control of variceal bleeding. When a surgical shunt is indicated, the choice depends on the surgeon's familiarity with a given procedure and on the importance of maintaining some portal flow to lower the risk of encephalopathy, particularly in patients with nonalcoholic liver disease.

Total portal systemic shunts are either a side-to-side portacaval shunt or an interposition shunt of the mesocaval type that is more than 10 mm wide. These shunts divert portal flow away from the liver and are excellent at controlling bleeding; they decompress the liver sinusoids, and thus control ascites.

Figure 1 illustrates a side-to-side portacaval shunt. The main technical components are as follows:

1. Adequate exposure of the portal vein and the subhepatic inferior vena cava (IVC)
2. Mobilization of sufficient length of the portal vein and IVC to allow approximation for direct anastomosis or safe placement of an interposition graft, if that is the choice

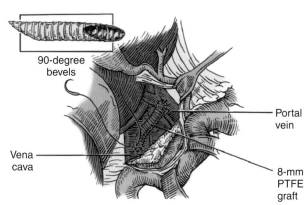

FIGURE 2 Partial shunt using an 8 mm PTFE-reinforced graft between the portal vein and the IVC. Beveling of the graft and its position at implantation are shown. *(From Bell RH Jr, Rikkers LF, Mulholland MW [eds]: Digestive tract surgery: a text and atlas, Philadelphia, 1996, Lippincott-Raven.)*

3. Completion of the anastomosis with running Prolene sutures, ensuring sufficient size for total decompression and no purse stringing

A *partial portal systemic shunt* is achieved with an 8 mm graft between the portal vein and the IVC. The operative exposure is similar to that for a side-to-side portacaval shunt, but the difference lies in the careful positioning of the 8 mm reinforced polytetrafluoroethylene (PTFE) graft between the IVC and the portal vein (Figure 2). The ends of the graft need to be beveled to double the size of the anastomosis relative to the graft diameter, and these are positioned at right angles to each other on the graft to avoid any kinking of the graft when it sits in the correct anatomic position.

A *mesocaval shunt* is a total or partial shunt that takes the dissection for the shunt away from the liver hilum. This may be advantageous in patients who may ultimately require liver transplantation. The dissection for a mesocaval shunt involves isolating the superior mesenteric vein in the root of the mesocolon, mobilizing it for a safe anastomosis, and identifying and clearing enough IVC below the third portion of the duodenum, which needs to be mobilized superiorly. An interposition, reinforced PTFE graft is placed between these two vessels (Figure 3).

A *distal splenorenal shunt* is the most widely used selective shunt for variceal decompression. The concept is different from the portosystemic shunts described above, in that varices are selectively decompressed through the short gastric veins, the spleen, and the splenic vein to the left renal vein, and portal hypertension is maintained to keep portal flow to the liver. The procedure is done by access through the lesser sac, taking down the splenic flexure of the colon. The pancreas is then mobilized so that the posterior surface is exposed, and the splenic vein is dissected out from the posterior surface. Sufficient vein is mobilized to allow the splenic vein to come down to the left renal vein without kinking. The anastomosis is made with a running suture to the posterior wall, but interrupted suture is used for the anterior wall so as not to narrow the opening (Figure 4). The operation is completed by ligating the coronary vein at its origin on the splenic or portal vein and again in the superior border of the pancreas.

PERIOPERATIVE PATIENT MANAGEMENT

One of the keys to the success of surgical shunts for portal hypertension is careful perioperative management. The role of the whole team and use of defined protocols are important. Fluid, electrolyte,

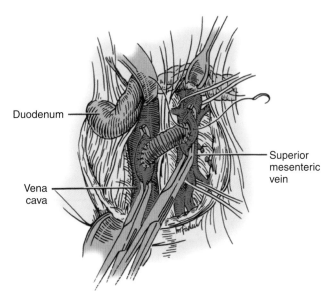

FIGURE 3 Mesocaval shunt uses a graft between the fully mobilized superior mesenteric vein (SMV) and the IVC. The pancreas is retracted superiorly off the SMV, and the duodenum is retracted superiorly off the IVC to optimize exposure and shunt placement. *(From Bell RH Jr, Rikkers LF, Mulholland MW [eds]: Digestive tract surgery: a text and atlas, Philadelphia, 1996, Lippincott-Raven.)*

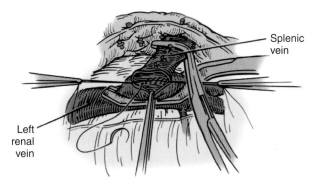

FIGURE 4 Distal splenorenal shunt requires dissection of sufficient splenic vein out of the pancreas and mobilization of the left renal vein. Those points are shown here as the posterior wall of the anastomosis is completed. *(From Bell RH Jr, Rikkers LF, Mulholland MW [eds]: Digestive tract surgery: a text and atlas, Philadelphia, 1996, Lippincott-Raven.)*

and blood product management is different in patients with liver disease than in the regular surgical patient, with an emphasis on sodium restriction and caution with narcotic and sedative management. Deterioration of liver function in the postoperative period is the major risk, and lab results showing liver function should be followed up with every second day.

CURRENT DATA COMPARING SHUNTS AND TIPS

Two randomized trials comparing surgical shunts with TIPS have been completed in the last decade. One compared TIPS and distal splenorenal shunt (DSRS) in CTP class A and B patients. The trial ran for over 7 years, with a median follow-up of 42 months. The re-bleeding rates were not significantly different (5.6% in the DSRS group and 11.5% in the TIPS group). Encephalopathy rates were not significantly different, with 50% of patients in each group having at least one clinical encephalopathy event by 5 years. The survival rates were not significantly different, with 85% survival at 1 year and 65%

survival at 5 years. What was significantly different was the reintervention rate, which was 82% in the TIPS group and 11% in the DSRS group (*P* < .001). It was the careful surveillance, protocol recatheterizations of TIPS at annual intervals, and completeness of follow-up that contributed to the low rebleeding rate in the TIPS group. This trial was conducted with uncovered stents. A European multicenter trial compared covered and uncovered TIPS, and the reintervention rate with covered stents reduced to 15% at 1 year.

The second trial compared TIPS to the 8 mm H-graft interposition portacaval shunt in an "all comers" population; 50% were Childe-Turcotte-Pugh class C, and 63% had alcoholic cirrhosis. At late follow-up, the rebleeding rate was significantly lower (*P* < .01) in the surgical shunt group (3%), compared with the TIPS group (17%), and fewer patients in the surgical shunt group came to transplant (*P* < .01). Mortality was not significantly different.

A cost effectiveness analysis of the DSRS versus TIPS trial showed the average yearly costs of managing patients after TIPS and DSRS over 5 years were similar, $16,363 and $13,492, respectively. Cost of TIPS for surviving patients exceeded the cost of DSRS at years 3 and 5 but not significantly. Incremental cost-effectiveness ratios per life saved favored TIPS at year 5.

A current review of the literature shows only 22 cited papers on surgical shunts in the past decade. These fall into the categories of the randomized studies cited above (seven reports), large series, or patients being shunted for specific circumstances. This paucity of recent publications on surgical shunts speaks to there being few indications for their current use.

SUMMARY

Surgical shunts should rarely be used, however they do play a role in a few highly selected patients. Plans for their use should be made proactively by the multidisciplinary team caring for patients with portal hypertension.

SUGGESTED READINGS

Boyer TD, Henderson JM, Heerey AM, et al: DIVERT Study Group: cost of preventing variceal rebleeding with transjugular intrahepatic portal systemic shunt and distal splenorenal shunt, *J Hepatol* 48:407–414, 2008.

Elwood DR, Pomposelli JJ, Pomfret EA, et al: Distal splenorenal shunt: preferred treatment for recurrent variceal hemorrhage in the patient with well-compensated cirrhosis, *Arch Surg* 141:385–388, 2006.

Henderson JM, Boyer TD, Kutner MH, et al: DIVERT Study Group: distal splenorenal shunt versus transjugular intrahepatic portal systematic shunt for variceal bleeding: a randomized trial, *Gastroenterology* 130:1643–1651, 2006.

Henderson JM, Rikkers LF: Atlas of liver surgery. In Bell RH, Rikkers LF, Mulholland MW (eds): *Digestive tract surgery, a text and atlas*, Philadelphia, 1996, Lippincott-Raven.

Livingstone AS, Koniaris LG, Perez EA, et al: 507 Warren-Zeppa distal splenorenal shunts: a 34-year experience, *Ann Surg* 243:884–892, 2006

Rosemurgy AS, Bloomston M, Clark WC, et al: H-graft portacaval shunts versus TIPS: ten-year follow-up of a randomized trial with comparison to predicted survivals, *Ann Surg* 241:238–246, 2005.

THE ROLE OF LIVER TRANSPLANTATION IN PORTAL HYPERTENSION

Nancy L. Ascher, MD, PhD, and John P. Roberts, MD

PORTAL VENOUS ANATOMY

An understanding of portal venous anatomy is important in appreciating the manifestations of portal hypertension (PHTN). Seventy percent of blood going to the liver comes through the portal vein, with the remaining flow coming via the arterial blood supply, derived from either the celiac axis or the superior mesenteric artery. The portal vein is formed via the confluence of the splenic vein and the superior mesenteric vein. The inferior mesenteric vein generally drains into the splenic vein, but its position may be variable. The portal vein receives drainage from the esophagus through the coronary vein, from the stomach and spleen via the splenic vein, and from the splanchnic circulation (superior mesenteric vein and inferior mesenteric vein). Any obstruction to portal venous flow results in increased pressure in the portal vein, which in turn is transmitted throughout the entire system.

Three main areas can be obstructed to portal venous flow: the areas 1) before the liver sinusoids (presinusoidal), 2) within the sinusoids (intrasinusoidal), and 3) after the sinusoids (postsinusoidal). An example of presinusoidal hypertension would be a thrombus in the portal vein. When this type of obstruction occurs with a normal liver, it is called *extrahepatic portal hypertension*. An example of this phenomenon can be seen in infants, in whom catheterization of the umbilical vein results in portal vein thrombosis. The principal manifestation of this obstruction is the development of varices, with ascites being a less common sequela.

Worldwide, a common form of presinusoidal hypertension is seen in schistosomiasis. In this disease, parasite eggs cause granulomatous inflammation of the portal tracts, leading to obstruction of the portal venules before the sinusoids. As with extrahepatic PHTN, liver function is usually maintained until the inflammation progresses beyond the portal tracts.

Intrahepatic or sinusoidal portal hypertension is by far the most common form of PHTN. Any disease that causes scarring of the liver that distorts the sinusoids results in obstruction to portal flow. Destruction of sinusoidal architecture leads to obstruction of portal venous flow in the liver, which is transmitted upstream and throughout the portal system.

Worldwide, viral hepatitis is the predominant cause of cirrhosis and PHTN. In the United States, adults with chronic active hepatitis C are those most commonly affected by PHTN. Posthepatic (postsinusoidal) PHTN reflects an obstruction distal to the parenchyma; etiologies falling into this category include the venous occlusive disease seen in allogenic bone marrow transplantation; Budd-Chari syndrome, which results from occlusion of the major hepatic veins; and the ultimate downstream cause—heart failure.

MANIFESTATIONS OF PORTAL HYPERTENSION

PHTN is manifested by a constellation of sequelae that can result in significant morbidity and mortality. Elevated pressure within the portal venous system is transmitted throughout the system and may result in the development of collateral circulation.

Varices

Varices are enlarged veins that develop when blood that normally passes through the liver meets increased resistance. The increased portal pressure results in a reversed direction of flow in the veins that typically carry blood toward the liver. These veins enlarge as more portal blood flow escapes through them. For example, increased pressure in the coronary vein results in varices developing in the esophagus and stomach, as the blood tries to make its way to the low-pressure azygous system.

Varices can occur anywhere in the portal vein drainage but are most commonly seen in the distal esophagus and gastric atrium. Bleeding hemorrhoids and peristomal bleeding in patients with stomas may also occur. Recanalization of the obliterated umbilical vein is another common event, in which blood from the left portal vein makes its way out to the systemic circulation via collaterals from the umbilicus to the systemic venous circulation. These veins can be seen on the abdominal wall, forming a *caput medusae*. An illustration of the importance of the pressure gradient in the development of varices is demonstrated by the lack of variceal formation in patients with PHTN from heart failure. While these patients develop ascites, they do not develop varices, because there is no gradient between the portal system and the azygous system.

Increased pressure transmitted through the splenic vein results in hypersplenism, which leads to trapping of platelets and white blood cells. The presence of thrombocytopenia in a patient with liver disease strongly suggests the presence of PHTN.

PHTN is also a factor in the development of ascites, which is associated with pooling of blood in the splanchnic circulation, retention of water, and sodium and fluid accumulation in the peritoneal cavity. The shunting of blood around the liver leads to hepatic encephalopathy.

PATHOPHYSIOLOGY OF PORTAL HYPERTENSION

Portal hypertension is defined as elevated pressure within the portal venous system. The pressure in the portal veins is measured relative to the pressure in the vena cava, referred to as the *portal pressure gradient*, or the *hepatovenous pressure gradient* (HVPG). Quantification of PHTN may be performed via indirect portal pressure measurement, though liver vein catheterization with wedging of the catheter in a small hepatic vein. This allows for measurement of the upstream pressure, analogous to the measurement of left heart pressure by wedging the balloon of the Swan-Ganz catheter in a pulmonary vein.

Most often the diagnosis of elevated portal pressure is made in the context of one of the complications of portal hypertension. The HVPG level may be more useful in determining response to treatment or for differentiating ascites secondary to PHTN from other causes of ascites, such as cardiac or renal disease. The hepatovenous pressure gradient is normally less than 10 mm Hg, but PHTN is quantified as a pressure differential greater than 10 mm Hg, which is the pressure differential that heralds the onset of ascites; variceal bleeding may be seen with pressure gradients greater than 12 mm Hg, and the mortality rate with bleeding significantly rises with gradients above 20 mm Hg. PHTN is also associated with an increased mortality rate for hepatic resection in patients with cirrhosis.

While the wedged hepatic vein pressure is increased in patients with sinusoidal causes of PHTN, presinusoidal causes are associated with a normal wedge pressure, as the upstream blockage results in a pressure that is not reflected in the sinusoids. Physiologic and metabolic derangements seen with PHTN are reflections of 1) changes in portal venous pressure, 2) autonomic effects, and 3) liver metabolism.

Regardless of the site or etiology of obstruction to portal vein flow, the result is the release of cytokines, which have important effects on circulation. Within the liver, there is also an active component to portal vein obstruction, with active contraction of portal/septal myofibroblasts, hepatic satellite cells, and vascular smooth muscle cells in the portal veins. This active process is in addition to the passive resistance associated with the scarring, which also increases resistance.

The vascular tone is the result of the balance between endogenous vasoconstrictors—including endothelin, leukotrienes, and angiotensin II—and the vasodilators, including nitric oxide and prostacyclin. The relative imbalance in these modulators, with a paucity of nitric oxide within the liver, favors vasoconstriction and further obstruction to portal vein flow.

In the splanchnic circulation, nitric oxide is produced, resulting in splanchnic arterial vasodilation and increased blood flow into the splanchnic circulation, which further increases portal pressure. The vasodilation in peripheral circulation results in hypotension and decreased effective circulatory blood volume. In turn, the decrease in systemic blood pressure leads to activation of neurohormonal systems and results in water and sodium retention. Accumulation of sodium and water further increases the splanchnic circulatory volume and leads to ascites.

Increased circulatory blood volume is manifested by hyperdynamic cardiac output because of increased stroke volume. Despite increases in total circulatory blood volume, renal compromise may be seen secondary to low effective perfusion pressure of the kidney and/or vasoconstriction of the renal circulation and the potential for hepatorenal syndrome.

ALTERNATIVE TREATMENT OF PORTAL HYPERTENSION

The ultimate treatment for PHTN is liver transplantation, but in the absence of other indications, PHTN alone does not constitute an indication for liver transplantation. As such, treatment for the manifestations of PHTN is based on the severity of symptoms. The most serious complication of portal hypertension is variceal bleeding. The first variceal bleed confers a mortality rate of 20% to 30%, and without therapy, there is a 60% chance of re-bleeding during the first 2 years.

Treatment for variceal bleeding may be categorized in four ways: 1) prevention in patients who have documented varices but have not bled (primary prophylaxis), 2) treatment of acute bleeding, 3) prophylaxis to prevent subsequent bleeding, and 4) re-bleed therapy. Once a patient has documented cirrhosis, they need to be screened for varices; this is best done with endoscopy.

In patients who have not bled from varices, two methods are used to prevent bleeding: 1) using β-blockers to decrease portal flow or 2) obliterating the varices. Recent studies indicate that empiric β-blockade without endoscopy for patients with medium to large varices for prophylaxis is cost effective, but β-blockade is frequently poorly tolerated at optimal dosing. When optimal dosing is achieved (heart rate less than 55, or 25% reduction in heart rate), β-blockade significantly reduces the chance of initial bleeding but does not affect mortality rate.

Endoscopic band ligation is effective therapy in preventing bleeding and is recommended in patients with large varices who do not tolerate β-blockers or in those who have contraindications for their use.

TREATMENT OF ACUTE VARICEAL BLEEDING

Mortality rates from acute variceal bleeding have decreased from 40% to 20%. Improvement in mortality is based on the following treatments: 1) replacement of blood volume, 2) correction of coagulopathy, 3) prevention of infection, and 4) remedies to control the bleeding and to decrease portal pressure. Therapies in this last category include use of pharmacologic agents such as terlipressin, somatostatin, octreotide, and vasopressin; transjugular intrahepatic portosystemic shunt (TIPS) and surgical shunts that decrease portal pressure; and endoscopic banding and tamponade therapy, which control bleeding but do not decrease portal pressure (Figure 1).

The resuscitation of a patient with massive variceal hemorrhage should progress using the basic principles of airway, breathing, and circulation. For massive hemorrhage in a cirrhotic patient, where endoscopy is not immediately available or when other therapies fail, balloon tamponade with a Minnesota tube is effective in 60% to

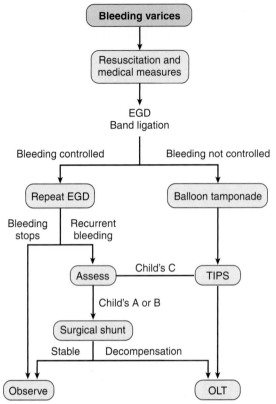

FIGURE 1   Management of acutely bleeding gastroesophageal varices. *EGD*, esophagogastroduodenoscopy; *OLT*, orthotopic liver transplantation.

90% of patients. For less dramatic bleeding, pharmacologic therapy, though not β-blockade, is used to decrease portal pressure. Octreotide is most commonly used to decrease portal pressure, because it has relatively few side effects and appears to be effective.

After resuscitation, endoscopic ligation of the esophageal varices is needed to stop the bleeding and prevent recurrent bleeding. This is done by placing rubber bands on the varices to cut off their blood flow, leading to necrosis. Ligation appears to be the safest and most effective method for immediate control of bleeding.

Bleeding gastric varices are difficult to treat with ligation; these are treated with vasoactive drugs, tube tamponade, and endoscopic therapy with cyanoacrylate, TIPS, and surgical shunt. For acute recurrent bleeding from varices, repeat endoscopy is necessary; if this fails, consideration should be given TIPS or surgical shunting.

Variceal hemorrhage in the setting of cirrhosis is accompanied by a significant risk of infection. These patients should be treated with broad-spectrum antibiotics such as a quinolone from the time of admission.

PREVENTION OF RE-BLEEDING

Endoscopy with variceal ligation is the treatment of choice to prevent re-bleeding. Endoscopic therapy is used in combination with β-blockade to prevent recurrent hemorrhage. The second line of therapy to prevent and treat re-bleeding esophageal varices is with the TIPS procedure. The procedure is more effective than ligation in controlling bleeding, but there is a higher risk of encephalopathy and hepatic decompensation, as the blood flow is diverted from the liver.

In the TIPS procedure, the hepatic vein is accessed via a jugular stick, and the liver is transversed with a needle to find a portal vein branch. A wire is passed through the needle from the hepatic vein branch (usually right system) to the portal vein branch (usually right portal vein), over which a stent is passed to effect an intrahepatic portosystemic shunt.

The main problems with the TIPS procedure are hepatic decompensation and TIPS occlusion. Hepatic decompensation is an early complication that may be seen days to weeks after insertion and is manifest by progressive coagulopathy and jaundice; its occurrence may be predicted by the patient's Model for End-Stage Liver Disease (MELD) score prior to insertion. Balloon occlusion of the TIPS may alleviate part of the hepatic insufficiency. Encephalopathy may occur independent of hepatic decompensation, and its severity varies. TIPS occlusion is progressive over time and relates to endothelial overgrowth. The management of patients after TIPS requires frequent ultrasonography to evaluate impending occlusion. TIPS revision is undertaken when shunt velocity increases or occlusion is identified. Shunts are covered with polytetrafluoroethylene, which decreases the risk of endothelial overgrowth and occlusion. In addition to treating bleeding, TIPS may be used to treat ascites.

In the settings of conserved hepatic function (Child's A or B cirrhosis), an open surgical shunt may be considered. Shunts may be nonselective, in that blood is totally diverted away from the portal circulation into the low-pressure venous circulation; this effectively decreases portal venous pressure but diverts blood flow from the liver parenchyma, which can lead to hepatic decompensation. A typical example of this type of shunt would be a mesocaval shunt.

A TIPS is also a nonselective shunt. With a selective shunt, blood flow to the liver is maintained. The distal splenorenal (Warren) shunt involves a disconnection between the splenic vein at its confluence with the portal vein. The end of the splenic vein is anastomosed to the left renal vein. Combined with coronary vein ligation and division of the veins along the greater curve of the stomach, this shunt attempts to decrease the pressure on the left side of the portal system to decompress the esophageal and gastric varices while maintaining the flow toward the liver.

Randomized trials of surgical shunts and TIPS have revealed similar rates of encephalopathy. Re-bleeding rates are either lower with the surgical shunt or the same. As the trials were done prior to the development of a covered TIPS stent, shunt thrombosis and stenosis were significant problems. A trial of a mesocaval shunt using an 8 mm graft compared to TIPS demonstrated no difference in survival for all patients treated, but there was increased survival for the surgical shunt patients, with well-preserved synthetic function compared with TIPS. A similar trial comparing distal splenorenal shunts to TIPS demonstrated similar survival and encephalopathy rates.

With the increase in the use of endoscopic ligation, TIPS, and transplantation, the need for surgical shunts has fallen dramatically. Few surgeons have enough long-term experience and ongoing surgical experience to maintain competency in this complex field.

In children with extrahepatic portal vein thrombosis, a mesoportal shunt (Rex shunt) may be used; in this method, a jugular vein graft is used to bypass the blockage between the superior mesenteric system and the intrahepatic portal vein.

Ascites is a common sequela of PHTN, and it is treated with fluid restriction and diuretics. A combination of furosemide and spironolactone is advised. A TIPS may be effective in alleviating ascites, but the risk of liver decompensation forces consideration of whether the risk/benefit ratio of the TIPS is favorable.

Spontaneous bacterial peritonitis is characterized by the finding of an abnormal quantity of polymorphonuclear white blood cells on a peritoneal tap; although culture of the peritoneal fluid may be negative, it is treated with intravenous antibiotics. The incidence of spontaneous bacterial hepatitis may be reduced with the prophylactic use of fluoroquinolone or trimethoprim and sulfamethoxazole.

Although liver transplantation resolves PHTN, the shortage of cadaveric donor organs and the need for chronic immunosuppression dictates that transplantation for PHTN is only done in the context of decompensation in hepatic function or in hepatocellular carcinoma. Deceased donor liver distribution the United States is based on the MELD system. This system calculates a score based on bilirubin, prothrombin, and creatinine and indicates how likely a patient with end-stage liver disease is to die without transplantation. Patients with the highest MELD score—that is, those most likely to die—are given first priority for liver grafts.

The use of this system has significantly decreased death on the waiting list. The calculation does not, however, take into consideration the presence of PHTN. Additional points are added to the MELD to accommodate patients with hepatocellular carcinoma, so they can receive a transplant prior to tumor spread outside the liver. Although patients with live donors may undergo transplantation at a lower MELD, this option may be more open to patients with PHTN but may in fact be more problematic.

Intraoperative consideration in patients with PHTN who are undergoing transplantation relate to the issues that may jeopardize the success of the transplant procedure. In patients undergoing transplantation, the risk of bleeding relates to the coagulopathy associated with decompensated liver disease and the presence of an extensive collateral circulation, which results from PHTN. Disruption of collaterals in the retroperitonum and bleeding from esophageal varices may be particularly hazardous during occlusion of the portal vein in the anhepatic phase of the procedure. Agents such as octreotide may be used to decrease splanchnic hypertension.

It may be necessary to employ venovenous bypass to relieve PHTN during the anhepatic phase. The piggyback technique is another strategy used to shorten the anhepatic phase. An important consideration is the size of the graft relative to the degree of PHTN. High flow through the portal system has the potential for damaging the graft endothelium, and endothelial damage in turn may lead to compromised graft function, or it may inhibit graft regeneration. This is an important consideration in the small graft, the split liver, or the live donor liver transplant.

To protect small-for-size grafts from additional endothelial injury, measures are taken to decrease the portal pressure gradient. This has been done with pharmacologic agents used in the postoperative period, TIPS, and portosystemic shunts, which direct some flow away from the liver.

In general, PHTN resolves with successful liver transplantation, though this process may take weeks to months to occur. Many patients continue to have esophageal and gastric varices, though recurrent bleeding is rarely a clinical problem. An enlarged spleen is frequent after liver transplant, and often thrombocytopenia and leukopenia persist. Whether these conditions are secondary to persistent hypersplenism or the result of immunosuppressive drugs is unclear.

In the case of small-for-size grafts (in the setting of live donor liver or split liver transplantation) manifestations of PHTN may persist for an extended time, with ongoing ascites, encephalopathy, and thrombocytopenia.

Any process that causes parenchymal scarring can result in recurrent PHTN; this includes fatty infiltration (recurrent alcohol abuse, recurrent nonalcoholic steatohepatitis), recurrent hepatitis, and chronic rejection. The reappearance of thrombocytopenia or esophageal varices many years after transplant may be the first sign of recurrent cirrhosis in the graft. These findings dictate endoscopy and liver biopsy to establish the status of the graft.

SUGGESTED READINGS

Abraldes JG, Angermayr B, Bosch J: The management of portal hypertension, *Clin Liver Dis* 9:685–713, 2005.

De Franchis R, Primignani M: Endoscopic treatments for portal hypertension, *Semin Liver Dis* 19:439–455, 1999.

Elwood DR, Pomposelli JJ, Ponfret EA, et al: Distal splenorenal shunt, *Arch Surg* 141:385–388, 2006.

Gazzera C, Rghi D, Valle F, et al: Fifteen years' experience with transjugular intrahepatic portosystemic shunt (TIPS) using bare stents: retrospective review of clinical and technical aspects, *Radiol Med* 114:83–94, 2009.

Helton WS, Maves R, Wicks K, et al: Transjugular intrahepatic portosystemic shunt vs. surgical shunt in good-risk cirrhotic patients: a case-control comparison, *Arch Surg* 136:17–20, 2001.

Klupp J, Kohler S, Pascher A, Neuhaus P: Liver transplantation as the ultimate tool to treat portal hypertension, *Dig Dis* 23:65–71, 2005.

Pek-Radosavijevic M: Portal hypertension: old problem, new therapeutic solutions, *Wien Med Wochenschr* 156(13-14):397–403, 2006.

Rosemurgy AS, Serafini FM, Zweibel BR, et al: Transjugular intrahepatic portosystemic shunt vs. small-diameter prosthetic H-graft portacaval shunt: extended follow-up of an expanded randomized prospective trial, *J Gastrointest Surg* 4:589–597, 2000.

ENDOSCOPIC THERAPY FOR ESOPHAGEAL VARICEAL HEMORRHAGE

Gregory V. Stiegmann, MD

OVERVIEW

Bleeding from esophageal varices occurs in up to 30% of patients with cirrhosis of the liver. Mortality associated with a first variceal hemorrhage has declined markedly over the past three decades but remains as high as 20% to 30%. Endoscopic therapy is the primary treatment for bleeding esophageal varices at most centers.

All patients with gastrointestinal (GI) hemorrhage should be rapidly resuscitated, and they must be hemodynamically stable before endoscopy for diagnosis and treatment is performed. Uncooperative patients and those with hepatic encephalopathy may benefit from endotracheal intubation, which protects the airway from aspiration and allows controlled ventilation. Vasoactive drugs such as octreotide (50 μg IV bolus, then 25 to 50 μg/hour IV) improve bleeding control in patients with variceal hemorrhage and should be administered prior to endoscopy if variceal bleeding is suspected. Vasoactive drugs are continued for 3 to 5 days after endoscopic treatment for acute bleeding if portal hypertension is the source of bleeding.

Cirrhotic patients who experience GI hemorrhage are at greatly increased risk for infection-related complications such as pneumonia and infected ascites. Such complications are associated with an increased risk of recurrent variceal bleeding, which can be mitigated by administration of broad-spectrum antibiotics (e.g., levofloxacin) given initially intravenously and continued orally for 5 to 7 days when oral intake resumes.

About 10% to 25% of patients with upper GI bleeding, known portal hypertension, and esophageal varices may not have esophageal varices as the source of bleeding. Gastritis, portal hypertensive gastropathy, peptic ulcer, Mallory-Weiss tears, and gastric fundal varices should be sought in a carefully performed diagnostic endoscopy in patients who lack clear evidence of bleeding from esophageal varices. In the patient with active or recent upper GI bleeding, detection of varices and identification of no other potential source of bleeding presumes a variceal source of hemorrhage.

SURGICAL THERAPY

Endoscopic Band Ligation

Diagnostic endoscopy is done prior to attaching the ligating device to the endoscope (Figure 1). Most endoscopists use multiple-fire banding devices that allow five to seven elastic bands to be deployed with

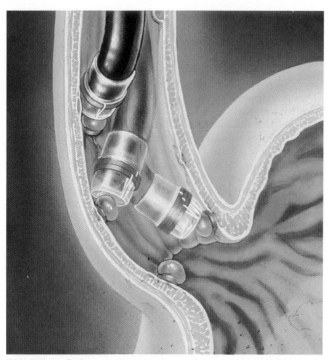

FIGURE 1 Endoscopic band ligation performed with a multiple-band ligating device. The endoscopist makes circumferential contact between the end of the ligating device and the varix to be ligated. Endoscopic suction draws the varix into the device, after which the elastic band is ejected to ensnare the varix. The ligated tissue sloughs after 3 to 5 days, leaving a shallow ulceration that generally heals within 1 week. *(Courtesy Bard Endoscopic Technologies, Billerica, Mass.)*

one insertion of the endoscope. Single-fire devices are best used with an endoscopic overtube that allows easy insertion and withdrawal of the endoscope for reloading and multiple-band applications.

After inserting the endoscope and attached ligating device, the target varix is identified, and the endoscope is advanced under direct vision until the banding cylinder is in 360 degree contact with the varix. Endoscopic suction is activated, drawing the varix into the banding cylinder. When the entrained varix fills the banding cylinder, the firing mechanism is activated, and a constricting latex O-ring is deployed around the base of the varix. Endoscopic suction is stopped, and the ligated tissue bolus is disengaged from the banding cylinder, and the process is repeated.

Band ligation of esophageal varices begins with ligation of the most distal varices at or just below the gastroesophageal junction. Subsequent ligations are performed at the same level or more cephalad. Patients with actively bleeding varices are treated similarly, except when the site of active bleeding is discretely identified. In this case, the actively bleeding varix is first ligated by placing a band either directly on the rent in the varix or by placing a band both caudal and cephalad to the rent. Subsequent ligations are performed until all varices have been ligated at least once. Repeat band-ligation treatments to eradicate varices from the distal 5 cm of the esophagus are performed at 10- to 14-day intervals. Eradication of varices usually requires three to four treatment sessions.

Endoscopic Sclerotherapy

Endoscopic sclerotherapy is performed using an injector needle passed via the working channel of the endoscope following the diagnostic examination. Sclerosant can be injected beside the varix (paravariceal) or into the lumen of the varix (intravariceal) or a combination of both. Most endoscopists use intravariceal injections of

1 to 5 mL of sclerosant per varix. Treatment is confined to the distal 5 cm of the esophagus, unless a discrete site of variceal bleeding is located elsewhere, and usually starts at or just below the gastroesophageal junction. A second injection several centimeters cephalad to the initial puncture may be done at the same treatment session if varices are large. Tetradecyl sodium (1% to 3% solution), sodium morrhuate (2.5% to 5% solution) and ethanolamine oleate (5% solution) are the most common sclerosing agents.

Patients with active bleeding from a discretely identified site on a varix should have this site treated first by injection of sclerosant below the site of active bleeding. After bleeding is controlled, injections are continued at or near the gastroesophageal junction beginning with the most gravity-dependent varix and proceeding in circumferential fashion to the least dependent. Three to five variceal channels are usually present, and all should be treated.

Injections should be made with caution in the mid- or proximal esophagus, because sclerosant may escape from a large varix into the azygos system and then into the pulmonary circulation. Total sclerosant volume per treatment session should seldom exceed 20 or 5 mL per individual varix. Retreatment after control of acute bleeding is aimed at eradicating varices from the distal esophagus and is usually initiated 7 to 14 days after the acute bleed. Three to five outpatient endoscopic treatment sessions are needed to obliterate varices in most patients.

Other Endoscopic Methods

Endoscopic injection of rapidly setting polymers (N-butyl-2-cyanoacrylate, Histoacryl; Braun, Melsungen, Germany) is effective for controlling active variceal bleeding. Almost all experience with this method has been outside the United States, because the glues have not been approved for this use by the U.S. Food and Drug Administration. The glue is mixed with radiopaque contrast (lipiodol) in 1:1 or 1:1.5 ratios to slow hardening and allow fluoroscopic monitoring to determine proper intravariceal location of the injected material and minimize risk of embolization. This mixture is injected in 1 mL aliquots, after which the injection catheter is flushed with saline or water. Care must be taken to avoid gluing the injector needle into the varix or the endoscope.

Patients treated with polymer injection should have repeat endoscopy 2 to 3 weeks afterward to determine whether varices were obliterated. In those with persistent varices, repeat polymer injection, conventional sclerotherapy, or band ligation can be done. The polymer cast of the obliterated varix is eventually extruded into the GI lumen and passed harmlessly.

Endoscopic ligation using one of several detachable endoscopic snare devices has been reported in several small series. The technique is similar to elastic band ligation. A ligation cylinder is attached to the end of the endoscope, and a detachable snare device is passed via the working channel of the endoscope. The open snare is positioned near the end of the ligation cylinder, and the varix is aspirated into the cylinder using endoscopic suction. The snare is tightened around the base of the varix and then detached, and the procedure may be repeated without removing the endoscope. When compared with elastic band ligation, this technique reportedly takes longer to perform, and it requires the presence of a skilled assistant.

RESULTS

Endoscopic sclerotherapy and band ligation control acute variceal hemorrhage in 80% to 95% of patients. Band ligation is the preferred treatment for acute bleeding because of a lower risk of treatment-induced complications, and it is superior to sclerotherapy when used in serial treatments aimed at preventing recurrent variceal bleeding by eradicating distal esophageal varices. Band ligation requires fewer endoscopic treatment sessions than sclerotherapy to eradicate varices, it results in fewer complications, and it is associated with a lower incidence of recurrent bleeding (~25%).

Recurrent varices following initial eradication are more common in patients treated with band ligation (30% to 40%) than in those treated with sclerotherapy (10% to 30%). These varices can generally be eradicated with one or two additional treatment sessions. Long-term administration of nonspecific β-adrenergic blocking agents to cirrhotic patients treated with endoscopic therapy results in a lower risk of recurrent bleeding from varices and other sources.

Endoscopic polymer injection results in control of active bleeding in 80% to 100% of patients. Comparison of polymer injection with conventional sclerosants found results from polymer injections equal or superior to other sclerosants. One trial found polymer injection associated with a substantial improvement in survival, and another trial compared snare ligation with elastic band ligation and found both techniques equally effective for control of bleeding, eradication of varices, and recurrence of varices after initial eradication.

Complications

Endoscopic sclerotherapy is associated with a high incidence of minor complications such as bacteremia, fever, pleural effusions, pulmonary infiltrates, deterioration of pulmonary function, and mediastinal enlargement, all of which usually resolve spontaneously. Ulceration at the site of sclerosant injection is common and is associated with recurrent bleeding (2% to 13%) and esophageal stricture formation (10% to 20%). Most strictures respond to bougienage.

Endoscopic band ligation is associated with a low incidence of treatment-related complications. Shallow ulcers occur at all treated sites and result in recurrent bleeding in 5% to 7% of patients. Most bleeding from band ligation–induced ulceration is self-limited. Transient chest pain caused by esophageal spasm may occur as a result of band ligation. Esophageal strictures are uncommon.

Endoscopic polymer injection is associated with a small but definite risk of systemic embolization of the hardened polymer. Several deaths and a number of serious complications associated with end-organ ischemia from polymer embolus have been reported. Complications associated with endoscopic snare ligation appear similar to those with endoscopic band ligation.

Prevention of a First Variceal Hemorrhage

Conventional endoscopic sclerotherapy is not effective for preventing a first variceal bleed. Endoscopic band ligation, β-adrenergic blocking agents, or a combination of both have been shown to diminish the risk of a first variceal hemorrhage in patients with large varices that have never bled. Prophylactic band ligation treatment reduces the risk of a first variceal bleed in such patients by up to 70% when compared with no treatment. Band ligation treatment to eradicate distal esophageal varices is equal or better at preventing a first variceal bleed than prophylactic administration of β-adrenergic blocking drugs.

SUMMARY

Endoscopic treatment is widely employed for treatment of patients with bleeding esophageal varices. Control of acute bleeding should be followed with serial treatments aimed at preventing recurrent bleeding by obliterating varices. Endoscopic ligation may be used to prevent a first episode of variceal bleeding in patients with large varices that have not bled. Endoscopic band ligation is associated with a lower incidence of complications and more efficient eradication of varices than sclerotherapy, although recurrence of varices after initial eradication is more common with ligation than sclerotherapy. Control of bleeding with either endoscopic treatment is enhanced by the long-term administration of nonspecific β-blocker therapy.

SELECTED READINGS

American Society for Gastrointestinal Endoscopy Technology Committee: Endoscopic banding devices, *Gastrointest Endosc* 68(2):217–221, 2008.
Dell'Era A, Cubero Sotela J, Fabris FM, et al: Primary prophylaxis of variceal bleeding in cirrhotic patients: a cohort study, *Dig Liver Dis* 40(12):936–943, 2008.
Gonzalez R, Zamora J, Gomez-Camarero J, et al: Meta-analysis: combination endoscopic and drug therapy to prevent variceal rebleeding in cirrhosis, *Ann Int Medicine* 149(2):109–122, 2008.
Park WG, Yeh RW, Triadafilopoulos G: Injection therapies for variceal bleeding disorders, *Gastrointest Endosc* 67(2):313–323, 2008.
Rengen MR, Adler DG: Detachable snares (endoloop), *Gastrointest Endosc* 8(1):12–15, 2006.

TRANSJUGULAR INTRAHEPATIC PORTOSYSTEMIC SHUNT

Christos S. Georgiades, MD PhD, and
Jean-Francois H. Geschwind, MD

OVERVIEW

The creation of a transjugular intrahepatic portosystemic shunt (TIPS) was put forth as a possible treatment for the symptoms of portal hypertension in the early 1970s. Over the ensuing two decades, the work of many pioneers—including Rosch, Uchida, Colapinto, Palmaz, and others, many of whom lent their names to relevant apparatus—culminated with the introduction of TIPS in mainstream clinical practice.

TIPS can be a life-saving procedure as well as one that alleviates severe symptoms related to portal hypertension. It is, however, a double-edged sword, demanding meticulous technique and stringent patient selection to keep what was once a high morbidity and mortality at a minimum.

INDICATIONS

The list for causes of portal hypertension is long; it is summarized in Table 1. Whatever the causative pathophysiology, TIPS can reduce or normalize the portal pressure and ameliorate the associated symptoms. As the technique for placing a TIPS became more refined and safer, and the technology became more adapted to the specific

TABLE 1: Causes of portal hypertension

Presinusoidal	Perisinusoidal	Postsinusoidal
Portal, splenic, or superior mesenteric vein thrombosis	Cirrhosis	Budd-Chiari syndrome
Idiopathic portal hypertension	Congenital hepatic fibrosis	Venoocclusive disease (Sinusoidal obstruction syndrome)
Mass effect (i.e., tumor)	Sarcoidosis	Chronic passive congestion (Nutmeg liver)
Schistosomiasis		Mass effect (i.e., tumor)
Precirrhotic stage, primary biliary cirrhosis		
Alcoholic central sclerosis		
Endothelitis (liver rejection, radiation injury)		
Arterioportovenous fistula (traumatic or Osler-Weber-Rendu)		
Hyperdynamic spleno-megaly (infectious or myelodysplastic)		
Nodular regenerative hyperplasia		

TABLE 2: Indications and contraindications for TIPS

INDICATIONS		CONTRAINDICATIONS	
Indication	Condition	Absolute	Relative
Portal variceal hemorrhage	Refractory to medical/ endoscopic management	Severely elevated right heart pressure	Hepatic vein thrombosis
Recurrent ascites	Refractory to medical management	Severe enceph-alopathy	Portal vein thrombosis
Recurrent hepatic hydrothorax	Refractory to medical management	Uncorrectable bleeding diathesis	Poor liver function reserve
Hepatorenal syndrome	May help in type II	Active infection	Polycystic liver disease
Hepatopul-monary syndrome	Scant evidence		Central liver mass
Budd-Chiari syndrome	Bridge to transplant		
Portal gastropathy	Refractory to β-blockers		

physiology and anatomy of a portosystemic shunt, the indications for TIPS have gradually expanded. Table 2 shows the indications and contraindications for TIPS.

Variceal Bleeding

Portal hypertension can cause varices along the entire GI tract, including the small bowel and colon (hemorrhoids). Varices are more apt to bleed through the mucosa of the gastroesophageal junction, where the coronary vein is particularly disposed to dilatation.

The primary treatment of bleeding gastroesophageal varices is medical management and/or endoscopic banding or sclerosis. Even though endoscopic management is often successful, because of the progressive nature of the liver disease, recurrent bleeding should be expected in more than 50% of patients. Unlike medical or endoscopic management, TIPS addresses the underlying cause of variceal bleeding (portal hypertension) and is therefore the only definitive treatment, with long-term efficacy of 90%. The primary indication for TIPS is to control portal variceal bleeding refractory to medical management and endoscopic interventions.

Ascites

Ascites is the most common complication of cirrhosis, and in addition to the severe limitations in lifestyle, it poses a risk for bacterial peritonitis and other infections, renal failure, and increased mortality. No single cause for ascites has been identified. However, it is likely that a combination of causes, including decreased plasma albumin levels, increased bowel permeability, and cirrhosis-related hemodynamic changes—such as increased cardiac output, vasodilatation, and increased plasma volume—factor together in the formation of ascites.

Initial management consists of sodium restriction and administration of loop diuretics and aldosterone antagonists. In advanced stages, ascites becomes refractory to medical management, and TIPS may be indicated. TIPS is very effective in eliminating ascites. Because the root causes are hemodynamic/hormone related, response to TIPS is not immediate. It may take 2 to 4 weeks after TIPS for ascites to resolve, during which time additional paracenteses may be necessary.

Hepatic Hydrothorax

Hepatic hydrothorax is defined as the accumulation of at least 500 mL of pleural fluid in a patient with cirrhosis without cardiopulmonary disease. Even though this definition is not 100% specific to hepatic hydrothorax, additional signs, such as isolated right-sided hydrothorax and concurrent ascites, help confirm the diagnosis. It occurs in less than 10% of patients with cirrhosis, as peritoneal fluid permeates via small diaphragmatic communications. Again, initial management is sodium restriction and diuretics. In nonresponsive patients, TIPS will eliminate hydrothorax in most and decrease the frequency of thoracenteses in the rest.

Hepatorenal Syndrome

Hepatorenal syndrome portends a poor prognosis for the cirrhotic patient, as it occurs during the late stages of the hemodynamic changes related to cirrhosis. Alterations in vasoactive hormones responding to these hemodynamic changes result in renal arterial vasoconstriction and the opening of small intrarenal arteriovenous communications. The end result is renal hypoperfusion and ensuing renal failure.

Two distinct forms of hepatorenal syndrome have been identified: *type I*, which is rapidly progressing, and *type II*, which is more chronic. Even though TIPS has been shown to provide moderate improvement in type II hepatorenal syndrome, it should be undertaken after serious consideration because of the contrast load and acute hemodynamic changes it involves.

Hepatopulmonary Syndrome

Hepatopulmonary syndrome is the presence of intrapulmonary vasodilatation and multiple small, right-to-left shunts that result in impaired gas exchange. Because of the lack of data, TIPS cannot be recommended as a standard treatment for hepatopulmonary syndrome. In selected cases, however, especially in severely compromised patients on the liver transplant list, TIPS may prove to be a life-saving bridge to surgery.

Budd-Chiari Syndrome

Budd-Chiari syndrome is caused by mechanical obstruction of the hepatic venous outflow and gradually results in cirrhosis and portal hypertension. Excluding the hepatic venous web, which can successfully be treated with simple balloon angioplasty, treatment for the fulminant form of Budd-Chiari syndrome is liver transplantation, although anticoagulation may help stave off disease progression. TIPS has proven to be a valuable tool to bridge such patients to transplantation.

Additionally, in a small percentage of patients, TIPS may permanently stabilize liver function and eliminate the need for liver transplantation. This has become evident recently, as a few Budd-Chiari patients bridged with TIPS were alive with stable liver disease years after TIPS placement. Nevertheless, the data are scant, and TIPS is still considered a bridge to transplant, not a substitute.

Portal Gastropathy

Portal hypertensive gastropathy (to be distinguished from vascular ectasia) is the diffuse dilatation of gastric veins that, along with the inflamed and fragile mucosa of the stomach, predispose the patient to bleeding. TIPS, which normalizes the portal pressure, and mucosal protection (avoiding nonsteroidal antiinflammatory drugs, alcohol) combine to minimize this risk.

TECHNIQUE

Patient Preparation

Many of the complications related to the placement of TIPS can be avoided by proper patient work up. Review of pertinent cross sectional imaging will confirm a patent (nonthrombosed) portal vein and reveal the relative orientation of the hepatic and portal veins. This minimizes the number of attempts to engage the portal vein and therefore minimizes the associated bleeding risk. Good hydration will minimize the risk of acute renal failure, and initiation of metronidazole (Flagyl) and/or lactulose mitigates the risk of encephalopathy. Type and cross of blood may prove life saving if a bleeding complication is encountered. Finally, all involved should be cognizant of related risks, especially the 30 day mortality, which ranges from less than 5% for elective procedures in well-compensated patients to 50% for emergent procedures in unstable patients with advanced liver disease.

Access

Access through the right internal jugular vein is preferred, although the left internal jugular vein can also be used. Access is maintained with a long, large vascular sheath parked in the intrahepatic inferior vena cava to allow multiple catheter-wire exchanges without recrossing the right atrium (Figure 1).

Diagnostic Assessment

Optimizing the TIPS outcomes requires not only anatomic assessment but also functional assessment of the patient's hemodynamic status. One of the contraindications of TIPS is elevated right heart

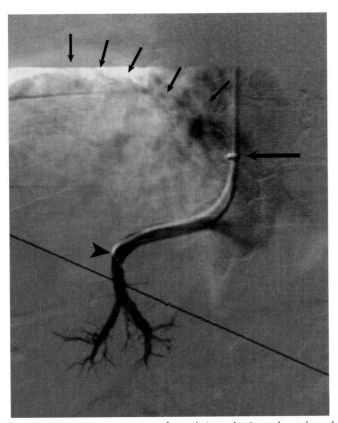

FIGURE 1   Subtracted right hepatic venogram performed via a selective catheter (*arrowhead*). The tip of the internal jugular sheath (*large arrow*) is below the diaphragm (*small arrows*) to avoid catheter/wire manipulations in the right atrium.

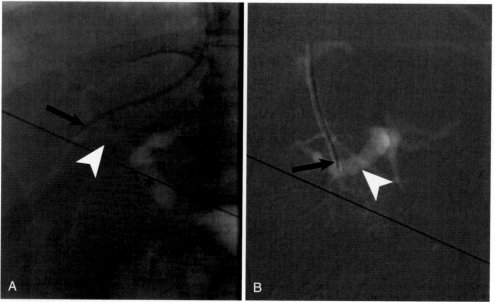

FIGURE 2   Frontal unsubtracted (**A**) and lateral subtracted (**B**) views of a CO_2 hepatic venogram. CO_2 is injected via a balloon occlusion catheter (*arrow*) to force the CO_2 back into the portal system. The right portal vein (*arrowhead*) and the main portal vein (asterisk in **A**) are easily visualized. The operator usually targets the right portal vein from the right hepatic vein with a long needle introduced via the right internal jugular sheath.

pressure. Ensuring the right atrial pressure is not severely elevated is mandatory prior to shunting the portal venous blood to an already overburdened right heart. Right atrial pressures below 15 mm Hg are generally safe, whereas pressures above 20 mm Hg predispose the patient to acute right heart failure. There are no specific guidelines, and sound clinical judgment is important. For example, a right atrial pressure of 16 mm Hg should not preclude a TIPS in a patient with ongoing variceal bleeding whose only chance for survival is a TIPS.

In the vast majority of patients, the TIPS is placed from the right hepatic vein into the right portal vein, thus the next step is selecting the right hepatic vein. Free and wedged hepatic venous pressures are measured at this point, which usually confirm portal hypertension. Normal corrected pressures should not necessarily terminate the procedure, as these are not terribly accurate in general and are wholly inaccurate in cases of presinusoidal portal hypertension.

Delineation of the portal venous system is accomplished by injection of CO_2 via a catheter wedged into the hepatic vein. Frontal and lateral views show the anatomical relationships, so that the right portal vein can be targeted for access (Figure 2). Another advantage of CO_2 is that it can be given in virtually unlimited quantity and is not nephrotoxic.

Shunt Placement

The next step is the cannulation of the right portal vein from the right hepatic vein. To accomplish this, a curved metallic sheath is advanced via the existing right internal jugular sheath in the right hepatic vein. The new catheter is rotated based on the anatomy revealed during CO_2 portography, so that it targets the right portal vein. When the operator judges the curved sheath to be directed toward the right portal vein, a long needle is advanced toward it. Aspiration of blood suggests intravascular location, and contrast injection confirms the tip to be in the portal vein (Figure 3).

Once it is confirmed that the tip of the needle is in the right portal vein, a wire is passed distally through the main portal vein into the superior mesenteric vein or splenic vein for security (Figure 4). The traversed liver parenchyma is fibrotic and difficult to cross unless predilated. A small caliber (4 to 6 mm diameter) balloon is used to predilate

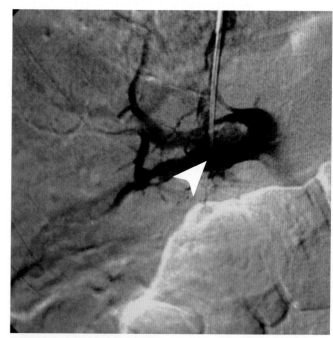

FIGURE 3   Frontal subtracted venogram via a needle (*arrowhead*) after it was advanced from the right hepatic vein toward the right portal vein. Contrast fills branches of the right portal vein with hepatopedal blood flow.

the liver parenchyma between the right hepatic and right portal vein now crossed by the wire (Figure 5). A marking catheter is then passed over the wire into the portal venous system. This allows for direct portal pressure measurement and a portal venogram. The venogram will be used to select the appropriate length stent to be placed (Figure 6).

If the direct portal pressure is within normal limits, the TIPS is abandoned irrespective of the clinical picture, because its creation will not offer any benefit. If a TIPS is not possible or is contraindicated, the gastroesophageal varices can be embolized via a catheter to stop the hemorrhage without placing a TIPS. Though this is very effective, it is nevertheless temporary; the ongoing portal hypertension will likely cause new varices to form. The stent is advanced through the larger sheath, which keeps it constrained and in position. The sheath is pulled back into the right atrium, uncovering the stent. The distal 2 cm of the stent is uncovered and flares out upon withdrawal of the sheath. The rest of the stent is ripcorded open once it is in the appropriate position (Figure 7).

Shunt Evaluation

Usually, a 10 mm diameter stent is used and initially plastied up to 8 mm in diameter. The direct portal pressure is measured again, and if it is not satisfactory, a 10 mm balloon is used to open the stent to capacity (Figure 8). The smaller the stent diameter, the lesser the chances for encephalopathy post procedure. A final portal venogram is performed to document flow and lack of variceal filling (Figure 9).

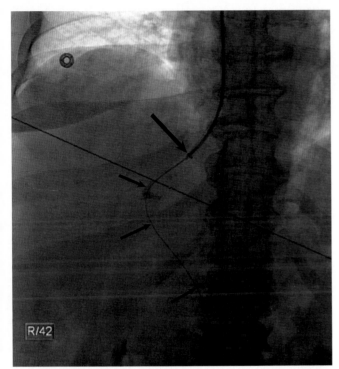

FIGURE 4 After the needle is confirmed to be in the targeted portal vein branch, a wire is advanced through it into the portal vein (*small arrows*), through the right internal jugular sheath (*large arrow*). The wire now crosses from the right hepatic vein through a short segment of liver parenchyma into the right portal vein.

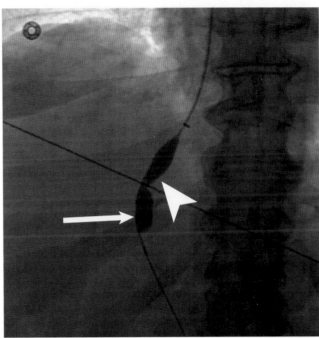

FIGURE 5 Because cirrhotic liver is difficult to cross, it is predilated with a small balloon (*arrow*) to facilitate the necessary sheath exchanges. The "waist" (*arrowhead*) in the middle of the balloon reveals just how hard the liver parenchyma can be.

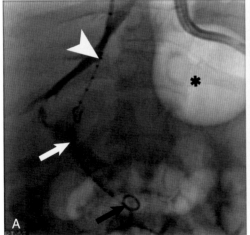
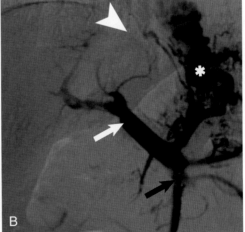

FIGURE 6 **A,** Frontal subtracted venogram with simultaneous contrast injection via the right internal jugular sheath (*arrowhead*). Marker catheter (*black arrow*) in the portal vein allows for calculation of the required length of the stent. Note the inflated Blakemore tube in the stomach (*asterisk*) used to tamponade bleeding gastroesophageal varices. **B,** In another patient, the ominous gastroesophageal varices (*asterisk*) are seen during a direct portal venogram. The *white arrow* shows the portal vein, and the *black arrow* shows the superior mesenteric vein.

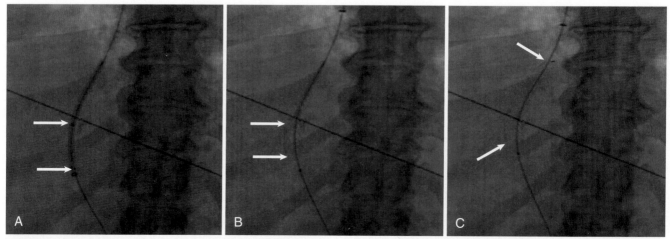

FIGURE 7 Frontal views of the deployment sequence of a TIPS stent. The stent is first advanced via a sheath through the right hepatic vein, across the liver parenchyma and into the portal vein (**A**). The stent's distal 2 cm (*arrow*) are constrained only by the sheath, and once the sheath is pulled back, it springs open (**B**). Once the operator judges the stent to be in proper position, the remainder of the stent (*arrows*) is opened by pulling on the ripcord (**C**).

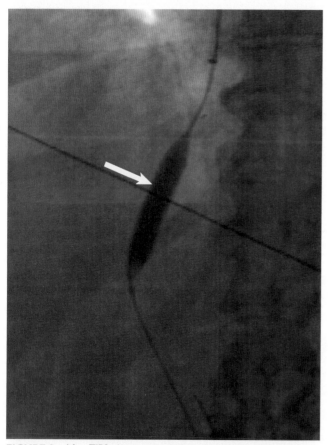

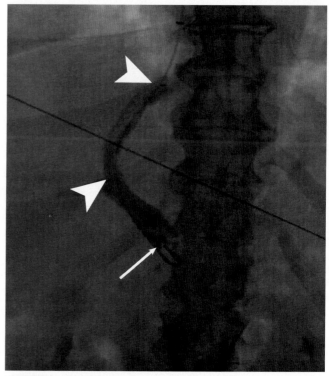

FIGURE 9 Frontal view of a portal venogram via a catheter (*arrow*) after TIPS placement (*arrowheads*). Note the antegrade flow of contrast into the right atrium and no contrast filling the varices.

FIGURE 8 After TIPS placement, a balloon (*arrow*) is used to open the stent to the desired diameter. The objective is to open the stent to the minimal diameter required to reduce the portal pressure to the desired level.

Special Cases

Budd-Chiari Syndrome

The placement of a TIPS in a patient with Budd-Chiari syndrome is especially challenging, because the hepatic veins are thrombosed. This shows as the classic spider vein appearance on a hepatic venogram

(Figure 10). Though it is best if the TIPS is placed from hepatic vein to portal vein, the lack of patent hepatic veins may necessitate an IVC to portal vein TIPS.

Parallel TIPS

Rarely, despite a previous TIPS, the patient's symptoms may not be completely alleviated. If portal hypertension and variceal bleeding are a persistent problem despite a TIPS, or if the first TIPS thromboses, a second TIPS may be placed utilizing the other hepatic portal veins (Figure 11).

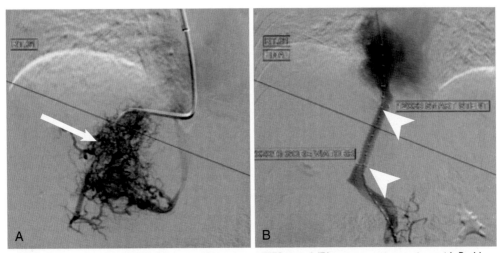

FIGURE 10 Frontal subtracted hepatic (**A**) and post-TIPS portal (**B**) venograms in a patient with Budd-Chiari syndrome. Hepatic venogram shows the spider-like appearance (*arrow*) of multiple small collateral draining veins. The stent (*arrowheads*) allows the venous drainage to bypass the thrombosed hepatic veins.

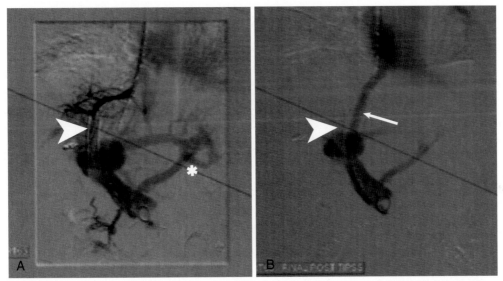

FIGURE 11 Frontal subtracted portal venogram (**A**) via a catheter placed through the middle hepatic vein shows the previously placed right hepatic to right portal vein TIPS (*arrowhead*) to be occluded. Because of this, the patient had recurrent bleeding from gastric varices (*asterisk*). Repeat portal venogram (**B**) after placement of a parallel TIPS (*arrow*) shows antegrade flow into the right atrium and lack of filling of the gastric varices.

Transumbilical or Direct Portal Access

When access into the portal vein is challenging due to anatomy, the operator has two other options. First, access into the umbilical vein, which is usually dilated, provides a conduit into the left portal vein. A catheter there allows opacification of the portal venous system, which provides a better target for TIPS (Figure 12, *A*). When the umbilical vein is not accessible, direct percutaneous access into the right or left portal vein can allow for contrast opacification and targeting (Figure 12, *B*).

TIPS Reversal/Revision

Occasionally a TIPS reversal or revision is necessary. Limited liver reserve and/or overzealous shunting may result in liver failure or intractable encephalopathy. In such cases the interventionalist has the option to decrease the shunting or shut down the TIPS altogether. Several maneuvers exists to reduce shunting, including placing a stent within the TIPS, or two stents side by side, or even a "waisted" (hourglass-like) stent. If these interventions are not possible or are inadequate, then the entire TIPS can be shut down. TIPS shut-down is a rarely performed and advanced procedure beyond the scope of this text.

CLINICAL OUTCOMES

Clinical Response to TIPS

TIPS is the most effective option for treating gastroesophageal variceal bleeding. The re-bleeding rate after TIPS placement is 4% per year—the lowest among all treatment options, including endoscopic management. TIPS is reserved after failure of endoscopic management only because of the greater risks associated with it. Cessation of bleeding is evident almost immediately after a TIPS.

TIPS has also been shown to be very effective in treating ascites, and it reduces the risk of ascites by 50% to 80% over the life of the patient. Additionally, TIPS has been shown to improve survival and transplant-free survival compared to other treatment options. Resolution of ascites may take up to 4 weeks after TIPS placement.

In patients with hepatorenal syndrome, TIPS improves renal function in 62% of patients. However, it is occasionally difficult to distinguish non-cirrhotic-related chronic renal insufficiency from hepatorenal syndrome.

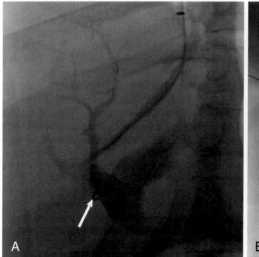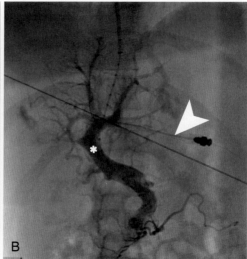

FIGURE 12   Frontal view of a portal venogram (**A**) via a percutaneously placed transumbilical vein catheter (*arrow*) opacifies the portal branches. In cases where no other option is available, direct percutaneous portal vein access (**B**) can be useful. A needle (*arrowhead*) is placed under ultrasound guidance into the portal venous system (*asterisk*), which is then opacified with contrast and targeted for TIPS from the right hepatic vein.

Complications and Management

The complications related to TIPS are shown on Table 3. The most feared complication is liver failure, which usually results from excessive portohepatic venous shunting in a liver with limited baseline reserve. If patients with no liver reserve are appropriately excluded, the risk of liver failure is 2% to 4%.

Encephalopathy can be seen in up to 12% of patients with compensated liver disease and in up to 50% of patients with noncompensated liver disease. Flagyl and/or lactulose provide significant relief for such patients, however, a small percentage (~4%) will not respond and may require TIPS reversal.

Death from sepsis is rare (~4%) but very difficult to treat. Bacteremia results in TIPS stent seeding, which can be very challenging or impossible to treat. Broad-spectrum antibiotics may clear the bacteremia, but in some cases it recurs after cessation of treatment, as the seeded stent elutes more bacteria. Active infection is an absolute contraindication to TIPS, and any infection must be cleared prior to intervention.

The overall post-TIPS 30 day mortality ranges from less than 10% to up to 40%. The higher mortality rate is seen in patients with poorly compensated liver disease who are having a TIPS placed on an emergent basis, usually for life-threatening variceal bleeding. For patients with compensated liver disease who are having a TIPS placed on an elective basis, mortality is less than 5%. It is therefore important to carefully select patients and refer for TIPS placement before it manifests into an emergency.

Follow-up

TIPS follow-up is mostly based on clinical signs and symptoms. Ultrasound surveillance can be useful. However, false positive reports (of occluded stent) can result if ultrasound is performed too early. The newly placed TIPS has air trapped within the material, which limits ultrasound penetration and can be read as occluded TIPS. Waiting at least 2 weeks after TIPS for the air to be absorbed is generally adequate to avoid this problem. Recurrent variceal bleeding or ascites is a very specific indicator of TIPS restenosis or occlusion and should prompt a diagnostic venogram and/or intervention. There is a 10% rate of reintervention for stenosed or occluded TIPS. The primary patency rate is 80% to 85% over 1 year with the ePTFE covered stents. There is no role for the use of noncovered stents for TIPS, as their restenosis rate is unjustifiably high.

TABLE 3: Complications related to TIPS

Complication	Predisposing Factors	Mitigating Factors
Liver failure	Limited reserve High bilirubin Overshunting	Reduce or close the TIPS
Encephalopathy	History of encephalopathy High ammonia levels Limited reserve	Reduce or close the TIPS Flagyl or lactulose
Bleeding	Difficult anatomy Abnormal coagulation profile	Correct coagulation profile
Sepsis	Active infection	Treat infection prior to TIPS
Renal failure	Elevated creatinine Dehydration High contrast load	Hydrate Bicarbonate Use CO_2

SUMMARY

The most important determinant of clinical outcomes after TIPS placement is proper patient selection and preparation. Cirrhotic patients with portal hypertension should be under surveillance and should be referred for TIPS after conservative management fails, but before the complications of portal hypertension manifest into an emergency. This, along with optimal patient preparation, can help reduce the morbidity and mortality related to TIPS to the lowest possible levels. Additionally, the introduction of expanded polytetrafluoroethylene stents has improved the efficacy and patency rate of TIPS, and many patients survive with a TIPS for many years. The benefits of a TIPS include reduced drop-off risk from the transplant list, improved lifestyle quality (i.e., resolution of ascites), as well as reduction in the many portal hypertension–related complications. But most importantly, TIPS often is a life-saving procedure for those with variceal hemorrhage.

REFERENCES

Lo GH, Liang HL, Chen WC, et al: A prospective, randomized controlled trial of transjugular intrahepatic portosystemic shunt versus cyanoacrylate injection in the prevention of gastric variceal rebleeding, *Endoscopy* 39(8):679–685, 2007.

Salerno F, Cammà C, Enea M, et al: Transjugular intrahepatic portosystemic shunt for refractory ascites: a meta-analysis of individual patient data, *Gastroenterology* 133(5):1746, 2007.

Silva RF, Arroyo PC Jr, Duca WJ, et al: Complications following transjugular intrahepatic portosystemic shunt: a retrospective analysis, *Transplant Proc* 36(4):926–928, 2004.

Charon JP, Alaeddin FH, Pimpalwar SA, et al: Results of a retrospective multicenter trial of the Viatorr expanded polytetrafluoroethylene-covered stent-graft for transjugular intrahepatic portosystemic shunt creation, *J Vasc Interv Radio* 15(11):1219–1230, 2004.

Hausegger KA, Karnel F, Georgieva B, et al: Transjugular intrahepatic portosystemic shunt creation with the Viatorr expanded polytetrafluoroethylene-covered stent-graft, *J Vasc Interv Radiol* 15(3):239–248, 2004.

REFRACTORY ASCITES

Jonathan M. Hernandez, MD, and
Alexander S. Rosemurgy, MD

OVERVIEW

Although a myriad causes can be responsible for the development of ascites, the practicing surgeon will most frequently care for this disease in the context of cirrhosis. The commentary following, therefore, is directed toward this patient population unless otherwise stated.

The onset of ascites marks a transition from compensated cirrhosis to decompensated cirrhosis, with an attendant increase in mortality from 1% to 3% to 20% to 57% at 1 year. In addition, the morbidity associated with ascites, and refractory ascites in particular, can be significant. Refractory ascites can dramatically impact quality of life through abdominal distension that results in early satiety, discomfort, progressive immobility, umbilical hernias, progressive renal insufficiency, sepsis, respiratory distress (often further exacerbated by pleural effusion from hepatic hydrothorax), and professional and social isolation. The optimization of medical therapy—as well as institution of more definitive procedures, such as transplantation, drainage procedures, or shunting procedures—is necessary to curb the morbidity associated with ascites, particularly medically refractory ascites, although admittedly no therapy outside of liver transplantation has been convincingly demonstrated to impact mortality.

DEFINITIONS

Ascites, or the pathologic accumulation of fluid in the abdominal cavity, is termed *refractory* when the condition is either diuretic resistant or diuretic intractable. *Diuretic-resistant ascites* is defined as either failure to respond to intensive diuretic therapy (loss of <0.8 kg over 4 days with sodium output less than intake) or recurrence of clinically detectable ascites within 4 weeks. We define *intensive therapy* as the combination of both spironolactone 400 mg/day and furosemide 160 mg/day with a 1 to 2 g sodium-restricted diet of at least 1-week duration. Of note, the preceding diuretic doses can be exceeded under appropriate supervision; in properly selected patients, however, it is advisable to maintain a 100 mg/40 mg ratio.

Diuretic-intractable ascites is defined as failure to respond to therapy or a recurrence of clinically detectable ascites within 4 weeks of initiation of therapy because of failure to achieve optimal diuretic dosing secondary to diuretic-induced complications. Diuretic-induced complications include the development of encephalopathy; renal impairment, defined as a doubling in serum creatinine to greater than 2 mg/dL; hyponatremia, defined as a decrease in serum sodium greater than 10 mEq/L to less than 125 mEq/L; and hyperkalemia, defined as a serum potassium level more than 6 mEq/L. In addition, aldosterone antagonists are known to cause painful gynecomastia and decreased libido.

PATHOPHYSIOLOGY

A thorough understanding of the physiologic aberrations that culminate in ascites formation provides the practicing surgeon with the rationale for the use of individual drugs, as well as an understanding of the currently unexploited therapeutic targets. Recall that aside from liver transplantation, there is no available treatment, medical or surgical, that has been shown convincingly to affect mortality.

For patients with cirrhosis, the initial insult is an increase in vascular resistance at the level of the hepatic microcirculation, resulting in a widening of the portosystemic pressure gradient (portal hypertension; specifically, *sinusoidal* portal hypertension). The increased intrahepatic vascular resistance is the result of both mechanical alteration of the hepatic architecture, as a result of the underlying liver disease, as well as a dynamic imbalance between local vasodilator and vasoconstrictor stimuli. A predominance of vasoconstriction results, at least in part, from a relative deficiency of local nitric oxide (NO) and leads to contraction of septal myofibroblasts, stellate cells, and vascular smooth muscle cells. Strategies to increase local NO concentrations, and thereby relieve portal congestion, include the use of NO donors, agents that enhance the activity of endothelial nitric oxide synthase (e-NOS), and antioxidants to increase NO bioavailability by limiting oxidative stress. Although a relative deficiency of NO and other vasodilatory agents exists in the liver, persistent portal hypertension results in an overproduction of vasodilatory stimuli (particularly NO) in the splanchnic arterial bed, causing increased inflow and further exacerbating portal hypertension. Interestingly, bacterial translocation to regional mesenteric lymph nodes and the ensuing cytokine production seemingly play an integral role in the overproduction of splanchnic vasodilatory agents, and may serve as potential therapeutic targets with antimicrobials.

The pooling of blood in the splanchnic circulation leads to a decrease in effective circulating volume, which results in baroreceptor-mediated activation of the sympathetic nervous system and the renin-angiotensin-aldosterone system (RAAS) and triggers the release of arginine vasopressin from the posterior pituitary gland. This neurohormonal compensation results in avid sodium and water retention in the kidneys in an attempt to restore circulating blood volume, although to the detriment of the liver.

Coupled with decreased oncotic pressure secondary to compromised hepatic synthetic function (decreased serum albumin and total protein), the culmination of increased inflow into a high-resistance system results in an increase in hepatic lymph formation. The increased hepatic lymph overwhelms the liver lymphatic system, and the excess lymph, a plasma ultrafiltrate containing the retained sodium and water, accumulates in the peritoneal cavity as ascites.

EVALUATION AND OPTIMIZATION OF MEDICAL THERAPY

The cirrhotic patient with ascites should be approached in a comprehensive manner with attention paid to the patient's entire constellation of problems. Several caveats are worth emphasis. Patients with ascites have decompensated cirrhosis and are therefore at risk for acute hepatic failure and extreme morbidity due to the liver's limited reserve. Acute exacerbations such as encephalopathy or variceal bleeding are often triggered by infection, particularly spontaneous bacterial peritonitis. Prompt intervention with antimicrobial agents is imperative and should be instituted prior to confirmation with laboratory tests or cultures. Additionally, avoidance of hepatotoxins (alcohol) and nephrotoxins (intravenous contrast, aminoglycosides, antibiotics, etc.) is desirable to avoid fulminant hepatic failure and/or progressive renal dysfunction.

The patient suspected of having refractory ascites should be approached with two initial questions: 1) Is cirrhosis the cause of ascites, or is cirrhosis the result of another etiology that is not likely to be responsive to diuretic therapy, such as malignant ascites (see below); and 2) Does the patient truly have refractory ascites? In other words, has medical therapy been maximized? Confirmation of refractory ascites requires demonstration of compliance with dietary restrictions and diuretic doses as previously outlined.

Confirmation is most readily accomplished with measurement of random urinary sodium and potassium. A ratio of Na/K greater than 1 is equivalent to a 24-hour sodium intake of greater than 2 g, demonstrating noncompliance. Additionally, a single 80 mg dose of furosemide can be given intravenously, followed by urine sodium measurement over the next 8 hours. Patients with diuretic-resistant ascites will have a sodium excretion of less than 50 mEq over this time period.

Following confirmation of compliance with dietary restrictions and verification of diuretic dosing with unsatisfactory responsiveness, the clinician should next consider the patient for candidacy for both adjunctive medications, which can increase the efficacy of diuretic therapy, and drainage and shunting procedures. Several drugs that interfere with the pathologic compensatory mechanism (see Pathophysiology above) have shown promise in improving the management of refractory ascites (Table 1). Octreotide causes splanchnic vasoconstriction via decreased glucagon secretion and inhibits the release of renin and aldosterone. Midodrine increases mean arterial pressure and decreases plasma renin and aldosterone activity. Of note, the combination of octreotide and midodrine is also effective in treating hepatorenal syndrome, which often complicates the management of patients with refractory ascites. Clonidine, by virtue of its ability to decrease sympathetic outflow, decreases sodium reabsorption and inhibits the RAAS, thereby increasing the effectiveness of spironolactone diuresis. Long-term albumin infusions can also increase responsiveness to diuretic therapy, although cost may be prohibitory. These measures may be instituted prior to or concomitantly with drainage or shunting procedures and, therefore, complete patient evaluation should also include duplex ultrasonography to document portal vein patency.

Interventional Treatment

The most effective and only curative treatment for refractory ascites is liver transplantation. However, ascites is rarely a sole indication for liver transplantation, and unfortunately, many patients with refractory ascites are not candidates for or will ultimately not receive a new liver because of psychosocioeconomic concerns. Nonetheless, hepatic transplantation should always be considered before other options are executed. Beyond transplantation, other interventional options are discussed below and provide varying degrees of relief from the morbidity of ascites. Each intervention is associated with its own unique set of issues, risks, and complications, and therefore the ultimate decision must be made on an individual basis. Our treatment algorithm is shown in Figure 1.

TABLE 1: Primary medical therapy and adjunctive medications used to increase the efficacy of primary therapy in the treatment of ascites

Class	Medication	Dosing	Relevant Action	Notes
Diuretics	Spironolactone	400 mg + QD*	Aldosterone receptor antagonist	Primary therapy
	Furosemide	160 mg + QD*	Inhibits Na-K-2Cl symporter	Primary therapy
	Mannitol	20%*	Osmotic diuresis	Give dose just prior to furosemide and spironolactone
Vasoconstrictors	Octreotide	300 µg BID*	Splanchnic vasoconstriction, inhibits RAAS	Also used in combination with midodrine to treat hepatorenal syndrome; given for first 5 days following variceal bleeding to decrease recurrence
	Midodrine	7.5 mg TID*	Inhibits RAAS	Also used in combination with octreotide and albumin to treat hepatorenal syndrome
α_2 agonist	Clonidine	0.075 mg BID*	Inhibits sympathetic outflow, inhibits RAAS	Increases sensitivity to spironolactone
Colloid	Albumin	25 g*	Increased oncotic pressure	Also utilized with LVP and in the treatment of hepatorenal syndrome
Aquaretics	None are FDA approved	?	Vasopressin receptor antagonist	May also treat hyponatremia

*The above doses have been derived from various studies and may not be suitable for all patients. Titration is always recommended.

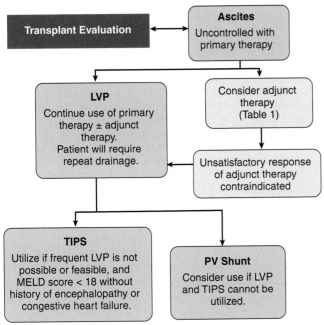

FIGURE I   Treatment algorithm for patients with refractory ascites.

Large Volume Paracentesis

Large volume paracentesis (LVP) is the draining of 5 L or more of fluid from the peritoneal cavity. Systemic hypovolemia can be an untoward consequence of LVP, as can events related to the procedure, such as bleeding and the introduction of infection into the peritoneal cavity. Systemic hypovolemia can be aided or even avoided by concurrent administration of albumin (6 to 8 g/L removed). Concurrent albumin administration should be particularly considered if 7 to 10 L or more of ascites are removed. LVP can also accentuate hyponatremia, which tends to manifest 24 to 48 hours after the procedure, and therefore LVP is always undertaken with optimized diuretic therapy.

Repeated LVP, with concomitant diuretic therapy, has been studied and compared with other therapies for refractory ascites with regard to many parameters, including complications, hospital days, time between hospitalizations, successful relief of tense ascites, and mortality. LVP has been shown to be effective, fast, and safe, albeit transient. The major detriment of LVP is, by its very nature, its dependence on repeated applications. Of note, in patients unable to excrete any sodium, drainage of 6 L of ascites removes 10 days of retained sodium, but drainage of 10 L of ascites removes 17 days of retained sodium. Therefore patients requiring more frequent LVP are noncompliant with dietary restrictions.

Limitations of LVP as definitive therapy include the need for repeat puncture, tense ascites during intervals between punctures, diuretic complications, bacterial peritonitis, intestinal violations from punctures, profound coagulopathy, renal insufficiency, and exacerbation of hepatorenal syndrome. However, LVP is an effective short-term fix that can provide long-term palliation with repeated applications, even if it is intermittently suboptimal.

LVP is performed with the patient supine, although positioning can be manipulated during the procedure to increase the amount of fluid drainage. Additionally, ultrasonography can aid in the identification of an optimal location for needle insertion, but it is generally unnecessary. Following identification of a suitable location for drainage—often the right upper quadrant, 2 finger breadths below the costal margin in the midclavicular line, or the left lower quadrant, 2 finger breadths cephalad and medial to the anterior superior iliac spine—the location should be prepped and draped using full barrier precautions. We recommend utilizing any number of the paracentesis/thoracentesis kits that provide an appropriately sized hollow-bore needle and sterile tubing, in addition to 1 L vacuum bottles. A nonlinear needle insertion course is desirable to minimize postprocedural ascites leakage, although nylon suture may be necessary.

Peritoneovenous Shunts

Peritoneovenous (PV) shunts palliate refractory ascites by removing fluid from the peritoneal cavity and transferring it into the circulating volume. By increasing circulating volume and by decreasing intraperitoneal volume, PV shunts improve renal function. Relative to diuretics, PV shunts provide faster resolution of ascites, fewer and shorter hospitalizations, and longer ascites-free intervals, but they do not improve survival. Although PV shunts do provide better long-term control of ascites, they do not provide indefinite control, as they are plagued by occlusion; however, PV shunts may best be positioned to control ascites for a finite time, for example, as a short-term "bridge" to transplantation. Unfortunately, shunt occlusion often leads to rehospitalization while patients await transplantation. Nonetheless, this approach can palliate more than three fourths of patients awaiting liver transplantation, while improving glomerular filtration rate and renal function.

While PV shunts may have some role in treating refractory ascites, it seems to be ever shrinking because of immediate concerns of disseminated intravascular coagulation (DIC), infection, congestive heart failure, limited duration efficacy, and procedural issues (e.g., pneumothorax) that can complicate placement. In addition, the shunts require continued compliance with diuretics, albeit at doses that are probably reduced. Our experience with PV shunts is extensive and telling. Despite vigilance, our mean patency with Denver shunts is near 6 months. Beyond occlusion, we found that infection, DIC, and other complications occurred in 25% of patients within 1 year. Because PV shunts have been shown to be a generally inferior option to transjugular intrahepatic portosystemic shunting (TIPS), they are now mostly reserved for patients intolerant and noncompliant with LVP and in patients who are poor candidates for TIPS because of portal vein occlusion.

PV shunting is undertaken in the operating room with the patient in supine position. Venous access is established using the right subclavian vein. Using an incision cephalad to the costal margin, the peritoneal cavity is catheterized in the right upper quadrant. The ascites are drained and replaced with saline at approximately half the volume to reduce the incidence of DIC. A subcutaneous tract is established between the venous catheterization site and the chest wall incision and is dilated along its caudal extent using a ring forceps to accommodate the peritoneovenous shunt. The venous end of the shunt is cut to length, so that it will ultimately lie in the right atrium. The shunt is sewn into place to avoid rotation or twisting, which can compromise function postoperatively. The wounds are closed in layers with absorbable suture followed by nylon skin sutures. The nylon sutures are removed once they have become loose, as wound contracture is the sine qua non of healing for these patients.

Portosystemic Shunting

Portal decompression treats the underlying sinusoidal hypertension that causes ascites. Portal decompression is particularly useful with refractory ascites and variceal bleeding not amenable to, or refractory to, endoscopic therapy when patients are not candidates for imminent transplantation. Portosystemic shunting treats refractory ascites well, with dramatic resolution and reductions in spontaneous bacterial peritonitis, hepatorenal syndrome, and hospitalizations. In our experience with small-diameter, prosthetic H-graft shunts, refractory ascites resolved in nearly 60% and required no adjunctive therapy after shunting. In the other patients, ascites improved with continued diuretic therapy. Encephalopathy accompanied relief of ascites in only 5% of patients.

Today, TIPS is the main portosystemic shunting vehicle to obtain portal decompression. TIPS has been compared to LVP and is equivalent with respect to mortality, GI bleeding, infection, and renal failure. However, TIPS is associated with increased rates of encephalopathy, and advanced liver disease can be prohibitive secondary to fulminant liver failure resulting from decreased nutrient hepatic blood flow. TIPS has also been compared to PV shunting and is superior in duration of efficacy; it seems to promote survival, with 25% of patients surviving 5 years with functioning shunts.

SPECIAL CONSIDERATIONS

Malignant Ascites

Malignant ascites is a collection of fluid containing cancer cells in the peritoneal cavity. It occurs secondary to direct invasion (peritoneal carcinomatosis) or from the biological effects of cancer cells. Malignant ascites portends an extremely poor prognosis if the underlying malignancy is of GI tract origin, with a median survival of 3 months. Consideration for treatment with chemotherapeutic agents directed against the primary tumor should be given on an individual basis. Currently no standard of care exists, as treatments have largely been adapted from those utilized in the care of patients with cirrhosis-related ascites, such as diuretic therapy (although highly resistant), paracentesis, and PV shunts. Of note, PV shunts will not promote dissemination of the malignancy and will not hasten demise, but they can palliate the mass effect of a protuberant abdomen. In addition, a number of investigational therapies are currently being evaluated, including intraperitoneal chemotherapy, cytokine therapy, and immunotherapy.

Postoperative Ascites Leak

Postoperative ascites leak carries a high mortality. Such leaks frequently lead to wound failure, sepsis, systemic collapse, and death. Prevention of ascites leaks is therefore a high priority if an operation is undertaken. Prevention begins preoperatively with optimization of medical therapy, and it is carried into the immediate postoperative period in association with judicious fluid administration. We use nylon skin sutures in a running, locking fashion, left in place until the sutures become loose. When ascites leak does occur, strong consideration should be given to early reexploration. Fascial disruption must be considered when an ascites leak develops. Early repair of the fascial dehiscence often prevents ongoing leakage, providing the best opportunity for the patient to survive the insult. Ascites should be drained prior to or during reexploration, with an intraperitoneal drain left in place for several days postoperatively. In our experience, this practice confers a survival advantage as opposed to observation, wound care, abdominal binders, or repeat paracentesis.

SELECTED READINGS

Rosemurgy AS, Statman RC, Murphy CG, et al: Postoperative ascetic leaks: the ongoing challenge, *Surgery* 111(6): 623–625, 1992.
Rosemurgy AS: *Small diameter interposition shunt, mastery of surgery* 3:1301–1307, 1998.
Rosemurgy AS, Zervos EE, Clark WC, et al: TIPS versus peritoneovenous shunt in the treatment of medically intractable ascites: a prospective randomized trial, *Ann Surg* 239(6): 883–889, 2004.
Saab S, Nieto JM, Lewis SK, Runyon BA: TIPS versus paracentesis for cirrhotic patients with refractory ascites, *Cochrane Database Syst Rev* 18(4) 2006, CD004889.

HEPATIC ENCEPHALOPATHY

Patricia Wong, MD, and H. Franklin Herlong, MD

OVERVIEW

Hepatic encephalopathy (HE) is a complex, potentially reversible, neuropsychiatric syndrome seen in patients with cirrhosis or acute liver failure. Patients with HE may have symptoms ranging from subtle abnormalities, detectable only through specialized psychological testing, to frank coma. Generally accepted stages for the broad spectrum of clinical manifestations of encephalopathy are based on level of consciousness, cognitive function, behavioral disturbances, and neuromuscular features (Table 1). In milder cases, the encephalopathic patient may be unaware of any deficits, and symptoms such as sleep pattern reversal, mild confusion, irritability, or personality changes may be apparent only to close contacts. Consequently, it is often helpful to obtain a history from a cirrhotic patient in the presence of family members.

HE remains largely a clinical diagnosis; there are no specific signs, symptoms, or laboratory tests that are diagnostic of this disorder. The symptoms commonly associated with HE can also be seen in other conditions, such as hypoglycemia, head trauma, or intoxication. Asterixis, a flapping tremor of the outstretched hands, is a common feature of HE but may also be seen in other metabolic encephalopathies. Elevated plasma levels of ammonia are common in HE but are not universal, and the level of blood ammonia concentration does not always correlate with the severity of encephalopathy. Electroencephalography testing is always abnormal in overt HE, but observed changes, such as triphasic waves, are not specific. Focal neurologic deficits such as hemiplegia or hemiparesis are observed in fewer than 20% of patients with HE, and seizures are rarely seen. Consequently, other causes of altered mental status must be excluded before making the diagnosis of HE, and any focal neurologic deficiency should prompt central nervous stystem imaging to exclude structural lesions.

PATHOPHYSIOLOGY OF HEPATIC ENCEPHALOPATHY

The pathogenesis of hepatic encephalopathy is multifactorial, and despite a large body of research in both humans and animals, it remains unclear. The basic tenet of most hypotheses is that the brain is exposed to toxic substances produced in the gut by the actions of bacteria on nitrogenous compounds, which are incompletely cleared from the blood by the compromised liver. Ammonia was the first substance described and has been the most extensively studied. There are compelling reasons to believe that ammonia is an important pathogenetic factor in HE: Most patients with overt HE exhibit elevated plasma levels of ammonia, and children with urea cycle enzyme deficits and otherwise normally functioning livers develop profound hyperammonemia and symptoms indistinguishable from HE.

Recent research suggests several mechanisms by which ammonia can affect central nervous stystem (CNS) function. After crossing the blood-brain barrier, ammonia enters CNS astrocytes and combines with the neurotransmitter glutamate to form glutamine through the action of glutamine synthetase. Astrocytic glutamine enters mitochondria, where it is converted back to ammonia and glutamate. Mitochondrial ammonia contributes to the production of reactive oxygen species and upregulates aquaporin 4. This results in astrocytic swelling that causes histologic changes known as *Alzheimer type II astrocytosis*. Adverse effects of ammonia on cerebral perfusion and glucose metabolism additionally contribute to CNS impairment.

There is evidence that γ-aminobutyric acid (GABA), the primary inhibitory neurotransmitter in the CNS, may also play an important role in the pathogenesis of HE. Increased GABA levels have been

TABLE 1: Clinical manifestations and severity of HE

Encephalopathy	Level of Consciousness	Cognitive Function	Behavioral Disturbance	Neuromuscular Feature
Stage I (mild)	Abnormal sleep pattern	Shortened attention span, mildly impaired computations	Euphoria, depression, irritability	Tremor, muscular incoordination, impaired handwriting
Stage II (moderate)	Lethargy, mild disorientation	Amnesia, grossly impaired computations	Overt change in personality, inappropriate behavior	Slurred speech, asterixis (flapping), hypoactive reflexes, ataxia
Stage III (severe)	Somnolence, semistupor	Inability to compute	Paranoia, bizarre behavior	Hyperactive reflexes, nystagmus, Babinski sign, clonus, rigidity
Stage IV (coma)	Stupor, unconsciousness	None	None	Dilated pupils, opisthotonus, coma

Modified from Conn H, Lieberthal M: *The hepatic coma syndromes and lactulose*, Baltimore, 1979, Williams & Wilkins.

TABLE 2: Proposed nomenclature of HE

Type	Nomenclature	Subcategory	Subdivisions
A	Encephalopathy associated with *a*cute liver failure		
B	Encephalopathy associated with portosystemic *b*ypass and no intrinsic hepatocellular disease		
C	Encephalopathy associated with *c*irrhosis and portal hypertension or portosystemic shunts	Episodic HE	Precipitated Spontaneous Recurrent
		Persistent HE	Mild Severe Therapy dependent
		Minimal HE	

From Frenci P, Lockwood A, Mullen K, et al: Hepatic encephalopathy—definition, nomenclature, diagnosis and quantification: final report of the working party at the 11th World Congresses of Gastroenterology, Vienna, 1998, *Hepatology* 35:716–721, 2002.

TABLE 3: Precipitating factors in HE

Gastrointestinal bleeding
Sedatives or analgesics
Dehydration
Renal failure
Hypokalemia
Metabolic alkalosis
Infection (spontaneous bacterial peritonitis, pneumonia, urinary tract infection)
Excessive dietary protein
Constipation

liver disease and the persistence and severity of symptoms (Table 2). This chapter will focus on the management of patients with type C hepatic encephalopathy complicating cirrhosis and type A hepatic encephalopathy complicating acute liver failure

Type C: Hepatic Encephalopathy Associated with Cirrhosis and Portal Hypertension

HE is a common complication of cirrhosis and can be *episodic,* developing over a short period of time with fluctuations in severity, or *persistent,* with continuous overt neurologic or behavioral abnormalities. In most patients with episodic encephalopathy, a precipitating factor other than liver disease can be identified (Table 3). Gastrointestinal (GI) bleeding is the most common precipitant. This occurs through a combination of decreasing hepatic and renal perfusion and a large protein load to the gut, which results in increased production of nitrogenous byproducts. Evaluation of GI blood loss and control of active bleeding must be performed in all patients with episodic HE.

A high prevalence of infection in patients with HE suggests a potential pathogenic link between the systemic inflammatory response and HE. Cytokines can exacerbate astrocytic swelling, and certain bacteria cell wall compounds can augment the effects of ammonia on compromising cerebral blood flow. Consequently, a careful search for occult infection is imperative. It is important to note that cirrhotic patients frequently have baseline neutropenia from hypersplenism and may not exhibit leukocytosis in response to bacterial infections. Similarly, patients with advanced liver disease, particularly fulminant hepatic failure, are often hypothermic and do not mount a fever in response to infection. All patients with HE and ascites should undergo a diagnostic paracentesis to exclude

associated with liver injury and hyperammonemia. Increased production of endogenous benzodiazepine ligands by gut bacteria can result in increased GABA-ergic transmission and altered CNS function. This explains why some patients with HE respond to the benzodiazepine antagonist flumazenil even in the absence of exposure to exogenous benzodiazepines.

Other substances, such as mercaptans, neurosteroids, and manganese toxicity may also contribute to neuronal and astrocytic injury in HE. In all likelihood, these factors have varying influences in individual patients depending on the etiology, acuity, and severity of the liver disease and hence the protean manifestations of HE.

CLASSIFICATION AND MANAGEMENT OF HEPATIC ENCEPHALOPATHY

In order to classify HE more precisely and aid in its investigation, a working group within the World Congress of Gastroenterology proposed a classification scheme based on the nature of the underlying spontaneous bacterial peritonitis, the most common bacterial infection in hospitalized patients with cirrhosis. If there is a high index of suspicion for infection, empiric antibiotic therapy should be started after cultures have been drawn and before results are known.

Cirrhotic patients with HE, particularly those with ascites, are often exposed to potent diuretics. Intravascular volume depletion from vigorous diuresis can reduce renal perfusion and result in azotemia and increased ammonia production. A hypokalemic alkalosis can enhance renal ammonia production and increase transport across the blood-brain barrier by favoring ammonia over ammonium ion. In these patients, reestablishing intravascular volume and correcting electrolyte imbalances can often reverse encephalopathy without any other specific therapy.

Exposure to sedatives and analgesics, especially benzodiazepines, can potentiate the effects of putative neurotoxins in HE and should be avoided. In a minority of patients, increased dietary protein intake can precipitate an episode of encephalopathy that can be reversed with simple changes in the diet.

In patients with persistent encephalopathy, or those with episodic encephalopathy whose symptoms persist after precipitating factors have been treated, *specific therapy* directed toward encephalopathy is indicated. A reduction in gut bacterial production of toxins derived from intraluminal nitrogenous substances is common to all proposed therapies over the past 5 decades. Based on our understanding of the pathogenesis of HE, this assumption seems reasonable. However, the efficacy of most of these therapies remains equivocal based on data from clinical trials and meta-analyses.

Oral Disaccharides

For many years, the nonabsorbable disaccharides lactulose and lactitol have been the mainstay of therapy for HE. Theoretically, lactulose increases ammonia clearance through its cathartic action and decreases ammonia absorption from the gut by "trapping" it in the acidic colonic lumen, which results from accumulation of short-chain fatty acids. Many patients have an improvement in symptoms of HE within hours of lactulose administration. However, a Cochrane systematic review concluded "there is insufficient evidence to determine whether nonabsorbable disaccharides are of benefit in patients with HE" and "nonabsorbable disaccharides should not be used as the comparator in randomized trials of HE."

Despite the absence of compelling evidence to support its use, lactulose remains the most commonly used agent for the treatment of HE. It may have the greatest efficacy in patients whose encephalopathy is precipitated by GI bleeding, because its cathartic action rapidly evacuates the colon of blood, thereby reducing bacterial protein load. For patients unable to take lactulose orally, it can be administered per rectum as a retention enema (300 mL lactulose with 700 mL water).

Lactulose is also given to most patients with persistent HE at a dose sufficient to produce three to five soft bowel movements per day. For most patients, 30 mL given twice a day is adequate; higher and more frequent dosing may cause bloating and excessive diarrhea that may compromise patient compliance. Lactulose has few adverse effects other than occasional hypernatremia.

Dietary Protein Restriction

The potential association between dietary protein intake and encephalopathy was first described decades ago. In theory, reducing dietary protein intake should reduce nitrogenous toxin production. While improvement may be seen in individual encephalopathic patients with dietary protein restriction, this benefit has been difficult to demonstrate in controlled trials. In fact, in several studies of severe acute alcoholic hepatitis, the administration of high protein/high calorie diets improved rather than exacerbated encephalopathy. In addition, protein restriction to less than 40 g/day can accelerate catabolism and contribute to malnutrition. During episodes of severe encephalopathy, dietary protein intake is negligible during the first few days in the hospital. Afterward, it is reasonable to modestly restrict dietary protein to 1.0 g/kg/day, and observe the patient for any clinical benefit. Some studies suggest that vegetable protein may be better tolerated than animal protein.

Low-Absorbable Antibiotics

Suppression of toxin production by gut bacteria provides the basis for the use of poorly absorbed antibiotics. Numerous clinical trials have assessed the efficacy of various antibiotics in patients with different classes of encephalopathy. The aminoglycoside neomycin is contraindicated in patients with HE due to the risk of ototoxicity and renal failure. Studies of metronidazole and vancomycin have yielded equivocal results. Rifaximin, a derivate of rifamycin, was originally developed to treat traveler's diarrhea and has broad-spectrum activity against gram-negative rods and gram-positive cocci. Several studies, including one meta-analysis, have suggested that rifaximin is superior to disaccharides in patients with both overt and minimal encephalopathy. Concerns about possible bacterial overgrowth or fungal colonization appear unfounded, as a recent study suggested that rifaximin can be given safely for prolonged periods. The recommended dose is 400 mg three times daily, however, its use may be limited by cost ($1200 to $2000 per month). FDA approval is pending.

Other Therapies

Used extensively in children with urea cycle deficits, *sodium benzoate* combines with ammonia to produce hippurate, which is renally excreted. In limited trials, it compares favorably with lactulose. *L-ornithine L-aspartate* increases hepatic conversion of ammonia and is better than placebo at lowering plasma ammonia and improving encephalopathy grade. *Flumazenil*, a benzodiazepine antagonist, showed improvement in encephalopathy grade but is not approved for this indication by the FDA. *Zinc* lowers plasma ammonia by increasing ornithine transcarbamylase activity, but its benefits in HE have been inconsistent. *Branched-chain amino acids* in several different formulations improve symptoms but not survival, and they are relatively expensive. Through fermenting potential, *probiotics* reduce substrate for other gut bacteria, and early trials suggested a possible benefit in minimal encephalopathy.

Type A: Hepatic Encephalopathy Associated with Acute Liver Failure

HE is a prominent component of acute liver failure, but it differs from that seen in cirrhosis and portal hypertension. Although marked hyperammonemia can be seen in both disorders, cerebral edema with intracranial hypertension is common in acute liver failure but is rarely seen in chronic liver disease. The risk of cerebral edema correlates with the encephalopathic grade. It is very low in grades 1 and 2 but progresses to 35% in grade 3 and 75% in grade 4. The reason for this association with acute liver failure is not entirely clear, because the consequences of hyperammonemia on cerebral function should be similar in acute and chronic liver disease. Some have proposed that markers of systemic inflammation commonly seen in acute liver failure may be a contributing factor. Excess free water with hyponatremia may exacerbate ammonia-induced cerebral edema.

Accurately assessing intracranial pressure (ICP) on clinical grounds is difficult. Physical findings such as papillary changes, abnormalities in the oculovestibular reflex, and decerebrate posturing are indicators of intracranial hypertension but often are apparent at an irreversible stage. Consequently, some medical centers advocate the use of invasive monitoring devices, which accurately measure ICP. However, one retrospective report from the U.S. Acute Liver Failure Study reported a 10% complication rate associated with invasive monitoring, of which 5% could have contributed to death.

There was also no significant improvement in outcomes in patients subjected to invasive monitoring.

Patients with acute liver failure who develop grade 2 HE should be admitted to an intensive care unit with integrated monitoring and multiorgan support. Patients with grade 3 encephalopathy should be ventilated for airway protection, and the head should be elevated to 30 degrees. Intravenous hypotonic solutions should be avoided because of the risk of hyponatremia-induced cerebral edema. Bolus infusions of mannitol (0.5 to 1 g/kg) or hypertonic saline should be given to those patients with objective evidence of increased ICP. Temporary hyperventilation, with a goal PaCO$_2$ of 25 mm Hg, may be helpful if the ICP cannot be adequately lowered with mannitol. Most patients require renal replacement therapy to lower ammonia levels, because lactulose is ineffective in acute liver failure. Intracranial hypertension refractory to medical management should prompt consideration for liver transplantation. More detailed instructions for the management of patients with acute liver failure can be found in recommendations published by the U.S. Acute Liver Failure Study Group.

Minimal Hepatic Encephalopathy

Minimal HE (MHE) is a milder form of HE in which impairment in cognitive function is only detectable through neuropsychological testing. The number-connection test and block-design test have reasonable specificities for MHE and are easy to administer. The deficits in MHE are primarily related to visuospatial orientation, attention problems, and impaired short-term memory. Oral and written skills show little impairment.

Neuroimaging studies have shown a correlation between MHE and changes in cerebral blood flow and abnormalities on neuropsychological testing. Although patients with MHE have no overt symptoms of encephalopathy, they may have a diminished capacity to work or drive. One study comparing physical requirements of employment with concurrent psychomotor and motor deficits concluded that over half of blue-collar workers and one quarter of white-collar workers with MHE were unfit to work. Studies assessing the effect of MHE on driving have yielded inconsistent results. Using a driving simulator and on-the-road testing, one study showed no impairment in driving ability, but another study with a similar assessment protocol suggested that over 40% of patients with MHE were unfit to drive. Other studies have shown that patients with MHE have more collisions and have difficulty with traffic rules and road signs. At present, there is no consensus as to whether driving restrictions should be mandated. Several recent controlled trials have suggested that both lactulose and rifaximin improve neuropsychological testing and quality of life in patients with MHE.

SUGGESTED READINGS

Als-Nielsen B, Gluud LL, Gluud C: Nonabsorbable disaccharides for hepatic encephalopathy: systematic review of randomized trials, *Cochrane Database Syst Rev* (2):CD003044, 2004.
Ferenci P, Lockwood A, Mullen K: Hepatic encephalopathy—definition, nomenclature, diagnosis, and quantification: final report of the working party at the 11th World Congress of Gastroenterology, *Hepatology* 35:716–721, 2002.
Munoz SJ: Hepatic encephalopathy, *Med Clin N Am* 92:795–812, 2008.
Norenberg MD, Jayakumar AR, Rama Rao KV, et al: New concepts in the mechanism of ammonia-induced astrocyte swelling, *Metab Brain Dis* 22:219–234, 2007.
Stravitz RT, Kramer AH, Davern T, et al: Intensive care of patients with acute liver failure: recommendations of the U.S. Acute Liver Failure Study Group, *Crit Care Med* 35:2498–2508, 2007.
Sundaram V, Shaikh OS: Hepatic encephalopathy: pathophysiology and emerging therapies, *Med Clin N Am* 93:819–836, 2009.

MANAGEMENT OF BUDD-CHIARI SYNDROME

Michael A. Zimmerman, MD, and Jeffrey Campsen, MD

OVERVIEW

Hepatic venous outflow occlusion, termed *Budd-Chiari Syndrome* (BCS), is the result of a spectrum of hypercoaguable illnesses and/or anatomic abnormalities. As the most common causes in the Western world center around myoproliferative disorders, including polycythemia vera and essential thrombocytosis, vascular webbing and stricture may provide an anatomic predisposition to acute thrombosis. Other causes include paroxysmal nocturnal hemoglobinuria, factor V Leiden mutation, antiphospholipid antibody, and deficiencies in proteins C and S. Although spontaneous resolution has been previously reported, the mortality rate for those left untreated is extremely high. As such, most patients require an aggressive multidisciplinary approach using medical, radiologic, and surgical intervention. Historically, portosystemic shunting has been employed to control symptoms and prevent disease progression. More recently, a combination of radiologic thrombolysis, angioplasty, and stenting has proven to be a valuable bridge to surgical therapy.

PRESENTATION AND DIAGNOSIS

The classic clinical presentation of BCS includes hepatomegaly, right upper quadrant pain, and ascites. However, up to 25% of patients are asymptomatic. The onset of disease ranges from acute to chronic. Not surprisingly, the onset of symptoms directly correlates with the rapidity of venous outflow occlusion. Patients with the chronic form of the disease progress to cirrhosis and severe portal hypertension. With an overall accuracy of nearly 70%, Doppler ultrasound is the initial study of choice in many centers to evaluate hepatic venous patency; in addition, it is relatively inexpensive and readily available.

Although hepatic venography is still considered the standard, second-line imaging in the form of computed tomographic (CT) scan or magnetic resonance imaging (MRI) has several distinct advantages. In addition to characterizing hepatic outflow, these modalities allow for the evaluation of parenchymal abnormalities, the degree of ascites, and the presence of caudate lobe hypertrophy (a compensatory mechanism following BCS with critical surgical implications; Figure 1).

Conversely, in addition to definitive characterization of the hepatic venous anatomy, venography affords the opportunity to measure caval pressures and perform liver biopsy. At our center the current protocol starts with Doppler ultrasound. If BCS is diagnosed or even suspected, the patient undergoes both a CT scan of the abdomen and venography to fully characterize the burden of thrombus in hepatic veins and inferior vena cava (IVC).

Pathologically, BCS demonstrates a continuum of histologic findings that range from sinusoidal congestion, inflammation, and fibrosis to cirrhosis. Additionally, with BCS the liver parenchyma may demonstrate characteristic "regenerative nodules." These nodules

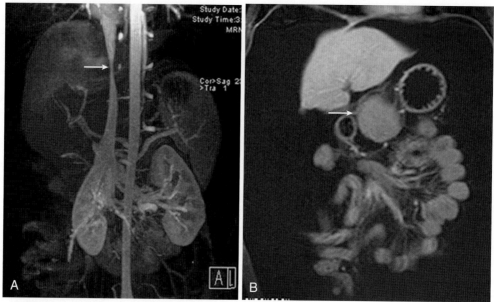

FIGURE 1   Magnetic resonance venogram. **A**, IVC obstruction (*arrow*) at the level of the caudate. **B**, Hypertrophic caudate lobe.

may represent hyperplasia and/or adenoma, and de novo hepatocellular carcinoma has been described in patients with hepatic venous outflow occlusion and end-stage liver disease. Importantly, portal vein thrombosis is frequently present and has important implications for future therapeutic strategies.

TREATMENT

Following an aggressive hypercoaguable workup, medical management is focused on the underlying cause and on controlling the dominant symptoms. Anticoagulation, control of daily sodium intake, and diuresis are the cornerstones of conservative medical therapy in patients who are otherwise asymptomatic or are high-risk with additional comorbidities. Although this approach can yield reasonable long-term results in select patients, the mortality rate at 2 years in patients treated by medical therapy alone is over 90%.

Importantly, Cameron and colleagues have clearly demonstrated progressive hepatocyte atrophy and impaired cellular regeneration in the setting of ongoing sinusoidal congestion. As such, BCS has evolved into a surgical disease with the primary goals of therapy focusing on the relief of venous outflow obstruction and debilitating symptoms and the prevention of recurrence. Unfortunately, these goals can be difficult to achieve, depending on the severity of disease and functional reserves of the patient.

Selection of Therapy

Selection of the appropriate therapeutic option is a multifactorial process that depends on the individual center's experience with liver disease and hepatic surgery, presence of cirrhosis, and availability of interventional radiology (Figure 2). In addition to aggressive medical management, it is our bias that transplantation is the most viable long-term treatment option. However, in the era of critical organ shortages, interventional radiology and surgical shunting techniques may provide short-term treatment alternatives, possibly slowing the onset of hepatocellular injury and subsequent disease progression.

At our center we initiate the decision process based on severity of disease and organ availability. In the presence of symptoms and/or absence of cirrhosis (subacute), we attempt a TIPS procedure to alleviate outflow obstruction, with close follow-up. If the occlusion

appears to be acute in onset, we will attempt to reestablish flow via thrombolysis, with angioplasty and stenting when technically feasible. Portosystemic shunting may be considered as an option in this situation.

Patients presenting with fulminant hepatic failure are candidates for orthotopic liver transplantation (OLT) with or without TIPS serving as a bridge. Patients with FHF are recognized by the United Network of Organ Sharing (UNOS) and are upgraded to the highest status on the liver transplant waiting list as a special exception. Finally, patients with cirrhosis and/or severe fibrosis are best served by OLT.

Thrombolytic Therapy and Interventional Techniques

The use of thrombolytic therapy is poorly studied and is generally limited to the acute setting with incomplete venous occlusion. Technical considerations mandate that the drug—a tissue plasminogen activator—be delivered directly to the site of thrombosis. Systemic therapy is of little or no value; however, over the last decade, modalities including a combination of balloon angioplasty, stent placement, and transjugular intrahepatic portosystemic shunting (TIPS) have emerged as effective adjuncts to medical therapy in the acute setting.

As the reocclusion rate in the setting of a hypercoaguable state is high, stent placement in one hepatic vein is recommended if technically feasible. Interestingly, the entire liver can be decompressed via a single vein stent, likely through patent collateral circulation. Concomitant stent placement in the inferior vena cava may prove effective in the face of severe caudate lobe hyperplasia and subsequent critical stenosis of this portion of the vena cava.

While balloon angioplasty and stenting provide a viable alternative to surgical intervention in the acute setting, the majority of patients do not develop symptoms or complications for months to years post occlusion. As a result, the ability to form a mechanical shunt between the portal and venous circulation via the TIPS procedure provides an effective method of splanchnic decompression in subacute and select chronic patients.

Not only does the TIPS procedure offer a relatively safe treatment option in high-risk patients, it can be applied in the setting of simultaneous hepatic and portal vein thrombosis. At the University of Colorado, success of stent placement was 100%, with over 80% of patients experiencing improved symptoms and/or better liver function in the short term. However, less than 50% of patients were clinically well at

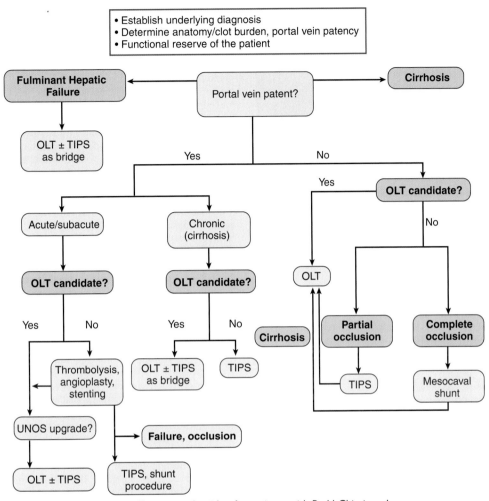

FIGURE 2 Treatment algorithm for patients with Budd-Chiari syndrome.

3 years post TIPS. Nearly one third of all TIPS patients required liver transplantation, and approximately 40% required a shunt revision or replacement. Furthermore, many TIPS patients are at risk of developing encephalopathy after TIPS placement. All patients also require long-term anticoagulation to help prevent occlusion of the stent. These observations underscore the fact that the majority of radiologic interventions serve effectively as a bridge to more definitive surgical therapy, providing a short-term window for optimization of hepatic function and overall functional reserve.

SURGICAL THERAPY

OLT certainly provides an effective therapy for all forms of BCS. However, the critical organ shortage inherently limits the availability of this procedure. As a result, portosystemic shunting has been developed as an alternate strategy over the last three decades, in parallel with transplantation. Importantly, portosystemic shunting provides a valuable bridge to OLT; previous shunt surgery does not technically preclude subsequent transplantation, nor does it have a negative impact on long-term outcome.

Portosystemic Shunting

After the first description of a surgical portocaval shunt was documented by Blakemore in the late 1940s, 3 decades passed before portosystemic shunting was recognized as more effective than medical

therapy alone (Figure 3). Several authors have noted excellent short-term results. In 2000, Orloff and colleagues reported an impressive prospective series of 50 patients undergoing portocaval shunting for BCS over a 27-year period. The overall survival rate for shunted patients was 94% with a mean follow-up of over 13 years. Using a side-to-side portocaval shunt in the majority of patients, less than 5% developed ascites, had encephalopathy, or required diuretics. The authors conclude that once the diagnosis of BCS is made, it is unnecessary to delay portal decompression in the absence of cirrhosis. They argue that if performed early in the process, portosystemic shunting can attenuate ongoing hepatocellular injury. A similar experience was reported by Xu in 2004, in documenting surgical shunting in over 1300 patients. An 89% success rate was noted, with a mean follow-up of nearly 7 years, when the type of shunt procedure was tailored to the specific anatomic defect.

Unfortunately, the data are conflicting with regard to long-term outcomes. Ringe and colleagues observed a 10 year survival of 69% following OLT versus a 29% success rate with portosystemic shunting. Furthermore, while Zeitoun reports 10 year survival of 57% with shunt surgery, the surgery had no statistical impact on survival compared to medical therapy alone.

The cumulative experience with these procedures is not definitive and faces several obstacles, which makes interpretation difficult. In general, the anatomic procedure performed varies by institution as well as by each individual patient, making this cohort a very heterogenous group. Also, the control groups against which these patients are compared range from those who received medical therapy to transplantation patients. Finally, most studies are limited to between 50 and 100 patients in either arm.

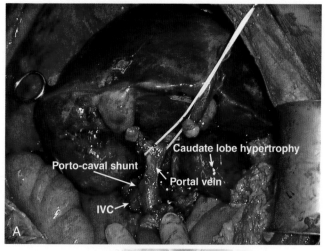

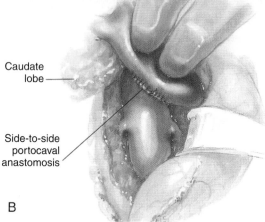

FIGURE 3   BCS with previous portosystemic shunt procedure at the time of OLT. **A,** Caudate lobe hypertrophy. **B,** Side-to-side portocaval shunt.

Overall, the experience with portosystemic shunt procedures suggests that a long-term benefit in the form slowing disease progression can be realized if performed early, and in select patients, at high-volume centers with proven success. However, several questions remain in this subset of patients, including questions about the appropriate follow-up regimen and timing to transplantation.

Orthotopic Liver Transplantation

Liver transplantation has clearly emerged as the preferred treatment option for most forms of BCS. In 1976, Putnam and Starzl reported the first case of OLT in a 22-year-old female with acute hepatic venous occlusion, noting excellent results at 16-month follow-up. Over the last 3 decades, experience with OLT in the setting of BCS has undergone a dramatic evolution. Early experience with OLT for BCS yielded inferior outcomes, with 3-year survival as low as 45%. In general, two factors have modified the approach and positively influenced outcomes: 1) aggressive initiation of medical and interventional therapy, and 2) anticoagulation. In the modern era of transplantation for BCS, actuarial 10-year survival approaches 70%. In the largest study of patients transplanted for BCS by Mentha and colleagues, from the European Liver Transplantation Registry, 248 patients had complete follow-up data. As 10-year survival approximated 70%, 27 patients developed venous thrombosis in the face of anticoagulation, 6 of which had recurrent venous outflow occlusion.

Liver transplantation in the setting of BCS poses several technical challenges. With acute or chronic disease, the liver may be markedly swollen and difficult to manipulate. Secondly, hyperplasia of the caudate lobe makes access and dissection of the IVC a difficult endeavor. Concomitant stenosis of the IVC makes suprahepatic and infrahepatic control equally difficult. Although a prior TIPS procedure does not preclude OLT, distal migration of the stent may complicate the portal vein anastomosis. Substantial migration may require transection of the stent and that the anastomosis be performed directly to the portal vein remnant of the stent in situ. Noted by many institutional experiences, isolation of the hepatic veins for a piggyback anastomosis can be difficult with active outflow occlusion.

As mentioned in previous editions of this textbook, portal vein thrombosis can be a difficult problem, and it requires a strategic plan prior to transplant. At present, we find that the portal vein can routinely be thrombectomized, and reasonable flow established, if the superior mesenteric vein (SMV) is patent. If this is not possible, a vein graft using donor iliac vein can be constructed between the donor portal vein and the SMV.

In the setting of complete mesenteric occlusion, two possibilities exist: First, many times these recipients have an extremely large and patent coronary vein because of severe portal hypertension; this vein can be used for portal inflow. Second, anastomosis of the recipient's portal vein to the recipient's IVC (caval hemitransposition) with partial or total occlusion of the IVC superior is an option. Unfortunately, this approach can have an extremely high morbidity and mortality.

Since performing the first right lobe, adult-to-adult, living-donor liver transplant (LDLT) in North America in 1996, we have used caval reconstruction with cryopreserved iliac vein grafts in multiple patients with large malignancies that anatomically precluded the use of the native IVC. Recently, several authors have reported using this technique in patients with BCS to facilitate LDLT. Due to caudate lobe hyperplasia and/or caval stenosis, the recipient IVC may not be usable for LDLT. In 2006, Yan and colleagues from Chendgu, China, reported the first case of an adult-to-adult LDLT for BCS using a cryopreserved iliac vein graft. The authors highlight several important technical issues. In this case, it was necessary to incise the diaphragm and expose the pericardium to the level of the right atrium secondary to hepatic venous outflow occlusion. The iliac graft was then sewn to the suprahepatic and infrahepatic vena cavae. The right hepatic vein of the right hepatic lobe allograft was then sewn to the iliac graft in end-to-side fashion.

Alternatively, a large series from Japan reports the long-term outcome in eight patients with BCS who underwent LDLT. Of these, five patients underwent cavoplasty using a replacement vein graft following extensive resection of the thrombosed anterior IVC wall. Although the combined experience with LDLT for BCS is small, the current data suggest living donation as an emerging treatment option for this patient population.

Treatment of Disease Recurrence

Recurrence of hepatic venous outflow obstruction has been observed in up to 10% of patients, ranging from months to years post transplant. As a result, lifelong anticoagulation is currently recommended. Early experience with recurrent BCS carried an extremely high mortality rate. Of three patients who had recurrence after OLT at the University of Pittsburgh, all died.

Over the last 2 decades, interventional techniques have provided some alternatives to retransplantation or death. In our experience, recurrent BCS can be approached in two ways: Primarily, retransplantation is an option in patients with mild to moderate thrombus burden in the hepatic veins and IVC refractory to an interventional approach. However, the anatomic features of the recurrent thrombus must be carefully delineated; recipients with a completely occluded IVC and portal vein are unlikely to be candidates for retransplant. In severe cases, TIPS can be employed to reestablish flow in one or more hepatic veins in the setting of preserved liver function.

Recently, we performed an open-assisted retrograde TIPS procedure, accessing the portal circulation through the inferior mesenteric vein. As a result, flow was reestablished in the middle hepatic vein with good anatomic stent placement. Despite limited options at this juncture, some grafts can be saved with this type of combined strategy.

SUMMARY

Orthotopic liver transplantation is clearly the most viable long-term treatment option for patients with all forms of BCS. However, in the era of severe organ shortages, alternate strategies have evolved to provide a bridge to transplantation via preservation, or at least attenuated progression, of hepatocellular injury and declining liver function. While select centers in North America have a robust experience with portosystemic shunt procedures, the majority of transplant institutions initially employ radiologic procedures for those with acute or subacute onset of disease.

SELECTED READINGS

Attwell A, Ludkowski M, Nash R, et al: Treatment of Budd-Chiari syndrome in a liver transplant unit, the role of transjugular intrahepatic portosystemic shunt and liver transplantation, *Aliment Pharmacol Ther* 20:867–873, 2004.

Mentha G, Giostra E, Majno PE, et: al: Liver transplantation for Budd–Chiari syndrome: a European study on 248 patients from 51 centers, *J Hepatol* 44:520–528, 2006.

Srinivasan P, Rela M, Prachalias A, et al: Liver transplantation for Budd-Chiari syndrome, *Transplantation* 73:973–977, 2002.

Yamada T, Tanaka K, Ogura Y, et al: Surgical techniques and long-term outcomes of living donor liver transplantation of Budd-Chiari syndrome, *Am J Transpl* 6:2463–2469, 2006.

Yan L, Li B, Zeng Y, et al: Living donor liver transplantation for Budd-Chiari syndrome using cryopreserved vena cava graft in retrohepatic vena cava reconstruction, *Liver Transpl* 12:1017–1019, 2006.

Zimmerman MA, Cameron AM, Ghobrial RM: Budd-Chiari syndrome, *Clin Liver Dis* 259–273, 2006.

GALLBLADDER AND BILIARY TREE

ASYMPTOMATIC (SILENT) GALLSTONES

Mouen Khashab, MD, and Samuel A. Giday, MD

OVERVIEW

Gallstone disease is one of the leading indications for surgery in the United States today, with approximately 500,000 cholecystectomies performed every year. As many as 10% to 20% of the population will develop gallstones at some stage of life, and the incidence increases with age. The advent of laparoscopic cholecystectomy has facilitated the management of this condition as symptoms or complications arise. However, when gallstones are found incidentally and are asymptomatic, management decisions have not been so clear-cut, and controversy exists in the medical and surgical literature.

NATURAL HISTORY OF ASYMPTOMATIC GALLSTONES

Natural history of "silent" gallstones does not appear to justify treatment with prophylactic cholecystectomy. Most studies, conducted mainly in the 1980s, demonstrated that nearly 80% of patients remain asymptomatic throughout their lives, with only 1% to 4% progressing to symptoms or developing complications from gallstones annually. Only 10% of those found to have asymptomatic gallstones develop symptoms within the first 5 years after diagnosis, increasing only to 20% at 20 years. This was first demonstrated by Gracie and Ransohoff in their landmark study of 123 patients followed prospectively over a 15 year period. They showed that 10% of patients progressed to symptomatic disease at 5 years, 15% by 10 years, and 18% by 15 years. Overall, patients developed symptoms or serious complications, such as acute cholecystitis, at a rate of 1% to 2% per year, with most patients developing symptoms within 5 years.

Critics of the study cited its homogenous population of primarily young white male patients. However, other investigators have shown similar results with more diverse patient populations. McSherry and colleagues studied 135 patients with asymptomatic gallstones and diverse ethnicity and gender. With a 58 month follow-up, 10% developed symptoms, and only 7% required cholecystectomy at annual rates of 2.2% and 1.5%, respectively. In their review of the literature, Friedman and colleagues looked at an ethnically diverse patient population as well. They showed that 3% to 4% of patients developed biliary symptoms in the first 10 years. Of these, nearly all patients who developed a complication had experienced previous symptoms; only

1% to 3% of patients with mild symptoms and 6% to 8% with severe symptoms progressed to a complication.

Several investigators have attempted to identify predictive factors for progression to symptoms or complications in patients with silent cholelithiasis. Generally, most studies have not shown gallstone size or nature, gallbladder wall thickness, or gallbladder contractility to be significant predictors of progression to symptoms or complications. A few studies have demonstrated that patients with gallstones larger than 2.5 cm have higher rates of acute cholecystitis and a higher risk for developing gallbladder cancer. Other studies have shown that smaller stones (≤5 mm) are associated with a higher risk of acute pancreatitis. In addition, patients with cholelithiasis who also happen to have porcelain gallbladder or large gallbladder polyps (≥10 to 15 mm) have higher rates of gallbladder cancer. Patient factors, such as age and sex, and comorbidities such as diabetes have also been generally nonpredictive of progression to symptoms or complications.

ROLE OF PROPHYLACTIC CHOLECYSTECTOMY

In their recent Cochrane review that aimed to assess the benefits and harms of surgical removal of the gallbladder in patients with asymptomatic gallstones, Gurusamy and Samraj found no randomized controlled trials comparing cholecystectomy to an expectant management strategy. They concluded that there was no evidence to recommend or refute prophylactic cholecystectomy for asymptomatic patients. Recently, Venneman and colleagues showed that small gallstones are associated with an increased risk of acute pancreatitis as compared with larger stones. They used a Markov model to study the benefit of prophylactic cholecystectomy in patients with small (≤5 mm) gallstones, and this decision analysis showed that although patients with small gallstones could theoretically benefit from prophylactic cholecystectomy, considering their apparently increased pancreatitis risk, under most scenarios life-years would be lost.

Ransohoff and colleagues also used a decision-analysis model to compare the consequences of prophylactic cholecystectomy with expectant management for silent gallstone disease. The former policy did not increase survival of patients and was substantially more expensive than an expectant management strategy. Nevertheless, some proponents of prophylactic cholecystectomy have proposed early operation. The argument is that the introduction of laparoscopic cholecystectomy, with its low morbidity and nearly zero mortality rates, may alter the risk/benefit ratio in favor of prophylactic cholecystectomy.

According to the National Institutes of Health (NIH) Consensus Conference report, however, the availability of laparoscopic cholecystectomy should not expand the indications for gallbladder removal. In fact, laparoscopic cholecystectomy for asymptomatic gallstones is reported to have a conversion to open laparotomy rate of 1.6% and morbidity of 5%.

Several authors have proposed criteria for patients with a relatively high risk for developing complications of asymptomatic gallstones who may benefit from a prophylactic cholecystectomy strategy (Table 1). Overall, the natural history of asymptomatic gallstones appears to be benign, and expectant management is the recommended course of action. On the other hand, some patients may be at a considerably higher risk for complications and may therefore require special consideration.

SPECIAL CASES

Diabetes

In the past, the management of diabetic patients with asymptomatic gallstones emphasized early cholecystectomy. The argument for prophylactic cholecystectomy was based on the assumption that these patients had diabetic autonomic neuropathy that masked the pain and signs associated with acute cholecystitis, and thus they presented with advanced disease and had more complications. Landau and colleagues found diabetics to have higher rates of infected bile, gangrene, gallbladder perforation, and surgical mortality than nondiabetics in the setting of acute cholecystitis (21% vs. 9%).

More recent evidence demonstrated that the prevalence and natural history of asymptomatic gallstones in diabetic patients are roughly the same as those reported for nondiabetic patients. The prevalence of gallstones in diabetics compared with nondiabetics (14.4% vs. 12.5%) was not significantly different. Symptoms or complications occurred in 15% of non–insulin-dependent diabetics who were initially asymptomatic after 5 years of follow-up. Since few patients with asymptomatic gallstones and non–insulin-dependent diabetes mellitus develop pain or complications over time, prophylactic cholecystectomy is not prudent for those patients.

Transplantation

The high prevalence (30% to 40%) of cholelithiasis in transplant patients has been attributed to cyclosporine and tacrolimus, both of which are prolithogenic due to decreased bile salt export-pump function. However, the incidence of gallstones and rate of progression to symptoms or complications varies among the organs transplanted.

Prophylactic cholecystectomy is not recommended in patients undergoing renal transplantation. Greenstein and colleagues followed renal transplant patients for 4 years and found only a 7% incidence of gallstones and a 3% incidence of sludge. Of these patients, 87% remained asymptomatic, with only 7% of patients developing acute cholecystitis requiring subsequent uncomplicated laparoscopic cholecystectomy. Others have supported this evidence and have shown that the presence of gallstone disease does not negatively affect graft survival.

On the contrary, heart transplant patients have been shown to have higher rates of gallstone formation and gallstone-related complications. Peterseim and colleagues showed a 42% incidence of silent gallstones,

TABLE 1: Proposed criteria for prophylactic cholecystectomy

Life expectancy >20 years
Calculi >2 cm in diameter
Calculi >3 mm and patent cystic duct
Radiopaque calculi
Gallbladder polyps >15 mm
Nonfunctioning or calcified gallbladder ("porcelain" gallbladder)
Women <60 years
Patients in areas with high prevalence of gallbladder cancer

with 58% of these patients developing symptoms within 2 years of heart transplant. Others have reported significantly increased mortality associated with the development of symptoms and complications and the need for emergent cholecystectomy. The Mayo Clinic reported that 36% of 178 heart-lung transplant patients had abnormal gallbladder ultrasound results, with 50% requiring intervention secondary to gallstone-related complications. The operative mortality rate was 29%. Milas and colleagues also showed a 30% incidence of gallstones, with nearly 50% of these patients going on to cholecystectomy secondary to symptomatic disease. However, they did not report any postoperative deaths in their study. This group concluded that screening ultrasound, followed by prophylactic laparoscopic cholecystectomy if stones are present, is prudent given the high incidence of gallstones and the subsequent risk of progression to symptomatic disease.

In a recent decision analysis by Kao and colleagues, prophylactic posttransplantation cholecystectomy resulted in less mortality than both pretransplantation cholecystectomy and expectant management in heart transplant patients with asymptomatic cholelithiasis (5:1000 vs. 80:1000 vs. 40:1000 deaths, respectively). On the other hand, expectant management in renal/pancreatic transplant patients was found to be a safer course of management than prophylactic cholecystectomy (2:1000 vs. 5:1000 deaths, respectively).

In short, prophylactic posttransplantation cholecystectomy is the preferred management strategy for cardiac transplant patients with incidental gallstones, and expectant management is the preferred strategy for pancreas and/or kidney transplant recipients with asymptomatic cholelithiasis.

Hemoglobinopathies

Patients with hemoglobinopathies are at a significantly increased risk for developing pigmented stones. Gallstones have been reported in up to 70% of sickle cell patients, 85% of hereditary spherocytosis patients, and 24% of thalassemia patients. In sickle cell patients, complications from asymptomatic gallstones have been reported to be as high as 50% within 3 to 5 years of diagnosis. This has been attributed largely to the diagnostic challenge of differentiating symptomatic cholelithiasis from abdominal sickling crisis.

Elective cholecystectomy should be considered in sickle cell anemia patients with symptomatic gallstones and in those with gallstone-related symptomatology that cannot be differentiated from sickle cell hepatic crises. Prophylactic cholecystectomy is otherwise not advocated in these patients because of the increased morbidity of surgical procedures. Haberkern and colleagues studied 364 sickle cell anemia patients who underwent cholecystectomy. The overall complication rate was 39%, and the death rate was 1%. In addition, the complication rate was similar in patients who underwent laparoscopic and open cholecystectomy. Notwithstanding, an incidental cholecystectomy should be considered in sickle cell anemia patients with asymptomatic cholelithiasis who are undergoing an abdominal operation (such as splenectomy) for other reasons.

Routine prophylactic cholecystectomy is not recommended for patients with hereditary spherocytosis and asymptomatic gallstones. These patients usually undergo splenectomy for symptoms of severe hemolysis; incidental cholecystectomy may be performed in these instances if gallstones are present. A decision analysis model by Marchetti and colleagues showed that a combined splenectomy and cholecystectomy is of benefit in hereditary spherocytosis patients who are under the age of 39 years and have mild hemolysis and asymptomatic gallstones.

Cirrhosis

Several studies have shown that cirrhotic patients with asymptomatic gallstones progress to symptoms at a rate similar to noncirrhotic patients. Castaing and colleagues reviewed gallstone disease in 64 cirrhotic patients and found that 17% had gallstones, with 14% of these patients going on to have symptoms or complications requiring cholecystectomy. There was one postoperative death and one postoperative complication secondary to variceal bleeding. Sleeman and colleagues studied 25 Child-Turcotte-Pugh class A and B cirrhotic patients who underwent laparoscopic cholecystectomy and reported the procedure to be feasible and safe. Despite a 32% morbidity rate (wound hematoma, pneumonia, and ascites), the mean length of hospital stay was 1.7 days, and there were no postoperative deaths.

Although the natural history of asymptomatic gallstones in cirrhotic patients does not significantly differ from that of the general population, there are certain important specific risks to consider. Cirrhotic patients do develop more severe symptoms from acute cholecystitis, and when severe symptoms do occur, they are often associated with increased morbidity and mortality. Furthermore, laparoscopic cholecystectomy, although safe and feasible, is more technically challenging in the context of cirrhosis and portal hypertension. The risk of hemorrhage from portal hypertension in the periumbilical area can affect trocar site placement, and varices in the perigastric and porta hepatis may affect dissection; therefore anatomic consideration and natural history of the clinical situation suggest that a course of expectant management is recommended in the cirrhotic patient.

Total Parenteral Nutrition

A well-documented relationship exists between prolonged total parenteral nutrition (TPN) administration and the formation of gallstones. This relationship has been shown to be secondary to multiple factors, such as gallbladder stasis and changed composition of bile. There may be a nearly 35% incidence of gallstone formation in these patients, among whom a larger than expected percentage will progress to symptomatic disease.

Roslyn and colleagues reported a retrospective review of patients who underwent cholecystectomy for TPN-induced gallbladder disease. Of the 35 patients included in the study, 40% required emergent cholecystectomy, with an overall operative morbidity of 54% and mortality rate of 11%. The authors concluded that those on long-term TPN should have ultrasound surveillance and that elective cholecystectomy should be performed when gallstones are detected. However, a delay in diagnosis was a major contributor to the high rate of complications in the study. In the modern era, practicing physicians are cognizant of biliary complications of TPN, and the results of this study likely do not pertain anymore. Expectant management is currently the preferred strategy in the treatment of patients with asymptomatic gallstones who are on long-term TPN.

Bariatric Surgery

Rapid weight loss increases the lithogenicity of bile. Cholelithiasis occurs in up to 40% of patients within 6 months after bariatric surgery, and 40% of those affected become symptomatic. It is debatable whether a prophylactic cholecystectomy should be performed during the operation, because there is no clear proof in the literature that such a strategy is beneficial. Actually, such an approach, although safe, increases the operative procedure time and the length of hospital stay. Pharmacologic prophylaxis with ursodeoxycholic acid, a synthetic bile salt, has been shown in two randomized double-blind and placebo-controlled trials to be effective for the prevention of gallstone formation. As few as 2% and 4.7% of patients developed gallstones or required cholecystectomy, respectively, after 6 months of therapy with ursodeoxycholic acid given twice daily. Given the limited available evidence, it seems reasonable to perform concomitant cholecystectomy when gallstones are documented, either preoperatively or intraoperatively, and to treat patients undergoing bariatric surgery without documented gallstones with a 6-month course of ursodeoxycholic acid.

Incidental Cholecystectomy

The management of cholelithiasis found incidentally during an abdominal or alimentary tract procedure is controversial. Although concomitant cholecystectomy eliminates the risk of gallbladder disease and its complications, it has the potential to increase patient morbidity and mortality. However, numerous authors have found concomitant cholecystectomy to be a safe and effective procedure. In a review of colorectal surgery patients, the Mayo Clinic found a 15% rate of symptomatic cholelithiasis over a 6-year period in patients with incidental cholelithiasis. They determined that the probability of requiring future cholecystectomy in this patient population was 12% at 2 years and 22% at 5 years.

Saade and colleagues also looked at patients undergoing colorectal, gastric, and gynecologic procedures over a 4-year period. In the 109 patients studied, 78 (72%) had incidental cholecystectomy, with only two postoperative complications. Thirty-one patients (28%) had their gallbladders left in situ; 12 remained asymptomatic, and 13 developed symptoms. Seven of these patients underwent open cholecystectomy 2 to 11 weeks later.

Thompson and colleagues followed 56 patients found to have incidental gallstones at the time of celiotomy; 33 underwent incidental cholecystectomy, with only one complication (3%). Twenty-three patients had their gallbladders left in situ, and 16 of them developed complications within 6 months, including 11 who had acute cholecystitis. Fifteen of the original 33 patients (65%) subsequently underwent open cholecystectomy, with 6 patients (40%) requiring common bile duct exploration.

McSherry and colleagues reviewed 137 patients undergoing incidental cholecystectomy for a variety of intraabdominal procedures. Only three patients in this cohort had postoperative complications directly attributable to cholecystectomy. In their review of 4072 patients above the age of 70 years who had asymptomatic cholelithiasis and underwent surgery for gastrointestinal malignancies, Watemberg and colleagues showed an increase in mortality, morbidity, and length of hospital stay when the gallbladder was left in situ; so incidental cholecystectomy seems to be most appropriate during abdominal or alimentary tract surgery in patients older than 70 years.

Management of incidental cholelithiasis during a vascular surgery procedure has been even more controversial because of the frequent use of prosthetic graft material. Concomitant cholecystectomy increases the risk for potential graft infection from bile spillage. However, despite this risk of potential contamination, several authors have reported data showing incidental cholecystectomy to be feasible during vascular surgery.

Ochsner and colleagues were among the first to show that concomitant cholecystectomy was safe during open abdominal aortic aneurysmectomies (AAAs). Fifty-one of 931 patients in their series underwent cholecystectomy at the time of AAA repair with no increase in mortality or morbidity. Ouriel and colleagues reported similar results in 42 of 845 patients found to have gallstones at the time of AAA repair. In the 18 patients who had simultaneous cholecystectomy during AAA repair, one graft infection occurred in a patient whose retroperitoneum was not closed before cholecystectomy. Furthermore, of the 11 patients who had aneurysmectomy without cholecystectomy, nine developed acute cholecystitis within 3 years, with one death due to biliary sepsis. Sonpal and colleagues reported on 113 patients who underwent a major abdominal vascular procedure with prosthetic graft placement; seven patients had incidental cholecystectomies with no complications. Therefore incidental cholecystectomy may be performed safely if necessary during AAA repair, provided that the graft is covered with peritoneum before proceeding with cholecystectomy.

SUMMARY

Most patients with asymptomatic gallstones remain asymptomatic. The advent of laparoscopy should not alter the indications for cholecystectomy; the optimal treatment for the vast majority of patients is expectant management, with laparoscopic cholecystectomy reserved for those who become symptomatic. Laparoscopic cholecystectomy may be performed for asymptomatic cholelithiasis in selective groups of patients who are at a particularly high risk for disease progression and thus require special consideration. Finally, intraoperative concomitant cholecystectomy should be directed by the clinical circumstance, largely technical, and the best judgment of the operating surgeon.

SUGGESTED READINGS

Gracie WA, Ransohoff DF: The natural history of silent gallstones: the innocent gallstone is not a myth, *N Engl J Med* 307:798–800, 1982.
Kao LS, Flowers C, Flum DR: Prophylactic cholecystectomy in transplant patients: a decision analysis, *J Gastrointest Surg* 9:965–972, 2005.
Marchetti M, Quaglini S, Barosi G: Prophylactic splenectomy and cholecystectomy in mild hereditary spherocytosis: analyzing the decision in different clinical scenarios, *J Intern Med* 244:217–226, 1998.
Ransohoff DF, Gracie WA, Wolfenson LB, Neuhauser D: Prophylactic cholecystectomy or expectant management for silent gallstones: a decision analysis to assess survival, *Ann Intern Med* 99:199–204, 1983.
Sugerman HJ, Brewer WH, Shiffman ML, et al: A multicenter, placebo-controlled, randomized, double-blind, prospective trial of prophylactic ursodiol for the prevention of gallstone formation following gastric-bypass–induced rapid weight loss, *Am J Surg* 169:91–96, 1995.
Watemberg S, Landau O, Avrahami R, et al: Incidental cholecystectomy in the over-70 age group: a 19-year retrospective, comparative study, *Int Surg* 82:102–104, 1997.

ACUTE CHOLECYSTITIS

Kyle J. Van Arendonk, MD, and Mark D. Duncan, MD

OVERVIEW

Acute cholecystitis is defined as symptomatic inflammation of the gallbladder. In cases of acute *calculous* cholecystitis, inflammation results from obstruction of the cystic duct by gallstones, which in the presence of continued mucosal secretion leads to gallbladder distension and eventual ischemia. The inflammation in acute cholecystitis is typically sterile, although secondary bacterial infection can occur. Untreated cholecystitis can therefore lead to perforation with peritonitis or intraabdominal abscess. When secondary infection with gas-forming organisms occurs, an especially severe form of cholecystitis can result in which gas is seen within the gallbladder wall and lumen, called *emphysematous cholecystitis*. Acute *acalculous* cholecystitis is thought to result from biliary sludge that causes obstruction of the cystic duct in the absence of gallstones. This less common entity is typically seen in the critically ill, in patients receiving long-term total parenteral nutrition, and in immunocompromised patients suffering from global ischemia or severe infections.

Cholelithiasis is present in approximately 10% of the general adult population. Less than one third of people with stones will ever develop symptoms, thus patients with incidentally discovered gallstones are not counseled for cholecystectomy. The risk of asymptomatic stones becoming symptomatic is about 1% to 2% per year.

CLINICAL PRESENTATION AND WORKUP

Patients with acute cholecystitis typically complain of fever and right upper quadrant pain accompanied by nausea and vomiting. In addition, referred pain to the right scapular region is also possible if the inflammation has caused irritation of the diaphragm. Patients may also report a history of preceding symptoms of biliary colic. In contrast to acute cholecystitis, biliary colic consists of intermittent or fleeting right upper quadrant pain in the absence of fever, often following fatty meals. Frequently there is a long-standing history of episodes of pain. If biliary colic is seen in a patient in the emergency department, the symptoms are often waning, and the patient has neither fever nor leukocytosis. This distinction is important, as patients with acute cholecystitis require immediate management, whereas those with episodes of biliary colic can be scheduled for cholecystectomy on an elective basis.

On physical examination, fever and tachycardia are often present. Right upper quadrant tenderness is a hallmark of cholecystitis. The finding of inspiratory arrest secondary to pain when the examiner performs deep palpation in the right subcostal area is known as *Murphy's sign*. Patients presenting at a late stage of the illness may demonstrate signs of peritonitis. Patients should also be examined for jaundice, which suggests the presence of choledocholithiasis leading to common bile duct obstruction. Less commonly, Mirizzi syndrome can occur, wherein a large gallstone in the cystic duct is able to cause compression of the common hepatic duct.

Workup of acute cholecystitis should include a complete blood count, which typically shows a mild leukocytosis, and a complete metabolic panel, which usually demonstrates normal liver function tests. Mild elevation of transaminases and alkaline phosphatase can occur. Hyperbilirubinemia must lead to consideration of common bile duct obstruction; however, severe necrotizing cholecystitis can show a mildly elevated bilirubin. Amylase and lipase levels should be obtained in any evaluation of abdominal pain.

The initial imaging study of choice is the right upper quadrant ultrasound, which can show gallstones, gallbladder wall thickening (considered 4 mm or greater), and pericholecystic fluid, the combination of which is highly suggestive of acute cholecystitis. Sonography will also allow evaluation of the common bile duct for dilatation or for the presence of stones. These findings can also be seen on computed tomography (CT) when completed to evaluate for other abdominal pathology or for the complications of cholecystitis. CT, however, is less sensitive for gallbladder abnormalities than ultrasound and should not be used as the initial study to evaluate for uncomplicated acute cholecystitis. We have found magnetic resonance cholangiopancreatography (MRCP) to be as accurate as sonography at demonstrating acute cholecystitis. MRCP is very sensitive to fluid stasis, which is seen with cystic duct obstruction in acute cholecystitis and in demonstrating pericholecystic fluid. MRCP is also highly effective at imaging common bile duct stones, and it is utilized in patients with elevated liver function tests or jaundice, both of which raise the suspicion for common bile duct obstruction (Figure 1).

We routinely use MRCP to rule out common duct stones when patients have dilated ducts seen on any imaging modality, or when the bilirubin is elevated, rather than proceeding to endoscopic retrograde cholangiopancreatography (ERCP). In these settings, more than half of all patients will have a negative ERCP, likely having already passed a stone. If the MRCP shows no stone, it obviates the need for ERCP and its attendant risks in these patients. Further benefits of MRCP are the speed of the test and that it is easy to read, so there is no need to wait for a skilled technician, which can hamper efforts to obtain sonographic imaging after hours or on weekends. The use of MRCP has not caught on in all centers, thus the sonogram still remains the standard.

When the ultrasound is equivocal or negative in the setting of the appropriate clinical symptoms, a hepatobiliary iminodiacetic acid (HIDA) scan can be undertaken. A HIDA scan that demonstrates nonfilling of the gallbladder is consistent with a diagnosis of acute cholecystitis due to obstruction of the cystic duct, but it is not diagnostic. We rarely find this test helpful, however, in part because a false-positive HIDA can often be seen, as most of the patients are fasting secondary to their illness at the time of the study.

DIFFERENTIAL DIAGNOSIS

Differential diagnosis of acute cholecystitis should include peptic ulcer, colitis, gastroenteritis, pancreatitis, renal colic, appendicitis, liver abscess, and pneumonia. Myocardial ischemia should also be ruled out in high-risk patients. Each year we see patients admitted to the cardiac intensive care unit (CICU) or evaluated in the emergency department to rule out myocardial infarction only to be found on reexamination to have acute cholecystitis.

MANAGEMENT

Upon diagnosis of acute cholecystitis, most patients should be scheduled for cholecystectomy. The appropriate timing of cholecystectomy in patients diagnosed with acute cholecystitis was previously a heavily debated topic. Early cholecystectomy, typically within the first 36 hours after onset of symptoms, has now been shown in multiple studies to have no higher morbidity, mortality, or rates of converting from laparoscopic to open approach than a cholecystectomy delayed several weeks after presentation. This was confirmed in a Cochrane analysis of five trials with 451 randomized patients. Surgery was performed on 222 patients in the early group and on 216 patients in the delayed group. There was no mortality in any of the trials, and no statistically significant difference was found between the two groups for any of the outcomes, including bile duct injury (odds ratio [OR], 0.63; 95% confidence interval [CI], 0.15 to 2.70) and conversion to open cholecystectomy (OR, 0.84; 95% CI, 0.53 to 1.34).

Additionally, early cholecystectomy allows for the disease process to be halted before progression of the inflammatory process to necrosis, gangrene, perforation, and/or abscess. Exceptions to the recommendation for prompt (same admission) cholecystectomy include critically ill patients with significant hemodynamic instability or other active problems that prohibit a safe operation. In these cases, a cholecystostomy tube should be placed either at the bedside or by interventional radiology. For those patients who survive their critical illness, the cholecystostomy tube should be maintained for 3 months. At that time, a contrast study should be completed to evaluate the patency of the cystic duct. If the duct is patent, the cholecystostomy tube can be removed. The patient's physiologic reserve can then be reevaluated to determine candidacy for an elective cholecystectomy.

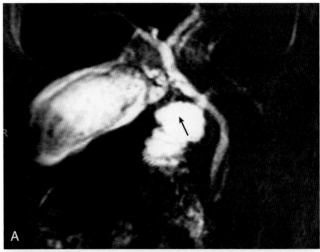

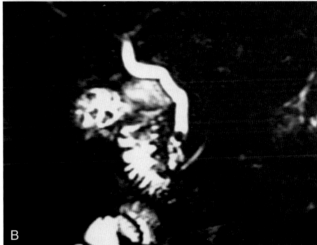

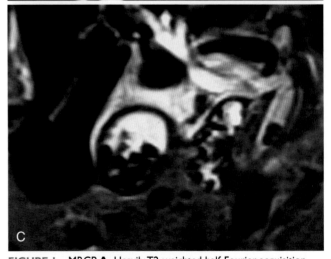

FIGURE 1 MRCP. **A,** Heavily T2-weighted half-Fourier acquisition single-shot turbo spin-echo (HASTE) MRI sequence demonstrating pericholecystic fluid and mild gallbladder wall thickening. **B,** Heavily T2-weighted HASTE MRI sequence demonstrating choledocholithiasis. **C,** Standard T2-weighted imaged demonstrating cholelithiasis, pericholecystic fluid, and choledocholithiasis (two stones in the common duct).

Although acute cholecystitis is usually sterile, inflammation and infection, typically poylmicrobial, can develop. Therefore patients are usually treated with broad-spectrum antibiotics, which should be started at the time of diagnosis of acute cholecystitis and continued until cholecystectomy has been performed. Only in severe cases of gangrenous or emphysematous cholecystitis should several days of additional postoperative antibiotic therapy be given. *Escherichia coli* and *Klebsiella*, *Enterococcus*, and *Enterobacter* species are the most commonly implicated bacteria. Antibiotics of choice are second or third generation cephalosporins, ampicillin-sulbactam, fluoroquinolones, or ertapenem. In patients with significant comorbidities, and in those with a high suspicion of nosocomial-acquired pathogens, piperacillin-tazobactam or meropenem can be used.

Laparoscopic Cholecystectomy

The laparoscopic approach to cholecystectomy is now the favored approach in the majority of cases of acute cholecystitis. The key to successful laparoscopic cholecystectomy is proper identification of the infundibulum–cystic duct junction, where further dissection must occur. Dissection inferiorly on the cystic duct risks injury to the common bile duct, and the surgeon should therefore deliberately avoid dissecting near the common bile duct during routine dissection. The gallbladder should be retracted superiorly and the infundibulum laterally to create a "critical view of safety" between the liver edge, gallbladder, and cystic duct. Attachments of the gallbladder serosa of the infundibulum to the liver are taken down on either side with electrocautery to facilitate the lifting of the infundibulum to provide the critical viewing angle. When the appropriate view is obtained, the cystic duct and cystic artery will be revealed as the only two structures entering the gallbladder (Figure 2). After their conclusive identification, the cystic duct and cystic artery are clipped. Any uncertainty should be handled by cholangiography, by use of the fundus-down technique, or by converting to an open procedure.

Occasionally. when the cystic duct cannot be safely dissected without potential risk to the common bile duct, a fundus-down approach can be taken in a manner similar to that used in open cholecystectomy. An EndoGIA 30 mm stapling device can then be used to divide the distal infundibulum, staying off the cystic duct and thus away from the common bile duct.

When common bile duct stones are discovered during a laparoscopic cholecystectomy, two operative options exist: The first, a laparoscopic common bile duct exploration, is technically difficult and feasible for very few surgeons. Another option is choledochoscopy with a 3 mm scope through an opening made in the cystic duct near the gallbladder. This approach allows basket retrieval of stones, but it can also be technically challenging. The advantage of this method is that the cystic duct can then be clipped in standard fashion, and use of a T-tube for closure can be avoided. The best practice would be to address common bile duct stones during the initial operation, given the small but significant chance of unsuccessful postoperative ERCP. However, completion of the laparoscopic procedure without addressing the common bile duct stones and then immediately referring the patient for postoperative ERCP is also considered to be within the standard of practice.

Approximately 15% to 20% of patients will have variations in their biliary anatomy. A short cystic duct is the most relevant anomaly, which can lead the surgeon to mistake the common bile duct for the cystic duct and thereby lead to the inadvertent transection of the common bile duct. Misidentification of anatomy can also result from the common hepatic duct appearing in the same plane as the distal common bile duct and cystic duct. Obtaining the critical viewing angle to see behind the apparent cystic duct is designed to prevent this potential error. Given the high morbidity associated with common bile duct injury, any uncertainty regarding anatomy during a laparoscopic cholecystectomy should be considered an indication for conversion to an open procedure.

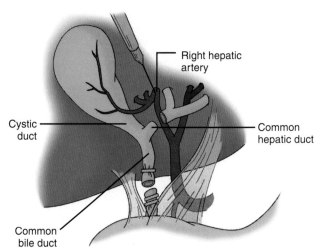

FIGURE 2   Classic laparoscopic bile duct injury. The common bile duct is mistaken for the cystic duct and transected. A variable extent of the extrahepatic biliary tree is resected with the gallbladder. The right hepatic artery, in the background, is also often injured. *(Reprinted from Lillemoe KD: Biliary injuries and strictures in sclerosing cholangitis. In: Mulholland MW, Lillemoe KD, Doherty GM, et al [eds]: Greenfield's surgery: scientific principles and practice, ed 4, Philadelphia, 2006, Lippincott Williams & Wilkins.)*

Alternatively, intraoperative cholangiography can also be used to better delineate anatomy, although cholangiography itself can injure the common bile duct if it is inadvertently cannulated instead of the cystic duct. Although in the past some surgeons advocated for the routine use of intraoperative cholangiography, almost all now prefer a more selective approach, using the modality only when common bile duct stones are suspected preoperatively (and have not yet been treated with ERCP), or when intraoperative anatomy is difficult to visualize. Inability of the patient to tolerate pneumoperitoneum or injury to a vital structure also mandates conversion to an open procedure. The rate of conversion from laparoscopic to open cholecystectomy has been reported in various studies to be between 0% and 20%.

Open Cholecystectomy

The open approach to cholecystectomy can be chosen initially based on surgeon preference with regard to patient comorbidities and previous abdominal operations that lead to high suspicion for significant intraabdominal adhesions. Open cholecystectomy can be performed through either a midline or subcostal incision. The use of two rolled laparotomy sponges is helpful in retracting the duodenum and hepatic flexure of the colon. A short Kocher clamp is placed on the fundus of the gallbladder, and a long Kocher clamp is put on the infundibulum. We use a fundus-down approach. The gallbladder is taken off the liver bed with electrocautery; as the dissection approaches the infundibulum, the cystic duct and cystic artery are separately encircled with 2-0 ties; after confirming that they are the only two structures entering the gallbladder, they are then divided. Care must be taken to avoid injury to the common hepatic duct when completing this fundus-down approach. Alternatively, the same direction of dissection used in laparoscopic cholecystectomy can also be used in the open procedure if preferred. One- or two-layered abdominal wall closure is performed.

There are no data to support the use of drains following routine laparoscopic or open cholecystectomy. Closed-suction drains can be placed intraoperatively when the surgeon perceives a significant risk of biliary leak. This is usually in circumstances of severe acute cholecystitis or in necrotizing/gangrenous cholecystitis, wherein the closure of the cystic duct stump may not be secure, or the hepatic parenchyma in the gallbladder fossa is severely inflamed.

Another minimally invasive option performed in some centers is the single-port laparoscopic cholecystectomy. This uses multiple flexible instruments that originate from a common, albeit larger, single port, and it otherwise follows the course of a standard laparoscopic procedure. This appears safe and appropriate in select patients. Natural orifice translumenal endoscopic surgery can be used to perform cholecystectomy with transgastric or transvaginal dissection and retrieval. Further evaluation is needed to validate the safety and outcomes of these newer approaches.

Postoperative care after a cholecystectomy should include rapid advancement of diet and appropriate pain control and prophylaxis for deep venous thrombosis. A brief in-patient stay is appropriate, and a slightly longer inpatient admission can be expected following an open cholecystectomy.

Complications

Complications from cholecystectomy include wound infection, bleeding, bile leak, hematoma, and incisional hernia. Abscesses can develop from intraoperative spillage of stones or bile, and therefore any stones or bile spilled during the operation should be retrieved or copiously irrigated and suctioned, respectively.

Minor and asymptomatic postoperative bile leaks are relatively common and typically resolve spontaneously. These minor leaks are thought to result from interruption of cholecystohepatic ducts (ducts of Luschka) when taking down the gallbladder's attachments to the liver. Abdominal pain and jaundice in the early postoperative period are concerning for a more significant bile leak from a common bile duct injury or from the cystic duct stump. Initial evaluation should include an ultrasound or CT scan to rule out intrahepatic biliary dilatation or a biloma, which would suggest a leak from the cystic or common bile duct. Neither CT nor ultrasound can definitively rule out an ongoing biliary leak. HIDA and ERCP can both visualize a leak from the cystic or common bile duct, but HIDA would be the initial test of choice, as it is a less invasive study. ERCP with sphincterotomy and stent placement is the treatment of choice for cystic duct leak.

A common bile duct injury should be repaired with a Roux-en-Y hepaticojejunostomy. When discovered intraoperatively, the repair should be completed immediately only if the surgeon is comfortable with advanced hepatobiliary surgery. If such a surgeon is not immediately available, the best approach is closure with drains followed by immediate referral to a tertiary center with surgical and radiological experience in biliary tract injuries.

Late complications of cholecystectomy include retained common bile duct stones or biliary stricture. A stone in the common duct postoperatively requires ERCP with sphincterotomy and possible stent placement. Postoperative biliary strictures are thought to result from ischemia of the bile duct caused by dissection and division of blood supply around the bile duct during cholecystectomy.

Special Populations

Several groups of patients deserve special mention. Elderly patients with acute cholecystitis may have minimal signs and symptoms. They may complain of vague symptoms, such as anorexia, but without complaints of pain; this makes diagnosis difficult. In critically ill patients under sedation or with altered consciousness, the usual signs and symptoms of acute cholecystitis are also frequently absent. More subtle findings, such as abnormal liver function tests, must therefore lead to investigation for acute cholecystitis in these patients. It is possible for an older patient to have a gangrenous gallbladder and yet still have no fever, a normal appetite, and few overt symptoms to suggest the severity of the illness. Urgent cholecystectomy in the elderly carries significantly higher mortality, whereas elective cholecystectomy in the elderly has the same low mortality as the general population, highlighting the importance of timely referral of symptomatic elderly patients with biliary colic for consideration of elective surgery.

In patients with cirrhosis, the morbidity and mortality of cholecystectomy is also increased. The reasons for this are multifactorial, including underlying coagulopathy or portal hypertension, possible thrombocytopenia from hypersplenism, and the potential for hepatic decompensation following surgery and general anesthesia. The firm character of the liver in these patients makes cephalolateral retraction of the liver difficult. For all of these reasons, there is an increased need for open cholecystectomy in patients with cirrhosis. In severe cases, significant bleeding can be limited by performing a partial cholecystectomy, in which the posterior portion of the gallbladder wall is left intact on the gallbladder fossa.

Acute cholecystitis that develops during pregnancy is best treated with laparoscopic cholecystectomy during the second trimester. Surgery during the first and third trimester is considerably more dangerous than during the second trimester. If acute cholecystitis develops during the first or third trimester, conservative treatment with intravenous antibiotics is therefore preferred, with delay of cholecystectomy until either the second trimester or the postpartum period, respectively. In severe cases of acute cholecystitis, however, management with immediate cholecystectomy is still required.

SUGGESTED READINGS

Bender JS, Duncan MD, Freeswick PD, et al: Increased laparoscopic experience does not lead to improved results with acute cholecystitis, *Am J Surg* 184:591–594, 2002.

Gurusamy KS, Samraj K: Early versus delayed laparoscopic cholecystectomy for acute cholecystitis, *Cochrane Database Syst Rev* (4):CD005440, 2006.

Kopetz ES, Magnuson TH, Duncan MD, et al: Complications of neglected cholelithiasis account for significant surgical mortality in the elderly, *Surg Forum* 51:489–491, 2000.

Magnuson TM, Bender JS, Duncan MD, et al: Utility of magnetic resonance cholangiography in the evaluation of biliary obstruction, *J Am Coll Surg* 189:63–72, 1999.

Marescaux J, Dallemagne B, Perretta S, et al: Surgery without scars: report of transluminal cholecystectomy in a human being, *Arch Surg* 142(9):823–827, 2007.

MANAGEMENT OF COMMON BILE DUCT STONES

Myriam J. Curet, MD

OVERVIEW

Choledocholithiasis occurs in approximately 10% to 15% of patients undergoing cholecystectomy. It is the second most common complication of cholelithiasis, and the incidence increases with age, being found in 30% to 50% of patients older than 70 years. Choledocholithiasis can lead to jaundice, cholangitis, and pancreatitis, and it represents a significant risk to patients.

The first successful common bile duct (CBD) exploration was performed in 1889, following several attempts that had all resulted in death. Some patients with choledocholithiasis (5% to 10%) may be completely asymptomatic with normal liver function tests. In these patients, if the stones are small and the ducts are not dilated, the stones can be left to pass spontaneously, although predicting which will pass successfully can be difficult. Some authors have stated that up to 30% of patients with CBD stones may pass them spontaneously with no intervention.

Some patients show signs and symptoms of CBD stones preoperatively, giving the patient and the surgeon the option of preoperative clearance of the CBD if desired. Evidence of possible choledocholithiasis includes enlarged CBD on ultrasound, imaging of a CBD stone on ultrasound, gallstone pancreatitis, or elevated levels of aspartate aminotransferase, alanine aminotransferase, lactate dehydrogenase, and bilirubin on liver function tests. A patient with two or more elevated liver function test results is more likely to have CBD stones.

Before surgery in patients with suspected choledocholithiasis, the surgeon may decide to image and potentially clear the CBD preoperatively with an endoscopic retrograde cholangiopancreatogram (ERCP) and endoscopic sphincterotomy. ERCP was first reported in 1974 and is now used widely for a variety of disease states. This approach requires a skilled endoscopist and coordination between the endoscopist and the surgeon. ERCP has a successful ductal clearance rate of 80% to 90%, although a normal exam can be found in 40% of patients with suspected CBD stones. The procedure does have risks (5% to 15% morbidity and 0% to 2% mortality) and significant costs associated with it. Alternatively, the surgeon also has the option of obtaining an intraoperative cholangiogram and clearing the CBD intraoperatively. Laparoscopic common bile duct exploration (CBDE) has not been adopted as rapidly and is not as widespread as laparoscopic cholecystectomy. Barriers to adoption include insufficient expertise, time constraints, and inadequate equipment.

Intraoperative cholangiogram (IOC) is helpful in determining whether choledocholithiasis is present. It can also be used to ensure proper identification of the anatomy and to identify bile duct injuries. Indications for IOC include suspected CBD stones and unclear anatomy. Some surgeons use IOC routinely during all laparoscopic cholecystectomies to decrease the incidence of inadvertent and unsuspected CBD transection. If used selectively, an IOC should be obtained in patients who have a history of jaundice, pancreatitis, or elevated liver function test results, as mentioned above. An intraoperative cholangiogram can be performed through an existing laparoscopic port or through a separate stab wound. Several catheters are available for this: some have a balloon at the tip, which can help hold the catheter in place, and others are stiffer, which may make them easier to insert.

After the cystic duct is identified and dissected circumferentially, a clip is placed across the cystic duct just below the gallbladder–cystic duct junction. A small ductotomy is then created below the

clip. A cholangiocatheter is inserted under direct visualization, either through one of the existing ports or through a percutaneously placed sheath in the right upper quadrant approximately at the midclavicular line; it is held in place either with a clamp, by inflating the balloon, or with a clip. The IOC is then obtained, preferably with fluoroscopy rather than with a static image.

It is critically important to identify both right and left hepatic ducts as well as the CBD. In addition, flow of dye into the duodenum should be demonstrated. If the left and right hepatic ducts are not immediately visualized, the patient can be placed in a Trendelenburg position and given morphine sulfate to spasm the sphincter of Oddi, which may help dye flow proximally. If these steps do not visualize the proximal ducts, the patient should be converted to an open procedure to make sure no ductal injury has occurred. If the proximal ducts are visualized, but dye does not flow into the duodenum freely, the patient can be positioned in a Trendelenburg position and given glucagon to relax the sphincter.

If a CBD stone is diagnosed, the surgeon can either obtain a postoperative ERCP or proceed with a CBDE, making sure that all the instruments needed for a CBDE are available, including the choledochoscope, helical stone baskets, biliary balloon catheters, syringes, and fluoroscopy. Because there are several ways to perform a CBDE, if the surgeon does not have the expertise and experience to do so laparoscopically, it is best to convert to an open procedure. If the surgeon chooses to proceed with a laparoscopic CBDE, then the CBD can be accessed via a transcystic approach or through a direct choledochotomy. In either case, use of a choledochoscope will be helpful; using separate monitor to display the choledochoscope image is much easier than switching the laparoscopic monitor back and forth.

A transcystic exploration is easier to perform than a direct choledochotomy, as it does not require suture repair. It is the preferred technique for most surgeons who perform a laparoscopic CBDE. The surgeon should use the IOC to help determine how many stones are present, their diameter, and the diameter of the bile ducts. The transcystic approach is most likely to be successful if the CBD is less than 6 mm in diameter, if the cystic duct is dilated, and if the CBD stones are small (less than 6 mm) and located in the CBD rather than in the common hepatic duct. The ductotomy used for the IOC is used for the CBDE as well. The surgeon can begin by flushing saline forcefully through the cholangiocatheter. This is often successful for small stones less than 2 to 3 mm. Relaxing the sphincter of Oddi with 1 to 2 mg of glucagon can improve success rates. The surgeon can repeatedly and forcefully flush the catheter until the small stones are cleared.

If flushing is unsuccessful, the surgeon can move on to transcystic insertion of a stone basket through the cystic duct into the CBD under fluoroscopic guidance (Figure 1). Passage of a biliary balloon catheter with an inflated diameter of 8 mm can also be attempted. Fluoroscopic insertion of a guidewire first may help facilitate insertion of the stone baskets or balloon catheters. The guidewires, baskets, and catheters can be inserted through the percutaneously placed sheath used for the IOC, through one of the laparoscopic ports, or through a 14 gauge angiocatheter placed in the right upper quadrant. Sometimes placement of a fifth trocar is necessary. This trocar should be placed close to the right costal margin lateral to the midclavicular line. Use of a balloon catheter can result in dragging stones into the common hepatic duct, which can make retrieval more difficult.

If these techniques do not work, or if the surgeon prefers, a 2.5 or 3 mm choledochoscope with a 1.2 working channel can be used via the cystic duct. The cystic duct may be too small and may need to be dilated. Dilation should begin with placement of a guidewire into the cystic duct. Generally, dilation up to 7 to 8 mm can be done with the passage of progressively larger ureteral bougies. Occasionally, dilation with a balloon catheter will be successful. The choledochoscope can be inserted through the fifth port, which allows the other ports to be used for retraction and guidance.

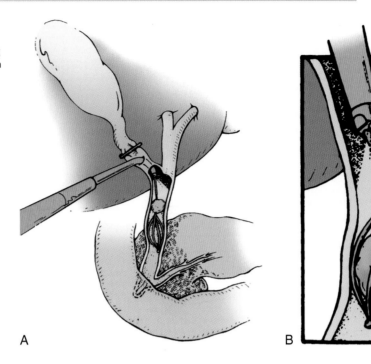

A   B

The scope is passed over the guidewire into the common bile duct under direct visualization, which is enhanced with continuous saline irrigation though the choledochoscope. The stones are retrieved with a helical stone basket passed through the choledochoscope, but occasionally the scope may be used to push stones through the ampulla of Vater. Visualization of the proximal ducts can be difficult with a choledochoscope passed through the cystic duct, however, it is critical to demonstrate a clear duct prior to completing the CBDE. This can be done with the choledochoscope by passing the scope through the ampulla of Vater into the duodenum. A completion IOC should be obtained to demonstrate clearance of the stones and dye in the duodenum. Following completion of the transcystic CBDE, the cystic duct is secured with endoloops or clips; endoloops and suturing offer a more secure closure.

This technique is highly successful and has been reported to be associated with a 70% to 90% success rate. Complication rates range from 0% to 10% and include cystic duct stump leaks, pancreatitis, or bile duct injury. Retained stones are found in 2% to 4% of patients, and the risks are higher in patients with stones in the proximal bile ducts.

If the cystic duct is too small or tortuous, the CBD stones are too large (>8 mm), or the stones are in the proximal ducts, a CBDE through a direct CBD ductotomy is a good option. It is a more technically difficult procedure than a transcystic approach and requires advanced laparoscopic and suturing skills. The technique is effective, and stones up to 10 to 15 mm can be successfully removed if the CBD is dilated. As with transcystic CBDE, the surgeon may need to place an additional port for adequate access.

First, the anterior surface of the CBD is exposed by following the cystic duct onto the CBD. Once the CBD is exposed, needle aspiration of bile can confirm its correct identification. The surgeon should begin by placing two stay sutures at 3 and 9 o'clock on the common bile duct for traction, as is done with open CBDE. The ductotomy is then created with scissors on the anterior surface along the vertical axis. The sides of the CBD should be avoided to preserve the blood supply. The ductotomy is generally 10 to 20 mm in length and should be at least as long as the diameter of the largest stone.

Once the CBD has been accessed, many surgeons begin by flushing it with a large, 14 Fr catheter, which is passed into the ductotomy through the fifth port (Figure 2). This maneuver often clears the duct, especially with smaller, mobile stones. If this is unsuccessful,

the surgeon can proceed with passage of the biliary balloon catheter, helical stone basket, and choledochoscope through the ductotomy as described above. Fluoroscopy should be used when passing guidewires, balloon catheters, or baskets, and it is often best to proceed directly to the use of a choledochoscope. In this case, a larger (5 mm) choledochoscope can be used; a larger scope provides better illumination and allows for use of larger instruments, which can improve success rates of ductal clearance.

The scope is inserted through the fifth port, as it is with the transcystic approach. Ensuring complete clearance of the duct is critical. Most surgeons will close the ductotomy over a T-tube, although reports of closing it without a T-tube in patients with a markedly distended CBD have been described. Generally a 10 to 14 Fr T-tube is used, cut to the appropriate length. Some surgeons open the T back, and others do not. The T-tube is placed through the fifth port and passed into the CBD, and the ductotomy is closed snugly around the T-tube with interrupted absorbable sutures (Figure 3). A completion T-tube cholangiogram is obtained to confirm no filling defects and no leak from the choledochotomy.

In experienced hands, success rates of 80% to 90% have been reported with this procedure. Complication rates range from 5% to 15% and include bile duct injury, pancreatitis, and bile leak around the T-tube. The T-tube can be removed approximately 10 days postoperatively, and some surgeons will obtain a T-tube cholangiogram prior to removal to ensure that no further CBD access is needed. There is a small risk of bile duct stricture following laparoscopic choledochotomy with both primary closure and T-tube closure.

If the surgeon is unable to successfully clear the CBD with either a transcystic approach or through a choledochotomy, there is still the option of completing the laparoscopic cholecystectomy and sending the patient for a postoperative ERCP or converting to an open CBDE and cholecystectomy. A single-stage laparoscopic approach to removing the gallbladder and clearing the CBD stones is preferred to combining a laparoscopic cholecystectomy with a postoperative ERCP and endoscopic sphincterectomy (ES). Data have proven that a single-stage procedure is less expensive and is associated with a shorter hospital stay. In addition, ERCP can fail to clear the duct in 5% to 10% of patients, and these patients may then need a second operation for an open CBDE. If the duct cannot be cleared laparoscopically, and the surgeon decides to proceed with

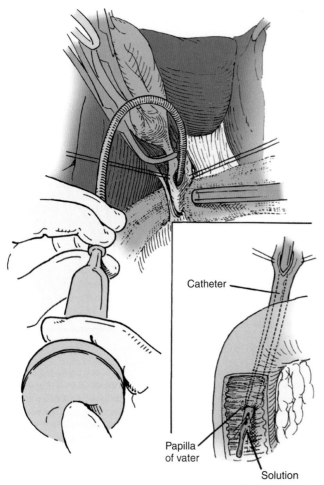

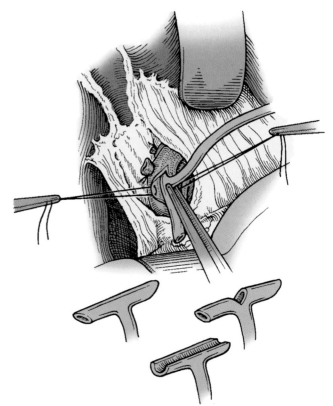

FIGURE 2   The CBD is irrigated with normal saline flushed through a rubber catheter. *(From Zollinger RM, Jr, Zollinger RM: Atlas of surgical operations, ed 7, New York, 1993, McGraw-Hill.)*

FIGURE 3   The T-tube is inserted into the CBD, and the choledochotomy incision is closed around it with fine absorbable sutures in a watertight fashion. *(From Zollinger RM Jr, Zollinger RM: Atlas of surgical operations, ed 7, New York, 1993, McGraw-Hill.)*

postoperative ERCP and ES, the surgeon could place a guidewire or stent through the sphincter of Oddi to facilitate identification and access during the postoperative ERCP.

With the widespread use of ERCP, open CBDE is an uncommon procedure. If the patient has a small duct (<5 mm), CBDE should be avoided; the small stones can be allowed to pass spontaneously, or the surgeon can proceed with a postoperative ERCP. If the surgeon decides to perform an open CBDE, the abdomen should be opened through a right subcostal incision. A self-retaining retractor should be used to help with exposure, and a wide Kocher maneuver should be performed to help identify and manipulate the CBD and the stones. As with laparoscopic choledochotomy, the surgeon follows the cystic duct to its junction with the CBD to help expose and identify the CBD, which can be aspirated with a small needle to help with identification. The surgeon then places two absorbable stay sutures in the CBD at the 3 and 9 o'clock positions.

Next, a 10 to 20 mm long ductotomy is created on the vertical axis, just opposite or slightly below the insertion of the cystic duct. The surgeon begins with flushing the CBD vigorously through a 14 Fr red rubber catheter (Figure 2). Stones palpated more distally can be milked to the ductotomy, and the surgeon can then proceed with use of biliary balloon catheters or with stone forceps to clear the duct. During insertion of catheters or forceps, the surgeon should place one hand behind the head of the pancreas to help guide the instrument into the duct to prevent bile duct injury. Most surgeons prefer to directly visualize the CBD with a 55 mm choledochoscope.

Saline should be infused continuously to keep visualization as clear as possible. If stones are visualized, they can be removed with passage of baskets through the working channel as previously described.

Although it is not done with a laparoscopic CBDE, most surgeons performing an open CBDE will make sure the ampulla is patent. This can be done with a biliary Fogarty balloon catheter, which is passed into the duodenum; the balloon is then inflated and pulled back through the ampulla. Alternatively, the surgeon can pass a Bakes dilator gently through the ampulla, while holding the head of the pancreas and the ampulla to help guide it safely. When it has passed through the ampulla, the Bakes dilator should be seen through the wall of the duodenum; complete clearance of the duct should be demonstrated with the use of the choledochoscope.

Finally, the duct is closed over a 14 Fr T-tube inserted through one of the port sites or through a separate stab wound. The T-tube is prepared as described above. Care should be taken to not insert the T-tube limb into the duodenum, as this can cause pancreatitis. The choledochotomy is closed with interrupted absorbable sutures in a watertight fashion. A completion T-tube cholangiogram should be obtained prior to completing the operation.

Occasionally, surgeons will encounter an impacted stone. Lithotripsy can be used to break up larger stones that are not amenable to extraction with the techniques described above. Small stones or stone fragments can be flushed into the duodenum after administration of glucagons, or the small fragments can be extracted with the techniques described above. Duodenotomy and sphincteroplasty have been described but are rarely performed and should only be attempted by an experienced surgeon. If the stone cannot be removed, a T-tube should be inserted and the cholecystectomy completed. The patient can then be referred for endoscopic or percutaneous extraction of the stone.

Suggested Readings

Bove A, Bongarzoni G, Palone G, et al: Why is there recurrence after transcystic laparoscopic bile duct clearance? Risk factor analysis, *Surg Endosc* 23:1470–1475, 2009.

Kroh M, Chand B: Choledocholithiasis, endoscopic retrograde cholangiopancreatography, and laparoscopic common bile duct exploration, *Surg Clin North Am* 88:1019–1031, 2008.

Phillips EH, Toouli J, Pitt HA, Soper NJ: Treatment of common bile duct stones discovered during cholecystectomy, *J Gastrointest Surg* 12:624–628, 2008.

Stromberg C, Nilsson M, Leijonmarck CE: Stone clearance and risk factors for failure in laparoscopic transcystic exploration of the common bile duct, *Surg Endosc* 22:1194–1199, 2008.

Tinoco R, Tinoco A, El-Kadre L, et al: Laparoscopic common bile duct exploration, *Ann Surg* 247:674–679, 2008.

Verbesey JE, Birkett DH: Common bile duct exploration for choledocholithiasis, *Surg Clin North Am* 88:1315–1328, 2008.

Acute Cholangitis

Sreenivasa Jonnalagadda, MD, and Steven M. Strasberg, MD

OVERVIEW

Acute cholangitis is a morbid condition characterized by acute inflammation and infection in the bile duct. It usually occurs in association with obstruction of the biliary tree. The clinical severity can range from mild disease to a potentially life-threatening state accompanied by septic shock and multiorgan dysfunction. Because of the propensity for rapid deterioration among patients with untreated acute cholangitis, expeditious diagnosis and therapy are essential to good patient outcome. The recent publication of the Tokyo Guidelines for the management of acute cholangitis and cholecystitis has brought an evidence-based approach to the definition, diagnosis, and management of this condition.

EPIDEMIOLOGY

The median age of patients diagnosed with acute cholangitis is reported to range from 50 to 60 years, and incidence increases with age. The most important risk factors are biliary stasis or obstruction, for which the most prevalent etiology is choledocholithiasis. In much of the world, secondary choledocholithiasis, caused by stones originating in the gallbladder, predominates; in Southeast Asia, however, where Oriental cholangiohepatitis is endemic, primary choledocholithiasis is an important cause of cholangitis. Other benign and malignant etiologies of acute cholangitis are listed in Table 1.

PATHOGENESIS AND RISK FACTORS

Mechanisms postulated to help maintain the normal sterility of the biliary tract include 1) an intact sphincter of Oddi that prevents reflux of duodenal contents into the common bile duct, 2) unimpeded *efflux* of bile from the common bile duct, 3) the presence of immunoglobulin A in bile, and 4) the bacteriostatic properties of bile salts. When one or more of these defenses is breached—or if a foreign body is present in the biliary tract, where it can serve as a nidus for infection—cholangitis may ensue. The presence of a foreign body such as a stone, fluke, or stent provides a protective niche for bacteria such as *Escherichia coli,* which secrete β-glucuronidase. This enzyme deconjugates bilirubin glucuronide and the resultant poorly soluble unconjugated bilirubin precipitates in bile, adding to the foreign body load and leading to brown pigment microstones. Eventually the

stage of contamination may evolve to frank infection, and repeated bouts of such infection lead to the end stage of stones, strictures, and parenchymal fibrosis and destruction (secondary biliary cirrhosis).

Most cases are thought to arise from direct ascent of bacteria from the duodenum into the common bile duct; hematogenous seeding of the biliary tract via the portal vein is likely to play only a minor role. Bacterial proliferation within the biliary tract, together with its entry into the systemic circulation via lymphatic and venous channels, results in the infectious manifestations of acute cholangitis. Biliary obstruction is typically a prerequisite for the development of suppurative cholangitis.

Cultures of bile, intraductal stones, or indwelling stents from patients with acute cholangitis indicate a polymicrobial infection in most patients, with bowel flora being the most common isolates. The most commonly identified gram-negative bacteria are *E. coli* (in 25% to 50% of patients), *Klebsiella* spp. (in 15% to 20%), and *Enterobacter* spp. (5% to 10%). The most commonly isolated gram-positive bacteria are *Enterococcus* spp. (10% to 20%).

The contribution of anaerobes such as *Bacteroides* and *Clostridium* spp. to the pathogenesis of acute cholangitis is controversial; however, they are commonly cultured in specimens obtained from elderly patients and in those who have undergone biliary tract instrumentation. Although bacteria are responsible for the great majority of cases of acute cholangitis, other pathogens—such as helminths,

TABLE 1: Etiologies of acute cholangitis

Noniatrogenic
Benign conditions
Choledocholithiasis
  Primary
  Secondary
Pancreatitis (chronic/acute), including pancreatic pseudocyst
Papillary stenosis
Mirizzi syndrome
Choledochal cysts (type V, Caroli disease)
Primary sclerosing cholangitis
Malignancies
Pancreatic cancer
Cholangiocarcinoma
Porta hepatis tumor/metastasis
Iatrogenic
Obstructed biliary endoprosthesis
Iatrogenic biliary stricture
  Direct surgical trauma
  Ischemia-induced stricture
Anastomotic stricture (biliobiliary/bilioenteric anastomosis)

fungi, and viruses (e.g., cytomegalovirus and Epstein-Barr virus)—can cause this syndrome. These organisms should be considered in the appropriate clinical setting, such as in areas where parasitic infections are endemic and among immunocompromised individuals.

Biliary instrumentation via an endoscopic or percuteneous route, choledocholithiasis, and benign and malignant biliary strictures all are risk factors for the development of ascending cholangitis. This is particularly the case when an indwelling biliary stent or drain gets obstructed and serves as a nidus for infection.

CLINICAL PRESENTATION

In 1877, Jean Charcot described the hallmarks of acute cholangitis: fever, jaundice, and right upper quadrant abdominal pain. All three features of this eponymous triad are present in only about 50% of patients with acute cholangitis (range in reports is from 15% to 75%). Jaundice is the most common symptom, present in 90% of patients, with fever and abdominal pain being less prevalent, present in 66%. Reynold's pentad, described by Reynold and Dargon in 1959, denotes the presence of mental status derangements and hypotension, in addition to features of Charcot's triad, and is suggestive of severe disease and systemic sepsis. It is present in only about 5% of patients.

DIAGNOSIS

Acute cholangitis is a clinical diagnosis that is based on the presence of the clinical features discussed earlier, together with supportive findings revealed by laboratory tests and radiographic studies. Because acute cholangitis can present without abdominal pain, particularly in elderly patients, absence of pain or of any of the individual symptoms and signs discussed earlier does not rule out this diagnosis. Acute cholangitis, therefore, should also be considered in septic patients without abdominal pain or tenderness who have attendant risk factors, such as choledocholithiasis or biliary strictures, with or without history of instrumentation. The diagnosis can be "suspected" or "definite" based on clinical presentation, laboratory tests, and imaging findings according to the Tokyo Guidelines (Table 2).

Along with the diagnosis, it is important to perform a severity grading of the condition, as that will affect management. The severity grading system proposed in the Tokyo Guidelines is shown in Table 3. It is based on response to initial treatment with antibiotics as well as on the presence or absence of infection-induced organ failure.

The differential diagnosis includes other conditions associated with right upper quadrant abdominal pain, jaundice, and fever; these include cholecystitis, liver abscess, and hepatitis. Laboratory test findings typically associated with acute cholangitis include leukocytosis with neutrophilia and liver function test abnormalities suggestive of cholestasis (e.g., increased serum alkaline phosphatase, γ-glutamyl transpeptidase, and conjugated bilirubin concentrations). Increased serum aminotransferase concentrations can also occur with acute liver injury resulting from cholangitis-induced hepatic microabscess formation, and serum amylase concentrations are elevated in up to 30% of patients with acute cholangitis.

Blood cultures should be performed in all patients suspected of having cholangitis. In addition, cultures of bile aspirated from percutaneous biliary catheters or obtained during endoscopic retrograde cholangiopancreatography (ERCP) and of any indwelling biliary prostheses that are removed may be useful.

Imaging studies play an important role in patients with suspected acute cholangitis: 1) they can confirm the presence of dilated bile ducts, a finding present in most cases of acute cholangitis; 2) they may reveal the specific etiology responsible for biliary obstruction, such as choledocholithiasis; 3) they can exclude other conditions in the differential diagnosis, such as acute cholecystitis; and 4) they can be used to guide therapeutic interventions, such as biliary drainage or removal of an obstructed biliary stent.

TABLE 2: Diagnostic criteria for acute cholangitis: Tokyo Guidelines

A. Clinical Context and Clinical Manifestations
   1. History of biliary disease
   2. Fever and/or chills
   3. Jaundice
   4. Abdominal pain (right upper quadrant or upper abdominal)
B. Laboratory Data
   5. Evidence of inflammatory response*
   6. Abnormal liver function tests†
C. Imaging Findings
   7. Biliary dilatation or evidence of an etiology (stricture, stone, stent, etc.)

Suspected diagnosis: Two or more items in A
Definite diagnosis:
   (a) Charcot's triad (2 + 3 + 4)
   (b) Two or more items in A + both items in B + C

*Abnormal white blood cell count, increased serum C-reactive protein level, and other changes indicating inflammation
†Increased serum alkaline phosphatase, γ-glutamyl transpeptidase, aspartate aminotransferase, and alanine aminotransferase levels.
From Tokyo Guidelines for the management of acute cholangitis and cholecystitis, *J Hepatobiliary Pancreat Surg* 14:1–126, 2007.

TABLE 3: Severity assessment criteria for acute cholangitis: Tokyo Guidelines

Mild (grade I) acute cholangitis, defined as acute cholangitis that responds to initial medical treatment*
Moderate (grade II) acute cholangitis, defined as acute cholangitis that does not respond to the initial medical treatment* and is not associated with organ dysfunction
Severe (grade III) acute cholangitis, defined as acute cholangitis associated with the onset of dysfunction in at least one of the following organs/systems:
1. Cardiovascular system: Hypotension requiring dopamine >5 µg/kg per min or any dose of dobutamine
2. Nervous system: Disturbance of consciousness
3. Respiratory system: PaO_2/FiO_2 ratio <300
4. Kidney: Serum creatinine >2.0 mg/dL
5. Liver: Prothrombin International Normalized Ratio >1.5
6. Hematologic system: Platelet count <100,000/µL

NOTE: Compromised patients (e.g., patients >75 years and patients with medical comorbidities) should be closely monitored.
*General supportive care and antibiotics.
From Tokyo Guidelines for the management of acute cholangitis and cholecystitis, *J Hepatobiliary Pancreat Surg* 14:1–126, 2007.

Transabdominal ultrasonography is the best initial imaging study in most patients with suspected acute cholangitis. It is noninvasive, rapid, cost effective, and highly sensitive in the detection of biliary tract dilation. However, the absence of biliary tract dilation does not rule out acute cholangitis, especially if the ultrasound is obtained soon after acute onset of biliary obstruction, before the bile ducts have had time to dilate. Remember also that transabdominal ultrasonography is associated with relatively low sensitivity in the detection of choledocholithiasis, particularly when small stones are present in the distal bile duct.

In most patients with acute cholangitis, ultrasonography should be followed by endoscopic ERCP, because it allows for both direct cholangiography and therapeutic intervention. Lack of availability or failure of ERCP should prompt percutaneous transhepatic cholangiography (PTC). Patients with indwelling biliary catheters (e.g., T-tubes or U-tubes) can undergo cholangiography with contrast instilled into these tubes, if they are externally accessible. The therapeutic roles of ERCP and PTC will be discussed.

Computed tomography (CT) scanning can reveal biliary tract dilation, and it allows for global assessment of intraabdominal pathology, but it has poor sensitivity in the detection of intraductal stones. Magnetic resonance cholangiopancreatography (MRCP) has greater sensitivity for choledocholithiasis than CT, however, the prolonged duration of MRCP examinations limits their application in unstable patients. MRCP is an excellent choice for the evaluation of the bile duct in patients with a low index of suspicion for biliary pathology. Endoscopic ultrasonography (EUS) is another imaging option with very high sensitivity for choledocholithiasis. Because CT, MRCP, and EUS do not offer therapeutic capability, ERCP should not be delayed to obtain these imaging studies unless diagnostic uncertainty or relative contraindications to ERCP exist.

THERAPY

Therapy for acute cholangitis consists of three main components: 1) *resuscitation,* 2) *antibiotics,* and 3) *biliary drainage* (Figure 1). Resuscitation with administration of intravenous fluids and correction of electrolyte abnormalities should be initiated without delay. Given that urgent interventional or surgical procedures are likely to be required, attention should be directed to identifying and correcting coagulopathies that may exist (e.g., those resulting from vitamin K deficiency or sepsis-induced thrombocytopenia). Vigilant monitoring to ensure adequacy of resuscitation and early recognition of clinical deterioration, such as shock or mental status abnormalities, is essential. High-risk patients with significant comorbidities are best monitored in a dedicated intensive care unit, where invasive monitoring and inotropic support can be instituted.

Antimicrobial agents should be administered to patients with suspected acute cholangitis as soon as possible, and treatment should be tailored appropriately once culture results become available. The antibiotics used initially should be effective against both gram-negative and gram-positive bacteria, especially *Enterococcus* spp. Factors to be considered in selecting antibiotics include the severity of the cholangitis, the agent's activity against potentially active bacteria, the presence or absence of liver and kidney disease, the patient's recent history of antimicrobial therapy, and culture results if available.

Activity against infecting isolates is of greatest importance; biliary penetration of the antibiotics is secondary. One useful first-line regimen for the empiric therapy of acute cholangitis is the combination of a fluoroquinolone (e.g., levofloxacin) with metronidazole. Metronidazole is used in this setting despite the low frequency with which anaerobes are isolated from bile cultures; this is because 1) standard culture techniques underestimate the true prevalence of anaerobic infections, 2) anaerobes are prevalent in cultures of bile obtained from some patient groups (e.g., those with prior biliary instrumentation), and 3) metronidazole has a favorable safety profile.

Other antibiotics appropriate for empiric therapy include the combination of ampicillin and gentamicin, carbapenems (imipenem and meropenem), extended-spectrum penicillins (piperacillin), and penicillin–β-lactamase inhibitor combinations (piperacillin-tazobactam, ampicillin-sulbactam, ticarcillin clavulanate). Given the substantial risk of aminoglycoside-induced nephrotoxicity, we prefer to avoid gentamicin-based regimens unless specific reasons for their administration exist. Although they provide excellent activity against gram-negative bacteria, second- and third-generation cephalosporins

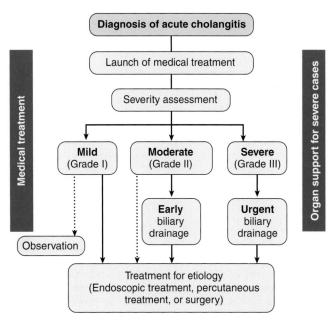

FIGURE 1 Flowchart for management of acute cholecystitis. Antibiotic treatment is commenced prior to staging. *Dashed lines* indicate that some patients with mild cholangitis require no definitve treatment (e.g., postopertative cholangitis). For some patients with moderate cholangitis, biliary drainage is the definitive treatment. *(From Miura F, Takada T, Kawarada Y, et al: Flowcharts for the diagnosis and treatment of acute cholangitis and cholecystitis: Tokyo Guidelines, J Hepatobiliary Pancreat Surg 14:27–34, 2007.)*

provide poor coverage against *Enterococcus* species and are therefore not recommended.

With resuscitation and empiric antibiotic therapy, up to 85% of patients with acute cholangitis improve, even in the absence of other interventions. The duration of antibiotic therapy should be based on clinical response; for patients documented to have bacteremia, antibiotic courses lasting 1 to 2 weeks are recommended.

Mild Acute Cholangitis

Patients with mild acute cholangitis are defined as those who respond to initial treatment with antibiotics. Unless they relapse such patients require no further treatment beyond that for the underlying condition, and some patients with mild postoperative cholangitis require no other treatment. However, relapse after initial good response requires biliary drainage.

Moderate Acute Cholangitis

By definition, patients with moderate acute cholangitis do not have a satisfactory response to initial treatment with antibiotics, and they require biliary drainage. In some cases the biliary drainage deals with the underlying cause, but when it does not, subsequent treatment of the underlying problem is required. Unsatisfactory responses include continuation or worsening of pain, fever, or leukocytosis over a 12 to 24 hour period or the onset of organ failure at any time.

Severe Acute Cholangitis

Patients with severe acute cholangitis require organ support, usually in an ICU setting, combined with administration of antibiotics and planned urgent biliary decompression. If necessary, treatment of the underlying cause is staged at a later date, after full recovery from the cholangitis.

Techniques of Biliary Drainage

Endoscopic Drainage

This is the first-line method for establishing drainage. ERCP is effective in establishing biliary drainage in 90% to 98% of patients. In procedures performed for acute cholangitis, bile should be aspirated from the common bile duct to decompress it before injection of contrast for cholangiography. Occlusive cholangiography performed before ductal decompression, particularly in cases of suppurative cholangitis, can induce bacteremia, sepsis, and rapid decompensation.

For patients in whom endoscopic sphincterotomy is contraindicated, such as those with persistent coagulopathy, temporizing biliary drainage can be achieved by placement of a nasobiliary drain or an internal biliary stent without sphincterotomy. For instance, a 10 Fr or smaller internal biliary stent can be safely placed across the major papilla without need for a biliary sphincterotomy. If biliary access at ERCP is unsuccessful, an additional modality in some centers is EUS-directed access of the biliary tree, followed by biliary drainage using this access. However, this is a consideration only in patients who are stable, and the same results can be achieved by PTC. Other therapeutic applications facilitated by ERCP in patients with acute cholangitis include replacement of obstructed biliary stents and stenting and/or dilation of benign biliary strictures.

Percutaneous Transhepatic Drainage

This somewhat more invasive approach is reserved for patients who fail ERCP or in whom there is no endoscopic access, or access is very difficult, to the biliary tree, as in patients who have had a hepaticojejunostomy, a proximal biliary obstruction caused by a hilar cholangiocarcinoma, or large periampullary duodenal diverticula. Intrahepatic biliary obstruction resulting from hepatolithiasis is another indication. When needed, percutaneous transhepatic drainage is also effective at providing biliary drainage.

Surgical Drainage

Surgical drainage, once the mainstay of treatment, fell out of favor because of poorer outcomes from this more invasive procedure in sometimes very ill patients. It is mainly of historical interest, but when needed, it involves a choledochotomy and placement of a large (16 Fr or greater if possible) T-tube in the bile duct. Definitive therapy should be delayed to a later time. In this context, surgery may play an important role in the definitive management of diverse conditions such as Mirizzi syndrome, cholelithiasis, and benign and malignant biliary strictures.

SUGGESTED READING

Tokyo Guidelines for the management of acute cholangitis and cholecystitis, J Hepatobiliary Pancreat Surg 14(1):1-126, 2007.

BENIGN BILIARY STRICTURES

Theodore N. Pappas, MD, and Eugene P. Ceppa, MD

OVERVIEW

Benign biliary strictures remain one of the more complex challenges facing general surgeons. The etiologies of benign biliary strictures are numerous; these include iatrogenic injury of the bile duct, inflammatory conditions, traumatic injuries, and congenital abnormalities. However, iatrogenic biliary strictures remain overwhelmingly the most common etiology. More than 750,000 laparoscopic cholecystectomies are performed annually in the United States, which accounts for 90% of all cholecystectomies; however, the inception of laparoscopic cholecystectomy has increased the occurrence of biliary stricture secondary to iatrogenic injury.

Common bile duct (CBD) injury has reached a plateau, evidenced by the frequency and distribution of bile duct injuries identified by endoscopic retrograde cholangiopancreatography (ERCP) at high-volume institutions; injury occurs at a rate of 0.4% to 0.6% following laparoscopic cholecystectomy, compared with a rate of 0.2% to 0.3% following open cholecystectomy. Some data suggest that the incidence of bile duct injury has decreased following improved laparoscopic experience, but it more likely depends on the individual surgeon's operative volume.

Other biliary tract surgeries make up the minority of iatrogenic injuries. A predisposition of bile duct stenosis can occur following other surgical procedures, including biliary reconstruction (choledochal cyst excision), extrinsic biliary duct inflammation (gastrectomy), or ischemic strictures from devascularization of the bile

duct (hepatic resection). Other well known but uncommon noniatrogenic etiologies of benign biliary strictures exist, such as chronic cholecystitis, chronic pancreatitis, trauma, and bacterial, parasitic, protozoal, or viral infections. Nevertheless, a CBD injury is a serious complication attributed to a technical misadventure during a laparoscopic cholecystectomy. The associated stress of this complication increases the emotional, financial, and health care burden to correct the problem.

MECHANISMS OF LAPAROSCOPIC CHOLECYSTECTOMY–INDUCED BILE DUCT INJURY

The incidence and mechanism of bile duct injuries have been investigated and summarized over the last two decades. Several technical factors appear to augment the risk of injury during laparoscopic cholecystectomy. The most convincing aspect appears to be the exaggerated cephalad retraction of the gallbladder fundus, resulting in a distortion of the plane between the cystic and common bile ducts. Specifically, the duct structures are parallel instead of perpendicular in orientation. This leads to the classic pattern as reported by Branum and colleagues, where the CBD is mistaken for the cystic duct and subsequently clipped and divided. The injury occurs just distal to the common hepatic duct–cystic duct junction (Figure 1). Several factors have been attributed as causes, including surgeon inexperience, inflammation, inadequate lateral inferior retraction, a short cystic duct, and use of a zero-degree laparoscope. The gallbladder is retracted superiorly to remove it from the gallbladder fossa of the liver. This maneuver elevates the common hepatic duct that is still attached via the cystic duct. The dissection is carried cephalad and posterior to the common hepatic duct until it is divided close to the hilar plate. Because of the plane of dissection, an injury of the right hepatic artery can also be seen.

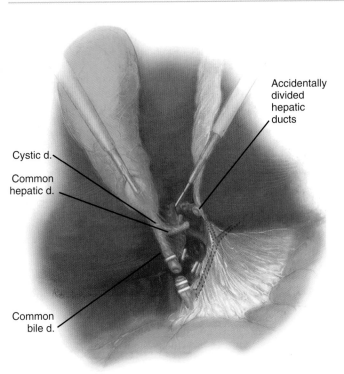

Cystic d.

Common
hepatic d.

Common
bile d.

Accidentally
divided
hepatic
ducts

FIGURE 1 Classic injury pattern during laparoscopic cholecystectomy. Mistaking the common duct for the cystic duct leads to excision of a length of common duct. *(From Branum G, Schmitt C, Baille J, et al: Management of major biliary complications after laparoscopic cholecystectomy, Ann Surg 217:532, 1993.)*

Another injury pattern consists of placement of proximal clips on the cystic duct and distal clips on the CBD. Upon division the gallbladder is removed, and the patient is left with a cystic stump leak and a distal CBD obstruction. An alternative and less common injury pattern includes excision of a segment of the CBD attached to the cystic duct, which presents with either biliary leak or biliary obstruction.

Neither routine nor selective intraoperative cholangiography has been proven to prevent bile duct injury during laparoscopic cholecystectomy. This remains a controversial topic. However, routine cholangiography does increase intraoperative recognition of a CBD injury. In patients with unclear anatomy, cholangiography via the gallbladder should assist in identifying the ductal anatomy. Otherwise, poor visualization is an indication for conversion to an open procedure.

ANATOMIC CONSIDERATIONS

Biliary anatomy has a wide variation due to the numerous abnormalities associated with both the extrahepatic biliary ducts and arterial vascular supply. Variation in ductal and vascular anatomy adds considerable operative risk. Upon inspection of the ductal anatomy, an anomalous low-lying segmental duct can be mistaken for the cystic duct. The right hepatic duct has a short extrahepatic course and a highly variable branching pattern of the right-sided sectoral ducts. During a repair of an injury to the right hepatic duct, multiple transected, small biliary radicals can be expected at the hepatic surface.

Bismuth and colleagues provided the first classification of extrahepatic biliary injuries as a descriptive and prognostic tool for open biliary duct injuries. A Bismuth level I injury is a CBD transection with a common hepatic duct stump greater than 2 cm; level II injuries possess a common hepatic duct stump less than 2 cm. Level III injuries consist of a hepatic duct stricture with preserved ductal continuity, and level IV injuries are those that disrupt the hepatic duct confluence. Bismuth level V injuries require transection of the right sectoral

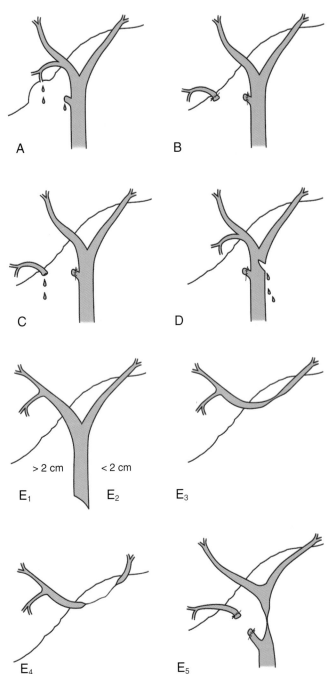

A

B

C

D

E₁ >2 cm   E₂ <2 cm   E₃

E₄   E₅

FIGURE 2 Strasberg-Soper classification of laparoscopic injuries to the biliary system. Type A injuries are leaks from the cystic duct or from ducts at the hepatic resection bed (ducts of Luschka). Types B and C involve injuries to aberrant right hepatic ducts. Type E injuries are chronic strictures resulting from occult laparoscopic biliary injuries; these are subclassified in a way similar to the original Bismuth scheme for benign biliary stricture. *(From Strasberg SM, Hertl M, Soper NJ, et al: An analysis of the problem of biliary injury during laparoscopic cholecystectomy, J Am Coll Surg 180:101, 1995.)*

duct. This classification served as a template for further classifications of laparoscopic biliary duct injuries.

Strasberg and colleagues developed a classification for laparoscopic biliary duct injuries (Figure 2). Type A injuries are bilomas due to leakage from either the cystic duct or minor hepatic ducts with no loss of biliary continuity. Type B and C injuries typically involve an aberrant right hepatic duct, misidentified as the cystic duct, draining into the

CBD. Type B (occlusion) and type C (transection) injuries are considered late (cholangitis) and early (biliary leak) presenting injuries respectively. These injuries frequently include an associated right hepatic artery injury. Type D injuries are defined as lateral damage to the CBD with a resulting biliary leak. Type E injuries are common hepatic duct injuries and are classified by the level of injury to the biliary tree.

Chronic biliary obstruction leads to anatomic and physiologic changes. Obstructed segments of liver eventually atrophy and become fibrosed; a concomitant hypertrophy of nonobstructed segments occurs as a compensation for the decrease in synthetic function. A single-lobe obstruction can result in rotation of the hepatic parenchyma and ductal structures toward the injured lobe. These deviations in anatomy can cause misinterpretation of intraoperative and radiologic findings.

PRESENTATION

CBD injuries are usually discovered 1) at the time of the initial procedure, 2) within a few days of surgery, and 3) weeks to months following surgery. Injuries discovered at the time of surgery are recognized by inspection of the specimen and by intraoperative cholangiography and persistent bile staining in the field. The symptoms of those injuries that occur a few days after surgery can include biliocutaneous fistula, bile peritonitis, jaundice, and abdominal pain. Patients who experience symptoms weeks to months later have a more insidious onset secondary to a less severe injury, resulting in preserved biliary function and the subsequent development of a stricture. Symptoms consistent with cholangitis—fevers, jaundice, and right upper quadrant pain—as well as weight loss are most common.

Inflammatory causes of CBD strictures are the most insidious; they lack the symptoms of cholangitis but rather mimic biliary obstruction. Traumatic injuries are recognized intraoperatively in the presence of concomitant injuries at the time of the exploratory laparotomy. Furthermore, major hepatic trauma can result in the formation of fistulas and strictures that occur as late injuries.

INJURIES DISCOVERED AT THE TIME OF SURGERY

The comparison between repair at the time of the surgery and repair postoperatively is untenable for two reasons: the successful repairs at the time of the injury are lost to follow-up, and elimination of the successful repairs results in an overestimation of the overall severity of injuries. The purported benefits of intraoperative repair include normal tissue planes, good physiologic conditions in the setting of an elective procedure, and one procedure overall. Late repair typically involves a dilated biliary duct to perform the repair, as well as allowing for referral to a high-volume tertiary care center.

When an intraoperative injury is encountered, the first step is to define the anatomy of the injury, so intraoperative cholangiography must be performed; any anatomic variation is an indication for cholangiography. Upon confirmation of an injury, the next step relies on the surgeon to decide whether to perform the repair or refer the patient to a tertiary care center. The decision relies on a self-assessment of competence to define the injury, perform the repair, and provide the appropriate postoperative care.

The hospital's ability to provide adequate support is an underappreciated component in the management of intraoperative injury. The necessary support consists of a quality intensive care unit, diagnostic imaging with interventional radiology, ERCP, and the prospect of chronic care and patient disability. This discussion is pertinent, because the majority of injuries are either a complete CBD transection or CBD excision, both of which require complex surgical repair. A complex repair at the time of injury commonly requires an anastomosis of the CBD or multiple segmental ducts of normal diameter. In addition, failure of a primary attempt at repair exacerbates the subsequent attempt at reconstruction.

The goals in managing a duct injury at the time of surgery are to preserve duct length and prevent postoperative biliary leak or obstruction. If the decision is made to refer the patient to another center, contacting the accepting surgeon prior to terminating the procedure is invaluable. If the gallbladder has not been devascularized, it should be left in place temporarily. If the classic injury pattern has occurred and been recognized, the second ductal incision should be avoided. The goal is to preserve CBD length; thus the procedure should be converted to an open exposure to facilitate the dissection of the gallbladder infundibulum. Upon identification of the gallbladder–cystic duct junction, the gallbladder can then be removed. A drain should be left in the area of the injury, and the fascia and skin are closed. Antibiotics with appropriate biliary coverage should be continued postoperatively, and all pertinent radiologic imaging should be included with the patient upon transfer.

In case a decision is made to repair at the time of injury, then the type of injury determines the appropriate management. Partial lacerations can be repaired primarily over a T-tube. However, the majority of laparoscopic injuries are CBD transections. If no loss of length is encountered, a primary repair can be attempted, unless there was cautery or clip-crush injury involved. A complete Kocher maneuver will loosen the duodenal end of the CBD and allow for approximation and a tension-free anastomosis. An end-to-end single layer of interrupted, fine caliber, absorbable suture is used, and a T-tube is placed. If there is any tension on the anastomosis after primary repair, the anastomosis should be revised with a Roux-en-Y hepaticojejunostomy instead. Other contraindications for primary repair include high biliary duct injuries and duct excision.

There are few successful primary repairs of duct injuries following laparoscopic cholecystectomy injuries. Longer segments of tissue loss require more definitive repair. Cystic stump and vein patches have been reported, yet the preferred repair is a Roux-en-Y hepaticojejunostomy.

DIAGNOSIS

The anatomy of the injury will alter the laboratory data findings. Liver function tests tend to show a cholestatic pattern, unless a biliary fistula has occurred following the biliary duct injury. An elevated bilirubin can suggest a biliary obstruction, yet a segmental obstruction can have a normal bilirubin. However, the alkaline phosphatase is typically elevated with any biliary obstruction.

Diagnostic studies are critical to defining the patient's biliary anatomy. ERCP is the preferred initial study, because it can define the anatomy, verify duct injury, and identify concurrent biliary pathology. Endoscopic cholangiography identifies a biliary leak after cholecystectomy in 95% of patients; it can identify the location of stones, strictures, and T-tubes. ERCP can also be therapeutic by readily allowing the extraction of stones or the deployment of biliary stents. If a common duct or cystic duct leak is found, placement of a stent may suffice as treatment in combination with adequate external drainage of any biloma. However, if a common duct transection, excision, or stricture is found at the level of the surgical clips placed during cholecystectomy, further management and surgical correction are necessary.

Percutaneous transhepatic cholangiography (PTC) and percutaneous biliary drainage (PBD) are performed for common duct stricture or transection. Bilateral lobar transhepatic cholangiogram and drainage catheters are necessary to define the injury and adequately decompress the liver prior to surgical repair. This specifically provides a thorough preoperative workup to avoid unrecognized concurrent biliary tract injuries. Axial computed tomography (CT) allows for the placement of drainage catheters to drain all intraperitoneal bilomas.

Surgery is planned once the patient is stabilized, the anatomy of the injury is visualized, and adequate biliary decompression and drainage exists. Recuperation from sepsis and medical optimization are paramount prior to surgery. Not all patients are evaluated and managed in the aforementioned diagnostic steps; some patients with cholangitis not adequately treated with antibiotics or high biliary duct transection proceed to PTC first, and some have intraabdominal sepsis, which requires CT scan and percutaneous drain placement as the first step. Those with sepsis and fluid collections not accessible by CT-guided drains require operative drainage, although simultaneous definitive repair is not recommended because of bile-stained tissues, hemodynamic instability, inflamed tissue planes, and undefined anatomy.

PRINCIPLES OF MANAGEMENT

The principles that guide the management of CBD injuries consist of sepsis control, physiologic support, definition of the injury anatomically, biliary drainage, and surgical repair. Bile duct injury can lead to dehydration, electrolyte abnormalities, intraabdominal sepsis, and malnutrition. Fluid resuscitation, biliary drainage, and medical optimization must be addressed prior to operative repair to provide optimal conditions for recuperation.

Presentation in the Early Postoperative Period

If the gastrointestinal continuity of the biliary tree is preserved, nonoperative therapy is effective. ERCP is recommended to define anatomy of the injury and treat cystic duct leaks and small ductal lacerations with stent placement alone. The stent traverses the ampulla of Vater and the injury site, diverting bile flow away from the injury, and it maintains a low-pressure environment within the duct. Transected segmental ducts may be associated with anomalous anatomy, such as a low insertion site or traversing the gallbladder fossa that results in biliary fistulas. These generally close spontaneously, yet a persistent fistula will require operative intervention. Cholangiography should confirm the leaking duct to be segmental or subsegmental; leaks larger than 2 mm require repair, but smaller ducts can be ligated safely.

If gastrointestinal continuity is not preserved, end-to-end bile duct reconstruction is not recommended. Difficulties arise from bacterial colonization, bile staining, and scar formation. These factors specifically alter compliance, tensile strength, and wound healing. Bilomas are converted into fistulas by the placement of external drains and are managed as described. In these cases, a Roux-en-Y limb reconstruction is the safest option.

Late Presentation

Injuries that show up weeks to months postoperatively occur in a manner similar to noniatrogenic biliary strictures, with an insidious onset of painless jaundice or cholangitis. The mechanism for stricture formation is due to partial clip occlusion or ischemic, electrical, or traumatic injury. Repair of a late-presenting biliary stricture requires exposure of the healthy proximal biliary duct. Dissection is difficult due to scar formation along the hepatoduodenal ligament, and a Roux-en-Y limb reconstruction is recommended.

Preoperative Therapy

The two critical aspects of preoperative treatment are drainage of the biloma and percutaneous transhepatic cholangiogram with biliary drainage. Either surgically placed external drains (injury recognized at time of surgery) or radiologic-guided percutaneous drains (injury recognized postoperatively) must be placed for sepsis control. Cholangiogram followed by placement of PBDs is mandated to prevent ongoing biloma formation and to define the anatomy for surgical repair. Other considerations should include tailoring preoperative antibiotics from bile or blood culture data, a process initiated several days in advance of the procedure.

Fistulas present an additional physiologic hurdle. The inability to absorb fat-soluble vitamins leads to vitamin insufficiency that results in prothrombin-time abnormalities; these can be addressed with parenteral vitamin K. Dehydration and electrolyte abnormalities, typically hypovolemic hyponatremia, can be addressed by fluid and electrolyte resuscitation. Anorexia and weight loss are common in late presenters with recurrent cholangitis. Nutritional support is successful with nasoenteric feeding tubes or, rarely, with parental nutrition in those who do not tolerate enteric feedings. Finally, additional comorbidities should be addressed preoperatively with the assistance of medical subspecialists for physiologic optimization. Otherwise peritonitis is the only indication for early surgical intervention that would preclude the preoperative workup and treatment.

Endoscopic Therapy

Some biliary duct injuries can be managed with endoscopic methods alone. The goal of endoscopic therapies is to reduce the transpapillary pressure gradient driving the bile flow preferentially away from a biliary leak. Biliary sphincterotomy can be sufficient for treatment of low-grade bile leaks, but many place stents due to technical simplicity. Bile leaks typically resolve quickly after sphincterotomy and stent placement, although previous biloma formation will typically require percutaneous drainage. Upon resolution of the biliary leak, the stents can be removed 4 to 6 weeks later.

On the other hand, more significant biliary duct injuries, including those with bile duct stricture, require more intensive therapies. Strictures are managed by serial incremental biliary dilations and side-by-side stent deployment. Endoscopic dilation and stent placement for strictures has been shown to be safe and effective for treatment of biliary obstruction over the short term. However, the limitation of these stents is frequent occlusion, requiring stent exchange every 3 to 6 months. Thus, sphincterotomy is commonly performed in addition, because of the necessity for numerous stent exchanges. Many gastroenterologists interrogate and exchange biliary stents every 3 months.

Dilation and stent deployment is discontinued as a therapy once cholangiography demonstrates resolution of the stricture, and 50% to 75% of patients require no further intervention or surgery. Recurrent strictures occur in 20% of patients after stent removal, most of which present in the first 6 months. About 10% to 15% of patients have complications, which include bleeding, cholangitis, pancreatitis, and stent migration that requires surgical intervention. A small percentage of patients die of biliary complications in the long term. Treatment of complete bile duct transections are considered not to be amenable to endoscopic therapies.

Operative Technique

Defining the anatomy of injured bile ducts is paramount for reconstruction. The left hepatic duct has a more predictable extrahepatic course and transverse orientation, thus it is more accessible compared with the right hepatic duct. The left hepatic duct is approached first if an injury is in proximity to the main duct confluence (Strasberg-Soper E). The other instance where this is applicable is in the presence of a nonvisualized, transected bile-producing duct; this occurs when the transected duct obliterates from scarring. In this instance, an incision is made 1 to 2 cm below and parallel to the Glisson capsule–peritoneal junction. The left lobular duct will be found adjacent and to the right of the umbilical fissure.

Devascularization of the bile duct leads to anastomotic failures and ischemic strictures, thus it is important to know that the blood supply of the bile ducts are located at 3 and 9 o'clock in the cross-sectional orientation. The anterior ductal surfaces are approached first, to spare the arterial supply. Circumferential dissection should be minimal, and a completely cleared duct length less than 5 mm is sufficient for enteric or primary reconstruction.

The dissection continues in a left-to-right approach to inspect the ductal confluence. If the injury is at the level of the confluence, a posterior remnant joining the left and right lobar ducts is commonly present. This is significant, because it identifies the right lobar duct and allows for a singular reconstruction of both ducts. However, if no confluence is evident, then the right lobar duct must also be dissected and exposed. Unlike the left lobar duct, the right lobar duct has a short, extrahepatic course and is known for its anatomic variance of the proximal segmental ducts. If the right hepatic duct is found with preserved right ductal confluence, then the superior surface should be dissected and exposed. If the right ductal confluence is injured, then dissection into the hepatic parenchyma along the gallbladder fossa may be necessary to acquire adequate length for repair.

Early branching of the segmental ducts should be anticipated, sought, and preserved in case a complex reconstruction of the right ductal system is necessary. A long segment of preserved common duct (Strasberg-Soper E_1, E_2) is reconstructed with a Roux-en-Y limb of jejunum. This is fashioned by an end-to-side single-layer anastomosis to the proximal end of the Roux-en-Y limb. Fine-caliber (4-0) interrupted absorbable sutures are preferred for the anastomosis. Drainage of the anastomosis is preferred through the liver or, less commonly, via a T-tube in patients with adequate CBD length. The construction of the Roux-en-Y limb is mindful of future evaluation and treatment; a 40 cm limb is created. The decision to stent the biliary-enteric anastomosis is controversial in the setting that good outcomes are seen if either is done. Thus, our preference is to leave the preoperatively placed PBD across the choledochojejunostomy or hepaticojejunostomy.

The left lobar duct can be fashioned if there is insufficient CBD length. The duct is opened along the long axis on the anterior surface, avoiding the vascular supply, to perform a side-to-side hepaticojejunostomy. If a posterior confluence of mucosa is preserved (Strasberg-Soper E_3), a single anastomosis can be created to include both lumens of the confluence to a single enterostomy. In this case, the left and right PBD are positioned across the anastomosis.

When a confluence is nonexistent (Strasberg-Soper E_4), a common channel is created by sewing together the medial walls of the left and right hepatic ducts. A single biliary-enteric anastomosis is performed, and each duct is drained individually. However, if the two lobar ducts cannot be united without tension, or if the right lobar duct possesses several discontinuous segmental ducts (Strasberg-Soper E_5), separate enterostomies are created to a single Roux-en-Y limb to reconstruct the segmental ducts. Closed suction drainage is left in the operative field prior to closure.

PROGNOSIS

The morbidity and mortality following bile duct injuries are pertinent. The morbidity is profound in that there are two phases at which the patient is at risk: after injury and after repair. Patients with unrecognized injuries are harmed by a delay in intervention to control biliary fistula and abdominal sepsis. Multisystem organ failure is a natural progression of persistent sepsis and can result in death even prior to repair. The data suggest that biliary reconstruction after biliary duct injury is associated with a major complication rate of 10% to 20%. The common complications include biliary anastomotic leak, cholangitis, cardiopulmonary failure, hemorrhage, and infection. The perioperative mortality has been reported to be 0.6% to 3%.

Both short-term and long-term results following repair of bile duct strictures have been published by numerous authors. Most of these studies report satisfactory results in 70% to 90% of patients. A satisfactory result is defined as a patient without symptoms of cholangitis or jaundice. Recurrent stricture formation is the most common late complication, and the stricture occurs at the site of the anastomosis. Two thirds of strictures present within 2 years of repair, and 90% are evident within 7 years, but strictures can occur as many as 20 years postoperatively. Factors that portend a favorable outcome include younger patient age at the time of repair, Roux-en-Y biliary-enteric reconstruction, the absence of infection and hepatic fibrosis, transhepatic stents, and a lower number of previous reconstructions.

NONIATROGENIC BENIGN BILIARY STRICTURE

Chronic Pancreatitis

Distal CBD strictures occur in the setting of long-standing intermittent inflammation of the pancreas. The stricture involves the entire intrapancreatic segment and is associated with dilatation of the biliary tree. Thus, jaundice is a common presenting symptom in this patient population. However, some patients may be asymptomatic, but they will have abnormal results on liver function tests. Serum alkaline phosphatase is the most sensitive indicator, and it is elevated in 80% of patients. ERCP is the preferred diagnostic study, because it demonstrates pancreatic ductal anatomy, identifies the stenosis, obtains tissue samples, and allows for stent placement. Benign CBD strictures are 2 to 4 cm long, smooth, and gradually tapered.

Most benign strictures can be managed successfully with medical, radiologic, and endoscopic techniques over the short term. Long-term benefits are not as rewarding, especially with endoscopic therapies. Sphincterotomy and balloon dilation of distal CBD strictures play a limited role in the treatment of chronic pancreatitis.

Symptomatic patients or those with a persistent elevation of alkaline phosphatase are candidates for biliary bypass to prevent the development of biliary cirrhosis from chronic obstruction. If pancreatic bypass is indicated for the chronic pain associated with chronic pancreatitis, a concomitant biliary bypass should be considered in patients with previous evidence of biliary obstruction. A Roux-en-Y limb reconstruction is the optimal repair in either side-to-side or end-to-side fashion, although some surgeons prefer a choledocho-duodenostomy. The latter has two advantages: biliary flow continues via the duodenum, which is technically easier, and the jejunum is left intact. Its disadvantage is that previous inflammation can leave the duodenum fibrotic and make mobilization to perform an anastomosis more difficult. Transduodenal sphincterotomy is insufficient, because the impediment is proximal to the ampulla, and the stricture is usually too long to be managed by this approach.

Periampullary neoplasms must be considered in patients with CBD stricture in the setting of chronic pancreatitis. Pancreatic cancer and chronic pancreatitis share symptoms and risk factors, making distinguishing the two a diagnostic dilemma. Even with the appropriate workup, repeated biopsy of the stricture may only be "suspicious" of a neoplasm. Pancreaticoduodenectomy is a treatment option in patients with a suspicious distal CBD stricture and abdominal pain, presumed related to chronic pancreatitis, although with good preoperative workup, this should be an unusual indication for treatment of chronic pancreatitis.

Mirizzi Syndrome

Chronic cholelithiasis can cause a benign stricture of the bile duct. Gallstones impacting the neck of the gallbladder can induce a narrowing of the common hepatic duct by mechanical compression and subsequent inflammation, scar formation, necrosis, and fistula formation. This form of biliary obstruction is known as *Mirizzi syndrome,* and it is a relative contraindication to laparoscopic cholecystectomy. Safe dissection depends on opening the triangle of Calot by lateral inferior retraction of the gallbladder infundibulum. However, in Mirizzi syndrome, the triangle no longer exists because of inflammation and scar formation that obliterate the triangle. The infundibulum is adherent to the CBD proximal to the cystic duct junction.

Patients who are initially seen with cholecystitis and jaundice uniformly warrant a preoperative contrast imaging study (ERCP vs. cholangiography). An open procedure is recommended, with careful dissection of the gallbladder wall from the hepatic duct. If a fistula is suspected between the gallbladder and hepatic duct, the gallbladder can be opened to prevent exacerbating the bile duct fistula. If the defect is small, the fistula can be primarily closed in the horizontal axis; if it is large, a Roux-en-Y hepaticojejunostomy reconstruction may be used. If the infundibulum is difficult to free from the hepatic duct, and no fistula is present, a small patch of gallbladder wall can be left behind to prevent hepatic duct injury. In the acute setting, the CBD returns to normal caliber following removal of the inciting stone and gallbladder. In the chronic setting, with strictures or large fistulas, Roux-en-Y hepaticojejunostomy may be more prudent.

RECOMMENDATIONS

The severity of bile duct injuries and strictures following cholecystectomy persists as a surgical dilemma. Management is dependent on preoperative investigation of the biliary anatomy with PTC or ERCP, as well as with the placement of biliary catheters for biliary tree decompression and adequate drainge of biliary fistulas. A Roux-en-Y hepaticojejunostomy remains the safest reconstruction, with a more than 90% success rate. The necessity of ample medical resources, medical subspecialties, and surgical experience to effectively treat bile duct injuries and strictures suggest that referral to specialized medical centers improves outcomes.

SUGGESTED READINGS

Bismuth H: Postoperative strictures of the bile duct. In Blumgard LH, ed: *The biliary tract*, Edinburgh, 1982, Churchill Livingstone, pp 209–218.
Branum G, Schmitt C, Baille J, et al: Management of major biliary complications after laparoscopic cholecystectomy, *Ann Surg* 217:532, 1993.
Strasberg SM, Hertl M, Soper NJ, et al: An analysis of the problem of biliary injury during laparoscopic cholecystectomy, *J Am Coll Surg* 180:101, 1995.
Stewart L, Way LW: Bile duct injuries during laparoscopic cholecystectomy, *Arch Surg* 130:1223, 1995.
Lillemoe KDL, Melton GB, Cameron JL, et al: Postoperative bile duct strictures: management and outcome in the 1990s, *Ann Surg* 232:430, 2000.

CYSTIC DISORDERS OF THE BILE DUCTS

Kamran Idrees, MD, and Steven A. Ahrendt, MD

OVERVIEW

Cystic disorders of the bile ducts, although rare, are well-defined malformations of the intrahepatic and/or extrahepatic biliary tree. These lesions are commonly referred to as *choledochal cysts*, which is a misnomer, as these cysts often extend beyond the common bile duct (choledochus). Classically, bile duct cysts are regarded as a disease of infancy and childhood. However, a higher proportion of patients with this diagnosis are being seen as adults. Although still a rare disease, it is important to recognize and treat this disease promptly because of associated high morbidity and mortality.

EPIDEMIOLOGY

Cystic disorders of the bile ducts account for approximately 1% of all benign biliary disease. The prevalence of this disease varies in different parts of the world. It is most common in East Asia, with an incidence of 1 in 13,000, compared with Western countries, where its incidence is 1 in 2 million. Interestingly, the incidence is not as high in Asian immigrants residing in Western countries as opposed to those residing in their native countries. Also, biliary cysts are four times more common in females than males. The majority of patients (60%) with bile duct cysts are diagnosed in the first decade of life, and approximately 20% are diagnosed in adulthood. The increasing number of cases diagnosed in adults is likely due to the increased utilization of diagnostic imaging, such as using CT scan to find the source of abdominal pain.

CLASSIFICATION

Cystic dilatation of the bile ducts occurs in various shapes—fusiform, cystic, saccular, and so on—and in different locations throughout the biliary tree. The most commonly used classification is the Todani modification of the Alonso-Lej classification (Figure 1 and Table 1). According to this classification, five types of cystic disorders are defined based on the site, shape, and extent of the biliary tree involvement. The prevalence of the different types of biliary cysts varies with the age at diagnosis and with patient nationality. The classification of choledochal cysts is also important in determining the management and prognosis of patients with this disease.

Type I choledochal cysts include dilatation of the common hepatic and common bile duct with a normal intrahepatic biliary duct. Type I cysts are the most common and are further classified as type IA (cystic), type IB (focal), and type IC (fusiform) based on shape. Type II cysts are a supraduodenal diverticulum of the common hepatic or bile duct, and they are rare. A type III cyst is a cystic dilation of the most distal intraduodenal segment of the common bile duct, also known as a *choledochocele*. Type IV choledochal cysts are defined as multiple and involving both the intrahepatic and extrahepatic biliary tract (type IVA), or they are limited to the extrahepatic bile duct (type IVB). Type V cysts, or Caroli disease, involves only the intrahepatic biliary tree, with either unilobar or bilobar involvement. The relative frequency of each type of choledochal cyst in decreasing order of frequency is shown in Table 1.

ETIOLOGY

The exact etiology of biliary cysts is unknown. Multiple theories have been proposed to explain the pathogenesis of these cysts; however, no single theory can clearly explain the formation of all types of cysts. An anomalous pancreatobiliary duct junction has been identified in a large number of patients with type I cysts. This anatomy increases the reflux of pancreatic juice into the bile duct and may lead to cystic dilatation of the duct wall. Increased ductal pressure may also produce cystic biliary dilatation. Abnormal sphincter of Oddi function

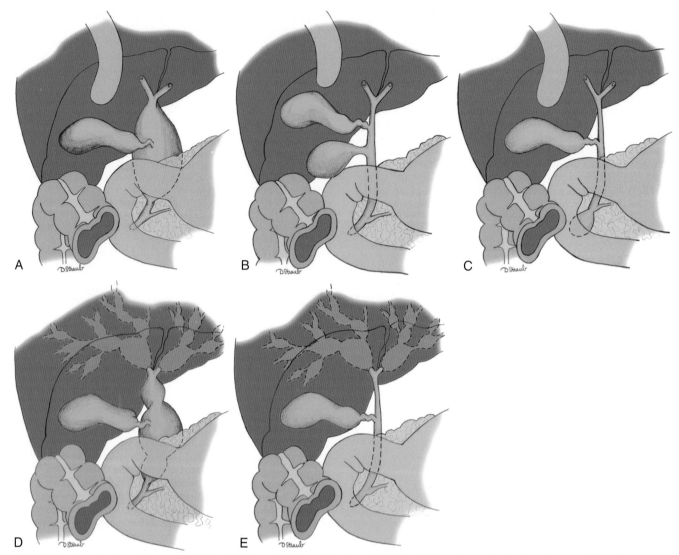

FIGURE 1   *Classification of biliary cysts.* **A,** Type I. **B,** Type II. **C,** Type III. **D,** Type IVA. **E,** Type V. *(From Lipsett PA, Pitt HA, Colombani PM, et al: Choledochal disease: a changing pattern of presentation, Ann Surg 220, 644, 1994.)*

has also been observed in patients with choledochal cysts. However, neither of these theories explains the preponderance of this disease in Asians, nor does it explain the decreased incidence of this disease in Asian immigrants in Western countries compared with Asians in their native countries. Although rare genetic predisposition (mostly autosomal recessive or infrequently autosomal dominant) also plays a role in the few familial cases of Caroli disease.

CLINICAL PRESENTATION

The initial clinical presentation varies significantly between children and adults. In children, the most common symptoms are intermittent abdominal pain, nausea and vomiting, mild jaundice, and an abdominal mass. The classical triad of abdominal pain, jaundice, and a palpable abdominal mass associated with choledochal cyst is observed in only 10% to 15% of children, and it is rarely seen in adults. Symptoms in adults often mimic those seen in patients with biliary tract disease or pancreatitis. Abdominal pain, nausea, and vomiting occur in the majority of adults with choledochal cysts. Seventy percent of adults with choledochal cysts also have gallstones, hepatolithiasis, or cystolithiasis. In addition, patients with biliary cysts may also develop cholangitis or pancreatitis. Not surprisingly, 40% of patients had

undergone a cholecystectomy prior to diagnosis of bile duct cysts in a recent large series from Johns Hopkins Hospital.

Biliary cirrhosis develops late in the disease and may occur with portal hypertension and its associated clinical stigmata of hepatosplenomegaly, varices, and ascites. Liver failure is seen especially with Caroli disease. Rarely, these cysts present with intrahepatic abscess or peritonitis from spontaneous cyst rupture. In the past 2 decades, bile duct cysts have been diagnosed with increasing frequency in adults in Western countries. Biliary cysts are often an incidental finding on radiological imaging performed for other reasons, and many of these patients are asymptomatic.

There is a well-established association between bile duct cysts and hepatopancreaticobiliary cancers. These cancers can arise either within the cyst itself or elsewhere within the hepatic or pancreatobiliary tree. Although the true incidence of cyst-associated cancer is difficult to ascertain, the reported incidence varies from 2.5% to 26%. The risk of malignancy increases with age, from 0.7% in the first decade to 2.3% in the third decade to as high as 75% in patients diagnosed with bile duct cysts in the ninth decade. A wide variety of cancers have been associated with bile duct cysts; these include squamous cell carcinoma, anaplastic carcinoma, cholangiosarcoma, hepatoma, pancreatic adenocarcinoma, and gallbladder carcinoma, but the most common cancer is cholangiocarcinoma. The incidence

TABLE 1: Cyst type: Alonso-Lej/Todani modification

Type	Description	% of All Cysts
Type I (choledochal cyst)	Cystic, fusiform, saccular extrahepatic biliary dilation	50%–80%
Mixed type I and II	Fusiform dilation of the extrahepatic biliary tree in combination with a separate diverticulum, midportion of the common bile duct, with cystic duct entering in the right of the diverticulum	1%
Type II	Extrahepatic biliary diverticulum	2%–3%
Type III (chole-dochocele)	Dilation of extrahepatic intraduodenal biliary tree	<10%
Type IVA	Intrahepatic and extrahepatic saccular/cystic dilation	30%–40%
Type IVB	Multiple extrahepatic cysts	<5%
Type V (Caroli disease)	Intrahepatic biliary cyst	<10%

of cholangiocarcinoma is 20 to 30 times higher in patients with bile duct cysts than in the general population. Among the five types of bile duct cysts, the risk is significantly greater in types I, IV, and V.

DIAGNOSIS

Adults are frequently diagnosed with cystic dilatation of their bile ducts during a workup for presumed cholecystitis or pancreatitis. Jaundice is common, and liver function tests usually reflect a pattern of mechanical obstruction, with elevations in bilirubin, alkaline phosphatase, and γ-glutamyl transferase being most common. Hyperamylasemia is often identified in patients presenting with acute pancreatitis.

Given recent advances in the antenatal diagnosis of choledochal cysts (type I), the differentiation between type I disease and biliary atresia is possible. Biopsy results can demonstrate the advanced liver disease associated with biliary atresia compared with the mild changes of early type I disease, identifying the need for earlier operation in the case of biliary atresia. Neonates, children, and young adults who are initially seen with jaundice and abdominal pain should be evaluated using abdominal ultrasound, because this is the most cost-effective method. In this patient population, biliary cysts are high on the list of differential diagnoses. In an older patient, however, a computerized tomographic (CT) scan may provide additional information, because the list of differential diagnoses is more expansive. A CT scan defines well the anatomy of the hepatobiliary and pancreatic regions in a jaundiced patient. Magnetic resonance cholangiopancreatography (MRCP) is increasingly used where available and frequently demonstrates the abnormal biliary anatomy, including an abnormal pancreaticobiliary union with a long common channel.

Precise definition of the biliary anatomy is necessary via cholangiography, which can be accomplished noninvasively via MRCP or invasively via ERCP or by percutaneous transhepatic cholangiography (PTC). The accuracy of MRCP is comparable to invasive cholangiography and often provides sufficient information to classify patients by choledochal cyst type to more effectively plan therapy. In adults, PTC and the placement of transhepatic stents may be considered in patients with a type IV cyst, in whom resection of the bifurcation may be necessary, and for whom postoperative stenting may be planned. Because long common channels are often present, and to avoid the development of periprocedural pancreatitis, placement of the stent through the ampulla should not be performed at the time of PTC. Similarly, during ERCP, care to avoid the pancreatic duct is important. ERCP may not define the most proximal biliary anatomy, which is often abnormal.

SURGICAL MANAGEMENT

The definitive treatment of bile duct cysts usually includes surgical excision of the abnormal extrahepatic bile duct with biliary-enteric reconstruction. This approach relieves biliary obstruction, preventing future episodes of cholangitis, stone formation, or biliary cirrhosis and thus interrupting the inflammatory liver injury cycle. It also stops pancreatic juice reflux, and more importantly, it removes tissue at risk of malignant transformation.

Patients should be medically optimized prior to operative intervention. Cholangitis should be adequately treated with broad-spectrum intravenous antibiotics and, if necessary, with biliary decompression. Severe portal hypertension, uncorrected coagulopathy, and end-stage liver failure are contraindications for operative intervention.

Type I: Extrahepatic Bile Duct Cyst

A midline or right subcostal incision is used to enter the abdomen, and the peritoneal cavity is explored for signs of malignancy. If the gallbladder is in place, it is dissected in a retrograde fashion from the liver bed with ligation of the cystic artery. Mobilization of the cystic duct to the common bile duct will lead to the choledochal cyst. The cyst is circumferentially dissected from the portal vein and hepatic artery with the gallbladder left in place to facilitate retraction. The duodenum is fully kocherized to allow access to the posterior pancreas and distal bile duct/cyst. The cyst is then dissected caudally, and the intrapancreatic portion of the common bile duct/cyst is separated from surrounding tissues.

Intraoperative ultrasound can be utilized as a useful adjunct to identify the anatomy and extent of the cyst, especially in cases with previous severe periportal inflammation. The duct/cyst is then transected as distally as possible with extreme care taken not to injure the pancreatic duct. Occasionally, the pancreatic duct can be visualized by opening the cyst. If dilatation of the bile duct is still present at the distal-most margin (duodenal), the mucosa must be stripped before closure. The cyst is then elevated anteriorly and dissected proximally, off the portal vein.

Care must be taken to identify aberrant or variant biliary or vascular anatomy. The cyst is usually transected just below the hepatic bifurcation. The hepatic bile ducts must be carefully examined for the presence of strictures, and separate left and right hepatic duct anastomoses must be performed if hilar strictures are present. Pathologic analysis of the resected specimen is obtained, along with frozen-section analysis of the proximal and distal margins, to exclude malignancy.

A standard 45 to 60 cm Roux-en-Y loop is used for an end-to-side hepaticojejunostomy. The anastomosis is constructed with a single layer of absorbable suture. If a bile stent is present, the stent is placed into the jejunum after the posterior suture line is completed. The anterior suture line stitches are then placed and tied. This resection and reconstruction may be completed laparoscopically or with robot assistance in selected patients; short-term results are equivalent to open surgery.

Occasionally, the inflammatory process surrounding the cyst is extensive, making excision seemingly hazardous. Because malignancy is always a concern, the cyst should be opened and the lining of the cysts excised. If this is technically difficult, injection of saline

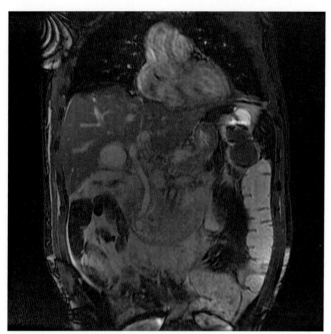

FIGURE 2   MRI demonstrating type III biliary cyst (choledochocele) in a patient presenting with acute pancreatitis.

into the cyst wall may facilitate dissection. A hepaticojejunostomy is then constructed as described earlier, leaving the cyst wall in place. However, as much as possible of the cyst wall should be removed. As a point of emphasis, leaving the cyst wall or any major part of it in place should be uncommon. Patients with a previous cystenterostomy can be approached in a similar fashion, if the cyst cannot be excised. However, cancer may be present in this patient population, and frozen-section analysis may be necessary to rule out the presence of malignancy.

Type II: Extrahepatic Biliary Diverticulum

Simple cyst excision is the treatment of choice for type II cysts. The common bile duct can be either primarily closed in transverse fashion or closed over a T-tube, depending on the size of the defect in the common bile duct after cyst excision; it is vital to avoid luminal narrowing. Occasionally Roux-en-Y hepaticojejunal reconstruction is required if there is significant risk of luminal narrowing.

Type III: Choledochocele

The malignant potential of type III cysts may be lower than types I, IV, and V. Endosocopic sphincterotomy (Figure 2) has been used to manage patients with choledochoceles without excising the cyst. Symptoms appear to be controlled in the majority of patients managed with sphincterotomy, although cases of cholangiocarcinoma following sphincterotomy have been reported. In a good surgical candidate, complete excision is recommended to eliminate the risk of malignancy. After kocherization of the duodenum, a lateral duodenotomy is performed, followed by identification of bile duct and pancreatic duct orifices. Cannulization of the ducts with silastic tubes is useful prior to cyst excision to avoid pancreatic duct injury. After cyst excision, interrupted absorbable sutures are utilized to perform a sphincteroplasty between bile duct mucosa and duodenal mucosa. Infrequently, the pancreatic duct is implanted into the duodenum in a similar fashion, if the pancreatic duct is draining into the cyst instead of into the duodenum directly. In rare instances

of suspected or established malignancy, pancreaticoduodenectomy is recommended.

Type IV: Bile Duct Cysts

The surgical management of type IV bile duct cysts differs from type I cysts in the presence of intrahepatic cystic disease. The operative treatment of type IVB entails complete extrahepatic ductal excision and Roux-en-Y hepaticojejunostomy, similar to type I cysts. The surgical decision making for type IVA cysts depends on the extent of intrahepatic cystic involvement and the presence of cirrhosis and/or portal hypertension. For unilateral cystic disease, hepatic lobectomy with hepaticojejunostomy suffices. In patients with bilobar disease, complete extrahepatic excision, biliary enteric bypass, and drainage of the intrahepatic biliary tree with bilateral, large-bore silastic stents is recommended. Adequate drainage of the biliary tree reduces the risk of biliary stasis, cholangitis, stone formation, and cirrhosis, which in turn can halt future liver injury; it also reduces the malignant risk.

In a patient with a type IV cyst, placement of a Hutson loop may be helpful to manage recurrent hepatic stones. This loop is fixed to the abdominal wall and marked along its course with metallic clips to facilitate identification of the limb for future percutaneous access to the biliary tree. The presence of cirrhosis or portal hypertension and failure of the previously mentioned operative intervention are indications for liver transplantation.

Type V: Caroli Disease

The clinical course of type V bile duct cysts is frequently complicated by biliary stasis, recurrent cholangitis, and intrahepatic abscesses. This chronic and recurrent inflammation eventually leads to cirrhosis and liver failure, thus early identification and intervention are warranted to slow down the progression to liver failure. The presence or absence of congenital hepatic fibrosis, biliary cirrhosis, portal hypertension, and the extent of intrahepatic bile duct cysts dictates the management of type V cysts.

Intrahepatic cystic involvement in Caroli disease varies from limited disease, restricted to a single segment or lobe, to diffuse disease involving the entire intrahepatic biliary tree. Unilobar cystic disease in the absence of cirrhosis and portal hypertension should be treated with hepatectomy and biliary enteric bypass. Contrary to limited intrahepatic cystic involvement, medical management should be instituted initially utilizing antibiotics, biliary drainage, and litholytic agents such as ursodiol in diffuse Caroli disease. Orthotopic liver transplantation is considered the treatment of choice in patients with diffuse Caroli disease with cirrhosis or portal hypertension and after a partial hepatectomy with biliary-enteric bypass has failed. It is crucial to meticulously manage these patients at first to slow or halt liver injury and avoid unnecessary operative interventions to increase the subsequent success of liver transplantation.

PROGNOSIS

In the postoperative period, early complications include anastomotic leak, postoperative bleeding, wound infection, acute pancreatitis, and pancreatic fistula. Late complications include anastomotic stricture, cholangitis, hepatolithiasis, cirrhosis, and malignancy. Anastomotic stricture and recurrent cholangitis are seen in 25% to 35% of patients and are associated with both intrahepatic and bile duct stone formation. These complications are greatest in patients with type IV cysts and should be managed aggressively. Occasionally, percutaneous dilation of a biliary stricture may be helpful. Choledochoscopy can be used to extract stones directly, and it may also be used to survey for the development of malignancy.

Although technically challenging, patients with a history of biliary cystic disease that was previously bypassed should be offered the option of resection. Resection reduces but does not eliminate the increase in cholangiocarcinoma risk present in patients with biliary cystic disease, therefore, all patients with choledochal cyst disease should undergo life-long surveillance.

SUGGESTED READINGS

Abbas HM, Yassin NA, Ammori BJ: Laparoscopic resection of type I choledochal cyst in an adult and Roux-en-Y hepaticojejunostomy: a case report and literature review, *Surg Laparosc Endosc Percutan Tech* 16(6):439–444, 2006.

Ammori JB, Mulholland MW: Adult type I choledochal cyst resection, *J Gastrointest Surg* 13:363, 2009.

Dhupar R, Gulack B, Geller DA, et al: The changing presentation of choledochal cyst disease: an incidental diagnosis, *HPB Surg*, 2009:103739. E-pub ahead of print.

Edil BH, Cameron JL, Reddy S: Choledochal cyst disease in children and adults: a 30-year single-institution experience, *J Am Coll Surg* 206:1000, 2008.

Lipsett PA, Pitt HA: Surgical treatment of choledochal cysts, *J Hepatobiliary Pancreat Surg* 10:352, 2003.

Lipsett PA, Pitt HA, Colombani PM: Choledochal cyst disease: a changing pattern of presentation, *Ann Surg* 220:644, 1994.

Metcalfe MS, Wemyss-Holden SA, Maddern GJ: Management dilemmas with choledochal cysts, *Arch Surg* 138:333, 2003.

Soreide K, Korner H, Havnen J, Soreide JA: Bile duct cysts in adults, *Br J Surg* 91:1538, 2004.

Wiseman K, Buczkowski AK, Chung SJ, et al: Epidemiology, presentation, diagnosis, and outcomes of choledochal cysts in adults in an urban environment, *Am J Surg* 189:527, 2005.

PRIMARY SCLEROSING CHOLANGITIS

Hiromichi Ito, MD, Michael A. Abramson, MD, and Edward E. Whang, MD

OVERVIEW

Primary sclerosing cholangitis (PSC) is a chronic and progressive disorder in which multifocal stricturing of intrahepatic and/or extrahepatic bile ducts leads to cholestasis and, ultimately, liver failure. The etiology of PSC is unknown, but prevailing hypotheses focus on genetic factors predisposing affected individuals to biliary inflammation, fibrosis, and stricturing induced by autoimmune, infectious, and/or ischemic insults.

The estimated prevalence of PSC in the United States ranges from 1 to 6 per 100,000 individuals. Seventy percent of affected patients are male, and the mean age at diagnosis is 40 years. There is a strong association between PSC and inflammatory bowel disease (IBD), particularly ulcerative colitis (UC); in some reports, up to 90% of patients with PSC have UC. Conversely, approximately 5% of patients with UC develop PSC.

CLINICAL MANIFESTATIONS

The clinical manifestations of PSC vary with disease stage (Table 1). Many patients are asymptomatic at the time of diagnosis; patients with IBD who are found to have unexplained liver function abnormalities comprise the majority of this group and therefore should be evaluated for PSC. Progressive biliary stricturing leads to cholestasis-related manifestations, particularly fatigue and pruritis, and to steatorrhea, deficiencies of fat-soluble vitamins (A, D, E, and K), and metabolic bone disease. Up to a third of patients with PSC develop cholelithiasis and choledocholithiasis. With onset of cirrhosis, liver failure and portal hypertension–related manifestations can emerge.

Although most patients with PSC have diffuse biliary stricturing, approximately 20% to 50% of affected individuals develop a dominant biliary stricture. These lesions have a propensity to develop at or near the hepatic duct bifurcation, but they can occur anywhere in the intrahepatic or extrahepatic biliary tree. Dominant strictures can be asymptomatic, or they can cause symptoms of mechanical biliary obstruction.

Cholangiocarcinoma (CCA) develops in 10% to 15% of patients with PSC. Some of these lesions present as dominant biliary strictures, and their radiographic appearance can be indistinguishable from that of their nonmalignant counterparts. Rapid clinical deterioration, weight loss, unremitting abdominal pain, and progressive biliary dilatation proximal to the dominant stricture should prompt concern for the presence of CCA. Unfortunately, these symptoms portend advanced disease; early lesions typically are asymptomatic or are associated with symptoms indistinguishable from those of PSC.

DIAGNOSIS AND EVALUATION

In most patients with PSC, the diagnosis is based on 1) identification of multifocal stricturing and dilation of the intrahepatic and/or extrahepatic biliary tree on cholangiography and 2) exclusion of other etiologies of biliary stricturing (secondary sclerosing cholangitis caused by conditions such as choledocholithiasis, iatrogenic biliary injury, bile duct neoplasm, Caroli disease, and IgG4-associated cholangitis).

Endoscopic retrograde cholangiopancreatography (ERCP) traditionally has been the preferred modality for diagnosing PSC; however, recent experience suggests magnetic resonance cholangiopancreatography (MRCP) has performance characteristics (>80% sensitivity and >95% specificity) approaching those of ERCP. Therefore MRCP is sufficient for diagnosis if it reveals findings characteristic of PSC; however, ERCP is still required if MCRP findings are equivocal, or if interventions are required.

TABLE 1: Staging of primary sclerosing cholangitis

Stage	Description
I—Portal	Portal edema, inflammation, ductal proliferation; abnormalities do not extend beyond the limiting plate
II—Periportal	Periportal fibrosis with or without inflammation extending beyond the limiting plate
III—Septal	Septal fibrosis, bridging necrosis, or both
IV—Cirrhotic	Biliary cirrhosis

Patients with the unusual PSC variant known as *small-duct PSC* require liver biopsy for diagnosis, as they typically are found to have no cholangiographic abnormalities. For most patients with PSC, however, liver biopsy is not required. However, biopsy can be helpful in defining disease stage and in predicting prognosis (although the current Mayo prognostic model does not include histology; see the link in the next section).

Laboratory test findings reflect cholestasis. Initially, elevations in serum alkaline phosphatase concentration may be the only abnormality, with serum total bilirubin concentration being normal until advanced disease develops. Serological abnormalities—the presence of antinuclear, antismooth muscle and anticardiolipin antibodies—may be found; however, antimitochondrial antibodies characteristic of primary biliary cirrhosis are usually absent.

Patients with PSC who are found to have a dominant stricture should be evaluated for the presence of CCA. Serum CA 19-9 concentration may be elevated with CCA, but its sensitivity is poor. Cytological examination of brushings obtained during ERCP is the most common modality; however, reported sensitivities of this technique vary widely (40% to 80%). Newer techniques, such as digital image analysis and fluorescence in-situ hybridization (FISH), may enhance sensitivity of cytology. For now, the most accurate modality for diagnosing CCA in dominant biliary strictures is endoscopic ultrasonography with fine needle aspiration (EUS-FNA; sensitivity >80%, specificity nearly 100%), which should be applied in patients with negative or equivocal brush cytological findings who are suspected of having CCA based on clinical features described above.

NATURAL HISTORY AND PROGNOSIS

PSC is a progressive disease that ultimately leads to liver failure, but the time course is variable among affected individuals. The median overall survival from the time of diagnosis is approximately 14 years, and the median survival in the absence of liver transplantation is approximately 10 years.

A prognostic model is available based on patient age, serum bilirubin concentration, serum aspartate aminotransferase concentration, serum albumin concentration, and the presence or absence of a variceal bleeding history (http://www.mayoclinic.org/gi-rst/mayomodel3.html). Survival estimates calculated using this model are well correlated with observed actual survival.

MANAGEMENT

A management algorithm is depicted in Figure 1. Numerous pharmacological agents—ursodeoxycholic acid, corticosteroids, and immunosuppressives—have been subjected to controlled clinical trials in patients with PSC. None of these agents, either alone or in combination, has been found to have any impact on disease progression, therefore observation alone is reasonable for asymptomatic patients.

Once symptoms develop, palliative therapy is initiated (e.g., cholestyramine and diphenhydramine for pruritis). Antibiotics can be used for treatment of and prophylaxis against cholangitis. Vitamin and calcium supplementation is given as appropriate.

Endoscopic and Percutaneous Interventional Therapy

Hilar dominant strictures and more distal strictures that are causing or exacerbating symptoms can be treated with endoscopic dilation with or without stenting. The reported technical success rates of these procedures at experienced centers approaches 80%, with good efficacy in short-term amelioration of laboratory value abnormalities and symptoms such as jaundice. Reported complication rates range

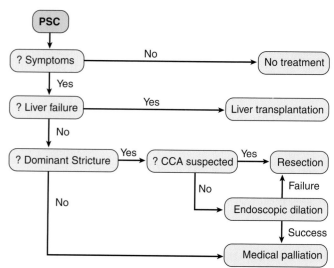

FIGURE I   Algorithm for management of PSC.

from 10% to 15%. For proximal (especially intrahepatic) strictures not amenable to endoscopic dilation, percutaneous dilation with or without stenting can be performed; however, success rates are lower, and complication rates are higher than those reported for endoscopic dilation of more distal strictures.

Whether asymptomatic dominant biliary strictures in patients with PSC should be subjected to endoscopic or percutaneous therapy is controversial. In some series, patients treated endoscopically were found to have longer median survival than predicted by the Mayo prognostic model. This finding has been interpreted by some investigators to suggest that endoscopic dilation of asymptomatic dominant strictures can impact the natural history of PSC. However, no data from randomized controlled clinical trials are available to guide decision making on this question.

Surgical Resection

Because dominant strictures associated with PSC have a propensity to develop at the hepatic duct bifurcation, surgical resection generally includes complete resection of the extrahepatic biliary tree and reconstruction using Roux-en-Y hepaticojejunostomy with or without stent placement. The best documented experience with this approach is from the Johns Hopkins Hospital, where outcomes are reported to be excellent.

Surgical resection provides durable relief of jaundice and recurrent cholangitis, and it may delay progression to cirrhosis and the need for liver transplantation. In the Johns Hopkins series of 146 patients with PSC, 5-year overall and transplant-free survival rates for noncirrhotic patients who underwent surgical resection were significantly higher (85% and 82%, respectively) compared with those for noncirrhotic patients who were contemporaneously managed by endoscopic or percutaneous balloon dilation (59% and 46%, respectively).

So far no randomized controlled trials have compared endoscopic therapy to surgical resection, and despite the relatively good outcomes reported in retrospective analyses of surgical resections, most centers are less enthusiastic about early surgical intervention that may complicate future liver transplantation. Most centers reserve biliary resection procedures to those rare symptomatic PSC patients with a dominant extrahepatic stricture in whom dilation by an endoscopic or percutaneous route is not feasible, or is unsuccessful, and in those with suspected CCA. Remember that these procedures are contraindicated in patients with cirrhosis because of high morbidity rates and poor long-term outcomes in these patients.

Orthotopic Liver Transplantation

Approximately 5% of adult orthotopic liver transplants (OLTs) in the United States are done in patients with PSC. The indications for OLT in PSC are similar to those in patients with other etiologies for end-stage liver disease. The outcomes are generally excellent, with 5-year overall survival of 85% after OLT in patients with PSC. However, 15% to 20% of these patients develop recurrent PSC, of which 30% require retransplantation.

Up to 10% of patients undergoing OLT for PSC are found to have a small, unsuspected CCA in their explanted livers. Although known CCA is a contraindication to OLT outside of study protocols, given the poor reported outcomes in such patients who have undergone OLT, this finding does not appear to impact overall survival. In addition, OLT following neoadjuvant chemoradiation therapy for patients with CCA and PSC is under investigation, with promising initial results.

For patients with PSC and concurrent IBD, there has been concern that immunosuppression regimens used after OLT may increase the risk of colorectal cancer developing. This concern has not been validated, therefore prophylactic total colectomy is not recommended in the absence of other indications; however, continued annual surveillance is warranted.

SUMMARY

OLT is associated with excellent outcomes in patients with PSC and end-stage liver disease. The role of nontransplantation resectional surgery in PSC is limited. These procedures may be indicated for patients suspected of harboring CCA and for those in whom nonsurgical interventional therapy fails.

SELECTED READINGS

Ahrendt SA, Pitt HA, Kalloo AN, et al: Primary sclerosing cholangitis: resect, dilate, or transplant?, *Ann Surg* 227(3):412–423, 1998.

Charatcharoenwitthaya P, Enders FB, Halling KC, et al: Utlity of serum tumor markers, imaging, and biliary cytology for detecting cholangiocarcinoma in primary sclerosing cholangitis, *Hepatology* 48(4):1106–1117, 2008.

Kim WR, Therneau TM, Wiesner RH, et al: A revised natural history model for primary sclerosing cholangitis, *Mayo Clin Proc* 75(7):688–694, 2000.

Lindor KD, Kowdley KV, Luketic VA, et al: High-dose ursodeoxycholic acid for the treatment of primary sclerosing cholangitis, *Hepatology* 50(3): 808–814, 2009.

Pawlik TM, Olbrecht VA, Pitt HA, et al: Primary sclerosing cholangitis: role of extrahepatic biliary resection, *J Am Coll Surg* 206(5):822–830, 2008.

Vera A, Moledina S, Gunson B, et al: Risk factors for recurrence of primary sclerosing cholangitis of liver allograft, *Lancet* 360(9349):1943–1944, 2002.

BILE DUCT CANCER

Reid B. Adams, MD, and Todd W. Bauer, MD

OVERVIEW

Bile duct cancers, also called *cholangiocarcinomas*, are rare; they account for only 2% to 3% of malignancies. In the United States, approximately 2500 cases of intrahepatic cholangiocarcinoma (IHC) occur each year, and an estimated 2000 to 3000 extrahepatic cholangiocarcinomas develop annually. Most extrahepatic tumors, 65% to 70%, arise in the perihilar region; they are commonly termed *Klatskin tumors*. The remaining 20% to 25% occur in the distal bile duct (periampullary). Less than 10% of patients present with multifocal or diffuse cholangiocarcinoma.

Epidemiological studies demonstrate an increasing incidence of IHC worldwide and a decrease in the incidence of extrahepatic tumors. The location-specific descriptive classification for these tumors—intrahepatic, perihilar, or distal—is based on the recognition that treatment differs significantly based on the tumor's site of origin. The time-honored Bismuth-Corlette system further classifies perihilar tumors by describing a detailed characterization of their position within the proximal biliary tract (Figure 1).

Most cholangiocarcinomas occur without any identifiable risk factors. Known risk factors include etiologies that cause chronic inflammation of the ducts: primary sclerosing cholangitis, with a lifetime risk of 10% to 15%; bile duct cysts (choledochal cysts), which have a 15% lifetime risk; chronic *Salmonella typhi* infection; and parasitic infections (e.g., *Clonorchis sinesis*). Most patients who develop cholangiocarcinoma are in their 60s and 70s, with the peak incidence in the 70s. However, patients with cholangiocarcinoma that occurs in the context of sclerosing cholangitis or bile duct cysts typically develop disease on average 20 to 30 years earlier.

Nearly all bile duct cancers are adenocarcinoma. Three morphologically distinct subtypes of cholangiocarcinoma are *sclerosing,* *nodular,* and *papillary.* More than 90% of tumors are sclerosing, characterized by an intense desmoplastic reaction. This feature makes the preoperative diagnosis of malignancy difficult, and intense desmoplasia also contributes to the technical challenges associated with resection of these tumors.

Growth patterns of the nodular, sclerosing subtypes play a part in the diagnostic and treatment dilemmas encountered with these tumors. These subtypes tend to infiltrate the periductal tissue, invade the perineural sheaths, and grow along the nerves; this results in unrecognized microscopic disease outside the clinical epicenter of the primary tumor, which can lead to unresectable disease or microscopically positive margins. More troublesome is the propensity of these tumors to grow subepithelially within the bile duct for distances up to 1 to 2 cm. Preoperative imaging typically underestimates the extent of the disease, which frequently is nonpalpable in the operating room. Again, these features result in persistent microscopic residual disease following resection. Finally, metastatic disease, particularly to the regional lymph nodes, is common (30% to 50%).

Papillary tumors, on the other hand, comprise fewer than 10% of cholangiocarcinomas but are important to recognize, as they have higher resection and survival rates compared to the other two subtypes. Papillary subtypes are recognizable on preoperative imaging; they tend to expand the bile ducts, rather than constricting them, as seen with the nodular or sclerosing subtypes. Despite the appearance of extensive involvement within the ducts, papillary tumors typically have a limited area of ductal involvement, allowing resection of seemingly extensive tumors.

INTRAHEPATIC CHOLANGIOCARCINOMA

Diagnosis

IHC often presents as an incidental finding during evaluation for an unrelated reason. Another common situation is discovery during evaluation of mild abnormalities in liver serum tests. When symptomatic, IHC most commonly causes pain and less frequently brings symptoms of fatigue, anorexia, and weight loss.

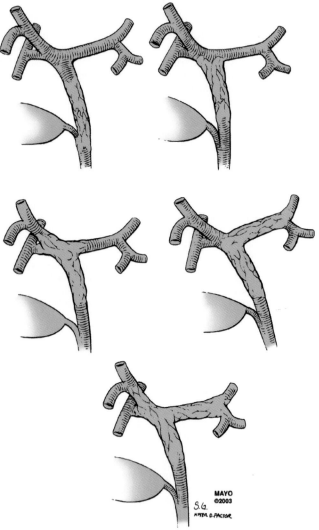

FIGURE I   The Bismuth-Corlette classification of perihilar cholangiocarcinomas. Type I tumors are located distal to the hepatic ductal confluence. Type II cancers involve the junction of the right and left hepatic ducts. Type IIIA bile duct cancers involve the confluence and the right hepatic duct, wheras type IIIB tumors involve the confluence and the left hepatic duct. Type IV cancers involve both the proximal left and right hepatic ducts to the segmental bile ducts. *(Courtesy Mayo Clinic.)*

The initial evaluation (Figure 2) typically discovers a liver mass with malignant features, based on the initial ultrasound or CT done under the circumstances indicated above. Because IHC occurs in an older population, initial suspicion is usually for metastatic disease (from colorectal, lung, breast, pancreatic primary, etc.) or hepatocellular carcinoma (HCC). We primarily see these patients when they are found to have an undefined liver mass on ultrasound or CT imaging. In this circumstance, we perform a contrast magnetic resonance imaging (MRI) and laboratory studies that include liver serum tests (alkaline phosphatase, aspartate aminotransferase, alanine aminotransferase, total bilirubin) platelet count, International Normalized Ratio, albumin, carcinoembryonic antigen (CEA), cancer antigen (CA) 19-9, α-fetoprotein, and hepatitis screening. Laboratory studies may be useful in supporting a specific diagnosis, such as elevated CEA or evidence of chronic liver disease, but they are rarely conclusive for a specific diagnosis. If the CEA or CA 19-9 is elevated preoperatively, they may be useful for surveillance following treatment.

MRI can evaluate the nature of the lesion and determine whether it has malignant features, those suggestive of HCC, or characteristics

confirming a benign lesion, such as hemangioma or focal nodular hyperplasia. Although high-quality CT imaging is a reasonable alternative, we prefer MRI for its superior performance characteristics in distinguishing hepatic lesions based on their imaging features. MRI also has advantages for treatment planning by providing details of the intrahepatic anatomy, including the vasculature and biliary tract. Finally, MRI provides excellent imaging of the pancreas, another potential primary tumor site.

If the MRI is consistent with a malignant lesion, and the patient has no evidence of chronic liver disease, metastatic disease remains the most likely diagnosis. Thus, we perform a chest CT, upper and lower endoscopy, and mammography (for women) to rule out a primary tumor at these common sites. In the absence of a primary tumor, consideration of positron emission tomography (PET)/CT is appropriate. Although its utility in this circumstance is unclear, we do PET/CT scans in patients at high risk for surgery to rule out an occult primary lesion and minimize the likelihood of a nontherapeutic hepatic resection. In addition, although currently not the standard of care, accumulating evidence demonstrates the utility of PET/CT for cholangiocarcinoma. Recent studies report discovery of additional disease in a significant minority of patients with cholangiocarcinoma, which affects the treatment approach in an estimated 25% of patients. Unless considering nonoperative therapy, biopsy of the mass is unnecessary. Although biopsy would appear to be a direct approach to the diagnosis, the pathology is rarely definitive for cholangiocarcinoma. Typically, the pathology is adenocarcinoma, leading to a diagnosis of metastatic disease.

While immunohistochemistry can support the diagnosis of IHC, rarely is it definitive. This is another common scenario we see for patients referred with a likely IHC: imaging of an unexpected liver mass followed by a biopsy showing adenocarcinoma. In this circumstance, we proceed with MRI of the liver, the laboratory and imaging studies noted above, and PET/CT.

Tumor Staging

IHC is staged the same as hepatocellular carcinoma (Table 1) by the American Joint Committee on Cancer (AJCC).

Preoperative Preparation

Because resection is the primary therapy for IHC, preoperative evaluation and preparation should evaluate tumor resectability, confirm the absence of extrahepatic disease, and assess the patient's ability to tolerate an operation. The MRI or CT scan defines the extent of the hepatectomy required for complete resection and thus the feasibility of resection. Because most patients with IHC are older, patients should receive treatment for correctable medical comorbidities, including cardiac, pulmonary, and renal disease and malnutrition. Unlike HCC, patients with IHC typically do not have chronic liver disease. Thus radiographic assessment of the future liver remnant (FLR) volume— that is, the liver remaining following resection—is sufficient to ensure adequate liver function following resection. Measurement of liver volumes from the preoperative MRI or CT scan is the simplest method.

Treatment and Outcomes

The only potentially curative therapy for IHC is complete resection, which is appropriate for medically fit patients without extrahepatic disease. The presence of metastases in the liver or within regional lymph nodes outside the hepatoduodenal ligament is a contraindication to resection. Local "satellite" tumors around the primary tumor, indicative of local portal vein invasion, are associated with a worse prognosis. If complete tumor clearance is achievable in this circumstance, we offer resection.

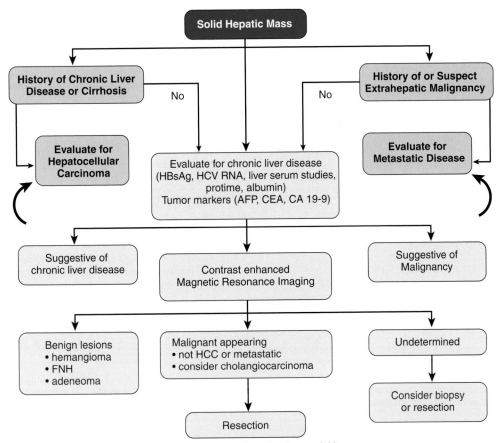

FIGURE 2   Evaluation algorithm for a solid liver mass.

The location and size of the tumor and its proximity to major vasculobiliary structures within the liver dictate the extent of resection. Segmental resections are reasonable for smaller, peripheral tumors, but a hemihepatectomy or extended hepatectomy is frequently necessary for tumor clearance. If satellite lesions are present, a formal segmentectomy or hemihepatectomy is appropriate to include the entire portal venous distribution for the affected segment.

If a hemihepatectomy or more appears necessary for resection, measurement of liver volumes allows assessment of the adequacy of the FLR. If the FLR is too small, portal vein embolization of the affected liver, the side of the resection, may allow sufficient compensatory hypertrophy of the FLR to allow safe resection. We begin all of these procedures with diagnostic laparoscopy. Small volume liver and peritoneal disease is discovered in 20% to 30% of patients, precluding nontherapeutic laparotomy. Overall resectability rates based on findings at laparoscopy or exploration are 50% to 70%. The 5-year survival for patients undergoing R0 resection is widely variable in the literature, but it approximates 30% to 40%. Most patients die of recurrence, typically within the liver remnant but less commonly with lung, lymph node, or bony metastases. Despite this, no data exist to support a role for adjuvant therapy following an R0 resection.

When patients are unresectable because of medical comorbidities or locally advanced disease, a number of palliative treatment options are available. Medically unfit patients with small tumors are candidates for percutaneous radiofrequency ablation (RFA). Palliation of unresectable, locally advanced IHC is feasible with RFA, chemoembolization, intraarterial radioembolization with yttrium-90–labeled microspheres, or external beam radiation. However, no evidence exists to support a significant survival benefit from any of these approaches.

Another approach for locally advanced disease or for patients with metastases is systemic therapy. A number of single-agent or combined regimens have demonstrated activity against cholangiocarcinoma. Again, this approach is palliative; none of the regimens

has improved survival beyond 8 to 15 months. The most common combination used is gemcitabine and cisplatin.

DISTAL CHOLANGIOCARCINOMA

Diagnosis

Distal cholangiocarcinoma shows symptoms similar to other periampullary neoplasms. The most common symptom is jaundice, and less common symptoms include anorexia, nausea, weight loss, and fatigue. The presentation is indistinguishable from other tumors of the periampullary region.

Typically, ultrasonography is the initial imaging test in patients with jaundice. Distal obstruction presents as dilated intrahepatic and extrahepatic ducts, down to the site of obstruction. Initially, pancreatic cancer is the most likely diagnosis, as distal cholangiocarcinoma represents less than 10% of periampullary tumors. Our preferred imaging modality is MRI/MRCP with contrast as the next step in evaluation; this allows assessment for choledocholithiasis, a pancreatic head mass, liver metastases, and vascular involvement. In addition, MRI can often identify a thickened duct and imaging findings suggestive of a cholangiocarcinoma. Unless treatment will be with nonoperative therapy, a tissue diagnosis is unnecessary. Although benign strictures can occur in the distal bile duct, definitive diagnosis short of resection is nearly impossible. Finally, CEA and CA 19-9 levels may be useful for surveillance following therapy if they are elevated before treatment.

Tumor Staging

Distal cholangiocarcinoma is staged the same as other extrahepatic cholangiocarcinomas by the AJCC (Table 1).

Preoperative Preparation

Resection is the primary therapy for distal cholangiocarcinoma. Preoperative evaluation and preparation, therefore, should evaluate tumor resectability, the absence of extrahepatic disease, and the patient's ability to tolerate operative care. The absence of extensive vascular involvement and metastatic disease by MRI or CT suggests the feasibility of resection. Because most patients are older, addressing correctable medical conditions will minimize perioperative morbidity.

Preoperative biliary decompression is not essential prior to resection, although practically speaking, most patients are referred with a stent already in place. If they are not decompressed at the time of presentation, we consider endoscopic stenting when the total bilirubin is greater than 10 mg/dL, or if the patient is unwell or malnourished and in need of nutritional repletion.

Treatment and Outcomes

Resection is the only potentially curative therapy for distal cholangiocarcinoma, and it is appropriate for medically fit patients without extensive vascular involvement or metastatic disease. Pancreaticoduodenectomy is necessary for adequate treatment of tumors from the level of the superior border of the pancreas to the ampulla of Vater. Tumors in the mid bile duct are rare. Occasionally, excision of the extrahepatic bile duct from the portal plate to the head of the pancreas is sufficient for tumors at this site. However, pancreaticoduodenectomy with excision of the bile duct to, or including, the confluence of the right and left ducts is necessary for adequate tumor clearance. For tumors above the head of the pancreas, we include a formal portal lymphadenectomy.

Similar to IHC, we begin all of these procedures with diagnostic laparoscopy to minimize the risk of nontherapeutic laparotomy.

Median survival following resection is reportedly 20 to 30 months with a 5-year survival of 15% to 40%. Lymph node involvement appears to be an important predictor of recurrence and cancer-related mortality. The role for adjuvant therapy following resection is undefined, but evidence suggests tumoricidal activity with fluoropyrimidine-based chemoradiotherapy; however, randomized studies are lacking. The most recent National Cooperative Cancer Network (NCCN) guidelines list consideration of fluoropyrimidine chemoradiotherapy and/or fluoropyrimidine- or gemcitabine-based systemic therapy for all resected distal cholangiocarcinomas regardless of margin or node status.

When patients are unresectable because of medical comorbidities or locally advanced disease, palliation of biliary obstruction by an endoscopic covered wallstent is optimal. These frequently remain patent for 6 to 12 months; because most unresected patients do not survive beyond a year, this approach maintains quality of life with minimal intervention and recovery. Palliative chemoradiotherapy is reasonable, albeit unproven, for the medically unfit or for locally advanced disease. A gemcitabine-based systemic therapy regimen is reasonable for metastatic disease.

PERIHILAR CHOLANGIOCARCINOMA

Diagnosis

Perihilar cholangiocarcinoma presents similar to distal cholangiocarcinoma with jaundice as the predominant finding. Weight loss, pruritis, anorexia, and pain are less common symptoms. Another

---

TABLE 1: AJCC staging of cholangiocarcinoma

Intrahepatic	Stage	Tumor	Node	Metastasis
	I	T1	N0	M0
	II	T2	N0	M0
	IIIA	T3	N0	M0
	IIIB	T4	N0	M0
	IIIC	any T	N1	M0
	IV	any T	any N	M1
Extrahepatic	**Stage**	**Tumor**	**Node**	**Metastasis**
	0	Tis	N0	M0
	IA	T1	N0	M0
	IB	T2	N0	M0
	IIA	T3	N0	M0
	IIB	T1-T3	N1	M0
	III	T4	any N	M0
	IV	any T	any N	M1

T1, Solitary tumor without vascular invasion; *T2*, solitary tumor with vascular invasion or multiple tumors <5 cm; *T3*, multiple tumors >5 cm or major vascular involvement; *T4*, direct invasion of adjacent organ (not gallbladder) or perforation of visceral peritoneum; *N1*, regional lymph node involvement; *M1*, distant metastatic disease; *Tis*, carcinoma in situ; *T1*, confined to bile duct; *T2*, beyond bile duct; *T3*, invades liver, gallbladder, pancreas, or unilateral hepatic artery or portal vein; *T4*, invades other adjacent organs or main hepatic artery or portal vein; *N1*, regional lymph node involvement; *M1*, distant metastasis
Modified from the American Joint Committee on Cancer: *AJCC staging manual*, ed 6, New York, 2002, Springer.

common presentation is unilateral biliary obstruction found during investigation of abnormal liver serum studies. This may be associated with significant unilateral biliary dilatation and/or lobar atrophy, as this can go undetected for a prolonged period due to the absence of symptoms.

Unlike distal cholangiocarcinoma, ultrasonography detects dilated intrahepatic, but not extrahepatic, ducts in patients with perihilar tumors. If done prior to any intervention, ultrasonography can detect the level of biliary obstruction, the absence or presence of vessel involvement, and evidence of a mass at the hepatic hilum. Usually, though, insufficient detail exists to allow operative decision making based on the ultrasound alone. Again, our preference is MRI/MRCP with contrast if perihilar cholangiocarcinoma is a concern. To obtain optimal results, this imaging should occur prior to any intervention of the biliary tract. MRI is the ideal study, as it gives detailed information regarding the status of the bile ducts, vascular involvement, hepatic metastases, and liver atrophy. Calculation of liver volumes permits determination of the adequacy of the FLR.

For diagnostic purposes, invasive cholangiography (endoscopic or transhepatic) is unnecessary. However, most patients already have had some intervention prior to referral. This often makes a difficult diagnosis more so. Furthermore, invasive cholangiography may contaminate isolated segments of the liver or an atrophied lobe, which can result in cholangitis that can be difficult to clear. This leads to the need for additional procedures to drain these isolated segments potentially delaying definitive treatment or affecting the ability to offer curative therapy. Thus, a clear plan should be formulated prior to any invasive cholangiography. Ideally, this decision is made following ultrasonography or MRI/MRCP and in the context of a multidisciplinary treatment team.

TABLE 2: Modified clinical tumor staging for perihilar cholangiocarcinoma

Stage	Criteria
T1	Tumor involving biliary confluence ± unilateral extension to the secondary biliary radicles
T2	T1 tumors and *ipsilateral* portal vein involvement ± *ipsilateral* hepatic lobar atrophy
T3	Tumor involving biliary confluence with bilateral extension to the secondary biliary radicles *or* unilateral extension to secondary biliary radicles with *contralateral* portal vein involvement *or* unilateral extension to secondary biliary radicles with *contralateral* hepatic lobar atrophy *or* main or bilateral portal vein involvement

From Jarnagin WR, Fong Y, De Matteo RP, et al: Staging resectability and outcome in 225 patients with hilar cholangiosarcoma, *Ann Surg* 234:507-519, 2001.

Unless treatment will be nonoperative therapy, a tissue diagnosis is unnecessary, particularly because it can be very difficult to obtain, and doing so frequently delays therapy. In the absence of a history of biliary tract intervention and gallstone disease, the primary differential diagnosis is primary sclerosing cholangitis and, less commonly, gallbladder carcinoma or an idiopathic benign stricture (malignant masquerade). Similar to cholangiocarcinoma at other sites, obtaining preoperative CEA and CA 19-9 levels may assist in postoperative surveillance. Finally, accumulating evidence supports the use of PET/CT for perihilar cholangiocarcinoma, with a utility similar to that discussed for IHC. Again, although not yet the standard of care, recent reports indicate the discovery of additional disease in a significant minority of patients with cholangiocarcinoma, ultimately altering their treatment and preventing nontherapeutic laparotomy.

Tumor Staging

Perihilar cholangiocarcinoma is staged the same as other extrahepatic cholangiocarcinomas by the AJCC (see Table 1). However, preoperative staging using the AJCC system is inadequate for guiding operative therapy. Recognition of this fact is behind the use of the Bismuth-Corlette classification for perihilar tumors (see Figure 1) and a clinical T-staging system based on local tumor features (Table 2). These systems combine preoperative data regarding biliary and portal venous involvement and the presence of hepatic lobar atrophy to determine resectability. These are critical determinants for gauging resectability, as most patients will require a major hepatectomy as part of their resection. Involvement of biliary or vascular structures on the side of the potential FLR precludes curative resection. Likewise, atrophy of the FLR precludes resection. Thus T1 and T2 tumors are potentially resectable, but T3 tumors are not. This staging system correlates well with resection rates and outcome (Table 3).

Conceptually, the treatment objectives for resection appear straightforward. However, from a practical perspective, the decision making for resection of perihilar tumors is among the most complex in hepatobiliary diseases. The difference between a successful resection and margin-positive disease is usually a matter of millimeters. This is critical, because a margin-positive resection confers little benefit compared with no resection in most series. Consequently, referral of patients with perihilar cholangiocarcinoma to a specialist center with extensive treatment experience is appropriate.

Preoperative Preparation

Similar to carcinoma in other locations, resection is the mainstay of treatment for perihilar cholangiocarcinoma. Preoperative evaluation and preparation is focused on tumor resectability, the absence of metastatic disease, and the patient's ability to undergo operative therapy. The MRI/MRCP findings define the extent of resection, the need for hepatectomy and its extent, and the volume of the FLR. If the FLR is

TABLE 3: Clinical T-staging system correlations with resectability and outcome

T Stage	N	Resected	R0 Resection	Hepatic Resection*	Metastatic Disease	Median Survival (Mo)†
1	87	51 (59%)	38 (44%)	33 (65%)	18 (21%)	20
2	95	29 (31%)	24 (25%)	29 (100%)	40 (43%)	13
3	37	0	0	0	15 (41%)	8
Total	219	80 (37%)	62 (28%)	62 (78%)	73 (33%)	16

*Hepatic resection percentages represent a proportion of all resections; remaining percentages represent proportion of total patients.

†Median survival includes all patients, resected and unresected.

Modified from Jarnagin WR, et al: Staging resectability and outcome in 225 patients with hilar cholangiosarcoma, *Ann Surg* 234:507-519, 2001.

inadequate, preoperative embolization of the portal vein on the side for resection is appropriate. A chest radiograph is sufficient evaluation for pulmonary metastases. The role of PET/CT was discussed previously; judicious use is reasonable based on the current data.

Preoperative biliary decompression remains controversial. In a healthy patient with resectable disease and a total bilirubin less than 10 mg/dL, ideal treatment would be resection without any biliary intervention. Patients rarely come in under these circumstances; usually, invasive biliary imaging and intervention takes place prior to consultation. If instrumentation occurs prior to operation, it is imperative to ensure the patient has patent stents and no evidence of cholangitis prior to resection. Fever, chills, or other evidence of cholangitis at the time of operation significantly increases the risk of morbidity and mortality in these patients.

Biliary imaging/stenting is appropriate in several circumstances: when the noninvasive cholangiogram is inadequate for preoperative planning, portal vein embolization is necessary, bilirubin is greater than 10 mg/dL, or the patient is unwell or malnourished and needs preoperative optimization. In addition, if there is a question regarding the function of the FLR, we stent the FLR side and observe the decline in the bilirubin to ensure adequate function of the FLR. Typically, an endoprosthesis is our choice for preoperative stenting, if feasible. Although endoscopic stenting can be difficult, experienced endoscopists can achieve adequate drainage in nearly all patients. If not, transhepatic drainage is obtained. If transhepatic stenting is done, biliary drainage should be internalized to restore bilioenteric continuity.

Treatment and Outcome

Patients with unresectable cholangiocarcinoma usually die within a year of the diagnosis. Most commonly the cause of death is liver failure or biliary sepsis due to biliary obstruction. Potentially curative therapy can be achieved only by complete resection, which typically requires en bloc hepatectomy. Thus, resection is appropriate for medically fit patients without extrabiliary disease.

The presence of metastases, either intrahepatic or within regional lymph nodes outside the hepatoduodenal ligament, is a contraindication to resection. Due to the high risk of undetected hepatic and peritoneal disease (20% to 30%), we begin all of these procedures with diagnostic laparoscopy to minimize the likelihood of nontherapeutic laparotomy.

Resection of perihilar cholangiocarcinomas is technically complex due to the intimate proximity of critical structures within the porta hepatis. The principles of resection include complete tumor excision with negative margins and restoration of bilioenteric continuity. Bismuth type I tumors and stage T1 tumors without unilateral extension to the secondary biliary radicles may be resectable by en bloc resection of the bile duct complex from the superior border of the pancreas to the hepatic hilum. This includes the gallbladder if present. Excision includes skeletonization of the portal veins and hepatic arteries, resulting in a complete lymphadenectomy of the hepatoduodenal ligament from the superior border of the pancreas to the hepatic hilum and the lymphatic tissues around the common hepatic artery.

Transection of the right hepatic duct occurs at the interface with the hepatic parenchyma; transection of the left duct is done at the base of the umbilical fissure, just after (distal to) the junction of the principle caudate lobe branch with the left hepatic duct. This results in at least two bile duct orifices requiring reconstruction. Frozen section analysis of the transected ducts is important to assess margin status. If a duct margin is positive, hemihepatectomy of the side with the involved duct is required. Thus, for any patient with a hilar cholangiocarcinoma, the surgeon should be prepared to perform a hepatectomy if necessary to achieve complete tumor resection.

Involvement of the distal common bile duct margin necessitates the addition of a pancreaticoduodenectomy. A Roux-en-Y hepaticojejunostomy brought into the right upper quadrant through a retrocolic mesenteric defect allows restoration of bilioenteric continuity. A single layer of interrupted 4-0 or 5-0 polydioxanone (PDS) suture approximates the end-to-side anastomosis with the right and left ducts reconstructed to separate enterotomies. We tack the mucosa to the serosa at each of the enterotomy sites with 6-0 PDS to ensure mucosa-to-mucosa approximation between the bowel and bile ducts. Stenting the anastomoses is unnecessary; closed suction drainage placed nearby remains until the patient resumes eating.

Most type II and all type III and stage T2 lesions require en bloc hepatectomy as part of the resection. This often includes resection of segment I, because the segment I ducts drain into the confluence of the right and left ducts. We selectively resect segment I based on the appearance of the cholangiogram or intraoperative findings suggesting involvement of one or more segment I duct.

Hepatectomy is an important component of resection. Multiple published series show a correlation between hepatectomy and the achievement of margin-negative resections and improved survival. En bloc segmental portal vein resection and reconstruction is reasonable if this allows complete resection. When multiple ducts are present following resection, we attempt to join these together by suturing the sidewalls in apposition in an effort to restore biliary continuity with a single enteric anastomosis.

Overall resectability rates for perihilar tumors at the time of laparotomy approximate 60% to 70%. Perioperative mortality is highest following resection of perihilar tumors, between 5% and 10%. For completely resected patients, 5 year survival ranges from 25% to 40%. Margin positivity and lymph node involvement are associated with worse survival.

As with distal cholangiocarcinoma, the role for adjuvant therapy following resection is undefined. In general, the guidelines for adjuvant therapy discussed for distal cholangiocarcinoma are the same used for perihilar tumors. Again, a number of uncontrolled series suggest a beneficial treatment effect from chemoradiotherapy. For patients with completely resected tumors and negative lymph nodes, we usually do not give adjuvant therapy. Patients with microscopically positive margins are offered chemoradiotherapy, and patients with perineural invasion or lymph node involvement are offered chemoradiotherapy with or without subsequent systemic therapy. Again, little data exist to support one approach over another.

Treatment of Unresectable Perihilar Cholangiocarcinoma

Liver Transplantation

Liver transplantation has been used for treatment of patients with locally advanced disease (Bismuth-Corlette type IV or stage T3). Except for reports from the Mayo Clinic of a highly select group of patients who underwent intensive preoperative staging and chemoradiation followed by liver transplant, little data exist to support this approach. A recent systematic review by the Agency for Healthcare Research and Quality (AHRQ) found little data to support this approach. Currently, liver transplant for unresectable cholangiocarcinoma is not standard of care, and its use is confined to a few transplant centers using clinical protocols to study this approach.

Palliation

Most patients with perihilar cholangiocarcinoma are not candidates for resection. Because liver failure and uncontrolled biliary sepsis are the most common causes of death in these patients, adequate treatment of both can prolong survival. Thus the primary goal in these patients is palliation by relief of biliary obstruction. A number of alternatives are available to achieve these goals.

Biliary Drainage

We prefer placement of endoprostheses, if feasible. The site of obstruction dictates whether plastic or metal wallstents are appropriate. Metal wallstents are preferred and can generally be used in most circumstances, as their patency rates are greater than plastic stents. When endoprostheses cannot be placed, percutaneous transhepatic stenting provides excellent palliation. If transhepatic stents are used, they should be internalized to restore enteric biliary drainage. Expandable metal wallstents also can be placed by a transhepatic approach.

Regardless of the approach, only 25% to 30% of the *functioning* hepatic parenchyma needs drainage to achieve adequate palliation. However, adequate drainage is not achieved if segments with portal vein occlusion or atrophy are stented, as these areas are not associated with functioning hepatic parenchyma. Additional stenting beyond relief of jaundice may be required when patients have cholangitis due to isolated, obstructed segmental bile ducts. Stenting is as effective as operative bypass, but it is associated with a lower morbidity. Thus operative bypass is unnecessary and rarely used, except on occasion, when an unresectable tumor is found at the time of laparotomy. In most circumstances, segment III bypass is an effective operative approach.

Chemoradiotherapy and Systemic Therapy

Patients with locally unresectable disease without metastases are candidates for palliative chemoradiotherapy. After adequate biliary decompression has been achieved, patients can be treated with fluoropyrimidine-based chemoradiation. Case series suggest a benefit for chemoradiation, and this approach is frequently used despite the lack of controlled studies demonstrating a benefit. A gemcitabine-based systemic therapy regimen is reasonable for patients with metastatic disease, although no randomized data that demonstrate a survival benefit are available.

Photodynamic Therapy

Patients with unresectable disease without metastases are candidates for photodynamic therapy. A photosensitizing agent, porphyrin, is given intravenously to patients. The porphyrin is retained in cancer cells longer than normal cells, and it is activated with a specific wavelength of light introduced via cholangioscopy. Light activation results in the release of reactive oxygen species and cell destruction.

Several randomized controlled trials demonstrate improved survival in patients treated with photodynamic therapy and stenting compared with stenting alone. Stenting and photodynamic therapy have become our standard approach for locally unresectable patients. Currently the addition of chemoradiotherapy to this approach is under study. A primary limitation of photodynamic therapy is its relatively limited availability.

SUMMARY

Cholangiocarcinoma represents a spectrum of disease, all of which share a high mortality rate despite complete resection. Adequate treatment is hampered by advanced disease stage at presentation and the lack of effective chemotherapy and radiotherapy. Long-term survival is best achieved by complete resection of early-stage disease. Recurrence is predicted by margin-positive resection and involvement of locoregional lymph nodes. An important component of care in these patients is adequate palliation of jaundice. Endoscopic stenting approaches are preferable, as is the use of transhepatic techniques when endoscopy is not successful. Photodynamic therapy is a relatively new approach that prolongs survival and improves quality of life in patients with unresectable extrahepatic cholangiocarcinoma.

SUGGESTED READINGS

Ito F, Cho CS, Rikkers LF, et al: Hilar cholangiocarcinoma: current management, *Ann Surg* 250, 2009:210-18l.

Kahleh M, Tokar J, Conaway MR, et al: Efficacy and complications of covered wallstents in malignant distal biliary obstruction, *Gastrointest Endosc* 61(4):528–533, 2005.

Kahaleh M, Mishra R, Shann VM, et al: Unresectable cholangiocarcinoma: comparison of survival in biliary stenting alone versus stenting with photodynamic therapy, *Clin Gastroenterol Hepatol* 6(3):290–297, 2008.

Li J, Kuehl H, Grabellus F, et al: Preoperative assessment of hilar cholangiocarcinoma by dual-modality PET/CT, *J Surg Oncol* 98(6):438–443, 2008.

Madoff DC, Abdalla EK, Vauthey JN, et al: Portal vein embolization in preparation for major hepatic resection: evolution of a new standard of care, *J Vasc Interv Radiol* 16:779–790, 2005.

National Comprehensive Cancer Network: Hepatobiliary cancers, v1.2010. Available at www.nccn.org/default.asp.

Weber SM, Jarnagin WR, Klimstra D, et al: Intrahepatic cholangiocarcinoma: resectability, recurrence pattern, and outcomes, *J Am Coll Surg* 193:384–391, 2001.

MANAGEMENT OF GALLBLADDER CANCER

Jason K. Sicklick, MD, and Yuman Fong, MD

OVERVIEW

Historically, surgeons have approached gallbladder cancer with fatalism. However, with improved surgical technique and knowledge about this disease, patient survival has been improved. This chapter will review data addressing the treatment of gallbladder cancer, beginning with a brief overview focusing on the epidemiology and natural history, followed by the results of surgical treatment. We will conclude by discussing an algorithmic approach to treating patients with gallbladder carcinoma, and we will provide evidence for this strategy.

EPIDEMIOLOGY

Gallbladder cancer is the most common biliary tract malignancy in the United States, and ranks as the fifth most common gastrointestinal malignancy. Moreover, gallbladder tumors will be found in 1% of cholecystectomy specimens. Annually, there are approximately 5000 new diagnoses, with a disease-specific mortality of approximately 2800 deaths. The annual incidence in females is 1.3 per 100,000; in males it is 0.8 per 100,000. The average incidence is 1.2 cases per 100,000 people per year.

NATURAL HISTORY OF DISEASE

Gallbladder carcinoma is most often associated with cholelithiasis and chronic cholecystitis. In fact, 75% to 98% of all patients with gallbladder cancer have cholelithiasis. Moreover, tumors will be found in 1% of presumed cases of gallstone disease.

Through numerous retrospective studies and large-scale surveillance programs, the natural history of gallbladder cancer has been well defined. The overall 5-year survival is consistently less than 5%, with a median survival of 5 to 8 months. Piehler and colleagues reviewed 5,836 cases in the world's literature from 1960 to 1978. For this 18-year study, they reported 1- and 5-year overall survival rates of 11.8% and 4.1%, respectively. In this cohort, only 25% of patients underwent resection with curative intent, and of those patients who underwent R0 resection, only 16.5% survived 5 years. Perpetuo and colleagues (1978) reviewed the M.D. Anderson Cancer Center experience with gallbladder cancer over 36 years and reported a 5-year survival rate of less than 5% and median survival of 5.2 months. Cubertafond and colleagues reported the results of a French Surgical Association Survey of 724 gallbladder carcinomas and found 1- and 5-year survival rates of 14% and 5%, respectively, as well as a median survival of 3 months. A review of gallbladder cancers from Australia revealed a 5-year survival rate of 12%, with all survivors having only stage I or II disease. In this study, the median survival for patients with stage III or IV disease was a mere 46 days. Finally, Surveillance Epidemiology and End Results (SEER) data from the United States demonstrated similarly dismal findings. Only marginal improvement over earlier studies was noted, with a median overall survival of 10 months (95% CI, 9 to 11 months), as well as 1-, 2-, 3-, and 5-year overall survival rates of 46%, 30%, 23%, and 17%, respectively, in 4180 patients.

THE ROLE OF RADICAL SURGICAL THERAPY

These data have led to a great deal of pessimism regarding the treatment of gallbladder cancer. However, a multiinstitutional review from Japan challenged this convention when researchers reported a 5-year survival of 50.7% for 984 patients who underwent radical resection versus 6.2% for 702 patients who underwent more conservative management. These results suggest that radical surgical therapy may play a role in altering the natural history of this disease. Based upon these and other data, it is now evident that radical liver resection, or extended liver resection, provides a survival benefit in the treatment of selected patients with gallbladder cancer.

The routine use of more radical resections, including those of hepatic segments IVb and V and the common bile duct (CBD), has gained some popularity despite a negative cystic duct margin. There are no randomized data in the literature to show that this is mandatory in patients with Tis, T1, or T2 disease, in which a negative margin is obtained. But despite the paucity of randomized data, recent experience has demonstrated that radical surgery may be a sensible and potentially curative option in the treatment of some of these patients. Together, the data demonstrate that surgical excision is the treatment option of choice for those patients whose gallbladder cancers are confined to the local region of the liver and porta hepatis.

PRESENTATION

The clinical presentation of gallbladder cancer is often identical to biliary colic and/or chronic cholecystitis, making it difficult to diagnose preoperatively. At early stages, gallbladder carcinomas are difficult to differentiate grossly from chronic cholecystitis. As a result, they are often found incidentally upon pathologic section. It is also difficult to distinguish gallbladder cancer from benign gallstone disease using blood tests. Elevated alkaline phosphatase and bilirubin levels are found in cases of advanced tumors, but they may also be found in patients with gallstones. A carcinoembryonic antigen (CEA) level greater than 4 ng/mL is 93% specific for the diagnosis of gallbladder cancer but only 50% sensitive. A serum CA 19-9 level greater than 20 units/mL has a 79.4% sensitivity and a 79.2% specificity, but neither test is routinely obtained in patients suspected of having benign gallstone disease. Therefore, vigilance in examining for cancers using preoperative sonograms or computed tomography (CT) scans is essential. Any mass or polyp associated with the gallbladder or the presence of a porcelain gallbladder should raise concern of gallbladder cancer.

Even at late stages, when the tumor can obstruct the CBD and produce jaundice, gallbladder cancer is often mistaken for benign disease associated with gallstones or Mirizzi syndrome. Therefore any long-term obstruction of the mid-CBD should be considered a gallbladder cancer until proven otherwise. Tumors that arise in the gallbladder neck or within a Hartmann pouch may also infiltrate the common hepatic duct, making them clinically and radiologically indistinguishable from hilar cholangiocarcinomas.

Approximately 60% of gallbladder tumors originate within the fundus; 30% originate in the body, and 10% start in the neck. Most commonly, such tumors grow in a diffusely infiltrative pattern and tend to involve the entire gallbladder by spreading in a subserosal plane. This is the same plane that is dissected for routine cholecystectomy. As a result, if the tumor is not recognized at the time of operation, it is unlikely that a simple cholecystectomy will completely excise the disease, and it may even lead to tumor dissemination. On the other hand, the nodular type of gallbladder cancer tends to have earlier invasion through the gallbladder wall and into the liver or adjacent structures. This type is often easier to treat surgically, because the margins are better defined. In contrast with the nodular growth pattern, the papillary growth pattern portends a better prognosis, because even large tumors often only have minimal gallbladder wall invasion.

The gallbladder lies on segments IVb and V of the liver. Consequently, these segments are often involved early in tumors of the fundus and body. Direct extension into the portal triad structures—the portal vein, hepatic artery, and bile duct—commonly occurs and is a frequent cause of symptoms. Moreover, lymphatic invasion is also common and most commonly involves cystic and pericholedochal nodes (Figure 1). Tumor cells may then metastasize to lymph nodes posterior to the pancreas, portal vein, and common hepatic artery. Advanced disease may ultimately reach the celiac axis, superior mesenteric artery, and aortocaval lymph nodes. Additionally, gallbladder cancers have an incredible propensity to seed and grow. This explains this tumor's ability to grow along needle biopsy tracts and laparoscopic port sites. Growth in these sites may be further exacerbated by bile spillage during laparoscopic cholecystectomy. Hematogenous spread is less common but will present most often as noncontiguous liver metastases (91%), and more rarely as lung (32%) or brain (5%) metastases, based upon postmortem examination.

STAGING

A multitude of systems have been used for staging gallbladder cancer. The most common system for evaluation worldwide has been the American Joint Committee on Cancer (AJCC) Tumor Node Metastasis (TNM) staging system (Table 1). In order to parallel the staging of other biliary cancers, the sixth edition of the AJCC staging system was created. Unfortunately, this system had many deficiencies. Thus the new seventh edition staging reverts to a system that is more congruent with the past staging system.

According to the seventh edition staging system, tumors without perimuscular invasion are considered stage I. Tumors with invasion into the perimuscular connective tissue but without extension beyond the serosa or into the liver are considered stage II. In the absence of regional lymph node metastasis, tumors that perforate the serosa and/or directly invade the liver and/or adjacent structures—such as the stomach, duodenum, colon, pancreas, omentum, or extrahepatic biliary tree—are stage IIIA. Stage IIIB tumors also have nodal metastases without vascular invasion, stage IVA includes those patients with vascular invasion, and stage IVB includes those patients with distant metastases or those with vascular invasion and distant nodal metastases.

RADIOLOGIC WORKUP

The radiologic investigation is often dictated by the disease, and it follows an initial set of investigations. Patients with laparoscopically discovered gallbladder carcinoma often have previously undergone

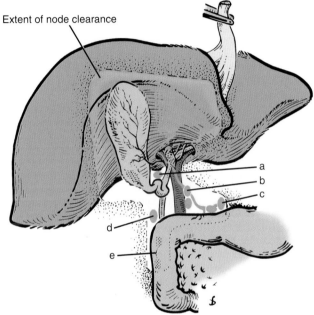

Extent of node clearance

FIGURE 1 Diagrammatic representation of lymph node dissection in an extended or radical cholecystectomy. *(From Blumgart LH, Fong Y: Surgery of the liver and biliary tract, ed 3, Philadelphia, 2000, WB Saunders.)*

an ultrasound. Review of this study is essential and may provide information concerning liver involvement by tumor, biliary extension, and/or vascular involvement. Additional cross-sectional imaging studies are often indicated for appropriate staging of disease. Together, CT and ultrasound make up the most frequently utilized combination for initial assessment. Magnetic resonance (MR) imaging may also be employed as a substitute for CT. If the initial laboratory or radiologic workup suggests evidence of biliary obstruction, additional imaging may be indicated. Endoscopic retrograde cholangiopancreatography (ERCP) and percutaneous transhepatic cholangiography (PTC) are the traditional methods for evaluating the biliary tree.

Over the last decade, MR cholangiopancreatography (MRCP) has improved and has become a suitable, noninvasive substitute for direct cholangiography. Doppler ultrasound and MR angiography also provide noninvasive substitutes for angiography and portography to determine resectability in patients in whom main portal vein or hepatic arterial involvement is suspected.

Recently, a role for fluorodeoxyglucose positron emission tomography (FDG-PET) in the management of patients with gallbladder cancer has been established. This test is useful in diagnosing nodal, peritoneal, and distant metastases. In a series of 31 patients with gallbladder cancer, 7 (23%) had therapy altered by staging with FDG-PET. Together, the radiologic workup will dictate which patients are candidates for operative intervention.

SURGICAL MANAGEMENT

A breadth of operations have been advocated for gallbladder cancer. These range from simple cholecystectomy to combined extended hepatectomy, CBD resection, and pancreaticoduodenectomy. Unfortunately, debate still exists regarding the appropriate extent of surgery. The most practical way of approaching gallbladder cancer is to base therapy upon clinical T stage because of the close correlation between T stage and prognosis. Knowing the likelihood of local, nodal, or peritoneal disease allows for a rational therapeutic approach.

For patients with the earliest stages of the disease, incidental Tis or T1A gallbladder cancer discovered in specimens following laparoscopic cholecystectomy, there is no need for further surgery if the disease is limited to the muscularis propria layer and the staging workup

TABLE 1: Summary of AJCC staging systems

Stage	Fifth Edition	Sixth Edition	Seventh Edition (Proposed)
I	Mucosal (T1N0M0)	IA: Mucosal or muscular invasion (T1N0M0) IB: Perimuscular invasion (T2N0M0)	Mucosal (T1N0M0)
II	Muscular invasion (T2N0M0)	IIA: Perforates the serosa and/or directly invades the liver and/or adjacent structures (T3N0M0) IIB: Tumors with regional nodal lymph node metastases but no invasion of the main portal vein, hepatic artery, or multiple extrahepatic organs/structures (T1-3N1M0)	Muscular invasion (T2N0M0)
III	Liver invasion <2 cm; lymph node metastases (T3N1M0)	Tumor invades the main portal vein, hepatic artery, or multiple extrahepatic organs/structures (T4NxM0)	IIIA: Transmural (T3N0M0) *or* IIIB: T1-3 with nodal involvement (T1-3N1M0)
IV	Liver invasion >2 cm (T4N0M0, TxN1M0) Distant metastases (TxN2M0, TxNxM1) N2 lymphadenopathy (peripancreatic [head only], periduodenal, periportal, celiac, superior mesenteric, or paraaortic nodes)	Distant metastases (TxNxM1)	

is negative. These patients have a 5-year survival rate ranging from 90% to 100%.

Historically, some surgeons have argued that T2 cancers with negative margins only required treatment with a simple cholecystectomy. Recent data from Memorial Sloan-Kettering Cancer Center (MSKCC) suggest that an improvement in survival can be achieved with extended or radical resection compared with simple cholecystectomy alone. Data would also indicate that liver resection with lymphadenectomy is a potentially curative approach for all other gallbladder cancers except those at the latest stages. It is clear from pathologic data that T2, T3, or T4 tumors are associated with more than a 50% chance of metastases to regional lymph nodes. As liver resections have become increasingly safer, increasing numbers of surgical centers are performing radical resections for this disease, and data are consequently accumulating results that justify such an aggressive approach.

Unless a patient has clear contraindications to resection, including medical comorbidities or unresectable disease, surgical exploration should be attempted. We will review the data supporting radical resection for gallbladder cancer at various stages of disease.

Tumors Confined to the Muscularis Propria (T1)

There is now an abundance of data that indicate that early stage gallbladder cancers that have not penetrated through the muscularis propria are adequately treated by simple cholecystectomy. Tsukada and colleagues (1996) demonstrated that in 15 cases with T1 lesions, there were no cases with lymph node metastasis. Following simple cholecystectomy, the 5-year survival was 78% to 100%. In a report of 56 patients treated with simple cholecystectomy alone, only 2 patients (3.6%) recurred and subsequently died of their disease. In retrospect, both patients had submucosal tumor spread that involved the cystic duct margin.

In patients with a pathologic diagnosis of T1 gallbladder cancer following laparoscopic cholecystectomy for suspected benign biliary tract disease, a careful review of the pathology is imperative. Care must be taken to verify negative margins, including the cystic duct. Areas of deeper invasion should also be ruled out. If the gallbladder wall margin is involved by tumor, a liver resection is required. If the cystic duct stump is involved, an excision of the CBD, including the confluence of the cystic duct, is indicated. No nodal dissection is necessary in these cases.

Tumor Invading into the Subserosal Layer (T2)

By definition, T2 tumors invade the muscular coat but do not penetrate the serosal plane. However, the recommended management for T2 disease is an extended (or radical) cholecystectomy that includes a liver resection and regional lymph node dissection. The latter would include removal of periportal, peripancreatic, and celiac nodes. Patients must be informed that the final pathology may not demonstrate residual tumor.

These recommendations are based upon the pattern of disease spread. In the most common infiltrative type of gallbladder cancer, the cancer grows in a subserosal plane, which is also the plane along which the lymphatics travel. When performing simple cholecystectomy for gallstone disease, the gallbladder is usually incompletely removed. The cystic plate, which is the gallbladder serosa on the liver side, is usually left behind, because the subserosal plane is the least bloody plane for dissection that does not enter the lumen of the gallbladder. For this reason, there is an increased likelihood of positive margins after simple cholecystectomy alone.

In a study by Yamaguchi and Tsuneyoshi, 25 patients with tumors extending into the subserosal layer were evaluated. In this group, 11 (44%) had positive microscopic margins after simple cholecystectomy. Furthermore, the likelihood of metastatic disease

to regional lymph nodes can exceed 50%. Indeed, it is perhaps patients within this group of T2 lesions who may have the best chance of benefiting from definitive, extended re-resection. The 5-year survival of stage II patients undergoing simple cholecystectomy is 20% to 57%, but the survival of patients undergoing radical resection is 70% to 100%.

Recommendations for liver resection for gallbladder cancer have ranged from a limited wedge excision of 2 cm of liver around the gallbladder bed to routine extended right hepatic lobectomy. We prefer an anatomic segment IVb and V resection when possible, because this anatomic operation allows the greatest chance of tumor clearance while minimizing the amount of functional liver removed.

For patients presenting with T2 gallbladder cancer discovered at laparoscopic cholecystectomy, a reexploration with the intent to perform a liver resection and regional nodal dissection is recommended. During this reexploration, inflammation from the previous operation may make it more difficult to determine the exact extent of disease. Thus a more radical resection may be necessary to ensure complete eradication of disease. It must be emphasized that complete excision of any suspicious areas must be performed, because any residual tumor will result in recurrence that is usually rapidly fatal. As a result, a right hepatic lobectomy or trisegmentectomy may be necessary.

In the past, recommendations for lymph node dissection have ranged from excision of the cystic duct node alone to en bloc portal lymphadenectomy with pancreaticoduodenectomy. However, combined liver and pancreatic resections have high operative mortalities of near 20% and are not justified by long-term results. On the other hand, portal lymphadenectomy for tumors penetrating the gallbladder beyond T2 is supported by our findings of positive nodes in over 50% of patients with T2, T3, or T4 gallbladder cancer. We believe that an adequate portal lymphadenectomy requires resection of the CBD. This is particularly the case in patients who have only undergone a cholecystectomy, because the periportal nodes are often intimately associated with the CBD. Moreover, resection of the CBD greatly facilitates nodal clearance. To that end, a full Kocher maneuver should be performed, and the lymphatic tissue behind the duodenum and pancreas should be dissected and swept superiorly. Any interaortocaval nodes or superior mesenteric nodes should be included in the specimen if possible.

The CBD should be transected as it courses posterior to the duodenum into the pancreas. The portal vein and hepatic artery should be skeletonized, and all tissue should be swept superiorly along with the transected duct. At the confluence of the right and left hepatic ducts, the CBD should be divided again (assuming the cystic duct does not enter the right hepatic duct). A Roux-en-Y hepaticojejunostomy should be performed to reestablish biliary-enteric continuity.

In addition, all of the laparoscopic port sites should be excised in a full-thickness manner. A number of studies have demonstrated the propensity of this cancer to recur in laparoscopic port sites, because gallbladder cancer has a great potential for peritoneal seeding and dissemination. In fact, the incidence of peritoneal metastases is higher now than was reported in the prelaparoscopic era. One report found a 32% recurrence rate, with the cancer reappearing as a new or enlarging abdominal wall mass on physical examination and/or CT scanning for follow-up of disease. Another study by Paolucci found 174 cases of port-site metastasis after laparoscopic cholecystectomy and 12 recurrences in the surgical scar after converted or open cholecystectomy. This report found a 14% incidence of port site metastases at 7 months after laparoscopic cholecystectomy for cancer. Therefore, it has become our standard practice to excise laparoscopic port sites at the reexploration. During that operation, care must be taken to perform a full abdominal inspection to rule out peritoneal disease. Whether such excision of port sites is useful requires further investigation, because port recurrence may be just a marker for diffuse peritoneal dissemination of disease.

Historically, it was thought that patients who undergo two operations have worse prognoses than those who are treated with a single procedure. Gall and colleagues reported a median survival of 42 months for patients undergoing a curative resection at the first operation versus 12.5 months for those undergoing a curative resection at a second operation. More recent data would suggest that there is no difference in outcomes in patients who have a radical resection after a previous laparoscopic cholecystectomy for unsuspected gallbladder cancer. Moreover, there appears to be no difference in survival or recurrence among patients who have a second operation after an initial open or laparoscopic cholecystectomy. What is also clear is that after a simple cholacystectomy for T2 gallbladder cancer, a subset of patients are later found to be unresectable because of peritoneal disease. Thus the summary of these data for gallbladder cancer treated with initial simple cholecystectomy are that 1) a subset of patients are rendered unresectable for cure because of cancer dissemination during a simple cholecystectomy; 2) if further workup does not find unresectable disease, and the patient successfully undergoes a second, radical resection with curative intent, they do well.

On the other hand, it is evident that an R0 resection significantly improves survival in patients undergoing re-resection. A study from the Johns Hopkins Hospital showed that there was no difference in survival among patients who underwent immediate conversion to an open resection for intraoperatively discovered gallbladder carcinoma (n = 6) versus those patients who underwent laparoscopic cholecystectomy followed by later reexploration for a tumor identified at histopathologic review (n = 33). To summarize, this study suggests that tumors incidentally discovered during laparoscopic cholecystectomy do not require conversion to an immediate open resection. Instead, patients should be referred to a tertiary care center for further evaluation and subsequent exploration.

Advanced Tumors (T3 and T4)

Patients with T3 or T4 gallbladder cancers are initially seen with advanced tumors. After laparoscopic cholecystectomy, not only will there be a pathologically positive margin, but there will also be a hepatic mass on cross-sectional imaging.

Historically, there has been some debate over the justification for more radical forms of surgery in patients with such advanced disease. But as radical resections have become increasingly safer, reports of long-term survivors after aggressive surgical management are now abundant in the literature. Onoyama and colleagues (1995) reported a 63.6% survival after 5 years for Japanese Biliary Surgical Society stage II disease and 44.4% for AJCC fifth edition stage III disease after extended cholecystectomy. They also reported a 5-year survival rate of 8.3% for stage IV disease, and they identified a 5-year survival rate of 60% for patients with N1 nodal disease. Shirai and colleagues (1992) reported a 5-year survival of 45% for patients with node-positive tumors, documenting nine patients surviving over 5 years after radical resection. Another group reported that four (50%) of eight patients undergoing curative resection for AJCC stage III and IV gallbladder carcinomas were alive 81, 50, 13, and 8 months after initial operation. Data from MSKCC (2008) revealed a median overall survival of 10.3 months for a 435 patient cohort. The median survival for those presenting with stage IA-III disease was 12.9 months, and it was 5.8 months for those presenting with stage IV disease. These results represented marked alterations in the natural history of this disease.

Together, these data would indicate that radical surgery for advanced gallbladder cancer may be potentially curative. Patients initially seen with T3 or T4 disease should undergo a staging workup that includes imaging studies to rule out signs of unresectable disease, including noncontiguous liver metastases or signs of carcinomatosis. Barring any contraindications to major abdominal surgery, such as cirrhosis or insufficient remnant liver volume to maintain adequate hepatic function, patients should be explored—or reexplored after laparoscopic cholecystectomy—for radical resection of the tumor, which usually requires a major liver resection and regional lymphadenectomy.

Complications

The operations described above are extensive procedures with substantial risks. In particular, most patients undergoing treatment for gallbladder cancer are in their seventh or eighth decade of life and may be at increased risk as a consequence of concomitant medical comorbidities. In a multiinstitutional review of 1,686 gallbladder cancer resections from Japan, a comparison of morbidity by procedure was made. A morbidity of 12.8% was reported for cholecystectomy, 21.9% for extended cholecystectomy, and 48.3% for hepatic lobectomy. The mortality rates were 2.9%, 2.3%, and 17.9%, respectively. There were 150 hepatopancreatoduodenectomies for gallbladder cancer, with a 54% morbidity rate and a 15.3% mortality rate.

The morbidity and mortality rates for major liver resections have been decreasing, even in the aged population. In our report of re-resection for laparoscopically discovered gallbladder cancer, all resected patients were subjected to some form of liver resection, and the operative mortality was 5%. Despite this fact, complications are real and potentially lethal. The most common complications are bile collections, liver failure, intraabdominal abscess, and respiratory failure. Therefore, the risks of surgical resection need to be weighed against the chances of benefiting from the procedure based on the stage of disease.

ADJUVANT THERAPY

Because of the rarity of gallbladder cancer and the infrequency of completely resected disease, only one prospective randomized trial has studied the utility of adjuvant therapy for gallbladder cancer. This trial evaluated the 5 year overall survival rate in patients following noncurative resection who received postoperative adjuvant chemotherapy using mitomycin C and 5-fluorouracil (5-FU). Survival was improved with adjuvant therapy (26% vs. 1%, P = .03). However, conclusive data do not support the routine use of chemotherapy.

Data regarding radiation therapy are more substantial but not conclusive. One group evaluated intraoperative radiation therapy after complete resection for stage IV gallbladder cancer and reported a 3-year survival of 10.1% for patients receiving radiation therapy versus 0% for surgery alone. Another study of seven patients showed that external beam radiation therapy after complete resection was a safe treatment, and 71.4% (five of seven patients) were alive at a median follow-up of 11 months. Hanna and Rider performed radiation therapy in 51 patients and reported survival to be significantly longer in those who received postoperative radiotherapy compared with those who had surgery alone. Finally, a study from the Mayo Clinic evaluated 21 patients following curative resection along with adjuvant external beam radiation therapy and 5-FU. These 21 patients had a 5-year survival rate of 64% versus 33% in a historical surgical cohort after R0 resection alone. Based on the above data, we advocate employing radiation therapy for patients with node-positive disease and suggest that chemotherapy only be used as a potential radiation-sensitizing agent following resection of disease.

Palliative Management for Unresectable or Metastatic Disease

Palliative therapy should be considered in the context that the median survival for patients initially seen with unresectable gallbladder carcinoma is 2 to 4 months. The goal of palliation should be relief of pain, jaundice, and bowel obstruction and the prolongation of life. These should be achieved as simply as possible given the aggressive nature of this disease.

Biliary bypass for obstruction can be difficult because of advanced disease in the porta hepatis. A segment III bypass is usually necessary if surgical bypass is chosen to relieve jaundice. However, such bypasses have a 30-day mortality rate of 12%. Therefore in the jaundiced patient with advanced, unresectable gallbladder cancer, a radiologic or endoscopic approach to biliary drainage is justified.

Systemic chemotherapy and radiation therapy have little effect on these tumors. Patients with unresectable disease and good functional status who desire therapy should be directed to investigational trials to determine whether any novel therapies may be of benefit.

SUMMARY

Gallbladder cancer is an aggressive disease with a dismal prognosis. It should not, however, be approached with a fatalistic attitude. Appropriate workup and extended resection can result in a cure. Gallbladder cancer will be encountered approximately once every 100 times that a gallbladder is removed for presumed benign gallstone disease. Because these tumors can present with an insidious course, any long obstruction of the mid-CBD is considered gallbladder cancer until proven otherwise.

Gallbladder carcinoma commonly disseminates by four modes: 1) direct extension and invasion of the liver and adjacent organs, 2) lymphatic spread, 3) shedding and peritoneal dissemination, and 4) hematogenous spread to distant sites. To radiologically investigate the extent of disease, the workup may include ultrasound, MRCP, CT, ERCP, and PTC. In addition to a rigorous radiologic workup to rule out locoregionally advanced or disseminated disease, selection for resection is based upon evaluation of the patient's general medical condition.

Based upon this workup, an algorithm has been developed for the surgical management of these tumors. For stage I (T1N0M0) disease, simple cholecystectomy alone is sufficient, if the cystic duct margin is negative; for stage II (T2N0M0) disease, a radical cholecystectomy should be performed. In cases of stage III (T3N0M0) with or without

hepatic invasion less than 2 cm in depth, a radical cholecystectomy is sufficient. For stage IV (T4N0M0) with or without liver invasion greater than 2 cm in depth and no evidence of dissemination, extended hepatectomy should be performed. Therefore those patients with resectable disease should undergo a standard extended cholecystectomy with an extensive nodal dissection to include the peripancreatic nodes, celiac axis nodes, and superior mesenteric artery nodes, as well as skeletonization of the porta hepatis. If the nodal dissection is compromised by the presence of the CBD, then this should be resected. In addition, a segment IVb and V resection of the liver or an extended hepatic resection should be included, as dictated by the location of the tumor as well as surrounding inflammation and scar tissue. Evidence of distant nodal (N2) disease on preoperative workup precludes a curative resection, as no long-term survivors have been reported with gross N2 disease. These patients should be treated for symptoms but should not be offered an operation with curative intent. In the presence of widespread dissemination, there are no surgical options.

SUGGESTED READINGS

Bartlett DL, Fong Y, Fortner JG, et al: Long-term results after resection for gallbladder cancer: implications for staging and management, *Ann Surg* 224:639–646, 1996.

D'Angelica M, Dalal KM, DeMatteo RP, et al: Analysis of the extent of resection for adenocarcinoma of the gallbladder, *Ann Surg Oncol* 16(4):806–816, 2009.

Fong Y, Wagman L, Gonen M, et al: Evidence-based gallbladder cancer staging: changing cancer staging by analysis of data from the National Cancer Database, *Ann Surg* 243(6):767–771, 2006.

Shih SP, Schulick RD, Cameron JL, et al: Gallbladder cancer: the role of laparoscopy and radical resection, *Ann Surg* 245(6):893–901, 2007.

GALLSTONE ILEUS

Parsia A. Vagefi, MD, and David L. Berger, MD

PATHOGENESIS

The first recorded case of a cholecystoenteric fistula with subsequent gallstone ileus is attributed to Dr. Erasmus Bartholin in 1654, originating from his postmortem studies. In 1890, Dr. Ludwig Courvoisier published the first article, citing 125 cases of gallstone ileus, which occurs when a gallstone lodges in the alimentary tract, most commonly the distal ileum, causing a bowel obstruction. For this to occur, however, there must be a cholecystoenteric fistula.

Formation of a cholecystoenteric fistula begins when cystic duct obstruction due to a gallstone causes inflammation of the gallbladder wall, which becomes adherent to a portion of the alimentary tract. Ischemia with subsequent erosion due to pressure necrosis between the gallbladder wall and the adjacent viscus surface leads to cholecystoenteric fistula formation. The mechanical obstruction that ensues is due to stone impaction at a site within the gastrointestinal (GI) tract following passage of a gallstone or gallstones through the fistula and into the lumen of the hollow viscus.

Biliary enteric fistulas occur in approximately 1% of patients with acute cholecystitis. Fistula formation most commonly occurs to the

duodenum (cholecystoduodenal), followed in decreasing incidence by fistulas to the stomach (cholecystogastric), colon (cholecystocolonic), duodenum and colon (cholecystoduodenocolic), and least commonly to the common bile duct (biliobiliary).

CLINICAL PRESENTATION

Gallstone ileus accounts for 1% to 3% of small bowel obstructions in the general population. There is a 5:1 female/male predominance, with elderly women in their sixth or seventh decade of life most commonly affected. Obstruction occurs more often with gallstones greater than 2.5 cm in diameter. It is reported that 80% of the time, enteric gallstones pass spontaneously.

The most common site of obstruction is approximately 6 to 12 cm from the terminal ileum because of its narrow caliber. Patients come in with clinical symptoms of small bowel obstruction—nausea, vomiting, obstipation, and abdominal pain—that have usually been present for a few days. Bilious vomiting is characteristic of a proximal obstruction, whereas feculent vomiting and abdominal distension are more commonly seen in more distal obstructions. Following cholecystocolonic fistula formation, impaction most commonly occurs in the sigmoid colon at an area of angulation with resultant large bowel obstruction. Gastric outlet obstruction caused by duodenal impaction of a large gallstone (Bouveret syndrome) occurs following passage of a gallstone into the duodenal bulb through a cholecystogastric or cholecystoduodenal fistula. Intermittent episodes of bowel obstruction have been termed *tumbling obstructions,* which describes

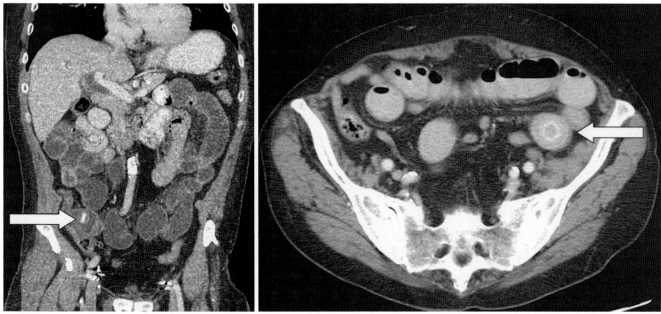

FIGURE I Coronal and axial images from a CT scan of the abdomen demonstrating gallstone ileus, with the gallstones (*arrows*) in the small bowel (photo shows two separate patients).

lodging of the stone at various points along the alimentary tract as the stone passes distally.

DIAGNOSTIC IMAGING

The roentgenographic findings of gallstone ileus were first described in 1941 by Rigler, and they consist of pneumobilia, intestinal obstruction, direct or indirect visualization of a stone within the alimentary tract, or migration of a previously observed gallstone. Unfortunately, these findings are present in only 30% of plain abdominal radiographs obtained in patients with gallstone ileus.

Abdominal computed tomography (CT) is increasingly being used in the assessment of the patient with abdominal complaints. In cases of gallstone ileus, CT scans demonstrate not only the ectopic gallstone with associated bowel obstruction (Figure 1) but also air or oral contrast within the gallbladder or biliary tree due to the cholecystoenteric fistula (Figure 2). Given their increased sensitivity and specificity for the diagnosis of gallstone ileus, CT scans have largely supplanted plain films in diagnosing gallstone ileus.

MANAGEMENT

The management of a patient with gallstone ileus begins with preoperative optimization. The majority of patients are elderly with associated medical comorbidities, thus initial preoperative therapy should include proximal decompression with a nasogastric tube, fluid resuscitation, and correction of electrolyte disturbances.

Once adequately resuscitated, the patient is brought to the operating room. Exploration is carried out through a midline laparotomy, which should allow for the entire bowel to be inspected, as well as the gallbladder. It is paramount that the entire bowel is inspected upon exploration, as multiple intraenteric stones can be present. Once the stone or stones have been identified, they are manually manipulated to a more proximal and unaffected segment of bowel. A longitudinal enterotomy is fashioned on the antimesenteric border of the bowel, with care taken to avoid peritoneal contamination from the proximal fluid-filled, dilated bowel. Following stone removal, the proximal bowel succus can be suctioned through the enterotomy, which is then

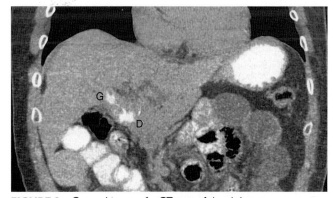

FIGURE 2 Coronal image of a CT scan of the abdomen demonstrating choloecystoduodenal fistula. The oral contrast from the duodenum (D) has filled the gallbladder (G) through the fistula.

closed in two layers in a transverse fashion to minimize narrowing. If full-thickness necrosis of the bowel wall is present at the impaction site, bowel resection is indicated.

Controversy still exists regarding the choice between stone extraction by enterolithotomy alone versus enterolithotomy and cholecystectomy with repair of the cholecystoenteric fistula. It has been suggested that enterolithotomy alone should be reserved for high-risk, unstable patients, and that a definitive one-stage procedure with repair of the biliary-enteric fistula should be performed to minimize the risk associated with a persistent fistula. However, persistent symptoms related to the biliary-enteric fistula—recurrent ileus, cholecystitis, cholangitis—that require reoperations have been documented in only about 20% of patients with a history of gallstone ileus. Indeed, in the absence of persistent cholelithiasis, spontaneous closure of the fistulous tract is noted to occur. The low incidence of recurrent disease, the associated inflammatory process in the right upper quadrant, which often requires an extensive dissection and repair of the cholecystoenteric fistula, and the commonly associated comorbidities in this elderly patient population have led to our support for enterolithotomy alone as the procedure of choice for the management of gallstone ileus.

In a 1994 review of 1001 cases of gallstone ileus, 80% of patients underwent enterolithotomy alone, with a mortality rate of 11.7%, and 11% of patients had an enterolithotomy, along with cholecystectomy and repair of the cholecystoenteric fistula, with a 16.9% mortality rate. In addition to a lower mortality, enterolithotomy alone is a safer operation for this elderly population; in addition, it is technically less demanding, and it is associated with shorter operative times. It should be noted that those patients treated nonoperatively had a mortality rate of 26.5%.

Due to the significant age and comorbidities afflicting this population, nonoperative strategies have been considered to relieve obstruction, as have minimally invasive approaches. For those patients seen initially with gastric outlet obstruction, endoscopic retrieval of stones has been reported for relief of obstruction. Given the size of the stones, the endoscopic approach has often required fragmentation prior to extraction, which has been accomplished with the use of laser lithotripsy. Care must be taken following fragmentation for complete fragment extraction, as the stone fragments have the potential to migrate distally and produce a more distal small bowel obstruction.

Laparoscopically assisted enterolithotomy has been reported with success; however, this approach should be reserved for surgeons with advanced laparoscopic experience. Safe entry into the abdominal cavity in the setting of a distended abdomen secondary to the bowel obstruction is of paramount importance. An open approach for trocar placement into the abdomen should be used in this setting. Although the site of obstruction can often be appreciated, a thorough inspection of the remainder of the bowel with atraumatic bowel graspers must be undertaken to exclude any additional stones. Longitudinal enterotomy with stone extraction, and subsequent transverse two-layer closure of the enterotomy, is carried out following exteriorization of a segment of bowel containing the gallstone through an enlarged laparoscopic port site.

RECURRENT DISEASE

Recurrent bouts of gallstone ileus have been reported in 5% of patients. More than half of the recurrences (57%) occur within 6 months of the initial operation. These early recurrences have been attributed to the presence of an additional intraenteric stone undetected during the initial operative exploration. This stresses the need for a thorough palpation of the entire bowel during initial exploration. It has been reported that 80% to 90% of the time, remaining gallstones pass spontaneously through the fistula without clinical consequence. In the absence of residual gallstones, the majority of cholecystoenteric fistulas will close spontaneously. The recurrence of gallstone ileus, or the persistence of symptomatic biliary tract disease (cholecystitis, cholangitis) in patients who have not had their gallbladder removed, should prompt consideration for cholecystectomy and cholecystoenteric fistula closure.

OUTCOMES

Courvoisier's original report in 1890 cited a 44% mortality rate for patients with gallstone ileus. The review from 1994, which analyzed many older reports, had an operative mortality rate ranging from 11% to 16%, depending on the operative approach. Unfortunately, due to the limited number of cases at individual institutions, it is difficult to obtain accurate morbidity and mortality rates for gallstone ileus over the last decade. With the increased use of CT scanning leading to earlier diagnosis, improved intraoperative anesthetic care, and improved perioperative ICU care, it makes sense to expect that the mortality rate would be significantly lower than the numbers quoted above.

SUMMARY

Gallstone ileus represents a relatively common cause of intestinal obstruction in the elderly female population. The diagnosis can be accurately determined by CT scanning. Operative intervention should be pursued following preoperative optimization of the patient. Enterolithotomy alone for relief of obstruction is the procedure of choice for this patient population, as such patients often carry significant comorbidities and are typically seen in a debilitated state. A laparoscopic approach should be reserved for surgeons who have advanced laparoscopic training.

If symptoms of biliary tract disease recur, consideration for cholecystectomy with repair of the biliary-enteric fistula is warranted, if the patient is healthy enough to undergo the operation. Enterolithotomy in combination with repair of the cholecystoenteric fistula and cholecystectomy should be undertaken with forethought, following careful consideration of the individual patient's suitability to undergo a more extensive operative intervention.

Selected Readings

Doko M, Zovak M, Kopljar M, et al: Comparison of surgical treatments of gallstone ileus: preliminary report, *World J Surg* 27(4):400–404, 2003.

Reisner RM, Cohen JR: Gallstone ileus: a review of 1,001 reported cases, *Am Surg* 60(6):441–446, 1994.

Rodriguez-Sanjuan JC, Casado F, Fernandez MJ, et al: Cholecystectomy and fistula closure versus enterolithotomy alone in gallstone ileus, *Br J Surg* 84(5):634–637, 1997.

Tan YM, Wong WK, Ooi LL: A comparison of two surgical strategies for the emergency treatment of gallstone ileus, *Singapore Med J* 45(2):69–72, 2004.

Vagefi PA, Ferguson CM, Hall JF: Recurrent gallstone ileus: third time is the charm, *Arch Surg* 143(11):1118–1120, 2008.

Transhepatic Interventions for Obstructive Jaundice

Anthony C. Venbrux, MD, Bhupender Yadav, MD, Rydhwana Hossain, MSIV, Shawn N. Sarin, MD, Elizabeth A. Ignacio, MD, Amy P. Harper, ACNP-BC, Jeffrey R. Gourley, MD, and Albert K. Chun, MD

OVERVIEW

The patient with obstructive jaundice is managed with a multidisciplinary team approach. This may involve the combined expertise of multiple healthcare providers and specialists to include primary care physicians, gastroenterologists, surgeons, and interventional radiologists. Although there are many causes for obstructive jaundice (Table 1), percutaneous transhepatic techniques used for such patients is the focus of this chapter.

The interventional radiologist is involved through use of advanced diagnostic imaging techniques, providing percutaneous image-guided access into the bile ducts and offering endoluminal therapies. Such therapies may include percutaneous management of benign biliary strictures, biliary duct biopsy, stone removal (using fluoroscopy or cholangioscopy), palliation of malignant biliary obstruction with endoprostheses, and occasional endoluminal therapies such as radiation, photodynamic therapy, and drug infusion. Therapy may also include application of physiological parameters, such as a biliary manometric perfusion test (BMPT), to help decide when a biliary drainage catheter may be removed (Figures 1 to 5). A dialogue among endoscopists, interventional radiologists, internal medicine specialists, oncologists, primary care physicians, nurses, and other team members is required to manage such patients effectively.

NONINVASIVE IMAGING

Biliary anatomy in the patient with obstructive jaundice is initially defined using noninvasive imaging techniques. Many centers utilize cross-sectional imaging techniques, and many have multidetector scanners that allow for rapid patient evaluation and reformatting of images in multiple anatomic projections. Ultrasound (US) is an inexpensive and generally available imaging modality that provides confirmation of dilated intrahepatic and extrahepatic ducts. It is operator dependent, but in skilled hands, it provides important information as to the possible etiology. For example, it is useful in confirming the presence or absence of dilated biliary ducts and detecting stone disease (cholelithiasis, choledocholithiasis, etc.) It is also advantageous in children, as it utilizes no ionizing radiation. It may also be used at bedside in the critically ill patient to drain the gall bladder (percutaneous cholecystostomy).

When using US to evaluate the liver, the addition of color-flow Doppler easily differentiates visualized tubular structures (dilated biliary ducts) from vessels (hepatic artery, hepatic vein, portal vein). Extrahepatic anatomy may not be adequately visualized in patients with extensive bowel gas (ileus or bowel obstruction), or it may not be technically feasible due to a limited "sonic window" for imaging, such as in a patient with multiple drains, wound dressings that cannot be removed, open abdominal incisions with a silo barrier, and so on.

As mentioned earlier, thin-section helical computed tomographic (CT) images, especially those taken with newer multidetector scanners, allow rapid evaluation of abdominal anatomy. Studies are reproducible, and axial images may be reformatted to provide anatomic detail of liver, biliary anatomy, and other adjacent organs, such as the pancreas and duodenum. CT is more expensive than US, and it utilizes ionizing radiation and generally requires administration of oral and intravenous contrast; however, initial images without contrast may be useful in detecting bile duct stones. Because of CT's greater sensitivity to density differences, poorly calcified or noncalcified stones on plain films may be readily detected on CT. On the downside, CT is not portable, hence ill patients must be transported to and from the scanner.

Magnetic resonance imaging (MRI) is useful, especially given the ability to reformat axial images and produce a MR cholangiogram. The technique requires a significant amount of time, but when performed well, it can result in a detailed representation of bile duct anatomy. In some centers, magnetic resonance cholangiopancreatography (MRCP) has replaced routine endoscopic retrograde cholangiopancreatography (ERCP) for defining bile duct anatomy. Because it utilizes no ionizing radiation, MR is useful in children. However, in such instances, sedation or anesthesia support may be required to complete the MR examination.

ENDOSCOPIC AND PERCUTANEOUS EVALUATION

After clinical evaluation, laboratory blood work, and cross-sectional imaging, the patient must be evaluated endoscopically. ERCP is often the first invasive procedure performed in patients requiring biliary surgery and/or intervention. An ERCP is especially useful in patients with coagulopathies, marked ascites, or in whom intrahepatic lesions,

---

TABLE 1: Etiology of obstructive jaundice

A. Benign
  1. Choledocholithiasis
  2. Papillary stenosis
  3. Choledochal cystic disease
  4. Postsurgical stricture
  5. Mirizzi syndrome
  6. Pancreatic pseudocyst
  7. Sclerosing cholangitis
  8. Parasitic disease
B. Malignant
  1. Pancreatic adenocarcinoma
  2. Cholangiocarcincoma
  3. Gallbladder carcinoma
  4. Ampullary/gastroduodenal carcinoma
  5. Periampullary/periportal lymphoma
  6. Metastatic disease
  7. Neuroendocrine tumors

From Mellinger J, MacFadyen B: Obstructive jaundice: endoscopic management. In Cameron J (ed): *Current surgical therapy,* ed 8, St Louis, 2004, Elsevier.

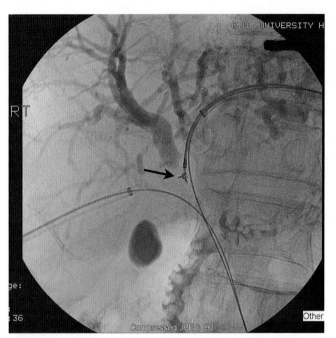

FIGURE 1   Digital spot fluoroscopic image in left anterior oblique projection showing "clam shell" biopsy (*black arrow*) being performed for a hilar mass lesion using the left-sided access. This patient presented with signs and symptoms of obstructive jaundice. Note the lack of contrast in the common bile duct.

such as multiple hepatic cysts, preclude a safe transhepatic approach. Limitations of ERCP in patients with obstructive jaundice include the inability to cannulate the biliary system because of surgically altered anatomy (biliary-enteric anastomosis) and technical limitations in treating intrahepatic or hilar lesions from an endoscopic retrograde approach.

For the patient to be considered an operative candidate for biliary reconstruction, such as with choledochoenterostomy, precise anatomic definition of the intrahepatic and extrahepatic bile ducts is essential in planning the surgical reconstruction. Therefore percutaneous transhepatic cholangiography (PTC) is the preferred procedure. PTC accurately depicts the intrahepatic biliary tree, lesion length, and lesion numbers, and it defines whether or not the biliary disease involves the bifurcation. Should a bifurcation be found, bilateral (right and left) PTC and biliary drainage procedures may be performed. At our institution, the placement of a transhepatic biliary drainage catheter facilitates biliary reconstruction, assisting the surgeon in creating a biliary-enteric anastomosis.

In a clinical situation in which the extrahepatic biliary system has been injured, such as with inadvertent complete clipping of the common hepatic or common bile duct, PTC alone may not fully define the distal extrahepatic bile duct anatomy. ERCP may be required to define distal anatomy up to the clip, and PTC and external percutaneous biliary drainage (PBD) may be used to define anatomy superior to the clipped duct. In this latter case, precise anatomic detail is delineated for eventual biliary reconstructive surgery.

PTC is the first step to PBD. The only absolute contraindication to PTC/PBD performed as a means of access into the biliary system for the treatment of patients with obstructive jaundice is a significant coagulopathy that cannot be corrected. PBD should also be avoided in patients with diffuse polycystic liver disease or in patients with hepatic cysts due to parasitic infections (e.g., *Echinococcus*). Occasionally, cross-sectional imaging and PBD under CT or US imaging guidance may be useful to find an appropriate safe "window" for access into the biliary system in those patients with multiple intrahepatic lesions.

Ideally, the patient with obstructive jaundice undergoing PTC/PBD should not have a coagulopathy. At our institution, PBD is generally not performed if the platelet count is below 100,000 or if the International Normalized Ratio (INR) is greater than 1.5. Should the platelet count or INR parameters be significantly altered, blood products—such as platelets, fresh frozen plasma, and vitamin K—may be administered to the patient for the biliary drainage procedure.

The presence of ascites presents a particular challenge for percutaneous transhepatic drainage. Should biliary drainage be required, ERCP with stent placement is the preferred means of drainage (i.e., "internal drainage"). The patient with significant ascites requiring a percutaneous transhepatic drainage catheter will often be plagued with leakage of ascitic fluid around the tube, which soaks dressings, causes skin irritation and inflammation, and theoretically places the patient at risk of bile leakage into the peritoneum (bile peritonitis).

PTC/PBD Technique Summary

The technique of PTC/PBD is well described and outlined below; it is an invasive procedure. Intravenous antibiotics are started immediately upon admission if a patient is seen with clinical signs and symptoms of biliary sepsis, cholangitis, and so on. In patients who are not septic, intravenous antibiotics are administered on the day of the procedure and are generally continued for 24 hours afterward. As mentioned above, the complete blood count (CBC), coagulation studies, and liver function tests are done as part of our routine preprocedure laboratory analysis.

After counseling as to the risks of the procedure informed consent is obtained. The patient is placed in the supine position. Intravenous sedation and analgesia are administered under an institutional conscious sedation protocol, and physiologic monitoring of blood pressure, pulse, and oxygen saturation is recorded frequently. Although some interventional radiologists prefer initial biliary access from the left subxiphoid approach, at our institution, a right mid-axillary approach is generally used.

The first step is to anesthetize the skin and subcutaneous tissues inferior to the level of the costophrenic angle and above the level of the hepatic flexure. A thin needle (Chiba; Cook, Inc., Bloomington, Ind.) is advanced under fluoroscopic guidance into the liver parallel to the tabletop and directed medially and superiorly. After removing the stylet, the hub of the needle is connected to tubing connected to a syringe containing diluted contrast (1:1 dilution of saline to contrast). As the needle is withdrawn slowly under fluoroscopic guidance, contrast is injected. If the tip of the needle is in a bile duct, contrast is seen to flow away from it. Upon opacification of the biliary anatomy, multiple images are obtained to accurately define anatomy.

Should PBD be considered, and if a peripheral duct has not been entered or the point of duct entry is unfavorable for advancement of a guidewire, a second skinny needle may be used to select a more peripheral right duct. Having placed the needle in a more peripheral location, a coaxial system consisting of a small-caliber, platinum-tipped, steerable guidewire and dilator/stiffening cannula is advanced and used to secure biliary access. Using this system, the initial small-caliber guidewire is exchanged for a larger guidewire, and a biliary drainage catheter may then be advanced to achieve drainage across a specific bile duct lesion.

In those patients with a high-grade biliary structure at the bifurcation isolating the right and the left ductal systems, a left PTC/PBD may be required. Anatomical depiction of the left biliary system requires access from a subxiphoid approach. As part of planning the left PTC/PBD approach, it is important that cross-sectional imaging studies be reviewed to determined whether or not major organs, such as the transverse colon, are interposed between the subxiphoid skin-entry site and the left lobe of the liver, and whether the left lobe is atrophic due to chronic left-sided biliary obstruction. If the left lobe is atrophic and requires drainage, an approach that is more medial than the standard left-sided subxiphoid percutaneous approach may be required.

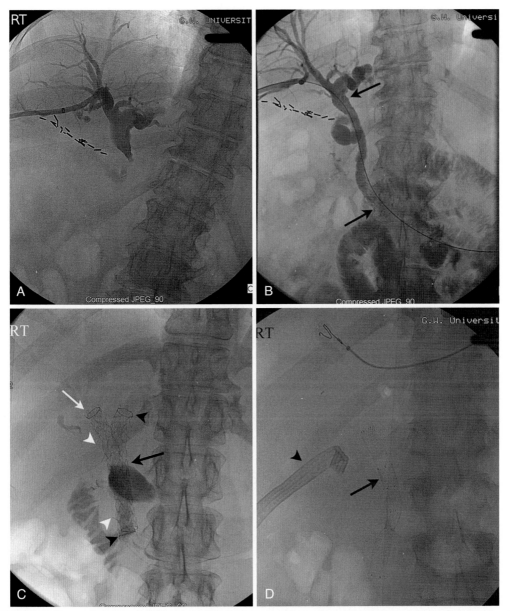

FIGURE 2 **A,** Digital spot fluoroscopic image of the right upper quadrant in right anterior oblique projection showing abrupt cutoff of contrast in the common hepatic duct. There is no opacification of the duodenum. Note the contrast injection via a preexisting right-sided external biliary drainage. **B,** Digital spot fluoroscopic image of the right upper quadrant in the same patient. Cholangiogram performed after placement of an expanded polytetrafluoroethylene (ePTFE) endoprosthesis (Viabil, W.L. Gore) shows rapid flow of contrast through the endoprostheses into the duodenum; *arrows* mark the extent of endoprosthesis. Because the pancreatic head mass was unresectable, an ePTFE endoprosthesis was placed. **C,** Another patient with cholangiocarcinoma who underwent bilateral ePTFE endoprostheses placement. Note the metallic stent "skeleton" (*black arrow*) and radiopaque rings indicating the edges of the ePTFE covering (*arrowheads*). Also seen are uncovered metallic ends adjacent to the radiopaque rings (*white arrow*) and anchoring. **D,** Another patient with a pancreatic head mass who underwent internal bare-metal stent placement for common bile duct obstruction. Note the three overlapping bare metal stents (*arrow*) outlining the common bile duct. Also seen is a Jackson-Pratt drain in the gallbladder fossa (*arrowhead*).

Having achieved percutaneous transhepatic access in the patient with obstructive jaundice, biliary catheter maintenance is required. Initially, the catheter is placed to external (bag) drainage. This is especially true for the patient with sepsis due to infected bile.

If the patient is critically ill and hemodynamically unstable, placement of an external drainage catheter alone will achieve biliary decompression (placement of a simple, locking, multisided pigtail-shaped perforated drainage catheter as an external drain). Once hemodynamically stable, the patient may return for conversion either to an external/internal biliary drainage catheter (biliary stent) or an internal drainage catheter of plastic or metal (internal biliary stent,

or *biliary endoprosthesis*). The latter is generally reserved for patients with surgically unresectable disease and limited life expectancy who are receiving palliative care. Specifics on the use of endoprostheses are covered later in this chapter.

Transhepatic external/internal biliary drainage catheter placement in the patient with obstructive jaundice requires crossing the lesions. The ultimate goal is to eventually reestablish the biliary-enteric "circulation." If left to external drainage alone—that is, given the inability to advance the multiple-sidehole drainage catheter into the small bowel—the loss of bile may result in significant morbidity to the patient, which includes dehydration and electrolyte disturbances.

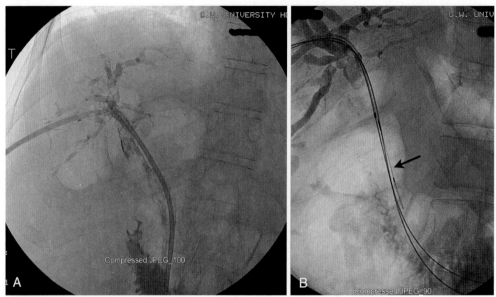

FIGURE 3   **A,** Digital spot fluoroscopic image of an adult patient who presented with obstructive jaundice. PTC/PBD revealed numerous intraluminal filling defects in both intrahepatic and extrahepatic bile ducts. **B,** Endoluminal brush biopsy (*arrow*) performed to confirm the diagnosis through a preexisting right-sided access. Pathologic analysis of the specimen later confirmed this to be metastatic colon adenocarcinoma.

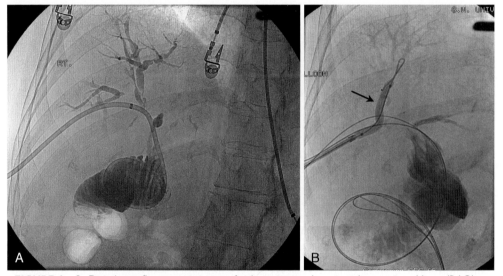

FIGURE 4   **A,** Digital spot fluoroscopic image of right upper quadrant in right anterior oblique (RAO) projection showing multiple intrahepatic biliary strictures in an adult patient who had undergone previous choledochojejunostomy. This patient has primary sclerosing cholangitis. **B,** Digital spot fluoroscopic image of right upper quadrant in RAO projection in the same patient. Patient underwent balloon cholangioplasty (*arrow*) for treatment of intrahepatic biliary strictures.

In such a patient, replacement is with intravenous electrolyte-rich fluid (e.g., Ringer's lactate) or orally with an electrolyte-rich sports drink if the patient is able to tolerate oral fluids.

Biliary drainage catheters are generally flushed once or twice a day, especially in patients with viscous or infected bile. The patient and health care providers must be instructed as to the technique. In the patient with an external/internal biliary drainage catheter, the importance of flushing *into* the tube, "forward flushing," taking care not to aspirate fluid *back* into the syringe must be emphasized. Forceful aspiration with a syringe may rapidly bring bacteria from the gastrointestinal (GI) tract into the biliary system (i.e., under pressure), and sepsis may result.

If left in place on a chronic basis, external/internal biliary drainage catheters require a periodic exchange. Generally, catheters are exchanged over a guidewire on an outpatient basis approximately every 2 to 3 months. For this procedure, the patient receives a single dose of intravenous antibiotics prior to the cholangiogram and biliary catheter exchange. If conscious sedation is required, the patient returns from the interventional suite to the recovery room usually for one hour. During this time, the newly exchanged biliary drainage catheter is connected to an external drainage bag. If the patient remains febrile during this time, the catheter is "capped" (i.e., the bag is removed) before discharge. Should the patient become febrile, a decision is made as to a subsequent course of therapy. The patient

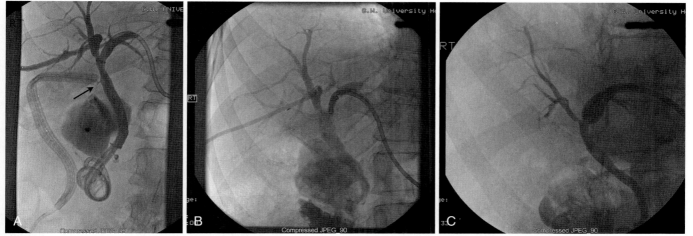

FIGURE 5 **A,** Digital spot fluoroscopic image of right upper quadrant in a patient who had undergone cholecystectomy. A postoperative cystic duct stump leak (*arrow*) was managed by bilateral percutaneous transhepatic internal/external drainage catheter placement to divert bile. The internal/external biliary drainage catheters were left in place for 6 weeks. Note contrast within the duodenal bulb (*asterisk*). **B,** Digital spot fluoroscopic image of right upper quadrant in right anterior oblique projection in the same patient. A trial was performed by keeping the catheter distal ends proximal to the confluence of right and left main ducts, allowing for internal drainage without assistance of drainage catheters across the site of postoperative bile leak. **C,** Digital spot fluoroscopic image of right upper quadrant in left anterior oblique projection showing adequate flow of contrast into the right main duct and common bile duct from a left-sided injection. External biliary drainage catheters were removed after 2 weeks. The patient remained asymptomatic at 6-month follow-up.

may be observed and later discharged on oral antibiotics with the biliary catheter left to external drainage for several more hours (or occasionally overnight) and then capped. The patient is told to return if symptoms worsen. Should an outpatient become septic, the patient should be admitted to the hospital and continued on intravenous antibiotics with the biliary drainage catheter left to external (bag) drainage. The clinical presentation of sepsis is fortunately infrequent after routine outpatient catheter exchanges.

Internal Drainage (Biliary Endoprostheses)

The patient who has undergone transhepatic biliary drainage for obstructive jaundice due to surgically unresectable malignant disease may receive a palliative biliary endoprosthesis (internal biliary stent). If clinically stable at the time of initial biliary drainage, the patient may have placement of the biliary endoprosthesis in a single step. This allows rapid treatment and reduces cost compared with placement of an external/internal drainage with later conversion to a completely internalized catheter system (i.e., a multistep procedure).

The endoprosthesis used is either polymer (plastic) or metallic (bare metal open mesh or a covered stent). The plastic endoprostheses are larger in caliber and require transhepatic tract dilation. This can cause considerable pain to the patient, and there is a theoretical risk of increased bleeding. In contrast, metallic endoprostheses are smaller in caliber at deployment but have significantly larger luminal diameters. For example, self-expanding bare metal stents used as biliary endoprostheses may be 6 or 7 Fr and expand to 1 cm in diameter. Thus for palliation, a patient could undergo PTC/PBD followed by placement of an endoprosthesis in a single step. Transhepatic access for the metallic stent does not require dilation to 10 or 12 Fr, the latter being required for plastic biliary endoprostheses. Although inexpensive compared to metallic endoprostheses, there are few manufacturers of plastic endoprostheses for transhepatic deployment. The majority of plastic endoprostheses are placed endoscopically.

After endoprosthesis placement, the patient's transhepatic access may be removed if there is no significant bleeding. Should bleeding occur, such as with a friable tumor, a temporary external drainage catheter should be initiated for the patient's transhepatic access tract.

This maintains access in the event that the endoprosthesis becomes acutely occluded with thrombus. Once thrombus has cleared, generally in 1 to 2 days, the catheter may be removed after a final cholangiogram confirms patency of the metallic endoprosthesis.

Biliary endoprostheses used for palliation are considered permanent implants, hence their use in patients with limited life expectancy. The patency is generally 6 to 12 months. Patients should be warned of this and told that should the endoprosthesis occlude, repeat endoscopic or transhepatic access may be required to relieve the obstruction.

More recently, covered biliary endoprostheses have been developed that have improved the long-term patency for palliation of malignant biliary obstruction. Percutaneous transhepatic placement of a stent-graft using expanded polytetrafluoroethylene (ePTFE) covered stents has been approved (Viabil biliary endoprosthesis; W.L. Gore & Associates, Flagstaff, Ariz.). These stent-grafts have been recently modified to include perforations or fenestrations in the ePTFE covering so as not to occlude biliary branches that may otherwise be obstructed by a continuous covering. Such stent-grafts also have anchor "barbs" that prevent migration. Greater long-term patency of such stent-grafts provides an additional therapeutic option to enhance the quality of life in patients with unresectable malignant biliary disease.

Early work suggests that in patients with benign disease, ePTFE covered stent-grafts used as biliary endoprostheses may be removed endoscopically. This is not the preferred treatment for benign disease, but it may be used as an alternative in patients who could otherwise not undergo biliary reconstructive surgery or percutaneous transhepatic catheters.

Complications of PTC/PBD

Technical success rates of the PTC/PBD are high, and major complication rates are generally low (5% to 8%). Some reported major complications include hemobilia or hemorrhage, sepsis, biloma, peritonitis, pancreatitis, pleural effusions, and, rarely, death. Another complication is cholangitis, which is found in 20% of patients. Fortunately, cholangitis is brief and often a result of catheter manipulation. Generally, outpatients are treated with oral antibiotic therapy.

Hemobilia/Hemorrhage

Hemobilia occurs when blood enters the bile duct during catheter exchange. This complication has been reported in 2% to 8% of patients undergoing PTC/PBD. It is usually a result of injury to one of the major vessels, either a hepatic artery or vein or portal vein. These patients generally are seen with bleeding from the biliary drainage catheter with right upper quadrant pain. The patient may also present with melena or hematochezia.

Hemobilia can occur from either the venous or arterial system. If it occurs from the hepatic or portal vein, it is generally nonpulsatile and dark in color; this sort is generally managed by either repositioning or upsizing the biliary drainage catheter.

If the bleeding occurs due to injury of an arterial branch, emergency consent should be obtained for hepatic arteriography. The bleeding is generally bright red and pulsatile and may be due to a hepatic artery–bile duct fistula or a pseudoaneurysm of the hepatic artery with communication to the biliary system. The treatment requires transcatheter arterial embolization, generally with embolic coils. Occlusion of the injured vessel is accomplished by advancing a catheter distal to the injury site and coiling it proximally. After hepatic artery branch embolization, the transhepatic access need not be abandoned.

Sepsis

If the patient develops a fever, rigors, and hypotension, sepsis should be suspected. Sepsis can arise even with prophylactic antibiotic treatment, and it can be treated with intravenous antibiotics, expansion of intravascular volume, and pressor support. Identification of the causative agent by bacterial culture is imperative to "tailor" the antibiotic use.

Pericatheter Leakage

Transhepatic access may result in leakage of bile around the catheter. This may also be due to occlusion of the lumen of the catheter, and the problem may be addressed by catheter exchange. Occasionally, ascites may also leak the around the catheter and may resemble bile leakage. The optimal way to treat ascites may be with an internal stent (endoprosthesis). If an endoprosthesis is not possible, the catheter maybe upsized in an attempt to temporarily tamponade the site, allowing time for tract maturation. A purse-string suture on the skin placed around the catheter may also be used to reduce leakage of ascitic fluid.

Biliary Catheter Removal

In addition to the routine biliary exchange every 8 to 12 weeks, the decision as to when to remove the biliary drainage catheter in a patient who has undergone treatment of benign biliary strictures is based on clinical and laboratory parameters and on biliary flow dynamics. As mentioned, the duration of stenting is controversial. If, for example, a focal benign biliary stricture has been stented for 3 to 6 months, a decision is made as to when to remove the tube.

Prior to losing transhepatic access, an "over the wire" cholangiogram is performed by pulling the biliary drainage catheter back over a guidewire. If the site of stented stricture looks patent based on an injection of contrast through the tube, a decision may be made to initiate a clinical trial. For this, a shortened biliary drainage catheter is reintroduced over the guidewire of the same caliber, but the tip is placed above the biliary stricture. Usually, multiple sideholes are cut off to achieve the shortened tube; this functions to maintain percutaneous access and to allow bile to flow across the nonstented, previously dilated stricture. The tube is capped for 1 to 2 weeks, and any signs or symptoms of cholangitis, right upper quadrant pain, fever, jaundice, or leakage around the biliary drainage catheter indicates

a probable failure of the trial. Since percutaneous access has been maintained, the stricture is redilated and restented, or the patient may require surgery.

If the patient remains asymptomatic during the trial, and there is documented evidence of flow across the stricture on follow-up cholangiography, a biliary manometric perfusion test may be performed. Stepwise infusions of dilute contrast are infused at each strictured site via the shortened percutaneously placed tube. Biliary pressures less than 20 cm of H_2O are considered normal. In patients with successful balloon dilation, an asymptomatic "clinical trail," and normal pressures during the biliary manometric perfusion test, a positive predicted value for biliary duct patency at 1 year approaches 90%. Patients are followed carefully with follow-up liver function tests obtained at periodic intervals after tube removal.

In the medical literature, published data for results of percutaneous balloon dilation and stenting indicate long-term patency of 55% to 76% with follow-up periods of 5 and 3 years, respectively. However, most of the data are retrospective in nature. Long-term patency rates for surgical repair of similar lesions are 89% at 72 months follow-up. The initial reports of percutaneous balloon dilation showed significant complications that included hemobilia. This, however, was primarily related to transhepatic access. A more recent multicenter review of cases revealed a 5% complication rate, primarily due to cholangitis with no hemobilia or significant mortality.

In patients with malignant biliary obstruction, the biliary drainage catheter may be removed after placement of an internal stent (endoprosthesis), either plastic or metallic. Patients with sclerosing cholangitis require a combined approached that may involve operative resection of the dominant strictures, PTC followed by drainage, and balloon dilation of intrahepatic strictures and periodic biliary catheter exchanges. If the disease progresses, the patient may ultimately require hepatic transplantation.

SUMMARY

Transhepatic access for obstructive jaundice provides several therapeutic options for patients with both benign and malignant obstructions. A range of therapeutic options is available, including emergent drainage, endoluminal biopsy, biliary stricture dilation, long-term stenting, and endoprosthesis for palliation (see Figures 1 to 5). In addition, direct visualization using endoscopic techniques (choloangioscopy) may assist in treatment of retained intrahepatic stones and may allow a significant reduction in radiation exposure to the patient, interventional radiologist, and personnel in the room.

Improvements in techniques of percutaneous transhepatic cholangiography, biliary drainage, and adjunctive biliary interventions provides the radiologist with ready access to the biliary system to assist in multidisciplinary management of patients with complex biliary disease. The team *approach* is warranted, as such patients often require management by surgeons, radiologists, gastroenterologists, and primary care physicians.

The nonsurgical treatment of patients using transhepatic interventions for obstructive jaundice continues to expand. It is hoped that the above information assists the reader in understanding some of the options available to such patients.

Suggested Readings

Braasch WJ, Warren KW, Blevens PK: Progress in biliary strictures repair, *Am J Surg* 129:34–37, 1975.

Burhenne HJ: Nonoperative retained biliary tract stone extraction: a new roentgenologic technique, *Am J Roentgenol* 117:388–399, 1973.

Burhenne HJ: The technique of biliary duct stone extraction, *Radiology* 113:567–572, 1974.

Gillman R, Alexander MS, Zucker KA, Bailey RW: The use of radionuclide imaging in the evaluation of suspected biliary damage during laparoscopic cholecystectomy, *Gastrointest Radiol* 16:201–204, 1991.

Krokidis M, Fanelli F, Orgera G, et al: Percutaneous treatment of malignant jaundice due to extrahepatic cholangiocarcinoma: covered Viabil stent versus uncovered wallstents, *Cardiovasc Intervent Radiol* 33(1): 97–106, 2009.

Lammer J, Deu E: Percutaneous management of benign biliary strictures. In Kadir S, editor: *Current practice of interventional radiology*, Philadelphia, 1991, Decker, pp 550–553.

Liapi E, Georigiades C, Geschwind JF: Transhepatic interventions for obstructive jaundice. In John Cameron (ed): *Current surgical therapy*, ed 9, St Louis, Elsevier, pp 456–467.

Lillemoe KD, Pitt HA, Cameron JL: Postoperative bile duct strictures, *Surg Clin North Am* 70:1355–1380, 1990.

Lillemoe KD, Pitt HA, Cameron JL: Current management of benign bile duct strictures, *Adv Surg* 25:119–174, 1992.

Mellinger J, MacFadyen B: Obstructive jaundice: endoscopic management. In Cameron J (ed): *Current surgical therapy*, ed 8, St Louis, 2004, Elsevier.

Osterman FA Jr, Venbrux AC: Obstructive jaundice: percutaneous transhepatic interventions. In Cameron JL (ed): *Current surgical therapy*, ed 5, St Louis, 1995, Mosby–Year Book, pp 394–399.

Picus D, Wyman PJ, Marx MV: Role of percutaneous intracorporteal electrohydraulic lithotripsy in the treatment of biliary tract calculi, *Radiology* 170:989–993, 1989.

Savader SJ, Cameron JL, Pitt HA, et al: Biliary manometry versus clinical trial: value as predictors of success after treatment of biliary tract strictures, *JVIR* 5:757–763, 1994.

Trerotola SO, Savader SJ, Lund GB, et al: Biliary tract complications following laparoscopic cholecystectomy: imaging and intervention, *Radiology* 184:195–200, 1992.

van Sonnenberg E, Casola G, Wittich GR, et al: The role of interventional radiology for complications of cholecystectomy, *Sugery* 107:632–638, 1990.

Venbrux AC, Robbins KV, Savader SJ, et al: Endoscopy as an adjuvant to biliary radiology intervention, *Radiology* 180:355–361, 1991.

Venbrux AC, Osterman FA Jr: Percutaneous biliary endoscopy. In LaBerge JM, Venbrux AC (eds): *Biliary interventions: Society of Cardiovascular and Interventional Radiology syllabus*, Reston, Va, 1995, SCVIR, pp 246–258.

Venbrux AC, Ignacio EA, Soltes AP, Washington SB: Malignant obstruction of the hepatobiliary system. In Baum S, Pentecost MJ (eds): *Abrams angiography and interventional radiology*, New York, 2006, Lippincott Williams & Wilkins.

Venbrux AC, Ignacio EA, Soltes AP, Chun AK: Imaging and intervention in the biliary system. In Klein AS, Pemberto JH (eds): *Shackelford's surgery of the alimentary tract vol II*, ed 6, Philadelphia, 2007, Saunders Elsevier.

ACKNOWLEDGEMENT

The authors thank Shundra Dinkins for her expertise in preparing this manuscript.

OBSTRUCTIVE JAUNDICE: ENDOSCOPIC THERAPY

Yongsik Kim, MD, PhD, and Anthony N. Kalloo, MD

OVERVIEW

Obstructive jaundice is caused by an interruption of bile drainage from the biliary system. It usually manifests as jaundice, dark urine, pruritus, nausea, and anorexia, as well as abdominal pain and fever when cholangitis is present. Biochemical tests of liver function show elevation of direct bilirubin, alkaline phosphatase, and serum transaminase.

Common causes of obstructive jaundice include choledocholithiasis, primary cancer of the pancreaticohepatobiliary system, metastatic cancer, and benign strictures of the bile duct. Choledocholithiasis and pancreatic cancer are the two most common causes of obstructive jaundice in the United States (Table 1).

Imaging studies such as ultrasonography (US), computed tomography (CT), magnetic resonance cholangiopancreatography (MRCP), endoscopic ultrasonography (EUS), and endoscopic retrograde cholangiopancreatography (ERCP) are useful for diagnosis. ERCP, first introduced in 1968, is an important diagnostic tool for obstructive jaundice, and it enables therapeutic interventions for relief of obstruction. However, ERCP is relatively invasive and is associated with risks of pancreatitis, perforation, and cholangitis. Hence if a nonobstructive cause of jaundice is suspected, or if the patient is at high risk for complications from underlying medical conditions, less invasive imaging diagnostic methods such as MRCP and EUS are indicated.

Endoscopic, percutaneous, and surgical approaches are effective for decompression of obstructive jaundice. These treatment options may be used alone or in combination. ERCP is less invasive but is as effective as other treatment options, therefore it is often selected as the first line of treatment for decompression of obstructive jaundice. Recently the development of new endoscopic technologies, such as self-expanding metal stents (SEMS) and direct cholangioscopy using the spyglass system, have expanded the role of endoscopy in the management of obstructive jaundice.

ENDOSCOPIC BILIARY DECOMPRESSION TECHNIQUES

Endoscopic nasobiliary drainage (ENBD) and endoscopic retrograde biliary drainage (ERBD) are common endoscopic biliary decompression techniques using ERCP. ENBD uses a long stent, which is placed proximal to the biliary obstruction at ERCP and brought out through the nares. There are several advantages to this approach. First, it allows the ability to measure and characterize biliary outflow.

TABLE 1: Causes of obstructive jaundice

Neoplastic	Pancreatic carcinoma
	Cholangiocarcinoma
	Ampullary carcinoma
	Gastric carcinoma
	Gallbladder carcinoma
	Hepatoma
	Metastatic disease
Benign	Choledocholithiasis
	Benign biliary stricture
	Postoperative stricture
	Posttraumatic stricture
	Pancreatitis
	Sclerosing cholangitis
	Mirizzi syndrome
	Parasites
	Bile duct web

Second, follow-up cholangiograms can be obtained without the need for repeat ERCP. Finally, it can be easily removed without repeating endoscopy. However, having a nasal tube in place may be uncomfortable for patients. Furthermore, because bile is externally drained, there may be loss of water, electrolytes, digestive enzymes, and bile salts.

With ERBD, the stents are placed internally just proximal and distal to the obstructive lesion. Unlike ENBD, there is no loss of body fluid and no extracorporeal bile bag, which is better tolerated by patients. However, endoscopy is needed for stent removal or repeat cholangiography.

Both plastic and SEMS are available. Plastic stents are commonly used because of their low cost and ease of removal. However, plastic stents may migrate and occlude early, within 3 to 6 months, as a result of bacterial colonization and development of a biofilm over the internal surface. When the stents are obstructed, plastic stents can be removed, and new stents can be reinserted. To prevent early occlusion, new stents coated with hydrophilic polymers, silver, or antimicrobial agents have been introduced. Furthermore, some reports show that placing distal ends of stents within the bile duct prevents proximal ascension of microorganisms and decreases bacterial overgrowth. However, none of these new stents or techniques has demonstrated clear benefit in improving stent longevity.

Recently a novel approach to stent design has made use of enhancing the surface area by creating wings and eliminating the traditional lumen. Although preliminary results are encouraging, long-term trials are needed to document efficacy. What is clear is that a larger lumen diameter ensures a longer patency.

The diameter of the SEMS is up to three times larger (8 to 11 mm) than plastic stents, and they have longer patency; however, they are more expensive and are difficult to remove. When the life expectancy of patients is more than 4 to 6 months, metal stents are more cost effective than plastic stents, because the SEMS has been shown to decrease the number of ERCPs needed for stent replacement caused by early stent occlusion. When a SEMS becomes obstructed, a second stent can be inserted through the obstructed stent.

To prevent the obstruction of metal stents by tumor ingrowth, covered metal stents were developed. Covered metal stents are removable and have shown a longer patency period than uncovered metal stents in a few reports. However, there are limitations to using a covered SEMS for hilar lesions, which have a higher risk of cholecystitis and pancreatitis due to the loss of interstrut space, and they have a higher risk of migration than uncovered metal stents.

Recently, new types of stents—such as self-expanding nonmetallic stents, stents with an antireflux valve, drug-eluting stents, and biodegradable stents—have been introduced, but long-term data are lacking for these novel stents.

In general, ENBD and ERBD with plastic stents are indicated for lesions needing temporary drainage or benign lesions, and a SEMS is usually used in patients with malignant biliary obstruction with a life expectancy of more than 3 months.

CHOLEDOCHOLITHIASIS

Choledocholithiasis refers to the presence of gallstones in the common bile duct, which may result in obstructive jaundice, pancreatitis, and cholangitis. ERCP is accurate for the diagnosis of choledocholithiasis with a sensitivity of 90% to 95%. However, ERCP is technically difficult and is associated with risks of pancreatitis. Therefore more noninvasive tests, such as ultrasonography or MRCP, should be performed initially instead of diagnostic ERCP. Transabdominal ultrasonography (TUS) is insensitive for choledocholithiasis with a sensitivity of 50% to 60%. Endoscopic ultrasonography (EUS) and MRCP have sensitivities of greater than 90% for bile duct stones, but MRCP is less accurate for sludge or stones less than 5 mm. EUS, which is more invasive than TUS or MRCP but less invasive than ERCP, is better at finding small stones than

ERCP. EUS could avoid unnecessary ERCP if it is taken before the ERCP in the same session.

CBD stones are found in about 15% of symptomatic gallstone patients and therefore should be considered in patients when planning a laparoscopic cholecystectomy. If CBD stones are detected by MRCP or other imaging tests, then preoperative ERCP is indicated, especially if there is acute cholangitis. The success rate of stone extraction through ERCP has been shown to be up to 90% when performed by experts. During ERCP, bile duct stones are removed by a basket or a balloon after endoscopic biliary sphincterotomy (EBS). Balloon dilation of the sphincter (EBD) to facilitate stone extraction as a sphincter-sparing procedure is associated with an unacceptably high rate of pancreatitis and is not recommended. Recently a few reports have shown that using EBS and EBD in combination made it possible to dilate the biliary sphincter to 20 mm to retrieve large stones without mechanical lithotripsy and without increasing the risk of complications.

Stones are extracted by baskets or balloons after EBS. Baskets are often used for the retrieval of large stones, because baskets have stronger traction force than balloons. Balloons are usually used for stones less than 1 cm or biliary sludge in nondilated bile ducts. Mechanical lithotripsy may be used to pulverize large stones (>15 mm) that cannot be extracted by baskets or balloons.

When extracting the stones with a basket, stones should be removed one at a time, from the distal to proximal bile duct, to avoid bleeding, perforation, and impaction of the basket in the ampulla of Vater. Stones are usually successfully retrieved with an open basket. If the stone is caught in the basket, attempts should be made to open the basket or gently squeeze through the ampulla of Vater. Using baskets that are compatible with an external lithotripsy system is important to prevent basket impaction because of large stones.

The success rate of mechanical lithotripsy is 70% to 80%, and the factors associated with failure are the size of the stone (>30 mm), impaction of the stone at the bile duct, a ratio of stone diameter to bile duct greater than 1, and the type of lithotripter used. Electrohydraulic lithotripsy, laser-induced shock-wave lithotripsy, and extracorporeal shock-wave lithotripsy can be used for pulverizing stones. The ability to perform direct endoscopic cholangioscopy has enhanced the success of electrohydraulic and laser-induced shock-wave lithotripsy. If stone removal is unsuccessful or partially successful, a biliary stent should be placed to prevent biliary obstruction while other therapies are considered.

MALIGNANT BILIARY OBSTRUCTION

Obstructive jaundice can be caused by intraductal or extrahepatic malignant tumors including cholangiocarcinoma, pancreatic cancer, ampullary carcinoma, gallbladder carcinoma, hepatocellular carcinoma, metastasis to the perihilar region or to the liver, and malignant lymphadenopathy.

ERCP is useful for both tissue sampling and palliative treatment. Brush cytology is the most common technique of tissue sampling with sensitivities of 30% to 70% and a specificity of 90%. Multiple sampling techniques, including the use of biopsy forceps, show sensitivity of 43% to 88%. In spite of many other techniques—such as predilation before bush cytology, sampling by a grasping basket, EUS with fine needle aspiration, and peroral cholangioscopy—the accuracy of endoscopic sampling techniques remains unsatisfactory.

Although surgery is the only cure for obstructive jaundice caused by a malignant tumor, most patients have locally extensive or metastatic disease at diagnosis, making curative resection improbable. For surgically unresectable patients, palliative treatment options—which include surgical bypass, percutaneous insertion of stents, and endoscopic insertion of stents—are effective in relieving jaundice and improving the quality of life by relieving pruritus, malaise, and cholangitis. The selection of the palliative method is made according to the location of the stricture, the patient's life expectancy and general condition, risk associated with the procedure, the cost, and patient preference.

TABLE 2: Outcome of endoscopic palliation of malignancy

	SUCCESS RATE (%)		MEAN TIME TO OBSTRUCTION (MO)		
				METAL	
Study	Plastic	Metal	Plastic	Covered	Uncovered
Yoon (2009)	—	—	3.3	—	9.3
Soderlund (2006)	98.0	95.9	1.8	3.6	—
Isayma (2004)	—	100	—	8.5	7.9
Schmassmann (1996)	88	95	4	—	10

When comparing endoscopic palliation methods with surgery, the survival and technical success rates were not different. Surgical palliation had lower rates of recurrent jaundice and better long-term palliation. Endoscopic techniques were more cost effective with lower procedure-related morbidity and mortality and shorter hospital stays.

The strategy for palliative treatment depends on the location of the obstruction. In distal common bile duct obstruction, commonly caused by pancreatic cancer, ERCP is the first choice for palliation. The success rates of endoscopic biliary drainage are around 95% with no differences between plastic and SEMS, however SEMS are reported to have twice as long a patency period as plastic stents. So when the life expectancy of patients is more than 3 months, SEMS should be considered (Table 2).

On the other hand, in hilar biliary obstruction caused by primary bile duct cancer, gallbladder cancer, and metastatic cancer, endoscopic stent insertion is more challenging. The success rate of drainage depends on the level of ductal obstruction. Bismuth type I or type II tumors showed better outcomes than Bismuth type III or IV tumors. When both hepatic ducts are occluded, unilateral stenting guided by MRCP is effective in most cases by targeting the stent to the most dilated ducts. Bilateral stenting should be considered in some selected cases of Bismuth type II cancers, or when there is underlying cholangitis.

Tumor ablation techniques, such as photodynamic therapy using an intravenous photosensitizer and laser and intraluminal brachytherapy, are other treatment options that can be delivered by endoscopy. These techniques complement stenting for palliation of patients with cholangiocarcinoma and are reported to be feasible, safe, and to increase the stent patency period.

BENIGN BILIARY OBSTRUCTION

The causes of benign biliary obstruction include strictures as a result of ductal injury from biliary surgery, such as laparoscopic cholecystectomy and liver transplantation. Other causes include chronic pancreatitis, primary sclerosing cholangitis (PSC), cholangitis, parasites, and external compression.

Surgical bypass procedure remains the definitive treatment for benign biliary strictures, but nowadays, ERCP and biliary stenting with or without endoscopic balloon dilation (EBD) is commonly used because of its minimal invasiveness, lower complication rate, and short hospital stay. The basic concept is to dilate the stricture and maintain patency of the duct by biliary stent until healing of the disrupted stricture occurs. Although plastic stents are easily occluded, they are commonly used, because they can be inserted in multiples and are easily removed. The use of uncovered SEMS has not been advocated because of lack of long-term patency and difficulty in removal because of epithelial hyperplasia. Their use may also make subsequent surgery difficult, when the stent extends into the intrahepatic duct. Recently, several reports using covered SEMS have been promising, but further studies are needed.

The success rate of EBD and stenting has been reported up to 90%. But without stent insertion, the recurrence of stricture approaches 50%. The success rate largely depends on the etiology of the stricture. Postcholecystectomy biliary strictures have been reported to have better outcomes than strictures caused by inflammatory conditions such as cholangitis. Treatment will depend on stricture length, location, severity, and etiology, as well as the patient's comorbidities and preferences.

POSTSURGICAL STRICTURES

Postsurgical strictures are the most common cause of benign biliary strictures, with laparoscopic cholecystectomy being responsible for more than 80%. The endoscopic treatment of postsurgical biliary stricture using biliary stenting shows early success rates of 74% to 90%. A recent study demonstrated a patency rate of 65% during 70 months of mean follow-up. The technique of sequential ERCPs at 3-month intervals with the goal of increasing the number and diameter of the stents with an endpoint of complete stent removal at 12 months appears to have the best outcome and should be considered as a first-line approach. The post–liver transplantation stricture also showed good results with endoscopic stent insertion treatment.

Biliary Stricture from Chronic Pancreatitis

Biliary strictures are present in 2.7% to 45.6% of patients with chronic pancreatitis and may lead to complications such as cholangitis and liver cirrhosis. Chronic pancreatitis accounts for 10% of all bile duct strictures.

Stricture from pancreatitis may resolve spontaneously or with simple biliary stenting as acute inflammation is resolving. But if dense fibrosis had already formed, endoscopic treatment may be difficult, and the patient may need bypass surgery. The single stent insertion showed various long-term outcomes ranging from 10% to 80%. But the recent report using multiple plastic stents with prior EBD revealed a 92% long-term success rate; using partially covered metal stents showed a 90% long-term success rate with fewer intervention numbers and a shorter duration of stent insertion than plastic stents. Endoscopic stenting seems effective for patients with obstructive symptoms and other comorbidities that may preclude surgery.

Primary Sclerosing Cholangitis

The rationale for an endoscopic approach to PSC is based on the stricturing disease causing extrahepatic ductal obstruction. Regardless of its etiology, the presence of significant extrahepatic strictures will contribute to patient symptoms and to decompensation of liver function. Some patients (15% to 20%) will experience obstruction from discrete areas of narrowing within the extrahepatic biliary tree known as *dominant strictures*. It is generally agreed that patients with symptoms from these strictures—such as cholangitis, jaundice, pruritus, right upper quadrant pain, or worsening biochemical indices—are appropriate candidates for endoscopic therapy.

Stricture dilation can be accomplished with balloons or coaxial dilators. At ERCP, a guidewire is placed in the stenotic bile duct, and a 4 mm to 10 mm balloon on a 5 or 7 Fr catheter is advanced across the stricture. Serial dilation is monitored under fluoroscopy to a maximum of 10 to 12 mm in the common bile duct and 6 mm in the hepatic ducts, and it is usually followed by cholangiography to confirm the therapeutic results. Balloon diameter is chosen to match the downstream duct diameter, and the balloon is inflated for 30 to 60 seconds, following the product recommendations, with a goal to improve the "waistline" or resolution of the stricture. Balloon dilation has been shown to be effective alone and may be performed periodically with or without stenting. However, biliary stenting has been shown to be associated with increased complications when compared to endoscopic dilation only and should be reserved for strictures that are refractory to dilation.

At this time, there has been no randomized controlled study to evaluate the effectiveness of endoscopic therapy. Still, much indirect evidence by large retrospective studies suggests that endoscopic therapy results in clinical improvement and prolonged survival. There are studies that show that endoscopic therapy may actually impact the natural history of the disease. Two studies evaluated patients with PSC and dominant strictures who underwent endoscopic balloon dilation and found that the observed 5-year survival rate was significantly better than that predicted by the Mayo risk score.

Complications of Endoscopic Retrograde Cholangiopancreatography

The overall complication rate of ERCP ranges from 4.0% to 15.9%. The most common and serious complication is acute pancreatitis, which occurs in 1.8% to 7.2%. Bleeding and perforation can occur in 1% to 2% and 1% respectively following sphincterotomy. The risk factors for acute pancreatitis include sphincter of Oddi dysfunction, female sex, young age, prior history of post-ERCP pancreatitis, history of recurrent acute pancreatitis, difficult cannulation, pancreatic duct injection, pancreatic sphincterotomy, failed attempts at placing a pancreatic duct stent, precut sphincterotomy, and low endoscopy volume. The risk factors for bleeding are coagulopathy, anticoagulation less than 3 days after endoscopic sphincterotomy, cholangitis prior to ERCP, bleeding during endoscopic sphincterotomy, and lower ERCP case volume.

SUGGESTED READINGS

Chapman R, Fevery J, Kalloo A, et al: Diagnosis and management of primary sclerosing cholangitis, *Hepatology* 51:660–678, 2010.

Cipolletta L, Rotondano G, Marmo R, Bianco MA: for the Italian Evidence-Based Gastroenterology and Hepatology Club: endoscopic palliation of malignant obstructive jaundice: an evidence-based review, *Dig Liver Dis* 39(4):375–388, 2007.

Farah M, McLoughlin M, Byrne MF: Endoscopic retrograde cholangiopancreatography in the management of benign biliary strictures, *Curr Gastroenterol Rep* 10(2):150–156, 2008.

Joyce AM, Heiss FW: Endoscopic evaluation and therapies of biliary disorders, *Surg Clin North Am* 88(6):1221–1240, 2008.

THE PANCREAS

ACUTE PANCREATITIS

David Fink, MD, and John C. Alverdy, MD

OVERVIEW

Despite improved imaging, better access to care, and an increase in the number of cholecystectomies performed as a result of early diagnosis and laparoscopy, acute pancreatitis continues to affect as many as 200,000 patients per year. The majority of new cases resolve with conservative management; however, severe acute pancreatitis (SAP) can develop in as many as 20% of patients and can be associated with infected necrosis, sepsis, and progressive organ failure with an attendant mortality rate approximating 15%. Thus it is important to be able to recognize the "severe" form of acute pancreatitis and monitor and treat those patients aggressively in an intensive care setting.

The most common causes of acute pancreatitis are alcohol use and choledocholithiasis. Less common causes include hyperlipidemia, drug induced pancreatitis, autoimmune disease, post-ERCP pancreatitis, and congenital abnormalities in pancreatic duct development. Despite the progress made in both imaging and laboratory studies to diagnose and stage pancreatitis—including abdominal ultrasound, CT scan, amylase, lipase, and CRP assays—many cases of acute pancreatitis (AP) remain idiopathic. Because there is no association between the etiology and severity of pancreatitis, identifying the cause of AP is important only in allowing the treating physician to remove any stimuli exacerbating the AP, such as a stone in the common duct or an offending pharmacologic agent.

Hospitalizations for AP in the United States have been slowly increasing, from approximately 170,000 per year in 1997 to 245,000 in 2003. Although it has been speculated that this increase may be related to an increase in alcohol consumption and an increase in the incidence of gallstone disease, a causal relationship in these trends has not been established. Over the same period, mortality from pancreatitis fell from 1.90% to 1.43%. This may be related to improvements in diagnosis and staging, earlier access to intensive care therapy, or improved treatment of the disease; no studies have identified specific factors responsible for the decreased mortality.

DIAGNOSIS AND RISK ASSESSMENT

The initial priorities in evaluating a patient with possible acute pancreatitis are to rule out alternative diagnoses and to identify patients with or at risk for progression to severe pancreatitis to manage those patients in an intensive care setting.

Acute pancreatitis most commonly occurs with acute onset of epigastric pain with radiation to the back and/or shoulder, nausea, vomiting, low-grade fever, and leukocytosis. The differential diagnosis includes gastric/duodenal ulcer, cholecystitis, small bowel obstruction, mesenteric ischemia, and abdominal aortic aneurysm. Physical exam is characterized by severe epigastric abdominal pain and the appearance of acute distress.

Laboratory evaluation should include a complete blood count to evaluate for anemia, volume depletion with hemoconcentration, and leukocytosis. Serum lipase is a more specific marker than amylase; a value greater than three times the upper limit of normal is 100% sensitive in diagnosing acute pancreatitis. Although lipase is a sensitive test for the presence of pancreatitis, neither lipase nor amylase levels predict disease severity or progression. Liver function tests may be useful in evaluating possible choledocholithiasis, and serum electrolytes may aid in evaluating volume depletion as a result of fluid sequestration from inflammatory stimuli. C-reactive protein (CRP) has been shown to be a relatively specific marker for severe disease, with values greater than 150 associated with progression to severe disease. Arterial blood gases or central venous oxygen saturation may be useful in patients with suspected sepsis or systemic inflammatory response syndrome.

Multiple scoring systems exist that are designed to predict the progression to SAP; although various scoring systems remain in use, no single system has been shown to be superior in its predictive value. The most well known is the Ranson Criteria, developed in 1974. Although sensitive but relatively nonspecific, a major drawback to the Ranson Criteria is that full evaluation requires data collected 48 hours after admission; this means that it is not an ideal test for early identification of those patient at risk for SAP who require intensive care. Subsequent testing has shown that the Acute Physiology and Chronic Health Evaluation II (APACHE-II) score, a tool designed to predict survival of any patient requiring intensive care, performs as well as the Ranson Criteria, however evaluation requires 24 hours of observation. The APACHE II score is more complicated than the Ranson Criteria and is not ideal for bedside use. As a result, the Bedside Index for Severe Acute Pancreatitis (BISAP) score was developed. This test is obtained at admission, it uses fewer data points, and it is easier to calculate than the APACHE II score. Finally, the computed tomographic scoring index (CTSI), also known as the *Balthazar score*, is another sensitive and specific test that utilizes differences in Hounsfield units on a CT scan performed with intravenous and oral contrast to quantify the percentage of pancreatic necrosis; it is an excellent test for predicting local complications but is less successful at predicting disease severity or mortality. Additionally, since pancreatic necrosis is radiographically indistinguishable from pancreatic edema/inflammation until 72 to 96 hours after the onset of symptoms, this test is the last to be available to the clinician. Table 1 lists some commonly used scoring systems and their relative advantages and disadvantages.

TABLE 1: Commonly used scoring systems: Advantages and disadvantages

System	Scoring	Advantages	Disadvantages
Ranson's criteria on admission: 1. Age >55 years 2. WBC >16 × 10⁹/L 3. LDH >350 U/L 4. AST >250 U/L 5. Glucose >200 mg/dL During initial 48 h: 1. Hgb falls below 10 mg/dL 2. BUN rises by >5 mg/dL 3. Ca <8 mg/dL 4. PaO₂ <60 mm Hg 5. Base deficit >4 mEq/L 6. Fluid sequestration >6 L	1 point for each factor listed; score >3 indicates severe AP	Well known, relatively easy to calculate	Requires 48 hours to complete evaluation
Apache II	Score >8 predicts SAP	Can be calculated within 24 hours of admission	Requires large dataset for processing
BISAP 1. BUN >25 mg/dL 2. Altered mental status 3. Presence of SIRS 4. Age >60 years 5. Pleural effusions	1 point for each factor listed; score >3 indicates severe AP	Ease of use, available within 24 hours of admission	Significantly lower sensitivity than either Ranson's or Apache II; results in greater likelihood of missing severe AP
CTSI	Based on radiographic data	Excellent predictor of local complications; can show infected pancreatic necrosis	Requires 72 to 96 hours, making it a poor test for guiding decisions at admission

WBC, White blood cell count; *LDH,* lactate dehydrogenase; *AST,* aspartate aminotransferase; *Hgb,* hemoglobin; *Ca,* Serum calcium; *SIRS,* systemic inflammatory response syndrome; *BUN,* blood urea nitrogen

GENERAL MANAGEMENT

Resuscitation and Initial Treatment

Once acute pancreatitis has been diagnosed, treatment is centered on maximizing tissue oxygen perfusion and pain control. Tissue perfusion is best improved with volume resuscitation and supplementary oxygen. The intense inflammatory response that accompanies pancreatitis can cause increased vascular permeability and dramatic fluid losses from the intravascular space. Adequacy of fluid resuscitation should be targeted to specific end-organ functional outputs such as blood pressure, heart rate, urine output, and mixed venous oxygen saturation. These endpoints will provide the best surrogate markers that tissue oxygenation has been achieved. In cases where baseline cardiac or renal dysfunction is present, central venous pressure and frequent mixed venous oxygen saturations may be used to guide fluid administration. Careful monitoring of fluid status is required, as fluid requirements can change rapidly and result in either underresuscitation and hypoperfusion or overly vigorous fluid administration that results in abdominal compartment syndrome, which can also impede tissue perfusion. In this latter case, using sequential bladder pressure measurements to gauge the degree of intraabdominal pressure can be useful. In some cases of aggressive fluid resuscitation, abdominal compartment syndrome may be unavoidable, and decompressive laparotomy may be necessary.

Nutrition

In mild disease, patients are often kept NPO until symptoms resolve; this is due to a concern that pancreatic stimulation may exacerbate the pancreatitis. There are no data to support the claim that feeding worsens the inflammatory process; however, it may produce pain and may be poorly tolerated due to ileus caused by the local inflammation. It is common practice to keep the patient NPO until the abdominal pain is resolving and then to slowly advance the diet to clear liquids, low fat foods, and then a more substantive diet as tolerated. However, if the patient tolerates a diet without nausea or significantly increased abdominal pain, many physicians will allow the patient with mild disease to eat a bland diet.

Similarly, the belief that a nasogastric (NG) tube is required to prevent gastric secretions from further pancreatic stimulation is not evidence based. NG tube decompression of the stomach is useful in cases of ileus to prevent aspiration but is not required in all cases of pancreatitis. Severe disease may require treatment with total parenteral nutrition, because nutrients cannot be taken by mouth, or because ileus precludes enteral feeding. However, there is a preponderance of data that demonstrate the benefits of aggressive enteral nutrition in patients with SAP who tolerate enteral feeding. Enteral feeding, either via NG tube or via direct enteral access, has been shown to enhance intestinal epithelial barrier function, reduce septic complications from SAP, and, in some series, reduce mortality. In cases of SAP, every attempt should be made to access the intestinal tract and enterally feed patients.

Endoscopic Retrograde Cholangiopancreatography

The precise role, timing, and complication rate of endoscopic retrograde cholangiopancreatography (ERCP) through the course of acute pancreatitis remains to be clarified. In each case the risks versus benefits must be assessed, and caution should be applied. Manipulation of the sphincter of Oddi and the use of contrast agents have the potential to dramatically worsen the course of the disease; some series have shown increased mortality rates when ERCP is deployed. Issues of timing may be critical, as obstruction may be treated after inflammation has subsided from supportive care. It is generally recommended that ERCP be reserved for patients in whom biliary obstruction is clearly identified and conservative measures are failing to attenuate inflammation.

Prophylactic Antibiotics

There is convincing evidence that morbidity and mortality from necrosis decrease significantly with increasing delay between the onset of pancreatitis and any debridement or intervention. There is also convincing evidence that morbidity and mortality increase significantly when necrotic tissue becomes infected. Although progression to infected necrosis occurs in 30% to 50% of those with necrosis, longer delays before surgical intervention result in lower morbidity and mortality. This has led some to advocate the use of prophylactic antibiotics to prevent or delay infection of necrotic tissue, including broad-spectrum, systemic antibiotic use and the use of nonabsorbable oral antibiotics to eliminate the intestinal microflora, termed *selective digestive tract decontamination*. This remains an area of active controversy; some prospective trials have shown benefits using prophylactic antibiotics, such as decreased infected necrosis and decreased mortality; other prospective trials have shown no benefit. Prophylactic antibiotics carry the risk of allergic reaction, antibiotic side-effect profiles (renal impairment), *Clostridium difficile* colitis, development of antibiotic-resistant bacterial infections, and fungal overgrowth. Individualized decisions regarding the appropriateness, timing, and duration of antibiotics must be tailored to each patient after considering the etiology and progression of the pancreatitis and suspicion of infection. We do not use prophylactic antibiotics in cases of mild pancreatitis, especially when patients can tolerate voluntary oral nutrition; also, when we choose to use prophylactic antibiotics, we use systemic antifungal agents in addition to broad antibacterial coverage to minimize fungal superinfection.

Probiotic Therapy

The same logic that leads some to routinely use prophylactic antibiotics to prevent infection of necrotic material has been applied to probiotic therapy to manipulate the microbiota of the gastrointestinal tract to prevent or delay infection. A recent randomized prospective trial showed increased mortality after such treatment. This experience has shed caution on the use of probiotic therapy in acute pancreatitis, and such therapy is not recommended outside of an approved clinical trial.

MANAGEMENT OF NECROSIS AND INFECTION

Management of Sterile Necrosis and Indications for Intervention

There is a recognized increase in morbidity and mortality in early versus late pancreatic debridement as well as infected versus sterile pancreatic necrosis. Thus, the goal is to delay any intervention as long as possible and to identify and promptly intervene in those patients who progress to infected necrosis. The keys to this conservative management were discussed in "General Management" above.

Although some continue to advocate aggressive surgical debridement in patients with extensive necrosis in the absence of documented infection, most experts advocate nonoperative management of the stable patient, and recent studies confirm this is both safe and successful. Controversy remains in managing patients with sterile necrosis who either fail to progress clinically or have symptoms

related to the presence of necrotic tissue, such as gastric outlet obstruction, persistent pain, fever, and tachycardia. We recommend that if such intervention is considered, surgery should be delayed to allow for demarcation and compartmentalization of the inflammatory and infectious process.

There is even a growing practice of delaying operative intervention in those patients with identified infected necrosis who remain stable. The fear that necrosis will progress to untreatable infection—or that when infection is recognized, a delay in surgery will lead to increased mortality rates—seems to be refuted by various observational studies, which suggest that waiting for demarcation of necrosis and compartmentalization of infection improves outcome. Optimization of physiologic parameters by achieving adequate volume resuscitation prior to imaging and intervention may require several days to achieve. Lower mortality rates for delayed necrosectomy versus early necrosectomy appear to reinforce this bias, although studies are not randomized and matched for severity of illness and underlying medical comorbidities. There is a tendency for most specialized centers to delay surgical intervention for 3 to 4 weeks until demarcation of necrosis and compartmentalization of infection become evident, prominent infectious sites are percutaneously drained, cardiopulmonary and renal function has been stabilized, and antibiotics have been adjusted relative to culture results and dosing parameters. Patients with significant sterile necrosis, or any infected necrosis, who deteriorate clinically and do not respond to conservative measures warrant intervention, albeit at the risk of incurring an increase in operative morbidity and mortality. As with most complex disorders of inflammation and infection, there is a trade-off to aggressive surgical intervention and a risk of delay to obtain adequate source control.

Another possible indication for intervention is abdominal compartment syndrome. Due to massive fluid sequestration and volume resuscitation, patients can have extremely positive fluid balances on the order of 15 L. This can produce elevated intraabdominal pressure leading to respiratory embarrassment and impaired visceral perfusion. Since the goal of treatment of acute pancreatitis is maintenance of adequate tissue perfusion, both to the pancreas and all vital organs, decompressive laparotomy may be required and should not be delayed when abdominal compartment syndrome is identified.

Diagnosing Infected Necrosis

Because infected necrosis is an indication for intervention, it is important to be able to identify the progression to infected necrosis. Fever, leukocytosis, and tachycardia are all common in patients with SAP, making the diagnosis of infected necrosis a challenge. Although many serum markers have been evaluated for their predictive value, none are routinely used in practice. Procalcitonin shows a great deal of promise, both as a predictor of progression to SAP and an identifier for infected necrosis, but specific threshold values and the timing of such assays remain areas of active study.

Without an accepted serum marker, imaging and microbial culture of necrotic tissue remain the primary diagnostic tools. Sequential imaging is often necessary to make the diagnosis of necrosis; clinicians should have a low threshold for imaging and reimaging in cases of SAP in which necrosis is documented or suspected. CT scanning can yield diagnostic clues, such as revealing the presence of extraluminal gas or highly septated and organized fluid collections that appear emphysematous. Preexisting renal impairment and pancreatitis-associated renal impairment are both common and present a challenge in a patient requiring repeated scanning with IV contrast. It is important to work closely with radiologists to develop protocols to minimize contrast dosing, and specific goals of each imaging study should be discussed with the radiologist to allow for individualized dosing of contrast material.

Ultimately the diagnosis of infection is made by the retrieval of tissue that is cultured positive for bacteria or fungi. The gold standard remains CT-guided fine needle aspiration (FNA). The possibility of sample error or sample contamination always exists, and patients who continue to display a fulminant course with no clinical improvement and persistent organ failure may require repeated FNA.

Pancreatic Debridement

Operative Planning

Considerable advances in technology and technique have expanded the potential therapeutic options for pancreatic debridement, including image-guided catheter drainage, endoscopic drainage, and laparoscopic drainage.

The patient's clinical condition guides the nature of the intervention. The timing of drainage, imaging, and surgical intervention are decisions based on the perceived immune status of the host, the aggressiveness of the infective organism, and the success or failure of source control with drainage and antibiotics. Concerns such as a severely immune compromised host, the presence of virulent and antibiotic resistant organisms, or an inaccessible infected collection should prompt a more aggressive approach.

In stable patients, using a step-up approach that starts with catheter drainage of infected collections may help minimize the morbidity associated with repeat procedures. Repeat imaging studies, improvements in critical care monitoring and management, tight glycemic control, catheter drainage, and new antibiotics all offer a degree of safety that has allowed this conservative approach to be more widely accepted. Mortality rates for SAP are still quoted as 10% to 15% by most authors, but a few academic centers have recently been reporting mortality of 5% to 10% using multidisciplinary teams in intensive care units. Despite this trend in improved outcome, the precise cause of decreased mortality relative to a specific management approach remains elusive.

Open Surgery

Pancreatic debridement can be achieved via various surgical approaches and incision strategies, including bilateral subcostal or midline incisions, intraperitoneal laparoscopy, or laparoscopic intracavitary dissection. Each has its own merits, and each is variably applied based on surgeon preference; previous abdominal surgery; location of necrosis, inflammation, or infection; time course from the onset of symptoms; and physiologic stability of the patient. In an early necrosectomy, tissues are inflamed, adherent, and hemorrhagic, and surgery is performed via open incision. This approach is associated with bleeding, adjacent organ injury, and difficulty in closing the abdomen, depending on the degree of dissection, blood loss, and volume resuscitation. Abdominal packing may be necessary and may temporarily provide damage control if abdominal closure is used. As a result, early debridement can be technically challenging and incomplete, as the risk to the normal pancreas and the risk for development of excessive bleeding and adjacent-structure injury is high. Late operative necrosectomy is easily facilitated by the ability to simply "scoop out" necrotic tissue that is loosely adherent to adjacent structures, including the pancreatic gland itself.

Standard open debridement can proceed along many routes; it can include direct access to the pancreas via division of the gastrocolic omentum or a lateral and inferior mesocolic approach to avoid the difficulties of entering an inflamed lesser sac, which can resist entry due to dense inflammatory adhesions. A primary survey of the entire upper abdomen to examine for bulging points of entry and potential sites of dense inflammation is warranted. Use of newer coagulation devices to address the highly friable and engorged omental and mesocolic vessels is also advisable. In many patients, suture ties are needed to control hemorrhage from these sites. Use of fibrin-soaked packs, collagen matrix sponges, and topical thrombin can be useful. Hemorrhage from raw, debrided structures, such as the pancreas itself and the retroperitoneal surface, may require packing, compression, and even packing closure for a second look within 24 to 48 hours with damage-control closure.

Depending on the extent of necrosis, full abdominal exploration may be necessary to include the deep recesses of the pelvis. Full exposure, irrigation, gentle debridement, and planned reexploration should be carried out in patients with severe inflammation. In some cases it may be necessary to carry out closed suction and irrigation when complete debridement is not possible because of the risk of excessive hemorrhage or adjacent-organ injury. There appears to be less enthusiasm for high-volume lavage.

Endoscopic Necrosectomy

Endoscopic methods utilizing both transgastric and transduodenal debridement of necrotic tissue have been described. Obviously this is a very specialized technique and should only be undertaken by experienced endoscopists; all techniques describe the use of endoscopic ultrasound to identify necrotic collections and avoid vascular structures when making enterotomies and debriding tissue.

Once the enterotomy has been established to provide access to the necrotic tissue, standard endoscopic tools—biopsy forceps, lavage, and suction—can be used to debride necrotic tissue. Because of the limited size of the available instruments and suction tubing, this technique will be more limited in its ability to debride thick fibrinous tissue. After removing as much necrotic tissue as is safely allowed, pigtail drains may be left in place for continued drainage through the enteronecrostomy. Alternatively, the endoscopic gastrotomy can be extended and left open to promote necroma evacuation, effectively functioning as a cyst gastrostomy.

Traditional Laparoscopic Necrosectomy

Traditional laparoscopic debridement using an established pneumoperitoneum and standard laparoscope, ports, and instruments has been described. Port placement is highly individualized; it should be well planned preoperatively and based on the location of the necrotic collections, with specific care devoted to avoiding major vascular structures. A CT scan is required to plan the operative strategy, and intraoperative ultrasound—either endoscopic, transcutaneous, or both—can be used to identify blood vessels and occult collections. Once ports have been placed and the necrotic tissue has been identified, tissue is debrided using a combination of blunt graspers, irrigation, and suction. An EndoCatch bag (USCC, Norwalk, Conn.) may be used for collecting larger pieces of necrotic tissue.

Laparoscopic Intracavity Debridement

Laparoscopic intracavity debridement is useful in patients who have had image-guided catheters placed with incomplete resolution of infected necrosis, usually related to insufficient drainage because of catheter size or thick necrotic material and tissue. The patient is taken to the operating room with interventional radiology assistance and fluoroscopy present. Using the existing small-bore catheters, a flexible wire is advanced under fluoroscopic guidance into the necrotic cavity. The drain is removed, and a blunt-tipped 5 mm port is carefully advanced into the necroma and then upsized to a 15 mm port using the Seldinger technique.

With the large-bore port in place, the diaphragm is removed from the port to allow direct access to the necroma, and evaluation of any liquefied material is carried out with irrigation and suction. Once the liquefied material has been evacuated, the diaphragm may be replaced to allow for gentle insufflation of the necrotic cavity and insertion of the laparoscope to visualize the entire cavity and possible internal septae/fibrous bands. A blunt grasper can be inserted through the same port coaxially with the camera (Figure 1) to allow for debridement and removal of tissue under direct visualization

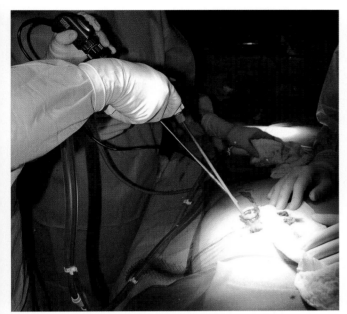

FIGURE 1 Intraoperative photo showing 15 mm single-port access allowing multiple instruments (camera, blunt grasper) to be used simultaneously. Debrided necrotic tissue is seen on the lap pad.

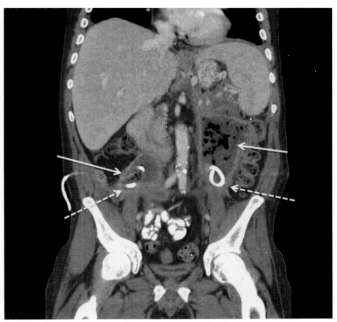

FIGURE 3 Coronal section of a preoperative CT scan showing extensive retroperitoneal emphysematous necrosis (*solid arrows*) despite the presence of interventional radiology-placed catheters (*dashed arrows*).

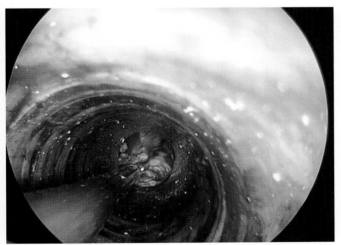

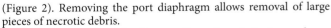

FIGURE 2 Intraoperative view from laparoscopic camera. Necrotic tissue at the base of the port is being manipulated and removed using the blunt grasper.

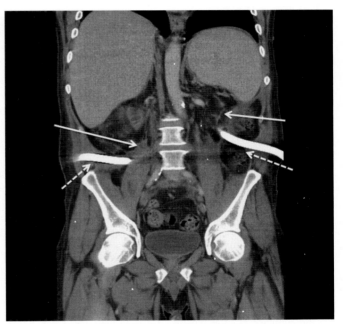

FIGURE 4 Coronal section of a postoperative CT scan showing resolution of inflammatory collections (*solid arrows*) and the up-sized large drains (*dotted arrows*).

(Figure 2). Removing the port diaphragm allows removal of large pieces of necrotic debris.

The large port allows for the use of large-bore irrigation and suction devices. One particularly useful instrument is a pulse-lavage device inserted through the port to break up the more densely adherent tissue. Once tissue has been debrided, a large (32 Fr) red rubber drain is fenestrated and placed in the cavity through the port; the port is then removed, and the site is closed around the drain, which is secured to the skin and placed to suction. Images are shown of preoperative coronal CT sections (Figure 3), revealing extensive emphysematous necrosis despite the presence of small-gauge, image-guided catheters in the collection; postoperative images show the much larger drains with complete resolution of the emphysematous tissue (Figure 4).

SUMMARY

Pancreatitis remains a relatively common condition that resolves with conservative treatment in the majority of cases, but it can progress to severe systemic disease in up to 20% of patients, requiring intensive care. Multiple algorithms for predicting disease severity exist, but no one, optimal system has been identified. The most effective decision aids at admission include APACHE-II, CRP, and BISAP criteria.

Procalcitonin is the most promising new marker being evaluated for prediction of SAP.

The focus of any care algorithm is to maximize tissue oxygen perfusion; fluid resuscitation and supplemental oxygen are also critical. CT scan is useful in quantifying necrosis and identifying infected necrosis, however, necrotic tissue is not radiographically distinguishable from inflamed viable tissue for 72 to 96 hours after onset of disease.

In mild disease, nutrition can be maintained through a diet as tolerated. In severe disease, early enteral nutrition has been shown to be beneficial. If enteral nutrition is poorly tolerated because of ileus, parenteral nutrition should be considered as a less effective alternative. Prophylactic antibiotic use remains controversial and is individualized based on severity of illness and suspicion of infection, and probiotic use remains unproven at this time.

Indications for intervention in severe disease include infected necrosis, sterile necrosis with prolonged failure to improve clinically (relative indication), and abdominal compartment syndrome requiring decompression. In SAP, delayed intervention/debridement is associated with decreased morbidity and mortality, and infected necrosis is associated with increased morbidity and mortality. The goals remain to maximize tissue oxygenation and identify potential infected necrosis via CT scan or FNA early.

Pancreatic debridement methods continue to evolve, with minimally invasive techniques emerging. Initial results are promising, but long-term follow-up and direct comparison between minimally invasive techniques and standard open debridement has yet to be completed. The gold standard remains open surgical debridement.

Suggested Readings

Dellinger EP, Tellado JM, Soto NE, et al: Early antibiotic treatment for severe acute necrotizing pancreatitis, *Ann Surg* 245:674–683, 2007.

Fagenholz PJ, Castillo CF, Harris NS, et al: Increasing United States hospital admissions for acute pancreatitis, 1988-2003, *Ann Epidemiol* 17:491–497, 2007.

Papachristou GI, Muddana V, Yadav D, et al: Comparison of BISAP, Ranson's, APACHE-II, and CTSI scores in predicting organ failure, complications, and mortality in acute pancreatitis, *Am J Gastroenterol* 105:435–441, 2010.

Petrov MS, van Santvoort HC, Besselink MGH, et al: Enteral nutrition and the risk of mortality and infectious complications in patients with severe acute pancreatitis, *Arch Surg* 143:1111–1117, 2008.

Rodriguez JR, Razo AO, Taragona J, et al: Debridement and closed packing for sterile or infected necrotizing pancreatitis: insights into indications and outcomes in 167 patients, *Ann Surg* 247:294–299, 2008.

Gallstone Pancreatitis

Timothy R. Donahue, MD, and Howard A. Reber, MD

OVERVIEW

The annual incidence of acute pancreatitis (AP) in the United States is 40 cases per 100,000 adults, a rate that is increasing. Despite improvements in critical care and interventional techniques, patients still experience high rates of morbidity and mortality. The severity of the disease varies widely, and there is still no specific treatment. Gallstone pancreatitis (GSP) is associated with gallstones, microlithiasis, and/or biliary sludge, and it is the most common type of AP in the Western world. Treatment of patients with GSP often differs from treatment of those with other types of AP and is dependent upon disease severity. Thus it is not only important to identify cases of GSP at the outset but also to predict the likely severity of disease. For example, patients with severe disease or concurrent cholangitis may benefit from early endoscopic retrograde cholangiopancreatography (ERCP) and endoscopic sphincterotomy (ES) to relieve biliary obstruction and clear the common bile duct (CBD). In contrast, patients with mild disease and no evidence of cholangitis do not need urgent ERCP, but they should have their gallbladder removed during the index hospitalization. This will prevent recurrent attacks of GSP if the gallbladder is left in situ. In this chapter we examine the etiology, pathogenesis, presentation, diagnosis, severity, and treatment of GSP.

ETIOLOGY AND PATHOGENESIS

Gallstones, including biliary sludge and microlithiasis, are the most common cause of AP in the Western world, and they account for 35% to 50% of cases. The second most common cause of AP is alcohol abuse (25% to 30% of cases). Patients with AP due to gallstones may have a history of symptomatic cholelithiasis. However, GSP is frequently caused by small, silent stones that cause transient pancreaticobiliary obstruction but have not previously caused symptoms of biliary colic. Alcoholic pancreatitis should be suspected when the patient has a history of alcohol abuse and prior episodes of AP that can be superimposed on a history of chronic pancreatitis. This is true even if they have coexistent gallstones. Numerous other, less common causes of AP also exist (e.g., pancreas divisum, various medications, ERCP, viral and bacterial infections).

Regardless of the etiology of AP, there probably is a common mechanism at the cellular level that initiates the acute inflammatory response. Normally, activation of the pancreatic proenzymes is delayed until the enzymes reach the lumen of the small intestine. There, enterokinase on the duodenal mucosa converts trypsinogen to its active form, trypsin, which in turn activates other pancreatic proenzymes. Indeed, multiple protective mechanisms prevent the intracellular activation of the pancreatic digestive enzymes within the acinar cells where they are formed. In pancreatitis at least one of those protective mechanisms appears to be overcome, and intracellular activation occurs. In experimental animal models of the disease, normal secretion of the digestive enzymes out of the cell is blocked, and the enzymes instead come into contact with certain intracellular lysosomal hydrolases (e.g., cathepsin B). These hydrolases activate the proteases, especially trypsinogen, and this causes acinar cell injury, which results in pancreatitis.

At the cellular level, this injury initiates the elaboration of proinflammatory cytokines that exacerbate the local pancreatic inflammation; if the inflammation is severe enough, it may become generalized and cause systemic inflammatory response syndrome (SIRS). The degree of local and systemic inflammation varies over a wide range, and patients with the most severe forms also experience other end-organ damage, including acute renal failure (ARF), acute respiratory distress syndrome (ARDS), gastrointestinal (GI) bleeding, and severe coagulopathy.

The precise mechanism that explains how *gallstones* initiate pancreatic autodigestion is not well established, but it appears to involve transient obstruction of the bile and/or pancreatic ducts by a stone. Indeed, gallstones are recovered in the stool of 85% of patients with GSP, compared with only 10% of patients with symptomatic cholelithiasis who do not develop pancreatitis. The obstruction of the main pancreatic duct is presumed to lead to the intracellular proenzyme activation already described.

PRESENTATION AND DIAGNOSIS

In clinical practice, a diagnosis of GSP is usually made in patients with AP who have radiologically confirmed cholelithiasis, gallbladder sludge, or choledocholithiasis and lack other potential causes for AP, especially alcohol abuse. Female and elderly patients develop GSP more frequently than males or younger patients. Typical symptoms include severe, acute, constant epigastric or generalized abdominal pain that radiates to the back with associated nausea and vomiting. It is rare that all symptoms are present, however. In patients with severe AP, the pain may be masked by other signs and symptoms of SIRS, including a depressed mental status. Patients with GSP also may have a history of biliary colic or may present with symptoms of acute cholangitis.

Findings on physical examination depend on the severity of the episode of pancreatitis. Patients with mild disease most often have mild abdominal tenderness. In contrast, patients with severe disease can have diffuse abdominal tenderness and evidence of peritonitis, rigidity, and guarding that mirrors a surgical abdomen. Such patients may also be seen in shock initially, because of large fluid sequestration in the extravascular space, with attendant hypotension, tachycardia, tachypnea, and lethargy. Despite aggressive resuscitation, over the first 24 to 48 hours, patients with severe disease can develop worsening abdominal signs with distension and tympany because of a paralytic ileus.

Serum amylase and lipase and liver chemistries that include transaminases, alanine aminotransferase (ALT) and aspartate aminotransferase (AST), alkaline phosphatase, total and conjugated bilirubin, calcium, and tryglycerides should be determined in patients who are suspected of having AP. The serum amylase can have a high false-positive rate because the pancreas is not the only source of amylase in the serum: 65% originates from the salivary glands. In contrast, the pancreas is the only source of serum lipase, so an elevated lipase has a much higher sensitivity (85% to 100%) and specificity (95% to 100%) for AP. An elevated serum ALT three times the normal value or total bilirubin at least twice the normal value has a positive predictive value (PPV) of 95% for gallstone-related AP as opposed to pancreatitis from other causes. Serum calcium and triglycerides should also be measured in these patients, because each can have an etiologic role.

Information from abdominal imaging complements the clinical history and laboratory results, and it aids in confirming the diagnosis of GSP. It also helps to assess the severity of disease. Ultrasound (US), contrast-enhanced CT scan, MRI with gadolinium contrast, and magnetic resonance cholangiopancreaticography (MRCP) are the studies most commonly used. In patients who are seen initially with symptoms of mild AP, a transabdominal US of the right upper quadrant should be ordered. US can identify gallstones in the gallbladder with a sensitivity of over 95%. It is less accurate in identifying choledocholithiasis (sensitivity 40% to 60%). US can also identify pancreatic parenchymal or peripancreatic edema, but it is not useful to assess the severity of pancreatitis. CT scan is more valuable in this regard. In addition, a CT scan may be less accurate than US in detecting gallbladder stones, but it is relatively sensitive (75% to 95%) in detecting choledocholithiasis or a dilated CBD.

Patients who have what is anticipated to be moderate or severe GSP and those who have mild pancreatitis whose clinical course worsens should have a contrast-enhanced CT scan early in their hospital course. This may show pancreatic and/or peripancreatic edema, which could help to confirm the diagnosis of AP. In addition, CT can be useful in patients who are seen initially with evidence of an acute abdomen, where the diagnosis is unclear. Early CT is the best test to gauge the severity of disease. Even if a CT is done at admission, a repeat CT scan usually after 3 days may be useful to evaluate disease progression.

The technique for the CT scan is important. Intravenous (IV) contrast-enhanced CT with so-called pancreas protocol provides the most detailed information about the pancreatic parenchyma. The protocol calls for 2 to 3 mm thin images of the pancreas following injection of IV contrast during the *pancreatic phase* with additional images obtained later during the *venous phase*. During the pancreatic phase, the pancreatic parenchyma, celiac axis, and superior mesenteric artery are enhanced with contrast; the venous phase shows the superior mesenteric, portal, and splenic veins.

Key information that can be obtained by the CT scan includes the degree of inflammation, parenchymal necrosis, fluid collections, and/or evidence of infection. Focal or diffuse pancreatic enlargement, irregularity of the pancreatic border, or peripancreatic stranding or fluid collections can be associated with inflammation. Evidence of gas bubbles within the pancreatic fluid collections can be a sign of superinfection, and parenchymal areas that do not enhance with contrast—a real value of less than 30 Hounsefield units, measured during the arterial or pancreatic phase—correlate well with pancreatic necrosis.

MRI with gadolinium contrast can be used as a substitute for a contrast-enhanced CT scan. Combined MRI with MRCP can provide detailed information about the pancreatic parenchyma; the CBD, including the presence of choledocholithiasis; and the main pancreatic duct. In addition, MRI is ideal for patients with renal insufficiency who are not yet on dialysis and for pregnant patients, as it does not require administration of nephrotoxic contrast agents or ionizing radiation.

PREDICTING DISEASE SEVERITY

Predicting the severity of pancreatitis early in patients with GSP is one of the most challenging and important aspects of their care: 80% of patients with GSP will have a mild or moderate course, and 20% will have severe disease. Overall, 5% of patients with AP, and up to 30% with severe AP, die of direct complications. Half of those who die do so during the first week from multisystem organ failure (MSOF); the rest die later from complications arising from infected pancreatic necrosis. Thus, it is important to accurately identify patients with severe disease at the time of admission to help guide their care, predict prognosis, and to anticipate and prevent complications. Multiple scoring systems—Ranson criteria, Acute Physiology and Chronic Health Evaluation (APACHE-II), Atlanta Classification of 2002, Glasgow score, and Balthazar CT Severity Index (CTSI)—have been developed to assess the severity of disease, but none have been universally accepted.

Patient demographics and signs and symptoms at the initial visit or early during the clinical course also help to predict severity. Older or obese patients with multiple comorbidities are more likely to have severe AP. Also, the presence of SIRS or organ failure at admission or early after admission as evidenced by shock, pulmonary insufficiency, renal failure, or gastrointestinal bleeding predicts severe disease.

Ranson criteria (Table 1) is the most commonly used pancreatitis staging system in the United States. Based on a combination of 11 different clinical and laboratory data points, each of which is assigned a score of 1 point, the Ranson scale was originally developed to predict severe disease, defined as disease resulting in death or the need for an intensive care unit (ICU) stay beyond 7 days. The 11-point scoring system is measured at two points: five initial data points are taken at admission, and six other data points are taken after 48 hours. The original system has been updated for use on patients with biliary pancreatitis, and in the modified system, the data point for arterial oxygen saturation (PaO_2) is omitted. To reflect this change, the disease-severity cutoff values are adjusted, and the total points are limited to 10. An initial Ranson score greater than 3 has been used as the cutoff to predict severe biliary pancreatitis. A recent meta-analysis

TABLE 1: Comparison of clinical and laboratory data used for Ranson criteria of severity in both biliary and nonbiliary acute pancreatitis

	Biliary Pancreatitis	Nonbiliary Pancreatitis
Admission		
Age	>70	>55
WBC (mm³)	>18,000	>16,000
Serum glucose (mg/dL)	>220	>200
Serum LDH (U/L)	>400	>350
Serum AST (U/L)	>250	>250
Within 48 Hours		
Hematocrit fall (%)	>10	>10
BUN increase (mg/dL)	>2	>5
Serum calcium (mg/dL)	<8	<8
PaO_2 (mm Hg)	—	<60
Base deficit (mEq/L)	>6	>4
Fluid sequestration (L)	>4	>6

TABLE 2: Atlanta criteria for severity (2002)

Feature	
Organ failure	Shock (systolic blood pressure <90 mm Hg) Pulmonary insufficiency (PaO_2 <60 mm Hg) Renal failure (serum creatinine level >2 mg/dL after rehydration) Gastrointestinal bleeding (>500 mL/24 h)
Local complications	Pancreatic necrosis (>30% of the parenchyma or >3 cm) Pancreatic abscess (circumscribed collection of pus containing little or no pancreatic necrosis) Pancreatic pseudocyst (collection of pancreatic juice enclosed by a wall of fibrous tissue or granulation tissue)
Unfavorable prognostic signs	Ranson score ≥3 APACHE-II score ≥8

estimated the accuracy for this cutoff level with a sensitivity of 75%, specificity of 77%, PPV of 49%, and negative predictive value (NPV) of 91%.

A frequently cited shortcoming of the Ranson criteria is that the clinician must wait 48 hours to complete the calculation and achieve the criteria's full predictive ability; however, an accurate prediction of disease severity at the time of presentation would better aid in initial treatment. The Glasgow criteria, primarily used in Europe and rarely in the United States, also requires 48 hours to complete.

In contrast, the APACHE-II score provides prognostic information and has the advantage of being able to be calculated at any time, which is particularly useful when the clinical picture changes, or when the patient is admitted to the hospital days after the beginning of the attack. Composite APACHE-II total scores of 5 to 10 have been used as cutoffs to predict severe AP at admission, after 24 hours, or after 48 hours. As the cutoff levels increase so do the sensitivity and specificity of the system. Cutoff levels of 5 yield a similar sensitivity and specificity, as does a Ranson score greater than 3. Calculating the APACHE-II composite score is cumbersome, which limits its widespread use; it includes 12 individual variable points, age points, and chronic health points.

The lack of precise, universally accepted definitions of disease severity and organ failure have limited the ability to compare scoring systems that predict prognoses of AP. Thus in 1992 an international symposium was held in Atlanta, Georgia, to address both of these issues (Table 2). *Severe AP* was defined as the presence of both organ failure and/or local pancreatic complications along with unfavorable prognostic signs as determined by either the Ranson criteria or the APACHE-II score.

Individual laboratory tests can also be used to predict severity. C-reactive protein (CRP) is used widely in Europe but not routinely in the United States, with a cutoff of 150 mg/L used to predict severe disease. Elevated CRP at the time of admission has little predictive value, but after 24 to 48 hours, it has a sensitivity of 80% and a specificity of 76%, both similar to the accuracy of the Ranson and APACHE-II scores. In addition, the degree of hemoconcentration,

as measured by the serum hematocrit (HCT), is associated with the amount of inflammation and intravascular fluid lost to the interstitium. Using the serum HCT to predict severity is theoretically useful, as more fluid is lost from the intravascular to interstitial space with worsening inflammation. However, a number of different retrospective analyses have found a wide range of sensitivities (35% to 79% and 80% to 95%) and specificities (35% to 90% and 70% to 90%) for serum HCT at the time of diagnosis and after 24 hours, thus calling its utility into question.

Contrast-enhanced CT scan or MRI with gadolinium contrast initially and/or after 48 to 72 hours can also help to predict disease severity. In fact, the CTSI (Table 3) combines a score for the degree of pancreatic and peripancreatic inflammation or fluid collections with a score based on the amount of pancreatic necrosis. The composite score is significantly associated with death, prolonged hospital stay, and need for necrosectomy. To calculate the composite score, the degree of pancreatic parenchymal or peripancreatic inflammation is assigned a score of 0 to 4 points, to which are added 2, 4, or 6 points that correspond to a less than 30% necrosis, 30% to 50% necrosis, or greater than 50% necrosis, respectively.

TREATMENT

Mild Disease

Patients with mild, acute GSP—as defined by a Ranson score less than 3, an APACHE-II above 8, or CTSI less than 2—initially require supportive care. At admission, they should be kept NPO and placed on maintenance IV fluids with electrolyte and fluid deficits aggressively replaced. Liver chemistries, amylase, lipase, electrolytes, and CBC should be determined at admission and followed daily. Routine use of prophylactic antibiotics does not improve morbidity or mortality rates for patients with mild disease. Appropriate triage is to the regular ward or to a monitored bed, depending on the patient's comorbidities and functional reserves.

The degree of resuscitation should be monitored closely, with *adequate* resuscitation defined by a urine output of 0.5 to 1 mL/kg/hr and resolution of tachycardia or hypotension. Serum hematocrit (HCT) and oxygen saturation (SaO_2) by pulse oximetry should also be measured frequently, as a progressive decrease in HCT and/or SaO_2 are early indicators of worsening systemic inflammation and interstitial fluid sequestration that may be present before lability of vital signs or oliguria. An arterial blood gas (ABG) level should be obtained with

TABLE 3: Balthazar CT score and CTSI

Balthazar CT Score

Grade	CT Findings
A	Normal
B	Focal of diffuse enlargement of the pancreas, including irregularities of contour and inhomogenous attenuation
C	Pancreatic gland abnormalities in grade B + peripancreatic inflammation
D	Grade C + 1 fluid collection
E	Grade C + ≥2 fluid collections and/or the presence of gas in or adjacent to the pancreas

CTSI

CT Grade	Points	Necrosis	Points	CTSI
A	0			
B	1	None	0	1
C	2	<30%	2	4
D	3	30% to 50%	4	7
E	4	>50%	6	10

worsening SaO_2 (<95%). There should be a low threshold to transfer the patient to the ICU with evidence of worsening disease.

A cholecystectomy, either laparoscopic or open, should be performed during the initial hospitalization in patients with mild GSP, because it decreases attacks of recurrent GSP to less than 10%, and it is safe. If the gallbladder is not removed, the risk of recurrent pancreatitis is as high as 90%, with a 90 day risk of recurrence of 50%, which supports cholecystectomy prior to discharge. The timing of cholecystectomy during the initial hospitalization has been the subject of much debate. We suggest waiting for evidence that the pancreatitis and peripancreatic inflammation is improving, as measured by resolving epigastric pain, which usually takes about 48 to 72 hours for mild disease; by waiting at least this long, the need to convert from a laparoscopic to open procedure and the chance for inadvertent CBD injury are decreased.

The best approach to managing the potential for CBD stones in patients with mild GSP is not well defined and is thus clinician dependent. Some clinicians image the CBD preoperatively with MRCP, ERCP, or endoscopic ultrasound (EUS); some image the CBD intraoperatively, with cholangiography or laparoscopic US, in all patients who come in with gallstone pancreatitis to identify those with persistent CBD stones, regardless of their initial US findings or laboratory results.

In contrast, most clinicians take a more selective approach, based on the observation that most of the stones (90% to 95%) will pass spontaneously. All patients with acute cholangitis, regardless of the severity of AP, should undergo urgent ERCP to decompress the CBD. Those who do have CBD stones visualized on US and those who have a persistently elevated total bilirubin (>3.0) during their initial hospital course should undergo ERCP/EUS, which is the most sensitive nonoperative method to detect or confirm choledocholithiasis.

Patients with GSP who undergo diagnostic US and have neither common duct dilation nor intraductal stones evident and who have a mildly elevated or down-trending total bilirubin or alkaline phosphatase may not require additional common duct imaging. Within this group, the subgroup of patients whose total bilirubin or alkaline phosphatase stays *mildly* elevated after 2 to 3 days may require MRCP prior to surgery, as they have a low but real probability of CBD stones that is not sufficiently high as to justify an invasive test (ERCP/EUS) that can be associated with complications such as perforation and bleeding, albeit at a very low frequency.

If a filling defect is identified in the patients who undergo MRCP, these patients should undergo ERCP before surgery. The advantages of MRCP include its noninvasive nature, which avoids the potential complications of ERCP. Its disadvantages are lower sensitivity at identifying CBD stones compared with ERCP/EUS. Moreover, if a stone is identified, the patient still needs an ERCP for stone removal. CBD exploration is reserved for the 5% of patients who have stones that cannot be retrieved by ERCP, or those with altered surgical anatomy that may not be approachable by endoscopic techniques. Alternatively, these patients could be managed by the interventional radiologist with transhepatic techniques.

Patients who are seen after multiple recurrent attacks of acute pancreatitis of unclear etiology, including lack of gallstones within the gallbladder, should have a cholecystectomy after all other potential causes of acute pancreatitis have been excluded. In these patients, sludge or microlithiasis that is undetectable by U/S and other imaging techniques may be present.

Severe Disease

Patients with severe GS—defined by a Ranson score above 3, APACHE-II above 8, or CTSI above 2—require aggressive critical care to maintain sufficient tissue oxygen delivery to minimize complications and avoid death. Patients should be urgently triaged to an ICU, given standard maintenance and aggressive replacement fluids to offset the fluid that extravasates from the intravascular space to the interstitium, and offered prompt treatment of electrolyte and metabolic imbalances. In addition to the routine labs obtained for patients with mild disease, an ABG should be drawn immediately at admission and followed closely thereafter. Low serum bicarbonate and base deficit are important signs of underresuscitation.

Consensus is emerging that restoration of normal acid-base status is the most reliable indicator of adequate resuscitation. In addition, a decreasing HCT or SaO_2/PaO_2 during fluid replacement can be an early sign of severe or worsening inflammation and extravascular fluid sequestration as already described. A nasogastric tube (NGT) and Foley catheter should be placed. A contrast-enhanced CT scan or MRI with gadolinium contrast can be obtained at admission for aid in diagnosis, but this is usually repeated after 48 to 72 hours to radiographically evaluate progression of disease.

The timing of ERCP in patients with severe GSP has been examined with a number of randomized controlled trials and meta-analyses, but the data are still somewhat controversial. For example, one recent trial randomized patients with severe GSP to either 1) early ERCP or 2) delayed ERCP and appropriately omitted patients with concurrent acute cholangitis. This trial failed to show any benefit of early ERCP. However, a subsequent meta-analysis found that in patients with severe GSP, early ERCP significantly decreased complications, with an odds ratio (OR) of 0.27, although it did not appear to decrease mortality (OR, 0.6). In patients with mild disease, neither mortality (OR, 0.62) nor complications (OR, 0.89) were significantly reduced. We believe that patients who do not respond to aggressive resuscitation during the first 24 hours and who exhibit signs of SIRS with persistent or worsening epigastric pain or elevated bilirubin have a high likelihood of an impacted biliary stone. They should undergo urgent ERCP, endoscopic sphincterotomy (ES), and stone extraction within 48 hours. All patients seen initially with acute cholangitis should be urgently decompressed with ERCP and ES.

Patients with severe GSP have at least a 50% risk of developing pancreatic necrosis that can become infected during their acute illness. A number of meta-analyses have evaluated the efficacy of prophylactic antibiotics in patients with severe GSP on various outcomes, including survival, with mixed results. Thus there is still no consensus statement that addresses prophylactic antibiotic administration. Regardless, if prophylactic antibiotics are chosen, drugs that have good pancreatic parenchymal penetration should be given. Imipenem, in particular, has been shown to significantly improve outcomes in patients with severe AP and should be used as a first-line treatment.

Clinical suspicion for the presence of infected pancreatic necrosis should be raised with significant leukocytosis (white blood cell count >15 × 10³/μL), fever (temperature >38.5° C), or other signs of sepsis. This clinical picture should prompt a contrast-enhanced CT scan done according to a pancreatic protocol. Areas of pancreatic parenchyma that do not enhance with IV contrast (<30 Hounsfield units) are likely necrotic. If small air bubbles are present within the nonenhancing areas, this indicates ongoing infection with gas-forming bacteria, and the patient should be taken to surgery after adequate resuscitation. In contrast, if no gas bubbles are present but there are nonenhancing areas or parenchymal or peripancreatic fluid collections, a fine needle aspiration (FNA) should be performed to determine whether infection is present. FNA is relatively precise (sensitivity 90%, specificity 100%) for detecting infection, but false negatives do occur. As a result, if infection is present, usually with intestinal flora, the patient should be taken to the OR for debridement. If infection is not present, but the clinical suspicion of infection continues, FNA should be repeated in a week or so. If the clinical suspicion is low, in the face of a negative FNA, the patient should continue to be treated nonoperatively until the acute SIRS resolves. Later debridement of necrotic tissue may still be advisable in some patients who do not recover promptly.

Deferring surgery as long as the clinical picture will allow is the best approach; with time, the necrotic area organizes, which decreases postoperative morbidity and the need for repeated interventions. The operative procedure performed depends on the intraoperative findings, and a preoperative CT scan that shows the involved areas (fluid collections, necrotic debris) provides an important roadmap: debridement of the necrotic pancreas with wide external drainage is required. If the degree of inflammation and infection allows the gallbladder to be removed safely, this should also be done.

Unlike patients with mild GSP, patients with severe GSP who do not require an operative debridement should have cholecystectomy delayed for at least several months or until much of the inflammation has subsided. A contrast-enhanced CT scan should be obtained to help with decisions about the timing of surgery and whether other complications of the pancreatitis (e.g., pseudocysts) also need to be addressed.

Special Situations

Patients Unfit for Surgery

Elderly patients or patients with mild to moderate GSP and comorbidities that preclude surgery can be managed by ERCP and ES alone under light sedation. The ES allows for free passage of stones, sludge, and debris through the sphincter of Oddi, which avoids pancreaticobiliary obstruction and repeated episodes of pancreatitis. Such patients have a low risk of recurrent AP (5% at 2 years' follow-up), but 20% still develop recurrent or persistent acute cholecystitis, cholangitis, or symptomatic cholelithiasis.

Pregnant Patients

Gallstone disease is common (25%) in pregnant patients, and cholecystectomy is the second most common surgery during pregnancy; appendectomy is the most common. If surgery is required, the best time is during the second trimester. Thus, patients who present with mild GSP in their first trimester should be managed conservatively until they reach their second trimester. If surgery is performed laparoscopically, insufflation of the abdomen should be limited to 10 mm Hg to minimize fetal loss. If CBD imaging is necessary, MRI/MRCP or EUS should be used, rather than CT scan, to minimize fetal radiation exposure.

Symptomatic patients who come in during their third trimester should be treated supportively and should undergo cholecystectomy in the immediate postpartum period. If open surgery is performed during the third trimester, preterm labor occurs in up to 40%; during pregnancy, the abdomen is inaccessible laparoscopically due to the enlarged uterus.

Suggested Readings

Forsmark CE, Baillie J, AGA Institute Clinical Practice and Economics Committee, AGA Institute Governing Board: AGA Institute technical review on acute pancreatitis, *Gastroenterology* 132:2022, 2007.

Ayub K, Slavin J, Imada R: Endoscopic retrograde cholangiopancreatography in gallstone-associated acute pancreatitis, *Cochrane Database Syst Rev* (4):CD003630, 2009.

Oria A, Cimmino D, Ocampo C, et al: Early endoscopic intervention versus early conservative management in patients with acute GSP and biliopancreatic obstruction, *Ann Surg* 245:10, 2007.

Petrov MS, van Santvoort HC, Besselink MGH, et al: Early endoscopic retrograde cholangiopancreatography versus conservative management in acute biliary pancreatitis without cholangitis, *Ann Surg* 247:250, 2008.

Hernandez V, Pascual I, Almela P, et al: Recurrence of acute GSP and relationship with cholecystectomy or endoscopic sphincterotomy, *Am J Gastroenterol* 99:2417, 2004.

Banks PA, Freeman ML: the Practice Parameters Committee of the American College of Gastroenterology: Practice guidelines in acute pancreatitis, *Am J Gastroenterol* 101:2379, 2006.

Pancreas Divisum and Other Variants of Dominant Dorsal Duct Anatomy

Thomas J. Howard, MD

OVERVIEW

Understanding pancreas divisum (PD) and other variants of dominant dorsal duct anatomy requires an appreciation of embryology and of the anatomic variants of pancreaticobiliary ductal development. The normal adult human pancreas is derived from a larger, dorsal pancreatic bud and a smaller, ventral pancreatic bud, which arise from opposite sides of the embryonic foregut (Figure 1, A). During the sixth to seventh week of gestation, the duodenum grows, elongates, and rotates toward the right (clockwise) along the long axis of the primitive gut (Figure 1, B). This movement carries the ventral pancreatic bud dorsally around the primitive foregut 180 degrees, where it fuses with the larger dorsal pancreatic bud to become the posterior pancreatic head and uncinate process (Figure 1, C). As these two separate pancreatic buds fuse, their respective drainage ducts merge.

The main pancreatic duct in the adult is thereby formed from the ventral bud duct in the pancreatic head and the splenic portion of the dorsal bud duct to create the duct of Wirsung. The duodenal portion of the dorsal pancreatic duct frequently persists as an accessory pancreatic duct (duct of Santorini). Anomalies and variations in this area of the upper digestive tract are relatively common because of this complex tissue migration and fusions that occur during normal development. Pancreas divisum (PD), in which the dorsal and ventral duct segments do *not* fuse during embryogenesis, is a common anomaly estimated to occur in approximately 10% of the general population, but other variants of dominant dorsal duct anatomy are also recognized (Figure 2).

Of the 10% of the general population with PD, it is estimated that only 5% will develop abdominal symptoms attributable to this anatomy. In patients with symptoms, the presumed pathophysiologic basis is a relative outflow obstruction of pancreatic secretions caused by a stenotic accessory papillary orifice, an egress site that presumably did not grow to handle the normal pancreatic juice flow (approximately 2 L/day), unlike the larger major papilla. This outflow obstruction produces ductal hypertension, which leads to abdominal symptoms and episodes of acute pancreatitis.

Despite the attractiveness of this theory, direct evidence to support it remains vague and imprecise, suggesting that other genetic, environmental, or physiologic factors may impact the ultimate clinical expression of disease in these patients. Because of these discrepancies, evaluation and management of patients with PD remains a complicated and vexing clinical challenge, perhaps more art than science.

CLINICAL PRESENTATION

Three clinical conditions are associated with PD and dominant dorsal duct anatomy: 1) acute recurrent pancreatitis, 2) chronic pancreatitis; and 3) pancreatic-type pain without evidence of pancreatitis (sharp, midepigastric pain with radiation to the back). Based on the results from collective clinical series, most patients with PD present in the third to fourth decade of life, and the majority are female. The main symptom that brings patients to a surgeon is midepigastric abdominal pain with radiation to the back or right upper quadrant. This pain is often of sufficient severity for the patient to have previously been seen in the emergency department for treatment, often more than once. Associated symptoms include nausea, vomiting, weakness, fatigue, and occasionally weight loss.

It is essential to establish the relationship of symptoms to objective criteria for acute pancreatitis early in the clinical course, either by serum amylase/lipase levels greater than three times the upper limit of normal or evidence of pancreatic inflammation on cross-sectional imaging, such as computed tomography (CT) or magnetic resonance imaging (MRI). Furthermore, in patients with objective evidence of pancreatic inflammation (pancreatitis), differentiating acute recurrent pancreatitis (ARP) from *early* chronic pancreatitis (CP) is critical. Having stated this, I recognize that making this distinction is a thorny issue often attainable only in hindsight. Pancreatic calcifications, endoscopic ultrasound (EUS) morphologic criteria, or subtle side-branch pancreatic duct abnormalities identified at endoscopic retrograde cholangiopancreatography (ERCP) are often helpful in this regard. These different clinical conditions—ARP, CP, and

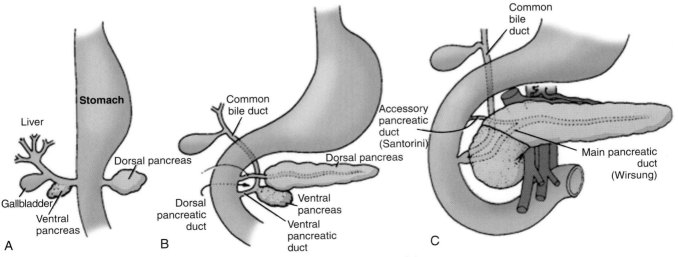

FIGURE 1 Embryologic development of the pancreas.

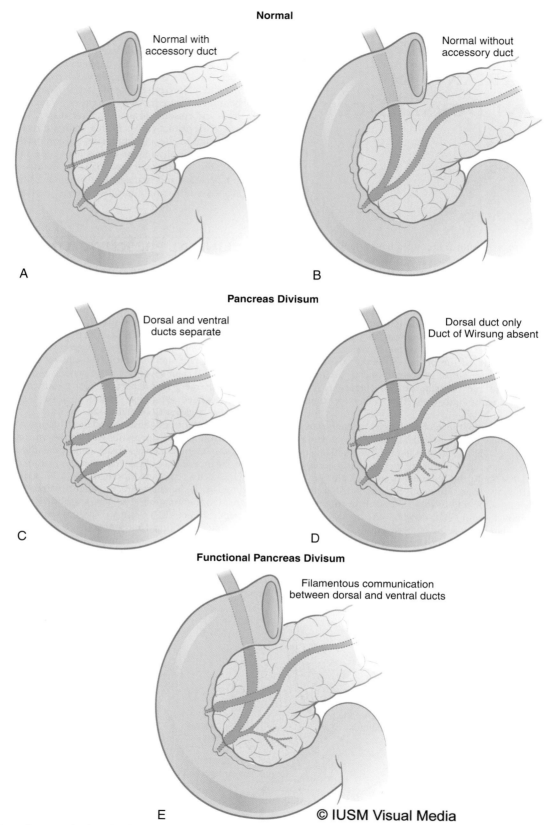

Normal

Normal with accessory duct

Normal without accessory duct

A

B

Pancreas Divisum

Dorsal and ventral ducts separate

Dorsal duct only
Duct of Wirsung absent

C

D

Functional Pancreas Divisum

Filamentous communication between dorsal and ventral ducts

E

© IUSM Visual Media

FIGURE 2   Normal pancreatic duct development and recognized variants of dominant dorsal duct anatomy. *(Courtesy Indiana University School of Medicine Office of Visual Media.)*

TABLE 1: Collective series of patients with PD from a systematic review and their response to endotherapy or surgery based on clinical subtypes

Clinical Subtype	Treatment Type	N	Response
Acute recurrent pancreatitis	Endotherapy	130	103 (79%)
	Surgery	125	104 (83%)
Chronic pancreatitis	Endotherapy	71	49 (69%)
	Surgery	9	6 (66%)
Pain	Endotherapy	68	37 (54%)
	Surgery	62	32 (52%)

Data from Liao Z, Gao R, Wang W, et al: A systematic review on endoscopic detection rate, endotherapy, and surgery for pancreas divisum, *Endoscopy* 41:439–444, 2009.

pancreatic-type pain without pancreatitis—are important to differentiate, because most clinical studies published on PD report significant differences in therapeutic outcome depending on the patient's clinical subtype (Table 1).

DIAGNOSIS

ERCP is the reference standard for the diagnosis of pancreas divisum and other dorsal duct variants, although recent improvements in imaging resolution have allowed several noninvasive techniques—EUS, magnetic resonance cholangiopancreatography (MRCP) with secretin stimulation, and multidetector-row CT with postprocessing reformations—to be extremely useful in making the diagnosis. In patients with PD, the ventral duct is typically from 1 to 4 cm in length and is formed by finely tapered normal ducts servicing the anatomic distribution of the posterior pancreatic head and uncinate process (remnant ventral pancreatic bud). This ductal morphology appears normal up to the point of prompt duct termination, always to the right side of midline.

When this anatomic relationship is recognized during ERCP, it is essential that cannulation of the minor papilla be pursued to demonstrate the presence of dominant dorsal duct anatomy and exclude possible secondary causes of ductal obstruction, such as tumor (*pseudo divisum*) or chronic pancreatitis (*false pancreas divisum*). EUS is a useful tool to make the diagnosis of PD as well as to evaluate the pancreatic parenchyma for small focal abnormalities (tumor or focal pancreatitis) or evidence of chronic pancreatitis. It seems both prudent and cost effective in the contemporary evaluation of patients with PD to include ductography (ERCP, EUS, MRCP), ductal response to intravenous secretin (EUS, MRCP), and a method of parenchymal evaluation (EUS, MRCP, CT) to fully characterize the disease process and type of intervention necessary.

In a patient with symptomatic PD, identification of a dominant dorsal duct system is necessary but not sufficient to establish candidacy for accessory papilla therapy. As previously mentioned, 10% of the general population has PD, and it is only in those patients with outflow tract obstruction, presumably because of accessory papillary stenosis, that endoscopic or surgical sphincteroplasty has a high likelihood of success. The dorsal pancreatic duct in most patients with PD has a normal, nondilated appearance. However, direct endoscopic visualization of accessory papilla size, degree of difficulty during endoscopic cannulation, or direct manometric measurements of accessory duct sphincter pressures are all undependable in patients with PD.

Indirect evidence of outflow obstruction, identified by duct imaging (EUS, MRCP) both before and after an IV bolus of secretin to stimulate

TABLE 2: Impact of a positive ultrasound secretin test on outcome following accessory papilla sphincteroplasty in patients with acute recurrent pancreatitis or chronic abdominal pain

Ultrasound Secretin Test	Acute Recurrent Pancreatitis	Chronic Abdominal Pain
Positive	90% (19/21)	94% (15/16)
Negative	64% (7/11)	21% (3/14)

From Warshaw AL, Simeone JF, Schapiro RH, et al: Evaluation and treatment of the dominant dorsal duct syndrome (pancreas divisum redefined), *Am J Surg* 159:59-66, 1990.

pancreatic secretions, has been advocated as effective in identifying those patients with PD who will most likely benefit from accessory sphincter ablation (Table 2). Stenosis of the minor papilla causing outflow obstruction is defined on secretin-stimulated MRCP as a persistent dilation (>3 mm) of the dorsal pancreatic duct above baseline 10 minutes after secretin injection in patients younger than 60 years of age.

A *santorinicele* is a cystic dilation of the distal dorsal pancreatic duct just proximal to the minor papilla that becomes more prominent during secretin stimulation. Speculation as to its etiology centers on a combination of both dorsal duct obstruction plus a weakness of the distal pancreatic duct wall leading to a circumscribed ductal dilation or bulge. In a small series of mostly elderly patients (mean age, 70 years), identification of a santorinicele during secretin-stimulated MRCP predicted a good symptomatic response following endoscopic sphincterotomy; however, questions remain regarding its actual prevalence in patients with PD, its association with elderly patients, and whether or not it represents a congenital or acquired abnormality.

As touched on previously, although a single structural mechanism (e.g., outflow obstruction) causing ARP in PD is appealing, to justify the benefit that occurs for certain patients following accessory duct therapy, a recent paper has identified abnormalities of the cystic transmembrane conductance regulator (CFTR) fibrosis gene in 22% patients with PD and idiopathic pancreatitis, implying a more complex disease phenotype than simple obstruction.

TREATMENT

The majority of therapeutic trials for both endoscopic and surgical treatment of PD are small, retrospective, single-institution case series. To date, only two randomized control trials have been completed evaluating endoscopic therapy in this disease, which studied only 19 and 33 patients. There have been no randomized controlled trials in surgery, nor have there been randomized trials comparing endoscopic therapy with surgical therapy. Because of these limited data, pooled results from selected series seem to be the best method to gauge overall treatment effects.

Endotherapy

The small accessory papilla orifice is difficult to identify, hard to cannulate, and anatomically indistinct. For these reasons, endoscopic therapy of the minor papilla *should not* be performed by all physicians who perform ERCP but rather by a subset with advanced skills and expertise with these techniques. In these experienced hands, successful cannulation of the minor papilla should be achievable in 90% to 95% of cases. Collective series of endotherapy over the last two decades have shown a substantial difference in outcome from treatment depending on the clinical indications for which it is applied (see Table 1). Endoscopic therapy historically encompasses a wide range of manipulations of the minor papilla including sphincterotomy, papillary dilation, stent insertion, or a combination of these techniques. Balloon dilation of the minor papilla was associated with a high rate of traumatic pancreatitis in most series and for this reason has been largely abandoned. Most patients receive some type of endoscopic sphincterotomy (ES) using either a needle-knife sphincterotomy (NKS) or the standard pull-type sphincterotomy (PTS). Both techniques utilize initial guidewire insertion through the minor papilla followed by a sphincterotomy, after which a small temporary stent is placed in the accessory pancreatic duct to protect against acute post-ERCP–induced pancreatitis.

Series of endoscopic sphincterotomy published in the 1990s were hampered by a high rate of recurrent papillary stenosis (20%) due to scarring at the sphincterotomy site. In response to this obstacle, most contemporary ES series have maintained dorsal pancreatic duct stenting, some for up to 18 months, in an effort to maintain sphincter patency. Heyries and colleagues retrospectively evaluated 24 patients with ARP and PD who underwent either sphincterotomy alone (*n* = 8) or sphincterotomy with dorsal duct stenting (*n* = 16). The dorsal duct stents varied in size from 5 to 11.5 Fr and were exchanged at 4 month intervals. More treatment-related complications occurred in the sphincterotomy-plus-stent group compared with the no-stent group (44% vs. 25%). At a mean follow-up of 39 months, only two documented episodes of recurrent pancreatitis were seen, both in the no-stent group (*P* < .01). Both groups had a decrease in chronic abdominal pain, and stenosis of the sphincterotomy site occurred in four patients (17%), three in the stent group.

Stent insertion in the pancreatic duct leads to numerous complications including acute pancreatitis, stent migration (either proximally or distally), stent occlusion, and, perhaps the most common and perplexing of all, stent-induced changes of the pancreatic duct that range from diffuse ductal enlargement to ductal stenosis and stricturing—changes often indistinguishable radiographically from those of chronic pancreatitis.

In the subgroup of patients with pancreatic-type abdominal pain but no objective evidence of pancreatitis, response to therapy has been highly variable. Sherman and colleagues conducted a randomized, controlled trial in 33 patients with PD and pain thought to be of pancreatic origin: 16 underwent minor papilla sphincterotomy, and 17 were randomized to the control group. A dorsal duct pancreatogram was obtained in all patients. Those randomized to therapy had a stent placed following a 3 to 5 mm sphincterotomy. Mean follow-up for the control and treatment groups were 1.2 years and 2.1 years, respectively. Complications were not reported. Improvement in pain scores was noted by 44% of patients in the treatment group versus 24% of those in the control group, a difference that failed to reach statistical significance. These poor results call into question the efficacy of minor papillary sphincterotomy in patients with abdominal pain without associated pancreatitis.

Surgical Therapy

The operative procedure in patients with dominant dorsal duct syndrome is strategically similar to the endoscopic approach, producing an enlargement of the dorsal duct outflow tract by enlarging the sphincter orifice. Unlike the uncertain single-cut sphincterotomy done endoscopically, the operative approach involves controlled, sharp sphincter ablation combined with a duct-to-mucosa reapproximation using fine, absorbable monofilament sutures (sphincteroplasty). Advantages to this approach over ES are definite sphincter ablation and the potential for greater long-term patency; the drawback is that to accomplish it requires general endotracheal anesthesia and a laparotomy.

Because of the exigencies of clinical practice, nearly all patients with nonsurgical abdominal pain are seen initially by gastroenterologists for evaluation. Perception that a minimally invasive approach is universally superior to an invasive procedure leads to endotherapy being the first line of treatment in the majority of patients with PD.

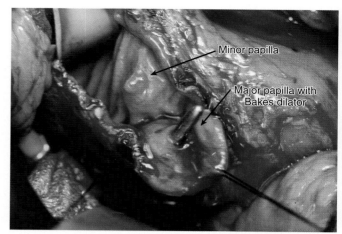

FIGURE 3   Facilitation of minor papilla identification with a Bakes dilator, through the cystic duct and into the duodenum. The minor papilla is approximately 2 cm proximal and 1 cm medial to the major papilla.

A corollary of this referral bias is that surgical sphincteroplasty is mostly relegated to patients whose symptoms recur following ES or to those who develop papillary stenosis. Of interest in this regard is the recent report by Morgan and colleagues on their surgical experience with transduodenal sphincteroplasty, in which they found that their surgical results were significantly better in those patients who had prior gastric surgery with Roux-en-Y reconstructions, presumably because this altered anatomy precluded routine endotherapy via the normal ERCP prograde approach.

My method of accessory duct sphincteroplasty is through an upper midline abdominal incision to gain access to the peritoneal cavity: The hepatocolic ligament is lysed using cautery, the right colon is mobilized inferiorly, and the omentum is taken off the colon and reflected medially to gain full access to the C-loop of the duodenum. A generous Kocher maneuver is then done to elevate and rotate the head of the pancreas and duodenum medially up out of the wound, so the antimesenteric wall of the duodenum is lying anteroposteriorly. Stay sutures of 2-0 silk are used to hold the duodenum in this position.

Next, a generous longitudinal duodenotomy is made, centered over the major papilla, which can usually be identified by careful palpation. Occasionally, this identification can be facilitated by placing a Bakes dilator through the cystic duct and manipulating it down into the common bile duct and duodenum (Figure 3). The accessory papilla is located approximately 2 cm proximal and 1 cm medial to the major papilla. This tiny papillary orifice is often difficult to identify, but its presence can be highlighted by a light spray of methylene blue, noting where the dye is removed from the duodenal mucosa by the flow of clear pancreatic juice. In challenging identifications, pancreatic juice flow can be accentuated by an intravenous dose of secretin. Once the accessory papilla is identified, the orifice is cannulated with a lacrimal duct probe, and fine tenotomy scissors are used to sharply cut through the superior-medial lip of the sphincter down to the wall of the underlying pancreatic duct (Figures 4). After sphincter ablation, the mucosa of the dorsal duct is reapproximated to the duodenum by closely spaced, fine monofilament absorbable sutures (Figure 5). These sutures augment hemostasis and facilitate wound healing with minimal scarring. The duodenotomy is closed longitudinally in layers without drainage (Figure 6.).

I do not routinely stent the pancreatic duct, but in patients with fibrous scarring, I use a 5 Fr pediatric feeding tube placed retrograde through the third portion of the duodenum, secured with a purse-string suture, to intubate the pancreatic duct through the sphincteroplasty. This feeding tube is then brought out through the anterior abdominal wall as a controlled pancreatic fistula while

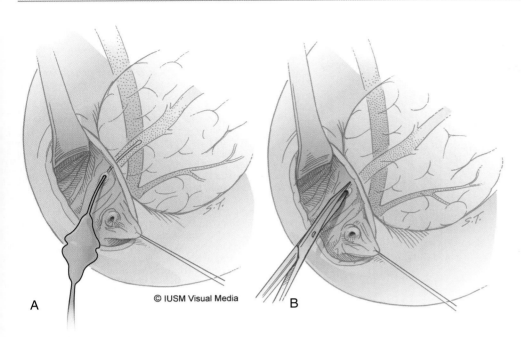

A   © IUSM Visual Media   B

FIGURE 4 Through a targeted duodenotomy, the accessory papilla is identified 2 cm superior and approximately 1 cm medial to the major papilla. A lacrimal duct probe is used to identify the sphincter (**A**), and the sphincter is divided sharply to the edge of the dominant dorsal duct using fine tenotomy scissors (**B**). *(Courtesy Indiana University School of Medicine Office of Visual Media.)*

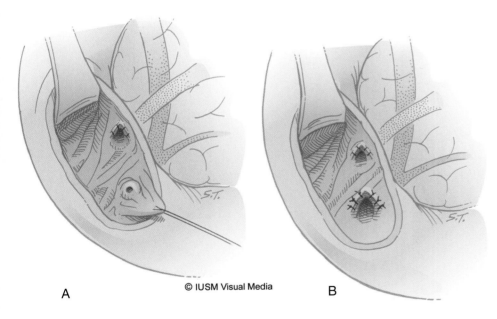

A   © IUSM Visual Media   B

FIGURE 5 Completion of the sphincteroplasty with a duct-to-mucosa approximation utilizing fine monofilament sutures. **A,** Minor papillary sphincteroplasty. **B,** Dual sphincteroplasty of both the major and minor papillas. *(Courtesy Indiana University School of Medicine Office of Visual Media.)*

the sphincteroplasty heals. The stent is removed 2 to 3 weeks postoperatively in the office.

Good to excellent results from accessory duct sphincteroplasty in patients with PD are closely associated with the clinical indications for which it is applied: ARP (~ 85%), CP (~67%), or pancreatic-type pain without evidence of pancreatitis (~50%). Mortality rates in published series are less than 0.5%, and morbidity rates are less than 25% (Table 3). The preponderance of morbidity for this operation is acute pancreatitis, surgical site infection, and pulmonary dysfunction. Duodenal leak is a serious but infrequent complication in most clinical series.

In those patients who develop postoperative sphincter stenosis with recurrent symptoms, reintervention, either endoscopically or operatively, is helpful less than 50% of the time. This observation implies that the initial sphincter ablation represents the best opportunity to achieve long-term benefit, and careful evaluation and patient selection are paramount. Symptomatic fibrous stenosis following sphincteroplasty, or in those patients who develop chronic pancreatitis following sphincteroplasty, is best treated by pancreatic head resection, either a duodenal-preserving or a Whipple-type procedure rather than revisional sphincteroplasty. Patients with PD who have established chronic pancreatitis and dorsal pancreatic duct dilatation are best treated by a longitudinal pancreaticojejunostomy (Puestow-type procedure) or by a Frey-type duodenal-preserving pancreatic head resection with longitudinal pancreaticojejunostomy to effectively decompress their entire dilated duct system.

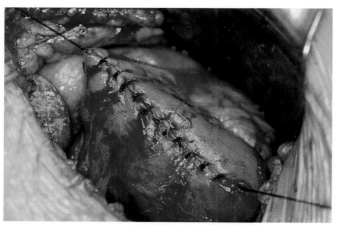

FIGURE 6   The longitudinal duodenotomy is closed in two layers utilizing an inner layer of absorbable synthetic sutures and an outer layer of seromuscular silk sutures.

TABLE 3: Morbidity, mortality, and response rate in four large surgical series of accessory papilla sphincteroplasty in patients with PD

Author	N	Morbidity	Mortality	Response (%)	Mean FU (Months)
Warshaw (1990)	88	NR	0	71%	53
Madura (2005)	74	25%	0	64%	NR
Morgan (2008)	17	10%	0	54%	43
Bradley (1996)	37	NR	0	84%	60

FU, Follow-up

Suggested Readings

Moore KL (ed): *The developing human: clinically oriented embryology*, ed 2, Philadelphia, 1977, WB Saunders.

Fogel EL, Toth TG, Lehman GA, et al: Does endoscopic therapy favorably affect the outcome of patients who have recurrent acute pancreatitis and pancreas divisum? *Pancreas* 34:21–45, 2007.

Liao Z, Gao R, Wang W, et al: A systematic review on endoscopic detection rate, endotherapy, and surgery for pancreas divisum, *Endoscopy* 41:439–444, 2009.

Matos C, Meten T, Devière J, et al: Pancreas divisum: evaluation with secretin-enhanced magnetic resonance cholangiopancretography, *Gastrointest Endosc* 53:728–733, 2001.

Heyries L, Barthet M, Delvasto C, et al: Long-term results of endoscopic management of pancreas divisum with recurrent acute pancreatitis, *Gastrointest Endosc* 55:376–381, 2002.

Morgan KA, Romagnuolo J, Adams DB: Transduodenal sphincteroplasty in the management of sphincter of Oddi dysfunction and pancreas divisum in the modern era, *J Am Coll Surg* 206:908–917, 2008.

Madura JA, Madura JA II, Sherman S, Lehman GA: Surgical sphincteroplasty in 446 patients, *Arch Surg* 140:504–513, 2005.

Warshaw AL, Simeone JF, Schapiro RH, et al: Evaluation and treatment of the dominant dorsal duct syndrome (pancreas divisum redefined), *Am J Surg* 159:59–66, 1990.

Bradley EL III, Stephan RN: Accessory duct sphincteroplasty is preferred for long-term prevention of recurrent acute pancreatitis in patients with pancreas divisum, *J Am Coll Surg* 183:65–70, 1996.

Schlosser W, Rau BM, Poch B, et al: Surgical treatment of pancreas divisum causing chronic pancreatitis: the outcome benefits of duodenum-preserving pancreatic head resection, *J Gastrointest Surg* 9:710–715, 2005.

MANAGEMENT OF PANCREATIC ABSCESS

Tjasa Hranjec, MD, and Robert G. Sawyer, MD

OVERVIEW

Pancreatic abscess (Figure 1) complicates approximately 5% of cases of acute pancreatitis and is invariably fatal if left untreated, resulting in progressive sepsis and multiorgan failure. It occurs on a natural continuum that ranges from infected pancreatic pseudocysts to pancreatic abscesses and infected pancreatic necrosis, with these entities often overlapping and blurring diagnostic boundaries. Even when it does not ultimately result in a cure, percutaneous drainage may be helpful to obtain a specimen for culture and to decrease the acute, systemic inflammation. In approximately 40% of patients, radiographic drain placement results in the resolution of symptoms (Figure 2), but frequently, the infected retroperitoneal space is honeycombed or contains necrotic debris that cannot pass though the catheter, and surgical debridement is necessary.

Like many other complex intraabdominal infections, pancreatic abscesses often require a multimodal approach. Appropriate care of a patient with a pancreatic abscess consists of four features: 1) treatment with broad-spectrum antibiotics, 2) resuscitation and supportive care, 3) nutrition, and 4) source control via radiographic and/or surgical interventions.

Patients should be treated with appropriate antibiotics when clinical signs and symptoms point to a septic focus within the pancreas and the CT scan reveals a peripancreatic fluid collection or extraluminal air in the retroperitoneum indicative of infected pancreatic necrosis or abscess. Bacteriologic cultures are often polymicrobial, commonly growing organisms such as *Escherichia coli*, *Enterococcus* spp., *Klebsiella pneumoniae*, *Pseudomonas aeruginosa*, *Staphylococcus aureus*, *Bacteroides fragilis*, or *Clostridium perfringens*. Broad-spectrum antibiotics such as imipenem or meropenem are often used for gram-negative and anaerobic coverage, with fluoroquinolones and metronidazole or piperacillin-tazobactam being substituted in

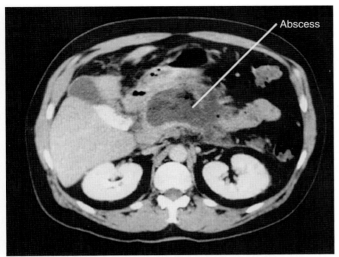

FIGURE 1   Pancreatic abscess with extraluminal air. *(From Sawyer RG, Barkun JS, Smith R, et al: Intra-abdominal infection. ACS surgery: principles and practice, WebMD, 2004, p 13. Available at http://www.acssurgery.com /acssurgery/institutional/tableOfContent.action.)*

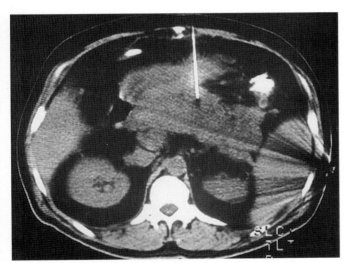

FIGURE 2   Radiographic drain placement via 20 gauge needle (inserted under CT guidance). *(From Mithofer Mueller PR, Warshaw AL, et al: Interventional and surgical treatment of pancreatic abscess, World J Surg 21[2]:162-168, 2008.)*

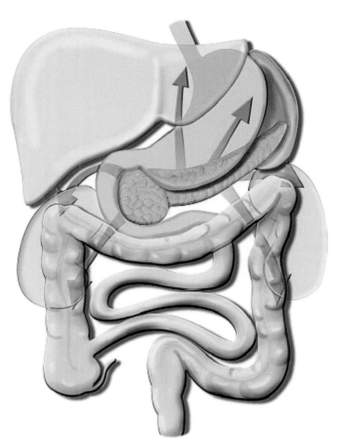

FIGURE 3   Extension routes of pancreatic necrosis (retroperitoneally). *(From Seewald S, Groth S, Omar S, et al: Aggressive endoscopic therapy for pancreatic necrosis and pancreatic abscess: a new, safe, and effective treatment algorithm, Gastrointest Endosc 62[1]:92-100; 2005.)*

patients who are intolerant to carbapenems. Occasionally, vancomycin is used for broader gram-positive coverage, especially if methicillin-resistant *Staphylococcus aureus* is isolated, and fluconazole is used for the treatment of yeast, particularly *Candida albicans*. In addition, critically ill patients require extensive nutritional and supportive care. But most importantly, source control via aspiration or open debridement of the septic focus established radiographically or surgically as soon as possible is the key to providing the appropriate treatment in a patient with a pancreatic abscess.

RADIOGRAPHIC DRAIN PLACEMENT

With or without drain placement, CT-guided aspiration of a peripancreatic fluid collection, including a potential abscess, offers several benefits. First, it provides culture material and confirms the diagnosis of a pancreatic abscess. The management of a sterile pancreatic necrosis or pancreatic pseudocyst is different than that of an infected

collection, and the differentiation between the two is important and can only be accomplished by direct sampling. Second, aspiration may be curative by eliminating the fluid collection completely and collapsing an abscess cavity. Third, it may halt and temporarily reverse the progression of severe sepsis in a patient who is unable to undergo open surgery secondary to medical comorbidities or high operative risk. This temporizing intervention can allow for the stabilization of critically ill patients in whom thick necrotic tissue and liquefied necrosis cannot be eradicated percutaneously, but who can improve enough to subsequently undergo open surgical treatment.

SURGICAL TREATMENT

At the height of an acute episode of pancreatic necrosis complicated by infection, complex pancreatic inflammation does not respect fascial planes. Occasionally, the exudate is confined to definitive spaces, surrounded by a capsule or pseudocapsule; more frequently, there is a diffuse retroperitoneal involvement, or the fluid can rupture into a hollow viscus or into free peritoneal cavity and spread throughout the abdomen. Approximately half of all patients with pancreatic necrosis have disease confined to the lesser sac; the other half have more than one retroperitoneal space affected. Figure 3 represents possible extensions of the pancreatic necrosis and purulent fluid into the thorax cranially and scrotum caudally, as well as into the left retroperitoneal, perihepatic, and peripancreatic spaces; transverse mesocolon; and gastrocolic omentum.

Most surgical techniques for the treatment of a pancreatic abscess in the setting of severe acute pancreatitis are associated with mortality of 10% to 20%; however, in patients with established multiple organ failure, mortality rates are even higher. Use of minimally invasive versus open procedures has been debated with the development of two contrasting philosophies. The first advocates a step-down approach in which open necrosectomy for peripancreatic infection plays the primary role, with less invasive methods used for residual or subsequent collections. The second, a step-up approach, relies initially on less invasive techniques with open necrosectomy used only as a last resort. The main impetus toward minimally invasive necrosectomy is the recognition that open surgery is associated with significant morbidity and mortality, especially early on in the disease. Since the interventional treatment should be combined with the desire to minimize physiologic insult in patients who are already critically ill, the step-up approach is now the one most commonly preferred.

Although percutaneous techniques may be favored for the initial management of infected peripancreatic collections, it is clear that these will not always be effective, and progression to an operative intervention will occur. For any given patient, it is useful to define goals and timelines to be followed when assessing the success of percutaneous drainage: for example, resolution of hypotension or respiratory failure within several days of intervention. In general, indications for surgery will include 1) progressive sepsis; 2) intermittent episodes of sepsis, especially during attempts at introducing an oral diet; 3) persistent symptoms—nausea, episodic emesis, or significant abdominal pain—after the onset of severe pancreatitis; 4) failure to tolerate an oral diet; and 5) failure to thrive. The balance of this chapter is dedicated to the various techniques that have been used to drain pancreatic abscesses and infected peripancreatic fluid collections.

Minimally Invasive Pancreatic Necrosectomy

Various techniques of minimally invasive necrosectomy, or surgical removal of infected necrotic material, include 1) endoscopic (transgastric) necrosectomy, 2) sinus tract endoscopy, and 3) laparoscopic necrosectomy. Each technique is classified by the type of scope used: a flexible endoscope, nephroscope, or laparoscope, and all of these generally necessitate multiple sessions and are occasionally regarded as an alternative approach to open debridement in highly selected patients with advantageous anatomy. The techniques have proven to be safe and highly effective, however, randomized trials comparing minimally invasive and open debridement and drainage have not yet been performed. The two most commonly used minimally invasive approaches utilize the endoscopic transgastric and nephroscopic retroperitoneal routes (sinus tract), probably because they are based on conventional operative procedures.

Endoscopic (Transgastric) Necrosectomy

Patients undergoing endoscopic necrosectomy (EN) are considered unfit for complex surgery requiring general anesthesia, either because they are too ill or because they have serious comorbid diseases. Most authors recommend at least 2 weeks of effective intravenous antibiotic therapy before EN is attempted.

The optimal drainage site, with interposed vessels excluded, is identified via a curvilinear echoendoscope and color-flow Doppler. On the initial day of the procedure, an endoscopic retrograde pancreatogram is performed, and transpapillary and/or transmural endoscopic ultrasound (EUS) is used to guide the drainage of the infected collection by puncturing the abscess cavity through the gastric or duodenal wall with a 22 gauge needle within a 6 Fr Teflon outer sheath. A successful puncture is confirmed via EUS and fluoroscopy. The needle is removed, and liquefied necrotic material is aspirated and sent for bacteriologic examination. Contrast is then injected into the cavity to evaluate its abdominal extension. Next, a guidewire is advanced through the opening, and the puncture site is dilated with an esophageal/pyloric balloon, as shown in Figure 4, creating a cystogastrostomy or cystoduodenostomy. At least one double-pigtail stent is left in place for continuing drainage of the cavity.

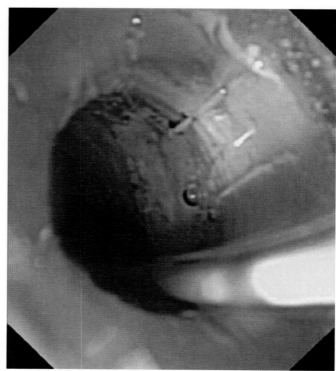

FIGURE 4   Balloon dilation of cystogastrostomy or cystoduodenostomy under direct endoscopic view. *(From Seewald S, Groth S, Omar S, et al: Aggressive endoscopic therapy for pancreatic necrosis and pancreatic abscess: a new, safe, and effective treatment algorithm, Gastrointest Endosc 62[1]:92-100; 2005.)*

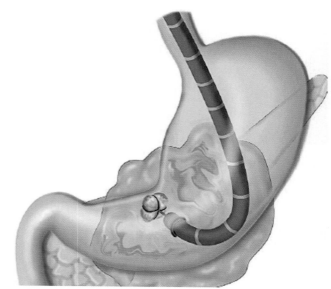

FIGURE 5   Insertion of a gastroscope directly into the abscess cavity. *(From Seewald S, Groth S, Omar S, et al: Aggressive endoscopic therapy for pancreatic necrosis and pancreatic abscess: a new, safe, and effective treatment algorithm, Gastrointest Endosc 62[1]:92-100; 2005.)*

Daily necrosectomy, lavage, and repeated balloon dilations are performed until the majority of the infected necrotic tissue is cleared. Endoscopic necrosectomy is performed using a Dormia basket introduced through a therapeutic gastroscope into the previously formed cavity under fluoroscopic guidance (Figures 5 and 6). Alternatively, a pediatric gastroscope or a gastroscope with a 6 mm channel may

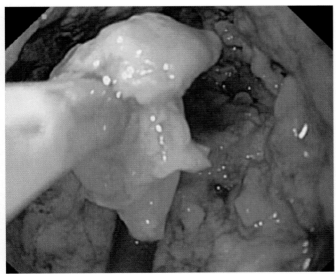

FIGURE 6   Large amount of necrotic material being extracted via Dormia basket. *(From Seewald S, Groth S, Omar S, et al: Aggressive endoscopic therapy for pancreatic necrosis and pancreatic abscess: a new, safe, and effective treatment algorithm, Gastrointest Endosc 62[1]:92-100; 2005.)*

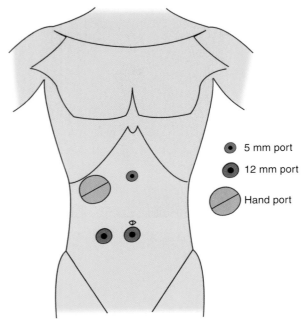

FIGURE 7   Port placement for hand-assisted laparoscopic pancreatic debridement.

be inserted directly to suction out the necrotic material. The cavity can also be continuously irrigated with standard peritoneal dialysis fluid. If there are multiple cavities, or if the cavity is septated and inadequately accessed during the initial drainage, further endoscopically guided drainages are recommended. Finally, the newly created cystogastrostomy or cystoduodenostomy may be sealed with *N*-butyl-2-cyanoacrylate.

Sinus Tract Endoscopy

Among the minimally invasive procedures, sinus tract endoscopy appears to be the most popular. The combination of radiographic drain placement and the least invasive surgical technique may potentially avoid complications associated with open surgical procedures. The original drain is placed under CT guidance with surgeons determining the most appropriate site and axis of the drain. Obviously, the appropriate anatomy to allow access is required. With the patient under general anesthesia in the operating room, the drain is removed, and a flexible or rigid endoscope is inserted along the preformed tract. The tract is dilated using a balloon dilator, and a twin-channel endoscope is passed through the skin opening to perform further antegrade dilation of the tract, until the entire length of the tract is visualized. Fluid collections are cleared using jet irrigation with a heater probe and suction, whereas adherent or solid necrotic material is teased away using a variety of endoscopic instruments, such as snares and stent-retrieval forceps. All necrosum need not be removed, and continuous cavity lavage may be provided through large-bore drains.

This procedure may be performed in patients with previous primary debridements (open or percutaneous) in whom residual sepsis is suspected and CT scan shows no satellite collections. Surgical preference guides the use of a flexible versus rigid endoscope, although a flexible endoscope can only remove small fragments of necrotic tissue with each pass. On the other hand, access to pockets of necrosis is limited with the rigid system, and flexible endoscopy remains valuable.

Laparoscopic Necrosectomy

Minimally invasive laparoscopic necrosectomy offers advantages over radiological drainage by enabling the debridement of infected peripancreatic tissue and abscesses while avoiding major laparotomies. Three common laparoscopic approaches to the pancreas for drainage

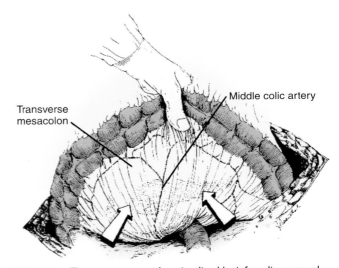

FIGURE 8   Transverse mesocolon visualized by infracolic approach. *(From Mithofer K, Mueller PR, Warshaw AL, et al: Interventional and surgical treatment of pancreatic abscess, World J Surg 21:162-168, 1997.)*

and debridement are used: 1) the direct route, through the gastrocolic ligament; 2) the infracolic/transmesocolic approach (described below); and, for right-sided collections, 3) a retroduodenal approach or dissection at the root of the mesocolon.

The patient should be placed in the left lateral position with the body tilted to 60 degrees for fluid collections or necrosis of the lesser sac or the left paracolic gutter. To access necrotic areas of the right paracolic gutter or retroduodenal area, patients should be placed in the right lateral position tilted to 60 degrees. A common technique includes three ports: two 10 to 12 mm standard laparoscopic ports and a hand-access device, as shown in Figure 7.

For the infracolic or transmesocolic approach (Figure 8), the omental pad is swept into the upper abdomen to identify the duodenojejunal (DJ) flexure. The area may appear discolored, thinned out, and

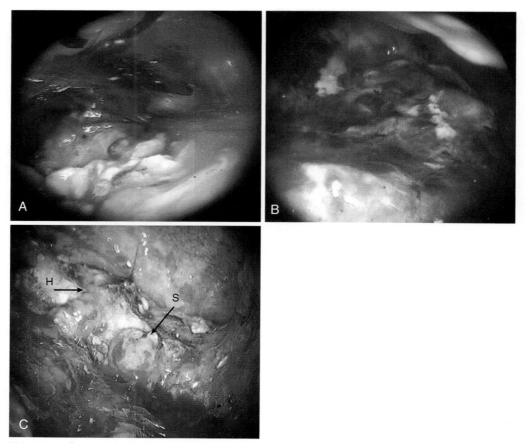

FIGURE 9 Perioperative view during the single-port laparoscopic necrosectomy. **A,** Necrotic cavity containing large amounts of pus and tail of the pancreas. **B,** Necrotic pancreatic tail. **C,** Necrosectomy cavity after completion of debridement. Note that the hepatic artery (*H*) and splenic artery (*S*) have been exposed during the procedure. (*From Bucher P, Pugen F, Morel P, et al: Minimally invasive necrosectomy for infected necrotizing pancreatitis, Pancreas 36[2]:113-119; 2008.*)

bulging into the infracolic compartment, as the fluid and necrotic tissue increase the pressure within the lesser sac. The area is often indurated and covered with small bowel adhesions that should be swept away using a 5 mm endodissector, allowing for visualization of the transverse mesocolon. A small incision is made in the transverse mesocolon just superolateral to the DJ flexure. Often, a gush of dark grayish material that is typical of pancreatic necrosis/abscess is seen. The opening in the transverse mesocolon is enlarged to accommodate debridement, carefully avoiding injuries to the middle colic vessels. All the necrotic material is removed via gentle dissection, and intraoperative bleeding is controlled through pressure. Visualization of bleeding within the lesser sac is excellent; however, bleeding from the disrupted omental adhesions is occasionally difficult to notice, especially in patients with rigid, thickened, or engorged omental pads, which may render such patients unsuitable for this technique. Large sump drains are routinely placed, and continuous irrigation can be performed postoperatively.

Single Large-Port Laparoscopic Necrosectomy

Similar to sinus tract endoscopy, single-port laparoscopic necrosectomy is conducted under general anesthesia, using drain tracts from radiologically placed drains. A 12 mm trocar is placed into the previously formed tract under direct laparoscopic visualization through a 30 degree, 5 mm scope. When the necrotic cavity is encountered, the drain is removed. Gas insufflation is set to a maximal pressure of 8 mm Hg to avoid bacterial translocation secondary to the high pressure within the abscess cavity, and lavage is performed using a jet-lavage irrigator/suction, core trumpet, and physiologic saline solution. The simultaneous use of 5 mm

instruments, such as atraumatic plate-shaped grasping forceps and a laparoscope, through the 12 mm trocar allow for debridement of the necrotic pancreatic tissue that is not possible using sinus tract endoscopy (Figure 9). When needed, hemostasis is maintained using monopolar coagulation connected to the grasping forceps. At the end of the procedure, a 10 mm laparoscope with a 30 degree optic is used to inspect the cavity for completeness of necrosectomy. Dual-lumen surgical drains are placed under laparoscopic visualization into the necrosectomy cavity prior to trocar removal, and continuous postoperative lavage can be employed if desired.

Open Abscess Drainage and Necrosectomy

When the expertise in minimally invasive surgery is unavailable, and percutaneous or endoscopic drainage has failed, open abscess drainage, often combined with necrosectomy, is indicated. Although simple, open pancreatic abscess drainage may be performed with minimal sequelae, extending the procedure to include pancreatic debridement results in significant morbidity, including gastrointestinal fistulas, incisional hernias, and local bleeding, with a mortality rate ranging from 15% to 65%.

When necessary, open surgical treatment that includes pancreatic debridement or necrosectomy should be performed as late as possible to allow sufficient demarcation between necrotic tissue and viable parenchyma, limiting the extent of necessary surgery. It is estimated that debridement after 12 days of nonoperative therapy for diffusely infected pancreatic disease carries a 27% mortality rate compared with 56% in cases of early open drainage and/or debridement (within 48 to 72 hours).

Furthermore, a delayed approach decreases the risk of bleeding and surgery-related loss of vital tissue, possibly preventing subsequent endocrine and exocrine pancreatic insufficiency.

SURGICAL TECHNIQUE

Open Necrosectomy

For assessment of the entire abdominal cavity and for versatility, a longitudinal midline incision creates the optimal access. Occasionally, for very well-localized collections, a smaller transverse or flank incision can be used if the entire abdomen does not need exploration. When wide exposure of an abscess or infected peripancreatic tissue is desired, gastrocolic and duodenocolic ligaments are divided close to the greater curvature of the stomach to expose the pancreas. Abscesses are drained, and any debridement that is required is carried out bluntly to avoid the removal of vital tissue and minimize bleeding complications. After all loose tissue has been debrided, the retroperitoneal cavity is irrigated with saline to further remove residual devitalized tissue.

Four methods following open abscess drainage and debridement have been advocated to control the focus of sepsis and cease progression of infection and the release of proinflammatory mediators: 1) open packing, 2) planned, staged relaparotomies with repeated lavage, 3) closed continuous lavage of the lesser sac and retroperitoneum, and 4) closed packing.

Open packing and planned, staged relaparotomies can lead to a high postoperative morbidity, including pancreatic and colonic fistulas, incisional hernias, and ongoing blood loss. Closed techniques utilizing continuous lavage or simple drainage allow for decreased morbidity when an adequate removal of infected tissue occurred with the initial procedure. The choice between these two techniques is a matter of surgeon preference, but both appear to be successful around 83% of the time. Currently, debridement with subsequent closed, continuous lavage of the lesser sac appears to be the most common open surgical treatment approach.

Open Packing

After open debridement and abscess drainage, the cavity is lined with nonadherent dressings and packed. The patient returns to the operating room every 48 hours for continuing debridement and repacking until inflammation resolves. The procedure may be eventually performed under sterile conditions and conscious sedation in the intensive care unit. Once healthy granulation tissue appears, the abdomen is closed over drains with or without lavage of the cavity.

Planned, Staged Relaparotomies with Repeated Lavage

Following the primary abscess drainage and debridement, the patient returns to the operating room every 48 hours for repeated laparotomy and debridement, and the abdomen is reclosed after every procedure. Similar to the open-packing process, after granulation tissue has developed, the abdomen is closed at the fascial level, but the pancreatic drains are left in place. For ease of repetitive surgical accesses and to conserve fascial integrity, a mesh that is split to allow repeat entry to the abdomen may be incorporated into the abdominal wall and removed at the time of definitive closure.

Continuous Lavage of the Lesser Sac and Retroperitoneum

After the initial abscess drainage and debridement, postoperative lavage is performed with two or more double-lumen Salem sump tubes (20 to 24 Fr) and single-lumen silicone rubber tubes (28 to 32 Fr) inserted from each side of the abdomen and directed to the left and right, terminating with the tip at the tail of the pancreas behind the descending colon, the head of the pancreas, and the ascending colon. The gastrocolic and duodenocolic ligaments are reapproximated to create a closed retroperitoneal space for postoperative lavage. The lavage inflow is connected with the smaller-lumen Salem drains, and larger-lumen drains are used for the evacuation of outflow that may include necrotic tissue. In the first few days, 35 to 45 L of lavage fluid (standard peritoneal dialysis fluid) are used and may be tapered as subsequent outflow becomes clearer. Drains are generally left in for 2 to 3 weeks.

Closed Packing

After abscess drainage and removal of devitalized tissue, the residual cavity is irrigated with saline and filled with multiple large closed-suction drains that are brought out laterally. Drains are removed over time as the drainage decreases.

A CT scan is performed around postoperative day 2 to evaluate the results of necrosectomy and drain placement. Lavage is stopped once the effluent becomes clear and bacteriologic cultures remain negative. Drain removal begins 2 days after lavage is terminated, ruling out pancreatic fistulas and excluding residual collections via the CT scan. Antibiotics should be continued until the drains are removed.

SUMMARY

Pancreatic necrosis and abscess formation are very serious surgical conditions, often life-threatening complications of acute necrotizing pancreatitis. Although they only occur in approximately 10% to 20% of patients with acute pancreatitis, with a clinical presentation that is late and indolent, the morbidity and mortality remain high. Any suspicion of this pathology should always lead to early diagnostic use of CT scans, where CT-guided fine needle aspiration of the suspicious collections may be necessary to confirm the infection. The strategy for management of pancreatic necrosis and abscess has significantly changed over the years, from open surgical debridement in all cases to a more conservative approach, through percutaneous drainage or less invasive methods, at least as a temporizing measure during a time when patients may be critically ill.

Over the past 2 decades, as treatment options have evolved, patient mortality rates have decreased substantially, from 50% in the 1970s to less than 20% at present. Although formal evaluation of all surgical, radiological, and minimally invasive techniques is ongoing, coordinated multidisciplinary care between surgery and radiology has shown significant promise.

SUGGESTED READINGS

Dambrauskas Z, Gulbinas A, Pundzius J, et al: Meta-analysis of prophylactic parenteral antibiotic use in acute necrotizing pancreatitis, *Medicina* 43(4):291–300, 2007.

Haan J, Scalea T: Laparoscopic debridement of recurrent pancreatic abscesses in the hostile abdomen, *Am Surg* 72:511–514, 2006.

Isaji S, Takada T, Kawarada Y, et al: JPN guidelines for the management of acute pancreatitis: surgical management, *J Hepatobiliary Pancreat Surg* 13:48–55, 2006.

Werner J, Hartwig W, Hackert T, et al: Surgery in the treatment of acute pancreatitis: open pancreatic necrosectomy, *Scand J Surg* 94:130–134, 2005.

Talreja JP, Kahaleh M: Endotherapy for pancreatic necrosis and abscess: endoscopic drainage and necrosectomy, *J Hepatobil Pancreat Surg* 16:605–612, 2009.

Management of Pancreatic Pseudocyst

Marisa Cevasco, MD, MPH, Servet Tatli, MD, and
Stanley W. Ashley, MD

OVERVIEW

Pseudocysts are chronic fluid collections associated with the pancreas. In contrast with true cysts, they lack an epithelial lining. They generally occur in the setting of pancreatitis or external trauma to the pancreas and are believed to result from disruption of major or minor pancreatic ducts. Although the majority of acute pancreatic fluid collections resolve spontaneously, some fail to do so, and the enzyme-rich secretions then incite a local inflammatory response. Fibroblasts accumulate and lay down a layer of extracellular matrix proteins that forms a wall or capsule. Traditionally, a *pseudocyst* was defined as any fluid collection that persisted more than 4 to 6 weeks and therefore had presumably matured enough to develop an inflammatory capsule that would permit internal surgical drainage. With modern imaging, particularly computerized tomography (CT), this wall can be identified to facilitate a more anatomic differentiation between pseudocysts and acute fluid collections.

This broad definition of pseudocysts encompasses a range of pancreatic and peripancreatic fluid collections; several classification schemes have been developed. In fact, a proposed revision of the Atlanta Classification of Acute Pancreatitis would relabel cysts that develop in the setting of pancreatic necrosis as "walled-off necrosis" rather than pseudocyst (personal communication, Peter A. Banks, MD). Acknowledging this, it still seems appropriate to consider management options in the context of the broader definition, which includes both asymptomatic and symptomatic pseudocysts that develop in the context of acute interstitial pancreatitis, pancreatic necrosis, or chronic pancreatitis. Distinction between these clinical entities based on differences in pathophysiology, presentation, and diagnostic evaluation is important in determining management options.

PATHOPHYSIOLOGY

Pancreatic pseudocysts typically develop from alcoholic or biliary pancreatitis or from iatrogenic or external trauma. In acute interstitial pancreatitis, the pancreas has not been previously injured; although these cysts often result from an acute disruption of a pancreatic duct, the pancreatic parenchyma itself recovers, and the ductal disruption may heal spontaneously. In the setting of necrosis, although collections do result simply result from the inflammatory response or from similar ductal disruptions, not infrequently they evolve as areas of necrosis, organize, and liquefy. These may also communicate with the pancreatic ductal system, either in the context of an intact main duct or, with more severe disease, a totally disconnected pancreatic tail; they may contain considerable necrotic debris that must be removed with drainage. In chronic pancreatitis, there is generalized loss of acinar cells and local collagen deposition. The pancreatic parenchyma becomes progressively fibrotic, and there is irregularity of the duct with areas of narrowing, dilatation, and often obstructing calculi. Elevated intraductal pressure ultimately results in disruption of an obstructed duct, which then produces the pseudocyst.

PRESENTATION

Pancreatic pseudocysts may occur singly or as small multiple cysts, and they may be intraparenchymal or adjacent to the pancreas. In acute pancreatitis, single pseudocysts form in or adjacent to the pancreas and are commonly retrogastric in the lesser sac, but they may also develop in the small bowel mesentery, transverse mesocolon, or behind the right and left colon. There are also rare reports of pancreatic pseudocysts in the mediastinum, scrotum, and thorax. Patients with chronic pancreatitis may develop multiple, small intraparenchymal pseudocysts. Pseudocysts that develop after blunt trauma often form anterior to the pancreatic neck and body, as the duct is injured where it crosses the vertebral column.

Many small pseudocysts are asymptomatic, discovered as incidental findings on CT scans or during ultrasonography. They are also discovered in the setting of acute pancreatitis, when a patient fails to improve after a week of treatment, or after improving for some time, the symptoms recur. Larger pseudocysts, typically greater than 6 cm, may be associated with abdominal pain, early satiety, nausea, vomiting, or back pain. Patients may also present with weight loss from gastrointestinal (GI) tract obstruction, pruritis and jaundice secondary to biliary obstruction, or even lower extremity edema due to compression of the inferior vena cava. Patients with infected pseudocysts may manifest fever, leukocytosis, and other signs of systemic illness. Other complications include duodenal stenosis and portal, superior mesenteric, or splenic vein thrombosis. In contrast with those that evolve in interstitial disease, in the setting of necrosis or chronic pancreatitis, it may be difficult to determine whether symptoms are related to the pseudocyst itself or to the necrosis or ductal obstruction respectively.

Pseudocysts occasionally rupture into surrounding structures or into the peritoneum; this is most common in the context of necrosis. Rupture into an adjacent organ occurs via erosion into the adjacent GI tract, which may lead to resolution of the pseudocyst or to fistula formation. Rupture into the peritoneum results in severe abdominal pain, pancreatic ascites, and rigidity from chemical peritonitis. Pseudocysts may lead to life-threatening hemorrhage from damage to GI tract mucosa or an adjacent vessel, such as the splenic, gastroduodenal, or middle colic vessels. Erosion into the splenic hilum may lift the capsule off the spleen and lead to intraabdominal bleeding, and aneurysm or pseudoaneurysm formation may precede a catastrophic bleed.

DIAGNOSTIC EVALUATION

Ultrasound (US) is a cost-effective and efficient means for detecting a large pseudocyst, and it may provide information about cyst content such as internal debris; however, US is limited in the evaluation of the pancreas and retroperitoneum. Contrast-enhanced CT has emerged as the primary means of imaging cystic lesions of the pancreas. A pseudocyst appears as a rounded, fluid-filled mass with a well-defined wall of uniform thickness adjacent to the pancreas (Figure 1). In addition to the size, location, and extent of a pseudocyst, CT allows comprehensive evaluation of the pancreas and other organs. The pancreatic parenchyma, the presence and extent of necrosis, the degree of pancreatic atrophy and calcification, and the presence of pancreatic duct dilatation are all important factors in determining patient management that can be readily evaluated with CT. Although the pancreatic duct and biliary system are easily visualized, the integrity of the pancreatic duct may be difficult to evaluate with CT. Infection is sometimes identified by the presence of gas within the pseudocysts (Figure 2), although in most patients this requires needle aspiration, Gram stain, and culture.

In the asymptomatic patient with no antecedent history of pancreatitis, CT may be inadequate to differentiate between pseudocyst and cystic neoplasm; in this instance, magnetic resonance imaging

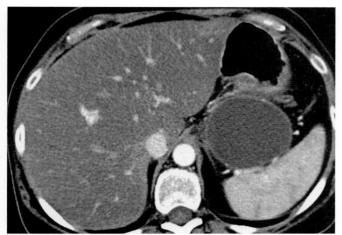

FIGURE 1   A single pseudocyst that arose in the setting of acute interstitial pancreatitis. An axial contrast-enhanced CT image shows a unilocular, low-density, fluid-filled mass encapsulated by a smooth, distinct, well-defined wall in the lesser sac in close relationship with the greater curvature of the stomach and the spleen. The cystic fluid is homogenous and of low attenuation. No visible intracystic septations or solid components are present, and the cyst wall is thin and uniform. All these imaging features are typical of a pancreatic pseudocyst. *(Courtesy Konraad J. Mortele, MD, Department of Radiology, Brigham and Women's Hospital.)*

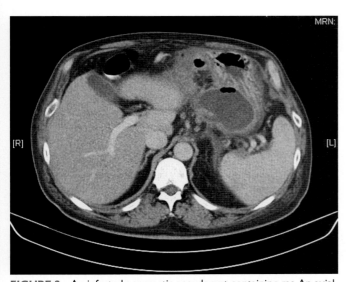

FIGURE 2   An infected pancreatic pseudocyst containing gas. An axial contrast-enhanced CT image shows a pseudocyst located in the lesser sac, closely attached to the stomach, associated with peripancreatic stranding; the thick wall and internal gas is suggestive of infection. Internal drainage to decompress the pseudocyst was achieved with endoscopic-guided cystogastrostomy *(Courtesy Konraad J. Mortele, MD, Department of Radiology, Brigham and Women's Hospital.)*

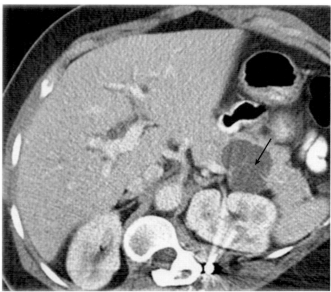

FIGURE 3   Pseudocyst versus mucinous cystic tumor. Axial contrast-enhanced CT image shows a cystic density mass with a thin wall and internal septations *(arrow)* in the body of the pancreas. The remaining pancreas is normal with no features of acute or chronic pancreatitis. A mucinous cystic tumor was suspected, but FNA revealed a CEA level of 2.5 ng/mL and amylase of 242,100 U/L, which is consistent with a pseudocyst. *(Courtesy Konraad J. Mortele, MD, Department of Radiology, Brigham and Women's Hospital.)*

(MRI) is helpful. Because of excellent soft-tissue contrast capability, MRI may demonstrate solid components, irregularity in the cyst wall, or septations, all of which are suggestive of neoplasm. The presence of internal dependent debris is a highly specific imaging finding for the diagnosis of pancreatic pseudocyst and is better appreciated with MRI or US.

Endoscopic retrograde cholangiopancreatography (ERCP) and magnetic resonance cholangiopancreatography (MRCP) are important tools in determining if a connection exists between the main pancreatic duct and the pseudocyst. Judicious use of ERCP is important;

it may exacerbate pancreatitis and could lead to infection through seeding of GI flora. For these reasons, it is ideally performed no more than 48 hours prior to a planned drainage procedure. MRCP confers the advantage of being noninvasive, although it lacks the sensitivity of ERCP. It may be particularly useful in distinguishing pseudocysts from cystic neoplasms.

If there is any concern for a neoplastic cyst (Figure 3), cyst fluid aspiration and analysis is essential. This may be obtained through endoscopic US with fine needle aspiration (EUS-FNA). Cyst fluid may be assessed for pancreatic enzymes, cells, tumor and genetic markers, and mucin. Pseudocyst fluid is typically acellular, with a low tumor-marker concentration, an absence of genetic alterations and mucin, and a significant elevation in amylase and lipase. This is in contradistinction to the fluid found within cystic neoplasms, characterized by high levels of mucin, genetic alterations, and carcinoembryonic antigen (CEA). Fluid should also be sent for Gram stain and bacterial culture to evaluate for infection. Pseudocysts are typically sterile in the absence of prior instrumentation.

MANAGEMENT

The management of pancreatic pseudocysts continues to evolve. Not only has their natural history been better defined, but newer imaging techniques have permitted a better definition of their anatomy and pathogenesis. These distinctions are important in selecting among therapeutic options.

Asymptomatic Pseudocysts

Traditionally, most pseudocysts were treated surgically based on data suggesting that those persisting longer than 6 weeks were unlikely to resolve and that the risk of complications if left untreated (up to 50%) outweighed the risk of intervention. With improvements in imaging, it has become clear that pseudocysts continue to spontaneously resolve for periods of up to a year and that the complication rate for asymptomatic disease may be even less than 10%. Although size greater than 6 cm was for a time considered an indication for intervention, several series suggest that even larger asymptomatic cysts can be safely observed. Although the availability of less invasive drainage procedures has reduced the morbidity of intervention, we do not believe that this should alter the indications. Even in the presence of documented ductal communication or stricture, we favor a conservative approach to the asymptomatic patient.

Serial imaging in the asymptomatic patient is appropriate, although little data exist on the appropriate interval. Following an acute episode of pancreatitis, we would typically reimage at 3 months with progressively longer subsequent intervals between studies. If the possibility of a cystic neoplasm remains a consideration, more frequent imaging is appropriate. Pseudocysts that seem to be enlarging are imaged more frequently; significant expansion may be an indication for intervention, although specific criteria have not been defined.

Symptomatic Pseudocysts

Although mildly symptomatic pseudocysts that are improving after a bout of pancreatitis may occasionally still be managed expectantly, symptoms are generally considered an indication for intervention.

Therapeutic Options

In addition to traditional open surgery, management options in the symptomatic patient include not only percutaneous and endoscopic drainage but also minimally invasive surgical approaches. To date, these interventions have not been compared in randomized trials, but accumulating experience would suggest that they might have a place in specific clinical settings. The availability of appropriate expertise continues to play a significant role in decision making.

Surgical drainage remains the most reliable means of achieving successful resolution of a pancreatic pseudocyst. Approaches include cystogastrostomy, cystoduodenostomy, Roux-en-Y cystojejunostomy, and distal pancreatectomy with or without splenectomy; each may be performed using minimally invasive techniques with reductions in wound-related morbidity and sometimes in length of stay. Cystogastrostomy is appropriate when the collection abuts the gastric wall. We employ a longitudinal anterior gastrostomy (Figure 4). Needle aspiration may be useful in locating the pseudocyst, if it is not immediately apparent upon exposure of the posterior wall of the stomach. The cautery is used to widely open the cyst wall, sometimes excising a button of gastric and cyst wall. A portion of the wall is sent for frozen-section analysis to rule out malignancy. To ensure hemostasis the opening is oversewn with a running, locking suture; we typically utilize 2-0 polydioxanone (PDS). Laparoscopic cystogastrostomy is performed in a similar fashion; laparoscopic US may facilitate identification of the cyst wall, which is then opened with the cautery. The opening is extended using several fires of the endoscopic gastrointestinal anastomosis (GIA) stapler.

Although it has been suggested that cystojejunostomy should be employed routinely for larger cysts, extending down the retroperitoneum to achieve dependent drainage, we believe that because of intraabdominal pressure relationships, most such collections can be drained successfully with cystogastrostomy, if they share a common wall with the stomach. Roux drainage, to prevent exposure of the cyst to GI contents, is appropriate in cases where the cyst wall is not directly adherent to the stomach. In this setting, a 40 to 60 cm limb is created and anastomosed to a generous opening in the mature cyst wall. All defects in the mesocolon and jejunal mesentery are closed. Cystoduodenostomy is occasionally indicated for patients with a pseudocyst in the head of the pancreas that closely adheres to the medial wall of the duodenum. Care must be taken to ensure that

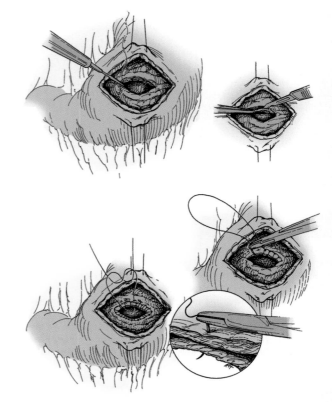

FIGURE 4   Surgical drainage of a pseudocyst through the posterior wall of the stomach. *(Reprinted from Zinner MJ, Ashley SW, editors: Maingot's abdominal operations, ed 11, New York, 2007, McGraw Hill.)*

the sphincter of Oddi and the intrapancreatic portion of the common bile duct are not injured during this operation; we have utilized this approach infrequently.

Resection, most commonly distal pancreatectomy to include the cyst, is typically reserved for unusual settings. Hemorrhage, usually from a pseudoaneurysm, is an appropriate indication; if the bleeding can be controlled by angiographic embolization prior to operation, it is preferable. Simple drainage of pseudocysts in the splenic hilum or dissecting beneath the splenic capsule may be associated with significant hemorrhage; we prefer resection in conjunction with splenectomy. Finally, if neoplasia remains a serious consideration, removal of the cyst with adequate margins seems appropriate.

Percutaneous drainage can be an effective approach to management. Although certainly less invasive than any surgical approach, it may require prolonged drainage and may be a source for bacterial colonization of the cyst. The benefits of octreotide to reduce drainage and speed healing have not been clearly established. Reported success rates vary from 40% to greater than 90%; this likely represents differences in patient selection. Patients with persistent ductal disruptions or strictures are unlikely to heal with this approach. Although transgastric percutaneous drainage followed by internalization has been applied successfully in these settings, endoscopic drainage is usually simpler.

Endoscopic approaches avoid a puncture wound to the abdominal wall. They are also less invasive than surgery, but they still achieve decompression by creating a connection between the pseudocyst and the lumen of the stomach or duodenum. Success rates of 60% to more than 90% have been reported. Endoscopic cystoduodenostomy is preferred by some endoscopists because of reduced vascularity and the relative dependency of the duodenum, although studies have not shown a difference in outcome. EUS can assist in localizing the site for drainage and in identifying vascular structures. In some instances, the tract is dilated with a balloon catheter to widen the opening and facilitate the insertion of the endoscope to permit direct visualization of the cavity, aspiration and debridement of cyst contents, and biopsy for histologic analysis. In situations where there is a demonstrated connection between the main pancreatic duct and the pseudocyst, endoscopic transpapillary stent placement across the defect or into the cyst may help establish definitive control. Stenting the sphincter of Oddi alone can help to lower ductal pressures and may also facilitate resolution.

Relative contraindications to endoscopic intervention include pseudocysts that contain extensive necrotic material, have a thin or immature wall, or are adjacent to a pseudoaneurysm or other vascular structure.

Treatment Recommendations

Selection among treatment options for symptomatic pseudocysts should be a multidisciplinary decision that includes interventional radiologists, endoscopists, and surgeons; such a decision must be based not only on the specific clinical setting but also on local expertise and the patient's comorbidities and preferences.

Pseudocysts Following Acute Interstitial Pancreatitis

These pseudocysts seldom contain much debris, and if they lie adjacent to the stomach or duodenum, they are most simply managed with endoscopic drainage. Persistent communication with the ductal system may be present in up to 60% of patients, although more conservative estimates place this at less at 10%. A transpapillary approach is useful for cysts in close proximity and with likely communication to the main pancreatic duct. Surgery is reserved for pseudocysts that fail to resolve with endoscopic drainage; we have been satisfied with the results of laparoscopic cytogastrostomy, although this is an increasingly unusual procedure in this setting.

For pseudocysts in more distant locations that cannot be easily drained internally, we use MRCP or ERCP to make an effort to determine whether there is ductal communication. Isolated cysts are drained percutaneously, whereas those with communication typically are treated with Roux-en-Y cystojejunostomy; we have found this cumbersome with the laparoscope.

Traditionally, all infected cysts were treated with external drainage, and this still seems appropriate in the setting of sepsis, although we have had success draining colonized cysts internally, either endoscopically or surgically.

Pseudocysts Following Pancreatic Necrosis

Intervention in the setting of pancreatic necrosis is seldom a question of resolving a symptomatic pseudocyst alone; typically, areas of adjacent necrosis are responsible for symptoms as well. Although occasionally pseudocysts represent simple peripancreatic collections, most often such cysts evolve from areas of pancreatic necrosis. Not only may these be associated with significant ductal disruptions, but the thickness of their contents may be considerable. Imaging can help to determine the quantity and nature of this debris.

Intervention in this setting must be tailored to the indications. Even in the symptomatic patient, we have generally attempted to delay operation for as long as seems reasonable after the initial episode, permitting areas of necrosis to organize. Early intervention is indicated in the presence of documented infection, demonstrated either by the presence of gas or by FNA. Depending on the content of the collections, percutaneous drainage under these conditions may resolve the sepsis, sometimes providing definitive therapy or temporizing until the necrosis is more fully organized; large-bore catheters with frequent irrigation may provide adequate drainage for even the thickest collections. Even in the patient with a well-organized collection, internal drainage is seldom appropriate in the context of infection.

Patients who are managed conservatively may continue to improve; in others, areas of necrosis and cystic collections produce

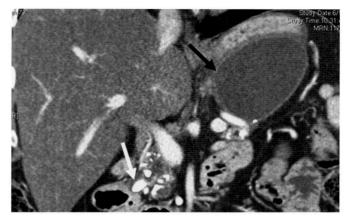

FIGURE 5   Pancreatic pseudocyst in the setting of chronic pancreatitis. Coronal contrast-enhanced CT image shows a pseudocyst in the tail of the pancreas (*black arrow*) compressing the adjacent stomach. The pancreas has diffuse, coarse calcifications (*white arrow*), and the pancreatic duct is dilated, which is consistent with chronic pancreatitis. (*Courtesy Konraad J. Mortele, MD, Department of Radiology, Brigham and Women's Hospital.*)

symptoms of pain and an inability to tolerate an oral diet. The timing of intervention is individualized based on the indications and the patient's general condition, which may or may not be compromised by multiorgan failure. Although endoscopic drainage of postnecrotic collections may be attempted, because of the viscous debris, this alone is frequently inadequate. Endoscopic and minimally invasive approaches to debridement have been described with increasing frequency; often these techniques require multiple staged procedures that may be less well tolerated than a single operative intervention. If operation is elected, open or laparoscopic approaches may be appropriate; although debridement through the posterior wall of the stomach is often successful, even with large areas of necrosis, our experience with laparoscopic debridement has not been as successful as that reported in the literature.

Pseudocysts Associated with Chronic Pancreatitis

Pseudocysts in the setting of chronic pancreatitis most often occur in the context of a strictured or abnormal pancreatic duct, ductal calculi, and parenchymal calcification (Figure 5). It is frequently impossible to distinguish symptoms related to the pseudocyst from those secondary to ductal stricturing, stones, and elevated parenchymal pressures.

Management directed at the pseudocyst alone is typically unsuccessful in resolving symptoms. Instead, an approach based on an understanding of ductal anatomy is most appropriate. A variety of transpapillary endoscopic approaches, including stenting and stone fragmentation, have been described with mixed results. If operation is elected, lateral pancreaticojejunostomy that incorporates pseudocyst drainage, and sometimes coring out the pancreatic parenchyma (Frey procedure), has been our preference. This approach may incorporate pseudocyst drainage, although pancreaticojejunostomy alone may be adequate in resolving the pseudocyst. In the setting of complications such as hemorrhage and biliary or duodenal obstruction, pseudocyst resection may be indicated.

SUMMARY

Pancreatic pseudocysts are peripancreatic or intraparenchymal fluid collections with a defined wall that have developed as a consequence of acute, traumatic, or chronic pancreatitis. Important considerations in the management of pancreatic pseudocyst include the etiology of the pancreatitis, the maturity of the pseudocyst wall, its anatomic relationship to adjacent solid organs and vasculature, and whether the main pancreatic duct communicates with the pseudocyst. Better definition of their natural history has suggested that asymptomatic pseudocysts can be observed expectantly. Symptoms that include pain, nausea, and early satiety and complications such as infection, rupture, hemorrhage, and GI obstruction are indications for intervention.

Management should be multidisciplinary, involving not only surgeons but interventional radiologists and endoscopists also. For simple cysts in the setting of interstitial pancreatitis and cysts adjacent to the stomach or duodenunum, endoscopic drainage is appropriate. For most other pseudocysts, establishing pancreatic ductal anatomy, including the presence of stricture or occlusion, prior to initiating treatment has emerged as an important consideration in selecting among percutaneous, endoscopic, and operative interventions.

SUGGESTED READINGS

Bergman S, Melvin WS: Operative and nonoperative management of pancreatic pseudocysts, *Surg Clin North Am* 18:447, 2007.
Bradley EL, Clements JL, Gonzalez AC: The natural history of pancreatic pseudocysts: a unified concept of management, *Am J Surg* 137:135, 1979.
Nealon WH, Bhutani M, Riall TS, et al: A unifying concept: pancreatic ductal anatomy both predicts and determines the major complications resulting from pancreatitis, *J Am Coll Surg* 208:790, 2009.
Yeo CJ, Bastidas JA, Lynch-Nyhan A, et al: The natural history of pancreatic pseudocysts documented by computed tomography, *Surg Gyn Obstet* 170:411, 1990.
Zinner MJ, Ashley SW, editors: *Maingot's abdominal operations*, ed 11, New York, 2007, McGrawHill, pp 961–970.

PANCREATIC DUCTAL DISRUPTIONS LEADING TO PANCREATIC FISTULA, PANCREATIC ASCITES, OR PLEURAL EFFUSIONS

William H. Nealon, MD

TERMINOLOGY

Ductal Disruptions

In general, the role of ductal disruptions in the various complications of pancreatitis is only recently being fully recognized and has been the basis of ongoing investigation by our clinical center. Ductal disruptions are predictably found after episodes of severe necrotizing pancreatitis, as we have recently reported and as reported, among others, by Howard and colleagues from the Pancreatitis Study Group at the University of Indiana. We have repeatedly demonstrated the presence of ductal disruption in the background of pancreatic pseudocysts, and their presence can be suspected in patients with persistent pseudocysts or in those with failed endoscopic or percutaneous cyst management.

Pancreatic ascites and *pancreatic pleural effusions* are manifestations of the same phenomenon. Enzyme-rich fluid spilling beyond the confines of the pancreas into any extrapancreatic site is clearly a representation of some element of disruption of the intraparenchymal ductal system. Although not always associated with main ductal injury, the presence of either pleural effusions or ascites should immediately raise suspicions that a ductal disruption has taken place, and we encourage the reader to immediately consider whether directly addressing the ductal pathology may provide a simple solution to what otherwise appears to be a very treacherous clinical challenge.

Decades of publications on the complications of pancreatitis have focused upon the epiphenomena of ductal injury. Peripancreatic debris after necrotizing pancreatitis; pancreatic ascites; *organized*

pancreatic necrosis, one of many terms applied to the rigid-walled fluid collections seen 4 to 8 weeks after an episode of necrotizing pancreatitis; pancreatic pseudocyst; pancreatic pleural effusions; and *pancreatic fistula,* whether post pancreatitis or postoperative, are all largely manifestations of the same phenomenon: active leakage of enzyme-rich fluid from the pancreatic ductal system. Although each of these manifestations requires unique timing and strategies for management, the complexity can be reduced by recognizing early in the course that the duct will elucidate and predict the behavior of each, so addressing the duct will likely be the solution. Thus some standard terms and their likely underlying ductal findings should be established.

Peripancreatic Fluid Collections

Peripancreatic fluid collections is a broad term applied to the combination of fluid with or without a component of semisolid debris seen in the aftermath of episodes of pancreatitis or of pancreatic trauma. The liquid elements of these collections are always composed of enzyme-rich pancreatic juice, thus we would stress that they are fed by some disruption in the pancreatic ductal system. What is not known is whether the disruption is in the peripherally located secondary and arborized tiny ductules, distributed throughout the pancreatic parenchyma, or if the fluid represents a major disruption of the main pancreatic duct (MPD), the ducts of Santorini and Wirsung. It is our postulate that the behavior of these early, disorganized collections can help predict which patients have sustained injury to the MPD and which patients have trivial leaks from tiny ductules, primarily by observing the resolution or persistence of the fluid; persistence suggests main ductal injury. Thus, for the sake of clarity we will restrict the term *pancreatic ductal disruption* to apply to those patients with documented injury to the MPD.

Pancreatic Pseudocyst

Pancreatic pseudocyst is perhaps the most highly recognized complication of both acute and chronic pancreatitis, with literally decades of documented clinical experience reported in large series. The International Symposium on Pancreatitis held in Atlanta in 1992 (reported in 1993) determined that the term *pseudocyst* was acceptably applied only to fluid collections that persist for more than 4 weeks. As the literature has progressed, rigorous adherence to this definition has largely been abandoned, and most now generally accept the definition of *pseudocyst* as a persistent postinflammatory fluid collection consisting of enzyme-rich fluid surrounded by a thick or "matured" wall and lacking an epithelial lining.

It is clear that establishing the transition from peripancreatic fluid collection to pseudocyst is vulnerable to individual interpretation, with different practitioners applying different terms to the same fluid collection. This distinction has unique importance in the surgical literature, in which we advocate delaying interventions until at least 4 weeks have elapsed since the initial episode of pancreatitis. The primary reason for the delay is the high likelihood of spontaneous resolution and the likelihood that persistence can then be traced to injuries or disruptions of the MPD.

Other entities that may be inappropriately called a *pseudocyst* are the fluid- and debris-filled structures we see after an episode of severe or severe necrotizing pancreatitis. Although some patients may develop pseudocysts in the aftermath of such an episode, the majority of these patients are noted to have persistent structures that typically have a thicker and less uniform wall, are clearly still composed of

debris, and at times have undergone surgical, endoscopic, or percutaneous interventions. They may also have persistent drainage from tubes placed in the bed of these structures. Although some controversy has surrounded the proper name for these entities, we favor the term *organized pancreatic necrosis,* but these structures are routinely called *pseudocysts* in the radiographic reading.

Organized Pancreatic Necrosis

An organized pancreatic necrosis is a residual structure that persists after an episode of severe necrotizing pancreatitis; it is composed of a rigid, thickened irregular wall, some amount of necrotic debris, and enzyme-rich pancreatic juice. An important feature of these collections is the fact that surgical decompression does not result in immediate collapse of the fluid collection. In contrast, drainage of pseudocysts will predictably result in immediate collapse of the cyst (Figure 1).

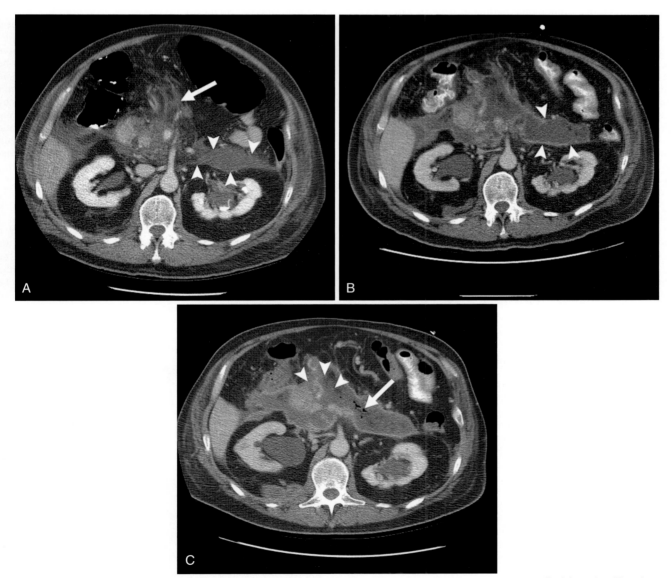

FIGURE 1   A 64-year-old male patient admitted with acute pancreatitis. **A,** The CT scan demonstrates peripancreatic fluid (*arrowheads*) and extensive inflammatory changes in the root of the mesentery (*arrow*). **B,** Follow-up CT scan 20 days later reveals evolution of the peripancreatic fluid with development of an enhancing wall (*white arrowheads*), confirming maturation of the collection. **C,** Fourteen days later, another CT scan reveals small pockets of gas within the collection (*arrow*), a powerful indication of infected necrosis.

Pancreatic Necrosis

The term *pancreatic necrosis* gained widespread use after the Atlanta Symposium, once the distinction was drawn between acute pancreatitis with or without identifiable necrosis and necrotizing pancreatitis with sterile or infected necrosis. These distinctions were made based upon available and subsequent data, which have established that patient outcomes, including survival, are profoundly altered when the populations are segregated on the basis of this one measure: infected versus sterile necrosis. An episode of acute pancreatitis without necrosis has a far less virulent course than acute pancreatitis in a patient with necrosis. Similarly the course of an episode of necrotizing pancreatitis with sterile necrosis is considerably less morbid, and has a measurably improved survival, compared with the course in individuals who develop infected necrosis.

Determination of the presence or absence of necrosis is made on the basis of opacification of pancreatic tissue during a CT scan with simultaneous infusion of intravenous contrast. Areas of the pancreas that fail to opacify are termed *necrotic*. After years of observation and correlation with operative findings, it is generally agreed that the radiographic finding of necrosis can be over-ascribed and that some tissue defined as necrotic proves to be subsequently viable. We do know that the constellation of cytokines released in an episode of severe acute pancreatitis includes substances that possess powerful vasoactive properties, and these may at times contribute to nonuniform opacification. There are, in spite of this fact, data to suggest that the degree of necrosis correlates with the likelihood of infected necrosis developing. In other words, more necrosis in the pancreas correlates with likelihood of infection.

The incidence of ductal disruption correlates with necrosis when compared with patients whose episode of pancreatitis is mild or moderate. Our data and others have elucidated several features of the course of necrotizing pancreatitis, which is dictated by the degree of ductal injury. Length of ICU stay, duration of system failure and of SIRS, likelihood of infected necrosis, and likelihood of recurrent pancreatitis after survival of an episode of necrotizing pancreatitis all have an increased frequency among those whose episode of necrotizing pancreatitis is found to have resulted in ductal injuries. Persistent drainage of pancreatic juice in survivors of debridement of pancreatic necrosis and in patients who have had percutaneous drains placed to treat necrosis are highly likely to have ductal injuries as the reason for that persistent drainage.

Pancreatic Fistula

In the context of this discussion, we will slightly broaden the terminology for describing fistula. In its strictest definition, *fistula* describes an abnormal communication between two epithelialized spaces. Our terminology will include the abnormal communication between the pancreatic duct and a pseudocyst, which is not epithelialized. Pancreatic fistulas will be found discussed in specific circumstances. They will be most commonly discussed as a complication of pancreatic resection, either pancreaticoduodenectomy or distal (tail) pancreatectomy. In each of these cases, the obvious source of drainage is the pancreatic duct. At times, particularly in tail resection, the fistula may manifest itself as a peripancreatic fluid collection or pseudocyst.

Pancreatic fistula is a recognized complication of pancreatitis that can manifest in a number of ways. The least common and perhaps most dramatic manifestations are seen when the inflammatory process associated with severe necrotizing pancreatitis leads to the development of drainage to another space, such as the pleural space, the mediastinum, or the skin. In a young man recovering from an episode of acute pancreatitis, we found drainage in the crease between the buttock and the lower extremity. The liquid was rich in pancreatic enzymes, which is consistent with fistula.

More common is pancreatic fistula seen after percutaneous or operative debridement of the necrotic pancreas in the background of severe acute pancreatitis. Persistent drainage, as previously mentioned, is essentially always a reflection of ductal disruption; the surgeon should promptly recognize that this circumstance exists, because this recognition will direct therapy. Similarly, persistent drainage after percutaneous management of a pseudocyst should prompt the same assumptions and strategies.

Pancreatic Ascites

As stated, *pancreatic ascites* is the term applied to the presence of abdominal fluid that is indistinguishable by imaging or by physical exam from any other form of ascites. I would caution the clinician that in patients with a long history of ethanol abuse, ascites and cachexia might be immediately dismissed as end-stage alcoholic cirrhosis, when in fact they may indicate pancreatic ascites. One distinguishing characteristic is an elevated serum amylase level, but this will not be seen in all patients; paracentesis and sampling for enzyme-rich fluid will confirm the diagnosis.

Generally speaking, free pancreatic juice within the peritoneal cavity rarely causes findings consistent with peritonitis. In the majority of circumstances, this phenomenon is seen in patients who have had a ruptured pseudocsyt. The term *pancreatic ascites* might be used early in the course of acute pancreatitis, when sufficient time has yet to elapse for the fluid to spontaneously resolve or to permit the formation of a fibrous wall surrounding the fluid, the process by which pseudocysts are created. Once again, any patient manifesting a collection of enzyme-rich pancreatic juice outside of the pancreatic parenchyma has a ductal or ductular disruption by definition. Main pancreatic ductal disruption is highly likely in the setting of persistent pancreatic ascites (Figure 2).

Pancreatic Pleural Effusions

The anatomic presence of pleuroperitoneal foramina is reflected by a number of clinical phenomena, including mediastinal or pleural air traversing these foramina to manifest as pneumoperitoneum. In the case of pancreatic pleural effusions, the direction of flow is from the peritoneal cavity to the pleural space. The enzyme-rich fluid may be seen in either side of the chest. The likely mechanism for this flow of fluid is a ductal disruption (Figure 3).

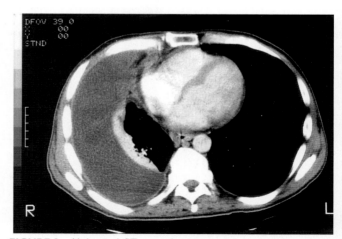

FIGURE 2 Abdominal CT scan of a patient with pancreatic ascites. The initial collection will accumulate in the lesser sac (*white arrowheads*) and then diffuse throughout the abdominal cavity (*arrows*).

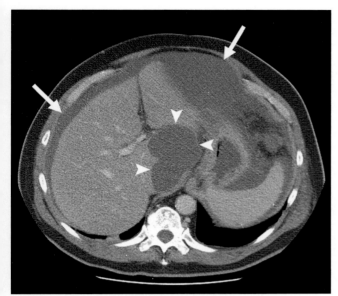

FIGURE 3 CT scan of the chest demonstrating a pancreatic pleural effusion on the right side. The likely channel of entry is via the documented tracts between the peritoneal and pleural spaces, although given the possibility that activated pancreatic enzymes play a role, there may be nonanatomic channels created by the disease process. *(From Cameron JL [ed.]: Current surgical therapy, ed 6, Philadelphia, 1998, Mosby Year–Book, p. 510.)*

CATEGORIES OF DUCTAL DISRUPTION

We have created a system to categorize the varieties of ductal disruptions seen as a consequence of pancreatitis (Figure 4). There are four categories: type I is a normal pancreatic duct; type II is a ductal stricture; type III is a complete occlusion of the duct, a phenomenon that has been termed *disconnected duct syndrome;* and type IV represents chronic pancreatitis. Each category includes a distinction for those with a radiographically demonstrable communication between the duct and the fluid collection or pseudocyst. Thus there is a type IIa and a type IIb duct: the subtype denoted by the lower case "a" denotes no radiographically demonstrable communication between the duct and the fluid collection, and subtype "b" denotes communication. A central premise in the development of this system was to facilitate the choice of modality to treat the disruption, pseudocyst, fistula, or fluid accumulation resulting from the disruption.

The impact of the pancreatic duct on the management of pancreatitis in general, and in ductal disruptions leading to pseudocyst in particular, is well demonstrated in patients with chronic pancreatitis. Ductal drainage for the treatment of chronic pain associated with this diagnosis has been durably demonstrated over decades of surgical literature. Recent reports on the placement of transpapillary stents to manage the pain of chronic pancreatitis support the same concept. In circumstances in which there is a coexistence of chronic pancreatitis and a pseudocyst, we have demonstrated that operative drainage of the ductal system alone is sufficient to result in resolution of the pseudocyst and of the ductal disruption associated with the pseudocyst, thus confirming the role played by the duct in the persistence of the pseudocyst.

Location of the Ductal Disruption

Kozarek and colleagues have confirmed that ductal disruptions occur in the duct in the head of the pancreas in 50% of patients, in the body in 30%, and in the tail in 20%. Howard and colleagues have described

Categories of Ductal Anatomy

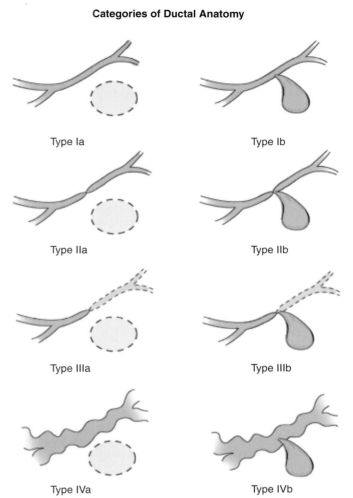

FIGURE 4 System to categorize the ductal anatomy seen in pancreatitis. Type I is a normal pancreatic duct, type II is a ductal stricture, type III is a completely occluded duct (disconnected duct syndrome), and type IV is chronic pancreatitis. The subtype denoted by the lower case "a" denotes no radiographically demonstrable communication between the duct and the fluid collection. Subtype "b" denotes communication. *(Modified from Nealon WH Bhutani M, Riall T, et al: A unifying concept: pancreatic ductal anatomy both predicts and determines the major complications resulting from pancreatitis, J Am Coll Surg 208[5]:790–801, 2009, American College of Surgeons.)*

what they have termed a *vascular watershed area* in the midbody of the pancreas and suggest that necrosis—and by inference, ductal disruptions—are more common in that region of the gland. Our position is that determining the location of the ductal injury offers little information regarding the final definitive management, with the possible exception that operative resectional therapy may be a viable option for patients whose ductal disruption is located in the tail of the pancreas; resection of the head of the pancreas should be implemented only under extraordinary circumstances.

One other aspect of the location of the ductal injury may prove to be pertinent. When a patient with an otherwise unexplained pseudocyst or with unexplained recurrent pancreatitis is found to have a midbody stricture or disconnection, consider the possibility of a posttraumatic ductal injury, and explore the patient's history for even remote episodes of trauma. In this case the location of the ductal injury is consistent with the classic site of injury, where the gland traverses the spine, and the body of the pancreas can be crushed by blunt force, such as from a seatbelt or a kick from a horse. In this setting the location of the disruption can assist in assigning etiology to the pancreatic pathology.

CLINICAL PRESENTATION

Ductal disruption may present during the index hospitalization or after discharge, which we have discussed. Patients whose course of acute pancreatitis fails to follow the standard of 3 to 5 days to complete recovery in all likelihood have a peripancreatic fluid collection. Failure to resolve the acute episode of pancreatitis is therefore one mode of presentation. Many claim that the management of complicated acute pancreatitis, after the resolution of SIRS and multiple organ dysfunction in severe cases, is the management of fluid collections. We would add that such patients also likely possess some element of ductal disruption. Although it is difficult to avoid broad use of CT scanning in patients admitted with pancreatitis, we recommend reserving this imaging modality for patients with severe, potentially necrotizing pancreatitis and for patients whose course fails to evolve in the predicted fashion; that is, those who have had persistent pain beyond the 3- to 5-day window. Many now advocate that even in episodes of severe, necrotizing pancreatitis, the optimal timing for the first CT scan is 48 hours after onset of symptoms, because the degree of necrosis and of fluid collections will be more reliably determined.

Persistent Fluid Collection

We should clarify that although we have repeatedly advocated obtaining information regarding ductal anatomy, we do not advocate indiscriminate use of ERCP in these patients until specific criteria have been met. Two significant issues should be considered: First, the acute fluid collections have a high potential for spontaneous resolution over a 3- to 6-week period of observation; early intervention may therefore simply be unnecessary. Second, it should be recognized that many studies have documented the fact that ERCP brings with it a considerable risk of postprocedure sepsis, because the injected contrast is not sterile. Even the more recently confirmed potential benefit in performing transpapillary stent placement in the pancreatic duct during an ERCP carries a risk of contamination of the peripancreatic fluid. We do not, therefore, advocate early ERCP in the management of these patients, and we do not subscribe to the theory that evacuating the enzyme-rich fluid from the lesser sac plays any role in reducing the degree of glandular necrosis. It should be understood that the fluid persisting after an acute attack, and certainly the fluid found at a time remote from the index attack, is composed of nonactivated enzymes. Most accept that one element in the pathogenesis of acute pancreatitis is the activation of enzymes by cytokines or by some other process. Decades of investigation have well established that bacteria possess enzymes that are capable of activating pancreatic enzymes. Thus one can acknowledge the seriousness of converting a sterile pancreatic collection to an infected one, particularly a postnecrotizing collection, with its combination of fluid and devitalized debris. The risk of causing infection in another sterile collection in the body, accompanied by the deleterious effects of activated enzymes, render the decision to perform ERCP potentially catastrophic, and it has been described as setting a "fire in a fireworks factory."

From the surgeon's point of view, an added disincentive for proceeding with ERCP early in the course of acute pancreatitis without necrosis is the fact that the pseudocyst wall has not matured, and therefore the only operative option if the surgeon is forced to proceed to surgery is external drainage with a high likelihood that subsequent surgery will be required. In the case of necrotizing pancreatitis, the accumulated data over the past 10 to 15 years clearly demonstrates that early operative intervention for this clinical diagnosis is associated with a considerably increased risk of mortality and morbidity.

Thus in the event that premature instrumentation results in infected collections and sepsis, the outcome, including the likelihood of survival for the patient, is negatively impacted.

Recurrent Pancreatitis and Recurrent Pain

Some patients who prove to have sustained ductal disruptions will not present with fluid collections. There are two additional patterns of presentation, both with approximately the same frequency. One is recurrent pancreatitis. This specific presentation may fail to be identified by the managing physician, particularly in the patient who has recovered from an episode of acute ethanol-induced pancreatitis. The assumption will readily be made that the patient simply continues to drink and thus has a well-explained recurrence. Even protestations by the patient that they have not continued alcohol consumption will be viewed as simply untrue. Suspicions should be raised if consumption can be accurately determined and in patients whose inciting cause of pancreatitis, such as gallstones after an episode of biliary pancreatitis, causes them to experience recurrent attacks even after the gallbladder has been removed and the bile duct has been cleared of any residual stones. The other manifestation that is not associated with fluid collections is the patient who returns with persistent pain, particularly postprandial pain. In both of these subsets of patients, ERCP can be performed promptly.

Finally, it is reasonable to wonder why MRCP cannot be useful in determining ductal disruption. There is certainly reason to be optimistic that improvements in technology may overcome current impediments. The most significant reason for the inadequacy of MRCP in evaluating ductal disruptions associated with peripancreatic fluid collections is the fact that the fluid collections contain pancreatic juice, and therefore they opacify and obliterate the visualization of the pancreatic duct. Further, some elements of the pancreatic ductal anatomy are currently not demonstrated with the degree of detail achieved by ERCP. One example we have seen repeatedly is the patient with ductal disconnection in the tail of the pancreas whose MRCP is read as normal but whose ERCP clearly demonstrates an abrupt cutoff of the duct in the tail, which is consistent with disruption.

PRINCIPLES OF MANAGEMENT AND THERAPEUTIC INTERVENTIONS

We have discussed the issue of timing of intervention. Early intervention in simple acute pancreatitis and in severe necrotizing pancreatitis is discouraged for the reasons stated. We completed and published a study that evaluated patients who survived an episode of moderate or severe acute gallstone pancreatitis with documented persistent fluid collections. This study was prompted by referrals of such patients who had undergone early cholecystectomy, apparently under the misconception that this intervention played any role in the resolution of the initial attack. The only purpose of cholecystectomy in that setting is to prevent recurrent attacks, which are documented to take place with a high frequency without that intervention, and it is therefore uniformly advised that cholecystectomy be performed during the initial hospitalization for patients with uncomplicated pancreatitis. We evaluated a modification of that current dogma in patients with significant fluid collections by recommending that these patients be managed with a period of follow-up imaging not to exceed 6 weeks. In our study nearly 40% had spontaneous resolution and underwent only cholecystectomy. Those whose fluid collections evolved into pseudocysts were treated with simultaneous management of the gallbladder and the pseudocyst, thus avoiding a need to for two procedures and two general anesthetics. No patient had an episode of pancreatitis during the follow-up period. More than 70% of those patients whose pseudocysts persisted had ductal disruptions found at the time of ERCP.

Urgent Operation

Early management will involve medical supportive measures while the acute event subsides. Although we have stated that our data and that of others have shown that complications of severe pancreatitis—including necrosis, infected necrosis, and the need for operative debridement of necrosis—are all associated with ductal disruption, we do not make use of this information when urgent operation is mandated by infected necrosis, hemorrhage, or by a suddenly plummeting clinical status. Our utilization of the evaluation of the status of ductal anatomy primarily comes into play when essentially elective procedures are being considered. In that setting our strategy is to partner with an experienced pancreatic surgeon and a practitioner skilled in interventional radiology techniques and in therapeutic ERCP, EUS, and advanced flexible endoscopic techniques.

The surgeon must decide, by some criteria, which circumstances mandate intervention. A first criterion is persistence, and by that we mean a minimum elapsed time since initial event of 4 to 6 weeks. The primary reason for delay is to permit spontaneous resolution. Be skeptical of the literature, particularly in the endoscopic or percutaneous management of fluid collections, when the procedures were performed shortly after the attack.

The belief remains prevalent that the size of a fluid collection influences the decision to intervene invasively. Certainly we would not advocate intervening for fluid collections less than 2 cm in diameter; but again, we would direct the reader to consider the symptoms and the possible role being played by an unrecognized pancreatic duct disruption. A stricture or a ductal disconnection can cause pain or recurrent pancreatitis, therefore a patient with an apparently trivial fluid collection should still be offered evaluation of their duct as a possible explanation of the persistent symptoms. Fluid collections or pseudocysts that cause symptoms, are larger than 4 cm in diameter, and have persisted beyond 4 weeks should be treated with invasive intervention.

The discussion of the management of *asymptomatic pseudocysts* has persisted for several decades. We generally discourage intervention for asymptomatic fluid collections, although collections larger than 6 or 7 cm are rarely asymptomatic in our experience, and the data from the original papers by Sarr and Yeo both found that patients with pseudocysts of that size were highly likely to ultimately require intervention and were also highly likely to develop life-threatening complications compared with patients with smaller collections.

We have not encountered patients with ductal disruptions, with or without fluid collections, who were asymptomatic. Patients with persistent fistulas in drains after percutaneous or operative intervention require further intervention. After deciding that intervention is reasonable, the question of which mode to use for managing the patient must be addressed. Once again, we advocate defining the pancreatic ductal anatomy at this point and not sooner. Figure 5 demonstrates the ERCP findings in a patient who had undergone operative debridement of necrosis and was found to have persistent drainage from her operatively placed drains. ERCP documented duct disconnection.

A retrograde *fistulogram* (Figure 6) demonstrates the duct in the remaining portion of the pancreas, the isolated pancreatic segment. This finding must be managed operatively, as the isolated segment will otherwise forever remain out of continuity with the intestinal tract, and stents (endoscopic or percutaneous) will be required indefinitely, bringing with them all the issues seen with long-term drains, including occlusion, sepsis, and the need for repeated procedures for management.

Modalities for Intervention

The three modes of treatment in the management of the complications of pancreatitis are *endoscopic, surgical,* and *percutaneous.* Similar to many other areas in which alternative nonoperative measures have been substituted for operative techniques, the primary advantage for the nonoperative technique is the possibility of avoiding

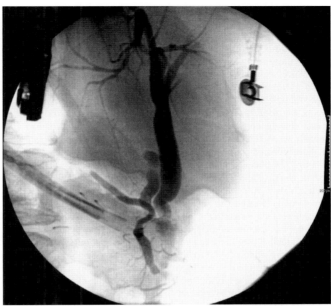

FIGURE 5   ERCP in a patient with a duct disconnection. The other structure that abruptly stops is a long cystic duct remnant after cholecystectomy.

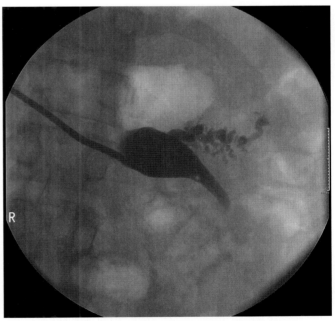

FIGURE 6   After contrast was injected through a percutaneous drainage catheter in a patient with ductal disconnection, contrast can be seen filling a small intraabdominal chamber and then filling the duct in the isolated segment of pancreas located in the tail of the gland.

operation; the trade-off is most often some level of reduced success rates or the requirement for multiple procedures instead of one operation. The distinction between the alternatives is rarely black and white, and the circumstances in the current discussion are similar.

Pseudocyst with Duct Disruption

The success rates for permanently resolving a pseudocyst with operation are reported to be between 90% and 95%. For endoscopic and percutaneous management, the achievement of permanent resolution of pseudocyst is more on the order of 70% to 80%. Multiple procedures and drain occlusion or sepsis are common in those whose drainage persists beyond 3 weeks. Advantages of percutaneous techniques compared with endoscopic therapies may be the fact that fistulograms can be obtained without sedation or an invasive procedure. Advantages of endoscopic therapy include the absence of an external drainage tube and the option to utilize transpapillary stents. Percutaneous management is limited to simple drainage of the pseudocyst, but endoscopic management includes either transmural placement of multiple stents into the fluid collection, frequently assisted by endoscopic ultrasound directing the access point, or placement of transpapillary drains. Transpapillary drains consist of 5 or 7 Fr plastic catheters placed across the sphincter of Oddi to reduce the resistance to flow and encourage pancreatic juice to drain preferentially into the duodenum, thus decompressing the pseudocyst. When effective, this technique can achieve prompt resolution. It should be recognized that under some circumstances, combined percutaneous and endoscopic transpapillary drainage may be required. Surgical techniques include cystogastrostomy and cystojejunostomy. We strongly advocate cystojejunostomy for a number of reasons. First, postoperative hemorrhage is considerably more common after cystogastrostomy. Second, the data reflect that cystogastrostomy employed for pseudocysts larger than 7 cm and those that extend for some distance inferior to the stomach are at considerably higher risk of sepsis, presumably as gastric contents empty into this space.

Pancreatic Necrosis with Duct Disruption

In the management of the liquid and solid material surrounding an area of necrosis, both endoscopic and percutaneous techniques are challenged because of the character of the targeted material. In spite of this fact, both methodologies have achieved a measure of success, but only by significantly expanding their repertoire of devices. Percutaneous techniques now routinely involve the use of extra-large-bore drains (18 to 24 Fr) and active mechanical debridement with manipulation of the tubes and aggressive irrigation with saline. Endoscopic management has now added the creation of a large rent in the stomach sufficient to pass the endoscope into the necrotic area, where active debridement can be performed over several sessions, and large transmural drains are left in place.

While operative debridement is a gold standard of sorts, the parameters and techniques employed for these procedures have evolved over time. As stated, intervention is delayed as long as possible and is dictated by the finding of infected necrosis after fine needle sampling or by suddenly plummeting clinical status. Operative debridement should be complete, and all nonviable tissue should be excised. Reoperation should be unusual, and open abdominal procedures are discouraged.

It has become our protocol to utilize percutaneous, large-bore drains for patients with infected necrosis in the first 4 weeks after the index event. In the event this fails to result in stabilization after 4 weeks, we preferentially resort to operation. It is in this relatively more elective setting that we would examine ductal anatomy before proceeding, as we believe this information can and should be broadly utilized to select the most appropriate modality.

Persistent Pancreatic Fistula and Duct Disruption

Persistent pancreatic fistula and duct disruption will often be seen in patients who have undergone percutaneous or operative interventions with drain placement, and the drain outputs remain at a high volume. These patients have nearly always reached a stable clinical status. ERCP evaluation of the ductal system should accompany the planned intervention. Depending upon the findings, a therapeutic endoscopic procedure may be suitable (transpapillary drain), or the information may direct the decision to proceed with percutaneous or operative intervention. We will discuss the use of this information to choose strategies.

Ductal Disruption Presenting as Pain, Recurrent Pancreatitis, or as Recurrent Abscess Formation

The final category of patient seen with ductal disruption is the patient who has been discharged home but returns complaining of pain and showing classic symptoms of pancreatitis or recurrent abscess. Our message is that the clinician should be immediately suspicious for ductal disruption even in the absence of a fluid collection, or when a fluid collection appears to be trivial based upon its size. The clinician should organize therapeutic plans based upon this suspicion. ERCP will be required to define anatomy and help with the choice of one of three available modalities—endoscopic, percutaneous, or surgical. These decisions will also be dictated by the specific expertise at a given institution. Some medical centers may not have experts in each modality. As a surgeon, I also perform ERCP, so that somewhat simplifies my decisions. Interventional radiologic support should be sought before proceeding if it is anticipated that such support may be required. In best circumstances a protocol has been defined for management.

Utilizing Ductal Categories to Determine Therapeutic Modalities

Type I ductal findings (Figure 4) suggest no disruption. We favor nonoperative techniques with these patients. We consider endoscopic or percutaneous techniques comparable in their success rates, and the choice between these two depends upon the skills and equipment available at your institution.

Type II ductal stricture can be managed by either transpapillary endoscopic techniques or by operation. We do not advocate percutaneous management when ductal stricture has been documented. It has been our experience that the degree of stricture plays a role in the success of transpapillary stents. The standard size of a pancreatic duct stent (5 or 7 Fr) may explain these limitations. Prolonged cannulation may be required for these strictures, and prolonged stent placement raises a host of potential negative outcomes, including stent occlusion. Obstruction of the duct with resulting upstream ductal dilatation has been documented after stent occlusion, and the existence of a clinical diagnosis of infected pancreatic duct comparable to cholangitis has been proposed. Operation is therefore our therapy of choice for Type II lesions with significant flow restriction shown by ERCP contrast injection.

With both type II and type III ductal disruptions, there are three operative strategies: 1) operative drainage of the collection or pseudocyst, 2) resection of the pancreas, or 3) operative drainage of the main pancreatic duct in the tail of the pancreas.

Operative Drainage of Fluid Collections/Pseudocyst

This option is employed when the pancreatic duct in the tail of the pancreas is not accessible due to the hostile intraabdominal condition resulting from the episode of pancreatitis or the changes resulting from prior operative procedures.

Operative Resection of the Pancreas

Pancreatic resection is primarily employed for lesions in the body and tail of the pancreas. We believe this choice is employed only in the event that no fluid collection is available for drainage, or the collection does not offer what is viewed as adequate drainage, and when the tissue planes for dissection are viewed as unacceptably hostile for exploration and identification of the pancreatic duct. Both the length of operation and the likelihood that it will require blood transfusion are elevated when resectional therapy is employed. In addition, the undesirable sequelae of insulin dependence, postoperative pancreatic duct leak, and postsplenectomy sepsis renders this choice our least acceptable option.

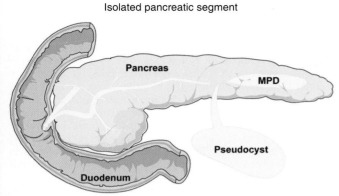

Isolated pancreatic segment

FIGURE 7   Illustration demonstrating the entire pancreas in a patient who has sustained a ductal disconnection associated with pancreatitis.

Operative Drainage of the Main Pancreatic Duct in the Tail of the Pancreas

Operative drainage of the main pancreatic duct in the tail of the pancrease is our preferred operative management. It is limited by the operative accessibility of the pancreas in the often hostile environment and the presence of a dilated duct. We have performed drainage procedures on small ducts, but we routinely perform a longitudinal incision along the anterior surface of the gland in a manner similar to a Puestow-type pancreaticojejunostomy. We have had success opening a fluid collection by incising the anterior wall and visualizing the pancreas within the cavity. It is not uncommon to find the pancreas fairly discretely identified within the pseudocyst itself. We also take advantage of the fistula tract created by operative or percutaneously placed drains, when operation is required for persistent drainage. In this case we have performed retrograde contrast injection either through the drain preoperatively or through a catheter placed in the tract intraoperatively. Once the operating surgeon reaches the retroperitoneum, there are two choices: to either suture a roux limb to that ostium or to use a probe in the tract as a guide. Either method will provide access to the pancreatic duct and thus will result in successful drainage of the pancreatic fistula.

Our results confirm that ductal drainage procedures offer the lowest likelihood of subsequent admissions for pain, recurrent pancreatitis, or recurrent fluid collections and pseudocysts. This approach also carries none of the negative outcomes documented after resection, and it has the advantage over the drainage of fluid collections of documenting adequate drainage of the pancreatic duct. We believe some patients with ductal disruption and a consequent fluid collection may have only a pinpoint drainage channel communicating between the duct and the pseudocyst, which provides the ideal environment for continued symptoms caused by the equivalent of a high-grade stenosis of the duct. In this case postoperative pain and recurrent pancreatitis are seen, particularly in patients with ductal disconnection.

Type III (Figure 7) ductal disruption, the *disconnected duct syndrome*, is in our opinion successfully managed only by operation. The pancreatic parenchyma upstream from the stricture will continue to secrete enzyme-rich fluid and will be forever clinically apparent with recurrent pain, pancreatitis, or abscess formation. Percutaneous drainage will not cease, endoscopic transmural drainage fails when the stents become dislodged or occluded, and transpapillary drains simply have no effect on the environment on the opposite side of the disruption. The three operative approaches just mentioned are the only available options in this setting.

Thus we strongly advocate making use of the ductal categories (see Figure 4) to drive the decision as to which modality to employ in managing these complex patients. I cannot stress enough the value of interdependence and partnering among the skilled endoscopist, the skilled interventional radiologist, and the skilled pancreatic surgeon. Each will play a role in the outcome.

Suggested Readings

Lau ST, Simchuk EJ, Kozarek RA, et al: A pancreatic duct leak should be sought to direct treatment in patients with acute pancreatitis, *Am J Surg* 181:411, 2001.

Nealon WH, Bhutani M, Riall TS, et al: A unifying concept: pancreatic ductal anatomy both predicts and determines the major complications resulting from pancreatitis, *J Am Coll Surg* 208:790–799, 2009.

Nealon WH, Walser E: Main pancreatic ductal anatomy can direct choice of modality for treating pancreatic pseudocysts (surgery vs. percutaneous drainage), *Ann Surg* 235(6):751–758, 2002.

Pelaez-Luna M, Vege SS, Petersen BT, et al: Disconnected pancreatic duct syndrome in severe acute pancreatitis: clinical and imaging characteristics and outcomes in a cohort of 31 cases, *Gastrointest Endosc* 68:91–97, 2008.

Nealon WH, Walser E: Duct drainage alone is sufficient in the operative management of pancreatic pseudocyst in patients with chronic pancreatitis, *Ann Surg* 237:614–622, 2003.

Howard TJ, Rhodes GJ, Selzer DJ, et al: Roux-en-Y internal drainage is the best surgical option to treat patients with disconnected duct syndrome after severe acute pancreatitis, *Surgery* 130:714–721, 2001.

Nealon WH, Bawduniak J, Walser EM: Appropriate timing of cholecystectomy in patients who present with peripancreatic fluid collections, *Ann Surg* 239(6):741–751, 2004.

MANAGEMENT OF CHRONIC PANCREATITIS

L. William Traverso, MD, and Richard A. Kozarek, MD

OVERVIEW

Principles for Treatment Based on Clinical and Anatomic Patterns

Almost every patient with chronic pancreatitis seen by a surgeon seeks relief of abdominal pain, although a few require treatment for chronic fistula or come with a clinical diagnosis of steatorrhea. Since the head of the pancreatic gland is the epicenter of the disease, any treatment for pain relief must be designed around this area. The head of the gland is frequently referred to as the *pacemaker of chronic pancreatitis*. If the head is not involved, the patient has an unusual pattern that deserves more thoughtful investigation. Our treatment decisions are based on an algorithm where surgery is used if endotherapy fails.

Severity Classification of Chronic Pancreatitis: Anatomic and Clinical

The Cambridge Image Severity Classification (CISC) system should be used as a guideline to select patients for treatment and to ensure almost 100% relief for *disabling* pain. In fact, an achievable outcome is *complete* pain relief in about 75% of patients, if patients are properly selected. The CISC is based on ductal imaging and is summarized in Table 1.

Indications for Treatment: Selection Criteria

The primary goal of any therapy for chronic pancreatitis is pain relief. Surgical decompression of the pancreatic ductal system has been shown to delay or even reverse exocrine insufficiency after long-term follow-up. This phenomenon has yet to be shown for decompressive endotherapy, but it is conceivable, because endotherapy is primarily a decompressive modality. Whether one uses surgical or endoscopic treatment to relieve pain, our best efforts will fail unless the selection criteria outlined in Table 2 are met. More specifically, the five criteria are described below.

1. *Chronic pancreatitis is really present.* Chronic pain syndromes, particularly in young women, are commonly mistaken for chronic pancreatitis when the pancreas is normal. A good starting point is to use the 1963 Marseilles definition of *chronic pancreatitis:* "residual pancreatic damage, either anatomical or functional, that persists even if the primary cause or factors are eliminated." The irreversible change in the pancreas is usually fibrosis, and functional changes are exocrine and/or endocrine insufficiency. With the recent availability of the elastase test, the presence of normal exocrine function is easily established. Checking diabetic status with HbA1C is a convenient way to test endocrine status.
2. *Imaging studies must show a* severe *anatomical defect.* The Cambridge classification category of "marked" is required before endotherapy can be effective and definitely before surgical resection or drainage procedures are indicated. To qualify as "marked," at least one main pancreatic duct stricture, with or without stones, is required, as shown Table 1.

3. *The "driver" (etiology) has been removed.* Pain relief cannot be achieved if the cause of the chronic pancreatitis—gallstones, alcohol use, or autoimmune pancreatitis—has not been remedied or eliminated. Good pain relief will not be sustained if patients continue to use alcohol, nor will it be sustained in the unfortunate patient afflicted with hereditary chronic pancreatitis.
4. *Pathologic anatomy fits a pattern.* The treatment is designed to address the pathological anatomy, which is almost always in the pancreatic head. It is unusual for the epicenter of the disease to be isolated in the tail. The symptoms must fit an anatomic pattern. Consider a neoplastic etiology or that the patient is currently ingesting any quantity of alcohol.
5. *Plans are made with only current anatomy from updated imaging.* If endotherapy has failed, surgical treatment will depend on the current anatomy and is also tempered by institutional bias.

Using the algorithm above, the patient considered for endotherapy or surgery is highly selected to ensure success. After long-term follow-up, the outcomes are promising; these highly selected patients will achieve a significant reduction in their disabling pain, and many will have complete pain relief, albeit with a mandatory amount of additional treatment and/or follow-up if endotherapy alone has been employed.

ENDOTHERAPY

Techniques

The evolution of endoscopic therapy to treat pancreatic disorders has moderated the need for resection in some centers. Although the results of pancreatic head resection in patients with multiple strictures and stones associated with pseudotumors of the pancreatic head cannot be duplicated, endotherapy can nevertheless improve pain and decrease relapsing attacks of pancreatitis by approaching *obstructing calculi* and isolated *inflammatory stenoses,* with or without upstream ductal disruptions, that manifest as pseudocysts, pancreatic ascites, or high-amylase pleural effusions. Treatment is not done by an endoscopist acting independently; it requires access to various forms of lithotripsy, interventional radiologic support, and surgical salvage when endotherapy fails. Head resection is the final option, the default after multiple sessions in patients where stone extraction is unsuccessful, or where the patient remains stent dependent despite repeated treatment of obstructing stenoses.

The endoscopic approach to strictures and stones presupposes access to the pancreas through the major or minor papilla, although transgastric or transduodenal access to an obstructed pancreatic duct is occasionally undertaken under endoscopic ultrasound (EUS). Sphincterotomy can either be done using a conventional or needle-knife sphincterotome, usually with a pure cutting current to minimize the chance of cautery transmission and iatrogenic PD stenosis from electrocautery transmission. When approaching the pancreatic duct through the major papilla, most endoscopists undertake an initial biliary sphincterotomy to expose the pancreaticobiliary septum and help define the length of the subsequent PD sphincter incision. Slick guidewires, such as the Tracer or Metro (Wilson-Cook, Winston-Salem, NC) or a Jagwire (Boston Scientific, Natick, Mass.) are used to provide access and orientation and to act as a "rail" for all subsequent treatment.

Prior to consideration of endotherapy, scans must ensure that the pancreatic stricture is benign. The patient will have already had an axial computed tomogram (CT) using a pancreas protocol, an endoscopic ultrasound (EUS), and brush cytology or direct biopsy of any stricture considered potentially malignant. These anatomic criteria will have been correlated with the signs and symptoms as well as with blood tumor markers such as CA 19-9. Clinical follow-up is also a mandatory part of endotherapy, as any neoplastic process can masquerade as chronic pancreatitis.

TABLE I: Cambridge classification of image severity for chronic pancreatitis

Cambridge Class	Main Pancreatic Duct	Abnormal Side Branches
Normal	Normal	0
Equivocal	Normal	<3
Mild	Normal	>3
Moderate	Abnormal	>3
Marked	Abnormal*	>3

*Main pancreatic duct (MPD) terminates prematurely (abrupt, tapering, irregular), multiple MPD strictures, MPD dilated >10 mm, ductal filling defects (stones), intrapancreatic or extrapancreatic "cavities" are observed, or contiguous organ involvement (stenoses of common bile duct or duodenum, arterial venous fistula)
(Modified from Axon ATR, Classen M, Cotton PB, et al: Pancreatography in chronic pancreatitis: international definitions, *Gut* 25:1107-1112, 1984.)

TABLE 2: Selection criteria summary

Selection Criteria for Pain Relief Must Be Inclusive

Chronic pancreatitis is really present.

Imaging studies show a *severe* anatomic defect.

The "driver" (etiology) has been removed.

Symptoms fit the anatomic pattern.

Plans are made based on current anatomy from up-to-date imaging.

Benign strictures may be dilated by 4 to 6, 5 to 7, or 7 to 10 Fr dilating catheters but are more commonly treated by 4 to 8 mm hydrostatic dilating balloons. Occasionally, extremely tight strictures, particularly those associated with an upstream stone, may need to be breached by a screw-like device called a *Soehendra stent extractor* (Wilson-Cook, Inc.). Following dilation to a size approximating the downstream pancreatic duct, most endoscopists attempt to place a 5 to 10 Fr prosthesis across the stricture. This stent is usually retrieved in 2 to 4 months, and if the stricture is persistent, it is retreated with additional dilation and replacement of one or multiple parallel prostheses, particularly for stenoses in the head of the gland.

If initial stent insertion is not helpful to relieve pain, most endoscopists seek surgical consultation. If the stent insertion is helpful, the process can be repeated several times over a year. If the patient becomes stent dependent for symptom relief, most endoscopists consider surgical referral. In contrast to placement of a single stent for a stricture, our practice has evolved into placement of multiple smaller prostheses (5 to 7 Fr) across the stenosis. Not only does this allow drainage between the stents at the time of inevitable stent occlusion, it has been demonstrated in the endoscopic treatment of biliary strictures that multiple stents appear to improve subsequent stricture patency rates.

The removal of obstructing pancreatic calculi is considerably more difficult than the endoscopic removal of bile duct stones. Not only are pancreatic stones frequently associated with downstream strictures, they may also lodge at acute angulations of the duct and result in upstream ductal disruption in the form of a pseudocyst or pancreatic ascites. Approximately half of main pancreatic ductal stones can be removed after PD sphincterotomy, with or without dilation of a concomitant stricture, using conventional biliary stone baskets or an extraction balloon over a guidewire. In the remaining cases, fragmentation is required.

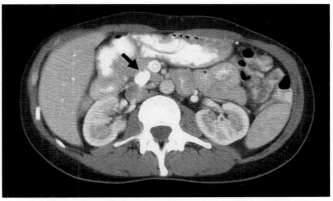

FIGURE I   CT demonstrates a calcified I cm calculus (*arrow*) with upstream PD dilation.

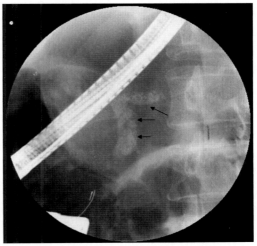

FIGURE 2   A fluoroscopic view is shown during stone retrieval after extracorporeal shock wave lithotripsy.

Extremely large, impacted, and irregularly shaped calculi require fragmentation prior to removal. Although this can take the form of mechanical, electrohydraulic, or laser lithotripsy, the fragmentation procedure can be undertaken with direct pancreatoscopy using Spy-Scope technology (Boston Scientific); most centers, including our own, prefer extracorporeal shock wave lithotripsy (ESWL). Stones can be targeted prior to ERCP if they are sufficiently calcified (Figure 1), or they may require a baseline ERCP with insertion of a stent or nasopancreatic drain for localization.

Once the stone or stones have been localized and fragmented (Figure 2), the fragments are usually removed via a transampullary approach during an additional endoscopic procedure to include balloon dilation of downstream strictures (Figure 3), although some investigators have used multiple ESWL procedures in lieu of repeat ERCP. Following fragment extraction, prosthesis placement is usually undertaken to minimize obstructive pancreatitis from edema at the site of previously impacted fragments or at the sphincterotomy site (Figure 4). Also, small side-branch calculi frequently migrate into the main pancreatic duct after decompression, and the prosthesis keeps the ductal system decompressed.

Results After Endotherapy for Stricture Without Stones

Multiple recent series have reported a 60% to 80% reduction in attacks of relapsing pancreatitis, as well as a comparable relief in chronic pain complaints, following endoscopic treatment of pancreatic strictures;

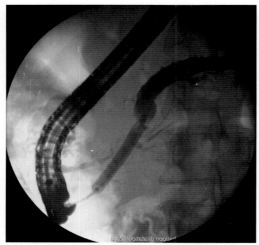

FIGURE 3 Fluoroscopic view during endotherapy depicts a 6 mm balloon used for dilation of a downstream stricture.

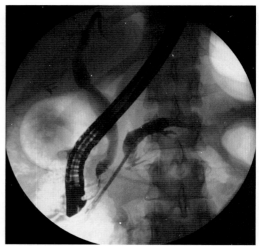

FIGURE 4 After balloon dilation, 2 to 7 Fr pancreatic duct prostheses are placed.

however, three to four treatment sessions may be required. These results are consistent with our experience.

Several caveats need to be mentioned. Stents themselves can cause ductitis and parenchymal injury as a consequence of side-branch occlusion or direct stent pressure by the upstream end or by side prongs. Additionally, stent placement invariably leads to bacterial colonization within the ductal system, and stent occlusion can occasionally result in upstream duct blowout or even pancreatic sepsis.

The results of endotherapy for pancreatic duct stricture have to be considered in two categories, persistence of stricture and symptom relief. Anatomically, stricture resolution approximates only 20% to 30% in published series, even when therapy has been undertaken for up to 1 year. Clinically, most series suggest that only 80% to 90% of patients achieve pain relief with initial stent placement, particularly those without upstream ductal dilation or those with multiple stones. A majority of the remaining patients will achieve a relatively asymptomatic level after stent removal, whereas a minority (15% to 20%) become stent dependent for pain relief. The reason for stent dependence is uncertain but may be related in part to location, because strictures in the pancreatic head are more pernicious, or to the original etiology; those strictures that are a consequence of severe pancreatitis with ductal disruption are often problematic.

Results After Endotherapy for Stones

About half of the patients considered for endotherapy will have strictures with stones. In contrast to some of the uncertainty associated with endoscopic treatment of pancreatic duct strictures, data reasonably confirm that endotherapy for calculi is associated with short- and long-term pain relief. This is obviously contingent upon successful clearance of stones from the main pancreatic duct, the treatment of concomitant biliary or pancreatic ductal stenosis, and patient selection; patients with multiple stones and strictures in the head of the pancreas (pseudotumor) have problems not necessarily related to stones and should be excluded from endotherapy.

Between 1995 and 2000, we did studies on pancreatic duct stone extraction. Half the patients required lithotripsy, and 35 of 40 patients required a single ESWL session, but a total of 86 ERCPs were required to completely clear the main pancreatic duct. There was a 20% rate of minor procedural complications. After a mean follow-up of 2.4 (± 0.6) years, 80% of the patients avoided surgery, and four of these patients died of a cause unrelated to chronic pancreatitis. A statistically significant decrease in pain scores, oxycodone-equivalent narcotic use, and yearly pancreatitis-related admissions were seen.

Since 2000, an additional 250 cases have been added with comparable results. The utilization of endoscopy to approach pancreatic strictures and stones in our institution has not been associated with an increase in operative drainage or resective procedures for pancreatic duct stones despite a relative increase in referrals for evaluation of chronic pancreatitis problems. The lack of an increase in surgical procedures may be due to endotherapy. However, as some have suggested, endotherapy might simply delay an inevitable and more effective drainage or resection procedure in a subset of patients who come in for treatment.

SURGICAL TECHNIQUES AND OUTCOMES

Surgical Drainage and Resection Techniques

The most common procedures for attempts at pain relief are illustrated in Figures 5 through 7. Table 3 outlines how the anatomy guides the surgeon in the choice of procedure. The longitudinal pancreaticojejunostomy (LPJ) originally described by Puestow was modified by Partington and Rochelle to extend into and over the head of the pancreas. However many still refer to it as a *Puestow procedure*. The Frey procedure, first reported in 1987, is a hybrid of resection and drainage. It combines a subtotal ventral head resection or local resection (LR) with a drainage procedure (LR-LPJ or Frey procedure). Frey and colleagues described the extent of resection as a partial head resection in a coronal (frontal) plane through the head of the pancreas. The depth of resection "involves excision of the pancreas overlying the ducts of Wirsung and Santorini and the duct to the uncinate process along with its tributary ducts, and opening of the main duct in the body and tail of the pancreas."

In 1972, the Beger procedure was first described, which involved removing almost all of the pancreatic head with preservation of the duodenum and bile duct, while the pancreatic remnant was drained into a jejunal limb. If a significant biliary obstruction was present, the jejunal limb could be also connected to the bile duct. In the order described, these three procedures progress from a simple drainage procedure to a drainage procedure with partial head resection to an almost complete head resection with a drainage procedure.

Finally, complete head removal with drainage is a pancreaticoduodenectomy, and in a noncancerous environment, the pylorus-preserving pancreaticoduodenectomy (PPPD) is usually preferred. Except for a variety of reconstruction methods, the pylorus-preserving technique is generally performed in the same manner throughout the world. The procedure removes all of the head of the pancreas and the duodenum except the duodenal bulb. Reconstruction is depicted in

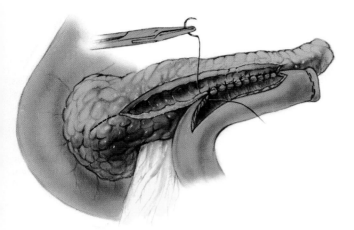

FIGURE 5 The Puestow procedure (lateral pancreaticojejunostomy) is depicted. Note the end of the limb is positioned toward the tail of the pancreas. If the Puestow procedure fails to relieve pain in long-term follow-up, and a head resection is required, this position of the jejunal limb allows for the preservation of the pancreatic anastomosis and also allows addition of the biliary connection to the jejunal limb. *(Reprinted from Pancreaticojejunostomy [Puestow] for Chronic Pancreatitis. In Scott-Conner CEH [ed.]: Chassin's operative strategy in general surgery: an expositive atlas, ed 3, New York, 2002, Springer-Verlag, p 722, With kind permission of Springer Science+Business Media.)*

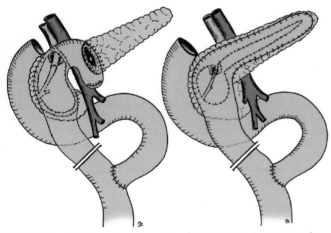

FIGURE 6 The Beger technique (duodenum-preserving pancreatic head resection) on the left is compared to the Frey procedure (LR-LPR, subtotal ventral head or local head resection combined with a lateral pancreaticojejunostomy). *(Reprinted from Köninger J, Seiler CM, Sauerland S, et al: Duodenum-preserving head resection: a randomized controlled trial comparing the original Beger procedure with the Berne modification, Surgery 143:490-498; 2008.)*

Figure 7. Note that the duodenojejunostomy is in an antecolic position, a position we believe minimizes delayed gastric emptying (DGE), which after PPPD in an antecolic position should be less than 10%; when it does occur, it will most often be associated with a pancreatic anastomotic leak.

Review of Randomized Controlled Trials After Endotherapy, Drainage, and Resection

In an ideal world, the surgeon could look at Table 3 and choose an operation that had been tested in randomized controlled trials (RCTs). A recent review using "evidence-based medicine" examined the RCTs completed for the surgical and endoscopic treatment of chronic

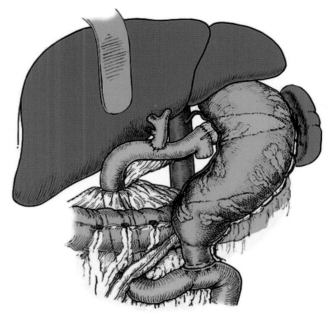

FIGURE 7 After pylorus-preserving pancreaticoduodenectomy (PPPD), reconstruction of the pancreatic duct and bile duct are in a retrocolic fashion. The pancreaticojejunostomy can be made in a side-to-side fashion if a chain-of-lakes ductal pattern exists in the pancreatic remnant. The end-to-side duodenojejunostomy is in an antecolic position to isolate the duodenal anastomosis from the pancreatic anastomosis and minimize delayed gastric emptying if the pancreatic anastomosis should leak. *(From Traverso LW: The surgical management of chronic pancreatitis: the Whipple procedure. In Cameron JL, editor: Advances in surgery, vol 32, St Louis, 1999, Mosby, p 33.)*

pancreatitis. These studies were difficult to compare because of the lack of standard selection criteria to initiate any therapy, particularly head resection. The five selection criteria, based on imaging studies listed in Table 2, offer a great opportunity to solve this problem.

After summarizing the highest level of evidence to treat the pain of chronic pancreatitis with surgical or endoscopic techniques, just eight RCTs have been reported since 1995 (Table 4). A review of these eight articles was summarized as they

> "do not have prognostic factors that predict pain relief following a large variety of treatment options—endotherapy with or without ESWL, surgical drainage, or the variety of head resection techniques. At this time we cannot provide guidelines in the treatment of this disease. Subsequent trials require a more international source of patients, a standardized set of inclusion and exclusion criteria based on objective criteria such as ductal anatomy (although the Amsterdam 2007 methodology would be a good template), and an adequate length of follow-up (5 years). Because of the paucity of patients in the available RCTs, physicians and surgeons must rely on their own experience with a variety of therapies and subsequent outcomes. Careful interpretation of case series still remains the bastion of our literature. These studies, as well as the RCTs, must be read carefully because of the lack of homogeneity of study design among them."

Many pancreatic head resections in Europe are done for an inflammatory "pseudotumor" of the head without mention of ductal anatomy (Figure 8). The severity of chronic pancreatitis preoperatively is difficult to evaluate without imaging studies that include ductal anatomy. Without imaging ductal anatomy, it is also difficult to make an inference on pretreatment endocrine and exocrine function, unless these are measured. The few prospective trials comparing the complete head resection to partial head resections have been small, with between 20 to 30 patients in each group. We believe our results after PPPD, of good to excellent pain relief after long-term follow-up, support head resection of any kind, with the proviso that the operation is

warranted using objective criteria and that it is performed safely and with few long-term sequelae.

In regard to patient safety, the morbidity and mortality for all of these operations are also similar. The Beger procedure appears to be practiced mainly in German-speaking countries, and the Frey operation appears to be gaining popularity in North America because of less surgical difficulty. Note that any limited head resection, like the Beger or the Frey operations, requires dissection through more pancreatic parenchyma than the PPPD procedure, where just the neck of the gland is transected. Rapid blood loss occurs from any cut surface of the pancreas. Paradoxically, blood loss would be expected to be higher during parenchymal resection of these "limited" head resections. The estimated blood loss (EBL) for the Beger procedure has not been reported. We found the average EBL for a Whipple procedure in 16 reports to be 964 mL, but our high-volume center's EBL was 204 mL.

The infrequency of chronic pancreatitis cases requiring head resection and the surgical difficulty of the Whipple or the Beger procedures has led many North American surgeons to stay with the more familiar Whipple operation rather than trying the Beger procedure or the Frey procedure. This case-volume infrequency is further compounded by the promising results of endotherapy for chronic pancreatitis; perhaps even fewer patients will require head resection.

TABLE 3: Choice of operation based on pattern of anatomy

Pattern	No Surgery	Puestow	Frey*	PPW*	Distal Resection
MPD obstruction† in the head					
No MPD dilation‡: body/tail				X	
MPD dilation: body/tail		X*	X*	X*	
No MPD obstruction in the head					
No MPD dilation: body/tail	X§				
MPD dilation: body/tail		X			
MPD obstruction in body/tail					X

MPD, Main pancreatic duct; *PPW*, pylorus-preserving Whipple procedure
*See text for description of surgery.
†*Obstruction of MPD* means any stricture with or without stones.
‡Main pancreatic duct dilation, as per the Cambridge conference, is >6.5 mm in the head and >5 mm in the body.
§Consider pancreatitis in evolution because of continued use of alcohol (usually denied) or chronic pain syndrome.

Outcomes of PPPD: Endotherapy First, then Head Resection with PPPD

Our institutional bias is to use PPPD preferentially for head resection, because it has a proven track record for pain relief, but we also are using the study of these cases to support other head resection techniques that remove almost as much pancreatic head. This information is important to support head resection in general. Each of our patients had failed to respond to conservative therapy as outlined in the introduction of this chapter.

The following indications for head resection were listed in Table 2. All patients had intractable abdominal pain, and we felt they had chronic pancreatitis, according to the Marseilles 1963 classification. All patients had the Cambridge image severity of "marked." In addition to main pancreatic duct obstruction or pancreatic head pseudocyst, all patients had multiple other elements of the Cambridge

TABLE 4: Comparison of pain relief observed in the RCTs for chronic pancreatitis treatments: All European studies

Year	Location	Group 1	Group 2	Pain Relief	Follow-up	Patients
1995	Bern/Ulm	PPPD (n = 20)	Beger (n = 20)	Beger better, 75% vs. 40%	6 mo	40
2006	Szeged, Hungary	PPPD (n = 20)	Beger (n = 20)	Same, ~85%	12 mo	40
1998	Hamburg	PPPD (n = 30)	Frey (n = 30)	Same, ~95%	24 mo	60
1995	Hamburg	Beger (n = 20)	Frey (n = 22)	Same, ~100%	36 mo	NA
2005	Hamburg	Beger (n = 38)	Frey (n = 36)	Same, ~90%	9 yr	74
2003	Brno, Czech Republic	Endo Tx, no ESWL (n = 36)	Mixed surgeries (36)	Surgery better, 85% vs. 61%	5 yr	72
2007	Amsterdam	ESWL then EndoTx (n = 19)	LPJ only (n = 20)	Surgery better, 75% vs. 53%	24 mo	39
2007	Brussels, Rome	ESWL then EndoTx (n = 29)	ESWL only (n = 26)	Same, ~55%	50 mo	55
TOTAL						380

From Deviere J, Bell RH, Beger HG: Treatment of chronic pancreatitis with endotherapy or surgery: critical review of randomized controlled trials, *J Gastrointest Surg* 12:640–644, 2008.

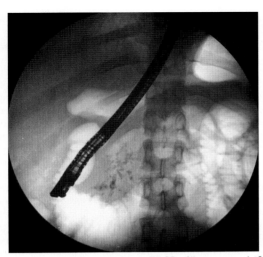

FIGURE 8 Fluoroscopic view during ERCP of "popcorn calcification" in pancreatic head associated with a pseudotumor; diagnosis was made from diffuse enlargement of the pancreatic head by CT. The use of just "pseudotumor" is made more objective with ductal imaging during ERCP. If the main pancreatic duct is filled with stones, thereby achieving Cambridge status of "marked," the patient will respond to head resection. Also, because of the diffuse nature of the calcifications, endotherapy would not be tried; head resection would be best.

Classification, as listed in the footer of Table 1, to support head resection. The role of endotherapy was prominent in these patients. Common bile duct obstruction was observed in 65%, and common bile duct stenting had been necessary in 47%. Pancreatic duct stricture was observed in 96%, main pancreatic duct blowout was documented in 39%, and pancreatic duct stenting that failed to achieve pain relief was seen in 35%. No hospital mortality or 30-day mortality occurred.

Follow-up was obtained in 98% of patients after a mean of 42 months. One third were diabetic before PPPD, but in the subset of patients not diabetic preoperatively, the actual 5 year diabetic occurrence rate was 32%. This diabetes was not a consequence of the resection, because no patient became diabetic sooner than 12 months after the resection, indicating that the criteria for surgery had been accurate enough to ensure that nonfunctional pancreatic tissue had been excised. This follow-up supports the concept that new diabetes after resection was a result of continued fibrosis in the pancreatic remnant.

Over 1 year after their Whipple operation, patients ($n = 43$) were questioned after a mean follow-up period of 55 months. Every patient indicated that they had a "good" response to surgery and that their pain was no longer disabling, and 76% of the patients indicated that their pain relief was "excellent," indicating they had become pain free. However, true to the human nature associated with those patients who develop alcohol-associated chronic pancreatitis, 14% were still taking some postoperative narcotic medication, even if they did not have pancreatic pain, and 24% had resumed drinking alcohol. In regard to activity, 93% of the patients had returned to work, school, or full activity. Exocrine enzymes use was 77%, and 14% indicated that they had diarrhea if they did not take exocrine enzymes. Marginal ulceration was observed in 14% and almost exclusively found in those with total pancreatectomy (44% had peptic ulceration). Since this study, we have avoided total pancreatectomy in almost all patients regardless of their diabetic status.

One final note about the often discussed need for total pancreatectomy for small-duct pancreatitis: The vast majority of patients we have seen for "small ductal pancreatitis" were found to be currently drinking alcohol or did not meet criteria for resective surgery. Resection is not indicated in these unfortunate cases.

SUMMARY

Endotherapy for chronic pancreatitis is being used more frequently at our institution. When it fails to relieve pain, and if the surgical indications are met, the patient can be salvaged with surgical drainage or pancreatic head resection. Good pain relief can be expected in almost all cases. The technique of endotherapy requires endoscopic access to the pancreatic ductal system, where pancreatic strictures can be dilated and stented, upstream pancreatic disruptions can be bridged or drained, and pancreatic stones can be removed with or without ESWL. Endotherapy works best for patients whose pancreatic duct stones are exacerbating the pain of chronic pancreatitis. Still the majority of patients with strictures and no stones will have pain relief sufficient to avoid surgery. Endotherapy has become so effective that the need for surgical drainage and resection has remained constant, even though the number of patients referred for problems associated with chronic pancreatitis has increased.

Resection after endotherapy is required for some patients. Generally they comprise two groups: the first group has recalcitrant stone disease behind a main pancreatic duct stricture; the second group has a main pancreatic duct stricture but no stones. Endotherapy either has had no effect on their pain, or they have become stent dependent for pain relief. These two groups form the new and more selected subset that might benefit from head resection. When endotherapy has failed, and if the patient meets the criteria for severe chronic pancreatitis centered in the head of the gland, we have observed good to excellent relief of pain after PPPD. Long-term follow-up, which has never been available with cancer patients after the Whipple procedure, has revealed few GI side effects from PPPD without predisposition for diabetes from the procedure. We avoid total pancreatectomy because of a higher marginal ulceration rate, even if the patient is diabetic.

From this personal experience, our understanding of this disease has improved. We can select patients who will benefit from endotherapy the majority of the time and, if endotherapy fails, these patients can be salvaged for pain relief by head resection. After long-term follow-up of almost 5 years, the benchmark for disabling pain relief should approach 100% if using anatomic selection criteria outlined in this chapter. It is hoped that this benchmark could be equaled by a variety of promising operations using a more limited head resection, such as the Frey and Beger operations. First, the patients should be selected with a standard list of reliable clinical and anatomic imaging criteria such as those used in this chapter. If the premise that the head of the pancreas is the "pacemaker" of chronic pancreatitis is correct, limited head resection should approach or equal the pain relief that we have observed after the pylorus-preserving Whipple procedure.

SUGGESTED READINGS

Deviere J, Bell RH, Beger HG: Treatment of chronic pancreatitis with endotherapy or surgery: critical review of randomized controlled trials, *J Gastrointest Surg* 12:640–644, 2008.

Kozarek RA, Brandabur JJ, Ball TJ, et al: Clinical outcomes in patients who undergo extracorporeal shock wave lithotripsy for chronic calcific pancreatitis, *Gastrointest Endosc* 56:496–500, 2002.

Traverso LW, Kozarek RA: Pancreaticoduodenectomy for chronic pancreatitis: anatomic selection criteria and subsequent long-term outcome analysis, *Ann Surg* 226:429–438, 1997.

PERIAMPULLARY CANCER

Harish Lavu, MD, and Charles J. Yeo, MD

OVERVIEW

Periampullary cancers are those that arise in the pancreaticoduodenal region near the ampulla of Vater. The most common of these tumors is pancreatic ductal adenocarcinoma, which accounts for nearly 85% of all periampullary cancers. Cholangiocarcinoma of the distal common bile duct (CBD), primary adenocarcinoma of the ampulla of Vater, and duodenal adenocarcinoma make up the remaining 15%. Taken together, these four cancers have an incidence of approximately 50,000 new cases per year in the United States.

Despite the differences in histologic type, these cancers share a similar clinical presentation, preoperative assessment, and surgical treatment strategy. It is not uncommon that the precise organ of tumor origin is unknown prior to surgical resection. Patient outcomes following surgery vary widely depending upon tumor origin, degree of differentiation, stage at diagnosis, and adequacy of surgical treatment (Table 1). Due to the complexity of the diagnostic and treatment decisions, a multidisciplinary approach to patient care is recommended.

Although we will not discuss them in this chapter, a host of other, less common cancers can arise from within the periampullary region; these include neuroendocrine carcinoma, pancreatic cystadenocarcinoma, acinar cell and squamous cell carcinomas, gastrointestinal (GI) stromal tumors, sarcomas, lymphomas, and metastatic tumors. After a brief overview of the four most common periampullary cancer types, this chapter will focus on the surgical management of pancreatic ductal adenocarcinoma, recognizing that the management strategies for the other periampullary malignancies follow closely.

PERIAMPULLARY CANCER TYPES

Pancreatic Ductal Adenocarcinoma

Pancreatic ductal adenocarcinoma is the tenth most common cancer and the fourth leading cause of cancer death in the United States. In 2008, an estimated 37,680 new cases were diagnosed, with 34,290 deaths from the disease. The peak incidence occurs in the sixth and seventh decades of life, and men and women are equally affected by this disease, which has an overall 5 year survival rate of 4%. Smoking and obesity are clear risk factors for the development of pancreatic ductal adenocarcinoma; industrial asbestos exposure, experimental radon exposure, alcohol abuse, and diabetes appear to be less clearly associated. Approximately 5% to 10% of patients are believed to have a familial form of pancreatic cancer most commonly associated with mutations in BRCA-2 (familial breast cancer), PRSS1 (hereditary pancreatitis), p16 (familial atypical multiple mole or melanoma), or HNPCC (hereditary nonpolyposis colorectal cancer).

Surgical resection via pancreaticoduodenectomy (PD) is the only potentially curative therapy; such resection improves the overall 5 year survival rate to 15% to 25%. Because of the presence of locally advanced disease, distant metastases, or significant medical comorbidities, only a minority (20% to 30%) of patients at the time of diagnosis are candidates for surgical resection, the lowest percentage among all of the periampullary malignancies.

Adenocarcinoma of the Distal Common Bile Duct (Cholangiocarcinoma)

Distal CBD cholangiocarcinoma is the second most common periampullary tumor. It is defined as an adenocarcinoma arising from the junction of the cystic duct and common hepatic duct proximally to the level of the ampulla of Vater distally. Two other forms of cholangiocarcinoma exist, *intrahepatic cholangiocarcinoma* and *proximal extrahepatic cholangiocarcinoma* (Klatskin tumor).

Cholangiocarcinoma has an incidence of 1 to 2 new cases per 100,000 persons per year, with 20% to 30% arising from within the distal common bile duct. These cancers are more common in the elderly, with peak diagnosis in the seventh decade, and they are slightly more prevalent in men. Risk factors include chronic inflammatory conditions of the biliary tree such as primary sclerosing cholangitis, choledochal cysts, and parasitic infestations. Prior to surgical resection, these tumors may be difficult to distinguish from pancreatic ductal adenocarcinoma. Surgical resection via PD is the most effective form of treatment, with 5-year survival rates postresection ranging from 15% to 40%. Approximately 10% of all PDs are performed to treat cholangiocarcinoma of the distal CBD. These distal tumors are thought to have a higher long-term survival rate than the more proximal (Klatskin) tumors, not because of an inherent difference in tumor biology, but rather because of increased rates of tumor resectability and margin-negative resections and a reduced risk of perioperative mortality. Hilar cholangiocarcinomas offer greater technical challenges to resection, because they generally require extensive hepatic resection to obtain negative margins, and they tend to be at a later stage at the time of diagnosis.

Adenocarcinoma of the Ampulla of Vater

Ampullary adenocarcinoma is the third most common periampullary malignancy, occurring with an incidence of six new cases per million persons per year. The peak incidence is in the sixth and seventh decades, and it is slightly more common in males. Patients typically develop steady or waxing and waning biliary obstruction, often leading to diagnosis at an early stage with consequently high resectability rates. This early stage at initial diagnosis, combined with a lower biological aggressiveness as compared with pancreatic ductal adenocarcinoma or distal cholangiocarcinoma, results in a relatively high 5-year survival rate (35% to 55%) following resection. Patients with benign ampullary adenomas may be candidates for endoscopic or surgical ampullectomy; however, patients who have biopsy-proven adenocarcinoma or tumors that penetrate into the muscularis layer of the duodenum are recommended to undergo PD in most circumstances.

Duodenal Adenocarcinoma

Duodenal adenocarcinoma is a rare disease, accounting for only 4% to 7% of all periampullary cancers. These tumors have an equal gender distribution and an average age at diagnosis in the sixth and seventh decades. Many of these tumors are thought to arise from duodenal polyps in a continuum that closely mimics the transformation of colonic polyps to colonic adenocarcinoma. Duodenal cancers tend to be larger than other periampullary neoplasms at the time of diagnosis due to significant intraluminal growth. Duodenal adenocarcinoma has a more favorable biologic profile than either pancreatic or distal CBD adenocarcinoma, and patients who undergo resection have the highest 5-year survival rate among those with the four periampullary tumors discussed, in the 30% to 60% range.

TABLE I: Approximate 5-year survival rates for patients with resected periampullary adenocarcinoma

Pancreatic adenocarcinoma	15% to 25%
Distal bile duct adenocarcinoma	15% to 40%
Ampullary adenocarcinoma	35% to 55%
Duodenal adenocarcinoma	30% to 60%

CLINICAL PRESENTATION AND PHYSICAL FINDINGS

The most common presenting sign of periampullary cancer is progressive obstructive jaundice (75%). Early on, patients may note dark urine and pale stools, followed by scleral icterus and yellow skin pigmentation. Pruritis secondary to the deposition of bile salts in the skin is common. Patients may also complain of anorexia, pain, and weight loss. Occasionally, the initial symptoms may be quite vague and may include upper GI discomfort, dyspepsia, and maldigestion or steatorrhea due to pancreatic exocrine insufficiency. Other nonspecific symptoms that may occur include nausea, early satiety, abdominal fullness, discomfort, malaise, weakness, fevers, and night sweats. A new diagnosis of adult onset diabetes is noted in a minority of patients. Those patients with ampullary or duodenal adenocarcinoma may have heme-positive stools or a microcytic anemia at their initial visit, given the tendency for these tumors to bleed. Patients often complain of a dull and constant midepigastric abdominal pain that radiates to the back and is the result of chronic biliary or pancreatic duct obstruction. The presence of more severe pain that responds poorly to analgesics may reflect neural invasion of the peripancreatic autonomic plexus, which portends a poorer prognosis.

Initial evaluation should include a complete medical history with special emphasis on a past history of chronic pancreatitis and a family history of pancreatic, colon, or breast cancer. Physical examination may be normal, with the exception of signs of obstructive jaundice. Scleral icterus typically precedes altered skin pigmentation. Sites of self-inflicted skin excoriation may be apparent due to the presence of intense pruritis. Enlarged left supraclavicular (Virchow node) or periumbilical (Sister Mary Joseph node) lymph nodes or a perirectal tumor mass (Blumer shelf) represent findings of disease dissemination. Hepatomegaly and a palpable gallbladder (Courvoisier sign) are both signs of chronic biliary obstruction. Ascites is uncommon, but when present it may signify disease dissemination, chronic obstructive biliary cirrhosis, or, rarely, locally advanced disease with portal venous obstruction.

DIAGNOSIS AND STAGING

Laboratory Studies

In evaluating patients with suspected periampullary malignancy, routine laboratory examination should include a complete blood count, electrolyte panel, liver function tests, coagulation profile, tumor markers (carbohydrate antigen [CA] 19-9 and carcinoembryonic antigen [CEA]), and serum albumin measurement to assess nutritional status. A hallmark finding is the presence of elevated liver function tests, and because the underlying pathology results in biliary obstruction, the alkaline phosphatase is generally more elevated than the alanine aminotransferase (ALT) or aspartate aminotransferase (AST).

Hyperbilirubinemia will have a significant conjugated component, with direct bilirubin being higher than indirect bilirubin. Malabsorption of fat-soluble vitamins from prolonged biliary obstruction may lead to vitamin K deficiency and abnormalities in the vitamin K–dependent clotting factors, with resultant prolongation of the prothrombin time (PT).

The tumor marker CA 19-9 is frequently elevated, however its sensitivity in detecting pancreatic ductal adenocarcinoma is only 80%, and its specificity is only 60% to 70%. CA 19-9 levels may be elevated with biliary inflammation and benign obstruction, such as in cases of cholangitis, choledocholithiasis, or benign biliary strictures; it may also be increased with malignancies such as ovarian, stomach, or colon cancer. CA 19-9 levels are dependent on the Lewis blood-group antigen phenotype and therefore are undetectable in Lewis AB– patients, roughly 7% of the population. In total, one in five patients will have a normal CA 19-9 level in the face of a subsequently proven pancreatic ductal adenocarcinoma. Therefore CA 19-9 has a limited usefulness in the diagnosis of periampullary malignancy when used alone, though it can aid in supporting such a diagnosis when used in the proper clinical setting. Perhaps the most significant role for tumor markers in the management of patients with periampullary malignancies is in monitoring for disease recurrence and progression after treatment.

Imaging and Preoperative Staging

The goal of preoperative staging of periampullary malignancy is to determine tumor resectability by excluding patients with locally advanced disease involving the mesenteric (visceral) vasculature and those with distant metastases. We find high-quality, contrast-enhanced, thin-section computerized tomography (CT) using a focused pancreas protocol to be the most valuable imaging modality in the evaluation of patients with periampullary cancer. CT offers detailed three-dimensional (3D) anatomic information that allows for the identification of tumors in the periampullary region and for delineation of the relationship of the neoplasm to the major visceral vessels (Figure 1).

Unresectable locally advanced pancreatic adenocarcinoma is generally defined by the presence of tumor abutment of the celiac trunk or superior mesenteric artery (SMA) of greater than 180 degrees or occlusion or encasement (greater than 270 degrees) of the superior mesenteric vein (SMV) and portal venous (PV) axis (Figure 2). Locally advanced disease of this extent limits the chances for a successful margin-negative resection, thus patients in this group are typically offered neoadjuvant chemoradiation in the hopes of downstaging the tumor.

Pancreas protocol CT also allows for the assessment of distant metastases to the liver or peritoneal cavity. Liver lesions as small as 1 cm can be reliably imaged, though lesions close to the liver capsule may be difficult to visualize; peritoneal and omental implants are subcentimeter in size and difficult to visualize. The presence of ascites on CT is a concerning sign for peritoneal metastasis. Despite sophisticated preoperative imaging, unsuspected distant metastases are identified at laparotomy 10% to 20% of the time. Arterial 3D reconstructions of the visceral vessels allow the surgeon to anticipate and plan for anatomic variants, such as a replaced right hepatic artery originating from the SMA or atherosclerotic celiac stenosis (Figure 3).

The use of magnetic resonance imaging (MRI) in the evaluation of periampullary malignancy has increased in recent years. The cross-sectional information derived from MRI is similar to that acquired by high-quality CT, with the added advantages of allowing imaging of the biliary and pancreatic ductal systems via magnetic resonance cholangiopancreatography (MRCP) and an improved safety profile compared with contrast-enhanced CT in patients with renal dysfunction. In the vast majority of patients, there is no need for both CT and MR imaging, and we discourage obtaining both studies.

Endoscopic ultrasound (EUS) is a procedure that images periampullary tumors in real time; it may determine their relationship to the visceral vessels (highly operator dependent), and it allows for the acquisition of a tissue sample via EUS-guided fine needle

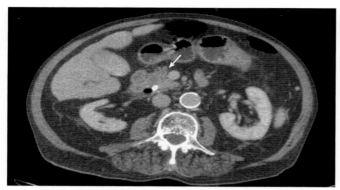

FIGURE 1   Pancreatic adenocarcinoma with abutment of less than 50% of the SMV (*arrow*). The patient underwent successful margin-negative resection. A metallic biliary endoprosthesis is visible.

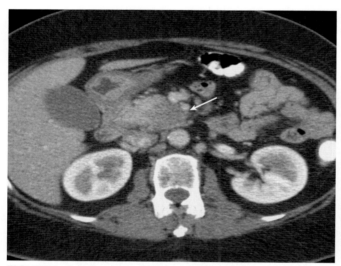

FIGURE 2   Locally advanced PDA in the uncinate process with loss of the SMA fat plane (*arrow*). This tumor was deemed unresectable, and the patient was referred for neoadjuvant chemoradiation therapy.

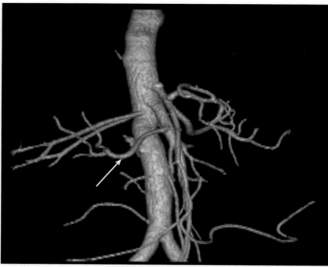

FIGURE 3   Replaced right hepatic artery (*arrow*) arising from the SMA. The vessel was carefully preserved during pancreaticoduodenectomy.

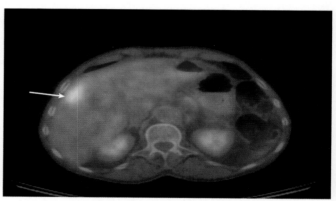

FIGURE 4   PET–CT demonstrates hypermetabolic focus within the right hepatic lobe (*arrow*), which represents metastatic PDA.

aspiration (FNA). EUS with FNA has a higher sensitivity (80%) in obtaining a tissue diagnosis than cytologic biliary brushings (roughly 30% to 50%) from endoscopic retrograde cholangiopancreatography (ERCP). EUS-FNA is particularly useful in patients with unresectable disease, as it may yield a tissue diagnosis prior to the commencement of chemotherapy or chemoradiation therapy. In patients who have resectable lesions, a preoperative diagnosis of cancer is not required prior to surgical therapy; preoperative biopsies have measurable false-negative rates and add cost to the workup.

The role of positron emission tomography combined with computerized tomography (PET-CT) as a diagnostic and staging tool for pancreatic cancer is still being defined. Normal pancreas tissue has low glucose uptake, whereas pancreatic ductal adenocarcinoma has a higher rate of glucose utilization, thus uptake of a fluorodeoxyglucose (FDG) tracer may be seen on PET imaging. The combination of CT with PET allows for further 3D tumor imaging.

Studies have shown the overall sensitivity and specificity of PET-CT for the diagnosis of pancreatic ductal adenocarcinoma to be in the range of 80% to 90%. The most useful role for PET-CT in the preoperative setting of periampullary malignancy is in ruling out distant disease in patients with suspicious hepatic lesions (Figure 4). We do not use PET-CT in routine cases of apparently resectable pancreatic or periampullary cancer, although it may have a role in postresection surveillance of dissemination or disease recurrence.

Preoperative Stenting and Biopsy

In patients who are seen initially with obstructive jaundice, endoscopic retrograde cholangiography (ERC) serves both a diagnostic and therapeutic function. Cholangiography can exclude certain benign causes of jaundice, such as choledocholithiasis, and it can help identify the presence of a distal CBD stricture; the characteristic appearance of the stricture noted on cholangiography can point to malignant disease (abrupt cutoff) versus inflammatory disease (smooth taper; Figure 5).

Direct endoscopic visualization at ERC may also provide information regarding the likelihood of duodenal or ampullary adenocarcinomas. Patients with pancreatic ductal adenocarcinoma may also have a pancreatic duct stricture, usually at the *genu* (knee) of the pancreatic duct because of tumor mass effect. When taken together with the distal CBD stricture, this so-called *double-duct sign* strongly suggests the presence of underlying malignant disease. Bile and pancreatic duct brushings and fluid cytologic analysis can be performed as part of the ERC procedure, and though these are associated with relatively low sensitivity and specificity, they may be useful in counseling a patient preoperatively when they do reveal malignancy.

In patients with cholangiocarcinoma, new techniques of analysis of tissue specimens, including digitized image analysis (DIA) of cell nuclei and fluorescence in situ hybridization (FISH) of specific chromosomal abnormalities, have increased sensitivity compared with standard cytologic assessment, but they are not typically needed. Preoperative biliary stenting is not mandatory in fit patients with periampullary malignancy who can undergo surgical resection in a timely fashion, as routine biliary stenting has been shown to increase the rates of postoperative wound infection and hospital stay. Patients with cholangitis, intractable pruritis, or major nutritional deficiency may benefit from preoperative stenting. When ERCP is unsuccessful, percutaneous transhepatic cholangiography and biliary drainage (stenting) may be performed, particularly in patients with a dilated intrahepatic biliary tree.

SURGICAL THERAPY

Pancreaticoduodenectomy (PD) is the operation of choice for patients with periampullary malignancy (Figure 6). The patient is prepared with a clear liquid diet on the day prior to surgery. Deep venous thrombosis prophylaxis with subcutaneous heparin is given, and a lower extremity hose and sequential compression devices are employed. Central venous and arterial monitoring lines are placed in many cases, and prophylactic antibiotics are given 30 minutes prior to the incision, and redosed 4 hours into the procedure.

Extirpative Phase

PD is performed in the supine position, through a midline incision from the tip of the xiphoid process to the umbilicus. The abdomen is thoroughly explored for occult metastatic disease, which means assessing the liver, base of the transverse mesocolon, intestines, and all peritoneal surfaces. A cholecystectomy is performed, and a wide

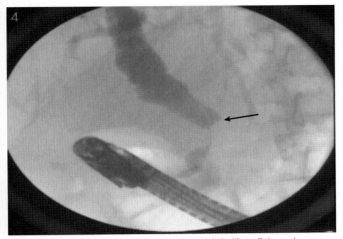

FIGURE 5   Malignant biliary stricture with "shelf sign" (*arrow*) secondary to PDA.

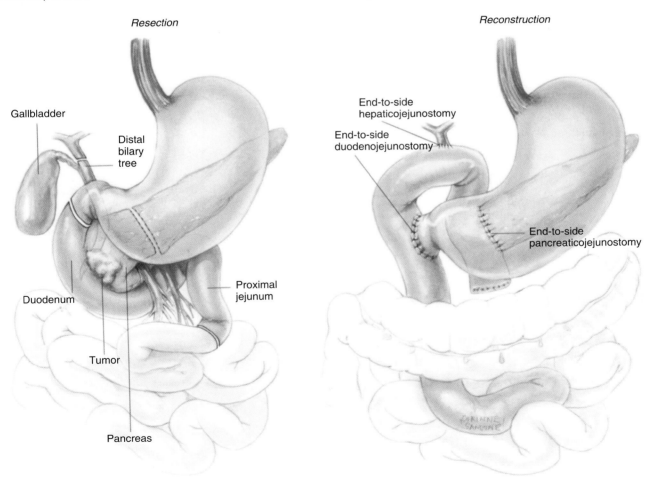

FIGURE 6   *Left,* Anatomy prior to pylorus-preserving pancreaticoduodenectomy, with lines of transection at the distal common bile duct, pancreas neck, and proximal jejunum shown. *Right,* Completed reconstruction showing end-to-side pancreaticojejunostomy (PJ), end-to-side hepaticojejunostomy (HJ), and end-to-side duodenojejunostomy (DJ). *(From Cameron JL, Sandone C: Atlas of gastrointestinal surgery vol 1, ed 2, Hamilton, Ontario, 2007, BC Decker, p 302.)*

Kocher maneuver is carried out by releasing the duodenum from its retroperitoneal attachments. Once the pancreatic head is mobilized, the tumor is palpated, and its relationship to the SMA and SMV are appreciated. Though this step is routinely carried out, it is important to recognize that preoperative contrast-enhanced cross-sectional imaging, most often via CT scan, offers the most accurate assessment of the tumor's proximity to the visceral vessels.

Dissection within the hepatoduodenal ligament allows for common hepatic duct or CBD isolation and transection. The gastroduodenal artery (GDA) is identified, but prior to transection, the vessel is test clamped to ensure that flow in the proper hepatic artery is not diminished. The GDA is ligated and divided, thus allowing for exposure of the portal vein at the superior aspect of the pancreatic neck. The duodenum is then divided 2 to 3 cm distal to the pylorus with a GIA stapler. Pylorus preservation is favored in the majority of patients undergoing PD (85%), however "classic" resection, which includes a limited distal gastrectomy, is still performed when the tumor encroaches upon the first portion of the duodenum or the pylorus.

Ligation of the right gastroepiploic artery and vein (downstream GDA) exposes the inferior aspect of the pancreatic neck overlying the SMV. Dissection in this area allows for identification of the SMV and the creation of a tunnel posterior to the pancreatic neck, overlying the SMV. After the placement of four 3-0 silk stay sutures that control intrapancreatic arterial arcades and allow for retraction, the pancreas neck is transected using electrocautery in the vertical axis of the SMV-PV (Figure 7). Care is taken to identify the pancreatic duct, which tends to lie in a posterior-superior location within the pancreatic neck remnant.

The ligament of Treitz is exposed and lysed at the base of the transverse mesocolon. At a distance approximately 15 cm distal to the ligament, the jejunal mesentery is divided, and the jejunum is divided using a GIA stapler. The proximal jejunum and fourth part of the duodenum are separated from their mesentery and passed posterior to the superior mesenteric vessels, toward the right side of the operative field.

The retroperitoneal soft tissue margin of the specimen and the uncinate process are dissected along the lateral border of the SMA,

beginning at the cranial end of the specimen and progressing distally, or vice versa. Care is taken to stay adjacent to the artery and to remove all pancreatic tissue from the perivascular plane (Figure 8). The specimen is then removed and marked to properly identify the pancreatic neck, bile duct, and retroperitoneal margins for intraoperative frozen-section analysis of the margins and for pathologic analysis of the primary tumor. In our institution most patients consent to have their tumor and blood banked for subsequent molecular analyses, following an IRB-approved protocol.

Reconstructive Phase

A defect is made in the transverse mesocolon to the right of the middle colic vessels. The proximal jejunum is delivered through this defect. The pancreatic remnant is mobilized for a distance of 2 to 3 cm off of the splenic vein to facilitate the creation of the invaginated pancreaticojejunostomy (PJ). The pancreatic duct is probed to ensure distal patency. An end-to-side invaginated pancreaticojejunostomy is constructed in two layers. The outer rows are constructed with interrupted 3-0 silk suture, and the inner rows are made with running 3-0 polyglactin suture. Care is taken to prevent inadvertent ligation of the pancreatic duct while placing these sutures (Figure 9).

An end-to-side hepaticojejunostomy (HJ) is begun by making a small jejunotomy on the antimesenteric aspect of the jejunum, approximately 10 cm distal to the PJ. This anastomosis is performed using 4-0, 5-0, or 6-0 polydioxanone suture, depending on the size and thickness of the common hepatic or bile duct. These sutures are

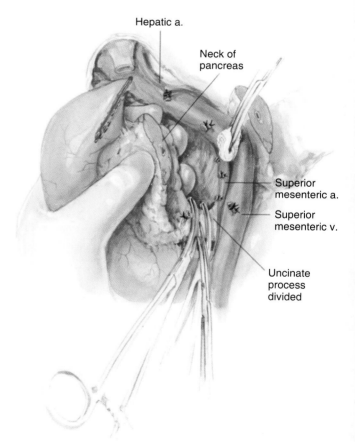

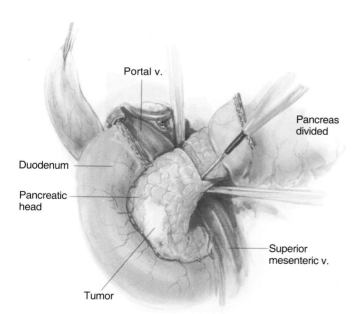

FIGURE 7   The pancreas neck is shown being transected with electrocautery. The duodenum has been previously divided 3 cm distal to the pylorus using a GIA stapler. *(From Cameron JL, Sandone C: Atlas of gastrointestinal surgery vol 1, ed 2, Hamilton, Ontario, 2007, BC Decker, p 291.)*

FIGURE 8   The final step in the extirpative phase of the pylorus-preserving pancreaticoduodenectomy. The last attachments of the uncinate process of the pancreas to the superior mesenteric artery are being divided. *(From Cameron JL, Sandone C: Atlas of gastrointestinal surgery vol 1, ed 2, Hamilton, Ontario, 2007, BC Decker, p 292.)*

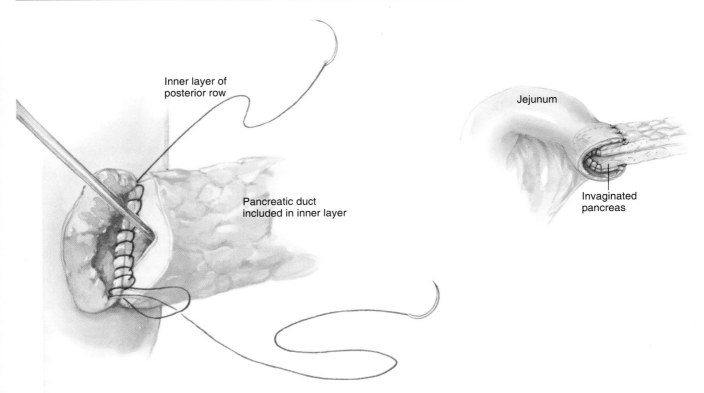

Inner layer of
posterior row

Pancreatic duct
included in inner layer

Jejunum

Invaginated
pancreas

FIGURE 9   *Left,* The posterior inner row of the end-to-side pancreaticojejunostomy is being completed using running 3-0 polyglactin suture. *Right,* The pancreas neck is shown invaginated into the side of the jejunum. *(From Cameron JL, Sandone C: Atlas of gastrointestinal surgery vol 1, ed 2, Hamilton, Ontario, 2007, BC Decker, pp 295-296.)*

placed in an interrupted fashion with the posterior row placed first and tied. The long limb of a transected T-tube (an "I-tube") is then placed into the anastomosis as a temporary stent to prevent backwall injury while placing the anterior row of sutures.

The duodenojejunostomy (DJ) is performed in a retrocolic position, about 10 to 15 cm downstream from the HJ. The previously placed I-tube is removed when the jejunotomy is made. The duodenojejunal anastomosis is performed in two layers, with an outer row of interrupted 3-0 silk sutures and an inner row of running 3-0 polyglactin suture.

The efferent limb of the DJ is tacked to the transverse mesocolon at its exit point 5 cm below the DJ. The defect at the ligament of Treitz is closed with interrupted 3-0 silk sutures. Two 3/16 Jackson-Pratt drains are placed exiting the abdomen on either side. The right-sided drain is placed in the subhepatic space and posterior to the right upper quadrant jejunal loops; the left-sided drain is placed through the gastrocolic ligament and a few centimeters cephalad to the PJ. No drains are placed posterior to the PJ or HJ, and care is taken to avoid having the drains come into contact with the PJ or HJ anastomoses directly. The fascia is closed with running #2 nylon suture, and the subcutaneous tissue and skin are closed with 3-0 and 4-0 polyglactin suture, respectively.

POSTOPERATIVE CARE

In high-volume centers of excellence, the use of critical pathways and a team-oriented approach speed post-PD patient recovery and improve outcomes. Patients are routinely monitored in an ICU setting in the initial postoperative period, with serial laboratory evaluation. On postoperative day (POD) 1, the nasogastric tube is removed, patients are given oral ice chips, intravenous fluids are reduced, and ambulation is encouraged. On POD 2 the diet is advanced to clear liquids, the Foley catheter is removed, and most patients are diuresed with furosemide. Patients begin a solid diet on POD 3, drains are routinely removed on POD 3 to 6, depending upon quantity and character of output. Patients are discharged home when they tolerate adequate oral intake, are ambulating, and have good pain control. This typically occurs by POD 6 to 8. Most patients are seen by oncology consultants prior to hospital discharge, to allow for planning of postoperative therapy.

SURGICAL OUTCOMES

Much progress has been observed following PD in recent years, such that an operation that in the 1960s and 1970s had a mortality of 20% to 40% is now associated with an operative mortality of 1% to 3% at most high-volume institutions. Ample evidence suggests that perioperative morbidity, mortality, and median survival are improved when the procedure is performed at high-volume institutions that carry out more than 20 PDs per year; several institutions in the United States perform over 100 PDs annually. Hospital stays that commonly lasted beyond 2 weeks are now 6 to 8 days in most cases. These remarkable improvements are due not only to advances in operative technique but also in management algorithms (Figure 10), perioperative critical care, standardized intervention for complications, the institution of critical pathways for postoperative treatment, improvements in endoscopic and interventional radiology techniques, and increasing experience of surgeons. Despite these advancements, PD still carries a high perioperative morbidity of 30% to 40%, with the most common postoperative complications being pancreatic fistula, delayed gastric emptying, intraabdominal abscess, wound infection, urinary tract infection, and cardiac arrhythmia.

A recent dual-institution randomized trial focused on techniques of pancreaticojejunal reconstruction during PD revealed that an

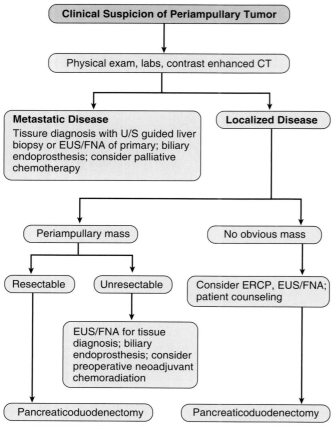

FIGURE 10 Periampullary cancer-management algorithm.

invaginated PJ leads to lower rates of pancreatic fistula formation compared with the duct-to-mucosa PJ technique. Several studies also suggest that preoperative diabetes has a preventive effect on the development of pancreatic fistula, whereas soft gland texture and high gland fat content are associated with higher rates of pancreatic fistula formation.

PROGNOSTIC FACTORS

The most important factors affecting long-term survival following the resection of periampullary adenocarcinoma include the site of tumor origin, tumor size, histologic grade, resected lymph node status, and resection margin status. The presence of lymphovascular and perineural invasion also have negative prognostic significance, although to a lesser degree. The most potent negative predictor of long-term survival is the presence of lymph node metastases within the resection specimen. As the ratio of positive nodes to total nodes examined increases, the median and long-term survival rates decrease. Patients who undergo an R0 resection for pancreatic malignancy who have the most favorable tumor characteristics—size less than 3 cm, well-differentiated tumors, and an absence of nodal metastasis—have the most favorable outcomes, with a median survival of 4 years and a 5-year survival rate exceeding 40%.

PALLIATION

Nonoperative Palliation

The majority of patients with periampullary malignancy will have locally advanced or distant metastases at the time of diagnosis, precluding curative surgical resection. This makes effective palliation a vital aspect in treatment strategies designed to improve the quality and longevity of life. In patients with suspected liver metastases, the diagnosis can be confirmed by tissue acquisition with ultrasound-guided liver biopsy; for patients with locally advanced disease, EUS-FNA may be an effective way to obtain a confirmatory tissue specimen. Patients are typically palliated with a biliary endoprosthesis to relieve jaundice. Self-expanding metal biliary endoprostheses, which have a larger luminal diameter and are more durable than their plastic counterparts, have increased the length of stent patency and have reduced the number of repeat procedures required to manage stent occlusion. Some patients who have gastric outlet or duodenal obstruction due to tumor growth and luminal compromise may require endoscopic duodenal stenting.

Surgical Palliation

Patients explored with curative intent and found to be unresectable generally benefit from palliative bypass of the bile duct and stomach to treat symptoms of jaundice or early satiety or to prevent future problems from disease progression. Patients are considered for palliative surgical bypass if they are found on exploration to have occult metastatic disease and evidence of impending or concurrent GI or biliary obstruction, or if their tumor is deemed locally advanced, preventing an attempt at surgical resection.

The technique we use for palliation of duodenal obstruction is a two-layered, hand-sewn, side-to-side, retrocolic isoperistaltic gastrojejunostomy. Biliary bypass is performed as a single-layer end-to-side Roux-en-Y hepaticojejunostomy; a cholecystectomy is performed if the gallbladder is present. Celiac plexus neurolysis (nerve block) has been shown to reduce the severity of tumor-associated abdominal pain; it is performed by injecting 20 mL of 50% ethanol on either side of the aorta, at the level of the celiac axis, in the area of the celiac plexus.

ADJUVANT THERAPY

Adjuvant therapy for pancreatic ductal adenocarcinoma (treatment given after resection) improves both median and long-term survival. In the past decade, gemcitabine in combination with 5-fluorouracil (5-FU) based chemoradiotherapy has become the adjuvant treatment of choice. This regimen has been shown to improve median and long-term survival when compared with surgery alone in the largest trial of resected patients in North America (RTOG 97-04). In contrast, the largest European trial has shown no benefit to the chemoradiotherapy (ESPAC-1), and thus in Europe, adjuvant treatment tends to utilize chemotherapy alone. The focus in recent years has been to study combination therapies by adding other cytotoxic agents—such as capecitabine, cisplatin, or mitomycin-C—to a gemcitabine-based regimen, or by combining gemcitabine with newer molecular targeted therapies that affect specific cellular pathways, such as topoisomerase-1 inhibitors, matrix metalloproteinase inhibitors, vascular endothelial growth factor inhibitors, or epidermal growth factor inhibitors. To date, the majority of these trials have shown limited clinical efficacy with drug combinations, except for the epidermal growth factor receptor (EGFR) inhibitor erlotinib, which has shown a modest survival benefit.

With the recent mapping of the pancreatic genome, more attention is being drawn to the specific genetic alterations and major signaling pathways underlying pancreatic ductal adenocarcinoma. This may allow for the accelerated identification and development of specific targeted agents. The newest trials under development include the use of specific targeted agents such as insulin-like growth factor 1–receptor inhibitors, poly (ADP-ribose) polymerase (PARP) inhibitors, and c-Met inhibition, as well as the use of immunotherapy for the adjuvant treatment of pancreatic ductal adenocarcinoma. Many laboratories are currently working on better defining the crucial intracellular signaling pathways that are abnormal in pancreatic and other periampullary adenocarcinomas, with the focus on defining a therapeutic target specific for each resected tumor. Given the complex nature of genetic alterations in pancreatic ductal adenocarcinoma, such a personalized treatment model may be critical to developing more effective adjuvant treatment strategies.

Selected Readings

Berger AC, Howard TJ, Kennedy EP, et al: Does the type of pancreaticojejunostomy after pancreaticoduodenectomy decrease the rate of pancreatic fistula? A randomized, prospective, dual-institution trial, *J Am Coll Surg* 208:738–749, 2009.

Constantino CL, Witkiewicz AK, Kuwano Y, et al: The role of HuR in gemcitabine efficacy in pancreatic cancer: HuR upregulates the expression of the gemcitabine-metabolizing enzyme deoxycytidine kinase, *Cancer Res* 69:4567–4572, 2009.

Kennedy EP, Brumbaugh JP, Yeo CJ: Reconstruction following the Whipple resection: PJ, HJ and DJ, *J Gastrointest Surg* 14:408–415, 2010.

Kennedy EP, Rosato EL, Sauter PK, et al: Initiation of a critical pathway for pancreaticoduodenectomy at an academic institution: the first step in multidisciplinary team building, *J Am Coll Surg* 204:917–924, 2007.

Kennedy EP, Yeo CJ: Pancreaticoduodenectomy with extended retroperitoneal lymphadenectomy for periampullary adenocarcinoma, *Surg Oncol Clin North Amer* 16:157–176, 2007.

Lavu H, Mascaro A, Grenda D, et al: Margin-positive pancreaticoduodenectomy is superior to palliative bypass in locally advanced pancreatic adenocarcinoma, *J Gastrointest Surg* 13:1937–1947, 2009.

Neoptolemos JP, Stocken DD, Friess H, et al: A randomized trial of chemoradiotherapy and chemotherapy after resection of pancreatic cancer, *N Engl J Med* 350:1200–1210, 2004.

Pawlik TM, Gleisner AL, Cameron JL, et al: Prognostic relevance of lymph node ratio following pancreaticoduodenectomy for pancreatic cancer, *Surgery* 141:610–618, 2007.

Regine WF, Winders KA, Abrams RA, et al: Fluorouracil vs. gemcitabine chemotherapy before and after fluorouracil-based chemoradiation following resection of pancreatic adenocarcinoma, *JAMA* 299:1019–1026, 2008.

Riall TS, Cameron JL, Lillemoe KE, et al: Resected periampullary adenocarcinoma: 5 year survivors and their 6 to 10 year follow-up, *Surgery* 140:764–771, 2006.

Schmidt CM, Glant J, Winter JM, et al: Total pancreatectomy (R0 resection) improves survival over subtotal pancreatectomy in isolated neck margin-positive pancreatic adenocarcinoma, *Surgery* 142:572–580, 2007.

Shirley LA, Yeo CJ: Pancreaticoduodenectomy: past and present. In Lowy AM, Leach SD, Philip PA, editors: *Pancreatic cancer*, New York, 2008, Springer, pp 313–327.

Showalter SL, Charles S, Belin J, et al: Future perspective—identifying pancreatic cancer patients for targeted treatment: the challenges and limitations of the current selection process and vision for the future, *Expert Opin Drug Deliv* 7:1–12, 2010.

Showalter SL, Huang Y-H, Witkiewicz A, et al: Nanoparticulate delivery of diphtheria toxin DNA effectively kills mesothelin-expressing pancreatic cancer cells, *Cancer Biol Ther* 7:1–7, 2008.

Showalter SL, Showalter TN, Witkiewicz A, et al: Evaluating the drug–target relationship between thymidylate synthase expression and tumor response to 5-fluorouracil: Is it time to move forward? *Cancer Biol Ther* 7:986–994, 2008.

Williams TK, Rosato EL, Kennedy EP, et al: Impact of obesity on perioperative morbidity and mortality following pancreaticoduodenectomy, *J Am Coll Surg* 208:210–217, 2009.

Winter JM, Cameron JL, Campbell KA, et al: 1,423 pancreaticoduodenectomies for pancreatic cancer: a single institution experience, *J Gastrointest Surg* 10:1200–1211, 2006.

Winter JM, Cameron JL, Yeo CJ, et al: Biochemical markers predict morbidity and mortality following pancreaticoduodenectomy, *J Am Coll Surg* 204:1029–1038, 2007.

Winter JM, Cameron JL, Yeo CJ, et al: Duodenojejunostomy leaks after pancreaticoduodenectomy, *J Gastrointest Surg* 12:263–269, 2008.

Witkiewicz AK, Costantino CL, Metz R, et al: Genotyping and expression analysis of IDO2 in human pancreatic cancer: a novel, active target, *J Am Coll Surg* 208:781–789, 2009.

Witkiewicz A, Williams TK, Cozzitorto J, et al: Expression of indoleamine 2,3-dioxygenase in metastatic pancreatic ductal adenocarcinoma recruits regulatory T cells to avoid immune detection, *J Am Coll Surg* 206:849–856, 2008.

Yeo CJ, Yeo TP, Hruban RH, et al: Cancer of the pancreas. In DeVita VT Jr, Hellman S, Rosenberg SA, editors: *Cancer: principles and practice of oncology*, ed 7, Philadelphia, 2005, Lippincott Williams & Wilkins, pp 945–986.

Yeo TP, Hruban RH, Brody J, et al: Assessment of "gene–environment" interaction in cases of familial and sporadic pancreatic cancer, *J Gastrointest Surg* 13:1487–1494, 2009.

Vascular Reconstruction During the Whipple Operation

Alysandra Lal, MD, MPH, Kathleen K. Christians, MD, and Douglas B. Evans, MD

OVERVIEW

Principles of Surgical Treatment

Portal vein (PV) resection at the time of pancreaticoduodenectomy (PD) was initially described as part of an en bloc resection of the pancreas and surrounding structures, termed *regional pancreatectomy*, with the intent of improving local tumor control. This application of vein resection did not confer a survival benefit, as it did not address the major variables associated with early tumor recurrence, namely, the absence of metastatic disease, a gross complete resection at the

level of the superior mesenteric artery (SMA), and the status of local-regional lymph nodes.

As computed tomography (CT) and magnetic resonance imaging (MRI) technology has improved, radiographically occult liver metastases have become less common; this finding, combined with the routine use of combined modality therapy, has improved the survival of patients who have their primary tumor successfully removed. However, based on the initial negative experience with regional pancreatectomy, surgeons have continued to classify patients with isolated tumor extension to adjacent vascular structures as unresectable. Considerable confusion remains on the part of surgeons, medical oncologists, and radiation oncologists regarding what defines an unresectable pancreatic head cancer and what vascular procedures can be safely performed. We describe our definitions of *resectable*, *borderline resectable*, and *locally advanced* (*unresectable*) pancreatic cancer in Table 1. These definitions are based on the following principles:

1. In most patients, pancreatic cancer is a systemic disease at diagnosis. The primary tumor has access to the systemic venous system long before it grows large enough to abut or encase the superior mesenteric vein (SMV) or SMV-PV confluence. Tumor extension to the SMV or SMV-PV confluence is a consequence of tumor location and size and does not reflect a more aggressive tumor biology.

TABLE 1: Clinical/radiographic staging system for adenocarcinoma of the pancreatic head and uncinate process

Clinical Stage	AJCC Stage	TUMOR-VESSEL RELATIONSHIP ON CT			
		SMA	Celiac Axis	CHA*	SMV-PV
Resectable (all four are required to be resectable)†	I/ II	Normal tissue plane between tumor and vessel	Normal tissue plane between tumor and vessel	Normal tissue plane between tumor and vessel	Patent (may include tumor abutment or encasement)
Borderline resectable (only one of the four required)	III	Abutment	Abutment	Abutment or short segment encasement	May have short segment occlusion if reconstruction possible
Locally advanced (only one of the four required)	III	Encasement	Encasement	Extensive encasement with no technical option for reconstruction	Occluded with no technical option for reconstruction

CHA, Common hepatic artery; SMV–PV, Superior mesenteric vein–portal vein confluence

Abutment refers to ≤180 degrees or ≤50% of the vessel circumference; encasement is >180 degrees or >50% of the vessel circumference.

*Assumes normal vascular anatomy; for example, encasement of the CHA is not a limitation in performing PD when there is an uninvolved replaced right hepatic artery arising from the superior mesenteric artery.

†Assumes the technical ability to resect and reconstruct the SMV, PV, or SMV-PV confluence when necessary. Others would consider tumor-vein abutment/encasement, which results in deformity of the vein as borderline resectable.

2. The SMV, PV, or SMV-PV confluence is not surrounded by autonomic nerves, as is the case with mesenteric arteries, thus there is no direct route on the venous side for tumor spread to the celiac ganglion, paraaortic nerves, or lymphatics, resulting in tumor infiltration into the retroperitoneum. Therefore, with venous resection and reconstruction, a complete resection is possible, in contrast to resection of the origin of the SMA or celiac axis, where a gross complete resection is usually not possible.
3. Resection of the SMA or circumferential skeletonization of this vessel with complete division of the surrounding autonomic nerve tissue will result in de-innervation of the midgut and hyperperistalsis with rapid gastrointestinal (GI) transit. This may result in nutritional depletion in patients of normal or thin body habitus.
4. The need for venous resection can usually be anticipated based on high-quality preoperative CT imaging. The type of venous reconstruction needed can also be planned prior to surgery based on accurate assessment of cross-sectional imaging studies.
5. For venous resection to be successful, mesenteric venous return must be maintained with preservation of at least one branch of the SMV. If the splenic vein is preserved (not divided), and the SMV is resected, an interposition graft will usually be necessary.
6. If the SMV-PV confluence is resected with ligation of the splenic vein, the anatomy of the inferior mesenteric vein (IMV) must be appreciated. In the setting of splenic vein ligation, the IMV, if it enters the splenic vein, will provide collateral venous return (retrograde) from the stomach and spleen. If the IMV enters the SMV and splenic vein ligation is required, there will be no remaining named vein draining the stomach and spleen if the splenic vein is divided (assuming the left gastric vein is divided, which is usually the case). In this situation, we will often sew the splenic vein into the left renal vein (splenorenal shunt) to prevent sinistral portal hypertension and gastric varices.
7. Arterial resection, when performed, is largely limited to the hepatic artery in situations in which no radiographic evidence of tumor extension to the celiac axis is found.
8. Patients with borderline resectable tumors because of tumor abutment of the SMA or hepatic artery are always treated with neoadjuvant therapy, including chemoradiation, in an effort to treat radiographically occult metastatic disease and to enhance the

likelihood of a margin-negative resection by creating a zone of cell kill at the tumor's periphery.

When venous involvement is an unexpected finding during PD, surgeons may attempt to separate the SMV, PV, or SMV-PV confluence from the pancreatic head. When this maneuver is unsuccessful, the surgeon is left with either a grossly positive margin or an inadvertent venotomy. Venous injury often results in uncontrolled hemorrhage and the necessity for rapid removal of the tumor without proper attention to the SMA dissection; it is easy to appreciate how this can result in a grossly incomplete (R2) resection. Therefore, anticipating such extended procedures preoperatively and obtaining adequate vascular control to allow for planned excision and reconstruction of the affected vascular structures is critical to performing vascular resection and reconstruction during PD.

Computed Tomographic Staging

Prior to surgery, contrast-enhanced pancreas-protocol CT is performed with vascular reconstructions. The CT aides in the identification of aberrant vascular anatomy, helps delineate the extent of vascular involvement, and allows classification of the tumor as resectable or borderline resectable. Identification of tumor involvement of the SMV or its first-order branches on preoperative CT images should prompt a thorough radiographic evaluation of the venous anatomy. As mentioned above, CT imaging with venous-phase contrast enhancement should accurately demonstrate the potential need for venous resection in the majority of cases. When the tumor is in direct contact with the SMV or PV, the need for vein resection should be anticipated. When the SMV or PV is distorted or narrowed, the need for venous resection should be expected. Current imaging studies allow for accurate preoperative planning with respect to tumor–vessel relationships; the need for venous resection should rarely be an unexpected finding at the time of laparotomy (Figures 1 through 5).

Surgical Anatomy of the Superior Mesenteric Vein

The SMV drains the midgut and joins the splenic vein to form the PV posterior to the pancreatic neck. The SMV is composed of jejunal and ileal branches, which join together inferior to the pancreatic neck to

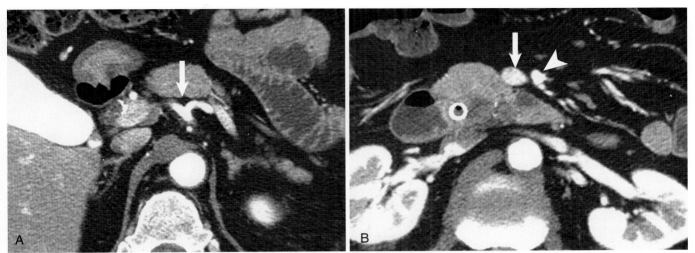

FIGURE 1   CT image of a resectable tumor that does not extend to the bifurcation of the celiac axis or the SMVs. **A,** *Arrow* identifies bifurcation of celiac axis. **B,** *Arrow* identifies SMV; *arrowhead* identifies the SMA. Note the metal stent within the bile duct.

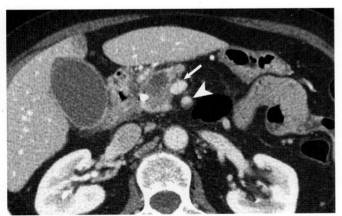

FIGURE 2   CT image of a resectable tumor that will likely require at least tangential resection of the SMV (*arrow*). Note the low-density tumor that abuts the SMV. There is a normal tissue plane between the tumor and the SMA (*arrowhead*).

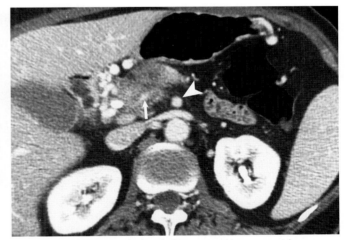

FIGURE 4   CT image of a borderline resectable tumor with more challenging vascular involvement. In this pretreatment CT image, the SMV (*arrow*) is nearly completely occluded. Note the very narrow tissue plane between the tumor and the SMA (*arrowhead*).

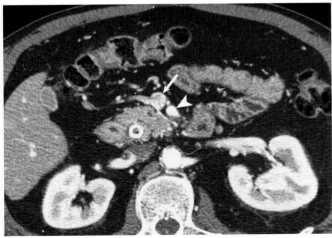

FIGURE 3   CT image of a borderline resectable tumor because of SMA (*arrowhead*) abutment. In this patient, the tumor does not extend to the SMV (*arrow*).

form the main trunk of the SMV. The middle colic vein and the gastroepiploic vein empty into the main trunk of the SMV and may be joined by a common trunk, often referred to as the *gastrocolic trunk*, or they may enter the SMV as separate vessels.

The jejunal branch (JB), sometimes referred to as the *first jejunal branch* of the SMV, usually travels behind the SMA after draining the proximal jejunum; it then enters the posterior-medial aspect of the ileal branch of the SMV to form the main trunk of the SMV. When the JB lies posterior to the SMA, the small venous branches from the uncinate process (to the JB) must be divided to separate the JB from the uncinate process and allow medial retraction of the SMV, which is necessary for the traditional approach to expose the SMA. When the JB lies anterior to the SMA, it is much easier to separate the uncinate process from the SMV, as the small venous branches from the uncinate usually enter the ileal branch rather than the JB. When an anterior JB exists, a high rate of associated anatomic variations may also be present, including the lack of a main SMV trunk and drainage of the IMV directly into the JB of the SMV.

The JB-SMV confluence is important, because the JB can easily be injured during dissection of the uncinate process from the vein,

FIGURE 5 CT image of the same patient as shown in Figure 4 after systemic chemotherapy followed by chemoradiation. **A,** The SMV (*arrow*) shows much less compression than on the pretreatment image (SMA is identified by the *arrowhead*). Not shown on this static image is complete occlusion of the splenic vein just proximal to the SMV-PV confluence. **B,** The IMV (*arrowhead*) is noted to enter the SMV (*arrow*). At the time of surgery, the splenic vein was anastomosed to the left renal vein to prevent sinistral portal hypertension. The SMV-PV confluence was resected en bloc with the tumor, and a primary end-to-end anastomosis was performed. **C,** The pancreatic head and associated Whipple specimen has been removed. *IVC,* Inferior vena cava; *HA,* Hepatic artery; *SplA,* Splenic artery; *SplV,* Splenic vein; *LRV,* Left renal vein.

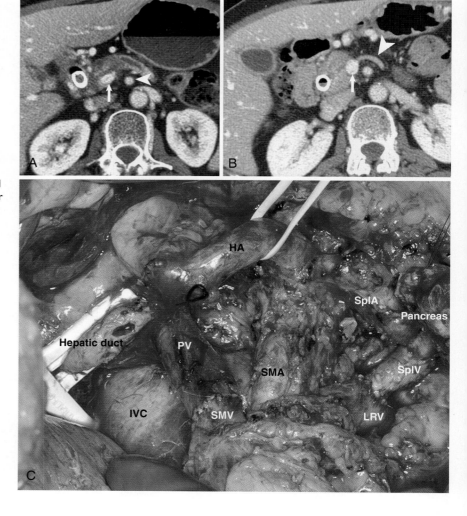

especially in the setting of an uncinate process tumor. Attempted suture repair of a tangential laceration in the JB can cause an SMA injury if the SMA is not completely exposed. Therefore, exposure of the SMA medial to the SMV by incising the root of mesentery should be accomplished prior to dissecting the JB from the uncinate process, whenever this dissection is difficult, or whenever the need for vein resection (tangential or segmental) is anticipated.

After exposing the SMA, the JB can be approached from the left of the SMV by slowly dividing the root of the small bowel mesentery to the right of the SMA. When performing a PD, although the surgeon cannot ligate the main trunk of the SMV and maintain normal venous return from the midgut, we have found that either of the two first-order branches of the SMV, the ileal and jejunal branches, can be safely ligated or resected along with the pancreatic tumor over a short distance, provided that the remaining branch is preserved and of sufficient caliber to allow for collateral mesenteric venous flow.

Surgical Technique

Five types of vein resection can be performed (Figure 6). When the tumor is adherent to a small aspect of the lateral or posterior wall of the SMV, PV, or SMV-PV confluence, a tangential resection with a vein patch is possible. We most commonly use the greater saphenous vein for this type of reconstruction.

Occasionally, a vein patch can be avoided if the tumor involves the lateral SMV-PV confluence across from the splenic vein insertion. In this case a pie-shaped defect in the vein can be repaired transversely

(analogous to a pyloroplasty). If the area of tumor involvement is at the level of the splenic vein confluence, necessitating splenic vein ligation, an end-to-end primary anastomosis of the SMV and PV can be performed. By dividing the splenic vein, the PV is then free (no longer tethered to the splenic vein) to bridge a fairly large gap, at least 3 to 4 cm, and it can still reach the divided end of the SMV.

Occasionally, an interposition graft will be needed even if the splenic vein is divided. We described the use of the internal jugular (IJ) vein as an interposition graft in 1994 (see Cusack et al in the Selected Readings), and it remains the most commonly used conduit for mesenteric venous reconstruction. When segmental resection of the SMV is performed and the splenic vein is preserved, a tension-free, primary, end-to-end anastomosis of the SMV to the intact PV-splenic vein confluence is rarely possible without an interposition graft.

Isolated tumor involvement of the first-order branches of the SMV does not represent a contraindication to resection, although it should alert the surgeon to the possibility of a more difficult technical operation, as the tumor extends into the root of mesentery. During PD, we prefer to identify the infrapancreatic SMV early in the operation when possible, but complete mobilization of this vessel does not occur until the retroperitoneal/mesenteric dissection is performed during the final step of the resection.

After transection of the neck of the pancreas, the head and uncinate process are separated from the SMV and PV by ligation and division of the small venous tributaries to the pancreas, including two or three small branches from the JB to the uncinate process. Isolated involvement of the JB of the SMV may be managed by division and

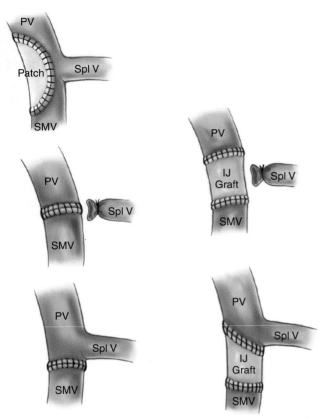

FIGURE 6   Illustration of the different forms of reconstruction of the SMV and SMV-PV confluence. *(Modified from Tseng JF, Raut CP, Lee JE, et al: Pancreaticoduodenectomy with vascular resection: margin status and survival duration, J Gastrointest Surg 8[8]:935-949; 2004.)*

segmental resection of this branch without reconstruction, as long as the ileal branch remains intact and is of sufficient caliber. As seen on axial CT images, the diameter of the ileal branch of the SMV is visibly larger than the SMA, at least 1.5 times its diameter. Exposure of the JB of the SMV in the root of mesentery is accomplished by developing the plane of dissection to the right of the SMA and medial to, or to the left of, the SMV (as discussed above). The soft tissue of the mesenteric root between these vessels is divided until the JB is identified posterior to the SMA. Involvement of the confluence of the ileal and jejunal branches in association with more proximal involvement of the common trunk of the SMV may be successfully managed by ligation of the JB of the SMV and segmental resection and reconstruction of the main SMV trunk (and proximal ileal branch) with or without an interposition vein graft.

As already discussed, when the splenic vein is left intact, the PV remains immobile, and an interposition graft is usually necessary to connect the ileal branch to the main SMV; an internal jugular vein interposition graft is most commonly used for this purpose. Reconstruction of the ileal branch is always preferred over the JB, as the JB is usually posterior in location, extending into the proximal left jejunal branch, and therefore technically difficult to access for an anastomosis. Moreover, the JB is rather delicate in nature with a very thin wall. Division of the JB and resection of the confluence of the jejunal and ileal branches with reconstruction of the ileal branch (caudal to the tumor) and the main SMV (cephalad to the tumor) should only be performed if the ileal branch is of adequate caliber. As a general rule and as mentioned above, we do not attempt resection and reconstruction of the ileal branch (in the setting of ligation of the jejunal branch) when the diameter of the ileal branch is not visibly larger than the diameter of the SMA as seen on the axial

CT images. This recommendation is based on the observation that long-term graft patency becomes a concern the farther out one proceeds into the small bowel mesentery and the smaller the diameter of the ileal branch.

If the area of venous abutment or encasement is distal (caudal) to the splenic vein confluence, it is preferable to preserve the splenic vein because of the potential for sinistral portal hypertension after splenic vein ligation. However, preservation of the splenic vein makes the vascular reconstruction much more difficult. With the splenic vein intact, one cannot complete the dissection of the specimen from the right lateral border of the SMA to the origin of this vessel in standard fashion. Therefore options include either placing the graft prior to specimen removal or separating the pancreatic head from the SMA by medial rotation of the specimen as was initially described in 1996 (see Leach et al in Selected Readings). Segmental resection of the SMV with splenic vein preservation adds significant complexity to PD but prevents the potential complications of hypersplenism, which may result in mild to significant thrombocytopenia, thereby possibly complicating the delivery of cytotoxic chemotherapy, and sinistral portal hypertension with the risk for gastroesophageal varices and hemorrhage. With splenic vein preservation, a vein graft is usually necessary for reconstruction, unless the segmental resection is less than 2 cm in length. The IJ is an ideal conduit for interposition grafting, and this vein is harvested after it is clear that the graft will be required but before any vascular clamps are applied.

When the SMV is occluded for reconstruction, inflow occlusion of the SMA is performed using a Rummel tourniquet to prevent bowel edema, which may complicate the pancreatic and biliary anastomoses. Prior to occluding the SMA, patients are systemically heparinized (2000 to 3000 U).

Preoperative CT imaging should also accurately identify tumor extension to the common or proper hepatic artery and aberrant hepatic arterial anatomy. Dissection of the hepatic artery should be performed with gentle, sharp dissection, especially in patients who have received prior external beam radiation therapy and in those with extensive scar formation from prior surgery. If a short segment of the hepatic artery needs to be resected, it can often be repaired with a primary anastomosis (the artery is often quite redundant) or with the use of a reversed saphenous vein graft.

The most common arterial variants include an accessory or replaced left hepatic artery, arising from the left gastric artery, and an accessory or replaced right hepatic artery, arising from the SMA. The aberrant right hepatic artery that arises from the SMA may be encased by the pancreatic head tumor. Intrahepatic communication between the right and left hepatic arteries should allow for ligation of the right hepatic artery in the setting of a normal serum bilirubin. However, the proximal bile duct receives most of its arterial supply from the right hepatic artery after the gastroduodenal artery is ligated. Therefore, when the right hepatic artery is divided or resected, it is usually revascularized. When the entire common hepatic artery arises from the SMA, it is necessary to recognize this anatomic variant and preserve or revascularize this artery. It is also important to assess the hepatic artery pulse after the GDA is ligated. If the pulse becomes diminished or is not palpable, it is necessary to dissect the common hepatic artery to the celiac axis. The surgeon must then either relieve extrinsic compression (median arcuate ligament syndrome, inflammatory entrapment) or, in the rare setting of atherosclerotic disease, proceed with revascularization of the celiac axis.

SUMMARY

Vascular resection during PD adds complexity to an already challenging operation with potential for significant morbidity and mortality. Patient selection is critically important and is largely based on CT imaging. Resectability should be defined by clear, consistent, objective anatomic criteria that must be accurately interpreted on cross-sectional imaging studies. For potentially resectable patients, the survival benefit of surgery is predicated on negative surgical margins and the successful delivery of multimodality therapy. Therefore, the surgeon must avoid inadvertent venous injury that will necessitate rapid removal of the tumor and increase the chances of an incomplete gross resection.

Preoperative planning is key; the surgeon must plan for possible vascular resection prior to surgery rather than discovering the need for revascularization in the operating room. The vascular dissection must be done in a careful fashion so that all of the relevant anatomy is clearly defined prior to attempted removal of the specimen. With adequate exposure and a controlled approach to vascular resection and reconstruction, PD with vascular resection can offer patients the chance for cure and a median survival identical to that of patients who undergo standard PD without the need for vascular reconstruction. Isolated involvement of venous structures is not a contraindication to PD, however, the procedure should be performed by experienced surgeons at high-volume centers as part of a multidisciplinary protocol-based approach to patients with pancreatic cancer.

SUGGESTED READINGS

Christians K, Evans DB: Pancreaticoduodenectomy and vascular resection: persistent controversy and current recommendations, *Ann Surg Oncol* 16(4):789–791, 2009.
Cusack JC, Fuhrman GM, Lee JE, et al: Management of unsuspected tumor invasion of the superior mesenteric–portal venous confluence at the time of pancreaticoduodenectomy, *Am J Surg* 168:352–354, 1994.

Evans DB, Varadhachary GR, Crane CH, et al: Preoperative gemcitabine-based chemoradiation for patients with resectable adenocarcinoma of the pancreatic head, *J Clin Oncol* 26(21):3496–3502, 2008.
Katz MH, Pisters PW, Evans DB, et al: Borderline resectable pancreatic cancer: the importance of this emerging stage of disease, *J Am Coll Surg* 206(5):833–846, 2008:discussion 846-848.
Katz MH, Fleming JB, Pisters PWT, et al: Anatomy of the superior mesenteric vein with special reference to the surgical management of first-order branch involvement at pancreaticoduodenectomy, *Ann Surg* 248(6):1098–1102, 2008.
Leach SD, Davidson BS, Ames FC, et al: Alternative method for exposure of the retropancreatic mesenteric vasculature during total pancreatectomy, *J Surg Oncol* 61:163–165, 1996.
Raut CP, Tseng JF, Sun CC, et al: Impact of resection status on pattern of failure and survival after pancreaticoduodenectomy for pancreatic adenocarcinoma, *Ann Surg* 246(1):52–60, 2007.
Scoggins CR, Lee JE, Evans DB: Pancreaticoduodenectomy with en bloc vascular resection and reconstruction for localized carcinoma of the pancreas. In VonHoff DD, Evans DB, Hruban RH, editors: *Pancreatic cancer*, Sudbury, Mass, 2005, Jones and Bartlett, pp 321–334.
Tseng JF, Raut CP, Lee JE, et al: Pancreaticoduodenectomy with vascular resection: margin status and survival duration, *J Gastrointest Surg* 8(8):935–949, 2004.

PALLIATIVE THERAPY FOR PANCREATIC CANCER

Jonathan C. King, MD, and O. Joe Hines, MD

OVERVIEW

Although important progress has been made in the understanding of pancreatic cancer biology during the past decade, this knowledge has not yet resulted in a substantial change in patient survival. The incidence of pancreatic cancer has been increasing over the same period, and the death rate mirrors this rise (Figure 1). For the estimated 42,270 patients diagnosed with pancreatic cancer this year, almost all will succumb to the disease within a year of diagnosis. Most patients with pancreatic cancer are seen initially with advanced disease and are not candidates for resection, and 5-year survival for all stages currently approaches 5% and has not changed substantially in the last 25 years. Consideration of these statistics is critical when establishing treatment plans and considering palliative intervention for patients with pancreatic cancer.

All patients fit enough for surgery should undergo resection of the primary pancreatic lesion, because they gain a significant survival advantage over those who are not resected. The appropriateness of resection can be reliably determined by high-quality preoperative imaging. Generally, a pancreatic cancer is deemed unresectable if there is evidence of hepatic, peritoneal, or extraabdominal metastatic disease; involvement of the celiac or superior mesenteric artery; or

disease identified in the lymph nodes, outside of the area normally included in the resection specimen (paraaortic or celiac nodes, see Table 1). Unfortunately this scenario represents the majority of patients who come in for evaluation.

The sixth edition of the AJCC staging guidelines for pancreatic cancer is provided in Table 2. Patients with stage 0, I, or II disease are generally considered resectable. Some surgeons consider tumors with venous invasion acceptable for resection, and surgeons familiar with the technique may attempt a vascular reconstruction. A recent meta-analysis reported that survival rates for resection of tumors with superior mesenteric or portal vein invasion was better than that for patients who underwent palliative chemotherapy. This was true as long as perioperative mortality and the likelihood of positive

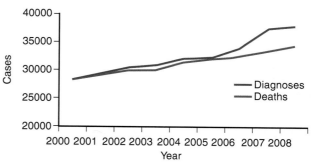

FIGURE I   New pancreatic cancer diagnoses and deaths in the United States, 2000 through 2008. *(Modified from American Cancer Society: Cancer Facts and Figures 2008, Atlanta, 2008, American Cancer Society.)*

TABLE I: Determinants of pancreatic cancer unresectablity

Vascular invasion*
Hepatic metastases
Peritoneal disease
Extraabdominal metastases
Metastases to lymph nodes outside of the resection area

*If cancer has invaded into the portal or superior mesenteric vein, a potentially curative resection may be attempted. Curative resections with or without venous resection carry similar prognoses.

resection margins (R1 or R2 resection) were low. These data must be viewed critically, however, as there is currently no level I evidence that venous resection and reconstruction will alter prognosis for pancreatic cancer patients.

For patients not eligible for resection, palliation of symptoms associated with locoregional tumor growth and invasion becomes the focus of therapy. Palliative therapy for pancreatic cancer includes treatments directed toward the prevention or relief of biliary obstruction, duodenal obstruction, and tumor-related pain. Although traditionally thought to be best managed by open operative approaches, less invasive endoscopic, laparoscopic, and radiologic methods are now accepted as preferred interventions.

■ INITIAL EVALUATION

Most patients who are thought to have pancreatic cancer undergo an initial evaluation by a primary care physician, and they are referred to a surgeon only if there is no obvious evidence of unresectability. This initial evaluation should include a detailed history and physical examination. The classic presentation of pancreatic cancer originating in the head or uncinate process of the pancreas is obstructive jaundice, weight loss, and abdominal pain. These signs and symptoms result from biliary obstruction, anorexia and possible duodenal obstruction, and local growth of the tumor, respectively. As part of an evaluation for pancreatic cancer, the physician may assay serum tumor markers such as CA 19-9. The serum level of CA 19-9 is related to the tumor burden, and values above 1000 U/mL have been considered to signal the presence of widespread and unresectable disease, although this is not always the case and should not be claimed as the sole reason to forgo exploration.

The single most valuable study used to stage patients with pancreatic cancer is the helical CT scan done according to a specific pancreatic protocol. This requires 2 to 3 mm collimation through the pancreas itself, intravenous (IV) contrast, and separate scans for both the pancreas and the liver during the arterial and venous phases. In our experience, the ability of CT to accurately predict resectability is approximately 85%. The accuracy of such a prediction is related to the expertise of the radiologist, the nature of the CT findings, and the experience and philosophy of the surgeon. Incorrect predictions are usually because of small liver or peritoneal metastases or cancer invading the superior mesenteric or portal veins.

Endoscopic ultrasound (EUS) also has the potential to provide information about resectability, but the quality of the information is highly operator dependent. The reliability of EUS predictions increases not only with the experience of the endoscopist, but also with the increasing collaboration between the endoscopist and surgeon. Furthermore, EUS can safely and reliably obtain fine needle aspirates of suspicious lymph nodes for cytologic examination. As indicated earlier, metastatic disease in lymph node basins outside of the area of resection—for example, in the celiac nodes—would preclude resection.

TABLE 2: AJCC TNM staging

Primary Tumor (T)

TX	Primary tumor cannot be assessed
T0	No evidence of primary tumor
Tis	Carcinoma in situ*
T1	Tumor limited to the pancreas, ≤2 cm in greatest dimension
T2	Tumor limited to the pancreas, >2 cm in greatest dimension
T3	Tumor extends beyond the pancreas but without involvement of the celiac axis or the superior mesenteric artery
T4	Tumor involves the celiac axis or the superior mesenteric artery (unresectable primary tumor)

Regional Lymph Nodes (N)

NX	Regional lymph nodes cannot be assessed
N0	No regional lymph node metastasis
N1	Regional lymph node metastasis

Distant Metastasis (M)

MX	Distant metastasis cannot be assessed
M0	No distant metastasis
M1	Distant metastasis

STAGE GROUPING

Stage 0	Tis	N0	M0
Stage IA	T1	N0	M0
Stage IB	T2	N0	M0
Stage IIA	T3	N0	M0
Stage IIB	T1	N1	M0
	T2	N1	M0
	T3	N1	M0
Stage III	T4	Any N	M0
Stage IV	Any T	Any N	M1

*This also includes the "PanInIII" classification.

From Greene FL, Page DL, Fleming ID, et al: *AJCC cancer staging manual,* ed 6, New York, 2002, Springer.

Some practitioners utilize MRI to evaluate patients' eligibility for surgery. Although data indicate that MRI is at least equivalent to CT for this purpose, most prefer the image quality of CT. For patients with severe iodine contrast allergy, MRI is the preferred study. Magnetic resonance cholangiopancreatography (MRCP) may help evaluate patients with main duct intraductal papillary mucinous neoplasm but otherwise is not necessary for evaluation.

Other factors that influence the decision to proceed with operation are tumor size and the age of the patient. Larger tumors should not be considered unresectable strictly on the basis of their size. In our own series, 65% of resections have been for tumors 1 to 4 cm in diameter, and 35% were for tumors greater than 4 cm. Additionally, several series have documented the safety of performing pancreatic resections in older patients. An assessment of the patient's general medical condition drives the decision for operation, not chronologic age.

PALLIATION FOR ADVANCED DISEASE

By the time most patients with pancreatic cancer come to a physician, many have locally advanced and/or metastatic disease (85% to 90%). Because of the inevitability of disease progression to gastric outlet or biliary obstruction and intractable abdominal pain, palliation of pain and obstructive symptoms becomes the most important consideration for improved quality of life. The majority of patients with unresectable pancreatic head lesions will experience biliary obstruction and jaundice and will therefore require palliative intervention. Furthermore, the incidence of gastric outlet obstruction because of tumor invasion of the duodenum likely ranges between 5% to 10%, and it necessitates palliation if the patient is to maintain a reasonable nutritional status during chemotherapy. Finally, most patients will experience pain, but when it is described to be located mostly in the patient's back, it is associated with tumor unresectability. Palliation of pain symptoms is critical for optimal quality of life for these patients.

NONOPERATIVE PALLIATION OF BILIARY OBSTRUCTION

The options for decompression of the obstructed bile duct include percutaneous, endoscopic, and laparoscopic methods. Endoscopic stent placement is the most efficient and least invasive method of biliary decompression. Occasionally, the biliary tract cannot be accessed endoscopically because of local tumor growth or anatomic considerations, including prior Roux-en-Y gastric bypass. In this instance, a percutaneous approach would be the next consideration. However, percutaneous techniques for placement of transhepatic biliary drains and stents are less favored because of the increased risks of infection, obstruction, and dislodgement. In addition, patients have poorer satisfaction because of pain and the inconvenience of the drain. In a staged procedure, drains can be internalized with a stent, and the percutaneous drain can be removed. Prospective randomized data confirm that endoscopic stenting has a significantly higher rate of jaundice relief and significantly lower 30-day mortality rate than percutaneous stent placement.

Endoscopically placed biliary stents are clearly effective at relieving biliary obstruction. The endoscopist may choose from a variety of metal or plastic stents that are effective at relieving jaundice, but metal stents are more durable and are less likely to be associated with recurrent biliary occlusion (Figure 2). Occlusion of plastic stents is related to bilioduodenal reflux that results in bacterial colonization and biliary sludge deposition in the luminal surface of the stent. Plastic stents require scheduled exchange every 2 to 3 months or on an emergent basis if obstruction or cholangitis are evident.

Studies have shown that elective plastic stent changes are superior to replacement at signs of stent obstruction in terms of symptom management and cost effectiveness. Patency rates of metal stents are longer (about 10 to 12 months), so metal stents should be used for patients with greater than 4 to 6 months of expected survival, and plastic stents should be used for patients with less than 4 months life expectancy (Figure 3). Patients with locally advanced disease who are being considered for neoadjuvant treatment and subsequent resection are probably best served by a metal stent, because most of these patients ultimately will remain unresectable, and treatment may last longer than the predicted life of a plastic stent. This recommendation is supported by recent series indicating that the presence of a metal

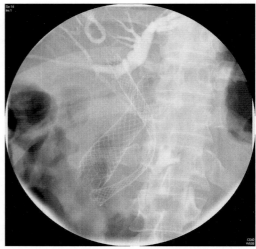

FIGURE 2   Plain abdominal radiograph showing metallic biliary and duodenal stents.

biliary stent does not preclude subsequent tumor resection. Finally, covered metal stents have been developed to prevent tumor ingrowth that may cause reobstruction of metal stents. Patency rates are 78% at 12 months, and there is less stent obstruction and more time before obstruction, which leads to fewer rehospitalizations and repeat interventions and lower costs compared with uncovered metal stents.

Generally, patients with biliary obstruction should not require surgical bypass unless endoscopic therapy is unsuccessful. However, in those patients who require operation, surgery is an effective alternative. Randomized controlled trials comparing endoscopic biliary stenting to surgery have generally found roughly equivalent early rates of technical success and long-term survival, but results favor endoscopic stenting in terms of shorter initial hospital stay and less postprocedural morbidity and mortality; however, surgical bypass is associated with superior long-term bypass patency (Table 3). Both open and laparoscopic techniques can be utilized to bypass distal malignant obstructions via anastomosis of the bile duct or gallbladder to the duodenum or jejunum.

NONOPERATIVE PALLIATION OF GASTRIC OUTLET OBSTRUCTION

Endoscopic stenting for duodenal obstruction has been shown to be as effective as gastrojejunostomy in terms of technical success, complication rates, persistence of obstructive symptoms, and overall survival for patients with unresectable periampullary cancer. A recent meta-analysis reviewed randomized controlled trials ($n = 2$) and comparative studies ($n = 6$) of duodenal stenting versus gastrojejunostomy, either open or laparoscopic. Of the 1,046 patients identified, stent placement was successful in 96%, versus a 99% technical success rate for gastrojejunostomy. Early clinical success measured by improvement in the Gastric Outlet Obstruction Scoring System was somewhat better in the duodenal stenting group (odds ratio [OR], 3.39), but this difference was not statistically significant. Major and minor complications were equivalent between the two groups, though reinterventions were more common in the stenting group because of stent occlusion resulting from tumor ingrowth, stent migration, bleeding, and perforation (Table 4).

Similar to biliary stents, coated metal duodenal stents have longer patency periods because of prevention of tumor ingrowth, though at the expense of increased risk of stent migration. Endoscopic stent placement may be better for patients with a relatively short life expectancy (<6 months), but gastrojejunostomy is preferable in patients with longer expected survival.

Review: Palliative biliary stents for obstructing pancreatic carcinoma
Comparison: 2 Metal versus Plastic Stents
Outcome: 6 Recurrent biliary obstruction prior to death/end of study

Study or subgroup	Metal n/N	Plastic n/N	Risk Ratio M-H, Fixed, 95% CI	Weight	Risk Ratio M-H, Fixed, 95% CI
Knyrim 1993	6/31	12/31		12.4%	0.50 (0.21, 1.16)
Davids 1992	16/49	30/56		28.9%	0.61 (0.38, 0.98)
Kaassis 2003	11/59	22/59		22.7%	0.50 (0.27, 0.94)
Prat 1998	6/34	24/33		25.2%	0.24 (0.11, 0.52)
Carr Locke 1993	11/86	10/78		10.8%	1.00 (0.45, 2.22)
Total (95% CI)	**259**	**257**		**100.0%**	**0.52 (0.39, 0.69)**

Total Events: 50 (Metal), 98 (Plastic)
Heterogeneity: $Chi^2 = 6.92$, df = 4 (P = 0.14); $I^2 = 42\%$
Test for overall effect: Z = 4.44 (P < 0.00001)

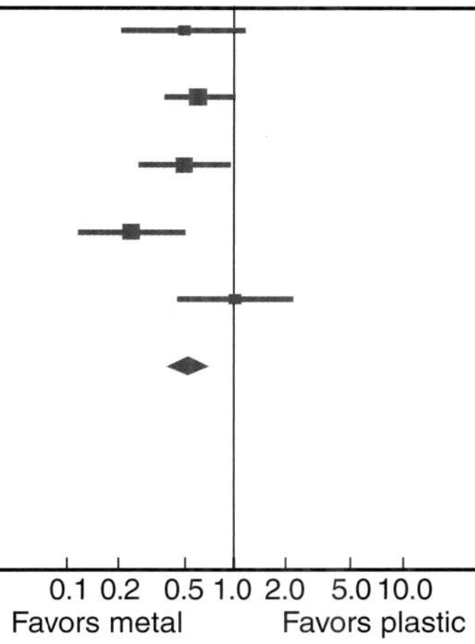

0.1 0.2 0.5 1.0 2.0 5.0 10.0
Favors metal   Favors plastic

FIGURE 3 Meta-analysis of prospective trials comparing recurrent biliary obstruction with self-expanding metal stents versus plastic stents. *(From Moss AC, Morris E, MacMathuna P: Palliative biliary stents for obstructing pancreatic carcinoma, Cochrane Upper Gastrointestinal and Pancreatic Diseases Group. Cochrane Database Syst Rev [2]:CD004200, 2006.)*

TABLE 3: Comparison between endoscopic stents and surgery for decompression of malignant biliary obstruction

	ENDOSCOPIC STENTS (n = 789)		SURGICAL BYPASS (n = 180)	
	Range	Mean	Range	Mean
30-day mortality	0–20	14	0–31	12
Hospital stay (days)	3–26	7	19–30	17
Success rate (%)	82–100	90	75–100	93
Early complications (%)	8–34	21	6–56	31
Late complications (%)	13–45	28	5–47	16

From Watanpa P, Williamson RCN: Surgical palliation for pancreatic cancer: developments during the past two decades, *Br J Surg* 79:1, 1992.

INTRAOPERATIVE PALLIATION

Despite the excellent diagnostic tools available, 10% to 15% of patients will be found to have metastatic or locally advanced disease at the time of operation. The surgeon must then determine if a palliative surgical procedure is warranted. Considerations include biliary and gastric bypass and the need for intraoperative celiac nerve block. The extent of disease identified at exploration partially drives the need for these procedures, and most patients who have been offered resection will tolerate any indicated palliative procedures.

Biliary Bypass

Our practice has been to perform a biliary bypass if the patient is obstructed and a stent has not been placed preoperatively. In this case the classic biliary bypass is a Roux-en-Y choledochojejunostomy. This approach is probably associated with the lowest incidence of reobstruction and cholangitis. Alternatively, a loop of jejunum can be used to perform the anastomosis, but this bypass may be complicated by reflux of enteric contents and food into the biliary tree. As long as the anastomosis is large enough, this should not be a concern. A patulous 2 to 2.5 cm anastomosis is made between the common bile duct and bowel in a side-to-side fashion with a single running absorbable monofilament suture. If the gallbladder is in place, a cholecystectomy is performed as well.

If the patient has not had a cholecystectomy prior to exploration, the gallbladder provides an alternate route for biliary decompression. However, cholecystojejunostomy is associated with a higher rate of recurrent obstruction because of variable insertion of the cystic duct into the common bile duct and local tumor growth. Preoperative imaging may help to delineate the biliary anatomy but, generally, if the gallbladder is distended, the surgeon can assume that the obstruction is downstream of the bile duct–cystic duct junction. A Roux-en-Y limb or simple loop of jejunum can be utilized, along with a side-to-side anastomosis with absorbable monofilament suture. Any gallstones should be cleared from the gallbladder at the time of the cholecystotomy.

Finally, bypass may be accomplished via the duodenum, though this approach is likely associated with a higher chance of failure because of local tumor growth as well. However, some retrospective reports suggest this approach may be as effective as hepaticojejunostomy. A choledochoduodenostomy is performed using a longitudinal 2 to 3 cm choledochotomy and a running single layer anastomosis to the duodenum with absorbable suture. A closed suction drain should be placed next to all biliary bypasses to control the potential complication of anastomotic leak.

Enteric Bypass

The decision to perform a gastrojejunostomy is based on the patient's symptoms at the time of surgery and the intraoperative findings. Patients complaining of nausea and vomiting or even early satiety will benefit from enteric bypass. At the time of exploration, assessment may reveal locally invasive tumor that predictably will lead to duodenal obstruction.

The gastrojejunostomy should be constructed utilizing a loop of jejunum and the posterior aspect of the stomach a few inches off the greater curvature. A Roux limb should not be used, because the emptying of this reconstruction is inferior to that of a loop construction. A side-to-side anastomosis is constructed in two layers with an outer layer of interrupted silk suture and a running inner layer of

---

TABLE 4: Outcomes of endoscopic duodenal stenting versus gastrojejunostomy (GJJ)

	Stent	GJJ
Technical success (%)	972/1012 (96)	203/204 (99)
Clinical success (%)	890/1000 (89)	79/110 (72)
Complications (%)		
Early major complications	43/609 (7)	6/159 (4)
Late major complications	171/950 (18)	34/201 (17)
Minor complications	66/732 (9)	66/201 (33)
Persistent obstructive symptoms	43/535 (8)	10/106 (9)
Reintervention	147/814 (18)	1/138 (1)
Mean hospital stay (days, [range])	7 (2–18)	13 (7–30)
Mean survival (days, [range])	105 (23–210)	164 (64–348)

From Jeurnink SM, van Eijck CH, Steyerberg EW, et al: Stent versus gastrojejunostomy for the palliation of gastric outlet obstruction: a systematic review, *BMC Gastroenterology* 7:18, 2007.

---

absorbable suture. Alternatively, the anastomosis may be performed with a stapler, and it may be positioned in an antecolic or retrocolic position. Either method is acceptable, and neither seems to offer a significant advantage over the other. Concerns regarding local tumor growth into a retrogastric anastomosis rarely materialize, and this position may allow for better emptying. If this approach is used, the anastomosis should be secured to the colonic mesentery through which it traverses, preventing the possibility of internal herniation.

Some controversy exists on the need for prophylactic enteric bypass in patients found to be unresectable at laparotomy. Multiple observational and retrospective studies have indicated that prophylactic gastrojejunostomy does not decrease the incidence of late gastric outlet obstruction; instead, it leads to increases in hospital stay, morbidity, and even death. However, three randomized controlled trials have found that between 19% and 41% of patients who do not receive prophylactic gastrojejunostomy go on to develop late gastric outlet obstruction and thus require a second procedure. In two studies, retrocolic gastrojejunostomies were performed in patients who did not have imminent duodenal obstruction (one study did not specify anticolic or retrocolic anastomosis). Operative morbidity and blood loss were similar between the two groups for all three studies, highlighting the fact that enteric bypass can be performed safely. A recent meta-analysis compiled these results and found the odds ratio for late gastric outlet obstruction in patients who undergo prophylactic gastrojejunostomy was 0.06 compared with patients who did not undergo enteric bypass (Figure 4).

Celiac Plexus Neurolysis

If the patient is discovered to be unresectable at laparotomy, celiac plexus block can be easily achieved. Using a 20 or 22 gauge needle, 20 mL of 50% absolute ethanol diluted in sterile saline is injected, 10 mL on either side of the aorta at the level of the celiac axis. Alternatively this can be performed percutaneously or transgastrically, utilizing endoscopic ultrasound. In randomized controlled trials comparing celiac plexus neurolysis with sham injection, significantly better pain control was observed in patients receiving ethanol injection.

A recent meta-analysis of randomized controlled trials comparing systemic opiate therapy with neurolytic celiac plexus block identified 302 patients, most of whom underwent percutaneous celiac plexus block. Pain scores were lower at 2, 6, and 8 weeks after randomization, as were systemic opiate use and constipation, for patients undergoing celiac plexus block. The meta-analysis was unable to reliably compile quality-of-life data because of differences in measurement (Figure 5).

LAPAROSCOPIC APPROACHES TO PALLIATION

Laparoscopy remains a viable tool for assessment of metastatic disease and locally advanced lesions. If the surgeon is familiar with laparoscopic techniques, laparoscopic gastrojejunostomy is the preferred method of

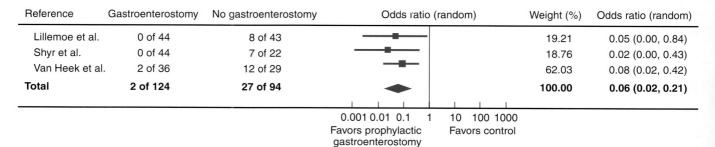

Reference	Gastroenterostomy	No gastroenterostomy	Odds ratio (random)	Weight (%)	Odds ratio (random)
Lillemoe et al.	0 of 44	8 of 43		19.21	0.05 (0.00, 0.84)
Shyr et al.	0 of 44	7 of 22		18.76	0.02 (0.00, 0.43)
Van Heek et al.	2 of 36	12 of 29		62.03	0.08 (0.02, 0.42)
Total	**2 of 124**	**27 of 94**		**100.00**	**0.06 (0.02, 0.21)**

0.001 0.01 0.1   1   10 100 1000
Favors prophylactic   Favors control
gastroenterostomy

FIGURE 4 Meta-analysis of prophylactic gastrojejunostomy versus no gastroenterostomy on development of late gastric outlet obstruction. *(From Hüser N, Michalski CW, Schuster T, et al: Systematic review and meta-analysis of prophylactic gastroenterostomy for unresectable advanced pancreatic cancer, et al: Br J Surg 96:711, 2009.)*

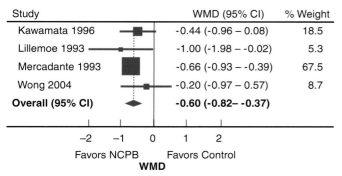

FIGURE 5   Meta-analysis of neurolytic celiac plexus block versus opiate therapy for relief of pancreatic cancer pain at 8 weeks. *(From Yan PM, Myers RP: Neurolytic celiac plexus block for pain control in unresectable pancreatic cancer, Am J Gastroenterol 102:430, 2007.)*

palliation for a patient with an unresectable pancreatic head mass. In a randomized-controlled trial of laparoscopic versus open gastrojejunostomy for patients with obstructing foregut tumors, less operative blood loss and shorter time to oral diet was reported in the laparoscopic group, and no patients experienced delayed gastric emptying in the laparoscopic group compared with 2 patients in the open group. Retrospective studies have also demonstrated that dual biliary and gastric bypass can be accomplished laparoscopically with good results. Finally, celiac nerve blockade can be easily performed at the time of laparoscopy.

PALLIATIVE PANCREATICODUODENECTOMY

Recently some centers have reported series of noncurative resections for locally advanced and metastatic pancreatic adenocarcinoma, suggesting a survival advantage to pancreaticoduodenectomy with positive margins (R1 resection) over leaving the tumor in situ. Some studies have concluded that the survival benefit is similar to that of complete tumor resection (R0 resection). Whether palliative pancreaticoduodenectomy offers a true survival advantage or if this simply reflects the rarity of a truly curative operation for R0 resections has not been determined. Currently no evidence justifies elective palliative pancreaticoduodenectomy, and thus it is not recommended.

PALLIATIVE CHEMORADIATION

Chemotherapy and radiation appear to offer a clear survival advantage for patients with unresectable pancreatic cancer. Some retrospective studies have reported tumor downstaging and subsequent resection with negative surgical margins in 10% to 20% of patients initially seen with signs of venous invasion, encasement, or limited arterial involvement but not metastatic disease. Median survival in one study was 20 months, approximately equal to that of patients who undergo resection followed by adjuvant chemotherapy.

A Cochrane review of the literature found that chemotherapy significantly reduced the 1 year mortality when compared with best supportive care, as did chemoradiation (0% vs. 58%, $P = .001$); the magnitude of effect was equivalent when comparing chemoradiation with chemotherapy alone. Combination therapy with 5-fluorouracil (5-FU) did not alter 1-year mortality, nor did combination therapy with gemcitabine. However, there may be a 6-month survival benefit to gemcitabine-platinum combinations when compared with gemcitabine alone. The study also found that radiation therapy alone was inferior to combination chemoradiation therapy, and it was associated with more toxicity. The authors concluded that chemoradiation therapy could not be recommended in place of chemotherapy alone, because they found no survival benefit.

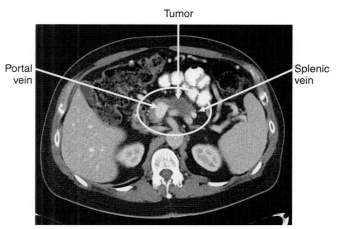

FIGURE 6   Abdominal CT scan showing splenic vein thrombosis and splenomegaly in a patient with unresectable pancreatic adenocarcinoma and thrombocytopenia.

Targeted therapies for pancreatic cancer including erlotinib (anti-EGFR) and bevacizumab (anti-VEGF) have been tested, with marginal results. Combination therapy with gemcitabine and erlotinib produced an overall survival benefit to patients compared with single-agent gemcitabine therapy in a phase III clinical trial, though the difference was small, at just under 2 weeks improved survival (6.0 vs. 6.4 months). Results of gemcitabine and bevacizumab combination therapy are less promising, as overall survival is unchanged. However, one recent phase III clinical trial combining gemcitabine, erlotinib, and bevacizumab did show improved progression-free survival versus gemcitabine and erlotinib alone.

SPLENECTOMY FOR HYPERSPLENISM

Locally advanced pancreatic cancer can lead to thrombosis or occlusion of the splenic, superior mesenteric, and portal veins, resulting in hypersplenism (Figure 6). Similar to patients with cirrhosis and portal hypertension, splenic sequestration often results in thrombocytopenia. Additionally, cytotoxic chemotherapeutic regimens, especially those containing gemcitabine, often induce bone marrow suppression and further reduce circulating platelet numbers. Considering that chemotherapy has been shown to provide a significant survival benefit for patients with unresectable pancreatic cancer, we believe that palliative splenectomy for patients with thrombocytopenia may be useful for extending treatment and thus improving disease-specific survival. In our experience, splenectomy for patients who have been forced to discontinue treatment because of thrombocytopenia significantly improves platelet counts, allows for the resumption of chemotherapy in all patients, and favorably impacts survival.

SUMMARY

Unfortunately, most patients diagnosed with pancreatic cancer will succumb to their disease within a year or two of diagnosis. For those who are candidates for resection, recent data suggest they can expect a 5-year survival as high as 35%. Until a new method for early detection and substantially improved targeted treatment is developed, pancreatic cancer will remain a uniformly lethal condition. Patients who are not candidates for curative resection often require intervention to address complications associated with local tumor growth, to achieve improved quality of life, and to maximize the benefits of medical therapy.

Despite the fact that most pancreatic cancer patients are not candidates for surgical resection, the surgeon plays an important role in their management. A clear understanding of the interventions

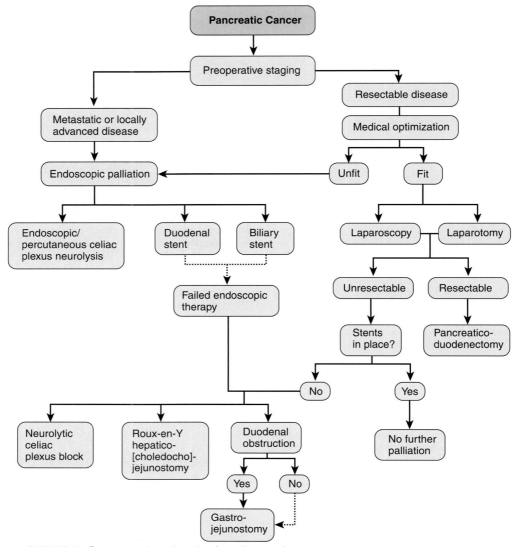

FIGURE 7   Decision-making algorithm for palliation of patients with unresectable pancreatic cancer.

available to mitigate the local effects of pancreatic cancer growth on the bile duct, duodenum, and celiac plexus helps to navigate the nonoperative and intraoperative approaches to palliate this group (Figure 7). When appropriate, nonoperative intervention should be the first line of treatment for unresectable patients. Biliary stenting, duodenal stenting, and percutaneous celiac plexus block are effective for palliation of patients with short life expectancies. Operative bypass can effectively address biliary and duodenal obstruction for patients who fail endoscopic therapy or who are identified as unresectable at the time of laparotomy or laparoscopy. Optimal palliation of these conditions improves quality of life, minimizes the need for hospitalization, and allows the patient to engage in palliative chemotherapy, thus maximizing survival benefit.

Suggested Readings

Artifon EL, Sakai P, Cunha JE, et al: Surgery or endoscopy for palliation of biliary obstruction due to metastatic pancreatic cancer, *Am J Gastroenterol* 101(9):2031–2037, 2006.

Hüser N, Michalski CW, Schuster T, et al: Systematic review and meta-analysis of prophylactic gastroenterostomy for unresectable advanced pancreatic cancer, *Br J Surg* 96:711–719, 2009.

Jeurnink SM, van Eijck CHJ, Steyerberg EW, et al: Stent versus gastrojejunostomy for the palliation of gastric outlet obstruction: a systematic review, *BMC Gastroenterology* 7:18, 2007.

Kazanjian KK, Hines OJ, Duffy JP, et al: Improved survival following pancreaticoduodenectomy to treat adenocarcinoma of the pancreas: the influence of operative blood loss, *Arch Surg* 143:1166–1171, 2008.

Moss AC, Morris E, MacMathuna P: Palliative biliary stents for obstructing pancreatic carcinoma, Cochrane Upper Gastrointestinal and Pancreatic Diseases Group, *Cochrane Database Syst Rev* (2):CD004200, 2006.

Mullen JT, Lee JH, Gomez HF, et al: Pancreaticoduodenectomy after placement of endobiliary metal stents, *J Gastrointest Surg* 9:1094–1104, 2005.

Yip D, Karapetis C, Strickland A, et al: Chemotherapy and radiotherapy for inoperable advanced pancreatic cancer, *Cochrane Database Syst Rev* (3):CD002093, 2006.

Adjuvant and Neoadjuvant Therapy of Pancreatic Cancer

John P. Hoffman, MD

OVERVIEW

The recommendations for adjuvant therapy (AT) for pancreatic cancer have undergone several changes since the first trials over 30 years ago. Back then, we had the almost universal certainty that postoperative radiation therapy (RT) along with bolus 5-fluorouracil (5-FU), both during and after the radiation therapy, was the preferred and optimal regimen. This first prospective randomized trial was published in 1985. Although the conclusions of the trial were accepted worldwide, critics have noted the extended time to perform the trial and the small number of patients, such that the conclusions of the trial have become less widely accepted.

There have been two other trials since then with a surgery-only control group: one from the European Organization for Research and Treatment of Cancer (EORTC), with an attenuated adjuvant program without postchemoradiation chemotherapy, and another from the European Study Group for Pancreatic Cancer (ESPAC 1), where four groups were compared: surgery only, surgery plus chemotherapy, surgery plus chemoradiotherapy, and surgery plus chemotherapy plus chemoradiotherapy. Unfortunately, we are left with more questions than answers, since the ESPAC 1 trial showed a definite superiority in survival for those treated with adjuvant chemotherapy alone and a definite disadvantage for those receiving chemoradiotherapy alone. Surprisingly, the group receiving chemoradiotherapy had inferior survival to those receiving no adjuvant therapy of any kind. The EORTC trial was not helpful because the conclusion, that chemoradiotherapy was no better than surgery alone, was not clear. The group with pancreatic cancer actually receiving adjuvant treatment was small, but the trend clearly favored the group receiving it (two-sided P value of .09). These two trials apparently have convinced European cooperative groups, because all further trials of adjuvant therapy regimens have included chemotherapy only.

Meanwhile, the only phase III trial in North America compared two chemotherapy regimens given before and after the same chemoradiotherapy regimen. The trial was unique for including intensive radiation therapy quality control. The initial concept was to test whether gemcitabine would be superior to 5-FU in the adjuvant setting, as it was in the metastatic setting. Initial results showed improvement in the gemcitabine arm, but the latest analysis shows no difference between 5-FU and gemcitabine.

The Charité Onkologie Hospital (CONKO) 001 trial has provided support for the findings of the ESPAC 1 trial, in that adjuvant chemotherapy alone proved superior to treatment without adjuvant therapy. The CONKO-001 study randomized patients who had pancreatic cancer resections to no further therapy or 6 months of gemcitabine. Most of those randomized to no further therapy were then given gemcitabine at recurrence. The initial reports found no overall survival differences between the groups, but a later report showed statistically significant differences in survival between the groups, favoring those receiving the drug in the immediate postoperative period. Formal, final publication of these results are still not in, a year after the verbal presentation. The trial was unique in that CA 19-9 levels less than 90 were used as an entry criterion, meaning that these patients were less likely to harbor residual cancer than those in prior trials. This criterion will most likely, and should, be used in all future trials of adjuvant therapy. In fact, a lower level would probably be even better.

There has been only one positive phase III (controlled randomized) trial for those with stage IV disease in the past decade, the phase III trial of gemcitabine versus gemcitabine plus erlotinib, which demonstrated a small survival advantage for the combination. RTOG 0848, a phase III Intergroup trial, is current testing it as well as chemoradiotherapy in the postoperactive adjuvant setting.

Many phase II trials of postoperative adjuvant therapy regimens have been conducted, by both institutional and cooperative groups (Table 1). The most striking aspect of such trials is that an inverse relationship is seen between the number of patients in a trial and the median survival. This emphasizes the importance of well-conducted, large trials (preferably phase III) upon which to base both present recommendations as well as future trial directions.

The best reported median survival rates for postoperative adjuvant therapy have been for the regimen of postoperative chemoradiotherapy with Interferon A, cisplatin, and 5-FU developed by Picozzi and colleagues. This has been tested both by an American College of Surgeons Oncology Group (ACOSOG) trial and a separate, single-institution trial at Barnes Medical Center, which confirmed good efficacy along with significant toxicity. However, the overall 5-year survivals have not reached the very high level (45%) originally reported by Picozzi and colleagues.

NEOADJUVANT THERAPY

Neoadjuvant therapy for pancreatic adenocarcinoma was first conceived and demonstrated in the late 1970s. Chemotherapy was added to the preoperative radiation therapy within the next decade. The sequencing of adjuvant chemotherapy or chemoradiation therapy before resection has two fundamental advantages: 1) the patient is assured adjuvant therapy (15% to 20% of those who have surgery first are not able to receive adjuvant therapy because of weakness, postoperative complications, or disease recurrence); and 2) patients who have aggressive micrometastatic disease at primary cancer discovery have a 3-month window in which to manifest metastases and thereby avoid a surgical resection that would not be helpful. The fundamental disadvantage is that the initial pathological stage of the tumor remains unknown because of the alteration of tumor, nodal, and margin status by the neoadjuvant therapy. Problems with biliary stent occlusion and consequent cholangitis are also a disadvantage, but they can be overcome, either by rapid stent replacement or by the initial placement of metal stents.

Several institutional and cooperative group phase II experiences of various neoadjuvant approaches have been reported (Table 2). The best of these was from Evans and colleagues from the M.D. Anderson Cancer Center (MDACC), where 86 patients with clearly resectable cancers determined by radiologic imaging were given both gemcitabine alone and radiation therapy with attenuated gemcitabine prior to surgical resection. Of these, one patient refused surgery, three had debilitation severe enough to disallow surgery, and eight displayed liver or peritoneal metastases during the preresection stage. Liver or peritoneal metastases were found in nine of the remaining 74 patients at laparoscopy (n = 1) or laparotomy (n = 8), and one patient refused to have surgery, leaving 64 patients who had a pancreatic resection. No patient was seen to develop locally unresectable disease during the preoperative treatment program, and one patient died of multiorgan failure after a pancreatic leak. Median survival for those 64 patients was 34 months, and their 5-year survival was 36%.

There are no mature phase II experiences with postoperative adjuvant gemcitabine and radiation therapy that can rival this MDACC

TABLE 1: Phase II trials of postoperative adjuvant therapy regimens

Author (Year)	n	Radiation Therapy	Chemotherapy Type	% Node+	% Margin+	Median OS (Mo)	5-Yr Survival
GITSG (1985)	21	Yes	5-FU	30	0	21	19%
ESPAC 1 (2004)	75	No	5-FU, leukovorin	N/A	N/A	21.5	29%
RTOG 9704 (2008)	221	Yes	Gemcitabine	68	35	20.6	N/A
CONKO 1 (2007)	179	No	Gemcitabine	70	19	22.1	22.5%
Picozzi (2004)*	43	Yes	IntA/CDDP/5-FU	84	19	44	45%
Linehan (2008)	53	Yes	IntA/CDDP/5-FU*	76	33	25	N/A

*Gemcitabine used after radiotherapy rather than infusional 5-FU (Picozzi protocol)
OS, Overall survival; 5-FU, 5-fluorouracil; IntA, interferon A.

TABLE 2: Institutional and Cooperative Group Phase II experiences of various neoadjuvant approaches

Author	n	RT?	Chemo Type	% Node+	% Margin+	Median OS (Mo)	5-Yr Survival
Hoffman (1995)	25	Yes	5-FU/MitoC	18	9	45	40%
Hoffman (1998)	53	Yes	5-FU/MitoC	21	68	15.7	N/A
Pisters (1998)	35	Yes	5-FU	65	10	25	N/A
Varadhachary (2008)	52	Yes	Gem/CDDP	60	23	31	28%
Evans (2008)	64	Yes	Gem	38	26	34	36%

RT, Radiation therapy; OS, overall survival; Gem, gemcitabine; 5-FU, 5-fluorouracil; MitoC, mitomycin-C

experience. However, this was a highly selected group of patients, and those with borderline resectable lesions were rejected from the study. This borderline resectable category of patients, with lesions intermediate between clearly resectable and clearly unresectable pancreatic cancers, has only recently been articulated. It is quite possible that the patient database for many of the past trials of adjuvant and neoadjuvant therapy comprised patients with borderline resectable lesions, which may account for much of the difference in outcome. In fact, there were many phase II trials for neoadjuvant therapy that allowed entry of patients with initially unresectable cancers. Accordingly, our conclusions regarding the type of adjuvant therapy, the types of drugs as well as the presence or absence of radiation therapy, and the sequencing strategy may be less certain than we had previously thought.

Borderline Resectable Category

This category, intermediate to clearly resectable and locally advanced unresectable, was first published early in the decade by the National Comprehensive Cancer Network (NCCN, see Table 3). It has since been refined by NCCN and the MDACC. Essentially, a lesion seen abutting the superior mesenteric artery (SMA) or hepatic artery for less than 180 degrees or one occluding a reconstructable, short segment of the superior mesenteric vein (SMV) or portal vein (PV) is determined by most surgeons to be not removable with clear margins unless presurgical adjuvant therapy is delivered. The NCCN and MDACC category A definitions for borderline resectable cancer consist entirely of imaging characteristics and differ only in that the NCCN category includes lesions that severely narrow the PV or SMV. A consensus panel of experts has offered a third definition, which varies by including those with any narrowing of the SMV

TABLE 3: NCCN classifications of resectability

Resectability Category	SMA, HA, Celiac Axis	PV, SMV
Clearly resectable	Clear fat plane around	No occlusion or near occlusion
Borderline resectable	<180 degree abutment	Near occlusion or occlusion, reconstructable
Locally advanced, unresectable	>180 degree abutment	Occlusion, not reconstructable

or portal vein by any tumor. Since the definitions vary, it will be important for any writer to express which is being used.

MDACC has defined two other categories of borderline resectability. Category B includes those with a high likelihood of harboring metastatic disease (patients with prior explorations, or needle biopsies that demonstrated positive regional nodal disease, or those with imaging characteristics with suspicious but unproven evidence for distant disease). Category C comprises patients who are not strong enough to undergo surgical resection initially, but who are believed to have the capacity to regain that strength after completion of neoadjuvant therapy.

This "borderline resectable" category needs to be studied and further refined. To make progress, there will need to be close cooperation among radiologists, surgeons, and pathologists so that close margins called by the radiologist can be resected and marked by the surgeon and inspected by the pathologist. Furthermore, biologic parameters such as CA 19-9 and other novel markers can and should be integrated into the category. However, at this time there is evidence that patients in this category have lower resectability rates than those with clearly resectable cancers, yet over one third can eventually attain significant long-term survival (36% 5-year survival) with neoadjuvant therapy and resection.

COMPARISONS BETWEEN ADJUVANT AND NEOADJUVANT THERAPY

No phase III trials have been performed that have attempted to compare results with neoadjuvant therapy to those with postoperative adjuvant therapy. An ongoing phase III trial in Europe is examining preoperative chemoradiotherapy versus surgery alone, and both groups receive postoperative chemotherapy, but there have been no intermediate publications.

Comparing phase II experiences is very risky. A phase III trial of sequencing alone would require hundreds of patients to be intensively studied from the time of registration by a large group of surgeons with equipoise (no bias toward either strategy). Even though doing such a study would be remotely possible, the question of finding better adjuvant regimens has greater priority. However, the very mature series from MDACC have by far the longest survival of any phase II experiences with gemcitabine-based chemoradiotherapy in adjuvant therapy for patients with clearly resectable pancreatic cancer. Moreover, those with borderline resectable cancers are best addressed with neoadjuvant approaches. Since the Picozzi regimen seems to be superior to other regimens in the postoperative setting, we eagerly await trials of the interferon A/cisplatin/5-FU/radiotherapy regimen in the neoadjuvant setting.

Current Trials and Plea for Accrual

There are a few recently closed, ongoing, or imminent phase III or randomized phase II trials examining postoperative adjuvant regimens. However, none meet all of the criteria suggested by Wolff for an optimal trial of adjuvant therapy (pretreatment high-quality CT or MRI, defined radiographic criteria for resectability, a standardized system for the evaluation of surgical margins, and postoperative imaging before enrollment). The ESPAC 3 trial has recently been completed and presented, showing no difference between postoperative adjuvant gemcitabine and postoperative 5-FU with folinic acid (median survival 23.6 months versus 23 months).

The latest intergroup trial of postoperative adjuvant therapy opened in the fall of 2009, a phase III trial of postoperative gemcitabine versus postoperative gemcitabine and erlotinib. A second randomization was used for chemoradiation therapy versus no chemoradiation after both completion of chemotherapy and another CT scan. ACOSOG is currently doing a phase II trial of preoperative gemcitabine and erlotinib for patients with clearly resectable pancreatic cancers. Those with borderline resectable cancers are ineligible.

At least one single-institution trial, in addition to the multiinstitutional ACOSOG Z5041 trial, is looking at preoperative therapy without radiation therapy ("A Phase II Study of Neoadjuvant Gemcitabine and Oxaliplatin in Patients with Potentially Resectable Previously Untreated Pancreatic Adenocarcinoma: Protocol 07-113," Memorial Sloan-Kettering Cancer Center). Unlike the ACOSOG trial, it accepts patients with borderline resectable lesions. Both of these may be premature in omitting RT, as there is only one (flawed) phase III trial, ESPAC 1, that showed a decrease in median survival for those treated with radiation therapy. Certainly, most experts recommend radiation therapy in a neoadjuvant setting for borderline resectable cancers.

Some may have inferred that since the median survival for patients treated by chemotherapy alone in the CONKO-001 trial was superior or equal to those treated in trials containing RT, that RT is unneeded or perhaps harmful. If so, there are two important

facts that they are overlooking: First, the eligibility requirements for CONKO-001 (postresection CA19-9 less than 90 units) selected patients with the most optimal prognoses; thus, their survival should have been superior. Second, resectional surgery for pancreatic cancer seldom achieves surgical margins of more than a few millimeters, thus radiation therapy would be expected to be helpful. The new intergroup trial will be very important in its examination of the role of RT in the modern adjuvant treatment of pancreatic cancer. Most of the studies of new agents in patients with stage IV disease have been discouraging. Bevacizumab and cetuximab have shown no benefit in phase III trials. The only trial showing progress was a European phase III trial of gemcitabine versus Folfirinox (5-FU, oxaliplatin, and irinotecan), which showed a near tripling of response rates and a near doubling of overall survival.

There are many single-institution phase II trials examining various chemotherapy plus RT regimens. It is hoped that they will transparently identify and stratify the clearly resectable, borderline resectable, and locally advanced, unresectable groups such that regimens that are superior can be identified so they can be brought to the forefront in phase III testing. The surgical community will be absolutely essential to the enterprise. First, surgeons must be involved in the ordering and reading of images that classify tumors according to resectability status. For those patients with borderline or locally advanced unresectable cancers, referral and accrual into clinical trials of neoadjuvant regimens is paramount. For those with clearly resectable lesions, prompt and expert resections and reconstructions are key, with swift referral after recovery from surgery into clinical trials of postoperative AT. Also crucial is the processing of the resected specimen such that surgical margins can be identified and examined by the pathologist, and appropriate tissue can be harvested for translational research studies.

SUMMARY

Advances in the adjuvant and neoadjuvant therapy of pancreatic cancer are sorely needed. Pancreatic surgeons will be essential for success in this endeavor.

SUGGESTED READINGS

Evans DB, Varadhachary GR, Crane CH, et al: Preoperative gemcitabine-based chemoradiation for patients with resectable adenocarcinoma of the pancreatic head, *J Clin Oncol* 26:3496–3502, 2008.

Kalser MH, Ellenberg SS: Pancreatic cancer. Adjuvant combined radiation and chemotherapy following curative resection, *Arch Surg* 120:899–903, 1985.

Katz MH, Pisters PW, Evans DB, et al: Borderline resectable pancreatic cancer: the importance of this emerging stage of disease, *J Am Coll Surg* 206:833–846, 2008.

Linehan DC, Tan MC, Strasberg SM, et al: Adjuvant interferon-based chemoradiation followed by gemcitabine for resected pancreatic adenocarcinoma: a single-institution phase II study, *Ann Surg* 248:145–151, 2008.

Neoptolemos JP, Stocken DD, Friess H, et al: A randomized trial of chemoradiotherapy and chemotherapy after resection of pancreatic cancer, *N Engl J Med* 350:1200–1210, 2004.

Oettle H, Post S, Neuhaus P, et al: Adjuvant chemotherapy with gemcitabine vs observation in patients undergoing curative-intent resection of pancreatic cancer: a randomized controlled trial, *JAMA* 297:267–277, 2007.

Wolff RA, Varadhachary GR, Evans DB: Adjuvant therapy for adenocarcinoma of the pancreas: analysis of reported trials and recommendations for future progress, *Ann Surg Oncol* 15:2773–2786, 2008.

Unusual Pancreatic Tumors

Charles M. Vollmer Jr, MD, Tara S. Kent, MD, and Mark P. Callery, MD

OVERVIEW

Historically, the vast majority of pancreatic operations have been performed for either malignant pancreatic ductal adenocarcinoma (PDAC) or for benign symptomatic chronic pancreatitis. However, in a contemporary specialty pancreatic surgical practice, other less prevalent lesions may comprise up to half of all resections performed. The inclusion of these lesions as valid surgical indications is justified by two phenomena: First, in the modern era of pancreatic surgery—that is, the last 30 to 40 years—considerable experience has been accrued to indicate which diseases will benefit from resection and which will not. This knowledge was garnered in an era in which preoperative diagnostics was not up to today's standards, so many "masses" were resected without a good idea of the actual diagnosis. Natural history of these processes was therefore understood through a trial-and-error basis. Second, the advent and refinement of state-of-the-art axial imaging and endoscopic diagnostics has ushered in the era of the *asymptomatic pancreatic lesion*, otherwise known as the "pancreatic incidentaloma." Through this technology, numerous lesions are being identified whose courses are less well defined, particularly cysts, and whose evaluation and treatment remain to be refined.

Although diagnostics have come a long way, obtaining an accurate and final diagnosis still frequently requires surgical resection in far too many circumstances. This chapter introduces some of these less appreciated lesions and discuss optimal diagnostic and therapeutic approaches to managing them.

PANCREATIC CYSTS

In the last decade, pancreatic cystic lesions have come to the forefront in pancreatic surgery; they account for a significant number of referrals and, ultimately, resections. Cysts cause consternation for surgeons due to inaccurate diagnostics, ill-defined natural histories, and significant consequences for inappropriately performed operations. Analysis of cysts should be approached systematically and categorically. Inflammatory pseudocysts are the most common cysts of the pancreas, and their management is outlined elsewhere in this text. On the other hand, the category of neoplastic cysts is now recognized to account for up to 50% of pancreatic cysts.

In general, three categories of pancreatic cysts exist: 1) mucinous cysts, 2) serous cysts, and 3) all others. Neoplastic cysts can further be classified into dysplastic (premalignant) and frankly malignant variants. Mucinous cysts can be broken down into *intraductal papillary mucinous neoplasms* (IPMNs), *mucinous cystadenomas* (MCAs), and *nondysplastic mucinous cysts* (NDMCs). Serous lesions are dominated by *serous cystadenomas* (SCAs) but also include the exceedingly uncommon *serous cystadenocarcinoma*. Most cysts in the "other" category are actually malignancies that uncharacteristically demonstrate cystic morphology. Many of the more commonly encountered cystic entities are delineated below, with the exception of IPMN, which is developed elsewhere in this text.

Serous Cystadenoma

Despite being the best-characterized pancreatic cystic neoplasm, which is readily identified by current axial imaging techniques, SCAs continue to vex surgeons, as these neoplasms are all too frequently misdiagnosed and removed unnecessarily. They account for only 1% of *all* pancreatic neoplasms but make up a far larger proportion (one third) of *cystic* neoplasms. They are ubiquitous throughout the entire gland and can show up in various sizes and morphologies. Most are completely innocuous and asymptomatic, but larger lesions have the capability of obstructing the bile duct and causing jaundice, obstructing the pancreatic duct and causing pancreatitis, or interfering with the outflow tract of the stomach, leading to gastric outlet obstruction. This occurs not by invasion but rather by space-filling, compressive impingement, or an associated local inflammatory effect. With larger lesions, epigastric abdominal pain can be a prelude to these more overt symptoms. Like many pancreatic cystic pathologies, SCAs are found more frequently in females but usually at a later age than other cystic pathologies, which are typically found from the seventh decade on.

SCAs are benign lesions with a true epithelium lined with glycogen-rich, clear, cuboidal cells that stain positive for periodic acid-Schiff (PAS). They do not communicate with the pancreatic ductal system. Imaging displays a characteristic thin-walled capsule with a microcystic pattern with thin-walled septa. Most SCAs are readily identified by one of two characteristic imaging findings (Figure 1): either a "starburst" pattern of a central scar, which is often calcified, or a more common "ground glass," "cluster of grapes," or honeycomb appearance. Fine needle aspirate (FNA) analysis of the cyst fluid yields a clear, serous fluid low in CEA and mucin content. However, cytology obtained from these lesions sometimes shows atypia, which leads to diagnostic uncertainty and operative intervention that unfortunately proves to be inappropriate.

A variant of the overwhelmingly benign SCA is serous cystadenocarcinoma, believed to represent a malignant degeneration of SCA. In the handful of such cases described in the literature (fewer than 10), this entity has been defined by the presence of metastatic carcinoma in the presence of a primary lesion that otherwise appears identical to an SCA. In that an SCA is a benign neoplasm that is not dysplastic, observation is the rule for asymptomatic lesions. Natural history studies indicate that some will increase in size over time (approx 0.5 cm/year), but cysts larger than 4 cm in diameter may progress at a greater pace (2 cm/year) and are more likely to eventually cause symptoms. In this case, growth indicates progressive fluid accumulation in the cyst as opposed to accumulating dysplastic tissue (solid components), as is the scenario in other cystic neoplasms of the pancreas.

Although most SCAs are simply observed, surgical intervention is indicated for certain SCAs, namely, any cyst that is clearly symptomatic and perhaps for larger cysts—on an individual, case-by-case basis—given their propensity for rapid growth. As mentioned earlier, far too often these lesions are disappointingly diagnosed after resection for what was presumed to be a more aggressive entity, such as MCA or side-branch IPMN. This is on account of the fact that a second, less distinct morphology exists for SCAs—the macrocystic form (Figure 1, D). Although preserving the same histologic epithelial features, these lack the classic features described above and have larger, more discrete cystic cavities separated by obvious septa. Often, these are smaller (1 to 4 cm) lesions that occur at a younger age (40s), found more frequently in the head of the pancreas and more often in males. Such features all add up to confusing these lesions with MCAs and IPMNs, which are more threatening lesions due to their premalignant propensities. Distinguishing SCAs from these lesions is a primary management dilemma, given the current epidemic of incidentally identified cysts. Often the distinction can be made by the identification of mucin and/or elevated CEA levels by FNA, along with careful scrutiny for any of the clinical and radiographic features suggested above.

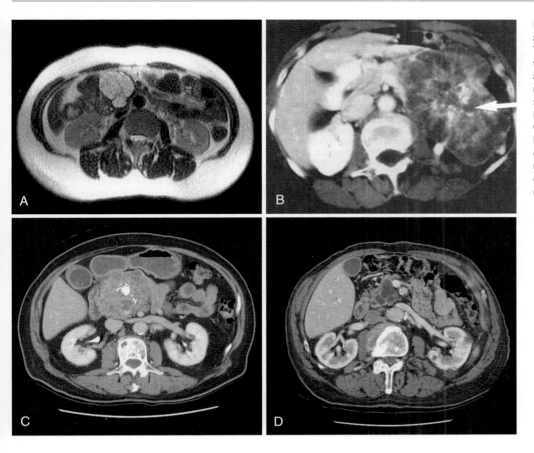

FIGURE 1 The variable appearances of SCAs. **A,** T2-weighted MRI image shows the most common "honeycomb" appearance from numerous microcysts. **B,** Classic "stellate scar" in a large lesion in the tail of the pancreas. **C,** Internal calcification. **D,** The less common but clinically challenging macrocystic morphology, which is commonly confused for a mucinous neoplasm.

Mucinous Cystadenoma

MCA is a dysplastic neoplasm with clear-cut malignant potential, and it represents 2% of all pancreatic neoplasms but up to a quarter of all cystic neoplasms. Classically, MCAs are single, large (<5 cm), thick-walled cysts lined with mucin-secreting columnar epithelium; they have no communication with the pancreatic ductal system, distinguishing them from IPMNs (Figure 2, A). Pathologically, they are defined by the distinct "ovarian" type stroma within their capsule, which can only be determined histologically after surgical resection (Figure 2, B). There is an outright female predilection, and tumors are most commonly situated in the body and tail of the organ; a mucinous cystic lesion situated in the head of the pancreas should be considered to be more likely an IPMN. The usual clinical scenario is of a younger woman in her 40s to 50s, although MCA is often seen in women in their teens and 20s, who complains of with vague abdominal pain. However, these tumors are more commonly identified incidentally, and sometimes they are giant, growing to over 10 cm.

Diagnosis is commonly made by axial imaging (CT or MRI) that reveals either a single unilocular lesion (more common) or a smaller, macrocystic multilocular lesion with septations. Sometimes the wall contains calcium, a finding that adds to diagnostic confusion with chronic pseudocysts, which also can be calcified. In general, MCAs are most often misdiagnosed as pseudocysts, and it is common to see patients in whom internal drainage operations were initially employed only to have persistent symptoms and cysts recur on account of neoplastic progression. To avoid this problem, begin with a careful consideration of the clinical history. EUS with cyst aspirate (FNA) is helpful, as it can demonstrate a viscous, string-like nature to the mucin-rich fluid. Furthermore, a CEA level over 200 from the cyst aspirate is strongly indicative of mucinous etiology but not necessarily malignant transformation, whereas pseudocyst fluid

is generally extremely high in amylase activity. Finally, cyst aspirate cytology can be obtained to determine whether invasive malignancy is present. Findings of "consistent with malignant cells" are reliable when present, whereas "atypical" or "nondiagnostic" descriptors are not as trustworthy.

As is the case for IPMN, its mucinous cystic cousin, MCA, is dysplastic and has been observed to follow an adenoma-to-carcinoma sequence of degeneration that ends in invasive malignancy. In fact, numerous series in the literature of MCA resections show that close to 50% of cases are either high-grade dysplasia or frankly invasive. The latter condition equates to the diagnosis of mucinous cystadenocarcinoma. Identification of mural nodules, calcifications, positive aspirate cytology, or distant metastatic spread should alert the surgeon to this possibility. For this reason, it is suggested that *all* suspected MCAs be surgically resected in suitable operative candidates, a policy supported by the International Association of Pancreatology through their Sendai Consensus Conference Guidelines. It should be emphasized, however, that the natural history of these mucinous cystic neoplasms is poorly defined, and, in particular, it is near impossible to predict the pace of the progression and if or when malignant degeneration will occur.

MCA is amenable to definitive surgical resection, usually accomplished by a distal pancreatectomy (now more commonly achieved laparoscopically in select cases), given their most common position in the pancreas. However, smaller lesions may be suited for "targeted" parenchymal-sparing pancreatectomy or even enucleation. If margins are completely clear, recurrence after resection of a noninvasive MCA does not occur, nor is there a threat of "another" MCA developing in the remnant pancreas. These are generally solitary lesions. However, mucinous cystadenocarcinomas follow an oncologic trajectory similar to invasive PDAC, and they should be considered for adjuvant therapy and close surveillance following resection.

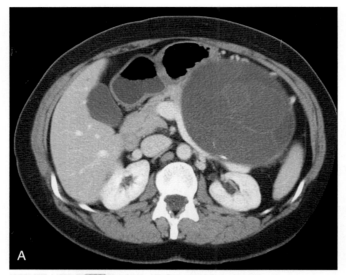

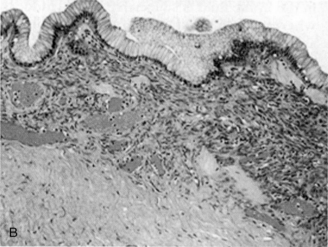

FIGURE 2   A, This large MCA situated in the tail of the pancreas showed up as a palpable mass in an otherwise healthy, asymptomatic 22-year-old woman. Notice the macrocystic appearance with internal septations. **B,** The classic histologic appearance of MCA demonstrating mucinous columnar epithelium with dysplastic features associated with characteristic "ovarian" type stroma.

Solid Pseudopapillary Tumor

Solid pseudopapillary tumor (SPT), a moniker defined by the World Health Organization (WHO) in 1996, is a unique entity that goes by many other names in the literature, including *Frantz tumor, Hamoudi tumor,* and *papillary* or *cystic tumor.* The third most prevalent cystic neoplasm of the pancreas (10%), it is yet another rare pancreatic neoplasm overall (1% to 2%), with fewer than 500 cases reported in the literature, and most single series include fewer than 25 patients. Although usually benign, SPT can be aggressive, with invasion of local structures, and it has certain malignant and even metastatic potential in around 5% of patients. Distant spread occurs most commonly to the liver and peritoneal cavity; lymphatic spread has also been recognized but is not consistent.

A diagnosis of SPT should be considered for young patients (40 and younger; mean age, 27 years) who show a large pancreatic mass (mean size, 11 cm), usually focused in the body or tail. Most reported cases have been female (10:1 ratio); and interestingly, there is a bimodal age distribution, with SPT occurring in young children

as well. The tumors are generally asymptomatic, but they can cause abdominal pain, nausea, vomiting, or palpable masses when they become excessively large. With so few tumors described, prognostic factors for malignancy and survival are lacking.

Due to their amorphous appearance, characterized by significant patchy areas of hypodensity on CT scans (Figure 3, *A*), SPTs are often categorized as cystic in etiology. This is, however, false. The cystic appearance reflects necrotic degeneration of the primary cytoarchitecture, solid papillary vascular stalks that slough and hemorrhage as the tumor progresses in size. Diagnosis by imaging is aided by attention to the four Cs: *c*ircumscribed, *c*ystic-appearing lesion with a *c*apsule that is often internally *c*alcified. There are no distinct tumor markers, and the tumor does not produce a paraneoplastic syndrome.

Because of this tumor's largely necrotic composition, FNA biopsies are usually unrewarding. Histologic analysis features sheets of polygonal epithelial cells with prominent stalks and an incohesive appearance (Figure 3, *B*). Foamy histiocytes and cholesterol crystals are common. The histologic progenitor cell is undefined, and there are lines of evidence to support genesis from each of the endothelial, epithelial, or mesenchymal lineages. However, a consistent immunophenotype is observed, with vimentin, neuron-specific enolase, and α_1-antitrypsinase expression being near universal.

Given their unpredictable but real metastatic potential, SPTs should be operatively resected. Although tumors may be extremely large, and they generally impinge on vital structures, they can invade critical vasculature but usually are completely resectable. Obviously, negative margins are desired, and they are typically attainable. Cure rates higher than 90% can be achieved following total resection with clean margins, which reflects the fact that many of these lesions are noninvasive. However, it is probably prudent to follow patients after resection with axial imaging, given the potential for distant spread.

An aggressive approach to both synchronous and metachronous metastatic disease to the liver and elsewhere is justified, especially because most patients are generally young and healthy. Adjuvant therapies that include 5-FU–cisplatin, streptozosin, or radiotherapy for advanced disease unamenable to surgical clearance have been applied in selected circumstances.

Lymphoepithelial Cysts

Lymphoepithelial cysts (LCEs) are exceedingly rare (less than 75 reported cases), totally benign lesions that cause diagnostic and therapeutic consternation. Despite their large size (usually more than 5 cm), they are generally asymptomatic and are discovered throughout the gland, most often through axial imaging performed for other reasons in 60- to 70-year-old patients. Unlike other cystic lesions, there is a definite fourfold male predominance.

Imaging features include either unilocular or multilocular morphology with an enhancing fibrous rim. Similar to MCAs, these cystic cavities are not in communication with the ductal system. The cyst contents are complex and contain keratin, cholesterol, and other debris that is sloughed from the epithelial lining. MRI can be useful in distinguishing these from other cystic lesions by identifying bright, high-signal keratin on T1-weighted images. This is the opposite scenario in most cysts, where static fluid exhibits a bright signal during the T2 phase. Furthermore, the lipid content of the cholesterol can be discerned by MRI.

Histology of these lesions is unique. As its name implies, there is a combination of lymphoid stromal tissue surrounding a stratified squamous epithelial lining. The cyst cavity is cluttered with keratinized debris. EUS analysis of the cyst fluid will often demonstrate high levels of tumor markers (CEA, Ca 19-9) and sometimes amylase. However, as opposed to mucinous lesions with dysplasia and malignant potential, analysis of the fluid aspirate from an LCE will not display mucin but rather may demonstrate the histologic hallmarks of this lesion: squamous cells, lymphocytes, and cholesterol.

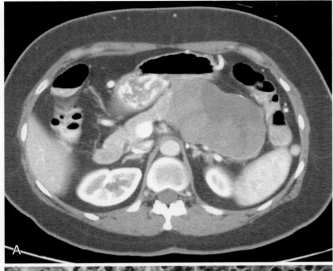

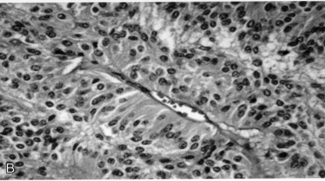

FIGURE 3   **A,** Solid pseudopapillary tumor of the distal pancreas in a 41-year-old woman. Note the typical large size and heterogenous appearance indicative of internal cystic degeneration from necrosis and sloughing of the pseudopapillas. **B,** Histologic appearance of a pseudopapilla showing crowded sheets of cells arranged around vascular stalks. As the tumor enlarges, these cells slough from their vascular supply and cause necrosis, which simulates cystic qualities on axial imaging.

If a diligent analysis yields any of this evidence in an asymptomatic scenario, observation is appropriate management. However, for LCEs that cause pain or obstruction, surgical options exist. Complete resection through partial pancreatectomy may be necessary based on individualized factors; yet given the benign nature and natural history of these particular cysts, internal drainage operations are a reasonable alternative, but only if the correct diagnosis is made.

Nonneoplastic Mucinous Cysts

Common dogma that *every* mucinous cyst of the pancreas is dysplastic, and therefore has a certain malignant potential, has lead to a general policy of resection for all such lesions. However, in our specialty pancreatic surgical practice, we have recently encountered a number of nonneoplastic mucinous cysts (NMCs) of the pancreas that have yet to be described in the literature. Over the course of two and a half years, 67 resections were performed for suspected cystic neoplasms at our institution, with IPMNs, SCAs, and MCAs predominating. Of these, six cases of mucinous cysts, devoid of dysplastic features, were identified, representing 9% of all resected cysts and 13.3% of the 45 cysts of mucinous etiology. Mean age was 71 years, and five of the six patients were women. Although two thirds of the cysts were

identified incidentally and their size was relatively small (2 cm average), preoperative clinical and radiographic features of these NMCs were indistinguishable from more onerous lesions. Fine needle aspiration cytology was *atypical* in all cysts that were analyzed in this fashion. Histologically, these NMCs demonstrated a simple columnar mucinous epithelium with a pancreatobiliary phenotype but lacked dysplasia, ovarian stroma, or papillary growths. Unfortunately, these lesions masquerade clinically, radiographically, and biochemically as true mucinous cystic *neoplasms* of the pancreas, which leads to surgical resection, perhaps unnecessarily. It is yet uncertain whether these cysts are entirely benign or whether they represent part of the suspected neoplastic spectrum of mucinous cysts.

Autoimmune Pancreatitis

Autoimmune pancreatitis (AIP) is a particularly important albeit unusual condition of the pancreas, in that when properly recognized, it is treated medically and not surgically. The primary dilemma is that it presents as a mass effect in the pancreas, which mimics adenocarcinoma both radiographically and clinically. At the advent of this disease, this fact led to most cases being diagnosed only through pathologic analysis of resected specimens following major pancreatectomy. More recently, other criteria that rely heavily on characteristic clinical, radiologic, and biochemical findings have allowed for less invasive diagnosis management.

Often referred to as *lymphoplasmacytic sclerosing pancreatitis* (LPSP), this condition reflects an autoimmune destruction of the pancreatic parenchyma that is likely mediated by both humoral and cellular components. It is common for the patient or their family members to suffer from other autoimmune conditions such as PSC, inflammatory bowel disease, Sjögren syndrome, psoriasis, retroperitoneal fibrosis, sarcoid, and others. The clinical picture is variable: some patients have overt symptoms—jaundice, pancreatitis, progressive pain, and endocrine or exocrine insufficiency suggestive of malignancy—others have more subtle findings such as weight loss, anorexia, fatigue, and lethargy. These symptoms may take months to develop and manifest, distinguishing LPSP from the more sudden presentations that occur with pancreatic malignancy. The clinical picture is distinctly different from generic acute pancreatitis from other causes; in fact, serum elevation of pancreatic enzymes, although possible, is not typical.

On imaging, AIP often appears as if the whole pancreas is "full" with a hypoenhancing mass effect that resembles a sausage with a characteristic enhancing rim, indicative of local edema. However, there can also clearly be focal hypoenhancing CT appearances that more often resemble pancreatic adenocarcinoma. Sometimes, evidence of autoimmune disease in other abdominal or thoracic organs is recognized (Figure 4). ERCP or MRCP will show structuring of the intrapancreatic, and sometimes extrapancreatic, common bile duct, as well as focal, segmental, or diffuse strictures of the pancreatic duct. Notably, the pancreatic duct usually seems diminutive and beaded and is rarely dilated.

Diagnostic suspicion by imaging studies should be confirmed by either serologic or histologic means. A specific subtype of serum immunoglobulin (IgG4) that is unique to AIP, as opposed to other pancreaticobiliary inflammatory processes, is often elevated (in 70% of patients) but not always. Other markers, such as anticarbonic anhydrase and antilactoferrin antibodies, are emerging as useful. Histologic confirmation is more troublesome, as EUS-based FNA sampling is notoriously inaccurate. In some patients we have performed laparoscopic ultrasound-guided core biopsies to obtain certainty in a minimally invasive fashion. The last resort, of course, is open biopsy or, ultimately, pancreatic resection. Plasma cell infiltration of the pancreas, frequently IgG4 positive, with ductocentric inflammatory destruction is characteristic of this diagnosis.

Optimal diagnosis of this heterogenous disease is in constant flux. The Mayo clinic has recently proposed advanced diagnostic

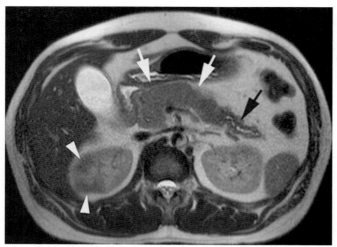

FIGURE 4   Axial T2-weighted image of the abdomen shows diffuse enlargement and loss of the normal acinar pattern in the head, neck, and body of the pancreas (*white arrows*). There is upstream dilatation of the pancreatic duct and atrophy of the gland in the tail (*black arrow*). Note the hypointense ill-defined lesions in the kidneys (*white arrowheads*) consistent with lymphoplasmacytic infiltrates. Both the pancreatic findings and renal infiltrative lesions improved with therapy.

TABLE 1: Mayo Clinic extended diagnostic criteria for autoimmune pancreatitis

Imaging

Pancreas mass/enlargement, focal pancreatic duct stricture, pancreatic atrophy, pancreatic calcification, or pancreatitis

Serology

Elevated serum IgG4 level

Histology

At least one of the following: periductal lymphoplasmacytic infiltrate with obliterative phlebitis and storiform fibrosis or lymphoplasmacytic infiltrate with storiform fibrosis *and* abundant IgG4 positive cells (>10 cells/high power field)

Other Organ Involvement

Hilar/intrahepatic biliary strictures, persistent distal biliary stricture, parotid/lacrimal gland involvement, mediastinal lymphadenopathy, retroperitoneal fibrosis

Response to Steroid Therapy

Resolution or marked improvement of pancreatic/extrapancreatic manifestation with steroid therapy

Modified from *Curbside consultation of the pancreas*, Thorofare NJ, 2010, Slack.

guidelines that incorporate not only the original classification system of the Japanese Pancreas Society (imaging, serology, and histology), but also other organ involvement and/or response to steroid therapy (Table 1). From this, three categories of patients seem to segregate: 1) those with characteristic histology, 2) those who satisfy classic imaging features along with elevated IgG4 titers, and 3) those whose disease process responds to therapy in the setting elevated IgG4 levels or unexplained pancreatic disease.

Treatment consists of high-dose systemic corticosteroids (prednisone 40 mg/day) until symptoms resolve, followed by a slow taper. If successful, repeat imaging at 4 to 6 weeks will demonstrate dramatic changes for the better. The natural history of AIP over the long term is, so far, poorly defined. Most patients can be totally weaned off their steroids, but clinical recurrence can occur in about 25%. For those patients, another cycle of treatment may be necessary, and some patients even require lifelong therapy or conversion to another immunosuppressant, such as azathioprine. In cases of jaundice, biliary strictures are treated first with temporary endobiliary stents and will often completely resolve within a few months of initiating steroid therapy. If no change is observed in either radiographic appearance, serum IgG4 levels, or stricture morphology, then a misdiagnosis of AIP should be entertained, and malignancy should be strongly considered instead. In certain cases of initial diagnostic uncertainty, inability to obtain an accurate histologic diagnosis, or failed medical treatment, surgical resection is required; however, this should be a rare event these days, unlike in the past, when this entity was less well defined.

Acinar Cell Carcinoma

Acinar cell carcinoma (ACC) has unique characteristics that distinguish it from other pancreatic tumors, both unusual and common. As more experience accrues with this rare (less than 2%) pancreatic tumor, it appears that its biology is more favorable than PDAC. It is diagnosed earlier (mid 50s) and is found more frequently in males; the tumors are larger at diagnosis (around 5 cm), and they lead to nonspecific symptoms such as weight loss, pain, and bloating. Jaundice is not as ubiquitous. On CT evaluation, these tumors mimic hypodense PDACs, but the tumor borders are often less discrete, sometimes showing hyperenhancement. On gross inspection they are fleshy, rather than infiltrative; upon histologic review they often resemble neuroendocrine tumors with clusters of cells and hemorrhagic and necrotic areas. Immunohistochemistry analysis can distinguish between the two entities: pancytokeratin stains strongly for both, but ACC does not express chromogranin or synaptophysin.

What makes ACC even more interesting is the regular generation and release of lipase by the tumor. This lipase expression can act as a tumor marker, as it regresses with surgical resection of the primary tumor; but similar to other tumor markers, it has no role in predicting ultimate survival. Alpha-fetoprotein is similarly expressed by some of these tumors and serves a similar role in postresection surveillance.

ACC is generally diagnosed postoperatively after thorough histologic review. Evidence continues to accrue indicating a more favorable prognosis when compared with PDAC. One multiinstitutional series of 17 patients showed 1- and 5-year survival rates of 92% and 53%, respectively, with a median survival of 61 months in resected cases. In another population-based review of 672 patients with ACC, 16% had localized disease, 26% had regional disease, and 58% had distant metastases; patients with locoregional ACC were more likely to be resectable when compared with PDAC. In this broader patient sample, the authors reported 5-year survival for ACC to be as high as 72%, markedly better than the survival for PDAC (17%); and even 22% of unresectable ACC cases lived 5 years. Given a clear propensity for metastases, adjuvant chemoradiotherapy might contribute to this improved survival, and there is even a report of neoadjuvant conversion from an originally unresectable to a resectable tumor; however, no uniform adjuvant therapy has emerged because of the rarity of this particular malignancy.

Pancreatic Lymphoma

Although the actual occurrence of pancreatic lymphoma may be a once-in-a-career event for most surgeons, it is necessary to consider it in any workup for a pancreatic mass, given its unique treatment requirements. Non-Hodgkin's lymphoma can certainly manifest in any non-nodal tissue throughout the body, but it is highly uncommon in the pancreas.

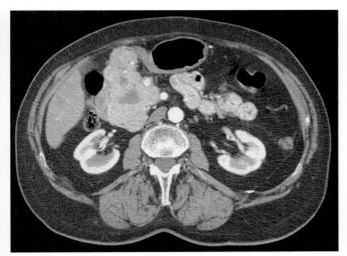

FIGURE 5   The typical appearance of a bulky, lobular primary lymphoma situated in the pancreatic head.

The clinical picture is vague and features weight loss, nausea and vomiting, pain, and sometimes other B symptoms (fever, sweats). Usually, the patient proceeds to axial imaging for workup of these nonspecific abdominal complaints, and the appearance is of a bulky lesion with considerable local lymphadenopathy, findings that exceed what can be expected for pancreatic adenocarcinoma (Figure 5). Jaundice and back pain are surprisingly absent, given the size of the observed mass. Laboratory values, including white blood cell count, are generally normal, but an elevated lactate dehydrogenase may provide a clue. Such an atypical lesion will usually proceed to EUS evaluation, and FNA is reliable in obtaining enough tissue to secure the diagnosis under a skilled cytopathologist's purview.

The primary and best therapy for this condition is systemic chemotherapy, not surgical resection. The prevalent regimen is cyclophosphamide, adriamycin, vincristine, and prednisone, or *CHOP*, which can literally disintegrate the bulky disease. Complete remissions occur in around 75% of patients with early-stage contained disease. Improved outcomes are now evident with the addition of targeted biologic therapies in addition to the CHOP approach, especially for more diffuse, advanced disease.

Surgeons will generally rue the decision to operate on bulky pancreatic lymphoma, as resection is both technically challenging and fraught with potential complications that can impair the patient's recovery. However, a report from the Johns Hopkins University describes a few cases of early, smaller lymphomas that were resected under the assumption that they were actually pancreatic adenocarcinomas. Interestingly, these have resulted in complete 5-year remissions.

Metastatic Lesions

Very few cancers metastasize to the pancreatic parenchyma, and this scenario represents well under 1% of all pancreatic resections performed. The best characterized of these is renal cell carcinoma (RCC), but melanoma, breast, lung, colon, and gynecologic malignancies have also been recognized. For the most part, metastatic tumors to the pancreas are indicative of advanced-stage disease of the primary tumor, with a dismal overall prognosis. Therefore complete and thorough staging appropriate for the specific primary tumor in question should be undertaken to determine if the pancreatic lesions are indeed isolated.

Most of these metastases characteristically present as *hypervascular* tumors rather than the more common hypoenhancing appearance of adenocarcinoma of the pancreas. Accordingly, these can be

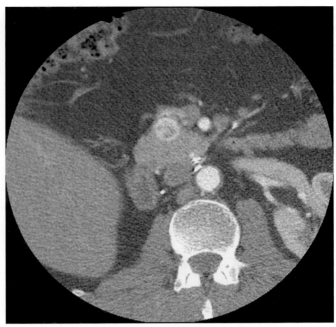

FIGURE 6   A solitary, well-circumscribed renal cell carcinoma (RCC) metastatic to the pancreatic head demonstrates characteristic hypervascularity. This asymptomatic lesion presented 8 years after the index nephrectomy through active cancer surveillance.

confused with other rare conditions in the pancreas, including ectopic splenules or primary neuroendocrine tumors. When in doubt, definitive tumor diagnosis may be obtained via EUS-guided FNA, but it is generally not required if there is an established cancer diagnosis of RCC, melanoma, or breast cancer already.

RCC is the most common and best understood of these metastatic tumors. Most are metachronous, and there is often a long disease-free interval, greater than 10 years in many cases, from the primary nephrectomy to discovery of metastases, which often occurs incidentally on serial cancer surveillance. What makes it even more unique, and validates aggressive surgical resection, is the fact that many patients achieve long survivals (more than 5 years) after pancreatectomy. RCC appears as discrete hypervascular masses (Figure 6), which may be situated anywhere in the pancreas and may even be multiple. In suitable operative candidates, it is reasonable to proceed with targeted pancreatectomy based on the extent and position of the lesions.

As a general rule for all metastatic lesions to the pancreas, as with RCC, surgical interventions are appropriate for instances where the disease is confined to the pancreas and there is no systemic burden otherwise in good candidates. More frequently, however, concurrent metastatic disease is found elsewhere in the body, thus surgical resection has little positive impact and more likely has negative consequences in light of a limited life span. However, these cases should be considered on an individual basis, as sometimes the lesions present in a symptomatic fashion, which requires pancreatic resection (such as transfusion-dependent upper gastrointestinal bleeding or frank hemorrhage). Furthermore, with the advent of new biological adjuvant therapies for RCC and melanoma, strategies that rely on surgical debulking of dominant large tumor burden are gaining favor.

Selected Readings

Sachs T, Pratt WB, Callery MP, et al: The incidental asymptomatic pancreatic lesion: Nuisance or threat? *J Gastrointest Surg* 13(3):405, 2009.
Tseng JF, Warshaw AL, Sahani DV, et al: Serous cystadenoma of the pancreas: tumor growth rates and recommendations for treatment, *Ann Surg* 242:413, 2005, discussion 419.

Tanaka M, Chari S, Adsay V, et al: International consensus guidelines for management of intraductal papillary mucinous neoplasms and mucinous cystic neoplasms of the pancreas, *Pancreatology* 6:17, 2006.

Wisnoski NC, Townsend CM Jr, Nealon WH, et al: 672 patients with acinar cell carcinoma of the pancreas: a population-based comparison to pancreatic adenocarcinoma, *Surgery* 144(2):141, 2008.

Vollmer CM, Dixon E, Grant DR: Management of a solid-pseudopapillary tumor of the pancreas with liver metastases, *HPB* 5:264-267, 2003.

Tenner S, Brown A, Gress FG: *Curbside consultation of the pancreas: 49 clinical questions*, Thorofare, NJ, 2009, Slack.

Reddy S, Edil BH, Cameron JL, et al: Pancreatic resection of isolated metastases from nonpancreatic primary cancers, *Ann Surg Oncol* 15(11):3199, 2008.

Demirjian AN, Vollmer CM, McDermott DF, et al: Refining indications for contemporary surgical treatment of renal cell carcinoma metastatic to the pancreas, *HPB* 11(2):150, 2009.

INTRADUCTAL PAPILLARY MUCINOUS NEOPLASMS OF THE PANCREAS

C. Max Schmidt, MD, PhD, MBA,
Joshua A. Waters, MD, and Keith D. Lillemoe, MD

OVERVIEW

Cystic lesions of the pancreas are a common clinical entity found at autopsy, and radiographic studies have demonstrated an incidence of up to 25% of the general population for such lesions. The increased frequency of detection of incidental pancreatic cystic lesions may in part be explained by technological advances and by the broad use of cross-sectional imaging, specifically, computed tomography (CT) and magnetic resonance imaging (MRI). This has led to an increased rate of referral to pancreatic surgical specialists reaching an almost epidemic rate over the last 5 years.

Paramount in the management of pancreatic cysts is accurate characterization and diagnosis, as the behavior and aggressiveness varies significantly with cyst type. Arguably the most threatening of the cystic neoplasms of the pancreas are intraductal papillary mucinous neoplasms (IPMNs). These lesions were initially described in the early 1980s by Ohashi and colleagues and were eventually characterized by the World Health Organization in 1996. More recently, in 2006, the *International Consensus Guidelines (ICG)* for Management of IPMNs of the Pancreas provided diagnostic and treatment recommendations for this disease. Today, IPMNs represent a relatively new clinical entity, so our approach continues to evolve and in many aspects remains poorly understood. The goal of this chapter is to highlight the current state of knowledge with respect to diagnosis and management of IPMNs.

DEFINITION AND PATHOLOGY

IPMNs are defined histologically as mucin-producing, papillary cystic lesions of the pancreatic ductal system. IPMNs are pathologically distinguished from the other pancreatic mucinous cystic neoplasm, mucinous cystadenoma, by lack of the characteristic ovarian-type stroma and by continuity with the pancreatic ductal system (Figure 1).

Topography

IPMNs may develop anywhere within the pancreatic ductal system but, by definition, they must be in continuity with the pancreatic ductal system. IPMNs are generally classified based upon the extent of

main pancreatic duct (MPD) involvement. *Branch*-type IPMNs lack MPD involvement and represent the most common variant, accounting for approximately 70% of all cases. Arguably, differentiation of main duct involvement is the single most important clinicopathologic feature with regard to oncologic risk stratification, as the probability of harboring invasive IPMNs is 30% to 50% when the MPD is involved.

The distribution of IPMNs may be diverse. Branch-type IPMNs may be unifocal or multifocal, segmental or diffuse and may involve all pancreatic regions: head, neck, body, and tail. They may be contiguous or discontiguous; they may skip regions, evidencing involvement of head and tail with a sparing of the neck and body. Branch-type IPMNs can also vary in shape from a tubular, broad-based branch to circular to grapelike clusters of small cysts associated with multiple minor pancreatic duct branches. Main duct IPMNs can be diffuse or segmental but have not been reported to be noncontinuous. They occur most commonly in the head of the pancreas (60% to 70%) but may occur in any region of the gland. Though very important with regard to operative planning, the role of cyst location and number has not consistently been associated with cyst behavior. Paradoxically, some authors have asserted that increased side-branch cyst burden is associated with decreased oncologic risk, and an increased cyst number may lead to earlier symptom presentation, earlier diagnosis, and a reduced rate of malignancy.

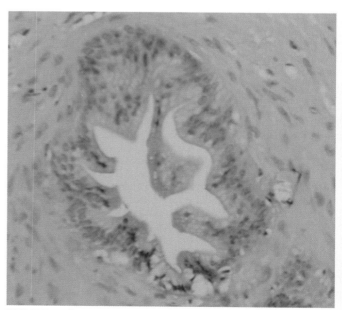

FIGURE 1 Permanent section of hematoxylin and eosin stained Whipple specimen demonstrating frondlike papillary epithelium consistent with IPMN.

Dysplasia

IPMNs are stratified based on degree of *dysplasia*. The grading schema used to classify IPMNs from a histologic standpoint has evolved over time. Currently, IPMNs are divided histologically into low-grade, high-grade, or invasive lesions. Low-grade lesions vary with regard to the presence of papillary epithelium, with the lowest grades having flat, columnar, mucinous epithelium. High-grade lesions (carcinoma in situ) are characterized by papillary epithelium, high mitotic activity, and loss of nuclear polarity. Invasive IPMNs can be divided into colloid (50%) and tubular (50%) adenocarcinomas. Invasive colloid (mucinous type) IPMNs are characterized by extensive pools of extracellular mucin and demonstrate less aggressive biology and an indolent course. In contrast, invasive tubular IPMNs are virtually identical pathologically and prognostically to typical ductal adenocarcinoma.

Genetics

Genetic abnormalities associated with IPMNs are similar to those seen in typical pancreatic ductal adenocarcinoma. Loss of heterozygosity in the *K-ras* oncogene is common, and disruption of p53 tumor suppression is seen more typically in high-grade dysplastic or invasive lesions. Alternatively, the *SMAD4* gene mutation commonly seen in pancreatic ductal adenocarcinoma is rarely seen in IPMN.

DIFFERENTIAL DIAGNOSIS

The diagnosis of IPMN is often difficult, largely because numerous other cystic lesions (inflammatory or neoplastic) arise within the pancreas, many of which have similar clinical and radiographic features. Differentiation of these lesions is important, as they each behave differently with regard to natural history and oncologic risk. Pseudocysts may mimic IPMNs in the setting of recurrent or severe pancreatitis. This may be problematic, as patients with IPMNs may present with symptoms of pancreatitis.

The neoplastic pancreatic cysts can be divided generally into benign or potentially malignant cysts. Benign lesions include serous cystadenoma, lymphoepithelial cyst, and simple pancreatic cysts. These lesions may cause symptoms and may warrant resection if they become large, but rarely do they present a cancer risk. Premalignant and malignant cystic lesions of the pancreas include solid pseudopapillary neoplasm (SPN), also known as *Hamoudi tumor;* mucinous cystic neoplasm (MCN), or mucinous cystadenocarcinoma; and cystic neuroendocrine tumors. All of these entities tend to show up at a younger age than IPMN, in the third and fifth decades of life for SPN and MCN respectively, and in both cases, the disease is predominant in females. In contrast to many other cystic lesions of the pancreas, IPMN appears to have slight male gender prevalence.

CLINICAL PRESENTATION

IPMN most commonly occurs in the sixth or seventh decade of life, and advancing age is associated with increased risk of IPMN malignancy. Male gender is also an independent risk factor associated with invasive IPMN.

The clinical manifestations of IPMN are variable. One of the most common presentations for IPMN (30% to 60%) is as an asymptomatic lesion found incidentally on cross-sectional imaging performed for another indication. The early symptoms of IPMN are commonly subtle and include vague pain, pressure, or tenderness in the epigastrum or back. Presumably this occurs either because of local compressive effects or mild pancreatitis from mucus plugging the pancreatic duct. Clinical acute pancreatitis, usually mild, or recurrent pancreatitis may also be a common initial occurrence. Patients may also demonstrate signs of endocrine or exocrine pancreatic insufficiency. Pancreatic endocrine insufficiency may manifest as new or worsening diabetes mellitus. Exocrine insufficiency may be present as bloating, flatulence, steatorrhea, weight loss (in the presence or absence of steatorrhea), or malnutrition. Finally, obstructive jaundice may be an initial symptom, but it is seen typically in patients with invasive IPMN. Although physical findings are generally absent in most patients with noninvasive IPMN, patients with advanced invasive IPMN have symptoms similar to those seen with advanced pancreatic adenocarcinoma: jaundice, profound weight loss, and cachexia (Table 1).

DIAGNOSIS AND PREOPERATIVE EVALUATION

Diagnosis and characterization of the malignant potential of cystic lesions of the pancreas may be facilitated by a thorough history, noninvasive imaging, and endoscopy. Due to the wide variability in behavior of these lesions and the considerable morbidity associated with pancreatectomy, accurate diagnosis of IPMN and characterization of its malignant potential are paramount in determining an optimal treatment or surveillance strategy.

CT Versus Magnetic Resonance Cholangiopancreatography

Following appropriate history and physical examination, the primary modality for the initial diagnosis and characterization of IPMN is cross-sectional imaging. CT and magnetic resonance cholangiopancreatography (MRCP) predominate with regard to diagnosis and characterization of IPMN. Although diagnosis of IPMN may be made by either modality, MRCP is superior in establishing certain diagnostic criteria, including multifocality and pancreatic ductal continuity (Figure 2). Both modalities are comparable in characterizing malignant radiographic features such as mural nodules, associated masses, vascular invasion, adjacent organ invasion, lymph node and distant organ metastases, and peritoneal carcinomatosis. MRCP, however, provides a more accurate assessment of MPD involvement and quantification of lesion numbers, both important factors in oncologic risk stratification and operative planning.

Endoscopy

Endoscopy has become a mainstay in IPMN diagnosis and in characterization of IPMN malignant potential. On endoscopic analysis, the presence of mucin extruding from a patulous, gaping ampulla of Vater is a pathognomonic finding of IPMN (Figure 3).

Endoscopic ultrasound (EUS) can be used to identify IPMN but is considered suboptimal imaging when compared with MRCP, and the quality is largely operator dependent. The most significant benefit of EUS, however, is the ability to perform fine needle aspiration (FNA) for cytologic sampling of cyst fluid and of any concerning areas of soft-tissue growth (mural nodules, associated mass) within or adjacent to the IPMN. EUS-guided FNA facilitates analysis of cyst fluid for markers such as CEA, amylase, *K-ras* mutation, and loss of heterozygosity (LOH). These may provide clues to the likelihood that a pancreatic cyst is intraductal (cyst amylase exceeds serum amylase), mucinous (CEA >250 ng/mL, *K-ras* mutation), or malignant (*K-ras* mutation and LOH). EUS-FNA may provide a definitive cytopathologic diagnosis of IPMN and may characterize its malignant potential (low-grade atypia, high-grade atypia, adenocarcinoma); it remains the single most predictive test for malignancy in IPMN. Although the presence of high-grade atypical or adenocarcinoma cells on EUS-FNA is highly specific for malignancy, it is not particularly sensitive for carcinoma in situ largely because of sampling error.

Endoscopic retrograde cholangiopancreatography (ERCP) and *pancreatic ductoscopy* may be employed selectively in the evaluation of

TABLE 1: Demographics and symptoms in noninvasive and invasive IPMN

	Noninvasive IPMNs	Invasive IPMNs	P Value
Demographics			
Mean age (yr)	63 (low grade) 67 (moderate to high grade)	68	.08
Gender (% male)	61	52	NS
Race (% white)	90	87	NS
Presenting Signs/Symptoms			
Nausea/vomiting	21%	2%	.002
Acute pancreatitis	13%	12%	NS
Abdominal pain	51%	54%	NS
Obstructive jaundice	7%	33%	<.001
Weight loss/cachexia	20%	44%	.002
Diabetes	20%	30%	NS

NS, not significant
Modified from Sohn TA, Yeo CJ, Cameron JL, et al: Intraductal papillary mucinous neoplasms of the pancreas: an updated experience, *Ann Surg* 239:788-797, 2004; and Schmidt CM, White PB, Waters JA, et al: Intraductal papillary mucinous neoplasms: predictors of malignant and invasive pathology, *Ann Surg* 246(4):644-654, 2007.

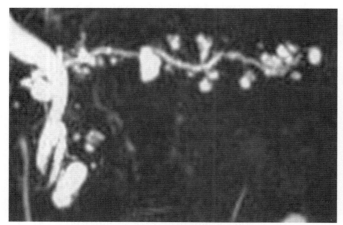

FIGURE 2   MRCP of a multifocal branch-type IPMN.

IPMN. These endoscopic modalities are very sensitive for detecting IPMN involvement of the MPD. With these modalities, direct visualization, duct brushings, and biopsies of the MPD epithelium may be performed (Figure 4). Limitations of ERCP include its inability to adequately fill contrast into branch pancreatic ducts and sometimes MPD during the ductogram, especially in the presence of significant mucin plugging, thereby reducing its sensitivity for detection of branch duct and MPD lesions, particularly those in the pancreatic tail. Pancreatic ductoscopy is limited in its inability to navigate smaller caliber MPDs.

Fluorodeoxyglucose Positron Emission Tomography

A few retrospective series have demonstrated high sensitivity and specificity of fluorodeoxyglucose positron emission tomography (FDG-PET) for predicting invasive cancer within cystic lesions and specifically IPMN. Patients with FDG-avid components within IPMN are highly likely to have high-grade dysplastic or invasive IPMN, though this remains investigational.

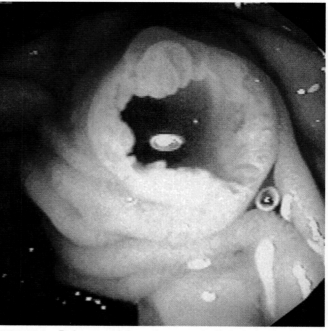

FIGURE 3   Endoscopy of the pathognomonic finding of mucin extruding from the ampulla of Vater.

Indications for Resection

Decisions regarding surgical intervention in IPMN should be driven primarily by patient symptomatology and oncologic risk stratification. Surgical resection may be indicated in patients to relieve symptoms such as abdominal pain and recurrent pancreatitis regardless of oncologic risk. In these patients, it is important to rule out etiologies other than IPMN (e.g., cholelithiasis, peptic ulcer disease,

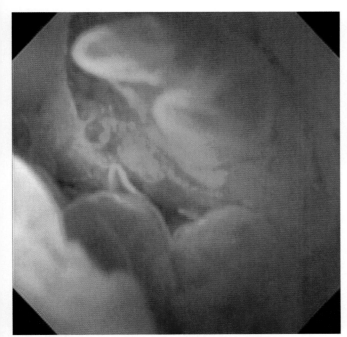

FIGURE 4 Peroral pancreatic ductoscopy demonstrating epithelial changes of IPMN in situ.

gastroesophageal reflux, and irritable bowel disease) for such non-specific and common symptoms.

More commonly, surgical resection is indicated in IPMN with high malignant potential regardless of symptom profile. Essentially all patients with MPD involvement who are suitable candidates for major surgery should undergo resection because of a high rate of malignancy, which can approach 50% (Figure 5). Resection should be strongly considered in patients without MPD involvement (Figure 6) who have any of the following: 1) symptoms attributable to IPMN, including steatorrhea, weight loss, new onset or worsening diabetes, and jaundice; 2) concerning radiographic features, including a mural nodule, thick (more than 2 mm) septa, pancreatic duct stricture, cysts so numerous that surveillance is difficult, or associated mass; 3) positive cytopathology (high-grade atypia or adenocarcinoma); or 4) a family history of pancreatic adenocarcinoma, such as two first-degree relatives with pancreatic cancer or one first-degree relative with pancreas cancer and one with IPMN (Table 2). Resection should also be strongly considered in patients with positive pancreatic cyst fluid markers (K-*ras* mutation and loss of heterozygosity both present, CEA more than 1000 ng/mL) or serum markers (progressive elevation of serum CA 19-9 with absolute value more than 100 ng/mL). Cyst size greater than 3 cm remains a relative indication for resection based on the ICG recommendations, though neither size alone nor increase in size over time has been consistently correlated with risk of malignancy (Figure 7).

For unfit patients, endoscopic ablation with alcohol or paclitaxel may be considered. Alternatively, meticulous surveillance may be performed until more definitive evidence of malignancy, such as positive cytopathology or positive FDG-PET, justifies operative intervention.

OPERATIVE MANAGEMENT

Operative management begins with a discussion regarding the unique aspects of IPMN including cancer risk, treatment, surveillance, postoperative progression or recurrence, and possibility of eventual completion pancreatectomy. Patients should be informed of the possibility of intraoperative conversion of segmental pancreatic resection to more extensive resection or even total pancreatectomy

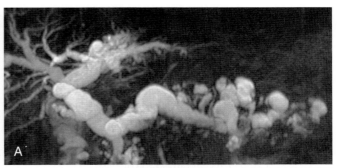

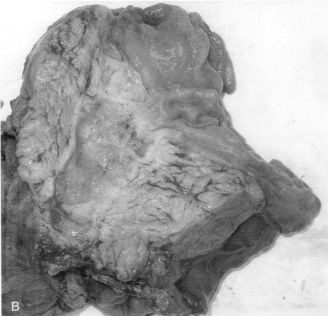

FIGURE 5 **A,** IPMN involvement of the main pancreatic duct as seen on MRCP. **B,** Surgical specimen showing invasive IPMN involving the main pancreatic duct.

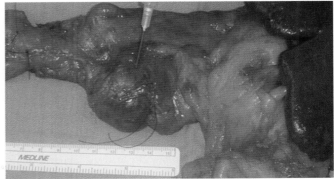

FIGURE 6 Distal pancreatectomy specimen demonstrating a large, branch-type IPMN.

based upon intraoperative margin status. Patients with a significant chance of total pancreatectomy should also be counseled in regard to exocrine pancreatic insufficiency and the importance of exogenous pancreatic enzyme supplementation. These patients should also undergo preoperative counseling with an endocrinologist to become familiar with a diabetic diet, glucometer technique, and glucose management. Social barriers to successful diabetic management

TABLE 2: Surveillance protocol: Low risk or high risk

Low Risk

No symptoms attributable to cyst

No concerning radiographic features

Family history of pancreatic cancer *without* an index pancreas lesion

Two first-degree relatives with pancreas cancer

One first-degree relative with pancreas cancer and one with IPMN

Baseline MRCP, EUS, serum Ca19-9, Ha1C

Surveillance annually with history/physical, MRI-MRCP, and serum CA19-9, Ha1C, alkphos (in head lesions)

High Risk*

Family history of pancreatic cancer *with* an index pancreas lesion

Two first-degree relatives with pancreas cancer

One first-degree relative with pancreas cancer and one with IPMN

Symptoms attributable to cyst (steatorrhea, weight loss, diabetes, jaundice, pain, pancreatitis)

Worrisome radiographic features

Main duct dilation ≥5 mm

Mural nodule(s) or thick (≥2 mm) septa

Pancreatic duct stricture

Quantity of cysts so numerous that surveillance is difficult

Size 3 cm or greater

Associated mass

Greatest diameter increase by ≥5 mm for lesions ≥1 cm since last surveillance

Doubling of size for lesions <1 cm since last surveillance

Concerning cytopathology or surgical pathology

High-grade atypia

Surgical pathology (prior resection): High-grade dysplasia or invasive disease

DNA analysis (KRAS mutation and loss of heterozygosity)

Rising serum CA19-9; absolute value serum CA19-9 >100 ng/mL

Rising alkphos or bilirubin total

Rising Ha1C (±)

Baseline MRCP, EUS, serum CA19-9, Ha1C, alkphos

Surveillance every 3 to 6 months with history/physical, MRI-MRCP, and serum CA19-9, Ha1C, and likely EUS-FNA every 1 to 2 years

*If fit, many will be offered surgery; if unfit or surgery averse, they may be offered cyst ablation.

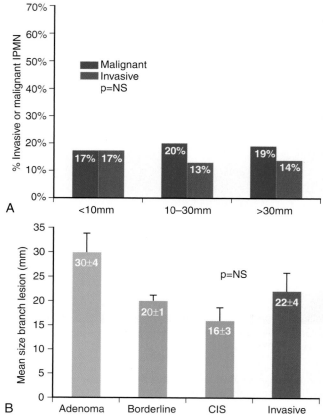

FIGURE 7 **A,** Incidence of branch-type IPMN with malignant (*gray bars*) or invasive (*black bars*) disease, according to International Consensus Guideline (ICG) size categories. **B,** Mean size of lesions according to dysplastic grade. *(From Schmidt CM, White PB, Waters JA, et al: Intraductal papillary mucinous neoplasms: predictors of malignant and invasive pathology, Ann Surg 246[4]:644-654; 2007.)*

Due to the high frequency of multifocal IPMN (50% to 60%), the dilemma of which lesion to remove often arises. In these cases, it is often appropriate to address the dominant or most threatening lesions and plan radiographic surveillance of the remaining gland. The dominant or most threatening lesion is typically the lesion with main duct involvement, mural nodularity, associated mass, pancreatic duct stricture, or positive cytopathology. If there is concern over multiple threatening lesions diffused throughout the pancreas, FDG-PET-CT may be helpful in discrimination. Total pancreatectomy under such circumstances may be reasonably considered.

Currently, a number of minimally invasive operations, such as laparoscopic pancreatectomy, are being utilized in highly selected patients at specialized pancreatic centers. Specifically, laparoscopic distal pancreatectomy is being implemented more commonly and has demonstrated a reduction in postoperative morbidity without compromising the adequacy of resection.

Parenchymal-sparing operations (central pancreatectomy and enucleation) may be used in carefully selected patients. Central or middle pancreatectomy has been employed for neck lesions to spare pancreatic parenchyma, compared with a more formal, distal pancreatectomy. Enucleation for isolated side-branch lesions may also be employed in selected cases to avoid more formal segmental pancreatectomy. Enucleation has a high risk of pancreatic fistula due to the typically small ductal connection with these lesions. The role of these parenchyma-sparing approaches remains unclear with respect to adequacy of resection, and close surveillance after resection is necessary.

Regardless of the type of pancreatectomy, margin assessment via frozen-section analysis is an important component of operative

should also be weighed in decisions to offer patients the option of total pancreatectomy.

Intraoperative management traditionally involves one of three approaches: 1) distal pancreatectomy, 2) pancreaticoduodenectomy, or 3) total pancreatectomy. The surgical approach to IPMN of the pancreas should focus on the type, location, and extent of disease. Operative planning relies heavily on preoperative imaging, and ultrasound may be employed intraoperatively to complement preoperative imaging. Total pancreatectomy is associated with increased perioperative mortality and significantly increased short- and long-term morbidity when compared to segmental pancreatectomy. For these reasons, this approach should be reserved for fit patients with extensive MPD involvement; extensive, multifocal, diffuse, branch-duct involvement with high suspicion of malignancy; or with invasive IPMN, where R0 resection cannot be achieved with segmental resection.

decision making. In patients undergoing segmental pancreatectomy, a reasonable effort should be made to achieve a negative pancreatic margin. Some authors have reported positive IPMN margins in up to 30% of noninvasive IPMN and 10% of invasive IPMN initial frozen-section margins. Invasive or high-grade dysplastic disease identified on frozen-section margin should result in re-resection, and potentially even conversion to total pancreatectomy, to achieve microscopically negative margins. Leaving low-grade IPMN at the surgical margin should be weighed against the potential increased morbidity of extending the resection on a patient-by-patient basis. Although achievement of negative margins should be strived for, leaving low-grade IPMN, particularly in branch ducts, has not proven to add significant cancer risk. Furthermore, the necessity of long-term surveillance is not obviated despite margin-negative resection, and the incremental oncologic risk does not justify such an aggressive approach.

Postoperative management should include all of the provisions for major abdominal surgery and is comparable to pancreatic resections for other conditions. Overall, perioperative mortality is comparable, and postoperative morbidity appears to be unchanged, with largely similar rates of pancreatic fistula, biliary leak, and delayed gastric emptying compared with similar resections for pancreatic adenocarcinoma. Not uncommonly, patients with IPMNs require pancreatic enzyme supplementation postoperatively, and patients routinely require exogenous insulin, administered intravenously or subcutaneously, to regulate serum glucose intraoperatively and postoperatively.

Follow-up and Surveillance

Because of the variable behavior of IPMN and significant differences with regard to malignant potential, the appropriate follow-up and surveillance of IPMN can be complex. Generally, surveillance can be subdivided into primary surveillance for those patients not undergoing initial resection and secondary surveillance of the pancreatic remnant in those patients undergoing subtotal pancreatectomies for IPMN.

The first group is primarily composed of patients who are asymptomatic and lack significant associated risk factors for malignancy (no MPD involvement) or patients in whom the risk of pancreatic resection exceeds the expected risk of malignancy in the lesion. In younger patients with low-risk IPMN, prolonged surveillance would result in a costly and burdensome approach, and early resection should be considered based on patient and surgeon discretion.

Given the indolent course of the disease, and the bias toward surgical resection, data regarding primary surveillance is limited. Salvia and colleagues observed 89 patients with low-risk branch-type IPMN based on ICG recommendations for 32 months. During this period 6% of the IPMNs increased in size and underwent resection, none of which ultimately had malignant pathology. Annual focused history and physical examination, measurement of serum CA 19-9, and cross-sectional imaging with either CT or MRCP is appropriate. In addition, EUS–FNA for those branch-type lesions that enlarge or develop a solid mass component is a useful adjunct to this approach.

Patients who have undergone resection for their IPMN should be closely followed postoperatively for recurrence or progression of disease. Patients with invasive disease must be followed for evidence of both metastatic and local recurrences, whereas the remnant gland must be followed in all patients for "new" lesions. The frequent multifocal and multicentric nature of IPMN raises the possibility that "benign" recurrences or new foci of disease are just a progression of small lesions that were not detected on preoperative imaging.

Postresection patients can be subdivided into those with known IPMN in the remnant (positive IPMN at the surgical margin or radiographically evident disease) and those with no disease evident in the remnant pancreas. The first group should undergo resection of the most concerning lesion and be generally left with histologically low-grade disease at the surgical margin or known low-risk disease, based on imaging characteristics, in the remaining pancreas. These patients can be followed similarly to those patients undergoing primary surveillance.

In patients with no evidence of remaining disease after a resection, the appropriate follow-up is controversial. A surveillance plan should be developed based principally on tumor pathology from the initial operation, and it should be modified based on patient factors such as age and potential to tolerate a completion pancreatectomy.

The rate of subsequent cancer development in patients with noninvasive initial pathology is 8% to 10% at 5 years. In contrast, patients with invasive initial lesions demonstrate recurrence, often in the form of metastatic disease, of 50% to 65% at 5 years. Consequently, patients with high-grade lesions (carcinoma in situ or invasive carcinoma) should be serially imaged at least every 6 to 12 months initially. If no evidence of recurrent disease arises by 3 years, this interval could be lengthened, though further prospective study is warranted to refine this approach.

PROGNOSIS

A favorable prognosis is seen in those patients with low- and high-grade dysplastic lesions, in which a resection encompassing all visible disease can be performed. Many series have demonstrated disease-specific survival at or approaching 100% at 5 years.

The prognosis following resection of invasive IPMN reflects the malignant nature of the disease, with 5 year survival following resection between 35% to 60% (Figure 8). Interestingly, invasive IPMN appears to have a significantly improved prognosis when compared with typical pancreatic ductal adenocarcinoma. Much of the difference has been attributed to IPMN-associated cancer being diagnosed at an earlier AJCC stage with a lower rate of lymph node metastases (30% to 50%). Additionally, IPMN uncommonly invades surrounding vascular structures, making vascular reconstruction a much less common component of the therapy. New observational data suggest that the biology of IPMN-associated carcinoma may be less aggressive with a more indolent course, even when factors such as pathologic stage, extent of disease, and lymph node involvement are taken into account. Currently, adjuvant chemotherapy or chemoradiation protocols mimicking regimens typically used for pancreatic cancer

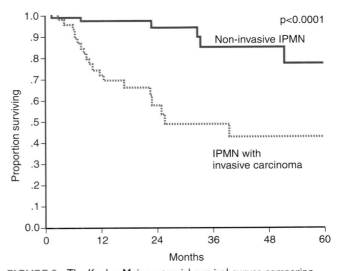

FIGURE 8 The Kaplan-Meier actuarial survival curves comparing patients with noninvasive intraductal papillary mucinous neoplasms (IPMNs, *n* = 84) to patients with IPMNs with invasive carcinoma (*n* = 52, *P* < .0001). *(From Sohn TA, Yeo CJ, Cameron JL, et al: Intraductal papillary mucinous neoplasms of the pancreas: an updated experience, Ann Surg 239:788-797; 2004.)*

are being offered to patients with invasive IPMN, though no prospective data exist to support this practice given the rarity of this disease.

Concomitant Extrapancreatic Malignancy

Several investigators have described a significant association between those patients with IPMN and subsequent development of other gastrointestinal malignancies, including gastric and colorectal cancers. This phenomenon has been described in up to one third of IPMN cases. Additionally, familial cohorts of patients have been described, suggesting a possible relationship to hereditary pancreatic cancer in these patients. Importantly, clinical suspicion for associated malignancy should be maintained in these patients, which may present an additional role for PET scans in evaluating for concomitant malignancy in IPMN.

SUGGESTED READINGS

D'Angelica M, Brennan MF, Suriawinata AA, et al: Intraductal papillary mucinous neoplasms of the pancreas: an analysis of clinicopathologic features and outcome, *Ann Surg* 239:400, 2004.

Katabi N, Klimstra DS: Intraductal papillary mucinous neoplasms of the pancreas: clinical and pathologic features and diagnostic approach, *J Clin Pathol* 61:1303–1313, 2008.

Sohn TA, Yeo CJ, Cameron JL, et al: Intraductal papillary mucinous neoplasms of the pancreas: an updated experience, *Ann Surg* 239:788–797, 2004.

Schmidt CM, White PB, Waters JA, et al: Intraductal papillary mucinous neoplasms: predictors of malignant and invasive pathology, *Ann Surg* 246(4):644–654, 2007.

Tanaka M, Chari S, Adsay V, et al: International Consensus Guidelines for management of intraductal papillary mucinous neoplasms and mucinous cystic neoplasms of the pancreas, *Pancreatology* 6:17–32, 2006.

Waters JA, Schmidt CM: Intraductal papillary mucinous neoplasm: when to resect, *Adv Surg* 42:87–108, 2008.

MANAGEMENT OF PANCREATIC ISLET CELL TUMORS EXCLUDING GASTRINOMA

Ellen H. Morrow, MD, and Jeffrey A. Norton, MD

OVERVIEW

Pancreatic neuroendocrine tumors (PNETs) include a diverse group of neoplasms originating from neuroendocrine-type cells. They are also referred to as *islet cell tumors,* and they are rare, with an annual incidence of 4.5 per million in the United States. In 2000, the World Health Organization (WHO) adopted a pathologic classification system for PNETs emphasizing histologic grade. Terminology then changed from "islet cell" to "neuroendocrine carcinoma." Most neuroendocrine tumors, up to 85%, are nonfunctional, but several types actively secrete hormones and have characteristic clinical syndromes. The majority of PNETs occur in a sporadic fashion, but 5% to 25% of cases are associated with genetic syndromes such as Multiple Endocrine Neoplasia type 1 (MEN1). The most common subtypes in MEN1 are gastrinoma and insulinoma, as in sporadic cases (Table 1).

FUNCTIONAL TYPES

Insulinoma
Presentation

Insulinomas are the most common functional neuroendocrine tumor. They present with *Whipple's triad* of hypoglycemia, neuroglycopenic symptoms, and relief of symptoms with administration of glucose. Neuroglycopenic symptoms may include fatigue, confusion, blurry vision, weakness, and even seizures.

Diagnosis

Symptomatic hypoglycemia (blood glucose level <45 mg/dL) with inappropriately elevated insulin levels (>5 mU/mL) is the mainstay of diagnosis. The study of choice is a 72-hour fast performed in a hospital setting, where patients have blood drawn every 6 hours for glucose and insulin levels. Once the patient develops neuroglycopenic symptoms, serum glucose, insulin, proinsulin, and c-peptide are measured, intravenous glucose is administered, and the fast is terminated. The intravenous glucose should ameliorate the symptoms.

Insulinomas are typically diagnosed at a small size (<2 cm in diameter). Distribution is even throughout the pancreas, and in the setting of MEN, insulinomas are often multiple. Only 10% of cases are malignant.

Imaging

Since insulinomas are usually very small in size, tumor localization may be problematic. First-line imaging is pancreatic protocol computed tomography (CT). PNETs are hypervascular, so they appear as a blush on the arterial phase of a CT. High-resolution thin-slice multidetector CT scanners timed appropriately with arterial contrast can have a sensitivity for insulinoma of 82%. Magnetic resonance imaging (MRI) is marginally superior to CT in some reports, so it is another valuable study, especially if CT is negative. Somatostatin receptor scintigraphy (SRS), which has a high sensitivity in most PNETs, is a poor method for imaging insulinomas. Most of these tumors fail to express type 2 somatostatin receptors. Endoscopic ultrasound (EUS) can also be useful, although it is operator dependent and may be less sensitive for lesions in the tail; tumors appear sonolucent compared to the more echoic pancreas. Tumors may also be biopsied, making the diagnosis unequivocal and eliminating false-positive results. Sensitivity of EUS is 80% to 90%. Intraoperative ultrasound (IOUS) is the most sensitive method of detection and localization. Further, the relationship of the tumor to vital structures, such as the pancreatic and common bile duct, can be delineated to allow safe routes for enucleation. More invasive preoperative localization procedures, such as calcium angiogram and portal venous sampling, were popular previously but now are less commonly used. Surgical exploration with IOUS is indicated when the diagnosis of insulinoma has been made biochemically, even if preoperative localization studies are uninformative. Blind pancreatic resection is no longer indicated. Precise preoperative and intraoperative tumor localization should guide surgical extirpation (Figures 1 through 7).

TABLE 1: Summary of gastrointestinal neuroendocrine tumor types

Tumor	Incidence	% in Pancreas	% in Duodenum	% Malignant	% MEN Associated	5-Year Survival
Insulinoma	4 in 5 million	>99		5–11	5	97
Glucagonoma	Rare	>99		>70	Occasional	50–60
VIPoma	Rare	85–90	10–15	50	Occasional	50
Somatostatinoma	<1 in 5 million	50	50	90	—	40
Nonfunctioning	1 in 5 million	>99		>50	—	30–50

Modified from Peterson DA, Dolan JP, Norton JA: *Surgery: basic science and clinical evidence,* ed 2, New York, 2008, Springer.

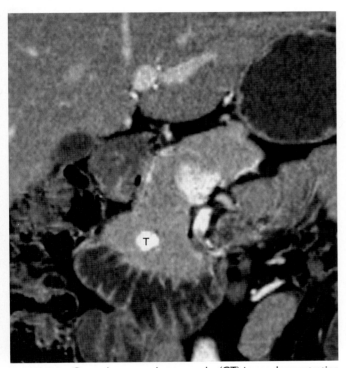

FIGURE 1   Coronal computed tomography (CT) image demonstrating a small, hypervascular insulinoma (T) in the head of the pancreas.

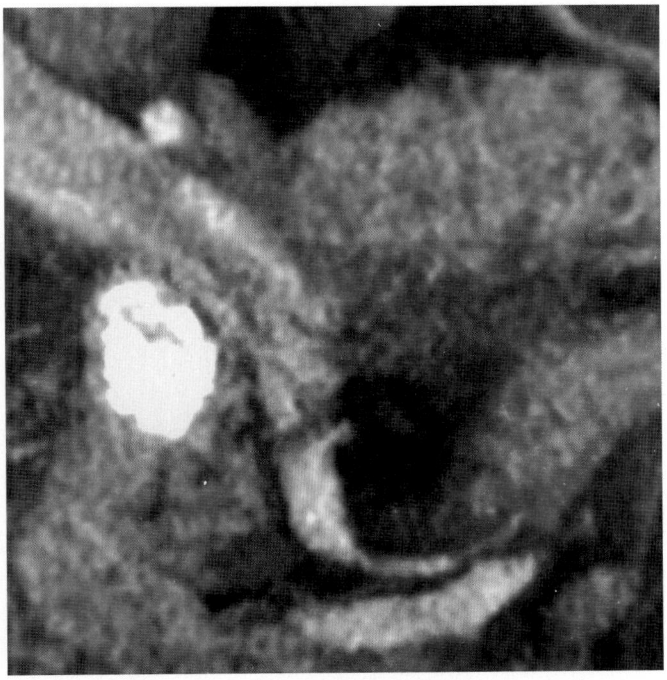

FIGURE 2   This coronal CT image shows a small, hypervascular PNET near the confluence of the superior mesenteric vein and the portal vein.

Preoperative Treatment

The goal of preoperative management is control of hypoglycemia. This is usually achieved with frequent small feedings, including awakening at night to take extra carbohydrates. Cornstarch can be used as a carrier to prolong the absorption of carbohydrate. About 60% of patients with insulinoma respond to either diazoxide or octreotide to suppress insulin secreted by tumors.

Pancreatic Polypeptide Secreting Tumor

Presentation

Excessive secretion of pancreatic polypeptide does not cause any signs or symptoms in humans, so pancreatic polypeptide-secreting tumors, or PPomas, are considered nonfunctional. PPomas may present with a pancreatic mass that causes weight loss, bleeding, bowel obstruction, or pain. Tumors are often diagnosed incidentally on a CT scan ordered for another reason.

Diagnosis

Fasting pancreatic polypeptide levels greater than 300 pg/mL are diagnostic. Most PNETs secrete pancreatic polypeptide, but the definitive diagnosis of PPoma is made with immunohistochemistry, when more than half the tumor stains positive for pancreatic polypeptide.

Preoperative Considerations

PPomas are large at presentation and thus are easily identified on cross-sectional imaging. They are also imaged by SRS.

VIPoma

Presentation

Oversecretion of vasoactive intestinal peptide (VIP) produces massive secretory diarrhea. The syndrome is named *Verner-Morrison syndrome* after the physicians who first reported it. It is also known as *WDHA* (watery diarrhea, hypokalemia, and achlorhydria) *syndrome.*

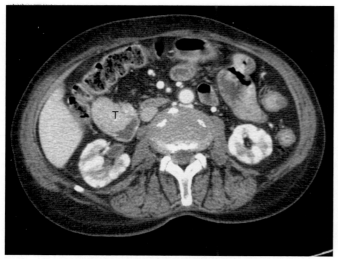

FIGURE 3   Axial CT image shows a large PNET in the duodenum.

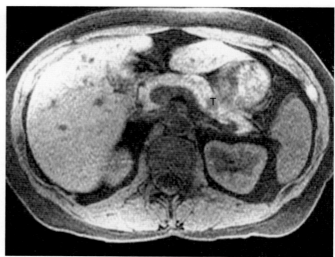

FIGURE 5   MRI shows an insulinoma (*T*) in the tail of the pancreas.

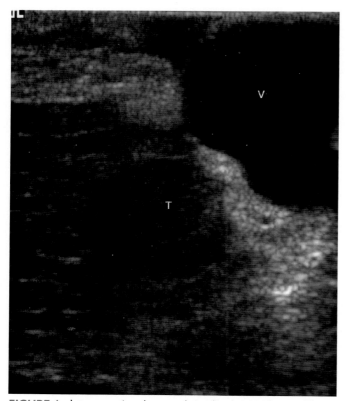

FIGURE 4   Intraoperative ultrasound visualized an insulinoma (*T*) near the SMV (*V*).

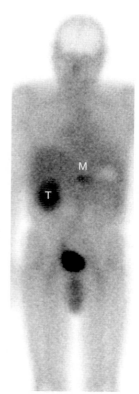

FIGURE 6   Somatostatin receptor scintigraphy demonstrates primary tumor (*T*) and liver metastasis (*M*).

The secretion of VIP induces a severe secretory diarrhea, approximately 5 to 10 L per day, with associated electrolyte abnormalities; it is one of the causes of hypercalcemia. VIPomas are very rare, and they may occur in either the pancreas or duodenum.

Diagnosis

VIPoma can be diagnosed with fasting plasma VIP levels greater than 500 pg/mL in the setting of secretory diarrhea, which is diagnosed if diarrhea persists when the patient is NPO.

Preoperative Considerations

Patients require proper fluid resuscitation and rehydration prior to surgery. Dehydration with secretory diarrhea is so severe that this had been nearly impossible to manage with intravenous fluids alone, before the advent of treatment with somatostatin analogs, either octreotide or somatuline, which can rapidly control the diarrhea and allow restoration of fluid and electrolyte balance.

These tumors may occur in the duodenum or pancreatic tail and are commonly malignant. VIPomas are usually greater than 3 cm in diameter, making them easily visualized by CT scan. SRS is also effective, especially for visualizing unexpected metastases.

Somatostatinoma

Presentation

Somatostatinomas are very rare tumors that produce a syndrome of steatorrhea, cholelithiasis, diabetes mellitus type 2, and hypochlorhydria. They are malignant tumors that often present with stage IV disease. About half are found in the pancreas and half in the duodenum. Duodenal somatistatinomas are associated with Von Recklinghausen disease.

Diagnosis

The diagnosis of somatostatinoma can be made with fasting plasma somatostatin assay. Serum somatostatin levels will usually be elevated.

Glucagonoma

Presentation

Glucagonomas are a rare PNET that causes a characteristic rash, called *necrolytic migratory erythema* (NME). It is an erythematous scaly rash affecting the perioral, pretibial, and intertriginous areas. The rash often precedes other symptoms by years. Patients scratch the rash incessantly, and dermatologists often diagnose glucagonoma as a result of searching for the cause of the rash. Glucagonoma causes severe hypoaminoacidemia, weight loss, type 2 diabetes, and cachexia. Patients with glucagonoma are also at high risk for deep venous thrombosis (DVT) and pulmonary embolus.

Diagnosis

Biochemical diagnosis is made with elevated serum levels of glucagon (usually >500 pg/mL) and low plasma levels of amino acids.

Operative Considerations

Because patients often present with severe malnutrition, they should be managed with total parenteral nutrition and insulin prior to any surgical intervention. Correction of the hypoaminoacidemia totally ameliorates the rash, and both TPN and octreotide have proven effective. Unfortunately, most patients have large (5 to 10 cm) locally advanced or metastatic tumors that may not be surgically curable.

Extremely Rare Functional Pancreatic Neuroendocrine Tumors

PNETs can rarely produce hormones other than those described above. These may include adrenocorticotropic hormone (ACTH), parathyroid hormone–related peptide (PTH-RP), serotonin, neurotensin, and growth hormone–releasing factor. These patients can present with Cushing syndrome, hypercalcemia, flushing, hypertension, and acromegaly, respectively.

Nonfunctional Pancreatic Neuroendocrine Tumors

Nonfunctional neuroendocrine tumors of the pancreas are the most common type. Since they do not produce hormone-related symptoms, they often present with symptoms of a mass. This means that they are usually large and malignant at the time of presentation. Initial signs and symptoms can result from biliary obstruction, bleeding, or bowel obstruction, but tumors may be seen on a CT scan ordered for another purpose.

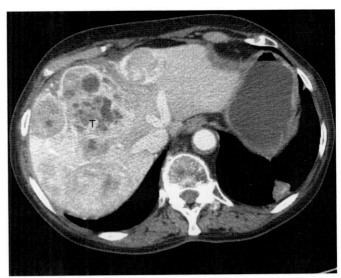

FIGURE 7   Axial CT image shows multiple liver metastases (*T*), which were resectable with a trisegmentectomy.

Diagnosis

Because these tumors are usually large at presentation, they are easily identified on cross-sectional imaging. Distant metastases should be excluded by four-phase imaging of the liver and SRS.

OPERATIVE CONSIDERATIONS

A more advanced tumor burden and disease stage at the time of diagnosis may more commonly require a major pancreatic resection, such as a Whipple pancreaticoduodenectomy or a subtotal pancreatectomy splenectomy, if the tumor is resectable. Concomitant liver resections may also be required.

INDICATIONS FOR SURGERY

Recent data indicate that surgical resection may be underutilized for PNETs, but surgical resection is the only potentially curative treatment modality for neuroendocrine tumors, all of which have some malignant potential. Some physicians may be biased against referring patients for surgery, given the relatively indolent course of many neuroendocrine tumors and the potential complications of pancreatic surgery. Pancreatic surgery, however, has become significantly safer over the past several decades, especially in high-volume centers. Given the relatively low rate of complications and deaths from modern pancreatic surgery, and the malignant potential of neuroendocrine tumors, surgical resection should be carefully considered for all patients. Specific considerations should include the extent of disease, the presence of MEN1, efficacy of medical management, and operative risk.

Even patients with metastatic disease may benefit from surgical resection. Patients with distant metastatic disease are less likely to benefit than patients with surgically curable disease, but debulking procedures can be palliative in the case of functional tumors. In one series, the 10 year survival rate for patients undergoing reoperation for pancreatic endocrine tumors was 72%.

SURGICAL APPROACH

The appropriate procedure for resection of a neuroendocrine tumor depends mostly on the location of the tumor in the pancreas. The surgical approach also varies based on the size and the likelihood of malignancy. For insulinomas, which are most likely benign, enucleation is favored. This approach preserves normal pancreas and spleen; palpation and intraoperative ultrasound should be used to facilitate the resection. Laparoscopic resection has been performed for most pancreatic neuroendocrine tumor types. The procedures performed to date include laparoscopic spleen-preserving distal pancreatectomy, laparoscopic distal pancreatectomy with splenectomy, and laparoscopic enucleation. Laparoscopic ultrasound has greatly facilitated the surgical procedure. Lymph node dissections have also been performed laparoscopically, and laparoscopic approaches appear to result in a shorter hospital stay and comparable complication rates.

When metastases are confined to the liver, metastatic disease may still be resectable. Liver metastases can be treated with wedge resections, lobectomy, radiofrequency ablation (RFA), or chemoembolization. In these patients, surgical resection may provide some survival benefit. Survival following resection of neuroendocrine tumor metastases to the liver is 60% to 70% at 5 years. Surgical resection is recommended when all gross tumor can be removed by the planned procedure with an acceptable risk of morbidity and mortality. It is also important to determine that the PNET is well-differentiated using SRS and Ki67 staining on pathology. Liver resection is not generally recommended for poorly differentiated tumors.

RESULTS OF SURGERY

Results of surgery vary by tumor type, but overall they are good, given the usually indolent course of PNETs. Large series have shown that more than 90% of patients with insulinoma can have successful surgery that results in complete correction of the hypoglycemia. Even in the case of an inability to remove all gross disease with more

malignant PNETs, patients may have significant amelioration of their symptoms after debulking surgery.

ADJUVANT THERAPY

Standard chemotherapy for metastatic neuroendocrine tumors has been used with modest effect. Older regimens include streptozotocin and doxorubicin or 5-FU. Depot octreotide has also been used. Tumors with high-affinity somatostatin receptors such as carcinoids, nonfunctional tumors, gastrinomas, glucagonomas, and VIPomas are most sensitive to this therapy. Somatostatin analogs can often stabilize disease but are unlikely to cause tumor regression. Recent protocols with xeloda, oxaliplatin, and avastin have shown some encouraging preliminary results.

SELECTED READINGS

Bilimoria KY, Tomlinson JS, Merkow RP, et al: Clinicopathologic features and treatment trends of pancreatic neuroendocrine tumors: analysis of 9,821 patients, *J Gastrointest Surg* 11(11):1460–1467, 2007, discussion 1467-1469.

Fendrich V, Langer P, Celik I, et al: An aggressive surgical approach leads to long-term survival in patients with pancreatic endocrine tumors, *Ann Surg* 244(6):845–851, 2006, discussion 852-843.

Fernandez-Cruz L, Blanco L, Cosa R, et al: Is laparoscopic resection adequate in patients with neuroendocrine pancreatic tumors? *World J Surg* 32(5):904–917, 2008.

Norton JA: Surgery for primary pancreatic neuroendocrine tumors, *J Gastrointest Surg* 10(3):327–331, 2006.

Strosberg JR, Nasir A, Hodul P, Kvols L: Biology and treatment of metastatic gastrointestinal neuroendocrine tumors, *Gastrointest Cancer Res* 2(3):113–125, 2008.

TRANSPLANTATION OF THE PANCREAS

David E.R. Sutherland, MD, PhD, Gideon A. Zamir, MD, and Kenneth L. Brayman, MD, PhD

OVERVIEW

The goal of pancreas transplantation is to induce insulin independence and euglycemia in insulinopenic diabetic transplant recipients by providing functioning β cells. Although the immediate benefit of improved quality of life by obviating the need for insulin injections and glucose monitoring to adjust the insulin dose is obvious, restoration of normoglycemic function can also prevent or halt the progression of some of the diabetic complications secondary to disordered glucose metabolism, including those involving the ocular, nervous, renal, and vascular systems that afflict more than 30% of individuals with insulin-dependent diabetes.

An alternative to β cell replacement by pancreas transplantation is transplantation of free grafts of isolated allogenic islets, usually embolized to the liver via the portal vein (PV). This minimally invasive surgical approach has been successful but remains investigational, and its application has been limited for logistical reasons, and in most islet programs,

by the need for multiple donors to achieve sufficient β cell mass to induce insulin independence. Thus pancreas transplantation remains the most common form of β cell replacement and is the focus of this chapter.

Studies in pancreas transplant recipients document improvement in metabolic parameters and an impact on secondary complications of diabetes. The drawback of pancreas and islet transplantation is the need for immunosuppression to prevent rejection. Thus the majority of pancreas transplants have been in diabetic renal allograft recipients who are obligated to immunosuppression to obviate the need for dialysis. It is clear that immunosuppression to sustain a kidney transplant is preferable to dialysis both from a quality of life and survival standpoint, but the nonuremic diabetic doing well on exogenous insulin may not be better off on immunosuppression given solely for a pancreas transplant to achieve insulin independence. Once immunosuppression is needed for a diabetic kidney transplant recipient, there is no reason, other than the surgical risk, not to add the additional benefit of a pancreas transplant. Nevertheless, there are nonuremic diabetics who are extremely labile metabolically, with hypoglycemic unawareness, who are at risk of sudden death from insulin reactions and whose quality of life is extremely low from the diabetes per se; in this subgroup, the trade-off of immunosuppression for becoming insulin independent and euglycemic is worthwhile.

The benefits of pancreas transplantation in selected recipients have resulted in a steady application of the procedure since the 1980s (the first cases were done in the 1960s). In the past decade, approximately 1500 transplants have been carried out annually in the United States (Figure 1).

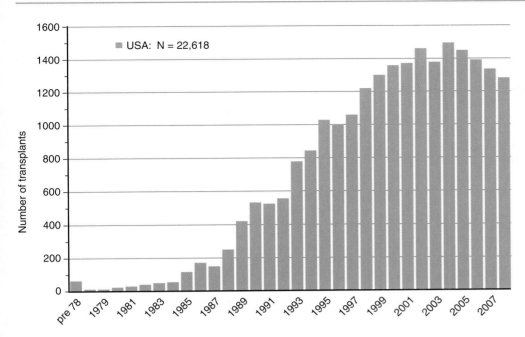

FIGURE 1 Annual number of pancreas transplants in the United States reported to the International Pancreas Transplant Registry (IPTR) and United Network for Organ Sharing (UNOS) from 1966 through 2008. *(Data from Gruessner AC, Sutherland DER: Pancreas transplant outcomes for United States (US) cases as reported to the United Network for Organ Sharing (UNOS) and the International Pancreas Transplant Registry (IPTR). In Cecka M [ed]: Clinical transplants 2008, Los Angeles, 2009, Terasaki Foundation Laboratory, pp. 45-56.)*

RECIPIENT CATEGORIES AND SELECTION CRITERIA

Table 1 shows the pancreas transplant recipient categories and selection criteria established by the University of Minnesota Pancreas Transplant Evaluation Committee. A nonobese insulin-dependent diabetic uremic patient who does not have a living donor (LD) for a kidney and who is thus a candidate for a deceased-donor kidney transplant should almost always be considered for a simultaneous pancreas and kidney transplant (SPK). Immunosuppressive management is no different for such patients than if they received a kidney transplant alone, and the surgical risk of adding the pancreas is relatively low (approximately 15% reoperation rate). A diabetic patient who received a previous kidney transplant, from either a related living or deceased donor, should be considered for a pancreas-after-kidney transplant (PAK). We advise all uremic diabetic patients that an LD kidney transplant followed by a PAK is preferable to waiting for a deceased-donor SPK transplant because of the long waiting time, usually years, and the high mortality rate of patients on dialysis awaiting transplant (about one in six die while waiting during the first year; by 4 years, it is nearly three in six). An LD kidney transplant can be done to preempt the need for dialysis, thus decreasing the mortality rate associated with end-stage diabetic nephropathy and more than compensating for the fact that the pancreas graft survival rate is slightly higher with SPK than PAK transplant.

It should also be noted that although few are done, LD segmental transplants can also be done simultaneously with a kidney from the same donor, thus allowing dialysis to be preempted while achieving insulin independence with one operation. LD PAK segmental transplants are also done, and if the donor for the pancreas is the same donor as for the kidney, pancreas rejection is very unlikely if there has been no rejection of the kidney.

The third category of recipients comprises those patients who receive a pancreas transplant alone (PTA). PTAs have largely been done in patients with very labile diabetes and hypoglycemic unawareness. In this situation pancreas transplantation is the most effective treatment, because it completely obviates insulin reactions. However, for patients who are not labile but who wish to obviate a lifetime need for insulin, as well as to eliminate the risk of secondary diabetic complications by taking the alternative risk of immunosuppression, PTA can reasonably be chosen.

SURGICAL TECHNIQUE

Pancreas Procurement

The general criteria for selection of deceased donors for pancreas procurement are similar to those for liver, renal, or thoracic organs. A history of type I diabetes is a contraindication to pancreas procurement. Relative contraindications include acute or chronic pancreatitis or pancreatic trauma. Hyperglycemia occurring after brain death is not a contraindication to pancreas procurement, because the cause is severe insulin resistance in the donor, a problem presumably not present in the recipient. An elevated serum amylase level by itself is not a contraindication to pancreas procurement, because it may be salivary; but if the serum lipase is elevated, it does indicate pancreas injury and is a contraindication. The standard multi-organ procurement is performed in most situations. Which of the abdominal organs to dissect first is a matter of surgeon preference and agreement among procurement teams, if there is more than one procurement team. The most efficient method of procurement is to have one team, so the various organs can be mobilized together, especially for the liver and pancreas, not necessarily one first and then the other, because dissection of part of one dissects the other by default via the shared origin of vessels and other structures (see Figure 2, A, for predissection anatomy).

A midline laparotomy is made and extended to join the midline thoracic incision. The distal and supraceliac aorta, the infrahepatic inferior vena cava (IVC), and the inferior mesenteric vein (IMV) are first isolated in preparation for cannulation. The gastrocolic ligament is divided next, from the pylorus to the greater curvature of the stomach, to facilitate exposure of the anterior surface of the pancreas through the lesser sac. The transverse colon is completely mobilized, from hepatic to splenic flexure, so that the pancreas may be adequately dissected from the surrounding retroperitoneal structures. Short gastric vessels are divided to the level of the gastroesophageal junction, and the lienocolic ligament is incised. The left gastric vessels are ligated and divided close to the stomach to preserve the blood supply to the liver via the celiac axis. The stomach is thus completely mobilized. The nasogastric tube is advanced into the duodenum, and 300 mL of amphotericin antibiotic solution is instilled into the duodenal segment. The stomach is then divided just distal to the pylorus with a GIA stapler and is then retracted into the left subdiaphragmatic space

TABLE 1: University of Minnesota pancreas transplant recipient categories and selection criteria

Uremic Diabetic Patients: Simultaneous Pancreas and Kidney (SPK) Transplant

Most candidates for a kidney transplant are candidates for a pancreas transplant. Obesity and age are relative contraindications. Screening for coronary artery disease is mandatory, along with corrective measures (angioplasty, stent, bypass) before transplant if significant lesions are present. If there is no living donor (LD) for a kidney alone (or in some cases an LD segmental pancreas and kidney transplant), the patient is placed on the waiting list for deceased-donor SPK transplant.

Previous Kidney Transplant (Functioning): Subsequent Pancreas Transplant (Pancreas after Kidney Transplant [PAK])

This is an option for diabetic patients who have undergone successful related-living–donor or deceased-donor kidney transplants. Sequential kidney and pancreas transplants are even preferred when an LD for a kidney alone is available to avoid the potentially long wait for a deceased-donor SPK transplant, with the attendant high mortality rate for patients on dialysis awaiting transplant.

Nonuremic, Nonkidney Transplant Patients: Pancreas Transplant Alone (PTA)

Patients with such severe difficulty with diabetes control that day-to-day quality of life is poor on exogenous insulin can be considered for this reason alone. The most common indication is hypoglycemic unawareness.

Patients with early but progressive secondary diabetic complications that are predictably more serious than the potential side effects of chronic immunosuppression with or without day-to-day management problems are candidates for PTA. Such patients usually have retinopathy and neuropathy. Early nephropathy would certainly be an indication if nephrotoxic calcineurin inhibitors were not the mainstay of antirejection treatment, because once nephropathy is present, the long-term survival probabilities of diabetics so afflicted compared to those not afflicted is much lower. In the absence of a randomized trial, at the University of Minnesota, we consider nephropathic diabetics with the following characteristics for PTA:
1. Albuminuria
2. Diabetic lesions on kidney biopsy
3. Mesangium 20% to 40% of glomerular volume (<20% is normal; >40% is severe nephropathy; need for kidney transplantation is inevitable, but we prefer to wait and add a pancreas when a kidney transplant is indicated, rather than precipitate the need with a pancreas transplant and introduction of calcineurin inhibitors.)
4. Creatinine clearance greater than 70 mL/min; calcineurin inhibitors for immunosuppression will likely be tolerated, but careful monitoring of kidney function over time is needed, and some PTA recipients may later need a kidney transplant.

to the hepatoduodenal ligament, where the common bile duct (CBD) is identified and incised. The gallbladder is incised, and the bile is flushed with saline solution through the cut CBD.

Next, the donor is systemically heparinized, cannulas are introduced into the infrarenal aorta and IMV, the suprahepatic IVC is cut to allow venting of blood into the right side of the chest, and the supraceliac aorta is cross clamped. The liver, pancreas, and kidneys are flushed with cold preservation solution, and the intraabdominal organs are cooled with ice slush. During the vascular flush, the mesenteries of the small bowel and colon are divided using a thoracoabdominal stapler, leaving sufficient distance between the pancreas and the staple line to permit safe religation of the mesenteric root on the back table. A limited dissection of the hepatoduodenal ligament is then performed. The gastroduodenal, common hepatic, and splenic arteries are identified, and the PV is divided in a manner that will allow safe use of both liver and pancreas grafts (approximately 1 cm cephalad to the superior margin of the pancreas). The liver, pancreas, and kidneys are then excised sequentially. The celiac axis on an aortic Carrel patch is retained with the liver after the splenic artery is divided close to its origin. The superior mesenteric artery (SMA) is procured on an aortic Carrel patch with the pancreas graft. If a replaced right hepatic artery comes off the SMA, it is carefully dissected free from the posterior surface of the pancreas. At the time of pancreas removal, the SMA is dissected just distal to the right hepatic artery takeoff. The aortic Carrel patch is left bearing the celiac axis, and the proximal SMA is left with the liver graft and the distal SMA with the pancreas graft.

The above description is of a combined procurement of pancreas and liver. If the liver is not procured, then neither the splenic nor the gastroduodenal arteries need to be divided, and the celiac axis and SMA can be included on a common Carrel patch (Figure 2, B). Although uncommon because most donors suitable for pancreas procurement are suitable for liver procurement, this method allows a single arterial anastomosis in the recipient. In either case, at the completion of the procurement, the pancreas remains attached to the duodenum and proximal jejunum with the bowel stapled at both ends.

When the liver is procured, which is the situation in most cases, the final anatomy of the excised pancreas appears as in Figure 2, C). The gastroduodenal artery has been ligated. The splenic artery and SMA, with the inferior pancreaticoduodenal artery intact, constitute the arterial inflow of the distal and proximal pancreas, respectively; the PV above the splenic-portal bifurcation provides the venous outflow, and the duodenal segment serves as a conduit for the exocrine secretions of the graft.

Back-Table Preparation of the Pancreas Graft

Back-table preparation of the combined pancreas-duodenum graft for transplantation consists of four steps:
1. Removal of the spleen
2. Trimming of excess distal and proximal duodenum and reinforcement of stump staple lines
3. Shortening, restapling, and suture reinforcement of colonic and small bowel mesenteries
4. Arterial reconstruction

The pancreas is immersed in a basin of cold preservation solution (Figure 3, A). The spleen is detached from the pancreas, ligating all vessels in the hilum so as not to injure the pancreas (Figure 3, B). If the bladder drainage technique is used, the proximal jejunum and distal duodenum are removed (Figure 3, C) to avoid excessive secretion of bicarbonate into the bladder that can result in metabolic acidosis in the recipient. If enteric drainage is to be used in the recipient, shortening does not need to be done, because the proximal jejunum can be used for anastomosis in the recipient. In either case, staple lines need to be reinforced (Figure 4) to prevent leakage after implantation in the recipient.

or is divided at the lower esophagus. The pancreas is further mobilized by dividing the lienophrenic ligament to free the pancreas from its posterior attachments to the left kidney and adrenal. The spleen remains attached to the pancreas allograft and serves as a handle when manipulating the pancreas. The jejunum at the level of the ligament of Treitz is divided with a GIA stapler. Attention is then given

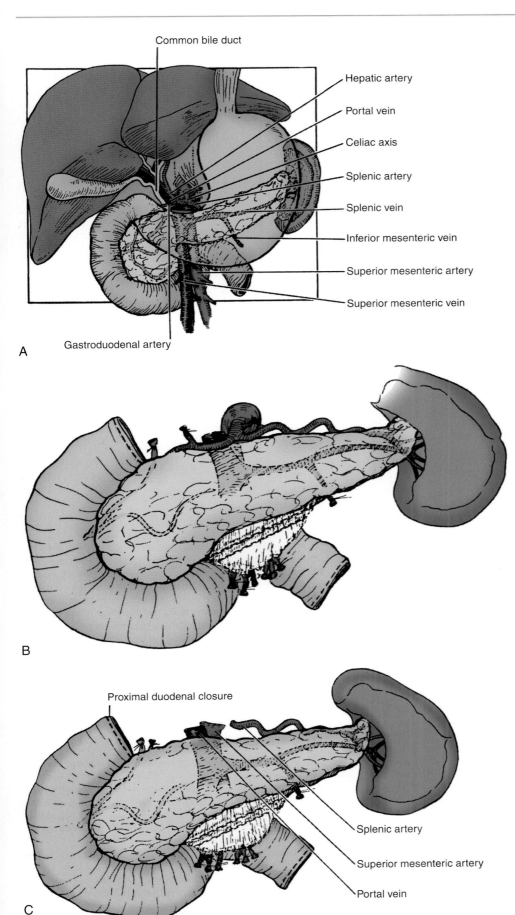

A

Common bile duct

Hepatic artery

Portal vein

Celiac axis

Splenic artery

Splenic vein

Inferior mesenteric vein

Superior mesenteric artery

Superior mesenteric vein

Gastroduodenal artery

B

C

Proximal duodenal closure

Splenic artery

Superior mesenteric artery

Portal vein

FIGURE 2 Procurement of the pancreaticoduodenal allograft. **A,** Vascular anatomy of the liver and pancreas. Note the gastroduodenal artery, which is divided during simultaneous procurement of the liver and pancreas but not the pancreas alone. **B,** Pancreaticoduodenal allograft after procurement (nonliver donor). Both the celiac axis and superior mesenteric artery are included in a Carrel patch of the aorta. Note that the proximal duodenum has been divided with the GIA stapler and that the mesentery to the small intestine, inferior to the inferior border of the pancreas, has also been ligated and divided after placement of two parallel rows of the TA 90 stapler. **C,** Pancreaticoduodenal allograft after procurement from a donor in which the liver was also procured. Note the splenic and superior mesenteric arteries, which required ex vivo reconstruction prior to implantation.

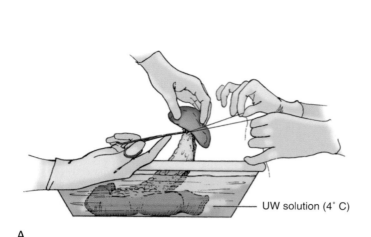

UW solution (4° C)

A

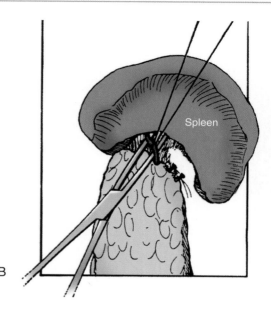

Spleen

B

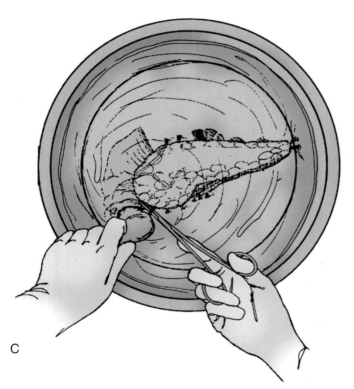

C

FIGURE 3   Ex vivo preparation of pancreaticoduodenal allograft I. Splenectomy and the distal duodenal segment. **A,** The spleen is removed ex vivo at 4° C with the pancreaticoduodenal allograft immersed in preservation solution. **B,** Technique for splenectomy: the splenic hilar vessels are ligated close to the spleen to prevent injury to the tail of the pancreas. **C,** The distal limb of the duodenal segment of the pancreaticoduodenal allograft is shortened to minimize bicarbonate loss, a problem with the bladder drainage technique. Note that the divided tissue on the pancreatic and duodenal sides has been ligated to prevent troublesome bleeding after revascularization.

The most common technique used to provide a single arterial inflow to the graft is Y-graft reconstruction using the donor iliac artery bifurcation (Figure 5). The external iliac artery of the extension graft is anastomosed to the SMA of the graft in an end-to-end fashion. The internal iliac artery of the extension graft is anastomosed end-to-end to the splenic artery of the graft, leaving the proximal common-donor iliac artery for anastomosis to the recipient inflow vessel. Alternatively, the splenic artery can be anastomosed directly end-to-side to the SMA or, more commonly, using an extension graft of iliac artery, so there is no tension. The latter technique may be useful when a Y graft is atherosclerotic, particularly at the bifurcation.

A short PV decreases the risk of venous thrombosis by kinking or impingement; therefore a portal extension graft is rarely needed and is dictated by the recipient anatomy and the site of placement of the graft.

RECIPIENT OPERATION

General Considerations

The main decisions facing the surgeon are how to manage the exocrine secretions (bladder or enteric drainage) and how to establish venous drainage (portal or systemic). Methods of restoring the exocrine drainage of the pancreatic graft have evolved through different technical stages. The two methods used commonly today are drainage of the duodenal segment via the bladder with bladder drainage (BD) or via the small bowel with enteric drainage (ED).

BD is safe and technically convenient, and if there are anastomotic problems, control of the situation and healing can occur by inserting a Foley catheter to relieve pressure in the bladder; BD avoids the microbial contamination that occurs with ED. BD also enables monitoring of pancreatic amylase activity in the urine, which is particularly

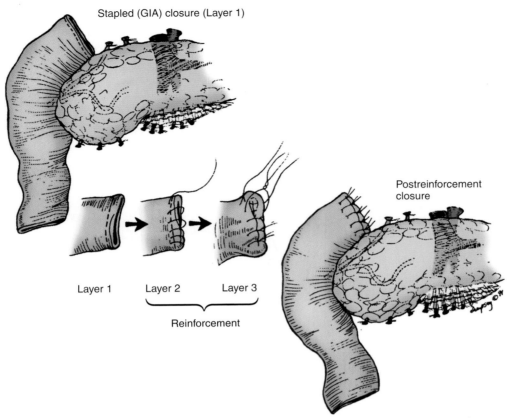

Stapled (GIA) closure (Layer 1)

Postreinforcement closure

Layer 1   Layer 2   Layer 3

Reinforcement

FIGURE 4   Ex vivo preparation of the pancreaticoduodenal allograft II. Management of the proximal duodenal stump. A three-layered closure is used to ensure a secure closure. The first layer is completed in the donor at the time of procurement (GIA staple line). Layers two and three (reinforcement layers) are performed ex vivo before transplantation.

advantageous in solitary pancreas transplants where there is no surrogate marker for pancreas rejection, as there is in SPK transplants, when the kidney and pancreas are from the same donor, and serum creatinine can be used for monitoring. In solitary (PAK and PTA) pancreas transplants, a rise in serum amylase and lipase secondary to rejection is only transient, sometimes lasting less than a week, as the rejection process decreases amylase and lipase production; but such a decrease is reflected in urine amylase in bladder-drained patients, and because the decrease is not transient, it is not missed by an arbitrary frequency of monitoring.

Nevertheless, drainage of pancreatic secretions via the lower urinary tract has associated complications. These can be metabolic, such as dehydration from fluid and bicarbonate loss, and urologic, such as dysuria, cystitis, and hematuria. Such complications necessitate conversion to ED in approximately 20% of recipients. With current immunosuppressive regimens, graft survival rates are comparable for ED and BD, and approximately 80% of pancreas transplants performed in the United States are now done with ED, slightly more in the SPK category, slightly less in the solitary pancreas transplant categories. A decrease in urinary amylase is a sensitive marker of rejection and always decreases before hyperglycemia ensues. A rise in serum amylase may precede a decrease in urinary amylase, but serum amylase does not always rise. Thus, for solitary pancreas transplants that use ED, rejection episodes may be missed until hyperglycemia ensues, decreasing the probability of reversal by an increase in immunosuppression. In the SPK category, isolated rejection of the pancreas is rare; rejection episodes affecting the transplanted kidney and pancreas are nearly always first manifested by a rise in serum creatinine and can be easily confirmed by kidney biopsy. Thus most transplant centers use ED for SPK transplants, and they would use

BD only when risk factors dictate avoidance of enteric contamination, or if the duodenum had characteristics that made BD safer at the time of transplantation.

A second consideration is whether to use the systemic or portal venous system for the graft's venous anastomosis. Although there is no evidence that the peripheral venous hyperinsulinemia associated with systemically drained grafts is detrimental in this setting, portal drainage is more physiologic and may result in a better lipid profile. Portal venous–drained transplants are nearly always done with exocrine ED, which is technically more convenient than BD in this setting.

Technical Details

Bladder Exocrine Drainage and Systemic Venous Drainage

The pancreas graft is usually placed intraabdominally through a midline laparotomy. The pancreas is also usually placed in the right side of the pelvis for two reasons: dissection of the right iliac vessels is easier compared with the left side, and the natural position of the right iliac vessels, which is the vein lateral to the artery, does not require vascular realignment when the graft is placed with the pancreatic head and duodenum pointing caudally.

In SPK transplants, the kidney is usually implanted first, on the left, while a second team performs the back-table preparation of the pancreas graft. Usually before but sometimes after completion of the kidney transplant, the common, external, and internal iliac arteries and veins and the ureter on the right are mobilized (Figure 6). The cecum is mobilized as necessary for exposure and to provide a lie without tension or twisting of the vessels to the pancreaticoduodenal graft.

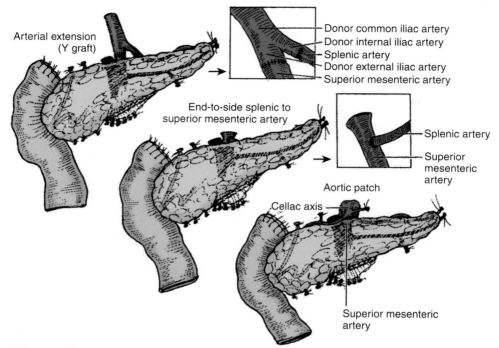

Arterial extension
(Y graft)

Donor common iliac artery
Donor internal iliac artery
Splenic artery
Donor external iliac artery
Superior mesenteric artery

End-to-side splenic to
superior mesenteric artery

Splenic artery

Superior
mesenteric
artery

Aortic patch

Celiac axis

Superior mesenteric
artery

FIGURE 5 Ex vivo preparation of the pancreaticoduodenal allograft III. Revascularization. An arterial extension (Y graft) is commonly used to revascularize the splenic and superior mesenteric arteries (SMAs) of the pancreas (see Figure 2, C). Alternatively, an end-to-side splenic-to-SMA reconstruction (no Y graft required) can be performed if adequate length and mobility of the arteries can be achieved. The aortic patch that includes the celiac and SMA of a pancreas procured from a nonliver donor requires no vascular reconstruction.

The internal iliac artery is preserved, but all posterior branches of the common and external iliac veins are ligated and divided, including the internal iliac vein (Figure 6, A). Complete mobilization of the iliac vein from the vena cava to the inguinal ligament is achieved. Because the PV of the graft is kept short, mobilization of the iliac vein facilitates the completion of the venous anastomosis and also prevents tension on the anastomosis. If the hypogastric veins are not divided, the iliac vein may remain sufficiently deep, so that an extension venous conduit to the pancreas graft PV is required; because we usually do not find hypogastric vein dissection and ligation particularly difficult, full mobilization and avoidance of an extension graft is our preference. The bladder is mobilized by dividing the lateral peritoneal attachments.

The recipient is systemically heparinized before clamping of the proximal and distal iliac artery and vein. The head of the pancreas is positioned in a caudal orientation, and the venous anastomosis is performed first in an end-to-side fashion to the iliac vein, with the vein kept lateral to the artery (Figure 6, B). The arterial anastomosis is performed next, between the stem of the pancreas arterial Y graft and the common iliac artery, unless no Y graft was used, in which case the Carrel patch encompassing the celiac axis and SMA is used, or the SMA if the graft splenic artery was attached to it during the bench work (Figure 6, C). The vascular clamps are sequentially removed, and the graft is reperfused.

Next, the duodenocystostomy is performed using either a hand-sewn or end-to-end anastomosis (EEA) stapling technique as illustrated in Figure 7. For the hand-sewn anastomosis, a horizontal cystostomy is made on the posterosuperior aspect of the bladder, and a two-layered anastomosis between the bladder and duodenum is performed. For a stapled pancreaticoduodenocystostomy, a circular EEA stapler is inserted through the distal end of the duodenum, and the anvil is placed in the bladder through an anterior cystostomy (Figure 7, A). The duodenum and posterior bladder wall are approximated without tension, and the stapler is applied. The exposed staples of the duodenocystostomy are then covered by mucosa with a running

absorbable suture within the bladder (Figure 7, B). The distal duodenal opening through which the EEA was inserted is then stapled closed (Figure 7, C), and the distal duodenal stump is reinforced with sutures placed in a fashion similar to the closure of the proximal stump.

For recipients of PAK transplants who have a functioning kidney graft on the right side, the pancreas graft is placed on the left side in a similar fashion, taking care not to disrupt the existing ureteroneo-cystostomy. When pancreas grafts are placed on the left side with the head and duodenum pointing caudally, it is advisable to divide the hypogastric artery so the iliac vein, after division of the hypogastric veins, can lie medial to the common and external iliac artery, because the PV coming off the pancreas graft will also lie medial to the artery. Crossing vessels predisposes to thrombosis in pancreas grafts, and small details such as this minimize the risk of such an event.

Enteric Drainage

In most patients the pancreas is oriented in the usual caudal manner, and the vascular anastomoses are fashioned as described for systemically drained BD transplants. The distal part of the C-loop of donor duodenum and proximal jejunum, if left intact, will actually point cephalic, making it easy to do the enteric anastomosis to the midportion of recipient jejunum. The antimesenteric side of the graft duodenal-jejunal segment, or the end of the segment, is anastomosed to the side of the recipient of jejunum. The enteric anastomosis can also be performed to a defunctionalized Roux-en-Y jejunal loop to reduce the severity of enteric leak, should it occur at the site of the graft intestinal component, but it entails a second anastomosis that has its own chance of a leak. A randomized controlled study comparing ED with or without the Roux-en-Y has not been done, but in registry analyses of outcomes, there is no discernable difference.

Alternatively, the graft can be oriented with the head and duodenal segment facing cephalic. The vascular anastomoses are again to the iliac vessels, but the vein and artery have to cross, which may

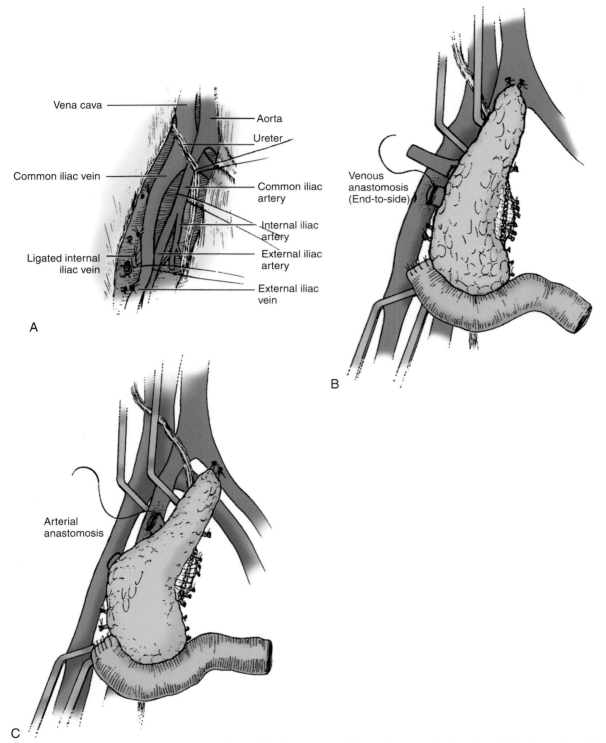

FIGURE 6　Transplantation of the pancreaticoduodenal allograft. **A,** Preparation of the recipient vessels. Note that all deep branches of the common and external iliac veins are ligated and divided. The vein is brought lateral to the artery. The ureter is mobilized and brought medial to the artery. **B,** The venous anastomosis is performed end-to-side with the portal vein of the pancreas graft anastomosed to the proximal external or distal common iliac vein. **C,** The arterial anastomosis is performed after the venous anastomosis and is placed superior to the venous anastomosis. The common iliac artery of the recipient is commonly used as the site for arterial anastomosis.

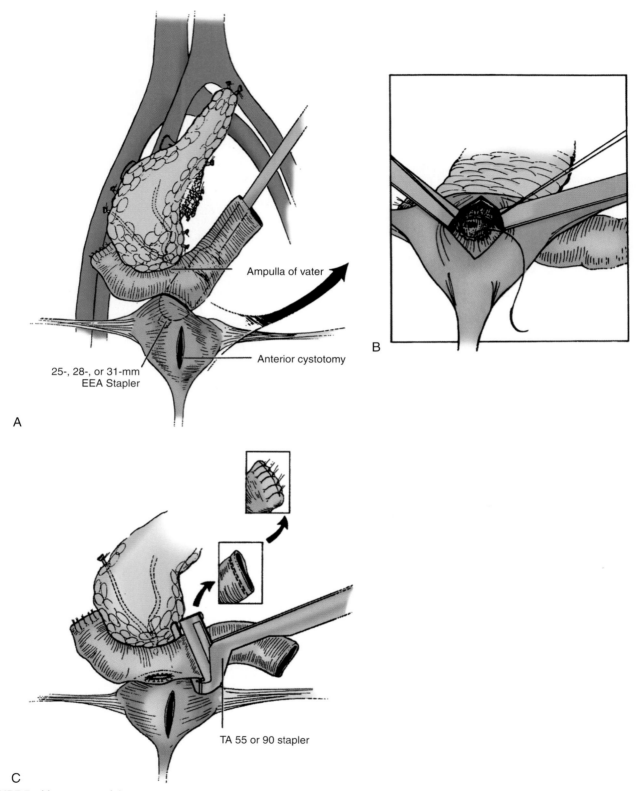

FIGURE 7   Management of the pancreatic exocrine secretions. The stapled duodenocystostomy. **A,** A 25, 28, or 31 mm EEA stapler is passed proximally through the open end of the distal duodenal segment to an area opposite the ampulla. Cystostomy is made on the anterosuperior aspect of the bladder to facilitate exposure and placement of the anvil of the EEA stapler. The anastomosis is performed between the antimesenteric border of the duodenum and the posterosuperior aspect of the bladder. **B,** The EEA staple line is reinforced with a whipstitch of 4-0 absorbable suture (PDA or Maxon) to facilitate hemostasis and ensure a watertight closure. **C,** The distal duodenal segment is closed with a TA 55 or TA 90 stapler. Excess distal duodenum is removed. The TA stapler places a parallel row of staples. The distal duodenal segment closure is reinforced in two layers similar to the proximal duodenal reinforcement shown in Figure 4.

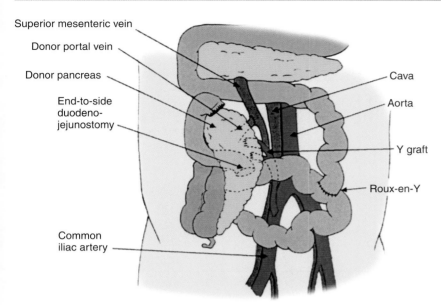

Superior mesenteric vein

Donor portal vein

Donor pancreas

End-to-side duodeno-jejunostomy

Common iliac artery

Cava

Aorta

Y graft

Roux-en-Y

FIGURE 8 Overall view of completed pancreaticoduodenal pancreas transplant with venous drainage to recipient portal system via the anterior superior mesenteric vein (SMV) and enteric exocrine drainage via a Roux-en-Y graft-to-recipient duodenojejunostomy In this illustration, a long arterial Y graft from the donor pancreas to the retroperitoneal recipient iliac artery traverses the bowel mesentery, because the pancreas graft lies anterior to the recipient bowel. An alternative method of portal–enteric drainage (see Boggi, Amorese, & Marchetti, 2010) is to place the graft under the mobilized right colon with the portal vein of the graft anastomosed to the posterior surface of the recipient SMV and the (shorter) arterial Y graft anastomosed directly to the common iliac artery without traversing the mesentery. A long Roux-en-Y limb of recipient jejunum is then brought through the mesentery for anastomosis to the graft duodenojejunal segment.

predispose to vessel thrombosis. An additional advantage of caudal orientation is that in patients in whom the duodenum appears dusky after reperfusion, the duodenum can be anastomosed to the bladder, rather than to small bowel, to minimize the consequences of a leak.

ED is usually necessary when portal venous drainage is performed (Figure 8). The venous anastomosis is usually established by reflecting the transverse mesocolon superiorly and exposing the anterior surface of the superior mesenteric vein (SMV) at the inferior margin of the native pancreas. The PV of the pancreas graft is anastomosed end-to-side to the SMV or to a major tributary of the SMV, usually the splenic vein. The donor iliac artery Y graft is brought through a window made in the small bowel mesentery and is anastomosed end-to-side to the right common iliac artery. The graft duodenal-jejunal segment is then anastomosed to a loop of recipient jejunum or, as illustrated in Figure 8, a Roux-en-Y limb of jejunum.

An alternative to portal drainage via the anterior surface of the SMV is to use the posterior surface, as described by the group at the University of Pisa in an illustration accompanying a journal article by Boggi et al (see Suggested Readings). The right colon and hepatic flexure are mobilized and reflected medially, and a Kocher maneuver is also done, exposing the SMV from below. The pancreas is oriented cephalad with its ventral surface turned dorsally, so the graft PV can be anastomosed to the recipient SMV. The arterial anastomosis of the Y graft is then made to the common iliac artery. A Roux-en-Y limb of jejunum is created and brought through the colonic mesentery for anastomosis to the graft duodenal–jejunal segment.

Currently, about 20% of pancreas transplants in the United States are done with portal venous drainage, all with ED of exocrine secretions. Thus systemic venous drainage continues to be the most common method, and most of these are done with ED of exocrine secretions.

Complications

The technical failure rate (approximately 8%) for pancreas transplantation is higher than that for any other routinely performed solid organ transplant. Several factors contribute to surgical complications after pancreas transplantation, which include 1) the transplanted organ itself, with its broad spectrum of potential surgical complications, such as pancreatitis, necrosis, infection, pseudocyst, and fistula (the pancreas is a low blood flow organ fed by large vessels, namely the SMA and splenic artery, without the normal runoff in the *in situ* situation, which predisposes to stagnation and thrombosis); 2) the transplant procedure, which requires connection of two hollow

viscera (duodenum to either bladder or intestine) and the inherent complications of contamination or leak; 3) the underlying disease of diabetes, predisposing to infection in addition to the increased risk of cardiovascular complications; and 4) increased incidence of rejection episodes (compared with kidney transplantation alone or liver transplantation), predisposing to more immunosuppression early on.

Surgical complications include graft complications and those related to the mode of exocrine drainage. Graft complications commonly lead to a second laparotomy and have a negative impact on the graft and on patient survival. The three most common indications for early laparotomy include 1) vascular graft thrombosis, 2) intraabdominal infection with or without graft pancreatitis, and 3) duodenal stump leaks. Thrombosis of the pancreas graft is more common than in other vascularized grafts and is more commonly venous than arterial.

BD is associated with an array of urologic complications. Most are a result of the irritating nature of pancreatic enzymes to the bladder and urethra that can lead to recurrent episodes of cystitis, hematuria, and dysuria. Dehydration and metabolic acidosis from fluid and electrolyte loss can also be a problem. Many of these complications are chronic, leading to conversion to ED in about 20% of patients. Acute problems also arise, most early on, but they can be late. Leak from the duodenal closures or from duodenocystostomy should be suspected with any elevation of serum amylase associated with pain, and this can be confirmed by cystogram. In selected patients the leak can be controlled by Foley drainage of the bladder, whereas in others prompt exploration should be performed and a decision made whether to repair the leak or convert to ED. Leak from the duodenojejunal anastomosis with ED is a complication of greater severity than a leak from a duodenocystostomy. Spillage of enteric and activated enzyme-rich pancreatic juice causes an extensive intraabdominal infection. Early exploration may allow repair or takedown of the anastomosis and conversion to BD. However, with extensive peritonitis, graft pancreatectomy is advised.

Up to a 30% incidence of surgical complications has been reported in large series. The complication rate can be decreased by careful identification of risk factors in prospective donors and recipients, meticulous surgical technique, and judicious use of immunosuppression.

Results

As of 2008 more than 30,000 pancreas transplants had been performed worldwide, including more than 22,000 in the United States (Figure 1). An analysis of outcomes for more than 5,300 primary, deceased-donor pancreas transplants done in the United States from

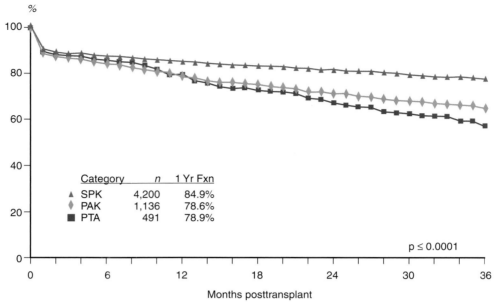

FIGURE 9   Pancreas graft functional survival (insulin independence) rates for primary deceased-donor transplants according to category for United States cases done between 2004 and 2008. *(Data from Gruessner AC, Sutherland DER: Pancreas transplant outcomes for United States (US) cases as reported to the United Network for Organ Sharing (UNOS) and the International Pancreas Transplant Registry (IPTR). In Cecka M [ed]: Clinical transplants 2008, Los Angeles, 2009, Terasaki Foundation Laboratory, pp. 45-56.)*

2004 through 2008 (Gruessner et al., 2008) showed patient survival rates to be higher than 95% at 1 year and higher than 90% at 3 years in all three categories (SPK, PAK, and PTA). About 75% of the pancreas transplants were in the SPK category, 20% were in the PAK category, and 10% were in the PTA category. In the PAK category, about three fourths of the recipients got their kidney from a living donor. Pancreas graft survival rates, as defined by insulin independence, in all three categories are shown in Figure 9. Pancreas graft survival rates continue to be higher in SPK (85%) than in PAK (79%) or PTA (79%) recipients at 1 year. The technical failure rate was slightly higher with ED than with BD in all three categories, but overall graft survival rates were not significantly different according to the method of exocrine (BD vs. ED) or venous (portal vs. systemic) drainage. The higher graft survival rate in SPK versus PAK recipients should not be taken as meaning SPK transplants should be the preferred procedure for the uremic diabetic. Unless waiting time is short (<1 year), the mortality rate while waiting is high, while an LD kidney can be used to preempt dialysis; the mortality while waiting for a PAK transplant is significantly less than while waiting for an SPK transplant.

Metabolic Effects

Restoration of normal metabolism is the immediate goal of pancreas transplantation. Most recipients become insulin independent immediately after transplant, and nearly all are euglycemic and have normal glycosylated hemoglobin. Recipient lipid profiles usually improve after successful pancreas transplantation; however, no randomized studies have been done to see if the improved lipid profile translates into lower risk for vascular disease versus a kidney transplant alone in uremic diabetics or continuing on insulin without immunosuppression in nonuremic diabetics. Microangiopathy can improve after pancreas transplantation, including retinopathy, if the intervention is early enough. Neuropathy has been shown to improve after pancreas transplantation, including autonomic features such as vesicopathy and gastropathy. Diabetic nephropathy does not recur in recipients with sustained insulin independence after SPK transplant. Furthermore, studies have shown improvement in histologic features of established nephropathy 10 years after successful PTA transplant,

though it is unclear whether this offsets the nephropathic effect of the calcineurin inhibitors currently necessary for immunusuppression.

FUTURE DIRECTIONS

A major advancement in the field of transplantation as a means to induce insulin independence in type I diabetes has been the clinical application of islet transplantation. The process involves pancreas procurement as described and extraction of islets by ex vivo intraductal perfusion of the pancreas with proteolytic enzymes. The human pancreas contains approximately 1 million islets, and about 10,000 islets per kilogram embolized to the liver via the portal vein—accessed percutaneously via a transhepatic approach or through a mesenteric tributary via a minilaparotomy—are required for allotransplantation to induce insulin independence; this is in contrast to islet autografts after total pancreatectomy for treatment of painful, chronic pancreatitis, in which 5000 islets per kilogram will suffice, though such a yield is obtained in only a third of patients. For islet allografts, more than one pancreas may be required to obtain a sufficient number of islets. Recent series of single-donor islet allografts with prolonged insulin independence have been reported, but such an achievement requires very careful donor and recipient selection.

Logistically, it is much easier to use deceased donors for the pancreas rather than using islet transplantation. Both require preservation, but for islet transplants, the long preservation commonly used for pancreas transplants, usually 12 to 18 hours, is detrimental to islet isolation. Even if this problem were solved, the number of pancreases available to treat diabetic patients in need is inadequate, and for that reason some groups are investigating islet xenotransplantation in preclinical models (pig to monkey) with some success. Stem cell differentiation into β cells suitable for transplantation is also being investigated. The future of β cell replacement probably lies in one or both of these modalities. Meanwhile, until such approaches are fully developed, pancreas transplantation remains the major method of β cell replacement for insulin-dependent diabetic patients.

SUGGESTED READINGS

Bellin MD, Kandaswamy R, Parkey J, et al: Prolonged insulin independence after islet allotransplants in recipients with type 1 diabetes, *Am J Transplant* 8:2463, 2008.

Blondet JA, Carlson AM, Kobayashi T, et al: The role of total pancreatectomy and islet autotransplantation for chronic pancreatitis, *Surg Clin North Am* 87:1477, 2007.

Boggi U, Amorese G, Marchetti P: Surgical techniques for pancreas transplantation, *Curr Opin Organ Transplant* 15:102, 2010.

Fiorina P, Shapiro AM, Ricordi C, Secchi A: The clinical impact of islet transplantation: a review, *Am J Transplant* 8(10):2008, 1990.

Fridell AJ, Mangus RS, Hollinger EF, et al: The case for pancreas after kidney transplantation, *Clin Transplant* 23:447, 2009.

Gruessner AC, Sutherland DER: Pancreas transplant outcomes for United States (US) cases as reported to the United Network for Organ Sharing (UNOS) and the International Pancreas Transplant Registry (IPTR). In Cecka M, editor: *Clinical transplants 2008*, Los Angeles, 2009, Terasaki Foundation Laboratory, pp 45–56.

Gruessner RWG, Sutherland DER, Gruessner AC: Mortality assessment for pancreas transplants, *Am J Transplant* 4:2018, 2004.

Gruessner RWG, Sutherland DE, Kandaswamy R, et al: Over 500 solitary pancreas transplants in nonuremic patients with brittle diabetes mellitus, *Transplantation* 85:42, 2008.

Humar A, Khwaja K, Sutherland DER: Pancreas transplantation. In Humar A, editor: *Atlas of organ transplantation*, London, 2006, Springer-Verlag, pp 133–196.

Kandaswamy R, Sutherland DER: Pancreas versus islet transplantation in diabetes mellitus: how to allocate deceased donor pancreata, *Transplant Proc* 38:365, 2006.

Kleinclauss F, Fauda M, Sutherland DE, et al: Pancreas after living donor kidney transplants in diabetic patients: impact on long-term kidney graft function, *Clin Transplant* 23:437, 2009.

Sollinger HW, Odorico JS, Becker YT, et al: One thousand simultaneous pancreas–kidney transplants at a single center with 22-year follow-up, *Ann Surg* 250:616, 2009.

Sutherland DER, Gruessner RW, Dunn DL, et al: Lessons learned from more than 1,000 pancreas transplants at a single institution, *Ann Surg* 233:463, 2001.

Sutherland DER, Gruessner RWG: History of pancreas transplantation. In Gruessner RWG, Sutherland DER, editors: *Transplantation of the pancreas*, New York, 2004, Springer–Verlag, pp 39–68.

Tan M, Kandaswamy R, Sutherland DE, et al: Laparoscopic donor distal pancreatectomy for living donor pancreas and pancreas–kidney transplantation, *Am J Transplant* 5:2005, 1966.

SPLENECTOMY FOR HEMATOLOGIC DISORDERS

Maakan Taghizadeh, MD, and Peter Muscarella II, MD

OVERVIEW

Although the most common indication for splenectomy is trauma, this procedure continues to play an important role in the management of a number of hematologic disorders. Indications for splenectomy in patients with hematologic disorders include splenomegaly-related symptoms, such as abdominal pain and distension, and cytopenias. Staging laparotomy for Hodgkin lymphoma is rarely, if ever, performed today because of the high accuracy of radiologic staging modalities such as computed tomography (CT) and positron emission tomography (PET) scanning.

Splenectomy for hematologic conditions rarely leads to a cure of the underlying hematologic disorder. However, it may be beneficial for resolving hematologic abnormalities and improving symptoms of splenomegaly. Furthermore, splenectomy may offer an overall reduction in the morbidity associated with these disorders, which may be broadly classified as *autoimmune/idiopathic disorders, red blood cell disorders, white blood cell disorders,* and bone marrow disorders (Table 1).

AUTOIMMUNE/IDIOPATHIC DISORDERS

Idiopathic Thrombocytopenia Purpura

Idiopathic thrombocytopenia purpura (ITP) is a condition in which platelets bind to circulating antiplatelet antibodies and are cleared by phagocytic cells. The splenic production of immunoglobulin G (IgG) leads to removal of platelets by macrophages, predominantly in the spleen and liver. Clinically, this results in thrombocytopenia, petechiae, purpura, and ecchymosis. Bleeding may occur from mucosal surfaces such as the gingivae, gastrointestinal system, vagina, and genitourinary system. The incidence of intracranial hemorrhage is 1%. Women are affected two to three times more commonly than men, but children are affected equally between genders.

The spleen is usually of normal size in ITP. Thrombocytopenia in the face of splenomegaly for suspected cases of ITP should prompt further workup for other diagnoses. The finding of megakaryocytes is consistent with a diagnosis of ITP, so bone marrow biopsy may be useful in patients who are initially seen with these symptoms. ITP is a diagnosis of exclusion, and other illnesses that can cause secondary ITP must be considered, such as human immunodeficiency virus

(HIV) infection, systemic lupus erythematosus (SLE), antiphospholipid antibody syndrome, hepatitis C, and lymphoproliferative disorders. Certain drugs may also elicit similar immune-mediated platelet destruction. A medication history that includes cocaine, gold, certain antibiotics, antihypertensives, antiinflammatories, heparin, quinidine, and abciximab may result in this immune phenomenon.

Children are often seen with ITP at a young age (about 5 years) with a sudden onset of petechiae or purpura, commonly occurring days to weeks after an infectious illness. ITP is usually self-limiting in children, with over 70% of patients achieving remission. Most cases of ITP in children are managed with observation and short-term medical therapy, although the risk of intracranial hemorrhage may be a concern when platelet counts are less than 20,000/mm³. Intravenous immunoglobulin (IVIG) therapy improves severe thrombocytopenia, and short courses of prednisone (4 mg/kg for 4 days) produce excellent results. Splenectomy is reserved for patients with thrombocytopenia persistent for more than 1 year, for failures of medical therapy, and for patients with severe thrombocytopenia. Splenectomy may rarely be indicated in children presenting with severe or life-threatening bleeding.

In adults, ITP displays a more insidious onset. Treatment is usually indicated once platelet counts are in the 20,000 to 30,000/mm³ range. Patients with platelet counts around 50,000/mm³ who have significant mucosal bleeding or risk factors for bleeding also require treatment. Again, the initial treatment is medical. Results of prednisone administration (1 to 1.5 mg/kg/day) are usually appreciated after 3 weeks. The prednisone dose can then be tapered after an adequate platelet response. Response rates for medical therapy are 50% to 75%, but only 15% to 20% of patients achieve a long-term response, and relapses are common.

If platelet counts remain low after 6 to 8 weeks of steroid therapy, or if thrombocytopenia recurs after steroid taper, splenectomy should be considered. IVIG (1 mg/kg/day for 2 to 3 days) is indicated for internal bleeding with platelet levels below 10,000/mm³. IVIG may also be used as an adjunct to steroid therapy, for extensive purpura, and preoperatively in patients at high risk for bleeding who have continued low platelet counts despite steroid therapy. Splenectomy is indicated in patients whose medical therapy has failed, in those who relapse, or when prolonged steroid use causes unwanted side effects. Splenectomy results in a 75% to 85% permanent response with no need for further therapy. If platelet transfusion is required perioperatively for bleeding or persistent platelet counts below 10,000/mm³, transfusion should be held until the splenic artery is ligated. Postoperatively, good responses are usually seen by the end of the first week.

Thrombotic Thrombocytopenic Purpura

Thrombotic thrombocytopenic purpura (TTP) is a rare disorder in which damage to the endothelium triggers platelet deposition in small arterioles and capillaries, leading to microvascular thrombotic episodes. TTP is characterized by a microangiopathic hemolytic

TABLE 1: Hematologic disorders for which splenectomy can be considered

Autoimmune/Idiopathic Disorders

Idiopathic thrombocytopenic purpura
Thrombotic thrombocytopenic purpura
Idiopathic autoimmune hemolytic anemia
Felty syndrome
Sarcoidosis

Red Blood Cell Disorders

Cell Membrane Deficiencies
Hereditary spherocytosis
Hereditary elliptocytosis
Hereditary pyropoikilocytosis
Hereditary stomatocytosis
Hereditary xerocytosis

Genetic Deficiencies

Thalassemia
Sickle cell anemia
Gaucher disease
Pyruvate kinase deficiency
G6PD deficiency
Amyloidosis

White Blood Cell Disorders

Hodgkin lymphoma
Non-Hodgkin lymphoma
Chronic lymphocytic leukemia
Chronic myelogenous leukemia
Hairy cell leukemia

Bone Marrow Disorders

Primary myelofibrosis
Myeloproliferative disorders

anemia, severe thrombocytopenia, fever, neurologic complications, and renal failure. TTP has been seen after ticlopidine or clopidogrel therapy, as well as during pregnancy and in the postpartum period. The clinical presentation of TTP includes petechiae, most commonly on the lower extremities, along with fever, myalgia, and fatigue. Neurologic symptoms include headache, mental status changes, seizures, and even coma. Patients may present with congestive heart failure or cardiac arrhythmias. Diagnosis is usually confirmed with a peripheral blood smear demonstrating schistocytes, nucleated red blood cells, and basophilic stippling. First-line treatment is with daily plasmapheresis and fresh frozen plasma (FFP) transfusions. Most patients will respond to therapy. Platelet transfusions are not generally recommended for use in TTP because of the risk of severe clinical deterioration that has been reported after their administration.

Splenectomy in TTP is reserved for patients who have frequent relapses. Along with high-dose steroid therapy, splenectomy can aid in prolonging the disease-free interval. The response rate for splenectomy in TTP has been reported to be only about 40%.

Autoimmune Hemolytic Anemia

Autoimmune hemolytic anemia (AIHA) is a disorder in which autoantibodies are formed and directed against red blood cell antigens. Patients show signs and symptoms of anemia, and red blood cells may be sequestered by tissue macrophages or destroyed in the periphery. The etiology may be idiopathic, or the condition may be related to infection, systemic lupus erythematosus, or leukemia.

AIHA is classified into two major types, *warm autoimmune hemolytic anemia* and *cold autoantibody syndromes,* most commonly cold agglutinin syndrome. In warm AIHA, IgG autoantibodies react optimally at 37° C. The peak incidence of warm AIHA is between the ages of 40 and 70 years, but it can occur at any age. In children it is often self-limited, occurring after a viral infection and resolving over 2 to 3 months. Diagnosis is made based on clinical findings and laboratory results, including a peripheral blood smear and direct antiglobulin test. First-line treatment is with corticosteroid therapy (1.0 to 2.0 mg/kg/day) with improvement in hemoglobin usually seen within several days; remission is achieved in 60% of patients.

Children generally respond better to steroid therapy than adults. The steroid dosage is tapered gradually to the lowest dose needed to control hemolysis. If remission cannot be achieved in 3 weeks, or if the hemoglobin concentration cannot be maintained by a low dose of steriods, then splenectomy is indicated. A 60% to 80% improvement in anemia can be expected within the first 2 weeks after splenectomy. Approximately 50% of patients will continue to require low-dose steroids (15 mg/day) to maintain hemoglobin concentrations after splenectomy.

Cold agglutinin syndrome compromises 15% to 25% of AIHA. This disorder is usually caused by an infectious process, such as Epstein-Barr virus (EBV) infection, or by a lymphoproliferative disorder. Signs and symptoms are of a more progressive nature. The IgM autoantibodies react optimally at 0° to 5° C, and patients may also complain of Raynaud phenomenon. Treatment consists of avoiding cold by staying indoors and wearing appropriate clothing, which can prevent an acute hemolytic crisis. Alkylating agents such as chlorambucil and cyclophosphamide have been used successfully for treatment, along with plasmapheresis. Steroids are usually not an effective treatment for cold agglutinin syndrome, and splenectomy is not indicated because the erythrocytes are destroyed in the liver and not the spleen. If patients require transfusions for supportive care, a blood warmer is recommended. Cross-matching blood products for transfusion can be a challenge in these patients.

Felty Syndrome

Felty syndrome consists of rheumatoid arthritis, otherwise unexplained neutropenia, and splenomegaly. The size of the spleen may be variable, and splenomegaly is not essential for the diagnosis, but 85% of patients will have the HLA-DR4 antigen. Patients may have severe or chronic infections due to neutropenia, especially with neutrophil counts below $0.5 \times 10^9/mm^3$. They may have spontaneous remissions of their neutropenia. First-line treatment is with low-dose methotrexate or disease-modifying antirheumatic drugs. Granulocyte colony stimulating factor (G-CSF) may be used for treatment failures in cases of increased infection risk, or prior to planned joint surgery. Splenectomy is indicated when medical treatment has failed, as evidenced by recurrent infections or severe neutropenia. Splenectomy results in an 80% hematologic response rate.

Sarcoidosis

Sarcoidosis is a noncaseating granulomatous disease. Although 90% of patients have primary lung involvement, the disease can affect every organ in the body. Primary splenic sarcoid is very rare, and splenic involvement is often found as part of a multiorgan sarcoidosis. Up to 40% of patients with sarcoidosis have splenomegaly, and 3% have massive splenomegaly. Splenic involvement occurs in 10% to 15% of patients with sarcoidosis. Treatment is primarily medical, with the use of corticosteroids or methotrexate. Indications for splenectomy include symptoms related to splenomegaly, intractable pain, exclusion of a neoplastic process, and hematologic abnormalities related to sequestration. Splenectomy does not alter the course of sarcoidosis, but it has been shown to aid in treatment of refractory hypercalcemia in case reports.

RED BLOOD CELL DISORDERS

Cell Membrane Deficiencies

Hereditary Spherocytosis

Hereditary spherocytosis (HS) is the most common red blood cell membrane disorder in Europe and North America. The majority of patients (75%) will have an affected relative. It is an autosomal-dominant inherited disease that results in a deficiency of the cytoskeletal protein spectrin and, to a lesser extent, ankyrin. A rare autosomal-recessive variant with a more severe hemolytic anemia has also been reported. The defect leads to a loss of the cell membrane surface area, resulting in sphering of the red blood cell. This leads to increased osmotic fragility and decreased deformability, and it impairs passage of the red blood cell through the splenic pulp. The spherocytes are then destroyed prematurely.

In milder forms of HS, patients may be asymptomatic, or they may suffer only mild jaundice. Commonly, patients present with anemia, jaundice, splenomegaly, and cholelithiasis with pigmented (bilirubin) gallstones. Splenomegaly usually develops after infancy, and approximately 50% of patients will develop gallstones after age 5 years. Diagnosis is made by family history, blood smear showing spherocytes and reticulocytosis, and the finding of splenomegaly.

Treatment by splenectomy is curative in almost all patients with common forms of spherocytosis, which is the most common indication for splenectomy in congenital anemias. Cholecystectomy is recommended at the time of splenectomy for patients with gallstones, but splenectomy is usually delayed until after age 5 years to prevent the risk of overwhelming postsplenectomy infection (OPSI).

Some controversy exists over whether patients with milder forms of spherocytosis should undergo splenectomy. Although there may be a role for partial splenectomy in children younger than 5 years, some studies have shown an improvement in anemia with potential maintenance of splenic immune function after partial splenectomy.

Hereditary Elliptocytosis

Hereditary elliptocytosis (HE) is a rare disorder that results from mutation of certain red blood cell membrane skeleton proteins (spectrin and protein 4.1R). In the United States, HE has a prevalence of approximately 3 to 5 cases per 10,000 population. It is most commonly an autosomal-dominant disorder and is more common in people of African and Mediterranean ancestries. The true incidence is unknown because of the wide variety of clinical presentations. Most patients with the dominant inheritance are asymptomatic with a mild compensated anemia or no anemia at all. Affected cells are morphologically characterized by biconcave elliptocytes or rod-shaped cells. These cells are much more deformable than spherocytes and have a less severe clinical course. There is, however, a rare autosomal-recessive form that can lead to severe hemolysis. If patients have a mild form of HE and are asymptomatic with no evidence of hemolysis, no treatment is needed. Patients with chronic hemolysis may require blood transfusions and folic acid daily. Splenectomy is indicated for severe hemolysis and its complications and is curative.

Hereditary Pyropoikilocytosis

Hereditary pyropoikilocytosis (HPP) has been described as an autosomal recessive, more severe hemolytic anemia with striking micropoikilocytosis and thermal instability of red blood cells. HPP represents a subtype of common HE, with the presence of the same molecular

TABLE 2: Guidelines for OPSI prophylaxis

Incidence of OPSI
First 2 years following splenectomy: adults (0.9%), children (5.0%)
Risk factors: age <18 years, hematologic disorders, immunosuppressive therapy

Vaccination and OPSI Prophylaxis Recommendations
Vaccinations
Haemophilus influenzae B, *Pneumococcus, Meningococcus* 2 weeks preoperatively (elective cases) *or* at discharge *or* 2 weeks postoperatively
If patient received immunosuppression therapy, vaccinate 3 months after treatment
Booster vaccinations for *Pneumococcus ± Meningococcus* every 5 years
H. influenzae AB titers can be followed to assess need for a booster dose
Consider monitoring *H. influenzae* AB titers of all three pathogens in immunocompromised patients

Antibiotic Prophylaxis
Less than 60 minutes prior to incision to cover skin flora
Continue prophylactic antibiotics for 2 years postoperatively in children

defect of spectrin. Patients with HPP usually have one parent with a common hereditary elliptocytosis mutation and one parent with a milder, subclinical defect in spectrin synthesis. The disease usually presents in newborns and infants with anemia and jaundice. Splenectomy is curative for patients with severe anemia.

Hereditary Stomatocytosis and Xerocytosis

Hereditary stomatocytosis (hydrocytosis) and xerocytosis are rare autosomal-dominant hemolytic anemias characterized by a variable clinical course, from asymptomatic to a mild hemolytic anemia. The underlying defect leads to increased erythrocyte cation permeability and an increased erythrocyte volume in stomatocytosis. Stomatocytes have a mouth-shaped area of central pallor, and xerocytes present as target cells. In xerocytosis, membrane cation permeability and cell volume are decreased.

In cases of severe hemolysis, splenectomy may improve the anemia but does not fully correct the hemolysis. In patients with stomatocytosis, the role for splenectomy should be carefully considered; such patients have developed hypercoagulability after splenectomy, leading to catastrophic thrombotic episodes and chronic pulmonary hypertension. Fortunately, the majority of patients with these rare forms of hemolytic anemia have a mild clinical course and do not require splenectomy.

Genetic Deficiencies

Thalassemia

Thalassemia describes a group of autosomal-dominant inherited hematologic disorders caused by a defect in the synthesis of one or more of the hemoglobin chains. As a group, the thalassemias represent the most common genetic disorder known worldwide. The clinical manifestations associated with thalassemia arise from quantitatively imbalanced accumulation of globin subunits and inadequate hemoglobin production. Each subtype is characterized by the globin chain affected (α, β, γ, or δ). The β subtype is the most common form of thalassemia in the United States and occurs mainly in patients of Italian and Greek descent.

Patients who have the heterozygous form (thalassemia minor) of β thalassemia are usually asymptomatic with a microcytosis and mild anemia. The homozygous form—thalassemia major, or Cooley anemia—is much more severe. Patients usually are asymptomatic until 6 months of age because of the presence of fetal hemoglobin. Patients then show signs and symptoms of severe hemolytic anemia: abdominal swelling, growth retardation, irritability, jaundice, pallor, splenomegaly, pigmented gallstones, and skeletal abnormalities. Laboratory values show a severe microcytic anemia with nucleated red blood cells, anisocytosis, and poikilocytosis. Patients may have a mild neutropenia and thrombocytopenia.

Treatment is with periodic, lifelong blood transfusion and iron chelation therapy. Splenectomy is indicated for severe splenomegaly, requiring increased blood transfusions. Massive splenomegaly is usually rare in appropriately transfused patients. A transfusion requirement of more than 180 to 200 mL/kg/year of packed red blood cells usually represents excessive red blood cell requirements and warrants splenectomy. A reduction of 25% to 60% in transfusion requirements can be expected after splenectomy, but patients may also develop a significant thrombocytosis. Splenectomy is usually delayed until age 4 or 5 to decrease the risk of infectious complications. Bone marrow transplantation is the only curative approach, however, most patients do not survive beyond the age of 30 years because of severe cardiac sequelae.

Sickle Cell Anemia

Sickle cell anemia is an autosomal-recessive hemoglobinopathy characterized by an amino acid substitution on the β chain of the hemoglobin molecule. This hemoglobin molecule, HgS, has the propensity to deform and take on a sickle shape when exposed to low-oxygen tension. The sickle cells cause stasis and vasoocclusion in microvasculature of the body, leading to tissue ischemia, severe pain, and chronic organ tissue damage. These episodes are referred to as *sickle cell crises*. Patients who are homozygous for the disorder have sickle cell disease, and many undergo autosplenectomy at an early age because of multiple infarcts. Treatment includes hydration, transfusions, and avoidance of situations that can precipitate a sickle cell crisis.

Splenectomy is rarely indicated in sickle cell disease because of autoinfarction of the spleen, but it can be indicated for splenic abcess and sequestration. Splenic abcess can be a complication of splenic infarction and is an indication for splenectomy. Acute splenic sequestration has a high mortality and is characterized by massive splenomegaly, acute exacerbation of anemia, and hypovolemia. This is initially treated with restoration of blood volume and red blood cell mass, but recurrence is common. Splenectomy should be considered to prevent further episodes of sequestration. It is important to maintain euvolemia and normothermia to prevent complications of an acute sicke cell crisis in the perioperative period.

Gaucher Disease

Gaucher disease is a glycolipid storage disease in which a deficiency in β-glucosidase (glucocerebrosidase) leads to deposition of glucocerebroside in the reticuloendothelial system. This deposition leads to severe organomegaly, pulmonary infiltrates, and bone marrow infiltration. Patients may experience bone pain and may show signs of anemia, thrombocytopenia, osteopenia, osteonecrosis, and massive hepatosplenomegaly. Splenectomy is indicated for severe and symptomatic splenomegaly and refractory cytopenia.

Partial splenectomy has been advocated in some children with Gaucher disease to preserve some splenic function. Splenectomy does not alter the disease progression of this disorder, but the thrombocytopenia will improve. Splenectomy for Gaucher disease can result in severe bone disease, a tenfold increased risk

of osteonecrosis, and worsening lung or kidney function. Careful patient selection is recommended prior to splenectomy in this patient population.

Pyruvate Kinase Deficiency

Pyruvate kinase deficiency (PKD) is the most common genetic defect to cause congenital enzymopathic hemolytic anemia. PKD is an autosomal-recessive disease, and a defect in the glycolytic pathway results in a deficiency of adenosine triphosphate (ATP). Red blood cells are less deformable and are often destroyed in the spleen, leading to splenomegaly. Hemolysis can be exacerbated by acute infections and pregnancy, and patients show symptoms of mild to moderately severe anemia with splenomegaly. Clinically, the effects of hemolysis are often milder than in other hemolytic anemias because of elevated levels of 2,3-diphosphoglycerate (DPG) in pyruvate kinase–deficient red cells. These red blood cells permit more efficient delivery of oxygen to the tissues for the same concentration of hemoglobin in the blood. Splenectomy is indicated in patients with the severe hemolytic variants of PKD or in patients who require frequent transfusions. As in the previous sections, splenectomy should be delayed in children until after the age of 4 or 5 years.

Glucose-6-Phosphate Dehydrogenase Deficiency

Glucose-6-phosphate dehydrogenase (G6PD) deficiency is the most common enzyme defect associated with hereditary hemolytic anemia worldwide. It is an X-linked disorder of the enzyme G6PD in the glutathione pathway that leads to damage of red cell macromolecules by toxic oxygen products. Hemolysis may be precipitated by acute infections, oxidant drugs such as sulfas and antimalarials, and fava beans. Treatment is directed at the inciting agent, and severe anemia is treated with transfusion. Splenectomy is rarely, if ever, indicated for the anemia associated with G6PD deficiency.

Amyloidosis

Amyloidosis is one of the most common hereditary or acquired disorders that involve extracellular deposition of insoluble fibrillar proteins in tissues and organs. Hepatosplenomegaly may occur in 25% of patients, and severe splenomegaly is seen in approximately 10%. These patients may develop functional hyposplenism, and splenectomy is indicated for signs and symptoms associated with a massively enlarged spleen. It does not, however, alter the ultimate course of the disease.

■ WHITE BLOOD CELL DISORDERS

Hodgkin Lymphoma

Hodgkin lymphoma is a malignant neoplasm of lymphoreticular cell origin that usually affects young adults in their second and third decades. The mainstay of treatment is with chemotherapy and radiation. Historically, splenectomy was performed as part of a staging laparotomy, including lymph node sampling, bone marrow biopsy, and liver biopsy. Staging laparotomy is rarely used today and has largely been replaced by imaging modalities such as CT scanning, lymphangiography, and PET scanning. Splenectomy is rarely indicated for patients who develop thrombocytopenia or symptoms related to splenomegaly.

Non-Hodgkin Lymphoma

Non-Hodgkin lymphoma (NHL) is the most common type of lymphoma and comprises a diverse group of lymphomas varying in prognosis based on histologic subtype and clinical features. NHL is the most common primary splenic neoplasm with splenic involvement occurring in 65% to 80% of patients. Splenectomy is indicated for symptoms related to anemia, massive splenomegaly, and thrombocytopenia, and neutropenia related to splenic sequestration.

There are some subtypes of NHL that involve the spleen more than others. Splenic marginal zone lymphoma (SMZL) is an indolent B-cell lymphoma seen in older patients (>50 years), with microvascular invasion of the spleen with marginal zone differentiation. The first-line treatment for SMZL is splenectomy, which has been shown to lead to partial remission in many patients and complete remission in some, because the spleen is the site of lymphoma origin. Recent studies have investigated the role of chemotherapy with some promise, but splenectomy remains the first-line treatment.

Hairy Cell Leukemia

Hairy cell leukemia (HCL) is a rare leukemia, representing only 2% of all leukemias. It is characterized by B-lymphocytes that possess cytoplasmic projections from the cell membrane ("hairy cells"). This is an indolent disease that presents in the fifth decade with splenomegaly (80% to 90% of patients), pancytopenia, and neoplastic mononuclear cells in the periphery and bone marrow. Pancytopenia is caused by hypersplenism and replacement of bone marrow by leukemic cells.

In the past, splenectomy was an essential component of standard of treatment, and it resulted in improvement in symptoms from massive splenomegaly and a 40% to 70% improvement in the hematologic cell lines for up to 10 years irrespective of splenic size. Treatment with the purine analogs pentostatin and cladribine has supplanted the use of interferon-α, other chemotherapeutic agents, and splenectomy as primary therapy. These agents have proven response rates of 92%, with complete remission rates of 80%, and 10 year survival rates greater than 90%. Splenectomy is rarely indicated for the treatment of HCL and is reserved for cases of pancytopenia refractory to medical therapy, splenic rupture, and severe bleeding from thrombocytopenia.

Chronic Lymphocytic Leukemia

Chronic lymphocytic leukemia (CLL) is a B-cell leukemia in which there is progressive accumulation of functionally incompetent lymphoctyes. CLL usually develops after the fifth decade of life and is more common in men than in women. Splenic infiltration is common in advanced stages and can lead to severe splenomegaly and substantial cytopenia, which results from hypersplenism.

Splenectomy is indicated to relieve symptoms associated with massive splenomegaly, such as abdominal pain, distension, and early satiety. Splenectomy for treatment of severe thrombocytopenia and anemia has a 60% to 70% hematologic response rate and has been shown to lead to improved survival. Some patients in the very advanced stages of CLL who have been refractory to medical treatment may not respond as well to splenectomy. Because this is a disease of the elderly, the risks and benefits should be fully weighed before undertaking splenectomy in critically ill patients.

Chronic Myelogenous Leukemia

Chronic myelogenous leukemia (CML) is a disorder of abnormal proliferation and accumulation of granulocytes; 95% of CML patients will have the characteristic Philadelphia chromosome with a reciprocal translocation between chromosomes 9 and 22. CML may occur in childhood, but it is mainly found in adults, with a mean age of 65 at diagnosis. Diagnosis is commonly made during the chronic phase, which is commonly asymptomatic, and 40% of patients in the chronic phase will be initially seen for splenomegaly. The disease can then progress to an accelerated phase with the development of fever, night sweats, weight loss, bone pain, increased white blood cell count, and increasing splenomegaly despite medical therapy. An acute blastic crisis can develop, which results in severe splenomegaly and hypersplenism that in turn leads to severe anemia, bleeding complications, and infection.

Current first-line therapy is with imatinib, a tyrosine kinase inhibitor. Bone marrow transplantation can be used in cases of poor response or relapse as can interferon-α. Splenectomy has not shown any survival benefit in the early chronic phase, or before bone marrow transplantation, but it may offer palliation in patients with severe symptoms of splenomegaly or hematologic disorders from hypersplenism.

MYELOPROLIFERATIVE DISORDERS

Primary Myelofibrosis (Myelofibrosis with Myeloid Metaplasia)

Primary myelofibrosis (PMF) is a chronic, malignant hematologic disorder that results in hyperplasia of abnormal myeloid precursor cells leading to marrow fibrosis and extramedullary hematopoiesis in the liver and spleen. This can lead to significant splenomegaly, cytopenias from splenic sequestration, and portal hypertension from venous thrombosis. PMF is prevalent in patients with a history of radiation or toxic industrial chemical exposure. It is more common in men than women, and the average age of diagnosis is 65 years.

Splenectomy is indicated in patients who develop thrombocytopenia, hemolysis requiring significant transfusions, pain from massive splenomegaly, recurrent splenic infarctions, and portal hypertension with refractory ascites and variceal hemorrhage. Splenectomy in PMF has a substantial risk of morbidity (15% to 30%) and mortality (10%) and should only be performed in a select group of patients. Splenectomy in patients with PMF has been associated with hemorrhage, infection, leukocytosis, severe thrombocytosis (18% to 50%), progressive hepatomegaly (12% to 29%), fatal hepatic failure (7%), and leukemic transformation (11% to 20%). Some studies have reported an increase in the complication rate with a laparoscopic approach versus an open approach in PMF.

The appropriate use of palliative splenectomy in can result in improved quality of life for patients who are unresponsive to less invasive approaches. Postoperatively, the use of platelet-lowering agents such as hydroxyurea, interferon-α, aspirin, and anagrelide has been shown to aid in reduction of thrombotic complications. Surgical technique involving ligation of the splenic vein flush at its confluence with the superior mesenteric vein has been described to improve laminar flow and decrease portal vein thrombosis. Compensatory massive hepatic enlargement can be treated with low-level radiation and multiple chemotherapeutic agents for patients awaiting possible autologous stem cell transplantation.

Bone Marrow Disorders

The myeloproliferative disorders are a group of disorders caused by abnormal proliferation of erythroid, megakaryocytic, or granulocytic myeloid cells beginning in bone marrow and extramedullary sites. These disorders include CML, polycythemia vera, PMF, essential thrombocytopenia, hypereosinophilic syndromes, mast cell disease, and chronic neutrophilic leukemia. Splenectomy can play a role in palliative treatment of some of these disorders. The indications are for symptoms of massive splenomegaly and cytopenias from splenic sequestration. Splenectomy is of little benefit in polycythemia vera in the early stages, but as myelofibrosis develops later, it can provide palliation similar to PMF. Splenectomy is rarely indicated in essential thrombocytosis.

PREOPERATIVE CONSIDERATIONS

Preoperative imaging is crucial for operative planning, and CT offers numerous advantages over ultrasound. CT images are excellent for determining splenic size, anatomic relationship with surrounding organs, and anatomy of the variable splenic blood supply, and it has the potential to locate accessory spleens (Figure 1). In cases of massive splenomegaly or portal hypertension, preoperative splenic arterial embolization can be considered to help reduce blood loss, and it can make laparoscopic surgery much more manageable. Appropriate perioperative antibiotics are given 60 minutes prior to making the skin incision and should cover skin flora. The use of an orogastric or nasogastric tube can reduce gastric distension and can improve visualization and dissection of the short gastric vessels along the greater curvature of the stomach.

Blood products should be available intraoperatively, especially in patients with thrombocytopenia. Platelets are transfused only as needed for bleeding after ligation of the splenic artery. If patients have been treated with chronic corticosteroids, stress-dose steroids should be administered with a rapid taper postoperatively. In elective cases, it is recommended to vaccinate patients against encapsulated organisms (*Haemophilus influenzae* B, polyvalent *Pneumococcus*, and *Meningococcus* vaccines) 2 weeks prior to splenectomy. If splenectomy is emergent, the patient should be vaccinated postoperatively (Table 2).

OPERATIVE CONSIDERATIONS

For open splenectomy, the surgeon can use a midline incision or a left subcostal approach. Midline incisions are preferable in cases of massive splenomegaly (Figure 2) or in patients with a narrow costal margin. The splenic hilum can be ligated first, or it may be ligated after mobilizing the spleen from the splenophrenic, splenorenal, and splenocolic ligaments. This is advantageous in patients with ITP to facilitate the transfusion of platelets if necessary once the splenic artery is ligated. It may also be preferred in patients with malignancy, massive splenomegaly, hilar lymphadenopathy, or with dense perisplenic adhesions to avoid bleeding related to tearing of the vessels or capsule. This approach involves entering the lesser sac and dissecting the vessels at the hilum (Figure 3) to gain control and thereby avoid injuring the tail of the pancreas.

The hilar vessels are commonly divided individually to prevent arteriovenous fistula formation. They can be ligated with a vascular load on a linear stapling device or with suture ligatures. In patients with enlarged splenic veins, a suture ligature can be used, either with a stapler or with ligation. The splenogastric ligament is divided, and the short gastric vessels are identified and are suture ligated or clipped. In laparoscopic splenectomy, an EndoGIA stapler (Covidien, Norwalk, Conn.) can be used for the hilar vessels, and Ligasure (ValleyLab, Boulder, Colo.), EndoClips (Covidien), or harmonic scalpel can be used to divide the short gastric vessels.

In laparoscopic splenectomy, the surgeon can use an abdominal or a right lateral decubitus approach, utilizing three trocars. The lateral approach allows better access to the splenic pedicle and pancreatic tail. The splenic flexure is mobilized followed by the lateral attachments. The splenic pedicle is dissected from the lower pole in a cephalad progression to the main vascular pedicle and short gastric vessels. These are ligated as described above. The splenophrenic ligament may be kept intact to allow placement of the spleen into the bag for extraction. The neck of the bag is pulled through the trocar site, and the spleen is fragmented within the sack and removed in a piecemeal fashion. Once the spleen is removed, careful inspection for hemostasis of the splenic bed, the inferior surface of the diaphragm, and the greater curvature of the stomach should be performed. Accessory spleens are present in 10% to 30% of patients, and the common locations should be explored prior to closure.

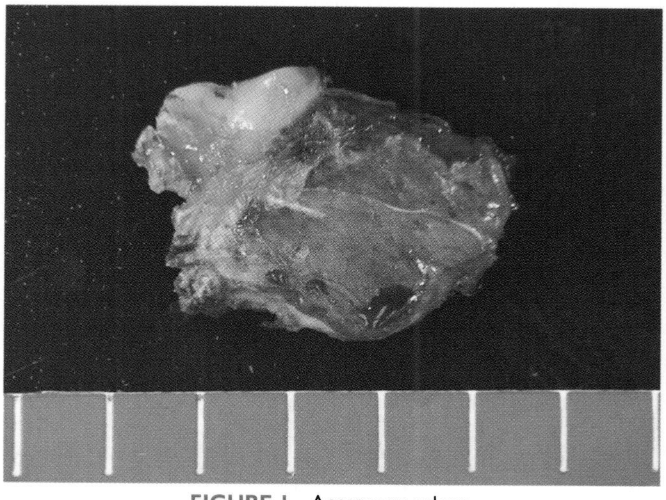

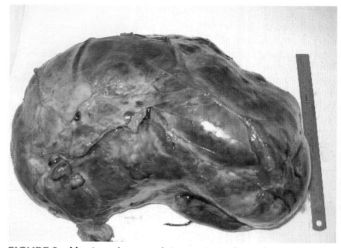

FIGURE 2 Massive splenomegaly in a patient who underwent splenectomy for complications of a lymphoproliferative disorder.

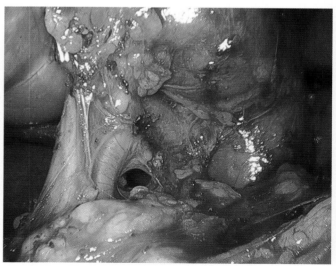

FIGURE 3 Laparoscopic view of splenic hilar vessels following dissection, prior to division with a vascular stapling device.

FIGURE 1 Accessory spleen.

LAPAROSCOPIC SPLENECTOMY

Laparoscopic splenectomy has become the standard approach in most cases of splenectomy. It is indicated in most cases of splenectomy for benign and malignant hematologic disorders, although there are still some areas of controversy. Laparoscopic splenectomy provides the advantage of shorter length of stay, decreased use of postoperative analgesia, and a potential decrease in morbidity. Recent studies have shown a trend toward shorter operative times that are comparable to open splenectomy in cases of normal or moderately enlarged spleens. Most data show comparable detection of accessory spleens, which can cause recurrence in cases of autoimmune hematologic disorders.

Much of the controversy surrounding laparoscopic splenectomy involves the size of the spleen. The normal adult spleen measures 11 cm on its long axis and weighs approximately 100 to 250 g. *Splenomegaly* is defined as a long axis measurement greater than 15 cm. *Massive splenomegaly* is defined as a measurement greater than 20 cm, and *megaspleen* indicates a size greater than 22 cm. Most authors state that laparoscopic splenectomy is still preferred in cases of splenomegaly. For massive splenomegaly or megaspleen, the laparoscopic approach becomes much more technically challenging with a much higher rate of open conversion. In our experience, the use of laparoscopic splenectomy is limited by the size of the bag used for retrieval. In cases of massive splenectomy with associated hematologic abnormalities, it may be prudent to proceed with open splenectomy as the planned procedure. A hand-assisted approach may be considered in some cases, but a laparoscopic approach should be avoided in patients with portal hypertension from cirrhosis because of the extremely high risk of hemorrhage.

POSTOPERATIVE MANAGEMENT AND COMPLICATIONS

Patients should be monitored for hemorrhage, atelectasis, and infection in the early postoperative period. The most common site of hemorrhage at reexploration is the undersurface of the diaphragm. Patients will usually have a physiologic increase in leukocytes postoperatively. Infectious complications include subphrenic abscess and OPSI. If the patient did not receive preoperative vaccinations, they should be administered 2 weeks after surgery. If compliance is a concern, they may be administered prior to discharge from the hospital. Vaccinations should be held for 3 months after surgery in patients who have been treated with immunosuppressive agents, and patients should receive booster vaccinations every 5 years for *Pneumococcus* and *Meningococcus*.

Prophylactic antiobiotics have been recommended for at least 2 years in children but are not generally used in adults. The risk for OPSI is highest in the first 2 years after surgery but does carry a lifelong risk. Risk factors for OPSI include age (chidren at 5% vs. adults at 0.9%), splenectomy for a hematologic disorder, and history of immunosuppressant therapy. OPSI has a reported fatality rate of 50%. *Streptococcus pneumoniae, Neisseria meningitides,* and *Haemophilus influenzae B* account for most of the severe infections. *Escherichia coli, Capnocytophaga,* and intraerythrocytic parasites also pose a risk. Patients typically come in with an upper respiratory infection that rapidly proceeds to sepsis and multisystem organ failure. A high index of suspicion for OPSI is required, and early and aggressive treatment with broad-spectrum antibiotics and supportive measures can be life saving.

Other postoperative complications include thrombocytosis, pneumonia, pleural effusions, pancreatitis, pancreatic fistula, venous thrombosis, injury to adjacent organs, and missed accessory spleens. Risk factors for postoperative complications include massive splenomegaly and myeloproliferative disorders, mainly PMF.

Thrombocytosis can occur in the immediate postoperative period, but it peaks at 3 weeks. Antiplatelet therapy is only indicated for thrombotic complications or as a prophylaxis when platelet counts reach 1 million. Patients with an accessory spleen will have an absence of Howell-Jolley bodies, Heinz bodies, and target cells and may require reexploration for accessory spleens or selective embolization.

Portal vein or mesenteric vein thrombosis can be a serious complication of splenectomy, and postsplenectomy venous thrombosis has been reported in up to 14% of patients, with some studies reporting a higher rate for laparoscopic splenectomy. Risk factors for thrombosis include myeloproliferative disorders, hemolytic anemias, a long splenic vein stump, postoperative thrombocytosis, hypercoagulable states, and splenomegaly. Patients complain of vague abdominal pain, distension, ileus, fever, and nausea, and they may develop intestinal infarction and portal hypertension. Systemic anticoagulation is required, with recannulation rates greater than 90% if treated promptly.

SUGGESTED READINGS

Crary SE, Buchanon GR: Vascular complications after splenectomy for hematologic disorders, *Blood* 114(14):2861–2868, 2009.

Feldman LS, Demyttenaere S, Polyhronopoulos GN, Fried GM: Refining the selection criteria for laparoscopic versus open splenectomy for splenomegaly, *J Laparoendosc Adv Surg Tech A* 18(1):13–19, 2008.

Friedman RL, Hiat JR, Korman JL, et al: Laparoscopic or open splenectomy for hematologic disease: which approach is superior? *J Am Coll Surg* 185(1):49–54, 1997.

Habermalz B, Sauerland S, Neugebauer E, et al: Laparoscopic splenectomy: the clinical practice guidelines of the European Association for Endoscopic Surgery (EAES), *Surg Endosc* 22(4):821–848, 2008.

Mourtzoukou EG, Pappas G, Peppas G, Falagas ME: Vaccination of asplenic or hyposplenic adults, *Br J Surg* 95:273–280, 2008.

Cysts, Tumors, and Abscesses of the Spleen

Hien T. Nguyen, MD, and Michael R. Marohn, DO

OVERVIEW

The spleen was first described by Hippocrates in 421 BCE, but it was not until the eighteenth and nineteenth century that the spleen's role in forming white blood cells and removing red blood cells was discovered. Controversy remains over when the first splenectomy was performed, whether by Zacarelli in 1549 or by Quittenbaum in 1826. But since Jules Pean described the first successful splenectomy for a splenic cyst in 1867, surgeons have encountered cysts, tumors, and abscesses of the spleen requiring surgical management with increasing frequency.

With improving imaging capabilities, incidentally discovered splenic lesions have increased the number of surgical requests for diagnosis and management. Definitions and classifications of splenic lesions, particularly cysts, have continued to evolve for over 100 years. Contemporary surgeons caring for disorders of the spleen need to be familiar with the incidence, classifications, evaluation, and management strategies for splenic cysts, tumors, and abscess following the broader principle of splenic preservation when possible.

Classifications of splenic cysts, tumors, and abscesses remain debated, but most classifications require pathologic information not available prior to treatment. Table 1 provides a broad framework for classifying splenic lesions.

Up to 80% of all splenic cysts are pseudocysts caused by trauma, infection, or infarct. Worldwide, 8% of splenic cysts are parasitic hydatid cysts, and 10% to 20% are epithelial-lined "true" primary cysts.

IMAGING

Preoperative ultrasound or computed tomographic (CT) imaging is critical for operative planning. As outlined above, imaging can not only help with patient selection based upon spleen size, it can also define useful anatomic relationships that impact the conduct of surgery, recalling that the spleen is positioned against the stomach, pancreas, colon, and kidney, and it has a rich and variable blood supply. The normal spleen measures about 11 cm in length. Moderate splenomegaly, from 11 to 20 cm, should be noted in preoperative planning. Massive splenomegaly, defined as a spleen greater than 20 cm length, may alter operative strategy.

Preoperative imaging may also identify accessory spleens, reported in from 10% to 20% of patients. Preoperative imaging can provide key information for deciding whether a partial or a complete approach is best, including size of lesions, their relation to splenic hilar vessels and parenchyma, and the amount of healthy splenic tissue remaining. CT may be the preferred imaging modality because of the additional information provided regarding intrasplenic and extrasplenic anatomic relationships, vasculature, and flow. Preservation of at least 25% of the spleen appears sufficient to preserve splenic function, and the volume of potential splenic parenchyma to be preserved can be estimated preoperatively.

STRATEGIC PRINCIPLES

Partial Versus Complete Splenectomy

Regardless of origin of the splenic lesion, the shift since the 1970s toward preservation of functioning splenic tissue remains a guiding principle. Treatment of most splenic lesions can be partial or complete splenectomy, depending upon the size, location, and preoperative assessment of the likely etiology of the lesion. Again, factors affecting decision making about partial versus complete approach include the size of the lesion, its relation to splenic hilar vessels and parenchyma, and the amount of healthy splenic tissue remaining.

Unroofing/Marsupialization

For selected lesions, unroofing and/or marsupialization of the splenic cyst may be an option that results in preservation of splenic function.

Laparsocopic Versus Open Surgery

Treatment of splenic lesions may be via an open, laparoscopic, or a hybrid hand-assisted approach. Factors impacting decision making about laparoscopic versus open splenectomy include spleen size, prior surgeries, and surgeon experience. Spleen size is the most important factor for patient selection in determining which approach to use. When outcome measures of conversion rates, length of stay, and complications were compared for patients with normal-sized spleens versus those with splenomegaly, with 500 mg as the criterion for a large spleen, no statistical differences were observed in outcomes. However, some authors use spleen weight greater than 1 kg as an exclusion criterion for laparoscopy, noting conversion rates from laparoscopic to open splenectomy approaching zero for small spleens and 60% for spleens weighing more than 1 kg. Other surgeons use 2 kg as a laparoscopic splenectomy exclusion criterion, citing similar outcome variables of higher conversion rates, greater blood loss, longer hospitalization, and increased morbidity with larger spleens. Weight criteria, however, are difficult to assess preoperatively. Spleen size based upon CT or ultrasound imaging measurements provides a more useful preoperative selection criterion.

As a guideline, spleen size on ultrasound or CT scan should be less than 20 to 25 cm in the craniocaudal axis. Larger spleens have been removed laparoscopically but are technically challenging and may require use of a hand-assist device. Spleens measuring more than 30 cm leave little room for favorable port placement, they limit working space, and they often require hand-assisted laparoscopic splenectomy (HALS); specimen removal may require either an incision comparable to the open technique or use of a morcellation technique, which may adversely impact pathologic analysis.

Robotic Splenectomy

Robotic-assisted laparoscopic splenectomy has been reported and may play a role in future minimally invasive surgery approaches to the spleen. The current benefit of robotic systems for general surgery remains a matter of debate. A retrospective review compared six laparoscopic splenectomies against six robot-assisted laparoscopic splenectomies performed for idiopathic thrombocytopenia purpura, with patients matched for age, ASA score, body mass index, and preoperative platelet levels. No conversions or complications were reported. In the robotic group, median postoperative stay was 1 day longer, mean average costs were almost one third higher, and operative times were about 20% longer. In this analysis, robot-assisted laparoscopic splenectomy resulted in prolonged operative time, length of stay, and procedural costs, and while feasible, no relevant benefit was demonstrated. However, with advancement of surgical robotic technology, robotic systems may play a more integral role in future minimally invasive surgery.

TABLE I: Classification of splenic cysts, tumors, and abscesses

Cysts

Primary (true)
Parasitic
Nonparasitic
Congenital
Epidermoid
Dermoid
Mesothelial (serous)
Transitional
Neoplastic
Secondary (false): pseudocysts
Traumatic
Degenerative
Inflammatory
Hemorrhagic

Tumors

Malignant
Lymphoproliferative disease
Non-Hodgkin lymphoma
Hodgkin disease
Hairy cell leukemia
Chronic lymphocytic leukemia
Myeloproliferative disease
Chronic myelogenous leukemia
Myelofibrosis
Primary tumors
Angiosarcoma
Metastatic tumors
Benign
Hemangiomas
Hamartomas
Lymphangiomas
Sclerosing angiomatoid nodular transformation (SANT)

Abscesses

Bacterial
Fungal

Modified from McIntyre T, Zenilman ME: Cysts, tumors, and abscesses of the spleen. In Cameron JL, editor: *Current surgical therapy*, ed 9, Philadelphia, 2008, Mosby Elsevier, p 552.

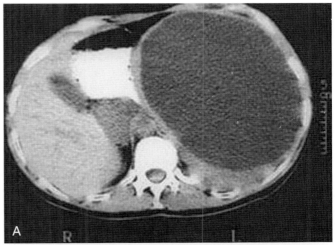

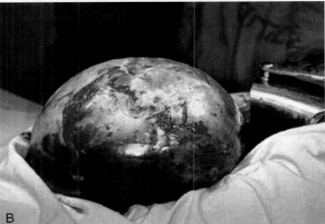

FIGURE I   CT image of the upper abdomen demonstrating a very large, homogenous splenic cyst (**A**) and intraoperative image of the enlarged spleen after initial mobilization (**B**). In **A**, a peripheral narrow rim of normal spleen is visible. In **B**, the spleen is still attached to its vascular root. *(From Avital S, Kashtan H: A large epithelial splenic cyst, N Engl J Med 349[2]:2173–2174, 2003.)*

CYSTS

A century ago, Fowler classified splenic cysts as parasitic and nonparasitic based upon etiology. Parasitic cysts of the spleen are almost always hydatid cysts formed by *Echinococcus*. Traditional classifications of splenic cysts were based upon the presence or absence of a cellular lining. Primary, or "true," cysts have an epithelial lining.

From a practical standpoint, because most parasitic cysts are echinococcal, early differentiation between parasitic and nonparasitic cysts can be helpful, guided by a careful history, imaging, and serology, which in most cases can then focus management strategies.

Among nonparasitic cysts, posttraumatic cysts are the most common, accounting for 70% to 80%. Most of these are secondary cysts, or pseudocysts, without a true epithelial cyst lining. Among true primary nonparasitic cysts, 90% are epidermoid.

Symptoms

Clinical presentation of splenic cysts commonly occurs with incidental discovery, especially for congenital and neoplastic cysts. Splenic cysts may grow quite large before they are diagnosed. Considerable growth can occur from the cell lining or from accelerated secretion from these cells. Additional splenic cyst enlargement can result from bleeding into the cyst or from an osmotic imbalance of the cystic fluid. Figure 1 displays a giant splenic epithelial cyst.

When splenic cysts are symptomatic, complaints are usually left upper quadrant–related symptoms, such as vague left upper quadrant abdominal discomfort, referred left shoulder pain from diaphragmatic irritation, early satiety, or nausea and vomiting. Symptoms can also occur when splenic cysts enlarge, cause a mass effect, become infected, or rupture. The mass effect of an enlarging splenic cyst can also impinge upon the adjacent left kidney, even resulting in kinking of the ureteropelvic junction and associated left renal dysfunction. Risk of splenic rupture increases with size and can exceed 25% when splenic cyst diameter exceeds 5 cm.

Parasitic Echinococcal Cysts

Hydatid disease can involve any organ of the body. Worldwide, 8% of splenic cysts are due to hydatid disease. In the United States, about 5% of splenic cysts are parasitic, and most are hydatid. A high suspicion for hydatid disease is warranted in endemic regions.

Hydatid cysts are caused by *Echinococcus granulosus, E. multilocularis,* and *E. vogeli,* which form larval cysts in mammalian tissue. *Echinococcus granulosus* causes cystic hepatic echinococcosis. This species occurs worldwide, typically in rural areas of Africa, the Middle East, southern Europe, Russia, China, Australia, and South America. *Echinococcus multilocularis* causes alveolar hydatid echinococcosis and occurs only in the northern hemisphere. *Echinococcus vogeli* causes polycystic echinococcosis and occurs in Central and South America. Dogs, cats, foxes, and coyotes are definitive hosts that harbor adult tapeworms in their intestines; these hosts are asymptomatic and are not harmed by the parasites. Ova pass in feces and are ingested by intermediate hosts such as cattle, sheep, rodents, and humans. Ova penetrate the intestine and pass via the portal vein to liver (75%), lung (15%), or other tissues, including the spleen (6%). Ovum develop into cysts, with capsules containing scoleces budding into the lumen. These "endocysts" may cause secondary intraperitoneal cyst formation if spilled into the peritoneal fluid.

Diagnosis of hydatid disease is based on medical history, imaging, and biochemical and serologic tests. Nonspecific upper abdominal pain is present in 75% of patients, and about 25% of patients are asymptomatic beyond vague symptoms of fullness or a mass effect.

Imaging is typically done by ultrasound and/or CT scan. Figure 2 is an example of a splenic hydatic cyst with a typical associated hepatic hydatid cyst. Imaging characteristics of splenic hydatid cysts are typical of most hydatid cysts, showing calcification of the cyst wall, the presence of daughter cysts, and membrane detachment.

Three types of serologic tests are used to diagnose echinoccal disease: indirect hemagglutination, indirect fluorescent antibody, and enzyme immunoassay/enzyme-linked immunosorbent assay (ELISA). Individual sensitivity ranges from 60% to 95%.

Because of the risk of spontaneous or traumatic rupture, splenic hydatid cysts are treated surgically. Standard therapy is total splenectomy with splenic-preserving surgery if feasible. Cyst fluid can be cautiously drained with puncture and aspiration to reduce the intracystic pressure to make a large, unwieldy spleen manageable or to improve operative exposure. Splenectomy without puncturing the cyst is preferable to prevent potential anaphylaxis from spillage of cyst contents into the abdominal cavity.

Spleen-preserving surgery is possible for splenic *Echinococcus,* but location of the lesion is key in operative strategy. Partial splenectomy is feasible for noncentral lesions, and spleen-preserving cystotomy and omentoplasty can selectively be performed. Total splenectomy is recommended for patients with large cysts located centrally or near the hilum. Both open and laparoscopic approaches have been reported for all of the approaches described, including use of hand-assist devices.

Benzimidazole carbamate compounds (albendazole and mebendazole) remain the cornerstone of medical therapy for echinococcosis hydatid disease and typically is administered in the preoperative and postoperative periods.

Nonparasitic Cysts

Nonparasitic splenic epithelial-lined cysts account for 10% to 20% of all cysts. Simple binary classification of nonparasitic cysts into "primary" or "true" and "secondary" or "false" is based upon presence or absence of cellular lining and may not always be helpful or accurate as classification criteria. "True" cysts may be only partially lined by epithelial cells. For example, if pressure degeneration has occurred, sampling error of a non–epithelial-lined section would result in false classification of a cyst as a secondary cyst.

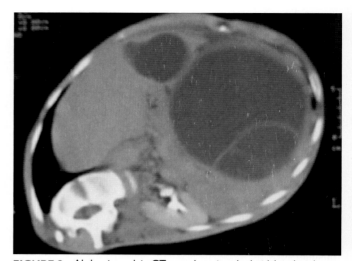

FIGURE 2   Abdominopelvic CT reveals a giant hydatid, loculated cystic mass originating from the spleen and a normal-sized cyst originating from the left lateral segment of the liver. *(From Karabicak I, Yurtseven I, Yuruker S, et al: Splenic hydatid cyst, Can J Surg 52[4]:E209–E210, 2009.)*

Beyond the true-false classification systems, more than 10 nomenclatures have been proposed in the past 50 years. Table 2 describes a classification proposed by Mirilas and colleagues of nonparasitic splenic cysts divided into primary and secondary based upon pathogenesis and on different macroscopic and clinical characteristics. For instance, a primary splenic cystic cavity can result from compaction of mesothelial cells during development (congenital), from aberrant germ cells (dermoid), or because of vessel malformation (angiomas). In secondary splenic cysts, the causative event—trauma, infarct, or inflammation—leads to secondary formation of the cystic cavity. Primary cysts can be congenital or neoplastic.

Primary Cysts

Congenital splenic cysts arise from invagination of the mesothelium-lined splenic capsule during development; they are either *dermoid* or *epidermoid* and typically are detected in children or young adults. Epidermoid cysts account for 90% of all nonparasitic true cysts. Neoplastic cysts are rare, but the most common types are angioma of blood vessels (hemangioma) or lymph vessels (lymphangioma). Splenic hemangiomas can be *capillary* or *cavernous.* Based upon pathogenesis, some authors differentiate angiomas as splenic cysts rather than cystic tumors. Angiomas are neoplastic cysts derived from maldeveloped blood or lymphatic vessels, whereas cystic tumors are derived from epithelial cells, usually glandular, that form cystic masses.

Secondary Cysts: Pseudocysts

Secondary cysts account for 70% to 80% of nonparasitic splenic cysts. Trauma is the most common cause of secondary splenic cysts. Hepatosplenic injury most commonly occurs following blunt abdominal trauma, hence most secondary splenic cysts are posttraumatic, frequently occurring in teenagers and young adult men. A traumatic impact results in formation of a cystic cavity, which then organizes circumferentially and results in a fibrous cystic wall, but without a cellular lining. Traumatic cysts have thick, collagenous walls with spotty calcification and a shaggy hemorrhagic interior with evidence of normal splenic architecture. Cyst fluid may be brown or greenish brown from breakdown of heme products. The fibrous cystic wall

TABLE 2: Classification of nonparasitic splenic cysts

Classification	Criteria
Primary	
Congenital	Cystic lining: mesothelial, transitional and/or stratified squamous
Neoplastic	
Angiomas	Cystic lining: endothelial
Hemangiomas	Blood content in cyst
Lymphangiomas	
Dermoid cysts	Cystic lining: ectopic, mature ectodermal tissues
Secondary	
Traumatic	Positive trauma history Gross appearance of cyst (interior): shaggy, hemorrhagic, normal splenic architecture Cystic wall: thick, collagenous
Necrotic	Infarct: left upper quadrant pain History or active bacterial infective endocarditis Nonspecific acute splenitis (e.g., typhoid fever, infectious mononucleosis, blood dissemination of hemolytic *Streptococcus,* generalized lymphadenopathy)

From Mirilas P, Menessidou A, Skandalakis JE: Splenic cysts: are there so many types? *J Am Coll Surg* 204(3):459–465, 2007.

that encapsulates the splenic hematoma persists after absorption of the hematoma.

Less common causes of secondary cysts are splenic infarct, often from emboli or bacterial infection. Both splenic infarct and bacterial inflammation can lead to liquefaction necrosis of splenic tissue resulting from hydrolytic enzyme activation. Necrotic debris and fluid form the cystic cavity, which is surrounded by fibrous tissue walls.

Treatment

Splenic cyst diameter and patient symptoms determine surgical treatment of splenic cysts. For asymptomatic patients, potential risks related to rupture increase with cysts larger than 5 cm. Conservative, nonoperative management is reasonable with interval imaging for splenic cysts less than 5 cm, because most will resolve. Cysts larger than 5 cm have an increased risk of spontaneous rupture or rupture associated with relatively minor trauma. Complications associated with splenic cyst rupture can include bleeding, abscess formation, peritonitis, hypersplenism, portal vein thrombosis, and portal hypertension. Surgery is recommended for splenic cysts larger than 5 cm, and operative strategy of partial splenectomy, unroofing, or complete splenectomy is based upon size, location, and preoperative characterization of the lesion, with the goal of preserving greater than 25% of the splenic parenchyma if feasible. Percutaneous drainage of splenic cysts is reported, but it is discouraged because of the high incidence of recurrence and associated inflammation, which can adversely limit future operative approaches.

OPERATIVE STRATEGIES

Splenectomy

In cases of multiple splenic cysts, polycystic spleens, or for large central/hilar lesions, complete splenectomy is recommended. When possible, splenectomy should be performed laparoscopically, with size, prior surgery, and surgeon experience as factors in operative decision making. Although laparoscopic approaches continue to evolve, the lateral/flank approach is typically preferred.

Unroofing, Fenestration, and Marsupialization

For superficial, peripheral, simple splenic cysts, unroofing or fenestration can be considered and may often be approachable laparoscopically. Unroofing of splenic cysts carries a slightly increased recurrence risk but preserves the most splenic parenchyma of any approach. Risk of recurrence can be mitigated by removal of as much cyst wall as possible and by placement of omentum in the cyst bed.

Partial Splenectomy

Key decision-making factors for partial splenectomy include size and location of the lesion with respect to the splenic hilum. Polar lesions are more amenable to partial splenectomy than central/hilar lesions. Operative principles include complete splenic mobilization and control of segmental blood supply prior to division of the splenic parenchyma. Several techniques have been described for division of the splenic parenchyma, including techniques that use staplers, electrocautery, harmonic scalpel, argon beam coagulation, finger-fracture technique, and a variety of hemostatic agents. Open, laparoscopic, and hand-assisted approaches have all been described for partial splenectomy.

TUMORS

Tumors of the spleen are categorized primarily as *benign* or *malignant,* with malignant splenic tumors further categorized as *lymphoid, myeloprolifiverative,* or *metastatic.*

Primary Splenic Tumors

Primary tumors of the spleen are rare and include lymphoma, sarcoma, hemangioma, and hamartoma. The most common benign splenic tumors arise from the red pulp of the spleen. They can become large, resulting in splenomegaly with associated left upper quadrant symptoms.

Splenic hamartomas can be cystic or solid, and they can be a source of diagnostic uncertainty at laparotomy or laparoscopy. Harmartomas can be confused grossly with lymphoma. Splenectomy may be considered to exclude tumor, but partial splenectomy and observation are reasonable options if the diagnosis is certain. Typically, these lesions are incidentally discovered at surgery in an asymptomatic patient. They rarely become large enough to be symptomatic.

Peliosis of the spleen is a rare disease characterized by multiple blood-filled cavities in the splenic parenchyma; these can be associated with spontaneous intraperitoneal hemorrhage, which can be fatal. Peliosis can occur in association with other disorders, such as tuberculosis, diabetes, or neoplasm.

Inflammatory pseudotumors are benign lesions with constituent inflammatory cells and granulomatous reaction, which can affect several different organs, including the spleen. Associated symptoms can include fatigue, vague left upper quadrant pain, and weight loss; symptoms are improved with splenectomy.

Sarcoidosis is a disease of unknown etiology that manifests as noncaseating granulomas found in tissues and organs with an affinity for the lymphatic system. The spleen is involved in 24% to 59% of patients with sarcoidosis, but it is usually asymptomatic. Rare patients with splenic involvement can develop hypersplenism-associated symptoms, with severe cases at risk for spontaneous rupture. Amyloidosis also involves the spleen, but rarely is the splenic component of amyloidosis clinically significant.

Vascular Tumors of the Spleen

Benign vascular tumors of the spleen, hemangiomas, can result in hypersplenism with attendant risk of spontaneous rupture and massive hemorrhage. Splenectomy is indicated for lesions larger than 5 cm.

Lymphangiomas are rare, benign, cystic tumors of the spleen that occasionally lead to hypersplenism. They may be solitary, or they may be found in association with hepatic, pulmonary, cutaneous, or bony counterparts. Splenectomy has a role only for palliation of symptoms or in a diagnostic dilemma.

Sclerosing angiomatoid nodular transformation (SANT) of the spleen is a rare, benign, peculiar vascular lesion characterized by marked stromal sclerosis and presence of plasma cells; it shares histopathologic features with IgG4-related sclerosing disease. SANT can be associated with abdominal calcifying fibrous tumors (CFT). Figure 3 is an example of an SANT lesion of the spleen. Each angiomatoid nodule is made up of slit-like vascular spaces lined with endothelial cells and interspersed ovoid cells. A spoked-wheel pattern seen on imaging studies can be diagnostic, representing the capsule with radiating septa.

Malignant Tumors of the Spleen

Malignant tumors of the spleen fall into four general categories: 1) *lymphoproliferative,* which includes non-Hodgkin lymphoma, Hodgkin disease, hairy cell leukemia, and chronic lymphocytic leukemia; 2) *myeloproliferative,* such as chronic myelogenous leukemia and myelofibrosis; 3) *primary splenic,* or the nonlymphoid and angiosarcomas; and 4) *metastatic* lesions. Most tumors of the spleen (70%) are related to lymphomas.

In lymphoproliferative and myeloproliferative disease, the spleen is rarely the primary site of malignancy, but the spleen is often secondarily involved. Angiosarcoma is the most common nonlymphoid malignant tumor of the spleen, characterized by rapid growth rate, early metastatic activity, and poor prognosis, even with splenectomy.

Lymphoproliferative Disorders

Non-Hodgkin lymphoma (NHL) is the most common malignancy with splenic involvement. While rarely the primary site, the spleen is involved in 40% of NHL patients. NHL therapy is multiagent systemic chemotherapy with or without radiation. Splenectomy is limited to managing complications of cytopenia or symptomatic splenomegaly, and it has no impact on disease survival.

Hodgkin disease stages I and II involve occult disease of the spleen in 35% of patients. These data provided the historic rationale for including splenectomy as part of routine staging for Hodgkin's disease. However, improvements in radiographic imaging for staging and in chemotherapy regimens have reduced the need for staging laparotomy to less than 5%. In the small group of patients needing traditional staging, it can be performed effectively laparoscopically to include inspection of the peritoneum, splenectomy, wedge and core liver biopsies, and sampling of paraaortic, iliac, portal, and mesenteric lymph nodes. Further, long-term data have shown that splenectomy and the number of courses of mustard + oncovin + procarbazine + prednisone (MOPP) chemotherapy courses are prognostic factors that increase the risk of secondary acute nonlymphocytic leukemia in Hodgkin's

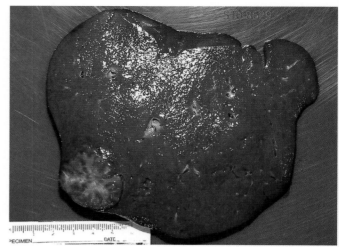

FIGURE 3   Sclerosing angiomatoid nodular transformation (SANT) of spleen. *(Courtesy Johns Hopkins Medical Center Pathology Department.)*

disease patients treated with combined modality therapy with splenectomy. Today, Hodgkin's disease has high cure rates with multimodal therapy, and the role of splenectomy is limited and ideally avoided.

Myeloproliferative Disorders

Splenomegaly is the most common physical finding in chronic myelogenous leukemia (CML), which accounts for 30% of adult leukemias. In more than 50% of CML patients, the spleen extends more than 5 cm below the costal margin at diagnosis. Splenic size correlates with peripheral blood granulocyte counts, and very large spleens predict transformation into acute blast crisis. Splenectomy in selected blastic or accelerated blast phases can improve quality of life and decrease transfusion requirements.

Primary or idiopathic myelofibrosis, also known as *myelosclerosis,* is a rare, fatal disorder that occurs when the bone marrow produces excess collagen or fibrous tissue within the bone marrow, reducing red cell production capacity. Splenectomy can play a palliative role by reducing transfusion requirements and improving quality of life.

Metastatic Disease of the Spleen

The spleen is a common site for metastatic disease in advanced cancers, particularly from lung, breast, and melanoma. At autopsy, splenic metastases are commonly found but are usually not clinically significant.

Treatment of Splenic Tumors

Whether complete, partial, open, or laparoscopic, splenectomy is a reasonable treatment option for nearly all splenic tumors to either manage symptoms or to provide definitive diagnosis. When malignancy is suspected, complete splenectomy is recommended. Outcomes for open versus laparoscopic series are comparable.

SPLENIC ABSCESS

Splenic abscesses are rare, but they are highly lethal. Traditional outcome data reported 100% mortality rates with untreated splenic abscess, but with appropriate therapy, mortality rates are less than 15%. The mechanism for most splenic abscesses is hematogenous spread to the spleen from another primary septic focus, such as endocarditis, intraabdominal abscess, diverticulitis, pyelonephritis, or direct circulating bacteria from intravenous drug abuse. Patients

The most commonly cultured organisms from splenic abscesses
include gram-positive *Staphylococcus* and *Streptococcus*, gram-negative *Salmonella*, and fungal agents such as *Candida* and *Aspergillus*, the latter being more common in immunocompromised hosts. Secondary infection of a splenic hematoma or infarct can be a cause of splenic abscess. Susceptible splenic infarct tissue can develop after a noninfectious embolic event or trauma that results in a demarcated segment of spleen; this infarcted splenic tissue is seeded with an infectious agent, which can evolve to a splenic abscess. Patients with abnormal spleens, such as those in immunocompromised states, are more susceptible to this process. Intravenous drug abuse can also be a source for embolic infectious involvement of an infarct or hematoma.

Direct penetration of splenic parenchyma can also result from an adjacent intraabdominal infectious process, most commonly from an adjacent pancreatic abscess, but it can also occur from a subphrenic, diverticular, or, rarely, a perinephric abscess. Splenic abscesses may be iatrogenic and may be complicated by mycotic pseudoaneurysm. In addition, systemic immunosuppression from chemotherapy, human immunodeficiency virus (HIV), or autoimmune disease and immunosuppression for organ transplantation pose an increasingly frequent risk factor for splenic infectious vulnerability.

Treatment of Splenic Abscess

Splenectomy can provide definitive treatment for splenic abscess. The surgical approach may be open or laparoscopic, although though the latter represents a challenging minimally invasive procedure. The foundation of medical treatment for splenic abscesses remains intravenous antibiotics, beginning with broad-spectrum coverage and then tailored to a culture-specific regimen. Percutaneous aspirates can be useful in guiding antibiotic therapy.

Imaged-guided percutaneous techniques continue to evolve as adjuncts to managing splenic abscess. Percutaneous splenic abscess drainage is increasingly popular and can be safe and effective in selected patients. Collections can usually be accessed by ultrasound guidance, and a single-wall 18 gauge needle can be used to obtain culture material, along with a 10 Fr drain placed over an 0.035 guidewire. Drain removal is determined by output and resolved collection on repeated imaging.

Failure rates for percutaneous splenic abscess drainage ranges from 50% to 60% with longer hospitalizations and longer treatment periods. Subphrenic abscesses are treated with drainage and intravenous antibiotics. Patients with persistent postoperative fevers, increased white blood cell count, and abdominal pain should undergo repeated CT scan of the abdomen.

OVERWHELMING POSTSPLENECTOMY INFECTION

Lifetime Risk and Immunization Against Overwhelming Sepsis

Patients who undergo splenectomy are at increased lifetime risk for overwhelming postsplenectomy infection (OPSI), reported by most experts at 3% to 5%; the annual incidence is reported between 0.23% to 0.42%. Groups at lowest risk for overwhelming postsplenectomy pneumococcal sepsis are those whose spleen was removed for trauma. Groups at highest risk include those requiring splenectomy for a hematologic disorder, immunocompromised patients, and patients at the extremes of age. Cases of overwhelming sepsis are emergencies that can be lethal; they require immediate parenteral antibiotics and intensive care, and they carry a mortality rate of 38% to 69%. Intravenous immunoglobulin may play a beneficial role.

The mechanism of OPSI may be due to decreased antigen clearance in postsplenectomy patients and decreased antigen response. *Steptococcus pneumoniae* is the most common infective agent, recovered in 50% to 90% of isolates from septic patients, followed by *H. influenzae B*, *Streptococcus B*, *Staphylococcus aureus*, *Escherichia coli*, and various other coliform bacteria. Increased susceptibility to parasites and malaria is noted in endemic areas, and a hypothesized increased risk of *Neisseria meningitidis* is unclear.

Optimally, immunization against encapsulated organisms should occur 14 days prior to surgery. Recommended immunizations include polyvalent pneumococcal, meningococcal, and *Haemophilus* vaccinations. Pneumovax provides protection against 73% of causative organisms. Data on revaccination remain unclear, but current consensus favors a pneumovax booster every 5 to 10 years, which may be protective against common pathogens. Hib/meningococcal/influenza vaccine benefit is unproven but recommended. For patients who do not receive recommended immunizations prior to surgery, immunization can be given just prior to hospital discharge.

Counseling, Antibiotics, and Treatment

All patients undergoing splenectomy should be counseled regarding their increased lifetime risk of overwhelming sepsis. Patients should be advised to seek medical care immediately if they develop any febrile illness.

The use of long-term prophylactic antibiotics after splenectomy remains controversial. Long-term antibiotic therapy risks selection of resistant microbial strains. Pediatric hematologists often recommend treatment for 2 years postsplenectomy with a penicillin-based regimen. Studies have demonstrated benefit from antibiotic prophylaxis in children with sickle cell disease, but no similar studies have been done in adults.

We discharge patients with a supply of oral antibiotics, with clear instructions to initiate therapy with the onset of symptoms of infection, as they simultaneously arrange to seek urgent medical attention.

SUGGESTED READINGS

Bodner J, Kafka-Ritsch R, Lucciarini P, et al: A critical comparison of robotic versus conventional laparoscopic splenectomies, *World J Surg* 29(8):982–986, 2005.

Culafic DM, Kerkez MD, Mijac DD, et al: Spleen cystic echinococcosis: clinical manifestations and treatment, *Scand J Gastroenterol* 45(1):186–190, 2010.

Carbonell A, Kercher K, Matthews B, et al: Laparoscopic splenectomy for splenic abscess, *Surg Laparosc Endosc Percutan Tech* 14:289, 2004.

Dawes LG, Malangoni MA: Cystic masses of the spleen, *Am Surg* 52:333–336, 1986.

Heniford BT, Park A, Walsh RM, et al: Laparoscopic splenectomy with normal-sized spleens versus splenomegaly: does size matter? *Am Surg* 67(9):854–847, 2001.

Losanoff JE, Richman BW, Jones JW: Nonparasitic splenic cysts, *J Am Coll Surg* 195:437–438, 2002.

Mirilas P, Menessidou A, Skandalakis JE: Splenic cysts: are there so many types? *J Am Coll Surg* 204(3):459–465, 2007.

Pedrosa I, Saíz A, Arrazola J, et al: Hydatid disease: radiologic and pathologic features and complications, *Radiographics* 20:795–817, 2000.

Recommendations of the Advisory Committee on Immunization Practices (ACIP): use of vaccines and immune globulins in persons with altered immunocompetence, *MMWR* 42(4):4–5, 1993.

Uranues S, Alimoglu O: Laparoscopic surgery of the spleen, *Surg Clin North Am* 85:75–90, 2005.

SPLENIC SALVAGE PROCEDURES: THERAPEUTIC OPTIONS

Philip A. Efron, MD, and David T. Efron, MD

OVERVIEW

The spleen is one of the most commonly injured abdominal organs. In a suitable, hemodynamically stable patient, the principle of organ preservation is preferred. With the advancement of technology and of trauma management and emergency systems, splenic salvage has increasingly become the standard of care for appropriate patients in hospital systems with adequate support mechanisms. Thus it is important for surgeons to have a broad knowledge of splenic salvage therapies.

The semantics of defining specific splenic salvage therapies can make negotiating the medical literature on this topic difficult. In addition, some authors would further separate the term "splenic salvage therapy" from "splenic preservation." In this chapter, *splenic salvage therapy* is defined as any intervention that is not an open splenectomy. This includes both nonoperative management and operative maneuvers to retain the organ, ideally with continued function.

NONOPERATIVE MANAGEMENT

Currently the majority of blunt splenic injuries are managed nonoperatively (NOM), although sufficient prospective randomized studies comparing nonoperative and operative management in hemodynamically stable patients are lacking. The Eastern Association for the Surgery of Trauma (EAST) has created guidelines for the treatment of blunt splenic injury based on the best clinical data available. Using these guidelines, overall success rates in excess of 90% with nonoperative management of splenic injuries have been reported. Advantages of nonoperative strategies include the immunologic benefit of splenic preservation, the prevention of nontherapeutic laparotomies, and reduced intraabdominal complications such as injury to the tail of the pancreas. Asplenia has its own inherent risk, which includes overwhelming postsplenectomy infection (OPSI), which, although rare, is lethal in adults. Although debated, the majority of the medical literature illustrates that nonoperative splenic injury management is associated with a relatively low morbidity.

Patient Selection

Hemodynamic status is the prime determinant of operative versus nonoperative intervention. Hemodynamically unstable victims of blunt trauma are rapidly evaluated by focused abdominal sonography for trauma (FAST) ultrasound or diagnostic peritoneal lavage (DPL). Evidence of intraabdominal fluid or blood by DPL criteria necessitates operative exploration. Alternatively, a stable patient with obvious peritonitis requires exploration. If the spleen is found to be injured, associated injuries, comorbidities, and physiologic status dictate whether the patient is a candidate for the operative salvage strategies described here. Similarly, victims of penetrating abdominal trauma require, at a minimum, hemodynamic stability and an evaluable abdomen (without peritonitis) to be considered for selective nonoperative management. Suitablity for operative splenic salvage following identification of splenic injury at laparotomy mirrors those identified with blunt splenic injury.

Patient selection is vital for the success of nonoperative splenic salvage therapy. Although there are few contraindications to nonoperative management in the setting of hemodynamic stability, adult blunt splenic injury patients must fulfill certain criteria. Nonoperative management requires the availability of computed tomography (CT) scanning as well as experienced physician interpretation of the results. CT scan with intravenous (IV) contrast is considered the diagnostic test of choice to determine the severity of splenic injury and hemoperitoneum. The use of both oral and IV contrast results in the best technical images; however, oral contrast is not required to diagnose splenic injury and may not be practical in the setting of an acutely injured patient. The addition of oral contrast potentially aids in the identification of concomitant hollow viscus injury.

CT scanning contributes important anatomic information, including confirmation and grading of splenic trauma as well as identification of concomitant injuries that contribute to management decisions (Figure 1). Using the Organ Injury Scale created by the American Association for the Surgery of Trauma (AAST), splenic injuries are classified by grade of anatomic disruption as seen on CT (Table 1). An additional advantage of CT scanning is the added anatomic information regarding other injuries.

In addition to hemodynamic instability, peritonitis, and the presence of intraperitoneal or retroperitoneal organs requiring an operation, the need for anticoagulation or the inability to correct a coagulopathy contraindicate an attempt at nonoperative management of splenic injury. This is classically of concern in a polytrauma patient with extraabdominal vascular injury.

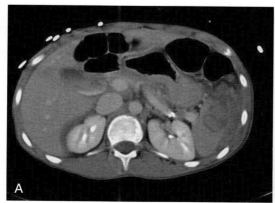 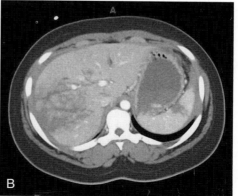

FIGURE I   A, Grade IV splenic injury in a 15-year-old following a bicycle accident. **B,** Grade III splenic and liver injuries in an 18-year-old following a fall from over 20 feet.

TABLE 1: American Association for the Surgery of Trauma Organ Injury Scale for the Spleen

Grade*	Injury Type	Description of Injury
I	Hematoma	Subcapsular, <10% surface area
II	Laceration	Capsular tear, <1 cm parenchymal depth
	Hematoma	Subcapsular, 10% to 50% surface area; intraparenchymal, <5 cm in diameter
	Laceration	Capsular tear, 1 to 3 cm parenchymal depth that does not involve a trabecular vessel
III	Hematoma	Subcapsular, >50% surface area or expanding; ruptured subcapsular or parenchymal hematoma; intraparenchymal hematoma ≥5 cm or expanding
	Laceration	Parenchymal depth >3 cm or involving trabecular vessels
IV	Laceration	Laceration involving segmental or hilar vessels producing major devascularization (>25% of spleen)
V	Laceration	Completely shattered spleen
	Vascular	Hilar vascular injury with devascularized spleen

*Advance one grade for multiple injuries up to grade III.
From Moore EE, Cogbill TH, Jurkovich GJ, et al: Organ injury scaling: spleen and liver, 1994 rev., *J Trauma* 38;323–324 1995.

Unlike in children, multiple transfusions in adult patients with splenic injury should be approached with caution. Blood transfusions should be limited, as transfusion is an independent risk factor for subsequent infections, especially in the injured patient, likely outweighing the risk of OPSI. Opinions vary as to the trigger for operative intervention, though most clinicians identify an absolute hematocrit or limit to transfusion beyond which nonoperative therapy is declared a failure. Figure 2 demonstrates a sample algorithm.

AAST injury grade, neurologic status, the presence of neurologic injuries, hemoperitoneum, and age greater than 55 years are not absolute contraindications to the nonoperative management of splenic injuries. Lengthy, emergent nonabdominal operations, such as open fractures, may be accompanied by significant blood loss and the inability to serially examine the patient, thus precluding an attempt at a nonoperative course. However, these factors should be considered on a case-by-case basis in determining the treatment algorithm for an individual patient. Some authors suggest that the admission systolic blood pressure, the amount of extraabdominal injury, and the requirement for blood transfusion can be used to predict the success of nonoperative therapy. The rate of failure of nonoperative management also appears to increase as the grade of injury increases. Significant hemoperitoneum has also been associated with an increase in failure rates.

Angioembolization

Angiography and angioembolization are important adjuncts for nonoperative splenic salvage, and their availability should be considered when determining the management algorithm for a specific patient. In the adult blunt trauma population, increased use of splenic artery angiography and embolization has been associated with a decrease in the failure rate of nonoperative management (for all grades of splenic injury), hospital mortality, and hospital length of stay. In addition, angiography and embolization are not associated with an increase in blood transfusions. Selective angiography is now proposed over mandated diagnostic angiography, and routine angiography for blunt splenic injury has been determined to be unnecessary. With the use of selective angiography and embolization, success rates for controlling ongoing bleeding and subsequent splenic salvage can exceed 80%. However, formal indications for angiography have not been established. Many would suggest that a high-grade lesion (greater than grade 2) or a contrast blush/vascular injury would be an indication for angiography. In addition, persistent tachycardia and a declining hematocrit may also be indications.

Embolization can be done proximally, distally, or both. Proximal embolization decreases pressure in the spleen to allow intrinsic hemostasis rather than directly inducing coagulation at the site of injury (Figure 3). Perfusion to the spleen continues through collateral vessels. Distal embolization involves direct hemostasis of the splenic parenchyma. Studies have not demonstrated superiority of either method or of the type of material used for embolization, however, the presence of an arteriovenous fistula on the initial CT scan is associated with an increased failure rate. In addition, authors have suggested that patients older than 55 years or those with hemodynamic instability may have greater failure rates.

It has not been determined how many trials of angioembolization can be attempted prior to the patient requiring splenectomy. Regardless, the patient must always meet the criteria for nonoperative therapy for each attempt, and increased consideration must be given to the risk of repetitive intravenous contrast use. Many surgeons would argue that the initial failure of angioembolization is an indication for splenectomy.

Monitoring and Progression of Care

It should be noted that nonoperative management does not free the surgeon from further responsibility. Regardless of whether angioembolization has been performed, patients should be initially admitted to an intensive care or immediate care unit, or some similar setting, so that vital signs are monitored continuously. If clinically appropriate, a urinary catheter should be placed; nasogastric decompression of the stomach is not mandated and should be determined on a case-by-case basis. Frequent physical examinations should be performed, and serial hemoglobin and/or hematocrit levels should be followed. Operative intervention should be immediately available should the patient's condition decline.

There are several facets of the nonoperative management of splenic injury that do not have strong enough evidence to provide specific guidelines. These include the length of intensive care monitoring, length of bed rest, use of chemical deep vein thrombosis (DVT) prophylaxis, length of hospital stay, timing of serial imaging, and resumption of normal activities. The decisions regarding each of these are often based on experiential evidence. The majority of failures secondary to delayed bleeds occur within the first 6 to 8 days, so the data on the grade of the splenic injury, concomitant injuries, and patient comorbidities will help to guide management.

Inpatient Monitoring

Patients are often kept in a monitored setting for 24 to 72 hours and then continue in an inpatient setting thereafter. Lengths of stay up to 1 week will likely capture failures of nonoperative management but are usually reserved for patients with higher grade injuries.

Deep Vein Thrombosis Prophylaxis

At the time of initial injury, chemical DVT prophylaxis is contraindicated. Although the absolute risk of bleed is as yet undefined, the use of prophylaxis is guided by common sense. In turn, the high risk of DVT

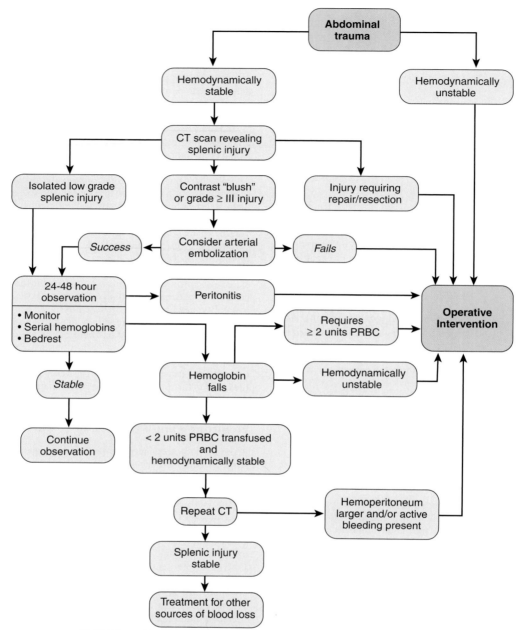

FIGURE 2 Algorithm for nonoperative management of blunt splenic injuries.

in trauma patients makes use of mechanical DVT prophylaxis, such as TED hose and sequential compression devices, imperative. Additionally, the comparative risk of DVT versus the theoretical benefit of bed rest to prevent delayed bleeding is undefined. The recent trend is toward early mobilization and shortened mandatory periods of bed rest. Again, the specific management is usually dictated by the severity of the injury, with high-grade injuries subject to more restricted early activity.

Serial Imaging and Resumption of Activities

Though many clinicians feel that serial imaging plays a role in the nonoperative management of splenic injury, optimal frequency and length of surveillance has not been established. As with other facets of management, this may be driven by the grade of injury.

At least half of surveyed trauma surgeons (EAST members) stated that for grades I and II splenic injuries, they would require the patient to wait 2 weeks prior to resuming normal activity and would not obtain a follow-up CT scan. However, in patients with high-risk occupations or high-grade injuries (grades III to V), patients would be required to obtain a repeat CT scan in 4 to 6 weeks, prior to granting the patient medical clearance for normal activity. Splenic capsule healing in experimental models does not achieve preinjury strength for approximately 8 weeks. Therefore the traditional conservative recommendation to avoid contact sports and other similar activities for 2 to 4 months carries some merit. Interval CT imaging for high-grade injuries (III or above) can assist the surgeon in making return to activity decisions, especially for patients with large focal hematomas or extensive capsular disruption.

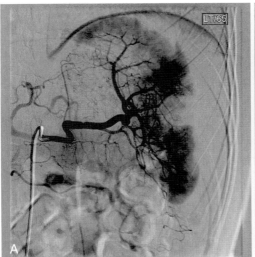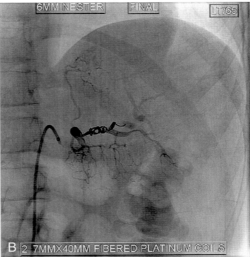

FIGURE 3   **A,** Selective angiography of the splenic artery in a patient with a grade IV blunt injury. Note the large areas of malperfusion throughout the spleen and concern for blush toward the upper pole. **B,** The same patient following proximal coil embolization of the main splenic artery.

Failure and Complications of Nonoperative Management

The most common cause of failure of NOM is bleeding within 4 days of therapy. Occasionally, an injured vessel will not be revealed on initial investigation due to spasm. Hemodynamic instability warrants immediate splenectomy, otherwise the algorithm for nonoperative management should be followed. Other complications of nonoperative therapy can include contrast-induced nephropathy, coil migration, splenic abscess, splenic infarct, OPSI, and impaired immune function due to asplenia. Complication rates can range from 6% to 27%. The rate of missed injury with nonoperative therapy is low, although morbidity will increase with a missed injury.

Vaccination

Vaccination for encapsulated gram-positive organisms, specifically *Streptococcus pneumoniae, Niesseria meningitidis,* and *Haemophilus influenzae,* are clearly required in the setting of operative splenectomy. Ideally these vaccinations are administered in the setting of functional splenic tissue—that is, prior to splenectomy—to maximize the immune response. For most trauma splenectomies, this is not an option.

Ensuring vaccination in a population that demonstrates a predictably poor postdischarge follow-up poses a challenge. This has led some centers to administer the vaccines in the operating room at the time of the splenectomy. We favor vaccination on the day of discharge after allowing a reasonable time for resolution of the perioperative inflammatory response, but we ensure administration prior to discharge.

Some clinicians favor immunization of all nonoperatively managed patients based on the idea that if the patients fail this management, they derive the greatest benefit from the vaccination. Given the very high success rates of nonoperative management of splenic trauma, this may not be warranted. There is additional concern that aggressive arterial embolization of the spleen results in compromise of splenic immunity. Recent reports assessing markers of immune response suggest that after embolization therapy, patients do not imunologically mimic those who are asplenic.

OPERATIVE SPLENIC SALVAGE PROCEDURES

Once the decision to explore the patient's abdomen is made, the principles guiding operative trauma are paramount. The ease and effectiveness of splenectomy for the control of hemorrhage ensures that

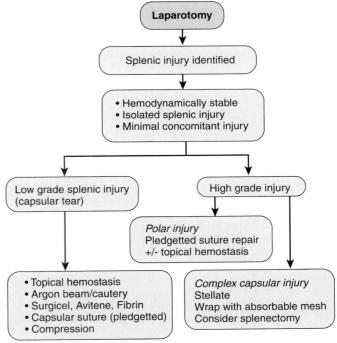

FIGURE 4   Algorithm for splenorrhaphy.

the patient meets the criteria of stability before any attempt at operative preservation of the injured spleen is made. The primary goal of all splenic salvage procedures is durable hemostasis, and techniques range from topical coagulation strategies to partial splenectomy with capsular pledgeted suture to enveloping compression of the splenic parenchyma with mesh material (Figure 4).

While low-grade superficial injuries to the surface of the spleen may be well managed in situ, complete mobilization and medialization of the spleen is often required to effect a successful repair. Mobilization of a spleen with a torn capsule with the intent of effecting a repair requires careful manipulation, and release of the retroperitoneal attachments can be challenging in the setting of ongoing blood loss. Firm cupping of the body of the spleen in the palm from the right side of the table allows compressive retraction toward the vertebral column, which avoids further avulsion of the capsule and facilitates

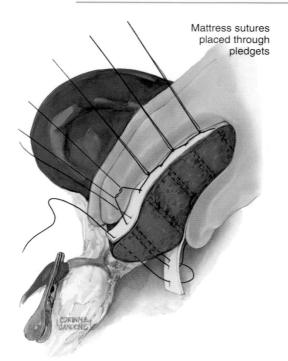

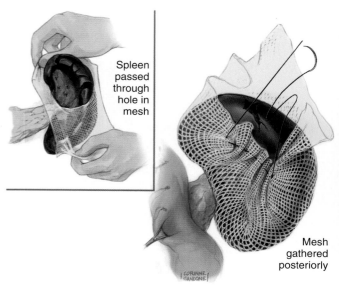

FIGURE 6   Mesh-wrap technique for repair of a shattered spleen. *(Courtesy C. Sandone, Johns Hopkins School of Medicine, Baltimore, MD. Reproduced with permission.)*

FIGURE 5   Pledgetted repair of splenic injury. *(Courtesy C. Sandone, Johns Hopkins School of Medicine, Baltimore, MD. Reproduced with permission.)*

hemostasis during the dissection. Release of these attachments, the lienophrenic and lienorenal ligaments, allows access to the avascular plane posterior to the tail of the pancreas. The spleen and tail of the pancreas, intimately juxtaposed at the splenic hilum, are then medialized with the main splenic artery and vein that course along the posterior aspect of the pancreas. This affords complete inspection of the splenic capsule, exposes the main splenic vessels for rapid control, and allows easy control and division of the short gastric vessels. The lienocolic attachments are essentially avascular and are also easily divided, either before or after mobilization, which completely frees the spleen from all but its hilar attachments.

Grade I and II injuries are often not the sole reason for abdominal exploration and are usually identified at laparotomy. Small linear tears are usually well managed with direct application of electrocautery or argon beam coagulation. This can be achieved without or with topical hemostatic agents such as Avitene (microfibillar collagen) and Surgicel (methylcellulose). We have had success with a combination of argon beam coagulation and applied Surgicel, followed with a short period of packing for these injuries.

Grade III or greater injuries or lower grade injuries that demonstrate persistent bleeding despite initial efforts warrant more aggressive intervention. Suture of the splenic capsule often requires the use of pledgets to prevent capsular tears. We favor the use of Surgicel as pledget material over polytetrafluoroethylene (PTFE), because Surgicel offers the benefit of hemostatic properties and ultimately will reabsorb without leaving a permanent material in place. Overlapping horizontal mattress sutures provide excellent hemostasis. For injuries at one or the other of the poles, partial splenectomy—that is, debridement of distally devitalized tissue—can be achieved by placing similar overlapping horizontal mattress sutures just proximal to

the cut edge. Ligation of a clearly identified pole vessel in the hilum also facilitates hemostasis (Figure 5).

Severe, blunt splenic injury—often characterized by deep, stellate lacerations encompassing much of the splenic body—do not provide adequate tissue for conventional suture splenorrhaphy. Patients with this type of injury who are hemodynamically stable enough to consider for splenic salvage are rare. Compression of splenic tissue and roughly reestablishing preinjury geometry can be accomplished by wrapping the spleen with an absorbable mesh and securing the open end with a purse-string suture to ensure compression of the mesh (Figure 6). Hemostatic agents can be added within the wrap to encourage coagulation and apply additional compression hemostasis. Additionally, the topical application of fibrin glue to the raw, injured edge has been described. These injuries are often the primary reason for exploration; however, because splenic repair takes some time and can be associated with significant blood loss, it is not appropriate in a true damage-control setting. Unlike emergent splenectomy, in which the distal tail of the pancreas is at significant risk of injury, the use of drains in the left upper quadrant following isolated operative splenic salvage procedures is not warranted.

SUGGESTED READINGS

Eastern Association for the Surgery of Trauma, Practice Management Guidelines Work Group: *Practice management guidelines for the nonoperative management of blunt injury to the liver and spleen,* 2003. Available at http://www.east.org/tpg/livspleen.pdf. Accessed march 8, 2010.

Haan HM, Biffl W, Knudson MM, et al: Splenic embolization revisited: a multicenter review, *J Trauma* 56:542, 2004.

Haan JM, Bochicchio GV, Kramer N, Scalea T: Nonoperative management of blunt splenic injury: a 5 year experience, *J Trauma* 58:493, 2005.

Jacobs L: The spleen and diaphragm in advanced trauma operative management: surgical strategies for penetrating trauma, *Woodbury, Conn* 70–106, 2004:Cine-Med.

INGUINAL HERNIA

Keith W. Millikan, MD

OVERVIEW

Inguinal hernia repair is one of the most common procedures performed by general surgeons in the United States, with more than 750,000 performed annually. The cost of health care related to the treatment of inguinal hernia and associated disability is substantial. Historically, hernias have been repaired by many different surgical methods without universal consensus as to the optimal type of repair. Introduction of different prosthetic meshes to relieve tension, different approaches to groin dissection, and various methods of anesthesia have complicated and confused both surgeons and patients as to which procedure to choose. This chapter will attempt to identify the disease process; describe the relevant factors that affect choice of repair; outline and describe pertinent repairs, approaches, and prosthetics available for repairs; and, lastly, outline results, complications, and cost to society for the treatment of this disease process.

DISEASE AND DIAGNOSIS

An inguinal hernia will develop in nearly 25% of men during their lifetime, but less than 2% of women will be afflicted. There are three types of inguinal hernias of surgical importance: *indirect, direct,* and *femoral.* A patent *processus vaginalis* is responsible for indirect hernias in infants and the pediatric population. Because most hernias occur de novo during adulthood, another mechanism must be responsible for indirect hernia formation. Most likely, a widening and weakening of the internal ring occurs during adulthood from an unknown or unexplained phenomenon.

Indirect hernias vary in size, as the defect at the internal ring enlarges, and it should be pointed out that an indirect hernia that destroys the posterior floor of the direct space or extends down into the scrotum should be considered different from the common indirect hernia that involves a peritoneal sac in the inguinal canal with an enlarged internal ring. A direct hernia occurs through the posterior wall of the canal (Hesselbach triangle), because this area is only composed of fascia (transversalis and aponeurotic fibers of transversus abdominis) with no true muscle covering. Direct inguinal hernias almost exclusively occur in men due to increased intraabdominal pressure from factors such as constipation, chronic cough, and difficulty in urination. Femoral hernias occur primarily in women with a broad, flat pelvis coupled with a medially shifted insertion of the iliopubic tract, thus creating a wide orifice of the femoral canal.

A bulge in the inguinal area remains the mainstay for diagnosis. The bulge is usually seen by the patient, although a number of hernias are detected by the patient's primary care physician or urologist. A physical exam with a finger invaginating the scrotal skin into the external ring, accompanied by a Valsalva maneuver while the patient is in the standing position, confirms the diagnosis for indirect and direct inguinal hernias. A bulge detected in the medial thigh or below the inguinal ligament confirms a femoral hernia.

Most bulges are asymptomatic at first but may develop pain over a period of months to years. A surgeon should be suspicious when the first presentation of the disease is pain without an obvious bulge on palpation. It is typical for referrals to be made to a surgeon based on pain alone. Reexamining these patients after long-term standing or exercising, using ultrasound or possibly computed tomographic scan to evaluate the groin, or, lastly, using diagnostic laparoscopy before hernia repair is performed for patients with pain and no palpable hernia. Operating for pain alone in these patients and finding a weak posterior floor or a small sac or lipoma of the cord and performing a definitive repair usually results in chronic pain and a workers' compensation claim for permanent disability. A bulge that has pain associated with it also deserves special attention with accurate documentation of the pain and also a search for the cause of pain at the time of repair, which will be elucidated on later in this chapter.

Inguinal hernias can occur bilaterally, but many patients will develop a hernia on the contralateral side subsequently during their lifetime. It is therefore important to examine both sides at initial presentation and to inform the patient about future contralateral occurrence. A thorough prostate exam for men over 40 years of age and documenting colon cancer screening in patients over 50 years of age should be done to ensure that simultaneous disease of the prostate or colon is not present.

When to Repair

During the past few decades, the recommendation has been to repair almost all inguinal hernias. As the population ages, more patients present with hernias and significant comorbid disease processes. Recent randomized studies have shown that the morbidity of watchful waiting in the asymptomatic hernia patient does not result in increased morbidity or mortality, especially with regard to the risk of strangulation. These studies also reveal that close to 25% of these patients will become symptomatic and will require repair in less than 2 years' time. These studies allow the surgeon some leeway in delaying or deferring asymptomatic hernia repair in patients with short life spans or severe comorbid conditions. Otherwise, elective hernia repair should proceed when it best fits into the patient's work or home schedule. Of course, the symptomatic hernia should be repaired earlier to alleviate pain or obstructive symptoms. The nonreducible, acutely incarcerated hernia obviously should be considered an emergency and must be taken to the operating room immediately.

SURGICAL OPTIONS

Nonmesh Repair

Tissue-to-tissue repairs were the mainstay of treatment before the 1990s. The Bassini, McVay (Cooper ligament), and Shouldice repairs are the three most common tissue-to-tissue repairs performed today. The Bassini repair is performed by suturing Bassini's triple layer—which includes the internal oblique and transversus abdominis muscles and the transversalis fascia—to the iliopubic tract/inguinal ligament with interrupted permanent sutures. The McVay repair is similar to the Bassini repair except that the medial portion of the repair utilizes the Cooper ligament rather than the inguinal ligament. These first few sutures narrow the femoral ring, eliminating the space between the inguinal ligament and the Cooper ligament. A transition stitch is used to transition back up to the inguinal ligament at the level where the iliac vein crosses the Cooper ligament. The remaining sutures are similar to the lateral superior Bassini repair sutures.

The Shouldice repair is also similar to the Bassini repair, only done in layers. The Shouldice method utilizes a continuous nonabsorbable suture for even distribution of tension. During dissection, the transversalis fascia is opened from the internal ring to the pubic tubercle, creating a medial flap along the internal oblique and transversus abdominis muscles. This flap is sewn from the pubic tubercle to the iliopubic tract until it reaches the cremaster muscle at the internal ring. The suture line is then reversed, creating a second suture line approximating internal oblique and transversus abdominis muscles to the inguinal ligament. The third suture line begins a new suture, which approximates the external oblique aponeurosis to the medial flap and ends at the pubic crest. This suture line is then reversed, creating a fourth suture line, which acts as a superficial reinforcing line over the top of the third line. A number of surgeons outside the Shouldice Clinic only perform the first two suture lines and document this variation as a Shouldice repair. All three of the tissue repairs can utilize a relaxing incision medially on the rectus fascia to relieve tension on the primary repair.

Mesh Repairs

The Lichtenstein repair, or onlay mesh repair, was first introduced in the mid 1980s and was coined the "tension-free repair." A prosthetic mesh is used, and the lower edge of the prosthesis is suture fixated to the inguinal ligament, overlapping the pubic tubercle by 2 cm and extending laterally beyond the internal ring. The superior portion of the prosthesis is fixated to the rectus sheath superiorly and medially and is then affixed to the internal oblique. A slit is made in the mesh for the cord structures. The lateral wings of the mesh created by the slit are overlapped and fixed to the inguinal ligament laterally, creating a new internal ring and shutter mechanism for the cord structures. Polypropylene mesh of approximately 8 ×16 cm is commonly used, and Prolene suture is usually the suture of choice.

The Kugel repair involves a minimally invasive approach to place a prosthesis into the preperitoneal space. A 2 to 3 cm incision is used, located inferior to the superior iliac spine but still above the internal ring, dissecting through the external oblique, internal oblique, and the transversalis fascia into the preperitoneal space. Indirect sacs are inverted into the preperitoneal space, and a preperitoneal pocket is developed medial to the inferior epigastric vessels. A Kugel patch is placed into the pocket underlying the femoral direct and indirect spaces. The Kugel patch has a semirigid outer ring that keeps the patch from invaginating into the hernia defect. The patch is also composed of two layers of polypropylene with a slit in one layer to allow a surgeon's fingers to be placed to aid in positioning of the patch. The patch is secured with a single suture, and the muscle-splitting incision is then closed.

The plug-and-patch repair, or PerFix repair, was first introduced in the early 1990s. The original description by Rutkow and Robbins involved placing a cone-shaped plug with inner petals into an indirect, direct, or femoral defect. The outer rim of the cone was sutured to the edge of the defect. For indirect and direct hernias, an onlay patch was placed over the entire inguinal floor from 2 cm over the pubic tubercle to 2 cm lateral to the internal ring. A slit for the cord structures was premade into the onlay patch. This was the first repair to utilize both the anterior and preperitoneal spaces. The modified technique was first introduced in 1997 and utilized the inner petals of the plug for fixation to the anatomical structures of the defect (internal oblique and inguinal ligament for indirect hernias and Cooper ligament, inguinal ligament, internal oblique, and transversus abdominis arch for direct hernias); utilizing the internal petals for fixation allows the outer umbrella (rim) of the cone to flatten out in the preperitoneal space and perform as an underlay preperitoneal repair. The patch is then placed in the traditional onlay position without sutures. The modification technique does not allow for the possibility of plug migration or for the plug balling up into a meshoma.

The Prolene Hernia System (PHS; Ethicon, Somerville, NJ) was designed in 1998 to replicate the advantages of the anterior and preperitoneal repairs similar to the plug-and-patch repair. The PHS comprises two layers of Prolene mesh attached together by a connector. One layer of the mesh is placed in the preperitoneal space; the top layer requires a slit to be cut in it for the cord structures and is then fixated as an onlay, similar to the Lichtenstein repair.

Laparoscopic repair can be performed by entering the peritoneal cavity (TAPP procedure) or by staying in the preperitoneal space (TEPP procedure). TAPP repairs are performed by entering the abdominal cavity with a 10 mm port placed in an infraumbilical position and two 5 mm ports placed in the left lower quadrant (LLQ) and right lower quadrant (RLQ) respectively. The hernia is identified, and a peritoneal flap is developed to reduce the hernia and identify the Cooper ligament, lateral border of the rectus, cord structures, iliopubic tract, and the iliac and inferior epigastric vessels. A large piece of mesh is placed over the hernia defect, including coverage of the femoral, direct, and indirect spaces. The mesh is then fixated in place with a tacking device to the Cooper ligament and the rectus muscle. To avoid major vessel injury and injury to the lateral branch of the genital femoral nerve, no tacks are placed below the iliopubic tract.

After mesh fixation, the peritoneal flap is closed over the mesh to prevent visceral attachment to the mesh. For the TEPP repair, a 10 mm port is placed in the infraumbilical position preperitoneally, after a balloon dissector has been placed to open this space. The preperitoneal space is then insufflated, and two lower midline 5 mm ports are placed. The preperitoneal space is dissected, reducing the hernia and again identifying the Cooper ligament, lateral border of the rectus muscle, inferior epigastric vessels, iliac vessels, and cord structures. A preformed mesh can then be placed over the hernia defect and the direct, indirect, and femoral spaces; the preformed meshes do not require tack fixation. The trocar sheaths are removed, and desufflation of the space keeps the mesh in place.

Outcome Measures

For the last century, hernia repair was judged by its associated recurrence rate. During the 1990s, with the advent of regional anesthesia, the safe introduction of prosthetic meshes, and the advances in minimally invasive approaches, other outcome measures emerged in the discussion of which procedure to choose. Surgeons now base the efficacy of a hernia repair on five measures: 1) recurrence rate, 2) technical difficulty, 3) rehabilitation time, 4) complication rate, and 5) cost to the healthcare system and work environment. A recurrence rate of less than 1% to 2% is now considered optimal for hernia repair.

Most tissue-to-tissue repairs have recurrence rates greater than 10% and have fallen out of favor by the majority of the surgeons in the United States. There are pockets around the world that still favor the Shouldice repair and report long-term recurrence rates of 1% or less. Proponents of the Shouldice repair also argue that the avoidance of mesh in young adults should be a priority. Most surgeons still agree that a tissue-to-tissue repair should be the procedure of choice for incarcerated or strangulated hernias in an effort to avoid the dreaded complication of mesh infection. A new yet unproven option to avoid mesh infections would be to use a biologic mesh or long-term absorbable mesh, which have recently been developed and introduced to the marketplace.

Another advantage purported by tissue-to-tissue repair advocates is that young surgeons in training need to learn the anatomy of the inguinal area to understand the utility of other repairs. This point does not withstand criticism if our patients are placed at risk for recurrence and long-term rehabilitation. The development of teaching models or the reinstitution of cadaver dissection should be able to teach our students groin anatomy.

The difficulty of some procedures has long been forgotten with new innovations in approaches to the groin and technological advances. The laparoscopic hernia repair advertised short recovery times with low recurrence rates once the learning curve was attained. Surgeons jumped on the laparoscopic bandwagon only to encounter a steep learning curve, high initial recurrence rates, increased cost of the procedure, and added complications of bowel and bladder injury, major vessel injury, and nerve injury different from open anterior approaches. The national study comparing onlay mesh repair to laparoscopic repair found a learning curve of 250 or more cases to become proficient and safe with low recurrence rates in the laparoscopic group. Despite laparoscopic repair being introduced in the early 1990s and the reported short recovery times, the laparoscopic TEPP and TAPP approaches still only account for less than 15% of all inguinal repairs nationally. At the present time, laparoscopic approaches should be limited to bilateral and recurrent hernia repairs.

The Kugel repair is another minimally invasive repair with a short recovery time that can be performed under regional anesthesia. Kugel has reported excellent results and has established a training center to educate surgeons. Unfortunately, surgeons have found the learning curve to be relatively long with recurrence rates higher than those reported. The procedure provides an excellent preperitoneal tension-free mesh repair when mastered but has only been adopted by a minority of surgeons in the United States.

The Lichtenstein onlay mesh repair, however, was easily mastered by surgeons performing open tissue-to-tissue repairs. Introduced in the mid-1980s, it was the only tensionless option for surgeons during this time. If a surgeon was willing to accept mesh placement in the groin, the anatomical dissection was similar to tissue-to-tissue approaches, and thousands of surgeons converted to the Lichtenstein technique. Well-documented reports of reduced recovery times, the use of regional anesthesia with low recurrence rates, and a short learning curve accounted for its popularity among surgeons in the United States in the 1990s.

In the early 1990s, the plug-and-patch repair was introduced as a method with a very short learning curve. Performed under regional anesthesia, it offers a shorter recovery than the Lichtenstein repair and is at least equal to laparoscopic repair, with a less than 1% recurrence rate. At first, the technique was severely criticized for the completely different configuration of the mesh. Surgeons feared that the conical configuration would ball up in the groin and cause migration and possibly meshomas. Modifications to fixation and the relative ease of placement while still conforming to exact identification of all anatomical structures of the groin has piqued the interest of many surgeons who perform inguinal hernia repair, and over 50% of surgeons use this technique. Over the last 5 years, the plug-and-patch repair has been the most commonly performed hernia repair in the United States. Over 350,000 repairs were performed in 2008. Also, our report of a 0.15% recurrence rate with a 3 day return to normal activities, a 99% return to manual labor in 14 days, and a chronic pain rate of less than 1 in 200 has established a standard by which other repairs should be judged.

The PHS repair introduced by Gilbert in the 1990s uses a similar concept to the plug-and-patch repair by placing mesh into both the preperitoneal space and the onlay position. The device is somewhat large, making the placement tedious and requiring a very large preperitoneal dissection. Therefore, the learning curve is somewhat lengthened compared with other open mesh repairs. Studies are few and have not shown significant advantages over the plug-and-patch or Lichtenstein repairs. The lack of evidence supporting the advertised claims may be responsible for the low use of this system.

With reported recurrence rates of less than 1% for mesh repairs performed properly, the topic of discussion these days is chronic pain. Hernia experts publish on and debate about this topic frequently. No one is sure of the etiology, but common causes are stated: inguinal nerve injury, pubic tubercle trauma, and the mesh itself. Proponents of each reported technique argue that the other techniques cause more chronic pain. The truth of the matter is that the cause is most likely multifactorial and is probably not completely known or identified. We can only stick to certain principles. First, document during initial examination whether the patient has pain associated with the palpable hernia. If a nerve is attached to the hernia sac by chronic inflammation, or pain is significant, dissection is required to separate the nerve from the sac; in this case, transection should be performed. Transection that is as proximal as possible is preferred, and some also advocate implantation of the nerve stump into the proximal muscle.

A chronic pain rate of 0.5% should be achievable. When a patient complains of pain postoperatively, a conservative approach is taken in most cases. Most pain will slowly resolve after a 6 to 12 month period of avoiding activity that produces the pain symptom and with use of anti-inflammatory drugs such as ibuprofen for pain relief. The exception to this rule is the patient with severe pain in the immediate postoperative period in the distribution of either the ilioinguinal, iliohypogastric, or genitofemoral nerves. For open procedures, or in the distribution of the lateral cutaneous branch of the genitofemoral nerve for laparoscopic repairs, patients should be taken immediately back to the operating room, as a suture or tack has entrapped one of these nerves during the initial repair. If pain starts after the immediate postoperative period and persists 6 to 12 months after a repair, a series of steroid injections with a local anesthetic should be injected into the painful area. If these injections are unsuccessful, then referral to a pain clinic for more intensive, specific medication or possible radiofrequency ablation (RFA) or cryoprobe should be performed to alleviate pain.

Persistent pain after these endeavors warrants groin exploration with triple neurectomy and possible mesh removal. Of course, before groin exploration occurs, a thorough search for other causes of pain should be undertaken. Most pain clinics recommend at minimum a bone scan to rule out pubic osteitis, a computed tomographic scan or magnetic resonance imaging (MRI) to rule out pelvic pathology and spinal diseases, and a referral to a spine surgeon for evaluation. Despite an aggressive and thorough approach to the treatment of chronic pain, many patients fail after all therapies have been tried. The best approach to the chronic pain patient is to not have it happen in the first place. Therefore, the procedure you choose for hernia repair should be the one with a low recurrence rate and low chronic pain rate in your hands.

Cost of hernia repair is becoming more and more important in today's health care environment. The cost of laparoscopic repair, including use of disposable instruments, longer recovery room stays due to general anesthesia, and the cost of treating severe complications should preclude the performance of laparoscopic repair for the initial unilateral hernia. All other open repairs can be performed under regional anesthesia with short ambulatory recovery room stays. We found that the recovery room stay was less than 1 hour for the modified plug-and-patch repair, with a 3-day recovery for normal activities. At our institution, the plug-and-patch repair is the most cost effective, as proven by evidence-based medicine.

Complications of open mesh hernia repair occur at a relatively low rate. Mesh infections with the single use of prophylactic antibiotics occur in less than 1% of patients. In fact, our series of more than 2000 patients had no reported mesh infections. We recommend a single dose of prophylactic intravenous antibiotic before incision and routine surgical preparation with the application of an adhesive sterile barrier placed on the skin to prevent mesh from coming in contact with the skin during placement. Urinary retention is less than 1% in open mesh repairs if a prostate exam or evaluation is done preoperatively and treated accordingly before going ahead with hernia repair. Hematomas and seromas do occur infrequently and usually resolve on their own if left to observation. Major vessel, bowel, or bladder injury can be reduced to a minimum if laparoscopic repair is limited to only bilateral and recurrent hernias, and surgeons privileged for these procedures have completed the learning curve (approximately 250 cases) with a preceptor. The overall complication rate for hernia repair should be lower than 2%, as shown in our large series over a 10-year period.

Special Circumstances

Groin hernias in women are uncommon but not rare. Although femoral hernias occur more commonly in women, the overall majority of groin hernias in women are indirect. Another fact of unknown etiology is that chronic pain occurs in women at a significantly higher rate. Since the treatment of chronic pain may require mesh removal, you may want to consider not placing mesh in the preperitoneal space. Also, the indirect sac is usually densely adherent to the round ligament. Round ligament ligation is required to reduce the sac into the preperitoneal space, and an onlay mesh can then be used as an efficient and long-lasting repair. Elective femoral hernias should be approached with an infrainguinal incision and a small plug placed into the defect. The plug can be sutured to the inguinal ligament superiorly and the Cooper ligament medially. The inguinal canal does not need to be opened or explored.

Bilateral or recurrent hernias should be approached laparoscopically as long as prostate surgery is not anticipated or already performed and provided that no mesh has been previously placed in the preperitoneal space. The multiple recurrent hernia with all spaces previously violated should either be approached with a TAPP procedure or a Lichtenstein repair with possible orchiectomy. The scrotal hernia with destruction of the entire posterior floor also requires a large onlay Lichtenstein repair. The distal sac should be left in place to avoid testicular ischemia and the formation of large hematomas. Strangulated and acutely incarcerated hernias require general anesthesia, reduction, and inspection of the strangulated or incarcerated tissue followed by tissue-to-tissue repair or biologic mesh repair.

The sports hernia is now a common topic of discussion among hernia experts, but it was first popularized by European surgeons and described as an injury or disease that occurs in professional soccer or hockey players. It should be noted that it is not a hernia but rather pain that is caused by a weak posterior floor and entrapment of nerves due to muscle tears, most commonly at rectus insertion on pubis or adductor insertion on the pubis, and pain will have been persistent after 6 to 8 weeks of rest and conservative physical therapy. MRI criteria are now available to make the diagnosis.

Whether to use an open or laparoscopic treatment is debated, and there is no consensus among experts. Neurectomy has also been proposed in open repairs. Also, the use of mesh is debated among open hernia experts. The majority of surgeons who do not perform these procedures doubt the existence of the disease. It is important to understand the controversy, because a number of nonprofessional athletes are being referred to surgeons as a sports hernia when persistent pain is present in the groin. We need to closely evaluate these patients, take a conservative early approach, and only consider sports hernia repair when there is MRI evidence of the injury; otherwise a number of unnecessary procedures will be performed on teenage to middle-aged adults with pain from another etiology. Remember, a diagnostic laparoscopy can always be done with a 5 mm scope to confirm the presence or absence of a hernia in the case of a negative MRI and physical exam.

SUMMARY

Inguinal hernia repair has become the most common procedure performed by the general surgeon. It should be noted that many procedures can be performed, and no one procedure should be considered the treatment of choice for all types of hernias. Also, in the patient who is considered at high risk for significant complications, with multiple comorbidities and a predicted short lifespan, it is within the standard of care to recommend watchful waiting. For the routine unilateral inguinal hernia, the modified plug-and-patch repair is recommended based on the long-term low recurrence rate (0.15%), short recovery (3 days), low overall complication rate (1.5%), low chronic pain rate (<0.5%), early return to manual labor (14 days), and low overall cost (using ambulatory surgery, basic instrumentation, and quick operating room and recovery room times). Laparoscopic repairs should be reserved for bilateral and recurrent hernias. Lichtenstein repairs should be recommended for large scrotal hernias, inguinal hernias in women, and recurrent hernias where the preperitoneal space has previously been violated or a TAPP repair is not advisable (multiple previous lower abdominal or pelvic surgeries).

Elective femoral hernias are efficiently repaired with an infrainguinal approach and a plug repair. Incarcerated and strangulated hernias require knowledge and expertise in tissue-to-tissue repairs or the utilization of biologic mesh. The near future and present will see the introduction of lightweight mesh repairs and either long-term absorbable mesh repairs or biologic mesh repairs. No clear data are available to recommend use of these prosthetics, and most likely it will take over a decade to see the long-term results of these new technologies.

In conclusion, the above statements summarize decades of information concerning inguinal hernia repair and, at the present time, a surgeon who can master the learning curve of a procedure and produce evidence-based results may perform any of the above-mentioned procedures for the treatment of an inguinal hernia.

SUGGESTED READINGS

Millikan KW, Doolas A: A long-term evaluation of the modified mesh-plug hernioplasty in over 2,000 patients, *Hernia* 12:257–260, 2008.

Millikan KW, Cummings B, Doolas A: The Millikan modified mesh-plug hernioplasty, *Arch Surg* 138:525–530, 2008.

Millikan KW, Deziel DJ: The management of hernia: considerations in cost effectiveness, *Surg Clin North Am* 76(1):105–116, 1996.

Neumayer L, Giobbie-Hurder A, Jonasson O, et al: Open mesh versus laparoscopic mesh repair of inguinal hernia, Veterans Affairs Cooperative Studies Program: 456 investigators, *N Engl J Med* 350:1819–1827, 2004.

Thompson JS, Gibbs JO, Reda DJ, et al: Does delaying repair of an asymptomatic hernia have a penalty? *Am J Surg* 195:89–93, 2008.

Takata MC, Duh QY: Laparoscopic inguinal hernia repair, *Surg Clin North Am* 88:157–178, 2008.

Woods B, Neumayer L: Open repair of inguinal hernia: an evidence-based review, *Surg Clin North Am* 88:139–155, 2008.

RECURRENT INGUINAL HERNIAS

Meghan Edwards, MD, Kerry Fisher, MD, and Leigh A. Neumayer, MD

OVERVIEW

Approximately 10% of the more than 700,000 inguinal hernia repairs in the United States annually are performed on patients with recurrent inguinal hernias. Recurrent inguinal hernia repairs are technically more difficult than primary repairs because of inflammation and scarring from the prior repair. Critical anatomy is more difficult to identify, operative complications are more frequent, and repair is less likely to be successful in the long term. Strategies for repair have been widely variable and are continuing to evolve in the era of mesh repair.

INDICATIONS FOR REPAIR

Risk for incarceration of asymptomatic inguinal hernias is low, so repair should generally be recommended only for symptomatic hernias. A large, randomized multicenter clinical trial published in 2006 compared patients with primary or recurrent inguinal hernias treated with surgery or watchful waiting. The results demonstrated no difference in outcomes or cost between groups and concluded that surgery can safely be delayed for patients who are asymptomatic.

Complications during and after repair of recurrent inguinal hernias are more frequent and more significant than complications after primary repair, so it is essential to select appropriate operative candidates. These complications include chronic pain, scrotal hematomas, injury to major structures, testicular atrophy (after 3% to 5% of recurrent repairs), as well as recurrences. Studies have shown a significantly higher recurrence rate after repair of recurrent inguinal hernias (22%) compared to primary repair (7.7%).

In selecting patients for repair, it is important to consider patient characteristics and comorbidities. Recurrences can be a direct result of technical errors, or they can be attributed to patient factors. Age older than 50 years, smoking status, cardiac/pulmonary disease, prostate disease, heavy work, obesity, retirement or unemployment, and the presence of two or more similarly affected relatives have been found to be independent risk factors for recurrence. Any of the above modifiable risk factors should be adjusted if possible prior to repair, and all should be considered when counseling patients preoperatively.

Another important factor to consider, particularly in women, is whether the recurrent hernia actually represents a missed primary femoral hernia. A large prospective analysis of hernia repairs in women was published in 2005 using data from the Swedish Hernia Registry. At the time of reoperation, more than 40% of women previously reported to have inguinal hernias were found to have femoral hernias. This number was less than 5% in men, suggesting the possibility that women were misdiagnosed at the time of primary repair. Due to the high incidence of femoral hernias found in women with recurrences, it is imperative that operation for recurrent hernias in women involve an exploration and reinforcement of the femoral space.

The diagnosis of recurrent inguinal hernia must also be distinguished from chronic groin pain prior to repair. Physical exam is the primary method of diagnosis and is sufficient in most instances. However, in some cases, a hernia bulge may not be appreciable on examination. Patients may have postoperative groin pain without recurrence, so reoperation for a presumed recurrence is not recommended. Alternatively, imaging may be used as an adjunct to physical exam. Ultrasound, computed tomography (CT) scan, and magnetic resonance imaging (MRI) have all been used with variable results, but none has been established as superior to the others. Radiographic studies should be obtained during a Valsalva maneuver if possible.

TIMING OF REPAIR

Inguinal hernia recurrences can occur anytime, from days to years after initial repair. Repair of reducible recurrent inguinal hernias should generally be delayed until at least 6 weeks after primary repair but can otherwise be scheduled whenever it is most convenient for the patient.

TYPE OF REPAIR

As with primary inguinal hernias, recurrent hernias can be repaired via an open or laparoscopic technique, with or without mesh reinforcement. Similar to repair of primary inguinal hernias, tension-free repair of recurrent hernias with mesh has been proven by multiple trials to be superior to tissue repair with regard to recurrence rates. The repair can be approached anteriorly or in the preperitoneal space.

The method of primary hernia repair should always be considered when selecting the type of repair for recurrent hernia. When approaching the patient with a recurrent hernia, every effort should be made to obtain the operative report of the prior repair. Other intervening operative procedures should also be considered, such as radical retropubic prostatectomy and open pelvic fixation, as these procedures may have led to scarring of the preperitoneal space.

Open repairs have withstood the test of time and have had high success rates reported in multiple trials. The most common open anterior mesh repair is the Lichtenstein procedure. An anterior abdominal wall incision is made, the external oblique aponeurosis is opened, and the cord structures are skeletonized. The hernia sac is identified and reduced or excised, and the defect is covered by a mesh onlay. The mesh is sutured to the conjoint tendon, inguinal ligament, and internal oblique aponeurosis. The external oblique aponeurosis is then closed over the mesh. This technique can be modified by the addition of a mesh "plug" into the hernia defect after reduction of the sac, prior to placement of the mesh onlay. Multiple trials worldwide have demonstrated the effectiveness of open anterior mesh repair for recurrent inguinal hernias.

Open preperitoneal repair can be performed with mesh as well. The advantage to a preperitoneal approach is the opportunity for dissection of virgin tissue planes if the prior repair was done anteriorly. A transverse incision is made in the abdominal wall two finger breaths above the pubic symphysis. This incision is extended through the external oblique, internal oblique, and transversus abdominis muscles and transversalis fascia, which is then dissected from the underlying peritoneum. The cord structures are dissected from the peritoneum and hernia sac, and a mesh patch is placed between the peritoneum and cord structures. The patch should be anchored with one suture during closure of the transversalis fascia. The open preperitoneal approach is less popular than other repairs, but at least one recent prospective study has reported low complication and recurrence rates when used for repair of recurrent hernias (Figure 1).

Though open repair has historically been the more common approach, recent randomized controlled trials have suggested some specific advantages with laparoscopic repair. As with many other laparoscopic surgeries, laparoscopic inguinal hernia repairs have been demonstrated to result in decreased postoperative pain and shorter recovery periods than open repairs. In addition, in the case of prior

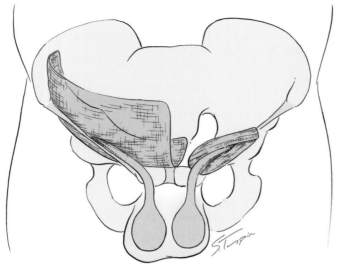

FIGURE I   A transparent view of the lower abdomen showing typical mash placement for open, tension-free (*left*) and laparoscopic (*right*) inguinal hernia repairs.

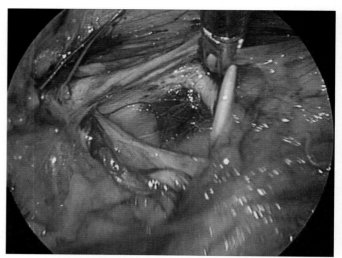

FIGURE 2   Reduction of the indirect hernia sac.

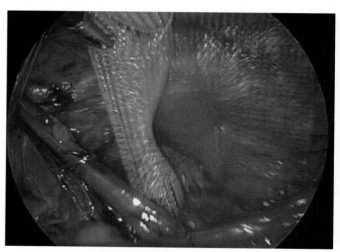

FIGURE 3   Mesh placement.

anterior repair, laparoscopic repair allows for dissection of virgin tissue planes in the preperitoneal space. This theoretically allows for decreased operative difficulty and fewer complications than a second open repair.

Options for laparoscopic repair include totally extraperitoneal repair (TEP) and transabdominal preperitoneal repairs (TAPP). For a TEP repair, an incision is made in the abdomen, the space anterior to the posterior rectus sheath is dissected, and a trocar or balloon-tipped trocar is inserted. The preperitoneal space is dissected bluntly, or the balloon is inflated to complete dissection of the preperitoneal space. Two additional trocars are then placed in this space, the cord structures are identified and skeletonized, and the hernia sac is reduced or excised. A large mesh is then placed over the defect and stapled if desired (Figures 2 and 3).

Many different types of mesh can be used, however, the mesh should be at least 13 by 15 cm to reduce the incidence of re-recurrence. TEP repairs are relatively contraindicated in patients with prior surgeries or radiation to the pelvis, due to scarring of the preperitoneal plane. This contraindication has been refuted by experts, however, and some studies have demonstrated safe TEP repair after prior pelvic surgeries and radiation.

For a TAPP repair, trocars are placed in the abdominal cavity. The peritoneum on the anterior abdominal wall is incised superiorly to the hernia, and a peritoneal flap is created and dissected inferiorly to identify the underlying anatomy. The cord structures are skeletonized, the hernia sac is reduced or divided, and a large piece of mesh is laid over the cord structures and hernia defect. The mesh can be stapled in place if desired, and the peritoneal flap is closed over the mesh. Similar to TEP repairs, multiple types of mesh are available, but the size of the repair appears to be the only significant factor affecting recurrence rates. If inflammation, scarring, or damage to the peritoneum makes closure of the peritoneal flap impossible, the mesh used should be designed for intraabdominal placement. A TAPP repair can be combined with another abdominal surgery if indicated.

During repair of recurrent inguinal hernias, mesh from prior repair is sometimes encountered. Frequently the hernia recurrence is around the edge of the mesh or through a slit in the mesh. Mesh removal can be extremely difficult and can increase operative complications, so in general, the prior mesh should be left undisturbed. Most defects can be adequately covered with a large piece of mesh that has 2 to 3 cm of overlap on each edge. Some studies have shown benefit of partial or complete mesh removal, particularly when an abscess surrounds the mesh or with chronic groin pain unrelated to hernia recurrence; these should be addressed on a case-by-case basis as opposed to adopting a standard policy of mesh removal at reoperation.

OPEN VERSUS LAPAROSCOPIC REPAIR

Several randomized clinical trials in the past few years have addressed the dilemma regarding open versus laparoscopic repair of recurrent inguinal hernias. These studies have shown similar success and recurrence rates between the two. Open repairs have been associated with shorter operative times but higher incidence of postoperative hematomas. Laparoscopic repairs have resulted in less postoperative pain and shorter recovery times. Many of these studies have been limited by exclusion of prior mesh repairs and/or prior laparoscopic repairs.

The majority of studies evaluating types of repair for recurrent inguinal hernias have excluded patients with prior mesh repairs. However, in 2008, more than 90% of primary inguinal hernias were repaired using mesh. Because of randomized controlled trials demonstrating the superiority of hernia repair with mesh, this number will likely continue to increase. The majority of patients with recurrent inguinal hernias in the future will have undergone primary repair with mesh. The inflammatory reaction from the mesh makes these repairs technically more difficult. For this reason, most experts in hernia surgery believe that laparoscopic repair is superior to open repair for hernia recurrences after primary mesh repair via an anterior approach. A recent large prospective study analyzed a subset of patients with recurrent hernias after primary Lichtenstein repair. Results confirmed higher recurrence rates after open repair of the recurrence when compared with laparoscopic repair.

SUMMARY

Repair of recurrent groin hernias is more difficult than primary repair and has higher complication and recurrence rates. Operative candidates should be carefully selected and counseled preoperatively. Multiple strategies have been used in the past for successful repair. The method of prior repair should be considered when planning an approach to recurrent hernia because traversing previously dissected planes, especially when mesh was used, can be difficult. As a result of the increasing number of primary repairs with mesh, laparoscopic repair is emerging as the favored repair for recurrent inguinal hernias.

SUGGESTED READINGS

Bisgaard T, Bay-Nielsen M, Kehlet H: Re-recurrence after operation for recurrent inguinal hernia: a nationwide 8-year follow-up study on the role of type of repair, *Ann Surg* 247:4, 2008.

Dedemadi G, Sgourakis G, Karaliotas C, et al: Comparison of laparoscopic and open tension-free repair of recurrent inguinal hernias: a prospective randomized study, *Surg Endosc* 20:1099, 2006.

Eklund A, Rudberg C, Leijonmarck C, et al: Recurrent inguinal hernia: randomized multicenter trial comparing laparoscopic and Lichtenstein repair, *Surg Endosc* 4:634, 2007.

Fitzgibbons R, Giobbie-Harder A, Gibbs J, et al: Watchful waiting vs repair of inguinal hernia in minimally symptomatic men, *JAMA* 295:285–292, 2006.

Kouhia S, Huttunen R, Silvasti S, et al: Lichtenstein hernioplasty versus totally extraperitoneal laparoscopic hernioplasty in treatment of recurrent inguinal hernia: a prospective randomized trial, *Ann Surg* 249:3, 2009.

INCISIONAL, EPIGASTRIC, AND UMBILICAL HERNIAS

Karl A. LeBlanc, MD, MBA

OVERVIEW

The hernias listed in the title of this chapter are some of the more common defects in the abdominal wall that surgeons are called upon to treat. The etiology varies with the specific entity. Incisional hernias result from the disruption of the integrity of the musculofascial layers of the abdominal wall after surgery. These will develop in up to 13% of patients who undergo a midline laparotomy, and in more than 28% if a wound infection develops. Epigastric hernias generally are acquired also and are especially frequent in obese individuals with attenuated tissues caused by obesity or the aging process. Umbilical hernias are usually considered to be congenital in origin. However, many occur later in life and could be considered to result from aging and increases in abdominal girth and pressure. The repair of all of these defects revolves around the strength of the tissues and more frequently requires the use of a prosthetic biomaterial to achieve a lasting repair.

There are a few technical considerations that apply to all of these hernias, whether they are repaired laparoscopically or via an open procedure. Complete dissection is necessary to identify all of the fascial edges. This dissection should remove much of the fat from the fascia so that the mesh will contact collagen tissues, rather than adipose tissues, to allow for more rapid and secure tissue ingrowth. The use of any energy source adjacent to any bowel is ill advised. The lateral spread of heat from electrocautery, bipolar cautery, or even ultrasonic devices can result in thermal burns that may not be recognized initially. Intestinal perforation can result within a few days and can result in devastating consequences. Therefore, only cold scissors should be used near the intestine in this dissection. In addition, patients should quit smoking prior to the repair, and medical conditions and nutritional status should be optimized.

INCISIONAL HERNIA

More than 90% of incisional hernias occur in the midline of the abdominal wall. Incisional hernias in other locations represent the relative infrequency of other approaches to operations in the abdominal cavity. The sutured closure of these defects has proven to be inadequate to provide a durable repair in the vast majority of patients. Any defect less than 4 cm could be considered for primary closure with permanent sutures. However, given predisposing factors for recurrence—such as obesity, smoking, steroid usage, or advanced age—the use of a prosthetic material is recommended even in smaller fascial defects, and defects larger than 4 cm should always be repaired with a prosthesis, unless an associated infection or other source of contamination is present.

The type of material to use is a matter of debate, but most of the products available today will support the intraabdominal pressures generated and will help reduce the recurrence rates. A large variety of meshes are currently available, which makes a choice necessary. When direct contact is required, we recommend using a product that contains a substance to separate the intestines from the mesh. Some biomaterials do not have this additional layer, as they themselves resist adhesion formation; these are considered to possess "tissue separating" properties (Table 1).

All of these products make various claims regarding effectiveness, ingrowth characteristics, resistance to infection, ease of use, ability to treat in an infection, and contraction or shrinkage to name a few. Clinical experience and results should dictate a preference. For the most part, mesh products can be used either laparoscopically or in the open technique, but there is increasing emphasis on the use of the laparoscopic method to repair these hernias. The open tissue repair has recurrence rates from 25% to 50%, but the addition of a mesh product reduces this to 10% to 25%. This latter figure is due, in part, to the placement of the mesh as a bridge over the fascial defect, in which the product is secured to the edges of the defect as an inlay repair. Because of the high recurrence rate, the use of any mesh as a bridge is contraindicated in most, but not all, instances (such as an infection in a septic patient or the open abdomen).

An underlay method that applies the biomaterial to the undersurface of the abdominal wall with strong fixation provides the most durable repair, and this requires the use of transfascial sutures. The Stoppa repair was the first to employ this concept, but it utilized uncoated polyester in the preperitoneal position. Currently, the availability of the meshes listed in Table 1 makes their use in the intraperitoneal position feasible. This "clock" repair mimics the laparoscopic repair in that transfascial sutures are placed.

The sublay position of the prosthetic biomaterial is the preferred location for an open hernia repair. In this repair, the posterior rectus sheath is opened and sewn together to close the midline. The mesh, which in this repair could be an "unprotected" product (i.e., non–tissue separating), is positioned between the rectus muscle and the posterior fascial closure, and the anterior sheath is closed over this to complete the repair. When the defect is too large to accomplish a closure, the hernia sac should be preserved to serve as a barrier between the mesh and the intestine. However, if the hernia should recur, one of the products in Table 1 is suggested.

The sublay method is limited in the overlap of the mesh by the confines of the rectus sheath. If one of the other techniques is used, it is generally accepted that a minimum overlap of the fascial defect by the prosthesis should be 3 cm. Over the last several years, however, this has been expanded to 4 to 5 cm, especially in the obese, elderly, and in smokers, diabetics, and multiply recurrent or other high-risk patients.

The application of the mesh in the open technique can sometimes be difficult, and transfascial sutures are required to adequately fixate the biomaterial. The laparoscopic method is becoming the procedure of choice for these hernias. Laparoscopy allows for the identification of multiple hernia defects and for the placement of larger sections of prosthetic biomaterials. It is also associated with a shorter length of stay, decreased costs, and a quicker recovery time. Additionally, the recurrence rates noted with the laparoscopic approach range from 3% to 11%, averaging about 5%.

The most challenging portion of the repair is the adhesiolysis that is virtually required in all of these patients and the ever-present risk of intestinal injury. Therefore the use of any instrument with an energy source attached—such as electrocautery, ultrasonic devices, and the like—are not recommended adjacent to any intestine at any time. The risk of bowel injury is less than 2% and is similar to the open procedure. However, the potential for an unrecognized enterotomy must be acknowledged, because it is the greatest factor in significant complications and death of these patients.

For a successful repair, complete dissection of all of the adhesions that involve areas the mesh will cover is important. It is best to provide prosthetic reinforcement to areas behind any incision where the incisional hernia originates to prevent new hernia development in areas not covered by the mesh. The 3 cm overlap mentioned above should be strictly adhered to in all cases. However,

hernias in the subxyphoid and subcostal areas and those at the suprapubic level are particularly difficult, and at these sites, an overlap of mesh of 7 to 10 cm is recommended because of the difficulty of fixation.

In the upper abdomen, the surgeon must be sure to avoid piercing the heart and diaphragm with any fixation method. In both the upper and lower abdomen, all fat, such as that near the falciform ligament and the preperitoneal fat in the pelvis, must be dissected off the abdominal wall to assure that the mesh will contact fascia and not fat; otherwise, tissue ingrowth into any biomaterial will be impeded. For those hernias that result in the overlap of the mesh onto the diaphragm, the mesh should be hand sewn to the diaphragm. A few interrupted permanent sutures suffice, as the liver assists in flattening out the product and holding its position. Placement of tacks might result in penetration into the pleural or pericardial cavity. In the pelvis, the mesh must be fixed to the Cooper ligament in the same manner as in the inguinal hernia repair to ensure adequate overlap and fixation.

Some surgeons believe that the hernia defect should be closed during the laparoscopic repair, if possible. Although this is seldom feasible, it might result in decreased seroma formation. It is not felt to reduce recurrence rates and could result in more pain for the patient, so most surgeons do not employ this option.

The fixation of biomaterials continues to be an area of controversy. Careful research of the issues has revealed that devices currently available are quite strong, such as the tacks that are permanent and even the newer absorbable ones. The use of transfascial sutures is disputed, but there is little disagreement when the hernia defect measures greater than 10 cm that the use of permanent transfascial suture fixation is preferred. Sutures should be placed no more than 5 cm apart. Smaller hernia defects, those less than 5 cm, could be adequately repaired without sutures if the patient is not significantly obese or a smoker, or if the hernia is not multiply recurrent. These sutures can be placed with a variety of suture-passing instruments. The argument against sutures is the fact that there may be a more frequent incidence of pain in patients with incisional hernias, but this represents only about 2% of this surgical population. If that occurs, usually injection of these sites with a local anesthetic will alleviate the symptoms.

Absorbable tacking devices are now available that will fix the product and then disappear after 3 to 12 months (Figure 1). The use of these products is appealing, but there are no long-term data on them. If these are chosen, it is best to place transfascial sutures to ensure a secure repair until such a time as data prove them unnecessary. There are many perceived benefits to the use of such devices, however, a challenge remains in their placement into the Cooper ligament.

The repair of hernias less than 15 to 18 cm in their widest dimension can be accomplished via an open or laparoscopic technique.

TABLE 1: Prosthetic biomaterials with tissue-separating properties

Product	Manufacturer
C-Qur	Atrium Medical, Hudson, NH
Composix EX	C.R. Bard, Providence, RI
Composix L/P	C.R. Bard, Providence, RI
Composix Kugel	C.R. Bard, Providence, RI
DualMesh, DualMesh Plus	W.L. Gore & Associates, Elkhart, Md.
Parietex	Covidien, Mansfield, Mass.
Proceed	Ethicon, Inc., Somerville, NJ
Sepramesh IP Composite	C.R. Bard, Providence, RI
Ventrio	C.R. Bard, Providence, RI

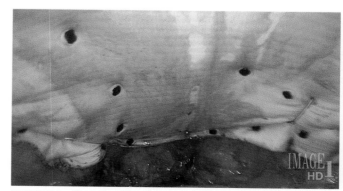

FIGURE 1   Completed laparoscopic incisional hernia repair with DualMesh Plus (W.L. Gore) fixed with sutures and SorbaFix tacks (C.R. Bard).

Hernias larger than this, especially in lateral dimension, are increasingly being seen. These present a particular challenge because of loss of domain and the effect on the respiratory function of the abdominal musculature. In these individuals, the use of the component separation technique is increasingly being used, in which an extensive lateral dissection of the space between the subcutaneous tissue and the fascia is performed that exposes the lateral edge of the rectus sheath and the external oblique insertion. The external oblique aponeurosis is incised 1 cm lateral to the rectus sheath and is then separated from the internal oblique aponeurosis. This allows the rectus sheath to slide medially as much as 10 cm from either side of the abdomen at the midportion of the abdominal wall. This can be aided with the use of the laparoscope. The laparoscope will be inserted below the eleventh rib, in between the tissue planes of the oblique muscles, to dissect them apart; this avoids the large dissection of the subcutaneous plane, which disrupts the perforating vascular supply. This technique has utility in the smaller of these complex hernias, but if the defects are 15 cm or greater, this may not result in enough of a tissue "slide" to reapproximate the rectus sheath. If this occurs with or without the use of the laparoscope, a prosthetic from Table 1 should be used as an underlay.

If the component technique is successful, the rectus sheath can be sutured primarily, as in the traditional procedure. However, many prefer to place a synthetic or biologic mesh in the intraperitoneal position (Figure 2, *A* and *B*) or as an onlay in addition to the primary repair. Others, myself included, place an intraperitoneal biologic mesh with transfascial suture fixation and use an onlay of a medium weight polypropylene product (Table 2). In any case, such techniques are proving to be effective to repair these very challenging hernias, however, there is a need for more studies to investigate the utility of these biologic products. As in the usual ventral and incisional hernia, the use of a prosthesis will reduce the recurrence rate from the 33% seen with primary repair to 0% to 17% in even the most complex of these defects.

Because of the metabolic effects of closure of the abdomen with significant loss of domain, careful preoperative evaluation must be undertaken. Pulmonary and cardiac status must be optimized, smoking should be stopped, and weight loss should be attempted. For extreme cases, the application of progressive pneumoperitoneum to increase the intraabdominal cavity may aid in the final closure, but this is not guaranteed in many patients.

It is quite interesting that there are so many new biologic products available today for the treatment of hernia defects. There are a paucity of data to support the use of these materials, but they seem to have a place in the repair of hernias. Although they were originally touted to be ideal in the treatment of contaminated and infected sites or in enterocutaneous fistulas, the success in these situations has not lived up to the claims that were made in the early introduction of these materials. Certainly, these can be considered in situations where the use of a synthetic product would be ill advised because of ongoing infection. However, the permanence of such a repair should be suspect.

Another point of contention is the use of biologic products as a "bridge" for a fascial defect. In other words, there is objection to these being used as an inlay in which they would be sewn to the fascial edges in the hopes that the tissue replacement will suffice to repair and/or replace the fascial absence at the hernia site. This has been shown to be unsuccessful, and it fails in almost all cases, therefore their use in this manner should be considered only as an interim step toward a permanent repair at some point in the future.

All biologic meshes consist of collagen. To effect the intended replacement and regeneration by native collagen, a vascular supply to the product must be assured, which is why their use as a bridge, with no underlying supply of blood vessels, results in universal failure. Therefore, if these products are used to effect a permanent repair, there must be a supply of blood. This sort of repair can be accomplished with complete closure of the fascia and the application of these materials as either an onlay or an underlay. This can be difficult in many cases, therefore this method of use is not advised. If this

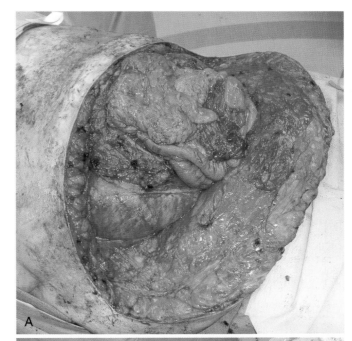

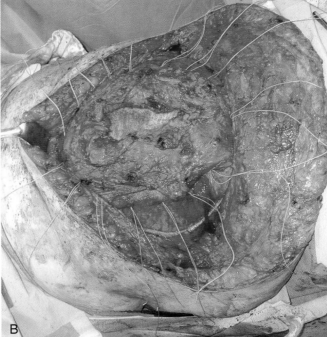

FIGURE 2   Component separation repair of a large recurrent incisional hernia. **B,** Placement of CollaMend (C.R. Bard) as an underlay. Note the transfascial sutures to fixate the product.

seems to be the only option, the hernia sac should be preserved and closed over the bioprosthesis. In that manner, it will serve as a source of vascularity to the collagen product.

Biologic products can also be placed laparoscopically, but they have limited applications in such situations because of the lack of closure of the fascial defects in most cases. These do have particular appeal, however, if used following intestinal operations such as gastric bypass. If the hernia opening is small enough to be closed primarily, reinforcement with a biologic material can lead to a lower recurrence rate.

TABLE 2: Biologic products for hernia repair

Product and Origin	Manufacturer
Alloderm (cadaveric dermis)	Lifecell, Branchburg, NJ
AlloMax (cadaveric dermis)	C.R. Bard, Providence, RI
CollaMend (porcine dermis)	C.R. Bard, Providence, RI
FlexHD (cadaveric dermis)	Ethicon, Inc., Somerville, NJ
Permacol (porcine dermis)	Covidien, Mansfield, Mass.
Strattice (porcine dermis)	Lifecell, Branchburg, NJ
SurgiMend (fetal bovine pericardium)	TEI Biosciences, Boston, Mass.
Surgisis (porcine small intestinal submucosa)	Cook Medical, Bloomington, Ind.
Veritas (bovine pericardium)	Synovis, St. Paul, Minn.
XenMatrix (porcine dermis)	C.R. Bard, Providence, RI

TABLE 3: Prosthetic products for umbilical hernia repair

Product	Manufacturer
Gore bioresorbable hernia plug	W.L. Gore & Associates, Elkhart, Del.
Perfix plug	C.R. Bard, Providence, RI
Prolene Hernia System (PHS)	Ethicon, Inc., Somerville, NJ
Proceed Ventral Patch (PVP)	Ethicon, Inc., Somerville, NJ
Ventralex mesh	C.R. Bard, Providence, RI

EPIGASTRIC HERNIA

Epigastric hernia is not an infrequent occurrence, especially in the male population. Because of its etiology, mesh reinforcement is nearly always recommended. The method of repair is similar to that of the incisional hernia; as this is generally a primary hernia, either an open or laparoscopic repair is possible. Considerations regarding the choice between the two are the level of skill of the surgeon, size of the hernia, fascial integrity, body mass index, and age of the patient. A small defect can be approached via an open method, but a large underlay of mesh (see Table 1) should be used to bolster the weakness that exists well beyond the identified hernia. Firm fixation with transfascial sutures is necessary. In hernias less than 4 to 5 cm, the use of the Ventralex mesh (C.R. Bard, Providence, RI) or PVP mesh (Ethicon, Inc., Somerville, NJ) will allow placement of a posterior mesh with tissue-separating properties, and it lets the surgeon primarily close the defect over the product in many cases. Other choices exist, but they are infrequently used in this application (Table 3).

Small hernias in obese patients and larger defects should be approached laparoscopically. This technique will allow the identification of any other areas of herniation that may not be identified on clinical examination and will provide for a larger overlap of biomaterial than is generally provided by the open method. The use of transfascial sutures is recommended in addition to the tacks, especially if the defect is larger than 10 cm. As with the incisional hernia, it is particularly important to dissect all of the fat that may contact the fascia during this repair.

Difficult situations occur when a patient is seen with a hernia that lies within an area of diastasis recti. Although repair can be done, the weakened fascial separation will result in an unsatisfactory cosmetic result. In these cases, the laparoscopic approach is preferred. With the laparascopic method, a very large area of the abdominal wall can be reinforced by the synthetic prosthesis. This will provide support of the entire area that is weakened. In many patients the cosmetic result will be better than anticipated because of the support by the biomaterial and the contraction of the tissues around the product.

Regardless of the repair method that is chosen if a diastasis exists, it is apparent that the use of an onlay mesh is not recommended in these patients because of frequent protrusion of the abdominal contents beneath the mesh used to repair the hernia over the fascial weakness. The long-term outcomes are much improved if the prosthesis is placed in the intraperitoneal position, preferably laparoscopically.

UMBILICAL HERNIA

The repair of umbilical hernias has undergone significant changes within the last few years, and numerous products have been introduced to repair these defects. Additionally, increasing evidence has shown that the use of a prosthetic biomaterial in these hernias is beneficial even in relatively small defects. If the patient is young and thin and the defect is small, the use of prosthetic material may be avoided. However, if the patient is older or obese and the defect is larger, a prosthetic repair of the hernia is preferred.

Several products can be used if a synthetic product is chosen. Table 3 lists only the prostheses that are designed for this repair. As noted, all of them will provide for the placement of a product beneath the fascia rather than above it. Of course, an onlay of one of the many flat sheets of a synthetic product can be used over a fascial closure for these hernias. The decision to place one of these should be based upon those findings noted above. Also, if the hernia is recurrent, a prosthesis should be placed. Generally, with defects smaller than 3 cm, the fascia can be reapproximated. A flat sheet of mesh can then be placed as an onlay, but an underlay product is preferred, as the recurrence rates are much lower.

All of the products listed above have a permanent component, but one exception is the Gore plug (Table 3 and Figures 3 and 4). This product is meant to resorb entirely over a 6 month interval postimplantation. The Proceed Ventra Patch (PVC; Ethicon) contains oxidized regenerated cellulose that will also resorb, but within 4 weeks, leaving behind a lightweight polypropylene mesh.

Generally, the first choice to repair these hernias should revolve around the open versus laparoscopic alternatives. If the hernia measures less than 3 cm, the open method is preferred unless the patient is morbidly obese. The final decision whether to use a mesh will occur at the operating table. If the defect is less than 1 cm, a primary closure can be done unless the patient has an associated diastasis recti, a condition indicative of a very weak or abnormal collagen matrix in the tissues. In that instance, a mesh should also be applied, and an underlay product should also be used, as this will provide the best cosmetic repair as well as a secure one. This is most easily accomplished with less morbidity with the laparoscopic method.

Defects that are 1 to 3 cm can be repaired with any of the products listed in Table 3. However, the Perfix plug and the Prolene Hernia System (Ethicon) are bare polypropylene material, which will predispose to adhesion formation even if placed in the preperitoneal space. A better choice may be one of the completely resorbable products, such as the Gore plug (Figures 3 and 4), the PVP, or the Ventralex mesh (C.R. Bard). The latter two prostheses are recommended if one violates the peritoneal cavity, as these products possesses a barrier layer that will be positioned between the fascia and the intestine.

Hernias larger than 3 cm in a thin individual may be considered for open mesh repair. These would be performed much the same as the repair for incisional and epigastric hernias. In the obese patient, however, the laparoscopic approach with the placement of a larger

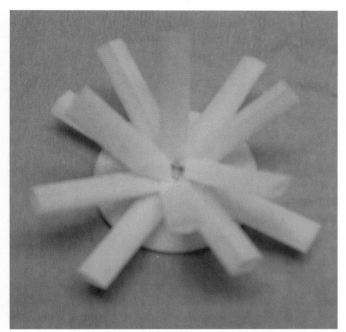

FIGURE 3   Gore bioresorbable hernia plug (W.L. Gore & Associates).

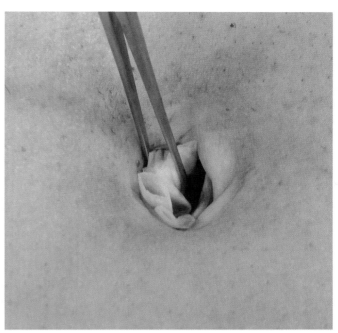

FIGURE 4   Insertion of the Gore plug (W.L. Gore) after it has been cut to size. The disk is placed into the preperitoneal space first. The tubes will be caught with the sutures used to close the fascia over the product.

prosthesis with firm fixation is the better choice, as intraabdominal forces will result in a high frequency of recurrence in these individuals. The biomaterial choices available for these patients are listed in Table 1. As with the incisional hernias, defects less than 5 cm may be repaired without the use of transfascial sutures, however, sutures are recommended for larger defects. Regardless of the method and mesh chosen, the placement of the product behind the musculature of the abdominal wall will provide for the most durable repair in these patients.

Suggested Readings

Dumont F, Fuks D, Verhaeghe P, et al: Progressive pneumoperitoneum increases the length of abdominal muscles, *Hernia* 13:183–187, 2009.

Elieson MJ, LeBlanc KA: Enterotomy and mortality rates of laparoscopic incisional and ventral hernia repair: a review of the literature, *JSLS* 11: 408–414, 2007.

LeBlanc KA: Laparoscopic incisional hernia repair complications: how to avoid and handle, *Hernia* 8(4):323–331, 2004.

LeBlanc KA: Incisional hernia repair: laparoscopic techniques, *World J Surg* 29:1073–1079, 2005.

LeBlanc KA: Laparoscopic incisional hernia repair: are transfascial sutures necessary? A review of the literature, *Surg Endosc* 21:508–513, 2007.

Martin DF, Williams RF, Mulrooney T, et al: Ventralex mesh in umbilical/epigastric hernia repairs: clinical outcomes and complications, *Hernia* 12:379–383, 2008.

Ziad TA, Puri V, LeBlanc KA, et al: Mechanisms of ventral hernia recurrence after mesh repair and a new proposed classification, *J Am Coll Surg* 201(1):132–140, 2005.

Spigelian, Lumbar, and Obturator Hernias

Charles M. Ferguson, MD, and Andrew J. Meltzer, MD

INTRODUCTION

Spigelian, lumbar, and obturator hernias are uncommon hernias that may present a diagnostic challenge. They are infrequently detected on physical examination, even by seasoned clinicians. Although uncommon and difficult to detect, these rare defects may result in intestinal obstruction and incarceration. Until recently, these hernias were frequently unrecognized prior to abdominal exploration for generalized peritonitis. Increasing utilization of computed tomography (CT) in the evaluation of patients with abdominal pain and symptoms of intestinal obstruction have led to increased recognition of these defects. Elective repair is usually warranted to prevent the serious sequelae of intestinal incarceration.

Recent contributions to the surgical literature include several reports describing the utilization of prosthetic material to effect tension-free hernia repairs in the setting of bowel ischemia and mild contamination. We advocate a more conservative approach and suggest primary repair of these defects in the setting of contamination. When elective repair is undertaken after clinical or radiologic diagnosis of these hernias, synthetic mesh is generally used. Laparoscopic repairs have been described for Spigelian, lumbar, and obturator hernias. Minimally invasive repairs have demonstrated decreased morbidity in small series and should be undertaken as indicated by the clinical setting and surgeon experience with these techniques.

Although abdominal wall defects are infrequently encountered in surgical training and clinical practice, surgeons should possess an understanding of the anatomy and evolving treatment (i.e., laparoscopy) of these.

SPIGELIAN HERNIA

The semilunar line, or line of Spiegel, marks the lateral border of the rectus sheath, from the pubic spine to the tip of the ninth costal cartilage. The region between the semilunar line and the medial borders of the external oblique, internal oblique, and transversus abdominis muscles is composed of the aponeuroses of these muscles. This region, known as the *Spigelian zone* (Spigelian fascia), represents the site of Spigelian hernias, which may contain preperitoneal fat or peritoneal sac, possibly containing abdominal viscus (Figures 1, 2, and 3).

Spigelian hernias may occur at any level of the abdominal wall. Most commonly, however, they are found in the so-called *Spigelian belt*, an approximately 6 cm region of the lower abdomen between the umbilicus and the anterior superior iliac spines. It is within this region that the arcuate line (semicircular line, line of Douglas) demarcates the presence (above) or absence (below) of the posterior rectus sheath. The increased width of the Spigelian fascia in this region, combined with the absence of the dorsal lamella of the rectus sheath in the inferior portion of this "belt," leads to more frequent hernia defects in this region.

Symptoms of Spigelian hernias include a painless lump in the aforementioned anatomic region, abdominal pain, incarceration, or intestinal obstruction. As with other hernias, symptoms may be exacerbated by elevations in intraabdominal pressure and are relieved by rest. The defects are often small in size, leading to a relatively frequent rate of incarceration.

Diagnosis may be made on physical examination in patients with a palpable mass in the correct anatomic region. The mass may disappear when the patient is supine and will increase in size with the Valsalva maneuver. In the obese patient, detection on physical examination may prove more difficult. Even in thin patients, however, the hernia may pass through the transversalis fascia only, possibly dissecting between planes of the body wall. In such cases, CT scan may prove beneficial, although these hernias may reduce with the patient in the supine position. In some cases, Spigelian hernias are only diagnosed at the time of laparotomy for obstructive symptoms.

The classically described repair of these defects is initiated by a transverse or vertical incision through the skin, subcutaneous tissue, and aponeurosis of the external oblique. The internal oblique muscle and hernia sac should be visible; the sac is opened to inspect contents and is ligated and reduced into the abdomen. The ring of Spigelian fascia must be freed from preperitoneal and peritoneal adhesions. Primary repair may be performed by approximation of the aponeurotic defect with interrupted, nonabsorbable suture. The aponerosis of the external oblique is closed in a similar manner. Alternatively, a prosthetic patch may be placed in the preperitoneal space below the fascia.

Although the low prevalence of Spigelian hernia is not conducive to large trials examining different techniques for repair, recently several reports and small series have advocated laparoscopic repair. In the intraperitoneal onlay mesh (IPOM) technique, the hernia contents are reduced laparoscopically, and adhesions are lysed to permit at least 5 cm of circumferential overlap of synthetic mesh around the defect. The mesh can be secured using transabdominal sutures and tacks, as has been well described for laparoscopic repair of ventral hernias.

A transabdominal preperitoneal (TAPP) repair can also be employed. After reduction of the hernia sac, the peritoneum is incised, and a 5 cm circumferential flap is raised. A nonabsorable mesh is placed anterior to the peritoneum, which is then closed. A total extraperitoneal repair (TEP) utilizing the laparoscopic balloon insufflator to "create" the extraperitoneal space has also been described.

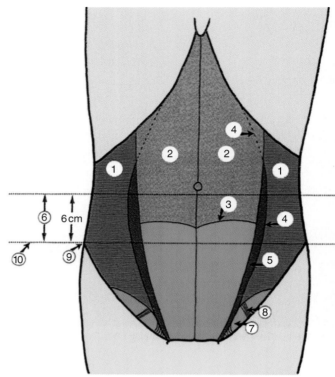

FIGURE 1 Diagrammatic representation of posterior view of the anterior abdominal wall. External oblique, internal oblique, and rectus abdominis muscles have been cut away. *1,* Transversus abdominis muscle. *2,* Dorsal lamella of the rectus sheath. *3,* Semicircular line (of Douglas). *4,* Semilunar line (of Spiegel). *5,* Spigelian aponeurosis. *6,* Spigelian hernia belt. *7,* Hesselbach triangle. *8,* Inferior epigastric vessels. *9,* Anterior superior iliac spine. *10,* Interspinal plane. *(From Skandalakis PN, Zoras O, Skandalakis JE, et al: Lumbar hernia: surgical anatomy, embryology, and technique of repair, Am Surg 27:42, 2006.)*

The risk of recurrence with a Spigelian hernia is low, provided a tension-free repair is performed and the basic tenets of hernia repair are followed. In the only randomized controlled trial comparing laparoscopic and traditional approaches, laparoscopic repair resulted in less morbidity and shorter hospitalizations.

LUMBAR HERNIA

Another uncommon entity, the lumbar hernia, occurs when intraperitoneal or extraperitoneal structures protrude through the posterior abdominal wall in the region bordered superiorly by the twelfth rib, inferiorly by the iliac crest, medially by the erector spinae muscles, and laterally by the external oblique. The overwhelming majority (95%) of lumbar hernias occur in two defined regions: the superior and inferior lumbar triangles (Figure 4).

The superior triangle (Grynfeltt triangle) is defined by the twelfth rib superiorly, the lateral edge of the quadratus lumborum medially, and the posterior free edge of the internal oblique muscle laterally. The inferior triangle (Petit triangle) is bordered at the base by the iliac crest, medially by the lateral border of the latissimus dorsi, and laterally from the posterior margin of the external oblique.

Typically, patients show an asymmetric bulge in the flank. Again, evaluation of the patient in different positions and attempts to provoke herniation by a Valsalva maneuver may aid in attempts to discriminate this finding from lipomas, hematomas, and other masses of the posterior abdominal wall. CT scan may better elucidate the presence of a defect and its contents.

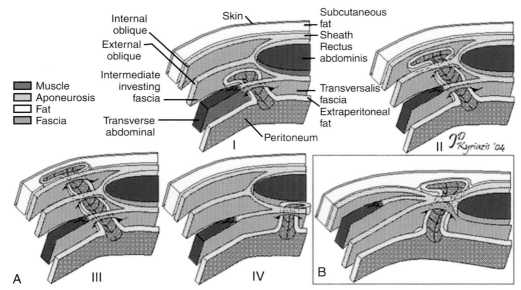

FIGURE 2 Three-dimensional schematic presentation of cross-section of the abdominal wall in vicinity of the left border of the sheath of the rectus abdominis muscle, posterior view. Spigelian hernia sac is shown at various surgical levels: **A,** Above the semicircular line (of Douglas). *(I)* Superficial to the aponeurosis of the transverse abdominal muscle; *(II)* superficial to the aponeurosis of the internal oblique; *(III)* superficial to the aponeurosis of the internal oblique muscle; *(IV)* penetrating the posterior lamina of the rectus sheath. **B,** Below the semicircular line (of Douglas). *(From Skandalakis PN, Zoras O, Skandalakis JE, et al: Lumbar hernia: surgical anatomy, embryology, and technique of repair, Am Surg 27:42, 2006.)*

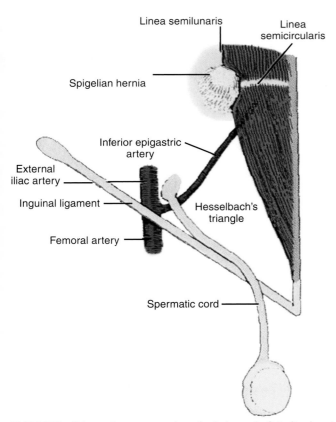

FIGURE 3 Schematic representation of relations of a Spigelian hernia to inguinal structures. *(From Skandalakis PN, Zoras O, Skandalakis JE, et al: Lumbar hernia: surgical anatomy, embryology, and technique of repair, Am Surg 27:42, 2006. Used with permission.)*

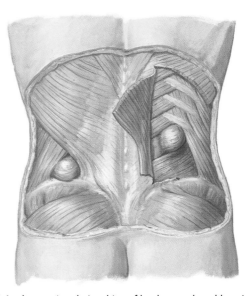

FIGURE 4 Anatomic relationships of lumbar or dorsal hernia. *Right,* Lumbar or dorsal hernia into space of Grynfeltt. *Left,* Hernia into Petit's triangle (inferior lumbar space). (Netter illustration from www.netterimages.com. © Elsevier Inc. All rights reserved.)

Lumbar hernias tend to slowly enlarge over time, and they carry a reported 25% risk of incarceration. Early repair is recommended in the medically stable patient. The hernia can be repaired via a posterior approach, with the patient positioned laterally, or via an anterior retroperitoneal approach. Small hernias may be amenable to primary repair, whereas synthetic mesh or a myoaponeurotic flap may be required to correct larger defects.

In the superior triangle, the hernia sac can be found below skin, superficial fascia, and the latissimus dorsi muscle. In the inferior triangle, there is no muscular layer covering the hernia sac. In either case, the hernia is freed from surrounding tissues and reduced into the abdominal cavity. A synthetic patch is placed over the defect and sutured to the latissimus dorsi, external oblique, and periosteum of the iliac crest. The external oblique and latissimus are approximated over the patch as closely as possible, and the residual defect is repaired with a flap of gluteal fascia that is turned superiorly (Dowd-Ponka repair). A laparoscopic approach has also been described in which mesh is secured to the costal margin, iliac crest, erector spinae investing fascia, and the external oblique fascia using a transabdominal approach.

OBTURATOR HERNIA

Although obturator hernias are also uncommon, they do represent the most common pelvic floor hernias, and they account for 0.1% of all hernias. The obturator foramen is formed by the rami of the ischium and pubic bones; it is nearly obliterated by the obturator membrane, although the obturator canal traverses the cephalad portion of the foramen and contains the obturator nerve, artery, vein, and fat pad.

Obturator herniation is believed to result from progressive laxity of the pelvic floor and is associated with advanced age, poor nutritional status, increased intraabdominal pressure, and multiparity. The prototypical patient is a thin, elderly woman.

The Howship-Romberg sign refers to hip and medial thigh pain exacerbated by external rotation and extension of the hip as the hernia sac compresses the obturator nerve against the pubic ramus. Although some reports suggest its presence in up to 50% of patients

with obturator hernia, it may easily be confused with osteoarthritis in this patient population. Both CT scan and ultrasound may be useful in establishing the diagnosis, and the majority of patients with obturator hernias present with bowel obstruction.

At laparotomy, obturator hernia may be diagnosed when a loop of small intestine is encountered in the pelvis. An attempt is made at reduction, which may require incision of the obturator membrane with careful attention to avoid the neurovascular bundle. The bowel is inspected for viability, and resection is performed as indicated. The small obturator defect may be repaired with one or more simple sutures. Larger defects may require mesh repair, which should be avoided in the setting of gross contamination from necrotic intestine. Although some authors advocate the use of autogenous tissue (omentum or hernia sac) to create a plug, we remain skeptical of the long-term efficacy. Laparoscopic approaches to repair of obturator hernia have been reported.

Suggested Readings

Chang SS, Shan YS, Lin YJ, et al: A review of obturator hernia and a proposed algorithm for its diagnosis and treatment, *World J Surg* 29(4):450–454, 2005.

Mittal T, Kumar V, Khullar R, et al: Diagnosis and management of Spigelian hernia: a review of literature and our experience, *J Minim Access Surg* 4(4):95–98, 2008.

Stamatiou D, Skandalakis JE, Skandalakis LJ, et al: Lumbar hernia: surgical anatomy, embryology, and technique of repair, *Am Surg* 75(3):202–207, 2009.

ATHLETIC PUBALGIA: "THE SPORTS HERNIA"

William C. Meyers, MD, MBA

OVERVIEW

Over the past 2 decades, we have learned a lot about the problem of athletic pubalgia, inaccurately called "sports hernia." These injuries are not hernias, nor are they just one problem as implied by that term. The lay press and even some medical literature continues to promote the term, which, unfortunately, puts pressure on general surgeons to do things about which they are unsure. Certainly, the problems are not life threatening, and there is time for a proper evaluation and a well-considered plan of care. Often, athletes with frustrating abdomen and pelvic pain are anxious to resume their sports as soon as possible. When general surgeons are asked to evaluate such patients, they should take a step back and consider the modern concepts and plan management accordingly.

These are injuries to a conceptually new joint that involves the attachments to the pubic bone plus bony and soft-tissue structures adjacent to it (see Meyers et al in Suggested Readings). Multiple parallels can be made to knee injuries; with the knee there are central attachments, and there are supportive structures that cross the center of activity or hinge. The same holds true for the pubic joint. Accurate diagnosis and management of athletic pubalgia requires a detailed understanding of the anatomy and biomechanics of the musculoskeleton of the pelvis. Like knee injuries, these are not life-threatening problems, but they can pose significant quality-of-life issues.

Let me dwell on the misnomer a bit longer: The term "sports hernia" is grossly misleading. First, the term suggests that the problem is

a hernia, which it is not, not even by the more generous definitions of *hernia*. The term misleads surgeons, physicians, patients, and the public into wrong operations. As a result, too many hernia repairs are being done for this set of problems, and the repairs are often unsuccessful. Second, the term suggests that the condition is a single problem, but it is not. It is a set of problems emanating from disruptions of a complex and hugely dynamic joint. Therefore, when surgery is indicated, it requires consideration of a variety of different surgical solutions.

In clinical practice today, patients with undiagnosed pain in the pelvis—lower abdomen, inguinal region, or groin (medial thigh, adductor or acetabular area)—are referred to a general surgeon. Before the patient arrives in the office, the patient may be labeled as having a "sports hernia" or "suspected sports hernia." The general surgeon sees the patient, rules out a conventional hernia, and then does one of two things: either the surgeon admits a disbelief in sports hernias or confesses little knowledge of the condition and refers the patient back, or the surgeon feels pressured—and some support may be found in the literature for this—and does a traditional or laparoscopic inguinal hernia repair. The patient may, in fact, get some short-term relief from the repair, thereby providing positive feedback to the surgeon, which may lead to a repeat scenario with another patient. Both courses of management are, in fact, wrong.

It is interesting to speculate whether we are stuck with the term. Certainly *sports hernia* is easier for the lay public and media to say than *athletic pubalgia*. Perhaps the public also wants to think that it has some understanding of this. The latter thought is particularly interesting considering that the average person on the street probably has no real understanding of a true hernia, either. In any event, the above set of circumstances should not dictate how medicine and surgery are practiced. Perhaps a catchier medical term will be coined. For the purposes of this chapter, the term *athletic pubalgia* is used and is defined as a set of persistent, disabling injuries involving the pubic joint. In addition, these injuries involve a distinct functional anatomy and pathophysiology.

ANATOMY, PATHOPHYSIOLOGY, AND DIFFERENTIAL DIAGNOSIS

The anatomy of this region is actually quite different than what was taught in anatomy courses in medical school. Subsequent to medical school, this region of the body has basically been a no-man's land for most physicians. General surgeons, orthopedists, gynecologists, and urologists almost never dissect the soft and bony tissue anatomy of this region, nor have they had much reason to do so; therefore it is understandable why there remains a paucity of anatomic information regarding the region.

Several recent papers have addressed this issue. Basically, the two pubic symphyses can be seen as together acting as a fulcrum, the center of many levers or forces (Figure 1). The symphyses are covered on either side by two plates of investing fibrous tissue or cartilage and are joined relatively tightly across the midline. The muscles and investing epimysia blend with the plates in various patterns, with considerable variability from one individual to another.

Hyperextension and hyperabduction, as well as some rotational forces, cause most of the injuries, which can be to both the soft tissue pubic attachments and the supportive soft tissue structures that cross the joint (e.g., psoas, rectus femoris). The injuries may also involve the bone. In a sense, the attachments act like the cruciate ligaments of the knee, and the crossing support structures act like the knee's collateral ligaments. Like the knee, when the attaching structures disrupt, the joint may become unstable. Disruption of enough support structures can also cause instability, and pain may occur at both at the primary site of disruption and at other sites, where there is compensation. The injuries may accumulate and eventually cause instability, or there may be one severe, disruptive event. In addition, the pubic symphyses or rami may be the primary sites of injury, but this is much rarer. Usually, osteitis pubis, or inflammation of the pubic bone, is only reactive to injuries of the attachments.

As one might imagine, because of the complexity of the anatomy, there is a long list of possible injuries. Nowadays, most of these injuries can be identified. Some require surgery, but some do not. However, from the standpoint of the differential diagnosis, three categories should be considered: 1) pubic bone joint problems (athletic pubalgia), 2) hip joint problems (the traditional ball-in-socket joint), and 3) "other" problems (a long list, such as gynecologic, urologic, musculoskeletal, neoplastic, and back problems and inflammatory bowel disease). The "other" category is perhaps the scariest because it involves such a large number of considerations, some of which can be life threatening. On the other hand, it may be obvious from history and physical examination whether the problem is musculoskeletal in nature.

MANAGEMENT

Getting the patient into the hands of someone experienced in the diagnosis of athletic pubalgia is probably the most important thing to do. Presently, there are very few such experienced surgeons. One possibility is to refer the patient to an experienced sports medicine orthopedist, physiatrist, or even a team trainer. Fortunately, the number of orthopedists and sports medicine physicians who understand the diagnoses are increasing. Because of a near 15% incidence of simultaneous hip and athletic pubalgia problems (annals), several experienced hip arthroscopists have also become very knowledgeable with respect to the soft-tissue problems. This also may be an appropriate route for referral.

Things to Do in the Office

Certainly, ruling out a traditional inguinal hernia or recurrence after a repair makes sense. If a hernia is found, care must be taken in attributing the pain to the hernia; the hernia could be purely coincidental.

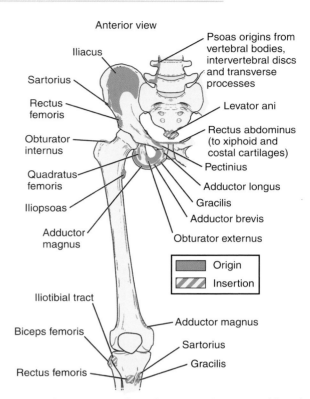

FIGURE 1 Anterior view of muscle origins and insertions. Note that all adductors originate in the pubic ramus and the relatively anterior location of insertion of the psoas tendon onto the lesser trochanter. *(From Meyers WC, Yoo E, Devon O, et al: Understanding "sports hernia" [athletic pubalgia] the anatomic and pathophysiologic basis for abdominal and groin pain in athletes, Op Tech Sport Med 15:165–177, 2007.)*

Hernia-related pain is in general very different from athletic pubalgia pain. Pain from a hernia is usually episodic and related to the appearance of a lump, or it may appear after standing or walking all day. Pubalgia pain is usually predictable and exertional, and it is related to certain specific descriptions of the exertion. The differential diagnosis includes a number of different gastrointestinal problems, so an appropriate history and physical examination should be undertaken.

The surgeon must also consider the pelvic diagnoses that involve other specialties, such as urology and gynecology. It may be appropriate to do rectal and pelvic examinations, and the male genitalia should certainly be examined, because testicular cancers are common in the age group that predominates with respect to pubalgia problems. The pain issue could also be related to previous surgery, most commonly, it seems, in hernia repairs using mesh. Local tenderness over the mesh, of course, may lead to specific diagnostic tests (e.g., regional block) and treatment. Good musculoskeletal pelvic and hip examinations are important for determining the precise musculoskeletal injury if one is present. The surgeon must also pay attention to the possibility of injuries to both the hip and soft tissues at the same time. Most general surgeons are probably not very experienced in this area, but it may be worth reviewing some of the basic tests and considering whether the pain is musculoskeletal in nature.

Beware of sending the patient on "wild goose chases" that involve multiple consultants and multiple imaging tests that waste time and money, as these can cause great frustration. If the history seems straightforward, and the pain occurs predictably, even though it may change with respect to side or site, the problem may be a straightforward athletic injury. Although the differential diagnosis may include many different possibilities, the diagnosis of a musculoskeletal injury may be straightforward, even though the precise injury may not be obvious.

Imaging

Imaging should be appropriate to what is suspected based on history and physical examination, and it may include plain films or computed tomography (CT) scan of the abdomen and pelvis. The value of pelvic ultrasound to look for hernias has been largely disproven, and history and physical examination remain the most important clues for diagnosis. Because occult hernias are not the cause of these problems, ultrasound is generally not helpful and is often misleading. Likewise, herniagrams do not make sense, except in select pediatric populations. New literature that suggests that ultrasound may be the way to go lacks validated diagnostic criteria and scientific scrutiny. A few physicians in Europe with good marketing skills seem to be trying to popularize ultrasonography for hernia. Considering the number of different injuries that occur in athletic pubalgia, ultrasonography as an initial test does not make sense.

Bone scan does have limited usefulness in the diagnosis of osteitis pubis. In a practical sense, history and physical examination, plain films, and magnetic resonance imaging (MRI) are generally better for that diagnosis. The way we think about osteitis pubis is that there are two types: *Primary osteitis* is a mysterious and debilitating problem that usually afflicts nonathletes and is very difficult to treat. By nature, it is not associated with an identifiable injury or cause. Fortunately, primary osteitis pubis seems to be quite rare, and some authors have suggested that it is a manifestation of a rheumatologic disease. *Secondary osteitis* is an inflammatory condition of the pelvic bones associated with another cause, such as athletic pubalgia injury or a soft tissue or bony injury as a result of giving birth. If secondary osteitis is suspected, the precise injury must be identified.

Fortunately, we have recently developed some magnetic resonance (MR) imaging techniques that can identify the specific pubic joint injuries with about 91% specificity. These techniques do take considerable set-up time, effort, and expertise on the part of the imaging center and radiologist. Several locales in the country can now do these. A conventional MR image of the pelvis may likely be read as normal or as showing some nonspecific changes of the pubic symphysis or edema patterns in adjacent soft tissues.

If the physician feels comfortable with the hip examination and believes the source of the patient's disability to be the hip, then it is reasonable to have an experienced musculoskeletal radiologist do MR arthrography of the hip. This needs to be done with a specific protocol and needs to be interpreted by a radiologist and/or orthopedist truly experienced in the subtleties of these examinations. One problem is that the MR arthrograms have gotten, in a sense, too good. They pick up a lot of pathology that may be circumstantial and not the cause of symptoms. To do a proper assessment, it is important for the radiologist to get into the joint on the first pass and with minimal trauma.

We usually combine MR arthrography with a "sensorcaine test" to see whether the patient's symptoms improve or worsen with this test. There are certain patterns of pain relief and/or worsening that correlate with pathology that is significant. We have also seen patients with normal architecture MR arthrography who get relief and subsequently had treatable pathology via hip arthroscopy.

Surgical Versus Nonsurgical Therapy

The vast majority of the injuries to the abdomen and groin do not need surgery. Most resolve without such therapy. Plus, many patients are able to tolerate the discomfort or necessary change of life pattern and deal with it easily. Physical therapy also plays a role as a primary treatment of several injuries.

The most important factor in terms of managing abdominal injuries successfully is precise diagnosis. Three categories of diagnosis must be considered: 1) athletic pubalgia, 2) hip problems, and 3) other problems. An intimate relationship between what goes on inside and outside the hip must be recognized, along with the fact that the first

two categories of injury can occur together. In fact, as stated above, about 15% of patients have simultaneous injuries involving the first two categories; injuries in the third category sometimes occur with either of the other two.

The next step toward deciding on operative or nonoperative management is to diagnose precisely the muscle attachments and/or supporting structures that are injured. A combination of variables must be considered including the precise pathology; importance of athletic participation; degree of diminution of performance; likelihood that injury will get better without surgery; contract issues; team, coach, and ownership considerations; and other factors. The decision whether to operate is based on consideration of all these. Short-term versus long-term results can be very important in the decision to operate, and the type of operation can also be important with respect to expectations regarding the length of recovery time. There is sometimes a role for staged operations, one for an earlier return to play and one for more definitive treatment.

Timing of Surgery

One way to think about this issue is to divide patients into four categories: 1) *high-performance athletes,* defined as those whose wish to continue to compete is their primary professional and/or personal consideration; 2) *general athletes,* who place a high priority on athletics but not so much so that they have strict deadlines with respect to the importance of return to play; 3) *nonathletes,* who view physical activity as not important; and 4) *military personnel and workmen,* those on active duty, with the ability to do physical work being the primary objective of either the individual or an organization.

Of course, decisions about surgery and its timing may be drastically different depending on which of the four categories the patient fits into. Again, the importance of short-term versus long-term considerations becomes important. For example, consider the baseball pitcher in a major league baseball pennant race who gets hurt near the end of the season. Does he continue to play, or does he have surgery? There are risks to both. Continuing to play with pain may be what is best for the team, but playing with pain may hurt the pitcher's mechanics and result in a career-threatening arm problem.

Technical Points

As mentioned above, because of the large number of injuries that athletic pubalgia, or "sports hernia," comprises, a large number of precise procedures designed to fix the various problems have evolved (Table 1). The procedures focus on different combinations of tightening and loosening attachments to supporting structures. However, the surgeon must be thoroughly familiar with the anatomy in this area to ensure a high success rate.

Again, these injuries are *not* hernias. Treating these problems as if they were hernias is therefore often ineffective. It is difficult to be sure of the failure rates of the traditional or laparoscopic operations being applied to these patients, but it must be high. On average, I operate on more than three patients per week who have had failed such attempts at repair. Most of the failed repairs involve mesh, and most patients experience persistent or recurrent pain. Sometimes, it is difficult to determine whether a component of the pain was due to mesh. In addition, we do not know the true incidence of failure for such procedures, as the aforementioned patients represent only a numerator; we do not know the total number of hernia repairs performed for this set of problems, because no short- or long-term outcomes analyses are reported for traditional hernia repairs.

For athletes, we must consider several additional factors related to hernia repair attempts: 1) potential harm from the mesh and accompanying fibrosis; 2) primary and compensatory pain from multiple attachments (e.g., adductors longus and brevis, pectineus, psoas, rectus femoris); 3) short-term versus long-term success; and 4) failure rates for the many different problems.

TABLE 1:   Clinical entities of athletic pubalgia

Structure/Clinical Syndrome	Defect	Possibly Indicated Procedure
Unilateral RA/unilateral AD AD longus (AL) Pectineus (P) AD brevis (AB)	Tears and compartment syndrome (CS)	Repair and release
Pure AD syndromes	Usual CS	Release
Bilateral RA/bilateral AD	Aponeurotic plate disruption; tear and CS	
Unilateral RA	Tear	Repair
Bilateral RA	Tears	Repair
Severe osteitis variant	Usually tears, CS, and bone edema	Repair, release, and steroid injection
Unilateral/bilateral	Combination tears and CS	Repair(s) and release(s)
Iliopsoas variant	Impingement and bursitis	Release
Baseball pitcher/hockey goalie syndrome	AD muscle belly tear and CS	Release
Spigelian variant	Tear	Repair
Rectus femoris variant	Impingement	Release
High RA variant	Tear	Repair
Female variant	Medial disruption with lateral thigh compensation	Repair and release(s)
Round ligament variant	Inflammation with tear	Excision and repair
Dancers' variants	Usually obturator externus/internus	Release(s)
Rowers' rib syndromes	Subluxation	Excision and mesh
Avulsions	Usually acute adductor injury	Repair and/or release(s)
AD/RA calcification syndromes	Chronic avulsion	Excision, release
Midline RA variant	Tear and muscle separation	Repair
Anterior ischial tuberosity variant	Posterior perineal inflammation, often gracilis/hamstring tear	Release
AD contractures	Often associated with hip pathology	Release and hip repair
More uncommon variants	Gracilis, quadratus, iliotibial band	Variable

RA, Rectus abdominis; *AD,* adductor
Modified from Meyers WC, McKechnie A, Philippon MJ, et al: Experience with "sports hernia" spanning two decades, *Ann Surg* 248(4):656–665, 2008.

SUMMARY

In summary, these problems are not hernias; instead, these injuries involve a distinct anatomy and pathophysiology. Proper evaluation and experience lead to effective management. The surgeon must understand the true anatomy, multiple injuries, and the multiple variables that enter into the decision-making process.

SUGGESTED READINGS

Byrd JWT: Gross anatomy. In Byrd JWT, editor: *Operative hip arthroscopy,* New York, 2005, Springer, pp 100–109.
Meyers WC, Greenleaf R, Saad A: Anatomic basis for evaluation of abdominal and groin pain in athletes, *Op Tech Sports Med* 13:55–61, 2005.

Meyers WC, Yoo E, Devon O, et al: Understanding "sports hernia" (athletic pubalgia): the anatomic and pathophysiologic basis for abdominal and groin pain in athletes, *Op Tech Sport Med* 15:165–177, 2007.
Meyers WC, McKechnie A, Philippon MJ, et al: Experience with "sports hernia" spanning two decades, *Ann Surg* 248(4):656–665, 2008.
Omar IM, Zoga AC, Kavanagh EC, et al: Athletic pubalgia and the "sports hernia": optimal MR imaging technique and findings, *Radiographics* 28:1415–1438, 2008.
Zoga AC, Kavanagh EC, Meyers WC, et al: MRI findings in athletic pubalgia and the "sports hernia", *Radiology* 247:797–807, 2008.
Zoga AC, Kavanagh EC, Meyers WC, et al: MRI of the rectus abdominis/adductor aponeurosis: findings in the "sports hernia," presented at the American Roentgen Ray Society, Annual Proceedings, Orlando, FL, 2007.

MANAGEMENT OF BENIGN BREAST DISEASE

Michele A. Gadd, MD

INTRODUCTION

Patients with breast problems are commonly referred to surgeons for evaluation. The most common problems are palpable breast masses, pain, nipple discharge, and abnormal radiologic findings that merit consideration of a breast biopsy. The underlying question in most cases is whether the problem requires a biopsy to rule out breast cancer. This chapter will outline the steps in evaluating these common breast problems, and it will offer guidance on how to decide when a breast biopsy is necessary.

EVALUATION OF COMMON BREAST PROBLEMS

History, Examination, and Radiologic Imaging

Evaluation of a breast problem begins with a focused history and physical examination. The history should include a full description of the problem, whether any changes have been noted since onset, whether the patient has experienced these symptoms in the past, and what makes the symptoms better or worse. It is often insightful to know who initially identified the problem, the patient or the physician, and whether the patient performs frequent self-examination and whether the patient perceives a mass as new. Also pertinent to the evaluation are the patient's age, menstrual status, timing of last menstruation if applicable, and family history of breast cancer.

The physical exam should include a visual inspection of the breast for asymmetries and skin lesions such as rash, retraction, or erythema. Palpation should include a thorough evaluation of both breasts and the axillary and supraclavicular nodal basins. If recent breast imaging has been performed, these images should be reviewed; imaging may need to be scheduled to further evaluate the area in question, and a two-field mammogram and/or breast ultrasound are the standard first lines of evaluation.

Radiologic imaging may further characterize a suspected abnormality and assist in determining the best method for performing a biopsy. Ultrasound is the best tool for evaluating a mass, and it can often clearly differentiate between a solid mass and a hollow lesion with cyst fluid. Breast magnetic resonance imaging (MRI) is used more commonly to evaluate patients with increased risk of breast cancer, but it may also be helpful for evaluating patients with dense breasts or patients who have had previous surgery. It is important to remember that negative breast-imaging studies should not deter one from a biopsy of a palpable mass or other suspicious finding.

Breast Masses

Breast masses remain the most common breast complaints and are generally accompanied by substantial patient anxiety. In the premenopausal years, most breast masses are benign, secondary to hormonal influences within the breast. The most common diagnoses are fibrocystic changes, cysts, fibroadenomas, and lipomas. Nonetheless, ruling out cancer is the most important part of the evaluation of all breast masses. In the postmenopausal years, the risk of breast cancer is increased, and generally the breasts are not changing as much. In these patients a needle or excisional breast biopsy should always be considered to determine the etiology of the mass or density. If a biopsy is not done for a breast mass, a follow-up exam within a few weeks to months should be scheduled.

A careful examination of the breast should allow the examiner to form an initial impression of whether the lesion is likely to be fibrocystic (vague thickening or rubbery, ill-defined mass or density), a cyst (discrete fluid-filled mass), fibroadenoma (smooth-margined solid mass in a premenopausal woman), lipoma (smooth, soft, mobile mass) or cancer (discrete solid mass with irregular edges). A palpable and discrete mass that is at least 7 mm in size can be evaluated for definitive diagnosis by fine needle aspiration (FNA) or core needle biopsy in the office. If the result does not clearly explain the finding—such as a cyst that resolves with aspiration, fibroadenoma, lipoma or cancer—or the mass is too small to approach with a needle biopsy, then an excisional biopsy should be considered to completely exclude an underlying breast cancer. These biopsies can generally be done with local anesthesia or local anesthesia plus intravenous (IV) sedation in the operating room or in an outpatient, minor-procedure setting. To help reduce the anxiety and pain associated with these procedures, the surgeon can offer the patient a mild antianxiety medication, such as lorazepam; the patient can also be asked to prepare the skin surface for the biopsy by applying a topical ointment, either eutectic mixture of local anesthetics (EMLA) or lidocaine, over the area at home and covering it with plastic wrap or tegaderm.

Nonpalpable masses should be evaluated by radiologically guided core needle biopsy. If the lesion is clearly visible on ultrasound, an ultrasound-guided core needle biopsy is the preferred technique. Alternatively, a stereotactically guided core needle biopsy can be done for masses not visible by ultrasound but visible by mammography. If the mass is deep in the breast and close to the chest wall, close behind the nipple, or if the patient has a small breast that compresses to less than 3 cm in thickness, a needle-localized excisional breast biopsy is the preferred technique for establishing a definitive diagnosis. In most cases the target lesion is small enough that it can be removed completely at the time of biopsy. Finally, it is important to compare the pathologic results of the biopsy with the target lesion and radiographic images to confirm concordance. This final review will help avoid the mistake of falsely assuming that the benign diagnosis is 100% accurate in situations where the site biopsied does not necessarily correlate with the intended target, and a cancer diagnosis is missed.

Vague densities and ill-defined masses on exam present a more challenging problem in establishing a clear diagnosis. Aspirating a vague density is not very helpful in planning, and the cytologic results are fraught with misinterpretation. It is best to avoid needle aspiration unless there is a clearly palpable and well-defined mass on exam or a radiologic abnormality that can be targeted. Vague densities on exam that are not seen on breast imaging should be followed up with a repeat exam. If the density persists or increases in size, an incisional biopsy should be considered to exclude an underlying breast cancer.

Breast Pain

Mastalgia, or breast pain, is common throughout life, especially during the reproductive years and usually related to hormonal and fibrocystic changes. This type of cyclical breast pain is generally diffuse and bilateral but may be more severe in one breast. The fact that the pain improves after the onset of menses is reassuring; so-called cyclical mastalgia is seldom associated with a cancer and almost never requires a biopsy.

The etiology of most noncyclical breast pain is unknown. Common benign causes of focal persistent breast pain may include cysts, fibroadenomas, mastitis, and abscess. There is also an association between noncyclical breast pain and some medications, including antidepressants and antihypertensives. Pain that is noncyclical or associated with a palpable breast lesion or a radiologic abnormality requires additional diagnostic evaluation, similar to the evaluation of a mass. An annual mammogram should be reviewed for women over 40 years, and it should be considered for younger women depending on the level of suspicion, if there is a family history of early-onset breast cancer, or if the patient has a known genetic factor that predisposes her to breast cancer. A breast ultrasound may be helpful if there is any question about an underlying mass based on exam or focal unilateral pain.

There are a two chest wall syndromes that may manifest as breast pain, *costochondritis* and *Tietze syndrome*. Both are associated with pain and tenderness in the costochondral or chondrosternal joints, and in Tietze syndrome, swelling of the cartilaginous articulations is also present. Nonsteroidal antiinflammatory agents and rest is the treatment of choice.

Relief of mastalgia generally occurs gradually, over a few months, without treatment. In some cases the pain may linger, or it may consistently become severe around the luteal phase of the menstrual cycle. This type of cyclical pain may be reduced by taking evening primrose oil tablets (1500 mg daily increased to 1500 mg twice daily after a month if once a day is ineffective). Antiinflammatory agents and heat may help relieve acute symptoms, and some pain may be increased with caffeine and chocolate consumption; reducing or eliminating caffeine or chocolate for at least 2 months may help. Additional interventions may include a low-fat diet or a 3- to 6-month trial of tamoxifen (10 mg/day). Reassuring the patient that pain is generally not a sign of breast cancer and that pain does not lead to an increase in breast cancer risk helps significantly alleviate the patient's anxiety, and frequently no treatment is necessary.

Nipple Discharge

Nipple discharge is common and is usually of benign etiology. Most premenopausal women can induce a small amount of discharge from one or both nipples with massage. This type of induced, nonspontaneous discharge is a normal finding; it may occur after a mammogram or warm shower and requires no specific evaluation.

Nipple discharge that requires surgical evaluation is spontaneous and recurrent, generally unilateral, and from a single duct. It may be sanguineous or serous. Testing for occult blood or cytology of nipple discharge is not recommended, because the results are confusing and are often misinterpreted. In most cases, the cytologic results of nipple discharge do not yield sufficient evidence to obviate the need for a surgical biopsy.

Evaluation begins with physical examination, a mammogram, and sometimes an ultrasound. If a specific, targetable lesion such as abnormal microcalcifications or a solid mass is found, a core needle biopsy or needle-localized biopsy should be done. If no suspicious lesion is found on imaging to correlate with the discharge, an excisional biopsy of the offending duct is necessary to make a specific diagnosis and rule out cancer. A ductogram (galactogram) is not generally needed for preoperative planning. Identifying a ductal filling defect with these imaging studies is painful for the patient and challenging for the radiologist, and the results are fraught with misinterpretation.

In most cases where a drop of discharge can be expressed on the day of the procedure, a narrow (000 or 0000) lacrimal duct probe can be used in the operating room to cannulate the offending duct, and excision is directed at this site. A subareolar incision is made, and dissection begins just under the nipple (papillomas may lie within the duct orifice directly beneath the skin surface) and continue along the duct down to the chest wall or terminal ducts. Ligating the duct beneath the nipple helps to prevent postbiopsy drainage through the ligated duct. If it is not possible to cannulate the duct from the nipple, sometimes the dilated duct can be identified just beneath the nipple/areolar complex and cannulated at this point. It is helpful to ask the patient not to express discharge between the last office visit and the biopsy; this increases the chances of identifying discharge on the day of the procedure. Most causes of nipple discharge are benign, especially in younger women; they include papillomas, duct ectasia, and fibrocystic changes. Bloody discharge is commonly due to a benign papilloma. The risk of cancer in patients presenting with nipple discharge increases with age but is still rare.

True galactorrhea is uncommon and is characterized by copious bilateral discharge that is spontaneous and persistent, milky, and from multiple ducts. It has an underlying physiologic cause—such as hyperprolactinemia related to a pituitary tumor, hypothyroidism, or drug side effect—and should be evaluated with prolactin and thyrotropin levels. No surgical intervention is needed, but these patients should be referred to an endocrinologist for management.

Breast Infection

Breast infections are common in premenopausal patients; they are painful, but they generally respond to oral antibiotics if treated early after onset to avoid abscess formation. Acute mastitis is divided into those cases associated with pregnancy and lactation and those secondary to a bacterial infection of unknown origin. The latter are more difficult to treat and may become a chronic problem. Acute mastitis in a lactating patient is usually secondary to a *Staphylococcus* infection. Oral antibiotics early on and warm packs followed by massage to decompress the plugged duct will eradicate most minor infections.

Incision and drainage may be necessary if conservative measures fail or if there is abscess formation. If incision and drainage is needed, lactation must cease on the affected side to allow healing. In the nonlactating patient, oral antibiotics early on also generally lead to complete resolution of the infection, but this may take several weeks. IV antibiotics may be needed in some cases due to the extent of systemic symptoms or comorbidities. In all cases where an abscess is identified on physical exam or confirmed by ultrasound, incision and drainage should be considered early on in the treatment. For abscesses larger than 2 cm in diameter, incision and drainage are best performed in an operating room with complete sedation. It is rarely possible to treat abscesses with a closed drain.

Breast Skin Changes

Skin changes associated with infection are generally accompanied by pain, erythema, and edema. These signs may suggest an underlying abscess or infected cyst. If there is a discrete fluid collection identified by palpation or ultrasound, aspiration for culture should be done prior to beginning antibiotics. If the changes in the skin do not resolve with antibiotics or a steroid ointment within a month, a punch biopsy of the skin, and often a core biopsy of the underlying breast tissue, should be done to exclude the diagnosis of an inflammatory breast cancer.

The second most common skin change resembles eczema and generally affects the nipple or areola. If these changes include persistent scaling or itching and do not resolve with application of a steroid ointment, a skin punch biopsy is recommended to rule out Paget disease.

Finally, small hypertrophic skin tags around the areola and plugging of the ducts as they exit the areola, leading to a dilated orifice, may prompt a patient to inquire about the etiology of these findings. All of these lesions are benign and do not require a biopsy. Elective excision is an option but is not medically necessary.

Abnormal Screening Mammograms

Many women seek a second opinion regarding the need for further evaluation of mammographic findings such as microcalcifications, vague densities, and suspicious masses. In these cases the patient generally has a normal breast examination. The films require careful evaluation with a radiologist and comparison with previous films if available. In most cases if the finding is new on imaging, either a radiologically guided core needle biopsy or a needle-localized excisional biopsy is recommended to establish a diagnosis. In some cases a 6 month follow-up mammogram or ultrasound can be done to establish stability or resolution of a likely benign group of calcifications or density.

▉ MANAGING BENIGN BREAST PROBLEMS

Fibroadenoma

Fibroadenomas are common throughout the reproductive years and after menopause. The majority are small, very discrete with smooth edges, mobile, and asymptomatic or minimally symptomatic. After menopause, fibroadenomas often present as a calcified density on mammogram, and they can fluctuate with menses and grow with the hormonal stimulation of oral contraceptives and pregnancy. Their identity can usually be confirmed by ultrasound-guided core biopsy, after which most can be left in place and observed over time with serial exams or ultrasound if a mass is not palpable. A fibroadenoma generally requires excision if it grows over time, is large (>2 or 3 cm) at diagnosis, or is painful. Overall there is little to no proven increase in the risk of developing breast cancer with the finding of a true fibroadenoma. However, if there is any doubt about the diagnosis—either because of atypia on the core biopsy, increased cellularity of the lesion, rapid growth of the mass, or questionable concordance with the exam—the mass should be excised to rule out a small associated cancer or a phyllodes tumor.

Breast Cysts

Cysts are a common cause of breast pain or a focal mass, and they are common in the reproductive years but can occur in postmenopausal women as well. A simple cyst, determined by imaging evaluation or resolution with aspiration, is not likely to be associated with a cancer. Simple cyst aspiration is appropriate for cysts that are large or symptomatic. Cyst fluid that is bloody should be sent for cytopathology, otherwise it should be discarded. Cytologic interpretation of cyst fluid, like nipple discharge, is fraught with confusion and is not necessary for management. A cyst that is complex on ultrasound or associated with a solid component must be biopsied. The best technique is a radiologically guided core biopsy, with a clip left in place, or a needle-localized excisional biopsy. If the aspirate is bloody or the solid component is atypical, an excision should be performed to rule out cancer.

Intracystic breast cancers are rare. In pregnancy, a complex cyst may be the result of a lactating adenoma and will resolve without treatment. Repeat imaging to document a decrease in size of the cyst and resolution over time may be considered in this situation and in other cases where the possibility of an underlying breast cancer is low. If a needle biopsy diagnosis is preferred during late pregnancy or lactation, a small-gauge needle can be used without much risk of forming a milk fistula. Performing an open breast biopsy during lactation often leads to milk fistula and may require cessation of breast-feeding.

Breast Lipomas

Lipomas are benign and generally nonpainful. If the clinical exam is consistent with a lipoma, excision is not mandatory. If the diagnosis is in question, excision or needle aspiration are necessary. Painful fatty tumors are likely to represent an underlying angiolipoma and should be excised to eliminate pain.

Benign Abnormalities Associated with Increased Breast Cancer Risk

Often a new finding on a screening mammogram or a change noted during a 6-month follow-up mammogram will prompt a radiologically guided core needle biopsy of a lesion. When the histologic examination of the lesion reveals atypical ductal hyperplasia, atypical lobular hyperplasia, lobular carcinoma in situ (LCIS), fragments of a complex sclerosing lesion, or a radial scar, a needle-localized excisional biopsy is recommended to exclude the approximate 5% risk of an associated small breast cancer at the target site.

▉ MALE BREAST MASSES

Gynecomastia is common in two age groups: between 20 to 30 years and after 60 years. Unilateral enlargement of the breast directly behind the nipple area is common in patients with gynecomastia. The enlargement is often painful and requires an evaluation to rule out breast cancer. A thorough breast exam, mammogram, and often a core or excisional biopsy are needed to rule out breast cancer in males with a breast mass or nipple changes. Breast cancer in males is rare, and therefore male patients more often present at a later stage due to delay in diagnosis. Causes of gynecomastia include drug interactions, alcoholism, loss of testosterone, elevation of estrogen levels due to thyroid or liver problems, or hormone-secreting tumors. A panel of blood tests should be done if the exam is consistent with gynecomastia, and a testicular examination should be performed to exclude an underlying hormone-secreting tumor.

▉ SUMMARY

Patients with breast problems are commonly referred to surgeons for evaluation. From a surgical standpoint, the key question is whether the problem requires a biopsy to rule out an underlying breast cancer. When a biopsy is not recommended, it is extremely important to reassure the patient that you do not feel that their problem represents an underlying breast cancer. An effective way to convey this message is by listening carefully to the patient and providing an explanation for the problem and why their symptoms do not suggest breast cancer as the cause. Generally this approach will leave the patient satisfied that their concerns were taken seriously and with information and a plan to deal with the problem when they leave the office. If a biopsy is not recommended, it is important to consider scheduling a follow-up exam and to provide clear instructions to call or return to the office if something changes.

Suggested Readings

Gray RJ, Pockaj BA, Karstaedt PJ: Navigating murky waters: a modern treatment algorithm for nipple discharge, *Am J Surg* 194:850–855, 2007.

Greenberg R, Skornick Y, Kaplan O: Management of breast fibroadenomas, *J Gen Intern Med* 13:640–645, 1998.

Narula NS, Carlson HE: Gynecomastia, *Endocrinol Metabol Clin North Am* 36:283–296, 2007.

Smith RL, Pruthi S, Fitzpatrick LA: Evaluation and management of breast pain, *Mayo Clin Proc* 79:353–372, 2004.

Screening for Breast Cancer

Amy C. Degnim, MD, and Judy C. Boughey, MD

OVERVIEW

Since breast cancer is such a significant health concern for women, screening for this disease is an important public health issue. Breast cancer is the most common malignancy occurring in women in the United States, and it is the second most common cause of cancer death in women. In 2009, the estimated number of new cases of breast cancer in women was 192,370, and 40,610 deaths due to breast cancer were estimated. However, from 1990 to 2000, breast cancer mortality declined approximately 25%.

In addition to improved treatments, screening is also judged to be a key factor in this reduction in breast cancer mortality, which is supported by the increasing proportion of breast cancers diagnosed at early stage. Before screening mammography, tumors presented only when they were palpable. Since annual screening mammography has been adopted in the United States, there has been a decrease in the T stage of the primary tumor and increased detection of ductal carcinoma in situ. Despite some trials showing reduced mortality with mammographic screening, controversy remains about some aspects of breast cancer screening. The preponderance of evidence supports breast cancer screening practices that have been endorsed as described below.

SCREENING RECOMMENDATIONS

The American Cancer Society (ACS) recommendations for breast cancer screening are maintained on the ACS Web site (http://www.cancer.org/docroot/CRI/content/CRI_2_4_3X_Can_breast_cancer_be_found_early_5.asp). For women of average risk, screening includes clinical breast examination, counseling to raise awareness of breast symptoms, and regular annual mammography beginning at age 40. Recommendations from the U.S. Preventive Services Task Force (USPSTF) (http://www.ahrq.gov/clinic/uspstf/uspsbrca.htm) were revised in November 2009 to recommend screening mammograms every 2 years for women between the age of 50 and 74 years. The decision to start regular screening mammography prior to age 50 years was recommended to be on an individual patient basis, taking into account the benefits and harms. These guidelines caused significant controversy, and the majority of centers in the United States and the American Cancer Society continue to recommend mammographic screening from age 40 years.

Family history of breast cancer, early detection, and the importance of regular mammography can be discussed at the time of clinical breast exam. Breast self-examination (BSE) has been deleted from recommended screening practices, but informing patients about the benefits, limitations, and harms of BSE is still recommended.

There is no set age at which mammography should be discontinued; it should continue as long as the woman is a candidate for breast cancer treatment. The USPSTF found insufficient evidence to assess additional benefits and harms of screening mammograms in women age 75 years and older. A common rule of thumb is that breast cancer screening may be omitted if a woman has a life expectancy of less than 5 years. Screening recommendations are based on disease incidence in the screened population; for this reason, routine screening mammography is not recommended for women younger than age 40 years, whereas more intensive screening that includes other, more sensitive imaging modalities is recommended for high-risk individuals.

Screening recommendations are adjusted for women whose risk is estimated to be higher than average. The ACS describes increased intensity of screening, depending on the estimated risk level. *High risk* is defined as a greater than 20% lifetime risk of breast cancer development. *Moderately increased risk* is defined as a 15% to 20% lifetime risk. These risk estimates can be obtained by one of several risk-prediction models, such as the Gail model, Claus model, Tyrer-Cuzick model, and Breast Cancer Program models. Women at high risk should have annual mammogram and annual MRI in addition to clinical breast examination every 6 months. Women with a strong family history, such as first-degree family member with premenopausal breast cancer, should initiate screening 5 to 10 years before the youngest age of diagnosis of breast cancer in a relative. Patients with known *BRCA* mutations should begin screening at the age of 25 years. Women at moderately increased risk should talk with their doctors about the benefits and limitations of adding magnetic resonance imaging (MRI) screening to their yearly mammogram.

SCREENING MODALITIES

Breast Self-Examination

BSE was advocated in the past, however recent updates have removed it from the screening guidelines. Large randomized trials failed to show any reduction in breast cancer–specific or all-causes mortality from regular BSE in large populations of average risk. Cochrane review concluded BSE offered no beneficial effect and that it increased the number of biopsies performed. Because of this the USPSTF judged the evidence insufficient to recommend for or against teaching or performing routine BSE.

Clinical Breast Examination

Clinical breast exam remains a key component of breast cancer screening, because approximately 10% to 20% of all breast cancers are not visible on screening mammography. Therefore, the only screening mechanism to identify breast cancer in those patients is clinical breast examination. Beginning at age 20 years, women should have a clinical breast exam every 2 to 3 years and then annually after age 40 years. Clinical breast exam should be performed before screening mammography, so that any concerns on clinical exam can be identified and the planned imaging studies converted from screening to diagnostic intent. All suspicious palpable lesions should be evaluated with an ultrasound and biopsy, even if the mammogram is normal. Women with a high risk of breast cancer (family history, *BRCA* mutation, atypia, lobular carcinoma in situ, history of radiation to the breast/chest wall) should have clinical breast examinations every 6 months.

Mammography

Mammography is the foundation of breast imaging and is used to screen asymptomatic women for breast cancer. Screening mammography has been shown to decrease the mortality from breast cancer by approximately 30%. The ACS recommends annual mammography starting at age 40 years, the USPSTF recommends it starting at age 50 years. For patients with a strong family history of breast cancer in first-degree relatives, screening mammography is usually initiated 10 years younger than the age at which the youngest relative was diagnosed with breast cancer. There is some concern regarding the decreased sensitivity of mammography in women between 40 and 50 years of age due to the increased breast density in this age group. In addition to the decreased sensitivity of mammography, density is also associated with an increased risk of breast cancer.

Screening mammography provides two views of each breast: the *craniocaudal (CC) projection* images the breast from a superior to inferior view, and the *mediolateral oblique (MLO) projection* images the breast from a medial to lateral approach. National standards of quality mammography are established and regulated by the Mammography Quality Standards Act (MQSA). Screening mammography should be differentiated from diagnostic mammography, which includes additional mammographic views for any palpable or screen-detected abnormality. These additional views can include spot compression, magnification views, exaggerated views, or true lateral views as well as diagnostic ultrasound of the area of concern.

Women with implants should undergo implant displacement views (Eklund views) in which the implant is pushed back against the chest wall, and the breast is pulled forward over it, improving the imaging of the anterior portion of each breast. This increases the amount of breast tissue visualized. Overall, less breast tissue is visualized in patients with implants, and the amount of breast tissue visualized varies with location of the implant and degree of capsular contracture.

Digital mammography has been widely embraced in the United States. The Digital Mammographic Imaging Screening Trial study compared film analog mammography and digital mammography in more than 40,000 women. In this study, film-screen mammography was found to be equivalent to digital mammography in all women except those older than 50 years, premenopausal or perimenopausal women, and those with increased breast density.

The use of computer-assisted diagnosis (CAD) with either digital or film-screen mammography has been shown to improve both sensitivity and specificity. This allows a computer algorithm to identify new lesions and flag them for review by the radiologist. The radiologist then reviews the films and determines whether the lesions identified by CAD are suspicious. A second mammographic read, whether by either CAD or a second radiologist, improves the diagnostic accuracy of mammography.

Mammography reporting is standardized with use of the Breast Imaging Reporting and Data System (BIRADS) classifications, shown in Table 1. The BIRADS categories classify mammographic findings by their level of suspicion. Each category is associated with guidelines for patient management to aid clinicians regarding the need for

TABLE 1: BI-RADS classification of breast imaging

Category	Assessment	Recommendation
0	Incomplete	Need additional imaging or prior studies for comparison
1	Negative	Resume routine screening mammography
2	Benign	Resume routine screening mammography
3	Probably benign	Risk of malignancy <2%; short-term interval follow-up at 6 months recommended
4	Suspicious abnormality	Intermediate risk of malignancy; biopsy recommended
5	Highly suggestive of malignancy	Chance of malignancy >95%, appropriate action should be taken
6	Known biopsy-proven malignancy	Treatment of known malignancy

biopsy as well as follow-up recommendations. The method of biopsy should be percutaneous core needle biopsy if at all possible. When breast biopsy is performed, pathologic and radiologic findings should always be correlated, and discordance requires additional evaluation. A BIRADS 5 lesion on imaging that has benign pathologic findings on core needle biopsy should still undergo surgical excision. Any lesion with radiologic and pathologic findings that are not concordant should be recommended for surgical excision. Clinically suspicious lesions in patients with negative mammograms and ultrasound should also undergo biopsy.

OTHER IMAGING MODALITIES

Other imaging modalities in screening are primarily considered to be supplemental to mammography and clinical breast examination at this time, other than MRI for screening high-risk women.

Ultrasonography

Whole breast ultrasound is not routinely used for breast cancer screening. In contrast, focused breast ultrasound does have an established role in diagnostic breast imaging, to characterize palpable or screen-detected lesions and to direct biopsy sonographically visible lesions. Any patient with a clinically suspicious palpable abnormality but normal mammography should have ultrasound to further characterize the abnormality. It is also increasingly used for further evaluation of areas of abnormality detected on MRI and other imaging modalities.

Ultrasound is the best imaging modality to differentiate a cystic from a solid lesion. Ultrasound characteristics of malignancies include lesions taller than they are wide and those with an irregular shape, ill-defined margins, posterior acoustic shadowing, hypoechogenicity, and increased vascularity. Although microcalcifications are usually not seen with ultrasound, sonographic evaluation may be considered to evaluate an area of mammographic calcification to determine whether a sonographically visible mass is present in conjunction with the calcifications.

The role of whole-breast screening ultrasound was evaluated by the American College of Radiology Imaging Network National Breast Ultrasound Trial (ACRIN 6666), which demonstrated that screening ultrasound in addition to screening mammogram increases detection of breast cancer at the cost of additional benign biopsies. Among more than 2800 high-risk women with dense breast tissue who underwent mammogram and whole-breast screening ultrasound, an additional 1.1 to 7.2 cancers per 1000 women were detected. Screening whole-breast ultrasound may improve detection of early breast cancer in the moderately increased risk group, who do not currently meet the recommendations for screening MRI.

Magnetic Resonance Imaging

In 2007 the American Cancer Society (ACS) issued guidelines regarding use of MRI for breast cancer screening in high-risk women. Annual screening MRI is recommended for women with an approximately 20% to 25% or greater lifetime risk of breast cancer, including women with a strong family history of breast or ovarian cancer and women who received radiation for Hodgkin disease. Data were insufficient to recommend for or against MRI screening in women with a personal history of breast cancer, carcinoma in situ, atypical hyperplasia, and extremely dense breasts on mammography. Table 2 summarizes the recommendations of the ACS regarding the use of screening MRI.

The ACS Web site recommends that women at moderately increased risk (15% to 20% lifetime risk) should talk with their doctors about the benefits and limitations of adding MRI to their screening regimen. Yearly MRI screening is not recommended for women whose lifetime risk of breast cancer is less than 15%. Screening MRI is in addition to, not instead of, a screening mammogram, as some cancers may be detected on mammogram that are not seen on MRI. Women who choose to undergo screening MRI should do this at a center with MRI-guided biopsy capabilities so that any abnormality detected can be biopsied as needed.

Molecular Breast Imaging

Molecular breast imaging (MBI) provides functional imaging of the breast by detecting uptake of technetium-99m sestamibi in breast lesions. In the 1980s, scintimammography consisted of a whole-body detection of radiotracer uptake, with the goal to detect lesions in the breast. Not surprisingly, this had poor detection of smaller breast lesions, and this approach was abandoned. Recently the development of small detectors positioned directly around the breast in a manner similar to mammography has led to a resurgence of molecular imaging of the breast as a clinically useful tool in the workup of breast lesions. In a screening study of over 1000 high-risk women with dense breast tissue, MBI with a dual-headed detector found three times as many cancers as mammography. The keys to adequate resolution of small breast lesions appear to be use of two detector heads and semiconductor technology in the detection plate. With these technological advances that afford improved resolution, the radiation dose of technetium-99m sestamibi can be reduced, making this technology a promising and feasible screening option for the future.

High-Risk Screening

Risk assessment is important to direct the appropriate screening for individual patients. The most commonly used risk-prediction tool is the Gail model, which is available on the National Cancer Institute (NCI) Web site (http://www.cancer.gov/bcrisktool). It estimates an individual woman's 5-year and lifetime risk of breast cancer development based on personal history of prior biopsies, age of menarche, age at first live birth, current age, and first-degree family history. A 5-year risk greater than 1.66% indicates high risk. Other tools

TABLE 2: ACS recommendations for breast MRI screening as an adjunct to mammography

Recommend Annual MRI Screening (Based on Evidence*)
BRCA mutation
First-degree relative of BRCA carrier but untested
Lifetime risk ~20% to 25% or greater, as defined by BRCAPRO or other models that largely depend on family history

Recommend Annual MRI Screening (Based on Expert Consensus Opinion†)
Radiation to chest between age 10 and 30 years
Li–Fraumeni syndrome and first-degree relatives
Cowden and Bannayan-Riley-Ruvalcaba syndromes and first-degree relatives

Insufficient Evidence to Recommend for or Against MRI Screening‡
Lifetime risk 15% to 20% as defined by BRCAPRO or other models that largely depend on family history
Lobular carcinoma in situ (LCIS) or atypical lobular hyperplasia (ALH)
Atypical ductal hyperplasia (ADH)
Heterogeneously or extremely dense breast on mammography
Women with a personal history of breast cancer, including ductal carcinoma in situ (DCIS)

Recommend against MRI Screening (Based on Expert Consensus Opinion)
Women at <15% lifetime risk

BRCAPRO, Breast Cancer Program
*Evidence from randomized screening trials and observational studies.
†Based on evidence of lifetime risk for breast cancer.
‡Payment should not be a barrier. Screening decisions should be made on a case-by-case basis, as there may be particular factors to support MRI. More data on these groups are expected to be published soon.
From Saslow D, Boetes C, Burke W, et al: American Cancer Society guidelines for breast screening with MRI as an adjunct to mammography, *CA Cancer J Clin* 57:75–89, 2007. © 2007 American Cancer Society. This material is reproduced with permission of Wiley-Liss, Inc., a subsidiary of John Wiley & Sons, Inc.

available include the Tyrer-Cuzick, Claus, and BRCAPRO models. Calculating the lifetime risk of breast cancer with these models is important when deciding which patients might benefit from screening MRI for breast cancer.

Generally, patients who would be found to be high risk using prediction models are individuals with a family history of breast cancer in a first-degree relative, patients with a prior breast cancer diagnosis, patients with germline mutations in the *BRCA-1* or *BRCA-2* genes, a prior radiation therapy field that included the breast, or a prior diagnosis of atypical hyperplasia or lobular carcinoma in situ. In this group of patients, modifications to the standard recommendations for screening apply as discussed above. Women with a strong family history of breast cancer in a first-degree relative at a premenopausal age should initiate screening 5 to 10 years before the youngest age of diagnosis of breast cancer in the family cohort. Individuals with *BRCA* mutation should begin screening at age 25 years.

The presence of a known mutation in the *BRCA-1* or *BRCA-2* genes in men is managed with monthly BSE, a semiannual clinical breast examination, and annual mammography. Men with a personal history of breast cancer are recommended to have clinical breast examination every 6 months and to consider genetic testing.

SUGGESTED READINGS

Berg WA, Blume JD, Cormack JB, et al: Combined screening with ultrasound and mammography vs mammography alone in women at elevated risk of breast cancer, *JAMA* 299:2151, 2008.

Hruska CB, Boughey JC, Phillips SW, et al: Molecular breast imaging: a review of the Mayo Clinic experience, *Am J Surg* 196:470, 2008.

Pisano ED, Gastonis C, Hendrick E, et al: Diagnostic performance of digital versus film mammography for breast-cancer screening, *N Engl J Med* 353:1773, 2005.

Saslow D, Boetes C, Burke W, et al: American Cancer Society guidelines for breast screening with MRI as an adjunct to mammography, *CA Cancer J Clin* 57:75, 2007.

Smith RA, Cokkinides V, Eyre HJ: American Cancer Society guidelines for the early detection of cancer, *CA Cancer J Clin* 56:11, 2006.

US Preventive Services Task Force: Screening for breast cancer: US Preventive Services Task Force recommendation statement, *Ann Intern Med* 151(10):716–726, 2009.

ROLE OF STEREOTACTIC BREAST BIOPSY IN THE MANAGEMENT OF BREAST DISEASE

Eric B. Whitacre, MD

OVERVIEW

Stereotactic breast biopsy is an invaluable tool for the breast specialist. The importance of percutaneous breast biopsy in the diagnosis and management of breast cancer is well established, and although many benign and malignant lesions are amenable to ultrasound-guided needle biopsy, stereotactic-guided needle biopsy remains important for diagnosis of microcalcifications and nonpalpable densities seen only on mammography. In addition, the stereotactic imaging platform is an important potential tool for emerging percutaneous therapeutic technologies for breast cancer. This chapter will review the basic principles of stereotactic breast biopsy, discuss difficult clinical scenarios, and outline steps to facilitate the practice of stereotactic biopsy by the surgeon.

HISTORICAL BACKGROUND

Although the first stereotactic table was brought to this country by a surgeon, its potential for the diagnosis of mammographically detected abnormalities was not generally accepted by the surgical community when it was first introduced. Its potential began to be recognized only after the development of spring-loaded core biopsy devices, which allowed stereotactic percutaneous biopsy to achieve an accuracy that made it an acceptable alternative to surgical biopsy (Table 1). Later development of directional rotating-cutter, vacuum-assisted biopsy tools (the "Mammotome" type biopsy) improved the diagnostic accuracy of the technique, and today percutaneous image-guided needle biopsy has become the preferred method to diagnose breast cancer. Indeed, there is general consensus among experts and professional organizations that malignancies of the breast should be diagnosed first using imaged-guided techniques, as this allows for better preoperative planning for the therapeutic surgical procedure and decreases the false-negative rate of sentinel lymph node biopsy

compared to open biopsy (Table 2). In addition, for the surgeon with stereotactic skill, placement of localization wires prior to local excision of cancer or atypical/high-risk lesions offers a real advantage in planning the surgical approach.

STEREOTACTIC EQUIPMENT AND BIOPSY DEVICES

Most stereotactic units in use today are tables upon which the patient is positioned prone with the breast suspended through a small aperture. Upright tables are also available and are occasionally useful in

TABLE 1: Accuracy of stereotactic percutaneous core needle biopsy

Investigator	Year	Number of Cases	Concordance with Surgical Biopsy
Parker	1991	102	96%
Dronkers	1992	53	91%
Elvecrog	1993	100	94%
Gisvold	1994	104	90%

TABLE 2: Organizations supporting percutaneous biopsy prior to surgical intervention for cancer

Organization	Year	Reference
National Comprehensive Cancer Network (NCCN)	2009	http://www.nccn.org
American Society of Breast Surgeons (ASBS)	2006	http://www.breastsurgeons.org
National Consortium of Breast Centers (NCBC)	2005	http://www.ncbcinc.org
National Accreditation Program for Breast Centers (NAPBC)	2005	http://accreditedbreastcenters.org
National Quality Forum (NQF)	2007	http://www.qualityforum.org

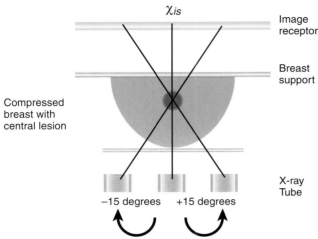

FIGURE 1 The computer calculates the position of the lesion in the breast based on the difference in the 15-degree offset views. *(Based on drawings courtesy Beth A. Boyd, RN.)*

patients whose underlying body habitus or medical problems prevent prone positioning. Whichever equipment is being used, it is essential that the surgeon be familiar both with the principles of stereotaxis as well as the actual mechanics of the table.

Stereotactic imaging depends on the principle of parallax to calculate the position of an imaged target using the relative shift of the image as seen on two 15-degree offset views, which is very simply using computer right-eye and left-eye views to calculate depth of the lesion in the compressed breast (Figure 1). Machines may use either polar or Cartesian coordinates for calculation of the needle position, and it is essential that the surgeon understand how the computer interface and mechanics of the machine translate into positioning of the needle in the breast. If there is any question about how the equipment works, it is best to review this ahead of time rather than try and problem solve during the procedure.

Similarly, because of a variety of biopsy tools are available, it is important to feel comfortable with the operation of the biopsy equipment. Most stereotactic biopsies are performed today using an 8 to 11 gauge vacuum-assisted rotating cutting device, usually referred to as a *Mammotome-type needle,* but each biopsy device has specific individual features that should be clearly understood to allow for optimal performance. Biopsy devices range from 18 gauge core biopsy devices to 1.5 cm biopsy devices to remove intact tissue specimens. The smaller needles might be used in a patient with coronary stents requiring ongoing anticoagulation; the larger devices are useful to achieve intact removal of mammographic densities or extensive calcifications. Also, the relative length of the biopsy aperture and the "throw" of the needle will impact how the needle will be positioned in the breast relative to the targeted lesion as discussed below. If stereotactic procedures are performed infrequently, or if you are using new equipment, it may be best to review this with a phantom biopsy before the actual procedure.

THREE IMPORTANT CONCEPTS: TARGETING, PULLBACK, AND STROKE MARGIN

The three critically important concepts in stereotactic biopsy procedure involve understanding how to assess the accuracy of targeting and the principles of *pullback* and *stroke margin* of the biopsy needle. Fortunately, the stereotactic equipment will generally calculate the needle biopsy parameters, which are input into the computer during initial setup of the equipment, so only the accuracy of targeting

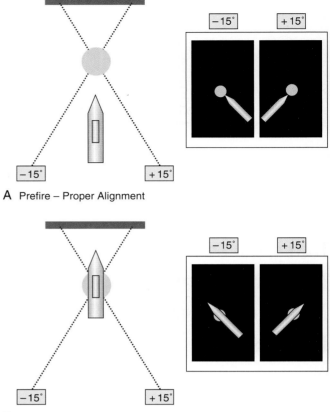

FIGURE 2 **A,** Prefire views of the biopsy needle properly aligned relative to the target. **B,** Postfire views. *(Based on drawings courtesy Beth A. Boyd, RN.)*

remains as the usual day-to-day issue. Still, it is important for the surgeon to understand these concepts well.

Targeting involves a visual interpretation of the stereotactic images to verify correct placement of the biopsy needle relative to the target. This becomes routine with experience, but early on it may seem confusing, as it involves interpretation of an image obtained at a 15-degree angle. Figure 2 shows proper placement of a vacuum-assisted biopsy needle in the prefire and postfire positions with corresponding stereotactic images. Figure 3 is an example of a needle positioned to the right of the target. Recognition of proper placement of the device is obviously critical to proper sampling, and if there is any question during the procedure, the images should be reviewed and the lesion and tip of the biopsy device retargeted.

Stroke margin and pullback of the biopsy device are not related to stereotactic imaging per se but are a function of the design and operation of the needle. Ideally, at the time of sampling during any needle biopsy, the biopsy device is designed to be positioned with the center of the biopsy aperture in the middle of the targeted density. The stereotactic machine actually calculates the final position of the needle to do just this, but it cannot account for location of the lesion relative to the image receptor/back plate or for the size and relative mobility of the lesion in the breast. The *stroke* of the needle is the distance it is advanced when "fired," and the *stroke margin* is the distance of the tip of the needle from the image receptor (back support for breast compression) after the needle has been fired. This is demonstrated in Figure 4. When the center of the biopsy aperture is optimally centered in the midportion of the lesion, the biopsy needle projects past the center of the lesion by half the length of the biopsy aperture plus the length of the needle tip.

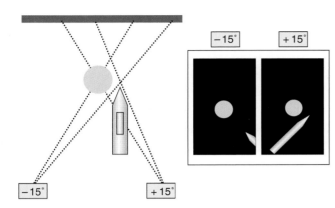

Prefire – Needle to the Right

FIGURE 3   Prefire view of the needle to the right of the target. Understanding the 15-degree offset projection will help interpret the location of a misaligned biopsy needle. *(Based on drawings courtesy Beth A. Boyd, RN.)*

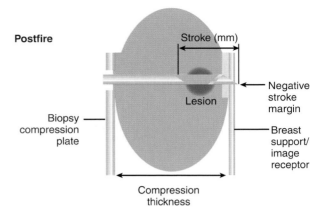

Negative Stroke Margin

FIGURE 5   Negative stroke margin. The fully deployed needle is accurately placed but damages the image receptor. *(Based on drawings courtesy Beth A. Boyd, RN.)*

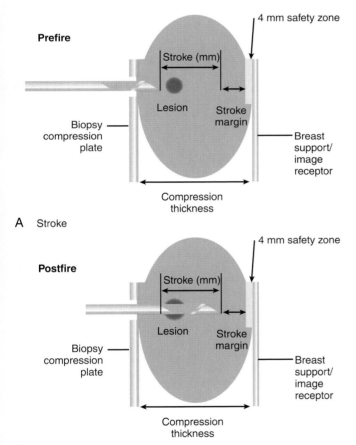

FIGURE 4   **A,** When fired, the needle will advance a preset distance, called the *stroke*. **B,** The distance of the tip of the needle from the back plate once the needle has been fired is the *stroke margin*. It should always be a positive number to avoid damage to the image receptor. *(Based on drawings courtesy Beth A. Boyd, RN.)*

With lesions located close to the skin touching the image receptor, it is possible for the stereotactic machine to calculate a position that projects the tip of the needle through the skin of the breast and into the image receptor. To prevent this, it is important to verify that the needle position allows for a *positive* stroke margin (Figure 5). This

is calculated for you in some machines, such as the Fisher/Siemens table (reported as the "adjusted depth"), but it must be manually adjusted with other equipment. It is important to mentally visualize the final location of the needle based on the coordinates displayed on your particular machine before deploying a specific biopsy device.

Pullback of the needle is related to the importance of centering the biopsy aperture in the midportion of the targeted lesion; this concept is valid for all needle biopsy procedures independent of the use of image guidance. For small lesions, a biopsy device with a long *throw,* if positioned too close to the target, can actually point past the lesion and result in poor sampling (Figure 6). This is sometimes visible during the biopsy, as the targeted tissue is visible only as a small piece of the core specimen, and it is located at the proximal end, away from the needle tip. Alternatively, the lesion may move during positioning of the needle. It is easy to recognize if the lesion moves off the axis of the biopsy device (up, down, right, or left); but if the lesion is pushed forward by the biopsy needle, that may be harder to recognize. It is sometimes necessary to retarget the lesion to confirm that the sampling portion of the biopsy device is properly positioned (Figure 7).

THE STEREOTACTIC BIOPSY PROCEDURE

A stereotactic biopsy is no different from any minor surgical procedure. It begins with a review of the history, a complete patient examination with attention to the area of concern on imaging, as well as a thorough review of the imaging studies. Complete preoperative imaging is important, as many mammographic nodular densities are evident on ultrasound, and are more readily biopsied using ultrasound guidance. In addition, it is important to perform a baseline physical examination in the event that cancer is detected or any complications occur following the procedure. A detailed review of the procedure with the patient will also help identify any additional issues that may interfere with the biopsy, such as an inability to lie prone for an extended period. As for any surgical procedure, it is important to stop any anticoagulation, including aspirin, warfarin (Coumadin), and clopidogrel (Plavix).

Before the procedure, the surgeon should personally review the films and understand the three-dimensional (3D) location of the lesion in the breast to readily locate the abnormality on the stereotactic machine (Figure 8). It is best to have already determined a probable optimal approach before beginning the procedure, and it is useful to have considered alternative approaches in the event that it is difficult to identify the abnormality or its location prevents ready access with the biopsy device. It is also important to be intimately

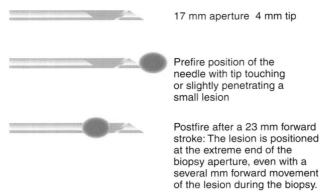

17 mm aperture 4 mm tip

Prefire position of the needle with tip touching or slightly penetrating a small lesion

Postfire after a 23 mm forward stroke: The lesion is positioned at the extreme end of the biopsy aperture, even with a several mm forward movement of the lesion during the biopsy.

Core Biopsy Needle—Without Pullback

FIGURE 6 The core biopsy needle is positioned too far into the lesion; when fired, it may pass too far to adequately sample the target. *(Based on drawings courtesy Beth A. Boyd, RN.)*

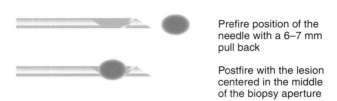

Prefire position of the needle with a 6–7 mm pull back

Postfire with the lesion centered in the middle of the biopsy aperture

The formula for the prefire pullback is:
Pullback = Stroke − (1/2 Aperture + Needle tip)

Core Biopsy Needle—With Pullback

FIGURE 7 Proper position of the core biopsy needle to center the biopsy aperture within the lesion. (Note that the stereotactic machine will calculate the proper position of the biopsy device including the required pullback.) *(Based on drawings courtesy Beth A. Boyd, RN.)*

familiar with the stereotactic and biopsy equipment being used. If necessary, a quick refresher with the technologist who will be assisting will facilitate the procedure considerably.

The Routine Stereotactic Biopsy Procedure

The patient is positioned on the stereotactic table, and based on pre-procedure imaging, the area in the breast is targeted. A scout film is obtained documenting the presence of the mammographic abnormality, and two 15-degree offset views are obtained. These are used to designate the location of the abnormality for the computer, which can then calculate the position in three dimensions. An appropriate biopsy device is selected, and the skin is sterilely prepared. Local anesthesia is administered, generally using a 30 gauge needle to inject lidocaine without epinephrine in the skin, followed by a 25 to 22 gauge needle to inject lidocaine with epinephrine for the deeper tissues.

The biopsy device is introduced through a small puncture in the skin, and appropriate location of the device is verified. This may include stereotactic images in the prefire as well as postfire views, documenting the abnormality in the appropriate location to the biopsy portion of the device. Specimens are obtained sufficient to adequately sample the abnormality (typically 10 to 15 samples for an 11 gauge device, six to eight for an 8 gauge), which is documented both by review of postbiopsy stereotactic views as well as by radiograph of the biopsy specimens to document the presence of the targeted abnormality. Placement of a biopsy marker is almost always advisable, unless the patient has strong objections and refuses placement, which should be discussed with the patient preprocedure. Appropriate location of the marker is then verified on additional stereotactic views

and/or a follow-up two-view mammogram. The puncture site is generally closed with adhesive tape followed by a dry gauze dressing held in place with an Ace wrap (tape alone may cause blistering of the skin). The technical portion of the procedure generally requires only 20 to 30 minutes, although the biopsy itself is not completed until the pathology is obtained and correlated with the imaging studies.

Difficult Clinical Scenarios

Lesions close to the chest wall require that the patient understand how to best accommodate a position to optimize imaging. Once patients understand the goal of the positioning, they are generally very helpful in suggesting small maneuvers that can help, whether it is padding a part of the table to decrease discomfort against the rib or turning slightly from the prone position to improve access to the posterior lateral breast. On occasion it may be necessary to actually bring the arm through the table aperture, in which case it is important to be conscious of axillary structures to avoid injury by the biopsy device. Some patients who are very anxious may require an oral anxiolytic, such as alprazolam (Xanax) or diazepam (Valium), but this is actually quite rare once the procedure is fully explained.

More frequently, problems are encountered based on location of the lesion within the breast. It is important to remember that the physics of the imaging will allow for better visualization of faintly seen lesions when they are placed close to the image receptor and farther from the beam source. For example, faint calcifications at the 6 o'clock position in the breast are better seen using the craniocaudal approach than the lateral or medial approach. This, however, may complicate the biopsy, as it would result in a calculated negative stroke margin. Several techniques can be used to overcome this problem. In general, once the targeted lesion has been identified, it is possible to alter the biopsy approach slightly to improve the stroke margin. If this does not work, it may still be possible to perform the biopsy by making an adjustment in the needle depth to avoid penetrating the skin close to the image receptor and still allow for the biopsy aperture to be under the targeted lesion. The Fischer/Siemens table allows for use of the "lateral arm" so that the imaging may be performed through one approach, and the biopsy needle introduced perpendicular to that. It is sometimes possible to place local anesthesia between the skin and the targeted lesion to improve distance from the skin. Finally, placement of a second compression paddle posterior to the breast may allow for offset of the target from the image receptor to permit biopsy. This is rarely required and does mean that the patient should be informed that the needle may traverse the entire breast and come out on the other side.

In planning the approach of the needle biopsy, any large vessels should be avoided, which may actually require slightly changing the imaging approach. The stereotactic table can be used to determine the depth of the vessels relative to the target. As with any surgical procedure, bleeding may occur during the course of the biopsy. If substantial bleeding is encountered following a single pass of the cutting device, and the patient is not in pain or otherwise in distress, it is generally best to use suction to evacuate the blood and to continue with the biopsy. This is important not only to obtain sufficient pathology for a definitive biopsy but also because a partially transected vessel will continue bleeding. Once a biopsy with significant bleeding has been completed, it is often useful to continue to suction the cavity for 5 to 6 minutes. This maintains a dry field, improves the quality of the postbiopsy stereotactic views, and allows the vessels to constrict so coagulation can begin. A postbiopsy hematoma will generally become apparent within 4 to 12 hours and manifests as severe pain with swelling and ecchymosis. It can usually be managed with aspiration and additional compression, and only very rarely is surgery required. Many surgeons use a compression dressing (Ace wrap or binder) following a stereotactic biopsy to help prevent this complication. Infection related to the procedure is extremely rare, and routine prophylactic antibiotics are not indicated.

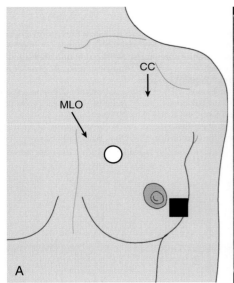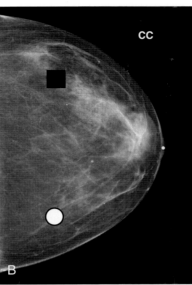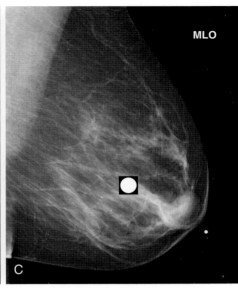

FIGURE 8 Interpreting anatomic location of lesions based on craniocaudal (*CC*) and mediolateral oblique (*MLO*) views. The CC view will accurately represent the location of the lesion; on the MLO view, however, medial lesions are higher in the breast than they appear on the mammogram, and lateral lesions are lower than they appear. A true lateral view will show the actual location.

Pathologic Correlation

One of the most important steps in the stereotactic biopsy procedure is correlation of the biopsy results with the anticipated pathology. The accuracy of a percutaneous needle biopsy depends on precise targeting, adequacy of the tissue sample, and the volume of intact tissue relative to the size of the actual lesion. A stereotactic biopsy may fail to satisfy any one or a combination of these factors. For example, a malignant-appearing lesion that shows only benign breast tissue may simply reflect poor targeting and would clearly require follow-up surgical biopsy to confirm the results. Other pathologies, such as atypical ductal and lobular hyperplasia, are known to be associated with a 10% to 20% risk of associated malignancy on follow-up surgical excision, even when the stereotactic biopsy appears technically accurate. Radial scars, especially those larger than 6 mm, have a similar increased risk of associated malignancy.

Diagnosing cancer in other lesions, such as papillomas, depends to a great degree on the ability to completely excise the lesion for review by the pathologist. As this can be difficult to confirm on stereotactic imaging, using a needle biopsy device that fragments the tissue, most experts recommend that papillary lesions be followed by open surgical biopsy. There is currently some controversy concerning management of lobular carcinoma in situ found on stereotactic biopsy, especially if noted incidentally with pathology concordant with the stereotactic target. As a rule, if any question remains about the accuracy or adequacy of the biopsy or the presence of unexplained additional pathology, follow-up surgical excision is indicated (Table 3). In patients older than 35 years, a unilateral diagnostic mammogram is generally obtained as a new baseline study within 4 to 6 months of the procedure.

Certification

Stereotactic breast imaging has been the unfortunate focus of turf battles between surgery and radiology. Both specialty groups have an interest in breast imaging and in using percutaneous image-guided techniques to diagnose breast cancer. It is important for anyone performing stereotactic biopsy to demonstrate appropriate training and skill and to document ongoing education. To that end, the American Society of Breast Surgeons has developed a formal certification program in stereotactic procedures for individual surgeons and a

TABLE 3: Needle biopsy pathology requiring surgical excision

Any pathologic finding that does not correspond to the breast imaging findings (discordance)
Atypical ductal hyperplasia, including atypical columnar cell hyperplasia
Atypical lobular hyperplasia
Radial scar (if >6 mm)
Papillary lesions
Vascular proliferations (not simple hemangiomas)
Pseudoangiomatous stromal hyperplasia

Management of incidentally detected lobular neoplasia and pseudoangiomatous stromal hyperplasia (i.e., when other documented pathologic findings explain the targeted lesion) remains controversial. When in doubt, surgical excision should be performed.

comparable accreditation program for facilities. These require board certification in surgery with documentation of appropriate training through recognized Council on Medical Education (CME) programs, as well as completion of a minimum number of stereotactic procedures. The certification program requires that the applicant complete a hands-on examination, exceptional among many professional certifications, to demonstrate safety and proficiency in stereotactic imaging and biopsy. In addition, CME has developed a Web-based database for surgeons interested in recording and tracking percutaneous breast procedures, which is also required for certification.

Future Directions

The stereotactic platform is not only useful for performing needle biopsy and needle wire localization but also provides a platform for breast interventions that require stabilization of the breast.

Stereotactic tables have been used for percutaneous placement of brachytherapy catheters for adjuvant radiotherapy following lumpectomy. In addition, selected patients have successfully undergone laser ablation of breast cancer using the stereotactic table to position the laser fiber and to monitor tissue temperature during the procedure to confirm the zone of ablation. Proficiency in stereotactic breast biopsy is the basis for acquiring more advanced skills and should be part of the routine skill set of all surgeons interested in breast disease.

ACKNOWLEDGEMENT

I am indebted to Beth A. Boyd, RN, who has helped countless surgeons learn stereotactic breast biopsy, for her work on graphics depicting stereotactic procedures.

SUGGESTED READINGS

American Society of Breast Surgeons Web site (http://www.breastsurgeons.org) for the statement on performance and practice guidelines for stereotactic biopsy, for information on stereotactic certification and accreditation programs, and for a Web-based program to track stereotactic procedures, "The Mastery of Breast Surgery Program."

Silverstein MJ, Recht A, Lagios MD, et al: Special report: Consensus Conference III. Image-detected breast cancer: state-of-the-art diagnosis and treatment, *J Am Coll Surg* 209(4):504–520, 2009.

Fajardo LL, Willison KM, Pizzutiello RJ, editors: *A comprehensive approach to stereotactic breast biopsy,* Cambridge, MA, 1996, Blackwell Science.

CELLULAR, BIOCHEMICAL, AND MOLECULAR TARGETS IN BREAST CANCER

Tari A. King, MD, and Monica Morrow, MD

OVERVIEW

High-throughput molecular technologies are reshaping our understanding of cancer. It is now quite clear that the term *breast cancer* encompasses a heterogenous group of diseases with a wide variety of clinical behaviors. Traditional histopathologic classification systems based on morphology are being combined with molecular data generated from expression profiling to provide robust prognostic information, and large-scale efforts are focused on using molecular technology to identify new predictive markers and novel therapeutic targets. As we move toward genomic biomarkers and more personalized medicine, the development of rational therapeutic approaches requires an understanding of the signaling pathways involved in carcinogenesis. This chapter focuses on cellular and molecular targets important in current clinical practice, those under investigation in clinical trials, and promising avenues for the future.

MOLECULAR PROFILING

The discovery that breast cancers can be classified based on their gene expression profile was first described in the seminal publications by Perou (2008) and Sorlie (2001). The five intrinsic breast cancer subtypes—*luminal A, luminal B, HER2, normal-like,* and *basal-like*—have now been validated by several groups and have been shown to have implications for both tumor biology and treatment.

The most robust distinction observed by microarray analysis is between the transcriptome of estrogen receptor (ER)-positive (luminal) and ER-negative breast cancers. Luminal tumors show expression patterns similar to normal luminal breast epithelial cells, including expression of low molecular weight cytokeratin 8/18, ER, and genes associated with an active ER signaling pathway. Luminal tumors are further classified into two subgroups. *Luminal A tumors* are usually a low histologic grade, and they have high levels of ER expression and

an excellent prognosis; *luminal B tumors* are more often a higher histologic grade, and they have higher proliferation rates and a poorer prognosis than luminal A tumors.

Human epidermal growth factor receptor-2 (HER2) tumors are usually ER negative and are characterized by overexpression of HER2 and genes associated with the HER2 pathway and/or the HER2 amplicon on chromosome 17q12. HER2 cancers tend to be more aggressive, although they are responsive to targeted therapies. A small proportion (10% to 15%) of HER2-amplified cancers are also ER positive and fall into the luminal B group by microarray analysis.

The basal-like group was named for the higher expression of genes characteristic of normal basal cells of breast epithelium, including high molecular weight cytokeratins 5/6, 14, and 17; HER1; and smooth muscle actin. Basal-like cancers are generally high-grade, poorly differentiated tumors with a poor prognosis. They are predominantly negative for ER, progesterone receptor (PR), and HER2; clinical adoption of this breast tumor classification uses immunohistochemical "triple negativity" as the most practical surrogate for the identification of basal-like tumors. In reality, however, triple-negative tumors likely encompass a more heterogenous group. Only about 70% of triple-negative tumors display basal-like expression patterns when classified by gene expression profiling; similarly, not all basal-like tumors from expression arrays display a triple-negative phenotype (~77% are triple negative). Basal-like tumors are more common in younger women and in women of African descent. They are also typically the tumors that arise in carriers of *BRCA1* germline mutations. The intrinsic breast cancer subtypes and their characteristics are summarized in Table 1.

Efforts to define more limited sets of genes for prognostic purposes include a 70-gene expression profile first described by Van de Vijver and colleagues in 2002. Commonly referred to as the *Amsterdam signature,* the expression profiles of these 70 genes were demonstrated to classify 295 patients with breast cancer into a good or poor prognosis group, as judged on the basis of distant relapse and overall survival. Interestingly, women with node-positive and node-negative disease were evenly distributed between the two groups, whereas other poor prognostic factors, such as ER negativity and high histologic grade, were clustered in the poor prognosis group. The 10-year disease-free survival was 94.5% in the good prognosis group and 50.6% in the poor prognosis group. This genomic assay, which requires fresh frozen tumor samples, is now commercially available as MammaPrint (Agendia, Amsterdam, The Netherlands) and is undergoing clinical validation as part of a multicenter trial.

Another gene-based approach is the 21-gene assay using reverse transcription polymerase chain reaction (RT-PCR) on RNA isolated from paraffin-embedded breast tumors (Oncotype DX, Genomic Health, Redwood City, Calif.). This assay provides individualized

TABLE 1: Intrinsic molecular subtypes of breast cancer

Type	Characteristics	Markers
Luminal A	Low grade, high ER, 50% of breast cancer	ER+, PR+, HER2−, CK8+, CK18+
Luminal B	Higher grade, lower ER, 10% of breast cancer	ER+, PR+/−, HER2+/−
HER2	High grade, p53 mutations 5% to 10% of breast cancer	ER−, PR−, HER2+
Basal	High proliferation CK5+, CK14+, CK17+, EGFR+ 30% of breast cancer	ER−, PR−, HER2−

CK, Cytokeratin

TABLE 2: Molecular targets in clinical breast cancer management

Target	Drug	Status
ER	Tamoxifen	Survival benefit, adjuvant treatment, and metastatic disease, premenopausal and postmenopausal women
	Aromatase inhibitors (anastrozole, letrozole, exemestane)	Survival benefit, adjuvant and metastatic disease, postmenopausal women
	Fulvestrant	Second-line therapy, metastatic disease in postmenopausal women
HER2	Trastuzumab	Survival benefit, adjuvant and metastatic disease
HER1+ HER2	Lapatinib	Second-line therapy, metastatic disease; phase II adjuvant trials ongoing
HER1 (EGFR)	Gefitinib, erlotinib	Benefit unclear after phase II trials
	Cetuximab	In trial
VEGF	Bevacizumab	Progression-free survival benefit, metastatic disease; phase III adjuvant trials ongoing
PARP1/PARP2	PARP1 inhibitor	Improved PFS, OS in phase II trial, phase III initiated

PFS, Progression-free survival; *OS,* overall survival

risk estimates, called a *recurrence score* (RS), based on measurements of 16 cancer-related genes and five reference genes. The 16 cancer-related genes comprise components of the ER pathway (*ER, PGR, BCL2,* and *SCUBE2*); proliferation (*Ki67, STK15, Survivin, CCNB1,* and *MYBL2*); *HER2* amplicon (*HER2* and *GRB7*); invasion (*MMP11* and *CTSL2*); and *GSTM1, CD68,* and *BAG1.* The assay was originally developed by retrospective analysis of available tumor tissue from 447 patients treated with tamoxifen with or without chemotherapy in three clinical trials. Independent validation was performed in 668 stage I and II, node-negative, hormone receptor–positive patients treated with tamoxifen in the National Surgical Adjuvant Breast and Bowel Project (NSABP) B-14 trial. In the validation study, the RS was superior to age, tumor size, and grade in predicting prognosis, and when subdivided into low-risk (RS <18), intermediate-risk (RS 18 to 30), and high-risk (RS >31) groups, the 10-year disease-free survival was 69% for the high-risk group and 93% for the low-risk group.

Further analysis of patients from NSABP-B20 demonstrated that patients in the high-risk group experienced a significant benefit from the addition of chemotherapy to tamoxifen, whereas those in the low-risk group derived little to no benefit from chemotherapy. The assay has been accepted as a clinical practice tool for appropriately selected patients. However, optimal therapy for patients in the intermediate-risk group remains unclear, and this question is being tested in a prospective trial (Trial Assigning Individualized Options for Treatment [Rx] [TAILORx]) in which Oncotype DX is being used to select hormone receptor–positive, node-negative patients with an intermediate RS for randomization to hormonal therapy or combined hormonal therapy and chemotherapy.

Subsequent studies have demonstrated similar prognostic and predictive value for the assay in patients with node-positive, hormone receptor–positive cancers, but the high residual risk of relapse after treatment with endocrine therapy alone in this group is problematic when considering omitting chemotherapy. Use of this assay in node-positive women has the potential to identify high-risk groups of node-positive women who would be excellent candidates for clinical trials of innovative therapeutic approaches.

ESTROGEN RECEPTOR SIGNALING PATHWAYS

The ER signaling pathway has been a therapeutic target in breast cancer since the report by Beatson in 1896 that oophorectomy could produce regression of metastatic breast cancer. In the 1950s, Jensen and colleagues demonstrated that estradiol binds to, and is retained by, the estrogen target tissues (uterus, vagina, and pituitary gland) but not by nontarget tissues, and that this effect could be blocked by the coadministration of a nonsteroidal antiestrogen, indicating the presence of an ER.

It is now recognized that there are two ERs: ER-α and ER-β. ER-α is the "classic" ER. Both are members of the steroid receptor superfamily and they share homology, but they are encoded on different chromosomes and have distinct patterns of distribution within tissues. The assays used for ER determination in clinical practice measure ER-α levels; approximately 75% of breast cancers express ER-α. It is estimated that approximately 60% of tumors coexpress ER-α and ER-β, but the role of ER-β in breast cancer management is uncertain at this time. Some evidence suggests that the ratio of ER-α to ER-β at a target site is important, and high ratios are associated with high levels of cellular proliferation and tamoxifen resistance.

PR is an estrogen-responsive gene that is expressed as a result of ER activation. Approximately 55% of ER-positive tumors are also PR positive, and PR positivity is not thought to occur in the absence of ER. The ER functions as a ligand-dependent transcription factor. The binding of a ligand to ER-α or ER-β results in the formation of a nuclear receptor complex (NRC), whose shape is influenced by the specific ligand. The NRC then interacts with either coactivators or corepressors to initiate estrogenic or antiestrogenic action, respectively.

The broad spectrum of ligands for the ER, coupled with the large number of coactivators and corepressors, result in a wide range of estrogenic or antiestrogenic responses. Once the NRC has bound to the promotor region of an ER-responsive gene to initiate transcription, additional molecules are bound to the NRC-promotor complex; these modulate exposure to DNA and prepare the complex for destruction. The recognition of the complexity of estrogen action at individual target sites offers the opportunity to develop new, targeted therapeutic agents.

The endocrine therapies in use today target the ER signaling pathway in several different ways. The selective ER modulators (SERMs) tamoxifen and raloxifene interact directly with the ER, binding to inhibit estrogen-dependent transcription in the breast but maintaining agonist activity at some sites, as discussed above. In contrast, the pure estrogen antagonist fulvestrant binds to the ER, induces degradation of ER protein, and has no agonist activity. The aromatase inhibitors and surgical or medical oophorectomy do not interact directly with the ER, but they reduce the amount of estrogen available as a ligand for the receptor, resulting in a reduction of ligand-activated signaling.

Endocrine therapy has proven to be a remarkably successful strategy for breast cancer management. Adjuvant therapy with 5 years of tamoxifen reduces the odds of breast cancer recurrence by 40% to 50% and lowers the odds of breast cancer death by 30%; similar benefit is seen with the aromatase inhibitors in postmenopausal women. The improved understanding of the molecular pathway of estrogen signaling is also providing greater insight into mechanisms of endocrine resistance, which should result in new approaches to overcoming it.

GROWTH FACTOR RECEPTORS AND DOWNSTREAM PATHWAYS

The epidermal growth factor receptors (EGFRs; erbB family) are transmembrane type 1 tyrosine kinase (TK) receptors. The erbB family consists of four closely related members: erbB1, erbB2 (HER2/neu), erbB3 (HER3), and erbB4 (HER4). Structurally, these TK receptors all have the same three basic features: 1) an N-terminus extracellular ligand-binding region, 2) a transmembrane domain, and 3) an intracellular region containing the TK domain. In the resting state, the receptors exist as monomers that form either homodimers or heterodimers with each other in response to ligand binding. Dimerization is accompanied by transphosphorylation of specific tyrosine residues within the cytoplasmic tail and leads to the activation of numerous signaling pathways.

Some members of the erbB family—erbB1, erbB3, and erbB4—can be activated by various growth factor ligands; however, no specific endogenous ligand for erbB2 (HER2) has been identified. Instead, ligand binding between HER2 and other members of the erbB family induces receptor dimerization and activation of HER2. The kinase domain of HER3 is inactive, and its signaling functions are mediated through the kinase of its heterodimeric partners. HER2 is the preferred partner for each of the HER receptors and has the strongest kinase activity. Activation leads to multiple transduction cascades through a wide variety of kinase pathways, resulting in protein synthesis, transcription, cell proliferation and survival, angiogenesis, invasion, and metastasis. The best characterized signaling pathways induced by the HER family are the phosphatidylinositol-3 kinase/AKT (PI3K/AKT), the *Ras*/mitogen-activated protein kinase (*Ras*/MAPK), and the phospholipase C/protein kinase C (PLC/PKC) pathways.

Overexpression of HER2

The *HER2* gene, also known as *HER2/neu* or *c-erbB2*, is located on chromosome 17q and is normally involved in regulation of cell proliferation. The *HER2* gene is a protooncogene, a normal gene with the potential to become an oncogene upon molecular alterations, such as mutation, amplification, or overexpression of its protein product. The HER2 protein is overexpressed, and/or its gene is amplified, in about 20% of invasive breast cancers. HER2 amplification is associated with a more aggressive phenotype and predicts for response to trastuzumab therapy, a recombinant humanized monoclonal antibody

specific for the external region of HER2, or to HER2 TK inhibitors. Immunohistochemistry for membrane-bound HER2 protein is most commonly used for semiquantitative analysis of staining (0, 1+, 2+, or 3+) followed by fluorescence in situ hybridization (FISH) for confirmation of gene amplification in cases scored as positive (2 or 3+).

The advent of trastuzumab (Herceptin) therapy in the adjuvant management of HER2-positive breast cancer in 2005 was a major breakthrough in the application of targeted therapy to breast cancer. Results from five studies that randomized 11,650 women with early stage HER2-positive breast cancer to trastuzumab versus non–trastuzumab-based adjuvant chemotherapy demonstrated that the addition of trastuzumab to adjuvant chemotherapy results in a significant improvement in both disease-free (50%) and overall (33%) survival. The clinical benefit of trastuzumab is clearly limited to tumors with HER2 amplification; however, the mechanisms of action of trastuzumab are not fully understood. Despite the remarkable survival benefits associated with trastuzumab, a significant proportion of patients with HER2-positive breast cancer will ultimately experience a recurrence or develop disease progression; therefore elucidating the mechanisms of de novo and acquired resistance to trastuzumab and identifying alternative mechanisms for disrupting HER2-mediated signaling are active areas of investigation.

Lapatinib is an oral, reversible, small-molecule dual inhibitor of both the EGFR (HER1) and HER2 kinases. In 2007 it was approved for use in trastuzumab-refractory HER2-positive metastatic breast cancer. Preclinical evidence suggests that lapatinib exerts its antitumor effects by inducing growth arrest and/or apoptosis, as well as by blocking downstream mitogen-activated protein kinase (MAPK) and AKT signaling pathways. Cell-line models indicate that the ability of lapatinib to specifically inhibit trastuzumab-resistant cell growth may reflect its inhibitory effects on insulinlike growth factor-1 signaling. These distinct features suggest that lapatinib may have a role in the treatment of both trastuzumab-naïve and trastuzumab-resistant HER2-positive breast cancer.

A large international phase III study is randomizing women with operable HER2-positive breast cancer to conventional chemotherapy with trastuzumab alone, lapatinib alone, or a combination of the two. The Adjuvant Lapatinib and/or Trastuzumab Treatment Optimization (ALTTO) study is expected to refine the treatment algorithm for HER2-positive breast cancer in the adjuvant setting.

Several other novel, small-molecule tyrosine kinase inhibitors of HER2, dual inhibitors of EGFR and HER2, and pan-HER inhibitors are currently in preclinical and clinical development. A second humanized monoclonal antibody against HER2, pertuzumab, is also being evaluated in a phase III clinical trial for patients with HER2-positive metastatic breast cancer.

PI3K/AKT Pathway

Even when HER2 is overexpressed and in its oncogenic state, it is dependent on its HER family partners, particularly HER3, for tumorigenesis. The primary oncogenic signaling pathway activated by the HER2-HER3 heterodimer is the PI3K/AKT pathway, activation of which is mediated through the tyrosine phosphorylation of HER3. Phosphorylated HER3 then directly interacts with the p85 regulatory subunit of PI3K, causing activation of the pathway and regulation of essential cell functions, such as proliferation, growth, apoptosis, angiogenesis, and invasion. The PI3K/AKT pathway can also be activated indirectly by loss of the tumor-suppressor gene *PTEN* or as a direct result of an activating mutation of the *PIK3CA* gene. It is currently accepted that activation of the pathway by these alternate events represents two of several potential mechanisms of de novo or acquired resistance to therapies that target HER2. Cross-talk between PI3K and ER-α has also been demonstrated, suggesting a role for the activation of this pathway in resistance to endocrine therapy.

Activating mutations in *PI3KCA* have been reported in 18% to 40% of breast cancers and are typically found at one of three hot spots—E542, E545, and H1047—in exons 9 and 20. A recent integrative genomic analysis demonstrated that the frequency of PI3K pathway mutational aberrations is markedly different among the most common breast cancer subtypes, being most common in hormone receptor–positive tumors and least common in basal-like (ER-/PR-/HER2-negative) cancers. This breast cancer subtype specificity suggests that *PI3KCA* mutations and other PI3K pathway aberrations may play a role in the pathogenesis of these different diseases, yet it remains unclear as to when and how PI3K activity mediates breast carcinogenesis. PI3K protein kinase inhibitors are currently under development for cancer therapy.

EGFR and MAPK

The HER2/EGFR heterodimer has been proposed to act as a master regulator of the signaling network that drives breast carcinoma epithelial cell proliferation. Although EGFR (HER1) gene status is not used to guide therapy, increased HER1 expression is present in about 40% of breast cancers, and the *HER1* gene is amplified in up to 14% of cases in nonselected series. Heterodimerization of EGFR with HER2 results in activation of the major signaling pathways, including the PI3K/AKT pathway mentioned above, and the *Ras*/MAPK pathway. Whereas trastuzumab inhibits the PI3K pathway in HER2-amplified breast cancer, it does not inhibit the MAPK pathway. This observation supports the rationale for dual kinase inhibitors such as lapatinib (Tykerb, Tyverb), an oral, reversible, small-molecule dual inhibitor of both the EGFR (HER1) and HER2 kinases described above.

Inhibition of EGFR alone using anti-erbB1 small TK inhibitors such as gefitinib (Iressa) and erlotinib (Tarceva) has shown mixed results in metastatic breast cancer. However, recent profiling studies and preclinical data suggest that this may be an important target in triple-negative breast cancer. Increased EGFR expression has been reported in up to 80% of triple-negative (basal) and metaplastic breast cancers, another group that demonstrates a high proportion of basal-like features, and the *HER1* gene is amplified in up to 28% of metaplastic cancers. EGFR dependence for growth and proliferation has also been demonstrated in basal-like breast cancer cell lines. Clinical trials are underway to investigate the efficacy of an anti-EGFR monoclonal antibody (cetuximab) either alone or in combination with chemotherapy in basal-like triple-negative breast cancer.

ANGIOGENESIS AND LYMPHANGIOGENESIS

Angiogenesis is the mechanism by which new vessels are formed from preexisting vessels. This process has a fundamental role in the development of cancer and is vital to both local tumor growth and metastasis. In contrast to the tightly regulated process of physiologic angiogenesis, tumor angiogenesis is highly disorganized. Tumoral microvessels frequently lack complete endothelial linings and basement membranes, they are irregular and tortuous, and tumor-associated capillaries are more permeable than those in normal tissues. Vascular endothelial-derived growth factor (VEGF) is the best studied target for antiangiogenic therapy. VEGF is synthesized inside tumor cells and secreted into the surrounding tissue, where it binds the VEGF receptor (VEGF-R). The interaction between VEGF and VEGF-R activates a protein cascade that ultimately leads to vascular endothelial growth, migration, and survival; it also plays a critical role in lymphangiogenesis.

Bevacizumab (Avastin, rhuMAb VEGF) is a recombinant humanized monoclonal antibody that recognizes all known isoforms of VEGF-A, thereby sequestering the ligand and inhibiting activation of the protein cascade. Bevacizumab proved disappointing in the refractory metastatic setting (heavily pretreated patients)

yet demonstrated improved progression-free survival when given as first-line treatment in metastatic breast cancer with chemotherapy. Supporting the notion that timing may be important, recent laboratory studies suggest that the initial events in the development of metastases are VEGF dependent. If this proves true in the clinic, then the most successful application of angiogenesis inhibitors may be in the adjuvant setting. Trials of bevacizumab in the adjuvant and neoadjuvant settings in combination with other chemotherapy agents are ongoing.

High-expression levels of VEGF-A and VEGF receptor 2 (VEGFR-2) have been observed in inflammatory breast cancer (IBC), and several angiogenesis-related genes are upregulated by RT-PCR in IBC compared with noninflammatory breast cancer, suggesting a potential role for antiangiogenic therapy in IBC. Therapies directed against molecular targets in angiogenesis and lymphangiogenesis have yielded promising results in preclinical studies. A small phase I trial investigating the efficacy of a small-molecule inhibitor of VEGFR2, SU5416 (semaxanib), in combination with doxorubicin in IBC demonstrated decreased tumor blood flow after treatment, as assessed by dynamic contrast-enhanced MRI. Further investigations are needed to determine whether angiogenesis is a clinically relevant unique target in IBC.

DNA REPAIR PATHWAYS

BRCA1 and *BRCA2* are two high-penetrance genes associated with hereditary breast and ovarian cancer syndrome; inherited mutations in these genes account for 5% to 10% of all breast cancer cases. Cells with mutated *BRCA1* or *BRCA2* are unable to properly sense DNA damage, transmit the damage response signal, or repair DNA by homologous recombination. Instead they must rely on single-strand annealing and nonhomologous end-joining mechanisms, which are particularly error-prone and lead to genomic instability. The association of *BRCA1* and *BRCA2* with DNA repair was first established by the seminal observation that *BRCA1* and *BRCA2* colocalize with the homologous recombinase RAD51 in subnuclear foci, and subsequent studies confirmed that *BRCA1* is an integral part of the repair process itself. While the inability of cells with mutated *BRCA1* or *BRCA2* to repair double-strand breaks in DNA is likely a factor contributing to carcinogenesis, a better understanding of *BRCA1* and *BRCA2* biology is also leading to tailored approaches for the treatment of *BRCA*-associated breast cancers.

PARP Inhibitors

Poly–ADP-ribose polymerase-1 (PARP1) is an enzyme that functions as a DNA damage sensor for both single- and double-strand breaks. PARP2 is a similar protein that plays an important role in base excision repair by homodimerization and heterodimerization with PARP1. Thus both PARP1 and PARP2 play critical roles in the maintenance of genomic stability by regulating DNA repair mechanisms.

It has recently been demonstrated that *BRCA1* and *BRCA2* familial breast cancers are highly sensitive to inhibitors of PARP1, and PARP1 inhibitors reduce repair of both single-strand breaks and double-strand breaks in *BRCA*-mutated tumors, resulting in increased sensitivity to DNA-damaging agents such as cisplatin. In normal cells heterozygous for *BRCA,* the wild-type *BRCA* allele is active, and its protein product can repair double-strand breaks by error-free, homologous recombination. Thus treatment of *BRCA* mutation carriers with PARP inhibitors is expected to be highly specific for cancer cells and nontoxic to healthy tissues. Two PARP1 inhibitors are currently in clinical trials as monotherapy for women with *BRCA*-associated breast or ovarian cancer.

There is a growing body of evidence to suggest that the *BRCA1* pathway is also dysfunctional in sporadic basal subtype breast cancers. Using triple negativity as a surrogate for basal subtype, gene expression studies have also demonstrated that PARP1 is upregulated in triple-negative breast cancers. These observations led to a randomized multicenter phase II trial of the PARP1 inhibitor BSI-201 given in combination with gemcitabine-carboplatin in patients with triple-negative metastatic breast cancer. Promising results demonstrating both prolonged progression-free and overall survival compared with a gemcitabine-carboplatin regimen alone have prompted the initiation of a phase III trial for this patient group.

In addition to their role in DNA repair, PARP1 and PARP2 also play a role in organization of chromatin domains, modulation of transcription, and control of cell division. In combination with DNA-damaging agents—such as DNA-methylating drugs, topoisomerase I inhibitors, and radiation—these agents may prove to be a valuable addition to the limited therapies available for triple-negative breast cancers.

Topoisomerase II

Topoisomerases are enzymes that catalyze the transient breaking and rejoining of DNA strands, thereby regulating transcription. The topoisomerase II gene, *TOP2A,* is located at chromosome band 17q12-21, close to the *HER2/neu* gene; it is a target for various chemotherapeutic agents such as anthracyclines, which inhibit *TOP2A* by trapping the DNA strand break intermediates, leading to persistent DNA cleavage. *TOP2A* was first associated with response to anthracyclines as a result of the retrospective observation that overexpression or amplification of *HER2* is associated with increased sensitivity toward anthracycline-containing therapy. *TOP2A* aberrations (amplification, deletion) are found in 30% to 90% of *HER2*-amplified breast cancer, with amplifications being more common than deletions; however, no correlation has been found between amplification and overexpression. Good response to anthracyclines is associated with *TOP2A* amplification, and deletion has been associated with a poor prognosis; however, study results are not uniform, and clarification of the mechanism of this effect requires additional study.

FUTURE DIRECTIONS

MicroRNAs

MicroRNAs (miRNAs) are a newly discovered class of non–protein-coding RNAs, 18 to 25 nucleotides in length, that modulate gene expression by targeting mRNAs for translational suppression or mRNA cleavage. MicroRNAs play a key role in the regulation of fundamental processes such as differentiation, proliferation, apoptosis, and metabolic homeostasis. With the advent of high-throughput technology for global measurement of microRNAs, these regulatory molecules are now emerging as a new class of cancer biomarkers, and a growing body of evidence suggests that miRNAs may play a role in breast tumorigenesis. Depending on whether miRNAs target tumor suppressor genes or oncogenes, they can act as oncogenes or tumor suppressors. Both normal and malignant tissues have been shown to have specific microRNA signatures, and microRNAs show differential expression across tumor types, with associations along lines of tissue development. Interestingly, miRNAs remain stable and retain reliable expression profiles when investigated in archival formalin-fixed, paraffin-embedded samples, providing an opportunity for use in routine diagnostic pathology. Ultimately, miRNAs may be used to classify breast cancers and predict prognosis, as well as to provide novel therapeutic targets for personalized treatment.

DNA Methylation

DNA methylation is an epigenetic modification that contributes to breast cancer progression by transcriptionally silencing certain tumor-suppressor genes. Although cancer cells exhibit global genome *hypo*methylation, aberrant cytosine *hyper*methylation occurs at discreet 5′-CG-3′ (CpG) dinucleotides, generally located in clusters termed *CpG islands,* which are often associated with the 5′ region of structural genes. How specific genes are targeted for CpG hypermethylation and consequential silencing during the process of tumorigenesis is not well understood; however, it is becoming increasingly clear that epigenetic silencing stems from a complex set of biochemical modifications that transform chromatin from a transcriptionally active to an inactive state.

Although epigenomic analysis has identified gene methylation profiles associated with molecular subtypes of breast cancer based on HR status, HER2 status, or both, it has proved limited in distinguishing between histologic subtypes of established invasive disease. Perhaps more promising is a subset of tumor-suppressor genes that are methylated in proliferative and in situ breast lesions, suggesting a role for epigenetic silencing in the initiation or progression of disease. Efforts to apply epigenetic analysis to cells collected from nipple aspirate fluid, ductal lavage, and fine needle aspiration are underway and may ultimately improve the diagnostic capabilities of these techniques. Patient blood samples are also being explored as a source of epigenetic biomarker detection with potential applications in cancer detection.

SUMMARY

Breast cancer is a complex disease caused by the progressive accumulation of multiple gene mutations combined with epigenetic dysregulation of critical genes and protein pathways. Recent advances in DNA microarray technology and other large-scale gene expression analyses have been adopted for both the biologic characterization and clinical management of breast cancer. The most successful examples of targeted therapy, endocrine therapy and trastuzumab, were realized after progress in cancer biology led to the characterization of ER and *HER2/neu.* Further understanding the molecular biology and genetic and epigenetic regulation of breast cancer is critical for identifying new biomarkers and novel therapeutic approaches. This is particularly important for women with triple-negative disease, for whom treatment options remain suboptimal and prognosis is poor.

SELECTED READINGS

Perou CM, Sorlie T, Eisen MB, et al: Molecular portraits of human breast tumours, *Nature* 406(6797):747–752, 2000.

Jordan VC: A century of deciphering the control mechanisms of sex steroid action in breast and prostate cancer: the origins of targeted therapy and chemoprevention, *Cancer Res 15;* 69(4):1243–1254, 2009.

Browne BC, O'Brien N, Duffy MJ, et al: HER-2 signaling and inhibition in breast cancer, *Curr Cancer Drug Targets* 9(3):419–438, 2009.

Dowsett M, Dunbier AK: Emerging biomarkers and new understanding of traditional markers in personalized therapy for breast cancer, *Clin Cancer Res* 14(24):8019–8026, 2008.

Breast Cancer: Surgical Therapy

Theodore N. Tsangaris, MD

OVERVIEW

As breast cancer care moves into the second decade of the twenty-first century, much has changed regarding diagnosis, staging, and treatment. However, in the multidisciplinary approach to breast cancer care, the surgeon remains the pivotal individual in orchestrating and delivering care to the patient.

PREOPERATIVE EVALUATION

The surgeon may or may not be the first person to see the woman with a breast problem, so it is imperative that the surgeon be able to come to an evaluation of the problem quickly and accurately. The basic workup for any problem includes a good history, clinical exam, and a diagnostic bilateral mammogram. Digital mammography provides many advantages over traditional film-screen images, and ultrasound and magnetic resonance imaging (MRI) continue to be important supplemental studies, particularly for the difficult breast. Nipple aspiration, duct lavage, and ductoscopy continue to be promising research tools.

Breast biopsy should be preformed by core or fine needle aspiration (FNA). Both can be performed in the office or clinic, however, FNA requires an experienced cytologist. Preoperative FNA of suspicious lymph nodes in the ipsilateral axilla seen on ultrasound is becoming more widespread. Core biopsy is the diagnostic procedure of choice for clinical or mammographically detected masses or mammographic calcifications because of the histologic information it provides, and because the specimen is suitable for prognostic assays. Because core biopsy and FNA preserve breast integrity, they are preferred over excisional biopsy and should be considered the standard of care for tissue diagnosis. Excisional biopsy should be considered only in situations in which core biopsy is unsuccessful in obtaining sufficient tissue, or if there is discordance between the clinical or mammographic findings from core biopsy. In fact, incisional biopsy should almost never be performed.

Workup

The extensive metastatic workup for the newly diagnosed breast cancer patient should be avoided, and it is not appropriate for most early stage breast cancer patients. A good oral history, physical exam, and appropriate age-related preoperative studies should suffice for most of these individuals. Clinical evidence of locally advanced or systemic disease or pathologic confirmation of positive lymph nodes should initiate appropriate testing.

INVASIVE BREAST CANCER

The surgical treatment of invasive breast cancer is much less controversial than the treatment of noninvasive disease. This is not to imply that defining an appropriate surgical treatment is not emotionally and intellectually challenging. Most early-stage breast cancers should be treated with breast conservation, lumpectomy, and radiation therapy.

Because of local recurrence concerns, rare is the individual with invasive breast cancer who is appropriately treated with lumpectomy alone. Exceptions would include individuals over the age of 70 years with estrogen-receptor–positive breast cancers. Relative contraindications to breast conservation include 1) large breast cancer relative to a small breast size, 2) inability to undergo radiation therapy, and 3) multicentric disease. The validity of breast conservation for the treatment of invasive breast cancer is well documented in the National Surgical Adjuvant Breast and Bowel Project (NSABP) B-06 and the many other similar and subsequent trials with extensive follow-up (Figure 1).

SURGICAL TECHNIQUE

Lumpectomy

For those patients who meet the criteria for breast conservation, the basic principles of lumpectomy are well defined. First, the incision should be placed directly over the site of the tumor and in most situations should be curvilinear in nature to reflect the skin tension lines of the breast. Radial scars may be used for tumors located in the medial or infraareolar aspects of the breast. Tunneling to the tumor should be discouraged. Accurate placement of the incision facilitates radiation therapy and short- and long-term follow-up, and it ultimately provides the best cosmetic result.

Excision of the tumor with adequate margins and preservation of cosmetic integrity are the primary goals of the surgeon performing lumpectomy. Hopkins defines minimally adequate margins as 2 to 3 mm of microscopically free tissue. Specimens should be handled carefully in the operating room so that the integrity and orientation of the specimen are maintained, and it is unacceptable practice to omit orientation of an excised specimen. I use a 2-point orientation system with suture; the pathologist is then able to use colored ink to designate the margins. I empirically take additional tissue from the tumor cavity, incorporating all margins that are submitted separately to the pathologist. This practice provides the pathologist with margin tissue that is not subject to crush artifact or dye irregularities. I have therefore been able to reduce reexcision rates significantly.

Before closure of the wound, microclips are placed to delineate the tumor cavity. This facilitates identification of the tumor bed radiographically for the radiation oncologist and the mammographer. Reapproximating breast tissue or the placement of drains to close dead space is usually undesirable. The closure I use consists of a two-layer skin closure, and the breast tissue is allowed to reapproximate naturally.

Mastectomy

The mastectomy is making a comeback of sorts. With the increased use of genetic testing and magnetic resonance imaging (MRI), more women are personally questioning breast conservation as an acceptable option. With the increased utilization of skin-sparing and nipple-sparing mastectomy, coupled with numerous reconstructive options, more women than ever are choosing ipsilateral and bilateral mastectomy.

When performing a mastectomy, oncologic and cosmetic principles should be considered simultaneously. It should be stressed again that the practice of core biopsy for diagnosis facilitates a superior cosmetic outcome in all mastectomies. Care should be taken to preserve the viability of the skin flaps, and the thickness of the flaps should be carefully considered. Remembering that skin, subcutaneous tissue, and fascia exist superficial to the glandular tissue, the flap thickness should reflect the breast size, body habitus, and weight of the patient. We dissect superficial to the fascial layer anteriorly and include the pectoralis fascia posteriorly with our dissection.

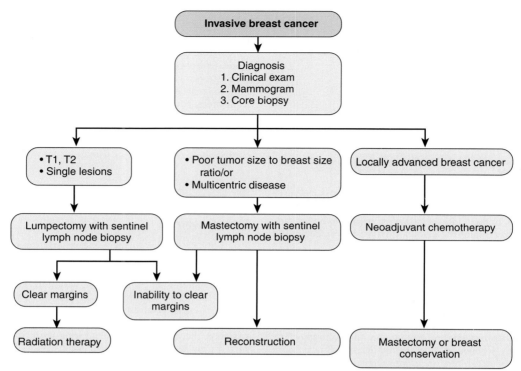

FIGURE I Algorithm for treatment of invasive breast disease.

It is important to respect the anatomic boundaries of the breast and in particular to not try to violate the inframammary fold, which adds little to the cancer operation but compromises the cosmetic outcome.

Nipple-Sparing Mastectomy

The evolution of the mastectomy procedure has brought us to the threshold of using another form of cosmetic enhancement, the nipple-sparing mastectomy (NSM). It should be noted that the nipple-sparing mastectomy is essentially the same operation as the subcutaneous mastectomy. A nipple-sparing mastectomy with reconstruction may alter the perceived loss to the patient while still providing an oncologically safe mastectomy that achieves a good cosmetic result (Figure 2).

The nipple-sparing mastectomy is essentially a skin-sparing mastectomy (SSM) with retention of the nipple areolar complex (NAC). The literature concerning the safety of SSM shows that the incidence of local recurrence is similar to conventional mastectomy, and after SSM it is most likely a manifestation of the tumor biology rather than preservation of the skin. Furthermore, local recurrence of breast cancer after SSM is not associated with systemic relapse. Similarly, NSM appears to be safe in selected patients in our series at Johns Hopkins. Our data also suggest that local and systemic recurrence after NSM are also secondary to tumor biology rather than preservation of the NAC.

Our current surgical technique for NSM is to remove the breast tissue through a lateral radial incision measuring 4 to 6 cm in length that is at least 2 cm from the edge of the areola. This incision may be extended medially above or below the NAC to access the internal mammary vessels for autologous free-flap anastomosis. A lateral inframammary fold incision may also be employed for the small- to medium-sized breast. Standard anatomic mastectomy borders are utilized. To assess the NAC base for tumor on permanent histologic evaluation, the NAC is inverted through the incision, and a thin slice of tissue is removed from the base to establish a true margin.

This ensures viability of the NAC while obtaining an adequate tissue sample.

We do not advocate coring out the nipple duct bundle. Evidence suggests that breast cancer originates in the terminal duct lobular unit (TDLU), and only 9% of nipples contain TDLU. Additionally, coring out the nipple duct could disrupt the vasculature, increasing nipple necrosis and diminishing cosmetic results. The sentinel node is obtained through a separate axillary incision in the usual standard fashion and is routinely done prior to the mastectomy. Immediate reconstruction ensues, either with an autologous free flap, tissue expander, or implant.

Our retrospective results, and those reported elsewhere in the literature, suggest that NAC preservation may be oncologically safe in patients with defined clinical and pathologic criteria. We propose the following criteria for NSM: tumors 4.5 cm in size or smaller, tumors located 2.5 cm or more from the areolar edge or 4 cm or more from the nipple center, and no gross involvement of the NAC, including bloody nipple discharge or Paget disease. The tumor-to-nipple or tumor-to-areolar distance is assessed clinically if possible and/or mammographically, with ultrasound, or with MRI to obtain precise distance. Tumors that are multicentric, mutifocal, or those that contain extensive ductal carcinoma in situ (DCIS) and otherwise meet the stated criteria can be included. Women who have undergone neoadjuvant therapy and subsequently meet the criteria for tumor size and location can also be considered, but inflammatory breast cancer is absolutely excluded.

Further studies at Johns Hopkins and other institutions are needed to further clarify the validity of our current criteria for NSM, long-term oncologic outcomes, and cosmetic and body image evaluation and satisfaction.

Reconstruction

At our institution, all patients who meet the requirements for mastectomy are considered for immediate reconstruction. Often this is just a temporizing tissue expander, but it starts the reconstructive

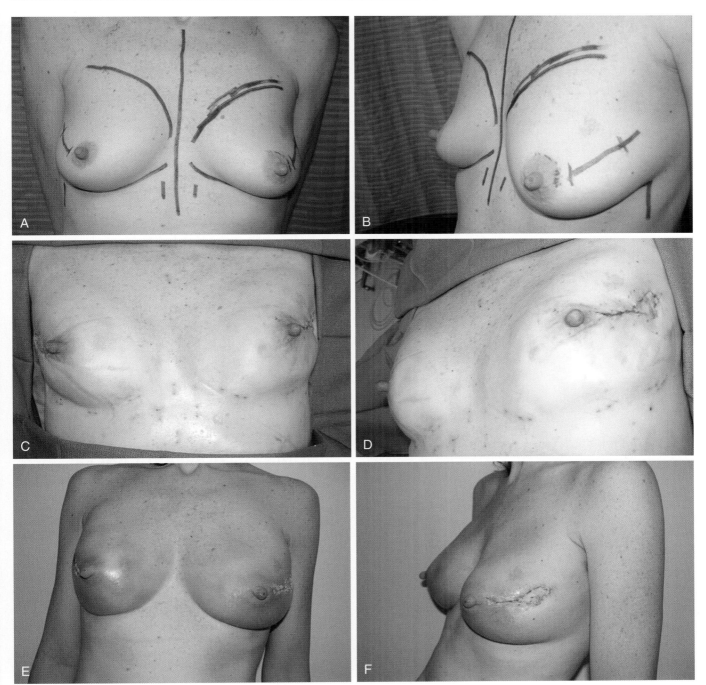

FIGURE 2 Nipple-sparing mastectomy.

process that all women deserve. Implants and autologous tissue transfers are the mainstay of breast reconstruction. Among autologous tissue transfers, utilization of the more technically demanding deep inferior epigastric perforator (DIEP) flap is preferred over its less sophisticated cousin, the transverse rectus abdominis muscle (TRAM) flap, as it provides superior cosmesis with limited abdominal wall morbidity. Ultimately the type of reconstruction should be based on the cosmetic and physiologic needs of the patient. Oncologic considerations should have little impact on the decision of the plastic surgeon except in those situations of locally advanced disease in which postmastectomy radiation will be used. Those with locally advanced disease should initially have a tissue expander placed until all treatments for the cancer have been completed.

THE AXILLA

Axillary sampling should be performed in most cases of invasive disease, and sentinel lymph node biopsy is the standard of care for determining the status of the ipsilateral axilla. In the absence of clinically worrisome lymph nodes, most women with stage I and II breast cancer should be considered for sentinel lymph node biopsy. Two methods are used today: one uses a vital dye injected into the breast, and the other uses a radioactive isotope. Individually or in combination, they share the same goal: to identify the sentinel lymph node. The surgeon's familiarity, experience, and confidence with a sentinel lymph node biopsy technique are more important than the method used.

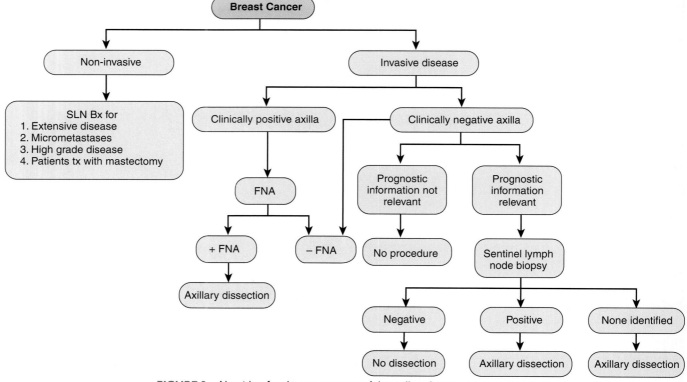

FIGURE 3 Algorithm for the management of the axilla in breast cancer patients.

In the vital blue dye technique, 5 mL of isosulfan blue dye are injected in the subareolar parenchyma of the ipsilateral breast, followed by 5 to 7 minutes of breast massage. The exact interval between injection and incision is somewhat variable. Large, dense breasts and breasts with recent surgeries may require longer times for the dye to travel. A standard axillary incision is made just beneath the hairline, and dissection is carried down to and through the clavipectoral fascia.

Recognizing a blue lymphatic or blue-tinged lymph node is the first objective. The lymphatic should be followed both proximally and distally to determine which lymph node is the most proximal. That lymph node should be harvested along with any intimately associated lymph nodes to ensure the accuracy of the procedure.

It is our practice to perform an intraoperative histologic examination of the sentinel lymph node. We have had excellent success with this approach with only a 5% to 6% discordance rate between frozen section and permanent section. Our sentinel lymph nodes are analyzed with standard hematoxylin and eosin (H&E) staining. The wound after a sentinel lymph node biopsy is closed primarily without a drain.

An axillary dissection should be performed for a positive sentinel lymph node or clinically suspicious axilla (Figure 3). A dissection limited to level I would seem justified in most cases, as there is a diminishing return on lymph nodes obtained and an increased morbidity when the surgeon moves into level II and level III. The boundaries of a level I dissection are as follows: anterior, clavipectoral fascia; posterior, subscapularis muscle; inferior, axillary tail (upper outer breast tissue); superior, just below the axillary vein; medially, lateral edge of pectoralis major; and laterally, anterior border of the latissimus dorsi muscle. Care should be taken so that the axillary vein is not skeletonized, as this only increases the risk for lymphedema. Care should also be taken to identify and preserve the long thoracic and thoracodorsal nerves, and the intercostal nerves may also be preserved when feasible. Drains are employed after axillary dissection through a separate stab incision, and the wound is closed primarily.

NONINVASIVE BREAST CANCER

Ductal carcinoma in situ (DCIS) remains a challenge for breast surgeons and patients alike. Controversies regarding biologic behavior, correct local control modalities, and even its legitimacy to be classified as a true cancer fuel the uncertainties. This brief discussion is founded on an acknowledgement of DCIS as a preinvasive cancer that is a highly curable local disease, which requires appropriate local therapy. Breast conservation with or without radiation therapy is the standard of care for most individuals. At our institution, we find that lumpectomy with radiation is appropriate for the majority of our patients. However, women with minimal disease and adequate margins may be offered lumpectomy alone in a clinical trial or off protocol. As it is with invasive breast cancer, women with extensive disease or diffuse calcification relative to a small breast or multicentric disease are offered mastectomy with immediate reconstruction.

Standard external beam radiation is currently the treatment of choice for those receiving radiation therapy after lumpectomy. Shorter courses of radiation based on the Canadian model are being utilized with more frequency, but partial breast radiation should still be considered investigational (Figure 4).

The incidence of positive nodes in DCIS is 1% to 3%, implying undiagnosed invasive disease. At our institution, we perform sentinel lymph node (SLN) biopsy in some DCIS patients. Our indications for employing this technique include 1) extensive disease with core biopsy diagnosis, 2) high-grade disease with or without a comedo component, 3) evidence or suggestion of microinvasion, 4) disease in the subareolar area or upper outer quadrant, and 5) treatment with mastectomy.

Adjuvant therapy for noninvasive breast cancer currently consists of hormonal therapy, specifically tamoxifen. The NSABP-B24 study suggests that for ER-positive noninvasive breast cancer, tamoxifen after lumpectomy and radiation will further reduce the rates of ipsilateral local recurrence and first-time events in the contralateral breast.

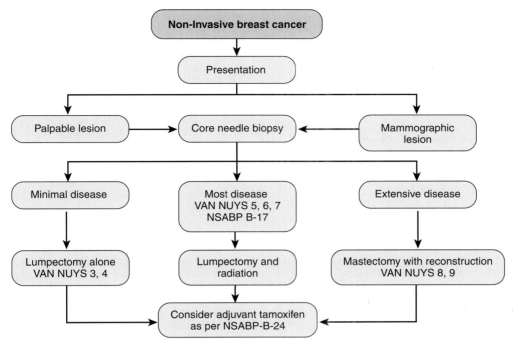

FIGURE 4   Algorithm for treatment of noninvasive disease.

ADJUVANT THERAPIES

Systemic adjuvant therapy should be considered for all women with invasive breast cancer. This might include chemotherapy, targeted therapy, hormone therapy, or various combinations of these. In addition to the patient's age, menopausal status, and general health condition, tumor prognostic factors are taken into consideration. These include tumor size, lymph node status, histologic grade, estrogen and progesterone receptor status, Ki67, and HER2/neu. Neoadjuvant therapy continues to be explored and utilized, especially for locally advanced breast cancers.

Radiation therapy should be considered standard of care for most invasive and noninvasive breast cancers treated with lumpectomy. Standard radiation therapy consists of 6 weeks of external whole-breast radiation with a boost to the tumor bed. New treatment regimens such as partial breast and accelerated radiation therapy are promising and should be conducted in a protocol setting. Postmastectomy radiation is still controversial but is finding greater utilization for tumors of a certain size and with nodal positivity.

PREVENTION

The NSABP-P1 and -P2 trials have shown that tamoxifen and raloxifene decrease the incidence of cancer in high-risk patients, which includes women who are *BRCA1* and *BRCA2* positive or those who have strong family histories. Women with the diagnosis of lobular carcinoma in situ or atypical ductal hyperplasia could also benefit from chemoprevention.

Prophylactic mastectomies are very effective in reducing the risk for breast cancer. Because of the extensive reconstructive options and the increased utilization of cosmetically friendly mastectomies, surgical prevention is an attractive option for many women. Open discussions between the patient at high risk and her breast health team should occur before this approach is initiated.

SUMMARY

The surgeon who treats breast cancer patients continues to work in the ever-changing landscape of a multidisciplinary approach. Even as old procedures, like the mastectomy, get facelifts and are rediscovered, some things remain constant. The surgeon's role in diagnosis, treatment, and management of breast cancer remains vitally important.

SUGGESTED READINGS

Bevers T, Anderson BO, Bonaccio E, et al: NCCN Clinical practice guidelines in oncology: breast cancer screening and diagnosis, *J Natl Compr Canc Netw* 7(10):1060–1096, 2009.

Zellars R, Stearns V, Frassica D, et al: Feasibility trial of partial breast irradiation and concurrent dose-dense doxorubicin and cyclophosphauride in early stage breast cancer, *J Clin Oncol* 27(17):2816–2822, 2009.

Voltura A, Tsangaris TN, Rosson GD, et al: Nipple-sparing mastectomy: critical assessment of 51 procedures and implications for selection criteria, *Ann Surg Oncol* 15(12):3396–3401, 2008.

Cao D, Lin C, Woo S, et al: Separate cavity margin sampling at the time of initial breast lumpectomy significantly reduces the need for reexcisions, *Am J Surg Pathol* 29:1625–1632, 2005.

Ablative Therapies in Benign and Malignant Breast Disease

Stefan S. Kachala, MD, and Rache M. Simmons, MD

OVERVIEW

Current strategies in the surgical treatment of breast cancer include resection of tumor while conserving breast tissue for optimal cosmesis. Lumpectomy, however, can necessitate multiple resections to obtain negative margins. Excision of significant breast volume can deform the breast, which is clearly contrary to the goals of breast-conservation surgery (BCS). Almost 50% of new breast cancer cases annually are stage I; thus, investigators are driven to evaluate new procedures that destroy cancer tissue, are well tolerated without extensive anesthesia, and provide excellent cosmesis.

Ablation has been employed in the treatment of lung and hepatic tumors, and percutaneous ablative techniques have great potential in their application to breast neoplasms. Several approaches to percutaneous ablation are currently under investigation, which include interstitial laser ablation (ILA), radiofrequency ablation (RFA), and cryoablation. The success of these methods holds the promise of office-based treatment with minimal anesthetic needs, less burden on operating rooms, decreased patient recovery times, and lower overall costs and complications.

Certain procedural prerequisites must be fulfilled prior to using any ablative technique. The surgeon must obtain a definitive biopsy, usually a large-core needle biopsy (LCNB), to provide pathologic concordance with imaging modalities. In addition, for malignant neoplasms, the biopsy will determine the presence of estrogen and progesterone receptors, *HER-2/neu*, and tumor grade. The neoplasm should be visualized in real time or by stereotactic images to effectively apply the ablative field and encompass the target lesion.

CRYOABLATION

Cryoablation uses argon gas to freeze and destroy tumor cells (Figure 1). The distribution of necrosis is uniform and symmetric around the cryoprobe. The mass is identified using ultrasound (US), and the path of cryoprobe entry from the skin to the mass is numbed using local anesthetic. The cryoprobe is guided via US and placed through the long axis of the target lesion (Figure 2).

The cryoprobe is insulated along its length except for 4 cm at its tip, which makes the maximum diameter of the freeze zone 4 cm. If the lesion is adjacent to skin, there are two methods of protecting the skin from cryopathic burn. Using US guidance, saline is injected subcutaneously to distance skin from the cryogenic zone. Alternatively, the skin is warmed with room temperature saline applied directly to the epidermis continually throughout the procedure.

When the gas is flowing during the freeze cycle, the target lesion is visualized in real time using US. The cryogenic zone is hypoechoic with a hyperechoic interface between frozen and unfrozen tissue (Figure 3). This allows for precise delineation of the margin of cryoablation, ensuring that the tumor is within the cryogenic zone. The patient is awake and alert during the procedure, and because extreme cold anesthetizes breast tissue, no further local or regional anesthesia is required; thus the procedure can be performed in an office setting. Typically two cycles of freeze and thaw are undertaken with removal of the probe after the second thaw cycle.

Cryoablation is currently FDA approved for treatment of breast fibroadenomas. The fibroadenoma cryoablation treatment (FACT) registry represents data on 444 treated fibroadenomas collected across 55 practice settings. In a report of interim results, follow-up at 1 year revealed that 35% reported palpability of the mass and 29% of cryoablated fibroadenomas remained visible on US. Kaufman and colleagues (2005) have reported on long-term follow-up of office-based cryoablation of fibroadenomas. Most patients reported complete resorption of their original mass. This reporting correlated with fibroadenoma size, with 94% of small (<2 cm) and 73% of large (>2 cm) fibroadenomas nonpalpable at follow-up. Median volume reduction was 99% when assessed with US and in most patients was indistinguishable from normal breast tissue. For patients who had mammograms performed, there was no artifact from cryoablation that would impair mammogram interpretation.

With the successful implementation of cryoablation for benign breast disease, several trials have begun to examine the role of cryoablation in breast cancer. Given the maximum diameter of the cryogenic zone of 4 cm, cryoablation appears to be optimally applied to lesions less than 2 cm in diameter. Table 1 lists the results of several clinical trials of cryoablation in breast cancer and their results. Of note is the absence of complications. Initial studies have identified the keys to successful cryoablation to include optimizing cryoprobe design and application, duration of freeze and thaw cycles, methods of protecting skin from cold injury, and use of US guidance. A pilot study by Sabel and colleagues (2004) confirmed the safety and efficacy of cryoablation for small invasive breast cancer and elucidated factors that precluded complete ablation of disease. They report that given current cryoprobe design, cryoablation was successful in tumors less than 1.5 cm without an extensive intraductal component.

Ablative therapy relies upon accurate assessment of disease by imaging and aggregate LCNB. Invasive lobular and colloid carcinomas are poorly defined by mammogram and US. In the 2004 study, three of five patients with invasive lobular or colloid carcinoma had residual disease after cryoablation, likely secondary to underestimation of disease from their preoperative assessment.

Other investigations of cryoablation have revealed that DCIS may be more difficult to identify on preoperative imaging by mammogram and US. This is consistent with Sabel and colleagues' results, where patients with an extensive DCIS component were not free of disease after cryoablation. These data have led to the efficient design of the American College of Surgeons Oncology Group (ACOSOG) Z1072 phase II clinical trial. In this trial patients are eligible who have unifocal invasive ductal carcinomas measuring 2 cm or less. All patients are evaluated before and after cryoablation with breast magnetic resonance imaging (MRI), which may prove more accurate in assessing appropriate eligibility and success of cryoablation. In this trial patients will undergo surgical resection of the cancer after cryoablation to evaluate the pathologic effectiveness of the cryoablation.

The biology of cryoablation is also an area of investigation. Compared with thermal ablation, cryoablation preserves tumor proteins and tumor-associated antigens within an inflammatory environment that can foster an antitumor immune response. There is anecdotal evidence of regression of distant disease after cryoablation of primary breast cancer, and animal studies have confirmed a T-cell response directed against tumor cells afterward. Preclinical animal models have attributed this immune response as precluding the reengraftment of tumor cells after cryoablation. Given the success of immunotherapy for other solid malignancies, these preclinical studies may lead to protocols for adjuvant adoptive cellular immunotherapy for breast cancer.

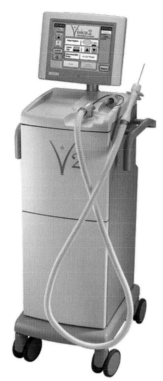

FIGURE 1   An argon-based cryoablation system. *(Courtesy Sanarus Technologies LLC, Pleasanton, Calif.)*

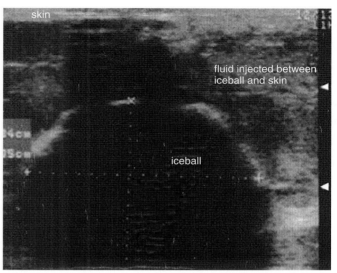

FIGURE 3   Ultrasound image of hypoechoic ice ball and protective saline injection. *(From Kaufman C, Bachman B, Littrup P, et al: Office-based ultrasound-guided cryoablation of breast fibroadenomas, Am J Surg 184[5]:394–400, 2002. Reprinted with permission.)*

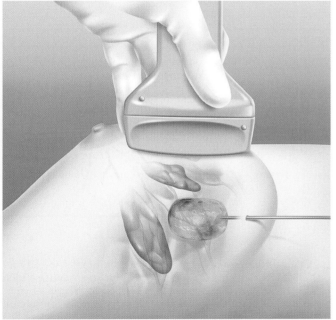

FIGURE 2   Ultrasound is used to monitor the developing cryogenic zone from the cryoprobe. *(From Kaufman C, Littrup P, Freman-Gibb L, et al: Office-based cryoablation of breast fibroadenomas: 12 month follow-up, J Am Coll Surg 198[6]:914–923, 2004.)*

RADIOFREQUENCY ABLATION

Radiofrequency ablation (RFA) is the application of thermal energy from a metallic multiarray probe that is generated by high-frequency alternating electric currents that create electromagnetic waves that agitate ions in adjacent tissue. The result is intense heat, which produces coagulation and denaturation of cellular proteins, leading to necrosis. The amount of energy transduced through the probe is gradually increased to a set level that allows for maximum tissue death within the target lesion.

RFA is currently approved for the treatment of unresectable tumors and is under investigation for its application in malignant disease of the breast. For treatment of lesions of the breast, local anesthesia and intravenous sedation are required for RFA. A grounding pad is placed on the patient's skin to prevent electric shock. There must be a minimum distance of 1 cm from the outer limit of the ablation zone to the skin to minimize the risk of thermal injury. Some studies also advocate the use of 5% glucose in water injected subcutaneously to increase the distance from the thermal zone to the skin; this solution of glucose is highly resistant to heating by RFA due to its high impedance.

The probe is introduced through the tumor using US guidance; the power is gradually increased, and the thermal zone is monitored with US. As the temperature of the tissue increases, the US will display a hyperechoic region. This provides a method of monitoring RFA to ensure that the tumor is within the ablative zone. Doppler US has been observed to be useful in determining tissue destruction with RFA, especially in hypervascularized tumors. When the tissue is completely ablated, the power delivered will drop, and impedance will rise rapidly. These parameters are monitored continuously during the procedure by the RFA device.

RFA in invasive breast cancer has been under intense study, as investigators seek to reproduce its successes in lung and hepatic tumors. Early phase I studies (Table 2) have delineated the safety and efficacy of RFA in breast cancer. Trials performed by Izzo and colleagues (2001) and at M.D. Anderson Cancer Center (MDACC) observed almost complete ablation of all tumors (Fornage, 2004). Izzo and colleagues accrued 26 patients, and histologic examination of the excised lesions after ablation revealed complete ablation of the index lesion in 96% of patients. MDACC reported complete ablation of the US-identified target lesion in all 21 patients. These encouraging results were accompanied by few complications and technical difficulties. Izzo reported one patient who sustained a full-thickness skin burn, which was excised at surgery. MDACC reported no thermal skin injuries, but one patient who had received neoadjuvant chemotherapy required redeployment of the RFA probe. This second attempt achieved complete ablation within the US target lesion,

TABLE 1: Trials of cryoablation in breast cancer

Trial	Tumor Size	N	Treatment	Results
Stocks et al. (2002)	IBC 7–22 mm; mean, 13 mm	11	Cryo → BCS	90% (10/11) complete ablation of index lesion
Pfleiderer et al. (2002)	IBC 9–40 mm; mean, 21 mm	16	Cryo → BCS or mastectomy	31% (5/16) without evidence of disease
Roubidoux et al. (2004)	IBC 8–18 mm; mean, 12 mm	9	Cryo → BCS	78% (7/9) without evidence of disease
Morin et al. (2004) (using MRI)	IBC 12–60 mm; mean, 29.8 mm	25	MR-guided cryo → partial or total mastectomy	52% (13/25) without evidence of disease 100% NED within cryozone
Sabel et al. (2004)	IBC 6–20 mm; mean, 12.2 mm	27	Cryo → BCS or mastectomy	85% (23/27) without viable tumor cells

IBC, Invasive breast cancer; *Cryo*, cryoablation; *BCS*, breast conservation surgery; *MR*, magnetic resonance; *NED*, no evidence of disease

TABLE 2: Trials of RFA in breast cancer

Trial	Tumor Size	N	Treatment	Results
Izzo et al. (2001)	IBC 7–30 mm; mean, 18 mm	26	RFA → partial or complete mastectomy	96% (25/26) complete ablation of index lesion 1 patient with full-thickness burn
Burak et al. (2003)	IBC 8–16 mm; mean, 12 mm	10	RFA → partial or complete mastectomy	90% (9/10) complete ablation of index lesion
Hayashi et al. (2003)	IBC 5–26 mm; median, 9 mm	22	RFA → partial or complete mastectomy	86% (19/22) complete ablation of index lesion
Fornage et al. (2004)	IBC 6–20 mm; mean, 12 mm	21	RFA → partial or complete mastectomy	100% complete ablation of index lesion
Khatri et al. (2007)	IBC 8–15 mm; mean, 12.8 mm	15	RFA → BCS or mastectomy	86% (13/15) complete ablation of index lesion 2 patients with skin burn
Oura et al. (2007)*	IBC 5–20 mm; mean 13 mm	52	RFA with XRT and chemo	100% complete ablation of index lesion 1 patient with full-thickness burn
Medina-Franco et al. (2008)	IBC 9–38 mm; mean 20.8 mm	25	RFA → BCS or mastectomy	76% (19/25) complete ablation of index lesion 3 patients with skin burn
Garbay et al. (2008)	IBC 10–22 mm; mean, 14 mm	10	RFA → mastectomy	60% (6/10) complete ablation of index lesion; trial stopped due to poor efficacy
Imoto et al. (2009)	IBC 9–24 mm; median 17 mm	30	RFA → partial mastectomy	92% (24/26) complete ablation of index lesion 2 patients with skin burn 7 patients with burn to pectoralis major

*Tumor assessed postprocedurally with LCNB and MRI.
XRT, Radiation therapy; *chemo*, chemotherapy

but histopathologic examination revealed extensive US and mammographically occult invasive carcinoma beyond the ablated target lesion. This corresponds with other percutaneous modalities that rely on imaging to identify the extent of the malignant lesion.

Oura and colleagues (2007) undertook the most progressive clinical trial of RFA to date. They enrolled 52 patients with a mean tumor size of 13 mm and performed percutaneous RFA under general anesthesia. The tumors were not resected after ablation. Instead, all patients underwent US-guided LCNB for cytological assessment and MRI, and they received 50 Gy radiation therapy and chemotherapy as appropriate. While LCNB is not equivalent to surgical excision for assessment of histopathology, they reported complete absence of viable tumor cells. Furthermore, postoperative MRI confirmed the absence of residual tumor. During a mean follow-up of 15 months (range, 6 to 30 months), 100% of patients were free of recurrent disease.

Although this encouraging study reports a large cohort of successfully treated patients, there are several criticisms. Administration of RFA under general anesthesia does not benefit the patient compared with the percutaneous approach, and the absence of a surgical resection hinders the assessment of the therapeutic efficacy of this method. And even though the patients' tumors in this study were imaged with US, mammography, and MRI, occult lesions may still be present. Finally, the short follow-up does not provide a meaningful determination as to the rate of local recurrence. In spite of these criticisms, this remains an important study with significant results and only one reported complication (skin burn).

More recent studies have had their difficulties. Medina-Franco (2008) enrolled 25 patients and reported a rate of 76% complete target lesion ablation as revealed by histopathology. This is likely due to the large range of tumors that were treated in the study, which also reported three patients with minor skin burn. Garbay and colleagues

TABLE 3: Selection of clinical trials of laser ablative therapy in breast cancer

Trial	Tumor Size	N	Treatment	Results
Dowlatshahi et al. (2000)	IBC 10–27 mm; mean, 18 mm	34	ILA → BCS or mastectomy	70% (24/34) complete necrosis of target lesion
Dowlatshahi et al. (2002)	IBC 5–23 mm; median, 13 mm	54	ILA → BCS	70% (38/54) complete necrosis of target lesion
Haraldsdóttir et al. (2008)	IBC 7–55 mm; mean, 23	24	ILA → BCS or mastectomy	12% (3/24) complete necrosis of target lesion
van Esser et al. (2009)	IBC 8–37 mm; mean, 17	14	LITT → BCS or mastectomy	50% (7/14) complete necrosis of target lesion

BCS, Breast conservation surgery; *IBC*, inflammatory breast cancer; *ILA*, interstitial laser ablation; *LITT*, laser interstitial thermal therapy

in 2008 reported a phase II clinical trial of RFA in recurrent breast cancer that was aborted after accrual of 10 patients secondary to poor efficacy. Only 60% of target lesions were completely ablated from the procedure. Garbay concluded that RFA was not sufficiently effective for treatment of recurrent breast cancer.

In 2009, Imoto reported a successful study of RFA in clinical stage I breast cancer patients. However, with an enrollment of 30 patients, they reported a complication rate of 30%, adverse events in nine patients, two patients sustained skin burn (one with severe necrosis of the nipple-areolar region). In addition, seven patients had burns to the pectoralis major muscle, and one patient required prolonged anti-inflammatory therapy to control severe chest wall pain. This study and others highlight that although RFA is a promising modality for percutaneous ablation of primary breast cancer, standardization of the approach is necessary for uniform therapy and patient safety.

INTERSTITIAL LASER ABLATION

Interstitial laser ablation (ILA) uses a fiber-optic probe to apply the photodynamic therapy from within the target lesion. Anesthesia requirements are typically field-block infiltration of local anesthetics along the probe tract and peritumorally with intravenous sedation. General anesthesia is unnecessary. The laser probe is a fiberoptic wire that only releases its energy at its exposed, 2 to 3 cm end. One or several probes are placed into the target lesion under US guidance or stereotactically using mammogram or MRI.

When ILA is used with US guidance, a release of air bubbles permeates the target. This is thought to be secondary to the tendency of the laser to vaporize target tissues and can obscure the surgeon's view, increasing the difficulty in monitoring the ablation zone. Some investigators have used a contrast-enhanced Doppler US to observe cessation of tumor blood flow, which can be a therapeutic end point for ILA. In addition, a temperature probe can be oriented several centimeters away from the ILA wire to monitor the energy delivery and ensure tissue necrosis. The amount of energy required for ILA therapy is calculated using the formula for a spherical volume ($V = 4/3\pi$ [radius]^3) and is delivered over time.

Several clinical trials (Table 3) have examined the use the laser ablative therapy in invasive breast cancer. Earlier studies by Dowlatshahi and colleagues (2000, 2002) reported a 70% success rate in complete ablation of target lesions. They attributed the incomplete ablation mainly to technical factors, such as inadequate delivery of energy and suboptimal target visualization. These elements can be

improved upon and minimized as the surgeon becomes more skilled with this technique. However, European groups have been unable to reproduce these results in their trials. Lund University Hospital of Sweden reported a dismal rate of only 12% complete tumor necrosis on histologic examination (Haraldsdóttir, 2008). In a trial from the University Medical Center of Utrecht in The Netherlands in 2009, led by van Esser, half of the tumors were completely ablated. The European groups used variants of the therapy employed by Dowlatshahi and colleagues; however, these results indicate that ILA and its variants require further standardization before application in a randomized controlled trial.

SUMMARY

There exist many forces driving surgery toward minimally invasive methods. Lower costs from decreased hospital stays and the feasibility of office-based procedures are attractive ways of decreasing health care spending. The promise of excellent cosmesis and decreased recovery time is appealing to patients, and percutaneous cryoablation, RFA, and ILA represent the future of early stage breast cancer therapy.

Advances in imaging will help overcome the pitfalls of occult disease, which can preclude effective therapy with these approaches. An already proven therapy for fibroadenomas, cryoablation is an excellent candidate for a randomized controlled trial to determine its role and effectiveness in the treatment of breast cancer. Its ease of use, minimal anesthesia requirements, and effective tumor ablation make it a practical alternative to breast conservation surgery if further studies confirm its efficacy.

SUGGESTED READINGS

Huston T, Simmons R: Ablative therapies for the treatment of malignant diseases of the breast, *Am J Surg* 189(6):694–701, 2005.

Kaufman C, Littrup P, Freeman-Gibb L, et al: Office-based cryoablation of breast fibroadenomas with long-term follow-up, *Breast J* 11(5):344–350, 2005.

Kontos M, Felekouras E, Fentiman IS: Radiofrequency ablation in the treatment of primary breast cancer: no surgical redundancies yet, *Int J Clin Pract* 62(5):816–820, 2008.

Sabel M, Kaufman C, Whitworth P, et al: Cryoablation of early-stage breast cancer: work-in-progress report of a multiinstitutional trial, *Ann Surg Oncol* 11(5):529–542, 2004.

Lymphatic Mapping and Sentinel Lymphadenectomy

Alice Chung, MD, and Armando E. Giuliano, MD

OVERVIEW

Patients with a diagnosis of invasive breast cancer require evaluation of the axillary lymph nodes for staging. Traditionally this was achieved by performing axillary lymph node dissection (ALND), which involves removal of level I and II axillary lymph nodes and level III nodes when those are grossly involved. This procedure has been associated with a risk of lymphedema, pain and paresthesias, and infection. As a result of screening mammography, 80% of breast cancers are discovered at an early stage, and only 25% to 30% will have lymph node involvement; only those with lymph node involvement are likely to receive any therapeutic value from ALND.

The sentinel node biopsy (SNB) was introduced as a less invasive means of evaluating the axilla with a much lower risk for the morbidities associated with ALND. This procedure has been validated in a number of large series and in randomized studies throughout the world, and it has become the standard of care for patients with clinically node-negative invasive breast cancer.

SNB is based on the concept that the lymphatics from the breast drain first to the "sentinel" nodes before draining into the more distal nodes. The concept was first introduced for penile carcinoma by Cabanas in 1977. In 1991, Morton and colleagues reported the SNB technique in melanoma, and Giuliano and colleagues began to apply this procedure to breast cancer patients. Multiple studies demonstrate that if the sentinel lymph node (SLN) is free of metastatic disease, the remaining lymph nodes in the axilla are usually tumor free, and additional ALND is not likely to be beneficial.

INDICATIONS AND PATIENT SELECTION

SNB is indicated in patients with clinically node-negative T1 to T3 invasive breast cancer. Initially, SNB was limited to patients with small, unicentric tumors because of concern that involvement of the lymph nodes in larger tumors might obstruct or alter the lymphatic drainage and lead to false-negative (FN) results. However, in several studies, the accuracy of SNB in T2 and T3 tumors has been shown to be comparable to that in T1 tumors. In addition, multicentric disease was considered a contraindication to this procedure in the past. However, a number of single-institutional reports and one multicenter validation study have demonstrated that SNB can be applied to patients with multicentric and multifocal breast cancer with acceptable FN rates.

In certain cases of ductal carcinoma in situ (DCIS), the SNB procedure can be helpful in identifying patients with microinvasion. It may also be helpful to do SNB in cases where there is suspicion that DCIS diagnosed by needle biopsy may be upstaged to invasive disease upon excision. Patients with palpable DCIS, high-grade DCIS, and extensive DCIS requiring mastectomy or suspicion of microinvasion have a reported incidence of SLN involvement ranging from 10% to 25%; therefore in these cases, SNB is recommended.

Controversy surrounds the appropriate timing of SNB in clinically node-negative patients undergoing neoadjuvant chemotherapy (NAC). Staging may be more definitive when SNB is performed before the potential downstaging effects of chemotherapy can occur. The data supporting SNB after NAC have demonstrated inferior SLN identification rates and higher FN rates, with reported mapping failure rates of 2.4% to 28% and FN rates ranging from 0% to 33%. This may be related to altered lymphatic patterns after chemotherapy and to the possibility that the effect of NAC on axillary metastases may not be uniform. Studies evaluating SNB before NAC consistently report FN rates of less than 5%.

Based on these data, we believe SNB should be performed prior to neoadjuvant chemotherapy in clinically node-negative patients. However, a recent study from M.D. Anderson Cancer Center performed a direct comparison of SNB before NAC (n = 575) with SNB after NAC (n = 3171). They found the SLN identification rates and FN rates to be similar between the two groups. The SLN identification rates for SNB before NAC were 97.4% compared to 98.7% for SNB after NAC, and the respective FN rates were 5.9% versus 4%. With a median follow-up of 47 months, the authors found no significant difference in disease-free or overall survival between the two groups of patients. The authors argue that SNB after NAC is accurate, results in fewer positive SLNs, and may spare some patients from unnecessary ALND. The American College of Surgeons Oncology Group (ACOSOG) Z1071 trial is currently accruing patients with T1 to T4, N1 to N2, M0 breast cancer who will undergo preoperative NAC for a clinical trial to address this controversy.

In the past, ALND without SNB was recommended for any patient with clinically palpable axillary lymph nodes. However, this recommendation does not account for lymph nodes that are clinically palpable secondary to reactive changes following breast biopsy. Furthermore, when clinical examination of the axilla suggests metastases, it is accurate in only 70% to 80% of cases. Axillary ultrasound has been shown to have sensitivities ranging from 51% to 62% for detecting metastatic lymph nodes and specificities ranging from 65% to 79%. Characteristics of suspicious lymph nodes on ultrasound (US) include lymph node enlargement, asymmetry of the cortex, and loss of the fatty hilum. We currently perform axillary US in patients with clinically palpable axillary lymph nodes or large primary tumors. If the axillary US identifies an abnormal lymph node, fine needle aspiration (FNA) or core biopsy is performed; if the needle biopsy identifies metastatic carcinoma, ALND is indicated. However, if the US or cytology is nondiagnostic or indeterminate, SNB is recommended. At the time of SNB, any clinically suspicious nodes should be removed, as an involved node may be the SLN.

SNB is usually not recommended for patients with T4 invasive tumors or inflammatory breast cancer. These patients should have level I and II ALND for axillary staging. In addition, the effects of pregnancy and lactation on lymphatic mapping and the safety of lymphazurin blue dye in this population are unknown. There is evidence that lymphatic mapping with radioisotope is safe in pregnant and lactating patients, suggesting that SNB with radioisotope may be safely performed in these women. However, there are insufficient data to determine the SLN identification rate or FN rate of SNB in this patient population.

Many have questioned the use of SNB in elderly and obese patients and in patients who have had previous excisional breast biopsy, prior nononcologic breast surgery—such as reduction mammaplasty, or augmentation—or previous axillary surgery, with concerns that lymphatic mapping may be inaccurate; however, studies show that SNB can be performed in all of these scenarios. The SLN identification rate may be lower in these situations, but if the SLN is identified, it has been shown to be reliable. In all cases of mapping failure, routine level I and II ALND should be performed.

SENTINEL LYMPH NODE BIOPSY TECHNIQUE

Lymphatic mapping has been successfully described using several agents, such as isosulfan blue dye, methylene blue dye, vital blue dye, technetium-99m sulfur colloid (filtered or unfiltered), or technetium-99m albumin. Allergic reactions and anaphylaxis have been reported with isosulfan blue dye in 0.1% of cases, and skin and nipple necrosis have been reported with intradermal injection of methylene blue dye. The most commonly used agents are isosulfan blue dye and filtered technetium sulfur colloid. These agents can be used alone or in combination, but an increased SLN identification rate with the use of the combination of blue dye and radio-isotope is well documented. However, in the only prospective randomized trial comparing blue dye alone with the combined use of isotope and blue dye in 92 patients, Morrow and colleagues showed no difference in SLN identification between the two groups. In addition the authors found that the number of cases performed by an individual surgeon was a significant predictor of successful SLN identification.

Given the learning curve associated with this procedure, experience is needed to achieve an acceptable failure rate of 5% or less. Surgeon experience has been shown to significantly impact the SLN identification and FN rates. The combined technique should probably be used while learning the SNB procedure; however, in experienced hands, single-agent mapping can be reliable, and the use of a second agent may not enhance the performance of SNB.

If using radioisotope, intradermal or subdermal injection of a single dose of 0.3 to 1.0 mCi of technetium-99m sulfur colloid is performed 3 to 24 hours prior to incision. Lymphoscintigraphy should be performed after injection to document migration of the radioisotope, but this procedure is not required. Intraoperative injection of the radioisotope has been reported with successful identification of the SLN. Intraoperative isotope injection is performed while the patient is anesthetized and is followed by SNB without a significant time delay. This method offers the advantage of avoiding the pain associated with radioisotope injection, as well as avoiding scheduling difficulties with Nuclear Medicine, but a lymphoscintigram cannot be obtained using this method; in addition, the license required to handle radioisotope is not easily accessible for surgeons in many locations.

There is no consensus on the optimal location of injection of either blue dye or radioisotope, but most data indicate that SLN identification is successful with peritumoral, subareolar, or subdermal injections. Methylene blue should not be injected intradermally because of the risk of skin necrosis, and isosulfan blue dye may result in skin tattooing. Once the patient is sedated or anesthetized, 2 to 5 mL of blue dye is injected approximately 5 to 10 minutes prior to incision. Many advocate gentle breast massage to encourage migration of the blue dye to the axilla with an interval of 3 to 10 minutes between dye injection and axillary incision to ensure adequate time for drainage of the dye to the SLN.

A 2 to 3 cm transverse incision is made in the axillary fossa slightly caudal to the line that is traditionally used for ALND. The SLN is often localized quite low in the axilla. Dissection is carried through the subcutaneous tissues and clavipectoral fascia, taking care to avoid transection of the afferent lymphatics. Gentle blunt dissection is used to localize and expose blue-stained lymphatics, which are further dissected along a parallel plane and traced proximally or distally to any blue nodes (Figure 1). In addition, the handheld gamma probe can be used to direct dissection and identification of radioactive or "hot" sentinel nodes. With dual-agent mapping, nodes may be blue, hot, or both. All are SLNs and should be surgically excised. Radioactive counts of the excised nodes should be noted, and the axilla should be assessed for residual radioactivity. Nodes with radioactive counts greater than 10% of the count of the "hottest" node should be excised. In addition, because lymph nodes blocked by tumor could divert the mapping agent to an alternative lymph node, the bed of dissection should be palpated for any suspicious palpable lymph nodes. These nodes should be considered SLNs and should also be excised. In the event that no blue or radioactive nodes are identified, ALND is warranted.

HISTOPATHOLOGIC EVALUATION

Depending on the preference of the surgeon, the SLN can be sent for intraoperative analysis or it can be evaluated with permanent sectioning alone. The benefit of performing intraoperative assessment is that ALND can be performed immediately in patients with a positive

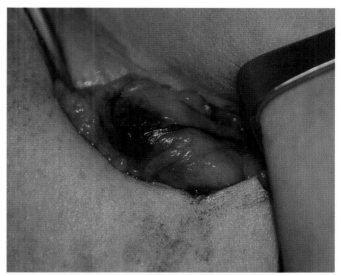

FIGURE 1   Sentinel node stained with blue dye.

TABLE 1: Techniques and sensitivity of intraoperative SLN analysis

Authors	Patients	Positive SLN Detected by H&E	Intraoperative Technique	Sensitivity (%)
Tillman et al.	247	68	TP	94.2
Quill et al.	13	39	TP	93.0
Motomura et al.	631	107	TP	84.6
Veronesi et al.	295	119	FS + SS	93.7
Flett et al.	56	21	FS	83.0
Turner & Giuliano	278	72	FS & TP	73.6

TP, Touch prep; *FS*, frozen section; *SS*, serial sectioning

SLN. Several methods of intraoperative examination have been described, including frozen section, imprint cytology, scrape cytology, and immunohistochemistry (IHC) staining. Multiple studies have shown similar sensitivities between frozen section and imprint cytology techniques, ranging from 74% to 94% for metastases that can be detected by hematoxylin and eosin (H&E) staining on permanent section (Table 1). The sensitivity for the detection of intraoperative micrometastases is lower, with reported rates ranging from 52% to 83%. The disadvantage of frozen section analysis is that as much as 25% of the nodal tissue may be lost during processing. The sensitivity of intraoperative lymph node examination is significantly higher in larger tumors because of the increased incidence of macrometastases in these patients, and intraoperative assessment in T1a and T1b tumors has been associated with a very low yield. Therefore, the clinical benefit of intraoperative nodal examination in smaller tumors may be limited, and some suggest selective use of intraoperative examination only in clinical situations likely to yield SLN metastases.

All SLNs that are negative by standard H&E analysis should be examined with multiple sections and IHC staining. This enhanced evaluation has been shown to increase detection of occult metastases,

TABLE 2: Propspective studies of complications in patients who underwent SLN biopsy without ALND

Study	N	F/U (Mo)	Pain (%)	Lymphedema (%)	Paresthesia (%)	ROM (%)
Swenson, 2002	247	12	28.7	3.5	24.9	6.4
Veronesi, 2003	100	24	8.0	7.0	1.0	0.0
Barranger, 2005	54	20	21.2	0.0	5.9	9.4
Ronka, 2005	43	12	28.0	13.0	19.0	31.0
Wilke, 2006	4160	6	—	6.9	8.6	3.8
Langer, 2007	449	31	15.3	3.5	10.9	3.5
Bianco, 2008	336	24	7.5	5.0	9.0	2.5
Madsen, 2008	164	18	18.0	7.0	15.0	14.0

F/U, Follow-up; *ROM,* range of motion

and a standard protocol is usually established by individual pathology departments. Typically, each node processed for permanent sectioning is blocked individually. The nodal tissue is sliced lengthwise at three levels at 100 micron intervals and stained with H&E. Any node that is negative by H&E staining is additionally sectioned and stained for cytokeratin. If intraoperative analysis is not performed, all SLNs will be subject to serial sectioning with H&E and IHC staining. Introduction of SNB and the enhanced pathologic evaluation of the SLN have resulted in improved axillary staging, leading to upstaging from node-negative to node-positive disease in 10% to 25% of cases.

CLINICAL IMPLICATIONS OF SENTINEL NODE BIOPSY

Multiple studies have demonstrated that in SLN-negative cases, the remaining axillary lymph nodes do not harbor metastases, and ALND is not warranted. In addition, the rate of axillary recurrence in SLN-negative patients is less than 2%, further supporting this recommendation. Currently ALND should be performed when the SLN harbors metastases. Additional involved lymph nodes will be identified by ALND in 50% of cases with SLN macrometastases. However, in cases of micrometastatic SLN involvement, only 10% to 15% of patients will have additional metastatic axillary lymph nodes. In cases of isolated tumor cells, approximately 5% will have nonsentinel node (NSLN) involvement, and ALND of negative NSLN offers no clinical advantage but brings potential morbidity. Because of this, there has been considerable controversy regarding completion ALND in patients with SLN involvement with micrometastases (0.2 to 2 mm) or isolated tumor cells (<0.2 mm).

Several clinicopathologic features have been associated with involvement of NSLNs, and these factors can be used in combination to determine the likelihood of NSLN involvement. Significant factors that have been identified include size of the primary tumor, tumor grade, size of the SLN metastasis, proportion of SLNs that are involved, estrogen receptor status, and presence of lymphovascular invasion. Many of these factors have been incorporated into nomograms that can calculate the risk of NSLN involvement to help clinicians determine the need for completion ALND. However, there is no threshold of risk for which ALND is recommended by the nomogram, and the predictive power of these tools varies with areas under the curve (AUC) ranging from 0.7 to 0.8.

The clinical trial ACOSOG Z10011 was initiated to address the value of completion ALND in SLN-positive patients by assessing the outcome of these patients following randomization to ALND or no further surgery. Unfortunately this trial was closed prematurely due to poor patient accrual and low event rate. However, over 900

node-positive patients were randomized, and valuable data may still be obtained.

The clinical significance of micrometastases is not well understood. Our group conducted a prospective study of 790 patients with clinical stage I to III invasive breast cancer who underwent SNB. Among these patients, 486 (61.5%) had no evidence of disease in the SLN, 84 (10.6%) had isolated tumor cells, 54 (6.9%) had micrometastases, and 166 (21%) had macrometastases. With a median follow-up of 72.5 months, the size of the SLN metastasis was found to be a significant predictor of disease-free and overall survival. However, there was no significant difference in 8-year disease-free or 8-year overall survival between the node-negative group, those with isolated tumor cells, or those with micrometastatic SLNs.

A group from the Netherlands recently reported a tumor registry study of outcomes in 2707 breast cancer patients who had SNB. The authors conducted a retrospective comparison of three groups of patients: 856 women with node-negative breast cancer who did not receive adjuvant therapy, 856 patients with isolated tumor cells or micrometastases who did not receive adjuvant therapy, and 995 patients with isolated tumor cells or micrometastases who received either adjuvant chemotherapy or hormonal therapy. After a median follow-up of 5.1 years, the authors found that among the patients who did not receive adjuvant therapy, those with isolated tumor cells and micrometastases had a worse disease-free survival compared to the node-negative cohort with a hazard ratio of 1.5 (CI, 1.15 to 1.94). However, disease-free survival was broadly defined to include contralateral breast cancer, other malignancies, and locoregional recurrence. There was no significant difference in overall survival. Among patients with isolated tumor cells or micrometastases, those who received adjuvant therapy had an improved disease-free survival over those who did not receive adjuvant therapy (HR of 0.57, CI, 0.45 to 0.73).

These studies suggest that the presence of isolated tumor cells or micrometastases in SLN of patients who have received adjuvant therapy may not be prognostically significant. However, there have been no published randomized data to address this question. At this time, we await the results of several multicenter randomized trials, such as the National Surgical Adjuvant Breast and Bowel Project (NSABP) B32 and ACOSOG Z0010, to achieve a better understanding of the prognostic significance of occult metastases.

COMPLICATIONS

Results from a large, prospective international cooperative group trial have reported a very low incidence of complications after SNB. Early and late complications include wound infection (1%), hematoma

(1%), seroma (7%), paresthesia (8%), decreased upper extremity range of motion (4%), and lymphedema (7%). There have been a number of prospective trials comparing the morbidity of SNB to ALND, and all studies clearly demonstrate decreased morbidity associated with SNB, although with long-term follow-up, the differences diminished over time. The most common symptoms of late morbidity associated with SNB include pain, lymphedema, paresthesias, and limited range of motion (Table 2).

SUMMARY

SNB is a safe and accurate procedure that has replaced ALND as the standard of care for axillary staging in patients with node-negative early breast cancer. SNB results in decreased morbidity, allows detailed nodal analysis, provides more precise regional staging, and identifies occult invasion. This procedure should be offered to most patients with T1 to T3 invasive breast cancer with few relative or absolute contraindications. Several issues remain to be resolved, including timing of SNB in the neoadjuvant setting and the prognostic significance of isolated tumor cells and micrometastases. We currently await results from several ongoing randomized multicenter trials to address these areas of controversy.

SUGGESTED READINGS

Coutant C, Olivier C, Lambaudie E, et al: Comparison of models to predict nonsentinel lymph node status in breast cancer patients with metastatic lymph nodes: a prospective multicenter study, *J Clin Oncol* 27(17): 2800–2808, 2009.

De Boer M, van Deurzen C, van Dijck J, et al: Micrometastases or isolated tumor cells and the outcome of breast cancer, *New Engl J Med* 361: 653–663, 2009.

Hansen N, Grube B, Xing Y, et al: Impact of micrometastases in the sentinel node of patients with breast cancer, *J Clin Oncol* 27(28):4679–4684, 2009.

Kim T, Giuliano A, Lyman G: Lymphatic mapping and sentinel lymph node biopsy in early-stage breast carcinoma: a meta-analysis, *Cancer* 106:4–16, 2006.

Lucci A, McCall L, Beitsch P, et al: Surgical complications associated with sentinel lymph node dissection (SLND) plus axillary dissection compared to SLND alone in the American College of Surgeons Oncology Group Trial Z0011, *J Clin Oncol* 25(24):3657–3663, 2007.

Lyman G, Giuliano A, Somerfeld M, et al: American Society of Clinical Oncology guideline recommendations for sentinel lymph node biopsy in early stage breast cancer, *J Clin Oncol* 23(30):7703–7720, 2005.

Wilke L, Giuliano A: Sentinel lymph node biopsy in patients with early stage breast cancer: status of the National Clinical Trials, *Surg Clin North Am* 83:901–910, 2003.

MANAGEMENT OF THE AXILLA IN BREAST CANCER

Elizabeth Min Hui Kim, MD, and Barbara L. Smith, MD, PhD

OVERVIEW

The pathologic status of the axillary lymph nodes remains one of the most important prognostic factors in patients with breast cancer. The presence of axillary node metastases indicates a poorer prognosis and often prompts a recommendation for more aggressive systemic and local therapies. As yet, no imaging technology provides a reliable alternative to surgical staging of the axilla.

In the past, axillary dissection was indicated for nearly all patients with breast cancer, providing both staging data and effective treatment of axillary disease. However, axillary dissection carries significant morbidity, including lymphedema, decreased range of motion, and acute and chronic pain. These negative aspects of axillary dissection have led to more selective use of axillary surgery and to investigation of less morbid options for staging and treatment.

A surgeon may now choose among a variety of options for axillary management based on tumor and patient characteristics. These options include sentinel node biopsy (SNB), standard axillary dissection, axillary radiation, and observation alone.

CLINICALLY NODE-NEGATIVE INVASIVE BREAST CANCER

Although results of prospective clinical trials evaluating SNB are not yet available, it has largely replaced axillary dissection for breast cancer patients with clinically negative nodes. This technique takes advantage of the intrinsic anatomy of breast lymphatic drainage, in which the dominant lymphatic channels of the breast converge to initially deliver tumor cells or injected dye particles to a small number of "sentinel" nodes. If the sentinel nodes show no evidence of tumor metastases, the chance that other axillary nodes will contain metastases is low enough that completion axillary dissection may be omitted.

Pilot studies of sentinel node biopsy with completion axillary dissection have shown acceptably low false-negative rates (0% to 11%) with the sentinel node approach. In practice, axillary recurrence rates are under 1% when the sentinel node is negative, and no additional axillary treatment is given.

Technical Aspects of Sentinel Node Biopsy

Sentinel node biopsy is accurate with lumpectomy or mastectomy. Radiolabeled particles and/or blue dye are injected adjacent to the tumor or in a subdermal, periareolar location, and the breast is lightly massaged to enhance dye transit. A gamma probe is used to identify the location of radiolabeled sentinel nodes and guide incision placement. Radioactive or blue-stained nodes and lymphatics are identified by inspection within axillary fat.

Sentinel nodes identified by dye uptake are excised for pathology analysis. Dye uptake may be reduced in nodes replaced by tumor or when afferent lymphatics become plugged by tumor emboli, leading to false-negative (FN) sentinel node mapping. Careful intraoperative palpation of axillary tissue can identify suspicious firm or enlarged nodes for excision and testing and can reduce FN rates.

Frozen section analysis intraoperatively allows completion axillary dissection during the same surgical procedure for positive nodes. Complete histologic analysis includes serial sectioning of the sentinel nodes with three to five sections per node examined. Many centers also add immunohistochemical staining for breast epithelial cytokeratins to facilitate identification of small tumor deposits. Axillary node metastases are classified by size as macrometastases (over 2 mm, N1), micrometastases (0.2 to 2 mm, N1mic), and isolated tumor cells (ITCs, N0[i+]), with prognosis inversely proportional to the size of the metastatic deposit.

Sentinel node mapping appears reliable in the majority of clinical situations, including in patients with prior biopsies, biopsy site seromas, and large or multifocal primary tumors. Repeat node mapping is possible after prior axillary SNB or dissection, with lower rates of mapping success, but reliable results, if a new sentinel node is identified.

SNB is contraindicated in patients with inflammatory carcinoma because results are unreliable, most likely because lymphatic tumor deposits impede dye mapping. It is also not appropriate for patients with clinically positive axillary or supraclavicular nodes, as nodal status is already known, or for patients with distant metastases, where axillary node status is irrelevant.

Ultrasound-Guided Axillary Node Biopsy

Axillary ultrasound is being used with increasing frequency for preoperative evaluation of axillary nodes and to guide fine needle biopsy for suspicious nodes. Patients with positive fine needle node biopsies may proceed directly to axillary dissection or neoadjuvant systemic therapy without sentinel node mapping. SNB is still required if the needle biopsy is negative, as axillary fine needle biopsy has a significant FN rate.

Management of a Positive Sentinel Node

Approximately 40% to 50% of all patients with a positive sentinel node will have additional positive nonsentinel axillary nodes. Since breast cancer staging and resulting adjuvant treatment recommendations are based on the total number of involved axillary nodes, completion axillary dissection is generally indicated when a sentinel node is positive.

Completion axillary dissection remains the standard of care of patients with sentinel node macrometastases and micrometastases, as these patients are at moderate to high risk for additional positive nodes. However, completion axillary dissection is often omitted for patients whose sentinel nodes contain only isolated tumor cells, because the risk of additional positive nodes is fairly low. Predictive models, such as the nomogram designed by Van Zee and colleagues, which estimates risk of additional positive nodes based on features of the primary tumor and sentinel nodes, may be useful in deciding whether completion axillary dissection is indicated.

Clinical trials addressing the use of axillary radiation, rather than completion dissection, have been conducted with results being evaluated.

Alternatives to Axillary Surgery

Axillary radiation without axillary node surgery provides effective local control for breast cancer patients with clinically negative nodes. Axillary recurrence rates are only 1% to 3% after 50 Gy of radiation to the axilla as a third field or as two-field-high tangents. Axillary radiation without surgical staging is reasonable for patients whose nodal pathology results will not change treatment plans, for example, for elderly women for whom systemic therapy decisions have been made. Endocrine therapy without surgery or radiation may be considered for elderly patients with estrogen receptor–positive tumors and clinically negative nodes.

CLINICALLY NODE-POSITIVE INVASIVE BREAST CANCER

Patients with grossly palpable nodes or axillary node involvement confirmed by needle biopsy should proceed directly to axillary dissection or neoadjuvant therapy. SNB may be considered for node-positive patients who become clinically node negative after neoadjuvant systemic therapy, although some favor axillary dissection for all patients whose nodes were initially positive.

Technical Aspects of Axillary Dissection

The standard level 1 and 2 axillary dissection removes node-bearing axillary fat deep to the axillary fascia in an area between the pectoralis and latissimus dorsi muscles. Level 1 axillary nodes are inferior to the axillary vein and lateral to the pectoralis minor muscle. Level 2 nodes are more superior and medial to level 1 nodes and lie posterior to the pectoralis minor muscle. The long thoracic, thoracodorsal, and medial pectoral motor nerves are preserved during axillary dissection, and every effort is made to preserve the intercostobrachial sensory nerve branches. A level 3 dissection, which adds axillary tissue medial to the pectoralis minor muscle, significantly increases risk of lymphedema and is performed only when palpable nodes are present in level 3.

The placement of magnetic resonance imaging (MRI)-compatible metal clips at the highest point of the surgical dissection may be helpful to delineate dissected versus nondissected areas in subsequent radiation planning. Most surgeons will place a closed suction drain in the axilla after dissection to collect the seroma fluid expected over the first 7 the 10 days following surgery. Some surgeons prefer to avoid drain placement and perform serial aspirations of axillary seromas if they become symptomatic.

Postoperative pain may be significantly reduced by injection of a long-acting local anesthetic such as bupivacaine into the axillary incision and through the axillary drain after the skin is closed. The drain is then clamped for 1 to 2 hours to bathe the axillary cavity with anesthetic before connecting the drain to suction. Pain relief will facilitate early postoperative mobilization of the arm, which may help reduce shoulder stiffness and reduce risk of lymphedema.

Early problems after axillary dissection include acute pain, the need for a drain in the surgical bed, the need for hospital admission, and reduced range of motion. Long-term problems resulting from axillary dissection include permanent lymphedema in 10% to 25% of patients, numbness, chronic pain, and reduced range of motion in the shoulder. Assessment of patients' subjective symptoms of arm problems show even higher rates of persistent arm symptoms with 25% to 50% of patients reporting arm swelling, pain, numbness, and/or decreased mobility.

Axillary Radiation after Dissection

Axillary and supraclavicular node irradiation is used after axillary dissection for patients at highest risk of local recurrence, including those with multiple positive axillary nodes and significant extranodal tumor deposits. A total dose of 45 to 50 Gy is given in daily 1.8 to 2.0 Gy fractions. Treatment of the entire axilla requires a separate radiation field that commonly includes the supraclavicular nodes and is matched to the breast and chest wall fields caudally.

The rate of brachial plexus injury after axillary radiation is approximately 1% with current techniques. Use of axillary radiation after axillary dissection increases risk for lymphedema, with lymphedema rates of 15% to 30% reported after radiation combined with a level 1 and 2 axillary dissection.

AXILLARY MANAGEMENT FOR DUCTAL CARCINOMA IN SITU

The use of axillary dissection was largely abandoned in patients with DCIS because of the very low risk of positive axillary nodes and the morbidity of dissection. Recently, the low morbidity of SNB has led to reconsideration of axillary staging in DCIS, particularly since DCIS is now frequently diagnosed by core needle biopsy, and invasive carcinoma is found at definitive excision in up to 20% of patients. Serial sections stained with hematoxylin and eosin identify sentinel node tumor deposits in 1% to 3% of patients with DCIS without invasion. Keratin immunohistochemistry staining will identify sentinel node tumor deposits in 9% to 13% of DCIS patients. The majority of positive sentinel nodes in DCIS patients are ITCs, with occasional micrometastases identified.

These high rates of sentinel node involvement are inconsistent with the established natural history of DCIS and have raised speculation that these small sentinel node deposits in DCIS patients represent tumor debris rather than viable metastatic tumor cells. Retrospective and prospective studies have found that sentinel node ITCs and micrometastases are not associated with increased local or distant recurrence in patients with pure DCIS or DCIS with microinvasion.

Given these results, SNB should be used selectively for patients with DCIS. Since mastectomy precludes subsequent sentinel node mapping, SNB is appropriate for DCIS patients undergoing mastectomy. This avoids the need for full axillary dissection if invasive carcinoma is found on final pathology. However, as sentinel node mapping is unaffected by lumpectomy, SNB should be reserved for those lumpectomy patients at highest risk of invasive tumor, such as those with palpable DCIS or DCIS on core biopsy but a suspicious mass on imaging studies.

AXILLARY MANAGEMENT IN THE ELDERLY

For many elderly patients with clinically negative nodes, surgical staging of the axilla should not be performed, because information from axillary surgery will not alter treatment decisions. For example, axillary surgery is usually omitted in elderly or otherwise frail patients with estrogen receptor–positive, clinically node-negative tumors, as chemotherapy is not under consideration, and endocrine therapy will be used regardless of nodal status. Axillary recurrences following lumpectomy and endocrine therapy are low for such patients, even without radiation or axillary surgery. The rate of axillary recurrence was approximately 1% at 5 years among women treated with lumpectomy and tamoxifen without radiation in the Cancer and Leukemia Group B trial (CALGB 9343), and many of these women did not have surgical staging of their axilla.

Axillary dissection should be performed in elderly patients with clinically positive nodes who are treated surgically. SNB should be performed for clinically node-negative elderly patients in whom chemotherapy may be considered or for estrogen receptor–negative tumors in patients at higher risk for positive nodes.

MANAGEMENT OF THE AXILLA IN PREGNANT PATIENTS

The use of radiolabeled dye for sentinel node mapping in pregnant women remains controversial, although the dose received by the fetus with standard Tc-99m sulfur colloid sentinel node mapping falls well below National Council on Radiation Protection and Measurements threshold guidelines for pregnant patients. Little data exist on the safety of isosulfan blue in pregnancy. Some centers use methylene blue mapping for pregnant women, and others favor use of Tc-99m sulfur colloid with hydration and placement of a bladder catheter to avoid accumulation of excreted isotope in the pelvis.

POSITIVE AXILLARY NODES WITH AN OCCULT BREAST PRIMARY TUMOR

Between 0.3% and 1.0% of breast cancers present as englarged axillary nodes with no detectable primary tumor in the breast on physical examination or mammography. Breast MRI will identify the breast primary in approximately 50% of such patients; these patients may be managed with standard breast-conserving surgery and neoadjuvant or adjuvant systemic therapy.

If no breast tumor is identified by physical examination or breast imaging, other primary tumor types must be considered, including lymphoma, melanoma, and occasionally lung, thyroid, or neuroendocrine tumors and tumors at other sites. Core or fine needle biopsy is the preferred approach for obtaining a tissue diagnosis, with excisional biopsy reserved for cases where needle biopsy is nondiagnostic. Additional imaging studies are performed to identify the primary tumor site, guided by histologic results, and a staging workup should be performed to rule out distant metastases.

If axillary node histology is consistent with a breast origin, but no primary breast lesion is identified, axillary dissection should be performed in operable patients. Patients with bulky or fixed axillary nodes should receive neoadjuvant systemic therapy followed by axillary dissection. Most patients may then be safely treated with whole-breast irradiation without mastectomy with low rates of subsequent local failure.

MANAGEMENT OF AXILLARY TUMOR RECURRENCE

Axillary node recurrences may appear as late as 5 to 10 years after initial treatment, most often as an asymptomatic mass in the axilla. Occasionally, patients will present with arm edema, neurologic impairment, or pain. The tissue diagnosis is established by fine needle aspiration (FNA), core biopsy, or surgical biopsy.

New axillary nodal disease ipsilateral to a previously treated cancer may be a recurrence of the prior cancer or metastases from a new primary tumor. A thorough search for a new breast primary tumor and a full metastatic workup is indicated at the time of regional node recurrence. Completion axillary dissection with resection of palpable disease is indicated, with consideration given to regional radiation and additional systemic therapy.

An isolated axillary recurrence has a favorable prognosis with 5-year survival in the 70% range. Prognosis is significantly worse for patients seen initially with disease in the supraclavicular, internal mammary node, or multiple sites of nodal disease.

SUGGESTED READINGS

Lyman GH, Giuliano AE, Somerfielt MR, et al: American Society of Clinical Oncology guideline recommendations for sentinel lymph node biopsy in early stage breast cancer, *J Clin Oncol* 23:7703–7720, 2005.

Van Zee KJ, Manasseh DM, Vevilacqua JLB, et al: A nomogram for predicting the likelihood of additional nodal metastases in breast cancer patients with a positive sentinel node biopsy, *Ann Surg Oncol* 10:1140–1151, 2003.

Murphy CD, Jones JL, Javid SH, et al: Do sentinel node micrometastases predict recurrence risk in ductal carcinoma in situ and ductal carcinoma in situ with microinvasion? *Am J Surg* 196:566–568, 2008.

Hughes KS, Schnaper L, Berry D, et al: Comparison of lumpectomy plus tamoxifen with and without radiotherapy (RT) in women 70 years of age or older who have clinical stage I, estrogen receptor–positive breast carcinoma, *N Engl J Med* 351:971–977, 2004.

INFLAMMATORY BREAST CANCER

Helen Krontiras, MD, and Marshall M. Urist, MD

OVERVIEW

Inflammatory breast cancer (IBC) is an aggressive and rare form of breast cancer, comprising only 1% to 6% of all cases of breast cancer in the United States. The prognosis has been uniformly poor, but with recent advances in multimodal treatment that combines chemotherapy, mastectomy, and radiation therapy, the outcome is improving. Current data from the National Cancer Institute's Surveillance, Epidemiology, and End Results (SEER) program database shows that the 5-year survival for IBC patients is 40% compared with 87% for all patients with invasive breast cancer.

Although breast cancer incidence and mortality in general is decreasing, including locally advanced breast cancer (LABC), the incidence of IBC appears to be increasing. It now occurs more frequently in younger women, with a mean age at diagnosis of 58 years, compared to 61 years of age for non-T4 breast cancer and 66 years for LABC. Data from the SEER program also demonstrate that IBC is found more frequently in black women than in white women. Black women with IBC have a poorer survival when compared with white women with the same presentation characteristics.

CLINICAL PRESENTATION

Lee and Tannenbaum in 1924 and Taylor and Metzler in 1938 described IBC as a distinct clinical entity. In 1956, Haagensen further defined the disease by outlining the specific criteria that characterize this deadly form of breast cancer (Table 1). The clinical hallmark of IBC is skin changes that include erythema, edema, peau d'orange, tenderness, induration, and warmth. These changes often arise quickly with erythema and edema covering more than a third of the surface of the breast. Sometimes there is a palpable border or ridge to the erythema, and the color ranges from a pink blush to a purple, almost ecchymotic appearance. The degree of color changes may vary over the breast and may extend to the skin of the other breast. Erythema is often accompanied by warmth or a sensation of heat, and the edema associated with IBC causes peau d'orange, which resembles the peel of an orange, with dimpling and pitting of the skin. These skin changes are due to plugging of the dermal lymphatics with subsequent edema of the tissues around exaggerated hair follicles. Other presenting symptoms include breast heaviness, burning, and or aching. Approximately 30% of the time an underlying mass is not palpable. Nipple changes that include retraction, inversion, or flattening may also be seen.

DIAGNOSIS

The diagnosis of IBC is a *clinical diagnosis* made by the physician based upon the entire clinicopathologic picture. A differential diagnosis includes mastitis, abscess, venous congestion of the breast, dermatitis, LABC, and primary breast lymphoma. All patient evaluations begin with a complete history and physical examination. Defining the duration of symptoms is important in distinguishing IBC from LABC, which commonly arises from the neglect of a slower growing cancer.

In IBC, erythema is often one of the earliest changes. Rapid enlargement of the breast is common and is often mistaken for an infection. Patients may report failed antibiotic trials, but most will have normal white blood cell counts and will be afebrile. The patient should be asked about symptoms of metastatic disease. The most likely sites of distant disease, in order of frequency of occurrence, are bone, lung, liver, and brain. Photographs may be helpful for documenting the extent of skin changes and assessment of response to chemotherapy.

A baseline mammogram is important in the evaluation of patients with IBC. However, the changes in the breast might be subtle; such changes include diffusely increased parenchymal density, trabecular distortion, and skin thickening. Ultrasound is useful for facilitating biopsy of parenchymal breast lesions and for evaluating regional nodal basins. Magnetic resonance imaging (MRI) of the breast with a dedicated breast coil may be selectively employed. MRI findings frequently include heterogeneous internal enhancement that is often masslike. These findings may assist the clinician with assessment of response to neoadjuvant therapy, but results should be cautiously interpreted.

A biopsy confirming the presence of cancer is necessary and can be performed with a percutaneous core biopsy of the breast parenchyma or a skin punch biopsy or both. A punch biopsy is typically taken from the most suspicious site of skin involvement. Pathologically, IBC is frequently of the ductal histologic type. On punch biopsy, IBC is characterized by the presence of tumor emboli within the dermal lymphatics. Although dermal lymphatic invasion is supportive of a diagnosis of IBC, it is not required for the diagnosis. Moreover, the presence of dermal lymphatic invasion without the clinical signs of IBC is often not IBC. Tissue obtained should be processed for determination of standard tumor markers, including estrogen and progesterone receptors and *HER2neu*.

Most IBCs are estrogen receptor (ER) and progesterone receptor (PR) negative. Breast cancers that do not express these receptors are associated with a worse prognosis than ER-/PR-positive tumors, and the same is true for IBCs. More than half will overexpress the epidermal growth factor receptor, including *HER2neu*. This may account for the early and aggressive spread seen in IBC.

STAGING

Once a diagnosis has been made, accurate staging is paramount to assure appropriate therapy commensurate with disease progression. Most patients with IBC will have spread to the axillary lymph nodes. IBC without distant metastasis is stage IIIB (T4d, N0-N3, M0) breast cancer based on the American Joint Committee on Cancer (AJCC) sixth edition *Cancer Staging Manual*.

Because approximately one third of patients will have distant spread at presentation, a thorough evaluation for metastatic disease is required for all patients with IBC. This workup includes a complete blood count, liver function tests, a whole-body bone scan, and computed tomography (CT) scans of the chest, abdomen, and pelvis with IV contrast. A fluorodeoxyglucose positron emission tomography (FDG-PET) CT scan may be helpful to assess indeterminate areas on the previous mentioned scans. Further testing should be ordered based on patient symptoms, and tissue biopsy to confirm spread is preferred whenever possible.

TREATMENT

Multimodal therapy is the mainstay of current treatment for IBC. Because of the ability of IBC to rapidly and frequently disseminate, preoperative or neoadjuvant chemotherapy is recommended before any local therapy is instituted (Figure 1). Although multiple studies utilizing neoadjuvant therapy have been performed to evaluate

TABLE 1: Common clinical characteristics of inflammatory breast cancer

Physical examination
- Erythema
- Edema or peau d'orange
- Ridging of the skin
- Lymphadenopathy common

Medical history
- Rapid onset
- Signs of bacterial infection absent

Biopsy
- Diagnosis of carcinoma confirmed
- Dermal lymphatic invasion common

Imaging Findings
- Skin thickening
- Diffuse increase in density
- Axillary adenopathy

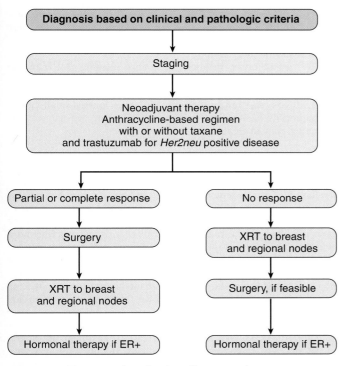

FIGURE 1   Treatment algorithm for inflammatory breast cancer.

patients with LABC, studies that specifically evaluate neoadjuvant therapy in IBC are limited. Regimens currently recommended are anthracycline-based treatments with or without a taxane. Trastuzumab, a monoclonal antibody directed at the *HER2neu* oncogene, is added if the tumor is *HER2neu* positive but it is not given with an anthracycline, because it can potentiate cardiotoxicity.

The response to chemotherapy should be periodically monitored during the course of treatment. A nonresponse or signs of progression should lead to consideration of an alternate regimen. Clinical response rates as high as 86% and pathologic complete response (PCR) rates of approximately 12% to 33% have been reported. PCR in the breast and/ or axilla is associated with an improved overall survival.

Because clinical examination may not accurately reflect treatment response, and residual disease may be underestimated, preoperative planning is important. If dermal lymphatic invasion is detected before therapy, mapping out the response with skin punch biopsies before surgery is useful for planning resection margins. If regression is not observed, additional systemic chemotherapy and preoperative radiation therapy should be strongly considered, because mastectomy is unlikely to provide a benefit in this situation.

If response is observed with systemic therapy, surgical therapy is warranted. The operative procedure is performed approximately 3 weeks after the completion of chemotherapy to allow the cytotoxic effects to normalize. The operation of choice is modified radical mastectomy or total mastectomy with complete axillary node dissection, including axillary levels 1 and 2, with level 3 reserved for gross involvement. Breast conservation therapy is not recommended for patients with IBC. Sentinel lymph node biopsy is also not recommended, because IBC is associated with an unacceptably high false-negative rate, which is thought to be due to the disruption of the lymphatic channels with tumor emboli.

Resection to negative margins should be attained if at all possible. Intraoperative assessment of skin margins may assist with adequate resection but may also underestimate residual disease. Care should be taken to avoid skin-flap tension during closure, because this may result in wound dehiscence and may delay the administration of radiation therapy. An autologous skin flap, such as a latissimus dorsi myocutaneous flap, may be necessary to facilitate wound closure. Tissue reconstruction of the breast, if the patient wants it, is delayed 6 to 12 months after radiation therapy has been completed.

Radiation therapy is recommended for local control regardless of response to chemotherapy. If systemic therapy fails to achieve a response amenable to surgical resection, radiation therapy should be delivered before surgery. After surgery, radiation therapy is directed to the chest wall, supraclavicular nodes, and in some instances the internal mammary chain nodes. The treatment is given daily for approximately 6 weeks. After completion of radiotherapy, the chemotherapy regimen may be resumed to deliver a full year of trastuzumab for patients with *HER2neu*-positive disease. Lastly, endocrine therapy is appropriate for women with ER-positive IBC after systemic chemotherapy and local therapy are complete. Tamoxifen is recommended for premenopausal women, and an aromatase inhibitor is indicated in postmenopausal women.

FUTURE THERAPY FOR INFLAMMATORY BREAST CANCER

Significant advances have been made in the overall therapy of IBC. Surgery remains an integral component of the multidisciplinary management of this disease, and research is ongoing to identify its pathogenesis. Molecular pathways in angiogenesis, lymphangiogenesis, vasculogenesis, proliferation, and motility may yield additional sites for targeted therapies that, in turn, may translate into improved patient outcomes.

SUGGESTED READINGS

American Joint Committee on Cancer: *AJCC cancer staging manual,* ed 6, Chicago, 2002, Springer-Verlag.

Carlson RW, Allred DC, Andersen BO, et al: Breast cancer: clinical practice guidelines in oncology, *J Natl Compr Canc Netw* 7(2):122–192, 2009.

Cristofanilli M: Inflammatory breast cancer: defining a new entity, *Semin Oncol* 35(1):6, 2008.

Hance KW, Anderson WF, Devesa SS, et al: Trends in inflammatory breast carcinoma incidence and survival: the surveillance, epidemiology, and end results program at the National Cancer Institute, *J Natl Cancer Inst* 97(13):966–975, 2005.

Ductal and Lobular Carcinoma in Situ of the Breast

Thomas N. Wang, MD, PhD, and Kirby I. Bland, MD

OVERVIEW

Ductal carcinoma in situ (DCIS) and lobular carcinoma in situ (LCIS) of the breast are noninvasive cancers with dissimilar implications. Whereas DCIS is a precursor lesion to invasive ductal carcinoma, LCIS is considered to be a marker of increased risk for breast cancer development. Malignant cell proliferation in both entities is confined to the basement membrane. Because the risk of systemic metastases is virtually nonexistent, the prognosis for DCIS and LCIS is excellent. The goal of treatment of in situ breast carcinoma is to prevent the development of invasive disease. The challenge in management is determining which patients are at risk for subsequent invasive breast cancer (IBC) and providing the appropriate therapy that minimizes recurrence without causing unnecessary morbidity. Personalization of treatment necessitates careful patient evaluation and multidisciplinary planning.

DUCTAL CARCINOMA IN SITU

DCIS is a clonal proliferation of malignant epithelial cells confined within the basement membrane of the mammary ducts. It represents a spectrum of pathological lesions with variable malignant potential predetermined by histologic architecture, presence of necrosis, and nuclear grade. Two major histologic subtypes of DCIS exist: *comedo* is evidenced by central necrosis, many mitotic figures, and large pleomorphic nuclei; *noncomedo* is evidenced by the absence of central necrosis and mitotic figures and the presence of specific papillary, micropapillary, or cribriform architecture carcinoma. Nuclear grade is classified as low, intermediate, or high as determined by nuclear morphology and mitotic index. High-grade DCIS is commonly associated with necrosis and has the most aggressive biological characteristics with the highest local recurrence rates. Regardless of nuclear grade or histologic subtype, the long-term prognosis of DCIS is excellent, with survival rates at 10 years exceeding 95%. Therefore, the challenge in the treatment of DCIS is to balance the risk for local recurrence with unnecessary surgical morbidity.

DCIS incidence rates have increased 7.2-fold from 1980 to 2001. In 2005, the incidence of DCIS was approximately 60,000 new cases in the United States, making it the fastest growing subtype of breast cancer. The growing incidence is a result of better detection through the increasing use of screening mammography. DCIS currently accounts for over 20% of all mammographically detected breast cancers, and it usually presents as microcalcifications detected by screening mammography with confirmation of the diagnosis by histologic examination of biopsy specimens. In the majority of women with DCIS that goes untreated, IBC develops at or near the same site as the index DCIS lesion. Therefore management of DCIS aims to rule out concurrent IBC (present in 10% to 25% of cases of DCIS) and prevent future development of IBC. The optimal treatment for DCIS remains complete surgical excision by either breast-conserving surgery (BCS) and adjuvant radiation therapy or mastectomy. Areas of controversy include adequate margin size of excision, the role of sentinel lymph node biopsy to assess for regional metastasis, the need for adjuvant radiation therapy after lumpectomy, and the need for systemic therapy with hormonal agents.

Diagnosis

The majority (90% to 95%) of DCIS cases show up as suspiciously grouped, pleomorphic, or fine, linear microcalcifications on mammograms. Rarely, patients with DCIS present with a palpable mass, a mammographically detected mass, Paget disease of the nipple, or suspicious nipple discharge. Indeterminate calcifications are further evaluated with magnification views of the breast. Breast cancer that is diagnosed by detecting incidental calcifications on mammography is pure DCIS in 65% of patients, DCIS with a focus of invasion in 32%, and IBC in 4%. The presence of invasive foci is more often associated with large areas of calcifications (>10 mm) and linear versus granular calcifications. All mammographically detected lesions are confirmed by pathologic evaluation of breast tissue obtained through biopsy. Stereotactic core needle biopsy has replaced needle-localized excisional biopsy as the optimal diagnostic tool, as it permits the acquisition of tissue for accurate strategic planning without an additional, potentially deforming operation. However, needle-localized breast biopsy is still necessary when lesions are not amenable to stereotactic core needle biopsy; that is, when they are adjacent to the chest wall, too superficial, too close to breast implants, or lacking sufficient breast tissue for compression.

The role of breast magnetic resonance imaging (MRI) in the diagnosis of DCIS is presently evolving. Currently, mammography remains the standard of care for the detection and diagnosis of noninvasive breast cancer. Because MRI often misses small, mammographically visible foci, it is not an adequate replacement for mammography in DCIS.

Treatment

Similar to IBC, management of noninvasive breast cancer has evolved with the application of multimodal therapy and less aggressive surgery. In the past, DCIS was often treated with simple mastectomy or even modified radical mastectomy. However, when overwhelming evidence demonstrated that BCS and adjuvant radiation therapy for IBC achieved similar survival rates to total mastectomy, investigators questioned whether mastectomy for DCIS was necessary. Unlike IBC, no randomized trials exist that compare total mastectomy to BCS for DCIS. Retrospective studies have shown that total mastectomy for DCIS is superior to BCS in terms of disease-free survival.

Silverstein and colleagues compared local recurrence among 227 patients with DCIS. They reported a disease-free survival rate of 98% in patients undergoing mastectomy versus 81% in those receiving BCS (P = .0004). Recently, Tunon-de-Lara and colleagues reported similar results in a review of 676 patients with DCIS. They reported a local recurrence rate of 2.6% for the mastectomy group, 7.5% for the group receiving lumpectomy plus radiation therapy, and 14.5% for the lumpectomy-only group. Involved surgical margins and young patient age were predictive of local recurrence after BCS. Nevertheless, no significant difference in survival in any subgroup comparison was seen, regardless of treatment. Thus, the standard therapy for DCIS is BCS followed by radiation therapy or mastectomy alone.

Surgical Therapy

The optimal management of DCIS needs to take into consideration the patient's risk of local recurrence associated with BCS. Although the long-term prognosis of DCIS is excellent, with low mortality rates regardless of treatment, the psychological impact of a local recurrence, especially an invasive recurrence, is devastating for any patient.

Therefore the aim of BCS for DCIS is complete excision with clear margins and a cosmetically acceptable result. Mastectomy should be considered for multicentric DCIS, large lesions, centrally located disease, and inadequate margins after repeated attempts at breast conservation, as well as in patients who prefer to have a mastectomy, or if adjuvant radiation therapy is contraindicated. Certainly, deciding between BCS and mastectomy involves extensive discussion among the patient, surgeon, radiologist, medical oncologist, and radiation oncologist. A multidisciplinary approach allows for the personalization of care. Finally, all patients requiring total mastectomy for DCIS should be offered the option of immediate breast reconstruction, which is associated with a psychological benefit and a similar oncologic outcome. In the United States, approximately one third of patients with DCIS undergo mastectomy.

The size of the negative margin remains controversial, because there are no prospectively acquired definitive data defining an adequate margin. Silverstein and colleagues retrospectively evaluated margin status in 469 patients with DCIS: 256 were treated with BCS alone, and 213 were treated with BCS and adjuvant radiation therapy. They acquired precise data on margin size by analyzing samples with three-dimensional reconstruction. The authors observed that with a margin width of 10 mm or more, the incidence of local recurrence was only 2.3%, and no added benefit from adjuvant radiation therapy was seen. Patients with margin widths between 1 to 10 mm benefited from adjuvant radiation therapy with an acceptable risk of recurrence. However, patients treated with a margin width of less than 1 mm had a suboptimal outcome with or without adjuvant radiation therapy. Although adjuvant radiation therapy significantly decreased the incidence of local recurrence from 58% to 30% in this group, such a recurrence rate is unacceptably high, suggesting that adjuvant radiation therapy is not adequate treatment. More recently, Neuschartz and colleagues also showed that margin width of less than 1 mm was associated with an increased rate of local recurrence despite adjuvant radiation therapy. Margin widths greater than 1 mm were associated with a 5 year recurrence rate of 10.9% for BCS alone and 4.6% for BCS plus adjuvant radiation therapy. Therefore, we recommend at least a 2 to 3 mm margin of excision for DCIS if adjuvant radiation will be administered. Further excision or possibly mastectomy may be indicated in patients with an excision margin of less than 2 mm.

Traditionally, axillary dissection and sentinel lymph node biopsy have had no role in the management of DCIS. The risk for nodal metastases in patients with DCIS is less than 3%. The low rate of nodal metastases, the high survival rate of DCIS, and the significant morbidity of an axillary lymph node dissection makes axillary nodal dissection unnecessary. However, the evaluation of axillary nodes by sentinel lymph node biopsy may be considered in certain situations, such as in the presence of large DCIS lesions (>4 cm), palpable breast lesions, high-grade disease, microinvasive disease, or suspicious appearing axillary lymph nodes on physical examination or on ultrasound. These particular features may increase the risk of finding an invasive cancer in the lumpectomy specimen by as much as 20%. Sentinel node biopsy performed at the same time as the lumpectomy may save the patient an additional operation. In addition, all patients undergoing a mastectomy for DCIS should undergo a concomitant sentinel node biopsy, because a sentinel node biopsy would not be possible after a mastectomy.

Radiation Therapy

Three prospective randomized controlled trials have investigated the role of adjuvant radiation therapy in DCIS after lumpectomy (Table 1). The National Surgical Adjuvant Breast and Bowel Project (NSABP) study B-17 enrolled 818 patients with DCIS between 1985 and 1990. The patients were randomized to undergo either lumpectomy alone or lumpectomy followed by breast irradiation to a total dose of 50 Gy. Through 12 years of follow-up, the investigators observed a 58% lower incidence of ipsilateral breast tumor recurrences associated with the use of adjuvant radiation therapy. Local recurrence rates were 17% in patients who did not receive radiation and 8% in patients who did. All subsets benefited from radiation therapy, regardless of the clinical or mammographic tumor characteristics. These data led to the recommendation that all patients with DCIS treated with BCS receive adjuvant radiation therapy. There was no difference in the distant metastatic disease-free survival or overall survival. Two other randomized controlled trials, the European Organization for Research and Treatment of Cancer (EORTC) study and the United Kingdom and Australia and New Zealand (UK/ANZ) study, demonstrated similar findings, as summarized in Table 1. Together, these three prospective trials show that adding radiation to lumpectomy for DCIS statistically decreases a patient's risk for developing recurrent breast cancer.

Although adjuvant radiation therapy significantly decreases local recurrence with BCS, it does not provide a clear survival advantage for patients with DCIS. In addition, radiation therapy is time consuming and condemns the patient to potential morbidities. Therefore, many clinicians are interested in identifying a subset of patients that could be treated with BCS alone. Silverstein and colleagues evaluated the effect of pathologic features—tumor size, margin width, nuclear grade, and the presence or absence of necrosis—on local recurrence. Patient age was later included to improve the accuracy of predicting local failure. By assigning a numerical score to each parameter, this group devised the University of Southern California-Van Nuys Prognostic Index (USC/VNPI, Table 2). In a retrospective review of a prospective database, which included a 12-year surveillance of 706 women who had BCS for pure DCIS, they found that USC/VNPI scores of 4, 5, and 6 had an average recurrence rate of 2%, of which 0% was invasive. USC/VNPI scores of 7, 8, and 9 had an average recurrence rate of 22%, of which 46% were invasive. USC/VNPI scores of 10, 11, and 12 had an average recurrence rate of 52%, of which 43% were invasive. Based on these findings, Silverstein and colleagues recommended lumpectomy alone for scores of 4, 5, and 6; lumpectomy and radiation for 7, 8, and 9; and mastectomy for 10, 11, and 12.

Wong and colleagues from the Dana Farber Cancer Institute conducted a single-arm prospective study of the use of wide excision alone for patients with favorable DCIS, defined as non–high-grade DCIS without necrosis, diameter less than or equal to 2.5 cm, and excision margins greater than or equal to 1 cm. From May 1995 to July 2002, they accrued patients who were treated with surgery alone and no radiation. The trial was terminated early, when the number of local recurrences met the predetermined stopping boundary. Only 158 patients had been enrolled (the initial target had been 200 patients). The rate of ipsilateral local recurrence was 2.4% per patient-year, corresponding to a 5-year recurrence rate of 12%. Thirty-one percent of these recurrences were IBC. Despite the use of margins greater than or equal to 1 cm, the local recurrence rate was substantial in patients with small, low- to intermediate-grade DCIS lesions treated with excision alone. These findings contradict Silverstein's evaluation and question the validity of the USC/VNPI.

TABLE 1: Clinical trials evaluating radiation therapy in DCIS patients after breast-conserving surgery

Trial	Follow-up (Years)	BREAST RECURRENCE RATE	
		No Radiation	Radiation
NSABP B-17	12	17%	8%
EORTC	4	16%	9%
UK/ANZ	5	14%	6%

NSABP B-17, National Surgical Adjuvant Breast and Bowel Project B-17 (*P* < .001); *EORTC,* European Organization for Research and Treatment of Cancer (*P* < .005); *UK/ANZ,* United Kingdom and Australia and New Zealand (*P* < .0001).

Criticisms of the Dana Farber study include the fact that this was a single-arm study that was not compared to treatment with adjuvant radiation therapy. In addition, the number of patients enrolled in the study was small, and the follow-up time was relatively short because of its required early termination. Undoubtedly, the USC/VNPI is a simple and reliable scoring system that has been confirmed by other groups to accurately identify a subset of patients who are at risk of local recurrence and who may benefit from radiation therapy or mastectomy. However, only prospective randomized trials can precisely predict the risk of local recurrence of conservatively treated DCIS. Except in a controlled trial adopting uniform criteria for margin evaluation, USC/VNPI should not be utilized to determine which patients can be treated with local excision alone. To date, no subset of patients from prospective randomized clinical trials has been identified that does not benefit from radiation therapy when undergoing BCS for DCIS.

Hormonal Therapy

Similar to the success of tamoxifen in the treatment of early invasive breast cancer, the NSABP B-24 trial demonstrated a benefit from tamoxifen for women with DCIS after treatment with BCS and adjuvant radiation therapy. Conducted from 1991 to 1995, investigators randomized 1,804 patients with DCIS treated with excision and radiation to receive either tamoxifen or placebo for 5 years. Tamoxifen and radiation were administered concurrently. In that trial, surgical margins were allowed to have tumor involvement. At 5 years, the women treated with tamoxifen had fewer breast cancer events, with a 5% reduction in absolute risk and a 37% reduction in relative risk. The cumulative incidence of all IBC events in the tamoxifen group was 4.1% (2.1% ipsilateral, 1.8% contralateral) versus 7.2% (4.2% ipsilateral, 2.3% contralateral) in the placebo treated group. Additionally, a retrospective analysis of estrogen receptor (ER) expression in the NSABP B-24 trial demonstrated that increased levels of ER expression predict a better tamoxifen benefit with respect to improved risk reduction for the development of breast cancer following BCS. Therefore, tamoxifen treatment should be considered as a strategy to reduce the risk of breast cancer recurrence in women with DCIS treated with BCS, especially in ER-positive DCIS.

Surveillance

Surveillance of patients previously treated with DCIS includes physical examination every 6 months for 5 years and then annually. A diagnostic mammogram should be performed yearly. Evaluation of both breasts is paramount with special attention to the ipsilateral breast following BCS. Most recurrences occur in close proximity to the site of prior disease. Mastectomy is often necessary in patients who present with a DCIS recurrence initially treated with BCS and adjuvant radiation therapy. Local recurrences following a mastectomy for DCIS should be treated with a negative margin resection followed by chest wall radiation if possible. Finally, local recurrences that present as IBC should receive the appropriate systemic therapy after the indicated surgical treatment. Figure 1 outlines our management algorithm of patients with DCIS.

LOBULAR CARCINOMA IN SITU

Foote and Stewart first coined the term *lobular carcinoma in situ* in 1941 to emphasize the similarity between cells of LCIS and invasive lobular carcinoma. In addition, they noted that the foci of neoplastic cells in LCIS were contained within the basement membrane, which is similar to DCIS. They believed that LCIS was a premalignant lesion to invasive lobular carcinoma and recommended mastectomy as the primary treatment. Later, the term *atypical lobular hyperplasia*

TABLE 2: USC/VNPI prognostic index scoring system for DCIS

	SCORE		
	1	2	3
Size	≤15 mm	16–40 mm	>40 mm
Margin	≥10 mm	1–9 mm	<1 mm
Pathology	Not a high nuclear grade, no necrosis	Not a high nuclear grade, necrosis	High nuclear grade with or without necrosis
Age	>60	40–60	<40

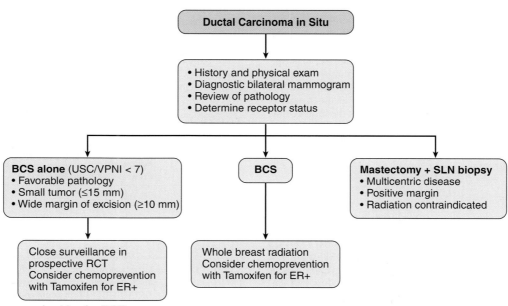

FIGURE 1   Management algorithm for DCIS.

(ALH) was introduced to describe morphologically similar but less well-developed lesions.

Over the past 60 years, it has become clear that LCIS and ALH are not precursor lesions for invasive carcinoma in the same way that DCIS is a precursor lesion to invasive cancer. The diagnosis of LCIS represents a marker for increased risk for subsequent carcinoma. Radical surgery for LCIS has fallen out of favor, but recommendations for treatment are not uniform; they vary from close surveillance with mammography to surveillance alone to bilateral mastectomy in some cases. Recently, new data suggesting that LCIS may be an obligate precursor lesion for IBC may have significant implications for the future management of patients with LCIS.

Pathophysiology

The histologic features of LCIS and ALH are well established. LCIS is divided into two specific subtypes: classic and pleomorphic LCIS. Classic LCIS consists of a monomorphic population of small, round, polygonal or cuboidal cells with a thin rim of clear cytoplasm and a high nuclear/cytoplasmic ratio. The cells are loosely cohesive and regularly spaced, and they fill and distend the acini. The nucleus is characterized by small nucleoli and few mitotic figures. Pagetoid spread, in which the neoplastic cells extend along adjacent ducts, is frequently seen. Pleomorphic LCIS exhibits cells with distinctly larger nuclei and prominent nucleoli with frequent mitotic figures. Central necrosis and calcification within lobules are common. For a diagnosis of LCIS, more than half the acini in an involved lobular unit must be filled and distended by the LCIS cells, leaving no central lumina. A lesion is regarded as ALH when the characteristic cells fill less than half the acini with no distension of the lobule, or there is mild distension of the lobule but the lumina are visible.

Natural History

Women with LCIS usually are diagnosed in the fifth decade of life with a mean age of diagnosis between 44 and 46 years of age, 10 years earlier than women with DCIS. Only 10% of women are seen with LCIS after menopause. The risk of developing IBC in patients with LCIS is 7 to 18 times higher than that of the general population. The SEER data between 1973 and 1998 revealed that the minimum cumulative risk of developing IBC after LCIS was 7.1% at 10 years, with a lifetime risk of 30% to 40%. It was once commonly believed that this increased risk is equal for both breasts. More recent studies, however, demonstrate that carcinoma is three times more likely to develop in the ipsilateral breast compared with the contralateral breast. Furthermore, the Surveillance, Epidemiology, and End Results (SEER) data gathered between 1988 and 2002 revealed that women with LCIS are also 5.3 times more likely to develop invasive lobular carcinoma and 0.8 times less likely to develop invasive ductal carcinoma. These new data suggest that LCIS may behave as both a precursor lesion to invasive lobular cancer and a risk indicator for IBC.

Diagnosis

The diagnosis of LCIS is often an incidental finding after a breast biopsy is performed for another reason. There are no specific clinical abnormalities that would alert a physician to LCIS based on breast examination or on patient symptomatology, and rarely is LCIS visible on mammography or other imaging modalities. Therefore the true incidence of LCIS in the general population is unknown. The incidence of LCIS in otherwise benign breast biopsies is between 0.5% to 3.8%. Similar to DCIS, LCIS rates have also increased in the last two and a half decades as a result of the increasing numbers of screening mammograms and biopsies being performed; in some series, as much as a threefold increase has been seen. Characteristically, LCIS is multifocal and bilateral in many patients; over 50% contain multiple foci in the same breast, and 30% will have LCIS in the contralateral breast. It is this multifocality in a clinically undetectable lesion that makes management of this disease a significant challenge.

Treatment

As previously mentioned, new epidemiologic data support the premise that LCIS may be a precursor lesion to invasive lobular carcinoma as well as a risk indicator for IBC. In addition, recent studies comparing the molecular signatures of LCIS and coexisting invasive lobular carcinoma also support the hypothesis that LCIS may act as a precursor. Therefore, advocates for the precursor role of LCIS suggest that a more definitive treatment strategy with BCS and adjuvant radiation may be necessary for patients with LCIS. Recently, Ciocca and colleagues challenged this premise and hypothesized that if LCIS were a precursor, its presence in the lumpectomy specimen, particularly at the margin, would increase local recurrence after BCS. They evaluated 2894 patients treated with BCS at the Fox Chase Cancer Center for DCIS stage I or stage II breast cancer, of which 290 patients also exhibited findings of LCIS, with LCIS present at the margin of excision in 84 patients. Among patients with LCIS at the margin, LCIS within the lumpectomy specimen but not at the margin, or no LCIS, the 5- and 10-year local recurrence rates were not statistically different. The presence of LCIS at the lumpectomy margin did not have an impact on local recurrence, unlike the increase in local recurrence rates found in patients with positive or close lumpectomy margins for DCIS. These findings do not support LCIS as a precursor to the development of IBC. In addition, their results also confirm that reexcision of a positive margin for LCIS is not necessary. Until further studies can definitively clarify its precursor function, we maintain that LCIS should still be managed as a risk indicator for the development of IBC.

Specimen Evaluation

Stereotactic core needle biopsy has become the most common method for breast tissue sampling after a suspicious mammogram. Controversy exists as to the need for surgical excision after the finding of LCIS or ALH on a core needle biopsy specimen. Elsheikh and colleagues prospectively studied 33 patients who had core biopsies and underwent follow-up surgical excision. Surgical excision of the tissue surrounding a core biopsy of LCIS revealed IBC in 4 (31%) of 13 patients and 5 (25%) of the 20 patients with ALH revealed carcinoma, including four with DCIS and one invasive lobular carcinoma. Underestimation of cancer when a core biopsy showed LCIS or ALH was seen in 28% of prospectively examined patients, including 20% of those with ALH and 38% of those with LCIS. The authors recommended surgical excision to rule out malignancy in all patients with core needle biopsy specimens exhibiting findings of LCIS or ALH.

We believe that the best strategy for the management of LCIS and ALH found on core needle biopsy is a multidisciplinary team approach to determine whether there is discordance between the radiologically identified abnormality and the pathologic findings. If LCIS is identified in a core specimen with other high-grade lesions, or the imaged abnormality has not been adequately explained by the pathology (radiologic-pathologic discordance), further surgical excision is necessary. If LCIS is a true incidental finding with no suspicious findings or discordance, further excision is not necessary.

Management of surgical excision specimens exhibiting LCIS is also an area of some controversy. If only LCIS is seen in an excisional biopsy, then no further excision is required. Finally, a finding of LCIS at the margin of an excisional biopsy in association with an IBC also does not warrant further excision, if the IBC has been completely excised.

Treatment Options

Counseling regarding LCIS necessitates informing the patient of their increased risk of IBC and the need for close follow-up. The risk of IBC is 0.5% to 1.0% per year. Because the risk is low, observation

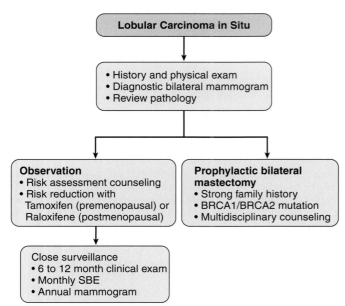

FIGURE 2 Management algorithm for LCIS. *SBE,* Self breast examination.

is the preferred treatment option for patients diagnosed with LCIS. In addition, the patient should understand that the biology of the potential IBC tends to be favorable, and death from an IBC detected early is unlikely. Prophylactic bilateral mastectomy should be considered in special circumstances, such as in women with a *BRCA1* or *BRCA2* mutation or a strong family history. Nevertheless, the decision to pursue prophylactic mastectomy for risk reduction should be made only after careful evaluation and multidisciplinary counseling. Women treated with bilateral mastectomy are appropriate candidates for breast reconstruction.

Two studies, the NSABP P-1 Breast Cancer Prevention Trial and the NSABP P-2 Study of Tamoxifen and Raloxifene (STAR) examined chemoprevention of invasive and noninvasive breast cancer for LCIS patients. The NSABP P-1 trial evaluated the use of tamoxifen for the prevention of breast cancer in 13,388 high-risk women. Risk was determined by the Gail model risk assessment based on the patient's age, age at menarche, age at first live birth, family history of breast cancer, and number of breast biopsies, including diagnosis of atypical hyperplasia and/or diagnosis of LCIS. Of the participants, 8.4% had a diagnosis of LCIS. The study found that tamoxifen decreased the risk for developing IBC by 49% in all enrolled high-risk

women. Subset analysis of patients with LCIS had an even greater risk reduction (56%). The STAR trial enrolled 19,747 women also determined to be at high risk by the Gail model. All of the women studied were postmenopausal, of which 9% had a diagnosis of LCIS. They were randomized to receive daily doses of tamoxifen or raloxifene. The two drugs were equally effective for the prevention of IBC in the postmenopausal women with a history of LCIS. Women taking raloxifene had a lower risk of thromboembolic events and fewer uterine cancers compared with those taking tamoxifen. However, unlike tamoxifen, which reduced the incidence of DCIS and LCIS by half, raloxifene had no effect in the prevention of noninvasive breast cancer occurrences.

The 2009 National Comprehensive Cancer Network guidelines recommend observation as the primary treatment of LCIS. The use of tamoxifen in premenopausal women or tamoxifen or raloxifene in postmenopausal women should be considered as a risk-reduction strategy in women with LCIS. Risk reduction or prophylactic bilateral mastectomy may be considered as an option for women with a history of LCIS, especially for women with *BRCA1 or BRCA2* mutation or a strong family history of breast cancer, only after following careful evaluation and counseling. Surveillance of LCIS patients should include interval breast examinations by a physician every 6 to 12 months and periodic breast self-examinations. All patients being followed by close observation should undergo annual diagnostic mammography (Figure 2). Finally, all LCIS patients should be offered the option of participation in clinical research protocols that evaluate screening or risk assessment.

Suggested Readings

Ciocca RM, Li T, Freedman MG, et al: Presence of lobular carcinoma in situ does not increase local recurrence in patients treated with breast-conserving therapy, *Ann Surg Oncol* 15:2263, 2008.

Fisher B, Land S, Mamounas E, et al: Prevention of invasive breast cancer in women with ductal carcinoma in situ: an update of the National Surgical Adjuvant Breast and Bowel Project experience, *Semin Oncol* 28:400, 2001.

Schwart GF, Allen KG, Palazzo JP: et al: Biology and management of lobular carcinoma in situ of the breast. In Bland KI, Copeland EM, editor: *The Breast,* ed 4, Philadelphia, 2009, Saunders Elsevier.

Silverstein MJ: Ductal carcinoma in situ: treatment, controversies, and oncoplastic surgeries. In Bland KI, Copeland EM, editors: *The Breast,* ed 4, Philadelphia, 2009, Saunders Elsevier.

Vogel VG, Constantino JP, Wickerham DL, et al: Effects of tamoxifen versus raloxifene on the risk of developing invasive breast cancer and other disease outcomes: the NSABP Study of Tamoxifen and Raloxifene (STAR) P-2 trial, *JAMA* 295:2727, 2006.

Wong JS, Kaelin CM, Troyan SL: Prospective study of wide excision alone for ductal carcinoma in situ of the breast, *J Clin Oncol* 24:1031, 2006.

Advances in Adjuvant and Neoadjuvant Therapy for Breast Cancer

Jennifer G. Reeder, MD, Barry C. Lembersky, MD, and
Nancy E. Davidson, MD

OVERVIEW

Recent advances in adjuvant and neoadjuvant systemic therapy have been an important component of the steady decline in breast cancer mortality rates over the past two decades. Innovations in various treatment modalities—including endocrine therapies, chemotherapeutic agents, and targeted biologic agents—have led to the delivery of less toxic and more effective treatment regimens. Additionally, gene expression profiling has revolutionized our ability to determine which patients are likely to benefit from specific types of therapy. Patients who have the highest chances of deriving benefit from chemotherapy or targeted biologic agents can be quickly identified, and those who will only benefit from endocrine therapy can be spared the adverse effects of cytotoxic therapy. A broader spectrum of treatment options and the advent of gene expression profiling have moved us into an era focused on providing increasingly more individualized cancer care.

ADJUVANT SYSTEMIC THERAPY

Endocrine Therapy

Approximately 75% of all invasive breast cancers will express some level of estrogen or progesterone receptors. The stimulation of these nuclear receptors by estrogen in the female body is believed to be a critical step in the process of breast cancer growth. Breast cancers that express these receptors are a highly heterogeneous group of tumors, with varying amounts of receptor expression. The higher the concentration of estrogen receptors (ERs), the more likely it is that adjuvant antiestrogen therapy will be beneficial. Although it is somewhat controversial whether patients with low levels of receptors derive benefit from endocrine therapy, the 2009 St. Gallen Consensus Panel defined *endocrine-responsive* tumors as those that have the presence of any detectable ER.

ER signaling is the process by which the biologically active form of estrogen, estradiol, binds to ERs within the cell and initiates the transcription of various genes that lead to cell proliferation, angiogenesis, and metastasis. Tamoxifen is a selective ER modulator (SERM) that has been the cornerstone of endocrine therapy for years based on its ability to target the ER signaling pathway. By competitively binding to the ER, tamoxifen blocks estradiol from initiating downstream signaling. Unfortunately, tamoxifen is associated with significant side effects in older women, including an increased risk of venous thromboembolism and endometrial cancer.

Aromatase inhibition was developed as an alternative method to reduce circulating estrogen in postmenopausal women. Aromatase inhibitors (AIs) inhibit the enzyme aromatase, which is responsible for the peripheral conversion of androstenedione to estrodiol. AIs have been shown to be more effective and less toxic than tamoxifen in postmenopausal women, but they cause a paradoxical increase in estrogen in premenopausal women. Therefore,

an accurate assessment of menopausal status is critical prior to initiating endocrine therapy in an ER-positive patient. The National Comprehensive Cancer Network (NCCN) defines *menopause* as prior bilateral oophorectomy, age 60 years or older, or age less than 60 years with amenorrhea for 12 or more months and follicle-stimulating hormone (FSH) and estradiol levels in the postmenopausal range.

Premenopausal Women

Approximately one fifth of all new cases of breast cancer occur in women younger than age 50 years, and 60% of these cases represent ER-positive disease. Compelling long-term data in support of tamoxifen have been recently reported by the Early Breast Cancer Trialists' Collaborative Group (EBCTCG) as part of their quinquennial international meta-analysis. With data from 15,000 women in this portion of the meta-analysis, the EBCTCG concluded that treatment of early stage ER-positive breast cancer with 5 years of adjuvant tamoxifen reduces the annual recurrence rate by 41% and the annual rate of breast cancer mortality by 34%. Further analysis revealed that these benefits occurred irrespective of age, menopausal status, or nodal status.

The role of ovarian suppression (OS) or ovarian ablation (OA) with or without additional adjuvant therapy remains controversial. The EBCTCG meta-analysis found that in nearly 8,000 women under age 50 years with early stage breast cancer, randomized into trials of OS/OA, recurrence risk and breast cancer mortality were reduced by 4.3% and 3.2%, respectively. The panel concluded that OS/OA clearly shows benefit for patients with early stage breast cancer in the absence of other treatments. Studies evaluating OS/OA in combination with chemotherapy, tamoxifen, and AIs are ongoing. Early results from the Austrian Breast and Colorectal Cancer Study Group Trial 12 (ABCSG-12) showed no difference in disease-free survival (DFS) between patients treated with OS plus tamoxifen versus OS plus anastrozole. The Suppression of Ovarian Function Trial (SOFT) is ongoing and will compare treatment with tamoxifen alone to OS plus either tamoxifen or exemestane.

Current guidelines for adjuvant endocrine treatment in premenopausal women with ER-positive breast cancer recommend the use of tamoxifen alone or in combination with OS/OA. AIs alone are contraindicated in premenopausal women. Their use in combination with OS/OA is considered experimental and should only be used in clinical trials or in situations in which tamoxifen is contraindicated.

Postmenopausal Women

Five years of adjuvant tamoxifen was the initial standard treatment for postmenopausal women with early stage breast cancer, but the increasing risk of venous thromboembolism and endometrial cancer in older women led investigators to explore the role of AI. Several large, randomized prospective studies have compared 5 years of tamoxifen to various strategies involving an AI (Table 1). All of the regimens—including up-front AI therapy, switching to an AI after 2 to 3 years of tamoxifen, or adding 5 years of an AI after 5 years of tamoxifen—appear to favor the use of an AI at some point in the treatment course.

Based on these data, current guidelines now recommend that AIs should be part of the standard endocrine therapy for postmenopausal women. The third-generation AIs in clinical use today, including the steroidal AI exemestane and the nonsteroidal AIs letrozole and anastrozole, are believed to be equivalent in terms of efficacy and safety. The optimal duration of adjuvant AI therapy is being evaluated in ongoing trials. For women who do not tolerate, have a contraindication to, or decline AI therapy, tamoxifen for 5 years is recommended.

TABLE 1: Aromatase inhibitors in the adjuvant setting

Trial	N	Standard Arm	Aromatase Inhibitor Arm	Median Follow-up (Mo)	DFS HR; P Value	OS HR; P Value
ATAC	9366	Tamoxifen for 5 yr	Anastrozole for 5 yr	100	0.85; P = .003	No difference
BIG 1-98	8010	Tamoxifen for 5 yr	Letrozole for 5 yr	51	0.82; P = .007	No difference*
IES	4724	Tamoxifen for 5 yr	Tamoxifen for 2 to 3 yr, then exemestane for 2 to 3 yr	55.7	0.76; P = .0001	0.83; P = .05
ABCSG-8/ ARNO 95/ITA	3672	Tamoxifen for 5 yr	Tamoxifen for 2 to 3 yr, then anastrozole for 2 to 3 yr	30	0.59; P < .001	0.71; P = .04
MA-17	5157	Tamoxifen for 5 yr	Tamoxifen for 5 yr, then letrozole for 5 yr	30	0.58; P = .00004	No difference*

*No survival difference was seen overall, but upon subgroup analysis a survival difference was found in the node-positive patients in BIG 1-98 (HR, 0.71; P < .001) and MA-17 (HR, 0.61; P = .04).
ATAC, Arimidex, Tamoxifen Alone or in Combination; *ABCSG-8/ARNO 95/ITA,* Antithrombotic Regimens aNd Outcome/Austrian Breast & Colon Cancer Study Group/Italian Tamoxifen Anastrazole; *BIG,* Breast International Group; *HR,* hazard ratio; *IES,* International Exemexane Study

Chemotherapy

Adjuvant chemotherapy has been an important part of the treatment plan for early stage breast cancer for three decades. Robust clinical research has led to sequential improvements in specific regimens and durations of therapy. One of the initial regimens—cyclophosphamide, methotrexate, and 5-fluorouracil (CMF)—was replaced in the early 1990s by anthracycline-based regimens, which were found to have improved efficacy and tolerability.

The preclinical and clinical development of the taxane class of cytotoxic agents was the next major advance in the management of early stage breast cancer. A number of large, multicentered, prospective phase III clinical trials evaluated the use of a taxane either concurrently or sequentially with an anthracycline-based regimen. Both methods of administration showed a statistically significant and clinically meaningful improvement in DFS and overall survival (OS). The optimal dosing and schedule of sequential taxane administration added to an anthracycline-based backbone was addressed by the recent Eastern Cooperative Oncology Group (ECOG) 1199 trial. Out of four possible dosing strategies, doxorubicin/cyclophosphamide (AC) followed by 12 weekly doses of paclitaxel proved to be the superior regimen in terms of both DFS and OS, at the cost of an increase in peripheral neuropathy.

Dose-dense chemotherapy is another strategy that has been proposed in the treatment of early stage breast cancer. This approach is based on theoretical modeling developed by Norton and others, which suggests that the administration of chemotherapy at shorter dosing intervals may be more effective at eradicating minimal residual disease. In Cancer and Leukemia Group B trial 9741, women who were randomized to receive four cycles of AC followed by four cycles of paclitaxel every 2 weeks, instead of the standard 3 weeks, benefited not only from an improvement in DFS and OS but also from a decrease in severe neutropenia. An important ongoing clinical trial is comparing dose-dense administration of AC followed by paclitaxel every 2 weeks with the concurrent administration of docetaxel, doxorubicin, and cyclophosphamide (TAC) given every 3 weeks. The current NCCN guidelines include AC followed by weekly paclitaxel, TAC every 3 weeks, and dose-dense AC followed by paclitaxel on their list of preferred adjuvant regimens.

One of the emerging controversies in the adjuvant treatment of breast cancer involves the role of anthracyclines. As patients are now living many years beyond their initial breast cancer treatment, the long-term toxicities associated with anthracyclines, such as cardiotoxicity and acute leukemia, are becoming more of a concern. In a large, prospective phase III trial, 1106 women with node-negative and node-positive breast cancer were randomized to receive four cycles of AC or four cycles of docetaxel and cyclophosphamide (TC). At a 7-year follow-up, women receiving TC had a statistically significant improvement in both DFS and OS, and they had a unique but acceptable toxicity profile.

The role of anthracyclines was further called into question by the results of the Breast Cancer International Research Group (BCIRG) 006 trial, in which patients whose tumors were positive for the *HER2/neu* gene were randomized to receive either an anthracycline-containing regimen with or without trastuzumab or a non–anthracycline-based regimen with trastuzumab. Both trastuzumab-containing arms had equal efficacy, but the anthracycline arm had significantly more critical adverse events, including grade III and IV cardiotoxicity and anthracycline-related leukemia. These results, along with the superiority of TC compared to AC, have led many clinicians to question the need for anthracyclines at all in the adjuvant treatment of breast cancer. In addition, preclinical and clinical research efforts are now focused on identifying potential markers of anthracycline sensitivity.

One important target for anthracycline cytotoxicity is the topoisomerase II gene (*TOPO II*). To date, conflicting results have been reported from a number of studies on whether amplification of the *TOPO II* gene is associated with enhanced anthracycline cytotoxicity and efficacy. Further results of this translational research, as well as an ongoing phase III clinical trial comparing the adjuvant use of TC versus TAC, are eagerly awaited.

Targeted Therapy

One of the most promising advances in modern oncology has been the development of therapeutic agents that target specific pathways in the process of tumorigenesis. HER2 is a transmembrane receptor tyrosine kinase that participates in the growth, differentiation, and survival of breast cancer cells. Overexpression of the HER2 protein occurs in approximately 25% of breast cancers and is associated with more aggressive tumor behavior. Trastuzumab is a humanized monoclonal antibody that binds to the extracellular domain of the HER2 protein and inhibits downstream signaling. In multiple recent phase III trials conducted in both the United States and Europe, trastuzumab in combination with standard chemotherapy has had an enormous impact on DFS and OS in early stage *HER2*-positive breast cancer (Table 2). Pooled results from a recent meta-analysis showed a significant reduction in mortality (P < .00001), recurrence (P < .00001), and rate of metastasis (P < .00001) in these patients

TABLE 2: Trastuzumab in the adjuvant setting

Trial	N	Standard Arm	Trastuzumab-Containing Arm	Median Follow-up (Mo)	DFS HR; P Value	OS HR; P Value
NSABP B-31/ NCCTG N9831	3351	AC × 4 → P × 4 q3wk	AC × 4 → P × 4 q3wk + trastuzumab weekly × 52 wk	24	0.48; P < .0001	0.67; P = .015
HERA	5090	Any chemo → observation	Any chemo → 1 or 2 yr trastuzumab	23.5	0.64; P < .0001	0.66; P = .0115
BCIRG 006	3222	AC × 4 → D × 4	Concurrent TCH + trastuzumab × 1 yr	36	0.67; P = .0003	0.66; P = .017
			AC × 4 → D × 4 + trastuzumab × 1 yr	36	0.61; P < .0001	0.59; P = .004
Fin HER	232	D or V × 3 → FEC × 3	D or V + trastuzumab × 3 → FEC × 3	36	0.42; P = .01*	0.41; P = .07

*Combined end point of DFS and OS.

AC, Adriamycin and cyclophosphamide; *BCIRG*, Breast Cancer International Research Group; *D*, docetaxel; *FEC*, 5-fluorouracil, epirubicin, cyclophosphamide; *Fin HER*, Finland Herceptin Study; *HR*, hazard ratio; *HERA*, Herceptin Adjuvant Study; *NCCTG*, North Central Cancer Treatment Group; *NSABP*, National Surgical Adjuvant Breast and Bowel Project; *P*, paclitaxel; *TCH*, docetaxel, carboplatin, trastuzumab; *V*, vinorelbine

compared with those who received chemotherapy alone. Grade III or IV cardiotoxicity occurred in 4.5% of patients receiving trastuzumab-containing regimens compared with only 1.8% in patients who did not receive trastuzumab, indicating that cardiotoxicity remains a significant concern with trastuzumab. The 2009 St. Gallen and NCCN guidelines both recommend one year of trastuzumab therapy in all patients with *HER2*-positive disease whose tumor is greater than 1 cm, regardless of hormone-receptor status. The use of trastuzumab without concurrent chemotherapy or for tumors less than 1 cm requires clinical judgment, as these scenarios have not been adequately studied.

Lapatinib is an oral tyrosine kinase inhibitor that also targets the HER2 receptor. Lapatinib differs from trastuzumab in its site of action on the HER2 receptor as well as in its unique side effect profile. Lapatinib has shown clinical activity in metastatic breast cancer, including in tumors refractory to trastuzumab. Lapatinib alone or in combination with trastuzumab is being compared to trastuzumab alone in the adjuvant setting in *HER2*-positive patients in the Adjuvant Lapatinib and/or Trastuzumab Treatment Optimization (ALTTO) trial.

Bevacizumab, another humanized monoclonal antibody, binds to vascular endothelial growth factor (VEGF), a protein that promotes the growth of blood vessels. One potential mechanism of action for bevacizumab involves altering the blood supply needed for tumor growth and spread. The addition of bevacizumab to paclitaxel in the metastatic setting has shown increased response rate and increased disease-free survival and OS. The combination of bevacizumab and chemotherapy is now being studied in the adjuvant setting in several ongoing clinical trials.

NEOADJUVANT SYSTEMIC THERAPY

Preoperative chemotherapy, commonly referred to as *neoadjuvant* or *induction chemotherapy,* has revolutionized the management of locally advanced breast cancer. Neoadjuvant therapy is now considered the standard of care for patients with bulky breast or axillary disease, and it has also become an option for operable tumors, if tumor shrinkage is expected to improve eligibility for breast-conserving therapy (BCT). Initial skepticism regarding the use of neoadjuvant therapy focused on whether preoperative therapy would increase surgical complication rates, alter the prognostic significance of axillary nodal status, diminish the accuracy of sentinel node biopsy, or worsen overall survival by delaying the time to surgery. In fact, several studies have shown that neoadjuvant chemotherapy has no adverse effect on surgical complication rates or delivery of operative care. McCready and colleagues showed that axillary nodal status following preoperative chemotherapy continued to correlate well with prognosis. Moreover, the accuracy of sentinel lymph node biopsy (SLNB) following neoadjuvant treatment in clinically node-negative patients participating in the National Surgical Adjuvant Breast and Bowel Project (NASBP) B-27 study was comparable to that seen in patients undergoing primary surgery. However, the timing of SLNB in relation to neoadjuvant chemotherapy remains controversial (Table 3).

Several large, randomized studies conducted in the United States and Europe have uniformly shown no difference in OS between adjuvant and neoadjuvant chemotherapy. However, patients treated with neoadjuvant therapy who have a pathologic complete response (PCR) at the time of surgery have been observed to have a statistically significant survival benefit compared with patients with partial or no response. Thus PCR serves as a surrogate endpoint for OS and establishes neoadjuvant systemic therapy as an important clinical research paradigm.

Endocrine Therapy

The use of endocrine therapy in the neoadjuvant setting has been slow to develop, because the PCR rate has been reported to be substantially lower with endocrine therapy than with chemotherapy. However, neoadjuvant studies have repeatedly shown that hormone receptor–positive patients have lower response rates to chemotherapy than hormone receptor–negative patients, indicating that there may be a population of strongly ER-positive patients who will benefit more from neoadjuvant endocrine therapy than chemotherapy.

The superior efficacy of AIs over tamoxifen in the adjuvant setting has revived interest in neoadjuvant endocrine therapy. The P024 study was a large multinational trial in which ER-positive women who were ineligible for BCT were treated with either letrozole or tamoxifen with overall response rates of 55% and 36% respectively. Conversion to BCT occurred in 45% of patients treated with letrozole compared with only 35% of patients treated with tamoxifen,

TABLE 3: Considerations in the timing of SLNB

Time	Advantages	Disadvantages
SLNB after neoadjuvant chemotherapy	• More studies have evaluated the use of SLNB after neoadjuvant chemotherapy. • Surgical sequence is consistent with conventional neoadjuvant regimens.	• False-negative rates are not yet well defined. • Drug-induced lymphatic drainage may interfere with SLNB. • Patients who are truly node negative may receive a more aggressive chemotherapy regimen than required.
SLNB before neoadjuvant chemotherapy	• Significance of nodal status is better understood when axillary staging is performed at presentation. • A more accurate prognosis can be determined up front and may help guide treatment decisions, such as type of chemotherapy.	• Potential for unnecessary ALND exists, as patients with a metastatic SLN before neoadjuvant chemotherapy are committed to undergoing ALND, and chemo will sterilize up to 25% to 35% of node-positive patients. • Treatment exposes patient to risks of an additional surgical procedure.

ALND, Axillary lymph node dissection

demonstrating a clear benefit with letrozole over tamoxifen in the neoadjuvant setting.

The Immediate Preoperative Anastrozole Tamoxifen or Combined with Tamoxifen (IMPACT) study was a phase III trial that randomized 330 ER-positive postmenopausal women to receive either anastrozole alone, tamoxifen alone, or a combination of both for 12 weeks prior to surgery. Although no statistically significant difference was seen in response rates among the three groups, 46% of women treated with anastrozole underwent BCT, compared with 22% with tamoxifen and 26% with the combination. Gene expression profiles may help further define the population of patients who will receive maximal benefit from neoadjuvant endocrine therapy, but this approach is still investigational.

Chemotherapy

In general, trials comparing adjuvant and neoadjuvant chemotherapy have shown that neoadjuvant treatment increases the number of women eligible for BCT but does not have an effect on DFS or OS. In the NSABP B-18 trial, 1493 patients were randomized to receive four cycles of AC either preoperatively or postoperatively. No statistically significant difference in DFS or OS was found between the two groups through 16 years of follow-up. Women participating in NSABP B-27 were randomized to receive neoadjuvant AC, neoadjuvant AC followed by docetaxel and then surgery, or neoadjuvant AC followed by surgery and then docetaxel. The addition of docetaxel did not significantly improve DFS or OS, but it did show an increase in PCR of 26%, compared with 13% for AC only. The ongoing NSABP B-40 trial is evaluating whether the addition of capecitabine or gemcitabine to standard preoperative chemotherapy will improve PCR rates. The optimal treatment of patients

who have residual disease after neoadjuvant chemotherapy remains controversial.

The treatment of patients who do not respond well to initial chemotherapy also presents a treatment dilemma. In the GeparTrio trial, patients who did not respond to two cycles of preoperative TAC were randomized to either continue with four more cycles of TAC or to switch to four cycles of vinorelbine and capecitabine. Patients receiving the non–cross-resistant regimen did not have any improvement in outcome compared with patients who completed six total cycles of TAC. The development of new treatment strategies and new agents remains a priority for this patient population.

Targeted Therapy

The success of trastuzumab in the adjuvant setting has led to a number of trastuzumab trials in the neoadjuvant setting. A trial by Buzdar and colleagues (2004) randomly assigned women with *HER2*-positive breast cancer to paclitaxel followed by a combination of 5-fluorouracil, epirubicin, and cyclophosphamide (FEC) with or without trastuzumab as neoadjuvant therapy. The addition of neoadjuvant trastuzumab yielded a PCR of 65.2% compared to 26.3% in patients with chemotherapy alone. These promising results were followed up by the results of the NeOAdjuvant Herceptin (NOAH) trial, which were presented at the 2008 San Antonio Breast Cancer Symposium. In this trial, 228 patients with locally advanced *HER2*-positive disease were randomized to neoadjuvant chemotherapy with or without trastuzumab. Patients receiving trastuzumab had a significant improvement in 3 year DFS compared to patients who received chemotherapy alone (HR 0.55, $P = .006$). In addition, nearly twice as many patients receiving trastuzumab achieved a PCR. The regimen was well tolerated with very few reports of cardiotoxicity. These data established neoadjuvant trastuzumab as a standard treatment option in women with *HER2*-positive disease. Bevacizumab is currently being investigated in the neoadjuvant setting in an arm of the NSABP B-40 trial.

Individualizing a Treatment Plan

The ultimate goal in developing an individualized treatment plan is to provide each patient with systemic therapy that offers maximal benefit and minimal toxicity. For many years, the primary determinants of prognosis and treatment decisions included ER, progesterone receptor (PR), and *HER2* status, histology, grade, tumor size, and axillary lymph node status. A computerized algorithm, Adjuvant! Online, is a well-validated software program that incorporates this clinico-pathologic data to produce an estimation of prognosis and treatment response. Despite the development of this sophisticated algorithm, our ability to accurately predict tumor behavior and response to treatment remains imperfect. One important step toward the goal of individualizing treatment has been the development of gene expression profiles. A number of genes that appear to play a significant role in promoting the growth, invasion, and metastatic spread of breast cancer cells have been identified. Based on various combinations of these genes, six different multigene assays have been developed (Table 4).

The two assays most commonly used in the clinical setting are the 21-gene recurrence score (Oncotype DX; Genomic Health, Redwood City, Calif.) and the Amsterdam 70-gene profile (Mammaprint; Agendia, Amsterdam, The Netherlands). Using paraffin-embedded tissue samples from node-negative, ER-positive patients who participated in NSABP B-14, the 21-gene recurrence score has been shown to correlate with an increasing risk of distant recurrence at 10 years of 6.8%, 14.3%, and 30.5% in the low-, intermediate-, and high-risk groups, respectively. This multigene assay also predicts benefit from chemotherapy in the same group of node-negative patients, emphasizing its potential to have a strong impact in the clinical setting. The Trial Assigning IndividuaLized Options for Treatment (TAILORx) is an ongoing prospective study examining whether the 21-gene recurrence score assists physicians in choosing the most appropriate and effective treatment for each patient with node-negative, early-stage

TABLE 4: Gene expression profile models

Assay	Commercial Name of Test	Tissue Type	Populations Studied	Proposed Predictive Indication
21-Gene recurrence score	Oncotype DX	Fixed	Node negative, node positive, ER positive	Risk of distant recurrence at 10 yr Benefit from chemotherapy
Amsterdam 70-gene profile	Mammaprint	Fresh	Node negative, node positive	Risk of distant metastasis
76-Gene prognostic signature		Fresh	Node negative	DFS, OS
Two-gene ratio		Fixed	Early stage, hormone receptor positive	Benefit from addition of chemotherapy to tamoxifen
Wound-response gene expression profile		Fresh	Node negative, node positive	DFS, OS
Intrinsic subtype model		Fresh	Locally advanced disease	DFS, OS

TABLE 5: Clinicopathologic considerations for patients with ER-positive, *HER2*-negative disease

Clinicopathologic Features	Consider Adding Chemotherapy	Factors not Useful for Decision	Consider Endocrine Therapy Only
ER and PR	Lower ER/PR levels		Higher ER/PR levels
Grade	Grade 3	Grade 2	Grade 1
Proliferation	Ki-67 >30%	Ki-67 16% to 30%	Ki-67 ≤15%
Nodes	Node positive (four or more nodes)	Node positive (one to three nodes)	Node negative
Peritumoral vascular invasion	Extensive PVI		Absence of PVI
Tumor size	>5 cm	2.1–5 cm	≤2 cm
Patient preference	Favors using all possible treatments		Favors avoiding side effects of chemotherapy

Adapted from highlights of the St. Gallen consensus panel.

breast cancer. In node-positive patients, the 21-gene recurrence score was again able to identify a subset of node-positive women who do not appear to benefit from chemotherapy. Based on these results, the 21-gene recurrence score has become a valuable tool in the clinical setting, although its use in node-positive patients is less widely accepted at this time.

The Amsterdam 70-gene profile has been shown to be prognostic in both node-negative and node-positive patients and to be superior to Adjuvant! Online in predicting distant recurrence. The ability of the 70-gene profile to predict clinical benefit from chemotherapy is being studied prospectively in an ongoing randomized European study, the Microarray in Node-Negative Disease may Avoid Chemotherapy Trial (MINDACT). The other gene expression profiles, which include the intrinsic subtype model, a 76-gene assay, a two-gene ratio model, and a wound-response gene expression profile have shown varying utility as prognostic markers and have not yet made it into clinical practice.

A retrospective study was conducted in 2006 to determine the level of concordance between these gene expression profiles. Although there was minimal overlap in the genes that were identified in each profile, a high degree of concordance was seen between four of the five profiles included in the study. The intrinsic subtype, 70-gene profile, wound-response profile, and 21-gene recurrence score all accurately predicted DFS and OS. Thus although few of the genes in each gene profile overlap, the four models all seem to identify a similar biologic phenotype.

SUMMARY

The most significant advances in adjuvant and neoadjuvant systemic therapy have revolved around our improved ability to deliver individualized treatment. An increasing array of agents—including endocrine, cytotoxic, and targeted therapies—has expanded treatment options to improve efficacy and minimize toxicity. The clinicopathologic features of each patient's tumor must be considered when choosing from this wide array of treatment options (Table 5 and Figure 1). In situations in which these conventional markers do not provide adequate information, validated multigene assays may be used. Patients with a low score on the assay can be spared the risks and inconvenience of chemotherapy in favor of more effective endocrine therapy, whereas patients with a high score will derive significant benefit from chemotherapy. The use of molecular profiling to guide treatment decisions in clinical practice remains an important goal in this new era of individualized cancer care.

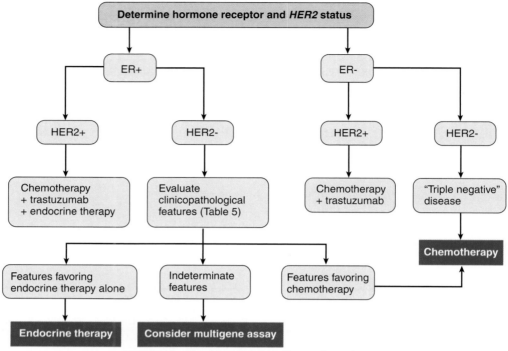

FIGURE 1 Considerations for adjuvant chemotherapy.

SUGGESTED READINGS

Early Breast Cancer Trialists' Collaborative Group (EBCTCG): Effects of chemotherapy and hormonal therapy for early breast cancer on recurrence and 15-year survival: an overview of the randomized trials, *Lancet* 365:1687–1717, 2005.

Goldhirsch A, Ingle JN, Gelber RD, et al: Meeting highlights—thresholds for therapies: highlights of the St. Gallen International Expert Consensus on the primary therapy of early breast cancer 2009, *Ann Onc* 20:1319–1329, 2009.

Kaufmann M, von Minckwitz G, Bear HD, et al: Recommendations from an international expert panel on the use of neoadjuvant (primary) systemic treatment of operable breast cancer: new perspectives 2006, *Ann Oncol* 18:1927–1934, 2007.

Lin NU, Winer EP: Advances in adjuvant endocrine therapy for postmenopausal women, *J Clin Onc* 26:798–805, 2008.

Viani GA, Afonso SL, Stefano EJ, et al: Adjuvant trastuzumab in the treatment of *HER2*-positive early breast cancer: a meta-analysis of published randomized trials, *BMC Cancer* 7:153, 2007.

MANAGEMENT OF RECURRENT AND METASTATIC BREAST CANCER

Gildy V. Babiera, MD, and Abigail S. Caudle, MD

OVERVIEW

Breast cancer is the most common cancer in women in the United States. According to the National Cancer Institute, there will be an estimated 192,000 new cases of breast cancer in 2009 and 40,000 deaths, accounting for 15% of all cancer deaths in women. The incidence of breast cancer is increasing; however, advances in therapy have improved survival rates and extended the life span of breast cancer patients. This expanding group of breast cancer survivors has made issues of surveillance and management of recurrent and metastatic disease of utmost importance.

Risk of relapse is directly related to tumor size and the presence of nodal metastasis, with 20% to 30% of node-negative patients and an estimated 50% to 60% of node-positive patients eventually having recurrence at some point. Long-term follow-up from the pivotal trials that established breast conservation as an acceptable surgical option confirms no differences in survival compared to mastectomy, but it does reveal different locoregional relapse patterns. In-breast recurrence based on data from the National Surgical Adjuvant Breast and Bowel Project (NSABP) B-6 trial demonstrated, although not with statistical significance, a local recurrence rate estimated to be 14% after breast-conserving therapy (BCT) at 20 years compared with 10% after mastectomy. Similar local failure rates were seen in the Milan III study, which used quadrantectomy instead of segmental mastectomy with recurrences of 9% after BCT versus 2.3% after mastectomy at 20-year follow-up. However, more contemporary series, although not randomized studies, suggest that with the more liberal use of systemic therapy, in-breast tumor recurrences after BCT may be lower compared with historic data. Therefore an understanding of risk stratification based on patient and tumor characteristics, treatment modalities, and time since initial diagnosis should guide management of these patients.

Although local recurrence is most common, distant disease makes up a significant number of those relapses with bone, lung, and liver being the most common sites. Twenty to thirty percent of all breast cancer patients will develop distant disease at some point. Approximately 155,000 women in the United States are currently diagnosed with metastatic breast cancer, although this number is estimated to rise to 162,000 by 2011. Although a small proportion of patients with distant metastasis will achieve a complete remission with currently available chemotherapy regimens, the goal is generally for palliation, disease control, and prolonged survival.

SURVEILLANCE FOR LOCOREGIONAL AND DISTANT RECURRENCE AND MAINTENANCE AFTER A BREAST CANCER DIAGNOSIS

History and Physical

After treatment for primary breast cancer, patients should be regularly evaluated for locoregional recurrence. The rate of relapse is highest in the first 5 years, with more than half occurring in the first 3 years; however, recurrences can be seen even 20 years after the primary tumor, so breast cancer survivors should be monitored for the rest of their lives. Although this evaluation is usually performed by a surgeon or medical oncologist in the first years after diagnosis, follow-up can be transitioned to a well-informed primary care provider as the disease-free interval increases. Patients should be evaluated by history and physical exam every 3 to 6 months for the first 3 years. After 3 years, this schedule can be lengthened to evaluations every 6 to 12 months. Patients should be asked about changes in their breasts, nipple retraction or discharge, and skin changes. Similar to the primary presentation, recurrences in an intact breast after BCT can be found by palpating masses, but they can also appear as skin thickening or erythema and nipple changes. Clinicians should have a high level of suspicion when examining patients after mastectomy, as recurrence can often present as a nodule or erythematous rash that may involve the postmastectomy scar and can be mistaken for fat necrosis, granuloma, or radiation change. In addition, patients should be encouraged to perform self-exams on a monthly basis and to seek medical attention immediately if they notice changes. In some studies, 80% of recurrences are discovered by patients.

Careful attention should also be made to screen for the presence of new primary breast cancers in the previously unaffected breast. Some studies suggest that as many as 1 in 25 breast cancer survivors will develop a second breast cancer in the contralateral breast with an estimated risk as high 0.5% to 1% per year. Routine self-examination in adjunct with clinician exams and screening mammography should be performed, especially in younger women who are at greater risk.

Breast Imaging

If the patient underwent BCT, a diagnostic mammogram should be performed 6 months after the completion of therapy. Screening mammogram should be done of the contralateral breast at this time. Mammography should be repeated annually thereafter if no abnormalities are detected. Ultrasound of the chest wall and nodal basins may be helpful after mastectomy to look for chest wall or regional recurrences if the patient is symptomatic, but it is not indicated for routine surveillance. The role of magnetic resonance imaging (MRI) of the breast in surveillance after treatment of breast cancer remains to be determined. When the American Cancer Society published recommendations for the use of MRI in various subsets of patients, data were insufficient to support the use of MRI in patients with a personal history of breast cancer.

Surveillance for Distant Disease

Patients should be questioned for symptoms of distant metastasis, such as bone pain or fracture, pleuritic chest pain, dyspnea, weight loss, anorexia, abdominal pain, headaches, seizures, or changes in mental status. These symptoms in a cancer survivor should always prompt further investigation to rule out metastasis. Routine imaging with chest radiograph, bone scans, or abdominal imaging should not be routinely performed in the asymptomatic breast cancer survivor. Likewise, routine laboratory testing of tumor markers, such as CEA and MUC1, is not warranted in these patients.

Health Maintenance

Routine health maintenance should be tailored to the patient. Patients on tamoxifen should undergo annual pelvic exams to screen for uterine cancer, and patients on aromatase inhibitors should have yearly bone-density scans. With the increasing survival from breast cancer, patients should be strongly encouraged to continue routine health screening for other diseases, such as hypertension and cardiac disease, as well as for other cancers.

Workup of Local Recurrences

If an abnormality is found either by physical exam or imaging, a biopsy should be performed to confirm the diagnosis. The pathologist should be asked to perform stains to determine estrogen receptor (ER), progesterone receptor (PR), and HER2 status, as these affect further therapy and may be used to determine whether this represents a true local recurrence or a new primary breast cancer. Mammography should be performed of both breasts along with ultrasound of the involved site and nodal regions. MRI may also be useful in the setting of inconclusive or disconcordant findings after mammography, ultrasound, or biopsy. While concurrent distant disease is found in 10% of patients who develop in-breast recurrences after BCT, local recurrences after mastectomy are associated with metastatic disease in over 60% of patients. Because of this high rate of distant disease, a full metastatic workup should be performed when a locoregional recurrence is identified. This includes chest radiograph (CXR), bone scan, and abdominal imaging, either by computed tomography (CT) or MRI. Positron emission tomography (PET) and biopsies should be considered if abnormalities are found.

Workup of Distant Disease

Similar to the workup for local recurrence, any patient presenting with metastatic disease should be fully evaluated to determine all sites of disease. This includes imaging of both breast and nodal regions, CXR, bone scan, and abdominal imaging. Brain MRI should also be performed in these patients. Between 10% and 15% of patients presenting with metastasis will have multiple sites of involvement.

MANAGEMENT OF LOCOREGIONAL RECURRENCE

Recurrence After BCT

Mastectomy is standard therapy for local recurrence in patients who undergo breast-conservation surgery and adjuvant radiotherapy. Salvage breast-conservation surgery can be considered in highly selected patients who did not receive postoperative radiotherapy after their first operation. If repeat BCT is attempted, however, adjuvant radiotherapy is definitely recommended. If regional lymph nodes are clinically positive, a lymph node dissection should be added to the operative plan. If the patient is clinically node negative by physical exam and/or ultrasound, sentinel lymph node biopsy (SLNB) can be considered, however the patient should be counseled that this approach is investigational and that the procedure may be technically impossible, especially if there has been previous radiotherapy or extensive axillary dissection. Several groups have reported that SLNB is possible in 65% to 75% of patients after BCT and in 40% to 50% after mastectomy or extensive nodal dissection. If an axillary dissection was previously performed, the sentinel lymph node is likely to be extraaxillary, so preoperative lymphoscintigraphy should be performed to guide dissection. Systemic therapy should be combined with surgical therapy in these patients after a recurrence.

After Mastectomy

Local recurrence after mastectomy is referred to as a *chest wall recurrence* (CWR), which can be found in skin, subcutaneous tissue, muscle, or even bone. CWR rates of 10% to 30% have been reported after mastectomy, even after adjuvant chemotherapy. Postmastectomy radiation can reduce this risk by two thirds in high-risk patients. As mentioned previously, the identification of CWR should prompt a thorough investigation for distant disease, as it is associated with metastasis and poor prognosis. Factors that predict a favorable prognosis after the diagnosis of CWR include initial node-negative status, CWR more than 2 years after primary surgery, and treatment of CWR. Median survival can vary as widely as 141 months in patients with favorable features to as little as 16 months in patients without these characteristics. For this reason, systemic chemotherapy is standard for patients. The surgeon should consider excision if the CWR is completely resectable, followed by chemotherapy. Neoadjuvant chemotherapy followed by resection can be considered in high-risk situations such as a short disease-free interval, multiple nodules, or a marginally resectable recurrence. If surgical resection is attempted, evaluation for nodal recurrence, and lymph node dissection if nodal metastases are found, should be considered. Radiotherapy to the chest wall and nodal basins should be considered if there has been no previous radiotherapy (Figure 1).

Nodal Recurrence

Nodal recurrence is rare (<1%) after axillary lymph node dissection, and it remains less than 1% in the sentinel node era, particularly for sentinel lymph node (SLN)-negative patients. This contrasts sharply to the nodal failure rates of 20% in patients who did not undergo axillary node dissection before the advent of SLN biopsy (SLNB). As with chest wall recurrence, nodal recurrence presents with a high probability of distant disease. If no other disease is found after breast imaging and complete metastatic workup, an axillary lymph node dissection should be performed with adjuvant systemic therapy. If other metastatic disease is found, systemic therapy should be the primary treatment.

▌ MANAGEMENT OF METASTATIC DISEASE

Metastatic Disease with an Intact Primary Tumor

A small percentage of women, less than 10%, present with metastasis at the time of initial diagnosis. The treatment algorithm for patients who present with a primary breast tumor and synchronous metastasis is evolving (Figure 2). In the past, because these patients were considered to have such poor survival, the primary tumor was usually left intact, unless it was removed for palliation in locally advanced disease. In addition, there were theoretical concerns that surgery released tumor growth factors and removed inhibitors of angiogenesis that worsened outcomes. This paradigm has shifted, and more groups are reporting a survival advantage with tumor excision; these studies are summarized in Table 1. Critics point to the fact that the results from these retrospective reviews could be confounded by stage migration bias and selection bias, because those patients undergoing surgical excision are more likely to have favorable prognostic features. While definitive prospective data are currently not available to determine survival advantage from surgical resection of the primary tumor, resecting the primary tumor in the setting of metastatic

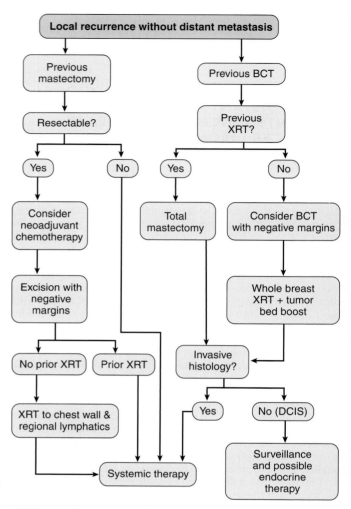

FIGURE 1   Treatment algorithm for local recurrence without distant metastasis.

disease can be considered in highly selected groups of patients, such as those with fewer metastatic sites, resectable primary tumors, stable disease, long disease-free interval, and high performance status.

Surgical Management of Distant Metastatic Sites

Stage IV breast cancer is not curable with currently available modalities, so disease control and palliation should be the primary goals of any therapy. Traditionally, metastasectomy was not offered, but with the improvements in systemic therapy, this may be an option in very highly selected patients; however, this should only be considered when complete resection could render the patient NED (no evidence of disease). In reported series of completely resected patients, median survivals can be as long as 44 to 79 months with pulmonary metastasis and 22 months with isolated liver lesions. In one series from Spain, patients who developed liver metastasis within 24 months of their primary diagnosis had 1 year overall survival rates of 0% after liver resection; survival rates for the group who presented with liver disease after 24 months were far better (1 year, 100%; 3 years, 83%; 5 years, 60%). The best candidates are those with a single site of disease, good performance status, and a long disease-free interval after treatment of the primary tumor. Systemic therapy should be a component of the treatment plan in all cases.

Contralateral axilla metastasis (CAM) is a rare occurrence. Differential diagnosis includes an occult primary tumor of the contralateral breast presenting as axillary metastasis, a primary breast cancer seen

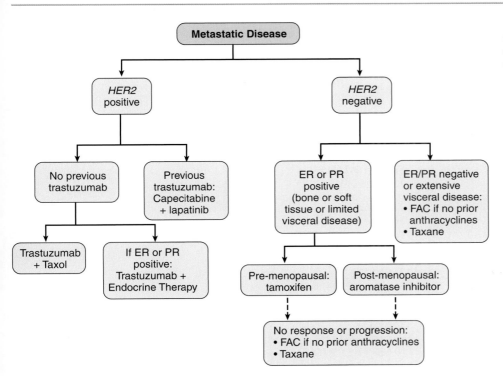

FIGURE 2 Treatment of metastatic breast cancer. This figure shows a treatment algorithm for the systemic therapy of metastatic breast cancer based on tumor receptor status, patient menopausal status, and site of metastasis.

in the axillary tail, or metastasis from another primary cancer such as colon, lung, ovarian, or thyroid. As prognosis and treatment will vary depending on the diagnosis, it is imperative that a firm diagnosis be established if at all possible. Clinical presentation, tumor markers such as ER and PR, *HER2* status, histopathology, and radiographic imaging may help to confirm the diagnosis.

Radiotherapy for Metastatic Disease

Radiotherapy can be an effective palliative modality for patients with metastatic disease. It is commonly used to treat bone and brain metastases as well as disseminated central nervous system disease. Although it is not curative, it can prevent fracture, help with bleeding and pain, and can control central nervous system symptoms such as seizures and paralysis. If life expectancy is longer than 12 weeks, patients with bone metastasis should also receive a bisphosphonate such as pamidronate to prevent future adverse events.

Chemotherapy

The systemic treatment of breast cancer is at the forefront of personalized cancer care, as agents are selected based heavily on tumor markers and patient menopausal status. Sites of metastasis are also important in devising treatment plans. In general, median survival for patients with metastatic breast cancer is approximately 24 months, although those with bone-only disease may have survivals as long as 60 months.

Systemic Agents

The systemic agents most commonly used can be roughly divided into three categories: 1) endocrine therapy, 2) cytotoxic chemotherapy, and 3) targeted therapy other than endocrine therapy. Targeting the endocrine system in breast cancer has been in practice since the late 1800s, when physicians noticed regression of breast tumors after oophorectomy. This has evolved into a number of agents, such as tamoxifen and the aromatase inhibitors, which are highly effective in patients with hormone receptor–positive tumors. Tamoxifen works

by blocking estradiol binding to the estrogen receptor. It is administered orally once or twice a day with side effects that include hot flashes, increased risk of endometrial cancer, and thromboembolic events. Aromatase inhibitors lower tumor and serum estrogen levels by blocking the conversion of androgen precursors to estrogen in peripheral tissues. Therefore these agents are used only in postmenopausal women, whose estrogen production is predominantly from nonovarian sources; they are associated with fewer thromboembolic events and a lower incidence of endometrial cancer, but they have higher rates of cardiac events and bone fractures.

Cytotoxic regimens are usually anthracyline-based or taxane-based. The anthracycline regimens usually consist of an anthracyline such as doxorubicin, 5-fluorouracil, and cyclophosphamide, also referred to as FAC or FEC. Anthracyclines inhibit topoisomerase and act as antimetabolites. This regimen is usually administered in four cycles by infusion. Because anthracylines have known cardiac complications, ejection fractions are evaluated by echocardiogram before initiation. Taxane-based regimens are also very effective in metastatic breast cancer and are usually added sequentially to the anthracyline-based regimens. Taxanes such as paclitaxal target microtubule formation and can have dose-limiting neutropenic effects. This complication has been lessened by changing the dosage schedule to smaller doses infused weekly.

Trastuzumab (Herceptin) is a monoclonal antibody that targets the HER2/neu receptor, which is overexpressed in approximately 25% of breast cancer patients. This is another excellent example of using tumor molecular markers to devise targeted therapy. While initially used as a single agent, trastuzumab has been approved by the Food and Drug Administration for use with paclitaxel; however, when added to doxorubicin, the rate of congestive heart failure may be as high as 15%. Clearly, clinicians must weigh the tumor molecular characteristics, disease burden, and risk profiles when devising chemotherapy regimens.

HER2-Negative Patients

In *HER2*-negative patients who are ER or PR positive or who have limited soft tissue disease, endocrine therapy should be the first-line therapy. Tamoxifen is the drug of choice in premenopausal women, and aromatase inhibitors are usually used in postmenopausal patients.

TABLE 1: Outcome after primary tumor removal in patients presenting with distant metastasis with a synchronous primary breast tumor

Author	Institution	No. Patients	Outcome Measured	Probability
Babiera et al. (2006)	M.D. Anderson Cancer Center	Total: 244 Surgery: 82 (37%) No surgery: 142 (63%)	Overall survival: RR = 0.50 (CI, 0.21–1.19) Progression-free survival: RR = 0.54 (CI, 0.38–0.77)	$P = .12$ $P = .0007$
Blanchard et al. (2008)	Baylor University	Total: 395 Surgery: 242 (61%) No surgery: 153 (39%)	Median survival with surgery: 27.1 mo No surgery: 16.8 mo	$P < .0001$
Khan et al. (2002)	National Cancer Data Base (NCDB)	Total: 16,023 Surgery: 9162 (57%) No surgery: 6861(43%)	3-year survival: Mastectomy: 32% Partial mastectomy: 28% No surgery: 17%	$P < .0001$
Gnerlich et al. (2007)	Surveillance, Epidemiology, and End Results (SEER)	Total: 9734 Surgery: 4578 (47%) No surgery: 5156 (53%)	Median survival: Surgery: 36 mo No surgery: 21 mo	$P < .001$
Rapiti et al. (2006)	Geneva Cancer Registry	Total: 300 Surgery: 127 (42%) No surgery: 173 (58%)	Disease-specific survival: HR, 0.6 (CI, 0.4–1)	$P = .049$
Fields et al. (2007)	Washington University	Total: 409 Surgery: 187 (46%) No surgery: 222 (54%)	Median survival: Surgery: 31.9 mo No surgery: 15.4 mo	$P < .0001$
Bafford et al. (2009)	Brigham and Womens' Hospital	Total: 147 Surgery: 61 (41%) No surgery: 86 (59%)	Median survival: Surgery: 3.52 No surgery: 2.56 Surgery group had survival benefit on multivariate analysis (HR, 0.47)	$P = .09$ $P = .003$
Leung et al. (2009)	Medical College of Virginia	Total: 157 Surgery: 5 (33%) No surgery: 105 (67%)	Median survival: Surgery: 25 mo No surgery: 13 mo Multivariate analysis showed chemotherapy as the only factor that improved survival	$P = .06$

If there is no response to endocrine therapy, the patient should be switched to conventional chemotherapy. Conversely, cytotoxic chemotherapy should be used first in ER- and PR-negative patients who are also *HER2/neu* negative. This usually consists of FAC if anthracyclines were not used previously, followed by a taxane-based regimen. Bevacizumab is sometimes added to the regimen.

HER2-Positive Patients

HER2-positive patients have markedly improved results when the HER2 antibody trastuzumab is used. If a patient has not been treated with trastuzumab in the past, it can be used as a single agent or with paclitaxal. Alternatively, in ER- and PR-positive patients, endocrine therapy can be combined with trastuzumab or lapatinib.

▮ SUMMARY

The improvements in breast cancer therapy have led to an expanding population of breast cancer survivors. Active surveillance and prompt treatment for local and distant recurrence are crucial to continue to improve mortality rates. These patients are best served by a thoughtful, multidisciplinary approach to disease relapse with attention to tumor biology, disease sites, and patient factors.

Selected Readings

Khatcherssian JL, Wolff AC, Smith TJ, et al: American Society of Clinical Oncology 2006 update of the breast cancer follow-up and management guidelines in the adjuvant setting, *J Clin Oncol* 24(31):5091–5097, 2006.

Singletary SE, Walsh G, Vauthey JN, et al: A role for curative surgery in the treatment of selected patients with metastatic breast cancer, *Oncologist* 8(3):241–245, 2003.

Ross JS, Slodkowska EA, Symmans WF, et al: The HER2 receptor and breast cancer: ten years of targeted anti-HER2 therapy and personalized medicine, *Oncologist* 14(4):320–368, 2009.

Carlson RW, Allred DC, Anderson BO: Breast cancer: clinical practice guidelines in oncology, *J Natl Compr Canc Netw* 7(2):122–192, 2009.

MANAGEMENT OF MALE BREAST CANCER

Catherine E. Pesce, MD, and Lisa K. Jacobs, MD

OVERVIEW

Carcinoma of the male breast accounts for only 0.8% of all breast cancers. Annually in the United States, 1500 new cases of male breast cancer are diagnosed, and 400 deaths occur due to the disease. Just as in female breast cancer, the goals of surgical management are local control and disease staging. Because the rarity of the disease precludes large randomized trials, optimal management of breast cancer in men is largely unknown. Treatment is therefore based on our understanding of the disease and its response to treatment in women.

RISK FACTORS

The median age at diagnosis is in the mid-60s, about 5 years later than the median age at diagnosis for women. However, breast cancer has been reported in male patients ranging in age from 5 to 93 years. As in females, the incidence has been increasing with a rise of nearly 26% over the past 25 years. Risk factors include abnormalities in estrogen and androgen balance. States of increased estrogen exposure such as cirrhosis and obesity, as well as states of decreased testosterone, have been associated with increased risk. Testicular abnormalities such as undescended testes, congenital inguinal hernia, mumps orchitis after age 20 years, orchiectomy, and infertility have also been associated. Klinefelter syndrome, in which men carry XXY chromosomes, affects 0.1% of the population and is characterized by underdeveloped secondary sexual characteristics, gynecomastia, and low testosterone levels. Patients with the disease have a 50-fold increased risk of male breast cancer over the general male population.

A family history of male breast cancer is seen in 15% to 20% of patients, and a male with a family history of breast cancer in a female relative is also at increased risk. The disease is more common in persons of Ashkenazi Jewish descent, and infection with hepatic schistosomiasis has also been associated. A history of radiation to the chest wall, employment in the soap and perfume industries, and prolonged exposure to electromagnetic fields have all been implicated in elevated risk of disease. Benign breast disease, including a history of breast trauma and nipple discharge, has been associated; however, gynecomastia has not been shown to be a risk factor.

BRCA2 mutations predispose men to breast cancer and may account for 4% to 16% of all cases. Such patients may present with breast cancer at a much younger age, they often have bilateral disease, and such mutations may be associated with a poorer survival. In families with one case of male breast cancer and one other case of breast cancer, the chance of a *BRCA2* mutation is as high as 60% to 75%. *BRCA1* gene mutations have also been implicated in male breast cancer but to a much lesser extent. In men known to carry either of these genes, there may be a role for prophylactic mastectomy. In addition, the presence of a genetic mutation may be used as a criterion to perform mammographic screening. Aside from these considerations, the benefits of genetic testing are largely for offspring or siblings of the affected individual and must be considered.

Other genes have been thought to be associated with male breast cancer, however further studies are needed to elucidate their role. Both *PTEN* (Cowden syndrome) and mismatch repair genes, such as *MLH1*, have been investigated for a potential role in male breast

cancer etiology, however, research to uncover a clear association is ongoing.

Histologically, 90% of male breast cancers are invasive ductal carcinomas. The remaining 10% are usually ductal carcinoma in situ, often of the papillary and cribriform type and of low to intermediate grade. Given the absence of terminal lobules in the normal male breast, lobular carcinoma, both invasive and in situ, is rarely seen. Paget disease and inflammatory carcinomas have both been described. Male breast cancers have high rates of hormone-receptor expression, and as in female breast cancer, the rates of hormone-receptor positivity increase with increasing patient age. Approximately 90% of male breast cancers are estrogen-receptor positive, and as in women, estrogen receptor positivity corresponds to better prognosis. Nearly 80% are progesterone receptor positive, but only 25% overexpress *HER2/neu*.

PRESENTATION

Most men present with a painless, subareolar breast mass. It is the job of the clinician to distinguish a primary cancer from gynecomastia and other possible lesions such as metastatic carcinoma of the breast, sarcoma, and breast abscess. In addition to local discomfort and axillary adenopathy, other initial symptoms may include nipple retraction, ulceration, bleeding, and nipple discharge. As in females, there is a slight preponderance of left-sided versus right-sided disease. Gynecomastia is the most common cause of a breast mass in a male, but it can be distinguished from the harder consistency often seen in breast cancers; gynecomastia is often more mobile, rubbery, and tender than cancers. Breast cancers also often directly invade the skin and muscle in males.

The physical exam in men should be executed just as in women patients. The primary lesion is examined, as well as the opposite breast, and regional lymph nodes are examined. A chest radiograph and liver enzymes are appropriate for initial staging evaluation of small- to moderate-sized tumors. Bone scans and computed tomography (CT) scans can be reserved for patients who present with more advanced lesions, with abnormalities found on x-ray films, or with abnormal liver enzymes.

Diagnostic mammography has been shown to have a sensitivity and specificity of 92% and 90%, respectively, for the diagnosis of male cancer. Ultrasound can also be useful to further characterize lesions and determine nodal involvement. Any discrete mass requires a biopsy to establish a definitive diagnosis, and a radiology-guided core needle biopsy is usually preferred. In addition, a patient who comes in with suspicious, palpable adenopathy should preoperatively undergo ultrasound-guided fine needle aspiration.

PROGNOSIS

Prognostic factors in male breast cancer are the same as in female breast cancer and include tumor size, nodal involvement, histologic grade, and hormone receptor status. The same staging system of the American Joint Committee on Cancer is used for both men and women, which considers tumor size, nodal involvement, and distant metastases. It has been shown that at the time of diagnosis, 60% of men have stage I or II disease, 30% have stage III disease, and 10% have stage IV disease. Men with tumors 2 to 5 cm in size have a 40% higher risk of death than men with tumors less than 2 cm in size, and men with lymph node involvement have a 50% higher risk of death than those without lymph node involvement. Poorer prognosis is also associated with extensive axillary lymph node involvement. In some reports, overall survival has been shown to be worse for men than for women, however, it is thought that these studies did not take into consideration the older age at diagnosis and more advanced disease at presentation in male study subjects. It has been concluded that when matched for stage and age at diagnosis, survival for men is similar to that in women.

TREATMENT

Most men are treated with mastectomy with axillary lymph node dissection. Sentinel node biopsy is also appropriate. Radical mastectomy is uncommon today, and it is reserved for disease that invades into the pectoral muscle. Axillary staging is an important component of surgery, for studies have shown that patients who underwent mastectomy without axillary dissection developed nodal recurrence and had poorer outcomes. Lumpectomy with postoperative radiotherapy remains an option for some patients; however, because the majority of male tumors are located deep in the retroareolar tissue, breast-conserving therapy can be difficult. Careful attention must be given to obtaining negative margins, and breast-preserving surgery should be followed with radiotherapy to decrease local recurrence.

Due to the rarity of the disease, sensitivity and specificity of sentinel node biopsy have not been established in male breast cancer. However, just as in female breast cancer, several case series have shown a benefit among men with clinically negative nodal disease. For patients found to have a positive sentinel node, axillary dissection for completion of staging and for regional control is appropriate.

Whether or not there is a benefit of postmastectomy radiotherapy on overall survival in men has been underpowered in most studies. Overall, similar general guidelines are used for both males and females, in that radiotherapy should be considered for patients with large tumors, microscopically positive margins, or four or more positive nodes. Men also tend to be treated with radiotherapy more often than women, because men are more likely to have nipple or skin involvement.

As in female breast cancer, adjuvant chemotherapy for males is used for those thought to be at increased risk of recurrence and death from breast cancer. These patients include men with tumors greater than 1 cm or with lymph node involvement. Because most breast cancers in men are receptor positive, hormonal therapy clearly has a role as adjuvant therapy. Many retrospective studies have investigated the role of tamoxifen and have shown clear benefit in reducing risk of recurrence and death. About 20% of male patients, however, discontinue tamoxifen because of hot flashes, decreased libido, mood changes, or venous thrombosis.

Given the high rates of receptor positivity in males, hormonal therapies are often used as first-line adjuvants. Tamoxifen remains the gold standard of adjuvant hormonal therapies; however, use of luteinizing hormone–releasing hormone agonists, with or without antiandrogens, has also been reported. The data on aromatase inhibitors are sparse, and these drugs are not currently used in the adjuvant setting. Because of testicular production of estrogen independent of the aromatase enzyme, the utility of aromatase inhibitors in the male population is in question. Other hormonal therapies including progestins, androgens, steroids, aminoglutethimide, estrogens, and letrozole have also shown responses in case reports. However, it is generally accepted that receptor-negative patients or those with receptor-positive disease refractory to hormonal agents are subsequently treated with chemotherapy.

Male breast cancer patients are at increased risk of developing subsequent primary cancers. Studies have shown that men with a history of breast cancer have a thirtyfold greater risk of developing contralateral breast cancer. A small increase in risk of melanoma and prostate cancer may also be present in male breast cancer survivors, and thus close follow-up for men with breast cancer is especially warranted.

SUMMARY

Care of the male breast cancer patient is modeled after that of female breast cancer patients, because little scientific and clinical data exist that specifically address male disease. However, there are areas where the recommendations vary. Genetic assessment is more strongly encouraged with a history of male breast cancer in a family, use of antiestrogens is modified because of the unique mechanism of actions of the drugs, surgical management is altered due to the generally small breast size and location of the primary tumor, and screening is modified based on risk of subsequent primary disease. Other aspects of care such as chemotherapy, nodal management, risk assessment, physical examination, and follow-up are all patterned after guidelines for management of female breast cancer.

Suggested Readings

Giordano SH: A review of the diagnosis and management of male breast cancer, *Oncologist* 10:471–479, 2005.

Goss PE, Reid C, Pintile M, et al: Male breast carcinoma: a review of 229 patients who presented to the Princess Margaret Hospital during 40 years, *Cancer* 85:629–639, 1999.

Ribeiro G, Swindell R, Harris M, et al: A review of the management of the male breast carcinoma based on an analysis of 420 treated cases, *Breast* 5:141–146, 1996.

Stalsberg H, Thomas DB, Rosenblatt KA, et al: Histologic types and hormone receptors in breast cancer in men: a population-based study in 282 United States men, *Cancer Causes Control* 4:143–151, 1993.

Breast Reconstruction after Mastectomy: Indications, Techniques, and Results

Maurice Y. Nahabedian, MD

OVERVIEW

The reconstructive options for women after mastectomy have evolved over the past decade. Traditional breast reconstruction included autologous tissue and prosthetic devices and was reserved for women who had undergone total mastectomy. However, recent advancements have resulted in an increased incidence and acceptance of partial mastectomy. Thus current concepts and options have changed based on our enhanced understanding of the biology and pathophysiology of breast cancer and ability to better target tumors with adjuvant therapies. As such, many women are electing to preserve more of their natural breast tissues and components when oncologically indicated and safe. Partial breast excisions, skin-sparing mastectomies, and total nipple/areolar conservation procedures have gained momentum, as clinical studies have demonstrated safety and efficacy in properly selected women. Sentinel lymph node biopsy has become commonplace and has essentially supplanted total axillary lymph node dissection during the initial partial or total mastectomy. As breast surgeons continue to modify traditional oncological approaches, plastic surgeons continue to evolve the reconstructive options. Much of this paradigm shift with regard to the management of breast cancer is because of advancements made by ablative and reconstructive surgeons to provide better outcomes.

This chapter highlights some of the recent innovations in breast reconstruction. It includes not only the basic techniques of prosthetic and autologous reconstruction but also some of the newer methods that use acellular dermal matrices and perforator flaps. In addition, this chapter reviews many of the advances in oncoplastic breast surgery with an emphasis on indications and techniques of adjacent tissue rearrangement, reduction mammaplasty, and local miniflaps. It also reviews the benefits of skin-sparing and nipple/areolar–sparing techniques as a means of improving outcomes while maintaining oncologic safety.

PROSTHETIC BREAST RECONSTRUCTION

The use of prosthetic devices remains the most common method of breast reconstruction after mastectomy. The typical patient has been and continues to be the woman with mild to moderate breast volume with minimal to moderate ptosis and early-stage breast cancer. In general, women who have received prior radiation therapy are not ideal candidates for prosthetic reconstruction because of the compromised local vascularity, the increased incidence of capsular contracture, and the increased risk of postoperative infection. However, in the nonradiated patient, prosthetic devices can result in excellent outcomes with high patient satisfaction.

Traditionally, prosthetic breast reconstruction has been performed in two stages using a temporary tissue expander followed by a permanent implant. The tissue expander is a textured and contoured saline device, whereas the permanent implant can be filled with saline or silicone gel. As a result of the safety and efficacy of these devices, many surgeons and patients are choosing to use them. All devices are usually placed in the total or partial subpectoral position. The expanders are partially filled in the operating room with a volume that typically ranges from 10% to 20% of the expander capacity. The advantage of the two-stage technique is that the skin is expanded during the first stage, and the contour, position, and volume of the breast are optimized during the second stage (Figures 1 and 2).

An alternative to the two-stage reconstruction is the single-stage reconstruction in which a permanent implant is placed immediately following the mastectomy. A requirement for the single-stage technique is that there must be ample breast skin available, such as following a skin-sparing mastectomy or mastectomy with nipple/areolar preservation. This technique is most appealing to women considering prophylactic mastectomy, because there is no cancer, and the thickness of the skin flaps can be optimized. In women with breast cancer, a single-stage technique may be considered but with some degree of caution, as the mastectomy skin flaps may be quite thin and predispose to postoperative complications such as skin necrosis or severe distortion. Although a single device is used, the reported revision rate with this technique has approached 20%.

Since about 2005, prosthetic reconstruction has been facilitated with the use of acellular dermal matrices. These materials are derived from several sources and include human, bovine, and porcine variants. Because of their acellular nature and lack of antigenicity, these materials are safe and readily incorporate into the host tissues. The properties of these biomaterials allow for total revascularization and for fibroblast ingrowth without rejection. The utility of acellular dermis is to extend the pectoralis major muscle and to compartmentalize the tissue expander and/or implant in the breast pocket. These materials can be used for one- and two-stage reconstructions.

When a tissue expander is used, it is often filled to 40% to 70% of its capacity; the exact amount will depend on the quality of the mastectomy skin flaps, the size of the implant, and the amount of skin remaining following the mastectomy. The advantage of intraoperative filling is that the number of postoperative expansions is reduced, and the effects of scar tissue are negated. Its clinical benefit is that women will wake up from anesthesia with some degree of a breast mound rather than a flat surface. Postoperative outcomes have generally been improved, because total expansion is usually complete before scar tissue or a capsule forms. When the postoperative expansion process is protracted, the development of scar tissue or capsule around the implant can impede optimal expansion of the device.

Complications associated with prosthetic reconstruction include but are not limited to capsular contracture, device rupture, implant distortion, pain, migration, and premature removal. The controversy regarding saline versus silicone gel devices has essentially been eliminated, as numerous studies have demonstrated that silicone gel implants do not cause connective tissue disorders, peripheral neuropathy, chronic fatigue syndrome, or cancer. The devices currently used for prosthetic reconstruction have a finite life span; they do not last forever but are generally good for 10 to 15 years. Following prosthetic reconstruction, patients have reported high satisfaction in terms of breast contour and volume and postoperative recovery.

AUTOLOGOUS BREAST RECONSTRUCTION

Autologous breast reconstruction is most commonly performed using musculocutaneous pedicle flaps that include the transverse rectus abdominis musculocutaneous (TRAM) flap and latissimus dorsi flaps. Both of these methods are capable of creating a beautiful breast mound, but they are limited in that they both usually require harvest of the donor site muscles, namely the rectus abdominis and the latissimus dorsi muscles respectively. The reason that the donor site

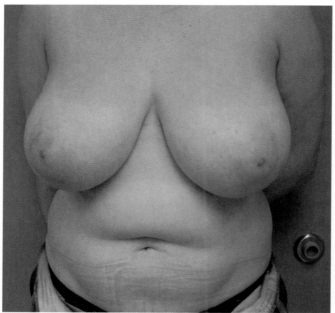

FIGURE 1 Preoperative image in a patient with stage I left breast cancer (*BRCA* positive).

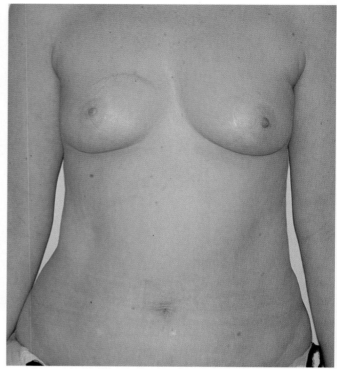

FIGURE 3 Preoperative image in a patient with cancer of the right breast.

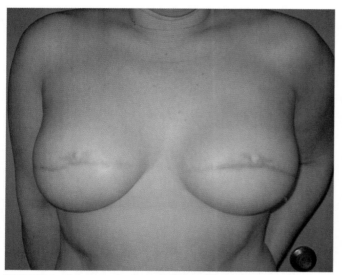

FIGURE 2 Postoperative image following bilateral mastectomy and two-stage prosthetic reconstruction using acellular dermal matrix.

muscle is harvested with the flap is not usually for the added volume, but rather because the vascularity of the important adipocutaneous component traverses within the muscle itself. Donor site morbidities with these musculocutaneous flaps have included donor site weakness, abnormal contour, and seroma. As a result of these potential morbidities, alternative options have evolved.

An alternative to the traditional pedicle musculocutaneous flap is free-tissue transfer. The advantage of free-tissue transfer is that the amount of donor site muscle harvested is usually minimized or eliminated. Several potential donor sites exist that include the abdomen, flanks, gluteal region, medial thigh, and posterior thorax. The two types of free flaps are musculocutaneous flaps and perforator flaps. Musculocutaneous flaps, by definition, will include some muscle, although they are often muscle sparing, as only a segment of muscle is usually removed. Perforator flaps, on the other hand, require

no muscle at all. Perforator flaps can originate from many potential donor sites that include the abdomen, gluteal region, anterior thigh, posterior thorax, medial thigh, and chest wall. Donor-site morbidity has improved, hernias and contour abnormalities are rarely observed, and weakness is minimal or absent.

The indications for autologous reconstruction can include but are not restricted to patient preference, complex reconstruction associated with prosthetic device failure, and prior radiation. Candidates must have adequate skin and fat at the donor site and must be provided a thorough understanding of the risks and benefits. The main advantages of autologous tissue are that the reconstruction will last forever and will generally improve with time when successfully performed. This is in contrast to prosthetic breast reconstruction, in which the devices do not last forever and will generally deteriorate over time.

There are several free flaps that can be used for breast reconstruction, of which only a few will be discussed. The three that I perform most often include the muscle-sparing free TRAM, the deep inferior epigastric artery (DIEP) flap, and the superior gluteal artery perforator (SGAP) flap. Of the three, the DIEP flap is performed most often, because it utilizes the adipocutaneous component of the lower abdomen without sacrificing the rectus abdominis muscle. It can be safely performed in the vast majority of patients in whom a dominant perforating artery and vein are present to adequately perfuse the flap (Figures 3, 4, and 5).

When suitable perforators are not present, or the patient's body habitus dictates that additional flap perfusion may be needed, a muscle-sparing free TRAM flap is usually performed. With this operation a small, central segment of the rectus abdominis muscle is harvested with the flap to include several smaller-perforating vessels. The advantages of including a segment of the muscle is that additional perforators can be captured that can optimize flap perfusion. In some situations, these perforators are small. When used individually, they would be insufficient to adequately perfuse the flap, but collectively they work well.

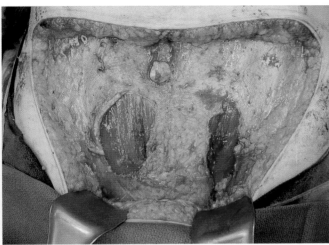

FIGURE 4   Intraoperative image after bilateral DIEP flap harvest. The continuity and volume of the rectus abdominis muscle is intact.

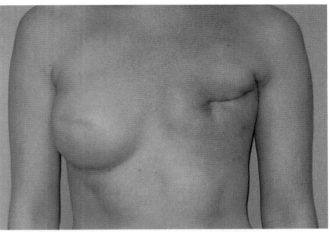

FIGURE 6   Preoperative image of patient with cancer of the left breast after mastectomy, radiation, and failed implant reconstruction. The right breast was successfully reconstructed with a prosthetic device.

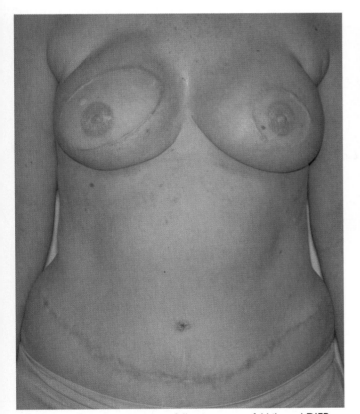

FIGURE 5   Postoperative image following successful bilateral DIEP flap and nipple/areolar reconstruction.

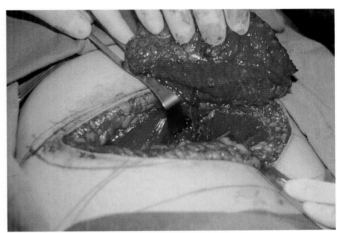

FIGURE 7   Intraoperative image of an SGAP flap.

artery perforator (TAP), and the transverse upper gracilis (TUG). In all of these free flaps, a microvascular anastomosis to recipient vessels is required and is usually the internal mammary artery and vein, although the thoracodorsal artery and vein can be used as well.

Complications associated with autologous reconstruction include but are not limited to partial or total flap failure, fat necrosis, asymmetry, donor-site weakness, and abnormal donor-site contour. With the pedicle flaps, the incidence of flap failure is approximately 1%, whereas for the free flaps, the incidence of flap failure ranges from 1% to 5%. Fat necrosis is due to a perfusion deficiency in a specific, small region of the flap, resulting in a firm nodule. Abdominal contour abnormalities include a bulge or a hernia. The distinction is based on a fascial defect with a true hernia and fascial laxity with the bulge. The pedicle TRAM flap results in abnormal contour in 10% to 20% of patients, whereas the DIEP flap results in abnormal contour in 5% to 10% of patients.

RECONSTRUCTION FOLLOWING MASTECTOMY WITH NIPPLE/AREOLAR PRESERVATION

Mastectomy with nipple/areolar preservation has traditionally been controversial and is considered relatively unsafe. However, recent data from several investigators has demonstrated that the technique

In some women, use of the lower abdominal donor site is not an option because of insufficient lower abdominal skin and fat or previous abdominal operations that have negated the ability to create a flap safely. In these cases, an SGAP flap is typically used, assuming the patient is either not interested or is not a candidate for prosthetic reconstruction (Figures 6, 7, and 8). The SGAP flap is considered a more complex flap, in that the vessels used for the anastomosis are smaller in caliber and length than the DIEP or free TRAM flaps. Other free flaps include the superficial inferior epigastric artery (SIEA), inferior gluteal artery perforator (IGAP), thoracodorsal

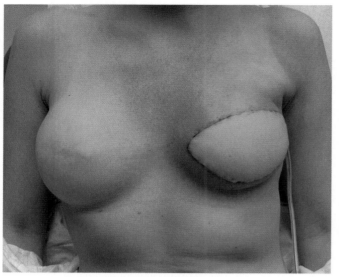

FIGURE 8   Early postoperative image after SGAP flap reconstruction.

is safe in properly selected women. These include patients with mild to moderate breast volume who are having prophylactic or therapeutic mastectomy. The indications for women without breast cancer include patient preference, mild to moderate breast volume, and relatively good health. The indications for women with breast cancer include small localized tumors (<2.5 cm), a distance of at least 3 cm away from the nipple/areolar complex (NAC), and no prior radiation therapy. Nipple sparing is not advised for women who will receive postoperative radiation therapy and for women with large breast volume, because the vascularity and perfusion of the remaining mastectomy skin flaps and NAC is often severely compromised.

Important considerations for nipple/areolar preservation include breast size, location of the incision, adequate breast removal, type of reconstruction, and timing of reconstruction. In general, NAC-sparing techniques are most effective in women with mild to moderate breast volume (A or B cup size) based on the vascularity issues. Incision location is variable and can be supraareolar, infraareolar, lateral to the areola, and along the inframammary fold. With all incisions, it is important to appreciate the subsequent vascularity of the mastectomy skin flaps. Certain locations may result in additional compromise, because they may disrupt the points of origin. Incision located around the periphery may diminish blood flow toward the apex, whereas incisions near the apex will not disrupt the peripheral origin. This is because the skin flaps following a mastectomy are perfused solely via the subdermal plexus, which originates around the periphery of the breast. With most nipple-sparing mastectomies, the incision length tends to be limited. Care must be taken to ensure adequate length to ensure adequate access to the breast parenchyma for complete removal. My preference is to create a supraareolar or infraareolar incision with a lateral extension. With these incisional approaches, the vascularity of the skin flaps is optimized, and the breast borders are easily defined to achieve adequate exposure to the breast parenchyma and to ensure adequate mastectomy margins to minimize the chances of local recurrence.

The reconstructive options following nipple/areolar preservation can include prosthetic devices or autologous tissues. The choice is often based on patient preference, surgeon experience, and anatomic considerations. In most cases the reconstruction is performed immediately following the mastectomy; however, in cases where there is a question about the viability of the mastectomy skin flaps, the reconstruction can be delayed a few weeks. This will allow the skin to heal without jeopardizing the reconstruction. In women having unilateral mastectomy, it is important to adequately fill the cutaneous envelope to maintain symmetry. In women having bilateral

mastectomy, symmetry is more easily achieved, and the results can be outstanding.

Outcomes following mastectomy with nipple/areolar preservation and reconstruction are generally good to excellent when proper patient selection protocols have been followed. In women with breast cancer, the incidence of local recurrence is less than 5% when appropriate oncologic parameters are followed.

Although aesthetic outcomes can be excellent, there are certain sequelae to this operation that should be explained and understood by patients. The incidence of delayed healing around the NAC can be problematic, which can result in areolar distortion and discoloration. Delayed healing can be managed via local wound care or surgical debridement. Sensory loss to the NAC has been reported in 50% of women. Other sequelae, such as asymmetry and poor cosmetic result, can also occur.

ONCOPLASTIC BREAST SURGERY

Oncoplastic breast surgery is defined as partial mastectomy with wide margins followed by partial breast reconstruction. The oncologic basis for this stems from the fact that a wider margin of resection will result in a reduced incidence of local recurrence that approaches that of mastectomy. The advantages of oncoplastic breast surgery are that contour abnormalities of the breast will be minimized, the number of operations for the patient will be reduced, women are usually able to preserve the NAC, and patient satisfaction is usually increased.

When evaluating a patient's candidacy for oncoplastic breast surgery, there are several salient factors that warrant consideration. The first is oncologic feasibility. Candidates include women with tumors less than 5 cm when breast volume is large and women with smaller tumors when breast volume is small. Women with stage I or II focal breast cancers are usually considered. Some women with large tumors who have had successful neoadjuvant chemotherapy may be candidates for oncoplastic resection when adequate tumor shrinkage has been achieved. The dilemma for many women is whether to proceed with total or partial mastectomy. Patients with recurrent breast cancer or women who have had previous breast radiation are usually not considered. It is important to adequately image these breasts using mammography, computed tomography (CT), and/or magnetic resonance imaging (MRI) to delineate the extent and orientation of the breast cancer. It is also important to anticipate the extent of the skin and parenchymal defects to facilitate the planning of the operation.

Reconstructive techniques following partial mastectomy include two categories: *volume displacement* and *volume replacement* techniques. Volume displacement techniques include adjacent tissue rearrangement, mastopexy, and reduction mammaplasty, whereas volume replacement includes use of local or remote flaps. Adjacent tissue rearrangement is reserved for smaller excisions, resulting in minimal distortion in women with large or small breasts. In some women with larger breasts, reduction mammaplasty techniques are considered and are completed by removal of the cancerous tissue with a generous rim of normal breast parenchyma (Figures 9 and 10). In women with smaller breasts who have a larger defect, autologous tissue reconstruction is considered. This is usually accomplished using a latissimus dorsi miniflap or a lateral chest wall perforator flap. These reconstructive procedures are usually performed immediately following the mastectomy but can be performed on a delayed basis as well.

The principal caveat of oncoplastic breast surgery is to ensure adequate margins. Cavity sampling of the resultant defect is recommended. The excised specimen should be imaged to ensure that the tumor and microcalcifications are included, and clips should be placed in the resultant breast cavity to delineate the location of tumor excision. When tumor margins are in question, a delayed oncoplastic reconstruction can be performed once final pathologic status has been confirmed. In the event that a margin is positive on final pathology, the options are to reexcise the defect if the breast has not been reconstructed or to perform a mastectomy if the breast has been reconstructed.

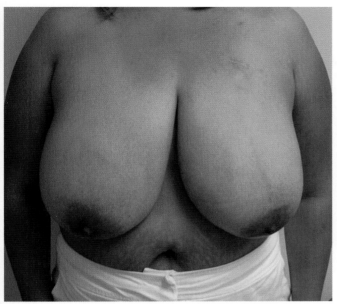

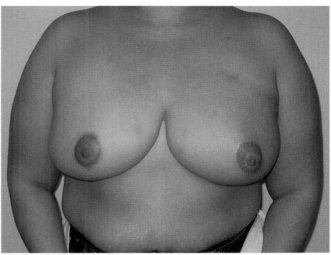

FIGURE 10   Postoperative image after left partial mastectomy and immediate bilateral oncoplastic reduction mammaplasty.

FIGURE 9   Preoperative image with bilateral mammary hypertrophy and left breast cancer.

Complications following oncoplastic breast surgery include but are not limited to infection, delayed healing, seroma, hematoma, breast asymmetry, nipple necrosis, loss of sensation, fat necrosis, tumor recurrence, secondary operations, and a poor cosmetic result. Despite these risk factors, patient satisfaction typically ranges from 80% to 100%. Comparing oncoplastic surgery to skin-sparing mastectomy with reconstruction, patients have reported improved breast and nipple sensation, equal self-examination, and less restriction in their activities of daily living.

SUMMARY

Reconstructive options for women following partial or total mastectomy have expanded. Many women are able to at least consider breast reconstruction rather than live with a permanent deformity. Reconstruction depends on a good collaborative effort between the ablative and reconstructive surgeons. Women should be provided the option of consultation with a plastic surgeon in the event of a partial or total mastectomy. In the end, our goal is to facilitate the transition from being a breast cancer victim to a breast cancer survivor.

SUGGESTED READINGS

Nahabedian MY: Breast reconstruction: a review and rationale for patient selection, *Plast Reconstr Surg* 124:55–62, 2009.

Nahabedian MY, Mesbahi AN: Breast reconstruction with tissue expanders and implants. In Nahabedian MY, editor: *Cosmetic and reconstructive breast surgery*, London, 2009, Elsevier.

Nahabedian MY, Momen B, Tsangaris T: Breast reconstruction with the muscle sparing (MS-2) free TRAM and the DIEP flap: is there a difference? *Plast Reconstr Surg* 115:436–444, 2005.

Losken A, Toncred M, Styblo TM, et al: Management algorithm and outcome evaluation of partial mastectomy defects treated using reduction or mastopexy techniques, *Ann Plast Surg* 59:235–242, 2007.

Nahabedian MY, Tsangaris TN: Breast reconstruction following subcutaneous mastectomy for cancer: a critical appraisal of the nipple–areolar complex, *Plast Reconstr Surg* 117:1083–1090, 2006.

Nahabedian MY: Secondary operations of the anterior abdominal wall following microvascular breast reconstruction with the TRAM and DIEP flaps, *Plast Reconstr Surg* 120:365–372, 2007.

ENDOCRINE GLANDS

ADRENAL INCIDENTALOMA

Peter J. Mazzaglia, MD, and Thomas J. Miner, MD

OVERVIEW

Because of the unprecedented number of cross-sectional imaging studies being performed, the detection of adrenal incidentalomas is skyrocketing. It is estimated that up to 5% of all abdominal and chest computed tomographic (CT) exams will identify such a lesion. For the most part, surgeons are seeing just the tip of the iceberg; many incidentalomas are being characterized as benign by radiologists and are followed by primary care providers and endocrinologists. However, for surgeons asked to consult on and manage these patients, it is essential to have a basic knowledge of adrenal neoplasms and an efficient algorithm for establishing tumor functionality, malignant potential, and indications for excision (Figure 1).

Today's definition of *adrenal incidentaloma* is any adrenal mass 1 cm or more in diameter discovered on a radiologic exam performed for indications other than adrenal disease. Traditionally, this excludes patients undergoing imaging procedures as part of the staging or workup of extraadrenal cancer, as well as those for whom the diagnosis of a symptomatic adrenal-dependent syndrome was missed because of insufficient suspicion. The prevalence of these lesions increases with age; it is less than 1% in people younger than 30 years and up to 7% in those older than 70 years. Therefore the concern for malignant potential is necessarily higher when larger lesions are found in younger patients.

The vast majority of adrenal incidentalomas are benign, nonfunctional adenomas. Because surgical series are inherently biased, the percentage of functional and malignant neoplasms is likely significantly higher than the prevalence in the general population. That said, a recent review of more than 2000 incidentalomas identified nonfunctioning adenoma to be the most likely diagnosis (82%), followed by subclinical Cushing syndrome (5.3%), pheochromocytoma (5.1%), adrenocortical carcinoma (4.7%), metastatic disease (2.5%), and aldosteronoma (1.0%). Other infrequent diagnoses include adrenal cyst, hemorrhage, lymphoma, sarcoma, and neuroganglioma.

The consulting surgeon will often have the dual responsibility of determining both the neoplasm's risk of being adrenocortical cancer (ACC) and whether it is biochemically active. Although some of these determinations will be straightforward, many are not, and these will require additional laboratory and/or imaging studies. It is paramount to have good working relationships with experts in the disciplines of radiology and endocrinology who can reliably assist with the interpretation of inconclusive data as well as assist with decisions regarding what additional studies will be helpful.

EVALUATION OF HORMONAL FUNCTION

Because a significant proportion of patients with hormone-secreting adrenal neoplasms are relatively asymptomatic, all incidentalomas should be evaluated for biochemical function. Upon investigation, some patients will reveal symptoms of adrenal hormone overproduction because of pheochromocytoma or aldosteronoma; symptoms include hypertension that is difficult to control despite multiple medications or unexplained weight gain and hyperglycemia caused by a cortisol-producing adenoma. It should be routine in the evaluation of these lesions to rule out the three most common secretory neoplasms: pheochromocytoma, cortisol-producing adenoma, and hyperaldosteronoma, which may be omitted in normotensive patients. However, because not all patients with hyperaldosteronism are hypokalemic, all hypertensive patients should be screened, especially in light of new evidence that upward of 12% of essential hypertension is due to hyperaldosteronism. The laboratory analysis should be kept as simple as possible, beginning with the most sensitive tests but also with those that are logistically the easiest to carry out for the patient (Figure 2).

For pheochromocytoma, the most sensitive markers are serum metanephrines and normetanephrines, which are the breakdown products of circulating catecholamines. If the serum metanephrines are twice the normal level or higher, the patient has a pheochromocytoma; if they are normal, there is virtually no possibility of a false-negative result. However, frequently the levels will fall somewhere in the middle. Certain antihypertensives, including beta blockers and angiotensin-converting enzyme (ACE) inhibitors, can contribute to these elevations and should be discontinued if at all possible prior to retesting. Do not make the mistake of ordering serum catecholamines, as their rapid fluctuations render them useless. If the result of the serum metanephrines leaves the diagnosis in doubt, a 24 hour urine collection for metanephrines, catecholamines, and vanillylmandelic acid should be ordered. While the sensitivity of this test remains above 95%, it also has better than 95% specificity.

In rare cases of patients who have bilateral incidentalomas, and biochemical testing is diagnostic of pheochromocytoma, it becomes essential to gather as much information about the functionality of each lesion prior to operation. Such patients should undergo further imaging with either metaiodobenzylguanidine (MIBG) or magnetic resonance imaging (MRI). Since 10% or fewer of pheochromocytomas are bilateral, there is a significant chance that one of the incidentalomas is a benign cortical adenoma that may not require adrenalectomy.

By definition, a cortisol-secreting adrenal incidentaloma should not yet have produced the full phenotypic manifestations of Cushing disease/syndrome. Rather a *forme fruste* that is found to be subclinical or preclinical Cushing syndrome might exist. More than 50% of these patients may have hyperglycemia, hypertension, osteopenia, obesity, and fatigue but have yet to develop the classic moon facies, buffalo

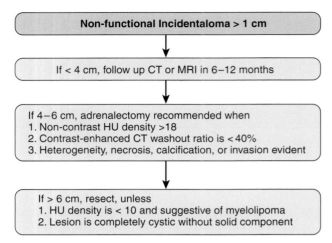

Non-functional Incidentaloma > 1 cm

↓

If < 4 cm, follow up CT or MRI in 6–12 months

↓

If 4–6 cm, adrenalectomy recommended when
1. Non-contrast HU density >18
2. Contrast-enhanced CT washout ratio is < 40%
3. Heterogeneity, necrosis, calcification, or invasion evident

↓

If > 6 cm, resect, unless
1. HU density is < 10 and suggestive of myelolipoma
2. Lesion is completely cystic without solid component

FIGURE 1 Overall strategy for adrenal incidentaloma (mind mapping).

hump, abdominal striae, and advanced proximal muscle weakness diagnostic of Cushing disease/syndrome. The risk for developing full-blown Cushing syndrome is elevated, and when this diagnosis is confirmed, patients should undergo adrenalectomy.

The simplest method of screening for hypercortisolism is a low-dose overnight dexamethasone suppression test, which is more than 95% sensitive. The patient is prescribed 1 mg of dexamethasone to be taken before bedtime on the night prior to a fasting morning blood sampling. The morning cortisol should suppress to less than 5 μg/dL. If it does not, confirmatory testing for elevated 24-hour urinary free cortisol should be performed. If hypercortisolism is confirmed, a serum adrenocorticotropic hormone (ACTH) level must be checked to confirm that the source of excess cortisol is indeed the adrenal gland and not a pituitary or ectopic source of ACTH production.

There is a low prevalence of bilateral macronodular adrenal hyperplasia in patients with subclinical Cushing syndrome. In patients with obvious bilateral adrenal incidentalomas and biochemical proof of excess adrenal cortisol production, bilateral adrenalectomy may be warranted. The patients who would most benefit from aggressive treatment are those with obvious end-organ effects of hypercortisolism, including diabetes and osteoporosis. Some studies have suggested that unilateral adrenalectomy in these patients may sufficiently decrease cortisol levels so as to have a beneficial effect. Planning surgery in such a patient is complex and requires the agreement of the patient, surgeon, and endocrinologist as to the most prudent approach.

Any patient with an adrenal incidentaloma who also has hypertension or documented hypokalemia should be screened for primary hyperaldosteronism. Typical aldosteronomas are small (1 to 2 cm) and benign in appearance. The evaluation for hyperaldosteronism should begin with measurement of serum aldosterone and plasma renin activity, followed by calculation of the aldosterone to plasma renin activity ratio. If the ratio is greater than 20, reflecting autonomous aldosterone secretion rather than hyperreninemia, it is considered positive for primary hyperaldosteronism. A confirmatory 24-hour urine aldosterone test should be performed. Patients should be instructed to consume a liberal salt diet during the laboratory testing for hyperaldosteronism to prevent volume depletion, which normally elevates serum levels of renin and aldosterone.

To complicate matters, approximately one third of hyperaldosteronism is caused by bilateral adrenal hyperplasia. So if the contralateral adrenal is slightly enlarged, it too may be hypersecreting, or it could even be the sole source of aldosterone excess. Therefore if there is any question as to the normality of the contralateral gland, adrenal venous sampling may be warranted, although it is technically challenging and inherently complex, as it requires the simultaneous

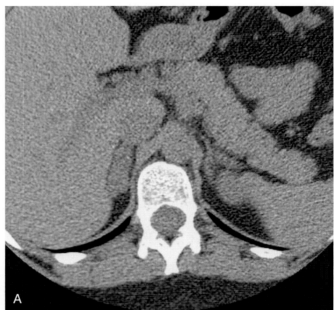

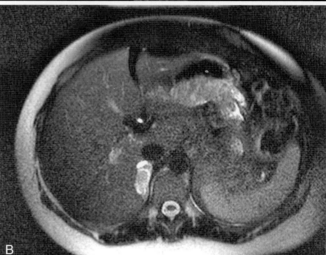

FIGURE 2 25-year-old female with typical-appearing 3.4 cm nonfunctional right adrenal incidentaloma on noncontrast CT (*left*) and MRI (*right*).

administration of intravenous ACTH while collecting aliquots of blood from both adrenal veins for aldosterone and cortisol levels. It should only be performed at centers of excellence with a highly skilled interventional radiologist interested in performing such time-consuming evaluations. If such analysis confirms unilaterality, an adrenalectomy is warranted; however, bilateral hyperplasia is treated pharmacologically.

Imaging Studies Used to Evaluate Adrenal Incidentalomas

Lesion size continues to play a major role in determining malignant potential. For lesions smaller than 4 cm, less than 2% will prove to be ACC, as opposed to more than 20% of lesions 6 cm in diameter or larger. An essential first step in the evaluation is to locate any previous imaging studies that would have included the adrenals. If such studies have been performed, and no significant change was seen over a

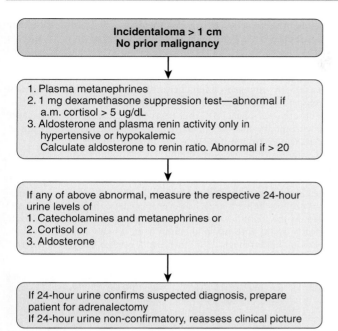

FIGURE 3   Hormonal evaluation of adrenal incidentaloma.

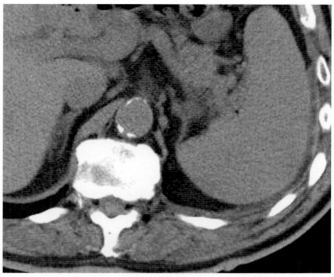

FIGURE 4   79-year-old male with serial noncontrast CT scans showing progressive enlargement of a nonfunctioning left adrenal mass. The left adrenal was reported as normal.

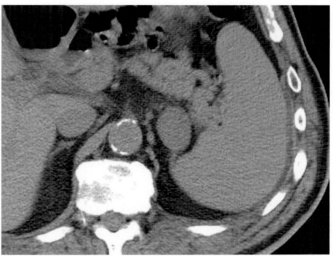

FIGURE 5   A 3.5 cm left adrenal mass.

2-year period or longer, the risk of malignancy is extremely low, even for lesions greater than 4 cm. Likewise, if an incidentaloma is evident that was not present on a scan obtained within the last 5 years, a high level of suspicion for malignancy should be raised, even for lesions less than 4 cm in diameter (Figures 3, 4, and 5).

While advances in cross-sectional imaging with CT and MRI have contributed to the growing numbers of adrenal incidentalomas, these technical improvements are also aiding radiologists' efforts to characterize incidentalomas as benign or malignant. Large, heterogeneous, irregular lesions and those that invade surrounding structures are suggestive of malignancy (Figure 6); benign adenomas are generally small, homogeneous, and well defined (Figure 7). The initial CT or MRI may not provide the complete imaging characteristics for the lesion in question, since the study was performed for another reason. However, much information will be available to begin a formulation of the incidentaloma's imaging phenotype. These include size, contour, complexity, presence of calcification and necrosis, and the Hounsfield unit (HU) density.

HU densities vary depending on the intracellular lipid concentration of a tissue. Lipid-rich benign adenomas generally have low HU densities (<18), whereas pheochromocytomas and malignancies contain few lipids and typically measure higher (Figure 8). Radiologists can predict with 98% specificity the benign nature of an incidentaloma if the unenhanced HU density is less than 10; if not biochemically active, such lesions can generally be followed radiographically. However, not all adenomas can be characterized using unenhanced CT alone, because lipid-poor adenomas can compromise 10% to 40% of all benign incidentalomas. In addition, some malignant lesions, especially adrenal metastases, will appear similar to nonfunctional adenomas on unenhanced CT.

When dealing with a small, relatively benign-appearing incidentaloma with a higher HU density, an adrenal protocol CT scan may be helpful. This scan is performed with and without intravenous contrast, taking 3 mm cuts through the lower chest and upper abdomen. The study compares immediate to 15 minute delayed images to take advantage of differences in the uptake and washout of contrast seen in benign adrenal adenomas compared with malignancies. The most commonly used criteria for establishing an adrenal neoplasm as a benign adenoma is a 15-minute delay washout ratio of 40% or more. Lesions demonstrating less than 40% washout should be considered suspicious for malignancy. Accuracy of this technique has

been confirmed for both lipid-rich and lipid-poor adenomas, with both sensitivity and specificity greater than 90% when evaluated by radiologists specializing in the interpretation of such scans. It is still recommended that most lesions greater than 4 cm be excised, however in older or high-risk patients, a benign appearance on contrast-enhanced CT scan with washout may allow for a nonoperative management approach. As radiographic characterization of incidentalomas continues to improve, this threshold for resection may change.

In some cases, an MRI will have been the study by which the incidentaloma was identified, and MRI has become a well-accepted diagnostic tool in the characterization of adrenal masses. MRI provides the advantages of imaging without radiation, is useful for patients with iodine contrast allergies, has excellent contrast resolution for tissue characterization, and is superior to CT for identifying invasion of adrenal carcinomas into adjacent organs. Although spatial resolution is less than with CT, it is adequate for detection of lesions as small as 0.5 to 1.0 cm. Both T1- and T2-weighted images are utilized to differentiate adrenal lesions. Generally, primary and metastatic adrenal malignancies are denser than benign adenomas because of their higher fluid content and therefore appear brighter on T2-weighted images. This is also true of pheochromocytomas (Figure 9). However, up to 30% of pheochromocytomas will have low signal intensity on T2-weighted images. Although there are reported exceptions, such as fat-containing metastases and lipid-poor adenomas, adenomas usually have low signal intensity on T2 imaging.

Fat suppression is used so that T2-weighted images are not degraded by artifact from the retroperitoneal fat that surrounds the adrenals. Since fat-containing areas in myelolipomas cannot be distinguished in signal intensity from retroperitoneal fat in all sequences, fat-saturated MRI can be used to test for fatty content. Metastases are usually hypointense compared with liver on T1 images and hyperintense on T2 images.

The administration of contrast helps to demonstrate enhancement patterns, which on postcontrast MRI series demonstrate washout curves similar to those observed on delayed postcontrast CT

imaging. After injection of contrast, metastases typically demonstrate strong enhancement with delayed washout. Further differentiation of adrenal neoplasm by MRI imaging sequences can be made with in-phase/opposed-phase chemical shift imaging. Adrenal lesions with high lipid content, such as adenomas, typically show loss of signal intensity on opposed-phase chemical shift sequences. Malignant lesions, however, do not show any appreciable loss of signal intensity on opposed-phase MRI, but necrosis is often observed. Because pheochromocytomas do not contain intracellular lipids, there are no signal changes from out-of-phase to in-phase images.

Certain specific imaging findings are pathognomonic for particular adrenal lesions. An MIBG nuclear medicine scan is highly sensitive and specific for identification of pheochromocytoma (Figure 10). Myelolipoma, a universally benign fatty adrenal lesion, can sometimes grow to be very large, however it can be definitively diagnosed based on the identification of macroscopic fat. If the incidentaloma is clearly cystic, with no solid component, it likely represents a congenital or hemorrhagic cyst, carrying a benign prognosis. In rare

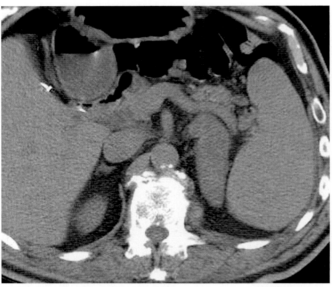

FIGURE 6   A 7.9 cm left adrenal mass. Given the rapid enlargement, the lesion was highly suspicious for ACC, which was confirmed after open left adrenalectomy.

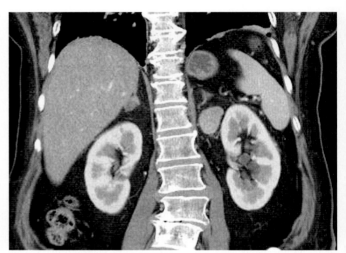

FIGURE 8   Abdominal CT with IV contrast showing bilateral enhancing adrenal incidentalomas (*left*, 4.5 cm; *right*, 1.5 cm) in a 68-year-old woman with hypertension and diabetes. Biochemical evaluation was diagnostic for pheochromocytoma.

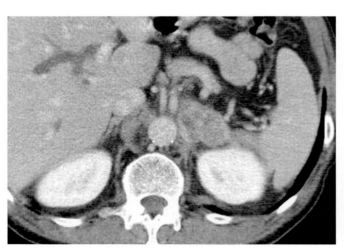

FIGURE 7   A previously healthy 54-year-old male with left upper quadrant pain was found on contrast CT to have a 4.6 cm heterogeneously enhancing left adrenal mass highly suspicious for malignancy. Open adrenalectomy with renal vein reconstruction because of tumor invasion was performed. Pathology showed a high-grade B-cell lymphoma, the patient's only site of disease.

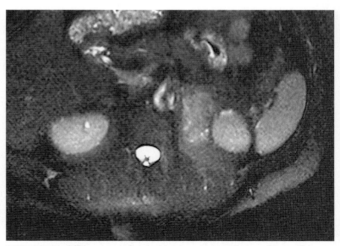

FIGURE 9   MRI scan performed in the same patient as Figure 8 to confirm pheochromocytoma was not bilateral. This T2-weighted image shows the characteristic brightness exhibited by the left pheochromocytoma. Signal dropout on out-of-phase imaging confirmed the mass on the right to be a benign adenoma.

instances, patients will hemorrhage into an adrenal neoplasm, and they may present acutely with flank and/or abdominal pain. Evaluation with contrast-enhanced CT and MRI may be helpful to determine whether such an event has occurred by differentiating perfused adrenal tissue from nonperfused periadrenal hemorrhage. Initially, however, there will be increased CT attenuation related to inflammatory change. Although the majority of such hemorrhagic events are not associated with malignancy, these lesions should either be excised or followed closely with CT or MRI in 3 to 4 months. Malignant neuroblastoma and benign ganglioneuroma (Figure 11) have no specific imaging features.

Role of Adrenal Biopsy

Adrenal biopsy is rarely helpful or indicated in the evaluation of adrenal incidentaloma despite its frequent recommendation within the text of a radiology report. For the consulting surgeon, news that an adrenal biopsy has been performed is unwelcome. It often will have produced periadrenal hemorrhage with associated inflammatory change and obliteration of the normal tissue planes, increasing the difficulty of dissection and potential for surgical morbidity. Despite their retroperitoneal location, which makes them easy targets for CT-guided percutaneous biopsy, tissue obtained is rarely sufficient to distinguish benign from malignant adrenal cortical neoplasms. Before such a procedure is ever considered, tumor functionality must be ruled out. A recent review of over 160 adrenal biopsies performed at a tertiary care center over a decade confirmed that the procedure has no utility in the workup of adrenal incidentalomas. Rather, the

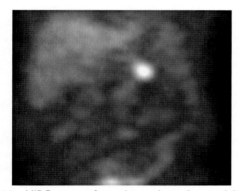

FIGURE 10   MIBG scan performed to evaluate the possibility of bilateral pheochromocytoma shows intense uptake on the left. Scan was interpreted as equivocal uptake on the right.

only clinical situations in which it proves helpful are in diagnosing adrenal metastatic disease in patients known to have, or suspected of having, melanoma, lymphoma, or extraadrenal cancer such as lung, renal cell, breast, or gastrointestinal cancer.

Adrenalectomy

In general, all hormone-secreting adrenal neoplasms require resection. Adrenalectomy for nonfunctional incidentalomas is performed to rule out or treat an adrenal malignancy (Figure 12). In the era preceding laparoscopic adrenalectomy, the generally accepted size threshold for adrenalectomy was 6 cm, with a risk for ACC approaching 20%. Today most endocrine surgeons who perform laparoscopic adrenalectomy employ a 4 cm size threshold, below which the risk for ACC is less than 2%. However, when the imaging phenotype can definitively characterize lesions as benign despite larger diameters, it may be acceptable to follow a nonoperative management strategy. Before proceeding with adrenalectomy, always confirm that the contralateral gland is normal.

Since the first reported laparoscopic adrenalectomy in 1992, the laparoscopic approach has become standard for the treatment of benign functioning and nonfunctioning adrenal neoplasms. Because the risk of primary adrenal malignancy is low, the laparoscopic approach is used for most incidentalomas 6 cm in diameter or smaller. Compared with open adrenalectomy, laparoscopic adrenalectomy is proven to result in less blood loss and decreased need for transfusion, fewer wound complications, decreased postoperative pain, and shorter hospitalizations. Although the technical difficulty of performing laparoscopic adrenalectomy increases with increasing tumor size, uncomplicated resection of lesions larger than 10 cm in diameter has been reported.

Although controversial and once considered an absolute contraindication to a laparoscopic approach, potentially malignant primary tumors and adrenal metastases are now being removed laparoscopically in some centers. Although laparoscopic removal of larger adrenal tumors is technically possible, it must be recognized that these lesions are more likely to be malignant. An open approach should be considered for any lesions that demonstrate features worrisome for malignancy, such as rapid growth, areas of necrosis, or possible invasion of adjacent structures. Open resection remains the gold standard for suspected adrenocortical carcinoma to ensure an oncologically correct operation that maximizes the chances of a margin-negative resection; avoids violation of the tumor capsule and tumor spillage; facilitates vascular control of the inferior vena cava, aorta, and renal vessels; and allows maximal exposure for en bloc resection of associated anatomic structures.

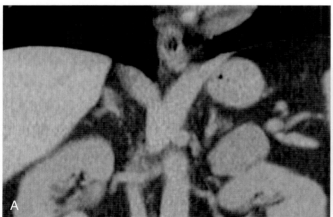
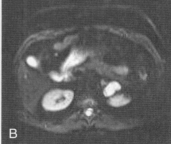

FIGURE 11   **A,** Paraganglioma situated between the left adrenal and kidney first identified on noncontrast CT. **B,** Subsequent MRI shows a 3.3 cm contrast-enhancing mass.

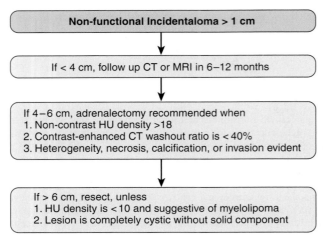

FIGURE 12   Resection algorithm for nonfunctional adrenal incidentaloma.

Patient Preparation

Once the decision is made to perform adrenalectomy, preoperative patient preparation will depend on whether or not the tumor is functional. For patients with pheochromocytoma, alpha blockade should begin with phenoxybenzamine 10 mg daily and be titrated to 10 mg three times daily over 3 weeks, after which time adrenalectomy can be safely performed via a laparoscopic approach. The main side effects of this treatment will be orthostatic hypotension, fatigue, and sinus congestion; and in some patients, dose titration can be difficult. Pheochromocytoma induces diuresis and volume depletion, so patients must be adequately hydrated before and during surgery. Beta blockade is not recommended, unless patients are persistently tachycardic. The importance of working with an experienced anesthesiologist cannot be overstated, as even the best prepared patients can demonstrate extreme hemodynamic instability intraoperatively.

Patients with cortisol hypersecretion will become adrenally insufficient in the immediate postoperative period, requiring perioperative stress-dose steroids and often a prolonged steroid taper at the time of discharge. The addisonian state can persist for upward of a year, and the involvement of an endocrine consultant is always recommended.

For aldosteronoma there is no special preoperative preparation. Usually the hypokalemia rapidly resolves, allowing for discontinuation of potassium-sparing diuretics. Many of these patients will continue to require antihypertensive medications; however, the number and dosage of medications can be reduced. Improvements in blood pressure control continue to be seen for up to a year following adrenalectomy.

Technical Aspects

Laparoscopic adrenalectomy can be performed via a transabdominal approach with the patient in the lateral decubitus position or via a retroperitoneal approach with the patient prone on a Wilson frame. The latter method is especially useful in patients with small tumors and in those who are expected to have significant peritoneal adhesions from previous operations. It avoids the need for mobilization of the colon, spleen, and liver that is employed in the transabdominal approach. It is also an excellent choice when bilateral adrenalectomy is required. However, because of the small retroperitoneal working space, limitations to its use include very large tumors and morbidly obese patients.

The transabdominal approach remains the most widely practiced; it is readily taught and learned, has low rates of complications, and can be performed safely by proficient laparoscopic surgeons. The

patient is placed on a beanbag in the lateral decubitus position, with the adrenal to be resected away from the table. An axillary roll is placed, and the bed is flexed at the level of the iliac crest to maximally open the space between it and the costal margin for trochar insertion. Next, the beanbag is firmed, and the patient is secured, ensuring excellent padding of all pressure points. A 12 mm OptiView trocar (Ethicon, Cincinnati, Ohio) is used to gain peritoneal access two fingerbreadths below the costal margin at the midclavicular line, and pneumoperitoneum is established. For both left and right adrenalectomies, two 5 mm ports are placed 6 cm apart lateral to the camera port, and an additional 5 mm port is placed medially on the right for liver retraction.

On the left, the lateral attachments of the spleen should be mobilized with the harmonic scalpel up to the level of the gastric fundus. Full mobilization allows the spleen to fall medially, pulling the tail of the pancreas with it, allowing for better adrenal exposure. Pancreatic tissue is similar in appearance to adrenal tissue and should be avoided. Judicious use of laparoscopic ultrasound will quickly clarify the borders of the adrenal, kidney, and pancreas on the left and the liver, kidney, and major vessels on the right, allowing for safe and expeditious dissection, especially when there is abundant retroperitoneal fat.

When mobilizing the right hepatic lobe, especially for very medial and cephalad adrenal tumors, always be cognizant of the proximity of the inferior vena cava. On both sides, avoid entering the plane lateral to the kidney, because its mobilization will obscure the field of dissection. During the actual mobilization of the adrenal, it is not essential to dissect and ligate the adrenal vein first, even in the case of pheochromocytoma. In fact, it is often easier and safer to mobilize the gland in a top-down approach, peeling it out of the retroperitoneum until it remains tethered only by the vein. Very often there exists a tail of adrenal cortical tissue that travels down along the vein in proximity to its junction with the renal vein on the left and vena cava on the right. Meticulous dissection in this region is essential to avoid leaving adrenal tissue behind.

Long-Term Follow-up for Small, Nonfunctional Incidentalomas

Few studies have documented the long-term evolution of the adrenal incidentaloma. The estimated 5 year risk of enlargement and hyperfunction can approach 20%. Patients should undergo annual screening for pheochromocytoma and cortisol secretion for 3 years after an incidentaloma is first detected. In a patient with a tumor less than 4 cm and no radiographic suggestion of malignancy, annual CT scan should be performed for 2 to 3 years. If there is no change, it is generally safe to assume that the lesion will remain benign. However, repeat CT is recommended at 3, 6, and 12 months if the radiographic characteristics raise suspicion of possible malignancy, as the growth rate for adrenocortical cancer is expected to be more than 2 cm per year. Lesions that enlarge more than 1 cm in follow-up should be removed.

SUGGESTED READINGS

Boland GW, Blake MA, Hahn PF, Mayo-Smith WW: Incidental adrenal lesions: principles, techniques, and algorithms for imaging characterization, *Radiology* 249:756, 2008.

Brunt LM, Moley JF: Adrenal incidentalomas, *World J Surg* 25:905, 2001.

Miner TJ: Mazzaglia P: The unexpected finding: adrenal incidentaloma, *Curr Prob Surg* 45:360, 2008.

Shen WT, Sturgeon C, Duh QY: From incidentaloma to adrenocortical carcinoma: the surgical management of adrenal tumors, *J Surg Oncol* 89:186, 2005.

Young WF Jr: Clinical practice: the incidentally discovered adrenal mass, *N Engl J Med* 356(6):601, 2007.

Management of Adrenal Cortical Tumors

Manish Parikh, MD, and H. Leon Pachter, MD

OVERVIEW

The adrenal glands are retroperitoneal paired organs that lie superior to the kidneys. The key surgical anatomic fact is that the adrenal vein is inferomedial to the gland on the left side and drains into the left renal vein, and it is superiomedial on the right side and drains directly into the inferior vena cava posterolaterally. About 80% of the adrenal gland consists of the adrenal cortex, which is subdivided into the zona glomerulosa, which produces aldosterone, the zona fasciculata, which makes glucocorticoids, and the zona reticularis, which produces sex hormones. Patients with adrenal cortical lesions should undergo a thorough history and physical followed by functional evaluation, including:

- Plasma renin activity (PRA)
- Plasma aldosterone concentration (PAC) and PAC/PRA
- 24-hour urinary free cortisol
- 24-hour urine catecholamines/metabolites

The adrenal cortical tumors of those patients who are referred for surgery typically fall into one of following four categories: 1) functional tumor causing a clinical syndrome due to hormonal excess, which includes aldosteronoma, Cushing syndrome, and virilizing/feminizing tumors; 2) adrenocortical cancer; 3) adrenal metastasis; and 4) incidentaloma (see Chapter 128).

ALDOSTERONOMA

Excess aldosterone production by the adrenal glands (primary hyperaldosteronism) should be suspected in any patient with hypertension and hypokalemia, persistent hypertension refractory to medical treatment, or hypertension and an adrenal mass. Recent data indicate that up to 12% to 15% of patients with hypertension may have primary hyperaldosteronism. Primary hyperaldosteronism is diagnosed by an elevated plasma aldosterone concentration (PAC >15 ng/dL) with a suppressed plasma renin activity (PRA <0.5 ng/mL/hr) and PAC/PRA of 30 or greater (Figure 1). Elevated urinary aldosterone levels (>14 g/day) during intravenous saline infusion confirm the diagnosis. Increased plasma renin activity and a PAC/PRA less than 30 may indicate secondary hyperaldosteronism, which is treated medically.

Further evaluation is required to differentiate between aldosteronoma—Conn syndrome, which accounts for 80% of primary hyperaldosteronism and is treated by adrenalectomy—and bilateral adrenal hyperplasia, which is treated medically with spironolactone or eplerenone and potassium (see Figure 1). Computed tomography (CT) scan with adrenal mass protocol (thin 2 mm cuts) through the adrenal gland is accurate in detecting adenomas larger than 0.5 cm. A benign adenoma is suggested by a nodule that is 10 to 15 Houndsfield units (HUs) or lower on unenhanced CT, a 10-minute delayed CT washout greater than 50%, or a 15-minute delayed CT washout greater than 60%. On MRI, the presence of intracellular lipid, diagnostic of adenomas, is reliably identified with the use of chemical shift imaging with an accuracy greater than 90%. Adrenal tumors that are not characterized by the above techniques include lipid-poor adenomas (up to 30% of all adenomas), pheochromocytomas, adrenocortical carcinoma, and metastases.

A radiographically apparent unilateral adenoma with biochemically proven hyperaldosteronism is not always an aldosteronoma. It is not uncommon to encounter the scenario of a patient with an incidentaloma (3% to 5% incidence overall in the general population) *and* a functioning contralateral microadenoma (seen in up to 20% of all aldosteronomas). Therefore we routinely use adrenal vein sampling to confirm that the adrenal mass is the source of hyperaldosteronism. An adrenal vein aldosterone/cortisol ratio on one side that is five times higher than the contralateral side is diagnostic of unilateral functioning adenoma.

Unilateral adenoma is best treated by laparoscopic adrenalectomy. Hypertension and hypokalemia should be managed preoperatively with a 3 to 5 week course of spironolactone (100 to 400 mg daily) and/or oral potassium. Preoperative normalization of blood pressure with spironolactone is a good predictor of a successful outcome after adrenalectomy. Adrenalectomy for aldosteronoma results in immediate resolution of hypokalemia in 98% to 100% of patients and significant improvement in blood pressure in 70% of patients. Spironolactone and potassium supplements should be discontinued postoperatively. Steroid replacement is not required for patients undergoing unilateral adrenalectomy for non-Cushing adrenal tumors.

CUSHING SYNDROME

Glucorticoid excess, or Cushing syndrome, has several associated manifestations (Table 1). Loss of diurnal variation in cortisol levels is one of the first signs of Cushing syndrome. Elevated 24-hour urinary free cortisol is the most sensitive and specific test for diagnosing Cushing syndrome. A low-dose dexamethasone suppression test can also diagnose Cushing syndrome, because cortisol levels in patients with Cushing syndrome are not suppressed by a single low dose (1 mg) of dexamethasone.

The most common cause of Cushing syndrome is exogenous steroid use. Endogenous excess cortisol production can be from a pituitary tumor or hyperplasia (Cushing disease, 60% to 70%); ectopic adrenocorticotropic hormone (ACTH)-producing tumor in paraneoplastic syndromes caused by bronchial carcinoids, small cell lung cancer, pancreatic islet cell cancers, and thymomas (10% to 20%); or an adrenal adenoma or adrenocortical carcinoma (10% to 20%). Basal ACTH levels using an immunoradiometric assay help differentiate between ACTH-dependent Cushing syndrome from pituitary or ectopic sources and ACTH-independent Cushing syndrome caused by adrenal lesions (Figure 2).

If Cushing syndrome is due to solitary adrenal adenoma, laparoscopic adrenalectomy is the procedure of choice; if it is due to adrenocortical carcinoma, en bloc surgical resection can be curative, usually via an open approach using a subcostal incision or anterior midline incision. Bilateral, pigmented, micronodular adrenal hyperplasia is a rare cause of Cushing syndrome and is treated by bilateral laparoscopic adrenalectomy. Staged bilateral adrenalectomy may be prudent if the patient has severe comorbidities as a result of the cortisol excess. Occasionally, patients with Cushing disease (pituitary source) may fail transsphenoidal pituitary resection or irradiation and may benefit from bilateral adrenalectomy.

Cortisol excess may be controlled preoperatively with cytochrome P-450 inhibitors such as ketoconazole (600 to 1200 mg daily). Patients undergoing surgery for Cushing syndrome should receive stress glucocorticoids perioperatively, usually 100 mg IV hydrocortisone preoperatively followed by 100 mg every 6 hours postoperatively. These doses are gradually transitioned to oral steroids, which are tapered once the ACTH-stimulation test normalizes, and the contralateral gland is no longer suppressed. Patients undergoing bilateral adrenalectomy will require lifelong replacement therapy.

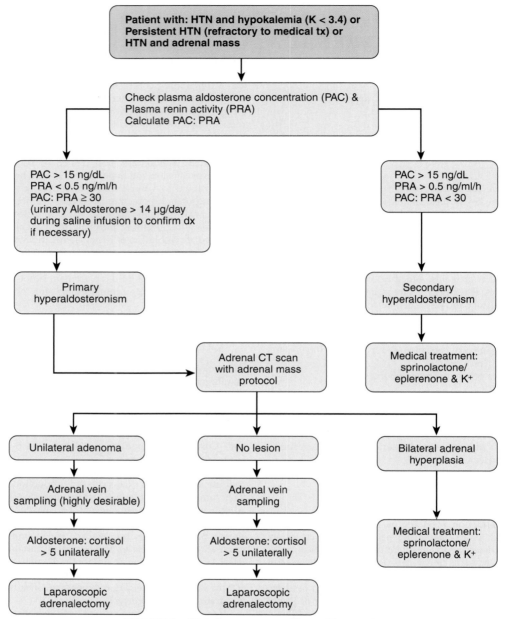

FIGURE I   Clinical management of hyperaldosteronism.

VIRILIZING/FEMINIZING TUMORS

Although virilizing and feminizing adrenal tumors are relatively uncommon, 80% of them are malignant. Women with hirsutism, alopecia, irregular menses, and other virilizing signs may have a hypersecreting adrenal tumor or a functioning ovarian tumor. Elevated serum testosterone, dehydroepiandrostenedione (DHEA-S), and 24-hour urinary 7-hydroxysteroids and 17-ketosteroids establish the diagnosis of a virilizing tumor. Abdominal CT scan with 3 mm cuts usually identifies the adrenal tumor. If an ovarian mass is present, a dexamethasone suppression test will suppress androgens and ketosteroids produced by ovarian tumors but not adrenal tumors.

Men with gynecomastia, gonadal atrophy, impotence, or loss of libido may have an estrogen-secreting adrenal tumor, which may be adrenocortical carcinoma, or a testicular tumor. Routine physical exam should identify the presence of a testicular tumor. Elevated serum estrogen levels with suppressed gonadotropins, follicle

stimulating hormone (FSH), and luteinizing hormones suggest a feminizing tumor. CT scan with 3 mm cuts should identify the adrenal mass. Generally these tumors can be safely removed laparoscopically, with a low threshold for converting to an open approach if features of malignancy are present.

ADRENOCORTICAL CARCINOMA

Adrenocortical carcinoma (ACC) is a rare adrenal malignancy that accounts for 1% of all adrenal masses and afflicts 1 to 2 individuals per million population. The median age at diagnosis is 44 years. Although it is potentially curable in its early stages, only 30% are confined to the adrenal gland at the time of diagnosis; lung and liver are the most frequent sites of metastasis. The majority of ACC patients (60%) are seen with signs and symptoms of Cushing syndrome with or without virilization. The remainder have large retroperitoneal

TABLE 1: Overlapping conditions and clinical features of Cushing syndrome*

Symptoms	Signs	Overlapping Conditions
Features that best discriminate Cushing syndrome (most do not have high sensitivity):		
	Easy bruising	
	Facial plethora	
	Proximal myopathy (or proximal muscle weakness)	
	Striae (especially if reddish purple and >1 cm wide)	
	In children, weight gain with decreasing growth velocity	
Cushing syndrome features in the general population that are common and/or less discriminatory:		
Depression	Dorsocervical fat pad ("buffalo hump")	Hypertension[†]
Fatigue	Facial fullness	Incidental adrenal mass
Weight gain	Obesity	Vertebral osteoporosis[†]
Back pain	Supraclavicular fullness	Polycystic ovary syndrome
Changes in appetite	Thin skin[†]	Type 2 diabetes[†]
Decreased concentration	Peripheral edema	Hypokalemia
Decreased libido	Acne	Kidney stones
Impaired memory (especially short term)	Hirsutism or female balding	Unusual infections
Insomnia	Poor skin healing	
Irritability		
Menstrual abnormalities		
In children, slow growth	In children, abnormal genital virilization	
	In children, short stature	
	In children, pseudoprecocious puberty or delayed puberty	

*Features are listed in random order.
†Cushing syndrome is more likely if onset of the feature is at a younger age.
From Nieman L, Biller B, Findling J, et al: The diagnosis of Cushing's syndrome: an endocrine society clinical practice guideline, *J Clin Endocrinol Metab* 93: 152-154, 2008.

masses without any evidence of hormone overactivity, although evidence suggests that sophisticated urinary steroid analysis reveals hormonal activity in almost all ACC cases. Incidentalomas account for 1% to 5% of ACC. Concern for malignancy should always be raised for any adrenal lesion larger than 6 cm.

Thorough preoperative endocrine workup is essential to establish the adrenocortical origin of the tumor and to guide perioperative and postoperative management (Table 2). Elevated hormones may serve as tumor markers during follow-up. Although CT and MRI are equally effective, MRI may be more useful than CT in determining extension of tumor into the renal vein and inferior vena cava (IVC). Invasion into the IVC and/or the presence of thrombus are considered regional involvement and are not contraindications to resection.

The two most important prognostic factors are completeness of resection and stage of disease (Table 3). Immunohistochemistry may also be important, specifically Ki67 expression, which has been associated with poor clinical outcome in the German ACC Registry. In all stage I and II ACC patients and most stage III patients, complete R0 resection (often en bloc with local organs, if necessary) is feasible in experienced hands. Because of the large size of these tumors—in most large series, average size ranges from 12 to 16 cm—a conventional open approach may offer the best chance at complete resection, via either a subcostal incision or anterior midline laparotomy. For tumors with invasion into the diaphragm or IVC, a thoracoabdominal approach may be necessary, with or without venovenous bypass.

Mitotane, a pesticide analog with adrenolytic activity, is the single most important drug for adjuvant ACC treatment for patients with residual, recurrent, or metastatic ACC. Some centers use mitotane after complete R0 resection if the tumor is large (>8 cm), or if it appears aggressive (Ki67 >10%). Prolonged mitotane treatment is limited by gastrointestinal and neurologic toxicity. Since mitotane can induce adrenal insufficiency, patients may need glucocorticoid and mineralocorticoid supplementation during treatment. Up to 80% of mitotane-treated patients with functioning tumors will show significant decreases in hormone production. Radiotherapy is recommended in patients with incomplete resection or, in some centers, with advanced local disease (stage III) or aggressive tumors (Ki67 >20%). Cisplatin has had beneficial effects in select patients with metastatic disease. Occasionally, local recurrences and select metastatic sites can be palliated surgically. Radiofrequency ablation of metastatic ACC lesions (<5 cm) is an alternative to surgical resection; chemoembolization is an option for metastatic ACC to the liver.

Overall 5-year survival depends on tumor stage, with reported rates ranging from 40% to 60% for stage I and II, 20% to 30% for stage III, and 10% 1-year survival for stage IV disease.

ADRENAL METASTASES

Any adrenal mass in a patient with a history of malignancy should be suspected of being an adrenal metastasis. The most common tumors to metastasize to the adrenal gland are lung carcinoma (especially small cell), renal cell carcinoma, melanoma, gastric adenocarcinoma, hepatocellular carcinoma, esophageal adenocarcinoma, and breast adenocarcinoma. CT or MRI characteristics of adrenal metastases include irregular borders, hemorrhage, tumor necrosis, and a region of interest (ROI) greater than 20 HU on unenhanced CT. 18-Fluorodeoxyglucose positron emission tomography (18F-FDG-PET) may help differentiate between metabolically active malignant disease and benign adenoma; however, in our experience, up to 40% of PET-positive lesions turned out to be benign in patients with lung, brain, and breast cancers. Fine needle aspiration may be required to confirm the diagnosis, but only after pheochromocytoma has been ruled out to avoid potentially life-threatening hypertensive crisis.

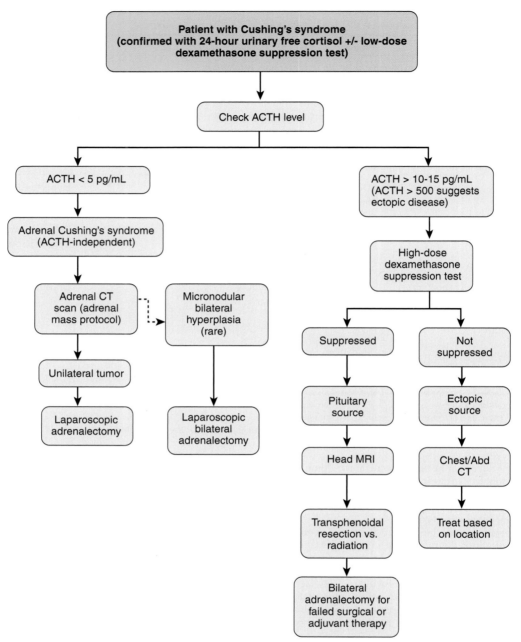

FIGURE 2 Clinical management of Cushing syndrome.

In carefully selected patients, especially with long-term disease-free intervals, laparoscopic or open adrenalectomy may be beneficial. Laparoscopic resection can be done safely in patients who do not have local invasion. Median survival for adrenalectomy for metastases ranges from 2 to 3.4 years.

LAPAROSCOPIC ADRENALECTOMY

First performed in 1992, the laparoscopic approach to adrenalectomy has evolved to become the standard of care for the removal of most adrenal tumors. Numerous comparative studies have shown the benefits of laparoscopic adrenalectomy over open adrenalectomy including decreased morbidity, shorter length of stay, reduced postoperative analgesic requirements, better patient satisfaction, and quicker return to work.

The most common laparoscopic approach is transabdominally via the flank, with the patient in the full lateral decubitus position and the table flexed to open up the flank (Figure 3). It permits gravity to retract the small bowel and colon out of the field of view and thus effectively exposes the adrenal gland, using easily recognized intraabdominal anatomic landmarks. This technique is reproducible and is the easiest to teach to inexperienced laparoscopic surgeons. The key surgical maneuvers for successful laparoscopic adrenalectomy are mobilization of the spleen for left adrenalectomy and mobilization of the right lobe of the liver for right adrenalectomy.

We routinely use prophylactic antibiotics (cefazolin 1 g); however, this is not standard. Sequential pneumatic compression devices are placed for deep venous thrombosis prophylaxis, and adequate large-bore intravenous access is established. Once general anesthesia has been administered, a Foley catheter is placed by the surgical team. The patient is then positioned as detailed below.

TABLE 2: Diagnostic workup in patients with ACC and suspected or proven adrenocortical carcinoma: Recommendation of the ACC Working Group of ENSAT (May 2005)

Hormonal Workup	
Glucocorticoid excess (minimum 3 of 4 tests)	• Dexamethasone suppression test (1 mg, 23 hr) • Excretion of free urinary cortisol (24-hr urine) • Basal cortisol (serum) • Basal ACTH (plasma)
Sexual steroids and steroid precursors	• DHEA-S (serum) • 17-OH-progesterone (serum) • Androstenedione (serum) • Testosterone (serum) • 17β-estradiol (serum, only in men and postmenopausal women)
Mineralocorticoid excess	• Potassium (serum) • Aldosterone/rennin ratio (only in patients with arterial hypertension and/or hypokalemia)
Exclusion of a pheochromocytoma (minimum 1 of 3 tests)	• Catecholamine excretion (24-hr urine) • Metanephrine excretion (24-hr urine) • Metanephrines and noretanephrines (plasma)
Imaging	• CT or MRI of abdomen and CT thorax • Bone scintigraphy (for suspected skeletal metastases) • FDG-PET (optional)

DHEA-S, Dehydroepiandrosterone sulphate; *ENSAT,* the European Network for the Study of Adrenal Tumours
From Fassnacht M, Eder E, Allolio B: Clinical management of adrenocortical carcinoma, *Best Pract Res Clini Endocrinol Metab* 23:273-289, 2009.

Left Adrenalectomy

The patient is placed in the lateral decubitus position with the left side up (see Figure 3). A beanbag is placed under the right flank, and a protective roll is placed under the right axilla. The left arm is extended. The table is flexed, and the left side is hyperextended to maximize the space between the left costal margin and iliac crest (the flank muscles should appear taut). The patient's torso and legs are secured to the table with 2 inch cloth tape.

The surgical prep extends from the nipple to the anterior superior iliac spine and from the umbilicus to the spine posteriorly. The surgeon and assistant stand on the right side of the patient. We prefer the open technique to access the abdomen 2 cm below and parallel to the costal margin, just medial to the left anterior axillary line (see Figure 3, C). Once the peritoneal cavity has been entered under direct vision, a 10 mm trocar is placed, and carbon dioxide is insufflated to 15 mm Hg. A 10 mm 30-degree laparoscope is introduced, and a diagnostic laparoscopy is performed. A second 10 mm trocar is placed under the eleventh rib at the midaxillary line, also parallel to the costal margin. A third 5 mm trocar is placed medial and anterior to the first trocar, along the midclavicular line and lateral to the rectus muscle. Ideally, all trocars should be at least 5 cm apart to avoid crossing of instruments. If needed, a fourth 5 mm trocar is placed at the costovertebral angle after the splenic flexure has been mobilized.

The laparoscope is then placed through the middle trocar, and the working instruments are placed through the two other ports. Our

TABLE 3: TNM staging for adrenocortical carcinoma

TNM	
• T1: <5 cm, no invasion	
• T2: >5 cm, no invasion	
• T3: Any size, locally invading (but not adjacent organs)	
• T4: Any size, locally invading adjacent organs	
• N0: No regional positive nodes	
• N1: Positive regional nodes	
• M0: No distant metastatic disease	
• M1: Distant metastasis present	

Stage	
• I: T1N0M0	
• II: T2N0M0	
• III: T1N1M0, T2N1M0, T3N0M0	
• IV: T3N1M0, T4N1M0, TXNXM1	

approach follows what many French surgeons emphasize: identify and divide the blood supply first. This approach avoids inadvertent distal pancreatectomy due to misidentification of the adrenal gland, particularly in situations where the gland is fatty and difficult to identify.

Using a laparoscopic peanut in the surgeon's left hand for retraction and the ultrasonic scalpel in the surgeon's right hand, the splenic flexure is mobilized inferomedially to open the retroperitoneal space between the spleen and lateral abdominal wall and to expose the splenorenal ligament (Figure 4, A). If needed for extra retraction, the fourth 5 mm trocar is placed dorsally at the costovertebral angle. The splenorenal ligament is incised until the stomach is visualized, thus liberating the diaphragmatic attachments and exposing the superior pole of the left kidney.

It is critical to mobilize the entire splenorenal ligament to the left crus to completely expose the adrenal gland. This maneuver allows the spleen to fall medially, exposing the retroperitoneal space, and exposing the avascular plane situated between the Gerota fascia and the pancreas. Next, the peritoneum along the inferior border of the pancreas is incised, and this dissection continues cranially to the level of the left crus (Figure 4, B). The pancreatic tail is retracted superiorly, facilitated by the mobilized spleen and the flexed table, to expose the left kidney and adrenal gland; the space between the kidney and the pancreas should open like pages in a book. It is important to differentiate between the tail of the pancreas and the left adrenal gland by dissecting inferiorly to identify the adrenal vein emptying into the left renal vein. The laparoscopic peanut dissector is an invaluable tool for retraction, rather than grasping the adrenal gland itself, which frequently creates oozing that obscures the operative field.

The next step is identification of the main adrenal vein. Retraction of the pancreas and spleen to the patient's right side will allow identification of the left renal vein. Dissection along the superior border of the renal vein will allow the surgeon to accurately identify the main adrenal vein (Figure 4, C). Retraction via the fourth trocar at the costovertebral angle of the kidney may help expose the vascular landmarks: the renal vein, adrenal vein, and phrenic vein. The adrenal vein is circumferentially dissected with a right-angled instrument and then divided between medium to large (10 mm) titanium clips (Figure 4, D).

Next, the accessory vein is divided, and the left middle arterial pedicle—which runs posterior to the accessory vein, usually directly from the aorta—is divided with the ultrasonic scalpel. The posterior diaphragm should now be visible; the remainder of the gland, including the superior arterial pedicle from the left inferior phrenic artery and the inferior arterial pedicle from the left renal artery, can be mobilized with the ultrasonic scalpel (Figure 4, E).

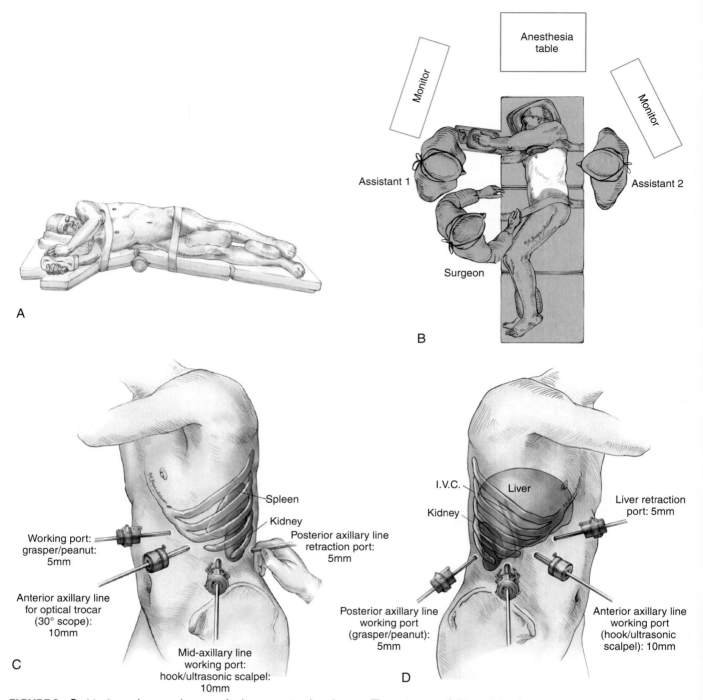

FIGURE 3   Positioning and trocar placement for laparoscopic adrenalectomy. The patient is in full lateral decubitus position, and the table is flexed to open up the flank. *(Courtesy Lianne Krueger Sullivan.)*

Particularly for adrenal glands smaller than 5 cm, it is safe and feasible to dissect and divide the adrenal vein first. For glands larger than 5 cm, the size of the tumor often precludes early identification of the adrenal vein, and frequently dissection proceeds superiorly and laterally first, dividing the arterial supply and then retracting the gland medially to expose the adrenal vein.

Once the gland has been freed, it is placed in an impermeable bag, and the bag is removed through the Hasson trocar site. Occasionally, the incision may need to be enlarged with a Kelly clamp to permit removal of the bag, especially if the lesion is larger than 4 cm.

Drainage is rarely required unless pancreatic injury is suspected. The 10 mm fascial incisions are closed with absorbable sutures, and all skin incisions are closed with 4-0 subcuticular sutures.

Right Adrenalectomy

The patient is placed in the lateral decubitus position with the right side up (see Figure 3). A beanbag is placed under the left flank, a protective roll is placed under the left axilla, and the left arm is extended. The table is flexed, and the right side is hyperextended to maximize

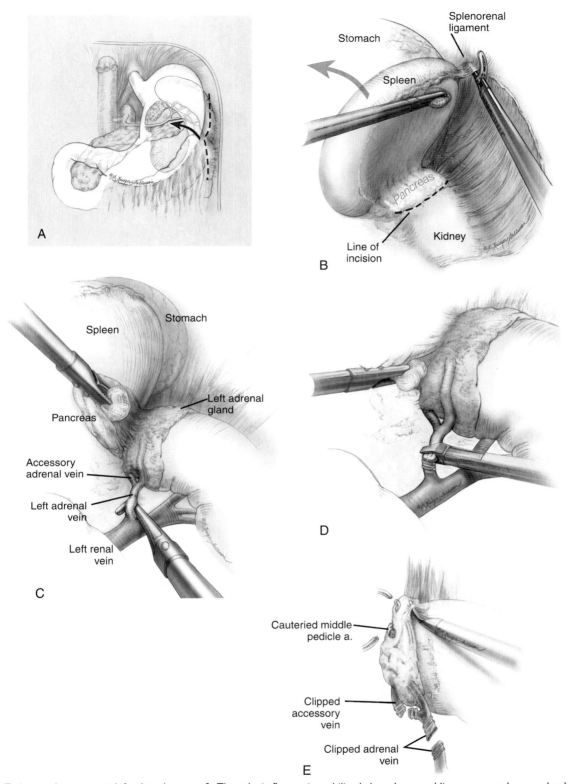

FIGURE 4 Technique: laparoscopic left adrenalectomy. **A,** The splenic flexure is mobilized; the splenorenal ligament must be completely mobilized to the left crus of the diaphragm. **B,** Incise the peritoneum along the inferior border of the pancreas to expose the adrenal gland. **C,** Dissect along the superior border of the renal vein to identify the main adrenal vein. **D,** Divide the main adrenal vein between 10 mm clips. **E,** Mobilize the remainder of the adrenal gland with the ultrasonic scalpel. *(Courtesy Lianne Krueger Sullivan.)*

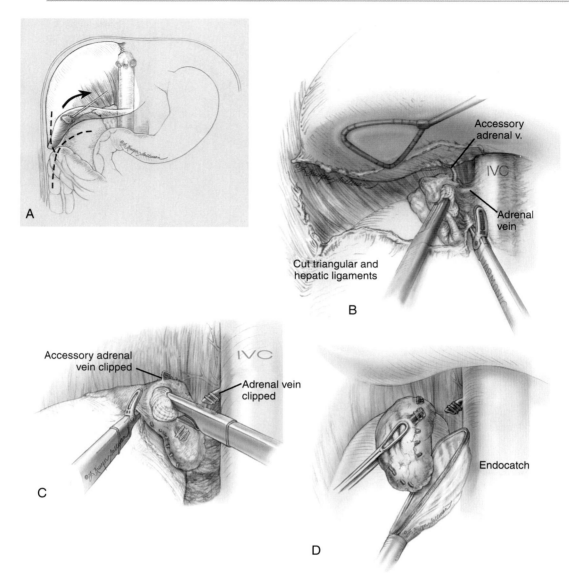

FIGURE 5   Positioning and trocar placement for laparoscopic right adrenalectomy. **A,** The right hepatic lobe must be completely mobilized to expose the right adrenal gland and vein. **B,** Dissect along the lateral wall of the vena cava until the right adrenal vein is identified. **C,** Mobilize the remainder of the gland with the ultrasonic scalpel. **D,** Remove gland with sterile impermeable bag. *(Courtesy Lianne Krueger Sullivan.)*

the space between the right costal margin and iliac crest (the flank muscles should appear taut). The patient's torso and legs are secured to the table with 2 inch cloth tape.

The surgical preparation extends from the nipple to the anterior superior iliac spine and from the umbilicus to the spine posteriorly. The surgeon and assistant stand on the left side of the patient. Open cutdown technique is done approximately 2 cm below the costal margin in the right anterior axillary line (see Figure 3, D). The 10 mm 30-degree laparoscope is used to conduct a diagnostic laparoscopy. Under direct vision, the remaining three trocars, usually two 5 mm and one 10 mm, are placed 2 cm inferior and parallel to the costal margin, at least 5 to 8 cm apart. Four trocars are necessary, because the right lobe of the liver must be retracted to expose the most medial aspect of the right adrenal gland.

The liver retractor is inserted in the most anterior trocar to lift the right hepatic lobe and reflect it anteromedially. The right lateral hepatic attachments and the right triangular ligament are divided with hook electrocautery or ultrasonic scalpel to permit medial retraction of the right hepatic lobe and to allow adequate visualization of the

right adrenal gland (Figure 5, A). *This is the key surgical maneuver to providing adequate exposure of the right adrenal vein and its entry into the IVC.*

Once the liver has been mobilized adequately, dissection begins on the lateral wall of the vena cava, just above the duodenum, until the right adrenal vein is identified (Figure 5, B). It is important to remember that compared with the left adrenal vein, which drains into the left renal vein, the right adrenal vein is more superomedial, because it drains directly into the vena cava posterolaterally. This vein is often short and broad. Gentle dissection superior and inferior to the vein going back to the adrenal can lengthen the vein and provide more room to place the clips safely. Minimal traction should be placed on the right adrenal vein to avoid tearing it off the vena cava. It is divided between two or three proximal titanium clips and two clips distally. Dissection continues along the inferior aspect of the liver to identify an accessory adrenal vein, if present, which usually joins a right subhepatic vein.

Next, the adrenal gland is retracted inferiorly and laterally using a laparoscopic peanut dissector to expose the medial arterial pedicle (from the aorta), which usually lies posteriorly or inferiorly to the main adrenal vein. Once this is divided, the posterior diaphragm should be visible, and the remainder of the gland can be mobilized in a medial-to-lateral fashion. The superior adrenal artery (from the inferior phrenic artery) and the inferior adrenal artery (from the renal artery) can be divided with the ultrasonic scalpel (Figure 5, C).

Once the gland has been completely mobilized, it is placed into a sterile, impermeable bag, which is removed through the most anterior trocar site (Figure 5, D). All incisions are closed as described for the left adrenalectomy.

Postopertive Care

Generally the postoperative care of these patients is similar to that of laparoscopic cholecystectomy patients. Oral fluids can be started on the same day of surgery. Nasogastric tubes are unnecessary and are almost never used, and the Foley catheter is removed the same day or the next morning; on the rare occasion that a Jackson-Pratt drain is used, it is removed within 48 hours. Oral analgesics adequately control postoperative pain in most patients; in some instances, parenteral analgesics are required for the first 12 hours. Patients are typically discharged by the second or third postoperative day, but length of stay may be longer in patients with functional adrenal tumors who require hormonal support and follow-up laboratory data. Usually, steroid replacement therapy is required only for those patients with overt or subclinical Cushing syndrome and patients undergoing bilateral adrenalectomy.

SUGGESTED READINGS

Fassnacht M, Allolio B: Clinical management of adrenocortical carcinoma, *Best Pract Res Clin Endocrinol Metab* 23:273–289, 2009.

Funder J, Carey R, Fardella C, et al: Case detection, diagnosis, and treatment of patients with primary aldosteronism: an endocrine society clinical practice guideline, *J Clin Endocrinol Metab* 93:3266–3281, 2008.

Gagner M, Pomp A, Heniford B, et al: Laparoscopic adrenalectomy: lessons learned from 100 consecutive procedures, *Ann Surg* 225:495–502, 1997.

Gumbs A, Gagner M: Laparoscopic adrenalectomy, *Best Pract Res Clin Endocrinol Metab* 20:483–499, 2006.

Lee J, El-Tamer M, Schiffttner T, et al: Open and laparoscopic adrenalectomy: analysis of the national surgical quality improvement program, *J Am Coll Surg* 206:953–961, 2008.

Nieman L, Biller B, Findling J, et al: The diagnosis of Cushing's syndrome: an endocrine society clinical practice guideline, *J Clin Endocrinol Metab* 93:152–154, 2008.

Thompson S, Hayman A, Ludlam W, et al: Improved quality of life after bilateral laparoscopic adrenalectomy for Cushing's disease: a 10-year experience, *Ann Surg* 245:790–794, 2007.

MANAGEMENT OF PHEOCHROMOCYTOMAS

Eric Silberfein, MD, and Nancy D. Perrier, MD

OVERVIEW

Pheochromocytomas are rare, usually slow-growing catecholamine-secreting tumors that arise from chromaffin cells. Approximately 90% of pheochromocytomas arise from the chromaffin cells of the adrenal medulla; and 10%, known as *paragangliomas*, arise from extraadrenal chromaffin tissue, found in the paraaortic sympathetic chain, the organ of Zuckerkandl at the origin of the inferior mesenteric artery, the sympathetic chain in the neck or mediastinum, and the wall of the urinary bladder. Males and females are equally represented, with peak presentation in the fourth and fifth decades of life. The annual incidence of these tumors ranges from only 0.005% to 0.1% of the general population. Prompt diagnosis is important, because untreated pheochromocytomas can be associated with significant morbidity, including myocardial infarction and cerebrovascular catastrophe, and they cause up to 1000 deaths annually. As the use of abdominal imaging has increased, and techniques have become more sensitive, a growing number of adrenal incidentalomas, including pheochromocytomas, have been reported in recent years. Furthermore, recent advances in the ability to detect germline genetic mutations have shown that up to 25% of pheochromocytomas are due to a genetic mutation, and consequently more than 10% of pheochromocytomas could be bilateral and extraadrenal. Malignant disease, defined by the presence of locoregional invasion or distant metastatic disease, is more commonly seen in extraadrenal sites and in women.

CLINICAL PRESENTATION

Because of excessive secretion of catecholamines, patients with pheochromocytomas classically experience the clinical triad of headache, sweating, and palpitations, the so-called *hypertensive spell*; but other debilitating symptoms such as anxiety, chest and abdominal pain, visual blurring, nausea and vomiting, and diaphoresis are frequently present and decrease quality of life. Individuals with paradoxical blood pressure responses during surgery or anesthesia, volatile or resistant hypertension, or sudden panic or anxiety attacks; asymptomatic patients with an adrenal incidentaloma; and individuals with a hereditary predisposition to pheochromocytoma should be considered for testing. Hypertensive spells can vary substantially among individuals and can be spontaneous or triggered by anxiety, exercise, defecation, medications, or changes in posture. Spells associated with urination may indicate a paraganglioma of the urinary bladder. The hypertension resulting from pheochromocytomas may be of new onset, refractory, paroxysmal, or recently exacerbated. About 20% of pheochromocytomas are asymptomatic and discovered incidentally during abdominal imaging. Asymptomatic pheochromocytoma is more likely in younger patients with a genetic predisposition.

Compared with sporadic pheochromocytomas, hereditary pheochromocytomas are frequently multiple, bilateral, and/or extraadrenal; are rarely malignant; and generally present at an earlier age. Pheochromocytomas occur in a number of familial syndromes associated with germline mutations: von Hippel–Lindau (VHL) syndrome, caused by the *VHL* gene; multiple endocrine neoplasia type 2 (MEN2), related to the *RET* protooncogene; neurofibromatosis type 1 (NF1), associated with the *NF1* gene; and familial paraganglioma/pheochromocytoma syndrome, recently linked to the genes encoding subunits B, C, and D of mitochondrial succinate dehydrogenase (*SDHB*, *SDHC*, and *SDHD*).

DIAGNOSIS

All patients with suspected pheochromocytoma or paraganglioma should undergo biochemical testing. The diagnosis of pheochromocytoma depends on demonstrating excessive production, especially increased metabolism of catecholamines; imaging studies are then performed for confirmation and localization.

Twenty-four hour measurements of urinary catecholamines, total and fractionated metanephrines, and vanillylmandelic acid have traditionally been used to *screen* patients for pheochromocytoma, but more recent studies suggest that measurement of plasma-free metanephrines is a superior test to *exclude* the diagnosis of pheochromocytoma. Most true-positive elevations in plasma-free metanephrines can be distinguished from false-positive results by the magnitude of increases above reference intervals. Most patients with pheochromocytomas have increases well above the upper limit of normal. Measurement of urinary fractionated metanephrines combined with plasma chromogranin A in patients with mildly elevated plasma-free metanephrines can significantly reduce the false-positive rate.

At the University of Texas M.D. Anderson Cancer Center, we prefer to measure both plasma-free metanephrines and urinary metanephrines for initial evaluation. Patients are asked to fast and abstain from caffeinated beverages and acetaminophen for 5 days before testing, as these drugs can interfere with the plasma normetanephrine assay. On the day of testing, patients rest supine for 20 minutes before their blood is drawn. Levels of plasma-free metanephrines greater than 57 pg/mL, plasma-free normetanephrines greater than 148 pg/mL, or total metanephrines greater than 205 pg/mL are considered abnormal. It should be noted that false-positive results can be seen with a number of foods and medications (Table 1).

After a biochemical diagnosis of pheochromocytoma has been established, the precise location of the tumor must be identified. Computed tomography (CT) or magnetic resonance imaging (MRI) of the adrenal glands and abdomen should be the first localization test. CT has the advantages of excellent sensitivity (95%) for detecting both adrenal and extraadrenal disease, surgeon familiarity with the cross-sectional images produced, and cost-effectiveness. On CT, pheochromocytomas usually have an attenuation higher than 10 Hounsfield units (HUs) and show much less washout of contrast material at 15 minutes than benign adenomas. CT using an adrenal imaging protocol can detect up to 95% of adrenal masses. The protocol includes non-contrast-enhanced CT followed by contrast-enhanced and delayed contrast-enhanced CT with contiguous 2 to 5 mm–thick scanning sections. The scans should extend from above the neck to below the aortic bifurcation to include possible extraadrenal sites of disease. On contrast-enhanced CT scans, pheochromocytomas appear irregular in shape, and the periphery of a pheochromocytoma is often more intense than the central portion. Occasionally, pheochromocytomas contain hemorrhagic, cystic, or calcified areas. Catecholamine excess may mobilize brown fat, resulting in changes in the CT appearance of the retroperitoneal fat (Figure 1). These diffuse changes, although they may appear infiltrative or highly vascularized in appearance, should be recognized as benign reactive changes rather than locally invasive or metastatic disease.

MRI is recommended in children, pregnant women, patients with documented allergy to CT contrast agents, and patients in whom no additional radiation exposure is desired. Pheochromocytomas are typically isointense to hypointense relative to the liver on T1-weighted MRI and hyperintense on T2-weighted MRI. Pheochromocytomas appear bright, with a "light bulb" appearance on T2-weighted images, and are typically heterogeneous. MRI is excellent in delineating the relationship between a tumor and the surrounding vasculature and thus can help identify vascular invasion.

CT and MRI are excellent for delineating the regional anatomy but have poor specificity for identifying pheochromocytomas. In contrast, nuclear scintigraphy using iodine-131 or ^{123}I-metaiodobenzylguanidine (MIBG) has excellent specificity (95% to 100%) while providing information on tumor function. Indications for

TABLE 1: Food and medications associated with false-positive elevations of plasma metanephrines

Foods
Cheese
Bananas
Wine
Soy sauce
Avocados
Fermented, smoked, or aged meat and fish

Drugs Used in Obesity Management
Phentermine
Phendimetrazine
Phenylethylamine
Sibutramine

Over-the-Counter Drugs
Pseudoephedrine
Acetaminophen

Antidepressants
Amitriptyline
Nortriptyline
Reboxetine
Duloxetine
Venlafaxine

Antibiotics
Linezolid

Antiemetics
Metoclopramide
Chlorpromazine
Prochlorperazine

MIBG scanning have drastically changed over the past 5 years and currently include localization of most cases of biochemically confirmed pheochromocytomas, when an adrenal mass is not identified, or in suspected metastatic disease. ^{123}I-MIBG is preferred over ^{131}I-MIBG because it results in more avid tumor uptake and shorter scan times and can be used in association with single photon emission CT to better identify the tumor. To prevent thyroid ablation when ^{131}I-MIBG is used, thyroid blockade is achieved by oral administration (4 drops) of saturated potassium iodide three times a day for a total of 5 days starting on the day before injection of the radiopharmaceutical. When ^{123}I-MIBG is used, oral administration of saturated potassium iodide can be reduced to three times a day for 3 days. Patients who are allergic to iodine may be given potassium perchlorate three times a day, starting 1 day before injection and continuing for a total of 4 days for ^{131}I-MIBG or 3 days for ^{123}I-MIBG.

Positron emission tomography (PET), with a number of different agents, has been used for localization of pheochromocytomas. PET with ^{18}F-fluorodeoxyglucose (FDG) and rubidium-82 has been successful, particularly in localizing metastatic disease, but is limited by its nonspecificity. It should be kept in mind that FDG uptake in the retroperitoneum may make the distinction between tumor and surrounding brown fat difficult with PET alone; PET-CT fusion is particularly helpful in this regard. Newer and more expensive agents including ^{11}C-hydroxyephedrine and 6-^{18}F-fluorodopamine show improved sensitivity and specificity but are limited by cost and availability.

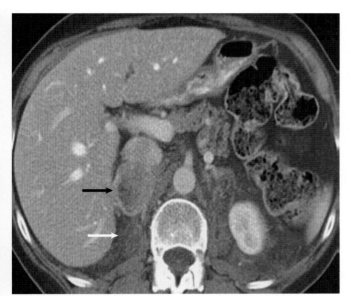

FIGURE 1 Contrast-enhanced CT scan shows right adrenal mass (*black arrow*) with significant stranding in surrounding fat (*white arrow*). (*From Perrier ND, Kennamer DL, Bao R, et al: Posterior retroperitoneoscopic adrenalectomy: preferred technique for removal of benign tumors and isolated metastases, Ann Surg 248[4]:666–674, 2008. Used with permission.*)

PREOPERATIVE MANAGEMENT

Surgical resection is the treatment of choice for pheochromocytoma. However, before surgery, drug treatment is necessary to normalize the blood pressure, the heart rate, and the function of other organs; to restore depleted intravascular volume; and to prevent cardiovascular collapse from surgery-induced catecholamine storm.

Adrenergic blockade is needed preoperatively in all pheochromocytoma patients; although there is no standard regimen, β-adrenergic antagonists, dihydropyridine calcium channel blockers, the competitive α- and β-receptor blocker labetalol, and metyrosine have all been successfully used for preoperative adrenergic blockade in patients with pheochromocytoma (Table 2). The selective α_1-adrenergic antagonists such as prazosin, doxazosin, and terazosin have the advantage of causing competitive α_1-receptor antagonism without rebound tachycardia.

At M.D. Anderson Cancer Center (MDACC), we typically begin nonselective alpha blockade at the time of diagnosis using phenoxybenzamine; the starting dosage of 10 mg orally twice daily is gradually increased over 10 to 14 days to 10 mg orally three times daily until effective blockade occurs, as evidenced by the development of postural hypotension or nasal congestion. The total dose should not exceed 2 mg/kg/day.

Because of the chronic vasoconstriction experienced by most patients with pheochromocytoma, volume contraction is often present, so liberal salt and fluid intake is encouraged to promote intravascular expansion. With appropriate nonselective α-blockade and restoration of intravascular volume, some patients will experience rebound tachycardia, which can be effectively treated with β-blockade. However, β-blockade should not be initiated before first documenting the efficacy of α-blockade, because a hypertensive crisis may ensue from unopposed α-adrenergic stimulation. This could lead to left-heart strain and congestive heart failure. The goal of β-blockade is a resting heart rate of 60 to 80 beats/min; this can usually be achieved with oral administration of a selective β-blocker such as atenolol or metoprolol (given once or twice daily). Alternatively, labetalol may be given at a starting dose of 100 mg orally twice daily and titrated every 2 to 3 days in 100 mg increments. In cases of refractory hypertension, metyrosine can be added at doses of up to 250 to 750 mg orally every 6 hours. The last oral doses of α- and β-blockers should be administered the morning of surgery.

INTRAOPERATIVE MANAGEMENT

Even with effective preoperative adrenergic blockade, a hypertensive crisis or tachyarrhythmia can occur intraoperatively, as manipulation of the tumor can cause a catecholamine surge. Patients should therefore have adequate peripheral and central venous access catheters, as well as a radial artery catheter, in place. Intravenous, titratable agents to control blood pressure should be premixed and available, should fluctuations in blood pressure occur. The dihydropyridine calcium channel blocker nicardipine, at a concentration of 0.5 to 1.0 mg/mL, and the direct acting vasodilator sodium nitroprusside, at doses of 0.5 to 3 µg/kg/min, are the agents of choice for rapid control of acute hypertension. Conversely, ligation of the adrenal vein in the case of pheochromocytoma, or of other draining vessels in the case of paraganglioma, can cause abrupt cessation of catecholamine release and subsequent acute hypotension. If hypotension occurs, epinephrine, norepinephrine, or phenylephrine should be administered and titrated, with crystalloids and blood products added as needed.

OPERATIVE TECHNIQUE

Pheochromocytomas can be resected by an open or laparoscopic approach, which can be performed by a transabdominal or retroperitoneal operation. Transabdominal laparoscopic adrenalectomy has become the procedure of choice for resection of pheochromocytomas. This approach is safe, and it is associated with comparable blood loss, less postoperative pain, shorter hospital stay, and quicker return to work compared with open adrenalectomy. Open surgery is reserved for larger pheochromocytomas and for paragangliomas in locations that make laparoscopic removal difficult. Conversion to open adrenalectomy may be necessary during laparoscopic adrenalectomy in cases of difficult dissection or uncontrolled bleeding. The posterior retroperitoneoscopic technique offers an alternative laparoscopic approach with minimal dissection and early access to the adrenal vein.

At MDACC, the surgical procedure chosen depends upon whether the tumor is spontaneous or hereditary and whether it is unilateral or bilateral. Retroperitoneoscopic adrenalectomy is used for unilateral spontaneous pheochromocytomas less than 5 cm in diameter. For patients with a unilateral hereditary pheochromocytoma and a normal contralateral gland, a laparoscopic or retroperitoneoscopic total adrenalectomy is performed. If bilateral hereditary disease is present, patients undergo an attempt at a unilateral cortex-sparing adrenalectomy and contralateral total adrenalectomy by an open approach. For patients with a metachronous contralateral pheochromocytoma after previous unilateral adrenalectomy, a cortex-sparing procedure is attempted.

Posterior Retroperitoneoscopic Adrenalectomy

Following the induction of general anesthesia with the patient supine, the patient is placed in the prone jackknife position on a Cloward table saddle (Cloward Surgical Saddle; Surgical Equipment International, Honolulu, Ha.). The hips and knees are carefully positioned at approximately 90 degree angles relative to the spine and femur, with proper padding at pressure points (Figure 2). It is essential to limit the pressure on the knees to prevent anterior displacement of the hips, which can limit instrument mobility, especially in large, overweight patients. The twelfth rib is identified by palpation, and a 1.5 cm transverse incision is made just beneath the tip of the rib. The soft tissues are divided with scissors or electrocautery, and the retroperitoneal space is entered. A small space is developed with the index finger deep to the ribs and diaphragm within the retroperitoneum. With the index finger in the retroperitoneal space, a 10 mm trocar, designated the medial trocar, is inserted along the paraspinal musculature and angled cephalad, at approximately 45 degrees, toward the anatomic location of the adrenal gland. A 5 mm trocar is inserted in a similar fashion 4 to 5 cm lateral

TABLE 2: Drugs used in the management of pheochromocytoma

Drug	Starting Dose	Maximum Dose	Notes
Phenoxybenzamine	10 mg PO BID at time of diagnosis	2 mg/kg/day	May increase to 10 mg PO TID over 10 to 14 days; goal is postural hypotension; nonselective α-blocker
Prazosin	1 mg PO BID at time of diagnosis	15 mg/day	May increase to TID dosing; goal is postural hypotension; selective α-blocker
Doxazosin	1 mg PO daily	16 mg/day	May increase weekly; at time of diagnosis, goal is postural hypotension; selective α-blocker
Terazosin	1 mg PO qHS at time of diagnosis	20 mg/day	May use BID dosing; goal is postural hypotension; selective α-blocker
Verapamil	80 mg PO TID	480 mg/day	Calcium channel blocker used for paroxysmal hypertension
Amlodipine	5 mg PO daily	10 mg/day	May increase after 1–2 weeks; calcium channel blocker used for paroxysmal hypertension
Nifedipine	30–90 mg PO daily	120 mg/day	May increase after 1–2 weeks; calcium channel blocker used for paroxysmal hypertension
Labetalol	100 mg PO BID	2400 mg/day	May increase in 100 mg increments every 2–3 days; used after α-blockade for rebound tachycardia with a goal of resting HR 60–80 beats/min; has α-blocking properties
Atenolol	50 mg PO daily	100 mg/day	May increase after 7–14 days; used after α-blockade for rebound tachycardia with a goal of resting HR 60–80 beats/min
Metoprolol	50 mg PO BID	450 mg/day	May increase dose 50 mg every week; used after α-blockade for rebound tachycardia with a goal of resting HR 60–80 beats/min
Metyrosine	250–750 mg PO QID	4 g/day	For refractory hypertension

PO, Orally; *BID,* twice a day; *qHS,* at bedtime; *TID,* three times a day; *HR,* heart rate; *QID,* four times a day

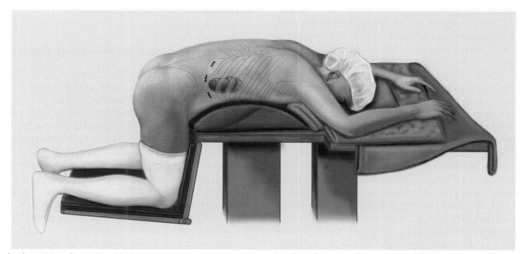

FIGURE 2   Standard position for right-sided posterior retroperitoneoscopic adrenalectomy. *(From Perrier ND, Kennamer DL, Bao R, et al: Posterior retroperitoneoscopic adrenalectomy: preferred technique for removal of benign tumors and isolated metastases, Ann Surg 248[4]:666-674, 2008. Used with permission.)*

to the initial incision and beneath the eleventh rib. A blunt trocar with an inflatable balloon for an anchor is then introduced between the medial and lateral trocars (Figure 3). Pneumoretroperitoneum is created and maintained at a pressure of 20 to 24 mm Hg.

A 10 mm, 30-degree videoscope is initially introduced into the middle trocar but is moved to the medial trocar after the retroperitoneal space is expanded. The retroperitoneal space beneath the diaphragm is developed using sharp and blunt dissection. The Gerota fascia is entered, and the superior border of the kidney is identified (Figure 4). The paraspinous muscles, the posterior surface of the liver or spleen as seen through the peritoneum, and the upper pole of the kidney are identified and serve as landmarks. The tissue superior to the kidney containing the lower aspect of the adrenal gland is completely separated from the kidney with blunt dissection. This is an important step in the operation, as the adrenal gland is still attached superiorly and medially. The upper pole of the kidney

usually needs to be retracted caudally by an instrument in the medial or lateral trocar.

After the inferior edge of adrenal gland is separated from the upper pole of the kidney, medial mobilization is completed (Figure 5). The adrenal (suprarenal) vein is identified, clipped, and divided. On the left side, the phrenic vein can often be preserved. On the right side, the posterior approach to the inferior vena cava greatly facilitates exposure, ligation, and division of the right adrenal vein. The posterior, lateral, and diaphragmatic dissection of the adrenal gland is completed using an EnSeal device (SurgRx Inc., Redwood City, Calif.) or Harmonic scalpel (Ethicon Endosurgery, Cincinnati, Ohio). When the adrenal gland is completely separated from its retroperitoneal attachments, it is placed in an EndoCatch device (Ethicon Endosurgery) and removed through the middle trocar site. In some cases, the middle trocar site incision needs to be enlarged to facilitate specimen removal. All trocar sites are then closed in layers with absorbable sutures.

Transabdominal Laparoscopic Adrenalectomy

Transabdominal laparoscopic adrenalectomy has been the gold standard for resection of small, solitary, unilateral pheochromocytomas. The procedure is performed with the patient in the lateral decubitus position, with the bed flexed at the patient's waist to maximize the distance between the iliac crest and ribs. An incision is made approximately 2 cm below and parallel to the costal margin to access the abdominal cavity. Three 10 mm trocars are placed under direct vision along the subcostal region two fingerbreadths below the costal margin. The trocars are equally spaced between the midclavicular line medially (lateral to the border of the rectus abdominis sheath) and the midaxillary line laterally, inferior and posterior to the tip of the eleventh rib. A 30-degree laparoscope is then placed through the middle trocar, and a fourth trocar is placed at the costovertebral subcostal angle, after the peritoneal reflection of the kidney has been dissected.

For a right adrenalectomy, the liver is mobilized medially by incising the right lateral hepatic attachments and the triangular ligament. A fan retractor is inserted through the most medial port to retract the liver, but the hepatic flexure of the colon may need to be mobilized for optimal exposure. The adrenal gland is identified at the medial aspect of the superior pole of the kidney. The Gerota fascia is incised, and dissection of the adrenal gland is performed circumferentially. The right adrenal (suprarenal) vein is identified, clipped, and divided. It is important not to avulse this vein from the vena cava. Often, multiple smaller veins are present; these need to be divided between clips, with

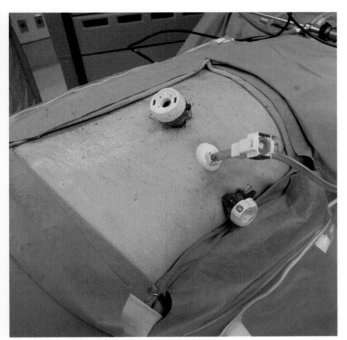

FIGURE 3 Trocar placement for right-sided posterior retroperitoneoscopic adrenalectomy.

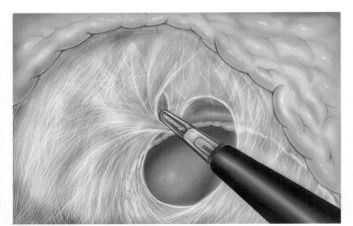

FIGURE 4 Right-sided posterior retroperitoneoscopic adrenalectomy depicting immediate visualization of retroperitoneal space upon entry with the videoscope and retractor.

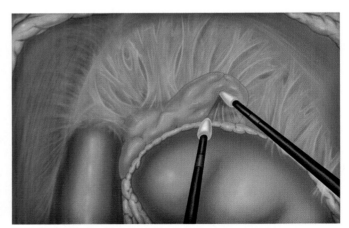

FIGURE 5 Right-sided posterior retroperitoneoscopic adrenalectomy depicting elevation of the inferior border of the adrenal gland while maintaining downward pressure on the right kidney.

an EnSeal device or Harmonic scalpel. The arterial branches can be divided using the same techniques.

For a left adrenalectomy, the splenic flexure is mobilized medially to move the colon away from the inferior portion of the adrenal and to expose the lienorenal ligament. The lienorenal ligament is incised approximately 1 cm from the spleen, and dissection is carried up to the diaphragm and stopped when the short gastric vessels are encountered behind the stomach. The tail of the pancreas and the spleen are allowed to fall medially to expose the underlying adrenal gland, which is often referred to as the "opening the book" technique. A fan retractor may be used to retract the spleen or kidney in obese patients. The lateral and anterior portions of the adrenal gland are dissected free by first grasping a small amount of periadrenal fat for retraction, leaving the adrenal capsule intact. The dissection can then proceed. The adrenal vein is identified and clipped, with attention to the fact that the vein drains into the left renal vein. The remainder of the dissection proceeds similar to the technique described for right adrenalectomy.

Open Cortex-Sparing Adrenalectomy

Accurate preoperative imaging is essential in planning a cortex-sparing adrenalectomy to identify the blood supply of the portion of cortex to be spared. The adrenal gland is supplied by blood from branches of the aorta, renal artery, and inferior phrenic artery. It has been our experience at MDACC that the most cephalad portion of the adrenal gland, based on the phrenic circulation, is most suitable for in situ preservation. Standard techniques for open adrenalectomy are performed. On the right side, the liver must be mobilized medially to expose the right hepatic vein and inferior vena cava to allow for complete visualization of the adrenal. On the left, the spleen and pancreas must be mobilized by medial visceral rotation to allow visualization of the junction of the left renal vein and left adrenal (suprarenal) vein. It is critical that the portion of the adrenal gland to be preserved in situ not be mobilized out of the retroperitoneum, especially when ligation of the adrenal vein is required.

POSTOPERATIVE MANAGEMENT

For the first 12 to 24 hours after surgery, patients should be monitored closely in a step-down or intensive care unit, because hemodynamic fluctuations can occur. It is important to keep patients well hydrated after resection of a pheochromocytoma, as hypotension is not uncommon. At times, small doses of vasopressors may be needed to maintain normotension. Acute adrenal insufficiency can occur if no functional cortical adrenal tissue remains. Adrenal insufficiency should be treated with hydrocortisone at a dosage of 100 mg intravenously every 8 to 12 hours as needed to maintain vascular tone. Hypoglycemia can also occur postoperatively, so blood glucose should be monitored to allow prompt detection and treatment of this condition. Although some surgeons measure plasma metanephrines immediately after surgery to confirm the absence of residual disease, that is not the practice at MDACC, because normal results at this time do not exclude the presence of microscopic residual disease.

Patients who undergo retroperitoneoscopic or transabdominal laparoscopic resection are usually discharged home on postoperative day 2, but those who undergo open resection are discharged upon return of bowel function. Most patients do not need to be prescribed antihypertensive medications at discharge, as blood pressure is usually normal within a few days after surgery. However, hypertension can persist through the postoperative period and into the short-term follow-up period because of the resetting of baroreceptors and altered sensitivity of blood vessel smooth muscle to circulating catecholamines.

MALIGNANT PHEOCHROMOCYTOMA

Several biochemical, pathologic, and molecular markers for distinguishing benign from malignant pheochromocytomas have been investigated, but none have been shown to reliably predict malignant behavior. A diagnosis of malignant pheochromocytoma requires documentation of local invasion, recurrence, or metastasis, with the most common sites of metastasis being the liver, lung, bone, and retroperitoneal lymph nodes. Overall, approximately 15% of pheochromocytomas are malignant, having metastasized at the time of presentation. However, the diagnosis of malignancy is frequently made after surgery, when distant metastases become apparent. Patients with an *SDHB* mutation have a high risk of malignancy (50%), whereas those with an *SDHD* mutation have a low risk (3%). Nondiploid tumors also confer an increased risk of malignancy. In contrast, almost all pheochromocytomas in patients with MEN2, and more than 90% in those with VHL and NF1, are benign.

Once the diagnosis of malignancy has been made, the overall survival rate is approximately 50% at 5 years, but the prognosis can vary. There is no difference in overall survival among patients with malignant pheochromocytomas and those with malignant paragangliomas; the outcome worsens with increasing tumor size in both groups.

Surgical resection is the treatment of choice in patients who have localized recurrence in the tumor bed or one or a few metastatic lesions amenable to resection. Unfortunately, most patients with malignant pheochromocytomas and paragangliomas are seen initially with multiple metastases. Palliative tumor debulking can be performed for extensive disease. Other palliative techniques such as radiofrequency ablation, cryoablation, and arterial embolization can help to alleviate symptoms and decrease complications.

For patients with unresectable disease or soft-tissue metastases, ^{131}I-MIBG has been shown to produce partial, temporary responses in approximately one third of patients. Patients are treated with ^{131}I-MIBG for 3 to 6 months, with reevaluation including biochemical analysis and MIBG imaging performed prior to each treatment. In patients with poor MIBG uptake or a poor response to MIBG therapy, cytotoxic chemotherapy can be used alone or in combination with MIBG and may have a therapeutic benefit in up to 65% of patients. The most common regimen is a combination of cyclophosphamide, vincristine, and dacarbazine, but other regimens exist. Newer targeted therapies, such as temozolomide, thalidomide analogues, imatinib mesylate, and everolimus have not shown as much promise. Some patients treated with the tyrosine kinase inhibitor sunitinib have shown clinical improvement. Currently, a clinical trial is underway to investigate the effects of sunitinib in patients with malignant pheochromocytoma. Identification of the overexpressed protein HSP-90 in malignant pheochromocytomas also makes it a target of ongoing research.

SUGGESTED READINGS

Adler JT, Meyer-Rochow GY, Chen H, et al: Pheochromocytoma: current approaches and future directions, *Oncologist* 13:779–793, 2008.

Mittendorf EA, Evans DB, Lee JE, et al: Pheochromocytoma: advances in genetics, diagnosis, localization and treatment, *Hematol Oncol Clin North Am* 21:509–525, 2007.

Pacak K, Eisenhofer G, Ahlman H, et al: Pheochromocytoma: recommendations for clinical practice from the First International Symposium, October 2005, *Nat Clin Pract Endocrinol Metab* 2:92–102, 2007.

Perrier NP, Kennamer DL, Bao R, et al: Posterior retroperitoneoscopic adrenalectomy: preferred technique for removal of benign tumors and isolated metastases, *Ann Surg* 248:666–674, 2008.

Yip L, Lee JE, Shapiro SE, et al: Surgical management of hereditary pheochromocytoma, *J Am Coll Surg* 198:525–535, 2004.

Young WF, Grant CS: Management of adrenal medullary neoplasms. In Pollock RE, Curley SA, Ross MI, Perrier NP, editors: *Advanced therapy in surgical oncology*, Hamilton, ON, Canada, 2008, BC Decker, pp 405–413.

MANAGEMENT OF THYROID NODULES

Jessica E. Gosnell, MD, and Orlo H. Clark, MD

INCIDENCE AND BACKGROUND

Thyroid nodules are common. They can be found on physical examination, on targeted neck ultrasound, or incidentally on imaging tests done for other reasons. Palpable thyroid nodules are present in 4% of the American population, according to data from the Framingham study. Nonpalpable thyroid nodules identified by ultrasound, or when autopsy studies are done, are generally less than 1 cm and are reported in up to 50% of Americans over 50 years of age. Thyroid nodules are four times more common in women, and they are more common with advancing age, radiation exposure, family history of goiter, and iodine deficiency.

Thyroid nodules can be solitary or multiple (multinodular goiter [MNG]), benign or malignant. Most thyroid nodules are benign, and their natural history over time is unknown. The differential diagnosis for thyroid nodules is extensive (Table 1) and includes benign colloid nodules, follicular adenoma, toxic nodules, toxic nodule within a multinodular goiter (Plummer disease), and thyroid cancer. Papillary thyroid cancer is the most common type of thyroid cancer (about 85%), followed by follicular (10%), medullary (5%), and anaplastic (1%) cancers. Rare forms of thyroid cancer include lymphoma, metastatic nodules, and teratomas.

MANAGEMENT

Because most thyroid nodules are benign, the main challenge in the management of thyroid nodules is to differentiate benign nodules from the small percentage of those that are malignant, about 3% to 5%. This requires a systematic approach that includes a thorough history and physical followed by the judicious use of labs, imaging, and biopsy and finally the integration of all the available data to develop a reasonable treatment plan.

CLINICAL EVALUATION

History

Several key historical components help to categorize thyroid nodules into low-, intermediate-, or high-risk groups. These components include general background about the patient and applicable risk factors, local symptoms in the neck, and systemic symptoms of thyroid function.

Demographics alone can be important. For example, cancer is more common in patients at the extremes of age (<20 or >60 years). In addition, although thyroid nodules are more common in women, a solitary nodule in men carries a greater risk of malignancy. History also provides two important risk factors for thyroid cancer: radiation exposure and a family history of thyroid cancer. Exposure to low-dose therapeutic ionizing radiation to the head and neck region and whole body irradiation for bone marrow transplantation can increase the risk of thyroid cancer, usually papillary thyroid cancer, to as much as 40% in patients with thyroid nodules. Patients may not understand what constitutes radiation exposure, so follow-up questions are important. For example, treatment of childhood cancers such

as Hodgkin lymphoma or neuroblastoma often includes radiation. Other benign conditions of the head and neck—ringworm, acne, enlarged tonsils, and hemangiomas—were once treated with radiation. This practice was abandoned in the early 1970s, when the link between radiation and thyroid cancer was recognized. Patients from Japan and Ukraine may have been exposed to fallout radiation from Nagasaki, Hiroshima, and Chernobyl, so patients should be questioned closely as to where they lived and when they emigrated. Children exposed to radiation before the age of 12 years are at greatest risk for the development of thyroid cancer. A family history of thyroid cancer also places patients at increased risk, either as an isolated familial thyroid cancer (papillary, follicular, or medullary) or as part of a familial cancer syndrome. Medullary thyroid cancer is one of the known components of multiple endocrine neoplasia 2 (MEN2A or 2B), and papillary thyroid cancer is associated with Cowden disease and familial adenomatous polyposis (Gardener syndrome). A personal or family history of other endocrine disorders such as primary hyperparathyroidism, pancreatic islet cell tumors, pituitary tumors, breast cancer, and adrenal tumors are also associated with a higher risk of thyroid cancer. A personal or family history of other cancers is also important. Malignant renal, pulmonary, and breast tumors can metastasize to the thyroid, as can melanoma.

Most thyroid nodules are asymptomatic, but when they are symptomatic, they may either cause local symptoms in the neck or systemic symptoms from thyroid hormone dysfunction. Local compression can occur with benign disease or by infiltration or invasion from aggressive cancers. Specifically, symptoms of dysphagia, dyspnea, and voice change should be elicited. Patients may describe the sensation of food sticking in their throat, with either liquids or solids, or a persistent and nagging cough. They may describe a choking sensation, or they may report having some trouble breathing. Some patients may only notice difficulties at night, when they are lying flat, and they may identify specific postures that alleviate the symptoms. Rapid growth of the thyroid nodule and neck pain can be worrisome signs. Our endocrine group recently reported that patients with medullary thyroid cancer are more likely to experience neck or tumor pain, so testing patients with this particular symptom should be considered. All patients should be specifically questioned as to whether they have noticed a change in the quality or character of their voice. Hoarseness may suggest tension, traction, or invasion of the recurrent laryngeal nerve. Patients with any voice change should have direct laryngoscopy as a part of their workup to document vocal-cord mobility and function of the recurrent laryngeal nerve. Eye symptoms such as dryness, diploplia, or protrusion can be manifestations of Graves disease. The majority of patients with thyroid nodules are asymptomatic and euthyroid. However, questions about thyroid function are important.

Weight gain, fatigue, depression, constipation, dry skin, and brittle nails are symptoms of hypothyroidism, and weight loss, weakness, anxiety, palpitations, and diarrhea are symptoms of hyperthyroidism.

Physical Examination

A complete physical examination of patients with thyroid nodules is critical, as it provides valuable information and allows interpretation of the laboratory and imaging results in the proper context. Thyroid-associated tachycardia and systolic hypertension can be found by determining the vital signs. Weight and recent changes in weight should be recorded. An ongoing qualitative assessment of the patient's voice can be made during the patient visit, and voice complaints or hoarseness should prompt direct laryngoscopy to evaluate vocal-fold mobility and thus the function of the recurrent laryngeal nerve. Important eye signs include stare, lid lag, or exophthalmos, all of which can suggest Graves disease with ophthalmopathy. The neck should be carefully examined both visually and by palpation. First, the thyroid should be inspected as the

TABLE 1: Differential diagnosis

Benign
Colloid nodule
Thyroid cyst
Thyroiditis
Follicular adenoma
Hurthe cell adenoma
Toxic adenoma
Plummer disease

Malignant
Papillary thyroid cancer
Follicular thyroid cancer
Hurthle cell thyroid cancer
Medullary thyroid cancer
Anaplastic thyroid cancer
Thyroid lymphoma
Distant metastases to the thyroid

patient extends his or her neck and swallows. Is there a visible goiter, or visible nodule? Are the midline structures of the neck, such as the laryngeal and cricoid cartilage, still in the midline, or have they shifted to one side? The neck should be carefully examined with an emphasis on thyroid size, symmetry, texture, presence of nodules, and tenderness. Are there palpable nodules, and do they move with deglutition? Is the inferior aspect of the nodule palpable? If not, the thyroid nodule or lobe may be extending in a retrosternal position. Patients should be tested for Pemberton sign by asking them to raise their arms overhead. A positive sign is when the maneuver is followed by facial discoloration and venous enlargement, which is seen in patients with large retrosternal goiters that narrow the thoracic inlet. Pertinent findings on physical exam more suggestive of cancer include fixation of the nodule, a gritty texture, and associated lymphadenopathy, usually ipsilateral. The cardiac examination is important as well, both as an assessment of the patient's overall fitness and as a sign of thyroid disease. Patients with Graves disease may have quite impressive cardiac exams, with tachycardia, a booming hyperdynamic precordium, and widened pulse pressure. Extremities should be examined. Tremor may be a sign of thyrotoxicosis. Pretibial myxedema and thyroid acropachy are uncommon signs of Graves disease.

Laboratory Analysis

The single best test of thyroid function is the thyrotrophin, or thyroid-stimulating hormone (TSH), test. A normal TSH value indicates a biochemical euthyroid state. An abnormal TSH indicates thyroid dysfunction and should prompt measurement of both T3 and T4. Patients with a low or suppressed TSH have either clinical hyperthyroidism, in which T4 levels are high, or subclinical hyperthyroidism, evidenced by isolated suppression of TSH with normal T4 levels. Both groups should have nuclear medicine thyroid scans to check for isolated, autonomously functioning nodules (toxic adenoma); autonomously functioning nodules with a multinodular goiter (Plummer disease); or diffusely hyperfunctioning tissue (Graves disease). Patients with a high TSH alternatively have subclinical or clinical hypothyroidism. These patients should have their thyroid autoantibodies measured to rule out Hashimoto thyroiditis. Patients with Hashimoto thyroiditis can rarely develop thyroid lymphoma, and such patients usually present with a rapidly growing thyroid mass.

There are no currently available blood tests to reliably distinguish between benign and malignant thyroid disease. Thyroglobulin is increased in both benign and malignant disease. Our group and others have therefore concluded that thyroglobulin levels cannot be used to either make the diagnosis of thyroid cancer or to reliably exclude it. It is useful as a postoperative tumor marker in patients with differentiated thyroid cancer, as a measure of how much remnant thyroid tissue is present after thyroidectomy and as a measure of disease recurrence following additional multimodal therapy for papillary and follicular thyroid cancer.

Finally, it is a good practice to check serum calcium levels in all patients with thyroid nodules who need surgery. The incidence of concomitant primary hyperparathyroidism in patients with thyroid disease is about 3% to 5%.

Imaging

Ultrasound

Ultrasound of the neck by an experienced ultrasonographer is one of the most useful imaging tests for the evaluation of thyroid nodules and adjacent lymph nodes. It is better than palpation or thyroid scintigraphy for the identification of thyroid nodules. Ultrasound is relatively inexpensive and noninvasive. It can provide information about the size and texture of the thyroid gland and about the presence and characteristics of thyroid nodules. It can differentiate between cystic nodules and solid nodules, with or without microcalcifications, and it can identify the presence of associated cervical lymphadenopathy and evaluate vascularity of thyroid nodules. Ultrasound is also an excellent tool for directing needles for biopsy.

Ultrasound generally cannot distinguish benign from malignant thyroid nodules. However, several characteristics of thyroid nodules are considered more worrisome; these include hypoechoic nodules, nodules with irregular borders, or those that are ill defined. Nodules with an absent colloid halo sign and those with microcalcifications are also suspicious, as they are more common in patients with papillary thyroid cancer. Finally, nodules that have increased vascularity may have a higher incidence of malignancy. All of these radiographic findings are useful but offer low specificity. Ultimately, ultrasound is a useful tool for identifying suspicious nodules that then need formal fine needle aspiration (FNA) biopsy.

Thyroid Scintigraphy

The role of thyroid scintigraphy is limited. Historically, its utility was to characterize thyroid nodules by their ability to take up isotope as a way to distinguish between benign and malignant nodules. Although up to 80% of thyroid nodules are "cold" (nonfunctioning), only 20% of those are malignant. Conversely, as few as 5% of nodules are "hot" (hyperfunctioning) nodules that can occasionally represent cancer (~1%). The chief utility of nuclear thyroid scintigraphy is in localizing hyperfunctioning tissue in patients with biochemical evidence of hyperthyroidism (Figure 1). Thyroid scan results can help differentiate between toxic thyroid adenoma, Plummer disease, and Graves disease.

Other Imaging Modalities

Retrosternal goiters are often diagnosed on routine screening chest radiographs (Figure 2). Computed tomography (CT) and magnetic resonance imaging (MRI) are useful in selected circumstances. They both can define the presence and extent of retrosternal goiters and whether there is associated tracheal compression and/or deviation. They provide additional anatomic information in patients with locally advanced thyroid cancer, specifically with regard to vascular and tracheal involvement. CT scans should be ordered without radiographic contrast in patients with thyroid nodules, in the event that radioiodine ablation will be used soon after thyroidectomy. Using iodinated contrast could potentially postpone treatment for up to 6 months.

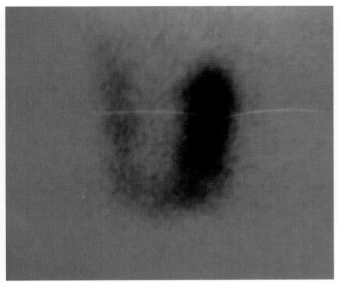

FIGURE 1 Thyroid scintigraphy of a patient with a toxic adenoma in the left superior pole.

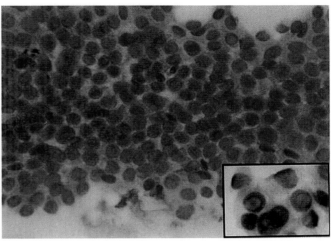

FIGURE 3 Typical FNA cytology findings for papillary thyroid cancer. Inset photograph shows cells with "Orphan Annie eye" changes (cytoplasmic clearing, nuclear grooves).

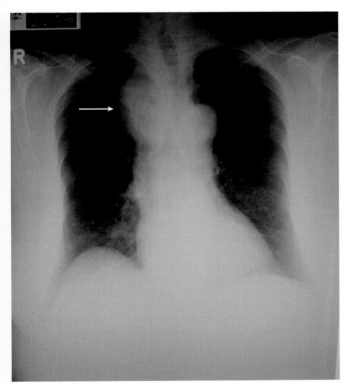

FIGURE 2 Screening chest radiograph of a patient with a retrosternal goiter.

Fine Needle Aspiration

Because clinical evaluation, laboratory assessment, and thyroid imaging are insensitive and nonspecific, FNA has emerged as one of the best tools for the evaluation of thyroid nodules. It has supplanted many of the previously used tests, such as nuclear scanning, for discriminating between benign and malignant thyroid nodules, and it has streamlined the workup. The cost is low, and it is associated with few local or systemic risks. The concern for FNA tract

seeding in cases of thyroid cancer has not been borne out in the literature.

Using either palpation or ultrasound guidance, a small needle, usually 23 or 25 gauge, is inserted into the thyroid nodule under direct vision. Cellular contents are aspirated and are placed on glass slides for cytologic review. A minimum of six groups of cells are considered sufficient for complete assessment. If cell-block preparations are done, immunohistochemical analysis can often confirm a cytologic diagnosis. False-negative results are approximately 3% to 5%, and false-positive results are rare, about 1%. FNA cytology can reliably diagnose many of the more benign conditions, as well as papillary, medullary, and anaplastic thyroid cancer. Papillary thyroid cancer is evidenced by classic cytologic findings, including nuclear crowding, cytoplasmic clearing with the so-called "Orphan Annie eyes," and nuclear grooves (Figure 3). Medullary thyroid cancers lack colloid, have spindle-shaped cells, and often have amyloid and apple-green birefringement under polarized light. Immunohistochemical staining with calcitonin is diagnostic. Anaplastic cancers have characteristic hypercellularity with necrosis and cellular pleomorphism.

Follicular and Hurthle cell thyroid cancers cannot be diagnosed using FNA. Follicular cancer is cytologically bland; it is not characterized by classic cellular changes. Cytology usually reveals clumps of follicular cells with a microfollicular pattern (Figure 4). The diagnosis of carcinoma is dependent on histology rather than cytology, with a full evaluation of the nodule capsule for evidence of vascular or capsular invasion. Follicular neoplasms are associated with about a 20% risk of malignancy, usually prompting the recommendation for a thyroid lobectomy.

FNA is generally not recommended for the evaluation of hyperfunctioning thyroid nodules, as the vast majority are benign (about 99%). FNA is also unreliable in the evaluation of toxic nodules. These nodules are hypercellular, usually monoclonal lesions of thyroid follicular cells. Like follicular neoplasms, these toxic nodules are cytologically bland and do not have cellular features that are diagnostic for malignancy.

The results from FNA biopsy are generally classified into four groups: 1) nondiagnostic, 2) benign, 3) indeterminate/suspicious, and 4) malignant. Nondiagnostic FNA should not be regarded as benign and should generally be repeated, perhaps best with the use of ultrasound guidance. In the absence of other high-risk red flags (historical, anatomic, or on imaging), benign FNA results can be followed with repeat ultrasound examination in 6 months to 1 year. Malignant results should prompt the appropriate thyroid cancer staging and treatment. Indeterminate or suspicious thyroid nodules need to be evaluated carefully within the context of the

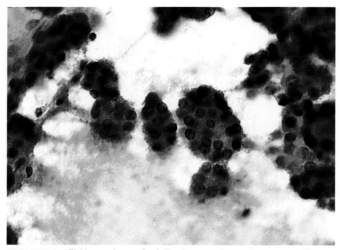

FIGURE 4 FNA cytology of a follicular neoplasm, showing small clusters of bland follicular cells.

specific clinical scenario. At a minimum, repeat FNA or thyroid lobectomy should be recommended; about 20% of follicular and Hurthle cell neoplasms are malignant, whereas about 60% of suspicious cells are malignant.

THE ROLE OF DIAGNOSTIC SURGERY

Despite a complete evaluation, there are situations that necessitate surgery for diagnostic and therapeutic purposes. The most common is when a thyroid nodule has FNA findings suggestive of a follicular or Hurthle cell neoplasm. As mentioned above, there is a 10% to 20% risk of malignancy associated with these nodules. In the absence of significant comorbid conditions or patient refusal, a thyroid lobectomy is reasonable. Diagnostic surgery should also be considered for thyroid nodules, when the aspects of the clinical evaluation remain worrisome, such as a growing nodule, even if the FNA result is benign.

Intraoperative frozen-section analysis is helpful for nodules suspicious for papillary thyroid cancer but not follicular or Hurthle cell nodules. It is also helpful to evaluate abnormal lymph nodes during thyroid operations. Frozen-section analysis should not be used for thyroid nodules that are definitively either benign or malignant on FNA.

Special Circumstances

Thyroid Nodules in Pregnant Women

Thyroid nodules in pregnant patients should be evaluated in much the same way as those in nonpregnant patients, with several important considerations. A careful history and physical exam, serum TSH, and neck ultrasound should be done. Radioisotopes must be avoided. According to recent Endocrine Society clinical practice guidelines, 1) FNA should be recommended for thyroid nodules larger than 1 cm; 2) when FNA reveals thyroid cancer, or when nodules rapidly grow, surgery can be offered in the second trimester; 3) suppressive doses of thyroid hormone can be given postoperatively; and 4) radioactive isotope administration with ^{131}I should not be given during pregnancy and lactation. Women treated postpartum with radioiodine should wait 6 months to 1 year before conceiving.

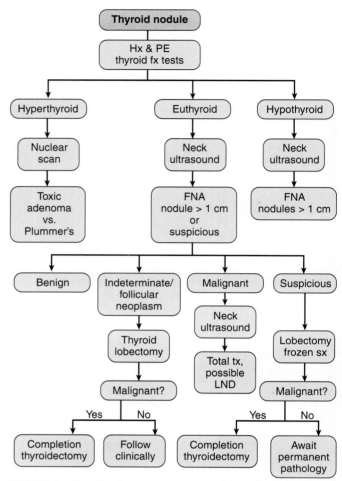

FIGURE 5 Algorithm for the management of thyroid nodules.

SUMMARY

Thyroid nodules are common and are usually benign. A thorough history, physical examination, and laboratory investigation are critical components of the workup and often reveal findings more worrisome for thyroid cancer. Selective laboratory tests can help determine thyroid function. FNA with the use of high-resolution ultrasound is the single best tool to definitively diagnose or exclude thyroid cancer. More specialized imaging is useful in cases worrisome for large and locally aggressive cancers. Figure 5 is an algorithm summarizing the recommended approach to thyroid nodules.

SUGGESTED READINGS

Abalovich M: Management of thyroid dysfunction during pregnancy and postpartum: an Endocrine Society clinical practice guideline, *J Clin Endocrinol Metab* 92(Suppl 8):S1–S47, 2007.

Clark OH, Duh QY, Kebebew E, editors: *Textbook of endocrine surgery,* ed 2, Philadelphia, 2006, Saunders Elsevier.

Gosnell JE, Clark OH: Surgical approaches to thyroid tumors, *Endocrinol Metab Clin North Am* 37(2):437–455, 2008.

Loevner LA, Mukherji S, editors: Thyroid and parathyroid glands: imaging, treatment, and beyond, *Neuroimaging Clin N Am* 18(3), 2008.

Nontoxic Goiter

Geoffrey B. Thompson, MD

OVERVIEW

A goiter, derived from the French *goitre*, meaning *throat*, refers to any enlargement of the thyroid gland. This may be due to a toxic multinodular goiter (Plummer disease), Graves disease, thyroiditis, or cancer; worldwide, it is most often associated with a nontoxic (colloid or nodular) goiter, which is the focus of this chapter.

Around the world, nontoxic goiters are often endemic due to iodine deficiency. It is especially common in high mountain regions, away from the ocean, in such places as the Andes and Himalayas. In the early 1900s, the concept of goiter prevention was first introduced in the United States and Switzerland with salt iodination.

PATHOGENESIS

A *nontoxic* (multinodular) goiter is defined as an enlargement of the thyroid gland containing follicles that are morphologically and functionally altered. The pathogenesis is multifactorial, including iodine deficiency, goitrogens (bamboo shoots, maize, and sweet potatoes), genetic factors, dyshormonogenesis, and excess circulating growth factors such as thyroid-stimulating hormone (TSH) and insulinlike growth factor (IGF).

CLINICAL FEATURES

Nontoxic goiters may remain totally asymptomatic, or they may give rise to compressive features such as dyspnea or dysphagia. A change in voice, albeit uncommon, may occur from the effects of pressure on the recurrent laryngeal nerve or larynx from large nodules or from sudden hemorrhage into a preexisting nodule. Stretching of the recurrent laryngeal nerve over a nodule may result in transient, intermittent, or permanent hoarseness. Thyroidectomy may or may not result in voice restoration. Hoarseness is more often associated with malignant infiltration of the nerve than with a benign, nontoxic goiter. Pain or sudden increase in the size of the goiter may indicate acute hemorrhage or malignant change within the gland, and clinical features of hypothyroidism or hyperthyroidism that may evolve over time should be monitored. A family history of nontoxic goiter may indicate dyshormonogenesis.

On physical examination, one should estimate the size of the gland and note whether there is diffuse enlargement or nodularity, tracheal deviation, retrosternal extension, or lymphadenopathy; the consistency of the gland, as well as any features of hypothyroidism or hyperthyroidism, should also be noted.

EVALUATION

TSH, free T4, and T3 levels should be checked to identify subclinical or overt thyrotoxicosis, hypothyroidism, or a euthyroid state. Fine-needle aspiration (FNA) biopsy should be performed under ultrasound guidance on any suspicious thyroid nodule; that is, a nodule evidencing hypoechogenicity, nodular hypervascularity, and microcalcifications. Plain chest films may demonstrate tracheal deviation, retrotracheal and retrosternal extension, incipient airway compromise, and calcifications. Computed tomography (CT) and/or magnetic resonance imaging (MRI) more precisely detail these findings.

Radioiodine scanning is less useful but may help delineate toxic nodules or Graves disease in a patient with subclinical or overt thyrotoxicosis, as well as the presence of substernal or lingual thyroid tissue (Figure 1). Pulmonary function tests, flow volume loops, and barium studies may better quantify the degree of airway or esophageal compromise in select cases.

INDICATIONS FOR TREATMENT

Goiters may give rise to local discomfort, such as tightness or a choking sensation, or they may cause mechanical obstruction of the upper aerodigestive tree. Goiters have an annual growth rate on average of about 20%. Patients may develop subclinical or overt thyrotoxicosis with its potential for atrial fibrillation and bone mineral loss in the aging population. The incidence of thyroid cancer (5% to 10%) in nodular goiter is no different than with solitary thyroid nodules. Cosmesis is rarely an isolated concern or indication for treatment in and of itself.

TREATMENT MODALITIES

Thyroxine-suppressive therapy has little role in the management of a euthyroid (nontoxic) goiter (Figure 2). Evidence is lacking from several prospective clinical trials to demonstrate the value of thyroxine in the management of multinodular goiter. Side effects that include bone mineral loss and cardiotoxicity negate any theoretical value, particularly in the elderly. Radioiodine, on the other hand, can cause goiter reduction in up to 40% to 60% of patients within 2 years, decreasing compressive symptoms. Complications include radiation thyroiditis and hypothyroidism (20% to 45%). Radiation-induced extrathyroidal malignancies are extremely rare. Recent studies have addressed the use of recombinant TSH to augment the uptake of radioiodine in an otherwise nontoxic goiter with low iodine uptake. Again, such interventions must be undertaken cautiously in the elderly. Percutaneous laser ablation and radiofrequency thermal ablation technologies are available for the treatment of symptomatic dominant nodules. Although safe in experienced hands, long-term follow-up data are limited.

Surgical management remains the mainstay of treatment for symptomatic, nontoxic goiters and is well tolerated even in the elderly and infirm. Median sternotomy and posterolateral thoracotomy are rarely indicated in first-time operations for substernal goiters given the cervical origin of the arterial anatomy in the majority of cases. In experienced centers, complication rates remain low (≤2%) with careful attention to detail, meticulous hemostasis, and liberal use of parathyroid autotransplantation. One of the most critical parts of the operation is safely securing the airway. Conscious fiberoptic intubation is often necessary when marked tracheal deviation and/or compression exists.

The thyroid gland is exposed by a generous collar incision (Figure 3); this is not the operation for a keyhole incision. Wide, subplatysmal fat flaps are created, and the strap muscles are separated in the midline. I often divide the sternothyroid muscle near the upper pole to facilitate exposure. The plane between the larynx and the upper pole is opened, exposing the superior thyroid artery, superior thyroid vein, and the external branch of the superior laryngeal nerve. Nerve stimulation is used to trace out the path of the external branch of the superior laryngeal nerve to avoid injury during ligation of the superior pole vessels. The superior thyroid artery and vein are individually ligated on the thyroid capsule, minimizing the risk of incorporating the external nerve into the vascular ligature.

Once the upper pole is fully mobilized, the thyroid is partially rotated up and out to expose the middle thyroid vein, which is then ligated in continuity or divided with ultrasonic dissecting shears. I do

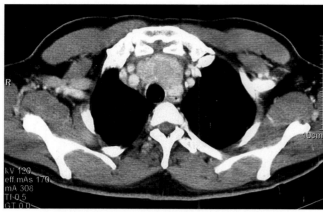

FIGURE 1   Goiter with significant substernal component.

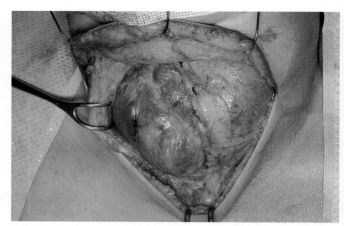

FIGURE 3   Operative photograph: nontoxic multinodular goiter.

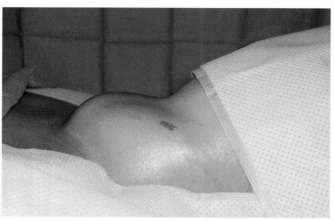

FIGURE 2   Nontoxic multinodular goiter.

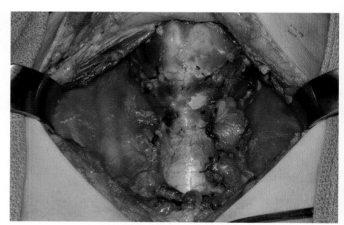

FIGURE 4   Dunhill procedure.

not use this device anywhere near the recurrent laryngeal nerve or external nerve, but I find it helpful for dividing inferior and middle veins, the thyroid isthmus, and the thyroid parenchyma when performing a less-than-total lobectomy. At this point, the proper fascial plane along the thyroid can be safely entered with gentle finger dissection. With gentle traction, the goiter, be it totally cervical or partially substernal, can be delivered into the wound in its entirety. The recurrent nerve and parathyroid glands are identified, and the inferior thyroid veins and rare thyroid inferior mesenteric arteries off the aortic arch are divided and ligated.

One important note of caution: in posteriorly displaced goiters (e.g., retroesophageal), the recurrent laryngeal nerve may actually pass over the gland between nodules. When this is evident on preoperative CT or intraoperatively, the surgeon should attempt to identify the nerve behind the upper pole, where it pierces the inferior constrictor, and then follow it back proximally. Preservation of the nerve may require piecemeal removal of the posterior component of the thyroid so as to avoid stretching or inadvertent injury to the recurrent nerve. With anteriorly displaced goiters, the recurrent laryngeal nerve and parathyroids are often displaced posteriorly, safely out of harms way. Transection of the isthmus early in the dissection can help mobilize the lobe out of the wound, facilitating exposure of the posterior and medial structures (recurrent laryngeal nerve and parathyroids).

Finally, the recurrent laryngeal nerve is traced to its insertion, and the terminal branches of the inferior thyroid artery are divided

and ligated between ligaclips. The nerve and parathyroids are gently separated from the thyroid and the ligament of Berry and are divided, freeing the lobe and isthmus from the trachea. A prominent tubercle of Zuckerkandl can make visualization of the recurrent laryngeal nerve more difficult during the final part of the dissection. Devitalized parathyroid should be cut into small (1 mm) pieces and autotransplanted into pockets of the sternocleidomastoid muscle, and the site should be marked with a permanent suture. If a parathyroid gland appears congested, one can nick its capsule with an iris scissors or number 11 blade. If bleeding persists and normal color returns, in situ survival can generally be expected.

On the contralateral side, a total or near-total thyroidectomy is performed; the choice depends on parathyroid viability. A small remnant can be left (<1 g), or even a 2 to 3 g remnant (Dunhill procedure; Figure 4), to ensure viability of at least one superior parathyroid gland. Bilateral subtotal thyroidectomy is generally not preferred because of an increased lifetime risk of recurrence. Utilizing recurrent laryngeal nerve monitoring, a normal and unchanged audible signal from the vagus nerves bilaterally at completion of the dissection indicates intact recurrent laryngeal nerve function. A small, closed-suction drain to obliterate dead space, along with a topical hemostatic agent, are placed in the thyroid bed. The layers are closed with absorbable suture, and the skin is closed with a running absorbable 4-0 subcuticular stitch.

The drain is removed the following day, and calcium supplementation is instituted based on symptoms, serum calcium and phosphorus levels, and serum parathyroid levels. Thyroid hormone replacement therapy is instituted prior to dismissal, and thyroid function tests are rechecked in 6 weeks' time.

SUMMARY

Symptomatic nontoxic goiters are best managed with either near-total or total thyroidectomy. Nonoperative treatment is less efficacious but can be considered in the rare situation of a high-risk surgical candidate.

Suggested Readings

Franko J, Kish KJ, Pezzi CM, et al: Safely increasing the efficiency of thyroidectomy using a new bipolar electrosealing device (LigaSure) versus conventional clamp-and-tie technique, *Am Surg* 72:132, 2006.

Gharib H, Mazzaferri EL: Thyroxine suppressive therapy in patients with nodular thyroid disease, *Ann Intern Med* 128:386, 2006.

Leenhardt L, Hejblum G, Franc B, et al: Indications and limits of ultrasound-guided cytology in the management of nonpalpable thyroid nodules, *J Clin Endocrinol Metab* 84:24, 1999.

Marqusee E, Benson CB, Frates MC, et al: Usefulness of ultrasonography in the management of nodular thyroid disease, *Ann Intern Med* 1339:696, 2000.

Medeiros-Neto G, Marui S, Knobel M: An outline concerning the potential use of recombinant human thyrotropin for improving radioiodine therapy of multinodular goiter, *Endocrine* 33:109, 2008.

Moli R, Wesche MF, Tiel-Van Buul MM, et al: Determinants of long-term outcome of radioiodine therapy of sporadic nontoxic goiter, *Clin Endocrinol (Oxf)* 50:783, 1999.

Papini E, Guglielmi R, Bianchini A, et al: Risk of malignancy in nonpalpable thyroid nodules: predictive value of ultrasound and color-Doppler features, *J Clin Endocrinol Metab* 87:1941, 2002.

Spiezia S, Garberoglio R, Francesco M, et al: Thyroid nodules and related symptoms are stably controlled two years after radiofrequency thermal ablation, *Thyroid* 19:219, 2009.

Management of Thyroiditis

**Catherine E. Pesce, MD, and
Martha A. Zeiger, MD**

OVERVIEW

Thyroiditis refers to a group of inflammatory diseases affecting the thyroid gland. The many different subtypes not only mimic other diseases but also mimic each other. Although some patients experience only occult or self-limited symptoms, others may suffer from local symptoms or systemic symptoms associated with hyperthyroidism or hypothyroidism. Differentiation of the subtypes of thyroiditis requires an understanding of their unique clinical presentations, radiologic findings, laboratory data, and indications for medical treatment, surgery, or both. Thyroiditis may be characterized as *chronic* (lymphocytic), *subacute* (granulomatous or lymphocytic), or *acute* (suppurative).

CHRONIC LYMPHOCYTIC THYROIDITIS

Chronic lymphocytic thyroiditis (Hashimoto thyroiditis) is the most common inflammatory condition of the thyroid gland and the most common cause of goiter and hypothyroidism in the United States. It is an autoimmune condition characterized by high titers of circulating antibodies against both thyroid peroxidase and thyroglobulin. It is also referred to as *chronic progressive thyroiditis, struma lymphomatosa,* and *autoimmune chronic lymphocytic thyroiditis.*

Epidemiology

Up to 95% of chronic lymphocytic thyroiditis occurs in women, usually between the ages of 30 and 50 years. Chronic lymphocytic thyroiditis is also the most common cause of sporadic goiter in children.

The incidence of Hashimoto thyroiditis has risen exponentially over the past 50 years, possibly related to an increase in dietary iodine intake in North America.

A genetic predisposition to Hashimoto thyroiditis exists and is inherited as a dominant trait. In addition, Hashimoto thyroiditis has been linked to many other autoimmune diseases including systemic lupus erythematosus, rheumatoid arthritis, pernicious anemia, diabetes mellitus, primary biliary cirrhosis, and Sjögren syndrome. A rare but serious complication believed to be associated with chronic autoimmune thyroiditis is thyroid lymphoma. These lymphomas, generally the B-cell non-Hodgkin type, tend to occur in women 50 to 80 years of age and are usually limited to the thyroid gland.

Presentation

Hashimoto thyroiditis is usually asymptomatic, but some patients may complain of a feeling of tightness or fullness in the neck. The disease is the most common cause of hypothyroidism in the United States; however, at the time of diagnosis, symptoms of hypothyroidism are present in only 20% of patients. Even fewer (~5%) will develop thyrotoxicosis during the early phase of the disease. Euthyroid patients with Hashimoto disease develop hypothyroidism at a rate of approximately 5% per year. Physical examination generally reveals a firm, irregular, nontender goiter with or without cervical lymphadenopathy. An enlarged pyramidal lobe is often characteristic of Hashimoto thyroiditis.

Diagnosis

When suspected clinically, diagnosis is confirmed by documenting elevated antibody titers to thyroid-specific antigens: thyroglobulin, thyroid microsomal antigen, thyroid peroxidase, and thyrotropin receptor. In contrast, other thyroid diseases, such as multinodular goiter and thyroid malignancy, have low levels of these antibodies. Antithyroid microsomal antibodies in titers greater than 1:6,400 or antithyroid peroxidase antibodies in excess of 200 IU/mL are strongly suggestive of chronic autoimmune thyroiditis. Radioactive iodine uptake (RAIU) is variable and can be depressed, normal, or increased depending on the extent of follicular destruction. Ultrasonography shows an enlarged gland with a diffusely hypoechogenic pattern in most patients; however, RAIU and thyroid ultrasonography are not essential for the evaluation of this disease. A dominant nodule in a patient with Hashimoto disease should prompt a fine needle aspiration (FNA) biopsy to exclude malignancy.

Management

Treatment of Hashimoto thyroiditis is nonsurgical; because it is usually asymptomatic, and the goiter is small, many patients do not require treatment. When hypothyroidism is present, treatment with levothyroxine (T4) is indicated. Thyroid hormone replacement therapy may also be indicated in patients with a TSH level in the normal range to reduce goiter size and prevent progression to overt hypothyroidism in high-risk patients. The role of the surgeon is to confirm the diagnosis and address any suspicious nodules in the thyroid gland with FNA biopsy or surgical resection if necessary. Enlarging or persistent goiters that result in local compressive and obstructive symptoms, cosmetic deformity, or suspicion of malignancy may require thyroidectomy.

SUBACUTE GRANULOMATOUS (DE QUERVAIN) THYROIDITIS

Subacute granulomatous thyroiditis is the most common cause of a painful thyroid gland. It is most likely caused by a viral infection and is generally preceded by an upper respiratory tract infection. Numerous etiologic agents have been implicated, including mumps virus, echovirus, coxsackievirus, Epstein–Barr virus, influenza, and adenovirus. It has also been associated with hepatitis B vaccination and interferon-α treatment for chronic hepatitis C. Subacute granulomatous thyroiditis is also known as *de Quervain thyroiditis, giant-cell thyroiditis, subacute painful thyroiditis,* and *pseudogranulomatous thyroiditis.*

Epidemiology

Women are three to five times more likely to be affected than men, and the average age of onset is 30 to 50 years of age. The disorder tends to occur most often in the summer and fall.

Presentation

Subacute granulomatous thyroiditis presents clinically with acute onset of thyroid pain. The pain is described as constant, starting in one lobe and extending bilaterally, and fever is common. Such pain may be exacerbated by turning the head or swallowing and may radiate to the ipsilateral jaw, ear, or occiput. The thyroid is firm, nodular, and exquisitely tender to palpation.

Thyroiditis can last from weeks to several months. The course of disease follows one of initial destruction of thyroid follicles, corresponding with symptoms of hyperthyroidism such as tachycardia, palpitations, heat intolerance, weight loss, and nervousness. Up to 70% of patients experience clinical signs and symptoms of thyrotoxicosis related to destruction of thyroid follicles and release of preformed thyroid hormone into the bloodstream, accompanied by enlargement of the thyroid gland. The thyrotoxic phase may last up to several weeks and is followed by a period of euthyroidism. In 20% to 30% of patients, biochemical hypothyroidism may subsequently ensue due to destruction of the gland. Approximately 5% of patients will go on to exhibit persistent hypothyroidism; however, most patients demonstrate complete resolution of the disease with return of normal thyroid function by 4 to 6 months.

Diagnosis

In addition to physical exam findings, biochemical studies are consistent with destruction of the thyroid gland, with elevated erythrocyte sedimentation rate (ESR), decreased RAIU, and elevated serum thyroglobulin and thyroid hormone levels. A normal ESR essentially rules out the diagnosis of subacute granulomatous thyroiditis, as does a normal thyroglobulin level. The serum T4 concentration is disproportionately elevated relative to T3 levels, and serum TSH concentrations are low to undetectable. In 10% to 20% of patients, thyroid antibody titers will be elevated and will become negative within 1 to 6 months after recovery. Biopsy is rarely necessary, and FNA sampling reveals characteristic destruction of follicles and giant cells.

Management

During the initial phase of acute thyrotoxicosis, therapy with antithyroid drugs is not indicated, because the disorder is caused by the release of preformed thyroid hormone rather than synthesis of new T3 and T4. Therapy with β-blockers may be indicated for the symptomatic treatment of thyrotoxicosis.

Most treatment for subacute granulomatous thyroiditis is aimed at controlling pain. Nonsteroidal antiinflammatory drugs are generally effective in reducing thyroid pain in patients with mild symptoms. Patients with more severe disease may require a tapering dose of prednisone (20 to 40 mg per day, given over 2 to 4 weeks), with relief of symptoms generally seen within 24 to 48 hours. If steroids do not significantly improve thyroid and neck pain within 72 hours, the diagnosis of subacute granulomatous thyroiditis should be questioned. Additionally, up to 20% of patients experience recurrence of thyroid pain on discontinuation of steroids and may require an additional month of treatment before complete resolution.

Because a smaller proportion of patients go on to develop hypothyroidism with the disease, levothyroxine therapy may be instituted to decrease the duration of disease or to prevent relapse. The literature is not clear on this issue. Fewer than 5% of patients will remain permanently hypothyroid and require ongoing thyroid hormone replacement therapy.

SUBACUTE LYMPHOCYTIC THYROIDITIS

Subacute lymphocytic thyroiditis is subdivided into two groups: *postpartum thyroiditis* and *sporadic painless thyroiditis.* These are considered variants of the same disorder, distinguished only by their relationship to pregnancy. Although the precise cause of subacute lymphocytic thyroiditis is unknown, the etiology is believed to be autoimmune in nature. Antithyroid peroxidase antibodies are present in nearly all patients, and antimicrosomal antibodies are present in 50% to 80% of patients. The disease starts with an initial hyperthyroid phase, followed by subsequent hypothyroidism and a subsequent return to the euthyroid state.

Epidemiology

Subacute lymphocytic thyroiditis comprises 30% to 50% of all cases of thyroiditis and occurs most often in women during the fourth and fifth decades of life. The severity of the hypothyroid phase correlates directly with the antimicrosomal antibody titer. A titer of 1:1600 or greater early in pregnancy is associated with a high risk of postpartum hypothyroidism. Approximately one third of patients who have the postpartum form develop chronic hypothyroidism.

Several observations point to an autoimmune etiology of the thyroiditis. Circulating antithyroid antibodies have been detected in most patients, with a higher incidence of antimicrosomal antibodies noted in the postpartum form (80%) compared with the sporadic form (50%) of the disease. Women who test positive for antithyroid antibodies during the first trimester of pregnancy are at high risk for development of postpartum thyroiditis at the time of delivery. In addition, postpartum thyroiditis has been reported more often in women with HLA-DR3, HLA-DR4, or HLA-DR5 phenotypes. A family history of autoimmune thyroid disease is also found in 50% of patients with the postpartum form of thyroiditis.

Presentation

Patients usually are seen initially with acute symptoms of hyperthyroidism. Unlike subacute granulomatous thyroiditis, however, systemic symptoms are less common, and thyroid tenderness and pain are unusual. In postpartum thyroiditis, the timing and nature of disturbances in thyroid function are variable, and thyrotoxicosis usually develops in the first 3 months following delivery and lasts for 1 or 2 months. A hypothyroid phase develops between 3 and 6 months after delivery, with normal thyroid function achieved by 1 year. This classic course, however, is seen in fewer than 30% of patients. Some patients (35%) experience only thyrotoxicosis, and some (40%) experience hypothyroidism alone. Patients with an initial episode of postpartum thyroiditis have a notably high risk of recurrence in subsequent pregnancies.

Diagnosis

A careful clinical and family history may alert the physician to risk factors for postpartum thyroiditis. Systemic symptoms noted with subacute granulomatous thyroiditis, such as fever and elevated erythrocyte sedimentation rate (ESR), are unusual in subacute lymphocytic thyroiditis. With an initial presentation of thyrotoxicosis, T4 and T3 levels are initially elevated with a disproportionate increase in T4 compared with T3. In the hyperthyroid phase of the disease, thyroglobulin levels are elevated, and serum TSH and RAIU are decreased. This situation contrasts markedly with Graves disease, in which there is an elevated RAIU; a larger, more diffuse goiter; and extrathyroidal manifestations.

Screening strategies are not universally agreed upon, although selected screening of women at risk may be reasonable. Such screening would include women with prior episodes of postpartum thyroiditis, type 1 diabetes, history of antithyroid peroxidase antibody positivity, autoimmune disorders, or family history of autoimmune thyroid disease.

Management

Acute symptoms of hyperthyroidism are managed primarily with β-blockers. Propranolol may be safely used in lactating females, but antithyroid drugs are not indicated, because symptoms are caused by the release of preformed T3 and T4 and not overproduction of thyroid hormone. Replacement of thyroid hormone in the hypothyroid phase is indicated if the patient's symptoms are severe or of long duration. If the hypothyroid phase lasts longer than 6 months, permanent hypothyroidism is likely. In addition, hypothyroidism can be associated with adverse effects on fertility, increased miscarriage rates, and a negative effect on the intellectual development of the fetus in subsequent pregnancies; thus hormone therapy is recommended.

ACUTE SUPPURATIVE THYROIDITIS

Acute suppurative thyroiditis is a rare thyroiditis subtype caused by bacterial, fungal, mycobacterial, or parasitic infection of the thyroid gland. The disorder is rare because of the intrinsic resistance of the thyroid gland to infection, and it is usually self-limited, lasting only weeks to months. Nonetheless, prompt recognition is critical, because infection can potentially be life threatening. The disease is also known as *infectious thyroiditis, bacterial thyroiditis,* and *microbial inflammatory thyroiditis.*

Epidemiology

The thyroid gland is intrinsically resistant to infection due to its rich blood supply and lymphatic drainage, the protective fascial compartments that separate the thyroid from structures in the neck, and the potential bactericidal activity of its high iodine content. Acute suppurative thyroiditis occurs most often in women 20 to 40 years of age, and infections are most often bacterial. Up to two thirds of patients have a preexisting thyroid disorder such as simple goiter, multinodular goiter, Hashimoto thyroiditis, or thyroid cancer. Evidence supports hematogenous, lymphatic, or direct mechanisms of infection. Infection after an upper respiratory tract illness or pharyngeal infection suggests seeding through a pyriform sinus fistula or patent thyroglossal duct. Studies have shown that up to 90% of patients with acute thyroiditis have a pyriform sinus fistula identified, most commonly on the left side.

Presentation

Acute thyroiditis and subacute granulomatous thyroiditis present similarly, with neck pain. Clinical features in acute thyroiditis, however, generally include higher fever, pharyngitis, dermal erythema, and local compressive symptoms resulting in dysphagia or dysphonia. A fluctuant mass may be palpated when an abscess is present.

Diagnosis

Also in contrast with subacute thyroiditis, thyroid function tests are normal with acute suppurative thyroiditis, including TSH, T4, and T3 levels. RAIU may be normal or may show "cold" (nonfunctional) nodules in areas of abscess formation. Radiographic imaging is useful for patients in whom the diagnosis is not clear. Neck ultrasonography, magnetic resonance imaging (MRI), and computed tomography (CT) are helpful in identifying anatomic changes such as a pyriform sinus tract, abscess, thyroid nodules, or soft-tissue changes consistent with infection. FNA cytology is the best test for determining cause of infection; in addition, Gram stain, culture, and sensitivity of samples must be obtained.

Management

Once the cause of the infection has been determined, appropriate antibiotics should be prescribed. Patients with abscess require surgical drainage and possibly a thyroid lobectomy. Heat, rest, and aspirin provide symptomatic relief, and steroids may offer additional benefit.

Bacterial infections are most common, with *Staphylococcus aureus* and *Streptococcus pyogenes* involved in 80% of cases, and α-hemolytic and β-hemolytic *Streptococcus* accounts for more than 50% of pediatric cases. Intravenous antibiotics are indicated based on culture results. When no definitive organism has been identified, broad-spectrum antibiotics are appropriate. In patients with a pyriform sinus fistula, surgical excision is indicated to prevent recurrence.

Fungal infection of the thyroid gland is unusual, however, it is the second most common cause of infection. Fungal infections usually affect immunocompromised patients. Disseminated aspergillosis is most common, as well as coccidiomycosis and histoplasmosis in endemic regions. Similar principles of treatment apply and include intravenous antifungal agents and abscess drainage if necessary.

Tuberculosis of the thyroid gland is usually associated with miliary or disseminated disease. Multiple-agent antituberculosis therapy is indicated. Recurrent laryngeal nerve damage and even death have been reported.

Parasitic infection is very rare and is best diagnosed by specific serologic testing to avoid spillage of cysts at the time of biopsy. *Echinococcus granulosus* infection is most common, and definitive surgery followed by adjuvant antiparasitic therapy is indicated. Infection by *Strongyloides stercoralis* has been reported in tropical climates, as well as in immunocompromised individuals, and mortality is high as a result of infection and immune status of affected patients.

Patients with AIDS require special attention in acute thyroiditis. Multiple opportunistic infections affect the thyroid, including cytomegalovirus and *Mycobacterium avium-intracellulare*. Extrapulmonary infection with *Pneumocystis carinii* can involve the thyroid, presenting as a painless nodule that increases in size and is cold on RAIU. Intravenous antibiotics, followed by a prolonged course of oral therapy, is usually curative.

INVASIVE FIBROUS THYROIDITIS (RIEDEL STRUMA)

First described by Riedel in 1898, invasive fibrous thyroiditis remains the rarest type of thyroiditis. In addition to the development of dense fibrosis of the thyroid gland itself, extracervical sites of fibrosis frequently occur with other inflammatory fibrosclerotic processes, including sclerosing cholangitis, retroperitoneal fibrosis, sclerosing mediastinitis, and orbital pseudotumor. Studies suggest that one third of patients with fibrous thyroiditis go on to develop a more generalized condition known as *multifocal fibrosclerosis* within 10 years of diagnosis.

Epidemiology and Presentation

The mean age at presentation is 50 years, and 80% of all cases occur in females. A stone-hard or woody mass involving the thyroid is common, but symptoms vary according to the structures involved: compression of the trachea can cause dyspnea, compression of the esophagus can cause dysphagia, and compression of the recurrent laryngeal nerve can result in hoarseness and even stridor. The thyroid mass can grow suddenly or slowly and is usually unilateral. Up to one third of patients may even develop hypothyroidism, and others may develop hypoparathyroidism if there is involvement of the parathyroid glands.

Diagnosis

Most patients remain euthyroid, and the ESR is frequently elevated. Antithyroid antibodies are present in 45% of patients, and RAIU is decreased in affected areas of the gland. Eosinophilia is also common. Because of the similarities between fibrous thyroiditis and thyroid carcinoma, diagnosis must be made using FNA or open biopsy. Biopsy reveals acellular material with fibrosis, lymphocytes, and plasma cells.

Management

The disease may be self-limited, however, in patients with significant compressive symptoms, surgical resection of the thyroid may be necessary. Long-term use of high-dose steroids has shown clinical benefit in some patients. Tamoxifen has also elicited a clinical response in some patients, although the antiestrogen mechanism is not largely understood. In patients who are found to be hypothyroid, thyroid replacement therapy is instituted.

SUGGESTED READINGS

Braverman LE, Utiger RD, editors: *Werner and Ingbar's the thyroid: a fundamental and clinical text*, Philadelphia, 1997, Lippincott-Raven, p 583.

Dayan CM, Daniels GH: Chronic autoimmune thyroiditis, *N Engl J Med* 335:99–107, 1996.

Farwell AP, Braverman LE: Inflammatory thyroid disorders, *Otolaryngol Clin North Am* 29:541–556, 1996.

Pasieka JL: Hashimoto's disease and thyroid lymphoma: role of the surgeon, *World J Surg* 24:966–970, 2000.

Roti E, Emerson CH: Clinical review 29: postpartum thyroiditis, *J Clin Endocrinol Metab* 74:3–5, 1992.

Singer PA: Thyroiditis: acute, subacute, and chronic, *Med Clin North Am* 75:61–77, 1991.

HYPERTHYROIDISM

Bruce Lee Hall, MD, PhD, MBA, and Jeffrey F. Moley, MD

OVERVIEW

Hyperthyroid states result from an excess of thyroid hormone, leading to characteristic hypermetabolic symptoms. Medical treatments for hyperthyroidism can be safe and effective. A surgical approach to hyperthyroid disease is reasonable when medical therapies have failed or are contraindicated, or when an informed patient chooses surgery based on its relative advantages and disadvantages compared with medical approaches. When surgery is selected, medical preoperative preparation of the patient is also critical to safety.

Surgery for hyperthyroidism is safe and effective when properly performed. Surgery is considered in several major disease scenarios, including Graves disease; toxic multinodular goiter (TMNG), or Plummer disease; solitary toxic nodule (STN); and amiodarone-associated thyrotoxicosis (AAT). These all have common themes but also significant differences, and recurrent hyperthyroidism after previous surgery, particularly for Graves disease or toxic multinodular goiter, poses special challenges.

HYPERTHYROID STATES: SYMPTOMS AND DIAGNOSIS

Hyperthyroidism refers to a state of excess production and secretion of thyroid hormone, and it has a prevalence of roughly 2% in women and 0.2% in men. Thyrotoxicosis refers to the characteristic hypermetabolic state caused by hyperthyroidism. Toxic symptoms, physical findings, and potential complications of thyrotoxicosis, or the hyperthyroid state, are shown in Table 1.

Hyperthyroidism with overt clinical thyrotoxicosis is confirmed by suppressed levels of serum thyroid stimulating hormone (TSH or thyrotropin) and elevated serum levels of free thyroxine (T4), free triiodothyronine (T3), or both T4 and T3. With subclinical hyperthyroidism, TSH levels are decreased, but T4 and T3 levels may remain normal. In Graves disease, thyroid-stimulating immunoglobulin (TSI) is often present, as are antimicrosomal, antithyroglobulin, and antithyroperoxidase (TPO) antibodies. Elevated anti-TPO antibodies can also characterize autoimmune thyroiditis (Hashimoto disease), but this condition is not always associated with hyperthyroidism, nor does it require surgical intervention.

Radioactive iodine uptake is diffusely, and more or less symmetrically, elevated in Graves disease, but it can be elevated or normal with hyperthyroidism related to TMNG or an STN. TMNG can be characterized by focal areas of increased uptake with intervening suppressed areas. STN typically reveals a solitary focus with the remaining gland suppressed. With AAT, typically low or undetectable uptake is seen, along with a history of amiodarone use. Low or undetectable uptake also characterizes autoimmune thyroiditis, which again is not always associated with hyperthyroidism and does not require surgical intervention. The differential diagnosis for hyperthyroidism is presented in Table 2.

MEDICAL TREATMENT OF HYPERTHYROIDISM

Most hyperthyroid patients are treated nonsurgically, either aiming for long-term control or in preparation for surgery. Nonsurgical treatments are safe and effective and are based on two main modalities, *thionamide inhibition* and *radiation*. Thionamide inhibition using propylthiouracil (PTU) or methimazole (Tapazole), and less commonly carbimazole, is effective, because thionamide drugs inhibit organification of iodine and coupling of iodothyronine. This inhibition decreases thyroid hormone synthesis and controls hyperthyroidism in most patients within several weeks, but relapse after discontinuation is common. Most pregnant women with Graves disease are treated medically, and in the United States, PTU is the drug of choice for thionamide therapy during pregnancy. Radioactive iodine (RAI, iodine-131) ablation treatment is generally highly effective at relieving hyperthyroidism, but it can be weeks to months for the full effect to be realized. In a minority of cases, additional rounds of treatment are required, and controversy persists over long-term risks of carcinogenesis and malignancy, especially for younger patients. Although major genetic or carcinogenic effects have not been observed, some evidence indicates a slight increase in certain malignancies after RAI treatment, namely, cancers of the stomach, kidney, and breast. RAI is contraindicated during pregnancy, and pregnancy should be avoided for 6 to 12 months after treatment.

Treatments are discussed in detail for each diagnostic category below. In conjunction with these, β-blockade is typically used to control the peripheral manifestations of hyperthyroidism quickly, and it can also be used alone in special circumstances; however, no long-term control of the disease is obtained. In addition, iodine supplementation can have certain beneficial effects when preparing for surgery, as discussed below. New treatments for Graves disease, including immunomodulatory agents such as rituximab and other biologics, are emerging and being investigated.

SURGERY FOR HYPERTHYROIDISM

Patients with known malignancy or suspicious findings on fine needle aspiration (FNA), patients with a history of neck irradiation, and patients with suspicious (growing), cold, nonfunctioning nodules are best treated with surgery without debate. In addition, patients with local compressive symptoms due to the goiter, or pending concerns of such, are most rapidly, definitively, and safely treated with total thyroidectomy, which is of course true also in the absence of hyperthyroidism. Apart from this, the hyperthyroid states of Graves disease, TMNG, STN, and AAT can each be considered for surgery; these are discussed separately below.

GRAVES DISEASE

Graves disease is an autoimmune, toxic, diffuse goiter. It most commonly develops during the second to fifth decades of life. It affects up to 2% of the female population, with a female to male preponderance of 5 to 10 to 1, and has a strong hereditary component. It is the cause of 50% to 80% of hyperthyroidism cases. Graves disease is caused by antibodies binding to and stimulating the TSH receptor, resulting in follicular hypertrophy and hyperplasia as well as excessive thyroid hormone synthesis and secretion. The thyroid gland enlarges, usually in a diffuse and symmetric fashion, and becomes firm.

Specific Notes on Medical Treatment

Thionamides

Thionamides (PTU three times a day or methimazole once daily) control hyperthyroidism for about 90% of Graves patients within 3 to 4 weeks. Treatment is often continued over 12 to 18 months in an attempt to induce remission, but after discontinuation, relapse will occur in 40% to 80% of patients. After relapse, most patients are

TABLE 1: Symptoms, findings, and complications of the hyperthyroid state

Symptoms

Fatigue
Weight loss
Diaphoresis
Palpitations
Heat intolerance
Muscle weakness
Diplopia, impaired vision, photophobia
Increased appetite
Dyspnea
Insomnia
Anxiety, nervousness
Restlessness
Irritability, emotional lability
Hair loss
Diarrhea, loose stools
Irregular menses

Clinical Findings

Goiter (firm, diffuse, possibly tender)
Thyroid bruit
Tachycardia (at rest)
Tremor
Stare, lid lag
Proptosis, exophthalmos
Keratitis, conjunctivitis
Chemosis
Periorbital edema
Ophthalmoplegia, strabismus
Hyperreflexia
Hyperpyrexia
Flow murmur
Gynecomastia
Splenomegaly
Warm, moist skin
Thin skin, dermopathy
Leg swelling, pretibial edema

Potential Complications

Thyroid storm
Cachexia
Psychosis, delirium
Cardiac arrhythmias
Congestive heart failure
Jaundice
Osteoporosis
Infertility, spontaneous abortion

TABLE 2: Differential diagnosis of hyperthyroidism

Toxic diffuse autoimmune goiter (Graves disease)
Toxic multinodular goiter (Plummer disease)
Solitary toxic nodule, adenoma
Amiodarone-associated thyroiditis, type I or type II
Other iodine-induced thyroiditis
Jod-Basedow effect with intravenous contrast
Betadine application (topical absorption)
Excess dietary iodine
Metastatic thyroid carcinoma
Painful, subacute thyroiditis
  • Radiation-induced
  • Granulomatous
  • Lymphocytic
  • Postpartum
  • Palpation-induced
Silent thyroiditis (lymphocytic, postpartum)
Ectopic thyroid hormone from *struma ovarii*
Excessive pituitary TSH (pituitary adenoma)
Pituitary resistance to thyroid hormone
Excessive trophoblastic TSH
Excess human chorionic gonadotropin from hydatidiform mole/
  choriocarcinoma
Ingestion of thyroid hormone (factitious)

should be obtained; prospective blood testing during therapy is not indicated. As the metabolic rate is reduced during treatment, weight gain can occur. Even when therapy is not aimed at remission, these treatments are commonly employed to achieve preoperative control of hyperthyroidism or for control of Graves disease during pregnancy; β-blockade is often added for symptom control, as discussed below (see "Preoperative Preparation in Graves Disease").

Radioactive Iodine

Radioactive iodine (RAI) treatment with ^{131}I is the therapy chosen for the vast majority of Graves disease patients in the United States. It is highly effective, with 80% to 90% of patients achieving control of hyperthyroidism with a single dose in a dose-dependent fashion. This is especially true for those with mild symptoms, small goiters, or Graves disease associated with Hashimoto lymphocytic thyroiditis, and it is a safe and effective choice for patients who are poor anesthetic risks. All women of reproductive age should have a pregnancy test immediately before treatment, as RAI is contraindicated during pregnancy. Patients commonly become hypothyroid, which is easily managed with thyroid hormone supplementation. Minor side effects can include neck pain from radiation thyroiditis, sialadenitis, and dry mouth. More concerning side effects can be temporary worsening of thyrotoxicosis and at times worsening of ophthalmopathy, which can be at least partially controlled with concomitant steroid therapy.

Achievement of a euthyroid or hypothyroid state can evolve over weeks or even months, which is a major limitation for some patients. In addition, some patients have a significant fear of any radioactivity, although long-term negative associations, such as with certain types of cancer, are quite limited. Treatment with ^{131}I is contraindicated during pregnancy and lactation. It is less commonly used in children and adolescents because of uncertainty over potential long-term effects but remains an option. Particularly in children under the age of 5 years, surgery is preferred because of uncertainty surrounding long-term RAI consequences. Recurrence or the need for repeated treatment (dose-dependent effects) may also be more common in these younger patients (children and adolescents), which might be related to dose reduction (secondary to fear of long-term consequences).

advanced to other treatments to seek definitive control. Minor side effects, such as rash and joint pain, can occur in about 5% of patients. Serious side effects include agranulocytosis (0.1% to 0.3% of patients) and allergic hepatitis (0.1% to 0.2%). Because of these, baseline blood counts and liver function tests are obtained prior to therapy.

Agranulocytosis is slightly more common in the elderly and with larger drug doses, and it can occur at any time during treatment. Patients are advised to monitor for rash, joint pain, liver inflammation, and symptoms of agranulocytosis—fever, sore throat, and mouth ulcers—during treatment. If these develop, the drug should be discontinued, and a white blood cell count and liver function test

Surgery for Graves Disease: Advantages

Rapidity of Resolution

Resolution of Graves hyperthyroidism is most rapid with surgery. Most patients can be prepared for surgery in less than 6 weeks, many within 2 weeks if necessary. In emergencies, surgery can be done almost immediately. If mass effects such as compression of the trachea or esophagus from thyroid enlargement are problematic, excision provides immediate relief. In contrast, response to thionamides can be measured in weeks, with treatment typically continuing for 6 months or more, involving multiple visits and blood tests. The full response to RAI takes 2 to 6 months.

Robust Cure

The surgical cure is definitive and long lasting for virtually 100% of patients. Recurrence rates are less than 1% with total thyroidectomy. In contrast, relapse after thionamide discontinuation can reach 75% at 5 years. Relapse is more likely with medium or large goiters or pronounced symptoms. Relapse is also greater when there are high initial T3 levels, high T3 to T4 ratios, high stimulating immunoglobulin levels, or high antithyroid antibodies. Relapse after RAI treatment is less common than after thionamides, but rates are proportional to RAI dose. More than one course can be needed.

Tissue Diagnosis

Only surgery provides substantial tissue for diagnosis. From 5% to 15% of Graves patients may have concerning or dominant nodules. The chance that a "cold" (nonfunctional) nodule is malignant is roughly the same as for patients without Graves, on the order of 15%. FNA can be used as in any other situation, but TSH suppression of nodules has no utility in these hyperthyroid patients. Occult carcinoma is discovered incidentally in about 2% of Graves specimens, and most are papillary carcinoma. This is not significantly different than in the general population, but at times it is reported as doubling the risk of papillary carcinoma; however, the finding is not clinically significant for the majority of patients.

No convincing support has been found for carcinoma in Graves being more aggressive or having a worse prognosis compared with matched controls. Therefore, *in the absence of a specific concern*, potential for occult malignancy does not drive treatment.

Compliance

Thyroidectomy can ameliorate problems with long-term medication compliance, but patients must still comply with preoperative preparation and often with postoperative calcium or thyroid supplements.

Concerns over Radioactivity

Some patients have a profound fear of radioactivity and are unwilling to undertake RAI treatment. This is despite the fact that major genetic or carcinogenic effects have not been observed. As mentioned above, some evidence indicates a slight increase in certain malignancies—specifically of the stomach, kidney, and breast—after RAI treatment, but surgery can resolve the fear of radioactivity and its long-term effects by obviating the need for RAI treatment.

Young Patients

Children and adolescents may be less responsive to thionamides, which have a 60% to 80% failure rate in the preteen population. RAI treatment is also problematic; recurrence and hypothyroidism are common, possibly related to RAI dose reductions. Rates of subsequent malignancy may be increased and are inversely related to age. This topic remains controversial, but particularly under the age of 5 years, surgery is preferred, and surgery is equally effective across age groups. Several experts favor surgery in the setting of concomitant Down syndrome.

Pregnancy

For women wishing to become pregnant, surgery provides rapid resolution and avoids exposure to radioactivity or antithyroid medications. In contrast, pregnancy should be avoided for 6 to 12 months after RAI treatment. During pregnancy, most patients are treated with antithyroid medication. When control is not achieved, and surgery is necessary during pregnancy, the second trimester is preferred; surgery in this interval is considered acceptably safe. However, because the immunologic process is not immediately halted, there does need to be a balanced management of both maternal and fetal hyperthyroidism; thyroidectomy and withdrawal of other management can result in isolated fetal hyperthyroidism. Surgery is also considered the safest option for lactating mothers.

Salvage

Some patients fail to achieve satisfactory resolution with medical therapy, often despite repeated courses. Others, particularly after previous treatments, become intolerant. They may develop rashes, urticaria, arthralgias, arthritis, fevers, nausea, vomiting, agranulocytosis, infections, hepatotoxicity, or vasculitis, all of which mandate cessation of therapy. These groups are effectively treated with surgery.

Ophthalmopathy

Manifestations of ophthalmopathy are clinically evident in 30% to 50% of Graves patients. Ablation of thyroid tissue with either surgery or RAI may decrease the incidence or halt the progression of Graves-related ophthalmopathy, but this remains controversial. Surgery might be slightly more effective, resulting in improvement in eye signs in as much as 85% of the population, but evidence is not conclusive. Total thyroidectomy may be more effective than the subtotal approach, perhaps on the basis of reducing the residual immunologic process. In some patients with severe ocular disease, RAI can incite a disease flare. Because of this, steroid treatments are often used in conjunction with RAI. In severe or difficult to manage cases, surgery to extirpate the thyroid may have a slight advantage for reducing risk of worsening ophthalmopathy or of Graves relapse. At times surgery is advocated, when there is a lack of other proven options. In fact, evidence is building that total thyroidectomy combined with subsequent RAI might be the most effective approach. Surgery on the orbit itself, which is a separate topic, has an important role in preserving sight and function in severe cases.

Thyroid Storm

Emergency surgical treatment of thyroid storm is reasonable and effective, particularly when the patient is not responding to medical therapy. Surgery itself probably does not stimulate release of T3 or T4. Patients should always be prepared with antithyroid medication, or should be controlled with β-blockade to the fullest extent possible.

Cosmesis

The cosmetics of a grossly enlarged goiter are quickly resolved in exchange for a scar 4 to 8 cm in length, which often can be concealed in a skin crease.

Cost

Surgery is believed by some to be less costly than thionamide therapy, which can involve 6 to 18 months of treatment, numerous office visits, and blood tests; but this issue has yet to be settled. Patients who relapse after thionamides frequently undertake surgery anyway, driving up costs of the intent to use thionamides. Similarly, surgery may cost somewhat more than RAI (~15% more), but recurrences after radiotherapy often require surgery driving up the costs of the intent to use RAI. Surgery typically entails only a single night of hospitalization, but the long-term costs of surgical complications can be difficult to assess. Other evidence suggests that both surgery and RAI treatment may cost slightly more than drug therapy. However, no high-grade evidence exists to definitively favor any of the three therapies based on cost benefit; each is viewed as acceptably cost effective for Graves disease.

Surgery for Graves Disease: Disadvantages

Rates of nerve injury, parathyroid compromise, and bleeding appear to be slightly higher for operations for Graves goiters and TMNG than for total thyroidectomies performed for other indications, possibly related to the enlarged thyroid, its firm consistency, venous engorgement, distortion of normal anatomy, or other specific factors. The hypervascularity of these goiters makes control of intraoperative bleeding important, and postoperative bleeding rates are somewhat elevated over other thyroid procedures, mandating caution.

Nerve Injury

Damage to laryngeal nerves results in permanent vocal cord dysfunction in up to 5% of patients. Transient dysfunction can also occur in a similar proportion of patients.

Parathyroid Compromise

Damage to parathyroids or their blood supply results in permanent hypoparathyroidism in up to 4% of patients, and temporary dysfunction occurs in another 8%. Temporary dysfunction is treated with calcium and calcitriol orally for 6 to 8 weeks or until function returns. These complications decrease with experience of the surgeon. Identification of parathyroids and meticulous reimplantation of compromised glands should be sufficient to completely avoid permanent hypoparathyroidism, and 70% to 80% of reimplanted glands should function after 4 to 6 weeks. Success rates can approach 100% if glands are finely minced (1 mm pieces) and carefully implanted into numerous intramuscular pockets.

Bleeding or Infection

Other surgical complications occur in less than 1% of "clean cases" despite being slightly more common in larger Graves or TMNG glands.

Hypothyroidism

Bilateral total thyroidectomy is expected to result in hypothyroidism. This is easily identified and effectively treated with thyroid hormone supplementation. Supplementation is inexpensive, is generally free of side effects at proper dosages, and is effectively monitored and managed with minimal blood testing. In comparison to surgery, thionamides rarely or never cause permanent hypothyroidism, but RAI commonly does, in up to 80% of patients.

General Anesthesia

Proper preparation of patients minimizes the risks of general anesthesia but does not eliminate them. Some ill patients will be at particularly high risk for anesthetic complications. These patients may be more safely treated medically.

Scar

Surgery results in a 4 to 8 cm scar on the anterior neck; cosmetic issues are minimized by careful technique and placement of the incision in a skin crease. Adjunct dressing materials help minimize scar formation and visibility.

Preoperative Preparation in Graves Disease

Surgery is chosen for about 10% of patients in the United States; the majority of the rest receive RAI; however, preoperative medical preparation significantly increases the safety of surgery when it is performed. Coexisting cardiac, respiratory, or renal disease must also be evaluated. Preparation controls existing hypermetabolic signs and symptoms, decreases risk of thyroid storm, and may diminish thyroid vascularity.

The most common preoperative regimen is based on thionamide inhibition using PTU, methimazole, or carbimazole. Since these drugs affect hormone levels and the results of thyroid scanning, diagnostic testing should be completed prior to initiation. Calcium should be checked to screen for concurrent hyperparathyroidism, and pregnancy should be ruled out.

A typical treatment initiates PTU at 50 to 100 mg by mouth three times a day. At the start of treatment, the patient should be educated about side effects of rash, joint pain, liver inflammation, and signs and symptoms of agranulocytosis (fever, sore throat, mouth ulcers). If the patient is euthyroid at 3 to 4 weeks based on T3 and T4 levels at or near normal (TSH need not normalize), surgery can proceed. Otherwise the dose is increased—up to 600 mg total dose per day, split into three or four doses by mouth per day—and the patient is monitored until a euthyroid state has been achieved. Alternately, methimazole can be used, typically a 10 to 45 mg total dosage by mouth per day (maximum dose 60 mg/day); given in a single daily dose (up to 15 mg for a single dose) or split into two doses or more per day. Hypothyroidism is to be avoided, so that the gland is not further stimulated by TSH. Levothyroxine can be used to prevent hypothyroidism if necessary, but this "block and replace" approach is controversial. Thionamides are discontinued at the time of surgery.

β-Blockade is used in conjunction with thionamides if the patient is symptomatic with tachycardia, hypertension, tremor, or diaphoresis. Hyperthyroid effects, mediated by the sympathetic nervous system, are usually controllable in this fashion. β-Blockade can be initiated early in the patient's diagnostic and therapeutic course. Atenolol or propranolol are often used. Propranolol has the added beneficial effect of inhibiting peripheral conversion of T4 to T3. Optimal propranolol doses vary by patient, from 40 to 320 mg/day, and half-life is just over 3 hours, mandating dosing three or four times daily. A stable heart rate of 80 beats per minute with mild exertion is desired. Continued judicious administration of intravenous β-blockade is essential to the safe conduct of surgery. Propranolol or esmolol are used intraoperatively.

If preoperative preparation consists solely of β-blockade because of previous intolerance of thionamides or emergent status, careful attention must be given to continued perioperative and postoperative β-blockade, because risk of thyroid storm is increased. Without antithyroid preparation, T3 and T4 levels will take 3 to 4 days to normalize postoperatively, and β-blockade should continue with the patient weaned off β-blockade over the course of 1 week.

Iopanoic acid is an alternate agent that can rapidly and effectively control hyperthyroidism perioperatively. It blocks conversion of T4 to T3, rapidly normalizing T3. Administration of concentrated iodine can also have beneficial effects on the thyroid preoperatively. Iodine initially inhibits the release of T4 and T3, decreasing the hyperthyroid state. This effect begins within 24 hours and peaks around 14 days. Thereafter, the iodine acts as a substrate, and hyperthyroidism returns. During the inhibition phase, thyroid vascularity may diminish, and the gland is believed to become firmer. It is best if the patient is euthyroid before iodine is administered, to diminish hyperthyroid rebound. Iodine is administered for 10 to 14 days prior to surgery and is discontinued at the time of the procedure. A supersaturated solution of potassium iodide (SSKI, 0.05 to 0.25 mL [50 to 250 mg] diluted in a full glass of water, fruit juice, milk, or broth three times per day for 10 days before surgery) or Lugol solution (iodine and potassium iodide, 8 mg iodide per drop: 3 to 5 drops by mouth three times a day) is given, used in conjunction with thionamides and β-blockade. Some authorities doubt the significance of iodine treatment as long as the patient is made euthyroid, therefore iodine treatment is considered optional.

Choice of Operation for Graves Disease

The surgeon can remove each of the thyroid lobes in either a total or subtotal fashion. At times confusion exists over the terms *total, near total,* and *subtotal.* Typically, "near total" acknowledges that even the well-intentioned "total" procedure leaves behind residual microscopic, if not gross, thyroid tissue. In addition, the term *near total* is used to describe preservation of small fragments of tissue adjacent to the parathyroids or to the recurrent laryngeal nerve, to protect these structures. Thus, *total* and *near total* descriptors are often equivalent for practical purposes. *Subtotal resection* refers to purposely leaving larger, gross remnants of thyroid tissue laterally or at the poles, often with the hope of avoiding hypothyroidism. Thus, for practical purposes, the surgical options comprise bilateral total or near-total, bilateral subtotal, or unilateral total or near-total thyroidectomy with contralateral subtotal thyroidectomy.

As mentioned, even total thyroidectomy rarely extirpates all traces of thyroid tissue. Tissue often remains at the superior poles, pyramidal lobe, or ligaments of Berry. However, such residual tissue is not usually sufficient to avoid hypothyroidism. If the goal of the subtotal approach is to avoid hypothyroidism, a vascularized remnant, or remnants, must be left large enough to support the patient but small enough to prevent hypertrophy or hyperfunction in the future. In practice, this is difficult to control based on a visual, intraoperative assessment. In general, remnant size is only poorly correlated with euthyroid outcome. This is partly because of the difficulty assessing 1) the vascular viability of the remnant; 2) the functional reserve of the tissue, particularly if there is lymphocytic infiltration; and 3) the absolute amount of tissue spared.

Unfortunately, recurrence after a subtotal approach is problematic: recurrence rates of 5% to 20% are common, depending on remnant size. In contrast, total thyroidectomy has less than 1% recurrence. Recurrence can occur from 1 to 30 years after surgery, and reoperation for recurrent disease carries significantly higher risk. For this reason, many experienced surgeons oppose a subtotal approach, accepting only the total or near-total approach of sparing very small remnants to protect parathyroids or nerves.

Hartley and Dunhill advocated a total thyroid lobectomy and isthmusectomy on one side with a subtotal resection on the other, leaving a remnant of 4 g or more. The posited advantage of this approach was that dissection was not carried far enough laterally on the subtotal side to disturb recurrent nerve or parathyroids, in theory reducing the risk of later reoperation if disease recurs. On the other hand, recurrence may be more common when leaving these larger remnants. Total thyroidectomy results in hypothyroidism, but recurrence of hyperthyroidism approaches 0%. For these reasons, the Hartley and Dunhill approach is now less favored. An additional disadvantage of the subtotal approach is that time can be required for the thyroid remnants to escape pituitary suppression. During this period, the patient is hypothyroid, but supplementation is withheld to maximize TSH stimulation. These patients also require long-term monitoring for onset of hypothyroidism.

With respect to recurrent nerve injury, accepted technique mandates identifying the nerve and tracing its course. It is incorrect to assume that leaving a remnant and not visualizing the nerve increases safety. In fact, when thyroid is transected without identifying the nerve, injuries may be several times more common. It can be reasonable to leave a small remnant of tissue in the ligament of Berry region, where the gland and nerve are often closely apposed. This should, however, be done with the nerve well visualized.

Parathyroid glands can be tightly adherent to the thyroid or even partly encased. Preservation of an adjacent rim of thyroid tissue can

TABLE 3: Summary of recommended surgical approaches

Condition	Preferred Approach
Graves disease	Bilateral total thyroidectomy with thyroid remnants only to protect nerves and parathyroids (total or near-total thyroidectomy)
Toxic multinodular goiter (TMNG)	Bilateral total thyroidectomy with thyroid remnants only to protect nerves and parathyroids (total or near-total thyroidectomy)
Solitary toxic nodule (STN)	Unilateral thyroid lobectomy with generous remnant to protect nerves and parathyroids as necessary (subtotal thyroidectomy) or Unilateral total lobectomy or Bilateral total thyroidectomy if additional concerns warrant such
Amiodarone-associated thyrotoxicosis (AAT)	Bilateral total thyroidectomy with thyroid remnants only to protect nerves and parathyroids (total or near-total thyroidectomy)

help preserve parathyroid perfusion. The parathyroids are typically vascularized from their anterior aspect, knowledge of which informs dissection. Furthermore, the superior parathyroids are generally more reliably located (behind the superior thyroid poles) than are the inferior parathyroids, which can be markedly displaced by goiter. Parathyroid devascularization can lead to serious and permanent hypocalcemia, a problem that can be difficult to manage. When there is any concern over the vascularity of a parathyroid, it should be removed, chilled, finely minced, and reimplanted in an intramuscular pocket (e.g., the sternocleidomastoid) without hesitation. A single, well-protected normal parathyroid can reliably support the patient with normal physiology.

Based on these considerations, bilateral total or near-total thyroidectomy is the favored approach to Graves hyperthyroidism. Table 3 summarizes the recommended surgical approaches for each of the hyperthyroid conditions. Direct laryngoscopy should be performed prior to anesthesia induction for patients with hoarseness to document preexisting vocal cord dysfunction. Some surgeons perform laryngoscopy on all patients. A substantial thyroid remnant is not purposely left to avoid hypothyroidism, but tissue can be left near the ligaments of Berry to protect the viability of nerves or near parathyroids (near-total thyroidectomy). Compromised parathyroids should be reimplanted. Postoperatively, hypothyroidism is expected, and patients should be immediately supplemented with thyroxine.

It should be noted that in certain situations, when traditional therapeutic options or surgical approaches have not been applicable, some success has been achieved treating Graves disease with arterial embolization, but experience with this modality remains limited.

TOXIC MULTINODULAR GOITER (PLUMMER DISEASE)

Toxic multinodular goiter (TMNG) was first described by H.S. Plummer in 1913, which is why STNs are also often described as Plummer disease. In contrast to Graves disease, TMNG often occurs after the age of 50 years and becomes more prominent with increasing age. It often develops in the setting of long-standing nontoxic multinodular goiter, and thus it can have a long subclinical phase before the appearance of overt symptoms. TMNG is more common in regions of dietary iodine deficiency. With large goiters complications from local pressure on the trachea, esophagus, or venous system arise. Jugular venous compression can lead to Pemberton sign, evidenced by facial plethora, inspiratory stridor, and venous congestion when arms are raised above the head.

A *hot nodule* is one that takes up radioactive tracer at higher than normal levels. Technetium will label many nodules hot that are not truly hypermetabolic, thus proper differentiation of nodules must be done with radioactive iodine (RAI). In addition, a hot nodule can be either autonomous—not responsive to TSH suppression, or showing abnormal TSH response to thyrotropin-releasing hormone—or not autonomous. Furthermore, an autonomous nodule can be either toxic, producing thyroid hormone in excess (clinically hyperthyroid), or nontoxic. Thyroxine suppression of TSH for multinodular goiter is viewed as generally ineffective and is not favored; but in any case, when multinodular goiter becomes autonomous and toxic (clinically hyperthyroid), suppression is no longer an option. Because the rate of malignancy in hot nodules is low, surgery has a role mainly for toxic hot nodules. The rate of occult malignancies in the remainder of the thyroid for TMNG is on the order of 2% to 3%, slightly elevated from other conditions; but as discussed for Graves disease, this is rarely a driving concern.

The same treatment options are available for TMNG as for Graves disease: thionamides, RAI, and surgery. For both thionamides and RAI, remission of TMNG is less common, and recurrence of hyperthyroidism is more common than in Graves disease. Life-long thionamide treatment is not considered acceptable, so these medications are seldom or never used as *definitive* treatment, although they remain important for preoperative preparation. An additional option for patients unfit for surgery is ethanol ablation of toxic nodules, but this is less proven and may be less successful than surgery or RAI.

The majority of patients in the United States are treated with RAI. However, RAI treatment may require large doses or repeated treatments in 15% to 20% of cases. Even when RAI controls hyperthyroidism, nodule or goiter size may not decrease—the average reduction in size is about 40%, which leaves compressive problems unaddressed. The full treatment effect evolves over 5 to 6 months. Radiation-induced thryoiditis can occur, but serious complications are rare; eventual hypothyroidism is not uncommon and is dose dependent. Therefore RAI is particularly favored for patients in poor health, for those who are not good surgical candidates, and for patients with mild disease.

Surgery is the preferred approach for large goiters and compressive symptoms in the absence of factors that make the patient a poor surgical candidate. However, surgery is also generally a reasonable option for most cases of TMNG. The surgical approach is similar to that for Graves disease, except that there may be even less concern about recurrence of disease in the small remnants left behind. If more tissue is left behind in these areas, the procedure becomes a bilateral subtotal approach, and the risk of recurrence rises. With surgery, resolution of hyperthyroidism is prompt and permanent (hypothyroidism is expected); recurrence is rare, tissue is obtained for pathology, and compressive or cosmetic issues are rapidly relieved. According to level V evidence, cost benefit may slightly favor surgery for this condition.

Preoperative preparation is the same as mentioned for Graves disease, except that supplementation with iodine is not believed to be beneficial, because the multinodular gland is not homogenously hypervascular. In fact, iodide supplementation of autonomous nodules can exacerbate hyperthyroidism, known as a *Jod-Basedow effect*.

SOLITARY TOXIC NODULES

Most solitary toxic nodules (STNs) are benign, monoclonal, follicular adenomas; probably 1% or less are carcinomas. The solitary nodule may have a life cycle of progression from a hot nodule to an autonomous hot nodule to an autonomous STN. The change to a toxic nodule is more common in nodules that have grown to 2.5 to 3 cm. There has been debate over suppression of hot nodules. Nonautonomous, nontoxic hot nodules can potentially be observed on or off thyroxine suppression; however, the autonomous STN, by definition, is not suppressible.

If a hot nodule being suppressed or observed continues to grow to 3 cm or more or other worrisome characteristics develop (e.g., tenderness, fixation, hoarseness, or other secondary or mass or pressure effects), lobectomy is reasonable; total thyroidectomy might be warranted for other concerns. This is despite the low probability of malignancy for hot nodules. After lobectomy most patients become euthyroid. FNA can be performed to assist in surgical planning but is unlikely to avert surgery. Despite the low risk of malignancy, provision of tissue for pathology remains an advantage of surgery. Recurrent hyperthyroidism after lobectomy is uncommon and much less frequent for solitary nodules than for Graves disease or TMNG, therefore remnants can be left to protect nerves or parathyroids without major concerns.

For nodules that are not otherwise worrisome, RAI remains an effective treatment option. It is favored for those who are poor surgical candidates or for those who are averse to surgery. Large doses are often required, and disease can relapse in 20% to more than 50% of patients; relapse rates are dose dependent. Hypothyroidism is less common after radiotherapy for nodular disease than for Graves disease. This is because only the nodules are autonomous, and surrounding tissues are suppressed. Ideally a treated nodule should disappear, regress, or at least persist without change; up to half of all nodules will regress. Persistence remains worrisome, and growth of the nodule mandates removal. Pregnancy and lactation are contraindications to RAI. In comparison, treatment with thionamides poorly controls the STN, remission does not occur, and therefore recurrent disease is inevitable when life-long thionamide medication is not accepted. Surgery or RAI are preferred over thionamides. As with TMNG, ethanol ablation remains an option for some patients, particularly for poor surgical candidates, but effectiveness is unproven.

Because STNs are monoclonal neoplasms, the preferred definitive treatment is unilateral total or subtotal lobectomy, with a conservative approach to protect parathyroids and the recurrent laryngeal nerve. Nodulectomy is not recommended, as this can compromise excision margin and pathologic evaluation of the tumor capsule. Frozen-section analysis of nodules is unreliable, and subsequent completion lobectomy for malignancy after nodulectomy alone carries higher risk of surgical complications. Capsular invasion defines carcinoma. Total or subtotal lobectomy is effectively a cure, and few patients will become hypothyroid. Unexpected well-differentiated carcinoma is discovered in 1% to 3% of patients and can be definitively diagnosed. This is an advantage of surgery, but in the absence of specific preoperative information, concern for this rarely drives choice of treatment. Vocal cord compromise with unilateral surgery is rare, and hypoparathyroidism should not occur. Disadvantages include the inconvenience of surgery, risk of anesthesia, and scarring. Lifetime costs associated with thyroidectomy appear somewhat lower (about $3000 lower) than with RAI, when surgery is performed by experienced surgeons who have achieved results with minimal morbidity and no mortality.

Preoperative preparation is the same as mentioned for Graves disease, except that supplementation with iodide is not believed beneficial, because the entire gland is not homogenously hypervascular.

AMIODARONE-ASSOCIATED THYROTOXICOSIS

Amiodarone is an iodine-rich, class III antiarrhythmic drug initially used for refractory arrhythmias and now more widely used because of its antiarrhythmic effectiveness. Use of the drug significantly expands the iodine pool. Amiodarone-associated thyrotoxicosis (AAT) can be a form of the Jod-Basedow effect, which describes hyperthyroidism following administration of iodine or iodide, whether as dietary supplement, contrast medium, topical agent, or drug. This form of AAT, referred to as *type I,* typically develops in patients with preexisting goiter, in whom the marked iodine excess results in excessive thyroid hormone production. It appears that amiodarone can also induce a second type of AAT, referred to as *type II,* which is the result of chemically induced thyroiditis and subsequent release of excessive thyroid hormone. Type II usually occurs in the absence of preexisting thyroid disease and is the more common type in the United States, affecting as many as 2% of amiodarone-treated patients. Both types of AAT are characterized by subsequent low iodine uptake.

Because of the patient population treated with amiodarone, AAT often occurs in those with significant cardiac dysrhythmias and underlying cardiac dysfunction, who poorly tolerate the cardiac effects of hyperthyroidism. Unfortunately, AAT is notoriously refractory to medical management. Given that AAT is characterized by low iodine uptake, it is not effectively treated with radioactive iodine. Cessation of amiodarone can help, but underlying cardiac arrhythmias may preclude this, and the drug's long half-life necessitates weeks to months for resolution of its effect. Antithyroid thionamide drugs have been employed with only very limited success for this scenario and seem most likely to be effective if amiodarone can be discontinued, and if hyperthyroidism is mild.

Surgical thyroidectomy offers prompt and permanent control of AAT. As with surgery for other thyrotoxic states, risk of recurrent laryngeal nerve compromise or permanent hypoparathyroidism is low, influenced mainly by the extent of underlying inflammation or preexisting goiter. The procedure is often followed by a short hospitalization and quick recovery, depending largely on the underlying cardiac conditions that necessitated amiodarone treatment. These underlying cardiac conditions are the primary drivers of operative complication risks for this population. Prior to surgery, these patients should have evaluation and optimization of underlying cardiac and associated conditions to whatever extent time allows. The procedure of choice is bilateral total or near-total thyroidectomy, just as would be recommended for Graves disease. The majority of these patients do well, and surgery is commonly the most efficacious treatment option. Table 3 summarizes recommended surgical approaches for hyperthyroid conditions.

RECURRENT HYPERTHYROIDISM: SPECIAL CONSIDERATIONS

Recurrent hyperthyroidism poses special challenges for the surgeon. At the time of initial lobectomy or total thyroidectomy, the neck is often extensively dissected, with mobilization of parathyroids and the recurrent laryngeal nerves. After healing and scarring, these important structures can have atypical relationships to other structures in the neck, and the normal blood supply to the parathyroids can already be partially compromised. Scarred and disturbed tissues also predispose to bleeding upon reoperation, further obscuring anatomy. This greatly increases the risk of injury to parathyroids and nerves during reoperative surgery. For instance, permanent recurrent nerve injury can occur in up to 12% of reoperations versus 0% to 3% of primary procedures. For this reason, recurrent hyperthyroid disease should be carefully considered for medical treatment before surgery is undertaken.

If medical treatment is not acceptable, surgery must be performed with extreme caution. One particular point of concern is the recurrent laryngeal nerve. After initial surgery and mobilization, recurrent hyperthyroid tissue can originate from behind this nerve rather than on top of it. This can result in the nerve being displaced anteriorly onto the anterior superficial surface of the recurrent thyroid tissue. As a result, the nerve might not be found in the tracheoesophageal groove and can be in any location, starting immediately under the strap muscles.

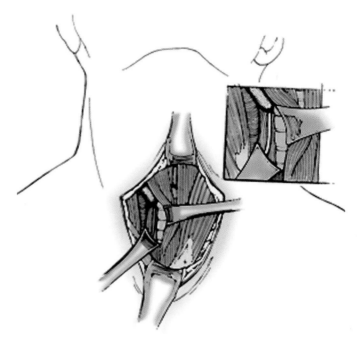

FIGURE I   Lateral or "backdoor" approach to identification of the recurrent laryngeal nerve. *(From Moley JF, Lairmore TC, Doherty GM, et al: Preservation of the recurrent laryngeal nerves in thyroid and parathyroid reoperations, Surgery 126:673-677, 1999.)*

Reoperative safety can be improved by using certain approaches. Direct fiberoptic laryngoscopy should be performed at the start of the surgery to determine whether the patient has preexisting vocal cord dysfunction. The surgical procedure should focus on early identification of the recurrent laryngeal nerve. This may safely be accomplished by a "backdoor" approach, in which the strap muscles are mobilized away from the sternocleidomastoid muscle, before the plane between the carotid artery and sternothyroid is developed (Figure 1). After the straps are mobilized off of the carotid artery, the nerve can be found in the space between the carotid and the trachea or posterior to the carotid distal to its meeting with the vagus nerve. This dissection should be done as low in the neck as possible to avoid areas of scarring from previous surgery. Once located, the recurrent laryngeal nerve may be dissected superiorly through areas of scarring and should be kept in view while the thyroid tissue is being resected. Intraoperative nerve monitoring can also be valuable in these settings.

SELECTED READINGS

Bartalena L, Tanda ML: Graves' ophthalmopathy, *N Engl J Med* 360:994–1001, 2009.

Brent GA: Graves' disease, *N Engl J Med* 358:2594–2605, 2008.

Hegedus L: Treatment of Graves' hyperthyroidism: evidence-based and emerging modalities, *Endocrinol Metab Clin N Am* 38:355–371, 2009.

Iraci GS, Fux-Otta C: Graves' hyperthyroidism, *N Engl J Med* 360(24):e31, 2009.

Moley JF, Lairmore TC, Doherty GM, et al: Preservation of the recurrent laryngeal nerves in thyroid and parathyroid reoperations, *Surgery* 126:673–677, 1999.

Porterfield JR, Thompson GB, Farley DR, et al: Evidence-based management of toxic multinodular goiter (Plummer's disease), *World J Surg* 32: 1278–1284, 2008.

Stalberg P, Svensson A, Hessman O, et al: Surgical treatment of Graves' disease: evidence-based approach, *World J Surg* 32:1269–1277, 2008.

MANAGEMENT OF THYROID CANCER

Christopher R. McHenry, MD, and Judy Jin, MD

OVERVIEW

Thyroid cancer comprises 95% of all endocrine malignancies and 1.5% of all cancers. It is categorized into follicular cell–derived and non–follicular cell–derived variants. Follicular cell–derived malignancies include papillary thyroid cancer (PTC), follicular cancer (FC), Hurthle cell cancer (HCC), and *anaplastic cancer* (ATC). PTC, FC, and HCC are also referred to as *differentiated thyroid cancer* (DTC). Non–follicular cell–derived malignancies include medullary thyroid cancer (MTC), lymphoma, and metastases. Thyroid cancer has the greatest annual percentage increase in incidence of any cancers in both men and women. From 1973 to 2002, the rate of thyroid cancer in the United States has more than doubled, yet the mortality rate has remained unchanged. This is in contrast to the age- and gender-adjusted mortality for other solid tumors, which have declined.

The lifetime risk of developing thyroid cancer in the United States is estimated to be 0.8% for women and 0.3% in men. The overall incidence of thyroid cancer is increasing, at a rate of 4% per year, and it has become the sixth most commonly diagnosed malignancy in women. Based on statistics from the National Cancer Institute, approximately 410,404 men and women alive in 2006 were treated for thyroid cancer. In 2009, there will be an estimated 37,200 new cases of thyroid cancer diagnosed, with 1630 thyroid cancer–related deaths. The median age of diagnosis for thyroid cancer is 48 years. The age-adjusted death rate is 0.6 per 100,000 individuals per year, and the mortality rate is the highest in individuals between the 65 and 74 years of age.

Thyroid malignancy can range from an incidentally discovered, occult PTC, which has a 30 year survival of almost 100%, to an aggressive, undifferentiated lesion that is uniformly fatal. Well-differentiated thyroid cancer, which comprises more than 90% of all thyroid cancer, has an overall good prognosis.

In recent years, major advances have been made in the diagnosis and treatment of thyroid cancer. Advancements in ultrasound technology with the addition of high-frequency transducers have led to the detection of thyroid nodules as small as 2 mm. The increased use of office-based ultrasound has resulted in the increased diagnosis of papillary cancers less than 2 cm. Ultrasound-guided fine needle aspiration biopsy (FNAB) has helped improved the diagnostic yield of FNAB. Genetic testing for MTC and the detection of new oncogene mutations involved in ATC have the potential to alter the clinical outcomes for affected patients.

DIAGNOSIS

Most patients with thyroid cancer are initially seen with a palpable thyroid nodule but are otherwise asymptomatic. Less commonly, patients are first seen for compressive symptoms that include dysphagia, dyspnea, hoarseness, or coughing or choking spells. Cervical lymphadenopathy may be the initial manifestation of thyroid cancer in some patients. Clinically inapparent or occult cancer may be detected incidentally on radiographic imaging studies, or when thyroidectomy is performed for benign disease. In the case of suspected multiple endocrine neoplasia (MEN) syndrome, MTC may be diagnosed as a result of genetic testing or serum calcitonin measurement.

Although thyroid nodules are common, only 5% are malignant. Risk factors for carcinoma include a prior history of head or neck radiation and a family history of thyroid cancer or other familial syndromes in which thyroid cancer is associated (Table 1). Children, men, adults over 60 years of age, anyone presenting with a rapidly growing thyroid nodule, and patients with a personal history of breast cancer have an increased risk of thyroid malignancy. A firm, fixed thyroid nodule, an enlarged cervical lymph node, and vocal cord paralysis are physical findings associated with malignancy.

The workup of a thyroid nodule (Figure 1) includes a routine serum thyrotropin (TSH) level to evaluate the functional status of the thyroid gland and a routine ultrasound examination of the neck to characterize the nodule and to evaluate the rest of the thyroid gland. Sonographic features of a thyroid nodule concerning for malignancy include ill-defined margins, irregular shape with an anteroposterior dimension greater than the transverse dimension, an intranodular vascular pattern, and microcalcifications. FNAB is performed for nodules 1 cm or larger and nodules smaller than 1 cm with suspicious sonographic features. In the case of multinodular thyroid disease, FNAB of the most suspicious nodule should be performed. Cytological analysis of FNAB specimens may be categorized as benign, *malignant, suspicious for thyroid carcinoma, indeterminate* (follicular or Hurthle cell neoplasm), or *persistently nondiagnostic*.

FNAB is accurate in identifying PTC and MTC, with a false-positive rate of 1% to 2%. If an MTC is identified on FNAB, a baseline serum calcitonin level should be obtained, and the patient should also be screened for pheochromocytoma and hyperparathyroidism. Patients with FNAB diagnosis of PTC can undergo definitive cancer operation without the need for intraoperative frozen-section analysis. Prior to operation, an ultrasound of the central and lateral neck should be performed to look for abnormal lymph nodes. A modified neck dissection and/or central neck dissection can be performed concurrently with thyroidectomy for patients with metastatic lymph nodes in the central or lateral neck.

A major limitation of FNAB is the inability to make a definitive diagnosis of follicular carcinoma or HCC, which requires the identification of capsular or vascular invasion from a tissue sample. In patients with an FNAB result that is consistent with a follicular or Hurthle cell neoplasm, serum TSH along with iodine-123 scintigraphy of the thyroid can help differentiate a hypofunctioing nodule from a hyperfunctioning nodule: a hyperfunctioning nodule has a greater uptake than the surrounding thyroid tissue and is associated with a less than 1% incidence of malignancy; a hypofunctioning nodule has a 20% risk of malignancy in a patient with an FNAB result consistent with a follicular or Hurthle cell neoplasm.

PAPILLARY THYROID CARCINOMA

Papillary thyroid carcinoma (PTC) accounts for 80% of all thyroid malignancies in iodine-sufficient areas but is less common in iodine-deficient areas. In general, PTC is an indolent cancer with an overall 10 year survival rate of 93%. It occurs more often in women, with a

TABLE 1: Inherited syndromes associated with thyroid cancer

Multiple endocrine neoplasia (MEN) 2A and 2B
Isolated familial medullary thyroid cancer
Gardner syndrome
Familial adenomatous polyposis
Carney complex
Cowden syndrome
Familial nonmedullary thyroid cancer

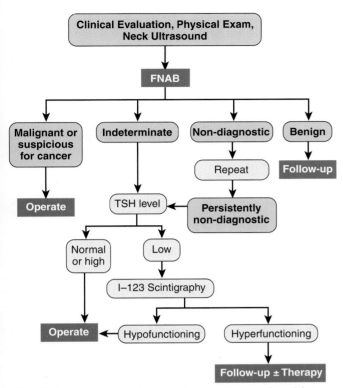

FIGURE 1 Algorithm for the evaluation of patients with nodular thyroid disease.

TABLE 2: American Joint Commission on Cancer Staging for well-differentiated thyroid cancer based on tumor, node, and metastases (TNM) descriptors

T1	Tumor ≤2 cm, limited to the thyroid
T2	Tumor >2 cm but ≤4 cm, limited to the thyroid
T3	Tumor >4 cm, limited to the thyroid
T4a	Tumor of any size extending beyond the thyroid capsule to invade subcutaneous soft tissues, larynx, trachea, esophagus, or recurrent laryngeal nerve
T4b	Tumor invades prevertebral fascia or encases carotid artery or mediastinal vessels
N0	No regional lymph node metastasis
N1	Regional lymph node metastasis
N1a	Metastasis to level VI (pretracheal, paratracheal, and prelaryngeal/Delphian lymph nodes)
N1b	Metastasis to unilateral or bilateral cervical or superior mediastinal lymph nodes
M0	No distant metastasis
M1	Distant metastasis

TABLE 3: Stage groupings for DTC

≤45 Years	>45 Years
Stage I any T, any N, M0	Stage I T1, N0, M0
Stage II any T, any N, M1	Stage II T2, N0, M0
	Stage III T3, N0, M0T1, N1a, M0T2, N1a, M0T3, N1a, M0
	Stage IVA T4a, N0, M0T4a, N1a, M0T1, N1b, M0T2, N1b, M0T3, N1b, M0T4a, N1b, M0
	Stage IVB T4b, any N, M0
	Stage IVC any T, any N, M1

female to male ratio of 2:1, and the mean age at diagnosis is approximately 30 to 40 years. The most common manifestation of PTC is a palpable thyroid nodule, 50% of which are discovered by the patient; the other 50% are discovered during routine physical exam or during imaging evaluation for some other disease process.

Multiple patient factors are associated with an increased risk of malignancy: age less than 15 years or greater than 45 years, male gender, prior head or neck irradiation, and a family history of thyroid cancer in a first-degree relative. PTC is the most common thyroid malignancy associated with a previous history of radiation. Thyroid nodules may develop within 5 years from the time of radiation exposure, with new nodules developing at about 2% per year. This rate peaks at 30 years following exposure, but the incidence remains high even after 40 years.

Most PTCs can be diagnosed with FNAB with an overall accuracy is nearly 100%. Supplemental genetic analysis for *BRAF* and *RAS* mutations, *RET* and *PAX-8-PPARγ* gene rearrangements may help improve the diagnostic accuracy in patients with FNAB that is indeterminate or suspicious for PTC. Cytology samples that stain positive for galectin-3 are five times more likely to have carcinoma on the final pathology. The presence of *BRAF* mutations in indeterminate fine needle aspirates results in a sevenfold to ninefold increase in the risk of PTC. Identification of *RET* rearrangements may also improve the sensitivity of FNAB. Although molecular markers may offer additional information on the potential for thyroid malignancy, none of them have a high negative predictive value.

Cervical lymph node involvement is common in PTC, occurring in up to 50% of patients. The preoperative identification of lymph node metastases in the central or lateral neck, by either palpation or ultrasonography, may alter the surgical management and allow the surgeon to plan for a lateral or central neck dissection. Stulak and colleagues identified nonpalpable lateral lymph nodes using ultrasound in 14% of patients who underwent initial surgery for thyroid cancer and 64% of patients who underwent reoperation for recurrent or persistent disease.

The American Joint Committee on Cancer staging for DTC is based on tumor size, extrathyroidal tumor spread, and the presence or absence of lymph node metastases and distant metastases (Table 2). The staging system for DTC (Table 3) is unique in that age is an important factor for determination of stage. In patients with DTC who are less than 45 years of age, stage II is used to categorize patients with metastatic disease and is the highest stage.

There are no prospective randomized studies addressing the extent of thyroidectomy necessary for treatment of thyroid cancer. As a result, the extent of thyroid resection for PTC is controversial, and recommendations for therapy are based on the results of retrospective analysis and expert consensus. Most experts agree that total thyroidectomy should be performed for all patients with high-risk papillary carcinoma (Table 4). Low-risk PTC may be treated with thyroid lobectomy, however, it may not be the optimal therapy. Total thyroidectomy is associated with the lowest incidence of local and regional recurrence. It also allows for the most effective use of serum thyroglobulin and radioiodine for detection of recurrent disease and high-dose radioiodine for treatment of metastatic disease. Total thyroidectomy also eliminates a 1% incidence of anaplastic dedifferentiation.

The National Comprehensive Cancer Network (NCCN) guidelines recommend total thyroidectomy for patients with papillary cancer and one or more of the following characteristics: age less than 15 years or greater than 45 years, prior head and neck radiation, tumor greater than 4 cm in diameter, cervical lymph node metastases, or an aggressive histologic variant (tall cell, columnar cell, insular, oxyphilic, or poorly differentiated). In patients who have undergone thyroid lobectomy and isthmusectomy who are subsequently diagnosed with PTC, completion thyroidectomy is indicated for PTC that is 1 cm or larger or PTC smaller than 1 cm when it is multicentric or associated with lymph node or systemic metastases.

TABLE 4: Criteria for distinguishing low- and high-risk well-differentiated thyroid carcinoma based on the AGES classification system

Low	High
Women <50 years	Women ≥50 years
Men <40 years	Men ≥40 years
Well-differentiated tumor	Poorly differentiated tumor (tall cell, columnar cell, or oxyphilic variants)
Tumor <4 cm in diameter	Tumor ≥4 cm in diameter
Tumor confined to thyroid	Local invasion
No distant metastases	Distant metastases

Completion thyroidectomy should be performed within 6 months of the initial procedure, as the risk of lymph node metastases is significantly lower, and the overall survival rate is increased when compared with patients whose completion thyroidectomy was delayed beyond 6 months.

Patients with extrathyroidal tumor spread should have an en bloc resection performed. Resection of a recurrent laryngeal nerve involved by tumor should be reserved for patients with a paralyzed vocal cord; the tumor should be shaved from a functioning recurrent laryngeal nerve, which underscores the importance of preoperative laryngoscopy in patients with hoarseness or other voice changes. Conservative procedures that maintain function are also preferred in patients with esophageal, tracheal, and laryngeal invasion.

A central or modified neck dissection (Figure 2) is indicated at the initial surgical procedure if macroscopic nodal disease is present in the central or lateral neck. A central neck dissection consists of removal of all lymph nodes and fibrous fatty tissue from the hyoid bone superiorly to the brachiocephalic artery inferiorly and between the common carotid arteries laterally. The prelaryngeal, pretracheal, and paratracheal lymph nodes, which comprise the level VI nodes, are removed (see Figure 2, *A*). A modified neck dissection consists of removal of the upper, middle, and lower cervical lymph nodes (levels II, III, and IV) and the posterior cervical and supraclavicular lymph nodes (level V; see Figure 2, *A* and *B*).

The American Thyroid Association (ATA) recommends that a routine central neck dissection be considered for patients with PTC, whereas the NCCN only recommends central neck dissection for grossly positive lymph node metastases. The rationale for prophylactic central neck dissection is that the likelihood of occult microscopic disease is high, and reoperation for a recurrence in the central neck may be associated with a high complication rate. The rationale against prophylactic neck dissection is the potential for an increased rate of hypoparathyroidism and recurrent laryngeal nerve injury and the lack of evidence that it has a beneficial effect on recurrence or mortality rates.

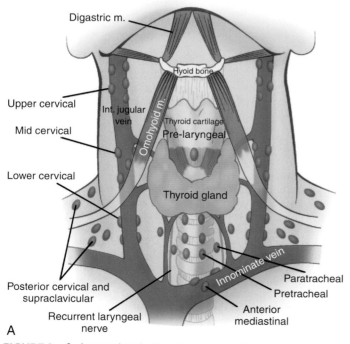

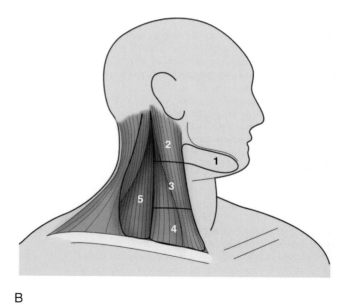

A   B

FIGURE 2   **A,** A central neck dissection consists of removal of prelaryngeal, pretracheal, paratracheal, and anterior mediastinal lymph nodes. **B,** Lymph nodes from level II, III, IV, and V are removed in a modified neck dissection. (**A** *From McHenry CR, Difficult problems in thyroid cancer surgery, Minerva Chirugica 65[1]:83–93, 2010;* **B** *From Mittendorf EA, McHenry CR: Thyroid cancer. In Cameron JL, editor: Current surgical therapy, ed 8, St Louis, 2004, Elsevier, pp 584–591.)*

FOLLICULAR THYROID CARCINOMA

Follicular thyroid carcinoma (FTC) accounts for approximately 11% of all cases of thyroid malignancy and 25% to 40% of cases in iodine-deficient areas; however, the overall incidence of FTC is decreasing as a result of the increased recognition and more accurate diagnosis of the follicular variant of PTC and the widespread efforts to correct iodine deficiency. Patients with FTC are older than patients with PTC; mean age at diagnosis is 60 years, and the female to male ratio is approximately 3:1.

Patients with FTC usually are initially seen with a thyroid nodule and FNAB consistent with a follicular neoplasm, and they undergo an initial diagnostic thyroid lobectomy and isthmusectomy. Intraoperative frozen-section analysis offers little additional help in differentiating a follicular adenoma from FTC. Approximately 20% of patients with FNAB consistent with follicular neoplasm will have FTC, the follicular variant of PTC, or a PTC, and most will need a total thyroidectomy. In patients with a follicular neoplasm who have nodular disease 1 cm or greater involving the contralateral lobe or a prior history of head or neck irradiation, an initial definitive total thyroidectomy should be performed.

FTC may be classified into one of two variants based on the final pathology: *Minimally invasive carcinoma* is defined as an encapsulated FTC with minor capsular invasion; *invasive carcinoma* refers to the presence of angioinvasion or extensive tumor invasion beyond the tumor capsule with diffuse infiltration of the affected lobe of the thyroid gland.

Minimally invasive FTC is indolent and can be treated with thyroid lobectomy and isthmusectomy alone. The disease-free survival in patients with minimally invasive disease is similar to patients with a benign follicular adenoma. All patients with invasive FTC should be treated with a total thyroidectomy, as the risk for vascular invasion and systemic metastases are much higher. The 10 year disease-specific mortality for invasive FTC is 28%.

Less than 10% of patients with FTC have lymph node metastasis. As a result, prophylactic central neck dissection is not indicated. Central neck dissection and modified neck dissection are reserved for patients with biopsy-confirmed lymph node metastases in the central and lateral neck. The overall 10 year survival rate for FTC is about 85%.

HURTHLE CELL CANCER

Hurthle cell cancer (HCC) is the least common of the well-differentiated thyroid cancers, accounting for approximately 4% of all thyroid malignancies. Although classified as a subtype of FTC by the World Health Organization, HCC is a distinct clinical entity. It is more often multifocal and bilateral and more frequently metastasizes to regional lymph nodes than FTC. About 10% to 20% of patients with HCC will present with metastases, and about one third of patients will develop metastases during their lifetime. Of all the histologic types of well-differentiated thyroid carcinoma, HCC has the highest incidence of metastases. Systemic metastases most commonly involve the lung, bone, or central nervous system. HCC is radioresistant and has a worse prognosis than PTC or FTC, with a 10 year survival rate of approximately 75%.

Patients with HCC usually present with a dominant nodule in the thyroid gland that is identified as a Hurthle cell neoplasm on FNAB. A thyroid lobectomy and isthmusectomy is performed to distinguish a benign Hurthle cell adenoma from HCC. Twenty percent of patients with FNAB consistent with a Hurthle cell neoplasm will be diagnosed with HCC, and a completion thyroidectomy is necessary for all patients. As such, all patients with HCC are treated with total thyroidectomy.

The ATA recommends that a central neck dissection be considered in all patients with HCC. This is because HCC is associated with a high rate of lymph node metastasis; because it is radioresistant

and surgical resection offers the best chance of cure. The benefit of prophylactic central neck dissection in the absence of macroscopic lymph node metastases, however, has yet to be established.

POSTOPERATIVE MANAGEMENT OF DIFFERENTIATED THYROID CANCER

Postoperative management of patients with DTC includes radioiodine ablation of remnant thyroid tissue in selected patients and the administration of thyroid hormone. Postoperative iodine-131 treatment is advocated to ablate residual normal thyroid tissue and to treat residual microscopic disease. It also helps to optimize the use of serum thyroglobulin (Tg) and radioiodine whole-body scanning for detection of recurrent disease. Radioiodine emits β-radiation over a 1 to 2 mm distance, which is cytotoxic to the follicular epithelia. Therapy with ^{131}I has been shown to reduce recurrence and cancer-specific mortality in patients with high-risk PTC and should be recommended for patients with incomplete tumor resection, extrathyroidal tumor spread, nodal or distant metastases, or aggressive histology (tall cell, columnar cell, or diffuse sclerosing carcinoma). Whether routine radioiodine ablation is of value for patients with low-risk PTC is controversial. Ablation therapy is not indicated for patients with unifocal PTC that is less than 1 cm without extrathyroidal tumor spread or metastases.

Radioiodine uptake is dependent on TSH stimulation and is inhibited by excess iodine from the diet or from the intravenous contrast used for computed tomography (CT). Patients are placed on short-acting triiodothyronine (T3) postoperatively, 25 µg twice a day, to minimize the period of hypothyroidism prior to ablation therapy. Alternatively, radioiodine ablation may be completed following the administration of recombinant human TSH, which avoids the development of hypothyroid symptoms associated with hormone withdrawal. Two weeks before receiving iodine, T3 is discontinued, and the patient is placed on a low-iodine diet to maximize the uptake and retention of radioiodine by the remnant tumor cells. Prior to proceeding with radioiodine ablation, the patient's serum TSH level should be greater than 30 µIU/mL to enhance radioiodine uptake by the residual normal follicular cells and tumor cells. A 30 mCi dose of ^{131}I can be given on an outpatient basis and is successful in ablating residual thyroid cells in 80% of patients. A whole-body scan is routinely performed 2 to 5 days after thyroid ablation to evaluate for residual uptake. If residual thyroid tissue remains following the first ablative therapy, a second dose of 30 mCi of ^{131}I may be given 6 to 12 months later.

Thyroid hormone is administered postoperatively for treatment of hypothyroidism and to reduce serum TSH, which has been shown to stimulate tumor growth, invasion, and angiogenesis. TSH-suppressive doses of thyroid hormone have been shown to reduce recurrence and cancer-specific mortality rates. Following radioiodine ablation, patients are started on levothyroxine at a dose of 2 µg/kg per day, and serum TSH is measured 5 to 6 weeks later. The goal is to maintain the serum TSH level between 0.1 to 0.5 µIU/mL, for patients with high-risk DTC who are free of disease, and between 0.3 to 2.0 µIU/mL for patients with low-risk DTC. In patients with metastatic disease, the levothyroxine dose is adjusted to maintain a serum TSH level less than 0.1 µIU/mL.

External beam radiation plays a limited role in the management of patients with DTC. It is indicated for patients in whom complete surgical excision is not possible and for tumors that do not concentrate radioiodine. It may also be used for patients with extrathyroidal tumor spread and extracapsular lymph node spread because of a high likelihood of residual disease, and it is used for palliation of bone pain in patients with skeletal metastases and for unresectable brain metastases. Chemotherapy has minimal benefit in the management of DTC and is rarely used.

Long-term follow-up of patients with DTC includes physical examination, serum TSH and basal thyroglobulin (Tg) levels, anti-Tg antibody measurement, and neck ultrasound. Surveillance should be performed every 6 months for 2 years and then annually, if the patient remains disease free. Neck ultrasound should be performed yearly after the initial resection. Tg is a glycoprotein produced by normal and neoplastic thyroid tissue, and its level should be undetectable after total thyroidectomy and radioiodine ablation. Tg production is also reliant on the serum TSH concentration; therefore Tg is a reliable tumor marker and, in the setting of a high TSH level, an undetectable Tg excludes residual or metastatic disease in 99% of patients. Anti-Tg antibodies, found in 25% of patients with DTC, can interfere with the accuracy of the Tg measurements and are a cause for both false-positive and false-negative results.

For patients with negative Tg levels, a negative radioiodine whole-body scan, and negative neck ultrasound, routine radioiodine scans are unnecessary. In patients with an elevated serum Tg level and a negative neck ultrasound, radioiodine whole-body scanning is indicated to help localize metastatic disease. We advocate whole-body scanning when the serum Tg is greater than 3 ng/dL while on thyroid hormone or greater than 10 ng/dL when a patient is off thyroid hormone. In patients who cannot tolerate withdrawal of thyroid hormone, recombinant human TSH is used to facilitate the measurement of Tg, avoiding the morbidity associated with hypothyroidism. Studies have found a 90% concordance for Tg measurement in patients following thyroid hormone withdrawal and measurement following recombinant human TSH administration.

DTC will recur in 20% to 40% of patients, and the incidence is generally the greatest in the first 2 years. Metastatic disease can occur in up to 10% to 15% of patients and most often will involve the lung or bone. Patients with metastatic disease are treated with radioiodine in therapeutic doses ranging from 150 to 200 mCi, and a response rate of 45% has been seen in patients with distant metastases that concentrate iodine. The 10 year survival rate for patients with DTC and metastatic disease ranges from 25% to 40%.

Patients with metastatic or locally unresectable DTC that does not concentrate radioiodine should be referred for appropriate clinical trials (http://www.clinicaltrials.gov). New molecular-based therapies are being investigated for metastatic thyroid cancer that is radioiodine unresponsive; these include multikinase inhibitors that target receptors for vascular endothelial growth factor and epithelial growth factor, nuclear receptor antagonists to restore radioiodine uptake, and celecoxib, thalidomide, proteasome inhibitors, histone deacetylase inhibitors, and DNA-methylation inhibitors.

MEDULLARY THYROID CANCER

Medullary thyroid cancer (MTC) is a neuroendocrine tumor that arises from the parafollicular or C cells of the thyroid gland. It accounts for 4% of all thyroid malignancies. Patients with MTC have elevated serum calcitonin levels and may also have elevated carcinoembryonic antigen (CEA) and calcitonin gene-related peptide (CGRP) levels. MTC is sporadic in 70% to 80% of cases. Sporadic MTC is usually confined to one lobe of the thyroid gland, however, multicentric or bilateral disease can be present in 30% of patients. MTC is familial in 20% to 30% of patients, occurring as part of the MEN2A, MEN2B (Table 5), or isolated familial MTC (FMTC) syndromes, all of which have an autosomal-dominant inheritance and result from germline mutations in the *RET* protooncogene. Germline DNA testing for *RET* gene mutations is recommended for all patients with MTC regardless of family history, because approximately 10% of patients with apparent sporadic MTC will have a de novo mutation in the *RET* protooncogene.

Patients with familial MTC have multicentric and bilateral disease, often with diffuse C cell hyperplasia. MEN2A is the most common familial syndrome, making up two thirds of all hereditary MTC. Patients usually present in the third or fourth decade of life, and 90% of gene carriers will develop MTC, 60% will develop unilateral or bilateral pheochromocytoma, and 15% to 30% will develop

TABLE 5: MEN2A and 2B

MEN 2A

Medullary thyroid carcinoma
Pheochromocytoma
Hyperparathyroidism
Lichen planus amyloidosis
Hirschsprung disease

MEN 2B

Medullary thyroid carcinoma
Pheochromocytoma
Muscuskeletal abnormality (*marfanoid habitus, pes cavas, pectus excavatum*)
Mucosal neuromas of the lips, tongue, and conjunctiva
Ganglioneuromatosis of the gastrointestinal tract
Medullated corneal nerve fibers

hyperparathyroidism. *Familiar medullary thyroid cancer (FMTC)*, a variant of MEN2A, is defined as the presence of MTC in four or more affected family members without other manifestations of MEN2A (see Table 5). Patients are typically diagnosed later in life than patients with MEN2A, and the penetrance of MTC is lower.

MEN2B is the rarest and most virulent of the hereditary MTC syndromes. It can be distinguished from MEN2A by the presence of developmental defects and the absence of hyperparathyroidism (see Table 5). The average age of onset of MTC for patients diagnosed with MEN2B is 10 years. All patients have neurogangliomas, and 50% develop pheochromocytoma. Fifty percent or more of MEN2B cases occur as a result of de novo germline *RET* mutations.

Most patients with MTC present with a thyroid nodule, however, only 0.3% to 1.4% of all patients with a thyroid nodule will have MTC. The diagnosis of MTC is established by FNAB with immunohistochemical staining for calcitonin. At the time of presentation, 75% of patients with a palpable MTC will have cervical lymph node metastases, and 5% of patients will have systemic metastases, which most commonly involve the lung, liver, or bone. Patients with advanced disease may also have diarrhea or facial flushing related to tumor secretion of calcitonin or Cushing syndrome related to secretion of corticotrophin. Patients with a known family history of MTC may present with an elevated screening calcitonin level before MTC is clinically evident.

Preoperatively, all patients diagnosed with MTC should undergo testing for mutations in the *RET* protooncogene. Serum calcitonin and CEA levels should be measured to determine if these are being produced by the tumor and to establish a baseline for comparison with levels after surgery. High preoperative serum calcitonin levels correlate with tumor bulk, lymph node metastases, and systemic metastases, and high CEA levels are associated with a poorer prognosis. Because of the possibility of MEN2 disease, all patients with MTC should have serum calcium level and either plasma free metanephrines or 24 hour urinary catecholamines and metanephrines measured prior to operation to screen for hyperparathyroidism and pheochromocytoma. A coexisting pheochromocytoma should be treated prior to the thyroidectomy.

Preoperative imaging is indicated in selected patients who are diagnosesd with MTC to determine the extent of local neck disease and the presence of systemic metastases, which may alter the surgical approach. An ultrasound of the neck is indicated to evaluate for abnormal lymph nodes in the central and lateral neck in all patients. Additional imaging studies are reserved for patients with lymph node metastases or a serum calcitonin level over 400 pg/mL, which raises concern for systemic metastases. CT of the neck, chest, and upper abdomen is useful to evaluate for possible tumor invasion of the upper aerodigestive tract and metastases to

TABLE 6: Stage groupings for MTC

Stage I	T1N0M0
Stage II	T2N0M0
Stage III	T3N0M0, T1N1aM0, T2N1aM0, T3N1aM0
Stage IVa	T4aN0M0, T4aN1aM0, T1N1bM0, T2N1bM0, T3N1bM0, T4N1bM0
Stage IVb	T4b, any N, M0
Stage IVc	Any T, any N, M1

the mediastinal lymph nodes, lungs, and liver. Magnetic resonance imaging (MRI) is the most sensitive imaging modality for detection of liver metastases, and it is complementary with bone scintigraphy for detection of bone metastases. Diagnostic laparoscopy has been advocated prior to initial operation in patients with marked hypercalcitoninemia (>1000 pg/mL) to document the presence of liver disease. Staging of MTC is based on tumor size, extrathyroidal tumor spread, local or regional lymph node metastases, and systemic metastases (Table 6).

The mainstay of treatment of MTC is surgical. Total thyroidectomy is the preferred treatment for all patients with MTC, because 30% of patients with sporadic MTC and all patients with familial MTC have multicentric or bilateral disease. MTC spreads to the lymph nodes in the central neck in 50% of patients with sporadic and hereditary MTC. The ATA recommends a total thyroidectomy and a routine central compartment (level VI) neck dissection for patients with clinically detectable MTC and no evidence of distant metastases. A modified neck dissection is performed in patients with metastatic lymph nodes in the central or lateral neck, removing lymph nodes from levels II, III, IV, and V (see Figure 2). The frequency of lymph node involvement is high in MTC, and the presence of lymph node metastases in the central neck is a risk factor for lateral node involvement. Unfortunately, patients with regional lymph node metastases are rarely biochemically cured, even with aggressive bilateral neck dissection.

Routine genetic testing is performed in children who have a parent with hereditary MTC. Prophylactic total thyroidectomy is recommended within the first year of life in patients with *RET* germline mutations for MEN 2B and within 3 to 5 years in patients with *RET* germline mutations for MEN 2A and FMTC. The goal is to treat the patient before serum calcitonin levels become elevated and prior to the development of lymph node or systemic metastases, so the patient can be cured. Furthermore, it obviates the need for a central compartment lymph node dissection and its risk of hypoparathyroidism, unless there is a thyroid nodule or clinical or radiologic evidence of lymph node metastases.

Postoperatively, patients are started on a replacement dose of thyroid hormone. In contrast to DTC, patients with MTC are not treated with TSH-suppressive doses of thyroid hormone or radioiodine, because the C cells of the thyroid gland are not responsive to TSH, and they do not concentrate radioiodine. Subsequent follow-up consists of periodic physical examination and measurement of serum calcitonin and CEA levels to detect recurrent disease. In patients with a calcitonin level less than 150 pg/mL, an ultrasound of the neck is often sufficient for further evaluation. Ultrasound is the most sensitive examination for identification of persistent disease in the neck. However, when serum calcitonin levels remain persistently high, especially in the case of patients with lymph node involvement, further imaging is necessary to locate other potential sites of metastases. The recommended imaging studies include CT of the chest, MRI of the liver, and bone scintigraphy.

Prognosis is related to disease stage. The 10 year survival is approximately 75% but decreases to 45% in patients with lymph node

involvement. External beam radiation therapy to the neck and upper mediastinum is not endorsed by the ATA as a substitute for surgery or as a general adjuvant therapy for patients with elevated calcitonin postoperatively. External beam radiation therapy, however, is an option for grossly positive or microscopically positive margins following surgery and for high-volume disease involving the central and lateral compartments of the neck.

ANAPLASTIC THYROID CARCINOMA

Anaplastic thyroid carcinoma (ATC) is a rare undifferentiated form of cancer that arises from the follicular cells of the thyroid gland. However, it does not retain any of the biological features of the follicular cells, including uptake of iodine and the synthesis of Tg. ATC may arise de novo, but most appear to arise from a preexisting, well-differentiated thyroid cancer. It accounts for approximately 2% of all thyroid malignancies and is almost always rapidly fatal. *BRAF* and *RAS* mutations commonly seen in PTC are also seen in patients with ATC.

Patients with ATC are older than patients with DTC, usually in their sixth to seventh decade at diagnosis. They often have a history of a multinodular goiter, and their primary symptom is a rapidly enlarging neck mass that is firm, tender, and fixed to surrounding structures. Patients have neck pain and compressive symptoms related to invasion of the aerodigestive tract, and they also may have systemic manifestations that include weight loss, anorexia, and fatigue. On physical examination, patients have marked bilateral thyroid enlargement that is nodular and hard with substernal extension and indistinct borders. The trachea is often not palpable because of the extent of the overlying tumor mass, and associated cervical lymphadenopathy is common. Vocal cord paralysis, facial edema, and venous dilation may be present as a result of invasion of the recurrent laryngeal nerve and the superior vena cava.

The diagnosis of ATC is established by FNAB or core needle biopsy. Open biopsy may be necessary, particularly when there is extensive necrosis. Ultrasound can be of help in identifying a nonnecrotic area for FNAB, and CT of the neck and chest is of value for determining the extent of disease and identifying invasion of the aerodigestive tract, retrosternal extension, superior vena cava syndrome, and pulmonary metastases. At the time of diagnosis, 90% of patients will have regional or systemic metastases. Systemic metastases occur in the lung in 90% of patients and less commonly in the bone and the brain.

Most patients with ATC present with advanced disease, and as a result, there is no role for surgery other than to establish a diagnosis. Thyroidectomy may be indicated for the rare patient with disease limited to the thyroid gland. Multimodal treatment that consists of external beam radiation and chemotherapy for local control of the disease is the conventional therapy for most patients with ATC. Radiosensitizing doses of doxorubicin are often combined with hyperfractionated radiation to improve the local response rate. Paclitaxel is the most effective chemotherapeutic agent for treatment of ATC, and tracheostomy may be performed in patients with impending airway obstruction.

All patients with ATC are classified as having stage IV (Table 7) disease. The median survival for ATC is approximately 5 to 6 months. Survival rates at 1 year are 20% to 35% and are 5% to 14% at 5 years. Patients ultimately die from asphyxiation as a result of airway obstruction and less commonly as a result of systemic metastases. Currently, there are three active clinical trials using molecular-based therapies for ATC. The agents being investigated include trials using gefitinib and axitinib, both of which are tyrosine kinase inhibitors, and combretastatin A4 phosphate, which inhibits tubulin polymerization. Patients who were treated with gefitinib showed reduction in tumor volume and a longer stable disease interval than untreated patients. Although these features did not meet the criteria for partial response, it does indicate that gefitinib has some biologic activity against anaplastic tumor cells. So far, none of these novel agents have been shown to have significant efficacy against ATC.

TABLE 7: Stage groupings for anaplastic thyroid carcinoma

Stage IVa	T4a, any N, M0
Stage IVb	T4b, any N, M0
Stage IVc	Any T, any N, M1

All anaplastic carcinomas are considered stage IV.

LYMPHOMA

Primary lymphoma of the thyroid gland accounts for only 2% of extranodal lymphomas and less than 1% of all thyroid malignancies. Most primary thyroid lymphomas are non-Hodgkin diffuse large B-cell type. Over 50% of thyroid lymphomas arise in a background of Hashimoto thyroiditis, which is the only known risk factor for primary thyroid lymphoma. Patients with Hashimoto thyroiditis are 60 to 80 times more likely to develop thyroid lymphoma than the general population. Lymphoma of the mucosa-associated lymphoid tissue (MALT) is the next most common subtype, and it is also generally associated with Hashimoto thyroiditis. T-cell lymphoma and Hodgkin disease have also been described.

The presenting signs and symptoms of lymphoma can mimic those of ATC. Patients are typically women in their seventh decade of life, who present with difficulty breathing and a rapidly enlarging neck mass. Patients may have dysphagia, dyspnea, hoarseness, stridor, or facial edema from compression of the esophagus, trachea, recurrent laryngeal nerve, or the superior vena cava. They may have a history of goiter and/or hypothyroidism. Systemic manifestations that include fever, night sweats, weight loss, and anorexia may also occur. A diagnosis of lymphoma should always be considered in a patient with known Hashimoto thyroiditis with an enlarging goiter.

On physical examination, patients typically have marked bilateral thyroid enlargements with substernal extension. The thyroid gland is hard and is often fixed to surrounding structures, and patients frequently have associated cervical lymphadenopathy. The initial workup consists of a serum TSH level, an antimicrosomal antibody titer, and an FNAB; to make a definitive diagnosis of lymphoma, FNAB with flow cytometry, and occasionally core needle biopsy, is necessary. An open biopsy with immunohistochemical studies is usually necessary to determine the specific cell type of lymphoma. CT of the neck, chest, and abdomen, FDG-PET scanning, and bone marrow biopsy are used to determine the stage of the disease (Table 8).

Thyroid lymphoma is highly responsive to both chemotherapy and radiotherapy. Patients with diffuse, large B-cell lymphoma of the thyroid gland are treated with a combination of cyclophosphamide, doxorubicin, vincristine, and prednisone. Patients usually experience a dramatic decrease in the size of their goiters within hours of initiation of prednisone therapy. Patients with MALT lymphoma may be treated with radiation alone; chemotherapy is added for more advanced disease. Thyroidectomy has a limited role in the management of lymphoma. It has been curative in rare patients with disease confined to the thyroid gland (stage IE), in whom the diagnosis was not established preoperatively. Surgical intervention is usually reserved for diagnostic biopsy alone.

Prognosis depends on the histologic grade of the tumor and the disease stage. Poor prognostic factors include advanced stage, a tumor greater than 10 cm, mediastinal involvement, age greater than 65, and dysphagia. Patients with primary thyroid lymphoma will have stage IE in 50%, IIE in 45%, and either IIIE or IV in 5% of cases. Overall 5-year survival for patients with thyroid lymphoma ranges from 50% to 70%. For patients with stage IE or IIE disease treated with combined modality therapy, 5-year survival rates as high as 90% have been reported.

TABLE 8: Staging classification for thyroid lymphoma based on the Ann Arbor classification for non-Hodgkin lymphoma

Stage IE	Localized disease within the thyroid gland
Stage IIE	Disease confined to the thyroid gland and the regional lymph nodes on one side of the diaphragm
Stage IIIE	Disease in the thyroid gland with involvement of lymph node regions on both sides of the diaphragm
Stage IV	Disseminated disease

All cases are subclassfied to indicate the absence or presence of systemic symptoms of unexplained fever, night sweats, and weight loss exceeding 10% of body weight during the 6 months prior to diagnosis.

TECHNIQUE OF THYROIDECTOMY

The patient is placed in a supine position with the arms tucked at the sides and a soft roll placed lengthwise beneath the shoulders to extend the neck. This will optimize the exposure of the thyroid gland. A soft foam headrest is used to stabilize the head. A transverse collar incision is made approximately two fingerbreadths above the sternal notch along a normal skin crease. The subcutaneous tissue and the platysma muscle are divided. Skin flaps are raised in a subplatysmal plane to the level of the thyroid cartilage superiorly, the sternal notch inferiorly, and the sternocleidomastoid muscles laterally. The strap muscles are separated in the midline along the median raphe from the prominence of the thyroid cartilage to the sternal notch. Division of the sternohyoid and sternothyroid muscles may be necessary in patients with very large cancers, or when these muscles are invaded by the cancer, but these are otherwise not routinely divided. The middle thyroid vein is divided, and the lobe of thyroid is mobilized anteromedially.

The superior pole vessels are identified by exerting downward traction on the upper pole of the thyroid gland. The superior thyroid vessels are individually ligated close to the thyroid gland to avoid injury to the external branch of the superior laryngeal nerve (Figure 3). Next, the areolar tissue between the common carotid artery and the thyroid lobe is dissected using a combination of blunt and sharp techniques, facilitating the anterior and medial rotation of the thyroid lobe.

With the lobe of the thyroid gland retracted anteromedially, the inferior thyroid artery is delineated, and the recurrent laryngeal nerve is identified and is traced through its entire course and preserved; routine exposure of the recurrent laryngeal nerve has been shown to reduce the rate of nerve injury. Intraoperative nerve monitoring is not necessary and should not be used in lieu of routine exposure of the recurrent laryngeal nerve.

Once the recurrent laryngeal nerve has been identified, the inferior pole of the thyroid gland is mobilized by ligating the tertiary branches of the arteries and veins close to the thyroid gland to preserve the blood supply to the inferior parathyroid gland (Figure 4). The anterior surface of the trachea is exposed; simultaneous anteromedial retraction of the superior and inferior poles of the thyroid lobe enhances the exposure of the recurrent laryngeal nerve cephalad to the inferior thyroid artery (Figure 5). The remaining branches of the inferior thyroid artery are ligated and divided close to the thyroid parenchyma, and the remaining thyroid lobe and ligament of Berry are separated from the recurrent laryngeal nerve, preserving the blood supply to the superior parathyroid gland.

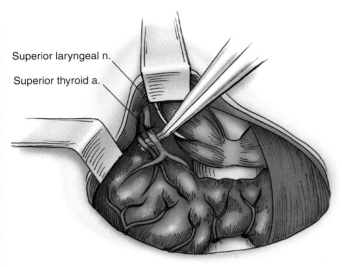

Superior laryngeal n.

Superior thyroid a.

FIGURE 3 Ligation of the superior pole vessels of the thyroid gland. *(Courtesy Michael T. Muster, Medical Illustrator, MetroHealth Medical Center. From McHenry CR: Thyroidectomy for nodules or small cancers. In Duh Q, editor: Atlas of endocrine surgical techniques, Philadelphia, 2009, Saunders Elsevier.)*

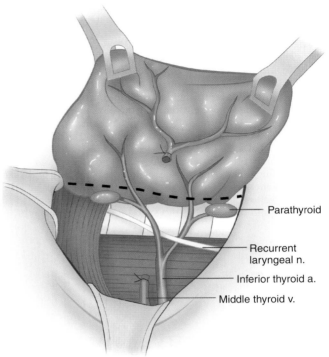

Parathyroid

Recurrent laryngeal n.

Inferior thyroid a.

Middle thyroid v.

FIGURE 5 Exposure of the recurrent laryngeal nerve. *(Courtesy Michael T. Muster, Medical Illustrator, MetroHealth Medical Center. From McHenry CR: Thyroidectomy for nodules or small cancers. In Duh Q, editor: Atlas of endocrine surgical techniques, Philadelphia, 2009, Saunders Elsevier.)*

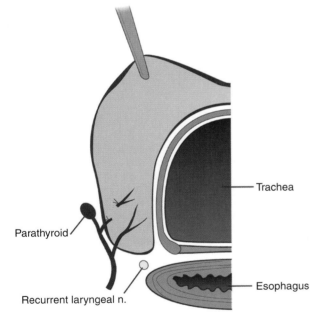

Trachea

Parathyroid

Recurrent laryngeal n.

Esophagus

FIGURE 4 Mobilization of the inferior pole of the thyroid gland, preserving the blood supply to the inferior parathyroid gland. *(Courtesy Michael T. Muster, Medical Illustrator, MetroHealth Medical Center. From McHenry CR: Thyroidectomy for nodules or small cancers. In Duh Q, editor: Atlas of endocrine surgical techniques, Philadelphia, 2009, Saunders Elsevier.)*

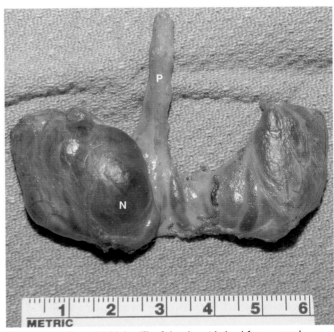

FIGURE 6 Pyramidal lobe (*P*) of the thyroid gland from a total thyroidectomy showing a nodule (*N*). *(Courtesy Vince Messina, Biomedical Photographer, MetroHealth Medical Center. From McHenry CR: Thyroidectomy for nodules or small cancers. In Duh Q, editor: Atlas of endocrine surgical techniques, Philadelphia, 2009, Saunders Elsevier.)*

Attempts should be made to visualize the parathyroid glands during thyroidectomy. It is usually possible to separate them from the surface of the thyroid gland and preserve them in situ. When it is not possible to preserve a parathyroid gland in situ, a small piece is sent for frozen-section analysis to confirm the presence of parathyroid tissue. The remainder of the gland is sliced into multiple sections and autotransplanted into the sternocleidomastoid muscle in patients with DTC, sporadic MTC, MTC of MEN2B, and FMTC. Devascularized parathyroid glands in patients with MEN2A and a *RET* mutation are associated with a high risk of hyperparathyroidism and should be autotransplanted into the brachioradialis muscle of the nondominant forearm. Parathyroid autotransplantation will minimize the risk of postoperative hypoparathyroidism.

Once the lobe of the thyroid gland has been separated from the recurrent laryngeal nerve, the remainder of the ligament of Berry can be divided sharply, separating the isthmus from the trachea. At this point, the pyramidal lobe of the thyroid gland should be resected (Figure 6). It is present in the midline in approximately 50% of patients, arising from the isthmus or the medial aspect of one of the thyroid lobes and extending to the hyoid bone. When it is not resected, it is the site for persistent radioiodine uptake after surgery and is a potential site for persistent disease.

The contralateral lobe of the thyroid gland is removed in an identical fashion. Once the thyroidectomy has been completed, the sternohyoid muscles are reapproximated in the midline, leaving the inferior aspect open over a distance of 3 to 4 cm to allow blood to decompress into the subcutaneous space if bleeding develops. This will help prevent or delay the onset of respiratory compromise in the rare patient who develops a neck hematoma. A drain is not used.

SUGGESTED READINGS

Chen AY, Jemal A, Ward EM: Increasing incidence of differentiated thyroid cancer in the United States: 1988-2005, *Cancer* 115(16):3801–3807, 2009.

Cooper DS, Doherty G, Haugen BR, et al: Management guidelines for patients with thyroid nodules and differentiated thyroid cancer, *Thyroid* 16(2):109–142, 2006.

Rosenbaum MA, McHenry CR: Contemporary management of papillary carcinoma of the thyroid gland, *Expert Rev Anticancer Ther* 9(3):317–329, 2009.

Kloos RT, Eng C, Evans DB, et al: Medullary thyroid cancer: management guidelines of the American Thyroid Association, *Thyroid* 19(6):565–612, 2009.

Phitayakorn R, McHenry CR: Follicular and Hurthle cell carcinoma of the thyroid gland, *Surg Oncol Clin North Am* 15(3):603–623, 2006.

PRIMARY HYPERPARATHYROIDISM

Herbert Chen, MD

DIAGNOSIS AND INDICATIONS FOR SURGERY

Primary hyperparathyroidism (HPT) is the most common cause of hypercalcemia. Most patients are diagnosed incidentally during routine laboratory screening or in the evaluation for other illnesses. Common symptoms and signs include bone pain or osteopenia/osteoporosis, kidney stones, constipation, urinary frequency and incontinence, pancreatitis, fatigue, muscle weakness, joint pain, difficulty concentrating, nausea, and vomiting. Patients with primary HPT typically show both elevated serum calcium and intact parathyroid hormone (PTH) levels, often termed *classic* disease (Table 1, patient 1). However, it is important to note that patients with primary HPT may only have a high calcium or PTH on any individual day of testing. Furthermore, a substantial number of patients will also have an elevated serum calcium and a normal but nonsuppressed PTH level (Table 1, patient 2). These patients definitely have primary HPT, because the PTH level should be undetectable when hypercalcemia is due to causes other than HPT. In addition, patients with primary HPT can also have serum calcium in the high normal range with an elevated PTH (Table 1, patient 3). After ruling out and/or treating vitamin D deficiency, if the PTH remains high, the individuals also have primary HPT. In the literature, patients 2 and 3 would often be categorized as having *mild* HPT. However, recent data suggest that, in fact, patients 2 and 3 may have more severe HPT and may benefit more from surgical intervention.

The most common cause of primary HPT is a single parathyroid adenoma (80%); other likely causes are double adenoma (5% to 10%), hyperplasia (5% to 10%), and parathyroid cancer (<1%). Any of these etiologies can be seen in individuals with familial HPT, however, HPT occurs in virtually all patients with multiple endocrine neoplasia type 1 (MEN 1) and in 25% of patients with MEN 2A.

Surgery remains the only curative therapy for primary HPT. All physicians agree that patients with overt symptoms and signs of HPT should be referred for surgery. In patients who are asymptomatic, some controversy exists as to the benefit of surgery. Consensus guidelines recommend surgery for asymptomatic patients with reduced renal function or osteoporosis (T score ≤−2.5, <50 years of age, and a serum calcium ≥1.0 mg/dL above the normal range). However, emerging data from multiple investigators have shown that surgical management of primary HPT is associated with several benefits (Table 2). Thus I strongly believe that all patients with primary HPT who do not have prohibitive operative risks should be offered parathyroidectomy as the definitive treatment.

Parathyroid Localization

After making the biochemical diagnosis of primary HPT, I usually proceed with a parathyroid localization study. In the past, it was often stated that the best localization study for an abnormal parathyroid gland is an experienced surgeon. Although that statement still may be true today, with the advent of focused or minimally invasive parathyroidectomy, I believe that virtually all patients should undergo parathyroid imaging prior to surgery. It is important to recognize that localization studies are meant to *localize* the abnormal parathyroid glands, not confirm the diagnosis; therefore, patients with negative localization studies *still* have the diagnosis of primary HPT.

I generally utilize the parathyroid imaging protocol shown in Figure 1, starting with a technetium-99m sestamibi scan with single photon emission computed tomography (SPECT). At our institution, about 70% to 75% of patients will have a positive SPECT scan finding, and we would then proceed with a minimally invasive parathyroidectomy. In patients with negative results from a SPECT scan, I usually obtain a cervical ultrasound; if results are positive for disease, I recommend a minimally invasive approach.

In patients with negative SPECT and ultrasound scan results, I perform bilateral internal jugular venous sampling in the operating room. With this technique, a 22 gauge needle under ultrasound guidance is used to sample blood from both internal jugular veins prior to surgical incision, and the samples are sent for intraoperative PTH levels. If there is more than a 10% difference between the PTH levels, the test is considered positive, or lateralizing, and a minimally invasive parathyroidectomy is attempted on the side with the higher PTH level. In cases of reoperative parathyroidectomy, I occasionally use magnetic resonance imaging scans to localize parathyroid adenomas, especially with equivocal results from a SPECT scan or an ultrasound examination.

TABLE 1: Diagnosis of primary hyperparathyroidism

Patient Laboratory Values	Diagnosis of Primary Hyperparathyroidism?
Serum calcium = 11.0 mg/dL Intact PTH = 92 pg/mL	Yes, classic disease
Serum calcium = 11.2 mg/dL Intact PTH = 49 pg/mL	Yes, mild disease
Serum calcium = 9.9 mg/dL Intact PTH = 81 pg/mL	Probably mild disease, but rule out vitamin D deficiency

Normal serum calcium = 8.5 to 10.2 mg/dL; normal intact PTH = 10 to 72 pg/mL.

TABLE 2: Benefits from surgical management of primary HPT

- Renal function and bone density improvement
- Resolution of neuropsychiatric symptoms
- Quality of life better
- Prolongs survival (10% reduction if untreated)
- Reduction in cardiovascular incidents
- Low complication rates
- Cost of parathyroidectomy at 5 years is less than the cost of surveillance

Intraoperative Adjuncts

I use the following two adjuncts for virtually all patients undergoing surgery for primary HPT: the γ-probe and intraoperative PTH testing. Radioguided parathyroidectomy utilizing the γ-probe is based upon the principle that hyperfunctioning parathyroid glands take up and retain sestamibi longer than surrounding tissues. Thus, a handheld γ-probe can be used to localize the parathyroid gland intraoperatively to confirm that it is hyperfunctioning. It is important to realize that *radioguided surgery is effective for all patients with HPT*, even those with results that are apparently "negative" on sestamibi scans.

For the procedure, the patient receives an injection of 10 mCi of sestamibi about 1 hour prior to surgery. In the operating room, a background count is set by scanning the thyroid isthmus with the γ-probe (Figure 2). After incision, the γ-probe is utilized to scan for in vivo counts that are higher than the background counts (Figure 3). Once the abnormal parathyroid gland has been resected, the tissue is placed on the probe for an ex vivo count (Figure 4). If the ratio of ex vivo to ex vivo background counts is 20% or greater, the resected mass is hyperfunctioning parathyroid tissue. We and others have previously reported that radioguided techniques during parathyroidectomy are associated with a shorter operative time; they also facilitate intraoperative localization and dissection and are useful in reoperative cases.

Intraoperative PTH testing is an important adjunct for parathyroid surgery, because it allows confirmation that all hyperfunctioning parathyroid tissue has been excised. It is based upon the principle that PTH has a half-life of 2 to 4 minutes; therefore 5 minutes after resection of a single adenoma, the PTH level in the bloodstream should fall by 50%. However, if a second hyperfunctioning gland is present, the PTH levels should not fall by 50%, prompting the surgeon to explore for an additional abnormal parathyroid. Intraoperative PTH can also be utilized for intraoperative localization (lateralization) of a hyperfunctioning parathyroid gland by sampling the internal jugular veins as described above. Several groups, including ours, have shown that intraoperative PTH sampling increases the operative success rate for parathyroid surgery.

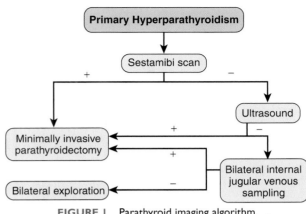

FIGURE 1 Parathyroid imaging algorithm.

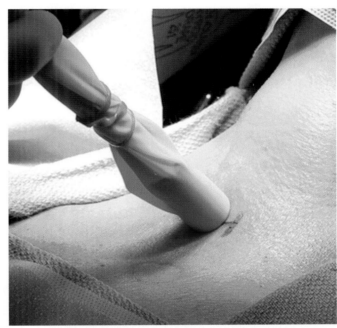

FIGURE 2 Background counting on the thyroid isthmus.

MINIMALLY INVASIVE OR FOCUSED PARATHYROIDECTOMY

Based upon positive localization studies (see Figure 1), we would begin our operation by targeting the lesion seen on the imaging study with a unilateral exploration. About an hour before the operation, the patient is given 10 mCi Tc-99m sestamibi intravenously to use with the γ-probe. In the operating room, the patient is placed in the beach-chair position with a head ring and an inflatable IV bag behind the shoulders to facilitate neck extension. A second peripheral IV is placed, and a blood sample is obtained for the baseline PTH level. A background reading with the γ-probe is made by obtaining the radiocounts on the thyroid isthmus (see Figure 2). A 1.5 to 3 cm incision is made transversely in a skin fold just below the cricoid cartilage, and the platysma is divided transversely; I do not raise any subplatysmal flaps for parathyroid surgery. The strap muscles are separated vertically in the midline, and the muscles are separated from the thyroid. The thyroid gland is rolled medially with a Kittner dissector, sometimes dividing the middle thyroid vein if the thyroid is enlarged, and the γ-probe is inserted to scan for in vivo counts above the background counts.

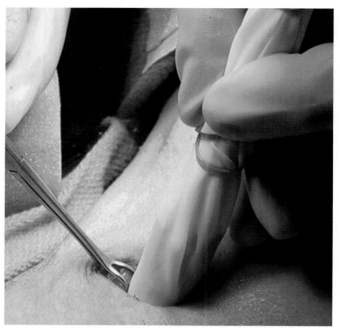

FIGURE 3   In vivo search for the enlarged parathyroid gland.

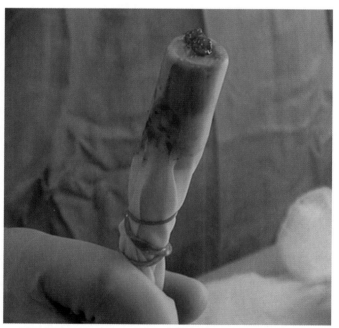

FIGURE 4   Ex vivo counting of the resected parathyroid gland.

Once the area of sustained radiocounts above the background is located, I dissect the enlarged parathyroid with a sharp clamp and divide its vascular pedicle with a small clip. The excised parathyroid gland is placed on top of the γ-probe, and an ex vivo count is obtained. If the ratio of ex vivo to ex vivo counts is 20% or greater, the resected mass is hyperfunctioning parathyroid tissue. PTH levels from the second peripheral IV are measured 5, 10, and 15 minutes after resection of the gland. A decrease in PTH by more than 50% from the baseline level indicates that all hyperfunctioning parathyroid tissue has been resected.

If the PTH falls by more than 50% at any of the time points, the strap muscles are closed with a running 2-0 vicryl suture, and the platysma is closed with a running 3-0 vicryl. Marcaine (0.25%) is injected

---

TABLE 3: Steps to find a missing parathyroid gland

1. Perform bilateral internal jugular venous sampling for PTH.
2. Look in the retroesophageal space.
3. Perform a cervical thymectomy.
4. Open the carotid sheath.
5. Search for an undescended gland, occasionally found in undescended thymic tissue.
6. Perform intraoperative ultrasound of the thyroid gland.
7. If the gland cannot be found, terminate the operation, leaving normal parathyroid gland intact.

---

locally, and the skin is closed with a 5-0 prolene suture, which is removed 1 week later. If the PTH does not fall by more than 50%, the other parathyroid gland is scanned with the γ-probe and visualized. If it is enlarged and has in vivo counts higher than the background, the second gland is resected, ex vivo counts are measured, and PTH levels are again obtained at 5, 10, and 15 minutes after removal of that gland. If the PTH falls by more than 50% from the original baseline level, then the operation is terminated. However, if the PTH does not fall, the procedure is converted to a bilateral exploration. The contralateral side of the neck is explored in a similar manner with the γ-probe.

Bilateral Neck Exploration

Open bilateral neck exploration was previously the preferred operation for patients with primary HPT. Today, the bilateral approach is still utilized when 1) the intraoperative PTH level did not fall after unilateral exploration; 2) parathyroid localization studies are negative; 3) suspected four-gland hyperplasia is suspected, such as when multiple endocrine neoplasia type 1 (MEN 1) is present; and 4) the surgeon or patient prefers it.

I perform this operation in a similar manner to unilateral exploration. I make the incision, typically less than 3 cm, in the same location. The γ-probe and intraoperative PTH testing are also employed in the same manner. All four parathyroid glands are identified but not biopsied. The inferior parathyroid glands are usually located just posterior to the inferior thyroid lobe and anterior and medial to the recurrent laryngeal nerve. Sometimes, the gland can be found within the thymus. The superior parathyroid is frequently found posterior to the upper pole of the thyroid just lateral to the insertion of the recurrent nerve into the larynx.

If four-gland hyperplasia is found, a subtotal parathyroidectomy (3.5 gland resection) or a total parathyroidectomy with forearm implantation is performed. In patients with MEN 1 and in young patients with nonfamilial four-gland disease, I prefer a total parathyroidectomy with implantation of 5 to 10 small pieces (1 by 3 mm) of parathyroid tissue to the nondominant forearm muscle. When performing a total parathyroidectomy, it is critical to cryopreserve nontransplanted parathyroid tissue, in case the forearm implant is not fully functional, thereby allowing implantation of additional tissue in the future if needed. Implanted parathyroid tissue typically does not function for 2 to 4 weeks, so patients must take oral calcium and calcitriol during this time. In older patients with four-gland disease, or in those patients who cannot tolerate transient hypocalcemia, I prefer a subtotal parathyroidectomy. It is important to perform the partial resection on the parathyroid remnant prior to resecting the remaining glands, in the event that the remnant becomes ischemic. If the remnant has questionable vascular flow, then another gland should be selected for the remnant, and the ischemic gland should be resected.

In the event that the abnormal parathyroid gland cannot be located, we generally go through the steps in Table 3. If the missing gland is not found, then it is important to document which parathyroid glands were identified and what areas were explored. Normal parathyroid glands should never be resected, and a median sternotomy should never be performed in the absence of definitive localization to the mediastinum.

Parathyroid cancer is rarely a cause of primary HPT, but parathyroid cancer should be suspected in patients who present with very high calcium (>14.0 mg/dL) and PTH (>300 pg/mL) levels. Intraoperatively, a cancerous parathyroid gland is rock hard and usually adherent to the thyroid gland. Definitive treatment is an en bloc resection with an ipsilateral thyroid lobectomy and central lymph node dissection if enlarged nodes are present.

FOLLOW-UP CARE

I normally see patients 1 week after parathyroid surgery to remove their skin prolene suture and obtain calcium and PTH levels. About 20% to 25% will have an elevated PTH in the setting of normal postoperative calcium. This may be due to vitamin D deficiency and/or a reactionary secondary HPT. Appropriate vitamin D and calcium supplementation will lead to resolution of the elevated PTH; we obtain a serum calcium and PTH after 6 months. Cure after parathyroid surgery is defined as a normal serum calcium more than 6 months postoperatively. We generally recommend that patients have yearly serum calcium levels after successful parathyroidectomy, because 2% to 3% of patients will develop recurrent HPT.

SUGGESTED READINGS

Adler JT, Sippel RS, Schaefer S, Chen H: Surgery improves quality of life in patients with "mild" hyperparathyroidism, *Am J Surg* 197:284–290, 2009.

Chen H, Mack E, Starling JR: Radioguided parathyroidectomy is equally effective for both adenomatous and hyperplastic glands, *Ann Surg* 238:332–338, 2003.

Chen H, Mack E, Starling JR: A comprehensive evaluation of perioperative adjuncts during minimally invasive parathyroidectomy: which is most reliable?, *Ann Surg* 242:375–383, 2005.

Chen H, Pruhs ZM, Starling JR, Mack E: Intraoperative parathyroid hormone testing improves cure rates in patients undergoing minimally invasive parathyroidectomy, *Surgery* 138:583–590, 2005.

Chen H, Sippel RS, Schaefer S: Is radioguided parathyroidectomy effective in patients with negative sestamibi scans? *Arch Surg* 144:643–648, 2009.

Ito F, Sippel RS, Lederman J, Chen H: The utility of intraoperative bilateral internal jugular venous sampling with rapid parathyroid hormone testing,, *Ann Surg* 245(6):959–963, 2007.

Ning L, Sippel RS, Schaefer S, Chen H: What is the clinical significance of an elevated parathyroid hormone level after curative surgery for primary hyperparathyroidism? *Ann Surg* 249(3):469–472, 2009.

Weigel TL, Murphy J, Kabbani L, et al: Radioguided thoracoscopic mediastinal parathyroidectomy with intraoperative parathyroid hormone testing, *Ann Thorac Surg* 80:1262–1265, 2005.

PERSISTENT OR RECURRENT HYPERPARATHYROIDISM

Jason D. Prescott, MD, PhD, and Robert Udelsman, MD, MBA

OVERVIEW

Persistent and recurrent hyperparathyroidism (HPT) have posed significant diagnostic and therapeutic challenges ever since Felix Mandel performed the first successful parathyroidectomy in 1925. The most famous example of this observation is that of Captain Charles Martell, an early twentieth-century sea captain who underwent six unsuccessful explorations for HPT, between 1927 and 1933, before dying from sepsis and hypocalcemia after his curative seventh operation. Normal tissue planes in the reoperative neck are absent, normal cervical anatomy is distorted by fibrosis, and aberrant parathyroid tissue is more commonly ectopic than in nonreoperative cases. These factors increase the technical difficulty of reoperative neck surgery and often necessitate more extensive exploration. Thus patients undergoing remedial surgery for recurrent or persistent HPT experience lower cure rates and higher complication rates. Nonetheless, nonoperative medical treatments for HPT offer inferior outcomes.

ANATOMY AND PATHOPHYSIOLOGY

Persistent HPT is defined as the continuation or redevelopment of HPT within 6 months of parathyroid exploration, and it is usually the result of inadequate resection during the previous operation. The incidence of persistent disease is low at high-volume centers, ranging between 1% and 6%, and this has been minimized by the employment of intraoperative adjuncts, most notably the intraoperative rapid parathyroid hormone (PTH) assay.

Recurrent HPT is defined as the development of HPT more than 6 months after successful parathyroid surgery, and it results from the development of hyperfunctioning parathyroid tissue. Causative lesions include recurrent parathyroid adenoma, hyperplasia, carcinoma, and parathyromatosis, a rare condition in which seeding and subsequent growth of aberrant parathyroid cells occurs after contamination of the operative field during previous parathyroid surgery. Recurrent HPT is less common than persistent disease; however, recurrence frequently occurs in the setting of familial HPT, a condition in which all residual parathyroid tissue is genetically abnormal.

Normal parathyroid gland distribution can be highly variable. Supernumerary glands are present in approximately 8% of the population, and normal parathyroid glands can occur in ectopic locations, including the mediastinum/thymus, carotid sheath, adjacent to the cervical vertebral bodies, and within the thyroid gland. Despite this positional variation, persistent HPT most often results from normally positioned (eutopic) aberrant parathyroid tissue left behind after failed previous cervical exploration (Figure 1).

DIAGNOSIS

Given the risk of recurrent or persistent disease in the patient with postoperative HPT, confirmation of cure is required in all cases following surgery. Serum intact parathyroid hormone (iPTH; normal range, 10 to 65 pg/mL, 1.1 to 7.6 pmol/L) and total serum calcium (normal range, 8.5 to 10.5 mg/dL, 2 to 2.5 mmol/L) should be measured within 1 week of parathyroidectomy; if they fall within normal limits, they should be remeasured annually thereafter. Elevation of either level within the first week of parathyroid surgery may represent persistent disease, and recurrent HPT should be suspected if serum iPTH and/or total serum calcium levels become elevated after 6 months. A cured postoperative patient will commonly demonstrate elevated iPTH levels in association with low serum calcium values. This represents physiologic adaptation to relative postoperative hypocalcemia and generally resolves when treated with oral calcium supplementation. In contrast, persistent early postoperative elevations in both serum iPTH and total calcium likely represent

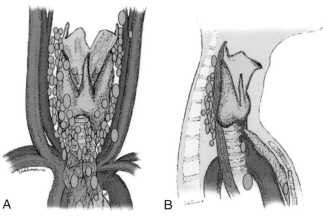

FIGURE 1 Anatomic localization of aberrant parathyroid glands found during reoperative parathyroid surgery. **A,** Anterior-posterior view. **B,** Lateral view. *(From Udelsman R, Donovan PI: Remedial parathyroid surgery: changing trends in 130 consecutive cases, Ann Surg 244[3]:474, 2006. Reprinted with permission.)*

persistent disease. Finally, all postoperative parathyroid patients with an elevated serum calcium level should undergo 24-hour urinary calcium measurements, as values less than 30 mg are suggestive of familial hypocalciuric hypercalcemia (FHH), a benign condition for which operative intervention is rarely indicated.

INDICATIONS FOR REOPERATION

Morbidity and mortality associated with HPT result from the chronic effects of excessive serum PTH and calcium. Hypercalcemia can produce nephrolithiasis and/or nephrocalcinosis, which can progress to end-stage renal disease. Osteopenia, osteoporosis, and associated bony fractures develop from hyperparathyroid-mediated bony resorption. Hypercalcemia is associated with pancreatitis, peptic ulcer disease, coronary artery disease, and premature death. In addition, HPT is associated with neurocognitive derangements that include depression, emotional lability, impaired cognition, and insomnia. Given the morbidity associated with HPT and the current lack of effective long-term medical interventions, all patients with symptomatic HPT should be referred for surgical intervention.

No clear consensus exists regarding the management of asymptomatic patients who demonstrate biochemical evidence of recurrent or persistent HPT. Furthermore, careful evaluation of "asymptomatic" HPT patients usually reveals evidence of bone resorption and/or subtle neurocognitive symptoms, both of which have been shown to improve following successful surgery. Therefore, resection is indicated in the majority of patients with persistent or recurrent disease.

Guidelines for the management of asymptomatic HPT in patients who have not undergone previous neck surgery have been established, and were recently revised, by an international panel of experts (Table 1). Although these experts focused primarily on nonremedial HPT, it is reasonable to consider their recommendations when evaluating reoperative patients for surgery.

PREOPERATIVE EVALUATION

A direct association exists between surgeon experience and favorable outcomes following endocrine surgery. Management of such cases by experienced endocrine surgeons results in decreased complication rates and costs.

A favorable surgical outcome following reoperation for HPT depends on a thorough preoperative evaluation. A meticulous history

TABLE 1: Indications for surgical treatment in asymptomatic hyperparathyroid patients

1. Total serum calcium greater than 1.0 mg/dL (0.25 mmol/L) above the upper limit of normal
2. Creatinine clearance less than 60 mL/min
3. Bone mineral density T score ≤2.5 at any site and/or previous fragility fracture
4. Age <50 years
5. Inability or unwillingness to comply with biannual biochemical surveillance

Modified from Bilezikian JP, Khan AA, Potts JT Jr, et al: Guidelines for the management of asymptomatic primary hyperparathyroidism 2008, Summary statement from the Third International Workshop on Asymptomatic Primary Hyperparathyroidism, *J Clin Endo Metab* 94(2):333–334, 2009.

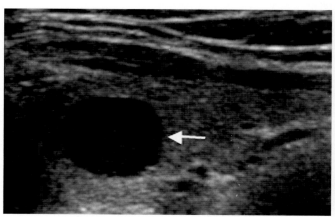

FIGURE 2 Ultrasonic identification of a parathyroid adenoma in remedial primary HPT (*arrow*). *(From Prescott JD, Udelsman R: Remedial operation for primary hyperparathyroidism, World J Surg 33[11]:2324–2334, 2009.)*

and physical exam is required, including assessment of personal and family history for evidence of HPT genetic susceptibility. The surgeon should also confirm the diagnosis by verifying the biochemical data, and all reoperative patients should undergo preoperative laryngoscopy to identify preexisting vocal cord dysfunction. Further, all previous relevant imaging studies, operative reports, and pathology must be carefully reviewed. Finally, often in collaboration with the referring endocrinologist, the surgeon must determine whether the patient requires remedial exploration.

Preoperative localization is essential to facilitate reoperative planning. Imaging is not diagnostic of remedial disease, as negative imaging studies do not rule out the presence of recurrent or persistent HPT. Initial imaging should be noninvasive, safe, and relatively inexpensive. As such, ultrasound (US) and sestamibi (MIBI) scans are the most common initial imaging modalities employed. Adequate preoperative localization of hyperfunctioning parathyroid tissue is possible using a single imaging study. However, equivocal or negative imaging data are not uncommon in remedial cases; and sequential preoperative imaging, using two or more separate modalities, is often necessary.

US findings (Figure 2) are reproducible intraoperatively and can identify comorbid thyroid disease. However, the positive predictive value (PPV) of US in remedial HPT cases is highly variable (52% to 92%), depending on body habitus and operator experience. Further, US cannot penetrate bony or cartilaginous structures, making localization of substernal and posttracheal lesions unlikely. Like US, the PPV of MIBI (Figure 3) for remedial HPT is also highly variable, ranging between 79%

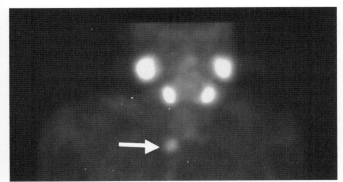

FIGURE 3 Sestamibi scan showing radiotracer uptake in the right inferior thyroid bed of a remedial primary HPT patient (*arrow*). Note the physiologic uptake of radiotracer in the normal salivary glands. *(From Prescott JD, Udelsman R: Remedial operation for primary hyperparathyroidism, World J Surg 33[11]:2324–2334, 2009.)*

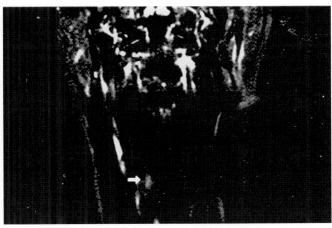

FIGURE 5 T2-weighted fat-saturation MRI demonstrating a right-sided parathyroid adenoma. *(From Prescott JD, Udelsman R: Remedial operation for primary hyperparathyroidism, World J Surg 33[11]:2324–2334, 2009.)*

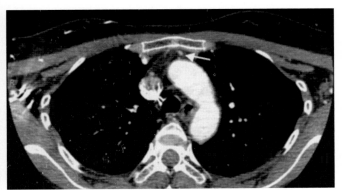

FIGURE 4 Contrast CT scan showing an anterior mediastinal parathyroid adenoma (*arrow*) in a patient with remedial primary HPT. *(From Prescott JD, Udelsman R: Remedial operation for primary hyperparathyroidism, World J Surg 33[11]:2324–2334; 2009.)*

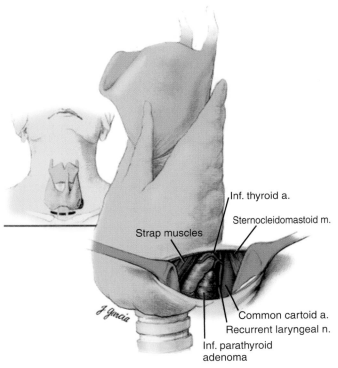

FIGURE 6 The lateral approach to cervical exploration in remedial primary HPT. The plane between the strap muscles and sternocleidomastoid muscle is opened using the previous Kocher incision. This facilitates posterior access to the thyroid and avoidance of scar tissue from previous medial neck explorations. *(From Wang T. Udelsman R: Remedial surgery for primary hyperparathyroidism, Adv Surg 41:1–15, 2007, with permission.)*

and 100%. MIBI can, however, detect substernal and posttracheal hyperfunctioning parathyroid tissue, and PPV may be significantly improved by coimaging with single photon emission CT (SPECT).

MRI and CT scans—and multiple-run, thin-slice, four-dimensional CT in particular—are also useful for parathyroid localization in remedial cases (PPV 51% to 100% and 36% to 100%, respectively; Figures 4 and 5). These modalities can identify mediastinal disease but are more expensive than either US or MIBI scans, and CT requires exposure to ionizing radiation. In addition, preexisting metal implants reduce CT scan sensitivity and may compromise safe performance of MRI. Finally, if noninvasive imaging studies are negative or equivocal, invasive modalities, including US-guided fine needle aspiration (FNA) and/or arteriography with selective venous sampling (SVS) should be considered.

Parathyroid FNA facilitates preoperative planning by confirming the presence of PTH, and thus parathyroid tissue, in suspicious lesions (aspirate PTH levels >1000 pg/mL); however, FNA requires image guidance, most commonly US. SVS involves selective sampling of cervical and mediastinal veins for PTH levels, but it is expensive and requires endovascular expertise; nonetheless, it can be very helpful in remedial cases.

The surgeon should exercise caution prior to exploring a reoperative HPT patient if preoperative imaging fails to identify the site of disease. A subset of patients can be maintained with nonsurgical interventions, and preoperative localization may be reattempted at a later date.

OPERATIVE TECHNIQUE AND INTRAOPERTIVE ADJUNCTS

Causative lesions in patients with remedial HPT are usually located in the cervical region. Reoperative cervical surgery involves either a standard medial or lateral approach (Figure 6). Although both approaches involve reincision of the preexisting Kocher incision, the medial approach requires dissection through the previously

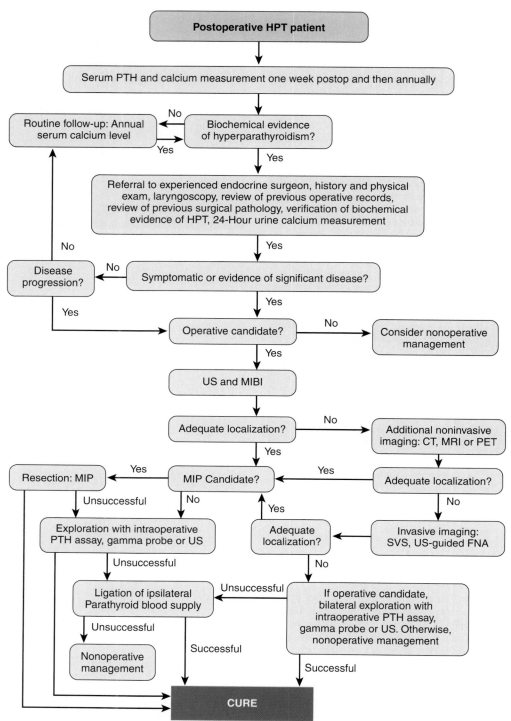

FIGURE 7   Algorithm for the diagnosis and management of recurrent and persistent HPT. *(From Prescott JD, Udelsman R: Remedial operation for primary hyperparathyroidism, World J Surg 33[11]:2324–2334, 2009.)*

explored operative field. Nonetheless, the medial technique is the most direct approach for anterior lesions. The lateral approach involves dissection of the plane between the carotid sheath and the strap muscles. This technique generally avoids the previous operative field and facilitates early identification of the ipsilateral recurrent laryngeal nerve (RLN). Employment of both techniques during the same operation is common in challenging remedial patients.

Patients in whom convincing preoperative localization is obtained may be candidates for minimally invasive parathyroidectomy (MIP). This technique is generally performed under cervical block anesthesia and involves focused exploration through a single small incision.

Recurrent and persistent HPT may be the result of mediastinal lesions. In such cases, the causative hyperfunctioning parathyroid tissue is typically retroesophageal or intrathymic and is often accessible via a cervical incision. Nonetheless, rare cases may require partial or complete median sternotomy or a transthoracic approach.

Curative resection of hyperfunctional parathyroid tissue in patients with remedial HPT is facilitated by employment of intraoperative adjuvants. Cervical exploration may be guided intraoperatively by high-resolution US or by a γ-probe in patients receiving preoperative radiolabeled sestamibi. Intraoperative US has the same limitations associated with preoperative US, however, and background signals from thyroid tissue and blood vessels can limit γ-probe specificity. The rapid intraoperative PTH assay, which monitors peripheral venous PTH levels, can verify adequate resection of hyperfunctioning parathyroid tissue. After resection of suspicious tissue, a PTH decrease of 50% relative to the initial intraoperative baseline is associated with cure in 94% to 96% of remedial cases.

A number of additional techniques designed to decrease the morbidity associated with remedial parathyroid surgery have also been proposed. Real-time electromyographic (EMG) nerve monitoring has been employed in hopes of reducing the rate of RLN injury during remedial surgery. Unfortunately, prospective data do not demonstrate improvement in the incidence of RLN injury when intraoperative EMG is used. Similarly, US-guided ethanol ablation of hyperfunctional parathyroid tissue has been proposed as a less invasive alternative to reexploration. This technique, however, has a much lower cure rate than remedial surgery and can cause RLN injury. For these reasons, ethanol ablation is generally limited to patients for whom surgery is contraindicated. Finally, because all normal parathyroid tissue may have been removed during previous surgery, and scarring in the reoperative field increases the risk of injury to remaining parathyroid tissue, intraoperative autotransplantation or cryopreservation of parathyroid tissue should be considered in patients with remedial HPT.

Occasionally, hyperfunctional parathyroid tissue will not be found despite adequate preoperative localization, appropriate use of intraoperative adjuncts, and meticulous operative technique. Such remedial cases are often characterized by normal-appearing parathyroid glands in all but one eutopic position or by previous resection of all but one parathyroid gland. In these cases, ligation of the relevant parathyroid blood supply may result in a durable cure.

POSTOPERATIVE MANAGEMENT

Patients with remedial HPT experience an increased risk of postoperative complications, including RLN injury and hypoparathyroidism. Unilateral RLN injury can result in hoarseness, and bilateral RLN dysfunction can cause airway obstruction. RLN injury should be anticipated, and the surgeon should be present during extubation to assist with airway management.

Transient hypoparathyroidism is common after reoperative HPT surgery, resulting from dysfunction of residual normal parathyroid tissue postoperatively. Eucalcemia generally redevelops within 2 or 3 days, but a short course of oral calcium and activated vitamin D is usually sufficient treatment. However, a subset of patients will develop permanent postoperative hypoparathyroidism; these patients may develop life-threatening hypocalcemia and may require intravenous calcium gluconate administration. Permanent hypocalcemia can be avoided by parathyroid autotransplantation in selected patients, either during reoperation or at a later date, if cryopreserved specimens are available.

Cure rates for remedial HPT range between 94% and 96% when the reoperation is performed by an experienced endocrine surgeon. All reoperative patients must receive careful follow-up, both for detection of complications and for assessment of cure. Patients found to have subsequent persistent or recurrent disease should undergo total reevaluation. Truly asymptomatic patients with borderline serum PTH and total calcium elevations may be treated medically, as complication rates rise with each repeat neck exploration. In contrast, symptomatic patients should undergo reoperation (Figure 7).

Suggested Readings

Prescott JD, Udelsman R: Remedial operation for primary hyperparathyroidism, *World J Surg* 33(11): 2324–2334, 2009.

Udelsman R, Donovan PI: Remedial parathyroid surgery: changing trends in 130 consecutive cases, *Ann Surg* 244:471–479, 2006.

Hessman O, Stålberg P, Sundin A, et al: High success rate of parathyroid reoperation may be achieved with improved localization diagnosis, *World J Surg* 32(5):774–781, 2008.

Udelsman R, Pasieka J, Sturgeon C, et al: Surgery for asymptomatic primary hyperparathyroidism: proceedings of the third international workshop, *J Clin Endo Metab* 94(2):366–372, 2009.

Secondary and Tertiary Hyperparathyroidism

Marlon A. Guerrero, MD, Reza Rahbari, MD, and Electron Kebebew, MD

OVERVIEW

Secondary hyperparathyroidism (SHPT) refers to increased parathyroid hormone (PTH) production due to external factors that stimulate the parathyroid glands to enlarge and secrete PTH. The most common condition causing SHPT is chronic renal failure. Less common causes of SHPT include gastrointestinal malabsorption, vitamin D deficiency, osteomalacia, rickets, malnutrition, osteoporosis, hypermagnesuria, and idiopathic hypercalciuria.

Tertiary hyperparathyroidism (THPT) refers to autonomous hypersecretion of PTH even after the cause of SHPT has been corrected (i.e., after kidney transplantation with normal renal function in patients with history of chronic renal failure), or when patients with SHPT develop refractory hypercalcemia. In this chapter, the pathogenesis of SHPT due to chronic renal failure, metabolic complications of SHPT, and medical therapy for SHPT is discussed; in addition, parathyroidectomy indications, perioperative management considerations, and the benefits of parathyroidectomy are reviewed.

PATHOPHYSIOLOGY OF SECONDARY HYPERPARATHYROIDISM

SHPT results from a compensatory hypersecretion of parathyroid hormone (PTH) in response to hypocalcemia, vitamin D deficiency, and/or hyperphosphatemia. Factors that contribute to hypocalcemia include increased blood phosphate levels, vitamin D deficiency, resistance in vitamin D metabolism, and skeletal resistance to the calcemic effects of PTH. Vitamin D deficiency can result from inadequate intake, insufficient sunlight, or more commonly from chronic renal failure resulting from the inability of the kidneys to hydroxylate 25-hydroxycholecalciferol to the active form 1,25-dihydroxycholecalciferol ($1,25(OH)_2D_3$). Chronic renal failure can also lead to decrease in the calcium-sensing receptors (CaSR) or vitamin D receptors, affecting blood levels of both.

Hyperphosphatemia results from the kidneys' inability to excrete phosphorus, retention of which potentiates hypocalcemia by lowering the levels of ionized calcium in the blood and interfering with the production of $1,25(OH)_2D_3$. But hypocalcemia can develop independently of hyperphosphatemia, indicating that the pathogenesis of hypocalcemia is multifactorial. Skeletal resistance to the calcimimetic effects of PTH is evidenced by failure of the elevated PTH levels to properly stimulate elevation in serum calcium levels. The skeletal resistance to PTH is due in part to deficiencies of vitamin D and the downregulation of the PTH receptors.

These metabolic abnormalities are the most common and important factors that contribute to the compensatory parathyroid gland hyperplasia and overproduction of PTH in SHPT. The hyperplasia that develops in SHPT differs from that of primary hyperparathyroidism in that enlargement of all glands is present in all cases of SHPT. This compensatory effect is usually reversible after renal transplantation. In 3% to 5% of patients with SHPT, parathyroid gland function becomes autonomous, and PTH hypersecretion persists despite normal renal function.

MEDICAL THERAPY

Chronic renal failure results in the inability of the body to excrete toxins from the body. The metabolic derangements associated with SHPT are hyperphosphatemia and deficiencies in calcium and vitamin D. Almost all patients with chronic renal failure have SHPT, but the majority can be medically managed successfully. Nonoperative treatment consists of dietary modifications and medical therapy. Dietary control entails restriction of phosphate intake to between 800 to 1000 mg/day when the serum phosphorus concentrations are elevated (>4.6 mg/dL for stages 3 and 4 and >5.5 mg/dL for stage 5), or when the PTH level is higher than the target range for the stage of renal failure (>70 pg/mL for stage 3, >110 pg/mL for stage 4, and >300 pg/mL in stage 5). Deficiencies in serum calcium and vitamin D are corrected by supplementing normal dietary intake (Table 1).

With worsening renal failure, dietary modification becomes insufficient to maintain adequate phosphorus concentrations. Hemodialysis is usually effective at decreasing the blood phosphate concentrations in the majority of these patients; however, phosphate binders are added when dietary phosphorus restriction and dialysis cannot effectively control the hyperphosphatemia. Due to the potential of developing aluminum toxicity, aluminum-based phosphate binders are infrequently used. Calcium-based phosphate binders are very effective in lowering serum phosphorus concentrations, however, there is a risk of hypercalcemia and soft-tissue calcification. This risk is higher in patients on dialysis, so the use of calcium-based phosphate binders is not recommended when the serum calcium concentration is above 10.2 mg/dL, or the plasma PTH is below 150 pg/mL. Non-calcium, non-aluminum–based phosphate binders are preferred in this situation. No single phosphate binder may adequately control hyperphosphatemia, so a combination of phosphate binders may be attempted.

Despite adequate dietary modifications, medical therapy, and hemodialysis, some patients with renal failure will develop progressively worsening bone disease. Vitamin D analogs have been used to effectively prevent or improve high bone turnover in this situation. The use of calcitriol or other vitamin D analogs is recommended for patients with persistently elevated PTH (>70 pg/mL for stage 3 or >110 pg/mL for stage 4) despite adequate dietary restriction or in patients with stage 5 renal failure and PTH over 300 pg/mL.

Recently, a new class of drugs, calcimimetics, has been utilized for the treatment of SHPT. Cinacalcet, a calcimimetics agent, targets the calcium-sensing receptor on the surface of the chief cells of the parathyroid gland. It acts as an allosteric modulator of the calcium-sensing receptor and decreases PTH secretion, leading to the reduction in serum calcium and phosphorus levels. It has been approved by the Food and Drug Administration for use in patients with SHPT who are on dialysis, and it can be used concomitantly with vitamin D sterols and phosphate binders. Patients on calcimimetics require initial close follow-up because of the risk of severe hypocalcemia. Calcimimetic therapy results in about a 50% reduction in the intact serum PTH concentration, but it may not be tolerated by some patients because of side effects, such as severe nausea and vomiting. Calcimimetics are quickly becoming an integral part of SHPT treatment, but further evaluation is required to assess its cost effectiveness and its effect on the metabolic complications associated with SHPT. It also remains to be seen whether calcimimetic therapy decreases the number of patients who require parathyroidectomy for treatment of their SHPT.

INDICATIONS FOR PARATHYROIDECTOMY

The majority of patients with SHPT are effectively treated nonoperatively. However, despite appropriate medical treatment, up to 30% of patients will eventually require a parathyroidectomy (Table 2). Surgery is indicated when SHPT is refractory to medical therapy that results in progressive worsening of bone disease and extraskeletal soft-tissue calcification. Persistent and uncontrolled SHPT can produce debilitating manifestations, such as bone pain, pruritus, and anemia, which are indications for surgical treatment. A calcium-phosphate product above 55 or a PTH above 600 pg/mL in patients with renal failure are also indications for surgery. The most common manifestations of medically refractory SHPT are described in Table 2.

Bone Disease

Renal osteodystrophy is defined as bone disease associated with renal failure. Renal osteodystrophy results from a combination of phosphate retention, bone resistance to the metabolic effects of PTH, and the inability of the kidneys to hydroxylate 25-hydroxy-vitamin D to $1,25(OH)_2D_3$. Persistent elevation of PTH produces increased osteoclast and osteoblast activity, resulting in high bone turnover and the haphazard deposition of collagen that ultimately replaces the bone marrow with fibrosis and cysts (*osteitis fibrosa cystica*). As a consequence, bone is severely weakened, increasing the risk of pathologic fractures. Worsening bone disease may also be associated with bone pain, and the presence of persistent debilitating bone pain that is refractory to medical therapy is also an indication for surgical intervention.

TABLE 1: Medical therapy for SHPT

Class	Drugs
Phosphate binders	Calcium based
	Calcium carbonate
	Calcium acetate
	Non-calcium, non-aluminum–based
	Sevelamer HCl
Vitamin D analog	Calcitriol
	Alfacalcidol
	Doxercalciferol
Calcimimetics	Cinacalcet (Sensipar)

TABLE 2: Indications for parathyroidectomy for SHPT

Calciphylaxis
SHPT refractory to medical therapy consistent with the following:
PTH >600 pg/mL
$(Ca^{+2} \times PO^{-4})$ >55
High-turnover bone disease
SHPT consistent with the above conditions and associated with one of the following:
- Subperiosteal resorption
- Bone pain
- Pathologic fractures
- Severe pruritus
- Persistent anemia
- Renal osteodystrophy
- Hypercalcemia
- Hyperphosphatemia
- Extraskeletal nonvascular calcification

TABLE 3: Indications for parathyroidectomy for tertiary hyperparathyroidism after kidney transplantation

Subacute severe hypercalcemia (Ca^{+2} >12.5 mg/dL)
Persistent hypercalcemia 2 years posttransplant associated with the following:
- Decline in renal function
- Nephrolithiasis
- Acute pancreatitis
- Progressive bone disease

Extraskeletal Calcification

Unregulated and persistent hypercalcemia results in the extraskeletal deposition of calcium, particularly in the blood vessels, periarticular surfaces, and soft tissue. Calcification of blood vessels develops in 20% of patients with renal failure and can result in hypertension, or worsen preexisting hypertension, and can increase the risk of cardiovascular or cerebrovascular events. Though vascular calcification can affect small, medium, and large blood vessels, it is the calcification of small and medium blood vessels that produce the ischemic damage. Periarticular calcium deposition can cause decreased mobility, joint effusion, and arthritic pain. Soft tissue calcification can develop in the myocardium, heart valves, lungs, and other organs. Parathyroidectomy can successfully reverse or ameliorate the effects of extraskeletal calcification; however, vascular calcifications rarely improve.

Calciphylaxis

Persistent refractory hypercalcemia resulting in disseminated vascular and soft-tissue calcification can produce severe tissue ischemia and necrosis. These end-stage sequelae of renal failure–induced SHPT are rare but can be extremely debilitating to patients, and it is associated with a high mortality. Patients develop painful, violaceous, erythematous lesions that progress to ulcers and subsequently to frank gangrene. Gangrene usually develops in the lower extremities, fingers, and abdomen. Calciphylaxis may also develop in THPT. Parathyroidectomy may slow the progression of ulcer formation and allow for proper wound healing, but calciphylaxis is associated with over a 50% mortality rate. The presence of calciphylaxis is an absolute and emergent indication for parathyroidectomy.

Posttransplant Hypercalcemia (Tertiary Hyperparathyroidism)

In patients who undergo a successful kidney transplant, SHPT usually resolves in over 95%, but hypercalcemia may persist for 2 years or more because of THPT. Surgery should be considered earlier if the function of the renal graft is declining or is at risk of being compromised, or when the patient has significant bone loss and will be on steroids for immunosuppression. Additionally, progressive symptoms in association with hypercalcemia, despite adequate renal function, are another indication for surgery in patients with THPT (Table 3).

PREOPERATIVE MANAGEMENT

Patients being considered for surgery should undergo a comprehensive medical workup to ensure that they are good surgical candidates, and surgery should be coordinated with hemodialysis so that the patient is metabolically optimized; the optimal timing for hemodialysis is no later than the day before surgery. Particular attention should be paid to ensure that hyperkalemia, acidosis, and hypervolemia are corrected.

Since SHPT results in the development of large, hyperplastic parathyroid glands, the standard surgical approach consists of a bilateral neck exploration. Localizing studies, therefore, are not used to plan a focused or minimally invasive parathyroidectomy (MIP) but rather to help determine the presence of ectopic or supernumerary glands. Ectopic glands should be suspected when large parathyroid glands are not seen on ultrasound. In this situation, a sestamibi scan and computed tomography (CT) or magnetic resonance imaging (MRI) can help localize the ectopic parathyroid gland.

SUBTOTAL VERSUS TOTAL PARATHYROIDECTOMY

The decision to perform either a subtotal parathyroidectomy (3.5 gland resection) or total parathyroidectomy with autotransplantation rests primarily on surgeon preference. Debate regarding which approach provides the optimal therapy centers on the risks and benefits of each approach. Proponents of a subtotal parathyroidectomy advocate its use primarily because of the lower risk of permanent hypoparathyroidism (HPT) while achieving high cure rates. On the other hand, advocates of a total parathyroidectomy with autotransplantation point out the potential for persistent or recurrent hyperparathyroidism with a subtotal resection. Debate in the literature persists, and studies support each method; both approaches are acceptable treatment for SHPT.

In the past, some surgeons used total parathyroidectomy without autotransplantation, which results in significant adynamic bone disease but may be a reasonable approach in patients who are not candidates for renal transplantation, who are at high risk of persistent or recurrent disease because of noncompliance with medical therapy, or for those who have had multiple episodes of recurrent disease.

Surgical Technique

The patient is positioned in supine position with both arms tucked in straight at the sides. The neck is hyperextended with the use of a shoulder roll or beanbag. After the neck is prepared, a 3 to 5 cm transverse Kocher cervical incision is made in a skin crease 1 cm below the cricoid cartilage; a skin crease is chosen to minimize tension and maximize the cosmetic outcome. Subplatysmal skin flaps are raised cephalad to the thyroid cartilage and caudal to the sternal notch, and a self-retaining retractor is placed for exposure. The median raphe of the strap muscles is divided, and the sternohyoid muscles are dissected from the sternothyroid muscles. Next, the sternothyroid muscle is dissected off the thyroid, and the strap muscles are retracted laterally. Care must be taken to maintain a bloodless field, because bloodstaining makes it difficult to differentiate the parathyroid glands from adipose tissue or thyroid nodules.

Exploration is performed in a systematic manner, and exposure of the glands is facilitated by medially rotating the thyroid lobe. Though often not necessary, the middle thyroid vein may be divided to allow better mobilization of the thyroid gland and optimize exposure. The parathyroid glands are explored, and if a subtotal parathyroidectomy is to be performed, all four glands should be visualized prior to excising any glands. The gland that is the most normal should be partially resected first, because any evidence that the remnant is not viable should prompt another gland to be chosen. A 40 to 60 mg remnant is left in situ and marked with a clip.

Knowledge of surgical anatomy is crucial. Superior parathyroid glands are usually situated posterior to the thyroid gland within 1 cm of the intersection of the inferior thyroid artery and recurrent laryngeal nerve (RLN) at the level of the cricoid cartilage. If the superior parathyroid gland cannot be located, the tracheoesophageal groove, retroesophageal space, posterior mediastinum, carotid sheath, and thyroid capsule should be explored. On the other hand, inferior glands are usually located posterior to the inferior pole of the thyroid lobe and ventral to the RLN. Ectopic inferior parathyroid glands are usually found in the thymus, but they may also be found within the thyroid gland, undescended in the carotid sheath, and in the anterior mediastinum. Though the majority of glands situated within the thymus can be removed through a cervical approach, a sternotomy may be required. Nearly 15% of patients have supernumerary parathyroid glands, the majority of which are found in the thymus. A bilateral cervical thymectomy should therefore be performed on all patients to minimize the risk of persistent or recurrent disease, as embryologic rests in the thymus may be present in up to 41% of patients.

Confirmation of parathyroid tissue can be performed by frozen-section analysis or by directly aspirating the parathyroid gland. The gland is aspirated with a 3 mL syringe filled with 1 mL of saline or water, and an aspirate with a PTH concentration above 1000 is confirmatory. Aspiration of the parathyroid gland can be helpful, because differentiation between follicular thyroid tissue and parathyroid glands is sometimes difficult on frozen section. Though the use of intraoperative PTH monitoring has been advocated in patients with SHPT or THPT, in our experience, it is not useful for indicating biochemical cure or persistent disease. Moreover, the use of intraoperative PTH monitoring does not supplant anatomical knowledge or meticulous operative technique, as patients should have a bilateral neck exploration and identification of all the parathyroid glands.

If a total parathyroidectomy is performed, the smallest, most normal gland is autotransplanted. A 40 to 60 mg portion of the smallest gland is sectioned into 1 mm pieces, and 10 to 20 pieces are inserted into several muscle pockets and marked with metal clips. Placing the pieces of parathyroid tissue into muscle allows for neovascularization and graft survival. Either the sternocleidomastoid muscle or the brachioradialis muscle in the nondominant forearm are the traditional sites of choice; however, the forearm is the optimal site, because reoperation for recurrent disease is associated with less morbidity in the forearm. Reoperative neck operation is associated with complication rates two to three times higher than the initial operation. A portion of the resected parathyroid glands should also be cryopreserved, in case the patient develops hypoparathyroidism. Autotransplantation of cryopreserved parathyroid tissue for hypoparathyroidism is successful in 50% to 60% of patients.

Postoperative Management

Patients with SHPT and renal failure have a high risk of experiencing hungry bone syndrome postoperatively, which results from increased skeletal calcium deposition and causes severe hypocalcemia. Transient hypocalcemia occurs in as many as 85% of patients, and permanent hypocalcemia occurs in approximately 10%. To prevent symptoms of hypocalcemia, patients are placed on 4 to 6 g/day of calcium postoperatively. Calcitriol (0.5 to 4 μg/day) is often necessary to prevent hypocalcemia. Despite these measures, some patients may require intravenous calcium gluconate for severe hypocalcemia. Intravenous replacement of calcium should be done through a well-positioned intravenous catheter to minimize the risk of infiltration, as it can result in severe skin necrosis. Magnesium levels should also be corrected, because low levels aggravate hypocalcemia and prevent resolution of the hypocalcemia. Careful control of hyperphosphatemia should be maintained, and hemodialysis should be scheduled per normal routine with high calcium dialyzate. We prefer that no heparin be used during hemodialysis for 1 week after parathyroidectomy, as some patients will develop a delayed neck hematoma, likely related to the effects of heparin.

BENEFITS OF PARATHYROIDECTOMY FOR SECONDARY HYPERPARATHYROIDISM

The benefits of parathyroidectomy in patients with SHPT can be dramatic and immediate. Pruritis improves early and in most patients. In up to 80% of the patients with bone pain, this symptom improves in a few days, and a third of patients report decreased muscle weakness. Symptoms of abdominal pain and ocular irritation are less likely to respond to parathyroidectomy. Improvement in anemia is also observed in over 50% of patients. In approximately two thirds, bone resorption is suppressed, and nonvisceral calcification decreases. Overall, parathyroidectomy improves many symptoms associated with SHPT, as well as metabolic sequelae, such as hypertension; it also reduces the rate of major cardiovascular events and results in reduced mortality.

SUMMARY

Medical management reduces most metabolic complications of SHPT associated with chronic renal failure, but many patients will develop significant symptoms and medical therapy–refractory disease that would benefit from parathyroidectomy. Surgical management of SHPT and THPT should include bilateral neck exploration with subtotal parathyroidectomy or total parathyroidectomy and autotransplantation. Parathyroidectomy for SHPT and THPT is associated with significant symptom relief, reversal of metabolic complications, and reduced cardiovascular events and mortality.

SUGGESTED READINGS

Andress DL, Coyne DW, Kalantar-Zadeh K, et al: Management of secondary hyperparathyroidism in stages 3 and 4 chronic kidney disease, *Endocr Pract* 14(1):18–27, 2008.

Dosanjh A, Kebebew E: Calciphylaxis: rare but fatal, *Curr Surg* 62(5):455–458, 2005.

Kebebew E, Duh QY, Clark OH: Tertiary hyperparathyroidism: histologic patterns of disease and results of parathyroidectomy, *Arch Surg* 139(9):974–977, 2004.

Shen WT, Kebebew E, Suh I, et al: Two hundred and two consecutive operations for secondary hyperparathyroidism: has medical management changed the profiles of patients requiring parathyroidectomy? *Surgery* 146(2):296–269, 2009.

SKIN LESIONS: EVALUATION, DIAGNOSIS, AND MANAGEMENT

Tim A. Iseli, MBBS, and Eben L. Rosenthal, MD

OVERVIEW

Nonmelanoma skin cancer (NMSC) is the most common cancer in the United States. The incidence continues to increase, and lifetime risk is estimated at 10% for whites. Most melanomas occur in the head and neck, and most (80%) are basal cell carcinomas (BCCs), with squamous cell carcinomas (SCCs) the next most common. The primary etiologic factor is cumulative sun exposure, especially exposure to ultraviolet B radiation.

EVALUATION AND DIAGNOSIS

Most cutaneous lesions can be diagnosed by visual inspection. Good lighting in a tangential direction improves the ability to discern features. Raised edges at the periphery commonly denote BCC. Palpation of the tumor determines infiltration into the subcutaneous tissue as well as fixation to deep structures. Patients complain of itchy or nonhealing wounds that bleed when traumatized; marked tenderness is uncommon.

There are three common scenarios requiring surgical management: 1) likely benign lesions (Figure 1), in which biopsy or excision is required to rule out malignancy or for aesthetic reasons (Table 1); 2) known or suspected nonmelanoma skin cancer; and 3) known or suspected melanoma (not discussed in this chapter).

For larger or recurrent tumors, or if perineural invasion is suspected, magnetic resonance imaging (MRI) may detect enhancement of a major nerve and may give an estimate of the proximal extent. A computed tomographic (CT) scan with contrast is preferred if the lesion clinically invades deep structures (bone or muscle), or if there is palpable lymphadenopathy. Fine needle aspiration (FNA) of regional lymphadenopathy is helpful if it is positive and is an indication for regional lymphadenectomy. A negative FNA with suspicious lymphadenopathy on CT does not rule out metastatic spread; in these cases, it is best to repeat the FNA or proceed to open biopsy. Because an open biopsy violates tumor lymphatics and may seed tumor, frozen-section analysis should be performed and, if positive, regional lymph node dissection should be performed immediately.

Cutaneous SCC staging is defined by the standard American Joint Committee on Cancer (AJCC) tumor node metastasis (TNM) staging system (Table 2). Because basal cells do not metastasize, only the tumor part of the system applies to this histologic diagnosis, however, SCC of the lip is included in the oral mucosal staging for its more aggressive behavior.

Screening for skin lesions is typically performed by full-body cutaneous exam. People with previous skin tumors are at highest risk (30% for a second SCC within 5 years). After treatment, patients should be seen at least every 3 to 6 months for 2 years, then every 6 to 12 months for the third year, then annually. Organ transplantation patients should also undergo regular screening regardless of previous skin cancers.

TREATMENT

Basal Cell Carcinoma

Basal cell carcinoma (BCC) typically appears as a slow-growing nodule (doubling time: ~1 year) with overlying telangiectasia on the head or neck in fair, sun-damaged skin, but histology is required for definitive diagnosis. Associated genetic abnormalities include tumor-suppressor gene mutations (*PTCH1* and *p53*) and oncogene mutations (*p21Ras* and *c-fFos*). Metastatic potential is very low for lesions less than 10 cm^2 (0.1%), but local recurrences may be seen. About 50% of local recurrences occur in the first 2 years, and 20% occur after 5 years. Classically defined subtypes include *nodular, superficial* (erythematous scaly lesions on legs and/or torso), *morpheaform* (scarlike with subtle edges), *basosquamous* (SCC-type appearance), and *pigmented* (appearance similar to melanoma on dark-skinned individuals). These types do not impact clinical management, with the exception of basosquamous pathology, which is more likely to metastasize and therefore is staged and treated as SCC.

More aggressive surgical management should be reserved for high-risk lesions. The primary prognostic factors for recurrence are site and size (Table 3). Surgical excision with a 4 to 5 mm margin with permanent section analysis achieves a local control of 95% for primary cases and 83% for recurrent cases. Consequently, this is the standard of care for low-risk BCCs. High-risk BCCs should be excised with a 10 mm margin, or the patient should undergo Mohs micrographic surgery. Frozen-section analysis or Mohs should be considered for recurrent tumors and lesions greater than 30 mm in high-risk site (e.g., around eyes, ears, nose, mouth, hands and feet >6 mm or other head and neck sites >1 cm). If pathologic analysis of the specimen on permanent analysis suggests involved margins, the patient should return for re-resection of the lesion. If clear margins cannot be obtained with acceptable morbidity, or if there is perineural invasion, radiotherapy should be offered.

Mohs has been advocated for high-risk or recurrent BCCs with quoted cure rates of 98% for primary cases and 95% for recurrences. This technique involves close excision of the tumor with frozen-section

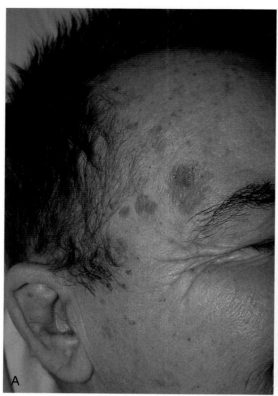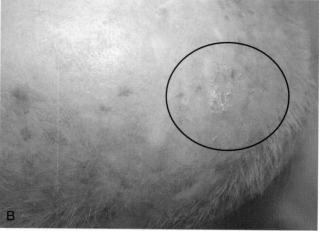

FIGURE 1 **A,** Extensive seborrheic keratosis is often seen, especially on the trunk, face, and arms of individuals older than 30 years of age. Seborrheic keratosis typically presents as a sharply circumscribed, waxy, papillomatous plaque with a friable, hyperkeratotic surface, most often described as having a "stuck on" appearance. **B,** AK is found primarily on exposed surfaces as rough, adherent hyperkeratosis that is skin colored, yellow-brown, or brown, possibly with a reddish tinge. AKs are often numerous in older adults.

TABLE 1: Common nonpigmented benign skin lesions for which surgical excision may be indicated

Lesion	Appearance	Reason for Surgery	Treatment
AK	Sun-damaged skin, adherent hyperkeratosis on red base, lacking the thickness of SCC	A 6% to 10% lifetime SCC risk Rule out SCC	Facial razor Biopsy/excision Topical 5-FU Cryotherapy
Keratoacanthoma	Similar to SCC, rapid growth for 1 or 2 months then involution for 1 or 2 months	Rule out SCC	Excisional biopsy
Bowen disease (SCC in situ)	Thin, erythematous plaque with scale	Rule out invasion	Excision preferred Topical 5-FU/ imiquimod or radiation therapy if very large
Nevus, sebaceous	Hairless plaque on face/scalp since birth, enlarges during puberty	10% develop BCC	Excise 1 mm margin
Acrochordon (skin tag)	Soft skin tag with narrow pedicle	Cosmetic	Scissor pedicle
Epidermoid cyst (tricholemmoma or pilar cyst on scalp)	Cyst attached to epidermis, often has punctum	Infection, cosmetic	Excision with small ellipse around punctum

analysis of margins mapped to a tumor diagram. A typical Mohs excision takes 2 to 4 hours. A randomized trial of Mohs compared with standard excision showed a 1% improvement in local control in primary cases, favoring Mohs and 3% in recurrent cases; in addition, Mohs may result in smaller defects compared with routine 4 mm macroscopic margins and may thereby spare adjacent vital structures.

Squamous Cell Carcinoma

SCC is the second most frequent skin cancer and usually arises within sun-damaged skin from a preexisting actinic keratosis (AK). SCCs can arise within any area of chronic irritation such as burns, radiotherapy fields, and chronic ulcers. Typically they appear as a

TABLE 2: AJCC staging of nonmelanoma skin cancer*

Stage	Criteria
T0/Tis	No primary, in situ
T1	<2 cm
T2	2 to 5 cm
T3	>5 cm
T4	Invades deep extradermal structures (cartilage, muscle, bone, nerves)
N0	No nodal disease
N1	Involved lymph nodes

*For multiple simultaneous tumors, use the highest individual stage with the number in parenthesis; for example, T2(5) for five lesions (maximum <5 cm).

From American Joint Committee on Cancer: *AJCC cancer staging manual,* ed 6, Philadelphia, 2002, Lippincott-Raven.

TABLE 3: Surgical margins for nonmelanoma skin cancers treated with standard surgical excision

Lesion	Margin (mm)
BCC	
Low risk • Trunk and extremities <2 cm • Head and neck <1 cm • Around eyes, ears, nose, mouth, hands, feet <6 mm	4–5
High risk • Site, size >6 mm • Recurrent tumor • Immunocompromised patient • In radiotherapy field • Morpheaform, sclerosing, micronodular • Perineural invasion	10
SCC	
Low risk • Site/size as per BCC	4–6
High risk • As per BCC and poorly differentiated • As per BCC and adenoid, adenosquamous, or desmoplastic types	10

keratinous crust over an erythematous base that has thickness to palpation, unlike an AK.

Similar to BCCs, primary risk factors for recurrence are location and size (see Table 3). High-risk patients should be assessed more frequently, and the surgeon should have a very low threshold for biopsy of any skin lesions. Precancerous lesions (AKs) in high-risk patients should be aggressively managed with shave excision or topical treatments such cryotherapy, photodynamic therapy, or topical 5-fluorouracil (5-FU, discussed below). Lesions resistant to nonsurgical therapy should undergo excision or biopsy. If the frequency and severity of skin tumors becomes life threatening, reduction of immunosuppression medications may be considered.

Excisional biopsy of low-risk cutaneous SCCs is the standard of care. Small, low-risk SCCs can be surgically excised with macroscopic 4 to 6 mm margins and permanent histologic analysis, which offers a 5-year local control rate of approximately 92%. If pathologic margins are found to be positive, the preferred option is reexcision. High-risk SCCs should be excised with a macroscopic 1 cm margin. If critical structures, such as eyelid or nasal ala, are included in this margin, Mohs is recommended to spare uninvolved tissue. If pathologic margins are involved as a permanent section, further excision with frozen-section analysis intraoperatively or Mohs is recommended. Alternatively, radiotherapy may be used for involved margins if surgery would have unacceptable morbidity (e.g., extensive eyelid resection), or if regional lymph nodes are at risk. Pathologically enlarged lymph nodes detected by exam or radiographs are managed with regional lymph node dissection for therapy and to direct postoperative adjuvant treatment. Postoperative radiotherapy is recommended for multiple involved lymph nodes or extracapsular nodal spread.

Technical Aspects of Surgical Excision and Reconstruction

Excision

The edges of the lesion should be marked to include the appropriate oncologic margin; the excision line may be injected with local anesthetic with epinephrine to reduce skin-edge bleeding. Excise the oncologic specimen before planning any closure, and orient the specimen for histologic analysis of margins. The incision should be carried down to the deep fascia using a scalpel, beveling the blade at a 90-degree angle or more to avoid undermining the oncologic

margins. Atraumatic tissue handling using toothed forceps will optimize healing.

Reconstruction and Closure

Closure of small defects is most commonly performed using an ellipse designed to excise excess skin that would otherwise result in a standing cutaneous deformity. A long elliptical incision should be avoided in excisional biopsies, as it will significantly enlarge the scar, which may need to be widely excised if margins are involved. An ellipse is fashioned along relaxed skin tension lines, which may be observed as underlying skin wrinkles; the ellipse is typically three times as long as it is wide. The deep dermis is closed with buried 3-0 vicryl sutures to reduce the tension on the closure, and the epidermis is closed with interrupted prolene monofilament sutures of appropriate size (5-0 or 6-0), which are removed 5 to 7 days later. To avoid a return visit early in the postoperative period, the surgeon may elect to use absorbable suture, which retains tensile strength for 5 to 7 days (5-0 or 6-0 fast-absorbing gut). Patients on chronic steroids or those with wound beds in a previous radiation field require epidermal suture closures with 10 to 14 days tensile strength.

Small, low-risk lesions are closed at the time of excision. However, for high-risk lesions where the margins are in doubt, healing by secondary intention, primary closure, or simple skin grafting is preferred, if histologic margins have not been assessed intraoperatively (by frozen section), as reexcision may be required. Local flap closures when the margins are in question are contraindicated, because they distort the margins relative to the original specimen. An alternative is to place a cadaveric dermis (e.g., AlloDerm, LifeCell, Branchburg, NJ) while awaiting definitive pathologic margin analysis, and plan reconstruction as a secondary procedure. Wide undermining may seed tumor into surrounding tissues and should be avoided unless intraoperative margins are negative.

Once clear margins have been confirmed, definitive reconstruction of large defects can be planned. Most cutaneous defects can be closed using a V-Y closure, rotation flap, transposition flap, or an advancement flap. Larger defects may require pedicled flaps or free-flap reconstruction. The pectoralis myocutaneous pedicled flap is widely used in the head and neck but is not well suited to reconstruct defects superior to the mandible. Free-tissue transfer techniques are recommended in previous radiotherapy fields, when separating skin from saliva or cerebrospinal fluid or when covering vital structures such as the carotid sheath.

Complications of Surgery

Unsightly scars should be allowed to mature for at least 3 months before considering revision. Incisions that cross relaxed skin tension lines can result in contracture and cosmetically unacceptable scars. The Z-plasty technique may be used to align the scar with skin tension lines (Figure 2). In addition, the use of early silicone pressure dressings for 6 to 12 weeks is helpful if patients have a history of hypertrophic scars and, after 3 months, dermabrasion may flatten raised scars. Patients with a

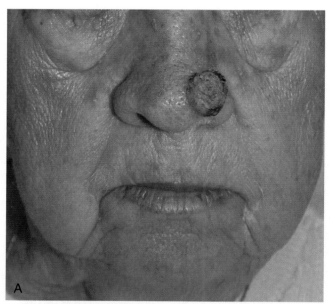
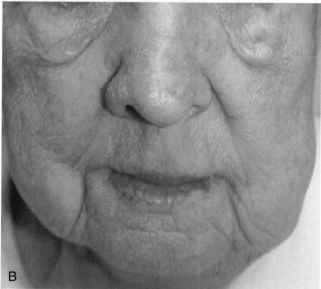

FIGURE 2 Full-thickness skin grafts are useful in older patients and may be taken from around the ear or clavicle. **A,** Squamous cell carcinoma of the left nasal ala. **B,** Cosmetic result of full-thickness skin graft reconstruction is satisfactory 6 months later.

history of keloid formation should be aggressively managed with silicone dressings and steroid injections (e.g., triamcinolone), which can be performed at the time of the initial resection and repeated.

Alternatives to Surgical Excision

Electrodissection and Curettage

Low-risk lesions less than 1 cm and superficial to the dermis are commonly treated with electrodissection and curettage, and multiple lesions may be quickly treated at a single sitting. Sequentially smaller curettes are used to remove tumor, using tension on the underlying dermal sling to delineate surrounding normal tissues. To control the subsequent bleeding, cautery (electrodissection) is applied. Use in hair-bearing sites is relatively contraindicated, because tumor may resist treatment by spreading down the follicles. The method is inexpensive, requires limited technical expertise, and results in acceptable scars. Local control is 95% at 5 years for lesions smaller than 6 mm but is lower in high-risk tumors (60% >2 cm), in which excision with margin analysis is more appropriate.

Cryotherapy

Cryotherapy is the application of liquid nitrogen, in this case, to small lesions less than 1 cm in diameter. Recurrence rates are approximately 8% to 13% with excellent cosmetic results.

Chemotherapy

Topical agents are appropriate for low-risk BCCs in patients refusing or not fit for surgical excision. Superficial BCCs and AKs can respond to topical 5% 5-FU cream applied twice daily for 4 to 8 weeks (use for Bowen disease is not FDA approved but is widely used). Patients develop a brisk inflammatory reaction with redness, serous oozing, and pain similar to a moderate sunburn that abates approximately 2 weeks after discontinuation of treatment. In addition, 5% imiquimod is an apoptosis promoter that is FDA approved for low-risk BCCs and AKs. It is applied with a 1 cm margin of normal tissue for 8 hours (apply at night, wash in the morning) 5 times a week for 6 to 12 weeks and cures approximately 80% of superficial BCCs and 66% of nodular BCCs. Skin reactions are even more brisk than with 5FU and may be associated with systemic symptoms such as fatigue and flulike illness. Photodynamic therapy for low-risk BCCs offers similar cure rates to other topical therapies. Oral retinoids such as isotretoin have proven effective for chemoprevention of AK and for skin cancers in high-risk patients. Few patients tolerate long-term treatment because of side effects such as fatigue, photosensitivity, dermatitis, and teratogenic effects, and the benefits cease when the medications are stopped.

Radiation Therapy

Radiotherapy may be used primarily for BCCs and SCCs or post-operatively as an adjuvant to surgery for very high-risk BCCs and SCCs. Primary radiotherapy is suitable for patients over 50 years old who hope to avoid surgery because of likely deformity (e.g., extensive nasal cartilage resection) or medical comorbidities. Most series report 5-year local control slightly below surgical excision: 91% to 93% for primary cases and 86% to 91% for recurrent cases. Primary radiotherapy tends to be more expensive than surgery and produces local tissue effects, most commonly dermatitis, telangiectasia, and alopecia. Tumors that occur after radiotherapy are very aggressive and make subsequent protection difficult. Less common severe side effects include marked dermal fibrosis, skin breakdown with chondronecrosis or osteoradionecrosis, and radiation-related malignancies. Radiation therapy is more commonly used as an adjuvant to surgical therapy. Common indications for postoperative radiation therapy include involved margins in which further excision has unacceptable morbidity, perineural invasion, and spread to multiple lymph nodes.

Rare Nonmelanoma Skin Malignancies

Merkel Cell Carcinoma

Merkel cell carcinoma (MCC) is a rare neuroendocrine skin cancer that typically shows up as a rapidly growing, firm, intradermal nodule in sun-exposed areas of older (median age, 53 years) white males; the male/female ratio is 3:1. MCC has recently been shown to be caused by a polyomavirus infection and is more common in immunosuppressed patients. After histologic diagnosis, CT or positron emission tomographic (PET) imaging should evaluate regional lymph nodes (involved in 15%) and distant metastases (2% at diagnosis, 40% eventually), especially to liver, bone, and brain and to exclude a lung primary. Treatment is wide excision down to fascia or pericranium, with 1.5 to 2.0 cm margins, or using Mohs to obtain negative margins; negative margins and size are prognostic. Lymph nodes may be evaluated with sentinel node biopsy or regional dissection, and adjuvant radiotherapy to the primary and lymph node sites improves local control and survival in the poor-prognosis group. Cisplatin and etoposide chemotherapy may also be used for regional or distant metastases. Failure is commonly local (30%) or in regional lymph nodes (50%), and most recurrences (90%) occur in the first 2 years. Overall 5-year survival is 70% for node-negative disease, 50% with involved nodes, and 20% for distant metastases.

Dermatofibrosarcoma Protruberans

The second most common sarcoma, dematofibrosarcoma protruberans (DFSP), typically shows up as a slow-growing red plaque on the trunk of patients in their 30s and 40s. Histology reveals a low-grade (90%) spindle cell tumor that stains for CD34, and an unbalanced gene translocation is often present on chromosome 22 related to *PDGFB*. Simple imaging with a chest radiograph is usually adequate, as distant metastases are uncommon. Subclinical disease extending outside visibly involved skin is classic for this tumor; therefore treatment with wide excision and frozen-section analysis of margins (typically 3 cm margins) or Mohs reduces local recurrence from 50% for simple excision to approximately 10%. Involved margins should ideally be reexcised. Radiotherapy is selectively used for close (<1 cm) or involved margins that cannot be reexcised. Although most local recurrences occur in the first 5 years, 25% will occur after 5 years, so long-term follow-up is required. Imitinib, a small molecular tyrosine kinase inhibitor, has shown promise in treating metastatic disease.

Kaposi Sarcoma

The most common skin sarcoma is related to HHV-8 infection and typically shows up as a slow-growing, painless, vascular-appearing lesion on the face or groin of HIV-positive or immunosuppressed patients. The surgeon's role is primarily to biopsy the area to confirm the diagnosis and exclude bacillary angiomatosis, which has a similar appearance. Solid organ disease is excluded with fecal occult blood testing and a chest radiograph. Treatment includes optimization of the underlying HIV with antiretroviral therapy and either intralesional vinblastine or radiotherapy for localized disease and systemic doxorubicin for advanced disease.

Angiosarcoma

Angiosarcoma is a rare skin tumor that typically presents as a rapidly growing, vascular-appearing lesion with ulceration and satellite nodules on the head and neck of elderly (median age, 70 years) male patients. Careful evaluation should be made for distant metastases, which occur most commonly in the lungs, to avoid aggressive treatment in terminal cases. Traditional treatment has been surgery with wide margins (2 cm) that usually require free-flap reconstruction and postoperative radiotherapy. Despite this, prognosis is poor (20% 5-year survival) with more local recurrences than distant metastases (30%). Because of the poor prognosis and the significant proportion of patients who are initially diagnosed with unresectable disease, many centers are now using induction chemotherapy (paclitaxel or doxorubicin) and following it with surgery and/or radiotherapy.

SUGGESTED READINGS

NCCN Clinical Practice Guidelines in Oncology v.1.2009, *Basal cell and squamous cell skin cancers.* Available at http://www.nccn.org. Accessed March 18, 2009.

Telfer NR, Colver GB, Morton CA: Guidelines for the management of basal cell carcinoma, *Br J Dermatol* 159:35–48, 2008.

Alam M, Ratner D: Cutaneous squamous cell carcinoma, *N Engl J Med* 344:975–982, 2001.

Smeets NW, Krekels GA, Ostertag JU, et al: Surgical excision vs. Mohs' micrographic surgery for basal cell carcinoma of the face: randomized controlled trial, *Lancet* 364:1766–1772, 2004.

Euvrard S, Kanitakis J, Claudy A: Skin cancers after organ transplantation, *N Engl J Med* 348:1682–1690, 2003.

CUTANEOUS MELANOMA

Marc K. Wallack, MD, John J. Degliuomini, MD, Jennifer E. Joh, MD, and Manijeh Berenji, MD

OVERVIEW

Melanoma is one of the most common forms of cancer in the United States. It is estimated that approximately 62,000 cases are diagnosed annually, and the mortality rate attributed to melanoma is approximately 8400 patients per year. The incidence of melanoma continues to increase dramatically. It is the most common form of cancer in young adults between the ages of 25 to 29 years and is the second most common cancer in adolescents and young adults between the ages of 15 and 29 years.

Risk factors for melanoma include family history of melanoma, prior blistering sunburn, prior melanoma, multiple clinically atypical moles or dysplastic nevi, inherited genetic mutations such as *xeroderma pigmentosa* and Wiskott-Aldrich syndrome, and chronic sun exposure. Individuals with fair skin that sunburns easily or light-colored hair and eyes are at a greater risk for developing melanoma. Chronic sun exposure secondary to military activity in the Middle East is expected to have significant implications for the incidence of melanoma in the United States. Lesions that should raise suspicion are those that are *a*symmetric, with an irregular *b*order, variegated with respect to *c*olor, and large (>6 mm) in *d*iameter (ABCD mnemonic).

BIOPSY TECHNIQUES

The goal of biopsy is to obtain enough tissue to make a complete evaluation of the lesion. Biopsy may be performed either as an excisional or incisional biopsy. When performing an excisional biopsy, consideration must be given not only to the radial diameter but to the entire depth of the lesion, because prognosis is in part related to the depth of penetration (Figure 1). A reexcision with margins may be necessary once the diagnosis is made, so thoughtful orientation of the incision is essential; axial orientation is preferable in the extremities.

An incisional or punch biopsy may be used with large lesions (>2 cm) or in areas that may be difficult to close primarily, such as the scalp, face, or extremities. These biopsies should include the darkest areas of pigmentation and the thickest palpable area; otherwise, our strong recommendation would be a complete excisional biopsy for proper evaluation of the lesion.

TREATMENT OF THE PRIMARY LESION

The goal in the treatment of the primary lesion is to achieve long-term local disease control and to cure patients who do not yet have micrometastases to lymph nodes or distant sites. This involves wide local excision (WLE) of the diagnostic biopsy site with a margin of skin and fat down to muscle fascia.

Traditional treatment of primary melanoma involved the use of margins greater than 2 cm. However, studies have shown no significant overall survival benefit with those margins; current recommendations for resection margins are summarized in Table 1. In the treatment of upper extremity subungual melanoma, WLE must observe the same margins; therefore recommendations generally consist of amputation of the digit to the midproximal phalanx with reimplantation of the flexor and extensor digitorum tendons. In the lower extremity, this amputation is taken to the metatarsal head.

TREATMENT OF ATYPICAL MELANOCYTIC LESIONS

Atypical melanocytic lesions can present a diagnostic dilemma and may require that specimen slides be sent for outside consultation with an expert dermatopathologist. When confusion exists as to the primary diagnosis, it is best to treat the lesion according to the diagnosis that carries the worst prognosis. Misdiagnosis is not uncommon, and local recurrence rates can be high.

Lentigo maligna represents a histologic subtype of in situ melanoma, whereas *lentigo maligna melanoma* implies that the primary lesion has an invasive component. These lesions occur on chronically sun-exposed areas that can be anatomically restrictive to conventional resection. Reconstruction of the defect may require flap closure, and therefore a delayed or staged reconstruction may be appropriate, until margin status can be verified by histologic analysis.

REGIONAL LYMPH NODE ASSESSMENT

Major changes have been made in the management of regional lymph nodes for melanoma patients over the past couple decades. With ongoing research and interest in this field, the management of melanoma will continue to evolve. Historically, all patients with melanoma once underwent elective regional lymph node dissection (ELND). However, a significant number of patients did not have involved lymph nodes at the time of dissection, and they were subjected to considerable morbidity from the procedure.

In 1992, a major advance was made when Morton and colleagues first described the technique of lymphatic mapping and sentinel lymph node (SLN) biopsy in the management of melanoma. This technique involved minimal risk and morbidity while properly identifying

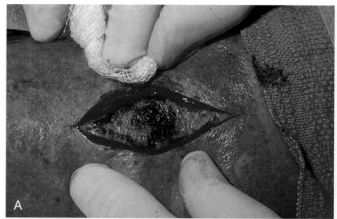

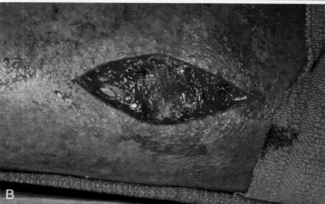

FIGURE 1   A, Excisional biopsy of suspicious lesion. **B,** Biopsy site extending down to muscle fascia.

TABLE 1: Recommended margins in the resection of primary melanoma

Thickness	Margin	Considerations
In situ	0.5–1 cm	Local recurrence may be present as invasive disease. Microscopically, *lentigo maligna* may extend beyond normal-appearing skin and may require wider margins.
<1 mm	1 cm	
1–2 mm	2 cm	A 1 cm margin may be acceptable in anatomic regions where obtaining a 2 cm margin would impact function.
2–4 mm	2 cm	
>4 mm	2 cm	Local recurrence rates can be as high as 11%, but no reported benefit in overall survival has been observed with wider margins.

occult metastatic disease. Currently, SLN biopsy is recommended in all melanoma patients with clinically and radiographically negative regional lymph nodes and the primary lesion either larger than 1 mm or 1 mm or smaller with ulceration or a mitotic rate less than 1 mm².

Evaluation of the SLN for metastasis is one of the most important prognostic factors in patients with melanoma. Results of the

Multicenter Selective Lymphadenectomy Trial (MSLT) demonstrated that those patients with tumor-negative SLN biopsies had a significantly higher 5-year survival rate compared with those found to have tumor-positive SLN biopsies.

Lymphatic Mapping and SLN Biopsy

The SLN is the first lymph node to receive lymphatic drainage from the primary tumor site. If the melanoma were to spread, malignant cells would be carried through draining lymphatic channels to the first, or sentinel, node in the lymphatic chain. Lymphoscintigraphy simulates lymphatic drainage from the primary tumor site. This is performed preoperatively on the day of surgery with an intradermal injection of technetium-labeled sulfur colloid around the primary melanoma site. Lymphatic mapping should image all areas, because there are instances where the drainage is uncertain, such as in primary lesions of the trunk, head, and neck. The patients are then placed as they would be in the operating room, and the skin is marked where the SLN is located.

Intraoperatively, a second lymphatic tracer, vital blue dye, is injected intradermally at the melanoma site. Only 1 or 2 mL of dye is needed, and the injection site is gently massaged for 1 or 2 minutes to increase lymphatic flow. Allergy-type complications from the vital blue dye may occur, including anaphylactic reactions, but these are extremely rare (<1%). If possible, the vital blue dye injection should be performed within the boundaries of the WLE, as it may be retained within the skin for several months. Patients should be advised beforehand of the presence of dye in urine and stool during the first 24 hours.

Before making the incision, a handheld γ-probe may be used to reconfirm the location of the SLN. Most of the time, only a small incision is needed to perform the biopsy. Consideration of incision location should take into account the possibility of eventual completion lymph node dissection, as excision of the old scar site is part of that operation. Continual scanning of the nodal basin during dissection of the area will help direct the surgeon to the SLN. Oftentimes, co-localization with a functional, radioactive node that has taken up the vital dye ("hot and blue") is common. The node is then removed from the surrounding fatty tissue with careful ligation of vessels and lymphatic channels, and ex vivo radiotracer counts are performed on the SLN. If the node appears grossly metastatic, and the possibility of completion lymph node dissection was discussed for the current operation, the SLN is sent to pathology for frozen-section analysis; otherwise, it is preserved in its entirety for permanent section. The remaining tissue basin is rescanned for other areas of increased radiotracer activity. Sometimes, more than one SLN may be present, and each subsequent node is handled in the same manner. The biopsy site is then irrigated and inspected for hemostasis, and the wound is closed in two layers.

Approximately 10% of all patients who undergo lymphoscintigraphy and SLN biopsy have complications. In the MSLT, wound infection, wound separation, and seroma/hematoma were reported as 4.6%, 1.2%, and 5.5%, respectively. Given the limited dissection in SLN biopsy, the rate of lymphedema is less than 1%.

Regional Lymphadenectomy

Regional lymphadenectomy should be undertaken for all patients with a positive SLN or macroscopic *metastatic nodal disease,* defined as clinically palpable nodal disease and a pathologically proven involved lymph node. Patients who have a positive SLN are at risk for additional involved lymph nodes within that nodal basin. In regard to microscopic metastatic nodal disease, there has been ongoing investigation into its management and indications for performing regional lymphadenectomy. However, it is our current view that those patients with metastatic nodal disease, whether microscopic or macroscopic, should undergo regional lymphadenectomy.

TABLE 2: Recommended number of regional nodes in lymphadenectomy

Region	Number of Nodes
Axillary	15
Inguinofemoral	8
Iliac/obturator	6
Cervical, anterior	15
Cervical, posterior	15
Supraclavicular	6
Suprahyoid	4
Parotid	3
Popliteal	2–3

Regional lymph node dissection offers the best chance for control and cure of locoregional disease. Approximately one third of patients with macroscopic nodal disease are cured with regional lymphadenectomy. For that reason, complete removal of the entire involved nodal basin is of paramount importance (Table 2).

Regardless of the anatomic location for lymphadenectomy, the first step is the creation of skin flaps. If possible, sharp dissection of the flaps is employed to reduce the incidence of thermal injury causing flap necrosis. This may be particularly important in the inguinal dissection, as these flaps tend to be more tenuous. The use of skin hooks at the onset may also be helpful. To reduce the incidence of lymphocele, all lymphatic channels should be ligated during the dissection. At the end of the procedure, closed-suction drainage is placed through a separate stab incision and is usually left in place for 2 to 5 days postoperatively, until the drainage is less than 20 to 25 mL per day. Strenuous exercise should be avoided until all drains are removed and wounds have healed; however, simple range-of-motion exercises may be employed.

Neck Dissection

The extent of lymphadenectomy in the neck is variable and takes into account the primary melanoma site and degree of nodal disease. Radical neck lymphadenectomy with resection of the sternocleidomastoid muscle, spinal accessory nerve, and internal jugular vein is rarely employed because of the functional deficits associated with its use. Melanomas associated with clinically apparent cervical disease require modified radical neck lymphadenectomy involving clearance of all ipsilateral cervical nodal tissue with preservation of one or more of the structures sacrificed in a radical neck dissection. Lymphadenectomy for a positive SLN typically does not require sacrifice of any of these functional structures. In patients with melanomas of the anterior face, scalp, and upper neck and clinically apparent cervical disease, superficial parotidectomy should be considered in conjunction with lymphadenectomy. Another consideration specific to neck lymphadenectomy includes the use of bipolar cautery during dissection for better control of current transmission and heat conduction.

Axillary Dissection

Unlike axillary lymph node dissection for breast carcinoma, removal of all three levels of axillary lymph nodes with skeletonization of the axillary vein should be accomplished. If the pectoralis minor must be sacrificed to accomplish this, it should be divided as close to the coracoid process as possible. During dissection, the long thoracic and thoracodorsal nerves should be found and preserved, if they are not grossly involved with tumor. Oftentimes, intercostobrachial nerves may need to be sacrificed and will lead to sensory changes on the posterior upper arm.

Groin Dissection

There are two nodal basins in the groin, the inguinofemoral and iliac/obturator, that may require lymphadenectomy. Inguinofemoral dissection, formerly referred to as *superficial inguinal dissection,* involves the lymphatic tissue over the lower external oblique and inguinal ligament and within the femoral triangle. Iliac/obturator dissection, previously called *deep inguinal dissection,* includes removal of nodal tissue adjacent to the iliac vessels, obturator nerve, and the node of Cloquet at the iliofemoral junction. Iliac/obturator inguinal dissection is only performed if preoperative radiologic staging demonstrates involvement of these deep nodes. Other possible indications include a positive Cloquet node, more than four positive nodes on inguinofemoral dissection, and palpable or extracapsular extension of femoral nodes. The term *radical groin dissection* is a combination of both superficial and deep inguinal dissections and is rarely performed.

Ectopic Nodal Sites

With the use of lymphoscintigraphy, detection of metastatic disease in ectopic nodal sites, including those located in the popliteal and epitrochlear regions, has increased. These sites may be considered extensions of their adjacent nodal basins, as some evidence suggests that metastatic disease at the ectopic nodal sites might indicate subclinical disease in the adjacent basin and therefore requires regional lymphadenectomy. However, ectopic nodal dissection is rarely performed, unless palpable disease is evident.

STAGING

Staging is useful for determining prognosis and survival in melanoma patients. It is based on TNM classification and may be further divided into *clinical* and *pathologic* staging (Table 3). The difference between clinical and pathologic staging is dependent upon whether the regional lymph nodes were staged by a clinical radiographic exam or by pathologic evaluation. Significant differences in survival rates are seen when comparing pathologic staging with clinical staging; this highlights the importance of determining nodal status with SLN examination. Poor prognostic factors in melanoma patients include thick tumors, ulceration, high mitotic rate, age over 60 years, truncal lesions, male gender, higher Clark level, macrometastases, increased number of positive nodes, and an elevated lactate dehydrogenase.

RECONSTRUCTION TECHNIQUES

Following WLE of the primary lesion, proper closure of the defect is essential to ensuring optimal wound healing. The goal of reconstruction after WLE is to achieve stable soft-tissue coverage and prompt healing, ideally in one step, while maintaining the contour, texture, color, and function of the region. Options for wound closure include primary closure, local and distant flaps, and skin grafting.

In the past, wide resection margins necessitated more complex solutions to wound closure. However, new recommended margin guidelines have allowed for wide undermining with primary closure in most cases (Figure 2). Primary closure requires that the longitudinal axis of the elliptical incision be at least three times the length of the short axis, with ensuing two-layer (dermal and subcuticular) closure. Although small lesions can be closed in this manner, the management of larger, more complex defects may require cooperative

TABLE 3: TNM classification of melanoma

Primary Tumor (T)	
TX: Primary tumor cannot be assessed	
T0: No evidence of primary tumor	
Tis: Melanoma in situ	
T1: Melanoma ≤1.0 mm in thickness	a: Without ulceration and mitosis <1 mm^2 b: With ulceration or mitoses >1 mm^2
T2: Melanoma 1.01–2.0 mm in thickness	a: Without ulceration b: With ulceration
T3: Melanoma 2.01–4.0 mm in thickness	a: Without ulceration b: With ulceration
T4: Melanoma >4.0 mm in thickness	a: Without ulceration b: With ulceration
Regional Lymph Nodes (N)	
N0: No regional metastases detected	
N1: One node	a: Micrometastasis* b: Macrometastasis†
N2: Two to three nodes	a: Micrometastasis* b: Macrometastasis† c: In-transit met(s)/satellite(s) without metastatic nodes
N3: Four or more nodes, matted nodes, or in-transit met(s)/satellite(s) with metastatic nodes	
Distant Metastasis (M)	
M0: No detectable evidence of distant metastasis	
M1a: Metastases to skin, subcutaneous, or distant lymph nodes	Normal LDH
M1b: Metastases to lung	Normal LDH
M1c: Metastases to all other visceral sites or distant metastases to any site	Normal LDH Elevated LDH

LDH, Lactate dehydrogenase
*Micrometastases are diagnosed after SLN biopsy and completion lymphadenectomy (if performed).
†Macrometastases are defined as clinically detectable nodal metastases confirmed by therapeutic lymphadenectomy or when nodal metastasis exhibits gross extracapsular extension.

interaction between the general surgeon and the plastic surgeon to yield a satisfactory closure. In such cases, if primary closure is not possible, local flaps provide good cosmetic and functional results for areas such as the face and distal extremities. Two types of local flaps may be employed: either a *rotational* or *transposition flap,* which revolves around a fixed point, or a *single-pedicle/bipedicle* or V-Y *advancement flap.* Distant or regional flaps are harvested from a site near the defect and are only used when sufficient tissue is not available for a local flap.

Skin grafting may also be used for wound closure. They may either be full- or split-thickness grafts. Split-thickness skin grafts are more likely to shrink and cause hyperpigmentation compared with full-thickness grafts; however, they are also more likely to survive. Full-thickness skin grafts require a well-vascularized recipient bed. If expertise is not available, we propose that the simplest form of closure for a WLE site is to use a split-thickness skin graft that is "pie-crusted" and stapled to the edges of the wound. A bolster dressing or negative-pressure wound management system may then be placed over the wound to promote graft success (Figure 3). Closed-suction drainage may be used to ensure proper wound healing in preparation for skin grafting.

IN-TRANSIT METASTASIS

Satellite and in-transit metastases are a form of intralymphatic locoregional disease that is thought to result from tumor emboli trapped within dermal and subdermal lymphatics. Satellite lesions are those lesions that occur within 2 cm of the primary melanoma. In-transit metastases occur at a distance greater than 2 cm from the primary melanoma, located between the primary site and the regional lymph node basin. In-transit lesions are usually multiple, they evolve over time, and they are usually associated with simultaneous and or subsequent distal disease.

The incidence of in-transit metastasis has been projected to range from 4.8% to 22% and is influenced by the initial stage of the primary lesion and its treatment. In-transit disease has been measured in various studies to occur as early as 13 to 24 months after surgery for the primary lesions. It is estimated that 70% to 80% of regional recurrences happen within the first 3 years after treatment of the primary melanoma.

Associated risk factors include tumor thickness and ulceration, lesions on the lower extremity, and positive lymph node status. The number of positive lymph nodes has also been correlated with increased risk for the development of in-transit disease: it is 11% in patients with one positive node and up to 33% in patients with three or more positive nodes. The location of the positive lymph node basin also has implications: patients with inguinal lymph node disease are at higher risk of developing in-transit metastases compared with those who have cervical or axillary lymph node disease.

Treatment options for in-transit disease can be classified into *local, regional,* and *systemic* therapies. The number of lesions, their location and size, and the presence of extraregional disease will factor into the optimal choice of therapy. These patients should be considered for enrollment in clinical trials. Local treatment options include surgery, intralesion injection, CO_2 laser, and external beam radiation.

Surgical excision with a negative margin may be an option for patients with a limited number of lesions. Wide margins are unnecessary, however, it should be noted that surgery alone does not usually control regional disease and further recurrence is the rule. Patients with multiple lesions may be candidates for injection with either bacillus Calmette-Guérin or dinitrochlorobenzene. Interferon-α has also been shown to have some effectiveness in conjunction with the above-mentioned therapies the treatment of these skin metastases.

CO_2 laser therapy is another form of local treatment for in-transit melanoma. There are no systemic effects and also no reported impact on overall survival. External beam radiation has been used in surgically unresectable regional recurrence with limited success. The rationale behind regional therapy is that patients treated with only local therapy have a high rate of subsequent regional failure. The goal in treatment is durable long-term control of clinical and subclinical regional disease.

Hypoxic isolated limb infusion and hyperthermic isolated limb perfusion are two regional modalities that can deliver chemotherapeutic and biologically active agents with minimal systemic toxicity. In an experienced center, where morbidity is low, hyperthermic isolated limb perfusion with melphalan would be considered to be the treatment of choice for those patients with unresectable in-transit melanoma. The patient selected for limb perfusion should have good peripheral arterial and venous circulation, and optimally most of the in-transit disease should be located in the distal two thirds of the extremity.

Systemic chemotherapy may be of use in patients with in-transit melanoma who are not candidates for local or regional therapy. Traditional single-agent regimens have utilized dacarbazine and temozolomide. Response rates have been low with most being partial and transient. The use of multiagent chemotherapy may promise improved response rates, however, this must be balanced with the increased risk of systemic toxicity and the poor expectation of durable long-term response. The results of regional chemotherapy may be improved when combined with resection of residual in-transit disease.

TREATMENT OF METASTATIC DISEASE

Once melanoma spreads to distant sites, the number of treatment options begins to dwindle. The decision to treat should be made in conjunction with the medical and radiation oncologist. Most patients at this advanced stage will have disease that is either too extensive to resect or is unresectable based on its location. Median survival for stage IV melanoma is 7 to 8 months, and 5-year overall survival rates for stage IV melanoma are 5% to 6%.

Surgical resection is most effective in patients exhibiting advanced disease limited to isolated accessible distant metastases, irrespective of whether the primary tumor has been identified. However, determining a patient's candidacy for such surgery involves evaluating the actual location of the metastases, the underlying tumor biology, the likely duration of survival, and the individual's overall performance status.

Although the majority of patients succumbing to melanoma will have multiple tumor-involved organ sites, nearly 90% will initially show involvement of only one metastatic site. The most common sites of metastasis, in descending order, are lung, skin, lymph nodes, brain, liver, bone, and gastrointestinal tract.

The behavior and operability of the metastatic lesion and the patient's chance of survival is a function of tumor growth kinetics based on tumor doubling time. If the metastatic tumor is slow to double during the period of observation, usually 3 to 6 months, and does not metastasize, the patient is a good candidate for resection. In this way, patients who would otherwise not be cured by metastatic resection are identified and spared noncurative resection.

Multiple retrospective studies have reported long-term survival in these patients, with several surviving for more than 10 years despite being considered incurable. Despite all of this, patients with brain and bony metastases have had less success with such interventions. Although previous data had demonstrated that melanoma was a relatively radioresistant tumor, recent data have shown that radiation therapy is beneficial as a palliative measure, helping 50% to 86% of patients alleviate bone pain and spinal cord compression.

IMMUNOTHERAPY

Since melanoma is an immunogenic solid tumor, the role of immunotherapy in eliciting the patient's immune system to target and potentially eradicate these tumors continues to be an area of active research interest. Such immunotherapeutic regimens are employed alone, in combination protocols, or with additional chemotherapy and radiotherapy.

TABLE 4: American Joint Committee on Cancer Staging

CLINICAL STAGING				PATHOLOGIC STAGING*			
Stage 0	Tis	N0	M0	Stage 0	Tis	N0	M0
Stage IA	T1a	N0	M0	Stage IIIA	T1–4a	N1a or 2a	M0
Stage IB	T1b or T2a	N0	M0	Stage IIIB	T1–4b	N1a or 2a	M0
Stage IIA	T2b or 3a	N0	M0		T1–4a	N1b or 2b	M0
Stage IIB	T3b or 4a	N0	M0		T14a	N2c	M0
Stage IIC	T4b	N0	M0	Stage IIIC			
Stage III	Any T	N ≥ N1	M0	Stage IV	Any T	N3	M0
Stage IV	Any T	Any N	M1		Any T	Any N	M1

*Pathologic stages I and II are the same as the clinical stages.
Based on the *AJCC Cancer Staging Manual,* ed 7, New York, 2009, American Joint Committee on Cancer.

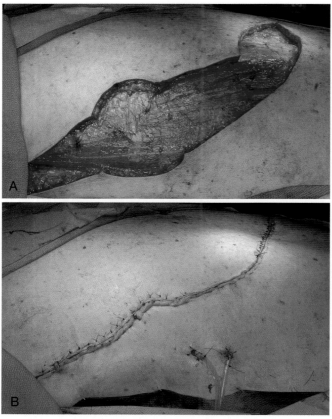

FIGURE 2   **A,** Surgical wound following en bloc wide excision of primary melanoma site and in-transit metastasis. **B,** Primary closure of complex wound accomplished over closed-suction drains.

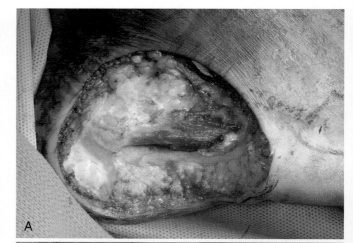

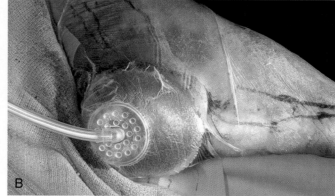

FIGURE 3   **A,** Open wound following wide excision of a melanoma of the lower extremity. **B,** Use of a negative-pressure dressing to facilitate wound healing and eventual closure with autologous tissue grafting.

- Cytokines: Currently, high-dose interferon α2b is the only FDA-approved agent in the treatment of resected stage IIb and III melanoma. Interleukin-2 (IL-2) at high doses has also been evaluated in advanced disease with noted tumor regression, but it is associated with significant toxicity.
- Antibodies: Monoclonal antibodies have been developed to target T-cell and melanoma cell surface antigens.

- Adoptive cell transfer: This treatment involves the infusion of expanded autologous T cells into the lymphodepleted melanoma patient.
- Vaccines: Melanoma vaccines offer a unique approach to tumor immunology. In a recent phase III randomized trial, patients with metastatic melanoma were immunized with a specific

melanoma peptide, followed by high-dose IL-2, then compared with patients given high-dose IL-2 alone. The patients who were given the peptide vaccine with IL-2 had improved response rates compared with those given IL-2 alone, a clear demonstration of the "proof of principle" that cancer vaccines can, and indeed, do work.

- Molecularly targeted therapy: Identification of gene mutations, such as *BRAF* and *NRAS,* in the cell-signaling pathway has become a prime area of interest for targeted drug therapy in melanoma.

Immunotherapy will become an even more potent therapeutic strategy in the treatment of advanced melanoma and in those patients at high risk for recurrence.

SUGGESTED READINGS

Balch CM, Houghton AN, Sober AJ, et al: *Cutaneous melanoma,* ed 5, St Louis, 2009, Quality Medical Publishing.

Cady B: The changing role of the surgical oncologist, *Surg Clin North Am* 80(2):459–469, 2000.

Jack A, Boyes C, Aydin N, et al: The treatment of melanoma with an emphasis on immunotherapeutic strategies, *Surg Oncol* 15:13–24, 2006.

Morton DL, Cochran AJ, Thompson JF, et al: and the Multicenter Selective Lymphadenectomy Trial Group: sentinel node biopsy for early-stage melanoma: accuracy and morbidity in MSLT-I, an international multicenter trial, *Ann Surg* 242(3):302–313, 2005.

Schadendorf D, Algarra SM, Bastholt L, et al: Immunotherapy of distant metastatic disease, *Ann Oncol* 20(Suppl 6):vi41–vi50, 2009.

MANAGEMENT OF SOFT TISSUE SARCOMAS

Sam S. Yoon, MD, and Francis J. Hornicek, MD, PhD

OVERVIEW

A soft tissue sarcoma (STS) is a malignant tumor that arises from the mesoderm-derived tissues—fat, muscle, connective tissue, and vessels—excluding bone and cartilage. In addition, malignant tumors of peripheral nerve sheaths are usually included as STS despite being ectodermal in origin. STS is an uncommon malignancy with only about 10,000 new cases and 3500 deaths in the United States per year. These tumors occur at any age, with a median age of about 50 years, and they are equally common in men and women.

STS constitutes a highly heterogenous group of tumors with respect to anatomical distribution, histologic subtype, and clinical behavior. They occur throughout the body, with nearly one half occurring in the extremities. Another one third of STS occurs in the abdomen and pelvis, and these are equally divided among intraabdominal visceral sarcomas, primarily gastrointestinal stromal tumors and leiomyosarcomas, and retroperitoneal sarcomas. Over 50 different histologic subtypes of STS exist, the most common of which are malignant fibrous histiocytoma (MFH), liposarcoma, leiomyosarcoma, synovial sarcoma, and fibrosarcoma. STS previously classified as MFH is now classified more commonly as myxofibrosarcoma or undifferentiated pleomorphic sarcoma.

Although each histologic subtype may have a certain unique clinical behavior, all STS can generally be categorized into *low-, intermediate-,* and *high-grade* tumors. Low-grade tumors generally grow more slowly, can recur locally after resection, but have a low risk of distant metastases (~5%). High-grade tumors tend to grow more rapidly, can also recur locally after resection, and have the added risk of distant metastasis that can approach 50% for large (>8 to 10 cm) tumors.

ETIOLOGY

The vast majority of STS occurs as sporadic tumors in patients with no identified genetic or environmental risk factors. However, certain genetic syndromes are associated with an increased risk of developing sarcomas. Neurofibromatosis 1 (NF1, or von Recklinghausen disease) is associated with an approximately 15% risk of developing malignant transformation of a neurofibroma into a malignant peripheral nerve sheath tumor (MPNST). Individuals with NF1 also carry an increased risk of gastrointestinal stromal tumors (GIST). Patients with Gardner syndrome, resulting from a defect in the *APC* gene, have an increased risk of developing intraabdominal/mesenteric desmoid tumors. Hereditary retinoblastoma and Li-Fraumeni syndrome are associated with a risk of both bone sarcoma and STS. Specific genetic abnormalities, as evidenced by nonrandom chromosomal aberrations, are well established in certain STS histologic subtypes and are often used in the definitive diagnosis. For example, synovial sarcomas usually have a translocation that fuses the *SSX1* or *SSX2* gene to the *SYT* gene.

Radiation is recognized as being capable of inducing sarcomas in soft tissue and bone. The incidence of radiation-associated sarcomas increases with radiation dose and with the postradiation observation period. Following breast irradiation, the most common radiation-induced sarcomas are angiosarcomas. The actuarial frequency of radiation-associated sarcoma at 15 to 20 years is approximately 0.2% in adults treated with radiation alone to full dose. The frequency is higher following treatment of children, especially those treated with both radiation and chemotherapy. Chemotherapeutic agents and exposure to a few select industrial chemicals are likewise associated with risk of sarcoma induction. Trauma is rarely a factor in the development of these tumors with the exception of desmoid tumors. The usual history is of a traumatic incident occurring shortly before awareness of the mass, suggesting that the trauma merely brought the patient's attention to the presence of the mass.

TREATMENT

Given that STS is uncommon, occurs throughout the body, and has over 50 histologic subtypes, each with variations in biologic behavior, the workup and treatment of these tumors can be confusing and quite challenging. Optimal treatment often requires multimodal therapy, so treating surgeons, radiation oncologists, and medical oncologists should be involved at the outset, and a treatment plan should be determined after multidisciplinary discussion. Certain complex tumors may be best treated at sarcoma referral centers.

The clinical workup and subsequent treatment of STS is often specific to the anatomic location of the primary tumor. Thus the treatment of extremity STS will be discussed, and much of the treatment of extremity tumors can be applied to truncal tumors. The treatment of retroperitoneal STS will be discussed separately, and treatment of gastrointestinal stromal tumors is reviewed in Section II.

EXTREMITY SOFT TISSUE SARCOMA

Clinical Evaluation

The most frequent initial complaint with extremity STS is that of a painless mass for a few weeks to several months, however, pain or tenderness can precede the detection of a mass. With progressive growth of the tumor, symptoms such as edema and neuropathy can appear secondary to infiltration of or pressure on adjacent structures. A complete history and physical examination should be obtained, with particular attention paid to the region of the primary lesion and the definition of size, site of origin (superficial or deep, mobile or fixed to deep structures), involvement or discoloration of overlying skin, functional status of vessels and nerves, and presence of distal edema. Laboratory studies need not go beyond a complete blood count and chemistry panel. There are no established tumor markers for STS.

For the primary site, the radiographic evaluation should include a computed tomographic (CT) and/or magnetic resonance imaging (MRI) scan. The most useful radiologic study to evaluate an extremity or trunk primary site is an MRI, but CT scans can provide supplemental information. A chest CT should be obtained for high-grade tumors to evaluate for lung metastases, and chest radiograph is probably adequate for low-grade tumors. The role of positron emission tomography scans has yet to be defined, but most primary and metastatic tumors do show increased fluorodeoxyglucose uptake.

An adequate biopsy is required to establish a histologic diagnosis (histologic subtype and grade) and to determine a definitive treatment strategy. In the majority of cases, the diagnosis can be established by core needle biopsy. Superficial lesions that are readily palpable can be directly biopsied without imaging in an outpatient clinic under local anesthesia. For deep tumors or tumors requiring a more precise biopsy, an image-directed core biopsy can be performed. Image-guided biopsy may be better than even an open biopsy, because the biopsy can be directed to a specific region in a typically heterogenous tumor. Open biopsies should be reserved for the uncommon patient, in whom core biopsy is not adequate. For small tumors (<3 to 5 cm), an excisional biopsy can be performed, and incisional biopsies can be performed for larger lesions. The incision for open biopsies should be oriented longitudinally, such that it can be easily incorporated in the definitive resection. Care should be taken to minimize bleeding and contamination of surrounding tissues. Fine needle aspiration (FNA) biopsy can be employed to confirm metastatic or recurrent tumor, when the primary diagnosis is already established, but it is usually not adequate to establish an initial diagnosis. All suspected STS cases should be reviewed by an experienced sarcoma pathologist, because about 10% of tumors originally designated as STS are in fact not STS, and about 20% are initially assigned the incorrect histologic subtype.

Staging

The Task Force on Soft-Tissue Sarcomas of the American Joint Committee on Cancer (AJCC) Staging and End-Result Reporting has established a staging system for soft-tissue sarcomas that is an extension of the TNM system to include G for histologic grade (Table 1). Grade, size, depth, and presence of nodal or distant metastases are the determinants of stage. Tumor grade is determined on the basis of the histologic features of the individual tumor, such as cellularity, differentiation, pleomorphism, necrosis, and mitotic activity. Some institutions assign grades 1 through 3: grade 1 lesions are considered low-grade lesions, with minimal metastatic potential; intermediate-grade (grade 2) and high-grade (grade 3) lesions are both considered to be capable of metastasis. Other institutions use a two- or four-tiered system.

Surgical Treatment

STS is generally surrounded by a thin layer of fibrous tissue known as the *pseudocapsule*. If STS is "shelled out" along the pseudocapsule, which is done for benign tumors such as lipomas, the local recurrence rates will be up to 90%. More radical resection of tumors with a margin of normal tissue can decrease the local recurrence rate to 10% to 30%. However, STS of the extremities can grow adjacent to major blood vessels, nerves, and bones; and until the early 1980s, the standard operation for many STS patients was amputation. In 1982 Rosenberg and colleagues at the National Cancer Institute (NCI) published a randomized trial of amputation versus limb-sparing surgery and radiation (both groups received chemotherapy) and demonstrated equivalent overall survival with a local recurrence rate of 0% for amputation versus 15% for limb-sparing surgery. Limb-sparing surgery can now be performed in over 90% of patients with extremity STS, and overall local recurrence rates with limb-sparing surgery and adjuvant radiation are often less than 10%.

Several surgical principles should be followed when resecting STS. First, the preoperative imaging studies should be carefully examined to identify the full extent of tumor penetration as well as the relationship of the tumor to adjacent vital structures. Second, the operative plan should be carefully considered, and additional consultants, such as plastic or vascular surgeons, should be arranged in advance if their assistance is anticipated. Third, an adequate incision and exposure are essential (Figure 1). Incisions should generally be oriented longitudinally and should extend beyond the proximal and distal extent of the tumor. Fourth, the skin and subcutaneous tissue overlying the STS should be resected if needed to gain an adequate superficial margin. The surgeon should not sacrifice an adequate margin by leaving skin and subcutaneous tissue adjacent to the tumor to avoid a skin graft or flap. Fifth, for subfascial tumors, subcutaneous flaps can be raised at the level of the Scarpa fascia both medially and laterally, until an adequate surgical margin beyond the edge of the tumor is reached, at which point the dissection can be taken deeper into the overlying fascia. It can be difficult to determine an adequate margin with a tumor that has an indistinct border. Sixth, tumors should be resected with an attempt to obtain a 2 cm margin of normal tissue, if this can be done without severe morbidity. Leaving the operating surgeon's nondominant hand at the edge of the tumor can give good tactile feedback regarding the apparent adequacy of the margin. Seventh, some normal tissues, such as fascia, provide a better quality margin than other tissues, such as fat and muscle; thus a close (1 mm) fascia margin is often acceptable, but the surgeon should be more concerned about a close margin of fat or muscle. Finally, STS does not usually invade the periadventitial tissue of arteries, the perineurium of nerves, or the periosteum of bone, and thus can often be dissected with incorporation of these barriers to obtain a negative margin.

Surgeons must use considerable judgment in resecting STS. Positive microscopic margins are associated with an increased risk of local recurrence, so the surgeon should strive for negative microscopic margins in all patients, unless this would create unacceptable morbidity. Local recurrence following surgical resection with negative microscopic margins and adjuvant radiation is 10% or less. Where there is a positive microscopic margin, the dosage of adjuvant radiation therapy is usually increased, leading to a higher risk of radiation-related side effects; but local recurrence can often be reduced to 20% or less.

In addition to good surgical judgment, the surgeon must also be familiar with the varying tumor biology of certain histologic subtypes when determining the optimal treatment strategy. For example, atypical lipomas of the extremity, also termed *well-differentiated liposarcomas* by some sarcoma pathologists, have a relatively low recurrence rate when excised with a positive microscopic margin; so surgical resection should not be overly aggressive, and adjuvant radiation is often not necessary. On the other hand, cutaneous angiosarcomas can have highly irregular and infiltrative margins, thus aggressive surgical resection and adjuvant radiation therapy are usually warranted.

TABLE 1: AJCC staging system for STS

Histologic Grade of Malignancy				
GX		Grade cannot be assessed		
G1		Grade 1		
G2		Grade 2		
G3		Grade 3		
Primary Tumor				
TX		Primary tumor cannot be assessed		
T0		No evidence of primary tumor		
T1		Tumor ≤5 cm or less in greatest dimension		
T1a		Superficial tumor		
T1b		Deep tumor		
T2		Tumor >5 cm in greatest dimension		
T2a		Superficial tumor		
T2b		Deep tumor		
Regional Lymph Nodes				
NX		Regional lymph nodes cannot be assessed		
N0		No regional lymph node metastasis		
N1		Regional lymph node metastasis		
Distant Metastasis				
MX		Distant metastasis cannot be assessed		
M0		No distant metastasis		
M1		Distant metastasis		
Stage IA	G1, GX	T1	N0	M0
Stage IB	G1, GX	T2	N0	M0
Stage IIA	G2–G3	T1	N0	M0
Stage IIB	G2	T2	N0–1	M0
Stage III	G3, any G	T2	N0	M0
Stage IV	Any G	Any T	Any N	M1

From American Joint Committee on Cancer: *AJCC cancer staging manual,* ed 7, Philadelphia, 2010, Lippincott-Raven.

Careful closure of extremity wounds following extirpation of tumors may result in lower wound complication rates. The skin and subcutaneous tissue should be handled carefully during the procedure to avoid unnecessary trauma. Closed-suction drains should be used liberally in the dissection bed, and they should be left in place until the output is low. Tissues should be closed in multiple layers to approximate as much dead space as possible. Ace wraps, extremity elevation, and limited activity all decrease the amount of tissue edema and fluid accumulation and thus may limit wound problems. For larger defects or defects located in areas with poor wound healing, rotational or free flaps and skin grafts can be used. The wound complication rate increases from about 17% to 35% when operations are performed following neoadjuvant radiation. Because preoperative radiation reduces the ability of the surrounding tissues to absorb fluid and delays wound healing, in patients who have received preoperative radiation, drains should be left in place until output is low, and external staples or sutures should be left in place for 3 to 4 weeks.

Adjuvant Radiation and Chemotherapy

The vast majority of extremity STS can be treated with limb-sparing surgery with low local recurrence rates when adjuvant radiation therapy is appropriately used. Several randomized trials have

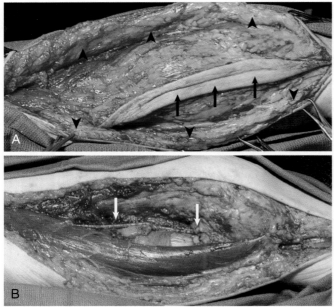

FIGURE I Operative photos of a 12 cm left anterior and medial thigh leiomyosarcoma involving superficial femoral vessels. **A,** Biopsy scar incision (*black arrows*) resected and subcutaneous flaps (*black arrowheads*) raised medially and laterally beyond tumor edge. **B,** Tumor has been removed along with portions of vastus lateralis, biceps femoris, superficial femoral artery, and superficial femoral vein. Reverse saphenous vein (*white arrows*) are used as conduit for superior femoral artery bypass graft. The patient received postoperative radiation therapy and remained disease free beyond 5 years.

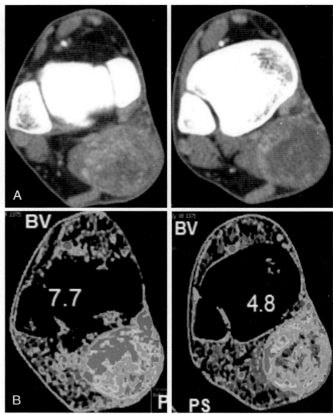

FIGURE 2 **A,** Perfusion CT scan of a 5.5 cm right ankle synovial sarcoma before and after a single dose of bevacizumab, showing a dramatic reduction in uptake of intravenous contrast. **B,** Computer-generated images demonstrate blood volume within the tumor decreasing from 7.7 to 4.8 mL/100 mg/min after a single dose of bevacizumab. This patient subsequently received 50 Gy of radiation therapy in combination with bevacizumab followed by surgical resection and rectus abdominis free-flap reconstruction. The patient remained disease free 2.5 years after surgery.

helped define the role of radiation therapy in the local control of STS. One NCI randomized trial published in 1998 compared limb-spring surgery alone to surgery and external beam radiation (patients with high-grade tumors all received chemotherapy) and demonstrated that radiation reduced local recurrence from 20% to 33% to 0% to 4%. The rate of distant recurrence was the same in both groups.

Brachytherapy has also been used to deliver radiation. For this modality, catheters are placed into the tumor bed following surgical resection and prior to closure. These catheters can also be placed by image guidance and may be anchored to the surrounding soft tissues. Iridium-192 seeds are then loaded into the catheters about 5 days after surgery and are left in place for another 5 days. In a randomized trial of surgery alone versus surgery plus brachytherapy, local recurrence for high-grade tumors was reduced from 30% to 5% with brachytherapy. At our institution, brachytherapy is usually reserved for patients who have a local recurrence after prior surgery and radiation, where brachytherapy allows the delivery of additional radiation while minimizing morbidity.

The timing of radiation therapy in relation to surgery is a subject of debate between major sarcoma centers. One randomized trial by the Canadian NCI examined preoperative and postoperative radiation therapy and found no difference in local recurrence rates. Wound complications were twice as high in the preoperative therapy group (35% vs. 17%), but tissue fibrosis and other late complications were more frequent in the postoperative radiation group. Small (<5 cm), superficial, and well-circumscribed STS resected with a wide margin (>1 cm) of normal tissue have a local recurrence rate of less than 10% and may not require adjuvant radiation therapy.

Patients with large (>8 to 10 cm), deep, high-grade sarcomas often present difficult problems in terms of local control and

additionally are at significant risk of distant metastasis. Several approaches to these difficult tumors have tended to be based on institutional biases and preferences. Our institution has employed a regimen of preoperative mesna, doxorubicin (Adriamycin), ifosfamide, and dacarbazine (MAID) chemotherapy interdigitated with radiation therapy (44 Gy) and followed by postoperative MAID chemotherapy for patients with lesions larger than 8 cm or high-grade STS. In a series of 48 patients, 5-year local control was 92%, and 5-year disease-free and overall survival (70% and 87%, respectively) were significantly better than historic controls. Currently, our institution is investigating whether bevacizumab, an inhibitor of tumor blood vessels, can augment the effects of radiation therapy (Figure 2).

Hyperthermic isolated limb perfusion (HILP) has been used in several centers, primarily in Europe. In this procedure, vascular catheters are placed into the main artery and vein of the involved extremity, and the extremity is further isolated using a tourniquet. The standard protocol involves tumor necrosis factor-α and melphalan infusion under mild hyperthermic conditions (38.5° to 40° C). In one multicenter study of 186 patients, an 82% response rate was obtained and limb salvage was achieved in 82% of patients.

Although surgery and radiotherapy achieve control of the primary tumor in the majority of patients, about 25% to 50% of patients with large, high-grade STS develop metastatic disease that is not evident at diagnosis, thus providing a rationale for adjuvant chemotherapy in such patients. Doxorubicin and ifosfamide are the most active chemotherapy agents in metastatic STS. For doxorubicin, objective response rates between 20% and 40% have been reported for overt metastatic disease. Several prospective studies using single-agent doxorubicin failed to show an improvement in disease-free or overall survival in patients receiving postoperative chemotherapy compared with surgery alone. A meta-analysis of 14 randomized trials of doxorubicin-based adjuvant chemotherapy versus no chemotherapy in STS was performed in 1997. The adjuvant chemotherapy group had a statistically significant higher rate of local recurrence-free survival (81% vs. 75%, $P = .016$), distant recurrence-free survival (70% vs. 60%, $P = .003$), and overall recurrence-free survival (55% vs. 45%, $P = .001$). However, overall survival differed only by 4% (54% vs. 50%), and this difference did not attain statistical significance. The European Organization for Research and Treatment of Cancer recently reported an interim analysis of a trial that randomized 351 patients to adjuvant doxorubicin and ifosfamide or no chemotherapy, and no difference in recurrence-free survival or overall survival was found. Thus at some institutions, adjuvant chemotherapy is generally reserved for relatively young and healthy patients who are at high risk of recurrence, but at other institutions, no adjuvant chemotherapy is recommended.

RETROPERITONEAL SOFT TISSUE SARCOMA

Approximately 15% of STSs arise in the retroperitoneum. These tumors are frequently asymptomatic until they become large, and they are often identified on imaging studies for unrelated complaints. The average size of tumors in large series is often greater than 10 cm. Patients may also come in with a palpable abdominal mass or with symptoms such as abdominal discomfort, early satiety, or lower extremity neurologic symptoms. Upon histologic examination, about two thirds of tumors are either liposarcomas or leiomyosarcomas, with the remaining tumors distributed among a large variety of other histologic subtypes.

Most unifocal tumors in the retroperitoneum that do not arise from adjacent organs will either be benign soft-tissue tumors, such as Schwannomas, or sarcomas. Other malignancies in the differential diagnosis include primary germ cell tumor, metastatic testicular cancer, and lymphoma. Following a careful history and physical examination, radiologic assessment of these tumors is usually performed with an abdominal and pelvic CT scan. Liposarcomas often have a characteristic appearance with large areas of abnormal-appearing fat (well-differentiated liposarcoma) sometimes containing higher density nodules (de-differentiated liposarcoma; see Figure 3). Patients with high-grade tumors should have a chest CT to evaluate for lung metastases, but a chest radiograph is adequate for low-grade tumors. If preoperative therapy is planned, then CT-guided biopsy is necessary to establish a diagnosis.

The primary treatment for local control of these tumors is surgical resection. The optimal goal of surgical resection is complete gross resection with microscopically negative margins, but this goal can be quite difficult to accomplish, and complete gross resection rates in large series are reported to be around 60%. In about three quarters of patients, complete gross resection requires removal of adjacent viscera. Even with complete gross resection, negative microscopic margins are frequently not achieved, and thus local recurrence is seen in 40% or more of patients. Unlike extremity STS, the primary cause of death in patients with retroperitoneal STS is local recurrence.

Some general principles can be followed when resecting retroperitoneal STS. First, as with extremity STS operations, the preoperative

imaging studies should be carefully examined to identify the full extent of tumor penetration as well as the relationship of the tumor to adjacent vital structures. Second, the colon should be prepped, and contralateral kidney function should be confirmed if resection of colon or kidney is a possibility. Third, the patient should be positioned, and the incision should be oriented, to optimize exposure and dissection of these generally large tumors. Often for lateral tumors, positioning patients in a modified lateral decubitus position and the use of midline or paramedian incisions provides the best exposure, and thoracoabdominal incisions provide good exposure for upper abdominal tumors abutting the diaphragm. Fourth, tumors and adjacent organs should be dissected circumferentially from anterior to posterior. Tilting the bed from side to side, or in a Trendelenburg or reverse Trendelenburg position, as one works circumferentially often helps significantly with exposure. It is tempting at times to continue working as deeply as possible in one area before moving on to the next area, but injuring a major blood vessel while working in a hole can have serious consequences. How aggressive one should be in the resection of retroperitoneal STS is a subject of significant controversy. We generally operate with the goal of aggressively resecting adjacent organs en bloc to obtain a negative anterior margin. The posterior margin is then sharply dissected under direct vision, and the best possible posterior margin is obtained by resecting retroperitoneal fat and muscle as needed. Fifth, to have an accurate assessment of margins, the surgeon should take the operative specimen to the pathology lab and orient the specimen, as well as indicate the closest margins, for the pathologist. It is often impossible for the pathologist to accurately assess the closest margins when a large, unoriented specimen is provided.

Controversy also exists as to the optimal role of radiation therapy for local control of retroperitoneal STS. Those who advocate radiation therapy usually prefer that radiation be delivered preoperatively. With the tumor still in place, normal organs are pushed away from the radiation field, the margin around the tumor at risk of local recurrence is more clearly defined, and the effective radiation dose required to control microscopic disease is likely to be lower. In the extremity, the local recurrence of sarcomas treated with total gross resection with positive microscopic margin and adjuvant radiation therapy is about 20% or less. Typically, positive microscopic margins are treated with a boost of postoperative radiation to a total dose of about 60 to 70 Gy.

It is reasonable to assume that total gross resection of retroperitoneal tumors, along with adequate doses of radiation, could achieve local control rates similar to those seen for extremity tumors resected with positive microscopic margins. However, unlike the extremity, it is difficult to deliver high doses of radiation to the abdomen. In a 2001 report from our institution, 29 patients were treated with preoperative radiation to a median dose of 45 to 50 Gy and then underwent complete gross resection. Intraoperative radiation therapy (IORT; 10 to 20 Gy) was delivered to 16 of the 29 patients. Local control at 5 years was 83% for patients who received both preoperative and intraoperative radiation therapy and 61% for those who received only preoperative radiation.

Radiation therapy techniques have recently been developed that allow for more accurate delivery of radiation to tumors located in challenging anatomic locations including the retroperitoneum. Intensity-modulated radiation therapy (IMRT) is one such technique in which normal tissue constraints are combined with tumor-dosage objectives in sophisticated computer planning algorithms to deliver radiation doses to the tumor in three dimensions while limiting doses to radiation-sensitive organs. Proton-beam radiation therapy (PBRT) involves the use of protons, or the nuclei of hydrogen atoms, rather than traditional photons. Because of the lack of an exit dose, protons reduce the dose to normal tissues by about 60%. Intraoperative electron radiation therapy (IOERT) involves the use of a linear accelerator in the operating room to deliver high doses of radiation to the tumor bed, while radiation-sensitive organs are retracted out of the field.

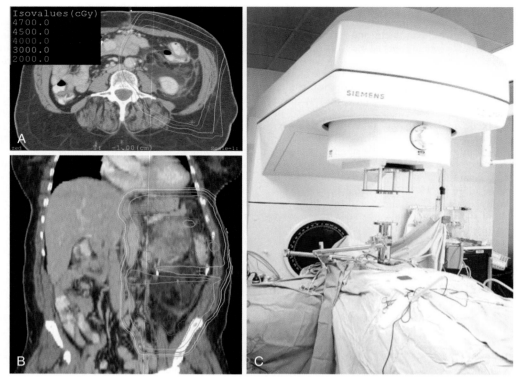

FIGURE 3   Images of right retroperitoneal, well-differentiated, and de-differentiated liposarcoma along with isodose lines that indicate the percent of the radiation prescription for preoperative proton-beam radiation therapy (PBRT). **A,** Axial images. **B,** Coronal images. **C,** Delivery of intraoperative radiation therapy (IOERT) to the tumor bed following resection of tumor along with distal pancreas, spleen, left kidney/adrenal, and left colon. The patient remained disease free after 4.5 years.

In 2003, our facility instituted a strategy for the treatment of retroperitoneal sarcoma that incorporated these radiation therapy modalities along with a synchronized surgical approach (Figure 3). Patients were treated preoperatively with PBRT and/or IMRT to a dose of 45 to 50 Gy. Aggressive surgical resection, often with removal of contiguous organs, was then performed with a goal of removing all gross residual disease and obtaining a microscopically negative margin along the *anterior* surface of the tumor. The tumor specimen was then analyzed by frozen section to determine the adequacy of the surgical margin, and IOERT was delivered to any close or positive *posterior* margin or any margin along an unresected contiguous organ or vital structure. For patients in whom a diagnosis of STS could not be obtained prior to surgery, or for those who were too symptomatic to tolerate preoperative radiation therapy, surgical resection was performed first along with IOERT to the tumor bed. An omental flap was placed over the tumor bed, and postoperative radiation was then delivered by PBRT. In the first 20 patients, who were first seen with primary tumors and were treated with this strategy, after a median follow-up of 33 months, only two patients (10%) had local recurrence (Figure 4).

METASTATIC DISEASE

Prognostic factors for the development of metastatic disease include high tumor grade and large tumor size (>8 to 10 cm). Median survival after the development of metastatic disease is about 12 months with 20% to 25% of patients alive at 2 years. The most common site of metastatic disease for extremity and trunk STS is the lung; intraabdominal and retroperitoneal sarcomas metastasize with about equal frequency to the lung and liver. STS uncommonly metastasizes to regional lymph nodes (~5%) except for certain histologic subtypes, including epithelioid sarcoma, clear cell sarcoma, and synovial sarcoma.

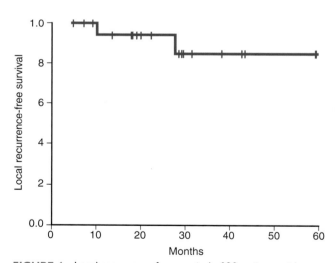

FIGURE 4   Local recurrence-free survival of 20 patients with retroperitoneal sarcoma treated with PBRT, IMRT, and/or IOERT at Massachusetts General Hospital.

As noted above, doxorubicin and ifosfamide have been demonstrated to be the most active chemotherapy agents in widely disseminated STS. These two agents carry significant risks of toxicity: doxorubicin dosage is limited by cardiotoxicity, and ifosfamide causes hemorrhagic cystitis and nephrotoxicity. Ifosfamide-induced hemorrhagic cystitis can be avoided by adding the protective agent mesna. Another agent with some activity against STS is dacarbazine (DTIC), with reported response rates around 20%. However for metastatic disease, complete responses are uncommon (<15% even with combination therapy); duration of response averages 8 months, and as yet the higher response rates seen with intense combination therapy have not been proven to provide a survival advantage over that conferred by sequential single-agent treatment. Ongoing trials are evaluating the use of other chemotherapy agents such as taxotere, gemcitabine, vinorelbine, and topotecan; certain histologic subtypes may be more responsive to particular chemotherapeutic agents.

Surgical resection has been performed for isolated STS metastases to the lung or liver. For patients with STS metastases isolated to the lung or liver, surgical resection can be performed, and 5 year survival can approach 20% to 30% in these highly selected patients.

SUMMARY

The treatment of STS has advanced significantly over the past few decades. Until the early 1960s, surgery offered the only serious prospect for cure. Radical surgery, particularly amputation, produced an impressive gain over simple local excision but at the cost of major functional loss and cosmetic disfigurement. Clinical studies over the last three decades have demonstrated that more conservative surgical approaches, combined with adjuvant radiation therapy, can be highly effective, and local recurrence rates are now often less than 10%. Although STS can occur in varied locations, several surgical principles should be followed as outlined above. For difficult extremity tumors, strategies such as neoadjuvant chemoradiation or HILP may increase response rates and limb-salvage rates. For retroperitoneal STS, newer radiation techniques such as IMRT, PBRT, and IOERT may allow for the delivery of adequate radiation doses and may reduce local recurrence rates. Adjuvant chemotherapy to eradicate occult metastatic disease is controversial, and more effective agents are clearly needed. Optimal results from more conservative local treatment strategies, especially for difficult tumors, require a multidisciplinary team approach that includes not only an experienced surgeon but also a radiation oncologist, medical oncologist, pathologist, and radiologist who are expert in this disease.

SUGGESTED READINGS

Brennan MF, Singer S, Maki RG, O'Sullivan B: Soft tissue sarcoma. In DeVita VT, Lawrence TS, Rosenberg SA, editors: *Cancer: principles and practice of oncology*, ed 8, Philadelphia, 2008, Lippincott Williams & Wilkins, pp 1741–1794.

O'Sullivan B, Davis AM, Turcotte R, et al: Preoperative versus postoperative radiotherapy in soft-tissue sarcoma of the limbs: a randomised trial, *Lancet* 359(9325):2235–2241, 2002.

Yang JC, Chang AE, Baker AR, et al: Randomized prospective study of the benefit of adjuvant radiation therapy in the treatment of soft tissue sarcomas of the extremity, *J Clin Oncol* 16(1):197–203, 1998.

Yoon SS, Chen YL, Kirsch DG, et al: Proton beam, intensity modulated, and/or intra-operative electron radiation therapy combined with aggressive anterior surgical resection for retroperitoneal sarcomas, *Ann Surg Oncol* 17(6): 1515–1529, 2010.

Yoon SS, Hornicek FJ, Harmon DC, DeLaney TF: Soft tissue and bone sarcomas. In Chabner BA, Lynch TJ, Longo DL, editors: *Harrison's handbook of medical oncology*, New York, 2008, McGraw Hill, pp 549–566.

MANAGEMENT OF THE ISOLATED NECK MASS

Suman Golla, MD, Umamaheshwar Duvvuri, MD, PhD, and Jonas T. Johnson, MD

OVERVIEW

Like other disease processes in the head and neck, the management of the isolated neck mass is heavily dependent on the etiology. The algorithm for the management of such masses differs tremendously for benign masses versus malignancies. The diagnosis, of course, relies on the history, physical exam findings, and radiologic characteristics. In concert, these modalities may provide clues to narrow the extensive differential diagnosis. Perhaps most important in honing in on this list is tissue acquisition. Medical and surgical treatments may ensue based on the identification of the mass.

EVALUATION

Isolated neck masses may be differentiated into many categories that include infectious, inflammatory, congenital, acquired, primary malignant, and metastatic malignant masses (Table 1). Duration and location of the mass, rate of growth, patient age, associated symptoms, and accompanying risk factors may provide clues to rapidly differentiate among these categories. Within the pediatric age group, neck masses often represent inflammatory, infectious, and congenital causes, but persistent masses in adults are concerning for malignancy. In adults, risk factors not only include tobacco and alcohol use but also sun exposure. Also important is inquiry into the presence of constitutional symptoms such as fevers, sweats, weight loss, or fatigue. These may implicate lymphoma or atypical bacterial or viral infections as the cause. Tender masses that grow rapidly may represent infectious or inflammatory processes.

Location of any neck mass is based either on descriptive terminology (jugulodigastric, posterior cervical) or neck-level nomenclature (Figure 1). The location of masses within the various levels or triangles of the neck may help to differentiate the etiology. The location of a metastatic lesion or neck mass may help to direct attention to the primary tumor site based on well-described lymphatic drainage pathways for the head and neck. An isolated cystic neck mass in an adult warrants a careful evaluation of the base of tongue and palatine tonsils, because an increase in the prevalence of herpes papilloma virus–associated cancer has been observed in the past decade.

Workup

The initial evaluation, of course, depends on a thorough examination of the head and neck. Knowledge of neck anatomy is critical in differentiating normal structures from pathologic lesions. The exam should include the size of the mass, documented with a tape measure, and the location of the mass in comparison to known anatomic landmarks within the neck. Normal anatomic structures that may show up as a neck mass include a prominent carotid bulb or bifurcation. In thin people, the transverse process of the second cervical vertebra may be palpable. A mass within the thyroid, submandibular, or parotid gland calls for a different differential diagnosis. Ptosis of the submandibular gland in the elderly patient may be mistaken for a pathologic process, and enlarged lymph nodes may represent reactive lymphadenopathy or a malignant mass. Visualization of the mucosal surfaces of the upper aerodigestive tract is essential, as is evaluation of the skin of the head and neck, including the scalp.

Flexible fiberoptic laryngoscopy (FFL) facilitates a more complete examination and can be especially helpful for patients in whom historic risk factors and suspicious symptoms exist. In those patients, special attention should be given to all of the aerodigestive mucosa, especially the lymphoid region of the nasopharynx, base of the tongue, and oropharynx (Waldeyer ring). Palpation, including bimanual examination of the floor of the mouth and the neck, can help identify abnormalities that exist deep beneath normal mucosa.

A neurologic exam of cranial nerve function is necessary. Examination of dentition is essential, because dental sources can contribute to both reactive lymphadenopathy and primary, unusual, and atypical infectious processes.

Imaging studies are helpful in further characterizing the location of the mass and delineating features not appreciated on physical exam. Studies that are often employed include ultrasonography, computed tomography (CT), or magnetic resonance imaging (MRI). Occasionally, a chest radiograph may be ordered. Posterior, anterior, and lateral views of a chest radiograph should be obtained if there is concern that the neck mass is related to an atypical infectious or granulomatous source. These studies should be obtained especially in cases of suspicious history of cough or travel. If the chest radiograph demonstrates suspicious lesions, a chest CT scan may be warranted.

CT and MRI are very useful modalities that help characterize the neck mass and localize the primary site responsible for metastatic disease. To differentiate the neck mass from normal anatomical and vascular structures, the study should be a contrast-enhanced scan using contiguous 3 to 5 mm slice intervals. In addition to allowing for the differentiation of bone, fat, and soft-tissue structures, advantages of the CT scan include availability and patient tolerance (Figure 2). MRI may be suited for evaluating soft tissue involvement of the mass and its surrounding areas. It may also be helpful in patients with significant dental artifact and in those with iodine contrast reactions. Gadolinium may help further differentiate masses, as may techniques such as fat suppression.

Certain paragangliomas display classic features, for example, splaying of the internal and external carotid artery with carotid body paragangliomas; these may be best noted with MRI. This imaging modality may also be beneficial in ascertaining the extent of vascular and lymphatic lesions in the pediatric population, especially since angiography is rarely employed for the characterization of neck masses in this population. It should be noted, however, that the experience and preference of the radiologist greatly impacts the quality of information obtained from any imaging study. Personal communication with the diagnostic radiologist is particularly important to make the decision

TABLE 1: Differential diagnosis of neck masses

Benign	Autoimmune
Developmental	Sjögren syndrome
Inclusion cyst	***Miscellaneous***
Thyroglossal duct cyst	AIDS-related disease
Congenital vascular malformation	***Benign Neoplasms***
Branchial cleft cyst	Hemangioma, lymphangioma
Cystic hygroma	Thyroid nodule or goiter
Laryngocele	Parathyroid adenoma
Teratoma	Lipoma
Bronchogenic cyst	Fibroma
Lymph nodes, infective	Neurofibroma
Benign reactive hyperplasia	Sebaceous cyst
Bacterial	Aneurysm
Bacterial lymphadenitis: *Staphylococcus aureus, Streptococcus pyogenes,* tuberculosis, cat-scratch fever (*Bartonella*), and *Brucella*, a typical mycobacteria in tuberculosis	Salivary gland tumor (parotid or submandibular)
	Tumefactive fibroinflammatory lesion
	Nodular fasciitis
Viral	**Malignant**
Viral lymphadenitis: Epstein-Barr virus, HIV/AIDS	***Malignant Neoplasms***
Protozoal	Metastatic carcinoma or melanoma in a lymph node
Toxolasmosis, leishmaniasis	Lymphoma
Fungal	Carotid-body tumor
Histoplasmosis, blastomycosis, coccidiomycosis	Soft tissue, bone, or cartilage sarcoma
Lymph nodes, granulomatous	Primary major salivary gland tumor
Sarcoidosis	Malignant melanoma
Foreign-Body Reaction	Adnexal carcinoma of the skin
Salivary gland (parotid or submandibular)	Thyroid cancer
Infective	Parathyroid cancer
Sialadenitis, sialolithiasis	Direct extension of a head and neck neoplasm into the neck
Sublingual gland obstruction	Histiocytosis
	Plasmocytoma
	Carcinoid

regarding which type of scan to order. It would be rare to obtain both types of scans, as this generally adds to unnecessary expense.

Positron emission tomography (PET) has been used in the identification of primary sources of cancer in patients with known neck malignancy despite inconclusive endoscopy. It has also been utilized to characterize recurrent neck masses in patients with a previous known history of head and neck malignancies. PET is performed with the isotope fluorodeoxyglucose. An increased rate of glycolysis of tumor cells indicates increased tumor cell activity. Fusion PET/CT is now a more useful tool, because it allows for improved anatomic localization of tumors and metastases. This dual modality has been found to be quite accurate in detecting occult cervical nodal metastases. The above imaging studies serve not only to narrow the differential diagnosis but also serve as an anatomical roadmap during surgical intervention.

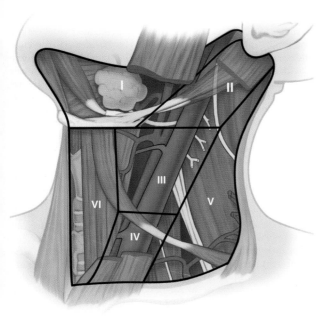

FIGURE 1   Levels in the neck. (*Courtesy Douglas Denys, MD. Reprinted from Cummings CW Haughey BH, Thomas JR, et al, editors: Cummings otolaryngology—head and neck surgery, ed 4, Philadelphia, 2005, Mosby Elsevier.*)

A PET scan is not appropriate when a malignancy has been diagnosed. If a neck mass is clearly palpable, tissue diagnosis can be obtained with fine needle aspiration (FNA). Especially in superficial lesions, this tool provides rapid cytopathologic diagnosis; this modality is especially helpful, because even an inconclusive but suggestive result may guide management of the mass. The presence of an isolated neck mass in an adult over the age of 40 years should be considered malignant until proven otherwise. We strongly recommend FNA biopsy of such masses before empiric therapy is initiated.

Contraindications to office aspiration would be masses thought to be vascular in nature. Suspicion would be based on the patient's history, physical exam findings, and presence of an enhancing lesion in contrasted imaging studies. Typically, the needle aspiration procedure can be performed in the outpatient setting. Local anesthetic is injected into the site of interest. The described technique by many authors emphasizes entering the mass under slight negative pressure with a 20 mL syringe using a small-diameter needle (21 gauge or smaller). Using the thumb and forefinger, the mass may be contained with the nondominant hand during the procedure. Multiple angled passes under negative suction, along with several aspirates (three to four), increase the likelihood of obtaining an adequate specimen. The suction on the syringe is removed prior to the removal of the needle, and blood should be discarded in hopes of ascertaining a few representative cells. While the air is expelled out of the syringe, the contents of the aspirate expelled from the needle lumen are placed on a slide, and that slide is smeared with another. Finally, prompt placement of the slides into formalin or ethanol prior to desiccation of the cells is essential. FNA may be facilitated by having a cytopathologist on site to assist with the procedure and to assess the adequacy of the specimen. For small or deep masses, or for those thought to be related to and within the thyroid parenchyma, accuracy can be improved by using ultrasonography to guide the FNA. For solid neck metastases, FNA cytology has a high yield for tissue diagnosis. In general, the sensitivity and specificity approach 90% and are highest for thyroid masses and solid carcinomas. If the node is cystic, care should be taken to biopsy the wall of the node with ultrasonographic guidance. If adequate, the results of the FNA are especially helpful with patient counseling, preoperative discussions, and surgical planning.

Although many primary cancer sites can be biopsied in the office, examination under anesthesia may be an important component of the evaluation of tumors of the upper aerodigestive tract, regardless of the adequacy of office or clinic assessment. Visualization of all mucosal surfaces before digital or instrumental manipulation allows

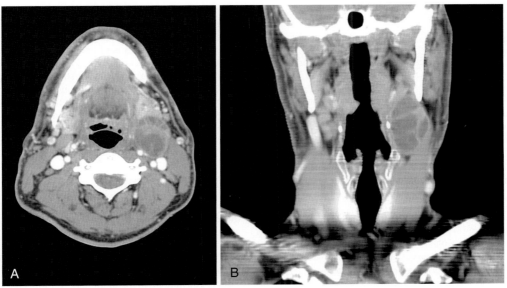

FIGURE 2   CT scan of a cystic neck mass.

important assessment of tumor extent. Biopsies can be obtained under a controlled setting, and the pathologist should be informed in advance if lymphoma is suspected. In those patients, care must be taken to obtain a sufficient amount of tissue, and the sample should be submitted fresh and in saline to allow for receptor typing.

Indications for Surgery versus Medical Management

As mentioned, the presence of an isolated neck mass in an adult over the age of 40 years suggests the presence of an occult malignancy until proven otherwise. With this paradigm in mind, the practitioner should order the appropriate imaging evaluations and FNA biopsy to provide the patient with the appropriate diagnosis. If the results of FNA biopsy suggest the presence of a malignancy, definitive therapy is indicated. However, the results of the FNA biopsy may be inconclusive. In this situation an open biopsy, either incisional or excisional, is the next appropriate step.

In summary, the first line of treatment for children and young adults under 40 years of age with an isolated neck mass is conservative therapy with medical management. FNA biopsy and radiologic evaluation is reserved for patients who do not respond to conservative therapy. Conversely, the first line of treatment for adults over the age of 40 years who come in with an isolated neck mass is FNA biopsy; the results of the biopsy should guide further treatment.

TECHNIQUES OF SURGERY

Surgical intervention for the isolated neck mass should be chosen on a patient-by-patient basis and should be guided by the results of laboratory investigations. When FNA is unsuccessful or tissue is required for tumor architecture or molecular characterization (lymphoma), an open biopsy may be required. Even though this can be performed under local anesthesia, many neck masses lie deep to the platysma and may involve major neurovascular structures. For these reasons, open biopsies are usually performed under general anesthesia, which can be safely administered via an endotracheal tube inserted transorally in the usual fashion. However, if the neck mass causes compression or deviation of the airway, fiberoptic intubation may be required. A tracheotomy is required when the airway is markedly compromised or when intubation and/or postoperative extubation could be dangerous. In these situations, a planned tracheotomy should be performed before the patient develops extremis. Also important is good communication with the anesthesia team to ensure the patient does not receive any paralytic anesthesia agents once the surgical procedure begins.

Incision Planning

Transverse skin incisions in relaxed skin tension lines are preferred for optimal cosmetic results. The incision should be placed so as to allow for larger incisions, should a comprehensive neck dissection be required. Incisions should allow for exposure and identification of critical landmarks, including the great vessels, digastric muscle, posterior border of the sternocleidomastoid (SCM) muscle, and the eleventh cranial nerve.

Risks and Complications after Surgery for the Isolated Neck Mass

The major risks and complications associated with neck surgery include neurovascular injury, chyle fistulas, and inadvertent injury to the laryngopharyngeal complex. Neural structures at risk in neck surgery include the spinal accessory (XI), hypoglossal (XII), and vagus (X) nerves, the marginal branch of the facial nerve (VII), and the phrenic nerve. Cranial nerves VII and XI are among those most commonly injured. The marginal branch of the facial nerve courses

from the main trunk of the nerve in the parotid gland over the mid-body mandible (at the area of the facial artery) onto the fascia of the submandibular gland. The nerve then courses superiorly to cross over the mandible and ultimately innervates the depressor of the lower lip. Avoiding the region of the body of the mandible can minimize chances of injury to this nerve. All incisions should be made at least two fingerbreadths below the inferior edge of the mandible.

The spinal accessory nerve exists in the cranial base at the jugular foramen and typically courses over the internal jugular vein as it travels to the trapezius muscle. This nerve can be identified as it innervates the sternocleidomastoid (SCM) muscle, if the anterior border of the muscle is skeletonized, and the fascia is followed to the SCM tendon. The nerve is deep to the posterior belly of the digastric muscle. Alternatively, the spinal nerve can be identified along the posterior border of the SCM muscle about 2 cm superior to the Erb point, the intersection of the greater auricular nerve with the posterior border of the SCM muscle. The nerve has a very superficial course in the posterior triangle of the neck and can be injured easily when lesions in this area are dissected. The only reliable method to avoid injury to the spinal accessory nerve (XI) is to identify it with meticulous dissection and a thorough knowledge of surgical anatomy. It is therefore best to avoid cutting any neural structure greater than 2 mm in size in the posterior triangle of the neck.

The hypoglossal nerve (XII) traverses levels I and II deep in the neck tissues. It descends between the internal jugular vein and the carotid artery before turning to innervate the tongue musculature. It runs under the posterior belly of the digastric muscle, where it is surrounded by the *venae comitantes* (the Ranine veins). Paragangliomas, metastatic squamous cell carcinoma, and large brachial cleft anomalies may reside in this area. Injury to this nerve often occurs when bleeding from the Ranine veins is being controlled, and the nerve is inadvertently clamped during hemostasis.

The lower neck contains the thoracic duct, which lies deep in the inferomedial aspect of the left supraclavicular region. The duct runs behind the common carotid artery and empties into the internal jugular vein near its junction with the subclavian vein. There are chyle-containing lymphatics in the right neck that must be controlled during dissection of this area. All tissue between the phrenic and vagus nerves should be carefully ligated to avoid an inadvertent chyle fistula. Chyle leaks are initially managed conservatively with a low-fat diet and medium-chain triglyceride supplementation. Somatostatin can also be used to augment closure of a delayed chyle leak. Rarely, surgical intervention is required to close persistent chyle leaks.

Resection of a carotid body paraganglioma is a challenging operation that is best performed by expert surgeons in tertiary centers. These tumors are highly vascular and can encapsulate the internal carotid artery. The diagnosis is made with CT or MRI. Biopsies of these lesions is discouraged, and the diagnosis is made on the basis of radiologic investigations. Cranial nerves X, XI, and XII are at risk in this procedure and should be identified with meticulous hemostatic dissection. Tumor resection is accomplished by a subadventitial dissection of the carotid system, and vascular reconstruction is rarely required. However, a skilled and experienced surgeon who can reconstruct the carotid artery if required should be available. Resection of tumors that encompass more than 270 degrees of the internal carotid artery is associated with a higher rate of vascular injury. We rarely perform embolization for these tumors, as it can obscure the subadventitial dissection plane.

MANAGEMENT

Discussion of treatment options is dependent on identification and the diagnosis. When an infectious or inflammatory lesion is suspected in the face of a lack of response to antibiotics, tissue diagnosis may be warranted. In the case of a metastatic lesion, identification of the cytology of the mass, as well as the primary source, is necessary. Occasionally, malignant neck masses have no identifiable primary source, and all patients with malignancy may benefit from discussion at a multidisciplinary tumor board.

SUGGESTED READINGS

Gor DM, Langer JE, Loevner LA: Imaging of cervical lymph nodes in head and neck cancer: the basics, *Radiol Clin North Am* 44(1):101–110, 2006.

Lin DT, Deschler DG: Neck masses. In Lalwani AK, editor: *Current diagnosis and treatment in otolaryngology—head and neck surgery*, New York, 2004, Lange Medical Books/McGraw Hill, pp 413–423.

Mehta VM, Lim J, Har-El G: Neck masses. In Lucente FE, Har-El G, editors: *Essentials of otolaryngology*, Philadelphia, 2004, Lippincott Williams & Wilkins, pp 277–289.

Pincus RL: Congenital neck masses and cysts. In Bailey BJ, Johnson JT, Newlands SD, editors: *Head and neck surgery—otolaryngology*, vol 1, Philadelphia, 2006, Lippincott Williams & Wilkins, pp 1209–1216.

HAND INFECTIONS

Thomas M. Brushart, MD

CASE REPORT

The Johns Hopkins Hand Surgery Service was consulted to evaluate a 55-year-old HIV-positive diabetic male with a lesion on the tip of his left thumb. The thumb tip was eroded and scabbed over but was not tender, and thumb flexion was present but reduced and did not cause discomfort. The patient's upper extremities were quite large but appeared symmetrical. During the course of the examination, the patient's nurse obtained his vital signs and noted that he was tachycardic and that his previous hypertension had resolved. Firm pressure over the volar forearm resulted in drainage of several milliliters of purulent material from the thumb tip. The patient was taken to the operating room emergently, where his entire deep flexor musculature was found to be necrotic and infected and was excised.

EVALUATION OF THE PATIENT WITH A HAND INFECTION

A thorough history and physical examination should be performed to evaluate a hand infection. Critical information includes the patient's hand dominance, occupation, the nature of any predisposing injury or illness, and the precise chronology of the hand infection. *Herpes simplex* infections are common in dental and health care workers, *Vibrio vulnificus* and *Mycobacterium* infections are common in fisherman and marine workers, and *Sporothrix schenckii* infection is common in gardeners. *Eikenella corrodens* is often the causative agent in infected human bites, and *Pasturella multocida* is more common after cat and dog bites. Comorbidities that include diabetes and immunosuppression should also be sought out, as illustrated in the above case report. With either or both of these conditions, infections are more serious and less symptomatic, which makes them far more dangerous.

Physical examination begins with comparison of the size and contour of the affected and unaffected hands to look for areas of focal swelling or changes in posture that could signal an infection. The skin surface is then examined for areas of erythema, blistering, ecchymosis, incipient necrosis, and for the presence of fresh or partially healed wounds. The entire hand surface is then palpated, working from uninvolved to involved areas, seeking to elicit focal tenderness over joints or tendinous structures, areas of crepitance, or any firmness or tenderness that could localize soft-tissue infection. A complete neurovascular and functional exam should be performed. Plain radiographs of the affected area should always be obtained to rule out the presence of a foreign body, bony pathology, or gas within the soft tissues. On rare occasion when the history and clinical examination are unreliable, additional radiological tests such as computed tomography, ultrasound, or magnetic resonance imaging may be helpful.

Laboratory tests should include a complete blood count, C-reactive protein, and erythrocyte sedimentation rate. Blood cultures may be obtained depending on the clinical scenario. If an open wound or purulent drainage is noted, cultures and Gram stain for aerobic and anaerobic bacteria, fungus, and *Mycobacteria* should be obtained prior to administering antibiotics. Tetanus prophylaxis should be given if tetanus status is unknown or not up to date.

The initial history and physical examination will help determine whether the infection is cellulitis, and if it has consolidated to form an abscess or has involved a joint or tendinous compartment. Cellulitis can usually be treated with elevation, splinting, and antibiotics; however, the late conditions require surgical drainage.

SURGICAL PRINCIPLES IN THE TREATMENT OF HAND INFECTION

Localized infections of the fingertip or superficial soft tissues can be treated effectively under local anesthesia. Digital anesthesia is obtained by blocking the digital nerves at the base of the finger. Lidocaine without a vasoconstrictor is infiltrated on the radial and ulnar aspects of the digit through a dorsal puncture just distal to the metacarpophalangeal joint. Complicated or deep-space infections are more effectively treated under general anesthesia.

As with other surgical procedures involving the hand, incision and drainage can be performed under tourniquet control with either a Penrose-type drain wrapped carefully around the base of the finger or a well-padded pneumatic tourniquet placed on the upper arm. Exsanguination of the affected limb is performed by elevation of the arm prior to inflation of the tourniquet. Use of an elastic bandage to exsanguinate the extremity runs the risk of spreading the infection proximally. General anesthetic is generally preferred, as infiltration of anesthetic around neurovascular structures can potentially interfere with lymphatic drainage from the limb.

Damage to neurovascular structures and tendons is avoided by careful dissection guided by detailed knowledge of hand anatomy (Figure 1). Incisions are planned to allow for easy proximal or distal

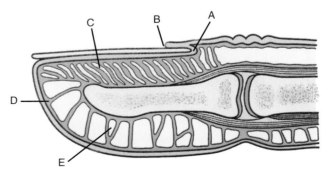

FIGURE I   Anatomy of the fingertip. **A,** Nail fold. **B,** Eponychium. **C,** Nail bed. **D,** Hyponychium. **E,** Vertical septa.

extension, should it be necessary. Once the infected space has been entered, adequate debridement should be performed, including tenosynovectomy when indicated. The wound is then irrigated with normal saline. Pulse lavage is not used in the hand, because it traumatizes and infiltrates previously undamaged soft tissues. Continuous irrigation may be used for specific infections such as suppurative flexor tenosynovitis.

When an infection involves a joint space, the articular surfaces and adjacent bone must be evaluated. When bone is found to be soft and spongy, it should be debrided and sent for pathologic examination to confirm the diagnosis of osteomyelitis, which may require 6 weeks of antibiotic therapy.

COMMON INFECTIONS OF THE HAND

Paronychia

Acute paronychia, the most common hand infection, occurs when the soft-tissue folds surrounding the lateral aspects of the fingernail become infected (Figure 2). The usual pathogen is *Staphylococcus aureus*. An infection of the proximal nail fold is referred to as an *eponychia*. Common causes of paronychia include minor trauma from nail biting or manicure.

Symptoms

An acute paronychia occurs with edema, erythema, and tenderness of the soft tissue surrounding the nail. Left untreated, a small abscess may form under the nail fold, and severe infections can spread proximally along the involved finger.

Treatment

Early paronychia can be treated with splint immobilization, warm soaks, and oral antibiotics if no purulence is present. For more advanced infections, drainage can be performed under digital-block anesthesia with a proximal digital tourniquet. The tourniquet should be placed just tightly enough to block blood flow to the finger and should be removed immediately after the procedure. The nail plate is carefully elevated from the nail bed adjacent to the infection, and a longitudinal strip of the nail is removed with small scissors (Figure 3). If this does not decompress the infection, it may be necessary to carefully open the lateral or proximal aspect of the nail fold by spreading it carefully with the scissors. After thorough irrigation, the finger is bandaged, splinted, and elevated for 24 hours before beginning daily soaks and dressing changes. Antibiotics are continued for

10 to 14 days, and the patient can be seen for follow-up in 3 to 5 days or sooner if needed.

Felon

A felon is a painful infection of the volar pulp of the fingertip (Figure 4). Fibrous septa that originate from the periosteum of the distal phalanx and insert on the dermis initially contain the infection, often resulting in a mini compartment syndrome (Figure 5). If a felon is not treated promptly, infection can track along these septa down to the phalanx, leading to osteomyelitis, fat necrosis of the fingertip, and eventually suppurative tenosynovitis. Felons are usually caused by penetrating trauma to the fingertip from a thorn, splinter, or needle. Radiographs of the fingertip are necessary to look for a foreign body and for evidence of osteomyelitis of the distal phalanx.

Symptoms

The patient is usually seen with pain and tense swelling a day or two after a penetrating injury to the fingertip. Felons are exquisitely tender to palpation because of the increased pressure within the septal compartments.

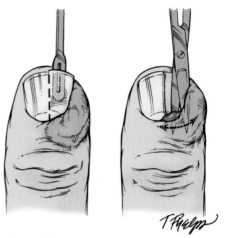

FIGURE 3   Surgical drainage of acute paronychia. The lateral nail on the affected side is gently elevated from the nail bed, and a longitudinal strip of nail is removed. If this does not decompress the infection adequately, the margins of the nail fold are opened gently to drain the adjacent soft tissues.

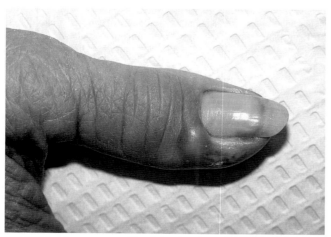

FIGURE 2   Acute paronychia of the thumb involving the inferior aspect of the thumb nail fold.

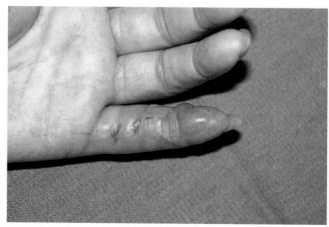

FIGURE 4   Acute felon. Blistering is evident distally, where tissue pressure is significantly elevated.

Treatment

Early felons can be treated with splinting, elevation, and antibiotics. If symptoms worsen or fluctuance is identified, the felon should be drained promptly. A digital block can be used for regional anesthesia. The risk of incomplete treatment can be minimized by providing free drainage for all of the compartments in the volar pulp. This is achieved by making bilateral incisions parallel to and 2 to 3 mm from the edges of the nail, then spreading with fine scissors to connect the incisions through the digital pulp just volar to the distal phalanx.

After incision and drainage, the cavity is irrigated, and a single drain is placed that runs through all of the released compartments (see Figure 5). Warm soaks are initiated after 24 hours, and the drain is removed after 48 hours. Antibiotics are continued for 10 to 14 days. The patient should be seen in 2 to 3 days, or sooner if needed, to make sure the abscess is adequately drained. The incisions will heal by secondary intention without the need for further surgical treatment.

Herpetic Whitlow

Herpetic whitlow is a painful infection of the hand usually involving one or more fingers. The infection, caused by herpes simplex virus 1 (HSV-1) and/or 2 (HSV-2), is transmitted by contact with infected body fluids. In adults, herpetic whitlow is most common in dental or health care workers but can also result from contact with lesions of genital herpes. Children usually obtain the infection from thumb sucking in the presence of primary oropharyngeal lesions.

Symptoms

The incubation period for herpetic whitlow is 2 to 14 days. Fever and malaise may precede pain, burning, or tingling of the affected digit. Within 7 to 10 days, small clear vesicles form and coalesce, and

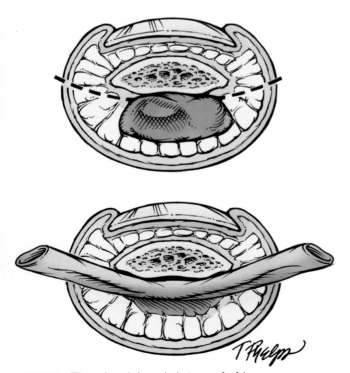

FIGURE 5   Through-and-through drainage of a felon ensures complete decompression and minimizes the risk of incomplete treatment. A drain is placed and maintained for 48 hours.

vesicles may rupture and ulcerate. Although this is a self-limiting infection, recurrence rates as high as 50% have been reported.

Treatment

It is important to distinguish between herpetic whitlow and paronychia, as the treatment of herpetic lesions is nonsurgical. With a Tzanck test, viral cultures or rapid immunoflourescent antibodies can confirm the diagnosis. As the disease is self-limiting, treatment is aimed at providing symptomatic relief. Although unroofing the blisters may reduce pain, it increases the risk of bacterial superinfection. Topical or oral acyclovir can shorten the duration of symptoms and prevent recurrence, and antibiotics are only used to treat superimposed bacterial infection.

Suppurative Flexor Tenosynovitis

The majority of patients with suppurative flexor tenosynovitis will seek treatment after having sustained a penetrating injury to the volar surface of the finger. Bacterial inoculation of the flexor tendon sheath between the first annular pulley (A1 pulley) at the metacarpal head and the insertion of the flexor digitorum profundus (FDP) tendon at the distal phalanx can infect this closed, potential space. The proximal aspect of the tendon sheath of the thumb and small finger communicate with the radial and ulnar bursas respectively, allowing for the proximal spread of infection. *Staphylococcus aureus* and *Streptococcus* species are the most common causative organisms.

Signs and Symptoms

In 1925, Kanavel described the following four cardinal signs of flexor tenosynovitis, which are still used to make the diagnosis today: 1) symmetric enlargement of the affected finger (fusiform swelling; Figure 6, *A*), 2) semiflexed position of the finger, 3) pain along the flexor tendon sheath, and 4) severe pain along the tendon sheath upon passive digital extension.

Treatment

Early diagnosis and treatment of suppurative flexor tenosynovitis is critical to prevent destruction and scarring of the gliding surfaces of the sheath and tendon. Early suppurative flexor tenosynovitis may be treated with splinting, elevation, and intravenous antibiotics targeted at *Staphylococcus aureus* and group A *Streptococcus*. Presentation beyond the day of onset or failure to improve after 24 hours of intravenous antibiotics necessitates surgical intervention. The flexor system is approached initially through a 2 cm transverse incision at the proximal end of the A1 pulley (Figure 6, *B*). If infection is encountered within the flexor sheath, a counterincision is made in the midlateral line of the digit just proximal to the distal interphalangeal (DIP) joint (Figure 7). A small catheter is threaded into the flexor sheath at this level and is used to irrigate the sheath, taking the finger through its range of motion several times, until the fluid draining through the palmar wound is clear. If only cloudy tenosynovial fluid is encountered initially, the catheter can be removed, and wounds can be left open.

If more substantial purulence is encountered, the catheter is sewn in place and is irrigated with 20 to 30 mL of saline every hour for the first 24 hours. When infection has progressed even further, and the tenosynovium is grossly involved, the finger is approached through a midlateral incision, and a thorough tenosynovectomy is performed. A Brunner incision should not be used, as extensive dissection in the face of potential vascular compromise often results in poor healing and tissue loss. Sutures at the level of the DIP and proximal interphalageal (PIP) creases will allow continued drainage and will provide apposition sufficient for healing. The hand is loosely wrapped and splinted; after 48 hours, the splint can be removed, and physical therapy can be initiated.

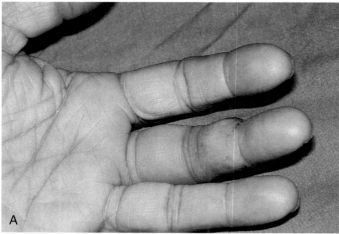

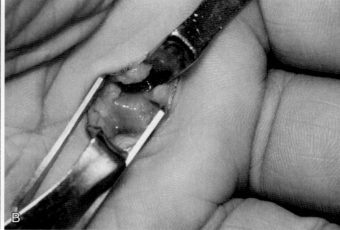

FIGURE 6   **A,** Early septic flexor tenosynovitis of the middle finger. Swelling and a slightly flexed posture are evident. **B,** A transverse incision over the proximal A1 pulley reveals purulent material within the flexor sheath.

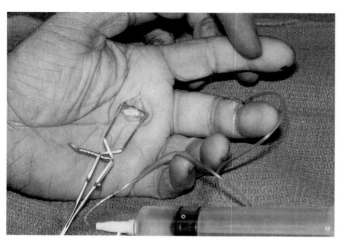

FIGURE 7   A pediatric feeding tube placed within the flexor sheath just proximal to the DIP joint is used for initial irrigation and for 24 hours thereafter.

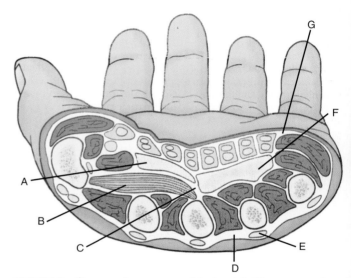

FIGURE 8   Cross-section anatomy of the hand. **A,** Thenar space. **B,** Adductor pollicis. **C,** Midpalmar septum. **D,** Dorsal subaponeurotic space. **E,** Extensor tendon. **F,** Midpalmar space. **G,** Hypothenar space.

DEEP INFECTIONS OF THE HAND

Deep infections involve the subfascial spaces of the hand and forearm. There are six such areas: the *thenar, hypothenar, midpalmar, interdigital,* and *dorsal subaponeurotic spaces* of the hand and the *Parona space* of the volar forearm (Figure 8). Deep space infections usually occur as a result of penetrating injury and are often caused by *Staphylococcus aureus* or *Streptococcus* species.

Interdigital Space (Web Space) Infection

Web space infections can occur through a break in the skin between the fingers, through a palmar callus that becomes secondarily infected, or from proximal spread of an infection in the subcutaneous area of the fingers. Those who frequently cut the hair of humans or animals are at increased risk for this infection.

Symptoms

The patient is frequently seen with painful swelling of the distal palmar region. Tenderness and fluctuance are usually present. The adjacent finger rests in an abducted position when there is a large volar web-space collection, and a "collar button" abscess forms when there is a volar and dorsal component to the web-space infection.

Treatment

Surgical incision and drainage can be performed through a volar, dorsal, or combined approach to the web space. Access to the palmar space should be performed using a zigzag incision that starts at the edge of the web space and ends just distal to the distal palmar crease (Figure 9, *A*). The subcutaneous tissue is bluntly dissected and retracted, and the palmar fascia is incised to drain the collection. The digital neurovascular bundle should be identified and protected. When additional dorsal drainage is needed, a longitudinal incision should be made from the metacarpal phalangeal joint level to the edge of the web space (Figure 9, *B*). The incisions should be loosely closed over a Penrose drain, and the hand should be splinted. The tissue of the web space itself should not be violated.

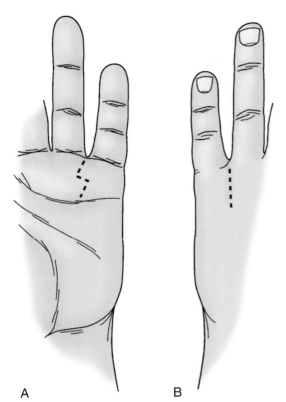

A   B

FIGURE 9   **A,** Palmar zigzag. **B,** Dorsal longitudinal incision for drainage of a web space infection.

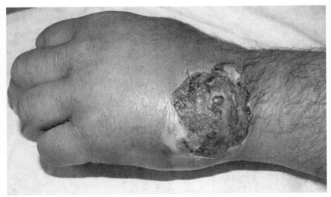

FIGURE 10   Infection of the dorsal subcutaneous and subaponeurotic space resulting from a puncture wound.

Dorsal Subcutaneous Space and Subaponeurotic Space Infections

The dorsal subaponeurotic space lies deep to the extensor mechanism and superficial to the periosteum of the metacarpal bones and fascia of the dorsal interosseous muscles. Infections of the subaponeurotic and subcutaneous spaces usually result from a local penetrating injury and are often seen in intravenous drug users.

Symptoms

Patients come in with pain, erythema, and marked edema of the dorsum of the hand (Figure 10). Because of the proximity of the extensor mechanism, tenderness will be elicited by finger extension.

Treatment

Cellulitis of the dorsum of the hand can be treated with antibiotics, elevation, and splint immobilization. When fluctuance is noted, surgical drainage is performed through a dorsal longitudinal incision. The fascia between the extensor tendons is incised to enter the subaponeurotic space. On occasion, two parallel incisions are needed to provide adequate drainage. Care should be taken when planning these insicions to ensure that the skin bridge has adequate blood supply. The wound can be left open or loosely closed over a Penrose drain. It is important to protect the extensor tendon paratenon from dessication to prevent subsequent tendon adhesions. The hand is splinted, and physical therapy is initiated when the edema begins to resolve.

INFECTIONS INVOLVING THE PALMAR SPACES

Thenar Space

The thenar space is a triangular space defined by the interosseous muscles and abductor pollicis longus, the midpalmar septum, and the thumb metacarpal bone.

Symptoms

Thenar-space infections are characterized by edema, pain with passive or active movement of the thumb, and exquisite tenderness to palpation of the thenar eminence and radial side of the palm; the thumb may be held in abduction when a large abscess is present (Figure 11). The infection can spread dorsally through the adductor pollicis and first dorsal interosseous muscle to create a "dumbbell" or "pantaloon" abscess.

Treatment

Surgical drainage can be performed by through a palmar incision along the thenar crease or a transverse incision proximal to the metacarpophalangeal crease, in the distal area of the thenar musculature. When necessary, dorsal drainage is achieved through longitudinal incision of the first web space (Figure 12).

Midpalmar Space

The midpalmar space is located deep to the palmar fascia. It is bordered radially by the oblique septum and ulnarly by the hypothenar septum. Infection of the midpalmar space is uncommon and may result from a penetrating injury, following rupture of a pyogenic flexor tenosynovitis or in association with a distal abscess that extends through the lumbrical canal.

Symptoms

Patients come in with edema of the volar and dorsal surfaces of the hand, and the normal palmar concavity may be effaced. The palm is tender to palpation, and pain occurs with passive flexion and extension of the fingers.

Treatment

Drainage of this space is performed through a longitudinal or transverse palmar incision over the most prominent portion of the abscess (Figure 13). The deep space is entered through blunt dissection while protecting the neurovascular bundles. As with other hand infections, the wound can be left open or loosely closed over one or more Penrose drains. The hand should be splinted and elevated postoperatively, and therapy can be initiated when pain and swelling improve.

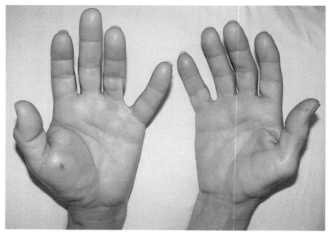

FIGURE 11   Thenar space infection resulting from a cat bite, showing thenar edema and abduction of the thumb.

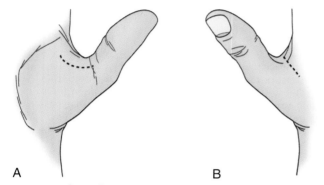

A   B

FIGURE 12   Surgical approach for incision and drainage of a thenar-space infection. **A,** Transverse incision. **B,** Dorsal longitudinal incision.

Hypothenar Space

The hypothenar space is located between the hypothenar fascia and the hypothenar musculature. Infections of the hypothenar space are rare.

Symptoms

Hypothenar-space infections present with edema and tenderness of the hypothenar eminence. Pain with flexion of the small finger often occurs.

Treatment

The hypothenar space is accessed through an incision along the ulnar aspect of the palm beginning proximal and ulnar to the midpalmar crease (Figure 14). The terms *radial* and *ulnar* are the standard convention for describing the hand. The incision should not cross the wrist flexion crease. Blunt dissection is used to enter the deep space while protecting the ulnar nerve and artery.

The Parona Space

The Parona space is found deep to the flexor tendons of the forearm and is bounded dorsally by the *pronator quadratus* muscle and the interosseous membrane. The space communicates with the radial and ulnar bursa and midpalmar space and thus may become infected following deep hand infections or pyogenic flexor tenosynovitis.

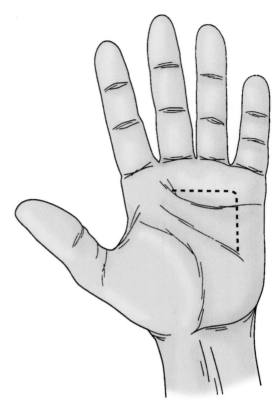

FIGURE 13   Combined longitudinal and transverse incision for drainage of midpalmar space abscess.

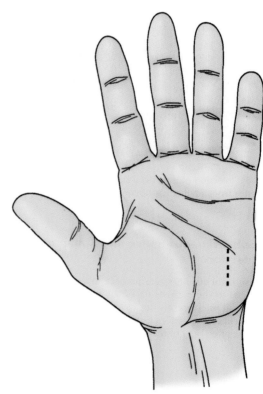

FIGURE 14   Longitudinal incision for drainage of a hypothenar space abscess.

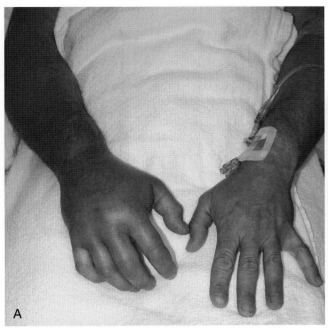

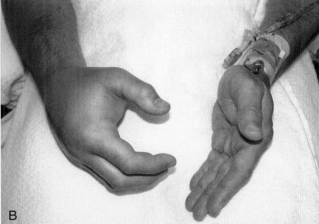

FIGURE 15 Two views of an infection involving the Parona space in an intravenous drug user. **A,** Dorsal view. **B,** Lateral view. This patient required volar and dorsal incisions to adequately drain and decompress the hand.

Symptoms

Edema, tenderness, and fluctuance will be noted on the volar distal forearm (Figure 15). Passive flexion of the wrist and fingers elicits pain.

Treatment

Access for drainage is provided by a longitudinal incision between the flexor tendons, ending proximal to the wrist crease.

SEPTIC ARTHRITIS

Septic arthritis is most often caused by penetrating trauma, bites, or contiguous spread from adjacent infection. Early diagnosis and treatment is important, as inflammatory reaction resulting from the infection can destroy the articular cartilage. Joint aspiration confirms the diagnosis.

Signs and Symptoms

The affected joint will be swollen and tender, and motion is restricted and painful. Fever and chills may also be present. In the digit, septic arthritis most often occurs with dorsal swelling and tenderness. When the wrist is involved, swelling may be subtle, but focal tenderness and pain with motion are usually severe. Gout may often present as septic arthritis, so aspiration should be undertaken in any patient with a history of previous gout attack.

Treatment

Dorsolateral arthrotomy lateral to the extensor tendon and dorsal to the collateral ligament is the preferred method of drainage for the digital joints. It may be necessary to excise a portion of the transverse retinacular ligament (at the PIP joint) or the sagittal band (at the metacarpophalangeal joint) to gain full exposure, though the functional integrity of both structures must be preserved. The wound is

closed over a Penrose drain, the hand is splinted, and physical therapy is initiated after the pain has resolved.

Septic arthritis of the wrist can usually be drained through a longitudinal incision between the third and fourth extensor compartments, taking great care to avoid damage to the extensor tendons. If adequate exposure is not possible, a second longitudinal incision can be made between the fifth and sixth compartments.

OSTEOMYELITIS

Osteomyelitis usually results from a penetrating injury or, rarely, from hematogenous spread. The most common pathogen is *Staphylococcus aureus;* infection is usually treated with debridement and long-term antibiotics, although certain cases may require amputation of the affected finger.

BITES

Human bites, usually the result of a clenched-fist blow to the mouth, are most commonly seen over the metacarpophalangeal joints (Figure 16, *A*). Communication with the joint space occurs in up to 60% of cases, resulting in septic arthritis. The most common organism cultured from this type of infection is *Eikenella corrodens.* It is mandatory to obtain radiographs of the involved area to identify bony injury and/or tooth fragments that sometimes remain in the wound.

Streptococcus viridans and *Staphylococcus aureus* are the two most common organisms found in infected dog-bite wounds. *Pasturella multocida* is often cultured from infected cat bites. Dog bites can be accompanied by significant tissue destruction from tearing or crushing. The wound from a cat bite is usually a small puncture.

Treatment

A detailed hand exam should be performed. Penetration of the joint, even when grossly evident at surgery, is rarely visible through the skin wound; the puncture occurs with the digits fully flexed, so skin,

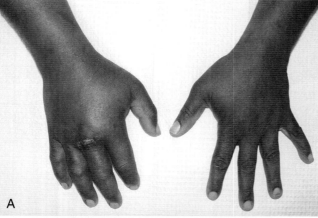

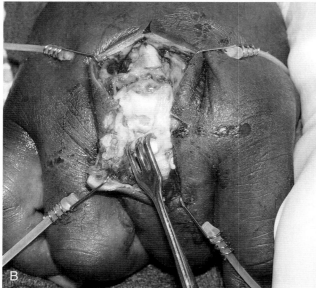

FIGURE 16 **A,** Human bite to the metacarpophalangeal joint of the right long finger following a fight. **B,** Surgery revealed a complete laceration of the extensor digitorum communis, violation of the joint space, and damage to the articular cartilage.

tendon, and capsule injuries will be out of register when the hand is relaxed.

If there is any question of joint involvement, the joint should be explored in a bloodless field and irrigated copiously. Fresh human bites can be irrigated clean, leaving the wound open, and should be treated with oral antibiotics and close follow-up. Human-bite joint infections are aggressive and should be treated accordingly with urgent incision and drainage and high-dose intravenous antibiotics. Advanced infections may require debridement of necrotic soft bone (Figure 16, *B*). The hand should be splinted and elevated, and physical therapy is initiated when pain begins to resolve. Tetanus prophylaxis should be considered if immunization status is unknown or outdated.

Many animal bites can be treated in the emergency department. Lacerations from a dog bite can usually be closed after thorough irrigation and debridement of devitalized tissue, but 40% of puncture wounds from a cat become infected. Oral antibiotics are given if indicated, and all human and animal bites should be followed closely to inspect the wounds for infection. Consider tetanus and rabies prophylaxis.

SUGGESTED READINGS

Weinzweig N, Gonzalez M: Surgical infections of the hand and upper extremity, *Ann Plastic Surg* 49:621, 2002.
Benson LS, Edwards SL, Schiff AP, et al: Dog and cat bites to the hand: treatment and cost assessment, *J Hand Surg* 31A:468, 2006.
Spann M, Talmor N, Nolan WB: Hand infections: basic principles and management, *Surg Infect (Larchmont)* 5:210, 2004.
Clark DC: Common acute hand infections, *Am Fam Physician* 68:2167, 2003.
Haussman MR, Lisser SP: Hand infections, *Orthop Clinic North Am* 23:171, 1992.

NERVE INJURY AND REPAIR

Marie-Noëlle Hébert-Blouin, MD, and Robert J. Spinner, MD

OVERVIEW

Nerve lesions can be traumatic, iatrogenic, neoplastic, or inflammatory in origin; they can be partial or complete, can involve any part of the body, and may lead to significant impairment and disability. The management of nerve injuries involves principles and techniques that differ from those used to treat other injuries. Answering five simple questions related to nerve injuries—what, when, how, why, and who—gives a medical care provider a platform on which to approach nerve injuries.

WHAT IS THE NERVE INJURY?

The first step for the treatment of nerve injuries is to determine *what* nerve injury has been sustained by the patient; this will in turn dictate the right treatment. The nerve injury is defined by the mechanism of injury, the degree of injury, and the nerve components affected by the injury. The mechanism of injury may be penetrating, such as a sharp or ragged laceration, or nonpenetrating, such as occurs with overstretching or blunt or compressive trauma. Nerve injuries caused by gunshots are considered nonpenetrating injuries, because the nerve damage is generally due to the shock wave along the tract of the projectile and not by the tract itself; contrary to common belief, the affected nerves are rarely severed.

The extent of nerve injury is determined by a careful neurologic assessment done by clinical and often electrophysiologic examinations to determine the severity of the injury. A detailed knowledge of the anatomy and expected deficits for each nerve or plexus element involved is therefore essential to document complete or partial motor and/or sensory loss

TABLE 1: Classification and expected recovery of nerve injuries

	CLASSIFICATIONS	NERVE COMPONENT INJURED					EXPECTED RECOVERY		
Seddon	Sunderland Degree (Modified)	Myelin	Axon	Endoneurium	Perineurium	Epineurium	Extent	Rate	Surgery Indicated
Neurapraxia	First	X					Complete	Fast	No
Axonotmesis	Second	X	X				Good	Slow	Not usually
	Third	X	X	X			Variable	Slow	Variable
	Fourth	X	X	X	X		None		Yes
Neurotmesis	Fifth	X	X	X	X	X	None		Yes
	Sixth	Combination of injury					Variable	Variable	Variable

X, Injury

of function in the nerve distribution. Finally, determining the degree of injury, either as neurapraxia, axonotmesis, and/or neurotmesis using the Seddon or Sunderland classifications of nerve injuries, may help determine if and when nerve injury requires surgical intervention (Table 1).

Nerves are composed of axons, myelin sheaths, and supporting connective tissues of the endoneurium, perineurium, and epineurium. Injuries involve these components to variable degrees. If the injury is limited, neurological function may recover—for example, if only the myelin is injured, recovery will occur. In contrast, if the injury involves all components, surgical repair is needed.

Treatment Options

Various options are available for the treatment of nerve injury and include observation; neurolysis; direct nerve repair; nerve graft; nerve transfer, which may be direct or via interpositional graft; nerve reimplantation; tendon and/or muscle transfer, including free-functioning muscle transfer; and bone or joint procedures. Each repair option has its own indications (Table 2). Inherent limitations include 1) speed of regeneration (1 mm/day or 1 inch/month), 2) distance from repair site, 3) muscle atrophy or neuromuscular junction degeneration, 4) limited availability of functional donors or graft materials, and 5) expected outcomes that may determine best use of resources. These limitations are reflected in the differences between the management of an individual injured nerve and the management of multiple injured nerves. Although a single nerve injury in the distal part of an extremity can be effectively reconstructed, multiple nerve injuries, such as from a brachial plexus lesion, may only be partially reconstructed, in which case functions requiring reconstruction must be prioritized, and expectations must be limited. For example, in severe injuries, reconstructive efforts are aimed at restoration of elbow flexion, shoulder stability, shoulder abduction and/or external rotation, hand sensibility, grasp, wrist and finger extension, and intrinsic hand function, in that order.

WHEN IS SURGERY INDICATED?

Deciding if and *when* a patient with a nerve injury would benefit from a surgical intervention is crucial. The window of opportunity for repair of a nerve injury is limited: early surgery or early referral is important.

Pathophysiology

Understanding the pathophysiology of nerve injury underscores the importance of the timing of nerve repair and will therefore be briefly discussed. Three broad scenarios are possible: First, when only the

TABLE 2: Treatment options and indications for the repair of nerve injuries

Options	Indications
Observation	Recovering nerve injury; partial nerve injury
Neurolysis	Neuroma-in-continuity with positive NAP
Direct repair	Laceration; short gap after resection of a neuroma-in-continuity with negative NAP
Nerve graft	Laceration with retracted stumps (delayed repair); larger gap after resection of a neuroma-in-continuity with negative NAP; direct repair without tension not possible
Nerve transfer	Avulsion (brachial plexus injury); alternative to nerve graft with transfer to distal targets
Nerve reimplantation	Under investigation
Tendon and/or muscle transfers	Delayed (>1 year) for improvement of function
Bony and/or joint procedures	Delayed (>1 year) for improvement of function
Amputation	Rarely indicated; sometimes desired by patients

NAP, Nerve action potential

myelin is injured, and the axon remains intact (neurapraxia), the neurologic deficit is secondary to a conduction block. As the myelin heals, functional recovery occurs, often within days. Usually by 6 weeks, recovery is complete. In this scenario, no surgical intervention is indicated. A common example is a wrist drop from radial nerve palsy due to pressure from prolonged compression in one position, so-called *Saturday night palsy*. Second, when the axon is injured (axonotmesis), its proximal portion, the part connected to the neuron cell body, remains intact and viable, but its distal portion, now disconnected from the neuron cell body, undergoes Wallerian degeneration. The proximal axon will attempt to regenerate by sprouting and growing at a rate of approximately 1 mm per day or 1 inch per month. If the supporting tissues of the nerve—the endoneurium, perineurium,

TABLE 3: "3 Plus 1" rule for timing of nerve repair

Timing	Time	Injury Type	Injury Classification
Early	3 days	Laceration	Neurotmesis
Subacute	3 weeks	Blunt transection Ragged transection	Neurotmesis
Delayed	3 months	Lesions-in-continuity	Axonotmesis
Late	>1 year	Salvage procedures	Neurotmesis or axonotmesis

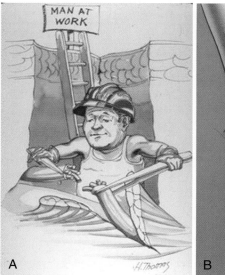
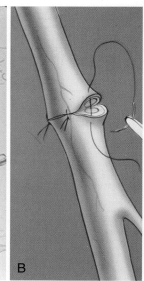

FIGURE 1   A, A transected or ruptured nerve cannot recover function spontaneously. This type of neurotmetic injury, a Sunderland grade V injury, requires surgical repair. **B,** If possible, direct nerve repair with end-to-end suture is the preferred technique. Epineurial sutures are shown; epineurial vessels are used to align nerve ends.

and epineurium—are sufficiently intact, the regenerating axons will be appropriately guided and will reach the distal target, the neuromuscular junctions or sensory receptors, within months or even years, depending on the distance from the zone of injury. If and when spontaneous recovery occurs, it usually gives better results than any surgical intervention. Third, when the axon and its surrounding tissues are injured—either partially (axonotmesis) or completely (neurotmesis), such as damage that occurs after a transection injury—the regenerating axon sprouts will not be able to be guided toward the end organ. They will create a neuroma, if the nerve is transected, or a neuroma-in-continuity, if the nerve is significantly injured but in continuity, as in more severe axonotmesis injuries. In these cases, surgery is required for return of function. Regeneration will start at the time of repair and proceeds at a rate of 1 mm per day from the repair site. However, with time, generally 18 to 24 months after the injury, the neuromuscular junctions start to undergo irreversible damage, and the muscles undergo irreversible atrophy and fibrosis. After this period, even if a functional axon would reach the muscle, little meaningful function will return. This explains why repair of nerve injury must occur early and why some injuries, if very proximal, may not substantially recover, even if repaired immediately (e.g., ulnar nerve injury in the proximal upper arm, supplying the distal hand muscles). Because sensory receptors do not undergo degeneration, sensory recovery can theoretically occur longer after injury, even after 5 years.

The timing of surgery is based on the above scenarios and can be simplified by the "3 plus 1" rule (Table 3) for early surgery, which occurs within 3 days; subacute surgery, occurring around 3 weeks; delayed surgery for chronic symptoms, which takes place within 3 to 6 months; and late surgery, which can occur after 1 year.

Early surgery, occurring within 3 days after the injury or at presentation if evaluated after 3 days, is indicated in cases of suspected transection with sharp injuries, when the transected nerve will not spontaneously recover function (Figure 1). It is also indicated in situations with vascular (e.g., hematoma, pseudoaneurysm) and/or bony injuries causing acute nerve compression, especially if it occurs in the vicinity of a closed compartment. If a neurologic examination worsens acutely under close observation, the nerve damage can potentially be reversed or reduced by immediate surgical intervention.

Subacute repair (around 3 weeks) is advocated by some for blunt or ragged transections (e.g., propeller blades, chain saws), but others still treat them acutely. Again, this situation is clearly one of neurotmesis. Those who advocate waiting for several weeks stress the importance of allowing the zone of injury to define itself with time, manifested by changes due to Wallerian degeneration that occur during this period. At the time of repair, the nerve endings can be resected back to healthy tissue, which would be difficult to evaluate if the injured nerve were to be explored immediately after the injury.

In contrast, advocates for earlier surgery feel that surgery is easier and more practical at an earlier time, especially when a surgical intervention is done by another team, such as a general, vascular, or orthopedic surgical team. Furthermore, the additional technical challenges of dealing with spontaneous or postoperative scarring can be avoided.

For example, if a patient with a fracture and associated nerve palsy is being explored by an orthopedist, it would be reasonable to explore the nerve at the same time. If the nerve is found to be in continuity but nonfunctional, observation for several months is indicated. If the nerve is found to be ruptured, some would repair it at the same time. Others would perform the surgery at a second stage, when the zone of injury can be better defined; nerve ends are tacked down under tension, so they do not retract, using radiopaque clips or staples, so they can be easily identified. At a later time, a subacute nerve repair can be done.

Delayed surgery (approximately 3 months, but up to 6 months) is indicated for lesions-in-continuity, such as the majority of stretching injuries, contusive injuries, and gunshot wounds. In these cases, it is difficult to predict with certainty which path the nerve injury will follow from those described above, and whether the injury will spontaneously recover or require surgical repair. Nonoperative treatment can be continued in patients with early signs of spontaneous recovery or in partial lesions. Note that 90% of nerve injuries that recover do so within 4 months. Surgery is indicated when there has been no evidence of clinical or electrophysiologic recovery after this period of observation. In theses cases, the delay will also allow lesions-in-continuity to be evaluated intraoperatively with nerve action potential (NAP) testing, described below, to distinguish between recovering lesions and nonrecovering lesions that require repair.

Late surgery that occurs after 1 year may be considered in patients presenting late or in those who have either not recovered or have recovered incompletely after spontaneous recovery or previous nerve surgery. Nerve repair typically does not work well after this period, which can be considered to be as short as 9 months by some authors, because of permanent changes at the muscular level. However, reconstructive options addressing muscles, tendons, bones, and joints may be useful.

HOW TO TREAT PATIENTS WITH NERVE INJURIES

The management and surgical treatment of nerve injury involves the application of general principles applicable to all nerve surgeries and of specific nerve repair techniques particular to each situation. Preoperative assessment of the nerve injury should include a detailed

TABLE 4: Key operative principles of nerve repair

Preparation for repair	Know the anatomy.
	Plan adequate exposure, and plan for the possible need for additional exposure.
	Plan for nerve graft harvest.
	Expose the normal segment of nerve first, then find the pathologic segment.
	Dissect down to the nerve, then dissect along the nerve.
	Dissect between the muscle groups.
	Preserve vascular structures.
Repair	Use NAP to evaluate neuroma-in-continuity.
	Prepare nerve endings.
	Employ microsurgical technique.
	Perform a tension-free nerve repair.
	Simpler is better.

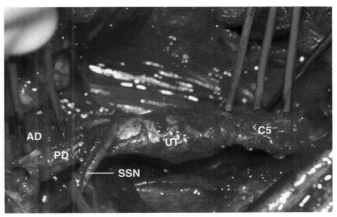

FIGURE 2 Intraoperative photograph showing a nerve action potential (NAP) being recorded. The NAP is tested across a neuroma-in-continuity at the level of the upper trunk (UT) of the brachial plexus. The C5 spinal nerve, the UT, the anterior (AD) and posterior (PD) divisions of the UT, and the suprascapular nerve (SSN) are seen. The C6 spinal nerve contributing to the UT is not seen in this view. The stimulating electrode (three prongs) is seen proximal to the neuroma-in-continuity; the recording electrode (two prongs) is seen distal to it.

history of the mechanism of injury and onset of the deficit; a physical exam (neurologic examination but also examination of the associated vascular and musculoskeletal elements); electrodiagnostic studies, such as electromyelogram and nerve conduction studies; and appropriate imaging, which may include radiographs, ultrasound, computed tomography, magnetic resonance imaging, and/or myelogram.

A sensory and motor-function grading system, such as the Medical Research Council (MRC) muscle grading system, should be used to document the initial physical examination and each subsequent exam. The grading system will help measure the outcomes of observation and surgical interventions. After determining the type of nerve injury and that surgery is indicated, patients should be adequately informed to ensure that they have realistic expectations of the surgical procedure.

At surgery, the steps to expose the injured nerve prior to the nerve repair itself are important (Table 4). Knowledge of the anatomy is crucial, especially when scarring from the injury is expected and will likely distort the anatomy. Adequate exposure should be planned, including the possibility of harvesting nerve grafts. Dissection is usually done between two muscle groups parallel to the long axis of the nerve. Ideally, a normal segment of the nerve is first identified both proximally and distally, before dissection is carried toward the injured segment. For practical purposes, there are two possibilities: the identification of a neuroma-in-continuity or nerve stumps.

If there is a neuroma-in-continuity (Figure 2), intraoperative NAP recordings can be performed to assess the degree of injury (recovery or no recovery). In our opinion, these are helpful, because gross inspection or palpation of a neuroma-in-continuity does not predict histology, recovery, or outcomes. Furthermore, NAP can determine recovery across a short segment of nerve (i.e., proximal and distal to an injury) before recovery can be seen by conventional electromyelogram or physical examination. When a NAP is present (+) across a lesion, the lesion should not be resected, as the outcome will generally be better with neurolysis alone. If an NAP is absent (−) across a lesion, then the outcomes are generally poor if the lesion is left intact; therefore, surgical repair is indicated.

If two nerve ends suggestive of a rupture or transection are identified, or if a nerve end suspicious for an avulsion is found, a nerve repair or reconstruction is indicated. The use of NAP recordings can still be helpful in these situations and can allow identification of the proximal location at which nerve grafting can be performed. Some use NAP in brachial plexus avulsion injuries to define preganglionic responses. Others use other techniques, including somatosensory-evoked potentials (SSEP) and motor-evoked potentials (MEP), to assess whether the proximal nerve stump is intact and can be used for reinnervation.

For the nerve repair, microsurgical techniques should be used, including the use of microinstruments and of a microscope or magnifying loupes (Figure 3). The nerve ends on both sides should be prepared by removing the neuroma and scar tissue, until normal fascicular structure is obtained. Optimal microsurgical technique will cause minimal surgical trauma and permit an end-to-end repair (see Figure 1) or interpositional grafting; it is further recommended that 8-0, 9-0, or 10-0 sutures be used, and using the fewest number of sutures to approximate the nerve accurately is preferred. The repair must be without tension to obtain good results. Fibrin glue may be used to reinforce the suture line, but other methods include the use of fibrin glue alone or with a variety of nerve conduits (entubulation).

Postoperatively, the nerve repair should be protected for 3 weeks. After this period, early protected mobilization is started to promote neural gliding. During the observation period, physical therapy should be continued. Careful sequential clinical and electrophysiologic examinations should be performed to assess neurologic function, and these can be compared to baseline examinations. The Tinel sign, which consists of a sensation of tingling in the distribution of the nerve caused by percussion over the nerve, is indicative of nerve regeneration. Percussion should be performed from a distal site to a more proximal one, and the exact location of the Tinel sign should be recorded using topographic landmarks. The Tinel sign should advance (move distally) in cases of recovery; with time, the Tinel sign at the distal site should be stronger than the one at the suture line.

Once reinnervation has started, sensory and motor reeducation can improve functional recovery. Follow-up of nerve repairs should continue for at least 2 years in children and up to 5 years in adults, because the regeneration distance is longer in adults. However, in some pediatric cases, such as with brachial plexus injuries, even longer follow-up is needed to ensure that secondary deformities—for example, shoulder deformities—that could be addressed are not developing.

Techniques for Nerve Surgery

Neurolysis

Neurolysis, defined as releasing scar tissue surrounding the injured nerve, is indicated when a neuroma-in-continuity conducting an NAP is found. Generally, external neurolysis, which is completed during the nerve exposure, is sufficient. In select instances, some

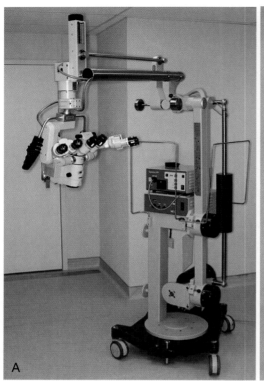
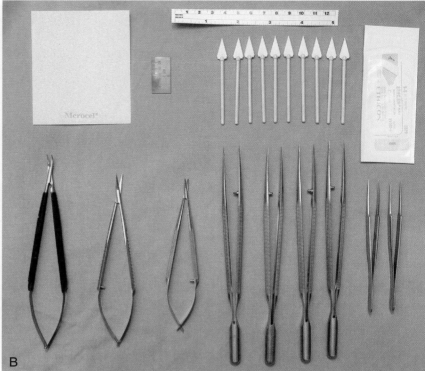

FIGURE 3   A, Microscope used for the repair of nerve injury. **B,** A basic microsurgical instrument tray for repair of nerve injuries.

advocate limited internal neurolysis, or removal of the scar tissue between the various nerve fascicles.

Direct Repair

Direct nerve repair is the end-to-end suture of nerve stumps (see Figure 1). It is indicated when a short nerve gap exists, either from a sharply transected nerve—such as a cut from glass, a knife, or a razor—or after removing a focal neuroma-in-continuity that did not conduct an NAP (Figures 4 and 5). Direct repair is the preferred method of nerve repair whenever possible, assuming that the damaged segment of the nerve has been resected and that the sutures are without tension. This method allows direct delivery of proximal axons to the distal stump via a single suture line. It also usually permits fascicular alignment, which increases matching between motor and sensory axons and their targets (Figure 6).

Epineurial or grouped fascicular repair can both achieve fascicular alignment. If a small nerve gap is present, several methods can be used to reduce the gap and achieve a direct repair. Commonly used methods include nerve mobilization (see Figure 5); nerve transposition, as with the ulnar and radial nerves; and joint positioning, such as flexion of the knee with gradual postoperative extension. In some cases, bone shortening, as with a comminuted fracture, may offer an opportunity for decreasing a nerve gap. Some innovative surgeons have applied nerve-elongation techniques. Intraoperatively, restoration of fascicular orientation can be facilitated by 1) epineurial alignment of the vessels; 2) knowledge of the serial cross-sectional topography; and 3) gross fascicular matching. Some surgeons use other techniques, such as fascicular stimulation and histochemical stains. Fascicular stimulation of the stumps allows mapping of motor and sensory fascicles: distally, motor fascicles can be identified by stimulation that produces muscle contraction if early exploration is done before Wallerian degeneration occurs; proximally, sensory fascicles can be identified by stimulation that produces dysesthesias, but the technique requires the patient to be awake, although sedated, and may be painful. Histochemical stains may be used to identify motor fascicles.

Nerve Graft

Nerve grafting is performed when nerve stumps on either side of a gap cannot be apposed for a direct end-to-end repair without tension (Figure 7). Often, this technique is necessary for neuromas-in-continuity of moderate or longer lengths with unrecordable (negative) NAP or for transected nerves with retracted stumps, which occurs when the initial surgery is delayed. Nerve grafts are not indicated for brachial plexus injuries, in which the nerves are avulsed because there is no "functional" proximal nerve stump (Figure 8).

The most frequent source for a nerve graft is the sural nerve (Figure 9). However, the medial or lateral antebrachial cutaneous nerves, superficial sensory radial nerve, superficial peroneal nerve, distal posterior interosseous nerve, great auricular nerve, and cervical plexus nerves are alternatives. The disadvantage of nerve grafting relates to the minor sequelae associated with donor morbidity from the nerve harvest, such as expected permanent sensory loss and small chance of neuropathic pain.

The graft length is calculated by measuring the nerve gap and adding 10% to account for some desiccation of the graft and to avoid tension. One graft or several "cable" grafts are placed to maximize the surface area at the repair sites and to prevent mismatch (Figure 10). Interposed grafts may be sutured individually at both ends or may be glued together and then sutured as a single unit.

Vascularized nerve grafts have been advocated by some to improve the speed and quality of regeneration compared with standard, nonvascularized nerve grafts; however, this practice is controversial. Autogenous or synthetic conduits may be used for short gaps (<3 cm) of small diameter, usually sensory nerves (e.g., digital nerves).

Nerve Transfers

Nerve transfers, also known as *neurotizations,* consist of the transfer of an expandable or redundant working nerve, branch, or fascicle to a nonfunctioning nerve. The donor functional nerve may be intraplexal or extraplexal, motor or sensory. Preferably, the donor nerve

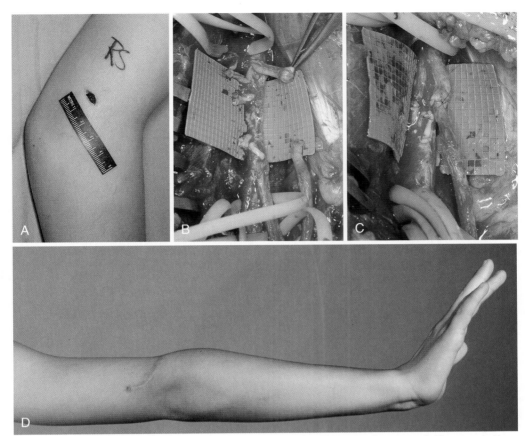

FIGURE 4   Patient with a partial laceration of the radial nerve treated at presentation 1 week after injury. **A,** The open knife-entry wound is seen in the right arm, slightly proximal to the elbow, near the interval between the brachioradialis and triceps. The knife blade had penetrated the arm to a depth of approximately 5 cm (2 inches). The patient had no thumb extension, partial weakness of the finger extensors and wrist extensors, and decreased sensation in the dorsum of his hand. **B,** At exploration, the radial nerve was found to be partially lacerated at its bifurcation into the deep and superficial radial nerve. The complete laceration of the superficial (sensory) radial nerve is seen, as is the partial injury to multiple fascicles of the deep (motor) branch of the radial nerve. **C,** The direct repair of the superficial sensory radial nerve and the fascicles of the deep branch of the radial nerve are shown; a 9.0 suture was used to perform this repair. **D,** After 6 months, the patient had already regained good (MRC grade 4) finger and wrist extension. His thumb extension (the most distal motor target) improved to MRC grade 3, although he still had sensory abnormality in the dorsum of the hand.

should be synergistic to the recipient, and relearning of a new function with independence is possible in many situations. The indications for nerve transfers include 1) irreparable brachial plexus nerves (avulsions); 2) specific cases of nerve injury, for which nerve transfer may lead to a more rapid or reliable recovery because of proximity of the end-organ (an alternative to nerve grafting); and 3) innervation of free-functioning muscle transfers.

The two main advantages of nerve transfers are that they are often closer to the end organ, thereby decreasing the distance, and by extension, the time to reinnervation; and they typically have a large number of relatively "pure" (motor or sensory) axons, because they are more distal. The cost/benefit ratio of neurotization needs to be evaluated for each patient and for each nerve transfer. Standard examples of extraplexal "donor" nerves are the spinal accessory nerve and the intercostal nerves; intercostal motor nerves are distinct from intercostal sensory nerves, and each may be used separately. Examples of intraplexal donor nerve branches are medial pectoral branches and triceps branches, and examples of intraplexal donor nerve fascicles are fascicles from the ulnar and median nerves (Figure 11).

Less common and potentially more risky examples of extraplexal nerve transfers include the use of the phrenic nerve, contralateral C7 nerve, and hypoglossal nerve. Because of improvements in

techniques and outcomes with newer nerve transfers, many surgeons are advocating nerve transfer in cases where more conventional nerve grafting could be done. Furthermore, wherever possible and feasible, many are advocating distal nerve transfers closer to the end organ as opposed to proximal nerve transfers farther from the end organ.

Muscle and Tendon Transfer and Bone and Joint Procedures

These various procedures are usually performed in a delayed fashion, sometimes more than a year after the injury. Muscle and/or tendon transfer is the transfer of a muscle and/or tendon that is working and is expendable to achieve a new function. This technique, similar to nerve transfer, requires a functional expandable innervated muscle in the vicinity. Examples of reliable tendon transfers include opponensplasty, anticlaw procedure, thumb adductorplasty, flexor to extensor transfers, elbow flexorplasty, transfers for shoulder external rotation, antiwing (scapular) transfers, transfers for pronation, and extensor-flexor transfers. An alternative is the transfer of a free-functioning muscle, such as the gracilis muscle from the lower extremity, which can be transferred at a late stage for elbow flexion and/or finger flexion. This requires the presence of an arterial and venous supply as well as a functioning nerve to reinnervate the muscle. Bone and joint procedures, such as osteotomies and arthrodesis, may also improve

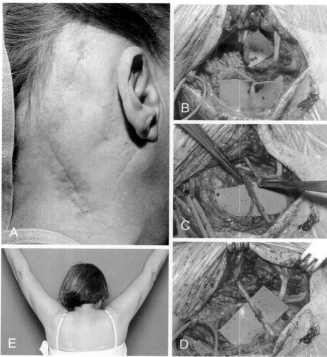

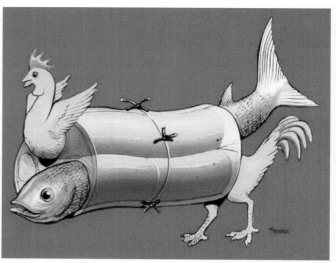

FIGURE 6   This schematic depicts fascicular mismatch. When a nerve is repaired, an attempt is made to restore the fascicular alignment to allow matching between motor and sensory axons and their targets. Restoration of fascicular orientation is easier in direct repair, but as the nerve gap increases, restoration becomes more difficult.

FIGURE 5   Patient with a spinal accessory nerve injury after a right retrosigmoid craniotomy for removal of a vestibular schwannoma. **A,** Photograph of the surgical incision used for the resection of the right vestibular schwannoma. Postoperatively, the patient developed prominent scapular winging, atrophy of the right trapezius muscle, and significant difficulty in abducting her right arm. Electromyography 3 months after surgery confirmed a right spinal accessory neuropathy affecting the motor branch to the trapezius (normal sternocleidomastoid) without evidence of reinnervation. **B,** At exploration soon thereafter, the great auricular nerve (at the right of the nerve stump) and the greater occipital nerve (in the blue vasoloop) were identified. The proximal and distal stumps (seen here clipped to a green background) of the spinal accessory nerve were found within the scar of the prior surgical exposure. **C,** To achieve a direct repair, the two nerve stumps were mobilized proximally and distally. **D,** A direct end-to-end repair was performed using an 8.0 suture. **E,** The patient regained excellent function, scapular stability, and range of motion, shown here at 15 months after the repair.

function. Shoulder fusion may be an option for patients with brachial plexus palsy and refractory instability with pain.

EXPECTED OUTCOMES FROM REPAIR AND RECONSTRUCTION

The main reason *why* surgeons perform nerve repair and/or reconstruction procedures is to improve outcomes for patients with nerve injuries. In general, the goals of surgical intervention—which include motor function, sensibility, sudomotor function, pain, patient satisfaction, and return to work—often can be achieved to varying extents. However, it is difficult to predict the outcome for an individual patient with a nerve injury because multiple factors influence nerve recovery (discussed later). It is also difficult to analyze and study these patients' outcomes because of several issues: 1) definition of a "good result" is lacking; 2) multiple variables exist, and data from a single surgeon using the same technique at the same time postinjury in the same population of patients with the same pattern of injury is often unavailable; and 3) examination and analysis is unfortunately often performed by the surgical team alone, creating a potential for bias.

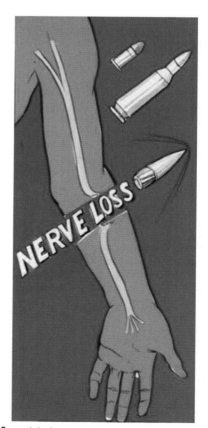

FIGURE 7   Some injuries may cause nerve tissue loss and create a nerve gap, which can occur in blunt or ragged transection, in sharp transection if the repair is done late, in nerve rupture (as can occur in brachial plexus injuries), and after resection of a nonconducting neuroma-in-continuity. In these instances, a graft is needed to bridge the gap and repair the nerve.

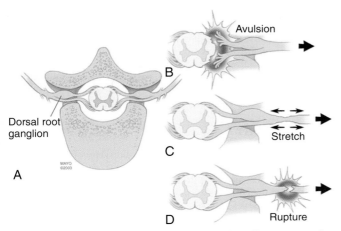

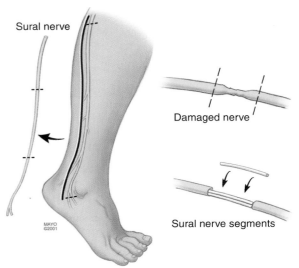

FIGURE 8 This schematic illustration depicts the different types of spinal nerve injuries seen in closed/traction injuries of the brachial plexus. **A,** Axial cross-section of a vertebral body showing the normal anatomy of the spinal cord, giving rise to the anterior and posterior spinal rootlets, which combine to form the spinal nerve. The dorsal root ganglion is seen in the intervertebral foramen. **B,** In brachial plexus injuries, the spinal roots can be directly avulsed from the spinal cord. These lesions are characterized as *preganglionic*. In this injury, the spinal nerves cannot be used and grafted, as there is no "functional" proximal nerve stump, and the reconstruction consists of nerve transfers. **C,** Spinal nerves and brachial plexus elements may be stretched by trauma. Although the nerve is in continuity, the nerve injury may be variable (axonotmesis, Sunderland grades II to IV). Some of these nerve injuries will spontaneously recover function, but others will not. At surgery, a neuroma-in-continuity (postganglionic) will be found, and NAP recording may help evaluate whether the nerve is recovering or if it will require repair. If repair is needed, the spinal nerve proximal to the lesion is generally available for grafting. **D,** The spinal nerves and brachial plexus elements can be ruptured by trauma and may be found in discontinuity at surgery (neurotmesis, Sunderland grade V). In these cases, spontaneous recovery is not possible; these lesions require repair. The rupture is generally *postganglionic*. The proximal spinal nerve stump found at surgery can be used for grafting; NAP, somatosensory-evoked potentials, and/or motor-evoked potentials can help to assess its integrity (i.e., its connection to the spinal cord). *(Courtesy Mayo Foundation for Medical and Educational Research. All rights reserved.)*

FIGURE 9 The sural nerve is the most common source of nerve graft. A purely sensory nerve, it supplies sensation to a small area of the dorsolateral aspect of the foot. The sural nerve is up to 40 cm long in each leg; nerve grafts may be harvested bilaterally, and sural nerve segments are used to bridge the nerve gap. *(Courtesy Mayo Foundation for Medical and Educational Research. All rights reserved.)*

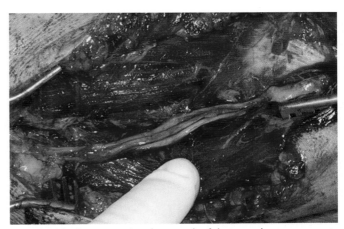

FIGURE 10 Intraoperative photograph of three sural nerve segments bridging a radial nerve gap in the distal arm following a humeral fracture.

Despite these issues, generalizations can be made. The best outcomes are achieved when there is evidence of early spontaneous neural recovery (i.e., when surgery is not indicated). Other factors influencing the recovery of nerve repair and/or reconstruction include the following:

1. Patient age: The younger the patient, the better the recovery because of inherent physiologic factors related to regeneration, limb length, and capacity for cortical reorganization and reeducation.
2. Level of injury: Distal injuries fare better because of the shorter distance to the end organ.
3. Type of nerve injured: Pure nerves fare better than mixed nerves, because there is less chance of fascicular mismatch.
4. Specific nerve involved: Radial nerve recovers better than median nerve, which recovers better than ulnar nerve; nerves C5 and C6 and those of the upper trunk recover better than nerves C8 to T1 and those of the lower trunk; and tibial nerve recovers better than peroneal nerve.
5. Mechanism of injury: Lacerations have better outcomes than low-velocity gunshot injuries, which in turn do better than high-velocity gunshot injuries; transections have better outcomes than crush or avulsion injuries; and stretch injuries generally have better outcomes than ruptures, which fare better than avulsions.

These variations in outcomes are related to the zone of injury and associated soft-tissue and vascular damage.

6. Timing of repair and reconstruction: The earlier the better; outcomes are typically best before 6 months, but they depend on the size of the gap, the status of the end plate, and the status of the α-motor neurons.
7. Type of repair or reconstruction: Patients in whom exploratory surgery is indicated, but in whom only neurolysis is performed because of a positive NAP, have good results 90% of the time. Patients in whom direct end-to-end nerve repair can be performed generally have better outcomes than patients who undergo conventional interpositional nerve grafting. Improved techniques with nerve transfers, especially distal nerve transfers, have improved outcomes in peripheral nerve surgery in recent years. Distal nerve transfers are now thought by some to be better than proximal nerve grafts in some situations, but there is still controversy. Direct nerve transfers have better outcomes than nerve transfers with interpositional grafts. In the future, other

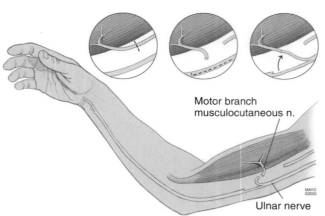

Motor branch
musculocutaneous n.

Ulnar nerve

FIGURE 11 Example of an intraplexal nerve transfer technique used for the repair of injury to the brachial plexus or musculocutaneous nerve leading to loss of biceps motor function. To perform this transfer, called an *Oberlin procedure*, the ulnar nerve function must be preserved. At the level of the middle or proximal third of the arm, a functioning ulnar nerve fascicle is used to reinnervate the biceps motor branch originating from the musculocutaneous nerve. Generally, ulnar motor function is preserved (deficit in <1%), but the patient may experience transient sensory changes in the distribution of the ulnar nerve. Patient series on this technique report that 85% recovered good elbow flexion after surgery. (*Courtesy Mayo Foundation for Medical and Educational Research. All rights reserved.*)

techniques and strategies may further improve outcomes for patients with nerve injuries. It is likely that other nerve transfer techniques will be developed. Nerve reimplantation, now experimental, may one day become an option. Techniques, growth factors, and materials that could accelerate axonal growth, promote regeneration, preserve end organs, and improve the interface between the nerve ends may also lead to improved outcomes.

WHO SHOULD OPERATE

By extrapolation based on data related to other surgical techniques, it seems reasonable to expect improved outcomes with centers performing high-volume practice. Timely referral to centers specializing in evaluation and management of these injuries is important and should be considered.

SUMMARY

The treatment and management of nerve injuries requires thorough knowledge of anatomy, the nerve injury process, and of the available repair and reconstructive options. It also requires specific microsurgical skills in the context of a multidisciplinary team able to address the peripheral nerves and associated muscle, tendon, and joint problems as well as concomitant injuries to the central nervous system (spinal cord and brain) and other systems.

SUGGESTED READINGS

Kline DG, Happel LT: Penfield lecture: a quarter century's experience with intraoperative nerve action potential recording, *Can J Neurol Sci* 20:3–10, 1993.

Midha R, Lee P, Mackay M: Surgical techniques for peripheral nerve repair. In Wolfa CE, Resnick DK, editors: *Neurosurgical operative atlas: spine and peripheral nerves,* ed 2, New York, 2007, Thieme, pp 402–408.

Midha R, Serrano-Almedia C, Mackay M: Harvesting techniques of sural and other cutaneous nerves for cable graft repair. In Wolfa CE, Resnick DK, editors: *Neurosurgical operative atlas: spine and peripheral nerves,* ed 2, New York, 2007, Thieme, pp 409–413.

Oberlin C, Durand S, Belheyar Z, et al: Nerve transfers in brachial plexus palsies, *Chir Main* 28:1–9, 2009.

Robert EG, Happel LT, Kline DG: Intraoperative nerve action potential recordings: technical considerations, problems, and pitfalls, *Neurosurgery (S)* 65:A97–A104, 2009.

Spinner RJ, Kline DG: Surgery for peripheral nerve and brachial plexus injuries or other nerve lesions, *Muscle Nerve* 23:680–695, 2000.

GAS GANGRENE

Jan K. Horn, MD

OVERVIEW

Gas gangrene, also known as *clostridial myonecrosis,* is a unique infection characterized by soft-tissue destruction and localized production of gas within the tissues. These infections spread within muscle tissue and subcutaneous fat, promoted by thrombosis of microvasculature and generation of an anaerobic environment. They are potentially lethal and can follow simple introduction of organisms into the soft tissues by puncture with contaminated objects; for example, following injury, contaminated surgical procedures, or injection of illicit parenteral drugs. Alternatively, they may result from internal necessitation of an intraabdominal abscess. On rare occasions, there is a lack of preceding tissue injury, and infections arise in association with comorbidities. Such patients are often very young and immunocompromised or older and more debilitated. Based on these etiologies, gas gangrene is generally classified as *posttraumatic, postoperative,* or *spontaneous.*

BACTERIOLOGY

Clostridium species, in particular *C. perfringens,* is a common pathogen responsible for gas gangrene. *Clostridium* species are gram-positive anaerobic bacilli that are found ubiquitously within the environment, particularly in soil or in decaying organic matter, but they also reside among the normal gastrointestinal flora of many animals. In humans, they cause a wide range of diseases, including botulism, tetanus, gas gangrene, and psuedomembranous colitis.

Virtually all of the known *Clostridium* species have been isolated from cases of gas gangrene. The majority of human disease is caused by *C. perfringens* (formerly *welchii*), although *C. novyi, C. septicum, C. histolyticum, C. sordellii, C. bifermentans, C. sporogenes, C. fallax,* and *C. tertium* are also capable of producing gas gangrene. *C. perfringens* displays a moderate amount of oxygen tolerance and a rapid growth rate. It is estimated that 25% of necrotizing soft tissue infections (NSTIs) are caused by *Clostridium* species.

Gas gangrene can also be caused by nonclostridial species. In some series such infections have been recorded in 60% to 85% of cases. One in particular showed that aerobic gram-negative bacteria predominated, and gram-positive *Clostridium* species were only cultured in 4.5% of patients. The predominant gram-negative species were *Pseudomonas aeruginosa, Escherichia coli, Klebsiella pneumoniae,* and *Proteus* species.

Clostridium species are capable of forming heat-resistant endospores, which can reside in the environment almost indefinitely and pose a potential threat when introduced into a host. A relative hypoxic tissue environment is critical for the induction of growth and proliferation from the endospore state. The typical incubation period following injection is 8 days with a range of 3 to 21 days; however, infection in as little as 6 hours has been reported.

The anaerobic growth is associated with production of gas within tissue planes, accounting for the characteristic radiographic findings. The production of gas is largely attributed to fermentation of glucose. Information obtained from cases of gas gangrene caused by *C. septicum* showed that the mixture of gases contained nitrogen (74.5%), oxygen (16.1%), hydrogen (5.9%), and carbon dioxide (3.4%). Late production of hydrogen sulfide and carbon dioxide leads to dissemination through less loose tissue planes and encourages spread of the infection.

C. perfringens has a particular predilection for muscle tissue, wherein microvascular thrombosis causes tissue necrosis. Further spread of infection by clostridial organisms is encouraged by suppression of host defenses. This was first recognized on examination of pathological specimens that displayed gram-positive bacilli and no evidence of neutrophil accumulation in the tissues. Studies have shown that this organism uniquely impairs diapedesis and suppresses neutrophil sequestration. Pathologically, what is observed is significant accumulation of neutrophils in the vessels supplying the infected sites (margination). This appears to be a consequence of pathological upregulation of endothelial cell adhesion molecules for neutrophils, an α-toxin–dependent phenomenon.

The virulent nature of clostridial infections is accounted for by the production of tissue-destructive enzymes, factors that suppress host immune defenses, and exotoxins that exert systemic effects. Following the sequencing of the entire genome, it was possible to appreciate how this organism is particularly capable of eliciting an array of products that account for these effects. There is remarkable duplicity of function, so that disabling mutations within one bacterial product are less crippling, as long as a similar alternative is produced. It is clear that the organism has also derived some of its virulent potential from other bacterial species through plasmid transfer.

C. perfringens has been subdivided into five biotypes, A through E, that each produce a variable array of different exotoxins, displayed in Table 1. Some toxins are considered lethal, and their distribution among the biotypes is displayed in Table 2. *C. perfringens* utilizes a two-component regulatory system to modulate gene expression of important virulence factors. Termed the *VirR/VirS system*, it relies on VirS, a histidine kinase, to respond to environmental signals and phosphorylate VirR. Phosphorylated VirR is a transcription regulator for some of the toxins. Although environmental factors have not been identified, α-toxin is upregulated in wounds; evidence from animal studies suggests that α-toxin production, the major factor thought to account for virulence and mortality in humans, is decreased when hyperbaric oxygen is utilized.

Etiology

The clinical presentation of patients with gas gangrene depends somewhat on the circumstances that contributed to the infection. Posttraumatic gas gangrene follows open fractures, generation of contaminated wounds, penetration by contaminated foreign bodies, crush injuries that damage nutrient blood supply, and frostbite. Injury precedes 60% of all cases of gas gangrene in nonmilitary series. Postsurgical wound infections that progress to gas gangrene often follow contamination by gastrointestinal or biliary contents and may be further encouraged by techniques of wound closure that produce ischemia within the tissues. Preceding intraabdominal infections may cause abscesses that burrow from intraperitoneal sites into adjacent soft tissues. Illicit drug injection may cause direct inoculation

TABLE 1: Common clostridial exotoxins

Exotoxin	Lethality*	Functions
Alpha (α)	+	Lecithinase, necrotizing, hemolytic, cardiotoxic
Beta (β)	+	Necrotizing
Epsilon (ε)	+	Permease
Iota (ι)	+	Necrotizing
Delta (δ)	+	Hemolysin
Phi (φ)		Hemolysin, cytolysin
Kappa (κ)	+	Collagenase, gelatinase, necrotizing
Lambda (λ)		Protease
Mu (μ)		Hyaluronidase
Nu (ν)	+	Deoxyribonuclease, hemolytic, necrotizing

*Tested by injection into mice.

TABLE 2: Distribution of lethal exotoxins in biotypes of *Clostridium perfringens*

Type	Alpha (α)	Beta (β)	Epsilon (ε)	Iota (ι)
A	+	–	–	–
B	+	+	+	–
C	+	+	–	–
D	+	–	+	–
E	+	–	–	+

of deep soft-tissue compartments and often occurs with a paucity of physical findings on the skin. Less commonly, therapeutic injections of vasoconstrictive medications have preceded cases of gas gangrene. Uterine gas gangrene is a well-described complication of nonmedical "back alley" abortions.

C. septicum associated with spontaneous gas gangrene is recognized in patients with advanced malignancy, diabetes, and immunosuppression. It carries a mortality of 60%, twice that of *C. perfringens*. The α-toxin of *C. septicum* acts as a hemolysin in a manner not dissimilar to that of *C. perfringens* by attaching to glycophosphatidylinositol-anchored membrane proteins. Patients with *C. septicum* infections have overt or occult malignancies approximately five times more often than patients with other clostridial infections. In a large series of nontraumatic *C. septicum* myonecrosis, malignant tumors were identified in 92% of patients; of these, 58% had colonic adenocarcinomas. Children receiving chemotherapy are also found with these infections. In children, neutropenia, either induced by chemotherapy or cyclic in nature, represents the single most important risk factor for spontaneous *C. septicum* infections. The remaining cases are associated with diabetes or neutropenic colitis. In many cases, no predisposing condition can be found. Although *C. perfringens* and *C. septicum* infections are commonly reported, *C. septicum* infection predominates.

CLINICAL PRESENTATION

Early symptoms of localized pain, characteristically severe and disproportionate to physical findings, should prompt immediate concern. With extremity infections, alert patients report heaviness within the limb. As infections spread, the zone of pain widens, and patients begin to experience systemic effects of the exotoxins. Lethargy, apathy, and depression from a sense of impending doom may occur.

Physical examination is notable for tachycardia that is often quite severe yet accompanied by only low-grade fever. Less than 5% of patients will have positive blood cultures, so chills and rigors are not common. Overlying the painful regions, the skin takes on a brawny character and progresses with patches of blue-black mottling, and hemorrhagic bullas begin to appear. Rapid progression of localized edema can follow. With extremities, marked disparity in circumference is observed. If open wounds are present, a sweet, mousy smell is apparent in some cases, but others have no odor. As gas accumulates, crepitus is sometimes present, however, brawny edema may make crepitus difficult to detect. Range of motion is severely restricted, and excruciating pain can be experienced with passive motion. Later systemic findings include hypotension, dehydration, oliguria indicating onset of renal failure, and paradoxical agitation and sharpening of mental acuity.

Illicit Parenteral Drug Injections

Injection drug use presents a formidable and growing problem for urban hospitals and contributes significantly to the problem of gas gangrene. Direct deposit of organisms into deep spaces with needles can bypass superficial layers and promote gas gangrene. Such infections are physically silent for a considerable period, until gas in the tissues or severe pain with passive motion becomes evident. These infections are most common in the deltoid, hip, and buttocks, preferred sites for self-injection that are concealed by clothing. Infections often occur in clusters of individuals, because illicit drug use is common among those who share paraphernalia for injection.

Some illicit preparations contain additive substances commonly used to "cut" or expand the quantity of the illicit material. This material may serve as an adjuvant promoter of infection. The use of heat to prepare material for injection can pyrolyze certain added chemicals and create nasty deposits of foreign-body material. So-called *black tar heroin* is associated with more serious infections. Clinical signs of pain and physical signs of hypovolemia can be altered by the illicit drugs themselves; opioids can blunt the painful nature of some infections or induce euphoria and altered perceptions of the need for intervention, which can cause an individual to delay seeking appropriate treatment. Concurrent use of sympathomimetic stimulants, such as methamphetamine or cocaine, can produce tachycardia and vasoconstriction, thereby altering the hemodynamic status or the physical findings on admission.

LABORATORY FINDINGS

Gram stain of the exudate or infected tissues reveals large grampositive bacilli without neutrophils. Alternatively, frozen-section microscopic examination by a trained pathologist is also reliable for diagnosis of gas gangrene. However, availability of pathology personnel should not delay the surgical debridement process.

Presentation with hemolytic anemia and increased lactate dehydrogenase levels is common in patients with gas gangrene. Disseminated intravascular coagulation is displayed by altered prothrombin time, low serum fibrinogen, and evidence of fibrin split products. With gas gangrene, despite serious infection, white blood cell counts may not show leukocytosis. Leukocytosis is more common in patients with toxic shock syndrome resulting from *C. sordellii* or *C. septicum*, wherein the red blood cell count may show hemoconcentration and extreme leukocytosis.

The use of specific laboratory parameters to help identify the presence of gas gangrene has not been reported, however, studies have been done of laboratory predictors of NTSIs in general. The chemistry profile may show significant metabolic abnormalities frequently associated with tissue injuries and hypotension, such as metabolic acidosis and renal failure. Efforts to identify quantitative measures that correlate with presence of infection were first introduced by Wall and colleagues. They reported that an admission white blood cell count above 14×10^9/L, serum sodium below 135 mEq/L, and blood urea nitrogen above 15 mg/dL identified patients more likely to have necrotizing infections.

A more elaborate analysis has popularized the Laboratory Risk Indicator for Necrotizing Fasciitis (LRINEC) score to identify patients at risk for necrotizing infections. It assigns weighted integer scores based on admission threshold values of C-reactive protein, leukocyte count, hemoglobin, sodium, creatinine, and glucose, the sum of which correlates with the presence of infection. The use of such laboratory data is supportive but by no means specific for gas gangrene.

Radiology

The use of radiologic techniques for diagnosis of NTSI has been reported and can provide adjunctive information regarding the extent of tissue involvement. Plain radiography is probably the most useful and rapidly obtainable study available for examination of gas gangrene. The presence of gas within tissues is highly predictive of gas gangrene, and in cases where physical findings are absent or equivocal, plain radiographic examination should always be obtained.

Computed tomography, magnetic resonance imaging, and ultrasound all provide specific information regarding the presence of edema and thickening of fascial layers, sometimes with enhancement. Such findings lend support to clinical impressions obtained from physical examination. Although these studies can be sensitive, they lack any greater specificity than the physical exam. Information regarding the spread of infection may be helpful in planning the positioning for surgical debridement. This is especially important in cases of perineal truncal gangrene, in which anterior and posterior extension can occur. However, delay of surgical debridement in a critically ill patient for a radiologic study should never occur.

MEDICAL MANAGEMENT AND CRITICAL CARE

Gas gangrene follows a typical pattern of localized tissue destruction followed by systemic derangement largely from the production of exotoxins, heralded clinically by septic shock, progressive organ failure, and death. Surgical debridement is often conducted hastily to prevent progression of the infection locally, and debridement constitutes a secondary traumatic insult to the system. Applying the concept of a two-hit theory of multiorgan injury, it is possible that the infection is the priming event, and the debridement is the secondary event. Therefore, treatment of early sepsis is an important initial step that may improve tolerance to the surgical debridement. This approach demands aggressive monitoring and treatment without delaying surgical therapy. It may be reasonable to consider 1 to 2 hours of medical therapy, considering that most patients will display a much greater interval of time from inoculation to arrival in the hospital. Studies that examine delay to surgical debridement are generally based on consideration of the interval from hospital arrival to surgery, and not on the longer interval of time from inoculation to surgery.

Following identification of patients suspected of gas gangrene infection, it is helpful to admit them to the intensive care unit for full assessment of their medical status prior to proceeding to the operating room. Taking an underresuscitated patient directly from the emergency room to the operating room can worsen the secondary insult. Initial resuscitation should include assessment of arterial blood gases, a coagulation profile, and some estimation of volume status with either central venous monitoring or echocardiography. Acidosis should be treated, and coagulation deficits should be corrected.

Attention to volume reconstitution should be addressed with goal-directed therapy. Systemic hypotension and sepsis can progress rapidly. Patients with gas gangrene may occasionally seek treatment in early, uncompensated septic shock, making the diagnosis of a local process even more difficult. In obtunded patients lacking clinically overt physical findings, diagnosis is often delayed. The use of adrenergic pressors is potentially deleterious and should only be employed in severe refractory shock. The use of vasoconstrictors should be avoided, as redistribution of blood flow could deprive the peripheral soft tissues injured by infection from achieving adequate perfusion and thereby enhance the spread of infection. Evidence from studies of host-bacterial interactions indicates that sympathomimetic agents are potential signals that may induce bacterial proliferation by indicating to pathogens that the host is in a more vulnerable, stressed state.

Patients with gas gangrene frequently have end-organ failure and other concomitant serious medical conditions that require intensive supportive care. More advanced infections that display systemic sequelae and septic shock prior to surgical debridement are at the highest risk for mortality. Patients become hypovolemic from overwhelming systemic microvascular extravasation and progressive acidosis; oliguria and escalating hypoxemia are followed by a status that is refractory to adrenergic support. This is a critically dangerous progression that can limit further operative debridement, and supportive care is the only option available. Onset of rapidly progressive septic shock following surgical debridement is not uncommon, with early death within 24 to 36 hours of presentation.

Antibiotic Therapy

The institution of antibiotics should be started before the patient arrives in the operating room, and these should be continued throughout the course. Initially, broad-spectrum antibiotic coverage is desirable, until positive identification of pathogens can be made. Early identification of organisms is sometimes possible from Gram stain of aspirates, swabs obtained from open wounds, or tissue obtained at debridement. This can help narrow the spectrum of antibiotic coverage long before positive culture results and sensitivity studies become available.

When initial Gram stain indicates clostridial infection, high-dose penicillin G (10 to 24 million U/day) is the drug of choice. It is a β-lactam antibiotic that interferes with synthesis of cell-wall mucopeptides during active multiplication, resulting in bactericidal activity against susceptible bacteria. It is now recognized that addition of clindamycin (15 mg/kg IV every 8 hours in adults and 10 mg/kg IV every 8 hours in children) is helpful, because this agent inhibits protein synthesis, possibly by blocking dissociation of peptidyl t-RNA from ribosomes. Although clindamycin is directly effective for eradication of anaerobic *Streptococcus* species, but not *Enterococcus*, when utilized in gas gangrene, clindamycin can blunt the production of exotoxins.

A recent murine study of gas gangrene demonstrated markedly improved survival with clindamycin, metronidazole, and rifampin compared with penicillin G. Alternatively, chloramphenicol (10 to 15 mg IV every 6 hours) and tetracycline (1 g IV every 12 hours) have the same potential effect but are used less frequently because of potential bone marrow toxicity with chloramphenicol and blunting of penicillin effectiveness with tetracycline. In the event of penicillin allergy, clindamycin and metronidazole (7.5 mg/kg IV every 6 hours or 15 mg/kg IV every 12 hours) are a good alternative. For nonspeciated gas gangrene, addition of gram-negative enteric coverage is certainly indicated.

Adjuvant Therapy

Specific adjuvant therapy for severe sepsis has been evaluated following introduction of recombinant human activated protein C (drotrecogin alfa activated) into the clinical arena. It is intended and approved for patients with severe sepsis who score 25 or more on the Acute Physiology and Chronic Health Evaluation (APACHE II). Use in patients with NTSI has not been rigorously evaluated. Conclusions regarding the use of drotrecogin alfa activated in surgical patients can only be derived from subset analysis of data obtained from two larger trials, Recombinant Human Activated Protein C Worldwide Evaluation in Severe Sepsis (PROWESS) and Administration of Drotrecogin Alfa (Activated) in Early Stage Severe Sepsis (ADDRESS). Comparing the specific group of patients who had both single-organ dysfunction and had undergone surgery within 30 days prior to treatment with drotrecogin alfa activated, the observed mortality rate was higher for the treatment group than for the control group. Consequently, this therapy is not recommended for treatment of gas gangrene. Further studies that specifically evaluate drotrecogin alfa activated in patients with gas gangrene could be designed with careful monitoring and control of tissue hemorrhage, along with a protocol for alternative rates of drug administration that would not interfere with periodic wound inspection and debridement.

Hyperbaric Oxygen

With the development of modern chambers and more widespread implementation of hyperbaric oxygen (HBO) therapy, application to patients with gas gangrene has become more common. Proponents of hyperbaric oxygen point to the advantages of hyperoxia, including improved phagocytosis of leukocytes, eradication of anaerobes, reduction of tissue edema, stimulation of fibroblast growth, and increased collagen formation.

Human studies, most reporting retrospective series, often suggest improved outcomes when HBO is added to antibiotics and surgery. Evidence-based support is lacking, however, and at best a multicenter retrospective review failed to demonstrate a survival advantage for treatment of truncal infections. Gas gangrene is relatively rare, and so the possibility of obtaining a randomized trial to examine its efficacy is unlikely. Its use is supported by a combination of largely uncontrolled clinical series and more carefully controlled animal studies. Table 3 displays results from a number of series for comparison.

HBO appears to have a direct bactericidal effect on clostridial species by inhibiting the production of the α-toxin. Oxygen in concentrations of two and one half to three times absolute atmospheres is typically administered for 90 to 120 minutes in divided treatments three times per day for 48 hours. Complications in general are related to barotraumas (otitis and pneumothorax) and oxygen toxicity (myopia and seizures). Since advanced infections can be lethal, and the risks are minimal, the adjunctive use of HBO is certainly indicated. Controlled studies are difficult to perform because of the relative paucity of cases overall, and evidence-based recommendations are not likely to emerge. One noted advantage of hyperbaric oxygen use is direct visual enhancement of the demarcated zones of necrosis, allowing for more accurate debridement. However, delay of initial debridement for application of HBO is felt by most clinicians to be unwise, and thus the enhancement effect has limited utility.

SURGICAL TREATMENT

Treatment strategies for gas gangrene have focused on surgical debridement as the mainstay of therapy. Medical therapy is far less effective, because the areas of tissue necrosis are poorly perfused

TABLE 3: Effect of hyperbaric oxygen treatment on survival of patients with necrotizing soft tissue infections

Study	N	HBO Treatment: No. Survived (%)	No HBO Treatment: No. Survived (%)
Gibson et al. (1986)	46	20/29 (69)	5/17 (29)
Riseman et al. (1990)	29	13/17 (77)	4/12 (33)
Brown et al. (1994)	54	21/30 (70)	14/24 (58)
Shupak et al. (1995)	37	16/25 (64)	9/12 (75)
Hollabaugh et al. (1998)	26	13/14 (93)	7/12 (58)
Wilkinson et al. (2004)	33	31/33 (94)	7/11 (64)
Summary	225	114/148 (77)	46/88 (53)

secondary to vascular thrombosis, and antibiotic penetration is poor. The aggressive progression of these infections has led to the mandate for prompt radical surgery, avoidance of delay, and the institution of early postoperative reexamination and continued debridement. The rates of extremity amputation for gas gangrene are high.

Operating rooms should be warmed to avoid hypothermia; maintenance of adequate oxygenation should be deployed with ventilators capable of delivering positive end-expiratory pressure. Fluid and ventilatory gas warmers can be used to protect the patient from hypothermia. Surgery can be therapeutic, as well as diagnostic, because early clinical differentiation of the entities encompassing NTSI can be difficult. Gram stain of affected tissues can be utilized for early diagnosis and institution of appropriate antimicrobial therapy. Debridement is performed radically to the level of viable tissue. If functionality is potentially impaired after extremity debridement, amputation may be the best alternative.

During operative debridement, necrosis is easily identified by the lack of normal bleeding from involved tissues and by fascial planes that separate easily with little resistance. Wide exposure is mandatory to allow for adequate examination of deeper tissues. Involved muscles often display overt edema, and if muscle relaxants are avoided, these tissues fail to respond to stimulation by electrocautery. Complete removal of nonviable tissue is mandatory. Superficial tissue and skin may not be initially gangrenous but are likely to become subsequently gangrenous as a result of interruption of their perforating blood supply with deeper tissue debridement. Because retained broken needles are common with illicit drug users, blunt digital dissection of tissues should be avoided. In general, wide-open wounds are preferred to avoid creation of anaerobic pockets that might encourage return of infection. Gram stain by slide touch preparation or frozen-section biopsy of the debrided tissue can be employed to confirm that margins are free of infection. Tissue and fluid samples should be submitted for culture of aerobic, anaerobic, and fungal organisms to assist in the refinement of antibiotic regimens. Some organisms are extremely sensitive to oxygen and temperature changes ex vivo; therefore rapid

delivery to the laboratory for initial processing assures the greatest chance for obtaining accurate results.

Reconstruction

Reconstruction is a secondary consideration during the initial debridement phase. Patients should be scheduled for a repeat exploration with possible further debridement within 6 to 24 hours, depending on the acuity of the systemic response. In general, this should be conducted in the operating room under general anesthesia, as bedside examination is generally too painful for the patient and may not allow for adequate wound inspection. Tissues and fascia should be carefully inspected with particular attention to wound boundaries and overlying skin, because areas of NSTI can persist after an inadequate initial debridement or with disease progression. Amputation may be necessary if tissue destruction predicts a useless extremity, or if infection threatens spread to the torso.

Chronic wounds should be allowed to heal by secondary intention. Application of vacuum-assisted sponge dressings can be efficacious in promoting contraction and removal of bacteria and chronic exudates and may promote earlier granulation tissue formation. Most conditions respond to split-thickness skin grafting alone. Alternatively, myocutaneous rotational flaps and free-tissue flaps may be deployed to provide more durable coverage where a skin graft alone would be considered inadequate. Coverage of exposed bone, weight-bearing surfaces, and those areas at risk for pressure necrosis require more elaborate reconstructive approaches. Such approaches should not be undertaken before the patient has resolved the infection and recovered from any septic sequelae, as successful repair requires adequate nutritional status and freedom from nosocomial infection.

Mortality and Morbidity

The reported mortality rates vary widely, with a rate of 25% in most recent studies. The mortality rate approaches 100% in individuals with spontaneous gas gangrene and in those in whom treatment is delayed. Although age is not a prognostic factor in gas gangrene, advanced age and comorbid conditions are associated with a higher likelihood of mortality. Identification of factors that predict mortality have been evaluated in a number of larger series of patients with NTSIs.

Statistical analysis with logistic regression has allowed identification of factors that predict mortality from necrotizing infections. Several larger series have attempted to identify factors that can be measured on admission. The presence of three or more predisposing risk factors—diabetes, illicit drug injection, age over 50 years, malnutrition or obesity, and hypertension—contribute to mortality in excess of 50%. Anaya and colleagues (2005) found that death was significantly more likely in patients with an admission leukocyte count over $30,000 \times 10^3/\mu L$, creatinine concentrations greater than 2 mg/dL, or the presence of heart disease. Furthermore, the presence of clostridial infection was a predictor of both mortality and need for amputation but is less valuable as a prognostic indicator, because the finding is not discernable on admission. In comparing surgical and nonoperated patients, abnormalities of the coagulation system and arrival in shock had a strong correlation with mortality independent of the treatment.

Elliot and colleagues (1996) found by logistic regression analysis that risk factors for death included age, female gender, extent of infection, delay in first debridement, elevated serum creatinine concentrations, elevated blood lactate level, and degree of organ-system dysfunction at admission. Recently, cytokine profiles have been examined, and elevated levels of proinflammatory cytokines, particularly interleukin-1 receptor antagonists, correlated with death.

Suggested Readings

Abraham E, Laterre PF, Garg R, et al: Administration of Drotrecogin Alfa (Activated) in Early Stage Severe Sepsis (ADDRESS) Study Group: Drotrecogin alfa (activated) for adults with severe sepsis and a low risk of death, *N Engl J Med* 353(13):1332–1341, 2005.

Anaya DA, McMahon K, Nathens AB, et al: Predictors of mortality and limb loss in necrotizing soft tissue infections, *Arch Surg* 140:151–157, 2005.

Bangsberg DR, Rosen JI, Aragon T, et al: Clostridial myonecrosis cluster among injection drug users: a molecular epidemiology investigation, *Arch Intern Med* 162:517–522, 2002.

Ba-Thein W, Lyristis M, Ohtani K, et al: The virR/virS locus regulates the transcription of genes encoding extracellular toxin production in, *Clostridium perfringens, J Bacteriol* 178:2514–2520, 1996.

Bentley S, Holden M, Thompson N, Parkhill J: Armed to the teeth, *Trends Microbiol* 10:163–164, 2002.

Bernard GR, Vincent JL, Laterre PF, et al: Efficacy and safety of recombinant human activated protein C for severe sepsis, *N Engl J Med* 344(10):699–709, 2001.

Bosshardt TL, Henderson VJ, Organ CH: Necrotizing soft-tissue infections, *Arch Surg* 131:846–854, 1996.

Brown PW, Kinman PB: Gas gangrene in a metropolitan community, *J Bone Joint Surg* 56(7):1445–1451, 1974.

Brown DR, Davis NL, Lepawsky M, et al: A multicenter review of the treatment of major truncal necrotizing infections with and without hyperbaric oxygen therapy, *Am J Surg* 167:485–489, 1996.

Callahan TE, Schecter WP, Horn JK: Necrotizing soft tissue infection masquerading as cutaneous abscess following illicit drug injection, *Arch Surg* 133:812–818, 1998.

De A, Varaiya A, Mathur M, Bhesania A: Bacteriological studies of gas gangrene and related infections, *Indian J Med Microbiol* 21(3):202–204, 2003.

Dellinger RP, Carlet JM, Masur H, et al: Surviving Sepsis Campaign guidelines for management of severe sepsis and septic shock, *Crit Care Med* 32(3):858–873, 2004.

Elliott D, Kufera JA, Myers R: Necrotizing soft tissue infections, *Ann Surg* 224:672–683, 1996.

Francis KR, Lamaute HR, Davis JM, Pizzi W: Implications of risk factors in necrotizing fasciitis, *Am Surg* 59:304–308, 1993.

Gibson A, Davis FM: Hyperbaric oxygen therapy in the management of Clostridium perfringens infections, *NZ Med J* 99:617–620, 1986.

Giuliano A, Lewis F, Hadley K, et al: Bacteriology of necrotizing fasciitis, *Am J Surg* 134:52–57, 1977.

Green RJ, Dafoe DC, Raffin TA: Necrotizing fasciitis, *Chest* 110:219–229, 1996.

Hart GB, Lamb RC, Strauss MB: Gas gangrene, *J Trauma* 23(11):991–1000, 1983.

Hollabaugh RS Jr, Dmochowski RR, Hickerson WL, et al: Fournier's gangrene: therapeutic impact of hyperbaric oxygen, *Plast Reconstr Surg* 101(1):94–100, 1998.

Hsiao GH, Chang CH, Hsiao CW, et al: Necrotizing soft tissue infections: surgical or conservative treatment? *Dermatol Surg* 24:243–247, 1998.

Larson CM, Bubrick MP, Jacobs DM, et al: Malignancy, mortality, and medicosurgical management of Clostridium septicum infection, *Surgery* 118(4):592–597, 1995.

Lungstras-Bufler K, Bufler P, Abdullah R, et al: High cytokine levels at admission are associated with fatal outcome in patients with necrotizing fasciitis, *Eur Cytokine Netw* 15:135–138, 2004.

Lyristis M, Bryant AE, Sloan J, et al: Identification and molecular analysis of a locus that regulates extracellular toxin production in Clostridium perfringens, *Mol Microbiol* 12:761–777, 1994.

Majeski J, Majeski E: Necrotizing fasciitis: improved survival with early recognition by tissue biopsy and aggressive surgical treatment, *South Med J* 90:1065–1068, 1977.

McGuigan CC, Penrice GM, Gruer L, et al: Lethal outbreak of infection with Clostridium novyi type A and other spore-forming organisms in Scottish injecting drug users, *J Med Microbiol* 51(11):971–977, 2002.

McNee JW, Dunn JS: The method of spread of gas gangrene into living muscle, *Br Med J* 1:727–729, 1917.

Nichols RL, Smith JW: Anaerobes from a surgical perspective, *Clin Infect Dis* 1918(Suppl 4):S280–S286, 1994.

Patrick DA, Moore FA, Moore EE, et al: Neutrophil priming and activation in the pathogenesis of postinjury multiple organ failure, *New Horiz* 4(2):194–210, 1996.

Riseman JA, Zamboni WA, Curtis A, et al: Hyperbaric oxygen therapy for necrotizing fasciitis reduces mortality and the need for debridements, *Surgery* 108:847–850, 1990.

Shimizu T, Ohtani K, Hirakawa H, et al: Genome sequence of Clostridium perfringens, an aerobic flesh-eater, *Proc Natl Acad Sci USA* 99:996–1001, 2002.

Shupak A, Shoshani O, Goldenberg I, et al: Necrotizing fasciitis: an indication for hyperbaric oxygen therapy? *Surgery* 118, 873-838: 1995.

Sperandio V, Torres AG, Jarvis B, et al: Bacteria-host communications: the language of hormones, *Proc Natl Acad Sci* 100(15):8951–8956, 2003.

Stamenkovic I, Lew PD: Early recognition of potentially fatal necrotizing fasciitis: the use of frozen-section biopsy, *N Engl J Med* 310:1689–1693, 1984.

Stevens DL, Bisno AL, Chambers HF, et al: Practice guidelines for the diagnosis and management of skin and soft-tissue infections, *Clin Infect Dis* 41(10):1373–1406, 2005.

Stevens DL, Bryant AE, Adams K, Mader JT: Evaluation of therapy with hyperbaric oxygen for experimental infection with Clostridium perfringens, *Clin Infect Dis* 17(2):231–237, 1993.

Stevens DL, Maier KA, Laine BM, Mitten JE: Comparison of clindamycin, rifampin, tetracycline, metronidazole, and penicillin for efficacy in prevention of experimental gas gangrene due to Clostridium perfringens, *J Infect Dis* 155(2):220–228, 1987.

Stevens DL, Maier KA, Mitten JE: Effect of antibiotics on toxin production and viability of Clostridium perfringens, *Antimicrob Agents Chemother* 31(2):213–218, 1987.

Stevens DL, Musher DM, Watson DA, et al: Spontaneous, nontraumatic gangrene due to Clostridium septicum, *Rev Infect Dis* 12(2):286–296, 1990.

Struk DW, Munk PL, Lee MJ, et al: Imaging of soft tissue infections, *Radiol Clin North Am* 39:277–303, 2001.

Tibbles PM, Edelsberg JS: Hyperbaric oxygen therapy, *N Engl J Med* 334(25):1642–1648, 1996.

Titball RW: Gas gangrene: an open and closed case, *Microbiology* 151:2821–2828, 2005.

Wall DB, De Virgilio C, Black S, Klein SR: Objective criteria may assist in distinguishing necrotizing fasciitis from nonnecrotizing soft tissue infection, *Am J Surg* 179:17–21, 2000.

Weed T, Ratliff C, Drake DB: Quantifying bacterial bioburden during negative pressure wound therapy: does the wound VAC enhance bacterial clearance? *Ann Plast Surg* 52:276–279, 2004.

Wilkinson D, Doolette D: Hyperbaric oxygen treatment and survival from necrotizing soft tissue infection, *Arch Surg* 139:1339–1345, 2004.

Wong CH, Khin LW, Heng KS, et al: The LRINEC (Laboratory Risk Indicator for Necrotizing Fasciitis) score: a tool for distinguishing necrotizing fasciitis from other soft tissue infections,, *Crit Care Med* 32:1535–1541, 2004.

Necrotizing Skin and Soft Tissue Infection

Eileen M. Bulger, MD

OVERVIEW

Necrotizing skin infections and necrotizing soft tissue infections (NSTIs) are the most severe form of bacterial infection in the soft tissues, and they represent a wide spectrum of disease. Common acronyms that have been applied to this disease process include *necrotizing fasciitis, Fournier gangrene, clostridial myonecrosis, gas gangrene, Meleney ulcers,* and *"flesh eating" infections.* What all these have in common is aggressive bacterial infection of the deep spaces of the soft tissue and/or muscle that result in tissue necrosis, which can be rapidly progressive and highly lethal. The blood supply to the fascia and subcutaneous fat is more tenuous than the skin or underlying muscle and is thus more vulnerable to an infectious process. Bacteria invade the soft tissues and track along either the superficial or deep fascial planes. The combination of the invading organisms and the infiltration of polymorphonuclear cells can lead to microvascular thrombosis, which results in tissue ischemia and necrosis. Some organisms, such as *Clostridium perfringens,* also produce toxins that can cause necrosis of otherwise well-perfused tissue, such as muscle. The average mortality for NSTI in recently published series is 22%, but this varies based on the patient population. The severity and progression of the disease depends largely on the site of infection, the medical comorbidities of the host, and the pathogenic organisms involved.

DIAGNOSIS

Because these infections can spread rapidly in the deep tissues, skin findings may be minimal, and there is frequently a delay in the diagnosis of NSTI. Several studies have associated a delay in diagnosis and treatment of NSTI of greater than 12 hours with increased mortality. Thus, it is paramount that clinicians maintain a high index of suspicion for this disease process, especially in high-risk populations. Patients at increased risk for the development of NSTI include those with a history of injection drug use, deep penetrating injuries, morbid obesity, diabetes mellitus, peripheral vascular disease, and immunosuppression. Common infections and sites involved include perineal or perianal infections, perirectal abscesses, foot or lower extremity ulcerations, penetrating wounds, bite wounds, injection drug sites, postsurgical wounds, pressure ulcers, and gastrointestinal pathology with perforation. In up to 10% of cases, however, there is no identifiable portal of entry for these organisms.

Clinical signs and symptoms include pain out of proportion to the physical exam, induration and edema with or without erythema, skin blistering or sloughing, patches of skin necrosis showing a blue-black discoloration, crepitus, and thin gray drainage from the wound (Figures 1 to 3). Plain radiographs may reveal evidence of gas in the soft tissues, but the absence of this finding does not rule out the disease. Evidence of systemic sepsis including tachycardia, hypotension, low urinary output, and high fluid requirements are generally late signs that suggest advanced disease. NSTI should also be considered in patients with soft tissue infections that continue to progress despite antibiotic therapy. Several authors have focused on the utility of basic laboratory studies to raise concern for NSTI in the setting of a soft-tissue infection. These include leukocytosis or leukopenia,

hyponatremia, and evidence of early renal insufficiency that includes elevated blood urea nitrogen or creatinine. Very high white blood cell counts have been associated with severe clostridial infections. In one study, a presenting white blood cell counts over 40,000 carried a 50% predicted mortality rate.

The diagnosis of NSTI should depend on the clinical presentation combined with the initial laboratory studies. Additional imaging with computed tomography or magnetic resonance imaging may be helpful in identifying deep abscesses in equivocal cases but should not delay operative exploration when there is high suspicion. In most cases these studies will merely show fat stranding in the subcutaneous tissue, which is nonspecific for infection. Tissue biopsies and frozen-section analysis has been described, but they are likely to delay surgical exploration and may not be definitive. When in doubt, the best course of action is to proceed to the operating room for exploration. The surgical incision should extend down to the deep muscle fascia with inspection of all tissue layers for necrotic tissue, and the wound should be probed to identify any tracking in the fascial planes. If necrotic tissue is encountered, the diagnosis is confirmed, and debridement can be initiated.

MICROBIOLOGY

To select appropriate antibiotic treatment strategies, it is important to understand the variety of pathogens involved in these infections. Most NSTIs are polymicrobial with an average of 4.4 organisms isolated per infection. These polymicrobial infections can cause significant local tissue necrosis but tend to be more indolent and carry a lower mortality than infections caused by a limited number of highly virulent pathogens, such as *Streptococcus pyogenes* (group A β-hemolytic *Streptococcus*), *Clostridium* species, and community-acquired methicillin-resistant *Staphylococcus aureus* (MRSA). Due to the unique nature of these infections, each will be individually addressed.

Polymicrobial Infections

Polymicrobial infections are commonly seen in the setting of perineal and perirectal infections, chronic diabetic ulcerations, pressor ulcers, and surgical-site infections. Organisms involved include both

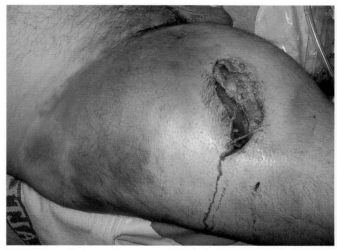

FIGURE 1   Patient with a penetrating thigh wound who developed skin discoloration and induration representing a severe underlying NSTI.

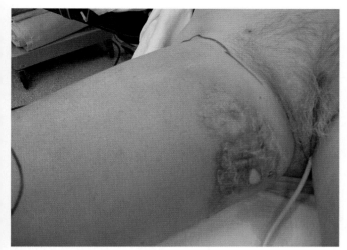

FIGURE 2 Patient with skin blistering and necrosis of the medial right thigh, representing an underlying NSTI.

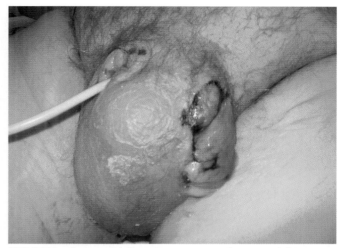

FIGURE 3 Patient with Fournier gangrene and an area of skin necrosis on the scrotum.

gram-positive and gram-negative organisms, which may be either aerobic or anaerobic. Infections arising from colonic pathology will involve the organisms frequently associated with peritonitis. Chronic wounds and surgical-site infections may involve highly resistant organisms as a result of hospital exposure (nosocomial infections) and prior antibiotic therapy. Bite wounds are also typically polymicrobial and may include two relatively unique pathogens: *Pasturella* species and *Capnocytophaga canimorsus*. In human bite wounds, *Haemophilus* species and *Eikenella corrodens* are also common. Water-associated infections are also typically polymicrobial and include unique pathogens such as *Aeromonas* species, *Vibrio* species, and *Micobacterium marinum*.

Group A β-Hemolytic Streptococcus

Group A β-hemolytic *Streptococcus* can produce a rapidly aggressive NSTI with systemic toxicity and high mortality rates. These organisms produce virulence factors and exotoxins, which contribute to the severity of disease. Such toxins allow the infection to spread rapidly through otherwise healthy tissue and induce shock and organ failure in the host.

Clostridial Infections

Among the clostridial species, *Clostridum perfringens* is the most common cause of NSTI. Other species have been reported, especially in patients with a history of injection drug use, and *C. septicum* has been reported in NSTI associated with gastrointestinal neoplasms. Under ideal conditions, *C. perfringens* has a germination time of only 8 minutes and produces potent extracellular toxins, including α-toxin (phospholipase C) and θ-toxin (perfringolysin). In addition to direct tissue injury, these toxins impede neutrophil migration and lead to hemolysis and microvascular thrombosis. As a result, clostridial infections can cause extensive necrosis of previously healthy muscle. In addition, α-toxin has also been shown to be a direct inhibitor of myocardial contractility, which can lead to rapid circulatory collapse. These infections are classically associated with traumatic puncture wounds, but in recent years, they have been seen most commonly in the injection drug use population.

Community-Acquired Methicillin-Resistant Staphylococcus Aureus

MRSA has traditionally been associated with nosocomial infections and prior antibiotic exposure, but recently the epidemiology of community-acquired *Staphylococcus aureus* infections has shifted to a predominance of MRSA in the general population. A recent Centers for Disease Control and Prevention (CDC) report indicated that 60% of community isolates of *S. aureus* are now methicillin resistant. Community-acquired MRSA (CA-MRSA) outbreaks have been reported in several populations including contact sports teams, prisoners, military recruits, injection drug users, institutional residents, and those who attend day care centers. CA-MRSA is seen primarily in skin and soft-tissue infections that result from a mutation in the Panton-Valentine leukocidin gene, and these organisms can now produce toxins that lead to direct tissue invasion and thus have resulted in cases of NSTI.

TREATMENT

Surgical Debridement

The cornerstone of treatment for NSTI is rapid and aggressive surgical debridement of all necrotic tissue. In some cases this may require emergent amputation of an extensive extremity infection. The extent of debridement will depend on the findings at the time of surgery. The fascial planes should be explored, because the ability to separate the fascia easily from its surrounding tissues suggests tracking of infection. In some critically ill patients with extensive edema, this can be difficult to distinguish. Debridement should be extended to include all frank necrosis and should ensure drainage of all fluid collections. The presence of normal bleeding at the edge of the wound, along with viable soft tissue and muscle, can guide the extent of debridement. Figures 4 to 6 illustrate typical surgical debridement.

Most authors recommend a scheduled return to the operating room within 24 hours for reexploration and further debridement as needed. Patients should continue to return to the operating room frequently, until there is no further progression of necrosis. The average number of operative procedures is three to four per patient. In those requiring extensive perineal debridement, subsequent diverting colostomy may be considered to facilitate wound management and healing. Cases of colonic perforation presenting as NSTI in the thigh compartments have been reported. In these cases, celiotomy is usually required to control the source of infection and for further debridement of the retroperitoneum.

Wounds should be managed by serial dressing changes, until the infection is clearly resolving with no further progression. At that point, negative-pressure therapy can be considered to facilitate wound healing. Application of negative-pressure therapy prior to resolution of the infection should be avoided, as it may result in

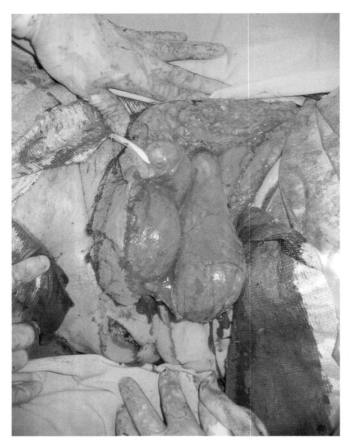

FIGURE 4 Typical wide debridement required for management of Fournier gangrene.

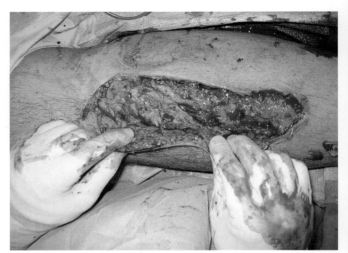

FIGURE 6 Fascial debridement of the thigh for NSTI.

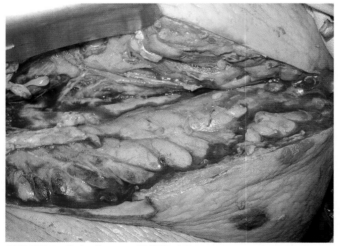

FIGURE 5 Debridement of NSTI of the pannus in a morbidly obese woman.

unrecognized progression of disease. A multidisciplinary team that includes a plastic surgeon can aid in ultimate reconstruction.

Antibiotic Therapy

Broad-spectrum antibiotics should be started empirically based on the suspected organisms involved. All wounds suspicious for NSTI should be cultured in the operating room to allow subsequent deescalation of antibiotic therapy if indicated. The choice of antibiotic coverage should be based on the anticipated microbiology of the wound, with consideration of the risk factors for antimicrobial resistance. In general, patients with polymicrobial infections require coverage for gram-positive, enteric gram-negative, and anaerobic organisms. Several agents can be used in this setting including imipenem-cilastatin, meropenem, piperacillin-tazobactam, ticarcillin-clavulanate, and tigecycline. Given the progressive emergence of CA-MRSA, additional coverage for this organism is recommended until sensitivities are known. The gold standard for MRSA is vancomycin, although a recent study suggests linezolid may be more effective. For patients with wounds suspicious for high-virulence organisms such as clostridial species, group A β-hemolytic *Streptococcus,* severe *Vibrio* and *Aeromonas* infections, and *Staphylococcus* species that produce the Panton-Valentine leukocidin (PVL) toxin, emerging data suggest that the use of protein synthesis–inhibiting agents such as clindamycin may be beneficial. These agents are thought to reduce toxin production in this setting. Thus the addition of high-dose clindamycin (1200 mg IV every 6 hours) has been recommended for these cases. Penicillin (24 million U/day) should also be added for suspected clostridial infection.

Adjuvant Therapies

A number of adjuvant therapies have been reported but with no definitive randomized controlled studies to support these options. It is important to remember that no adjuvant therapy that would delay or impair surgical debridement should be considered. Some options for adjuvant therapy include hyperbaric oxygen (HBO) therapy, intravenous immunoglobulin, and extracorporeal plasma exchange. HBO therapy has several theoretical advantages to limit progression of NSTI, but there are insufficient data to support its routine use, and the logistics of transporting critically ill patients and potential delays in surgical debridement limit its use in most cases. Intravenous immunoglobulin has been reported as an effective adjunct, especially in cases of staphylococcal toxic shock syndrome, in which binding of superantigens may reduce systemic toxicity. Whether this will be effective with other toxin-producing organisms is unknown, and data are insufficient to support routine use. Also, extracorporeal plasmaphersis and plasma exchange have been described for management of severe sepsis and in some cases for management of NSTI. Whether these therapies effectively reduce the toxin and inflammatory cytokine load is unknown, and further study is warranted in these areas.

SUMMARY

NSTIs are rare but devastating infections that carry a high morbidity and mortality. The key points to remember include the following:

- Skin findings may be subtle, and thus a high index of suspicion must be maintained, especially in high-risk populations.
- Diagnosis is based on clinical signs and symptoms combined with initial laboratory abnormalities. Gas in the soft tissues is not always present.
- When in doubt, proceed to surgery for exploration. Plan on scheduled returns to surgery for reexploration, until there is no more progression of infection.
- Delays in operative debridement have been associated with increased mortality.
- Broad-spectrum antibiotics should be initiated, including coverage for MRSA and protein synthesis inhibitors (e.g., clindamycin) when toxin-producing organisms are suspected.
- Adjuvant therapies can be considered but should not delay operative management.

SUGGESTED READINGS

Anaya DA, Dellinger EP: Necrotizing soft-tissue infection: diagnosis and management, *Clin Infect Dis* 44:705–710, 2007.

Anaya DA, McMahon K, Nathens AB, et al: Predictors of mortality and limb loss in necrotizing soft tissue infections, *Arch Surg* 140:151–157, 2005.

King MD, Humphrey BJ, Wang YF, et al: Emergence of community-acquired methicillin-resistant *Staphylococcus aureus* USA 300 clone as the predominant cause of skin and soft-tissue infections, *Ann Intern Med* 144: 309–317, 2006.

May AK, Stafford RE, Bulger EM, et al: Surgical Infection Society guidelines for the treatment of skin and soft tissue infections, *Surg Infections* 10(5):467–499, 2009.

Patel M: Community-acquired methicillin-resistant *Staphylococcus aureus* infections: epidemiology, recognition, and management, *Drugs* 69: 693–716, 2008.

Stevens DL, Bisno AL, Chambers HF, et al: Practice guidelines for the diagnosis and management of skin and soft-tissue infections, *Clin Infect Dis* 41:1373–1406, 2005.

MANAGEMENT OF ABDOMINAL WALL DEFECTS

Nelson H. Goldberg, MD, and Ronald P. Silverman, MD*

OVERVIEW

The abdominal wall functions as a multilayered structure that keeps us waterproofed on the outside and leak proof on the inside, as well as assisting with breathing, coughing, rotation and flexion of the trunk, posture, emesis, urination, and defecation. Defects of the abdominal wall can compromise these functions, cause pain, or lead to herniation of the viscera. The components of the abdominal wall include the skin and subcutaneous fat layer, fascia, muscle, and peritoneum. The loss of each component or combination of components requires specific techniques for reconstruction.

ABDOMINAL WALL DEFECTS

Skin and Subcutaneous Fat

The skin layer is of course important in retaining fluids, regulating temperature, and as a barrier to infection, and the fat layer underneath acts as insulation and allows the skin to glide over the muscles in the many different vectors that the trunk can move. Defects of the skin and fat layers can occur from burns, large cutaneous tumors (e.g., giant congenital nevi), sarcomas, avulsion-type traumatic injuries, and infections.

Reconstruction of skin and fat layer defects is relatively straightforward in that in most cases, a split-thickness skin graft will solve the problem. There is no issue with hernia in these patients, and there is a healthy, vascularized fascial layer beneath the defect that can easily support a skin graft. Skin grafts alone do have some disadvantages, such as contraction over time, causing contractures and compromising the skin's ability to glide over the fascia, which can restrict motion and cause pain. Furthermore, skin grafts are unattractive, and patients often feel that the appearance is unacceptable. Therefore, secondary procedures that occur later, such as serial excision or the use of tissue expanders under the adjacent skin, can be used to remove the skin grafts and replace them with normal-appearing skin and subcutaneous fat. These defects generally do not warrant the added donor site morbidity created when using more distant flaps from the back or thighs (Figure 1).

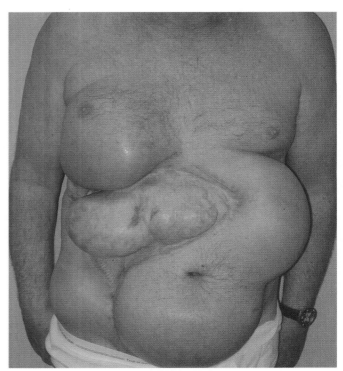

FIGURE 1 A 61-year-old male with a skin graft on bowel after developing necrotizing fasciitis following a cholecystectomy, shown here with tissue expanders in place.

*Dr. Ronald P. Silverman is Senior Vice President and Chief Medical Officer of KCI Corporation, San Antonio, Texas.

Fascia

Fascial defects are uncommon and usually occur when a subcutaneous tumor that is fixed to the fascia is being removed. Of course many incisional hernias are failures of the fascia to heal at the linea alba. Incisional hernias, however, ultimately show up as composite defects of both fascia and muscle, because the failure of healing at the linea alba results in unopposed action of the lateral muscles of the abdominal wall, which gradually shorten and pull the rectus muscles apart to create a progressively larger defect of both the fascia and rectus abdominis muscle in the midline.

True fascia-only defects that leave healthy muscle behind are generally not of significant consequence, because in most of the abdominal wall, fascial layers are redundant. These redundant layers include the anterior and posterior rectus fascia above the arcuate line and the three layers of fascia lateral to the rectus abdominis muscle, the external oblique, internal oblique, and transversus abdominis. Sometimes the underlying muscle can bulge through a small fascial defect, creating the appearance of a mass that may be bothersome to some patients, which is a reason to repair small fascia-only defects. One exception to this is when the anterior rectus sheath is resected below the arcuate line. Because there is no posterior rectus fascia below the arcuate line, located at a position approximately 2 cm superior to a horizontal line drawn between the two anterior superior iliac spines, an anterior rectus fascia defect in this area will ultimately result in a hernia and should be repaired.

Muscle

Muscle-only defects are also very rare, but defects of muscle and fascia are very common. The myofascial defect is the standard defect seen in routine incisional hernias, which generally are not a result of a true lack of tissue, but rather a shortening of the lateral muscle elements, as they pull in an unopposed fashion against the failed linea alba closure. The management of the standard incisional hernia was covered earlier in this section.

Peritoneum

The peritoneum is a flimsy layer of vascularized tissue that is inconsequential from a standpoint of biomechanical strength. The presence of peritoneum is only of concern when it is missing in combination with the myofascial layer, because it then allows some type of fascial replacement implant to be in contact with the bowel. Certain types of adhesiogenic prosthetic materials, such as polypropylene mesh, should generally not be placed in contact with the bowel out of concern for a robust inflammatory response, which can result in adhesions and, in a worst case scenario, enterocutaneous fistulas. Strategies to prevent this horrific complication include using omentum or muscle flaps to protect the bowel from the synthetic mesh. Our group tends to avoid the use of synthetic mesh altogether in this scenario and instead utilizes acellular dermal matrices, which can safely contact the bowel and tend to be resistant to adhesion formation.

COMPOSITE TISSUE DEFECTS OF THE ABDOMINAL WALL

Composite tissue defects of the abdominal wall present a major challenge to surgeons. Composite defects generally include a defect or inadequacy of both the skin and the myofascial layer. Examples include extreme cases of tissue loss such as in necrotizing fasciitis, which necessitates debridement of both the skin and the myofascial layer; blast wounds, such as from a shotgun; or large oncologic defects. More common composite abdominal defects include myofascial defects in combination with a cutaneous wound. Often the

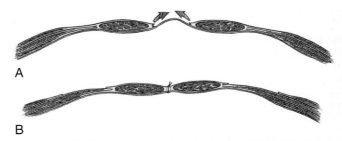

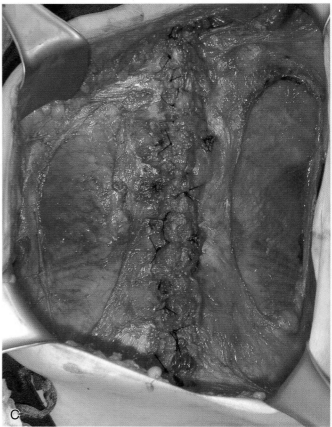

FIGURE 2 **A,** Schematic cross-sectional diagram of the abdominal wall musculature with a midline hernia. **B,** The two rectus abdominis muscles sutured together with the external oblique fascia having been divided laterally. **C,** An intraoperative photograph of a patient after component separation with the rectus abdominis muscles sutured together in the midline. (**A** and **B** *from Karp NS: Abdominal wall reconstruction. In McCarthy JG, Galiano RD, Boutros SG, editors: Current therapy in plastic surgery, Philadelphia, 2006, Saunders Elsevier.*)

wound is not large, but the presence of a contaminated or infected wound precludes the use of standard synthetic materials.

Closure of the Fascia

Simple primary repair of fascial defects is not recommended, even when possible, because of unacceptably high recurrence rates (Luijendijk, 2000), and the use of synthetic materials is also not recommended when there is inadequate skin coverage or contamination. Options for fascial closure in these complex defects include component separation, fascial grafts, flaps, tissue expansion, and biologic materials.

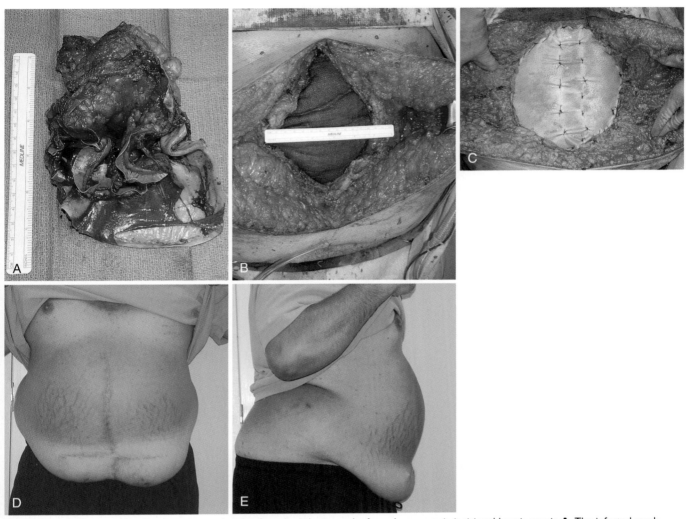

FIGURE 3   A 36-year-old male who presented with infected synthetic mesh after a laparoscopic incisional hernia repair. **A,** The infected mesh shown here was excised with the overlying contaminated tissue and sinus tract. **B,** Intraoperative photograph showing the hernia defect after removal of infected mesh. **C,** Intraoperative photograph showing Strattice (LifeCell Corporation, Branchburg, NJ) after primary closure obtained using component separation. **D,** A year later, no recurrence was seen. **E,** Lateral view.

Component Separation

The component separation technique takes advantage of the multiple myofascial layers in the lateral abdominal wall. First, any intraabdominal adhesions should be taken off the underside of the abdominal wall to prevent tethering of the fascia to the viscera. Next, undermining of the skin is performed. Wide undermining of the skin does allow some fascial advancement, but it is done at a cost: the further the undermining, the higher the risk of fat necrosis and even skin-edge necrosis. To allow for the external oblique incision, we often undermine only 1 or 2 cm beyond the rectus and no farther, unless more undermining is necessary to obtain skin closure. The external oblique fascia is then incised 1 cm lateral to the lateral edge of the rectus abdominis muscle for its entire vertical length. It is important to carry this incision all the way over the costal margin (at this level it is often necessary to divide the external oblique muscle fibers in addition to fascia) and several centimeters below the hernia, being careful not to violate the inguinal ligament.

Once the external oblique has been divided, the rectus abdominis myofascial complex can be advanced toward the midline (Figure 2). If this does not allow enough advancement, the external oblique can then be elevated off the internal oblique all the way to the anterior axillary line; and finally, for an additional 1 or 2 cm of advancement,

the posterior rectus sheath can be separated from the underside of the rectus abdominis muscle. Performing this technique bilaterally can achieve primary fascial closure in the vast majority of patients with midline fascial defects, about 85% of the cases in our group, by allowing 8 to 10 cm of advancement on each side at the level of the umbilicus.

Once primary fascial closure is achieved, it is important to strengthen the repair with an over or under layer, otherwise, the closure is simply a primary, edge-to-edge repair that carries an unacceptable recurrence rate. Many groups advocate placing an implant as an "underlay" intraperitoneally and then closing the fascia over top of the implant. In our group, we place an implant as on onlay, and we do so only when primary fascial closure has been achieved. The onlay spans all the way from the laterally released external oblique fascia, and it is pulled tight across the midline. The material is then quilted down to the abdominal wall with multiple sutures so as to obliterate the space between the implant and the fascia and to encourage vascular ingrowth (Figure 3). This technique allows reinforcement not only of the midline but also of the relatively weakened lateral areas, where the external oblique was divided. When primary fascial closure is not achieved, despite having done component separation, we place our implant as an underlay, tucking the implant 3 to 5 cm under the fascial edge and fixing it with transfascial sutures (Figure 4). In extreme cases, where the tissues are particulary weak and the patient is multiply recurrent, we have performed both an underlay and

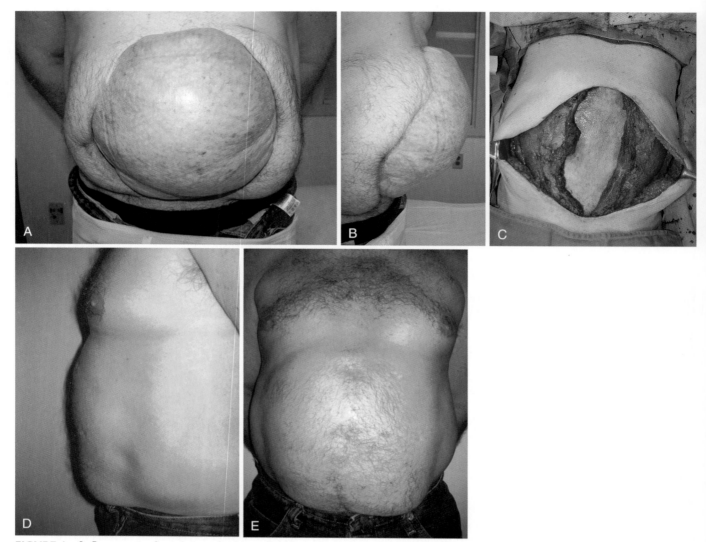

FIGURE 4   **A,** Preoperative frontal view of a skin graft on bowel in a 44-year-old male one year after a small bowel volvulus, managed with bowel resection and open abdomen with skin graft on the bowel. Note the tremendous loss of domain. **B,** Lateral preoperative view. **C,** Intraoperative view showing component separation with an underlay placement of Alloderm (LifeCell Corporation, Branchburg, NJ). The underlay technique was used in this case because primary fascial closure was not obtainable. **D,** Postoperative lateral view 18 months after the repair with no recurrence. **E,** Postoperative frontal view.

an overlay (also referred to as the "sandwich technique"), but whether this proves to be helpful has yet to be determined (Figure 5).

It should be noted that when dealing with trauma patients with acute loss of domain resulting from abdominal compartment syndrome, or in patients treated with damage-control laporatomies and left open, our group does not advocate the use of component separation during the initial hospital stay. Instead, maintenance of domain with the use of negative-pressure wound therapy combined with early, progressive primary fascial closure is preferred, potentially using a biologic material to bridge any fascial defect that cannot be closed during the first 2 weeks of the initial hospitalization and generally closing the skin. This leaves the component separation technique available as an option if needed in the future rather than burning this valuable bridge at a time when the patient is not likely optimized.

Implant Selection

The choice of an ideal implant material is complex, controversial, and still evolving. In general, our group avoids the use of synthetic material when there is active infection, lack of reliable skin coverage, bacterial

contamination (such as violation of the bowel wall during the procedure), or substantial comorbidities such as obesity, diabetes, smoking history, immunosuppression, radiation, chronic obstructive pulmonary disease, and malnutrition; these place the patient at an increased risk for infection or wound complications. In the rare situation that calls for the use of a synthetic material such as in a large sterile abdominal wall malignancy resection, we prefer polypropylene mesh for its excellent incorporation, provided an adequate barrier between the mesh and the bowel can be established; this barrier could be omentum or even peritoneum. If this is not possible, we prefer acellular dermal matrices to prevent bowel adhering to the synthetic mesh. In those cases in which we would avoid synthetic material but would still need a material for implantation, a few good options are still available. Fascia lata grafts, harvested from the thigh and sutured into the defect, were the mainstay in our group for many years for their reliability, ease of harvest, and ability to revascularize and therefore resist infection (Figure 6). Since good biologic materials have become commercially available, the use of the fascial graft has been limited so as to avoid any donor site morbidity. Our current preference is for acellular dermal matrix.

It is important to note that a number of acellular dermal matrices, as well as other types of biologic fascial replacement materials,

SKIN AND SOFT TISSUE

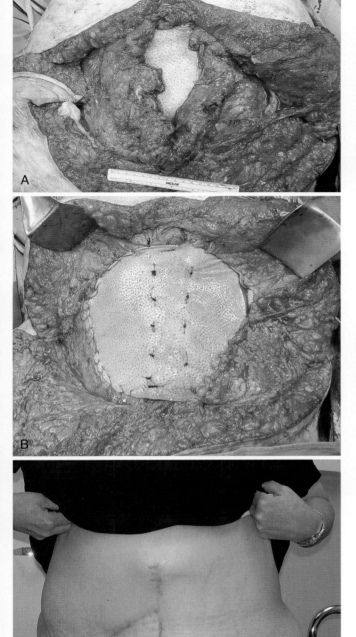

FIGURE 5 The "sandwich" technique in a 61-year-old female with a multiply recurrent incisional hernia. **A,** Intraoperative photograph showing the underlay with Alloderm (LifeCell Corporation, Branchburg, NJ). **B,** Intraoperative photograph showing the onlay with Strattice (LifeCell Corporation, Branchburg, NJ) after primary fascial closure was obtained. **C,** Appearance 1 year after surgery.

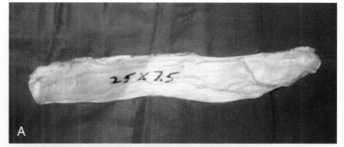

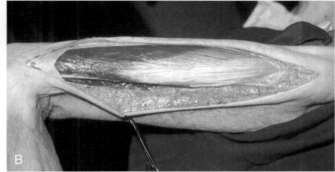

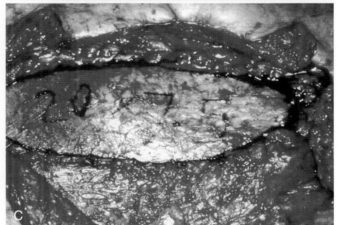

FIGURE 6 **A,** A free fascia lata graft after harvest. **B,** Fascia lata thigh donor site. **C,** An intraoperative photograph with the fascia lata graft shown in position just prior to inset.

are commercially available; these are supported by various data, and the field is rapidly evolving. The surgeon should use caution when selecting a product and should base the decision on the best available peer-reviewed literature.

Closure of the Skin

Closure of the skin is absolutely critical when using synthetic mesh. One of the advantages of the use of autologous tissue, as well as acellular dermal matrices, is that they can, in our experience, tolerate exposure and go on to heal by secondary intention. Therefore inadequate or tenuous skin closure is yet another reason to avoid the use of synthetic materials. In general, the skin can be closed in the majority of cases with aggressive undermining. At times, it is necessary to perform local skin flaps, such as rotational flaps, to achieve closure. In some cases, it is necessary to leave the skin open; in these situations, we tend to use negative-pressure wound therapy. We find that the negative-pressure wound dressings tend to increase granulation tissue and facilitate contraction of the wound as well as helping to

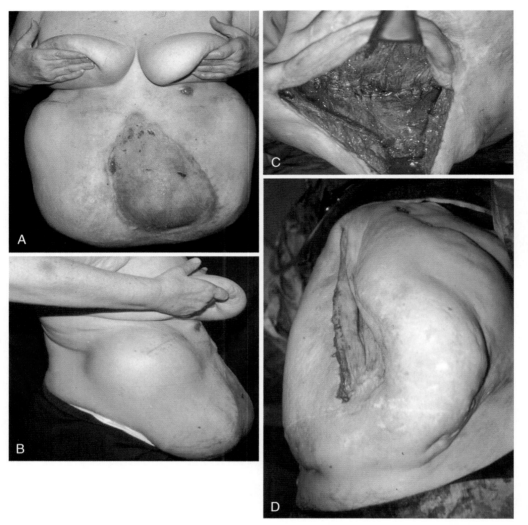

FIGURE 7 A, Trauma patient treated with an open abdomen and skin graft on bowel 1 year after skin graft placement, shown with tissue expanders in position between the external and internal oblique fascia lateral to the rectus abdominis. The expanders have been sufficiently expanded, and the patient is ready for the second-stage closure procedure. **B,** Lateral view. **C,** Intraoperative view showing a low-tension primary fascial graft after removal of expanders. **D,** Intraoperative photograph showing an excess of tissue after primary fascial repair, allowing for a second-layer repair with the expanded external oblique fascia.

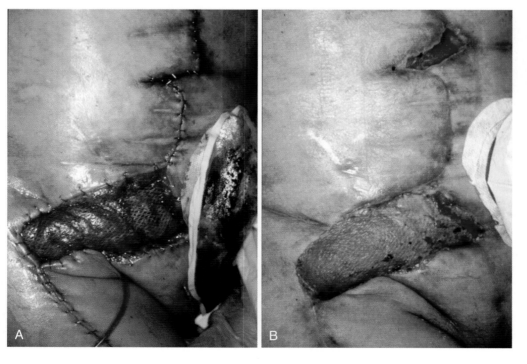

FIGURE 8 A, Immediate postoperative photograph of a rectus femoris pedicled muscle flap with an overlying skin graft used to close the inferior portion with an abdominal wall defect. **B,** After 4 weeks; a successful take of the split-thickness skin graft on the muscle flap.

remove exudates and edema from the wound. Once healthy granulation tissue is observed, the decision can be made to either skin graft the wound or allow it to heal secondarily.

Tissue Expansion

Tissue expansion remains an option for fascial replacement and is particularly warranted when there is an extreme lack of both fascia and skin. By placing the tissue expander between the external and internal oblique fascia lateral to the rectus and expanding to very large volumes, the fascia below (internal oblique and transversus abdominis) and the external oblique and skin above become expanded. This allows primary approximation of the fascia (rectus to rectus) followed by a second layer of external oblique to external oblique (with overlying skin) as a second layer (Figure 7). This is an excellent option but has the considerable downside of requiring a second operation and multiple office visits for expansion. Tissue expansion also has a relatively high complication rate in the abdomen with risk of infection, exposure, and hematomas. Because of these factors, it is a less commonly used option and is generally reserved for extreme cases.

Flaps

Pedicled flaps such as latissimus dorsi, rectus femoris, and tensor fascia lata myocutaneous flaps have been used in the past in our group. The main limitation of these flaps is their arc of rotation, which is limited by the vascular pedicle (Figure 8). Delay incisions, particularly for the tensor fascia lata myocutaneous flap, can extend the reach of these flaps; however, because of the donor site morbidity and the availability of biologic fascial replacements, these options are less commonly used. Free flaps have been described for the abdominal wall but are also only rarely used because of the considerable increase in operative time and technical complexity associated with microsurgical free-tissue transfer, in comparison to the other available techniques.

SUGGESTED READINGS

Cunningham SC, Rosson GD, Lee RH, et al: Localization of the arcuate line from surface anatomic landmarks: a cadaveric study, *Ann Plast Surg* 53:129–131, 2004.

Disa JJ, Goldberg NH, Carlton JM, et al: Restoring abdominal wall integrity in contaminated tissue-deficient wounds using autologous fascia grafts, *Plast Reconstr Surg* 101(4):979–986, 1998.

Disa JJ, Klein MH, Goldberg NH: Advantages of autologous fascia versus synthetic patch abdominal wall reconstruction in experimental animal defects, *Plast Reconstr Surg* 97:801–806, 1996.

Itani K, Awad SS, Baumann D, et al: Prospective clinical study evidence of safe, single-stage repair of infected/contaminated abdominal incisional hernias using Strattice reconstructive tissue matrix, *Hernia* 13(S1):S28, 2009.

Jacobsen WM, Petty PM, Bite D, et al: Massive abdominal wall hernia reconstruction with expanded external/internal oblique and transversalis musculofascia, *Plast Reconstr Surg* 100:326–335, 1997.

Karp NS: Abdominal wall reconstruction. In McCarthy JG, Galiano RD, Boutros SG, editors: *Current therapy in plastic surgery*, Philadelphia, 2006, Saunders Elsevier.

Luijendijk RW, Hop WC, van den Tol MP, et al: A comparison of suture repair with mesh repair for incisional hernia, *N Engl J Med* 343:392–398, 2000.

Menon NG, Rodriguez ED, Byrnes CK, et al: Revascularization of human acellular dermis in full-thickness abdominal wall reconstruction in the rabbit model, *Ann Plast Surg* 50(5):523–527, 2003.

Milburn ML, Holton LH, Chung TL, et al: Acellular dermal matrix compared with synthetic implant material for repair of ventral hernia in the setting of perioperative *Staphylococcus aureus* implant contamination: a rabbit model, *Surg Infect (Larchmont)* 9(4):433–442, 2008.

Ramirez OM, Ruas E, Dellon AL: "Components separation" method for closure of abdominal wall defects: an anatomic and clinical study, *Plast Reconstr Surg* 86:519, 1990.

Silverman RP, Li EN, Holton LH III, et al: Ventral hernia repair using allogenic acellular dermal matrix in a swine model, *Hernia* 8:336–342, 2004.

Silverman RP, Singh NK, Li EN, et al: Restoring abdominal wall integrity in contaminated tissue-deficient wounds using autologous fascia grafts, *Plast Reconstr Surg* 113:673–675, 2004.

PRIMARY TUMORS OF THE CHEST WALL

Maurice A. Smith, MD, and Stephen C. Yang, MD

OVERVIEW

Primary chest wall tumors are rare and only constitute 1% to 2% of all primary neoplasms and 5% of all thoracic neoplasms. Estimated to account for only 0.04% of all new cancers diagnosed in the United States, they can be categorized into two dominant types based on the tissue of origin: *bony and cartilaginous tumors* and *soft tissue tumors.* Sixty percent of primary chest wall tumors are malignant.

CLINICAL EVALUATION

Primary chest wall tumors show up as slow-growing masses, 75% of which are painless. Painful tumors are more often malignant or originate in bone. Pain usually represents expansion into cortex or periosteum, destruction of cortex, or a fracture.

After performing a history and physical examination, imaging studies are required. A plain chest radiograph is typically done first, as many of these tumors have characteristic radiographic appearances. Computed tomography (CT) yields the most useful information concerning site, size, and bony involvement, and it is the best modality for screening the lungs for metastases. Magnetic resonance imaging (MRI) provides further insight into the relationship of the mass to vascular structures, nerves, and spine and chest apex. Positron emission tomography (PET) can help better differentiate benign from malignant tumors and delineate tumor grade. Studies are ongoing to provide parameters for analysis, but currently PET is a complement to biopsy, not a replacement.

After developing a differential diagnosis based on the workup described above, an initial biopsy may be necessary, unless surgical resection is planned irrespective of diagnosis. Excisional biopsies should be used for lesions smaller than 2 cm or lesions suspected of being benign. Core biopsies with evaluations of cellular aspirates with monoclonal antibodies, immunochemistry, and electron microscopy are used for larger tumors. These core biopsies are 95% accurate. Incisional biopsy is reserved for tumors larger than 5 cm, where core biopsies do not provide diagnosis. The incision size and orientation should not compromise subsequent resection. Extensive dissection and flap creation should be avoided, as local spread into soft tissues has been documented. Treatment and outcomes are tumor dependent. We discuss the presentation, diagnosis, and treatment for some of the more common lesions in this chapter, and a complete list can be found in Table 1.

Benign Soft Tissue Tumors

Desmoid Tumors

Desmoid tumors arise from fibroblasts of deep muscle and connective tissue, and 50% occur in the abdomen. Among the extraabdominal sites of origin, the chest wall is the most common. Desmoid tumors are often seen in the teen years to age 30 years with complaints of pain (62%) and are associated with a history of trauma, prior thoracotomy, and Garner syndrome. They are slow growing along tissue planes and have a high rate of recurrence. Wide local excision, optimally with 4 cm margins, is the primary treatment. Radiation has been used to decrease local recurrence rates with both negative and positive margins. A report from Mayo Clinic demonstrates an 89% 5-year probability of local recurrence after resection with positive margins versus 18% with negative margins.

Hemangiomas and Lymphangiomas

Hemangiomas occur in children, and treatment is indicated for cosmetic reasons or for complications that include bleeding and ulceration. Otherwise, these lesions do not warrant aggressive resection. Lymphangiomas likewise mostly occur in children and are different from hemangiomas in that they lack blood cells within their channels. Traditional treatment has been surgical excision to prevent recurrence. Meta-analysis has shown nonsurgical therapies such as OK-432 and acetic acid sclerotherapy to be safe and efficacious, and these do not alter future surgical therapy should that become necessary.

Malignant Soft Tissue Tumors

Malignant Fibrous Histiocytomas

Malignant fibrous histiocytomas are the most common chest wall sarcomas, and they are more common in men. These are seen later in life, in the 50s to 70s, as a painless, slow-growing mass that originates from musculature and grows along fascial planes and between muscle fibers. Despite wide local resection as the treatment of choice, there is a high local recurrence rate. Postoperative radiation is used for tumors where resection margins were inadequate or in tumors with a high histologic grade. Re-resection of low-grade tumors can be performed as an alternative to radiation. These tumors metastasize 30% to 50% of the time and have a 5 year survival of 38%.

TABLE 1: Primary chest wall tumors

Benign	Malignant
Soft Tissue	
Lipoma	Malignant fibrous histiocytoma
Hemangioma	Rhabdosarcoma
Lymphangioma	Liposarcoma
Fibroma	Neurofibrosarcoma
Rhabdomyoma	Leiomyosarcoma
Neurofibroma	
Desmoid tumor	
Bony and Cartilaginous	
Fibrous dysplasia	Chondrosarcoma
Osteochondroma	Osteogenic sarcoma
Chondroma	Ewing sarcoma
Askin tumor	
Plasmacytoma	

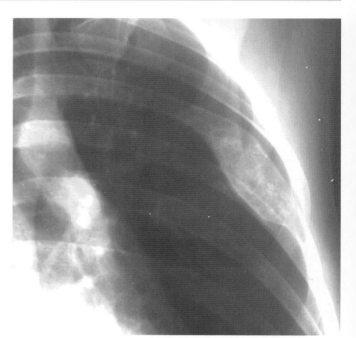

FIGURE 1   Chest radiograph of fibrous dysplasia with classic ground-glass appearance of rib. *(From Levine BD, Motamedi K, Chow K, et al: CT of rib lesions, Am J Roentgenol 193:5-13, 2009.)*

Liposarcoma and Rhabdomyosarcoma

Rhabdomyosarcoma most often affects children and adolescents. Treatment is wide local excision and multidrug chemotherapy. Neoadjuvant chemotherapy protocols followed by excision have survival rates of 75% compared with 25% for surgery alone. Liposarcoma occurs more frequently in men in their 40s to 60s. These tend to be large encapsulated tumors, and primary treatment is wide excision to prevent local recurrence; the 5-year survival for patients with liposarcomas is 60%.

Benign Bone and Cartilaginous Tumors

Fibrous Dysplasia

Fibrous dysplasia represents the most common bony chest wall tumors, accounting for 30% of all benign chest wall tumors. It usually occurs on the posterior or lateral aspect of the ribs as an asymptomatic incidental finding; less commonly, it is associated with Albright syndrome with the presence of skin lesions and precocious sexual maturity in girls. It is usually seen in those aged 20 to 30 years, usually as a slow-growing, painless mass. Typical radiographic characteristics are a ground-glass appearance in the central area of the rib with thinning of the cortex and irregular calcification in the medulla (Figure 1). The treatment is local excision for painful lesions, but excision of asymptomatic lesions usually is not necessary, unless the diagnosis is in doubt. Needle or incisional biopsies are of very little yield.

Osteochondromas

Osteochondromas are cartilage-capped growths arising from cortical bone, usually anteriorly at the costochondral junction along the sternum. The peak incidence is at 20 years of age, and they are usually three times more common in men. If the lesion is on the external aspect of the bone, it can be palpated; otherwise, radiographic findings are of a pedunculated protuberance with intact cortex and stippled calcification in the area of the tumor. Malignant

degeneration is rare. For lesions that are symptomatic or enlarging, if the diagnosis is in doubt, or if the patient is an adult, treatment is local excision.

Chondromas

These benign lesions present in both genders equally and occur between the ages of 20 and 40. Chondromas are typically asymptomatic, slow-growing tumors. On radiographs, the tumor appears as a periosteal mass that is lytic in nature with a thinning cortex but sclerotic borders. Radiographically it is hard to distinguish a chondroma from a malignant, degenerate chondrosarcoma, so treatment is excision with wide margins, especially when such a distinction cannot be made clinically.

Malignant Bone and Cartilaginous Tumors

Ewing Sarcoma and Primitive Neuroectodermal Tumors

Askin tumors, which are primitive neuroectodermal tumors (PNETs), belong to the Ewing sarcoma family of tumors. These are small, round-cell tumors, and both have translocations between chromosomes 11 and 22.

Ewing sarcomas are rapidly enlarging, painful masses that occur between the ages of 10 and 15 years and happen twice as often in males. The characteristic radiographic finding is the onion-peel appearance that occurs from bony destruction and the reactive multiple layers of new periosteal formation. Core biopsies are useful in making a definitive diagnosis for accurate reverse-transcription polymerase chain reaction analysis of gene locations. Treatment is neoadjuvant chemotherapy followed by wide local excision, and radiation is added for additional local control and for positive margins. Survival rates are 56% to 65% at 5 years and 43% at 10 years.

An Askin tumor is a rare tumor in the thoracopulmonary region, and it shares the same characteristics as Ewing sarcomas. The workup and treatment are also the same, but these tumors are more aggressive, with a 5-year survival of 16%.

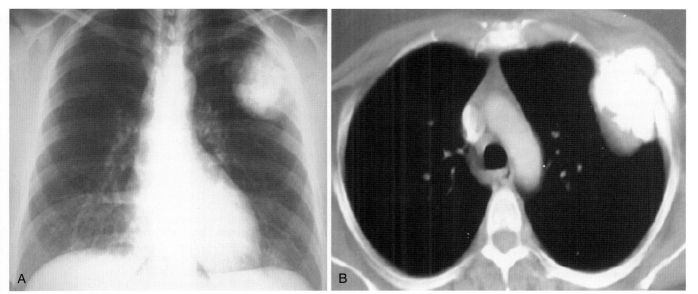

FIGURE 2   Osteosarcoma. **A,** Chest radiograph. **B,** CT scan. Osteosarcoma is more densely calcified than chondrosarcomas. *(From O'Sullivan P, O'Dweyer H, Flint J, et al: Malignant chest wall neoplasms of bone and cartilage: a pictoral of CT and MR findings, Br J Radiol 80:678–684, 2007.)*

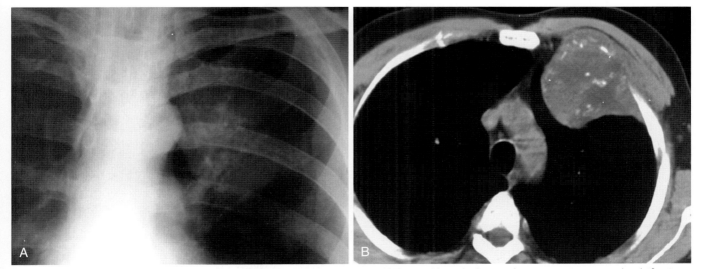

FIGURE 3   Chondrosarcoma. **A,** Chest radiograph. **B,** Computed tomography (CT) scan. Note the large soft tissue component with calcifications and the lytic nature of the tumor. *(From Cakir O, Tapal U, Bayram S, et al: Sarcomas: rare primary malignant tumors of the thorax, Diagn Interv Radiol 11:23–27, 2005.)*

Osteogenic Sarcomas

Mostly seen in long bones, osteogenic sarcomas make up 6% of primary chest wall malignancies. They are seen as a rapidly expanding painful mass with elevated alkaline phosphatase levels. A classic sunburst pattern is sometimes seen on radiograph, which represents calcifications at right angles to the cortex. A second radiographic sign is a Codman triangle, where the tumor lifts the periosteum; the shadow between the cortex and the raised periosteum forms the triangle. Evidence of the density of the calcifications is seen in Figure 2. Osteogenic sarcomas are mostly seen in teenagers, but in the adult population, these can be seen in Paget disease or with prior radiation or prior bone infarction. Osteogenic sarcomas are also associated with mutations in the RB gene *p53*. Twenty percent of patients are seen with metastasis, of which the lung is the primary site. Treatment is neoadjuvant chemotherapy and wide local excision, and the overall survival is 14% to 20%.

Chondrosarcoma

Chondrosarcoma is the most common malignancy of the anterior chest wall, usually seen between the ages of 30 and 60, and 80% arise from the costochrondal angle; the other 20% arise from the sternum. Chondrosarcoma has been associated with trauma and presents as a painful, hard, fixed mass. Radiographically it appears as a mixed lytic and sclerotic pattern (Figure 3). An ovulated mass is seen originating from the medulla with cortical lytic lesions as well as some areas of thickened cortex. All localized lesions should be resected with wide local excision, and they usually require concomitant reconstruction. Low-grade tumors of mild hypercellularity have been reported to have 10-year survival rates up to 96% with few reported metastasis. Tumors that are high grade with marked hypercellularity have metastases 75% of the time and a 5-year survival of 20% to 30%. Poor prognostic factors include high tumor grade, large tumor size, incomplete resection, local recurrence, metastasis, and patient age over 50 years.

These tumors are relatively chemoresistant and radioresistant; therefore excision is the primary treatment. Radiation is reserved for positive margins.

Plasmacytoma

Plastocytoma occurs in men in their 60s and 70s and is associated with multiple myelomas. It is usually accompanied by pain with no palpable mass. Diagnosis is made from the presence of Bence-Jones proteinuria, abnormal protein electrophoresis, and hypercalcemia; bone marrow biopsy confirms the diagnosis. The characteristic radiographic appearance is of a multicystic expansile mass. Surgery is indicated only for tissue diagnosis, often by incisional biopsy, which can be quite bloody. Treatment consists of high-dose radiation, and 35% to 55% of patients progress to multiple myelomas, with an overall 5-year survival of 25% to 35%.

SURGICAL TECHNIQUE

Chest Wall Resection

Appropriate resection is the key to improving survival in many circumstances. In an effort to allow patients the best chance of cure, wide resection guidelines consist of at least 4 cm margins. This includes the rib above and below the tumor and taking skin, especially from previous incisional biopsy sites, and parietal pleura if they are involved. One study reported a 5-year freedom from recurrence of 56% in patients with malignant primary chest wall tumors resected with 4 cm margins compared with a 5-year freedom from recurrence of 25% in a cohort resected with 2 cm margins.

Planning for chest wall tumor resection includes identifying superior and inferior margins of resection. A periosteal elevator is used to free the intercostal musculature and neurovascular bundles from upper and lower ribs. Electrocautery clears the periosteum 1.5 cm from each border, and a periosteal elevator separates the rib from the underlying pleura. A sheer rib cutter is used to cut the rib. After resection, additional 1 cm posterior and anterior margins of the ribs are sent separately and marked appropriately. Any soft tissue margin with questionable involvement should be sent for pathologic frozen section to assess whether wider margins are required. Tissue adherent to the tumor—including superficial chest wall muscles, lung, thymus, pericardium, or diaphragm—should be resected en bloc.

If the sternum is involved, it may require partial or total sternectomy along with excision of the contiguous bilateral costal margins. It is best to maintain the circumferential integrity of the chest wall for pulmonary function reasons, even if only a small section remains intact. When only the lower sternum is involved, the manubrium can be preserved; if the sternal body is involved, a subtotal sternectomy is performed, preserving the upper 2 cm of manubrium and clavicles; finally, if the manubrium is involved, the lower half of the sternum can be spared.

Chest Wall Reconstruction

Reconstruction should be considered for defects greater than 5 cm, resection of three or more ribs, or removal of two or more ribs if baseline pulmonary compromise exists. Also, consider reconstruction for resection of the sternoclavicular junction, entire sternum, or upper part of the manubrium.

In general, skeletal reconstruction is achieved by suturing prosthetic mesh to the chest wall under tension. A variety of materials have been used, including Prolene mesh and polytetrafluoroethelyne. Other biologic materials, such as bovine pericardium or processed cellular matrix (Alloderm), could be used, especially in an infected or irradiated field. A Marlex "sandwich" is used when more rigid support is needed for sternal or anterolateral resections. This consists of measuring a mesh to fit the defect, then pouring a 2 to 3 mm layer of methylmethacrylate within 5 mm of the mesh edge. A second layer of mesh is then placed over the methylmethacrylate to make a "sandwich," and the mesh edges are sutured to the edge of the wound defect

TABLE 2: Various flaps used to cover thoracic wall defects after resections for chest wall neoplasms

Type of Flap	Arterial Supply	Indications
Latissimus	Primary: thoracodorsal Secondary: perforating vessels from posterior intercostal vessels	Covers defects anterolaterally and posteriorly
Pectoralis major	Dominant: thoracoacromial artery Turnover flap: internal mammary perforators	Covers anterior chest wall defects
Serratus	Subscapular artery	Covers the intrathoracic area
Rectus abdominus	Deep superior or inferior epigastric	Covers lower sternal wounds
External oblique	Segmental blood supply from posterior intercostal arteries	Covers defects at the inframammary fold

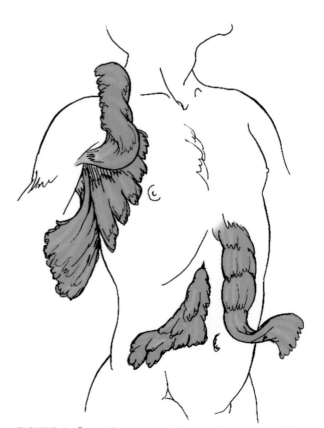

FIGURE 4 Pectoralis, serratus, latissumus dorsi, rectus abdominis, and external oblique can be used to provide soft tissue coverage for chest wall reconstruction.

with permanent suture. Prosthetic reconstruction is contraindicated in infected wounds, in which case skeletal reconstruction should be delayed, or biologic material should be used.

When there is less concern for skeletal instability of the rib cage, soft tissue reconstruction alone is sufficient. These techniques include split-thickness skin grafts, muscle grafts, and musculocutaneous grafts, both free and with pedicles. Some of the most commonly used flaps are summarized in Table 2 and Figure 4. The greater omentum can be used in infected sites and has the potential to cover areas often larger than what can be covered by muscle flaps, and omentum has been utilized in both pedicle and free flaps.

SUMMARY

Chest wall tumors comprise a heterogenous group of lesions that require a fairly consistent diagnostic and therapeutic approach. Diagnostic approach consists of careful history and imaging followed by a histologic diagnosis when indicated, obtained via biopsy without compromise of future treatment. Most benign lesions can be observed, and common malignant lesions are treated surgically. Appropriate excisional margins must be obtained to minimize the chance of local recurrence. A subsequent reconstruction may use simple prosthetic placement or more complex tissue transposition techniques.

SUGGESTED READINGS

Athanassiadi K, Kalavrouziotis G, Rondogianni D, et al: Primary chest wall tumors: early and long-term results of surgical treatment, *Eur J Cardiothorac Surg* 19:589–593, 2001.
LaQuaglia MP: Chest wall tumors in childhood and adolescence, *Semin Pediatr Surg* 17(3):173–180, 2008.
Skoracki RJ, Chang DW: Reconstruction of the chest wall and thorax, *J Surg Oncol* 94(6):455–465, 2006.

MEDIASTINAL MASSES

Aaron M. Cheng, MD, and Douglas E. Wood, MD

OVERVIEW

The mediastinum extends from the thoracic inlet superiorly to the diaphragm inferiorly, from pleural space to pleural space laterally, and from the sternum anteriorly to thoracic spine posteriorly. Disease of the mediastinum can originate from structures that reside in the mediastinum, invade the mediastinum from an adjacent structure, or involve the mediastinum secondarily from metastases.

The mediastinum can be divided into three compartments: the *anterosuperior, middle,* and *posterior* or *paravertebral.* The anterosuperior compartment extends from the manubrium and first ribs down to the diaphragm; its posterior boundary is the anterior pericardium and great vessels. Contained within this compartment are the thymus, lymph nodes, fat, and connective tissue. Lesions commonly found in this compartment include thymomas, lymphomas, and germ cell tumors. Substernal thyroid goiter, thyroid malignancy, or displaced parathyroid glands can also be found in the anterosuperior compartment.

The middle component is also referred to as the *visceral component,* and its boundaries are the anterior border of the pericardium and the anterior border of the vertebral bodies. The middle mediastinum contains the heart and pericardial sac, the trachea and major bronchi, the esophagus, the hilar pulmonary vessels, and also lymph nodes. A variety of foregut cysts, as well as primary and secondary tumors of the lymph nodes, can be found in this compartment.

The posterior compartment extends from the first thoracic vertebra to the diaphragm and from the anterior border of the vertebral bodies to the most posterior curvature of the ribs. The sympathetic chain, vagus nerves, thoracic duct, descending aorta, and also lymph nodes are located within the posterior compartment.

Although this is a common division of the mediastinum, it is important to know that other divisions are commonly used; some surgeons differentiate the superior mediastinum, a region cephalad to an imaginary line drawn between the sternomanubrial junction and the inferior aspect of the T4 vertebral body, and they use the posterior aspect of the pericardium, rather than the anterior aspect of the vertebral bodies, as the dividing line between the middle and posterior mediastinum.

CLINICAL PRESENTATION

Nearly half of the patients identified with mediastinal masses are asymptomatic, and their lesions are detected on radiological imaging taken for unrelated reasons. The most common symptoms of those who are symptomatic are cardiorespiratory—specifically, chest pain and cough—but symptoms can include dysphagia, the sensation of chest heaviness, and dyspnea. Compression or invasion of mediastinal structures by a mediastinal neoplasm can lead to signs of superior vena cava obstruction, Horner syndrome, and vocal cord paralysis. Recurrent respiratory infections are also common complaints. Several mediastinal lesions are also associated with paraneoplastic syndromes: thymoma with myasthenia gravis, red cell aplasia, and hypogammaglobulinemia; Hodgkin lymphoma with recurrent fevers; and von Recklinghausen disease with neurofibromas.

DIAGNOSIS

Imaging

Although patient history and physical examination may help the surgeon narrow the differential diagnosis of a mediastinal mass, computed tomography (CT) is the most important tool in the workup of a patient with a mediastinal lesion. Chest CT provides excellent imaging of the mediastinum; in many instances, certain lesions can be diagnosed with sufficient certainty, such as aortic aneurysms and pericardial fat pads, so that additional diagnostic workup is unwarranted. Additionally, CT is the most common modality used to assist with fine needle aspiration (FNA) or core needle biopsies, when a tissue sample is required.

Magnetic resonance imaging (MRI) can supplement CT imaging to aid in preoperative determination of a tumor's invasion into neural or vascular structures. Particularly for posterior mediastinal tumors or those close to the thoracic inlet, MRI is useful to identify invasion of the vertebral foramina and brachial plexus respectively.

Patients with anterior mediastinal masses, and particularly young men, should have levels of α-fetoprotein (AFP), β-human chronic gonadotropin (β-HCG), and lactate dehydrogenase (LDH) measured.

Serum levels of AFP and β-HCG can increase in the presence of nonseminomatous malignant germ cell tumors or some teratomas and carcinomas. If a mediastinal mass is suspected to be a thymoma, and the patient has clinical symptoms suggestive of myasthenia gravis, measurement of antiacetylcholine antibodies may aid in establishing a diagnosis.

Invasive Techniques

The decision to proceed with biopsy should be based on the most likely tumor pathology, the location and extent of the lesion and local symptoms, and tumor markers. Performing an invasive biopsy on a patient with a mediastinal mass in many cases is not necessary, and in some cases, it is potentially detrimental. Particularly, biopsy of a clinically suspected, well-encapsulated, early-stage thymoma is unnecessary and may be associated with tumor dissemination within the mediastinum or pleural space. Asymptomatic lesions confined to the anterior mediastinum that show no evidence of local invasion, associated adenopathy, or tumor markers can usually be primarily resected for both diagnostic and therapeutic purposes. Likewise, posterior mediastinal tumors that appear benign and resectable on preoperative diagnosis can undergo primary resection without biopsy. If a mediastinal mass represents a cyst, it should be resected rather than biopsied.

Bulky lymphadenopathy should undergo biopsy, as surgical resection is usually not the primary means of treatment. If lymphoma is suspected, biopsy is warranted for adequate tissue typing and for flow cytometric studies. Tissue should also be obtained in the patient with a mediastinal mass in whom serum concentrations of AFP or β-HCG are elevated, suggesting a germ cell tumor. Primary treatment of these tumors is achieved systemically with chemotherapy, and surgical resection is usually reserved for treatment of residual disease.

Invasive Biopsy Procedures

The primary purpose of FNA biopsy is to prevent unnecessary surgical intervention. Conversely, it does not stage patients with mediastinal or pulmonary malignancies; therefore in the patient who is a surgical candidate, undergoing FNA biopsy may be superfluous, as it does not obviate the need for surgery when an operation is required for staging or resection. However, in patients in whom lymphoma is suspected, FNA should not be performed, as it does not provide a sufficient tissue sample for flow cytometric and phenotypic characterization. Although it can be diagnostic in approximately 75% of mediastinal masses appropriately chosen for biopsy, overall the FNA biopsy for diagnosis of mediastinal masses is inconsistent and limited.

Likewise, core biopsy may provide more tissue for diagnosis of mediastinal masses, but a more invasive surgical approach is often needed for definitive tumor diagnosis. Surgical approaches to obtain tissue from the mediastinum include cervical mediastinoscopy, anterior mediastinotomy (Chamberlain procedure), and video-assisted thoracoscopy (VATS).

Cervical mediastinoscopy, performed through a small suprasternal incision, allows the surgeon to sample masses and lymph nodes in the paratracheal and subcarinal portion of the middle mediastinum. It does not allow access to lesions in the anterior mediastinum, a common misunderstanding of many medical specialists and inexperienced surgeons. Biopsies of tumors in this region can usually be performed safely and with minimal morbidity by core needle biopsy via a parasternal approach. If core needle biopsy is unavailable or tissue obtained is insufficient, an anterior mediastinotomy on either the left or right can be performed. These surgical procedures can be performed in the outpatient setting and do not delay chemotherapy or radiotherapy treatment.

VATS approaches to either the left or right side of the mediastinum are relatively straightforward and can be used to provide access to all mediastinal compartments for tissue sampling. However, in most cases a mediastinoscopy or anterior mediastinotomy can provide excellent access with less operative time and less morbidity and hospitalization. Because of the risk of tumor seeding in the pleural space, VATS biopsies of some mediastinal masses, such as suspected thymoma, are contraindicated.

ANTERIOR MEDIASTINAL TUMORS

Anterior mediastinal masses comprise the most common tumors of the mediastinum. Over 90% of the tumors of the anterior compartment include thymic neoplasms, teratomas or germ cell tumors, lymphoma, and thyroid goiter or neoplasm.

Thymomas

Thymomas are the most common of the thymic malignancies and the most common isolated anterior mediastinal tumor. These tumors occur with equal frequency in men and women, most often in those 40 to 70 years of age.

The cellular classification of thymomas is largely based on the World Health Organization (WHO) classification scheme published in 1999. Thymoma is a thymic epithelial tumor in which the epithelial component commonly exhibits no overt cellular atypia and maintains the histologic features specific to the normal thymus. Because of this, small-volume tissue samples obtained by FNA or core needle biopsy are often nondiagnostic. Immature nonneoplastic lymphocytes are present in variable numbers, depending on the histologic type of thymoma. In distinction, thymic carcinoma, also known as the *type C thymoma*, exhibits cytological atypia and histologic features similar to those observed in other carcinomas rather than the regular features of the normal thymus. Thymic carcinomas lack the immature lymphocytes seen in thymomas. Thymic carcinomas are usually advanced when identified and have a higher recurrence rate and poorer survival prognosis than thymomas, with 5-year and 10-year survival of 38% and 28%, respectively. In contrast to thymomas, the association of autoimmune disorders with thymic carcinomas is rare.

Surgical resection remains the mainstay of treatment for thymic tumors, and most surgeons would advocate median sternotomy over VATS for the procedure. Resectable thymomas are generally histologically diagnosed and staged at the time of surgical resection. The staging system proposed by Masaoka in 1981 is widely employed (Table 1). A total thymectomy with complete resection can usually be achieved in nearly all patients with stage I and stage II thymomas but in only 27% to 44% of patients with stage III disease.

Radiologic suggestion of an unresectable stage III or IV thymoma warrants tissue diagnosis, usually by anterior mediastinotomy, to initiate chemotherapy and/or radiation. Locally advanced (stage III) thymomas are usually best treated by induction chemotherapy

TABLE 1: Masaoka staging system for thymoma

Masaoka Stage	Disease Extent
I	Totally encapsulated
II	Capsular invasion and/or invasion of surrounding fat or pleura
III	Invasion into organs (pericardium, lung, great vessels)
IVa	Pleural or pericardial implants
IVb	Hematogenous metastases

followed by surgery and adjuvant radiation. The local recurrence rate after complete surgical resection of a stage I thymoma is less than 2%, and no adjuvant therapy is warranted; radiation after thymectomy for stage II disease is controversial, with consideration given to a variety of histologic factors (Figure 1). Patients who have stage IVa disease can rarely be completely resected; such patients are usually offered chemotherapy and adjuvant radiotherapy, and debulking surgery may also be considered. Radiation therapy has been reported to achieve local control in 60% to 90% of patients with residual macroscopic disease after attempted surgical resection. Because of the slow growth of thymic neoplasms, survival is often expressed in terms of both 5 and 10 year survival. Overall 5- and 10-year survival after resection are 90% and 90% for stage 1, 80% and 70% for stage II, 65% and 55% for stage III, and 60% and 35% for stage Iva, respectively.

Recurrence after treatment is usually local, either in the pleural space or in the mediastinum; recurrent disease is sometimes curable with repeat surgical resection along with other therapeutic modalities. Distant recurrences are less common, usually occurring with bone metastases. Combination chemotherapy regimens have been reported to achieve complete or partial remission in patients with stage IV or locally progressive recurrent disease; however, the number of patients who have been treated is small.

Paraneoplastic Syndromes Associated with Thymomas

Myasthenia gravis is the most common autoimmune disorder associated with thymomas; it can be present in approximately one third of patients with thymomas. Although thymectomy may provide marked clinical improvement in patients with myasthenia gravis and thymoma, improvement or remission is variable and cannot be predicted.

Pure red cell aplasia occurs in 5% of patients with thymomas, whereas 33% to 50% of patients with red cell aplasia have thymomas; thymectomy can produce remission in up to 40% of these patients.

Hypogammaglobulinemia has been associated with 5% to 10% of patients with thymomas and is more frequent in those who also have rheumatoid arthritis, ulcerative colitis, cytopenia, or extrathymic malignancy. Up to 20% of patients with thymomas will develop extrathymic cancers, most commonly lymphomas, bronchogenic carcinomas, and thyroid cancers.

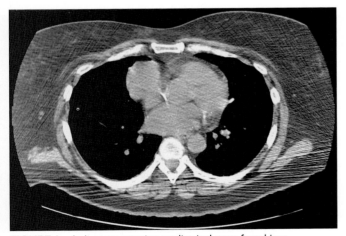

FIGURE I A discrete anterior mediastinal mass found in a 65-year-old woman during a workup for anemia. The radiographic features suggested thymoma, and the patient underwent a median sternotomy for a radical thymectomy. The thymoma was found to extend through the tumor capsule into the adipose tissue (Masaoka stage II), and the patient was referred for adjuvant radiotherapy to improve local control.

Germ Cell Tumors

Germ cell tumors are the fourth most common mediastinal tumor in adults, and such tumors can be either benign or malignant. Malignant germ cell tumors can be classified as *seminomas*, which occur almost exclusively in men in their 20s to 40s, or *nonseminomatous germ cell tumors* (NSGCTs), which include teratocarcinomas, choriocarcinomas, embryonal carcinomas, and yolk sac or endodermal sinus tumors. NSGCTs typically produce high levels of AFP or β-HCG. Serum levels of AFP and β-HCG are usually low in patients with pure seminomas, although a small percentage (10%) may have slight increases in these serum markers. In general, if these levels are increased, it suggests that nonseminomatous elements are likely present. Serum LDH usually is elevated in seminomas.

Benign teratomas consist of disorganized elements derived from all three germinal embryological layers: ectoderm, mesoderm, and endoderm. These benign germ cell tumors most often occur in adolescents or adults and with equal frequency in males and females. Approximately one third of patients with a benign teratoma are asymptomatic.

Tissue diagnosis is generally necessary before initiating treatment. Tissue can be obtained via needle biopsy or by open biopsy when necessary. Open biopsy is usually performed through a small anterior parasternal incision under general anesthesia. Because these tumors are frequently large and bulky, airway compression can make intubation difficult, and strict airway maintenance is required. Rigid bronchoscopy should be promptly available.

Benign mediastinal teratomas are the only germ cell tumor in which surgical resection is the indicated primary treatment. The tumor should be resected in its entirety without violation of the capsule. Most commonly this is performed via a median sternotomy; however, the VATS approach has been increasingly used for benign teratoma resection.

Seminomas are exquisitely radiosensitive, therefore radiotherapy is usually the primary therapy. Surgical resection can be appropriate in early stage lesions confined to the anterior mediastinum without evidence of regional or distant metastatic disease. Only complete resection can contribute to cure, but surgical excision as primary treatment is often precluded, as these tumors are frequently bulky and unresectable, or they show evidence of intrathoracic metastases at the time of diagnosis. Additionally, even after complete resection in early stage seminomas, mediastinal radiotherapy is indicated.

Cisplatin-based chemotherapeutic agents are used for the primary treatment of malignant mediastinal NSGCTs. Surgical resection is advised when radiographic studies show residual mediastinal disease after primary treatment with chemotherapy (Figure 3). In cases of seminoma, controversy exists regarding the role of resection for residual posttreatment tumor.

Lymphoma

Lymphoma comprises 20% of the masses found in both the anterior mediastinum and the middle mediastinum but is rare in the posterior compartment. Diagnosis of primary mediastinal lymphoma requires a significant tissue sample, therefore FNA biopsy samples are insufficient. Although radiographic-guided core biopsies may provide enough tissue sample for a diagnosis, cervical or anterior mediastinoscopy is often needed to provide sufficient tissue for lymphoma subclassification. Seventy-five percent of patients with Hodgkin lymphoma present with mediastinal disease, in contrast to only 5% of patients with non-Hodgkin lymphoma (Figure 2). Mediastinal B cell lymphoma, a subset of diffuse large B-cell lymphoma, can arise primarily in the mediastinum. It is an aggressive disease, primarily of younger patients in their 30s and 40s, with greater prevalence in women. Mediastinal B-cell lymphoma is often seen with symptoms of compression of intrathoracic structures, such as SVC syndrome. Mediastinal lymphoma is frequently bulky and clearly unresectable.

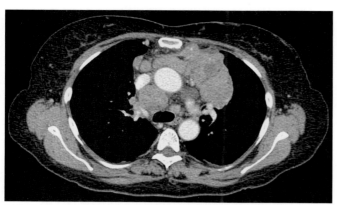

FIGURE 2 A bulky anterior mediastinal mass with associated lymphadenopathy found in a 62-year-old woman on chest CT during a workup for chest pressure. The patient underwent a left anterior mediastinotomy for tissue biopsy and was diagnosed with Hodgkin lymphoma, nodular sclerosis subtype, and the patient underwent treatment with chemotherapy.

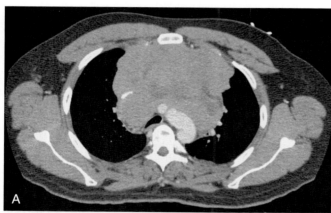

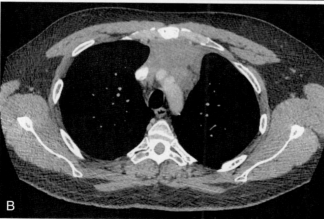

FIGURE 3 **A,** Massive anterior mediastinal mass found on CT scan of a 38-year-old patient seen for cough and shortness of breath. CT core biopsy demonstrated seminomatous histology; however, AFP and β-HCG serum tumor markers were slightly elevated, suggesting occult nonseminomatous germ cell tumor components. **B,** The patient underwent chemotherapy and had significant tumor reduction with normalization of the serum markers. Resection of the residual tumor mass and pathology demonstrated predominantly mature teratomatous elements; no evidence of residual seminomatous or malignant germ cell tumor elements was identified.

It often has other areas of lymphadenopathy, which allows it to be distinguished from early-stage (resectable) thymoma. However, it is still appropriate to obtain a biopsy when lymphoma is suspected to confirm the diagnosis.

The treatment of localized lymphoma consists of combination chemotherapy with or without radiotherapy. As with other aggressive lymphomas, stem cell transplant is the preferred treatment option after relapse. Surgical resection does not play a role in the treatment of mediastinal lymphoma.

Thyroid

Substernal goiters represent 7% of mediastinal masses, and essentially all descend from the neck; primary mediastinal thyroids are extremely rare, therefore mediastinal thyroid can usually be reliably diagnosed by CT imaging for the characteristic appearance of a multinodular goiter and continuity with the cervical thyroid gland. Substernal goiters can remain asymptomatic for several years, but when symptoms do arise, they are usually related to compression of adjacent structures within the thoracic cavity. The occurrence of symptoms does not indicate malignancy, as most substernal thyroid masses represent benign goiter; however, most surgeons would consider the presence of a substernal goiter an indication for removal.

There is no role for medical therapy in treating patients who have compressive symptoms, and such an operation may become more technically difficult if surgery is delayed until a patient with a substernal goiter develops symptoms. Substernal goiters can often be resected through a low collar incision without the need for a sternotomy. Should greater exposure become necessary, a partial sternal split down to the second intercostal space via a T-incision from the initial collar incision is usually sufficient, and a full sternotomy can be avoided. Airway management in these patients is crucial, as many patients have some degree of airway compression. Conscious fiberoptic intubation may be considered, and rigid bronchoscopy for airway control should be readily available.

DISEASES OF THE MIDDLE MEDIASTINAL COMPARTMENT

Lymphadenopathy is the most frequently encountered abnormality noted in the visceral mediastinum. It can stem from both malignant and nonmalignant causes. Frequent malignant causes of lymph node enlargement include secondary metastases from lung tumors, esophageal cancer, and head and neck cancer. Lymphadenopathy from lymphoma is often associated with the disease process involving the anterior mediastinal compartment as well.

Granulomatous infections may also manifest with mediastinal lymphadenopathy, and lymph node calcifications are common findings. Histoplasmosis and coccidiomycosis are most commonly found among residents of the Ohio River Valley and southwestern United States, respectively.

Sarcoidosis often presents with mediastinal or hilar lymphadenopathy and is characterized by noncaseating granulomas. Frequently, sarcoidosis is seen in asymptomatic patients in their 30s to 40s who are found to have bilateral hilar and mediastinal lymphadenopathy. Patients who do have symptoms often are seen with cough and dyspnea, and they may complain of fatigue and malaise. The diagnosis is one of exclusion and may require a biopsy of lung or of mediastinal lymph nodes.

Castleman disease, also known as *giant lymph node hyperplasia*, is a rare disease that can be confused with lymphoma; over time, it can evolve into lymphoma. The etiology is unclear, but it may be related to lymphoid hyperplasia or inflammatory lymph node reactivity. The mass is usually a vascular lymphadenopathy, and CT scan is very useful, typically revealing an encapsulated mass surrounded by lymphadenopathy that enhances brightly. Surgical excision is the usual treatment for localized lesions. Multicentric Castleman disease, however, is usually treated with steroids.

Lymphadenopathy in the middle mediastinum can be diagnosed with needle biopsy via a transbronchial or transesophageal approach, which is now possible using endobronchial ultrasound (EBUS) and/or esophageal ultrasound (EUS). However, when more diagnostic tissue is required, a mediastinoscopy can provide a sufficient sample from the paratracheal and subcarinal regions. Alternatively, a VATS approach, usually from the right side, can be performed to obtain a tissue sample.

Mediastinal cysts comprise 20% of all mediastinal masses, with bronchogenic cysts making up nearly 60% of all mediastinal cysts. Patients who are diagnosed with bronchogenic cysts are frequently asymptomatic. When symptoms do occur, they typically result from compression of adjacent structures or infection of the cyst. Diagnosis can be based on CT scan, which usually reveals a smooth rounded or oval structure of soft tissue density that is associated with the tracheobronchial tree, most commonly in the subcarinal region. Symptoms and suspicion of malignancy are an indication for resection. Most surgeons also recommend resection of asymptomatic bronchogenic cysts because of the concern of enlargement or development of infection, although little data regarding the long-term natural history of bronchogenic cysts is available, leading others to recommend observation rather than surgery.

Esophageal cysts are much less common than bronchogenic cysts. These periesophageal lesions have a gastroesophageal epithelial lining and are frequently attached to the esophagus but rarely communicate directly with the esophagus. Both esophageal ultrasound and chest CT can be used for diagnosis, but obtaining a transesophageal biopsy should be avoided because of resulting infection. Resection is the preferred treatment for esophageal cysts, but in the absence of symptoms, the same considerations exist as outlined above for asymptomatic bronchogenic cysts.

Pericardial cysts are usually located at the right cardiophrenic angle or along the diaphragm. They also may be found along the heart border and can be confused with the pericardial fat pad. Rarely are patients symptomatic from pericardial cysts, which are not associated with malignant potential. Pericardial cysts do not have to be resected, and percutaneous aspiration alone may be therapeutic if necessary.

Resection of cysts can be performed either by a VATS approach or by open thoracotomy. All epithelialized tissue should be removed to avoid recurrence, and when this is technically impossible, the secreting epithelial tissue that remains should be fulgurated.

POSTERIOR MEDIASTINAL TUMORS

Neurogenic tumors comprise approximately 15% of all mediastinal masses found in adults; they arise from the peripheral nerves, the sympathetic ganglia, or the paraganglionic cells (Table 2). In adults, these tumors are usually benign, arising most frequently from the nerve sheath; but in children, half of these lesions are malignant and arise from autonomic ganglia. Patients are usually asymptomatic, but some will complain of chest wall pain, cough, dyspnea, or hoarseness related to local compression, and some will show signs of spinal cord compression.

The posterior mediastinum along the paravertebral sulcus is the most common site for neurogenic tumors (Figure 4). CT scanning can be used to define tumor characteristics and anatomical relationships. When intraspinal extension of the tumor is a concern, a MRI should be done. Up to 10% of patients with neurogenic tumors may have invasion into the neural foramen.

Surgical resection is the mainstay of treatment for virtually all neurogenic tumors. Discrete tumors in the paravertebral sulcus may be removed using a VATS technique or a by an open thoracotomy approach. Complete surgical resection is required to prevent local recurrence, and with malignant tumors, complete resection is

TABLE 2: Neurogenic tumors

Origin	Benign Tumors	Malignant Tumors
Nerve sheath	Neurilemmoma (benign schwannoma) Neurofibroma Granular cell tumor	Neurofibrosarcoma Malignant schwannoma
Autonomic nervous system ganglia	Ganglioneuroma Chemodectoma Pheochromocytoma	Ganglioneuroblastoma Neuroblastoma

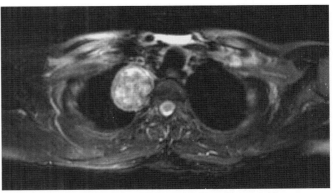

FIGURE 4 A mediastinal mass discovered in a 61-year-old man on routine chest radiograph. On MRI, the mass was determined to be an encapsulated heterogenous tumor in the posterior mediastinum, arising from the costovertebral gutter. The patient underwent surgical resection, and the tumor was determined to be a benign schwannoma (neurilemmoma).

essential for long-term survival. If intraspinal extension is present, it should be identified preoperatively, and operative planning should include a consultation with a spine surgeon to allow complete resection at the time of primary surgery. Adjuvant chemoradiation may be administered to patients with malignant tumors originating from the nerve sheath or sympathetic ganglion.

Tumors that originate from the ganglia of the autonomic nervous system also should be resected whenever feasible. Pheochromocytomas can be localized using iodine-131 metaiodobenzylguanidine (MIBG) scintigraphy in combination with CT scanning. Pheochromocytomas tend to be resistant to chemotherapy and radiotherapy, and they are treated by complete excision with preoperative control of blood pressure in metabolically active tumors. Chemodectomas can be highly vascular, therefore angioembolization before resection may be advocated. These tumors can undergo radiotherapy for tumor control if surgical excision is not feasible.

SELECTED READINGS

Detterbeck FC, Parson AM: Thymic tumors, *Ann Thorac Surg* 77:1860–1869, 2004.
Duwe BV, Sterman DH, Musani AI: Tumors of the mediastinum, *Chest* 128:2893–2909, 2005.
Ribet ME, Copin MC, Gosselin BH: Bronchogenic cysts of the mediastinum, *J Thorac Cardiovasc Surg* 109:1003–1010, 1995.
Takeda S, Miyoshi S, Minami M, Matsuda H: Intrathoracic neurogenic tumors: 50 years' experience in a Japanese institution, *Eur J Cardiothorac Surg* 26:807–812, 2004.
Wright CD, Kesler KA: Surgical techniques and outcomes for primary mediastinal nonseminomatous germ cell tumors, *Chest Surg Clin N Am* 12:707–715, 2002.

Primary Tumors of the Thymus

Marc Sussman, MD

OVERVIEW

The thymus is located in the anterior mediastinum adjacent to the posterior surface of the sternum and the anterior pericardium. Thymic tumors are the most common anterior mediastinal neoplasms. About half of thymic tumors are initially asymptomatic and found on radiographs obtained for other reasons. Patients with symptomatic tumors typically report chest pain, but less commonly compression of the airway or venous return is seen, or compromise of the phrenic or recurrent laryngeal nerves is evident. Patients may also show symptoms and signs of paraneoplastic syndromes. A computed tomographic (CT) scan of the chest with intravnous contrast is the most valuable diagnostic procedure (Figure 1), although magnetic resonance imaging can be helpful in evaluating invasion of the chest wall and vascular structures.

In addition to thymic neoplasms, the differential diagnosis of an anterior mediastinal mass includes intrathoracic thyroid, parathyroid tumors, lymphoma, and germ cell tumors. It is most important to separate those lesions that will primarily be treated by resection from those that will be primarily treated with chemotherapy. Frequently, these lesions can be differentiated by their radiographic appearance. Thymic tumors tend to originate in the area of the thymus itself, rarely extend into the neck, and usually do not have associated adenopathy. The coexistence of one of the parathymic syndromes would be highly suggestive of a thymoma. Elevated levels of β-human chorionic gonadotropin (HCG) or α-fetoprotein (AFP) can be diagnostic of germ cell tumors.

For small lesions it is often most appropriate to forego needle biopsy and proceed to complete resection to make the diagnosis. For those lesions that cannot be resected easily, a diagnostic biopsy should be obtained. This can be done with a CT-guided needle or an incision via an anterior mediastinotomy or thoracoscopic approach. For an anterior mediastinotomy, or Chamberlain procedure, an incision is made over the second rib, and the second costal cartilage is excised. Adequate biopsies can usually be obtained without excision of the cartilage, and a video mediastinoscope can be inserted into the wound to allow for visualization. If the pleural space is entered, the pneumothorax can be aspirated with a red rubber catheter that is pulled out as the incision is closed, or a chest tube can be placed. A needle biopsy may yield insufficient tissue to fully characterize a lymphoma, particularly if flow cytometry is needed. If the mass compresses the airway, great care must be used in proceeding with a general anesthetic.

Thymoma, which arises from the thymic epithelium, is the most common primary thymic neoplasm. A number of different staging systems have been proposed for thymomas. At this time, two systems are used in conjunction: the World Health Organization (WHO) histologic classification and the Masaoka system, which describes invasion and metastasis. The WHO classification is outlined in Table 1. Tumors with A, AB, and B1 histology have a better prognosis. The Masaoka classification is shown in Table 2. Most patients are initially seen with early stage disease, and these patients have an excellent overall prognosis when treated. The incidence of distant metastasis is very low.

The primary treatment for thymoma is surgical resection. Patients who have resectable disease without distant spread should undergo resection, and complete R0 resection is correlated with improved survival. Patients with unresectable Masaoka stage III or IV disease can sometimes be rendered resectable with multimodal therapy, therefore they should be considered for neoadjuvant chemotherapy or radiation therapy. Unresectable tumors can be treated with platinum-based chemotherapy and radiation.

Adjuvant therapy is not recommended for patients with Masaoka stage I lesions that have been completely resected. Adjuvant radiation therapy has been recommended for completely resected stage II and III tumors, although some have questioned the benefit of additional therapy. Patients with less than a complete resection should be referred for adjuvant therapy, and those with recurrent disease that is resectable should undergo surgery.

The surgical approach to early stage thymomas is usually through a partial or complete median sternotomy. This is done to allow complete resection of all thymic tissue and improve the chances of a complete resection of the tumor, which is critical to a good outcome. After sternotomy the chest is evaluated for unanticipated metastatic disease. The tumor is evaluated to be sure it can be completely resected and to see what if any structures will need to be removed en bloc. Although dissection can begin at the inferior pole of the thymus, I prefer to begin by freeing the more easily identifiable superior horns of the thymus and then dividing and ligating the thyrothymic ligament. With the superior horns freed, it is easier to dissect around the innominate vein and divide the large veins that drain the thymus. In an adult the thymic tissue will have involuted, so it can be difficult to distinguish from mediastinal fat. The dissection should extend laterally to the phrenic nerves on both sides. If the tumor does not involve the nerves, it is important to preserve them. The arterial blood supply from the internal mammary arteries can usually be divided with

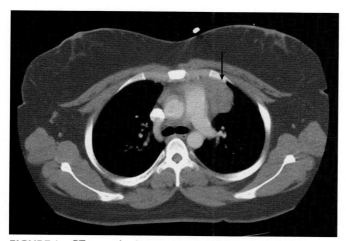

FIGURE 1 CT scan of a thymoma in the left anterior mediastinum.

TABLE 1: World Health Organization histologic categories

A	Spindle cell or medullary thymoma
AB	Mixed thymoma
B1	Lymphocyte-rich or predominately cortical thymoma
B2	Cortical thymoma
B3	Epitheleal thymoma
C	Thymic carcinoma

TABLE 2: Masaoka staging system and survival

Stage	Definition	Frequency at Presentation	5-Year Survival	10-Year Survival
I	Macroscopically encapsulated, no microscopic invasion of the capsule	40%	92%	88%
II	IIa: Macroscopic invasion into mediastinal fat or pleura IIb: Microscopic invasion of the capsule	25%	82%	70%
III	Invasion into neighboring organs	25%	68%	57%
IVa	Pleural or pericardial metastasis	10%	61%	38%
IVb	Lymphatic or hematogenous metastasis	1% to 2%		

Data summarizing the results from multiple large studies; from Detterbeck FC, Parsons AM: Thymic tumors, *Ann Thorac Surg* 77:1860–1869, 2004.

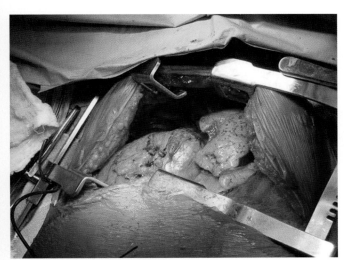

FIGURE 2 View of both pleural spaces and the mediastinum through a clamshell incision.

electrocautery. Usually the thymus and tumor can be bluntly peeled off of the pericardium; however, if the tumor invades the pericardium, it can be resected without consequence.

Recently, the use of minimally invasive thoracoscopic approaches for resecting small thymomas has increased. Invasive or locally disseminated thymomas, Masaoka stage III or IV, should be approached through a sufficiently large incision. Most commonly this is done via median sternotomy. If greater exposure is needed, particularly laterally into the pleural space, a bilateral transverse thoracotomy ("clamshell incision"; Figure 2) may be useful. Another incision that can give improved exposure in the pleural space is a partial median sternotomy that is extended into the fourth or fifth intercostal space (referred to as a J incision).

Thymomas can be associated with a wide variety of systemic syndromes. The neuromuscular disease myasthenia gravis is the most commonly associated syndrome. Myasthenia gravis is caused by autoantibodies blocking acetylcholine receptors in the neuromuscular junction. This manifests as weakness that tends to worsen with activity, and it can be seen in the muscles that control speech, respiration, the eyes, and limbs. It is estimated that 30% to 50% of patients with a thymoma will have myasthenia, but only 15% of myasthenics will have a thymoma. Thymectomy will improve the symptoms in up to 60% of patients with myasthenia, but this improvement occurs slowly over time. Because the improvement in symptoms is not immediate, thymectomy is not undertaken in the midst of myasthenic crisis. Patients with severe neurologic symptoms should be treated with plasmapheresis or intravenous γ-globulin prior to surgery. Serum levels of antiacetycholine receptor antibodies can be measured if the diagnosis of myasthenia is unclear. Patients with severe symptoms should be managed in conjunction with a neurologist.

Thymomas are also associated with hematologic abnormalities, especially red cell aplasia, immunodeficiencies, and collagen vascular diseases. Resection of the thymoma does not reliably improve the symptoms in these patients.

Unlike thymoma, thymic carcinoma is an aggressive tumor with a poor prognosis. There are two histologic types, *squamous* and *lymphoepithelioma*. Median survival of all patients is only 2 years, but this can be improved when complete surgical resection is accomplished. Aggressive resection is warranted, but overall results remain poor. Partial responses to chemotherapy and radiation therapy have been reported.

Thymic carcinoid is a rare tumor. It can be associated with multiple endocrine neoplasia type 1 (MEN1) and Cushing syndrome. Many patients have nodal metastases at the time of presentation. Even with complete resection, the recurrence rates are high, and survival rates are difficult to estimate because of the low incidence of the tumor. Other rare thymic neoplasms include small cell tumors and sarcomas.

SUGGESTED READINGS

Detterbeck FC, Parsons AM: Thymic tumors, *Ann Thorac Surg* 77:1860–1869, 2004.

Kondo K: Optimal therapy for thymoma, *J Med Invest* 55:17–28, 2008.

Thomaszek S, Wigle DA, Keshavjee S, Fischer S: Thymomas: review of current clinical practice, *Ann Thorac Surg* 87:1973–1980, 2009.

MANAGEMENT OF TRACHEAL STENOSIS

Stacey Su, MD, and Joel D. Cooper, MD

OVERVIEW

The management of tracheal stenosis is a logistic and technical exercise requiring the multidisciplinary input of thoracic surgeons, pulmonologists, otolaryngologists, experienced anesthesiologists, and intensivists at different stages of the patient's care. Patients with acquired tracheal stenosis often present with comorbidities that require medical optimization prior to surgical resection. In carefully selected patients, however, surgical resection of tracheal stenosis offers a definitive treatment with excellent outcomes and low perioperative risk. The management of tracheal stenosis encompasses diagnosis, initial assessment and often management of a critical airway, temporizing maneuvers, and ultimate definitive treatment.

Tracheal resections can be broadly divided into three different types, each of which requires a specific operative approach and technique, depending on the location and extent of tracheal involvement. The most straightforward of these is a segmental resection with end-to-end anastomosis of a stenosis located in the proximal to mid-trachea. Resections at either end of the trachea, namely a laryngotracheal resection at the upper end or a carinal resection at the other end, may require unique release maneuvers, different approaches, and more complicated anastomotic procedures.

ETIOLOGY

Characterization of tracheal stenosis is based on the etiology of the stenosis, its location and length, whether the stenosis is evolving or mature in nature, and whether the stenosis is limited to a single segment or separate segments in series. Each of these factors is considered in planning the most appropriate intervention.

Benign conditions for which tracheal resection is considered include traumatic injury, inhalation injury, postintubation and post-tracheostomy stricture, postintubation tracheoesophageal fistula, and a variety of inflammatory conditions. One such cause is idiopathic subglottic stenosis, which occurs primarily in young women. Idiopathic subglottic stenosis requires unique attention in terms of management. The division of the airway and reconstruction must be performed in a way that spares the recurrent laryngeal nerves. Benign tracheal stenosis may also occur as part of a constellation of systemic inflammatory diseases, for example Wegener granulomatosis, relapsing polychondritis, sarcoidosis, or amyloidosis.

The most common benign cause of tracheal stenosis is acquired stenosis as a result of prolonged endotracheal intubation or as a complication related to a previous tracheostomy. Although these two acquired forms both represent postintubation strictures, they are explained by different pathophysiologies. Whether from endotracheal or tracheostomy tubes, cuff strictures typically become symptomatic 6 to 10 weeks after extubation, when the damaged tracheal segment undergoes cicatricial contraction. The etiology of cuff strictures was initially attributable to the ill-suited design and physical properties of high-pressure cuffs. The inflation of the highly elastic, relatively rigid balloon to create an adequate seal within the elliptical cross section of the trachea often led to transmural ischemic injury to the tracheal wall with ulceration and dissolution of the adjacent cartilaginous rings. This pattern of stricture manifests as a tight circumferential stenosis with surrounding tissue inflammation. With the introduction of low-pressure, high-volume cuffs on endotracheal and tracheostomy tubes, the incidence of cuff stricture decreased significantly; but it persists today, in spite of improved cuff design.

Cuff stricture is caused in part by choosing a cuffed tube that has too small a resting diameter or by overinflation of the cuff. In general, for an adult patient, the cuff should have a minimum diameter of 2.5 cm in the resting state, so that inflation achieves a seal without having to stretch the cuff. If not, inflation can transform a soft, deformable cuff into a rigid, high-pressure cuff. Furthermore, cuff pressures must be closely monitored to avoid cuff overinflation. The minimum cuff pressure required to achieve an adequate seal around the cuff is defined as the patient's peak airway pressure at any given time. Factors that increase peak airway pressure, such as obesity and poor lung compliance, may require a higher cuff pressure, which in turn results in pressure necrosis to the tracheal wall, especially with a prolonged period of ventilatory assistance.

In contrast to cuff strictures, stomal stenosis is characterized by less severe and less progressive symptoms, which may first be detected years after the tracheostomy was placed. The etiology behind stomal strictures is due to loss of anterior tracheal wall support and inward collapse of the lateral walls. This can result from excessive removal of cartilage to accommodate an inappropriately large tracheostomy tube, relative to the tracheal lumen, and to excessive tension on tracheostomy tubing, which leads to erosion of the cartilage around the tracheostomy stoma. This pattern of stricture is characterized by an upside-down, V-shaped stenosis anteriorly with preservation of the anteroposterior diameter but side-to-side narrowing, which leads to loss of cross-sectional area. Stomal stenosis can sometimes lead to airway obliteration, especially in cases of high placement of tracheostomies, at the level of the cricoid cartilage (Figure 1).

Airway obstruction from malignant tumors may result from extrinsic compression, local transmural invasion, or endoluminal obstruction. Indications for tracheal resection for malignant tumors include adenoid cystic carcinoma, locally invasive thyroid cancer, and primary squamous carcinoma of the trachea. Adenoid cystic carcinoma is characterized by extensive microscopic involvement of the tracheal wall well beyond the visible borders of involvement. Resection in these cases may be of value, even if the final margins show microscopic involvement, as subsequent postoperative radiation may be associated with survival of 10 years or more. Resection for primary squamous

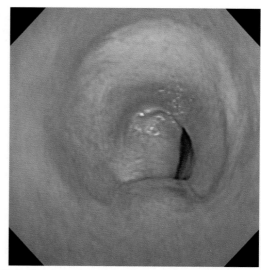

FIGURE 1 This bronchoscopic view shows a nearly obliterated upper airway, which may result from postintubation stenosis or high tracheostomies incorrectly placed near the cricoid.

carcinoma of the trachea is rare because of the advanced stage at the time of diagnosis and likelihood of mediastinal nodal involvement.

PREOPERATIVE WORKUP

Routine preoperative assessment includes a history, physical exam, radiographic imaging, and bronchoscopic evaluation. Whenever possible, patients undergo pulmonary function tests, including a flow-volume loop, which shows a decrease in both maximal inspiratory and expiratory flows. Standard radiographs include anteroposterior and lateral cervical views. Fluoroscopy, which was previously used to evaluate dynamic features such as tracheomalacia, has been replaced by spiral computed tomographic (CT) imaging performed during inspiration and expiration. A three-dimensional (3D) reconstruction using CT of the airway yields measurements of the length of the stenosis and its relationship to the rest of the airway. These measurements serve as a guide before proceeding to more precise confirmation by bronchoscopy. Although the 3D reconstruction may be somewhat misleading, depending on the technique of acquisition—that is, whether the images are reconstructed from the soft-tissue images or from the air column—it is nonetheless helpful to demonstrate the thickness of the tracheal wall above and below the stenosis, as well as the luminal dimensions (Figure 2).

As part of the thoracic surgeon's diagnostic armamentarium, the use of bronchoscopy is essential to show the anatomy of the larynx and glottis, the function of the vocal cords, and the configuration of the stenosis and remaining trachea. It is important to note the distance from the stenosis to anatomic landmarks (vocal cords, carina, tracheal stoma) in addition to the length of the stenotic segment and the health of the surrounding mucosa.

PRE-RESECTION AIRWAY MANAGEMENT

Management of critical tracheal stenosis requires close cooperation among the surgeon, anesthesiologist, and nursing staff. The immediate objectives of operative intervention in the acute setting are to safely evaluate the anatomy and establish a patent airway. Examination through a flexible bronchoscope with a laryngeal mask in place allows access to and complete evaluation of the larynx, vocal cords, and the extent of the entire airway. Especially in the case of critical stenosis, it is important to avoid muscle relaxants, until a safe airway has been established. The equipment for an emergent tracheostomy should be readily available in case it is needed.

General anesthesia is usually administered through a combination of inhaled and intravenous forms. Although not an ideal general anesthetic, dexmedetomidine is a sedative that produces minimal depression of respiratory drive, and it can be used to maintain spontaneous breathing in a patient during bronchoscopy.

As a therapeutic modality, bronchoscopy may be utilized to initially establish an adequate airway or to dilate tracheal stenosis on repeated occasions. Dilations are achieved by balloon or rigid bronchoscopy. The Alliance CRE balloon dilator system (Boston Scientific, Natick, Mass.) applies radial pressure dilation to the entire stenosis throughout the length of the balloon. Under direct visualization, it can also be used over a guidewire in areas that are difficult to intubate, such as nearly obliterated airways. However, balloon dilations often do not lead to as significant an increase in the diameter as expected; this is because of the "hourglass" indentation that the inflated balloon assumes within a tight stricture. For this reason, dilations achieved in this manner are not as effective as those achieved by rigid bronchoscopy.

Rigid bronchoscopy capitalizes on the beveled tip of the scope, which is used as a leading edge to intubate tight stenoses. Available in various sizes from various manufacturers, rigid bronchoscopes can be serially used, starting with pediatric sizes and increasing in diameter. This allows for safe, successive dilation while maintaining

the ability to ventilate, visualize, and suction at the same time. When using small diameter scopes, a laryngoscope can assist with the introduction of the scope into the airway.

The inflammatory process underlying conditions such as postintubation strictures and idiopathic subglottic stenosis often leads to recurrence of granulation tissue at the site of previous dilations. This is one reason why the use of laser ablation or electrocautery to treat strictures usually leads to recurrent stenosis. On the one hand, performing repeated dilations allows the clinician to witness the benefit gained by the patient in the postdilation period and to delay resection until the patient's medical condition is optimized. This permits strategic timing of surgery and selective treatment of patients whose symptoms are directly attributable to tracheal stenosis, as opposed to other confounding conditions such as chronic obstructive pulmonary disease (COPD) and cardiopulmonary deconditioning.

Most cases of critical stenosis can be initially managed for 7 to 10 days with a single dilation, after which an overall plan for long-term management of the airway should be formulated. This takes into consideration the patient's overall medical condition and surgical candidacy. The options include serial dilation, elective referral for surgical resection, or placement of an airway prosthesis (stent, tracheostomy, or T tube). If tracheal resection is planned in the ensuing few weeks, dilation alone may be adequate to carry the patient until this time. If internal tracheal stents are to be used, only silicone stents or T tubes should be utilized since expandable metal stents potentially lead to further mucosal damage and complicate a subsequent surgical resection.

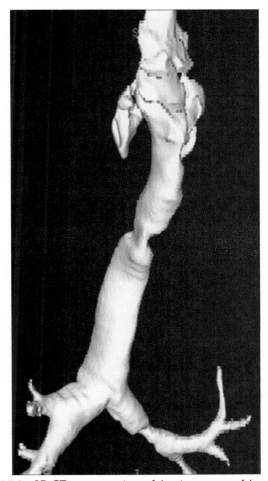

FIGURE 2 3D CT reconstructions of the airway are useful to assess the configuration of tracheal stenosis before precise measurements are obtained by bronchoscopy.

T tubes offer an alternative to the use of internal tracheal stents in maintaining a patent airway across a stenosis. Made of silicone that can be custom sized, the T tube has a horizontal limb that exits the airway from a tracheal stoma and effectively stents across a stenosis through its proximal or distal vertical limb. Its advantages are manifold: it offers patients a more comfortable solution compared with rigid tracheostomy tubes, allows phonation when capped, and provides easy access to the proximal and distal airway for pulmonary toilet. However, T tubes should only be used if the patient can breathe comfortably with the horizontal limb capped, as otherwise the upper vertical limb becomes inspissated with mucus.

Finally, tracheal strictures can be treated with tracheostomy, with the tip of the tube extending beyond the stenosis. Although it is a commonly performed procedure, tracheostomy is not without its disadvantages and can itself lead to stomal stenosis. The tracheal stoma should be situated if at all possible through the damaged portion of the airway with the objective of preserving as much length of normal trachea as possible. In some cases, a T tube or tracheostomy affords a long-term solution to airway stenosis, either in patients with multiple segments of affected trachea or in those who are poor surgical candidates for resection.

TRACHEAL RESECTION

The last few decades have seen a shift in clinical practice, as data on tracheal resection and reconstruction has yielded excellent outcomes with tolerable morbidity and mortality rates. Tracheal resection carries multiple benefits. Primary reconstruction offers immediate decannulation. The question of which patient characteristics make up a good surgical candidate requires a consideration of risk factors for poor outcomes in tracheal resection. As there is seldom a situation that requires emergent tracheal resection and reconstruction, careful patient selection and appropriate timing of surgery are central to successful outcomes of resection. The routine use of steroids and any ongoing requirement for ventilatory support set the stage for a higher rate of anastomotic dehiscence and other complications of tracheal resection. Any patient with reversible medical conditions should have resection deferred, until they are optimally conditioned and deemed best equipped from a cardiopulmonary standpoint. After a failed tracheal resection, reoperation is associated with increased risk and complexity, and it may produce an inferior result compared to an initial, successful reconstruction.

Principles of Tracheal Resection

The principles of tracheal resection are derived from elementary surgical tenets: a healthy anastomosis will result from meticulous mucosal apposition between well-vascularized tissues approximated without undue tension. To that end, the following corollaries hold 1) the limits of tracheal resection must extend to healthy, normal tissues, and 2) circumferential dissection beyond the resected ends should be minimized so as not to jeopardize the segmental nature of tracheal blood supply. Up to half of the trachea (about 6 cm) may be resected with primary end-to-end anastomosis. However, if more than three to four cartilaginous rings are resected, tension-releasing maneuvers beyond flexion of the head and mediastinal mobilization within the avascular pretracheal plane must be employed. Such maneuvers include the suprahyoid release, as described by Montgomery, and the hilar release; each of these permits an additional 1 to 2 cm of resection. Important landmarks include the posterior cricoid plate, behind which the recurrent laryngeal nerves ascend to enter the cricoarytenoid joint on either side. Excepting this area, dissection immediately adjacent to the tracheal wall will prevent injury to the recurrent laryngeal nerves and esophagus. When the condition to resect back to healthy tissue cannot be met—for example, in many inflammatory conditions, where there are multiple affected segments in series or

globally inflamed mucosa—surgical candidacy for tracheal resection must be questioned.

Important Landmarks

The cartilaginous skeleton of the larynx, which houses the vocal cords, consists of the thyroid, cricoid, and arytenoid cartilages. Here the external diameter is narrowest at the cricoid cartilage and the internal diameter is narrowest at the level of the vocal cords. The recurrent laryngeal nerves lie in the tracheoesophageal groove and enter the larynx at the level of the inferior cornu of the thyroid cartilage. The cricoarytenoid joints lie at the back of the larynx and rotate with vibration of the vocal cords. Injury to the cricoarytenoid joints during posterior dissection of the cricoid plate may lead to restricted excursion of the vocal cords and airway obstruction.

Incisions

The surgical approach is dictated by the location and extent of diseased trachea. Malignant lesions involving the upper and middle thirds of the trachea and benign conditions extending down to within three rings of the carina may be managed through a cervical incision but may also require a partial sternotomy for adequate visualization. Malignant lesions involving the distal third and benign conditions extending within three rings of the carina may be accessed via a right thoracotomy, although a transsternal approach can also be considered. The latter approach allows an exposure of the carina by incising the posterior pericardium while retracting the superior vena cava to the right and the ascending aorta to the left.

Operative Steps

Management of the airway requires close communication between the surgeon and anesthesiologist. At the start of the procedure, assessment by bronchoscopy guides whether initial dilation is required to permit the passage of an endotracheal tube beyond the stenosis. In the setting of nearly obstructive lesions, induction without use of paralytic agents should be employed to preserve spontaneous ventilation. If possible, intubation across the lesion is preferred, unless a preexisting tracheostomy is in place. Sterile anesthesia tubing and connectors are handed to the anesthesiologist for use across the operative field.

Upon tracheal division, the endotracheal tube is retracted out of the field, and a sterile, cuffed 6-0 flexible armored endotracheal tube is intermittently inserted into the distal trachea to provide cross-table ventilation. Alternatively, a jet ventilation catheter can be directly placed into the distal airway from the field, or a separate jet catheter can be advanced from within the lumen of the partially withdrawn oropharyngeal endotracheal tube. This is our preferred method whenever possible. Once the anastomotic sutures for the posterior wall are complete, the original orotracheal tube is advanced into the distal airway, until the procedure is complete.

With an eye toward upholding the above principles of tracheal resection, the steps of tracheal resection and reconstruction can be reduced to the following: 1) localize the diseased segment, 2) mobilize the trachea, 3) transect the trachea, 4) resect the affected area, 5) and reconstruct.

The patient is placed supine with a roll beneath the upper back to extend the neck. An esophageal bougie (size 30 Maloney) or nasogastric tube can be placed to facilitate later dissection of the trachea from the esophagus. A cervical incision centered at the cricoid cartilage is made. Skin flaps are elevated in the subplatysmal plane, extending from the superior extent of the larynx to the sternal notch inferiorly (Figure 3). The larynx and upper trachea are partially mobilized by bluntly developing the plane between the superficial and deep layers of the strap muscles. The strap muscles are retracted laterally, and the

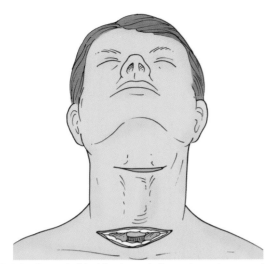

FIGURE 3   A cervical incision is made 2 cm above the sternal notch. Through the cervical incision, skin flaps are elevated, extending from the larynx superiorly to the sternal notch inferiorly. In laryngotracheal resections, a suprahyoid release may be performed through a separate transverse incision over the hyoid bone. *(From Urschel HC Jr, Cooper JC: Atlas of thoracic surgery, New York, 1995, Churchill Livingstone, p 121.)*

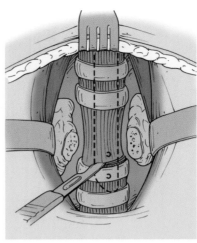

FIGURE 4   Once the thyroid isthmus is divided, the tracheal stenosis is evident through the outward appearance of a narrowing, dense scar and surrounding inflammation. A circumferential tracheal dissection is carefully performed, and the trachea is transected through the stenotic segment. *(From Urschel HC Jr, Cooper JC: Atlas of thoracic surgery, New York, 1995, Churchill Livingstone, p 113.)*

thyroid isthmus is divided in the midline. The pretracheal plane is bluntly developed with a finger toward the carina.

The level of the tracheal stenosis is usually evident through the outward appearance of narrowing, dense scarring, and surrounding inflammation (Figure 4). The tracheal stenosis can also be localized with the use of a flexible bronchoscope inserted through the endotracheal tube and is identified with a transtracheal 25 gauge needle inserted through the tracheal wall under bronchoscopic control. The tracheal wall at this point is then marked with a fine stitch. After mobilization is complete, circumferential tracheal dissection at the level of the affected segment is performed sharply, taking care to remain close to the tracheal wall to minimize risk of injury to the recurrent laryngeal nerves and to avoid airway devascularization.

Before the trachea is incised, proximal and distal 2-0 silk traction sutures are placed 1 to 2 cm away from the proposed line of resection on either side in the midlateral position, and the trachea is partially transected anteriorly through the stenotic segment. Subsequent incisions can be extended distally, until the airway lumen is sufficient to allow direct tracheal intubation and cross-table ventilation. Transection of the posterior wall of the trachea is performed under direct vision from the luminal, as well as external, aspects with the esophageal bougie used as a guide to help avoid esophageal injury when separating the membranous wall of the airway from the esophagus. The caliber and thickness of the airway wall at the distal extent of the resection is evaluated. If the distal end is not free of disease, further resection is done, incising 1 to 2 mm at a time in a "bread loaf" fashion to avoid removing normal airway.

Attention is then turned to the proximal end of the stenosis, which is gradually incised in stepwise fashion, until normal airway is encountered. With the head in flexion and the shoulder roll removed, the traction sutures are approximated to determine whether adequate mobilization has been achieved to allow a tension-free anastomosis, or whether a release maneuver will be required. If no release maneuvers are needed, a single layer of interrupted 4-0 vicryl sutures lubricated with mineral oil is placed along the posterior membranous wall in an end-to-end fashion. Sutures are placed 3 to 4 mm apart and 3 to 4 mm away from the edge. The armored tube is removed and replaced as needed to allow the meticulous placement of sutures.

Alternatively, a jet catheter into the distal airway can be used, either through the partially withdrawn endotracheal tube or across the field directly into the distal end of the trachea (Figure 5). Folded blankets are placed under the head to maintain it in a flexed position, while the posterior wall sutures are tied. Once the posterior wall is complete, the anesthesiologist advances the jet catheter within the oropharyngeal endotracheal tube and continues ventilation in this manner, while the sutures for the anterior anastomosis are placed. Before the anterior wall sutures are tied, the oropharyngeal endotracheal tube is advanced past the anastomosis. With the endotracheal tube cuff desufflated, the anesthesiologist tests the anastomosis for a leak by insufflating to 20 cm H_2O airway pressures.

If the airway damage involves the cricoid cartilage, as in the case of idiopathic subglottic stenosis, the anterior cricoid ring can be removed to the midpoint of its lateral aspect on either side. The posterior cricoid plate can be partially reamed out with a pituitary rongeur or a diamond burr, but its posterior perichondrium must be preserved to protect the recurrent laryngeal nerves. The perichondrium and mucosa anterior to the cricoid plate form the subsequent posterior portion of the anastomosis to the membranous portion of the distal trachea. Fine stainless steel wire may be used to provide a strong, inert suture line and decrease the formation of granulation tissue, which can result from the use of absorbable sutures.

To protect it from erosion into surrounding structures, such as the innominate artery, the anastomosis may be buttressed by reapproximating the thyroid isthmus or strap muscles. If necessary a pedicled strap muscle may be used. A Penrose drain is placed in the subplatysmal plane prior to reapproximating the platysma and skin. At the end of the procedure, a "guardian" chin stitch is placed between the submental crease and the skin of the anterior chest wall at the level of the sternomanubrial junction. The stitch serves as a reminder to the patient to keep the neck flexed and thus avoid excessive tension on the anastomosis. As the patient resumes spontaneous ventilation and slowly awakens from general anesthesia, a final bronchoscopy is performed via a laryngeal mask to observe vocal cord function, glottic edema, and anastomotic patency.

Release Maneuvers

When residual tracheal length is deemed inadequate for the creation of an end-to-end anastomosis without tension, it is advisable to perform a release maneuver to release the larynx from its superior attachments. As a guideline, a release is usually anticipated if 4 cm or more of tracheal length is resected. Because of the decrease in associated pharyngeal dysfunction and risk for aspiration in the early postoperative interval, the suprahyoid release described by Montgomery is

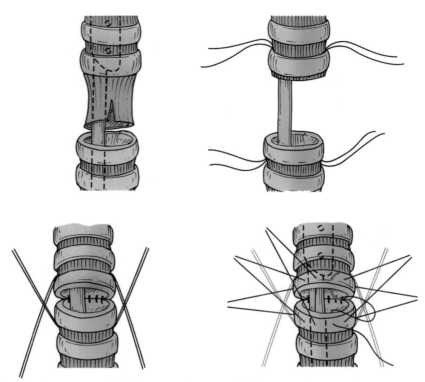

FIGURE 5 While the trachea remains transected, the airway may be managed with a jet ventilation catheter placed in the distal airway, either across the field or through the lumen of a partially withdrawn oral endotracheal tube. The posterior wall of the anastomosis is performed with the jet catheter in position. Before the anterior wall sutures are secured, the endotracheal tube is carefully advanced over the jet catheter and past the anastomosis. *(From Urschel HC Jr, Cooper JC: Atlas of thoracic surgery, New York, 1995, Churchill Livingstone, p 115.)*

preferred to the infrahyoid release described by Dedo, Fishman, and Ogura. The suprahyoid release may be carried out through a separate, short transverse incision over the hyoid bone and is ideally performed prior to tracheal transection. The subplatysmal plane between the two incisions is fully developed so as to maximize the descent of the larynx. Once the hyoid bone is exposed, the muscle attachments to its superior surface are sharply divided, and the lesser cornu of the hyoid bone are transected. The hyoid bone is vertically divided on either side lateral to the transected lesser cornu, allowing the central portion of the released bone to descend along with the larynx. The preepiglottic tissue is then incised with a scalpel down to the mucosa.

In the case of a laryngotracheal resection, a vertical laryngofissure may improve access to the posterior mucosa along the subglottic region. With the thyroid alae separated, careful coring out of the cricoid plate superiorly toward the level of the vocal cords can be performed while preserving the cricoarytenoid joints intact. If posterior scar tissue extends between the arytenoids, collaboration with an otolaryngologist will allow the advancement of a supraglottic mucosal flap to cover the posterior portion of the anastomosis. The posterior and lateral aspects of the anastomosis are completed before the laryngofissure is closed. After closure, the anterior portion of the anastomosis to the inferior rim of the thyroid cartilage anteriorly can be completed. Usually a portion of the cricothyroid membrane is preserved along the lower edge of the thyroid cartilage to facilitate the anterior portion of the anastomosis.

A postoperative protective tracheostomy should be considered when a laryngotracheal tracheotomy has been performed. At the completion of the resection, a cuffless minitracheostomy (Portex #4 OD, ID) can be placed a couple of rings below the anastomosis through the inferior skin flap. The decision to place a tracheostomy postoperatively is determined based on expected vocal cord edema rather than by anticipation of an ongoing need for positive-pressure ventilation. The tracheostomy assures airway patency prior to resolution

of perioperative edema and also facilitates pulmonary toilet. Minitracheostomies require additional nursing education for safe, informed handling.

POSTOPERATIVE MANAGEMENT

There is no role for routine use of prolonged postoperative systemic steroids. A dose of methyl prednisolone sodium succinate (Solu-medrol 250 mg) may be administered at the end of the procedure, followed by one or two doses in the first 24 to 36 hours. To further decrease glottic and supraglottic edema and to improve airflow, a variety of concurrent maneuvers may be employed; these include voice rest, racemic epinephrine nebulizers, humidified air, maintaining an upright position, gentle diuresis, and heliox administration. To decrease the movement of the larynx and avoid aspiration, patients are maintained NPO for the first few days, with a longer interval prescribed the closer the anastomosis lies relative to the glottis. Bedside swallow evaluations are initially performed by the staff, starting with jello and followed by oral intake monitored for cough or other signs that accompany aspiration. Patients are slowly advanced in their diet accordingly.

Laryngotracheal resections are associated with a higher rate of transient pharyngeal dyscoordination with the potential risk of aspiration attributable to postoperative pain and regardless of the status of glottic sensory feedback. Physical restrictions against hyperextension are initially reinforced through the maintenance of the chin stitch for the first 5 to 7 days after resection.

One week postoperatively, a surveillance bronchoscopy is performed to evaluate the health and patency of the anastomosis. Patients are subsequently scheduled for outpatient visits at established intervals and monitored for symptoms that might herald the development of anastomotic strictures or excessive granulation tissue at the anastomosis.

OPERATIVE RESULTS

The rationale behind rigorous planning of the timing and selection of surgical candidates before tracheal resection is to avoid complications that can be life threatening, if an adequate airway is compromised. Temporizing maneuvers, including tracheostomy, may be used for as long as a year to reduce or eliminate comorbidities that could compromise the surgical outcome. Grillo and colleagues were among the first to publish their experience with complications after tracheal resection. They demonstrated a progressive rise in tension with increasing length of resection and suggested a safe limit of 4.5 cm, corresponding to 1000 g of tension, to avoid anastomotic failure. Airway complications can be divided into those that involve the anastomosis and those that do not. Airway-related complications that do not involve the anastomosis include glottic edema, aspiration, vocal cord paralysis, and the need for a temporary tracheostomy. These are more common after a laryngotracheal resection than with simple segmental tracheal resection.

Anastomotic complications are uncommon but can lead to severe morbidity when they do occur. They result from infection or excessive tension across the suture line and manifest along a spectrum of severity that ranges from granulation tissue to stenosis to airway disruption. The incidence of complications varies according to the underlying pathology of tracheal stenosis, and whether the anastomosis involves the larynx. In the largest series of tracheal resections, examining 901 cases over 28 years, Wright and colleagues reported that the highest rate of anastomotic complications occurred in diagnoses such as tracheoesophageal fistula and postintubation stenosis rather than idiopathic subglottic stenosis and tracheal tumors.

Successful results following resection were identified in 95% of patients, anastomotic complications occurred at a rate of 9%, and overall perioperative mortality rate was 1.2%. A multivariate analysis identified certain risk factors to be associated with anastomotic complications; these include diabetes, reoperation, longer resections (>4 cm), young age (pediatric patients <17 years), need for tracheostomy before the operation, and laryngotracheal resection. Some of these factors—such as preoperative tracheostomy, longer resections, and laryngotracheal resection—are surrogate markers of more complicated injuries with greater severity of tracheal involvement. In patients who had anastomotic complications, the mortality was 7.4%; in those without them, it was 0.01%.

This series established the excellent outcomes of surgical resection and the associated low mortality rate that can be achieved in the hands of experienced surgeons. It also emphasizes the value of routine bronchoscopy before hospital discharge in the early detection of anastomotic complications. Depending on the severity, anastomotic complications may be managed by bronchoscopic interventions such as debridement and dilation, placement of an airway stent, tracheostomy, or reoperation. Limited separation may heal over temporary silicone stents or T tubes without further intervention. If deemed necessary, reoperation is usually deferred for at least 6 months to a year, until peritracheal inflammation resolves maximally.

SUGGESTED READINGS

Ashiku SK, Kuzucu A, Grillo HC, et al: Idiopathic laryngotracheal stenosis: effective definitive treatment with laryngotracheal resection, *J Thorac Cardiovasc Surg* 127(1):99–107, 2004.

Grillo HC, Mathisen DJ, Wain JC: Laryngotracheal resection and reconstruction for subglottic stenosis, *Ann Thorac Surg* 53(1):54–63, 1992.

Grillo HC, Donahue DM, Mathisen DJ, et al: Postintubation tracheal stenosis: treatment and results, *J Thorac Cardiovasc Surg* 109(3):486–492, 1995.

Grillo HC: *Surgery of the trachea and bronchi*, ed 1, Hamilton, Ontario, 2004, BC Decker.

Mathisen DJ: Surgery of the trachea, *Curr Probl Surg* 35(6):453–542, 1998.

Montgomery WW: The surgical management of supraglottic and subglottic stenosis, *Ann Otol Rhinol Laryngol* 77(3):534–546, 1968.

Pearson FG, Cooper JD, Nelems JM, et al: Primary tracheal anastomosis after resection of the cricoid cartilage with preservation of recurrent laryngeal nerves, *J Thorac Cardiovasc Surg* 70(5):806–816, 1975.

Urschel HC Jr, Cooper JD: *Atlas of thoracic surgery*, ed 1, New York, 1995, Churchill Livingstone.

Wright CD, Grillo HC, Wain JC, et al: Anastomotic complications after tracheal resection: prognostic factors and management, *J Thorac Cardiovasc Surg* 128(5):731–739, 2004.

MANAGEMENT OF ACQUIRED ESOPHAGEAL RESPIRATORY TRACT FISTULA

Ashok Muniappan, MD, and Douglas J. Mathisen, MD

OVERVIEW

Acquired esophageal respiratory tract fistulas are encountered in a variety of benign and malignant disorders. In all cases, patients typically present with signs and symptoms of aspiration and difficulty with oral intake, and they are often on the verge of a precipitous decline in clinical status. Although the management of malignant fistulas has evolved from an operative approach to a largely endoscopic approach, the management of benign fistulas relies on established and trusted operative techniques.

BENIGN ESOPHAGEAL RESPIRATORY TRACT FISTULA

Benign esophageal respiratory tract fistulas are most commonly associated with prolonged mechanical ventilation via an orotracheal or tracheostomy tube. They can also arise in the setting of trauma or inflammatory conditions that include mediastinal granulomatous disease, caustic injuries of the airway or esophagus, and mediastinal infection. Although there are isolated reports of spontaneous closure of very small, benign esophageal respiratory tract fistulas, in general, operative closure should be undertaken.

POSTINTUBATION TRACHEOESOPHAGEAL FISTULA

Postintubation tracheoesophageal fistula (TEF) is a well-known complication of prolonged mechanical ventilation that has been mitigated, but not eliminated, by the use of low-pressure, high-volume cuffed tubes. An indwelling, hard nasogastric tube that presses against the inflated tracheal cuff is also thought to contribute to the development of TEF. The problem is commonly diagnosed while the patient is still being ventilated, and it is recognized usually due to an acute difficulty with ventilation or gross aspiration of gastric contents.

Bronchoscopy with movement or removal of the orotracheal or tracheostomy tube is necessary to confirm the diagnosis and manage immediate complications, such as aspiration. The length of the fistula, distances from the vocal cords and carina, and other tracheal pathology, such as stenosis, should be assessed. Immediate operative intervention is avoided in mechanically ventilated patients. Repair is most likely to succeed in patients who are spontaneously breathing at the conclusion of the operation. A long tracheostomy tube (a variety of vendors supply nonstandard or custom tube lengths), in which the cuff resides distal to the TEF, should be used while the patient is weaned from ventilatory support. The nasogastric tube is removed, a gastrostomy tube is placed for drainage, and a jejunostomy tube is placed for nutritional support. When the patient has been weaned completely from mechanical ventilation, and their condition has improved, definitive repair may be undertaken. Although there are a variety of approaches to repair postintubation TEFs, the anterior cervical approach is the most common and is very successful.

any tracheal stoma, and subplatysmal flaps are developed cephalad and caudally. A partial sternotomy to just below the angle of Louis may be performed to enhance access to a TEF that is relatively distal. The strap muscles are separated in the midline, and the thyroid isthmus is divided.

If there is no tracheostomy stoma, the trachea is exposed anteriorly from the cricoid cartilage to the carina. The proximal and distal extents of the fistula are identified by introducing a 25 gauge needle anteriorly under bronchoscopic vision. When a stoma is present, a decision must be made as to whether the tracheal stoma should be encompassed by the planned resection; if it is far enough away from the fistula, it may be left intact.

Circumferential dissection around the trachea is performed at the site of the planned division or resection, with care taken to dissect directly on the trachea; to avoid nerve palsy, no attempt should be made to visualize the recurrent nerves. The trachea is divided, typically at the distal extent of the fistula, and intermittent cross-field ventilation is established by intubating the distal trachea. The orotracheal tube is withdrawn into the proximal trachea, and the esophagus is dissected away from the membranous aspect of the trachea above and below.

TRACHEAL RESECTION AND RECONSTRUCTION WITH ESOPHAGEAL FISTULA CLOSURE

Grillo promulgated the anterior cervical approach (Figures 1 through 4) to repair postintubation TEFs. This approach recognizes that associated tracheal stenosis and malacia at the fistula is often present that is best managed with concomitant tracheal resection and reconstruction. Even if tracheal resection is unnecessary in patients with relatively normal tracheal anatomy, division of the trachea in the anterior approach greatly facilitates the dissection and repair of the esophageal defect. The trachea is then simply reanastomosed without any tracheal resection.

The patient is positioned supine, with the back elevated and the neck extended. A low cervical collar incision is used that encompasses

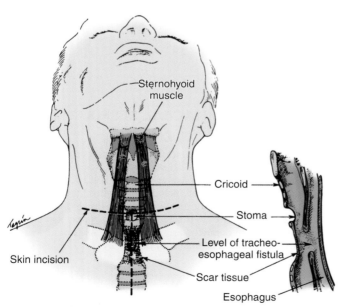

FIGURE 1 Anterior approach for postintubation tracheoesophageal fistula. Most high fistulas can be repaired through a simple collar incision. For lower fistulas, the manubrium can be divided in the midline to give excellent exposure. *(From Mathisen DJ, Grillo HC, Wain JC, et al: Management of acquired nonmalignant tracheoesophageal fistula, Ann Thorac Surg 52:759, 1991.)*

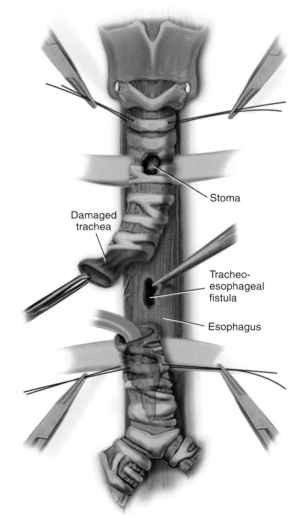

FIGURE 2 The trachea is divided below the fistula, providing excellent exposure to the esophageal fistula. The distal trachea is intubated with a sterile endotracheal tube for ventilation. *(From Mathisen DJ, Grillo HC, Wain JC, et al: Management of acquired nonmalignant tracheoesophageal fistula, Ann Thorac Surg 52:759, 1991.)*

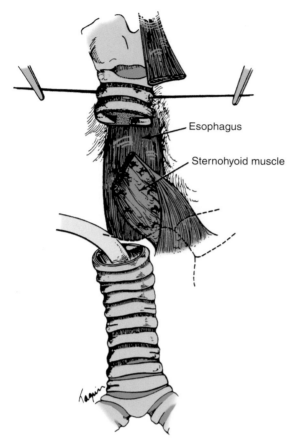

FIGURE 3 The esophagus is closed, and a pedicled strap muscle is carefully sutured around the edges to provide a reinforcing layer and to separate the two suture lines. *(From Mathisen DJ, Grillo HC, Wain JC, et al: Management of acquired nonmalignant tracheoesophageal fistula, Ann Thorac Surg 52:759, 1991.)*

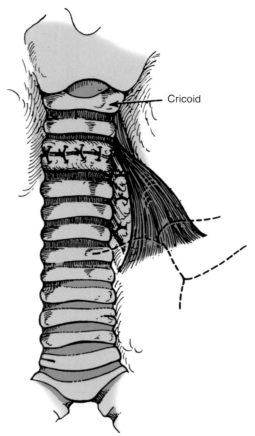

FIGURE 4 The tracheal repair is complete; the pedicled strap muscle is seen separating the two suture lines. *(From Mathisen DJ, Grillo HC, Wain JC, et al: Management of acquired nonmalignant tracheoesophageal fistula, Ann Thorac Surg 52:759, 1991.)*

Next, the edges of the esophagus are freshened, the mucosa is identified, and a two-layered longitudinal repair is performed over a nasogastric tube. The inner layer is a series of inverting, interrupted 4-0 silk sutures through the full thickness of the mucosa, with the knots lying within the esophageal lumen. The outer layer is a series of interrupted 4-0 silk sutures that approximate the esophageal muscle over the mucosal closure. The sternohyoid muscle, which is the muscle flap that is used most often, is mobilized and based inferiorly to cover the esophageal repair and to separate it from the tracheal reconstruction.

The tracheal reconstruction is performed in our standard fashion. Stay sutures (2-0 Vicryl; Ethicon, Somerville, NJ) are placed laterally in the proximal and distal trachea. Interrupted sutures using 4-0 Vicryl are then placed in a circumferential fashion, starting with the posterior membranous wall. After placement of the sutures, the orotracheal tube is advanced across the anastomosis, and the neck is flexed to reduce tension once the sutures are tied. The stay sutures are tied together first, followed by the finer anastomotic sutures. The anterior tracheal suture line is also covered with a strap muscle, the cervical incision is closed in layers over a suction drain, and the patient is extubated in the operating room.

When the length of the tracheal involvement is too long for resection and reconstruction, repair of the fistula should still be performed. The esophagus is repaired in two layers as described and covered with a strap muscle. The trachea may then be closed over a T tube (Figure 5). Intraoperative management of the airway is facilitated by placing a pediatric endotracheal tube through the side arm of the T tube once it is in place. The correct length of the tube is determined and confirmed intraoperatively by bronchoscopy.

REPAIR OF ACQUIRED BENIGN BRONCHOESOPHAGEAL FISTULA

Benign causes of bronchoesophageal fistula (Figure 6) include histoplasmosis, silicosis, foreign-body impaction, caustic injury, and postoperative complication, such as from esophagectomy. The diagnosis is confirmed by barium swallow and endoscopy. Almost all patients should have operative repair, and the approach is typically through a right thoracotomy, which permits division of the fistula. The bronchus and esophagus are repaired primarily, and resection of either is typically unnecessary. As with tracheoesophageal fistulas, we prefer a two-layered closure of the esophagus, and the repairs are separated by vascularized tissue. The intercostal muscle flap is an excellent option for this purpose, and 12 out of 13 patients who underwent this procedure at our institution had excellent results.

Important Considerations

Although benign esophageal respiratory tract fistulas are relatively uncommon, when they do occur, careful patient preparation and operative planning are required. It is critical that patients be weaned from mechanical ventilatory support before operating to abrogate the possibility of positive pressure on the airway suture line. Once the patient is ready, an operation is performed that not only eliminates the fistula but also corrects any airway pathology. We also are diligent about interposing vascularized tissue between the esophageal and airway suture lines to avoid a recurrence.

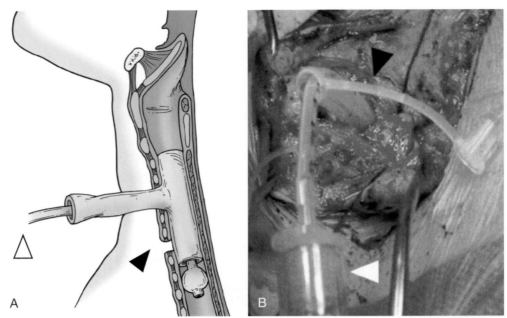

FIGURE 5 Tracheal repair performed over a T tube. When the tracheal disease is too long to resect, the esophageal fistula should still be repaired; the trachea may be closed over a T tube (*black arrowhead*) without any resection. The patient may be ventilated with a pediatric endotracheal tube placed within the T tube (*white arrowhead*). *(Illustration courtesy Edith Tagrin.)*

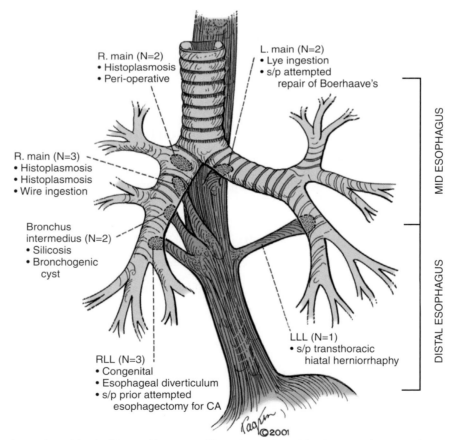

FIGURE 6 Benign bronchoesophageal fistula. Observed locations of bronchoesophageal fistula in a single series of patients. *CA,* Cancer; *LLL,* left lower-lobe bronchus; *L. MAIN,* left main stem bronchus; *RLL,* right lower-lobe bronchus; *R. MAIN,* right main stem bronchus; *s/p,* status post. *(From Mangi AA, Gaissert HA, Wright CD, et al: Benign broncho-esophageal fistula in the adult, Ann Thorac Surg 73:911–915, 2002.)*

MALIGNANT ESOPHAGEAL RESPIRATORY TRACT FISTULA

Although a variety of malignant disorders within the thorax may lead to an esophageal respiratory tract fistula, esophageal cancer followed remotely by lung cancer is responsible for the majority of cases. It cannot be emphasized enough that a patient presenting with esophageal cancer and an airway fistula has an extremely poor prognosis and a median survival that is between 4 and 10 weeks in most series. Prompt intervention is necessary to palliate symptoms secondary to aspiration and to possibly prolong life. The procedural management of malignant esophageal respiratory tract fistula has evolved from esophageal diversion or exclusion to esophageal intubation with a plastic stent to contemporary placement of a self-expanding metallic stent (SEMS). Placement of a SEMS is a relatively easy and very effective technique to relieve dysphagia and prevent aspiration via the fistula (Table 1).

Esophageal Stents

There are a variety of thin-walled, self-expanding covered stents that may be used to manage esophageal airway fistulas. They typically are formed on a metal frame composed of steel or nitinol. At least one self-expanding covered stent is built on a plastic frame, but its use is predominantly in benign esophageal pathology; it is remarkable for being fully retrievable. The various stent models are distinguished by differences in diameter, length, intrinsic expansile force, foreshortening with deployment, delivery systems, and deployment patterns. In spite of this, most reports that describe the use of stents to manage malignant esophageal airway fistulas rely on one or at most two stent models.

Stent Placement Technique

Although esophageal stents may be placed with only local anesthesia and sedation, we prefer to perform this procedure with general anesthesia. This ensures patient comfort and facilitates simultaneous evaluation and management of pulmonary complications with bronchoscopy. The patient is positioned on a bed that permits fluoroscopy. Esophagoscopy is performed to establish landmarks, identify the fistula, and evaluate the stricture in terms of severity and length. The least amount of dilation necessary to permit the placement of a guidewire and the stent delivery system is performed with a balloon designed for esophageal dilation. The esophagus is intentionally underdilated, because the stricture holds the stent in place and maximizes the probability of sealing the fistula.

Under fluoroscopic and esophagoscopic guidance, the proximal and distal extents are marked with radiopaque safety pins taped to the surface of the thorax. A guidewire is placed with the tip in the stomach, and the esophagoscope is withdrawn. A stent that is at least 3 to 4 cm longer than the length of the stricture should be chosen, and the stent and delivery system are threaded over the guidewire and positioned across the stricture and fistula under fluoroscopic guidance using the previously placed safety pin markers. Esophagoscopy is repeated, and stent position and fistula sealing are verified. Balloon dilation may be performed to treat any significant stenosis that remains, and the stent is expected to continue to expand beyond the initial result. We typically have the patient undergo a barium swallow study to confirm that the fistula is sealed before allowing the patient to eat.

Complications of Esophageal Stents

Most reports of stent placement for malignant fistulas describe successful closure of the fistula and effective relief of dysphagia in more than 90% of patients. However, the procedure is associated with several specific complications that should be anticipated, including esophageal perforation, chest pain, hemorrhage, distal stent migration, and stent occlusion (Box 1). The likelihood of complications and need for reintervention will increase the longer the stent remains in place.

Airway Stents

Some malignant esophageal respiratory tract fistulas will require tracheobronchial stenting to relieve airway obstruction and seal the fistula. This is the case with primary lung cancer that presents with a fistula. The absence of a malignant esophageal stricture makes placement of an esophageal stent more difficult. Moreover, the airway stricture would not be relieved and in fact may be exacerbated by esophageal stenting. In other patients, concurrent esophageal and tracheobronchial stenting is necessary to provide adequate lumens and proper sealing of the fistula. As with esophageal stents, a variety of models are available to choose from.

Stent Placement Technique

We choose to perform tracheobronchial stenting under general anesthesia to maximize patient comfort and provide the most options and time to deal with secretions and the anatomy. Fluoroscopy can be used, but typically we deploy tracheobronchial stents under direct endoscopic vision, with either flexible or rigid bronchoscopy. Flexible bronchoscopy is first performed to study the anatomy, measure the lengths of the stricture and fistula, and to deal with secretions. The airway may then be dilated if necessary. A guidewire may be used, but it is typically unnecessary. The stent is partially deployed, repositioned appropriately, and then fully deployed. Balloon dilation is then performed within the stent to ensure proper apposition of the stent wall. A chest radiograph is obtained to document the position of the stent, to assess lung volumes, and to assess for a possible

TABLE 1: Management of esophageal respiratory tract fistula with SEMS

Author	Patients	Effective Palliation (%)	Median Survival (Days)	Complications (%)	Journal
Ross et al. (2007)	22	90	72	37	*Gastrointest Endosc*
Murthy et al. (2007)	12	100	55	8	*Dis Esophagus*
Shin et al. (2004)	61	80	94	43	*Radiology*

BOX 1: Complications of SEMS placement for esophageal respiratory tract fistula

Chest pain
Stent migration
Airway compression
Hemorrhage
Gastroesophageal reflux disease
Food impaction
Stent overgrowth
Persistent or recurrent fistula
Perforation

pneumothorax. Again, we have patients undergo a barium swallow study to document proper sealing of the fistula.

SUMMARY

The rapid evolution of esophageal and airway stent technology has facilitated the management of malignant esophageal respiratory tract fistulas. Prompt if not immediate intervention is mandatory given the extremely short expected survival of the patients. It should be emphasized that although stents are usually easily placed, a number of complications and the need for reintervention should be expected, and close patient follow-up is necessary.

SELECTED READINGS

Dua K: Stents for palliating malignant dysphagia and fistula: is the paradigm shifting? *Gastrointest Endosc* 65:77–81, 2007.

Macchiarini P, Verhoye J, Chapelier A, et al: Evaluation and outcome of different surgical techniques for postintubation tracheoesophageal fistulas, *J Thorac Cardiovasc Surg* 119:268–276, 2000.

Mangi A, Gaissert H, Wright C, et al: Benign broncho-esophageal fistula in the adult, *Ann Thorac Surg* 73:911–915, 2002.

Mathisen D, Grillo H, Wain J, et al: Management of acquired nonmalignant tracheoesophageal fistula, *Ann Thorac Surg* 52:759–765, 1991.

Ross W, Alkassab F, Lynch P, et al: Evolving role of self-expanding metal stents in the treatment of malignant dysphagia and fistulas, *Gastrointest Endosc* 65:70–76, 2007.

VASCULAR SURGERY

OPEN REPAIR OF ABDOMINAL AORTIC ANEURYSMS

Virendra I. Patel, MD, and Richard P. Cambria, MD

OVERVIEW

Aneurysmal dilatation of the abdominal aorta, defined as a 1.5-fold increase in normal aortic diameter or an aortic diameter greater than 3 cm, is typically isolated to the infrarenal aorta (>80%). An increasing incidence and prevalence of abdominal aortic aneurysms (AAAs) has been noted in recent years with rates as high as 10% to 15% in certain high-risk populations, such as those with a family history of aneurysms or long-term smokers. The natural history of aneurysmal disease is that of progressive enlargement and eventual rupture, with up to 20,000 deaths occurring annually as a result. Aneurysm rupture risk is increased in patients with chronic obstructive pulmonary disease (COPD), hypertension, family history of AAA, rapid AAA expansion, and most notably increasing with aneurysm size. Effective management of abdominal aortic aneurysms relies upon timely diagnosis and graft replacement.

Since Parodi's initial 1991 report, endovascular aneurysm repair (EVAR) has dramatically altered the technical management of AAA. For many, perhaps for most patients, the manifest benefit of a minimally invasive procedure, which has been abundantly documented, is an appropriate exchange for an approximately 10% risk of a secondary intervention. This is reflected in our own practice, wherein 70% of AAAs are repaired using EVAR. Accordingly, conventional surgical repair is utilized in patients with anatomy unfavorable for EVAR; in emergency situations, where stent grafts may not be readily available; and most notably and frequently in patients with complex aortic neck anatomy, such as pararenal and suprarenal aneurysms.

Pararenal AAAs are defined by an infrarenal aneurysm neck of 1 cm, and the term *pararenal* is often used interchangeably with the term *juxtarenal*. Suprarenal aneurysm occurs when one or both main renal arteries arise from the aneurysm itself, implying that separate renal artery reconstruction will be required. In instances of complex proximal anatomy, the cross clamp will need to be applied in a suprarenal or supraceliac position to permit proximal aortic reconstruction (Figure 1).

INDICATIONS FOR REPAIR

Symptomatic Aneurysm

The majority of abdominal aortic aneurysms are asymptomatic; however, some may occur with signs and symptoms of thrombosis, embolization of mural debris, compression of adjacent organs, aortic dissection (rare), rapid expansion, and impending or frank rupture. The presence of associated symptoms warrants early repair independent of aneurysm size. Distal embolization can present with digital ischemia or gangrene, often referred to as "trash foot" or "blue toe syndrome." Although rare, compression of the duodenum and stomach can result in gastric outlet obstruction, in which symptoms are seen along a spectrum from early satiety and fullness to nausea and vomiting with dehydration and malnutrition. Compression of other surrounding structures may be seen with symptoms referable to the structure involved, such as hydronephrosis with ureteral compression. Dissection within an aneurysmal aorta is seen with acute onset severe abdominal or back pain, often described as tearing in nature, and it is associated with a significant increase in rupture risk. Acute dissection within an AAA should therefore be promptly repaired. Up to 25% of AAAs occur with symptoms of rapid expansion or impending rupture that include mild to severe abdominal, back, or flank pain; in cases of frank rupture, disease may be seen initially in association with hemodynamic instability. On spiral computed tomographic (CT) angiography, the findings of heterogenous mural thrombus with intraplaque hemorrhage, loss of fat planes around the aorta, periaortic inflammation, and retroperitoneal hematoma are suggestive findings that call for urgent AAA repair. Hemodynamic instability suggestive of rupture in patients with known AAA should prompt emergent exploration and repair; however, in most cases, rapid CT scan is appropriate to facilitate operative planning.

Asymptomatic Aneurysm

The majority of AAAs are asymptomatic, therefore natural history data are needed to balance aneurysm rupture risk with that of surgical morbidity and mortality. Rupture risk correlates directly with aneurysm size and is very low for aneurysms smaller than 5 cm in diameter. Based on level 1 studies, an AAA diameter of 5.5 cm is typically used as a threshold for open repair. Other predictors of rupture include female gender, family history of AAA, a history of smoking, and concomitant hypertension or COPD.

Recently, two randomized controlled trials have been performed to evaluate the role of early repair of small aneurysms. The results of these trials echo similar recommendations of earlier retrospective data for the repair of AAA. The U.K. Small Aneurysms Trial randomized 1,090 patients 60 to 76 years old who were found to have AAAs 4.0 to 5.5 cm in diameter to early open AAA repair or surveillance. The early-surgery group included 563 patients, with 92% having open

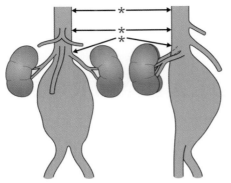
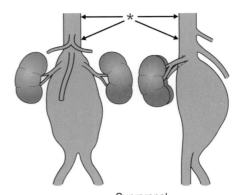

Pararenal/Juxtarenal
(less than 1cm neck)

Suprarenal
(including at least 1 renal artery)

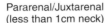

* Potential cross-clamp sites

FIGURE 1   Classification of complex abdominal aortic aneurysms. **A,** Pararenal aneurysms with an infrarenal neck of less than 1 cm. **B,** Suprarenal aneurysm with at least one renal artery involved in the aneurysm. *(Modified from Hallett JW, Mills JL: Comprehensive vascular and endovascular surgery, New York, 2004, Mosby Elsevier, p 446.)*

AAA repair with an operative mortality of 5.8%. The surveillance group included 527 patients, of which 73% underwent AAA repair by the end of the study. The annual rupture rates in the surveillance group were 1% overall, 0.3% for AAAs smaller than 4 cm, 1.5% for those 4.0 to 4.9 cm, and 6.5% for those 5.0 to 5.9 cm. The results of the study showed no significant improvement in survival for patients undergoing elective repair of a small AAA. The study authors concluded that patients should undergo surveillance in the surveillance group of AAA until the diameter exceeds 5.5 cm; they also noted that women were more likely to seek medical treatment, and they were more likely to die as a result of AAA rupture.

The Aneurysm Detection and Management (ADAM) trial was performed within the Veterans Affairs (VA) medical system and presented similar results. A total of 1,136 patients aged 50 to 79 years with aneurysms 4.0 to 5.4 cm were randomized to undergo immediate open surgical repair or routine surveillance; repair was performed for AAAs 5.5 cm or larger, symptoms attributable to the AAA, or an annual increase of more than 1 cm. The immediate repair group consisted of 569 patients, of which 93% underwent aneurysm repair; the 30 day mortality rate was 2.7%. The annual aneurysm rupture rate in the surveillance group was 0.6% and was not stratified based on aneurysm size. A total of 350 (61.6%) patients in this group underwent aneurysm repair during a mean follow-up of 4.8 years, and repair rates increased as aneurysm diameter at enrollment increased; of these, 27% of AAAs 4.0 to 4.4 cm required repair, compared with 81% of AAAs 5.0 to 5.4 cm. Long-term survival was similar in both groups, and the authors concluded that elective AAA repair should be reserved for aneurysms at least 5.5 cm in diameter.

The decision to proceed with AAA repair is complex and involves assessment of the patient's life expectancy and perspective. Current data support open aneurysm repair at a threshold size of 5.5 cm in men and 5.0 cm in women. The natural history of patients under surveillance is such that 70% to 80% of patients eventually undergo aneurysm repair.

PREOPERATIVE PATIENT PREPARATION

Patients undergoing elective aneurysm repair should be appropriately risk stratified from a cardiovascular standpoint in accordance with published American College of Cardiology/American Heart Association guidelines. Open AAA surgery is considered high risk; despite this, initial clinical profiling should guide the decision to obtain further cardiac testing. Even patients with significant cardiovascular risk can safely undergo aortic reconstruction with optimal

medical therapy, as recently highlighted by the Coronary Artery Revascularization Prophylaxis (CARP) trial, which showed no significant benefit in preoperative revascularization in patients with coronary disease, excluding patients with left main coronary artery disease, low ejection fraction (<20%), and valvular disease. CARP trial patients were noted to have similar rates of cardiovascular complications and cardiovascular mortality at 30 days and 2 years in both revascularized and nonrevascularized patients undergoing vascular surgical procedures.

OPERATIVE PLANNING

Accurate and complete preoperative imaging is of utmost importance to assess the extent of proximal and distal aortic resection and the desirability and mode of possible concomitant visceral/renal artery reconstruction. In contemporary practice, the detail available with contrast-enhanced thin-slice CT angiography provides the surgeon with an adequate preoperative map. As the proximal aortic anatomy becomes more complex, or the need to investigate potential renovascular or aortoiliac occlusive disease arises, arteriography may be added; the information from these two studies is complementary with respect to the important operative decisions. Given the current level of sophistication with three-dimensional reconstructions of fine-cut CT scans, the need for aortography is rare in our practice.

A thorough evaluation of preoperative imaging aids in the development of an operative plan, which should include 1) the extent of resection; 2) location of aortic cross-clamp application; 3) qualitative assessment of the aortic lumen, intended to minimize the risk of atheroembolism; 4) evaluation of visceral vessel topography and patency; 5) identification of aneurysmal or occlusive iliac disease; and 6) the need for concomitant renovisceral reconstructions.

SURGICAL APPROACHES

Abdominal aortic surgery can be readily performed using transperitoneal/transabdominal (TP) or retroperitoneal (RP) approaches, and the merits of both have been espoused by randomized and uncontrolled studies (Figure 2). The transperitoneal approach may be performed with a longitudinal midline (xiphoid to pubis) incision or a generous transverse incision extending from flank to flank. The latter has the advantage of keeping the incision away from the epigastrium, possibly decreasing postoperative pain and respiratory compromise. The retroperitoneal approach is through the left flank and can vary

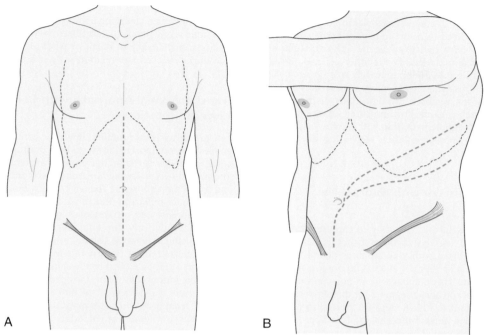

A   B

FIGURE 2   Surgical approaches for abdominal aortic aneurysm repair. **A,** The anterior transabdominal approach via a midline xiphoid-pubis incision (*dashed line*). **B,** The lateral approach with low thoracoabdominal (*upper dashed line*) or retroperitoneal (*lower*) incision. (*Modified from Hallett JW, Mills JL: Comprehensive vascular and endovascular surgery, New York, 2004, Mosby Elsevier, p 427.*)

from a total retroperitoneal to thoracoabdominal exposure. Depending on body habitus, aneurysm anatomy, a number of other anatomic factors, and the surgeon's experience, either approach can be used for the majority of infrarenal and juxtarenal AAAs, whereas suprarenal aneurysms are best approached by one of the left flank approaches. Irrespective of the benefits or the approach used, certain anatomic and clinical circumstances clearly dictate preferential use of a particular approach in individual patients. These variables are considered below in the individual descriptions of each surgical technique.

Anterior Transperitoneal Approach

The transperitoneal anterior midline approach, performed through a vertical xiphoid-pubis incision, is commonly employed and remains favored by most surgeons. Exposure for the majority of infrarenal AAAs is quite satisfactory and allows the surgeon to explore the remainder of the abdomen and provides superior exposure for dealing with the vagaries of iliac aneurysmal and/or occlusive disease. With the usual inframesocolic exposure, the root of the mesentery and small bowel is retracted to the right, generally with evisceration, and the transverse colon is retracted superiorly. Following division of the ligament of Treitz and the retroperitoneal tissues over the aneurysm itself, exposure and mobilization of the left renal vein is straightforward. Division of the inferior mesenteric vein generally allows for lateral retraction of the left mesocolon and superior retraction of the pancreas. The latter should be well padded to minimize the chance of perioperative pancreatitis. Depending on the length of the aneurysm neck, wide mobilization of the left renal vein may be desirable by ligation of its adrenal, gonadal, and lumbar branches, thus allowing cephalad retraction of the left renal vein (Figure 3). Division of the left renal vein is to be avoided, as it may increase the risk of postoperative renal failure; more importantly it will contribute to local venous hypertension, leading to increased venous bleeding.

Additional proximal exposure on the aneurysm neck and/or visceral aortic segment can be obtained by sharply dissecting off the dense neural and splanchnic tissue enveloping the aorta at the

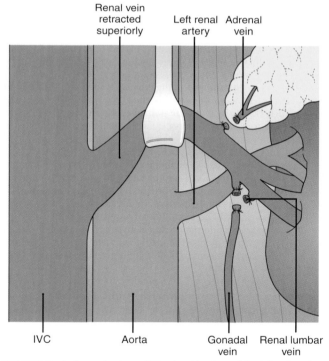

FIGURE 3   Left renal vein mobilization. Ligation of the left adrenal, gonadal, and renal-lumbar veins results in exposure of the left renal artery and suprarenal aorta. (*Modified from Hallett JW, Mills JL: Comprehensive vascular and endovascular surgery, New York, 2004, Mosby Elsevier, p 455.*)

level of the origin of the superior mesenteric artery (SMA). This will frequently allow placement of a suprarenal clamp below the origin of the SMA without the need to resort to clamping the supraceliac aorta. In patients who have had prior aortic surgery, suprarenal aneurysms, and extensive juxtarenal aortic atherosclerotic disease, modifications of the transabdominal approach will be needed for more proximal aortic cross-clamp placement and/or partial exposure of the visceral aortic segment. Modifications of the anterior transabdominal approach include 1) transcrural supraceliac aortic control and clamping, 2) supplementation with a right-sided medial visceral rotation, and 3) supplementation with a left-sided medial visceral rotation.

Transperitoneal Approach with Supraceliac Clamping

This maneuver is most useful in the setting of ruptured AAA, juxtarenal aortic aneurysm, infected aortic graft/tissue, or when the AAA neck is heavily involved with atheromatous debris, such that clamping in the infrarenal or suprarenal location poses a significant threat of atheroembolism. This maneuver does not permit continuous "exposure" of the visceral aortic segment for direct operation.

A number of important technical steps are crucial to achieving control of the supraceliac aorta from the midline approach. The proximal extent of the abdominal incision must be carried well onto the xiphoid. Depending on the anatomy of the costal arch, it may be necessary to split the lower sternum or at least its cartilaginous portion. The triangular ligament of the left lobe of the liver must be taken down to facilitate retraction of the left lobe for the majority of patients. Adequate retraction of the underside of the diaphragm on either side of the midline is necessary, and the left hepatic lobe should be folded upon itself, padded, and retracted to the right of midline along with the diaphragm.

A nasogastric (NG) tube should be placed next, and its location should be confirmed within the stomach by palpation. With gentle traction on the stomach and gastroesophageal (GE) junction, the lesser omentum (gastrohepatic ligament) is divided. Evaluation of preoperative imaging for the existence of a replaced left hepatic artery, which travels beneath the gastrohepatic ligament, will assist in preventing injury to this vessel. Using tactile orientation of the esophagus by palpating for the NG tube, the esophagus is mobilized to the patient's left at the level of the GE junction, and the right diaphragmatic crus is divided to facilitate access to the aorta (Figure 4). This is mandatory if the aorta is to be clamped in this region, but it may be unnecessary if temporary proximal control is being obtained with an aortic compressor. In elective circumstances, we prefer to dissect out the aorta in this region and surround it with a vessel tape for easy subsequent manipulation and clamping. The surgeon should avoid the temptation to incise the median arcuate ligament from the anterior approach, as this may result in injury to the celiac axis.

Transperitoneal Approach with Right Medial Visceral Rotation

The usual midline incision in the retroperitoneal tissues is extended over the right pelvic rim, and the entire right colon is mobilized in continuity with the duodenum. The small bowel and right transverse colon are eviscerated and placed superiorly on the patient's chest. The root of the mesentery and the origin of the SMA are thus exposed, and the orientation of the SMA is now straight up and down at 90 degrees to the aorta rather than the usual 45 degrees (Figure 5).

Next, the dense splanchnic autonomic nervous tissue that envelops the aorta at and onto the origin of the SMA is sharply dissected away. It will be necessary to divide the insertions of the diaphragmatic crus posteriorly to achieve exposure of the posterolateral aspects of the aorta. After all of these maneuvers have been performed,

suprarenal clamping is easily achieved; if the SMA and renal origins are close together, clamping above the SMA can be carried out. This technique is one that is underutilized; however, it can be very helpful for juxtarenal aneurysm repair or when right renal artery bypass or transaortic renal endarterectomy are necessary.

Transperitoneal Approach with Left Medial Visceral Rotation

Left medial visceral rotation allows for continuous exposure of the entire abdominal aorta; however, when continuous exposure of visceral aortic segments is required, we prefer a lateral approach (Figure 6). The small bowel is wrapped in moist towels and is reflected superiorly and to the patient's right. The left colon is mobilized by dividing the left peritoneal reflection (line of Toldt). This is continued on to divide the splenorenal and phrenocolic ligaments superiorly and the sigmoid colon inferiorly. The sigmoid colon, descending colon, splenic flexure, distal transverse colon, stomach, spleen, and pancreas are then mobilized in continuity; this mobilization can include the left kidney, which is facilitated by incision of the Gerota fascia. Mobilization of the kidney allows for unimpeded access to the visceral aorta. Alternatively, if extensive dissection and exposure of the SMA and/ or right renal artery is necessary, the left kidney is left in situ. The decision as to whether the left kidney will be reflected anteriorly also depends upon the anatomic variants of the left renal vein. Splenic and pancreatic injury are a potential complication of this exposure.

Lateral Retroperitoneal and Thoracoabdominal Approaches

The term *retroperitoneal approach* has been used to refer to incisions at the level of the eleventh rib or below; incisions higher than the tenth interspace, implying division of the costal margin, are referred to as *thoracoabdominal*. The main considerations when using this type of exposure are the level of the flank incision necessary and whether the left kidney is to be left in situ. Infrarenal and pararenal aneurysms can readily be approached through a retroperitoneal incision; for more extensive aneurysms or for supraceliac exposure, an eighth or ninth interspace incision with partial division of the diaphragm and entry into the left thoracic cavity is necessary. The lateral approaches are advantageous in obese patients and with complex proximal aortic anatomy, however, access to right-sided aortic branches is limited.

There are two ways to perform a lateral approach to the abdominal aorta. For a truly retroperitoneal aortic exposure, the patient is positioned in the right lateral decubitus position with the shoulders and torso at angles 60 to 70 degrees from the table and the hips rotated back as close to horizontal as possible. The operating table is jackknifed to open the flank, and the patient's position is held by a vacuum beanbag and an armrest for the left arm. Appropriate padding of the legs, arms, and pressure points is applied.

The retroperitoneal approach starts with an incision overlying the eleventh rib, from the posterior axillary line to the lateral rectus border, that is carried through the abdominal wall musculature onto the rib. The eleventh rib is mobilized, and the distal 6 to 8 inches of the rib are excised. The more posterior the surgeon brings this incision, the higher the likelihood of pleural cavity entry. The incision is carried through the transversalis fascia, and the retroperitoneal space is entered laterally. The peritoneal sac is swept anteromedially, further defining the retroperitoneal space. This is continued medially, until the aneurysmal segments are identified. As above, a plane anterior or posterior to the left kidney may be developed, and in most circumstances, the retrorenal plane is chosen. The aorta is thus approached on its left posterolateral aspect, and the aortic origin of the left renal artery is an important point of anatomic reference. Depending on the patient's body habitus and the nature of the pathology, it is possible to carry the dissection proximally, divide the median arcuate ligament

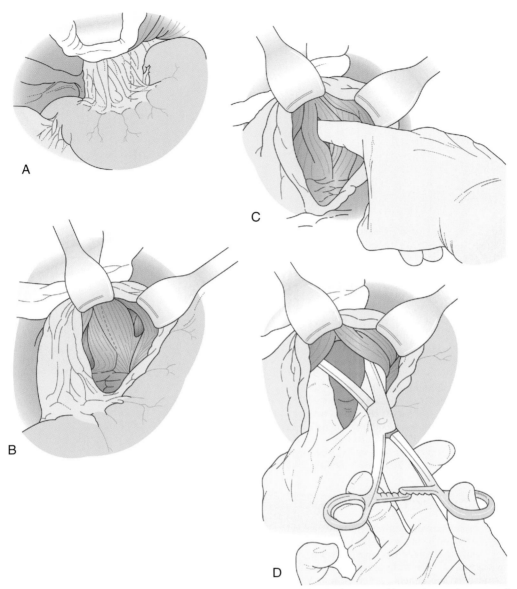

FIGURE 4 Exposure and supraceliac aortic clamping. **A,** Appropriate retraction of the diaphragm and liver adequately expose the gastrohepatic ligament. **B,** Following division of the gastrohepatic ligament, the right crus of the diaphragm is exposed. **C,** Division of the crus or dissection with a fingertip identifies the aorta. **D,** Further dissection on either side of the aorta allows for placement of the aortic cross-clamp with its tips against the vertebral body. *(Modified from Hallett JW, Mills JL: Comprehensive vascular and endovascular surgery, New York, 2004, Mosby Elsevier, p 454.)*

and left diaphragmatic crural muscle fibers, and expose and control the suprarenal aorta.

Although frequent references are made in the literature to the undue morbidity of a two-cavity approach, this has been greatly overestimated. We believe a formal thoracoabdominal approach with pleural and peritoneal cavity entry and sharp division of the costal margin is the preferred approach for the majority of lesions, when the surgeon will be working on the visceral aortic segment. The proximal extent of the incision is dictated by the nature of the pathology, the patient's body habitus, and the nature of the surgery to be carried out.

Although advocates of a retroperitoneal approach to the aorta frequently refer to this incision as a *thoracoretroperitoneal approach* when the abdominal portion is kept retroperitoneal, we have found this to have no specific advantage; however, the inability to directly inspect intestinal contents and/or palpate visceral vessel pulses on the other side of the transverse mesocolon is a valid reason to enter the peritoneal cavity. Following entry into the left thoracic and abdominal

cavities, the costal margin is sharply divided, and a limited radial, lateral incision in the diaphragm will allow the surgeon to preserve the phrenic nerve and retract and work entirely below the diaphragm.

The abdominal dissection then proceeds as described for left medial visceral rotation. Although the entire operation is conducted in the retroperitoneum, patient positioning is such that evisceration is generally not necessary. The position and handling of the left kidney is as discussed, and in the majority of patients, the left kidney is elevated out of its bed. Direct and continuous exposure of the aorta from the posterior mediastinum to the bifurcation is therefore possible with this approach. We have found this approach most useful with 1) suprarenal aneurysms, 2) extensive redo or otherwise difficult aortic surgery, 3) Linton splenorenal venous shunt or splenorenal arterial anastomosis, 4) transaortic multiple visceral vessel endarterectomy, and 5) ruptured abdominal aortic aneurysms in patients with extensive prior intraabdominal surgery. In our opinion, this is the preferred approach for the majority of suprarenal aortic pathology.

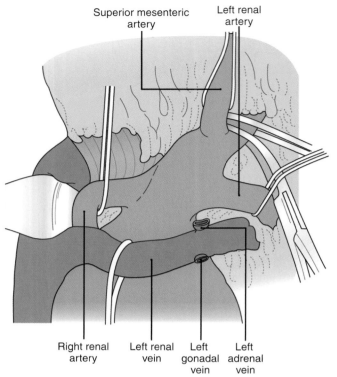

FIGURE 5 Suprarenal aortic exposure with right medial visceral rotation. The suprarenal aorta is easily accessible following medial visceral rotation, mobilization of the left renal vein, and division of periaortic splanchnic tissue. Note that the superior mesenteric artery (SMA) is perpendicular to the aorta, and clamp placement superior to the SMA is feasible. *(Modified from Hallett JW, Mills JL: Comprehensive vascular and endovascular surgery, New York, 2004, Mosby Elsevier, p 456.)*

OPERATIVE CONDUCT

For elective AAA repair, preoperative planning should dictate patient positioning and an approach such that a complete resection of the aneurysm and occlusive disease, rather than partial resection of a more diffuse disease process, is achieved to prevent late aneurysmal degeneration and the need for subsequent reintervention. Anatomic dissection such that deliberate attempts to confine either clamping or resection to the infrarenal aorta are inappropriate, when this represents a compromise in resection of the aneurysmal process. However, in emergent surgery with patient instability and extensive comorbidities, surgical objectives must be tailored to fit the clinical circumstances.

A number of clinical adjuncts aimed at improving patient outcomes apply to all patients. Besides technical considerations, perioperative bleeding complications may occur as a result of dilutional coagulopathy resulting from large blood turnover and inadequate repletion of blood products. Blood turnover by necessity may be excessive, especially in circumstances of complex aneurysm repair; therefore except in cases of suspected infection, a cell saver is used during all aortic reconstructions. Blood component replacement with fresh frozen plasma and platelets during surgery alleviates coagulopathic bleeding. Infusion lines and monitoring lines appropriate for the anticipated complexity of aneurysm repair and planned level of aortic cross clamping should be placed in conjunction with the anesthesia team. Fluid and external warmers should be applied with the intention of maintaining normothermia throughout the procedure. Use of an epidural for intraoperative anesthesia and postoperative analgesia has been associated with increased pain control, decreased ileus, and improved pulmonary toilet, and it aids in rapid recovery.

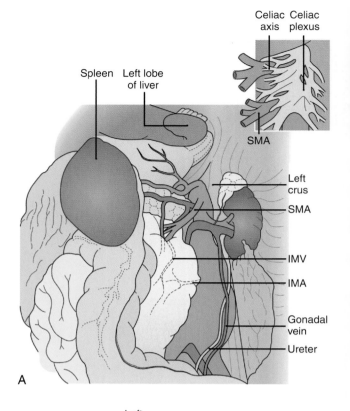

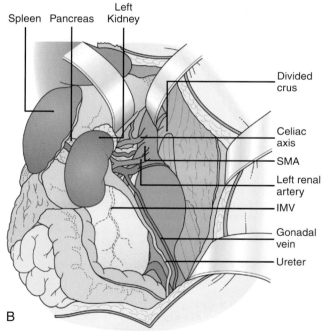

FIGURE 6 Left lateral retroperitoneal or thoracoabdominal approach. **A,** Various levels of incision depend on the extent of aneurysmal disease. The abdominal portion is not carried to midline to keep the viscera intraperitoneal and to decrease evaporative and heat losses. **B,** Excellent contiguous exposure to the visceral aortic segment is obtained, as division of the left crus at the aortic hiatus facilitates supraceliac aortic exposure. Note the renal-lumbar vein at the level of the left renal artery. Identification of the left renal artery serves as a point of reference for further dissection of the visceral aorta. *(Modified from Hallett JW, Mills JL: Comprehensive vascular and endovascular surgery, New York, 2004, Mosby Elsevier, p 455.)*

During the conduct of the operation, a number of technical principles contribute to surgical efficiency and success. Continuous and adequate exposure of the involved portions of the aorta is necessary, implying the routine use of a fixed, self-retaining retractor system. Gentle dissection on and around an AAA should be performed, as atheroembolism is just as likely to occur during dissection of the aneurysm as during application of cross clamps. This concern is particularly appropriate in patients with a preoperative history of blue toe syndrome. Careful conduct of dissection with emphasis on hemostasis reduces blood turnover and decreases the likelihood of bleeding complications. Except in cases of rupture, all patients are judiciously anticoagulated prior to application of cross clamps or occlusion of branch vessels, and systemic anticoagulation is reversed following completion of all distal anastomoses.

Locations for aortic clamping should be such that an adequate aortic "cuff" is available for anastomosis. Additionally, in planning the location of proximal or distal cross clamps, it is imperative to avoid clamping a heavily diseased aorta, particularly where extensive mural atherothrombotic debris is demonstrated on preoperative imaging studies. This principle is specifically intended to avoid atheromatous embolization to renal, visceral, or outflow vessels. Accordingly, visceral vessel clamps and distal outflow vessel clamps are applied prior to proximal aortic cross clamping.

Following clamp application, the aortic sac is longitudinally opened, and mural thrombus/debris is evacuated with care, such that pushing of debris into outflow iliac vessels is avoided. Retrograde bleeding from lumbar vessels is controlled by suture ligatures and may require local endarterectomy and removal of calcific plaque for successful control of the bleeding vessels.

Aortic reconstructions are typically performed with appropriately sized Dacron or polytetrafluoroethylene (PTFE) tube grafts with use of bifurcated grafts in instances where distal reconstruction should require iliac or femoral level outflow anastomoses (Figures 7 and 8). The main body of a bifurcated graft should be short (~4 cm) to prevent kinking of the iliac limbs. For a suprarenal AAA, or when significant left renal artery stenosis is present, our preferred construct is a beveled proximal suture line, whose inferior aspect begins at or into the right renal artery origin. Superiorly, the graft extends for a variable distance, depending on the pathology. As shown in Figure 8, B, this can be extended cephalad to the level of the celiac artery for an extent IV thoracoabdominal aneurysm. This reconstructive strategy implies that the "heel" of the anastomosis will be coursing around the right renal artery orifice from the 3 to 9 o'clock positions. When the suture line potentially compromises the right renal artery origin, or when significant right renal artery stenosis exists, direct placement of a balloon-expandable stent (as opposed to right renal orificial endarterectomy) both facilitates and simplifies the reconstruction (Figure 9). More proximal clamp placement is associated with increased cardiac strain, hemodynamic compromise, and the potential for coagulopathy; however, with appropriate exposure and planning, the proximal reconstruction can be performed with clamp times of less than 30 minutes in most instances.

Aortic grafts can be prefashioned with side arms for visceral vessel reconstruction prior to cross-clamp application to expedite reperfusion of the reconstructed vessels. In instances of suprarenal clamp application, renal preservation is achieved through direct instillation of renal preservation fluid (4° C Ringer's lactate solution with 25 g/L of mannitol and 1 g/L of methyl prednisolone) into the renal artery ostia following opening of the aorta.

Following completion of the distal anastomosis, hemodynamic shifts associated with reperfusion should be coordinated and managed in conjunction with the anesthesia team. Reimplantation of the inferior mesenteric artery (IMA) is rarely needed but should be considered in patients with occluded hypogastric arteries, poor back-bleeding from the IMA, and in those with previous colon surgery, such that normal collateral pathways have been significantly altered. Following aortic reconstruction, and in cases of TP exposure, coverage of the graft by closing the aneurysm sac over the reconstruction and closure of the retroperitoneum, augmented with omental

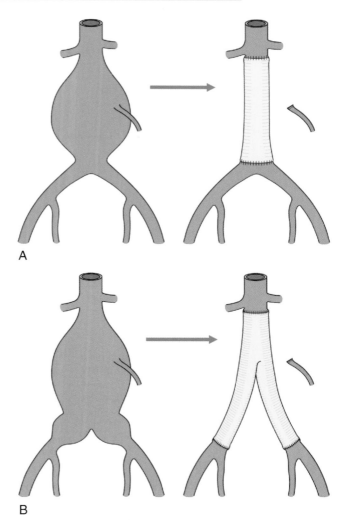

A

B

FIGURE 7   Constructs for common infrarenal aneurysm repairs. **A,** Tube grafts. **B,** Bifurcated grafts. *(Modified from Hallett JW, Mills JL: Comprehensive vascular and endovascular surgery, New York, 2004, Mosby Elsevier, p 431.)*

flap coverage, reduces the likelihood of late graft-enteric erosion and attendant graft infection or fistulas (Figure 10).

Prior to wound closure, inspection of the viscera, Doppler evaluation, palpation of reconstructed vessels, and pulse-volume recording analysis of the distal circulation are performed. Postoperative splenic bleeding and undetected bleeding from intercostal or lumbar vessels are principle sources of postoperative hemorrhage. A careful search for bleeding vessels and a low threshold to perform splenectomy in the setting of splenic injury prevent such complications. All AAA patients are transferred to the surgical intensive care unit for postoperative monitoring and treatment.

An expeditious operation is to be emphasized in all patients. We reviewed a series of 200 consecutive aortic operations at Massachusetts General Hospital, 80% of which were conducted for AAA, and evaluated a variety of preoperative and intraoperative technical variables to assess their impact on operative complications and mortality. Among these, only a prolonged operation (>5 hours) was statistically and independently associated with death or major cardiopulmonary complications after abdominal aortic surgery (odds ratio [OR], 5.11; 95% confidence interval [CI], 1.69 to 15.52; $P < .004$). Technical factors of significance in predicting perioperative complications also include urgency of procedure, body core temperature (≤35° C), volume of blood loss, perioperative fluid requirements, and duration of suprarenal and supravisceral clamping.

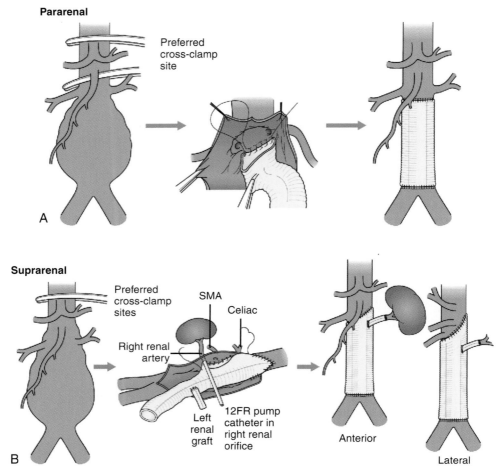

Pararenal

Preferred
cross-clamp
site

A

Suprarenal

Preferred
cross-clamp
sites

SMA

Celiac

Right renal
artery

Left
renal
graft

12FR pump
catheter in
right renal
orifice

Anterior

Lateral

B

FIGURE 8   Preferred methods for pararenal and suprarenal aneurysm repair. **A,** Pararenal aneurysm. Cross-clamp: supraceliac or suprarenal inframesenteric, depending upon aortic disease and renovisceral artery spacing. *Center,* Sewing proximally to the "cuff" of the aorta at the renal artery orifices. **B,** Suprarenal aneurysm. Cross-clamp: supraceliac. *Center,* Beveled proximal anastomosis with 12 Fr perfusion catheter to stent open the right renal artery to inhibit orificial compromise. Left renal artery reconstruction with 6 mm polytetrafluoroethylene preattached to aortic prosthesis. *(Modified from Hallett JW, Mills JL: Comprehensive vascular and endovascular surgery, New York, 2004, Mosby Elsevier, p 457.)*

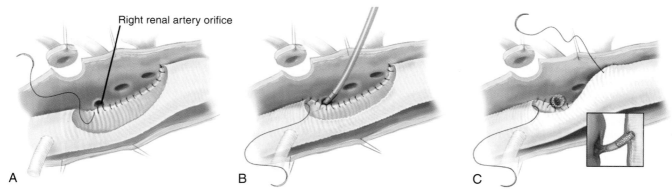

Right renal artery orifice

A   B   C

FIGURE 9   Open right renal artery stenting. **A,** For more complex aneurysm repair, the proximal anastomosis is often beveled and courses directly below the right renal artery orifice. **B,** In the presence of renal artery stenosis, or if the suture line compromises the right renal artery orifice, open right renal artery stenting is performed under direct visualization with the stent delivery catheter advanced into the right renal artery manually. **C,** The stent is deployed so as to extend into the aortic lumen for 1 to 2 mm. *Inset,* The final construct is shown. *(From Patel R, Conrad MF, Paruchuri V, et al: Balloon expandable stents facilitate right renal artery reconstruction during complex open aortic aneurysm repair, J Vasc Surg 51[2]:310–315, 2004.)*

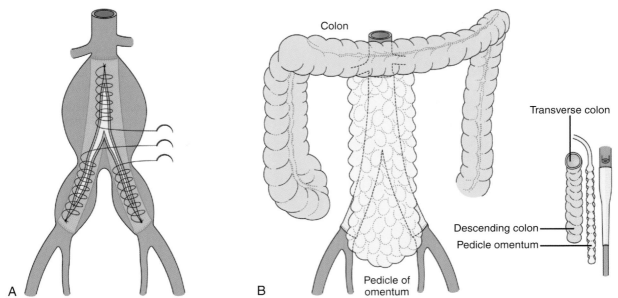

FIGURE 10   Aneurysm sac closure and coverage. **A,** Closure of the aneurysm sac over the aortic graft following aneurysm repair. **B,** Use of an omental flap to separate the synthetic graft material from the gastrointestinal tract. *(Modified from Hallett JW, Mills JL: Comprehensive vascular and endovascular surgery, New York, 2004, Mosby Elsevier, p 446.)*

RESULTS

Irrespective of operative conduct, perioperative morbidity and mortality of AAA repair are dependent upon and influenced by patient characteristics and circumstances of clinical presentation. Patient age, number and type of comorbid conditions, and complexity of aneurysm repair have all been reported to increase operative risk. Mortality rates associated with elective pararenal or suprarenal AAA repair approach 5% to 10%, but patients undergoing infrarenal AAA repair have mortality rates of less than 5%. In circumstances of symptomatic or ruptured AAA repair, mortality rates ranging 20% to 70% have been reported with an equally high incidence of major morbidity. In a recent report of our own experience with open AAA repair in the era predating the widespread use of endovascular aneurysm repair (EVAR), we reported an operative mortality rate of 3% and major morbidity of 10%. In this series of 540 patients, 25% required suprarenal clamp application for AAA repair. Independent predictors of both perioperative morbidity and mortality included previous myocardial infarction (OR, 2.0; 95% CI, 1.2 to 3.6; $P = .01$) and renal insufficiency (OR, 2.5; 95% CI, 1.2 to 5.3; $P = .02$).

Many series, including our own, demonstrate increased operative risk in patients with coronary artery disease, COPD, and renal insufficiency, with dysfunction in these respective organ systems increasing the risks of organ-specific postoperative complications. Variables predictive of cardiac complications include recent myocardial infarction, advanced age, diabetes, functional status, history of arrhythmia, and congestive heart failure. Cardiac complications can be prevented with appropriate risk stratification and optimizing of perioperative medical management, such that patients are treated with statin medications, aspirin, and β-blockade (target HR <60 beats/min and systolic blood pressure <100 mm Hg).

Variables predictive of postoperative pulmonary complications include active cigarette smoking, COPD, clinical presentation, and extent of operation. Respiratory complications are avoided by preoperative smoking cessation and can be managed in the postoperative setting with optimal bronchodilator therapy and aggressive pulmonary toilet in conjunction with a pulmonary specialist. Factors related to development of renal failure include preoperative renal insufficiency (most relevant), duration of renal ischemia, failure of renal artery reconstruction, and cholesterol embolization from surgical manipulation.

Transient decreases in renal function are inevitable as a result of the obligatory periods of ischemia, resulting in nonoliguric renal insufficiency that is easily managed with maintenance of intravascular volume and hemodynamic support. The use of adjuncts such as cold crystalloid renal perfusion, renal-dose dopamine infusion, and fenoldopam infusion may prevent postoperative renal insufficiency; however, minimizing renal ischemia time is the most important factor in avoidance of this complication. In addition to predicting perioperative morbidity, the presence of cardiopulmonary and renal comorbidities is also associated with significant decreases in long-term patient survival.

Long-term (5-year) survival in patients after complex abdominal aortic aneurysm repair is reported to be 40% to 75%. The majority of late mortality is related to cardiovascular events, and some groups have reported improved late outcomes in patients who have undergone previous coronary revascularization. Our own experience noted late survival of about 71% and 44% at 5 and 10 years, respectively. Predictors of late mortality included age at operation, history of myocardial infarction, congestive heart failure, and preoperative renal insufficiency. In the same patient cohort, freedom from aneurysm-related mortality rate was 95% at both 5 and 10 years. Graft-related complications were identified in 2% of patients, and additional aneurysmal disease in noncontiguous aortic segments was found in 13% of patients at a mean follow-up of 7.2 years. Thus patients undergoing open AAA repair are afforded good long-term survival and excellent durability of the reconstruction.

SELECTED READINGS

Cambria RP, Brewster DC, Abbott WM, et al: Transperitoneal versus retroperitoneal approach for aortic reconstruction: a randomized prospective study, *J Vasc Surg* 11:314–325, 1990.

Cambria RP: Simultaneous aortic reconstruction and renal artery revascularization. In Dean RH, editor: *Modern management of renovascular hypertension and renal salvage*, Philadelphia, 1996, Williams & Wilkins, pp 203–221.

Clouse WD, Cambria RP: Complex aortic aneurysm: pararenal, suprarenal, and thoracoabdominal. In Hallett JW, Mills JL, editors: *Comprehensive vascular and endovascular surgery*, New York, 2004, Mosby Elsevier, pp 445–478.

Conrad MF, Crawford RS, Pedraza JD, et al: Long-term durability of open abdominal aortic aneurysm repair, *J Vasc Surg* 46:669–675, 2007.

Dardik A, Lin JW, Gordon TA, et al: Results of elective abdominal aortic aneurysm repair in the 1990s: a population-based analysis of 2,335 cases, *J Vasc Surg* 30:985–995, 1999.

Green RL, Ricotta JJ, Ouriel K, et al: Results of supraceliac aortic clamping in the difficult elective resection of infrarenal abdominal aortic aneurysm, *J Vasc Surg* 9:125, 1989.

Lederle FA, Johnson GR, Wilson SE, et al: Rupture rate of large abdominal aortic aneurysms in patients refusing or unfit for elective repair, *JAMA* 287:2968–2972, 2002.

Lederle FA, Wilson SE, Johnson GR, et al: Immediate repair compared with surveillance of small abdominal aortic aneurysms, *N Engl J Med* 346:1437–1444, 2002.

Nevitt MP, Ballard DJ, Hallett JW Jr: Prognosis of abdominal aortic aneurysms: a population-based study, *N Engl J Med* 321:1009–1014, 1989.

O'Hara PJ: Abdominal aneurysm—open repair. In Hallett JW, Mills JL, editors: *Comprehensive vascular and endovascular surgery*, New York, 2004, Mosby Elsevier, pp 425–444.

Parodi JC, Palmaz JC, Barone HD: Transfemoral intraluminal graft implantation for abdominal aortic aneurysms, *Ann Vasc Surg* 5:491–499, 1991.

Patel R, Chung TK, Paruchuri V, et al: Balloon expandable stents facilitate right renal artery reconstruction during complex open aortic aneurysm repair, *J Vasc Surg* 51:310–316, 2010.

Reilly L, Ramos T, Murray J, et al: Optimal exposure of the proximal abdominal aorta: a critical appraisal of the transabdominal medial visceral rotation, *J Vasc Surg* 19:375–390, 1994.

The UK Small Aneurysm Trial Participants: Mortality results for a randomized controlled trial of early elective surgery or ultrasonographic surveillance for small abdominal aortic aneurysms, *Lancet* 353:1649–1655, 1998.

ENDOVASCULAR TREATMENT OF ABDOMINAL AORTIC ANEURYSMS

Paul J. Foley, MD, and Ronald M. Fairman, MD

OVERVIEW

The Centers for Disease Control and Prevention estimates that over 13,000 deaths in the United States in 2006 were related to aortic aneurysms. The natural history of aortic aneurysms is that of gradual expansion on average of 0.3 to 0.4 cm/year and eventual rupture, which carries with it a high mortality of nearly 50%. The annual risk of rupture increases along with aneurysm diameter, and this risk significantly increases in aneurysms larger than 5 cm. Specific variables such as the presence of hypertension, chronic obstructive pulmonary disease (COPD), smoking, and an eccentrically shaped aneurysm also increase the risk of rupture. Altering the natural history of aortic aneurysms to prevent rupture and death is the driving force behind surgical intervention.

Surgical repair is considered for abdominal aortic aneurysms (AAAs) that have reached 5.5 cm in diameter; for those that demonstrate rapid expansion, defined as growth of more than 0.5 cm within a 6-month interval; or for those patients that manifest signs or symptoms. In general, intervening on smaller aneurysms does not improve outcomes. Long-term follow-up data from two large, randomized prospective trials, the U.K. Small Aneurysm Trial and the Aneurysm Detection and Management Trial, showed no survival benefit with prophylactic open surgical repair for aneurysms less than 5.5 cm in diameter. Perioperative mortality from these trials was 5.8% and 2.7%, respectively. Higher morbidity and mortality rates are expected in the presence of comorbidities such as coronary artery disease, COPD, and renal insufficiency. This highlights the importance of considering individual patient variables in the risk–benefit analysis when deciding on the appropriate timing of surgery.

Introduced in 1991 by Parodi, endovascular aneurysm repair (EVAR) of abdominal aortic aneurysms involves the placement of a graft across the aneurysm, within the aortic lumen, via a transfemoral or transiliac approach. Proximal and distal fixation of the graft excludes the aneurysm sac from blood flow and systemic blood pressure, thereby reducing the risk of expansion and rupture. EVAR evolved from the desire to reduce the morbidity and mortality from open repair and to provide a minimally invasive alternative for select patients. The endovascular approach has gained widespread acceptance, and recent data reveal that nearly 60% of all intact aneurysm repairs nationwide were performed this way. Current recommendations from a subcommittee of the Joint Council of the American Association of Vascular Surgery and the Society for Vascular Surgery state that EVAR should be limited to patients with suitable anatomy who are at high risk for conventional open repair.

ENDOGRAFTS

The first endografts were fashioned from Dacron tube grafts and fixed to the aorta by using balloon-expandable stents. Since that time, endograft technology has evolved considerably. Five devices have been approved by the Food and Drug Administration (FDA) for use in EVAR in the United States (Table 1). Several basic components are common to all of these devices: an expandable stent attached to a fabric component to serve as a conduit, a mechanism that seals the endograft in position, and a delivery system to allow deployment via a transarterial approach.

The main body of the endograft has either a modular or unibody design (Figure 1). A unibody device is deployed as a single, symmetric, bifurcated unit. The contralateral iliac limb is pulled down via access from the contralateral groin, and the device rests on the aortic bifurcation. Proximal and distal extension cuffs are then deployed as needed. Modular devices consist of a main body component that has a short contralateral limb segment. Contralateral limb assembly is completed in vivo.

PREOPERATIVE IMAGING AND ANATOMIC CONSIDERATIONS

Less than 50% of AAAs are suitable for endovascular repair because of unfavorable anatomy. Obtaining precise diameter and length measurements at various levels along the abdominal aorta and iliac arteries is therefore of vital importance when considering a patient for endovascular repair, and these measurements serve as a template to determine the feasibility of endovascular repair and to appropriately size the endograft. One established method for obtaining such measurements is the combination of preoperative axial imaging with angiography. Computed tomography angiography (CTA) with reformatted three-dimensional reconstruction using software such as M2S (West Lebanon, NH) has now emerged as an accurate preoperative imaging assessment tool (Figure 2).

TABLE 1: FDA-approved devices for endovascular repair of aortic aneurysms

Device	Talent Abdominal Stent Graft System	Endologix Powerlink System	Zenith AAA Endovascular Graft	Excluder Bifurcated Endoprosthesis	AneuRx Stent Graft System
Manufacturer	Medtronic (Minneapolis, MN)	Endologix (Irvine, CA)	Cook Medical (Bloomington, IN)	W.L. Gore & Associates (Flagstaff, AZ)	Medtronic (Minneapolis, MN)
Composition	Woven polyester over nitinol	over cobalt-chromium alloy	Woven polyester over stainless steel	ePTFE over nitinol	Woven polyester over nitinol
Main body design	Modular	Unibody	Modular	Modular	Modular
Fixation	Passive suprarenal (uncovered stent)	Anatomic fixation*	Active suprarenal (uncovered stent with barbs)	Active infrarenal (hooks)	Passive infrarenal
Year approved	2008	2004	2003	2002	1999

ePTFE, Expanded polytetrafluoroethylene
*The Powerlink device rests on the aortic bifurcation. Suprarenal and infrarenal proximal extension cuffs are available.

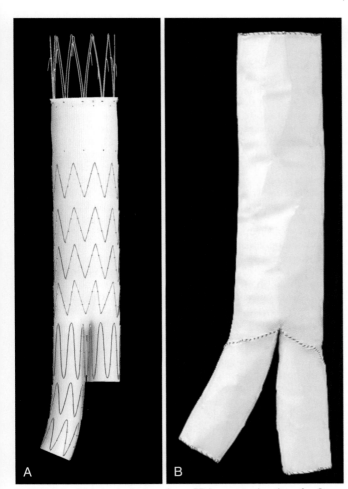

FIGURE 1　Main body design of two FDA-approved endografts. **A,** The Zenith endograft (Cook Medical) is an example of a modular main-body device with active fixation to the suprarenal aorta from an uncovered stent with barbs at the top of the graft. **B,** The Powerlink device (Endologix) has a unibody design and rests on the aortic bifurcation after deployment.

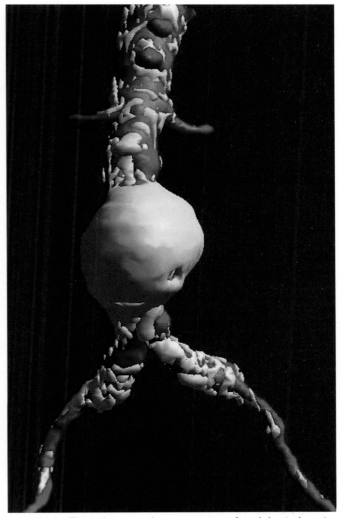

FIGURE 2　Three-dimensional reconstruction of an abdominal aortic aneurysm as demonstrated with software from M2S (West Lebanon, NH). Precise measurements of the aorta and iliac arteries can be obtained from these reconstructions and are essential to a successful endovascular repair.

Proximal Aortic Neck Anatomy

The *proximal neck* of an aneurysm is the length of normal aorta, measured from the lowest renal artery to the most superior extent of the aneurysm; this neck serves as the proximal attachment site of the endograft. The minimum length needed varies slightly among devices but is typically 15 mm. Grafts that allow for suprarenal fixation can be placed in patients with a shorter proximal neck length. The neck should be a normal-appearing segment of aorta, without abundant thrombus or heavy or circumferential calcification.

Accessory renal arteries are present in up to 30% of the population and are a relative contraindication to EVAR. Exclusion of an accessory renal artery by an endograft can result in partial renal infarction. Current data suggest that segmental renal infarction, as a result of covering an accessory renal artery during EVAR, is well tolerated and does not result in accelerated renovascular hypertension. Alternatively, in diabetic patients with an elevation of baseline creatinine above normal, coverage of an accessory renal artery during EVAR may result in further reduction in renal function postoperatively.

The diameters of the proximal and distal attachment sites for the endograft are measured preoperatively. Typically the graft is oversized by approximately 10% to 20% relative to the diameter of the aneurysm neck. Undersizing the diameter of the endograft may lead to an inadequate seal and failure to exclude the aneurysm, and oversizing may result in fabric pleats and a similar outcome. Currently, the largest neck diameter that can be treated with an FDA-approved device is 32 mm.

Angulation

The *angulation* of an aneurysm is the angle formed between the vertical plane and a line that transects the long axis of either the neck or the aneurysm. Angulation in an AAA of 60 degrees or more leads to difficulties in implantation, kinking, endoleaks (see below), and the possibility of downward migration of the device; thus it is considered a contraindication to EVAR with commercially available devices.

Iliac Artery Attachment Site

Most patients with AAAs do not have a normal distal aortic neck to allow for the placement of a tube endograft. Therefore, the distal site to seal the endograft is within the iliac arteries. The common iliac artery (CIA) is the preferred distal attachment site, although the external iliac artery (EIA) may be used in the case of aneurysmal dilatation of the CIA. Ideally, 1 to 2 cm of distal fixation length is necessary.

Each device has various lengths and diameters available for the iliac limbs, depending on measurements made on preoperative imaging. The largest iliac limb diameter currently approved by the FDA is 24 mm for modular devices and 25 mm for the unibody device. Severe tortuosity, heavy calcification, or diffuse narrowing of the iliac arteries may preclude an endovascular approach.

When the EIA must be used as the distal attachment site, the endograft will cover the origin of the internal iliac artery (IIA). Embolization of the IIA prior to EVAR will prevent backward flow of blood into the aneurysm sac. Bilateral embolization of the IIA has been described in the literature, with a low incidence of serious ischemic complications; however, buttock and thigh claudication were frequently reported.

Femoral Artery Diameter

A minimum common femoral artery diameter of 7 mm is required to accommodate the smallest delivery system available. Diffuse narrowing and heavy calcification can pose significant problems when introducing the endograft. A challenging delivery via the femoral artery can be overcome by sewing a synthetic conduit to the distal CIA in an end-to-side fashion and using this to introduce the device.

Inferior Mesenteric Artery

Preoperative imaging is also important to demonstrate arterial flow through the mesenteric vessels. Patients with significant stenosis or occlusion of the superior mesenteric artery (SMA) rely on limited collateral circulation to the intestine. In such patients, covering a patent inferior mesenteric artery (IMA) with an endograft may compromise blood flow to the large intestine, possibly resulting in bowel ischemia. Endograft placement in this setting is contraindicated.

POSTOPERATIVE SURVEILLANCE

Postoperative imaging is essential to both follow changes in the size of the aneurysm sac following EVAR and to assess for device migration and endoleak. After successful placement of the endograft, the aneurysm sac will eventually thrombose, and approximately 50% of aneurysm sacs will decrease in size by 12 months. The integrity of an endograft may be sensitive to the changing configuration of the aneurysm. Changes in the aneurysm may lead to angulation, kinking, thrombosis, or migration of the endograft. Patients with larger preoperative aneurysms tend to have greater aneurysm sac shrinkage. Patients with endoleaks (see below) and preprocedure neck thrombus or plaque tend to have less sac shrinkage.

Abdominal radiographs are inexpensive and offer a gross picture of the position of the endograft and the integrity of the stent framework but fail to give specific information regarding aneurysm sac size or the presence of an endoleak. After an uncomplicated EVAR, a common practice is to obtain a CTA at 1, 6, and 12 months. Beyond 12 months, patients with shrinking or stable aneurysm sacs and no evidence of migration can be monitored with yearly scans. If complications develop, the interval between scans should be shortened to help determine when an intervention is necessary. Evidence-based protocols for long-term surveillance are lacking, and the hazardous effects of serial CT scans over many years can be anticipated but are not well established.

Gadolinium-enhanced magnetic resonance angiography (MRA) is an alternative to CT and spares the patient from exposure to radiation and iodinated contrast, but its use depends on the composition of the stent. Stents composed of either nitinol (e.g., Talent [Medtronic, Minneapolis, Minn.], Excluder [W.L. Gore & Associates, Inc., Flagstaff, Ariz.], and AneuRx [Medtronic]) or cobalt-chromium alloy (e.g., Powerlink; Endologix, Irvine, Calif.) are compatible with the magnet; however, the device lumen in cobalt-chromium alloy stents may be obscured on MRA. Stainless steel grafts (e.g., Zenith; Cook Medical, Bloomington, Ind.) cause extensive image artifact and have the possibility to migrate or deform in a strong magnetic field. As such, MRA should not be performed as a means of endograft surveillance in patients with these devices. However, MRI has been performed safely on other regions of the body in patients with stainless steel endografts under specific conditions, and the Zenith device now carries an FDA-approved label of MR conditional.

In patients without evidence of endoleak within the first month or in those with stable or shrinking aneurysm sacs, limited data support yearly abdominal duplex ultrasonography for routine postoperative surveillance. However, ultrasound has limitations, including operator dependence, and it has not gained widespread acceptance in this application. Angiography is performed for the evaluation of specific problems, such as limb flow abnormalities or a documented endoleak. When an enlarging aneurysm sac is identified on imaging in the absence of an endoleak, angiography is useful to measure sac pressures. An implantable device to remotely measure aneurysm sac pressures for postoperative surveillance is currently being investigated in clinical trials.

TABLE 2: Types of endoleaks

Type	Description
I	Inadequate seal at the proximal (Ia) or distal (Ib) attachment site
II	Flow into the aneurysm sac from an aortic branch vessel (e.g., inferior mesenteric artery or lumbar artery)
III	Endograft fabric tear or failure of seal between graft components
IV	Endograft fabric porosity

Complications

Complications associated with EVAR include arterial injury during endograft deployment or during removal of the delivery system, endoleak, endograft migration, stent fractures, separation of endograft components, and breakdown of the graft material.

Endoleaks

An *endoleak* refers to a persistent flow of blood into an aneurysm sac after endograft placement. Failure to completely exclude the aneurysm from the systemic circulation exposes the sac to elevated pressures and puts the patient at risk for continued aneurysm expansion or rupture. Endoleaks are the most common cause of secondary interventions and aneurysm-related morbidity following EVAR. Four types of endoleaks have been defined, based on their proposed etiology (Table 2).

Type I

A type I endoleak results from an incompetent seal at either the proximal (type Ia) or distal (type Ib) attachment site. Undersizing or oversizing the endograft, severe aortic neck angulation, or deploying a device to seal to a vessel wall that is heavily calcified or lined with circumferential thrombus leads to this type of endoleak. Type I endoleaks can be visualized on angiography immediately after deployment, but delayed or late type I endoleaks may also be encountered and are thought to be due to changes in the configuration of the aorta, as the sac diameter decreases over time.

Type I endoleaks are repaired as soon as they are discovered. These leaks rarely if ever close spontaneously. If discovered at the time of initial endograft placement, repair may consist of reballooning of the attachment site and reversal of anticoagulation. These leaks may also be obliterated by the use of proximal or distal extension grafts. In rare situations when endovascular techniques fail to seal a type I endoleak, conversion to an open surgical repair and explantation of the endograft may be necessary, although this is associated with a mortality as high as 30% in some series.

Type II

Type II endoleaks are the most common type, occurring in up to 25% of endovascular aortic aneurysm repairs. These leaks occur from retrograde flow into the aneurysm sac from a patent aortic branch vessel such as the inferior mesenteric artery (IMA) or a lumbar artery. They are most often identified during postoperative surveillance imaging. On CTA and MRA they appear as collections of contrast within the aneurysm sac but outside of the endograft wall. Delayed images are often necessary, because the sac fills retrograde through a collateral network, and the endoleak may not be visualized during the arterial phase.

The significance and management of type II endoleaks is somewhat controversial. Spontaneous resolution can occur in 30% to 90% of cases, so close observation with short interval serial imaging may be appropriate. However, the presence of elevated sac pressures places the patient at higher risk for aneurysm growth and rupture. Percutaneous translumbar or transarterial coil embolization of type II endoleaks is considered in the setting of an enlarging aneurysm sac. In experienced hands, laparoscopic clipping of the feeding vessel is an alternative strategy.

Type III and Type IV

Type III and type IV endoleaks are much less common. Type III endoleaks are due to separation between modular endograft components or because of erosion or tears in the endograft fabric. Treatment with additional stents to cover the leak is indicated as soon as they are discovered to exclude the sac from systemic pressure. Type IV endoleaks result from the egress of blood through the pores in the fabric. They are sometimes noted on the completion arteriogram following EVAR and generally resolve spontaneously with reversal of anticoagulation.

Endotension

Sometimes referred to as a *type V endoleak, endotension* is the term for elevated aneurysm sac pressure leading to sac expansion in the absence of a radiographically documented endoleak. The exact mechanism is likely multifactorial, and possible explanations include a low-flow endoleak leading to thrombus accumulation, accumulation of protein-rich fluid in the aneurysm sac after exclusion as the result of a hyperosmotic state within the sac from fibrinolysis of sac thrombus, and transmission of systemic pressure through the endograft wall to thrombus lining the sac. The original endograft was associated with more aneurysm sac growth than other devices, even in the absence of endoleaks. This was thought to be due to movement of fluid into the aneurysm sac across the expanded polytetrafluoroethylene (PTFE) material, and it prompted a modification of the device in 2004 to decrease graft permeability. Treatment of endotension is a difficult problem and is largely undefined. Fenestration of the aneurysm sac has been described with some success, and secondary conversion to an open repair is sometimes necessary but carries a high mortality rate of 20% to 30% in some series.

Device Migration

Migration of an endograft following successful placement can lead to complications that include endoleak, stent fracture, aneurysm expansion, and rupture. Rates of migration seem to be device specific and may be related to the mechanism of fixation. Risk factors for migration include short proximal aortic neck length, dilation of the aortic neck over time, severe proximal neck angulation, endograft oversizing (>30%), and the presence of thrombus at the proximal aortic neck.

Brewster and colleagues published their 12-year EVAR experience in 2006, including over 800 patients using 10 different devices. Clinically significant device migration was observed in 2.9% of patients over the study period. In 2005, Tonnessen and colleagues published long-term data for the AneuRx and Zenith devices. With the AneuRx device, freedom from device migration, defined as a movement greater than 10 mm or a clinical event, was 96.1%, 89.5%, 78%, and 72% at 1, 2, 3, and 4 years, respectively. The Zenith device had significantly lower rates of migration, with 100%, 97.6%, 97.6%, and 97.6% of patients free from device migration at 1, 2, 3, and 4 years, respectively. Higher migration rates with the AneuRx device may relate to the fact that many physicians were inexperienced and performed their first EVAR cases using this device. Since the AneuRx endograft was one of the first commercially approved devices, longer term follow-up data are available, but lack of active fixation and suprarenal fixation within the aortic lumen may play a role. Wang and colleagues (2008) published 6 year results with the Powerlink device, and device migration was observed in 4.2%. Interestingly, all patients who demonstrated migration had the device secured at the renal arteries rather than resting on the aortic bifurcation.

Outcomes

Short Term

Multiple nonrandomized clinical trials have demonstrated a significant early postoperative survival benefit in EVAR compared to open repair. Furthermore, the incidence of serious postoperative complications is reduced in patients undergoing EVAR compared with the open approach.

Two randomized controlled trials were published in 2004 that firmly established the short-term benefits of endovascular repair over the conventional open approach. EVAR-1 was a multiinstitutional trial that randomized 1,082 patients age 60 or older with aneurysms at least 5.5 cm in diameter to undergo either EVAR or open AAA repair; all patients included in this trial were healthy enough to undergo open repair. At 30 days, mortality was significantly lower with endovascular repair (1.6% vs. 4.6%; adjusted odds ratio, 0.35; 95% confidence interval [CI], 0.15 to 0.78). In-hospital mortality rate was reduced by 75% with endovascular repair and was associated with a significantly shorter hospital stay (7 vs. 12 days), although more secondary interventions were required with endovascular repair than with the open repair (9.8% vs. 5.8%).

The DREAM trial randomized 345 patients with aneurysms at least 5 cm in diameter to undergo either open or endovascular repair. Again, patients included in this trial were determined to be healthy enough to undergo open repair. When compared with open repair, EVAR resulted in significant decreases in operative time, blood loss, transfusion requirements, duration of mechanical ventilation, duration of intensive care unit stay, and duration of hospitalization. Operative mortality was higher in the open-repair group compared with the EVAR group, but this was not statistically significant (4.6% vs. 1.2%; risk ratio, 3.9; 95% CI, 0.9 to 32.9; $P = .1$). Moderate and severe systemic complications were more frequent with open repair (26% vs. 12%; $P < .001$), but moderate and severe local vascular or implant-related complications were more frequent with endovascular repair (16% vs. 9%; $P = .03$).

The OVER trial was conducted at 42 Veterans Affairs Medical Centers across the United States. This trial randomized 881 patients who had aortic aneurysms of at least 5 cm in diameter (or 4.5 cm with rapid expansion) to open or endovascular repair. Thirty-day perioperative mortality rate was significantly higher in the open repair group (2.3% vs. 0.2% $P = .006$). Patients in the endovascular group had reduced median duration of procedure (2.9 hours vs. 3.7 hours, $P < .001$), time on mechanical ventilation (3.6 hours vs. 5.0 hours, $P < .001$), estimated blood loss (200 mL vs. 1000 mL, $P < .001$), transfusion requirement in the first 24 hours following repair (0 units vs. 1 unit, $P < .001$), time in the intensive care unit (1 day vs. 3 days, $P < .001$), and hospital stay (3 days vs. 7 days, $P < .001$).

Long Term

Whereas the early advantages of EVAR versus open repair are clear, its durability and long-term benefits are not well established. Limited data are available on survival in patients who underwent EVAR compared with both open repair and no surgery.

Survival

EVAR Versus Open Repair

The early survival benefit seen with endovascular repair is lost between 1 and 4 years, after which survival appears equivalent. Two-year follow-up data from the DREAM trial demonstrated no difference in cumulative survival between EVAR and open repair (89.7% vs. 89.6%, respectively). This observation was noted as early as 12

months following EVAR or open repair. Aneurysm-related death was lower with endovascular repair (2.1% vs. 5.7%), but this was entirely because of a lower rate of perioperative mortality and was not statistically significant. Lower rates of severe events in the EVAR patient population at 2 years were noted, but this was again because of the lower incidence of in-hospital events in the perioperative period. Survival free from moderate or severe postoperative events was not significantly different between the two groups at 2 years, and there were no documented postoperative aneurysm ruptures. Reintervention rates at 9 months were nearly three times higher with endovascular repair (11% vs. 4%; hazard ratio, 2.9; 95% CI, 1.1 to 6.2; $P = .03$) but were parallel thereafter.

Follow-up data from the EVAR-1 trial provided similar results, with no difference in all-cause mortality between the two groups at 4 years. Patients treated with endovascular repair had lower aneurysm-related mortality (4% vs. 7%; $P = .04$) but experienced significantly more postoperative complications (41% vs. 9%) and had a high secondary intervention rate.

The OVER trial observed no significant difference in all-cause mortality both after 30 days or hospitalization (6.1% vs. 6.6%, $P = .74$) and at 2 years (7.0 vs. 9.8%; hazard ratio, 0.7; 95% CI, 0.4 to 1.1; $P = .13$). Over a mean follow-up period of 1.8 years, there were no significant differences in procedure failures, secondary therapeutic procedures, or 1-year major morbidity. The difference in outcomes with respect to secondary interventions between the OVER trial and previous trials can partly be explained by how these interventions were defined. The EVAR-1 trial included secondary interventions only if they were directly related to the graft. However, the OVER trial included any secondary procedures that were related to the original procedure, such as incisional hernia repairs.

Long-term survival was also evaluated in nearly 23,000 Medicare beneficiaries who underwent elective repair with either EVAR or open repair between 2001 and 2004. A significantly lower rate of perioperative mortality was observed with endovascular repair (1.2% vs. 4.8%), a benefit that was more pronounced with increasing age. Long-term survival seemed to be age dependent and largely a result of differences in perioperative mortality. In patients 65 to 74 years old, the initial survival benefit was lost after 1 year. The survival curves for patients between 75 and 84 years old converged between 3 and 4 years. Patients 85 years and older continued to demonstrate improved survival beyond 4 years. At 4 years, the rate of rupture was three times higher in the endovascular group, albeit still uncommon (1.8% vs. 0.5% with open repair). Secondary intervention was more common after endovascular repair (9.0% vs. 1.7% with open repair).

Additional data regarding the long-term durability of EVAR compared with open repair is forthcoming from a multicenter French study, Aneurysme de l'aorte abdominale, Chirgurie versus Endoprothèse (ACE) trial.

EVAR Versus No Surgery

Patients who were excluded from the EVAR-1 trial because they were deemed to be unfit for open repair were included in the EVAR-2 trial, which randomized 338 patients (≥60 years old; AAA ≥5.5 cm) to undergo endovascular repair or observation. At 4 years, no difference was seen in all-cause or aneurysm-related mortality. Perioperative mortality was significantly higher in the EVAR-2 patients compared with those studied in EVAR-1 (9% vs. 1.7%; $P < .0001$); however, the EVAR-2 patients had significantly worse health.

FUTURE

Appropriate timing for surgical intervention on aortic aneurysms must weigh the risk of rupture against the risks of the procedure. As mentioned, open repair of aneurysms less than 5.5 cm in diameter is not associated with a survival benefit. The diameter threshold for

EVAR has not been clearly established, but data suggest that patients with smaller aneurysms (<5 cm) have more favorable long-term outcomes compared with those who have larger aneurysms (>6 cm). Lower perioperative morbidity and mortality associated with EVAR may make this approach superior to surveillance in patients with smaller aneurysms. Two multiinstitutional randomized prospective trials are ongoing to evaluate this: the Positive Impact of endoVascular Options of Treating Aneurysms earLy (PIVOTAL) trial in the United States and the Comparison of Surveillance versus Aortic Endografting for Small Aneurysm Repair (CAESAR) trial in Europe.

Advances in endograft design have been significant since the introduction of endovascular approaches in the early 1990s. Continued improvement in endograft technology will allow for greater ease in device deployment and positioning. The Anaconda device (Vascutek/Terumo, Ann Arbor, Mich.) allows for repositioning of the proximal ring stents and has a unique magnetic guidewire to facilitate cannulation of the contralateral gate, one of the most challenging aspects of EVAR. In addition, modifications to the mechanism of proximal fixation may provide an improved proximal seal and even lower rates of device migration. For example, the Aptus endograft (Aptus Endosystems, Sunnyvale, Calif.) uses screws, or endostaples, to fix the graft to the proximal neck. Lower profile delivery systems for existing endografts will facilitate deployment through smaller and more diseased access vessels.

Many patients are excluded from endovascular repair because of unfavorable proximal neck anatomy. The Aorfix endograft (Lombard Medical Technologies, Oxfordshire, UK) is a flexible device that can be used to treat aneurysms with severely angulated proximal necks up to even 90 degrees. Customized branched and fenestrated endografts are currently being investigated for the treatment of juxtarenal AAAs and thoracoabdominal aneurysms involving visceral segments. These endografts can be placed at more favorable sites in the proximal aorta while maintaining flow to visceral arteries. The Zenith fenestrated device is only available in the United States on an investigational device exemption from the FDA but is available for sale in both Australia and Europe. Branched iliac grafts are also in development to further broaden the applicability of EVAR to patients with complex vascular anatomy.

SUGGESTED READINGS

Cowan JA Jr, Dimick JB, Henke PK, et al: Epidemiology of aortic aneurysm repair in the United States from 1993 to 2003, *Ann N Y Acad Sci* 1085: 1–10, 2006.

Brewster DC, Cronenwett JL, Hallett JW Jr, et al: Guidelines for the treatment of abdominal aortic aneurysms: report of a subcommittee of the Joint Council of the American Association for Vascular Surgery and Society for Vascular Surgery, *J Vasc Surg* 37:1106–1117, 2003.

Brewster DC, Jones JE, Chung TK, et al: Long-term outcomes after endovascular abdominal aortic aneurysm repair: the first decade, *Ann Surg* 244:426–438, 2006.

Drury D, Michaels JA, Jones L, et al: Systematic review of recent evidence for the safety and efficacy of elective endovascular repair in the management of infrarenal abdominal aortic aneurysm, *Br J Surg* 92:937–946, 2005.

EVAR Trial Participants: Endovascular aneurysm repair and outcome in patients unfit for open repair of abdominal aortic aneurysm (EVAR trial 2): randomised controlled trial, *Lancet* 365:2187–2192, 2005.

Giles KA, Pomposelli F, Hamdan A, et al: Decrease in total aneurysm-related deaths in the era of endovascular aneurysm repair, *J Vasc Surg* 49:543–551, 2009.

Greenhalgh RM, Brown LC, Kwong GP, et al: Comparison of endovascular aneurysm repair with open repair in patients with abdominal aortic aneurysm (EVAR trial 1), 30-day operative mortality results: randomised controlled trial, *Lancet* 364(9437):843–848, 2004.

Lederle FA, Wilson SE, Johnson GR, et al: for the Aneurysm Detection and Management Veterans Affairs Cooperative Study Group: Immediate repair compared with surveillance of small abdominal aortic aneurysms, *N Engl J Med* 346:1437–1444, 2002.

Powell JT, Brown LC, Forbes JF, et al: Final 12-year follow-up of surgery versus surveillance in the UK Small Aneurysm Trial, *Br J Surg* 94:702–708, 2007.

Prinssen M, Verhoeven EL, Buth J, et al: for the Dutch Randomized Endovascular Aneurysm Management (DREAM) Trial Group: a randomized trial comparing conventional and endovascular repair of abdominal aortic aneurysms,, *N Engl J Med* 351:1607–1618, 2004.

Schermerhorn ML, O'Malley AJ, Jhaveri A, et al: Endovascular versus open repair of abdominal aortic aneurysms in the Medicare population, *N Engl J Med* 358(5):464–474, 2008.

MANAGEMENT OF RUPTURED ABDOMINAL AORTIC ANEURYSMS

Guillermo A. Escobar, MD, and Gilbert R. Upchurch Jr, MD

EPIDEMIOLOGY

Thirty years ago, autopsy studies revealed that individuals with abdominal aortic aneurysms (AAAs) die more often when not treated. Currently, surveillance programs for AAAs have successfully decreased the rate of rupture and its attendant substantial mortality, particularly in male smokers aged 65 to 79 years. This notwithstanding, aortic disease is still the thirteenth leading cause of death in adults in the United States. The nationwide mortality rate for elective operative repair of AAAs is between 4% and 8% in multiinstitutional

reports and about 2% in high-volume centers. This is substantially less than the overall 40% to 50% death rate of open repair of ruptured AAAs (rAAAs), which still underestimates the lethality of a rupture, because nearly half of patients never reach the operating room alive.

The size of the AAA is the factor most often linked to rupture risk; however, the diameter "threshold" for repair remains somewhat elusive, given the ever-changing impact of endovascular technology. The timing of operation is determined by considering the risk of rupture of the aneurysm versus the risks of repair—death, organ failure, and loss of quality of life—as well as by balancing the short-term complications and costs versus the potential long-term consequences: hernias and bowel obstruction after open repair and life-long surveillance imaging after endovascular repair.

The Large Aneurysm Study from the VA Cooperative Group demonstrated a 1 year incidence of rupture of about 10% for AAAs 5.5 to 5.9 cm in diameter, 20% for those 6.5 to 6.9 cm, and 30% for those 7.0 cm or larger; at 8 cm, more than one fourth ruptured within 6 months. Conversely, smaller aneurysms have a low risk of rupture based on the results of the Aneurysm Detection and Management (ADAM) trial and the U.K. Small Aneurysm trial. Thus small aneurysms are generally observed with serial imaging until either they become symptomatic or grow to a size greater than 5.5 cm.

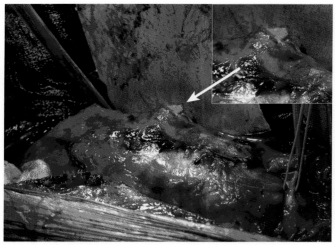

FIGURE 1   Retroperitoneal exposure of a ruptured abdominal aortic aneurysm, showing the protruding mural thrombus plugging the rupture (*inset*) and effectively containing the patient's circulating volume. An orange vessel loop surrounds the left renal artery.

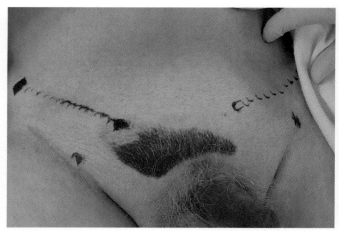

FIGURE 2   Patient with an abdominal aortic aneurysm that ruptured into the right retroperitoneal space presented to the emergency department 3 days later with unrelenting back pain. Note the ecchymosis spreading to the suprapubic space and penis, confirming the prolonged time between rupture and treatment. Black marks on the skin indicate the inguinal ligament.

The high mortality rate of open repair for rAAA has stimulated many to try to predict the patient's outcome with direct management. In this manner, the question of whether the care of patients with rAAA should be regionalized to centers with the best outcomes could be addressed. A review of elective AAA repair in the state of Michigan demonstrated that centers that perform over 30 elective aortic repairs a year had about half the overall operative mortality than those that did fewer repairs. There was also a small but statistically significant improvement in the outcome of open repair of rAAA in high-volume centers, especially in patients over the age of 65. Additional factors that predict poor outcome include age greater than 65 years and female gender, both of which double the mortality rate after open repair of rAAA. Also, among patients with rAAA who underwent emergent endovascular repair from a national cohort, the mortality rate was higher when the repair was done at nonteaching hospitals (55% vs. 21%).

DIAGNOSIS

Patients with rAAA are typically white, male smokers older than 50 years who nearly always are seen for acute onset of back pain that becomes progressively worse. The pain is secondary to sudden dissection of the retroperitoneum that accompanies aneurysm rupture. It is presumed that patients who survive long enough to make it to the hospital do so because bleeding is successfully contained by a plug formed by ejected aortic mural thrombus (Figure 1), or it may simply be due to the equilibrium of tissue pressure and the patient's resultant blood pressure. For this reason, patients who are stable but hypotensive should be left as such, and not aggressively resuscitated. Some patients may even come in several days after the AAA rupture with cutaneous stigmata of contained retroperitoneal bleeding (Figure 2). Those with free intraperitoneal rupture may have peritonitis, but survivors with this clinical presentation are rare; thus the constellation of a pulsatile abdominal mass with hypotension should immediately be treated as a ruptured AAA until proven otherwise. Other nonspecific clinical findings associated with progressive hypovolemic shock from a rAAA include tachycardia, hypotension, fainting, chest pain, dizziness, nausea, vomiting, and altered states of consciousness. A complete physical examination should include evaluation of the patient's carotids for significant bruits and an evaluation for other aneurysms in the femoral and popliteal fossas, as these may be relevant in the repair of the rAAA. Care should be taken to note whether the patient's

pulses are present at the feet to compare with the pulse exam after repair to rule out embolic complications after surgery.

Although the patient's survival is first determined by spontaneous containment of the rupture, a high clinical suspicion will help avoid progressive decline in organ function and subsequent death. Once patients present with hypovolemia, they will manifest with secondary ischemic complications such as myocardial infarction, coagulopathy, multiple organ failure, and death. There is no good laboratory marker for rAAA, as these patients can present with signs of systemic inflammatory response syndrome and lactic acidosis; however, this is not specific to this abdominal catastrophe but may be useful if evaluating the patient for intestinal ischemia.

Historically, when the diagnosis of a rAAA was made in a hypotensive patient, aggressive hydration to raise the blood pressure was initiated. However, most now believe that unless the patient is in shock, intravenous fluids should be minimized. Large-bore peripheral venous catheters should be placed, blood should be cross matched, and resuscitation goals should be limited to maintain a systolic blood pressure of 80 to 90 mm Hg or lower, as long as the patient has normal mentation. Elevating the blood pressure of a contained rupture and subsequently diluting coagulation factors with overexuberant administration of fluids may precipitate more bleeding and accelerate the abdominal compartment syndrome many of these patients get from bleeding into the retroperitoneum. Liberal use of short-acting intravenous antihypertensives can help achieve the above-mentioned goals and reduce cardiac afterload.

Although the act of obtaining imaging on patients with rAAAs may have been heresy in the past, studies have documented that after admission to the hospital, untreated patients with rAAA survive 11 hours on average, and most will survive at least 2 hours. Given the present rapid nature of most computed tomography (CT) scanners, appropriate imaging to help determine which type of repair a patient with a rAAA should undergo is indeed indicated for most patients. Some proponents of an endovascular "stent grafting first" approach have championed taking the patient directly to a fixed-imaging, hybrid operating room and evaluating the aorta there without a CT angiogram (CTA). This strategy may be useful if the patient is truly too unstable to perform a CTA, and aortic bleeding can be controlled by inserting a percutaneous intraaortic occlusion balloon. In general, however, this approach is less than ideal, because a thrombus-laden aorta can be mistaken for a normal aortic neck, if angiography is the sole imaging technique used. In addition, anatomical landmarks, such as the level of the main renal arteries along with localization of accessory renal arteries, and other anatomical factors—patency of the inferior mesenteric artery, aneurysmal involvement of the iliac arteries, aberrant anatomy of the veins, and so on—are useful even when a primary open repair is contemplated. Thus, we prefer to obtain a CT, even without contrast, whenever possible prior to operating on patients with a suspected rAAA.

If an endograft is planned, careful measurements need to be obtained from the CT scan to accurately determine the size of the graft needed. We always calculate linear distances on axial CT scans by subtracting the collimator positions that are reported in the axial cuts and thus negating the need to determine the thickness of the cuts in scans from outside institutions. We also recommend using the zoom function on the software when doing diameter measurements to avoid mistakes in choosing the appropriate endograft. Finally, choosing a stent graft that is intentionally shorter but can be extended to fit the patient's anatomy is prudent if a bifurcated endograft is planned.

OPEN REPAIR

Multiple studies have documented that the patient should be kept warm using forced-air warmers during rAAA repair to avoid coagulopathy. The patient is positioned such that both arms are accessible to the anesthesiologists for access if necessary. An indwelling bladder catheter is placed, and the patient is cleansed from chin to feet. Approaches to the abdominal aorta include a transabdominal laparotomy or retroperitoneal exposure. Most ruptures can be approached via a laparotomy, which offers the fastest access to the abdominal aorta and both iliac and femoral arteries.

The greatest limitation of this approach is that if the extent of the aneurysm enters the thorax, exposing the aorta in the chest will potentially require another incision, which makes for a suboptimal exposure; this again highlights the usefulness of a CT scan prior to operating on an rAAA. Retroperitoneal exposure allows access to the entire descending aorta by rotating the patient's pelvis slightly to the left with the thorax turned almost 45 degrees, limiting exposure to the right iliac artery and the right renal artery. Retroperitoneal dissection must be done carefully to avoid entry into the peritoneum and prevent injury to the spleen and other organs from erroneous or forceful placement of retractors. Another drawback to the retroperitoneal incision is that if bleeding or ischemic colitis occurs, they may go unrecognized, as the intestine cannot be examined directly during the procedure. Detecting this complication is critical, because patients with rAAA have a 35% incidence of colonic ischemia, with a subsequent doubling of mortality.

Regardless of exposure, the aorta is dissected remotely from the site of rupture to obtain proximal control. This is performed first by dissecting the supraceliac aorta free from the esophagus and crus of the diaphragm. Placement of a nasogastric tube aids in dissecting the esophagus away from the aorta. Once an aortic clamp can be positioned proximally, it is left open around the aorta; the rest of the dissection proceeds to the lowest portion of healthy aorta, before the aneurysm starts to minimize splanchnic and renal ischemia from a supraceliac clamp. This will ensure rapid control of the aorta should bleeding occur during the dissection. The surgeon should avoid the ruptured area, and expeditious dissection of the iliac arteries should follow. If the patient is actively bleeding and unstable, an intraaortic occlusion balloon can be placed proximal to the rupture percutaneously via a femoral or brachial technique, which can be done in the emergency room or on the operating room table; in lieu of this, an aortic cross clamp may be expeditiously placed across the supraceliac aorta, until it can be replaced distally. If the aorta has unstable bleeding and has not been sufficiently exposed to allow a cross-clamp, a sponge stick can be used to compress the proximal aorta against the spine. This can be done by an assistant until exposure for a clamp is obtained, or it may also allow the aorta to be opened and occlusion balloons can be inserted. Placing vascular clamps blindly can injure

iliac veins, renal veins, mesenteric veins, the vena cava, ureters, or the bowel; injury to these structures are all life threatening.

Choosing the aortic graft configuration should allow for the minimum length necessary to repair the rupture. Tube grafts should be placed whenever possible, but bifurcated grafts should be used only if the patient's iliac aneurysmal or occlusive disease is severe. Repairing these aneurysms at a later date in the elective setting is more reasonable than extending the dissection and ischemia time. A strip of felt incorporated into the proximal suture line, a technique we use on all elective and emergent repairs, reinforces the strength of the suture lines and reduces the number of repair sutures required following release of the aortic clamp.

The main benefit to open repair of rAAA is the longevity of the repair, which may last for decades. However, when compared to endovascular repair, open rAAA repair increases the physiologic strain on a patient who is already very ill. General anesthesia uniformly decreases systemic blood pressure and may worsen hypotension and hypoperfusion. Sudden decompression of the retroperitoneal space and the attendant decrease in intraabdominal pressure may result in free aortic rupture with subsequent hypotension, myocardial infarction, and death. The extensive retroperitoneal exposure needed to repair the aorta inherently leads to dehydration, hypothermia, blood loss, and the need for additional blood transfusions. More patients develop abdominal compartment syndrome following open repair when compared with endovascular repair; thus the surgeon should have a low threshold for leaving the fascia open to prevent compartment syndrome, covering it with a negative-pressure dressing, and closing the abdomen when the intraabdominal pressure has normalized.

Abdominal compartment syndrome in open rAAA repair is secondary to extensive blood loss, transfusions, and volume shifts during repair. Abrupt changes in blood pressure should be avoided when the vascular clamps are placed or removed. This can best be accomplished by maintaining close communication with the anesthesia team and coordinating the rate of clamp removal with the patient's hemodynamic state. If the patient becomes hypotensive after a clamp is removed, gentle or intermittent digital pressure on the graft will allow time for the anesthesiologist to buffer the blood pressure drop and still maintain distal perfusion.

The most common cause of death in patients who survive rAAA repair is acute myocardial infarction, but multiple other complications can also occur. Small bowel ischemia may occur after clamping the aorta above the superior mesenteric artery (SMA), particularly if mural thrombus is embolized into the SMA or celiac artery (CA). The large bowel may also become ischemic from the above mechanism or, more commonly, from ligating the inferior mesenteric artery (IMA). If the sigmoid colon is found to be ischemic after completion of the aortic anastomosis, then the IMA should be implanted into the aortic graft either directly as a Carrel patch, if it will reach, or with a separate interposition graft from the aortic graft to the IMA.

Renal failure poses a particular risk, as it is not only morbid but also directly linked to a higher mortality. Renal malperfusion can occur upon admission in the hypotensive rAAA patient and is only aggravated by the events that follow. Particular care must be taken not to allow mural thrombus to embolize into the renal arteries when a suprarenal aortic clamp is placed. Avoidance of this can be achieved by occluding the renal arteries prior to clamping the aorta and/or by first placing an aortic clamp proximally in an area of healthy infrarenal aorta before replacing it near the renal arteries.

The only therapy documented in a randomized controlled fashion to improve renal outcome during aortic surgery is infusion of the kidney with cold (4° C) crystalloid solution (Ringer's lactate). However, this can be cumbersome to deliver into some renal arteries, as the os may be difficult to cannulate. In addition, the cannula may fall out periodically and distract the surgical team, prolonging the overall ischemic time. Unfortunately, there have been no drug therapies shown to protect or reverse ischemic renal failure in any large trial in patients with rAAA. Ongoing trials using a perioperative infusion of human atrial natriuretic peptide (ANP) are being performed.

ENDOVASCULAR REPAIR

Endovascular repair of abdominal aortic aneurysms in the elective setting is currently the most common technique used. Since the first report of endovascular repair of an rAAA in 1994 by Yusuf and colleagues, the use of stent grafts for emergent repair quickly became more and more popular. Stent grafts have the advantage that they can be performed with local anesthesia and sedation alone in up to 70% of patients, thus eliminating the complications associated with general anesthesia. Mortality rate following endovascular repair of rAAA has been reported in a number of series to be less than 20%, with discharge from the hospital as early as 2 days after repair and an average of less than 10 days. In contrast, open repair of rAAA has an average length of stay of 2 weeks and double the mortality.

The factors that limit placement of aortic endografts are often related to arterial anatomy but also include hospital-specific characteristics. The anatomic considerations that may prevent placement of an aortic endograft include 1) aortic neck diameter greater than 32 mm at or directly below the renal arteries; 2) aortic neck less than 10 to 15 mm in length below the renal arteries, the most common exclusion criteria; and 3) inadequate access to the AAA, as seen in cases with iliac artery diameters less than 6 mm. Facility limitations may also prevent aortic endograft placement, including 1) the lack of a rapidly available image intensifier, such as a C-arm or fixed-imaging room; 2) an inadequate stock of stent grafts; and 3) lack of an experienced team cross trained in endovascular and open techniques.

When patient is deemed to be an endovascular candidate by CT or angiogram, the patient is transferred to an operating room with fluoroscopic capabilities. Incisions to expose both common femoral arteries are made using local or general anesthetic. Once femoral sheaths are placed, stiff guidewires are inserted and advanced to the thoracic aorta. A multihole catheter is then placed at about L2, and an aortogram and bilateral iliac artery runoff angiograms are obtained. We prefer to use carbon dioxide (CO_2) as a contrast agent, primarily to reduce the contrast load, but also because it gives us sufficient landmarks to place endografts. In lieu of this, or if CO_2 does not demonstrate the landmarks we are looking for (renal or iliac arteries), then iodinated contrast is used sparingly. If the patient is unstable, an aortic occlusion balloon may be placed. In this setting, a single aortouniiliac endograft may be placed rapidly from the infrarenal aorta to one iliac artery to exclude the majority of antegrade flow into the ruptured aortic sac. When using this type of graft configuration, endovascular occlusion of the uncovered common and/or internal iliac arteries results, and a femoral-femoral bypass is performed to restore flow to the contralateral leg and pelvis (Figure 3). The long-term patency of the femoral-femoral bypass in these patients is nearly 100% at 5 years, making this technique an attractive option. If the patient remains hemodynamically stable, a bifurcated graft is placed, and no extraanatomic bypass is needed.

EVAR shares many of the complications of open rAAA repair, but usually to a lesser degree, as the patient's abdomen is closed, and the aorta is not cross clamped, unless an intraaortic occlusion balloon is used. The use of iodinated contrast dye administered during CTA and angiography can induce renal failure. To ameliorate this, we use CO_2 aortography whenever possible, as it has no consequence to the patient's renal function and is inexpensive. Persistent perfusion into the ruptured sac (endoleak) after rAAA repair is often detected during completion aortography at the initial procedure and is managed at the time of repair. Our rAAA protocol includes obtaining a CTA during the initial hospitalization to ameliorate or treat all endoleaks prior to discharge.

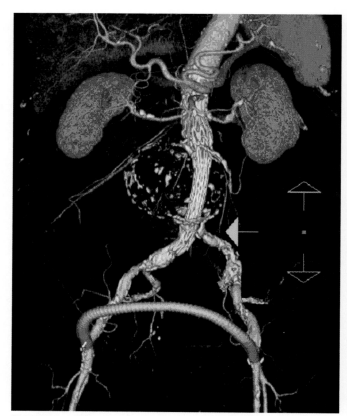

FIGURE 3   CTA of a patient treated with an aortouniiliac endograft and femoral-femoral bypass for a ruptured abdominal aortic aneurysm. The patient also had his calcified left common iliac artery occluded (*yellow arrow*) to eliminate retrograde flow into the aneurysm sac from the left femoral artery, while maintaining flow into the left internal iliac artery.

SUMMARY

After almost 60 years of experience in the open repair of AAA and following dramatic improvements in emergency medical transportation and critical care, the mortality of open rAAA repair is still unacceptably high. Repair of rAAA at high-volume centers and by surgeons with subspecialty training, open or otherwise, offer significantly improved short- and long-term survival with a greater likelihood of being discharged home, all of which argues in favor of regionalization.

Endovascular rAAA repair is dramatically changing the outcome of this lethal disease. Although current endografts anatomically accommodate only 40% to 60% of rAAAs, and not all centers have the capability of performing endovascular rAAA repair, it is likely that this will become the primary paradigm by which these patients are managed. Fenestrated and multibranched endografts, available outside the United States or in select centers in investigational trials, may become more widely available, and the percentage of patients who undergo rAAA endovascular repair will increase.

When questions arise as to the longevity and surveillance of aortic endografts, most patients and caregivers would agree that survival is the primary concern. Paradoxically, as more endografts are placed to improve patient outcomes, training in open repair in both the elective and emergent setting will gradually diminish and potentially worsen the outcome of open AAA repair. Therefore, as the algorithm (Figure 4) for the proper treatment of these complex patients evolves, it is imperative that surgeons who perform this operation be familiar with both open and endovascular repair to deliver optimal patient care.

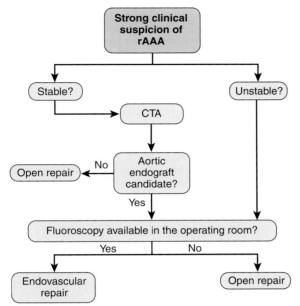

FIGURE 4 Algorithm documenting the approach to ruptured abdominal aortic aneurysms (rAAAs) at the University of Michigan. Unstable patients may still undergo endovascular repair if imaging has confirmed them as candidates. Until the patient is stabilized or repaired, percutaneous aortic balloon occlusion will replace aortic cross clamping, and it can be used for either repair technique.

SUGGESTED READINGS

Boyle JR, Gibbs PJ, Kruger A, et al: Existing delays following the presentation of ruptured abdominal aortic aneurysm allow sufficient time to assess patients for endovascular repair, *Eur J Vasc Endovasc Surg* 29(5):505–509, 2005.

Cosford PA, Leng GC: Screening for abdominal aortic aneurysm, *Cochrane Database Syst Rev* (2):CD002945, 2007.

Darling RC, Messina CR, Brewster DC, Ottinger LW: Autopsy study of unoperated abdominal aortic aneurysms: the case for early resection, *Circulation* 56(Suppl 3):II161–II164, 1977.

Egorova N, Giacovelli J, Greco G, et al: National outcomes for the treatment of ruptured abdominal aortic aneurysm: comparison of open versus endovascular repairs, *J Vasc Surg* 48(5):1092–1100, 2008.

Lederle FA, Johnson GR, Wilson SE, et al: Relationship of age, gender, race, and body size to infrarenal aortic diameter: the Aneurysm Detection and Management (ADAM) Veterans Affairs Cooperative Study Investigators, *J Vasc Surg.* 26(4):595–601, 1997.

Lederle FA, Johnson GR, Wilson SE, et al: Rupture rate of large abdominal aortic aneurysms in patients refusing or unfit for elective repair, *JAMA* 287(22):2968–2972, 2002.

Lesperance K, Andersen C, Singh N, et al: Expanding use of emergency endovascular repair for ruptured abdominal aortic aneurysms: disparities in outcomes from a nationwide perspective, *J Vasc Surg* 47(6):1165–1170, 2008.

Mayer D, Pfammatter T, Rancic Z, et al: Ten years of emergency endovascular aneurysm repair for ruptured abdominal aortoiliac aneurysms: lessons learned, *Ann Surg* 249(3):510–515, 2009.

Mehta M, Taggert J, Darling RC III, et al: Establishing a protocol for endovascular treatment of ruptured abdominal aortic aneurysms: outcomes of a prospective analysis, *J Vasc Surg* 44(1):1–8, 2006.

Upchurch GR Jr, Eliason JL, Rectenwald JE, et al: Endovascular abdominal aortic aneurysm repair versus open repair: why and why not? *Perspect Vasc Surg Endovasc Ther* 21(1):48–53, 2009.

Yusuf SW, Whitaker SC, Chuter TA, et al: Emergency endovascular repair of leaking aortic aneurysm, *Lancet* 344(8937):1645, 1994.

ABDOMINAL AORTIC ANEURYSM AND UNEXPECTED ABDOMINAL PATHOLOGY

David Kuwayama, MD, Umair Qazi, MD, MPH, and Mahmoud B. Malas, MD, MHS

OVERVIEW

Abdominal aortic aneurysm (AAA) is a common, typically asymptomatic, potentially life-threatening condition. Management revolves around excluding the dilated segment of aorta from blood flow to prevent further growth and eliminate the risk of rupture. Currently, two major approaches exist for treating AAA: open surgical repair, via either anterior or retroperitoneal approaches, and minimally invasive endovascular aneurysm repair (EVAR).

Open repair remains the gold standard for treating AAA, with proven long-term efficacy. However, EVAR is quickly replacing open AAA as the first-line treatment in suitable candidates because of the significantly decreased risk of perioperative morbidity and mortality. Continued evolution of stent grafts and delivery systems has made endovascular repair feasible in progressively more unfavorable aneurysm anatomy. As EVAR grows in popularity, fewer patients are undergoing laparotomy for repair of their aneurysms; thus the discovery of unexpected, coincident intraabdominal pathology at the time of operation has become less common. Furthermore, the frequent preoperative use of noninvasive imaging modalities—including computed tomography (CT), Doppler ultrasound, and magnetic resonance imaging (MRI)—has increased the likelihood of discovering coexisting conditions well before the patient ever sees the operating room. Nevertheless, indications for open AAA repair still exist, and surgeons who subsequently make unexpected discoveries at the time of repair must still know how to prioritize their findings so as to develop an operative strategy that minimizes the overall risk to the patient.

Clinical scenarios involving aortic aneurysms and coincident intraabdominal pathology may be generally separated into four distinct categories: 1) elective operation for aortic pathology with incidental finding of asymptomatic nonvascular pathology, 2) emergent operation for presumed symptomatic aortic pathology with incidental findings of nonvascular pathology, 3) emergent operation for abdominal pathology with incidental finding of an aortic aneurysm, and 4) elective operation for abdominal pathology with incidental finding of an aortic aneurysm.

This chapter describes each of these scenarios, focusing on those clinical entities most commonly encountered.

ELECTIVE ABDOMINAL AORTIC ANEURYSM REPAIR AND ASYMPTOMATIC ABDOMINAL DISEASE

Virtually every patient undergoing an elective aneurysm repair, either EVAR or open, has undergone a preoperative CT scan. When asymptomatic intraabdominal disease is discovered on CT scan prior to planned EVAR, the surgeon is generally able to choose whether to proceed with EVAR or to treat the concomitant pathology first. Because EVAR is so well tolerated and causes minimal physiologic derangement, the aneurysm can typically be repaired without significantly delaying the subsequent treatment of other time-sensitive pathology, such as cancer. Furthermore, the peritoneal cavity is left untouched by EVAR, permitting a clean laparotomy for other intraabdominal interventions.

At the time of elective open AAA repairs, pathology that went unrecognized during the prescreening process is often discovered. Frequently this discovered pathology will have either been too small to appear on CT scan or will have been of a nature making it unlikely to appear. At this point the surgeon has three options: 1) continue the open AAA without any other concomitant surgical procedure; 2) abandon the AAA and treat the concomitant condition first; or 3) attempt simultaneous treatment of both AAA and the unexpected pathology. The decision depends upon the type and severity of abnormality found. If the surgeon elects to continue the AAA repair without synchronous treatment of concomitant disease, it must be recognized that the patient may not have another opportunity for the secondary disease process to be safely addressed for quite some time, because of the need for the patient to recover from the physiologic insult of a major open vascular procedure in the immediate postoperative period, and the well-recognized risk of reoperative laparotomy because of adhesion formation in the intermediate term. If the surgeon elects to treat only the concomitant pathology without treating the AAA, the increased risk of aneurysmal rupture caused by delay in repair must be accepted. Because open AAA repair is almost always reserved only for those aneurysms large enough to exhibit an elevated risk of rupture, this risk should not be considered insignificant. If the surgeon chooses to address both problems simultaneously, he or she must be willing to accept the potentially increased morbidity of putting a patient through two procedures instead of one, lengthening anesthetic time and increasing blood loss. Furthermore, resection of the concomitant pathology may require opening the gastrointestinal or biliary tracts, thereby risking the potentially devastating complication of an aortic prosthetic graft infection. The most commonly encountered abnormalities include cholelithiasis, appendix and Meckel diverticulum, gastrointestinal malignancies, genitourinary malignancies, and solid organ tumors.

Cholelithiasis

Cholelithiasis is found in up to 20% of AAA laparotomies. When noted, the surgeon must choose whether to leave the gallstones alone, as simultaneous treatment may increase the chances of graft infection, or to perform a cholecystectomy to avoid the risk of postoperative cholecystitis or choledocholithiasis. Since cholecystectomy can generally be performed quickly with a minimum of blood loss, the greatest factor at play is the elevated risk of graft infection associated with opening the biliary tract.

This topic was once a subject of much debate in the literature, with some citing an elevated risk of cholecystitis in the postoperative period. However, as advances in minimally invasive and interventional radiologic techniques have improved our ability to treat gallbladder disease, the weight of opinion has shifted away from synchronous cholecystectomy. Laparoscopic cholecystectomy, transhepatic biliary stenting, and endoscopic retrograde cholangiopancreatography (ERCP) have permitted symptomatic cholelithiasis and choledocholithiasis to be safely treated almost always without the need for second laparotomy.

Because any AAA repair, open or endovascular, requires close postoperative follow-up, the patient may be screened in the postoperative period for any signs or symptoms suggestive of symptomatic cholelithiasis and referred for elective laparoscopic cholecystectomy when indicated. Patients with recognized gallstone disease should be educated in dietary modification and should be considered for treatment with ursodiol.

Appendix and Meckel Diverticulum

Because of the significant risk of aortic prosthetic infection associated with opening the gastrointestinal tract, asymptomatic appendices and Meckel diverticula should unequivocally be left alone during an open AAA repair. Incidental discovery of acute appendicitis during an open AAA repair would be a rare occurrence indeed, but if discovered, it would certainly need to be resected. A more challenging dilemma arises if evidence of a chronically inflamed appendix or Meckel diverticulum is discovered. In our opinion, the risk–benefit ratio would still argue against synchronous resection, unless the inflammation clearly appears to be acute. Advances in laparoscopic management of appendix and Meckel diverticula have made resection following AAA repair, even in the immediate postoperative period, quite feasible, with a low likelihood of need for repeat laparotomy.

Gastrointestinal Malignancies

Gastrointestinal (GI) malignancies are notoriously difficult to identify on CT scans. Furthermore, aortic aneurysms and GI malignancies tend to occur in the same patient populations: in smokers and in those older than age 50 years. Thus the discovery of previously unrecognized colorectal or small bowel malignancies at the time of laparotomy for AAA repair is a relatively common occurrence. Colorectal cancers (CRCs) are most common, with an estimated frequency of concurrence with AAA of between 0.5% and 1.4%. Therefore the occasional discovery of synchronous GI malignancies would most certainly be encountered in high-volume vascular centers.

Concomitant surgical correction of both CRC and AAA is considered controversial because of the magnitude of a combined operation. Generally, a staged procedure is recommended, with the order of treatment depending upon the judged severity of each condition; a 4- to 6-week period of convalescence between operations is required to maximize the patient's physiologic reserve. Unfortunately, during this period, the untreated pathology may worsen or become symptomatic. Repairing the AAA first postpones colectomy and risks metastasis of colorectal cancer, and starting with colectomy leaves the patient at risk of death from rupture of the aneurysm. Synchronous treatment, on the other hand, avoids the need for a second operation, which may not be well tolerated in the frail vascular surgical population; postoperative recovery may be faster from a psychological point of view as well.

Baxter (2002) published a retrospective review of 83 patients with AAA and concomitant CRC. Among the 64 cases in which CRC was treated first, Baxter observed no ruptures among patients with aneurysms less than 5 cm, but he observed a 10% rupture rate among patients with aneurysms larger than 5 cm. Among the seven patients who underwent AAA repair first, the time to subsequent colectomy averaged 122 days. Baxter's results support the idea of concomitant AAA repair with CRC treatment in patients with aneurysms 5 cm or larger.

Velanovich and Andersen (1991) performed an applied decision analysis and concluded that patients with aneurysms larger than 5 cm, a colonic tumor that has a greater than 75% chance of obstruction or perforation, and a projected mortality of less than 10% would benefit from a combined operation rather than a staged one. Conversely, in patients with small aneurysms, tumors unlikely to perforate or obstruct in the near term, or a poor American Society of Anesthesiologists classification, Velanovich and Andersen recommended a staged approach.

Shalhoub and colleagues recently published a review of 24 cases from prospectively maintained databases of patients with concurrent colorectal malignancy and abdominal aortic aneurysms. In

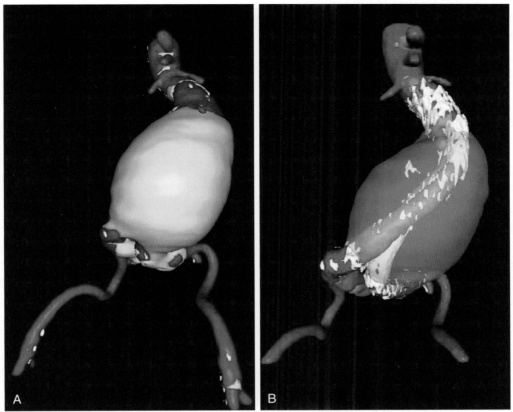

FIGURE 1   **A,** Three-dimensional model of the aneurysm preoperatively. **B,** The model of the aneurysm at 2-year follow-up CT scan. Note the complete endograft exclusion of the aneurysm with no evidence of endoleak. *(Courtesy M2S Medical Images and Data Management Services, West Lebanon, NH.)*

patients undergoing staged management with colectomy first, they documented no interval aneurysm ruptures. However, in their series, patients with large aneurysms underwent EVAR prior to colectomy. The authors concluded that staged management is a reasonable approach with a low risk of aneurysm rupture. They also stressed the usefulness of EVAR in preventing delay of CRC management. It may be preferable to perform EVAR first for a large aneurysm: the patient is discharged home within 24 hours and is able to undergo colectomy, usually via laparascopic approach, in the next 2 to 4 weeks. In one case, an 8 cm AAA was discovered incidentally on preoperative CT scan for colon adenocarcinoma in a 72-year-old man. He underwent EVAR followed by laparoscopic hemicolectomy 3 weeks later and was cancer free with a stable aneurysm at his 2-year follow-up (Figure 1).

Should the surgeon opt to proceed with synchronous resection, excellent surgical technique with control of peritoneal contamination is a must if graft infection is to be avoided. Preoperative administration of antibiotics and aggressive bowel preparation should also be performed, if the cancer was recognized preoperatively.

Discoveries of small bowel and gastric tumors have also been reported, with patients undergoing simultaneous enterectomies or gastrectomies. In such cases, we feel a management algorithm similar to that described above for colorectal malignancies is best followed. Patients should be staged when possible, unless the acuity of each condition individually is felt to be so high as to mandate synchronous intervention.

Genitourinary Malignancies

Renal carcinoma, unless large or invasive, may go unrecognized if aneurysms are approached via midline laparotomy. The chance of discovering a synchronous renal mass is increased with the retroperitoneal approach.

Synchronous repair of AAA and nephrectomy have been described, with a low risk of bacterial graft contamination. Although synchronous treatment avoids necessitating a second retroperitoneal exploration, a staged approach should be used if theAAA repair is particularly difficult, or if intraoperative blood loss is significant. Additionally, patients with known reduced preoperative kidney function may benefit from a staged approach with more meticulous operative planning.

In cases of bladder or prostate cancer, the risk of urinary bacterial contamination is higher. Although there are reports of simultaneous resection of aggressive bladder cancer and aneurysm repair, a staged approach would be considered most prudent to minimize the risk of bacterial graft contamination.

A prospective study by Grego (2003) compared simultaneous aneurysmectomy and radical cystoprostatectomy with a staged procedure and found no statistically significant difference in the outcome and morbidity. Preoperative renal function must be assessed before a concomitant operation, as an early trend toward increased mortality was found by Grego in those patients with preoperative moderate renal insufficiency. Again, aneurysm size matters here: an AAA greater than 5 cm may undergo a simultaneous operation, and smaller AAAs may be staged, also considering EVAR if possible.

Solid Organ Tumors

Solid tumors of the spleen, liver, and adrenal gland have also been documented and successfully resected at the time of AAA repair. Giventhe typically sterile nature of these organs, simultaneous resection appears reasonable, so long as the patient can physiologically tolerate the blood loss and additional anesthetic time associated with the second procedure.

EMERGENT ABDOMINAL AORTIC ANEURYSM REPAIR AND CONCOMITANT DISEASE

Emergent AAA repair is indicated in two situations, with symptomatic AAA and ruptured AAA (rAAA). Imaging studies are usually available in the first case but not necessarily in the latter because of the extreme urgency of the condition and need for prompt transport to the operating room. In either case, the first priority is aneurysm repair, after which the major goal should be for prompt and aggressive resuscitation in the intensive care unit. Pursuing other intraabdominal findings at this time would be ill advised unless they were deemed to be life threatening in nature.

Among patients with a symptomatic but unruptured AAA and a synchronous intraabdominal lesion, the prioritization of conditions should depend upon the severity and related mortality risk of each. Symptomatic AAAs are felt to represent aneurysms in the initial stages of rupture, suggesting that the risk of leaving them untreated would be significant. However, if a concomitant intraabdominal condition is considered life threatening or extremely urgent, aneurysm repair could conceivably be temporarily delayed. If the AAA is massive or is demonstrating early signs of rupture on visual inspection, synchronous open repair would be necessary. Thankfully, the concurrence of two such unrelated yet life-threatening conditions is a rare event.

The treatment of ruptured AAAs is gradually shifting away from open repair toward EVAR when technically possible, with studies indicating a 30% mortality rate reduction in EVAR cohorts. Unexpected concomitant disease may be evident on preoperative imaging conducted for EVAR planning but is otherwise unlikely to be discovered. Even if other pathology is noted preoperatively, treatment of the aneurysm always takes first priority. However, if suspicion develops during EVAR of a synchronous intraabdominal catastrophe, aneurysm repair may need to be followed by diagnostic laparoscopy or exploratory laparotomy prior to transport to the ICU.

Unfortunately, patients in whom control of aneurysmal bleeding has been achieved and aortic continuity restored may nevertheless have suffered enough visceral ischemia during the procedure to develop bowel necrosis. In such cases, clearly nonviable bowel should be resected prior to returning the patient to the ICU for resuscitation, and the abdomen should be left open for marginal bowel to be inspected 24 to 48 hours later.

EMERGENT LAPAROTOMY FOR SYMPTOMATIC ABDOMINAL PATHOLOGY WITH INCIDENTAL ASYMPTOMATIC ABDOMINAL AORTIC ANEURYSM

A broad spectrum of emergent intraabdominal pathologies may bring a patient to the operating room without prior CT imaging. Possible scenarios include blunt or penetrating abdominal trauma, severe lactic acidosis of suspected intraabdominal origin, obvious bowel obstruction in a virgin abdomen, or clear perforation with peritonitis, to name only a few.

Clearly, acute intraabdominal pathology must be prioritized and treated first, and any life-threatening conditions should be addressed promptly. If the aneurysm is found to be exceedingly large or at imminent risk for rupture, either an intraoperative or prompt postoperative vascular surgical consult should be sought.

Operations for intraabdominal infectious conditions, such as perforated viscus or infected necrotizing pancreatitis, make open aneurysm repair in the near-term time frame prohibitively dangerous given the high likelihood of graft infection. If at all possible, the patient should be considered for endovascular repair, as this prevents infected peritoneal contents from ever coming into contact with prosthetic material.

If the patient did not undergo preoperative imaging or was taken for laparotomy based solely upon clinical impression, it is important to ascertain whether the patient's acute presentation (e.g., abdominal pain) was actually a result of the anticipated nonvascular pathology or was rather stemming from the aneurysm. If laparotomy is otherwise negative for findings explaining severe abdominal pain, a symptomatic aneurysm in the early stages of rupture should be added to the differential diagnosis, and a vascular surgeon should be consulted intraoperatively for prompt assessment.

Necrotic small bowel with superior mesenteric artery (SMA) compromise in the setting of AAA should also prompt an urgent vascular surgical consultation. Aneurysmal thrombus or dissection could account for a sudden SMA ostial thrombosis. This life-threatening condition would require emergent revascularization, with or without concomitant aneurysm repair, if the patient is to survive.

ELECTIVE LAPAROTOMY FOR ABDOMINAL PATHOLOGY WITH INCIDENTAL ASYMPTOMATIC ABDOMINAL AORTIC ANEURYSM

With the frequent use of preoperative imaging studies in preparation for elective intraabdominal surgeries, the unexpected discovery of AAA at laparotomy is rare. The discovery of an unexpected aneurysm may be alarming, especially to an operating surgeon who in all likelihood is not a vascular specialist. Unless the aneurysm is exceedingly large or appears to be at imminent risk for rupture, it is probably reasonable for the surgeon to proceed with the planned abdominal operation. A vascular surgeon should be consulted either intraoperatively or promptly following the conclusion of the operation to assess the aneurysm and the patient's suitability for repair. Given the need for high-quality preoperative CT angiography, as well as specialized equipment including fluoroscopy, synchronous EVAR in such a situation is generally not feasible. However, patients with aneurysms larger than 5 cm may be considered for prompt endovascular repair in the perioperative period. Patients necessitating open repair of an aneurysm may do better with a more extended convalescent interval.

SUMMARY

Although several case series and theoretical models do exist in the literature addressing the topic of AAA repair and synchronous disease management, much of the decision making boils down to basic surgical principles of infection control and minimization of patient morbidity.

Several general recommendations may be followed:

1. Emergent AAA repair takes priority over any concomitant disease.
2. Any nonlethal, nonvascular pathology discovered during elective AAA repair may be left alone at that time.
3. Incidental AAA found during emergent or elective laparotomy should be promptly evaluated by a vascular surgeon in the perioperative period; if large enough to represent a rupture risk, it should be addressed soon thereafter, preferably via EVAR.
4. Meticulous surgical technique must be followed if the gastrointestinal or biliary tracts are to be violated during a synchronous aneurysmectomy, as aortic graft infection is a highly lethal complication.

SUGGESTED READINGS

Baxter NN, Noel AA, Cherry K, et al: Management of patients with colorectal cancer and concomitant abdominal aortic aneurysm, *Dis Colon Rectum* 45:165, 2002.

Bickerstaff LK, Hollier LH, Van Peenen HJ, et al: Abdominal aortic aneurysm repair combined with second surgical procedure, *Surgery* 95:487, 1984.

Grego F, Lepidi S, Bassi P, et al: Simultaneous surgical treatment of abdominal aortic aneurysm and carcinoma of the bladder, *J Vasc Surg* 37(3):607–614, 2003.

Ouriel K, Ricotta JJ, Adams JT, et al: Management of cholelithiasis in patients with abdominal aortic aneurysm, *Ann Surg* 198:717, 1983.

Prusa AM, Wolff KS, Sahal M, et al: Abdominal aortic aneurysms and concomitant disease requiring surgical intervention: simultaneous operation versus staged treatment using endoluminal stent grafting, *Arch Surg* 140:686, 2005.

Shalhoub J, Naughton P, Lau N, et al: Concurrent colorectal malignancy and abdominal aortic aneurysm: a multicentre experience and review of the literature, *Eur J Vasc Endovasc Surg* 38(1):137, 2008.

String ST: Cholelithiasis and aortic reconstruction, *J Vasc Surg* 1:664, 1984.

Swanson RJ, Littooy FN, Hunt TK, et al: Laparotomy as a precipitating factor in the rupture of intra-abdominal aneurysm, *Arch Surg* 115:229, 1980.

Thomas JH, McCroskey BL, Lliopoulos JI, et al: Aortoiliac reconstruction combined with nonvascular operations, *Am J Surg* 146:784, 1983.

Valanovich A, Andersen CA: Concomitant abdominal aortic aneurysm and colorectal cancer: a decision analysis approach to the therapeutic dilemma, *Ann Vasc Surg* 5:449, 1991.

MANAGEMENT OF DESCENDING THORACIC AND THORACOABDOMINAL AORTIC ANEURYSMS

Peter I. Tsai, MD, Scott A. LeMaire, MD, and Joseph S. Coselli, MD

OVERVIEW

Aneurysms of the descending thoracic and thoracoabdominal aorta, in which the aorta is dilated to a diameter at least 1.5 times greater than normal, can be caused by medial degenerative disease, aortic dissection, connective tissue disorders, aortitis, infection, and trauma. Descending thoracic aortic aneurysms (DTAAs) involve the segment of aorta bounded by the origin of the left subclavian artery and the diaphragm. Thoracoabdominal aortic aneurysms (TAAAs) are characterized by dilatation of the aorta at the diaphragmatic hiatus and varying degrees of extension into the chest and abdomen (Figure 1).

As the population ages, and as the number and sophistication of diagnostic modalities increases, so does the number of incidentally identified DTAAs and TAAAs in need of surgical intervention. Hemodynamic factors clearly contribute to the process of progressive aortic dilatation and eventual dissection, rupture, or both. The vicious cycle of increasing diameter and wall tension, as characterized by Laplace's law: Tension = (Pressure × Radius)/Wall thickness, is well established. Many patients are asymptomatic at diagnosis, but without treatment, eventual dilation can lead to a variety of manifestations, including compression and erosion of adjacent structures that can lead to back pain, hoarseness, stridor, wheezing, cough, hemoptysis, dysphagia, gastrointestinal bleeding or obstruction, distal embolism, and rupture. This chapter describes indications for surgical treatment of DTAAs and TAAAs, open surgical and endovascular approaches to repair, and techniques used to decrease the risk of ischemic complications.

INDICATIONS FOR SURGERY AND PREOPERATIVE RISK ASSESSMENT

In asymptomatic patients, the decision to consider surgical repair is based primarily on the diameter of the aortic aneurysm. Treatment decisions in cases of thoracic aortic aneurysm are guided by our current understanding of the disease's natural history and the inherent risks of rupture or dissection. Elefteriades's analysis of data from 1600 patients with thoracic aortic disease has helped quantify these well-recognized risks. Aortic aneurysms were shown to

continuously increase, and the average expansion rate for DTAAs was 0.19 cm/year. For DTAAs greater than 6 cm in diameter, annual rates of catastrophic complications were 3.6% for rupture, 3.7% for dissection, and 10.8% for death. At 7 cm, the incidence of expected complications for DTAA significantly increased, including a 43% risk

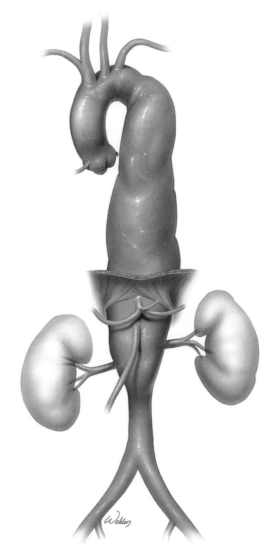

FIGURE 1 Anatomy of a thoracoabdominal aortic aneurysm. *(From Coselli JS, LeMaire SA: Descending and thoracoabdominal aortic aneurysms. In Cohn LH [ed]: Cardiac surgery in the adult, ed 3, New York, 2007, McGraw-Hill, pp 1277–1298. Used with permission of McGraw-Hill Companies.)*

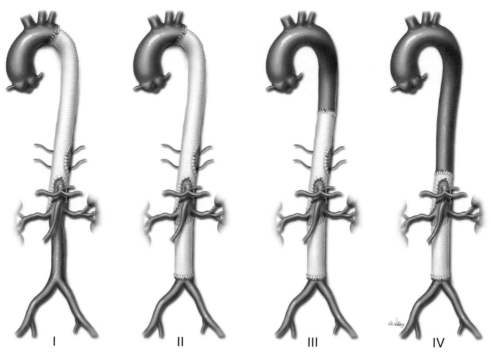

I   II   III   IV

FIGURE 2   The Crawford classification system for thoracoabdominal aortic aneurysm repairs. *(From Coselli JS, Bozinovski J, LeMaire SA: Open surgical repair of 2,286 thoracoabdominal aortic aneurysms, Ann Thorac Surg 83:S862, 2007.)*

of rupture. Elective operation is, therefore, recommended for distal thoracic aortic aneurysms exceeding 6.5 cm in diameter, or when the rate of expansion exceeds 1 cm/year. In patients with a connective tissue disorder (e.g., Marfan syndrome, Loeys-Dietz syndrome), the threshold is lower for both absolute size and rate of growth. Otherwise, strict blood pressure control, cessation of smoking, and at least annual surveillance with imaging studies are warranted.

Symptomatic DTAAs or TAAAs are treated with surgical repair. When the symptoms are acute, patients undergo emergent repair. Immediate operation is also warranted in patients presenting with acute dissection superimposed on an existing chronic aneurysm—a particularly dangerous situation.

The Crawford classification is used to convey the extent of repair needed and to also provide an indication of associated risks (Figure 2). Extent II TAAA repairs are traditionally considered highest risk, because they involve replacing the longest segment of aorta and are associated with the longest periods of spinal and visceral ischemia. It is generally assumed that the greater the extent of descending thoracic aortic replacement, particularly repairs encroaching on the T8 to L1 segment, the greater the assumed risk of spinal cord injury. In general, mortality in emergency or urgent operations is essentially double that in elective repairs.

Despite the variety of operative approaches employed in DTAA and TAAA repair, there are consistent themes with regard to clinical variables that influence both the overall risk of death and the specific risk of spinal cord injury. An adequate preoperative assessment of physiologic reserve is critical in evaluating operative risk. With the exception of patients who require emergent operation, patients undergo a thorough preoperative evaluation with emphasis on cardiac, pulmonary, and renal function. Because aortic aneurysms are considered to be markers of coronary atherosclerotic disease, preoperative cardiac testing is recommended in elective cases. Impaired myocardial contractility and reduced coronary reserve are common among elderly patients undergoing aortic reconstruction.

Given the prevalence of preoperative cardiac disease and the physiologic strain of aortic clamping, it is not surprising that cardiac complications are a major cause of postoperative mortality. Reports indicate that cardiac disease is responsible for 49% of early deaths and

34% of late deaths after TAAA repair. Echocardiography, whether transthoracic or transesophageal, is important to assess valvular and biventricular function, which may be adversely affected by afterload increases that occur during aortic cross-clamping. Dipyridamole-thallium myocardial scanning identifies regions of myocardium that have reversible ischemia, and this test is more practical than exercise testing in older patients with concomitant lower-extremity peripheral vascular disease. Cardiac catheterization and coronary arteriography are performed in patients with evidence of coronary disease, found either in the patient's history or on noninvasive studies, or in patients with an ejection fraction of 30% or less. Patients who have asymptomatic aneurysms and severe coronary artery occlusive disease undergo myocardial revascularization before aneurysm repair. In appropriate cases, percutaneous transluminal angioplasty may be considered before surgery. If clamping proximal to the left subclavian artery is anticipated in patients in whom the left internal thoracic artery has been used as coronary artery bypass graft, a left common carotid-subclavian bypass is performed to prevent cardiac ischemia when the aortic clamp is applied.

Pulmonary function testing is recommended to assess respiratory reserve. Patients with a forced expiratory volume in 1 second (FEV_1) greater than 1.0 L and a partial pressure of carbon dioxide (PCO_2) less than 45 mm Hg are considered satisfactory surgical candidates. In suitable patients, borderline pulmonary function can be improved by implementing a regimen that includes smoking cessation, weight loss, exercise, and treatment of bronchitis for a period of 1 to 3 months before surgery. Although surgery is not withheld from patients with symptomatic aortic aneurysms and poor pulmonary function, adjustments in operative technique, such as foregoing complete division of the diaphragm, are made to maximize these patients' recovery.

Preoperative renal insufficiency has been a major risk factor for early mortality throughout the history of TAAA repair. It was among the predictive variables selected in Svensson's multivariate analysis of Crawford's complete experience with TAAA surgery in 1509 patients treated between 1960 and 1991. The reports by Acher (2010) and our group confirm that preoperative renal impairment remains an important predictor of early death. Renal function is assessed preoperatively by measuring serum creatinine level. Information about kidney size and perfusion can be obtained from the computed tomography (CT) scan used to evaluate the aorta.

Because of the nephrotoxic effects of vascular contrast agents, surgery is delayed if possible for 24 hours or longer after CT scanning or aortography has been performed. This is especially important in patients with preexisting renal impairment. Strategies to reduce the risk of contrast-induced nephropathy include periprocedural administration of acetylcysteine and intravenous hydration. If renal insufficiency occurs or is worsened after contrast administration, the surgical procedure is postponed until renal function returns to baseline or is satisfactorily stabilized. Patients with severely impaired renal function frequently require at least temporary hemodialysis after surgery; these patients also have a significantly higher mortality rate than other patients. Patients with TAAAs and poor renal function secondary to severe proximal renal occlusive disease undergo renal artery endarterectomy, stenting, or bypass grafting during aortic repair.

ANESTHESIA MANAGEMENT AND CONSIDERATIONS

The anesthetic management technique used during the repair of DTAA and TAAA varies among institutions, but standard approaches include invasive hemodynamic monitoring with arterial lines and pulmonary artery catheters, double-lumen endobronchial tubes for single-lung ventilation, and rapid infusion systems for volume resuscitation. Choice of anesthetic may be influenced by the need to maintain basal motor function for neuromonitoring of motor-evoked potentials (MEPs).

Cerebrospinal fluid (CSF) drainage is perhaps the best studied and most widely accepted strategy for preventing paraplegia in patients who undergo thoracic aortic surgery. The body of evidence supports using CSF drainage to reduce the risk of ischemic spinal cord injury in patients undergoing extensive TAAA repairs. In our study of 145 patients undergoing extent I or II TAAA repair, patients were randomized to CSF drainage or no CSF drainage. Postoperatively, paraplegia or paraparesis developed in 9 patients (13%) in the control group but only in 2 patients (3%) in the CSF-drainage group. For this reason, we routinely use CSF drainage in patients undergoing Crawford extent I or II TAAA repairs. The use of CSF drainage does carry risks, including intracranial bleeding, perispinal hematoma, and meningitis; therefore, we do not routinely use CSF drainage during less extensive repairs, such as open DTAA or extent III or IV TAAA repairs, because the risks may outweigh the benefits in these cases. However, we do advocate using CSF drainage during selected high-risk DTAA and extent III and IV TAAA repairs, such as those in patients with acute dissection or contained rupture and DTAA repairs after previous infrarenal AAA repair.

After induction, an 18 gauge intrathecal catheter is placed through the second or third lumbar space. The catheter permits CSF pressure monitoring and aspiration of fluid throughout the operation and for 2 to 3 days postoperatively. The CSF is allowed to drain passively from the catheter and is aspirated with a closed collection system as needed to keep the CSF pressure between 8 and 10 mm Hg during the operation, between 10 and 12 mm Hg during the early postoperative period, and between 12 and 15 mm Hg after patients have confirmed that they are able to move their legs.

OPEN SURGICAL MANAGEMENT OF DESCENDING THORACIC AND THORACOABDOMINAL AORTIC ANEURYSMS

Adjuncts for Organ Protection

Organ ischemia is a major source of the morbidity related to DTAA and TAAA repair. We currently employ a multimodal approach (Box 1) in an attempt to maximize organ protection during these

---

BOX 1: Current strategy for spinal cord and visceral protection during descending thoracic and thoracoabdominal aortic aneurysm repair

All Extents

Moderate heparinization (1 mg/kg)
Permissive mild hypothermia (32° to 34° C, nasopharyngeal)
Aggressive reattachment of segmental arteries, especially between T8 and L1
Perfusion of renal arteries with 4° C crystalloid solution when possible
Sequential aortic clamping when possible

Extent I and II Thoracoabdominal Repairs

Cerebrospinal fluid drainage
Left heart bypass during proximal anastomosis
Selective perfusion of celiac axis and superior mesenteric arteries during intercostal and visceral anastomosis

---

operations (Figure 3). To preserve the microcirculation and prevent thromboembolization, heparin (1 mg/kg) is administered intravenously before aortic clamping or the start of left-heart bypass (LHB). By inhibiting the clotting cascade, the use of heparin may help to reduce the incidence of disseminated intravascular coagulation.

Hypothermia's protective effects are largely presumed to be secondary to decreased tissue metabolism and a general reduction in energy-requiring processes in the cell. We routinely use mild passive systemic hypothermia during DTAA and TAAA repairs, allowing the patient's nasopharyngeal temperature to drift down to 32° to 33° C. Warm water is used to irrigate the operative field and to slowly rewarm the patient after the aortic repair is complete. In addition, whenever possible during TAAA repairs, renal protection is achieved by perfusing the kidneys with cold (4° C) crystalloid (Figure 3, G). We conducted a randomized trial in patients who underwent Crawford extent II TAAA repair comparing two types of renal artery perfusion: cold lactated Ringer's solution and isothermic blood from the LHB circuit. This study showed that the use of cold crystalloid perfusion reduced the incidence of acute renal dysfunction.

Profound systemic hypothermia (typically below 20° C) and circulatory arrest is an alternative method of exploiting the protective effects of hypothermia. Because of the associated risks of coagulopathy and pulmonary dysfunction, we avoid this approach in routine cases. Hypothermic circulatory arrest is useful when rupture, an enormous aneurysm, or involvement of the arch makes proximal aortic clamping impossible.

We routinely use LHB during extent I and II repairs, as well as in other high-risk situations (e.g., acute dissection). Distal aortic perfusion is achieved by using a centrifugal pump to deliver blood from the left atrium via the inferior pulmonary vein to either the left femoral artery or the distal descending thoracic aorta at the level of the diaphragmatic hiatus. Flows between 1500 and 2500 mL/min are generally used to provide organ perfusion beyond the aortic clamp. Because LHB effectively unloads the left ventricle, it is useful in patients with suboptimal cardiac reserve. Using LHB facilitates rapid adjustment of proximal arterial pressure and cardiac preload, thereby reducing the need for pharmacologic intervention.

After the aorta is opened adjacent to the visceral branches during TAAA repairs, selective visceral perfusion can be delivered through separate balloon perfusion catheters placed within the origins of the celiac and superior mesenteric arteries; these catheters are attached to the LHB circuit by a Y line from the arterial perfusion line (see Figure 3, B). This provides oxygenated blood to the abdominal viscera while the intercostal and visceral branches are being reattached to the graft (see Figures 3, G and H). With this technique, the total

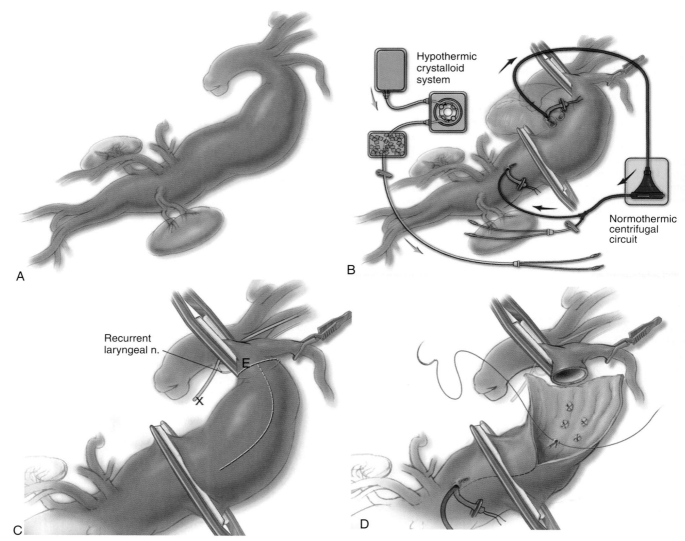

FIGURE 3   An extent II repair of a thoracoabdominal aortic aneurysm. **A,** Repair extends from the left subclavian artery to the aortoiliac bifurcation. **B,** Perfusion systems used during the repair are a left-heart bypass circuit to provide distal aortic perfusion and a cold renal delivery system to provide selective renal hypothermia. The proximal portion of the aneurysm is isolated between clamps placed on the aortic arch (between the left common carotid and left subclavian arteries), the mid-descending thoracic aorta, and the left subclavian artery. **C,** The phrenic, vagus (indicated by the *X*), and recurrent laryngeal nerves are ideally preserved during the repair. The isolated segment of aorta is opened longitudinally and divided circumferentially a few centimeters beyond the proximal clamp. **D,** Patent intercostal arteries in this region are oversewn.

mesenteric ischemic times are reduced to just a few minutes during even the most complex aortic reconstructions. Reducing hepatic ischemia in this fashion may decrease the risk of coagulopathy, and reducing bowel ischemia may decrease the risk of bacterial translocation.

Motor-evoked potential (MEP) monitoring, usually done at the calf muscle after transcranial stimulation, requires special anesthetic techniques. The results of several studies suggest that monitoring MEP to guide the use of spinal perfusion-enhancing measures—such as reattaching more segmental arteries, increasing distal and proximal perfusion pressures, and enhancing CSF drainage—improves the outcome of DTAA and TAAA repair.

Operative Techniques for DTAA and TAAA Repair

A fundamental principle of surgical DTAA and TAAA repair is the importance of adequate exposure, which is optimized when the patient is placed in a modified right lateral decubitus position with the shoulders placed at 60 to 80 degrees and the hips flexed to 30 to

40 degrees from horizontal. The patient is stabilized in this position with a beanbag, and double-lumen intubation and selective right-lung ventilation are used. This allows left-lung deflation to provide optimal exposure, reducing retraction trauma and cardiac compression from an otherwise inflated lung.

DTAA Repairs

Descending thoracic aortic aneurysms are exposed through a posterolateral thoracotomy in the fifth or sixth intercostal space (Figure 4, *A*). Whenever possible, the aortic clamp site is prepared immediately distal to the left subclavian artery. In patients with aneurysms that directly encroach upon the distal aortic arch, clamp sites are prepared at the arch between the left common carotid and left subclavian arteries (this is facilitated by division of the ductus arteriosus), as well as on the proximal left subclavian artery. Care is taken to preserve the vagus and recurrent laryngeal nerves. After heparin is administered, the aorta is clamped and the aneurysm is opened (Figure 4, *B*). Alternatively, LHB may be used in select cases (Figure 4, *C*).

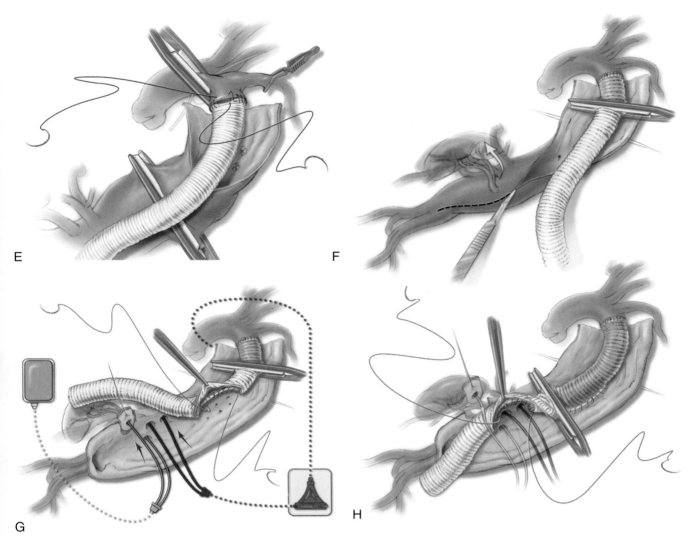

E

F

G

H

FIGURE 3, cont'd   E, Proximal anastomosis is performed with continuous polypropylene suture. **F,** Left-heart bypass is stopped, the proximal clamp is repositioned onto the graft, flow is restored to the left subclavian artery, and the remainder of the aneurysm is opened longitudinally. **G,** Balloon perfusion catheters are inserted into the celiac and superior mesenteric arteries to deliver selective visceral perfusion from the left-heart bypass circuit and into the renal arteries to deliver cold crystalloid intermittently. Patent lower intercostal arteries are reattached to an opening in the graft. **H,** The aortic clamp is repositioned to restore intercostal perfusion. The celiac axis and superior mesenteric and right renal arteries are reattached to an opening in the side of the graft. *(From Coselli JS, LeMaire SA: Descending and thoracoabdominal aortic aneurysms. In Cohn LH [ed]: Cardiac surgery in the adult, ed 3, New York, 2007, McGraw-Hill, pp 1277–1298. Used with permission of McGraw-Hill Companies.)*

In patients with aortic dissection, the dissecting membrane is excised. Upper intercostal arteries are ligated, and the aorta is prepared for the proximal anastomosis by transecting the aorta a few centimeters beyond the clamp and separating the resulting stump from the underlying esophagus. A polyester graft—usually 20, 22, or 24 mm in diameter—is then anastomosed to the proximal aortic stump with 3-0 polypropylene suture. If the aortic arch and left subclavian artery have been clamped, these clamps can be removed after the anastomosis is complete and the graft is clamped, thereby restoring blood flow to the left subclavian artery. Patent distal intercostal arteries are then selectively reattached to an opening in the side of the graft, especially in patients at increased risk for spinal cord ischemia, such as those with prior AAA repair. The graft is then anastomosed to the distal descending thoracic aorta, flushed of air and debris, and unclamped. Protamine sulfate is administered to reverse the heparin. After hemostasis is achieved, two pleural drainage tubes are placed, and the thoracotomy is closed in standard fashion.

TAAA Repairs

A posterolateral thoracotomy starting between the scapula and the spinal processes is performed through the sixth intercostal space for extent I and II TAAA repairs and through the seventh or eighth intercostal space for extent III TAAA repairs; the upper or lower ribs may be cut posteriorly for further exposure. Anteriorly, the incision is curved gently past the costal margin (Figure 5, A) toward the umbilicus. For extent IV TAAA repairs, a straight oblique incision is made through the ninth or tenth interspace (Figure 5, B). The incision is extended toward the pubis if iliac aneurysms also require repair.

With table-mounted retractors providing consistent static exposure, the diaphragm is divided in a circular fashion down to the diaphragmatic crus, leaving a 3 to 4 cm rim laterally, thereby protecting the phrenic nerve and preserving as much diaphragm as possible. The abdominal aorta is exposed retroperitoneally by reflecting the left colon, the spleen, and the left kidney medially. If a left retroaortic renal vein is encountered, division and subsequent repair or

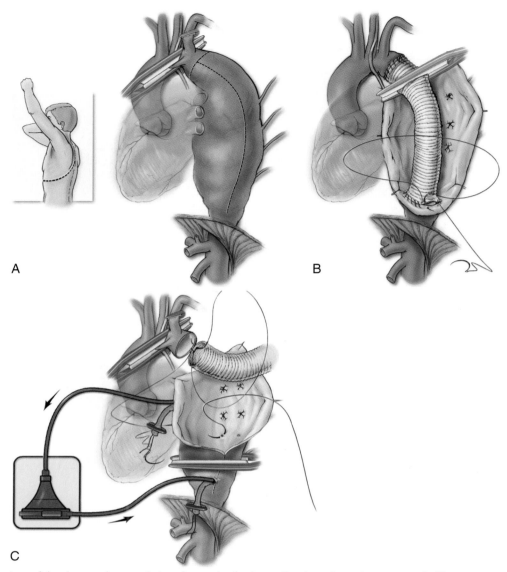

FIGURE 4   Illustrations of the clamp-and-sew technique for repair of a descending thoracic aortic aneurysm. **A,** The operation is performed through a posterolateral thoracotomy (*inset*). Clamps are placed on the aortic arch between the left common carotid and left subclavian arteries and directly on the left subclavian artery. The aorta is opened longitudinally and divided circumferentially a few centimeters beyond the proximal clamp. **B,** After the proximal anastomosis is complete, the aortic clamp is repositioned onto the graft, flow is restored to the left subclavian artery, and the remainder of the aneurysm is opened longitudinally. An open distal anastomosis completes the repair. **C,** As an alternative to the clamp-and-sew technique, left-heart bypass can be used to provide distal aortic perfusion during the repair. *(From Coselli JS, LeMaire SA: Descending and thoracoabdominal aortic aneurysms. In Cohn LH [ed]: Cardiac surgery in the adult, ed 3, New York, 2007, McGraw-Hill, pp 1277–1298. Used with permission of McGraw-Hill Companies.)*

reimplantation might be necessary, if the aortic repair extends below the vein.

For extent I or II repairs, a proximal aortic clamp site is prepared near the left subclavian artery as described above for DTAA repairs. For extent III repairs, the clamp site is prepared just above the mid-descending thoracic aorta (near T4 or T5); for extent IV repairs, the site is prepared immediately above the diaphragm. Heparin is administered and, in extent I and II repairs, cannulas are placed, LHB is initiated, and a distal aortic clamp is applied between T4 and T7 (see Figure 3, *A* and *B*).

After the aorta is opened, patent upper intercostal arteries are oversewn, and the aorta is transected in a manner that leaves a 2 to 3 cm proximal cuff. A 22 or 24 mm gelatin-impregnated woven polyester graft is used to reconstruct the aorta, and a 3-0 polypropylene suture is used for the aortic anastomoses. After the proximal anastomosis is completed, the entire remaining aneurysm is opened longitudinally (see Figure 3, *F*). Patent lower intercostal arteries are selected and reattached to an opening cut in the side of the graft (see Figure 3, *G*). The distal anastomosis is then performed open without a distal clamp (see Figure 3, *H*).

After aortic unclamping, protamine sulfate is administered to reverse the effects of heparin. Hemostasis is secured in all anastomotic suture lines. The renal, visceral, and peripheral circulations are then assessed, and the aortic aneurysm wall is loosely wrapped around the aortic graft. Two posteriorly placed thoracic drainage tubes and a closed-suction retroperitoneal drain are placed before closure. The diaphragm is closed with continuous #1 polypropylene suture.

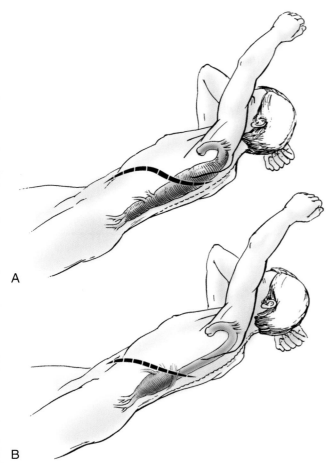

A

B

FIGURE 5 Typical incisions used in thoracoabdominal aortic aneurysm repairs. **A,** Curvilinear incision used to approach extent I, II, and III thoracoabdominal aneurysms. **B,** Straighter oblique incision used to approach extent IV thoracoabdominal aortic aneurysms. *(From Coselli JS, LeMaire SA: Descending and thoracoabdominal aortic aneurysms. In Cohn LH [ed]: Cardiac surgery in the adult, ed 3, New York, 2007, McGraw-Hill, pp 1277–1298. Used with permission of McGraw-Hill Companies.)*

RESULTS OF OPEN REPAIR OF DESCENDING THORACIC AND THORACOABDOMINAL AORTIC ANEURYSMS

Since 1986, we have performed more than 3000 open repairs of DTAAs and TAAAs. During this time, there has been tremendous innovation in the adaptation of surgical adjuncts to mitigate the most serious adverse events long associated with these repairs, namely death, paraplegia, and renal failure. Other common complications have included impaired pulmonary function, cardiac events, and bleeding that necessitates reoperation. To enable better comparison of the current risks associated with open surgical repair versus endovascular repair, it is preferable to report contemporary outcomes rather than outdated historical data. In this context, we present our contemporary experience regarding 519 patients who underwent DTAA and TAAA repair since May 2006 (Table 1). In the group of 406 patients who underwent open repair, 30-day mortality was 5.4% (n = 22) and ranged from 3.4% in extent I TAAA repairs to 7.0% in extent IV TAAA repairs. After open repair, overall rates of permanent paraplegia, paraparesis, and renal failure were 1.5% (n = 6), 7.4% (n = 30), and 5.2% (n = 21), respectively.

Postoperative Surveillance

Patients who have undergone DTAA or TAAA repair remain at risk for the development of new aneurysms in other aortic segments or in reattachment patches. Also, progressive weakening of aortic tissue at suture lines can lead to pseudoaneurysm formation. We recommend that all patients undergo annual CT of the chest and abdomen, and this strategy of follow-up is particularly important in patients with connective tissue disorders. Subsequent aortic repairs can be performed with surprisingly low risk of mortality and morbidity, particularly when done electively.

ENDOVASCULAR REPAIR OF DESCENDING THORACIC AORTIC ANEURYSMS

Stent graft repair of DTAA has recently become an accepted treatment option for selected patients. In 1994, Dake and colleagues reported performing endovascular DTAA repair with "homemade" stent grafts in 13 patients. First-generation stent grafts for thoracic endovascular aortic repair (TEVAR) were bulky, handmade devices that employed pressed polyester material hand sewn onto expandable metallic stents. These stent grafts required large-diameter sheaths (26 Fr) and stiff delivery systems that made accurate delivery and deployment difficult. In addition, the large-caliber devices required conduits to be sewn to the iliac artery or abdominal aorta to facilitate delivery of the devices. Newer generation devices are streamlined to provide improved flexibility and allow the use of smaller introducer systems. The Food and Drug Administration (FDA) approved the first TEVAR stent for treatment of degenerative DTAA in 2005.

The first endovascular device approved for use in the United States was produced by W.L. Gore & Associates (Flagstaff, Ariz.); the FDA approved the device in March of 2005. Both the Zenith TX2 device by Cook Medical (Bloomington, Ind.) and the Talent thoracic device by Medtronic (Minneapolis, Minn.) were FDA approved in 2008 (Figure 6). The currently available Gore device, the TAG, consists of a series of self-expanding nitinol stents affixed to a polytetrafluoroethylene (PTFE) membrane. The outer diameter of the sheath that delivers the largest diameter endoprosthesis (40 mm) is 9.2 mm; the latest 45 mm endoprosthesis is investigational. The TAG device is available in lengths of 10, 15, and 20 cm, and diameters range from 26 to 45 mm. The device is constrained in a PTFE membrane that is released by withdrawing a "rip cord" to deploy the device from the middle toward the ends. The Gore TAG system adds a soft, flexible tip to the leading end of the delivery system. The soft tip improves flexibility at the wire-catheter interface to facilitate tracking through challenging aortic anatomy. The hub component has also been modified to improve ease of use and durability.

The Zenith TX2 uses woven polyester affixed by suture to stainless steel Z stents. Barbs are oriented off the ends of the device to promote fixation to the aortic seal zone. Device diameters range from 28 to 42 mm, custom lengths range from 12.7 to 20.7 cm, and delivery sheath systems range between 6.4 to 7.0 mm in diameter.

The Talent graft features an uncovered proximal stent to cross arch vessels and aid fixation. The device is deployed by withdrawing the introduction sheath to allow self-expansion of the endograft into the aorta. The endograft is composed of a self-expanding, serpentine-shaped nitinol endoskeleton inlaid in a woven polyester graft. Device diameters range from 22 to 46 mm, covered lengths range from 11.0 to 11.6 cm, and delivery sheath systems range between 7 and 8 mm in diameter.

Patient Selection and Preoperative Planning

At this time, TEVAR is primarily used to treat degenerative DTAA. However, many authors have reported using this new, less invasive option in patients with aortic dissection or with traumatic or ruptured

TABLE 1: Outcomes of 519 contemporary descending thoracic and thoracoabdominal aortic aneurysm repairs

Extent/Type of Repair	Number of Patients	Death at 30 Days	Permanent Paraplegia	Permanent Dialysis
DTAA, open	57	3 (5.3%)	0	4 (7%)
DTAA, endovascular	113	6 (5.3%)	1 (0.9%)	3 (2.7%)
TAAA I	88	3 (3.4%)	0	2 (2.3%)
TAAA II	101	6 (5.9%)	2 (2%)	5 (5%)
TAAA III	74	4 (5.4%)	3 (4.1%)	2 (2.7%)
TAAA IV	86	6 (7%)	1 (1.2%)	8 (9.3%)
Total	519	28 (5.4%)	7 (1.3%)	24 (4.6%)

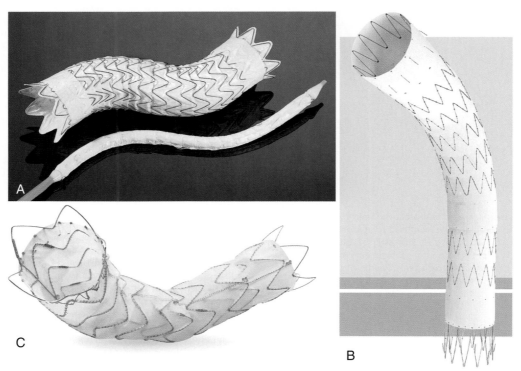

FIGURE 6 Endovascular devices approved for use in the United States for thoracic aortic aneurysm repair. **A,** The Gore TAG stent graft. *(Photo courtesy W.L. Gore & Associates.)* **B,** The Zenith TX2 stent graft. *(Photo courtesy Cook Medical.)* **C,** The Talent stent graft. *(Photo Courtesy Medtronic.)*

aneurysms of the descending thoracic aorta. An obstacle in using TEVAR in patients with blunt aortic injuries has been the lack of an approved device with a small enough diameter for use in relatively young patients who have normal aorta adjacent to the injury. In elderly patients with severe comorbidity and in patients who have undergone previous complex thoracic aortic procedures, endovascular repair is a particularly attractive alternative to standard open surgical procedures.

Preoperative planning, including analysis of the axial imaging data from CT or magnetic resonance angiography (MRA)—ideally with three-dimensional reconstruction, which can provide valuable aortic topographic information—is of utmost importance (Figure 7). The planning process requires a thorough understanding of the aortic diameters at the proximal and distal sealing sites as measured from outer wall to outer wall. Appropriate devices are selected according to their features, including sealing-zone configuration and delivery device properties. The graft is oversized by 10% to 20% to prevent

graft migration or collapse. The proximal fixation should be at least 20 mm in length, and there should be an acceptable aortic diameter throughout this seal zone. The distal aortic seal zone is usually cephalad to the celiac axis. If excessive tortuosity is encountered in either fixation zone, a longer seal length of up to 30 mm may be necessary to prevent an endoleak. When multiple devices are required to cover long lengths of diseased aorta, each piece should be made to overlap 30 to 50 mm with the adjacent piece.

Obtaining an adequate proximal landing zone commonly necessitates covering the left subclavian artery with the stent graft. However, doing so without revascularizing this vessel carries several risks, including arm ischemia, stroke, and paraplegia. To prevent these complications, left carotid–left subclavian bypass is performed in selected patients to maintain subclavian and branch artery blood flow. Left carotid–left subclavian bypass is also performed in patients with patent left internal thoracic artery grafts supplying the coronary circulation.

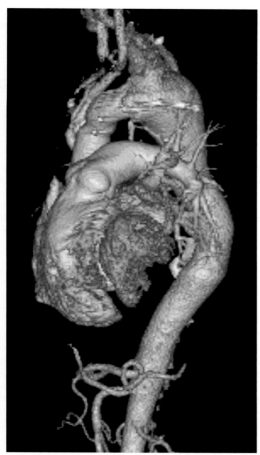

FIGURE 7   Three-dimensional reconstruction of aortic anatomy from CT imaging data shows the first stage of a combined open and endovascular repair. Detailed imaging indicates replaced ascending aorta and aortic arch; brachiocephalic circulation has been partly rerouted. This type of image is used to plan the second-stage endovascular repair, during which the use of the newly replaced aortic arch will be used as the proximal landing zone for the thoracic endoprosthesis.

Endovascular Aortic Repair Technique

Endovascular repair of the thoracic aorta is best performed in a hybrid suite that includes a high-resolution digital imaging system and radiolucent table. The setting should allow for immediate conversion to an open procedure, even if that procedure requires cardiopulmonary bypass should it become necessary. To protect patients against spinal cord ischemia during the endovascular repair, CSF drainage is performed to maintain a CSF pressure of 12 to 14 mm Hg.

The first step in the repair procedure is to obtain appropriate vascular access via a cut-down on the intended access vessel, most commonly the right common femoral artery. If the femoral artery will not accommodate the necessary sheath, an iliac artery is exposed. A conduit can be sewn to the iliac artery in an end-to-side fashion to facilitate deployment of the endograft. After 5000 to 10,000 U heparin are administered to maintain an activated clotting time greater than 250 seconds, a guidewire and the delivery sheath are inserted into the access artery under fluoroscopic guidance. An angiographic catheter is then inserted percutaneously via the opposite common femoral artery or brachial artery to the level of the aortic arch. Digital subtraction angiography of the aortic arch or thoracic aorta is performed to determine the appropriate positioning of the endoprosthesis. The endograft is then advanced into the aorta and suitably positioned after careful review and confirmation of its position under fluoroscopy. To

view the landing areas in the arch, it is often necessary to view the arch with a 45- to 90-degree left anterior oblique projection. "Road mapping" techniques or "fluorofade" may improve operator accuracy in proximal fixation. Maneuvers used to minimize stroke during device deployment in proximity to the great vessels include carefully flushing all air from the device sheaths and lumens. Manipulation of stiff wires into and through the arch should also be performed carefully under fluoroscopic guidance to prevent embolization and dissection.

The device is then deployed, after which a large-diameter, compliant occlusion balloon is used to fix the proximal and distal landing zones to maximize apposition of the stent graft to the aortic wall and seal any stent overlap regions if more than one device is used. A completion aortogram is then performed to rule out endoleak and to confirm the landing zones before protamine is administered to reverse the heparinization. The sheath is then removed, and primary repair of the access site is performed. Complications at this stage of the procedure are mostly due to iatrogenic injury to the iliac vessel; as a measure to mitigate against severe hemorrhage, the guidewire is left in the artery until the sheath has been removed and vascular control is ensured. If necessary, an occlusion balloon can be passed proximal to the injury and inflated to stop the bleeding. Small tears or dissections can be treated with endovascular stent placement, whereas severe tears in the vessel require a flank incision and reconstruction.

Complications and Outcomes

Patients undergoing TEVAR are vulnerable to many of the same complications associated with open DTAA repair, including paraplegia and renal failure. As experience with descending thoracic aortic stent grafts continues to accumulate, so do reports of complications specifically related to inadequate sealing and problems with device deployment. Endoleaks are characterized by persistent blood flow into the aneurysm sac; this blood flow can usually be seen on radiologic imaging. Type I endoleaks are those in which blood enters the sac because of an incomplete seal at the landing zones. These endoleaks are not benign because they lead to continual pressurization of the sac that can cause further expansion and eventual rupture over time. In type II endoleaks, the sac is filled by retrograde flow from branch vessels, such as patent intercostal arteries; these endoleaks are generally considered benign and often do not require surgical intervention because the majority of the culprit branch arteries will thrombose with time. Type III endoleaks are caused by a defect in the stent graft wall or an incomplete seal between two devices; these endoleaks require aggressive treatment. Type IV endoleaks are extremely rare and result from the porosity of the stent graft, which usually seals with time. Type V endoleaks are characterized by endotension and are treated by deploying another stent graft within the existing stent.

Many complications are directly related to manipulation of the delivery system within the common femoral and iliac arteries and the aorta. Therefore if an intended access vessel is less than 8 mm in diameter, severely calcified, or both, alternative approaches should be considered, such as anastomosing a 10 mm polyester graft to the common iliac or abdominal aorta via a flank incision with retroperitoneal exposure of the vessel. This avoids avulsion of the femoral or iliac artery upon withdrawal of the sheath at the end of the procedure if the access vessel turns out to be too small.

An equally deadly complication is acute iatrogenic aortic dissection into the aortic arch and ascending aorta. There are already several reports of this complication, which most often necessitates emergency open repair of the ascending aorta and aortic arch. Although not all complications related to stent grafts are fatal, endovascular repairs should be performed by expert teams qualified to address the variety of problems that may arise. Also, because late graft-related complications are common, close radiologic imaging surveillance is crucial.

Accumulating data support that TEVAR is associated with better early outcomes than traditional open DTAA repair. Because TEVAR is often used in patients who are unsuitable candidates for open

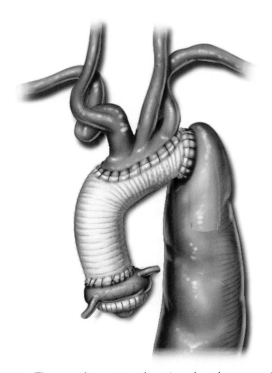

FIGURE 8 The ascending aorta and aortic arch replacement with island reattachment of the brachiocephalic vessels by the elephant trunk technique. *(From LeMaire SA, Carter SA, Coselli JS: The elephant trunk technique for staged repair of complex aneurysms of the entire thoracic aorta,* Ann Thorac Surg 81:1561, 2006.)

surgery, unadjusted rates for morbidity and mortality are often similar after endovascular and open DTAA repair (Table 1); risk-adjusted rates, however, generally favor TEVAR.

FUTURE DIRECTIONS OF THORACIC AND THORACOABDOMINAL AORTIC ANEURYSM REPAIR: HYBRID PROCEDURES

Hybrid repairs can be performed in patients with aortic arch aneurysms that extend into the descending thoracic aorta. The arch can be replaced by using the "elephant trunk" technique (Figure 8), after which the descending thoracic aorta can be excluded with a stent graft by using the "trunk" as the proximal landing zone. Conversely, the arch can be debranched by constructing bypass grafts off of the ascending aorta, if it is of normal caliber, then placing stent grafts across the arch and descending thoracic aorta.

The application of stent graft repair to TAAAs has been limited because the aneurysm involves the aorta at the origin of the visceral vessels. To address this challenge, several groups have reported using hybrid repairs on such TAAAs. This approach has primarily been used in patients at high surgical risk with limited physiologic reserve because of advanced age or significant comorbidities.

Hybrid procedures use open surgical techniques that reroute blood supply to the visceral arteries, so that their aortic origins can be covered by stent grafts without causing visceral ischemia (Figure 9). Endovascular methods are then used, either as part of the same procedure or at a later stage, to exclude the aortic aneurysm. Several reports of small series suggest that among patients with elevated surgical risk, these hybrid repairs produce acceptable outcomes that compare favorably with those of open TAAA repairs. For low-risk

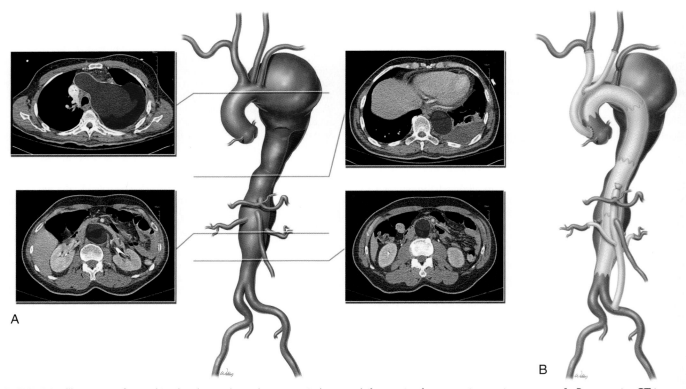

FIGURE 9 Illustration of a combined endovascular and open surgical approach for repair of an extensive aortic aneurysm. **A,** Preoperative CT images indicate an enormous aortic arch and a thoracoabdominal aneurysm. **B,** The brachiocephalic and visceral vessels have been debranched, facilitating extensive coverage with the endoprostheses. *(From LeMaire SA, Sharma K, Coselli JS: Thoracic aneurysms and aortic dissection. In Brunicardi FC, Andersen D, Billiar T, et al. [eds]: Schwartz's principles of surgery, ed 9, New York, 2009, McGraw-Hill, pp 665–700. Used with permission of McGraw-Hill Companies.)*

surgical patients, it is likely that open surgical repair will remain the gold standard, until the durability of hybrid repairs has been established.

ACKNOWLEDGMENTS

The authors express gratitude to Stephen N. Palmer, ELS, and Angela T. Odensky, MA, of the Texas Heart Institute; Susan Y. Green, MPH, for editorial assistance; and Scott A. Weldon, MA, CMI, for creating the illustrations and assisting with image selection.

SUGGESTED READINGS

Coselli JS, Bozinovski J, LeMaire SA: Open surgical repair of 2,286 thoracoabdominal aortic aneurysms, *Ann Thorac Surg* 83:S862, 2007.
Coselli JS, Green SY, Bismuth J, LeMaire SA: Current management of thoracoabdominal aortic aneurysms: patient-based selection strategy, *J Vasc Endovasc Surg* 14:231, 2007.

Coselli JS, LeMaire SA: Tips for successful outcomes for descending thoracic and thoracoabdominal aortic aneurysm procedures, *Semin Vasc Surg* 21:13, 2008.
Coselli JS, LeMaire SA, Conklin LD, Adams GJ: Left heart bypass during descending thoracic aortic aneurysm repair does not reduce the incidence of paraplegia, *Ann Thorac Surg* 77:1298, 2004.
Coselli JS, LeMaire SA, Köksoy C, et al: Cerebrospinal fluid drainage reduces paraplegia after thoracoabdominal aortic aneurysm repair: results of a randomized clinical trial, *J Vasc Surg* 35:635, 2002.
Köksoy C, LeMaire SA, Curling PE, et al: Renal perfusion during thoracoabdominal aortic operations: cold crystalloid is superior to normothermic blood, *Ann Thorac Surg* 73:730, 2002.
Svensson LG, Kouchoukos NT, Miller DC, et al: Expert consensus document on the treatment of descending thoracic aortic disease using endovascular stent grafts, *Ann Thorac Surg* 85(Suppl 1):S1, 2008.

ACUTE AORTIC DISSECTIONS

Tomas D. Martin, MD, and Philip J. Hess Jr, MD

OVERVIEW

Acute aortic dissection, defined as an aortal dissection that has occurred within the past 14 days, is seen by a vast array of primary care physicians and medical and surgical specialists and remains a medical, and many times a surgical, emergency. Left untreated, the mortality rate of a dissection involving the ascending aorta is greater than 90% at 14 days.

Definitive diagnosis of an acute dissection may be difficult in some cases but readily made in most, as long as dissection remains in the differential diagnosis, and contrast-enhanced computed tomographic (CT) scanning is available. The key is to have a high index of suspicion in most patients with acute chest or back pain. Management algorithms remained constant for many years; however, over the last decade, advances in medical knowledge and surgical techniques, particularly endovascular techniques, have changed the algorithms significantly.

CLASSIFICATION

Two classification systems of aortic dissections are used worldwide, the DeBakey and Stanford (Figure 1) systems. The Stanford classification system is the most commonly used, as it is easier for most to remember. Type A dissections include all those involving the ascending aorta, whether or not the arch and descending aorta are involved; type B dissections include all those that do not involve the ascending aorta. The original classification system by DeBakey is a more complete system in that it inherently gives the aortic surgeon information that relates to both acute and long-term management. Type 1 dissections have their point of origin in the ascending aorta with the dissection extending throughout the arch and into the descending aorta. Type 2 dissections are technically limited to the ascending aorta; however, many surgeons today will extend that to include the aortic arch but not the descending aorta. Type 3 dissections originate in the descending thoracic aorta. Neither system addresses

retrograde dissection with or without intramural hematoma, nor do they address intramural hematoma without flow in the false lumen.

PRESENTATION AND DIAGNOSIS

The classic description of the initial symptoms and presentation is that of acute sudden onset of what patients often describe as stabbing, ripping, or searing chest pain with radiation of the pain from front to back and centered between the scapulas. However, the presentation can be extremely variable, ranging from the classic symptoms just described to no symptoms at all. Pain of some kind is typical, including chest pain that mimics angina, neck pain, arm pain, back pain, midepigastric pain, low back pain, and even groin or lower extremity pain. Other symptoms may include syncope, stroke, seizure, myocardial infarction, congestive heart failure, or even acute paraplegia.

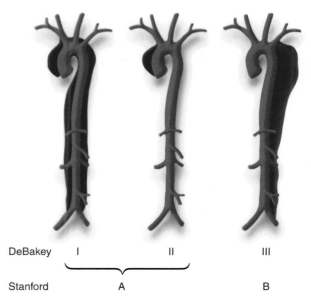

FIGURE 1 Anatomy and classification of aortic dissection: DeBakey and Stanford systems. *(Modified from Cambria RP, Brewster DC, Gertler J, et al: Vascular complications associated with spontaneous aortic dissection, J Vasc Surg 7:199, 1988.)*

Aortic dissection is a well-recognized emergency, and the classic presentation usually triggers a rapid and focused evaluation; however, for patients with a nontypical presentation, the diagnosis often is delayed. The key to a proper diagnosis is to at least have acute dissection included in the differential diagnosis. Acute dissection may be suspected by the symptoms outlined above and by initial physical exam, but it must be confirmed by some type of aortic imaging. Thin-slice, contrast-enhanced computed tomographic (CT) scanning is the imaging study of choice, as it is readily available in most hospitals. Arterial-phase images are mandatory, and delayed venous-phase images are good to have to document delayed flow into the false lumen from distal reentry sites. A high-quality CT scan of the chest, abdomen, and pelvis (Figure 2) provides not only an initial diagnosis but also prognostic information, particularly when evaluating malperfusion syndromes (Figure 3).

Contrast administration even in patients with renal insufficiency or contrast allergy is preferred, as long as they are treated appropriately with hydration and acetylcysteine (Mucomyst) and diphenhydramine (Benadryl) and steroids, respectively. Patients with previously documented life-threatening contrast allergy should be considered for transesophageal echocardiography, which is an excellent second choice and may also be used if the patient is not hemodynamically stable enough for transport to CT, or if a CT scan that has been done is equivocal. Magnetic resonance angiography (MRA) is an excellent choice but plays little role in the acute setting. Conventional angiography combined with cardiac catheterization, the previous gold standard, also plays little role in the acute setting. Cardiac catheterization is only requested if the patient is stable with no significant pericardial effusion and has a history of coronary disease or previous coronary bypass grafting.

MANAGEMENT

Management of acute aortic dissections as a whole is changing; however, the vast majority of DeBakey 1 and 2 and Stanford A dissections with active flow in the false lumen should still be considered for emergent surgical treatment, as the natural progression points to a poor prognosis. There are some patients, however, who could be considered for nonoperative treatment only, such as patients in whom medical management only may be indicated; these include the extremely elderly or frail, those with acute stroke secondary to the acute dissection, and patients with multiple comorbidities or previous cardiac surgery.

For definitive therapy, medical management of ascending dissections in the initial presurgical period should include 1) close observation in an ICU, 2) intraarterial pressure monitoring, 3) aggressive blood pressure management, 4) pain and anxiety control, and 5) β-blockade. The goal of medical management should be to halt progression of the dissection and prevent rupture. Pharmacologic treatment is meant to

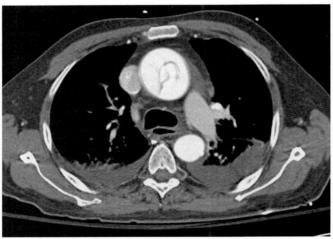

FIGURE 2 Thin-slice CT image of a classic ascending dissection with aneurysmal dilation.

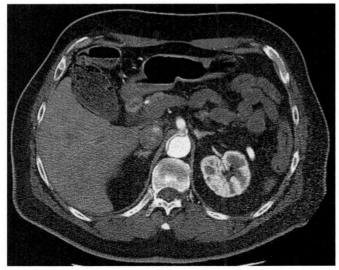

FIGURE 3 Classic anatomy of a patient with visceral malperfusion. Thin-slice CT image showing abdominal dissection with near occluded abdominal aorta, true lumen, and superior mesenteric artery.

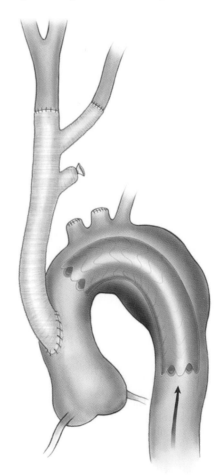

FIGURE 4 Debranching procedure with ascending aorta to innominate and left common carotid bypass, followed by endograft placed in the newly created landing zone (distal ascending and arch).

not only decrease blood pressure but to also reduce left ventricular ejection (dp/dt). We cannot emphasize enough the need for aggressive pain and anxiety control early in the course of treatment, because pain and anxiety in the acute setting are two of the leading causes of tachycardia and hypertension. By simply controlling these two factors, the incidence of acute rupture and extension will be reduced.

Once these two factors are controlled, pharmacologic treatment of blood pressure is paramount. The goal should be a systolic blood pressure of less than 120 mm Hg with a mean pressure of at least 60 mm Hg. Nitroprusside is the initial drug of choice in the monitored setting, as it has such a rapid onset and short half-life; in addition, β-blockade with IV metroprolol tartrate (Lopressor), esmolol, or labetalol should also be instituted, as long as the patient is not hypotensive or bradycardic. Patients treated medically as their definitive form of treatment should be weaned from IV medications to oral agents over a 2 to 5 day period, and they should be hospitalized and monitored for a minimum of 7 to 10 days.

SURGICAL MANAGEMENT OF ASCENDING DISSECTIONS

Stanford A and DeBakey 1 and 2 Dissections

Unless a patient is deemed a nonoperative candidate as described previously, emergent/urgent surgical treatment should be undertaken for Stanford A and DeBakey 1 and 2 dissections, given the high mortality associated with nonoperative treatment. In today's era of centers of excellence, it is not unusual for patients with aortic dissections to be transferred from one hospital to another, one city to another, or even one state to another based on surgical expertise and availability. Once the patient arrives at the surgical facility and a definitive diagnosis is made, surgical treatment should be undertaken on an emergent/urgent basis. Certainly exceptions to the rule exist, and treatment is patient specific: those with significant hemodynamic compromise, large pericardial effusions, moderate to severe aortic insufficiency, ischemic electrocardiographic changes, or malperfusion syndromes should proceed to surgery without delay.

Intraoperative techniques vary from institution to institution and from surgeon to surgeon. Arterial cannulation strategies are controversial and patient dependent and include central aortic, axillary, and femoral approaches. Resection of the entire ascending aorta and proximal aortic arch is recommended, using profound hypothermia with or without complete circulatory arrest. Management of the aortic root and arch are patient dependent. Most aortic valves can be salvaged; however, aortic root or aortic valve replacement are options if deemed necessary. Complete arch replacement with or without individual grafts to the arch branches (Figure 4) has been recommended by some, but this adds significantly to the complexity and length of the procedure.

In the past several years, a technique referred to as a "frozen elephant trunk" technique (Figures 5 and 6) has been reported, in which an endograft is deployed antegrade into the distal arch and proximal descending aorta via an open aorta. Early results suggest that patients with type 1 dissections may have a higher incidence of distal false lumen obliteration and thrombosis with this technique. Despite improvements in medical and surgical management, ascending aortic dissections still carry significant morbidity and mortality.

Stanford B and DeBakey 3 Dissections

Aggressive medical management of the uncomplicated B/3 dissection remains the recommended treatment, and all aspects of medical management previously described in this chapter apply. The management of the complicated dissection, however, is controversial and changing. A complicated dissection is defined by 1) suspicion or evidence of leak or rupture; 2) visceral, renal, spinal, or peripheral malperfusion; 3) significant aneurysmal dilation; 4) hypertension despite aggressive pharmacologic management; and 5) persistent pain despite aggressive pain management.

Open surgical management via left thoracotomy remains the definitive treatment for these patients in most institutions. In the majority of patients, the entry site will be at or just distal to the subclavian artery, making the proximal anastomosis or repair difficult using a cross-clamp technique, leading to the recommendation of femoral-femoral cardiopulmonary bypass with profound hypothermia

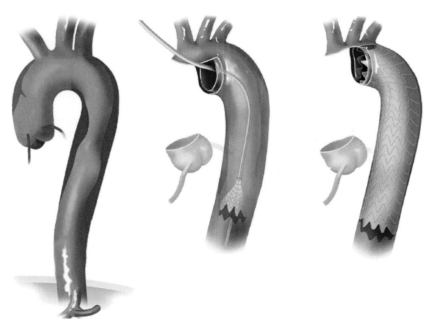

FIGURE 5 Antegrade deployment of stent graft in detail. *(From Pochettino A, Brinkman WT, Moeller P, et al: Antegrade thoracic stent grafting during repair of acute DeBakey I dissection prevents development of thoracoabdominal aortic aneurysms, Ann Thorac Surg 88[2]:482–490, 2009. Copyright 2009, The Society of Thoracic Surgeons.)*

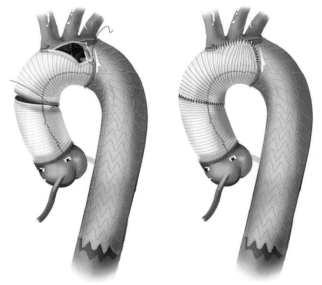

FIGURE 6 Proximal and distal anastomoses of Dacron arch graft. *(From Pochettino A, Brinkman WT, Moeller P, et al: Antegrade thoracic stent grafting during repair of acute DeBakey I dissection prevents development of thoracoabdominal aortic aneurysms, Ann Thorac Surg 88[2]:482–490, 2009. Copyright 2009, The Society of Thoracic Surgeons.)*

and circulatory arrest with an open proximal anastomosis in most patients. Again, this is patient and anatomy specific, and a combination of these techniques may be a viable option. Unless the patient has frank rupture with significant bleeding, some type of distal perfusion is recommended along with spinal fluid drainage.

The amount of aorta replaced is purely patient specific with the goal being to eliminate the primary entry site and any aneurysmal

dilatation. In most patients this can be accomplished by resecting the upper one third to one half of the descending aorta. Eliminating the primary entry into the false lumen, repairing any large thoracic reentry tears, and sandwiching the true and intimal and adventitial layers together at the distal anastomosis redirects flow into the true lumen and corrects visceral, renal, and peripheral malperfusion in the vast majority of patients; this is true unless the distal branch vessels themselves are dissected, and the malperfusion is secondary to flap occlusion inside the vessel itself. In most patients this can be predicted from the preoperative CT scan (see Figure 2).

Institutions with aggressive treatment programs and experienced thoracic endovascular surgeons are using a variety of endovascular techniques as their primary form of treatment for complicated dissections, as the open approach has carried such a very high morbidity and mortality. These techniques cannot be carried out, however, without access to high-quality, very thinly sliced (≤2.5 mm) contrast-enhanced CT scans with axial, coronal, and sagittal images and preferably three-dimensional reconstruction. Intraoperatively, intravascular ultrasound is tremendously helpful but not absolutely mandatory.

In all patients the primary goal is to cover the primary entry site and redirect flow into the true lumen. In patients with malperfusion, this corrects the problem in the vast majority. Covering the left subclavian artery is necessary in most of these patients, so preoperative knowledge of vertebral anatomy and dominance is mandatory. Patients with a dominant left vertebral artery, vertebral occlusive disease, or a previous coronary bypass with a patent left internal mammary artery require a left carotid to subclavian bypass or transposition prior to placement of the endograft. Preoperative knowledge of the origin of the visceral, renal, and iliac vessels and whether they are dissected is also mandatory. Intraoperative angiography combined with preoperative CT scans will determine whether any distal reentry sites need to be covered or stented. Fenestration of the septum as a primary or even secondary treatment is no longer used, unless a proximal endograft cannot be deployed for technical reasons.

CAROTID ENDARTERECTOMY

Bruce A. Perler, MD, MBA

OVERVIEW

Stroke is one of the most significant health care problems in the United States in terms of mortality, morbidity, and cost. Approximately 700,000 new strokes occur each year in this country. More than 80% of strokes are ischemic, and atherosclerosis of the extracranial carotid arteries is the most common preventable cause of ischemic stroke, responsible for 20% to 60%. It is therefore not surprising that carotid endarterectomy (CEA) is the most frequently performed peripheral vascular operation in the United States.

CLINICAL PRESENTATION

In formulating a treatment plan for the patient with carotid artery disease, the two most critical issues are the patient's clinical status and the degree of stenosis in the internal carotid arteries. The vast majority of individuals with significant carotid artery disease are completely asymptomatic, and most are identified by the presence of

a bruit in the neck. Although the cervical bruit is the only physical finding suggestive of carotid artery disease, it cannot be overemphasized that it is an insensitive and very nonspecific finding. Among individuals with a cervical bruit, no more than 30% to 50% will be found to have a clinically significant stenosis in the ipsilateral internal carotid artery. Conversely, among individuals with significant carotid stenoses, a bruit will be found in no more than 20% to 50% on the affected side.

A minority of patients with significant carotid artery disease may be identified after seeking care after a *transient ischemic attack* (TIA), defined as an abrupt interruption of focal neurologic function, usually with very rapid resolution. Symptoms consistent with a TIA include weakness, paralysis, numbness or paresthesias of an arm and/or leg on one side of the body (hemiparesis or hemianesthesia), difficulty speaking or finding words (aphasia or dysphasia), or acute loss of vision in one eye or a part of the eye (amaurosis fugax). The average duration of a TIA is about 14 minutes, but most last less than 5 minutes, and more than 80% of TIAs resolve within 2 hours. In other words, if symptoms have lasted longer than 2 hours, it is likely that the patient is in the process of evolving a completed stroke; to be considered a TIA, the symptoms must completely resolve within 24 hours. Formerly, if symptoms lasted longer than 24 hours but resolved within 48 hours, the event was classified as a *reversible ischemic neurologic deficit* (RIND), although this terminology is falling out favor. Finally, if symptoms persist, and if there is evidence of an infarct on cerebral imaging, the patient has had a stroke. Although the majority of patients who experience a stroke will have experienced at least one warning TIA, in as many as 50% of patients, an ischemic stroke may be the first clinical manifestation of significant carotid artery disease.

Crescendo TIA refers to a clinical scenario in which the patient is experiencing repeated neurologic events, often at increased frequency, with complete symptomatic resolution between attacks. A *stroke-in-evolution* refers to the manifestation of ongoing symptoms and often a worsening over a short period of time, ultimately culminating in a completed stroke.

The differentiation of patients into the proper clinical class is critical, because the risk of subsequent stroke, and thus the threshold for and risk of CEA one would be willing to accept, will depend on the clinical status. For example, among asymptomatic patients with a significant internal carotid stenosis, the risk of stroke over the subsequent 5 years is approximately 10% to 15%. On the other hand, among patients who have experienced a TIA, the incidence of stroke is approximately 25% within the first year; most of those strokes occur early, within the first few weeks or months after the TIA with a decreasing incidence over time. The 5 year incidence of stroke among individuals who have experienced a TIA is 35% to 45%. Finally, among individuals who have experienced an ischemic stroke secondary to carotid artery disease, the 5 year stroke incidence is roughly 50%, and nearly 50% of those second strokes may be fatal.

Imaging Studies

Carotid duplex ultrasound has emerged as the diagnostic modality of choice for evaluating patients with suspected carotid disease. Duplex evaluation provides both anatomic B-mode ultrasound imaging information about the carotid arteries and an assessment of flow velocities (spectral analysis). This allows the health care provider to predict the degree of stenosis in the carotid arteries. In the hands of experienced sonographers, duplex evaluation is more than 90% accurate in depicting significant carotid stenoses when compared with contrast angiography.

When further anatomic information is required—for example, in assessing a potentially high bifurcation or unusual lesion, or when previous duplex scans provide conflicting information—magnetic resonance angiography (MRA) or computed tomography (CT) arteriography may be obtained. On occasion, MRA may overestimate the degree of stenosis. CT arteriography can provide more anatomic information than MRA, but it requires contrast administration.

In light of its invasiveness, risks, and costs, contrast arteriography is very infrequently performed today prior to CEA. It might play a role if there are ongoing concerns about the underlying anatomy, such as a high carotid bifurcation; prior to reoperative CEA, to assess vertebrobasilar insufficiency; or in the case of possible intracerebral arterial disease.

In the symptomatic patient, CT or magnetic resonance imaging (MRI) should be obtained to asses for cerebral infarction and its extent. MRI is more accurate in the early hours after a stroke, and previous studies have demonstrated that as many as 10% of asymptomatic patients and 30% of those who have experienced TIAs will have evidence of cerebral infarctions on CT or MRI studies.

INDICATIONS FOR CAROTID ENDARTERECTOMY

The indications for CEA have been established by level I evidence derived from several randomized prospective clinical trials (Table 1). The North American Symptomatic Carotid Endarterectomy Trial (NASCET) demonstrated a clear benefit of CEA and best medical management compared with best medical management alone for symptomatic patients with high-grade (70% to 99%) carotid stenoses. The same year, the European Carotid Surgery Trial (ECST) demonstrated a similar but smaller benefit in symptomatic patients with high-grade stenoses. Analysis of a second cohort of symptomatic patients with moderate (50% to 69%) stenoses in the NASCET trial demonstrated a smaller but statistically significant benefit as well.

TABLE 1: CEA: Randomized trials

Trial	Indication	Perioperative CVA/Death	Risk Reduction	P value
NASCET	Sx: >70%	5.8%	16.5% at 2 yr	<.001
	Sx: 50%–69%	6.7%	10.1% at 5 yr	<.05
ECST	Sx: 70%–99%	7.5%	9.6% at 3 yr	<.01
ACAS	Asx: >60%	2.3%	5.9% at 5 yr	.004
ACST	Asx: >60%	3.1%	5.4% at 5 yr	<.0001

Sx, Symptomatic; *Asx,* asymptomatic; *NASCET,* North American Symptomatic Carotid Endarterectomy Trial; *ECST,* European Carotid Surgery Trial; *ACAS,* Asymptomatic Carotid Atherosclerosis Study; *ACST,* Asymptomatic Carotid Surgery Trial

Interim and late analysis of patients in the ECST trial did not show a benefit of treating patients with moderate stenoses, owing to higher perioperative morbidity and mortality rates.

The Asymptomatic Carotid Atherosclerosis Study (ACAS) demonstrated a significant benefit from CEA and best medical management compared with best medical management alone for patients with asymptomatic stenoses of 60% to 99%. These findings have been confirmed in the Asymptomatic Carotid Surgery Trial (ACST) in Europe.

The most recent published clinical practice guidelines of the Society for Vascular Surgery recommend CEA and optimal medical therapy for patients with symptomatic disease (stroke or TIA) and a greater than 50% internal carotid stenosis, and for asymptomatic patients with a greater than 60% internal carotid stenosis. These recommendations mirror earlier guidelines from the American Heart Association (AHA), which recommends CEA for patients who have experienced a TIA or stroke within 6 months and ipsilateral 70% to 99% internal carotid stenoses, when the surgeons' perioperative stroke/death rate is less than 6%. For symptomatic patients with a 50% to 69% ipsilateral internal carotid stenosis, CEA is recommended after consideration of patient-specific factors such as age, comorbidity, and severity of symptoms. For asymptomatic patients, the AHA recommends CEA for patients with a 60% to 99% stenosis, when the surgeons' perioperative stroke/death rate is less than 3%.

CAROTID ENDARTERECTOMY: OPERATIVE TECHNIQUE

Anesthesia

CEA may be performed under general anesthesia, regional anesthesia with deep or superficial cervical block, and even pure local anesthesia. Although early reports suggested a reduced length of stay associated with CEA performed under regional anesthesia, comparable lengths of stay are routinely documented today among patients who undergo operation under general anesthesia. The majority of studies comparing the two techniques have reported improved perioperative cardiac stability with regional anesthesia, but this does not necessarily result in a reduced incidence of myocardial infarction. Disadvantages of regional anesthesia include potential patient discomfort or anxiety, risk of seizure or allergic reaction, anxiety for the operating surgeon, and compromise of technique.

Patient Positioning

Careful positioning of the patient is important to ensure patient comfort and adequate operative exposure. Positioning begins with placing a roll behind the scapula to achieve some hyperextension of the neck.

A padded ring is placed under the head to prevent neck injury from extreme hyperextension. If general anesthesia is employed, the endotracheal tube should be taped to the corner of the mouth opposite to the surgical field. If local or regional anesthesia are used, a Mayo stand is placed over the patient's head to suspend the surgical drapes away from the patient's face to prevent sensations of claustrophobia.

Skin Incision

The standard incision used is a longitudinal incision parallel to the medial border of the sternocleidomastoid muscle. The upper portion of the incision is angled posterior to the earlobe, if cephalad exposure above the angle of the jaw is required. An alternative is to place the incision transversely in an appropriately located skin crease, usually 1 to 2 cm inferior to the angle of the jaw. This incision provides excellent cosmesis postoperatively; however, if the incision is made in a suboptimal location, it may be more difficult to obtain more cephalad and/or caudal exposure in the wound.

Operative Exposure

Meticulous surgical technique is paramount to a successful operation. Manipulation of the carotid artery should be minimized, as intraoperative embolization can result from careless handling. The dissection is begun by dividing the platysma and mobilizing the medial border of the sternocleidomastoid muscle. The external jugular vein lies deep to the platysma and should be sought out in this plane to avoid injury, or in the event it is needed for patching. It is more commonly encountered with an oblique skin-crease incision than with a longitudinal incision. The other structure located at this level is the greater auricular nerve, injury of which leads to numbness of the earlobe.

Next, the carotid sheath is entered, and the medial border of the internal jugular vein is dissected. The facial vein is identified crossing medially in the base of the wound and divided; sometimes it has an early bifurcation or trifurcation, and multiple branches must be ligated. The jugular vein is then retracted laterally. The vagus nerve is identified at this point in the carotid sheath, usually located posteriorly between the jugular vein and carotid artery; in a minority of patients, it may lie anteriorly. The common carotid artery (CCA) is controlled circumferentially with an umbilical tape and Rummel tourniquet, if a shunt is to be used. At this point the ansa cervicalis nerve should be identified; it usually lies medial to the distal CCA. Identifying this nerve facilitates the safe dissection of the carotid bifurcation and avoids injury to the hypoglossal nerve, which crosses medially from a superior to inferior location.

The superior thyroid artery is identified coming off the medial border of the carotid bifurcation or proximal external carotid artery (ECA), and it is controlled with a tie or vessel loop. The ECA and internal carotid artery (ICA) are encircled with vessel loops, making certain to control the ICA beyond the disease process. During the dissection of the carotid bifurcation and its branches, the surgeon should avoid dissecting in the crotch of the carotid bifurcation to avoid injuring the carotid body, because this can result in hemodynamic instability and troublesome bleeding. If hemodynamic instability results, the carotid body can be injected gently with 1% lidocaine.

Prior to clamping, the patient is administered 70 to 100 U/kg of heparin, and it is allowed to circulate for 3 minutes. The ICA is clamped first to prevent embolization that can result when the CCA or ECA is clamped. Care should be taken to make sure the ICA is clamped on a normal portion of the artery distal to the plaque.

If local anesthesia or intraoperative electroencephalogram (EEG) are used for selective shunting, a test clamp on the distal ICA should be applied for at least 3 minutes to check for changes in the neurologic exam or EEG pattern. If such changes occur, the artery should be unclamped to allow for reperfusion before reclamping and opening the carotid bifurcation, because opening the bifurcation and placing a shunt may take 2 to 3 minutes, so this should not be done while the brain is already ischemic; however, unclamping the ICA introduces the potential for embolization from a disrupted plaque.

If carotid stump pressure is to be measured, clamps are placed on the CCA and ECA, and a needle connected to a pressure line is placed into the distal CCA below the carotid bifurcation. A stump pressure greater than 50 mm Hg is generally indicative of adequate perfusion, but this is not foolproof. Clamping the CCA and placing the needle into the artery both introduce the potential for embolization.

Conventional Endarterectomy

The conventional technique for CEA consists of a vertical arteriotomy and closure with a patch angioplasty. The arteriotomy is begun in the CCA and is continued through the carotid bifurcation into the ICA. The surgeon should avoid making the incision too close to the flow divider at the ECA origin, because this can distort the anatomy and make the closure more difficult. If a shunt is used, it is first placed in the distal ICA and back-bled, before the proximal end is placed into the CCA. Two commonly used shunts are the Pruitt-Inahara (LeMaitre Vascular, Inc., Burlington, Mass.) and the Javid (Bard Peripheral Vascular, Inc., Tempe, Ariz.) shunts. A third shunt, which I prefer, is a simple vinyl tube that lies entirely within the artery; it allows the surgeon to almost completely finish closing the arteriotomy, before the shunt is removed. Its small diameter allows atraumatic placement in even small ICAs, and its short length offers less resistance to blood flow, such that physiologic flow in the ICA is maintained.

The endarterectomy is begun in the CCA in the plane between the media and the adventitia. The proximal end point in the distal CCA is established, and the plaque is trimmed at that location in a beveled manner. The endarterectomy is continued into the orifice of the ECA, first with a Freer elevator and then with a fine clamp that is passed up into the external carotid artery in the plane of the endarterectomy. The vessel loop on the ECA is released transiently, while the plaque is everted from within the external carotid. The end point of the plaque is inspected: a gradually tapering, feathered end point is ideal.

The endarterectomy is then continued up into the ICA. A technically perfect end point in the ICA is absolutely critical to avoid perioperative stroke and recurrent stenosis. It is virtually always possible to achieve a satisfactory end point in the ICA, although this may require special maneuvers to expose the distal ICA, with extension of the arteriotomy to facilitate extraction of a long endarterectomy specimen.

Tacking sutures at the distal end point should be avoided unless absolutely necessary; these are associated with increased perioperative stroke and are indicative of a problematic end point. The endarterectomy should be terminated in a normal ICA with a gradual, tapered transition to normal intima, which is best accomplished by pulling the plaque transversely away from the artery with lateral traction. The surgeon should avoid pulling out or down on the plaque, which is more likely to result in a step-off that can be difficult to correct.

The preponderance of evidence indicates that the arteriotomy should be closed with a patch. A variety of patch materials are available, including autologous vein, polytetrafluoroethylene, woven polyester (Dacron), and bovine pericardium; I prefer Dacron and running 6-0 polypropylene suture.

Next, the vessels are bled, and the endarterectomy site is vigorously irrigated with heparinized saline and inspected again for debris or intimal flaps, before the arteriotomy is finally closed. The clamp on the ICA is briefly released to fill the vessel with blood. It is then replaced, while the clamps on the CCA and ECA are released, so that any remaining air or debris will be flushed up the territory of the ECA rather than the ICA. At this point the ICA clamp is removed.

Eversion Endarterectomy

Eversion endarterectomy represents an excellent alternative technique. The ICA is amputated obliquely at the carotid bifurcation, and the adventitia is rolled back, until normal intima is encountered at the distal end point. Residual plaque in the common and/or external carotid arteries is removed, and the ICA is reanastomosed to the common carotid artery with 6-0 polypropylene suture.

The advantages of this technique are that the anastomosis can be performed rapidly, and it is not prone to restenosis, and therefore patching is not required. The disadvantages are that a more extensive dissection is sometimes necessary to mobilize the vessels during the eversion, and the procedure does not lend itself readily to shunting, although shunting is not precluded by this technique. It can also be difficult to visualize the end point in the ICA after the plaque has been removed, because the artery tends to retract as soon as the plaque pulls away from the adventitia, and it can be difficult to expose and reinspect this area of the artery again.

Cerebral Protection and Monitoring

One of the long-standing debates related to the performance of CEA concerns the use of intravascular shunts, specifically the routine nonuse of shunts, selective use of shunts, and routine use of shunts. The simplest method is to clamp the carotid bifurcation and perform the CEA without a shunt, and several large series have documented excellent results of CEA without shunts. However, all of these studies demonstrate at least a small incidence of stroke, and in at least some cases, the etiology of the stroke is intraoperative cerebral ischemia during carotid artery clamping.

Alternatively, some routinely shunt in all cases of CEA, and excellent results have been reported in several large series. However, all of these studies document an increased incidence of stroke, and in some of these cases, the stroke was attributed to technical problems related to the use of the shunt.

A third option is to shunt selectively, and several techniques have been utilized to identify the patient who truly needs a shunt. In the patient who is under general anesthesia, these include intraoperative measurement of carotid "stump pressure," after the common and external carotid arteries have been clamped; intraoperative neurologic monitoring of the patient's electroencephalogram or somatosensory evoked potentials; measurement of middle cerebral artery flow by transcranial Doppler, and monitoring of cerebral oximetry. The most accurate method is to perform CEA under regional anesthesia, whereby the selection of patients for shunting is based on alterations in the neurological exam that develop after the carotid artery is clamped.

Completion Studies

Although several potential etiologies of perioperative stroke exist among patients who undergo CEA, one preventable cause is thromboembolism or carotid artery thrombosis resulting from a technical imperfection in the carotid artery repair. To minimize this risk, intraoperative completion studies have been utilized, including continuous wave Doppler, duplex ultrasound, and intraoperative angiography.

Continuous wave Doppler analysis is a purely qualitative method by which an experienced operator can also identify areas of stenosis by the high pitch associated with a stenosis; however, it is insensitive to small intimal flaps or more subtle stenoses, and it is quite operator dependent. Duplex ultrasound is a much more sensitive tool that provides detailed anatomic imaging and real-time physiologic information regarding blood flow through the carotid vessels. However, data yielded from studies are still operator dependent, and there can be technical limitations with placing the Doppler probe in the wound

---

BOX 1: Options to facilitate high carotid exposure

Nasotracheal intubation
Division of posterior belly of digastric muscle
Resection of styloid process
Anterior subluxation of mandible
Vertical osteotomy ramus of mandible

---

to achieve an adequate examination. Intraoperative angiography has been considered the gold standard of completion studies.

Exposure for High Lesions

Several methods may be used to gain additional cephalad exposure of the high carotid bifurcation (Box 1). The easiest of these, and the initial approach, is to start the operation with nasotracheal intubation: with the patient's mouth closed, the vertical ramus of the mandible is displaced anteriorly 1 to 2 cm compared with when the mouth is open with an oral endotracheal tube in place. The additional few millimeters of exposure afforded by this maneuver will often be the difference in achieving a suitable endarterectomy end point in the distal ICA.

The next step to enhance distal exposure is to divide the posterior belly of the digastric muscle. This muscle takes the same diagonal course through the wound as the hypoglossal nerve but is located superficial to it. Therefore this nerve should be carefully identified and protected before the muscle is divided. Two other nerves that can be injured high in the neck are the spinal accessory nerve, which enters the tendinous portion of the sternocleidomastoid muscle, usually in the upper third of the muscle, and the glossopharyngeal nerve, which lies deep to the digastric muscle.

The next maneuver that can be extremely effective at gaining cephalad exposure is resection of the styloid process. The insertions of the muscles on the styloid process are excised, and it is carefully resected with a rongeur. This maneuver will permit exposure of the internal carotid artery all the way to the skull base.

Two other options are available to improve distal exposure of the high bifurcation, both of which require preoperative planning and coordination with an oral or plastic surgeon. Anterior subluxation of the mandible requires placing the mandible in temporary intermaxillary fixation. An even more aggressive approach utilizes a complete vertical osteotomy through the vertical ramus of the mandible, with separation of the mandible to expose the ICA.

PERIOPERATIVE MEDICAL MANAGEMENT

In addition to risk-factor control, the patient should be on an antiplatelet medication, aspirin, or clopidogrel (Plavix) at the time of the CEA. I prefer a continuous infusion of low molecular weight dextran for the first 24 hours postoperatively or until hospital discharge. In addition to its overall cardioprotective effects, data from my institution has demonstrated improved perioperative outcomes following CEA among patients taking a statin medication at the time of the procedure. Antiplatelet and statin therapy should be continued long term in the CEA patient.

RESULTS

Perioperative mortality has become exceedingly uncommon following CEA, averaging less than 1% and generally around 0.5%. Cardiac disease is the most common cause. The incidence of perioperative stroke ranges from 1% to 5% in contemporary practice, and it correlates directly with the clinical indication for operation.

The perioperative stroke incidence should be no more than 1% to 2% among asymptomatic patients, and it ranges from 2% to 6% among symptomatic patients.

Carotid artery disease is an excellent marker for underlying coronary artery disease, and perioperative myocardial infarction occurs in 2% to 4% of patients. Systemic blood pressure instability is seen in at least 60% of patients following CEA; it generally resolves within 4 to 8 hours in most patients, although it often requires close hemodynamic monitoring and aggressive pharmacologic treatment. The incidence of postoperative bleeding requiring reexploration is 1% to 4%. Wound infections are extremely uncommon following CEA and have been reported in less than 1% of patients.

One of the most frequent complications of CEA is cranial nerve injury, which relates to the anatomic location of these nerves with respect to the carotid arteries. The incidence ranges from roughly 5% to 17% in reported series (Table 2). The majority of these injuries result from traction or minor trauma and are quite transitory, often resolving in a few days or weeks.

Recurrent Carotid Stenosis

The incidence of recurrent stenosis has been estimated to range from 5% to 22% of patients in several published institutional series, although only about 3% of these lesions were symptomatic. Within the first 36 months after CEA, recurrent stenosis usually results from intimal hyperplasia. Evidence from serial duplex evaluations suggests that at least some of these lesions regress with time, and in part, this may be responsible for some variability in the reported rates of recurrent stenosis. An occasional "recurrent" stenosis in fact represents residual arteriosclerotic disease after the endarterectomy. Lesions that develop more that a few years after CEA usually result from progressive or new arteriosclerotic disease.

Recurrent stenoses develop more frequently in women, in patients who continue to smoke, and in hypercholesterolemic, diabetic, and hypertensive individuals. It has also been suggested that intraoperative injury secondary to arterial clamping, placement of an intraluminal shunt, or the placement of tacking sutures within the vessel may also predispose to early myointimal hyperplastic lesions. As noted above, there is compelling evidence that closure of the arteriotomy with a patch will reduce the incidence of recurrent stenosis, although the optimal patch material remains to be identified.

REOPERATIVE CAROTID ENDARTERECTOMY

Reoperative CEA presents additional challenges in the dissection and reconstruction, which can increase the risk compared with a primary procedure; but with careful planning and technique, excellent results can be achieved in this situation as well. An early recurrent stenosis usually develops within 2 years of CEA and typically results from intimal hyperplasia, an inflammatory response that produces a firm, rubbery plaque rich in fibroblasts and smooth muscle cells, surrounded by dense accumulations of collagen and acid mucopolysaccharide; it typically develops within the endarterectomy bed, but later restenoses typically have features of atheromatous plaques and are more widely distributed along the carotid artery. There are no

TABLE 2: Incidence of cranial nerve injury

Nerve	Incidence (%)
Hypoglossal	4.4–17.5
Recurrent laryngeal	1.5–15
Superior laryngeal	1.8–4.5
Marginal mandibular	1.1–3.1
Glossopharyngeal	0.2–1.5
Spinal accessory	<1.0

prospective randomized trials to support repeat CEA, but most available evidence supports treating symptomatic and very high-grade, asymptomatic recurrent stenoses.

Scarring typically makes the dissection more technically difficult, such that a higher incidence of cranial nerve injury and hematoma can be anticipated. In addition, more extensive disease within the carotid artery may necessitate carotid artery replacement with an interposition graft, which is technically more difficult; it also may preclude shunting and may be associated with longer periods of cerebral ischemia, possibly leading to higher perioperative stroke rates. However, endarterectomy is often possible, even with eversion endarterectomy.

SELECTED READINGS

Barnett HJM, Taylor DW, Eliasziw M, et al: Benefit of carotid endarterectomy in patients with symptomatic moderate or severe stenosis, *N Engl J Med* 339(20):1415–1425, 1998.

Endarterectomy for asymptomatic carotid artery stenosis: Executive Committee for the Asymptomatic Carotid Atherosclerosis Study, *JAMA* 273(18):1421–1428, 1995.

European Carotid Surgery Trialists' Collaborative Group: MRC European Carotid Surgery Trial: interim results for symptomatic patients with severe (70-99%) or with mild (0-29%) carotid stenosis, *Lancet* 337(8752):1235–1243, 1991.

European Carotid Surgery Trialists' Collaborative Group: Endarterectomy for moderate symptomatic carotid stenosis: interim results from the MRC European Carotid Surgery Trial, *Lancet* 347(9015):1591–1593, 1996.

Halliday A, Mansfield A, Marro J, et al: Prevention of disabling and fatal strokes by successful carotid endarterectomy in patients without recent neurological symptoms: randomised controlled trial, *Lancet* 363(9420):1491–1502, 2004.

Hobson RW III, Mackey WC, Ascher E, et al: Management of atherosclerotic carotid artery disease: clinical practice guidelines of the Society for Vascular Surgery, *J Vasc Surg* 48:480–486, 2008.

North American Symptomatic Carotid Endarterectomy Trial Collaborators: Beneficial effect of carotid endarterectomy in symptomatic patients with high-grade carotid stenosis, *N Engl J Med* 325(7):445–453, 1991.

Perler BA: Carotid endarterectomy: the "gold standard" in the endovascular era, *J Am Coll Surg* 194(suppl 1):S2–S8, 2002.

Perler BA: The effect of statin medications on the perioperative and long-term outcomes following carotid endarterectomy or stenting, *Semin Vasc Surg* 20:252–258, 2007.

MANAGEMENT OF RECURRENT CAROTID ARTERY STENOSIS

Benjamin S. Brooke, MD, PhD,
and Mahmoud B. Malas, MD, MHS

OVERVIEW

Atherosclerosis of the common and internal carotid arteries accounts for approximately one third of the etiologies of transient ischemic attacks (TIA) and strokes. Surgical procedures aimed at reducing the risk of these cerebrovascular events have been practiced at an increasing rate over the past half-century. Carotid endarterectomy (CEA), first introduced back in the 1950s, has steadily increased in frequency following the publication of multiple randomized clinical trials (RCTs) during the 1990s that demonstrated the superiority of CEA to medical management alone for the prevention of TIA and strokes. It is estimated that over 150,000 CEA procedures are performed annually in the United States alone. Moreover, carotid artery stenting (CAS) has recently emerged as a less invasive alternative to CEA in high-risk patients. Although the role of CAS in carotid revascularization in still being determined by ongoing RCTs, the popularity and acceptance of this endovascular therapy has benefited from ongoing innovations in devices and technology over the past decade.

As the increasing numbers of patients undergoing CEA and CAS have been followed in study cohorts and clinical practice, it has become apparent that a clinically significant subset of these patients will develop recurrent carotid stenosis. Long-term follow-up results of several published studies have shown the risk of restenosis following CEA to range between 7% and 15%, but restenosis following CAS is reported in up to 15% to 20% of patients. For both CEA and CAS, recurrent stenosis usually presents as an asymptomatic lesion during routine clinical or radiologic follow-up examination, but it may be associated with recurrent ipsilateral cerebrovascular symptoms. Evidence shows that the risk of suffering recurrent ischemic events with recurrent lesions increases over time.

The management of recurrent carotid stenosis presents a unique surgical challenge. Although a recurrent lesion is associated with an increased risk of stroke or TIA, this must also be balanced against the increased risk of perioperative complications associated with reoperation. It is important to review the pathogenesis and diagnosis of carotid restenosis, as well as understand the available treatment options, risks, and goals associated with reintervention.

NATURAL HISTORY AND PATHOGENESIS

The development of recurrent carotid stenosis may occur during different phases of the postoperative period, and it may be associated with several different etiologies. In general, these causative factors are categorized into three groups based on the length of time that has passed since the initial operation. The first phase occurs from the immediate perioperative period through the initial days to weeks following surgery; the second phase occurs from approximately 3 months up to 2 years after surgery; the third phase of restenosis occurs more than 2 years following surgery. It is essential to understand the pathogenesis of recurrent carotid stenosis as it occurs within each of these temporal phases of development.

Carotid occlusive disease that develops in the immediate or early postoperative period almost always results from a technical error that occurred during the procedure. During CEA operations, it is critical to use meticulous surgical techniques and established methods for arteriotomy closure. Specifically, the use of vein or Dacron patch angioplasty has been shown to maintain the arterial lumen diameter and reduce restenosis by 76% versus primary closure alone in a recent Cochrane review. In addition, careful attention should be paid to ensure that residual carotid disease does not lead to perioperative complications. A dissection flap or residual shelf of the atherosclerotic plaque may be left behind during the procedure that disrupts blood flow or provides an intraluminal nidus for thrombosis. Clamp trauma may also contribute to the generation of these vessel wall irregularities. Intraoperative duplex ultrasonography and completion angiography are standard techniques for assessing the presence of residual carotid lesions, irregularities, or thrombosis after CEA. Consequently, if surgical complications are detected in the operating room or during the early postoperative period, the arteriotomy can be reopened and repaired with minimal risk to the patient.

The second temporal phase of restenosis begins to appear between 3 to 6 months following CEA or CAS. These recurrent lesions typically consist of hyperplastic vascular smooth muscle cells along with collagen, mucopolysaccharides, and other extracellular matrix components. Also known as *myointimal hyperplasia*, this pathogenic sequence is thought to develop as an exaggeration of the arterial wall's normal repair process in response to injury. The resulting neointimal carotid lesions are found on routine histologic examination to contain a dense, fibrous core underlying an intact endothelial surface. Correspondingly, these lesions appear smooth on follow-up angiography and have a low clinical potential for thromboembolism. Although the majority of patients remain asymptomatic during the early stages of these lesions, symptoms may subsequently develop if the lumen diameter becomes progressively narrowed (>80%), or if an unstable fibrous plaque develops.

The last phase of recurrent carotid stenosis occurs more than 2 years after the initial surgical procedure and is generally attributed to progression of atherosclerotic disease within the region of the prior endarterectomy site. This may represent progression of disease from the borders of the prior endarterectomy or de novo formation of atherosclerotic plaque. And although these lesions may contain a component of fibrous neointimal hyperplasia as described above, they are differentiated by the presence of inflammatory cell infiltration and lipid cores comparable to the primary disease process. Progression of atherosclerosis may reflect the presence of both modifiable and unmodifiable risk factors that persist within each individual patient, such as smoking, hypercholesterolemia, and/or hypertension. Similar to the pathogenesis associated with primary carotid disease, these recurrent lesions may present with neurological symptoms, depending on characteristics of the occlusive plaques.

SURVEILLANCE AND DIAGNOSIS

Following successful CEA or CAS procedures, it is imperative that patients be followed closely to assess for recurrent stenosis and for disease in the contralateral carotid artery. A series of postoperative surveillance examinations are justified to provide baseline and interval evaluations within the first 12 months. In general, noninvasive duplex ultrasonography (DUS) is the follow-up study of choice given the combination of diagnostic yield, procedural cost, and low risk to the patient. A DUS study should include a careful examination of the endarterectomy site and contiguous vessel areas in B-mode and color flow analysis to assess for any lumen narrowing or flow irregularities.

The degree of restenosis is commonly estimated by measuring the peak systolic velocity (PSV), the end diastolic velocity (EDV), and the PSV ratio of the endarterectomized segment of internal carotid artery (ICA) to the mid common carotid artery (CCA). A recent study showed that PSV of 213 cm/sec or more and an EDV of 60 cm/sec or more were optimal for detecting a greater than 50% restenosis after CEA by patch closure, with a sensitivity and specificity of 99% and 100%, respectively. Moreover, an ICA/CCA PSV ratio of 2.25 or more was found to be most accurate for detecting 50% or greater restenosis.

In the same study, a PSV of 274 cm/sec or more and an EDV of 80 cm/sec or more could be used as a cutoff for diagnosing greater than 70% restenosis after CEA, with a sensitivity of 99% and specificity of 91%. The optimal ICA/CCA PSV ratio for detecting 70% or more restenosis was found to be 3.35 or greater. If the initial baseline DUS study is normal, the frequency of subsequent follow-up examinations should be determined by the status of the contralateral nonoperated carotid artery or the development of new neurologic symptoms. Conversely, the early detection of high PSV in an asymptomatic patient may warrant more frequent examinations, at 6 to 12 month intervals, to assess for progression of carotid disease. Our preference is to do intraoperative DUS and repeat it at 1, 6, and 12 month intervals and then yearly thereafter, unless there is a significant increase in the velocities.

The diagnosis of carotid restenosis by duplex ultrasound among patients undergoing CAS is more difficult, given that the biomechanical properties of the vessel wall are severely altered by the stent. Consequently, PSV criteria established for native carotid arteries tend to overestimate the degree of stenosis in angiographically normal stented arteries. Revised DUS criteria for in-stent restenosis have been proposed, including a recent study showing that a PSV of 220 cm/sec or more was optimal for DUS diagnosis of 50% or greater restenosis with a sensitivity of 100% and specificity of 96%. Furthermore, this same study showed that a PSV of 340 cm/sec or more and an ICA/CCA PSV ratio of 4.15 or more was the best cutoff for determining 80% or greater restenosis following CAS, with a sensitivity of 100% and specificity of 98%.

Digital subtraction angiography may still be warranted following CAS to estimate and validate the presence of recurrent stenosis, although it is associated with a small but nonnegligible risk of stroke and/or death. Alternate noninvasive diagnostic modalities to evaluate carotid restenosis include computed tomography angiography (CTA) and magnetic resonance angiography (MRA). Although most stents are MRA safe, the artifact generated by both of these modalities renders them less optimal for diagnosing carotid artery restenosis.

INDICATIONS FOR REOPERATION

Once a patient is diagnosed with recurrent carotid artery stenosis, the decision to pursue surgical intervention must take into account a host of clinical factors. This includes the time elapsed from the original operative procedure, most likely cause of restenosis, presence of neurological symptoms, individual patient comorbidities, and risks associated with reoperation. As stated previously, the presence of severe narrowing within an endarterectomized arterial segment in the early postoperative period is likely a result of technical error or residual carotid disease, and the patient should be taken back to the operating room for revision.

In comparison, the diagnosis of recurrent stenosis in asymptomatic patients between 6 to 18 months following CEA is likely because of progression of neointimal hyperplasia. The natural history of these recurrent lesions suggests that most will not progress to complete carotid occlusion, nor will they be associated with the onset of neurological symptoms. Therefore, when balanced against the risks of reoperation, the threshold is set higher for intervention with these lesions than with primary disease. Asymptomatic patients are generally not candidates for reoperation, until the recurrent stenosis reaches a threshold of greater than 80%. For symptomatic carotid

artery restenosis, however, the indications for reoperation are similar to those for the primary disease. Interventions are normally undertaken for recurrent carotid lesions with greater than 50% restenosis that are associated with ipsilateral symptoms of stroke or TIA. Nevertheless, it is important to first confirm that neurologic symptoms are originating from the ipsilateral carotid artery restenotic lesion.

When a patient with recurrent stenosis meets the clinical criteria for reintervention, the next step is to select the best procedure for operative management. This requires a thorough understanding of each patient's unique comorbidities and the inherent risks associated with a repeat procedure. Reoperative CEA with patch angioplasty has traditionally been the standard operative treatment for recurrent carotid stenosis following endarterectomy. This procedure, however, generally carries a higher risk of perioperative complications than the initial operation because of dense scar tissue surrounding the carotid artery and resulting difficulty in obtaining tissue dissection planes. Difficulty with dissection predisposes to a high incidence of cranial or cervical nerve injury, found to be 21% following CEA for restenosis by one prospective cohort study.

Further technical challenges when performing repeat CEA for restenosis resulting from neointimal hyperplasia stem from the fact that tissue planes between the fibrous stenotic tissue and native vessel wall are usually not well demarcated. Overall, combined perioperative stroke and mortality rates have historically ranged between 5% and 10% following repeat CEA, although some contemporary studies report rates as low as 2%.

As techniques and devices for carotid angioplasty and stenting have improved over the past decade, the utilization of this procedure for the management of recurrent carotid stenosis has increased in popularity. CAS can be carried out safely in patients with high medical and anatomic risk profiles, particularly when their recurrent stenosis has resulted from neointimal hyperplasia. This includes fibrous lesions that develop following CEA as well as in-stent restenosis following CAS. In general, these types of lesions are thought to be less prone to distal embolization during CAS than restenotic plaques formed later by the progression of atherosclerosis. This is supported by evidence showing that the rate of perioperative complications associated with CAS performed for restenotic lesions are at least equivalent or lower than when undertaken for primary carotid atherosclerosis.

The safety and efficacy of CAS for high-risk patients with recurrent carotid stenosis is supported by a growing number of randomized and nonrandomized studies. In a large multicenter cohort study of 338 CAS procedures for recurrent stenosis, the 30 day stroke and death rate was reported as 3.7% with a 3-year rate of freedom from fatal or nonfatal strokes of 96%. This was supported by data from 334 high-risk patients randomized to CAS in the Stenting and Angioplasty with Protection in Patients at High Risk for Endarterectomy (SAPPHIRE) trial, which revealed a 30 day composite of death, stroke, or myocardial infarction (MI) of 3.8%. The multicenter, single arm BEACH (Boston Scientific EPI: A Carotid Stenting Trial for High-Risk Surgical Patients) study reported a 30-day rate of stroke, MI, and death of 4.4%, 1.0%, and 1.5%, respectively, among high-risk patients with recurrent stenosis. After 1 year, this composite end point was reported to occur in 8.9% of patients. In the recent nonrandomized single-arm CABARET trial (Coronary Artery Bypass and REactivity of Thrombocytes), patients at high surgical risk with carotid artery stenosis treated with CAS were found to have a 30 day composite end point of death, stroke, or MI of 4.7%. The Carotid ACCULINK/ACCUNET Post-Approval Trial to Uncover Rare Events (CAPTURE) is a prospective postmarket single-arm surveillance study of the RX ACCULINK carotid stent system required by the FDA and sponsored by the Guidant Corporation (Indianapolis, Ind.). It included 3,500 patients at high surgical risk and with high-grade stenosis of the ICA. This study demonstrated a combined risk of stroke, death, and MI of 5.7% at 30 days. Taken together, these results demonstrate that CAS can be successfully undertaken in high-risk patients with recurrent stenosis who are not good candidates for repeat CEA.

OPERATIVE MANAGEMENT AND TECHNIQUES

Repeat Carotid Endarterectomy

A thorough preoperative patient assessment must be completed prior to repeat CEA. This includes careful review of the operative note or report from the initial CEA procedure to determine the extent of dissection, type of arteriotomy closure, and any complicating factors associated with the prior procedure. It is also important to ensure that patients are medically optimized, including an assessment of cardiopulmonary function, as well as ensuring that they are maintained on standard medical therapies during the perioperative period. All patients should be on aspirin 81 mg (or 325 mg) during the perioperative period, and they should continue taking β-blocker and statin medications if they were on these agents preoperatively. Finally, the patient should undergo a detailed informed consent process to ensure that they are aware of the increased risks of morbidity and mortality associated with repeat CEA, including the spectrum of potential cranial nerve injuries.

The operative technique for repeat CEA is similar to that of the initial operation, with the addition that even greater need for attention to surgical detail is required, and there is a lower margin for error. The patient is positioned supine in a slightly flexed position with a shoulder roll and the head turned away from the side being operated. The scar from the prior skin incision is used as a landmark and is carefully reopened with a 15 blade scalpel (Figure 1, A). The incision is carried down through the platysma using cautery, until the medial border of the sternocleidomastoid muscle is identified. Dissection should be carried out along the superior and inferior aspect of this muscle to define the extent of scarring from the prior surgery. The greater auricular nerve may cross over at the superior aspect of this dissection, and it should be preserved if possible.

Next, the internal jugular vein should be identified and partially mobilized to prevent inadvertent injury and bleeding. Dissection lateral to the vein, however, should be limited to prevent injury to the spinal accessory nerve. Partial mobilization of the vein should facilitate identification of the common carotid artery and help define a plane for the anterolateral dissection of the vessel. A proximal segment of the CCA that is not within scar tissue is identified first and secured with vessel loops prior to continuing the dissection along the lateral aspect of this vessel up to the carotid bifurcation. The vagus nerve is normally located deep to the artery in this lateral plane, but it may be more superficial as a result of scarring, and it should be identified if possible to prevent transection. Dissection should continue along the lateral border of the ICA to identify the distal border of this vessel, as it exits the plane of the prior surgical scar. Distal control of the ICA is obtained using careful circumferential dissection away from scar tissue, and it is secured with vessel loops. Given that this dissection needs to be carried out in a more cephalad direction during repeat CEA, care must be taken to prevent injury to the glossopharyngeal nerve as it crosses the distal ICA near the styloid process.

The next step involves a careful dissection of the anterior surface of the prior endarterectomized vessel, moving from a lateral to medial direction. Identification of the hypoglossal nerve above the carotid bifurcation is critical at this step, given that it is commonly enveloped within existing scar tissue. If dissection is maintained at the adventitial surface of the artery, this nerve may be moved superiorly and medially and thus spared injury. Occasionally, division of the digastric muscle may also be necessary to facilitate dissection in the caudal direction to prevent injury to either the hypoglossal or glossopharyngeal nerves.

Once the endarterectomized segment of common and internal carotid arteries is safely exposed and mobilized from scar tissue, proximal and distal control of the vessel should be secured with the use of atraumatic vascular clamps (Figure 1, B). Prior to applying clamps, a weight-based systemic heparin bolus (70 U/kg) is given. An attempt should be made to reopen the vessel along the prior endarterectomy site if possible (Figure 1, C). Depending on surgeon preference, a shunt may be routinely placed or selectively placed based on electroencephalography and somatosensory evoked potentials. Thereafter, surgical management will vary depending on the type of restenotic lesion encountered.

Atherosclerotic lesions can usually be treated to the same as in a primary operation, with plaque dissection carried out where a natural cleavage plane exists between intimal disease and the vessel wall media and closed using Dacron or saphenous vein patch angioplasty (Figure 1, D). When the restenotic lesion is caused by neointimal hyperplasia, however, this plane between the fibrous intimal lesion and medial wall is not defined. In general, the best treatment for this situation is to apply a generous patch angioplasty, using either a Dacron or saphenous vein patch without attempting endarterectomy.

Finally, when a long segment of concentric, high-grade carotid stenosis from neointimal hyperplasia is not amenable to patch angioplasty, the patient should be treated using an interposition graft of either polytetrafluoroethylene or a segment of saphenous vein harvested from the thigh. This is performed after ligating the external carotid artery and following complete resection of the carotid bifurcation (Figure 2). The interpositional graft should have a good size match, and the anastamoses should be performed in an end-to-end fashion to beveled ends of the native artery.

Carotid Angioplasty and Stenting

Prior to CAS, patients should undergo a thorough workup and preoperative assessment. This should include a detailed cardiovascular history and review of all invasive and noninvasive imaging studies to assess for severe occlusive disease or anatomic irregularities that may make carotid access difficult from a remote puncture site. In addition, consideration should be given to anatomic criteria that might increase the incidence of atheroembolism or complications and be a contraindication to CAS (Figure 3). All patients should be maintained on dual antiplatelet therapy consisting of 81 mg of aspirin and 75 mg of clopidogrel or 81 mg aspirin and 250 mg ticlopidine twice daily for at least 1 week before the procedure.

The percutaneous technique for carotid angioplasty and stenting undertaken in patients with recurrent stenosis is similar to that used for treating primary carotid occlusive disease. Under local anesthetics and minimal conscious sedation, arterial access is typically achieved through percutaneous access of the common femoral artery, although an approach through the brachial, radial, or very proximal common carotid artery (CCA) may also be used in cases with severe tortuosity and atherosclerosis of the aortic arch and the proximal CCA and/or ileofemoral arteries. After placing a 5 Fr femoral sheath, a long marker pigtail catheter is advanced into the aortic arch over a guidewire, and a diagnostic angiogram (at a 45-degree left anterior oblique angle) is undertaken to assess the aortic arch and any anatomic irregularities (Figure 4, A). We prefer to give systemic heparin (80 to 100 U/kg) prior to performing the angiogram to reduce the risk of embolization, with the activated clotting time (ACT) maintained at 250 to 300 seconds throughout. The pigtail catheter is removed over a stiff guidewire, and the 5 Fr sheath is exchanged for a long, 6 Fr shuttle sheath placed in the proximal descending aorta. A 260 cm angled-tip Glidewire (Terumo Medical Corporation, Somerset, NJ) is used for selection of the CCA, using a 125 cm long JB1 or V-Tek catheter (Cook Medical, Bloomington, Ind.) or vertebral catheter. Once the catheter is in the mid to distal CCA, the sheath can be advanced over the catheter and up the CCA to within a few centimeters of the restenotic lesion.

An anteroposterior and lateral angiogram are performed to assess length of the carotid lesion and the diameter of the normal vessels proximal and distal to the lesion. This helps determine which size of filter, stent, and balloon catheter to use. A calibrating ruler is placed externally on the ipsilateral neck to obtain an accurate measurement of the distal ICA diameter (a) and the narrowest segment of the ICA

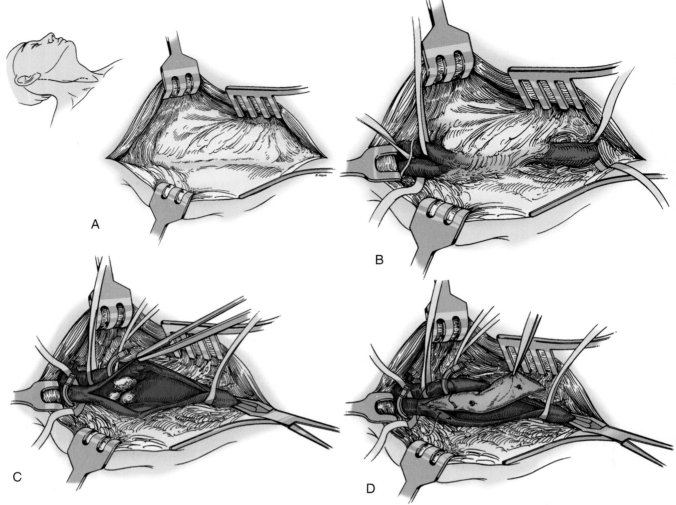

FIGURE I   Operative exposure and technique for repeat carotid endarterectomy. **A,** The prior skin incision is used, with dissection carried out proximally and distally to define the extent of scarring from prior surgery. **B,** Proximal and distal control of the vessel is obtained after circumferential dissection away from scar tissue. **C,** The vessel is opened along the site of prior endarterectomy repair, and plaque dissection is carried out. **D,** Repeat endarterectomy is closed using patch angioplasty sewn in with 6-0 Prolene suture in a running fashion. *(From Awad A: Tech Neurosurg 3[1]:61, 1997. Used with permission.)*

(b). The degree of stenosis should be confirmed in accordance with the NASCET (North American Symptomatic Carotid Endarterectomy Trial) and ACAS (Asymptomatic Carotid Atherosclerosis Study) criteria $(1 - a/b \times 100)$.

Once these measurements are taken, and the lesion is deemed suitable for CAS, an appropriately sized filter is advanced through the restenotic lesion and deployed into a relatively straight segment of the distal cervical ICA, just proximal to the petrous portion and at least 2 cm distal to the expected landing zone of the stent to prevent tangling (Figure 4, *B*). Next, a 2 to 4 mm diameter by 2 cm long rapid-exchange angioplasty balloon is advanced over a 0.014 filter wire up into the stenotic lesion and inflated briefly to ensure safe passage of the stent (Figure 4, *C*). Self-expanding nitinol stents are typically used, varying in diameter from 6 to 10 mm and in lengths up to 40 mm, deployed under direct fluoroscopic visualization. We prefer a tapered stent, oversized by about 20% of the diameter of the normal segment of the CCA, that extends from the CCA to the ICA beyond the actual angiographic length of the lesion by at least 0.5 cm proximally and distally (Figure 4, *D*). Attention is given to preventing movement of the filter during the exchange of the balloons and stents.

After the stent is deployed within the stenotic lesion, the delivery system is removed, and a completion angiogram is performed to assess residual narrowing and the need for poststenting angioplasty. If further dilation is necessary, an angioplasty balloon is selected that is undersized by 20% to 40% of the nonstenotic carotid arterial diameter. Gentle ballooning of the stent and slow deflation of the balloon is performed, as this is likely to cause the highest load of shower emboli during the entire procedure (Figure 4, *E*). We tend to balloon the stent only when the residual stenosis is greater then 30%.

Treating patients with atropine (0.5 to 1.0 mg) after balloon insufflation may be necessary if significant vasovagal events occur after stenting. Our preference is not to use atropine, because almost all events are self-limiting. A follow-up angiogram is performed following stent ballooning, with residual stenosis of up to 30% considered acceptable, given the significant embolic risk of further stent ballooning (Figure 4, *F*).

Finally, the filter is carefully removed using the retrieval catheter, and a completion angiogram is performed to visualize the extracranial/intracranial circulation and document the absence or presence of distal emboli (Figure 5). The long, 6 Fr Shuttle Select sheath (Cook Medical) is replaced with a short, 6 Fr sheath to allow systemic heparin to subside. The sheath is removed when the ACT is less than 150 seconds; alternatively, a percutaneous arterial closure device can be used to allow immediate patient mobilization.

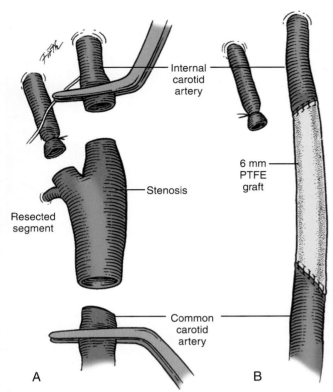

FIGURE 2 Surgical repair of carotid restenosis using interpositional graft. **A,** The diseased segment at the carotid bifurcation is resected after ligating the external carotid artery and obtaining proximal and distal control with vascular clamps. **B,** An appropriately sized segment of vein or polytetrafluoroethylene (PTFE) graft is anastamosed in an end-to-end fashion using 6-0 Prolene suture.

We strongly recommend use of embolic protection devices in all cases because of the strong evidence of stroke reduction in protected carotid stenting. When the lesion is nearly occlusive and prohibitive of passing a filter, a reverse-flow protection device is another option. Neurologic salvage procedures include mechanical emboli debris retrieval and systemic and intracranial thrombolysis (Figure 6).

Following CAS, patients should be monitored in a subacute ICU setting overnight. Occasionally, hemodynamic instability can be encountered postprocedure with hypotension (treated with intravenous hydration and pressers) resulting from stent pressure on the carotid body. Patients are typically discharged home within 24 hours and maintained on 75 mg of clopidogrel for 4 to 6 weeks and 81 mg aspirin indefinitely. A duplex scan and physical exam are obtained at 1-, 6-, and 12-month intervals and yearly thereafter.

MEDICAL MANAGEMENT

The secondary prevention of carotid stenosis following CEA and CAS can be augmented through optimization of medical management. Standard postoperative therapy includes the routine use of antiplatelet medications, such as aspirin or clopidigrel, to prevent clot formation during the process of reendothelialization. The prevention of platelet activation and aggregation with chronic use of these agents has also been suggested to play a role in reducing the stimuli for smooth muscle hyperplasia and neointimal formation.

Postoperative management should also involve efforts to control or reduce modifiable risk factors associated with atherosclerosis—such

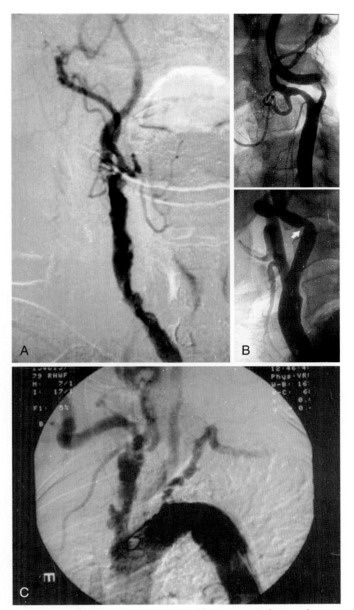

FIGURE 3 Contraindications to carotid artery angioplasty and stenting. **A,** Severe atherothrombosis and calcification in both the common and internal carotid arteries. **B,** Significant tortuousity in the internal carotid artery. Stenting of this lesion would result in a critical bend in the artery (*arrow*). **C,** Severe atherothrombosis and calcification in type III aortic arch and proximal major vessels.

as hypertension, smoking, and hyperlipidemia—with the use of medical agents and/or behavioral modifications. The perioperative and postoperative use of statin medications during CEA and CAS in particular has gained notoriety in recent years, given compelling evidence emerging from both observational and randomized trials. These studies suggest that statin therapy likely has a significant effect in stabilizing or even reducing carotid lesions though a combination of lipid-lowering and lipid-independent (*pleiotrophic*) mechanisms. Moreover, these benefits are attained among patients with normal cholesterol levels, further suggesting that statin medications should be part of the routine short- and long-term medical management prescribed to the majority of patients undergoing CEA or CAS procedures.

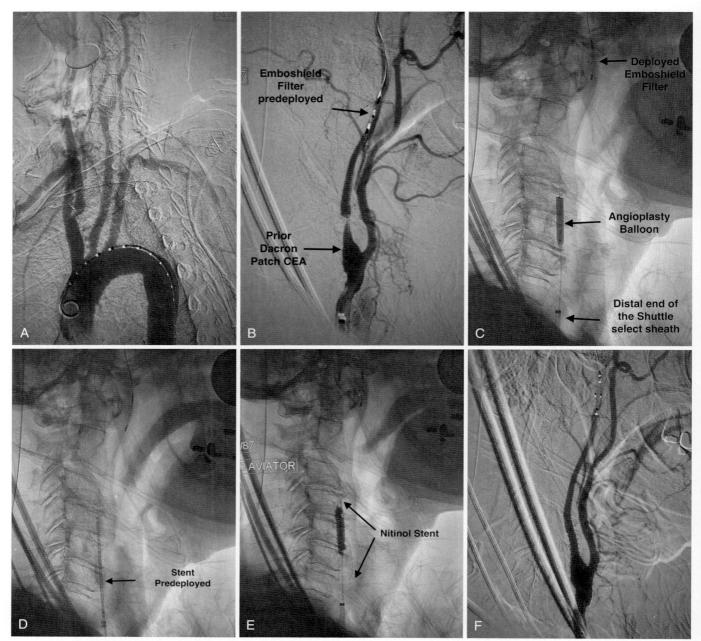

FIGURE 4   Carotid artery stenting. **A,** Arch aortogram showing minimal atherosclerosis and proximal major vessels free of significant stenosis. **B,** Near occlusive lesion in the distal patch repair of prior CEA. The filter is placed in a straight segment of the distal ICA, taking into consideration the landing zone of the stent. **C,** Angioplasty of the lesion after deployment of the filter. The tip of the sheath should be always visualized in the field. **D,** Self-expanding nitinol stent after passing through the sheath. **E,** Poststent dilatation. **F,** Completion angiogram shows patency of the stent.

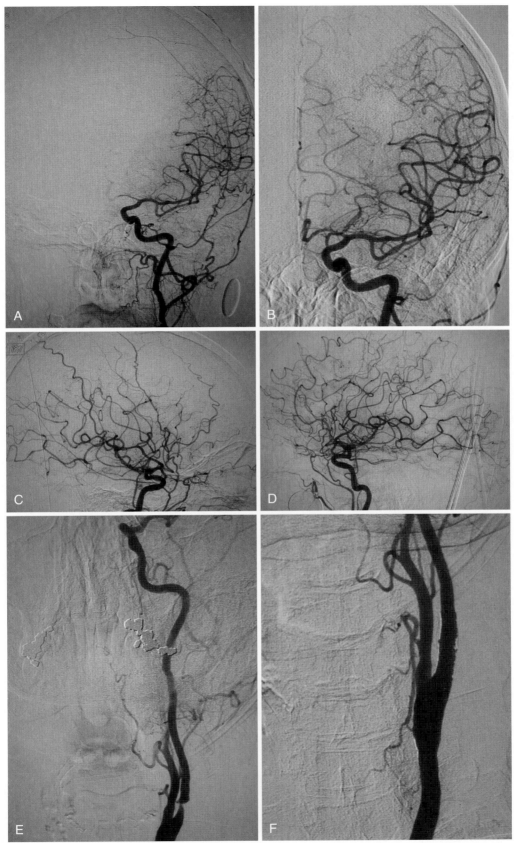

FIGURE 5 Prestenting and poststenting angiogram of the cerebral vessels. **A,** Anterior view before stenting. **B,** Anterior view after stenting. **C,** Lateral view before stenting. **D,** Lateral view after stenting. Significant improvement in cerebral perfusion is noted with opacification of the anterior cerebral artery that was absent prior to stenting. Also note the complete resolution of the near occlusive lesion in the ICA. **E,** Prestenting. **F,** Poststenting.

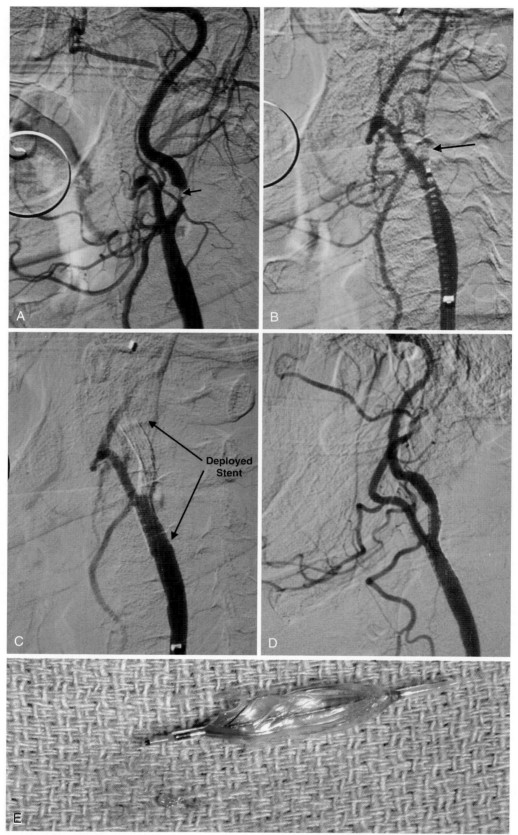

FIGURE 6 Neurologic salvage techniques. **A,** Near-occlusive symptomatic lesion in the ICA. **B,** After angioplasty and advancement of the stent revealed a complete occlusion of the ICA. **C,** After deployment of the stent, complete thrombosis of the ICA portion of the stent with no distal flow. **D,** After rapid-rescue measures, including mechanical suctioning with rapid-exchanged Export catheter and intraarterial thrombolysis, complete resolution of the occlusion with no neurological sequelae. **E,** An embolic protection device (Emboshield filter; Abbott Vascular, North Chicago, Ill.) with large debris retrieved from it.

SUMMARY

The management of recurrent carotid stenosis presents a unique challenge for the surgeon. It is critical to have a comprehensive understanding of the pathogenesis, diagnosis, and indications for treatment, along with the options for surgical and endovascular intervention. Each patient much be approached individually before making a decision between repeat CEA versus CAS. Repeat CEA can be successfully achieved in a subset of patients with favorable risk profiles, but it is associated with a high risk of cranial nerve injuries. In patients with increased anatomic and medical risks for repeat CEA, however, CAS has become a valuable and reliable technique with good short- and long-term results. Finally, it is important to optimize each patient's medical therapy as a complementary tool to surgical interventions for the long-term management of carotid artery restenosis.

Suggested Readings

AbuRahma AF, Stone P, Deem S, et al: Proposed duplex velocity criteria for carotid restenosis following carotid endarterectomy with patch closure, *J Vasc Surg* 50:286, 2009.

Bonati LH, Ederle J, McCabe JH, et al: Long-term risk of carotid restenosis in patients randomly assigned to endovascular treatment or endarterectomy in the Carotid and Vertebral Artery Transluminal Angioplasty Study (CAVATAS): long-term follow up of a randomized trial, *Lancet Neurol* 8:908, 2009.

Bowser AN, Bandyk DF, Evans A, et al: Outcome of carotid stent-assisted angioplasty versus open surgical repair of recurrent carotid stenosis, *J Vasc Surg* 38:432, 2003.

Hellings WE, Moll FL, De Vries JPM, et al: Atherosclerotic plaque composition and occurrence of restenosis after carotid endarterectomy, *JAMA* 299:547, 2008.

Lal BK, Hobson RW, Tofighi B, et al: Duplex ultrasound velocity criteria for the stented carotid artery, *J Vasc Surg* 47:63, 2008.

Lal BK: Recurrent carotid stenosis after CEA and CAS: diagnosis and management, *Semin Vasc Surg* 20:259, 2007.

Malas MB, Qazi U, Freischlag JA: Minimally invasive endovascular surgery. In Frezza EE, Gagner M, Li MKW, editors: International principles of laparoscopic surgery, Woodbury, CT, 2010, Cine-Med.

White CJ, Iyer SS, Hopkins LN, et al: Carotid stenting with distal protection in high surgical risk patients: the BEACH trial 30 day results, *Catheter Cardiovasc Interv* 67:503–512, 2006.

Endovascular Treatment of Carotid Artery Occlusive Disease

Martin G. Radvany, MD, and Philippe Gailloud, MD

BACKGROUND

According to the Centers for Disease Control (CDC) data, stroke was the third leading cause of death in the United States in 2008, and approximately 795,000 strokes occur in the United States each year. Of these, approximately 610,000 are first strokes. Nearly three quarters of all strokes occur in people over the age of 65 years, and the risk of stroke more than doubles each decade after the age of 55 years. The American Heart Association estimates that the direct and indirect costs of treating stroke patients reached $68.9 billion for the year 2009. Atherosclerosis of the internal carotid artery (ICA) is an important cause of stroke.

The efficacy of carotid endarterectomy (CEA) for the treatment for carotid artery stenosis was confirmed in the early 1990s by large multicenter trials comparing CEA to medical therapy, including the North American Symptomatic Carotid Endarterectomy Trial (NASCET) and the Asymptomatic Carotid Atherosclerosis Study (ACAS). The clinical benefit of CEA was found to be related to three main factors: 1) the degree of stenosis, 2) the presence or absence of symptoms, and 3) the rate of perioperative stroke and death.

Following the development of endovascular techniques and the introduction of self-expanding stents, carotid artery stenting (CAS) was proposed as a possible alternative to CEA, especially in high-risk patients. CAS is a less invasive procedure that eliminates the need for neck incision and its associated risks (i.e., cranial nerve injury, wound infection, hematoma). Although most CEAs are still done under general anesthesia, CAS can be performed under local anesthesia, avoiding the risks associated with CEA, especially when treating fragile patients. This is a relative advantage, however, as CEA can also be safely carried out under local anesthesia; although many operators, ourselves included, prefer to perform CAS under general anesthesia. Despite these advantages, the use of angioplasty and stenting to treat carotid artery stenosis remains controversial. The reason behind this partial failure lies principally in the contradictory and often poor results reported by several recent studies evaluating CAS (Table 1).

The Carotid Revascularization using Endarterectomy or Stenting Systems (CaRESS) study is a prospective, nonrandomized comparative cohort study of a broad-risk population of symptomatic and asymptomatic patients with carotid stenosis. This study found no significant differences in a broad-category population but did find a 4 year composite end point of death, stroke, and myocardial infarction that favored CAS (25% CEA vs. 14% CAS) in patients under 80 years of age. However, the risk of restenosis in the CAS group was two times higher than in the CEA group.

The Endarterectomy Versus Angioplasty in Patients with Symptomatic Severe Carotid Stenosis (EVA-3S) trial was stopped early because of the significantly higher stroke rate in the CAS arm of the study (9.6% vs. 3.9% in the CEA arm). This study concluded that CAS was as effective as CEA for midterm prevention of ipsilateral stroke, but CAS had a higher periprocedural risk for any stroke. However, this study has been criticized for the inclusion of less experienced operators, a problem that has unfortunately plagued most CAS studies so far, and for the lack of use of embolic protection devices (EPDs) in 8% of cases and a technical failure rate of 5%. It is also unclear whether some patients received only one antiplatelet agent rather than the dual therapy (aspirin and clopidogrel) now considered standard.

TABLE 1: Randomized multicenter carotid stenting versus endarterectomy trials

Trial	Year	N	30-Day M&M CAS	30-Day M&M CEA
CAVATAS	2001	504	10%	9.9%
CaRESS	2003	397	2.1%	NA
SAPPHIRE	2004	334	5.8%	12.6%
EVA-3S	2006	527	9.6%	3.9%
SPACE	2008	1214	6.8%	6.3%

CAVATAS, Carotid and Verterbral Artery Transluminal Angioplasty Study; *M&M*, Morbidity and mortality; *CAS*, carotid artery stenting; *CEA*, carotid endarterectomy; *NA*, not applicable; *SAPPHIRE*, Stenting and Angioplasty with Protection in Patients at High Risk for Endarterectomy

During the same period, the Stent-Protected Angioplasty versus Carotid Endarterectomy (SPACE) trial found no difference in the incidence of recurrent ipsilateral ischemic strokes or death between the CAS and CEA groups (6.8% vs. 6.3%) but failed to prove the non-inferiority of CAS versus CEA. The study was criticized for several weaknesses, including the lack of EPD use in 73% of patients, the variability in the types of stent platforms used, and the fact that it was statistically underpowered. In addition, the study did show a higher incidence of restenosis in the CAS group at 2 years, although the restenosis was asymptomatic in most patients.

These published trials have clearly increased our knowledge concerning CAS, especially in regard to patient selection, endovascular technique, and operator experience. Higher complication rates have been reported in patients who are older than 80 years and in patients with hemispheric symptoms. However, CAS seems to be more beneficial in asymptomatic patients and in those with recurrent carotid stenosis or a history of neck irradiation. In addition, patients with severe medical comorbidities, such as three-vessel coronary artery disease or chronic obstructive pulmonary disease (COPD), have better outcomes with CAS.

Finally, it has become apparent that loose inclusion criteria for endovascular operators compared to highly skilled and experienced surgical operators have influenced the result of most of the studies published so far. As it is suspected that a large fraction of embolic complications occur at the time of the initial vessel catheterization, prior to the placement of an EPD and/or stent, the experience of operators who have placed only a few stents, often under the supervision of a proctor, cannot match those of angiographers who have catheterized hundreds if not thousands of aortic arches. Sadly, this misconception has harmed the respectability of CAS as a potential alternative to CEA, even in selected clinical situations. The results of the randomized, prospective Carotid Revascularization Endarterectomy versus Stent Trial (CREST) will hopefully provide level I data to help clinicians select patients for CAS and CEA.

CAROTID ANGIOPLASTY: TECHNICAL OVERVIEW

Endovascular treatment of carotid arterial stenosis was pioneered with devices not designed for this purpose. This initially led to significant complications in the form of periprocedural strokes. The introduction of endovascular platforms specifically designed for carotid angioplasty and stenting—along with greater operator experience and the introduction of EPDs, whose usefulness remains somewhat controversial—has allowed a steady decrease in the rate of periprocedural strokes. With the endovascular equipment currently available,

CAS has become a conceptually and technically straightforward procedure.

Prior to treatment, patients should have a complete neurologic examination, optimally by a neurologist, and they should be placed under appropriate presurgical medication with dual antiplatelet therapy. Our regimen typically consists of 5 days of aspirin (325 mg) and clopidogrel (75 mg). For emergent situations, we use a bolus of 600 mg of clopidogrel and 650 mg of aspirin. If needed, these can be administered via a nasogastric tube. Aspirin may also be administered transrectally (i.e., two 300 mg suppositories). A 150 to 300 mg loading dose of Plavix may also be administered in patients who have been taking antiplatelet therapy on a chronic basis.

It should be noted that the degree of platelet inhibition has now been shown to be quite variable in patients taking antiplatelet therapy. The impact of aspirin and/or clopidogrel "resistance" on long-term stent patency and restenosis rates remains to be determined. In addition, the validity and significance of the currently available tests evaluating for aspirin and clopidogrel efficacy remain unclear (reported rates for aspirin resistance range from 5% to 60%). However, once the notions of aspirin and clopidogrel resistance are clearly defined, and the validity of the related tests are established, routine point-of-care testing will become a useful tool to adapt antiplatelet regimens for individual patients.

Preprocedure imaging with computed tomography angiography (CTA) or magnetic resonance imaging and angiography (MRI/MRA) offers important information about the condition of the brain parenchyma and the presence of additional intracranial or extracranial vascular anomalies, such as saccular aneurysms, vascular malformations, and so on. Preprocedure imaging can also document the type of aortic arch and the presence of anatomic variations that can directly affect the conduct of the procedure, such as supraaortic branching-pattern anomalies. When this information is not available, an aortic arch arteriogram can be performed at the time of treatment.

Knowledge of the aortic arch anatomy allows selection of the appropriate endovascular equipment. Complete four-vessel cerebral digital subtraction angiography (DSA) should be performed before initiating the stenting procedure, to document the baseline appearance of the cerebral vascular anatomy, as well as to distinguish the type and importance of the recruited collateral pathways (Figure 1, A and B). This initial angiogram will be used at the end of the procedure as a reference, to which the poststenting angiogram will be compared. The severity and morphology of the lesion itself also remains best analyzed by DSA, and the angiographic appearance of the plaque sometimes requires a modification of the treatment strategy. Finally, the initial diagnostic angiogram allows the surgeon to evaluate for the presence of additional cerebrovascular anomalies that may have escaped detection by noninvasive imaging techniques. Not infrequently, additional lesions discovered at the time of angiography, such as an intracranial carotid stenosis (i.e., tandem stenoses) or intracranial aneurysm, will alter the therapeutic plan.

After arterial access has been secured, heparin is administered intravenously to reach an activated clotting time (ACT) ranging between 250 and 300 seconds, although some manufacturers recommend even higher ACT values for specific devices. A guiding catheter or a long flexible sheath large enough to support the stent deployment system (6 or 7 Fr sheath or 8 or 9 Fr guide catheter) is advanced into the common carotid artery over a 0.035 inch guidewire. In most situations, the targeted carotid artery can be selected directly with the stent delivery platform.

In rare instances, the long sheath or guide catheter may have to be advanced over an exchange-length guidewire that has been previously placed in the carotid artery with a diagnostic catheter; although useful when facing extreme arterial tortuosity, this technique adds to the risk of a cerebral embolic complication by carrying forward small clots that form on the body of the exchange wire. In less experienced hands, exchange-length wires may also be advanced inadvertently into small branches or across the carotid plaque, potentially resulting in vessel perforation, arterial dissection, hemorrhage, and embolic stroke.

Depending on which EPD system is used, the stenosis is initially crossed with the wire tip of the EPD system itself, or with the EPD fitted over a separate microwire, from which the EPD is later advanced. Very tight stenoses that cannot be safely negotiated with the tip of the EPD device may require the use of a different technique that involves the use of a low-profile microcatheter (e.g., 1.7 Fr microcatheter) and a highly torqueable microwire (Figure 1, C and D). In this approach, the microcatheter is brought immediately below the stenosis, which is crossed with the microwire. The microcatheter is then advanced over the wire across the stenosis, and the microwire is withdrawn and replaced by a soft-tipped, exchange-length microwire, which is then used to advance either a predilation balloon or an over-the-wire EPD device. All these manipulations are performed under careful fluoroscopic guidance using the "road map" technique, a mode of live fluoroscopy in which an image of the targeted vascular tree is laid over the live subtracted fluoroscopy image. Presenting balloon angioplasty is performed when the degree of stenosis does not allow for primary passage of the stent delivery platform (Figure 2, A and B). It is important to undersize the balloon used for prestenting angioplasty to avoid plaque fracture, especially when treating a heavily calcified lesion.

Several measurement options are available when selecting the size of the devices to be used. Because the carotid artery is in a very superficial location, the simplest, and perhaps still the most reliable technique is to calibrate the angiographic image with an external marker, typically a United States quarter measuring 24.5 mm. It should be remembered that three-dimensional angiographic reconstructions of any imaging technique—MRA, CTA, and DSA—are prone to significant sizing variations in relation to image windowing. Self-expanding stents are typically oversized by 1 to 2 mm relative to the diameter of the normal vessel proximal to the lesion, and they must be long enough to cover the entire stenosis.

When placing the stent, covering the origin of the external carotid artery with the stent is not contraindicated. On the contrary, it is believed that the remodeling of the carotid bifurcation produced by the stent placement may improve local hemodynamic conditions and decrease the risk of restenosis. The stent is deployed under the "road map" guidance described earlier, and control angiography is performed. If the stent is adequately expanded, the EPD can be recovered. If a residual stenosis of more than 30% is present, poststenting angioplasty can be performed with a new angioplasty balloon prior to the recovery of the EPD. The balloon used for poststenting dilation is slightly undersized, according to the expected diameter of the artery, not to the diameter of the deployed stent, which is oversized 1 to 2 mm (Figure 2, C and D).

It should be remembered that nitinol stents continue to slowly expand after delivery, and that the final result should not be evaluated immediately after deployment. As it is believed that a significant percentage of embolic events occur during postdilation, allowing the stent to expand on its own as much as possible may help avoid the additional risk associated with poststenting angioplasty. Angioplasty and stenting, especially when treating tight stenoses, exposes prothrombogenic wall components to the bloodstream that can initiate clot formation and result in acute in-stent thrombosis. Performing a second control angiogram 10 to 15 minutes after stent delivery can readily identify this potential problem (Figure 2, E). This angiogram is optimally obtained before removing the EPD, which is possible when a filter-type EPD is used. Acute in-stent thrombus formation can be treated with abciximab (Reopro).

Carotid Stent Designs

Endovascular stents come in two basic configurations, *balloon-expandable stents* and *self-expanding stents*. Although appropriate for ostial lesions at the aortic arch, balloon-expandable stents are not adequate for the treatment of cervical carotid lesions, as they lack the ability to spontaneously reexpand after external compression. Self-expanding

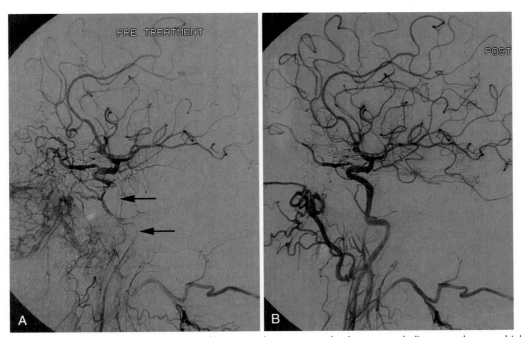

FIGURE I   A 55-year-old man with a past history of ruptured intracranial aneurysm and pulmonary embolism now shows multiple watershed-like strokes in his left cerebral hemisphere. **A,** Digital subtraction angiography (DSA; left common carotid injection, lateral cranial projection) obtained at the beginning of the procedure. This baseline angiogram shows a diminutive appearance of the cervical internal carotid artery (ICA), suggesting a string sign (*arrows*), and extensive external-to-internal carotid collaterals through the skull base and the orbit, revascularizing the distal ICA. The left anterior cerebral artery and both divisions of the left middle cerebral artery are, however, well delineated. **B,** DSA (left common carotid injection, lateral cranial projection) performed at the end of the procedure, showing that the cervical ICA has in fact a normal diameter and documenting the patency of all the cerebral branches opacified before stenting. Note the slightly increased capillary blush in the left temporal lobe, a finding that may indicate a local increase in the cerebral blood volume, emphasizing the need for tight control of the blood pressure.

Continued

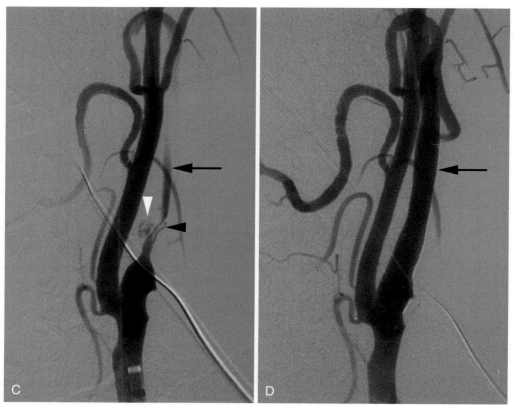

FIGURE 1, cont'd   C, DSA (left common carotid injection, lateral neck projection) showing a tight proximal ICA stenosis. Note the complex pattern of the lesion, with a narrow true lumen, a blind-ended false lumen (*black arrowhead*), and penetration of contrast agent into the soft, ulcerated portion of the atheromatous plaque (*white arrowhead*). The ICA distal to the stenosis fills with significant delay (*arrow*), while the external carotid artery is fully opacified. Visualization of these important anatomic characteristics requires obtaining an image in the right projection with good quality angiographic equipment. In this case, the optimal angiographic projection will help negotiate the passage of the tip of the wire through the patent lumen, while avoiding getting caught in either the false lumen or the soft component of the plaque. Note the presence of additional plaques proximal to the principal lesion. These lesions with a smooth appearance and resulting in minor lumen stenosis were not included in the treatment plan, as coverage of all the diseased segments would have required the use of two stents. This lesion was considered too tight and irregular for the passage of an EPD but was easily negotiated with a 1.7 Fr microcatheter (Prowler 10; Cordis Neurovascular, Miami Lakes, Fla.) advanced over a 0.010-inch microwire (Transend 10; Boston Scientific, Natick, Mass.). Once the microcatheter was across the stenosis, the microwire was replaced by an exchange-length, soft-tipped wire (Luge; Boston Scientific) and predilation was performed with a 2.5 mm by 15 mm angioplasty balloon. A tapered 6 to 8 mm by 40 mm stent was then deployed (Acculink; Abbott Vascular, Santa Clara, Calif.), followed by postdilation using a 5 mm by 20 mm angioplasty balloon (Aviator; Cordis Endovascular, Bridgewater, NJ). The procedure was uneventful, and the patient has had no new neurologic event after 2.5 year follow-up). **D,** DSA (left common carotid injection, lateral neck projection) after placement of a self-expandable stent in the proximal ICA. Note that the ICA distal to the lesion immediately recovers a normal caliber in spite of its diminutive appearance before treatment. This misleading presenting appearance is likely the result of two phenomena: partial opacification of the patent lumen, with contrast layering along the posterior wall of the vessel, and physiologically reduced lumen size distal to a tight stenosis. This latter mechanism can be difficult to distinguish from a true string sign, in which the narrow residual lumen resulting from chronic arterial remodeling is unlikely to reexpand after treatment of the lesion.

stents come in *open-cell* or *closed-cell* designs. Each design has advantages and disadvantages. The open-cell design has more flexibility, which allows for better vessel wall apposition and better navigability through tortuous vascular anatomy. However, open-cell stents have a lower radial force, which may result in a weaker scaffold and may compromise stent expansion due to recoil, especially in heavily calcified lesions. Open-cell design may also be more prone to in-stent restenosis, and the open-cell stent mesh may assume a spiked appearance in curves (see Figure 6, *D*). Closed-cell stents have more radial force, but they are less flexible, and they are more likely to produce arterial kinks and stenoses when used in tortuous vessels. Data from the SPACE trial suggests a higher rate of embolic complications with open-cell designs (11%) compared with closed-cell carotid stents (5.6%, $P = .029$).

Embolic protection devices (EPDs) are relatively new additions to the endovascular armentarium, based on the concept developed by Jacques Théron in the mid-1990s. Although their use is currently

mandatory in the United States, their positive effect on procedure safety remains to be clearly established. There are two types of EPD: those that provide cerebral protection by either blocking or filtering the blood flow in the ICA distal to the treatment site and those that stop the flow into the common carotid artery and external carotid artery proximal to the treatment site, causing reversal of flow in the internal carotid artery (i.e., flow-reversal devices; Figure 3).

Devices that must be placed distal to the treatment site consist either of a balloon, as in the initial experience with the Théron technique, or of a filter attached to a wire, which is now the most common variety. With the balloon technique, the balloon is attached to the working hypotube (or microcatheter), advanced distally to the stenosis, and inflated. After stenting and angioplasty are completed, a catheter is advanced across the treatment site and used to aspirate debris prior to deflating and recovering the balloon (Figure 3, *A*). The Théron technique also used forced flushing of the dead space below the balloon

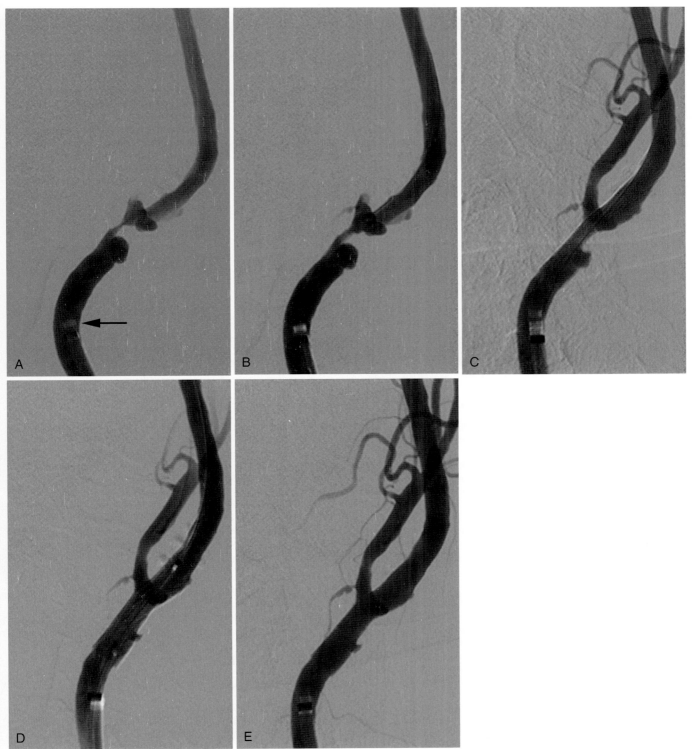

FIGURE 2 A 78-year-old man presenting with recurrent episodes of left-sided amaurosis fugax and facial numbness. Comorbidities included radical neck dissection and radiotherapy for laryngeal cancer 30 years earlier and COPD. Imaging used was digital subtraction angiography (DSA), left common carotid artery injection, left anterior oblique neck projection. **A,** Initial angiogram documenting a stenosis of the distal common carotid artery (CCA), measured at 85% in regard to the internal carotid artery (ICA), 90% in regard to the CCA. Note the tip of the 6 Fr, 90 cm long guiding sheath (Shuttle Select; Cook Medical, Bloomington, Ind.) in the distal CCA. **B,** Angiogram obtained after placement of an embolic protection device (Accunet; Abbott Vascular, Santa Clara, Calif.) in the distal ICA and predilation of the stenosis with a 2.5 mm by 15 mm angioplasty balloon (Powersail; Abbott Vascular). **C,** Angiogram performed after deployment of a tapered 6 to 8 mm by 30 mm self-expandable stent (Acculink; Abbott Vascular). Note the presence of a 35% residual stenosis. **D,** Control angiogram after dilation of the stent with a 4.5 mm by 20 mm angioplasty balloon (Aviator; Cordis Endovascular, Bridgewater, NJ). **E,** A final angiogram is obtained about 15 minutes after completion of the stenting procedure. This angiogram documents the stent diameter after slow continued expansion, especially if no dilation was performed afterward, and it checks for the presence of acute in-stent clot formation. The procedure was uneventful.

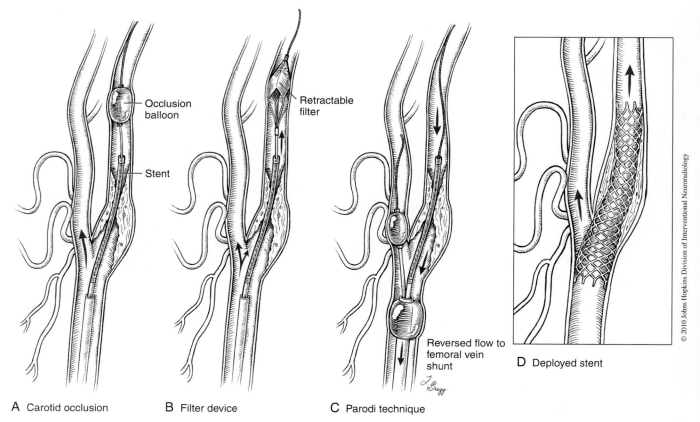

A Carotid occlusion   B Filter device   C Parodi technique   D Deployed stent

FIGURE 3   Schematic representation of the different types of embolic protection devices (EPDs). Black arrows indicate the direction of the blood flow. **A,** The Théron technique: the procedure is performed under flow interruption obtained by inflating a balloon within the internal carotid artery (ICA). After placement of the stent—and after postdilation, if performed—the delivery guide is advanced through the stent and placed immediately below the inflated balloon. The blood stagnating below the balloon, which may contain plaque debris, is aspirated forcefully. After aspiration, the space below the balloon is flushed with a bolus of saline solution that chases the reminder of the dead-space content into the external carotid artery (ECA). **B,** EPD, filter type: In this technique, the filter is advanced through the stenosis, using either its built-in wire tip or an over-the-wire technique with a wire selected by the operator. The filter is deployed in the ICA and is kept open for the duration of the procedure. At the end, a special recovery catheter is used to retrieve the filter and its contents. **C,** EPD, flow-reversal type: The blood flow through the lesion is reversed during this procedure, carrying the potential debris away from the cerebral circulation. Flow reversal is created by inflating two balloons, one in the common carotid artery and one in the ECA; blood leaving through the device is reinfused via a femoral vein catheter. **D,** A schematic representation of a deployed stent. *(Illustration courtesy Lydia Gregg, © 2010 Johns Hopkins Interventional Neuroradiology.)*

into the external carotid circulation. When using the filter-type EPD, the filter is attached to the working wire and is deployed distal to the stenosis (Figures 3, *B*, and 4, *A* and *B*). After the procedure, the filter is recovered, bringing along plaque debris trapped in its mesh. Several types of filter devices come paired with their individual stent platforms, and they should not be mixed. Several systems are available; ideally, an operator should become familiar with one or two stent/EPD systems.

One flow-reversal device based on the concept developed by Parodi is currently being tested (Figure 3, *C*). The idea of flow reversal is quite appealing, as it does not require crossing the lesion with the protection device. The early results appear promising; however, only patients with sufficient collateral flow, via the circle of Willis or via external to internal carotid anastomoses, can tolerate occlusion of antegrade carotid flow for the duration of the procedure. As with any type of occlusion device, intolerance to total carotid occlusion occurs in about 10% of patients, a factor limiting the application of the technique to a carefully selected group of patients.

The flow-reversal device necessitates the inflation of two balloons, a first one in the external carotid artery, and a second one, which is attached to the guiding catheter, in the common carotid artery. A closed circuit is then established between the guiding catheter and the venous system via the femoral vein to create retrograde flow.

There is a filter in the tubing connecting the guiding catheter and the femoral vein, which traps any embolic debris.

PERIPROCEDURAL MANAGEMENT

Antiplatelet Agents

As mentioned above, adequate antiplatelet therapy is essential to the success of CAS. Dual antiplatelet therapy with aspirin (325 mg/day) and clopidogrel (75 mg/day) is the current standard. Patients should be premedicated for at least 3 days prior to the procedure, although we prefer in our practice a 5 day preparation. Ticlopidine (250 mg bid) can be used in patients unable to tolerate clopidogrel. If a patient cannot stand a dual antiplatelet therapy, carotid stenting may need to be reconsidered, as the postprocedural stroke risk will be unacceptable. It is essential that patients remain on dual antiplatelet therapy for at least 3 months following the stent procedure, and they must continue on daily aspirin for life.

Glycoprotein IIb/IIIa inhibitors are no longer routinely used in CAS procedures; they have been associated with an increased risk of intracranial hemorrhage during the postprocedural period. Their role is now

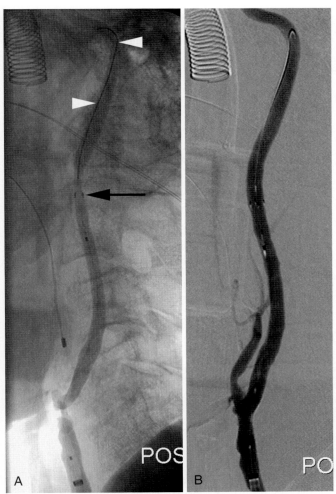

FIGURE 4 Same patient as in Figure 2, showing deployment of an embolic protection device (EPD) of the filter type. **A,** Digital subtraction angiography (DSA; left common carotid artery, unsubtracted lateral neck projection) after predilation, showing an EPD deployed in the midcervical segment of the left internal carotid artery (ICA). The metallic markers indicate the base of the device (*arrow*); the built-in wire tip is densely radioopaque (*arrowheads*). It is important to keep the tip of the wire constantly in sight. When using biplane angiography equipment, it is convenient to keep one plane magnified on the lesion to guide the angioplasty and stenting procedure (see Figure 1), while the other plane allows monitoring of the EPD and its wire. Mild vasospasm that can at times occur at the site of deployment of the EPD, as seen in this case, usually resolves spontaneously over a period of 5 to 10 minutes. **B,** DSA (left common carotid artery, lateral neck projection) after stenting and postdilation shows complete spontaneous resolution of the vasospasm.

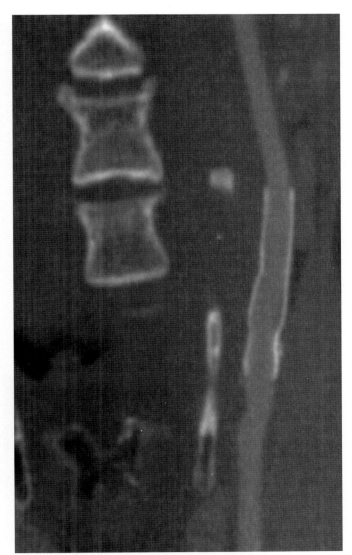

FIGURE 5 Follow-up of carotid stenting with CT angiography (same patient as Figure 1). Although digital subtraction angiography (DSA) remains the gold standard technique for precise evaluation of the cervical and cranial vasculature, CT angiography (CTA) has become the principal modality for the follow-up of patients after carotid stenting in our practice. Multiplanar reconstructions of the data set (here a 0.5 mm thick coronal image) not only shows patency of the artery but also documents the absence of significant endothelial hyperplasia and the integrity of the stent structure.

confined to the treatment of acute thrombus formation during the periprocedural or immediate postprocedural periods. In our practice, when facing acute in-stent thrombosis, abciximab is administered both intraarterially near the clot (half of the bolus dose) and intravenously (second half of the bolus dose), followed by a 24-hour maintenance dose.

Hemodynamic Instability

Periprocedural bradycardia can be seen in up to 25% of patients undergoing CAS. It occurs most commonly during balloon angioplasty, which may even precipitate hypotension and asystolic cardiac arrest. This issue is less common in patients who have previously undergone CEA, probably because their carotid bulb is denervated.

Periprocedural bradycardia is managed with atropine (0.5 to 1.5 mg intravenously) and with cardiac pacing if bradycardia is refractory. As a prophylactic measure, some operators choose to place a transvenous pacer prior to initiating the carotid stenting procedure.

The arterial hypotension that may accompany periprocedural bradycardia is usually treated with colloid and crystalloid fluid boluses, but intravenous administration of phenylephrine may be required in severe cases. Periprocedural arterial hypotension is believed to be secondary to continued expansion of the stent, which stretches the carotid baroreceptors.

Postprocedural hypertension is seen in up to 35% of patients who undergo CAS, and combined with impaired cerebral autoregulation, it can lead to the development of cerebral hyperperfusion syndrome (CHS). Patients with CHS typically are seen with headache, hypertension, seizures, and focal neurological deficits. CHS can result in severe brain edema, intracranial hemorrhage, and death. The incidence of CHS is slightly higher in patients undergoing CAS versus patients treated with CEA, likely in relation to antiplatelet therapy. The risk factors for CHS are still debated but seem to include female gender, advanced age (>75 years), a history of hypertension, a previous ipsilateral or recent contralateral CEA, previous cerebral ischemic damage, a high-grade carotid stenosis, and the development of periprocedural and postprocedural hypertension. Management relies on rapid control of the blood pressure using intravenous antihypertensive agents—such as labetalol, hydralazine, nicardipine, and/or a nitroglycerine drip—anticonvulsive therapy, and osmotic agents in case of significant cerebral edema.

Periprocedural Neurologic Assessment

Embolic events obviously represent one of the main complications that can occur during CAS, but the consequences of a cerebral embolic event vary widely. A small stroke may remain clinically silent, or it may be devastating, depending on the function of the cerebral tissue that has been damaged. Major strokes are generally associated with long-term disabilities and can at times be fatal. Although the risk of embolic events has supposedly been reduced by the introduction of EPDs, perioperative stroke remains a significant issue in CAS,

as has been shown in the various clinical trials described above. It is therefore important that operators eager to perform CAS are familiar with the normal anatomy of the brain and its vascularization, as well as with the clinical presentation and management of cerebrovascular disorders.

Follow-up

Patients who undergo CAS need to be closely followed up. Our practice typically includes follow-up visits at 2 weeks, 1 month, 6 months, and annually thereafter, or any time in between in the case of new or recurrent symptoms. Follow-up should include a complete neurological examination, and the 6 month follow-up visit should include a CT angiogram (Figure 5). Significant in-stent restenosis can usually be treated with angioplasty alone, but new stent placement may be required in selected situations (Figure 6).

Patients with atherosclerotic carotid arterial disease need a global assessment of their cardiovascular system; in particular, they should be evaluated for coronary artery disease and other comorbidities, including hypercholesterolemia and arterial hypertension. Statin medications have been shown to be beneficial in the long-term treatment of patients with carotid arterial stenosis, and smoking cessation should be strongly emphasized as well.

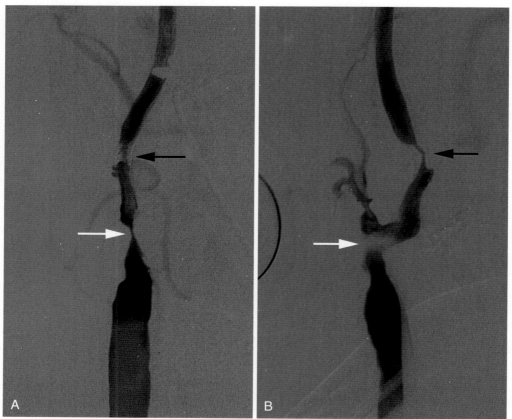

FIGURE 6 68-year-old man with a past history of right carotid endarterectomy and restenosis treated with a balloon-expandable stent, presenting with new symptoms on maximum medical therapy. Comorbidities include COPD, arterial hypertension, hypercholesterolemia, diabetes mellitus, chronic renal insufficiency, coronary artery disease (double bypass), and following repair of an abdominal aortic aneurysm. **A,** Digital subtraction angiography (DSA; right common carotid artery injection, right anterior oblique neck projection) showing the previously placed stent (*black arrow*) with in-stent restenosis and new, more proximal critical stenosis (*white arrow*). **B,** DSA (right common carotid artery injection, lateral neck projection) shows that both lesions appear slightly different in this projection: the in-stent lesion is better delineated and shows a higher degree of stenosis; the proximal lesion is more difficult to appreciate because of its tight but flat morphology. This emphasizes the importance of obtaining several angiographic projections when analyzing a vascular lesion.

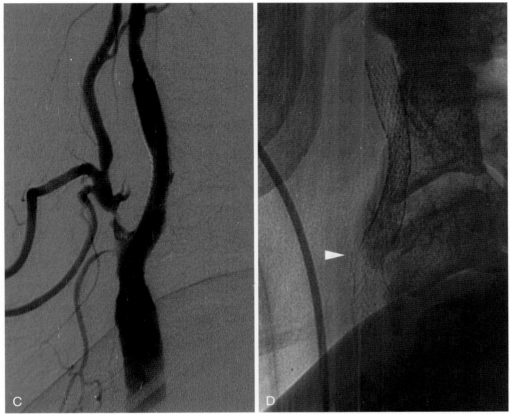

FIGURE 6, cont'd   C, DSA (right common carotid artery injection, lateral neck projection) after treatment. The procedure included predilation of both stenoses with a 2.0 mm by 15 mm angioplasty balloon (Voyager; Cordis Endovascular, Bridgewater, NJ), deployment of an EPD (Accunet; Abbott Vascular, Santa Clara, Calif.), and placement of two overlapping, self-expandable stents: a 5 mm by 30 mm stent distally (Precise; Cordis Endovascular) and a tapered 6 to 8 mm by 40 mm stent proximally (Acculink; Abbott Vascular). Postdilation was performed using a 4 mm by 20 mm balloon (Maverick; Boston Scientific, Natick, Mass.) in the distal stent and a 6 mm by 15 mm balloon in the proximal stent (Maverick; Boston Scientific). Note the mild vasospasm at the cranial tip of the distal stent. The procedure was uneventful. **D,** Right neck film, lateral projection, obtained after the placement of two overlapping stents. Note the slight protrusion of the stent mesh into the stem of the external carotid artery (*arrowhead*), a phenomenon typical of the open-cell stent design.

SUMMARY

Since the introduction of carotid angioplasty as a palliative treatment for inoperable patients with carotid arterial stenosis, technological improvements have revolutionized the endovascular management of this complex disease and have led to improved patient outcomes. Self-expandable stents and angioplasty balloons designed specifically for the purpose of treating the cervical carotid arterial system are now available, as well as various types of embolic protection systems that aim at decreasing the risk of stroke resulting from migration of plaque debris. Although these technological improvements have precipitated a decrease in the morbidity and mortality rates associated with the procedure, CAS remains a challenging procedure that necessitates adequate training and a specialized technological environment to be performed safely. Further information gathered through ongoing clinical trials will help refine patient selection criteria for CAS and CEA, and it will continue to improve the quality of care and outcomes for patients with atheromatous carotid artery disease.

SUGGESTED READINGS

Brott TG, Hobson RW, Howard G, et al: Stenting versus endarterectomy for treatment of carotid artery stenosis, *N Engl J Med* 363(1):11–23, 2010.

Carotid Endarterectomy Trial Collaborators: Beneficial effect of carotid endarterectomy in symptomatic patients with high-grade carotid stenosis, *N Engl J Med* 325:445–453, 1991.

Eckstein H, Ringleb P, Allenberg J, et al: Results of the Stent-Protected Angioplasty versus Carotid Endarterectomy (SPACE) study to treat symptomatic stenoses at 2 years: a multinational, prospective, randomised trial, *Lancet Neurol* 7(10):893–902, 2008.

Mas J-L, Chatellier G, Beyssen B, et al: Endarterectomy versus stenting in patients with symptomatic severe carotid stenosis, *N Engl J Med* 355: 1660–1671, 2006.

Management of Aneurysms of the Extracranial Carotid and Vertebral Arteries

Bashar Ghosheh, MD, and Charles S. O'Mara, MD

OVERVIEW

Aneurysms of the extracranial carotid and vertebral arteries are rare. Recent reports suggest that only 0.2% to 5% of all carotid procedures are performed for aneurysms. Therefore only small-series single-institution studies are available to guide treatment options.

CAROTID ARTERY ANEURYSMS

Etiology

The majority of extracranial carotid artery aneurysms (CAAs) are atherosclerotic or degenerative in nature. This etiology accounted for one third to one half of all cases reported by the two largest published series of CAAs from Houston's Texas Heart Institute (THI, 67 cases) and Baylor College of Medicine (BCM, 42 cases). Pseudoaneurysm following carotid endarterectomy (CEA) was also responsible for a large number of patients in both studies, but only about 15% of all reported extracranial carotid aneurysms are pseudoaneurysms. Other etiologies include fibromuscular dysplasia, infection, local injury, and dissection following blunt, penetrating, and iatrogenic trauma. Rare cases include radiation injury, Behçet syndrome, and collagen vascular disease.

Presentation

Patients with CAA are frequently asymptomatic, but most are seen with a pulsatile neck mass, which was found in more than 90% of patients in the BCM study (Figure 1). Most CAAs involve the carotid bulb, which is normally 40% larger in diameter than the more distal internal carotid artery (ICA). The definition of *aneurysm* is generally accepted to be a 50% increase in diameter of the normal artery, therefore aneurysms at the carotid bulb exist only when the bulb diameter is dilated to more than twice the ICA diameter, or more than 150% of the common carotid artery diameter. These relationships are helpful in determining the presence of CAA.

When symptoms of CAA do occur, they vary depending on the size, location, and etiology of the aneurysm. Neurologic symptoms include transient ischemic attack (TIA), stroke, and amaurosis fugax; these are caused by embolization from the aneurysm to the brain or retina on the side of the lesion. Compressive symptoms can result in cranial nerve palsy, Horner syndrome, headache or facial pain, hoarseness, and dysphagia. Infected pseudoaneurysms may occur with fever, leukocytosis, peritonsillar abscess, or cervical cellulitis. Rupture with frank hemorrhage, although rare, may occur into the pharynx or to the exterior through a draining sinus, usually associated with infected pseudoaneurysm following CEA. Concomitant abdominal aortic aneurysm or peripheral artery aneurysm occurs in about 20% of patients with CAA.

Differential Diagnosis

A coiled or redundant common carotid artery—typically on the right side in obese, hypertensive, elderly women—is the most common condition confused with CAA. A kinked or redundant common carotid artery produces a pulsatile mass at the base of the neck, which often can be distinguished on physical examination by the presence of pulsations parallel to the normal orientation of the long axis of the artery; these masses are not expansile in character, as are those found with an aneurysm. Carotid duplex ultrasound (DUS) readily defines the lesion and distinguishes it from CAA. Excessive length and redundancy of the ICA, which cause sigmoid curves and loops higher in the neck, are usually discovered by arteriography. A prominent carotid bifurcation in a patient with a thin neck can also be mistaken for a carotid aneurysm. Carotid body tumors, branchial cleft cysts, cystic hygromas, and enlarged lymph nodes should also be in the differential diagnosis.

Diagnostic Studies

Carotid DUS is the recommended initial diagnostic modality. This study readily defines those aneurysms in the middle and lower neck, but it can fail to detect aneurysms higher in the neck. Ultrasonography can determine the size, location, and flow characteristics of the aneurysm, as well as the presence of thrombus or dissection. Computed tomography (CT) and magnetic resonance imaging (MRI) are useful to image the lesion and surrounding structures and to identify preoperatively the presence of prior cerebral infarction. CT angiography (CTA) and MR angiography (MRA) with three-dimensional reconstruction now provide high-quality detailed images that define the arterial anatomy and help to plan intervention. These studies are done without risk of stroke, an inherent potential complication of conventional cerebral arteriography. Nevertheless, catheter-based cerebral arteriography remains an important modality for providing anatomic detail of the CAA and the aortic arch and its branch vessels. This information is especially useful for considering endovascular aneurysm repair, which can be done along with the arteriographic procedure.

Indications for Intervention

Intervention for CAA is indicated for relief of symptoms caused by local compression—such as pain, dysphagia, and cranial nerve compression—and for the treatment of rupture, which is associated with high morbidity and mortality. A CCA that is greater than 2 cm in diameter generally warrants consideration for repair; however, the most common indication for intervention is prevention of new or recurrent neurologic deficits caused by embolization of aneurysm contents. In a classic publication by Winslow in 1926, nonoperative management resulted in 70% mortality rate due to thrombosis, embolism, and rupture. Some small distal internal carotid aneurysms resulting from trauma or spontaneous dissection may remain stable, or they may even resolve over time, but close monitoring of such patients is essential. Most CAAs require treatment to relieve local symptoms, to prevent the development of new or recurrent neurologic events, and to avoid rupture.

Treatment

The treatment of extracranial carotid aneurysms has evolved over time. Wrapping of the aneurysm, the use of fascia lata or prosthetic material, and endoaneurysmorrhaphy are of historic interest and are no longer used. The current choice of treatment depends on the

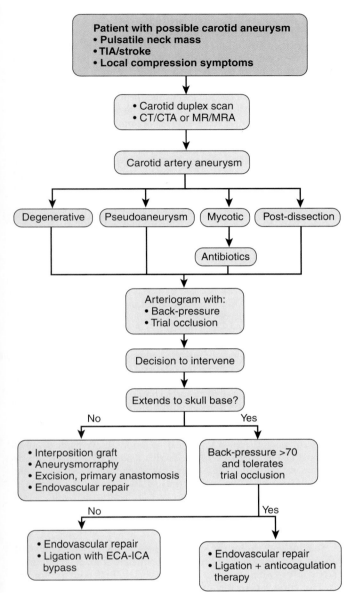

FIGURE 1   Algorithm for diagnosis and treatment of carotid aneurysms. *(Modified from Rothstein J, Goldstone J: Carotid artery aneurysm. In Cronenwett JL, Rutherford RB [eds]: Decision making in vascular surgery, Orlando, FL, 2001, WB Saunders, p 54.)*

Within the algorithm (Figure 1):

- **Patient with possible carotid aneurysm**
  - **Pulsatile neck mass**
  - **TIA/stroke**
  - **Local compression symptoms**

- Carotid duplex scan
- CT/CTA or MR/MRA

- Carotid artery aneurysm
  - Degenerative
  - Pseudoaneurysm
  - Mycotic → Antibiotics
  - Post-dissection

- Arteriogram with:
  - Back-pressure
  - Trial occlusion

- Decision to intervene

- Extends to skull base?
  - No:
    - Interposition graft
    - Aneurysmorraphy
    - Excision, primary anastomosis
    - Endovascular repair
    - No:
      - Endovascular repair
      - Ligation with ECA-ICA bypass
  - Yes:
    - Back-pressure >70 and tolerates trial occlusion
    - Yes:
      - Endovascular repair
      - Ligation + anticoagulation therapy

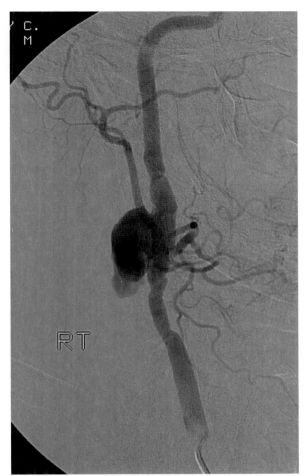

FIGURE 2   DSA of right carotid artery aneurysm at the site of carotid endarterectomy done 26 years previously.

size, location, and etiology of the aneurysm and the overall condition of the patient. Regardless of the choice of treatment, findings of a baseline neurologic examination should be documented. Patients with atherosclerotic CAA have an increased risk for having coronary and pulmonary disease, thus cardiopulmonary status should be thoroughly evaluated and optimized preoperatively.

Open surgical approaches require consideration of intraoperative cerebral perfusion monitoring and protection, because prolonged carotid artery clamp times are often required for reconstruction. Electroencephalography, transcranial Doppler, carotid backpressure measurement, and use of routine carotid shunts during operation have all been advocated. Local anesthesia has been used successfully for performance of carotid endarterectomy, but most surgeons prefer general anesthesia for CAA repair because of the potential for difficult dissection through inflamed periarterial tissue, extensive distal cervical exposure, or the need for complex arterial reconstruction. The location of the CAA varies with etiology and strongly impacts the treatment

approach. Atherosclerotic CAAs are commonly located at or near the carotid bifurcation, as are pseudoaneurysms that develop after carotid endarterectomy (Figure 2). Aneurysms resulting from blunt trauma injuries and dysplastic lesions typically occur more distally, often near the base of the skull (Figure 3). Operative exposure of the common carotid artery, the carotid bifurcation, and the proximal ICA can be achieved using a standard oblique cervical incision along the anterior border of the sternocleidomastoid muscle (SCM). More distal exposure requires extension of the incision to the level of the mastoid bone.

Care should be taken during dissection to avoid injuring the cranial nerves, particularly the vagus and its recurrent laryngeal branch, and the glossopharyngeal and hypoglossal nerves. The usual anatomic features of these nerves can be distorted by adherence to and compression by the aneurysm. The distal clamp should be applied after systemic heparinization but before any manipulation of the aneurysm, so that distal embolization is avoided. Extreme distal exposure of the ICA is facilitated by division of the posterior belly of the digastric muscle; anterior traction, subluxation, or division of the mandible; division of the styloid process; or division of the SCM from the mastoid bone. These maneuvers are facilitated by nasotracheal, rather than orotracheal, intubation. Subluxation and wiring of the mandible prior to initiation of the operation should be done by an oral surgeon experienced in this technique. If high exposure to the base of the skull is required for reconstruction, removal of the petrous temporal bone with division of the mastoid and external auditory canal may be necessary and should be undertaken with assistance from a neurosurgeon or otolaryngologist experienced in skull-base surgery.

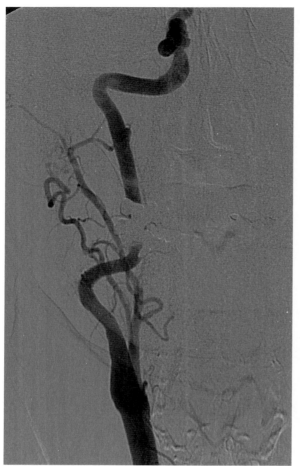

FIGURE 3   DSA of right internal carotid aneurysm at the skull base.

Current options for open reconstruction include ligation, resection with patch angioplasty repair, and resection with reconstitution of arterial continuity using a conduit. Sir Astley Cooper first described ligation for treatment of a CAA in 1805, and his patient developed postoperative stroke and subsequently died. Nevertheless, ligation continues to be a technically less demanding option that may be the only choice for a high lesion, for which distal access to the ICA cannot be achieved, or for rapid control of exsanguinating hemorrhage from aneurysm rupture. Unfortunately, ligation is associated with a high rate of stroke and/or death (30% to 60%). Ligation results in thrombosis of the ICA from the level of the interruption to the first major intracranial collateral artery, usually the ophthalmic artery, and thereby obliterates the aneurysm.

Selection of patients who will tolerate ligation may be accomplished by performing a balloon occlusion test with measurement of carotid backpressure at the time of cerebral angiography. Other methods for preoperative determination of the adequacy of cerebral collateral perfusion after carotid ligation are unreliable, such as carotid compression tests and observation of intracerebral crossfilling on angiography or transcranial Doppler. In the balloon occlusion test, the patient is heparinized, and a balloon on the distal end of a catheter positioned in the ICA is inflated to occlude antegrade cerebral flow for approximately 30 minutes. The patient's neurologic response is closely monitored, and carotid artery back-pressures are recorded. Carotid backpressures of 70 mm Hg or higher usually correlate with adequate cerebral collateral perfusion to allow reasonably safe carotid ligation if required. Patients with inadequate backpressure or unfavorable neurologic response to temporary balloon occlusion should be considered for extracranial–intracranial carotid bypass before

ligation. Anticoagulation should be considered after carotid ligation to prevent stroke caused by propagation of thrombus into the cerebral circulation beyond the first major intracranial collateral artery.

The aneurysm is repaired, and flow is restored, with either patch angioplasty or complete resection coupled with reconstruction of arterial continuity. Patch angioplasty is appropriate for small-necked, saccular aneurysms or pseudoaneuryms. The use of greater saphenous vein (GSV) and prosthetic material for patches and conduits has been well described. If infection is suspected, autogenous material must be used. Complete resection of the aneurysm with reconstruction of arterial continuity is the preferred method of open repair for fusiform or wide-based aneurysms. In this approach, ICA redundancy can be mobilized to permit reimplantation, but caution must be used to avoid creation of arterial kinking or angulation by straightening of a tortuous ICA. Another option is interposition grafting with GSV or a prosthetic graft. In some patients, the external carotid artery can be transposed a short distance to the end of the resected ICA.

Principles of cerebral protection during carotid artery repair are the same as those that apply to carotid endarterectomy. We favor routine shunting, but the technique of shunt placement for CAA repair may prove challenging and must be individualized according to specific anatomic features. Use of a shunt is facilitated by placing it through the interposition graft, performing the distal anastomosis around the shunt, and removing the shunt just prior to completion of the proximal anastomosis. For infected aneurysms, broad-spectrum intravenous antibiotics should be started before surgery. Wide debridement of infected and nonviable tissue should be done along with reconstruction of arterial flow through uninvolved tissue planes, using autologous conduits along with coverage by healthy tissue such as the SCM. Intraoperative cultures should be obtained, and long-term antibiotic therapy must be administered according to cultured organism sensitivity, especially if methicillin-resistant *Staphylococcus aureus* (MRSA) is the offending agent.

Recent advances in endovascular techniques have made some of the most challenging carotid aneurysms amenable to endovascular therapy. In the BCM series, 70% of patients in the recent treatment group (1995–2004) were managed using an endovascular approach. This method of treatment requires an experienced staff, a high-resolution imaging suite, and appropriate equipment, which includes embolic protection devices (EPDs) and a full array of catheters, wires, sheaths, and monitoring devices.

Suitable patients for this approach have aortic arch anatomy that can safely accommodate stable selective catheterization of the common carotid artery with a long, large-caliber sheath. Preferential consideration for endovascular treatment may be given to a surgically inaccessible lesion, a hostile operative field (prior neck irradiation or carotid surgery), or a patient who is medically unfit for general anesthesia.

Treatment techniques usually employ a transfemoral approach for access, although transaxillary and transcarotid approaches have been described. Following heparinization and selective catheterization of the common carotid artery with a long sheath over a supportive wire, an EPD is ideally deployed in the ICA distal to the aneurysm. A stent graft (covered stent) can then be placed across the aneurysm to exclude it from arterial flow, thus preventing expansion, rupture, and distal embolization.

Accurate sizing of the landing zones proximal and distal to the aneurysm is critical for achieving adequate seal. A bare metal stent can be used to close a dissection entry point (intimal flap), to treat associated arterial stenosis, or to cover a small pseudoaneurysm so that flow into the aneurysm is impeded, and the aneurysm sac thromboses (Figure 4). Thrombogenic agents such as coils, detachable balloons, glue, and synthetic particles can be injected directly into the aneurysm sac to cause thrombosis; however, care must be taken not to allow the escape of such materials into the parent artery, which could lead to thrombosis or distal embolization. A technique that has been described to ensure sac thrombosis is to place a bare metal stent across the aneurysm neck and deliver coils through a microcatheter directed into the sac across the struts of the bare metal stent.

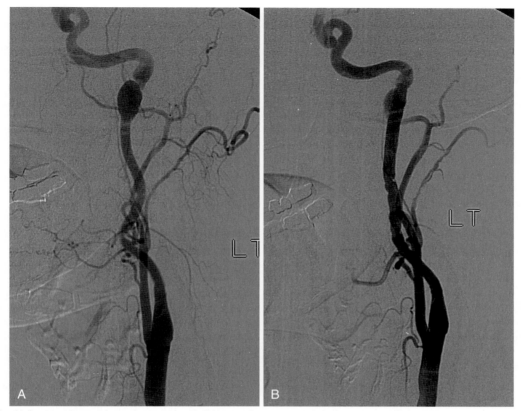

FIGURE 4   DSA of left internal carotid aneurysm at the skull base with associated web-like stenosis. **A,** Before treatment by bare-metal stent placement. **B,** After treament. Note absence of residual stenosis and presence of small residual aneurysm sac, which subsequently closed completely.

Results

The results of observation with and without anticoagulation follow the natural history of the disease, with stroke and mortality rates as high as 50% to 70%. Results of open surgical treatment vary widely depending on the type, size, and location of the aneurysm. Operative results tend to be worse for aneurysms located near the skull base and for infected aneurysms. Among the 67 cases reported by El-Sabrout and Cooley, death occurred in 6% and stroke in 7.5%, with a combined stroke and death rate of 10.4%; cranial nerve deficits occurred in 6%. These authors included a review of data from 13 single-center series reported from 1950 to 1995, which encompassed a total of 392 patients. Those patients treated nonoperatively had a combined stroke and death rate of 21%, but those treated with surgical reconstruction had a combined major stroke and death rate of only 9%. These data suggest that open surgical treatment of CAA can be performed with acceptably low morbidity and mortality rates. Long-term results from these series are generally favorable, with most deaths occurring from cardiovascular disease or diagnoses not related to the carotid aneurysm repair. Surgical reconstructions remained patent in most patients who had subsequent imaging, and late occlusion of the arterial repair was often asymptomatic.

The initial technical success rate for endovascular treatment of CAA is high. Periprocedural stroke and mortality are acceptably low in several small series reported to date. Cranial nerve injury and wound complications are avoided, the risk of femoral artery puncture-site issues is low, and the length of hospital stay is less with endovascular treatment compared with open surgical reconstruction. Short- and mid-term results up to 5 years after treatment are encouraging, with persistent exclusion of the aneurysm and patency of the reconstruction commonly noted on follow-up examination. With increasing use of endovascular techniques for treatment of carotid aneurysm, more data should accumulate regarding long-term results.

VERTEBRAL ARTERY ANEURYSMS

Aneurysms of the extracranial vertebral artery are extremely rare. Blunt and penetrating traumas are the most frequently cited causes, resulting in pseudoaneuryms or true aneurysmal dilatation after intimal dissection. Iatrogenic manipulation (chiropractic, vascular catheterization), fibromuscular dysplasia, prior neck irradiation, and collagen vascular disease have been described as causes of vertebral artery aneurysm. Patients may present with a pulsatile neck mass or with symptoms of vertebrobasilar insufficency. Contrast angiography remains the gold standard for imaging; however, CTA and MRA are also useful to define the aneurysm anatomy in relation to surrounding structures. More than 80% of lesions resolve spontaneously, therefore patients are often managed nonoperatively with anticoagulation. Intervention is indicated in cases of hemorrhage, aneurysm enlargement, neurologic symptoms, and contralateral vertebral artery absence or insufficiency.

Surgical exposure of the vertebral artery can prove difficult, because the artery lies deep in the posterior neck, and it courses through the transverse processes of the cervical vertebrae. Surgical exposure of the proximal vertebral artery is achieved through a transcervical incision, giving access from the vessel origin at the subclavian artery to the transverse process of C6 (V1 segment of the vertebral artery). Repair options include ligation, resection with repair, transposition onto the carotid artery, and bypass from the subclavian artery. The distal portions of the vertebral artery—which include the V2 segment (intraosseus course from C6 to C2), the V3 segment (from C2 to the atlantooccipital membrane), and the V4 segment (intracranial portion)—are all more difficult to expose. A posterior cervical approach may be feasible for exposure of the V2 and V3 segments. For surgically inaccessible lesions, endovascular access and use of stent grafts for embolization techniques have been reported with reasonable success to cover aneurysms in all segments of the vertebral artery.

Ligation or endovascular sacrifice of the vertebral artery is well tolerated in the presence of a normal contralateral vertebral circulation. Imaging of the contralateral vertebral artery preoperatively by CTA, MRI, or conventional arteriography is useful in planning treatment. An aneurysm of a dominant vertebral artery is best treated by a method designed to maintain patency of the involved artery.

Suggested Readings

Bush RL, Lin PH, Dodson TF, et al: Endoluminal stent placement and coil embolization for the management of carotid artery pseudoaneurysms, *J Endovasc Ther* 8:53, 2001.

Choudhary AS, Evans RJ, Naik DK, et al: Surgical management of extracranial carotid artery aneurysms, *ANZ J Surg* 79(4):281, 2009.

DuBose J, Recinos G, Teixeira PG, et al: Endovascular stenting for the treatment of internal carotid injuries: expanding experience, *J Trauma* 65:1561, 2008.

El-Sabrout R, Cooley DA: Extracranial carotid artery aneurysms: Texas Heart Institute experience, *J Vasc Surg* 31:702, 2000.

Rosset E, Albertini JN, Magnan PE, et al: Surgical treatment of extracranial internal carotid artery aneurysms, *J Vasc Surg* 31:713, 2000.

Rothstein J, Goldstone J: Carotid artery aneurysms. In Cronenwett JL, Rutherford RB, editors: *Decision making in vascular surgery*, Orlando, FL, 2001, WB Saunders, p 54.

Zhou W, Lin PH, Bush RL, et al: Carotid artery aneurysm: evolution of management over two decades, *J Vasc Surg* 43:493, 2006.

BRACHIOCEPHALIC RECONSTRUCTION

Jerry Goldstone, MD

OVERVIEW

Diagnosis and treatment of lesions of the three branches of the aortic arch have always been challenging. When compared with operations on the carotid bifurcation, surgical treatment of the more proximal portions of the aortic arch branch vessels is performed much less frequently, comprising less than 10% of the total revascularizations of the upper extremities and brain. Nevertheless, the occlusive and embolizing lesions that affect the brachiocephalic (innominate), common carotid, and subclavian arteries can produce serious symptoms, and their treatment can challenge even the most experienced surgeon.

The *supraaortic trunks*, as these vessels are collectively known, can be affected by degenerative, inflammatory, traumatic, dissecting, and aneurysmal diseases and disease combinations. By far the most common disease of these vessels that requires treatment is atherosclerosis. As in other locations, atherosclerosis primarily affects the orifices and proximal portions of the vessels. Thus lesions are most often located in the superior mediastinum at the level of the aortic arch rather than in the more distal portions of the vessels in the neck. This supports the concept that these lesions represent primary disease of the aortic arch that spills over into the orifices of the branch vessels. Similarly, aortic dissections frequently extend into the supraaortic trunks, but this is not the situation with other disease entities that occur here, such as the inflammatory arteritides, including Takayasu arteritis and radiation-induced stenoses. These vessels are also susceptible to injury by both penetrating and blunt trauma, and the principles of treating nontraumatic lesions can be employed in the treatment of trauma. Suffice it to say that the use of endovascular procedures has become a significant addition to the standard, open-surgical armamentarium for trauma patients.

Multivessel involvement is common, ranging from 24% to over 80% in reported series; but of all the vessels and disease processes affecting the arch vessels, atherosclerotic stenosis and/or occlusion of the origin of the left subclavian artery is by far the most common (Figure 1). Most occlusions are asymptomatic and are discovered by noting a supraclavicular bruit or blood pressure differences of over 20 mm Hg between the arms. It is very unusual for these lesions to produce effort-induced upper extremity symptoms, although distal embolization is one of the most common causes of digital ischemia. However, these lesions have assumed increased interest and importance because of their effect on blood flow in the internal mammary artery. Widespread use of the internal mammary artery for coronary revascularizations and treatment of subclavian stenoses is now a well-recognized cause of recurrent angina after coronary artery bypass graft (CABG). This has led some authors to recommend prophylactic treatment of even asymptomatic left subclavian stenoses in anticipation of future use in coronary revascularization.

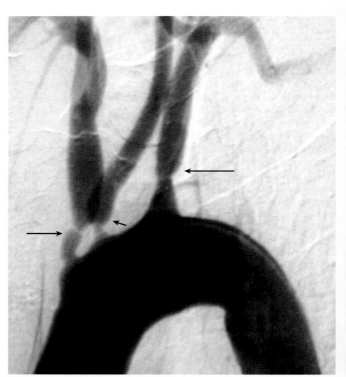

FIGURE I   Digital subtraction angiogram showing multivessel atherosclerosis involving brachiocephalic (*bold horizontal arrow*), left common carotid (*short arrow*), and left subclavian (*thin black arrow*) arteries.

Anomalies of the arch vessels are not infrequent. The most common is the origin of the left common carotid from the brachiocephalic artery (the now-preferred term for the *innominate artery*), the so-called bovine arch (Figure 2). In about 10% of patients, the left vertebral artery, rather than being the first branch of the subclavian, arises directly off the transverse arch, usually between the left common carotid and left subclavian arteries. A much less common anomaly is the origination of the right subclavian artery from the arch distal to the left subclavian, from where it courses across the upper mediastinum toward the right axilla; this can compress the esophagus and cause dysphagia (*dysphagia lusoria*). There seems to be a higher than expected incidence of aneurysmal degeneration of the origin of these anomalous right subclavian arteries (*Kommerell diverticula*).

There are a myriad other possible congenital anomalies, many associated with a right-sided aortic arch. All of them are important for the surgeon to be aware of, because they can cause confusion in the interpretation of diagnostic imaging studies. Thin-slice computed tomographic (CT) scans with reformatted multiplanar reconstruction can be particularly helpful for anatomic definition in these situations.

CLINICAL MANIFESTATIONS

Lesions of the arch vessels are more common than the symptoms they produce, because a substantial proportion of patients with such lesions are asymptomatic. When symptoms do occur, they can be typical of carotid territory, vertebrobasilar, or upper extremity ischemic syndromes, and they can be caused by either hypoperfusion or embolization. Thus focal transient hemispheric or retinal ischemic attacks, indistinguishable from those caused by carotid bifurcation lesions, can be caused by lesions of the brachiocephalic or left common carotid arteries. Multivessel occlusive lesions can produce global hypoperfusion, characterized by nonlateralizing symptoms such as light headedness, giddiness, or dizziness. A combination of right brain and right upper extremity symptoms can be caused by lesions in the brachiocephalic artery alone.

Proximal subclavian occlusion can produce reversal of flow in the ipsilateral vertebral artery. Known anatomically as *subclavian steal,* it is frequently seen on duplex ultrasound (DUS) and angiographic studies but is infrequently symptomatic (Figure 3). When symptoms of hind brain ischemia are associated with arm exercise, it is known as *subclavian steal syndrome,* admittedly a rare clinical entity. In general, flow reduction is thought to be the most frequent pathophysiologic mechanism in arch vessel disease, but embolization has also been well documented. Because of the extensive collateral circulation at the base of the neck, effort fatigue of the upper extremity is rare even in the face of occlusion of the subclavian artery. But digital ischemia can occur as a result of microembolization, and the proximal portions of the arch vessels are frequently overlooked as the embolic source. This causes delays in establishing the correct diagnosis and has been found to be one of the most common causes of ischemic

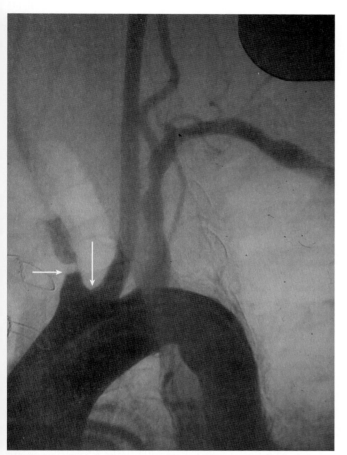

FIGURE 2 Digital subtraction angiogram showing brachiocephalic stenosis (*short arrow*) and common trunk of the brachiocephalic and left common carotid arteries (*long arrow*).

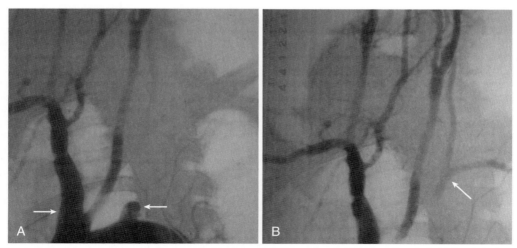

FIGURE 3 **A,** Digital subtraction angiogram showing so-called *bovine arch* (*left arrow*) and cul de sac of occluded left subclavian artery (*right arrow*). **B,** Later phase of the same angiogram, showing retrograde filling of subclavian artery from left vertebral artery (*arrow*).

tissue loss of the hand. However, it must be remembered that digital ischemia is far more commonly caused by collagen vascular diseases than by atheroembolism.

DIAGNOSIS

Lesions of the arch vessels can coexist with lesions in the carotid bifurcation, and it can sometimes be difficult to determine which is the symptom-causing lesion. A careful physical examination is essential, including bilateral blood pressure measurements, examination of the hands for signs of microemboli, determination of pulse lag at the wrist, and a careful search for supraclavicular and parasternal bruits. Any of these should suggest the presence of lesions of the aortic arch branches. A blood pressure difference of more than 20 mm Hg between the arms suggests the presence of a hemodynamically significant subclavian or brachiocephalic stenosis on the side of lower pressure. This is fairly common in elderly patients, most of whom have no symptoms attributable to this finding. As elsewhere, however, bruits are neither sensitive nor specific predictors of the severity of stenotic lesions. DUS is well established for the evaluation of the carotid bifurcation and cervical portion of the common carotid artery but is of limited value for direct assessment of the intrathoracic portions of the arch branch vessels, although abnormal velocity waveforms in the ultrasound-accessible segments of these vessels indicate the presence of significant stenosis. Reversal of flow in the vertebral arteries is strong evidence of proximal subclavian stenosis or occlusion (see Figure 3). Magnetic resonance angiography (MRA) may provide adequate imaging of the aortic arch and its branches, and computed tomographic angiography (CTA) can do the same; but in spite of its invasive nature and well-documented complications, the most definitive diagnostic method remains intraarterial digital subtraction catheter angiography. Multiplanar views and selective catheterization of each of the branches are usually necessary to fully evaluate the arch, its branches, and their relationships. If brain symptoms are present, thorough visualization of at least the cervical portions of these vessels in at least two projections should also be performed. Measurement of central aortic and translesion pressure gradients at the time of angiography can add valuable physiologic information when necessary. With the increasing utilization of endovascular techniques to treat these lesions, catheter angiography is once again becoming essential to therapeutic planning.

TREATMENT

Selection of Patients for Treatment

Most treated patients have been symptomatic, and despite the lack of data from randomized clinical trials, the indications for treatment of symptomatic arch branch vessels are usually logical and appropriate. Among these indications are clearly described symptoms that are entirely explainable by an appropriate stenotic or embolizing lesion or lesion combination in the artery or arteries supplying the affected body part. For example, focal right hemispheric symptoms associated with a severely stenotic brachiocephalic artery, and no lesions in the right common carotid artery or carotid bifurcation, can be safely assumed to arise from the brachiocephalic lesion.

Unfortunately, tandem lesions are often present in both the carotid bifurcation and the more proximal arch vessels, which can make it difficult to determine which is the causative lesion. Prior to the availability of angioplasty and stenting, such lesion combinations caused considerable debate about the prioritization of treatment, with the carotid bifurcation usually the initial choice because of its lower magnitude of risk and probably also because most surgeons have far more experience with carotid bifurcation operations than with operations on the arch vessels. Patients with nonfocal symptoms indicative of global hypoperfusion may also be appropriate

candidates for revascularization, particularly because they usually have multivessel involvement. Treatment of one lesion is usually sufficient to relieve the symptoms. Asymptomatic patients with lesions of the subclavian artery, either right or left, should generally not be operated on, even if there is documented reversal of flow in the ipsilateral vertebral artery. The same is true for asymptomatic stenosis of the common carotid arteries, because recommendations regarding such lesions cannot be based upon the extensive data available for treating carotid bifurcation lesions. However, there is an increasing need to treat even asymptomatic subclavian lesions to provide adequate hemodynamics to support upper extremity dialysis access, internal mammary–coronary bypass, and occasionally an axillofemoral bypass graft. Nonatherosclerotic conditions affecting the supraaortic trunks are being diagnosed with increasing frequency, including dissections, trauma, and arteritis (Takayasu arteritis, radiation-induced arteritis); and although we have only treated a small number of symptomatic patients with these conditions, the treatment principles outlined below are the same, and encouraging results have been achieved.

Treatment Options

There are many open surgical and endovascular options for the treatment of aortic arch branch vessels. Open surgical approaches can be categorized as *direct* or *indirect*. Direct approaches involve operations on the diseased vessels at the level of the aortic arch and result in nonturbulent, in-line antegrade flow in the normal direction. They require median sternotomy for lesions of the brachiocephalic and left common carotid arteries and left thoracotomy for proximal left subclavian lesions. For some lesions a direct approach has been mandatory—for example, aneurysms or traumatic disruption—but the availability of stent grafts has eliminated the need for open repair in many patients. Open repair is preferable when there is extensive calcification in the vessel that requires treatment. In addition, if coronary revascularization is required or anticipated in the near future, doing both procedures at the same time using a median sternotomy should be considered. Either prosthetic bypass or endarterectomy can be performed with very acceptable and durable results.

Because early publications reported relatively high morbidity and mortality rates for these transthoracic operations, the *indirect* or *extraanatomic* procedures have become far more common, particularly for the typical elderly patient with diffuse atherosclerosis and other surgical risk factors. These are performed through supraclavicular and cervical incisions and are very well tolerated by even the highest risk patients.

Some authors recommend performing these procedures under local anesthesia for selected high-risk patients, but we have not found this necessary. And although the indirect operations have excellent results and low morbidity and mortality rates, contemporary anesthetic and surgical techniques and advances in postoperative management have made direct repairs nearly equally safe. This is especially true for nonatherosclerotic diseases, such as Takayasu arteritis, which occur in a younger age group. Median sternotomy incisions are very well tolerated even in elderly patients with advanced atherosclerosis. The choice between direct and indirect approaches depends upon a number of factors, including the vessel or vessels involved, the pathologic process, the nature of the symptoms and their cause (embolic or perfusion), the status of other vessels supplying the brain and arm, the patients' medical comorbidities, whether they require other operations (e.g., carotid endarterectomy), and the surgeon's experience. In addition, the need for coronary revascularization and/or a previous sternotomy are important considerations in some patients.

The availability of a wide selection of angioplasty balloons, stents, and stent grafts has augmented and, in a significant percentage of cases, replaced both direct and indirect surgical approaches (Figure 4). In some patients, catheter-based and open surgical techniques are

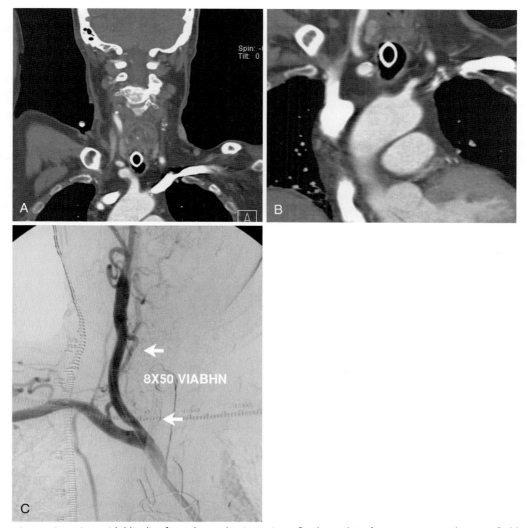

FIGURE 4 MR angiogram in patient with bleeding from the tracheoinnominate fistula resulting from recurrent malignancy. **A,** Note tracheostomy and region of artery effacement against trachea. **B,** Magnified view. **C,** Digital subtraction angiogram after transfemoral placement of an 8 mm diameter covered stent, which controlled the bleeding.

used together to treat lesion combinations. Because all of the treatment methods are useful, it is important for surgeons, and other interventionalists who treat such patients, to be thoroughly familiar with all of them.

Brachiocephalic (Innominate) Artery

Stenosis, aneurysms, dissections, and traumatic injuries of the brachiocephalic artery usually require a direct, open surgical approach, most often via a full-length median sternotomy. Attempts to limit the sternotomy to the portion from the sternal notch to the second or third interspace often result in fracture of the sternum at the lower level, especially in elderly patients, although a possibly improved technique that includes transection of the sternum in the third interspace has recently been reported. Other than the reduction in postoperative pain, we see little advantage in possibly compromising exposure of the great vessels by limiting the incision.

Atherosclerotic lesions of the brachiocephalic artery are usually confined to the proximal one third of the vessel and are amenable to treatment by endarterectomy or bypass grafting. Endarterectomy usually must extend proximally onto the aortic arch itself to remove all of the plaque that extends out from the aorta. This requires the use of a strong, partially occluding aortic clamp with deep jaws, so that

the clamp can exclude the entire innominate orifice from blood flow. Plaque removal is accomplished through a longitudinal arteriotomy that can be closed primarily without a patch. Occasionally the plaque extends distally into the proximal portion of the right subclavian or common carotid arteries, both of which are readily exposed and controlled by extending the sternotomy incision up into the neck, along the anterior border of the sternocleidomastoid (SCM) muscle.

To safely perform brachiocephalic endarterectomy without compromising flow to the left side of the brain, there must be enough room (1 to 1.5 cm) between the brachiocephalic and left common carotid origins to permit clamping the brachiocephalic artery without impinging on the left common carotid. The same limitations exist in the presence of the so-called bovine arch, wherein the brachiocephalic and left common carotid arteries arise as a common trunk (see Figure 2).

Extensive calcification of the aortic arch at the base of the brachiocephalic artery is another situation in which endarterectomy should not be attempted, because it may not be possible to adequately exclude the brachiocephalic orifice with the vascular clamp, along with the added risk of fracturing the plaque and causing distal embolization. Endarterectomy is also best avoided for inflammatory lesions, because the desired endarterectomy plane is usually not present.

Bypass grafting is performed more commonly than endarterectomy by most surgeons, and it permits revascularization of two or more distal arteries. These grafts should originate as far proximally as possible from the lateral aspect of the ascending aorta, which requires opening the pericardial reflection. Depending on the vessels being revascularized and the amount of retrosternal space for the graft, either a bifurcated or single-limb graft, with side arms as needed, can be used with the distal anastomosis made to the brachiocephalic, subclavian, or common carotid arteries.

Careful sizing and positioning of the graft is important to prevent kinking and graft compromise when the sternum is closed. The graft should pass posterior to the left brachiocephalic vein, which should be preserved if at all possible. It is almost unheard of for cerebral ischemia to occur from clamping the arch branches near their origins, even in the presence of multivessel occlusive disease; thus temporary shunts are rarely necessary. If maintenance of cerebral perfusion is required or desired, however, it can be accomplished by first sewing one limb of a bifurcated graft to the right subclavian artery before doing the brachiocephalic repair; this limb can then be dismantled after flow is reestablished in the brachiocephalic artery. Similarly, when debranching is being performed to permit proximal thoracic aortic stent grafting, a side-arm graft can be used for access for the endograft deployment. Atheroembolization can cause stroke, and digital ischemia can occur, so all of these vessels must be handled gently. The brachiocephalic territory can also be revascularized with indirect grafts from the left common carotid, axillary, or subclavian arteries or even in a retrograde manner using a femoroaxillary bypass.

Occasionally a patient with right cerebral or retinal symptoms will have severe tandem stenoses of both the brachiocephalic and right carotid bifurcation. It is not desirable to perform a carotid endarterectomy (CEA) with a flow-restricting lesion proximally; in these cases, treating both lesions together is prudent. Here again, extension of the sternotomy incision up into the neck, or a separate transverse cervical incision, will enable both arteries to be treated during the same operation. Combining standard CEA with angioplasty and stenting of the brachiocephalic is an alternative that avoids the need for median sternotomy. The brachiocephalic portion of the procedure is performed in a retrograde fashion, through an arteriotomy in the distal common carotid, which can then be extended farther distally for the bifurcation endarterectomy.

Tight lesions usually require predilation with a small angioplasty balloon (3 to 4 mm) before stent deployment, and balloon-mounted stents are preferable for the orificial lesions, because they are more rigid and offer more precise deployment. One major advantage of this retrograde stenting approach is that cerebral emboli can be prevented by flushing atheroembolic debris out the arteriotomy, avoiding the need for cerebral protection devices. Even in the absence of carotid bifurcation stenosis, we now prefer to treat most brachiocephalic lesions via the retrograde common carotid approach. This requires only a small cervical incision to expose the mid common carotid artery. Local anesthesia can be used, although we prefer general anesthesia, because it allows better control of the patient's breathing, which is important for optimizing the fluoroscopic images.

Endovascular treatment of brachiocephalic lesions can also be performed via an antegrade transfemoral approach analogous to the performance of carotid stenting, except that larger devices are used (see Figure 4). Unfavorable arch anatomy or difficult iliofemoral access favors the retrograde transcervical approach. The use of embolic protection devices (EPDs) is controversial, because none are designed for use in the common carotid artery, and their positioning and deployment in the internal carotid artery can be difficult and hazardous alongside the larger devices needed for treating the brachiocephalic lesion.

All patients treated for brachiocephalic arterial disease should take aspirin indefinitely after the procedure, and clopidogrel therapy should be added for at least 3 to 6 months following endovascular treatment. There are advantages and disadvantages to each of these approaches. All have been associated with successful and durable outcomes in most patients, but the endovascular approach has become the primary treatment strategy for the majority of patients.

Common Carotid Artery

Stenotic lesions affecting the proximal left common carotid artery are second only to those of the left subclavian in frequency, and like those of the left subclavian, most are asymptomatic. Surgical treatment is appropriate for symptomatic lesions, as well as for asymptomatic lesions proximal to a carotid bifurcation lesion that requires treatment, or when the lesion is thought to be the cause of thrombosis of the entire common carotid in the presence of a patent downstream internal carotid artery.

The proximal left common carotid can be approached directly through a median sternotomy similar to the approach described for treating brachiocephalic lesions. However, indirect methods employing supraclavicular incisions have proven to be safer and as durable as transthoracic approaches. Our preference here is for a prosthetic bypass between the left subclavian artery, if it is free of stenotic lesions, and the left common carotid artery near the base of the neck; the procedure is performed through a single transverse supraclavicular incision (*subclavian-carotid bypass*). Adequate exposure requires division of the clavicular portion of the SCM, the omohyoid, and the anterior scalene muscles. Care must be taken to avoid injury to the cervical lymphatics; several adjacent nerves, including the vagus, phrenic, and brachial plexus nerves; and, on the left, the thoracic duct.

Sometimes an additional incision along the anterior border of the SCM is necessary, when the anastomotic site on the common carotid is farther downstream. Subclavian-carotid bypass can be combined with ipsilateral carotid endarterectomy, and if the common carotid is occluded proximally, the distal anastomosis can be made at the level of the bifurcation. A very short graft of only a few centimeters in length is all that is usually needed. Because of this and their resistance to kinking and external compression, prosthetic grafts are preferable to autologous vein grafts, and they have a higher long-term patency rate. Both ePTFE and knitted polyester work well, although no good rationale exists for the use of externally supported grafts in this location. If the common carotid is patent, it can be safely occluded for the duration of the anastomosis without the need for temporary shunting. The use of a partial occluding clamp makes this anastomosis more difficult and usually restricts flow in the common carotid so much that it is largely ineffective at maintaining the desired level of cerebral blood flow.

Flow dynamics cannot be relied on to prevent recurrent embolization, so for common carotid lesions that are thought to be the source of emboli, the embolic focus must be eliminated by either proximal transection or ligation. Stenotic atherosclerotic lesions in the mid portion of the common carotid can be treated by endarterectomy, using the usual techniques with or without patch angioplasty, whereas radiation-induced lesions are usually best managed by graft replacement. Occlusion of the common carotid can be due to critical lesions at the level of the carotid bifurcation, with retrograde thrombosis, or the result of an orificial stenosis, with antegrade thrombosis to the level of the bifurcation. These lesions are often associated with patency of the internal and/or external carotid arteries, and reestablishment of flow in these vessels may be indicated for symptomatic patients and even in some asymptomatic patients with contralateral carotid occlusion. Reestablishment of antegrade flow in the common carotid can be accomplished by retrograde thrombectomy (not endarterectomy) of the common carotid with balloon catheters through the typical incision in the carotid bifurcation. For severe orificial stenosis of the common carotid, retrograde angioplasty can likewise be performed. This obviously requires adequate angiographic facilities in the operating room.

An alternative approach to a proximal common carotid lesion is *carotid-subclavian transposition,* which requires more extensive mobilization of the common carotid and subclavian arteries. It is possible to mobilize both of these vessels beneath the clavicle, almost to their origin off the aortic arch, through a supraclavicular incision, making it possible to bring them together in a tension-free anastomosis. The anatomic alignment can be challenging, and particular care must be taken to avoid injury or kinking of the vertebral and internal mammary arteries. One obvious advantage of this procedure is the avoidance of a prosthetic graft and its small attendant risk of infection. If the ipsilateral subclavian artery is not suitable as an inflow site, alternative sources of inflow are the contralateral common carotid or subclavian arteries. Prosthetic grafts are preferably tunneled in a retropharyngeal/esophageal, rather than subcutaneous, location, and dysphagia has been reported after this procedure. All of these grafts are easily monitored with follow-up duplex scanning.

Short-segment stenotic lesions of either common carotid artery are also treatable with catheter-based methods, either percutaneously or via open exposure, as described above for treatment of brachiocephalic lesions. For nonorificial lesions, self-expanding stents are preferable because of their flexibility and resistance to kinking.

Subclavian Artery

As previously noted, these are the most frequently encountered lesions, and they occur much more commonly than their symptoms. The natural history of asymptomatic subclavian stenosis and occlusion is generally quite favorable. Nevertheless, subclavian revascularization is indicated to treat symptoms of arm or hand ischemia resulting from hypoperfusion or embolization, as well as symptoms of vertebrobasilar insufficiency, when there is retrograde flow in the vertebral artery.

The rapid evolution of stent graft treatment for thoracic aortic aneurysms (TEVAR) has created considerable interest in, and debate about, how to deal with the left subclavian artery in terms of arm ischemia, endoleak, and adequacy of proximal stent graft attachment sites. This has led to a relatively large number of left subclavian revascularization procedures as a component of TEVAR (Figure 5).

With the increased utilization of the internal mammary artery for coronary revascularization, the patency of the subclavian artery has assumed increased importance, and treatment has increased accordingly. Several case series of recurrent myocardial ischemia due to subclavian stenosis proximal to a left internal mammary artery graft have been reported, with relief of symptoms after elimination of the subclavian lesion. Endovascular techniques are preferable because of their minimally invasive nature, and because they limit the duration of flow interruption to the internal mammary–coronary bypass. Either transfemoral or transbrachial approaches are appropriate, depending on a number of anatomic factors. The transbrachial approach is clearly better when the subclavian artery is occluded, the lesion is flush with the aortic wall with no cul-de-sac for guidewire access or the thoracic aorta is severely diseased and distorted (see Figure 3). In addition, a transfemoral approach to the right subclavian artery is often more difficult, and has increased risks of cerebral complications, because of the guidewire and catheter manipulations across the brachiocephalic artery that are required for successful treatment. Hematoma formation and nerve compression are potential hazards that are particularly worrisome after brachial approaches, because the brachial artery is relatively smaller than the femoral with respect to the devices used, and it is more vasoreactive.

The uncertainty of knowing preoperatively whether the subclavian artery is occluded or stenotic influences treatment planning. This distinction cannot always be made with even good quality CT or MR angiograms. Thorough definition of the vascular anatomy with digital angiography then becomes a crucial early step in endovascular procedures and often requires multiple image sequences taken at different angles. Most proximal subclavian lesions that require treatment are relatively short and calcified, and stent placement must be accurate to avoid stent protrusion into the aorta or impingement on the vertebral or internal mammary orifices. For these reasons, the radial strength and precision of deployment favor the use of balloon-mounted stents in this location, whereas self-expanding stents are

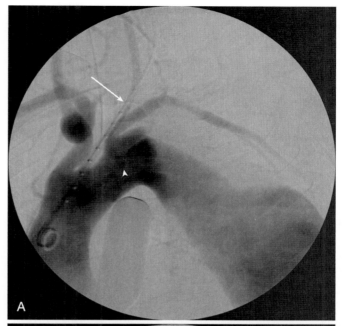

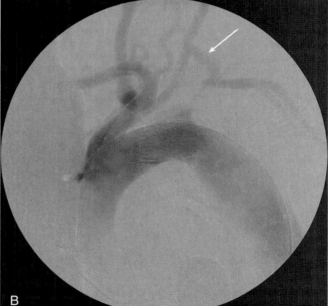

FIGURE 5 Digital subtraction angiogram during thoracic endograft procedure showing insufficient proximal attachment zone as a result of proximity of left subclavian artery (*arrowhead*). **A,** Note calibrated angiogram catheter in left common carotid artery (*arrow*). **B,** Angiogram after left carotid-subclavian bypass (*arrow*) shows satisfactory deployment of endograft at expanded landing zone.

favored in the more distal portions of the subclavian artery, where there is more motion, and where the possibility of compression by the clavicle and/or first rib is present.

Endarterectomy of the left subclavian orifice through a posterolateral thoracotomy is a technically elegant and challenging procedure that has largely been replaced by the less morbid extracavitary and endovascular techniques. *Carotid-subclavian bypass* and *subclavian-carotid transposition,* essentially identical to that described above as subclavian-carotid bypass and carotid-subclavian transposition, are the most frequent open surgical methods used, and the same precautions must be taken to prevent kinking. Both of these indirect surgical approaches have excellent and durable success rates.

When the diseased arterial segment is more distal, in the mid portion of the subclavian, as occurs with thoracic outlet syndromes, it may be necessary for the distal anastomosis to be made to the infraclavicular portion of the subclavian artery; in these cases, the graft can be tunneled beneath the clavicle. Subclavian-subclavian and axillary-axillary bypasses have also been used to restore pulsatile flow into the subclavian and vertebral arteries. They can also be used to restore flow in the right common carotid artery, when there is a proximal occlusion of the innominate artery. Here again, however, retrograde flow may not be effective in preventing recurrent embolization from a proximal atherothrombotic lesion in the innominate or proximal common carotid artery. Subclavian-subclavian grafts are usually tunneled across the suprasternal notch or retrosternally, whereas axilloaxillary grafts, which originate from the infraclavicular portion of the axillary artery, are tunneled subcutaneously across the front of the manubrium. Both of these types of reconstruction tend to be reserved for high-risk patients or those with unusually adverse anatomic or pathologic circumstances, such as radiation, infection, or extensive scarring from previous procedures. These grafts can be problematic if subsequent sternotomy is needed for myocardial revascularization.

SUMMARY

In-line antegrade arch vessel reconstruction is possible in almost all patients, but morbidity and mortality rates remain higher than for both subcutaneous bypass and endovascular techniques. The better durability of open repair may be an important factor for younger patients who require brachiocephalic reconstruction, but the evolving preferred treatment strategy is to attempt endovascular therapy first, reserving open surgery for those in whom this fails.

Endovascular techniques are appropriate for most proximal subclavian lesions, especially on the left side. Stenotic and totally occluded arteries can be recanalized using balloons, thrombolytic agents, and stents through either a retrograde brachial or antegrade femoral approach. Stent grafts are also useful to treat some traumatic lesions, especially those that pose major problems with exposure and bleeding, such as at the thoracic inlet behind the clavicle. Technical success rates approaching 95% have been reported in several series, although if the arteries are occluded, rather than stenotic, successful treatment occurs in only about 50%. No large series of such procedures have been published, and long-term durability is not known, but catheter-based techniques give the surgeon additional therapeutic options. Whether or not these less risky techniques should be used to expand the indications for treatment of asymptomatic lesions is a very controversial topic.

SELECTED READINGS

Berguer R, Morasch M, Kline R, et al: Cervical reconstruction of the supra-aortic trunks: a 16-year experience, *J Vasc Surg* 29:239–248, 1999.

Bountzos EN, Malagari K, Kelekis DA: Endovascular treatment of occlusive lesions of the subclavian and innominate arteries, *Cardiovasc Intervent Radiol* 29:501–510, 2006.

Fields CF, Bower TC, Cooper LT, et al: Takayasu's arteritis: operative results and influence of disease activity, *J Vasc Surg* 43:64–71, 2006.

Hassen-Khodja R, Kieffer E: Radiotherapy-induced supra-aortic trunk disease: early and long-term results of surgical and endovascular reconstruction, *J Vasc Surg* 40:254–261, 2004.

Ogino H, Matsuda H, Minatoya K, et al: Overview of late outcome of medical and surgical treatment for Takayasu arteritis, *Circulation* 118:2738–2747, 2008.

Rapp JH, Reilly LM, Goldstone J, et al: Upper extremity ischemia: the significance of proximal arterial disease, *Am J Surg* 152:122–126, 1986.

Rhodes JM, Cherry KJ Jr, Clark R, et al: Aortic-origin reconstruction of the great vessels: risk factors of early and late complications, *J Vasc Surg* 31:260–269, 2000.

Rodallec MH, Marteau V, Gerber S, et al: Craniocervical arterial dissection: spectrum of imaging findings and differential diagnosis, *Radiographics* 28:1711–1728, 2008.

Takach TJ, Ruel GJ, Cooley DA, et al: Brachiocephalic reconstruction. I. Operative and long-term results for complex disease, *J Vasc Surg* 42:47–54, 2005.

Tracci MC, Cherry KJ Jr: Surgical treatment of great vessel occlusive disease, *Surg Clin North Am* 89:821–836, 2009.

UPPER EXTREMITY ARTERIAL OCCLUSIVE DISEASE

Juan Carlos Jimenez, MD, and Peter F. Lawrence, MD

OVERVIEW

Revascularization of the upper extremity for symptomatic ischemia is less commonly performed than for lower extremity arterial disease. Fewer patients use their upper extremity for repeated activities, as they do the lower extremities, such as when walking. Consequently, upper extremity claudication disability is much less common. In addition, the presence of extensive collateral arteries demanding blood flow, as well as decreased muscle mass in the arm and hand, make symptoms less frequent, even in the face of significant arterial occlusion. Many patients remain asymptomatic until critical limb ischemia occurs, despite the presence of flow-limiting arterial lesions. However, when ischemic symptoms of the hand and digits do occur, they can lead to significant disability and functional impairment.

ETIOLOGY

The many causes of symptomatic upper extremity ischemia are listed in Table 1. Atherosclerosis and inflammatory arteritides are frequent causes of upper extremity arterial occlusive disease and are more commonly present in the proximal segments of the supraaortic trunks. Patients with diabetes, autoimmune disease, and renal failure often manifest ischemic symptoms in the more distal radial and ulnar arteries and particularly in the small arteries of the hand. When an iatrogenic arterial injury from a catheter or angioaccess procedure is superimposed on one of these preexisting arterial diseases, ischemic symptoms may be created.

Systemic Diseases

Takayasu arteritis and temporal arteritis are both large-vessel vasculitides that can affect the proximal upper extremity vasculature. Both are associated with an initial inflammatory stage—with myalgias, arthralgias, elevated erythrocyte sedimentation rate, and so on—and both produce characteristic smooth, tapering stenoses. Takayasu arteritis is most commonly encountered in young Asian females and frequently affects the larger branches of the supraaortic trunk. Temporal or giant cell arteritis is generally found in patients over 60 years of age

TABLE 1: Causes of upper extremity ischemia

Vasospasm

Raynaud disease
Medication induced–vasopressors, β-blockers
Ergot poisoning

Intrinsic Arterial Disease

Atherosclerosis
Radiation arteritis
Azotemic arteriopathy
Spontaneous dissection
Fibromuscular dysplasia

Inflammatory Diseases

Connective tissue disorders
Buerger disease
Takayasu arteritis
Temporal (giant cell) arteritis
Hypersensitivity angiitis

Noninflammatory Medical Disease

Thrombophilic states
Myeloproliferative disorders
Cold injury
Hepatitis-associated vasculitis
Cryoglobulinemia
Vinyl chloride exposure

Embolism

Cardiac (most common)
Proximal aneurysm
Arterial thoracic outlet syndrome
Atheroembolism
Paradoxic embolus (with accompanying septal defect)

Trauma

Iatrogenic
Blunt arterial injury
Penetrating arterial injury
Hypothenar hammer syndrome
Vibration

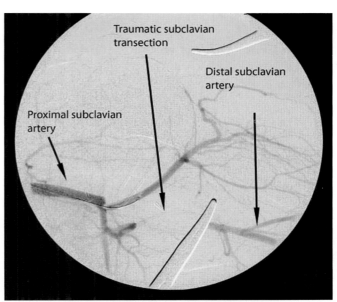

FIGURE 1   Upper extremity angiography reveals an acute occlusion of the left subclavian artery after penetrating trauma.

and usually affects more distal segments of the axillary and brachial arteries, as well as the superficial temporal and ophthalmic arteries.

A number of autoimmune, inflammatory, and rheumatologic disorders cause occlusive disease of the more distal upper extremity arteries. Scleroderma, CREST (*c*alcinosis, *R*aynaud phenomenon, *e*sophageal dysmotility, *s*clerodactyly, and *t*elangectasia) syndrome, lupus, and rheumatoid arthritis are frequently associated with small artery occlusive disease affecting the palmar and digital arteries. These diseases invariably affect the vessels in both upper extremities, making it easier to differentiate them from other occlusive diseases that cause unilateral hand ischemia.

Embolic Diseases

Embolic diseases typically cause unilateral arm or hand ischemia, which can help differentiate them from other systemic diseases. Cardiac emboli secondary to arrhythmias are the most common source of emboli to the upper extremity arteries, and proximal arterial aneurysms, ulcerated plaques, and paradoxical emboli from a deep venous thrombosis (DVT) through a septal defect are less frequent etiologies. Patients with embolic disease to the upper extremity often are seen with acute ischemic symptoms of the forearm and hand. When no arrhythmia or cardiac thrombus is identified, an aneurysm or ulcerative lesion in the subclavian artery associated with thoracic outlet syndrome is the most common etiology. Mural thrombus in the area of poststenotic dilatation is the common source of these distal emboli. Posttraumatic aneurysms (crutch-induced axillary artery aneurysms) and pseudoaneurysms secondary to trauma or infection are also potential sources.

Trauma

Both blunt and penetrating trauma to the upper extremity arteries can cause symptoms of acute ischemia. Traumatic injury to the vessel can lead to transection, dissection, or acute arterial thrombosis (Figure 1). Iatrogenic injuries from interventional procedures are the most common cause of upper extremity arterial trauma; brachial artery occlusion following cardiac catheterization is a well-recognized complication, which may remain undiagnosed in the acute setting because of abundant collaterals around the elbow. Forearm and hand claudication may develop later, after resumption of normal activities.

Hypothenar hammer syndrome results from repetitive blunt trauma to the terminal portion of the ulnar artery in the Guyon tunnel. This injury is caused by repetitively striking objects with the base of the palm. Segmental occlusion or aneurysm formation in the ulnar artery, with or without distal digital artery embolism, can result.

EVALUATION

History and Physical Examination

A detailed history and physical examination is the first step in diagnosing the correct etiology of the upper extremity ischemia symptoms. Symptoms can range from color changes, coolness, numbness, weakness, and claudication to ischemic resting pain and tissue loss. Exercise induced fatigue in the arm usually indicates disease of the large arteries. Symptoms in the hand and digits may be due to

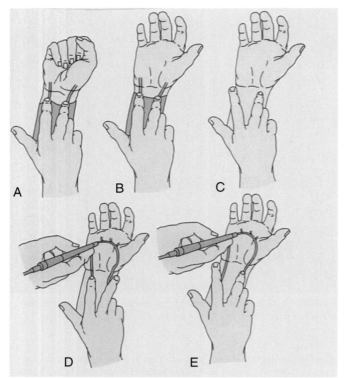

FIGURE 2   The Allen test may be performed to assess hand perfusion with or without the use of a handheld Doppler. *A,* Digital occlusion of radial and ulnar arteries. *B,* Patient is instructed to open and close hand. *C,* Digital occulsion of the ulnar artery is released and reperfusion of the hand is assessed to confirm the presence of a complete palmar arch. *D and E,* A handheld Doppler may also be used to evaluate signals in the palmar arch during an Allen test. *(From Wolcott, MW [ed]: Ambulatory surgery and the basics of emergency surgical care, ed 2, Philadelphia, 1988, Lippincott.)*

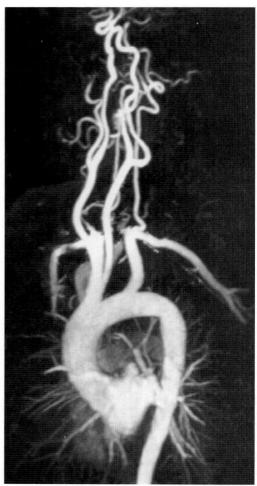

FIGURE 3   MRA of the supraaortic trunks and upper extremity arteries.

occlusion at multiple levels, including the small arteries. Digital tissue loss is nearly always associated with occlusive disease of the small arteries of the hand, with or without more proximal involvement. Associated dizziness, ataxia, and diplopia suggest ischemia of the posterior cerebral circulation, and an occlusive lesion of the proximal subclavian or innominate artery, proximal to the origin of the vertebral artery, should be suspected. Unilateral symptoms suggest a mechanical cause of the occlusive disease, and bilateral symptoms suggest the presence of a systemic cause.

A complete pulse examination of neck and upper extremities should be performed. Pulses documented should include the superficial temporal, carotid, subclavian, axillary, brachial, radial, and ulnar pulses. An irregular pulse should prompt a more detailed cardiac examination to identify atrial fibrillation or other arrhythmias that may predispose to cardioembolism. An electrocardiogram and echocardiogram should be performed to evaluate cardiac sources of emboli, such as cardiac mural thrombus. Auscultation should be performed at the level of the carotid and subclavian arteries to identify bruits, and the hand and digits should be inspected carefully for changes in color or temperature, trophic changes, and tissue loss.

The Allen test, first described in 1929, is used to evaluate the perfusion to the hand by the radial and ulnar arteries (Figure 2). The examiner occludes both the radial and ulnar arteries digitally after the patient opens and closes the hand. The ulnar and radial arteries are then released sequentially, and return of color to the hand indicates normal filling of the palmar arch by that artery. If equivocal, a Doppler placed over the palmar arch can substitute for visual inspection.

Noninvasive Evaluation

Handheld Doppler evaluation, segmental arterial pressures (digital-brachial index [DBI]), arterial duplex scanning, and digital plethysmography are all useful noninvasive modalities to evaluate occlusive disease of the upper extremity. In general, a DBI greater than 0.9 is considered normal, and a DBI greater than 0.7 indicates adequate perfusion; values less than 0.7 are indicative of hemodynamically significant lesions that produce symptoms. Calcified arteries, often associated with longstanding diabetes or renal failure, will yield falsely elevated DBI values. Color duplex combined B-mode imaging and color Doppler evaluation and can provide even more detailed information regarding arterial anatomy and blood flow. Digital plethysmography uses pulse volume recordings to measure digital volume changes. They should be used in conjunction with the other noninvasive tests described to assess overall upper extremity perfusion.

Computed tomography angiography (CTA) and magnetic resonance angiography (MRA) have emerged as powerful alternatives to catheter-based invasive angiography for evaluating the upper extremity arteries. The advantages of CTA are increased speed and accessibility compared with MRA, and CTA reliably images arterial calcification and is more useful for visualization of more proximal arteries, including the aorta and supraortic trunks. MRA (Figure 3) has better resolution of medium and small arteries than CTA. Disadvantages of MRA include longer imaging times to complete the study and inability to image calcification of vessel walls.

MEDICAL THERAPY

Conservative medical therapy is the first line of treatment for many patients with upper extremity occlusive disease. Abstinence from tobacco and cold avoidance are mandatory treatment for patients with severe Raynaud phenomenon. Calcium channel blockers are the initial medication of choice for patients with symptomatic Raynaud disease, and nifedipine is the most commonly used because of its relatively low cost and oral absorption. Other commonly used medications include α-blockers, angiotensin II receptor antagonists, prostaglandins, phosphodiesterase inhibitors, and endothelin receptor antagonists.

Patients with systemic vasculitides—temporal arteritis, Takayasu arteritis, and giant cell arteritis—generally manifest an early acute inflammatory phase with attendant fever, myalgias, night sweats, fatigue, and malaise. Corticosteroids are the mainstay of treatment during this phase. Alternative treatments include cyclophosphamide, methotrexate, azathioprine, infliximab, and mycophenolate mofetil. Percutaneous and/or surgical revascularization should be avoided during this acute inflammatory phase if possible.

Aggressive risk-factor modification should be implemented in patients with atherosclerotic upper extremity occlusive disease prior to revascularization. Lipid-lowering medications, antiplatelet agents, β-blockers, angiotensin-converting enzyme inhibitors, and aggressive blood glucose management should be used to reduce the progression of atherosclerotic disease prior to intervention.

ANGIOGRAPHY AND ENDOVASCULAR TREATMENT

Angiography remains the gold standard for imaging the upper extremity arteries for occlusive disease, but often it is reserved for therapeutic interventions rather than diagnosis. In recent years, endovascular interventions have become standard therapy for many upper extremity arterial occlusive diseases, and they are the initial treatment of choice for many embolic and thrombotic problems. However, the success of percutaneous interventions depends on the etiology of the occlusive disease and the extent of arterial involvement. Endovascular therapy is particularly indicated as initial therapy for short-segment stenoses and occlusions, such as subclavian artery stenosis, but longer segment arterial occlusions are often best treated with open surgical revascularization. Atherectomy of the brachial artery has been described in isolated reports with successful outcomes; however, the use of this technique for occlusive disease of the upper extremity remains controversial. Percutaneous revascularization for arterial disease related to inflammatory disorders in the acute phase yields poor results with high restenosis rates.

Endovascular therapy can also significantly decrease morbidity in selected patients with acute proximal injuries of the subclavian or innominate arteries, because thoracotomy and sternotomy would otherwise be required for proximal vascular control (Figures 4 and 5). Balloon angioplasty, embolization of pseudoaneurysms, and bare metal and covered stents can all be used for both acute and chronic pathology that leads to stenosis and occlusions.

Thrombolysis may also be used in certain patients with mild to moderate ischemia and proximal disease who do not require more urgent thromboembolectomy. Thrombolytic therapy also often works better than surgery for acute thrombosis of the small arteries of the forearm.

Endovascular Technique

For lesions of the proximal subclavian artery, a brachial, axillary, or femoral puncture may be performed. A brachial puncture from the ipsilateral arm is often the most direct approach for lesions of the subclavian artery. When using covered stents, a brachial artery cutdown, followed by arterial closure, may be required because of the larger diameter sheaths required to deploy these devices. We prefer the use

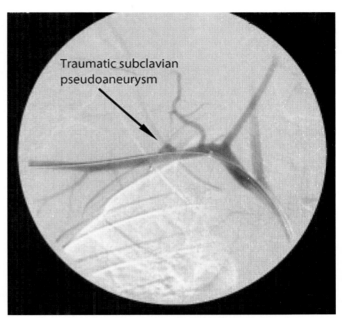

FIGURE 4 Pseudoaneurysm of the right subclavian artery following blunt trauma.

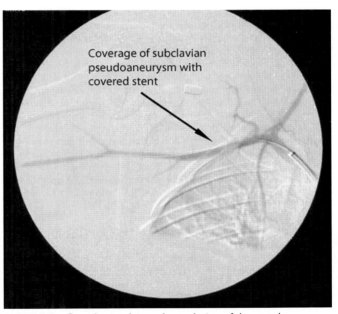

FIGURE 5 Complete endovascular exclusion of the pseudoaneurysm was performed using a covered stent.

of a stiff, 0.35 inch angled guidewire to traverse the stenosis or occlusion. A long destination sheath may be used for increased wire support and may be used to facilitate the crossing of longer, complete occlusions. Once the lesion is crossed with the guidewire, systemic heparin is administered, and an activated clotting time (ACT) is measured and maintained at greater than 250 seconds. A stiff catheter is used to follow the wire through the true lumen. Angiography should be performed at this time to ensure location of the wire and catheter in the true lumen.

Balloon angioplasty may be used to dilate stenosed or occluded subclavian and axillary arterial segments. We employ the use of self-expanding bare metal stents when residual stenoses 30% or greater are present, or when arterial dissection occurs following angioplasty. Covered stents may be used following penetrating trauma with extravasation, traumatic pseudoaneurysms, or when arterial rupture occurs following balloon angioplasty. Because covered stents usually require a larger diameter sheath for introduction into the artery, femoral cannulation may be the preferred access route to eliminate the need for surgical closure.

Catheter-directed thrombolysis of the upper extremity is useful for treatment of acute thrombosis that extends into the distal radial and ulnar arteries of the forearm and the deep and superficial palmar arches and their branches. These arteries are not generally accessible by surgical embolectomy catheters because of their small size and tendency for spasm. The preferred approach is through a femoral artery puncture. Following angiography to confirm the presence of thrombus in the upper extremity arteries, a 0.14 inch or 0.18 inch guidewire is used to traverse the thrombosed artery. Pulsed-spray thrombolysis (2 mg tissue plasminogen activator over 20 minutes) can be performed after placement of a thrombolysis infusion catheter or wire into the thrombus. If follow-up angiography reveals persistent arterial thrombosis, continuous thrombolytic infusion can be performed over the next 24 to 72 hours. Care must be taken to monitor the patient's fibrinogen levels and hemoglobin and to assess for any external signs of bleeding. Follow-up angioplasty is sometimes required following clot lysis for residual arterial stenoses.

For patients with severe ischemia and/or tissue loss due to acute thrombosis or embolism, surgical balloon embolectomy may restore perfusion to the distal arm and hand more rapidly than thrombolysis; however, this technique is less effective than thrombolysis for small arteries of the hand. Patients with severe or prolonged ischemia lasting longer than 6 hours are at risk for compartment syndrome and may require fasciotomy of the forearm and hand.

Several recent studies have supported the use of endovascular techniques for upper extremity arterial occlusive disease. De Vries and colleagues reviewed the results of 110 patients who underwent *percutaneous transluminal angioplasty* (PTA) of the subclavian artery over a 6 month period. The initial technical success rate was 93%, and primary clinical patency at 5 years was 89%. The local complication rate was 4.5%, and the combined stroke and death rate was 3.6%.

AbuRahma and colleagues compared the results of subclavian artery PTA with carotid-subclavian bypass for symptomatic lesions. PTA and stenting was performed in 121 patients, and bypass was performed in 51 patients over a 10-year period. No significant differences were seen in the survival rates between both groups at any time. Primary patency at 1 year was 100% for the bypass group and 93% for the PTA group. Carotid subclavian bypass had superior primary patency rates at 5 years compared with PTA (96% vs. 70%).

SURGICAL REVASCULARIZATION

The success of upper extremity surgical revascularization depends largely on the etiology of the arterial occlusive disease, the extent of disease, and location of the lesions.

Operative Exposure of the Subclavian Artery

Because the left subclavian artery travels posteriorly from its origin on the aortic arch, proximal control through a median sternotomy is challenging. The preferred approach for proximal control of the left subclavian artery is left anterolateral thoracotomy. The patient is positioned supine, and a rolled towel is placed beneath the scapula to position the chest wall slightly anteriorly. A transverse curvilinear incision is performed at the level of the fifth rib, extending from the lateral border of the sternum to the anterior axillary line. Dissection is performed through the pectoralis fascia. The intercostal muscles overlying the fifth rib are divided, the parietal pleura is exposed and incised, and the chest cavity is entered using a self-retaining rib spreader. Inferior retraction of the superior lobe of the left lung will reveal the aortic arch through the mediastinal pleura. Incising the mediastinal pleura exposes the origin of the left subclavian artery. Care should be taken to avoid injury to both the vagus nerve and the

thoracic duct in this region; the vagus nerve passes anterolateral to the artery, and the thoracic duct lies posteromedial in this approach.

The proximal right subclavian artery is best exposed through a median sternotomy. Cervical extension of the sternotomy allows for exposure of the carotid sheath. Mobilization of the left innominate vein allows visualization of the proximal right subclavian artery and the innominate artery, which is then followed to the bifurcation of the right common carotid artery. Care must be taken to avoid injury to the right recurrent laryngeal nerve, which wraps around the inferior border of the proximal right subclavian artery and ascends medially between the esophagus and the trachea.

Surgical Reconstruction for Subclavian Artery Lesions

Subclavian Transposition

The most frequently performed operations for occlusive disease of the subclavian artery are carotid-subclavian bypass and subclavian transposition. Both procedures have been described extensively in the surgical literature with excellent long-term patency and low morbidity. Patencies for subclavian transposition and carotid-subclavian bypass have been reported as 75% to 90% at 5 years. Noninvasive testing should be used prior to surgery to ascertain that the common carotid artery is free of flow-limiting lesions. Advantages of subclavian transposition for proximal subclavian artery occlusions include autogenous reconstruction, avoidance of prosthetic materials, and performance of only one vascular anastomosis (Figure 6).

The patient is placed supine with the head of the bed elevated to 20 to 30 degrees. A rolled towel may be placed under the shoulders to allow for optimal neck extension. A short transverse cervical incision is made approximately 2 cm above the clavicle and parallel to it. Division of the platysma muscle is performed, and the dissection is extended to the sternocleidomastoid (SCM) muscle; the clavicular head of the SCM may be transected for increased exposure. The scalene fat pad is mobilized superiorly and retracted to allow division of the anterior scalene from its tubercle on the first rib. The phrenic nerve, which usually courses from lateral to medial along the surface of the anterior scalene muscle, must be spared.

Next, the internal jugular vein is mobilized and retracted laterally, and the common carotid artery and the vagus nerve are mobilized from surrounding tissues and gently retracted medially. For left-sided exposures, the thoracic duct may be divided to enhance visualization of the arteries. Division of crossing veins allows the subclavian artery and its proximal branches to be identified posterior to the clavicle. Silastic tapes are then placed around the thyrocervical trunk,

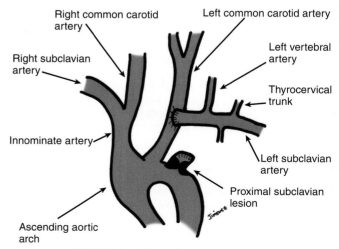

FIGURE 6 Left subclavian transposition.

proximal vertebral artery, and internal mammary artery. If a patient has had a previous internal mammary-coronary bypass, it is critical to avoid occlusion of this vessel with tapes and to not clamp the subclavian artery proximal to the internal mammary artery.

Once systemic heparin has been administered, small vascular clamps are used to control the proximal and distal subclavian artery. The subclavian artery is divided sharply as far proximal as safely possible. Care must be taken to oversew the proximal stump immediately to prevent retraction into the chest. Angled vascular clamps are used to control the proximal and distal common carotid artery; a shunt is not necessary. A longitudinal arteriotomy is performed on the posterolateral wall of the common carotid artery, and an end-to-side anastomosis with running Prolene suture is fashioned between the transected end of the subclavian artery and the common carotid artery. If the subclavian artery is too short, further mobilization of the carotid artery may be performed for lateral mobilization. Division of the internal mammary artery may be done to mobilize additional length of the subclavian artery for a tension-free repair. To identify lymphatic leaks, we routinely use suction drains to collect lymphatic fluid; we remove them after the patient has begun a regular diet.

Cina and colleagues reviewed the results of 27 patients who underwent subclavian–carotid transposition over an 11 year period. There were no perioperative deaths or strokes. Primary patency at a mean follow-up of 25 ± 21 months was 100%. Complications included hematoma (4%) and lymphatic leaks (9%), and all patients remained free of symptoms throughout the study period.

Carotid-Subclavian Bypass

Carotid-subclavian bypass (Figure 7) is superior to subclavian transposition in patients with a very proximal vertebral artery origin; patients with extension of plaque beyond the origin of the subclavian artery may also be better candidates for bypass. Another indication for this procedure is the presence of a patent internal mammary–coronary bypass graft. In this instance, a clamp may not be placed proximal to the internal mammary artery because of a high risk of myocardial ischemia.

Dissection is performed lateral to the clavicular head of the SCM, and the anterior scalene muscle is divided to expose a more distal segment of the subclavian artery. Phrenic nerve injuries are more likely with this more lateral exposure, and extra care must be taken to identify the nerve. Our conduit of choice is prosthetic polytetrafluoroethylene or Dacron, which in our experience has demonstrated improved long-term patency over saphenous vein. The graft is tunneled posterior to the internal jugular vein, and both anastomoses are performed using running Prolene suture in an end-to-side fashion. The proximal end of the graft should be beveled 20 to 30 degrees to promote a slightly downward course to the graft.

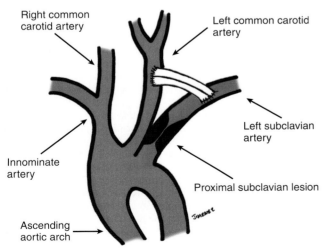

FIGURE 7   Carotid-subclavian bypass.

AbuRahma reviewed the results of 51 patients who underwent carotid-subclavian bypass over a 20-year period for symptomatic subclavian artery occlusive disease. Immediate relief of symptoms was achieved in 100% of patients, and 8% developed late recurrent symptoms. Primary patency rates at 1 and 10 years was 100% and 92%, respectively. Symptom-free survival rates at 1, 3, and 5 years were 100%, 96%, and 82%, respectively, and no perioperative strokes or deaths occurred.

Surgical Exposure of the Axillary Artery

Atherosclerotic lesions of the axillary artery are rare, and symptomatic occlusive disease is most commonly due to emboli and trauma. The axillary artery is traditionally categorized into three segments: the first portion extends from the lateral border of the first rib to the pectoralis minor muscle; the second is located behind the pectoralis minor muscle; and the third extends from the lateral border of the pectoralis minor muscle to the teres major. The first and second portions of the axillary artery are exposed optimally with the arm outstretched on an arm board. An infraclavicular incision is made 2 cm from the lateral clavicular border to the deltopectoral groove, the fibers of the pectoralis major muscle are split, and the underlying clavipectoral fascia is incised. The head of the pectoralis minor muscle may be divided for better exposure of the second portion of the axillary artery; the axillary vein lies inferior and slightly anterior to the artery, and several branches may require division for optimal exposure of the artery. Care should be taken to avoid injury to the lateral pectoral nerves, which may lead to postoperative atrophy of the pectoralis muscles.

Surgical Revascularization of the Axillary Artery

Surgical revascularization of the axillary artery is rare. Harris and colleagues reviewed the results of 30 upper extremity bypass procedures over a 10 year period. During this same period, over 2000 infrainguinal bypass procedures were performed. Most reports of surgical bypass across the shoulder joint for symptomatic occlusive disease of the axillary artery consist of retrospective series with limited patient numbers.

Contrary to findings described for carotid-subclavian bypass, saphenous vein has demonstrated improved long-term patency over prosthetic grafts for revascularization procedures distal to the subclavian artery and particularly in this location. The superior patency of autogenous vein for these upper extremity bypass procedures may be due to the longer lengths of graft required in this location. Vein grafts are usually tunneled anatomically. The distal anastomosis should be performed to the most proximal patent artery in direct continuity with the hand, because shorter autogenous grafts have higher patencies.

Carotid-axillary, carotid-brachial, subclavian-brachial, and axillobrachial bypasses have all been described with low patient morbidity and excellent long-term patency using autogenous vein grafts. Jain and colleagues performed 13 bypass procedures to the brachial artery over a 10-year period. Donor arteries were axillary (n = 7), carotid (n = 4), and subclavian (n = 2). Life table analysis demonstrated 100% patency at 3 years and 88% at 7 years. No neurologic complications and no perioperative deaths were noted. Mesh and colleagues performed 74 upper extremity arterial bypass procedures over a 15-year period. Autogenous conduits were superior at all sites compared with prostheses (70.9% vs. 37.7%), and the overall patency rate was 61.2% at 5 years. All distal forearm prosthetic bypasses failed within 1 year.

Surgical Exposure of the Brachial Artery

Similar to the axillary artery, symptomatic atherosclerotic lesions of the brachial artery are uncommon. Embolism and trauma account for the majority of lesions requiring revascularization for symptomatic ischemia. Optimal arm position is 90 degrees abduction on an arm board attached to the operating table. A longitudinal incision is made between the biceps and triceps muscle in the medial arm along the bicipital groove. Dissection through the subcutaneous tissues and the deep fascia of the biceps brachii muscle is performed. The basilic vein is usually found traveling medial to the brachial sheath, and the median nerve usually lies adjacent the artery during the surgical approach, in a more superficial location, and should be preserved. Paired brachial veins are frequently encountered surrounding the brachial artery. They may be divided to allow sufficient mobilization of the brachial artery for surgical revascularization. Alternatively, the distal brachial artery and its bifurcation into the radial and ulnar arteries can be exposed by making a longitudinal incision in the antecubital fossa just distal to the elbow crease and dividing the bicipital aponeurosis. If more exposure is required, a standard "lazy S" incision across the elbow crease will prevent scar contracture.

Surgical Revascularization of the Brachial Artery

For bypass procedures, a segment of proximal, disease-free artery and the most proximal portion of the distal artery continuous with the hand should be mobilized through two different longitudinal incisions. Duplex ultrasound can be used to precisely identify those segments in the operating room. Autogenous vein is the conduit of choice for surgical bypass at this level.

Following traumatic injury, mobilization of the brachial artery should be performed to expose uninjured proximal and distal segments. If the extent of injured brachial artery is relatively short, as frequently happens with cardiac catheterization injuries, adequate mobilization may allow for excision of the lesion and for a primary, tension-free anastomosis. Reversed interposition saphenous vein grafts harvested from the ankle are frequently useful for brachial artery reconstruction because of the comparable size match. Prosthetic material should be avoided in contaminated trauma cases because of a higher graft infection risk and lower patency. Penetrating injuries to the brachial artery are frequently associated with median nerve injuries because of their close proximity, and care must be taken to perform a detailed sensory and motor examination before and after revascularization.

Roddy and colleagues reviewed the results of 51 bypass grafts used for brachial artery reconstruction over a 12 year period. Life table analysis revealed a patency of 90.5% for all bypass grafts at 1 year, and limb salvage was 100%. Late occlusion was associated with PTFE bypass grafts across the shoulder. Although patency rates between PTFE grafts and autogenous vein were not statistically significant, a trend toward increased patency (90% vs. 70%) was seen with vein bypass grafts. Bypass grafts across joints had worse patency than those that did not.

Hughes and colleagues reported the results of 20 patients who underwent upper extremity bypass for brachial artery lesions over a 13 year period. Patency at 1 and 3 years was 85%. Autogenous vein was used in 90% of the bypasses. Mean survival after bypass was 62 months, and the limb-salvage rate was 100%. No perioperative deaths were noted. Thus the surgical literature supports the use of upper extremity bypass for lesions of the brachial artery, with acceptable morbidity and patency rates.

Surgical Exposure of the Radial and Ulnar Arteries

Exposure of the radial artery at the mid-forearm is best achieved with a longitudinal incision following a line from the antecubital crease to the styloid process of the radius. The fascia is dissected along the medial border of the brachioradialis muscle. In the proximal forearm, the radial artery lies beneath the medial fibers of the brachioradialis muscle. In the distal forearm, the radial artery lies deep to the antebrachial fascia between the tendons of brachioradialis and the flexor

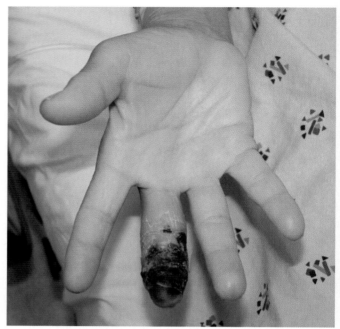

FIGURE 8   Patient with interval development of digital gangrene following placement of upper extremity AV graft.

carpi radialis muscles. At the wrist, the radial artery is exposed by incising the antebrachial fascia just medial to the radius.

The ulnar artery in the proximal forearm may be exposed by dissecting through a plane between the flexor carpi ulnaris and flexor digitorum superficialis. In the middle third of the forearm, the artery lies deep to the flexor carpi ulnaris muscle adjacent to the ulnar nerve. In the distal forearm, dissection through the antebrachial fascia exposes the ulnar artery just beneath the antebrachial fascia.

Bypass to the forearm arteries is rarely necessary and is most often used for trauma and neglected embolic occlusions. Sympathectomy, both cervicothoracic and digital, can lead to temporary improvement in skin blood flow, but its poor durability has limited it to highly selected patients who cannot be revascularized.

Angioaccess-Induced Steal Syndrome

Hand ischemia following creation of arteriovenous access is a rare but potentially debilitating condition (Figure 8). Patients with diabetes mellitus and renal failure frequently develop atherosclerotic narrowing in the medium and small arteries of the forearm and hand and are particularly susceptible to ischemia, when flow is diverted through a proximal arteriovenous (AV) fistula or graft. The most common symptoms include pain and paresthesias. Motor weakness, digital ulceration, and gangrene are signs of more advanced ischemia.

Ligation of the AV access causing *ischemia steal* is indicated for some symptomatic patients. Banding, plication, application of luminal clips, and partial suturing have all been described as techniques to improve distal perfusion, but they have high thrombosis and failure rates. In patients with limited sites for new hemodialysis access placement, *distal revascularization and interval ligation* (DRIL) can be performed (Figure 9). The procedure involves placement of a bypass conduit, preferably saphenous vein, around the AV access from the proximal brachial artery to either the distal brachial, radial, or ulnar arteries. The proximal anastomosis must be placed at least 5 cm proximal to the AV fistula or graft, and the native artery is then ligated immediately proximal to the distal anastomosis of the bypass conduit.

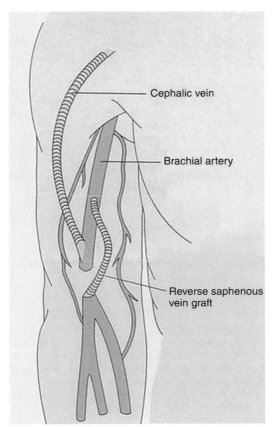

FIGURE 9   Diagram of the DRIL procedure. *(Modified from Knox R, Berman S, Hughes J, et al: Distal revascularization-interval ligation: a durable and effective treatment for ischemic steal syndrome after hemodialysis access, J Vasc Surg 36[2]:250–256, 2002.)*

Several authors have reported good results with this procedure. Berman and colleagues performed 21 DRIL procedures for symptomatic ischemia. Limb salvage and maintenance of a functional fistula were achieved in 100% and 94% of patients respectively at 18 months. Huber and colleagues performed 64 DRIL procedures.

Primary patencies were 77%, 74%, and 71% at 1, 3, and 5 years, respectively. The procedure relieved symptoms in 78% of patients; however, perioperative mortality was 3% and the complication rate was 22%.

SUMMARY

Symptomatic upper extremity ischemia due to occlusive disease remains an uncommon but potentially debilitating and lifestyle-altering condition when left untreated. Optimal medical management should be ensured prior to revascularization, especially in patients with systemic disorders. Improved endovascular techniques have limited the role of surgical bypass to patients who have failed percutaneous revascularization or those who demonstrate longer, more complex occlusive lesions. Excellent long-term patency can be achieved with surgical revascularization in these patients. Patients requiring AV access for renal failure are at risk for development of symptomatic ischemia steal. DRIL may be used to preserve the AV access site and improve distal perfusion.

SUGGESTED READINGS

AbuRahma AF, Robinson PA, Jennings TG: Carotid-subclavian bypass grafting with polytetrafluoroethylene grafts for symptomatic subclavian artery stenosis of occlusion, *J Vasc Surg* 32:411–418, 2000.

Berman SS, Gentile AT, Glickman MH, et al: Distal revascularization-interval ligation for limb salvage and maintenance of dialysis access in ischemia steal syndrome, *J Vasc Surg* 26:393–404, 1997.

Chloros GD, Smerlis NN, Li Z, et al: Noninvasive evaluation of upper extremity vascular perfusion, *J Hand Surg* 33A:591–600, 2008.

Huber TS, Brown MP, Seeger JS, et al: Midterm outcome after the distal revascularization and interval ligation (DRIL) procedure, *J Vasc Surg* 48:926–933, 2008.

Hughes K, Hamdan A, Schermerhorn M, et al: Bypass for chronic ischemia of the upper extremity: results in 20 patients, *J Vasc Surg* 46:303–307, 2007.

Jain KM, Simoni EJ, Munn JS, et al: Long-term follow up of bypasses to the brachial artery across the shoulder joint, *Am J Surg* 172:127–129, 1996.

Mesh CL, McCarthy WJ, Pearce WH, et al: Upper extremity bypass grafting: a 15 year experience, *Arch Surg* 128:795–802, 1993.

Roddy SP, Darling C III, Chang BB, et al: Brachial artery reconstruction for occlusive disease: a 12 year experience, *J Vasc Surg* 33:802–805, 2001.

AORTOILIAC OCCLUSIVE DISEASE

Christopher J. Abularrage, MD, and Mark F. Conrad, MD

DIAGNOSIS

Peripheral arterial disease (PAD) is part of a broad spectrum of atherosclerotic cardiovascular disease that affects multiple vascular beds including the coronary, cerebrovascular, visceral, aortoiliac, and infrainguinal circulations. Aortoiliac occlusive disease (AIOD) can be divided into three types (Figure 1): type I disease is confined to the infrarenal aorta and proximal common iliac arteries and is more common in young smokers and female patients; type II disease is similar

to type I but has more diffuse disease of the iliac arteries; and type III disease is AIOD in conjunction with infrainguinal occlusive disease or multilevel disease. Single-level AIOD in its early stages (type I disease) typically presents with calf claudication and the symptoms of Leriche syndrome—buttock claudication, impotence, and diminished or absent femoral pulses—may manifest in its advanced stages (type II disease). Approximately 13% to 42% of patients with AIOD will progress to multilevel (type III) disease, which can be seen anywhere along the spectrum of intermittent claudication to rest pain to tissue loss.

With the advent of endovascular surgical techniques, the options for aortoiliac reconstruction have become numerous. Selection of the most appropriate method of revascularization depends on the extent of occlusive disease and the patient's surgical risk. Evaluation of the patient begins with a thorough history and physical exam. The history should include a detailed assessment of coronary risk factors, including previous coronary events and functional status, to determine the need for further coronary evaluation. On physical exam, patients typically have diminished or absent femoral pulses and, consequently, diminished or absent distal pulses. Signs of impaired lower

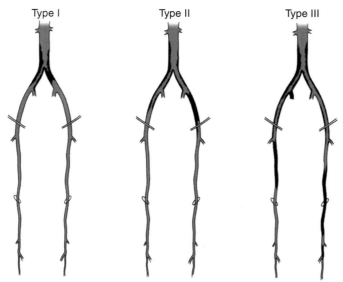

FIGURE 1 Patterns of aortoiliac occlusive disease. Type I is confined to the aortoiliac and common iliac arteries, type II is more extensive abdominal disease, and type III is multilevel disease. *(From Brewster DB: Direct reconstruction for aortoiliac occlusive disease. In Rutherford RB [ed]: Vascular surgery, ed 6. Philadelphia, 2005, Elsevier, p.1106.)*

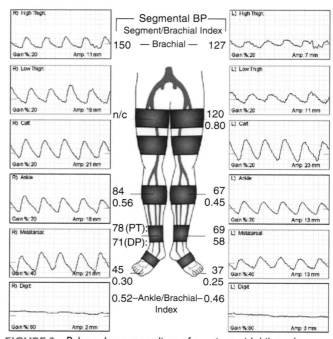

FIGURE 2 Pulse volume recordings of a patient with bilateral aortoiliac occlusive disease. Note the lack of augmentation from the brachial to the left high-thigh pressure as well as blunting of the bilateral high-thigh waveforms. Also note the pressure difference between the right and left brachial arteries, likely signifying left subclavian stenosis.

extremity perfusion include coolness, pallor, dependent rubor, and loss of pretibial skin turgor and hair.

Noninvasive laboratory evaluation is imperative to confirm the diagnosis, define the location and extent of disease, and provide a baseline for assessing revascularization results. This can include ankle-brachial indexes (ABIs), segmental pressures, and pulse volume recordings (Figure 2). Exercise testing can supplement the evaluation and elicit subtle but hemodynamically significant disease.

Further anatomic delineation of disease can be accomplished with Duplex ultrasound and either CT angiography (CTA) or MR angiography (MRA). Duplex ultrasound can interrogate specific lesions of the arterial tree, defining occlusions with B-mode and color mapping and defining stenoses based on velocity changes; however, this modality is often limited in the aortoiliac segment by overlying bowel gas and operator experience. High-resolution CTA has supplanted traditional angiography for diagnostic evaluation of AIOD, and it can be performed with a minimal amount of intravenous contrast to provide detailed anatomic pathology sufficient for both open and endovascular operative planning (Figure 3). MRA may be useful in patients with chronic renal insufficiency, in whom the risks of an intravenous dye load are significant. Non–gadolinium-enhanced MRA is limited by overestimation of the degree of stenosis. Digital subtraction angiography (DSA), the gold standard for assessing anatomic disease, is most frequently performed as part of a planned endovascular intervention.

MEDICAL THERAPY

The first line of treatment for patients with claudication should be medical therapy, which has three goals: 1) decrease the risk of cardiovascular morbidity and mortality, 2) improve symptoms, and 3) prevent limb loss. The guidelines for risk-factor modification are summarized in Table 1. Although not directly shown to improve PAD, strict control of hypertension and diabetes mellitus with intensive therapies decreases the risk of cardiovascular events. Treatment of hypercholesterolemia with 3-hydroxy-3-methylglutaryl coenzyme A reductase inhibitors and statins has been associated with stabilization and regression of PAD symptoms and angiographic lesions. The addition of niacin has been shown to increase high-density lipoprotein (HDL) levels and

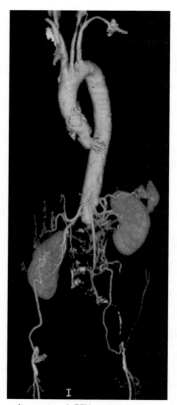

FIGURE 3 Three-dimensional CTA reconstruction demonstrating infrarenal aortic occlusion with reconstitution of the bilateral common femoral arteries.

TABLE 1: American College of Cardiology/ American Heart Association guidelines for the management of patients with peripheral arterial disease

Parameter	Target Goal	Therapy
Blood pressure	Systolic <130 to 140 mm Hg Diastolic <80 to 90 mm Hg	β-Blockers, ACE inhibitors
Diabetes mellitus	Hemoglobin A1c <7%	Insulin, ↑ insulin sensitivity
LDL cholesterol	<100 mg/dL	Diet, statins
HDL cholesterol	Men, ≥35 mg/dL Women, ≥45 mg/dL	Diet, fibric acid derivative
Tobacco cessation	Complete abstinence	Nicotine replacement, antidepressants, behavioral therapy
Exercise therapy	All patients	Supervised program three or more times a week
Antiplatelet therapy	All patients	Aspirin (81 or 325 mg/day), clopidogrel (75 mg/day)
Pharmacologic therapy	Trial in all patients with claudication in the absence of heart failure	Cilostazol

ACE, Angiotensin-converting enzyme; *LDL,* low-density lipoprotein; *HDL,* high-density lipoprotein.
From Hirsch AT, Haskal ZJ, Hertzer NR, et al: ACC/AHA guidelines for the management of patients with peripheral arterial disease: summary of recommendations, *J Vasc Interv Radiol* 17(9):1383–1397, 2006.

decrease triglyceride levels. Finally, smoking cessation is an integral part of medical therapy, as it has been shown to not only prevent progression of disease, it also improves symptoms in certain cases.

Exercise regimens have long been at the center of medical therapy for claudication, resulting in improvement in walking distance, quality of life, and community-based functional capacity. The mechanisms by which exercise regimens improve symptoms of PAD are unclear, but they are thought to be related to enzyme induction and adaptation of muscle cells to the low levels of oxygen delivery in ischemic conditions (i.e., tolerance). The type of exercise regimen utilized, whether supervised or unsupervised at-home exercises recommended by a physician, does not seem to make a difference, although supervised regimens may have slightly better results because of improved patient compliance.

Antiplatelet therapy has not been shown to improve symptoms of PAD directly, and it is associated with a decreased risk of cardiovascular events. In the Physicians' Health Study, aspirin was associated with a 54% risk reduction in the need for peripheral arterial surgery compared with placebo. Thus, aspirin is recommended for all patients with PAD. Clopidogrel was associated with an 8.7% to 24% risk reduction in cardiovascular events in the CAPRIE (Clopidogrel versus Aspirin in Patients at Risk of Ischemic Events) trial, and it is considered an effective alternative to aspirin in patients with PAD. Treatment with oral anticoagulation, such as warfarin, has not been shown to improve symptoms related to PAD, nor does it alter the risk of adverse cardiovascular events.

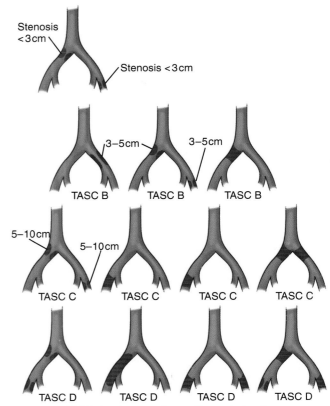

FIGURE 4   TASC classification of aortoiliac occlusive disease.

Cilostazol is a phosphodiesterase inhibitor that induces vasodilation through smooth muscle cell relaxation, inhibition of platelet aggregation, and improvement in lipid profiles. Cilostazol was superior to both pentoxifylline and placebo in a randomized controlled trial and is therefore indicated as a therapy for intermittent claudication. Absolute walking distance has been shown to improve by approximately 50% in patients taking cilostazol, however, in practice this may delay the onset of symptoms from 50 yards to 100 yards, which is often not sufficient to improve patient lifestyle. Pentoxifylline, a rheologic agent that decreases blood viscosity and platelet aggregation, may be used as a second-line, alternative therapy to cilostazol, but its clinical effectiveness has not been established.

INDICATIONS FOR TREATMENT AND LESION CLASSIFICATION

Although many patients with AIOD are asymptomatic, patients with lifestyle limiting claudication, rest pain, and tissue loss are candidates for either endovascular or open surgical revascularization. Less common indications include atheroembolism, inflow procedure for infrainguinal graft preservation, and access for coronary interventions.

Aortobifemoral bypass is considered the gold standard surgical therapy for patients with AIOD. With the advent of newer endovascular techniques, the line between open surgical and endovascular appropriate lesions has become blurred by patient risk factors, procedure durability, and life expectancy. In 2000 and again in 2007, the TransAtlantic Inter-Society Consensus (TASC) stratified AIOD lesions based on anatomic morphology in an effort to define which lesions do better with endovascular versus open surgical therapy (Figure 4, Table 2). Type A lesions are short and focal, and type D lesions represent more extensive, diffuse disease of the aortoiliac

TABLE 2: TASC morphologic stratification of aortoiliac occlusive disease

Class	Definition	Endovascular Revascularization 3-Year Primary Patency, Secondary Patency, Limb-Salvage Rates	Recommendation
Overall	—	76%, 90%, 97%	—
TASC A	Unilateral or bilateral stenoses of CIA Unilateral or bilateral single, short (≤3 cm) stenosis of EIA	>80%, >90%, >95%	Endovascular revascular-ization
TASC B	Short (≤3 cm) stenosis of infrarenal aorta Unilateral CIA occlusion Single or multiple stenosis totaling 3 to 10 cm long involving the EIA, not extending into the CFA Unilateral EIA occlusion not involving the origins of the internal iliac or CFA	78%, 95%, 100%	Endovascular revascular-ization
TASC C	Bilateral CIA occlusions Bilateral EIA stenoses 3 to 10 cm long, not extending into the CFA Unilateral EIA stenosis extending into the CFA[†] Unilateral EIA occlusion that involves the origins of the internal iliac and/or CFA[†] Heavily calcified unilateral EIA occlusion with or without involve-ment of the origins of the internal iliac and/or CFA[†]	73%, 93%, 97%	Endovascular or surgical revascularization
TASC D	Infrarenal aortic occlusion* Diffuse disease involving the aorta and both iliac arteries requiring treatment Diffuse multiple stenoses involving the unilateral CIA, EIA, and CFA[†] Unilateral occlusion of both the CIA and EIA Bilateral EIA occlusion Iliac stenoses in conjunction with AAA requiring treatment and not amenable to endograft placement or other lesion requiring open aortic or iliac surgery*	80%, 83%, 95%	Surgical revasculariza-tion, except in patients with prohibitive risk

*Endovascular treatment is not intended for these lesion types.
[†]Lesions involving CFA with severe stenosis are excluded in these lesion types.
CIA, Common iliac artery; *EIA*, external iliac artery; *CFA*, common femoral artery; *AAA*, abdominal aortic aneurysm

segment. Endovascular intervention was recommended for type A lesions, but most type D lesions are better managed with open repair.

The TASC committee suggested that type B lesions might be best treated with endovascular therapy and type C lesions by open surgi-cal therapy, but that more evidence was necessary to determine the best overall modality. Since that time, multiple studies have compared outcomes for TASC type B and C lesions treated by both endovas-cular and open surgical techniques. Independent predictors of poor outcomes of endovascularly treated type B and C lesions include poor infrainguinal runoff, external iliac artery disease, female gender, and chronic renal insufficiency.

Furthermore, technological advances and a better understand-ing of catheter-based techniques have led vascular surgeons and interventionalists to begin treating type D lesions with endovascular therapies (Figure 5). A recent study found that although primary patency of endovascular revascularization was less than that of open surgical revascularization, secondary patency, limb salvage, and long-term survival were similar between the two. Diabetes mellitus and the requirement of distal bypass were associated with decreased patency.

Based on the TASC recommendations and the results of these studies, the determination of endovascular versus open surgical

therapy for AIOD should be patient specific, with an understanding that endovascular therapies fare worse with increasing severity based on the TASC classification.

ENDOVASCULAR THERAPY

Diagnostic Angiography

Endovascular therapy for AIOD has become the first-line method of revascularization in our practice. DSA is a necessary component of endovascular revascularization, as it precisely delineates disease and allows for the assessment of lesion hemodynamic significance. How-ever, this is usually performed at the time of intervention, and it is common for patients to undergo preprocedure CTA or MRA to plan intervention and evaluate access vessels. With preprocedure knowl-edge of a long-segment iliac occlusion, the typical ipsilateral femoral retrograde access may not be ideal, and a contralateral femoral retro-grade or brachial retrograde access could be used.

We generally start with a bright-tipped 5 Fr sheath to obtain our initial angiographic images via a 5 Fr flush catheter in the aorta. The aortic bifurcation and common iliac arteries are best imaged in the anteroposterior views, and the origins of the hypogastric arteries

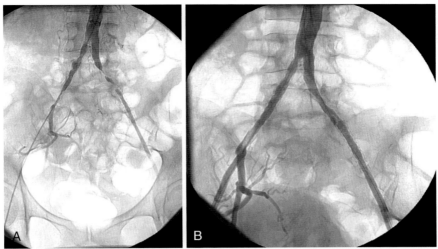

FIGURE 5   DSA demonstrating TASC type D aortoiliac occlusive disease. **A,** Before endovascular revascularization. **B,** After endovascular revascularization. This patient was deemed high risk for open surgical therapy.

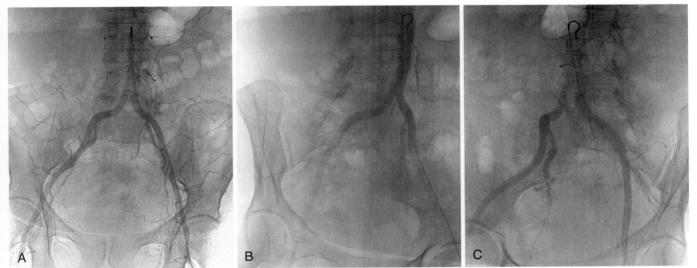

FIGURE 6   Views of the pelvis, demonstrating the ability of the oblique view to accurately identify the origin of the contralateral hypogastric artery. **A,** Anteroposterior view. **B,** Right anterior oblique view. **C,** Left anterior oblique view.

can be seen with the image intensifier in the opposite, oblique position. These oblique views prevent overlap of the contrast in the hypogastric and external iliac arteries, thus "opening" the contralateral iliac bifurcations and allowing accurate assessment of disease (Figure 6).

A 50% to 60% reduction in the transluminal diameter represents a hemodynamically significant lesion. If it is unclear on DSA alone, intravascular ultrasound and translesional pressure gradients can be measured. A gradient can be determined by comparing the pressure in the aorta above the lesion to that in the external iliac artery below the lesion, which necessitates the use of a catheter that is 1 Fr smaller than your sheath. A "pullback" gradient over a wire can also be performed, in which the pressure is documented on each end of the lesion by pulling the catheter across the lesion over the wire, thus not losing access. A resting gradient of 5 mm Hg can be hemodynamically significant, and activity can be simulated by injecting 200 mg of nitroglycerine or 30 mg of papaverine intraarterially, with a difference of 15 mm Hg considered hemodynamically significant. These vasodilators cause a pressure drop distal to a hemodynamically significant lesion because of the inability of the lesion itself to dilate.

Iliac Angioplasty and Stenting

Once the decision has been made to perform an endovascular revascularization, patients are therapeutically heparinized with a goal activated clotting time (ACT) of 200 to 250 seconds. We often cross lesions with a hydrophilic wire, but we will exchange that for a platinum-tipped wire for interventions, to avoid injury to other vessels outside of the field of view. Most lesions of the aortoiliac segment are highly calcified, so we routinely predilate with an undersized balloon, which facilitates the passage of stents and allows the operator to determine the appropriate stent size. The decision of when to stent is based upon lesion location and severity.

Aortic Bifurcation/Common Iliac Angioplasty and Stenting

Lesions of the aortic bifurcation characterize a special entity in the endovascular management of AIOD. These lesions typically represent spillover of atherosclerotic disease from the aorta into both common

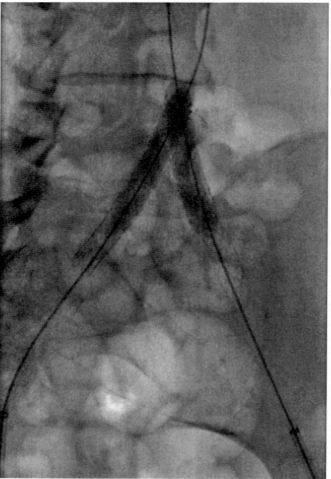

FIGURE 7 "Kissing balloon" angioplasty of the bilateral common iliac arteries performed to prevent contralateral plaque dissection.

iliac arteries. In this circumstance, simultaneous angioplasty is performed with a "kissing balloon" technique, in which the balloons are placed in parallel into the terminal aorta. This prevents shifting of the plaque to the contralateral iliac artery (Figure 7). These lesions are usually stented in a "kissing" manner as well. Because of the typically heavy calcification of these lesions, balloon-expandable stents are preferred over self-expanding stents (Figure 8).

More recently, balloon-expandable covered stents have been utilized in the common iliac arteries with good results. In one study, covered stents had improved 5-year primary patency compared with bare stents (87% vs. 53%, respectively). When deploying covered stents, care must be taken to avoid covering the origin of the hypogastric artery or any significant collateral vessels.

External Iliac Angioplasty and Stenting

The external iliac arteries can be treated with a primary stenting or selective stenting method. Some studies have shown that primary stenting improves outcome in patients with TASC type C and D lesions. We recommend selective stenting for TASC type A and B lesions based on the results of the initial angioplasty. The external iliac artery is highly mobile in the pelvis, therefore self-expanding stents are generally used in this artery.

Hypogastric Angioplasty and Stenting

Hypogastric endovascular revascularization is rarely performed but may be indicated in patients with severe buttock claudication, impotence, or as an inflow procedure in cases of bilateral diseased external iliac arteries. These lesions are typically found at the origin of the hypogastric arteries. The procedure can be performed from contralateral femoral or brachial access. Ipsilateral femoral access is possible but more challenging because of the sharp angle between the external iliac and hypogastric arteries. The hypogastric lesions are crossed with a wire, and a "buddy" wire is placed across the external iliac artery in case of plaque shift or dissection (Figure 9). Angioplasty is then performed as above. This is a fragile artery, and we avoid oversizing of the balloon to prevent injury. The hypogastric arteries are

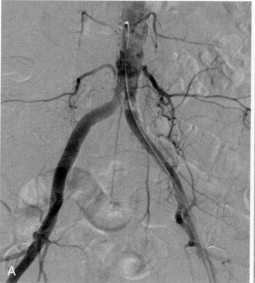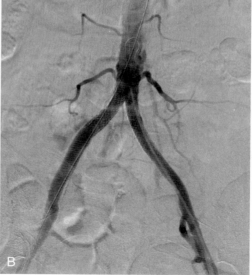

FIGURE 8 **A,** Aortoiliac angiography of a patient with bilateral common iliac disease. **B,** Completion angiogram after balloon-expandable "kissing" stents were placed for heavy calcific disease.

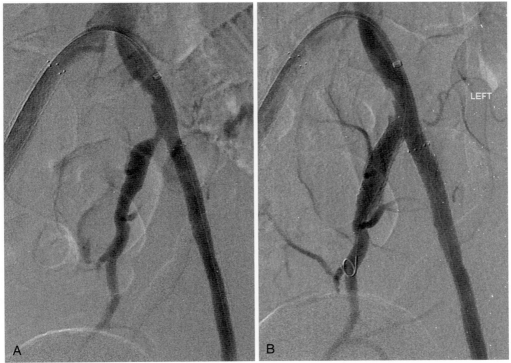

FIGURE 9   Endovascular revascularization of the left hypogastric artery. **A,** Before the procedure. **B,** After the procedure. Note the use of buddy wires to protect the external iliac artery during angioplasty.

also typically calcified, and we now stent these lesions, as angioplasty alone has been associated with poor patency.

Infrarenal Aortic Stenosis Angioplasty and Stenting

Atherosclerotic disease isolated to the infrarenal aorta is less common than disease involving the iliac arteries, and it is seen mostly in women who are heavy smokers. The traditional therapy for these lesions has been open surgical revascularization because of its excellent long-term results. Aortic angioplasty alone has been associated with excellent immediate success but poor long-term patency. More recently, primary stenting of infrarenal aortic stenoses has been performed with immediate technical success rates of 90% to 100% and 5 year primary and assisted patency rates of up to 77% and 83%, respectively. In theory, primary stenting may be associated with a decreased risk of distal plaque embolization.

The technique of aortic angioplasty and stenting is similar to that in the iliac system. Both self-expanding nitinol stents and balloon-expandable stents may be used, although balloon-expandable stents are favored for heavily calcified lesions. The limitation of using stents designed for peripheral use is that they are often too small to effectively treat the aorta. Giant Palmaz stents can be mounted on an angioplasty balloon and dilated to profile after placement. Finally, covered stents may be used in lesions that are thought to be at high risk for rupture after angioplasty, such as concentric, heavily calcified lesions in a small aorta, although the efficacy has not been proven.

Concomitant Femoral Disease

If a lesion in the external iliac artery extends into the common femoral artery, or if concomitant occlusive disease of the femoral arteries exists, this can be approached with a hybrid procedure consisting of an open common femoral endarterectomy or iliofemoral bypass followed by endovascular treatment at the same setting. These

procedures are associated with improved results compared with angioplasty alone. Furthermore, stents should not be placed across the inguinal ligament because placement across areas of increased flexion is associated with a high incidence of fracture and failure.

Complications of Aortoiliac Angioplasty and Stenting

The most common complications associated with endovascular therapy of AIOD include access-site issues, contrast nephropathy, and cardiopulmonary events. In most series, the overall incidence of any complication is less than 5%. Access-site complications such as thromboembolism, atheroembolization, dissection, pseudoaneurysm, bleeding, and arteriovenous fistula are the most common, and they occur in 1% to 2% of the population. Contrast nephropathy occurs in 1% of patients, and it can be minimized with preprocedure and postprocedure intravenous hydration as well as oral *N*-acetylcysteine. Periprocedure hydration with sodium bicarbonate (150 mEq/L normal saline) may also help prevent contrast nephropathy in patients with underlying renal insufficiency. Finally, cardiopulmonary complications occur less than 1% of the time and are less frequent than after open surgical therapy.

In-stent restenosis or recurrent disease at an angioplasty site occurs in approximately 25% of patients within 2 years. Therefore it is imperative that patients who undergo aortoiliac endovascular revascularization have some type of postprocedure surveillance. This is usually accomplished with noninvasive studies, such as rest and exercise pulse volume recordings, ankle brachial indices, or duplex ultrasonography.

SURGICAL THERAPY

Surgical therapy has long been the gold standard treatment of AIOD. Long-term patency of surgical revascularization is excellent with 5-year patency rates of aortobifemoral bypass exceeding 85% (Table 3).

TABLE 3: Patency and complication rates for surgical revascularization of aortoiliac occlusive disease

Bypass Type	5-Year Patency	Complication Rate	Mortality Rate
Aortobifemoral bypass	85%–90%	5%–8%	2%–5%
Axillobifemoral bypass	50%–80%	5%–15%	5%–10%
Femorofemoral bypass	70%–80%	5%	0%–5%
Iliofemoral bypass	80%–85%	—	0%–5%

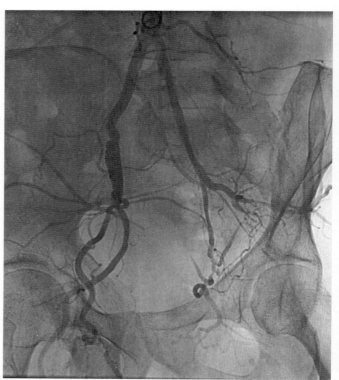

FIGURE 10   Preoperative angiography, via brachial access, of a patient with bilateral external iliac artery occlusions who underwent aortobifemoral bypass for aortoiliac occlusive disease. Delayed images demonstrate reconstitution of the common femoral arteries.

Surgical therapy is, however, associated with an increased risk of cardiopulmonary complications compared to endovascular therapy. Therefore surgical therapy is recommended in patients with appropriate anatomy and adequate surgical risk. Anatomic pathology best treated with open surgical revascularization comprises most TASC type C and D lesions, including flush aortic occlusions at the level of the renal artery, diffusely diseased vessels of diminutive caliber, and severe disease with heavy concentric calcification (Figure 10). Cardiopulmonary risk should be assessed by noninvasive means, including a coronary stress and pulmonary function test. Patients with concomitant coronary disease should have coronary revascularization prior to aortoiliac reconstruction. Patients with prohibitive risk who have failed endovascular intervention should be considered for extraanatomic bypass.

Aortobifemoral Bypass

Aortobifemoral bypass performed for extensive AIOD is associated with 5-year patency of 85% to 90%. Operative complications are seen in 5% to 8% of patients and death in 0% to 2%.

The procedure begins with exposure and control of the femoral arteries to minimize the time the peritoneal cavity is open and thus minimize evaporative fluid and heat loss. Side branches are encircled with vessel loops and preserved. If any significant occlusive disease of the profunda femoris artery is identified on preoperative imaging, division of the profunda vein that typically overlies the anterior surface of the artery and control of the vessel more distally is performed to facilitate profundaplasty at the time of distal anastomosis.

The abdominal aorta can then be exposed via a transabdominal approach through a vertical midline incision. A retroperitoneal approach may be advantageous in obese patients and those with hostile abdomens or previous aortic surgery. The bowel is retracted laterally and caudally, the ligament of Treitz is divided, and the fourth portion of the duodenum is mobilized to expose the left renal vein. In male patients, the retroperitoneal tissue surrounding the aorta from the renal arteries to the distal aorta below the inferior mesenteric artery (IMA) is divided, with care being taken to avoid the autonomic nerves that course along the left anterolateral aspect of the aorta and the proximal left common iliac artery; this is done to reduce the postoperative incidence of sexual dysfunction.

Retroperitoneal tunnels using blunt finger dissection are then created for passage of the graft. It is important to stay just anterior to the iliac vessels to ensure that the graft is placed posterior to the ureters, thus avoiding ureteral obstruction and hydronephrosis. When creating the retrograde tunnel underneath the inguinal ligament, care must be taken to avoid tearing the crossing venous branches anterior

to the external iliac artery; we routinely ligate these venous branches prior to creating the tunnel. Once complete, a blunt-tipped clamp is used to pass Penrose drains from the abdomen to the groins.

A Dacron graft is then chosen based on aortic caliber. Polytetrafluoroethylene or coated Dacron grafts are also available, although no data have shown one being superior to the other in terms of patency. For most patients an end-to-end anastomosis is preferred to decrease the risk of competitive flow through the native system and to reduce perianastomotic turbulence and distal atheroembolization (Figure 11). End-to-end anastomoses are also easier to cover with retroperitoneal tissue at the end of the case, theoretically decreasing the late complication of aortoenteric fistula.

Patients are heparinized, and aortic clamps are placed just distal to the left renal vein and proximal to the IMA. We place the proximal anastomosis as close to the renal arteries as possible to avoid failure secondary to progression of disease. A short-body, long-leg technique is used to avoid kinking of the limbs as they enter the tunnels. Thus the main body of the bifurcated graft is trimmed proximally to 2 to 3 cm (Figure 11). The infrarenal segment of the aorta is resected to the aortic bifurcation to allow the graft to sit low in the retroperitoneum and facilitate coverage to avoid a future aortoenteric fistula. The distal aortic stump is oversewn. Any thrombus or atheromatous debris is removed from the proximal aorta. The body of the graft is tailored to facilitate situating it in the bed of the previously resected aortic segment. This diminishes the take-off angle of the graft, making it easier to cover with retroperitoneal tissue and to reduce limb kinking. The proximal anastomosis is then performed in running fashion. If an aortic thromboendarterectomy has been performed, the proximal anastomosis is performed with interrupted pledgeted mattress sutures.

In cases of external iliac disease or sizable infrarenal accessory renal arteries, the proximal anastomosis should be performed in an end-to-side manner, retaining antegrade pelvic perfusion through the hypogastric arteries (Figure 12). Another advantage of an end-to-side

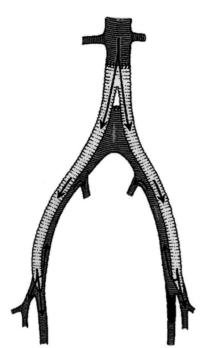

FIGURE 11 Aortobifemoral bypass performed with an end-to-end proximal anastomosis. Note the short body and long legs of the graft, created to avoid kinking of the limbs as they enter the retroperitoneal tunnels. *(From Brewster DB: Direct, open revascularization for aortoiliac occlusive disease. In Zelenock GB, Huber TS, Messina LM, et al [eds]: Mastery of vascular and endovascular surgery, Philadelphia, 2006, Lippincott, Williams, & Wilkins, p 260.)*

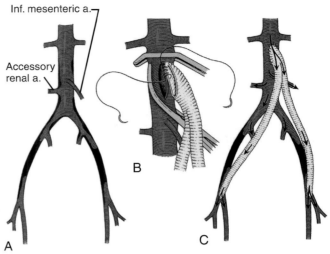

FIGURE 12 **A,** Aortoiliac occlusive diease with bilateral external iliac artery occlusion. **B,** A longitudinal arteriotomy is made in a segment of the proximal infrarenal aorta, and a running suture is used for the beveled body of the bifurcated graft. **C,** Complete end-to-side aortobifemoral bypass preserving flow to the accessory renal, inferior mesenteric, and hypogastric arteries. *(From Brewster DB: Direct, open revascularization for aortoiliac occlusive disease. In Zelenock GB, Huber TS, Messina LM, et al [eds]: Mastery of vascular and endovascular surgery, Philadelphia, 2006, Lippincott Williams & Wilkins, p 361.)*

anastomosis is that aortic flow returns to baseline should the graft occlude, thus reducing the risk of impotence, colonic ischemia, and paraplegia. The aorta may be clamped with a side-biting clamp or cross clamp. A small segment of the anterior aortic wall is resected to produce a slightly elliptical arteriotomy, and a thromboendarterectomy is performed. The graft is beveled 60 degrees, and the anastomosis is completed in running fashion.

The femoral anastomoses are then performed in standard fashion to the common femoral artery. In the presence of superficial femoral artery or profunda femoris orificial disease, the femoral arteriotomy is carried onto the profunda origin beyond its stenosis. In most circumstances, a profundaplasty can also be performed with interrupted mattress sutures on the long beveled toe of the graft. Carrying the limbs onto the profunda femoris artery also decreases the risk of limb occlusion in the presence of femoral disease progression (Figure 13). Once all anastomoses are complete, and the graft is flushed, the retroperitoneal tissue is reapproximated.

Aortobiliac bypass may be performed in patients with type I AIOD or in those with scarred groins from previous surgeries or infection. This may also be useful in morbidly obese patients, who have an increased risk of groin wound complications.

Finally, cases of juxtarenal aortic occlusion necessitate several important modifications. First, to avoid milking of atheromatous debris superiorly into the renal arteries by the clamp, the infrarenal aorta should not be clamped. Instead, a suprarenal clamp can briefly be placed just inferior to the superior mesenteric artery. Second, just prior to clamping, the renal arteries should be occluded with vessel loops or atraumatic bulldog clamps to prevent atheroembolization. The aortic thrombus is then teased out with an endarterectomy spatula without getting into a deep endarterectomy plane to avoid dissection of the endarterectomy plane into the renal arteries. Lastly, the aortic clamp is repositioned at the infrarenal level, and the remainder of the procedure is performed as above. Total renal ischemic time should be less than 15 minutes.

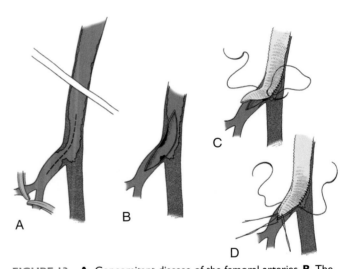

FIGURE 13 **A,** Concomitant disease of the femoral arteries. **B,** The distal arteriotomy is carried from the common femoral artery onto the profunda femoris artery. **C,** The heel of the distal limb of the graft is then sewn onto the common femoral artery. **D,** The toe of the distal limb of the graft is sewn to the profunda femoris artery with three interrupted stitches. *(From Brewster DB: Direct reconstruction for aortoiliac occlusive disease. In Rutherford RB [ed]: Vascular surgery, ed 6, Philadelphia, 2005, Elsevier, p 1117.)*

Aortoiliac Endarterectomy

Although endovascular revascularization has largely supplanted aortoiliac endarterectomy, it may be appropriate in the 5% to 10% of patients who have truly localized type I aortoiliac disease. Advantages of aortoiliac endarterectomy include improved inflow to the hypogastric arteries and minimal infection rate because of the lack of prosthetic material. Disadvantages include poor patency rates in patients with external iliac disease.

Aortoiliac endarterectomy can be performed via the transperitoneal or retroperitoneal approach (Figure 14). Two arteriotomies are performed; one from the infrarenal aorta onto a common iliac artery and the other confined to the contralateral common iliac artery. An endarterectomy plane is then established, and the plaque is removed. The distal points of the endarterectomy should terminate no more than 1 to 2 cm into the external iliac arteries. If necessary, tacking sutures may be placed. Primary closure of the arteriotomy is then performed, although patch closure may be required in smaller vessels. Alternatively, pledgets can be used to support the closure of the thin, endarterectomized aorta.

Complications

The mortality of aortobifemoral bypass should be less than 5%; in several single-center studies, it has been found to be as low as 1%. Complications related to surgical therapy for AIOD include wound, graft, and cardiopulmonary complications. Wound complications such as seroma, hematoma, and infection and graft complications such as infection, thrombosis, and anastomotic pseudoaneurysm can typically be avoided with meticulous operative technique.

Although many of the systemic risks are inherent to the procedures themselves, certain precautions can be taken to minimize the complications. Coronary risk can be assessed preoperatively with noninvasive stress testing. Optimization of cardiac function with pharmacologic therapy, perioperative β-blockade, and careful monitoring of postoperative volume status can reduce cardiac morbidity. Pulmonary complications can be decreased with incentive spirometry and early mobilization, and renal complications can be minimized with hydration, avoidance of hypotension, shorter cross-clamp times, and renal artery protection during manipulation of an occluded infrarenal aorta to avoid atheroembolization.

Pelvic ischemia is a rare complication after revascularization of AIOD, but it can be devastating. Pelvic ischemia manifests as colonic ischemia, buttock infarction, or lumbar plexopathy with neurologic deficit. In patients with early diarrhea, acidosis, or sepsis, immediate flexible sigmoidoscopy should be performed to rule out colonic ischemia and allow for early treatment. Pelvic ischemia can be avoided, for the most part, with end-to-side aortic anastomoses. Alternatively, one or both of the hypogastric arteries can be revascularized.

Distal atheroembolism can occur at any point during vessel manipulation. The degree of morbidity related to this depends on the size of the particles. Macroscopic particles can cause major vessel occlusion, requiring thrombectomy. Microscopic particles are not amenable to surgical therapy and can lead to blue toe syndrome, organ failure, and extensive tissue loss. Atheroembolism can be minimized with the techniques outlined above and with careful flushing of graft limbs prior to anastomosis completion.

NONATHEROSCLEROTIC AORTOILIAC OCCLUSIVE DISEASE

Less common causes of AIOD are frequently seen in younger patients who are nonsmokers. These include hypercoaguable states, fibromuscular dysplasia, mid aortic syndrome, radiation arteritis, and trauma-induced intimal fibrosis. Endovascular and surgical therapy should be performed with an understanding of outcomes in these unique patient populations.

Prospective studies evaluating younger patients with PAD have found an increased incidence of natural anticoagulant deficiencies, defective fibrinolysis, antiphospholipid antibodies, and oxidized low-density lipoprotein. Initial treatment is aimed at control of primary disease with endovascular and surgical therapy reserved for failure of medical therapy.

Mid aortic syndrome occurs through developmental faults during embryogenesis and is characterized by adventitial or periadventitial

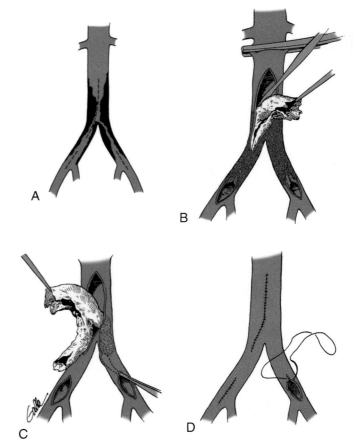

FIGURE 14 **A,** Aortoiliac occlusive disease confined to the aorta and common iliac arteries in a patient who underwent aortoiliac endarterectomy **B,** Arteriotomies are made. **C,** The plaque is removed. **D,** The arteriotomies are closed primarily. *(From Brewster DB: Direct reconstruction for aortoiliac occlusive disease. In Rutherford RB [ed]: Vascular surgery, ed 6, Philadelphia, 2005, Elsevier; p 1114.)*

fibrosis. When seen in association with an inflammatory cell infiltrate, the lesions, which are smooth and tapered, are typically caused by Takayasu arteritis. When confined to the abdominal aorta, treatment entails patch aortoplasty or aortobiiliac bypass. In cases of Takayasu arteritis, surgical therapy should be postponed until the inflammatory component of the disease is controlled. Endovascular therapy has been met with less-favorable results because of recoil of these lesions from excess elastic tissue.

Radiation arteritis may be observed after pelvic radiation for gynecologic, urologic, or rectal malignancies. Lesions are characterized by accelerated atherosclerosis and long-segment fibrosis, and they are better treated with open surgical bypass. In the rare case, a patient with a short stenosis may benefit from endovascular therapy.

Fibromuscular dysplasia typically occurs with serial stenoses and intervening mural aneurysms involving the proximal third of the external iliac artery. It can be treated by both open surgical and endovascular revascularization, although the long-term results of angioplasty are unknown.

Professional and avid cyclists may develop endofibrosis of the external iliac artery from repeated trauma. The mechanism is due to tethering of the iliac artery by the psoas arterial branch, muscle hypertrophy, and fibrous tissue. There are few studies evaluating the long-term results of open and endovascular revascularization, but open iliac artery release seems to provide the most symptomatic relief. Endovascular therapies include traditional balloon angioplasty and cutting balloon angioplasty. Stents should be avoided because of the high risk of stent fracture in these specific cases.

SUMMARY

AIOD may be caused by a wide range of pathologies but is most frequently associated with atherosclerosis. The treatment of AIOD is rapidly evolving, as new tools and techniques are introduced into the vascular surgical armamentarium. Although open surgical revascularization is the gold standard, endovascular revascularization is becoming more common, even for complex TASC type C and D lesions.

Suggested Readings

Chaer RA, Faries PL, Lin S, et al: Successful percutaneous treatment of gluteal claudication secondary to isolated bilateral hypogastric stenoses, *J Vasc Surg* 43(1):165–168, 2006.

Chang RW, Goodney PP, Baek JH, et al: Long-term results of combined common femoral endarterectomy and iliac stenting/stent grafting for occlusive disease, *J Vasc Surg* 48(2):362–367, 2008.

Hirsch AT, Haskal ZJ, Hertzer NR, et al: ACC/AHA guidelines for the management of patients with peripheral arterial disease (lower extremity, renal, mesenteric, and abdominal aortic): a collaborative report from the American Associations for Vascular Surgery/Society for Vascular Surgery, Society for Cardiovascular Angiography and Interventions, Society for Vascular Medicine and Biology, Society of Interventional Radiology, and the ACC/AHA Task Force on Practice Guidelines (writing committee to develop guidelines for the management of patients with peripheral arterial disease)—summary of recommendations, *J Vasc Interv Radiol* 17(9):1383–1397, 2006.

Kashyap VS, Pavkov ML, Bena JF, et al: The management of severe aortoiliac occlusive disease: endovascular therapy rivals open reconstruction, *J Vasc Surg* 48(6):1451–1457, 2008.

Laxdal E, Wirsching J, Jenssen GL, et al: Endovascular treatment of isolated atherosclerotic lesions of the infrarenal aorta is technically feasible with acceptable long-term results, *Eur J Radiol* 61(3):541–544, 2007.

Leville CD, Kashyap VS, Clair DG, et al: Endovascular management of iliac artery occlusions: extending treatment to TransAtlantic Inter-Society Consensus class C and D patients, *J Vasc Surg* 43(1):32–39, 2006.

Levy PJ, Gonzalez MF, Hornung CA, et al: A prospective evaluation of atherosclerotic risk factors and hypercoagulability in young adults with premature lower extremity atherosclerosis, *J Vasc Surg* 23(1):36–43, 1996.

Morse SS, Cambria R, Strauss EB, et al: Transluminal angioplasty of the hypogastric artery for treatment of buttock claudication, *Cardiovasc Intervent Radiol* 9(3):136–138, 1986.

Timaran CH, Prault TL, Stevens SL, et al: Iliac artery stenting versus surgical reconstruction for TASC (TransAtlantic Inter-Society Consensus) type B and type C iliac lesions, *J Vasc Surg* 38(2):272–278, 2003.

Valentine RJ, Kaplan HS, Green R, et al: Lipoprotein (a), homocysteine, and hypercoagulable states in young men with premature peripheral atherosclerosis: a prospective, controlled analysis, *J Vasc Surg* 23(1):53–61, 1996.

FEMOROPOPLITEAL OCCLUSIVE DISEASE

Peter Brant-Zawadzki, MD, and K. Craig Kent, MD

OVERVIEW

Peripheral vascular disease (PVD) is prevalent in the United States, affecting up to 20% of the population. As our population ages, and the incidence of diabetes, hypertension, and hyperlipidemia continue to increase, the frequency of PVD will continue to increase. Femoropopliteal occlusive disease is an anatomical subset of PVD that affects the vasculature between the inguinal ligament and the tibial vessels. The involved vessels are primarily the superficial femoral and popliteal arteries, and the etiology of the stenotic plaque is usually atherosclerosis. Patients with femoropopliteal occlusive disease may have no symptoms, or they may develop limb-threatening ischemia or pain with ambulation (claudication).

The majority of patients with PVD are asymptomatic, and treatment is not required. However, because lower extremity vascular disease is a marker of generalized atherosclerosis, patients found to have PVD are prime candidates for risk-factor modification, such as smoking cessation and exercise and dietary improvements, and/or medical therapy with statins, antiplatelet agents, and antihypertensives. In fact, routine screening for PVD in individuals over age 65 has been recommended by some to identify a target group in whom cardiovascular risk factors should be more aggressively managed.

Symptomatic patients may seek care for various complaints, but these are typically manifestations of either claudication or limb-threatening ischemia. Patients who experience claudication resulting from femoropopliteal disease usually describe calf pain that develops with ambulation and is relieved by rest. These symptoms are often quantified as the maximal distance that an individual can walk before needing to stop (e.g., one-block claudication). Diminished perfusion of the lower extremities must be severe to threaten limb viability. Symptoms and signs of limb threat include rest pain, usually in the forefoot or toes, nonhealing ulceration, or gangrene. Untreated, this disease process ultimately leads to amputation.

EVALUATION

Evaluation should begin with a thorough history. Does the patient have pain with ambulation? Is there pain at rest? Where is the pain? Are ulcers or necrotic tissue present? Particularly for patients with claudication, it should be determined how these symptoms affect the patient's quality of life. A young individual with half-block claudication who is actively employed may require intervention to maintain both employment and a reasonable lifestyle. Alternatively, an elderly patient with three-block claudication may not be sufficiently limited to warrant the risk of intervention. The natural history of claudication is relatively benign, and thus intervention is required only for individuals whose lifestyle or livelihood are impaired. Moreover, before intervention is advised, a trial of smoking cessation, exercise therapy, risk-factor modification, and sometimes medical treatment with cilostazole should be considered.

Limb-threatening ischemia mandates rapid assessment and intervention to relieve rest pain or promote wound healing with the ultimate goal of limb salvage. Physical examination, particularly the pulse exam, is critical in localizing the vascular lesion. The most common location for femoropopliteal occlusive disease is in the distal superficial femoral artery (SFA) as it passes through the adductor (Hunter) canal. The femoral pulse (common femoral artery) is usually easily palpable just below the inguinal ligament, however, popliteal and pedal pulses are either diminished or absent. A thorough examination also identifies the location and extent of nonhealing wounds or necrosis. Patients with severe ischemia will develop pallor upon elevation of the leg as well as rubor when the foot is placed in a dependent position.

Noninvasive vascular laboratory studies are a useful adjunct to history and examination in the evaluation of patients with PVD. Ankle-brachial indexes (ABIs) allow for an inexpensive, noninvasive measurement of the degree of vascular insufficiency. This test involves the creation of a ratio of the blood pressure at the ankle over the blood pressure in the arm. In general, an ABI greater than 0.9 is considered normal, and decreasing values are associated with worsening degrees of vascular insufficiency. An ABI less than 0.5 is often associated with critical limb ischemia. Some patients, usually diabetics, have noncompressible vessels, making it impossible to obtain an accurate ankle blood pressure. These patients can be evaluated with alternative techniques, including toe plethysmography, pulse volume recordings (PVRs), or measurement of transcutaneous oxygen (TcO_2).

Imaging and Disease Classification

Imaging studies should be obtained in patients who require surgery or intervention. Options for imaging include duplex ultrasound (DUS), computed tomographic angiography (CTA), magnetic resonance angiography (MRA), or conventional contrast arteriography. Each study has its own advantages and risks, which can include contrast toxicity and radiation exposure. Contrast arteriography remains the gold standard and has a unique advantage in that diagnosis and therapeutic endovascular intervention can be accomplished in the same setting. However, less invasive tests such as DUS, CTA, or MRA can provide adequate preoperative information for surgical intervention without the need for contrast arteriography. Moreover, these tests can assist in deciding whether to utilize surgery or a catheter-based intervention.

Femoropopliteal lesions are categorized by their location and severity using the TransAtlantic Inter-Society Consensus (TASC) guidelines (Figure 1). Type A lesions are short-segment stenoses or occlusions, and type D lesions are long-segment occlusions. Type B and C lesions are intermediate-complexity stenoses or occlusions. Traditionally, short lesions have been considered amenable to endovascular therapy, but more complex and longer occlusions have been treated with surgical bypass. However, with improvements in technology and skill, some interventionalists are now recommending treatment of long-segment (type D) occlusions involving the entire superficial femoral artery with endovascular therapy.

ENDOVASCULAR MANAGEMENT OF FEMOROPOPLITEAL DISEASE

In the last decade, there has been a tremendous increase in the utilization of endovascular procedures to treat patients with PVD. This has been driven by technological advances, patient demand, and in part by the nature of the patient population treated by vascular specialists. Elderly individuals with substantial comorbid conditions have proven to be an ideal group in which to pursue less invasive endovascular treatments because of their shortened life expectancy and their inability to tolerate the stress of surgical bypass. There is little doubt that endovascular options are generally less durable than open surgical bypass. However, in an elderly cohort of patients who develop PVD, the goal is to maintain the difficult balance between durability of an intervention versus its invasiveness and risk. The long-term patency of a reconstruction is not always the most critical factor. For example, in patients with nonhealing ulcers or necrosis, an angioplasty may need to remain patent only long enough for the wound to heal or for the necrosis to be surgically removed.

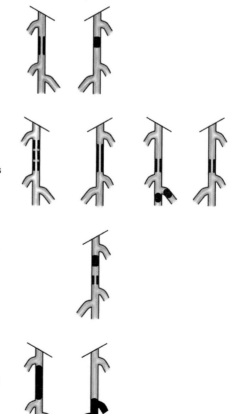

Type A lesions
- Single stenosis ≤10 cm in length
- Single occlusion ≤5 cm in length

Type B lesions
- Multiple lesions (stenoses or occlusions, each ≤5 cm)
- Single stenosis or occlusion ≤15 cm not involving the infrageniculate popliteal artery
- Single or multiple lesions in the absence of continuous tibial vessels to improve inflow for a distal bypass
- Heavily calcified occlusion ≤5 cm in length
- Single popliteal stenosis

Type C lesions
- Multiple stenosis or occlusions totaling >15 cm with or without heavy calcification
- Recurrent stenoses or occlusions that need treatment after two endovascular interventions

Type D lesions
- Chronic total occlusions of CFA or SFA (>20 cm, involving the popliteal artery)
- Chronic total occlusion of popliteal artery and proximal trifurcation vessels

FIGURE I TASC classification of femoral popliteal lesions. *CFA,* Common femoral artery; *SFA,* superficial femoral artery. *(From Norgren L, Hiatt WR, Dormandy JA, et al: Inter-Society Consensus for the Management of Peripheral Arterial Disease (TASC II), J Vasc Surg 45(suppl 1):S5–S67, 2007.)*

From the standpoint of technique, the fundamental steps in peripheral endovascular interventions include the following: 1) obtain access to the arterial system; 2) identify the lesion with angiography; 3) cross the lesion with a guidewire; 4) treat the lesion using one of a variety of techniques including balloon angioplasty, atherectomy, or stent placement; and 5) perform completion angiography to confirm resolution of the lesion. Arterial access is most frequently obtained via a common femoral artery puncture, but alternative sites may be utilized, including the brachial and occasionally the popliteal arteries. When treating the SFA, a retrograde puncture of the contralateral common femoral artery is often used, with access to the affected side gained by placing the guidewire up and over the aortic bifurcation. Alternatively, an antegrade or downward common femoral artery puncture on the affected side offers a somewhat straight shot into the ipsilateral SFA and popliteal arteries.

Once arterial access has been obtained, a sheath is placed to facilitate interventions through the puncture site, which allows the operator to introduce the various wires, catheters, balloons, and stents necessary to perform angiography as well as intervention. There are multiple versions of catheters, guidewires, and balloons, all with varying purposes and handling characteristics. Often the choice of which tool to use is related to personal experience and preference. Anticoagulation is initiated prior to the intervention.

Advanced techniques for crossing complex lesions or total occlusions include the use of subintimal angioplasty, reentry devices, or lasers. Once guidewire access across a lesion is obtained, a balloon can be introduced over the wire and inflated to dilate the lesion. Figure 2 demonstrates a TASC type B superficial femoral artery occlusion before and after angioplasty. Stent placement in the femoropopliteal system should be considered if a residual flow-limiting stenosis remains after angioplasty, or if there is a complication of angioplasty, such as a flow-limiting dissection.

Some authors recommend primary stent placement for treating SFA lesions, citing improved patency rates; others endorse a policy of selective stenting. The debate regarding the utility of SFA stenting has triggered multiple trials, some of which are ongoing. Specialized SFA and proximal popliteal stents have been developed, but it remains to be seen whether routine utilization of these devices will prove advantageous. Stenting of the popliteal artery across the knee joint should generally be avoided, because movement of the knee joint results in mechanical trauma that can lead to stent fracture and occlusion. For similar reasons, stent placement should be avoided across the groin crease at the junction of the external iliac and common femoral arteries.

Outcomes of endovascular treatment of femoropopliteal lesions vary with respect to the indication for treatment and the TASC classification. In general, patients with limb-threatening ischemia and more extensive lesions have diminished patency rates compared with those with claudication. Repeat interventions are commonly employed to treat recurrent stenosis or occlusion. Contemporary results for the endovascular treatment of lesions in the femoropopliteal system are maturing. In general, technical success is achieved in more than 95% of appropriately selected patients. Two year primary patency rates range from 30% to 70% and are universally higher in claudication patients compared with those who have limb-threatening ischemia. Assisted 2-year patency rates for both groups has approached 80% in some series, but this is highly influenced by the TASC classification of the lesions treated. Patients with type D lesions have reported 2 year assisted patency rates of 55% versus combined type A, B, and C lesions of 70% in one large series. Two year limb salvage rates for patients with limb-threatening ischemia have eclipsed 80% in most contemporary series.

SURGICAL MANAGEMENT OF FEMOROPOPLITEAL DISEASE

Surgical management of femoropopliteal occlusive disease usually involves a bypass (Figure 3), although endarterectomy can occasionally be used for selected isolated lesions, such as those in the common

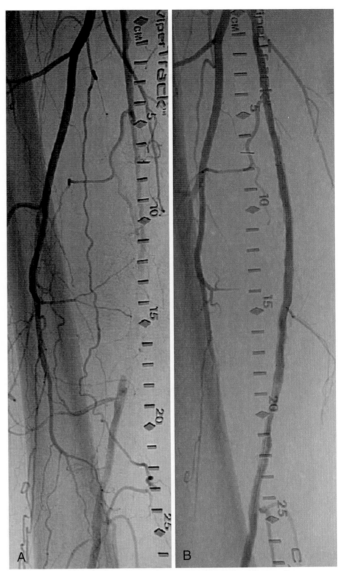

FIGURE 2 Angiogram of a TASC type B superficial femoral artery occlusion. **A,** Before angioplasty. **B,** After angioplasty.

femoral artery. Exposure of the common femoral artery is performed through a vertical or oblique skin incision. Distal exposure, usually of the popliteal artery above or below knee, is usually performed through a medial incision of the distal thigh and/or the proximal lower leg.

The bypass conduit should be determined preoperatively, but alternative plans should be in place if the conduit initially chosen is suboptimal. Preoperative vein mapping is invaluable to confirm the availability and adequacy of a vein conduit. The greater saphenous vein is the conduit of choice, if it is available and of suitable size. Alternative venous conduits include arm veins (cephalic or basilic) or the short saphenous vein. Other available biological grafts include cryopreserved autogenous vein or human umbilical vein. Prosthetic conduits include those created from polytetrafluoroethylene (PTFE) or Dacron.

Following anticoagulation, a proximal anastomosis, usually end to side, is performed between the conduit and the common femoral artery. A tunnel connecting this wound with the site of the distal anastomosis is then created, and the graft is passed through the tunnel. Great care must be taken when tunneling the graft to avoid twisting or kinking. In the case of an in situ saphenous vein bypass,

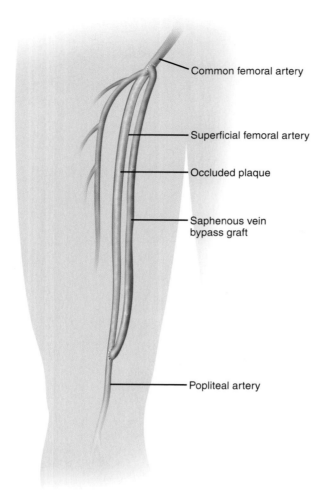

Common femoral artery

Superficial femoral artery

Occluded plaque

Saphenous vein
bypass graft

Popliteal artery

FIGURE 3 Femoral-popliteal bypass for occlusive disease.

the vein is left in its original anatomic plane. A distal anastomosis is then created to the popliteal artery below the disease. After the bypass is complete, angiography, DUS, or continuous wave Doppler may be used to assess the adequacy of graft function.

Robust data are available to document the expected outcomes following surgical bypass for femoropopliteal occlusive disease. Primary patency rates for femoral-popliteal bypass range from 30% to 90% at 5 years. Variations in outcomes depend upon the indication (claudication or limb threat); the conduit (autogenous vs. prosthetic); quality of the vein, if a vein is used; the distal extent of the bypass (above or below the knee); and runoff (patency of the tibial vessels). Patency at 5 years for saphenous vein femoral–popliteal bypasses above or below the knee range from 70% to 90%, whereas patency for prosthetic bypass below the knee at 5 years can be as low as 30%. For patients with limb-threatening ischemia, salvage rates of 90% at 5 years have been reported in multiple series, but varying degrees of resource utilization are necessary to achieve these results: expanded inpatient stays, reoperation, and diminished quality of life related to prolonged wound healing may accompany treatment.

DISCUSSION

The last decade has been a time of unprecedented evolution in the treatment of patients with femoropopliteal occlusive disease. In many patients, surgical bypass, once the mainstay of therapy, has been replaced by a host of endovascular interventions. However, the optimal treatment of patients with femoropopliteal occlusion (endovascular vs. surgical intervention) remains unresolved. It is relatively well accepted that endovascular intervention is preferable for TASC type A and B lesions. However, controversy remains over the most appropriate treatment of more extensive type C and D lesions. In the absence of level I randomized data, a number of differing philosophies exist. We practice a percutaneous first approach with the belief that in all patients, with occasional exceptions, the initial approach should be percutaneous, with either repeat percutaneous interventions or surgical bypass for those who develop recurrent disease. This philosophy is predicated on several principles: First, this group of patients, who are in general elderly, fares better with a minimally invasive approach with regard to mortality, morbidity and quality of life. Second, patients tolerate reinterventions relatively well, particularly if such reinterventions are percutaneous. Third, the life expectancy of this population of patients is diminished, thus durability is not always the critical issue. Fourth, percutaneous interventions can be performed without jeopardizing target vessels, thus allowing a subsequent surgical bypass to be as effective as if it were the initial intervention. Alternatively, those that would support surgical bypass as the primary approach would remind us that the 2-year patency of percutaneous intervention for long-segment occlusions can be as low as 20% to 30%, and although minimally invasive, percutaneous interventions can also produce mortality and morbidity, and the cost associated with endovascular technology is substantial.

Eventually, prospective data should help resolve many of these issues, but in the interim, each patient must be approached individually. For example, a relatively young patient with disabling claudication and complete occlusion of both the SFA and proximal popliteal artery might be best served with a durable saphenous vein bypass. Alternatively, an elderly patient with multiple comorbidities and a nonhealing ulcer might benefit greatly from a percutaneous intervention that will sufficiently increase circulation long enough to allow healing of the wound. Obviously there are many patients who fall somewhere between these two scenarios, and thus, the debate rages on.

SUMMARY

Disease in the superficial femoral artery is the most common manifestation of lower extremity vascular disease. It is essential that surgeons have the ability diagnose, evaluate, and treat patients who present with symptomatic femoropopliteal disease that produces either claudication or limb-threatening ischemia. Endovascular therapies to treat PVD will become more prevalent as the technology continues to evolve. Surgeons should be at the forefront of developing and testing new and minimally invasive approaches that will allow more optimal treatment of this complex group of patients. Surgical bypass will remain an important option in patients who fail endovascular therapy or in those with complex disease patterns not amenable to endovascular treatments.

SELECTED READINGS

Adam DJ, Beard JD, Cleveland T, et al: Bypass versus angioplasty in severe ischaemia of the leg (BASIL): multicentre, randomised controlled trial, Lancet 366:1925–1934, 2005.

DeRubertis B, Faries P, McKinsey J, et al: Shifting paradigms in the treatment of lower extremity vascular disease: a report of 1,000 percutaneous interventions, Ann Surg 246(3):415–422, 2007.

Goodney PP, Beck AP, Nagle J, et al: National trends in lower extremity bypass surgery, endovascular interventions, and major amputations, J Vasc Surg 50:54–60, 2009.

Lee LK, Kent KC: Infrainguinal occlusive disease: endovascular intervention is the first line of therapy, Adv Surg 42:193–201, 2008.

Norgren L, Hiatt WR, Dormandy JA, et al: for the TASC II Working Group: Inter-Society Consensus for the Management of Peripheral Arterial Disease (TASC II), J Vasc Surg 45(Suppl S):S5–S67, 2007.

MANAGEMENT OF TIBIOPERONEAL OCCLUSIVE DISEASE

Erin H. Murphy, MD, and Christopher K. Zarins, MD

GENERAL CONSIDERATIONS AND INDICATIONS FOR TREATMENT

The management of tibioperoneal occlusive disease is among one the most medically and surgically challenging problems in vascular surgery. Important factors to consider when approaching patients with this disease include the patient's general health, coexisting medical conditions, and overall functional status. Arterial occlusive disease in any one location is rarely an isolated entity and instead is usually associated with varying degrees of generalized atherosclerotic disease. Medical comorbidities are also common in this patient population. As a result of atherosclerotic disease in other locations and medical comorbidities, patients with tibioperoneal disease are predisposed to increased operative risk and poor medical outcomes. Diabetes mellitus, which coexists in approximately 60% of patients with tibioperoneal disease, results in calcified vessels that increase the difficulty of interventions. Multilevel disease further augments the complexity, because extensive infrapopliteal collateralization prevents earlier disease recognition. Lastly, the treatment options for this disease are accompanied by the frequent need for reintervention.

The medical and surgical complexity of this disease and the high risks of intervention should mandate conservative surgical decision making. Although patients with tibioperoneal disease may present with claudication, the ultimate decision to intervene should be reserved for patients with signs of impending limb loss manifested by ischemic rest pain, nonhealing soft-tissue ulceration, and gangrene. In this subset of patients who otherwise maintain a functional status, avoidance of amputation is paramount. Amputation in the elderly is associated with significant consequences, including loss of independence and decreased quality of life. Furthermore, the medical costs of amputation rival even the most extensive interventions for tibioperoneal disease, making avoidance of amputation a worthy undertaking, not only for the patient but also for society.

Patient Assessment

The goals of preoperative evaluation include identification of patients who are likely to benefit from tibioperoneal intervention, development of interventional plans individualized to each patient's disease extent, and consideration of comorbidities to allow medical optimization prior to surgery.

Assessment should always begin with a thorough history and physical examination that includes assessment of functional status. The mean age for patients presenting with this disease is over 70 years. Medical comorbidities in this patient population are the rule, not the exception. Patients are often seen with apparent or occult diabetes, renal insufficiency, cardiovascular disease, and cerebrovascular disease. Preoperative optimization of medical comorbidities is advised whenever possible. We do not routinely perform full cardiac evaluation in otherwise asymptomatic patients prior to intervention, as it has been demonstrated that these operations can be performed safely without it. In fact, delay for cardiac evaluation has been shown to result in higher amputation rates secondary to progression of ischemia and infection in patients who may have benefited from limb-salvage interventions. Monitoring of renal function is essential, as temporary worsening of renal function associated with contrast nephropathy after angiography is a frequent occurrence. With proper management, however, most renal insufficiency is transient.

Physical exam should include assessment of bilateral lower extremity pulses, wounds, extent of lower extremity infections, and coexistent venous disease. If intervention is planned, diligent control of foot sepsis with surgical debridement of infected tissue and treatment with antibiotics should be attempted before intervention. Toe amputations may be required and should, in most cases, be left open to drain. Final foot reconstruction can be performed postoperatively, after blood flow is restored.

Noninvasive vascular imaging, including ankle-brachial indexes (ABIs) and toe pressures, should be used to objectively document the degree of ischemia and to serve as a baseline for comparison postoperatively. An ankle pressure below 50 mm Hg with a flat pulse waveform indicates that the patient is unlikely to heal foot wounds without prior revascularization. More detailed imaging that includes conventional angiography, computed tomographic angiography (CTA), or magnetic resonance arteriography (MRA) should be completed and reviewed prior to consideration for intervention. Delayed images may be helpful in patients with poor runoff, and CTA and MRA may provide more detailed imaging of the distal circulation than routine angiography, thus it is our preferred method for preoperative assessment. Imaging should be obtained from the aorta distal to the renal arteries through the pedal vessels, with attention paid to the quality of inflow vessels, degree of multifocality of disease, vessel calcification, and vessel runoff. The number of patent tibial vessels is associated with improved success of revascularization. At a minimum, restoration of blood flow for wound healing or resolution of rest pain typically requires at least one continuous vessel to provide in-line flow to the foot. If this is not possible, revascularization is indicated to restore the vessel most likely to provide flow to the wound.

If the patient is a potential distal bypass candidate, noninvasive evaluation of the bilateral lower extremity venous systems should be done to evaluate for bypass conduits. Upper extremity duplex ultrasonography (DUS) may also reveal suitable veins for bypass procedures, should the greater or lesser saphenous veins prove unusable.

During the evaluation it should be remembered that primary amputation may be more advisable in patients who are nonambulatory, of limited functional status, or in those who have severe flexion contractures, predetermined prohibitive medical risks, and unsalvageable lower extremity infections. However, advanced age, most medical problems, incurable malignancy, and a contralateral amputation are not absolute contraindications for tibioperoneal intervention.

TREATMENT

Acutely threatened limbs may benefit from systemic heparinization or thrombolytics prior to either operative or endovascular intervention. This is a judgment call and depends on the acuity of symptoms and the severity of ischemia. Aspirin and an adenosine diphosphate receptor inhibitor, either clopidogrel or dipyridamole, should also be initiated at least 5 days prior to all elective endovascular interventions. We preferentially use clopidogrel in our patients. In those patients who require more urgent intervention, or in those who did not complete their course of clopidogrel as instructed, clopidogrel loading can be done the same day. When elective circumstances prevail, we also routinely start our bypass patients on aspirin and clopidogrel preoperatively. However, it is not our routine practice to use clopidogrel loading on bypass patients who have not already been taking this medication.

Tibial Artery Bypass

Outflow: Distal Bypass Target

Distal bypasses may be performed to the posterior tibial, anterior tibial, or peroneal arteries. Alternatively, bypass may be performed to the pedal vessels of the foot. All things considered, the most disease-free proximal vessel that can provide in-line flow to the foot is chosen.

Inflow Vessels

Choice of inflow vessel is determined by prior surgical interventions, characteristics of the inflow vessel, and length of available autogenous vein. The common femoral artery is a popular location for the inflow anastomosis. If this vessel is heavily calcified or scarred in from prior surgery, the surgeon can alternatively utilize the distal external iliac, profunda femoris, superficial femoral, or above-the-knee popliteal arteries. The profunda femoris, superficial femoral, and popliteal arteries may also be used if the length of the available conduit is limited. It is paramount to construct a tension-free anastomosis to avoid future pseudoaneurysms. Alternatively, a previous bypass conduit used for a femoral-femoral, axillofemoral, or aortofemoral bypass may be used for a proximal anastomosis.

Conduits

Autogenous vein is the preferred conduit for distal bypasses. The order of preference is greater saphenous vein, lesser saphenous vein, followed by arm vein. Although the cephalic and basilic veins are definite options for bypass, we have listed them last, because they are generally thin walled, often have fibrotic segments from previous venipuncture, and have lower patency rates compared to lower extremity veins. The venous segment may be used in a reversed (Figure 1) or in situ fashion. Regardless of the vein source, distended vein diameters of at least 3 mm are recommended. Both techniques require ligation of venous side branches, and the in situ technique requires lysing of venous valves. Veins with a single kink or twist can still be used, but they require intraoperative repair prior to bypass.

Use of expanded polytetrafluoroethylene (ePTFE) below the knee is discouraged when alternatives exist, because both patency and limb-salvage rates using this material lag significantly behind bypasses performed using autogenous vein. Segments of vein may be pieced together if a single, long, continuous vein is unavailable. However, patency rates using such multisegment bypass grafts appear to be decreased, and it is unclear how much benefit is gained over the use of a long prosthetic graft. Thus, if autogenous vein is compromised or unavailable in patients with critical limb ischemia, distal bypass with

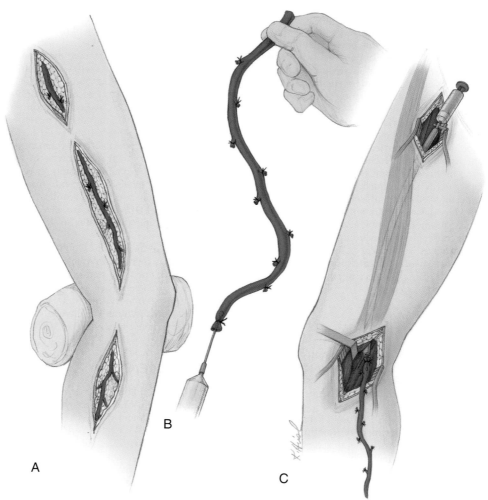

A

B

C

FIGURE 1   A, Reversed saphenous vein grafts. The wound morbidity associated with harvesting vein segments, which can be seen in up to 25% of patients, may be reduced by the use of skip incisions. Venous side branches are identified, ligated, and transected during harvest. **B,** The vein is flushed with heparinized saline, clearing blood from the lumen and confirming ligation of all venous branches. **C,** The vein graft is soaked in papaverine solution until the surgeon is ready to tunnel the graft and begin the bypass. *(From Zarins CK, Gewertz BL: Atlas of vascular surgery, ed 2, Philadelphia, 2005, Elsevier.)*

PTFE should be considered, because it is still superior to a primary amputation. Another consideration includes a composite distal bypass using a proximal ePTFE graft joined to a patent popliteal segment with a venous segment extended to a tibial artery. However, the benefit of composite grafts over PTFE alone has not been proven. Cryopreserved vein and umbilical vein allografts may be used, but their patency rates are no better than with ePTFE bypass. Other alternatives to autogenous vein are currently under investigation, but no evidence is available that advocates their use over either autogenous vein or PTFE at this time.

Procedural Details

Procedures may be performed under general, spinal, or epidural anesthesia with adequate monitoring that includes an arterial line. Preoperative antibiotics are given 30 minutes prior to skin incision.

Inflow and outflow vessels should be exposed, and the vein graft prepped, prior to anticoagulation and arterial clamping.

Surgical exposure varies depending on the target vessel and location of the distal anastomosis. The tibioperoneal trunk and proximal tibial vessels are exposed through a medial approach below the knee, avoiding injury to the greater saphenous vein during the skin incision. The muscular fascia is incised, and the medial head of the gastrocnemius muscle is retracted posteriorly. If exposure is insufficient, the medial head of the gastrocnemius may be divided at the medial femoral condyle. The proximal tibial arteries are exposed by separation of the soleus muscle from the tibia. The mid posterior tibial artery, the preferred target for distal bypass, runs between the tibialis posterior and the flexor digitorum longus muscles (Figure 2). Distally the posterior tibial artery is exposed through a longitudinal incision posterior to the medial malleolus, splitting the distance between the

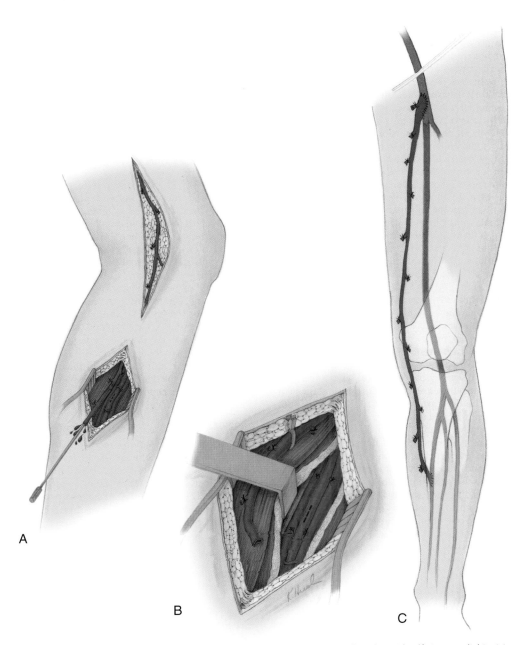

FIGURE 2   Exposure of the posterior tibial artery. **A,** The posterior tibial artery is exposed at the mid calf via a medial incision posterior to the tibia. **B,** The soleus muscle is retracted posteriorly. **C,** After tunneling the vein to the artery, the distal anastomosis completes the bypass. *(From Zarins CK, Gewertz BL: Atlas of vascular surgery, ed 2, Philadelphia, 2005, Elsevier.)*

malleolus and the Achilles tendon. The flexor retinaculum must be divided to expose the posterior tibial artery at this location. Exposure may be continued to the medial and lateral plantar arteries in the foot by continuing the dissection of the flexor retinaculum distally.

The anterior tibial artery may be exposed along its length by an incision 2 cm lateral to the tibia. The anterior tibial artery is found by dividing the fascia overlying the anterior compartment and bluntly separating the tibialis anterior muscle and the flexor digitorum longus. The anterior tibial artery is usually associated with two overlying veins and the deep peroneal nerve. The dorsalis pedis artery is a continuation of the anterior tibial artery after crossing the ankle joint. This artery is exposed via a 2 cm incision lateral to the extensor hallucis longus tendon on the dorsum of the foot.

The peroneal artery can be exposed through a medial or lateral incision on the calf. A medial approach is best suited for access of the superior two thirds of this vessel. The distal peroneal artery is exposed though a lateral incision over the fibula, with excision of a segment of the fibula to reveal the underlying peroneal artery, which is on the flexor hallucis longus muscle posterior to the intramuscular septum.

After target vessel exposure and vein harvest, intravenous heparin is given prior to arterial clamping, at a dose of 70 to 100 U/kg, and is redosed at 45-minute intervals as needed to maintain an activated clotting time (ACT) of 250 to 300 seconds. Gentle clamping techniques should be employed using atraumatic vascular clamps to minimize the possibility of clamp injury. Anastomoses are performed using small diameter (6-0 or 7-0) monofilament suture with good lighting and magnification. The proximal anastomosis is usually performed first. When using the nonreversed in situ technique, the saphenous vein is left in place, and the most proximal valve is lysed under direct vision; after the proximal anastomosis is complete, the remainder of the valves are lysed using a valvulotome. Reversed saphenous vein bypasses are usually tunneled in the subcutaneous plane but may be tunneled in the deeper anatomic plane. Regardless of the plane chosen, attention must be paid to avoid graft twisting or kinking.

A number of techniques can be used to enhance the distal anastomosis to improve outflow. The Linton patch enlarges the distal anastomosis by sewing a vein patch onto the tibial artery and then anastomosing the bypass graft onto the vein patch in an end-to-side fashion. Miller described a method of constructing a vein cuff secured to the distal target vessel, thus allowing the bypass graft to be anastomosed to the vein cuff end-to-end. This method is particularly useful for prosthetic ePTFE tibial artery bypasses. The Taylor patch utilizes a vein patch to widen the distal graft anastomosis. Alternatively, Dardik has described the creation of a side-to-side fistula between the distal target vessel and adjacent vein by opening both, sewing the back wall of the vein and artery together, and then anastomosing the vein graft to the anterior wall of both the artery and vein. These techniques should be considered when the tibial arteries are small, and the outflow is poor with high arterial resistance.

After completion of the anastomoses and flow restoration, the adequacy of perfusion is assessed by inspection of the foot and toes, palpation of distal pulses, and Doppler flow assessment in the bypass graft and outflow artery. We also perform intraoperative angiographic evaluation of the bypass and distal anastomosis to ensure there are no technical defects. Noninfected foot wounds greater than 2 cm may be debrided at the end of the operation after arterial reconstruction. Debridement may include toe amputations, which may be loosely closed. Skin grafts should be postponed until wounds are granulating.

Endovascular Treatment

General Considerations

The indications for endovascular interventions for tibioperoneal occlusive disease are similar to those for surgical bypass. Significant advances in imaging and endovascular technology and improved proficiency of interventionalists have resulted in improved outcomes after peripheral vascular endovascular interventions. Although some advocate extending the indications to intervene earlier in the course of tibioperoneal disease, evidence suggests that infrapopliteal procedures should be reserved for limb salvage in appropriate candidates. Endovascular treatment of tibioperoneal disease for claudication should be avoided. Early intervention may place patients with underlying medical comorbidities at risk from complications associated with intervention and early treatment failure. Unsuccessful endovascular treatment may result in worsening of symptoms and may lead to critical limb ischemia and a potentially unsalvageable acute limb-loss situation.

Despite the aforementioned concerns, the growing armamentarium of endovascular options provides excellent alternatives for patients who are not suitable candidates for bypass. Patients with inadequate vein conduits or patients at high risk for bypass surgery may benefit from endovascular procedures with good limb-salvage rates and low morbidity and mortality compared with open procedures. Endovascular procedures may also be used to temporize patients in preparation for bypass or supplemental bypass procedures by augmenting inflow or outflow. These procedures may also allow for healing of ischemic ulcers and toe amputations with long-term limb salvage, even if the endovascular intervention eventually fails. It is well known that limb-salvage rates exceed the patency rates for endovascular interventions. During the past decade, we have witnessed a dramatic increase in the number of endovascular treatments performed for lower extremity ischemia, and this has been accompanied by a decrease in the overall major amputation rate.

Access

Endovascular interventions are typically performed under epidural, spinal, or local anesthesia combined with sedation. Access for tibioperoneal disease may be obtained from the contralateral common femoral artery using a 5 or 6 Fr sheath. After diagnostic angiographic imaging, a crossover sheath is advanced over the aortic bifurcation into the ipsilateral external iliac artery. A long guide sheath, or a 6 Fr multipurpose catheter, is introduced into the ipsilateral superficial femoral or popliteal artery to provide support for infrapopliteal interventions. The crossover technique is best suited for angiographic evaluation or treatment of short, straight stenoses. More advanced complex interventions to treat long stenoses, calcified lesions, or very distal lesions may require antegrade access from the ipsilateral common femoral or popliteal artery. This approach allows more direct access for interventions and allows the operator to achieve maximal opacification of the distal circulation with smaller amounts of potentially nephrotoxic contrast.

Imaging

Infrapopliteal interventions require high-resolution imaging. The use of low-osmolar contrast will be less painful in a patient under sedation and local anesthesia. Imaging of the trifurcation is usually obtained using a straight anterior-posterior view with a 4 or 5 Fr diagnostic catheter. Additional views using a 30-degree ipsilateral oblique or a true lateral view may better delineate the proximal anterior tibial artery and distal popliteal arteries.

Procedural Details

Heparin is administered at the start of intervention at doses to maintain an activated clotting time of 250 to 300 seconds throughout the procedure. Most tibial interventions for stenotic lesions can be performed over a 0.014 inch guidewire. A 0.018 inch or 0.035 inch guidewire may be required for occlusive lesions, and catheter support may be used to traverse calcified or long lesions. On occasion, retrograde crossing of an occluded tibial artery can be achieved using a distal cutdown, followed by snaring and externalization of the wire from above, allowing antegrade performance of the remainder of the procedure.

Balloon angioplasty of stenotic lesions is the most common tibioperoneal endovascular intervention. Balloon angioplasty alone is most successful in the treatment of single, short-segment stenoses (<1 cm). Lesions less likely to respond to angioplasty include occlusive disease, long-segment stenosis, multiple lesions, and heavily calcified plaques. Stents may be used when the results of balloon angioplasty are suboptimal, and stents are useful to correct abnormalities such as hemodynamically significant vessel recoil and arterial dissection. Although the literature is inconsistent, the endovascular treatment of short-segment stenoses has been reported to be successful in up to 98% of patients (Figure 3). More challenging lesions, such as occlusions, have a reported technical success rate nearing 80%. Although long-term patency is uncertain, clinical resolution of symptoms exceed patency rates. Limb salvage, the ultimate goal of intervention, ranges from 50% to 84% at various intervals from 2 to 5 years.

Other endovascular treatment options include the use of cutting or scoring balloons, cryoplasty balloons, rotational atherectomy, and laser angioplasty. Although early success with these technologies has been reported, the literature contains conflicting and anecdotal reports and limited long-term follow-up. In our practice we have used cutting or scoring balloons for heavily calcified vessels with some success (Figure 4). Overall, results with rotational atherectomy appear disappointing but may be improved with use of glycoprotein IIb/IIIa inhibitors. Cryoplasty has shown little benefit over routine angioplasty and adjunctive stenting, but investigation into the use of this technology in the tibial vessels is currently underway. Some encouraging results have been demonstrated with laser atherectomy, but these reports are early.

POSTINTERVENTION TREATMENT AND SURVEILLANCE

Aspirin and ADP-receptor inhibitors should be continued after lower extremity endovascular interventions and should strongly be considered after distal bypass. The use of clopidogrel compared with aspirin alone has been demonstrated to decrease the incidence of vascular events in patients with peripheral artery disease. Antiplatelet drugs have further been shown to improve the patency of infrapopliteal grafts. Warfarin therapy should be considered in patients after bypass with prosthetic conduits, because this may improve patency rates, particularly in patients with failed previous bypass. Finally, statins should be considered for all patients unless contraindicated. In addition to the medical benefits of statins, recent trials indicate a cholesterol-independent improvement in graft patency after bypass.

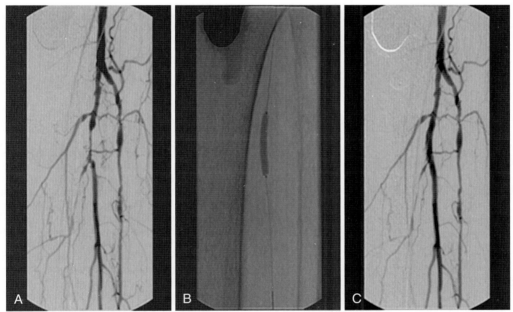

FIGURE 3 Angioplasty of the posterior tibial artery. **A,** Patient with critical limb ischemia. **B,** Angioplasty of the mid posterior tibial artery. **C,** Result was resolution of stenosis and rest pain.

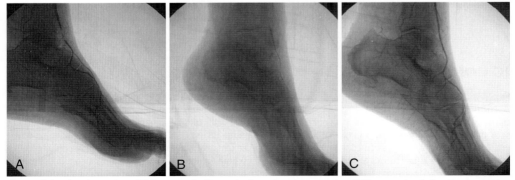

FIGURE 4 Angioplasty of the distal anterior tibial artery. **A,** Preangioplasty imaging reveals a 95% stenosis of the distal anterior tibial artery in a patient with critical limb ischemia. **B,** Angioplasty of the artery. **C,** Result was less than 10% residual stenosis and healing of ischemic foot ulceration.

Surveillance of patients with saphenous vein bypass grafts should include DUS of the bypass along with measurement of ABIs postoperatively at 1 month, 3 months, 6 months, 1 year, and annually thereafter. Patients with prosthetic grafts are followed at similar time frames with the exception of biannual follow-up after the first year, instead of continuing with annual follow-up. A decrease in the ABI of 0.15 or greater, increased focal velocity at the anastomoses or within the bypass, or increases in mean graft velocity are suggestive of early graft failure and should prompt further imaging with CTA, MRA, or angiography.

Early failures after open interventions are usually the result of technical errors, which can result in vessel recoil, dissection, and periprocedural plaque embolization. Early failures may be prevented by intraoperative imaging and recognition of the defect before leaving the operating room. Most patients with early graft failure will require surgical reintervention and reconstruction, typically with vein patch angioplasty. However, short-segment stenoses of less than 1.5 cm may be amendable to percutaneous angioplasty provided the vein diameter is of adequate caliber (>3 mm).

Treatment failures after 1 month but before 2 years are most often attributable to neointimal hyperplasia. Failures after more than 2 years are most often secondary to progression of atherosclerotic disease. In either case, these later failures are best treated with early recognition and reintervention. Early reintervention is often much simpler than the treatment required for complete thrombosis and is associated with improved long-term outcomes.

Patients treated with endovascular interventions should be followed with clinical examination, DUS imaging of the treated artery, and ABIs. Reintervention for these patients is reserved for recurrence of critical limb ischemia.

SUMMARY

The management of tibioperoneal occlusive disease should be focused on the primary goal of limb salvage. Patients with claudication should be managed conservatively, but patients with critical limb ischemia most often require intervention. Treatment options include tibial artery bypass and endovascular therapy. Good judgment is essential in patient and procedure selection, choice of operative and interventional techniques, postoperative surveillance, and decisions for reintervention. With optimal care the majority of patients can attain limb salvage, resulting in improved quality of life for the patient and overall cost savings for society.

SUGGESTED READINGS

Zarins CK, Gewertz BL: *Atlas of vascular surgery*, ed 2, Philadelphia, 2005, Elsevier.

Valentine RJ, Wind GG: *Anatomic exposures in vascular surgery*, Philadelphia, 2003, Lippincott Williams & Wilkins.

Gupta SK, Veith FJ, Samson RH, et al: Cost analysis of operations for infrainguinal arteriosclerosis, *Circulation* 66(suppl 2):II-9, 1982.

CAPRIE Steering Committee: A randomized, blinded trial of clopidogrel versus aspirin in patients at risk of ischemic events (CAPRIE), *Lancet* 348:1329-1339, 1981.

Henke PK, Blackburn S, Proctor MC, et al: Patients undergoing infrainguinal bypass to treat atherosclerotic vascular disease are underprescribed cardioprotective medications: effect on graft patency, limb salvage, and mortality, *J Vasc Surg* 39:357-365, 2004.

PROFUNDA FEMORIS RECONSTRUCTION

Evan C. Lipsitz, MD, and Amit Shah, MD

OVERVIEW

The importance of adequate profunda femoris flow in the setting of lower extremity occlusive disease cannot be underscored enough. Although the primary function of the profunda femoris artery is to provide blood flow to the large muscles of the thigh, it also provides flow to the lower leg via numerous collateral vessels. When there is occlusion or extensive stenotic disease of the superficial femoral artery, the profunda femoris provides flow to the entire lower extremity.

ANATOMIC CONSIDERATIONS

The profunda femoris originates at the femoral bifurcation, which is generally located from 3 to 5 cm below the inguinal ligament (Figure 1). However, the bifurcation may be located at the level of the inguinal ligament or more than 5 cm below it. It is useful for operative planning to note the location of the profunda femoris origin preprocedurally, based on any imaging studies that have been performed. The profunda femoris branches off the femoral bifurcation in a posterolateral direction, forming an acute angle with the superficial femoral artery. When dissecting the femoral vessels from the anterior approach, the location of the profunda origin can be identified by the change in caliber from the larger, common femoral to the smaller, superficial femoral artery. The profunda femoris then courses posterolaterally, deep to the sartorius and vastus medialis muscles. It is crossed anteriorly by the circumflex femoral vein at the level of the femoral bifurcation. This vein is a potential site of arteriovenous fistula development following percutaneous endovascular procedures, when the puncture is located at the level of the femoral bifurcation. When there is femoropopliteal occlusive disease, the profunda femoris provides collateral flow to the lower leg via numerous collaterals that anastomose with geniculate collaterals (Figure 2). The profunda also serves as an important source of retrograde collateral flow to the pelvis, when there is hypogastric occlusion via the medial and lateral circumflex arteries.

The profunda femoris can be divided into three zones relating to anatomic landmarks. The *proximal zone* begins at the profunda femoris takeoff and extends to the lateral femoral circumflex artery origin. The *middle zone* begins at the lateral femoral circumflex and extends to the takeoff of the second perforating artery; this portion lies posterior to the adductor longus muscle and anterior to the adductor brevis and magnus. The *distal zone* begins at the second perforating artery and extends to the fourth perforating artery (Figure 3).

EVALUATION AND IMAGING

It is difficult to evaluate the status of the profunda femoris by physical exam alone. The presence of a femoral pulse does not ensure patency of the profunda femoris. This is especially true in the acute setting, in which a femoral pulse may be palpable, even where there is an acute thrombus occluding the femoral bifurcation. Rarely, reconstitution via profunda femoris collaterals will allow for a palpable distal pulse in the setting of a superficial femoral artery occlusion.

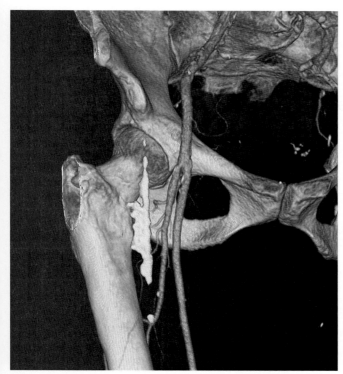

FIGURE 1   The profunda femoris artery originates from the common femoral artery in the groin and courses posterolaterally to supply the muscles of the thigh. *(Courtesy Dr. Dominik Fleischmann.)*

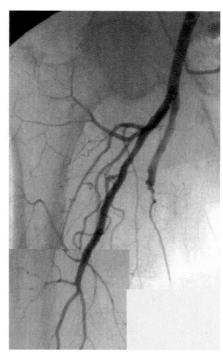

FIGURE 2   Angiogram of the common femoral, superficial femoral (with occlusion), and profunda femoris arteries. Note the separation of the superficial and profunda arteries in the oblique projection, as well as the extensive network of collateral vessels from the profunda femoris, in the setting of superficial femoral artery occlusion.

As noted above, it is important to evaluate the status and position of the profunda femoris during all imaging evaluations. In the case of a focal profunda femoris stenosis, input from multiple modalities may be beneficial. Findings may be confirmed with a number of diagnostic modalities. Pulse volume recordings (PVRs) are a plethysmographic evaluation of lower extremity arterial circulation that evaluates the total flow from both main vessels and collaterals at various segments of the lower extremity. As such, when superficial femoral occlusive disease is present, PVRs may provide an estimate of the adequacy of profunda femoris collateral flow to the lower leg. Duplex ultrasound may image the profunda femoris well, because most lesions are found in the proximal portion of the vessel. Color-flow imaging of the common femoral artery is performed in cross section and followed distally until the bifurcation is observed. Velocities are determined in the longitudinal view from the common femoral, superficial femoral, and profunda femoris arteries. Peak systolic velocities should be measured in all vessels, and it is helpful to have an estimation of adequate profunda flow distal to its origin. Flow reversal in the profunda may be seen in cases of acute thrombosis of the common femoral artery, when the profunda provides flow to the lower extremity via a patent superficial femoral artery. The first 5 cm of the artery is scanned, as the vessel size decreases with branching, and disease is less likely to be present. The presence of severe calcification may make duplex scanning more complex and less reliable.

Computed tomography (CT) is a useful examination for the diagnosis of common femoral and femoral bifurcation disease. It not only provides an evaluation of the degree and location of stenoses and occlusions, it also provides an anatomic road map of vessel calcification that allows for operative planning. Magnetic resonance angiography (MRA) is also a useful modality for defining the femoral anatomy but does not provide as detailed an evaluation of the degree and extent of calcification, and it is dependent on the magnet strength of the imaging device. Traditional angiography provides a dynamic imaging of the femoral vessels, where the flow can be evaluated in real time; it does not provide a detailed evaluation of vascular calcifications. Typically, an ipsilateral anterior oblique projection of anywhere from 15 to 45 degrees is required to offset the origin of the profunda femoris from the superficial femoral artery and optimize visualization of both vessels (see Figure 2).

Presentation and Indications for Intervention

Isolated atherosclerotic disease in the profunda artery is quite rare, and intervention is not usually undertaken in the absence of other, significant lower extremity atherosclerotic disease. Profunda femoris disease most commonly occurs at the orifice and in the proximal portion as a continuation of common and superficial femoral artery disease. Patients with lower extremity occlusive disease and profunda femoris involvement may have symptoms anywhere along the spectrum of peripheral vascular disease, from minimally symptomatic claudication to disabling claudication, rest pain, and tissue loss. Although determining the degree of symptoms attributable to the profunda femoris component is important and helpful, the profunda femoris disease should be addressed when possible to improve the immediate and long-term outcomes of therapy.

Profundaplasty may be performed as an isolated procedure or as an adjunct to either inflow or outflow procedures in patients suffering from varying degrees of lower extremity occlusive disease. Having noted the above concepts, isolated profundaplasty is often all that is required to relieve or ameliorate symptoms in medically and/or anatomically high-risk patients, such as those without a distal outflow site for a bypass, or with multiple reoperations. Patients who have disabling claudication, or even rest pain, with superficial femoral disease and profunda femoris stenosis may experience a marked improvement in walking distance or resolution of rest pain after profundaplasty alone. This procedure has the added advantage that it may be performed under local or regional anesthesia. Patients with a history

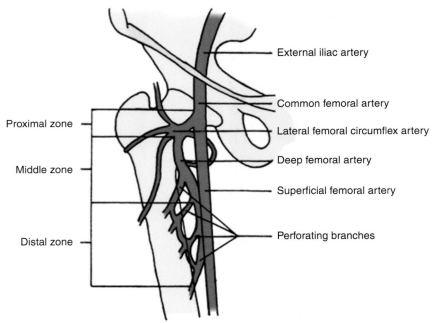

FIGURE 3 Anatomy of the profunda femoris artery. *(From Bertucci WR, Marin ML, Veith FJ, Ohki T: Posterior approach to the deep femoral artery, J Vasc Surg 29:741, 1999.)*

of claudication on the basis of superficial femoral artery disease may progress to limb threat if they develop profunda femoris disease.

Profundaplasty as an adjunctive procedure is performed for all degrees of chronic lower extremity ischemia. The goal and rationale of adjunctive profundaplasty is to increase the effectiveness and durability of the intervention. More importantly, if the bypass fails, a patent profundaplasty generally ensures adequate perfusion and obviates the need for further intervention in a dissected field.

Profunda Femoris as Inflow

The profunda femoris may be used for inflow with or without adjunctive profundaplasty. When there is no stenosis at the profunda femoris orifice, and the vessel is of good quality, it may be used as a source of inflow for a more distal bypass including femoropopliteal, femorotibial, or femoropedal bypass. Use of the profunda femoris as inflow has the advantages of shortening the length of autogenous conduit that is required to complete the bypass and/or avoiding a scarred, previously dissected field. These grafts may be tunneled in a standard fashion.

Profunda Femoris as Outflow

The profunda femoris may also be used as outflow for a variety of procedures including aortofemoral, axillofemoral, or femorofemoral bypass. In general, when the profunda femoris is used for outflow, it is the proximal or origin of the vessel that is used. Again, adjunctive profundaplasty may or may not be required. Where the common femoral bifurcation has been dissected, the distal anastomosis of any of the above-mentioned bypass grafts may be placed distally, usually a few centimeters past the bifurcation of the profunda femoris. In some cases it may be hazardous or impossible to tunnel through the scarred groin, and the grafts must be tunneled more laterally than normal. In addition, it may not be possible to tunnel under the inguinal ligament, and the graft must be brought out through a direct, more anterior puncture of the ligament. Care must be taken in these reoperative situations to avoid inadvertent tunneling through the viscera.

Isolated profundaplasty provides the greatest benefit in cases of rest pain and disabling claudication in the presence of significant stenosis in the proximal profunda femoris, in the absence of inflow disease, and with no treatable superficial femoral or popliteal disease. Patients with severe rest pain and ulceration with minor tissue necrosis can derive some benefit from only having profunda reconstruction, especially when other possibilities of distal revascularization are impossible. More extensive tissue loss is unlikely to be resolved by isolated profundaplasty.

TECHNIQUE

Surgical

The profunda femoris may be exposed through a variety of approaches, and each approach should be tailored to the clinical scenario and the goals of revascularization. The most common approach is performed through a vertical groin incision. In general this incision extends at the level of the inguinal ligament to a few centimeters below the groin crease. The surface landmark for the inguinal ligament is a curved line extending from the anterior-superior iliac spine to the ipsilateral pubic tubercle with the convexity toward the foot; however, this may become somewhat distorted in an obese patient.

The transition in the diameter of the common to the superficial femoral artery marks the origin of the profunda femoris. This transition usually occurs 5 cm below the inguinal ligament. Vessel loops are placed around the common and superficial femoral arteries, which are gently retracted medially. The dissection is continued along the anterior surface of the profunda femoris. Exposure is facilitated by ligating the lateral femoral circumflex vein, which crosses anterior to the profunda at its origin. Careful dissection is crucial, because multiple second-order branches of the profunda femoris may be encountered. Depending on the length of the profunda femoris to be exposed, multiple branches may require control, some of which will also take off in a posterior direction.

The profunda and its branches are delicate arteries that should be handled gently. Failure to do so may result in laceration of the artery or disruption of the intima. The profundaplasty is classified as *proximal* if it extends down to the second perforating branch; it is classified as *extended* if it passes beyond this point. In extremely obese patients, when a lengthy profundaplasty is not anticipated, and the location of the femoral bifurcation is known, the surgeon may consider an oblique groin incision for exposure to reduce the incidence of wound complications. This approach is not advisable when it appears that a more extensive profunda femoris or common femoral artery dissection are required.

When a more distal profunda femoris dissection is desired, when the groin has been previously dissected, or if there is an active groin wound infection, a lateral approach to the profunda may be utilized. A slightly oblique incision is made along the lateral border of the sartorius muscle a few centimeters inferior to the groin crease; the sartorius is mobilized along its lateral aspect and retracted medially, while the rectus femoris muscle is retracted laterally. The artery should be found between the adductor longus and the vastus medialis (Figure 4).

Finally, in rare cases where extensive previous dissection has been performed, the profunda femoris may be exposed via a posteromedial or even a direct posterior approach. In the posteromedial approach, the incision is placed more medially than the standard groin incision, and the dissection is carried out inferior to the adductor longus and superior to the gracilis, adductor magnus, and adductor brevis. This approach is closer anatomically to the standard approach and therefore may not achieve the greatest benefit in terms of facilitating dissection through an unscarred field.

The posterior approach is carried out with the patient in a prone position. A vertical incision is made beginning approximately 6 cm superior to 10 cm inferior to the gluteal crease extending along the lateral border of the hamstring muscles. The inferior portion of the gluteus maximus is mobilized, and the sciatic nerve is gently retracted. The dissection is carried between the adductor magnus and the vastus lateralis, and the insertions of the adductor magnus and brevis onto the linea aspera should be incised carefully. The profunda femoris should be found after this maneuver.

Three basic techniques are used for profunda femoris reconstruction. In the first, the vessel is opened, and a patch angioplasty alone is performed. This technique may be utilized where there is not excessive plaque burden, or when it appears that an attempt at endarterectomy may jeopardize the integrity of the vessel. The patch may be either autogenous saphenous vein or endarterectomized superficial femoral artery, a biologic material such as bovine pericardium, or a prosthetic material such as Dacron or polytetrafluoroethylene (PTFE). Autogenous saphenous vein is rarely used for profunda reconstruction, because it is usually reserved for use in coronary artery or lower extremity bypass. When autogenous material is used, proximal (thigh) saphenous vein is preferred to more distal (ankle) vein, because distal vein tends to have thinner walls. Although endarterectomized superficial femoral artery may be used as a patch for repair, it is not preferred, because it increases the amount of dissection required and is prone to restenosis. Prosthetic materials such as Dacron and PTFE can be used to successfully patch even long segments of the profunda femoris and are the most commonly used materials. The patch is generally secured to the artery with 6-0 polypropylene sutures in various configurations, depending on the anatomy (Figure 5).

In the second technique, an endarterectomy is performed, followed by patch closure of the vessel. This technique is utilized where there is a large plaque burden, and simple patch repair is unlikely to achieve satisfactory resolution of the stenosis. Because the disease frequently extends from the common femoral artery, a long-segment endarterectomy extending from the level of the inguinal ligament to the secondary profunda branches may be required. It is advisable to expose the profunda femoris to the level of the first perforating branch, because the disease frequently extends to this level, and control of branch vessels is more easily obtained prior to arteriotomy. This may also be the case when a simple patch is employed. In these cases the arteriotomy must be carefully carried across from the common femoral artery onto the profunda femoris. If a smooth, tapered end point is not achieved, the distal intima is tacked with interrupted

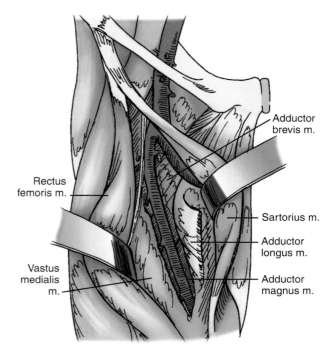

FIGURE 4   Operative exposure of the distal profunda femoral artery. *m,* Muscle. *(From Valentine RJ, Wind GG: Anatomic exposures in vascular surgery, ed 2, Baltimore, 2003, Lippincott Williams & Wilkins, p 429.)*

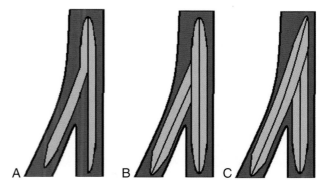

FIGURE 5   Patch configurations that may be used in profundaplasty when patch placement is performed over the profunda femoris and superficial femoral arteries. **A,** The distal patch is split longitudinally with half applied to the profunda femoris and half to the superficial femoral artery. **B,** The patch is sewn in continuity from the common to the superficial femoral artery, and an additional patch is sewn onto from the profunda femoris obliquely to the existing patch. **C,** The patch is sewn in continuity from the common femoral artery to the profunda femoris, and an additional patch is sewn from the superficial femoral artery obliquely to the existing patch.

6-0 or 7-0 polypropylene sutures. Branch vessels along the endarterectomized segment should be inspected to ensure orifice patency.

In either of these techniques, if the proximal superficial femoral artery is involved, the patch—and endarterectomy, if required—may be extended onto both the superficial femoral and profunda femoris arteries. In this case, greater care in performing the arteriotomy is required. The patch may be sewn either from the common onto the superficial femoral, with an extension onto the profunda femoris, or from the common onto the profunda femoris, with an extension onto the superficial femoral artery. Alternatively, the patch may be split in a longitudinal direction, with half secured to the superficial femoral and half secured to the profunda femoris artery.

The third technique is simply to use the hood of the graft being placed as a patch. This technique is used where there is minimal to no stenosis at the profunda femoris orifice, and there is no significant proximal common femoral or distal profunda femoris disease. It is commonly used in the setting of an inflow procedure to the profunda femoris with superficial femoral stenosis or occlusion. Reconstruction in combination with an inflow procedure is usually accomplished by extending the arteriotomy onto the profunda femoris and placing the hood of the graft across any potential stenosis at the orifice. Rarely, when there is occlusion of the entire common femoral and superficial femoral artery, end-to-end anastomosis to the profunda femoris of an inflow graft can be performed, as long as collateral branches are preserved.

Short-segment profunda femoris bypass is an alternative to endarterectomy, where there is a long occlusion, heavy calcification, or dense scarring. Inflow can be obtained from the common femoral or distal external iliac arteries. The major disadvantage is that fewer outflow collaterals are opened as compared with a long-segment endarterectomy.

Endovascular

The role of percutaneous profundaplasty is generally limited because of the presence of associated common femoral artery disease. When a significant lesion is identified by angiography in the profunda, it can be treated through an endovascular approach. Access is obtained by performing a contralateral common femoral arterial puncture. An angled guidewire and sheath are tracked over the aortic bifurcation and antegrade into the profunda. The patient is systemically anticoagulated, and the lesion is crossed with the wire. Isolated balloon angioplasty can be done for proximal lesions, and the "kissing balloon" technique can be done for orificial lesions; in this technique, a balloon is placed in the superficial femoral orifice and inflated simultaneously with the balloon in the profunda. This is done so as not to compromise the diameter of the superficial femoral orifice during profunda angioplasty. Stenting is not usually performed, especially for orifice lesions, unless a dissection or residual gradient is present.

RESULTS

Surgical

The improvement seen with isolated profundaplasty is modest, with documented improvement in ankle-brachial index (ABI) seen in up to 50% of patients. The procedure is associated with a low morbidity and is frequently employed in high-risk patients with limited anatomic options for revascularization. Kalman (1990) reported cumulative success rates of 83% at 30 days, 67% at 1 year, 57% at 2 years, and 49% at 3 years. The cumulative limb-salvage rate was 76% at 3 years. As expected, clinical success was greater when the operative indications were disabling claudication, and the tibial runoff was good. Overall, the change in ABI was significant though small (average of 0.12) in the immediate postoperative period. In patients with long-term clinical success, there was a significant increase in ABI early postoperatively as compared with those patients in whom the procedure was considered a clinical failure. Fugger (1987) reported success with symptomatic relief achieved in 75% of patients when two tibial arteries were patent, 64% when one was patent, and only 31% when none were; patency of the popliteal artery was not essential. The most frequent reported complication was related to the groin wound. Patients should be selected with consideration for not only the degree of profunda femoris stenosis or occlusion but also on the basis of the collateral circulation seen on preprocedural imaging.

The profunda popliteal collateral index (PPCI) was developed to help select patients for isolated profundaplasty. The formula developed was PPCI = AKSP − BKSP/AKSP, where *AKSP* is above-knee segmental pressure and *BKSP* is below-knee segmental pressure. PPCI is an objective measure of the collaterals between the profunda femoris and the distal vascular bed. A PPCI greater than 0.5 suggests poor geniculate collateral flow with a prediction of isolated profundaplasty failure. Boren and colleagues (1980) believed that PPCI could be used to accurately evaluate patients for profunda femoris revascularization.

Isolated profundaplasty is most effective where there is good collateralization, and tibial runoff is adequate. Profundaplasty for limb salvage has disappointing results and should be considered only in patients who are poor operative candidates for distal bypass. Some suggest that profundaplasty may provide sufficient perfusion to preserve the knee joint to permit healing of a below-knee amputation.

In an 18 year experience with 281 aortofemoral bypass grafts, Moore (1978) found that the primary cause of late graft failure was profunda femoris disease, which was believed to be the primary factor in limb occlusion in 54 patients. These patients were treated with thrombectomy and profundaplasty. When combined with an aortic inflow procedure, Kalman (1990) reported a 5-year cumulative patency of 97% for aortofemoral bypass when combined with profundaplasty. Similar improvements in patency have been observed, when profundaplasty was combined with other inflow procedures such as axillofemoral, iliofemoral, and femorofemoral bypass.

Endovascular

Endovascular therapy is an appealing option in high-risk patients with limited options. Because of the relative ease of access and durability of profundaplasty, the impetus for endovascular intervention is not as great as it is in other lower extremity disease. Silva (2001) has reported on 31 consecutive patients with critical limb ischemia treated with percutaneous profundaplasty with an immediate success in 91% of patients. These patients experienced an increase in ABI from 0.5 to 0.7. At 34 months no additional amputations were required, three patients required repeat revascularization, and five patients died. The majority of the lesions treated in this study were of the proximal profunda before the lateral circumflex takeoff. The use of cutting balloon angioplasty has also been recently applied to focal stenoses at the femoral bifurcation with some success.

SUMMARY

Profunda reconstruction is an important adjunct to maintaining limb viability, and it can be performed with low morbidity and mortality. Optimal candidates have a significant profunda stenosis or occlusion, a patent and disease-free good distal profunda, and abundant collaterals to the distal vascular bed. Critical limb ischemia may be treated with isolated profundaplasty but is best treated with a distal bypass and adjunctive profundaplasty if indicated. Profunda stenosis should be corrected wherever possible in patients undergoing either inflow or outflow procedures.

SUGGESTED READINGS

Bertucci WR, Marin ML, Veith FJ, Ohki T: Posterior approach to the deep femoral artery, *J Vasc Surg* 29:741, 1999.

Boren CH, Towne JB, Bernhard VM, Salles-Cunha S: Profundapopliteal collateral index: a guide to successful profundaplasty, *Arch Surg* 115:1366, 1980.

Kalman PG, Jolustor KW, Walker PW: The current role of isolated profundaplasty, *J Cardiovasc Surg* 31:107, 1990.

Silva JA, White CJ, Ramee SR, et al: Percutaneous profundaplasty in the treatment of lower extremity ischemia: results of long-term surveillance, *J Endovasc Ther* 8:75, 2001.

Valentine RJ, Wind CG: *Anatomic exposures in vascular surgery*, ed 2, Baltimore, 2003, Lippincott Williams & Wilkins, p 429.

POPLITEAL AND FEMORAL ARTERY ANEURYSMS

Ryan Messiner, DO, and David C. Han, MD

OVERVIEW

Popliteal and femoral artery aneurysms are the most common peripheral arterial aneurysms. Although popliteal artery aneurysms are typically true aneurysms, involving all three histologic layers of the arterial wall, true femoral artery aneurysms are uncommon. Most commonly, femoral artery aneurysms are false aneurysms (pseudoaneurysms), involving fewer than three layers, and they can occur as a result of penetrating trauma or anastomotic breakdown. True popliteal and femoral artery aneurysms are typically degenerative aneurysms, occurring as a result of atherosclerosis. True aneurysms of the popliteal artery occur predominantly in men, with the highest prevalence during the sixth and seventh decades of life. Patients with a popliteal artery aneurysm often have aneurysms elsewhere in the arterial tree, including the contralateral popliteal artery, the abdominal aorta, or the iliac arteries. Estimates of the incidence of coexistent aneurysms vary but range as high as 50% or more, with the highest incidence in those with bilateral peripheral artery aneurysms. Given the high likelihood of contemporaneous multiple aneurysms, screening in this patient population appears to be justified.

POPLITEAL ARTERY ANEURYSMS

Clinical Presentation

Diagnosis and treatment of popliteal artery aneurysms is directed toward preventing the most typical complication: thromboembolism. Rupture of popliteal artery aneurysms is rare, causing bleeding into the confined popliteal space leading to limb-threatening, but not life-threatening, hemorrhage. Thromboembolism may manifest as *blue toe syndrome* from digital artery emboli or as acute limb-threatening ischemia. Other symptoms of a popliteal artery aneurysm include compression of adjacent structures, leading to either neurological deficits or venous congestion, and deep venous thrombosis. Because up to half of popliteal artery aneurysms are asymptomatic when discovered, a high level of suspicion is necessary, particularly in patients with aortic, iliac, or femoral arterial aneurysms. Other risk factors for atherosclerotic disease, including smoking, hypertension, and diabetes, are often present. A thorough physical examination is mandatory, although palpation for an aneurysmal popliteal artery may be a specific but not very sensitive finding.

Diagnosis

Duplex ultrasound is particularly useful, given the amount of information that can be obtained noninvasively. Diameter, presence of thrombus, and flow characteristics can all be obtained in most vascular labs (Figure 1, *A*). Computed tomography (CT) and magnetic resonance imaging (MRI) can give similar information but do not compare favorably with duplex ultrasound in terms of portability or the avoidance of contrast media and ionizing radiation (Figure 1, *B*). Contrast arteriography is helpful for preoperative planning, as well as endovascular intervention with either thrombolysis of acutely thrombosed popliteal aneurysms, or definitive treatment with endoluminal stent grafting (Figure 1, *C*).

Treatment

Popliteal artery aneurysms that present with limb-threatening ischemia should undergo immediate operative treatment. Although clearly this would preferably include vascular reconstruction and restoration of flow, in some cases of severe ischemia and multiple significant comorbidities, immediate guillotine amputation may be indicated; in rare cases, functional amputation with external cooling and subsequent staged amputation may be done. As in other situations with limb-threatening ischemia, individualization of therapy is necessary, taking into account the amount of time required to initiate either endovascular or open therapy and the patient's condition and available resources. Patients with minimal or mild symptoms, such as claudication or compressive symptoms, should undergo operative repair. Thrombosed asymptomatic popliteal artery aneurysms can be managed nonoperatively.

Because the natural history of popliteal artery aneurysms is not well defined, management of asymptomatic popliteal artery aneurysms remains somewhat controversial. One of three approaches can be taken, with an emphasis on observational care, surgical care, or selective management. Observational management is recommended based on the reduced life expectancy compared with age- and sex-matched controls and high success rates of thrombolytic therapy and subsequent surgical reconstruction for patients with acutely thrombosed popliteal artery aneurysms and acute ischemia.

Proponents of early surgical therapy point to the eventual development of symptoms in a third or more patients, as well as what appears to be a higher incidence of symptoms developing early, within 1 to 2 years after diagnosis. Additionally, bypass patency and limb-salvage rates are higher in asymptomatic patients than in symptomatic patients. A selective approach would take into account patient comorbidities, the presence of available adequate autogenous conduit, and potential risk factors for subsequent complications from the aneurysm. A variety of these risk factors have been proposed, including size greater than 2 cm, presence of mural thrombus, loss of runoff vessels, and distortion within, above, or below the aneurysm; however, none of these have been evaluated in a prospective fashion.

Operative Technique

As with all vascular reconstructions, the decision tree in approaching the patient with a popliteal artery aneurysm that requires repair involves inflow, outflow, and conduit. Autogenous vein is preferable to prosthetic vein, as in other below-knee reconstructions. Determination of inflow can be made by physical exam but is perhaps best done with contrast arteriography in the event of a diminished ipsilateral femoral pulse. Outflow can be assessed by duplex ultrasound but is again probably best suited to evaluation by contrast arteriography. In the setting of an acutely thrombosed popliteal artery aneurysm, a patient whose neurovascular findings suggest tolerance of the time required for catheter-directed thrombolysis is best treated using that technique, with determination of outflow based on the outcome. When time is insufficient for percutaneous thrombolysis, intraoperative balloon catheter embolectomy is indicated, potentially supplemented by intraoperative intraarterial instillation of thrombolytic agents.

In the elective setting, repair can be performed through either a medial or posterior approach. The medial approach is preferred by many, given its familiarity and that it affords the surgeon the opportunity to extensively expose the femoral, popliteal, and tibial vessels. Additionally, access to the saphenous vein in the thigh is convenient and allows a more appropriately sized conduit in these patients, who often have diffuse arteriomegaly. For this approach, the guiding principles include exclusion of the aneurysmal portion of the artery, while constructing as short a bypass as feasible. End-to-end or end-to-side

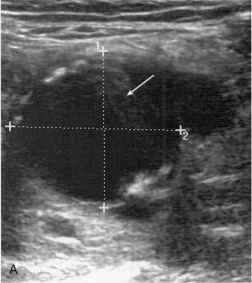

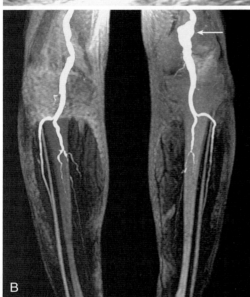

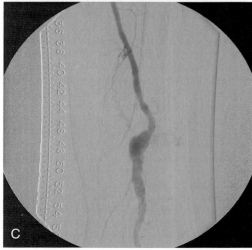

FIGURE I   **A,** DUS of popliteal artery aneurysm (*transverse view*) with intraluminal thrombus (*arrow*). **B,** Magnetic resonance angiogram showing left popliteal artery aneurysm (*arrow*). **C,** Contrast arteriogram showing left popliteal artery aneurysm.

anastomoses are acceptable, with an end-to-side anastomosis preferred when size is mismatched between artery and conduit. Proximal and distal ligation are performed to prevent both competitive flow through the native artery and distal thromboembolization. Exploration along the outer wall of the popliteal artery can be hazardous because of adherence to adjacent veins, but it should be done to the extent possible to ligate side branches and prevent retrograde flow into the aneurysm sac, which is analogous to a type II endoleak from endovascular repair of an aortic aneurysm.

A posterior approach to the popliteal artery limits the proximal and distal extent of arterial exposure and limits access to the greater saphenous vein in the thigh. Nonetheless, this is the preferred approach when the popliteal artery aneurysm is large, or when it is causing compressive symptoms. Through this approach, the aneurysm can be incised and decompressed, with oversewing of branches from within and repair performed through a standard endoaneurysmorrhaphy technique. The saphenous vein in the thigh can be harvested initially, and the patient can then be turned in a prone position. In some cases, the small saphenous vein may be used; preoperative vein mapping using duplex ultrasound is very helpful in this setting.

Endovascular techniques using covered stent grafts are gaining in popularity, with multiple successful case reports. Advantages include the less invasive nature of a percutaneous approach and attendant decreases in wound complications and recovery time. Prospective studies, however, are lacking, and the concern of placing a prosthetic into a position across and below the knee joint continues to hamper enthusiasm for widespread acceptance of this method for those who are suitable candidates for open reconstruction.

Results

Patients who undergo elective repair of asymptomatic popliteal artery aneurysms enjoy excellent outcomes with regard to perioperative mortality, patency, and limb-salvage rates. Indeed, patency rates are generally better than those grafts done for atherosclerosis, with 10 year patency rates approaching 94%. For those who undergo repair for symptomatic aneurysms, however, 10-year patency rates drop to approximately 50%. Similarly, perioperative morbidity and mortality rates are higher in patients undergoing repair for symptomatic aneurysms.

Particular attention should be given to longitudinal follow-up of these patients. Up to one third of patients can develop additional aneurysms (aortoiliac, femoral, and contralateral popliteal). Additionally, for patients who have undergone interposition grafting with aneurysm ligation, the risk of retrograde bleeding and persistence of the aneurysm sac is present. This can occur in as many as 33% of patients, with the risk of subsequent compression of the adjacent vein and nerve. When this occurs, an attempt at endovascular coiling is reasonable (Figure 2), but these patients can be easily treated through a posterior approach, with direct visualization and ligation of the back-bleeding branch vessels (Figure 3).

FEMORAL ARTERY ANEURYSMS

Aneurysms of the femoral artery are either true or false aneurysms. When considered together, the femoral artery is the most common location for peripheral arterial aneurysms, although true aneurysms are more common in the popliteal artery than the femoral artery. Because the femoral artery is a common site for percutaneous access for diagnostic, therapeutic, and recreational use, as well as a useful site for bypass grafting as an outflow or inflow vessel, false aneurysms can occur in the setting of direct trauma, infection, or breakdown of an anastomosis. True aneurysms, as in the popliteal artery, are often degenerative and are more strongly associated than popliteal aneurysms with bilaterality and aneurysms in other arterial beds.

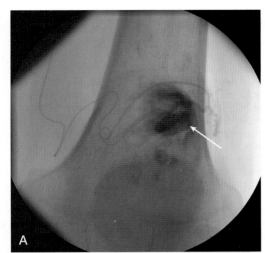

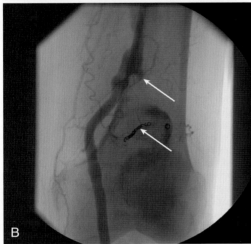

FIGURE 2   **A,** Angiogram demonstrating persistent filling of popliteal aneurysm sac (*arrow*) through collateral vessels. Initial bypass and ligation was performed 3 years prior. **B,** Coil embolization of collateral vessel causing persistence and growth of popliteal artery aneurysm (*bottom arrow*). The ligated native popliteal artery is seen proximally (*top arrow*).

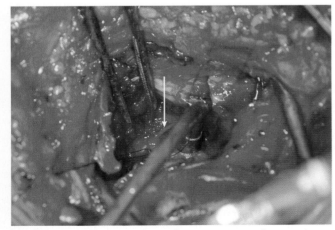

FIGURE 3   Intraoperative photo of posterior approach to persistent enlarging popliteal artery aneurysm sac. Active backbleeding is noted (*arrow*).

Femoral aneurysms typically involve the common femoral artery. Aneurysms localized only to the deep femoral or superficial femoral artery are rare. A common classification scheme denotes type I aneurysms as those limited to the common femoral artery; type II are those that involve the orifice of the deep femoral artery, which is helpful in recognizing that type II aneurysms will generally require more complex reconstruction. Aneurysms of the external iliac artery are rare.

Clinical Presentation

Femoral artery aneurysms may be asymptomatic and discovered on physical exam. Because CT scans done for abdominal aortic aneurysms routinely acquire images through the femoral arteries to assess eligibility for endovascular grafting, femoral artery aneurysms may be found incidentally as well. Symptoms of a femoral aneurysm often are due to their size, with a pulsatile palpable mass, local discomfort, or compression of the adjacent vein and/or nerve evident. Pain, swelling, bruising, or a new bruit are suggestive of an iatrogenic femoral pseudoaneurysm. Traumatic aneurysms should be thoroughly assessed, as significant bleeding can occur into the retroperitoneal space with few physical findings until the onset of hypovolemic shock. As with popliteal aneurysms, femoral aneurysms are much more common in men than women. Thromboembolism is the most concerning complication, although superficial and deep femoral aneurysms appear more prone to rupture.

Diagnosis

Beyond physical examination, duplex ultrasound provides a reliable, noninvasive method of diagnosis. CT arteriography can also supply the necessary information for both diagnosis and treatment, although contrast angiography is still considered by many a necessary step to evaluate reconstruction options. Ultrasound findings consistent with an iatrogenic false aneurysm include a back-and-forth flow in the pedicle leading to the pseudoaneurysm, as well as swirling within the false aneurysm itself, consistent with inflow and outflow through a common pedicle (Figure 4).

Treatment

Operative repair is indicated for symptomatic femoral artery aneurysms, regardless of size. For asymptomatic aneurysms, as with popliteal aneurysms, decisions to intervene should be determined by the risk of development of complications balanced by the patient's comorbidities. There is no consensus as to the size at which a femoral artery aneurysm is likely to cause symptoms, although a rapid expansion of the aneurysm or the presence of intraluminal thrombus would suggest that surgical intervention should be considered.

Iatrogenic Femoral Pseudoaneurysms

The advent of ultrasound-guided compression and ultrasound-guided thrombin injection has allowed a less invasive method of treating these lesions. Although many small (<1 cm) pseudoaneurysms will spontaneously thrombose, many patients remain anticoagulated as a result of their original percutaneous intervention. Contraindications to thrombin injection include a short and/or wide pedicle, where thromboembolic complications are more likely, or an indication for open surgical repair, such as the presence of a large hematoma or skin necrosis. In experienced hands, however, the incidence of complications from ultrasound-guided thrombin injection is low, and thus it should be considered in appropriate patients.

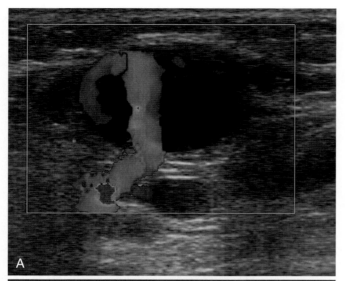

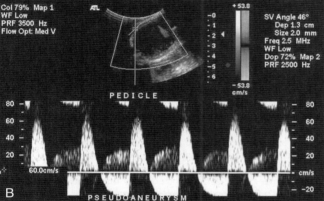

FIGURE 4 **A,** DUS of femoral pseudoaneurysm. **B,** Back-and-forth flow in pedicle of femoral pseudoaneurysm.

Infected Femoral Pseudoaneurysms

As with symptomatic aneurysms, infected femoral aneurysms should be repaired regardless of size. Overtly infected aneurysms, with associated drainage and cellulitis, and evidence of remote infection, such as septic arthritis or endocarditis, represent management challenges but not necessarily a diagnostic dilemma. More challenging is the anastomotic false aneurysm with no clinical signs of infection, in which as many as 60% are positive on culture for low-virulence staphylococcal organisms such as *Staphylococcus epidermidis*. Although in situ repair can generally be accomplished, preferably with autogenous conduit, an operative plan that includes ligation, wide debridement, and extraanatomic bypass must be prepared.

Operative Technique

The same principles for repair of other aneurysms apply to femoral artery aneurysms: exclusion of the aneurysm and restoration of arterial flow. Similarly, the operative plan is formed around inflow, outflow, and conduit. Variable involvement of the superficial and deep femoral arteries, as well as the potential for the presence of infection, requires a preoperative plan that can adapt intraoperatively as needed to any unexpected findings. For most femoral aneurysms, the presence of multiple branches in an area that crosses a joint makes endovascular repair less attractive than open repair. In the case of traumatic or iatrogenic aneurysms, however, less invasive methods may be available, and in many cases, they are preferable.

Degenerative True Aneurysms

The approach to the uninfected femoral aneurysm that has not had prior surgical exposure is relatively straightforward. Inflow is typically obtained from the distal external iliac artery, given that aneurysms of the external iliac artery are extremely rare. In some cases, such as a large femoral aneurysm in a very thin patient, proximal control may be required through a transplant-type flank incision, with retroperitoneal control of the external iliac artery. Intraluminal balloon control via the contralateral femoral artery is also an option but is probably unnecessary.

Outflow is constructed to the distal common femoral artery in type I femoral aneurysms, when the superficial femoral and deep femoral arteries are normal. For type II aneurysms, depending on the orientation of the vessels, an end-to-end anastomosis to one vessel is appropriate, with either a separate jump graft to or reimplantation of the other vessel. In some cases the adjacent walls of the superficial and deep femoral arteries can be sewn together, creating a common orifice for the outflow target. Prosthetic material is acceptable, given the high flows and no demonstrated improvements in patency with saphenous vein; although if reconstruction beyond the most proximal superficial femoral artery is required, autogenous conduit should be considered.

Anastomotic Femoral Aneurysms

Because of the previous surgical dissection, reoperative surgery is often challenging and tedious. Again, the operative plan requires an assessment of inflow, outflow, and conduit. As much direct control of the graft and the native vessels and branches should be obtained as possible. Intraluminal control with balloon catheters is helpful but can become quite cumbersome if multiple catheters are required. In some patients, proximal and distal control are best obtained through incisions remote to the groin. Retroperitoneal control of the inflow graft or the native external iliac artery is helpful, particularly if the aneurysm extends up to or above the inguinal ligament. An incision in the proximal to mid thigh, to identify the superficial and/or deep femoral artery, and then subsequent dissection back into the groin is also a useful technique.

After obtaining proximal and distal control, the patient is systemically anticoagulated, and the aneurysm is entered. In many cases, the suture line has dehisced, and the fibrous capsule of the false aneurysm is holding the anastomosis together. Debridement of the involved artery may allow preservation of enough of the native vessel to allow its use again for anastomosis, and either the graft limb can be reattached to the native artery or, more commonly, an interposition graft from the graft limb to the native artery is performed. More extensive resection may be required, particularly if damage to the native vessels occurs during the reoperative dissection. In particular, the vessels should be closely examined to ensure that the adventitia is intact, as aggressive dissection in a reoperative field can often lead to dissection in the subadventitial plane. In these cases the vessel with the stripped adventitia must be resected and replaced.

Infected Femoral Aneurysms

Primarily infected femoral aneurysms occur as a result of direct injection without aseptic technique. Femoral aneurysms can also become secondarily infected from a remote source, such as endocarditis. Both require an appreciation of the standard principles of ligation of the involved vessels, wide debridement, and reconstruction as necessary through uninvolved tissue planes. Such bypasses can be constructed as an axillary to superficial femoral artery bypass or an obturator bypass, both of which avoid tunneling through the infected groin. Our preference has been to perform the reconstruction and the excision at the same time, with the reconstruction performed first, thus avoiding both prolonged ischemia and the need to reprep and change instruments prior to beginning the "clean" portion of the procedure.

Staging of these procedures runs the risk of allowing the extraanatomic bypass to become secondarily infected. An alternative approach is to ligate and excise the infected vessels, and then assess the circulation. This is a reasonable approach when extraanatomic bypass is not feasible or is relatively contraindicated, such as in a patient with ongoing drug abuse, where placement of a subcutaneous graft would not address the underlying cause.

A less appealing alternative is treatment with in situ graft replacement, which is best done with autogenous conduit, although polytetrafluoroethylene (PTFE) and rifampin-soaked Dacron have been used with limited success. But the same attendant risks as in aortic replacement apply in these patients, including anastomotic blowout. The likelihood of success is increased with less virulent organisms, and several studies have attempted to assess the timing of infection relative to the original graft implantation, as it relates to the identification of the causative organism. Rotational muscle flaps are often helpful to provide vascularized tissue coverage of the repair.

Iatrogenic Femoral Aneurysms

Although less invasive methods for repair that include thrombin injection and compression using ultrasound guidance have become widely used, open surgical repair is the gold standard against which these methods should be compared. If the pseudoaneurysm is sufficiently large to cause compressive effects, or if there is significant skin distension or necrosis, thrombin injection will not relieve these symptoms, and open repair is indicated.

Open Surgical Repair

Wide skin preparation is essential to allow the surgeon access for proximal and distal control in areas remote from the injury. A retroperitoneal approach may be required to obtain control of the external iliac artery for injuries to the common femoral artery at the groin. Additionally, preparation of an uninjured limb for vein harvesting is preferable. After obtaining proximal and distal control, the aneurysm is entered, and the site of the injury is identified. In many cases, simple suture repair is all that is necessary, but in those vessels with significant underlying atherosclerotic occlusive disease, endarterectomy and patch angioplasty may be required. In these patients, thromboembolic complications are likely to be encountered. In patients with an injury near the femoral bifurcation and a chronically occluded superficial femoral artery (SFA), profundaplasty using an endarterectomized segment of the SFA is a good option. Interposition grafting, if required, can be performed with autogenous vein, Dacron, or PTFE. In these more complex cases with underlying occlusive pathology, the primary goal is to restore the circulation to the preinjury state; attempts to make significant circulatory improvements, such as extensive endarterectomy or concomitant bypass, are generally ill advised in this setting.

Ultrasound-Guided Repair

The goal of ultrasound-guided treatment is to induce thrombosis of the pseudoaneurysm without causing thrombosis or introducing thrombus in the underlying feeding vessel. Ultrasound-guided compression has been used with moderate success but should be considered a second-line therapy to thrombin injection. Compression therapy uses ultrasound imaging to guide the operator, such that the aneurysm is compressed, but the underlying vessel remains patent. Although no standard protocol has been defined, most reports and most experienced operators suggest compression for up to an hour, with repeated episodes of compression sometimes required to achieve success. Because of the significant discomfort, conscious sedation of the patient may be needed, and this procedure can be very tiresome for the operator. Success rates are variable, and with the availability of thrombin injection, compression should not be considered as an initial therapy.

Ultrasound-guided thrombin injection is a safe, rapid, effective, and durable method to treat iatrogenic femoral aneurysms. After localization

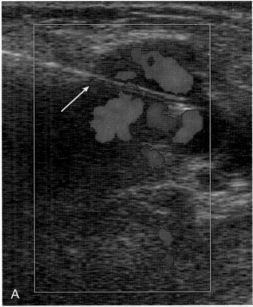

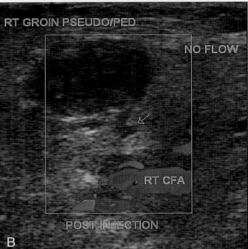

FIGURE 5 **A,** Placement of needle (*arrow*) into pseudoaneurysm. **B,** Successful thrombosis of femoral pseudoaneurysm.

with ultrasound, either a 21 or 18 gauge spinal needle is introduced with the stylet in place. Although a 21 gauge needle can be used without the need for local anesthetic, the larger 18 gauge needle is more easily seen (Figure 5, *A*). Turning off the color flow will allow optimal visualization of the needle. As the needle is seen to enter the aneurysm, the stylet is withdrawn. If there is no return of pulsatile blood, the needle is not in the aneurysm. Color flow is turned back on, and a prepared solution of thrombin (1,000 U/mL) in a 1 mL tuberculin syringe is then injected slowly over 2 to 3 seconds. Cessation of flow is seen as the color flow disappears (Figure 5, *B*). Typically, 600 to 800 units of thrombin are required, however, with larger or multilobulated aneurysms, more may be needed. Great care should be taken to avoid injecting directly in or around the neck or pedicle of the pseudoaneurysm, as this will increase the chances of thrombus entering the underlying artery.

Endovascular Repair

Although traumatic injury to the visceral and pelvic vessels can lead to pseudoaneurysms that are best treated with percutaneous methods, such as microvascular coils or thrombotic agents or particles,

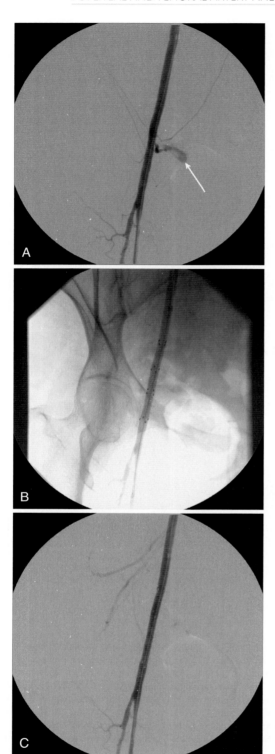

injuries to the femoral vessels, where thrombosis of the vessel is not an option, are more suited to treatment with commercial, investigational, or homemade covered stents. In these patients, treatment must be individualized. Iatrogenic injury to the femoral vessels may be treated quickly using a covered stent, with rapid cessation of hemorrhage (Figure 6). This is highly advantageous in the morbidly obese patient, in whom rapid proximal and distal control would be difficult in an open setting. This also avoids the potential morbidity from large incisions. These solutions, although rapid, may be temporary, given that placement of a stent across a joint often leads to occlusion and subsequent open revision.

Results

Results of repair of femoral artery aneurysms depend on the underlying cause and comorbid factors. For open repair of degenerative aneurysms, results are excellent, and long-term patencies approach 100%. For repairs done under urgent or emergent circumstances, results are less favorable, as would be expected. Outcomes from iatrogenic femoral aneurysms often depend on the underlying condition, such as coronary artery disease, that led to the need for femoral access. Infected femoral aneurysms have a much higher likelihood of wound complications, subsequent graft infection, and thrombosis. Major amputations may be required in up to 25% of these patients.

SELECTED READINGS

Calton WC, Franklin DP, Elmore JR, Han DC: Ultrasound-guided thrombin injection is a safe and durable treatment for femoral pseduoaneurysms, *Vasc Surg* 35(5):379–383, 2001.

Diwan A, Sarkar R, Stanley JC, et al: Incidence of femoral and popliteal artery aneurysms in patients with abdominal aortic aneurysms, *J Vasc Surg* 31(5):863–869, 2000.

Michaels JA, Galland RB: Management of asymptomatic popliteal aneurysms: the use of a Markov decision tree to determine the criteria for a conservative approach, *Eur J Vasc Surg* 7(2):136–143, 1993.

FIGURE 6   **A,** Contrast arteriogram demonstrating extravasation into false aneurysm sac from distal external iliac artery/proximal common femoral artery. **B,** Percutaneous stent placement across area of injury. **C,** Completion arteriogram demonstrating resolution of the pseudoaneurysm.

Treatment of Vasculogenic Claudication

Spence M. Taylor, MD

OVERVIEW

Lower extremity peripheral arterial disease (PAD) affects more than 10 million individuals in the United States, including an estimated 4.3% of adults older than 40 years and 14.5% older than 70 years. Clinically, patients with PAD have one of these three symptoms: 1) asymptomatic chronic subclinical ischemia, 2) intermittent claudication, or 3) critical limb ischemia (CLI). In turn, CLI can occur with either rest pain or tissue loss.

When considering lower extremity PAD, any patient older than 40 years who is found to have an ankle-brachial index (ABI) of less than 0.9 has significant PAD. Interestingly, more than 50% of patients with an abnormal ABI have no appreciable symptoms, a condition referred to as *asymptomatic chronic subclinical ischemia* (ACSI). When a patient is identified as having ACSI, initiation of cardiovascular risk-factor modification is indicated. In contrast, patients with CLI are generally offered surgical revascularization for the concern that the severity of the vascular disease will result in major limb amputation if left untreated.

Patients with vasculogenic claudication fall in the middle of the spectrum. Consequently, its treatment has been controversial. Conventional wisdom, founded on evidence from the 1960s and 1970s, has recommended nonoperative management for the vast majority of patients with intermittent claudication. This recommendation was based on the benign natural history of untreated claudication and the substantial risk of morbidity and mortality associated with operative intervention. Recently, however, that wisdom has been challenged, and a more liberal approach toward operative intervention for patients with claudication has emerged. The basis of this approach rests on the growing popularity of endovascular intervention and the reappraisal of treatment goals from "physician-oriented" to "patient-oriented" end points. Regardless of whether operative intervention is chosen, an understanding of the medical treatment of claudication is essential.

MEDICAL TREATMENT OF CLAUDICATION

Treatment recommendations for intermittent claudication have traditionally balanced the risk of intervention against the natural history of the disease. The natural history of lower extremity PAD has been well studied and is summarized in Figure 1. It has long been appreciated that claudication is more a marker of systemic atherosclerosis and less a predictor of limb loss. The American College of Cardiology/American Heart Association (ACC/AHA) guidelines suggest that the risk of major limb amputation for a patient with intermittent claudication is approximately 1% per year, and the risk of cardiac death is approximately 3% to 5% per year. Treatment strategies have therefore stressed cardiovascular risk-factor modification and medical therapy as the best initial treatment for patients with intermittent claudication.

Revascularization is recommended only in cases of severe claudication and only after medical therapy has failed. As well, the conservative treatment of claudication has been further rationalized by the belief that revascularization can negatively impact the benign natural history of the disease. Intervention opens a Pandora's box of therapy manifested by a series of revascularizations, failures, repeat revascularizations, and eventual limb amputation. Although this is unproven, it dovetails with the premise that surgical morbidity, such as the leg edema after open infrainguinal bypass, often offsets the palliative advantages of revascularization. Therefore, the current accepted initial treatment of vasculogenic claudication is nonsurgical and includes cardiovascular risk-factor modification, smoking cessation, supervised exercise, and pharmacologic therapy.

Cardiovascular Risk Factor Modification

Other than advanced age, which has been shown to increase the incidence of PAD by 150% to 200% for every decade of life, the most common risk factors for the development of PAD include smoking, diabetes mellitus, hypertension, and hyperlipidemia. All patients with the diagnosis of PAD should pursue risk-factor modification, regardless of whether intervention is being contemplated.

Smoking Cessation

For the good of their overall cardiovascular health, patients with intermittent claudication should be encouraged to abstain from all tobacco products. However, the benefit of smoking cessation in the relief of claudication is not clear. Although studies have shown that smoking cessation can improve walking distances in some cases, these findings are not universal. However, the association between tobacco cessation and the reduction of subsequent cardiovascular events is undisputed. The role of the physician in smoking cessation is to educate patients about the consequences of this high-risk behavior, to provide emotional support, and to prescribe pharmacologic aids aimed at treating the addiction. While structured smoking-cessation programs have demonstrated 22% cessation rates at 5 years, compared with 5% in patients who attempt to stop smoking independently, a recent meta-analysis has shown that long-term smoking cessation is successful in as few as 6% of patients. Pharmacologic agents such as bupropion, and more recently varenicline, have increased smoking-cessation rates in randomized studies of patients with PAD, but they have no documented long-term track record. Despite the promise of these new pharmacologic agents, tobacco addiction tends to be characterized by frequent relapses and poor long-term (>1 year) success, and the best hope for prevention is to avoid initial exposure.

Control of Diabetes

The association between diabetes mellitus and atherosclerotic vascular disease is well documented. Diabetes is widely prevalent among patients with lower extremity ischemia. It has been estimated that each incremental 1% increase in glycosalated hemoglobin is associated with a 28% increase in risk for PAD. In addition, diabetes is associated with a variety of microvascular complications, such as diabetic retinopathy and nephropathy, which appear to be a direct consequence of poor blood glucose control. Although the role of tight glucose control on the prevention of macrovascular complications is less clear, experts continue to believe that strict glucose control in PAD patients is important to prevent further atherosclerotic complications. The current American Diabetes Association (ADA) guidelines recommend hemoglobin A1c of less than 7.0% as a global goal for treatment of patients with diabetes. The ADA further suggests that the goal of therapy should be to maintain serum glucose as close to normal as possible (A1c less than 6%) in patients with atherosclerosis without inducing significant hypoglycemia.

Hypertension Therapy

Multiple studies have confirmed that hypertension is associated with a twofold to threefold increased risk of PAD. Hypertension is also a risk factor for stroke, coronary artery disease, congestive heart failure, and

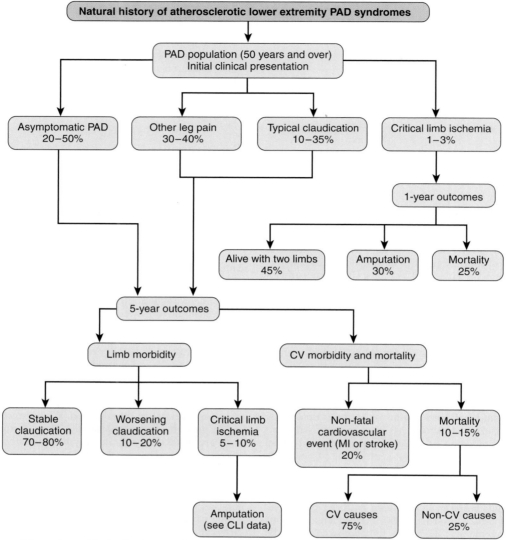

FIGURE 1   The fate of the patient with claudication over 5 years. *(From Norgren L, Hiatt WR, Dormandy JA: Inter-Society Consensus for the Management of Peripheral Arterial Disease (TASC II), J Vasc Surg 45[suppl S]:S10A, 2007.)*

chronic renal insufficiency. Current guidelines recommend achieving a target blood pressure less than 140/90 mm Hg in high-risk groups, such as those with documented PAD, and less than 130/80 mm Hg in patients who also have diabetes or renal insufficiency.

Cholesterol Reduction Therapy

Elevated total serum cholesterol levels greater than 200 mg/dL are associated with an increased risk of cardiac-related events, especially when found in combination with a low level of high-density lipoprotein (HDL) (<40 mg/dL in men, <50 mg/dL in women) and an elevated level of low-density lipoprotein (LDL) (>130 mg/dL). Lipid-lowering agents, specifically 3-hydroxy-3-methylglutaryl coenzyme A (HMG-COA) reductase inhibitors, also known as *statins,* have been shown to be beneficial by reducing cardiac-related events in multiple well-designed studies. Recently, PAD-specific benefits have been shown to occur with statin therapy. These include improvements in ABI, walking performance, symptoms of claudication, and perioperative and long-term mortality. Currently the ACC/AHA guidelines recommend an LDL cholesterol level below 100 mg/dL in patients with PAD and an even lower level in high-risk patients with more generalized atherosclerosis.

Supervised Walking Programs

Multiple reports have clearly demonstrated improvements in pain-free ambulation and overall walking performance with structured walking exercise training. The benefits of exercise extend beyond symptomatic improvement of claudication. Regular aerobic exercise reduces cardiovascular risk by lowering cholesterol and blood pressure and by improving glycemic control. The current ACC/AHA guidelines regarding the management of PAD support supervised exercise for the treatment of intermittent claudication as a level IA recommendation. The guidelines suggest exercise training, in the form of walking, for a minimum of 30 to 45 minutes per session, three to four times per week, for a period of not less than 12 weeks. Unfortunately, although exercise therapy appears easy to implement, effectiveness is often limited by poor patient compliance. Effective exercise training is not possible in up to 34% of patients because of other comorbid medical conditions, and an additional 30% of patients simply refuse to participate in exercise training. Although studies have shown the superiority of clinic-based exercise programs to home-based programs, supervised exercise training programs are not usually covered by most third-party insurance plans, including Medicare. Therefore, although exercise therapy in motivated patients offers proven benefits, its effectiveness is only applicable to approximately one third of patients with intermittent claudication.

Pharmacologic Therapy

There are currently two Food and Drug Administration (FDA) approved drugs for the treatment of vasculogenic claudication. The first drug, pentoxifylline, was approved in 1984 and is important not because of its clinical impact, but because it demonstrated that claudication could be successfully treated with pharmacologic intervention. Although its definitive mechanism of action is poorly understood, pentoxifylline is thought to improve oxygen delivery through its rheolytic effect on red blood cell wall flexibility and deformability, ultimately reducing blood viscosity. The second FDA-approved drug for the treatment of claudication is cilostazol, approved in 1999; an oral phosphodiesterase-3 inhibitor, it increases cyclic adenosine monophosphate and results in a variety of physiologic effects felt to enhance walking muscle performance. Several controlled clinical trials, including a meta-analysis, have shown cilostazol to increase maximum walking distances up to 50% and to significantly improve quality-of-life measures. Unfortunately, cilostazol has a significant adverse-effect profile that includes headache, diarrhea, and gastrointestinal discomfort. Its use is contraindicated in patients with congestive heart failure. Although ACC/AHA guidelines recommend a therapeutic trial of cilostazol as an effective method for increasing overall ambulation, its impact in my clinical practice has been minimally significant.

Patients with vasculogenic claudication should be started on an HMG-CoA reductase inhibitor, which has been shown to improve walking distance in patients with PAD, and an antiplatelet agent. Despite what may be directly marketed to the public, antiplatelet agents, including clopidogrel, do not relieve the symptoms of claudication, but they do reduce overall cardiovascular morbidity.

SURGICAL MANAGEMENT OF VASCULOGENIC CLAUDICATION

Although few would argue the importance of risk-factor modification in all patients with PAD, the ability of such measures to improve ambulatory pain has drawn increased scrutiny in recent years. Smoking cessation is successful long term in fewer than 20% of patients despite the latest and best pharmacologic aids. Supervised exercise therapy, though effective, is not tolerated in as many as 60% to 70% of patients because of associated comorbidities and patient noncompliance. Although pharmacologic therapy has been shown to increase walking distance, it is associated with side effects severe enough to stop the medication in 15% of patients. Thus current assessment of medical therapy for claudication can be summarized by saying that, at best, it is effective in relieving ambulatory leg pain in only one third of patients. Despite this, medical therapy has traditionally been considered the best initial therapy, chiefly due to the morbidity associated with open surgery. These perspectives, however, are changing, largely because of the emergence of endovascular intervention and the reorientation of our treatment goals to patient-centered, functional outcomes.

Endovascular Intervention and Its Impact on Therapy

Although the basic tenants of balloon angioplasty for the treatment of arterial stenoses have been present since the 1970s, surgeons initially favored open bypass to treat symptomatic PAD, citing dismal patency rates after angioplasty. Outcome results published by interventional radiology in the 1980s were largely ignored, and angioplasty was used infrequently, because the surgeons usually controlled the flow of patients to the radiologists. This radically changed with

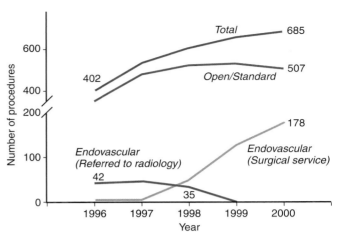

FIGURE 2 The impact of integrating an endovascular surgery program in which angioplasty is performed by vascular surgeons into a mature vascular practice.

the development of the endovascular stent graft for the treatment of aneurysmal disease. In a fairly unprecedented manner, vascular surgeons retooled themselves to incorporate endovascular therapy into their treatment armamentarium. The impact of this proved to be substantial. Technology previously dismissed as ineffective by most vascular surgeons quickly became integrated into the mainstream management of PAD almost overnight. In data published from our institution shortly after establishment of an endovascular service, wherein vascular surgeons who had previously referred cases to interventional radiology began performing their own peripheral interventions, open surgical volume dropped 5%, endovascular therapy increased by more than 400%, and referrals to interventional radiology essentially ceased (Figure 2). Thus the integration of endovascular skills into our practice resulted in a fourfold increase in peripheral angioplasty.

Although the mitigating factors influencing this rapid transition can be debated, the impact on the care of the vascular patient cannot. Percutaneous angioplasty is easier on the patient, the surgeon, and the health care delivery system. Angioplasty can be performed with lower morbidity and mortality than open surgical bypass. And although interventional patency rates are often inferior to open bypass, restenosis is often well tolerated and does not preclude the subsequent performance of a surgical bypass. These characteristics are particularly applicable to patients with intermittent claudication. Open bypass operations and their associated inpatient stay, wound-healing issues, and chronic lower extremity edema have been replaced by percutaneous outpatient angioplasty, with return to work in 48 hours and an almost instantaneous relief of ambulatory leg pain. It can safely be said that the incorporation of endovascular therapy into the treatment mix has substantially altered the risk/benefit ratio toward the interventional treatment of claudication.

Patient-Oriented Versus Physician-Oriented Outcomes

The traditional measures of success after lower extremity revascularization—namely, reconstruction patency, limb salvage, and mortality—often do not fully address the broad concerns of most patients with lower extremity PAD. These measures of success are physician-oriented endpoints. For instance, bypass patency after revascularization, the champion of physician-oriented outcomes, matters little to the patient if progressive disability, limb loss, or death occurs over the ensuing months. A better understanding of patient-oriented outcomes, characterized by patient expectations after treatment, is clearly needed. In the case of claudication, evidence is conspicuously absent. Not only are the traditional end points of success, limb salvage, and patency too insensitive, observational studies consisting exclusively of patients with claudication are almost nonexistent. Critical inspection of the current literature shows that published reports typically combine patients with claudication and critical limb ischemia. Outcomes, therefore, are usually a blend of results from both groups. This is particularly incriminating for claudication, because patients with claudication typically make up the minority of the study cohort, and outcomes predominantly reflect the relatively inferior results achieved when treating critical limb ischemia.

It is important to understand what patient-oriented goals after intervention might be. In the case of claudication, an obvious goal should be relief of the patient's chief complaint: exercise-induced leg pain. In 2000, Feinglass and his colleagues from Northwestern University published an important study that challenged our traditional view of success after treatment for claudication. They used SF-36 quality-of-life questionnaires to measure physical well-being and emotional improvement after revascularization. They found that intervention for claudication improved patients' quality-of-life scores considerably. Improvements varied directly with interventional patency but were similar to those found after coronary artery bypass surgery for angina and one half as beneficial as hip-replacement surgery. In a report from our institution that used SF-36 questionnaires to assess quality of life after angioplasty for claudication and critical limb ischemia, similar findings were obtained. However, findings were strikingly dissimilar between patients with critical limb ischemia and patients with claudication. Patients with critical limb ischemia achieved little or no measurable quality-of-life improvement after intervention, but patients with claudication improved in almost every category. Survival was markedly worse, as expected, for critical limb ischemia as well. Our findings suggest that PAD represents a broad clinical spectrum. Patients with critical limb ischemia tend to be chronically ill individuals, often near the end of life; patients with claudication are more akin to healthy people who have ambulatory leg pain. Our data suggest that patients with claudication expect relief of walking discomfort, a patient-oriented end point, as a goal of treatment, and they may not be satisfied by risk-factor modification alone, a physician-oriented priority.

With this in mind, we recently examined a contemporary series of over 1700 patients treated for PAD. We sought to examine both physician-oriented outcomes (primary and secondary patency and limb salvage) and patient-oriented outcomes (symptom relief, maintenance of ambulation, and maintenance of independent living status). We also sought to test the hypothesis that patients treated for claudication perform vastly differently from patients with ischemic rest pain and ischemic tissue loss. Indeed, we found a declining spectrum of performance outcomes, from claudication to rest pain to tissue loss, for both physician-oriented (Figure 3) and patient-oriented (Figure 4) outcomes. The findings suggested that claudication, ischemic rest pain, and ischemic tissue loss represent three different clinical syndromes of a single pathologic process. We concluded that treatment outcomes for lower extremity PAD depend on presentation, and therefore treatment regimens should be tailored accordingly. We also concluded that surgical revascularization is probably underutilized for patients with claudication and overutilized for patients with critical limb ischemia.

The outcomes for claudication were particularly noteworthy. Of the 999 limbs treated, angioplasty was utilized in 65% of cases, and 70% involved the treatment of aortoiliac occlusive disease. Periprocedural mortality was 0.7%, morbidity was 7%, and only 9 amputations were performed for the entire series, none of which occurred early. Primary reconstruction patency at 5 years was 71%, secondary patency was 94%, limb salvage was 99%, and survival was 77%. Symptom relief was reported in nearly 80% of patients treated. Symptom recurrence happened in only 18% of patients who achieved initial symptom relief, and maintenance of ambulation and independence occurred in more than 96% of patients.

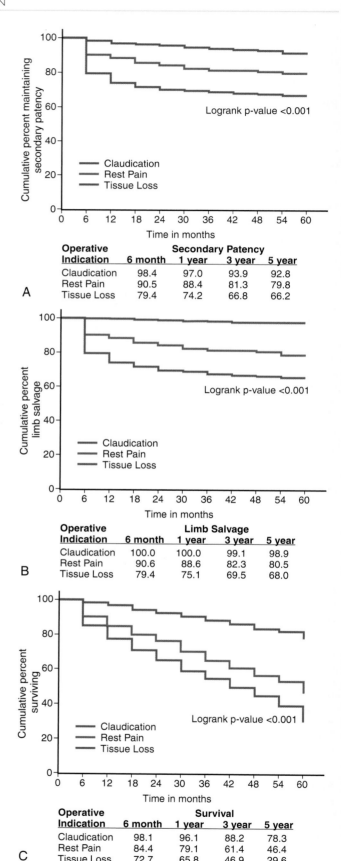

Operative	Secondary Patency			
Indication	6 month	1 year	3 year	5 year
Claudication	98.4	97.0	93.9	92.8
Rest Pain	90.5	88.4	81.3	79.8
Tissue Loss	79.4	74.2	66.8	66.2

A

Operative	Limb Salvage			
Indication	6 month	1 year	3 year	5 year
Claudication	100.0	100.0	99.1	98.9
Rest Pain	90.6	88.6	82.3	80.5
Tissue Loss	79.4	75.1	69.5	68.0

B

Operative	Survival			
Indication	6 month	1 year	3 year	5 year
Claudication	98.1	96.1	88.2	78.3
Rest Pain	84.4	79.1	61.4	46.4
Tissue Loss	72.7	65.8	46.9	29.6

C

FIGURE 3 A comparison of patients treated for claudication, ischemic rest pain, and ischemic tissue loss using the physician-oriented outcomes. **A,** Secondary interventional patency. **B,** Limb salvage. **C,** Survival.

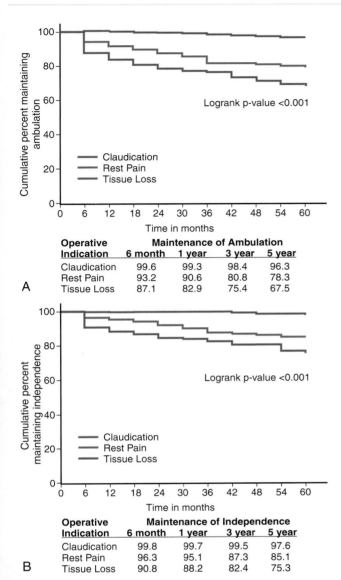

Operative	Maintenance of Ambulation			
Indication	6 month	1 year	3 year	5 year
Claudication	99.6	99.3	98.4	96.3
Rest Pain	93.2	90.6	80.8	78.3
Tissue Loss	87.1	82.9	75.4	67.5

Operative	Maintenance of Independence			
Indication	6 month	1 year	3 year	5 year
Claudication	99.8	99.7	99.5	97.6
Rest Pain	96.3	95.1	87.3	85.1
Tissue Loss	90.8	88.2	82.4	75.3

FIGURE 4 A comparison of patients treated for claudication, ischemic rest pain, and ischemic tissue loss using patient-oriented outcomes. **A,** Ambulation maintenance. **B,** Independent living status.

Our experience suggests that treatment of claudication is not dangerous; death and amputation are exceedingly rare, and intervention does not appear to alter the benign natural history. To the contrary, amputation rates at 5 years (1%) were less than what have been reported in natural history studies for untreated patients (up to 5% at 5 years). Lastly, the vast majority (80%) of patients achieve symptom relief with intervention. If the primary goal of therapy is to address the patient-oriented priorities of functional palliation, our findings support the concept that intervention should assume a more significant role in patients with claudication.

SUMMARY

Because the threat to the affected limb over time is relatively insignificant (0.5% to 1% per-year amputation rate), and the risk of systemic cardiovascular complications are quite substantial (5% per-year mortality rate), medical treatment aimed at cardiovascular risk-factor modification—such as smoking cessation, cholesterol-reducing therapy, control of diabetes, and hypertension—should be a treatment priority in all patients with vasculogenic claudication. Supervised exercise aimed at increasing walking distance should be employed as well. Recent data, influenced by the popularity and safety of percutaneous transluminal angioplasty, suggest that intervention for patients with claudication is associated with improved quality of life and enhanced functionality. Therefore, although patients should be carefully individualized, a more liberal use of surgical revascularization is justified for motivated patients who desire symptom relief from medically refractory vasculogenic claudication, especially when the anatomic pattern of disease is amenable to endovascular intervention.

SELECTED READINGS

Norgren L, Hiatt WR, Dormandy JA, et al for the TASC II Working Group: Inter-Society Consensus for the Management of Peripheral Arterial Disease (TASC II), *J Vasc Surg* 45(suppl S):S5–S67, 2007.

Hirsch AT, Haskal ZJ, Hertzer NR, et al: ACC/AHA 2005 guidelines for the management of patients with peripheral arterial disease (lower extremity, renal, mesenteric, and abdominal aortic): executive summary, *J Am Coll Cardiol* 47:1239–1312, 2006.

Taylor SM, Kalbaugh CA, Healy MG, et al: Do current outcomes justify more liberal use of revascularization for vasculogenic claudication? A single center experience of 1,000 consecutively treated limbs, *J Am Coll Surg* 206(5):1053–1064, 2008.

Taylor SM, Cull DL, Kalbaugh CA, et al: Comparison of interventional outcomes according to preoperative indication: a single-center analysis of 2,240 limb revascularizations, *J Am Coll Surg* 208:770–780, 2009.

FALSE ANEURYSMS AND ARTERIOVENOUS FISTULAS

Michael T. Watkins, MD, and Glenn M. LaMuraglia, MD

DEFINITIONS

False aneurysms (FAs), or pseudoaneurysms, are differentiated from true aneurysms specifically because they lack all three normal elements of the arterial wall. The most common etiology of FA is trauma, related to either catheter-based interventions or injury (Table 1). Vascular trauma to the artery wall that can result in FA can be either penetrating or blunt in nature. Infection can complicate the clinical course of pseudoaneurysms, when there is inadvertent puncture of arteries associated with drug abuse, contamination or secondary seeding after percutaneous interventions, or as a consequence of bacterial seeding in the presence of a prosthetic vascular anastomosis. In patients afflicted with vasculitides such as polyarteritis nodosa or Behçet disease, spontaneous nonbacterial pseudoaneurysms may arise at the aortic root, the ascending aorta, or the visceral and peripheral vessels. Arteriovenous fistulas (AVFs) are abnormal direct communications between an artery and vein. These communications can be iatrogenic, congenital, or acquired (see Table 1). In this chapter, discussion of AVFs will be confined to the iatrogenic and acquired variety.

TABLE 1: Etiology of FAs and AVFs

FA	AVF
Acquired	**Congenital**
Penetrating	Kawasaki disease
Gunshot	Osler-Rendu-Weber syndrome
Stab wound	**Acquired**
Needle wound	Aneurysmal erosion
Nonpenetrating	**Iatrogenic**
Blunt proximity injury	Vascular access
Stretch	
Iatrogenic	
Anastomotic	
Patch	
Bypass graft	
Vascular access	
Spontaneous	
Vasculitis	
Behçet disease	
Polyarteritis	

TABLE 2: Risk factors for the development of FAs

Catheter Associated	Perianastomotic
Sheath size	Hypertension
Anticoagulation	Endarterectomy
Female gender	α-Antitrypsin deficiency
Inadequate manual compression	Arteriosclerosis
Obesity	Perioperative complications
Calcified vessels	Technical errors
Improper puncture site	History of aneurysm disease
Hypertension	
Chronic steroid use	
Aortic valvular insufficiency	

RISK FACTORS

Risk factors for the development of iatrogenic FAs associated with catheter interventions and vascular reconstructions are listed in Table 2. Major perioperative complications, technical errors, and α-antitrypsin deficiency can contribute to the development of perianastomotic pseudoaneurysms. The incidence of these types of pseudoaneurysms ranges from 1.7% to 4.8% per anastomotic site, and this increases over time. The presence of a prosthetic bypass or an aortobifemoral or femoropopliteal graft does not contraindicate femoral access for cannulation. A relative contraindication for femoral access is the presence of a femorofemoral bypass graft because of the orientation of the graft and the single inflow source for both lower extremities.

When planning percutaneous access through a prosthetic graft, it is important to be certain that there is no preexisting anastomotic pseudoaneurysm; this is usually done with duplex ultrasound imaging. When there is a prosthetic graft in the femoral access site, ultrasound-guided puncture may be useful to ensure puncture of the graft rather than the anastomosis. Although catheters up to 14 Fr (4.4 mm) in diameter have been used to percutaneously access the femoral artery, the complication rate is correlated to the size of the introduced device. The incidence of complications after percutaneous diagnostic procedures is 0.7%, whereas the incidence of those requiring larger sheaths for percutaneous interventional procedures, and more aggressive anticoagulation, is approximately 3%. Other risk factors for iatrogenic pseudoaneurysms include advanced age, cannulation of the profunda or superficial femoral arteries, severe arterial calcification, increased body mass index (BMI), female gender, concurrent anticoagulation, combined arterial and venous puncture, and failure to provide appropriate postoperative compression. In an assessment of risk factors for AVF, female gender and arterial hypertension significantly increased the risk for this complication, but BMI and age had no impact. Procedure-related risk factors for AVF were puncture of the left groin and the intensity of anticoagulation (>12,500 units of heparin).

PREVENTION

It is essential to avoid multiple unsuccessful punctures of the artery, particularly when the pulse is not palpable. Fluoroscopic visualization of the femoral head may be very useful for accurate location of the common femoral artery, especially when some calcifications can be identified. Use of ultrasound guidance or the use of a Doppler needle is highly recommended in patients whose pulse is not palpable due to obesity, severely diseased vessels, scarring, or low perfusion pressure. Use of the smallest sheath size possible is desirable to limit the size of the arterial defect with respect to the arterial diameter. This factor plays a role in female patients, who have smaller arteries, and when the superficial femoral or profunda femoral artery are inadvertently accessed instead of the common femoral. When heparin is used during the course of the procedure, it is essential to keep the activated clotting time (ACT) to less than 160 seconds and to ensure that the patient's blood pressure is well controlled before the sheath is removed to avoid excessive bleeding.

A number of closure devices have been developed to replace manual compression and ambulate patients sooner after sheath removal. Despite their growing popularity, closure devices have their limitations and are not always successful. In the randomized trial leading to Food and Drug Administration (FDA) approval of the StarClose nitinol clip system (Abbott Laboratories, North Chicago, Ill.) for diagnostic cardiac catheterization, the list of angiographic and clinical exclusions included obesity, small femoral artery diameters, bleeding diatheses, femoral arterial disease, and non–femoral artery sheath insertion. These factors often exclude the precise patients who would optimally be candidates for a closure device. In addition, there are concerns that femoral closure devices may cause increased rates of complications. The introduction of a foreign body can lead to or complicate an infection in the arterial wall. Other complications associated with closure devices are artery lumen compromise, arterial laceration, uncontrolled bleeding, pseudoaneurysm, and device embolism down the leg leading to limb ischemia. Recent ongoing multicenter trials of closure devices using bioabsorbable materials appear to be applicable to a wider patient population with fewer complications, but ongoing analysis is essential before widespread use is recommended.

DIAGNOSIS

False Aneurysm

Suspicion of an iatrogenic pseudoaneurysm should arise when a swollen groin, excessive pain at the insertion site, or soft-tissue hematoma at the puncture site occur. The presence of a bruit and ongoing pulsatile bleeding are highly suggestive of a pseudoaneurysm.

Physical exam can be highly inaccurate for identifying pseudoaneurysms, but arterial duplex examination is associated with nearly 100% diagnostic accuracy. The test is simple, quick, and has excellent sensitivity and specificity. Duplex ultrasonography can be performed at the bedside at any location in the hospital, although it may be difficult to perform in morbidly obese patients, or when a very large hematoma is present. The location of certain vessels—including the

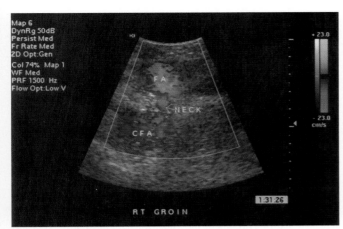

FIGURE 1   Duplex ultrasound examination. *CFA,* Common femoral artery.

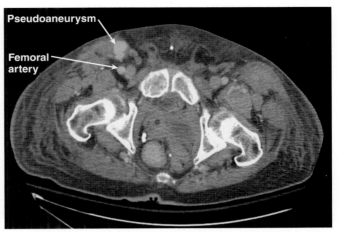

FIGURE 2   CT image of femoral pseudoaneurysm. This CT scan was performed to exclude the diagnosis of a retroperitoneal hematoma, however this femoral pseudoaneurysm was identified.

subclavian, profunda femoris, and visceral arteries—can make imaging by duplex ultrasound challenging because of vessel depth, overlying bone, or bowel gas. Duplex evaluation in the longitudinal and transverse planes is essential to identify the neck of the pseudoaneurysm, confirm flow outside the femoral artery, and accurately measure the size of the pseudoaneurysm (Figure 1).

The typical characteristics of a pseudoaneurysm noted on duplex imaging include swirling of color flow in a mass distinct from the underlying artery, color-flow signal through a tract leading to a sac, and a back-and-forth Doppler waveform in the pseudoaneurysm neck. Precise definition of the FA size and neck is one of the most important parameters for determining treatment options. The length and width of the neck are equally important to record, because a wider neck often directly correlates with larger arterial defects, which are generally more refractory to minimally invasive techniques. Multilobulated femoral aneurysms are more difficult to treat conservatively.

In the setting of a significant drop in blood pressure or in hematocrit—or in an obese patient, in whom duplex exam is technically difficult—a computed tomography (CT) scan with contrast may be useful to confirm the diagnosis of a pseudoaneurysm and exclude the presence of a large retroperitoneal hematoma that may have arisen from anticoagulation or antiplatelet therapy (Figure 2).

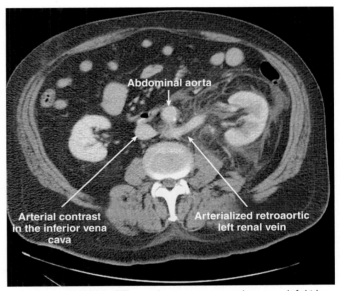

FIGURE 3   AVF. This CT scan demonstrates an edematous left kidney and equal contrast density in the aorta, the retroaortic left renal vein, and the inferior vena cava.

Arteriovenous Fistula

Although physical examination alone is not diagnostic for femoral pseudoaneurysm, it can be highly accurate and specific for detecting the presence of an AVF. A back-and-forth holosystolic/diastolic bruit at the puncture site is diagnostic and pathognomonic for an AVF. There are no other diagnoses that can be entertained when this particular bruit is identified. In addition, the intensity of the sounds correlates with the size of the fistula. An ultrasound is unlikely to improve upon this diagnosis or better characterize the extent of arteriovenous flow. In the acute setting, femoral AVFs after groin interventions tend to be small and have significantly less flow than AVFs constructed for patients requiring hemodialysis. In certain situations, days, months, or years after trauma or a groin intervention, the insidious onset of heart failure, limb swelling, or claudication can be the initial presentation for an AVF. The diagnosis of AVF can be made by duplex ultrasound, when the characteristic physical findings are not clearly present. Strict duplex ultrasound criteria for establishing a diagnosis of AVF are 1) a colorful, speckled mass at the level of the fistula with turbulent flow in the arteriovenous connection; 2) increased venous flow in the proximal common femoral vein compared with the contralateral side of the fistula; 3) no augmentation of

venous flow with Valsalva, and 4) decreased arterial flow distal to the suspected fistula.

CT scanning has no advantage in confirming the diagnosis of a femoral AVF in most patients. However, in patients who may have a more central lesion, such as an aortocaval or iliac artery–iliac vein AVF, imaging with CT is essential to delineate the arterial location of the connection and adjacent structures. In Figure 3, a CT scan demonstrates a retroaortic renal vein AVF.

Mycotic Pseudoaneurysms

These aneurysms can result from an infectious process, usually either from drug abuse or contamination of a catheter intervention. When these aneurysms develop in regions of previously placed prosthetic arterial reconstructions, remote sources such as a urinary tract infection, tooth abscess, or pneumonia must be identified as the possible source of seeding; both the source and the aneurysm must be treated aggressively in all patients except those who have limited life expectancy. Imaging with CT scanning is indicated to determine whether fluid collections or contiguous involvement of other organs is present.

Anastomotic Pseudoaneurysms

The potential diagnosis of femoral, carotid, or brachial artery anastomotic pseudoaneurysms is often brought to a surgeon's attention by physical exam, or it is noticed by the patient. Duplex ultrasound is useful for diagnosis of these peripheral anastomotic pseudoaneurysms. In the setting of femoral anastomotic aneurysms associated with aortobifemoral grafts, preoperative assessment with CT scanning is essential to determine the vascular inflow and outflow and to identify clinically silent areas of infection in continuity with the pseudoaneurysm. In patients who have aortofemoral bypass grafts, a FA in the groin may be associated with relatively silent proximal breakdown of the graft at the level of the aortic anastomosis (Figure 4).

TREATMENT OPTIONS

Nonanastomotic False Aneurysms

In the absence of impending cutaneous necrosis, femoral nerve compression symptoms, and bleeding unresponsive to local compression, most pseudoaneurysms can be observed. In a strict protocol in which patients' femoral aneurysms were less than 3 cm in diameter, not associated with severe pain, and the patient was not on ongoing anticoagulation, 82 patients were observed over a 12-week interval. In these patients an 89% spontaneous thrombosis rate was seen with no complications. The mean time for thrombosis was 23 days with a mean number of 2.6 duplex examinations per patient. Loss of distal circulation or impending necrosis of overlying skin from the expansion of a femoral artery pseudoaneurysm requires emergent surgical intervention.

Ultrasound-Guided Compression

To limit the risk of aspiration due to a vagal response, direct compression should usually be performed in an unfed patient whose tissue is infiltrated with copious amounts of xylocaine 1% or 2%. A FemoStop (St. Jude Medical, St. Paul, Minn.) or C clamp can be applied to the apex of the FA for 30 to 40 minutes and released over time. If these maneuvers fail, the next step usually involves ultrasound-guided thrombin injection.

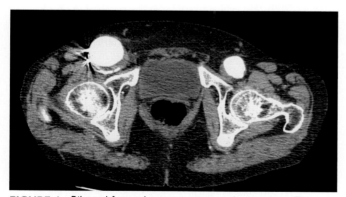

FIGURE 4 Bilateral femoral anastomotic pseudoaneurysms. This patient underwent bilateral common femoral endarterectomies and an aortobifemoral bypass for aortoiliac occlusive disease 15 years prior to presentation. There are no fluid collections or edematous streaks within the tissue surrounding the pseudoaneurysms, which suggests no evidence of infection. On physical exam and laboratory testing, no clinical evidence of infection was found.

Thrombin Injection

Ultrasound-guided thrombin injection is currently the method of choice in many centers. Bovine and human preparations are available, but the bovine form should be used with caution in patients with a history of previous exposure because of the risk of immunoglobulin-E–mediated anaphylaxis. Multilobulated FA may require several injections, and some evidence suggests that considerably lower doses of human thrombin are needed to treat pseudoaneurysms, thus risk of complications is reduced.

The procedure for injecting thrombin involves inserting a 22 gauge needle under direct ultrasound visualization through the superficial aspect of the pseudoaneurysm. With the needle tip lying centrally within the sac, thrombin, usually 50 to 1000 units, is injected until blood flow ceases on color Doppler ultrasound. Recurrence rates range from 0% to 9%; therefore ultrasounds are usually repeated within 24 hours of the initial injection. Intraarterial occlusion with thrombosis or embolization is estimated to be 2% and can be managed expectantly, depending on the clinical situation. Thrombin injection is contraindicated in the presence of an AVF or a very short, broad FA neck that would be concerning for thrombin or clot extravasating into the artery and embolizing down the leg.

Endovascular Repair

Traumatic injury to visceral and pelvic vessels can lead to FAs that are best treated with percutaneous methods including microvascular coils, thrombotic agents, and covered stents. In many instances prostheses developed to treat aneurysms can be modified to treat traumatic rupture and pseudoaneurysms of vessels on an individualized basis. To date, these endovascular repairs have been durable; in the absence of life-threatening bleeding, they require serious consideration for the prioritizing of the arterial injury in light of many other significant associated injuries. Endovascular repair of iatrogenic injury to femoral vessels can be achieved quickly but could inadvertently occlude the common femoral artery due to kinking. The groin is an area of repetitive flexion, which can lead to stent fracture and thrombosis.

Surgical Intervention

In patients with impending skin necrosis or compression of the adjacent nerve or vein, urgent open repair is indicated. In nonobese patients, the procedure could be done under local anesthesia. On rare occasions, especially when the presentation is delayed or an infectious process is suspected, access to the retroperitoneum may be necessary to achieve proximal control of the lower extremity inflow at the level of the iliac vessels. In most cases, simple suture repair of the defect is all that is needed to repair the vessel. The artery is exposed above and below the puncture site, and digital control of the bleeding can be obtained. Judd-Allis clamps can be used to approximate the edges of the arterial wall. Simple interrupted 5-0 polypropylene sutures are used to close the artery, while sequentially removing the Judd-Allis clamps. It is essential to check the back wall of the artery to be sure no other source of bleeding is present. Rarely, when considerable injury is present in a significantly diseased artery, a patch may be required to avoid compromising the lumen. Continuous suture repair may be preferable to interrupted suture, as it allows precise placement of individual sutures and avoids excessive tension on the repair of the arterial suture line.

Arteriovenous Fistulas

Femoral AVFs tend to persist in patients on steroids who have chronic renal insufficiency. Implantation of covered stents in the femoral artery has been reported but appears to be contraindicated. As previously mentioned, considerable concern exists regarding complications of this approach, which include risks for restenosis, stent fracture resulting from frequent flexion in the groin region, and possible limitations for future femoral intervention. Only time and ongoing investigations will provide definitive understanding of the utility of this technique for managing femoral AVFs.

In contrast to healthy concern about the durability of covered stent repairs in common femoral AVFs, the use of covered stents to manage iliac vein–iliac artery or aortocaval fistulas have been very effective. Operative repair of a chronic AVF can be hazardous because of the friable nature of the vessels and the risk for considerable bleeding. Proximal and distal control of the artery and vein are necessary. Optimal treatment requires obliteration of the fistula and restoration of arterial and venous flow. At times, interposition grafting or patch angioplasty are needed to preserve flow without narrowing vessels. With large vein defects, preoperative placement of arterial or venous balloons for intraoperative occlusion may help decrease hemorrhage during repair of the vessels feeding the fistula. Given the potential for large-volume blood loss, cell-saver and rapid-infusion devices are needed.

Anastomotic False Aneurysms

For uninfected paraanastomotic aortic or femoral artery FAs associated with reconstructions for infrarenal aortic vascular disease, the diagnosis itself represents an indication to treat because of the unpredictable evolution and high incidence of rupture of these pseudoaneurysms. For these, expectant strategy is justified only in patients with a short life expectancy and/or exorbitantly high surgical or anesthetic risk. Ultrasound compression does not play a role in the setting of a perianastomotic or mycotic pseudoaneurysm.

Open surgical repair is the procedure of choice for groin aneurysms, which can result from occult infection (see the Mycotic False Aneurysms section below) or arterial degeneration in a previously endarterectomized artery. Reoperation in the area of the groin may be hazardous and tedious. In the case of late presentation of femoral anastomotic aneurysms without gross sepsis or infection, it is common to be able to extend the incision into the retroperitoneum to get proximal control of the graft. It is important to consider potential outflow sites, such as the superficial femoral artery or the profunda femoris artery. In most instances, the superficial femoral artery can be identified outside of the dense groin scar by its proximity to the medial aspect of the sartorius muscle. Identification of the profunda is much more difficult, but it can often be found with the aid of a handheld Doppler probe. The surgeon should be prepared to control branch vessels off the common femoral artery intraluminally with balloon catheters, such as Fogarty or Pruitt inflatable balloon catheters. Usually an interposition graft, such as expanded polytetrafluoroethylene or Dacron, is needed to reestablish blood flow to the limb by creating a new anastomosis in an area where there is healthy arterial tissue. Because of the short distances needed for interposition grafting in most of these cases, it is easier to perform the distal anastomosis first, leaving a flushing hole in the anastomosis prior to performing the end-to-end anastomosis with the proximal section of graft. In selected circumstances when there is no clinical or laboratory evidence of infection, endovascular repair of proximal infrarenal aortic anastomotic pseudoaneurysms may be considered. The predominant anatomic requirement for such a repair is an adequate landing zone for anchoring the device proximally and distally. In the proximal region of aortic anastomotic aneurysms, endovascular repairs must avoid compromising renal blood flow.

Mycotic False Aneurysms

In cases of severe inflammation or tissue contamination, management requires wide debridement of the wound and ligation of the inflow and outflow vessels. In many instances, coverage of the stumps of ligated vessels requires mobilization of a muscle flap such as the sartorius, gracilis, or the rectus abdominis. Culture and Gram stain of fluid or tissue from the wound is necessary to guide specific postoperative treatment with antibiotics. Restoration of blood flow usually requires extranatomic reconstruction, although on occasion, in situ repair can be performed with vein and proper graft coverage. When in situ reconstruction appears inadvisable due to extensive tissue contamination, an obturator bypass from the external iliac artery to the superficial femoral vessel may be appropriate. In the rare patient with a relatively hostile abdomen, the external iliac artery may be approached through an oblique lower quadrant muscle–splitting incision.

Alternatively, an axillary artery to profunda, superficial femoral artery, or popliteal artery bypass with prosthetic graft can be attempted. With this bypass option, however, the subcutaneous location of the graft may provide another injection site for the IV drug abuser. If the infectious process involves the proximal anastomosis of an aortofemoral bypass graft, proximal control of the aorta at the diaphragmatic hiatus through the lesser sac is essential. Reconstructive options include in situ reconstruction using a rifampin-soaked prosthetic graft to protect against *Staphylococcus* species pathogens. A graft composed of superficial femoral veins harvested from both thighs has been used to reconstruct an infected aorta. If the residual aortic tissue is friable and precludes an attempt at creating another anastomosis, the aortic stump should be closed in two layers with interrupted, horizontal polypropylene mattress sutures. If the tissue is friable, fascia lata harvested from the lateral thighs can be used as pledgets for the sutures. It is important to mobilize a segment of omentum and approximate it directly over the aortic stump using absorbable suture in a manner similar to techniques used to create a Graham patch.

SUGGESTED READINGS

Applegate RJ, Sacrinty MT, Kutcher MA, et al: Trends in vascular complications after diagnostic cardiac catheterization and percutaneous coronary intervention in the femoral artery, 1998 to 2007, *J Am Coll Cardiol Cardiovasc Interv* 1(3):317–326, 2008.

Kelm M, Perings SM, Jax T, et al: Incidence and clinical outcome of iatrogenic femoral arteriovenous fistulas: implications for risk stratification and treatment, *J Am Coll Cardiol* 40(2):291–297, 2002.

Nigri GR, LaMuraglia GM: Management and complications from arterial access, *Adv Vasc Surg* 8:111–124, 2000.

Stone PA, AbuRahma AF, Flaherty SK, Bates MC: Femoral pseudoaneurysms, *Vasc Endovascular Surg* 40(2):109–117, 2006.

Toursarkissian B, Allen BT, Petrinec D, et al: Spontaneous closure of selected iatrogenic pseudoaneurysms and arteriovenous fistulae, *J Vasc Surg* 25(5):803–808, 1997.

Vagefi PA, Kwolek CJ, Wicky S, Watkins MT: Congestive heart failure from traumatic arteriovenous fistula, *J Am Coll Surg* 209(1):150, 2009.

AXILLOFEMORAL BYPASS

Alexander D. Shepard, MD

OVERVIEW

Axillofemoral bypass and its more commonly performed counterpart, axillobifemoral bypass, have been appropriately described in the literature as operations of compromise performed on compromised patients. Studies have clearly documented that the hemodynamic performance and long-term patency of this extraanatomic procedure is significantly inferior to other forms of open revascularization for aortoiliac disease. Standard 5-year patency rates quoted in the literature for axillobifemoral bypass remain in the 50% to 60% range compared with 80% to 85% for aorto(bi)femoral bypass, the gold standard open procedure for aortoiliac occlusive disease. In certain patients, however, aortofemoral grafting is not an option because of associated high medical risk or, increasingly in my experience, technical factors (e.g., aortic infection or severe intraabdominal scarring). By avoiding the physiologic stress associated with celiotomy and aortic cross clamping, axillofemoral bypass provides aortoiliac revascularization in such patients at an acceptable operative risk; the tradeoff is decreased hemodynamic improvement and reduced long-term patency. Axillofemoral bypass is therefore usually reserved for high-risk patients with limited life expectancy or those in whom a transabdominal approach is contraindicated.

The main indications for axillofemoral bypass are severe aortoiliac occlusive disease associated with critical limb ischemia or an aortoiliac infection of a native vessel or prosthetic graft. For patients with occlusive disease, axillofemoral bypass is usually considered only in patients at prohibitive risk for standard aortic reconstruction, including those unable to tolerate celiotomy and aortic clamping and those with a "hostile" abdomen. Factors most commonly associated with high risk include advanced age, severe cardiopulmonary disease, such as advanced chronic obstructive pulmonary disease or nonreconstructable coronary disease, and other concomitant disease states associated with a life expectancy of less than 2 years, such as malignancy. In my practice, profoundly depressed left ventricular function (ejection fraction ≤20%) is considered a relative contraindication to axillofemoral grafting because of particularly dismal patency in these patients. A hostile abdomen can result from multiple previous celiotomies (including prior aortic reconstruction), malignancy, radiation, stomas, or concomitant intraabdominal infection. Infection involving the native aortoiliac vessels or a prosthetic graft is another technical indication for performing this extraanatomic bypass, and at least in my experience, it is now the most common indication. This procedure can also be useful in patients with aortic dissection that causes isolated lower extremity malperfusion not amenable to endoluminal revascularization.

Careful patient selection is important; continuing advances in endoluminal techniques have allowed an increasing number of patients with severe aortoiliac disease to avoid open revascularization all together. In addition, we have found that patients with a hostile abdomen can frequently undergo standard infrarenal aortic reconstruction safely through a left-flank extraperitoneal approach. My utilization of axillofemoral bypass has been fairly conservative: I reserve it for high-risk patients with critical limb ischemia and for patients with aortoiliac (graft) infection. Inferior hemodynamic performance and poor long-term patency make this bypass a poor choice for patients with lifestyle-limiting claudication only.

PREOPERATIVE ASSESSMENT

Preoperative assessment requires a careful evaluation of the arterial system in the donor (proximal) arm to ensure that it is free of hemodynamically significant occlusive disease. Although some authorities have recommended arteriography, we have found the presence of a triphasic brachial artery Doppler waveform to be a reliable indicator of normal inflow. Contrast imaging of the aorta and its runoff vessels—most commonly via standard arteriography, to at least the tibial level—is required to define the extent of the patient's lower extremity occlusive disease. If one iliac artery has relatively discrete disease amenable to angioplasty or stenting, consideration should be given to treatment of this lesion with subsequent femorofemoral bypass rather than axillobifemoral grafting. Oblique views of the femoral bifurcations should be obtained to detect the presence of occlusive plaque, particularly at the profunda femoris origins; correction of this disease at the time of bypass is critical to optimizing long-term graft patency. Patients undergoing axillofemoral bypass because of significant comorbidities require careful evaluation of their overall medical status with close attention given to the factors contributing to their high risk.

OPERATIVE TECHNIQUE

Selection of the donor arm depends on the side of the ischemic lower extremity; with axillounifemoral bypass, the donor arm is always on the same side as the ischemic extremity. The same rule usually applies to axillobifemoral bypass, which is usually preferred to unifemoral bypass because of its superior patency, presumably related to increased flow (two outflow tracts vs. one). In most circumstances the right arm is used, because the right subclavian artery is less often affected by occlusive disease than the left. Light general anesthesia is preferred, because it facilitates creation of the subcutaneous tunnels, though local anesthesia can be used in very high-risk patients. Prophylactic antibiotics, usually a first-generation cephalosporin, are administered preoperatively.

The donor arm is placed on a narrow arm board at the patient's side to avoid significant abduction and stretching of the axillary artery. If required, an arterial line can be placed in the contralateral radial artery. The upper half of the donor arm and shoulder, the chest wall from the midline to just above the table and from just above the clavicle caudally, the lateral abdomen, and both groins to the mid thighs are prepped and draped into the field. If available, two teams can be utilized to perform this procedure more expeditiously; while one team performs the axillary dissection, the other can expose the femoral arteries.

The axillary artery is exposed through an incision running parallel to the fibers of the pectoralis major, one fingerbreadth below the clavicle and extending from the midclavicular line laterally to the deltopectoral groove. The pectoralis major is divided along its fibers to expose the underlying clavipectoral fascia. Incision of this fascia exposes small venous tributaries that can be traced back to the axillary vein, which lies just anterior and slightly caudal to the artery. Exposure of the axillary artery requires division of these small veins, along with a branch or two of the artery's thoracoacromial trunk, and mobilization of the upper border of the vein. The first portion of the axillary artery—the segment bounded by the lower margin of the clavicle proximally and the medial edge of the pectoralis minor distally—is dissected free for a distance of 4 to 5 cm and controlled with vessel loops. Care should be taken to avoid injury to the brachial plexus, which tracks just above and behind the artery. Lateral exposure can be facilitated by dividing the medial portion of the head of the pectoralis minor, although the second portion of the axillary artery—that segment lying directly behind the pectoralis

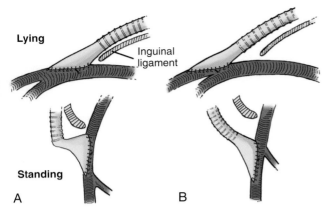

FIGURE 1 Location of axillofemoral anastomosis on femoral artery. **A,** Distal anastomosis placed on femoral artery immediately adjacent to inguinal ligament is prone to angulation and kinking when the abdominal wall pannus drops when the patient stands. **B,** This problem can be minimized by placing the anastomosis more distally on the artery, usually at the level of the bifurcation, sometimes crossing over it onto the origin of either the superficial femoral or profunda femoris artery.

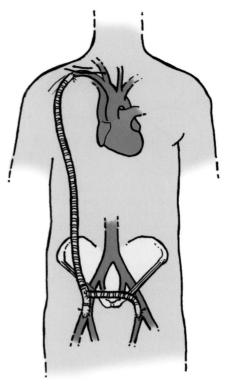

FIGURE 2 Configuration of typical right-sided axillobifemoral graft.

minor—should never be used to originate the graft because of the increased risk of anastomotic disruption when this segment is used. Posterior branches of the axillary artery in the region selected for anastomosis should usually be divided when encountered to avoid subsequent inadvertent injury and/or troublesome back-bleeding during performance of the axillary anastomosis.

Femoral artery exposure is performed through standard vertical groin incisions placed more distally than normal, because there is usually no need to expose the inguinal ligament. The femoral artery bifurcations are dissected free, and the most proximal superficial femoral artery (SFA) and profunda femoris are controlled as necessary. Meticulous care should be taken to ligate any crossing vessels or lymphatic structures; wound complications with a subcutaneously tunneled prosthetic graft can be potentially catastrophic. The sites of the femoral artery anastomoses should be chosen carefully to minimize problems with graft kinking and angulation. The femoral artery immediately adjacent to the inguinal ligament should be avoided because of the tendency of grafts anastomosed to this segment to kink, as the abdominal wall pannus drops when the patient stands up (Figure 1). Graft angulation can also occur with routine hip flexion during sitting or stair climbing. For this reason we usually place any femoral anastomoses at the level of the femoral bifurcation, crossing over the origins of either the profunda femoris or SFA. With very proximal bifurcations, it may be necessary to place the entire anastomosis on one of these two trunks.

Once the anastomotic sites on the femoral arteries have been selected, subcutaneous tunnels are created from the axillary incision to the ipsilateral groin and between the two groins. The upper portion of the axillary–groin tunnel passes between the two pectoral muscles laterally into the subcutaneous tissues of the lateral chest wall. This tunnel then follows a gentle arc across the lower chest and abdominal wall approaching the midaxillary line posteriorly in its most dependent portion before passing medial to the anterior superior iliac spine into the groin (Figure 2). This configuration reduces the risk of kinking when the patient bends over. A long tunneling device is used to create this tunnel, utilizing a small counter incision just above the costal margin in tall or obese patients. The subcutaneous tunnel between the two groins is more easily created, tracking just above the deep fascia of the lower abdominal wall. The course of the cross-femoral graft depends on the type of graft (see below); in most situations, a gentle inverted-C configuration is used. A tunneling device or a large curved aortic clamp can be helpful in creating this tunnel.

Some resistance is usually encountered in the midline, where the skin is frequently tethered to the fascia. Care should be taken in patients with previous lower midline incisions to avoid violating the fascia or peritoneal cavity.

A variety of graft materials, sizes, and configurations are available for axillofemoral grafting. We prefer external ring–supported extruded polytetrafluoroethylene (ePTFE). There is good evidence to suggest that supported grafts perform better than unsupported grafts, presumably by reducing the risk of compression and kinking. The literature suggests using a 10 mm axillofemoral graft limb coupled with an 8 mm cross-femoral limb as needed in large individuals, or an 8 mm axillofemoral limb with a 6 mm femorofemoral limb in smaller patients. Prefabricated 8 and 10 mm grafts with an attached cross-femoral limb in either a T or Y configuration are commercially available and are my preference for practical reasons.

Following graft placement in the tunnels, the patient is systemically anticoagulated. The first portion of the axillary artery is controlled proximally and distally, and a short arteriotomy is created on the anteroinferior surface of the artery. Again, a medial location on the axillary artery is chosen to reduce the risk of anastomotic disruption with arm abduction postoperatively. The graft is positioned in a gentle arc over the axillary vein, leaving only a few centimeters of unsupported graft. The most proximal graft is purposely left slightly redundant to avoid excessive tension during ipsilateral arm abduction and/or contralateral torso flexion. The proximal end of the graft is trimmed at a 30-degree angle and sewn end-to-side to the axillary artery with a running 5-0 polypropylene suture, beginning on the back wall (Figure 3, *A*). An alternative, more acutely angled proximal anastomotic configuration with concomitant tunneling of the graft parallel to the artery for 8 to 10 cm *below* the pectoralis minor has been advocated by some authors to further reduce the risk of anastomotic disruption (Figure 3, *B*). If a two-team approach is utilized, the left femoral anastomosis can be constructed simultaneously.

Graft tunneling and orientation should be double-checked prior to construction of a distal anastomosis to prevent kinking that could

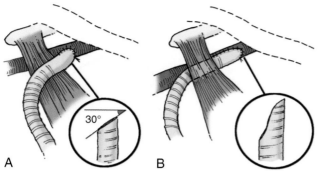

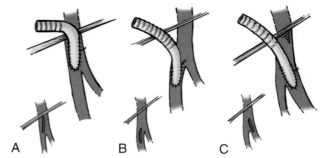

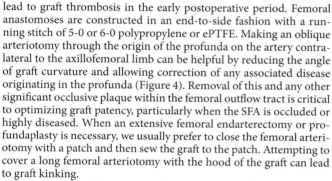

FIGURE 3   Construction of proximal anastomosis for axillofemoral graft. **A,** Standard technique with graft cut at a 30-degree angle; the proximal graft is passed under the pectoralis major and over the origin of the pectoralis minor muscle to reach the lateral chest wall tunnel. **B,** Alternative technique with a more traditional "cobra head" anastomosis; graft is passed below the pectoralis minor muscle, parallel to the axillary artery, for a distance of 8 to 10 cm before beginning subcutaneous lateral chest wall tunnel. This configuration is purported to reduce the risk of anastomotic disruption.

FIGURE 4   Configuration of contralateral femoral anastomosis for axillobifemoral bypass. **A,** Longitudinal arteriotomy confined to proximal common femoral artery can sometimes lead to angulation or kinking of the graft, particularly in the presence of a high bifurcation. **B,** Placing the arteriotomy more distally, crossing over the bifurcation onto the superficial femoral artery, alleviates this problem. **C,** Oblique femoral arteriotomy carried down on to the proximal profunda femoris lessens the angle of curvature of the graft further and allows correction of any occlusive disease present at the origin of this critical outflow artery.

lead to graft thrombosis in the early postoperative period. Femoral anastomoses are constructed in an end-to-side fashion with a running stitch of 5-0 or 6-0 polypropylene or ePTFE. Making an oblique arteriotomy through the origin of the profunda on the artery contralateral to the axillofemoral limb can be helpful by reducing the angle of graft curvature and allowing correction of any associated disease originating in the profunda (Figure 4). Removal of this and any other significant occlusive plaque within the femoral outflow tract is critical to optimizing graft patency, particularly when the SFA is occluded or highly diseased. When an extensive femoral endarterectomy or profundaplasty is necessary, we usually prefer to close the femoral arteriotomy with a patch and then sew the graft to the patch. Attempting to cover a long femoral arteriotomy with the hood of the graft can lead to graft kinking.

Construction of the proximal anastomosis of the cross-femoral limb of an axillobifemoral bypass was the subject of a great deal of discussion in the older vascular surgical literature. A variety of configurations have been advocated. Whether the cross-femoral limb is piggybacked onto the axillofemoral limb or vice versa, or simply sewn into the side of the axillofemoral limb, is probably immaterial in terms of graft patency (Figure 5, *A* to *C*). The important technical point is to place the proximal anastomosis of the cross-femoral limb as far distally as possible on the axillofemoral limb; this configuration maximizes flow through the longest possible segment of the axillofemoral limb, which as a long, small-caliber prosthetic graft is already at considerable risk for thrombosis. We prefer the convenience of prefabricated grafts utilizing a T or Y configuration for this connection (Figure 5, *D* and *E*). Meticulous hemostasis and wound closure are critical to avoiding wound complications.

POSTOPERATIVE MANAGEMENT

Because of the extracavitary nature of this procedure, recovery is usually fairly rapid. Good groin hygiene, particularly in obese patients, is critical to avoiding wound complications. Because of the subcutaneous location of these prosthetic grafts, any wound morbidity is potentially catastrophic. Strict bed rest is maintained until groin incisions have been bone dry for 24 hours. All patients are treated with low-dose aspirin, and unless strong contraindications exist, we have utilized long-term warfarin anticoagulation in most patients to enhance the patency of these hemodynamically "challenged" grafts. At discharge, patients are advised to avoid sleeping on the side their

grafts are on to prevent graft compression, though this concern has diminished considerably since the introduction of externally supported grafts. To protect against axillary anastomotic disruption, patients are also warned about strenuous activities that involve significant abduction of the donor arm.

Patients are followed in the outpatient clinic with ankle-brachial indexes (ABIs) and graft duplex scanning within 6 weeks postoperatively and at 6-month intervals thereafter. Because of inferior hemodynamics that result from the smaller size of the donor artery and the higher resistance of the long, small-diameter prosthesis, axillobifemoral grafts are associated with a lower rise in ABIs compared to aortobifemoral grafts. Duplex surveillance should include imaging of anastomostic sites for narrowing and measurement of graft flow velocities. A peak systolic flow velocity below 80 cm/sec in the mid portion of the axillofemoral limb has been associated with increased rates of graft thrombosis and should prompt a search for correctable causes of a failing graft.

Two rare but well-documented complications of axillofemoral grafting require mention: Disruption of the axillary anastomosis has been previously mentioned. This complication usually occurs during the first few weeks postoperatively following an episode of forceful abduction of the donor arm, such as might occur in opening a garage door. It is felt to result from too much tension on the axillary anastomosis. The best prevention is to place the proximal anastomosis as far medial as possible on the axillary artery and to leave the segment of graft just beyond this anastomosis slightly redundant. The other unusual complication of axillofemoral grafting is perigraft seroma, which can occur following any operation involving placement of a prosthetic graft; however, this seems to occur more frequently following axillofemoral grafting. Although the cause is unknown, the porosity of the graft leads to a collection of fluid surrounding the distal limbs of the graft; some authors have surmised that this may be due to the subcutaneous location of these grafts. Patients complain of a painless lump in the groin area, which on occasion can extend up the flank (Figure 6).

Management is conservative except when the diagnosis is in question, or when the patient is truly bothered by expanding masses. Aspiration can be diagnostic and at least temporarily therapeutic; repetitive aspirations should be avoided, however, because of the risk of introducing infection. In rare cases, graft replacement through fresh tissue planes with a different type of graft material, such as exchanging PTFE for Dacron, has been advocated as a successful treatment.

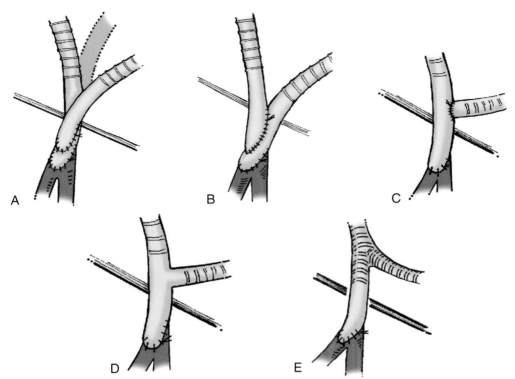

FIGURE 5   Different configurations of the proximal anastomosis for the cross-femoral limb of the axillobifemoral bypass. **A,** Proximal end of the cross-femoral limb piggybacked onto the hood of the axillofemoral limb. **B,** Distal end of axillofemoral limb piggybacked onto the hood of proximal cross-femoral limb. **C,** Cross-femoral limb sewn into the side of the axillofemoral limb. **D,** Prefabricated graft with cross-femoral limb originating at 90 degrees. **E,** Prefabricated graft with a Y-shaped cross-femoral limb origin.

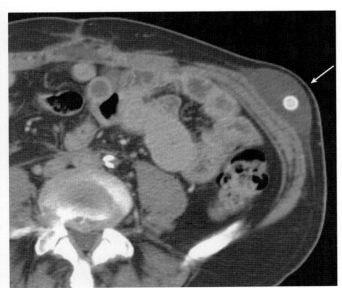

FIGURE 6   CT scan demonstrating a large perigraft seroma around a left axillofemoral graft limb.

RESULTS

Axillofemoral grafting is associated with widely variable results in the literature, which are largely dependent on patient selection criteria. When utilized in the higher risk patients for whom it was designed, the operative mortality rate is around 7% to 8%; inclusion of better risk patients has lowered the mortality to 3% to 4% in several series. Patency rates are clearly inferior to those of aortofemoral grafting; but again, these vary depending on patient selection. In high-risk patients, 3-year patency rates average 60%, but in low-risk patients with good runoff, 3-year patency rates of 75% to 80% have been reported. Several factors are reported to affect patency. Indication is one significant factor: patients who undergo axillofemoral grafting for nonocclusive disease, such as aortic infection, fare better than those who undergo bypass for occlusive disease. Patients undergoing axillofemoral bypass following a previous failed inflow operation fare worse. Graft material is another important factor: PTFE appears to work better than Dacron, and externally supported grafts do better than unsupported grafts. Distal runoff status figures in significantly, because patency is better with an open SFA versus an occluded one; the number of affected limbs is also a factor, given that axillobifemoral graft patency is superior to axillounifemoral graft patency. It is important to realize, however, that data supporting some of these conclusions are limited; in the absence of large-scale comparison trials, it is difficult to draw definitive conclusions.

SUMMARY

Axillofemoral bypass is a compromised revascularization procedure that should be reserved for patients unfit for direct aortic reconstruction or in the setting of technical factors that preclude aortofemoral bypass. The hemodynamic outcome and long-term patency of this bypass are clearly inferior to aortofemoral bypass, making axillofemoral bypass most suitable for older, debilitated patients with limited life expectancy. Despite these limitations, axillofemoral grafting can be extremely useful in treating certain subsets of patients with aortoiliac occlusive disease, aortoiliac (graft) infection, and aortic dissections in which direct aortic reconstruction is deemed unsafe or impossible.

SUGGESTED READINGS

Angle N, Dorafshar AH, Farooq MM, et al: The evolution of the axillofemoral bypass over two decades, *Ann Vasc Surg* 16:742–745, 2002.

Martin D, Katz SG: Axillofemoral bypass for aortoiliac occlusive disease, *Am J Surg* 180:100–103, 2000.

Passman MA, Taylor LM, Moneta GL, et al: Comparison of axillofemoral and aortofemoral bypass for aortoiliac occlusive disease, *J Vasc Surg* 23:263–271, 1996.

Schneider JR, McDaniel MD, Walsh DB, et al: Axillofemoral bypass: outcome and hemodynamic results in high-risk patients, *J Vasc Surg* 15:952–963, 1992.

Taylor LM, Park TC, Edwards JM, et al: Acute disruption of polytetrafluoroethylene grafts adjacent to axillary anastomoses: a complication of axillofemoral grafting, *J Vasc Surg* 20:520–528, 1994.

MANAGEMENT OF PERIPHERAL ARTERIAL EMBOLI

Zachary M. Arthurs, MD, and Sean P. Lyden, MD

OVERVIEW

Peripheral arterial embolization obstructs the arterial circulation typically at branch points, where diameter reductions occur. If left untreated the embolization leads to thrombosis of the native circulation. This process typically produces a cold, painful extremity that prompts the patient to seek medical evaluation. Restoration of circulation is the ultimate goal and can be accomplished by open thromboembolectomy, percutaneous mechanical thrombectomy pharmacologic thrombolysis, and peripheral arterial bypass. Understanding of the etiology of the peripheral arterial embolism will guide preoperative preparations and intraoperative and postoperative management.

ETIOLOGY

Eighty percent of peripheral arterial emboli arise from the heart. Figure 1 illustrates the distribution of peripheral embolic occlusions. Whereas rheumatic heart disease was the most common etiology, atrial fibrillation now accounts for half of cardiogenic emboli. Patients in atrial fibrillation with a dilated left atrium who are not treated with therapeutic anticoagulation are at an exceedingly high risk of embolism. The next most common etiology is myocardial infarction (MI) secondary to abnormal wall motion, ventricular scar, or ventricular aneurysm formation. Patients may or may not have a clear history of antecedent MI, but a history of chest pain or worsening shortness of breath may be elicited. In diabetic patients, a "silent" MI may be the etiology of peripheral embolization.

Other less frequent cardiac etiologies include valvular abnormalities, vegetations on prosthetic valve replacements, and cardiac tumors (most commonly atrial myxomas). In addition, paradoxical embolization can occur when there is an associated right-to-left cardiac shunt, most commonly through a patent foramen ovale. Paradoxical embolization should be considered when no embolic source has been identified, or when peripheral embolism occurs in the setting of deep venous thrombosis (DVT) or pulmonary embolism.

Noncardiac etiologies account for 20% of peripheral artery embolization, and unlike cardiac etiologies, noncardiac etiologies are more likely to cause microembolization. *Macroembolization* refers to complete occlusion of a named peripheral vessel, and *microembolization* refers to occlusion of terminal vessels. The most common source of microembolization is atheromatous debris from aortoiliac occlusive

disease. The next most common culprit is an aortic aneurysm. Interestingly, small abdominal aneurysms (3.5 to 4.0 cm) have a higher propensity of atheroembolization than larger abdominal aortic aneurysms. One possible explanation for this clinical finding is that larger abdominal aortic aneurysms have decreased blood flow velocity and may not create enough kinetic energy to dislodge debris. Peripheral artery aneurysms can also embolize debris. Popliteal artery aneurysms are the most common peripheral artery aneurysm, but femoral artery and subclavian artery aneurysms can also be the source of embolization. Unlike abdominal aortic aneurysms, which typically have microembolisms, peripheral artery aneurysms embolize thrombus, which leads to macroembolization and extensive tissue ischemia.

Infrainguinal occlusive disease can be the source of distal embolization. The most common location is an ulcerated plaque in the superficial femoral artery at the adductor canal. Rarely, a diffusely atherosclerotic or aneurysmal thoracoabdominal aorta may embolize

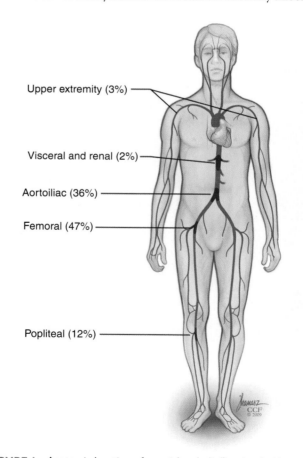

Upper extremity (3%)

Visceral and renal (2%)

Aortoiliac (36%)

Femoral (47%)

Popliteal (12%)

FIGURE 1 Anatomic location of arterial emboli. *(Reprinted with permission, Cleveland Clinic Center for Medical Art & Photography © 2009. All rights reserved.)*

atheromatous debris. Thoracic outlet syndrome and associated subclavian artery pathology is implicated in nearly half of patients with noncardiogenic upper extremity embolization. In addition, cases of iatrogenic emboli are increasing, as the number of percutaneous interventions has increased. Balloon angioplasty of occlusive lesions has the highest risk of embolization, but any catheter manipulation in the arterial tree can lead to atheroembolization.

CLINICAL PRESENTATION

A peripheral artery embolus most commonly presents with acute limb ischemia (Table 1). Classic symptoms of acute limb ischemia are categorized by the "six P's": *p*ain, *p*allor, *p*ulselessness, *p*oikilothermia, *p*arasthesias, and *p*aralysis. Pain is the most common symptom to prompt the patient to seek care, and the determinants of the pain syndrome are directly correlated to location of embolus, degree of ischemia, and extent of collaterals. Pallor is also common but less reliable as an indicator. Cool, pale, waxy skin may be observed, with decreased cutaneous perfusion, but these signs may not be present at rest. If the embolus is partially occlusive, elevation of the extremity will produce distal pallor, and lowering the foot to the floor will create dependent rubor (reactive hyperemia).

A careful pulse examination should be performed in all four extremities, including palpation for an abdominal aortic aneurysm. The uninvolved extremity should be referenced as the patient's baseline examination for determining the level of occlusion in the threatened limb. Acute embolism will cause a hyperdynamic "water hammer" pulse just proximal to the occlusion with no pulses below the occlusion. In addition, a temperature gradient can be felt distal to the occlusion. When the common femoral bifurcation is occluded with an embolus, a water-hammer femoral pulse is palpable, with no pulses distal and a temperature gradient across the thigh. In the setting of popliteal embolic occlusion, a water-hammer pulse is felt in the popliteal fossa, no pedal pulses are present, and a temperature gradient is present across the calf.

Doppler examination is critical for assessing distal vessel patency. Monophasic arterial signals in a pedal vessel documents small vessel patency and preservation of runoff. Loss of arterial Doppler signals in the foot suggests severe ischemia and should prompt immediate treatment. Assessment of venous filling should be performed by manually decompressing the veins of the forefoot to observe for venous return. Any venous filling confirms some inflow to the foot; a severely ischemic foot will have flat decompressed veins with no filling. In addition, venous filling can be assessed with Doppler examination of the veins. Ankle-brachial indices (ABIs) can be performed bed side with a handheld Doppler and blood pressure cuff. A bedside ABI reproducibly documents the degree of flow impediment; a low ABI in the nonischemic limb may suggest underlying atherosclerotic disease or bilateral lower extremity embolization.

Because neural tissue is the most sensitive to ischemia, the patient's neurologic status is a sensitive marker for the degree of ischemia and need for intervention. With mild ischemia, the patient may complain of numbness and tingling in the toes or the first web space. The anterior compartment of the lower extremity is most sensitive to neurologic ischemia that results in initial forefoot numbness; with progressive ischemia, numbness will progress more proximally and may evolve to complete loss of sensation. Once complete anesthesia has occurred, the patient's pain may subside, a sign of advanced ischemia. Motor function follows a similar pattern as ischemia progresses. Initially, symptoms of stiffness may prevail followed by progressive weakness until frank paralysis occurs. Pain on passive dorsiflexion should imply more advanced ischemia and potential concomitant compartment syndrome. Signs of advanced ischemia include rigor mortis, stiffness of the extremity, palpable firmness of the muscle compartments, paralysis, anesthesia, and diffuse mottling of the skin. Revascularization of a nonsalvageable limb will not restore lower extremity function and may increase the systemic morbidity and mortality of the patient. In the case of a nonviable extremity, amputation should be performed without attempts at revascularization.

Differentiation between acute native vessel thrombosis versus embolism can be challenging; however, the majority of cases can be differentiated by history and examination. Patients with peripheral vascular disease may have an antecedent history of claudication. Risk factors for atherosclerosis—hypertension, diabetes, smoking, and hyperlipidemia—plus a history of coronary artery disease, cerebrovascular disease, and previous peripheral artery bypass grafts may be present in native vessel occlusions. Patients with native vessel thrombosis may note a history of recent worsening of claudication symptoms or new-onset rest pain prompting medical evaluation. This process may occur over several days or even weeks leading to up to the patient seeking care.

In contrast, a patient with an embolic event can usually report the exact time of pain onset without any prodromal symptoms. Likewise, the degree of ischemia and resultant progression of symptoms is much worse in embolization, owing to the lack of peripheral collateralization. These patients typically seek medical attention within hours of pain onset. Patients with unilateral embolism may have palpable pulses in the unaffected extremity, whereas patients with thrombosis will generally have bilateral underlying vascular disease and nonpalpable pulses in the asymptomatic limb. In patients with popliteal artery aneurysm thrombosis, a palpable popliteal mass should suggest the diagnosis.

Thus far, clinical findings have referred to macroembolism and its sequelae, but some patients may present with isolated microembolism or a combination of the two. Microembolism occurs most commonly with atheroembolism from an arterial source. The emboli that occlude terminal arteries and arterioles are composed of cholesterol crystals, platelet aggregates, and fibrin. The patient will complain of severe, sharp pain localized to the digits. Embolization typically occurs to more than one digit and is frequently bilateral, when the source is proximal

TABLE 1: Clinical stratification of an ischemic extremity: Rutherford classification

| Category | DOPPLER SIGNALS | | NEUROLOGIC EXAM | | Capillary Return | Management |
	Arterial	Venous	Motor	Sensory Loss		
I. Viable	Present	Present	None	None	<4 sec	Elective angiography
IIa. Threatened (urgent)	Absent	Present	None	Mild	Delayed	Urgent angiography
IIb. Threatened (immediate)	Absent	Weak	Any	Present	Delayed	Emergent revascularization
III. Irreversible	Absent	Absent	Paralysis	Anesthetic	None	Amputation if duration >3 hr

From Rutherford RB, Baker JD, Ernst C, et al: Recommended standards for reports dealing with lower extremity ischemia: revised version, *J Vasc Surg* 26: 517, 1997.

to the aortic bifurcation, such as an abdominal aortic aneurysm. On exam, the macrocirculation may be intact, but the distal skin will have web-like areas of poor perfusion intermixed with normal skin. The characteristic pattern of purple skin (dermal necrosis) is termed *livedo reticularis,* and when it is extensive, it is called *blue toe syndrome.*

Patients with peripheral arterial embolism are also at risk for emboli to the cerebral, upper extremity, visceral, and renal arteries. Cerebral emboli will present with signs of transient ischemic attacks (TIAs) or stroke. Upper extremity emboli will shows symptoms similar to those of lower extremity emboli. Hepatic and splenic emboli are usually asymptomatic, whereas superior mesenteric artery emboli usually present with severe abdominal pain from intestinal ischemia or infarction. Renal artery emboli are typically silent, unless total infarction of the kidney occurs, causing flank pain and microscopic hematuria. In evaluating patients with peripheral artery embolism, the vascular territories discussed above should be investigated.

CLASSIFICATION

The Rutherford classification categorizes degrees of acute limb ischemia (Table 1), which guides timing of revascularization. Category I describes a viable limb that can be managed electively. Peripheral artery embolism usually presents with category II or III ischemia, and category IIa is marked by sensory deficits, representing a threatened extremity that should undergo urgent revascularization; these patients may stabilize or slightly improve with heparin therapy, allowing time for preoperative planning or the use of thrombolysis. Category IIb is marked by motor loss, and patients with ischemia in this category should undergo immediate revascularization to salvage function. Differentiation of category IIa and IIb ischemia is important for determining therapy; signs of motor loss should prompt immediate intervention. Category III represents a nonviable extremity. If the patient presents with rigor mortis of the affected extremity, they should not undergo revascularization but rather proceed directly to amputation.

DIAGNOSTIC EVALUATION

The category of ischemia and the urgency of revascularization will dictate the extent of diagnostic evaluation. In patients with category IIb or III ischemia, a rapid preoperative evaluation should be performed, and time-consuming diagnostic studies should be avoided. In all patients, the primary goal is to localize the site and source of embolization. Based solely on the history and physical examination, it is usually possible to diagnose the location and severity of the occlusion.

A standard 12-lead electrocardiogram is done to assess for cardiac dysrhythmias, signs of acute cardiac ischemia, or prior infarct. Blood work should include a complete blood count, blood type, chemistry, prothrombin time, and activated partial thromboplastin time. If prolonged ischemia exists, a creatinine phosphokinase level and urine myoglobin test may identify patients needing hydration to avoid acute tubular injury and nephrotoxicity. In patients suspected of having a clotting disorder, a comprehensive hypercoagulable panel should be drawn, which should include anticardiolipin antibodies, antiphospholipid antibodies, antiplatelet factor IV antibodies, and fibrinogen. The acute-phase response of some of the proteins and tests may necessitate confirmatory levels several months after the acute event.

Patients with category I and IIa ischemia have time to undergo contrast-enhanced computed tomographic angiography (CTA) to identify the source of the embolization and image the effected arterial distributions. The imaging protocol should include axial slices from the diaphragm to the toes. CTA will define inflow, demonstrate the level of vascular occlusion, and help to assess the outflow below the occlusion. In addition, CTA may provide information about the underlying atherosclerotic burden and identify any occult emboli

to the other beds, such as the visceral and renal vessels. In the case of isolated microembolization, CTA should be performed from the thoracic inlet through the femoral heads to assess the thoracic and abdominal aorta for sources of atheroembolization. Evaluation of the heart with transthoracic echocardiography may demonstrate an enlarged atrium, an enlarged atrial appendage, abnormal wall motion, intracardiac thrombus, and tumors. If transthoracic echo imaging does not reveal any abnormalities, transesophageal echocardiography (TEE) with bubble studies may be helpful, as it is more specific at diagnosing cardiac abnormalities. If available, intraoperative TEE can be performed at the time of revascularization.

MANAGEMENT

Initial Medical Therapy

The patient with suspected embolization should undergo immediate anticoagulation, most commonly with weight-based heparinization (80 to 100 U/kg bolus, followed by 10 to 15 U/kg/hr infusion); this will prevent distal arterial propagation of thrombus beyond the site of occlusion, reduce continued embolization, and prevent venous thrombosis. Low molecular weight heparin has also been successfully used, but inability to titrate and reverse the anticoagulation is a major limitation. Patients allergic to heparin may be anticoagulated with direct thrombin inhibitors such as bivalirudin, argatroban, and lepirudin. Patients will then be taken for angiography, catheter-directed thrombolysis (pharmacologic or mechanical), surgical embolectomy, or surgical bypass.

Operative Preparation and Initial Angiogram

The patient should be taken to an operative suite with an imaging table and fluoroscopic capabilities. The patient's chest, abdomen, and both lower extremities should be prepped into the field. In the case of suprainguinal occlusion (no femoral pulses), the surgeon should be prepared for an extraanatomic bypass if needed (axillofemoral or femorofemoral bypass). For patients who have not undergone preoperative imaging or in those with severe ischemia, the first stage of the procedure is to obtain an angiogram from the contralateral, uninvolved extremity; in the case of suspected aortoiliac occlusion, the angiogram should be performed from left brachial access. In patients with normal distal pulses in the contralateral extremity, without antecedent claudication symptoms and acute onset of limb ischemia, an angiogram may not be necessary before operative embolectomy.

The angiogram will help to determine the process that led to acute limb ischemia. Patients with embolic occlusion have relatively normal vessels with a sudden cutoff at the level of occlusion. The classical "meniscus" sign may be seen, and the embolus may be partially mobile within the lumen. In addition, embolic lesions have typically poor visualization distal to the occlusion, owing to the lack of developed collaterals. In contrast, patients with thrombotic occlusion have signs of atherosclerotic disease throughout their vessels, and varying levels of collaterals typically arise proximal to the occlusion. Imaging of the uninvolved extremity should always serve as a reference and can be very important in discerning etiology, especially in upper extremity limb ischemia.

Pharmacologic and Mechanical Thrombolytic Therapy Versus Surgery

Catheter-directed mechanical and pharmacologic thrombolysis can be an alternative or an adjunct to surgery. The utility of pharmacologic thrombolytic therapy is limited by the severity and duration of ischemia, extent of embolic or thrombotic clot, and the time to achieve clot resolution. Benefits of pharmacological thrombolytic therapy include noninvasive flow restoration, gradual reperfusion,

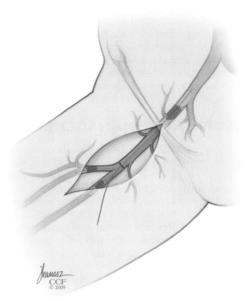

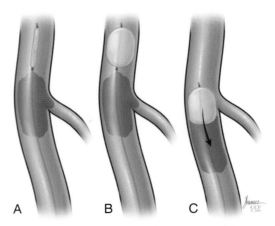

FIGURE 3 Technique of embolectomy. **A,** Passage of the embolectomy catheter through the clot. **B,** Gentle inflation to oppose without injuring the native vessel wall. **C,** Removal of the embolic debris. *(Reprinted with permission, Cleveland Clinic Center for Medical Art & Photography © 2009. All rights reserved.)*

FIGURE 2 Exposure of the femoral vessels for embolectomy. Arteriotomy is done just proximal to the profunda femorus origin. *(Reprinted with permission, Cleveland Clinic Center for Medical Art & Photography © 2009. All rights reserved.)*

and clearance of runoff and microvascular thrombosis. Pharmacologic thrombolysis works well with acute thrombosis (<2 weeks) but may have varied success on an embolic clot from the heart, which may have been organized over several weeks. Patients with category I or IIa ischemia can tolerate the 24 to 48 hours needed to achieve pharmacologic thrombolysis and allow identification and endovascular treatment of the underlying causative lesions. This is most common when native atherosclerosis or graft thrombosis is the underlying etiology. To expand treatment when more profound ischemia is present, and to address concerns regarding the time needed for dissolution of thrombus by pharmacologic means, mechanical thrombolytic devices have been used with success. Most percutaneous mechanical thrombectomy devices work by aspiration based on the Venturi effect, however, large particulate debris and well-organized emboli are still problematic for most devices.

Patients with category IIb ischemia represent more severe ischemia. After angiography, patients require rapid restoration of blood flow to the extremity. If percutaneous aspiration or mechanical thrombectomy with pulse-dose thrombolysis does not restore normal blood flow, the patient should proceed to open surgical thrombectomy or bypass. Continued pharmacologic thrombolysis may require an additional 24 to 48 hours to restore flow, which limbs with ischemia of this degree will not tolerate.

For suprainguinal or femoral occlusions, a vertical incision is made over the common femoral artery (Figure 2). The proximal common femoral, superficial femoral, and profunda arteries are controlled individually with elastic vessel loops. The patient's activated clotting time (ACT) should be maintained at twice baseline, or greater than 250 seconds. If the vessels are relatively free of atherosclerotic disease, a transverse arteriotomy is utilized to open the common femoral artery just above the profunda femorus origin; otherwise, a longitudinal arteriotomy should be utilized. Any free clot should be removed and sent to pathology as a specimen to evaluate for potential tumor.

Individually, each vessel should be assessed for flow; if a vessel proves inadequate, it should be treated with balloon-catheter embolectomy. Balloon embolectomy catheters consist of a balloon at the distal tip of a catheter with a proximal inflation port. A nondirected embolectomy catheter passed from the superficial femoral artery distally will usually cross into the peroneal vessel but not the anterior

tibial or posterior tibial arteries. Through-lumen embolectomy catheters provide a central port that can be utilized to pass over a guidewire that can be directed down into selected vessels under fluoroscopy. This is integral for performing selective tibial embolectomies from a femoral approach. Size 4 to 6 Fr embolectomy catheters are typically utilized in the iliac vessels; size 3 and 4 Fr are used for the superficial femoral, profunda, and popliteal arteries; and size 2 and 3 Fr catheters are used for tibial vessels. The balloon catheter is passed through the clot, and the operator inflates the balloon while simultaneously withdrawing the catheter (Figure 3). The pressure in the balloon is adjusted so that the balloon opposes the vessel wall, capturing the clot while avoiding overinflation, which would damage the intima of the vessel.

When performing suprainguinal embolectomy from the groin, contralateral pressure can be placed over the common femoral artery to limit the potential for displacing clot down the uninvolved extremity. After clearance of the femoral arteries, the arteriotomy should be closed; physical exam of the foot, Doppler exam, and completion angiogram dictate whether further groin embolectomy or more distal embolectomy is required. If distal clot burden still exists in the popliteal or tibial vessels, a below-the-knee popliteal approach should be undertaken.

A medial below-knee popliteal incision is utilized for popliteal and tibial embolectomy (Figure 4). The soleus muscle is divided from the tibial insertion proximally to expose the popliteal artery and tibial peroneal trunk. Isolation of the anterior tibial artery often requires division of the anterior tibial vein. The anterior tibial, posterior tibial, and peroneal arteries are individually controlled with elastic vessel loops. The arteriotomy should be placed just proximal to the anterior tibial origin, as this is the most challenging area to cannulate with the embolectomy catheter. Directed embolectomy should be performed on the inflow and all three tibial vessels.

Upon completion, a repeat exam and angiogram should be performed. After embolectomy has been completed, the macrovasculature may be eradicated of thrombus, but pedal vessels may still have residual thrombus. In this situation, intraarterial thrombolytic agents (e.g., tissue plasminogen activator in doses of 1 to 10 mg) and vasodilators (e.g., nitroglycerin or papaverine) can be used to improve outflow. Direct thrombectomy from a cutdown over the dorsalis pedis artery and posterior tibial arteries can be of benefit when a clot cannot be removed via the popliteal approach. If the tibial vessels appear tapered on the angiogram, and they do not respond to vasodilator therapy, the surgeon should suspect elevated compartment pressures as a potential etiology. Patients may require a period of heparin

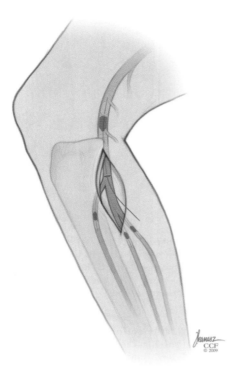

FIGURE 4   Exposure of the tibial vessels for embolectomy. Arteriotomy is done adjacent to the anterior tibial artery origin. *(Reprinted with permission, Cleveland Clinic Center for Medical Art & Photography © 2009. All rights reserved.)*

cessation in the intraoperative period to achieve hemostasis, but the patient should be continued on anticoagulation in the postoperative period to prevent recurrent embolization.

Fasciotomy

Patients who present with embolic occlusion typically suffer severe ischemia, and they may manifest signs of sensory or motor loss. With extremity reperfusion, tissue swelling increases secondary to

capillary leak. Four-compartment fasciotomy should be strongly considered following revascularization in patients whenever compartment syndrome is suspected, or when prolonged severe ischemia was present (generally >6 hours). Presentation of compartment syndrome in the postoperative period can be difficult to differentiate from normal postoperative pain without measuring compartment pressures, and this can result in a delayed diagnosis.

POSTOPERATIVE MANAGEMENT

Peripheral artery embolism carries a perioperative mortality of 10% and a limb amputation rate of 10%. The immediate metabolic consequences of returning perfusion to an acutely ischemic limb include hyperkalemia, myoglobinuria, acidosis, and hypotension. The potassium can be controlled with diuresis, insulin, and glucose, but in extreme cases, hemodialysis is required. Sodium bicarbonate is utilized to alkalinize the urine to minimize the risk of myoglobin-induced renal failure, and it is utilized to offset profound acidosis. In addition, hydration and mannitol can induce a brisk diuresis to combat acute renal failure.

During the postoperative period, anticoagulation should be continued to prevent recurrent embolization. Over the ensuing days, the etiology of the embolus should be ascertained. The evaluation should be focused on cardiogenic etiologies to include a 24-hour Holter monitor and echocardiogram. If this is negative for the aforementioned abnormalities, a CT scan should be performed of the chest, abdomen, and pelvis. Depending on the etiology of the embolus, the source should be treated if possible. If the source of the embolism cannot be eliminated, the patient should remain on lifelong anticoagulation to reduce the risk of recurrent embolization.

SUGGESTED READINGS

Rutherford RB, Baker JD, Ernst C, et al: Recommended standards for reports dealing with lower extremity ischemia: revised version, *J Vasc Surg* 26:517, 1997.

Norgen L, Hiatt WR, Dormandy JA, et al: TransAtlantic Inter-Society Consensus for the Management of Peripheral Arterial Disease (TASC II), *J Vasc Surg* 45(1):S5A–S67A, 2007.

Abbott WM, Maloney RD, McCabe CC, et al: Arterial embolism: a 44-year perspective, *Am J Surg* 143(4):460–464, 1982.

Sobel M, Verhaeghe R: Antithrombotic therapy for peripheral artery occlusive disease: American College of Chest Physicians Evidence-Based Clinical Practice Guidelines, ed 8, *Chest* 133:815S, 2008.

ACUTE PERIPHERAL ARTERIAL AND BYPASS GRAFT OCCLUSION: THROMBOLYTIC THERAPY

Frank K. Wacker, MD, and Thomas Keane, MD

OVERVIEW

Patients with acute limb ischemia as a result of nontraumatic vascular occlusion can show a wide variety of symptoms, and an accurate assessment is essential for effective treatment to be chosen. This chapter describes how to select appropriate therapy for acute limb ischemia, with an emphasis on the role of catheter-directed thrombolysis (CDT). Acutely ischemic limbs may be revascularized with surgery, endovascular treatments, and thrombolysis. These methods are complementary and often need to be combined to treat limb ischemia most effectively. According to a Cochrane review, last assessed as up to date in 2009, there is no difference in limb-salvage rate or mortality rate between thrombolysis and surgery for acute limb ischemia at 30 days, 6 months, and 1 year.

PATIENT PRESENTATION AND WORKUP

Clinical Assessment

When patients present with an acutely ischemic limb, a history helps to immediately determine whether the patient has baseline atherosclerotic disease—evidenced by a history of claudication, stroke, myocardial infarction, hypertension, high cholesterol, prior vascular surgery, and diminished contralateral ankle-brachial indexes (ABIs). It also helps to determine whether an embolic occlusion is likely—suggested by a history of atrial fibrillation, aortic aneurysm, or MI—and whether a nonatherosclerotic etiology is a contributing factor, such as in the case of systemic lupus erythematosus and with the use of vasospastic drugs such as ergot alkaloids. The physical exam should assess for the dominant signs of limb ischemia, conventionally known as the "Six P's": *p*ain, *p*ulselessness, *p*allor, *p*oikilothermia, *p*aresthesias, and *p*aralysis. Other variables that should be assessed in the history and physical examination are listed in Table 1.

Of particular note, the condition of the contralateral limb is used to make a "best guess" assessment of the baseline state of the vasculature in the ischemic limb. The initial test, which should be performed on all patients with limb ischemia, is Doppler sonography that evaluates signals at the level of ischemia and at the ankle. At the completion of the history, physical, and Doppler studies, the physician should immediately categorize the limb threat according to the Society for Vascular Surgery/International Society for Cardiovascular Surgery (SVS/ISCVS) classification: class I is *not immediately threatened;* class IIa is *marginally threatened;* class IIb is *immediately threatened;* and class III is *irreversibly damaged,* with major tissue loss and permanent nerve damage. This initial categorization determines whether time is available for additional workup, such as imaging, or if emergent therapy is to be initiated.

In addition to triaging the limb threat, the aim of the initial assessment described above is to identify the likely cause of ischemia, so that an appropriate therapeutic approach may be undertaken. To aid in this determination of cause, it is helpful for the physician to classify the limb ischemia as acute, chronic, or acute-on-chronic; the last category represents an acute ischemic exacerbation that occurs in a chronically vasculopathic limb. Most nontraumatic or iatrogenic cases of acute limb ischemia are caused by vascular thrombosis or embolism. Table 2 summarizes the entire differential.

After the history, physical exam, Doppler imaging, and determination of chronicity of the ischemia, the next step is to use ABI, pulse volume recordings (PVRs), and invasive or noninvasive angiography to select the optimal treatment. Angiography in particular is often instrumental in differentiating between ischemic etiologies and allowing for optimization of treatment.

Imaging Assessment

Imaging is done to confirm the clinical assessment, to determine the extent of blood flow compromise, to localize the lesion, and to reveal the extent of more general etiologies such as dissections, aneurysms, cardiac thrombi, or vasculitis. An acutely ischemic limb may be imaged with magnetic resonance (MR), computed tomography (CT), digital subtraction angiography (DSA), or ultrasound (US) prior to treatment.

Although a fair amount of literature suggests that US can be a used as a comprehensive, noninvasive evaluation tool for limb ischemia, no clear scientific consensus exists as to this assertion. In the hands of an experienced sonographer, Doppler US (DUS) has a reported sensitivity of 88% and specificity of 95% in the detection of arterial stenoses greater than 50%. US provides a picture of the patient's anatomy by displaying a map of how a particular tissue reflects a sound wave. DUS has the advantage of being the least invasive of the vascular imaging modalities, as it does not require the injection of a contrast agent. It is the method of choice for routine surveillance of bypass grafts. However, the speed and accuracy of DUS is contingent upon the skills and availability of the sonographer; the anatomic evaluation is more focused and usually does not include the aorta and pelvic arteries; in addition, interpretation is not as intuitive as with DSA, CT angiography (CTA), and MR angiography (MRA). Therefore DUS is only recommended for evaluation of acute limb ischemia at facilities where DUS is routinely used for nonemergent evaluation of ischemic limbs.

TABLE 1: Key variables for clinical evaluation of a patient with an acutely ischemic limb

History	Physical
Six P's: *p*ain, *p*ulselessness, *p*allor, *p*oikilothermia, *p*aresthesias, *p*aralysis	Skin quality (ulcers, mottling)
Pain abruptness and time of onset, location, and intensity over time	Skin temperature
Chronic ischemic symptoms in any limb (claudication, rest pain)	Skin color
Coronary, carotid, or aortic disease (MI, atrial fibrillation, stroke, aortic aneurysm)	Capillary refill
Risk factors: hypertension, hyperlipidemia, diabetes, smoking, family history	Sensory/neuromotor examination
Prior revascularization with attention to indication for procedure and revascularization technique	Check popliteal fossa
	Heart rhythm
Vasculitis, Raynaud syndrome, trauma, vascular procedures	ABIs of both limbs
Medication with attention to indications; compliance with anticoagulants	Doppler pulses of both limbs

---

TABLE 2: Causes of nontraumatic acute limb ischemia

Atherosclerotic	Nonatherosclerotic	Mimics
In situ thrombosis	Embolism from cardiac thrombus (atrial fibrillation, post-MI akinesis)	Phlegmasia cerulea dolens
Atheroembolism from TAA/AAA	Graft thrombosis, graft aneurysm	Acute neuropathy
Femoral/popliteal aneurysm ± compression	Mycotic emboli	Hypovolemia
Dissection	Raynaud syndrome	Systemic shock
	Arteritis with thrombosis	
	Inherited and acquired hypercoagulable states	
	Drug-induced vasospasm	
	External compression (Baker cyst, popliteal entrapment)	

TAA/AAA, Thoracic aortic aneurysm/abdominal aortic aneurysm; *MI,* myocardial infarction

Time-resolved, contrast-enhanced MRA provides a detailed and accurate assessment of ischemic limbs with sensitivity of up to 98% and specificity of up to 96% for detecting stenoses greater than 50%. MR provides a view of the patient's anatomy by displaying a map of the intrinsic magnetic properties of the patient's tissues. These properties are discerned by magnetizing the patient's body in the MR gantry with a large electromagnet and observing how the tissues react when the induced magnetization is disrupted by radiofrequency pulses—the "buzzing" heard during MRI. The standard protocols for angiographic imaging rely on time sensitive, gadolinium-contrast–enhanced, spoiled-gradient echo sequences. MR is particularly useful when an endovascular treatment is contemplated, because the modality does not require the administration of additional iodinated contrast. Noncontrast MRA—"time-of-flight" or phase contrast sequences—does not provide a sufficiently comprehensive assessment of the ischemic limb; furthermore, it takes longer to acquire than contrast-enhanced angiography. These noncontrast methods do have some value in determining residual flow, which is difficult to visualize with contrast-enhanced angiography. However, residual flow determinations are not recommended or required when a timely diagnosis is essential, such as in cases of acute limb ischemia. Contraindications to MRI include implantable pacemakers, certain other metallic implants, claustrophobia, and risk for NSF. We recommend the Web site http://www.mrisafety.com to check whether an implantable device is MR compatible.

CTA is the first-choice noninvasive imaging modality for patients with acute limb ischemia. Its sensitivity and specificity for detecting stenoses greater than 50% is similar to MRA. It is readily available in most hospitals and requires only minutes for an acquisition, making it ideally suited for emergency evaluations. CT provides a view of the patient's anatomy by displaying a map of tissue densities, determined by measuring the extent to which a particular tissue attenuates an x-ray beam. A timed bolus of isoosmolar iodinated contrast is given, and a multirow scanner is needed to acquire and reconstruct angiographic-quality images, with a minimum of 16-slice CT for favorable image quality. The high speed at which CT imaging is performed allows the physician to acquire images of the patient's entire vascular anatomy, which allows for evaluation of the ischemic limb and of potential cardiac and arterial sources of emboli. Curved multiplanar reconstructions and three-dimensional, maximum-intensity projections (MIP) should be created from the acquired helical dataset. We recommend consultation with a radiologist when interpreting the images, particularly when findings are ambiguous.

DSA remains an excellent choice for imaging of patients with acute limb ischemia, and it is still considered the gold standard for angiography, particularly when the assessment of small vessels is required. Recent data suggest that MRA and CTA are of similar or superior quality to DSA when modern imaging equipment is used. The chief benefit of DSA is that endovascular therapies may be initiated immediately after diagnostic angiography, using the same arterial access. DSA should be considered in all patients for whom endovascular interventions are anticipated. Although DSA is a more invasive technique than MRA or CTA, the risks associated with the size 4 Fr access required for imaging are minimal. More significantly, the performance of invasive angiography requires the availability of an angiography team and suite, and it is thus less readily available than CT. As such, CT is still preferred for the evaluation of the acutely ischemic limb (Figures 1 and 2).

Selection of Therapy

To provide patients with the best possible outcomes, and for medicolegal reasons, the assessment of the ischemic limb should be completed as quickly as possible. Once a diagnosis is made, treatment should be initiated immediately. Regardless of etiology, all patients without contraindications should receive intravenous fluids, supplemental oxygen, an 81 mg dose of aspirin, and a 100 to 150 U/kg bolus

of heparin followed by a continuous heparin infusion to keep the partial thromboplastin time at 2.0 to 2.5 times normal. The length of time a limb can endure ischemia varies with cause and severity. The previously described SVS/ISCVC classification, based on sensory motor and Doppler evaluations, is used to triage initial limb treatments; choices are restaged for longer ischemic durations. Level I patients should be treated with heparin and observation, followed by more definite therapy once comorbidities, functional status, and activity level are determined. Level II patients should be treated soon (IIa) or immediately (IIb) after imaging. Endovascular or operative interventions are equally efficacious in such patients, the choice being contingent upon the availability of a surgeon experienced in a particular technique and its practice at a particular institution. Patients with more severe ischemia (IIb) have traditionally been sent to surgery, but the recent advent of fast-acting lysis drugs, sprayed-pulse infusion techniques, and mechanical thrombolysis allow endovascular techniques to have a wider application. Level III patients who seek care shortly after symptom onset are candidates for surgical revascularization and fasciotomy; those presenting some time after symptom onset require amputation. Attempts to revascularize ischemic limbs late in the progression of disease are not only likely to fail but frequently result in severe pain, myoglobinemia, renal failure, and sepsis.

Recommended Interventions for Disease in Native Arteries

Ever since the Surgery versus Thrombolysis for Ischemia of the Lower Extremity (STILE) trial demonstrated that limb-loss rates were lower with CDT than with surgery, CDT has been the first-line treatment for thrombotic occlusions of bypass grafts. Less well known is the conclusion drawn from STILE trial, that CDT produces outcomes similar to surgery when used to treat thrombosed native arteries presenting within 2 weeks of the onset of symptoms. Patients presenting later than 2 weeks received greater benefit from surgery. The Thrombolysis or Peripheral Arterial Surgery (TOPAS) trial added the insight that CDT may be attempted—and then abandoned when ineffective in favor of more localized surgery—without increasing mortality or amputation rate. Nonrandomized trials have also demonstrated that attempting CDT and angioplasty before surgery can reduce the number of patients who ultimately require bypass grafts. Although these trials do not provide definitive answers as to a preferred treatment in all cases, they do suggest that trials of CDT may improve outcomes without compromising the efficacy of subsequent surgery. As such, we recommend CDT, if readily available, as the first-line therapy for acute native artery occlusion, with endovascular or surgical intervention to treat underlying lesions once unmasked.

Prior to starting CDT, the treating physician should assess the extent of disease in the affected limb, not only in the thrombosed segment, but also in the vasculature proximal and distal to the occlusion. This assessment is often complicated by the fact that imaging does not always reveal the state of runoff vessels, as outflow may be completely blocked at the level of the acute occlusion. Recent prior imaging studies, if available, can be consulted to assess runoff. If these are not available, the state of the contralateral limb can be used as a "best guess" estimate of the state of the vasculature in the affected limb, allowing a determination as to whether CDT would unmask a treatable short-segment stenosis in an artery with otherwise decent runoff. According to the Trans-Atlantic Inter-Society Consensus Document on Management of Peripheral Arterial Disease (TASC II) guidelines, such focal stenoses are best treated with percutaneous transluminal angioplasty (PTA) and stenting once the artery is opened with thrombolytics. In contrast, recent imaging and contralateral limb assessment showing long-segment stenosis, diffuse disease, or limited runoff in the affected vessel should dissuade the surgeon from using CDT. In diffusely diseased vessels, thrombolysis serves only to consume time, as it does not open the vessel up to treatment with PTA and stenting; vessels with more extensive disease require surgical bypass.

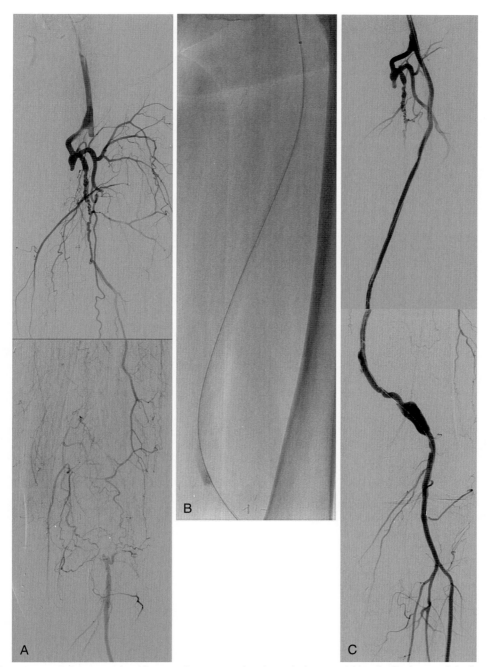

FIGURE 1   DSA of a patient with femoropopliteal bypass who presented with a pulseless, painful leg. **A,** Occlusion of the bypass. **B,** Overnight thrombolysis using a 40 cm infusion catheter followed by angioplasty of the proximal anastomosis. **C,** The procedure resulted in an open prosthetic graft with aneurysm at the distal anastomosis and excellent runoff.

In patients with native vessel occlusions from cardiac emboli, the lack of collateral flow results in dramatic, poorly tolerated symptoms; as such, patients usually come in early in the course of ischemia. When a patient assessment suggests minimal baseline atherosclerotic disease, or when history points to an embolic occlusion (i.e., a cardiac embolus), the patient should undergo transfemoral percutaneous Fogarty embolectomy. CDT in combination with mechanical or aspiration embolectomy is also an option. These endovascular techniques are especially efficacious below the knee, where fluoroscopic guidance allows for evaluation and selective intervention in small arteries.

Recommended Interventions for Disease in Bypass Grafts

In patients with thrombosed bypass grafts, the timing of the graft failure determines which treatment is preferred. If the patient presents within the first 30 days after bypass, graft failure is most often a result of technical problems with the graft, assuming the patient is not hypercoagulable. If the bypass is partially open, imaging usually reveals the causative lesion; the most common finding is a distal anastomotic stricture. In native vessel conduits, a surgeon will occasionally see a stenosis that results from the use of too small a caliber venous conduit, or even more uncommonly, a perivascular hematoma is seen,

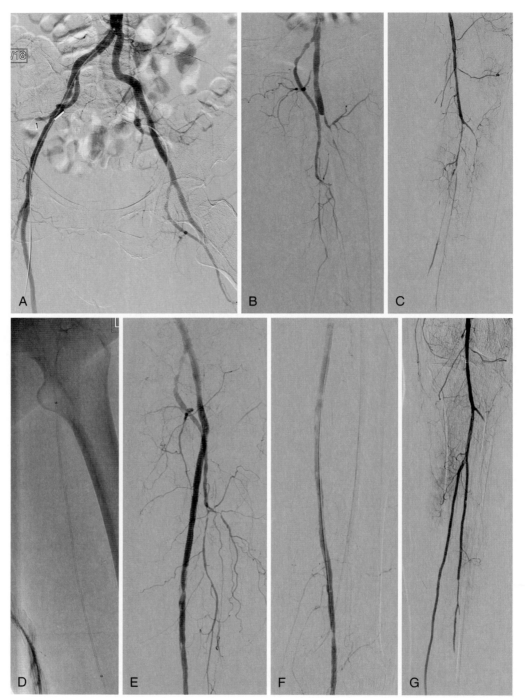

FIGURE 2 Patient with chronic kidney disease, acute onset of pain, and nonpalpable pulses in left lower extremity. **A,** DSA shows severe atherosclerosis of profunda femoris branches. **B,** Occlusion of left superficial femoral artery (SFA). **C,** Poor runoff. **D,** With a 20 cm infusion catheter in place, 12-hour thrombolysis was started. **E,** Angioplasty and placement of 6 mm diameter, 17 cm long stent in SFA. **G,** Angioplasty of posterior tibial and peroneal arteries showing improved outflow.

resulting from improper vein preparation. Patients with early bypass failure should undergo a revision surgery. An endovascular treatment is only recommended in the rare case of an isolated angiographic lesion that appears amenable to angioplasty. More often, thrombolysis serves only to open the bypass temporarily. The underlying technical problem quickly reasserts itself, and the limb again becomes ischemic.

If the bypass goes down outside of the 30-day perioperative window, the assessing physician should first consider the severity of the ischemia and the indication for the original surgery. If the ischemia does not threaten the viability of the limb, as it did in 30% of patients in the STILE trial, and the original bypass was performed to treat limb-threatening ischemia, a hands-off approach may be appropriate. It is unlikely that any revision of the graft will provide long-term improvement in the limb's vascularity, but it is possible that further surgery will make things worse. In these cases, noninvasive imaging and DSA are appropriate to assess whether distal target vessels are available for a secondary bypass and to assess whether endovascular treatments could improve perfusion of the poorly functioning bypass.

In cases of limb-threatening ischemia occurring outside of the 30-day perioperative window, the most common causative lesion is focal intimal hyperplasia, typically at a valve or anastomosis. Thrombolysis is the treatment of choice in these instances, because it allows for identification of the treatable lesion. CDT also restores flow through thrombosed collaterals, thus reperfusing the at-risk limb. Thrombolysis should be followed by angioplasty or minimal access surgery once the focal lesion is identified. If a correctable lesion can be found and treated, the 1-year patency rate is more favorable than if there had been no lesion. Grafts maintained exclusively by CDT and PTA have been found to have an excellent working life, especially if ABIs are high after treatment. There are two caveats, however: first, the outcomes of thrombolysis are much better in venous grafts than in synthetic grafts; second, the beneficial effect of thrombolysis is short-lived in diabetic patients, and 1-year patencies are very low. In these patients, if imaging reveals a suitable distal target vessel, secondary bypasses are a superior treatment choice because of higher patency rates.

Patients with vein grafts more than 1 year old are excellent candidates for CDT, as the conduit has proven itself over a length of time. The failure is usually a result of progressing atherosclerosis in the inflow or outflow vessels. CDT will most commonly unmask a normal-looking graft with poor inflow or outflow vessels, which themselves can be treated to maintain graft function.

Investigations have attempted to stratify the efficacy of bypass CDT by anastomotic site and bypass type. Data from these investigations allow no clear-cut conclusions to be drawn regarding recanalization and patency. However, one study drew the contrarian conclusion that venous grafts were *less* amenable to CDT than prosthetic grafts, suggesting that vein wall ischemia is the major factor in graft failure, which cannot be corrected by recanalization. As indicated earlier, however, the majority of studies conclude that venous bypass grafts respond *well* to CDT. Most studies of CDT in bypasses have concluded that the proximal anastomotic location has no influence on efficacy. Individual studies have asserted that CDT is less efficacious in bypasses with 1) tibial or pedal anastomoses, 2) short times to first failure, 3) poor runoff, and 4) bypasses in diabetics, as mentioned above.

CATHETER-DIRECTED THOMBOLYSIS

Systemic intravenous thrombolysis has been completely supplanted by CDT, in which an agent is delivered locally to the clot. As mentioned earlier, the role of thrombolysis is to 1) restore flow, 2) reveal an underlying causative lesion, and 3) improve perfusion of the outflow vessels. The unmasked lesion is then treated by angioplasty and stenting or surgery.

Preoperative Planning

If CDT is to be used as part of the ischemic limb treatment plan, the preprocedural consent should describe the risk of hemorrhage, limb loss, renal failure, anaphylaxis, stroke, and death. Bleeding is the most frequent significant complication of CDT. An intracranial bleed, the most feared and significant potential complication of CDT, occured in 1.2% (STILE) to 2.1% (TOPAS-I) of patients in prospective randomized clinical trials. Absolute contraindications to CDT include active bleeding, aortic dissection, recent intracranial or intraspinal surgery or trauma, intracranial arteriovenous malformation, and intracranial aneurysms. Relative contraindications include major operative procedures within the preceding 4 weeks, uncontrolled hypertension, gastric ulcers, recent eye surgery and stroke, pregnancy or the first 10 days postpartum, and intracranial neoplasms.

Patients should have aspirin and heparin started before arriving for CDT, and any previous noninvasive imaging should be available in the procedure suite. Pulses in both limbs should be documented,

and an operating room should be available in the event that conversion to open surgery becomes necessary. Isoosmolar contrast should be used throughout, and the procedure is usually performed under conscious sedation.

Technique

Retrograde femoral access should be obtained in the contralateral limb with the arterial puncture occurring over the femoral head. Ultrasound-guided 21 gauge micropunture access is advisable, to minimize risk of puncturing the femoral vein or the profunda. A 5 Fr Omni Flush catheter (AngioDynamics, Latham, NY) or pigtail catheter should be advanced through a 5 Fr vascular sheath to the level of the renal arteries, and an aortogram and bilateral lower extremity runoff should be obtained. Typically, one station is used for the abdomen and pelvis, and three stations are used for the lower extremities, for a total of four acquisitions.

Once the thrombosed vascular segment is identified, the wire-catheter combination should be maneuvered into the external iliac artery on the affected side. An Omni Flush catheter, with its reverse-curve tip, is specifically designed to facilitate "up and over" iliac access from the disease-free side. After a wire is placed into the external iliac artery, the access catheter and 5 Fr sheath are exchanged for a 7 or 8 Fr "up and over" sheath, which is positioned with its tip in the common or external iliac artery.

Next, the thrombosed segment must be traversed. We prefer two wire-catheter combinations: a combination 4 Fr angled glide catheter and hydrophilic guidewire (e.g., Glidewire [Terumo, Somerset, NJ], Magic-Torque [Boston Scientific, Natick, NJ], Roadrunner [Cook Medical, Bloomington, Ind.]); this is usually our first choice for a targeted recanalization, using the maneuverability of both catheter and wire. In arteries with significant atherosclerotic disease, a 4 Fr straight-glide catheter and 0.035 inch Rosen wire (Cook Medical) combination can be used to traverse the clot; the Rosen wire is configured such that it barely protrudes from the catheter, with its distal curve hugging the lip of the straight catheter. This wire-catheter combination assures that the blunt tip of the wire leads in the lumen of the vessel, minimizing the possibility of dissection. Gentle attempts should be made to traverse the thrombus, with focal hand injections of 50-50 contrast made whenever the catheter-wire combination does not advance easily. The goal is to push gently through the soft clot. Occasionally, a microwire (<0.016 inch) and microcatheter (<3 Fr) may be passed coaxially to aid successful clot traversal.

Once the clotted segment is traversed, the length of the occlusion should be measured, and an appropriate multiple side-hole infusion catheter should be advanced over the wire through the occlusion. For effective CDT, the catheter length should be as close as possible to the length of the thrombosed segment, erring on the side of a shorter infusion length. The goal is to deliver thrombolytics to the entire length of the occlusion, without having any of the catheter side holes lying outside of the clot. If some of the holes are in open artery, the infused drug will take the path of least resistance and will squirt out the holes and end up outside the clot.

After the infusion catheter is suitably positioned, the guidewire is removed, and the end hole of the infusion catheter is plugged up with an occlusion wire. The up-and-over vascular introducer sheath should be sutured to the skin, and the infusion catheter should be secured to the sheath with Steri-Strips and suture to ensure that the catheter does not move from its carefully selected position.

Infusion

Limited data are available to compare the efficacy of various fibrinolytic agents for use in CDT. In the United States, streptokinase, anistreplase, alteplase (a recombinant tissue plasminogen activator [tPA]), reteplase, and tenecteplase are available. Thrombus dissolution and bleeding rates are comparable among the various agents, with few direct comparison trials available. There is currently no convincing evidence of the superiority of one agent over another for CDT. Adjunctive agents such as glycoprotein IIb/IIIa platelet-receptor inhibitors may speed up thrombolysis (Platelet Receptor Antibodies in Order to Manage Peripheral Artery Thrombosis [PROMPT] trial), but they do not result in lower amputation rates or a decreased need for endovascular or surgical treatment. The intravenous heparin infusion should be discontinued once thrombolytics infusion begins, to reduce the risk of bleeding.

After an initial lacing of the thrombus with a high dose of the agent, low-dose continuous infusion is the least labor-intensive technique. We typically lace the clot with an initial 5 mg bolus of tPA then initiate a 0.25 to 0.5 mg/hr continuous infusion. A 150 to 300 U/hr *intraarterial* infusion of heparin via the vascular sheath is used prevent thrombus from forming around the tip of the sheath. Fibrinogen, platelets, hematocrit, and partial thromboplastin time should be checked at baseline and every 4 to 6 hours, with the tPA infusion rate halved for every fibrinogen measurement greater than 150 mg/dL. If the fibrinogen level drops below 100 mg/dL, conventional wisdom says to stop infusion because of the increased risk of bleeding. Alternatively, cryoprecipitate can be administered to raise the fibrinogen level and allow for continued infusion of tPA. No more than 10 bags of cryoprecipitate should be administered in any 24-hour period.

Patients should be admitted to a monitored bed, and clinical checks of the limb, including ABIs, should be performed every 2 hours. Paradoxically, reports of increased pain in the treated limb may indicate successful thrombolysis, with pain occurring as a result of distal microemboli showering. Other clinical variables such as temperature, color, pulse, and capillary refill should all point toward improving perfusion. If at any point the limb appears to be growing more ischemic, the catheter position should be checked in the angio suite. If the limb becomes critically ischemic, CDT should be aborted, and surgical revascularization should be attempted. If the limb ischemia is stable or improving, reevaluation with angiography is indicated every 12 to 24 hours until flow is restored.

Multiple new devices purport to shorten thrombolytic time, therefore decreasing the risk of hemorrhagic complications. Pulse-spray catheters, mechanical lysis catheters, aspiration catheters, rheolytic catheters, and ultrasound-accelerated devices are all currently available or under investigation. Use of these devices requires some experience and training, and angio suite table time is increased by their use. As more clinical experience with the devices accrues, a more accurate assessment of their efficacy can be made.

Once an occlusive clot is lysed in an appropriately selected patient, an underlying atherosclerotic lesion is typically revealed (except in patients with embolic occlusions). The reperfused limb should be assessed with DSA, and corrective treatment should be initiated.

Follow-up

The goal of the CDT is to provide timely, safe, effective, and durable revascularization of the affected limb. After successful revascularization of the ischemic limb, the patient should be kept on an 81 mg daily dose of aspirin for life. Underlying vascular risk factors should be addressed with antihypertensives, glycemic control, statins, smoking cessation, and so on. Additional antithrombotic drugs may be administered, depending on the nature of the revascularization procedure. In revascularized patients with a high risk for reocclusion, a vitamin K antagonist may be initiated in addition to the aspirin regimen. The value of dual antiplatelet therapy comprising aspirin plus clopidogrel or ticlopidine, which is well established in coronary stenting, remains controversial in peripheral revascularizations, and evidence-based guidelines do not recommend routine use. ABIs should be used to monitor patency after revascularization. If the ABI decreases by more than 0.2, angiography (invasive or noninvasive) is indicated.

SUGGESTED READINGS

Berridge DC, Kessel DO, Robertson I: Surgery versus thrombolysis for initial management of acute limb ischaemia, Cochrane Database Syst Rev (1):CD002784, 2002.

Comerota AJ: Development of catheter-directed intrathrombus thrombolysis with plasmin for the treatment of acute lower extremity arterial occlusion, *Thromb Res* 122(Suppl 3):S20–S26, 2008.

Earnshaw JJ, Whitman B, Foy C: National Audit of Thrombolysis for Acute Leg Ischemia (NATALI): clinical factors associated with early outcome, *J Vasc Surg* 39(5):1018–1025, 2004.

Hirsch AT, Haskal ZJ, Hertzer NR, et al: ACC/AHA 2005 practice guidelines for the management of patients with peripheral arterial disease (lower extremity, renal, mesenteric, and abdominal aortic): a collaborative report, *Circulation* 113:e463, 2006.

Kessel DO, Berridge DC, Robertson I: Infusion techniques for peripheral arterial thrombolysis. Cochrane Database Syst Rev (1):CD000985, 2004.

Norgren L, Hiatt WR, Dormandy JA, et al: TransAtlantic Inter-Society Consensus for the Management of Peripheral Arterial Disease (TASC II), *J Vasc Surg* 45(Suppl S):S5, 2007.

Rutherford RB: Clinical staging of acute limb ischemia as the basis for choice of revascularization method: when and how to intervene, *Semin Vasc Surg* 22(1):5–9, 2009.

ATHEROSCLEROTIC RENOVASCULAR DISEASE

John Byrne, MCh,
and R. Clement Darling III, MD

OVERVIEW

For many, management of renal artery atherosclerosis (RAS) is easy: severe stenosis mandates treatment. As a result, the number of patients undergoing endovascular renal artery therapies has grown steadily each year. From 1996 to 2000, claims for Medicare beneficiaries undergoing stent placement with an indication of RAS rose from 7660 to 18,520. Such an aggressive policy is based on published natural history data with regard to renal artery stenoses. Schreiber and colleagues (1984) reported angiographic progression of renal artery disease in 44% of vessels. Stenoses of greater than 75% went on to occlude 39% of the time, whereas only 5% of lesions less than 50% went on to occlude. Zierler and colleagues (1994) also documented a 5% annual occlusion rate for lesions greater than 60%. However, more recent data, such as the 2007 Agency for Healthcare Research and Quality (AHRQ) executive summary document on renal revascularization was equivocal on its benefits. Also, the Angioplasty and Stenting for Renal Artery Lesions (ASTRAL) trial published in 2009 has questioned whether renal revascularization offers any benefit compared with best medical therapy. A major National Institutes of Health (NIH) study, the Cardiovascular Outcomes in Renal Atherosclerotic Lesions (CORAL) trial, is also

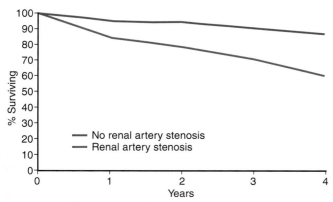

FIGURE 1   Life expectancy of patients with renal artery stenosis compared to those with nonrenal artery stenosis. *(From McLaughlin K, Jardine AG, Moss JG: ABCs of arterial and venous disease: renal artery stenosis, BMJ 320:1124–1127, 2000.)*

awaited. Unfortunately, the decision to intervene is not as clear as in most vascular diseases.

INCIDENCE AND SIGNIFICANCE

Renal artery stenoses are usually atherosclerotic (90%), and they occur in 0.1% of the general population. Up to 4% of all hypertensive patients will have RAS, and its incidence rises to between 10% and 20% in patients with concomitant hypertension and coronary artery disease. Among patients undergoing cardiac catheterization, 15% will have renal artery stenoses, with luminal compromise in over 50%; patients with symptomatic peripheral artery disease have a prevalence that rises to over 30%. Extrapolating from this, it appears that ischemic nephropathy due to RAS is probably responsible for 5% to 22% of end-stage renal disease in patients older than 50 years. As of 2004, according to the United States Renal Data System, 335,963 patients were receiving dialysis treatment at a cost of $18.1 billion per year. The annual mortality rate for patients on dialysis in the United States is high (23%), and few survive 10 years.

Renal artery stenosis is a negative predictor for long-term survival and particularly for cardiovascular events. In patients identified as having greater than 75% renal artery stenosis at the time of coronary angiography, only 57% were still alive at 4 years compared with 89% of those with normal renal arteries (Figure 1). Predictably, patients with bilateral RAS fared worst, with only 47% still alive at 4 years. Population-based studies confirm this. In 1999, a Swedish study compared 164 patients with RAS (<50%) with normal age-matched Swedish control subjects. Those with RAS had a 3.3 times increased mortality risk and a 5.7 times increased risk for cardiovascular mortality.

NATURAL HISTORY

Symptomatic Renal Artery Stenosis

Renal artery stenosis is implicated in the pathogenesis of hypertension, recurrent pulmonary edema, and deteriorating renal function (*ischemic nephropathy*). However, all these conditions are multifactorial; association does not imply causality. As far back as 1956, it was shown that nephrectomy lowered blood pressure in only 35% of patients with hypertension and RAS. Renal revascularization *rarely cures* hypertension, and established ischemic nephropathy is *rarely reversed*. The goals are to improve blood pressure control and end-organ damage and to avert dialysis. It is not clear why RAS produces hypertension in some, causes ischemic nephropathy in others,

generates flash pulmonary edema in a minority, and remains asymptomatic for the majority.

Renovascular hypertension generally does not occur until the renal artery stenosis exceeds 70% to 80%. Most of the changes fueling hypertension occur at the level of the juxtaglomerular apparatus by stimulating an excessive renin secretion. Atherosclerosis of the renal arteries is common but, in itself, it does not usually cause hypertension. On the other hand, a large number of normotensive individuals older than 60 years have RAS, with the number approaching 50% in some studies. *Ischemic nephropathy* is impairment of renal function beyond occlusive disease of the main renal arteries. The goal is usually to limit further damage rather than to resurrect terminally damaged nephrons. The outlook for patients with progressive, untreated ischemic nephropathy due to RAS is grim; the mean survival time of these patients on dialysis is 25 months, with a 5-year survival rate of only 18%. The question, of course, is whether renal revascularization improves prognosis. *Flash pulmonary edema* develops rapidly over a matter of minutes. It is a rare manifestation of RAS and usually is found in patients with significant bilateral renal artery stenosis or severe stenosis in a solitary kidney. The majority have some degree of ischemic nephropathy, although most have normal baseline left ventricular function.

"Asymptomatic" Renal Artery Stenosis

RAS frequently is an incidental finding. Patients are not particularly hypertensive and have normal creatinine levels. So what is its significance? In 1998, a cohort study of 170 patients with RAS affecting at least one renal artery, monitored with serial Duplex scanning for 33 months, reported disease progression in 35%. However, only 3% of all the arteries surveyed progressed to occlusion, and all these arteries had a 60% or greater stenosis to start. At 2 years, renal atrophy and loss of parenchyma only occurred in 20% of those patients with a greater than 60% stenosis, suggesting that asymptomatic renal artery stenosis is relatively innocuous for the majority of patients (80%).

In 2000, Iglesias showed that renal artery stenosis is an uncommon cause of progressive renal disease. Asymptomatic patients with renal atherosclerosis had the same risk of decline in renal function as matched controls with normal renal arteries. Also in 2000, a Mayo Clinic study looked at the outcome for 68 patients with high-grade (>70% stenosis) lesions who were treated medically over a mean of 39 months. Only 4 (5.8%) of the 68 patients required revascularization. By the end of the study, 28% of patients had died of nonrenal causes, and 7.4% were on dialysis for reasons unrelated to RAS. Most patients, however, did not require dialysis and remained normotensive. Most at risk were those with bilateral RAS or a single functioning kidney. In 2002, the United Kingdom Joint Vascular Research Group also confirmed that patients with renal artery stenosis and peripheral vascular disease had a poor prognosis, but this was not directly attributable to renal failure. Finally, in 2006, a study of 834 "free-living elderly Americans" in North Carolina showed that asymptomatic renal artery stenoses are relatively harmless in patients older than 65 years, only 4% progress to significant renal artery stenosis and none progress to occlusion. The strong advice from this study was that, based on its benign prognosis, incidental asymptomatic RAS in older patients should not be treated.

INDICATIONS FOR TREATMENT

Renovascular Hypertension

Even in the best series, no more than 60% to 70% of patients with hypertension improve after renal revascularization, and only 5% to 30% of patients are actually "cured." However, these results are still better than those for best medical treatment in the several small, randomized controlled trials to date. Poor patient selection and inadequate workup will produce poor results. However, it can be difficult to pick winners—improved blood pressure control is not dependent on age, sex, ethnicity, severity of stenosis, number of vessels treated, or baseline creatinine. The only variable that seems to be important is degree of hypertension. Patients with a mean arterial blood pressure over 110 mm Hg prior to revascularization fare better. The best advice in selecting patients is that those with *severe* hypertension and clearly documented renal artery stenosis have the best chance of responding to renal revascularization.

Ischemic Nephropathy

The goal of any treatment is to prevent disease progression. However, endovascular techniques carry risks of renal artery atheroembolism and contrast nephropathy with worsening of renal function. A meta-analysis in 1999 confirmed this possibility: creatinine levels improved in 25%, stabilized in 50%, and worsened in 25%. Patients who derive the most benefit are those with the most aggressive disease and most rapidly declining renal function.

Flash Pulmonary Edema

Patients with flash pulmonary edema are the rarest and the unhealthiest, and repeated hospitalizations in such patients should prompt the search for renal artery lesions. The finding of bilateral renal artery stenoses in these patients, or of a stenosis in a solitary functioning kidney, should prompt revascularization. The goal is not cure, but rather to reduce these patients' admissions to a medical center for acute congestive heart failure and to improve quality of life. Successful renal artery revascularization (open or endovascular) can reduce the need for further hospitalizations in 70% of patients.

Asymptomatic Disease

Asymptomatic renal artery stenoses are far more common than symptomatic lesions. Often these are discovered incidentally. The impetus for liberal application of intervention for asymptomatic RAS has come from two sources: first, the development of renal artery stenting; second, the suggestion in the 1980s that progression of renal artery stenosis was relentless and occurred at a rate of 20% per year. This had huge cost implications for both insurers and treating physicians, given the potential pool of patients.

More data are clearly needed on this issue. The best advice at present, besides optimizing atherosclerotic risk factors, is to treat lesions that are high grade (>80% stenosis), rapidly progressing on serial Duplex scanning, or significant (>60% stenosis) in a solitary kidney. Additionally, the physician must be more circumspect about intervening in the elderly.

Both surgery and stenting have high technical success rates (over 95%) and a 5-year patency of 90% in many series. However, technical perfection does not imply benefit. Good patient selection is imperative, and it is useful to devise a logical algorithm. The outcomes of major trials are awaited to fully define the role of revascularization.

MEDICAL THERAPY

What is the best medical therapy? Combination therapy is frequently prescribed: two or more *antihypertensive agents*, including angiotensin-converting enzyme (ACE) inhibitors or angiotensin receptor blockers, calcium channel blockers, and β-blockers to mitigate end-organ damage; *statins* to decrease low-density lipoprotein (LDL)

cholesterol levels; and *antiplatelet agents*, such as aspirin or clopidogrel, to reduce risk of thrombosis. However, good randomized controlled trials comparing medical therapy with intervention are few. Randomized control trials in 1998 and 2000, and two meta-analyses in 2003, concluded that renal angioplasty is superior to medical therapy for patients with renal artery disease. The British Angioplasty and Stenting for Regional Artery Lesions (ASTRAL) trial, published in 2009, randomized 806 patients to revascularization with medical treatment or medical therapy alone. Study end points were renal function (creatinine levels), blood pressure, major renal events, cardiovascular events, and death. Outcomes were measured at 5 years and showed no difference between those patients who received revascularization and those who received medicine alone. These results applied to all patient groups: patients with asymptomatic or "incidentally discovered" renal artery stenoses were considered, as were those with ischemic nephropathy and renovascular hypertension. However, the investigators accepted that further analysis of their data was needed, using post hoc methodology, to see if there were subgroups that might benefit. As this study contradicts established practice in many centers, as well as contradicting all previous randomized trials and meta-analyses, more data are needed before a consensus document can be drafted.

ENDOVASCULAR THERAPY

Most interventionalists have their own tricks. What is described here is our way of doing renal intervention. It works in our hands, but other techniques are equally effective.

Balloon Angioplasty

Balloon angioplasty of the renal arteries was first performed by Grüntzig in 1978. It is effective for nonatheromatous renal artery lesions, such as fibromuscular dysplasia. Renal artery ostial lesions are really an extension of aortic plaque into the renal artery origins, and balloon angioplasty is subject to elastic recoil, dissection, and residual stenosis. More effective for atherosclerotic stenoses in the mid and distal renal artery, it is still of use in patients with in-stent restenosis. For 90% of patients, the femoral artery is the preferred access method; only in 10% or so will the renal arteries be sufficiently angulated to make a transbrachial approach necessary.

To begin, we use a 6 Fr guiding sheath after administration of 70 IU/kg of heparin. A diagnostic catheter and guidewire are then used to selectively access the renal artery. The diagnostic catheter is removed, and an angioplasty balloon is advanced over the wire and through the guiding sheath. "Waisting" of the balloon should be seen as it is deployed. Following removal of the balloon over the guidewire, a completion angiogram is performed.

Renal Artery Stenting

Renal artery stenting is more difficult than simple balloon angioplasty but more effective for ostial and proximal renal artery stenoses. A diagnostic aortogram is performed, and the patient is given 70 U/kg of heparin, but the standard 5 Fr diagnostic sheath is exchanged for a 6 Fr guiding sheath. Through the guiding sheath, the renal artery is selected using a diagnostic catheter. The renal ostium and stenosis is then crossed with a stiff 0.014 inch or 0.018 inch guidewire, and the guiding catheter is advanced over the diagnostic catheter, in a "telescoping" technique, to the renal ostium. A 0.014 inch or 0.018 inch guidewire may reduce the risk of atheroembolization.

Next, a renal angiogram is performed to look for distal branch vessel disease and to indicate the site of the lesion. The diameter of the nondiseased renal artery proximal and distal to the stenosis is measured, and the appropriate stent is chosen. The stent is then carefully advanced over the guidewire, until it lies in the correct position, and then it is deployed with the 6 Fr guiding catheter "parked" at the renal ostium. The goal is to leave 1 to 2 mm of stent protruding into the aortic lumen. Following stent deployment, the delivery system is withdrawn over the 0.014 inch wire, and a completion angiogram is performed through the guiding catheter. Any residual stenosis is corrected by balloon angioplasty.

Unfortunately, manipulation of the renal artery origin and an atheromatous aorta has its problems. Despite careful attention to technique, renal function may worsen in patients after intervention. In experimental settings, angioplasty and stenting of renal arteries causes significant atheroemboli. Distal embolic protection devices (EPDs) are used in the carotid arteries. The thought has occurred to use EPDs in the renal arteries, but embolization often occurs upon advancing wires and catheters across the renal artery origin in addition to the percutaneous therapy, which is a prerequisite for deployment of filters. Renal anatomy may also play a role in deterring their use, given the branching, tortuosity, and short length of the typical renal artery. Despite this, encouraging reports of EPDs trapping debris that otherwise would have occluded smaller parenchymal vessels have been circulated.

Morbidity, Mortality, and Patency Rates of Endovascular Therapy

In 1993, prior to renal stenting, a Swedish study compared balloon angioplasty with mainly renal endarterectomy in 58 patients. The technical success rate was higher in the surgical groups (97% vs. 83%); however, secondary patency rates were similar. The authors suggested balloon angioplasty as the first-line treatment, provided adequate surveillance was performed. In 1999, a randomized controlled trial compared renal stents with balloon angioplasty. Stents had a superior technical success rate (88% vs. 55%), and 6-month primary patency was also significantly better (75% vs. 29%). The trial was stopped early following an interim analysis of the data. Trials performed since that time are shown in (Table 1).

SURGICAL THERAPY

Surgery for renal artery stenosis can be divided into three basic categories: *anatomic bypass, extraanatomic bypass,* and *nephrectomy* (Table 2). *Anatomic bypasses* arise from the aorta or from aortic bypass grafts but also include thromboendarterectomy and renal artery reimplantation. These reconstructions have both high flow and excellent patency, which is the reason we use them as our first-line choice in therapy. An alternative to bypass is ex vivo renal artery reconstruction. *Extraanatomic bypasses* are hepatorenal, splenorenal, and rarely iliorenal or mesorenal revascularizations. These are secondary procedures reserved for high-risk individuals, challenging anatomy, and patients with significant comorbidities. Ultimately, there is *nephrectomy*, which still plays a limited role even today.

Anatomic Bypass

Aortorenal Bypass as an Adjunct to Aortic Reconstruction

The most common scenario for aortorenal bypass in our practice is as part of aortobifemoral bypass or repair of an abdominal aortic aneurysm (Figure 2). Addition of left renal artery reconstruction to aortic surgery through a left retroperitoneal approach has not increased the incidence of adverse outcomes in our hands. However, we have experienced a significantly higher morbidity when bilateral renal artery reconstructions are performed. The aorta is exposed by a left-flank incision through the tenth intercostal space. Division of the lumbar branch of the left renal vein is required, as is division of the left crus

of the diaphragm to facilitate exposure of the left renal artery. The proximal 1 to 2 cm of the right renal artery can also be exposed from this approach, although it is difficult prior to division of the aorta. Limbs of 6 mm expanded polytetrafluoroethylene (ePTFE) are sewn onto the aortic graft prior to suprarenal or infrarenal artery clamping. The patient is given a bolus of 3000 units of heparin.

We do not routinely flush the kidney with cold saline, nor do we ice pack the kidney to prolong warm ischemia time during in situ revascularization. After clamping the aorta proximally and transecting it, the right renal artery can be accessed more readily if needed. The renal artery or arteries are clamped prior to aortic clamping. The proximal aorta–graft anastomosis is completed and suture line tested by repositioning the clamp distally. The ePTFE graft limb is now sewn end-to-end onto the appropriate renal artery; the clamp is repositioned below the origin of the renal artery bypass graft, and the renal artery is perfused. Introperative continuous wave Doppler is used to confirm blood flow. The distal aortic, iliac, or femoral anastomoses are then completed.

Primary Aortorenal Bypass

For primary aortorenal bypass, the infrarenal aorta is used, if possible, as the inflow (Figure 3). Reversed greater saphenous vein or 6 mm ePTFE is the conduit and it is usually sewn end-to-side onto the renal artery. Occasionally, the *suprarenal aorta* may be required as the inflow source, which makes the bypass more anatomic but translates into a more difficult exposure; this is not commonly used for bilateral primary renal artery bypasses. Instead, a laparotomy incision is made, and the supraceliac aorta is exposed, either through a medial visceral rotation or by traversing the lesser sac. A bifurcated graft can be used for reconstruction of both renal arteries.

Alternatively, if the abdominal aorta is healthy, an infrarenal aorta-renal artery bypass can be performed, either through a bilateral subcostal incision, a transverse abdominal incision, or a conventional laparotomy exposure. Exposure of the left renal artery and proximal right renal artery is accomplished by incising the posterior peritoneum overlying the aorta and dividing the ligament of Treitz to allow reflection of the duodenum downward and to the right. The incision in the peritoneum is then continued along the inferior border of the pancreas to the patient's left. By entering an avascular plane at the inferior border of the pancreas, the left renal hilum can be exposed. The left renal artery lies deep to the vein. It is necessary to divide the lumbar branch of the left renal vein to safely retract the vein and allow exposure of the left renal artery. Division of the suprarenal and gonadal veins may also be required. Exposure of the origin of the right renal artery will require division of two to three lumbar veins and retraction of the left renal vein superiorly, while the inferior vena cava (IVC) is retracted to the patient's right. To approach the distal right renal artery, the hepatic flexure of the ascending colon is taken down, and the right colon is retracted inferiorly. Next, the duodenum is reflected medially to expose the IVC and right renal vein. The right renal artery, usually inferior to the renal vein, is carefully mobilized and retracted superiorly to expose the artery.

Thromboendarterectomy

We perform thromboendarterectomy through a retroperitoneal incision through the tenth intercostal space, dividing the lumbar branch of the left renal vein and the left crus of diaphragm to facilitate exposure (Figure 4). The left kidney is mobilized and reflected anteriorly, and the aorta is clamped above the celiac axis and below the renal arteries. Clamps are placed on both renal arteries and the mesenteric vessels. A "trapdoor" incision is made in the aorta, along the anterolateral portion, and the aorta is endarterectomized to include the renal artery origins. Endarterectomy of the visceral vessels requires an "eversion" technique to ensure an adequate end point. Others use a transperitoneal approach. In this case, a medial visceral rotation must be performed to allow exposure to the visceral artery origins before

TABLE 1: Morbidity, mortality, and patency rates of endovascular renal therapy*

First Author	N	Bilateral Treatment (%)	Preoperative Renal Dysfunction (%)	RENAL FUNCTION RESPONSE (%)			HYPERTENSION RESPONSE (%)			PERIOPERATIVE OUTCOME (%)	
				Improved	Unchanged	Worsened	Cured	Improved	Failed	Death	Morbidity
Burket (2000)	127	NR	29	43	57		NR			2	4
Lederman (2001)	300	41	37	9	78	14	70		30	<1	2
Bush (2001)	73	16	68	23	51	26	NR			1.4	9
Rocha-Singh (2002)	51	55	100	77	18	5	91		9	0	14
Kennedy (2003)	261	NR	36	61		39	NR			NR	NR
Gill (2003)	100	26	75	31	38	31	4	79	17	2	18
Zeller (2003)	215	23	52	52	48		76		24	0	5
Henry (2003)	56	14	32	14	66	0	18	59	23	1.8	NR
Zeller (2004)	456	NR	52	34	39	27	46		54	<1	NR
Nolan (2005)	82	NR	59	23	53	24	NR	81	NR	0	7
Kashyap (2007)	125	36	100	42	23	25	NR			1.6	6
Holden (2006)	63	32	100	97		3	0	55	45	NR	NR
Corriere (2008)	99	11	75	28	65	7	1	21	78	0	5.5
Mean %†		30	55	31	38	31	18	54	28	1	6.2

NR, Not reported

*Series selected based on publication in 2000 or later, use of angioplasty and stenting, inclusion of ≥50 patients, and categoric reporting of renal function and/or hypertension responses.

†Weighted mean based on number of patients with reported data categorized according to column headings; references where data were not reported, or where categoric response categories were combined, were not included in the calculation.

From Edwards MS, Corriere MA: Contemporary management of atherosclerotic renovascular disease, *J Vasc Surg* 50(5):1197–1210, 2009.

TABLE 2: Anatomic and extraanatomic options for "open" renal revascularization

Anatomic	Extraanatomic	Other
Transaortic renal endarterectomy	Hepatorenal bypass	Nephrectomy
Aortorenal bypass	Splenorenal bypass	
Synchronous aortic/renal artery bypass	Iliorenal bypass	
Renal reimplantation (ex vivo surgery)	SMA-renal bypass	

SMA, Superior mesenteric artery

proceeding to endarterectomy. This involves mobilization of the left colon, spleen, and tail of the pancreas and their rotation to the right side of the abdomen, which then results in adequate access to the aorta. An alternative to a conventional trapdoor incision is a transverse aortotomy, carried across the origins of both renal vessels; in theory, this allows more distal endarterectomy of both renal arteries.

Renal Artery Reimplantation

Occasionally, with adequate dissection and mobilization of the renal arteries, they may be sufficiently redundant to allow division of the renal artery distal to the orificial renal artery stenosis, leaving enough length for reimplantation of the renal artery directly into the infrarenal aorta.

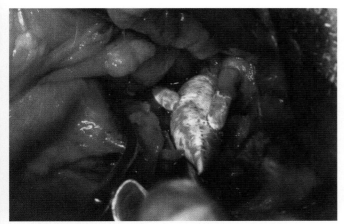

FIGURE 2 Renal artery bypass with aortic reconstruction.

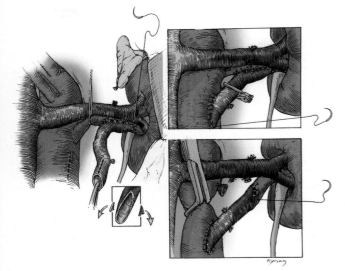

FIGURE 3 Aortorenal bypass grafting with end-to-side and end-to-end anastomoses. An end-to-end anastomosis between the graft and the native renal artery is generally preferred. *(From Benjamin ME, Dean RH: Techniques in renal artery reconstruction: part 1, Ann Vasc Surg 10:306, 1996. Used with permission.)*

Ex Vivo Reconstruction

This is usually required when previous renal artery stents or bypasses have failed, or when the distal renal branches are severely diseased. It is rarely used in our practice. The warm ischemia time of a kidney undergoing in situ revascularization is 30 minutes. With ex vivo reconstruction and cooling of the kidney to a core temperature of 10° to 15° C, the operating time can be comfortably prolonged to 2 to 3 hours. A standard flank nephrectomy incision is made, the Gerota fascia is divided, and a nephrectomy is performed with a cuff of IVC. Reversed saphenous vein is used, and the kidney is perfused with chilled preservation solution. After completion of the arteriovenous anastomoses, the kidney is returned to its fossa, and the renal vein is reanastomosed. Finally, the vein graft to aorta anastomosis is completed.

Extraanatomic Bypass

Splenorenal Bypass

Splenorenal bypass is performed in select cases. It is used in patients for whom renal stenting is not an option due to severe aortic

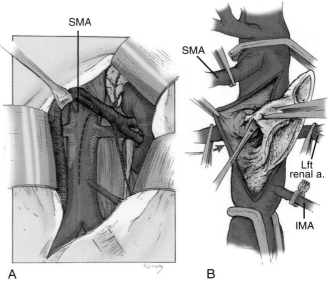

FIGURE 4 Transperitoneal approach for a longitudinal transaortic endarterectomy. **A,** Dashed line shows the location of the aortotomy. **B,** The plaque is transected proximally and distally, and the renal arteries are everted to remove the atherosclerotic plaque from each renal ostium. The aortotomy is closed with a running 4-0 or 5-0 monofilament polypropylene suture. *IMA,* Inferior mesenteric artery; *SMA,* Superior mesenteric artery. *(From Benjamin ME, Dean RH: Techniques in renal artery reconstruction: part 1, Ann Vasc Surg 10:306, 1996. Used with permission.)*

atherosclerosis (Figure 5). It is important to confirm the presence of an undiseased celiac axis prior to surgery by mesenteric angiography with both an anteroposterior and a lateral contrast injection. We usually employ a left subcostal incision; however, a laparotomy incision can also be used. The peritoneal cavity is entered (this is *not* an extraperitoneal operation), the colon is identified, and the splenic flexure is mobilized to reveal the tail of the pancreas.

Next, the pancreas is reflected superiorly by mobilizing its inferior border. A retropancreatic plane is developed, and the splenic artery is mobilized as far distally as the splenic hilum. The left renal artery lies above and behind the left renal vein, so the left suprarenal vein is divided, and the renal artery is carefully separated from the vein. A note of caution: These vessels reside deep within the abdominal cavity, even in slim patients, so good lighting and retraction is a necessity. The splenic artery is mobilized and divided as far distally as possible. The renal artery is also divided and spatulated. It is then sewn end-to-end with the left renal artery. After completion of the anastomosis, it is important to ensure no kinking occurs, especially in an excessively redundant splenic artery. Intraoperative continuous wave Doppler interrogation will confirm normal flow to the left kidney.

Hepatorenal Bypass

Hepatorenal bypass is performed via a right subcostal incision or a midline laparotomy approach. Again, a patent, disease-free celiac axis is a prerequisite. The lesser omentum is incised to expose the hepatic artery proximal and distal to the gastroduodenal artery. Then the duodenum is mobilized and retracted medially to identify the IVC. The right renal vein is located; the right renal artery crosses the right crus of the diaphragm and psoas muscle behind the IVC and the right renal vein. It is carefully separated from the renal vein. Reversed greater saphenous vein is used as the conduit, and the proximal anastomosis is created end to side on the hepatic artery (Figure 6). The vein graft is laid anterior to the IVC and is sutured end to end with the transected right renal artery.

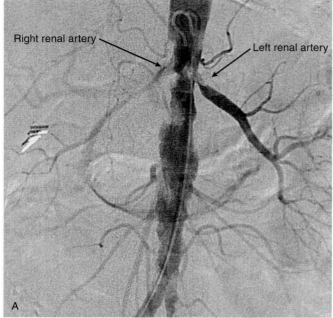

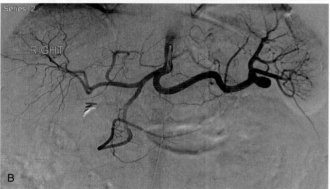

FIGURE 5 Angiogram demonstrating severe atherosclerosis of the aorta with severe stenosis of both renal arteries (**A**). The right kidney was atrophic, and the patient had significant comorbidities that made her a good candidate for splenorenal bypass. It is also important to assess inflow by selective celiac angiography (**B**).

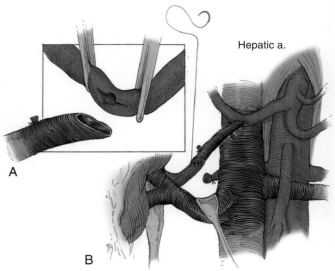

FIGURE 6 Extraanatomic approaches to renal revascularization include hepatorenal and splenorenal bypass grafts. **A,** Vein graft is anastomosed end-to-side to the hepatic artery. **B,** Graft is anastomosed end-to-end to the right renal artery. *(From Benjamin ME, Dean RH: Techniques in renal artery reconstruction, part 1, Ann Vasc Surg 10:409, 1996. Used with permission.)*

Iliorenal Bypass

Iliorenal bypass is rarely performed, though it has seen resurgence with recent "debranching" procedures that accompany endovascular treatment of complex aortic aneurysms. It requires a relatively disease-free common iliac artery. Classically, a midline abdominal incision is made, and the right or left colon is reflected medially to expose the ipsilateral renal and common iliac arteries. Either a reversed saphenous vein graft or a synthetic graft can be used. The inflow requires an end-to-side technique onto the common iliac artery, while employing an end-to-end anastomosis on the recipient renal artery. Alternatively, a right or left retroperitoneal incision can be made to access the appropriate renal artery for unilateral reconstruction.

Mesorenal Bypass

Mesorenal bypass is often described but rarely performed, as evidenced by the paucity of reports in the literature. The superior mesenteric artery (SMA) is exposed either by a retroperitoneal approach or by a medial visceral rotation. Conventional wisdom is

that manipulation of this vessel should be reserved only for hypertrophic SMAs to reduce the risk of steal and subsequent bowel ischemia; however, recent reports dispute this. In our experience, a reversed vein graft is sutured end to side onto the proximal SMA and end to end to the renal artery. Published series are small but report good patency rates and low mortality.

Morbidity, Mortality, and Patency Rates of Surgical Bypass

To date no randomized trials have directly compared surgery with stenting, but there have been large series done on renal artery reconstruction. In 2002, Cherr reported the results of operative management of 500 patients (776 kidneys) undergoing renal artery surgery for atherosclerosis (384 aortorenal bypass, 267 endarterectomy, 56 nephrectomy, 56 reimplantation, 13 splanchnorenal bypass). Perioperative mortality was 4.6% (Table 3). Of the 24 deaths that occured, 23 followed bilateral renal artery reconstruction combined with aortic or mesenteric repair. Mortality for isolated renal artery repair was 0.8%, and the authors reported an 85% improvement in blood pressure control and 58% improvement in ischemic nephropathy.

NEPHRECTOMY

For atrophic kidneys, those less than 8 cm in length, renal revascularization is pointless, as there is little or no chance of better blood pressure control or resurrection of renal function. Nephrectomy is therefore reserved for patients with renovascular hypertension in whom the kidney has no excretory function (less than 10% on radionuclide renography) and an occluded artery. In this situation, sacrifice of the kidney will not affect renal function but may potentially cure or improve hypertension. Removal of a functioning kidney is seldom performed today. Historically, it only resolved hypertension in a little over one third of patients, but it halved renal excretory function in all patients. Nephrectomy is still occasionally employed, usually for atrophic, nonfunctioning kidneys that are felt to be driving high blood pressure.

TABLE 3: Morbidity, mortality, and patency rates of surgical bypass*

Reference (Year)	N	Bilateral Repair (%)	Preoperative Renal Dysfunction (%)	RENAL FUNCTION RESPONSE (%)			HYPERTENSION RESPONSE (%)			PERIOPERATIVE OUTCOME (%)	
				Improved	Unchanged	Worsened	Cured	Improved	Failed	Death	Morbidity
Fergany (1995)†	175	2.3	92.3	35	47	18	46	54	0	2.9	NR
Cambria (1996)	139	13	77	73	—	27	8	71	21	8	7.2
Darling (1999)	568	18	NR	26	68	6	NR	—	—	5.5	15.9
Hansen (2000)	232	64	100	58	35	7	11	76	13	7.3	30
Paty (2001)	414	NR	4	97	—	3	NR	—	—	5.5	11.4
Cherr (2002)	500	59	48.8	43	47	10	73	12	15	4.6	16
Marone (2004)	96	27	100	42	41	16	NR	—	—	4.1	NR
Mean %†		31	38	38	47	14	12	73	15	5.4	21

NR, Not reported

*Renal function and hypertension responses expressed percentage of patients surviving operation. Series selected based on publication in 1995 or later, inclusion of ≥50 patients, and categoric reporting of renal function and/or hypertension responses.

†Weighted mean based on number of patients with reported data categorized according to column headings; references where data were not reported or categoric response categories were combined were not included in the calculation.

From Edwards MS, Corriere MA: Contemporary management of atherosclerotic renovascular disease, *J Vasc Surg* 50(5):1197–1210, 2009.

SUMMARY

Atherosclerosis of the renal artery is a difficult subject, because technical success and clinical benefit do not necessarily go hand in hand, and the conclusive role of intervention has yet to be determined. Renal artery revascularization should be applied judiciously. Patency rates are high for all reconstructions, but renal artery stenting has demonstrable advantages over simple balloon angioplasty. Although renal artery reconstruction has been practiced for decades, only now are its indications and role becoming established with well-designed randomized control trials. In this regard, it is not so different from carotid surgery prior to the North American Symptomatic Carotid Endarterectomy Trial (NASCET) and Asymptomatic Carotid Atherosclerosis Study (ACAS) trials, and aneurysm surgery prior to the United Kingdom and United States "small aneurysm" trials. In the next year or two, the role of revascularization should be clarified.

SUGGESTED READINGS

Balk EM, Raman G: *Comparative effectiveness of management strategies for renal artery stenosis: 2007 update, comparative effectiveness review no. 5 (update),* Rockville, MD, 2007, Agency for Healthcare Research and Quality.

Cooper CJ, Murphy TP: Is renal artery stenting the correct treatment of renal artery stenosis? The case for renal artery stenting for treatment of renal artery stenosis,, *Circulation* 115(2):263–269, 2007.

Dworkin LD, Jamerson KA: Is renal artery stenting the correct treatment of renal artery stenosis? The case against angioplasty and stenting of atherosclerotic renal artery stenosis,, *Circulation* 115(2):271–276, 2007.

Edwards MS, Corriere MA: Contemporary management of atherosclerotic renovascular disease, *J Vasc Surg* 50(5):1197–1210, 2009.

Fenstad ER, Kane GC: Update on the management of atherosclerotic renal artery disease, *Minerva Cardioangiol* 57(1):95–101, 2009.

Textor SC: Atherosclerotic renal artery stenosis: overtreated but underrated? *J Am Soc Nephrol* 19(4):656–659, 2008.

RAYNAUD SYNDROME

Ying Wei Lum, MD, and Glen S. Roseborough, MD

OVERVIEW

In 1862 Maurice Raynaud published a series describing 25 patients with varying degrees of intermittent digital pallor and cyanosis that was frequently associated with digital gangrene. He originally proposed that vasospasm was the underlying mechanism responsible for the condition. Hutchinson and others subsequently recognized that episodic digital ischemia commonly occurs in the setting of fixed organic vascular disease. Patients with isolated vasospasm were referred to as having *Raynaud disease,* whereas patients with underlying obstructive disease were referred to as having *Raynaud phenomenon.*

Today we refer to these two groups of patients as having *Raynaud syndrome* (RS); it is classified as *primary* if no disease or inducing factors are associated and *secondary* if either of these is present. The primary form is more common, tends to affect people at a younger age, is often reversible, takes a milder course, and rarely leads to ulceration or gangrene.

Epidemiologic studies suggest that RS is surprisingly common, with an incidence between 3% and 18% of the general population. Women are more commonly affected than men—between 70% and 90% of patients are female—and the syndrome is more commonly encountered in cold climates, such as those of northern Europe. Occupational disease has been documented in workers who handle cold materials regularly and in those who use vibrating machinery such as chainsaws and jackhammers; up to 50% of people who regularly use these devices ultimately develop RS. An interesting finding of longitudinal studies of patients with RS is that approximately 60% ultimately develop occlusive disease of the palmar and digital arteries. Half of these patients develop connective tissue disease, whereas the rest may experience one of a number of angiopathies (Table 1). Numerous studies have demonstrated that the risk of developing a connective tissue disorder is predicted by the presence of one or more signs of connective tissue disease at the time of diagnosis of RS. These signs include positive serology for antinuclear antibody (ANA); rheumatoid factor (RF); double-stranded DNA; single-stranded DNA; or clinical signs such as sclerodactyly, dysphagia, arthralgia, xerostomia, or abnormal nail-fold microscopy.

PRESENTATION AND DIAGNOSIS

The classic triad of symptoms and color variation is seen in fewer than 20% of patients; this triad consists of *pallor* from digital artery spasm, followed by *cyanosis* from slow reperfusion of desaturated blood, and ending in *reactive hyperemia* of the skin from reflex dilation of arterioles (Figure 1). RS usually occurs in the hands but can occasionally involve the feet. In addition, the symptoms can be accompanied by mild pain, numbness, or dysesthesia. These events are often precipitated by exposure to cold or emotional stimuli. Between attacks, the fingers appear normal. The history should elucidate symptoms of dysphagia, arthralgia, xerostomia, xerophthalmia, smoking, and cold and vibration exposure. The physical examination should focus on finding evidence of associated disease. Pulse deficits may be evident in atherosclerosis and Buerger disease; joint effusions, rashes, contractures, and pleural or pericardial rubs may be found in connective tissue disorders. Routine blood work includes a complete blood count, serum chemistry, urinalysis, erythrocyte sedimentation rate, RF, and ANA. Additional serologic examination may be required in select cases.

In the past, arteriography was often used to confirm the diagnosis. Hand arteriograms were obtained before and after immersing the hand in ice water and before and after intraarterial infusion of reserpine. This technique has documented impressive vasospasm induced by cold exposure that is then relieved by reserpine infusion. Arteriography is mainly used today to rule out other pathology, such as hypothenar hammer syndrome or an ulcerating lesion that can be found in thoracic outlet syndrome, which could be causing atheroembolism. This is usually in cases of unilateral symptoms, otherwise arteriography is rarely used today.

Most confirmatory testing for RS is performed in the noninvasive vascular laboratory. The hand–ice water immersion test measures fingertip temperatures every 5 minutes after a patient's hand is placed in ice water for 20 seconds; the temperature returns to normal within 10 minutes in a normal person, whereas this time is much delayed in patients with RS, often 20 minutes or longer. Similarly, the occlusive digital-hypothermic challenge test measures blood pressure in the fingertip with a mercury strain gauge, after the finger has been subjected to 5 minutes of hypothermia and ischemia with a special tourniquet. A decrease in digital blood pressure of 20% or more on reperfusion is positive for RS. Of those tests available for RS, this test is the most accurate; sensitivity is 100%, specificity is 80%, and overall accuracy is 97%. Finally, recently published studies have shown that capillaroscopy is of particular value for diagnosis and differentiation of primary and secondary RS. It involves examination of the nail-fold capillaries under a light microscope with cold-light illumination. Nail-fold capillaries are usually horizontal and appear enlarged in patients with connective tissue diseases such as scleroderma, mixed connective tissue disease, and dermatomyositis.

TABLE 1: Reported causes of secondary Raynaud syndrome

Autoimmune Disorders	Obstructive Arterial Disorders
Dermatomyositis	Atherosclerosis
Henoch-Schönlein purpura	Buerger disease
Hepatitis B virus antigen–induced vasculitis	Peripheral embolization
Mixed connective tissue disease	Thoracic outlet syndrome
Polyarteritis nodosa	**Environmental Exposure**
Polymyositis	Frostbite/chilblains
Reiter syndrome	Vibration injury
Rheumatoid arthritis	Repetitive trauma
Scleroderma/CREST syndrome	**Drug Induced**
Sjögren syndrome	Ergot alkaloids
Systemic lupus erythematosus	β-Blockers
Myeloproliferative Disorders	Nicotine
Leukemia	Oral contraceptives
Myeloid metaplasia	Chemotherapy agents
Polycythemia vera	**Miscellaneous Disorders**
Thrombocytosis	Chronic renal failure
Hematologic Disorders	Hypothyroidism
Cold agglutinins	Vinyl chloride toxicity
Cryglobulinemia	Polyneuropathy
Malignancy	Neurofibromatosis
Macroglobulinemia	
Multiple myeloma	

CREST, Calcinosis, Raynaud phenomenon, esophageal involvement, sclerodactyly, and telangiectasia

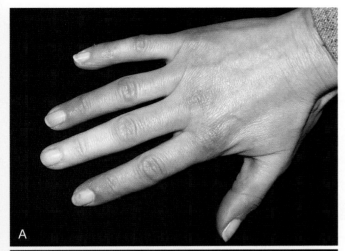

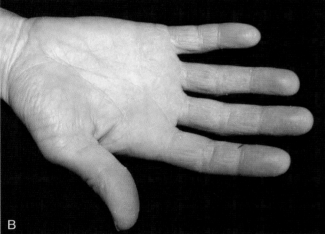

FIGURE 1   Ischemic and hyperemic phase of RS. *(From Gayraud M: Raynaud's phenomenon, Joint Bone Spine 74[1]:e1-e8, 2007.)*

TREATMENT

Conservative Therapy

Conservative therapy is the mainstay of management in all patients with RS. Patients should be instructed to avoid cold exposure, wear warm clothes and gloves, and stop smoking. Battery-powered electric gloves can be purchased. Medications with vasospastic properties should be avoided, and ergot alkaloids should also be discontinued; however, many RS patients take these medicines because they often have migraine headaches. Many authors recommend discontinuing β-blockers because of the potential for adverse peripheral β₂ effect, but in 1985 Coffman and Rasmussen found no effect of either propranolol or metoprolol on the number of vasospastic attacks in 16 patients with RS, nor did they note an effect on their overall evaluation of the patients' condition. Similarly, based on the Framingham study, the use of oral contraceptives has been cautioned against. However, the new low-dose oral contraceptives do not cause vasomotor disturbances and do not need to be stopped. In fact, treatment with estrogens of patients with systemic sclerosis has been found to cause vasodilation instead.

A change in occupation is recommended if a patient's work involves the use of vibrating tools or exposure to extremes of temperature. Many patients respond to these simple conservative measures; however, if symptoms persist or digital ulcers develop, medical therapy is appropriate.

Pharmacologic Therapy

Pharmacologic therapy plays an important role in the treatment of RS (Figure 2). In the last 20 years, more than 150 trials have been published in the literature regarding the effectiveness of various drugs in RS (Table 2). Most of these trials are small, placebo-controlled crossover studies consisting of only 10 to 20 patients. The results of these trials are often confusing, with many different studies looking at a particular drug and producing conflicting results. In addition, some drugs that have been found to have a clinical effect are not found to have any effect when peripheral blood flow is measured objectively. The reverse situation also holds for many drugs that have been found objectively to promote increased blood flow but that have no clinical effect. Several different classes of medicines have been advocated, corresponding to the numerous pathophysiologic mechanisms thought to be responsible for RS. These mechanisms include altered activity of the sympathetic nervous system, changes in the number or activity of α- and β-adrenergic receptors, abnormalities in the control or release of various vasoactive substances, and altered inflammatory or immune responses.

As mentioned previously, most patients will not need pharmacologic treatment for RS; however, if they do, calcium channel blockers are considered the drug of choice because of their favorable effect on peripheral vasodilation. Nifedipine and its analogs have been shown in multiple controlled, randomized studies to result in a decrease in frequency and severity of attacks, and it is considered the drug of choice in both primary and secondary RS. Benefit is usually obtained with dosages of 10 to 30 mg three times daily. Two recent studies have shown similar benefit using the long-acting form of nifedipine at 30 to 60 mg once daily. Patients generally tolerate the long-acting preparation better. Several of the nifedipine analogs, as well as diltiazem, have been shown to be useful in other studies and may be useful if nifedipine is not tolerated. Verapamil has not been shown to be effective in RS in any study.

Angiotensin-converting enzyme (ACE) inhibitors and angiotensin receptor blockers (ARBs) have also been studied in the treatment of RS. The pharmacologic effects of ACE inhibitors have been attributed to the prevention of bradykinin degradation, which promotes nitric oxide release from the endothelium and hence promotes vasodilation. However, limited evidence is available to suggest any clinical effectiveness in the routine use of ACE inhibitors to treat patients with RS. On the other hand, ARBs—in particular, losartan 50 mg daily—has been studied in a comparative study with 40 mg of nifedipine daily. The study concluded an improvement of symptoms in the group treated with losartan compared to the group treated with nifedipine, and a decrease in frequency of attacks in the group treated with losartan was also seen.

Other vasodilators have been studied in RS with variable degrees of success. Naftidrofuryl is a mild peripheral vasodilator with serotonin antagonist effect that has been shown in a large double-blind study to shorten the duration of attacks, reduce the severity of pain, and improve symptoms that interfere with daily activities. Another serotonin antagonist, ketanserin, was shown to be useful in RS in a large, multicenter international study involving 222 patients with primary and secondary RS. This study found a 16% reduction in frequency of attacks compared with placebo but no significant difference in duration or intensity of attacks. This drug also has a mild α-adrenergic antagonist effect. In a meta-analysis of three studies performed by Pope and colleagues (2000) in patients with RS secondary to scleroderma, ketanserin was not found to be useful. Its only benefit in these patients was a small decrease in the duration of attacks, which was offset by significant side effects of the drug. In another study by Coleiro and colleagues (2001), 26 patients with primary RS and 27 patients with secondary RS were randomized to treatment with either fluoxetine (20 mg daily) or nifedipine (40 mg daily). The severity and frequency of vasospastic attacks were significantly decreased in the patients who received fluoxetine. Subgroup analysis showed that this effect was most pronounced in females and in primary RS.

Symptomatic Raynaud's

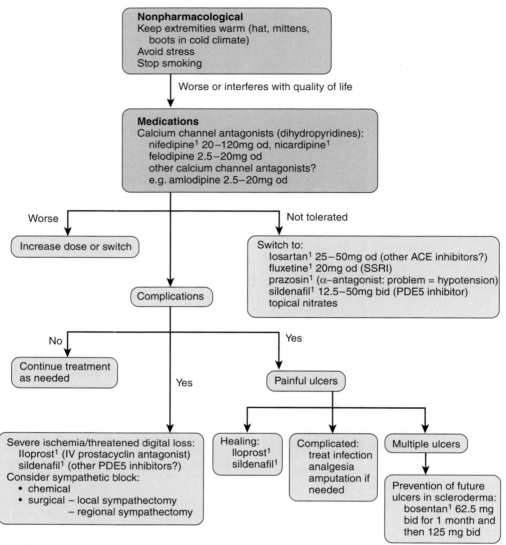

FIGURE 2   Treatment algorithm for RS. *od,* Once daily; *PDE5,* phosphodiesterase 5; *SSRI,* selective serotonin reuptake inhibitor. [1]Randomized, controlled trial evidence exists. *(From Pope J: The diagnosis and treatment of Raynaud's phenomenon: a practical approach, Drugs 67[4]:517–525, 2007.)*

TABLE 2:   Long-term outcome of Raynaud syndrome patients as classified by initial presentation

Initial Classification	Initial Presence of Connective Tissue Disease (%)	Final Presence of Connective Tissue Disease (%)	Presence of Digital Ulceration (%)	Requirement for Digital or Phalangeal Amputation (%)
Spastic, negative serology	0	2.0	5.2	1.6
Spastic, positive serology	48.6	57.0	15.5	1.4
Obstructive, negative serology	0	8.5	48.2	19.0
Obstructive, positive serology	72.9	81.2	55.6	11.6

From Oregon Health Sciences University

Sildenafil, a phosphodiesterase inhibitor, increases guanosine monophosphate levels in vascular smooth muscle to induce vasodilation. It has been successfully evaluated in patients with both primary and secondary RS and particularly in scleroderma, and the results suggest a dose of 12.5 to 50 mg of sildenafil two to three times daily is effective in decreasing the frequency and duration of attacks.

Similarly, the topical administration of nitrates, such as nitroglycerin creams and glyceril trinitrate patches, can also decrease severity and frequency of attacks in both primary and secondary RS by inducing local vasodilation through nitric oxide synthase activation.

In patients with RS, various rheologic abnormalities have been demonstrated, including increased plasma viscosity, abnormal platelet aggregation, decreased fibrinolysis, and increased von Willebrand factor levels. Prostaglandins have therefore been tested in RS, because they are known to alter some of these abnormalities. After original studies with prostacyclin and alprostadil (PGE_2) showed some promise, researchers focused on iloprost (PGI_2), because this compound is more stable. Several studies with intravenous infusions of iloprost have shown benefit in RS, and intravenous infusions given for 3 to 5 consecutive days will produce lasting effects for 6 weeks to 6 months. Infusions of 0.5 to 2 ng/kg/min are given for 6 hours at a time. When compared with nifedipine in one trial, both drugs were effective at reducing attacks, but iloprost was more effective at healing ulcers and had fewer adverse effects. Unfortunately, the need to administer iloprost intravenously limits its use. An oral preparation of iloprost has been found to be effective but so far is not licensed for use in RS. Another oral preparation, cisaprost, failed to show any benefit in RS secondary to scleroderma. Limaprost, an oral analog of alprostadil, is currently under investigation, and preliminary results are encouraging.

The most recent class of drugs to be evaluated in the treatment for RS are endothelin receptor antagonists. Endothelin, released by endothelial cells, induces vasoconstriction and competitively acts on two types of receptors: *type A*, found on vascular smooth muscle cells, and *type B*, found on endothelial cells. Stimulation of type A receptors mediates vasoconstriction, and stimulation of type B receptors mediates both vasoconstriction and vasodilation. Bosentan, a nonselective endothelin receptor antagonist to both receptors, has a higher affinity for type A receptors; as a result, it has been proven in double-blind, randomized controlled trials in patients with scleroderma to prevent the development of additional ulcers.

Alternative Therapies

Nonpharmacologic medical therapies that have been tested on patients with RS include acupuncture, temperature biofeedback, and plasmapheresis. A randomized trial in Germany showed that a 2-week course of acupuncture, consisting of seven treatments, reduced attacks by 63% in 17 patients with RS over a subsequent 12-week period in the winter. Evidence supporting biofeedback is anecdotal, and a recent randomized study that compared biofeedback with nifedipine demonstrated biofeedback to be ineffective in the treatment of primary RS. Plasmapheresis affects multiple rheologic parameters of the blood, including blood viscosity, red blood cell (RBC) velocity, and RBC aggregation. English and Dutch investigators documented improved symptoms and ulcer healing in 26 patients treated with four weekly sessions of plasmapheresis. Improvement was associated with a temporary decrease in blood viscosity and RBC aggregation; symptoms recurred in 14 patients after 6 to 9 months, when these values returned to baseline. Both research groups documented increased digital artery or capillary blood flow after plasmapheresis.

Surgical Therapy

Surgical therapy for RS consists of debridement, sympathectomy in select cases, and amputation when necessary. The likelihood of developing ulceration or requiring amputation is predicted by presence of abnormal serology findings indicating connective tissue disease, as well as obstructive pathology causing secondary RS (see Table 2). Unilateral upper extremity symptoms of RS should prompt a thorough search for arterial pathology of the thoracic outlet, which can cause symptoms secondary to ischemia or embolization.

Cervicothoracic sympathectomy of the upper extremity has been the primary surgical treatment for RS, through a supraclavicular, transaxillary, or thoracoscopic approach. All procedures have been demonstrated to be safe, with a small incidence of pneumothorax and Horner syndrome being the most serious complications reported.

In the last 15 years, the transthoracic approach has become the preferred approach. This operation is performed through one or two 2 cm incisions in the third intercostal space. Although a few surgeons report good long-term results in selected series—mostly for patients with primary, vasospastic RS—the worldwide experience is generally that at least 60% of patients who undergo upper extremity sympathectomy have recurrent symptoms within 1 year. The worst results are seen in patients with obstructive pathology. In a recent survey of RS patients in England, only 15% of 140 patients who had undergone sympathectomy obtained long-term benefit. However, lumbar sympathectomy seems to have a more lasting effect in patients with RS that affects the lower extremities. In two published series, all patients with primary vasospastic RS had long-term benefit from lumbar sympathectomy.

Despite the discouraging results seen with surgical cervicothoracic sympathectomy, investigators have attempted to apply alternative means of sympathectomy to patients with RS. Percutaneous ablation of the upper sympathetic ganglia has been attempted with phenol injection and radiofrequency energy. Dondelinger and Kurdziel (1987) reported good results in only seven of 14 limbs in nine patients with RS treated with phenol injection, with follow-up ranging from 4 to 33 months. Despite the "noninvasive" nature of the procedure, one third of patients experienced transient Horner syndrome or pneumothorax. Wilkinson (1996) achieved good results beyond 1 year in 69% of 247 limbs treated with percutaneous radiofrequency ablation. Although his results were not superior to surgery, he performed the procedure largely as an outpatient procedure with minimal morbidity.

Hand surgeons perform distal sympathectomies on RS patients, usually in the setting of rest pain or ulceration. This operation involves excising, through palmar incisions, variable lengths of adventitia from the common and proper digital arteries that supply affected fingers. The same procedure occasionally is performed on the radial and ulnar arteries at the wrist. Five separate surgical series representing experience with 47 patients have been reported. All but one of these patients had good relief of pain and healing of ulcers on long-term follow-up, and minor recurrent ulcers were seen in 4 others. In most of these studies, improved blood flow or skin temperature postoperatively was documented. This operation is favored in patients with scleroderma, in whom periarterial fibrosis occurs. Much of the benefit of this operation is attributed to releasing the artery from the fibrosis in addition to the sympathectomy. Finally, Spanish and French investigators have used spinal cord stimulation to treat RS patients who experience chronic pain. They report good relief of pain in most patients, but the overall experience is small.

A paper published by vascular surgeons at Oregon Health Sciences University contends that sympathectomy in any form is contraindicated in RS. They have published their experience with conservative treatment of a large series of patients who developed finger ulceration and gangrene associated with small-vessel disease. This consisted of a strict regimen of gentle soap scrubs, debridement of necrotic tissue, fingernail removal, culture-directed antibiotic therapy, and length-preserving digital amputation as required. In 88% of patients, ulcer healing was achieved with conservative therapy alone; the authors argue that these results cannot be improved upon with sympathectomy. However, only 52% of patients in the series had RS; in addition, the authors do not document their success at alleviating chronic pain and discomfort, which is a significant cause of morbidity in these patients.

SUMMARY

RS is a vexing problem that exists in a primary, vasospastic form and a secondary form that is associated with a multitude of medical disease, most commonly connective tissue disease. Many patients who initially are seen with primary RS ultimately develop one of these systemic disorders years later. The diagnosis is made on the basis of history, physical examination, noninvasive vascular testing, and serologic testing. It is important to distinguish between primary and secondary RS, because the natural history of the two disorders is considerably different with respect to progression to chronic pain and tissue loss. In addition, the response to both medical and surgical therapy varies in the two types of RS, with poorer results seen in secondary RS with obstructive features. Most patients respond to conservative and pharmacologic therapy, the mainstays of treatment. However, in select patients sympathectomy may be indicated for lower extremity symptoms or severe symptoms in the upper extremity. The efficacy of alternative therapies, such as acupuncture and spinal cord stimulation, remains to be proven.

SUGGESTED READING

Gayraud M: Raynaud's phenomenon, *Joint Bone Spine* 74(1):e1–8, 2007.
Dziadzio M, Denton CP, Smith R, et al: Losartan therapy for Raynaud's phenomenon and scleroderma: clinical and biochemical findings in a fifteen-week, randomized, parallel-group, controlled trial, *Arthritis Rheum Dec* 42(12):2646–2655, 1999.
Landry GJ, Edwards JM, Porter JM: Current management of Raynaud's syndrome, *Adv Surg* 30:333, 1996.
Pope J: The diagnosis and treatment of Raynaud's phenomenon: a practical approach, *Drugs* 67(4):517–525, 2007.

THORACIC OUTLET SYNDROMES

Harold C. Urschel Jr, MD

OVERVIEW

Thoracic outlet syndromes (TOS) is a term that refers to compression of one or more of the neurovascular structures in the superior aperture of the chest. Previously the syndromes were designated by the cause of compression, such as scalenus anticus or cervical rib syndromes. Most compressive factors operate against the first rib and produce a variety of symptoms, depending on which of the neurovascular structures are compressed. Figure 1 demonstrates the causes as well as the symptomatologies.

NERVE COMPRESSION

There may be multiple areas of compression of peripheral nerves between the cervical spine and the hand in addition to the thoracic outlet. In the instance of multiple compression sites, less pressure is required at each site to produce symptoms. Therefore a patient may have TOS, ulnar nerve constriction at the elbow, and carpal tunnel syndrome concomitantly; this is known as the *multiple crush syndrome.*

Diagnostic and Objective Tests

A careful history and physical examination are critical for accurate diagnosis. The primary objective test is the reduction of normal conduction velocities (85 m/sec) of the ulnar and median nerve across the thoracic outlet. The electromyogram should be normal. With nerve conduction velocities greater than 60 m/sec, the patient is usually improved with conservative physical therapy, which includes 1) improving posture, 2) strengthening the shoulder girdle, and 3) loosening of the neck muscles.

Indications for Surgery

Failure of conservative therapy with a significantly reduced nerve conduction velocity (less than 60 m/sec) and the elimination of other possible causes of the symptoms are the usual surgical indications.

Arterial aneurysm, emboli, or occlusion of the artery or vein are indications for surgery without conservative therapy.

SURGICAL THERAPY

Transaxillary Approach

Initial therapy involves anterior scalenectomy, resection of the first rib and costoclavicular ligament, and neurolysis of C7, C8, and T1 nerve roots and the brachial plexus (Figure 2) for nerve and vein compression (Table 1). Transaxillary first-rib resection, neurovascular decompression, and dorsal sympathectomy for TOS are performed for nerve and venous compression. The advantage of this approach is that the rib can be removed, and the thoracic outlet decompressed, without working through or retracting the brachial plexus and blood vessels. A double-lumen tube is employed to collapse the lung on the operative side, minimizing the chance for an unplanned pneumothorax. A lighted right-angle breast retractor and a narrow Deaver retractor are used for optimal exposure. The video thoracoscope is used for its magnification, as an excellent light source, and to facilitate teaching.

The patient is placed in a lateral position with an axillary roll under the "down" side. The "up" side arm is wrapped and elevated over a traction apparatus with a 2 lb weight. Two arm holders are used to hold the arm at 90 degrees from the chest wall, avoiding hyperabduction or hyperextension of the shoulder. Care is taken to relax the arm every 2 minutes. The arm, axilla, and chest wall are prepared and draped. The incision is transaxillary below the hairline and transverse between the pectoralis major muscle anteriorly and the latissimus dorsi muscle posteriorly (Figure 2, *A* and *inset*), and it is carried directly to the chest wall without angling up toward the first rib.

When the chest wall is encountered, the dissection is carried superiorly to the first rib, identifying the intercostal brachial nerve that exits between the first and second ribs. The brachial nerve is preserved by retracting it anteriorly or posteriorly. (Division produces 6 months to 1 year of paresthesias on the inner surface of the upper arm.) The first rib is dissected subperiosteally with a Shaw-Paulson periosteal elevator, and the scalenus anticus muscle is identified. A right-angle clamp is placed behind the muscle, being careful not to injure the subclavian artery or vein. The scalenus anticus muscle is divided near its insertion on the first rib to avoid injury to the phrenic nerve, which courses away from the muscle at this level.

After the scalenus anticus muscle is divided, the first rib is dissected free subperiosteally and is separated from the pleura (Figure 2, *B*). A triangular piece of the rib is removed in the avascular area with the vertex of the triangle at the scalene tubercle. The anterior part of the rib is removed by dividing the costoclavicular ligament and resecting the rib subperiosteally back to the costocartilage of

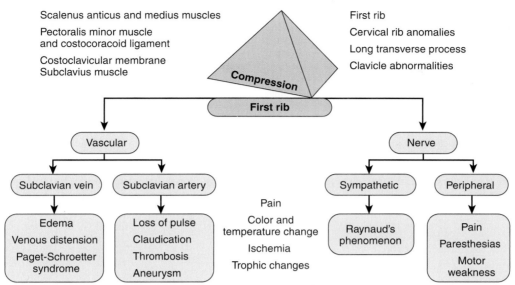

Scalenus anticus and medius muscles

Pectoralis minor muscle
and costocoracoid ligament

Costoclavicular membrane
Subclavius muscle

First rib
Cervical rib anomalies
Long transverse process
Clavicle abnormalities

Compression

First rib

Vascular

Nerve

Subclavian vein

Subclavian artery

Sympathetic

Peripheral

Edema
Venous distension
Paget-Schroetter
syndrome

Loss of pulse
Claudication
Thrombosis
Aneurysm

Pain
Color and
temperature change
Ischemia
Trophic changes

Raynaud's
phenomenon

Pain
Paresthesias
Motor
weakness

FIGURE 1   Schematic diagram showing the muscle, ligament, and bone abnormalities in the thoracic outlet that may compress neurovascular structures against the first rib. *(Modified from Urschel HC, Kourlis H: Thoracic outlet syndrome: a 50-year experience at Baylor University Medical Center, Bayl Univ Med Cent Proc 20[2]:125–135, 2007.)*

the sternum. The posterior part of the rib is dissected subperiosteally to the transverse process, removing the scalenus medius muscle, where it is divided by a pair of rib shears (Figure 2, *C*). The rib may be resected posteriorly with an Urschel-Leksell reinforced rongeur. Care is taken to avoid injury to the C8 and T1 nerve roots as the scalenus medius muscle is dissected from the rib. After visualizing the transverse process articulation, the head and neck of the rib are carefully removed with an Urschel reinforced pituitary rongeur (Figure 2, *D*). It is important to remove the complete head and neck of the rib to minimize regeneration. Care is taken not to injure the T1 nerve root below or the C8 nerve root above.

Following complete removal of the first rib, neurolysis of the C7, C8, and T1 nerve roots and the middle and lower trunks of the brachial plexus is performed. A video thoracoscope is used for this purpose because of its magnification and light. The scalenus medius and scalenus anticus muscles are resected up into the neck so that they will not reattach to the Sibson fascia or the pleura. Bands and adhesions are removed from the axillary-subclavian artery and axillary-subclavian vein so that they are completely free, and hemostasis is secured.

If a dorsal sympathectomy is indicated for Raynaud phenomenon or sympathetic maintained pain syndrome, the same incision is used (Figure 2, *E*). After the rib has been removed, the pleura and lung are retracted inferiorly with a sponge stick, the plane of separation being just below the T1 nerve root. The stellate ganglion and dorsal sympathetic chain are identified in the extrapleural plane. The stellate ganglion, which consists of C7, C8, and T1 ganglia, lies in a slightly transverse position in contrast to the up-and-down position of the chain between the T1 and T3 ganglia. Clips are placed on each of the gray and white rami communications to the intercostal nerves (Figure 2, *F*).

Next, the chain is resected, removing T2 and T3 ganglia. Cautery is used to control bleeding and also to scar the area so that sprouting or regeneration of the sympathetic chain is discouraged. Frozen pathologic sections are taken to ensure that ganglion cells are present. A #20 chest tube is placed through a separate stab wound into the axillary area; if the pleura is open, it is placed in the pleura. After antibiotic solution is lavaged in the wound, methylprednisolone (Depo-Medrol) and hyaluronic acid (SepraSeal) are injected over the areas of neurolysis. The wound is closed with 3-0 Vicryl interrupted and running sutures, and a subcuticular 3-0 Vicryl suture is used for skin

closure. The lung is reexpanded before closure. Postoperatively, an intercostal block posteriorly of T1, T2, and T3 intercostals is carried out by the anesthesiologist.

Supraclavicular Approach

The first rib with the compressive elements for arterial lesions is removed through the supraclavicular approach (Figure 3) to gain proximal control of the artery. This has the disadvantage of working through and retracting the brachial plexus as well as leaving an obvious scar.

Supraclavicular first-rib resection and neurovascular decompression plus dorsal sympathectomy is used for arterial aneurysm insufficiency or emboli (Figure 3). The supraclavicular approach to decompress the brachial plexus and excise the first rib releases soft-tissue compressive structures in the region of the interscalene portion of the brachial plexus. The lower trunk and C8 and T1 can be completely identified and protected, as the most posterior aspect of the first rib is resected under direct vision. Any cervical ribs or prolonged transverse processes are easily removed from this approach. The disadvantages include the necessity of brachial plexus and blood vessel retraction to expose the first rib. Loupe magnification, micro-bipolar cautery, and, frequently, a portable nerve stimulator are used throughout the procedure. A sandbag is placed between the scapula and the neck extended to the nonoperative side. Long-acting paralytic agents are avoided, and a double-lumen endotracheal tube expedites adjunctive sympathectomy, according to Mackinnon and Patterson (1995). A curvilinear incision in a neck crease parallel and 2 cm above the clavicle is made in the supraclavicular fossa (Figure 3, *A*). The supraclavicular nerves are identified beneath the platysma muscle (Figure 3, *B*), the omohyoid muscle is divided, and the supraclavicular fat pad is elevated (Figure 3, *C*). The lateral portion of the clavicular head of the sternocleidomastoid muscle is divided (it is repaired later). The scalenus anticus and scalenus medius muscles and the brachial plexus are easily visualized and palapated. The phrenic nerve is seen on the anterior surface of the scalenus anticus muscle. Similarly, the long thoracic nerve is noted on the posterior aspect of the scalenus medius muscle.

The scalenus anticus muscle is divided at its insertion into the first rib (Figure 3, *D*). The subclavian artery is noted immediately behind this, and an umbilical tape is place around the subclavian artery. The phrenic nerve is mobilized and encircled with the VessiLoop. The upper, middle, and lower trunks of the brachial plexus are easily visualized and gently mobilized. The scalenus medius muscle is divided from the first rib (Figure 3, *E*). It has a broad attachment to the first rib, and care is taken to avoid injury to the long thoracic nerve.

In this position the long thoracic nerve may have multiple branches and may come through and posterior to the scalenus medius muscle. With division of the scalenus medius muscle, the brachial plexus is easily visualized and mobilized. The lower trunk and the C8 and T1 roots are identified above and below the first rib, and congenital bands and thickening in the Sibson fascia are divided. The brachial plexus is gently retracted, and the first rib is visualized (Figure 3, *F*). Where it is easily visible, the first rib is encircled and divided with bone-cutting instruments (Figure 3, *G*). The posterior segment of the first rib is removed back to its spinal attachments with Urschel-Leksell reinforced and Urschel pituitary rongeurs (Figure 3, *H*). Using a fine elevator, the soft-tissue attachments to the first rib are separated; finally, the posterior edge of the first rib is grasped firmly with a rongeur, and using a rocking and twisting motion, the entire aspect of the first rib is removed. The cartilaginous components of the articular facets of the first rib, with both the costal vertebral and costal transverse joints, can be identified (Figure 3, *I*). The anterior portion of the first rib is removed in a similar fashion to the costochondral junction of the sternum to decompress the neurovascular elements.

Posterior Thoracoplasty Approach

The posterior thoracoplasty approach (Figure 4) for first-rib resection is preferably reserved for reoperation and neurolysis of the brachial plexus but may also be used for initial therapy. The posterior

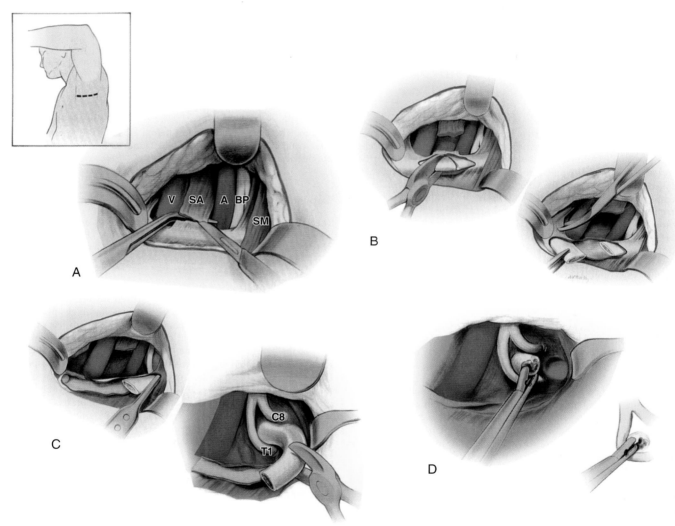

FIGURE 2 Transaxillary first-rib resection, neurovascular decompression, and dorsal sympathectomy. **A,** The incision is transaxillary below the hairline and transverse between the pectoralis major muscle anteriorly and the latissimus dorsi muscle posteriorly *(inset)*. The first rib is dissected subperiosteally, and the scalenus anticus muscle is identified. A right-angle clamp is placed behind the muscle, being careful not to injure the subclavian artery or vein. The scalenus anticus muscle is divided near its insertion on the first rib. **B,** After the scalenus anticus muscle is divided, the first rib is dissected free subperiosteally and separated from the pleura. A triangular piece of the rib is removed in the avascular area with the vertex of the triangle at the scalene tubercle. The anterior part of the rib is removed by dividing the costoclavicular ligament and resecting the rib subperiosteally back to the costocartilage of the sternum. **C,** The posterior part of the rib is dissected subperiosteally to the transverse process, removing the scalenus medius muscle, where it is divided by a pair of rib shears. The rib may be resected posteriorly with an Urschel-Leksell reinforced rongeur. **D,** After visualizing the transverse process articulation, the head and neck of the rib are carefully removed with an Urschel reinforced pituitary rongeur.

Continued

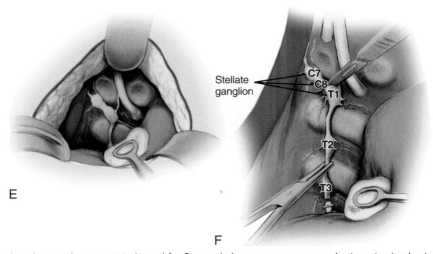

Stellate ganglion

C7
C8
T1
T2
T3

E

F

FIGURE 2, cont'd   E, If a dorsal sympathectomy is indicated for Raynaud phenomenon or sympathetic maintained pain syndrome, the pleura and lung are retracted inferiorly with a sponge stick, the plane of separation being just below the T1 nerve root. The stellate ganglion and dorsal sympathetic chain are identified in the extrapleural plane. The stellate ganglion consists of C7, C8, and T1 ganglia and lies in a slightly transverse position in contrast to the up-and-down position of the chain between the T1 and T3 ganglia. **F,** Clips are placed on each of the gray and white rami communications to the intercostal nerves. The chain is resected, removing T2 and T3 ganglia. *(Modified from Urschel HC Jr, Cooper JC: Atlas of thoracic surgery, New York, 1995, Churchill Livingstone.)*

TABLE 1: Surgical approaches for different types of TOSs

Type	Surgical Approach
Nerve compression	Transaxillary
Arterial compression	Supraclavicular and infraclavicular
Venous compression	Transaxillary
Recurrent	Posterior high thoracoplasty

high-thoracoplasty approach with dorsal sympathectomy for recurrent TOS is preferred for reoperation. It may also be used for primary large first- or cervical-rib resection. The transaxillary or supraclavicular route is usually preferred for the initial procedure, because rib stumps or regenerated ribs can be removed more easily from a "virgin" posterior approach, and because the nerve roots, as well as the brachial plexus, are easy to identify and access from the back.

Reoperation for recurrent compression usually incorporates a dorsal sympathectomy for causalgia-like symptoms, sympathetic maintained pain syndrome, or Raynaud phenomenon. The patient is placed in the lateral position with an axillary roll under the "down" side (Figure 4, *A*), and the upper arm is placed as for a thoracotomy. An incision is made approximately 6 cm in length with the midpoint at the angle of the scapula, halfway between the scapula and the spinous processes *(inset)*. The incision is carried through the skin and subcutaneous tissue down to the trapezius muscle, and the trapezius and rhomboid muscles are split. The posterior superior serratus muscle is resected, and the first rib stump is identified by retracting the sacrospinalis muscle medially (Figure 4, *B*).

Cautery is used to expose the first rib remnant (stump) and to open the periosteum. A periosteal elevator, or "joker," is employed to remove the stump subperiosteally. The head and neck of the rib usually have not been removed in the initial operation. The rib shears are used to divide the rib remnant, and the Urschel-Leksell reinforced and Urschel pituitary rongeurs are used carefully to remove the head

and neck of the rib. The T1 nerve root is identified grossly or with the nerve stimulator.

Once the T1 nerve root is identified, neurolysis is carried out using a ring-angle clamp, magnification, a knife, and special microscissors (Figure 4, *C*). A nerve stimulator may be helpful if extensive scarring is present. Neurolysis is extended to the C7 and C8 nerve roots and to the brachial plexus. All the scar is removed as far forward as necessary so that the nerve roots and the upper, middle, and lower trunks of the brachial plexus lie free. Care is taken not to injure the long thoracic nerve or any other brachial plexus branch. The axillary-subclavian artery and vein are decompressed through the same incision.

Next, the second rib is dissected free, and cautery is used to open the periosteum linearly (Figure 4, *D*). A 2 cm segment of the rib is resected posteriorly, medial to the sacrospinalis muscle, to perform the dorsal sympathectomy; this exposure may also help identify the T1 nerve roots. The lower third of the stellate ganglion is incised sharply (T1), and the gray and white rami communicans are clipped and divided (Figure 4, *E*). The T1, T2, and T3 ganglia are removed, along with the sympathetic chain, using clips on all the branches. Cautery is employed to effect hemostasis and to char the area so that sprouting and regeneration of the sympathetic chain are discouraged. Methylprednisolone and hyaluronic acid are left on the areas of neurolysis. The wound is closed in layers with interrupted #1 Neurlon in a figure-8 fashion ("Tom Jones" stitch) in each of the muscle layers. Running and interrupted 2-0 Vicryl sutures are used in the subcutaneous tissue and skin clips in the skin. A large, round Jackson-Pratt drain is placed in the area of neurolysis through a separate stab wound 2 cm below the inferior part of the incision, and care is taken not to incorporate the drain while closing the muscle layers over the top.

Summary of Approaches

Cervical rib and first rib can be removed through any of the approaches described. Dorsal sympathectomy may also be performed with neurovascular decompression through any of the above incisions for sympathetic maintained pain syndrome (reflex sympathetic dystrophy), causalgia, and Raynaud phenomena and disease (see Figures 2 and 4).

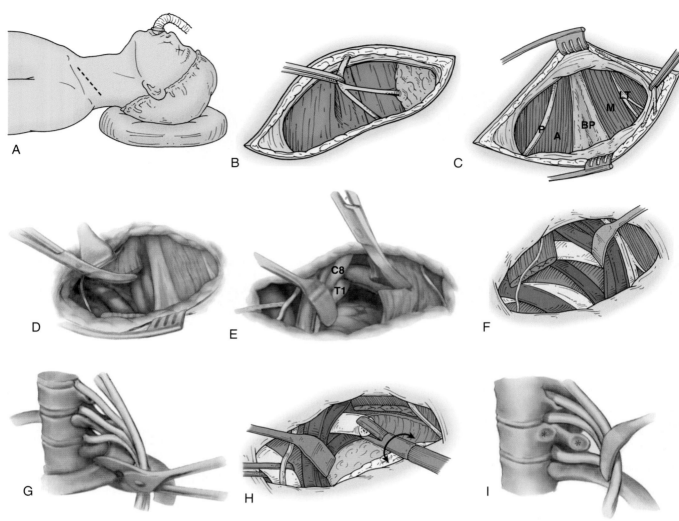

FIGURE 3   Supraclavicular first-rib resection and neurovascular decompression plus dorsal sympathectomy. **A,** A curvilinear incision in a neck crease parallel and 2 cm above the clavicle is made in the supraclavicular fossa. **B,** The supraclavicular nerves are identified beneath the platysma muscle. **C,** The omohyoid muscle is divided and the supraclavicular fat pad is elevated. The lateral portion of the clavicular head of the sternocleidomastoid muscle is divided. **D,** The scalenus anticus muscle is divided at its insertion into the first rib. The subclavian artery is noted immediately behind this, and an umbilical tape is placed around the subclavian artery. The phrenic nerve is mobilized and encircled with the VessiLoop. **E,** The scalenus medius muscle is divided from the first rib. It has a broad attachment to the first rib, and care is taken to avoid injury to the long thoracic nerve. **F,** The brachial plexus is gently retracted, and the first rib is visualized. **G,** The first rib is encircled and divided where easily visible with bone-cutting instruments. **H,** The posterior segment of the first rib is removed back to its spinal attachments with Urschel-Leksell reinforced and Urschel pituitary rongeurs. Using a fine elevator, the soft-tissue attachments to the first rib are separated; finally, the posterior edge of the first rib is grasped firmly with a rongeur, and using a rocking and twisting motion, the entire aspect of the first rib is removed. **I,** The cartilaginous components of the articular facets of the first rib, with both the costal vertebral and costal transverse joints, can be identified (*asterisks*). (*Modified from Urschel HC Jr., Cooper JC: Atlas of thoracic surgery, New York, 1995, Churchill Livingstone.*)

Previously, first-rib resection alone was not considered adequate therapy for upper plexus (median nerve) TOS. It was felt that the combined approach, with upper plexus dissection through a supraclavicular incision in addition to the transaxillary approach, was necessary. However, with better understanding of anatomy—specifically, that the median nerve receives fibers from C8 and T1, as well as the upper plexus, and that the muscles that compress the upper plexus attach to the first rib—it is now recognized that first-rib removal through the transaxillary approach alone can relieve upper plexus compression, and the transaxillary approach alone is satisfactory.

Although several routes have been described to remove the first rib, including posterior, transaxillary, supraclavicular, infraclavicular, transthoracic, and through the bed of the affected clavicle, the least morbidity results from the transaxillary approach (see Table 1).

ARTERIAL COMPRESSION

Diagnosis is confirmed by history, physical examination, Doppler studies, and arteriography. Therapy for arterial compression depends on its degree of involvement. An asymptomatic patient with cervical- or first-rib arterial compression producing poststenotic dilatation of the axillary-subclavian artery should undergo rib resection, preferably through the transaxillary approach, removing the ribs, both first and cervical, but not resecting the artery, which usually returns to normal following removal of compression. Patients experiencing compression from first and/or cervical ribs, producing aneurysm with or without thrombus, should undergo rib resection and aneurysm excision with graft through the supraclavicular and infraclavicular combined approach. Thrombosis of the axillary-subclavian artery or distal emboli secondary

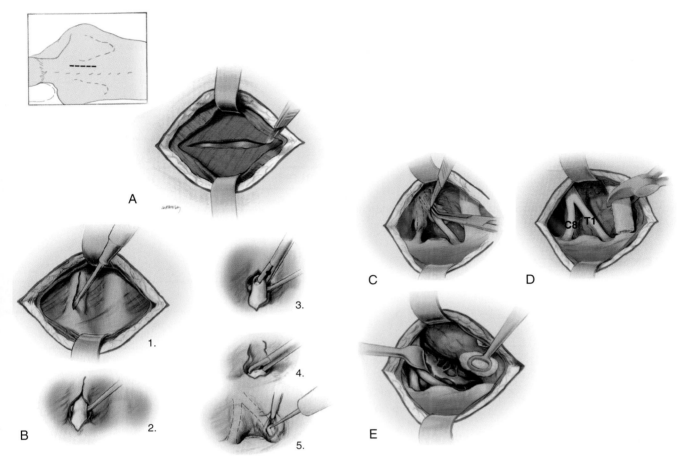

FIGURE 4   Posterior high-thoracoplasty approach with dorsal sympathectomy for recurrent thoracic outlet syndrome. **A,** The patient is placed in the lateral position with an axillary roll under the "down" side. The upper arm is placed as for a thoracotomy. An incision is made approximately 6 cm in length with the midpoint at the angle of the scapula, halfway between the scapula and the spinous processes (*inset*). The incision is carried through the skin and subcutaneous tissue down to the trapezius muscle, and the trapezius and rhomboid muscles are split. **B,** The posterior superior serratus muscle is resected, and the first-rib stump is identified by retracting the sacrospinalis muscle medially. **B1,** Cautery is used to expose the first-rib stump and to open the periosteum. **B2,** A periosteal elevator, or joker, is employed to remove the stump subperiosteally. **B3, B4,** The head and neck of the rib usually have not been removed in the initial operation. The rib shears are used to divide the rib remnant, and the Urschel-Leksell reinforced and Urschel pituitary rongeurs are used to carefully remove the head and neck of the rib. **B5,** The T1 nerve root is identified grossly or with the nerve stimulator. **C,** Once the T1 nerve root is identified, neurolysis is carried out using a ring-angle clamp, magnification, a knife, and special microscissors. **D,** The second rib is dissected free, and cautery is used to open the periosteum linearly. A 2 cm segment of the rib is resected posteriorly, medial to the sacrospinalis muscle, to perform the dorsal sympathectomy. **E,** The lower third of the stellate ganglion is incised sharply, and the gray and white rami communicans are clipped and divided. *(Modified from Urschel HC Jr, Cooper JC: Atlas of thoracic surgery, New York, 1995, Churchill Livingstone.)*

to compression should be treated with first-rib resection, arterial repair or replacement, and embolectomy with dorsal sympathectomy.

EFFORT THROMBOSIS OF AXILLARY-SUBCLAVIAN VEIN (PAGET-SCHROETTER SYNDROME)

Effort thrombosis of the axillary-subclavian vein, or Paget-Schroetter syndrome (PSS), is usually secondary to unusual or excessive use of the arm, in addition to one or more compressive elements in the thoracic outlet and a congenitally abnormal insertion of the costoclavicular ligament laterally. In most cases the costoclavicular ligament congenitally inserts much further laterally than normal, (Figure 5) and with hypertrophy of the scalenus anticus muscle, the vein clots. The diagnosis is established by a careful history and physical examination, Doppler studies, and a venogram. Intermittent obstruction and PSS should be treated with first-rib removal through the transaxillary approach, with

resection of the costoclavicular ligament medially, the first rib inferiorly, and the scalenus anticus muscle laterally. The vein is decompressed, and all the bands and adhesions are removed. The clavicle is left in place.

For many years, acute thrombosis (in PSS) was treated by elevation of the arm and the use of anticoagulants, with subsequent return to work. If symptoms recurred the patient was considered for a first-rib resection, with or without thrombectomy, as well as resection of the scalenus anticus muscle and removal of any other compressive elements in the thoracic outlet, such as the cervical rib or abnormal bands. Recent availability of thrombolytic agents combined with prompt surgical decompression of the neurovascular compressive elements in the thoracic outlet has reduced morbidity and the necessity for thrombectomy and has substantially improved clinical results, including the ability to return to work. The patient should be treated with intravenous urokinase through a localized antecubital catheter and, after thrombolysis, should be taken immediately to the operating room for first-rib resection and decompression of the external obstruction. Intravenous stents always clot, and these are contraindicated, as are bypass grafts in this low-flow, low-pressure system.

RECURRENT THORACIC OUTLET SYNDROME

Recurrent symptoms, primarily neurogenic, should be documented by objective nerve conduction velocities. When velocities are depressed in a symptomatic patient and remain unrelieved with conservative therapy, the patient should undergo posterior reoperation (see Figure 4) with removal of any rib stumps or regenerated fibrocartilage and neurolysis of C7, C8, and T1 nerve roots and the brachial plexus. Methylprednisolone and hyaluronic acid are indicated to minimize recurrent scar.

RESULTS

The results for the primary operation and reoperation for recurrent disease are presented in Tables 2 through 6.

ACKNOWLEDGEMENT

The contribution of Mrs. Rachel Montano was of immeasurable value for her dedication and commitment to the completion of this publication.

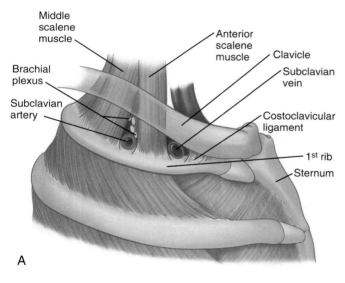

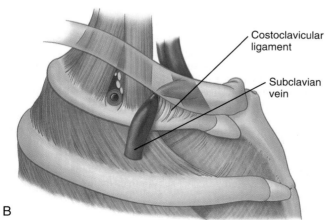

FIGURE 5   Congenital anatomic lateral insertion of the costoclavicular ligament. *(From Urschel HC Jr: Anatomy of the thoracic outlet, Thorac Surg Clin 17:4:511–520, 2007.)*

TABLE 2: Definition of results

Result Evaluation	Symptom Relief	Employment Limitation	Recreation
Good	Complete	Full	None
Fair	Partial	Limitation	Moderate
Poor	None	No return	Severe

TABLE 3: Results for initial TOC operation

Surgical Results: First Operation	5102 Patients
Good	4337 (85%)
Fair	612 (12%)
Poor	153 (3%)

TABLE 4: Results of first operation of different patient classification

TOS Results	% IMPROVEMENT	
	Early	Late
Classical syndrome	95	90
Traumatic TOS	75	60
Therapeutic trial	70	50

TABLE 5: Results of reoperation for recurrent TOS

Surgical Results: Reoperation	2305 Patients
Good	1729 (75%)
Fair	369 (16%)
Poor	207 (9%)

TABLE 6: Morbidity and mortality of TOS

	7407 Patients
Deaths	0
Complications	
Infections	22
Bleeding	4
Injury	
Nerve	4
Arterial	0
Venous	1
Horner syndrome	6

SUGGESTED READINGS

Urschel HC Jr, Razzuk MA: Current concepts: management of the thoracic outlet syndrome, *N Engl J Med* 286:1140, 1972.

Urschel HC Jr, Razzuk MA: The failed operation for thoracic outlet syndrome: the difficulty of diagnosis and management,, *Ann Thorac Surg* 42:523–528, 1986.

Urschel HC Jr, Razzuk MA: Neurovascular compression in the thoracic outlet: changing management over 50 years, *Ann Surg* 228:609, 1998.

Urschel HC Jr, Kourlis H Jr: Thoracic outlet syndrome: a 50-year experience at Baylor University Medical Center, *Bay Univ Med Cent Proc* 20:125–135, 2007.

Urschel HC Jr, Patel AN: Surgery remains the most effective treatment for Paget-Schroetter syndrome: 50 years' experience, *Ann Thor Surg* 86: 254–260, 2008.

Urschel HC Jr, Cooper JD: *Atlas of thoracic surgery*, New York, 1995, Churchill Livingstone.

DIABETIC FOOT

John E. McDermott, MD, and Timothy C. Fitzgibbons, MD

OVERVIEW

Recalcitrant ulcerization and infection of the foot represent a common surgical challenge. Type 2 diabetes, a common affliction in the United States for decades, is rapidly becoming epidemic in Asia and in the developing countries of Latin America and Africa. The sequelae of diabetes are now the most common cause of amputation in the world. It is now generally accepted that Joslin's original theory of a "thrifty gene," noted in its epidemic spread in Southwest Native Americans in the 1930s, has become manifest since World War II worldwide, secondary to "Americanization" of the diet. The challenge of successful treatment of these patients has led to the development of specialty clinics in surgical centers in the United States and now throughout the developed world.

PATHOPHYSIOLOGY

Diabetes affects the nerves and vascular tissues of the body through the more apparent destruction and cellular compromise of these tissues, compared with its affect on general cell metabolism. Patients with type 2 diabetes are prone to progressive atherosclerotic compromise and claudication. The metabolic disease process attacks neurologic tissue, resulting in loss of normal sensory and proprioceptive protection. The combination of vascular and neurologic compromise leads to further change in soft tissue and other muscular, osseous, and dermal structural systems. The net effect of this is the manifest skin breakdown and subsequent ulceration and musculotendinous compromise, followed by loss of underlying osseous support. The subsequent infection in the diabetic patient is further complicated by immunologic dysfunction secondary to impaired leukocyte activity. Once skin penetration and ulceration develops, infections are usually of the polymicrobial type, which are difficult to treat and often methicillin resistant.

EVALUATION

Confronted with a diabetic wound problem, the classic ankle-brachial indexes (ABIs) are the primary screening evaluation. This should be coupled with a complete neurovascular evaluation including Semmes-Weinstein monofilament sensory testing. The workup should include vascular studies, arteriogram, and, with respect to the wound itself, magnetic resonance imaging to provide insight to the depth and extent of the infectious process. Particularly in the mid and hind foot, radiographs are needed to determine the existence of occult Charcot bone and joint destruction and collapse.

Many authors have attempted to classify diabetic ulcers as an adjunct treatment decision. Most are variations of the classic Wagner classification on which the basic treatment plan is based (Table 1). Global classification, however, must be tempered with respect to specific locations on the foot. Ulceration over bony prominences, metatarsal heads, malleoli, and os calcis require addressing the "rock and a hard place" concept. Particularly, recalcitrant ulceration of the heel will often require extensive resection of the calcaneus to facilitate debridement and skin closure. Ulceration below the collapsed midfoot in Charcot-type deformity is best treated by reduction of the internal pressure to the skin through subfascial, direct resection of the bone, avoiding the superficial ulcer below the plantar fascia.

Confronted with plantar ulceration of the sole of the foot, evaluation should look for tarsal cuboid collapse. Resection of bony prominence may expedite treatment and healing. In the forefoot, ulcerations are frequently under metatarsal pressure areas, which need to be addressed in any surgical debridement or closure effort. Microbiologic evaluation of the ulcer's concurrent infections, of course, is necessary to provide accurate antibiotic infection management in conjunction with planned debridement surgery.

PROCEDURE

Two-stage surgical technique consists of deep surgical resection followed by soft tissue mobilization and then a delayed primary closure.

Stage One

The initial surgical effort is directed at deep, wide resection and debridement of the ulcer and underlying soft tissue and infected or pressure-producing osseous structures or nonviable digits. During this stage, cultures and deep biopsies are obtained for laboratory analysis and appropriate antibiotic identification for the postsurgical period and second-stage effort. All necrotic, avascular, and devitalized tissue is excised. Wounds are irrigated with commercially available dental water-jet devices. The wound is then loosely closed over drains. When possible, suction vacuum-type drains improve tissue viability and deep wound compression (Figure 1).

Postoperatively, the patient is placed on a non–weight-bearing regimen and treated with limb elevation. Antibiotics are given during surgery and are continued and modified 4 to 7 days later, based on deep surgical cultures.

Stage Two

At the second stage, the patient is returned to the operating room, and debridement and pulsatile irrigation is again carried out. Deep cultures are repeated, and appropriate adjustments are made in

TABLE 1: Wagner classification scheme of diabetic foot and recommendations

Grade	Definition	Treatment
Depth Classification		
0	The at-risk foot: previous ulcer or neuropathy with deformity that may cause new ulceration	Patient education Regular examination Appropriate shoe wear and insoles
1	Superficial ulceration, not infected	External pressure relief Total contact cast, walking brace, special shoe wear
2	Deep ulceration exposing tendon or joint (with or without superficial infection)	Surgical debridement → wound care → pressure relief if wound closes and converts to class 1 (prn antibiotics)
3	Extensive ulceration with exposed bone and/or deep infection (osteomyelitis or abscess)	Surgical debridement → ray or partial foot amputation → intravenous antibiotics → pressure relief if wound converts to class 1
Ischemia Classification		
A	Not ischemic	Adequate vascularity for healing
B	Ischemia without gangrene	Vascular evaluation (Doppler, $tcpO_2$, arteriogram, etc.) → vascular reconstruction prn
C	Partial (forefoot) gangrene of foot	Vascular evaluation → vascular reconstruction (proximal or distal bypass or angioplasty) → partial foot amputation
D	Complete foot gangrene	Vascular evaluation → major extremity amputation (BKA, AKA) with possible proximal vascular reconstruction

BKA, Below-knee amputation; *AKA,* above-knee amputation; *tcpO_2,* transcutaneous partial pressure of oxygen.

postoperative antibiotic management. Delayed primary closure is performed using a double-tension suture technique. We prefer #00 wire and #000 nonabsorbable synthetic suture for wide tension technique. A protective dressing is applied to the wound, and the patient is kept on a non–weight-bearing regimen until healing allows. Sutures are often left in for 4 to 6 weeks, as these patients are extremely compromised in tissue healing. Efforts to maintain tissue tension and position, including casting, are suggested. Again, wound vacuum technique can be helpful (Figure 2).

Following the two-stage procedure, the dressings are changed at 4 days, then followed with daily dry dressings. Laser Doppler velocimetry and transcutaneous oxygen studies of the extremity are predictors of success with the two-stage closure technique.

Amputation

Successful surgical treatment of neuropathic ulcers is, unfortunately, often not achievable. Thus, the diabetic patient represents a high risk for amputation. In dealing with the foot, any amputation proximal to the metatarsals is best treated by an ankle procedure followed by prescriptive prosthesis. We prefer the Syme technique, which allows preservation of leg length. When performed with two-stage technique, it will result in a stump shape easily accommodated by prescription shoe wear.

When dealing with toe metatarsal amputation, unless more than two toes can be salvaged, the complete forefoot amputation is easier to rehabilitate postoperatively. Resection of first and fifth metatarsals is well tolerated and will leave a relatively balanced foot. The forefoot amputation will not usually result in satisfactory gait when compared to an ankle amputation. Not only does it have a high failure rate, it is difficult to manage prosthetically.

Hyperbaric oxygen does not have universal availability and admittedly has some detractors. However, definitive studies have shown that there is a high success rate when properly used. The author's recommendation is 5 to 6 days a week of treatment in, of course, a true hyperbaric chamber, as oxygen is not well absorbed through skin tissue, but oxygen saturation levels in tissue are increased by an increased oxygen blood saturation in both cells and plasma.

The diabetic foot ulcer is principally a vascular complication. Thus, prior to any direct management of the ulcer problem, an appropriate vascular workup is indicated. The workup must focus on small vessel disease as well as global limb perfusion. The gross determination with blood pressure measurements and equal arm indexes should be augmented with PCP O_2 transcutaneous oxygen saturation level determination. A value less than 30 mm Hg is a predictor of healing.

MANAGEMENT OF COMPLICATIONS

Successful surgical management of diabetic ulcers requires assessment and management of the underlying metabolic disorder. Blood glucose levels must be brought into relatively normal range to allow tissue healing. A deep-seated ulcer with chronic infection cannot be expected to heal with direct resection and closure. This has led to the popularity of the two-stage technique described by Fitzgibbons and colleagues.

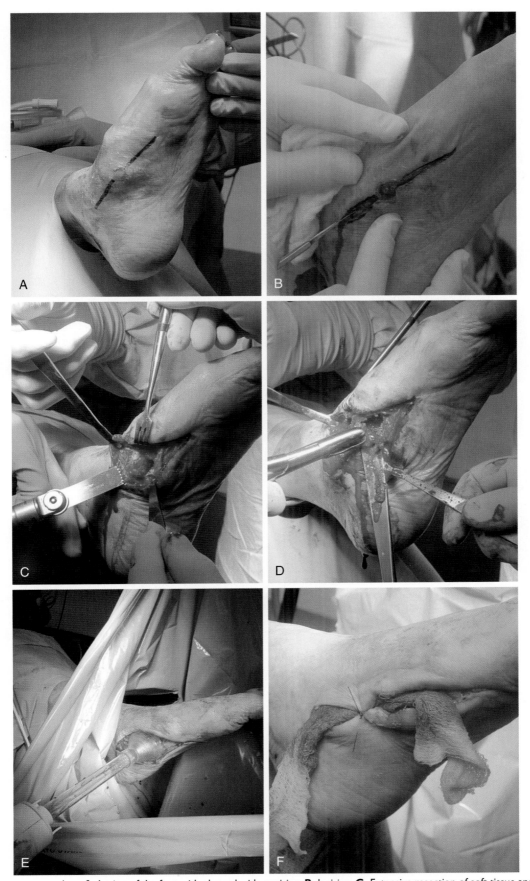

FIGURE I   Stage-one procedure. **A,** Lesion of the foot with planned wide excision. **B,** Incision. **C,** Extensive resection of soft tissue and sharp resection of bone. **D,** Debridement of all compromised tissue. **E,** Extensive pressure irrigation of wound. **F,** Loose closure with full extensive drainage allowed.

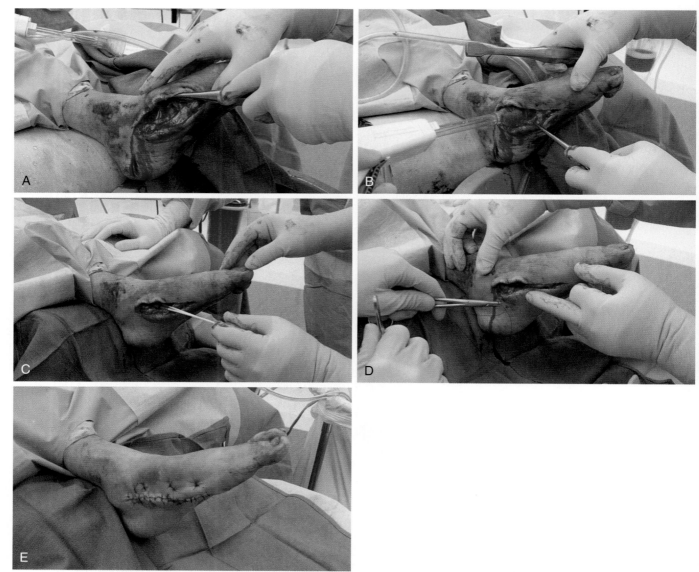

FIGURE 2   Stage-two procedure. **A,** Secondary debridement. **B,** Repeat pressure irrigation and microdebridement. **C,** Repeat culture followed with further careful debridement of all compromised tissue. **D,** Primary skin closure. **E,** Retention layer closure followed by dressing and/or cast.

Suggested Readings

Brodsky JW: Outpatient diagnosis and care of the diabetic foot, *Instr Course Lect* 42:121–139, 1993.

Karanfilian RG, Lynch TG, Lee BC, et al: The assessment of skin blood flow in peripheral vascular disease by laser Doppler velocimetry and transcutaneous oxygen tension determination in predicting healing of ischemic forefoot ulcerations and amputations in diabetic and nondiabetic patients, *J Vasc Surg* 4:511–520, 1986.

Khouri RK, Cooley BC, Kunselman AR, et al: A prospective study of microvascular free flap surgery and outcome, *Plast Reconstr Surg* 102:711–721, 1998.

Kumagai SG, Mahoney GR, Fitzgibbons TC, et al: Treatment of diabetic (neuropathic) foot ulcers with two-stage debridement and closure, *Foot Ankle Int* 19:160–165, 1998.

McDermott JE: *Diabetic foot,* Rosemont, IL, 1995, American Academy of Orthopedic Surgeons.

GANGRENE OF THE FOOT

Rachel J. Santora, MD, and Heitham T. Hassoun, MD

OVERVIEW

Gangrene is a consequence of critical limb ischemia, infection, or any process causing arterial occlusion. Subsequent oxygen deprivation leads to localized coagulative or liquefactive necrosis, respectively. With a superimposed bacterial infection, the rate of tissue decay is accelerated. Although gangrene can affect any part of the body, the distal extremities, particularly the digits and foot, are most susceptible.

Gangrene is commonly classified as either "dry" or "wet" gangrene. Both occur in the presence of arterial occlusion, however, dry gangrene occurs in the absence of bacterial infection and is characterized by mummification and demarcation of the necrotic tissue (Figure 1, A). In wet gangrene (Figure 1, B), the affected area becomes acutely infected and swollen, and rapid tissue decay is accompanied by systemic symptoms and significant pain. Any patient presenting with gangrene should undergo emergent evaluation to ensure adequate source control of the infected area or to optimize the chance of successful revascularization for limb salvage. Conversely, dry gangrene does not require immediate amputation; instead autoamputation may occur, negating the need for elective amputation. Autoamputation is characterized by spontaneous detachment of nonviable tissue after demarcation is complete. This process may take months to occur, while epithelization occurs under the existing eschar.

RISK FACTORS AND EPIDEMIOLOGY

Over the past two decades, the rate of lower extremity amputations in the United States has increased from 19 to 30 per 100,000 patient years, secondary to advancing patient age and critical limb ischemia. The associated mortality rate in patients who have undergone primary amputation is approximately 15%. A majority of patients with distal limb gangrene have chronic microvascular or macrovascular disease and advanced atherosclerosis as a result of diabetes, smoking, and/or chronic kidney disease.

The number of people with diabetes is increasing worldwide. The Centers for Disease Control and Prevention reports that over the past 20 years, the number of Americans with diabetes has tripled, from 5.6 million to 16.8 million. The prevalence of diabetes is expected to grow to over 24.5 million in the next 15 years. Diabetic foot infections that progress to ulceration and gangrene are frequently encountered in today's patient population. Prospective studies have shown that peripheral neuropathy and peripheral arterial disease (PAD) are independent risk factors for lower extremity amputations in diabetic patients. It is estimated that more than 60% of nontraumatic lower extremity amputations are a result of diabetic complications. The amputation rate for diabetic patients with severe foot infections is approximately 25%.

Smoking is also an important risk factor in the progression of PAD to critical limb ischemia. The TransAtlantic Inter-Society Consensus report (TASC-I) identifies smoking as a greater risk factor for the development and progression of PAD than coronary artery disease. Heavy smokers with intermittent claudication are more likely to require more revascularization attempts and major amputations compared to nonsmokers.

In most cases, gangrene is a unilateral phenomenon because of the conditions described above; however, an important cause of symmetrical gangrene in critically ill patients is disseminated intravascular coagulation (DIC). Other conditions leading to peripheral gangrene in the critically ill also include other hypercoagulable states and use of vasoactive drugs. The mortality rate associated with symmetrical peripheral gangrene is estimated to be approximately 35%, with almost half of patients requiring amputation of at least one lower extremity. In the absence of other ischemic arterial disease, other conditions that cause arterial occlusion leading to peripheral ischemia and gangrene include myeloproliferative disorders and vasculitides or vasospastic conditions such as Raynaud syndrome.

EVALUATION

Clinical Presentation

Initial patient evaluation begins with a thorough history and physical examination. The clinician should identify preexisting comorbidities that may complicate medical and surgical management. An imperative part of the initial assessment is to determine the severity of the infection. Patients with life-threatening infection often have significant metabolic and hemodynamic instability that requires immediate hospitalization and resuscitation.

The level of amputation can often be determined empirically by a thorough physical exam and the clinical judgment of an experienced surgeon. Physical examination findings—such as changes in skin temperature or color, muscle atrophy, presence of aortic or femoral bruits, or diminished pulses—are suggestive of significant arterial disease. Examination of the peripheral vascular system in the lower extremity should include palpation of the femoral, popliteal, posterior tibial, and dorsalis pedis pulses. Palpable pulses proximal to the anticipated level of amputation are a good prognostic indicator of successful postoperative healing, however, absence of palpable pulses is not a contraindication to amputation. A number of noninvasive tests are recognized as important adjuncts to clinical exam to determine the adequacy of tissue perfusion and oxygenation of the affected extremity.

Diagnostics

In patients with a propensity to develop vascular disease, both the microcirculation and macrocirculation should be evaluated to determine the likelihood of postoperative healing. A number of indices exist that can be used to predict the adequacy of circulation to support successful wound healing and to identify the need for adjunctive revascularization. Noninvasive arterial testing can be divided into two groups, which include assessment of the *macrocirculation* and *microcirculation*. Commonly used modalities include ankle-brachial index (ABI), segmental systolic pressures, skin perfusion pressures, and transcutaneous measurement of partial pressure of oxygen (Table 1).

Assessment of Macrocirculation

The integrity of the macrocirculation is most commonly assessed by measuring the ABI or segmental systolic pressures. The ABI is measured by comparing the pressure in the anterior tibial, peroneal, or posterior tibial artery with the brachial artery Doppler pressure. An ABI value less than 0.4 is a prognostic indicator of poor postoperative wound healing. In patients with abnormal ABIs, segmental systolic pressures and the respective indices are used to better localize arterial insufficiency. Segmental limb pressures (SLPs) are obtained by using a series of pneumatic cuffs positioned at different levels on the lower extremity to compare gradients among the respective segments.

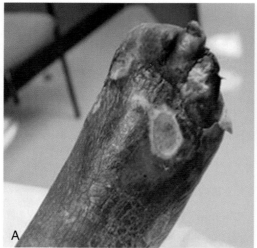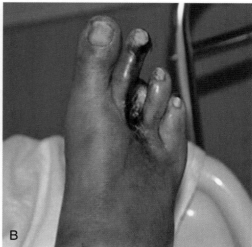

FIGURE 1   Dry vs. wet gangrene. **A,** Dry gangrene with evidence of autoamputation. **B,** Acute wet gangrene.

TABLE 1: Noninvasive Arterial Tests

	Critical Values
Macrocirculation	
ABI	<0.4
Microcirculation	
Toe-brachial index	<0.7
Toe systolic pressure	<50 mm Hg*
Pulse wave amplitude	<4 mm
Transcutaneous oxygen pressure	<30 mm Hg
Skin perfusion pressure	<40 mm Hg

*A toe pressure <50 mm Hg is a critical value in patients with active gangrene or ulceration.

In diabetic patients, both ABI and segmental pressures may be falsely elevated (ABI >1.4 or ankle pressure > 50 mm Hg) due to arterial calcification. In these instances, pulse volume recordings (PVRs) may also be obtained in conjunction with SLP measurements to more accurately diagnose peripheral artery disease. PVRs are obtained through a brachial cuff and limb cuffs, which are connected to a plethysmograph that measures changes in limb volume with respect to cardiac output. The waveforms obtained by the lower extremity cuffs are standardized to those from the brachial cuff. In this manner, low-amplitude waveforms secondary to poor cardiac function are not misinterpreted as lower extremity arterial insufficiency. Used together, SLPs and PVRs are approximately 95% accurate in diagnosing PAD.

Assessment of Microcirculation

Although the principal cause of critical limb ischemia is underlying macrovascular disease, the inability to heal after revascularization or amputation is determined by the status of the microcirculation. Therefore, the preoperative assessment of patients with peripheral ischemia and gangrene also mandates noninvasive tests to assess the microcirculation. The toe-brachial index (TBI) is an extremely useful tool in patients with arterial calcification; it uses photoplethysmography (PPG) to measure great toe pressure, which is then compared to the brachial artery pressure. Under normal conditions,

the great toe systolic pressure is about 30 mm Hg less than the highest brachial pressure, and a TBI greater than 0.7 is considered normal. A toe pressure less than 50 mm Hg in a patient with active gangrene or ulceration, or a value less than 30 mm Hg under nonulcerative conditions, satisfies the TASC-II criteria for critical ischemia.

In addition to using absolute toe pressures to assess the severity of PAD, the amplitude of the PPG waveform can be used to complement the TBI. It is also used as an index of successful wound healing. Pulse wave amplitudes less than 4 mm are associated with an increased risk of amputation.

Transcutaneous measurement of partial pressure of oxygen (TcPO$_2$) is another noninvasive diagnostic test that provides important prognostic information in patients with severe ischemia. TcPO$_2$ probes are used to determine the oxygen supply to microcirculation by measuring the partial pressure of oxygen at the surface of the skin. A number of studies have shown that a TcPO$_2$ level greater than 40 is a good prognostic indicator of wound healing after amputation or revascularization. An alternative to measuring TcPO$_2$ levels is to determine the skin perfusion pressure (SPP), which is obtained by deflating an external compression cuff and utilizing one of three modalities—radioisotope clearance, photoplethysmography, and laser Doppler. The minimal pressure above which skin blood flow ceases is defined as the SPP. Some retrospective studies suggest that SPP can more accurately predict the severity of limb ischemia and wound healing than other commonly used noninvasive tests. An SPP value of 40 mm Hg or higher predicts successful wound healing with a sensitivity of 72% and specificity of 88%.

Imaging

For patients with critical limb ischemia, a number of imaging modalities are used to determine whether the affected area is amenable to revascularization. The most commonly utilized modalities include digital subtraction angiography (DSA), multidetector computed tomography angiography (MDCTA), magnetic resonance angiography (MRA), and/or duplex ultrasound (DUS). While angiography is still considered the gold standard, this technique is invasive and is associated with potential complications and patient morbidity. Color-assisted DUS is an alternate modality that is safer and more cost effective than traditional angiography, with high sensitivity (95%) and specificity (88%) for detecting hemodynamically significant lesions. The sensitivity of detecting significant lesions is further improved by using gadolinium-enhanced MRA or MDCTA.

MDCTA and MRA are emerging as preferred imaging modalities for diagnosis and preoperative planning in most institutions. Both modalities are advantageous in their ability to provide rapid, high-resolution, three-dimensional images. Some drawbacks exist with both modalities, however; the degree of spatial resolution of small vessels achieved by MRA is significantly less than with MDCTA, but MRA does not require the use of ionizing radiation. One major disadvantage in MDCTA is that arterial calcification generates artifact that interferes with vessel assessment.

MANAGEMENT

Antibiotics and Medical Management

Initial antibiotic therapy is usually empirical and based on the patient's history and clinical appearance. Patients with chronic ulceration tend to have polymicrobial infections, with Gram-positive and Gram-negative cocci and anaerobic organisms. With increasing severity of infection, the number of potential pathogens and the prevalence of antibiotic resistance rise exponentially. Definitive antibiotic therapy is modified based on microbial culture and sensitivity results obtained from an appropriate specimen. Deep-tissue samples are the most meaningful culture samples.

The route of administration and duration of treatment are determined by the extent of the infection and the clinical response to treatment. For severe infections, intravenous therapy is usually preferred over oral or parenteral therapy for the initiation of treatment. Diabetic foot infections are a major factor leading to lower extremity amputations. The colonizing flora of patients with underlying metabolic alterations tends to be more virulent and complex than normal skin flora. Virulent, aerobic, Gram-positive cocci, such as *Staphylococcus aureus* and β-hemolytic *Streptococcus* are more likely to thrive in diabetic foot wounds, therefore initial antibiotic therapy should target these more virulent organisms to arrest infection and prevent progressive tissue loss.

Debridement

Debridement of devitalized tissue that is poorly vascularized and provides a surface for adherence of bacteria is essential for antibiotic therapy to be effective and to limit the duration of treatment. The most commonly used method of debridement is sharp, surgical debridement. Alternative techniques to surgical debridement involve mechanical or pharmacologic debridement by using wet-to-dry dressings or topical enzymes. To ensure removal of all necrotic tissues, repetitive debridement of nonviable tissue is often required. In addition to sharp debridement, a number of biologic therapies exist to promote healing in severe foot infections: these therapies include topical growth factors, protease scavengers, and biologic wound matrices that promote cellular ingrowth. In conjunction with local wound care, these agents have been shown to reduce healing times and increase overall healing rates, which leads to reduced amputation rates.

Revascularization

In most patients with limb-threatening ischemia, vascular intervention is often required to optimize the potential for limb salvage. The need for revascularization is determined by patient factors and noninvasive assessment of the underlying circulation. Endovascular procedures are being increasingly utilized for the initial management of inadequate perfusion. Short arterial occlusions and stenoses are usually amenable to percutaneous intervention, whereas longer arterial occlusions often require peripheral bypass procedures. Regardless of the techniques utilized, adequate perfusion must be achieved to ensure wound healing before soft-tissue reconstruction can be attempted.

Improvements in endovascular techniques have allowed for increases in attempted limb salvage in high-risk patients, who would have otherwise only been candidates for primary amputations. With these improvements, there have been decreasing rates of primary amputation; however, the incidence of limb loss despite patent revascularization is increasing in this patient population. Patients at high risk for limb loss after revascularization are those with diabetes, renal insufficiency, and gangrene. In such patients, inability to control primary or recurrent infection and inability to reverse ischemia are major factors contributing to limb loss despite intervention. Even with improved techniques and early intervention, a number of studies have demonstrated that the clinical durability of limb salvage in the setting of significant soft-tissue infection is often limited.

AMPUTATIONS

The most important aspects regarding lower extremity amputation for gangrene are 1) adequate source control through aggressive debridement of necrotic tissue and bone and 2) preservation of the greatest amount of viable tissue. The level of amputation must also maximize the rehabilitation potential of each individual patient. This is based on the health status of the patient and ambulatory status prior to amputation. The energy required to ambulate after lower extremity amputation increases significantly with more proximal amputations and may be a significant impedance to postoperative ambulation in patients with preexisting comorbidities.

Toe Amputation

Gangrene that is limited to the middle or distal phalanges, not involving the metatarsal head, is often amenable to simple toe disarticulation. It leaves the patient with limited disability and deformity. Digit amputation should not be performed if ischemia of the forefoot is present, or if infection involving the metatarsal head is present.

Great Toe Amputation

If amputation of the great toe is required, it is advantageous to preserve the base of the proximal phalanx rather than perform a complete metatarsophalangeal disarticulation. The first metatarsal head is important for balance and gait, and preservation of the proximal phalanx allows for better distribution of weight and pressure. This is particularly important in diabetic patients, who are susceptible to development of malperforans ulcers. A curvelinear incision at the base of the toe is carried down to the level of the bone in a circumferential manner. Skin incisions can be created in a "fish mouth" configuration, which utilizes dorsoplantar or mediolateral skin flaps, or in a racquet-like fashion. The choice of incision is based on viable tissue that is available to cover the remaining end of the proximal phalanx. An oscillating power saw is used to transect the distal phalanx, while preserving the proximal phalanx (at least 1 cm). Bone edges are smoothed to a bevel using a rongeur. Finally, full-thickness skin flaps are approximated in an interrupted fashion with nonabsorbable sutures.

Lesser Toe Amputation

The metatarsophalangeal joint is identified by flexing and extending the toe. A circumferential racquet-like or fish-mouth incision is made at the midpoint of the proximal phalanx. The incision is carried down to the level of the bone, and the joint capsule is opened. Resection of the cartilage at this time is not recommended; however, if viable skin flaps are present, cartilage ischemia is rarely a problem. Using an oscillating power saw, the distal end of the affected phalanx is resected. Dorsoplantar or mediolateral skin flaps are then reapproximated using interrupted nylon sutures.

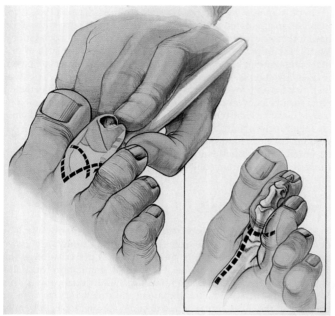

FIGURE 2   Ray amputation. Skin incision for a ray amputation with equal sagittal or dorsal and plantar flaps to ensure adequate blood supply. A racquet-like incision encircles the base of the toe and extends proximally over the dorsum of the metatarsal head. *(Modified from Barnes RW, Cox B: Amputations: an illustrated manual, Philadelphia, 2000, Hanley and Belfus, p 17.)*

Ray Amputation

Ray amputations involve complete resection of the phalanx and partial resection of the corresponding metatarsal. Ray amputations are indicated when there is not enough viable tissue to provide coverage for a disarticulation as described above. First and fifth ray amputations are often referred to as *border amputations* and are the easiest to perform. However, ray amputation to remove two adjacent toes may also be performed.

For border ray amputations, a racquet-like incision is carried out in a circumferential manner and extended onto the dorsal aspect of the foot. For amputation of the second, third, or fourth toe, a racquet-like incision that extends over the metatarsal is also used (Figure 2). Nerves and tendons are resected under tension, and the distal aspect of the metatarsal is transected with an oscillating saw, leaving the metatarsal head intact. The skin incision is closed with nonabsorbable sutures.

Transmetatarsal Amputation

Transmetatarsal amputation is indicated for gangrene that results in significant forefoot tissue loss. A slightly curved dorsal skin incision is made in a mediolateral fashion (Figure 3). The medial and lateral aspects of the dorsal skin excision are extended distally to ensure adequate skin coverage over the bone ends. The corresponding plantar flap is created slightly longer than the dorsal flap, and the tendons are resected under tension to the proximal edge of the wound and are allowed to retract.

Next, the metatarsals are resected using a power saw with a 15-degree bevel with respect to the transverse axis. Each metatarsal should be cut successively shorter than the adjacent metatarsal in a mediolateral fashion. Next, the amputated forefoot is resected away from the plantar flap. Prior to approximation of the plantar and dorsal skin flaps, the plantar flap often requires thinning to avoid undue tension on the closure, which threatens viability. Primary

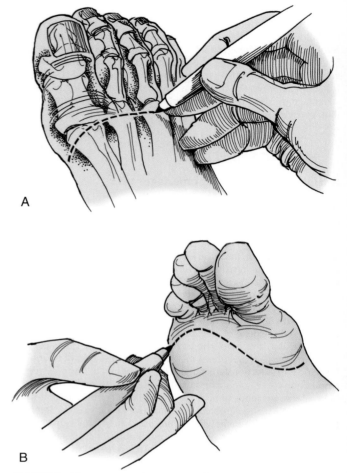

A

B

FIGURE 3   Transmetatarsal amputation. A transverse dorsal incision is made proximal to the metatarsal heads, and a curvilinear plantar incision is made at the base of the toes to create a long plantar flap. *(Modified from Barnes RW, Cox B: Amputations: an illustrated manual, Philadelphia, 2000, Hanley and Belfus, p 39.)*

closure is completed in an interrupted fashion using nonabsorbable sutures.

Syme Amputation

The chief indication for a Syme amputation is forefoot necrosis not amenable to a transmetatarsal amputation, while neuropathy and poor vascularity of the heel pad are absolute contraindications. The advantages of a Syme amputation are preservation of limb length and a partially weight-bearing residual limb. The sole vascular supply to the heel pad is the posterior tibial vessels, which should be carefully preserved. A transverse anterior incision that connects the anterior points of each malleolus is carried down to the bone. The corresponding dorsal incision is made down to the level of the calcaneus. The anterior tendons are identified and dissected under tension and allowed to retract (Figure 4).

The anterior tibial artery is identified and ligated, and the collateral ligamentous attachments of the talus are divided. After identification of the medial neurovascular bundle, the calcaneus is dissected away from the surrounding soft tissues, while applying traction on the talus to facilitate dissection. During this aspect of the dissection, careful attention is made to avoid any injury to the subcutaneous attachment of the Achilles tendon, which would compromise the integrity of the heel pad and cause the amputation

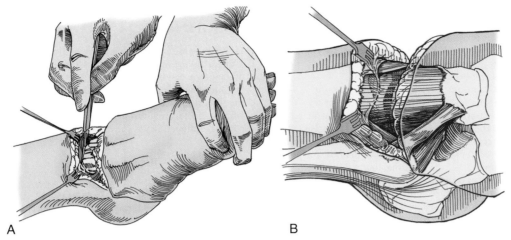

FIGURE 4   Syme amputation. *(Modified from Barnes RW, Cox B: Amputations: an illustrated manual, Philadelphia, 2000, Hanley and Belfus, p 53.)*

to fail. Subperiosteal dissection is carried out until the calcaneus is completely free from the soft tissue. Next, the malleoli are dissected flush with the joint surface, and the remaining bones are trimmed to avoid potential pressure points. The remaining soft tissue envelope is reapproximated using a three-layer closure. The plantar and deep fascias are approximated over the anterior portion of the tibia, followed by closure of the subcutaneous tissue in an interrupted fashion. The skin edges are reapproximated with nylon or other nonabsorbable sutures.

Below-Knee Amputation

In patients whose necrotic tissue is not amenable to foot salvage, a below-knee amputation (BKA) is indicated; however, prior to major lower extremity amputation, certain considerations must be taken into account, and the first is whether to use a tourniquet. Although some advocate the use of a proximal tourniquet when amputation of an infected hyperemic limb is required, there are no trials that support improved healing rates with intraoperative tourniquet use. A tourniquet may be used to control blood loss while removing the affected limb, but it should be released later to ensure adequate perfusion and viability of the skin flaps.

One important consideration when applying a pneumatic tourniquet for any lower extremity amputation is the presence of an underlying vascular graft. Another major consideration is what constitutes adequate debridement of necrotic tissue with maximal soft tissue preservation. In a gangrenous extremity, the initial incision site should be no more than 5 mm from the edge of the necrotic tissue to preserve maximal viable tissue for flap formation. Creation of inadequate tissue flaps may mandate a more proximal amputation than originally planned.

The most commonly performed procedure for BKA utilizes a long posterior flap technique. If the extent of gangrenous tissue precludes creation of a viable long posterior flap, numerous alternative techniques can be employed including equal anteroposterior flaps, unequal anteroposterior flaps, and sagittal flaps. The anterior skin incision to create a long posterior flap is made approximately 10 cm distal to the tibial tuberosity and extended medially and laterally approximately two thirds of the way across the circumference of the calf (Figure 5). The incision is extended distally to create a posterior flap that extends 9 to 13 cm beyond the anterior flap. The distal aspects of the medial and lateral incisions are created in a curved fashion and joined on the posterior surface of the calf, and the skin incision is carried down to the level of the fascia.

Next, the muscles of the anterior compartment are dissected sharply with a scalpel or electrocautery. As the muscle is further

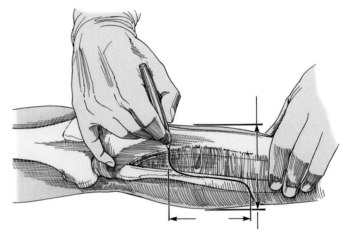

FIGURE 5   BKA. The anterior skin incision is made at the level of maximal girth of the calf, approximately 3 to 4 fingerbreadths distal to the tibial tuberosity. *(Modified from Barnes RW, Cox B: Amputations: an illustrated manual, Philadelphia, 2000, Hanley and Belfus, p 68.)*

divided, the anterior tibial artery and vein are often encountered in the more posterior aspect of the anterior compartment; these vessels should be ligated and transected. The tibia and fibula are circumferentially cleared of the periosteum and are transected with an oscillating power saw. The tibia is transected at a 45-degree angle approximately 1 cm proximal to the skin incision, and the fibula is transected 1 cm proximal to the tibia. A bone hook is used to apply traction on the tibia, and the muscles of the posterior compartment are carefully divided, until the posterior tibial and peroneal neurovascular bundles are encountered, which are then suture ligated and divided. The remaining muscles in the deep and superficial posterior compartment are divided, and the crural fascia is left in place with the posterior flap. At this time, the thickness of the posterior flap is evaluated and debulked as necessary to achieve a tension-free closure when approximated to the anterior flap. A 2-0 nonabsorbable suture is used to approximate the anterior and posterior fascia, and the skin is closed with a 3-0 nonabsorbable suture.

Above-Knee Amputation

An above-knee amputation (AKA) is indicated for patients with nonreconstructable ischemia or with extensive infection that precludes healing at a more distal amputation site. In addition, patients with a fixed knee contracture or a nonfunctional distal limb should also be considered for AKA. In these patients, the postoperative energy cost of ambulation increases 60% to 100% compared with 30% to 60% in patients who have undergone BKA. Increased energy costs have been shown to reduce postoperative ambulation to approximately 40% in patients with diabetes and occlusive arterial disease.

A suprapatellar "fish mouth" incision is carried down to the level of the deep subcutaneous fascia, creating equal anterior and posterior skin flaps. The skin and subcutaneous tissue are retracted in a proximal fashion, and the deep muscle fascia is sharply incised. After division of the quadriceps muscle, proximal traction is placed on all mobilized skin, subcutaneous tissue, and muscle to allow for periosteal elevation of the femur 2 to 3 cm proximal to the skin incision. The femur is transected with an oscillating or manual saw at the proximal level of the periosteum. The transected femur is retracted anteriorly, and the posterior muscle bundle is sharply divided. As major vessels and nerves are encountered, they should be clamped, transected, and ligated with an absorbable 2-0 suture. Wound closure is performed in multiple layers by approximating the anterior and posterior deep subcutaneous and muscle fascia to a cuff of periosteum. This myoplasty effectively stabilizes the anterior and posterior muscle bundles. Subcutaneous tissue and skin are approximated under uniform tension, and the stump is dressed with a bulky dressing of fluffed gauze and a light compression bandage.

SUMMARY

Lower extremity gangrene is a devastating condition that accounts for a majority of nontraumatic lower limb amputations. The morbidity of gangrene can best be reduced using a multidisciplinary approach, beginning with local wound care and source control. Vascular assessment is critical for preoperative planning and attempted limb salvage, when suitable. Finally, rehabilitation is vitally important to restore the patient's independence and sense of well-being.

SUGGESTED READINGS

Armstrong DG, Lipsky BA: Diabetic foot infections: stepwise medical and surgical management, *Int Wound J* 1:123–132, 2004.
Lipsky BA, Berendt AR: Principles and practice of antibiotic therapy of diabetic foot infections, *Diabetes Metab Res Rev* 16(suppl 1):S42–S46, 2000.
Lumsden AB, Davies MG, Peden EK: Medical and endovascular management of critical limb ischemia, *J Endovas Ther* 16(Suppl 2):II31–II62, 2009.
Zgonis T, Stapleton JJ, Girard-Powell VA, Hagino RT: Surgical management of diabetic foot infections and amputations, *AORN J* 87:935–946, 2008.

BUERGER DISEASE

**Natalia Glebova, MD, PhD,
and James H. Black III, MD**

OVERVIEW

Thromboangiitis obliterans (TAO) or Buerger disease, described by Leo Buerger in 1908, is a nonatherosclerotic segmental inflammatory disease that affects small- and medium-sized arteries and veins of the extremities. It is an autoimmune disease strongly associated with tobacco smoking. Patients are mostly young male tobacco smokers who present with distal extremity ischemia, ischemic ulcers, or gangrene. Buerger disease has a worldwide distribution, but it is more prevalent in the Mediterranean, the Middle East, and Asia. Recently, the prevalence of disease seems to have declined in the United States and Europe, however, an increased incidence has been seen in women, who constitute up to 20% of patients in some series. This relative rise in incidence in women is likely due to the increase in cigarette smoking among women.

Although the etiology of Buerger disease is unknown, the condition is strongly associated with heavy tobacco use. Smoking is considered by most to be an absolute requirement for diagnosis, and progression is closely linked to continued use. However, a causal relationship has not been conclusively demonstrated. There have been reports of the presence of TAO in cigar smokers and in users of smokeless tobacco products, such as chewing tobacco and snuff. Hence, the etiology is likely multifactorial, with an unknown intimal antigen thought to be the initiating factor, supported by certain human leukocyte antigens being associated with the development of disease. The pathologic hallmark is perivascular inflammation involving small and medium-sized arteries, veins, and nerves along with thrombus formation. Interestingly, markers of systemic inflammatory response are not usually present in Buerger disease patients.

PRESENTATION

Buerger disease typically presents with ischemic symptoms related to pathology of distal small arteries and veins. More proximal arteries may be involved when the disease progresses, but involvement of large arteries is unusual. The onset of symptoms usually occurs before the age of 40 to 45 years. Patients may present with paresthesias and claudication of the feet, legs, hands, or arms. Two or more limbs are always involved; all four limbs are affected in approximately 40% of patients. In patients with TAO, intermittent symptoms are initially localized to the forefoot or the arch of the foot because of the distal nature of the disease, as opposed to patients with typical peripheral atherosclerotic disease with classic calf claudication. Progression of the inflammatory disease leads to development of ischemic rest pain and ulcerations in the distal portion of toes or fingers. In most series, approximately three quarters of patients are seen initially with ischemic ulcers. Raynaud phenomenon and superficial migratory thrombophlebitis are commonly encountered.

Although Buerger disease predominantly affects the vessels of the extremities, a few instances of aortic, cerebral, coronary, mesenteric, pulmonary, and renal involvement have been reported in the literature. Mesenteric Buerger disease is extremely rare and is associated with a poor prognosis. Patients with known Buerger disease presenting with gastrointestinal manifestations should be urgently evaluated for bowel ischemia, and early surgical intervention is recommended.

DIAGNOSIS

Physical examination often reveals cyanotic and erythematous extremities. Paresthesias caused by ischemic neuropathy are common, as is cold sensitivity that may be related to ischemia or to increased sympathetic nerve activity. Absent distal pulses in the presence of normal proximal pulses are typical in patients with the disease. Involvement of both the upper and lower extremities is common. Dry, punctate ischemic lesions are often seen on both the hands and feet.

BOX 1: Angiographic findings in TOS (Buerger disease)

Involvement of small and medium-sized vessels; palmar, plantar, tibial, peroneal, radial, and ulnar arteries; and digital arteries of fingers and toes

Normal extremity arteries proximal to the popliteal and distal brachial levels

Absence of proximal atherosclerosis and vascular calcification

No source of thrombus

Abrupt transition from a normal and smooth proximal artery to an area of occlusion

Symmetrical and segmental arterial involvement

Tortuous "corkscrew" collaterals are suggestive, but not pathognomonic, of Buerger disease

Attempts have been made to establish a set of criteria for the diagnosis of Buerger disease, but to date no one set is widely used in clinical practice. The definitive diagnosis of TAO can be made with a vessel biopsy showing cellular thrombus and the classic acute-phase lesion involving all layers of the vessel wall. However, the history and physical evaluation are often enough to reveal the diagnosis. As a consequence, biopsies are rarely necessary unless a patient presents with unusual characteristics, such as large-artery involvement or an age older than 45 years.

Other vasculitides, as well as autoimmune and hypercoaguable disorders, may mimic Buerger disease, therefore several laboratory studies are useful in the workup of possible Buerger disease: a complete blood count with differential, electrolytes, renal and liver function tests, fasting blood glucose, urinalysis, erythrocyte sedimentation rate and C-reactive protein, and a hypercoagulability screen that includes antiphospholipid antibodies, antinuclear antibody, rheumatoid factor, complement measurements, SCL-70, and anticentromere antibody.

Standard arteriography is usually revealing but is not essential for the diagnosis. Noninvasive imaging, such as gadolinium-enhanced magnetic resonance angiography (MRA) and computed tomographic angiography (CTA), are good alternatives. Four-limb segmental arterial pressures and digital plethysmography—waveform, digital pressure measurement, or both—are useful to document the typically distal occlusive disease. When suggested by unilateral involvement, a proximal source of emboli should be excluded with echocardiography.

Arteriography should be performed in patients with threatened limb loss. A number of angiographic findings are suggestive of TAO, but there are no pathognomonic findings (Box 1 and Figure 1). The angiographic appearance of TAO may be identical to other types of small-vessel vasculitis or toxic arterial responses related to amphetamine, cannabis, or cocaine abuse. If a nonsmoking patient presents with signs consistent with Buerger disease, it is advisable to obtain a toxicology screen for these drugs.

Given the relatively young age of most patients, the possibility of popliteal artery entrapment syndrome, cystic adventitial disease, or popliteal artery aneurysm should be considered. The presence of diabetes mellitus, end-stage renal disease, or significant risk factors for atherosclerosis argues against a diagnosis of Buerger disease.

TREATMENT

Medical Therapy

The main and most effective treatment for Buerger disease is complete abstinence from tobacco products. Smoking or even using smokeless tobacco or nicotine replacement is closely related to exacerbation of the disease. There is a correlation between continued smoking and limb amputation. If patients discontinue tobacco use, they can be reassured that the disease will often remit, and amputation can be avoided as long as ischemic ulcers have not already occurred. That said, patients with already significant occluded arterial segments may continue to experience intermittent claudication or Raynaud phenomenon.

In patients whose disease progresses despite smoking cessation, effective therapeutic options are limited (Box 2). Initial enthusiasm for infusion of the prostaglandin analogue iloprost has not been borne out by further trials or experience. Other prostaglandins are currently undergoing investigation. Anticoagulants, antiplatelet drugs, and rheologic agents seem to be ineffective. Calcium channel blockers are only helpful if significant vasospasm is present, and intraarterial thrombolytic therapy has not been useful.

More recent experimental therapies aimed at inducing therapeutic angiogenesis with gene- or cell-based technologies, including intramuscular gene transfer of vascular endothelial growth factor or autologous bone marrow mononuclear cells, are showing promising results. Larger randomized studies are needed to evaluate the effectiveness of these therapies.

Surgical Therapy

Revascularization for critical limb ischemia usually involves femorodistal bypass with autologous vein and is associated with poor outcomes because of the diffuse segmental involvement and distal aspect of the disease. Moreover, the concomitant inflammatory venous disease often renders the saphenous veins unsatisfactory for use as conduits. However, if conservative treatment fails in patients with severe ischemia and nonhealing ischemic ulcers of the lower extremities, revascularization should be considered. The distal arteries must be thoroughly evaluated by arteriography for optimal preoperative planning. If surgical exploration reveals a diminutive receiving vessel, bypass should be abandoned.

Limb-salvage rates usually exceed graft patencies. Although patency for distal bypass is no more than 50% even in the small number of patients with Buerger disease who are able to undergo bypasses, limb-salvage rates frequently exceed 75%. In these well-selected patients, even limited periods of revascularization provide a sufficient interval to heal ischemic ulcers in the feet.

Other surgical approaches that have been used include sympathectomy and omental transfer. Sympathectomy as a primary or adjunctive treatment option has been used in a large number of patients with Buerger disease, with varying success. Implantable spinal cord stimulators have also been used, with ensuing pain reduction and ulcer healing. Omental transfer has also been utilized with successful ulcer healing. Unfortunately, many patients with Buerger disease undergo amputations for extensive gangrene or sepsis. The goal is to remove all nonviable tissue, preserve optimal residual function, and minimize surgical morbidity. Application of these principles may result in unconventional amputation levels with a preponderance of multiple digital or distal amputations.

Endovascular Therapy

Although less invasive endovascular approaches might be attractive in this population, the diffuse, distal, and segmental involvement of the lesions currently exceeds the available catheter-based technologies. For the patient presenting with advanced ulceration and gangrene, angiography may define a more proximal femoropopliteal lesion, which may also contribute to the arterial insufficiency. We consider treatment of such lesions extremely important to maximize the infrapopliteal flow into the collaterals seen in patients with Buerger disease.

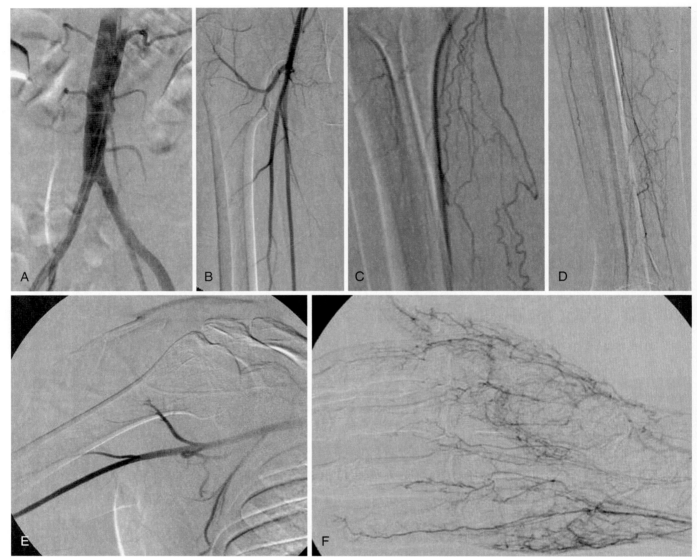

FIGURE 1 Angiograms of a patient with Buerger disease. **A,** Abdominal aortogram shows a normal aorta and iliac arteries. **B,** The appearance of proximal lower extremity vessels is also unremarkable. **C** and **D,** Distal runoffs show severe peripheral occlusive disease with corkscrew-appearing collaterals. **E,** Upper extremity angiogram also reveals normal proximal vasculature. **F,** Distal occlusive disease with many collaterals. *(Courtesy Dr. Thomas Reifsnyder.)*

BOX 2: Treatment options in TOS (Buerger disease)

Cessation of tobacco products
Local wound care
Arterial reconstruction with vein graft
Prostaglandin analog iloprost or treprostinil sodium
Cilostazol
Hyperbaric oxygen therapy
Calcium channel blockers (e.g., amlodipine or nifedipine for vasospasm)
Intermittent pneumatic compression pump
Implantable spinal cord stimulator
Therapeutic angiogenesis
Amputation

PROGNOSIS AND FOLLOW-UP

Buerger disease is characterized by periods of remission and exacerbation, with disease intensity peaking at 30 to 40 years of age and diminishing thereafter. The morbidity of extremity amputation is significant, and it approached 25% at 5 years and 50% at 20 years after diagnosis in one study. TAO historically has not been associated with increased mortality, although recent data dispute this view. Overall, repeated hospitalizations and major amputation markedly influence the quality of life for these patients.

SUMMARY

TAO, or Buerger disease, is a nonatherosclerotic segmental inflammatory disease characterized by the development of segmental thrombotic occlusions of the medium and small arteries and veins of the extremities. It occurs in young smokers who present with distal extremity ischemia, ulcers, or gangrene. The most important disease processes to exclude are atherosclerosis, emboli, and autoimmune diseases. The only effective treatment is complete and permanent abstinence from tobacco products. Several medical and surgical therapies are palliative.

SUGGESTED READINGS

Espinoza L: Buerger disease: thromboangiitis obliterans 100 years after the initial description, *Am J Med Sci* 337(4):285, 2009.

Malecki R, Zdrojowy K, Adamiec R: Thromboangiitis obliterans in the 21st century: a new face of disease, *Atherosclerosis* 211(1): 24, 2009.

Mheid IA, Quyyumi AA: Cell therapy in peripheral arterial disease, *Angiology* 59(6):705, 2009.

Mills JL Sr: Buerger disease in the 21st century: diagnosis, clinical features, and therapy, *Semin Vasc Surg* 16:179, 2003.

Ohta T, Ishioashi H, Hosaka M: Clinical and social consequences of Buerger disease, *J Vasc Surg* 39:176, 2004.

Olin JW: Thromboangiitis obliterans (Buerger disease), *N Engl J Med* 343:864, 2000.

Olin JW, Shih A: Thromboangiitis obliterans (Buerger disease), *Curr Opin Rheumatol* 18:18, 2006.

Paraskevas KI, Liapis CD, Brianna DD, et al: Throbboangiitis obliterans (Buerger disease): searching for a therapeutic strategy, *Angiology* 58:75, 2007.

ACUTE MESENTERIC ISCHEMIA

Andrew J. Meltzer, MD, Nicholas Melo, MD, and James H. Balcom IV, MD

OVERVIEW

Despite advances in technology and diagnostic modalities, acute mesenteric ischemia (AMI) remains a challenging clinical dilemma. The mechanism may be acute or chronic occlusion of the arterial supply, mesenteric venous thrombosis, or from multifactorial causes that contribute to nonocclusive mesenteric ischemia. Thirty-day mortality ranges from 32% to 80%; the wide variation can be attributed to diversity in presentation, delayed diagnosis, and comorbidities. Two thirds of patients are women in their early 70s with a history of systemic atherosclerotic disease, cardiac arrhythmias, or recent vascular instrumentation.

Cellular and molecular mechanisms related to bowel ischemia and reperfusion contribute to the increased mortality, as immediate ischemia causes mucosal ischemia. The splanchnic circulation receives 25% of the cardiac output, which is increased to 35% postprandially; 70% of this blood flow is to the mucosa and submucosa, and lack of blood flow to these layers is grave. Because injured mucosa compromises an immune barrier, even after reperfusion this allows for bacterial translocation, cellular degradation, reactive oxygen species, and intravascular thrombosis. The products resulting from these processes are released into the portal circulation and further propagate an inflammatory process unique to this ischemia-reperfused organ system.

The key to decreasing mortality is prompt diagnosis and treatment, as the presentation is nonspecific. Classically described as pain out of proportion to exam, this is usually an early presentation. As ischemia worsens, so does the pain; but symptoms progress to vomiting, diarrhea, distension, rebound, and eventually peritonitis. A thorough history aids in diagnosis, as the treatment differs if it is a chronic process. Resuscitation is paramount, and a variety of laboratory tests will help with the diagnosis, although none are specific. Leukocytosis, metabolic or lactic acidosis, and amylasemia may be present, although none are diagnostic; furthermore, all are usually late findings.

Plain films of the abdomen are not diagnostic but may be useful in the late stages, if air is demonstrated in the wall of the intestine or portal venous system. Because the majority of patients possess dilated, air-filled loops of bowel, duplex ultrasonography is of limited use. An aortogram is the gold standard for diagnosis, but in many clinical settings, a computed tomographic angiogram (CTA) has become a useful adjunct (Figure 1). In a patient with normal renal function, CTA can make the diagnosis and can be invaluable in planning a mesenteric revascularization.

ACUTE SUPERIOR MESENTERIC ARTERY EMBOLISM

The most common site of acute embolism of the superior mesenteric artery (SMA) is several centimeters distal to the SMA origin, in the region of the origin of the middle colic artery. Common etiologies include left atrial thrombi, left ventricular thrombi, and lesions of the cardiac valves. Classically the embolus arises in the heart in the setting of atrial fibrillation or myocardial infarction.

Symptoms are typical of acute mesenteric occlusion, including severe pain with acute onset. Spontaneous evacuation of the

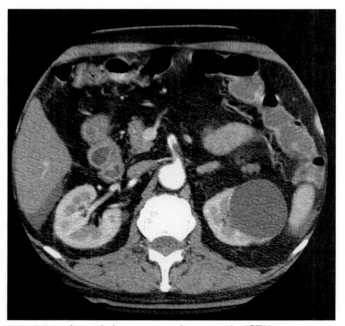

FIGURE 1 Arterial-phase computed tomography (CTA) in a patient with abdominal pain. Embolic material is present within the superior mesenteric artery just distal to its origin.

gastrointestinal tract may occur. The classic presentation is sudden onset of abdominal pain out of proportion to examination. As ischemia progresses, symptoms intensify and progress accordingly. There are no laboratory studies or routine diagnostic studies that clearly identify patients with SMA embolism in the early course of the disease. As the sequelae of bowel ischemia occur, examination and diagnostic studies change to reflect developing ischemia.

Patients with evidence of peritonitis on exam are taken urgently to the operating room for exploration. Once the diagnosis is confirmed, treatment with intravenous heparin is initiated. Recently, thrombolytic therapy has been utilized in patients presenting within 8 hours of the onset of symptoms, without peritonitis or evidence of bowel ischemia, after examination and laboratory evaluation. This approach is not recommended without significant local expertise and experience.

At laparotomy, the abdomen is explored through a generous midline incision, and the bowel is evaluated for viability. Following this initial assessment, restoration of inflow is the primary objective. The SMA is identified and palpated, and a proximal pulse is frequently present. Some debate surrounds the use of transverse and longitudinal arteriotomies in the SMA; if the latter is chosen, a patch angioplasty is generally used to facilitate closure. We tend to recommend a longitudinal arteriotomy, as it facilitates passage of embolectomy catheters in both directions under direct vision, especially in obese patients and those with deep abdomens. A balloon-tipped catheter is passed proximally to dislodge the embolus then distally to retrieve embolic fragments. In the presence of bowel necrosis requiring resection, patch angioplasty can be performed with saphenous vein or bovine pericardium. Restoration of inflow is confirmed with palpation and Doppler ultrasound. Bowel resection is then performed as required. A second-look operation in 24 to 48 hours is mandatory in our practice.

ACUTE SUPERIOR MESENTERIC ARTERY THROMBOSIS

Acute thrombosis of the SMA usually occurs in the most proximal portion. Clinically, it may be difficult to distinguish acute thrombosis of the SMA from embolus. Two patient populations generally at risk are elderly patients with diffuse atherosclerotic disease who present after plaque rupture or in those patients with a low-flow state. A second group of patients are young female smokers with chronic mesenteric angina underlying an acute presentation.

Angiography—specifically, lateral aortography—confirms the diagnosis. Therapy is directed primarily at the prompt reconstitution of visceral blood flow. This can be accomplished by a variety of measures such as antegrade or retrograde conduits; venous bypass grafts, particularly in the setting of a contaminated field; or synthetic conduits. Despite ongoing debates regarding the merits of different approaches, as in many emergent surgical situations, the best approach is the one that can be executed expeditiously by the surgeon faced with the situation. Thrombolysis and angioplasty of the SMA has been utilized in a select group of patients. However, concern for bowel viability frequently necessitates abdominal exploration, often making catheter-based interventions an adjunct to a necessary laparotomy.

The initial exploration is performed as described for acute SMA embolism. In the case of thrombosis, however, the SMA is controlled near its origin. A visceral bypass procedure is then performed, utilizing either antegrade or retrograde inflow. Antegrade bypass is performed from the distal thoracic or proximal abdominal aorta. Retrograde bypass is performed from a soft portion of the distal aorta or common iliac artery. Synthetic material may be used, but given concern for bowel viability, autologous vein graft is preferable. As in the case of acute embolism of the SMA, a second-look procedure is performed at 24 to 48 hours.

NONOCCLUSIVE MESENTERIC ISCHEMIA

Nonocclusive mesenteric ischemia is a clinical syndrome that does not result from a fixed stenosis or occlusion but is the result of hypoperfusion of the intestinal viscera. The patient is usually in the intensive care unit, and it may be a result of hypovolemia, underresuscitation, or vasopressor therapy, which all may cause poor perfusion. The presentation is varied and often difficult to diagnose, but it can be definitively diagnosed by angiography, which may demonstrate spasm of the SMA and branches without a focal occlusion. Treatment is directed at the underlying illness, and sometimes papaverine infusion and discontinuation of vasopressors may be employed. If signs of shock or peritonitis persist, operative exploration is warranted to determine intestinal viability and evaluate for possible resection.

MESENTERIC VENOUS THROMBOSIS

The underlying ischemia in mesenteric venous thrombosis is from vascular congestion due to poor venous outflow, which may be precipitated by an intraabdominal inflammatory process such as appendicitis or diverticulitis. Depending on the clinical condition of the patient, the initial treatment may be nonoperative (bowel rest, resuscitation) with anticoagulation. A hypercoaguable workup should be part of the diagnostic process. If signs of peritonitis develop, operative exploration is indicated, and all nonviable bowel is resected. Second-look laparotomies should be performed within 24 to 48 hours, and the decision to perform these should be made at the initial operation.

SUGGESTED READINGS

Schoots IG, Levi MM, Reekers JA, et al: Thrombolytic therapy for acute superior mesenteric artery occlusion, *J Vasc Interv Radiol* 16(3):317–329, 2005.

Kougias P, Lau D, El Sayed HF, et al: Determinants of mortality and treatment outcome following surgical interventions for acute mesenteric ischemia, *J Vasc Surg* 46(3):467–474, 2007.

Park WM, Gloviczki P, Cherry KJ Jr, et al: Contemporary management of acute mesenteric ischemia: factors associated with survival, *J Vasc Surg* 35(3):445–452, 2002.

MANAGEMENT OF CHRONIC MESENTERIC ISCHEMIA

Grace J. Wang, MD, and Andrew S. Resnick, MD, MBA

OVERVIEW

Chronic mesenteric ischemia is a rare clinical syndrome marked by atherosclerotic stenosis or occlusion of at least two of the three arteries—the celiac, superior mesenteric, and inferior mesenteric arteries—supplying the intestine. Common presenting symptoms include postprandial abdominal pain, weight loss, and intermittent diarrhea. Because of its rarity, the optimal treatment strategy has not been clearly defined. Open approaches have included endarterectomy and mesenteric bypass. In addition, the introduction of endovascular therapies has challenged traditional open approaches to mesenteric vessel revascularization. The presence of comorbid factors in this often frail and elderly population underscores the importance of determining the optimal revascularization strategy while minimizing morbidity and mortality.

INDICATIONS FOR INTERVENTION

Mesenteric revascularization should be undertaken when clinical symptoms of mesenteric ischemia are present in conjunction with occlusive disease, defined as greater than 70% occlusion affecting two of the three visceral arteries. Angiographic evidence of atherosclerotic occlusions can be detailed through CTA, MRA, or formal diagnostic angiography. Angiography is performed in a lateral orientation to demonstrate the takeoff of the anteriorly oriented mesenteric vessels (Figure 1). Patients with long-standing mesenteric ischemia have a classic history of angina brought on by ingesting food; as a result, they have "food fear" and are often severely malnourished, which should be taken into account in determining the appropriate revascularization strategy.

SURGICAL REVASCULARIZATION

The first successful open surgical procedure performed for chronic mesenteric ischemia was performed by Shaw and Maynard in 1958. In the ensuing three decades, open surgical revascularization was established as the preferred approach for treatment of patients with chronic mesenteric ischemia because of its excellent long-term durability. Open revascularization is typically approached via a midline laparotomy, although a bilateral subcostal incision may also be used for the antegrade bypass. The celiac axis or the common hepatic artery and the superior mesenteric artery (SMA) are the usual outflow sites. The decision to bypass to one or two vessels depends on the extent of disease and the ability of the patient to tolerate a more lengthy operation. The common hepatic artery is located parallel to the superior wall of the pyloroduodenal junction. The SMA can be exposed either anteriorly, by elevating the transverse colon and incising its mesentery, or laterally, by incising the ligament of Treitz and retracting the inferior border of the pancreas. The supraceliac aorta, infrarenal aorta, or common iliac artery can be chosen for inflow. The supraceliac aorta or antegrade bypass provides the most flow, but the morbidity of a supraceliac aortic cross clamp is not well tolerated by the typical vasculopath who presents with this condition, which should be taken into consideration. Theoretically, a side-biting clamp

on the aorta in this position would produce less hemodynamic and physiologic derangement, but it does not always provide good visualization of the inside of the aorta when performing the anastomosis, particularly if the aortic diameter is small.

Next, the left triangular ligament of the liver is divided, and the left lobe of the liver is gently retracted. The lesser sac is entered by dividing the gastrohepatic ligament. With a nasogastric tube in place, the esophagus is retracted to the left, and the diaphragmatic crura are divided to expose the supraceliac segment. The graft then needs to be tunneled in a retropancreatic orientation (Figure 2), which needs to be done carefully, in a blunt fashion, to avoid injury to the splenic and superior mesenteric vein.

The two retrograde types of bypasses involve the infrarenal aorta and the common iliac artery. The infrarenal aorta also provides good inflow but is not always an option, as there is often extensive occlusive disease present. The infrarenal clamp may be poorly tolerated by the patient, but probably not as poorly tolerated as the supraceliac clamp. The common iliac artery is a viable alternative, provided there is no occlusive disease present; this approach lends itself to less physiologic perturbation, less blood loss, and a relatively easy-to-construct anastomosis. Retrograde bypasses need to be constructed in a "lazy C" configuration to prevent graft kinking (Figure 3). There does not appear to be a difference in conduit patency among prosthetic grafts. Dacron grafts 6 to 8 mm in size or comparably sized externally supported PTFE grafts have been used with success. Either transaortic or

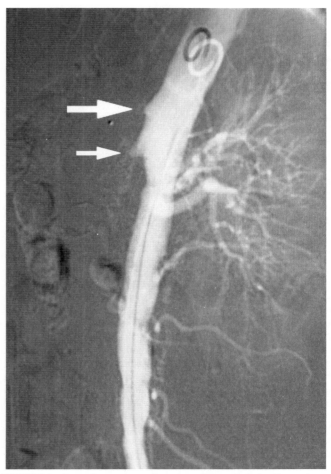

FIGURE 1 Lateral aortogram demonstrating occluded celiac and superior mesenteric arteries. *(From Rutherford RB: Vascular surgery, ed 6, Philadelphia, 2005, Saunders Elsevier.)*

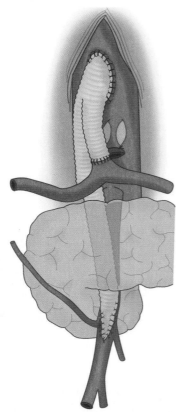

FIGURE 2   Antegrade bypass to celiac access and to the superior mesenteric artery (SMA). Note the retropancreatic tunnel for the SMA bypass. *(From Rutherford RB: Vascular surgery, ed 6, Philadelphia, 2005, Saunders Elsevier.)*

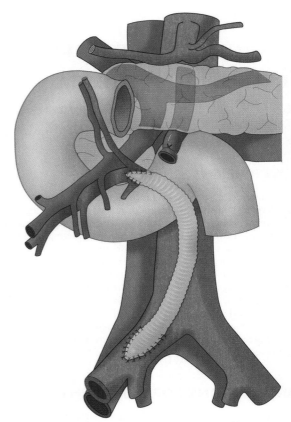

FIGURE 3   Retrograde bypass from right common iliac artery to the superior mesenteric artery. *(From Rutherford RB: Vascular surgery, ed 6, Philadelphia, 2005, Saunders Elsevier.)*

local endarterectomy of the outflow vessel may need to be performed to ensure adequate inflow and outflow for any contemplated surgical bypass. Indeed, the series by Mell and colleagues (2008) suggests improved overall graft patency and symptom-free survival when concurrent endarterectomy is performed (79% for bypass alone vs. 92% for combined procedures). Following completion of the bypass, the retroperitoneal tissue overlying the aorta and the mesenteric tissue overlying the SMA should be used to cover the prosthetic graft to exclude contact with the intestine.

ENDOVASCULAR THERAPY

Endovascular therapy consisting of percutaneous angioplasty with and without stenting has been increasingly applied to treat chronic mesenteric ischemia. Its attractiveness as a modality has been underscored by the perioperative morbidity of the open revascularization approach. It has a high initial technical success rate of 93% to 100% reported in recent series. The patency rate cited in the literature varies somewhat, depending on the duration of follow-up and the definition of patency; however, endovascular therapy has not shown the same durability as open bypass (88% to 96%), although the durability of endovascular therapy is respectable (70% to 95%). For patients who are deemed high risk for open revascularization, endovascular therapies are an attractive initial approach. These therapies may also help a subset of patients to gain weight and become more robust candidates for open surgery.

For endovascular therapy, a femoral or brachial access approach is chosen. The steep downward angulation of the SMA is often better cannulated from above, from the arm. The brachial approach is associated with a high rate of puncture-site related complications (12% to 15% in published series), but pseudoaneurysms or thrombotic

complications can be easily repaired if need be. The left-brachial approach is preferred as more direct than the right-brachial approach.

An abdominal aortogram in a steep lateral configuration is performed to demonstrate the origins of the celiac artery, SMA, and inferior mesenteric artery (IMA). Special attention is paid to the collateral connections between the celiac artery and SMA, via the gastroduodenal artery and pancreaticoduodenal arteries, and between the SMA and IMA, via the arc of Riolan and the marginal artery of Drummond. Delayed views are imperative to demonstrate these collateral pathways, and a glidewire is typically used to steer and maneuver past the orificial lesion. A guide catheter is traversed through the lesion and pulled back once the balloon-mounted stent is in position, taking care to extend the stent slightly into the aorta, as these are often spillover lesions of aortic disease. We favor a 6.0 or 7.0 mm diameter stent ranging from 15 to 30 mm in length on a 0.014 inch wire system. The procedure is performed with systemic anticoagulation, and all patients are maintained on clopidogrel (Plavix), in addition to aspirin, for 6 to 12 weeks following the procedure.

THERAPEUTIC DECISION MAKING

Chronic mesenteric ischemia (CMI) is an uncommon clinical entity, and few large series of patients undergo surgery for this disease. Revascularization is typically performed in patients with extensive atherosclerotic disease with severe malnutrition. The complication rate for operative revascularization is higher than that for endovascular treatment, with one recent series reporting 36% versus 18% morbidity rates, respectively. As expected, cardiac (10% vs. 2%) and pulmonary (15% vs. 1%) complications remain important causes of morbidity in the open bypass group. Technical complications include graft thrombosis (2%) in patients undergoing operative revascularization and dissection or stent dislodgment (10%) in those undergoing endovascular treatment. Results from relatively high-volume centers of excellence have reported operative mortality rates of up to 12%. This is in contradistinction to endovascular therapy, with a reported mortality rate of 2% to 3.7%. The repeat intervention rate for PTA and stenting is 25% to 28% at 2 years, but the assisted primary patency has been excellent, as high as 95.2% in one series.

Patients who clearly are not candidates for open surgery may be considered for endovascular therapy. Although not a durable solution, PTA and stenting may provide the patient with an interim period of better nutrition before a planned open operative intervention. Recent studies have suggested that revascularization of two vessels provides better relief from symptom recurrence than one vessel intervention. Further study that includes longitudinal follow-up is required to determine whether this is true.

Repeat interventions are likewise approached from the left brachial artery. Angioplasty, cutting-balloon angioplasty, and angioplasty with stenting have all been utilized.

SURVEILLANCE

Abdominal duplex imaging has previously been validated for the diagnosis of mesenteric arterial stenosis and is probably the best method for radiographic surveillance. Other noninvasive modalities may also be used, including CTA and MRA.

SUMMARY

Chronic mesenteric ischemia is a rare and difficult clinical entity to treat. The overall status of the patient and the relative morbidity of the strategy contemplated should be kept in mind when planning any operative intervention. Although not as durable as open surgery, endovascular therapy has a much decreased periprocedural morbidity and mortality rate—but it may be the only option in some of the moribund vasculopath patients who come in for treatment with this condition. Surveillance and close follow-up are required in these patients, as the need for reintervention is high. If the patient is a good operative candidate, open surgery is associated with a high patency and success rate. Inflow and outflow targets should be selected based on the ability of the patient to tolerate the associated hemodynamic sequelae of clamping and reperfusion of these vessels.

SUGGESTED READINGS

Cho JS, Carr JA, Jacobsen G, et al: Long-term outcome after mesenteric artery reconstruction: a 37-year experience, *J Vasc Surg* 35(3):453–460, 2002.
Cunningham CG, Reilly LM, Rapp JH, et al: Chronic visceral ischemia: three decades of progress, *Ann Surg* 214(3):276–287, discussion 287-288, 1991.
Mell MW, Acher CW, Hoch JR, et al: Outcomes after endarterectomy for chronic mesenteric ischemia, *J Vasc Surg* 48(5):1132–1138, 2008.
Oderich GS, Bower TC, Sullivan TM, et al: Open versus endovascular revascularization for chronic mesenteric ischemia: risk-stratified outcomes, *J Vasc Surg* 49(6):1472–1479, 2009.
Park WM, Cherry KJ Jr, Chua HK, et al: Current results of open revascularization for chronic mesenteric ischemia: a standard for comparison, *J Vasc Surg* 35(5):853–859, 2002.
Peck MA, Conrad MF, Kwolek CJ, et al: Intermediate-term outcomes of endovascular treatment for symptomatic chronic mesenteric ischemia, *J Vasc Surg*, 2009.
Schermerhorn ML, Giles KA, Hamdan AD, et al: Mesenteric revascularization: management and outcomes in the United States, 1988-2006, *J Vasc Surg* 50(2):341–348, 2009.

MANAGEMENT OF INFECTED VASCULAR GRAFTS

Colin M. Brady, MD, and Elliot L. Chaikof, MD, PhD

OVERVIEW

In an era of rapid advances in endovascular alternatives for the treatment of aneurysmal and occlusive peripheral vascular disease, prosthetic vascular implants remain a prominent and necessary therapeutic modality. With just under half a million vascular grafts implanted annually in the United States, vascular graft infection remains a relevant challenge for the contemporary vascular surgeon. In addition to considerable health care costs, such infections can engender significant morbidity and mortality for the patient, as they may serve as a prelude to hemorrhage, thrombosis, sepsis, associated embolic phenomena, multisystem organ failure, and amputation.

Despite an improved understanding of biomaterials and fabrication modalities designed to better mimic autogenous vessel structure and mechanics, the incidence of vascular graft infection has changed little over the last several decades. Infection is most common in femorotibial grafts for critical limb ischemia and in vascular access grafts for hemodialysis. Predisposing factors can be related to patients or to procedural elements (Table 1). In particular, inguinal incisions have long been deemed a risk factor for graft infection secondary to a combination of groin-crease contamination and bacterial seeding from lymphatic drainage at the site of incised femoral nodes. Although the true incidence of this potentially devastating complication remains difficult to establish, as it varies with anatomic position (e.g., aortofemoral vs. infrainguinal) and the graft material (polytetrafluoroethylene [PTFE] vs. Dacron), most series document a range between 1% and 5%. Given the increasing prevalence of advanced peripheral vascular disease requiring major vascular reconstruction, the number of patients presenting with vascular graft infection will likely increase.

BACTERIOLOGY

The presence of a foreign body reduces the required bacterial inoculum required to induce local infection. The most common organism responsible for prosthetic graft infection is *Staphyloccocus aureus*. In an era of increased bacterial resistance, virulence, and nosocomial transmission, methicillin-resistant *S. aureus* (MRSA) along with *Escherichia coli, Enterobacter, Klebsiella, Proteus,* and *Pseudomonas* have become increasingly common etiologic agents for early graft infection. Those more virulent organisms, such as *Pseudomonas*, produce proteases that are responsible for vein graft necrosis of autogenous grafts or anastomotic disruption of prosthetic implants.

Late infections are most commonly caused by the less virulent pathogen *S. epidermidis*. These organisms produce a polysaccharide biofilm, allowing adherence to the surface of the graft while serving

TABLE 1: Risk factors for vascular graft infection

Patient-Related Risk Factors	Procedural-Related Risk Factors
Diabetes mellitus	Anatomic bypass location (femoral-distal > aortoiliofemoral)
Tobacco use	Conduit type (prosthetic > autogenous)
Body mass index >30	Groin incision
Chronic renal failure	Overlying wound infection
Immunosuppression	Lymphorrhea
Malnutrition	Emergency surgery
	Reoperative intervention
	Prolonged operative time
	Incision-site fluid collection (hematoma, seroma, lymphocele)
	Local skin necrosis

TABLE 2: Signs and symptoms of vascular graft infection

Early (<4 Months)	Late (>4 Months)
Fever	Fever
Leukocytosis	Erythema
Lethargy	Fluid collection
Mental status change	Elevated erythrocyte sedimentation rate and C-reactive protein
Cellulitis	Impaired graft incorporation
Purulant drainage	Draining sinus tract
Lymphorrhea	Pseudoaneurysm
Anastomotic hemorrhage	Retained perigraft fluid collection
Pseudoaneurysm	

as a protective barrier from host immunity and the bacteriocidal effects of systemic antibiotic administration. The result is an indolent infection presenting 1 to 5 years postoperatively. Local tissue destruction limits the infection to the immediate area surrounding the graft and may present as a sinus tract, perigraft fluid collection, anastomotic pseudoaneurysm, or aortoenteric fistula. Given the decreased virulence of *S. epidermidis* and its characteristic adherence, culture can be difficult with aspiration alone and may require ultrasonic disruption. Unlike *S. aureus* and the Gram-negative species, which are accomplished colonizers (10^5 to 10^7 colony-forming units per gram [CFU/g]), *S. epidermidis* is usually associated with 10^2 to 10^3 CFU/g in the infected tissue.

PREVENTION

Given the recent increase in nosocomial infections, attention has been directed to guidelines for the prevention of surgical-site infections, including preoperative and intraoperative preparation methods to strict perioperative antibiotic strategies. It is accepted that the preponderance of graft infections, whether early or late, results from bacterial seeding at the time of implantation. Attention to antiseptic procedure is thus crucial to the prevention of postoperative infection.

Some advocate patient self-cleansing with a chlorhexidine scrub the night prior to elective admission. Given that commensurate skin flora are an important source of graft contaminants, the operative field should be sterilized with a bacteriocidal preparation, such as 10% povidone-iodine solution, and the skin should be prepped with an iodine impregnated drape. Skin flora can further be diminished with the administration of prophylactic antibiotics prior to skin incision. A cephalosporin, such as cefazolin, is typically selected, and vancomycin is commonly chosen as an alternative in patients with penicillin allergy. Antibiotics should be redosed every 3 to 4 hours during lengthy procedures. Patients who have received recent long-term broad-spectrum antibiosis, those who are immunosuppressed, and documented carriers of MRSA should undergo nasal swab and mupirocin eradication prior to elective surgery. Postoperative antibiotics should be continued for 24 hours unless otherwise indicated for treatment of concomitant infection.

Operative planning dictates that when feasible, clean-contaminated or other gastrointestinal (GI) procedures should be deferred

at the time of vascular reconstruction. Diligent attention to proper hemostasis and ligation of incised lymphatics is also important, to reduce the risk of hematoma and lymphocele formation, respectively. At closure, placement of a drain should be avoided if feasible.

In the setting of reoperative surgery, an operative approach that avoids the previous incisional site should be used to minimize infective complications whenever possible. In the management of aneurysmal or aortic occlusive disease, anecdotal evidence suggests that distal anastomosis to the iliac arteries reduces risk when compared with femoral anastomoses. Other potential measures to reduce graft infection include antibiotic-bonded Dacron or PTFE grafts (e.g., rifampin-gelatin impregnated). In animal studies, polycationic peptides and liposome-encapsulated amikacin bonded to Dacron grafts have shown promising results; however, their clinical utility has yet to be determined. Lastly, strict adherence to antiseptic technique should be observed in both the operating room and angiographic suite.

CLINICAL PRESENTATION

The clinical signs and symptoms associated with vascular graft infection vary depending on their categorization as an early or late presentation and by their anatomic location and causative organism. Early graft infections are generally defined as those presenting within the first 4 postoperative months. Late infections occur more than 4 months after graft implantation (Table 2).

Because of the more virulent causative organisms implicated, early graft infections are often associated with clinical signs and symptoms of systemic sepsis. Patients often present with fever, leukocytosis, lethargy, and mental status changes. Wound infections are commonly heralded by the presence of cellulitis, purulent drainage or lymphorrea, anastomotic hemorrhage, and pseudoaneurysm. Graft thrombosis or septic emboli are less common. It is important to remember that perigraft fluid in the first 3 months of implantation is normal and is not to be considered an absolute indication of graft infection; however, abdominal tenderness, fever, leukocytosis, and persistent ileus after recent abdominal graft implantation should be considered a graft infection until proven otherwise.

Late infection with the less virulent *S. epidermidis* organism is often indolent and can present a significant diagnostic challenge. Erythema, pseudoaneurysm, or a palpable fluid collection may be present; but presentation is often more subtle, and systemic manifestations are typically absent. Acute-phase reactants such as erythrocyte sedimentation rate and C-reactive protein may be elevated. Incomplete graft incorporation is common in late infection and may manifest as a draining sinus tract, false aneurysm, or as a perigraft fluid collection.

In the patient presenting with GI hemorrhage and systemic signs of sepsis in the presence of an intraabdominal graft, the presumed diagnosis is an aortoenteric fistula. The anatomic location of the fistula can be anywhere within the bowel, but the third and fourth portions of the duodenum are the most common sites. Hemorrhage may be accounted for by 1) erosion of the intact graft into the adjacent bowel, resulting in a mucosal bleed, or 2) direct communication of the graft anastomosis with the intestinal lumen. The high mortality associated with this infective complication is due to hemorrhage and to the virulence of the infective organisms.

DIAGNOSIS

A number of modalities can be used to help confirm the diagnosis of graft infection and assist in planning the surgical approach to operative reconstruction. Duplex ultrasonography is often considered the best initial screening modality for infection, especially in the infrainguinal region. Ultrasound facilitates detect perigraft fluid and anastomotic pseudoaneurysms while evaluating conduit patency, although it is ineffective in assessing graft infection in the chest, and its sensitivity for detecting perigraft fluid in the abdomen may be reduced due to poor depth of penetration in the obese patient and the potential for obfuscation by bowel gas.

Computed tomography (CT) is the most commonly utilized modality for assessment of graft infection given its high sensitivity (>95%) and specificity (85% to 90%) and its ability to image the entire graft. Perigraft air or fluid, phlegmon along normal tissue planes, and anastomotic pseudoaneurysm are suggestive of infection. The potential for concomitant CT-guided aspiration of a fluid collection for culture may be of value when diagnosis remains uncertain. Given its superiority in discrimination of tissue planes and subtle fluid collections, magnetic resonance imaging (MRI) has also been of value in the diagnosis of intrathoracic and intraabdominal graft infections.

Nuclear imaging has also been used to image sites of inflammation by identifying leukocytes in the region of an infected graft. Indium-111 emits gamma radiation and can be used to label white cells, which are removed from a patient and then reinjected. Gallium-67 is also a gamma radiation emitter, and it identifies sites of inflammation by binding directly to leukocyte lactoferrin, bacterial siderophores, and neutrophils' cell membranes. Both [111]I and ^{67}Ga are imaged by γ-scintigraphy. Recently, ^{18}F-2-fluoro-2-deoxy-D-glucose (^{18}F-FDG) has been used to identify sites of high metabolic activity associated with leukocyte infiltration. ^{18}F-FDG is a positron-emitting radioactive isotope imaged by positron emission tomography (PET), which may be combined with CT or MR scanning to superimpose both physiologic and anatomic information. These scans are of limited value in discerning an early graft infection in the acute postoperative setting given the characteristic inflammatory response that typifies normal wound healing.

In the setting of upper GI hemorrhage in a patient with a prosthetic aortic graft, upper GI endoscopy should be promptly performed. Because the site of an aortoenteric fistula may be located beyond the reach of the endoscope, a negative study does not exclude this diagnosis, and empiric surgical exploration may be warranted.

PRINCIPLES OF MANAGEMENT

Graft Excision and Extraanatomic Bypass

Treatment regimens should ultimately be patient specific. However, management strategies in the treatment of vascular graft infection should address the following fundamental tenets: 1) eradication of culture-specific infection and 2) preservation of distal perfusion. Resolution of the infective process requires complete or partial graft excision, wide soft tissue debridement, and long-term culture-specific antibiosis. Graft salvage may be appropriate in limited circumstances, but total graft excision and extraanatomic bypass should remain the convention in the setting of systemic sepsis or emboli, anastomotic disruption, infection of the body of an aortoiliofemoral bypass, or when the entirety of an infrainguinal prosthetic graft is involved. In the presence of an autogenous vein, the approach is often dictated by the type of contaminating organism.

When complete excision is required, the surgeon has a number of options for extraanatomic revascularization. In the management of an aortoiliofemoral graft infection, considerations for reconstruction include 1) axillobifemoral bypass, 2) bilateral axillary-superficial femoral bypass, 3) bilateral axillary–profunda femoris bypass, and 4) bilateral axillopopliteal bypass. Management of an infected femoropopliteal or femoral distal graft is complex. If feasible, extraanatomic reconstruction may consist of an obturator bypass from the iliac artery to the below-knee popliteal or other infrageniculate vessel.

In an occasional patient in whom the original bypass was performed for occlusive arterial disease that presented as claudication, the preexisting collateral blood supply may be sufficient to sustain distal perfusion in the absence of simultaneous revascularization. This option should be assessed by the presence of Doppler signals in the pedal vessels after excision of the infected graft. In this instance, subsequent revascularization can be performed following resolution of the primary infection.

Aortic Graft Infections

Historically, intraabdominal aortic graft infection has carried significant mortality (36% to 79%) and risk of limb loss (25% to 50%). To minimize the duration of distal ischemia, most surgeons advocate extraanatomic revascularization prior to graft excision as either a staged procedure or under a single anesthetic administration. Recent series have demonstrated significant improvement in both mortality (10% to 15%) and limb salvage rates (4% to 12%). In the septic patient with hemodynamic instability, single-stage graft excision and revascularization should remain the primary mode of management.

Extraanatomic reconstruction should be tunneled through uninvolved tissue planes. The axillary arteries serve as inflow, and distal anastomoses are performed to the superficial femoral artery at the mid thigh, the profunda femoris, or the popliteal artery depending on outflow anatomy. When possible, the common femoral artery should be preserved to maintain retrograde flow to the pelvis. Grafts of intraabdominal origin should be tunneled through the obturator canal. Autogenous saphenous or superficial femoral vein, endarterectomized occluded superficial femoral artery, and PTFE are all acceptable conduits in this setting.

Aortic stump blowout after aortic graft resection is almost universally fatal and may occur at any interval postoperatively. The risk of stump blowout can be minimized by adhering to a few basic tenets: 1) the aortic suture line should be resected to viable aortic tissue, 2) the stump should be oversewn in two layers with polypropylene suture, 3) the suture line should be reinforced with omentum or prevertebral fascia, and 4) the periaortic tissue should be aggressively debrided. Depending on the extent of stump destruction, sacrifice of one or both renals may be required to obtain a plane of viable tissue. In this situation, the surgeon should be prepared to perform hepatorenal or splenorenal bypass.

Infrainguinal Graft Infections

Despite a lower associated mortality, the risk of limb loss is higher in the management of an infected infrainguinal prosthetic graft when compared to an infected intraabdominal graft. Amputation rates range from 12% to 70%, with the risk primarily influenced by the inability to perform an effective secondary revascularization. Although most infected femoropopliteal grafts will require total excision and revascularization, total or partial graft preservation has been considered as an alternative, when the patient is free of systemic sepsis, anastomotic involvement, graft thrombosis, or septic emboli. The success of graft preservation is improved by aggressive local debridement and use of rotational muscle flap coverage. Because of significant risk of persistent or recurrent infection, graft preservation should not be attempted when a virulent gram-negative organism, such as *Pseudomonas,* is present.

As in the case of the infected aortic graft, secondary revascularization through uninvolved tissue planes is undertaken as the first stage in the stable patient. The proximal anastomosis is performed to the iliac artery, and the graft is tunneled through the obturator foramen, psoas tunnel, or through a superficial lateral plane to the site of distal anastomosis. The infected graft is subsequently excised, and the original anastomotic site is repaired with vein patch angioplasty in the absence of a gram-negative infection. Autogenous vein is the preferred conduit for revascularization, but PTFE or Dacron can be used if vein is not available.

Graft Excision and in Situ Bypass

Although conventional management with graft excision and extraanatomic bypass allows the surgeon to circumvent revascularization in an acutely infected field, it carries with it several disadvantages that include 1) prolonged operative time, 2) the potential for multiple surgeries, 3) prolonged hospital convalescence, 4) a revascularization that engenders the risk of early and recurrent thrombosis, 5) a less than satisfactory limb-salvage rate ranging from 11% to 29%, and 6) a significant risk of aortic stump blowout following graft excision in the patient with an infected aortic graft. Therefore, considerable enthusiasm exists for in situ replacement of infected grafts.

A number of potential conduits are available for in situ bypass, including autogenous arteries and veins, cryopreserved allografts, and venous and arterial homografts. Use of autogenous femoral vein, with preservation of the deep femoral vein, has been practiced extensively for both abdominal and lower extremity revascularization. In the setting of an infected infrainguinal graft, an occluded superficial femoral artery may be endarterectomized and used for in situ revascularization. Cryopreserved vein or arterial allografts have been advocated for in situ bypass in both the aortoiliac or infrainguinal positions. Short-term complication rates approaching 20% have been noted, including persistence of infection, graft thrombosis, hemorrhage, and pseudoaneurysm at the anastomotic site. Although autogenous vessel remains the preferred choice for in situ bypass, an ePTFE prosthesis and grafts impregnated with silver or antibiotics may be used when autogenous alternatives are not available, and when contamination is limited.

Graft Salvage

Graft salvage may be considered in patients who do not have systemic sepsis, thrombosis, septic emboli, or the presence of a virulent causative organism, such as *Pseudomonas aeruginosa.* The conventional approach to graft salvage has been aggressive local debridement, intravenous and local antibiotic therapy, and a variety of muscle flaps for coverage, but such treatment carries with it a reported reinfection rate of up to 35%.

Rotational Muscle Flaps

The use of muscle flaps is predicated on the notion that wound coverage with well-vascularized tissue raises the local oxygen tension and facilitates delivery of antibiotics to the infected region. Sartorius

TABLE 3: Options for rotational muscle flaps for wound coverage

Wound Location	Pedicled Muscle Flap
Groin	Rectus abdominis
	Rectus femoris
	Tensor fascia lata
	Gracilis
Knee	Gastrocnemius
	Soleus
Chest	Pectoralis major
	Latissimus dorsi
Head and neck	Sternocleidomastoid

muscle transfer remains a simple option for coverage of exposed graft in the groin; the rectus abdominis, rectus femoris, tensor fascia lata, and gracilis can be used for more extensive groin infection (Table 3). In the popliteal region, the gastrocnemius and soleus are commonly used, and for graft infections in the chest and neck, the pectoralis major or latissimus dorsi and the sternocleidomastoid may be employed.

Vacuum-Assisted Closure System

The vacuum-assisted closure (VAC) system has been commonly used as an adjunct to debridement with or without subsequent muscle-flap coverage. The VAC system has been reported to reduce bacterial content of the wound and accelerate the formation of oxygen-rich granulation tissue, facilitating the host's bactericidal oxidative burst.

Endovascular Stent Grafts

Although controversial, the risk of graft infection after endovascular aortic repair may be lower than after open surgery, perhaps because of the delivery of the endoprosthesis through a completely enclosed system or decreased dissection around the viscera. However, several recent analyses have reported a nearly identical incidence of graft infection of less than 0.2% to 0.4% up to 4 years after repair. Endograft infection may present in isolation or in association with a fistula to a neighboring viscus, most commonly the duodenum. The majority of patients require graft excision and surgical revascularization.

SUMMARY

Despite continued advances in medical therapeutics, the diagnosis and management of the patient with vascular graft infection remains an ongoing challenge. The clinical presentation of vascular graft infection may vary, but the goal of therapeutic intervention remains the eradication of the infective process while maintaining limb viability. Excision and extraanatomic revascularization remains the conventional strategy. Nonetheless, in situ revascularization with a variety of autologous conduits and allografts, and graft salvage with or without muscle-flap coverage, can provide an alternative approach, with the potential for reduced morbidity and mortality. Further advances in biomaterial science, wound care, enhanced periprocedural technique, and delivery of surgical care will be required to provide meaningful improvements in outcome.

SUGGESTED READINGS

Firoani P, Speziale F, Calisti A, et al: Endovascular graft infection: preliminary results of an international enquiry, *J Endovasc Ther* 10:919, 2003.

Noel AA, Gloviczki P, Cherry KJ Jr, et al: Abdominal aortic reconstruction in infected fields: early results in the United States cryopreserved aortic allograft registry, *J Vasc Surg* 35:847, 2002.

Pinocy J, Albes JM, Wicke C, et al: Treatment of periprosthetic soft-tissue infection of the groin following vascular surgical precedures by means of a polyvinyl alcohol-vacuum sponge system, *Wound Repair Regen* 11:104, 2003.

Seify H, Moyer HR, Jones GE, et al: The role of muscle flaps in wound salvage after vascular graft infections: the Emory experience, *Plast Reconstr Surg* 117:1325, 2006.

Stewart AH, Eyers PS, Earnshaw JJ: Prevention of infection in peripheral arterial reconstruction: a systematic review and meta-analysis, *J Vasc Surg* 45:148, 2007.

VASCULAR ACCESS SURGERY: AN EMERGING SPECIALTY

A. Frederick Schild, MD, Patrick S. Collier, BS, and Joseph C. Fuller, BS

OVERVIEW

At present, there are approximately 300,000 patients on hemodialysis in the United States. End-stage renal disease (ESRD) is growing by approximately 15% each year and doubling every 4 to 6 years. Total annual costs were projected to exceed $28 billion by 2010.

HISTORY

Dialysis was first described and used in 1854 to separate substances in aqueous solutions based on different rates of diffusion through a semipermeable membrane. Hemodialysis was first carried out on humans in Holland by Willem Kolff during World War II. Soon afterward, Kolff came to the United States to share the discoveries from his experiments. Dialysis in this fashion could only be achieved once or twice on a patient until 1960, when the external arteriovenous shunt described by Quinton, Dillard, and Scribner led to the establishment of chronic hemodialysis (Figure 1).

In 1966 Brescia, Cimino, and Appel proposed to surgically create an internal arteriovenous fistula (AVF) in the forearm. In this procedure, the vein would be made easily accessible for percutaneous puncture due to enlargement and increased flow secondary to the anastomosis with an artery. Within a decade of its creation, the internal AVF replaced the external shunt for the preferred mode of vascular access (Figure 2).

Interestingly enough, there was no Medicare to pay for dialysis, therefore a selection committee decided who would and would not be placed on this life-saving treatment. It was decided that patients had to be rehabilitatable and between the ages of 18 and 50 years. Fortunately, after some time, Medicare announced that they would pay for long-term hemodialysis, but only after the patient had been on dialysis for 90 days. Now all ESRD patients are eligible for dialysis despite any comorbidities.

The use of saphenous vein was also quite popular in the 1970s and 1980s. They are no longer in common use; the literature shows that after 2 years, only 20% to 60% of these fistulas are still functioning. We try to reserve the saphenous veins for later coronary artery bypass. In 1973, polytetrafluoroethylene (PTFE) grafts were introduced. Now PTFE is the most commonly used artificial material for vascular grafts in hemodialysis. Other types of grafts include bovine grafts, umbilical vein grafts, and polyetherurethane urea grafts. In 1980, a double-lumen catheter was designed. It has slowly evolved, and now the double-lumen catheter is a commonly used access for hemodialysis, while patients await maturation of an AVF. Although the catheter has evolved into a better and safer design, a great risk of complications of central vein stenosis and infection still exist.

VASCULAR ACCESS REQUIRES A MULTIDISCIPLINARY APPROACH

American Medical News, April 21, 2003, reported, "Patients with chronic illnesses must navigate a complex regimen of multiple physicians and medications. Coordination of the medical team supports patients by improving care and avoiding hospitalizations."

A structured and well-organized multidisciplinary team approach appears to be the most practical and efficient way to achieve quality care for ESRD patients. Patients receiving this standard of care have earlier access to surgeons and therefore a higher incidence of AVF, because veins are not destroyed. The use of temporary catheters is also decreased. Further, complications are identified and corrected in a timely fashion, leading to increased long-term patency, fewer hospitalizations, and less repeat surgery. However, early access care continues to be a challenge, as most patients wait until they have a catheter before they see a surgeon. Participating specialties include primary care physicians, nephrologists, interventional nephrologists, interventional radiologists, anesthesiologists, surgeons, and especially a coordinator, which may be a nurse; the coordinator is critical to the success of a multispecialty team.

PREOPERATIVE WORKUP

Prior to vascular access surgery, it is imperative that the patient undergo a complete workup that includes history and physical and evaluation of the veins and arteries in the extremities being considered

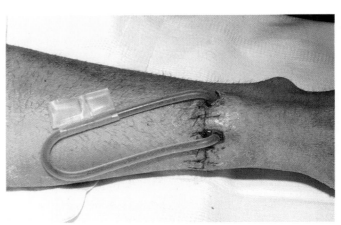

FIGURE I   Scribner shunt.

for placement of the access. Bilateral duplex Doppler study of the arteries and veins should be performed. If this does not produce enough information, bilateral arteriograms and venograms should help determine the best limb for access. The surgeon should make sure no proximal venous stenosis is present and that there is adequate blood supply to the lower arm and hand. Attention should be paid to the patient's cardiac, pulmonary, and liver function tests and bleeding and clotting times. Also, the patient's medications—particularly aspirin, clopidigrel, warfarin, and heparin—should be clearly noted.

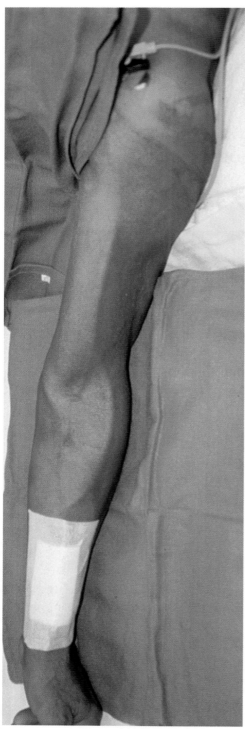

FIGURE 2   Immediate postoperative arteriovenous fistula.

It is helpful to refer patients to surgery prior to the need for chronic hemodialysis. With this early referral, it is likely that they will not need a double-lumen cuffed catheter and will not have had veins damaged by multiple IVs and blood draws. As a result, patients will be more likely to receive a fistula instead of a graft.

SURGICAL TECHNIQUE

In creating a vascular access, the surgeon must try to place the anastomosis as distally as possible; doing so provides more territory for revisions as surgery progresses up the arm. Most distally, a radial-cephalic AVF (Brescia-Cimino-Appel fistula) may be accomplished. If the veins are not available for a fistula in the wrist, the surgeon may create a brachial-cephalic fistula or brachial-basilic transposition. Ultimately, the decision as to where to place an access is based primarily on the preoperative workup as described above.

Figure 3 illustrates a good technique for the venous arterial anastomosis site. Usually, there is a branch in the vein where the anastomosis is planned. By ligating the two branches and excising the bottom, you can create a very nice aperture for the anastamosis. We have found that this technique helps to create an excellent flow through the fistula to help with early maturation.

Over the years, data have shown that an interrupted anastomosis has superior patency to a running anastomosis. However, the majority of surgeons stopped using the interrupted anastomosis because tying all of the sutures was time consuming. In the recent past, some surgeons have used titanium clips in an interrupted fashion, but use of these clips requires a short learning curve; if they are not placed correctly, you will have problems with the anastomosis, such as bleeding and thrombosis. Most surgeons still prefer to use a running monofilament suture for their anastomosis, with acceptable results.

In closing the incision, we have had great success using a small, absorbable, subcuticular suture followed by placement of Steri-Strips on the skin. We have found this to be very successful in many non-compliant patients who do not come back for suture removal in a timely fashion; this tends to reduce the incidence of wound infection.

In patients who do not have veins available for a primary autologous fistula, a nonautologous graft should be placed. The best graft in the lower arm is a loop graft from brachial artery to cephalic vein. If the cephalic vein is not available, the surgeon can create a brachial artery-basilica vein loop graft, or a graft can de done from the brachial artery over the biceps to the axillary vein.

At the conclusion of the procedure, before the wound is closed, it is very important to check the hand, as well as the distal pulses, to make sure there are no signs of steal syndrome. This can be done

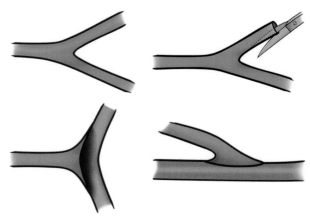

FIGURE 3   One technique for the venous arterial anastomosis site. Usually, there is a branch in the vein at the point where the anastomosis is to take place. By ligating the two branches and excising the bottom, an aperture for the anastomosis is created.

manually or with the use of the latest technology. If the hand is cool to the touch or radial and ulnar pulses are absent, this must be remedied as soon as possible with banding, a standard or modified distal revascularization-interval ligation (DRIL) procedure, or, as a last resort, ligation of the fistula.

Vascular access surgery should be performed in a very meticulous manner, using the finest monofilament suture available. It is also best performed by experienced surgeons, as it has been shown that surgeons who do many AV accesses a year have a better result than those who perform fewer than five per year.

COMPLICATIONS OF VASCULAR ACCESS

Thrombosis

Thrombosis is the most common complication of vascular access. If thrombosis occurs, the proximal vein should be evaluated to determine type of revision, as it may be treated by endovascular repair, such as angioplasty or stent, or by surgical revision consisting of a local patch graft or interposition graft to a more proximal open vein. Regardless of treatment type, all thrombi must be removed, with emphasis on the arterial plug. In some instances, the proximal vein above the graft anastomosis has developed to a point that an autologous fistula can be created.

Infection

Long-term cannulation of any vessel carries significant risks, and vascular access is no exception. The establishment of the AVF by Brescia, Cimino, and Appel reduced the risk relative to older methods; but over the past 30 years, the accelerating incidence of diabetes and hypertension has led to increased need for vascular access procedures and to a corresponding increase in infection rates. Infection is now the second most common complication in vascular access. The development of sepsis can lead to further complications, such as subacute bacterial endocarditis, spinal abscesses, and in some instances brain abscesses. Death secondary to infection in dialysis patients is estimated at 36%.

The definition of *infection* of a vascular access can vary depending on the physician, but it is important to have a consistent approach to diagnosis and treatment. Usually, infection is diagnosed when there are local signs of inflammation or purulence requiring intravenous antibiotics and removal of the access. Once infection in an AVF or graft is identified, it is important to understand the cause and the typical time involved and the course of its development. Studies have shown that infections attributable to access operations had a low prevalence, and the largest number of infections occurred in patients undergoing routine dialysis. When *postoperative complication* is defined as a complication occurring within 30 days after surgery, retrospective review has shown that the overall postoperative infection rate was 0.51% (n = 1574). Breakdown of this result reveals that the AVF has a virtually perfect track record, at 0% (n = 521). For an AV graft, the infection rate was found to be slightly higher, at a rate of 0.86% (n = 921). It is important to understand that infections most often are a result of chronic cannulation and not from postoperative complications.

Schild and colleagues reviewed the medical records of 1574 consecutive vascular access procedures performed on 850 patients over a 60-month period. This review included 443 new grafts, 478 graft revisions, and 521 new fistulas. Of the 963 new procedures, 54% were autologous fistulas, and 46% were prosthetic grafts. In addition, 132 procedures were performed for infection in 87 patients; this can be interpreted as an 8% overall infection rate. Of those, 86 were infected grafts and 1 was an infected AVF—2 years following access surgery, which was complicated by a pseudoaneurysm (see Table 1).

In this study, much of the blame is placed on dialysis centers, which were found to be responsible for 50% of all infections

TABLE 1: Sources of vascular access infection

Source of Infection	Percentage of Grafts Operated on for Infection
Operative (within 30 days)	6%
Interventional radiology (post-thrombectomy)	5%
Dialysis center (>30 days after surgery)	50%
Spontaneous in nonfunctional graft	23%
Remaining stump of previously excised graft	17%

TABLE 2: Organisms most often cultured from vascular access infections

Organism	Percentage of Total Infections Cultured
Staphylococcus aureus	26.32%
Negative cultures	22.81%
Methicillin-resistant *Staphylococcus aureus*	21.05%
Pseudomonas aeruginosa	5.26%
Staphylococcus epidermidis	3.51%
Streptococcus viridans	3.51%
Enterobacter cloacae	3.51%
Acinetobacter baumannii	1.75%
Alcaligenes xylosoxidans	1.75%
Corynebacterium	1.75%
Enterococcus spp.	1.75%
Enterobacter faecalis	1.75%
Mycobacteria chelonae	1.75%
Serratia marcescens	1.75%

identified. Multiple organisms were cultured as the cause of infection, the most common being *Staphylococcus aureus* and methicillin-resistant *Staphylococcus aureus* (Table 2). Possible reasons may include poor hygienic practice, including improper use of sterile gloves during cannulation of the fistula. These data suggest that infection can be easily avoided, or rates reduced at least, based on simple, inexpensive changes in employee habits. Given these statistics, close observation in dialysis centers is strongly advised.

In addition, there should be a high index of suspicion for thrombosed grafts as a source of bacteremia even in the absence of local signs of infections. It is recommended that when infection is identified in nonfunctional grafts, they should be removed immediately. Delay due to antibiotic therapy is not warranted, as the presence of a foreign body will not allow complete eradication of infection with antibiotics alone. Previously, when removing an infected graft, it was common to leave a graft stump at the arterial anastomosis, when the artery was very small and no vein was available for a patch. Since it was shown that 17% of these procedures were performed because the stumps became infected, it is now highly recommend that when grafts are infected, they be totally removed. If the infection in a graft is localized, however, in some cases it can be bypassed, and the infected area can be removed. Infection is a major cause of vascular access failure (Figure 4).

Other Complications

Other complications of vascular access procedures include seromas (Figure 5), aneurysms (Figure 6), pseudoaneurysms, proximal vein occlusion secondary to central vein stenosis (Figure 7), and bleeding; ultimately, death may result if the problem goes untreated.

MATURATION AND FAILURE RATES IN ARTERIOVENOUS FISTULAS

With the number of vascular access procedures nearing 500,000 per year, the National Kidney Foundation Dialysis Outcome Quality Initiative (KDOQI) guidelines recommend an aggressive approach to the creation of AVFs, in contrast to prosthetic accesses. However, it is clear that not all patients are candidates for this type of vascular access procedure. In certain subpopulations of patients, fistulas may never mature or function, requiring additional surgeries to establish a means for dialysis.

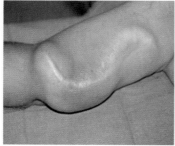
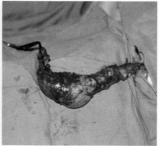

FIGURE 4   A 20-year-old infected arteriovenous fistula.

Previously, surgeons in the United States were creating more grafts than fistulas. The KDOQI now recommends at least 66% of all vascular access procedures be AVFs, thus switching the trend and beginning a fistula-first movement. However, some surgeons have adopted a fistula-only mentality. Now the question becomes, Have we gone too far to the other side by trying to create fistulas in 100% of ESRD patients?

In 2004 Schild and colleagues published a retrospective review of 374 consecutive fistulas in the *Journal of Vascular and Endovascular Surgery*. Of these fistulas, 31.3% either never matured or were not able to be cannulated, requiring patients to have further surgery. The failure rate for females was higher than in males (41.2% and 27.2%, respectively), but increasing comorbidity did not result in major changes in failure rate. Additionally, it was shown that the brachiocephalic position matures at a higher frequency than the radiocephalic position.

Other studies show even higher failure rates for AVFs. Miller and colleagues reported, "Of the 101 fistulas for which adequacy could be determined, 54 (or 53.5%) did not develop adequately, as defined by our prospective criteria." Biuckians and colleagues state, "Even in the best of circumstances in which a patient is undergoing a first-time access procedure, many AVFs [57%] failed, and of those functioning, only two thirds are working at the end of 1 year" and "[KDOQI] does not necessarily translate into high AVF utilization."

Findings like these bring up several questions. Should KDOQI guidelines be revisited in terms of developing more focused criteria for AVF, or should we be more meticulous in our preoperative workup? In light of published AVF failure rates. ranging from 20% to 50%, are we submitting patients to an unnecessary second operation, namely, AVF followed by prosthetic access? Some patients do not have the vasculature necessary to create a successful fistula. These patients can often be identified by physical examination and radiographic studies, and such patients would be better served by a nonautologous graft.

AVFs require 4 to 12 weeks or longer to mature, but on average, AV grafts may be used within 10 to 14 days. Furthermore, newer grafts have been developed that can be cannulated safely within 24 to 72 hours. While waiting for the fistula to mature, patients must be dialyzed through double-lumen cuffed catheters, which can be quite detrimental to patient health. Double-lumen cuffed catheters come with a great deal of danger from central venous stenosis and, especially, infection. It is estimated that infection with central venous catheters will cost over $30,000 per patient per admission secondary to prolonged hospitalization and expensive antibiotics. Lee and

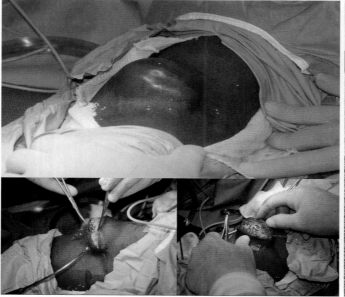
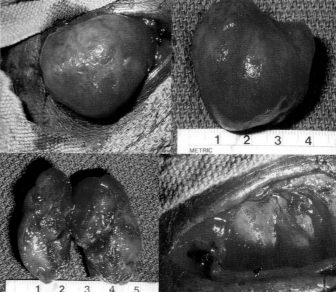

FIGURE 5   Surgical removal of seroma.

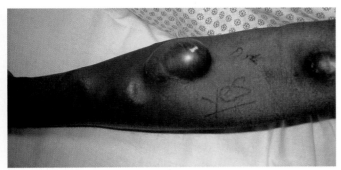

FIGURE 6   Aneurysm in a 9-year-old fistula.

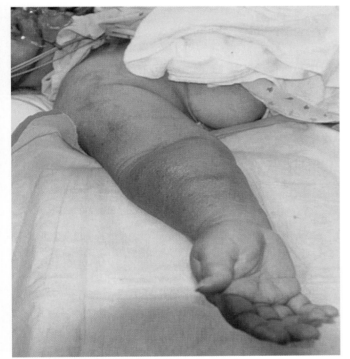

FIGURE 7   Markedly edematous upper extremity secondary to central venous obstruction.

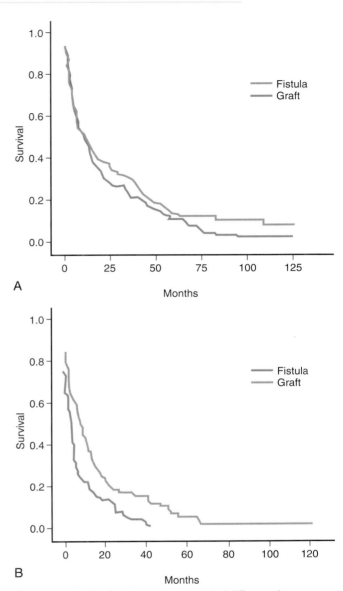

FIGURE 8   **A,** Timeline showing no statistical difference between survival of primary AV fistula and primary AV graft. **B,** Comparison of revised AV fistula and revised AV graft at 120 months. *(Data from Schild et al: Arteriovenous fistulae vs. arteriovenous grafts: a retrospective review of 1,700 consecutive vascular access cases, J Vasc Access [4]:231–235, 2009.)*

colleagues found 50% catheter bacteremia at 6 months, and Allon and colleagues reported that relative risk of death was 3.43 times greater over 1 year with a catheter compared with an autologous fistula.

Recently, at the University of Miami, Miller School of Medicine, a retrospective review of access procedures comparing fistulas and grafts was performed. A total of 1700 consecutive cases performed by one surgeon at a single institution between 1997 and 2005 were reviewed. Patients were classified according to demographics and comorbidities. Fistula and graft survival were independently calculated from time of surgery to last contact date or loss of access (Figure 8). Primary, primary assisted, and secondary patencies of grafts and fistulas were calculated.

It is apparent that grafts are most often placed in patients with the largest number of comorbidities, previous failed fistulas, and the worst vasculature. Infection, thrombosis, aneurysms, female gender, and black race are independent prognostic factors of a worse outcome by multivariate analysis; however, the type of access is not a prognostic indicator of worse outcome.

AV fistulas and grafts are equivalent in providing vascular access for chronic hemodialysis as proven by univariate and multivariate analysis. Although grafts have a higher rate of thrombosis, revisions are more successful when compared with revisions of thrombosed fistulas. It is clear that there is no indication for attempting 100% fistulas in chronic hemodialysis patients; nonautologous grafts also have a place in chronic renal failure. Finally, when fistulas fail, a graft is always a superior option to a double-lumen cuffed catheter.

FUTURE DEVELOPMENTS

Data have shown that interrupted anastomosis is superior to a running suture anastomosis. Currently, there are three clips produced for interrupted anastomosis: Anastoclip (LeMaitre Vascular, Burlington, Mass.), VCS (Vascular Closure System; Covidien, Dublin, Ireland), and U-Clip (Medtronic, Minneapolis, Minn.). Also, some companies are presently trying to develop a glue to anastomose arteries and veins. In addition, studies are being done to change the genes in the vein at the venous anastomosis to prevent neointimal hyperplasia.

So far, this has shown favorable results in animal studies. Another company has developed Vascugel, a product that causes a change in the cells in the vessels when wrapped around an anastomosis, again to prevent neointimal hyperplasia and stenosis.

New developments in the manufacture of grafts show considerable promise in lowering the incidence of infection, pseudoaneurysms, and seromas. Many companies are also trying to develop early cannulation grafts, and research is being done on a particular graft, Flixene, in which cannulation has been done within the first 24 to 72 hours with excellent results. It is also predicted that there will be fewer seromas and pseudoaneurysms as well.

DO'S AND DON'TS OF VASCULAR ACCESS

Top 10 DO's of Vascular Access

1. Always obtain a complete history and physical on the patient.
   - It is essential that every new patient have a complete workup, or you will certainly miss some important irregularities.
2. Get vein mapping when indicated.
   - Doing vascular access surgery without an excellent knowledge of the patient's veins may be analogous to flying an airplane blindfolded.
   - When a patient has excellent veins and no previous catheter dialysis, vein mapping may not be indicated.
3. Remain open to using a PTFE early cannulation graft as an alternative to a double-lumen cuffed catheter.
   - This should be done when there are no adequate veins on physical exam or vein mapping that will allow creation of an AVF.
4. Obtain early referrals.
   - As a surgeon, it is very beneficial to have an early referral before the patient's veins have been mutilated by multiple hospitalizations, previous IVs, and IV medications.
   - Patients referred earlier are more likely to have a functional fistula created.
5. Explain the operation to the patient in detail.
   - It puts patients at ease if you make them aware of exactly what you are going to do.
   - Establishing good rapport with patients may hold you in good stead in the future.
6. Use the most distal site available for access in the upper extremity.
   - Since we only have two arms, it is paramount to place the access as distal as possible in each arm.
   - This may ultimately maintain the patient on chronic hemodialysis longer.
7. Place access in the upper extremity when possible.
   - Our experience with thigh grafts has not been as good as those in the upper extremity because of a higher incidence of infection.
   - If a thigh graft suffers a blowout, it becomes a very difficult problem, because it is almost impossible to get proximal and distal control easily.
8. Follow up with patients after surgery.
   - It is extremely important to see the patient postoperatively.
   - Patients should be seen early on after surgery to determine whether the wounds are healing and access is maturing.
   - Patients should be seen a second time to determine if the access is ready for dialysis.
9. Communicate with the referring physician before and after surgery.
   - There is no question that communication is very important.
   - You should write a letter and/or call the referring physician after you have seen and evaluated the patient.
   - After surgery, you should make the referring physician aware of what procedure you did to allow the best care for the patient on dialysis.
10. Provide an in-service to dialysis nurses and technicians regarding sterile technique.
    - In some dialysis centers, there is very poor sterile technique.
    - In a recently published retrospective study of 1574 consecutive patients, the most common infections (50%) were from the dialysis center.

Top 10 DON'Ts of Vascular Access

1. Don't operate on patients with HIV or hepatitis C under local anesthesia.
   - Operating on patients with HIV and hepatitis C under general anesthesia is safer, because some patients under local anesthetic and sedation become restless and move an arm or leg, which could cause you to cut or stick yourself with a needle.
2. Don't prolong the use of double-lumen cuffed catheters.
   - Everyone knows that prolonged use of double-lumen cuffed catheters has a high infection rate and often leads to central vein stenosis.
3. Don't always rely on the vein-mapping report; see the films yourself.
   - • We have had reports of vein mapping that were not exactly correct, and at the time of surgery, veins were found to be different than the report.
   - Films are often read by residents or fellows, and key issues are overlooked.
4. Don't operate on a patient that you have not seen and examined yourself.
   - There is great danger in operating blindly, even if you have been informed by the referring physician.
   - You may find problems that you did not know existed, such as poor veins or sclerotic arteries.
   - Operating blindly would be very hard to defend in court.
5. Don't forget to tell every patient the all complications that can occur and document this when obtaining consent for surgery.
   - If you don't, you may be very sorry when the subpoena arrives.
6. Don't place an AVF in a patient when you know it probably will not work.
   - A professor once told me, "Don't ever do anything that you think *might* work because 99% of the time, it won't."
   - If you are meticulous with your preoperative workup, you should have very successful access surgery, and the patient will not need a second operation.
7. Don't be surprised if a fistula fails to mature.
   - Because of "fistula first," many surgeons are attempting fistulas that for many reasons will never mature.
   - Sometimes, even though the vein and artery look good, the fistula will fail for causes unknown.
   - Fistula failure rates are now being reported at 30% to 50%.
8. Don't operate on patients taking aspirin, clopidogrel (Plavix), or warfarin (Coumadin).
   - Although some surgeons will operate on patients taking these drugs, the platelet abnormalities of ESRD and the combination of these drugs cause bleeding that is difficult to control during surgery.
   - I advise my patients not to take aspirin and/or clopidogrel for at least 10 days prior to surgery and to discontinue warfarin at least 5 days prior to surgery.
9. Don't let the dialysis center cannulate the access until you feel it is ready.
   - We have had a number of cases in which cannulation was carried out without the surgeon's permission, the access was blown, and a large hematoma followed that caused considerable morbidity.
   - You may have to do a second or even a third operation, prolonging the double-lumen cuffed catheter time.

10. Don't schedule your access patients at the end of your surgery schedule.
    - You may be prone to making errors that might otherwise be easily avoided. At the end of the operative schedule, your brain may not be as sharp as your scalpel.

SUMMARY

Vascular access procedures are becoming the most common surgery performed in the United States, and it should be a multidisciplinary effort. Vascular access surgery encompasses many difficult problems and should be only done by those dedicated to its success. Although a greater effort should be made to create more AVFs than prosthetic grafts, to comply with KDOQI guidelines, grafts still have a place in chronic renal failure and should always be the first alternative over a double-lumen cuffed catheter. Studies show that up to 50% of infections may be attributable to dialysis centers. Therefore, an in-service should be provided to dialysis nurses and technicians regarding sterile technique.

SUGGESTED READINGS

Allon M, Daugirdas J, Depner TA, et al: Effect of change in vascular access of patient mortality in hemodialysis patients, *Am J Kidney Dis* 47(3):469–477, 2006.

Bennion RS, Wilson SE: *Vascular surgery: a comprehensive review*, ed 6, Philadelphia, 2002, Saunders Elsevier, p 652.

Biuckians A, Scott EC, Meier GH, et al: The natural history of autologous fistulas as first-time dialysis access in the KDOQI era, *J Vasc Surg* 47(2):415–421, 2008.

Landa A: Collaborating for care: when joining forces helps patients, *Am Med News* 45(15), 2003.

Lee T, Barker J, Allon M: et al: Tunneled catheters in hemodialysis patients: reasons and subsequent outcomes, *Am J Kidney Dis* 46(3):501–508, 2005.

Miller PE, Tolwani A, Luscy CP, et al: Predictors of adequacy of arteriovenous fistulas in hemodialysis patients, *Kidney Int* 56(1):275–280, 1999.

Ronco C, Levin NW, editors: Hemodialysis, vascular access, and peritoneal dialysis access, *Contrib Nephrol* 142, 2004, pp 1–13.

Schild A, Pruett CS, Newman MI, et al: The utility of the VCS clip for creation of vascular access for hemodialysis: long-term results and intraoperative benefits, *J Cardiovasc Surg* 9(6):526–530, 2001.

Schild A, Simon S, Prieto J, et al: Single-center review of infections associated with 1,574 consecutive vascular access procedures, *J Vasc Endovasc Surg* 37(1):27–31, 2003.

Schild A, Prieto J, Glenn M, et al: Maturation and failure rates in a large series of arteriovenous dialysis access fistulas, *J Vasc Endovasc Surg* 38(5):449–453, 2004.

Schild A, Perez E, Gillaspie E, et al: Arteriovenous fistulae vs. arteriovenous grafts: a retrospective review of 1,700 consecutive vascular access cases, *J Vasc Access* 9(4):231–235, 2008.

Shenoy S, Miller A, Petersen F, et al: A multicenter study of permanent hemodialysis access patency: beneficial effect of clipped vascular anastomotic technique, *J Vasc Surg* 38(2):229–235, 2003.

Uribarri J: Past, present and future of ESRD therapy in the United States, *Mount Sinai J Med* 66(1):14–19, 1999.

Work J: Fistula first: Has the pendulum swung too far? The unintended consequences, *Vasc Access Practicum*, 2007.

VENOUS THROMBOEMBOLISM: DIAGNOSIS, PREVENTION AND TREATMENT

Peter K. Henke, MD

EPIDEMIOLOGY AND RISK FACTORS

Venous thromboembolism (VTE) has become better recognized as a major cause of morbidity and mortality in both surgical and medical patients. The incidence has not significantly decreased over the last 20 years, and estimated treatment costs are in the billions per year. The estimated incidence of VTE is 200,000 new cases in the United States, of which the mortality rate may be 30%—mostly due to pulmonary embolism (PE). Up to a third of patients develop a recurrent VTE within 10 years of their first deep vein thrombosis (DVT), and this more commonly occurs in the elderly, those with hypercoagulable states, obesity, and malignancies. Venous thromboembolism may be considered related to a proximate event (e.g., surgery or trauma; provoked) or idiopathic (unprovoked).

Recent studies have better clarified the incidence of clinical VTE after major surgical procedures. In a large administrative database review of different surgical procedures over 4 years, the overall incidence was 0.8%, of which approximately 40% had a PE. Predictors of VTE included advanced age, presence of malignancy, and prior VTE. Of note, about one half were diagnosed 30 days after discharge, which suggests that the risk of VTE extends well beyond the perioperative hospital course. In a review of patients undergoing cardiovascular procedures, VTE occurred in 1%, increased the risk of death by more than 200%, and raised the cost of hospitalization by 75%.

A more detailed study evaluated the risk of VTE after the 10 most common operations performed in the Veterans Health System. The overall incidence of VTE was approximately 1%, varying directly with procedure type, and the risk of death doubled. By multivariate logistical regression, low albumin, postoperative infections, and other complications were associated with an increased risk of VTE. Infection was also shown in a community study to be a significant risk of VTE, with a twofold increase within the first several months after the index pneumonia or urinary tract infection. These series suggest that certain preoperative factors and systemic inflammation create a prothrombotic physiologic state. These series also confirm the significant negative impact VTE has on patients.

The primary risk factors may be inherited, acquired, or a combination of both (Table 1). Heritable hypercoagulable disorders are relatively common, varying from 1% to 20% prevalence. Categorically, these are primarily anticoagulant deficiencies, abnormal procoagulant proteins, or increased levels of procoagulant proteins. These thrombophilias increase the risk of recurrent VTE by as much as 150% to 400%. Consistent with other pathobiologic processes is the "two hit" hypothesis; for example, a person with Factor V Leiden deficiency without prior VTE undergoes a major surgery and then develops a postoperative DVT. Testing for an inherited hypercoagulable disorder is recommended for those under 50 years of age with an unprovoked VTE, unusual sites of VTE, and multiple recurrent unprovoked VTE (Box 1).

Obesity has become epidemic, and bariatric procedures are now commonly performed. The risk of VTE in bariatric surgery patients is low with appropriate prophylaxis that includes pharmacologic prophylaxis, pneumatic compression devices (PCDs), and early ambulation. Several studies show the incidence of DVT to be about 1%, excluding those who had a prior history of VTE. Preoperative weight was the single most significant predictor of VTE.

TABLE 1: Risk factors associated with venous thromboembolism

	Factors	Comments
Acquired	Advanced age	Increases significantly at age 70 years
	Surgery	Abdominal, pelvic, and orthopedic are highest risk
	Malignancy	Solid tumors > hematologic
	Prior VTE	Consistently high risk factor
	Family history	Often forgotten on history intake
	Immobilization	Spinal injury
	Systemic infection	Pneumonia, urinary tract infection; sepsis significantly increases risk
	Venous catheters	Upper and lower extremity
	Estrogen/oral contraceptive use	Depends somewhat on formulation
	Inflammatory bowel disease	Crohn's disease, ulcerative colitis
	Antiphospholipid antibodies	Lupus
Inherited	Deficiency of anticoagulants	Protein C, protein S, antithrombin deficiency
	Additional genetic coagulation protein	Factor V Leiden, prothrombin 20210A
	Increased coagulation protein	Factor VIII/IX elevation
	Hyperhomocysteinemia	Not common

BOX 1: Hypercoagulable screeningadjuncts

Coagulation tests (activated partial thromboplastin time, International Normalized Ratio) and platelets
Antithrombin antigen and activity
Protein C antigen and activity
Protein S antigen
Factor V Leiden genetic test
Prothrombin 20210A genetic test
Homocysteine level
Antiphospholipid/anticardiolipin antibody
Factor VIII levels

DIAGNOSIS AND RISK STRATIFICATION

History and Physical Examination

Postsurgical patients may not have the classic symptoms—limb pain, swelling, and fever—and physical exam findings of DVT. Clinical factors associated with DVT include presence of malignancy, prior DVT, recent immobilization, and difference in calf diameter; absence of calf swelling is associated with a lower risk of DVT. Postsurgical conditions may mask these common factors, thus a high index of suspicion is warranted. Note that these same factors are associated with PE.

Other conditions may be confused with DVT, including leg swelling due to systemic illness, lymphedema, and muscle strain. Iliac vein obstruction can lead to unilateral leg edema and can predispose to DVT (May-Thurner syndrome), and the presence of a cyst behind the knee may produce unilateral leg pain and edema. Other causes of leg swelling, which is usually bilateral, include cardiac, renal, or hepatic abnormalities. Upper body jugular, axillary, subclavian, and brachial DVT also needs to be considered in patients with fever of unknown origin, neck or arm swelling, or those with indwelling catheters.

Biomarkers and Imaging

The use of D-dimer is now standard for stratifying patients into a low or high likelihood of DVT. D-dimer has excellent sensitivity (>95%) but poor specificity for DVT, and it may be elevated for numerous reasons in the postsurgical setting. However, it is still a useful test to help exclude DVT. There are two types of D-dimer assays, either *latex agglutination* or *enzyme-linked immunosorbent assay* (ELISA). The timeliness of the test is also important, and now most major hospitals have rapid return of this test, making it practical to order and use.

The use of venous compression duplex ultrasound is the gold standard for diagnosing proximal vein DVT, and it has good sensitivity for infrapopliteal DVT as well, depending on the vascular lab (Figure 1). Two caveats apply: First, variations in lower extremity venous anatomy are common, including duplicated popliteal veins. Second, an Intersocietal Commission for the Accreditation of Vascular Laboratories (ICAVL) accredited vascular laboratory is associated with better test accuracy. Other advantages of duplex imaging include that it is painless, requires no contrast, can be serially repeated, and is safe during pregnancy. The test also identifies other potential causes of a patient's symptoms.

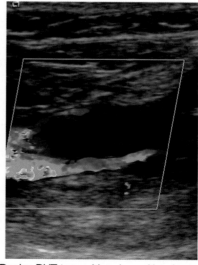

FIGURE 1 Duplex DVT image. Note large dilated vein with limited flow around the thrombus.

TABLE 2: VTE group risk stratification by age and comorbities

Risk	Example
Low	Minor surgery in patients <40 years Surgery <30 minutes
Moderate	Major surgery in patients <40 years Minor surgery in patients >40 years with risks
High	Major surgery in patients >60 years Major surgery in patients >40 years with risks
Very High	Major spinal or orthopedic surgery Spinal cord or major orthopedic injury Major surgery in patients >40 years with malignancy, prior VTE, hypercoagulable states

Modified from Geerts WH, Bergqvist D, Pineo GF, et al: Prevention of venous thromboembolism: American College of Chest Physicians evidence-based clinical practice guidelines (ed 8), *Chest* 133(suppl S):381S–453S, 2008.

The diagnosis of PE has evolved with computed tomographic angiography (CTA), essentially replacing ventilation/perfusion scintigraphy in many institutions. The Prospective Investigation of Pulmonary Embolism Diagnosis (PIOPED II) study compared CTA–CT ventriculography with other imaging modalities and concluded a positive predictive value of 96%, a sensitivity of 90%, and a specificity of 95% in patients with a high pretest clinical probability based on history and physical examination. The use of pretest probability with D-dimer testing and CTA for PE diagnosis is particularly efficacious. Diagnostic adjuncts to better classify severity of PE include echocardiography and troponin and brain natriuretic protein levels. These tests can visualize and reflect right heart strain, respectively. If strain is present, more aggressive measures may be necessary.

Magnetic resonance venography (MRV) is useful for imaging pelvic and vena cava thrombosis pathology. A comparison study of MRV with contrast venography showed very high sensitivity and specificity, nearly 100%. However, MRV is expensive, and patients with metallic implants or claustrophobia are excluded from this treatment. Currently, MRV is used infrequently and even less often for evaluating anatomic abnormalities for interventions.

Often, differentiation of recurrent DVT from chronic DVT by duplex ultrasound is not possible. In these cases, the D-dimer assay can reliably exclude recurrent DVT. The risk of a missed VTE if heparin is withheld based on a negative D-dimer is low (<1%). Thus measurement of D-dimer provides a reliable method for determining initial risk and helps rule out recurrent DVT.

Risk Stratification

VTE risk stratification is a national quality of care measurement emphasized by the Centers for Medicare & Medicaid Services and the National Quality Forum. Assessment of risk can be done by categorizing broad group risk (Table 2) or by using a scoring system based on individual patient factors (Figure 2). Regardless of the system used, the important point is to determine each patient's risk and implement risk appropriate prophylaxis. At our institution, we use the Caprini risk-assessment scoring sheet, a checklist that has been adapted for risk stratifying all admitted patients. High-risk patients generally have a Caprini score of 5 to 7, which correlates with increased VTE risk. The specific risk factor weights have not yet been fully validated prospectively.

Developing the habit of VTE risk assessment is important for surgeons. A computer-based physician order entry reminder is beneficial and has been shown to significantly reduce VTE at 90 days.

VENOUS THROMBOEMBOLISM PROPHYLAXIS

Methods for VTE prophylaxis include pharmacologic, mechanical, and combination prophylactics. The goal is to prevent VTE while minimizing bleeding.

Pharmacologic and Mechanical Prophylaxis

Evidence-based pharmacologic prophylaxis includes low-dose unfractionated heparin (UFH), low molecular weight heparins (LMWHs), fondaparinux, and warfarin. Enoxaparin and dalteparin are the LMWHs used in the United States. Prophylactic dosages for enoxaparin are either 30 mg subcutaneously every 12 hours or 40 mg once daily, whereas the dalteparin dosage is either 2500 or 5000 anti–Factor Xa units subcutaneously once daily, and the fondaparinux dosage is 2.5 mg subcutaneously once daily. Bleeding complications associated with pharmacologic prophylaxis are quite low, generally less than 3%. Aspirin alone is not recommended for prophylaxis.

Mechanical methods of prophylaxis include PCDs and graded elastic stockings, often applied together. Mechanical prophylaxis with a PCD reduces the incidence of DVT, although this has not been proven with the same rigor as with pharmacologic agents. The effectiveness of PCDs is based on overcoming venous stasis, increasing lower extremity blood flow, and possibly by increasing native fibrinolytic activators. Compliance with these devices is a primary issue, as they need to be physically on the limb to provide protection, and some clinical conditions prevent this.

The estimated VTE risk dictates the prophylaxis, ranging from no specific VTE prophylaxis outside of early ambulation to both pharmacologic prophylaxis and PCDs (Figure 3). Specific surgeries have various levels of evidence with different pharmacologic agents and clinical conditions. The consensus recommendations in general, vascular, urologic, and gynecologic surgeries are that prophylactic low-dose heparin (LDH) (5000 units three times daily) is as efficacious as LMWH for VTE prophylaxis, although bleeding risk and heparin-induced thrombocytopenia (HIT) risk may be higher.

In trauma patients without prophylaxis, DVT may occur in up to 50% of high-risk patients, and PE is the third most common cause of death in those surviving beyond the first day. In several series LMWH has been found to be more efficacious than LDH. In trauma patients at high bleeding risk who are not receiving pharmacologic prophylaxis, duplex ultrasound screening is appropriate when dictated by clinical indications. Placement of a vena caval filter is often done in this group of patients, but this is not supported by evidence.

Other Issues with Prophylaxis

It is unclear whether presurgical (on call to operating room) or early postsurgical (<6 hours after surgery) pharmacologic agent administration is best, and no clear consensus exists about general surgery patients; but it is reasonable to proceed with either. The institution of PCDs should be started before surgery begins so they can be functioning throughout the procedure.

Prolonged posthospital prophylaxis (1 month) may decrease overall VTE rates, as up to one third of episodes of VTE may occur after discharge. Specific patient groups that benefit include hip and knee replacement orthopedic patients and those with abdominal or pelvic malignancies. Fondaparinux is also effective for extended prophylaxis after hip fracture.

Pharmacologic prophylaxis, especially LMWH, in the presence of spinal and epidural catheters may increase the risk of epidural

Venous Thromboembolism Risk Factor Assessment

Patient's Name: _____ Age: _____ Sex: _____ Wgt: _____lbs. Hgt: _____ inches

Choose All That Apply

Each Risk Factor Represents 1 Point

- ☐ Age 41-59 years
- ☐ Minor surgery planned
- ☐ History of prior major surgery
- ☐ Varicose veins
- ☐ History of inflammatory bowel disease
- ☐ Swollen legs (current)
- ☐ Obesity (5 MI > 30)
- ☐ Acute myocardial infarction (< 1 month)
- ☐ Congestive heart failure (< 1 month)
- ☐ Sepsis (< 1 month)
- ☐ Serious lung disease incl. pneumonia (< 1 month)
- ☐ Abnormal pulmonary function (COPD)
- ☐ Medical patient currently at bed rest
- ☐ Leg plaster cast or brace
- ☐ Central venous access
- ☐ Other risk factor _____
- ☐ Blood transfusion (< 1 month)

For Women Only (Each Represents 1 Point)

- ☐ Oral contraceptives or hormone replacement therapy
- ☐ Pregnancy or postpartum (< 1 month)
- ☐ History of unexplained stillborn infant, recurrent spontaneous abortion (≥ 3), premature birth with toxemia or growth-restricted infant

Each Risk Factor Represents 2 Points

- ☐ Age 60-74 years
- ☐ Major surgery (> 60 minutes)*
- ☐ Arthroscopic surgery (> 60 minutes)*
- ☐ Laparoscopic surgery (> 60 minutes)*
- ☐ Previous malignancy
- ☐ Morbid obesity (BMI > 40)

Each Risk Factor Represents 3 Points

- ☐ Age 75 years or more
- ☐ Major surgery lasting 2-3 hours*
- ☐ BMI > 50 (venous stasis syndrome)
- ☐ History of SVT, DVT/PE
- ☐ Family history of DVT/PE
- ☐ Present cancer or chemotherapy
- ☐ Positive Factor V Leiden
- ☐ Positive Prothrombin 2021DA
- ☐ Elevated serum homocysteine
- ☐ Positive Lupus anticoagulant
- ☐ Elevated anticardiolipin antibodies
- ☐ Heparin-induced thrombocytopenia (HIT)
- ☐ Other thrombophilia Type _____

Each Risk Factor Represents 6 Points

- ☐ Elective major lower extremity arthroplasty
- ☐ Hip, pelvis or leg fracture (< 1 month)
- ☐ Stroke (< 1 month)
- ☐ Multiple trauma (< 1 month)
- ☐ Acute spinal cord injury (paralysis)(< 1 month)
- ☐ Major surgery lasting over 3 hours*

Total Risk Factor Score ☐

*Select only one from the surgery category

FIGURE 2   VTE risk factor assessment.

hematoma. Factors that contribute to this problem include coagulopathy, traumatic catheter or needle insertion, use of continuous epidural catheters, concurrent administration of medications that increase bleeding, vertebral column abnormalities, older age, and female gender. A logistical problem also arises from discontinuation of the epidural catheter and starting and stopping pharmacologic prophylaxis. Timing of prophylaxis dosing should be kept in mind. Our practice is to allow about 2 hours between prophylaxis administration and catheter removal. It is imperative to make sure that the prophylactic agent is not fully discontinued around the time of catheter removal.

THERAPY FOR UNCOMPLICATED VENOUS THROMBOEMBOLISM

The primary treatment of VTE is systemic anticoagulation, which reduces the risk of PE, extension of thrombosis, and recurrence of thrombosis (Figure 4). Immediate systemic anticoagulation should be achieved, as recurrence rates for VTE are approximately four to six times higher if anticoagulation is not therapeutic in the first 24 hours. This is less of an issue with LMWH compared with UFH.

Traditionally, systemic intravenous UFH (loading dose ~80 U/kg; adjusted drip to maintain an activated partial thromboplastin time of approximately 2 to 2.5 times normal) has been administered for 5

days, during which time oral anticoagulation with a vitamin K antagonist, usually warfarin, is instituted. Because the International Normalized Ratio (INR) is slightly prolonged by heparin preparations, and most of the liver coagulant factors have long half-lives, therapeutic INRs for 2 consecutive days are recommended before stopping heparin. However, because of the need for intravenous administration, frequent monitoring, and the bleeding risks, UFH is less commonly used.

LMWHs, derived from the lower molecular weight range of standard heparin, are now primary therapy for VTE, because they demonstrate less direct thrombin inhibition and more anti–factor Xa inhibition. LMWH is equivalent to UFH if not slightly superior regarding thrombus recurrence, with a lower risk for major hemorrhage. LMWH may be administered subcutaneously; doses are weight based (e.g., 1 mg/kg or 100 U/kg twice daily); they do not require monitoring except in certain circumstances, such as renal failure, morbid obesity, and during pregnancy; and they may be given in the outpatient setting. There is also some evidence that LMWH may decrease the incidence of postthrombotic syndrome. Lastly, once a day as compared with twice a day dosing regimens are of equivalent efficacy.

Fondaparinux is also efficacious for the treatment of both DVT and PE, and it also is administered in a weight-based fashion (5 mg/kg body weight <50 kg; 7.5 mg/kg body weight 50 to 100 kg; and

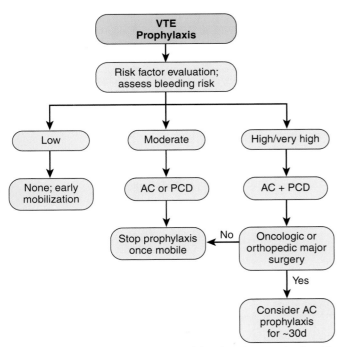

FIGURE 3 VTE prophylaxis algorithm. Note broad categories for risk because options of prophylaxis are relatively limited. *AC,* Anticoagulation.

10 mg/kg body weight >100 kg). Treatment for at least 5 days with concurrent administration of oral anticoagulation is recommended until the INR is therapeutic at a level of 2 to 3.

Warfarin should be begun after anticoagulation is therapeutic to prevent warfarin-induced skin necrosis, which can occur due to transient hypercoagulability, as warfarin inhibits protein C and protein S before the other coagulation factors. Typical doses are 5 mg per day until therapeutic level is reached and then adjusted. The therapeutic level of anticoagulation for warfarin is usually an INR between 2.0 to 3.0.

Duration of Anticoagulation and Other Treatment Issues

The recommended duration of anticoagulation after a first episode of VTE with an identifiable risk factor is 3 months. Calf-level thrombi may be treated with 6 to 12 weeks of warfarin. Isolated intramuscular vein thrombi may be observed, as few propagate to the tibial or popliteal level. The current recommendation is for a follow-up duplex scan and active ambulation if possible. However, if the patient has multiple risk factors for VTE, a limited duration of anticoagulation is reasonable.

After a second episode of VTE or an unprovoked VTE, the usual recommendation is prolonged warfarin, unless there are modifying factors, such as a high bleeding risk. VTE recurrence is increased in the presence of homozygous factor V Leiden and prothrombin 20210A mutation, protein C or protein S deficiency, antithrombin deficiency, antiphospholipid antibodies, and unresolved cancer. However, heterozygous factor V Leiden/prothrombin 20210A does not carry the same risk as their homozygous counterparts, and the length of oral anticoagulation may be shortened. Thus the optimal duration of warfarin is quite variable.

Two additional tests can be helpful to determine the length of anticoagulation. First, follow-up duplex ultrasound that shows residual (chronic) thrombus is associated with a significantly increased recurrent DVT risk. The second and better validated criterion involves D-dimer levels, obtained 1 month after warfarin is stopped. If the

D-dimer level is significantly elevated above normal, the patient is still prothrombotic, and warfarin should be continued. A large study demonstrated a fourfold decrease in recurrent VTE if the D-dimer assay is positive and the patients remains on warfarin compared with placebo at more than 1.4 years of follow-up.

The safety of LMWH compared with warfarin has led to selective long-term use of LMWH as a replacement for warfarin. Furthermore, rates of vein recanalization have been reported to be higher in certain venous segments using LMWH versus VKA agents. Additionally, when LMWH was used for 6 months in certain cancer patients, it has been associated with decreased rates of VTE recurrence and even decreased mortality rates, without differences in major bleeding.

For the perioperative management of anticoagulation, a patient with a recent (<3 months) VTE should be bridged with LMWH or UFH, offered surgery with prophylactic-dose anticoagulation, and then be restarted on anticoagulation after the operation. Occasionally, an IVC filter is indicated for very high-risk patients.

It is important that patients with a newly diagnosed DVT be placed in graduated compression stockings, generally at 30 to 40 mm Hg and knee high. This significantly reduces long-term PTS. But this is often forgotten, and no evidence shows that compression stockings (within 24 to 48 hours after anticoagulation has begun) increase the risk of "milking" a DVT to cause a PE. Rather, the evidence suggests that this early compression decreases the venous distension and subsequent vein wall injury. Similarly, early ambulation is important and may decrease the risk of subsequent PE.

Complications

The most common complication of anticoagulation is bleeding. With UFH, bleeding occurs in approximately 10% of cases over the first 5 days; with warfarin at an INR of 2 to 3, the incidence of major bleeding is approximately 6% per year. Reversal of heparin is with protamine, and reversal of warfarin is with vitamin K and/or fresh frozen plasma.

Another complication of UFH and LMWH is HIT, which occurs in 0.6% to 30% of patients in whom heparin is administered. HIT occurs when a heparin-dependent antibody immunoglobulin binds and activates platelets, leading to thrombocytopenia and thrombosis. It usually begins 3 to 14 days after heparin is begun but may occur earlier, if the patient has been exposed to heparin in the past. Routine platelet counts are needed approximately every 3 days after initiating therapy for those on either LMWH or UFH. Even small exposures to heparin, such as heparin coating on indwelling catheters, can cause the syndrome.

The diagnosis of HIT should be suspected when a patient experiences greater than a 50% drop in platelet count, when there is a drop in platelet count below 100,000/μL during heparin therapy, or when thrombosis occurs during heparin therapy. The most frequently used rapid test to make this diagnosis is an enzyme-linked immunosorbent assay (ELISA), which detects the antiheparin antibody in the patient's plasma. Another test that can be used is the serotonin release assay, which is more specific but less sensitive than the ELISA test.

Once the diagnosis is made, or even strongly suspected, cessation of heparin is the most important step. Warfarin should not be started until an adequate alternative anticoagulant has been established, to prevent paradoxic thrombosis. The direct thrombin inhibitors hirudin, lepirudin (Refludan), and argatroban are the treatments now approved by the Food and Drug Administratin, although other agents such as fondaparinux have been used to treat this syndrome. Lepirudin is excreted renally, and argatroban is metabolized by the liver, and this metabolism should be kept in mind when prescribing for patients with renal or liver disease. Lastly, the direct thrombin inhibitor bivalirudin has the advantage of a short half-life, and it is also effective for patients with HIT.

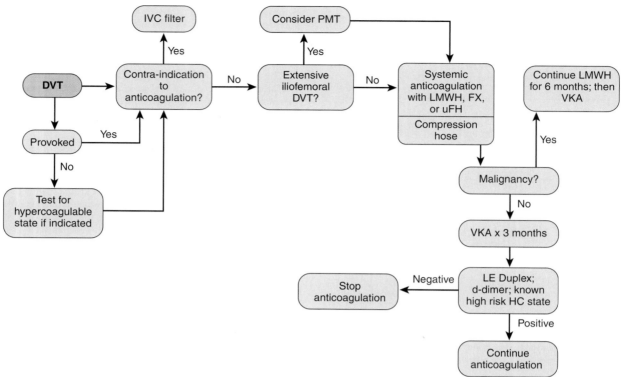

FIGURE 4 VTE treatment algorithm. Consideration of whether the DVT is provoked or unprovoked is important. If no contraindication to anticoagulation exists, and the DVT is not extensive, standard anticoagulation and compression are recommended. *VKA,* Vitamin K antagonist; *HC,* hypercoagulable condition; *Fx,* fondaparinux; *PMT,* pharmacomechanical thrombolysis.

THERAPY FOR COMPLICATED VENOUS THROMBOEMBOLISM

The use of thrombolytic and catheter (mechanical) extraction methods to rapidly decrease thrombus load may decrease PTS, especially in those with extensive iliofemoral DVT. In limb-threatening cases, with phelgmasia cerulea dolens or phlegmasia alba dolans, the thrombus burden must be rapidly cleared to salvage the limb. Examples of catheter devices include the EKOS catheter (EKOS Corporation, Bothell, Wash.), the Trellis device (Bacchus Vascular, Santa Clara, Calif.), and the AngioJet and the Possus catheters (MEDRAD, Inc., Warrendale, Pa.). Less commonly, active thrombus removal also includes an operative thrombectomy.

Pharmacomechanical thrombus clearance is generally more successful the earlier it is undertaken (<14 days), such that those with acute DVT and no history of prior DVT have better success. Complications include bleeding, but intracranial hemorrhage is rare (<0.5%), and mortality is less than 1%. Vein segment patency at 12 months is about 80% but is less with incomplete initial lysis. Valve reflux also correlates with complete or partial lysis, being generally absent with a complete response. More broadly, these aggressive therapies have been found to improve quality of life by follow-up survey methods.

Catheter-directed thrombolysis is well accepted for axillary and subclavian venous thrombosis, particularly effort thrombosis, in young patients. More rapid thrombolysis decreases long-term risk of swelling and dependence of venous collateralization for outflow. Subclavian vein angioplasty can be used as a temporizing method, but stenting should not be done, as stents may crimp, migrate, or erode through the vein. A thoracic outlet decompression procedure is efficacious, as thoracic outlet compression most often causes the underlying venous stenosis. Whether immediate or after a delay to allow the vein wall inflammatory response to subside, operative timing is

controversial. In cases of secondary axillary-subclavian DVT due to indwelling catheters, anticoagulation along with removal of the catheter is indicated. The duration of anticoagulation is usually 3 months, but it should be individualized to reflect the patient's thrombotic risk.

Thrombolytic therapy via catheter infusion for PE remains controversial, but in massive PE with hemodynamic compromise, it is reasonable. Recent data suggest that thrombolysis may be useful in patients with right ventricular dysfunction without significant hemodynamic instability. Results are optimal when patients are young, and the embolus is fresh (<48 hours old) and large. Lytics rapidly dissolve clot, but after 7 days, the advantage as compared with heparin decreases.

Surgical approaches for PE are indicated for patients with massive PE with hypotension who require large doses of vasopressors. These are often patients in whom thrombolysis has been unsuccessful. The technique of open pulmonary embolectomy is still associated with high rates of morbidity and mortality.

ALTERNATIVE AND FUTURE MEDICAL ANTICOAGULANT TREATMENTS FOR VENOUS THROMBOEMBOLISM

Two classes of agents for VTE treatment being developed include the oral direct thrombin inhibitors and direct factor Xa inhibitors. Dabigatran etexilate is an oral direct thrombin inhibitor currently undergoing phase III studies in the prophylaxis and treatment of VTE, and it has met a noninferiority target compared with enoxaparin in prophylaxis for orthopedic procedures. Importantly, there have not been elevations in liver enzymes or acute coronary events thus far.

New oral anti–factor-Xa agents include rivaroxaban and apixaban. Rivaroxaban has mainly renal excretion, but apixaban has less

25% renal excretion. Rivaroxaban is in phase III trials, showing good results in the prophylaxis and treatment of DVT, and apixaban is in phase II trials for patients with proximal DVT. These new agents hold promise for improved prophylaxis, as well as the potential to replace warfarin for long-term oral anticoagulation, but none of these have direct antidotes.

VENA CAVA FILTERS

The primary indications for inferior vena cava (IVC) filters include a complication of anticoagulation, a contraindication to anticoagulation, and/or failure of anticoagulation. As the IVC filter has achieved success, its indications have widened. Softer indications include a free-floating thrombus tail longer than 5 cm, excessive anticoagulation risk (e.g., in an older patient with full risk), or when the risk of PE is very high. The use of IVC filters strictly for prophylaxis in the highest risk patients requires prospective study, as does the proper use of retrievable versus permanent filters.

Protection from PE has been greater than 95% using cone-shaped, wire-based, permanent IVC filters over the past 30 years. Devices can be either permanent or optional retrievable. Vena cava filters are generally placed at the level of L2/L3 for the infrarenal location and T12/L1 for suprarenal IVC filter placement. However, they may be placed in the superior vena cava in rare situations. Indications for suprarenal placement include IVC clot, pregnancy or use in women of childbearing age, a previous filter filled with clot, or a previous filter that has failed. Filters are either placed under radiographic guidance or using either external ultrasound or intravascular ultrasound. External ultrasound may be ineffective in the face of morbid obesity, overlying bowel gas, or in the presence of open abdominal wounds. A large IVC (>28 mm diameter) needs to be imaged before the filter is placed, and either bilateral iliac venous filters or a "bird's nest" IVC filter should be used.

Complications

Misplacement of the filter may occur if cavography or ultrasound imaging is not used. If misplacement is evident, and the filter's efficacy is thought to be compromised, the decision whether to place a more proximal filter needs to be made on an individual basis. No increase in direct thrombotic complications has been observed in patients with two filters.

Filter migration is less common than previously thought, as respiratory variation may account for as much as 20 mm of movement on plain abdominal radiographs. Excessive filter tilt is another potential complication. This may occur with strut deployment into a vessel orifice or misplacement of the sheath device at the time of placement.

Device failure, defined as recurrent PE despite a technically good placement, may occur in 2% to 5% of patients. Various rates of IVC occlusion have been documented with all filter types. Several strategies are available to treat IVC occlusion. For an acute thrombus, full anticoagulation with heparin followed by catheter-directed thrombolysis may alleviate the problem. If the thrombus is older, catheter suction embolectomy and dissolution by a mechanical thrombus fragmentation device may be performed.

Less common filter complications include ensnared guidewires, either at the time of placement, which is more common with a jugular approach, or at a remote time, with a wire for another procedure or device (e.g., central venous access). Filter strut fracture may be demonstrated at late follow-up by duplex ultrasonography or by CT scan but rarely causes a complication, as the struts and the device are well incorporated via attachment sites.

SUMMARY

VTE is common in surgical patients, and the tools are available to prevent most occurrences by applying risk stratification and prescribing appropriate prophylaxis. Certain groups benefit from prolonged prophylaxis. VTE diagnosis should include a good history and physical, D-dimer and duplex compression ultrasonography for DVT, and CTA for PE. Rapid treatment with LMWH or fondaparinux and transition to a vitamin K antagonist for 3 months is standard for most patients with uncomplicated VTE. Adjuncts to determine anticoagulation duration include follow-up duplex ultrasound and D-dimer. Timely application of compression hose are essential. Aggressive thrombus removal should be considered for those with iliofemoral DVT and effort thrombosis and for those with PE and significant right heart strain.

SELECTED READINGS

Gangireddy C, Rectenwald JR, Upchurch GR, et al: Risk factors and clinical impact of postoperative symptomatic venous thromboembolism, *J Vasc Surg* 45(2):335–341, discussion 341-332, 2007.

Geerts W: Antithrombotic and thrombolytic therapy (ACCP Guidelines, ed 8), *Chest* 133(suppl):381s–451s, 2008.

Osborne NH, Wakefield TW, Henke PK: Venous thromboembolism in cancer patients undergoing major surgery, *Ann Surg Oncol* 15:3567–3578, 2008.

Meissner MH, Wakefield TW, Ascher E, et al: Acute venous disease: venous thrombosis and venous trauma, *J Vasc Surg* 46(suppl S):25S–53S, 2007.

Tooher R, Middleton P, Pham C, et al: A systematic review of strategies to improve prophylaxis for venous thromboembolism in hospitals,, *Ann Surg* 241(3):397–415, 2005.

Acute Pulmonary Embolism

Thomas Reifsnyder, MD, Charles Galanis, MD, and Andrew Reifsnyder, MD

OVERVIEW

The pulmonary circulation acts as a near-perfect filter for particulate matter in venous blood. Thrombus, fat, air, and foreign bodies all have been documented to cause pulmonary embolism (PE). Thrombus, particularly from an acute deep vein thrombosis (DVT), is by the far the most common. Generally, *acute PE* refers to venous thrombi breaking loose from their site of origin, traversing the right side of the heart, and lodging in a pulmonary artery. With an incidence as high as 1 per 1000 hospitalizations, it is estimated that as many as 300,000 people die annually from acute PE in the United States. PE is clearly a major cause of in-hospital morbidity and most likely the number one cause of preventable nosocomial mortality. PE has been implicated as the sole cause of death in 25% of postoperative deaths and as a contributing factor in 35%. Left untreated, PE carries a mortality of 30% to 35%. Considering these sobering statistics, all surgeons should be adept in the diagnosis and rapid treatment of PE.

RISK FACTORS

Because 80% of patients presenting with PE can be found to have evidence of DVT, and conversely, 50% of patients with acute DVT can be found to have had a PE, the risk factors are the same for both. Despite the age of the Virchow triad, it best summarizes the risk factors for thromboembolism: stasis of venous blood, endothelial trauma, and hypercoaguable states. Table 1 lists the more common acquired and hereditary risk factors for venous thrombosis and therefore PE.

PRESENTATION

The clinical picture of PE encompasses a spectrum from the asymptomatic incidental finding to cardiopulmonary collapse and immediate death. The presentation depends not only on the thrombus burden but also on the cardiac and pulmonary reserves of the patient. The etiology of symptoms involves two processes: 1) the obstruction of the pulmonary arteries leading to decreased oxygenation and right heart strain and 2) platelet activation in the pulmonary circulation, with its inherent release of vasospastic and bronchospastic substances, such as serotonin. The latter process is particularly noteworthy, as symptoms of PE may mimic those of reactive airway disease. Symptomatic patients most commonly complain of shortness of breath (75%), chest pain (60%), or cough (30%). The most common clinical sign is tachypnea. Other findings may include hypotension, tachycardia, distended neck veins, and unilateral lower extremity swelling. Although the classic picture of a massive PE may be hard to miss, the presentation of small pulmonary emboli may be quite subtle. Therefore, a high index of suspicion must be maintained at all times, particularly in postoperative patients.

EVALUATION

Initial Testing

The initial evaluation of a patient with respiratory distress includes an electrocardiogram (ECG), arterial blood gas measurement, and chest radiograph. The ECG screens the patient for myocardial ischemia, and occasionally with PE, evidence of right heart strain may be seen with an S wave in lead I, a Q wave in lead III, and T waves in leads III and V1 through V3. The arterial blood gas measurement helps assess the patient's respiratory status, and patients with PE may exhibit hypoxemia with a respiratory alkalosis. However, in up to 15% of cases, the Pao_2 will be near normal. The chest radiograph is nonspecific but is essential in excluding other causes of respiratory distress such as pulmonary edema, pneumonia, or pneumothorax. In patients with PE, atelectasis and pleural effusion are seen half the time. Uncommon findings include a Hampton hump, a peripheral wedge-shaped opacity at the costophrenic angle representing a pulmonary infarct; a Westermark sign, an area of focal oligemia; or a (Fleischer) knuckle sign, enlargement of the central pulmonary artery. In patients with a high clinical suspicion of PE, obtaining a chest radiograph should not delay the definitive imaging.

Diagnostic Imaging

Multidetector Computed Tomography

Intravenous contrast-enhanced multidetector computed tomography (MDCT) of the chest has supplanted pulmonary angiography as the gold standard imaging modality for the diagnosis of acute PE. Pulmonary angiography is now largely reserved for those cases in which percutaneous intervention is anticipated. The continued advances in CT technology have led to dramatic improvement in image quality, resulting in fewer indeterminate studies and high interobserver agreement. MDCT has both a high positive and negative predictive value, especially when there is a concordant clinical assessment. The negative predictive value has been shown to equal pulmonary angiography. The sensitivity and specificity have been reported to be as high as 100% and 97% respectively. The Prospective Investigation of Pulmonary Embolism Diagnosis (PIOPED) study showed increased sensitivity when combined CT angiography/venography was performed,

TABLE 1: Acquired and hereditary risk factors for the development of PE

Acquired	Hereditary
Trauma	Antithrombin deficiency
Major surgery	Protein C or S deficiency
Cancer	Plasminogen deficiency
Advanced age	Factor V Leiden mutation
Paralysis	Activated protein C resistance
Obesity	Prothrombin gene mutation
Hormone replacement therapy (including birth control)	Dysfibrinoginemia
Pregnancy	
Polycythemia vera	
Chemotherapy	
Venous catheterization	
Bed rest or immobilization	

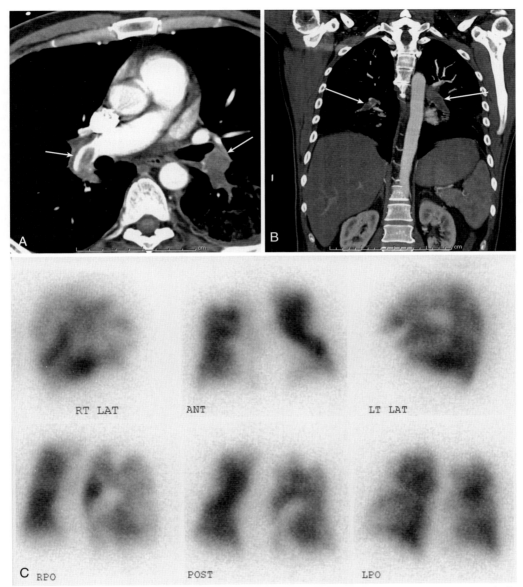

FIGURE 1   **A,** Large PE involving bilateral pulmonary arteries. **B,** Coronal view of large PE. **C,** V/Q scan demonstrating multiple wedge-shaped perfusion defects.

although the combined exam is not routinely performed in clinical practice. CT studies also allow for the global assessment of the thorax and frequently provide additional or alternative diagnoses when PE has been excluded. The classic finding on MDCT is that of a central, low-density filling defect within the lumen of the pulmonary arteries (Figure 1, *A* and *B*). Other findings include vessel cutoff, vessel enlargement, and clot in the right ventricle. Secondary findings include atelectasis, pleural effusion, and occasionally pulmonary infarct. Radiation exposure is a concern, but the risk/benefit ratio of CT still strongly favors the exam, even in pregnant patients, for whom there is a high index of suspicion of PE.

Ventilation/Perfusion Scanning

With the improvements in CT imaging, ventilation/perfusion (V/Q) scintigraphy has become the second-choice modality and is now mostly reserved for patients who should not receive iodinated contrast media because of severe allergy or impaired renal function. Nuclear medicine imaging is safe and widely available. A negative

V/Q scan essentially excludes the diagnosis of PE, which is shown as a wedged-shaped perfusion defect with normal ventilation—the classic mismatched defect (Figure 1, *C*). The studies are interpreted and categorized as normal or low, intermediate, or high probability. A scan showing low probability of PE with a low-probability clinical assessment showed PE in only 4% of patients; a scan showing a high probability of PE with a high-probability assessment showed PE in 96%. However, the majority (75%) of patients will fall into an indeterminate category of imaging/clinical assessment. Scintigraphy also provides little alternative imaging information. Moreover, the interobserver variability in the interpretation of the study is high. Therefore, except in patients with strong contraindications, MDCT is the diagnostic modality of choice.

Magnetic Resonance Imaging

Even though some studies have shown high sensitivity and specificity for MR imaging, the modality is rarely used in routine clinical practice for the diagnosis of PE.

Venous Duplex Ultrasound

Venous duplex ultrasound is the modality of choice for detecting DVT in the lower extremity, which is where most emboli originate. The study is easily performed, may be done bedside, and uses no ionizing radiation or contrast. In the hemodynamically stable patient, it is a reasonable initial study. If positive, it may obviate the need for additional testing, as the management strategies for DVT and PE in the acute setting are the same. However, if negative, it does not rule out PE, as the entire thrombus may have originated from another site or may have already migrated. In the patient with confirmed PE, a venous duplex scan should be obtained when the patient is stable; this acts as a baseline study for future comparison to ease the assessment for recurrent DVT.

Echocardiography

Echocardiography is a useful diagnostic tool for the critically ill patient. Like duplex ultrasound, it may be obtained bedside. In the hemodynamically compromised patient, it assesses for ventricular function, pericardial effusion, tamponade, and acute dissection. In patients with PE,

hypokinesis of the right ventricle is an independent predictor of mortality and may mandate more aggressive means of therapy (Figure 2).

TREATMENT

Preventing DVT, and therefore PE, should be second nature for any active surgeon. All patients undergoing surgical procedures should receive prophylaxis against DVT except those in the lowest risk category (Table 2). The mainstay of DVT prophylaxis is subcutaneous heparin. However, an equivalent dose of low molecular weight heparin (enoxaparin, dalteparin) is at least as effective and is superior for total knee and hip replacements, trauma, and spinal cord injury patients. Fondaparinux and warfarin have also been shown to be effective prophylactic agents and are frequently used for high-risk orthopedic patients. For those patients at high risk of DVT, prophylaxis should begin prior to surgery. Although surgeons frequently resist initiating DVT prophylaxis preoperatively, this is the most effective way to prevent DVT, with scant evidence of increased major bleeding. In the postoperative period, DVT prophylaxis should be

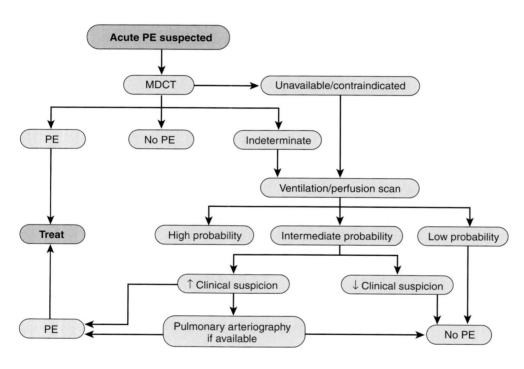

FIGURE 2 Treatment algorithm for the diagnosis of pulmonary embolism. *(Modified from Tapson VF: The diagnosis of venous thromboembolism, Dis Mon 51[2]:86-93, 2005.)*

TABLE 2: Classification of risk

Level of Risk	Calf	DVT (%), Proximal	PE (%), Clinical	Fatal
Low risk: Minor surgery in patients under age 40 with no additional risk factors	2	0.4	0.2	<0.001
Moderate risk: Minor surgery in patients with additional risk factors; surgery in patients 40 to 60 years with no additional risk factors	10–20	2–4	1–2	0.1–0.4
High risk: Surgery in patients >60 years or between 40 and 60 years with additional risk factors (prior DVT/PE, cancer, molecular hypercoagulability)	20–40	4–8	2–4	0.4–0.1
Highest risk: Surgery in patients with multiple risk factors (age >40 years, cancer, prior VTE); hip or knee arthroplasty, hip fracture/major trauma, spinal cord injury	40–80	10–20	4–10	0.2–0.5

Modified from Clagett G, Anderson F, Heit J, et al: Prevention of venous thromboembolism, *Chest* 108(4 suppl):312S–334S, 1995.

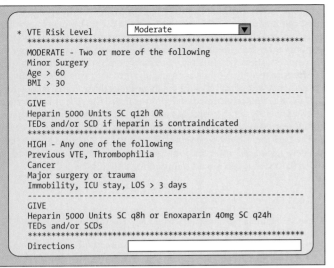

FIGURE 3   Simplified risk stratification in electronic physician order set.

continued until discharge and only withheld if replaced by another anticoagulant or if there is a strong contraindication to medicinal DVT prophylaxis.

At our institution, to help with physician compliance, the electronic physician order sets have a simplified pop-up box to stratify DVT risk (Figure 3). The order set then requires an input action to bypass ordering the standard subcutaneous heparin (5000 U every 8 hours).

The use of lower extremity sequential compression devices and elastic stockings (thromboembolic deterrent [TED] hose) has been shown in large studies to decrease the incidence of DVT and PE. However in high-risk patients, these should be considered as adjuvant therapy and not used in lieu of appropriately dosed prophylactic anticoagulation.

The acute treatment of patients with PE depends on the degree of clot burden and the resulting clinical picture. Patients with minor PE or major PE with adequate cardiopulmonary reserves can be adequately treated with anticoagulation alone. Hemodynamically compromised patients and those with insufficient cardiopulmonary reserves may be candidates for thrombolysis, catheter-directed therapy, or surgical thromboembolectomy in addition to anticoagulation. In patients with high clinical suspicion of having a PE, anticoagulation should be initiated prior to performing the necessary confirmatory diagnostic tests. Prompt therapy is crucial, as patients who do not survive most commonly die within the first hour after massive PE.

Anticoagulation

Anticoagulation with heparin stops propagation of the thrombus, thus allowing autogenous thrombolytic enzymes to begin dissolution of the embolus. With appropriate treatment the mortality associated with PE decreases from 30% to 2%. Low molecular weight heparins (LMWHs) and unfractionated heparin (UFH) have been shown to be equally efficacious, although UFH has a greater risk of heparin-induced thrombocytopenia. LMWH has gained popularity given its ease of administration and lack of need to monitor therapeutic levels. However, its use in patients who are obese or significantly edematous should be approached cautiously if not abandoned, as weight-based dosing makes the prediction of the degree of anticoagulation difficult. Patients with renal insufficiency also present difficulties, as drug clearance is reduced leading to unpredictable duration and extent of effect. With the advent of weight-based algorithms for UFH, therapeutic levels are rapidly reached while minimizing the potential

bleeding complications. At our institution, a UFH bolus of 80 U/kg is followed by an infusion rate beginning at 18 U/kg/hr and subsequently titrated to achieve a partial thromboplastin time ratio (PTTr) of 2.0 to 2.5.

In the postoperative patient, special consideration must be given to the risk of bleeding. Generally, the morbidity of a major PE outweighs the bleeding risk except in those patients who have had recent neurosurgery or those who have religious objections to the use of blood products. All postoperative patients with significant PE should be monitored in an intensive care unit to follow their cardiopulmonary status and to assess for any signs of hemorrhage upon the institution of anticoagulation. After the acute phase of treatment, patients should be transitioned to the oral anticoagulant warfarin. Ideally, the heparin infusion is only discontinued once the warfarin level is therapeutic, as indicated by an international normalized ratio (INR) of 2.0 to 2.5. We prefer to maintain warfarin therapy for 6 months. In patients with poor compliance or with significant bleeding complications, 3 months may be considered adequate. Following the course of anticoagulation therapy, if the major risks for DVT have dissipated, warfarin may be discontinued and generally replaced with standard aspirin therapy. Long-term LMWH is an option for those patients who cannot take oral anticoagulants, but the considerable additional expense outweighs any potential therapeutic benefit to warrant routine use. Lastly, in the occasional patient with heparin-induced thrombocytopenia and PE, treatment should be initiated with a direct thrombin inhibitor such as argatroban or lepirudin.

Inferior Vena Cava Filters

The development of inferior vena cava (IVC) filters adds an additional modality for the prevention of PE. As the ease of placement has simplified, use has increased. However, complications such as migration, thrombosis, and caval perforation are well documented, so strict indications for placement of filters should be maintained. The classic indication is the patient with confirmed DVT or PE who is at high risk of major bleeding with anticoagulation. Additionally, those patients who have had a significant PE and most likely will not tolerate an additional insult should be considered for an IVC filter. Although IVC filters are effective in preventing PE, their placement does not abrogate the need for anticoagulation, when it may be safely administered.

Thrombolytic and Catheter-Directed Therapy and Surgical Thromboembolectomy

The acute care of the patient with massive PE and hemodynamic compromise frequently requires more than just prompt anticoagulation. Currently there are no level I data to direct subsequent decision making, but the most commonly recommended next intervention is systemic intravenous infusion of a thrombolytic agent. Although streptokinase and urokinase have been used in the past, tissue plasminogen activator (tPA) is now the standard agent. Thrombolytics can rapidly dissolve clot, thus improving the patient's hemodynamic status. These agents, however, require at least 2 hours to become effective and are frequently contraindicated in the early postoperative period due to the possibility of initiating major bleeding. Since systemic thrombolysis for massive PE carries a risk of up to 5% for intracranial hemorrhage and 20% for major bleeding, it should only be initiated in those patients who demonstrate persistent hemodynamic instability.

Patients in extremis who are not candidates for systemic thrombolysis should undergo immediate catheter-directed therapy. This employs low-profile catheter-based techniques to mechanically break up the thrombus in the main pulmonary arteries. In addition, thrombolytics may be directly infused into the thrombus for more rapid dissolution. There are no randomized trials to evaluate the various techniques that have been employed. The most common technique is to place a simple pigtail catheter into the thrombus and rotate the catheter to break the thrombus up into smaller pieces, thereby relieving the pulmonary outflow tract and dramatically improving the patient's hemodynamics. However, there is a risk of sending small emboli out into the peripheral pulmonary arteries, thereby compromising oxygenation. Further, if the distal emboli do not dissipate, they may expose the patient to a risk of developing pulmonary hypertension and may negatively impact long-term survival. Although catheter-directed thrombolytic agents are often added to this procedure, they are not mandatory. Catheter-infused thrombolytics have a lower complication rate than systemically infused thrombolytics, and they clearly help dissolve the thrombus. If the hemodynamic response has been positive to the physical breakup of the clot, no further therapy other than anticoagulation is mandatory. Lastly, the Angiojet device, which is frequently used to emulsify thrombus in bypass grafts and lower extremity veins, is contraindicated for use in the pulmonary circulation.

The alternative to catheter-directed therapy is surgical pulmonary thromboembolectomy. Clearly, this is a major invasive undertaking in patients on the verge of death, and in many major institutions, it has been supplanted by catheter-directed therapy. The classic candidate has a massive PE with hemodynamic instability. This includes the hypotensive patient not responding to thrombolysis or the patient in whom thrombolysis is contraindicated. There have not been, and probably never will be, any randomized trials comparing catheter-directed therapy to surgical thromboembolectomy, but the minimally invasive nature of catheter-directed therapy and how quickly it can be performed make it an attractive choice at this time. However, patients with significant clot burden confirmed by imaging may be better suited for surgical intervention given the previously mentioned potential pitfalls of catheter-directed therapy. An additional group of patients who have done relatively well with open embolectomy are those uncommon patients found to have pulmonary embolus in transit, free-floating thrombus seen in the right atrium and/or ventricle. All patients who undergo surgical thromboembolectomy should have an IVC filter placed immediately to minimize the risk of recurrence.

Massive PE can be rapidly fatal, so a successful outcome may at times seem serendipitous. The rapid diagnosis by a physician versed in the treatment options, combined with the availability of an appropriately equipped interventional suite or operating room, and an experienced surgeon are all required for a successful outcome.

SUGGESTED READINGS

Dalen JE: Pulmonary embolism: what have we learned since Virchow? *Chest* 122:1801–1817, 2002.

Kuo WT, Gould MK, Louie JD, et al: Catheter-directed therapy for the treatment of massive pulmonary embolism: systematic review and meta-analysis of modern techniques, *J Vasc Interv Radiol* 20:1431–1440, 2009.

Stein PD, Fowler SE, Goodman LR, et al: for the PIOPED II Investigators: Multidetector computed tomography for actue pulmonary embolism, *N Engl J Med* 354:2317, 2006.

Stein PD, Woodard PK, Weg JG: Diagnostic pathways in acute pulmonary embolism: recommendations of the PIOPED II investigators, *Radiology* 242:15–21, 2007.

Tapson VF: Medical progress: acute pulmonary embolism, *N Engl J Med* 358:1037–1052, 2008.

VENA CAVA FILTERS

Ronald F. Sing, DO, and A. Britton Christmas, MD

INDICATIONS

The indications for vena cava filters (VCFs) continue to evolve. With continued design improvements, the use of VCFs has grown dramatically over the past decade. Surgical exposure and even laparotomy to insert a VCF was once required, but all modern devices can be percutaneously inserted, some even via a peripheral vein (e.g., antecubital vein). These advancements, and the portability of imaging equipment (e.g., C-arm), have facilitated the safe insertion of VCFs outside of the operating room or radiology suite or at the bedside in the intensive care unit. The most significant advancement with the greatest impact on the expanded use of VCFs has been the development of "optional retrievable" devices. An *optional VCF* refers to a device with a permanent indication but with the option of being retrieved when the patient's thromboembolic risk has abated (Figures 1 and 2).

The classic indications for VCF insertion are the presence of venous thromboembolism with a contraindication to or failure of therapeutic anticoagulation. Other relative indications include the presence of a free-floating thrombus in the inferior vena cava (IVC) or iliac veins, during thrombolysis of venous thrombosis, or in critically ill patients with limited cardiopulmonary reserves, those most likely unable to tolerate even the smallest pulmonary embolism (PE). A paucity of data regarding any of these indications exists, and level I data will likely never exist (large, prospective randomized trials) in light of the financial and ethical constraints of inserting or not inserting VCFs in patients with high thromboembolic risk.

The mid-1990s saw rapid growth of VCF use in severely injured patients without a diagnosed deep vein thrombosis (DVT) or PE who were believed too high a bleeding risk for even prophylactic anticoagulants (i.e., heparin). Based on level III evidence, the Eastern Association for the Surgery of Trauma recommended that the insertion of a VCF should be "considered" in very high-risk trauma patients who cannot receive anticoagulation because of increased bleeding risk, who have one or more of the following injury patterns: severe closed head injury (Glasgow Coma Scale <8), incomplete spinal cord injury with paraplegia or quadriplegia, complex pelvic fractures with associated long-bone fractures, and multiple long-bone fractures. Since these patients do not have an identified DVT or PE, the term *prophylactic filter* was coined. In actuality, all VCFs are prophylactic in that they do not treat DVT or PE, rather they prevent the next venous embolism from reaching the lungs. Therefore, the indication for VCF insertion is in a patient at high risk for PE who cannot receive anticoagulation. Unnecessary application of this technology is not recommended because of the complication risk (see Complications section below).

High-risk surgical patients, such as those with total joint replacements (knees and hips) and patients undergoing bariatric surgeries with additional risk factors, such as a prior PE or chronic venous stasis, are populations being examined for "prophylactic" VCF. Also, in therapeutically anticoagulated patients being treated for DVT and/or PE who require discontinuation of their anticoagulation, an optional VCF can be used as a bridge to anticoagulation.

The decision to insert a VCF should include a detailed risk/benefit analysis that includes the duration of thromboembolic risk, consideration and timing for retrieval, underlying coagulopathy, prior history of venous thromboembolism, and underlying venous disease (chronic venous stasis).

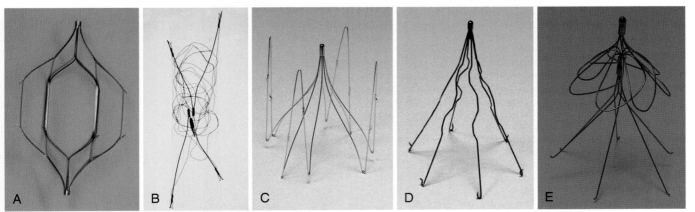

FIGURE 1   Permanent vena cava filters. **A,** TrapEase (Cordis). **B,** Bird's Nest (Cook Medical). **C,** Vena Tech LP (B. Braun, Bethlehem, Pa.). **D,** Titanium Greenfield (Boston Scientific, Natick, Mass.). **E,** Simon Nitinol (Bard Peripheral Vascular, Tempe, Ariz.).

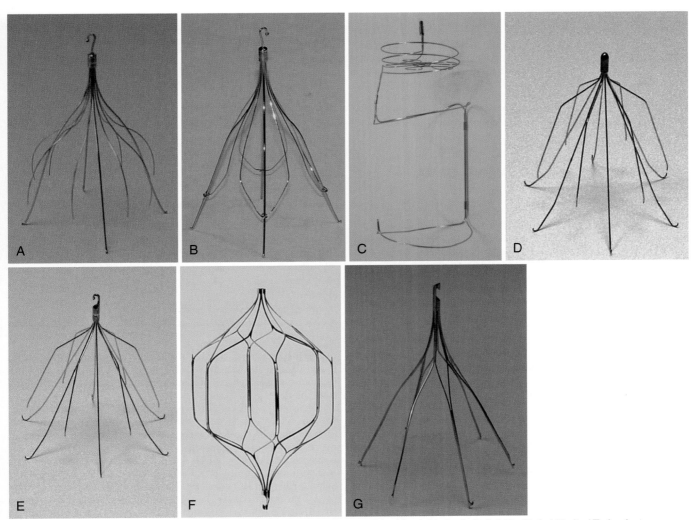

FIGURE 2   Optional vena cava filters. **A,** Celect (Cook Medical). **B,** Günther Tulip (Cook Medical). **C,** SafeFlo (Rafael Medical Technologies, Dover, Del.). **D,** G2 (Bard Peripheral Vascular, Tempe, Ariz.). **E,** G2 Express (Bard Peripheral Vascular). **F,** OPTEASE (Cordis). **G,** Option (Angiotech, Vancouver, BC, Canada).

SUPRARENAL INFERIOR VENA CAVA FILTERS

The long-term outcome of suprarenally inserted VCFs is essentially equivalent to infrarenally inserted devices. Initial concerns centered on the potential impact on renal function if cava thrombosis occurred; however, the extensive collateralization via the retroperitoneum obviates this. The ability to ligate the renal vein during aortic surgery illustrates this point. When inserting a VCF, it is important to avoid deploying the anchoring struts into a renal vein, which causes the filter to tilt significantly. The efficiency of filtration is based on the orientation of the filter within the vena cava lumen. Poor orientation of a filter impairs filtration, increases PE risk, and potentially interferes with blood flow, leading to an increased risk of caval occlusion.

Suprarenal insertion should be considered in women of childbearing age and may be necessary, provided an inadequate "landing zone" exists in the infrarenal position, such as in the presence of caval thrombus or short infrarenal IVC, a duplicated IVC, or PE from gonadal veins.

SUPERIOR VENA CAVA FILTERS

Although less often compared with lower extremity thrombosis, DVT of the upper extremities—including proximal veins such as the innominate, subclavian, and jugular veins—still carries risk of PE, including fatal PE. The true incidence of PE from the upper extremity veins has not been quantified. Proposed indications for a superior VCF are analogous to VCF insertion in the inferior vena cava with regard to the presence of DVT and/or PE with contraindication or failure of anticoagulation or the presence of free-floating thrombus. There are no "high risk" populations that warrant a superior VCF without an identified DVT. There are no VCFs approved by the Food and Drug Administration (FDA) for deployment into the superior vena cava (Figure 3).

COMPLICATIONS OF VENA CAVA FILTERS

Complications can be divided into *acute* (perioperative) and *chronic* types (Box 1). Acute complications can result from the technical aspects of the procedure and from the venous access. Similar to central venous catheter-line insertions, early complications include insertion-site hematomas, pneumothorax, arterial injuries, arteriovenous fistula, and insertion site thrombosis. The insertion site thrombosis rates are greater from the femoral access route (3% to 12%) compared with the jugular access (0% to 3%). This is an endovascular procedure, and similar to the placement of large-bore central venous catheters with sheaths and dilators (Hickman catheters), vessel wall perforation and even cardiac perforation is a potential risk. Excess force should be avoided during the insertion of catheters, because guidewires do not guarantee the direction of the dilator if it is inserted with too much vigor. Contrast nephropathy from iodinated contrast can result from the preinsertion cavagram. In addition, misplacement during deployment of VCFs is not uncommon, but such misplacements are greatly diminished when insertion is guided by preinsertion caval imaging.

Caval occlusion, the most dreaded complication of VCF, can occur acutely or chronically. In our opinion, acute caval occlusion (<60 days) likely is due to thrombus trapping a large clot, whereas chronic occlusion is due to intimal overgrowth. Acute caval thrombosis can result in hemodynamic instability as a result of the abrupt decrease in venous return.

Chronic complications include filter migration, which has been seen less often in the past decade because of a combination of better strut design and more emphasis on preinsertion caval imaging to

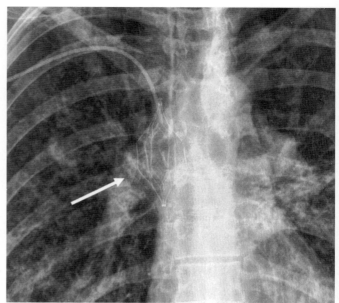

FIGURE 3   OPTEASE vena cava filter (Cordis) in superior vena cava (*arrow*).

BOX 1: Complications of vena cava filters

Procedural (Acute) Complications

Hematoma
Arterial puncture
Arteriovenous fistula
Pneumothorax
Malposition
Venous perforation or cardiac perforation with hemorrhage
Contrast nephropathy
Insertion-site deep vein thrombosis

Long-Term (Chronic) Complications

Thrombosis of vena cava
Postphlebitic syndrome
Strut fracture
Perforation
Migration
Fistula
J-tipped guidewire entrapment

---

determine caval diameter. The majority of currently used filters are recommended for caval diameters up to 28 to 30 mm; only the bird's nest filter (Cook Medical, Bloomington, Ind.) is recommended for a caval diameter up to 40 mm.

Recurrent PEs have been reported in only 1% to 3% of patients with most filters, and fatal PEs after VCF insertion are very uncommon. Perforations seen on imaging after VCF insertion are in part the result of intimal overgrowth of the struts. Therefore the struts are visualized outside the contrast column during cavography; some are true perforations. In any case, the majority of these are asymptomatic. Symptomatic fistulas or perforations into intestinal structures are rare.

A strut fracture is an incidental finding, and we are not aware of any clinical significance of this. Infection of a VCF is likely not an infection of the filter itself but an infection of the thrombus within the filter. Treatment is essentially with long-term antibiotics and anticoagulation, which would be the treatment for any intravascular infection.

Chronic caval occlusion can be asymptomatic, or it can result in chronic leg swelling and postphlebitic syndrome, a life-long debilitating problem, hence the development of optional retrieval devices.

Guidewire entrapment is likely underreported and results from J-tipped guidewires used for central venous catheter insertions with an in situ VCF. These occurrences can displace the filters themselves, or the disengaging of the wire may actually require endovascular intervention. The use of straight guidewires for central venous manipulations (central venous catheterization) or fluoroscopy avoids this complication.

TECHNIQUE OF VENA CAVA FILTER INSERTION

The successful insertion of VCFs necessitates an appropriate degree of expertise and caution. Familiarity with guidewires, catheters, venous access sites, anatomy, and the filters themselves is essential for appropriate deployment. Preferred access points for venous cannulation are either the right internal jugular or the right femoral vein unless contraindicated by existing injury or thrombosis. Certain devices can be used for the subclavian veins and even the antecubital veins for access. Venous cannulation should be performed using the Seldinger technique, and the guidewire is advanced into the distal IVC under fluoroscopic guidance.

All dilators, introducer sheaths, and imaging catheters are first flushed with heparinized saline. Our practice uses 2 U/mL of normal saline, unless there is a contraindication to heparin, such as heparin-induced thrombocytopenia. A digital subtraction/fluoroscopy unit is used to identify the twelfth thoracic and lumbar vertebrae. Guidewire placement, insertion of catheters, and deployment of the VCF are all fluoroscopically guided. Preinsertion imaging of the IVC is mandatory to appropriately determine the position within the vena cava for deployment of a VCF. The majority of complications related to VCFs can be avoided with preinsertion imaging.

The contrast venacavagram is performed using intravenous nonionic iodinated contrast medium (Figure 4). Although we prefer the use of a power injector, a handheld injection will suffice if an injector is not available. Caval diameter, the location of the iliac bifurcation, the location of the renal veins, the presence of caval thrombus, and any anomalies are determined. The VCF can then be deployed in an infrarenal position. A completion cavagram should be performed to confirm orientation and position of the VCF. The introducer catheter is removed, and direct pressure is applied to the insertion site for 10 minutes to ensure hemostasis.

Special Considerations for Imaging

Carbon Dioxide

Although the nonionic iodinated contrast agents have significantly reduced the incidence of pain and adverse reactions, the risk of contrast nephropathy and subsequent renal failure has not diminished. Furthermore, the risk of contrast nephropathy rises exponentially with the level of the serum creatinine. In patients with elevated serum creatinine, carbon dioxide (CO_2) can be used as a contrast agent, as it exhibits no hepatic or renal toxicity and is nonallergenic. Carbon dioxide imaging is performed using a hand-injection system (Angio-Dynamics, Latham, NY) with digital subtraction enhancement. This system is composed of a tubing system that has a series of one-way valves to prevent the introduction of air into the system and a 1,500 mL reservoir bag that can be filled from a tank of vascular grade CO_2 (99.99% pure). Multiple injections of 60 mL can be repeated with a breath hold if the first cavagram is suboptimal. There is very little cumulative effect of multiple boluses of CO_2 until several hundred milliliters are injected.

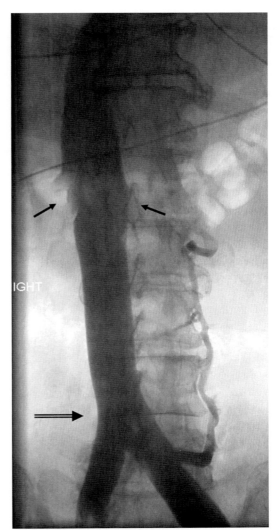

FIGURE 4 Contrast cavagram. Both renal veins (*solid arrows*) and iliac bifurcation (*open arrow*) are identified.

Intravascular Ultrasound and Duplex Ultrasonography

Increased experience with color-flow duplex scanning and intravascular ultrasound (IVUS) over the past decade has demonstrated these modalities to be safe and efficacious for preinsertion caval imaging and guidance of VCF insertion. However, it has not been determined whether these techniques can identify more subtle abnormalities (caval anomalies, such as a duplicated system). Furthermore, few general surgeons possess duplex or IVUS expertise to perform VCF insertion using these modalities.

VENA CAVA FILTER RETRIEVAL

The decision to retrieve or not to retrieve a VCF is multifactorial. The primary criteria for retrieval is that the patient's PE risk has returned to an acceptably low level or that the patient can be therapeutically anticoagulated. It is important that the patient be able to demonstrate compliance and tolerance with anticoagulation for at least 1 to 2 weeks. It is not absolutely necessary to discontinue anticoagulation for retrieval. Furthermore, the life expectancy of the patient should be at least 6 months from the time of planned retrieval. Filters that have migrated, tilted, or fractured should be removed and, if necessary, replaced. Device-specific recommendations on the time to retrieval

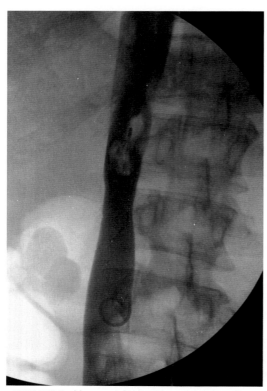

FIGURE 5   Vena cava filter with trapped thrombus.

may impact the decision to retrieve or not retrieve a filter. If a patient remains at significant PE risk beyond the recommended window of retrieval for a specific device, it should be left as a permanent implant.

Trapped Thrombus at the Time of Retrieval

Thrombus in a filter identified at the time of the retrieval denotes *venous thromboembolism,* and if the patient is not anticoagulated, the procedure is aborted, and the patient is begun on therapeutic anticoagulation, if no contraindications exist. This patient can return in 8 to 12 weeks for retrieval, allowing for autolysis of the thrombus. If there are device-related time constraints, the filter may be left as a permanent device.

Small trapped thrombi seen during retrieval in anticoagulated patients may be removed (<25% of the depth of the cone) with the filter. Again, later retrieval may be considered, or the device may be left in as a permanent device (Box 2 and Figure 5).

Filter Retrieval Technique

A preoperative lower extremity duplex ultrasonography is performed to exclude the occurrence of a new DVT or the extension of an existing DVT. Anesthesia is provided as local (1% lidocaine), local with sedation, or general anesthesia depending on the patient. Venous access is device specific. The majority of available optional VCFs are retrieved via the jugular approach; however, the OPTEASE (Cordis, Bridgewater, NJ) is retrieved via a femoral approach. Prior to attempted retrieval, imaging of the filter within the vena cava is performed. This is done to identify the presence or absence of trapped thrombus and to determine the orientation of the filter to aid in the retrieval technique.

The filter is either snared using a gooseneck or other type snare (Figure 6), or it is grasped with a cone-type device and withdrawn into an introducer sheath and removed from the field. It is important to document whether the filter is intact. A postremoval contrast image of the vena cava is performed to examine the integrity of the vena cava.

SUMMARY

VTE continues to impact health care providers of all disciplines. Much deserved attention has been directed to this disease as highlighted by its incorporation as a process measure of the Surgical

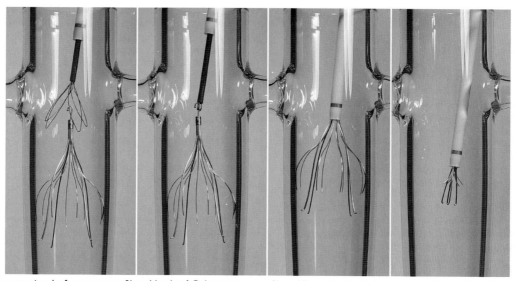

FIGURE 6   Snare retrieval of a vena cava filter. Hook of Celect vena cava filter (Cook Medical) snared and collapsed by advancement of sheath.

Care Improvement Project (SCIP) sponsored by the Centers for Medicare and Medicaid Services. Although the standard treatment and prevention of DVT and PE remains systemic anticoagulation, vena cava filters have proven efficacy in the reduction of VTE-related mortality.

SUGGESTED READINGS

Kaufman JA, Kinney TB, Streiff MB, et al: Guidelines for the use of retrievable and convertible vena cava filters: report from the Society of Interventional Radiology multidisciplinary consensus conference, *World J Surg* 31:251–264, 2007.

Paton BL, Jacobs DG, Heniford BT, et al: Nine-year experience with insertion of vena cava filters in the intensive care unit, *Am J Surg* 192:795–800, 2006.

Schmelzer TM, Christmas AB, Taylor DA, et al: Vena cava filter retrieval in therapeutically anticoagulated patients, *Am J Surg* 196:944–947, 2008.

Sing RF, Camp SM, Heniford BT, et al: Timing of pulmonary emboli after trauma: implications for retrievable vena cava filters, *J Trauma* 60:732–735, 2006.

Sing RF, Rogers FB, Novitsky YM, Heniford BT: Optional vena cava filters for patients with high thromboembolic risk: questions to be answered, *Surg Innov* 12:195–202, 2005.

Stefanidis D, Paton BL, Jacobs DG, et al: Extended retrieval of vena cava filters is safe and may maximize protection against pulmonary embolism, *Am J Surg* 192:789–794, 2006.

THROMBOSIS PROPHYLAXIS IN GENERAL SURGERY

Joseph A. Caprini, MD

OVERVIEW

Venous thromboembolism (VTE) is a serious problem that has been unrecognized by the public and medical profession alike. It is not widely known that the Surgeon General announced a call to action against VTE in 2008. It has been estimated that as many as 300,000 people die each year in the United States from pulmonary embolus (PE), which is astonishing compared to the 40,000 deaths each year from breast cancer and the 15,000 patients who die from AIDS yearly. One third of the deaths from PE present as sudden death, and one third of these occur after hospital discharge. PE is associated with a 1-year mortality rate of 39% in the elderly; deep vein thrombosis (DVT) has a 1-year mortality rate of 21% in the elderly. It has been estimated that VTE is the number one preventable cause of death in hospitalized patients. At least 4% of patients who survive PE will have pulmonary hypertension that may limit their physical activities and lifestyle.

THE MANY FACES OF VENOUS THROMBOEMBOLISM

The incidence of VTE in general surgery averages 20% to 40% depending upon various risk factors, the most important being malignancy. The vast majority of these factors (90%) are asymptomatic, which can create a false sense of security among surgeons and lessen their zeal for providing anticoagulant prophylaxis perioperatively. Most surgeons are much more aware of and fearful of postoperative hemorrhage, which can result in serious consequences including reoperation, infection, or rarely a fatality. Actual statistics about bleeding in over 13,000 patients from approximately 70 clinical trials worldwide involving surgical patients treated with heparin or assigned to a placebo group show no difference in bleeding deaths. On the other hand, the incidence of fatal PE in these patients is reduced by 60% in those receiving anticoagulants compared to the control group. Almost 60% of those who die from massive PE have no preliminary warning signs or clinically evident DVT.

Although the prevention of clinically evident or fatal VTE is an important issue, it is by no means the only reason why thrombosis prophylaxis in surgical patients is so important. Postthrombotic syndrome (PTS) is a significant health condition that can affect the quality of life of patients months or years after a DVT. It is estimated that 25% to 30% of those with a past DVT will develop some form of this syndrome, and 7% will be permanently disabled with this disorder. It is a life-long problem that affects over 10 million Americans, and it cannot be cured, only controlled. The clinical manifestations of this disorder may include leg pain, aching, tiredness, and swelling. Typically these symptoms increase as the day progresses, and the signs and symptoms worsen over time. Varicose veins and chronic skin changes, including ulceration, can develop. In advanced cases, lymphedema can also occur, making these limbs very susceptible to infection; the resulting cellulitis often requires hospitalization and intravenous antibiotic treatment.

Lifelong treatment involving heavy compression stockings, bandages, and other appliances is required to control the symptoms and prevent the progression of this disorder. A common treatment error is to treat these symptoms with antiembolism stockings with a pressure of 18 mm Hg at the ankle. Effective treatment includes the prevention of swelling and often requires compression pressures of 40 mm Hg or more. The use of effective stockings beginning when the DVT is diagnosed can decrease the incidence of postthrombotic syndrome by 50%. It would be very unusual for a surgeon to see postthrombotic changes in patients previously operated on, because the lag time may be great between the DVT and the onset of PTS symptoms. Surgeons working in large referral centers rarely even see the VTE cases because the majority of events occur following hospital discharge. A large, worldwide database recently reported that over 70% of VTE events occur following hospital discharge, and 55% of these events occur after the anticoagulants are stopped.

Another frequently overlooked manifestation of VTE is paradoxic stroke resulting from temporary enlargement of a patent foramen ovale (PFO) between the right and left atria. Such strokes occur when a clot breaks off from the legs or pelvis and travels to the right heart, producing dilatation of the atrium. This temporarily enlarges a PFO, and the clot enters the systemic circulation, commonly traveling to the brain and resulting in a nonhemorrhagic stroke. Once the clot travels into the systemic circulation, the heart and PFO return to normal size. Autopsy studies have indicated that 25% of the population have a nonfunctioning PFO, and the incidence in those with nonhemorrhagic stroke is 50% or more.

Patients having general surgical procedures often have silent thrombi, and statistics show that if such a person undergoes a subsequent surgical procedure, the risk of developing another DVT is over 60%. On the basis of these data, it is imperative that the surgeon inquire about a past VTE history or family VTE history as an essential part of the preoperative evaluation. With the advent of advanced imaging techniques in recent years, it has been popular to place less emphasis on the history and physical exam. This is a dangerous practice, and every surgeon is urged to develop their investigation skills. When these facts are uncovered, further preoperative studies may be necessary, and the approach to prophylaxis must be intensified according to the situation. Most of all, informing the patient about increased risks in the face of a past or family history of VTE is an important facet of the informed-consent process. An occasion may arise when the decision whether to perform a procedure that improves quality of life may rest on the relative risk of serious or fatal VTE.

RISK ASSESSMENT AS A GUIDE TO THROMBOSIS PROPHYLAXIS

It has become popular to classify the VTE risk according to patient groups and according to the type of surgery. This approach is favored by the CHEST consensus guidelines that summarize the results of clinical trials and make recommendations for thrombosis prophylaxis. Their conclusions only apply to patients that fit the inclusion and exclusion criteria used in the trials. Unfortunately, many of the common clinical situations seen in practice do not fit the guidelines. In these cases the unique individual risk factors of a given patient need to be identified, and prophylaxis is selected based on the relative VTE risk for that situation. A low-risk laparoscopic procedure in a patient with multiple risk factors can be associated with a degree of risk comparable to that of a patient undergoing a major cancer operation. The level of risk will dictate the choice of modalities—physical, pharmacologic, or both—and the onset, strength, and duration of prophylaxis.

The degree of risk may justify sending the patient home with injectable anticoagulants for a month or more, depending on the level of risk. One system to aid in this process is the use of a risk assessment tool that was derived by assigning a relative weight to each risk factor based on the likelihood of that factor to result in a thrombotic event. A study was recently completed in 8216 surgical patients using this tool to compare the admission risk score with the 30-day clinically relevant VTE incidence. A linear relationship was found between the score and the 30-day VTE incidence. Based on these data, a thrombosis prophylaxis plan can be tailored for each patient.

In the past these data have been hard to collect, but the current research indicates that administrative data in conjunction with the electronic medical record can be used to calculate the score. The approach was further validated by individual questioning of 1500 patients by physician assistants preoperatively. Both approaches agreed, showing the linear relationship between score and proven VTE; Figure 1 shows this relationship.

A 35-year-old having a routine laparoscopic cholecystectomy for biliary colic without other risk factors has a score of 2 with an expected VTE incidence at 30 days of 0.70%. The risk of any bleeding using an anticoagulant for this patient is 1%. The use of appropriately fitted and properly used intermittent pneumatic compression devices (IPC) for the legs is associated with a 95% efficacy and no bleeding risk. The clinican may choose the mechanical method (IPC), because the risk of bleeding exceeds the risk of clinically significant VTE. On the other hand, if a 42-year-old patient with a past history of VTE, body mass index of 32, and taking birth control pills has the same operative procedure, the score is 8, which is associated with an anticipated 2.5% VTE incidence at 30 days. This patient should receive anticoagulant and mechanical prophylaxis during hospitalization and 30 days of postoperative anticoagulant prophylaxis.

METHODS OF PROPHYLAXIS

Mechanical methods of prophylaxis include antiembolism stockings that may be thigh- or calf-high with an average ankle pressure of 18 mm Hg. They were once widely used in the early days of prophylaxis, and some studies demonstrate their efficacy compared with no prophylaxis. No venographic data are available to demonstrate efficacy, and a recent trial in the stroke population failed to demonstrate any VTE differences compared with usual care without any prophylaxis. On the other hand, a recent prospective randomized controlled trial demonstrated the effectiveness of IPC alone, as well as IPC in combination with an anticoagulant, in general surgery patients. This trial was conducted at 40 U.S. centers, and the end point was a bilateral venogram at day 7 or sooner if clinical symptoms of DVT appeared. More than 800 evaluable patients were available for the final analysis, and only one clinical event occurred in each group. Of patients in the IPC-only group, 5.3% had positive venograms compared with 1.7% in the combination-prophylaxis group. This study demonstrated the value of IPC both alone and in conjunction with fondaparinux. These results can be used to justify IPC alone in low-risk patients and combined prophylaxis in the highest risk patients. There are no venographic data for stockings, and on this basis, I do not agree with the CHEST guidelines that fail to differentiate among the physical

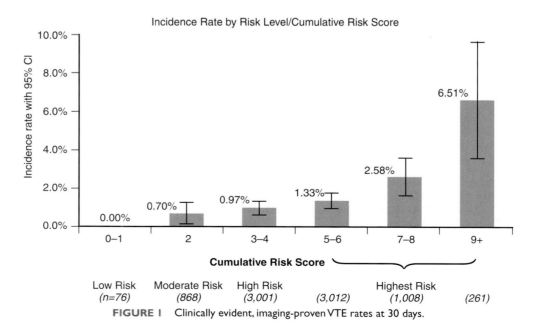

FIGURE I   Clinically evident, imaging-proven VTE rates at 30 days.

methods. Similar vein studies have shown the foot pump to be inferior to IPC when tested in a randomized trial. There is no evidence to suggest that long leg stockings or IPC is superior to the equivalent calf device. There is also no evidence to suggest that adding stockings to IPC increases efficacy. Finally, for IPC to be effective, it has to be properly used, and compliance must be ensured.

The use of small doses of unfractionated heparin (UFH) to prevent VTE was first demonstrated in a trial involving 4,000 patients in 28 medical centers in the United Kingdom over 35 years ago. The use of heparin cut the DVT rate from nearly 30% in the controls to less than 10% in the treated group. Fatal pulmonary emboli were reduced by 50% in the treated group compared with the controls. What is remarkable is the meta-analysis by Collins 15 years later, in which he analyzed 70 more trials in over 13,000 patients and found results equivalent to the original trial from the United Kingdom.

The refinement of UFH over the past 25 years has resulted in a number of low molecular weight heparins (LMWHs) that have a longer half-life and greater bioavailability than UFH. They require no routine monitoring and have an incidence of heparin-induced thrombocytopenia of 0.2% compared with 2.6% with UFH. A number of studies have shown these compounds to be beneficial in cancer patients and under certain circumstances to prolong survival in these patients. Furthermore a recent trial of more than 23,000 patients has shown that UFH and LMWH both reduce the rate of fatal PE in surgical patients to 0.15%. There also have been three trials that show the reduction of VTE when patients having abdominal surgery for cancer are given 30 days of LMWH compared to 7 days of prophylaxis. On this basis, 30 days of LMWH prophylaxis is advised for patients following abdominal surgery for cancer.

The issue regarding initiation of anticoagulation preoperatively or postoperatively is an ongoing debate. In general the bleeding risk is increased with preoperative compared with postoperative start of anticoagulation. Efficacy is similar for both approaches, and some feel that administration of the first dose is the most important factor—using prophylaxis for the entire time the patient is at risk appears to be the most important concept, which means continuing the anticoagulation following hospital discharge in many cases.

SUMMARY

Individual risk assessment is the key to providing the best thrombosis prophylaxis for all patients. This is critical, because VTE is the number one preventable cause of death in the hospital setting. Capturing all of

the VTE risk factors and scoring them provides a guide for selection of the type, duration, and intensity of prophylaxis. The score reflects the anticipated 30-day clinical VTE incidence. These data can be used by the clinician to provide appropriate informed consent, particularly for operations to improve quality of life. The score can also be used to recommend the use of combined modalities for inpatients. Most importantly the score can identify patients likely to benefit from extended out-of-hospital prophylaxis. Finally, in patients with low scores, the 30-day VTE incidence is less than the clinically significant bleeding rate using anticoagulants. In these situations the use of appropriate leg IPC devices may provide efficacy as shown in the recent clinical trial using IPCs. Attention to the proper use of these devices, including compliance, is mandatory if this option is selected.

Postoperative VTE remains an important cause of morbidity and mortality. Pharmacologic prophylaxis with LMWH or fondaparinux is effective and safe, but it is underused in many high-risk surgical patients. The burden of postoperative VTE outweighs the risk of bleeding complications, and the use of the validated-risk score can indicate which patients require prophylaxis and which should be continued for 7 to 30 days, depending upon the level of risk.

SUGGESTED READINGS

Bahl V, Hu H, Henke PK, et al: A validation study of a retrospective venous thromboembolism risk-scoring method, *Ann Surg* 251:344–350, 2009.

Borow M, Goldson HJ: Prevention of postoperative deep venous thrombosis and pulmonary emboli with combined modalities, *Am Surg* 49:599–605, 1983.

Collins R, Scrimgeour A, Yusuf S, Peto R: Reduction in fatal pulmonary embolism and venous thrombosis by perioperative administration of subcutaneous heparin: overview of results of randomized trials in general, orthopedic, and urologic surgery, *N Engl J Med* 318:1162–1173l, 1988.

Geerts WH, Pineo GF, Heit JA: Prevention of venous thromboembolism: the Eighth ACCP Conference on Antithrombotic and Thrombolytic Therapy, *Chest* 133:381S–453S, 2008.

Kakkar V, Corrigan TP, Fossard DP, et al: Prevention of fatal postoperative pulmonary embolism by low doses of heparin: an international multicentre trial, *Lancet* 2:45–51, 1975.

Prandoni P, Lensing AW, Prins MH, et al: Below-knee elastic compression stockings to prevent the postthrombotic syndrome: a randomized, controlled trial, *Ann Int Med* 141:249–256, 2004.

Turpie AG, Bauer KA, Caprini JA, et al: Fondaparinux combined with intermittent pneumatic compression vs. intermittent pneumatic compression alone for prevention of venous thromboembolism after abdominal surgery: a randomized, double-blind comparison, *J Thromb Haemost* 5:1854–1861, 2007.

LYMPHEDEMA

**Mazen I. Bedri, MD, Gedge D. Rosson, MD,
Ariel N. Rad, MD, PhD, and Jaime I. Flores, MD**

PATHOPHYSIOLOGY

Lymphedema is a therapeutically challenging condition caused by lymphatic dysfunction that results in the accumulation of protein-rich fluid in the interstitium of extremities or other anatomic regions. The high content of protein distinguishes lymphedema from other etiologies of edema and contributes to the often progressive nature of the disease. Whereas the venous capillary system is responsible for

90% of the return of interstitial fluid into circulation, the lymphatic system handles the return of the largest macromolecules and their associated fluid. Reduced lymphatic uptake capacity causes a net increase in the amount of interstitial proteins and fluid.

As the condition progresses, increasing dilatation of the remaining functional lymphatics causes valvular incompetence and reversal of flow; lymphatic walls undergo fibrosis, and fibrinoid thrombi ultimately obliterate the remaining patent channels. Stasis of interstitial proteins leads to an inflammatory response, with macrophages and fibroblasts replacing supple, elastic interstitium with fibrosclerotic, thickened, congested tissues. Soft, pitting edema gives way to induration, hypertrophy of adipose deposits, acanthosis, hyperkeratosis, and skin breakdown. Infectious complications often ensue, with recurrent bouts of cellulitis and lymphangitis. Rarely, chronic lymphedema degenerates into a highly aggressive lymphangiosarcoma, known as *Stewart-Treves syndrome*. A consensus on the staging of lymphedema has been published by the International Society of Lymphology (Box 1).

ETIOLOGY

Lymphedema may be classified as either primary or secondary by etiology. *Primary lymphedema* is the result of a developmental abnormality, although often with delayed manifestations. *Secondary lymphedema* is acquired and results from disease, trauma, or iatrogenic causes.

Primary etiologies are further divided into categories according to the age of onset of symptoms. *Congenital lymphedema,* or Milroy disease, includes all forms that present within the first 2 years of life, representing 10% to 25% of all primary cases. Typically, it affects females, with bilateral lower extremity involvement. Often the lymphedema is not progressive, and it may improve spontaneously with age. *Lymphedema praecox,* or Meige disease, typically presents at puberty (by definition, before age 35 years) and represents 65% to 85% of primary lymphedema cases. Females are predominantly affected, with unilateral lower extremity involvement. *Lymphedema tarda* presents spontaneously after the age of 35 years and is the rarest form of primary lymphedema, again typically affecting females. Table 1 describes demographics and typical presentations of the three forms of primary lymphedema.

Secondary lymphedema represents an acquired dysfunction of normally developed lymphatics. Worldwide, the most common cause is infection by the nematode *Wuchereria bancrofti,* spread by mosquitoes. Adult filarial worms reside in and obstruct lymphatic channels, causing irreversible scarring and fibrosis and often massive edema. In the United States and other developed nations, nearly all causes of secondary lymphedema are related to malignancies and their therapies. Mainstays of cancer treatment—such as tumor extirpation, radiation therapy, and lymphadenectomy—are related to higher rates of lymphedema. Other risk factors including trauma, infection, and obesity are considered to contribute to secondary lymphedema (Figure 1).

DIAGNOSIS

The workup for lymphedema starts with thorough history and physical examination. Other causes for edema must be ruled out, including cardiac, venous, renal, and hepatic etiologies and compressive or occlusive vascular syndromes. Lymphangioscintigraphy is currently

the imaging gold standard for patients in whom these secondary etiologies are not suspected. Magnetic resonance imaging and computed tomography are also useful in lymphatic visualization and may help to rule out suspicions of associated malignancy. Although imaging studies may be of some value, the majority of patients can be diagnosed without additional confirmatory testing.

TREATMENT

Conservative Management

This discussion of lymphedema treatments focuses on nonparasitic etiologies. Conservative therapies are directed at the reduction of proteinaceous interstitial fluid, thereby stemming the cycles of edema, inflammation, and fibrosis. Mainstays of conservative modalities include hygiene management, compression and elevation, physical therapy, and long-term compliance. Treatments are often time intensive and inconvenient, and patient compliance is a necessary component of any regimen.

Basic lifestyle modifications are essential in managing the sequelae of lymphedema. Hygeine and skin care are important to reduce skin breakdown and resulting infection. Patients should be encouraged to lose weight if obese, to address minor skin traumas and breakdown appropriately, and to avoid constrictive clothing.

Compression therapies range widely and include graduated compression garments, multilayered inelastic bandaging, and controlled compression therapy, and compression garments are refitted as swelling decreases. These methods reduce the volume of excess edema by approximately 30% to 45%. External sequential compressive devices have also been used with variable success. Compression therapies are typically combined with elevation of the affected extremity whenever feasible.

Physical therapy, specifically decongestive lymphatic therapy, is a more time-intensive treatment strategy. This modality emphasizes manual lymphatic drainage via massage, compressive garments, and exercise. Numerous protocols exist for such therapies, which operate on the belief that these methods reduce edema by augmenting lymphatic contractility and increasing lymphatic flow. Studies vary as to whether lymphatic massage therapy leads to improved outcomes as compared to compression garments or bandaging alone.

The success of conservative strategies varies widely, in part because of differences among patient populations and individual patients. However, patient compliance plays a significant role in outcomes as well; discomfort or embarrassment associated with compression garments or the inconvenience of physical therapy may limit outcomes. Thus it is important to communicate with the patient, to stress that individual investment and long-term compliance in therapies is central to managing this chronic, incurable condition.

Pharmacologically, antibiotics are valuable in treating recurrent infections that range from superficial infections to more serious cases of cellulitis or lymphangitis. Beyond antibiotics, however, pharmacologic therapies play a limited role in the management of lymphedema. Benzopyrenes are thought to increase lymphatic uptake of peptides through proteolysis of interstitial proteins, facilitating absorption into the bloodstream. Literature demonstrates conflicting results with respect to benzopyrene usage, and documented hepatotoxicity limits long-term therapy. Diuretics have been used historically, but with only limited benefit, and they may actually lead to increased interstitial protein accumulation and fibrosis. Studies examining the use of nutritional supplements, such as sodium selenite or vitamin E with pentoxifylline, have not demonstrated any significant benefit in patients with lymphedema.

Surgical Treatment

Surgery is an adjunct to primary conservative therapy in refractory cases, but the surgical indications for lymphedema are not absolute. Surgery is usually reserved for moderate to severe lymphedema, and

TABLE 1: Primary lymphedema classifications

Classification	Age of Onset	Gender Predilection	Presentation	Genetics
Congenital (Milroy disease)	Birth to 2 yr	F/M = 2:1	Predominantly lower extremity involvement, usually bilateral	Autosomal dominant inheritance
			May involve GI tract, intestinal lymphagiectasias, cholestasis	*FLT4*, tyrosine receptor kinase signaling pathway in lymphatics
			Anaplastic lymphatic trunks	
Praecox (Meige disease)	15 to 35 yr	F/M = 4:1	Predominantly lower extremity involvement, usually unilateral	Autosomal-dominant inheritance
			Associated anomalies may include vertebral defects, cerebrovascular malformations, distichiasis, yellow nails, sensorineural hearing loss, cleft palate	*FOXC2*, involved in adipocyte metabolism
			Hypoplastic peripheral lymphatics	*FLT4*
Tarda	>35 yr	F > M	Spontaneous onset	*FOXC2*
			Typically lower extremity involvement	
			Hyperplastic histologic pattern, large tortuous lymphatics with absent/incompetent valves	

F/M, Female/male ratio

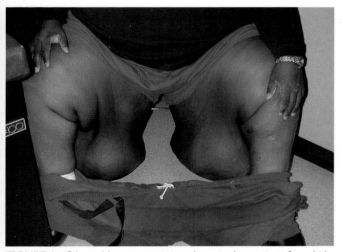

FIGURE 1 Bilateral lower extremity edema in the setting of morbid obesity.

its goal is long-term remission and improvement in quality of life. A number of variables are taken into account during assessment. Relative indications include size and weight of the patient, extent of lymphedema, recurrent lymphangitis, lymphorrhagia, abscess, fistula, diminished quality of life, worsening comorbidities, and, most importantly, failure of conservative management. Documentation with photographs, limb measurements, functional assessments, and radiology is paramount. Patient compliance and overall health are crucial to the success of any operation.

There is no single surgical procedure for all classifications of lymphedema. The two general categories of surgical therapy are *debulking* and *physiologic procedures*. It is critical to remember that conservative therapy such as lifestyle modifications, proper hygiene, and compressive therapies should be continued immediately following any surgical procedures, as these surgical procedures are clearly adjuncts to the above.

BOX 2: Charles procedure

1. Mark the lymphedematous area both proximally and distally.
2. Make an incision both medially and laterally down to the muscle fascia.
3. Excise all the tissue superficial to this plane.
4. Remove the skin of the affected area with a dermatome for a split-thickness graft or with a knife for a full-thickness graft. If a full-thickness graft, make sure to remove all the fat from the skin.
5. Use this graft to cover the exposed area.
6. Apply petroleum gauze or other nonadherent dressing over the graft.
7. Apply a pressure dressing via a vacuum-assisted device, bolster, or cotton.
8. Splint the extremity in the proper anatomic position.
9. Remove dressing after 3 to 5 days for a split-thickness graft or after 7 to 12 days for a full-thickness graft.

Debulking Procedures

The Charles procedure (1912), a radical excision technique, removes all skin and subcutaneous tissue down to the muscle fascia. Excised skin is used for grafting on the fascia. Refer to Box 2 for description of the procedure. The Van der Walt modification allows for negative-pressure dressing with grafting done in a delayed fashion. The surgery is indicated for severe cases and carries a high risk of complications, including but not limited to infection, ulceration, hyperpigmentation, dermatitis, and a severe altered aesthetic outcome (Figure 2).

The Sistrunk procedure (1918) is a planned, staged excision of affected subcutaneous tissues. This technique has been modified over the last 80 years and incorporates burying dermal flaps within the skin flaps. Refer to Box 3 for description of the procedure. Long-term

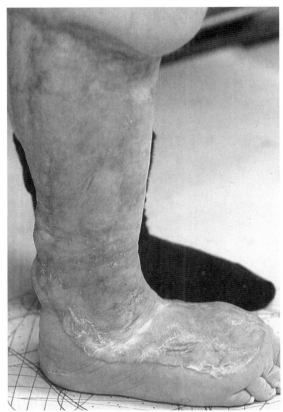

FIGURE 2   Lower extremity after Charles procedure.

BOX 3: Sistrunk procedure

1. Mark out the affected area.
2. Plan to excise and debulk sufficient tissue, leaving dermal flaps to bury beneath the skin in the closure. A variation of this is carried out in the Thompson procedure, in which dermal flaps are buried beneath the muscle.
3. Close the incision over drains.
4. Allow 12 weeks to heal before the next serial excision.

BOX 4: Liposuction

1. Mark out affected area and 2 cm beyond.
2. Choose port sites to effectively reach all areas, both proximally and distally.
3. Inject tumescent solution (1 L Ringer's lactate mixed with 1 mL ampule of epinephrine 1:1000 and 30 mL of 1% lidocaine). until blanching is achieved and a moderate amount of turgor is seen.
4. Wait 30 to 45 minutes.
5. Suction with a 4 to 6 mm canula in a deep plane in all areas, followed by a 2 to 3 mm canula in a more superficial plane for a smoother contour.
6. Close port sites with absorbable suture.
7. Apply sterile dressings and a pressure garment.
8. Advise the patient not to shower or remove the pressure garment for 72 hours, and encourage the patient to walk at least three times a day.
9. After 3 days, the patient can shower daily and may begin massaging the affected areas.
10. The pressure garment should be worn for 6 to 10 weeks.

BOX 5: Microsurgical lymphovenous shunt

1. Begin with lymphatic and venous scintigraphy.
2. Inject lymphozurin into the web space in the distal extremity.
3. Take postobstruction dissection down to venous and lymphatic channels.
4. Use microsurgical connection to reestablish lymph flow directly or using a vein graft.
5. Insert a Penrose nonsuction drain.
6. Evaluate postoperative flow and imaging studies.

BOX 6: Vascularized nodal transplantation

1. Palpate femoral pulse and design skin paddle lateral to pulse, inferior and parallel to the inguinal ligament.
2. Take dissection of the flap from distal to proximal, harvesting the superficial fibronodal tissue with the superficial circumflex iliac vessels.
3. Make a transverse incision on the wrist, and perform microvascular anastomosis to the radial artery and vein.
4. Use a skin paddle for monitoring.

results can achieve a reduction of at least half of the affected tissue in 75% of patients. It is safe, reliable, and predictable. Complications include nerve damage in the affected area, epidermolysis secondary to poor blood supply, wound dehiscence, and infection.

Liposuction was first used for brachial lymphedema in 1987 and was refined in 1993; it is now a useful adjunct for treatment. Liposuction is safe, quick, and allows for an immediate decrease in volume and pressure of the lymph fluid, promoting better lymphatic flow. Brorson of Sweden reports a complete reduction with no recurrence in his 15 year experience. Risks include lidocaine toxicity, thrombotic and fat emboli, hematoma, seroma, and contour irregularities. It has been used alone or in addition to other debulking procedures. Refer to Box 4 for a description of the procedure.

Physiologic Procedures

The main aim of physiologic procedures is to improve lymphatic flow and drainage. Omental flaps, enteromesenteric bridging, dermal flaps, and lymphangioplasty have all been attempted with minimal to no success. Microvascular lymphovenous shunts and nodal transplantation are new therapies that are showing promising results.

Microvascular lymphovenous shunts were first introduced in 1953 by Sherman and colleagues. Over the decades microsurgery has evolved and is now being used more to relieve postobstructive lymphedema. A more recent study describes Campisi's experience in treating over 800 patients who had failed previous conservative therapies, with an average follow-up of 7 years. Over 80% of patients undergoing microsurgical lymphovenous shunting experienced significant reduction of excess volume (67% on average), with an even greater reduction in the incidence of cellulitis. Results were stable by both volumetric assessment and lymphoscintigraphy. Refer to Box 5 for a description of the technique.

Vascular nodal transplantation has had several successful animal studies, those in rats by Shesol in 1979 and again by Chen in 1990. This technique harvests vascularized fat and nodal tissue from the groin and transplants it to the distal upper extremity via microvascular anastomoses to the radial artery and vein. This technique demonstrates improvements including decreased size, increased skin elasticity, decreased infection, increased lymphatic flow, increased lymphatic pathways toward the flap site, and most importantly, discontinued use of physiotherapy. Refer to Box 6 for a description of the technique.

SUMMARY

Lymphedema remains a challenging clinical problem with significant morbidities. Treatment includes early implementation of long-term conservative measures along with surgical procedures for more difficult cases. Patient commitment and lifestyle modifications are central to the success of any therapeutic regimen.

SUGGESTED READINGS

Becker C, Assouad J, Riquet M, Hidden G: Postmastectomy lymphedema: long-term results following microsurgical lymph node transplantation, *Ann Surg* 243(3):313–315, 2006.

Brorson H, Ohlin K, Olsson G, et al: Controlled compression and liposuction treatment for lower extremity lymphedema, *Lymphology* 41(2):52–63, 2008.

Campisi C, Davini D, Bellini C, et al: Lymphatic microsurgery for the treatment of lymphedema, *Microsurgery* 26(1):65–69, 2006.

International Society of Lymphology: The diagnosis and treatment of peripheral lymphedema: 2009 Consensus Document of the International Society of Lymphology, *Lymphology* 42(2):51–60, 2009.

Warren AG, Brorson H, Borud LJ, Slavin SA: Lymphedema: a comprehensive review, *Ann Plast Surg* 59(4):464–472, 2007.

TRAUMA AND EMERGENCY CARE

INITIAL EVALUATION AND RESUSCITATION OF THE TRAUMA PATIENT

Philbert Y. Van, MD, and Martin A. Schreiber, MD

PREHOSPITAL

Care of trauma patients begins well before their arrival in the emergency department. Regionalization of trauma care to specialized hospitals and the creation of an efficient transport system that delivers patients to the most appropriate facility have been shown to improve mortality after trauma. These are the most important characteristics of effective trauma systems. Care starts with the first responder, emergency medical technician, or paramedic at the scene. These prehospital providers must be adequately trained in airway management, control of hemorrhage, and rapid patient transport. In addition, critical information regarding the mechanism of injury and details from the scene—such as a bent steering wheel, significant vehicle intrusion, starred windshield (Figure 1)—should be communicated to the receiving hospital and can help with the process of triage and mobilization of resources that may include a neurosurgeon, orthopedic surgeon, interventional radiologist, and operating room staff.

IN THE HOSPITAL

Once the patient arrives in the emergency department, he or she should be evaluated in a designated resuscitation area, which should be stocked with all necessary equipment for expeditious evaluation and treatment of trauma patients. At a minimum, airway and intubation equipment, warmed intravenous fluids, and monitoring and basic imaging capabilities should be available (Figure 2). Personal protective gear should be worn by all personnel who come in contact with patients.

Primary Survey

Life-threatening conditions are identified and treated during the primary survey. Treatment priorities are established in a logical and sequential fashion designed to maximize the likelihood of survival. Problems that are most likely to result in death are addressed first. The ABCs of trauma begin with *airway, breathing, circulation, disability,* and *exposure.*

Airway

If the patient is able to communicate verbally, the airway is patent and not likely to require urgent intervention to maintain. Frequent reassessment should be performed, as patients with head injury may undergo a progressive decline in mental status, placing the airway in jeopardy. If the patient has an altered level of consciousness or a Glasgow Coma Score (GCS) of 8 or less, more definitive airway management is required. Because of possible injury to the cervical spine (C-spine), the airway must be managed with in-line immobilization. The jaw-thrust maneuver should be used to open the airway by moving the mandible forward, avoiding hyperextension of C1/C2 and hyperflexion of C5/C6. In cases where there is low suspicion of basilar skull fracture, an oropharyngeal or nasopharyngeal airway or, more definitively, an endotracheal tube can be placed. Rapid-sequence intubation is most commonly performed in trauma patients because of the risk of aspiration secondary to a full stomach. Succinylcholine and etomidate are commonly used for this purpose. In some situations, endotracheal intubation may not be possible, and a surgical airway must be provided (Figure 3). Cricothyroidotomy is performed by making a midline vertical incision directly over the cricothyroid membrane, between the thyroid and cricoid cartilage. The incision is carried through the underlying fat, fascia, and cricothyroid membrane, and a cuffed 6.0 mm endotracheal tube can be placed.

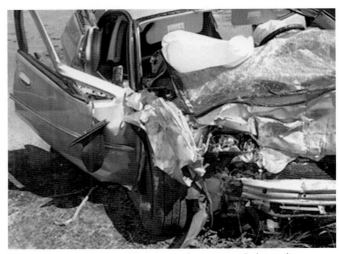

FIGURE 1   Information from the crash scene can help predict potential injuries and help the trauma team prepare for the incoming patient.

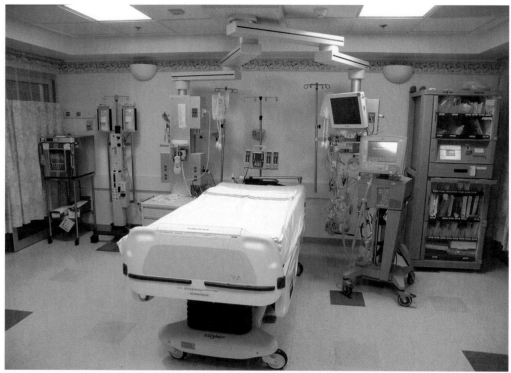

FIGURE 2   Resuscitation area with basic monitoring equipment, ventilator, prewarmed intravenous fluids, and rapid infuser.

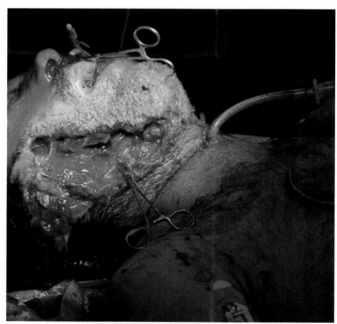

FIGURE 3   Severe facial injuries requiring cricothyroidotomy to secure airway.

Breathing

The establishment of a definitive airway does not ensure adequate ventilation, which can be assessed during the primary survey by noting the number and depth of chest wall movements. Auscultation, percussion, and palpation of the chest wall in conjunction with visualization of the neck veins will allow for the diagnosis of tension

pneumothorax, open pneumothorax, and flail chest. The presence of decreased breath sounds, contralateral deviation of the trachea (late sign), and distended neck veins are signs of a tension pneumothorax. Tension and open pneumothorax should be treated immediately with tube thoracostomy placement. If tension pneumothorax is suspected, and a chest tube cannot be placed immediately, a large-bore needle should be placed in the second intercostal space in the midclavicular line. In patients with hemothorax, if greater than 1,500 mL of blood is immediately evacuated with tube thoracostomy placement, the patient should be taken to the operating room emergently for a thoracotomy to locate and repair the source of hemorrhage. Ongoing output of 200 mL per hour for 2 to 4 consecutive hours is also an indication for thoracotomy.

Circulation

Because hemorrhage is the leading cause of preventable death after injury, it is important to identify and control external bleeding during the primary survey. Rapid bleeding should be controlled by direct compression. Advanced hemostatic dressings that contain kaolin (derived from clay) or chitosan (derived from shrimp shells) can be used in conjunction with direct compression to stop bleeding. (Figure 4). These dressings have been used in the military setting and are available for civilian use. Bleeding from extremities that cannot be controlled with direct compression or hemostatic dressings should be treated with a tourniquet for temporary control prior to definitive repair in the operating room.

Another aspect of evaluating circulation is to ensure the patient has adequate blood volume to restore and maintain tissue perfusion. Intravenous access with two large-bore peripheral intravenous lines should be achieved. Hypotension, hypothermia, weak or absent peripheral pulses, and decreasing level of consciousness are all signs of hypovolemic shock. The volume of fluid infused should be adequate to restore perfusion. Excessive crystalloid resuscitation prior to definitive hemorrhage control is associated with displacement of established clots, dilution of coagulation factors, hypothermia,

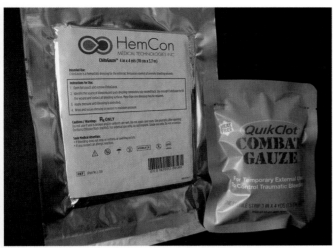

FIGURE 4 Chitosan-impregnated and kaolin-impregnated gauze dressings used to accelerate hemorrhage control.

TABLE 1: Glasgow Coma Scale

Eye Opening	Points	Verbal Response	Points	Motor Response	Points
Spontaneous	4	Oriented	5	Obeys commands	6
To voice	3	Confused	4	Purposeful movements	5
To pain	2	Inappropriate words	3	Withdraws (pain)	4
None	1	Incomprehensible	2	Flexion (pain)	3
		None	1	Extension (pain)	2
				None	1

activation of dysfunctional inflammation, abdominal compartment syndrome, multiple organ failure, and increased mortality. Mounting evidence suggests that early high-ratio transfusion of plasma and platelets to packed red blood cells is beneficial in patients who subsequently require massive transfusion.

Disability

During this portion of the primary survey, a rapid neurological assessment should be performed. Pupillary size and reaction should be recorded. The patient's spontaneous actions and responses to verbal and painful stimuli should be noted, and a GCS score should be recorded (Table 1). A decreased level of consciousness may have a variety of etiologies, which may include decreased oxygenation or perfusion, brain injury, hypoglycemia or hyperglycemia, and drug or alcohol use.

Exposure

The patient should be undressed and assessed for additional sites of injury. To assess the back, the patient should be logrolled while maintaining spine precautions.

Resuscitation

Resuscitation and management of life-threatening injuries occur simultaneously as they are discovered during the primary survey. If a patient's mental status is declining, or if the airway is compromised, a definitive airway must be secured and maintained, either with an endotracheal tube or surgically. All injured patients should receive supplemental oxygen. As discussed previously, a patient who is hypotensive with decreased breath sounds and suspected pneumothorax should have a chest tube placed without delay.

Flow rate through a tube is directly proportional to the radius of the tube to the fourth power, and it is inversely proportional to tube length; therefore peripheral intravenous (IV) catheters that have a short length and large diameter will provide the highest flow rates. Ideally, a minimum of two large-bore IVs are placed, preferentially in the upper extremities. Advanced Trauma Life Support guidelines advocate initial administration of 1 to 2 L of warmed crystalloid with consideration of blood products if the patient does not respond. Ringer's lactate is the preferred resuscitation fluid, because it is a balanced salt solution that does not contribute to acidosis. The minimal amount of fluid to restore and maintain end-organ perfusion should be infused.

Surrogates to measure end-organ perfusion include the character of the radial pulse and the patient's mental status in the absence of traumatic brain injury. Attempts to resuscitate patients beyond adequate perfusion risk elevating the blood pressure, which may "pop the clot." In combat casuality care, if the patient is alert and has a pulse of normal character, IV fluids are withheld. If the pulse character is weak and thready, or the patient is not alert in the absence of head injury, a 500 mL bolus of IV fluid is given, and the response is assessed.

Next, a decision must be made regarding whether to proceed to the intensive care unit for continued resuscitation, to the operating room for further assessment and treatment, or to the radiology suite for imaging studies.

Secondary Survey

After the primary survey is complete, and resuscitation has begun, a more detailed head-to-toe physical examination should be performed. In this portion of the survey, placement of a urinary catheter, gastric catheter, and radiographic imaging of the chest and pelvis should be considered. During the secondary survey, focused assessment with sonography in trauma (FAST) can also be performed for assessment of abnormal fluid in the peritoneal cavity, pelvis, and pericardium. If the patient decompensates at any time during the primary or secondary survey, the primary survey should be repeated with particular attention given to any intervention that has been performed.

History

Next, a brief history including allergies, medications, past medical and surgical history, last meal, and events/environment related to the injury should be obtained. Prehospital providers are a good source of information regarding the mechanism of injury and can often provide details about the scene. Seat belt use, steering wheel deformation, passenger compartment intrusion, and ejection from the vehicle are all details from the scene that can be used to help predict injury patterns. In penetrating trauma, information about the caliber and velocity of the projectile can help predict the severity of injury.

Head

Inspection and palpation of the head should be performed to assess for lacerations and hematomas that may be obscured by hair. The midface and mandible must also be palpated for instability, as fractures in these areas may contribute to airway compromise. Examination of the

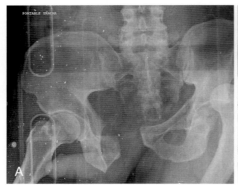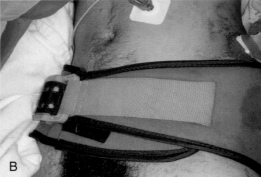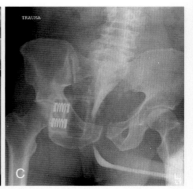

FIGURE 5   Application of external compression device to an open-book pelvic fracture. **B** and **C** show a significant reduction of the fracture with application of the device.

pupils and tympanic membranes should be performed, as abnormalities may suggest intracranial hypertension or basilar skull fracture.

Neck

In-line immobilization should be maintained during examination of the neck. If present, the cervical collar should be removed temporarily during this portion of the examination. Jugular vein distension, tracheal deviation (suggesting tension pneumothorax), and/or presence of ecchymosis and hematoma (suggesting vascular injury) are important findings. Ultrasound or computed tomographic angiography (CTA) should be ordered if a blunt cerebrovascular injury is suspected. The posterior neck can be examined when the patient is logrolled. If maxillofacial instability is discovered during the head examination, the patient should be presumed to have a cervical spine injury. Those with suspected cervical spine injury should receive a CT scan of the neck. Not all patients with cervical spine injury exhibit neurologic deficits. The location of penetrating injuries of the neck are characterized by zones I, II, and III. Zone I includes the horizontal area of the neck from above the clavicles to the level of the cricoid cartilage. The area from the cricoid cartilage to the angle of the mandible is zone II. Zone III begins at the angle of the mandible and ends at the base of the skull. Management is determined by the zone of injury and the stability of the patient. Zone II injuries are more amenable to a surgical approach, because the critical structures in this zone are readily accessible. Access to zone I requires a median sternotomy and may require extension of the incision along the sternocleidomastoid muscle. Zone III exposure may require division of the omohyoid, digastric muscles, and detachment of the sternocleidomastoid from the skull base. Distal control of zone III vascular injuries may be difficult to obtain because of the intracranial location. For these reasons, evaluation of zone I and zone III injuries typically includes esophagoscopy and bronchoscopy with laryngoscopy limited to zone III injuries.

Chest

A variety of chest injuries—rib fractures, flail segments, pneumothorax, and penetrating wounds—can be diagnosed with simple inspection, palpation, and auscultation. A chest radiograph is also helpful in diagnosing aortic injury (widened mediastinum), pulmonary contusion, and confirmation of endotracheal tube, chest tube, and/or central venous catheter placement. Use of ultrasonography during the FAST examination can reveal cardiac injury and possible tamponade. The chest CT is the current gold standard for diagnosis of chest injuries. The sensitivity and specificity are very high for injury to the aorta, heart, lung, and musculoskeletal structures.

Abdomen

It is important to remember that a normal initial examination of the abdomen does not exclude significant injury. The presence of distracting injuries (extremity, rib, and/or pelvic fractures) or a depressed level of consciousness secondary to head injury or intoxication may make it difficult to perform an accurate abdominal examination.

If tenderness accompanied by peritoneal signs is discovered, the patient should be taken to the operating room for exploratory laparotomy. If peritonitis is not found, and the patient is hemodynamically stable, evaluation by CT scan or serial abdominal examinations can be done. Hemodynamically unstable patients with a positive FAST examination or diagnostic peritoneal lavage (DPL) should proceed directly to the operating room for an exploratory laparotomy to locate and repair the source of intraabdominal hemorrhage.

Back

An assessment of the spine and back should be performed with the assistance of a minimum of four people: one to maintain the head and cervical spine alignment, two to logroll the patient, and one to palpate the entire length of the spine for deformities and tenderness. A digital rectal examination should also be considered at this time to assess for rectal injury, pelvic injury (high-riding prostate), and rectal muscular tone. The long backboard can now be removed prior to returning the patient to the supine position.

Pelvis

Rapid identification of pelvic injury is important, as it can be a significant source of hemorrhage. Mobility and tenderness of the pelvis with anterior to posterior compression of the anterior iliac spines on examination suggests the presence of a pelvic ring disruption. Pelvic fractures can also be identified by the presence of ecchymosis and leg-length discrepancy. A pelvic radiograph should be ordered if any of the above findings are present or index of suspicion is high because of the mechanism of injury. If an open-book fracture is seen on pelvic radiograph, and the patient is hemodynamically unstable, there may be a benefit from external compression of the pelvis with a commercially available device or a sheet wrap (Figure 5). These patients may need angioembolization to stop acute hemorrhage. The perineum and vagina should also be examined during this portion of the secondary survey. Hemodynamically stable patients can be evaluated with CT scan, especially if examination of the abdomen is indicated.

Musculoskeletal

All extremities must be inspected and palpated for blunt and penetrating injuries. Each extremity must also be assessed for neurovascular integrity, especially if an obvious deformity is present. Splinting and immobilization of unstable fractures should be performed, followed by reassessment of neurovascular integrity. Splinting increases patient comfort, minimizes secondary injury, and, with restoration of normal anatomy, can restore perfusion of the extremity. Severely injured or ischemic extremities should be assessed for signs and symptoms of compartment syndrome, which include pain out of proportion to injury, palpable tenseness of the compartment, asymmetry, and pain on passive stretch of the muscle. If the patient is hemodynamically stable, radiographs of the injured extremity should be performed.

SUMMARY

The evaluation, treatment, and resuscitation of the trauma patient is a multidisciplinary process that requires a wide spectrum of health care providers and technicians in addition to the trauma surgeon. It is vital that the examination of the injured patient should proceed in a logical, organized fashion as outlined, to discover and treat life-threatening injuries expediently and to avoid missing injuries.

SUGGESTED READINGS

Advanced Trauma Life Support for Doctors, ed 8, Chicago 2008, American College of Surgeons.

Bickell WH, Wall MJ Jr, Pepe PE, et al: Immediate versus delayed fluid resuscitation for hypotensive patients with penetrating torso injuries, *N Engl J Med* 331:1105–1109, 1994.

Holcomb JB, Wade CE, Michalek JE, et al: Increased plasma and platelet to red blood cell ratios improves outcome in 466 massively transfused civilian trauma patients, *Ann Surg* 248:447–458, 2008.

Kreig JC, Mohr M, Ellis TJ, et al: Emergent stabilization of pelvic ring injuries by controlled circumferential compression: a clinical trial, *J Trauma* 59:659–664, 2005.

AIRWAY MANAGEMENT IN THE TRAUMA PATIENT

Kent A. Stevens, MD, MPH, and Elliott R. Haut, MD

OVERVIEW

Evaluation of the airway is the first step in the management of the trauma patient. Airway management, the *A* of the widely used mnemonic *ABCDE*, is critical in the initial evaluation of the trauma patient as outlined in the Advanced Trauma Life Support (ATLS) guidelines. Concomitant injuries, such as cervical spine (C-spine) and traumatic brain injuries found commonly in trauma patients, often complicate the care provider's ability to secure a definitive airway. The trauma care provider must be vigilant in evaluating and, if needed, securing the airway to ensure good patient outcomes.

Failure to secure an adequate airway has been shown to be a significant contributor to mortality in the trauma patient population. In a review of 64 trauma patients with errors that contributed to their death, Gruen and colleagues found airway management errors in 16% of cases the most common cause of preventable death. Traditional means of securing the airway using rapid-sequence induction (RSI) and intubation using the laryngoscope are usually successful in securing the trauma patient's airway. We will review the tools and techniques that the practitioner should be prepared to utilize expeditiously in the patient with a compromised airway.

CLINICAL ASSESSMENT OF THE AIRWAY

The primary survey is used to initially evaluate the trauma patient. The first step in this survey is the evaluation of the airway. In the awake, nonintubated patient, this can be accomplished easily by asking the patient, "What is your name?" If the patient is able to respond, the airway is likely unobstructed. The presence of upper airway stridor, hoarseness, other speech abnormalities, a breathless response, and/or direct facial trauma may indicate an airway problem that may need to be addressed urgently. The chest physical exam basics of *look, listen,* and *feel* should be employed to help determine whether the patient has adequate respiratory effort, and pulse oximetry should be used to monitor oxygen saturations.

In the initial assessment, injuries to the face and neck should be noted. Although officially part of the secondary survey in ATLS, noting the presence and type of injury can raise clinician suspicion for possible airway compromise and can assist in the decision of the type of definitive airway to provide, if one is needed. Both blunt and penetrating trauma can result in direct injury to the airway but also can result in neck hematomas, which can cause airway compromise by extrinsic pressure. Penetrating trauma, particularly if located between the cricoid and the angle of the mandible, is associated with injury to the trachea and larynx. Additionally, most trauma patients arrive with initiation of C-spine precautions and a cervical collar in place. Although spine precautions must be followed, the presence of a cervical collar and possible C-spine injury can limit the evaluation of the airway. In patients with penetrating trauma, it is imperative to remove the collar and carefully examine the underlying neck, as collars have been known to obscure important physical exam findings, such as gunshot wounds, direct airway injuries, and expanding hematomas. Newer literature has shown that C-spine immobilization is not necessary in penetrating trauma patients and may actually cause harm, likely by delaying definitive diagnosis and treatment of otherwise survivable injuries.

Some physical features should be identified, as they may complicate securing a definitive airway if needed. These include the presence of a beard, the outward appearance of the neck and whether it is short or wide, surgical scars in the face and neck, and the geometry of the jaw. A short mandible, poor dentition, extensive tooth loss, the inability to open the mouth, and oropharyngeal bleeding also portend difficulty with intubation. The Mallampati classification grades the oropharyngeal anatomy from 1 to 4 to predict a difficult intubation. However, it is less useful in the trauma setting, as it was designed to evaluate a conscious patient who is sitting up. When it can be used, a class 3 or 4 may indicate a difficult standard intubation that will necessitate other options for securing the airway.

In concert with the evaluation of the airway, the remaining steps of the primary survey should be completed. Breathing should be evaluated by listening for bilateral breath sounds and observing chest rise. Exsanguinating hemorrhage is identified and controlled, pulses are palpated, and adequate intravenous access is established.

AIRWAY INTERVENTION DECISION MAKING AND PHYSIOLOGIC CONSIDERATIONS

The decision to intervene to provide a definitive airway should be driven by the patient's presentation and ability to protect the airway. Box 1 lists some indications for definitive airway control in trauma patients. Although hypoventilation is somewhat detrimental in the injured patient, hypoxia has much greater consequences and is rapidly fatal if not corrected. Airway compromise can result in the

BOX 1: Indications for definitive airway control in trauma patients

Respiratory insufficiency
Airway obstruction
Glasgow Coma Scale score of ≤8
Severe maxillofacial injury
Thermal airway injury
Persistent agitation
Large and/or expanding neck hematoma
Penetrating airway injury

BOX 2: Key airway decision-making questions from the Johns Hopkins Emergency Airway Course

1. Does the patient need to be intubated?
2. How rapidly does the patient need to be intubated?
3. Will the intubation be difficult?
4. What is the chosen method to control the airway?
5. What are my back-up plans?

inability to maintain SaO_2 greater than 90%, and it can be manifested by agitation, confusion, and combativeness. The later should not be attributed to a patient's inappropriate affect until anatomic or physiologic causes are ruled out. Airway obstruction can be caused by facial trauma; foreign objects, including broken teeth; or vomitus. In both blunt and penetrating trauma, direct injury to the oropharynx or larynx and hematoma and soft-tissue damage with swelling can lead to airway obstruction.

A Glasgow Coma Scale (GCS) score of 8 or less is a well-accepted indication for obtaining a definitive airway and can be remembered by the simple rhyming mnemonic, "GCS of 8 means intubate." Intoxicated or medicated patients, without other signs of injury (i.e., "found down"), present a unique problem, as their mental status may be chemically altered by drugs or alcohol, thus limiting their response to voice and stimuli. However, they may be oxygenating and ventilating without difficulty. If the decision is made to not obtain definitive airway control, these patients must be closely observed so that immediate intervention can be undertaken if decompensation occurs.

Severe maxillofacial trauma can lead to acute compromise of the airway. Fractures and soft-tissue swelling may cause severe respiratory distress and can make airway control difficult. Bleeding in the oropharynx and into the distal airway can lead to hypoxia and loss of airway control. Attempts to obtain a secure airway can also be made difficult by significant facial trauma, specifically midface injuries, where loss of normal anatomy can lead to loss of airway protection and can complicate intubation.

Thermal and inhalation injuries to the airway should be suspected in all burn victims, and early intubation should be considered even in patients protecting their airway on presentation. Singed facial or nasal hairs, carbonaceous sputum, and/or facial burns are clues to possible airway injury and should prompt rapid airway control. Waiting for progression of edema to result in voice changes and stridor will make intubation difficult. Patients who come in with a history of smoke inhalation or confinement in a smoke-filled space who do not have a clear indication for airway control should undergo bronchoscopy for evaluation of the airway with the potential for immediate intubation if severe findings are noted.

Agitated trauma patients present a major risk to themselves and to those providing their care. Agitation can be caused by brain injury, hypoxia, shock, and both drug—prescribed and illicit—and alcohol intoxication. Initial patient evaluation can be very difficult in these cases. The "rule of three" is an often quoted but rarely documented understanding: a patient who physically or verbally assaults the care team three times has declared their need for endotracheal intubation to allow rapid, safe, and proper evaluation and management.

Although the decision to obtain a definitive airway is straightforward in some patients, the decision of how and when to intubate other patients may not be so clear. For this reason, we have instituted a multidisciplinary emergency airway course for all residents from surgery, anesthesiology, emergency medicine, and otolaryngology at Johns Hopkins. The mechanical techniques of intubation are relatively easy to teach and master, but the complex decision making that often

precedes the actual intubation is much more difficult and is the mainstay of the course. Box 2 outlines a series of questions that we teach the residents, and these can be utilized in airway management decisions. If the need for a definitive airway is not immediately necessary, frequent reassessments should always be done. This is particularly true in the patient with a traumatic brain injury (TBI), where even one short period of hypoxia can lead to significantly worse outcomes. By frequently reassessing the patient, the deterioration of airway protection can be detected earlier, a plan can be formulated, and intubation can proceed in a timely fashion if needed. Once the decision has been made to obtain a definitive airway, an appropriately skilled member of the team should promptly initiate the planned method of airway control. This individual may be a physician—anesthesiologist, emergency medicine physician, or surgeon—a nurse anesthetist, or a respiratory therapist, depending on the local practice. At least one but preferably two or more back-up plans should be in place and explicitly stated for all members to hear, as the window of opportunity to obtain a definitive airway is short.

AIRWAY MANAGEMENT: NONINVASIVE TECHNIQUES

Many methods have been described for airway management in the trauma patient. These interventions range from noninvasive techniques, such as a chin lift and use of a bag-valve-mask, to the more invasive techniques of endotracheal intubation and creation of a surgical airway. Familiarity with multiple techniques is absolutely necessary to safely manage the airway in the trauma patient.

On presentation, all injured patients should be placed on a 100% nonrebreather mask. This simple intervention may benefit trauma patients by providing adequate oxygenation and beginning the preoxygenation process for those who may be intubated. Although not representing definitive airway management, noninvasive adjunctive techniques can be used to improve oxygenation and ventilation, and their implementation requires less training and experience. They include chin lift and jaw thrust maneuvers, oropharyngeal and nasopharyngeal airway insertion, and bag-valve-mask ventilation.

Chin Lift and Jaw Thrust Maneuvers

In the trauma patient with altered mental status, the tongue falling backwards can obstruct the hypopharynx. Chin lift and jaw thrust maneuvers can be performed to assist in airway protection by elevating the attached tongue anteriorly. The chin lift is performed by placing the fingers under the anterior mandible and lifting upward, while placing the thumb in the open mouth and lifting the lower teeth. Alternatively, in the jaw thrust, the angles of the lower jaw are grasped on each side and the mandible is displaced forward. The later technique is particularly useful when using bag-valve-mask ventilation, and it can facilitate obtaining a better mask seal. In all patients with potential for C-spine injury, implementation of in-line traction, collar placement, or manual stabilization of the C-spine is mandatory.

Oropharyngeal and Nasopharyngeal Airway

The placement of an oropharyngeal or nasopharyngeal airway displaces the tongue anteriorly, away from the posterior pharynx, increasing airway patency. Although they do not provide definitive airway management, both are compatible with and may improve the use of the bag-valve-mask. Care should be taken when inserting these devices in an awake patient, as placement may result in emesis, aspiration, and additional airway compromise. Nasopharyngeal insertion is contraindicated in the patient with known or suspected facial fractures, because the brain may be at risk of injury as a result of disruption of the normally protective skull base.

Bag-Valve-Mask

The bag-valve-mask is a commonly used method for providing positive-pressure ventilation in trauma patients and many other types of patients. The technique may seem simple and straightforward to the untrained eye; however, it is remarkably difficult to master and requires extensive practice to do well. The system consists of a flexible air chamber connected to a facemask via a one-way valve, usually attached to a high-flow oxygen source. When performed by one person, the mask is held in place over the patient's nose and mouth using the thumb and index finger, while performing a jaw thrust with the remaining three fingers. The second hand is used to deliver breaths by squeezing the attached bag. This technique can prove difficult, if not impossible, if the patient has facial hair, mandible or midface fractures, or is combative. It is also quite physically demanding for the relatively weak forearm and hand musculature. If possible, the two-person technique is much preferred, as it can be very effective in overcoming these obstacles and provides better airway management. One practitioner controls the mask with both hands to obtain the optimal seal, while a second provides breaths with the attached bag.

If bag-valve-mask ventilation or any of the noninvasive techniques is unsuccessful in maintaining oxygen saturation, then a more definitive control of the airway must be secured. This decision should be made early, and the intervention must be performed expeditiously to maintain adequate patient oxygenation and ventilation.

AIRWAY MANAGEMENT: INVASIVE METHODS

Endotracheal Intubation

Orotracheal intubation is the most common method for securing the airway in trauma patients. Using RSI and in-line mobilization of the C-spine as appropriate, placement of an endotracheal tube to secure the airway can be safe and timely. Prior to RSI, elements of the patient's medical history—such as prior difficult intubations, medications, allergies, and comorbid conditions—should be obtained if possible. Time permitting, the patient should be preoxygenated for 3 minutes with 100% oxygen.

Equipment needed to perform RSI includes a bag-valve-mask, laryngoscope, endotracheal tube (ETT), stylet, functioning suction, end-tidal CO_2 detector (either colorimetric or electronic), and stethoscope. The Macintosh (curved) or Miller (straight) blade can be used, and a functioning light source and bulb should be verified prior to use. The size of ETT used in adults usually ranges from 7.0 to 8.0; in pediatric patients, the width of the tube should be the same as the width of the patient's fifth finger, or it can be estimated using a formula: Tube size = (4 + Age in years)/4.

Intravenous access is necessary for nearly all sedatives, induction agents, and paralytic medications, although some, such as ketamine and succinylcholine, may be given intramuscularly. A commonly used combination is etomidate (0.3 mg/kg IV) and succinylcholine (1.5 mg/kg IV) as induction and paralytic agents, respectively. Other agents include ketamine (2 mg/kg IV) for induction and rocuronium (0.6 mg/kg IV) for paralysis. Propofol is commonly used for sedation and intubation in the operating room but is not ideal in the trauma situation, as it usually causes hypotension. The use of these rapid-onset, short-acting medications allows them to wear off quickly after administration in the patient who cannot be intubated. Cricoid pressure (Sellick maneuver) should be started before the administration of medications.

In-line spine stabilization should be maintained by a dedicated individual during placement of the ETT. The mouth is opened using the thumb and index finger of the right hand, while the laryngoscope is held in the left hand and introduced into the mouth on the right, sweeping the tongue to the left. When using the curved blade, the tip of the blade is placed in the vallecula anterior to the epiglottis; when using the straight blade, the epiglottis is lifted directly with the blade (Figure 1). Once positioned, the laryngoscope should be lifted along the axis of the handle, rather than levering against the teeth or mandible, resulting in decreased visualization and a broken tooth.

Once the vocal cords are visualized, the right hand is used to pass the endotracheal tube through the cords and into the trachea. A stylet can be used to shape the ETT into an L or "hockey stick" configuration, which may aid placement. An airway bougie may also be used to facilitate intubation, and some models allow short-term oxygenation through the bougie. The appropriate depth of the ETT is approximately 22 cm at the incisors for most adults. Proper placement should be verified using an in-line capnometer for detection of exhaled CO_2 and by auscultating for chest breath sounds bilaterally, noting an absence of gurgling over the epigastrium, which is a sign of inadvertent esophageal intubation. With proper placement, the chest should have equal bilateral rise and fogging of the ETT.

A frequent but minor complication is a mainstem intubation. This occurs when the tube is inadvertently placed past the carina into one of the mainstem bronchi, more frequently the right, which can be detected on physical exam by absence of breath sounds on the left. This is corrected by pulling the ETT back a few centimeters until bilateral breath sounds resume. A postintubation chest radiograph should be obtained with the ETT located 2 to 5 cm above the carina. Of special note, a simple pneumothorax may be converted to a tension pneumothorax after intubation and initiation of positive-pressure ventilation; this life-threatening condition needs to be identified and treated promptly to avoid an untoward outcome.

Other Airway Rescue Techniques

Although RSI followed by endotracheal intubation is the most commonly used method to secure a definitive airway, other techniques are available and may be used at the discretion of the trauma care provider. Often, they can be used in the anticipated difficult airway, before RSI is attempted, or more frequently as a back-up maneuver, if the initial RSI is unsuccessful. These techniques include use of a supraglottic airway, such as the laryngeal mask airway (LMA), and video laryngoscopes or flexible bronchoscopes to aid in placement of an ETT.

Supraglottic Airway (Laryngeal Mask Airway)

Now commonly used in the operating room for airway control, the laryngeal mask airway (LMA) is a supraglottic device that consists of a soft flange at the end of a tube. Use of the LMA is usually reserved for trauma patients as a temporizing measure, when initial attempts at endotracheal intubation have proven unsuccessful. Once inserted, the LMA provides a seal around the laryngeal inlet to allow ventilation. Before insertion, the cuff should be tested and lightly lubricated with water-soluble lubricant. Extending the head and neck facilitates LMA placement, but in trauma, this maneuver is often not possible because of the implementation of spine precautions. The mask is inserted into the open mouth and pressed against the posterior pharyngeal wall, until it becomes seated in the

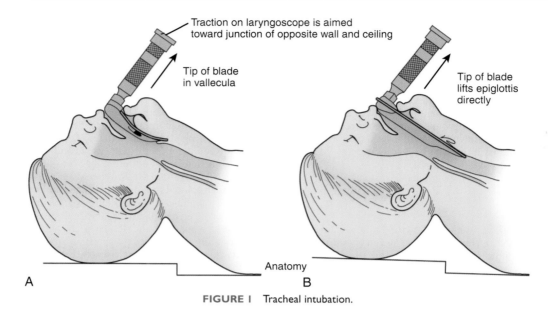

FIGURE 1   Tracheal intubation.

laryngeal inlet, where it can be inflated to allow oxygenation and ventilation using a bag-valve-mask. Placement is verified by end-tidal CO_2 detection and by auscultating bilateral breath sounds over the lungs with an absence of breath sounds over the epigastrum. The LMA does not protect well against aspiration. Contraindications for use of an LMA include pregnancy beyond 16 weeks and massive maxillofacial trauma.

Video Laryngoscopes

Fiberoptic visualization allows direct visualization of the airway and oral pathway and may require less movement of the head and cervical spine. The goal is to make visualization and recognition of airway structures easier, allowing intubation in the difficult airway. The video setup also permits multiple users to visualize the anatomy, allowing for enhanced collaboration as well as teaching (Figure 2). Inadvertent injury to oropharyngeal structures has been reported with some models, and the users must be properly trained and familiar with the model they are using. Video laryngoscopy has been shown to be particularly useful in morbidly obese patients and in those with limited neck and jaw mobility. It has also shown utility in the prehospital setting and should be considered as an airway rescue technique in the trauma patient with a difficult airway. Some ongoing trials are looking at its usefulness in routine trauma intubations, although this is certainly not a suggested standard of care at this time.

Flexible Fiberoptic Bronchoscopic-Assisted Intubation

Flexible fiberoptic bronchoscopic-assisted intubation is frequently applied to patients with known or suspected difficult airways as a result of their body habitus, airway tumors, or swelling and in patients with limited mouth opening or decreased neck mobility. In certain cases, it can be lifesaving. However, its use is somewhat limited in trauma, because it requires a provider with the advanced technical skill set to perform the intubation and the additional time to assemble the equipment and put it to use. This technique is not often used for emergent intubation, but it can be an adjunctive maneuver when time is less critical. The ETT is preloaded over a flexible bronchoscope, the scope is placed through the vocal cords, and the tube is slid off into the correct position. This is often done through the nose; however, the oral route is an option as well. This technique can be used to place an ETT for definitive airway control when an LMA has been placed as a temporizing measure.

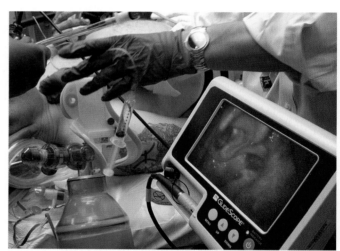

FIGURE 2   The use of a GlideScope (Verathon, Bothell, Wash.) makes visualization and recognition of airway structures easier.

Surgical Airway

If oxygenation and ventilation are inadequate, or endotracheal intubation cannot be secured using the techniques described, a surgical airway should be performed. A surgical airway provides timely and definitive airway control and is done through two commonly described methods, *cricothyroidotomy* and *tracheostomy*.

Cricothyroidotomy

To perform a surgical cricothyroidotomy, the operator stands on the patient's right side. The neck is quickly prepped and draped if time permits. The neck anatomy should be palpated, identifying the thyroid cartilage, cricoid cartilage, and cricothyroid membrane. The nondominant hand is used to immobilize the neck structures, while the other makes a 2.0 to 2.5 cm vertical skin incision over the cricothyroid membrane (Figure 3). Rapid blunt dissection is carried down to the membrane, which is then entered horizontally. A tracheostomy tube is then placed and secured; an endotracheal tube can be used if necessary. Elevating the thyroid cartilage upward using a tracheal hook can help facilitate tube insertion. The procedure is one more of feel, rather than sight, as it is most frequently performed in the suboptimal

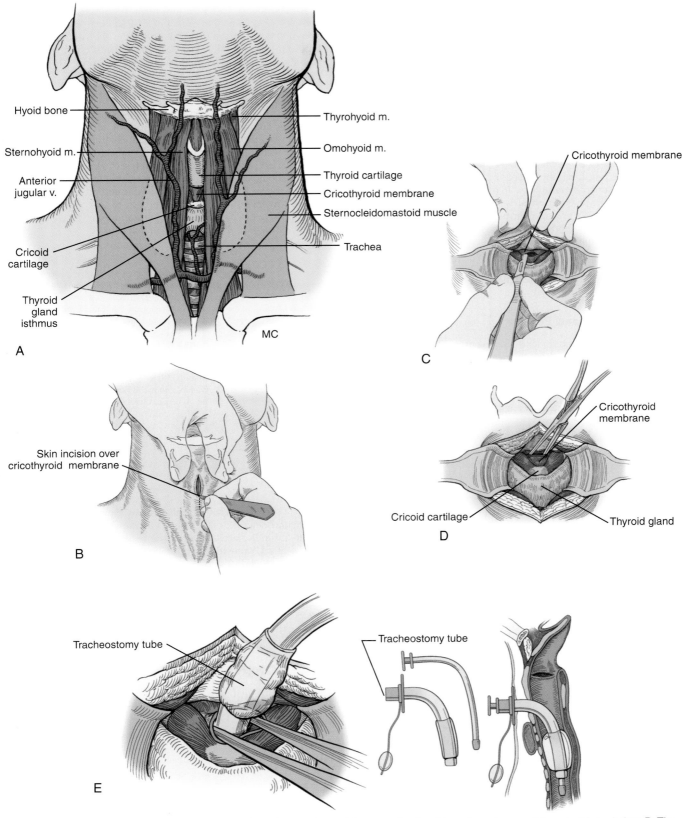

Hyoid bone

Sternohyoid m.

Anterior jugular v.

Cricoid cartilage

Thyroid gland isthmus

Thyrohyoid m.

Omohyoid m.

Thyroid cartilage

Cricothyroid membrane

Sternocleidomastoid muscle

Trachea

MC

A

Cricothyroid membrane

C

Skin incision over cricothyroid membrane

B

Cricothyroid membrane

Cricoid cartilage

Thyroid gland

D

Tracheostomy tube

Tracheostomy tube

E

FIGURE 3   Cricothyroidotomy. **A,** The cricothyroid membrane is located between the thyroid cartilage above and the cricoid ring below. **B,** The operator's nondominant hand holds the thyroid cartilage, while the other hand performs the procedure. A vertical skin incision avoids the anterior jugular veins to minimize bleeding. **C,** The cricothyroid membrane is incised transversely. **D,** The opening is widened with a small hemostat. **E,** The tracheostomy tube is placed into the airway, and the cuff is inflated. *(From Haut ER: Evaluation and acute resuscitation of the trauma patient. In Evans SRT [ed]: Surgical pitfalls: prevention and management, Philadelphia, 2009, Saunders Elsevier, pp 757-771.)*

conditions of minimal light, no suction, and a single operator. We have standardized the use of the vertical incision, because it avoids the anterior jugular and allows better exposure by retracting laterally with one hand or extending the incision vertically in either direction. Bilateral chest rise should be visualized, bilateral breath sounds should be auscultated, and end-tidal CO_2 should be detected; proper placement is verified using chest radiograph. Kits are available to aid in performing a Seldinger-type percutaneous cricothyroidotomy, but we prefer the open surgical technique, as the required tools—scalpel and hemostat—are always available, and minimal practice and set-up are necessary.

Tracheostomy

Although rarely utilized, an emergent tracheostomy is sometimes preferred to a cricothyroidotomy. It may be necessary in patients with tracheal disruption, direct airway injury, or laryngeal fracture. Tracheostomy is also preferred in pediatric patients, because performing a cricothyroidotomy may lead to larynx damage and postoperative airway complications. The use of percutaneous tracheostomy is increasing in the ICU setting and has been reported as a possibility in selective emergent cases, but it should only be used by those with significant experience with the technique.

Troubleshooting and Pitfalls

During the initial evaluation, and after securing a definitive airway, the trauma patient should be frequently reevaluated using ATLS guidelines and the ABC mnemonic. If the patient begins to decompensate, the airway must be reevaluated immediately. In the intubated patient, causes of acute respiratory decompensation include right mainstem ETT position, tension pneumothorax, and an obstructed, kinked, or dislodged ETT. In any event, the positioning should be reverified, suctioning and auscultation should be performed, and a follow-up chest radiograph should be obtained. Continuous monitoring of the patient will help ensure quick identification of the problem and provide information directing intervention.

SUMMARY

Delayed or complete lack of airway control and management is a known, preventable cause of early mortality in trauma patients. There are many techniques for obtaining and managing the airway in the trauma patient, a few of which have been reviewed here. The trauma provider should be familiar with many techniques and, more importantly, providers must become comfortable and proficient with their preferred interventions. Close adherence to ATLS guidelines and quick, decisive evaluation and intervention to secure the airway are crucial first steps in the care of the trauma patient.

SUGGESTED READINGS

American College of Surgeons: *Advanced trauma life support (ATLS)*, ed 8, Chicago, 2009, American College of Surgeons.

Haut ER: Evaluation and acute resuscitation of the trauma patient. In Evans SRT, editor: *Surgical pitfalls: prevention and management*, Philadelphia, 2009, Saunders Elsevier, pp 757–771.

Hsiao J, Pacheco-Fowler V: Orotracheal intubation, *N Engl J Med* 358(22):e25, 2008: Available online at http://www.nejm.org/doi/full/10.1056/NEJMvcm063574. Accessed October 29, 2010.

Kabrhel C, Thomsen TW, Setnik GS, Walls RM: Cricothyroidotomy, *N Engl J Med* 356(17):e15, 2007: Available online at http://www.nejm.org/doi/full/10.1056/NEJMvcm0706755. Accessed October 29, 2010.

THE SURGEON'S USE OF ULTRASOUND IN THORACOABDOMINAL TRAUMA

Scott A. Dulchavsky, MD, PhD,
and Andrew W. Kirkpatrick, MD

OVERVIEW

Traumatic injury remains a significant cause of death and a worldwide burden on health. The major causes of preventable death continue to be primarily represented by a discrete number of injury complexes predominantly located in the thoracoabdominal region. The general surgeon is often the only point-of-care provider for critical patients who arrive at the hospital after hours, therefore proficiency in using bedside ultrasound (US) to rapidly determine critical anatomy and physiology is both an opportunity and a responsibility of the acute-care surgeon. Fortunately, surgeons and emergency medical providers have shown that non–radiologist-performed, point-of-care US can provide rapid and reliable information to guide treatment decisions. Point-of-care US provides a targeted assessment to answer specific questions in the trauma patient: Is there a hemoperitoneum? Does the patient have a hemothorax or pneumothorax? Is there a nondisplaced fracture in a clinically equivocal situation? Point-of-care US provides an additional physical sense that links the physical exam and diagnostic imaging, making US complementary, rather than competitive, to computed tomography (CT) or magnetic resonance imaging (MRI). US is noninvasive, safe, inexpensive, and immediate; clinicians can utilize it to enhance many caregiver-patient interactions, creating a digitized depiction of internal function and structure that can only be inferred from a physical examination.

ABDOMINAL ULTRASOUND

Hemorrhage is the single most important cause of preventable death; the *focused assessment for sonography with trauma* (FAST) examination is an important component in the early evaluation of abdominal trauma patients, which can markedly reduce the time to determine what is wrong with a patient and guide appropriate therapy. The FAST exam is most useful in unstable patients, especially Advanced Trauma Life Support (ATLS) "nonresponders" who require immediate identification of the site of bleeding.

The right upper quadrant hepatorenal fossa is the most sensitive location to detect intraabdominal blood in trauma patients, where free fluid will be seen in 80% of patients in shock as a result of intraabdominal bleeding, followed by the left upper quadrant splenorenal view (60%), and the pelvis (40%). It is possible to score the positivity of the examination by indexing the number of positive sites and the amount of fluid at these sites for a gross estimation of the severity

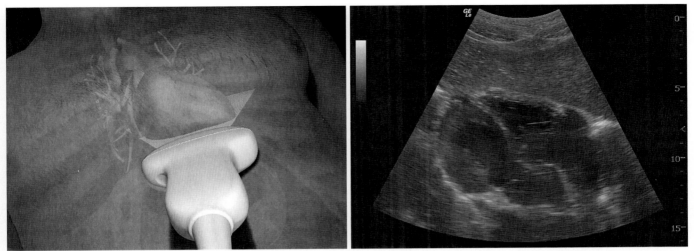

FIGURE 1   The ultrasound probe is placed in a subxiphoid location and directed toward the apex of the left chest; moderate pressure is required to obtain an image of the inferior portion of the heart and pericardial sac. Fluid will be seen as a darkened area in the dependent portion of the image.

of intraabdominal bleeding. Repeating the examination after a time interval and placing the patient in the Trendelenburg position, if tolerated, may be helpful in equivocal examinations.

A positive FAST exam in a stable patient should mandate a CT scan to further delineate injuries that may be appropriate for selective nonoperative management; a positive FAST in a hypotensive patient warrants immediate transfer to the operating room.

US can be used to evaluate abdominal trauma patients for the presence of free intraperitoneal air. The visceral and parietal peritoneum produces a to-and-fro sliding of the peritoneal surfaces with abdominal contraction or respiratory movements in patients without free air. The surfaces are separated in patients with pneumoperitoneum, which results in a loss of peritoneal sliding that can be reliably used to infer pneumoperitoneum with US. The examination should be repeated in dependent and superior locations to ensure accuracy in patients with a limited amount of free air.

US can also provide important information about the trajectory of a penetrating injury to the abdominal or thoracic cavity. This technique evaluates the wound tract for the presence of soft tissue, air, and fluid or blood using tissue US. Limited studies have suggested that US can provide useful information about the direction and depth of a wound tract to guide treatment decisions in patients with penetrating injuries to the abdomen and chest.

There are several limitations to abdominal US in the trauma patient. The FAST examination infers rather than proves injury; if no solid-organ injury is detected in the presence of free fluid, a high suspicion for either a hollow viscus or mesenteric injury should mandate further investigation. Injuries that do not typically produce a significant amount of free intraperitoneal fluid—such as diaphragmatic, intraparenchymal, and retroperitoneal injuries—will not produce a positive scan. Image generation can also be limited by patient factors, such as obesity or subcutaneous emphysema; indeterminate studies should prompt another diagnostic modality, such as CT or diagnostic peritoneal lavage, rather than repeat US.

Technique

The FAST technique consists of a rapid, sequential examination of the abdominal area to determine the presence of fluid, either blood or enteric contents, rather than individual organ injuries. The exam routinely begins by assessing the pericardial sac for free fluid using a lower frequency probe in a subxiphoid position. The transducer is directed toward the left shoulder to visualize the pericardial sac and heart; this

first view should also be used to optimize the US gain settings to ensure that intracardiac blood is anechoic (Figure 1). The probe is rapidly moved to the right upper quadrant (Figure 2) to visualize the interface between the liver and the right kidney; a dark, anechoic fluid density in this location is a sensitive indicator of intraabdominal bleeding.

This sonographic window is often located in the right inferior chest and requires orientation of the probe between the ribs to obtain the optimal image. The left upper quadrant is evaluated by visualizing the splenorenal fossa, which is often the most difficult view to obtain. The probe should be placed over the lower left ribs in a posterior location; cooperative patients can help with this view by holding a deep inspiration during the exam (Figure 3).

The final FAST image evaluates the presence of pelvic bleeding by visualizing the bladder and pelvic region in a transverse and longitudinal plane (Figure 4). These images are facilitated by having a full bladder, which can be obtained by either instilling sterile fluid or by clamping the Foley catheter after insertion.

THE PLEURAL SPACES AND ULTRASOUND

Thoracic injuries cause at least a quarter of all traumatic deaths, many of which are easily treatable with simple interventions. US provides a rapid method to determine the presence of blood or air in the chest and helps determine which body cavity mandates early intervention. US can also be used to guide performance of thoracic procedures, such as directed insertion of a chest tube, pleural drainage, and intercostal nerve block.

The healthy lung is essentially impervious to US due to the reflectance of air (high acoustic density). However, the most common life-threatening thoracic injuries are pleural, and US provides easy visualization. The visceral and parietal pleura slide in a physiologic movement known as *pleural sliding* or *lung sliding* during normal respiration. The sonographic confirmation of pleural sliding can be used to exclude pneumothorax as well as demonstrate respiration. The parietal pleura–air interface produces a recognizable pattern of a dominant hyperlucent line, called the *A line* or *batwing sign* (Figure 5), deep to the chest wall with multiple, regularly spaced lines in a step ladder pattern resulting from reverberation artifact. When small amounts of air separate the pleural surfaces, the US wave is reflected without detecting the underlying visceral pleura, and no sliding will be seen—the visual equivalent of absent breath sounds.

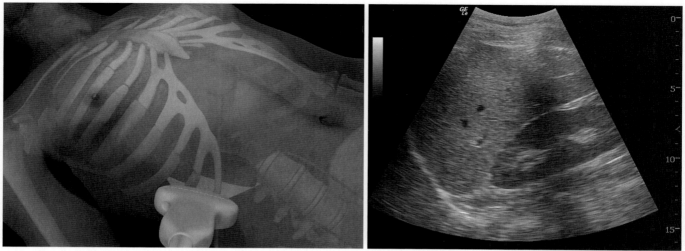

FIGURE 2   The FAST exam Morison pouch view is obtained by placing the probe in the posterior axillary line overlying the lower ribs and upper abdominal area. Fluid will be seen at the junction of the kidney and the liver on this long-axis view.

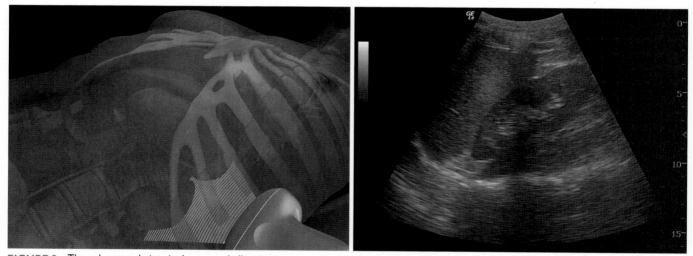

FIGURE 3   The splenorenal view is the most challenging image to acquire during the FAST examination. The probe should be placed over the inferior left chest just behind the posterior axillary line.

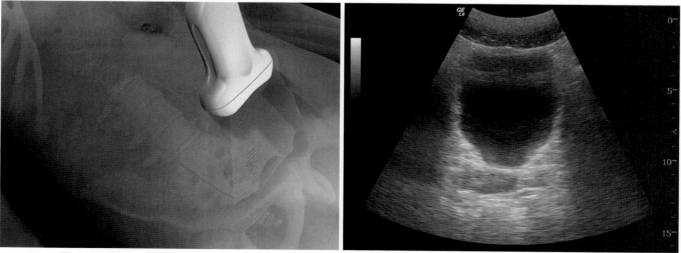

FIGURE 4   The pelvic FAST view can be done with the probe oriented in the short or long axis; a full bladder improves image quality and diagnostic accuracy.

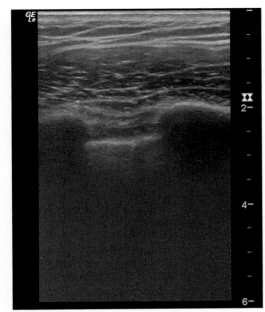

FIGURE 5   The visceral-parietal pleural interface is seen as a hyperechoic line between adjacent ribs, known as a *batwing sign or A line*. Sliding of the visceral and parietal pleura is a sensitive marker to exclude pneumothorax.

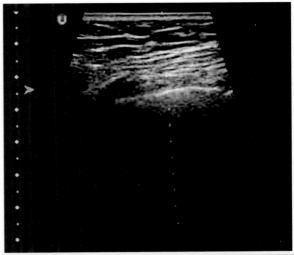

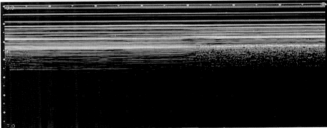

FIGURE 6   The *lung point* sign occurs when the US beam is placed at the contact point of a partially collapsed lung with the chest wall. The lung point is seen to slide through the US image, as the patient breathes and the lung moves.

The diagnosis of pneumothorax can be quickly inferred with US and may present a diagnostic advantage over chest radiography in trauma patients. Routine supine chest radiography frequently overlooks small apical pneumothoraces. Thoracic US appears to have a detection advantage over chest radiograph for small pneumothoraces in trauma patients. The extended FAST exam or thoracic US focuses on the most common location of radiographically occult pneumothoraces, the anterior and apical chest, allowing small areas of pleural separation to be visualized.

The absence of pleural sliding is relatively nonspecific and can represent apnea, pleural fusion, bullous emphysema, or death. When pleural sliding is absent, the chest wall should be progressively scanned laterally toward the midaxillary line in an attempt to detect the location on the chest wall where sliding alternates with absent sliding, known as the *lung point* (Figure 6). This finding confirms the presence of a pneumothorax and provides an index of the size of the air collection.

The visceral pleura should be examined for comet-tail artifacts, which are linear reverberation artifacts that emanate from the visceral pleura and radiate into the US field (Figure 7). Comet-tail artifacts are not normally present and can be associated with a variety of pathologies that increase lung water or edema, such as pulmonary contusion, aspiration, or fluid overload. The presence of multiple comet-tail artifacts on a thoracic US examination is the visual correlate to lung crepitations; alveolar comet tails appear closer together (3 mm or less), and interlobular comet tails are spread more widely (approximately 7 mm). The finding of comet-tail artifacts is an important US finding in the trauma patient. Comet-tail artifacts enhance the recognition of lung sliding, and because they originate at the lung surface, their presence excludes the diagnosis of pneumothorax.

Experienced investigators have also shown US to be extremely sensitive and specific for detecting intrathoracic fluid collections with a speed advantage over chest radiograph. This experience has led many investigators to augment the standard FAST exam with routine views of the pleural space to exclude hemothorax.

US can be used to determine the position of an endotracheal tube, which can be seen as a hyperechoic band in the lumen of the trachea

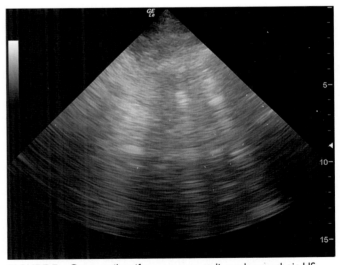

FIGURE 7   Comet-tail artifacts are seen as linear hyperechoic US signals that emanate from the visceral pleura. Comet-tail artifacts occur because of increased lung water, and they can be used to quantify edema and exclude pneumothorax.

(Figure 8). Vigorous, bilaterally symmetric lung sliding after intubation ensures that the endotracheal tube is positioned in the mainstem trachea. Dyssynchrony between right- and left-sided pleural sliding should suggest that the endotracheal tube is not in a mainstem bronchial position, which is particularly useful in environments where the stethoscope cannot be heard.

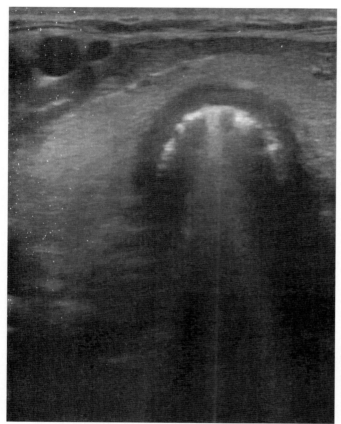

FIGURE 8 This image confirms appropriate placement of an endotracheal tube, which is seen as a rounded, hyperechoic structure in the lumen of the trachea.

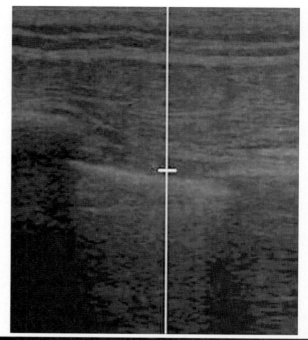

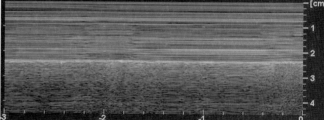

FIGURE 9 The *seashore sign* is demonstrated by using M-mode ultrasonography during a pulmonary exam. The bottom grainy portion of the image, the "sandy beach," is produced by the motion of lung sliding and can be used to exclude a pneumothorax.

Technique

A linear transducer and low-frequency phased-array transducer both produce excellent visualization of the pleural surfaces (pneumothorax) or diaphragmatic sulcus (hemothorax). The examination should begin in the uninjured chest cavity of the supine patient in the midclavicular line at the fourth or fifth interspace. The US probe should be placed to allow visualization of the superior and inferior rib with the focal zone at the hyperechoic pleural interface. Lung sliding should be confirmed as a to-and-fro gliding with normal respiration. The examination is then repeated in the contralateral chest with special emphasis on nondependent areas of the chest to provide the greatest sensitivity to detect small, localized pneumothoraces.

Color flow or power Doppler can be used to demonstrate and document pleural sliding on static images. The sensitivity of this dynamic scanning modality should be set to the proper level to readily demonstrate pleural sliding and exclude motion artifacts from intercostal muscle movement. The M-mode function provides a single image that also captures and documents lung sliding as a granular pattern of the pleural interface deep to the linear pattern of the stationary chest wall structures (Figure 9).

Hemothorax or pleural effusion can be readily detected in trauma patients through an extension of the FAST examination (EFAST). The transducer is placed in the midaxillary line over the lower ribs to demonstrate the liver or spleen and overlying diaphragm, which can be seen as a bright, hyperechoic line. Dependent pleural fluid collections are seen as darker, hypoechoic areas superior to the diaphragm. A "mirror" artifact can occasionally be seen secondary to echoic mismatch between the diaphragm and the subdiaphragmatic organ, which can be confused with a fluid collection; true fluid collections are consistently demonstrated on multiple views. The position of the probe on the chest wall also provides a guide to the appropriate window for insertion of a chest tube or drainage catheter.

Cardiac Evaluation

Although cardiac function is not a component of the standard FAST examination, clinicians can use US to determine intravascular volume status and cardiac functionality. A targeted cardiac trauma examination can quickly discern the presence of pericardial tamponade, a dilated versus empty heart, a flat vena cava (volume status), or gross cardiac contractility. Recent studies have shown that physicians with limited, focused training in echocardiography can estimate ventricular function with acceptable accuracy. US can also be used to distinguish pulseless electrical activity (PEA) from pseudo-PEA in arrest situations, which confers a survival advantage.

Chest Wall

The high acoustic density of bone allows US to accurately assess the integrity of bony structures including the ribs, clavicle, and sternum. Routine radiographic evaluation of the sternum is associated with a high rate of false-negative examinations. Musculoskeletal US is a useful technique to determine the presence of a sternal fracture by demonstrating a cortical irregularity, often associated with soft-tissue trauma in patients following anterior chest trauma. Sternal US can be

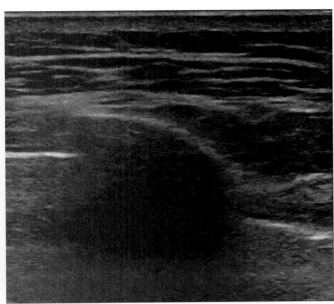

FIGURE 10 A disruption in the cortex of a rib and overlying soft-tissue edema is seen in this patient following blunt trauma.

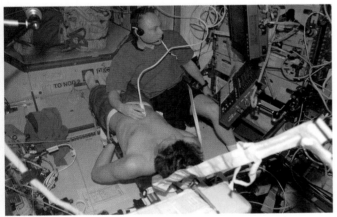

FIGURE 11 Astronauts on the International Space Station have performed over 100 hours of complex ultrasound examinations using a combination of just-in-time training and remote expert guidance. *(Courtesy National Aeronautics and Space Administration, Washington, DC.)*

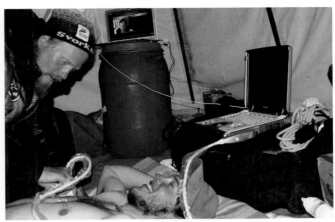

FIGURE 12 Ultrasound was used at Advanced Base Camp on Mt. Everest to investigate high-altitude pulmonary edema. A fellow climber performed the scan using a cue card and remote expert guidance via satellite phone. *(Courtesy Christian Otto.)*

rapidly performed with a high-frequency linear transducer; the accuracy of this test in patients with sternal fractures may exceed routine radiography. Care must be taken to contrast the normal cortical discontinuity seen at the sternomanubrial junction with a true fracture.

A targeted US examination can be used to confirm the presence of a rib or clavicular fracture. A generous amount of US gel should be placed over the point of maximal tenderness to provide bridging of irregular areas on the chest and to reduce the amount of pressure necessary to obtain a good image. Small cortical irregularities or discontinuity, associated with overlying soft-tissue trauma and hematoma formation, allow the diagnosis to be made with relative ease (Figure 10).

ULTRASOUND-ENHANCED TRAUMA CARE IN REMOTE ENVIRONMENTS

Advances in US technology, combined with surgical leadership in trauma care, have extended the role of point-of-care US for trauma patients to remote locations on and off the earth. US is increasingly being used on the front lines of conflict, at accident scenes, during aeromedical transport, and to provide research and medical capabilities on the International Space Station. NASA researchers have developed robust, just-in-time training methodologies and remote expert-guidance tele-US techniques, which enable nonexpert astronauts and cosmonauts to perform advanced US applications with minimal training (Figure 11). These techniques have been modified for use on Earth in divergent areas including the Olympic Games, Mt. Everest, and the North Pole (Figure 12). The verification of the accuracy and utility of abdominal and thoracic US for trauma care—combined with newer applications, such as musculoskeletal US and ocular US to detect elevated intracranial pressure—highlight the necessity of US proficiency for the trauma care provider. Support for didactic and hands-on US training through national organizations such as the American College of Surgeons, and by developing vertical programs in medical schools, ensures the place of US in the care of patients with abdominal and thoracic trauma in the future.

SUGGESTED READINGS

Chun R, Kirkpatrick AW, Sirois M, et al: Where's the tube? Evaluation of handheld ultrasound in confirming endotracheal tube placement, *Prehosp Disaster Med* 19(4):366–369, 2004.

Dulchavsky SA, Schwarz K, Hamilton DR, et al: Prospective evaluation of thoracic ultrasound in the detection of pneumothorax, *J Trauma* 50(2):201–205, 2001.

Kirkpatrick AW: Clinician-performed focused sonography for the resuscitation of trauma, *Crit Care Med* 35:S162–S172, 2007.

Lichtenstein DA: Ultrasound in the management of thoracic disease, *Crit Care Med* 35:S250–S261, 2007.

Scalea TM, Rodriguez A, Chiu WC, et al: Focused assessment with sonography for trauma (FAST): results from an international consensus conference, *J Trauma* 46:466–472, 1999.

EMERGENCY DEPARTMENT THORACOTOMY

Nicholas J. Spoerke, MD, and Donald D. Trunkey, MD

OVERVIEW

Few situations in surgery present as much potential for immediate lifesaving intervention as an emergency department thoracotomy (EDT). Because of this potential, EDT has been used in a wide variety of settings since its introduction in the 1960s. EDT is not without controversy, particularly in patients with blunt trauma. Effective use of EDT therefore requires a thorough understanding of current indications and contraindications, the common pathology and pathophysiology potentially encountered, and the appropriate surgical judgment and skill to achieve a good outcome.

DEFINITIONS AND INDICATIONS

The decision to perform an EDT is based on the mechanism of injury, the patient's physiologic status, and timing of the events leading up to their presentation in the emergency department. Put simply, EDT is best indicated to repair a simple injury in the thoracic cavity that is causing a serious physiologic insult. Unfortunately, the actual cause of the injury is often unknown until the EDT has been performed, thus certain specific surrogate criteria are used when deciding whether EDT is likely to be beneficial or futile. These criteria differ somewhat based on the mechanism of injury but can be broadly classified into *presence of vital signs* or *signs of life*. Vital signs include a palpable pulse, measurable blood pressure, and spontaneous respiratory activity. Signs of life include cardiac electrical activity, spontaneous respiratory effort, pupillary reflex, and extremity movement (Table 1).

Indications and contraindications for EDT are listed in Table 2. Indications include cardiac arrest after trauma and persistent severe postinjury hypotension. Contraindications to EDT include more than 15 minutes of cardiopulmonary resuscitation (CPR) and no signs of life for penetrating trauma, or more than 5 minutes of CPR and no signs of life for blunt trauma. An algorithm for EDT is diagrammed in Figure 1. In addition, we would consider EDT in a patient with blunt trauma, cardiac arrest, or severe hypotension if there is no evidence of severe head injury, such as a depressed skull fracture or obvious open wound with brain tissue exposed, and no step-off of the cervical spine or atlanto-occipital dislocation.

Basic Injury Patterns

Similar to trauma laparotomy, EDT is a general technique that is undertaken to rapidly correct a few basic injury patterns. Specifically, EDT is performed for release of pericardial tamponade, control of intrathoracic vascular or cardiac hemorrhage, correction of a bronchovenous air embolism, open cardiac massage, or temporary occlusion of the descending thoracic aorta.

Release of Pericardial Tamponade

Pericardial tamponade can be difficult to diagnose. Beck's classic triad of muffled heart sounds, hypotension, and jugular venous distension are not always present, and a high index of suspicion is key

to accurate diagnosis. Increasingly, ultrasound (US) is being used to confirm the diagnosis. The physiologic compromise that results from tamponade becomes increasingly more severe as the tamponade worsens. Initially, the pericardial pressure is moderately increased, and subendocardial blood flow and diastolic filling are decreased. Systemic perfusion is generally accomplished by a compensatory increase in systemic vascular resistance and tachycardia. As the pericardial pressure increases, diastolic filling and stroke volume are further compromised, and coronary artery flow is decreased. Aggressive volume loading will often temporarily maintain relative hemodynamic stability. Eventually, as the pericardial pressure continues to rise, compensatory mechanisms fail, and hemodynamic collapse ensues. If tamponade is recognized in its early stages, evacuation in the operating room is appropriate. However, if a patient presents in the final stages of tamponade, EDT is appropriate.

Control of Intrathoracic Vascular or Cardiac Hemorrhage

Due to the lack of surrounding solid organs, intrathoracic great vessel injury and cardiac injury are universally lethal unless surgically corrected. Timely recognition and control of bleeding are absolutely essential. EDT is performed in this setting for temporary control of major intrathoracic hemorrhage until definitive repair can be accomplished in the operating room. Cardiac injuries can

TABLE 1: Classification of signs of life and vital signs required for EDT

Vital Signs	Signs of Life
Palpable pulse	Pupillary response
Measurable blood pressure	Spontaneous ventilatory effort
Spontaneous respiratory activity	Palpable pulse
	Extremity movement
	Cardiac electrical activity

TABLE 2: Indications and contraindications for EDT

Indications	Contraindications
Clearly Indicated	
• Penetrating thoracic injury with SOL in patient not responding to fluids and losing vital signs in the ED or within 10 minutes of arrival to ED	• No field SOL in penetrating and blunt trauma • Blunt trauma with >5 minutes prehospital CPR • Penetrating trauma with >15 minutes CPR
Possibly Indicated	
• Penetrating abdominal injury with at least one field SOL and <15 minutes CPR • Blunt trauma patients who initially have field SOL and lose SOL within 5 minutes of arrival to ED	

SOL, Signs of life

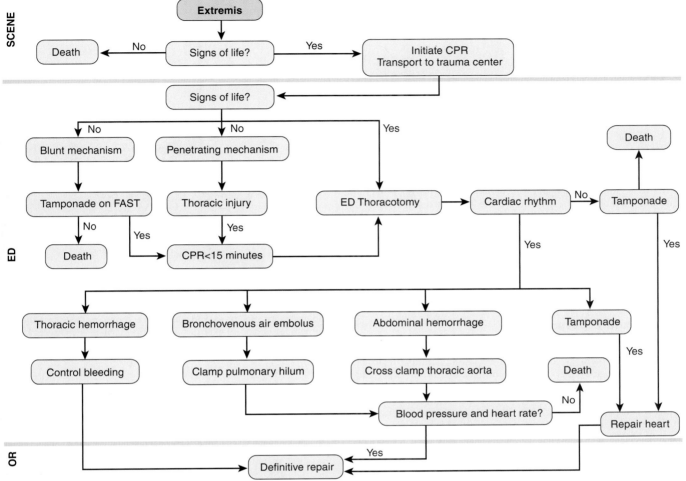

SCENE

FIGURE I   Decision-making algorithm when considering EDT. *FAST,* Focused assessment with sonography for trauma.

be temporarily controlled with suture ligature, finger occlusion of the injury, or skin-stapling devices. Chest wall bleeding can be controlled with vascular clamps or direct packing. Lung lacerations can be controlled with staples, sutures, or temporary clamping of the hilum of the lung.

Temporary Occlusion of the Descending Thoracic Aorta

Reducing blood loss below the diaphragm and shunting blood to the heart and brain during resuscitation are the main goals of occlusion of the thoracic aorta. The risks of cross clamping include acute cardiac failure resulting from ventricular dilation, injury to the esophagus, and reperfusion acidosis. We prefer temporary occlusion with the thumb of the surgeon's nondominant hand, which can be removed if a cardiac rhythm is restored. This prevents dilation of the left ventricle and minimizes reperfusion injury. The surgeon's dominant hand is used to massage the heart against the underside of the sternum.

Open Cardiac Massage

Closed chest compressions in patients with cardiopulmonary arrest generate approximately 25% to 40% of baseline cardiac output. Although this reduced percentage may provide some reasonable

perfusion of the heart and brain in cardiopulmonary arrest, trauma patients with hemorrhagic shock receive far less benefit from closed chest compressions because of their critically low blood volume. Open cardiac massage during EDT remains the only option for effective postinjury cardiopulmonary resuscitation.

Evacuation of Bronchovenous Air

Systemic, or left-sided circulatory air embolism occurs in approximately 4% of all penetrating or blunt thoracic injuries. It represents a fistula between the pulmonary bronchus and the pulmonary vein. The majority of systemic air embolism is due to penetrating trauma (65%); the remaining are lacerations to the lung caused by rib fractures or shear injury. Some of these patients will be seen with hemoptysis (25%); more often they are in hemodynamic collapse and cardiac arrest, and positive-pressure ventilation aggravates the condition. Often, the first indication that air embolism exists is when the pericardium is opened, and the anterior descending coronary artery is observed to have bubbles within the lumen. Other clinical signs include a penetrating injury to the chest but with focal or lateralizing neurologic signs and no obvious head injury; the patient initially has stable vital signs and then has sudden, unexplained cardiovascular collapse, usually following endotracheal intubation; fundoscopic examination reveals air bubbles in the retinal vessels, and Doppler monitoring of the peripheral pulses reveals a continuous machinery-like murmur.

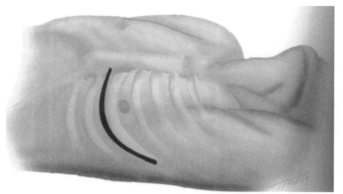

FIGURE 2 Incision at the fourth or fifth intercostal margin. A left anterolateral thoracotomy is initiated at the level of the fourth or fifth intercostal space. Generally, the incision is just inferior to the nipple in the male and the inframammary fold in the female. It is the preferred incision for resuscitation of the acutely injured patient in extremis. It provides the best access to the heart and great vessels.

PROCEDURAL TECHNIQUES

Incision and Exposure

Once the decision is made to undergo EDT, the surgeon should ensure that all members of the multidisciplinary trauma team are simultaneously activated, including notification of the operating room, initiation of massive transfusion protocols, and airway control. The patient should be positioned supine with the left arm raised above the head. After a splash prep, the skin incision should be initiated just to the right of the sternum, in case the thoracotomy must be extended bilaterally, and should proceed in the fifth intercostal space to the left midaxillary line, following the same gentle, natural curve as the underlying ribs (Figure 2). Intercostal muscles should be divided with scissors or the scalpel, and the pleura should be sharply incised. A Finochietto retractor is then placed with the handle directed laterally and toward the feet. Extension across the sternum, if indicated, can be accomplished with the Lebsche knife (Figure 3) or rib shears. A "clamshell" thoracotomy can be subsequently accomplished by creating a similar incision on the right side.

Pericardotomy

Once exposure has been established, the pericardium should be incised longitudinally from the aortic root to the apex, avoiding the phrenic nerve (Figure 4), and any blood clot should be removed. The myocardium should be thoroughly inspected, and any bleeding should be controlled with digital pressure. If injury to the heart is identified, temporary, rapid repair of any laceration should be performed using sutures or a skin stapler. Inserting a Foley catheter for control of bleeding should be avoided to prevent tearing and extension of the defect or injury to the papillary muscles and chordae tendineae. If cardioversion is necessary, it should be delayed until cardiac lacerations have been repaired. Emphasis should be placed on rapid repair of injuries to restore vital signs and allow expeditious transport to the operating room for definitive repair.

Aortic Cross-Clamping

The thoracic aorta can be accessed by retracting the lung medially and sliding a hand along the left lateral thoracic wall to feel the thoracic vertebral body. The aorta is on the anterior lateral surface, and immediate occlusion with the thumb is easily achieved. In some instances,

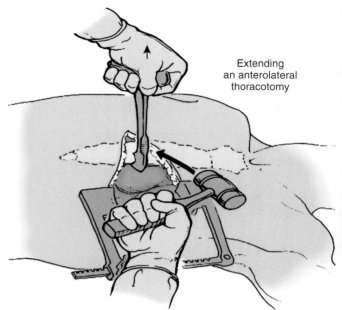

Extending an anterolateral thoracotomy

FIGURE 3 Extending anterolateral thoracotomy. A Lebsche knife and mallet are used to extend a left lateral thoracotomy across the sternum for additional exposure. When the sternum is transected, the internal mammary vessels must be ligated. Extension into the right thoracic cavity, a "clamshell" thoracotomy, gives wide exposure to both pleural cavities.

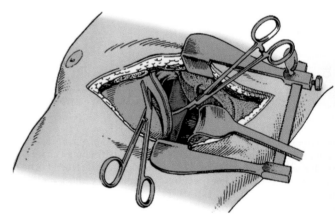

FIGURE 4 Opening the pericardium. Pericardial tamponade cannot be excluded using visual inspection alone. The pericardium is opened anterior to the phrenic nerve using a longitudinal incision.

sharp dissection with scissors or blunt dissection with the surgeon's fingers can be used to isolate a short segment of aorta to facilitate placement of an occluding clamp. Failure to dissect the pleura off the aorta can lead to ineffective cross clamping and risks damage to the esophagus and intercostal arteries.

Open Cardiac Massage

As noted above, it is often necessary for the surgeon to simultaneously control the descending thoracic aorta and, at the same time, initiate cardiac massage. This requires both hands to be in the chest, and the pericardium has to be open. Initially, the right hand is used to lift the posterior heart and gently push it against the underside of the sternum. This can achieve far better cardiac output than closed chest massage. For obvious reasons, the bimanual technique is preferred

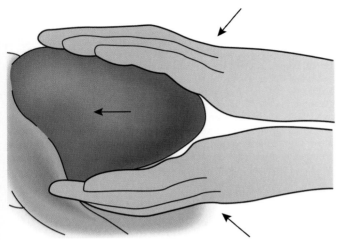

FIGURE 5 Bimanual cardiac massage. Open cardiac massage using the preferred bimanual technique. The palmar surfaces of the fingers act in a clapping motion compressing the heart. Fingertip pressure should be avoided at all times.

for open cardiac massage whenever possible. Both hands should be cupped and opposed at the wrist, and the heart should be gently compressed from the apex toward the aortic root (Figure 5). Internal cardiac defibrillation is often indicated, and the surgeon must be mindful that the 15 to 30 J of energy required for internal defibrillation is considerably less than for external defibrillation.

Evacuation of Bronchovenous Air Embolism

Once the clinical scenario of bronchovenous air embolism has been recognized, and EDT has been initiated, the following measures can be undertaken. If the patient has no cardiac activity, the immediate steps in resuscitation include isolating the injured lung by taking down the inferior phrenic ligament and clamping the hilum of the lung with a vascular clamp or a soft bowel clamp, such as a Doyen. The surgeon should then grasp the ascending aorta with the thumb and index finger and institute cardiac massage with the other hand to empty the coronary vessels of air. Using an 18 gauge needle, air should be aspirated from the left ventricle, left atrium, and rarely from the arch of the aorta. Epinephrine should be administered 1:10,000 down the endotracheal tube to drive the air bubbles out of the cerebral circulation and vital organs. Once cardiac activity is achieved, the lung injury should be oversewn or stapled; in a minority of cases, a lobectomy should be performed.

Other Useful Adjuncts

If the patient has no cardiac activity, the surgeon should instruct other members of the team to immediately obtain blood gases and initiate cardiac massage. If the blood gas pH is below 7.0, the first priority is to achieve fibrillation, which can be done by correcting the acidosis with bicarbonate. If fine fibrillation is obtained, the next priority is to convert this to coarse fibrillation, which is best achieved with epinephrine injected into the endotracheal tube or into a central line. We would avoid direct cardiac puncture, since patients are often coagulopathic, and bleeding from the ventricle can be problematic. Once a pH of 7.2 is achieved, it is then possible to defibrillate the coarse fibrillation. The surgeon should be mindful that once an effective cardiac output is achieved, the consequence to the patient will often be hypothermia, coagulopathy, and ongoing acidosis. The patient should be transported to the operating room as soon as possible, where proper lighting and instrumentation are available and anesthesia colleagues can continue resuscitation while the surgeon carries out repair of the injuries.

Clamping the Pulmonary Hilum

Massive bleeding from the central pulmonary vasculature requires rapid control of the pulmonary hilum. To access the hilum, ventilations are momentarily paused, the left lung is retracted superiorly and medially, and a curved clamp, such as a Satinsky, is placed around the pulmonary hilum.

OUTCOMES

Outcomes after EDT vary significantly based on the mechanism and pattern of injury. Survival rates are often slightly misleading, because the ultimate goal for EDT is survival with fully intact neurological function. The overall survival for penetrating trauma ranges from 5% to 50% in most series but generally averages approximately 20%. Isolated penetrating cardiac injury generally has the best overall prognosis, with survival rates in the range of 15% to 20%. Blunt trauma has the lowest overall survival rate (from 0% to 2%).

SUGGESTED READINGS

Cothren C, Moore E: Emergency department thoracotomy for the critically injured patient: objectives, indications, and outcomes, *World J Emerg Surg* 24(1):4, 2006.

Mejia J, Steward R, Cohn S: Emergency department thoracotomy, *Semin Thorac Cardiovasc Surg* 20:13–18, 2008.

TRAUMATIC BRAIN INJURY

Bryan A. Gaspard, MD, and Domenic P. Esposito, MD

OVERVIEW

Patients with traumatic brain injury (TBI) contribute to the approximately 1.4 million reported cases of head injury each year, with estimates of hospitalization reaching over 200,000 at a cost of $4 billion annually to society. Men are at highest risk, as are people between the ages of 15 and 29 years. The impact on medical institutions around the globe is significant, but great strides have been made to improve the initial management and long-term care of patients with TBI.

In 1995, the Brain Trauma Foundation published the first edition of "Guidelines for the Management of Severe Traumatic Brain Injury," which is now in its third edition, published in the *Journal of Neurotrauma* in 2007. "The Prehospital Management of TBI" is now in its second edition (2007), preceded by "Guidelines for the Acute Medical Management of Severe Traumatic Brain Injury in Infants, Children, and Adolescents" (2003), "Surgical Management of Penetrating Brain Injury" (2001), and "Guidelines for the Field Management of Combat-Related Head Trauma" (2005). *Neurosurgery* released a supplement in 2006 with "Guidelines for the Surgical Management of Traumatic Brain Injury."

With these and other numerous publications, and the ongoing clinical experiences of physicians around the globe, physicians have been able to better care for patients with TBI and to improve overall outcomes for many patients who suffer from these injuries.

PREHOSPITAL AND EMERGENCY DEPARTMENT MANAGEMENT

Most patients with TBI will come through an emergency department setting. Trauma surgeons are usually the initial consulting physicians, and after the initial "ABCs"—airway, breathing, and circulation—are assessed, the patient's clinical exam is reported, which should include a Glasgow Coma Scale (GCS) score. The GCS was published in 1974 by Teasdale and Jennett, both physicians at the University of Glasgow, and was originally designated for use with traumatic brain injury (Table 1). Ranging from 3 to 15, the scale provides a uniform way to describe the patient with a head injury that can be communicated effectively within the health care setting. A GCS score of 8 or less indicates a severe TBI, a score of 9 to 12 indicates a moderate TBI, and a score of 13 to 15 is considered a minor TBI.

For the patient with a possible or confirmed head injury, blood pressure and oxygenation should be monitored closely, as it is with all patients involved in trauma. Specifically, systolic pressures should be maintained at or above 90 mm Hg, oxygenation saturation should remain at or above 90%, and arterial blood gas should have a PaO_2 at or above 60 mm Hg. Patients who are allowed to drift below these parameters during both prehospital and in-hospital management have been shown to have worse outcomes overall. The preferred fluid for resuscitation of the patient with a head injury is normal saline, as hypotonic fluids can contribute significantly to worsening of brain edema.

Once in the emergency department, the patient will need imaging completed, which should include computed tomography (CT) of not only the head but also the cervical spine (C-spine), as many traumatic accidents occur with such force as to make it likely that the C-spine would be injured as well. In the United States, CT scan has become the imaging modality of choice for spine assessment given its ready availability, rapid scanning, and more detailed imaging compared with plain radiographs. Any other scans deemed appropriate for the mechanism and clinical exam should be obtained at this time as well. In the emergency room, if a patient is found to have sustained a head injury, a neurosurgeon should be consulted for management of the injury.

MEDICAL MANAGEMENT OR NONSURGICAL MANAGEMENT OF TRAUMATIC BRAIN INJURY

The initial management of most head-injured patients (90% or more) will be nonsurgical. The nonsurgical and surgical management of the TBI patient is aimed at protecting the brain and preserving brain function above all else. Much of what is done is aimed at preventing secondary injury or insults that could further damage neurons of the brain parenchyma. It is important to understand and relay to family members that the initial damage of the injury cannot be reversed, whatever the mechanism. Hence, the physician becomes concerned with parenchymal swelling and resultant intracranial pressure (ICP), cerebral perfusion pressure (CPP), and oxygenation of neural elements.

Management of ICP associated with TBI is divided into primary-tier and secondary-tier therapy. Primary-tier therapy includes the use of sedation and paralytics, external ventricular drains, parenchymal monitors, controlled hyperventilation, and mannitol and other hypertonic solutions. Secondary-tier therapy includes controlled hypothermia, surgical decompression, and pentobarbital-induced coma.

A TBI patient with or without polytrauma will be assessed by the neurosurgeon for the use of ICP monitoring. The clinical exam, neural imaging, the significance of the patient's other injuries, and the possible need for surgical intervention are factored into this decision.

In general, any patient with a severe TBI (GCS score of 3 to 8 after resuscitation) requires ICP monitoring if there are abnormalities depicted on CT scan. If the CT scan is read as normal, and the patient has two or more significant risk factors—age over 40 years, motor posturing on exam, or hemodynamic instability—the patient will very likely require ICP monitoring as well, but this is left up to the judgment of the neurosurgeon to decide on a case-by-case basis.

In general, a patient with abnormalities seen on CT scan would be more likely to have elevated ICP from mass lesions and swelling. Ventricular access in such a patient would allow for the primary-tier therapy of draining the space-occupying cerebrospinal fluid (CSF). Another patient may not have elevated ICP and thus will have no need for draining of CSF. Because of the advances in technology, both ICP monitoring and ventricular access are available in one device.

Once a patient has been assessed and is found to be a candidate for ICP monitoring, the neurosurgeon will place a monitor, with or without ventricular access, through a twist drill or burr hole over the right or left frontal bone. The location of the monitor depends on CT findings. For example, if a contusion is seen over the left frontal lobe, the monitor would be placed on the right to avoid the damaged parenchyma. Management of the patient begins according to the ICP readings and CPP, which are related by the equation CPP = MAP − ICP, where *MAP* is mean arterial pressure. A CPP of at least 60 is considered necessary to maintain the adequate homeostasis of the neural elements. If ICP is high (>20 mm Hg), and the patient is not adequately sedated or paralyzed, begin by adding sedation and paralytics to appropriate levels to effect. Once appropriate levels are reached, and ICP remains high, start draining CSF through the system.

TABLE 1: Glasgow Coma Scale

	Point Value
Eye Opening	
Spontaneous	4
To speech	3
To pain	2
No response	1
Motor Response	
Follows commands	6
Localizes	5
Withdraws	4
Flexor posturing	3
Extensor posturing	2
No response	1
Verbal Response	
Oriented	5
Confused conversation	4
Inappropriate words	3
Incomprehensible sounds	2
No response	1

If ICP remains elevated, the next step in management is that of controlled hyperventilation. With controlled hyperventilation, the physician is most concerned with controlling the autoregulatory mechanism of cerebral perfusion by controlling the level of carbon dioxide (CO_2) in the patient's bloodstream, monitored by arterial blood gas (ABG). The brain's autoregulatory mechanism of blood and oxygen supply to the brain is most influenced by the content of CO_2 dissolved in the bloodstream. High levels of CO_2 result in vasodilation, as the brain sees the need for more oxygen; an increase in ICP follows, as the intracranial vault volume is thus increased. Lower levels of CO_2 result in vasoconstriction of the smooth muscle surrounding the cerebral vasculature, resulting in less volume within the cranial vault and thus a decrease in the ICP. It is imperative that the ABG be followed closely and frequently during this time, as CO_2 levels less than 30 mm Hg are associated with a poor outcome and risk of stroke as the vasculature constricts. The target goal of controlled hyperventilation is a pCO_2 of 30 to 35 mm Hg.

Lastly, the patient who has had sedation, paralytics, ventricular drainage, and controlled hyperventilation can still have intermittent bouts with elevated intracranial pressures. Within the arsenal of primary-tier therapies lies mannitol and hypertonic solutions. Mannitol is a sugar alcohol that acts as an osmotic diuretic, as it decreases the extracellular volume and is excreted through the kidneys along with sodium. It has its most profound effects when used intermittently in a bolus of 0.25 to 1 g/kg, up to 100 g intravenously using the lowest effective dose. Mannitol's mechanism of action as it relates to ICP is related to rheology with a decrease in hematocrit and thus blood viscosity by plasma expansion. Through this mechanism it increases cerebral blood flow and thus oxygen delivery. The osmotic effect is caused by the increase in serum tonicity, which allows the drawing of sodium and water from the cerebrum. Mannitol's effect can last up to 6 hours.

Some studies advocate the use of 3% and 7.5% saline solutions to do the same with varying results, but mannitol is by far the most accepted and used for the effect of reducing ICP. Note that saline and mannitol can be used simultaneously; treatment with both has the effect of raising the serum sodium level, which ultimately assists in controlling cerebral edema through an osmotic effect.

In certain cases, when the above efforts are unsuccessful at reducing and controlling intracranial pressures and thus protecting the neural elements, secondary-tier therapies may be instituted. Such therapies include controlled hypothermia, surgical decompression, and pentobarbital-induced coma.

With controlled hypothermia, the aim is to bring the metabolism of the neural elements to a minimum, thus reducing oxygenation needs and therefore blood flow. The target temperature is between 33° and 35° C. During this controlled hypothermia, it is imperative that the patient be sedated and paralyzed to avoid the shivering response, as the body would try to combat the decreasing core temperature.

With pentobarbital-induced coma, the aim is again at decreasing the requirements for oxygen and decreasing other metabolic needs of the neural elements. Pentobarbital is a barbiturate and thus has an affinity to γ-aminobutyric acid (GABA) receptors. GABA is the main inhibitory neurotransmitter in the central nervous system (CNS); when attached to this receptor, it assists in activation of chlorine channels, thus decreasing the excitation of neurons. Pentobarbital also blocks a subset of receptors for glutamate, which is the main excitatory neurotransmitter in the CNS.

It is important to understand that not all patients with TBI are candidates for the therapies described above. Second-tier therapies are used sparingly, as each has an associated multitude of complications, such as coagulopathies, dysautoregulation, and increased infections. Individual patient needs and comorbidities must be weighed with each intervention. It is also important, in our opinion, that the family members understand the magnitude and limitations of each intervention as it relates to the patient's overall outcome.

SURGICAL MANAGEMENT OF TRAUMATIC BRAIN INJURY

For the use of surgical intervention, there must generally be a localized mass lesion that can be targeted by the surgeon. In other words, a diffuse injury involving bilateral cerebral hemispheres cannot be treated effectively with this method. The surgical management of TBI is aimed at removing a localized insult to the CNS, which is associated with up to 45% of severe TBI patients with up to 100,000 patients requiring surgical intervention. The insults are labeled according to their anatomical position in the brain: an *epidural hematoma* (EDH), for instance, lies above the dural covering of the brain; a *subdural hematoma* (SDH) lies below the dural covering of the brain; a *parenchymal hematoma,* or contusion, is a lesion within the brain parenchyma; and lastly, a *subarachnoid hemorrhage* (SAH) is a layering of blood along the surface of the brain within the subarachnoid space—the most common abnormality found on CT scan among TBI patients.

Each of these lesions has different indications for surgical intervention, and each and every patient must be treated on a case-by-case basis, remembering that not all patients may be salvageable. The neurosurgeon's decision will be based on various medical factors, such as timing of injury, time since clinical decline, CT findings, location of injury, extent of other injuries, and so on, including the patient's quality of life and the patient's known desires as well as those of the remaining family.

Surgical Management of Epidural Hematoma

The classic scenario of the lucid interval, wherein a patient is injured and progressively deteriorates, can and does exist in up to 50% of cases, but many other patients present along a continuum of neurologically intact and without deficit to comatose. EDHs are present in up to 4% of TBI patients; however, not all EDHs require emergent surgical evacuation, nor is arterial bleeding always the cause (Figure 1). EDH sources range from arteries, veins, and sinuses, as well as dural bridging between veins and bone.

The surgical indications for EDH are a hematoma volume greater than 30 cm^3 regardless of the patient's clinical presentation. Of course, a hematoma of this size can and usually does cause clinical deficits. As such, the less time that is allowed to elapse between when the patient deteriorates or is injured and the surgical intervention, the

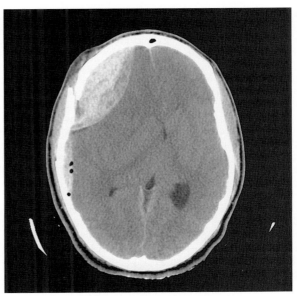

FIGURE I Epidural hematoma.

better the outcome. The method of choice is a craniotomy that allows for visualization of any ongoing bleeding.

A hematoma volume of less than 30 cm³ may still require surgery if the midline shift is 5 mm or more, or the shear thickness of the lesion is 15 mm or more. Clinically speaking, a lesion may warrant evacuation if the patient's GCS score is less than 8 with no other known injury that might to contribute to such a finding.

Surgical Management of Acute Subdural Hematomas

SDH is seen in up to 30% of severe TBIs (Figure 2). Venous bleeding or sinus bleeding is most often the cause of a SDH. The surgical indications for the management of acute SDH are a hematoma thickness greater than 1 cm or an MLS greater than 5 mm. These measurements are regardless of the patient's clinical exam or GCS score. Hematomas measuring less than these thicknesses and MLS should undergo evacuation if the patient's condition declines or the patient's GCS score deteriorates by 2 points following the initial insult. The preferred method is a craniotomy allowing for visualization of ongoing bleeding and a more complete evacuation of the acute hematoma. The timing of such surgery is as soon as possible after deterioration or initial presentation, depending on the situation.

Surgical Management of Traumatic Parenchymal Lesions

Parenchymal lesions are the most common lesions associated with TBI (Figure 3). They constitute anything from small, punctate contusions to large intracranial hemorrhages of lobular origin. They are most intimately associated with neuronal destruction, and they have great tendency to create mass effect with surrounding edema. Parenchymal lesions have been controversial in the past, when judging whether to evacuate, because of the possibility of further insult to an already taxed neural system.

Through a multitude of studies, the indications for the surgical evacuation of such an injury have been compiled to include any patient with a GCS score of 6 to 8 with contusions located in the frontal or temporal lobes greater than 20 cm³ with MLS greater than or equal to 5 mm and/or obliterated cisterns on CT scan. Furthermore, the indications for surgery include any patient with a contusion of 50 cm³ regardless of GCS score or clinical exam. However, this particular patient population may often have devastating neurological damage that may preclude any surgical intervention at all.

The phenomenon of *delayed traumatic intracerebral hematoma*, which is important to note but not fully understood, is still an area of research interest among neurosurgeons. It is thought to arise in an area of contused brain, and the mechanism seems to be linked to loss of autoregulation around the area of contused brain that in turn can lead to venous congestion and hypoxia of the surrounding tissue and subsequent development or enlargement of a preexisting hematoma. In a patient, this syndrome may manifest as deterioration or, for those with monitors in place, as an elevation of ICP, resulting in the repeating of CT scan to confirm the diagnosis. The timing of surgery is based on the patient's condition, ICP parameters, and the failure of medical therapy to adequately control the ICP. The method of choice, if surgery is chosen, is craniotomy for excision of the mass lesion.

Within this subset of injuries are included lesions of the middle and posterior fossas of the cranial vault. These regions are smaller within the cranial vault: the middle fossa, which houses the temporal lobes, and the posterior fossa, which houses the cerebellum and occipital lobes, are both in close proximity to the brain stem. Because of this, smaller mass lesions can significantly affect the clinical exam and overall outcome of this subset of patients. Therefore indications for surgical intervention when considering the

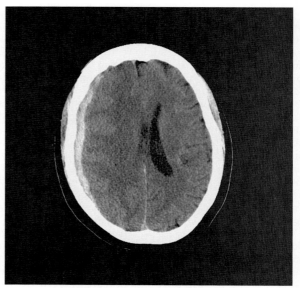

FIGURE 2   Acute subdural hematoma.

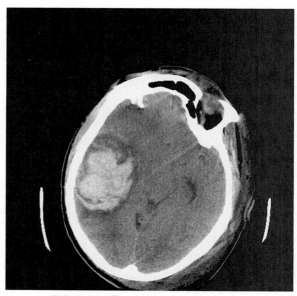

FIGURE 3   Traumatic parenchymal lesion.

middle and posterior fossas are less tolerant of even smaller mass lesions. Lesions in the area of the middle fossa (temporal lobe) and posterior fossa (cerebellum) measuring 20 cm³ or greater in volume may require evacuation in patients with poor clinical exams and GCS scores less than 8.

Decompressive Craniectomy

Decompressive craniectomy (DC) has become a useful tool in the armamentarium of the neurosurgeon battling TBI and elevated ICP. Decompressive craniectomy is the removal of the skull bone flap as in a craniotomy but then leaving it off. The next step in such a procedure includes duraplasty or dural expansion using pericranium or biologically engineered products. The main purpose of DC is to provide room for the swelling edematous brain to expand without placing undue pressure on other critical neural structures within the cranial vault. DC may be used to treat any of the lesions described above in the patient with TBI, provided that the lesion can be localized

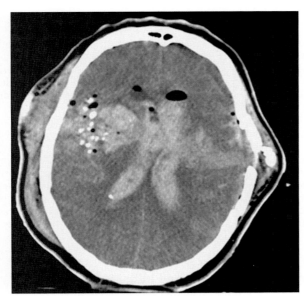

FIGURE 4   Penetrating brain injury.

to a specific side or lobe. If performing a one-sided DC, the size of the bone flap removed should be between 12 and 15 cm. If targeting diffuse cerebral edema, the method of choice is the bifrontal craniectomy with duraplasty, removing bilateral frontal bones and expanding the dura.

MANAGEMENT OF PENETRATING BRAIN INJURY

Much of the information known and applied to penetrating brain injury (PBI) has been gathered through military studies as far back as World War I. However, the practices of caring for these injuries do have a place within the civilian population, and this has served physicians caring for these injuries well over the years.

The physics of kinetic energy, related through E = {1/2}MV², where E is kinetic energy, M is mass of the projectile, and V is the velocity of the projectile, demonstrates that the energy of a projectile is much more influenced by its velocity than its mass. This information can be helpful when prognosticating about the effects of an injury, especially when the injury is the result of a gunshot, and the caliber of weapon used and distance fired can be ascertained from police or bystanders. The management of PBI, such as from a gunshot, begins a clinical exam and inspection of entrance and exit wounds (Figure 4). It is during this initial evaluation that control of any major bleeding sites must be addressed, and during this process, be mindful of possible forensic evidence that may be discovered. In the setting of PBI, the health care provider must take care not to be deceived by the obvious. Although the PBI may be the most pronounced injury, the physician must diligently inspect the patient's entire body for the possibility of other wounds that may have been suffered, whether from an explosion or gunfire.

Once the patient's exam is complete, the workup begins with a CT of the head and plain films. CTs and plain films of other areas of the body may also be warranted, depending on what is found during the initial examination and inspection. Once the initial CT is conducted, the physician should be on hand to review these studies. Evidence of diffuse SAH, intraparenchymal hematoma, or the trajectory of the missile may warrant a CT angiogram to evaluate for traumatic aneurysms or other injury to cerebral vasculature. If an injury is found, it usually requires medical or surgical management during the acute hospital stay. Depending on the patient's exam, early ICP monitoring is recommended, considering that many projectile injuries to the brain result in diffuse cerebral edema; therefore ICP is elevated.

Beyond the local treatment of the entrance and exit wounds, the treatment of the more extensive debris field depends on the extent of bone fractures, bone fragments, and local intraparenchymal injury. Current recommendations are not to debride bone or missile fragments extending some distance from the entrance site; however, repair of any air sinus injury or CSF leak by repairing dural defects as soon as the patient is medically stable is recommended.

Through the use of broad-spectrum antibiotics, physicians have seen a significant decrease in meningitis and brain abscesses following PBI and a decrease in the mortality associated with such infections. Currently no agreed upon recommendation exists to dictate the length of time antibiotics should be given, but it typically is 1 to 6 weeks. In regard to seizure prophylaxis, as with TBI, early use of antiepileptic drugs has been shown to reduce the incidence of posttraumatic seizures, but long-term use has not been shown to decrease the incidence of posttraumatic epilepsy.

SUGGESTED READINGS

Badjatia, Carney N, Crocco TJ, et al: Guidelines for prehospital management of traumatic brain injury, *Prehosp Emerg Care* 12(suppl 1), 2007.

Bullock MR, Chestnut R, Ghajar J, et al: Guidelines for the surgical management of traumatic brain injury, *Neurosurgery* 58(3 suppl 1), 2006.

Bullock MR, Chestnut R, Ghajar J, et al: Guidelines for the management of severe traumatic brain injury, *J Neurotrauma* 24(suppl 1), 2007.

Gudeman SK, Kishore PR, Miller JD, et al: The genesis and significance of delayed traumatic intracerebral hematoma, *Neurosurgery* 5(3):309–313, 1979.

Marion D: *Traumatic brain injury*, New York, 1999, Thieme.

Narayan R, Wilberger J Jr, Povlishock J, et al: *Neurotrauma*, New York, 1996, McGraw-Hill.

Narayan RK, Maas A, Servadei F, et al: Progression of traumatic cerebral hemorrhage: a prospective observation study, *J Neurotrauma* 25(6):629–639, 2008.

Polin R, Shaffrey M, Bogaev C, et al: Decompressive bifrontal craniectomy for the treatment of severe refractory posttraumatic cerebral edema, *Neurosurgery* 41(1):84–94, 1997.

Pruitt, et al: Management and prognosis of penetrating brain injury, *J Trauma* 51(2 suppl 1), 2001.

Reilly P, Bullock R, et al: *Head injury: pathophysiology and management of severe closed head injury*, London, 1997, Chapman and Hall.

Siddiqi J: *Neurosurgical intensive care*, New York, 2008, Thieme.

Valadka A, Andrews B, et al: *Neurotrauma: evidence-based answers to common questions*, New York, 2005, Thieme.

Young H, Gleave J, Schmidek H, et al: Delayed traumatic intracerebral hematoma: report of 15 cases operatively treated, *Neurosurgery* 14:22–25, 1984.

Chest Wall Trauma, Hemothorax, and Pneumothorax

R. Stephen Smith, MD, and
Jonathan M. Dort, MD

OVERVIEW

The chest wall, comprised of the bony thorax and associated soft tissues, provides protection for underlying vital structures—the heart, great vessels, and lungs—and it provides an airtight cylinder that makes respiration possible. *Pneumothorax,* the abnormal presence of air in the pleural space, is commonly encountered in trauma care and surgical practice. It may occur spontaneously or as the result of blunt or penetrating trauma, or it may be due to complications of surgical and medical treatment, such as with barotraumas or central line placement. *Hemothorax* is the presence of blood in the pleural space, which occurs most commonly as a result of blunt or penetrating injury. Injury to an intercostal or internal mammary artery is the most common source of intrathoracic bleeding.

INCIDENCE AND ETIOLOGY

Thoracic injury is second only to traumatic brain injury as the leading cause of death secondary to trauma. Thoracic injury is responsible for at least 25% of deaths resulting from trauma, and it is a contributing factor in another 25%. Associated extrathoracic injuries are common when significant chest wall injury is found. Rib fractures, one of the most common manifestations of thoracic wall injury, are frequently encountered in victims of trauma. For example, 94% of severely or fatally injured seat belt wearers in motor vehicle crashes are found to have rib fractures.

Spontaneous pneumothorax typically occurs in tall, slender, male cigarette smokers who are younger than 40 years; it occurs secondary to distal airway inflammation and obstruction, which produces emphysematous changes. Patients with underlying pulmonary disease such as chronic obstructive pulmonary disease, malignancy, tuberculosis, idiopathic pulmonary fibrosis, cystic fibrosis, and sarcoidosis are at greater risk for spontaneous pneumothorax. In addition, pneumothorax most commonly develops after blunt chest injury, and the risk of hemothorax following chest wall injury is directly proportional to the number of ribs fractured; patients with two or more rib fractures have an incidence of hemothorax as high as 80%. Nontraumatic hemothorax is uncommon and results from associated intrathoracic pathology, such as tumors or severe pulmonary infections, which may cause erosion of thoracic vessels. Medical anticoagulation or coagulopathy makes hemothorax more likely to occur following minor injury.

CHEST WALL INJURY

Associated Injuries

Up to 25% of patients with chest wall injuries have one or more associated injuries. Fractures of the first and second ribs, scapula, and sternum have long been associated with significant intrathoracic injury. This association is less prominent than previously thought, but fractures of these robust structures indicate that a great deal of kinetic energy has been transmitted to the thorax. Underlying pulmonary contusion is frequently associated with blunt chest wall trauma, and sternal fractures may be associated with cardiac contusion.

The geriatric patient tolerates chest wall injury poorly. Concomitant cardiorespiratory comorbidities and reduced physiologic reserves make this population ill equipped to handle the stress of chest wall injury. Elderly patients with minor chest wall injury may develop respiratory compromise soon after injury. Such patients should be closely observed in a monitored area for respiratory deterioration. In the pediatric population, the rib cage is extremely pliable. Therefore, pediatric patients may have significant intrathoracic injury in the absence of rib or sternal fractures, and the severity of their intrathoracic injuries may be missed.

Physical Examination and Initial Management

Inspection of the chest wall should be carried out during the initial evaluation of an injured patient. Auscultation is a mandatory component of initial evaluation, and pulse oximetry should be used during the evaluation of all seriously injured patients. Special attention should be paid to abrasions, contusions, lacerations, or any deformity of the chest wall; asymmetric chest wall motion during respiration, paradoxical movement of the chest wall, and splinting are indicative of flail chest. Palpation of the chest wall may reveal crepitance or point tenderness associated with rib or sternal fractures. The presence of fractures in ribs 9 through 12 should raise the suspicion of liver or spleen injury. Respiratory decompensation associated with flail chest and pneumothorax may present in a delayed fashion, and pulmonary contusion may not be recognized until 48 hours after injury.

Patients with chest wall injuries should undergo rapid evaluation of the airway, breathing, and circulation the same as with any injured patient. Supplemental oxygen is universally beneficial to all patients with a suspected chest wall injury. If a pulmonary contusion is present, judicious volume resuscitation should be carried out; overly aggressive resuscitation with crystalloid solutions is common in trauma and will worsen the severity of pulmonary contusion.

Radiographic and Laboratory Evaluations

An anteroposterior chest radiograph remains standard in the evaluation of patients with chest wall injury. It should be recognized, however, that a plain chest radiograph will miss significant pathology. As many as 7 of 10 rib fractures will not be diagnosed by a plain chest radiograph. Computed tomography (CT) of the chest wall with three-dimensional reconstruction is a major advance in the evaluation of chest wall injuries. Although this study is not indicated for patients with minor chest wall injury, it is the best method of demonstrating the presence of severe chest wall deformity associated with flail chest. Additionally, CT scan is important for the evaluation of patients with pulmonary contusion or suspected great vessel injury.

Evaluation of chest wall injury includes laboratory assessment. Measurement of arterial blood gases is an important method of determining the degree of respiratory compromise. Cardiac enzymes are not routinely indicated and are not directly associated with clinically significant cardiac contusion, but electrocardiographic changes may suggest cardiac contusion. If the initial electrocardiogram is abnormal, observation and cardiac monitoring for 24 to 48 hours are warranted.

Operative Treatment of Flail Chest

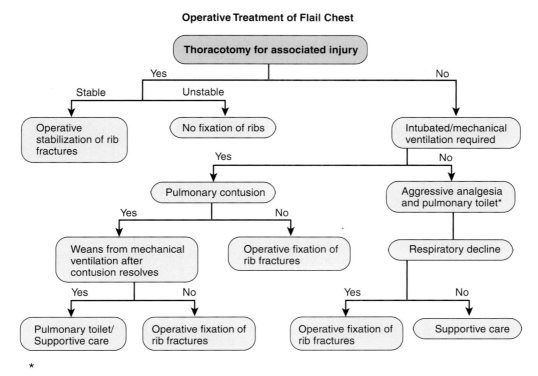

* • Thoracic epidural anesthetic
  • P.C.A.
  • Incentive spirometery
  • IPPR

FIGURE 1   Operative treatment of flail chest.

Specific Injuries

Open Chest Wound

An open (sucking) chest wound will cause the preferential movement of air through the chest wall as opposed to through the tracheobronchial tree at the initiation of negative intrathoracic pressure associated with inspiration. Initial treatment involves coverage of the wound with an impervious dressing secured on three sides. This type of dressing will make respiration possible while also serving as a flutter valve to permit the efflux of air in the pleural space. Chest wall injury involving significant tissue loss must be treated operatively as quickly as possible.

Flail Chest

Flail chest is the result of significant kinetic energy applied to the thorax. The definition of *flail chest* is the fracture of three or more consecutive ribs in at least two locations. Any patient with multiple consecutive rib fractures may exhibit the respiratory compromise and pulmonary dysfunction classically associated with flail chest. The associated respiratory failure is primarily a result of underlying pulmonary contusion, but the adverse biomechanical impact of multiple rib fractures, severe pain, splinting, and atelectasis are contributing factors. The biomechanical deficits created by flail chest may prevent adequate ventilation.

Treatment should be aggressive, and it must be initiated at the earliest opportunity. Therapy should include an emphasis on pain management and pulmonary toilet. Mechanical ventilation may be required in more than 50% of patients with flail chest, even with optimal analgesia and pulmonary toilet. The best method of providing pain relief for these patients is thoracic epidural analgesia, which should be initiated as soon as possible. All too often, this vital therapy is delayed past the initial 24 hours after injury. Alternatively,

intercostal nerve blocks may be useful if long-acting local anesthetics are used. The percutaneous placement of long catheters that permit the instillation of local anesthetic adjacent to the site of rib fractures may be useful, but this is an unproven technique. Application of external patches or dressings containing long-acting local anesthetic agents is unproven. Narcotic use is almost always necessary for analgesia. Patient-controlled analgesia devices are useful, but are inferior to epidural analgesia. Operative fixation of rib fractures in flail segments is gaining popularity and may be considered in a subset of patients (Figures 1, 2, and 3).

Simple Rib Fracture

Simple rib fractures are frequently encountered in patients with blunt chest injury. Methods of radiographic evaluation, such as chest radiograph and CT scan, are similar to patients with flail chest. Bedside ultrasound may be used to determine the specific location of a rib fracture. Management of simple rib fractures is focused on pain control and pulmonary toilet, and pain associated with rib fractures may continue for months and may become chronic and disabling. Many patients with rib fractures are unable to return to normal activity, which is particularly true if a pseudoarthrosis develops at the site of rib a fracture. Operative fixation of these areas of fracture nonunion may be indicated in a small subset of patients.

Sternal Fractures

Sternal fracture occurs in 5% of patients with blunt chest wall injury, which is most commonly found in an unrestrained driver after a crash that has caused rapid and sudden deceleration. Sternal fractures most commonly occur at the manubrium and are frequently missed on plain chest radiographs; such fractures are better delineated by CT scan. Clinically significant cardiac contusion is rarely associated with

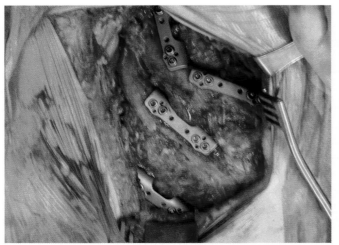

FIGURE 2 Operative fixation of flail chest with a U plate specifically designed for rib fractures.

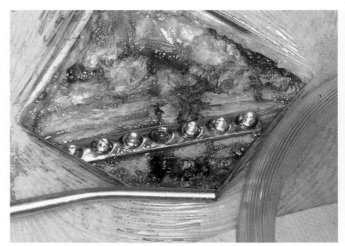

FIGURE 4 Titanium plate and screws used for fixation of a displaced transverse sternal fracture.

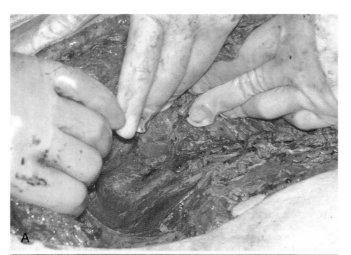

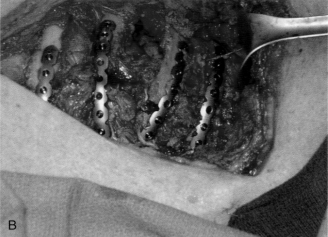

FIGURE 3 Operative fixation with a novel system specifically designed for the treatment of rib fractures.

sternal fracture, but rib fractures are associated with sternal fractures in up to 40% of patients. Treatment usually involves adequate analgesia. Rarely, a patient with severe sternal fracture, marked displacement, and instability may benefit from operative fixation (Figure 4).

Clavicle and Scapula Fractures

Clavicular fractures are quite common, with the majority occurring in the middle third of the bone. The vast majority of these injuries may be managed by a simple splint and oral analgesia. There is increasing enthusiasm for operative treatment of fractures with severe displacement or nonunion. Scapular fractures are indicative of significant kinetic energy transmitted to the thorax. These fractures are managed nonoperatively in the majority of cases but may require open reduction and internal fixation.

Sternoclavicular dislocation is uncommon. It occurs with very high kinetic energy injuries to the chest wall. Anterior dislocations are best managed with closed reduction. Posterior dislocation can be associated with injury to the great vessels and should be treated operatively.

PNEUMOTHORAX

Etiology and Presentation

Pneumothorax is the abnormal presence of air in the intrapleural space that results in lung collapse, and it has several etiologies. *Primary spontaneous pneumothorax* occurs in the absence of underlying lung disease and most commonly presents in young, thin males; it has a strong, dose-dependent association with smoking. *Secondary spontaneous pneumothorax* occurs in the presence of underlying lung disease and is typically seen in older patients. *Traumatic pneumothorax* occurs in the presence of injury, either by a penetrating or blunt mechanism. *Occult traumatic pneumothorax* is defined as pneumothorax seen only on CT scan and not chest radiograph, whereas *nonoccult traumatic pneumothorax* is seen on chest radiograph. *Iatrogenic pneumothorax* occurs as a complication of a procedure or therapeutic intervention, most commonly mechanical ventilation, placement of a central venous catheter, or invasive procedures that traverse the pleural space or bronchial spaces.

The presentation of pneumothorax can range from asymptomatic to imminently life threatening; when symptoms do occur, the most common are chest pain and dyspnea, but other complaints include cough and anxiety. The most common findings on physical exam are tachycardia, tachypnea, alteration or loss of breath sounds, and hyperresonance on chest wall percussion. In the setting of *tension pneumothorax,* where the air in the pleural space is under pressure and expanding, findings can also include hypotension, jugular venous distension, and diminished cardiac output.

Diagnosis

The standard method of confirming the presence of a pneumothorax is chest radiograph. The most reliable views are erect posterioanterior and lateral views. Studies have shown that inspiratory and expiratory films are equally sensitive. CT scan is usually not required for diagnosis but can reveal occult pneumothorax. Recent studies have shown the effectiveness of ultrasound for diagnosis of pneumothorax, which matches the sensitivity and specificity of other imaging techniques. Loss of "lung sliding" at the pleural interface and the absence of a comet-tail or ring-down artifact confirm the diagnosis.

Management

Appropriate management of pneumothorax ranges from simple observation to surgical intervention. This algorithm is determined by size, symptoms, etiology, and number of occurrences. Observation is most often used for asymptomatic patients and patients whose pneumothorax is occult or occupies less than 20% of the pleural space on chest radiograph. Observation includes close monitoring for the onset of symptoms as well as repeat chest radiograph approximately 6 hours after the initial films. Supplemental oxygen is often employed to increase the rate at which pleural air is absorbed. The onset of symptoms or an increase in occupied pleural space should prompt a reevaluation for the necessity of more invasive therapy.

Beyond observation, several methods have been employed to evacuate pleural air, with resultant lung reexpansion. The least invasive of these is simple aspiration after placing an 8 to 12 Fr catheter. This technique has been described as effective in the setting of primary spontaneous pneumothorax and iatrogenic pneumothorax. It is not as reliable as conventional tube thoracostomy and is not commonly used as the primary treatment method in most centers.

Heimlich valves and other flutter-valve devices have been utilized in the treatment of spontaneous pneumothorax and iatrogenic pneumothorax. Such devices allow for the outpatient treatment of these conditions and are effective 85% of the time. Follow up with repeat exam and chest x-ray is usually arranged within 48 hours.

Tube thoracostomy still remains the most widely used method of pneumothorax management. A variety of tube sizes can be employed, but a size equal to or greater than 36 Fr should be utilized for any traumatic mechanism or other mechanisms in which concern for associated hemothorax exists. Because the procedure is painful, appropriate analgesia and sedation should be employed. Tube thoracostomy carries infection risk, and therefore every effort to provide appropriate sterile precautions should be made. The prophylactic use of antibiotics is controversial, but the literature supports the option of perioperative prophylaxis; however, prolonged administration of antibiotics is not warranted.

Once these steps have been performed, and adequate local anesthesia of the skin, muscle, and periosteum is accomplished, a small skin incision is made at the nipple line, in the fifth intercostal space, between the anterior and midaxillary lines. Blunt dissection is then carried through the muscle, and a Pean or Kelly clamp can be used to penetrate the pleura. Tunneling to an intercostal space cephalad to the skin incision is often utilized but is not required. The tube is then directed to the apex for simple pneumothorax; if necessary, it can be directed posteriorly for hemothorax. Digital identification of the pleural cavity, as well as condensation of water vapor in the tube, can help to confirm the proper placement of the tube, which should be secured to the skin with sturdy, nonabsorbable suture and connected to a suction drainage system. An occlusive dressing is used, and chest radiograph confirms the appropriate placement of the tube. The drainage system, typically attached to wall suction, has an in-line water-seal chamber. Complications of tube placement include infection, bleeding, empyema, malpositioning, and occlusion.

Tension pneumothorax requires immediate decompression. This determination is made clinically; no imaging study is required or warranted. Immediate decompression can be achieved by placing a large-bore (14 to 16 gauge) needle or catheter in the second intercostal space at the midclavicular line. A rush of air should be appreciated. This intervention converts a tension pneumothorax to a simple pneumothorax, and standard tube thoracostomy can be performed as definitive therapy.

Thoracostomy tube removal can be considered when the pneumothorax has resolved without suction, and tube drainage is minimal; 24 hour totals of 75 to 200 mL have been described as the maximum output for tube removal. Optimal methods of removal have been debated to minimize pneumothorax recurrence, and these rates appear to be equivalent when performed at end inspiration or end expiration.

Certain clinical scenarios merit the use of surgical intervention for the ultimate resolution of pneumothorax. This can be accomplished with thoracotomy or minimally invasive thoracoscopic techniques. A second episode of primary spontaneous pneumothorax doubles the recurrence rate to 50%, whereas a first episode of secondary spontaneous pneumothorax has a recurrence rate approaching 50%. Because of this, the recommendations for surgical intervention include these scenarios, as well as the failure of a pneumothorax to resolve, or persistent air leak after 4 days. Other indications for surgical intervention can include bilateral pneumothorax, patients in high-risk professions, and patients with AIDS.

Thoracoscopic techniques continue to increase in prevalence and have been shown in multiple studies to be as effective and safe as thoracotomy but with shorter recovery. Therefore the minimally invasive technique is now considered the procedure of choice. Reexpansion may be accomplished in several ways: Pleurodesis involves the invocation of an inflammatory response of the pleura, either by chemical or mechanical means. The mechanical method is most often utilized surgically by abrading the pleural surfaces. Chemical pleurodesis has also been utilized most commonly with talc. Due to the availability of minimally invasive surgical techniques, the nonoperative chemical methods are used much less frequently, as these are painful procedures with recurrence rates up to 25%.

Video-assisted thoracoscopic surgery requires appropriate training and experience. With general anesthesia and single-lung ventilation, the patient is positioned in the lateral decubitus position. A single trocar is inserted inferior to the scapular tip at roughly the sixth intercostal space. After visual inspection, two additional ports are placed under direct vision in a triangulated fashion. Mechanical abrasion is then achieved. If a bleb is responsible for the pneumothorax, an endoscopic linear stapler is utilized for resection. Saline injection into the cavity with subsequent ventilation can reveal any further parenchymal leak, and chest tube placement completes the procedure, with lung reexpansion. Thoracoscopy is contraindicated in unstable patients.

HEMOTHORAX

Etiology and Presentation

Hemothorax is defined as the presence of blood in the pleural cavity. The most likely mechanism is penetrating or blunt trauma. Other less common sources can be seen, such as infections, tumors, rupture of blebs, pancreatitis, and ruptured aneurysm. Hemothorax can present in a wide clinical spectrum from small, asymptomatic collections to massive hemothorax in an unstable patient. The diagnosis of hemothorax by physical exam can be difficult, with findings that include diminished breath sounds, dullness to percussion, and hemodynamic changes. Unilateral opacification may be appreciated on chest radiograph, but CT is more sensitive in revealing a small or moderate hemothorax, and ultrasound will reliably identify fluid in the pleural space.

Management

The initial management of a suspected hemothorax is tube thoracostomy. It is important to remember to do this in the context of the standard resuscitation scheme of injured patients, to include airway control, ventilatory assistance, and circulatory resuscitation. Indications for immediate thoracotomy include an initial output greater than 1500 mL or an output greater than 200 mL per hour over 4 hours. Close monitoring of patients who do not reach these thresholds is also important, as clotting of the thoracostomy tube may require placement of a second tube, and hemodynamic changes or ventilatory difficulty may warrant more immediate surgical intervention.

If thoracotomy is required, it is best achieved in the lateral decubitus position through a posterolateral approach under general anesthesia. Hemodynamically unstable patients are best approached through an anterolateral thoracotomy incision. With single-lung ventilation, if tolerated, and appropriate prepping and draping, an incision at the fifth intercostal space provides the best exposure. Exposure may be improved by the removal of a rib.

Although the most common source of traumatic hemothorax is an intercostal or internal mammary artery injury, bleeding frequently results from injury to lung parenchyma or the great vessels. In this case, intercostal vessels may be suture ligated or clipped. Tractotomy or wedge resections, which may both be achieved with stapling devices, may be adequate to expose, seal, or resect the source of hemorrhage from lung parenchyma. With more significant parenchymal injury, formal lobectomy or pneumonectomy may be required. Vascular control of the hilum can be achieved by incising the inferior pulmonary ligament and grasping the hilar vessels, either with digital pressure or with a large vascular clamp. Twisting the hilum 180 degrees may be helpful. Once the hilum is controlled, the source of bleeding can be identified, and the extent of resection can be determined. Once the procedure is complete, the chest wall is closed, and chest tubes are left in place to assist in lung expansion and evacuation of residual fluid.

In very rare instances, with an exsanguinating patient who is coagulopathic, hypothermic, and acidotic, a damage-control procedure may be required. In this setting, packing may be employed to achieve control of hemorrhage and air leak, taking care not to affect cardiac function and venous return adversely. The patient is returned to the operating room after those physiologic conditions are improved. In the stable patient with ongoing hemorrhage, the thoracoscopic approach may be considered, but the procedure must be converted to thoracotomy at any sign of instability or if adequate visualization, evacuation, or hemorrhage control is not possible.

Patients who have persistent hemothorax as a result of delayed diagnosis or failure to evacuate with thoracostomy tube drainage are at risk for fibrothorax, which can result in chronically diminished pulmonary function, pain, and dyspnea. Avoidance of this complication requires aggressive therapy, when the retained hemothorax is identified. CT scan is most sensitive for diagnosis, and a hemothorax that occupies more than a third of the pleural space should be evacuated. Video-assisted thoracoscopic surgery is indicated for these patients, as second chest tubes placed more than 24 hours after injury fail to drain the hemothorax in almost 50% of patients.

Suggested Readings

Knudtson JL, Dort JM, Helmer SD, et al: Surgeon-performed ultrasound for pneumothorax in the trauma suite, *J Trauma* 56(3):527–530, 2004.
Smith RS: Cavitary endoscopy in trauma: 2001, *Scand J Surg* 91(1):67–71, 2002.
Baumann MH, Strange C, Heffner JE, et al: and the AACP Pneumothorax Consensus Group: Management of spontaneous pneumothorax: an American College of Chest Physicians Delphi consensus statement, *Chest* 119(2):590–602, 2001.
Casos SR, Richardson JD: Role of thoracoscopy in acute management of chest injury, *Curr Opin Crit Care* 12(6):584–589, 2006.
Tanaka H, Yukioda T, Yamaguti Y, et al: Surgical stabilization or internal pneumatic stabilization? A prospective randomized study of management of severe flail chest patients, *J Trauma* 52:727–732, 2002.
Kent R, Woods W, Bostrom O: Fatality risk and the presence of rib fractures, *Ann Adv Automot Med* 73–92, 2008 (Oct).
Flagel BT, Luchette FA, Reed RL, et al: Half-a-dozen ribs: the breakpoint for mortality, *Surgery* 138:717–725, 2005.
Solberg BD, Moon CN, Nissim AA, et al: Treatment of chest wall implosion injuries without thoracotomy: technique and clinical outcomes, *J Trauma* 67:8–13, 2009.
Nirula R, Allen B, Layman R, et al: Rib fracture stabilization in patients sustaining blunt chest injury, *Am Surg* 72:307–309, 2006.

Blunt Abdominal Trauma

Greta L. Piper, MD, and Andrew B. Peitzman, MD

OVERVIEW

Management of patients with blunt abdominal trauma is often challenging. Intraabdominal injuries generally occur in the multiply injured patient with competing threats to life and limb. If clinicians relied solely on physical examination, abdominal injury would be missed in as many as 45% of patients. Missed intraabdominal injury is one of the most common causes of preventable death for trauma patients who arrive alive at the hospital. Similarly, safe practice of nonoperative management and optimal management of abdominal injury requires exquisite judgment. The recognition of specific injury patterns is crucial for diagnosis, and the standardization of operative and nonoperative treatment options allows for an organized approach to the trauma patient with abdominal injury. The major metamorphosis over the past two decades has been toward less invasive approaches of diagnosis and management.

PATTERNS OF INJURY

The most common mechanisms of blunt abdominal injury are motor vehicle collisions, motorcycle crashes, pedestrians struck by motor vehicles, falls, and assaults. Following blunt trauma, the hemodynamically unstable patient is presumed to have active bleeding that must be recognized and promptly controlled. Potential sources of blood loss from blunt injury include external (open) wounds and fractures, the chest, abdomen, pelvis/retroperitoneum, and long bones. Mortality and morbidity from intraperitoneal bleeding increase with any delay to control of hemorrhage.

Injuries are determined by the body's velocity at the time of impact, but more important is the rate of deceleration (change in velocity). More rapid deceleration produces more energy dissipation on impact. In addition, where the body absorbs that force and the vectors of impact will also determine injury patterns. Unrestrained motor vehicle passengers are injured by frontal impact with the windshield, steering wheel, dashboard, and floorboard. Common abdominal injuries in unrestrained victims are to solid organs such as spleen, liver, kidney, and retroperitoneum. Restrained front-seat occupants have a 50% lower risk of mortality compared to unrestrained occupants but are at an increased risk of abdominal injury. Lap-belt injuries are associated with small and large bowel injuries,

Algorithm for Evaluation of Blunt Abdominal Trauma

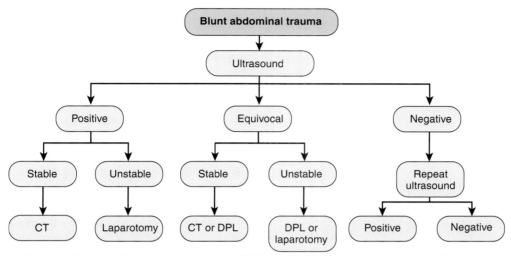

FIGURE I   Algorithm for the evaluation of blunt abdominal trauma. FAST is used as the initial screening test. *Stable* and *unstable* refer to hemodynamic status.

as well as mesenteric tears, and 25% of patients with a lap-belt mark will have associated intestinal or mesenteric injury. This is especially true with ill-fitting lap belts, commonly seen in children or petite adults, where the lap belt sits across the soft tissue of the abdomen rather than across the pelvic bones. The lateral impact from T-bone collisions results in twice the mortality of frontal impacts, because less space and material absorb the force. Most of these patients will present with thoracic and abdominal injuries, generally on the side of impact. Head injury is more common with lateral impact as well, whereas rear-end collisions result in so-called *whiplash injuries* and seat belt–related abdominal injuries.

Motorcycle drivers and passengers are at risk for less predictable injury patterns because of the lack of protection from impact. Although cranial injuries are the most common cause of mortality in motorcycle crashes, abdominal injuries from handlebars, such as duodenal tears and pancreatic injuries, are common.

Pedestrians struck by automobiles frequently present with a pattern of injuries known as *Waddell's triad*: tibiofibular or femur fracture, truncal injury, and craniofacial injury. Those with torso trauma are likely to have intraabdominal injuries as well.

Injuries from falls depend on the height of the fall, the surface struck, and the position of the patient on impact. Falls from a height greater than three stories have a mortality of 50%, and impact with harder surfaces results in more severe injuries. If the victim lands on his or her feet, the pattern of injury may include calcaneus, lower extremity, pelvis, and spine fractures. Associated visceral injuries may be related to fall impact or to the specific bony fractures.

Assault victims may also present with a variety of injuries, depending on the weapon used and the position of the victim. Torso and intraabdominal injuries are common from stomping and kicking injuries inflicted on a victim lying on the ground.

INITIAL EVALUATION

All trauma patients, regardless of injury mechanism, are evaluated according to Advanced Trauma Life Support (ATLS) protocols starting with the ABCs: airway, breathing, and circulation. Based on their hemodynamic status on arrival to the trauma bay, patients are triaged into one of three categories: *stable, unstable,* or *in extremis.* The basic blunt abdominal trauma algorithm accounts for stable and unstable patients (Figure 1). Patients in extremis are managed differently, as such patients have completely decompensated, and these physiologic

abnormalities must be immediately reversed for any chance of survival. All procedures performed for patients in extremis must be therapeutic, as their condition will not allow procedures that are simply diagnostic. For example, rather than obtaining a chest x-ray in such patients, bilateral chest tubes are empirically placed. If present, a tension pneumothorax is relieved. If the patient has a hemothorax, it is diagnosed, and the blood is drained. Thus, the management plan for trauma patients in extremis is intubation, placement of bilateral chest tubes, securing of venous access, and fluid resuscitation.

First, any source of blood loss must be promptly found, and bleeding must be controlled. If a blunt trauma patient loses vital signs in the trauma bay, a thoracotomy is performed. If no source for the hemodynamic collapse is evident at this point, and the patient has vital signs, he or she should be taken to the operating room immediately for a laparotomy, assuming a right chest tube has been placed and that the pericardium has not been infiltrated by blood.

For patients who are stable hemodynamically, the secondary survey includes a complete physical exam. The abdominal exam, although often nonspecific for traumatic injuries, should start with inspection of the entire abdomen, flanks, and back for external signs of trauma such as abrasions or bruises. A *seat belt sign* is a bruise caused by the impact of a shoulder or lap belt, which should raise concerns for bowel injury. A flank hematoma may indicate a kidney or spleen injury. A *Kehr sign* is shoulder pain referred from hemidiaphragmatic irritation, which may point to a splenic injury; abdominal tenderness should also be noted. It is important to note, however, that the absence of any or all of these signs does not exclude intraabdominal injury, and physical exam alone will miss up to 45% of injuries. Thus, adjunctive tests are essential in the evaluation of blunt abdominal trauma.

Although nonspecific, the chest radiograph and pelvic radiograph performed in the trauma bay may raise concerns for specific abdominal injuries. Lower rib fractures are often associated with spleen or liver injuries on the ipsilateral side, and abdominal contents seen in the chest indicate a diaphragmatic rupture. Up to 20% of pelvic fractures are associated with visceral injuries, most commonly to the bladder or urethra. Lumbar fractures seen on pelvic x-ray may be *Chance fractures,* forceful flexion fractures associated with duodenal or other bowel injury in 30% of patients.

Focused abdominal sonography for trauma (FAST) involves the use of ultrasound to look for blood in the peritoneal cavity and pericardium. Four ultrasound windows are interrogated: epigastrum/pericardium, Morison's pouch, splenorenal space, and pouch of Douglas

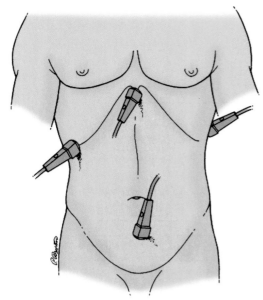

FIGURE 2 The four transducer positions for FAST: pericardial, right upper quadrant, left upper quadrant, and pelvis.

(Figure 2). In the diagnosis of hemoperitoneum, the FAST exam has a sensitivity of 86% and a specificity of 98% in blunt trauma patients. A hypotensive patient with hemoperitoneum on FAST should undergo prompt laparotomy. The false-negative rate of FAST—especially in patients with chest injury, rib fractures, spine fractures, or pelvic fractures—may be as high as 30%. FAST is insensitive in children because of the frequency of solid-organ injury without associated hemoperitoneum. In addition, the FAST provides information about the presence of hemoperitoneum but not about specific organ injury in most hands. A negative FAST exam is always followed by a more definitive test: CT scan in stable patients and laparotomy in unstable patients. McKenney and colleagues (2001) defined an ultrasound score based on the depth of free fluid identified and determined that the majority of patients with a score of 3 or higher will require a laparotomy.

Diagnostic peritoneal lavage (DPL) is aspiration followed by infusion and return of fluid from the peritoneal cavity to detect evidence of solid or hollow visceral injury. After placement of a nasogastric tube and urinary catheter, a periumbilical incision is made, and a catheter is placed in the peritoneal cavity. Although infraumbilical catheter placement can be performed in patients without pelvic fractures, this concern is eliminated with the supraumbilical incision. The catheter is then aspirated, with aspiration of 10 mL of frank blood or obvious gastrointestinal contents grossly positive lavage. If the initial aspirate is negative, 1 L of normal saline can be infused and allowed to drain. The lavage is considered to be positive if greater than 100,000 red blood cells/mm^3 of fluid are seen. White blood cell count, bilirubin, and amylase determinations are less specific. Although the sensitivity and specificity have been reported to be as high as 98% to 100% and 90% to 96%, respectively, the disadvantages include the risk of iatrogenic injury and missed retroperitoneal injuries. FAST has largely replaced DPL for use in unstable patients, but DPL is useful in unstable patients in whom the FAST is negative or inconclusive.

Computed tomography (CT) is the mainstay for diagnosis of intraabdominal injury. CT is sensitive and specific in the diagnosis of solid-organ injury, and it quantifies hemoperitoneum. CT is excellent for the diagnosis of solid visceral injuries to the liver, spleen, and kidneys with sensitivities of 99%, 90%, and 94%, respectively. It also shows intraperitoneal and retroperitoneal blood. The accuracy of CT has allowed the evolution of nonoperative management of solid-organ injury; however, sensitivity for blunt pancreatic injury is only

76%. Detection of hollow visceral injuries, such as to the small intestine and colon, remain difficult, even when CT is performed.

CT is most sensitive and specific when performed with IV contrast. This is essential to differentiate normal solid-organ parenchyma from injury such as splenic injury. The use of IV contrast is also essential to detect active extravasation, which has a high risk of failure of nonoperative management—24 times greater than injury without active extravasation. Realizing that the accuracy may not be ideal, a noncontrasted scan may be used on a particular patient with renal impairment, for whom we have a negative FAST and suspect low probability for intraabdominal injury. Any suspicious finding, including free fluid or unsuspected bony injuries, warrants special attention with either a contrasted scan or serial exams in a reliable patient. As mentioned, noncontrasted scans fail to show intraparenchymal hemorrhage and pseudoaneurysms. It is also crucial to remember that unstable patients should not leave the trauma resuscitation bay to undergo CT; only stable patients are taken to CT for imaging.

Initial laboratory data drawn from the trauma patient are often nonspecific, but they are useful as a baseline for future comparisons. A normal hematocrit is likely even in the bleeding patient, if the interval between injury and presentation is short. Knowing a patient's coagulation status is helpful when surgical intervention is a possibility. An admission International Normalized Ratio greater than 1.5 is predictive of higher mortality in trauma patients and indicates a more severe physiologic insult. Similarly, an arterial blood gas measurement that demonstrates a large base deficit raises concern for global ischemia, and follow-up labs should be drawn to confirm resolving acidosis with resuscitation. Failure to correct acidosis predicts patients with higher mortality. Base deficit on admission correlates with the degree of hypoperfusion and mortality. Base deficits that are normal (0), moderate (1 to 6), and severe (>6) in blunt abdominal trauma patients older than 65 years are associated with 14%, 27%, and 40% mortality rates, respectively. Some evidence exists to support the use of liver function tests, amylase, and lipase as adjuncts for determination of severity of liver, pancreatic, or small bowel injury; in general these lab values are also nonspecific. Drug and alcohol screening can help explain lab abnormalities and may also determine the reliability of a patient's abdominal exam.

MANAGEMENT

Following initial evaluation of the patient, the key decision involves recognizing patients who require prompt laparotomy. The decision to perform prompt laparotomy is generally based on hemodynamic instability and a positive FAST or DPL. In patients who are unstable or transient responders, do not leave the trauma bay until you have evaluated all possible sources for cavitary bleeding: chest radiograph or bilateral chest tubes for thoracic bleeding, and FAST in conjunction with DPL for intraperitoneal bleeding. Although some rely almost exclusively on FAST to exclude abdominal bleeding in this setting, the false-negative rate has been reported to be as high as 42%. Thus we would perform a DPL prior to leaving the trauma bay in an unstable patient. The next stop after the trauma bay—operating room, intensive care unit (ICU), or angiography—is driven by degree of instability and findings on diagnostic studies.

With the evolution of nonoperative management, positive findings on diagnostic studies no longer mandate laparotomy. The key factor is hemodynamic stability; in general, if the patient is stable enough for CT, he or she is appropriate for nonoperative management. About 85% of hepatic injuries and 75% of splenic injuries in adults can be observed, and these numbers are higher in children. A patient without a clear-cut indication for intervention should be admitted for observation and serial examinations. It should be noted that a single normal blood pressure does not define a stable patient; rather a stable patient is one in whom a continuum of prehospital and in-hospital heart rate and blood pressure measurements are normal or immediately responsive to a fluid challenge. Nonoperative management requires exquisite surgical judgment and should be reserved for the stable patient with a reliable exam. Patients with unreliable exams include elderly patients with dementia, intoxicated patients, and morbidly obese patients. Changes in a patient's vital signs or exam warrant further or repeat imaging versus operative intervention. Nonoperative management avoids the short-term risks of laparotomy and general anesthesia, as well as the long-term problems associated with adhesions, but it increases the risk of delayed or missed diagnoses.

CONDUCT OF THE LAPAROTOMY

Once the decision has been made to explore the abdomen, the operative approach should follow a standardized and organized set of sequential steps. Preoperative antibiotics should be given if potential exists for intestinal injury. A nasogastric or orogastric tube is placed for gastric decompression, and a bladder catheter is placed for bladder decompression and urine output monitoring. The patient should be prepped in sterile fashion, from the chin to the knees, and table to table laterally to allow for rapid exploration of any body cavity.

A midline incision is the best incision for trauma operations. The peritoneal cavity is entered, and after rapid examination, all four quadrants should be packed. Realize that with blunt trauma, the common sources for blood loss are the spleen, liver, and mesentery. Less common sites of major bleeding are the pelvis and kidney. Once packing has achieved some tamponade, the operation can be slowed to allow anesthesia to catch up in the underresuscitated patient. After the initial packing, the two main goals of the damage-control operation are hemostasis and control of gross contamination. The most active bleeding must be addressed first. The individual quadrants should be inspected in a serial fashion, looking for clots or active bleeding, and the liver and spleen should be visualized and carefully palpated and inspected. The lower quadrants are evaluated for retroperitoneal hematomas, and the bowel mesentery is inspected for tears that may be bleeding; significant mesenteric bleeding should be oversewn. The bowel can be inspected later in the operation for possible ischemia from the mesenteric injury.

Once hemostasis is achieved, the focus turns to control of contamination. The bowel is quickly examined from the gastroesophageal junction, over the stomach and duodenum, and from the ligament of Treitz to the terminal ileum, one segment at a time. The entire colon is also inspected, and any perforations are oversewn or stapled to control spillage. Definitive repair is not necessary, until the patient has been stabilized, and the entire abdomen has been assessed. Once hemostasis and control of contamination have been accomplished, the entire abdomen must be meticulously examined in a systematic fashion. In the right upper quadrant, the liver should be fully examined, and the right hemidiaphragm must be palpated. Diaphragmatic injuries, especially posteriorly, can be missed if not carefully sought. Suspensory hepatic ligaments should be divided as necessary, and the second portion of the duodenum should be visualized; if a hematoma or bile staining are seen, a wide Kocher maneuver should be performed. The right perinephric area should be evaluated for hematoma.

The left upper quadrant should be fully evaluated, including palpation of the entire left hemidiaphragm and examination of the stomach. The spleen may need to be mobilized for full inspection, and if so, the tail of the pancreas can be evaluated at this time; opening of the lesser sac allows for inspection and bimanual palpation of the body and duct of the pancreas. The left perinephric area should be examined as well.

The lower quadrants are primarily evaluated for retroperitoneal hematomas, which may represent large vessel injury. The entire gastrointestinal tract, from the gastroesophageal junction to the peritoneal reflection, is evaluated again to look for any signs of blood or bile in the bowel wall or in the mesentery. If either of these is seen, the root of the mesentery should be fully mobilized with a right medial visceral rotation, and the ligament of Treitz should be taken down to visualize the third and fourth portions of the duodenum. The colon should again be carefully examined and mobilized further if needed, and the bladder is inspected for intraperitoneal injury and hematoma, which may suggest extraperitoneal injury or pelvic fracture. The contribution of a pelvic fracture to blood loss can be estimated based on the size of the pelvic hematoma and whether it is expanding.

Once the entire abdomen has been examined, definitive bowel and bladder repairs may be performed in the stable patient. The abdomen of the unstable patient should be left open and packed, once surgical bleeding is stopped, GI contamination is controlled (damage control), and the patient is taken to the ICU. The criteria for truncating the laparotomy and applying damage control include acidosis, hypothermia, and coagulopathy. A pH less than 7.1, a body temperature less than 34° C, or generalized oozing from all peritoneal surfaces (coagulopathy) are all indications that the laparotomy should be truncated as soon as possible to allow for correction of this lethal triad. Common injury patterns necessitating damage control include major vascular injury, high-grade hepatic injuries, and pelvic fractures. On the other hand, do not leave the operating room if you have failed to control surgical bleeding.

SPECIFIC ORGAN INJURIES

Spleen

The spleen and liver are the most commonly injured organs from blunt abdominal trauma. Splenic injuries are most commonly diagnosed by CT, and the American Association for the Surgery of Trauma (AAST) has created a grading system for splenic injuries based on the CT findings. The majority of grade I to III spleen injuries can be managed nonoperatively in a stable patient with ICU monitoring and serial abdominal exams and hematocrits. Grade IV and V spleen injuries are usually seen in hemodynamically unstable patients, requiring laparotomy and splenectomy. The presence of a blush of parenchymal contrast extravasation on CT scan (active extravasation) is associated with a high rate of failure of observation. In a stable patient with a blush, angioembolization is an option. However, grade IV and V injuries have a 50% to 75% rate of failure of nonoperative management, requiring splenectomy. Increasing amounts of hemoperitoneum with splenic injury in adults also increases the likelihood of failure of nonoperative management. Remember that the patient's hemodynamic status drives treatment decisions far more than the grade of splenic injury. Vaccinations for *Haemophilus influenzae* and *Pneumococcus* and *Meningococcus* species should be given to the nonoperatively managed patient on admission. Postsplenectomy vaccines are given to patients prior to discharge from our hospital, rather than waiting for follow-up visits, to increase the likelihood of administration in the trauma patient.

Liver

Liver injuries are also diagnosed by CT scan and are also defined by an AAST grading system. The vast majority of liver injuries (85%) can be managed nonoperatively. The key decision point is the patient's hemodynamic stability. If the patient with hepatic injury is stable for CT scan, that patient can generally be observed irrespective of the grade of the liver injury and the amount of hemoperitoneum. Grade IV and V hepatic injuries should be followed in an ICU setting with serial exams and labs, because 25% of hepatic injuries will have a complication that requires intervention, and the majority of these are grade IV and V injuries. Selective hepatic angioembolization may be employed for contrast extravasation. In the unstable patient, laparotomy is warranted, and operative exposure with self-retaining retractors and subcostal incision extensions is often necessary. Compressive packing and hemostatic agents will control most low-grade liver injuries. Larger injuries are more apt to require packing, followed by second-look laparotomy once resuscitation has been optimized. If the bleeding is refractory to simple maneuvers, the liver can be mobilized by dividing the falciform and triangular ligaments, and the portal triad can be occluded with a Pringle maneuver. Major liver resection, usually resectional debridement or nonanatomic resection when necessary, should be performed expeditiously to limit blood loss. Mortality increases proportionately with red cell transfusion.

Duodenum and Pancreas

With their anatomic proximity and shared blood supply, injury to either the duodenum or pancreas should prompt concern for injury to the other. The second portion of the duodenum is injured in blunt trauma either by a crushing mechanism or a closed-loop blowout, and the fourth portion of the duodenum is injured secondary to traction. The pancreas can be injured when crushed against the vertebral column.

Diagnosis of these injuries by CT scan can be difficult. Although laboratory values may be nonspecific, steady increases in amylase and lipase are consistent with an injury. An oral contrast study is sometimes helpful for the diagnosis of duodenal injury, and contrast extravasation diagnoses a perforation that requires exploration. Intramural duodenal hematomas can be managed nonoperatively, and endoscopic retrograde cholangiopancreatography or magnetic resonance cholangiopancreatography can then be used to evaluate for pancreatic ductal injury if CT is nondiagnostic. The definitive test for pancreatic duct injury is full exposure, mobilization, and bimanual inspection of the pancreas in the operating room.

Stomach, Small Bowel, Colon, and Rectum

Injuries to hollow viscera are not easy to recognize, although findings of free fluid on the initial FAST ultrasound or CT scan should raise suspicion for such injuries. Stomach injuries occur in less than 1% of blunt abdominal trauma patients. Most perforations occur along the greater curvature, and these can be debrided and closed in two layers. The incidence of small bowel injury is 5% in blunt abdominal trauma patients undergoing laparotomy. Surgeons must maintain a high index of suspicion, as delay in diagnosis of small bowel injuries increases associated morbidity and mortality. The proximal jejunum and distal ileum are the most commonly injured areas, because they are areas of transition between fixed and mobile bowel.

In general, partial-thickness injuries and full-thickness injuries that are less than 50% of the bowel circumference may be repaired with clean edges. Full-thickness injuries greater than 50% circumference, devascularized bowel, and multiple, large, full-thickness defects in a short segment are indications for surgical resection of the injured bowel. Blunt colonic injuries are the result of significant force and are often more extensive than a simple perforation. When resection is required, the decision to primarily repair or divert must be made carefully with consideration for the patient's hemodynamic stability and other associated injuries. In a damage-control laparotomy, the bowel should be left out of continuity until a future exploration to determine ultimate viability of the bowel. Rectal injuries as a result of blunt trauma are rare and are most often diagnosed by proctoscopy. Intraperitoneal rectal injuries may be repaired or resected in the same manner as those in the colon, and extraperitoneal injuries should be treated by diversion with or without presacral drainage.

Kidney and Bladder

Blunt injuries to the kidney and bladder collecting systems are usually minor contusions that are managed nonoperatively. Isolated microscopic hematuria is common and alone does not warrant further investigation. However, gross hematuria or microscopic hematuria in a patient with flank pain, abdominal pain, or hypotension should trigger evaluation of the hematuria. Conversely, absence of hematuria does not exclude a urologic injury, but gross hematuria should always prompt further imaging that includes a retrograde urethrogram and a cystogram. A bladder catheter should not be placed in patients with blood at the urethral meatus until a retrograde urethrogram has been found to be normal.

CT is the modality of choice for diagnosis of renal injuries. The majority of renal injuries are low grade and can be observed, but more severe injuries to the kidney parenchyma or collecting system with a large hematoma, blush, or urine extravasation are treated operatively. Unilateral absence of contrast uptake may indicate a renal artery injury, which also requires operative intervention. Renal injuries discovered during laparotomy are usually nonexpanding hematomas; an expanding perinephric hematoma must be explored. Nephrectomy, although uncommonly necessary, should be performed for the unsalvageable kidney or in the unstable patient with associated injuries. The bladder may be ruptured extraperitoneally or intraperitoneally: extraperitoneal bladder injuries may be managed nonoperatively, but intraperitoneal rupture must be repaired in two layers and protected by prolonged maintenance of a Foley catheter or placement of a suprapubic catheter.

Retroperitoneal Hematoma

Management of a retroperitoneal hematoma is determined by location of the hematoma and stability of the patient. The retroperitoneum is divided into three zones (Figure 3). Zone I is the *central-medial retroperitoneal region,* which extends from the diaphragm to the aorta and vena cava bifurcations and bilaterally to the renal hila. It contains the aorta, vena cava, celiac trunk, the superior and inferior mesenteric arteries, and the renal pedicle vessels. A zone I retroperitoneal

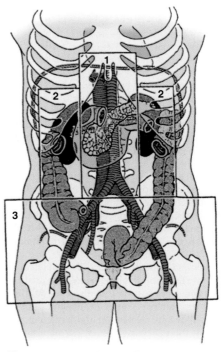

FIGURE 3 The retroperitoneal zones. Zone I is central, zone II is lateral, and zone III is the pelvis. *(From Kudsk KA, Sheldon GF: Retroperitoneal trauma. Blaisdell FW, Trunkey DD (eds): Trauma management—abdominal trauma, New York, 1982, Thieme Medical Publishers, p 281. Reprinted with permission.)*

hematoma from blunt injury requires laparotomy because of the high incidence of visceral or vascular injury. Zone II is the *lateral retroperitoneal region*, containing the kidneys, adrenal glands, ureters, and the renal hila. These are explored if very large or expanding, or to exclude possible colonic injury if suspected. Zone III is the *retroperitoneal pelvis*, including the distal ureters and the colon. Following blunt injury, zone I and expanding zone II hematomas require exploration. Nonexpanding zone II and zone III hematomas need not be explored.

SUMMARY

Management of the patient with blunt abdominal trauma is often complex because of the difficulty in diagnosis and high incidence of associated injuries. Certain injury patterns can be expected and should prompt further evaluation, although initial evaluation always begins with standard ATLS protocols. Once abdominal injuries are identified, nonoperative and operative options of solid-organ injury depend most prominently upon hemodynamic status. Hollow viscus and most pancreatic injuries require laparotomy.

SUGGESTED READINGS

Peitzman AB, Ferrada P, Puyana JC: Nonoperative management of blunt abdominal trauma: have we gone too far? *Surg Infect (Larchmt)* 10:427–433, 2009.

Lee JC, Peitzman AB: Damage control laparotomy, *Curr Opin Crit Care* 12(4):346–350, 2006.

McKenney KL, McKenney MG, Cohn SM, et al: Hemoperitoneum score helps determine need for therapeutic laparotomy, *J Trauma* 50(4):650–654, 2001.

Peitzman AB, Harbrecht BG, Rivera L, et al: Failure of observation of blunt splenic injury in adults: variability in practice and adverse consequences, *J Am Coll Surg* 201(2):179–187, 2005.

Watts DD, Fakhry SM: Incidence of hollow viscus injury in blunt trauma: an analysis from 275,557 trauma admissions from the East multi-institutional trial, *J Trauma* 54(2):289–294, 2003.

PENETRATING ABDOMINAL TRAUMA

David B. Hoyt, MD, and Allen Kong, MD

OVERVIEW

The cornerstone of management of penetrating trauma has been early intervention. As diagnostic and interventional options increase, the decision tree for penetrating abdominal trauma management has evolved considerably.

The history of penetrating abdominal trauma management has generally coincided with the history of wartime surgery. In the nineteenth century, gunshot wounds to the abdomen were managed nonoperatively. As shown in Box 1, the international community advocated supportive care for this type of injury. During World War I, a high mortality rate was associated with nonoperative management; following implementation of mandatory exploration, a precipitous decline was seen in both morbidity and mortality rates. This management paradigm was adopted in the civilian setting also, with routine laparotomies being performed for both stabbings and gunshot wounds to the abdomen.

This standard of care changed in 1960, when the concept of *selective conservatism* was initially introduced by G.W. Shaftan and was subsequently endorsed by Carter Nance. This radical departure from what was considered the gold standard of management of penetrating abdominal injuries initially received limited approval in the surgical community. The selective approach was eventually embraced for stab wounds to the abdomen, and the debate over the role of more selective management of patients with gunshot wounds continues today. Most advocate mandatory exploration for gunshot wounds penetrating the abdomen because of the findings of a 90% risk of significant intraabdominal injury.

INITIAL MANAGEMENT

The principles of initial assessment in Advanced Trauma Life Support (ATLS, American College of Surgeons) are as applicable to penetrating abdominal injuries as for any other injury. The primary survey, with its mandatory emphasis on the "ABCs"—airway, breathing, and circulation—in addition to resuscitation and a secondary survey are imperative in the optimal management of penetrating abdominal injuries.

A definitive airway, preferably a translaryngeal endotracheal intubation, should be performed where doubts about airway stability arise. Associated life-threatening complications—such as hemothorax, pneumothorax, and especially tension pneumothorax—can occur with penetrating wounds in the thoracoabdominal region. Such injuries necessitate prompt recognition and pleural space decompression. Circulatory assessment and stabilization are required after appropriate airway and ventilatory management.

In the case of a hemodynamically unstable patient with abdominal injury, assessment and stabilization should be performed in the operating room as soon as possible. It is likely that injury involves a vascular structure that will require expedient exposure. With a team approach, lifesaving measures can often be performed simultaneously. Fluid resuscitation should be prudent, while focusing on surgical control of the bleeding. For the hemodynamically stable patient, expeditious physical examination should be conducted during the secondary evaluation to detect any occult injuries or other penetrating wounds. At no time should wounds be probed, except in the operating room under direct visualization.

All knife and bullet wounds should be identified and marked with a paper clip or some other radiopaque marker before radiographs to

---

BOX 1: Management of gunshot wounds to the abdomen: Historical perspective

1800s: Surgical dogma dictates nonoperative management of gunshot wounds to the abdomen.

1880: Dr. J. Marion Sims, a southern surgeon, advocates operative management.

1881: President James A. Garfield is shot through the abdomen, and no surgical exploration is performed ("Garfield's death watch"); Dr. Sims openly criticizes this nonoperative approach.

1890: Sir William McCormick, chief army surgeon for the British troops, comments: "If a man undergoes surgery after being shot, he dies and lives if left in peace."

determine localization and possible trajectory. Two bullet wounds detected on abdominal inspection could represent a through-and-through injury or two entry wounds from two missiles. With a penetrating wound, nonvisualization of a foreign body and no evidence of an exit wound is suggestive of a bullet embolism. Pertinent history should always include the mechanism and time of injury, whether loss of consciousness occurred, and whether significant blood loss was noted at the scene. Sustaining penetrating trauma does not preclude blunt trauma as well.

Indications for Immediate Laparotomy

Patients who present with penetrating injuries to the abdomen with hemodynamic instability or peritonitis should undergo immediate laparotomy (Box 2). Centers with high volumes of penetrating trauma may benefit from a system in which these patients are triaged directly to the operating room from the field. Patients with penetrating abdominal injuries who do not have hemodynamic instability or peritonitis are candidates for further workup and may be able to avoid unnecessary laparotomy (Figure 1).

Anterior Abdominal Wall Stab Wounds

A variety of strategies have been described for the management of abdominal stab wounds. Admission with serial physical examinations has been shown in many studies to be safe and effective. Although this has been postulated to lead to a delay in diagnosis, outcomes in patients sustaining bowel injury are comparable. Hemodynamically stable patients who sustain anterior stab wounds can undergo local wound exploration (LWE) in the emergency department under local anesthesia. In obese patients or in patients who sustain multiple stab wounds, LWE may not be viable. If anterior fascial penetration is excluded on LWE, the patient can be discharged home after irrigation and wound care.

If fascial penetration is confirmed, or fascia integrity cannot be determined, a diagnostic peritoneal lavage (DPL) can be performed.

BOX 2: Penetrating abdominal injuries: Indications for emergency laparotomy

Peritoneal signs
Hemodynamic instability
Evisceration
Blood from any natural orifice
Extensive bleeding from the wound
Positive radiologic sign (e.g., pneumoperitoneum)
Impaled object
High-velocity missile injury

Penetrating Abdominal Trauma

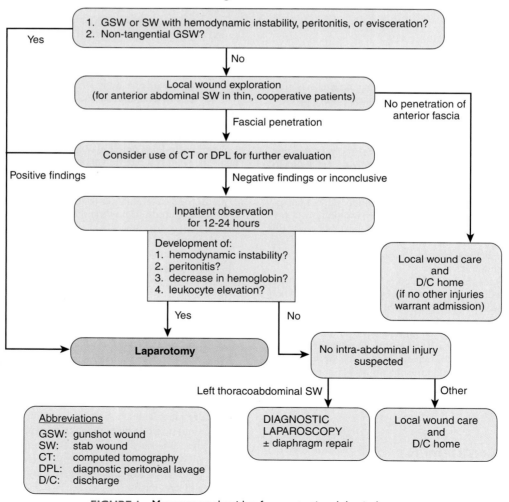

FIGURE 1   Management algorithm for penetrating abdominal trauma.

Thresholds that indicate the need for laparotomy are red blood cell counts over 1000 to 10,000 cells/mm³ and white blood cell counts above 500 cells/mm³. A negative DPL should be followed by 24 hours of observation.

Alternatives to DPL include focused assessment for sonographic evaluation of trauma (FAST), CT scan, or serial exams. FAST will detect fluid but is not reliable for bowel injury or for detecting patients who can be managed nonoperatively. Recently, anterior stab wounds have been comprehensively evaluated with CT without LWE or radiopaque markers. Only suspected bowel injury or major bleeding were critical for an operation; all other patients were clinically observed for the development of peritonitis or hemorrhage. The results were comparable to observation alone.

Thoracoabdominal Stab Wounds

Stab wounds below the nipples and above the costal margin, although theoretically thoracic, often penetrate through the diaphragm and create abdominal injury (Figure 2). If the injury is on the right side, the defect in the diaphragm is generally protected by the liver and is unlikely to allow bowel herniation. If the patient remains hemodynamically stable, the liver injury may be managed nonoperatively. A CT scan will usually illustrate the wound tract.

If the wound is on the left side, diaphragmatic injury must be ruled out. For wounds anterior to the posterior axillary line, laparoscopy is useful. If the diaphragm is uninjured, intraabdominal injury is effectively ruled out. If the laparoscopy is positive, the abdomen must be evaluated for associated injuries. Laparoscopic evaluation for penetrating bowel injury may lack sensitivity. Open laparotomy may be most prudent, allowing for an open diaphragm repair and complete abdominal evaluation. An alternative strategy is to delay the laparoscopy for 12 to 24 hours, until a bowel injury is ruled out by physical exam; then the diaphragm can be approached laparoscopically, and if an injury is discovered, it can be repaired laparoscopically, and open laparotomy can be avoided.

Back and Flank Stab Wounds

Stab wounds to the back have a low incidence of producing an intraabdominal injury requiring operative repair. Evaluation is usually with a triple-contrast CT scan, as laparoscopy and DPL are both inaccurate for evaluation of retroperitoneal injuries. CT scan can help rule out specific injuries, if the wound tract is of little concern for injury. Organs of specific concern include the diaphragm, spleen, liver, pancreas, duodenum, aorta, kidneys, ureters, and retroperitoneal colon. CT is suggestive of injury in this situation but is not always definitive; concern for injury is best evaluated by laparotomy.

Gunshot Wounds

Patients sustaining a gunshot wound (GSW) with a trajectory that potentially traverses the peritoneal cavity would traditionally undergo urgent laparotomy. The rationale for this relates to the thought that 90% of patients who sustain intraperitoneal penetration from a GSW will have injuries that require operative repair. Increasing evidence shows that selective nonoperative management may decrease the rate of nontherapeutic laparotomy after abdominal GSW. If peritonitis is absent, and the patient is hemodynamically stable, a CT scan can be considered. This is particularly true if the trajectory is suspicious for being transhepatic or tangential to the abdomen. Bullet tracts through the liver are illustrated quite well on modern CT scanners. These injuries may be addressed nonoperatively, as is done with blunt trauma.

GSWs suspicious for being tangential to the abdomen and extraperitoneal may be managed either by diagnostic laparoscopy or by CT scan, but CT scans have the significant advantage of being less invasive. The possibility of blast injury must be considered with high-velocity weapons. Adequate resources, especially personnel, to closely follow the physical exam of patients are essential if nonoperative management is followed.

Management of shotgun wounds to the abdomen (SGWA) is not well standardized. The magnitude of injury is closely related to the distance between the gun and the victim. The greater the distance, the wider the scatter of pellets. A scoring system divides patients into three different management groups: *type 1* has a greater than 25 cm scatter type, *type 2* scatters between 10 and 25 cm, and *type 3* scatters less than 10 cm. Two thirds of patients with type 1 injuries to the abdomen do not require laparotomy. Clinical judgment based on the pellet scatter and physical examination should be considered in determining whether to perform a laparotomy. DPL may be helpful when this is unclear, but CT will be difficult to interpret due to pellet scatter and as such is infrequently used.

Operative Approach

The patient should be placed supine on the operating room table, and the entire anterior torso, from the sternal notch to the middle thighs, should be prepared and draped; this will allow for maximum exposure and harvesting of the saphenous vein, should that become necessary for vascular repair. A midline incision is preferred, with few reasons to deviate from this course. The incision also allows extension into a median sternotomy in the event that more proximal control of the aorta or vena cava is needed, or if the patient is found to have cardiac injury. In any event, the surgical approach should be systematic (Box 3).

After the abdomen is opened, obvious blood and clot are removed, and packing of the four quadrants is continued as indicated by

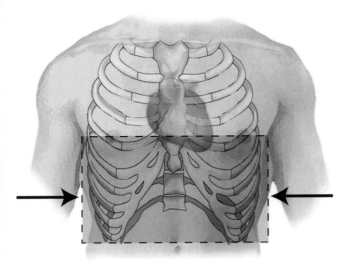

FIGURE 2 Areas of concern for thoracoabdominal injuries.

BOX 3: Surgical approach

1. Control hemorrhage
2. Control gross spillage and cross-cavity contamination
3. Meticulous exploration
4. Mobilization techniques
5. Adequate assessment of all holes/hematomas
6. Damage control*
7. Definitive repair of intraabdominal injuries

*Damage control will likely preclude all aspects of this specific operative plan being performed at the original operation.

ongoing bleeding. If the peritoneal cavity is full of blood, the location of clot is often a clue to the site of bleeding. Inflow occlusion can be accomplished if needed by clamping the aorta at the diaphragmatic hiatus adjacent to the esophagus. Obvious hollow viscus wounds should be rapidly controlled by sutures, clamps, or staples. This initial closure does not need to be definitive and is done primarily to minimize contamination during the course of the operation. Retroperitoneal bleeding may be the source of exsanguinating hemorrhage, if rupture into the free peritoneal cavity has occurred. Retroperitoneal hematomas are classified in zones that are central (zone I), perinephric or lateral (zone II), or pelvic (zone III). Retroperitoneal hematomas resulting from penetrating injuries are major, vascular (zone I), or renal injuries (zone II) unless proven otherwise. Even if the retroperitoneal hematoma is not pulsatile or expanding, zones I and II in the hematomas should be explored.

After packing has controlled hemorrhage, and ongoing contamination has been stopped, allow time for resuscitation of the patient's circulating blood volume. Warming is necessary if massive blood loss has occurred, and sustained periods of hypotension should be avoided at all costs. A complete and thorough exploratory laparotomy is performed methodically to investigate the entire contents of the abdomen for all injuries.

Specific Injuries

When abdominal exploration is required, it is imperative to be knowledgeable about the full spectrum of operative options and the potential outcomes. Specific diagnostic and management principles are shown in Table 1.

TABLE 1: Penetrating abdominal trauma

Organ	Incidence	Diagnosis	Specific Management	Results
Small Bowel	Highest incidence of injury of the intraabdominal organs	Physical examination: Cannot rely on tenderness or peritoneal signs in the early stage of injury	Perioperative antibiotics	Good outcome
		Radiography: Free air	Primary closure of simple lacerations	Negligible leak rate, even in a contaminated field
		FAST: Free fluid with CT scan demonstrating no solid-organ injury	Segmental resection of complex injuries with functional end-to-end tensionless anastomosis	
		CT: High false-negative rate; pneumoperitoneum; extravasation of enteral contrast; free fluid	One- (or double-) layer closure, anastomosis, or stapled anastomosis	
			Exploration of large, expanding mesenteric hematomas	
Colon	Stab wounds = 5%	Physical examination: Tenderness/peritoneal signs; gross blood on rectal examination	Perioperative antibiotics	Overall favorable outcome
	Gunshot wounds = 25%		Primary closure of simple injuries (avoid narrowing the lumen)	Complications: Low leak rate, wound infection, intraperitoneal abscess
			Segmental resection and fecal diversion of complex colonic wounds	
Liver	Most commonly injured solid organ	Physical examination: Right upper quadrant tenderness	Perioperative antibiotics	Variable outcome depending on the degree of hepatic injury (grade I–VI)
		Radiography: Nonspecific; pneumothorax if there is associated pleural space entry as a result of the penetrating injury	Depending on the severity of the injury (grade) and the hemodynamic status of the patient: • Expectant (observation) • Drainage • Hepatorrhaphy (including argon beam coagulation) • Debridement/resection • Packing • Angiography/embolization	

TABLE 1: Penetrating abdominal trauma—cont'd

Organ	Incidence	Diagnosis	Specific Management	Results
		FAST: Can be unreliable		
		CT: If necessary for diagnostic study; should only be performed in the hemo-dynamically stable patient		
Spleen	Less common injury rate than with blunt trauma	Physical examination: Left upper quadrant tenderness/peritoneal signs; referred pain to left shoulder (Kehr sign)	Perioperative antibiotics	Overall good outcome with all the management choices
		Radiography: Nonspecific; occasional associated pneumothorax	• Expectant (observation) • Splenorrhaphy (including argon beam coagulation) • Partial splenectomy • Splenectomy • Angioembolization	Infrequent complications: Pleural effusion, pneumonia, subphrenic abscess, thrombocytosis
				Overwhelming post-splenectomy infection (rare)
		FAST: Can be unreliable	Postsplenectomy immunization vaccines: *Streptococcus pneumoniae, Haemophilus influenzae, Neisseria meningitidis*	
		CT: If necessary for diagnostic study; should only be performed in the hemo-dynamically stable patient		
Diaphragm	6% of all intraabdominal injuries resulting from penetrating trauma	Physical examination: Chest pain and shortness of breath, scaphoid abdomen, bowel sounds on auscultation of hemithorax	Perioperative antibiotics	Associated injuries dictate morbidity and mortality and need for open approach
		Radiography: Hollow viscus noted in the left hemithorax; nasogastric tube in left hemithorax	Primary closure is preferred definitive management	
		FAST: Can be unreliable	With documentation of a diaphragmatic laceration, may use laparoscopic approach vs. open treatment	
		CT: May demonstrate diaphragm rupture or free fluid on either side of diaphragm		
		DPL: Inconclusive		
		Laparoscopy: Diagnostic modality of choice		
Stomach	More common injury in penetrating trauma than blunt trauma	Physical examination: Epigastric tenderness, peritoneal signs, bloody gastric aspirate	Perioperative antibiotics	Associated injuries affect morbidity and mortality

Continued

TABLE I: Penetrating abdominal trauma—cont'd

Organ	Incidence	Diagnosis	Specific Management	Results
	10% of penetrating injuries of the abdomen	Radiography: Free air under the diaphragm	Debridement when necessary	
		FAST: Can be unreliable	Primary closure (two layers)	
		DPL: Positive lavage (red blood cells, white blood cells, gross contamination)		
		CT: Pneumoperitoneum		
		Laparoscopy: Operator dependent		
Duodenum/ pancreas	Isolated injuries uncommon	Physical examination: Abdominal tenderness, peritoneal signs	Perioperative antibiotics	Highly lethal due to associated injuries
	High percentage of associated injuries	Radiography: Free air, retroperitoneal air	Duodenum: • Primary repair • Primary repair with gastrostomy, retrograde jejunostomy, feeding jejunostomy • Pyloric exclusion	Increased mortality with delayed diagnosis of duodenal injury
		FAST: Nonspecific	Pancreas: • Drainage • Debridement • Partial resection • Pancreaticoduodenectomy	
		DPL: Nonspecific		
		CT: Nonspecific		
Biliary	Extrahepatic biliary injury infrequent	Physical examination: Abdominal tenderness, peritoneal signs	Perioperative antibiotics	Cholecystectomy: Negligible mortality
		Radiography: Nonspecific	Cholecystectomy (for gallbladder injuries)	Biliary duct reconstruction: Bile leak
		FAST: Nonspecific	Biliary duct reconstruction (e.g., choledochojejunostomy)	Possible stricture
		DPL: Nonspecific		
		CT: Nonspecific		
Kidney	20% of renal injuries are from penetrating trauma	Physical examination: Penetrating wound or trajectory in close proximity to the kidney, hematuria	Perioperative antibiotics	Mortality related to associated injuries
		Radiography: Nonspecific	Primary repair with viable tissue buttress	
		FAST: Nonspecific	Nephrectomy or partial nephrectomy	
		DPL: Nonspecific		

Continued

TABLE 1: Penetrating abdominal trauma—cont'd

Organ	Incidence	Diagnosis	Specific Management	Results
		CT (if peritoneal penetration not suspected in a gunshot wound): Perinephric hematoma, extravasation		
Bladder	Usually occult injury found during intraoperative abdominal exploration	Physical examination: Penetrating wound or trajectory in close proximity to the bladder, hematuria	Perioperative antibiotics	Excellent outcomes
		Radiography: Nonspecific	Multilayer closure with absorbable sutures with indwelling bladder catheter	Morbidity and mortality relate to associated injuries
		FAST: Nonspecific		
		DPL: Nonspecific		
		CT (if peritoneal penetration not suspected): Extravasation of contrast agent		
Ureter	Infrequent injury in penetrating trauma	Usually an intraoperative diagnosis	Perioperative antibiotics	Good outcome if no major associated injuries
			Primary repair/stenting	
			Delayed repair and suprapubic cystostomy	
			Diverting nephrostomies	

SUMMARY

With advancing technology and surgical expertise in both the open and minimally invasive arena, the management of penetrating abdominal trauma will continue to evolve. Evidence-based practice should be the paramount driving force to guide decision making.

SUGGESTED READINGS

Biffl WL, Kaups KL, Cothren CC, et al: Management of patients with anterior abdominal stab wounds: a Western Trauma Association multicenter trial, *J Trauma* 66(5):1294, 2009.

Brown CV, Velmahos GC, Neville AL, et al: Hemodynamically "stable" patients with peritonitis after penetrating abdominal trauma: identifying those who are bleeding, *Arch Surg* 140(8):767, 2005.

Como JJ, Bokhari F, Chui WC, et al: *Practice management guidelines for nonoperative management of penetrating abdominal trauma: EAST guidelines,* 2007:Available online at http://www.east.org/tpg/nonoppene.pdf. 2007.

Cothren CC, Moore EE, Warren FA, et al: Local wound exploration remains a valuable triage tool for the evaluation of anterior abdominal stab wounds, *Am J Surg* 198(2):223, 2009.

Demetriades D, Hadjizacharia P, Constantinou C, et al: Selective nonoperative management of penetrating abdominal solid organ injuries, *Ann Surg* 244(4):620, 2006.

Kaban GK, Novitsky YW, Perugini RA, et al: Use of laparoscopy in evaluation and treatment of penetrating and blunt abdominal injuries, *Surg Innov* 15(1):26, 2008.

Nance FC, Wennar MH, Johnson LW, et al: Surgical judgment in the management of penetrating wounds of the abdomen: experience with 2212 patients, *Ann Surg* 179(5):639, 1974.

Shaftan GW: Indications for operation in abdominal trauma, *Am J Surg* 99:657, 1960.

Sugrue M, Balogh Z, Lynch J, et al: Guidelines for the management of haemodynamically stable patients with stab wounds to the anterior abdomen, *ANZ J Surg* 77(8):614, 2007.

Velmahos GC, Demetriades D, Toutouzas KG, et al: Selective nonoperative management in 1,856 patients with abdominal gunshot wounds: should routine laparotomy still be the standard of care? *Ann Surg* 234(3):395, 2001.

DIAPHRAGMATIC INJURIES

Gregory J. Jurkovich, MD

OVERVIEW

In 1541, Sennertus first detailed the postmortem finding of a strangulated stomach associated with a diaphragmatic hernia. Thirty-eight years later, Ambrose Paré reported the death of a patient from colonic strangulation in a diaphragmatic hernia caused by a gunshot wound. Over four centuries later, recognition and management of diaphragmatic injuries remains a challenge to the trauma surgeon. Traumatic diaphragmatic ruptures occur in 3% to 4% of patients with significant blunt abdominal trauma, yet only about 25% are diagnosed on the initial chest radiograph. Prior to widespread use of computed tomography (CT), studies have reported that 12% to 69% of diaphragmatic ruptures were not detected during the initial evaluation. Although CT scanning with three-dimensional reconstruction and magnetic resonance imaging (MRI) have been added to the armamentarium of noninvasive diagnostic techniques, the current standard for the definitive diagnosis of diaphragmatic rupture is video-assisted direct visual inspection. Both video-assisted thoracoscopy (VATS) and laparoscopy play a role in the diagnosis of diaphragmatic injury and can also be employed in the repair of select injuries. However, without suspecting the possibility of a diaphragmatic injury, the clinician will often overlook subtle signs and will fail to make the diagnosis acutely, subjecting the patient to the possibility of delayed bowel strangulation and its attendant morbidity and mortality.

EPIDEMIOLOGY

The incidence of traumatic diaphragmatic rupture following thoracoabdominal trauma is generally reported as 0.8% to 5%. Relatively small case studies provide this information, in part because so many diaphragmatic injuries have previously gone unrecognized in the acute phase, with as many as 30% of diaphragmatic ruptures presenting with late hernias with or without strangulation. The incidence of penetrating thoracic or upper abdominal wounds traversing the diaphragm is of course entirely dependent on trajectory, but it is generally felt that penetrating mechanisms of injury are responsible for an even higher incidence of injury. Diaphragmatic injury is estimated to occur in 0.4% of penetrating wounds to the thorax and upper abdomen or flank, but it occurs in up to 20% of penetrating wounds to the lower chest. These

injuries are evenly divided between the right and left sides, are usually shorter than 2 cm, and are most commonly diagnosed during laparotomy for other reasons. Increasingly, diagnostic thoracoscopy and/or laparoscopy are being utilized to diagnose and treat isolated and smaller diaphragmatic injuries from these mechanisms.

The most common cause of blunt diaphragmatic injury is motor vehicle crashes, although falls are an increasingly recognized injury mechanism. Blunt torso injury severe enough to warrant trauma center evaluation probably means there is a 1% incidence of diaphragm injury. At my institution, we have diagnosed 118 blunt diaphragmatic ruptures out of 28,412 blunt trauma admissions over the past 7 years, an incidence of less than 1%. Blunt diaphragmatic injuries are larger, usually greater than 10 cm, and they are more common in those wearing lap-type seat belts and in victims of lateral-impact collisions. The more widespread use of three-point restraints and airbags probably has decreased the incidence. Postmortem studies demonstrate an equal prevalence of right- and left-sided injuries, although a preponderance of left-sided injuries are recognized acutely, with some studies suggesting 75% to 90% of blunt diaphragmatic injuries occur on patients' left sides. Hence, although each hemidiaphragm is equally susceptible, the liver appears to either obscure the diagnosis on the right side or to perhaps buffer the forces, thereby producing the clinically evident left-sided predominance. A prompt and correct diagnosis is made in less than 50% of all cases, a pitfall attributed to the nonspecific signs and symptoms, lack of definitive noninvasive diagnostic measures, and the high incidence of concomitant injuries, which are distracting and at least initially appear more urgent in the diagnostic triage. Table 1 and Table 2 detail the association between diaphragmatic injury and other organ injuries and emphasize both the frequent occurrence of associated injuries, as well as the injuries most likely to be associated with blunt (Table 1) or penetrating (Table 2) injury mechanisms.

Although the natural course and history of unrecognized diaphragmatic injury are not well known, the majority of case reports of delayed diagnosis reveal that perhaps 18% of blunt and 32% of penetrating injuries are diagnosed in a delayed fashion, generally more than 3 years after the initial trauma, and sometimes as many as 40 years later.

ANATOMY AND EMBRYOLOGY

The human diaphragm develops from four embryonic sources: the transverse septum, mediastinum, pleuroperitoneal membranes, and muscles of the body wall. In the adult, the muscle fibers originate peripherally from the chest wall, upper lumbar vertebrae, and sternum arch centripetally to insert into the central tendon. The arterial supply stems from the phrenic arteries, direct branches of the abdominal

TABLE 1: Associations between diaphragmatic injury and specific associated organ injuries in blunt thoracoabdominal trauma

Injury	Diaphragm Rupture (%)	No Diaphragm Rupture (%)	OR (95% CI)	Sensitivity (%)	Specificity (%)
Pulmonary contusion	3770 (44.9)	87,183 (22.4)	2.8 (1.9-4.2)	44.9	77.6
Rib fracture	5368 (63.9)	209,940 (54.0)	1.5 (0.9-2.5)	63.9	46.0
Thoracic aorta	1294 (15.4)	13,083 (3.4)	5.2 (2.2-12.5)	15.4	96.6
Spleen	4483 (53.4)	46,844 (12.1)	8.4 (3.9-17.8)	53.4	88.0
Liver	3048 (36.3)	46,740 (12.0)	4.2 (1.7-10.6)	36.3	88.0
Pelvic fracture	3565 (42.5)	52,960 (13.6)	4.7 (2.7-8.0)	42.5	86.4

OR, Odds ratio; *CI,* confidence interval

From Reiff DA, McGwin G Jr, Metzger J, et al: Identifying injuries and motor vehicle collision characteristics that together are a suggestion of diaphragmatic injury, *J Trauma* 53:1139, 2002.

TABLE 2: Associated injuries of diaphragmatic rupture in penetrating abdominal trauma

Organ	Gunshot Wound	Stab	Blunt	Total
Liver	57	21	7	85
Stomach	18	22	5	45
Spleen	18	6	5	29
Lung	19	9	1	29
Colon	19	5	4	28
Kidney	12	6	2	20
Small bowel	10	4	2	16
Heart	2	6	3	11
Other	103	38	6	147
Total	258	117	35	410
Average	2.9	1.8	3.2	2.5

From Wiencek RG, Wilson RF, Steiger Z: Acute injuries of the diaphragm, *J Thorac Cardiovasc Surg* 92:989, 1986.

aorta; venous drainage is to the inferior vena cava. Motor innervation is provided by the phrenic nerve, which is also sensory to the central tendon, parietal pleura, and peritoneum; sensation wherein the peripheral circumference is carried by intercostal nerves.

The anatomy of the phrenic nerve termination at the diaphragm warrants special consideration. According to G.S. Muller Botha and a detailed anatomical dissection paper published in *Thorax* in 1957, the two phrenic nerves branch above the diaphragm, varying from a few millimeters to 2 cm above the diaphragm. Both nerves divide into a variable number of branches, from two to seven. The classical impression of only three or four branches is erroneous. The branches vary in size and thickness, with no particular relation to the area served, although the posteromedial branch is usually the largest. The most common branching pattern is best described as an anterior (toward the sternum), lateral (most variability), and posteriomedial (crural) branching. The branches diverge, enter the muscle or central tendon, and run obliquely within its substance for a varying distance. They then appear on the undersurface of the diaphragm and radiate deep to the subphrenic fascia, with numerous filaments innervating the muscle fibers (Figure 1). The lateral branches differ on the two sides. Right-side lateral branches are short, thick, and always pass posterior to the vena cava. Left-side lateral branches are long, slender, and directed toward the vertebral column, piercing the diaphragm and running along the inferior surface of the central tendon to the left hiatal margin.

During any repair of a diaphragm injury, the surgeon should try to avoid injuring or entrapping the phrenic nerve, but this may be particularly difficult with radial-type injuries originating near the central tendon and vena cava foramen or esophageal hiatus.

The natural history of unrepaired, small diaphragmatic tears is unknown, although the incidence of intestinal strangulation when diaphragm injuries appear after a latent period is reported to be as high as 20%. Most penetrating injuries are small and may heal without sequelae. Similarly, there is little evidence that right-sided rupture is associated with significant morbidity or mortality, a benefit perhaps imposed by the sealant effect of the liver. Nevertheless, the combination of the constant motion of the diaphragm, its thinness, and the pressure gradient between the pleural space and peritoneal cavity, favoring movement of viscera from abdomen to the thorax, may retard healing and predispose to the development of chronic diaphragmatic hernias, regardless of the size of the injury.

During normal respiration, the intrapleural pressure fluctuates between −5 and −10 cm H_2O, but the intraabdominal pressure is between +2 and +10 cm H_2O. This results in a +2 to +20 pressure gradient from the abdomen into the chest, encouraging the displacement and herniation of abdominal contents. With mechanical ventilation this pressure gradient difference is abolished, and diaphragmatic hernias, even with large lacerations, are usually not seen.

Diaphragmatic injuries are graded in severity from grades I to V, as described by the American Association for the Surgery of Trauma Organ Injury Scale (Table 3). It is important for billing, coding, and subsequent clinical care to specify the length and location of the laceration or rupture, the location of phrenic nerve branches, and any associated tissue loss.

DIAGNOSIS

The physical findings classically associated with acute diaphragmatic injury include audible bowel sounds in the lower thorax, unilateral absence of breath sounds, respiratory distress, and scaphoid abdomen. Unfortunately, these are frequently absent; in multisystem trauma, such findings are often overlooked. Most series have reported normal physical examinations in 20% to 45% of patients with diaphragmatic injury, with one larger series reporting normal physical findings in 53% of patients with a diaphragm rupture caused by blunt mechanism and 44% of patients with a penetrating mechanism of diaphragm injury. At one time, exploratory laparotomy for suspected diaphragmatic injury was considered the best diagnostic modality, but it carried the price of a 20% to 30% negative laparotomy rate with an attendant 10% incidence of significant morbidity. Video-assisted endoscopic inspection has largely supplanted exploratory laparotomy in this regard, but noninvasive techniques have also greatly improved the preoperative diagnosis.

Chest Radiograph

As the principal screening method for thoracic injury, early chest radiography (CXR) only occasionally (20% to 34%) makes the diagnosis of diaphragmatic injury. Although the reported incidence of a totally normal CXR in the face of diaphragmatic injury ranges from 5% to 20%, most abnormalities are nonspecific but suggestive of the diagnosis. Initial chest radiographs allow the diagnosis of 27% to 60% of left-sided injuries but only 17% of right-sided injuries. Differentiation of a herniated liver through a diaphragmatic tear from other causes of elevated diaphragm—such as atelectasis, pleural effusion, or pulmonary contusion—is difficult. Pathognomonic CXR findings are present in less than half of patients; these include air- or fluid-containing viscera or the tip of the nasogastric tube above the left hemidiaphragm (Figure 2). An elevated diaphragm, obscuration of a nonelevated hemidiaphragm, and a shift in the mediastinum away from the injured side are also suggestive of diaphragmatic injury. Serial CXR may improve the accuracy, as herniation may be delayed.

It is tempting to be lured into a false sense of security by a normal radiograph in the mechanically ventilated patient; the positive pressure ventilation reverses the abdominal-pleural pressure gradient and may reduce visceral herniation. Hence, it is prudent to maintain a high index of suspicion and to obtain a postextubation CXR and carefully inspect it for signs of diaphragm injury. The rate of missed diaphragmatic rupture on initial chest radiography ranges from 12% to 66%, emphasizing the need for awareness of the possibility of this injury and the need for subsequent investigations in high-risk patients.

Contrast Studies

Barium enema or upper gastrointestinal series may improve the diagnostic accuracy, although they also rely on the presence of visceral herniation and are now rarely used in the acute setting for the

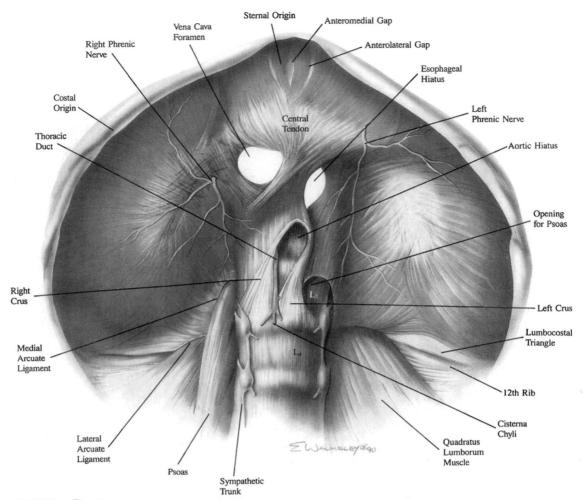

FIGURE I   The diaphragm, as viewed from below. *(Illustration courtesy Elise Walmsley. Copyright Romaine Pierson Publishers.)*

TABLE 3: American Association for the Surgery of Trauma organ injury scale for diaphragmatic injuries

Grade	Description
I	Contusion
II	Laceration ≤2 cm
III	Laceration 2–10 cm
IV	Laceration >10 cm with tissue loss <25 cm^2
V	Laceration with tissue loss >25 cm^2

purpose of diagnosing diaphragm injury. A focal constriction of bowel at the level of the hemidiaphragm and an obvious displacement of bowel into the thorax are pathognomonic signs. Such findings are demonstrated in the minority of patients, however, and even less so in the presence of mechanical ventilation.

Computed Tomography

CT of the abdomen is frequently used in stable blunt trauma patients, and a growing number of studies have attempted to define the role of CT in identifying diaphragmatic injury. Since the 1990s,

the introduction of helical CT, array-detector technology, and three-dimensional reconstruction has improved the accuracy of CT in detecting diaphragm injury. Helical CT has a sensitivity of 70% (78% for left sided and 50% for right sided), a specificity approaching 100%, and an overall accuracy of 88% for left-sided injuries and 70% for right-sided injuries. Several major findings should be identified on CT that are diagnostic or suggestive of diaphragm injury. These include direct discontinuity of the hemidiaphragm or a diaphragm defect and intrathoracic herniation of abdominal contents, with the stomach and colon the most common viscera to herniate on the left side, and the liver the most common to herniate on the right side; herniated omentum should be visualized because of its high fat content. The *collar sign,* a waist-like construction of the herniating hollow viscus at the site of the diaphragm tear, is another positive finding, along with *dependent viscera sign,* in which the herniated viscera are no longer supported posteriorly by the injured diaphragm, causing them to fall to a dependent position against the posterior ribs. On CT, the abdominal contents lie central to the diaphragm, and the thoracic contents lie peripheral. Hence, intrathoracic herniation of fat or organs can be identified by means of the abnormal position of these structures relative to the diaphragm. The use of intravenous contrast is generally recommended to more clearly reveal the vascular supply of organs. Reconstruction images on sagittal or coronal planes and three-dimensional reconstructions may provide additional useful information, but the formatting does take time.

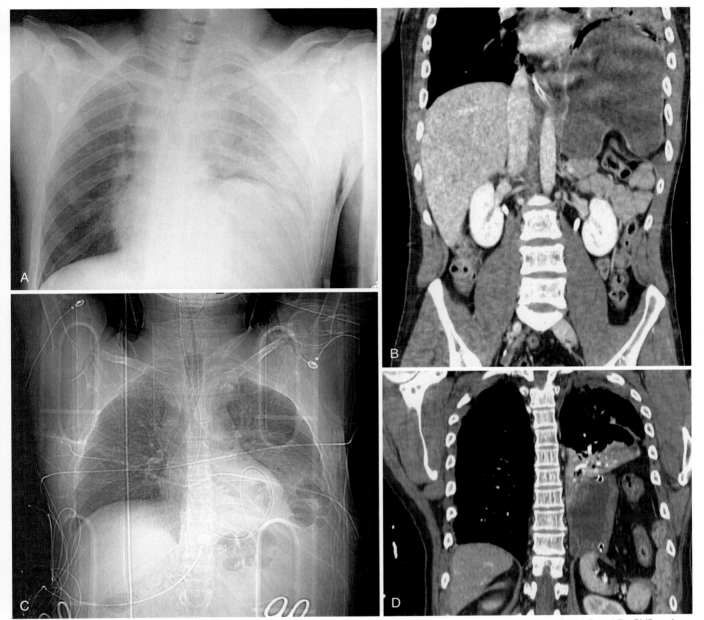

FIGURE 2 **A** and **B,** CXR and coronal CT imaging of the same patient. Note the subtle signs of diaphragm injury on CXR. **C** and **D,** CXR and coronal CT imaging of another patient. Note the signs of diaphragm injury, the coiled nasogastric tube, and intestinal gas bubble in the chest.

Pitfalls in the use of CT to diagnose diaphragm injuries include the fact that the dome of the diaphragm is difficult to discern, as the plane of the CT scan is tangential to the diaphragm, and frequently the thickness of the diaphragm is less than the thickness of the CT slices. Also, the diaphragm is difficult to distinguish from liver, spleen, and stomach unless separated by fat, fluid, or air; it is also difficult to discern from superimposed effusions or atelectasis. Furthermore, posterolateral defects are detected at CT in approximately 6% of asymptomatic adults, and they may mimic diaphragmatic tears and lead to a false-positive CT findings because these are thought to represent congenital, asymptomatic Bochdalek hernias. In addition, diaphragmatic eventration can mimic a rupture, and motion artifacts due to respiratory movement decrease the quality of multiplanar reformation and can mimic a diaphragmatic rupture. In combination with a normal increase in diaphragmatic defects with age, these characteristics limit the reliance on CT as a definitive diagnostic tool.

Magnetic Resonance Imaging

MRI is not useful in most traumatic diaphragm rupture cases because of its relatively long duration, sensitivity to motion artifact, and the strict requirement of no iron-metallic materials in the room. However, MRI can provide direct coronal and sagittal images that are well suited for optimal visualizations of the entire hemidiaphragm, if motion can be limited by respiratory and cardiac gating. The whole diaphragm is more clearly revealed on T1-weighted sagittal MRI showing anterior and posterior portions of diaphragm and the hernia orifices. Specific techniques of MRI are developing that may be more suited to the acute setting, with faster imaging sequences and better synchrony between the MR image capture, physiologic monitoring, and life-support equipment such as ventilators and intravenous pumps. Currently, however, MRI is less suited to the acute trauma setting and should be reserved for stable, cooperative, alert patients with uncertain CT diagnosis or delayed signs of a diaphragmatic tear.

Ultrasound

Ultrasound has gained wide acceptance in the initial evaluation of blunt abdominal trauma, and it has been reportedly used to evaluate right-sided diaphragmatic injury after blunt trauma; however, experience is limited, and interpretation is highly operator dependent. Furthermore, limitations imposed by subcutaneous emphysema and acoustic shadowing from the ribs, overlying bandages, and visceral intraluminal gas add to its unreliability. Findings to look for on abdominal ultrasound are direct visualization of the diaphragm defect, herniated organs and their vascular supply detected on Doppler ultrasound, or paracardiac hernia mass.

Diagnostic Peritoneal Lavage

The widespread use of CT and abdominal ultrasound in the acute evaluation of abdominal trauma for acute injury has supplanted the use of diagnostic peritoneal lavage (DPL) in most situations, but not all. DPL remains the most sensitive method of detecting intraabdominal hemorrhage in the hemodynamically unstable patient, in whom CT imaging is not appropriate. The sensitivity and specificity of DPL in identifying intraabdominal injury is largely determined by the red blood cell (RBC) threshold deemed necessary for surgical intervention. A DPL criteria of more than 1000 RBC/mm^2 will detect small amounts of blood in the abdomen and hence has been used to diagnose diaphragm injuries following stab wounds to the lower chest, flank, or back. False-negative DPL was noted in 14% and 40% of patients, respectively, with isolated diaphragmatic injuries in two series using higher RBC criteria; but even low RBC criteria have failed to detect isolated diaphragmatic stab wounds when the bleeding is nominal or primarily into the chest rather than the abdomen. Hence DPL is not recommended as an accurate determinant of diaphragm injury.

Laparoscopy

Video-assisted laparoscopy and thoracoscopy have proven highly accurate, as well as occasionally therapeutic, in the evaluation of diaphragmatic injury. Their role in detecting what might be called *occult* diaphragmatic injuries in stab or gunshot wounds to the lower chest may be particularly useful, and they appear to offer a clear advantage in diagnosing the more common blunt, left-sided injuries in the hemodynamically stable patient in whom the injury is suspected but unproven by noninvasive imaging studies. Laparoscopy requires a 35- or 45-degree laparoscope, visceral mobilization, retraction, and steep Trendelenburg positioning to afford adequate visualization of the entire diaphragm. Because standard CO_2 gas insufflation is required, the risk of a tension pneumothorax is significant, so the insufflation pressure should be limited to less than 12 mm Hg; this precludes the use of this technique in the unstable patient. In addition to visualizing the entire left hemidiaphragm, other potentially injured intraabdominal structures can also be visualized but to a more limited degree.

Thoracoscopy

Video-assisted thoracoscopy (VATS) is perhaps the most accurate means of identifying diaphragmatic rupture on either side, with all series to date reporting near 100% sensitivity and specificity. This modality also enables the evaluation of mediastinal structures and the remainder of the chest cavity, as well as allowing for the possibility of therapeutic intervention by either intracorporeal sewing or stapling of small diaphragm lacerations that have no tissue loss and are fairly central in location. Gas insufflation is not utilized, but exposure is greatly facilitated by bronchial occlusion and collapse of the lung

on the side of visualization, a maneuver that is poorly tolerated in the inadequately resuscitated patient or in someone with acute lung injury. Experience with thoracoscopic repair of the diaphragm is, however, limited; no long-term follow-up on the durability of these repairs is available.

Diagnostic Algorithm

Penetrating Trauma

Most diaphragmatic injuries due to penetrating trauma are identified during surgical exploration for intraperitoneal penetration; hence the surgeon must always inspect and palpate the diaphragm. Patients without indications for laparotomy, but who possess the possibility of diaphragmatic injury, require diagnostic evaluation. As with all thoracic trauma, patients are screened with an anteroposterior CXR with the full awareness that an injury may still exist in the presence of a normal study.

Independent predictors of diaphragmatic injury after penetrating chest trauma are noted in Table 4. Included are abnormal chest radiograph, lower thoracic penetrating wounds—such as a gunshot or stab wound caudal to the fourth intercostal space anteriorly, sixth intercostal space laterally, and tip of the scapula posteriorly (Figure 3)—and those with evidence of intraabdominal injury.

In the absence of an indication for laparotomy or thoracotomy, those suspected of harboring a diaphragmatic injury generally will undergo a contrast-enhanced (usually intravenous only) CT scan of the lower chest and abdomen. Clear tangential wounds can be safely observed for injuries presenting in a delayed fashion. Debate surrounds the need to repair a right-sided small diaphragm and liver injury in the hemodynamically normal patient with minimal blood loss, no hollow viscus injury, and no bile leak. I would favor thoracoscopic repair of the diaphragm in this setting if laparotomy is clearly not warranted. Other patients might be observed to exclude concomitant intraabdominal injury presenting in a delayed fashion, leading to a laparotomy.

When penetrating left hemidiaphragm injury is suspected, patients need to be more directly evaluated. Patients with radiographic findings suggestive of this diagnosis, and even those with normal results yet a mechanism and trajectory highly suggestive of such an injury, need further evaluation. Although DPL was once commonly used in this setting, a greatly expanded role for diagnostic laparoscopy is emerging, and it is preferable to thoracoscopy for the very same reasons that the best acute approach to most diaphragm injuries is via the abdomen. Although both thoracoscopy and laparoscopy are equally efficacious for evaluating the left hemidiaphragm, laparoscopy also enables a limited inspection of potential intraabdominal injuries and has the patient appropriately positioned for laparotomy, which is often required. Although thoracoscopy avoids the risk of tension pneumothorax and enables simultaneous evaluation of the mediastinum, the incidence of intraperitoneal injury is significant in penetrating trauma, and exclusion of concomitant abdominal injury needs to be made with exploration of the abdomen regardless of the thoracoscopic findings.

Blunt Trauma

Patients sustaining blunt trauma sufficient to cause diaphragmatic injury usually have significant concomitant trauma. Pathognomonic findings on the initial chest radiograph should prompt celiotomy. In the setting of a suggestive radiograph and negative abdominal evaluation by ultrasound or CT, further workup of the diaphragm is warranted. This setting is in fact the one most commonly encountered. As previously noted, the noninvasive diagnostic tests are often unclear and nondefinitive in the recognition and diagnosis of a diaphragmatic injury. Surgeons have the option of sequential radiologic examinations, diagnostic laparoscopy, or

TABLE 4: Independent predictors of diaphragmatic injury after penetrating chest trauma

Variable	Odds Ratio	95% CI	P Value
Abnormal chest radiograph	21.3	5–91	<.01
Entrance wound inferior to nipple line	7.0	2–24	<.01
Intraabdominal injuries	6.1	3–13	<.01
High-velocity mechanism	2.9	2–6	<.01
Right-side entrance wound	2.5	1–5	<.01

From Freeman RK, Al-Dossari G, Hutcheson KA, et al: Indications for using video-assisted thoracoscopic surgery to diagnose diaphragmatic injuries after penetrating chest trauma, *Ann Thorac Surg* 72:342, 2001.

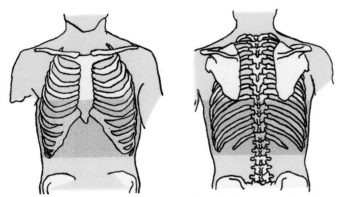

FIGURE 3 Topographic zone of risk: anterior (*left*) and posterior (*right*).

VATS to directly inspect the diaphragm. However, the expense, effort, and risk from the performance of thoracoscopy and laparoscopy are significant, and the incidence of injury to the diaphragm is low (less than 1%); hence the problem of delayed recognition of diaphragmatic injuries continues. The role of positive-pressure ventilation in masking the diagnosis must be emphasized, and it argues for a prehospital discharge CXR in patients with high potential injury mechanisms.

Chronic Hernia

Patients with chronic diaphragmatic hernia often present with signs and symptoms attributable to visceral incarceration, strangulation, or displacement of thoracic structures by herniated abdominal organs. Dyspnea, pleuritic chest pain, bloating or early satiety, abdominal pain, or frank sepsis can all be presenting symptoms and signs. Unlike the acute setting, the diagnosis of chronic hernia is usually made on screening posterior-anterior and lateral chest radiographs with findings mentioned above. CT with three-dimensional reconstruction can also be helpful to demonstrate intrathoracic herniation of visceral contents, most frequently the stomach, followed in descending order by colon, small bowel, and spleen. With the diagnosis confirmed, surgical intervention is always indicated because of the high incidence of strangulation.

THERAPY

Therapeutic intervention is tailored according to whether the diaphragmatic injury is acute or chronic and whether it is the result of penetrating or blunt trauma. In most circumstances, the preferred approach to the repair of an acute diaphragmatic rupture is via a laparotomy; visualization of the diaphragm is good, positive-pressure ventilation can be maintained without difficulty, and the commonly associated intraabdominal injuries can be addressed.

Exploratory Laparotomy

For exploratory laparotomy, the patient is draped and prepped in the supine position; arms should be extended to the sides, and the chest is prepped should the need for thoracotomy arise. A nasogastric tube to decompress the stomach should be inserted but with great care, as occasionally the esophagogastric junction is distorted by injury and herniation. Any pneumothorax of any size should be decompressed with a tube thoracostomy as soon as it is recognized, but again with great care and direct digital examination of the insertion site to ensure pleural space placement. Excellent exposure is achieved through a generous midline laparotomy, often with the aid of a mechanical retracting device.

The entire abdomen is routinely evaluated for concomitant injury, and the first priorities are hemorrhage and contamination control. Attention is then directed toward the diaphragmatic injury. It is not infrequent that viscera have herniated into the thorax so as to necessitate careful reduction. Passage of a red rubber catheter alongside the viscera resolves any vacuum and facilitates reduction. Should resistance persist, extending the phrenotomy may help. These should be carefully located so as to minimize damage to the phrenic nerve branches (see Figure 1). Rarely, a thoracotomy is needed to effect reduction; though this is more commonly needed with chronicity, in which adhesions between bowel and pleura have become established.

Exposure of the left diaphragm is accomplished by dividing the lienophrenic ligament to allow full mobilization of the splenic flexure inferiorly. The spleen, splenic flexure of the colon, and the body of the stomach are moved inferiorly and medially, which is best done by direct hand exposure. The left lateral segments (segments 2 and 3) of the liver will need to be mobilized medially to expose the central tendon and gastric hiatus. The right side of the diaphragm is, of course, largely buttressed by the liver. Mobilization of the falciform ligament should generally be accomplished in all blunt trauma inspections of the diaphragm, but the triangular ligament need only be taken down if injury is apparent, or with penetrating injuries with a high likelihood that the path of the offending agent is through the bare area of the liver. Division of the right triangular ligament and the posterior hepatic attachments will allow the liver to be pulled inferiorly to provide good exposure of most of the right diaphragm, along with the inferior vena cava, right adrenal, and right kidney.

Now, with the lesion well visualized, one may ascertain the method of repair. For most lesions, particularly those secondary to penetrating trauma, primary closure can be achieved. Allis clamps are initially used to isolate the edges of the tear and enable manipulation of the defect so as to facilitate repair. The defect is closed using interrupted horizontal mattress, figure-eight, or running sutures of 2-0 or 0 size permanent suture, ensuring adequate incorporation of viable tissue and exclusion and debridement of nonviable tissue. There is debate on the type of suture (monofilament vs. braided) and the technique of closure (running vs. interrupted mattress), but there is uniformity on the need to use permanent suture. I prefer braided nylon for easy tying and the ability to withstand repeated movement of the diaphragm. I use interrupted horizontal mattress sutures to avoid any ischemia and to allow exact closure if there has been any tissue loss or disruption, and it affords confidence in the repair holding that multiple sutures provide. The tail of the previously placed suture is used as a handle, similar to Allis clamps, to provide exposure and permit careful suture placement. Teflon pledgets may be employed if the repair is tenuous, but these add a greater foreign-body burden. Some recommend a two-layer closure with the inner layer an interlocking

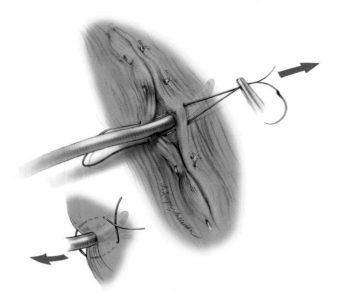

FIGURE 4   Evacuation of residual pneumothorax with a 24 Fr red rubber catheter. The catheter, which is connected to continuous suction, is removed as the final mattress suture is tied.

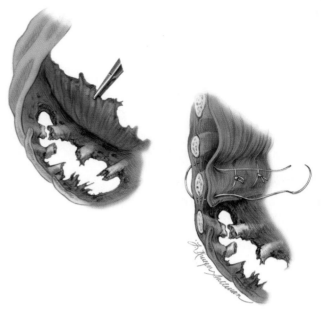

FIGURE 5   Reattachment of diaphragm. The diaphragm is resutured with interrupted mattress sutures encircling the entire rib.

horizontal mattress suture that everts the edges, reinforced with a running 3-0 polypropylene or silk closure.

An issue of consideration is the need for postoperative tube thoracostomy. If tube thoracostomy has not been performed preoperatively, and there is no indication for it postoperatively, the residual air and fluid can be aspirated from the pleural space with a 24 Fr red rubber catheter placed through the final mattress suture (Figure 4). However, should any doubt exist as to the presence of pulmonary injury or retained hemothorax, tube thoracostomy should be performed.

Larger wounds, specifically those exceeding 25 cm², can prove challenging. It is essential that any repair be accomplished with minimal tension to provide adequate diaphragmatic excursion for ventilation. Hence, these injuries may require transposing the insertion of the diaphragm to higher ribs, thereby decreasing the radius of span and minimizing tension (Figure 5). Alternatively, successful repair may require the placement of a bridging nonporous mesh material such as a biological mesh (pig or human dermis products) or Gore-Tex. In this instance, the mesh is sutured to the free edges with a 2 cm overlap of synthetic material and healthy diaphragm. Allis clamps are initially used to isolate the edges of the defect.

On occasion the diaphragm is avulsed from the chest wall. Repair can be accomplished by approximating the free edge to the rib with a 2-0 or 0-0 mattress suture that encircles the rib. Frequently, it is necessary to reattach the diaphragm one or two ribs higher than its insertion to permit closure without tension (see Figure 5).

Laparoscopy

The move toward nonoperative management of abdominal solid-organ injuries has led to a reduction in the number of urgent laparotomies in patients with a suspected diaphragm injury but no other indication for laparotomy. This development, together with the advanced laparoscopic instrumentation and skill training, has resulted in more diaphragmatic injuries being detected after the acute event is resolved and via laparoscopy in a semielective setting. Positioning of the surgeon and the equipment is depicted in Figure 6. Although the diagnosis of a left-sided injury is relatively straightforward as described above, the repair can be challenging. The surgeon

should be skilled in intracorporeal suturing, as the use of stapling instruments has not been verified as an acceptable method of repair. The risk of a tension pneumothorax during laparoscopic repair of a diaphragm injury is significant, requiring awareness and diligence in monitoring, as well as careful evacuation of the hemithorax prior to final closure.

Thoracoscopy

Thoracoscopy is more commonly used for the diagnosis of acute injuries. The patient is placed in the lateral decubitus position, and a 10 mm port for the camera is placed in the fifth intercostal space at the midaxillary line. The entire hemidiaphragm can be visualized, especially with a double-lumen endotracheal tube to enable deflation of the lung. Small injuries may be repaired transthoracically; however, for penetrating injuries, intraabdominal injury must be excluded; injuries resulting from blunt trauma are usually too large for endoscopic repair. Hence, after identifying an injury, laparotomy should be performed.

Chronic Diaphragm Hernia

Most chronic diaphragmatic hernias present long after the initial injury with symptoms attributable to visceral incarceration with or without incarceration; they are invariably on the left side. The workup proceeds as for acute injury, although these can frequently be diagnosed preoperatively with a combination of CXR complemented with contrast studies or with a CT scan. Unlike in the acute trauma setting, most surgeons favor the exposure afforded by a thoracic approach for the repair of chronic diaphragmatic hernias, where concern for associated intraabdominal injury is minimal, and the lung can be deflated without difficulty. The lack of a peritoneal sac can allow bowel to adhere to lung and diaphragm edges, leading to a tedious dissection and making reduction through a celiotomy difficult. Again, the surgeon must avoid injury to the phrenic nerve. The repair itself is similar, as described in acute injuries, although the use of biological mesh to buttress or bridge a large defect is becoming more prevalent.

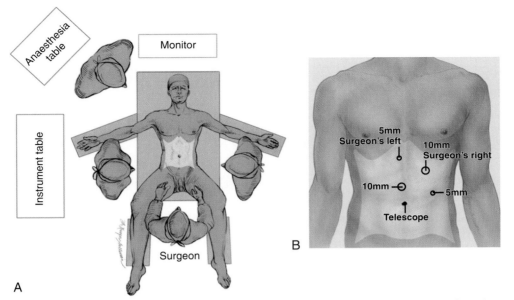

FIGURE 6 Explorative laparoscopy for suspected diaphragmatic injury. **A,** Operating room layout. **B,** Port placements.

SUGGESTED READINGS

Asensio JA, Petrone P, Demetriades D: Injuries to the diaphragm. In Moore EE, Feliciano DV, Mattox LK, editors: *Trauma*, ed 5, New York, 2004, McGraw-Hill, p 613.

Eren S, Kantarci M, Okur A: Imaging of diaphragmatic rupture after trauma, *Clin Radiol* 61:467, 2006.

Freeman RK, Al-Dossari G, Hutcheson KA, et al: Indications for using video-assisted thoracoscopic surgery to diagnose diaphragmatic injuries after penetrating chest trauma, *Ann Thorac Surg* 72:342, 2001.

Hanna WC, Ferri LE, Fata P, et al: The current status of traumatic diaphragmatic injury: lessons learned from 105 patients over 13 years,, *Ann Thorac Surg* 85:1044, 2008.

Iochum S, Ludig T, Walter F, et al: Imaging of diaphragmatic injury: a diagnostic challenge? *RadioGraphics* 22:S103, 2002.

Rashid F, Chakrabarty MM, Singh R, Iftikhar SY: A review on delayed presentation of diaphragmatic rupture, *World J Surg* 4:32, 2009.

LIVER INJURY

Nicholas Jaszczak, MD, and David T. Efron, MD

OVERVIEW

The management of liver injuries continues to pose difficult challenges for surgeons. Over the past few decades, many diagnostic and therapeutic advances have facilitated diagnosis and management of these injuries, thereby improving patient outcomes. Despite these changes, severe liver injury remains a life-threatening problem. The expanding options in nonoperative and interventional radiologic techniques have only served to reinforce the importance of a thorough understanding of all treatment modalities and a systematic approach to each patient.

The liver is injured in approximately 5% of all trauma admissions. Because of its size and its location directly under the right costal margin, the liver is at risk from both penetrating and blunt mechanisms of injury. The past few decades have brought about the acceptance of nonoperative management as the treatment of choice for 80% to 90% of all patients with blunt hepatic trauma. Increasing evidence also suggests that appropriately selected patients with penetrating trauma can be successfully managed with a nonoperative approach. As an adjunctive strategy, a subset of patients will benefit from

interventional radiology procedures, and these tools have markedly increased the success of nonoperative strategies. It is crucial for the surgeon to understand when each of these treatment strategies is indicated and when it is contraindicated.

Beyond these approaches, the surgeon must still operate on the group of patients who have either failed or are not candidates for nonoperative management. Within the operating room, the surgeon must be skilled at a variety of techniques to control hemorrhage. Of course, the surgeon must be coordinating and or cognizant of the ongoing resuscitation. In association with this, it is always important to consider the need to use damage-control techniques to prevent the patient from becoming hypothermic, coagulopathic, and acidotic.

Multiple technical options are available to control hemorrhage, including direct compression of the liver, mobilization and packing, portal triad occlusion, total hepatic vascular occlusion, finger fracture, direct suture repair, omental packing, balloon tamponade, and topical sealants. As hepatic surgery may not be a part of a surgeon's typical practice, consideration should always be given to calling for consultation from the most experienced hepatobiliary surgeon available. The additional expertise and wisdom can be invaluable in these potentially life-threatening injuries.

The expansion of available management options has underscored the importance of good clinical judgment. Although technology has expanded treatment options and has made increasingly precise diagnosis possible, decisions must still be guided by sound principles of hemodynamic stability, repeated physical exam findings, and serial lab values. It must be remembered that nonoperative management is an active treatment decision that requires vigilant surveillance and quick response to changes to be an effective therapy.

INITIAL EVALUATION AND MANAGEMENT

As with all acute trauma victims, initial management must begin with attention to airway, breathing, and circulation. Advanced Trauma Life Support (ATLS) protocols must be followed to guide the initial care and resuscitation efforts. A thorough and systematic trauma evaluation is always necessary to rule out other associated intraabdominal injuries and to identify injuries to the head, chest, and extremities. Consideration of liver injury is necessary in all trauma victims, as the liver is at risk from both blunt and penetrating mechanisms of injury. Blunt liver injuries occur most commonly in association with motor vehicle crashes but are also commonly associated with pedestrian-car collisions, falls, assaults, and motorcycle crashes. Penetrating liver injuries occur in up to 30% to 40% of penetrating thoracoabdominal trauma cases.

After the primary survey is complete and resuscitation has begun, further evaluation of liver injuries will depend on the hemodynamic stability of the patient. Hemodynamically unstable trauma victims should be evaluated for the presence of intraperitoneal blood by either focused abdominal sonography for trauma (FAST) or diagnostic peritoneal lavage (DPL). FAST exam has been shown to have a sensitivity of 97% for detecting hemoperitoneum greater than 1 L, although the exact location of the injury often cannot be reliably identified. This sensitivity is decreased when less than 400 mL of intraperitoneal fluid is present. Specific to liver injury, FAST has also been shown to have a sensitivity of 98% for detecting hemoperitoneum in grade III or higher liver injury.

Although FAST exam has become the preferred diagnostic modality in the unstable patient, diagnostic peritoneal lavage (DPL) is still an option for determining the presence of hemoperitoneum. DPL has a sensitivity of greater than 95% for detecting intraperitoneal hemorrhage. The DPL is considered positive if 10 mL of blood is aspirated initially. After peritoneal lavage, the return of lavage fluid with red blood cell (RBC) counts greater than 100,000 RBCs/μL is also considered positive in blunt trauma. The red cell count considered positive in penetrating trauma is controversial, but 10,000 to 50,000 RBCs/μL can be used to establish penetration of the abdominal wall. Additionally, the lavage fluid can be examined for white blood cells, particulate matter, bilirubin, and amylase to determine the need for laparotomy. Of course DPL does have limitations. It cannot help to determine the hemorrhagic source or evaluate the retroperitoneum, and it may be too sensitive, as the test can be positive with minimal hemoperitoneum. Any positive FAST or DPL in a hemodynamically unstable patient warrants immediate operative exploration. Specific characterization of the liver injury is accomplished in the operating room, and rapid control of bleeding is lifesaving.

The hemodynamically stable patient should undergo a thorough radiographic exam to diagnose all associated injuries. High resolution computed tomography (CT) with intravenous contrast enhancement is used to provide a detailed evaluation of the liver injury. Hepatic trauma can be graded based on CT findings according to the American Association for Surgery of Trauma Liver Injury Scale (Table 1). In addition to establishing the grade of injury, CT may demonstrate a contrast blush from the liver parenchyma or adjacent vessels (Figure 1). The use of FAST in hemodynamically stable patients can also be considered, but caution must be exercised when interpreting negative FAST exam findings. Not all hepatic injuries produce hemoperitoneum. The sensitivity of FAST exam for all grades of liver injury based on detection of free fluid alone is only 67%, and it does not identify signs of ongoing bleeding, such as the blush seen on CT scan. Although some question the clinical significance of injuries that do not result in hemoperitoneum, an associated risk of bleeding does remain.

TABLE 1: American Association for the Surgery of Trauma liver injury scale

Grade	Injury	Description
I	Hematoma	Subcapsular: <10% of liver capsule surface area
	Laceration	Capsular tear: <1 cm parenchymal depth
II	Hematoma	Subcapsular: 10%–50% surface area Intraparenchymal: <10 cm in diameter
	Laceration	1–3 cm parenchymal: depth >10 cm long
III	Hematoma	Subcapsular: >50% surface area or expanding; ruptured subcapsular or parenchymal hematoma Intraparenchymal: hematoma >10 cm or expanding
	Laceration	Parenchymal: depth >3 cm
IV	Laceration	Parenchymal disruption involving 25%–75% of hepatic lobe or one to three Couinaud segments within a single lobe
V	Laceration	Parenchymal disruption involving >75% of the hepatic lobe or more than three Couinaud segments within a single lobe
	Vascular	Juxtahepatic venous injuries (retrohepatic vena cava, central major hepatic veins)
VI	Vascular	Hepatic avulsion

From the American Association for the Surgery of Trauma. Available online at http://www.aast.org.

An additional diagnostic modality that can be considered for the evaluation of liver injuries is laparoscopy. Diagnostic laparoscopy can be used to avoid an unnecessary laparotomy in those patients with penetrating wounds that may or may not have entered the peritoneal cavity. The role of diagnostic laparoscopy in patients with blunt hepatic injury remains less clear. Additionally, although positive identification of liver injury may be easily confirmed, laparoscopically ruling out hollow viscus injury in the setting of even minimal hemoperitoneum remains a challenge.

NONOPERATIVE MANAGEMENT

Patient Selection

After the diagnostic evaluation is complete, further management must still be directed by the hemodynamic status of the patient. Patients who remain hemodynamically stable should be considered for nonoperative management regardless of the grade of injury found on CT. Appropriate candidates for nonoperative management will have no peritoneal signs on physical exam and no other injuries identified on CT scan that would indicate a need for laparotomy. These patients are admitted to a monitored setting and followed with frequent serial exams and hematocrit assessments. The onset of hemodynamic instability denotes a failure of nonoperative management and requires operative intervention. As such, a surgeon must be immediately available as part of a nonoperative management strategy. A falling hematocrit alone, especially in the setting of polytrauma, does not mandate operative intervention; however, it may be a trigger

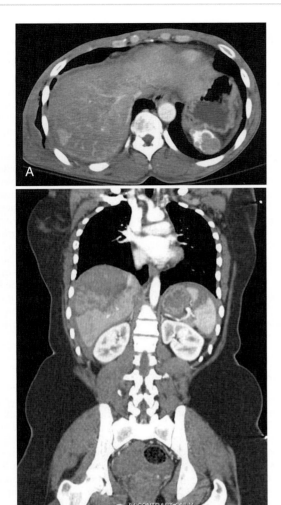

for angiographic evaluation and possible intervention. Angiography extends the potential for successful nonoperative management by adding the ability to selectively embolize arterial bleeding within the liver parenchyma. Those hemodynamically stable patients who are found to have a contrast blush on CT scan should also undergo emergent angiography and possible embolization of the bleeding source (Figure 2). Embolization is effective for managing bleeding from an arterial source, but venous bleeding is most effectively managed by tamponade. Ongoing blood loss following angiography necessitates operative intervention.

Patient Monitoring

The length of time required to keep patients monitored for successful treatment will depend on the severity of injury. Although practices vary, most grade I and II injuries can be watched in a monitored bed (intensive care unit [ICU] or step-down facility) for 24 hours; higher grade injuries require 48 to 72 hours or longer. Patients are often kept on bed rest for 2 to 5 days or more, depending on clinical judgment and the severity of injury. The risk of deep vein thrombosis (DVT) remains high in these patients, so graded elastic stockings and sequential compression devices must be used, as the bleeding risk will contraindicate chemical DVT prophylaxis.

Patients should be observed for delayed bleeding in the hospital for at least 24 hours after they are removed from bed rest restrictions. Routine repeat imaging after recovery is not recommended, unless clinical changes indicate a need for imaging. Return to full activity is allowed in 1 to 3 months, depending on injury severity and good clinical judgment.

Successful nonoperative management is reported in 80% to 90% of hemodynamically stable victims of blunt hepatic trauma. Nonoperative management has resulted in lower transfusion requirements, fewer abdominal infections, and decreased lengths of hospital stay. Failure does occur more frequently in higher grade injuries, with a 3% to 7.5% failure rate in minor injuries but a 14% failure rate for grade IV and a 23% failure rate for grade V blunt injuries. This increased rate of failure still should not be seen as a contraindication, if the patient is otherwise a candidate for nonoperative treatment. It must also be remembered that lower grade injuries can still bleed significantly, and decisions regarding management must be made based on hemodynamic stability and physical exam, not radiologic findings.

Four independent risk factors for failure of nonoperative management were identified in a prospective study of blunt abdominal

FIGURE 1 The advantages of CT scanning include identification of contrast exstravasation and identification of other intraabdominal injuries. **A,** CT scan of a large grade IV right lobe injury with active contrast blush toward the dome. **B,** A grade III liver and concomitant grade III splenic injury.

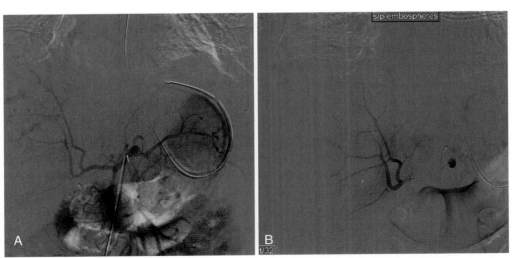

FIGURE 2 Angiography in a 40-year-old man following a blunt hepatic injury. **A,** Selective angiogram of right hepatic artery branch showing contrast blush in the upper left of picture. **B,** Status after bead embolization with resolution of blush.

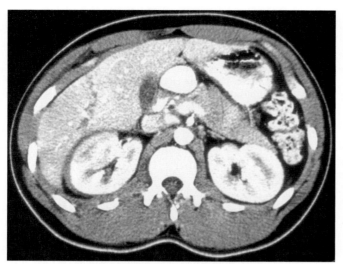

FIGURE 3 Hemondynamically stable 19-year-old man with a transabdominal gunshot wound without peritonitis. The track of the bullet is seen on CT scan; no contrast blush was noted. He successfully managed nonoperatively without complication.

trauma. These were injury to solid organs other than the liver (spleen and kidney); positive FAST exam; hemoperitoneum in excess of 300 mL, usually correlating with blood in multiple intraperitoneal areas; and the need for transfusion. The absence of all four of these correlated with a 98% success rate for nonoperative management. The presence of all four predicted a 96% rate of failure for nonoperative management.

Penetrating Injuries

Nonoperative management can also be considered in highly selected patients with penetrating trauma, although this is less widely accepted. Criteria for consideration of nonoperative management include hemodynamic stability, lack of peritoneal signs or other indications for laparotomy, and an intact level of consciousness to allow for serial abdominal exams. As in blunt trauma, consideration for nonoperative management is not based upon CT grade of injury (Figure 3). At most only about a third of all penetrating trauma patients will be candidates for nonoperative management. The majority who fail to qualify do so as a result of other organ injuries necessitating operative intervention. Of those properly selected candidates for nonoperative management, success rates of greater than 90% are reported. As described with blunt trauma, nonoperatively managed patients must be followed closely for any changes, and adjustments must be made to management strategies as indicated.

OPERATIVE MANAGEMENT

The operative management of liver injuries requires a systematic disciplined approach. Even prior to entering the operating room, the surgeon must be planning the operation to ensure that all available resources have been mobilized. Early consideration should be given to calling for help from an experienced hepatobiliary surgeon. The operating room should be warmed, and those parts of the patient not in the operative field should be covered to combat hypothermia. Blood products, a rapid infuser, and a warmer should be available. Multiple suction setups should be ready, and if no enteric spillage occurred, use of a cell saver unit should be considered. The skin is widely prepped from the chin to the knees to facilitate exposure. A

large self-retaining retractor, such as an Omni or Thompson retractor, can be key to allowing maximal exposure and free hands for the operative work. Ancillary treatment modalities, such as the argon beam coagulator and topical hemostatic agents, should also be made available early.

The incision of choice for trauma is a midline celiotomy, which can be extended to a median sternotomy or right thoracotomy if adequate vascular control cannot be obtained, or if further evaluation of the chest should become necessary. Control of the suprahepatic inferior vena cava (IVC) is often only possible from above the diaphragm. Massive hemorrhage may be encountered immediately upon entering the peritoneal cavity, as the tamponading effect of the peritoneum is lost. Manual compression of the injured liver over laparotomy pads and four-quadrant packing of the abdomen should be performed immediately in this situation. This allows placement of retractors, planning of resuscitation with the anesthesia team, and time for systematic evaluation of the abdomen for other injuries.

Once the patient has received adequate resuscitation, a thorough exam of the rest of the peritoneal cavity is performed. Sources of enteric contamination are rapidly controlled. Associated injuries to the intraabdominal vasculature and organs are identified and addressed as indicated, and attention then can be focused on the liver injury. The manual compression is slowly released to allow an accurate assessment of the degree of injury. Management will then depend on the severity of the injury encountered.

Minor Injuries

Patients with minor liver injuries can be managed with simple hemostatic techniques. Bleeding from superficial lacerations will often be controlled with 5 to 10 minutes of direct compression, topical agents, and electrocautery or argon beam coagulation. Diffuse bleeding from raw surfaces of the liver exposed by capsule disruption may respond well to topical agents such as fibrin glue, hemostat fabric, or topical collagen. After application of the topical agent, the liver is compressed for another 5 to 10 minutes and reassessed. If bleeding is controlled and bile leakage is not seen, no further treatment is necessary.

If continued bleeding is seen from superficial lacerations, direct suture hepatorrhaphy can be performed. We favor transcapsular liver sutures of size 0 chromic with blunt-nosed needles. Caution must be exercised with this technique, as sutures that are tied too tight may result in further tearing of the liver capsule. This can be prevented with pledgets, although in the setting of contamination, we favor the use of Surgicel (Ethicon, Somerville, NJ) to pledgets for these sutures, given the eventual dissolution of this material. Sutures should be placed reasonably close to the edge of the injury to prevent large areas of necrosis.

Moderate to Severe Injuries

If a slightly larger laceration is found, the wound can be managed by packing it with a tongue of omentum and using transcapsular liver sutures to hold the omentum in place. Prior to closing the defect, the wound must be entered, and any bile duct or vascular injuries must be ligated with figure-8 sutures. If bleeding is more significant, this technique may not be successful in controlling bleeding from an injury to larger branches of the hepatic artery or portal system deep within the liver parenchyma. In this situation, the finger-fracture technique is used. The injury is enlarged by pinching the parenchyma between the thumb and index finger to expand the wound, until the larger bleeding vessels deep within the wound can be identified. These vessels are then controlled with clips, ligation, or direct repair.

Patients who have significant bleeding when direct hepatic compression is released require different techniques to control the ongoing hemorrhage. First, direct compression should be reapplied, and efforts should be made to rapidly control inflow and mobilize the liver. The Pringle maneuver is performed by placing the surgeon's nondominant index finger through the foramen of Winslow and using the thumb to compress the portal vein and hepatic artery. The gastrohepatic ligament is then opened bluntly or with electrocautery, remembering to be aware of a possible replaced or accessory left hepatic artery located here. At this point, a vascular clamp or an umbilical tape and Rummel tourniquet can be substituted for the surgeon's thumb and finger. This maneuver will result in temporary control of bleeding in over 85% of complex liver injuries, allowing further evaluation of the injury. This also suggests hepatic artery or portal vein origins of bleeding.

The length of time the Pringle maneuver is applied remains controversial. Although many surgeons advocate cross clamping for 20 minutes followed by reperfusion for 5 minutes, evidence suggests that longer normothermic ischemic times may produce similar results. Severe liver injuries managed with up to 75 minutes of continuous cross clamping of the porta hepatis have been reported without adverse sequelae. Continued bleeding that is not affected by the Pringle maneuver is diagnostic of bleeding that is primarily from the hepatic venous system.

With hepatic inflow controlled, the liver must be mobilized to allow identification and management of the injury. The ligamentum teres and falciform ligament are divided and followed back to the suprahepatic vena cava. The right and left triangular and coronary ligaments are then mobilized. Care must be taken when this is performed to evaluate for a hematoma within the triangular ligaments; if a hematoma is present, this area should not be entered prematurely. This likely represents a vena cava or hepatic vein injury, and mobilization may disrupt a stable hematoma, which could result in rapid exsanguination.

After full mobilization of the liver is complete, the extent of the injury can be delineated. Visualized intrahepatic vessels that are bleeding are ligated directly, as are bile ducts that can be identified. A decision is made regarding the need to continue efforts to surgically control bleeding or pack the liver and employ a damage control strategy. Because much of the liver bleeding is from the venous systems, it is often well controlled by packing to tamponade the bleeding. Ongoing bright-red blood likely represents continued arterial bleeding. If the packing provides reasonable control, the patient may then be taken to angiography for selective embolization of suspected injured intrahepatic arterial arcades. If this bleeding remains uncontrolled to the point that it threatens hemodynamic stability, selective ligation of the left or right hepatic arteries outside of the liver parenchyma may be considered. Ligation of the common hepatic artery is the ultimate damage control maneuver, although it has the highest risk of massive liver ischemia and should be reserved for the most severe cases.

Most injuries are not along anatomic lines, and as such, attempts at formal hepatectomy are hazardous and will result in excessive blood loss and mortality. It should be remembered that although the defect may appear extremely large, further intervention is usually not required if the major vascular pedicles are intact. In rare circumstances, the injury itself will have devascularized a significant peripheral segment of the liver. In this case, completion of the resection of this segment may be performed.

Liver Packing

With full mobilization of the liver complete, packing can be effectively performed. The left lateral segment can now be rotated to the right, with packs placed posteriorly. Superiorly, packs can be placed between the diaphragm and liver. The right lobe is rotated medially, and laparotomy pads are packed along the vena cava between the liver and diaphragm. This allows compression of the liver between the anterior chest wall, diaphragm, and retroperitoneum, resulting in tamponade of bleeding.

Once packing is complete, the abdomen is closed with a temporary closure, and the patient is brought to the ICU for aggressive resuscitation and warming. Patients managed with this strategy must be monitored closely for abdominal compartment syndrome, as packing can result in intraabdominal hypertension and can also adversely affect venous return to the heart. Patients should return to the operating room within 24 to 72 hours of their original surgery after correction of their metabolic derangements for removal of packs. Timing of pack removal is somewhat controversial. Prolonged packing is associated with an increased risk of perihepatic sepsis, but early removal may result in higher rates of rebleeding that requires repacking.

If a decision is made to definitively close the abdomen, drains should be considered. Although some question the use of drains, as they could predispose to infection, others suggest a benefit in complex liver injuries. If closed-suction drains are placed and removed in a timely fashion, bleeding and bile leaks may be detected earlier, and management can be adjusted accordingly.

Penetrating Injuries

Penetrating injuries can produce unique surgical challenges because of the creation of long, narrow wounds that bleed significantly from deep within the wound tract. A useful technique for this situation is to use a red rubber catheter and Penrose drain to create a balloon to tamponade bleeding. The red rubber catheter is placed into the Penrose catheter, with extra holes cut in the red rubber catheter within the Penrose; the proximal and distal ends are secured over the red rubber catheter (Figure 4). The device is then inserted into the injury tract, and saline is use to inflate the device. A clamp is applied to the end of the catheter to keep the balloon inflated (Figure 5). As with external packing techniques, the abdomen is temporarily closed, and the patient is taken to the ICU for resuscitation. Deflation of the balloon can be done during a second-look laparotomy (Figure 6). If bleeding does occur, the balloon is reinflated, and further surgical management is planned to allow for elective total hepatic isolation and more formal anatomic exploration.

Extrahepatic vascular and biliary injuries also must be managed surgically. Exposure is vital, and mobilization of the hepatic flexure and wide Kocher maneuver should be performed to better expose the portal structures. Primary repair with lateral venorrhaphy should be performed for portal vein injuries when possible. When confronted with exsanguination, portal vein ligation is possible, with varying reports in the literature for survivability. These patients must be resuscitated aggressively, and second-look laparotomy should be performed to assess bowel and hepatic viability. Hepatic artery injuries should also be repaired primarily if possible. If not possible, hepatic artery ligation can also be considered, especially if the portal vein remains intact. These patients must also be followed closely to assess liver viability. All patients who have ligation of the right hepatic artery will need to have a cholecystectomy.

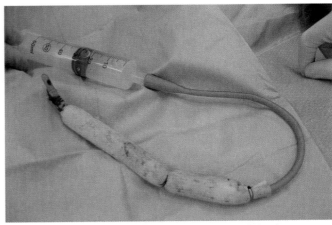

FIGURE 4   Catheter constructed for tamponade of bleeding transhepatic gunshot track.

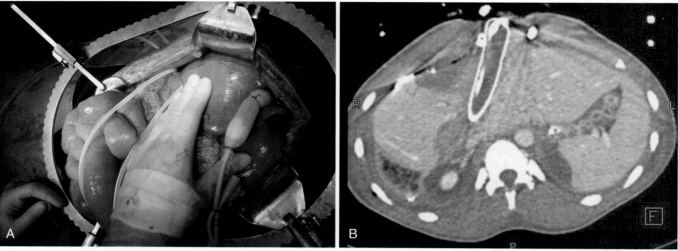

FIGURE 5   Intraoperative placement. **A,** Patient's head is to the right. **B,** CT images of intrahepatic tamponade balloon. Note the addition of horizontal mattress sutures pledgeted over Surgicel at the superior edge of the bullet track in the liver, placed to reinforce a stellate crack from the gunshot blast.

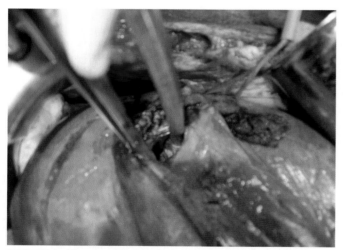

FIGURE 6   The same gunshot track at 60 hours, following deflation and removal of the tamponade device. Complete hemostasis is noted.

Injuries to the bile duct can be addressed after life-threatening hemorrhage is under control. Drains can be placed in the area of the injury, and definitive treatment can be delayed in the unstable patient. Minor injuries can also be addressed with primary repair or placement of a T tube. More extensive injuries are addressed with drainage and delayed Roux-en-Y biliary-enteric anastomosis.

One of the most difficult injuries to manage is the retrohepatic vena cava injury or hepatic vein injury. Several methods of management have been described with packing and tamponade showing the most favorable results. As mentioned previously, care must be taken when mobilizing the triangular ligaments of the liver. If right upper quadrant bleeding is not controlled with the Pringle maneuver, and a hematoma is seen in the triangular ligament, further mobilization in this area should be discontinued. Perihepatic laparotomy pads and/or intraparenchymal omental packing should be used to tamponade bleeding. After packing, resuscitation and adjunctive interventional radiologic techniques are considered.

Multiple other techniques have been described to manage these devastating injuries, which all present significant technical challenges. Direct repair of injuries with a prolonged Pringle maneuver, medial rotation of the liver, and finger fracture to the site of injury has shown only a 43% survival rate in experienced hands. Total hepatic vascular

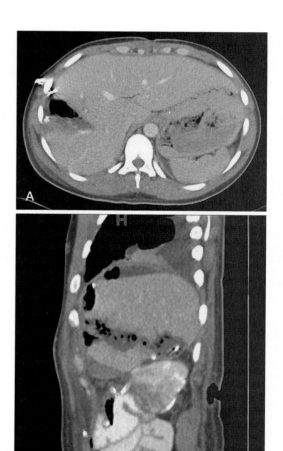

FIGURE 7   Abscesses indentified in the postoperative setting of gunshot wounds to the liver. **A,** Intrahepatic abscess. **B,** Suprahepatic abscess. Both patients had concomitant injuries to the right colon. Note the clear track of injury with small residual necrotic liver in **B.**

occlusion can also be performed with a Pringle maneuver and clamping of the suprahepatic and infrahepatic vena cava to allow direct repair.

Atriocaval shunting is technically difficult, and a decision to use this technique must be made early if there is to be any chance of a favorable outcome. The chest is opened, and a chest tube or endotracheal tube with the proximal end clamped is inserted through the right atrium down into the infrahepatic vena cava. An additional hole is cut in the tube, which will sit in the right atrium. The tube is then secured with a purse-string suture to the right atrium, and the umbilical tapes are passed around the vena cava, above and below the liver (above the renal veins). Rummel tourniquets are applied to allow blood to be shunted past the injury. Mortality rates of 60% to 100% have led many surgeons to abandon this technically challenging technique. Emergent venovenous bypass has been described, and reported survival rates are high, but this modality may not be widely available. Finally, liver resection and delayed transplantation has been described in extreme situations, but this option is also not widely available, and it comes with significant morbidity and mortality.

ADJUNCTIVE TECHNIQUES

In addition to operative and nonoperative management, interventional radiologic techniques have shown promise in improving outcomes for patients with liver injuries. As always, decisions are guided by hemodynamic stability, but appropriately selected patients will benefit from a closely monitored trip to the interventional radiology suite. Hemodynamically stable patients who have a contrast blush from the liver parenchyma or adjacent vessels should be evaluated with emergent angiography, if they do not otherwise have an indication for emergent surgical intervention. Injuries to the hepatic arterial tree can be treated by embolization. Hemodynamically unstable patients should first be stabilized with operative management. After operative management, further management in the interventional radiology suite is considered.

COMPLICATIONS

Although a majority of liver injuries heal without complications, this is not always the case. Therefore, the surgeon must maintain a high index of suspicion for complications and must be prepared to respond appropriately to problems when they occur. Bleeding, bile leaks, bilomas, biliary strictures, biliary fistulas, abscesses, devascularization of liver parenchyma, and hemobilia all may be seen in the management of the injured liver.

Early Hemorrhage

Bleeding can occur at any time after liver injury, although it usually occurs early. The surgeon must always reevaluate the treatment strategy and adapt to the current clinical situation. Regardless of what treatment strategy was initially used, patients who are hemodynamically unstable following liver injury must be evaluated in the operating room. Those patients who are stable with signs of bleeding can be further evaluated with repeat CT scan or angiography, and most patients with delayed bleeding will be successfully managed nonoperatively. Although practice varies widely, injuries to the liver contraindicate early use of chemical thromboprophylaxis.

Bile Leaks

Bile leaks are another frequent complication of both blunt and penetrating liver injuries due to disruption of the biliary system. Early signs of a significant bile leak may include abdominal distension, intolerance of feeding, and abnormal liver function tests. Evaluation

of symptomatic patients proceeds with high-resolution CT scan with oral and intravenous contrast. CT-guided percutaneous drainage of any significant fluid collections is often the only treatment necessary. Continued bile leakage can be documented by hydroxy iminodiacetic acid scan, although this may not be needed, as most leaks will close with percutaneous drainage alone. If percutaneous drains have persistently high output that is not resolving (>50 mL/day for more than 14 days), the patient has a biliary fistula. Cholangiographic evaluation of the biliary tree should be performed, which can be done by magnetic resonance cholangiopancreatograpy or by endoscopic retrograde cholangiopancreatography (ERCP). Because ERCP is both diagnostic and potentially therapeutic, it is the preferred test.

After identification of the injury, interventions can be performed endoscopically to treat the injured biliary system. A stent can be placed across the injury, or a sphincterotomy can be performed. This decreases the backpressure on the biliary system by disrupting the sphincter of Oddi, improves drainage of the biliary system, and allows the injury to heal. Percutaneous transhepatic cholangiography and percutaneous biliary drainage are another option if ERCP is unsuccessful in controlling or diagnosing the injury. Rarely, operative intervention may be required for resection or biliary enteric anastomosis for drainage related to biliary strictures.

A rare and difficult to manage complication sometimes seen in penetrating trauma is a thoracobiliary fistula due to injury of the liver and diaphragm. Early intervention is important to prevent the harmful effects of bile on the pleura. These can usually be managed by percutaneous chest tube drainage and endoscopic sphincterotomy. The negative inspiratory pressure during breathing efforts often will preferentially pull the bile toward the pleura, and as such, these injuries frequently take a long time to heal. Occasionally, large persistent fistulas need to be addressed with an operation to address the entrapped lung, close the diaphragmatic rent, and establish drainage below the diaphragm.

Abscess

Abscess is another frequent problem related to both operative and nonoperative management (Figure 7). Signs of abscess include fever, increasing white blood cell count, hemodynamic instability, abdominal distension, abdominal pain, food intolerance, and abnormal liver function tests. Risk of abscess formation is increased in those patients with associated enteric injuries, extensive parenchymal injury with inadequate debridement, and large transfusion requirements. Management is usually also successfully accomplished by percutaneous drainage. Rarely, patients who fail to improve with percutaneous interventions still may require operative drainage and debridement.

Necrosis

Necrosis due to devascularization of a portion of the liver can also occur following liver injuries. This can be related to the injury or to the interventions used to control bleeding. Patients may present with abdominal pain and tenderness, feeding intolerance, coagulopathy, elevated liver enzymes, and sepsis. CT scan can be used to identify devascularized segments of liver, and significant areas of necrosis may need to be resected.

Hemobilia

Hemobilia can occur following liver injuries, although this has become less common in the era of nonoperative management. In the past, large parenchymal sutures created iatrogenic connections between the hepatic arteries and bile ducts. Still, when patients have upper gastrointestinal bleeding following liver injury, hemobilia must be ruled out. The classic triad of hemobilia is right upper quadrant pain, jaundice, and upper gastrointestinal bleeding, although this may not be present in all patients. Appropriate management of these patients is with hepatic angiography and embolization. Rarely, operative intervention may be required for debridement or resection of large intrahepatic pseudoaneurysms.

SUGGESTED READINGS

Asensio JA, Demetriades D, Chahwan S, et al: Approach to the management of complex hepatic injuries, *J Trauma* 48:66, 2000.

EAST Practice Management Guidelines Work Group: *Practice management guidelines for the nonoperative management of blunt injury to the liver and spleen, Eastern Association for the Surgery of Trauma,* 2003. Available online at <http://www.east.org/tpg/livspleen.pdf>.

Jurkovich GJ, Hoyt DB, Moore FA, et al: Portal triad injuries: a multicenter study, *J Trauma* 39:426, 1995.

Kozar RA, Moore JB, Niles SE, et al: Complications of nonoperative management of high-grade blunt hepatic injuries, *J Trauma* 59:1066–1071, 2005.

Navsaria PH, Nicol AJ, Krige JE, Edu S: Selective nonoperative management of liver gunshot injuries, *Ann Surg* 249:653–656, 2009.

Velmahos GC, Toutouzas KG, Radin R, et al: Nonoperative management of blunt injury to solid abdominal organs, *Arch Surg* 138:844–851, 2003.

PANCREATIC AND DUODENAL INJURIES

David V. Feliciano, MD

OVERVIEW

Because of the retroperitoneal location of the pancreas and duodenum, diagnosis of an injury by physical examination alone is uncommon in the first several hours after *blunt* trauma to the abdomen has occurred. For this reason, many diagnoses of injuries to these organs in such patients will be made by contrast-enhanced computed tomographic (CT) scanning. In patients with *penetrating* trauma, injuries to both organs may be diagnosed during emergency laparotomies performed for hypotension, peritonitis, or evisceration.

Nonoperative management is appropriate for minor injuries of either organ diagnosed on contrast-enhanced CT. As with other visceral and vascular injuries in the abdomen, operative management is based on magnitude of injury, presence of associated injuries, and the patient's hemodynamic/metabolic state.

PANCREAS

Epidemiology

Injuries to the pancreas are present in only 6% to 7% of patients admitted after suffering blunt abdominal trauma and in those undergoing emergency laparotomies for either gunshot or stab wounds. Isolated injuries after blunt abdominal trauma occur in only 20% of patients, and the most common associated injuries are to the duodenum, liver, and spleen. Associated injuries are almost always present in patients undergoing laparotomy for penetrating wounds, and such injuries depend on the location of the wound. Wounds of the head of the pancreas are most commonly associated with injuries to the liver, duodenum, and major vascular structures; injuries to the body are frequently associated with perforations of the stomach and transverse colon.

Blunt Mechanism of Injury

A direct blow with compression of the upper abdomen and its viscera and vessels against the spine is the most common blunt mechanism of injury. Examples would include compression from the lower rim of the steering wheel in an unrestrained driver in a deceleration-type motor vehicle crash or compression by a misplaced lap-type restraint device in a child.

Diagnosis

As noted above, a delay in diagnosis of a blunt pancreatic injury was common in the past. The retroperitoneal location of the organ (peritonitis absent) with its tamponading effect, which prevents significant blood loss, is the major reason for this. Therefore, the surgeon cannot often rely on serial physical examinations, diagnostic peritoneal lavage (DPL), or surgeon-performed ultrasound to make an early diagnosis.

In similar fashion, the laboratory finding of hyperamylasemia on admission is not a precise marker for injury to the pancreas. Salivary rather than pancreatic amylase elevations are present in 30% to 40% of patients admitted with trauma secondary to acute alcohol intoxication. Also, approximately a third of patients with blunt transection of the pancreatic duct will have a normal amylase level on admission. Therefore the presence of hyperamylasemia—although it raises suspicion of a pancreatic, duodenal, or enteric injury—does not mandate an exploratory laparotomy in the absence of the aforementioned hypotension, peritonitis, or evisceration. A progressive rise in the amylase level over the first 24 to 48 hours of hospitalization is, however, strongly suggestive of injury to the pancreas or duodenum or for the development of the rare entity of posttraumatic pancreatitis.

Contrast-enhanced CT using a 64-slice scanner is the current diagnostic modality of choice in hemodynamically stable and asymptomatic patients with possible or suspected injuries to the pancreas. This would include patients who have sustained blunt abdominal trauma or those who are asymptomatic or modestly symptomatic after sustaining penetrating injuries to the flank or back. In the latter groups, triple-contrast—intravenous, oral or nasogastric, and rectal—CT has been performed for nearly 25 years. CT findings *suggestive* of injury to the pancreas include hematoma of the transverse mesocolon; thickening of the left anterior renal fascia; fluid in the lesser sac or between the pancreas and splenic vein; duodenal hematoma or laceration; injury to the left kidney, adrenal gland, or spleen; and Chance (transverse) fracture in the lumbar spine. CT findings *diagnostic* of injury to the pancreas are listed in Box 1 (Figure 1).

BOX I: CT findings diagnostic of injury to the pancreas

Parenchymal hematoma or laceration
Obvious transection of the parenchyma with fluid in the lesser sac
Disruption of the head of the pancreas
Diffuse swelling characteristic of posttraumatic pancreatitis

Pitfalls in diagnosing pancreatic injuries on CT include the presence of minimal extraperitoneal fat in some patients, artifacts from dense oral contrast, and nonopacification of adjacent duodenum or small bowel, so that the edges of the pancreas are difficult to define.

In the presence of an equivocal CT with or without associated hyperamylasemia, or when CT is not available, endoscopic retrograde cholangiopancreatography (ERCP) is appropriate to rule out an injury to the main pancreatic duct.

Grading System

The American Association for the Surgery of Trauma published the Pancreas Organ Injury Scale (OIS) in 1990 (Table 1). A separate classification system of pancreatic injuries diagnosed by ERCP is also available (Takishima et al, 2000).

Nonoperative Management

In the absence of hypotension, peritonitis, evisceration, and CT evidence of significant injuries to other organs or vessels, grade I and II pancreatic injuries are managed nonoperatively. Although a rare

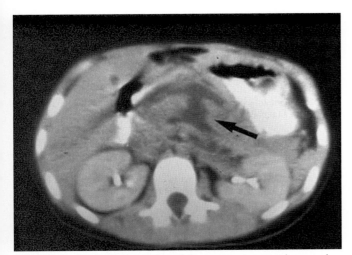

FIGURE 1   Grade III transection of the pancreatic parenchyma and duct with fluid in the lesser sac. *(From Feliciano DV: Abdominal trauma. In Schwartz SI, Ellis H [eds]: Maingot's abdominal operations, ed 9, Norwalk, CT, 1989, Appleton & Lange, p 494. Used by permission.)*

grade II injury, a major contusion or laceration, may progress to a parenchymal pseudocyst, it is very uncommon to have to intervene for a peripancreatic fluid collection during the period of observation with this low magnitude of injury. A follow-up abdominal CT at 5 to 7 days after injury is appropriate, when a significant grade II injury is present, or earlier whenever new symptoms in the upper abdomen or increasing hyperamylasemia develop.

Operative Management

Operative management of pancreatic trauma is determined by complete visualization of the organ to see whether a ductal injury is present. During a damage control laparotomy in the patient with associated injuries and intraoperative hypothermia, acidosis, and a coagulopathy, detailed inspection of the pancreas is delayed until reoperation, once peripancreatic hemorrhage is controlled. In more stable patients, a Kocher maneuver is necessary to properly visualize an injury to the head or neck of the pancreas, and the body of the pancreas is approached by dividing the gastrocolic omentum and the retroperitoneum on the inferior edge of the pancreas to allow for circumferential palpation of the gland. Injuries to the distal body and tail of the pancreas are evaluated by division of the gastrocolic omentum and elevation of the spleen and tail of the pancreas, as in distal pancreatectomy. All hematomas surrounding the pancreas or under the thin mesothelial capsule of the pancreas are explored after either blunt or penetrating trauma.

Injuries to the main pancreatic duct away from the head of the gland are usually characterized by extensive fat necrosis in the lesser sac, even if the patient's exploratory laparotomy has occurred shortly after trauma. A gunshot wound traversing the area of the duct in the midpancreas is considered to be presumptive evidence of an injury to the main duct by some surgeons. Others will evacuate the clot from the area of injury, cauterize or suture any local bleeding, put on magnifying lenses, and observe the laceration or penetrating wound for 3 to 5 minutes. The presence of clear fluid draining from the area of trauma documents that an injury to the main duct is present. On occasion, it may be necessary to inject the patient with secretin (1 mg/kg intravenously) to stimulate pancreatic secretion during the period of observation. However, finding this drug in the hospital at night is often a challenge.

In the absence of a ductal injury, no convincing data support drainage of a grade I (minor contusion/superficial laceration) or grade II (major contusion/major laceration) pancreatic injury noted at a laparotomy for other injuries. Some surgeons will tack a pedicle of viable omentum into a grade I or II laceration to plug any small

TABLE 1: The American Association for the Surgery of Trauma Pancreas OIS

Grade*	Type of Injury	Description of Injury	ICD-9†	AIS-90
I	Hematoma	Minor contusion without duct injury	863.81–863.84	2
	Laceration	Superficial laceration without duct injury		2
II	Hematoma	Major contusion without duct injury or tissue loss	863.81–863.84	2
	Laceration	Major laceration without duct injury or tissue loss		3
III	Laceration	Distal transection or parenchymal injury with duct injury	863.92–863.94	3
IV	Laceration	Proximal transection or parenchymal injury involving ampulla‡	863.91	4
V	Laceration	Massive disruption of pancreatic head	863.91	5

*Advance one grade for multiple injuries up to grade III.
†863.51, 863.91, head; 863.99, 862.92, body 863.83, 863.93, tail.
‡Proximal pancreas is to the patient's right of the superior mesenteric vein.
ICD, International Classification of Diseases; *AIS,* Abbreviated Injury Scale
Data from Moore EE, Cogbill TH, Malangoni MA, et al: Organ injury scaling II: pancreas, duodenum, small bowel, colon, and rectum, *J Trauma* 30:1427–1429, 1990.

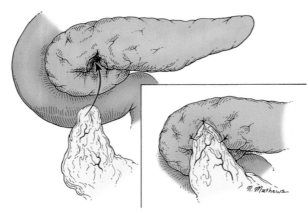

FIGURE 2 A pedicle of viable omentum may be tacked to a grade I or II pancreatic laceration to plug any leak from a small duct. *(From Cushman JG, Feliciano DV: Contemporary management of pancreatic trauma. In Advances in trauma and critical care, vol 10, St Louis, 1995, Mosby—Year Book, p 322.)*

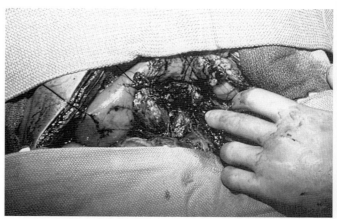

FIGURE 3 Grade IV transection of the pancreatic parenchyma and duct to the right of the superior mesenteric vessels. In a hemodynamically stable patient, a distal Roux-en-Y pancreatico-jejunostomy should be considered. *(From Feliciano DV: Abdominal trauma. In Schwartz SI, Ellis H [eds]: Maingot's abdominal operations, ed 9, Norwalk, CT, 1989, Appleton & Lange, p 497. Used by permission.)*

ductal leak and bring macrophages to the area of injury (Figure 2). On rare occasions, the size and location of a parenchymal laceration, rather than a through-and-through gunshot wound, are suggestive of a ductal injury, but neither fat necrosis nor clear fluid are present. Some surgeons will open the duodenum at this point, creating a combined pancreaticoduodenal injury, to cannulate the papilla and perform a retrograde pancreatogram. An easier option is to place an omental pedicle into the laceration and place a closed-suction drain nearby.

One option to manage a ductal transection in the tail, body, or neck of the pancreas is distal pancreatectomy, with splenic salvage in a child or adolescent or without in an adult. When splenic salvage is to be performed, fine ties are placed on pancreatic vessels on the splenic artery and vein side, and small metal clips are placed on the pancreatic segment to be resected. If the pancreatectomy is to include a splenectomy, the splenic artery and vein are suture ligated with 4-0 polypropylene suture 2 cm proximal to where the pancreas is to be divided. This maneuver, along with coverage of the vessels by a viable omental pedicle, isolates the vessels from any distal leak of the pancreatic stump in the postoperative period. Suturing of the proximal end of the remaining pancreas often results in necrosis, and many surgeons use 3.5 mm staples on a thin pancreas or 4.8 mm staples on a thicker pancreas to seal off the distal end. There are no clear-cut data that individual ligation of a visible pancreatic duct in the distal remnant before stapling changes the incidence of postoperative pancreatic fistulas from this site.

Another option to manage a ductal transection in the body or neck of the pancreas is to oversew or staple the proximal end of the transection and perform a distal Roux-en-Y end-to-end or end-to-side pancreaticojejunostomy. As this option is appropriate in only the most stable patients with more proximal transections (to the right of the superior mesenteric vessels; Figure 3), but without hypotension or significant associated injuries, it is not commonly performed in adults—only five times in my 32-year experience. The advantage is preservation of 70% to 80% of the pancreas, depending on the level of the transection, for the rest of the patient's life. The operative technique includes completion of the parenchymal transection; oversewing of the proximal end, if it is approaching the thicker head of the pancreas; and a cuff-type pancreaticojejunostomy in one of the conformations listed above. Because this operation is usually performed on a normal (soft) pancreas, one option is to place a polyethylene tube stent through the anastomosis to attempt to lower the incidence of a postoperative pancreatic fistula. The tube stent is passed through the abdominal wall in the right upper quadrant and then through the Roux

limb approximately 5 cm from the pancreaticojejunostomy *after* the posterior suture has been completed. Finally, it is placed into the pancreatic duct for a distance of 2 cm and secured in place with a 3-0 absorbable suture attached to the end of the duct. The anterior anastomosis is completed, and one or two closed-suction drains are placed nearby.

Ductal transections in the head of the pancreas adjacent to the neck are difficult to manage because of the thickness of the pancreas. Either of the two options described above for transections more to the left is appropriate but more technically challenging. There is *no* indication to perform an anterior Roux-en-Y pancreaticojejunostomy over both ends of the transection to "sump" the area as illustrated in older textbooks.

In the rare patient with combined pancreaticoduodenal destruction, maceration of the head of the pancreas, or destruction of the ampulla of Vater, a Whipple procedure is indicated. In hemodynamically stable patients, it is appropriate for an experienced surgeon to complete the procedure immediately. In some patients with blunt trauma, much of the dissection has been completed by the injury itself. When patients have associated injuries, hypotension, and signs of intraoperative "metabolic failure," bleeding from the area of injury is controlled, and peripancreatic or periduodenal packs are placed. Closed-suction drains may be placed underneath the packs to aspirate any bile or pancreatic juice not absorbed by the packs. As patients undergoing such damage-control procedures after abdominal trauma usually have marked distension of the midgut (perhaps less with the new blood-banking paradigm using 1 RBC: 1FFP:1 platelets), choosing the time of reoperation is difficult.

In general, once the patient's hypothermia, acidosis, and coagulopathy have resolved, oxygenation and ventilation are reasonable; and with appropriate urine output, reoperation is indicated. In borderline patients, the Whipple operation should be performed in two stages: first resection, then reconstruction. A Witzel jejunostomy should be performed in all of these patients to allow for early postoperative enteral feeding, once the patient is stable and edema of the midgut starts to resolve. Some surgeons use postoperative subcutaneous injections of somatostatin analog to lower the incidence of pancreatic fistulas after Whipple resections and after distal pancreatectomies performed in injured patients. Prospective data using this agent in large numbers of patients are lacking.

TABLE 2: The American Association for the Surgery of Trauma; Duodenum OIS

Grade*	Type of Injury	Description of Injury	ICD-9	AIS-90
I	Hematoma	Involving single portion of duodenum	863.21	2
	Laceration	Partial thickness, no perforation	863.21	3
II	Hematoma	Involving more than one portion	863.21	2
	Laceration	Disruption <50% of circumference	863.31	4
III	Laceration	Disruption 50%–75% of circumference of D2	863.31	4
		Disruption 50%–100% of circumference of D1, D3, D4		4
IV	Laceration	Disruption >75% of circumference of D2	863.31	5
		Involving ampulla or distal common bile duct	863.31	5
V	Laceration	Massive disruption of duodenopancreatic complex	863.31	5
	Vascular	Devascularization of duodenum	863.31	5

AIS, Abbreviated Injury Scale; *D1,* first portion of duodenum; *D2,* second portion of duodenum; *D3,* third portion of duodenum; *D4,* fourth portion of duodenum; *ICD,* International Classification of Diseases
*Advance one grade for multiple injuries up to grade III.
Data from Moore EE, Cogbill TH, Malangoni MA, et al: Organ injury scaling II: pancreas, duodenum, small bowel, colon, and rectum, *J Trauma* 30:1427–1429, 1990.

Overview of Operative Management and Results

Including all 1000 patients with pancreatic injuries described in one review, simple drainage was used in 72.6%, subtotal resesection in 16.9%, an exclusion procedure (to be described) in 1.7%, a Whipple procedure in 1.8%, and "other" in 7.1%. The most common postoperative intraabdominal complications were a pancreatic fistula in 6% (range, 3% to 17 %), intraabdominal abscess in 5% (range, 5% to 18%), and postoperative pancreatitis in 2% (range 1% to 13%). Mortality obviously depends on the mechanism of injury, magnitude of the pancreatic injury, and the presence of associated injuries to the gastrointestinal (GI) tract, liver, and abdominal vessels. Overall mortality in review articles is approximately 20% and has a wide range (stab wounds, 2.8% to 5%; gunshot wounds, 15.4% to 22%; blunt trauma, 16.9% to 19%; shotgun wounds, 46.1% to 50%).

DUODENUM

Epidemiology

Injuries to the duodenum are present in only 6% of patients admitted after suffering blunt abdominal trauma and in 10% to 11% and 1.6% of patients undergoing emergency laparotomies for gunshot or stab wounds, respectively. Associated intraabdominal injuries occur in 50% to 70% of patients with blunt injuries to the duodenum, and the most common associated injuries in patients undergoing laparotomies for penetrating wounds are injuries to the pancreas, liver, and inferior vena cava.

Blunt Mechanism of Injury

As with blunt injuries to the pancreas, a direct blow to the upper abdomen, possibly combined with tangential or shearing forces and a closed-loop blowout, is the most common mechanism of injury. The second portion of the duodenum is the anatomic area most commonly injured in most series.

Diagnosis

The retroperitoneal location of the duodenum, its low bacterial content compared with the small bowel or colon, and the ability of pancreatic juice to neutralize the pH of gastric chyme make diagnosis of a blunt injury to the duodenum difficult. In older series, patients with delays in diagnosis leading to an attempted operative repair more than 24 hours after injury have had a 40% to 50% mortality rate.

Aside from upper abdominal pain, a patient with a direct blow to the upper abdomen resulting in an intramural hematoma of the second or third portion of the duodenum will often have persistent vomiting within several hours after injury. Gastric dilatation, an airfluid level in the duodenum, and absence of the right psoas muscle shadow on an abdominal radiograph have been noted in an occasional patient with this injury. Diagnosis of a hematoma, rather than a full-thickness perforation, is confirmed by performing an upper GI radiograph series with water-soluble contrast with the patient turned on his or her right side. In the modern era, a 64-slice CT with oral or nasogastric tube contrast is the diagnostic test of choice. An intramural hematoma appears as a complete obstruction or as a "coiled spring" appearance of contrast just proximal to the obstruction.

In patients with full-thickness perforation of the duodenum, abdominal radiographic findings include retroperitoneal air outlining the duodenum in the right upper quadrant; obliteration of the upper psoas muscle border on the right; scoliosis of the lumbar spine to the left; and air in front of the first lumbar vertebra on a lateral radiograph. The routine abdominopelvic film taken to rule out a pelvic fracture in many patients with blunt trauma may not extend superiorly enough to visualize the air shadows or bubbles characteristic of a duodenal rupture in the retroperitoneum. Contrast-enhanced CT with a 64-slice scanner is used to rule out a duodenal rupture in asymptomatic or modestly symptomatic patients with blunt trauma or with penetrating injuries to the flank or back.

Grading System

The American Association for the Surgery of Trauma published the duodenum OIS in 1990 (Table 2).

Nonoperative Management

In the absence of hypotension, peritonitis, evisceration, and CT evidence of significant injuries to other organs or vessels, a grade I duodenal injury (hematoma in single portion/partial-thickness laceration) is managed nonoperatively. Patients with a duodenal wall hematoma are maintained on nasogastric suction and intravenous alimentation as the fusiform mass resolves over 2 to 4 weeks. Success rates without operation are approximately 90%, but the in-hospital time is substantial for any patient. A less commonly used approach is to take the patient to surgery shortly after diagnosis with the plan to evacuate what is most commonly a submucosal hematoma. The extent of the hematoma, difficulty in evacuating adherent clot, and the risk of creating a full-thickness injury make this approach somewhat unappealing. Without resolution of the hematoma at 3 to 4 weeks of nonoperative management, or with an inability to evacuate the hematoma at operation at any time, an open or laparoscopic antecolic gastrojejunostomy is performed. The patient should be screened for the presence of *Helicobacter pylori* in the perioperative period and, if screening is positive, the patient should undergo standard oral antibiotic treatment once feedings resume.

Operative Management

When a duodenal blowout or perforation needs to be ruled out in a patient with a periduodenal hematoma, or when it must be treated in a patient with a known injury, an extensive Kocher maneuver is performed from the porta hepatis to the superior mesenteric vessels. In a patient with a penetrating wound that might involve the third or fourth portions of the duodenum, the ligament of Treitz is divided as in performing a Whipple procedure, and the entire posterior aspect of these areas can be visualized as well.

A duodenal perforation or blowout is inspected to verify that the ampulla of Vater has not been injured. If it has not, the perforation is closed in a transverse or oblique fashion using an inner continuous suture row of 3-0 absorbable suture and an outer interrupted suture row of 3-0 absorbable or nonabsorbable suture. Through-and-through bullet holes in proximity to one another and away from the head of the pancreas are connected and closed in a similar fashion. Drains are not usually inserted when routine repairs are performed. When the perforation is quite large, and the adjacent wall of the duodenum is contused, some surgeons will buttress the underlying duodenal repair with a viable omental pedicle. The insertion of a closed-suction drain adjacent to the latter repair is appropriate.

Through-and-through missile holes, where one is on the mesenteric side of the duodenum, in association with an injury to the head of the pancreas mandate ruling out an injury to the adjacent distal common bile duct. In the absence of an overt leak of bile from the pancreatic injury, the common bile duct should be exposed in the porta hepatis. A 2 cm segment of a 5 Fr pediatric feeding tube is advanced into the common bile duct through a small choledochotomy and fixed in place with a U stitch. A standard choledochogram is performed after injecting 7 to 10 mL of an iodine contrast agent through the pediatric feeding tube. If the common bile duct is intact, the defect in the medial wall of the duodenum can be closed from within the lumen, using a row of interrupted 3-0 absorbable sutures followed by closure of the more lateral perforation. A #10 closed-suction drain should be placed adjacent to the duodenum. Also, consideration should be given to adding one of the duodenal diversion procedures.

Loss of a portion of the antimesenteric wall of the duodenum secondary to a penetrating wound is easily managed by bringing up a retrocolic, short Roux-en-Y–jejunal limb and performing a side-to-end duodenojejunostomy (Figure 4). A jejunal serosal patch applied to the duodenal perforation as illustrated in older textbooks is *never* indicated.

Whenever a duodenal repair is felt to be somewhat tenuous because of narrowing of the lumen, severe contusions of the duodenal wall, or the presence of an associated injury to the head of the pancreas, the addition of a diversion procedure must be considered. *Pyloric exclusion with gastrojejunostomy* (Figure 5) is the easiest and most commonly performed. Through a dependent gastrotomy, the pyloric muscle ring

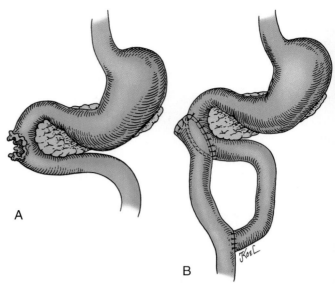

A

B

FIGURE 4 A short retrocolic Roux-en-Y duodenojejunostomy is appropriate when a portion of the antimesenteric wall of the duodenum is lost.

(not the prepyloric antrum) is grabbed with Babcock clamps at the 12 and 6 o'clock positions. A 1-0 polypropylene suture in two layers is used to close the longitudinal slit in the pylorus created by separating the Babcock clamps. An antecolic gastrojejunostomy is then performed to allow for postoperative feeding. The pylorus will stay closed for 2 to 3 weeks and then reopen in 94% of individuals, thereby protecting the injured duodenum as it heals. Should a duodenal fistula occur from breakdown of the repair, it will be an end rather than a side fistula, as the pylorus is closed. As previously noted, all patients in whom the gastrojejunostomy is performed should be screened for the presence of *H. pylori* in the stomach before discharge.

A second diversion procedure is the *duodenal diverticulization* originally described in 1968. This procedure includes a truncal vagotomy, antrectomy, gastrojejunostomy, tube duodenostomy, choledochostomy, and external drainage of the duodenal repair. Although accomplishing diversion of esophageal and gastric secretions away from the duodenal repair, it sacrifices normal vagus nerves and the gastric antrum/pylorus. In addition, the insertion of a choledochostomy tube into a normal 4 to 6 mm common bile duct would be considered to be unwise technically by most surgeons.

The third diversion procedure is the *triple-tube approach* described in 1978. Some combination of decompressive tubes is inserted, such as a Stamm gastrostomy, tube duodenostomy, or retrograde jejunostomy and a standard Witzel jejunostomy for enteral feedings. Decompression of the healing duodenum is obviously achieved by proximal, local, or retrograde tube decompression, which comes with a risk of associated GI leaks from the numerous new tubes inserted for decompression or feeding.

Complete devascularization of the second and third portions of the duodenum can occur from a direct blow to the right upper quadrant. Such injuries almost always occur in association with severe injuries to the head of the pancreas. A Whipple procedure is indicated, with timing based on the patient's hemodynamic and metabolic state, much as with maceration of the head of the pancreas.

Results

The major complication of a duodenal repair is a postoperative fistula, the incidence of which ranged from 2% to 14% with a mean of 6.6% in large series reported from 1968 through 1990. Because

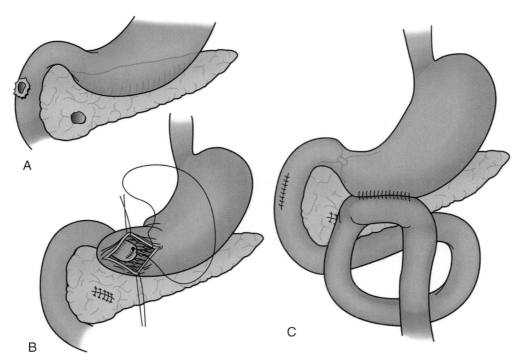

FIGURE 5 **A** and **B,** The first step in a pyloric exclusion procedure is a dependent gastrotomy and oversewing of the pyloric muscle ring with a 1-0 polypropylene suture. **C,** The second step is suturing or stapling an antecolic gastrojejunostomy at the site of the gastrotomy. *(From Schwartz et al: Principles of surgery, ed 7, New York, 1999, McGraw-Hill.)*

of the addition of diversion procedures and the availability of percutaneous drainage and nutritional support, deaths due directly to the duodenal injury have occurred in only 0.7% to 3.9% of patients in large series over the years. The overall mortality rate in patients with a duodenal injury in 17 series reported from 1968 through 1990 was 17%.

COMBINED PANCREATICODUODENAL INJURIES

Combined pancreaticoduodenal injuries are more common in patients who have suffered penetrating wounds. When one of these organs is severely injured and the other is not, the general principles of management call for the surgeon to perform an appropriate repair for each and consider adding a diversion procedure. If the injuries in both organs are serious and in proximity to one another, a major resection is indicated, either a Whipple procedure or distal pancreatectomy and resection of the third or fourth portions of the duodenum. Major postoperative complications in one series included

pancreatic fistula (26%), intraabdominal abscess (17%), and duodenal fistula (6.5%), and the overall mortality rate was 29.5%.

SUGGESTED READINGS

Asensio JA, Feliciano DV, Britt LD, et al: Management of duodenal injuries, *Curr Probl Surg* 30:1021–1100, 1993.

Asensio JA, Petrone P, Roldan G, et al: Pancreaticoduodenectomy: a rare procedure for the management of complex pancreaticoduodenal injuries, *J Am Coll Surg* 197:937–942, 2003.

Cushman JG, Feliciano DV, et al: Contemporary management of pancreatic trauma. In Maull KI, Cleveland HC, Feliciano DV, editors: *Advances in trauma and critical care,* vol. 10, St Louis, 1995, Mosby–Year Book, pp 309–336.

Feliciano DV, Martin TD, Cruse PA, et al: Management of combined pancreatoduodenal injuries, *Ann Surg* 205:673–680, 1987.

Subramanian A, Dente CJ, Feliciano DV: The management of pancreatic trauma in the modern era, *Surg Clin North Am* 87:1515–1532, 2007.

Takishima T, Hirata M, Kataoka Y, et al: Pancreatographic classification of pancreatic ductal injuries caused by blunt trauma to the pancreas, *J Trauma* 48:745–752, 2000.

INJURIES TO THE SMALL AND LARGE BOWEL

Panna A. Codner, MD, Todd Neideen, MD, and
John A. Weigelt, DVM, MD

OVERVIEW

Bowel injuries occur iatrogenically or secondary to external trauma. Management methods range from simple closure or resection with primary anastomosis to resection with diversion or damage-control procedures with later reconstruction. Although diagnosis is straightforward in most cases, small and large bowel injuries after blunt trauma remain a diagnostic challenge.

MECHANISM OF INJURY

Gastrointestinal injuries following gunshot wounds to the peritoneal cavity occur in over 80% of patients. The incidence of hollow viscus injury after stab wounds to the abdomen is approximately 20%. Injuries to the small bowel from blunt abdominal trauma vary from 5% to 15%. Although it is easy to understand how penetrating wounds cause small bowel injuries, a number of mechanisms are postulated for blunt injuries to the bowel. These include shearing of the bowel from its mesentery secondary to deceleration, referred to as a *bucket handle injury*, or bursting of a closed loop of bowel. This latter mechanism is associated with a seat-belt injury and lumbar spine fractures. The seat belt traps a loop of bowel against the retroperitoneum or spine, and the increased intraluminal pressure results in bursting of the small bowel along the antimesenteric border. This mechanism is commonly associated with anterior abdominal wall ecchymosis, known as a *seat-belt sign,* and possibly traumatic hernia. Also occurring with these injuries can be flexion compression fractures to the lumbar spine, called *Chance fractures.* Injury can occur with a lap belt only or with a lap-and-shoulder belt. Patients with a seat-belt sign or lumbar fractures have an increased probability of bowel injury. The incidence of small bowel injury is higher in patients wearing a seat belt; however, the incidence of total abdominal trauma is not changed, whether a seat belt is worn or not.

A final mechanism to mention is iatrogenic bowel injury. This is an Agency for Healthcare Research and Quality (AHRQ) quality indicator for hospital care, reported as patient safety indicator #15, for all surgical and medical discharges; it includes bowel injuries and other accidental punctures and lacerations to patients during medical care. This quality indicator is reported as a rate per 1000 discharges. AHRQ acknowledges that this indicator has a risk of being underreported or overreported and is not always considered preventable. A validation study placed this rate at two to three accidental punctures or lacerations per 1000 discharges. Bowel injuries were particularly common during operations for lysis of adhesions.

DIAGNOSIS

Because the majority of patients with blunt abdominal trauma do not have a bowel injury, a diagnostic approach is necessary to identify the minority of patients who require surgical intervention. Many centers still operate on all patients with anterior abdominal gunshot wounds because of the high incidence of associated injury. A more selective approach is used with stab wounds to the anterior abdomen because of the lower incidence of hollow viscus injuries. This approach includes local wound exploration (LWE) and, if positive, diagnostic peritoneal lavage (DPL) or computed tomographic (CT) scan. However, the patient with blunt abdominal trauma presents the greatest diagnostic challenge.

An LWE is performed after a surgical prep and infiltration with a local anesthetic. The original length of injury is used, and it is extended only for exposure. In the abdomen, an LWE is considered positive if the posterior fascia or peritoneum is violated. A DPL begins with decompression of the stomach and urinary bladder with a nasogastric (NG) tube and Foley catheter. Next, using sterile technique, an infraumbilical vertical incision is made. A percutaneous, open, or semiopen technique may be used. Fascia is visualized and divided, and peritoneum is entered sharply. The DPL catheter is placed intraperitoneally and directed toward the pelvis along the anterior abdominal wall. The catheter has openings along its length, and all openings must be intraperitoneal to prevent an airlock. A 10 mL syringe is attached to the catheter, and if there is return of blood, the patient is taken to the operating room for a positive DPL. Otherwise, intravenous (IV) tubing is used, and a scant 1 L of saline is infused via the catheter as quickly as possible; the full liter is not infused, otherwise air will enter the system. The IV bag is then dropped to the floor, and return of at least 300 mL is adequate for analysis. The catheter may need to be manipulated to dislodge omentum or blockage and maximize fluid return. The fluid is then sent to the laboratory for analysis and is considered positive if 100,000/mm^3 or more red blood cells, 500/mm^3 or more WBCs, or bile, fecal, or vegetable matter is found.

Abdominal tenderness is the most common finding in patients with perforated bowel injuries after blunt abdominal injury. Early peritonitis is usually not present in more than a third of these patients and should not be relied upon as an indication for surgical intervention. However, the presence of peritoneal signs mandates exploration. Another indication for early operation is hypotension in a patient with blunt abdominal trauma and no other obvious injuries. More commonly these patients are hemodynamically normal and are evaluated with an abdominal and pelvic CT scan. As CT scanning techniques have improved, a number of CT findings have become helpful in identifying patients with a possible bowel injury. These include intraperitoneal fluid with no solid-organ injury, pneumoperitoneum, bowel wall thickening, mesenteric fat streaking, mesenteric hematoma, and extravasation of luminal contrast or a vascular blush in the mesentery. Small amounts of intraperitoneal fluid can be normal. Intraperitoneal fluid collections extending for 3 cm in one location or the presence of fluid in multiple locations without a solid-organ injury are associated with hollow viscus injury in 50% to 67% of patients. Intraluminal contrast with extravasation is not a reliable sign, and our recommendation is to not use oral contrast for emergent CT scans in patients with blunt abdominal trauma. Bowel wall thickening also does not necessarily mean bowel injury, although when present early, and with other signs of bowel injury, it should not be ignored. Mesenteric hematomas and vascular blushes within the mesentery are commonly associated with a "bucket handle" injury, which occurs when the mesentery is stripped away from the bowel, causing bleeding and eventually an ischemic piece of small bowel.

SURGICAL MANAGEMENT OF BOWEL INJURIES

A number of principles can be applied to the management of small or large bowel injuries. These principles are identified in Box 1 and can be followed whether you are repairing a simple laceration or performing a resection and primary anastomosis. Little evidence exists to suggest that one repair technique is better than another. A single-layer technique is appropriate for both small and large bowel injuries;

BOX 1: Operative principles for managing small and large bowel injuries

1. Completely define all injuries with proper dissection.
2. Decide on the type of repair: simple repair, resection and repair, or damage control.
3. Debride all devitalized tissue.
4. Establish clean bowel edges in the area of the repair.
5. Use absorbable suture if a stapling technique is not employed.
6. Close mesenteric defects.

TABLE 1: Evaluation of severity of injury

	Mild	Severe
Agent	Stab	Blunt or missile
Size	<75% wall	≥75% wall
Site*	3, 4	1, 2
Injury repair interval	<24 hr	>24 hr
Adjacent injury	No CBD	CBD

*Site is duodenal location for the injury.
CBD, Common bile duct

however, a double-layer closure is advocated by some, particularly for large bowel injuries.

A controversy continues to swirl around the issue of stapled versus hand-sewn repairs. Some evidence suggests that emergent stapled repairs are associated with more complications, but other studies refute these findings. Care should be taken when using a stapling device if the bowel is extremely edematous, in which case a larger staple size should be considered.

Alternatively, it may be best to perform a damage control operation and leave the bowel in discontinuity. Damage control procedures stop the bleeding, control the contamination, and shorten the surgical procedure, permitting resuscitation of the patient to establish normal perfusion and organ function. Once organ function is restored, a return trip to the operating room is scheduled to definitively repair all injuries.

Injuries to the duodenum are often treated differently from other small bowel injuries. Suspicion is high in the presence of retroperitoneal hematoma, crepitus, or bile staining along the lateral margin of the duodenum. If these signs are present, exploration is warranted with complete duodenal mobilization via a Kocher maneuver and reflection of the mesentery of the right colon, if exposure of the third or fourth portions of the duodenum are required.

Most duodenal injuries can be managed by duodenorrhaphy or resection and anastomosis, especially if the injury is in the third or fourth portion of the duodenum. This will be successful in 75% to 80% of cases. However, when a destructive injury to the duodenum or an associated pancreatic or common bile duct injury is present, a complex repair will be required. Primary repair is not possible in the second portion of the duodenum because of the ampulla of Vater. If a complex repair is necessary, we favor using a piece of jejunum as a Roux-en-Y over the duodenal defect in either a side-to-side or end-to-side fashion. A side-to-side anastomosis is preferred when there is a large duodenal defect. A 35 to 40 cm defunctionalized length of jejunum is constructed and brought up in a retrocolic manner. This configuration has less tension and better blood supply. An-end-to-side anastomosis can be used if there is a large portion of distal duodenum missing, and the distal end can be oversewn. Complex repairs that alter gastroduodenal physiology are not recommended.

The high incidence of marginal ulcers in patients after pyloric exclusion procedures dissuades us from using this procedure for duodenal decompression and drainage, especially in younger individuals without preexisting peptic ulcer disease. Pyloric exclusion provides temporary diversion to allow healing of the duodenal injury and is performed through a gastrotomy. Absorbable suture may be used if the duodenal lumen is adequate, and pyloric patency is later desired. The pylorus will reopen in 2 to 3 weeks in 90% to 95% of patients. Nonabsorbable sutures or staples are used if the duodenal lumen is not adequate, but caution should be used when using a stapler to place the closure over the pylorus and prevent retained antrum. Drains are often used when a duodenal injury is present, although if a simple closure is accomplished, we rarely use drains.

Tube decompression for simple closures remains controversial. Moderate to severe injuries likely require tube decompression, but repairs with decompression have a 2.3% fistula rate compared with 11.8% without decompression. The tube can be placed antegrade via

a transnasal sump or retrograde via a jejunostomy. The decision for complex repair or tube decompression is difficult. Synder and colleagues (1980) identified five factors that might influence the choice for complex repair over simple closure (Table 1). Pancreaticoduodenectomy is rarely indicated for these injuries, although massive bleeding and ampullary destruction are the two indications that have stood the test of time. Pancreaticoduodenectomy can be done in a damage control manner with resection done in one setting, followed by reconstruction after the patient stabilizes.

Small bowel injuries are usually closed primarily. If multiple holes are present in close proximity, resection of all injuries may be accomplished with a single end-to-end or side-to-side anastomosis. Obviously, care must be taken not to resect excessive lengths of small bowel and create a short bowel syndrome. Most commonly a single-layer anastomosis is used to accomplish this repair (Figure 1).

Colon injuries have undergone a dramatic change in management approaches in the past 20 years. We have moved from routine colostomy to primary repair of most colon injuries. Simple laceration from either a gunshot wound or stab wound can be debrided and closed primarily with either a suture or stapling technique. Destructive wounds can also be resected, and an anastomosis can be performed. Again, damage control techniques may be necessary to control bleeding and correct coagulopathy in some patients. The injured colon is resected in such patients, and no attempt at repair is made. The patient's abdomen is left open, resuscitation is completed, the coagulopathy is corrected, organ function is improved, and negative fluid balance is achieved; negative fluid balance is important for decreasing edema to facilitate bowel anastomosis and abdominal wall closure.

Next, the patient returns to the operating room, where colon continuity is restored with either sutures or staples. We often prefer a side-to-side anastomosis, particularly if there is adequate colon length. We usually accomplish this as a hand-sewn anastomosis with either one or two layers. The side-to-side anastomosis may be better vascularized, but proper mobilization of the bowel is necessary to avoid undue tension on the repair. We also do an end-to-side anastomosis for the same reason, especially when performing a right hemicolectomy. Our choice of anastomosis is end-to-side for an ileocolic anastomosis.

A colostomy is still indicated when other injuries or the severity of injuries does not allow early anastomosis and abdominal closure. Persistence in attempting to reestablish bowel continuity in severely injured patients increases the opportunity for surgical complications such as enteric fistula. If closure cannot be accomplished in 72 hours, it may be best to divert the patient and close the abdomen before closure becomes impossible. The other area where a colostomy is still strongly considered is for rectal injuries.

Rectal wounds continue to be challenging for surgeons. The infectious complications and high mortality associated with these injuries make treatment difficult. Given its location deep in the pelvis, the rectum is usually spared from traumatic injuries. Most rectal injuries result from penetrating gunshot wounds (96%), but blunt injuries associated with pelvic fractures have been described. Rectal injury should be suspected with trauma to the lower abdomen,

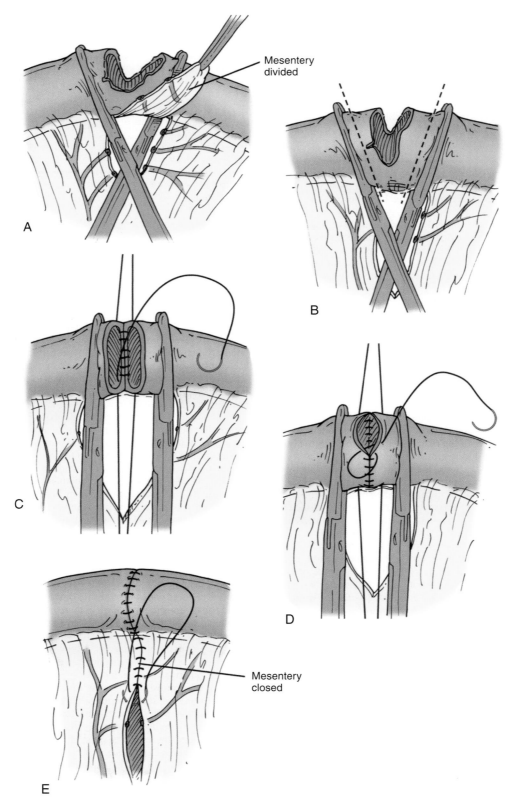

Mesentery
divided

Mesentery
closed

A

B

C

D

E

FIGURE 1   Small bowel injury requiring resection. Bowel is debrided, and bowel clamps are used proximally and distally. Single-layer anastomosis performed with a running absorbable 3-0 Lembert suture technique. *(Modified from Thal ER, Weigelt JA, Carrico CJ [eds]: Operative trauma management, an atlas, ed 2, New York, 2001, McGraw-Hill, p 207. Reproduced with permission from the McGraw-Hill Companies.)*

buttocks, perineum, upper thigh, and especially sacrum. Digital rectal examination is not very sensitive in detecting rectal injuries, and the absence of blood does not exclude injury. Rigid proctoscopy or sigmoidoscopy may be added to help diagnose injury.

Standard management of extraperitoneal rectal injuries should adhere to the "three D's": *d*efine the injury, *d*ivert the fecal stream, and *d*rain the pelvic space. Defining the injury is done by imaging or proctoscopy, but primary repair of the injury is usually not done. Diverting the fecal stream is the primary therapeutic component to prevent further pelvic soilage, and it allows the rectal wound to heal. Drainage of the retrorectal space is commonly used to remove blood and fecal contamination that could cause pelvic sepsis. Drainage or washout of the distal rectal stump is advocated for the same reason.

Each of these steps has been questioned. Recent suggestions imply that primary repair of rectal injuries can be done safely, especially if the wound is close to the peritoneal reflection. We still prefer to divert these patients with a sigmoid colostomy. Retrorectal drains should be used when the retrorectal space is severely contaminated, but their routine use is probably not indicated. Washout of the distal stump has little supporting data for civilian injuries, and we rarely employ it as part of our management approach.

Septic complications impact the morbidity and mortality associated with rectal injuries. This association makes initial management, repair, diversion, and drainage key to a successful outcome. Death rates for sepsis have improved, from 90% at the beginning of the century, but they continue to be high at 15% to 20%. Appropriate supportive measures include blood replacement, correction of fluid and electrolyte deficits, antibiotics, and tetanus prophylaxis.

Technique of Suture Anastomosis

When performing a hand-sewn anastomosis, we have switched completely to absorbable sutures. We use a 4-0 Vicryl suture for the inner layer in a running fashion. This stitch includes a small amount of serosa and an even smaller amount of mucosa, and it essentially approximates the mucosa and serosa. We follow this with a running Lembert stitch using polydioxanone suture. We find that the running technique speeds our repair and produces a secure closure. We sometimes also use the Lembert suture as a single layer, especially when repairing small bowel. Although we have nothing against a stapled anastomosis, the sutured anastomosis is easier to use in many locations within the abdomen. Although nonabsorbable suture material such as silk can be used for bowel anastomosis, we believe absorbable materials provide adequate strength, and their absorbable nature removes any concern for long-term suture complications. Our use of absorbable suture also extends to wound closure for the anterior abdomen.

Use of a Penrose drain instead of a bowel clamp is another technique that is especially useful for containing bowel contents during bowel resection and anastomosis. We use a cigarette drain placed proximally and distally around the bowel to prevent bowel contents from soiling the operative field. A small hole is made in the mesenteric side of the bowel, avoiding mesenteric vessels, and the Penrose drain is used to encircle the bowel. The cigarette drain is secured with one tie and is used as traction on the bowel if necessary. Although bowel clamps could certainly be used to prevent bowel contents from leaking into the field, using the Penrose drain avoids clamping the bowel, reduces the number of instruments in the operative field, and easily controls leakage. One must remember to remove the drain after the anastomosis is complete.

Mesenteric defects are closed with absorbable sutures, usually in an interrupted fashion. Drains are not typically required when we are repairing bowel injuries, and we do not normally place an NG tube in these patients unless there are associated injuries.

Perioperative care includes preoperative antibiotics for no more than 24 hours. Wounds are commonly closed with staples and dressed dry. We favor a subcuticular closure if time permits to avoid the need for staples. When a suture closure is used, we seal the wound with a liquid skin adhesive and avoid a dressing altogether. Early ambulation and diet are consistently attempted, as with any abdominal operation, along with chemical deep venous thrombus prophylaxis.

SUGGESTED READINGS

Brasel KJ, Olson CJ, Stafford RE, Johnson TJ: Incidence and significance of free fluid on abdominal computed tomographic scan in blunt trauma, *J Trauma* 44:889–893, 1998.

Chandler CF, Lane JS, Waxman KS: Seat-belt sign following blunt trauma is associated with increased incidence of abdominal injury, *Am Surg* 63:885–888, 1997.

Demetriades D, Murray JA, Chan LS, et al: Hand-sewn versus stapled anastomosis in penetrating colon injuries requiring resection: a multicenter study, *J Trauma* 52(1):117–121, 2002.

Henriksen K, Battles JB, Marks ES, Lewin DI, editors: *Advances in patient safety: from research to implementation. Vol. 2, concepts and methodology*, AHRQ Pub. No. 05-0021-2, Rockville, MD, 2005, Agency for Healthcare Research and Quality.

Maxwell RA, Fabian TC: Current management of colon trauma, *World J Surg* 27:632–639, 2003.

Snyder W 3d, Weigelt JA, Watkins WL, et al: Surgical management of duodenal trauma: precepts based on a review of 248 cases, *Arch Surg* 115:422–425, 1980.

Weigelt JA: Duodenal injuries, *Surg Clin North Am* 70(3):529–539, 1990.

Weigelt JA, Brasel KJ: Damage control in trauma surgery, *Curr Opin Crit Care* 6(4):276–280, 2000.

MANAGEMENT OF RECTAL INJURIES

Aurelio Rodriguez, MD, and
Vicente Cortes, MD

OVERVIEW

Rectal injuries are rare, and they may not be readily apparent; when overlooked, they often result in significant morbidity and mortality. An untreated rectal injury that results in a continued septic source is associated with almost 100% mortality rate.

The general principles of treatment of rectal injuries were established based on the military experience acquired during World War II, the Korean War, and the Vietnam War from treating high-velocity firearm injuries and mine-related injuries. Over the past 40 years, those principles have been challenged when applied to the less severe injuries seen in the civilian population.

ETIOLOGY, MORBIDITY, AND MORTALITY

Rectal injuries may be the result of penetrating or blunt external accidental trauma; iatrogenic trauma during diagnostic, endoscopic, or electrosurgical interventions in the rectum; or during surgical interventions in adjacent organs. Finally, the introduction of rectal foreign bodies in cases of autoeroticism, sexual assault, or criminal impalement may also result in rectal injuries.

Firearm wounds are the most frequent cause of rectal injuries in the civilian population (82% to 94%). Stab wounds to the lower abdomen, pelvis, and buttocks may rarely injure the rectum. Major pelvic fractures and perineal avulsion injuries are frequently associated with rectal injuries in victims of blunt trauma. Iatrogenic injuries are usually diagnosed early or may occur in the setting of a prepared bowel, and this may have an impact in the treatment selection. Accidental impalement in straddle falls may produce severe but usually obvious anorectal injuries. The same is true for injuries resulting from criminal impalement and sexual assault.

Burch and colleagues (1989) reported a series of 100 patients with extraperitoneal rectal injuries with an overall mortality of 4%. The overall complication rate of rectal trauma is greater than 50%. Rectal injury–related septic complications occur in 11% of patients and include intraabdominal and pelvic abscesses, rectocutaneous fistulas, rectovesical fistulas, wound infections, and missile tract infections.

CLINICAL DIAGNOSIS

The most frequent types of rectal injuries are not readily apparent by history and physical, and a high index of suspicion must be maintained to avoid missing these potentially lethal injuries.

During the primary survey of penetrating trauma victims, complete exposure and detection of all gunshot wounds, both entrance and exit, and stab wounds is essential. Carefully inspecting the groins, perineum, external genitalia, buttocks, gluteal folds, and proximal thighs avoids missing additional gunshot or stab wounds in the victims of penetrating trauma.

The simple anteroposterior pelvic film as an early adjunct to the primary survey of the blunt trauma victim identifies all severe pelvic fractures, and it identifies the need to look for perineal wounds and injuries to the outlets of the genitourinary and gastrointestinal (GI) tracts that require further investigation; as a result, this simple film may significantly change the prognosis and management of the skeletal injury. In the same fashion, biplanar abdominal films and pelvic films with markers in stable penetrating trauma victims may show the location of retained projectiles and point to transpelvic trajectories.

The digital rectal exam focuses attention to the perianal region, allowing the evaluation of sphincter function and the identification of gross blood in the rectum or a palpable anorectal wall defect. Testing for occult blood is neither helpful nor recommended. Rigid proctoscopy is the preferred bedside diagnostic investigation to rule out rectal injuries. In an unprepared bowel, the large caliber of the scope allows better visualization of the rectal wall and evacuation of stool if necessary. It must be performed whenever rectal bleeding is present, blood is found on digital rectal examination, or if injury is strongly suspected. IV sedation may be used to facilitate the exam in the trauma room or in the emergency department. Clear-cut rectal lacerations or surrogate markers of injury, such as gross blood or rectal wall or submucosal hematomas, may be observed. Recently, Johnson and colleagues (2008) have used and reported spiral computed tomographic (CT) scan in combat casualties with gunshot wound or blast and fragmentation injuries to screen those at high likelihood for rectal injuries and decrease the number of rigid proctoscopies performed.

Rectal injury should be suspected in any patient taken for abdominal exploration with transabdominal or transpelvic gunshot wounds, based on the greater than 90% probability of significant visceral injury. Since the extraperitoneal rectum may not be examined at laparotomy, it is advisable in the hemodynamically normal patient to perform preoperative rigid proctoscopy under anesthesia to exclude or confirm the diagnosis, and then to position the patient in low lithotomy to facilitate the surgical treatment of the injury.

In male patients with pelvic fractures and signs of urethral injury— blood at the urethral meatus, scrotal hematoma, and boggy or nonpalpable prostate on digital rectal exam—a retrograde urethrogram must be performed in the trauma bay, before insertion of the Foley catheter, followed by CT evaluation and CT cystogram or conventional cystogram.

In female patients with pelvic fractures, urethral injury is very rare, but bimanual pelvic and digital rectal exams should be done in the trauma room to rule out vaginal or rectal perforation by bone

TABLE 1: The American Association for Surgery of Trauma rectum injury scale

Grade*	Injury
I	Contusion or hematoma without devascularization or partial-thickness laceration
II	Full-thickness laceration <50% of the circumference
III	Full-thickness laceration ≥50% of the circumference
IV	Full-thickness laceration with extension into the perineum
V	Vascular: complete devascularization

*Advance one grade for multiple injuries up to III.

shards, followed by CT evaluation and CT cystogram or conventional cystogram. Careful review of the CT scan will determine whether rigid proctoscopy is necessary.

Iatrogenic injuries during diagnostic or therapeutic endoscopy occur more frequently at the rectosigmoid junction. The patient will report increasing abdominal pain and tenderness after the endoscopy, biopsy, or electrosurgery. Pneumoperitoneum may be seen on upright chest films, and a water-soluble enema may confirm the diagnosis and location. Nelson and colleagues (1982) reported an incidence of perforation of 0.18% for rigid proctoscopy, 0.24% for colonoscopy, and 0.16% for barium enema.

Classification According to Severity and Anatomic Location

The Committee of the American Association for the Surgery of Trauma created an organ injury grading severity scale in 1990 (Table 1). For purposes of surgical treatment, it is particularly important to establish the anatomic location as either *intraperitoneal, extraperitoneal,* or *anorectal.*

MANAGEMENT

Military experience has mandated a specific precept for the treatment of rectal injuries: Use primary repair when possible, followed by the "three D's": *d*iversion, *d*rainage, and *d*istal washout. Civilian experience with less severe injuries and major advances in prehospital and perioperative care, including antibiotics, have resulted in modifications, discussed below.

Intraperitoneal Rectum

The intraperitoneal rectum is a pelvic extension of the colon, without appendices epiploicae, haustra, or taenia coli. The surgical management of injuries in this location follows the principles of treatment of colonic injuries in general. The Eastern Association for the Surgery of Trauma Practice Guidelines Group recommends primary repair for all nondestructive colon wounds in the absence of peritonitis. They found level II evidence to recommend resection and primary anastomosis for destructive injuries in the absence of circulatory shock, significant comorbidities, and minimal associated injuries (Penetrating Abdominal Trauma Injury score <25, Injury Severity Score <25). On the other hand, based on a multicenter study of 297 patients, Demetriades and colleagues (2001) suggested that destructive colon injuries should be managed by resection and primary anastomosis without colostomy, regardless of risk factors.

In 2003 a Cochrane review was conducted to investigate the role of operative management for colonic injuries and concluded that compared with diversion, primary repair was associated with a significant decrease in overall complication rate; total infectious complications; abdominal complications, including dehiscence; and wound complications (excluding dehiscence). Based on this available level I evidence, routine primary repair should be attempted in the initial surgical management of all traumatic colon injuries, and diversion should only be considered if the colon itself is inappropriate for anastomosis: for example, in the case of massive contamination, severe edema, or ischemia after damage control procedures or overt peritonitis. Therefore all nondestructive and destructive intraperitoneal rectal injuries may be repaired primarily or may be treated by resection and primary anastomosis without mandatory colostomy.

If the surgeon, based on his/her judgement, elects to establish fecal diversion, the options include 1) primary repair with diverting loop colostomy, 2) resection and a Hartmann procedure, or 3) primary anastomosis with protecting diverting sigmoid-loop colostomy. The caveat here is that it is easier to close a diverting-loop colostomy than to take down a Hartmann procedure.

Iatrogenic perforations are treated using the same principles. Small perforations secondary to biopsy or polypectomy in the absence of peritoneal signs may be treated by nothing by mouth, intravenous antibiotics, and observation with serial abdominal examinations. Colonoscopic perforations are usually larger, located at the rectosigmoid junction, and they require abdominal exploration, surgical debridement, and primary repair.

Extraperitoneal Rectum

Simple, nondestructive, and easily accessible extraperitoneal rectal injuries (grades I and II) may be repaired and diverted with sigmoid-loop colostomy at laparotomy. Attempts at primary repair of extraperitoneal rectal injuries should be tempered by the need to violate an intact pelvic peritoneum, by the risk of causing neurovascular or genitourinary injuries during the pelvic dissection, and by the possibility of missing an injury in cases of through-and-through gunshot wounds. Small, nondestructive, distal rectal injuries may also be approached for repair via the transanal route.

Only in the presence of combined rectal and genitourinary injuries is it recommended to expose and repair both injuries, interposing omentum between the repairs and diverting the fecal and urinary streams to minimize the occurrence of rectovesical and rectourethral fistulas.

Navsaria and colleagues (2001 and 2004) have repeatedly reported the use of diagnostic laparoscopy to confirm isolated extraperitoneal rectal injuries due to low-velocity gunshot wounds. Having confirmed the absence of intraperitoneal injuries, they perform a trephine diverting sigmoid-loop colostomy without the need for drainage or distal washout. Others have added a laparoscope-assisted colostomy creation to this concept. Complex and destructive extraperitoneal injuries (grades III and V) require resection and a Hartmann procedure or resection and primary anastomosis with protecting diverting-loop colostomy.

In summary, the recent literature supports fecal diversion and presacral drainage of destructive extraperitoneal rectal injuries when the injury cannot be repaired or identified, or when the injury is extensive and communicates with the presacral space. The role of primary repair without fecal diversion is currently the subject of investigation.

Colostomy in Rectal Trauma

The main principle of the colostomy in rectal trauma is to completely divert the fecal stream from the injury. Although an end colostomy and mucous fistula achieve the goal, they result in additional difficulties at the time of eventual colostomy takedown. A properly constructed sigmoid-loop colostomy over a plastic or silicone bridge has been proven to be completely diverting but more difficult to care for with an appliance. Other alternatives include stapling the distal limb of the loop colostomy or constructing an end-loop colostomy as described by Prasad and colleagues (1984). All types may be closed using a peristomal incision without the need for formal relaparotomy, usually 3 to 4 months following the injury, when the patient has completely recovered. It must be stressed that colostomy closure is associated with a 15% complication rate, and that should be considered when diversion is entertained.

Renz and colleagues (1993) introduced the concept of same admission colostomy closure (SAAC). All patients underwent hydrosoluble contrast (diatrizoate) enemas 10 days after the injury. Those who showed no evidence of radiological leakage, no perirectal sepsis, and no concerns about continence were considered for colostomy closure. Sixty percent of the cases were deemed candidates, and approximately half of them underwent colostomy takedown without rectal injury–related complications. Two prospective randomized studies have shown that SAAC is safe and cost effective in appropriately selected groups.

Presacral Drainage in Rectal Trauma

The original rationale for the placement of presacral drains was to open the presacral space, allowing a point of egress of any perirectal infection that may result from an extraperitoneal rectal injury inaccessible to primary repair. This would halt the progression of the infection in a closed space and avoid extension up into the retroperitoneum.

Some investigators believe that the failure to drain the presacral space is the only statistically significant factor associated with septic complications, but others report that low-velocity rectal wounds may be treated without such drainage, and they have not observed an increase in the incidence of septic complications. Still others believe that whenever an extraperitoneal rectal injury is left unrepaired, drainage of the presacral space must be strongly considered.

Presacral drainage is performed in the lithotomy position. A curvilinear incision is made posterior to the anus, crossing the anococcygeal raphe, and is carried down on both sides of the raphe. It is not necessary to divide the anococcygeal ligament or to resect the coccyx as once proposed. The presacral space is entered, and two Penrose drains are left behind and secured in place (Figure 1). Drains are left in place for approximately 7 days.

When deciding whether or not to establish presacral drainage, its minimal morbidity should be balanced with the consequences of an uncontrolled retroperitoneal necrotizing infection.

Distal Rectal Washout in Rectal Trauma

Routine removal of the stool from the rectum reduced the incidence of septic complications in rectal injuries during the Vietnam War. Distal rectal washout was undertaken in the usually dehydrated and chronically constipated soldiers who had sustained high-velocity firearm injuries.

Shannon and colleagues (1988) reported in a series of civilian injuries a lower incidence of pelvic abscesses (8% vs. 40%), rectal fistulas (7% vs. 23%), and sepsis (8% vs. 15%) with the use of distal rectal washout, and the only death was reported was in the non–distal washout group. All subsequent studies have failed to demonstrate any benefit of distal rectal washout in improving outcomes or preventing septic complications. Some claim that distal washout, when performed without primary repair of the injury, may result in additional contamination of the perirectal tissues.

We believe the lack of popularity of distal rectal washout is mainly based on the aesthetic factor; however, proper setup may facilitate this process. Following the induction of anesthesia and completion of

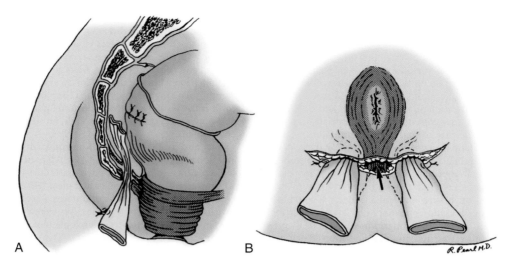

FIGURE 1   Presacral drainage. **A,** Lateral view. **B,** Interior view. *(From Fazio VW, Church JM, Delaney CP [eds]: Current therapy in colon and rectal surgery, ed 2, Philadelphia, 2005, Mosby Elsevier, p 145.)*

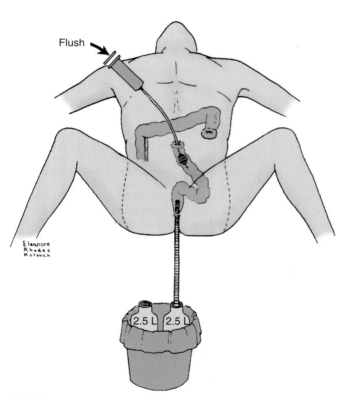

FIGURE 2   System of distal rectal washout. *(From Jacobs LM, Plaisier BR: An efficient system for controlled distal colorectal irrigation, J Am Coll Surg 178:305–306, 1994.)*

the rigid proctoscopy, the anus is digitally dilated, and the end of corrugated respiratory care tubing or a corrugated anesthesia machine circuit is inserted in the anal canal and is used to keep the sphincter open and to direct the rectal effluent into collection bottles or a large-capacity container. A purse-string suture is placed on the exteriorized sigmoid colon loop before maturation, and a colotomy is made in the center of the purse string; a large-bore Foley catheter is inserted downstream, and the balloon is inflated. Continuous gravity-driven warm saline irrigation is accomplished using 3 L urology irrigation bags (Figure 2). Once the effluent becomes clear, usually after 2 or 3

bags of irrigation, the Foley is removed, and the purse-string suture is tied down. The ostomy may then be matured in the usual fashion, stapling off the distal limb, depending on the surgeon's preference. Distal washout should still be considered an option in cases of high-velocity firearm destructive injuries.

Anorectal Injuries

The most common injuries to the anus and anal sphincters occur during vaginal deliveries with the use of midline episiotomies or with obstetrical instrumentation, such as forceps. Other injuries are iatrogenic, related to the use of enema tips and rectal thermometers or misadventures during anorectal surgical procedures. Overlapping sphincteroplasty, the preferred method of reconstruction, is generally performed by the colorectal specialist.

Blunt or penetrating trauma may result in rectal injuries extending into the perineum and involving the rectal sphincter (grade IV). There is controversy as to whether primary repair of the sphincter mechanism should be undertaken, or if delayed reconstruction should be left for the colorectal specialist, limiting the initial management to the diversion of the fecal stream and the meticulous debridement and irrigation of the injured tissues with the goal of maximal sphincter muscle preservation. Some of these cases may even require creation of neosphincters by transposition of the gracilis or gluteal muscles. The most severe, destructive, or traumatic anorectal injuries may even call for abdominoperineal resection and permanent colostomy.

Complex perineal wounds with or without pelvic fractures generally result from high-speed motorcycle crashes. These should be managed following some of the precepts of rectal trauma, including complete diversion of the fecal stream, distal washout, and aggressive and frequent surgical debridement utilizing pulsatile irrigation devices. These wounds should be allowed to close by secondary intention or by using a delayed primary closure technique to minimize the incidence of septic complications.

Patients with open pelvic fractures and perineal wounds involving the anorectum, ischiorectal fossa, and genitalia should be managed with fecal diversion. Patients with open pelvic fractures with nonperineal wounds involving the pubis, iliac crests, groins, and anterior thighs may be managed without fecal diversion with the use of occlusive vaccum-assisted closure dressings following initial pulsatile irrigation and surgical debridement. In patients with open pelvic fractures stabilized with external fixators, the left lower quadrant may become too crowded to allow the creation of a diverting sigmoid-loop colostomy, and occasionally a diverting transverse-loop colostomy may be more appropriate and easier to fit with an appliance without risking contamination of the pin sites.

Additional Therapy

In cases of colorectal injuries, all laparotomy incisions are best treated by delayed primary closure. All patients should receive broad-spectrum antibiotic coverage that includes agents with broad Gram-negative, aerobic, and anaerobic coverage. Antibiotic therapy should be initiated as soon as the diagnosis is entertained, and it should be continued during the perioperative period for no more than 24 hours. In their multicenter study of destructive colon injuries, Demetriades and colleagues (2001) reported an increased incidence of septic complications in those patients who received only single second-generation cephalosphorin coverage or ampicillin–sulbactam versus those who received combination therapy. This may indicate the need to use combination therapy in all destructive colorectal injuries to minimize the incidence of septic complications.

SUMMARY

We maintain a high index of clinical suspicion to identify all rectal injuries from penetrating or blunt mechanism. There is no substitute for the complete exposure of the patient, the diligent search for all injuries, and the digital rectal examination. Rigid proctoscopy remains our diagnostic aid of choice to directly identify rectal injuries or their surrogate markers. However, in hemodynamically normal victims of penetrating or blunt trauma, we found CT scan useful in the determination of missile trajectories and in screening candidates for rigid proctoscopy. When in doubt we presume an injury is present, and we manage it accordingly.

We usually identify intraperitoneal rectal injuries at exploratory laparotomy and treat them by primary repair for nondestructive injuries in the same fashion as for colonic injuries. For intraperitoneal destructive injuries, we attempt primary repair or resection and anastomosis, whenever a damage control approach is not indicated due to circulatory shock, hypothermia, and coagulopathy.

We manage extraperitoneal rectal injuries by diversion of the fecal stream and presacral drainage, leaving distal rectal washout at the discretion of the surgeon. Diverting sigmoid-loop colostomy is our preferred diversionary procedure. It may be easily created and easily closed without the need for laparotomy or relaparotomy. In patients with suspected isolated extraperitoneal rectal injury, we use laparoscopy to exclude peritoneal violation that would mandate formal exploratory laparotomy and to facilitate the creation of a laparoscope-assisted diverting sigmoid-loop colostomy.

In anorectal injuries, sphincter preservation and eventual repair are of the utmost importance to achieve continence. Sphincter repair by overlapping sphincteroplasty is preferred and is generally performed electively, after the associated soft-tissue injuries have healed and the disrupted sphincter has fibrosed.

For combined rectal and genitourinary injuries, we use a more aggressive approach that includes primary repair of both GI and genitourinary tract injuries, interposition of viable tissue between the repairs, and diversion of the fecal and urinary streams.

In open pelvic fractures with perineal injuries and traumatic perineal injuries, we use diversion of the fecal stream with loop colostomy and distal washout to eliminate continued fecal soilage and septic complications.

SUGGESTED READINGS

Cleary RK, Pomerantz RA, Lampman RM: Colon and rectal injuries, *Dis Colon Rectum* 49:1203–1222, 2006.
Herr MW, Gagliano RA: Historical perspective and current management of colonic and intraperitoneal rectal trauma, *Curr Surg* 62:187–192, 2005.
Herr MW, Warscher RA, Gagliano RA: Historical perspective and current management of traumatic injury to the extraperitoneal rectum and anus, *Curr Surg* 62:625–632, 2005.
Johnson EK, Judge T, Lundy J, et al: Diagnostic pelvic computed tomography in the rectal-injured combat casualty, *Mil Med* 173:293–299, 2008.
Navsaria PH, Edu S, Nicol AJ: Civilian extraperitoneal rectal gunshot wounds: surgical management made simpler, *World J Surg* 31:1345–1351, 2007.

INJURY TO THE SPLEEN

Stepheny D. Berry, MD, and Martin A. Croce, MD

OVERVIEW

Splenic injuries are among the most common solid-organ injuries identified after trauma. The great majority of splenic injuries come as a result of blunt trauma, with as many as 77% resulting from motor vehicle collisions. Penetrating splenic injuries are less common and more frequently require operative intervention for associated injuries. Historically, adult blunt splenic injuries have also been managed operatively. More recently, splenic preservation has become standard in hemodynamically stable patients in light of the high success rate in the pediatric population. Regardless of the mechanism or patient age, hemodynamic status of the patient now dictates management.

DIAGNOSIS

Initial management of all patients seen for trauma should be consistent with the American College of Surgeons Advanced Trauma Life Support (ATLS) guidelines. It is well recognized that patients with splenic injuries often have confounding injuries that make physical examination unreliable. The diagnosis of splenic injuries, therefore, relies on a high index of suspicion. Some associated findings that should increase the index of suspicion include lower left-sided rib fractures and generalized abdominal and/or left upper quadrant pain. Referred pain to the left shoulder (Kehr sign) may be present, but it may be unreliable in the multiply injured patient.

Because history and physical examination are neither sensitive nor specific, other diagnostic modalities should be employed to diagnose splenic injuries. The hemodynamic status of the patient dictates the diagnostic algorithm. A hypotensive, tachycardic patient requires rapid assessment of the cause of hemodynamic instability and immediate intervention. The focused assessment by sonography for trauma (FAST) is a quick examination that is sensitive for intraabdominal fluid, but it is not specific for injury pattern. A positive FAST in the unstable patient should prompt immediate operative exploration. An equivocal or negative FAST in the unstable patient requires further investigation. A diagnostic peritoneal lavage (DPL) is a bedside procedure that provides adjunctive information to the FAST, and a positive DPL should also prompt operative exploration. Computed tomography (CT) is the diagnostic test of choice for the hemodynamically stable patient.

FAST employs four windows of examination: Morison pouch, splenorenal fossa, pelvis near the bladder, and pericardium. Peritoneal fluid, which is typically hemoperitoneum in the face of trauma, appears hypoechoic (a dark stripe) on ultrasound when compared with adjacent structures. FAST has a sensitivity of 80% to 95% for intraperitoneal fluid, but it does not provide specificity regarding which organ is injured. Ultrasound also has limitations in that it is operator dependent, does not provide information about retroperitoneal structures, and can also be limited by patient body habitus or the presence of subcutaneous emphysema.

DPL is another rapid bedside procedure that provides helpful information for the hemodynamically unstable polytrauma patient. A small incision is fashioned under local anesthesia in either the supraumbilical or infraumbilical position, and access is gained to the peritoneal cavity in an open, semiopen, or percutaneous technique. A small, blunt catheter is placed into the peritoneal cavity and guided toward the pelvis. The return of 10 mL of gross blood or enteric contents indicates a positive result, which should prompt surgical exploration. If the DPL is grossly negative, 1 L of normal saline is instilled into the abdominal cavity and allowed to drain by gravity. The returned fluid is then sent for laboratory evaluation, and 500 white blood cells/mm^3 or 100,000 red blood cells/mm^3 also represents a positive DPL. The sensitivity of DPL for hemoperitoneum approaches 100%; however, as little as 30 mL of hemoperitoneum can cause a microscopically positive DPL and a nontherapeutic laparotomy in up to 30% of patients. A microscopically positive DPL is unlikely to be the cause of hemorrhagic shock. DPL, like ultrasound, is sensitive for hemoperitoneum, but it is not specific for which organ is injured and does not evaluate the retroperitoneum. Thus a true DPL is not beneficial for diagnosis or management of patients with blunt splenic injury. The lavage is beneficial for diagnosis of hollow-organ injury due to the leukosequestration following bowel injury. However, a microscopic positive DPL for red cells will not account for hemodynamic instability. In such patients, the peritoneal aspiration of at least 10 mL blood is much more beneficial.

Contrast-enhanced CT has become the standard diagnostic tool for hemodynamically stable patients. With the current generation of CT scanners, the diagnostic accuracy for both intraabdominal and retroperitoneal injuries is approximately 91% to 97%. In addition, advancements in CT technology have allowed for a grading system to be developed by the American Association for the Surgery of Trauma to help quantify splenic injuries and their subsequent treatment modalities (Table 1).

MANAGEMENT

Penetrating Splenic Injury

Penetrating abdominal injuries are typically managed by laparotomy, especially injuries due to gunshot wounds. When faced with a penetrating splenic injury, splenectomy is usually the appropriate procedure, especially if the patient is hemodynamically labile or persistently hypotensive. Penetrating wounds will violate intraparenchymal anatomic planes, and patients are thus more likely to sustain an intraparenchymal arterial injury. Thus observation of these wounds will likely lead to pseudoaneurysm formation and subsequent delayed rupture. The safest procedure, then, is splenectomy.

An exception to this rule involves wounds to the lower pole of the spleen. After complete mobilization of the spleen and careful inspection of surrounding viscera, especially the colonic splenic flexure, the lower pole may be resected by using a stapling device. Topical hemostatic agents may be used to control minor troublesome bleeding along the staple line.

Blunt Splenic Injury

The key to the successful management of patients with blunt splenic injury is recognition of hemodynamic instability. Hemodynamically unstable patients with either suspected or confirmed splenic injuries require prompt operative intervention, although the decision tree

TABLE 1: Spleen injury scale (1994 revision)

Grade	Injury	Description
I	Hematoma Laceration	Subcapsular, >10% surface area Capsular tear, <1 cm parenchymal depth
II	Hematoma Laceration	Subcapsular, 10%–50% surface area Intraparenchymal, <5 cm in diameter Capsular tear, 1–3 cm parenchymal depth that does not involve a trabecular vessel
III	Hematoma Laceration	Subcapsular, >50% surface area or expanding; ruptured subcapsular or parenchymal hematoma; intraparenchymal hematoma ≥5 cm, expanding Parenchymal depth >3 cm or involving trabecular vessels
IV	Laceration	Laceration involving segmental or hilar vessels producing major devascularization (>25% of spleen)
V	Laceration Vascular	Completely shattered spleen Hilar vascular injury with devascularized spleen

Modified from Moore EE, Cogbill TH, Jurkovich GJ, et al: Organ injury scaling: spleen and liver (1994 revision), *J Trauma* 38:323–324, 1995.

becomes a bit more complex when a patient is hemodynamically stable. The majority of hemodynamically stable patients with blunt splenic injury can be managed nonoperatively. If the patient develops hemodynamic instability at any time in the face of a known splenic injury, operative intervention should be considered, unless other reasons for hemodynamic compromise are identified.

Nonoperative management (NOM) can be used successfully in 60% to 80% of patients with blunt splenic injuries, and success rates for hemodynamically stable patients should exceed 90%. To achieve such rates, patient selection is paramount. A number of relative contraindicators to NOM have been described, including hypotension upon hospital admission, associated brain injury, advanced age, extensive hemoperitoneum, and advanced grade of injury, but these are certainly debatable. Admission hypotension does not appear to matter, providing the patient's hemodynamics are quickly returned to normal. Associated brain injury is not a contraindication either, because it does not alter overall failure rates. Although brain injury can eliminate physical examination as a tool while observing these patients, abdominal physical examination is notoriously inaccurate in a multiply injured patient anyway. Intuitively, it seems that increased hemoperitoneum would be a relative contraindication to NOM. Although some studies have demonstrated slightly higher failure rates in patients with large amounts of hemoperitoneum, others have disputed this finding. The maintenance of hemodynamic stability is more important than the amount of hemoperitoneum, but patients with extensive hemoperitoneum should still be observed very closely; patients older than 55 also have a slightly higher failure rate (~10% to 15%). Although these patients are at higher risk for failure, close observation and maintenance of hemodynamic stability can be successful.

Failure of NOM is more frequent in patients with higher-grade splenic injuries; however, the presence of a higher grade injury (grades III to V) is not an absolute contraindication for NOM. Patients with higher grade injuries, especially those with extensive hemoperitoneum and/or age over 55 years, warrant very close observation. These

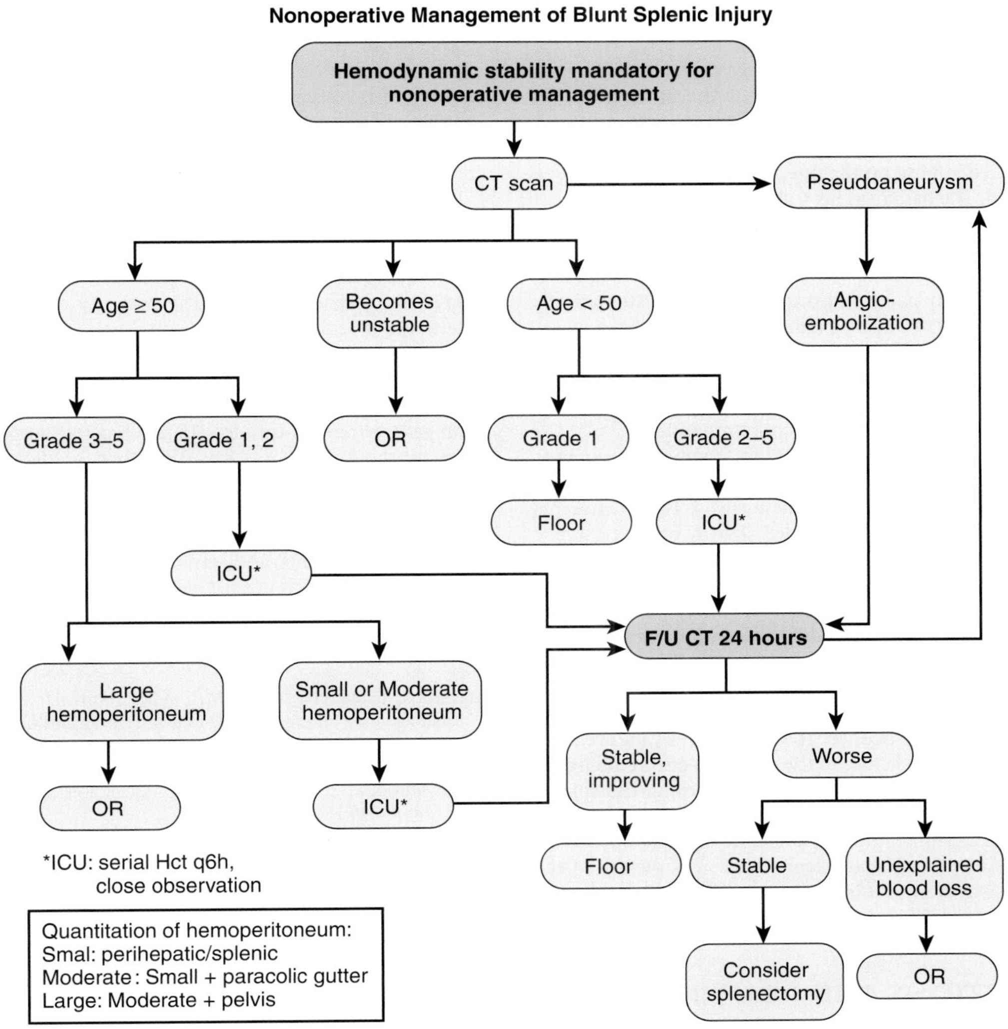

Nonoperative Management of Blunt Splenic Injury

FIGURE 1   Nonoperative management of blunt splenic injury.

patients should be monitored in a trauma center. If the ability to rapidly transport the patient to the operating room following failure of NOM is not available at a particular institution, perhaps the prudent management would be splenectomy, before giving the patient an opportunity to fail NOM.

In the multiply injured trauma patient, it is often difficult to know whether a patient is hemodynamically unstable from splenic bleeding because of his or her injury or if bleeding is from other associated injuries. It is helpful to assign amounts of blood loss for each injury. We use the following as a rough estimate of blood loss from various injuries: femur fracture, 2 units packed red blood cells; tibia fracture, 1 unit; multiple rib fractures and associated hemothorax, 2 to 4 units; humerus fracture, 1 to 2 units; facial trauma, 1 to 2 units; soft tissue injuries, 2 to 6 units; and pelvic fractures, 2 to 50 units. The estimate is doubled for open fractures. Once we have accounted for the associated injuries and have appropriately resuscitated the patient, hemodynamics are reassessed. If the patient has ongoing blood loss attributed to the spleen that requires further transfusion, the patient is taken to the operating room for splenectomy.

Angiographic embolization of splenic injuries when pseudoaneurysms or contrast blush are identified on initial and/or subsequent CT images has been debated in the literature. It has been found most beneficial for hemodynamically stable patients with pseudoaneurysms on CT imaging. When pseudoaneurysms can be

selectively coil embolized, the failure rates for NOM are decreased. Indeed, success rates when this scheme is followed exceed 95%. Some have advocated nonselective splenic artery embolization for management of splenic trauma. However, we believe that unstable patients should be managed in the operating room, not the angiography suite.

Another controversial discussion in the literature surrounds routine follow-up imaging. We have found that a significant number of pseudoaneurysms are not identified on the initial CT scan. Because pseudoaneurysms correlate with failure of NOM, we believe serial imaging 24 to 48 hours after admission is warranted to identify late pseudoaneurysms. These injuries may then be managed with selective angiographic embolization. Figure 1 illustrates an algorithm for the management of hemodynamically stable patients with blunt splenic injury.

Another injury that warrants specific mention is the subcapsular hematoma. Even seemingly small subcapsular hematomas can enlarge significantly and eventually rupture. This leaves a large, raw surface area of the spleen that bleeds. Once the subcapsular hematoma has ruptured, splenectomy is necessary. For this reason, this patient population requires close surveillance, serial hematocrit measurements, and sometimes repeat imaging. Enlargement of the subcapsular hematoma, even in hemodynamically stable patients, warrants consideration for splenectomy.

OPERATIVE MANAGEMENT

As stressed throughout, hemodynamically unstable patients with splenic injuries belong in the operating room. Other indications for operative management include ongoing hemorrhage, peritonitis, or suspected hollow viscus injury. These patients are taken to the operating room and placed supine on the operating table, where general anesthesia is induced. The patient's chest, abdomen, pelvis, and upper thighs are then prepped and draped in a sterile fashion. A midline incision is fashioned from the xiphoid to the pubic symphysis, and the abdominal cavity is entered. The hemoperitoneum is quickly evacuated with laparotomy pads, and the abdomen is systematically evaluated to identify areas of ongoing hemorrhage. Temporary packing can be used to control ongoing blood loss; however, if packing is not adequate to control the bleeding, the source should be identified and controlled. The rest of the abdomen is then inspected systematically to ensure control of obvious enteric contamination.

The spleen must be adequately mobilized for complete evaluation. The splenocolic ligament should be carefully divided, taking care to avoid injury to the colon and to ensure hemostasis. The splenorenal and splenophrenic ligaments may be divided sharply or with cautery. Exposure may be facilitated by grasping the spleen with the nondominant hand, pressing posteriorly and then medially for countertraction. After division of the ligaments, the surgeon's dominant hand can hold and compress the spleen to control bleeding. The index finger can then expose the gastrosplenic ligament and the short gastric vessels. These vessels should be ligated individually near the spleen, taking care not to injure the stomach. Once this maneuver is complete, the spleen should be freely mobile on its vascular pedicle. The splenic artery and vein are then individually suture ligated close to the spleen to ensure no injury to the tail of the pancreas. Once the spleen is removed, the splenic bed is carefully inspected to ensure hemostasis. In addition, the tail of the pancreas is inspected for injury. If pancreatic injury is suspected, a closed-suction drain is left in the splenic fossa near the tail of the pancreas. Routine use of drains is discouraged, as they have been associated with an increased incidence of subphrenic abscess formation.

IMMUNIZATIONS AND ROUTINE FOLLOW-UP

The spleen has immunologic function against encapsulated organisms, such as *Streptococcus pneumoniae*, *Neisseria meningitidis*, and *Haemophilus influenzae*. Patients who require splenectomy after trauma should be vaccinated against these organisms before discharge from the hospital. The *Streptococcus pneumoniae* vaccine should be repeated every 3 to 5 years. The indication for readministration of the *Neisseria meningitidis* and *Haemophilus influenzae* vaccines is still unknown.

Follow-up for patients who are successfully managed nonoperatively is still debated. As mentioned previously, we routinely repeat CT scans on our patients who have grade II to V injuries in 24 to 48 hours to identify late pseudoaneurysms. Once patients are discharged from the hospital, follow-up is still debated. Up to 1.4% of patients undergoing NOM of splenic injuries will return for splenectomy after discharge home. The majority of these patients require intervention within 3 weeks of discharge. Certainly, patient education regarding the risk of outpatient rupture is warranted. Routine activity restrictions are the practice in both the adult and pediatric population. We found that mild injuries (grades I or II) healed faster than severe injuries (grades III to V) using outpatient CT scans to evaluate the healing process. Therefore, graded activity restriction based on injury severity is recommended. The majority of splenic injuries demonstrated healing in 8 to 10 weeks; therefore patient and care giver education, close outpatient observation with imaging for symptomatic patients, and activity restriction are recommended during this time.

SUGGESTED READINGS

Davis KA, Fabian TC, Croce MA, et al: Improved success in nonoperative management of blunt splenic injuries: embolization of splenic artery pseudoaneurysms, *J Trauma* 44:1008, 1998.

Peitzman AB, Heil B, Rivera L, et al: Blunt splenic injury in adults: multi-institutional study of the Eastern Association for the Surgery of Trauma, *J Trauma* 49:177, 2000.

Savage SA, Zarzaur BL, Magnotti LJ, et al: The evolution of blunt splenic injury: resolution and progression, *J Trauma* 64:1085, 2008.

Zarzaur BL, Vashi S, Magnotti LJ, et al: The real risk of splenectomy after discharge home following nonoperative management of blunt splenic injury, *J Trauma* 66:1531, 2009.

RETROPERITONEAL INJURIES: KIDNEY AND URETER

Douglas J.E. Schuerer, MD, and Steven B. Brandes, MD

OVERVIEW

Trauma to the kidneys occurs in 1% to 5% of all trauma injuries, with no predisposition for either side. Across all trauma centers, the proportion of blunt to penetrating injuries is 80% to 20%, although penetrating injuries may be more common in urban trauma centers. Blunt trauma includes falls from heights, motor vehicle and motorcycle crashes, bicycle crashes, and direct blows to the renal area. Children younger than 16 years are more prone to renal injury because they have relatively large kidneys, less perirenal fat, an underdeveloped Gerota fascia, and incomplete ossification of the lower ribs.

Penetrating injuries result from stab wounds and gunshot wounds to the upper abdomen. Kidneys are injured in approximately 10% of all abdominal penetrating injuries. More than 77% of patients with penetrating renal injuries have associated abdominal injuries. Recent validation of the American Association for the Surgery of Trauma (AAST) injury scores for the kidney revealed that the majority (78% to 82%) are grades I and II, and only about 3% to 5% of those injuries will require operative intervention. The remainder are grades III through V, which will require operation 15% to 69% of the time, yielding an organ-specific operative rate of 11%. As renal injuries occur frequently in conjunction with other abdominal injuries, exploration of another organ may require intervention on a kidney that otherwise would not have required operation. Radiographic staging of

TABLE 1: American Association for the Surgery of Trauma: Injury scale for the kidney

Grade*	Type	Description
I	Contusion	Microscopic or gross hematuria, urologic studies normal
	Hematoma	Subcapsular, nonexpanding, and without parenchymal laceration
II	Hematoma	Nonexpanding perirenal hematoma confirmed to renal retroperitoneum
	Laceration	<1 cm parenchymal depth of renal cortex without urinary extravasation
III	Laceration	<1 cm parenchymal depth of renal cortex without collecting-system rupture or urinary extravasation
IV	Laceration	Parenchymal laceration extending through renal cortex, medulla, and collecting system
	Vascular	Main renal artery or vein injury with contained hemorrhage
V	Laceration	Completely shattered kidney
	Vascular	Avulsion of renal hilum, which devascularizes kidney

*Advance one grade for bilateral injuries up to grade III.
Modified from Moore EE, Shackford SR, Pachter HL, et al: Organ injury scaling: spleen, liver, and kidney, *J Trauma* 29:1664–1666, 1989.

renal injuries is essential to determine which can initially be treated nonoperatively. Table 1 shows the AAST injury scale for the kidney.

INITIAL EVALUATION

Hematuria is a standard marker for renal injury, although bladder or ureter injury may also have this presentation. Unfortunately, the degree of hematuria is not an indicator for extent of disease. Standard testing for microscopic hematuria should be performed in those at risk for renal injury. *Microhematuria* is commonly defined as greater than 5 red blood cells per high power field (RBC/hpf). Hematuria may not occur with injuries to the proximal renal vasculature in up to 50% of cases.

Blunt Trauma

It is important to obtain a thorough history that includes the mechanism of injury; this should include the speed of the car or the height of the fall to better determine whether deceleration injury is a component of the injury pattern. Also, the history should determine whether any direct blows occurred to the flank that could contribute to renal injury, especially from objects such as bike handles. If deceleration injury is suspected, this warrants evaluation for renal pelvis and ureteropelvic junction injury (UPJ).

All patients with severe trauma to the flank, abdomen, or lower chest warrant investigation for renal injury, regardless of the presence or absence of hematuria. Indicators of renal injury on physical exam include flank ecchymoses, lower rib fractures, and transverse process fractures. Minor trauma can also create significant injury in the congenitally abnormal kidney.

Penetrating Trauma

Information about the type of firearm may help with determination of injury extent, but this information is often unreliable. As with all penetrating injuries, all wounds should be identified with radiopaque markers to help with imaging. High-velocity bullet wounds cause blast effect and often will develop delayed tissue necrosis. Low-velocity missiles cause less damage and are not as devastating, unless they penetrate the renal hilum or collecting system.

The location of a stab wound is important when evaluating for injury. Any abdominal stab wound anterior to the anterior axillary line that causes renal injury is typically associated with concomitant abdominal injuries. Injuries posterior to the anterior axillary line are less likely to have other associated injuries except for the ascending and descending colon. Anterior stab wounds between the nipples injure abdominal contents 30% of the time; in patients with a concomitant renal injury, the likelihood of associated injuries is high, and exploration is likely necessary. It is helpful to note the size of the blade and the size of the patient to understand the depth of the injury.

Hemodynamically Stable Patients

Indications for Renal Imaging

1. *Blunt trauma and gross hematuria.* Hematuria is the hallmark of renal or bladder injury, but it does not predict the extent or location of the injury.
2. *Blunt trauma, microscopic hematuria, and shock.* Microscopic hematuria is greater than 5 RBC/hpf, and *shock* is defined as a systolic blood pressure of less than 90 mm Hg on arrival to the hospital or during transport.
3. *Major acceleration or deceleration injury.* This may be a fall from height, a high-speed motor vehicle crash, or a pedestrian–motor vehicle accident.
4. *Any hematuria after penetrating injury.* Specific concern is for flank, back, or abdominal trauma, or when the bullet path may be in line with the kidney.
5. *Pediatric trauma (younger than 16 years) with any degree of significant hematuria.*
6. *Associated injuries and physical signs.* Injuries such as flank ecchymosis or tenderness, lumbar spine fractures, or lower rib fractures may suggest underlying renal injury.

Imaging Studies

Computed Tomography

Computed tomography (CT) is the imaging study of choice for evaluating the stable abdominal trauma patient, and it is the gold standard for identifying kidney contusions, parenchymal infarcts, parenchymal lacerations, urinary extravasation from renal pelvis injuries, size and location of retroperitoneal injuries, and any associated injuries. The arteriographic phase of CT accurately identifies renal hilum arterial or venous injuries, including great vessel injuries. Any "blush," or extravascular contrast extravasation, seen around the renal vessels suggests an arterial injury that will require an intervention, whether open or endovascular.

Renal vein injuries are identified by a hematoma medial to the kidney that displaces the renal vasculature but does not contain a blush. Renal artery occlusion resulting from dissection, thrombosis, or renal infarcts is noted by lack of parenchymal enhancement or by a persistent *cortical rim sign.* Unfortunately, the classical rim sign is not usually seen until 8 hours after injury. As scanning rates increase, accurate imaging of the kidney must include arterial images with nephrogenic enhancement, as well as delayed images 2 to 10 minutes after, to identify collecting-system injuries.

Medial extravasation of contrast suggests UPJ injury, whereas lack of contrast distal to the UPJ suggests avulsion injury. Detection of injury continues to improve with increasing scanner capability and resolution.

Ultrasound

Ultrasound (US) is a safe, effective, and rapid tool for noninvasive imaging of the abdomen. The *focused assessment by sonography for trauma* (FAST) is well proven to identify occult blood in the abdomen, which is especially useful in the unstable patient. With renal injuries, though, the blood or urine is often contained in the Gerota fascia, so abdominal free fluid is not seen up to half of the time. US is further limited by obesity, subcutaneous air, and previous abdominal operations; it also cannot differentiate between urine leak and hematoma. Formal US of the kidneys may provide more clarity, but such examinations require more training and are usually not available acutely in the trauma resuscitation area. Although US is an effective tool for those with abdominal trauma and instability, it is not an effective tool for renal imaging.

Intravenous Urography

CT scanning, where available, has replaced intravenous urography (IVU) for imaging of the kidney in the acute setting. However, when a urogram is obtained, it is most useful to identify a nonenhancing kidney and the presence of a kidney contralateral to the site of injury. An IVU may identify an obscured renal outline, loss of the ipsilateral psoas margin, or displacement of the bowel or ureter suggestive of perirenal hematoma. It is often difficult to obtain a well-timed IVU in the trauma patient, as hypoperfusion is common in this population. Any abnormality found on IVU should be followed by further imaging or exploration.

Arteriography

Arteriography is used less in the initial evaluation of renal trauma, as CT angiography has largely replaced it for diagnostic use. However, arteriography with coil embolization has proven valuable in the treatment of arterial extravasation and arteriovenous fistulas. Endoluminal stent placement has also become an effective tool in managing renal artery tears or intimal flap injuries.

Hemodynamically Unstable Patients

The unstable trauma patient likely needs no further renal imaging prior to proceeding to laparotomy. Often the instability is due to associated injuries, but it may be secondary to renal injury. Although a one-shot IVU has been advocated in the past to evaluate the function of the noninjured kidney, the evidence now shows that such a study often adds little additional information and delays definitive treatment. An effective method to evaluate for the presence of a functioning contralateral kidney is to palpate the contralateral retroperitoneal space for a kidney of normal size and caliber. Another method to use is to loop and occlude the ipsilateral ureter of the injured kidney and then give indigo carmine intravenously. The presence of blue urine then identifies a functioning contralateral kidney.

Injury Scaling

The AAST has classified five grades of traumatic renal injuries, ranging from the least to the most severe (see Table 1). Grade I and II injuries are considered minor and are most often managed nonoperatively, unless the patient proceeds to laparotomy for another indication. Grade III injuries are those with deep parenchymal lacerations that do not involve the collecting system. Grade IV injuries comprise

deep parenchymal lacerations, urinary extravasation, or confined renal arterial and venous injuries. Grade V injuries are life threatening—the result of a totally shattered kidney or complete avulsion of the renal hilum.

Indications for Renal Exploration

The vast majority of renal injuries can be managed nonoperatively; this is due to the fact that most injuries are blunt, and there is little or no disruption of the Gerota fascia, which keeps most hematomas contained to the retroperitoneum. Injuries not confined to the retroperitoneum, those decompressed into the abdomen, typically require operation. Penetrating injuries more frequently disrupt the retroperitoneum; because of this, 75% of gunshot wounds and 50% of stab wounds require exploration, but less than 2% of blunt injuries do.

Absolute Indications

Persistent and life-threatening renal bleeding is an indication for renal exploration. Often this decision is made after celiotomy for another associated injury. Signs of continued renal bleeding are the presence of a pulsatile, expanding, or uncontained retroperitoneal hematoma, which should be explored. Stable and contained hematomas can be observed, as long as proper preoperative radiologic studies document a renal injury that can be observed safely. By definition grade V injuries require exploration, unless the kidney is already felt to be lost, and no instability or bleeding from the kidney is observed. Penetrating injuries with an opening to the abdomen typically require exploration, because the containment by Gerota fascia has been disrupted.

Relative Indications

Devitalized Parenchyma

A major devitalized renal segment greater than 50% is a relative indication for exploration, especially when associated with other injuries. With associated colon or pancreas injuries, urinary extravasation, or a large retroperitoneal hematoma, the subsequent abscess rate is higher for a large devitalized segment; thus the threshold for renal exploration should be lower.

Urinary Extravasation

Urinary extravasation will resolve spontaneously more than 75% of the time. If extravasation worsens, or if a urinoma develops, this can often be managed by percutaneous drainage or by placing a ureteral stent endoscopically. UPJ avulsion injuries usually require prompt surgical repair, although they may be temporized with percutaneous nephrostomy and a delayed, staged repair. Delayed imaging is vital in blunt trauma victims to visualize contrast extravasation presence and location to prevent understaging of grade IV injuries. Contrast noted distal to the UPJ in the ureter rules out complete avulsion.

Arterial Thrombosis

Renal artery occlusion usually occurs from a major deceleration injury in which the main renal artery is stretched, the less elastic intima is torn, the vessels thrombose, and the kidney infarcts. Renal salvage is remote after 6 hours of ischemia. If the contralateral kidney is normal, and if the diagnosis is prompt, it is controversial to attempt revascularization, because chances are poor that any significant renal function can be preserved. In only 20% to 56% of such cases is more than 17% of differential function preserved. In such circumstances, it has not been our practice to attempt revascularization or exploration. We typically leave the devascularized kidney in situ, because it rarely leads to late complications and usually just involutes. Blood pressure should be periodically monitored, however, for rare, persistent, renally induced hypertension. Revascularization should be reserved for bilateral renal artery occlusion or unilateral occlusion in a solitary kidney, regardless of the ischemic time. More recently, success has been reported in patients with intimal flaps using endoluminal techniques and stent placement.

Penetrating Renal Injuries

Theoretically, grade for grade, renal injuries should be managed the same, regardless of mechanism. This is particularly true for penetrating AAST grade I and II renal injuries, which can be managed conservatively. Penetrating AAST grade III and IV renal injuries are typically managed surgically because of the high rate of delayed bleeds (24%) and the necessity to explore for associated abdominal injuries. Also, the penetrating wound disrupts the Gerota fascia significantly. If the injury is isolated, however, and no major intraabdominal structure has been injured, it is safe to manage these injuries nonoperatively. Percutaneous, endoscopic, and endoluminal techniques may be necessary to control complications of these injuries. Stab wounds to the kidney posterior to the posterior axillary line are less likely to have visceral injuries and thus are more likely to undergo successful conservative management. The conservatively managed penetrating trauma patient must undergo frequent serial abdominal examinations, particularly for the first 24 hours. Any changes to the physical examination, including new tenderness or abdominal guarding, warrant abdominal exploration.

Incomplete Staging

Complete staging of the renal injury by appropriate imaging studies permits the selection of nonoperative management. Incomplete staging demands either further imaging or renal exploration.

SURGICAL MANAGEMENT

Retroperitoneal Exploration

The injured kidney is best exposed through a standard trauma laparotomy midline incision from the xiphoid process to the symphysis pubis. In the stable trauma patient, associated intraabdominal injuries should be systematically examined and repaired before the kidney injury is exposed. However, when renal bleeding is massive or persistent, as it is in renal hilar injury, the kidney should be explored first.

The location of the retroperitoneal hematoma often dictates the operative approach. Retroperitoneal hematomas are identified by their location (Figure 1). Zone I midline hematomas demand exploration. Zone II or lateral perinephric hematomas should be selectively explored in penetrating injury, but the threshold should be low when retroperitoneum is disrupted. Zone II hematomas in blunt injury are typically observed.

In the stable patient with a zone I injury, the approach is a medial visceral rotation of either the left or right colon, depending on the location of the hematoma. If more centered over the aorta, a Mattox maneuver should be performed, and the left colon and spleen should be mobilized to expose the left kidney and aorta. This provides access to the anterior and posterior kidney if required. Conversely, if the hematoma seems to be more over the inferior vena cava (IVC), the right colon should be mobilized with a Catell maneuver, and a Kocher maneuver should be performed to mobilize the duodenum. This provides access to the right kidney and the IVC. It is helpful to also obtain supraceliac aortic access to have proximal control, if a proximal renal arterial injury is found. Zone I injuries may also include an aortic injury, which is often devastating. In some conditions, especially with a high-velocity missile injury, the initial exploration of the injury may be through the missile tract.

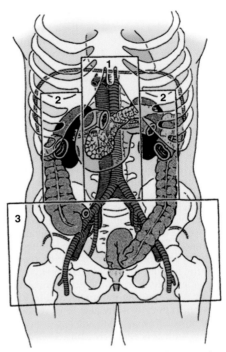

FIGURE 1   The retroperitoneal zones. Zone I is central; zone II is lateral; zone III is the pelvis. *(From Kudsk KA, Sheldon GF: Retroperitoneal trauma. In Blaisdell FW, Trunkey DD [eds]: Trauma management—abdominal trauma, New York, 1982, Thieme Medical Publishers, p 281.)*

BOX 1: Methods for managing massive retroperitoneal bleeding

1. Manually compress the aorta at the hiatus, potentially using a T bar.
2. Scoop and sponge blood from the peritoneal cavity.
3. Locate and manually compress sources of uncontained hemorrhage.
4. Resuscitate the patient with manual control in place.
5. Obtain proximal vascular control of the aorta or proximal renal artery if feasible.
6. Open the Gerota fascia and deliver the kidney.
7. Ensure control of the bleeding with manual compression or a renal hilar clamp.
8. Prove the function of the opposite kidney.
9. Repair or resect the damaged structures.

Exsanguinating Retroperitoneal Injuries

Two conditions are generally required for exsanguination from a retroperitoneal wound: 1) a full-thickness injury of a significant blood vessel, usually an artery or major vein; and 2) failed spontaneous containment or tamponade of the bleeding. As previously mentioned, this occurs most frequently in penetrating injury, particularly with high-velocity gunshot wounds or the most extreme blunt traumas. Clinical scenarios in which exsanguination from a renal artery or renal injury is present will also have patterns and mechanisms likely to be associated with hemorrhage from other vessels and viscera.

Because of these general facts, uncontained renal artery or hilar injuries are the most dangerous wounds that can involve the kidney and the proximal collecting system. Immediate manual control of hemorrhage and vigorous resuscitation are the keys to saving the life of the exsanguinating patient (Box 1). All maneuvers to get clamps on vessels and to expose renal or other injuries for resection or repair should be deferred until the patient has been properly resuscitated. After anesthesia has caught up with resuscitation, time can be taken to place a clamp on the proximal aorta if necessary and to perform further mobilization.

Much debate surrounds the next stage of control. Prior to renal exploration and opening of the Gerota fascia, some have mandated obtaining renal artery and venous control proximal to the site of injury. They argue that proximal and primary vascular control avoids a potentially massive bleed from release of the tamponade effect of the Gerota fascia. More recent evidence suggests that approaching the kidney and mobilizing it from the Gerota fascia laterally before proximal control yields equivalent blood loss and renal salvage rates. We use both methods of control, depending on the injury site. Most commonly, persistent parenchymal kidney bleeding can be controlled with manual compression and, if need be, a Satinsky clamp can be placed on the renal hilum. The more aggressive the bleeding, the more likely we are to approach the kidney laterally first.

In either scenario, a lateral approach to the kidney involves mobilizing either the left or right colon medially and exposing the Gerota fascia and the retroperitoneal kidney. When opening the fascia, it is essential to open laterally to avoid accidently dissecting the kidney subcapsularly, to avoid injuring the ureter, and to leave behind the perinephric fat. The capsule is essential in renal reconstruction as the strength layer that will prevent repair stitches from pulling through. Prior to opening the fascia, the perinephric hematoma often performs the dissection in the appropriate pericapsular plane, freeing the kidney from its perinephric fat. After opening the fascia, the kidney can often be easily mobilized medially and anteriorly. The kidney can then be manually compressed, and a clamp can be placed around the hilum at this point. Care must be taken not to further damage the kidney so as to make it unsalvageable, although higher grade injuries often require nephrectomy after function of the opposite kidney has been proven. In the unstable patient, a damage-control nephrectomy is often warranted, as any attempt at salvage risks further blood loss and development of the fatal triad of coagulopathy, hypothermia, and acidosis.

Renovascular Injuries

Injuries to the renal hilar vessels are less common and more challenging than most literature would suggest. A penetrating injury to the right renal hilum often has associated injuries to the pancreaticoduodenal complex, the right renal artery, the right renal vein, and the IVC. The right renal vein is short, and injury to it is equivalent to an IVC side hole. On the left, if the injury is proximal to the gonadal and adrenal branches, the renal vein can be ligated, unlike the uncollateralized right renal vein. If the patient is stable, we intermittently perfuse the kidney with iced, heparinized saline when repairing an injured renal artery, and we perform the simplest repair possible to limit ischemic time. Grafts are infrequently used, but polytetrafluoroethylene can be used to speed up the repair, if no bowel spillage is present and the artery is replanted to the aorta.

Stable Retroperitoneal Injuries

For the stable trauma patient without an exsanguinating bleed, there is more opportunity for obtaining proximal control. As with exsanguinating bleeds, debate still exists on when to obtain proximal renal vascular control, which can be time consuming, especially for the surgeon who encounters this infrequently. Although some literature has suggested improved renal salvage rates, more recent data have differed. If the bleeding is obviously from the lateral kidney, proximal control is likely not necessary, as parenchymal bleeding can be controlled with manual compression after mobilizing the kidney from the Gerota fascia.

If proximal control is to be obtained in those with a zone I inframesocolic retroperitoneal hematoma, the classic description of

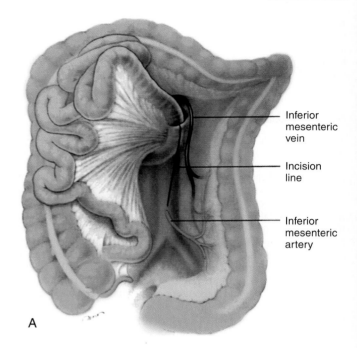

Inferior mesenteric vein

Incision line

Inferior mesenteric artery

A

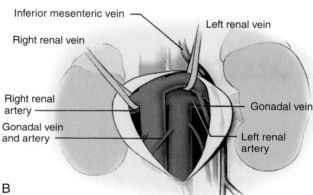

Inferior mesenteric vein — — Left renal vein

Right renal vein

Right renal artery

Gonadal vein and artery

Gonadal vein

Left renal artery

B

FIGURE 2 Technique of exposure of renal vessels. **A,** Exposure of the root of the mesentery to visualize the aorta. **B,** Relationship of the renal veins and arteries after incision of the posterior peritoneum over the aorta. *(From McAninch JW: Surgery for renal trauma. In Novick AC, Streem SB, Pontes JE [eds]: Stewart's operative urology, Baltimore, 1989, Williams & Wilkins.)*

proximal vascular control requires displacing the small bowel along the root of the mesentery to the right and laterally. The important anatomic landmarks are the inferior mesenteric vein (Figure 2) and the ligament of Treitz. Begin by taking down the ligament of Treitz, reflect the fourth portion of the duodenum laterally, and then dissect between these two structures onto the infrarenal aorta. Regardless of the size of the hematoma, the inferior mesenteric vein is a constant landmark, and the aorta can at least be palpated. Dissect up along the aorta, until the left renal vein is identified crossing the aorta. Note that in less than 5% of patients, the renal vein will run retroaortic, so this important landmark will be missing. Gentle traction on the left renal vein with a vein retractor will permit access to the left renal artery, which is slightly cephalad to the vein and coming off the lateral aspect of the aorta.

The right renal artery is more difficult to identify. With cephalad retraction of the left renal vein and interaortocaval dissection, the right renal artery can be identified and controlled. The origin of the right renal artery is slightly cephalad to the left renal artery, which can make it particularly time consuming to control. If the inframesocolic hematoma extends cephalad and totally obscures the ligament of Treitz, instead of obtaining vascular control at the level of the superior mesenteric vein, it is safe to obtain supraceliac control through the lesser omentum above the stomach, either by manually compressing the aorta against the spine or by clamping through the crus of the diaphragm.

Renal Reconstruction

In the absence of persistent hemodynamic instability or coagulopathy, kidney reconstruction is safe and effective. The method of kidney reconstruction is dictated by the degree and location of the injury and not by the associated intraabdominal and extraabdominal injuries. Even a concomitant pancreatic or colonic injury with frank fecal contamination is not an absolute contraindication to renal reconstruction. However, the resulting complication rates are slightly increased.

Reconstruction Principles for Renal Injuries

1. Broad exposure of the kidney and injured area
2. Temporary vascular occlusion for brisk renal bleeding, when bleeding is not well controlled by manual compression of the parenchyma
3. Sharp excision of all nonviable parenchyma
4. Meticulous hemostasis
5. Watertight closure of the collecting system
6. Parenchymal defect closure by approximation of the capsular edges over a hemostatic dissolvable bolster, such as Surgicel (Ethicon, Somerville, NJ), or coverage with omentum, perinephric fat, or peritoneum; wrapping with polyglycolic acid mesh to help with hemostasis of a shattered kidney (Figure 3)
7. Interposition of an omental pedicle flap among associated vascular, colonic, or pancreatic injuries and the injured kidney (Figure 4)
8. Ureteral stent placement for a renal pelvis or ureteral injury
9. Retroperitoneal drain

DAMAGE CONTROL

Damage-control surgery is now a mainstay in the care of the trauma patient. Once exsanguinating hemorrhage is controlled and bowel contamination is limited, it may be feasible to leave a nonexpanding and contained zone II retroperitoneal injury alone. If there is active oozing from the Gerota fascia, the area can be packed with laparotomy pads and left for future exploration. At times, the kidney bleeding may even be addressed by angiography after the patient has been resuscitated. If the kidney is massively injured, and the patient unstable, a quick damage control nephrectomy can be lifesaving.

NONOPERATIVE CONSERVATIVE MANAGEMENT

Nonoperative management of renal injuries is safe and effective and has increased as surgeons have incorporated nonoperative management of spleen and liver injuries. Properly staged and selected renal injuries can be conservatively managed, and strict bed rest has been suggested until the urine visibly clears. However, recent evidence suggests that bed rest can be avoided unless bleeding (hematuria) appreciably increases or resumes after ambulation. Patients should be monitored in an environment suitable for close hemodynamic monitoring, and serial hematocrit or hemoglobin levels should also be followed, more frequently for higher grade injuries with significant

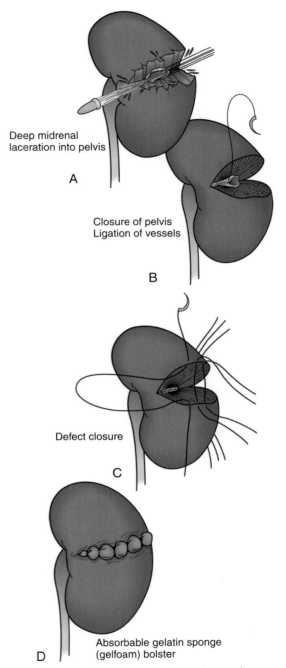

Deep midrenal laceration into pelvis

A

Closure of pelvis Ligation of vessels

B

Defect closure

C

D   Absorbable gelatin sponge (gelfoam) bolster

FIGURE 3   Suture repair of the renal pelvis and parenchyma over bolsters. *(From Armenakas NA, McAninch JW: Genitourinary tract. In Ivatury RR, Cayten CG [eds]: The textbook of penetrating trauma, Media, PA, 1996, Williams & Wilkins.)*

hematuria. Transfusions can be given as needed, but intervention may be required if serial transfusions are required. Routine antibiotic prophylaxis is not required.

As described before, the confined space of the Gerota fascia can tamponade and limit bleeding. Transfusion requirements of more than 6 units or hemodynamic changes demand repeat imaging and possible arteriography and embolization or surgical reexploration. Aggressive evaluation of any CT blush in the kidney should be performed in those patients not requiring laparotomy by angiography, and selective embolization should be used as needed.

FIGURE 4 Partial nephrectomy with omental patch. *(From Armenakas NA, McAninch JW: Genitourinary tract. In Ivatury RR, Cayten CG [eds]: The textbook of penetrating trauma, Media, PA, 1996, Williams & Wilkins.)*

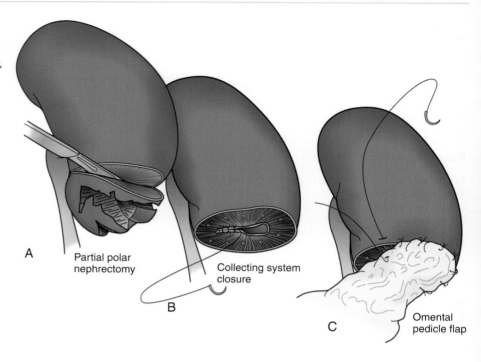

A Partial polar nephrectomy

B Collecting system closure

C Omental pedicle flap

Conservative measures are becoming more common in the care of renal injury, and they may improve renal salvage for higher grade injuries. For grade IV and V injuries, the kidney should be reimaged 3 to 5 days after the initial injury; this should be done by CT scan, with intravenous contrast to assess for persistent urinary leakage. Worsening or unimproved leaks warrant ureteral stent placement and possible urinoma drain placement. If the ureter cannot be stented from below, percutaneous nephrostomy and eventual antegrade stents can be employed.

COMPLICATIONS AFTER RENAL TRAUMA

Complications are dependent on the grade of the initial renal injury and the method of management. They usually occur within 1 month of injury.

Early Complications

Prolonged urinary extravasation is the most common complication after renal trauma. Urinomas occur in less than 1% of renal trauma cases. Small, uninfected, and stable collections do not require intervention. Large collections greater than 4 cm are prone to abscess formation and sepsis and should be managed by percutaneous catheter drainage. Other potential complications include shock from massive blood loss, renal infarction, and abscess formation, usually within 2 weeks of injury.

Late Complications

Other complications include delayed bleeding, arterial pseudoaneurysm, abscess, urinary fistula, and hydronephrosis. Most complications are limited and can be treated by minimally invasive means. For higher grade renal injuries, a follow-up CT should be obtained 3 to 6 months after injury to evaluate for delayed hydronephrosis, vascular compromise, or renal atrophy.

Hypertension

Vascular hypertension after renal trauma is usually transient. It can be secondary to a small amount of residual renal blood flow, possibly from an intimal flap in a renal artery. Sustained or delayed hypertension is renin mediated and relatively rare. Perinephric hematomas are not associated with hypertension, in contrast to subcapsular hematomas, which can compress renal parenchyma and result in a Page kidney. The resulting hypertension is usually controlled medically, and blood pressure monitoring should be routinely performed for several months after injury.

Hydronephrosis

Perinephric fibrosis that involves the UPJ is usually seen after a lower-pole kidney injury, and it can result in hydronephrosis. To prevent such occurrences, interposition of vascularized tissue (omentum or perinephric fat) between the injured kidney and the ureter is effective.

URETERAL AND RENAL PELVIS INJURIES

Mechanisms of Injury

External Trauma

Penetrating injuries to the ureter are rare, as only 2.5% of abdominal gunshot wounds involve the ureter. Blunt injuries are even more infrequent; thus 95% of ureteral injuries are from penetrating injuries, and 5% are from blunt injury as a result of severe acceleration and deceleration injuries. Even if a projectile missile does not directly injure the ureter, any proximity to the tumbling bullet can cause severe blast injury, sometimes resulting in severe ureteral contusion and delayed necrosis of the tissue fragments. High-velocity projectiles are more likely to cause blast injury. The rare blunt injury from extreme deceleration occurs at points of fixation, namely the UPJ and hilar vasculature. Another mechanism for blunt injury is hyperextension of the back, where stretching by the lumbar and lower thoracic vertebral bodies avulses the ureter. This most often occurs in motor vehicle accidents involving children, because children are limber.

Iatrogenic Trauma

Intraoperative iatrogenic ureteral injuries occur during difficult or bloody pelvic operations, particularly in reoperative surgery. The ureter is only injured in approximately 0.5% to 1% of pelvic operations. The most common surgeries in which ureteral injuries occur are urologic surgeries (ureteroscopy, vesicourethral suspension, radical prostatectomy); gynecologic surgery (transabdominal hysterectomy, salpingooophorectomy, cystocele repair); colorectal surgeries, such as abdominal perineal resection; and vascular surgery, including aortic and iliac graft surgery.

Of all surgeries, iatrogenic ureteral injury most commonly occurs during transabdominal hysterectomy. Sites of common ureter injury are at the uterine vessels and the cardinal and uterosacral ligaments. During reoperative surgery, preoperative ureteral stents are often employed. Data show that such stents do not decrease the incidence of ureteral injury, but they are effective in identifying injuries that do occur.

Diagnosis of Ureteral Injury

Successful surgical management of collecting-system injuries requires a high index of suspicion, early diagnosis, a low threshold for urinary tract imaging, and an intimate knowledge of ureteral anatomy and blood supply.

Preoperative Diagnosis

Neither gross nor microscopic hematuria is a reliable sign of ureter injury, as these are absent in up to 43% of penetrating ureteral injuries and 67% of blunt injuries. Without hematuria, a high index of suspicion and knowledge of missile trajectory are required to reliably diagnose ureter injures.

Intraoperative Diagnosis

Most penetrating ureteral injuries are diagnosed intraoperatively. Direct exploration is the most accurate method for diagnosis, but this may be difficult because of overlying hematoma. The surgeon must be careful not to devascularize the ureter during exploration. Ureteral peristalsis is not a reliable indication of viability or of adequate vascularity; the most reliable way to assess viability is by incision and monitoring for a bleeding edge. Intravenous indigo carmine is also helpful in identifying ureteral injury by searching for extravasation of blue dye from the injury site. Cystotomy and retrograde injection of indigo carmine by pediatric feeding tube is another method of testing ureteral integrity.

Missed Ureteral Injury Diagnosis

Delayed presentation of unrecognized ureteral injuries is a potentially lethal and morbid complication. Clinical signs of a missed injury may be delayed for several days after the injury and may include prolonged ileus, persistent flank or abdominal pain, palpable abdominal mass, prolonged drainage from drain sites, urinary obstruction, abscess, and sepsis. Laboratory values indicative of a urine leak are elevated blood urea nitrogen, elevated serum creatinine, elevated serum potassium, and a systemic metabolic acidosis.

Imaging

Intravenous Urography

Until recently, IVU was the primary imaging study used to evaluate ureteral integrity. However, CT urography has replaced IVU in most centers. Furthermore, IVU accuracy in diagnosing a ureteral injury is variable and unreliable. Findings on IVU that are suggestive of ureteral injury are incomplete visualization of the entire ureter, ureteral deviation or dilatation, urinary extravasation, and hydronephrosis. One-shot IVU has little utility in identifying ureteral injuries.

Computed Tomography

Contemporary evaluation of ureteral trauma frequently uses CT urography with delayed cuts, especially with the newer generations of scanners with high resolution. Medial perirenal extravasation of contrast is the most common finding of renal ureteropelvic injury and is often accompanied by no filling of the ipsilateral ureter. Lacerations of the UPJ also produce medial contrast extravasation; however, contrast is seen in the ipsilateral ureter distal to the UPJ. Hematomas around the ureter can also be identified with modern CT imaging, and the presence of a hematoma should result in increased scrutiny for possible ureter injury or delayed ureteral leak. When concerned for collecting-system injury, the rapid scan time of spiral CT imaging demands that imaging be delayed several minutes to ensure opacification of the entire ureter tract. Hypotension or significant renal injury may delay contrast excretion and decrease the sensitivity for detecting ureteral injury.

Retrograde Pyelography

Although accurate in demonstrating the site, presence, and location of extravasation, retrograde pyelography is time consuming and cumbersome. Thus it has almost no role in the acute trauma setting.

Percutaneous Nephrostomy

Percutaneous access to the renal pelvis is an invasive procedure often done by radiology interventionalists. After access, antegrade imaging can be performed to evaluate for renal pelvis and ureteral injury. At that point, treatment maneuvers such as antegrade stent placement can also be performed if necessary.

Classification of Ureteral Injury

Ureteral injuries are typically classified by location of the ureteral injury as well as the mechanism and manner of the injury, such as by avulsion, contusion, transection, devascularization, crush, ligation, resection, or fulguration. Table 2 shows the AAST injury scale for the ureter.

TABLE 2: American Association for the Surgery of Trauma injury scale for the ureter

Grade*	Type	Description
I	Hematoma	Contusion or hematoma without devascularization
II	Laceration	Transection <50%
III	Laceration	Transection <50%
IV	Laceration	Complete transection with <2 cm of devascularization
V	Laceration	Avulsion with >2 cm of devascularization

*Advance one grade for bilateral up to grade III.
Modified from Moore EE, Shackford SR, Pachter HL, et al: Organ injury scaling: spleen, liver, and kidney, *J Trauma* 29:1664–1668, 1989.

Associated Injuries

Patients with penetrating ureteral injuries also have associated multiorgan system injuries. More than 90% of such injuries are seen with concomitant injuries of the bowel, iliac vessels, liver, aorta, and vena cava. Patients with blunt ureteral trauma also commonly suffer from associated injuries due to the force required to create a ureteral injury.

Management of Ureteral Injuries

General considerations before ureteral repair are the patient's overall physical condition, presence of associated injuries, any delay in diagnosis, and the level and extent of ureteral injury. Promptly diagnosed ureteral injuries should be explored and reconstructed through a midline incision. Lack of bleeding from the cut edge suggests ischemia and warrants debridement until viable tissue is reached.

When a ureteral contusion is found, the minimal intervention should be ureteral stent and a retroperitoneal drain in the area of the contusion. If the contusion is severe, the ureter should be segmentally resected, debrided, and reanastomosed over a stent. In major crush injuries, which are usually iatrogenic, the affected segment should be excised, and formal reconstruction should be performed, depending on the location of the injury. Minor crush injuries require a stent to be placed either endoscopically or through a cystotomy.

The surgical principles for successful ureteral repair include 1) careful ureteral mobilization and preservation of the adventitia; 2) debridement of nonviable tissue to a bleeding edge; 3) mucosa-to-mucosa, spatulated, tension-free, and watertight anastomosis; 4) ureteral stenting or urinary diversion; 5) isolation of repair from associated injuries with vascularized tissue; and 6) placement of a retroperitoneal drain.

Ureteral Injuries Below the Iliac Vessels

Ureteroneocystostomy

For low injuries without significant ureteral loss after debridement, a simple refluxing ureteral reimplantation into the fixed area of the bladder (floor/trigone), rather than the mobile dome area, is preferred. A tunneled nonrefluxing reimplant is generally unnecessary and increases the chances for ureteral stenosis. Stents should be placed for 4 to 6 weeks.

Psoas Hitch

In lower injuries with greater distal ureter loss, the gap can be bridged by "hitching" (suturing) the apex of the bladder to the ipsilateral psoas minor tendon (Figure 5). The contralateral superior vesicle pedicle is often divided to improve bladder mobilization, and care is taken not to injure or entrap the genitofemoral nerve. The ureter is then reimplanted over a ureteral stent, and a Foley catheter or suprapubic tube is placed. The psoas hitch is relatively quick to perform but is only appropriate in the stable acute trauma patient. If the patient is unstable, the procedure should be delayed until the planned and staged repair, when the patient is fully resuscitated.

Transureteroureterostomy

Transureteroureterostomy (TUU) is rarely if ever needed in the acute trauma setting. As an alternative, the ureter can be treated in a damage-control approach by temporarily diverting the urine over a ureteral stent to the abdominal wall, with planned definitive reconstruction in a staged fashion, typically done by a urologist. TUU seems particularly useful when there are associated rectal, major pelvic vascular, or extensive bladder injuries. Relative contraindications to TUU are a history of urothelial cancer, genitourinary tuberculosis, nephrolithiasis, pelvic irradiation or infection, retroperitoneal fibrosis, or chronic pyelonephritis.

Midureteral and Upper Ureteral Injuries

Ureteroureterostomy

The majority of midureter complete transections, regardless of mechanism, can be repaired by primary ureteroureterostomy. Both ureteral segments are spatulated, and a watertight, tension-free anastomosis is performed over a double-J ureteral stent (Figure 6). Injuries to the upper third of the ureter are best repaired by primary ureteroureterostomy.

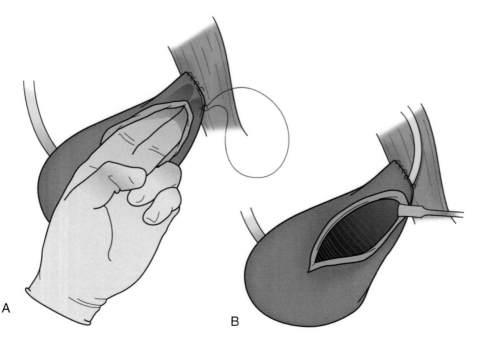

FIGURE 5 Psoas hitch provides additional length for low uretal injuries for creation of a tension-free reimplantation of the ureter. (*From NE Peterson: Genitourinary trauma. In Feliciano DV, Moore EE, Mattox KL [eds]: Trauma, ed 3, Stamford, CT, 1996, Appleton & Lange.*)

A

B

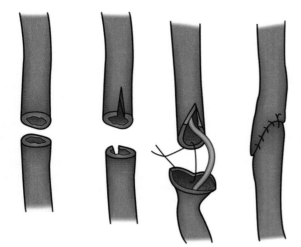

FIGURE 6   Ureteroureterostomy requires debridement, spatulation, stenting, and anastomosis with absorbable interrupted sutures. *(From NE Peterson: Genitourinary trauma. In Feliciano DV, Moore EE, Mattox KL [eds]: Trauma, ed 3, Stamford, CT, 1996, Appleton & Lange.)*

Ureteropelvic Junction Injuries

UPJ injuries are usually avulsions after blunt trauma. Avulsion of the UPJ is the most common blunt ureteral injury, and it occurs primarily in children younger than 16 years. Complete UPJ avulsion will not resolve spontaneously; it requires primary surgical repair, ureteral stenting, and a retroperitoneal drain. Incomplete UPJ lacerations can often be managed expectantly.

Large Ureteral Loss

The loss of large segments of ureter requires aggressive and time-consuming surgical reconstruction that is best performed in a staged fashion and not during an acute, multiorgan surgery for trauma injuries. Ileal interposition, Boari flap, renal displacement, urinary ileal conduit, and autotransplantation are complex procedures that are best performed by urologists in a staged and delayed setting.

The Unstable Patient and Damage Control

When the patient is too unstable, or if the decision is to proceed with an open abdomen for other reasons, a damage-control approach with a temporary cutaneous ureterostomy over a single-J ureteral stent or a pediatric feeding tube should be performed. No extra time should be spent mobilizing the ureter to bring it up to the skin, but rather a tie should be placed around the ureter and stent, and the stent should

be brought out through the skin. Alternatively, as a method of last resort, the ureter can be ligated proximal to the injury, followed by a percutaneous nephrostomy tube when the patient becomes stable. Intraoperative placement of a nephrostomy tube is time consuming and difficult and should not be performed. Definitive reconstruction is delayed until the patient has stabilized from his or her other injuries. Delayed ureteral reconstructions are time consuming and best left to urologists.

Improved minimally invasive techniques are used more frequently in ureteral injuries, especially in damage control. Techniques such as percutaneous nephrostomy followed by antegrade stents, if needed, and endoscopic ureteral stents fitted over thin wires and fluoroscopically placed past the injury can temporize or treat such injuries without further need for laparotomy. Any urine fluid collection or abscess can usually be drained by percutaneous drainage catheter, and any delayed complications from these methods can be treated when the patient has stabilized or recovered from the other acute injuries.

Management of Complications and Delayed Diagnosis

Delayed recognition of ureteral injuries is common, occurring in up to 60% of patients. Significant morbidity that includes sepsis, abscess formation, hydronephrosis, and loss of renal function occurs in up to 50% of such patients. Other complications include ureteral stricture and fistula and urinary extravasation with urinoma formation.

Ureteral injuries diagnosed within 2 weeks of initial trauma that have no significant infection should be explored and repaired, unless the patient otherwise has a hostile abdomen. If iatrogenic ligation of the ureter is found, the suture should be removed, and the ureter should be stented. Injuries that are identified after 2 weeks should undergo proximal urinary diversion by percutaneous nephrostomy tube; percutaneous drainage of any urinoma or abscess; and, when possible, antegrade stent placement across the injured ureter. Definitive ureteral reconstruction is usually delayed for at least 3 months.

SUGGESTED READINGS

Brandes SB, McAninch JW: Reconstructive surgery of the injured urinary tract, *Urol Clin North Am* 26:183, 1999.

Davis KA, Reed LR, Santaniello J, et al: Predictors of the need for nephrectomy after renal trauma, *J Trauma* 60:164, 2006.

Knudson MM, Harrison PB, Hoyt DB, et al: Outcome after major renovascular injuries: a Western Trauma Association multicenter report, *J Trauma* 49:1116, 2000.

Tasian GE, Aaronson DS, McAninch JW: Evaluation of renal function after major renal injury: correlation with the American Association for the Surgery of Trauma injury scale, *J Urol* 183:196, 2010.

Tinkoff G, Esposito TJ, Reed J, et al: American Association for the Surgery of Trauma Organ Injury Scale I: Spleen, Liver, and Kidney, Validation based on the National Trauma Data Bank, *J Am Coll Surg* 207:646, 2008.

DAMAGE CONTROL OPERATION

George C. Velmahos, MD, PhD, and Hasan B. Alam, MD

BASIC PRINCIPLES

The concept of damage control was described in the early 1990s as a method to save patients with severe injuries, accepting that definitive surgical management would not be achieved at the first operation. This was drastically different from previous practice, which usually called for prolonged operations and repair of all injuries at the expense of ongoing bleeding and physiologic deterioration. Damage control has three phases. In the first phase, an abbreviated operation aims to control bleeding and contamination by rapid surgical maneuvers, including packing, vessel ligation, vessel shunting, bowel resection without anastomosis, and open abdomen. In the second phase, the patient is transferred to the ICU for aggressive resuscitation, rewarming, and correction of coagulopathy. The third phase includes return to the operating room to definitively repair the injuries by reconstituting vascular and bowel continuity, completing the resection of injured organs, unpacking, and closing the abdomen. This third phase may require more than one operation.

The principles of damage control have been applied to almost any trauma operation, including laparotomies, thoracotomies, peripheral explorations, and orthopedic procedures. As a concept it has also been used in resuscitation, angiographic embolization, and organization of surgical combat support.

PHYSIOLOGY AND INDICATIONS

Severe injuries requiring operative intervention are almost always associated with the lethal triad of hypothermia, acidosis, and coagulopathy. Each of the three elements fuels the other two, creating a self-perpetuating vicious cycle that leads to death if left unbroken. Hypothermia develops because of a multitude of factors. Lying on the ground at the trauma scene, particularly in cold weather or in wet clothes, being unclothed in the emergency room, having viscera exposed in the operating room, transfusion of cold fluids and blood products, vasoconstriction due to blood loss, and the use of vasopressors all contribute to hypothermia. Acidosis is a result of hypoperfusion caused by all of the above factors, and coagulopathy is a result of hemodilution resulting from the infusion of acellular fluids and aged blood products, consumption of coagulation factors during the inflammatory process, and secretion of fibrinolytic agents.

In an attempt to interrupt the progress of the lethal triad, many authors have set criteria for damage control. Among the various numbers used are a temperature lower than 35° C, a base deficit greater than 14 mmol/L, a systolic blood pressure persistently lower than 80 mm Hg, a pH less than 7.2, and a blood transfusion volume greater than 10 units or an estimated blood loss greater than 4 L (Box 1). The numbers fluctuate according to the individual center's experience. It is probably true that when some of these numbers are recorded, it is already too late. In the elusive quest for the correct balance between performing a lifesaving but imperfect procedure versus a definitive but unnecessarily prolonged operation, experience and team preparedness counts more than absolute numbers.

Damage Control Laparotomy

The abdomen is the most common site for damage control procedures. As mentioned, the principal goal is control of the bleeding. Although four-quadrant packing has prevailed as the first operative maneuver upon opening the abdomen, we believe that random placing of packs does little to control the bleeding or guide the surgeon to the correct site. We favor the rapid evacuation of blood and blood clots, gross identification of the location responsible for the bleeding, and targeted packing of that area. In this way, the laparotomy pads are placed meaningfully, in direct contact with the bleeding site, and on the appropriate vector that ensures adequate compression.

Following this initial move, attention is turned to controlling contamination. Hollow visceral perforations can be temporarily controlled by atraumatic clamps (e.g., Babcock) or rapid suturing with any type of suture material already available on the table.

The third move consists of unpacking the area and assessing the bleeding site. A rapid determination needs to be made about the potential of definitive repair or temporary control, and it is exactly at this point that an early decision must be made about abbreviating the operation based on the extent of the injuries and physiology of the patient. The following organ-specific surgical maneuvers aim to control the damage.

Liver

Large retrohepatic hematomas are best left unexplored if not bleeding dramatically. Uncovering a retrohepatic inferior vena cava or major hepatic vein injury is associated with a mortality of 60% to 90%. There is little reason to risk a fatal outcome by opening the hematoma, if it can be left alone or controlled by packing. Laparotomy pads placed over the liver will effectively compress the hematoma. However, this may result in compression of the inferior vena cava and cessation of venous return to the heart. A couple of pads may be rolled and placed in the undersurface of the liver to prevent it from overexerting pressure on the cava.

Large lacerations, particularly of the posterior segments, are also hard to control. A variety of extraordinary techniques have been described, but simple hepatorrhaphy and packing are adequate for the majority of the cases. Although hepatorrhaphy is not universally accepted for the fear of hepatic necrosis, our experience with it has been very favorable. Deep bites with horizontal mattress sutures, usually with 0-0 chromic catgut on a large blunt-tipped needle, can effectively control bleeding. The sutures must be placed on healthy liver tissue away from the edges of the wound to avoid tearing through the wound and producing more bleeding (Figure 1).

BOX 1: List of proposed indications for damage control, including range of values reported in various articles

1. Core temperature <35° C (34°–35° C)
2. pH <7.2 (7.1–7.3)
3. Base deficit >14 mmol/L
4. Systolic blood pressure persistently <80 mm Hg (70–90 mm Hg)
5. Blood transfusion >10 units
6. Estimated blood loss >4 L
7. Operating room fluid replacement >10 L
8. Associated life-threatening injuries in a second anatomic location
9. Vascular injuries in inaccessible locations
10. Inability to close the abdomen due to visceral edema
11. Clinical evidence of coagulopathy (nonsurgical bleeding)

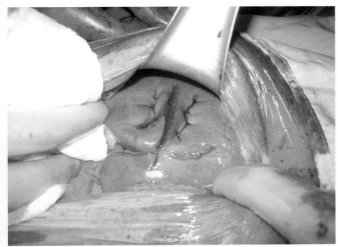

FIGURE 1   A deep laceration of the liver reapproximated with horizontal mattress sutures.

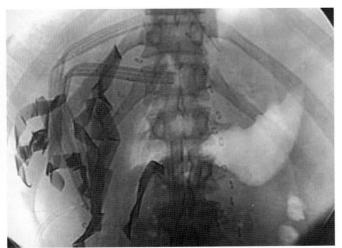

FIGURE 2   Packs placed to concentrically compress the liver. Two drains monitor bleeding in the immediate postoperative period.

It is possible that even if placed appropriately, the sutures will not completely close the cavity or reach a deep bleeding vessel. However, by closing the tissue over it, the hematoma self-tamponades. Concerns about hepatic necrosis, intrahepatic abscess, or hemobilia are valid but should be secondary to saving a patient's life. We have used the technique on many patients and have rarely seen hepatic necrosis that requires debridement. Abscesses and hemobilia are usually managed by minimally interventional techniques.

With or without hepatorrhaphy, packing has saved more lives than any complex liver operation for trauma (Figure 2). The packs must compress the liver concentrically and in this way reapproximate the edges of the laceration and apply pressure on the wound. Random placement of packs may achieve the exact opposite result; the wound edges are split apart rather than being pushed against each other. Packs should never be placed inside the laceration. As explained before, a delicate balance must be struck between adequately compressing the bleeding vessels and avoiding compression of the inferior vena cava. Communication with the anesthesiologist is important during placement of the packs to ensure that cardiac preload is still adequate. If the hemodynamics deteriorate rather than improve after pack placement, the packing must be rearranged, as the cava may be compressed.

Another bleeding control technique relates to gunshot wound tracts. It is hard to control bleeding from the tract through the narrow entry and/or exit sites. A hepatotomy to open up the tract may create more damage by incising healthy tissue. Compression of the bleeding site can be achieved by inserting a Foley catheter and inflating the balloon. Multiple trials of balloon inflation and deflation may be needed along the tract, until the responsible vessel is compressed, and the bleeding stops. If the tract is long, a Penrose drain can be inserted over a catheter and distended with water instilled through the catheter. The catheter can be left in place, until reexploration.

Kidney

Saving the kidney is a laudable goal, but such a goal is not always consistent with damage control principles. A patient who needs an abbreviated laparotomy because of multiple injuries is better served by a nephrectomy. If this decision is made, the contralateral kidney should be palpated to assess its location and size. Renal function tests are unnecessary, as it is extremely unlikely that a normal-size, normal-site kidney is not functional. However, when in doubt about the functionality of the contralateral kidney, the ureter of the injured kidney can be clamped, and methylene blue can be injected intravenously, so excretion of the blue dye in the urine collection bag can be observed.

Although it is usually preferable to control the hilar vessels before opening the Gerota fascia, in cases of damage control, we open the fascia first, deliver the kidney rapidly to the field while manually compressing it, and apply clamps to the hilum and ureter last. Nephrectomy by this maneuver should not take more than a few minutes. In cases of ureteral but not renal injury, a tube is inserted in the ureter and exteriorized through the skin as a ureterostomy.

Pancreas

In damage control operations, the pancreas is only packed and drained, not resected. In experienced hands and in highly selected cases, a quick distal pancreatectomy could be considered. In such cases, the spleen should always be resected at the same time to minimize the duration of the procedure. For proximal injuries, a pancreaticoduodenectomy should never be considered; wide drainage is the only maneuver needed.

Hollow Viscera

Perforations can be rapidly closed by running sutures in one layer. We have essentially abandoned two-layer repairs or anastomoses, because almost all gastric perforations are amenable to simple closure. Duodenal perforations occupying less than 50% of the lumen's circumference should also be closed primarily. A case-by-case decision must be made for larger perforations; some can still be closed primarily, whereas others need a more complex procedure, such as a serosal (Thal) patch, duodenojejunostomy, or pyloric exclusion. Closure of the duodenal perforation around a large-bore drainage tube is another temporary alternative.

Most small bowel and colon perforations should also be closed primarily. If a resection is necessary, it should be performed with staplers to minimize operative time. Depending on the urgency to "bail out," an anastomosis could be performed, or the resected ends could be left in the abdomen until bowel continuity is restored at a second operation. Although we use staplers for the resection, we typically hand sew the anastomotic line in one layer with two running absorbable sutures going in opposite directions. The time is essentially the same between stapling and hand sewing an anastomosis, and there is evidence that hand sewing produces better outcomes in trauma. We almost never do colostomies because creating a colostomy is as time consuming and has similar morbidity as creating an anastomosis. Additionally, having a colostomy next to an open abdomen is not ideal. Although in pressing situations we "resect and drop" the

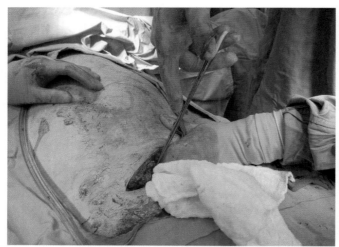

FIGURE 3 Placement of packs through a Pfannenstiel incision in the retroperitoneal pelvic space.

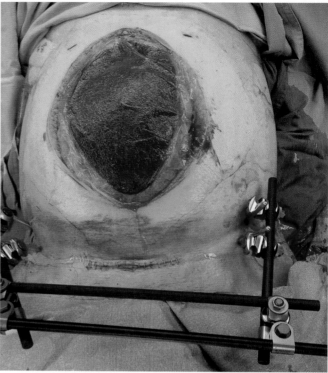

FIGURE 4 Note the separate incisions for laparotomy and preperitoneal pelvic packing. In this way, the pelvic peritoneum remains intact.

stapled ends, we typically take a few minutes to do a rapid end-to-end, single-layer anastomosis. Only in large injuries of the extraperitoneal rectum do we avoid a primary repair.

Retroperitoneum and Pelvis

If there is diffuse bleeding from the retroperitoneal space, packs can be applied, but the compression effect is questionable. A variety of hemostatic agents can be used, ranging from special gauzes to granular material and fibrin glue products. We have used these products with mixed results and little evidence of why they are effective in some cases and not in others.

In the presence of a large pelvic hematoma that is not leaking in the intraperitoneal space because the peritoneum is intact, invasion of the hematoma is not advisable, unless a major vascular injury is suspected, as may happen if the lower extremity pulses are absent. It is best to leave the hematoma undisturbed and seek control by postoperative angiographic embolization. However, in unusual cases, the hematoma is actively expanding, which may leave no other option besides surgical intervention. A retroperitoneal approach is preferable. This can be achieved by a subrapubic incision, either a midline or a Pfannenstiel (Figure 3). If a laparotomy has already been done, it is best to perform a separate incision for the retroperitoneal pelvic packing and not extend the midline laparotomy incision (Figure 4).

After incising the fascia in the midline, the hematoma is entered, and packs are placed deep into the retroperitoneal pelvis on both sides of the bladder. In this way, the peritoneum is not opened, and the retroperitoneal space does not become continuous with the intraperitoneal cavity. On occasions, a separate incision is not possible, and packing through the peritoneal cavity after incising the peritoneum is necessary. Typically, brisk bleeding from numerous unnamed vessels is encountered, and attempts to ligate or suture are rather futile. Packing is the best solution, but it is less effective when done through the abdomen rather than retroperitoneally.

Vessels

Most veins in the abdomen—except the suprarenal inferior vena cava, portal vein, and superior mesenteric vein—can be safely ligated. Ligation of the splenic vein may need a splenectomy, and ligation of the renal vein may also need a nephrectomy, if it is not close to the inferior vena cava. Ligation of the infrarenal inferior vena cava is usually well tolerated, although temporary edema is common, and extremity fasciotomies may be required on occasion. The same is true with ligation of the common and external iliac veins.

Splenic, hepatic, left gastric, and renal arteries can also be ligated, but others should not, such as the aorta and superior mesenteric artery. Successful ligation of the iliac arteries has been reported, but we do not recommend it. Shunting is an effective temporary way to maintain blood supply distal to the injury without ligation. A variety of shunts have been used for this purpose, but we typically use either an Inahara-Pruitt shunt or a simple carotid shunt. A piece of a nasogastric tube could be equally effective, if a shunt is not readily available. No consensus exists regarding the use of heparinization when a shunt is inserted, but given that these patients are usually bleeding and coagulopathic, we typically do not use heparinization. The shunt can stay in place for many hours, with reports of shunts being left in place for up to 4 days.

Open Abdomen

In almost all patients managed by a damage control procedure, the abdomen is left open at the end of the first operation. In the past we used a simple Bogota bag, typically part of a large saline bag or x-ray cassette drape, to cover the abdomen. Following that, we applied a vacuum-pack technique by placing a Silastic drape, perforated manually on numerous locations by the scalpel, and then laying multiple laparotomy pads over the drape, placing two suction catheters among the pads, and laying an adhesive drape over the entire system. Currently, we use the abdominal VAC system (KCI Inc., San Antonio, Tex.), consisting of a preperforated drape, large sponge, adhesive drape, and disk connected to a suction device.

Countless techniques are available to manage the open abdomen following the initial operation, and not a single one of them has emerged as the universally accepted standard. We typically change the vacuum dressing every 48 hours and close the wound gradually from the top and bottom, if the edematous bowel will allow it. If not, we seek abdominal closure with a mesh by the tenth posttraumatic day.

Because the field is contaminated, we always use a biologic mesh placed as an underlay to the fascia and secured with interrupted horizontal mattress sutures. We then undermine the skin to create large flaps that will allow skin closure over the mesh. Leaving the skin open requires a vacuum dressing on the mesh, which may cause desiccation of the mesh and an enterocutaneous fistula. In the unlikely event that we are not able to close the skin after adequate undermining, other techniques to close the open abdomen are considered, ranging from skin grafting over granulated bowel to the use of innovative devices to reapproximate the fascia. In addition, patients are educated about the high likelihood of developing a recurrent ventral hernia and need for reoperation in the future.

Damage Control Thoracotomy

Thoracic damage control operations are rather infrequent, as the two most commonly used elements of damage control, packing and leaving the cavity open, are harder to apply in the chest. The focus is on rapid bleeding control without extensive surgical maneuvers.

Position and Induction

Patients taken to the operating room should not be placed in the lateral position. This is time consuming and prevents access to the contralateral chest and abdomen, cavities that may need to be explored in blunt polytrauma or penetrating trauma with unclear trajectory. The patient should be placed supine with a pillow under the involved hemithorax. An anterolateral rather than posterolateral thoracotomy should be used, and time should not be spent to perform and confirm a double-lumen endotracheal intubation; a straightforward, single-lumen intubation is preferable, and a bronchial blocker can be used to exclude one lung if needed.

Lung

Upon entering the chest, severe bleeding from the lung can be controlled by clamping the hilum. The inferior pulmonary ligament should be cut, and a Satinsky clamp should be placed around the hilum. Another technique to achieve the same result is twisting of the lung by 180 degrees, which occludes the inflow and outflow but makes the anatomical identification and exploration of injuries more awkward.

If the injury is parenchymal, a stapled tractotomy is the fastest way to open the tract and individually ligate bleeding vessels. A gastrointestinal anastomotic stapler is applied through the bullet trajectory and fired. The tract then opens, and bleeding sites can be controlled by sutures. A stapled pulmonary resection can be safely done, whether it is the lobe or the entire lung that needs removal. A thoracoabdominal stapler is applied at the hilar structures en masse and fired (Figure 5). We recommend that it be fired twice, so that two staple lines are placed on the hilum. Typically, the hilar stump retracts in the mediastinum after resection, and control of bleeding from any misfired staples would be hard to achieve. Compared to meticulous dissection and individual ligation of the hilar elements, a resection stapled en masse is faster and equally safe, although large series and long-term results are unavailable.

It must be specifically mentioned that in contrast to the liver, deep sutures of an entry and exit wound from a gunshot to the lung is not advised. Because of the presence of open vessels and bronchi in the tract, there is a potential for air entering into the vessels (air embolism) or blood entering into the airway (aspiration); both are complications that can lead to death.

Heart

The placement of skin staples has been suggested as a method of rapid closure of a cardiac laceration. This may be an adequate technique

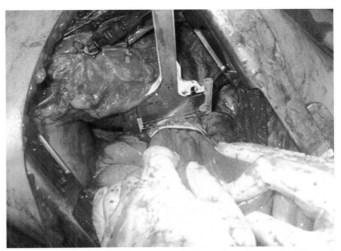

FIGURE 5 Application of a thoracoabdominal stapler on the hilum of the lung for a rapid pneumonectomy, following a gunshot wound to the hilum. Note the intravenous line inserted into the atrium of the heart for resuscitation.

for temporary control of bleeding in the emergency department if a qualified surgeon is not present or adequate tools are missing. The staples should be removed in the operating room and replaced with proper sutures.

Complete occlusion of cardiac inflow can be achieved by manual compression of the atrial orifices of the superior and inferior vena cava. This will cause a cardiac arrest and make a complex repair easier on a nonbeating heart; the heart may be restarted by compressions or electric shock. This maneuver should obviously last for a very short time and be reserved only for desperate situations. The atria can also be used to infuse fluid rapidly, if other venous access is not available. A small Foley catheter secured by a purse-string suture can provide a lifesaving fluid-infusion line.

Thoracic Wall

Packing of the thoracic cavity has been done, but the experience is too limited to draw any conclusions about its efficacy. It is hard to apply appropriate compression or even ensure that the packs will stay in place. Similarly, although some case reports describe leaving the thoracic wall open, the benefits are rather limited. It is mostly the rigid rib cage, not the closed surgical wound, that contributes to the lack of compliance and the development of a thoracic compartment syndrome.

Damage Control Orthopedics

One of the significant evolutions of orthopedic trauma surgery over the past few decades was the sense of urgency for repairing long-bone fractures. No longer was splinting for days acceptable; most fractures were repaired within hours after injury. This useful concept had limitations in the presence of severe polytrauma. Internal fixation is associated with long operative times, extensive blood loss, and a systemic inflammatory insult. If this is done shortly after the injury, and while the inflammatory cascade is rampant, the physiologic condition of the patient may be compromised rather than optimized. Damage control orthopedics aim to stabilize the bone effectively while avoiding a major secondary inflammatory insult.

Operative repairs on fractures that can be otherwise stabilized (e.g., splints, traction) should be delayed until the completion of resuscitation. Following that, external fixation is advisable over internal fixation, if the patient remains physiologically labile. External fixation may be used as the definitive approach, or the repair may be converted to internal fixation at a later stage, when the patient is stable. Although each patient should be considered individually, it is generally not advisable to proceed to internal fixation within 24 to 48 hours of severe injury.

The combination of orthopedic and vascular injuries presents a unique challenge. Delaying vascular restoration until the bone is fixed prolongs ischemia to the distal extremity. Repairing the vessel before orthopedic fixation subjects a tenuous anastomotic line to major manipulation and the possibility of damage. However, temporary shunting is the solution. The first step is to identify the vessel and insert a shunt to provide distal blood supply. The second step consists of the orthopedic repair. Finally, the operation is completed on the third step, which includes the removal of the shunt and definitive repair by primary vascular repair or with the use of a native or artificial graft.

Damage Control Angiographic Embolization

Angiographic embolization has become an indispensable method of controlling pelvic and other organ bleeding. We will only consider this option when patients are bleeding acutely, and urgent embolization is required as a lifesaving intervention. In such patients the principles of damage control—rapid, effective, temporary—apply exactly as they do in the operating room.

Under these principles, pelvic embolization should almost routinely involve the main stems of both internal iliac arteries by injecting gelatin sponge particles (Figure 6). Subselective embolization by coils is time consuming and likely to fail, as it is rare that only one site is responsible for life-threatening bleeding from a major pelvic fracture; usually, it is the entire pelvic vascular plexus that bleeds. By embolizing both internal iliac arteries with a temporary agent, the blood pressure in the pelvic vessels decreases, allowing clotting to occur. The procedure takes only a few minutes. Usually, there is still sufficient blood supply to ensure organ viability; and although in some case reports, gluteal muscle necrosis or rectal sloughing has been observed, it is very rare that significant complications occur according to our experience. The vessels typically recanalize within 5 to 14 days after embolization, although we have seen a few patients with either earlier recanalization or permanent occlusion. It should be remembered that approximately 15% of patients subjected to embolization may rebleed and require reembolization.

Embolization of other organs, such as the liver or kidney, requires a higher degree of selectivity and is usually performed by placing coils in the bleeding branch. Splenic bleeding is usually controlled by embolizing the main splenic artery, but this should never be done on an unstable patient, as such patients are much better served by a splenectomy.

On many occasions, both an operation and an embolization should be performed. Many authors recommend that the patient be routinely transferred to the angiography suite for embolization following a damage control operation to the liver or pelvis.

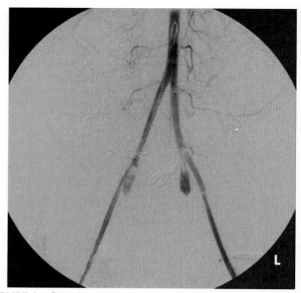

FIGURE 6   Complete truncation of both internal iliac arteries during angiographic embolization for major pelvic bleeding. The patient had no complications related to the embolization, and the bleeding was effectively controlled.

Other Applications

The concept of damage control can be applied on every part of the human body. Whether packing a large neck wound with spinal bleeding or inserting a Foley catheter inside a hole to control bleeding, the principles of rapid, effective, and temporary control of bleeding and contamination have seen numerous applications. These principles have been extended to methods of resuscitating civilians and soldiers in austere environments (damage control resuscitation) and to the development of systems of staged care in the battlefield (combat damage control). Damage control has introduced a new way of thinking about the management of devastating trauma and has allowed many lives to be saved by accepting that, on occasion, "better is the enemy of good."

SUGGESTED READINGS

Giannoudis PV: Aspects of current management: surgical priorities in damage control in polytrauma, *J Bone Joint Surg* 85-B:478–483, 2003.

Loveland JA, Boffard KD: Damage control in the abdomen and beyond, *Br J Surg* 91:1095–1101, 2004.

Phelan HA, Patterson SH, Hassan MO, et al: Thoracic damage control operation: principles, techniques, and definitive repair, *J Am Coll Surg* 203:933–941, 2006.

Shapiro MB, Jenkins DH, Schwab W, et al: Damage control: a collective review, *J Trauma* 49:969–978, 2000.

Velmahos GC, Chahwan S, Hanks SE, et al: Angiographic embolization of bilateral internal iliac arteries to control life-threatening hemorrhage after blunt trauma to the pelvis, *Am Surg* 66:858–862, 2000.

PELVIC FRACTURES

Lewis M. Flint, MD

OVERVIEW

Pelvic fracture is encountered in approximately 10% of patients admitted to urban trauma centers in North America. Reported overall mortality rates for these patients vary, but most agree that death as a direct result of the pelvic fracture occurs in less than 1% of the patients admitted with this injury and in less than 15% of patients who sustain pelvic fracture as a component of a severe multiple injury pattern. Most patients with pelvic fractures are injured by blunt force impacts from motor vehicle crashes. Patients with heavy force transfer causing displaced pelvic fractures, which carry an associated increase in risk for pelvic fracture bleeding, are more likely to be injured from auto-pedestrian collisions, motorcycle crashes, and falls from heights greater than 15 feet. Important risk factors for increased mortality and morbidity resulting from pelvic fractures are increased patient age, at least in part because of osteoporosis; female gender, probably because of decreased resistance of pelvic bones and ligaments to forced disruption; and increased impact forces. Certain vehicle crash characteristics are also associated with pelvic fracture. These include lateral impacts, particularly when the striking vehicle is larger and heavier than the impacted vehicle. Lack of restraint use also predisposes to pelvic fracture.

IMPORTANT ANATOMIC CONSIDERATIONS

The pelvic ring is a major supporting structure in humans that permits bipedal upright ambulation. The ring is made up of three bones—the *right ilium, left ilium,* and *midline dorsal sacrum*—held together by strong ligaments (Figure 1). The iliac bones are formed by the fusion of the embryonic iliac, ischium, and pubic bones.

The sacrum is an important component of the dorsal axial skeleton. The acetabula, bony complexes where the hip joints articulate bilaterally, are anatomically part of the pelvis, but fractures of these structures will not be discussed in this section. Major neural, vascular, and visceral structures reside within the bony pelvis and within the sacrum. These include the rectum and bladder; vessels of the iliac, obturator, and femoral arterial and venous systems; internal reproductive organs in women; and portions of the lower urinary tract in men.

The distal branches of the spinal motor, sensory, and autonomic nerves are located within the sacrum and enter the pelvic visceral space via the sacral foramina. Pelvic fracture hemorrhage can occur because the arteries and veins of the internal iliac system, as well as the presacral venous plexus, are located just anterior to the ligaments that bind the iliac bones to the sacrum and are, therefore, subject to injury by forces that disrupt these ligaments (Figure 2). Motor and sensory nerves—particularly the sciatic, femoral, and obturator nerves—are vulnerable to injury because of the proximity to the pelvic bones and ligaments. Autonomic nerves that supply the reproductive organs are found in these same areas. It is not surprising, therefore, that neurologic injury that gives rise to painful ambulation, paresthesias, muscle weakness, and sexual dysfunction are the most important sources of long-term disability following pelvic fracture. The proximity of the bladder and urethra to the anterior components of the pelvic ring exposes these structures to injury when there are fractures of the pubic bones.

PELVIC FRACTURE CLASSIFICATION

The most frequently used pelvic fracture classification system is the one published by Young and Burgess in 1986 (Table 1). This system grades pelvic injury based on the estimated direction of the major force vector—lateral compression, anterior compression, vertical shear, or combined force—and the degree of bony displacement. Displacement of pelvic skeletal elements is a function of fracture of the bones and disruption of the ligaments of the pelvis.

In general, vascular injuries that produce pelvic hemorrhage tend to cluster in the groups of fractures associated with the largest degree of bony displacement as determined by plain pelvic radiograph or computerized tomography (CT) imaging. A report by Eastridge and coauthors in 2002 presented data in support of this observation. However, fracture classification has limited utility in predicting the risk

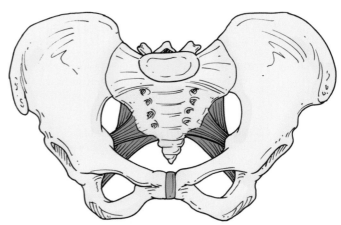

FIGURE 1 Inlet view of the pelvic ring showing posterior ligamentous complexes. *(Modified from Flint LM, Wayne MJ, Schwab CW, et al: Trauma: contemporary principles and therapy, Philadelphia, 2008, Wolters Kluwer/Lippincott Williams & Wilkins, p 523. Used with permission.)*

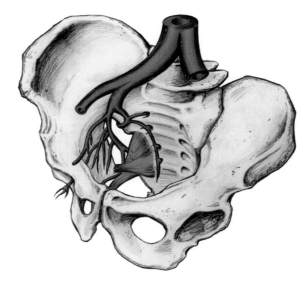

FIGURE 2 Pelvic vascular anatomy showing proximity to posterior ligaments. *(Modified from Flint LM, Wayne MJ, Schwab CW, et al: Trauma: contemporary principles and therapy, Philadelphia, 2008, Wolters Kluwer/Lippincott Williams & Wilkins, p 524. Used with permission.)*

TABLE 1: Burgess and Young modification of the Pennell and Sutherland classification of pelvic fractures

Fracture	Description
Anteroposterior Compression	
Type I	Disruption of pubic symphysis <2.5 cm of diastasis, no significant posterior pelvic injury
Type II	Pubic symphysis disruption >2.5 cm with tearing of anterior sacroiliac, sacrospinous, and sacrotuberous ligaments
Type III	Complete disruption of pubic symphysis and posterior ligament complexes with hemipelvic displacement
Lateral Compression	
Type I	Posterior compression of sacroiliac joint without ligament disruption or oblique pubic ramus fracture
Type II	Rupture of posterior sacroiliac ligament, pivotal internal rotation of hemipelvis on anterior sacroiliac joint, with crush of sacrum and an oblique pubic ramus fracture
Type III	Findings in type II with evidence of anteroposterior compression injury to contralateral hemipelvis
Vertical Shear	Complete ligament or bony disruption of hemipelvic associated with hemipelvic displacement

Modified from Young JW, Burgess AR, Brumback RJ, et al: Pelvic fractures: value of plain radiography in early assessment and management, *Radiology* 160(2):445–451, 1986.

of bleeding for individual patients, because, as noted by Sarin and coauthors, a significant proportion of patients with high-grade pelvic fracture do not have pelvic fracture hemorrhage. For the surgeon evaluating and setting management priorities for patients with pelvic fracture from high-impact trauma, a composite approach that includes assessment of injury mechanism, physical examination, physiologic data indicative of significant ongoing bleeding, and imaging will be necessary to predict patients who are at risk for pelvic fracture bleeding.

INITIAL ASSESSMENT OF PATIENTS WITH PELVIC FRACTURES

As mentioned previously, most patients who sustain pelvic fractures have minor injuries. As understanding of the risk for significant pelvic fracture has become more refined, data have been presented that support a selective approach to imaging of the patient who is awake, alert, and able to cooperate in a physical examination. The pelvic physical examination includes assessment of the lower spine and pelvic ring for pain, tenderness, and abnormal motion. Lateral and anterior–posterior compression of the iliac crests and assessment of the pubic symphysis for separation and pain are combined with evaluation of the urethral orifice for bleeding and a digital rectal examination. The plain anteroposterior (AP) pelvic radiograph has been a time-honored addition to this examination, and clear data demonstrate the dependable negative predictability of the normal

physical examination of the lower back and pelvis. An elevated blood alcohol level does not reduce the accuracy of the physical examination, if the patient is alert and able to cooperate. A few pelvic fractures are discovered in patients with unremarkable physical examinations who undergo detailed CT imaging, but these essentially never require specific intervention. Thus plain AP pelvic radiographs can be safely omitted in patients who have unremarkable physical examinations; imaging may be performed later if symptoms arise.

CT imaging has been shown to be a very sensitive means of detecting pelvic fractures. In recent experience using rapid, multislice helical scanners, head-to-pelvis images could be obtained in intervals of 5 to 7 minutes. Computer-assisted reconstructions of these images can provide high-resolution views to guide plans for operative interventions needed for pelvic reconstruction. Recent data from an analysis of patients in a European trauma registry suggest that incorporation of whole-body CT imaging into the initial resuscitation of severely injured patients is associated with improved survival. Certainly, careful clinical judgment and a full understanding of the imaging capabilities of each individual institution are necessary to support the decision to transport a potentially unstable patient to the CT scanner. The message for surgeons is that the plain AP pelvic film may be selectively omitted in patients who are going to have CT imaging of the torso.

Detection and Management of Injuries to the Lower Urinary Tract

Fractures of the pubic bones are associated with injuries to the lower urinary tract. These usually occur because of anterior compression forces transmitted in a ventral to dorsal direction, causing bladder rupture from compressive forces, or from lateral compressive forces that displace the pubic bone in a lateral–medial direction, catching the bladder wall on the bone ends. Straddle injuries and forces that produce thigh abduction are important causes of perineal trauma and urethral injury.

Important features of the evaluation and management of patients whose pelvic fractures put them at risk for lower urinary tract injury include careful physical examination to search for signs of injury. The examination should seek out suprapubic pain and tenderness, perineal ecchymosis, laceration and/or tenderness, blood at the urethral meatus, and blood or periprostatic hematoma discovered on digital rectal examination. Urethral injury is not confined to male patients only; in women with suspected pubic bone fractures, vaginal examination to examine the urethra for blood or laceration is necessary. The physical examination, though valuable, is not foolproof. A significant proportion of patients found to have urethral injury will not have positive physical findings.

A cautious attempt to place a bladder catheter is indicated with any suspected urethral injury. If resistance is felt, a retrograde urethrogram is performed. In patients with urethral disruption, realignment of the urethra with endoscopic assistance is the preferable approach. Although suprapubic cystostomy and delayed repair of the urethral disruption is a time-honored approach, clinicians now understand that the suprapubic catheter delays or prevents definitive open reduction and internal fixation (ORIF) of the pelvic fracture. If ORIF of the pelvic fracture is delayed or cannot be done, significant disability due to pain on ambulation is the result. Data are also clear that early realignment of the disrupted urethra in men and early definitive repair of the injured urethra in women are both associated with improved long-term urinary and sexual function. For these reasons, early expeditious diagnosis and realignment of urethral disruptions with avoidance of suprapubic catheterization is preferred.

Gross hematuria discovered after spontaneous voiding or following insertion of a Foley catheter is the most common sign of bladder injury. Traditionally, patients at risk for bladder injury have had AP, lateral, and oblique plain radiograph images of the bladder following instillation of at least 250 mL of contrast material in adults (20 mL/kg body weight in children). Adequate bladder filling is important to prevent missed injuries. Therefore the volumes mentioned are just estimates; the bladder should be filled by gravity until contrast will no longer flow in. Repeat views are obtained after bladder drainage. However, this approach also has been supplanted by CT imaging. Distended bladder and postemptying views are obtained during the course of CT imaging, and adequate bladder distension and careful postemptying views remain important features of an accurate bladder assessment. Extraperitoneal bladder ruptures can usually be managed with bladder drainage only, unless the patient will have abdominal exploration for other reasons, in which case accessible bladder tears may be directly sutured. Intraperitoneal rupture of the bladder is an indication for abdominal exploration and suture repair of the bladder. Laparoscopic bladder repair has been reported, but insufficient data are available to determine the real value of this approach.

Perineal Injury and Open Pelvic Fracture

In addition to predisposing to urethral injury, perineal lacerations may communicate with the pelvic fracture site. Contamination of the fracture is possible because of transmural laceration of the rectum or fecal soiling of the laceration. Careful digital rectal examination with selective sigmoidoscopy, either rigid or flexible, will often disclose the extent of injury and allow an estimate of the risk for fecal soilage. Diverting colostomy may be necessary to prevent septic complications. Open pelvic fractures with lacerations in the groin or pubic area carry a much lower risk of fecal soilage, and colostomy will usually not be needed in this situation.

Detection and Management of Pelvic Fracture Hemorrhage

Significant blood loss from pelvic fracture is possible because of the rich arterial and venous channels within the pelvis, the plentiful blood supply of the pelvic bones, and the fact that tissue pressure within the pelvic retroperitoneum is low, permitting accumulation of substantial volumes of blood before tissue pressure rises sufficiently to tamponade bleeding. Life-threatening hemorrhage can occur due to disruption of the branches of the internal iliac artery within the pelvis. Branches of the internal pudendal artery are commonly the source of bleeding in these patients. Detection of bleeding sufficient to justify intervention is based upon physiologic variables indicative of ongoing bleeding, the fracture pattern disclosed on pelvic imaging, and the presence of associated significant injuries.

Pelvic fracture hemorrhage occurs in the setting of major force transfer. This usually means that the surgeon is confronted with several potential bleeding sites necessitating rapid assessment. Major cavitary bleeding in the chest and abdomen can usually be excluded with plain AP chest radiograph, focused assessment by sonography for trauma (FAST), and/or rapid CT imaging. If FAST discloses intraabdominal fluid in a patient with signs of ongoing blood loss—variable blood pressure, tachycardia alternating with intervals of bradycardia, hematocrit below 30%, arterial pH below 7.2 that is resistant to blood and fluid therapy—abdominal exploration is chosen as the primary intervention, and pelvic fracture bleeding is approached when abdominal sources have been controlled and/or the pelvic hematoma is expanding. When the FAST or CT images disclose no intraabdominal bleeding site, the pelvic bleeding is controlled first. Later, repeat FAST imaging can be done if no pelvic bleeding site is discovered, or if signs of ongoing bleeding persist even after pelvic bleeding is controlled.

The approach to pelvic bleeding is chosen based on the type of pelvic fracture, the resources available in the individual institution, and the rapidity of bleeding. The available approaches to pelvic fracture bleeding include measures to decrease pelvic volume and thus increase pelvic retroperitoneal tissue pressure (pelvic C clamp, external fixator, or compression device), angiography with embolization, and pelvic gauze packing.

Significant pelvic fracture bleeding can occur from veins, bone edges, lacerated arteries, or combinations of these. Injuries to major pelvic arterial or venous trunks are unusual, but they occur occasionally; these can be effectively managed with endovascular approaches. The more typical patient presents with anterior compression, vertical shear, or a combined pelvic fracture with disruption of one or both sacroiliac ligamentous complexes. Separation of the pubic symphysis by more than 1 to 2 cm is the rule. The recognition that reapproximation of the separated pubic symphysis with a bed sheet placed around the pelvis just caudal to the anterior superior iliac spines reduced pelvic volume and controlled bleeding in a significant proportion of patients stimulated efforts to permanently achieve this with devices such as the pelvic C clamp and external fixators. The pelvic C clamp is applied to the dorsal iliac bones, and the external fixator is applied anteriorly. These devices are variably favored by orthopedic trauma surgeons; they can be applied in the emergency department, but many prefer to place these in the operating room.

The need to transfer the patient to the operating room without assurance that the device will control bleeding has stimulated trauma surgeons to attempt other means of reducing pelvic volume. The simplest of these approaches is the bed sheet described above. Recently, however, a pelvic compression device (T-Pod; Pyng Medical, Richmond, BC, Canada) has proven valuable for its ease of placement, lack of displacement with patient movement, and effective reduction of pelvic volume. A satisfactory response to pelvic volume reduction is signaled by stabilization of blood pressure and heart rate and improvement of acidosis. If these do not occur within 30 minutes of device placement, alternate approaches are indicated. Complications of pelvic compression include pressure injury to the skin and fracture overcorrection. Pressure injury to the skin can be avoided by removing the device within the first 36 hours after application or by periodically inspecting the skin for injury. Follow-up imaging will disclose overcorrection.

In most North American trauma centers, angiography with embolization is the approach preferred for patients with rapid pelvic fracture bleeding and/or an inadequate response to pelvic volume reduction. Guidance as to the general location of the pelvic bleeding site can be gained by observing contrast extravasation on the pelvic CT images. Pelvic contrast extravasation is associated with an angiographically demonstrated bleeding site in approximately 75% of patients. The choice of angiography and embolization means that the patient has to be transported to the angiography suite. This choice is not easily made by most trauma surgeons, but the alternative, transporting the patient to the operating room for pelvic packing (discussed below), is not attractive either. It is critical that all of the resources available within the trauma operating room be available in the angiographic facility during the procedure. These include anesthesiology support, devices for the rapid infusion of blood and blood products, monitoring devices, and surgeon presence. Fortunately, this challenge is becoming less burdensome in many institutions thanks to a move to equip angiographic suites for elective and emergency endovascular procedures. If one or more bleeding sites can be demonstrated, embolization will usually control these, and patient stability will result. Complications of embolization include gluteal muscle necrosis, which is infrequent but may prevent or delay ORIF, and rectal necrosis is a rare complication resulting from bilateral internal iliac embolization.

Gauze packing of the pelvic retroperitoneum is an alternative for patients when angiographic embolization is not readily available. This approach has been described in two reports from Smith and Cothren from the Denver Health Trauma Center. In their approach, a midline incision is made, the bladder is retracted, and gauze packs are positioned in the dorsal and lateral pelvic retroperitoneum (Figure 3). It is likely that similar exposure and access to the dorsal pelvic retroperitoneum could be achieved by unilateral or bilateral transverse incisions in the infraumbilical lower abdomen. A reduction in pelvic fracture mortality from 40% (historic comparison group) to 25%, using an approach that uses retroperitoneal gauze

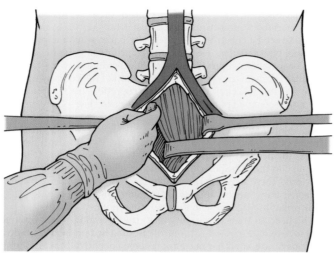

FIGURE 3 Exposure of pelvic retroperitoneum via midline incision for pelvic gauze packing. *(Modified from Smith WR, Moore EE, Osborn P, et al: Retroperitoneal packing as a resuscitation technique for hemodynamically unstable patients with pelvic fractures: report of two representative cases and a description of technique, J Trauma 59[6]:1510–1514, 2005. Used with permission.)*

packing complemented by angiography and embolization, has been reported by this group. Additional confirmatory clinical experience has not been forthcoming from other centers to date, but a multidisciplinary approach to pelvic fracture bleeding has been shown to improve attributable mortality.

DEFINITIVE FIXATION OF PELVIC FRACTURES

Severe pelvic fractures will usually require open reduction and internal fixation using approaches that effectively restore pelvic stability in both anterior and posterior elements of the pelvic ring. Early definitive fixation is a key component in the effort to effectively rehabilitate injured patients, maximize the prospect for pain-free ambulation, and return patients to productive lives.

Suggested Readings

Cothren CC, Osborn PM, Moore EE, et al: Preperitonal pelvic packing for hemodynamically unstable pelvic fractures: a paradigm shift, *J Trauma* 62(4):834–839, 2007.

Croce MA, Magnotti LJ, Savage SA, et al: Emergent pelvic fixation in patients with exsanguinating pelvic fractures, *J Am Coll Surg* 204(5):935–939, 2007.

Demetriades D, Karaiskakis M, Toutouzas K, et al: Pelvic fractures: epidemiology and predictors of associated abdominal injuries and outcomes, *J Am Coll Surg* 195(1):1–10, 2002.

Duane TM, Tan BB, Golay D, et al: Blunt trauma and the role of routine pelvic radiographs: a prospective analysis, *J Trauma* 53(3):463–468, 2002.

Eastridge BJ, Starr A, Minei JP, et al: The importance of fracture pattern in guiding therapeutic decision making in patients with hemorrhagic shock and pelvic ring disruptions, *J Trauma* 53(3):446–450, 2002.

Flint LM, Wayne MJ, Schwab CW, et al: *Trauma: contemporary principles and therapy*, Philadelphia, 2008, Wolters Kluwer/Lippincott Williams & Wilkins.

Huber-Wagner S, Lefering R, Qvick LM, et al: Effect of whole-body CT during trauma resuscitation on survival: a retrospective, multicentre study, *Lancet* 373(9673):1455–1461, 2009.

Mouraviev VB, Coburn M, Santucci RA, et al: The treatment of posterior urethral disruption associated with pelvic fractures: comparative experience of early realignment versus delayed urethroplasty, *J Urol* 173(3):873–876, 2005.

Sarin EL, Moore JB, Moore EE, et al: Pelvic fracture pattern does not always predict the need for urgent embolization, *J Trauma* 58(5):973–977, 2005.

Smith WR, Moore EE, Osborn P, et al: Retroperitoneal packing as a resuscitation technique for hemodynamically unstable patients with pelvic fractures: report of two representative cases and a description of technique, *J Trauma* 59(6):1510–1514, 2005.

Young JW, Burgess AR, Brumback RJ, et al: Pelvic fractures: value of plain radiography in early assessment and management, *Radiology* 160(2):445–451, 1986.

SPINE AND SPINAL CORD INJURIES

Robert R. Quickel, MD, and Thomas A. Bergman, MD

OVERVIEW

The most common causes of spine and spinal cord injury are motor vehicle crashes and falls. Spinal injury is diagnosed in approximately 20% to 25% of trauma patients, and 20% to 25% of those patients suffer spinal cord injury. The incidence of spinal cord injury is between 15 and 40 cases per million people. This translates to approximately 11,000 cases of spinal cord injury each year in the United States and 300,000 people living with spinal cord injuries. These patients are overwhelmingly male, with percentages as high as 80% in some studies. The average age at injury is approximately 33 years and is gradually rising over time. Cervical injuries are most common, followed by thoracolumbar injuries, with thoracic injuries occurring least often, presumably because of the rigidity of the thorax. The estimated yearly cost of treatment of spinal cord injury is $9.7 billion in the United States.

EVALUATION

Initial treatment of the trauma patient includes stabilization of the spinal column to prevent further spinal cord injury; this immobilization should remain in place until the spine is "cleared" of any injury. Airway, breathing, and circulation are addressed and disability is evaluated, which includes assessment of spinal cord function and Glasgow Coma Scale scoring, accomplished by a quick neurologic exam during the trauma primary survey. A more thorough neurologic exam is part of the secondary trauma survey.

Examination of the motor and sensory system depends on the patient's overall condition and whether a head injury is present, and evaluation can be difficult in the comatose patient with a severe head injury. In this situation, motor function is evaluated by determining the response to painful stimuli in both the upper and lower extremities. In patients who are posturing because of a cerebral injury, the spinal cord can be assumed to be at least partially functioning.

Patients with a severe cord injury will be flaccid secondary to spinal shock, even if they have a cerebral injury that might otherwise have resulted in decorticate or decerebrate posturing. Sensory level or function is extremely difficult to obtain in the comatose patient and is assessed by the response to pain with either a posturing or withdrawal response. For patients who have been intubated and paralyzed prior to the physician's assessment, information from the initial responders may be the only available means of assessment of spinal cord integrity. History of the traumatic event is important to obtain if possible, as mechanisms of injury may provide clues to the type and severity of the injury.

The neurologic exam is more straightforward for patients who are not intoxicated and those who are without head injury. Motor exam should emphasize the major muscle groups of the lower and upper extremities. Sensory exam is likewise performed with determination of sensory level–based dermatomal patterns. It is extremely important to include light touch, deep sensation, and position sense, as these functions depend on different spinal cord tracts that can be involved separately, depending on the type of injury. Cervical dermatomes are assessed by a careful examination of the upper extremities. As shown in Figure 1, the dermatomes skip from approximately C4 or C5 to T2 in the upper chest, with the remainder of the cervical dermatomes represented in the arms.

Bowel and bladder function and the integrity of the sacral system are assessed by determining rectal tone, cremasteric/bulbocavernosus reflex, and by careful pinprick examination of the perirectal area. Retention of the sacral reflexes, with the exception of rectal tone, does not necessarily imply an incomplete spinal cord injury because of lower sacral reflex arcs, which can be preserved and can quickly recover after injury. A complete injury is one in which there is no neurologic function below the level of the injury. In an incomplete injury, there is some preservation of neurologic function below the level of the injury to the spinal column. The differentiation of complete versus incomplete neurologic injury is straightforward in the majority of cases, and it is important because patients with incomplete injury have a better prognosis for recovery of spinal cord function. This can affect treatment and prognostic decisions.

It is important to remember that sensory function can be preserved for one or two dermatome levels below the injury to the spinal cord because of the multisegmental ascending and descending anatomy of the lateral spinal thalamic tract. Motor function deficit should begin at the level of cord injury plus or minus one segment, depending on how much contusion and internal cord injury is present.

Radiologic evaluation should be undertaken as soon as feasible with regard to the cardiovascular and respiratory stability of the patient. In totally conscious, neurologically intact patients not intoxicated and without painful distracting injury, the decision to obtain radiographic images can be based on symptoms and exam. Spinal injury is unlikely without significant pain or midline tenderness, and radiographs may be deferred unless there are other indications to obtain them.

In the 2009 Eastern Association for the Surgery of Trauma (EAST) practice management guidelines for the identification of cervical spine injuries following trauma, computerized tomography (CT) has replaced plain radiography for those patients requiring imaging of the cervical spine. In the patient with polytrauma, CT of the entire spine is obtained along with sagittal and coronal reconstructions. Thoracic and lumbar plain films are appropriate for patients who require those segments to be imaged but who do not require CT for other reasons. Lateral images, CTs, and sagittal reconstructions provide information about the alignment of the spine and the possibility of hyperflexion injury. Flexion-extension films are useful in assessing spinal instability in awake patients. Patients who have cervical spine fractures extending into the transverse foramen should be screened for vertebral artery injury.

There is considerable debate about appropriate evaluation of the spine in patients who remain obtunded. Flexion-extension films are no longer recommended for obtunded patients. Some studies and institutions recommend magnetic resonance imaging (MRI) to rule out ligamentous injury to the spinal column causing instability in obtunded patients. The criticisms of this approach are that MRI almost never identifies injuries requiring surgical stabilization when CT results are negative, and in most institutions, MRI is remote from the trauma intensive care unit, requiring transport and prolonged monitoring of the critically injured patient. In our institution, patients who remain obtunded and have a negative CT scan of the spine may have the cervical collar removed and spinal precautions relaxed. If pain is present when a patient awakens, assessment for dynamic stability is undertaken. A study by Stelfox and colleagues (2007) indicates that this approach to cervical collar removal results in fewer complications, fewer days of mechanical ventilation, and shorter stays in the ICU and hospital.

In most patients with major trauma and spinal cord injury, the information needed for treatment planning is obtained by a combination of an initial CT scan for spinal column evaluation followed by an MRI scan for spinal cord information. Decisions regarding imaging of patients who are neurologically normal and without major deformities are made on an individual basis. Special attention should be given to the role of dynamic flexion-extension radiographs to evaluate conscious patients with symptoms of spinal cord injury without radiographic abnormality (SCIWORA). Flexion-extension films should be used when the dynamic stability of the patient's spine is in question.

INITIAL MANAGEMENT

Patients with disruption of the upper thoracic or subaxial cervical spine may have hemodynamic instability due to interruption of sympathetic outflow. After hemorrhage has been ruled out as a source of hypotension in the trauma patient, the diagnosis of neurogenic shock may be entertained. Hypotension in neurogenic shock is due to vasodilation related to a lack of sympathetic vasomotor tone. Neurogenic shock must be differentiated from hypovolemic shock, as therapies are different. In neurogenic shock, extremities are typically warm and pink, appearing to be well perfused as a result of peripheral cutaneous vasodilation, and relative bradycardia is usually present. Patients with hypovolemic shock have cutaneous vasoconstriction and are usually tachycardic. Treatment of neurogenic shock involves judicious fluid resuscitation and intravenous pressors to avoid fluid overload and restore vasomotor tone.

The first step in the treatment of severe spinal column displacement and subluxation is realignment of the spine, which can be accomplished either nonoperatively or surgically. MRI is subsequently obtained to assess injury to the spinal cord.

FRACTURES

Upper Cervical Spine Fractures

Fractures of the cervical spine can be categorized as upper and subaxial (Box 1). Upper cervical fractures involve the top two cervical vertebrae and the occipital cervical junction. Included in the group are occipital cervical dislocation, C1 burst or Jefferson fractures, odontoid fractures, hangman's fractures, and atlantoaxial rotatory subluxation. Occipital cervical dislocations are almost uniformly fatal. These injuries disrupt the cervical medullary junction and cause loss of respiratory function and cardiovascular instability. C1 ring or Jefferson fractures are axial-load compression injuries and are best identified on axial CT scanning. The integrity of the transverse and atlantoaxial ligaments is important for treatment decisions. An anteroposterior cervical or open-mouth odontoid plain film can provide information about the integrity of the transverse ligament by the *rule of Spence,* which states that patients with greater than 7 mm of

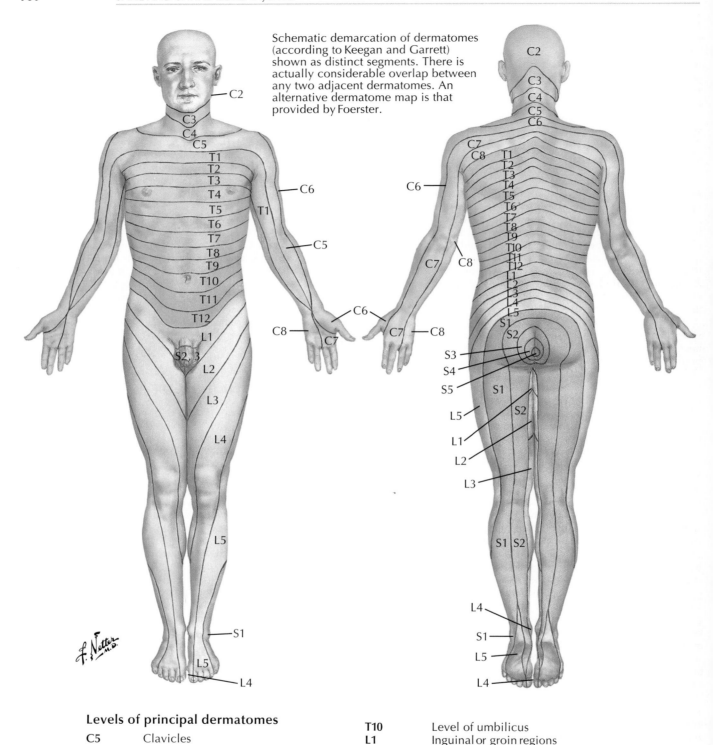

Schematic demarcation of dermatomes (according to Keegan and Garrett) shown as distinct segments. There is actually considerable overlap between any two adjacent dermatomes. An alternative dermatome map is that provided by Foerster.

Levels of principal dermatomes

C5	Clavicles
C5, 6, 7	Lateral parts of upper limbs
C8, T1	Medial sides of upper limbs
C6	Thumb
C6, 7, 8	Hand
C8	Ring and little fingers
T4	Level of nipples

T10	Level of umbilicus
L1	Inguinal or groin regions
L1, 2, 3, 4	Anterior and inner surfaces of lower limbs
L4, 5, S1	Foot
L4	Medial side of great toe
S1, 2, L5	Posterior and outer surfaces of lower limbs
S1	Lateral margin of foot and little toe
S2, 3, 4	Perineum

FIGURE 1 Dermatomal map of the human body. Each level of the spinal cord has spinal nerves that innervate and provide sensation to specific areas of the skin. Sensory dysfunction of the spinal cord can be determined by testing sensation in these areas. Motor function should also be assessed when injury to the spinal cord is suspected. It is useful to remember that C5 innervates the deltoid, C6 the biceps and wrist extensors, C7 the triceps, C8 the finger flexors, and T1 the fifth finger abductor. Lumbar spine segments innervate the leg: L2 innervates the hip flexors (psoas), L3 the knee extensors (quadriceps), L4 the quadriceps and ankle dorsiflexors (anterior tibialis), L5 the long toe extensors (hallucis longus) and ankle dorsiflexors, and S1 the ankle plantar flexors (gastrocnemius). *(Netter Illustration Collection at* http://www.netterimages.com © *Elsevier, Inc. All Rights Reserved.)*

BOX 1: Common fractures

Cervical Spine

Upper Cervical
- Occipitocervical dislocation
- Jefferson fracture (C1 burst)
- Odontoid fracture
- Hangman's fracture (C2 pars fracture)
- C2 extension-avulsion fracture

Lower Cervical
- Burst fracture
- Wedge compression fracture
- Unilateral or bilateral locked facets
- Facet/laminar fracture
- Clay-shovelers fracture
- Extension injuries

Thoracolumbar Spine
- Compression fracture (wedge)
- Burst fracture
- Chance fracture (seat-belt injury)
- Translational/shear fracture (flexion, distraction, rotation)

Sacral Fracture

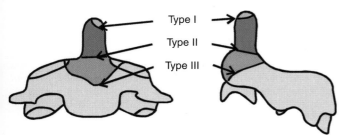

FIGURE 2 Odontoid fractures. Type I fractures are near the tip of the odontoid process, type II fractures occur at the base of the odontoid, and type III fractures extend into the vertebral body. *(From Grauer JN, Shafi B, Hilibrand AS, et al: Proposal of a modified, treatment-oriented classification of odontoid fractures, Spine J 5[2]:123–129, 2005.)*

lateral displacement of the C1 lateral mass on C2 have rupture of the transverse ligament, making the C1/C2 complex unstable.

Odontoid fractures are becoming more common as the population ages. These fractures typically occur with falls in elderly patients (Figure 2). Type I fractures are relatively unusual but are stable. Type II fractures are most common but can be difficult to treat. The amount of displacement and age of the patient are factors that affect eventual treatment decisions. Type III fractures involve the C2 body and are less frequent, and typically more stable, than type II fractures.

Hangman's fractures are hyperextension fractures where the pars interarticularis and/or pedicle of C2 are fractured, resulting in displacement of the posterior elements of the C2 body. Patients with hangman's fractures are usually either neurologically normal or present with severe injury or death. Essentially, the fracture opens up the spinal canal and allows protection of the spinal cord, as long as the distraction and displacement are not too severe.

There is one other fracture that occurs at C2 that is important to note, because it is inherently stable. This is an extension-type injury, which results in avulsion of the anterior inferior tip of either C2 or C3. The anterior longitudinal ligament avulses the edge of the vertebral body during hyperextension. These fractures can sometimes be mislabeled *teardrop fractures,* which typically describes a lower cervical flexion injury. It is important to distinguish between these two types of injuries, because the classic flexion-type teardrop fracture in the lower cervical spine is extremely unstable.

Subaxial Cervical Spine Fractures

Subaxial cervical spine fractures include wedge compression fractures, burst fractures, facet fractures, laminar fractures, and a combination of the above with ligamentous injury resulting in unilateral or bilateral locked facets and subluxation. The main difference in mechanism between burst fractures and wedge compression fractures, with or without facet subluxation, is the degree of hyperflexion and ligamentous damage at the time of the injury.

The spectrum of injury for flexion mechanisms ranges from a simple anterior wedge fracture without ligamentous injury to bilateral locked facets with severe subluxation of the superior vertebrae. Significant subluxation of a vertebral body indicates a severe flexion component to the mechanism of injury. Unilateral locked facets typically have a lateral rotation component to their flexion mechanism, which results in the inferior facet of a vertebra riding up and subluxing in front of the superior facet of the inferiorly involved vertebra. Bilateral locked facets (Figure 3) involve a pure flexion mechanism, in which both inferior facets slip up over the superior facet of the inferior vertebra, eventually perching on top of that facet and then slipping down anterior to it. Unilateral locked facets typically have subluxation of 25% of the vertebral body or less, whereas bilateral locked facets will result in 50% or greater subluxation in the majority of cases. Subaxial cervical spine fractures can result in cord injury, radicular or nerve root injury, or a combination of both.

Thoracolumbar Spine Fractures

The original principles outlined by Denis (1983) continue to be important in analysis of thoracic and thoracolumbar fractures. Dennis and colleagues define three separate columns in the spine. The anterior column includes the anterior vertebral body and the anterior longitudinal ligament. The middle column includes the posterior vertebral body and the posterior longitudinal ligament. The posterior column includes all of the posterior supporting structures and, most importantly, the facet joints. In its simplest interpretation, injury to two or more of the vertebral columns implies instability and the need for treatment.

Fractures in the thoracic spine are relatively uncommon because of the stability that is provided by the thoracic rib cage and sternum. In general, fractures and injuries to the thoracic spine have a higher rate of neurologic injury because of the forces that are necessary to cause such injuries. The *thoracolumbar spine,* defined as T10 to L2, has a higher rate of injury, because it represents the junction between the relatively fixed thoracic spine and the more mobile lumbar spine.

Thoracolumbar fractures are similar to subaxial cervical fractures with regard to type and mechanism. They include burst fractures, wedge or compression fractures, flexion-rotation injuries with secondary translation (Figure 4), and rarely extension injuries. The Chance fracture, or seat-belt fracture, secondary to a flexion injury with the axis of rotation anterior to the spine is unique. The vertebral body will split horizontally either between the disk space or through the pedicle.

Fractures due to axial-load mechanisms include compression and burst fractures. In compression fractures, a loss of height of the anterior vertebral body results in anterior wedging, whereas in burst fractures, loss of height of the entire vertebral body is seen with a characteristic burst pattern. The posterior superior aspect of the vertebral body is retropulsed back into the spinal canal in a characteristic "anvil" pattern (Figure 5). The degree of spinal canal compromise can

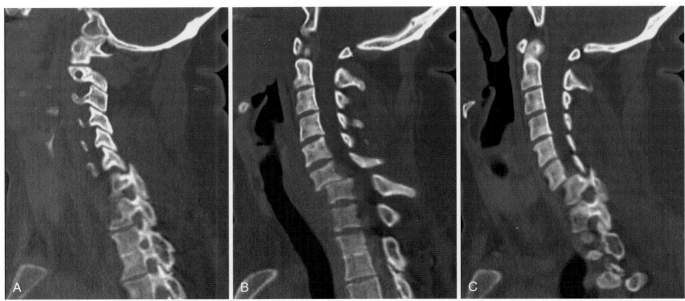

FIGURE 3   Bilateral locked facets, C6 on C7, with anterolisthesis and resultant spinal canal compromise.

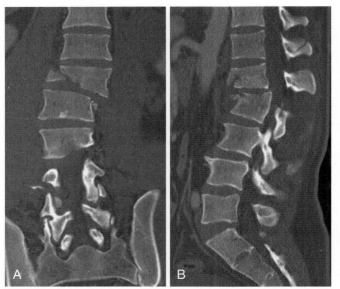

FIGURE 4   L1 and L2 fractures: this is a "translational injury" caused by rotational vector of force. Note the loss of vertebral height at L2.

be estimated with CT scanning, but the degree of actual spinal cord compression can only be estimated with either MRI or myelogram CT scanning. Transverse process fractures are commonly seen with a number of different types of injuries and frequently are not associated with significant vertebral body or facet/laminar fractures.

Sacral Fractures

Isolated sacral fractures are relatively uncommon, and most sacral fractures occur in patients with severe pelvic injuries. Most sacral fractures are stable. An exception to this rule is the fracture with bone displacement affecting the tip of the spinal canal or the S1 nerve root foramen. These are typically linear fractures that pass through the sacrum, crossing the nerve root foramina.

Spinal Cord Syndromes

A subset of patients with incomplete spinal cord injury have one of the six spinal cord injury syndromes. These patients may or may not have a bony spinal column injury, but the neurologic injury patterns are related to specific portions of the spinal cord that are injured. *Brown-Sequard syndrome* accounts for 1% to 4% of all traumatic spinal cord injuries and consists of ipsilateral loss of motor and proprioceptive function and contralateral loss of sensitivity to pain and temperature below the level of the spinal cord lesion. *Central cord syndrome* produces motor impairment that is more pronounced in the upper than lower extremities as well as bladder dysfunction and variable sensory loss below the level of the spinal cord lesion. It classically occurs in older patients with cervical spondylosis and a hyperextension injury causing cord compression. *Anterior cord syndrome* produces complete paralysis along with hyperesthesia and hypoalgesia below the level of the spinal cord lesion but with preserved touch, proprioception, and vibratory sense. *Posterior cord syndrome* is the least common of the spinal cord injury syndromes; it produces selective loss of only proprioceptive and vibratory sense below the level of the injury. *Conus medullaris syndrome* occurs as a result of an injury of the conus, or sacral cord, and lumbar nerve roots within the spinal canal; it produces saddle anesthesia, a reflexic bladder and bowel, and variable lower extremity weakness. *Cauda equina syndrome* is clinically similar to conus medullaris syndrome but is characterized by asymmetric lower extremity weakness.

TREATMENT

For emergency room personnel and general trauma surgeons, the main goal of initial treatment of injuries to the spine and spinal cord is to immobilize the spine to prevent further neurologic injury. After a thorough neurologic examination that includes radiologic documentation of the fractures and assessment of the patient's neurologic status, major treatment decisions regarding spinal injury will be made in conjunction with a neurosurgeon or orthopedic spine surgeon.

Evaluation and management of spinal injuries is complex, and a multitude of factors must be taken into account when formulating a treatment plan. The two major objectives are to provide the best opportunity for spinal cord recovery and to ensure skeletal stability for both the immediate and long term. These two objectives are not independent and can often be achieved with one treatment plan.

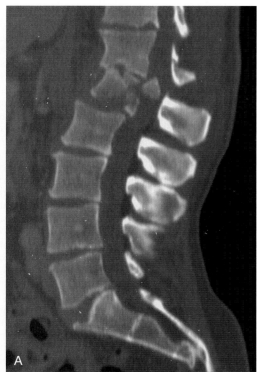

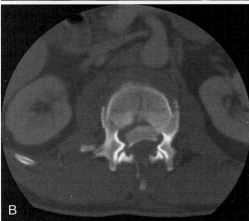

FIGURE 5 Unstable L1 burst fracture with retropulsed fragment of the vertebral body forming a characteristic "anvil" shape and resulting in spinal canal compromise.

Spinal stabilization operations are extensive with potentially significant blood loss and risk, and they should be undertaken during reasonable hours, when the spinal surgical team is available and prepared for every contingency. In patients with acute neurologic deterioration or incomplete injury and spinal canal compromise, decompression can and should be accomplished quickly. If the spine cannot be adequately stabilized at the initial operation, a subsequent formal stabilization may be required.

In patients with spinal cord injury, the primary physical injury is a result of contusion, compression, or stretching; in most cases, it is not from a transection of the spinal cord. Secondary injury, or degeneration, is a complex biochemical process that begins rapidly after the primary mechanical injury and may be attenuated by administration of corticosteroids. Current opinion is that the minor neurologic benefits of steroid therapy are greatly outweighed by the increase in infectious complications and subsequent morbidity and mortality, and most institutions no longer administer corticosteroids to patients with acute spinal cord injury.

Cervical Spine

Patients with upper cervical spine fractures are usually neurologically intact at presentation, because injury to the cervical medullary cord causes cessation of breathing and is rapidly fatal, unless endotracheal intubation and resuscitation are immediately provided. The need for decompression of the neural elements is unusual with fractures in this area, in part because the spinal canal is generous at the C1/C2 level. A hangman's fracture results in auto decompression of the spinal canal due to the laying open of the spinal canal from the fracture. Patients with odontoid fractures who present for evaluation are usually neurologically intact because spinal injury at this level is typically fatal. Therefore the major goal of treatment in patients with upper cervical spine injuries is to realign the spine as best possible and to stabilize it to allow healing either with bracing or surgical intervention.

Occipital cervical dislocations are also infrequently seen because of the generally fatal nature of this injury. If the patient does survive, occipital cervical fusion and instrumentation is the only method of definitive stabilization. These patients should not have traction administered in the early treatment stages because of the extremely unstable nature of occipital cervical dislocation; any type of traction may only exacerbate the stretching on the cervical medullary junction. Straightforward immobilization with sandbags or a carefully applied cervical collar is the treatment of choice until operative stabilization can be accomplished.

Jefferson fractures, or C1 burst fractures, can usually be treated with halo immobilization. If the degree of fracture displacement is minimal, patients with this injury may be treated with a cervical collar if they can be relied on to wear it as prescribed. At our institution, the preference is halo immobilization for these patients.

Treatment decisions are extremely complicated for patients with odontoid fractures. Type I fractures are rare and can be treated with a cervical collar. Type III fractures uniformly need immobilization and tend to heal well if proper alignment can be attained. Most patients with type III odontoid fractures at our institution are treated with halo immobilization with excellent fusion results.

Type II odontoid fractures are much more difficult to treat, and they are increasing in number due to the aging of the population. Once initial realignment is achieved, definitive stabilization can be accomplished via either halo immobilization or surgical stabilization. Halo immobilization is chosen if there is good alignment of the fracture fragment. Elderly patients or patients with displacement greater than 5 to 6 mm have a high failure rate with halo treatment. Elderly patients may have difficulty tolerating halo immobilization, and tracheostomy is used liberally in this population at our institution. Frail and elderly patients with type II odontoid fractures can occasionally be treated with only a cervical collar for comfort and may survive and end up with fibrinous healing that seems to suffice.

Patients who have adequate alignment of a type II odontoid fracture with an intact transverse ligament are candidates for odontoid screw placement. This obviates the need for halo immobilization and can be useful in elderly patients who will not tolerate halo vest immobilization. If all of these other treatment modalities fail, the standard surgical treatment is a C1/C2 posterior fusion. A number of techniques can achieve this goal, ranging from sublaminar cable techniques to atlantoaxial screw fixation. For patients with severely displaced type II fractures, fusion should be considered as an early treatment option.

Hangman's fractures can usually be treated with external immobilization if there is close approximation of the fracture fragments after reduction. With appropriate alignment, hangman's fractures show excellent healing, and it is unusual to require cervical fusion. Our institution typically uses halo immobilization for treatment of hangman's fractures, but many institutions use cervical collars to treat less significant fractures and obtain good results.

Patients with acute subaxial spine (C3/C7) injuries should have spine alignment restored as close to normal as possible and as quickly as is feasible. A major trial is currently under way to better understand the role of timing of fracture reduction and spinal cord decompression in patients with spinal cord injury. In the emergency room, the standard method of realigning the cervical spine is traction, utilizing Gardner-Wells tongs placed approximately 1 to 1.5 inches above the ear and screwed into the skull. Contraindications include skull fracture in the area where the tongs will be applied.

Most institutions now have a ready supply of halo ring devices that can be applied quickly to the cranium, and they allow a good platform for both traction and subsequent halo immobilization treatment. Once the halo ring device is placed on the skull, traction can be delivered in a straight-line fashion, beginning with approximately 3 to 5 pounds of traction for each injured level, such that a patient with a C3/C4 injury is started with 10 to 15 pounds of traction. Maximal weight that should be applied with traction is approximately 8 to 10 pounds per level. Fluoroscopy or sequential radiographs should be used to assess the results of traction as it is being administered, and to make sure that overdistraction is not occurring. Neurologic exam must be followed closely during the process to detect acute neurologic deterioration that may result from the applied traction. On occasion, reduction of a unilateral locked facet or bilateral locked facets requires a variety of maneuvers while the patient is in traction. These maneuvers include manual reduction with or without anesthesia, and they should only be performed by physicians experienced in these specialized techniques.

If reduction of a subaxial cervical spine fracture is not achieved with traction and manual attempts, operative intervention is required. A variety of techniques are used, and a general rule of thumb is to approach the problem through the avenue that exposes the most affected part of the vertebrae directly. In other words, most surgeons prefer to approach locked facets through a posterior approach, in which the facets can be unlocked, the nerve root foramina checked, and successful fusion accomplished, replacing the injured posterior structures with solid bony fusion and instrumentation.

Anterior burst fractures with retropulsed bone fragments are approached through an anterior approach, in which decompression of the spinal canal can be accomplished, followed by successful fusion. Techniques that are utilized include corpectomy with strut graft fusions and anterior cervical plating that utilizes a variety of different implants to replace the vertebral body. These implants range from fibular allograft bone struts to titanium cages and expandable constructs. A wide variety of posterior fusion techniques are available, ranging from sublaminar cables and bone graft and/or titanium rings versus lateral mass or pedicle screw-and-rod fixation. All of these techniques work well and may or may not need to be accompanied by halo immobilization or a cervical collar postoperatively.

Patients who have their subaxial cervical fracture reduced may be candidates for halo or collar immobilization, depending on the type of fracture. In general, cervical collars do not support the upper cervical spine well and do not provide rotational stability, whereas a halo vest provides good immobilization of the upper and lower cervical spine. Straightforward axial compression fractures—with no significant retropulsed bone and intact posterior elements, including the facet joints—can potentially be treated with a cervical collar. If significant compression of the vertebrae is present, or any evidence whatsoever of significant facet or lateral mass disruption, halo immobilization should be considered. Patients with foramen involvement and secondary radiculopathy may need surgical decompression and fusion if symptoms persist after fracture reduction.

Thoracic and Lumbar Spine

Choices for treatment of thoracolumbar fractures include bed rest, bracing, and surgery. Bed rest is not typically prescribed, but it is the mainstay of therapy for the occasional patient with such confounding injuries that surgery is not possible in the early stages of treatment, such as major pelvic or lower extremity fractures. Bracing of thoracolumbar fractures is frequently performed using a variety of different devices, ranging from hyperextension braces for less severe fractures to thoracolumbar sacral orthosis, used for more severe fractures or postoperative

patients. Thoracolumbar spine fractures, unlike cervical spine fractures, are not treated with traction, because it is not possible to provide enough force to reduce significant thoracolumbar fracture dislocations.

Patients with over 50% height loss of the vertebral body, greater than 30% kyphosis, or injury to two out of the three columns of the Dennis classification have unstable fractures that should be surgically stabilized. The integrity of the posterior support structure is very important in treatment decision making. Patients with wedge compression fractures that do not fit any of these criteria are treated with bracing and followed as they start to ambulate. Patients with kyphosis noted to be increasing along with continued pain are considered for surgery as well.

The specific operation performed for thoracolumbar fractures depends on the fracture type. Anterior approaches are useful for patients who have retropulsed bone fragments in the canal causing significant spinal canal compromise. These transthoracic, combined thoracoabdominal or retroperitoneal approaches to the vertebral column are typically accomplished with the assistance of a cosurgeon for exposure. Tables 1 and 2 list the incisions and complications of anterior spine exposure surgery. Corpectomy and decompression of the spinal elements is performed, followed by internal stabilization with a variety of strut grafts and anterior support with anterior lateral instrumentation. Posterior approaches use a variety of techniques including laminectomy, transpedicular decompression, and lateral extracavitary technique to decompress the spinal canal, provide anterior column support if necessary, and perform a solid posterior arthrodesis with internal stabilization. Occasionally, patients need both an anterior and posterior approach for their fractures.

Thoracolumbar burst fractures can be managed nonoperatively, if the patient is neurologically intact with a fracture deemed to be mechanically stable using the rules stated above. It is possible to have normal neurologic function in the presence of major spinal canal compromise from retropulsed bone fragments, and patients with retropulsed bone will have remodeling of the spinal canal over time, if the spine is stable and immobilized with appropriate bracing. The degree of retropulsed bone that compels the spine surgeon to operate on the neurologically intact patient is arbitrary. In general, if the canal is compromised by 50% or greater, surgical decompression is felt to be required, and compromise less than 50% can be managed without operation. Also important to consider is that a 50% spinal

TABLE 1: Anterior spine exposure incisions

Spine Anatomic Region	Incision
Cervicothoracic (C7/T2)	Oblique neck to median sternotomy High posterolateral thoracotomy
Thoracic (T3/T12)	Lateral thoracotomy Transpleural Retropleural Thoracoscopic
Thoracolumbar (T6/S1)	Thoracoabdominal Transpleural-retroperitoneal Retropleural-retroperitoneal Thoracoscopic
Lumbosacral (L2/S1)	Paramedian retroperitoneal Oblique anterolateral retroperitoneal Minilaparotomy retroperitoneal Open transabdominal (e.g., Pfannenstiel) Endoscopic transabdominal Endoscopic retroperitoneal

Data from Ikard RW: Methods and complications of anterior exposure of the thoracic and lumbar spine, *Arch Surg* 141:1025–1034, 2006.

TABLE 2: Complications of anterior spine exposure

Spine Anatomic Region	Complications
Thoracic	Pulmonary (atelectasis, pneumonia, respiratory insufficiency)
	Technical (hemothorax, pneumothorax, pleural effusion, infection, wound disruption)
	Chylothorax
	Spinal cord ischemia
	Miscellaneous (cardiopulmonary, stroke, ileus, urinary tract infection, renal failure)
Lumbar	Vascular
	Arterial injury (thrombosis, hemorrhage)
	Venous injury (hemorrhage, thrombosis)
	Neurogenic (retrograde ejaculation, groin nerve injury, warm leg)
	Wound problems (infection, disruption, hernia, muscle denervation)
	Ureteral injury
	Miscellaneous (cardiopulmonary, stroke, ileus, urinary tract infection, renal failure)

Data from Ikard RW: Methods and complications of anterior exposure of the thoracic and lumbar spine, *Arch Surg* 141:1025–1034, 2006.

canal compromise may not be as well tolerated in the thoracic spinal canal as in the lumbar spine due to the larger relative size of the thoracic cord in the spinal canal compared to the lumbar roots and canal.

Patients with incomplete injuries and thoracolumbar fractures causing significant spinal canal compromise warrant surgical decompression and stabilization as soon as reasonably possible. Factors that need to be considered include stability of the patient, the type of surgical procedure, and potential intraoperative complications. Patients with lumbar fractures with incomplete injuries tend to have a much better prognosis. Because the involved cauda equina nerve roots are lower motor neuron structures, patients with incomplete lesions and lumbar fractures can have significant recovery of neurologic function.

The prognosis for patients with complete injuries in either the thoracic, cervical, or lumbar spine is much more guarded and should be taken into account when considering the risk/benefit ratio before proceeding with urgent decompression.

OUTCOME

Patients with complete spinal cord injury are faced with a multitude of lifelong challenges. Patients with higher cord injuries obviously have poorer functional outcomes than those with lower injuries. Each segmental level that can be preserved can be important for function. For example, retaining thoracic trunk support can help a patient maintain good posture in the sitting or wheelchair position; and having a simple function, such as biceps function, can be extremely beneficial for a quadriplegic patient.

Patients with incomplete injuries have a significant chance for recovery. It is impossible to predict each individual patient's recovery level at the early stages of injury, but it is safe to assume that the more function patients have when they are first evaluated, the better their prognosis for recovery of function.

SUGGESTED READINGS

American Association of Neurological Surgery: Guidelines for the management of acute cervical spine and spinal cord injuries, *Neurosurgery* 50(suppl 3):S1–S199, 2002.
Dennis F: The three-column spine and its significance in the classification of acute thoracolumbar spine injuries, *Spine* 8:817–818, 1983.
Eastern Association for the Surgery of Trauma Practice Management Guidelines Committee: Practice management guidelines for identification of cervical spine injuries following trauma, 2009 update. Available at http://www.east.org/tpg/cspine2009.pdf.
Ikard RW: Methods and complications of anterior exposure of the thoracic and lumbar spine, *Arch Surg* 141:1025–1034, 2006.
Lindsey RW, Gugala Z, Pneumaticos SG: Injury to the vertebrae and spinal cord. In Feliciano DV, Mattox KL, Moore EE, editors: *Trauma*, ed 6, New York, 2008, McGraw-Hill.

EVALUATION AND MANAGEMENT OF FACIAL INJURIES

Michael P. Grant, MD, PhD, and
Paul N. Manson, MD

OVERVIEW

Facial injuries consist of damage to bone and soft tissue and disruption of the attachments between the two. The facial injury may be isolated or part of a multiple-system injury pattern. Multiple-system injuries that include facial injury often require a coordinated effort by general surgeons, trauma surgeons, and specialty teams. Even apparently isolated high-energy maxillofacial injuries warrant a complete evaluation by a trauma team.

EMERGENCY TREATMENT OF MAXILLOFACIAL TRAUMA

The presence of a facial injury implies a geographic (simultaneous) injury to the head, face, and neck region. Evaluation for brain injury, skull fracture, and cervical spine injury is mandatory in any patient with a maxillofacial injury to exclude serious injuries in adjacent anatomic regions. Maxillofacial trauma presents three life-threatening emergencies: 1) airway obstruction, 2) hemorrhage, 3) and aspiration.

Airway Obstruction

Airway obstruction is expected in patients with comminuted fractures of the upper and lower jaws and injuries that result in swelling or bleeding into the airway spaces (neck, pharynx, mouth, floor of the mouth, and nose). The onset of stridor, hoarseness, drooling, inability to swallow, and noisy respirations should prompt an alert clinician to urgently intubate the patient or in some cases perform a tracheostomy. Cricothyroidotomy is an emergency maneuver to access the airway through the cricothyroid membrane, and it should always be converted to tracheostomy as soon as feasible.

Life-Threatening Hemorrhage

Life-threatening hemorrhage results from two categories of injury: 1) facial and scalp lacerations and 2) closed fractures of the sinus and midface.

Facial Lacerations

Bleeding from facial lacerations is usually the result of partially or fully transected major arteries. These are controlled by direct ligation, carefully avoiding branches of the facial nerve. The partially transected artery cannot retract and will continue to bleed until effectively controlled.

Closed Fractures, Sinus Injuries, and Midface Injuries

Midface and orbital fractures produce hemorrhage from lacerations of arteries and veins in the walls, the sinus cavities, or adjacent structures. In the majority of cases, manual repositioning of the maxilla combined with anteroposterior nasal packing controls the bleeding. The maxilla is best put at rest in intermaxillary fixation (IMF). Angiographic embolization is the usual method of control in those few patients (<5%) who continue to bleed. Selective ligation of the internal maxillary artery, accessed through the posterior wall of the maxillary sinus, or bilateral external carotid and superficial temporal artery ligation can be performed, but these are seldom necessary.

Aspiration

Aspiration of oral secretions, gastric contents, or blood frequently accompanies fractures of the middle and lower face, especially with cerebral injury or depressed mental status secondary to drug or alcohol ingestion. Rapid, noisy respirations, low arterial oxygen content, and a decrease in pulmonary compliance are seen. Intubation prevents aspiration and should be performed immediately, when it becomes evident that the airway is not being protected.

Occult Injuries

The possibility of occult injuries demands a thorough, multisystem examination in every patient. Observations of other organ systems must be continued throughout the entire period of facial injury treatment. In patients with multisystem injuries, the contribution of distracting injuries must be assessed.

EARLY MANAGEMENT OF MAXILLOFACIAL TRAUMA

The early management of maxillofacial trauma comprises 1) clinical examination, 2) appropriate diagnostic imaging, and 3) definitive wound and/or fracture management.

Clinical Examination

The diagnosis of most facial injuries is accomplished by a thorough clinical examination, noting the pattern of contusions, bruises, discoloration, crepitus, pain, localized tenderness, numbness, paralysis, malocclusion, diplopia, visual acuity loss, facial asymmetry, deformity, and changes in eye position and facial contour. The care provider should assume that a fracture or foreign body underlies any soft tissue laceration, and a significant contusion or bruise marks the location of a fracture until proved otherwise.

The physical examination should be both sequential and direct, starting with an orderly examination of the facial structures in sequence from top to bottom, followed by a careful, redirected examination to those areas obviously injured. A double examination of the critical areas is thus performed. Palpation of all bony surfaces begins at the supraorbital rims around the orbit and extends to the infraorbital rims, includes the zygomatic arches and malar prominences, and concludes with an examination of the mandible, intraorally and externally in movement. Any malocclusion, crepitus, bone irregularity, or tenderness is noted.

An evaluation of facial nerve and trigeminal motor nerve function compares the two sides of the face. Facial sensation is documented in the supraorbital, corneal, infraorbital, and mental distributions (anesthesia or hypoesthesia). A search for occult lacerations in the ear canal, nose, mouth, and pharynx should be conducted. The excursion of the jaws, the relation of the teeth in occlusion, and the ability of the teeth to occlude are noted, looking for irregular arch forms and abnormalities of intercuspation of the teeth. Fractured or missing teeth, intraoral and gingival lacerations, and gaps or level discrepancies in the maxillary and mandibular dentition indicate the possibility of fractures. Lacerations of the lips, chin, and floor of the mouth often accompany anterior jaw fractures.

Visual sensory function should be evaluated in all patients with orbital trauma. Visual acuity and range of extraocular motility should be evaluated, and the presence of a relative afferent papillary defect, visual field defect, diplopia, hyphema (bleeding in the anterior chamber), periorbital ecchymosis, or subconjunctival hematoma imply the possibility of an orbital fracture or globe injury.

Alginate impressions of the dentition are taken, and stone models are prepared to provide a dental record. At the close of the physical examination, any grossly displaced midfacial or mandibular fractures can be manually repositioned, and if desired, IMF can be applied to the jaws to stabilize any fractures. The airway must be protected at all times.

Radiographs

Plain radiographs are of little value in radiographic evaluation of facial injuries, except when they may be necessary to exclude the presence of a radiopaque foreign body. The ideal examination is computed tomography (CT). Multiply injured patients should not be sent unmonitored for extensive radiographic evaluation, and such studies supplement, but do not replace, the findings of a physical examination. For most fractures, the best radiographic evaluation consists of images in all three axes—axial, sagittal, and coronal plane CT scans, including the frontal sinus, nasoethmoid, orbital, maxillary, and mandibular regions. If the patient cannot be positioned for direct coronal images, coronal images may less ideally be reconstructed from the axial CT format. A CT examination of the head or skull does not replace the need for a specific maxillofacial CT.

WOUND AND FRACTURE MANAGEMENT

Soft Tissue Injuries

Soft tissue injuries include lacerations, bruises, contusions, and hematomas. Cutaneous wounds are inspected for foreign material and assessed for depth and direction to predict deep structure involvement (probing with a cotton-tipped applicator, no sharp instruments) and to detect contamination or foreign material. Lacerations require inspection for damaged structures, followed by cleansing by scrubbing, gentle irrigation, and minimal, judicious sharp debridement of the contused tissue edge on rare occasions. A millimeter or two is usually a sufficient edge resection. A layered repair achieves a flat wound, resulting in minimal scar formation. Antibiotics are indicated when a clean wound (defined by surgical debridement) cannot be created, especially in the presence of contamination, such as an animal bite. Direct primary closure of facial wounds is always preferred, with second-look procedures at 48-hour intervals, when concern about infection or further devitalized tissue is an issue, as in the case of large degloving or avulsive wounds.

Open wound management is not used, with the possible exception of human bites. Debridement should be quite conservative in the region of the vermillion, oral commissures, eyelids, eyebrows, and distal nose. All foreign material must be meticulously removed at the time of the initial examination, because it cannot be satisfactorily removed after healing. Postoperative wound hygiene is accomplished four times daily with a 50/50 peroxide-saline solution on cotton-tipped applicators and the application of either bacitracin (facial sutures) or a combination steroid-antibiotic ophthalmic ointment (periorbital sutures). Intraoral repairs are cleansed with mouthwash and standard oral hygiene three times daily.

Any localized facial hematoma should be drained by incision, and a soft compressive dressing should be applied. Localized hematomas most commonly occur in the ear region and may involve the forehead or buccal areas. Laceration of the lacrimal system should be suspected in any wound on the nasal aspect of the upper or lower eyelids. Eyelid or periorbital lacerations raise the possibility of globe rupture or penetrating injury.

Lacerations of the facial nerve and parotid duct are managed by direct repair using loupe magnification. Parotid duct lacerations are diagnosed by inserting a #22 Angiocath sleeve (Becton Dickinson, Franklin Lakes, NJ) into the duct orifice intraorally and irrigating with saline. The presence of saline in the wound implies duct laceration.

The *Stensen duct* is a short structure that extends from the anterior margin of the parotid gland, 1 inch anterior to the tragus on a line between the tragus and floor of the nostril, to the second maxillary bicuspid. Ductal lacerations are almost always accompanied by buccal-branch facial paralysis, because the two structures are adjacent.

Cerebrospinal Fluid Rhinorrhea

Fractures involving the frontal or basilar skull may lacerate the dura, allowing cerebrospinal fluid (CSF) to exit from the nose (rhinorrhea), or fractures may allow air to enter the intracranial area (pneumocephalus). Either condition permits entry of organisms through the meninges with the possibility of meningitis. Generally, prophylactic antibiotics are used in a pulse rather than a prolonged basis in these conditions; perioperative antibiotics will accompany operative treatment when indicated. CSF rhinorrhea is detected by the presence of clear fluid exiting from the nose or pharynx. Often CSF is mixed with blood, making its detection difficult. The double-ring sign, absorption of blood and CSF onto a paper towel, produces a small, central blood ring with a large, peripheral, clearer fluid ring surrounding it. A detailed CT scan is mandatory if CSF leak or pneumocephalus is suspected.

Definitive Fracture Management by Region

Nasal Fractures

Nasal fractures produce dislocation either laterally or posteriorly or both. The diagnosis is suggested by epistaxis, bruising, swelling, lateral deviation, retrusion, and flattening of the nose in frontal impact injuries of the nasal pyramid (Figure 1). Intranasal inspection shows dislocation, deviation, or laceration of the septum with difficulty breathing. Nasal and periorbital hematomas generally accompany nasal fractures, and at least one third have a small laceration over the nasal bridge.

Classically, the radiographic evaluation consists of plain films: a nasal series, a Waters view, and sinus films. These are not particularly definitive, and again a CT scan is the best examination, making plain

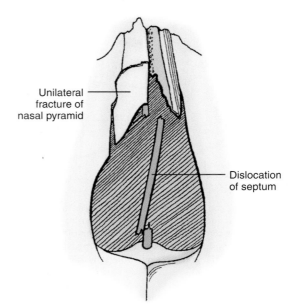

Unilateral fracture of nasal pyramid

Dislocation of septum

FIGURE I   Nasal fractures are characterized by lateral or posterior displacement, sometimes both. Both deformities require specific reduction maneuvers.

radiographs of little utility. The value of nasal radiographs in isolated low-energy injuries is both medicolegal and clinical. Adjacent bony injuries are excluded, and the exact displacement of structures, including the septum, is identified.

Treatment

Closed reduction of the septum and nasal pyramid is performed under anesthesia: less ideally, an external field block and intranasal topical Afrin (Schering-Plough, Kenilworth, NJ) are used. Laterally deviated nasal fractures are first completed by intranasal mobilization of the nasal pyramid and septum, restabilizing them in the midline and supporting them with external and internal nasal splints. The septum is straightened and centralized with an Asch forceps and supported with antibiotic-impregnated gauze packing. Frontal-impact nasal injuries produce varying degrees of nasal retrusion and may require open reduction and bone or cartilage grafting to restore projection and achieve the nasal support necessary to produce an adequate aesthetic result.

Zygomatic Fractures

The *zygoma* constitutes the malar prominence and forms the lateral and inferior walls of the orbit. The zygoma has five attachments to adjacent structures: laterally to the temporal bone, superiorly to the frontal bone, medially to the maxilla, inferiorly to the maxillary alveolus, and in the lateral orbit to the greater wing of the sphenoid (Figure 2). The diagnosis of a zygomatic fracture is suggested by the combination of a periorbital and lateral subconjunctival hematoma. These are sensitive but nonspecific signs that may accompany any orbital fracture. If the frontal process of the zygoma is dislocated inferiorly, the lateral canthus is inferiorly displaced by its attachment at the Whitnall tubercle. Depression of the malar eminence accompanies posterior displacement of the zygoma. Steps or level discrepancies may be palpated in the bone forming the inferior orbital rim or at the zygomaticofrontal suture. Intraorally, a hematoma is present in the upper buccal sulcus, and intraoral irregularity of the maxillary buttress may be palpated. Unilateral epistaxis is secondary to hemorrhage exuding through the ipsilateral maxillary antrum. If

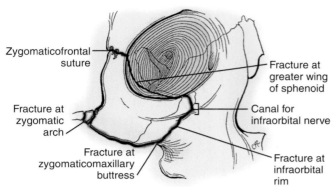

Zygomaticofrontal suture

Fracture at greater wing of sphenoid

Canal for infraorbital nerve

Fracture at zygomatic arch

Fracture at zygomaticomaxillary buttress

Fracture at infraorbital rim

FIGURE 2 The zygomatic bone constitutes the lateral and inferior portion of the orbit and malar eminence. It attaches to the frontal bone superiorly, the temporal bone posteriorly, and the maxilla medially and inferiorly. In the orbit, the alignment of the orbital process of the zygomatic bone with the greater wing of the sphenoid provides an accurate clue to reduction.

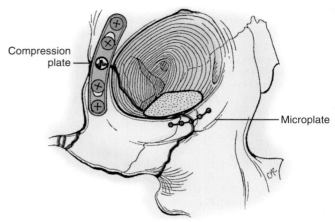

Compression plate

Microplate

FIGURE 3 Rigid internal fixation of a zygomatic fracture has been performed by applying plates and screws to the junction of the zygoma with the frontal bone and maxilla. The bone is maneuvered into position and temporarily secured with interfragment wires before rigid internal fixation is applied.

the zygoma is posteriorly or medially dislocated, difficult or painful chewing or difficulty bringing the teeth into occlusion may result from impingement of the zygomatic body or zygomatic arch on the coronoid process of the mandible, from bruising in the temporalis muscle, or from hemorrhage into the temporomandibular joint.

Orbital extraocular muscle entrapment symptoms (diplopia) result from the orbital floor fracture component and depend on the degree of involvement of extraocular muscles, with restriction of their motion by incarceration and/or entrapment in the fracture. Infraorbital nerve numbness accompanies most zygomatic fractures and is related to bruising or injury of the infraorbital nerve at the infraorbital foramen. In the case of a significant orbital fracture, globe dystopia, enophthalmos, and double vision may be present. The definitive radiographic examination of the zygomatic fractures is an axial, sagittal, and coronal CT scan with bone and soft tissue windows.

Indications for surgery include the functional symptoms produced by bone displacement, which include deformity, enophthalmos, double vision resulting from incarceration of an extraocular muscle or its surrounding fat, vertical malposition of the globe, loss of malar prominence, anesthesia of the infraorbital nerve (in medially dislocated zygomatic fractures that compress the nerve at the infraorbital foramen), radiographically extensive orbital floor fracture, and interference with the excursion of the coronoid process.

Treatment

Displaced fractures isolated to the zygomatic arch are treated by elevation through a "Gilles" approach. An incision in the temporal hair permits insertion of an elevator under the deep temporal fascia on the temporalis muscle to elevate the zygomatic arch. Because of periosteal continuity, medially displaced arch fractures are generally stable following closed reduction. Displaced zygomatic fractures not isolated to the arch are managed by open reduction and internal plate-and-screw fixation (Figure 3). Incisions for zygomatic fracture reduction consist of lower eyelid incisions (subciliary, midtarsal, or transconjunctival); gingivobuccal intraoral sulcus incision; and, in extensive fractures, a coronal incision. Simple fractures may often be reduced with a single approach. Comminuted zygomatic fractures, especially those with lateral displacement of the zygomatic arch, require three incisions, including a coronal incision.

Temporary alignment is initially achieved by placing interfragment wires at the zygomaticofrontal suture and infraorbital rim. The zygomaticomaxillary buttress, exposed through an intraoral gingivobuccal sulcus incision, is then stabilized by plate-and-screw fixation. The orbital floor is explored, and following retrieval of soft tissue

contents of the orbit from the antrum, the orbital floor is reconstituted with either alloplastic material or a thin, curved bone graft.

Nasoethmoid-Orbital Fractures

Nasoethmoid-orbital fractures are comminuted fractures of the central upper midface. They result either directly—from a blow to the glabella and upper nasal area that shatters the medial orbital rims, nose, and frontal sinus—or indirectly, by the extension of other midface or frontal fractures. One third of these fractures are unilateral. Commonly, a nasoethmoid fracture exists with a midface Le Fort fracture. The sine qua non of this fracture is the presence of breaks that isolate the lower two thirds of the medial orbital rim with the attached medial canthal ligament from adjacent bones, which allows migration (Figure 4).

The diagnosis of nasoethmoid fracture is suggested by the presence of a depressed, comminuted, frontal-impact nasal fracture. Pain and tenderness are present with direct finger pressure over the medial canthal ligament. Unilateral or bilateral eyelid (spectacle) hematomas are usually present. Nasal lacerations are present in 50% of patients, and epistaxis invariably accompanies this injury. A foreshortened, depressed nose is usually accompanied by telecanthus. Crepitation is present on palpating the nose, and a CSF leak, pneumocephalus, or orbital emphysema may be present.

Traumatic telecanthus is measured by an increase in the distance between the medial commissures of the eyelids. This distance normally equals the length of a palpebral fissure. A high index of suspicion is necessary to confirm the diagnosis of traumatic telecanthus in patients with minimal displacement or impacted fractures. Mobility of the medial orbital rim may also be detected on "bimanual examination" with simultaneous intranasal-extranasal examination. A palpating finger placed externally against the bone bearing the medial canthal ligament attachment detects movement of the bone produced by the tip of a clamp placed in the nose under the canthal ligament. Movement of the medial orbital rim confirms the presence of a fracture that will require open reduction. The definitive radiographic examination consists of axial, sagittal, and coronal CT scans.

Treatment

Treatment should generally be accomplished as soon as reasonably possible because of the high frequency of associated CSF leaks, frontal sinus fractures, and pneumocephalus. The fracture is exposed with coronal lower eyelid and gingivobuccal sulcus incisions, so

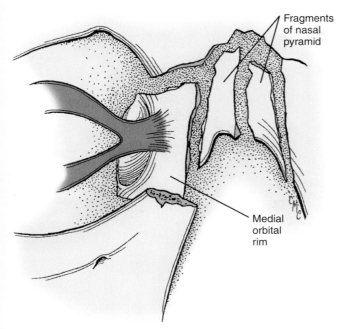

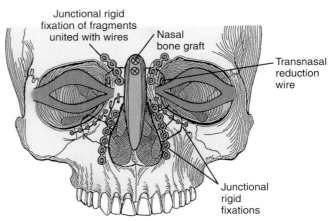

FIGURE 5 Scheme for open reduction and internal fixation of a nasoethmoid orbital fracture. Initially, the fracture fragments are maneuvered into position and temporarily held with interosseous wires. Plate-and-screw fixation is then applied. The two frontal processes of the maxilla are linked by a transnasal reduction wire and passed from one frontal process of the maxilla to the other at the posterior and superior edge of the lacrimal fossa.

FIGURE 4 The central segment of a nasoethmoid orbital fracture is the lower two thirds of the medial-orbital rim. Here the medial canthal ligament attaches to the frontal process of the maxilla. Dislocation of the frontal process of the maxilla dislocates the canthal ligament, producing canthal instability.

that the entire frontal-nasomaxillary buttress is visualized. Initially, fracture fragments are linked together with interosseous wires and then stabilized by plate-and-screw fixation (Figure 5). Reconstruction of the integrity of the internal orbit and nose is accomplished by inserting bone grafts in the nose and either bone graft or alloplastic material to replace orbital wall defects. The repair will reconstitute the orbital volume, nasal height, contour, and projection. Bone grafts replace critical areas of structural bone loss. If the medial canthus is detached from the frontal process of the maxilla, it is reattached by a transnasal canthopexy posterior and superior to the lacrimal fossa.

Frontobasilar Fractures

Frontobasilar fractures include fractures of the frontal bone, frontal sinus, supraorbital rims, and anterior cranial base. Anterior cranial base fractures often accompany frontal vault skull fractures and supraorbital, nasoethmoid, and frontal sinus fractures. High Le Fort (II or III) fractures are often accompanied by a fracture of the frontobasilar region.

The diagnosis of frontobasilar fracture is suggested by frontal contusions and lacerations, periorbital hematomas or swelling (the spectacle hematoma is a classic symptom of an anterior cranial base fracture), the presence of CSF leak, pneumocephalus, hemotympanum, frontal lobe injury symptoms (confusion, coma, and somnolence), epistaxis, anosmia, and visual impairment. The definitive radiographic examination is an axial and coronal CT scan of the frontal bone, frontal sinus, and anterior cranial fossa.

Frontal Sinus Fractures

The frontal sinus consists of two asymmetric cavities separated by one or more bony partitions. The size of the frontal sinus is quite variable, from almost nothing to pneumatization of the entire frontal bone and orbital roof. The most common symptoms of a frontal sinus fracture are lacerations, contusion, or bruises in the forehead area. Often these are the only physical signs of a fracture, and their presence should prompt a CT scan. Epistaxis is usually present. In severe

cases, a deformity or depression of the glabellar area may be seen, especially after resolution of the swelling. A CSF leak, pneumocephalus, or orbital emphysema may be noted. Radiographic examination consists of axial and coronal CT scans.

Treatment

Nondisplaced fractures without duct obstruction require only observation if they are confined to the anterior wall. Depressed fractures of the anterior wall that do not obstruct patency of the nasofrontal duct (Figure 6) can be treated by elevation and conservative mucosal debridement. Fractures blocking the nasofrontal ducts are treated either by obliteration with bone or cranialization of the sinus cavity after removing the mucosa. Posterior wall fractures imply the possibility of a dural laceration. Nondisplaced posterior wall fractures can be observed if duct obstruction is not present; however, posterior wall fractures displaced more than the thickness of the inner table may require surgical exploration. If the posterior wall of the frontal sinus is fractured, the integrity of the dura must be confirmed.

When enough of the sinus is destroyed, and there is a chance that it will not function, sinus mucosa may be removed both by stripping and light abrasion of the bony walls of the sinus cavity to eliminate microscopic invaginations of mucous membrane into the bone. Both nasofrontal ducts are then plugged with "formed to fit" calvarial bone grafts. The remainder of the sinus may then be obliterated with bone shavings or allowed to sclerose by the process of osteogenesis, a slow formation of scar tissue in the frontal sinus cavity containing small amounts of bone. The procedure of cranialization implies removal of the posterior wall, sealing the ducts with calvarial bone grafts following thorough removal of the mucosal membrane, and reconstruction of the anterior wall. In effect, the procedure of cranialization converts the sinus to a portion of the intracranial cavity (Figure 7). The anterior bony wall of the sinus may be reconstructed by bone grafts where appropriate.

Supraorbital Fractures

Supraorbital fractures are suggested by the presence of bruises or lacerations in the area, a depression of the supraorbital region, a downward and outward protrusion of the globe, ptosis, components of the superior orbital fissure or orbital apex syndromes, and in some

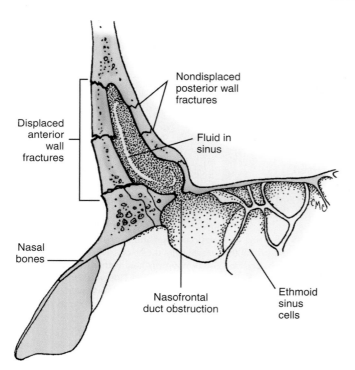

FIGURE 6 Depressed fractures of the anterior wall of the frontal sinus are treated by evaluation following mucosal debridement. Fractures blocking the duct are treated by obliteration of the sinus cavity, as absence of duct function would create an abscess. Fractures of the posterior wall of the frontal sinus imply the possibility of a dural laceration. Generally, displaced fractures of the posterior wall of the frontal sinus require surgical exploration.

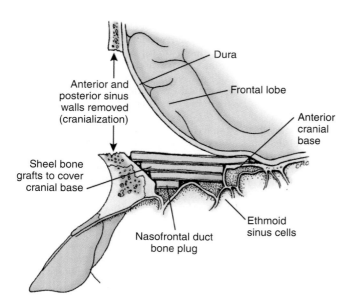

FIGURE 7 The procedure of cranialization of the frontal sinus involves removal of the posterior wall and all of the mucosa, sealing the nasal frontal ducts with bone grafts, and using bone grafting to fix defects in the anterior cranial fossa (floor of the frontal sinus). The anterior wall of the sinus is then reconstructed, either with the preserved fracture fragments of the anterior wall or with the bone grafts. Here, the sinus is being cranialized with the reconstruction of the anterior wall to follow.

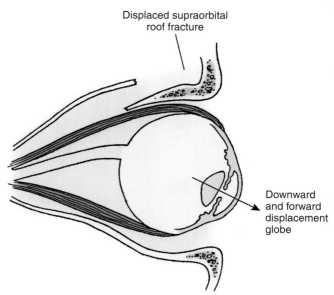

FIGURE 8 Displaced supraorbital fractures produce a downward deformity of the orbital roof. The globe is dislocated downward and forward, producing exophthalmos; reduction of the fracture corrects the eye position.

cases a superior gaze paresis that may mimic inferior rectus entrapment (Figure 8). A "step" or bone discontinuity may be palpated in the supraorbital rim, and numbness may occur in the distribution of the supraorbital or supratrochlear nerves. Radiographic examination consists of axial, sagittal, and coronal CT scans.

Treatment

The treatment of displaced supraorbital fractures involves confirmation of the integrity of the dura, replacement of bone pieces into the proper position, and direct stabilization by interosseous wiring or plate-and-screw fixation. Damaged segments of the orbital roof are replaced by repositioning or bone grafting. Frontal sinus involvement is frequent in supraorbital fractures and is managed as described. Exposure for operative reduction may occasionally be accomplished through a local laceration, but it generally requires a coronal incision.

Fractures of the Orbit

Isolated fractures of the internal portion of the orbit are accompanied by globe injury in 30% of patients. The minimal visual sensory examination consists of an assessment of visual acuity, confrontation fields, extraocular motility, examination of the anterior and posterior chambers, and a determination of intraocular pressure. The pupillary size and reaction must be assessed and compared bilaterally to exclude the presence of a relative afferent papillary defect. Subtle physical signs of an optic nerve injury are a decreased red saturation test and decreased color vision; with more significant injuries, an obvious reduction in central visual acuity may be observed.

Orbital Floor Fractures

The diagnosis of an orbital floor fracture is suggested by periorbital and subconjunctival hematomas. Anesthesia is invariably present in the infraorbital sensory nerve distribution, which produces cutaneous anesthesia of the ipsilateral nose, cheek, and upper lip and anesthesia of the anterior maxillary teeth on the affected side. Diplopia can be present in primary central gaze or in looking up or down or left or right, by virtue of contusion or entrapment of the fascial system of the rectus muscles. Exophthalmos is often present initially, because of swelling, and it is followed by enophthalmos when enlargement of the orbital cavity allows retrusion of the globe into the orbit as the swelling resolves. Acute posttraumatic enophthalmos implies a significant injury that will require a surgical repair. Inferior and medial displacement of the globe accompanies posterior displacement. Orbital emphysema and ipsilateral epistaxis are usually present. Topical anesthesia, instilled into the conjunctival sac, allows the performance of a forced-duction examination when indicated: the globe is manually rotated after grasping the insertion of the inferior rectus muscle through the conjunctiva with a forceps. More difficult rotation implies incarceration of the muscle or its ligament system, which would benefit from operative reduction.

The radiographic examination consists of axial, sagittal, and coronal CT scans with soft-tissue and bone windows. Indications for surgery are enophthalmos, entrapment of a muscle (diagnosed by restrictive strabismus producing double vision in a field of gaze controlled by the muscle), forced-duction examination and/or CT confirmation, and vertical or anterior-posterior malposition of the globe. Anesthesia of the infraorbital nerve usually resolves without treatment. If massive destruction of an orbital floor is seen on CT scan in the absence of globe malposition, reconstruction of the orbit is indicated to prevent late globe malposition.

Treatment

Surgical treatment consists of an exposure of the defect through a lower eyelid incision (subciliary, midtarsal, or transconjunctival) with dissection of the orbital floor and removal of any incarcerated tissue from the maxillary sinus. The orbital floor is then reconstituted with alloplastic material (Supramid [S. Jackson, Alexandria, Va.] and Medpor [Porex Surgical Products, Newnan, Ga.]) or curved bone grafts harvested from the calvarium, rib, or iliac region; the calvarium is preferred, because the head is a "self-contained reconstructive unit" (after Tessier).

Medial Orbital Wall Fractures

Medial orbital wall fractures are suggested by the presence of periorbital and subconjunctival hematoma, diplopia when looking laterally or medially, orbital emphysema, epistaxis, enophthalmos, and medial displacement of the globe. The radiographic examination consists of axial and coronal CT scans with both bone and soft-tissue windows.

The indications for surgery are radiographic entrapment of the medial rectus muscle with positive forced duction (rare medial-to-lateral rotation of the globe) and the presence of enophthalmos, either on physical examination or the prediction of such an occurrence on the basis of radiographic evidence of an extensive medial orbital wall fracture (Figure 9).

Treatment

Surgical treatment is accomplished by a medial conjunctival or coronal incision with removal of incarcerated tissue from the crushed ethmoid sinuses and reconstruction of the medial orbital wall with alloplastic material or bone grafts. Patients with orbital fractures should refrain from blowing their noses for 1 month.

Le Fort (Maxillary) Fractures

Le Fort, or maxillary, fractures are classified according to a pattern described by Rene Le Fort in 1901 (Figure 10). A Le Fort I fracture is a horizontal or transverse maxillary fracture separating the maxillary alveolus from the upper midfacial skeleton. A Le Fort II (pyramidal fracture) separates a central, pyramid-shaped nasomaxillary segment from the zygomatic and orbital portions of the facial skeleton. A Le Fort III fracture is a craniofacial dysjunction separating the facial

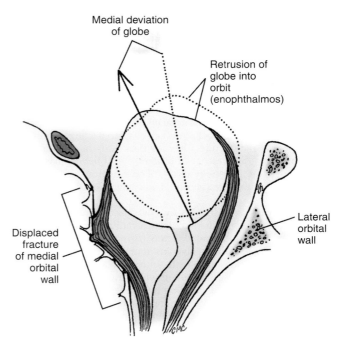

FIGURE 9 Displaced fractures of the medial orbital wall crush the ethmoid sinus and expand the orbital volume. The surgical treatment consists of inserting bone grafts to narrow the volume of the orbit. The soft tissue is removed from its prolapsed position into the fracture site.

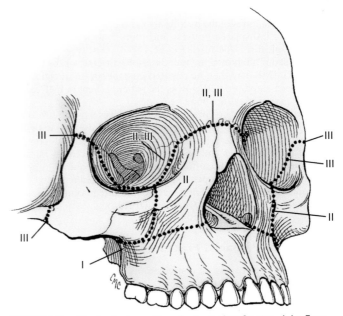

FIGURE 10 The Le Fort maxillary fracture classification. A Le Fort I fracture is a horizontal fracture separating the maxillary alveolus from the upper midfacial skeleton. The Le Fort II, or pyramidal fracture, separates a central, pyramid-shaped nasomaxillary segment from the upper midfacial skeleton. The Le Fort III fracture is a craniofacial disjunction in which the midface is fractured through the upper portion of the orbits. Generally, Le Fort II and III fractures do not exist as single segments but display comminution.

bones from the cranial skeleton through the upper portion of the nose and the lateral and medial orbits.

Most Le Fort II and III fractures are comminuted and consist of combinations of lesser Le Fort fragments, such as simultaneous fractures at the Le Fort I, II, and III levels. The injury is usually worse on one side than the other; commonly, a Le Fort III superior-level fracture is seen on one side with a Le Fort II superior-level fracture on the other. Single-fragment Le Fort III fractures are unusual and frequently are accompanied by bilateral eyelid hematomas, no maxillary mobility, and a slight malocclusion (half cusp), reflecting the minimal displacement of the fracture. They are thus easily missed on physical examination. The presence of bilateral eyelid hematomas should always suggest the possibility of a Le Fort fracture. Also, if fluid is seen in both maxillary sinuses on CT scan, a Le Fort fracture should be suspected.

The physical diagnosis of a Le Fort fracture rests on malocclusion and mobility of the maxillary alveolus in reference to the lower midfacial craniofacial skeleton. This mobility is confirmed by grasping the maxillary alveolus and testing for movement, holding the cranium stable with the contralateral hand. Upper Le Fort fractures possess signs of zygomatic, orbital, nasal, and nasoethmoid fractures, depending on the level and extent of the injury. When Le Fort fractures are not treated, midfacial proportions change, and midfacial elongation and retrusion follow. Profuse nasopharyngeal bleeding initially accompanies Le Fort fractures; marked facial and eyelid swelling also occur. CSF leak, pneumocephalus, and orbital emphysema occur less frequently in Le Fort II and III fractures, and 10% to 15% of Le Fort fractures are accompanied by palatal alveolar fractures that divide the maxillary alveolus in an anteroposterior plane ("sagittal fracture" of the maxilla), making treatment more complicated. The radiographic examination consists of axial and coronal CT scans with bone and soft-tissue windows.

Treatment

Treatment is accomplished by placing the patient in IMF in occlusion. Sagittal fractures of the maxilla are managed by plate-and-screw fixation at each displaced buttress, including the roof of the mouth and at the piriform aperture. The Le Fort I fracture is treated by plate-and-screw fixation at the four anterior buttresses of the maxilla (Figure 11). IMF may then be released postoperatively if rigid fixation has been employed. Otherwise, the patient is kept in IMF for a 6 to 8 week period to ensure bone healing.

The treatment of a Le Fort II fracture involves exposure through a lower eyelid incision (subciliary, midtarsal, or lower orbital rim), with a reduction of the orbital floor or medial orbital wall components of these fractures and open reduction of the central midface and nasoethmoid area. A coronal incision may be required in upper Le Fort II fractures for an open reduction and internal fixation of the nasofrontal area. Upper Le Fort fractures are often accompanied by simultaneous fractures in the frontobasilar region.

Complex or Panfacial Fractures

Panfacial fractures consist of combinations of frontal, midface, and mandibular fractures. The treatment consists of reconstructing the lower face as one unit and reconstructing the upper face as a separate unit, relating both units to the cranial base in their proper relationship. The upper face is then reconstructed to the lower face at the Le Fort I level, and both the horizontal and vertical portions of the mandible are stabilized with open reduction. The upper midface, the orbits and nasoethmoid area, is stabilized to the frontal bone and cranial base and then linked to the stabilized lower face (mandible and Le Fort I segment) at the Le Fort I level. Previously, as an initial step, the maxilla is aligned with the mandible and the dental arches through IMF.

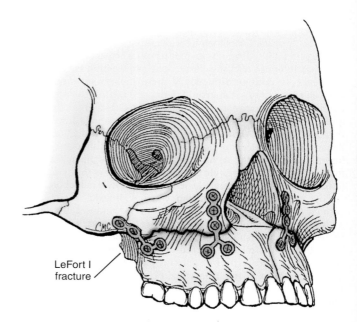

FIGURE 11 A Le Fort I fracture has been treated by plate-and-screw fixation at the four anterior buttresses of the maxilla at the Le Fort I level. The patient is initially placed in IMF. The fracture fragments are aligned, and fixation is applied to stabilize the reduction. Postoperatively the IMF can be released because of the stability of plate-and-screw fixation.

Mandibular Fractures

Mandibular fractures are one of the most common facial injuries. In the horizontal mandible and the tooth-bearing area, they are usually compounded into the mouth; less commonly, they are compounded through the skin. Fractured, loose, or broken teeth, bleeding from a tooth socket, and intraoral lacerations imply the presence of a mandible fracture. One third of such fractures occur in the condylar-subcondylar area, one third occurs in the region of the angle, and the other third occur in the body, symphysis, and parasymphysis areas (Figure 12), which represent weaker areas of the mandible. The angle is weakened by the presence of the third molar tooth and, anteriorly, the parasymphysis by the long root of the cuspid tooth and the mental foramen.

The subcondylar area represents a thin region in the mandible. More than 50% of mandibular fractures are comminuted; therefore the presence of a single mandibular fracture prompts a thorough search for a second or third fracture, often present contralaterally. Known combinations such as parasymphysis and contralateral subcondylar, parasymphysis and contralateral angle, or symphysis with unilateral or bilateral subcondylar fractures are frequent. The diagnosis of a mandibular fracture is suggested by pain; swelling; abnormal occlusion; numbness in the distribution of the mental nerve (lower lip); swelling; bruises; extraoral or intraoral lacerations; bleeding from a tooth socket; fractured or missing teeth; trismus, or pain on moving the jaw; inability to bring the teeth into occlusion, which may occur anteriorly, laterally, or bilaterally; abnormality or irregularity in dental arch form; malocclusion of the teeth; steps or level discrepancies in bone; or gaps detected either in the dentition or by palpating the mandible. Bleeding from the ear canal implies the possibility of a condylar fracture. In some cases, a segment of the dental alveolus is separated from the lower portion of the mandible and constitutes an alveolar fracture, which may occur alone or in the presence of more extensive mandibular fractures. An unpleasant odor in the mouth is present soon after mandibular fractures occur.

The plain radiographic examination includes posteroanterior (PA), lateral oblique, and Towne films of the mandible. Seldom are

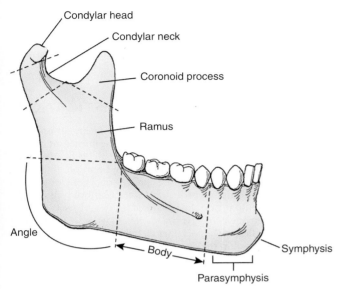

FIGURE 12 The anatomic region of the mandible includes the condylar and subcondylar areas, the angle, and the body; the symphysis and parasymphysis areas lie anteriorly. Weak areas are the subcondylar region; the angle, weakened by the third molar; and the parasymphysis area, weakened by the long root of the cuspid.

plain radiographs taken, but a CT scan for the condylar, coronoid, and ramus areas and horizontal portion of the mandible is routine. The Panorex examination is the one helpful "plain film," but it requires a cooperative patient who is able to stand, and often it cannot be obtained urgently. Occlusal and apical dental films are sometimes required to visualize specific areas of the teeth to examine for root fracture and apical or tooth root pathology.

Treatment

The treatment of mandibular fracture includes the application of arch bars to the teeth, placing the teeth of the mandible in IMF in occlusion with the maxilla. IMF is continued for 4 to 8 weeks, unless rigid internal fixation or the ability to spontaneously bring the jaws into proper occlusion permits immediate mobilization. Closed reduction is appropriate for many condylar, coronoid, and ramus fractures and those stable fractures in the angle that are not displaced. Displaced fractures in the horizontal mandible require open reduction with plate-and-screw fixation. Exposure is obtained intraorally, the preferred exposure for the anterior portion of the horizontal segment of the mandible. Angle fractures may be treated intraorally if simple and extraorally if comminuted. Condylar and subcondylar fractures that require open reduction, those that would result in mechanical interference with mandibular motion or a loss of ramus height, are exposed with a preauricular, upper mesh or intraoral ramus incision for fixation.

Patients who require IMF are given a blenderized diet, and the average patient with IMF loses 15 to 20 lb in 4 to 6 weeks. The use of rigid internal fixation (plate-and-screw fixation) allows many patients to immediately move the mandible, to have better oral hygiene, and to take a soft diet. Occlusion must be observed at least weekly in these patients to detect any displacement.

Gunshot and Shotgun Wounds

Gunshot wounds of low velocity may be managed as facial fractures with overlying lacerations. The soft-tissue injury is carefully excised and closed. High-velocity gunshot or close-range shotgun wounds produce extensive damage to, and loss of, soft-tissue and bone. A zone of soft-tissue and bone loss and a separate zone of soft-tissue and bone injury are characteristic. The bones are immediately stabilized in anatomic position in all regions by rigid internal fixation. Areas of bone loss are stabilized, preserving the length-of-bone defects to achieve anatomic reconstruction of the bone fracture to normal dimensions. Soft-tissue closure is obtained either by advancement or skin-to-mucosa closure after conservative debridement.

Serial second-look procedures are required at 48 hour intervals, until no further devitalized tissue is seen. Soft tissue reconstruction may then be completed, and distant flap transfer is usually required for intraoral lining and sinus obliteration. At the time of flap transfer, composite replacement of bone and soft tissue may be considered, or soft-tissue reconstruction may be accomplished first and then bone reconstruction secondarily. The bone defects resulting from missing bone are maintained by rigid internal fixation, until bone grafting can be performed.

Late Scarring from Wounds

Generally, it takes 1 to 2 years for a cutaneous scar to fully mature. A red, raised scar that is initially quite prominent and shows some soft-tissue contracture may resolve satisfactorily with time. Patients who understand the course of scar maturation can be patient through the healing process. Early scar revisions are not indicated; in fact, they are discouraged except in the cases of malalignment of tissues or contracture of the type that causes functional problems, such as ectropion and corneal exposure or oral incompetence.

SUMMARY

The face is of supreme importance in communication, nutrition, perception, and interpersonal relationships. The aesthetic attractiveness of an individual's facial features influences his or her personality and success. Although there are few facial emergencies, the literature has consistently underemphasized the advantage of prompt, definitive reconstruction of facial injuries and the contribution of early anatomic skeletal reconstruction to superior aesthetic results. It is not unusual for a victim of a multiple injury to be principally concerned about residual facial deformity after life-threatening injuries have been resolved. The early definitive care of maxillofacial injuries is safe and possible and will repay the surgeon with superior results and grateful patients. A coordinated reconstruction is accomplished by interspecialty communication. All patients require counseling and rehabilitation, and psychological dividends result from these efforts.

SUGGESTED READINGS

Clark N, Manson P: Complication in maxillofacial trauma. In Maull KI, Rodriguez A, Wiles CM, editors: *Complications in trauma and critical care*, Philadelphia, 1996, WB Saunders.

David DJ, Simpson DA: *Craniomaxillofacial trauma*, New York, 1995, Churchill Livingstone.

Dufresne C, Manson P: Facial injuries in children. In Mathes S, editor: *Plastic surgery*, vol 3, part 2, New York, 2005, Elsevier, p 381.

Fonseca R, Walker R: *Oral and maxillofacial trauma*, Philadelphia, 1991, WB Saunders.

Manson P: Facial injuries. In Mathes, editor: *Plastic surgery*, vol 3, part 2, New York, 2005, Elsevier, p 77.

Manson P, Vander Kolk C, Dufresne C: Facial trauma. In Oldham K, Columbani P, Foglia R, editors: *Surgery of infants and children*, Philadelphia, 2005, Lippincott-Raven.

Manson PN: Reoperative facial fracture surgery. In Grotting J, editor: *Reoperative plastic surgery*, St Louis, 2006, Quality Medical Publishing.

Mueller RV: Soft tissue injuries. In Mathes S, editor: *Plastic surgery*, vol 3, part 2, New York, 2005, Elsevier.

Williams JL, editor: *Rowe and Williams maxillofacial injuries*, Edinburgh, 1994, Churchill Livingstone.

Wolf A, Baker SA: *Facial fractures*, New York, 1993, Thieme.

Penetrating Neck Trauma

Charles E. Lucas, MD, and Anna M. Ledgerwood, MD

OVERVIEW

The neck may be divided into bilateral anterior and posterior triangles by the sternocleidomastoid (SCM) muscles. Wounds to the posterior cervical triangles require operative management only for the control of bleeding and repair of wounds; there are no hidden structures that lead to late complications when not treated promptly.

Consequently, the challenges regarding care of penetrating neck wounds relate to injuries in the anterior triangles. These challenges include 1) emergent airway control, 2) immediate control of active bleeding, 3) urgent operative treatment of major injuries not causing acute airway compromise or life-threatening bleeding, 4) urgent diagnostic investigations for patients not requiring emergent or urgent operation, 5) deciding whether to explore or observe stable patients, 6) optimal exposure for patients requiring operation, and 7) care of specific injuries.

EMERGENT AIRWAY PROBLEMS

Potentially life-threatening airway injuries may be caused by tracheal or cartilaginous rupture, soft-tissue compression of the airway from adjacent arterial injury, or active hemorrhage into the tracheobronchial tree due to a vascular-airway fistula. Air escape through the skin wound, dyspnea, stridor, hoarseness, or significant subcutaneous emphysema points toward airway disruption. The stable patient with hemoptysis wishes to sit up and lean forward in order to efficiently expectorate blood that enters the airway. Forcing the patient to lie down should be avoided until all preparations have been made for a rapid sequence intubation (RSI).

Ideally, the intubation is performed in the operating room by experienced anesthesia personnel. When excessive bleeding into the oral cavity is not present, an oral intubation should be successful; when bleeding obscures the passages, a fiberoptic nasotracheal intubation may be accomplished by experienced personnel. Although a coniotomy (cricothyroidotomy) is usually not needed in this circumstance, the resuscitation team should be mentally prepared to utilize this approach in patients suspected of having airway rupture.

Significant hemoptysis portends an arterial tracheal fistula; when the endotracheal tube is inserted, the balloon should be inflated at or below the site where the fistula is most likely located. Likewise, when a coniotomy is needed, the tracheostomy tube balloon should be positioned to occlude the fistula. After airway control, immediate neck exploration is performed.

EXTERNAL BLEEDING

Major external bleeding or a pulsatile hematoma are indicative of an artery injury. Direct digital pressure with the gloved finger is the optimal way to provide temporary control of bleeding while the patient is taken to the operating room. Wraps and compression dressings are ineffective and potentially dangerous. The digital control of bleeding is maintained during RSI and the preoperative prep of the operative field.

URGENT OPERATION

Patients without life-threatening signs of airway injury or compromise and without uncontrolled external bleeding require urgent operation when hard signs indicate major injury. These signs include a large hematoma, pulsatile hematoma, continued oozing, cervical crepitus, hoarseness, dyspnea, and large wounds with severance of soft tissues that need reapproximation.

URGENT DIAGNOSTIC INVESTIGATION

Patients without the above needs for emergent or urgent operative intervention need to have diagnostic studies performed to exclude a subtle injury to important structures. These patients may have soft signs following a penetrating wound in the mid portion of the neck such as superficial bleeding from the skin or subcutaneous tissue, a history of bleeding prior to arrival, hoarseness, a bruit, dysphagia, blood-streaked sputum, or mild neck swelling.

The first component of this urgent investigation is a thorough physical examination of the neck that includes an intraoral examination to look for blood in the oral cavity and the hypopharynx. Chest auscultation and examination for trachea deviation help identify a pneumothorax from a thoracic outlet injury. Chest radiographs will confirm or rule out a pneumothorax or hemothorax, and tracheal or esophageal penetration may be identified by combined endoscopy of the trachea and esophagus. However, small injuries may be missed with these procedures. Barium swallow, which is potentially hazardous and fails to identify some injuries, is not recommended. CT angiogram, formal angiography, or color-flow duplex ultrasound will help identify arterial injury. All these procedures should be promptly available in the trauma center to provide care for patients with penetrating neck wounds.

NECK EXPLORATION VERSUS OBSERVATION

The decision to explore a penetrating neck wound in a stable patient without the so-called hard signs depends upon the diagnostic findings and the zone in which the injury occurred (Figure 1). The anterior cervical triangles can be divided into three zones. Zone 1 is sometimes referred to as the *thoracic outlet* and extends from the clavicle to the cricoid cartilage. A decision to explore zone 1 injuries would be made on the basis of confirmed injury to the named vessels, trachea, or esophagus. Zone 2 of the anterior triangles extends from the cricoid to the angle of the mandible. Formerly, all patients who had penetration of the platysma muscle in zone 2 underwent mandatory exploration. Most surgeons would now explore zone 2 injuries only for patients who have evidence of organ injury, hematoma, continued bleeding, or high suspicion for tracheal or esophageal injury. Zone 3 of the anterior triangles extends from the mandible to the base of the skull. The decision to explore zone 3 injuries would be based upon angiographic evidence of arterial injury.

OPERATIVE EXPOSURE

Most penetrating cervical wounds are best explored through an ipsilateral incision along the anterior border of the SCM muscle (see Figure 1). The incision is extended through the platysma into the deeper planes; the trachea and thyroid gland are retracted anteriorly, and the neurovascular bundle and esophagus are displaced posteriorly. This exposes the tracheoesophageal groove and allows the operator to identify when further dissection is needed anteriorly or posteriorly. Superficial crossing veins are divided and ligated along with the omohyoid muscle, thus facilitating deeper dissection.

When a zone 3 injury requires repair of the internal carotid artery at the base of the skull, the mandible can be detached posterior to the angle and subluxated anteriorly to facilitate a direct primary repair. When the injury involves zone 1 structures in the thoracic outlet,

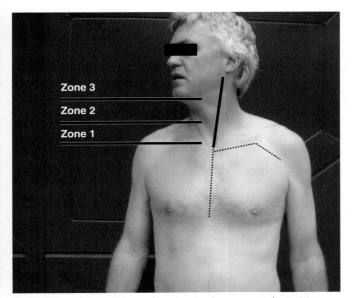

FIGURE I   Zones of the neck and optimal exposures. An incision along the anterior border of the sternocleidomastoid muscle provides access to zone 1 and zone 2 injuries. Extension of this incision inferiorly as a median sternotomy exposes anterior mediastinal injury. A lateral extension along the medial half of the clavicle and then over the cephalic vein gives access to the subclavian vessels.

the incision can be extended as a median sternotomy, thereby giving excellent exposure of the trachea, innominate artery, left common carotid artery, subclavian artery, subclavian veins, innominate vein, and superior vena cava. When the injury involves the subclavian vessels as they pass laterally, the incision can be tied off over the medial half of the clavicle and then over the basilic vein, where it passes posterior to the mid-clavicle (see Figure 1). Resection of the medial head of the clavicle facilitates exposure, control, and repair of the subclavian arteries and subclavian veins. Rarely, a bilateral incision along the anterior border of the SCM muscles is required for bilateral injuries. We prefer not to combine bilateral incisions by joining them just superior to the manubrium.

REPAIR OF SPECIFIC INJURIES

Venous Injuries

Venous injuries are the most common cause of non–life-threatening hemorrhage from penetrating neck wounds. Small veins, including the external jugular vein, are best ligated. The internal jugular vein often can be repaired primarily using a running, nonabsorbable fine suture. When there are large through-and-through wounds to the internal jugular vein, the vein should be ligated, which is well tolerated by trauma patients.

Arterial Injuries

After proximal control is obtained, dissection should begin just above the clavicle and proceed distally. Digital pressure of the area of injury is maintained while distal control is obtained. Once exposure is obtained, most arterial injuries can be treated by a primary lateral repair using a running 5-0 nonabsorbable suture. When there is more extensive arterial injury from a gunshot wound, the segment is resected. When the gap is 1 cm long or less, an end-to-end anastomosis can be accomplished. Resection of longer segments requires a reversed saphenous vein graft interposition. Prosthetic grafts should

be avoided, unless the patient has no saphenous vein. We prefer to instill a local heparin solution proximally and distally without using total body heparinization. A temporary arterial shunt should be used when the arterial repair cannot be performed promptly (within 30 minutes) because of higher treatment priorities elsewhere.

For zone 2 injuries, the branches of the external carotid artery can be safely ligated. When there is disruption at the carotid bifurcation, the intact external carotid artery can be anastomosed to the internal carotid artery distal to the area of irreparable damage. The distal stump of the external carotid artery is ligated.

Primary carotid arterial repair in patients with a neurologic neural deficit is controversial. This concern, in part, reflects the fear that a primary repair will convert an ischemic stroke into a hemorrhagic stroke. The authors recommend repair in this setting, because patients who subsequently succumb have diffuse cerebral edema without hemorrhage at the time of the postmortem examination. Control of intracerebral pressure in these patients may lead to survival.

Esophageal Injuries

Exposure of the esophagus through the anterior SCM approach permits the esophagus to be freed up from the trachea anteriorly and the prevertebral fascia posteriorly, where it can be surrounded with a Penrose drain. The presence of a nasogastric (NG) tube facilitates identification and safe digital mobilization of the esophagus. Once mobilized, most unilateral stab wounds can be repaired in two layers, being certain to incorporate the full-thickness mucosal and muscular wall in the inverted inner layer with an absorbable suture. The second layer of the muscular esophagus can be performed with interrupted 4-0 permanent sutures. With bilateral injury, the esophagus can be rotated to facilitate bilateral simple repair. Alternatively, the injury on the ipsilateral side of the esophagus can be slightly extended to permit the contralateral wound to be closed from the intraluminal approach. The ipsilateral wound can then be closed as described above. It is essential to identify all injuries to prevent an esophageal cutaneous fistula from a missed injury.

Following closure, a paraesophageal drain should be left in place. If any drainage exudes, it should be monitored for amylase. The likelihood of an esophageal cutaneous fistula is low for patients who have early operative intervention. Once a fistula is confirmed, NG tube feedings are instituted, while the fistula closes within the ensuing three weeks. The NG tube is left in place to allow immediate feeding postoperatively.

Pharyngeal Injuries

Perforations of the pharynx and hypopharynx are often suspected when blood is seen on the deep oral examination, and it may be confirmed at operation by following the penetrating wound tract to the perforation. Primary closure with full-thickness inverted bites of tissue using absorbable suture provides both hemostasis and a secure closure.

Tracheal and Cartilaginous Injuries

Through the anterior SCM approach, the trachea is freed up posteriorly by blunt dissection in the tracheoesophageal groove. Perforations of the posterior wall can be repaired with running or interrupted 3-0 absorbable sutures with the knots tied on the outside. Identification of a posterior wound is essential to be certain there is no adjacent esophageal injury. Closure of perforations of the anterior wall often require that sutures be placed in the inner space above the superior tracheal ring and below the inferior tracheal ring at the site of injury; the knots are tied on the outside. Cartilaginous injuries, likewise, can be repaired with sutures heavy enough to go through the cartilage and to provide apposition. Some cartilaginous injuries are best left alone. Significant tracheal ring injuries often require a formal tracheostomy to ensure airway control and circumvent airway resistance from the glottis. High tracheostomy insertion at the second tracheal ring is preferred, even when the actual injury is located more distally.

Thyroid Injuries

Most wounds that cause tracheal injury will also cause injury to the thyroid. When the injured thyroid gland is not directly over the tracheal injury, it may be made hemostatic with simple sutures or electrocoagulation. When the thyroid injury occurs in the absence of tracheal injury, simple hemostasis by the above techniques is required. When the injury goes through the thyroid gland into the trachea, that portion of the thyroid is best resected. Alternatively, the thyroid may be divided at the isthmus and rotated off the trachea to facilitate a primary tracheal repair.

Miscellaneous Injuries

Injuries to the recurrent laryngeal nerve from a penetrating neck wound are rare. If the injury is the result of a gunshot wound, the nerve is unlikely to be completely severed and is best left alone. If the surgeon identifies a stab wound with complete severance of the recurrent laryngeal nerve, a primary approximation is indicated using fine sutures. The results of such repairs are unknown.

Injuries to the thoracic duct may be recognized by the presence of lymph within the operative field. The duct should be freed up, isolated, and divided with each end appropriately ligated.

SUGGESTED READINGS

Azuaje RE, Jacobson LE, Glover J, et al: Reliability of physical examination as a predictor of vascular injury after penetrating neck trauma, *Am Surg* 69:804–807, 2003.

Demetriades D, Theodorou D, Cornwell E, et al: Evaluation of penetrating injuries of the neck: a prospective study of 223 patients, *World J Surgery* 21:41–48, 1997.

Ledgerwood AM, Mullins RJ, Lucas CE: Primary repair vs ligation for carotid artery injuries, *Arch Surg* 115:488–493, 1980.

Meyer JP, Barrett JA, Schuler JJ, et al: Mandatory vs selective exploration for penetrating neck wounds: a prospective assessment, *Arch Surg* 122:592–597, 1987.

BLUNT CARDIAC INJURY

Louis R. Pizano, MD, MBA, and Gerd D. Pust, MD

OVERVIEW

Blunt cardiac injury (BCI) is the general term used for injury that occurs from blunt trauma to the heart. The wide range of pathophysiologic changes that result from this type of trauma may be asymptomatic, or they may lead to death from ventricular wall rupture. Older terminology includes *blunt cardiac trauma, cardiac concussion,* and *cardiac contusion.* Cardiac injury is subclassified by pathologic mechanisms into BCI with 1) complex arrhythmia, 2) minor electrocardiogram (ECG) or enzyme abnormality, 3) cardiac failure, 4) coronary artery thrombosis, and 5) septal or 6) free wall rupture. Treatment of these different subclasses of BCI varies from ECG monitoring to complex surgical repair.

INCIDENCE

The true incidence of BCI in patients with chest and abdominal trauma is unknown. Because it includes a wide spectrum of injury, from minor myocardial contusion with or without cardiac arrhythmias to severe structural damage, it is difficult to measure an accurate incidence. Because of the varied presentation of signs and symptoms, the appropriateness of the diagnostic workup, including the use of ECG and other imaging studies, such as echocardiography, will influence the incidence in clinical studies. This is reflected in the wide range in the reported incidence in different case series—from 8% to 71%.

The incidence of BCI in patients with chest and abdominal trauma is significantly lower in clinical studies as compared with autopsy series, as many patients with BCI die in the field from either cardiac or other associated traumatic injuries. Schultz and colleagues (2004) found that the most common BCI identified in clinical studies is myocardial contusion (60% to 100%), followed by right ventricular injury (17% to 32%) and right atrial injury (8% to 65%) because of the anatomic anterior positioning in the chest.

The left heart is less commonly involved, with left ventricular injury (8% to 15%) and left atrial injury (0% to 31%) somewhat more rare. Septal, valve, and coronary artery injuries appear rarely in clinical studies and are documented only as case reports. These injuries are often lethal and are found primarily at autopsy with studies showing atrial septal defects (7%), ventricular septal defects (4%), valve injuries (5%), and coronary artery injuries (3%).

The largest autopsy series published by Parmley and colleagues reviewed 207,548 cases from the Armed Forces Institute of Pathology. The study showed a 0.1% incidence and identified 546 cases of blunt traumatic injuries. The most common chamber rupture was the right ventricle (66 cases), followed by the left ventricle (59 cases), right atria (41 cases), and left atria (26 cases). Of these, 106 cases had combined chamber ruptures, and 80 had an associated aortic injury. Turk and Tsokos (2004), however, reported that blunt atrial injuries are more common than ventricular injuries, with the most frequently injured cardiac chambers being the right atrium, followed by the right ventricle.

MECHANISM OF INJURY AND PATHOPHYSIOLOGY

The heart is well protected by the sternum and rib cage; therefore it requires significant kinetic energy to the chest to cause a BCI. The most common causes are motor vehicle collisions and pedestrians struck by vehicles. Events that lead to acute deceleration and torsion, such as falls, as well as thoracic crush injuries are also common causes of BCI. Other blunt mechanisms include blast injuries, assaults, and sports-related trauma, which can cause direct precordial impact. Severe abdominal compression can lead to rupture of the right atrium and ventricle secondary to increased hydrostatic pressure. Hydraulic effects from a sudden increase in blood return via the inferior vena cava leads to rupture of these chambers from rapidly increasing pressure.

Blunt coronary artery injuries are extremely rare, but direct impact can lead to intimal disruption and subsequent thrombosis of the coronary vessel; this is typically seen in conjunction with severe myocardial contusion, most commonly occurring along the distribution of the left anterior descending artery, as it lies beneath the sternum. In rare cases the right coronary artery can also be injured, usually within 2 cm of its origin. Sequelae of these injuries can lead to severe myocardial infarction, production of emboli, arrhythmia, ventricular failure, and possible delayed ventricular rupture.

Valvular injury is infrequent and is often diagnosed by the clinical findings of acute left ventricular dysfunction with cardiogenic shock and pulmonary edema. The most commonly affected valves are the aortic followed by the mitral. The rapid displacement of blood secondary to compressive forces during ventricular diastole results in laceration of the valve leaflets, chordae tendineae, and papillary muscles.

Blunt pericardial rupture can occur from high-energy chest and abdominal trauma. Both direct impact of the chest wall and a sudden rise in intraabdominal pressure can lead to laceration of the pericardium on both the pleural and diaphragmatic surfaces that usually occurs parallel to the left phrenic nerve. Evisceration of the heart into the thoracic or abdominal cavity can cause torsion of the great vessels and result in cardiac arrest. Chest radiographs may reveal displacement of the cardiac silhouette, pneumopericardium, or an abdominal gas pattern secondary to herniated hollow viscera.

More than 75% of all patients with BCI will have other associated thoracic injuries, including rib and sternal fractures, pulmonary contusions, pneumothorax, hemothorax, and great vessel injuries. The presence of a sternal fracture does not predict the presence of BCI and thus does not necessitate monitoring and further evaluation. Penetrating trauma can be the result of blunt mechanism, when fractured ribs or the sternum come in contact with the heart. Schultz and colleagues (2004) showed that extrathoracic injuries are also commonly found in patients with BCI, and the incidence of head injury (20% to 73%), extremity injury (20% to 66%), abdominal solid-organ injury (5% to 43%), and spinal injury (10% to 20%) is extremely high.

The American Association for the Surgery of Trauma (AAST) Organ Injury Scale for cardiac injuries describes six injury grades, from minor ECG abnormalities to avulsion of the heart (Table 1).

CLINICAL DIAGNOSIS AND EVALUATION

A high index of suspicion, along with a proper evaluation of the mechanism of trauma, is very important for the treating physician to diagnose possible BCI early. The most common complaint in patients with BCI is chest pain, which can be difficult to distinguish from pain associated with chest wall injuries such as rib and sternal fractures. A thorough physical examination is the most important initial step. After verifying a patent airway and appropriate respiration, the evaluation for possible cardiac injury is performed during the cardiovascular assessment of the patient. Although the majority of patients with BCI are asymptomatic, with only ECG abnormalities, those who make it to the hospital with more life-threatening types of BCI usually present with signs and symptoms of shock. It is essential to rapidly distinguish hemodynamically stable patients from those in shock. The cause of the shock state needs to be established by differentiating cardiogenic shock secondary to BCI from the more common causes, including tension pneumothorax, neurogenic shock from spinal cord injury, and hypovolemic shock secondary to bleeding.

Cardiac tamponade presents clinically with hypotension, muffled heart sounds, and jugular venous distension (Beck's triad). Diagnosis can be difficult, as jugular venous distension may be diminished due to hypovolemia secondary to blood loss from other injuries, and cardiac auscultation may be less conclusive in conjunction with coexisting injuries such as hemomediastinum, hemothorax, or pneumomediastinum.

TABLE 1: American Association for the Surgery of Trauma organ injury scale: Cardiac injuries

Grade*	Cardiac Injury
I	Blunt cardiac injury with minor ECG abnormality (nonspecific ST- or T-wave changes, premature atrial or ventricular contraction, or persistent sinus tachycardia)
	Blunt or penetrating pericardial wound without cardiac injury, cardiac tamponade, or cardiac herniation
II	Blunt cardiac injury with heart block or ischemic changes without cardiac failure
	Penetrating tangential cardiac wound, up to but not extending through endocardium, without tamponade
III	Blunt cardiac injury with sustained or multifocal ventricular contractions
	Blunt or penetrating cardiac injury with septal rupture, pulmonary or tricuspid incompetence, papillary muscle dysfunction, or distal coronary artery occlusion without cardiac failure
	Blunt pericardial laceration with cardiac herniation
	Blunt cardiac injury with cardiac failure
	Penetrating tangential myocardial wound, up to but not through endocardium, with tamponade
IV	Blunt or penetrating cardiac injury with septal rupture, pulmonary or tricuspid incompetence, papillary muscle dysfunction, or distal coronary artery occlusion producing cardiac failure
	Blunt or penetrating cardiac injury with aortic or mitral incompetence
	Blunt or penetrating cardiac injury of the right ventricle, right or left atrium
V	Blunt or penetrating cardiac injury with proximal coronary artery occlusion
	Blunt or penetrating left ventricular perforation
	Stellate injuries, less than 50% tissue loss of the right ventricle, right or left atrium
VI	Blunt avulsion of the heart
	Penetrating wound producing more than 50% tissue loss of a chamber

*Advance one grade with multiple penetrating wounds to a single chamber or multiple chamber involvement.
From Moore EE, Malangoni MA, Cogbill TH, et al: Organ injury scaling. IV: thoracic vascular, lung, cardiac, and diaphragm, *J Trauma* 36(3):299-300, 1994.

There is no single definitive test to diagnose BCI. Often a series of tests are required, and it is crucial to know the sequence in which they should be obtained. Focused assessment with sonography for trauma (FAST) performed by the trauma physician assists in the early evaluation and detection of possible cardiac tamponade with high sensitivity. Cardiac filling and contractility can also be estimated during FAST. However, for a more detailed anatomic and cardiac function evaluation, formal echocardiography—either transthoracic (TTE) or transesophageal (TEE)—is indicated. Echocardiography is the imaging tool of choice to detect early structural damage, including ventricular or atrial rupture leading to cardiac tamponade, septal and valvular injuries, and papillary muscle and chordae tendineae injuries. Chest radiographs, which are routinely obtained in almost all trauma patients, may detect the presence of a globular-shaped

BOX 1: EAST practice management guidelines for blunt cardiac injury workup

Recommendation Level I

1. An admission ECG should be performed on all patients in whom a BCI is suspected.

Recommendation Level II

1. If the admission ECG is abnormal (arrhythmia, ST changes, ischemia, heart block, unexplained ST changes), the patient should be admitted for continuous ECG monitoring for 24 to 48 hours. Conversely, if the admission ECG is normal, the risk of having a BCI that requires treatment is insignificant, and the pursuit of diagnosis should be terminated.

2. If the patient is hemodynamically unstable, an imaging study (echocardiogram) should be obtained. If an optimal transthoracic echocardiogram cannot be performed, the patient should have a transesophageal ECG.

3. Nuclear medicine studies add little when compared with ECG; thus they are not useful if an ECG has been performed.

Recommendation Level III

1. Elderly patients with known cardiac disease, unstable patients, and those with an abnormal admission ECG can be safely operated on provided they are appropriately monitored. Consideration should be given to placement of a pulmonary artery catheter in such cases.

2. The presence of a sternal fracture does not predict the presence of BCI and thus does not necessarily indicate that monitoring should be performed.

3. Neither creatinine phosphokinase with isoenzyme analysis nor measurement of circulating cardiac troponin T are useful in predicting which patients have or will have complications related to BCI.

From Pasquale, MD, Nagyk, Clarke J: *Practice management guidelines for screening of blunt cardic injury,* Chicago, 1998, Eastern Association for the Surgery of Trauma.

cardiac silhouette. In hemodynamically stable patients with suspicion for blunt cardiac trauma, an ECG to evaluate for potential arrhythmias should immediately follow the FAST.

The Eastern Association for the Surgery of Trauma (EAST) established practice guidelines for blunt cardiac trauma after Pasquale and colleagues (1998) performed a thorough literature review of 56 articles published from 1986 to 1997 (Box 1). All patients with suspicion for blunt cardiac trauma should have an ECG on admission (level 1 recommendation). ECG is helpful in diagnosing BCI; however, there is no one specific or classic finding that confirms the diagnosis. The most common finding is sinus tachycardia, which is very nonspecific, as it is commonly found in trauma patients with a multitude of injuries and is often associated with bleeding or pain. The next most common abnormality is premature atrial or ventricular contractions followed by a spectrum of findings, including nonspecific T-wave changes, ST-segment elevation or depression, atrial fibrillation or flutter, ventricular dysrhythmias, conduction delays, bundle branch and heart block, and the presence of Q waves. If the ECG reveals any of these findings or other evidence of ischemia, BCI should be ruled out, and the patient should be admitted to an intensive care unit (ICU) for continuous ECG monitoring for 24 to 48 hours (level 2 recommendation). However, if the ECG shows no abnormality, the chances of having a clinically significant BCI requiring treatment are negligible, and pursuit of the diagnosis should be terminated (level 2 recommendation).

There are however, reported cases of BCI with the clinical presentation delayed for as much as 24 hours after injury. It is recommended that patients older than 55 years of age and those with a known history of cardiac disease, both at risk for BCI, be admitted for continuous cardiac monitoring even if the initial ECG shows no abnormalities.

The EAST guidelines for screening of BCI also indicate that neither creatinine phosphokinase with or without isoenzyme analysis nor measurement of circulating cardiac troponin T is useful in predicting which patients will have complications related to BCI. However, several newer studies have shown an increased sensitivity in detecting BCI by combining ECG and cardiac troponin I. The combination of cardiac troponin I and ECG has been shown to have benefit in not only diagnosing but also ruling out clinically significant BCI. Velmahos and colleagues (2003) showed that the combination of a normal ECG and negative troponin I on admission and at 8 hours after suspected injury has a 100% negative predictive value and rules out clinically significant BCI.

If the patient is hemodynamically unstable from a suspected BCI, the FAST is the initial form of echocardiography to be conducted, because it can be performed rapidly at the bedside. The findings are obtained and immediately interpreted by the providing surgeon or emergency physician and are used to guide further treatment of the trauma patient. The FAST does not evaluate cardiac function but is highly sensitive for determining pericardial effusion and tamponade except in the rare cases of combined chamber and pericardial rupture with hemorrhage into the pleural cavity, which prevents the accumulation of blood in the pericardial space.

A formal TTE offers significantly more information than the initial FAST examination. It better defines pericardial tamponade and evaluates valvular and wall motion abnormalities as well as overall cardiac function. In trauma patients, however, studies have shown that there are often significant barriers to performing successful TTEs, and nearly 20% are suboptimal or nondiagnostic. In addition, TTE cannot detect the electrical instability that is commonly found in BCI, and although it may identify structural defects and wall motion abnormalities, it has not been found to correlate with complications or eventual outcome in BCI.

If an optimal, noninvasive TTE cannot be performed because of pain, pleural tubes, subcutaneous emphysema associated with pneumothorax, or other chest injuries, a TEE is indicated. TEE is recommended secondarily to an unsuccessful TTE, as it is an invasive, operator-dependent procedure that requires sedation and possible intubation, and it is not always available. TEE does, however, have a higher sensitivity and specificity for BCI than TTE and is better at diagnosing septal and valvular lesions, wall motion abnormalities, and cardiac performance. It also has the added benefit of providing visualization of most of the thoracic aorta to help diagnose or rule out blunt aortic injury.

Nuclear medicine studies—multigated acquisition scans, single-photon emission computed tomography, thallium 201, and radionuclide angiography—are not sufficiently sensitive or specific to reliably establish the diagnosis of BCI. They do not add additional information to echocardiography and therefore are rarely indicated in the early evaluation. The authors have never used these tests in the evaluation of BCI, and they appear to be of historic interest only. Even pericardiocentesis, which had been the definitive test to diagnose pericardial effusion in most cases, has been replaced by user-friendly, rapid, sensitive, and noninvasive echocardiography.

TREATMENT

The treatment of BCI varies greatly depending on the patient's hemodynamic status (Figure 1). Unstable patients need immediate treatment and diagnostic evaluation in parallel. The cause of hemodynamic shock must be determined quickly. If shock results from hypovolemia or hemorrhage, tension pneumothorax and neurogenic mechanisms are addressed and excluded, and the patient needs to be

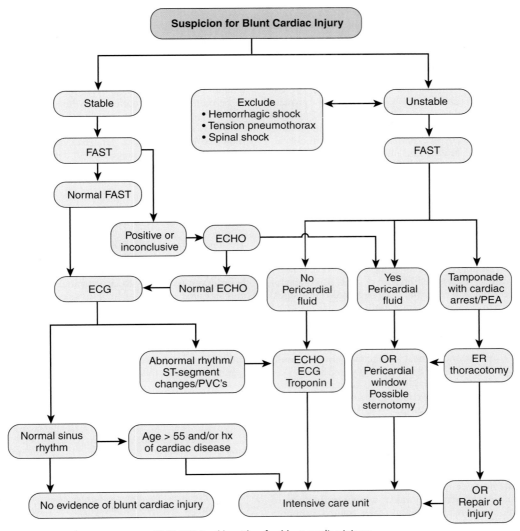

FIGURE 1   Algorithm for blunt cardiac injury.

evaluated for cardiogenic shock. If the source of cardiogenic shock is cardiac tamponade and BCI, all efforts must be made to immediately drain the pericardial space. Subxiphoid needle pericardiocentesis should be performed to temporarily decompress the pericardial space, if a surgeon is not immediately available.

In cases of witnessed or impending cardiac arrest, a left anterolateral thoracotomy performed by an experienced surgeon in the emergency department for rapid access to the heart is indicated. Even when the arrest is witnessed, and no time is lost intervening in a patient with a known or suspected BCI, survival is rare. Patients with prehospital cardiac arrest have nearly 100% mortality even with emergency department thoracotomy; therefore, the procedure is not indicated under these circumstances.

When a patient arrives with vital signs and then progresses to pericardial tamponade, diagnosed with a FAST examination, and goes into cardiopulmonary arrest, a thoracotomy in the emergency department is indicated. A left anterolateral thoracotomy is performed using the same technique as for a penetrating thoracic injury. Evacuation of the cardiac tamponade can easily be performed by pericardiotomy, opening the pericardium in a cephalad to caudal orientation with care taken to prevent injury to the phrenic nerve. Vital signs may be restored upon evacuation of the cardiac tamponade, once the atria are able to fill; however, BCI leading to tamponade may be very difficult to temporize in the emergency department. Pericardiotomy

exposes the heart and makes it possible to identify the source of bleeding. The descending thoracic aorta should be clamped to preferentially send any forward blood flow to the coronary vessels and the brain. The defect in the heart must be temporarily occluded with a finger, until the wound can be surgically repaired. Patients with return of vital signs should be taken directly to the operating room.

Hemodynamically unstable patients who present with a palpable pulse should be immediately transferred to the operating room for intervention, once the FAST examination demonstrates pericardial effusion/tamponade. If blood pressure permits, and to confirm that blood is the source of the pericardial effusion, a pericardial window followed by median sternotomy should be performed. In the event of impending cardiopulmonary arrest, as in the emergency department, a left anterolateral thoracotomy is indicated. Under these circumstances, however, the procedure occurs in the operating room, where definitive repair of the injury can be immediately performed after release of the pericardial tamponade.

Patients with BCI and a FAST or echocardiogram indicating pericardial fluid should, under stable hemodynamic conditions, be taken to the operating room for a pericardial window. Once hemopericardium is confirmed, a median sternotomy for optimal cardiac exposure should be performed. In the population of patients who maintain stable vital signs, the most commonly injured structures found upon entering the pericardium are the right atrium, right ventricle, and the atriocaval junction. Temporary occlusion of the defect should once again be accomplished with a finger, as it is a very easy maneuver. Allis clamps can temporarily pull the wound edges together to control a laceration of the atria, or a Satinsky clamp can be placed to occlude the opening. Bleeding from ventricular wounds should be controlled by digital compression, followed by running or interrupted suture repair. Horizontal mattress or single interrupted sutures using 3-0 Prolene with or without felt pledgets can be effective. Wounds in close proximity to a coronary artery should be repaired with horizontal mattress sutures to avoid ligating the vessel and infarcting the myocardium. These injuries can be repaired by an experienced surgeon without cardiac bypass. Cardiothoracic surgical consultation and cardiac bypass are necessary in patients with internal cardiac injuries. Valve disruption, which is most commonly found in the aortic area, followed by the mitral valve, septal rupture, and papillary muscle rupture diagnosed by echocardiography require urgent, not emergent, repair.

Injury to the coronary vessels is extremely rare in BCI. Coronary artery contusion, spasm, plaque rupture, dissection, and laceration present with signs and symptoms of myocardial infarction, and primary repair utilizing microvascular techniques by a cardiothoracic surgeon is necessary. Nonoperative management of coronary artery injuries, including cardiac catheterization with possible percutaneous angioplasty and stent placement by the interventional cardiologist, may be a viable alternative to restore blood flow.

In patients who sustain pericardial tears with or without cardiac herniation, the pericardium may be repaired using simple interrupted 2-0 polyprolene sutures. Pericardial laceration as an isolated injury, however, is usually of no clinical significance unless complicated by hemorrhage from a lacerated pericardiophrenic artery.

Patients with stable vital signs who have ECG changes or cardiac arrhythmias require 24 to 48 hours of continuous cardiac monitoring. Patients with BCI who have only minor ECG abnormalities should be observed in a monitored setting, as most of these findings will resolve within 24 hours with no intervention. An ICU admission is ideal for patients with BCI and complex arrhythmias, as they often require antiarrhythmic medications to manage the rhythm and control heart rate. The rhythms resulting from BCI are varied and occur so infrequently that there are no evidence-based recommendations as to how to treat them. Lethal ventricular arrhythmia, usually in the form of ventricular fibrillation after relatively minor chest trauma, is known as *commotio cordis*. These injuries are rare, but when they do occur, they are usually seen in contact and ball sports and can lead to sudden cardiovascular collapse. The underlying pathology is often ventricular tachycardia or ventricular fibrillation. Early defibrillation is the only lifesaving treatment and has been found to be successful in up to 25% of patients if performed within 3 minutes of injury. Survival is extremely rare if treatment is initiated beyond this time period.

ICU admission is a necessity for patients with BCI who develop cardiac failure, as they require aggressive management. Resuscitation of the patient with BCI and other concomitant injuries can be very challenging and often requires a pulmonary artery catheter to further diagnose and guide management. Preload to the injured heart needs to be monitored and optimized, while undergoing volume resuscitation. Inotropic support (e.g., dobutamine) is indicated in patients with a low cardiac index, and vasopressors (e.g., epinephrine) may be indicated in patients with persistent cardiogenic shock who are not responding to fluid management. If hypotension persists, the placement of an intraaortic balloon pump, or even a ventricular-assist device, may be necessary to improve cardiac function.

OUTCOMES AND FOLLOW-UP

The long-term outcome of BCI is not well studied. However, the outcome of minor cardiac injury in patients who arrive with arrhythmias is excellent, and patients' symptoms usually resolve within 24 to 48 hours. Even patients with structural injuries have a good long-term outcome after surgical repair, if they survive the initial event. Chronically impaired cardiac function after BCI with myocardial damage is uncommon but can occur. Long-term follow-up with Holter cardiac monitoring and nuclear medicine studies for a period of at least 1 year are necessary in this patient population to reduce the risk of sudden cardiac death. Patients with injuries to the coronary system require long-term follow-up with a cardiologist.

SUGGESTED READINGS

Mattox KL, Flint LM, Carrico CJ, et al: Blunt cardiac injury (editorial), *J Trauma* 33:649–650, 1992.

Moore EE, Malangoni MA, Cogbill TH, et al: Organ injury scaling. IV: thoracic vascular, lung, cardiac, and diaphragm, *J Trauma* 36(3):299–300, 1994.

Pasquale MD, Nagy K, Clarke J: *Eastern Association for the Surgery of Trauma (EAST): practice parameter workgroup for screening of blunt cardiac injury.* Available at: http://www.east.org/tpg/chap2.pdf.

Seguin A, Fadel E, Mussot S, et al: Blunt rupture of the heart: surgical treatment of three different clinical presentations, *J Trauma* 65(6):1529–1533, 2008.

Velmahos GC, Karaiskakis M, Salim A, et al: Normal electrocardiography and serum troponin I levels preclude the presence of clinically significant blunt cardiac injury, *J Trauma* 54(1):45–50, 2003.

Abdominal Compartment Syndrome and Management of the Open Abdomen

Joseph F. Sucher, MD, Zsolt J. Balogh, MD, PhD, and Frederick A. Moore, MD

OVERVIEW

Intraabdominal hypertension (IAH), defined by an intraabdominal pressure (IAP) exceeding 12 mm Hg, can result in local and systemic physiologic derangement. IAH that causes new end-organ dysfunction is termed *abdominal compartment syndrome* (ACS). As its name suggests, the abdomen is a compartment bound by the peritoneum, diaphragm, abdominal wall (muscle, fascia, and skin), ribs, and bony pelvis, all of which have limited compliance. However, unlike compartments of the extremities, elevation of the pressure within the abdomen can directly result in systemic pathophysiology. As abdominal pressure increases, there is corresponding impairment to the cardiac, respiratory, renal, neurologic, and musculoskeletal systems; if not recognized early and treated promptly, these result in unrecoverable multiple organ failure (MOF) and death. This chapter serves as a brief review of the current knowledge concerning the historic perspective, etiology and pathophysiology, diagnosis, and management of ACS and management of the open abdomen.

HISTORIC PERSPECTIVE

The deleterious effects of elevated IAP were recognized by pediatric surgeons in the 1960s, following repair of diaphragmatic hernias and omphaloceles. Further laboratory investigations into the pathophysiology of increased IAP continued into the 1970s. Sporadic clinical and laboratory reports documenting the pathophysiology of increased IAP began to appear in the 1980s. However, the term *abdominal compartment syndrome* was not coined until 1989 by Fietsam and colleagues. Since then, tremendous activity has been directed at defining an otherwise elusive and controversial clinical pathophysiology.

ACS is now understood to exist as a deadly entity across a spectrum of critically ill patients, requiring aggressive resuscitation in both medical and surgical intensive care units (ICUs). An epidemic of ACS emerged in the early 1990s in trauma centers worldwide as a result of four significant advances in trauma and surgical critical care. First, the development of trauma systems with high-volume level I trauma centers improved survival of the catastrophically injured patient, thus increasing the population most at risk for this entity and concentrating them in specialized shock trauma ICUs. Second, early empiric administration of isotonic crystalloids in the early management of injured patients was endorsed by Advanced Trauma Life Support (ATLS). Third, *damage control surgery* was embraced as a strategy to save patients who otherwise were exsanguinating in the operating room secondary to "the bloody vicious cycle," characterized by uncontrolled bleeding associated with hypothermia, acidosis, and coagulopathy. Finally, with the widespread availability of pulmonary artery catheters, trauma surgeons became champions of the concept of goal-directed shock resuscitation to achieve supranormal oxygen delivery as first advocated by Shoemaker (1988). This practice led to further excessive infusion of isotonic crystalloids. In 2006 and 2007 the World Society of Abdominal Compartment Syndrome (WSACS) published expert consensus for the diagnosis and management of IAH and ACS. They also defined the terminology, thus providing a basis for improved communication and comparison of current and future work.

ETIOLOGY AND PATHOPHYSIOLOGY

Abdominal compartment syndrome (ACS) is defined as sustained IAP greater than 20 mm Hg with associated new organ dysfunction. Primary ACS occurs with injury or disease in the abdominopelvic region. Etiologies include but are not limited to ruptured abdominal aortic aneurysms, abdominal trauma, and retroperitoneal hemorrhage from pelvic fractures. Secondary ACS occurs as a result of critical illness originating outside the abdominopelvic region, requiring large-volume resuscitation. Etiologies include mangled extremities, burns, severe systemic inflammatory response syndrome (SIRS), septic shock, and severe pancreatitis. Recurrent ACS is defined by redevelopment of ACS after previous medical or surgical therapy for primary or secondary ACS. In all cases, the physiologic derangements can culminate in MOF and death.

IAH exerts its effects through multiple mechanisms. Deleterious effects on cardiac, pulmonary, renal and splanchnic function are seen at pressures as low as 15 mm Hg. Mechanisms include expansion of intraabdominal contents via direct hemorrhage or bowel swelling and third-space fluid sequestration. Compression of abdominal viscera leads to impairment of intraabdominal organ and abdominal wall perfusion. Cardiopulmonary embarrassment occurs due to compression of the inferior vena cava, which decreases venous return, and intrathoracic displacement of the diaphragm that leads to pulmonary hypertension and right-heart failure with subsequent septal deviation to the left, causing decreased left-heart compliance.

Similar to the concept of pericardial tamponade, the acuteness of onset plays a role in how the abdominal compartment can adapt to the volume expansion. It has the ability to expand over a chronic period, as in pregnancy and cirrhotic ascites. However, in the acute setting, there is a point at which the abdominal wall and diaphragm (dynamic components) lose the ability to accommodate increases in volume. Therefore, although pressures can initially rise slowly, as the IAP reaches 20 mm Hg, this rate can increase significantly. The WSACS defines grades of intraabdominal hypertension based on risk of developing ACS (Table 1). There is no definitive IAP at which ACS occurs. Patients may have IAP greater than 30 mm Hg and still not

TABLE 1: World Society of Abdominal Compartment Syndrome grades of intraabdominal hypertension

Grade	Intraabdominal Pressure (mm Hg)
I	12–15
II	16–20
III	21–25
IV	>25

Data from Malbrain MLNG, Cheatham ML, Kirkpatrick A, et al: Results from the International Conference of Experts on Intraabdominal Hypertension and Abdominal Compartment Syndrome. I. Definitions, *Intensive Care Med* 32(11):1722–1732, 2006.

have ACS, but others can have IAP less than 20 mm Hg and potentially have ACS. It can be challenging to determine with certainty whether critically ill patients have ACS, because they frequently have a variety of organ dysfunctions for other reasons. Therefore, maintaining a high index of suspicion is necessary.

Sustained IAH can lead to ACS and is manifested by one or more of the following: 1) increased intracranial pressure; 2) impaired oxygenation with elevated peak inspiratory pressures secondary to decreased lung and chest wall compliance, with lowered functional residual capacity; 3) cardiac failure as a result of decreased preload and diastolic dysfunction along with elevated intrathoracic pressure, creating right ventricular impairment and increased afterload that is unresponsive to volume loading; 4) oliguric renal failure from direct effects on the renal parenchyma and renal veins, as well as indirectly, secondary to decreased cardiac output with increased systemic vascular resistance; 5) gastrointestinal ischemia due to decreased splanchnic perfusion; and 6) abdominal wall musculocutaneous ischemia, potentially resulting in surgical wound complications.

DIAGNOSIS

Identifying at-risk patients and preventing ACS is paramount to achieving optimal patient outcomes. However, ACS occurs across a heterogeneous group of patients; thus identifying at-risk patients will depend on the local patient population and maintaining a high index of suspicion. At-risk patients include, but are not limited to, those with major abdominal or thoracic operations requiring crystalloid

fluids greater than 5000 mL/day, trauma or burn patients in severe shock who fail to adequately respond to ongoing volume loading or require a massive transfusion (>10 units of blood in 6 hours), and patients with severe pancreatitis, severe SIRS, or septic shock who require more than 40 mL/kg of crystalloid volume in the first 24 hours. At-risk patients should then have objective intraabdominal pressure (IAP) measurements as recommended by the WSACS, shown in Figure 1.

Relying on physical examination, whether performed by use of simple subjective palpation or objective abdominal girth measurements, has been clearly shown to be nonspecific and poorly correlative with IAP. Therefore patients at risk for ACS, or those who are suspected to have IAH or ACS, should have IAP monitoring performed via the urinary bladder as described by Kron and colleagues and modified by Cheatham (Figure 2). Briefly, IAP can be assessed via Foley catheter with a pressure-transducer system by instilling 25 mL of sterile saline into the empty bladder and recording the pressure as leveled at the midaxillary line. Today, multiple commercial products are available to aid in performing IAP monitoring.

MANAGEMENT OF ACS

Balogh and colleagues (2003) showed that the mortality rate remains high despite early aggressive surgical abdominal decompression in patients with severe blunt trauma that progress to ACS. Balogh's prediction models suggest that patients with IAP greater than 20 mm Hg who require *ongoing* volume loading are those at highest risk. Early decompressive laparotomy based solely on elevated IAP would result

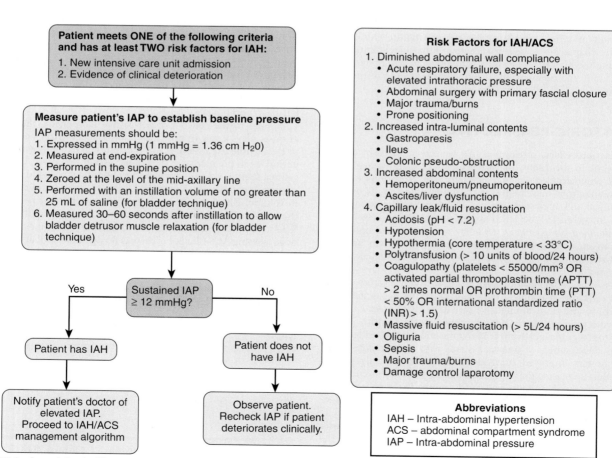

FIGURE 1 Intraabdominal hypertension assessment algorithm. *(From Cheatham ML, Malbrain MLNG, Kirkpatrick A, et al: Results from the International Conference of Experts on Intra-abdominal Hypertension and Abdominal Compartment Syndrome. II. Recommendations, Intensive Care Med 33[6]:951–962, 2007.)*

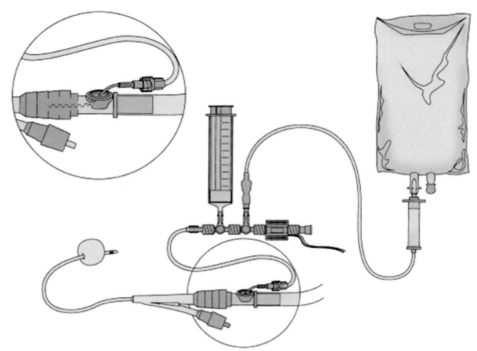

FIGURE 2   A closed, needle-free system for measurement of intravesicular pressure. Normal saline (1000 mL), a 60 mL Luer-lock syringe, and a segment of pressure tubing are attached to a disposable pressure transducer connected to two stopcocks. An 18 gauge angiocatheter is inserted into the culture aspiration port of the urinary drainage tubing, and the needle is removed, leaving the plastic infusion catheter in place. The infusion catheter is connected to the pressure tubing, and the system is flushed with normal saline. The infusion catheter may be taped to the urinary drainage tubing for added security. *(From Cheatham ML, Safcsak K: Intraabdominal pressure: a revised method for measurement, J Am Coll Surg 186[5]: 594–595, 1998.)*

in too many open abdomens. Therefore patients at high risk for ACS should have their shock resuscitation strategy altered, from conventional crystalloid volume loading, or have early surgical decompression before full-blown ACS ensues. Already, changes in resuscitation management for traumatic shock by employing massive transfusion protocols with early fresh frozen plasma directed at hemostatic control, along with judicious use of crystalloid volume early in the course of postinjury management, has attenuated the incidence of ACS in trauma. For those patients at high risk for development of ACS who require damage control laparotomy, we recommend leaving the abdomen open with an appropriate temporary abdominal closure (TAC) system.

In our experience, it is best to employ a modified Bogotá bag technique at the initial procedure, as it is quick, inexpensive, and effective. The simple Bogotá bag, a 3 L sterilized IV bag, sewn to the abdominal wall skin, not to the fascia, is modified to collect fluid leakage by placing flat Jackson-Pratt drains over the bag and sealing the system by placing a large Ioban cover over the abdomen (Figure 3). We have experienced recurrent ACS in patients who have had other closure techniques, such as conventional towel clipping or placement of commercial vacuum-assisted closure devices at the outset. The use of the Bogotá bag TAC technique and leaving ample room for visceral swelling helps reduce the risk of recurrent ACS. An alternative is to use the Vac-Pack technique as initially described by Barker and colleagues (1995). The key to optimizing patient outcomes is prophylaxis.

Recommendations for the monitoring and treatment of patients with IAH exhibiting signs of ACS are shown in Figure 4. This guideline, modified from the WSACS recommendations, provides new strategies for reversing IAH in patients with secondary ACS. That is, patients with conditions such as severe pancreatitis, septic shock, or thermal injury may benefit from noninvasive interventions prior to formal surgical abdominal decompression. These include placing

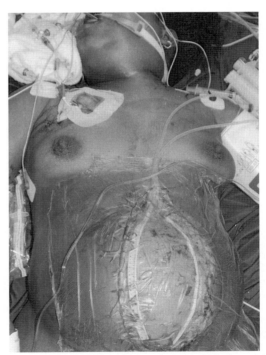

FIGURE 3   Patient after abdominal decompression with modified Bogotá bag temporary abdominal closure. The bag is sutured to the skin, Jackson-Pruitt drains are placed over the bag, and Ioban is placed over the entire abdomen to gain a seal that prevents abdominal fluid drainage.

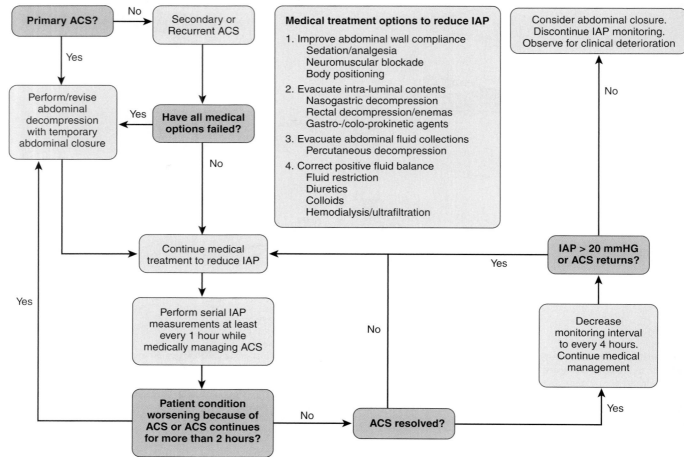

FIGURE 4 Intraabdominal hypertension/intraabdominal compartment syndrome management algorithm. *(Modified from Cheatham ML, Malbrain MLNG, Kirkpatrick A, et al: Results from the International Conference of Experts on Intra-abdominal Hypertension and Abdominal Compartment Syndrome. II. Recommendations, Intensive Care Med 33[6]:951–962, 2007.)*

the patient in full supine position and initiating muscle relaxation therapy; gastrointestinal decompression via nasogastric suctioning and rectal tube placement; diuretic therapy, if clinically applicable; or hemodialysis/hemofiltration to remove excess fluid.

Some have advocated maintaining abdominal perfusion pressure (APP) greater than 60 mm Hg, similar to maintaining cerebral perfusion pressure in patients with brain injury. Perfusion pressure is derived by the calculation APP = Mean arterial pressure (MAP) − IAP. Therefore, to achieve an APP greater than 60 mm Hg, either the MAP must be increased, or the IAP must be decreased. Traditional volume loading to increase MAP in the face of impending ACS can lead to futile crystalloid loading or the so-called *saltwater vicious cycle,* which precipitates the full-blown ACS that treatment was meant to prevent. Alternatively, the use of vasopressors such as norepinephrine or vasopressin may certainly increase MAP and thus APP but at the expense of decreasing an already compromised splanchnic perfusion. At this time, we are skeptical of this practice and recommend it be used only under scrutinized study protocols.

Less invasive measures such as escharotomy for burn patients, subcutaneous release of the linea alba fascia, and percutaneous drainage of peritoneal ascites have all been described in the literature. Burn patients in particular appear to develop ascites more often than the bowel edema seen in traumatic shock patients. We recommend the early employment of abdominal ultrasound to identify those patients in whom ascites may be the major cause of ACS, for the benefits derived from using the less invasive peritoneal catheter drainage management strategy. Less invasive techniques may be reasonable

and effective but should be used with caution, understanding that their ability to completely decompress the abdomen is less than that of a formal decompressive laparotomy. Patients with high predicted mortality based on Injury Severity Score (ISS) or Acute Physiology, Chronic Health Examination (APACHE), and documented ACS should undergo abdominal decompression immediately. If the patient is hemodynamically unstable, this lifesaving maneuver should not be delayed, and it can be performed safely in the ICU with the appropriate support staff. Decompressive laparotomy with subsequent management of the open abdomen is a safe and effective standard of care.

MANAGEMENT OF THE OPEN ABDOMEN

There are significant variations in the management of the open abdomen following damage control or decompressive laparotomies based mainly on personal preference, institutional biases, and the patient population. Techniques include: 1) vacuum-assisted closure techniques such as the commercial Wound VAC (Kinetic Concepts, San Antonio, Tex.) and the noncommercial vacuum pack (Vac-Pack) technique described by Barker (1995); 2) "zipper" closures, including the Wittmann artificial burr patch (StarSurgical, Burlington, Wis.) as well as other mesh with zipper mechanism techniques as originally described by Leguit in 1982; 3) placement of temporary absorbable or nonabsorbable mesh; 4) plastic silo technique (Bogota bag); and 5) temporary skin closure with towel clips or sutures.

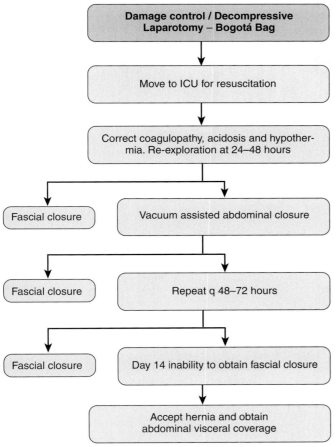

FIGURE 5   Management algorithm for the open abdomen.

used to bridge the remaining open fascial defect (Figure 6). This process should continue at repeat laparotomies, until complete fascial closure is obtained.

We reported the use of this technique in two publications that involved 53 trauma patients who required damage control or decompressive laparotomies. In this combined series, we were able to achieve primary fascial closure in 48 patients (90%) at a mean of 7 days. These results are very similar to those of the Wake Forest group. An ongoing debate surrounds how long the surgeon should persist in doing repeat laparotomies every 48 to 72 hours in hopes of achieving definitive fascial closure. Similar to the Wake Forest group, we have achieved delayed closures in a number of patients beyond 21 days; however, this approach requires significant ongoing resource utilization and increases the risk of GI fistula formation.

Our practice has evolved to the point that we now attempt progressive fascial closure with the Wound VAC for 14 days. We then proceed with closing the fascial defect and providing protective coverage of the viscera, accepting the delayed hernia. We use one of three techniques, depending upon the size of the defect and general condition of the patient. First, for smaller defects regardless of patient condition, simple full-thickness abdominal skin closure can be performed over the midline, as long as excessive tension is not an issue. We use 2-0 nylon sutures in an interrupted vertical mattress fashion. These sutures remain for at least 21 days to ensure complete healing of the midline skin. For larger defects in patients who are progressing toward hospital discharge, we will bridge the defect with acellular dermal matrix products. This technique may potentially reduce the incidence of clinical hernia formation and has the additional benefit of decreasing the risk of evisceration in the event of surgical wound dehiscence. We employ a Stoppa-like technique of circumferentially suturing thick, acellular dermal matrix as an underlay (Figure 7) using an interrupted U stitch and 1-0 monofilament absorbable sutures on a CT-X needle. At this point, the skin can be closed over Jackson-Pruitt drains. The timing of drain removal is controversial and is left to the reader's particular practice to dictate this timing. If the skin cannot be closed over the midline, it is safe to employ the continued use of vacuum-assisted wound closure systems on top of the acellular dermal matrix. The wound will granulate and contract over the following 6 to 8 weeks, depending on its size and the patient's nutritional status. Third, in patients with large defects and ongoing critical illness, we cover the abdominal defect with a split-thickness skin graft, once granulation tissue has adequately matured. However, this technique results in a grotesque abdominal wall defect that is associated with a higher incidence of fistula formation compared with the first two techniques. If this technique is to be undertaken, we recommend affixing expanded polytetrafluoroethylene (ePTFE) mesh to the fascia to cover and protect the viscera, because ePTFE has a very low fistula rate owing to its innate lack of the ability to incite an inflammatory response.

Over the next 14 days, the viscera will become "frozen" within the abdomen and will form a granulation bed underneath the ePTFE, which can then be removed, and we use wet-to-dry gauze dressing to allow the granulation tissue to mature. An STSG is then applied over the healthy granulation bed (Figure 8). Others advocate the use of absorbable mesh, such as Polyglactin 910 (Vicryl) mesh, to bridge these large defects and prevent evisceration until granulation tissue matures. However, the fistula rate associated with these absorbable meshes in most series exceeds 20%. Finally, we do not advocate performing myofascial advancement techniques (*component separation*) to achieve midline fascial closure during this acute stage. These patients are acutely ill and malnourished, and the fascial wound failure rate under the best conditions can be significant; this technique is the surgeon's last good tool in the toolbox, and it should be reserved for when the patient recovers from the original insult and returns under more optimal conditions for formal, definitive abdominal wall reconstruction.

Choosing one technique over another based on the current literature remains challenging; the use of such techniques is based on a heterogeneous patient population, and there is significant practice variation among the various authors. We therefore describe our successful approach to the management of the open abdomen.

At the initial damage control or decompressive laparotomy, we use the modified Bogotá bag described above as a TAC. It is imperative to recognize that ACS can occur with any TAC technique, and we recommend routine monitoring of IAP during ongoing resuscitation. The decision concerning timing of the second laparotomy is based on the indications of the first operation. In damage control situations, we focus on correcting acidosis, hypothermia, and coagulopathy within the first 24 hours, and we return at that point for planned reexploration and definitive operative repair. For decompressive laparotomies, we initially focus on correcting the deranged physiology, and we delay the second laparotomy until 48 hours. During this period, we will attempt to diurese the patient if clinically appropriate. If abdominal closure is not possible at the second laparotomy, we will place the Wound VAC and return to the operating room at 48 to 72 hour intervals to perform sequential fascial closure (Figure 5). Factors that prevent these goals include ongoing visceral edema and gross contamination. However, these processes will abate as the patient recovers from the pathologic insult. Additionally, we recommend the use of aggressive diuresis, if clinically possible, between laparotomies to decrease bowel edema. Moreover, at each subsequent laparotomy, intestinal adhesions are gently lysed, and the abdominal cavity is lavaged to ensure that it remains accessible and decontaminated. If definitive fascial closure is unobtainable, superior and inferior partial fascial closure should be done as much as possible utilizing simple interrupted sutures, and the Wound VAC should be

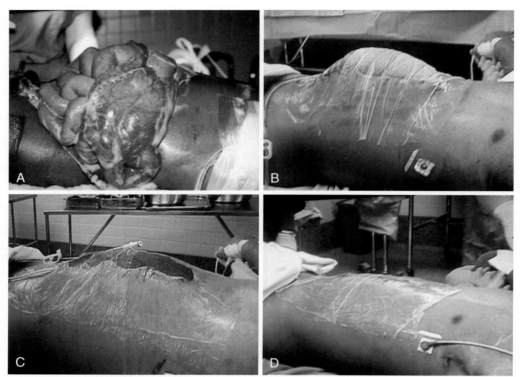

FIGURE 6 **A,** Postinjury day (PID) 1, after massive volume resuscitation and correction of coagulopathy. Extensive visceral edema is noted with inability to close abdomen. Wound VAC is applied at end of this operation. **B,** PID 2, after Wound VAC application. **C,** PID 5, significant reduction in visceral edema is evident. **D,** PID 7, visceral edema is resolved with ability to achieve midline fascial closure. Skin is left open with Wound VAC applied over fascia to assist with further open soft-tissue wound management.

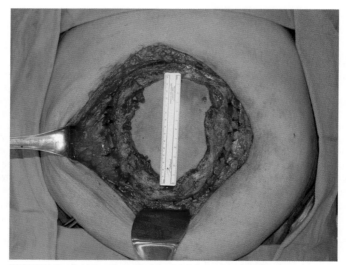

FIGURE 7 Bridging abdominal fascial defect with acellular dermal matrix.

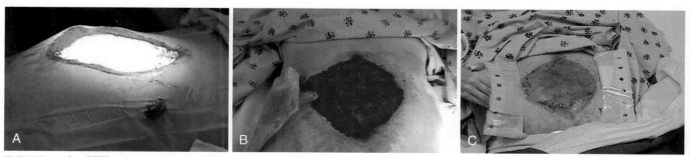

FIGURE 8 **A,** ePTFE covering abdominal viscera. **B,** The ePTFE is removed on day 14. Abdominal viscera are "frozen" with granulation bed. **C,** Three weeks after split-thickness skin graft.

SUGGESTED READINGS

Balogh Z, McKinley BA, Cocanour CS, et al: Secondary abdominal compartment syndrome is an elusive early complication of traumatic shock resuscitation, *Am J Surg* 184(6):538–543, 2002.

Balogh Z, McKinley BA, Cocanour CS, et al: Patients with impending abdominal compartment syndrome do not respond to early volume loading, *Am J Surg* 186(6):602–607, 2003.

Balogh Z, McKinley BA, Cocanour CS, et al: Supranormal trauma resuscitation causes more cases of abdominal compartment syndrome, *Arch Surg* 138(6):637–642, 2003.

Balogh Z, McKinley BA, Holcomb JB, et al: Both primary and secondary abdominal compartment syndrome can be predicted early and are harbingers of multiple organ failure, *J Trauma* 54(5):848–859, discussion 859–861, 2003.

Barker DE, Kaufman HJ, Smith LA, et al: Vacuum-pack technique of temporary abdominal closure: a 7-year experience with 112 patients, *J Trauma* 48(2):201–206, 2000.

Cheatham ML, Malbrain MLNG, Kirkpatrick A, et al: Results from the International Conference of Experts on Intra-abdominal Hypertension and Abdominal Compartment Syndrome. II. Recommendations, *Intensive Care Med* 33(6):951–962, 2007.

Cheatham ML, Safcsak K: Intraabdominal pressure: a revised method for measurement, *J Am Coll Surg* 186(5):594–595, 1998.

Fietsam R, Villalba M, Glover JL, Clark K: Intra-abdominal compartment syndrome as a complication of ruptured abdominal aortic aneurysm repair, *Am Surg* 55(6):396–402, 1989.

Garner GB, Ware DN, Cocanour CS, et al: Vacuum-assisted wound closure provides early fascial reapproximation in trauma patients with open abdomens, *Am J Surg* 182(6):630–638, 2001.

Kron IL, Harman PK, Nolan SP: The measurement of intra-abdominal pressure as a criterion for abdominal re-exploration, *Ann Surg* 199(1):28–30, 1984.

Malbrain MLNG, Cheatham ML, Kirkpatrick A, et al: Results from the International Conference of Experts on Intra-abdominal Hypertension and Abdominal Compartment Syndrome. I. Definitions, *Intensive Care Med* 32(11):1722–1732, 2006.

Miller PR, Meredith JW, Johnson JC, et al: Prospective evaluation of vacuum-assisted fascial closure after open abdomen: planned ventral hernia rate is substantially reduced, *Ann Surg* 239(5):608–614, 2004.

Miller PR, Thompson JT, Faler BJ, et al: Late fascial closure in lieu of ventral hernia: the next step in open abdomen management, *J Trauma* 53(5):843–849, 2002.

Moore EE, Thomas G: Orr memorial lecture: staged laparotomy for the hypothermia, acidosis, and coagulopathy syndrome, *Am J Surg* 172(5):405–410, 1996.

Richardson JD, Trinkle JK: Hemodynamic and respiratory alterations with increased intra-abdominal pressure, *J Surg Res* 20(5):401–404, 1976.

Suliburk JW, Ware DN, Balogh Z, et al: Vacuum-assisted wound closure achieves early fascial closure of open abdomens after severe trauma, *J Trauma* 55(6):1155–1160, discussion 1160–1161, 2003.

BLOOD TRANSFUSION THERAPY

Robert C. McIntyre Jr, MD, and Frederick A. Moore, MD

OVERVIEW

Blood transfusion therapy is an integral component of the practice of almost all fields of medicine. It is a critical part of the practice of all surgical specialties and surgical critical care. Safe practices have had a significant impact on errors leading to transfusion reactions. Bloodborne infectious disease transmission risk has also been significantly curtailed to a very low rate. Recently, more attention has been focused on noninfectious complications such as transfusion-related acute lung injury (TRALI). Changes in blood bank practices and recent technologic advances have improved the immunologic side effects of blood products. Further refinement of the indications for transfusion has made transfusion therapy safer by eliminating many unnecessary transfusion practices. Recent research has provided more evidence that governs the practice of transfusion therapy, and this chapter will focus on evidence-based transfusion practices, including recent emerging guidelines for massive transfusion. The chapter will also discuss the infectious and noninfectious risks of transfusion.

ALLOGENEIC BLOOD PRODUCTS

Current transfusion practice provides specific components of blood: red cells for oxygen-carrying capacity, plasma for coagulation factors, and platelets for microvascular bleeding. Whole blood is rarely used today; however, it may be appropriate in certain settings, particularly in massive trauma with ongoing hemorrhage. The component therapy approach allows for optimal use of a limited resource (Table 1).

Whole Blood

A unit of whole blood is collected into a bag with an anticoagulant without any further processing and is approximately 500 mL with a shelf life of up to 35 days (storage at 2 to 6° C). Fresh, unrefrigerated (20° to 24° C) whole blood has a shelf life of only 24 hours. Whole blood has limited indications, primarily symptomatic oxygen-carrying deficit and hypovolemic shock. However, components such as red cells and fresh frozen plasma (FFP) are usually used in preference to whole blood. Platelet and plasma coagulation factor activity in whole blood declines within 24 hours of collection. The primary advantage of whole blood is that it does not expose the recipient to packed red blood cells (PRBCs), plasma, and platelets from multiple donors. Given these characteristics, fresh whole blood is primarily used in military settings in field emergencies.

Packed Red Blood Cells

The primary purpose of transfusion of PRBCs is to provide oxygen-carrying capacity to the tissues. General rules for transfusion are problematic and usually are not appropriate. Factors that influence the decision to give PRBCs for acute blood-loss anemia include the presence of shock, control of ongoing hemorrhage, volume status of the patient in the absence of shock, associated symptoms, age, and comorbidity. The hematocrit of one unit of PRBCs is close to 60% and, as a rule, one unit of PRBCs increases the hemoglobin level by 1 g/dL or increases the hematocrit by 3%. The arbitrary transfusion trigger of 10 g/dL hemoglobin or 30% hematocrit, the *10/30 rule,* was first proposed by Adams and Lundy in 1942. They recommended transfusion in the perioperative period to decrease risk of complications. Despite the lack of data, this trigger was used widely, and further support for it in clinical practice came from multiple studies in the 1990s of resuscitation strategies to increase the oxygen delivery in the critically ill patient population to supraphysiologic levels. Blood loss of 10% or less does not require transfusion; loss up to 20% can be replaced with crystalloid; but loss of more than 30% generally requires RBC transfusion.

TABLE 1: Summary of blood components

Component	Indications	Storage Time	Disadvantage
Whole blood	Volume deficit, oxygen-carrying capacity, massive transfusion	35 days (2° to 6° C) Fresh: 24 hours	Short shelf life if fresh
PRBCs	Volume deficit, oxygen-carrying capacity	42 days	Immunomodulation
Leukocyte-reduced PRBCs	Reduced febrile reactions and alloimmunization, cardiac surgery patients, prevent CMV infection in transplant patients	42 days	Cost
Washed PRBCs	Prevention of allergic reactions	24 hours	Plasma depletion
FFP	Congenital or acquired coagulopathy, reverse warfarin	1 year	
Cryoprecipitate	Fibrinogen deficiency, von Willebrand disease	1 year	
Platelets	Microvascular bleeding, thrombocytopenia	5–7 days	Highest risk of transfusion-associated sepsis

Transfusion should be administered as clinically indicated for patients with acute, ongoing blood loss and for those with symptomatic anemia despite a euvolemic state. Symptoms of anemia include significant tachycardia without other etiology, orthostatic hypotension, dizziness, shortness of breath, and chest pain. Signs and symptoms of anemia are not likely when the hemoglobin level is above 7 to 8 g/dL; however, the hemoglobin level at which a patient manifests the signs and symptoms relates to underlying health status, cardiorespiratory reserve, and activity level.

The Transfusion Requirements in Critical Care Trial (TRICC) found that a more restrictive transfusion trigger of 7 g/dL hemoglobin, with the goal of maintaining the hemoglobin level between 7 and 9 g/dL, is as safe as 10 g/dL in a critically ill population of patients who are euvolemic and not bleeding. Overall 30-day mortality rate was similar in the two groups (18.7% vs. 23.3%). However, mortality rates were significantly lower with the restrictive transfusion strategy among patients with an Acute Physiology and Chronic Health Evaluation II (APACHE-II) score of less than 20 and in patients who were younger than 55 years. Other important subgroup analysis included patients with clinically significant cardiac disease, in whom mortality rate did not differ between the two groups. This study has lead to widespread adoption of a transfusion trigger of Hg 7 g/dL in asymptomatic, euvolemic patients.

Despite the data from TRICC suggesting that a restrictive transfusion trigger is safe in patients with cardiac disease, this topic remains controversial. Several nonrandomized studies provide conflicting results in patients with acute myocardial infarction or acute coronary syndrome. Wu and colleagues (2001) found that anemia on admission in Medicare patients was associated with increased 30-day mortality rate, and transfusion of patients with hematocrit less than 30% was associated with improved survival. Rao and colleagues (2004) used the databases of three large international trials of patients with acute coronary syndromes and found that transfusion was associated with an increased rate of death and myocardial infarction (MI) at 30 days. The predicted probability of death at 30 days was higher with transfusion at nadir hematocrit values above 25%. Lastly, analysis of a national quality-improvement database for patients with unstable angina showed a greater risk of death and reinfarction if the patient received a transfusion. These studies do not provide clear results to guide therapy; therefore a prospective trial of transfusion among patients presenting with acute coronary syndromes needs to be done.

In cardiac surgery patients, advanced age, preoperative anemia, small body size, noncoronary artery bypass surgery, urgent operation, preoperative antithrombotic drugs, coagulation disorders, and multiple comorbidities indicate high-risk patients for transfusion. Several retrospective studies show that morbidity and mortality are associated with a hematocrit of 14% to 22%; however, these studies do not review the effect of transfusion on outcome. On the other hand, some studies show that infection, stroke, and death are increased in association with transfusion. One prospective randomized trial that compared a transfusion trigger of 8 g/dL versus standard practice (hemoglobin < 9 g/dL) in 428 coronary artery bypass graft surgery patients found no difference in clinical outcome. Based on these data, the Society of Thoracic Surgeons Clinical Practice Guidelines recommend that transfusion is "reasonable in most postoperative patients whose hemoglobin is less than 7 g/dL."

Transfusion of PRBCs to maintain an hematocrit above 30% was part of the supraphysiologic resuscitation strategy promoted by Shoemaker and others. Multiple studies failed to reproduce a favorable outcome, and one study even showed that this strategy of resuscitation could be harmful. A recent randomized trial of early goal-directed therapy for the treatment of sepsis and septic shock was done by Rivers and colleagues, who randomized septic patients to either standard resuscitation or a goal-directed protocol. PRBCs were given if the hematocrit was below 30%, and the central venous oxygen saturation ($ScvO_2$) was below 70%. Patients in the early goal-directed therapy arm had a better overall mortality rates compared with those who received standard resuscitation (30.5% vs. 46.5%). It is difficult to isolate the effect of transfusion because it was among multiple interventions.

Leukocytes present in blood products are responsible for a number of complications associated with transfusion. Leukocyte reduction lowers the risk of these complications and is indicated in patients who need multiple transfusions, who have had febrile transfusion reactions, who are immunosuppressed, or are transplant recipients. Randomized trials show leukoreduction in cardiac surgery decreases mortality; however, a large randomized study in 2780 patients without established medical indications for leukocyte-reduced blood showed no benefit other than a decrease in febrile reaction. The added cost of leukocyte reduction has limited its widespread adoption. Washing RBCs removes plasma proteins and is indicated in patients who have allergic reactions (mediated by immunoglobulin E), such as immunoglobulin A–deficient patients. Radiation eliminates T lymphocytes and reduces the risk of graft-versus-host disease in bone marrow transplantation and certain immunodeficient states.

Plasma

Plasma provides coagulation factors that include fibrinogen, von Willebrand factor (vWF), the vitamin K–dependent coagulation factors—II, VII, IX, and X—factor VIII, and factor XIII. Plasma is frozen at −18° C and can be stored for up to 1 year. FFP is indicated for congenital or acquired coagulation defects and rapid reversal of anticoagulants. It is not indicated solely for volume expansion. Transfusion should be guided by clinical assessment of bleeding combined with coagulation test results or point-of-care testing, such as for thromboelastographic (TEG) changes. FFP may be used before procedures, depending on the risk of bleeding, if the international normalized ratio is greater than 1.6; however, FFP is not indicated for the stable, nonbleeding patient. FFP is also not indicated for a single coagulation factor deficiency. One unit of FFP is about 250 mL and provides approximately 7% of the coagulation factors necessary for a 70 kg patient.

Cryoprecipitate

Certain factors precipitate out of plasma at cold temperatures and are provided by cryoprecipitate; these include fibrinogen, fibronectin, factors VIII and XIII, and vWF. Cryoprecipitate is indicated for patients with fibrinogen deficiency, factor XIII deficiency, massive transfusion, and platelet dysfunction secondary to renal disease if resistant to desmopressin and estrogens. It is important to obtain fibrinogen measurements because levels less than 100 mg/dL cause prolongation of the prothrombin time (PT) and partial thromboplastin time (PTT), despite adequate clotting-factor replacement. Ten units of cryoprecipitate contains 2 g of fibrinogen and raises the fibrinogen by about 60 g/L. Cryoprecipitate should be given if the fibrinogen level drops below 100 g/L in the setting of bleeding or ongoing transfusions.

Platelets

Platelets are collected from either whole blood donations (platelet concentrates) or by apheresis (single-donor platelets). Each platelet concentrate contains approximately 5.5×10^{10} platelets suspended in a plasma volume of approximately 50 mL. An apheresis platelet unit contains a minimum of 3×10^{11} platelets, a dose equivalent to six pooled platelet concentrates. Platelets should be given for bleeding associated with platelet counts less than 50,000. Platelets are also indicated if the count is less than 50,000 prior to a major operation, less than 20,000 prior to an invasive procedure, or less than 10,000 even if stable without bleeding. The platelet count should increase 5000 to 10,000 per unit transfused or 30,000 to 60,000 per apheresis unit delivered.

AUTOLOGOUS BLOOD

Preoperative blood donation came into practice in the mid 1980s and reached a peak in 1992, during which time 6% of all transfused blood in the United States was autologous. Since then its use has declined, but it still remains a viable option for patients scheduled to have an operation that is likely to require transfusion. Autologous blood donation may be particularly useful in patients who have rare blood types or alloantibodies that make cross matching difficult, and many patients are interested in autologous blood donation as a way to reduce the risk of transmission of infectious diseases despite the reduction of risk with modern testing.

Autologous blood transfusion prevents transfusion-related disease transmission and sensitization to antigens, and it limits immune modulation. The typical volunteer allogeneic blood donor is allowed to give 1 U of blood no more than once every 8 weeks to avoid iron deficiency. On the other hand, autologous blood donation is usually started 3 to 5 weeks before an elective surgical procedure, and donation is done once a week. Sufficient time should be allowed for the patient to make a full recovery between the time of the last donation and the operation. Autologous donors should have a starting Hg above 11 g/dL and be free of significant cardiovascular or hematologic diseases. In general, autologous donors are not as healthy as allogeneic blood donors. Although the shelf life of refrigerated red blood cells is limited to 42 days, frozen storage for up to 10 years is possible at less than −65° C, using glycerol as a cryopreservative. Other options to autologous donation are hemodilution, intraoperative blood salvage, and postoperative blood salvage. Oral iron therapy can be used to maintain sufficient supplies. Erythropoietin is usually not necessary, and its cost effectiveness is uncertain; its use is approved in Japan and Canada but not in the United States. Forty-four percent of autologous donations are unused by the autologous donor, and these units are discarded for safety reasons.

MASSIVE TRANSFUSION

Hemorrhage is the most common cause of death in the first hour after trauma. Initial care of patients presenting in shock includes an empiric volume load to restore heart rate and blood pressure; however, deliberate hypotension may have advantages in penetrating torso trauma patients until hemostasis is achieved. Limiting crystalloid infusion may decrease bleeding, avoid hemodilution, and prevent problematic edema. Measurement of arterial blood gases with base deficit, serum lactate levels, and serial Hg guides resuscitation.

A significant percentage (25% to 50%) of trauma patients who require massive transfusion (more than 10 units of PRBCs in 24 hours) arrive at the emergency department with coagulopathy. The lethal triad of trauma consists of coagulopathy, hypothermia, and acidosis. *Hypothermia*, defined as a core body temperature below 35° C, is due to heat loss during resuscitation and use of room temperature or cold IV solutions. Hypothermia impairs both platelet and coagulation factor function. Acidosis from inadequate tissue perfusion and resuscitation with high-chloride-content crystalloid solutions also impair coagulation factor function, and dilutional coagulopathy results from replacement of blood losses with fluids that do not contain coagulation factors. Transfusion of less than 10 U of PRBCs alone rarely causes a significant coagulopathy.

Standard tests of coagulation function, such as the PT and PTT, do not detect all pathophysiologic changes in posttraumatic coagulopathy. The PT and PTT are run in platelet-poor plasma; thus the interactions of platelets and the coagulation factors are not evaluated. Furthermore, these coagulation tests are typically run at 37° C and do not reflect the patient's actual temperature. Point-of-care testing allows for a more rapid assessment of the clotting of whole blood and is useful in trauma resuscitation as well as in hepatic and cardiovascular surgery. Available point-of-care tests include the activated clotting time (ACT), viscoelastic methods such as TEG, and various bedside tests of platelet function. Despite its advantages TEG is not uniformly used in trauma centers because of the significant regulatory burden and training issues involved in point-of-care testing. With increased understanding of the early development of trauma-induced coagulopathy, greater attention to its correction has resulted in a number of protocols to deliver FFP and platelets more rapidly, without the delay of waiting for results of standard tests of coagulation function.

Military experience reveals that resuscitation with a high FFP/PRBC ratio in patients who need massive transfusion is associated with improved survival. This experience has also been shown in multiple studies of the civilian trauma population. These retrospective data suggest that resuscitation using an FFP/PRBC ratio greater than 1:1.5 is associated with improved outcome; however, the exact ratio of PRBC/FFP is not well established. A wide variability remains in massive transfusion protocols (MTP), but most require early recognition of a massively injured patient in uncontrolled hemorrhagic shock to initiate the protocol. Protocols are designed to immediately deliver aggressive component therapy in patients at risk of needing massive transfusion. Risk factors include penetrating mechanism, positive

TABLE 2: Massive transfusion protocol

Package	PRBC (Units)	FFP (Units)	Platelets (Units)	Other
1	6	6		
2	6	6	1 apheresis	
3	6	6		Cryoprecipitate, rFVIIa
4	6	6	1 apheresis	
5	6	6		
6	6	6	1 apheresis	Cryoprecipitate, rFVIIa

Data from O'Keeffe T, Refaai M, Tchorz K, et al: A massive transfusion protocol to decrease blood component use and costs, *Arch Surg* 143:686-691, 2008.

TABLE 3: Risk of transmission of four viruses per unit of blood component

Virus	Risk per Unit
HIV	1:2,135,000 to 1:4,700,000
HBV	1:31,000 to 1:205,000
HCV	1:1,935,000 to 1:3,100,000
HTLV	1:3,000,000

Data from Dodd RY, Notari EPT, Stramer SL: Current prevalence and incidence of infectious disease markers and estimated window-period risk in the American Red Cross blood donor population, *Transfusion* 42(8):975-979, 2002; and Kleinman S, Chan P, Robillard P: Risks associated with transfusion of cellular blood components in Canada, *Transfus Med Rev* 17(2):120-162, 2003.

TABLE 4: Incidence rates of viruses in repeat blood donors

	RATE PER 100,000 PERSON-YEARS			
	HIV	HBV	HCV	HTLV
United States (American Red Cross, 2000–2001)	1.55	1.27	1.89	0.24
Canada (2001–2005)	0.41	2.98	1.63	0.14
England (1999–2001)	0.30	0.20	0.23	NR

Data from O'Brien SF, Yi QL, Fan W, et al: Current incidence and estimated residual risk of transfusion-transmitted infections in donations made to Canadian Blood Services, *Transfusion* 47:316–325, 2007.

results from a focused assessment by sonography for trauma (FAST), arrival systolic blood pressure *less than* 90 mm Hg, arrival heart rate above 120 beats/min (BPM), unstable pelvis fracture, base deficit, and pH below 7.25. A blood sample should be obtained as early as possible to allow blood typing.

Components are delivered in packages of PRBC, FFP, and platelets. One example protocol's first package contains 6 units of group O PRBCs and 6 units of FFP (Table 2). As soon as the patient's blood type is known, type-specific products are delivered. The second package consists of 6 units of PRBCs, 6 units of FFP, and 1 unit of apheresis platelets. The third package contains the same products as the first, and the packages alternate thereafter until deactivation of the protocol. Variability in protocols among centers includes the use of cryoprecipitate and recombinant activated factor VII (rFVIIa). Cryoprecipitate may be given with the third package, after 12 units of PRBCs. Busy trauma centers may also use thawed plasma in the ER to prevent delay in obtaining plasma. Thawed plasma contains all of the clotting factors that FFP contains with some exceptions; it has lower levels of factor V and factor VIII, and it has a shelf life of 4 to 5 days.

Factor VIIa is an initiator of thrombin generation, and rFVIIa complexes with tissue factor (TF) at the site of tissue injury and binds platelets independent of TF. In a military study, rFVIIa given at 8 U of PRBCs decreased transfusion requirements. The current recommended dose is 90 to 120 μg/kg. This dose should be repeated at 1 to 2 hours if required. Multiple reports of thromboembolic events in patients receiving rFVIIa have surfaced, but randomized, controlled trials (RCTs) do not reveal an increase in risk, except in patients with hemorrhagic stroke. The drug is very expensive, approximately $5000 per dose, and its cost effectiveness has not been established.

Although multiple retrospective studies suggest that an MTP using a ratio of 1:1 FFP/PRBC improves mortality, there are numerous limitations to these studies. One study suggests that there may be a "survivor bias" in these retrospective studies. This bias may exist if early deaths that occur before initiation of the MTP are included in the cohort that does not receive a high FFP/PRBC ratio. The higher survival rate in patients who received a higher ratio may be a reflection that they lived long enough to receive the MTP. These concerns, plus the risk of TRALI, are certainly part of the justification for a large, multicenter prospective randomized trial.

COMPLICATIONS

Advances in blood bank practices have made transfusion very safe. Testing for infectious diseases has made transmission of pathogens such as human immunodeficiency virus (HIV) or hepatitis C virus

(HCV) on the order of 1 in 2 million units. As these advances have decreased the concern about infectious complications, awareness of immune-modulating effects of transfusion has increased.

Infectious Complications

A variety of bloodborne infectious agents can be transmitted through transfusion of infected blood donated by apparently healthy and asymptomatic blood donors. The spectrum of agents are shown in Table 3 and include those that are the typical concerns of doctors and patients: HIV, HCV, hepatitis B virus (HBV), human T-cell lymphotropic viruses (HTLV-I and HTLV-II), and cytomegalovirus (CMV). However, emerging infectious diseases are also of concern, including parvovirus B19, West Nile virus (WNV), dengue virus, trypanosomiasis, malaria, and variant Creutzfeldt-Jakob disease (vCJD).

Several strategies are implemented to reduce the risk of transmitting infectious agents: donor deferral for a history of risk factors, screening for the serological markers of infections, and nucleic acid testing (NAT) by viral gene amplification for direct and sensitive detection of the known infectious agents, first introduced in 2000 for HCV, then in 2003 for HIV-1, and finally in 2006 for HBV. NAT screening for viral DNA covers the *window period,* which is the time between acute infection and seroconversion in the donor. For current incidence rates of viruses in repeat blood donors and risk of transmission of viruses per unit of blood component, see Table 4.

Approximately 50% of blood donors in the United States have antibodies to CMV, which infects a variety of cell types but predominantly the monocyte-macrophage lineage. Thus leukocyte depletion largely eliminates the risk of transmission. The risk of CMV infection in immunocompetent seronegative patients who receive nonleukoreduced cellular blood components is approximately 1%. On the other hand, CMV infection in immunocompromised recipients receiving CMV-unscreened, nonleukoreduced blood components has been reported in various studies from 15% to 50%. Thus CMV-seronegative or leukocyte-reduced blood components are recommended for at-risk patients. Even with these precautions, 1% to 5% of at-risk patients have CMV infection after transfusion.

Epstein-Barr virus (EBV) is the etiologic agent of infectious mononucleosis and is closely associated with Burkitt lymphoma, nasopharyngeal carcinoma, and posttransplant lymphoproliferative disease (PTLD). Transfusion transmission is unlikely due to the greater than 90% incidence of previous exposure in the adult population. Human parvovirus B19 is ubiquitous in humans, but the prevalence of viremia in donors is rare; however, patients who receive pooled, plasma-derived products involving thousands of donors have a significant risk. As such, plasma manufacturers use NAT to detect plasma sources with high B19 titers. Despite very few cases of West Nile virus infection as a result of transfusions, blood-collection agencies conduct WNV RNA testing on every donation.

Classic CJD is a rare, fatal, degenerative neurologic disease caused by a prion protein. There are no reported cases of transmission of classic CJD by blood transfusion. Variant CJD is caused by the same agent as bovine spongiform encephalopathy (BSE), and four cases of transfusion-related vCJD have been reported in the United Kingdom. No screening tests are available, so development of pathogen reduction and inactivation methods (PRIM) such as filtration holds the most promise for prevention. A wide variety of PRIMs are either available or are undergoing testing, but these methods are not in widespread clinical use.

Transfusion-associated sepsis (TAS) is one of the top three causes of transfusion-related mortality. Bacterial contamination can occur through contamination at the time of donation from the skin, a break in sterile technique, or disruption of the storage container. Contamination is a much bigger problem in the room-temperature storage of platelets than it is in cold storage of red blood cells. Bacterial contamination is a higher risk in autologous than allogeneic donation. The frequency of contamination of PRBCs is 1 in 30,000 units with a prevalence of clinically significant events of 1 in 500,000 units. The rate of contamination of platelets is in the range of 1 in 1000 to 3000 units with clinically significant sepsis in 1 in 100,000. General precautionary methods to prevent contamination, as well as screening for affected units by culture and nonculture methods, are the current preventative techniques to decrease risk. Sepsis due to transfusion should be evaluated if a patient experiences fever, rigors, tachycardia, or hypotension within 1 to 4 hours of transfusion. Evaluation begins with recognition, cessation of the transfusion, blood cultures from the patient and from the blood component bag, and antibiotic administration. Febrile, nonhemolytic transfusion reactions are easily confused with transfusion-associated sepsis.

Febrile Nonhemolytic Transfusion Reaction

A febrile transfusion reaction is the most common transfusion reaction and results from donor leukocytes or cytokines. The cause of cytokine release is due to recipient antibodies against donor leukocytes or platelets. It is suspected when a temperature increase of 1° C or more occurs during or after transfusion, when no other cause can be found. Hemolysis, TAS, and anaphylaxis must be ruled out. Treatment consists of supportive care, acetaminophen, and diphenhydramine. Leukocyte-reduced blood products are useful to avoid repeated febrile reactions.

Hemolytic Transfusion Reactions

Hemolytic transfusion reactions occur due to immune-mediated lysis of red blood cells. Hemolysis may be early or delayed, and it can be intravascular or extravascular. Acute hemolysis is due to

---

BOX 1: Workup of acute hemolysis transfusion reaction

1. Stop transfusion.
2. Resuscitate with fluids.
3. Induce diuresis.
4. Return the unit to the blood bank along with the paperwork.
5. Obtain blood and urine for transfusion reaction workup.
   a. Direct Coombs
   b. Repeat cross match
   c. Hemoglobinemia
   d. Hemoglobinuria
   e. Blood urea nitrogen, creatinine
   f. Coagulation parameters
   g. LDH, haptoglobin
   h. Blood cultures (if sepsis is suspected)

---

transfusion of incompatible red blood cells into a patient with preformed antibodies. ABO-incompatible blood transfusions are the most common cause, but other antigen systems can also produce these reactions, such as the Kidd or Duffy blood group systems. In addition to the antibody effect, complement and cytokine activation occurs, which is a true medical emergency. The transfusion should be stopped immediately, and the component should be sent to the blood bank along with a new tube of patient blood for repeat cross matching (Box 1).

Fluid resuscitation to maintain renal blood flow and to prevent renal tubular necrosis is critical. Diuretics may be necessary to improve urine flow after fluid administration. On the other hand, excessive crystalloid should be avoided to prevent pulmonary edema and congestive heart failure. Laboratory evaluation includes urine analysis for hemoglobinuria, lactate dehydrogenase (LDH), haptoglobin, and indirect bilirubin. A direct Coombs test will be positive and is considered diagnostic. Patients should be monitored for disseminated intravascular coagulation (DIC) and acute renal failure.

An extravascular hemolytic transfusion reaction results in an antigen-antibody reaction without the complement activation of the acute intravascular reaction. The extravascular reaction occurs because the antibody-coated cells are cleared by the IgG receptors in the spleen or in the liver. Red cell lysis does not occur in the intravascular space. An extravascular hemolytic transfusion reaction is usually not an emergency. It is characterized by a positive direct Coombs test, an increase in indirect bilirubin and LDH, a decline in hematocrit and haptoglobin, and an increase in colorless urine urobilinogen. Hemoglobinuria and hemoglobinemia are rarely present. The patient often has a low-grade fever but does not have the toxic presentation of an intravascular hemolytic reaction.

Delayed hemolytic transfusion reactions occur 3 to 10 days after transfusion. The same diagnostic and treatment considerations are important; however, the reactions are usually milder than the acute reactions. Therefore the therapeutic interventions are not as aggressive.

Transfusion-Related Acute Lung Injury

TRALI was first recognized in the 1950s with the first publication of a case series in 1966. TRALI is now recognized as the leading cause of transfusion-related death. By consensus, TRALI is an acute lung injury temporally related to a transfusion of any blood product that contains plasma, and it is not physiologically different from other forms of lung injury, including acute respiratory distress syndrome (ARDS). To meet the definition of classic TRALI, there must be no

TABLE 5: Risk of noninfectious complications

Event	Risk per Unit of PRBCs
Febrile reactions	1:15 to 1:1400
Acute hemolytic reaction	1:250,000 to 1:1,000,000
Delayed hemolytic reaction	1:1,000 to 1:10,000
Major allergic reaction	1:23,000
TRALI	1:5,000 to 1:400,000

Data from Kleinman S, Chan P, Robillard P: Risks associated with transfusion of cellular blood components in Canada, *Transfus Med Rev* 17(2):120–162, 2003; and Goodnough LT, Brecher ME, Kanter MH, et al: Transfusion medicine, *N Engl J Med* 340:438–437, 1999.

other risk factor for acute lung injury, and the injury must occur within 6 hours of transfusion. Recent data suggest that transfusion in critically ill patients and trauma patients can cause a delayed TRALI that can occur 6 to 72 hours after transfusion. Delayed TRALI occurs in the setting of other risk factors for acute lung injury in up to 25% of patients, with a mortality of 35% to 45%. The incidence of TRALI in various studies depends on definitions and methods of detection, but it ranges from 1 in 432 to 1 in 88,000/U of platelets, from 1 in 4400 to 1 in 557,000/U of PRBCs, and 1 in 2000 U plasma-containing components (Table 5).

Two mechanisms of TRALI have been proposed: The first hypothesis is that TRALI is an antibody-mediated event that involves passive infusion of donor antibodies against recipient leukocyte antigens or infusion of donor leukocytes into a recipient who has antibodies directed against donor leukocytes. The second hypothesis is that TRALI is caused by two events: The first is the underlying clinical condition of the patient, which causes pulmonary endothelial activation and sequestration of neutrophils. Transfusion is the second event, involving infusion of antibodies against the adherent polymorphonuclear neutrophils in the lung. Activation of primed neutrophils causes pulmonary endothelium damage, neutrophil migration, capillary leak, and TRALI. Prevention of TRALI will include following restrictive transfusion practices to decrease unnecessary transfusion. Washing blood components to remove antibodies, leukocyte reduction, and using fresh PRBCs with less than 14 days shelf life have all been proposed as methods to decrease TRALI. Some have proposed excluding donations from females and from donors with previously demonstrated white blood cell (WBC) antibodies. Treatment is generally supportive and involves supplemental oxygen for mild cases and mechanical ventilation with a lung-protective strategy for patients who need intubation.

TRANSFUSION-RELATED IMMUNOMODULATION

Ever since Opelz discovered in 1973 that transfusions improved renal allograft success, the immune consequences of transfusion have been recognized. Interestingly, even in the age of cyclosporine, patients who receive donor-specific blood transfusion have an improved living renal allograft success rate compared with those who have not had a transfusion. This effect appears to be dependent on viable leukocytes in the PRBCs, as there is less immunologic benefit in transfusions that are leukocyte reduced, washed, or frozen-thawed. *Transfusion-related immunomodulation* (TRIM) has traditionally been defined as the immune suppression related to allogeneic blood. However, recent experience suggests that transfusion has additional effects that are proinflammatory, and it may have an effect on short-term outcomes. Other possible beneficial effects of this immunomodulation include

a decrease in the risk of Crohn's disease recurrence and a reduction in risk of spontaneous abortion. Other immunomodulating effects of transfusion are detrimental to the surgical patient, including an increase in perioperative infectious complications and an increase in cancer recurrence. In transplant patients, transfusion may activate latent CMV or other viral infections. TRIM may also be due to allogeneic mononuclear cells, WBC-derived soluble mediators, and soluble human leukocyte antigen (HLA) peptides. Thus many of the deleterious effects of allogeneic transfusion could be reduced by prestorage, but not poststorage, leukocyte-reduction methods, or autologous transfusion. Canada and several Western European countries use universal leukocyte reduction by prestorage filtration; however, this practice has not been adopted in the United States.

Perioperative Infectious Complications

Over 40 observational studies have examined the risk of infection in patients who receive blood transfusion compared with untransfused patients encompassing trauma, colon cancer, hip replacement, spine fusion, head and neck cancer, various gastrointestinal (GI) operations, and cardiac surgery. These studies are especially prone to confounding variables that make the results hard to interpret, although the results are remarkably consistent in showing an increase in perioperative infection in transfused patients; however, the effect appears to be small. The risk appears to be greater in trauma compared with other surgical procedures. Further, a dose-response relation has been identified, such that the higher the number of units transfused, the higher the risk. As an independent predictor of postoperative infection, the number of units transfused varied in the studies, from more than 4 units to more than 11 units of PRBCs transfused. This effect may be due to a combined or additive effect of blood transfusion on the immune system, with the immune hyporesponsiveness a result of trauma. Although multiple studies demonstrate this association, they have not established a cause-effect relation, nor has the mechanism of such an effect been established by preclinical or clinical studies. Multiple RCTs have compared infection in patients receiving either leukocyte reduction or autologous blood to non–leukocyte-reduced blood. Results have been conflicting, and too much heterogeneity in the studies precludes meta-analysis. Thus these studies do not provide conclusive evidence of a TRIM effect.

Cancer Recurrence

Prompted by observations in renal transplantation, Gannt (1981) suggested that immunosuppression as a result of transfusion could lead to an effect on cancer immune surveillance and thus increase recurrence risk. Over 100 observational studies and three prospective randomized trials have been done on the effects of transfusion on cancer recurrence. The most extensively investigated area is colorectal cancer, but studies have also examined recurrence rates in head and neck, breast, gastric, lung, prostate, and cervical cancer. The results of the observation studies have been subjected to three meta-analyses, and a statistically significant effect was found for all cancer sites except the cervix.

A recent meta-analysis focused on colorectal cancer found 36 studies on 12,127 patients, and 23 studies involving 8029 patients showed a detrimental effect of perioperative blood transfusion; 15 studies showed no difference in 4098 patients. In 23 studies multivariable analysis was used to control for confounders, and 14 found transfusion to be an independent prognostic factor; no effect was found in eight investigations. Pooled estimates of transfusion effect on colorectal cancer recurrence yielded an overall odds ratio of 1.42 (95% confidence interval, 1.20 to 1.67) against transfused patients in RCTs. The three trials compared transfusion with prestorage leukocyte reduction to buffy coat–prepared PRBCs—a process that removes approximately two thirds of donor leukocytes without filtration—in patients with colorectal cancer. These studies failed to find a significant effect on cancer recurrence.

Multiple Organ Failure

Several observational studies have found that transfusion is associated with an increase in the systemic inflammatory response and multiple organ failure (MOF) in trauma patients. When controlled for the potentially confounding variables of shock and injury, the Denver trauma group found blood transfusion to be an independent predictor of the incidence of MOF. Further, there appears to be a dose–response relationship between the amount of transfused blood (more than 6 units in the first 12 hours after injury) and MOF. The prevailing hypothesis is that PRBC storage leads to an increase in cytokines (interleukin (IL)-1b, IL-6, IL-8, and tumor necrosis factor-α) and lipids in the plasma fraction, and this causes priming and or activation of vascular endothelium and neutrophils. Some data suggest that fresher blood products (PRBCs <21 days old), washed units, and prestorage leukoreduction may decrease proinflammatory mediators and lead to improvements in rates of infection, MOF, and death. However, data are not sufficient to warrant universal application of these processes. Further, preparation time, cost, and the short outdating of units make these approaches impractical in most blood banks.

Red Cell Storage Duration

During storage, PRBCs undergo a series of changes that reduces their survival and function. Accumulation of biological by-products during PRBC storage may be harmful to recipients of blood transfusions. Five studies report a correlation between RBC age and development of infection, multiple organ dysfunction, and mortality in trauma patients. One recent study reported an association between red cell storage length and adverse outcome in cardiac surgery patients. Multivariate analysis in another recent study, which also looked at cardiac surgery patients, showed no effect of storage time on survival or ICU stay. Studies in colorectal surgery patients and in the critically ill have yielded conflicting results; thus it is difficult to draw firm conclusions about the association of the age of stored blood and outcomes. A large, prospective, RCT would be helpful in determining the true clinical significance of the effect of red cell storage duration on patient outcomes.

Leukocyte Reduction

Since deleterious immunomodulation related to transfusion is thought to be largely related to the WBCs in blood products, there have been several randomized trials comparing risk in recipients of non–leukocyte-reduced allogeneic blood versus autologous or leukocyte-reduced allogeneic PRBCs. If leukocytes are important mediators of TRIM, prestorage leukocyte reduction would prevent the accumulation of biologic response mediators, but poststorage reduction would not. Further, the autologous transfusion would exclude HLA peptides, but only prestorage leukocyte reduction would prevent accumulation of biologic response mediators. Alternatively, only fresh (and not stored) autologous blood that is not leukocyte reduced would determine whether soluble mediators were important.

There are 17 RCTs of autologous or leukocyte-reduced PRBCs versus non–leukocyte-reduced PRBCs, but significant heterogeneity in the trials precludes meta-analysis. Outside of cardiac surgery, combining subsets of the trials that are homogeneous fails to establish that leukocyte reduction decreases postoperative infection. Further, a large randomized study showed no benefits to patients without specific indications in a short-term analysis. Five studies involving cardiac surgery demonstrate lower mortality in patients who receive leukocyte-reduced PRBCs. Based on these results, leukocyte reduction of all blood components is recommended for cardiac surgery patients, but thus far it has not been recommended for other patients. Three other proven benefits of leukocyte reduction are the prevention of febrile transfusion reactions, HLA alloimmunization, and CMV infection.

BLOOD SUBSTITUTES

Over the past decade, several trials have been carried out on hemoglobin substitutes, otherwise known as *hemoglobin-based oxygen carriers* (HBOCs). Theoretically, these could offer several advantages including availability, an abundant supply, universal compatibility, prolonged shelf life, storage at room temperature, and safety compared to allogeneic blood. The ideal substitute would expand circulating volume, deliver oxygen to tissue beds, and be devoid of adverse immunologic and infectious problems. Eight commercially available products have now been tested, but questions of safety in these studies have prevented FDA approval.

The similarity of adverse events among the various HBOCs raises questions of a common mechanism of toxicity despite differences in the molecular characteristics of these products. The toxicity appears to be related to Hg oxidation, reactive oxygen species, and scavenging of the nitric oxide (NO) mediator, which maintains a relaxed vascular tone. Adverse events include renal toxicity, pancreatitis, hepatocellular injury, esophageal spasm, myocardial ischemia and infarction, and pulmonary hypertension. Future progress must include further modification of the molecular and biologic properties of HBOCs to improve the rate of NO scavenging and resistance to oxidation. Clinical trial design will need to define clinical benefit with meaningful, readily measureable efficacy end points.

FUTURE DIRECTIONS

Several clinical trials are currently recruiting patients and will yield results in the near future. These are focused on further refinement of the transfusion trigger in critically ill patients, those with GI bleeding, and those undergoing major orthopedic and cardiac surgery. Ongoing studies seek to better define the optimal ratio of blood products in massive transfusion in trauma patients. The Transfusion Medicine/Hemostasis Clinical Trials Network Platelet Dose (PLADO) trial seeks to compare three doses—a low, medium, and high dose—for prophylactic platelet transfusions in patients with thrombocytopenia. Ongoing studies should provide more data on the effect of PRBC storage duration and leukocyte reduction.

Methods to improve the safety of components include increasing the spectrum of NAT and fully automating lab systems. A number of methods for the detection of bacteria in components exist and are in use, but none seems to ensure complete safety. Progress has been made in the development of pathogen-reduction technologies, and a synthetic psoralen, is available and in use in parts of Europe. The method has been shown to readily inactivate the levels of relevant bacteria present in platelets around the time of their preparation. A second approach based upon the use of a photoinactivating agent, riboflavin, is also under development and appears to have the potential for improving safety. The epidemiology of infectious diseases in any given country or region has the most important impact on blood safety. The National Institutes of Health funded the Retrovirus Epidemiology Donor Study (REDS) in 1989, and REDS-II is now under way to monitor the appearance of newly discovered infectious pathogens in the blood supply.

Suggested Readings

Bracey AW, Radovancevic R, Riggs SA, et al: Lowering the hemoglobin threshold for transfusion in coronary artery bypass procedures: effect on patient outcome, *Transfusion* 39(10):1070–1077, 1999.

Dodd RY, Notari EPT, Stramer SL: Current prevalence and incidence of infectious disease markers and estimated window-period risk in the American Red Cross blood donor population, *Transfusion* 42(8):975–979, 2002.

Ferraris VA, Ferraris SP, Saha SP, et al: Perioperative blood transfusion and blood conservation in cardiac surgery: the Society of Thoracic Surgeons and the Society of Cardiovascular Anesthesiologists clinical practice guidelines, *Ann Thorac Surg* 83(suppl 5):S27–S86, 2007.

Hebert PC, Wells G, Blajchman MA, et al: and the Transfusion Requirements in Critical Care Investigators, Canadian Critical Care Trials Group: A multicenter, randomized, controlled clinical trial of transfusion requirements in critical care, *N Engl J Med* 340(6):409–417, 1999.

Kleinman S, Chan P, Robillard P: Risks associated with transfusion of cellular blood components in Canada, *Transfus Med Rev* 17(2):120–162, 2003.

Rivers E, Nguyen B, Havstad S, et al: Early goal-directed therapy in the treatment of severe sepsis and septic shock, *N Engl J Med* 345(19):1368–1377, 2001.

Sperry JL, Ochoa JB, Gunn SR, et al: An FFP: PRBC transfusion ratio ≥1:1.5 is associated with a lower risk of mortality after massive transfusion, *J Trauma* 65(5):986–993, 2008.

Toy P, Popovsky MA, Abraham E, et al: Transfusion-related acute lung injury: definition and review, *Crit Care Med* 33(4):721–726, 2005.

COAGULOPATHY OF TRAUMA: PATHOGENESIS, DIAGNOSIS, AND TREATMENT

Michael B. Streiff, MD, and Elliott R. Haut, MD, FACS

OVERVIEW

Each year over 5 million people die as a result of major trauma. It is the fifth most common cause of death worldwide and the leading cause among individuals aged 5 to 44 years. Current trends indicate that trauma will become the second leading cause of death by the year 2020. Despite dramatic improvements in acute trauma care, the number of deaths resulting from injury has not changed substantially in over a decade. Hemorrhage is the second leading cause of injury-related death, resulting in at least 20% to 40% of trauma-related mortality, and it has been reported as the second leading cause of preventable death, after airway-management problems, even in mature trauma centers. Therefore rapid assessment and treatment of traumatic hemorrhage are essential to reducing trauma-associated mortality. This chapter reviews the pathogenesis, diagnosis, and treatment of the coagulopathy associated with major trauma.

NORMAL HEMOSTASIS

Normal hemostasis involves the coordinated, synergistic, and balanced interactions of the vascular system, platelets, procoagulant factors, endogenous anticoagulant proteins, and the fibrinolytic system. At baseline, in the absence of vascular injury, each component exists in a relatively quiescent state such that the blood remains fluid but with the potential to rapidly form an insoluble coagulum/platelet plug. In the event of vascular injury, each of these elements springs into action: vascular disruption results in vessel-wall contraction in arteries, which reduces the loss of blood from the injured vessel and shunts the blood volume to intact vessels. Injury exposes subendothelial collagen to circulating von Willebrand factor (VWF), which initiates the adhesion of platelets to the site of injury and leads to the formation of a platelet plug.

Simultaneously, the coagulation cascade is activated by the exposure of subendothelial tissue factor, which forms a complex with activated factor VII (factor VIIa). This event ultimately triggers the formation of small amounts of thrombin, which activates factors XI, VIII, and V and leads to a burst of thrombin generation that triggers platelet activation, fibrin formation, and stable, covalently cross-linked fibrin clot formation through activation of factor XIII. The coagulation cascade and platelets synergize to promote more efficient clot formation (Figure 1).

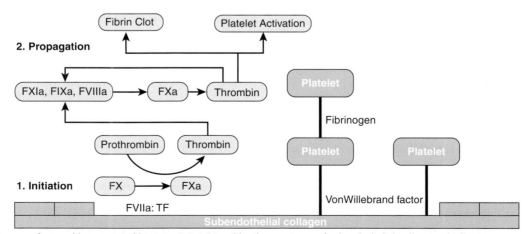

FIGURE 1   Diagram of normal hemostasis. Hemostasis is initiated by the exposure of subendothelial collagen, which initiates activation of the coagulation cascade through tissue factor and factor VIIa. Subsequent production of small amounts of thrombin results in propagation/amplification of the coagulation response leading to fibrin clot formation and platelet activation. Collagen exposure also triggers platelet adhesion and aggregation through interactions with von Willebrand factor (adhesion) and fibrinogen (aggregation).

These prothrombotic forces are balanced by the activity of endogenous antithrombotic proteins—including protein C, protein S, antithrombin III, and thrombomodulin—which prevent excessive clot formation in a necessary negative-feedback loop. The fibrinolytic system also plays a key role in limiting the extent of clot formation outside the immediate area of tissue injury and maintains vascular patency by digesting fibrin clot. Plasminogen is the primary fibrinolytic enzyme; it circulates in an inactive form until activated by tissue plasminogen activator (TPA), which is released by intact endothelial cells.

THE PATHOGENESIS OF TRAUMA-ASSOCIATED COAGULOPATHY

The "lethal triad" of trauma is classically conceived to include hypothermia, acidosis, and coagulopathy that contribute to a "bloody vicious cycle" (Figure 2). In this well-accepted paradigm, individual trauma-associated derangements of normal physiology synergize to trigger a spiral of progressively worsening bleeding that contributes to the high mortality rates from bleeding in trauma victims. The coagulopathy associated with trauma is a key factor in this pathway and has many potential causes, including extensive microvascular damage, hypotension, dilution, acidosis, and hypothermia. The contribution of each of these factors likely varies from patient to patient depending upon the type, severity, and mechanism of the injury.

Recent data suggest that genetic variation may play a role in the heterogeneity of the coagulopathic response to injury. For instance, individual differences in the fibrinolytic system may also contribute to the hemostatic defect associated with trauma. Patients with more robust activation of the fibrinolytic system or inadequate levels of fibrinolytic inhibitory proteins may develop a more severe bleeding diathesis.

Trauma results in extensive disruption of endothelial cells, exposing tissue factor and collagen and triggering widespread activation of coagulation and platelets. Depending upon the extent of injury, endothelial disruption may activate the hemostatic system to such a degree that consumption of coagulation factors and platelets exceeds the production capabilities of the liver and bone marrow, which results in a consumptive coagulopathy, when the supply of clotting factors cannot keep up with the demand. Patients who suffered extensive blunt-force trauma, which often results in more diffuse endothelial damage to many body regions, may be at higher risk for developing a consumptive coagulopathy than patients with more localized penetrating trauma. Patients with disease states that affect the bone marrow or liver function (cirrhosis) are at higher risk for development of a severe coagulopathy. A significant number of patients, especially the elderly, are taking antithrombotic agents; these include antiplatelet agents, such as aspirin and clopidogrel, and anticoagulants such as vitamin K antagonists (e.g., warfarin) or low molecular weight heparin. Taking such agents puts such individuals at an even greater risk for coagulopathic bleeding in the event of traumatic injury.

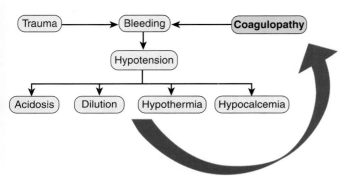

FIGURE 2 The lethal triad: the pathogenesis of the coagulopathy of trauma.

The severity of posttrauma coagulopathy is also influenced by the degree and duration of hypotension. Prolonged hypotension results in acidemia that impairs the function of coagulation factors. Previous studies have demonstrated a direct correlation between tissue hypoperfusion and the severity of coagulopathy on admission, as reflected in screening coagulation tests such as the prothrombin time (PT) and activated prothrombin time (aPTT). Using a porcine trauma model, Martini demonstrated that acidosis primarily impairs the propagation phase of coagulation and promotes accelerated degradation of fibrinogen. Activation of thrombin is reduced by 50% at pH 7.2 and 90% at pH 6.8, and fibrinogen degradation is increased by 180% in an acidic environment. In a prospective study of trauma patients, Brohi and colleagues demonstrated that hypoperfusion was associated with increases in soluble thrombomodulin and decreases in protein C activity, suggesting that the coagulopathy of trauma is also a result of the endogenous anticoagulant activity of activated protein C and hyperfibrinolysis associated with consumption of plasminogen activator inhibitor 1.

Hypothermia is also strongly associated with trauma-associated mortality and coagulopathy. Because the coagulation cascade is a series of enzymatic reactions optimized to perform at normal body temperature, it is not surprising that colder temperatures can precipitate a coagulopathy. Even in the presence of normal coagulation factor levels, temperatures below 33° C reduce clotting factor activity by 50%. Core body temperatures of 34° C or higher are associated with a mortality rate of only 7% compared with a mortality rate of 40% for core temperatures less than 34° C, 69% for temperatures below 33° C, and nearly 100% for patients with core temperatures below 32° C.

Postoperative blood loss is also correlated with lower perioperative body temperatures. Hypothermia impacts bleeding via alternative pathways, including a reduction in initiation of coagulation through the factor VII tissue factor pathway and decreases in the synthesis of fibrinogen. Hypothermia also decreases platelet activation and adhesion by reducing the rate of thromboxane B2 production and inhibiting interactions of platelet surface glycoproteins with VWF.

Hemodilution occurs both prior to and during resuscitation after major trauma. During hypotension, the body attempts to maintain intravascular volume by shifting protein-poor extravascular fluid into the intravascular space, thereby diluting coagulation proteins. The negative hemostatic effects of this endogenous maladaptive response is compounded by the routine administration of large volumes of crystalloid during field resuscitation, which further dilutes coagulation factors and platelets. Some colloid solutions, such as hydroxyethyl starch (Hespan), have been demonstrated to have a detrimental effect on coagulation activation.

Severe anemia can also have a negative effect on hemostasis. As the hematocrit declines from 40% to 10%, a fivefold decrease in platelet adhesion is observed; in the normal state, red cells typically push platelets toward the periphery, increasing the opportunity for interactions with the vessel wall. Red cells also enhance platelet function by serving as a rich source of adenosine diphosphate and adenosine triphosphate, which augment platelet reactivity. The impact of hematocrit on platelet function is reflected in the inverse correlation between hematocrit and bleeding time. Removal of 2 units of red cells is associated with a 60% increase in the bleeding time. Excessive red cell transfusion unaccompanied by platelet concentrates or plasma also has negative effects on hemostasis, as red cells can reduce the concentration of coagulation factors and platelets and induce a dilutional coagulopathy. Recognition of this phenomenon has lead to the recent emphasis on transfusion of plasma and platelets at predetermined ratios to avoid iatrogenic transfusion-associated dilutional coagulopathy.

Hypocalcemia is very common among trauma patients and is another contributor to the coagulopathy of trauma. Calcium is an essential cofactor in several reactions in the coagulation cascade. It is necessary for the formation of the tenase and prothrombinase complexes on activated platelets, for the generation of fibrin by thrombin, and the stabilization of polymerized fibrin clot. Hypocalcemia also impairs platelet activation, and it occurs in many trauma patients because of intrinsic physiologic responses to shock, as well as crystalloid and colloid-induced hemodilution, and the infusion of blood products containing a citrate anticoagulant. A retrospective study found that 58% of trauma patients had hypocalcemia (ionized calcium <1.16 μmol/L) on presentation, and 3.3% had severe hypocalcemia (ionized calcium <0.90 μmol/L). Mortality was greater than 30% for patients with ionized calcium concentrations between 0.90 and 1.09 μmol/L and more than 60% for patients with ionized calcium less than 0.90 μmol/L.

DIAGNOSTIC TESTING TO ASSESS TRAUMA-ASSOCIATED COAGULOPATHY

All trauma patients should have blood drawn for baseline coagulation tests upon arrival. The standard coagulation tests should include PT, aPTT, and fibrinogen. The PT provides information on the functional status of the extrinsic pathway, factor VII, and the common pathway, factors X, V, prothrombin, and fibrinogen. The aPTT measures the function of the intrinsic factors—XII, XI, IX, and VIII, prekallikrein, and high molecular weight kininogen—and the common pathway.

One limitation of the aPTT is that deficiencies of factor XII, high molecular weight kininogen, and prekallikrein are associated with abnormal aPTT results but do not impair hemostasis in vivo. Although both the PT and the aPTT assess fibrinogen function, direct measurement of fibrinogen is a much more sensitive and specific assessment of this crucial clotting protein. Several studies have demonstrated that abnormal coagulation test results on admission predict worse outcomes in trauma patients. MacLeod and colleagues found that 28% of trauma patients have an abnormal PT, and 8% have an abnormal aPTT on presentation. Abnormal PT and aPTT results were independent predictors of death, increasing it by 36% and 326%, respectively. The tight correlation between trauma-associated coagulopathy and increased mortality has been shown by other investigators as well. Platelet counts should also be routinely determined, although the absolute number does not give definite information regarding their function. Some patients will have qualitative defects in platelet function, either from medications such as aspirin and clopidogrel or from physiologic abnormalities such as renal failure, yet they will have normal quantitative platelet counts.

Although abnormalities in standard coagulation tests are associated with mortality, these tests have a number of limitations when applied to the diagnosis of trauma-associated coagulopathy. The PT and the aPTT are relatively insensitive to individual factor deficiencies. A factor VII activity of less than 30% is generally necessary to generate an abnormal PT. Therefore these screening tests generally do not become abnormal until significant reductions in factor levels have occurred. Another major limitation is the fact that these tests are performed in a clinical laboratory on platelet-poor plasma at room temperature; therefore they may not accurately reflect impairments in hemostasis in vivo. Furthermore, in the rapidly changing clinical situation of major trauma, central hospital laboratory coagulation testing can be too slow to inform clinical decision making and therapy. In addition, conventional coagulation tests do not reflect the contribution of fibrinolysis to trauma-associated bleeding.

Use of accurate bedside point-of-care (POC) tests avoids a number of the pitfalls associated with conventional laboratory-based hemostasis testing. POC coagulation tests such as the thromboelastograph (TEG; Hemoscope, Niles, Ill.) and rotational thromboelastometry (ROTEM; Pentapharm, Munich, Germany) have been demonstrated to be useful in management of patients undergoing liver transplantation and cardiac surgery. Their use is increasing in trauma centers as well, with many early reports showing potential benefits; both tests provide a more global measure of hemostasis and functional assessments of coagulation factors including fibrinogen, platelets, and the fibrinolytic system.

The principle behind both testing systems is similar. In TEG, whole blood is placed in a sample cup that contains a stationary pin suspended in the center of the cup. The cup oscillates through an angle of 4 degrees 45′ once every 10 seconds. Coagulation is initiated in the sample by the addition of calcium. Activators of the intrinsic pathway, such as kaolin, can also be used to accelerate reaction kinetics. Initial formation of a fibrin clot pulls the pin toward the side of the sample cup, a motion detected by a mechanical-electrical transducer attached to the pin (Figures 3 and 4). In the ROTEM device, clot formation is detected by an optical detector system. Unlike traditional coagulation assays, the TEG and the ROTEM measure the time to initial clot formation as well as fibrinogen and platelet function and fibrinolysis. The devices have been shown to be more accurate than conventional laboratory testing in identifying patients with hyperfibrinolysis, and their results appear to correlate with patient outcome and could be used to guide transfusion therapy (Figure 5).

These devices, as they are currently deployed, do have several limitations. Both devices analyze samples at 37° C; therefore they do not assess the contribution of hypothermia to coagulation dysfunction. In addition, they require up to 30 minutes to measure coagulation and fibrinolysis. Furthermore, adequate quality control and operator training are essential to ensure that the results are reliable. Finally, large prospective randomized controlled studies to

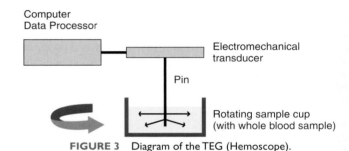

FIGURE 3 Diagram of the TEG (Hemoscope).

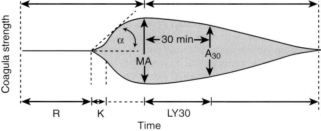

FIGURE 4 TEG tracing. The strength of a clot is graphically represented over time as a characteristic cigar-shaped figure. There are five parameters of the TEG tracing shown: *R, k, α angle, MA* (maximal amplitude), and *LY30* (lysis at 30 minutes), which all measure different stages of clot development. *R* is the period of time from the initiation of the test to initial fibrin formation, a measure of coagulation factor function. The *k* represents a measure of time from the beginning of clot formation until the amplitude of the thromboelastogram reaches 20 mm; this represents the dynamics of fibrin clot formation and is a measure of fibrinogen function. The *α* angle is the angle between the line in the middle of the TEG tracing and the line tangential to the developing "body" of the tracing. The alpha angle represents the acceleration (kinetics) of fibrin buildup and cross linking, another measure of fibrinogen function. *MA* reflects the strength of the clot, which is dependent on the number and function of platelets and their interaction with fibrin. *LY30* measures the reduction in the area of the curve 30 minutes after achieving MA, another measure of fibrinolysis. *(Adapted from Reikvam H, Steien E, Hauge B, et al: Thromboelastography, Transfus Apheres Sci 40:119–123, 2009.)*

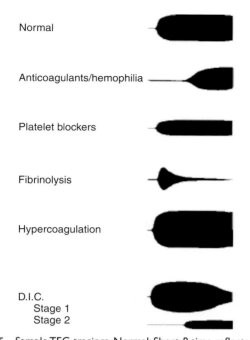

Normal

Anticoagulants/hemophilia

Platelet blockers

Fibrinolysis

Hypercoagulation

D.I.C.
 Stage 1
 Stage 2

FIGURE 5 Sample TEG tracings. Normal: Short *R* time reflects rapid formation of fibrin clot associated with normal amounts of all coagulation factors. Short *k* time and large α angle reflect rapid fibrin build up. The large maximal amplitude (MA) reflects normal platelet function and its interaction with fibrin. The small degree of lysis at 30 minutes reflects normal fibrinolytic function. Anticoagulants/hemophilia: Prolonged *R* time reflects reduced coagulation factor function typical of the impact of anticoagulants or hemophilia on the coagulation system. Platelet blockers (e.g., glycoprotein IIb/IIIa inhibitors) are medications that interfere with platelet function, so there is a reduction of the MA, but *R* time is normal. Fibrinolysis: The rapid reduction in the MA over time reflects the rapid lysis of clot. Hypercoagulation: Hypercoagulation is manifested in an abnormally short *R* time and *k* time as well as a large α and MA, reflecting more rapid fibrin clot formation and exuberant platelet-fibrin clot formation. Disseminated intravascular coagulation (DIC) stages 1 and 2: In stage 1 of DIC excessive thrombin generation and fibrin clot formation and platelet activation shortens the *R* time and the *k* time and increase the α and the MA. In stage 2, consumption of fibrinogen, other coagulation factors, and platelets and activation of fibrinolysis result in longer *R* and *k* times and a reduction in the α and the MA as well as a larger degree of lysis at 30 minutes (LY30). (*Modified from Winter PM, Kang YG, editors: Hepatic transplantation, New York, 1986, Praeger Publishers, p 151.*)

definitively demonstrate that TEG, ROTEM, and other POC coagulation tests improve transfusion management and patient outcome are lacking.

TREATMENT OF TRAUMA-ASSOCIATED COAGULOPATHY

Hemorrhage remains one of the most frequent causes of trauma-induced death, even at well-functioning, mature trauma centers. Temporary cessation of bleeding in the field may take the form of direct pressure, or it may be achieved through the rapidly expanding use of tourniquets. The definitive control of bleeding is most often accomplished via direct surgical control or percutaneous interventional techniques. Trauma surgeons should never assume that ongoing bleeding is related solely to coagulopathy; surgical bleeding must

always be considered and stopped rather than relying upon adjunctive noninvasive measures alone. The techniques of *damage control surgery* in trauma, whether applied to the abdomen or other body regions, are an absolutely necessary complement to the techniques of coagulopathy management. Successful execution of one without the other will not suffice.

The mainstay of treatment for the severe acute anemia of trauma is the transfusion of packed red blood cells (PRBCs). Other blood products available to replace trauma-associated losses include whole blood, fresh frozen plasma, cryoprecipitate, and platelets. The use of fresh whole blood—which contains physiologic amounts of red cells, plasma, and platelets—has risen dramatically in the military setting, where large numbers of young donors are readily available to provide whole blood for trauma victims. The results of the use of fresh whole blood are very encouraging; however, it is rarely used in the civilian setting, so we will not dwell further on whole-blood transfusion therapy in this chapter.

PRBCs are essential for adequate oxygen transport to the tissues. They optimize hemostasis by providing ADP and ATP for platelet activation, and they displace platelets to the periphery of the bloodstream, thereby increasing platelet-endothelial interaction. In actively bleeding patients, time may not be sufficient to perform pretransfusion testing. In these instances, blood group O red cells should be provided until testing can be performed. Women of childbearing age should be prioritized to receive Rh-negative group O red cell products to minimize their chances for forming Rh antibodies that may result in Rh sensitization. If this exposure cannot be avoided, timely administration of Rh immunoglobulin (RhoGAM) is essential to prevent fetal alloimmune hemolytic anemia during future pregnancies.

The benefits of red cell transfusion are often clear, and in the acutely bleeding patient, PRBC transfusion can be lifesaving. However, the use of PRBCs must be balanced against the associated risks, which have become more widely understood in the past few years. The immediate drawbacks to PRBCs include dilution of coagulation factors and platelets, transfusion-related acute lung injury (TRALI), hemolytic and febrile transfusion reactions, and hypocalcemia that results from the citrate anticoagulant used to preserve PRBCs. The delayed detrimental effects include increased risk of multiorgan failure, systemic inflammatory response syndrome (SIRS), sepsis, and transfusion-transmitted infections.

Higher mortality has been associated with red cell transfusion in trauma patients, and this risk appears to be higher with the use of older, as compared with younger, blood products (<14 days of storage). To avoid these adverse effects, many techniques to minimize the amount of blood transfused have been suggested in the trauma setting. These strategies include intraoperative salvage of spent red cells, hypotensive resuscitation to minimize bleeding until hemorrhage is controlled, and ICU-based treatment protocols for appropriate transfusion triggers (hemoglobin 7 mg/dL in nonbleeding ICU patients), once the immediate hemorrhage has been stopped. Identification of safe and effective blood substitutes, such as hemoglobin-based oxygen carriers and/or perfluorocarbons, remains an active area of ongoing research.

Plasma is derived from whole blood during the standard donor and apheresis collection process, and it contains normal concentrations of each of the coagulation factors. Fresh frozen plasma (FFP) and FP24 are frozen within 8 hours and 24 hours of collection, respectively, and they can be stored for up to a year without losing their coagulant activity. Because FFP and FP24 require 30 minutes to be thawed, many medical centers with active trauma services maintain a ready supply of thawed, type-specific plasma for emergency use, thereby allowing more rapid transfusion in an emergency setting.

Each 250 mL unit of plasma contains approximately 2 mg/mL of fibrinogen (500 mg total) and 1 U/mL of each of the other coagulation factors. Traditionally, the trigger for FFP transfusion in trauma patients has been a PT or aPTT ratio greater than 1.5 or a fibrinogen level below 100 mg/dL. However, given the rapid evolution of trauma-associated coagulopathy, recent guidelines increasingly recommend transfusion according to predetermined ratios prior to the availability of test results. The early empiric transfusion of FFP has been shown to decrease overall PRBC transfusions and may be associated with lower mortality in trauma patients. Although the ideal ratio of FFP to PRBCs has not yet been clearly defined, the data supporting the early use of FFP, before coagulopathy is definitively identified, are quite persuasive. Some military advocates suggest a 1:1 ratio, whereas data from the civilian sector suggest a ratio closer to 1:1.5. The term *damage control resuscitation* has been coined to describe the strategy of early factor repletion according to a prespecified ratio. Many trauma centers now use standardized massive transfusion protocols to assist providers in obtaining the large volumes of blood products necessary to resuscitate trauma victims using prespecified transfusion ratios.

Cryoprecipitate is the cold-soluble precipitate generated during the FFP thawing process. Since cryoprecipitate contains only factor VIII, factor XIII, VWF (1 U/mL), and fibrinogen (250 mg/U), it should be reserved primarily for patients requiring fibrinogen replacement, particularly when volume is an issue. Although cryoprecipitate is also a rich source of factor VIII and VWF, factor VIII concentrates are the preferred source for these factors, because they are virally inactivated, much less likely to transmit infectious illnesses, and can provide large quantities of these factors in small volumes. Cryoprecipitate has been used routinely as an adjunct to massive transfusion; however, this practice is becoming less common as other blood products are becoming available.

Adequate numbers of functional platelets are key to ensuring hemostasis in the early management of bleeding after injury. Yet platelets have only recently been suggested as a key component of trauma resuscitation to prevent and treat coagulopathy. The conventional laboratory trigger for platelet transfusions during trauma resuscitation has been a platelet count of less than $50,000/\mu L$. However, some centers now advocate a 1:1:1 ratio of PRBCs, FFP, and platelets in their massive-transfusion protocols. Platelet transfusion has also been advocated for patients with significant bleeding, especially intracranial bleeds, and for pateints taking antiplatelet agents such as clopidogrel. Platelets are harvested by centrifugation from whole-blood donations or donations from individuals during apheresis; a unit of blood from apheresis is equivalent to 6 to 10 units of random-donor platelets derived from blood donation. After transfusion of 6 random donor units or a single apheresis unit, the expected increment in the platelet count is approximately 30,000 to $50,000/\mu L$. The average platelet lifespan in the circulation after transfusion is 3 to 4 days.

Hypothermia is a major contributor to trauma-associated coagulopathy. Management of hypothermia falls into two main categories: *prevention* and *treatment via active patient warming*. Hypothermia prevention begins immediately after the onset of injury. Of the initial ABCDEs of trauma resuscitation, *E* stands for *e*xposure/*e*nvironment, a crucial aspect that mandates rapid removal of wet clothes as the first step to prevent further heat loss. Warmed rooms, both trauma bays and operating rooms, are necessary: the greater the temperature gradient, the quicker patients become hypothermic. Simple warming measures that include providing warm blankets, heat lamps, warm intravenous fluids, and Bair Hugger (Arizant, Eden Prairie, Minn.) warming devices can be initiated in all patients. Further advanced techniques include heated ventilator circuits and other proprietary temperature-management devices, such as the Arctic Sun Temperature Management System (Medivance, Louisville, Colo.) for active warming, and use of warm saline lavage via gastric, urinary, or intraperitoneal catheters. The most invasive methods, such as venovenous extracorporeal circuits or cardiopulmonary bypass, are only rarely used in the trauma setting.

Recombinant activated human factor VIIa (rh FVIIa, marketed under the brand name NovoSeven by Novo Nordisk, Princeton, NJ) is a lyophilized concentrate that is FDA approved for treatment of bleeding in hemophilia patients with factor inhibitors; rh FVIIa has been tested in a wide variety of settings associated with bleeding in patients without hemophilia, including trauma patients. Many researchers felt that this agent was going to be highly effective for trauma-associated coagulopathy, because it acts only at sites of injury. However, the ideal patient population in which to use it has not yet been determined. In a parallel double-blind randomized controlled trial, Boffard and colleagues enrolled patients with blunt and penetrating trauma to receive rh FVIIa or placebo after receiving 8 units of PRBCs. In blunt trauma patients, rh FVIIa reduced the 48 hour transfusion requirement by 2.6 units ($P = .02$) and reduced the frequency of massive transfusion (more than 20 units of RBCs) from 33% to 14% of patients. No differences in transfusion requirements were noted in the penetrating-trauma group, and mortality was similar in both groups.

Spinella and colleagues conducted a retrospective review of FVIIa use for combat-related trauma in Iraq, comparing outcomes for patients who received 120 µg/kg of rh FVIIa after transfusion of 4 to 6 units of blood with those for patients who did not receive rh FVIIa. Mortality rate was lower in rh FVIIa recipients. Reductions in transfusion end points, but not in mortality, have been noted in other studies using a variety of doses, and increases in thromboembolic events also have been seen; therefore routine use of rh FVIIa is not recommended for patients with major trauma. Some civilian trauma patients may benefit from this new blood product; however, the precise subgroups most likely to benefit from its use remain to be identified. It is likely that a well-designed randomized clinical trial would be hard to conduct because of the heterogeneity of the civilian trauma patient population and the wide variety of other adjunctive treatments employed in trauma management. Until such a study is conducted, rh FVIIa use will likely continue on a case-by-case basis, as its use is supported by a large amount of anecdotal evidence, and many trauma surgeons have patients whom they feel have benefited from its use.

RECOMMENDED APPROACH TO TRAUMA-ASSOCIATED BLEEDING

Evolving guidelines to manage trauma-associated coagulopathy suggest that initial resuscitation of trauma patients in the field should employ volumes of crystalloid necessary to maintain adequate perfusion pressures so as to limit the dilution of coagulation factors and platelets. Upon arrival in the emergency department, the initial clinical trauma evaluation should proceed, while laboratory studies that include screening coagulation studies, complete blood counts, and a type and cross match are being drawn, and radiographic studies are ordered. Until a type and cross match are available, type O blood and AB plasma can be used for replacement. Maintenance of a ready pool of thawed plasma in the blood bank facilitates rapid replacement therapy. Satellite blood banks in the emergency department can also speed blood product transfusion. To limit dilution of coagulation factors and platelets, PRBCs, FFP, and platelets should be transfused in a 1:1:1 ratio, while damage control surgery proceeds. Hypothermia should be limited by administering warmed fluids and blood products and keeping the patient in a warm environment. Serial laboratory testing can assist in tailoring blood-product component therapy to the patient's clinical situation. Although POC testing with TEG or ROTEM and blood components such as rh FVIIa may earn a place in routine trauma surgery, their application in this setting remains to be demonstrated.

SUGGESTED READINGS

Hess JR, Brohi K, Dutton RP, et al: The coagulopathy of trauma: a review of mechanisms, *J Trauma* 65:748–754, 2008.

Ketchum L, Hess JR, Hiippala S: Indications for early fresh frozen plasma, cryoprecipitate and platelet transfusion in trauma, *J Trauma* 60:S51–S58, 2006.

Lier H, Krep H, Schroeder S, Stuber F: Preconditions of hemostasis in trauma: a review—the influence of acidosis, hypocalcemia, anemia, and hypothermia on functional hemostasis in trauma, *J Trauma* 65:951–960, 2008.

Reikvam H, Steien E, Hauge B, et al: Thromboelastography, *Transfus Apheres Sci* 40:119–123, 2009.

Shaz BH, Dente CJ, Harris RS, et al: Transfusion management of trauma patients, *Anesth Analg* 108:1760–1768, 2009.

Tieu BH, Holcomb JB, Schreiber MA: Coagulopathy: its pathophysiology and treatment in the injured patient, *World J Surg* 31:1055–1064, 2007.

THE ABDOMEN THAT WILL NOT CLOSE

Adil H. Haider, MD, MPH

OVERVIEW

Over the past 20 years, the concept of an abbreviated laparotomy and leaving a patient's abdomen "open" has revolutionized the management of critically ill trauma and general surgery patients. In the 1980s surgeons began to acknowledge the perils of closing the abdomen under tension. As the pathophysiology of intraabdominal hypertension (IAH) and its sequela, abdominal compartment syndrome (ACS), were understood, it became acceptable to leave a patient who had ACS, or was at risk of developing it, with an open abdomen. At the same time, the advantages of abbreviating a laparotomy in a severely injured patient with profound shock—who would otherwise become cold, acidotic, coagulopathic, and die on the table before the operation could be completed—became apparent.

In 1993, Rotondo and Schwab coined the term *damage control surgery* (DCS), borrowing from a Navy term that described containment of severe damage, followed by stabilization of the ship—or in this case, the patient—before proceeding with definitive repairs. Today, the standard of care for patients with ACS or patients requiring DCS is to leave the abdomen open with a temporary abdominal closure (TAC). This chapter reviews TAC techniques, management of patients with an open abdomen, subsequent definitive closure of the abdomen, and long-term reconstruction of patients who develop hernias from their open abdomens.

INDICATIONS FOR LEAVING THE ABDOMEN OPEN

Initially described by trauma surgeons, DCS is the most common reason for leaving an abdomen open. It was originally reserved for a *maximally injured subset* of patients, defined as those with 1) at least one major vessel injury (e.g., inferior vena cava), 2) at least two visceral injuries, and 3) profound shock. Early results from DCS were very impressive. Survival for such maximally injured patients jumped from 11% to 77%, and use of DCS spread to less severely injured patients. However, many now believe that the pendulum has swung too far, and in some cases the risks associated with leaving the abdomen open outweigh the benefits. Thus patient selection is vital. In general, there are five distinct groups of patients in whom the abdomen should be left acutely open:

1. **Patients with or at risk of IAH and subsequent ACS.** This group includes patients undergoing major elective operations; those who subsequently require massive resuscitation are at risk for (primary) ACS. Similarly, patients who require substantial resuscitation because of severe medical illness or trauma that requires abdominal decompression (secondary ACS) are included in this group.
2. **Patients undergoing DCS.** This group includes patients undergoing DCS for massive abdominal trauma, such as a patient with a gunshot wound through a major vessel (e.g., renal artery), a solid organ (e.g., kidney), and multiple segments of bowel. Once the major vessel injury and solid-organ injury have been controlled, and spillage from the bowel injury is contained, the patient may be too unstable for reconstruction of the bowel injuries and closure of the fascia. In this case, DCS allows rapid truncation of

laparotomy before the patient enters the lethal triad of hypothermia, acidosis, and coagulopathy. Once the damage has been controlled, the patient can be taken to the intensive care unit (ICU) for resuscitation and stabilization. It is important to decide on the need to perform DCS early on in the operation. Predictors of DCS include temperature below 34° C; pH less than 7.2; serum bicarbonate level less than 15 mmol/L, and total operative fluid replacement—blood products, crystalloid, and so on—greater than 15 L. It may also be required in patients undergoing elective general surgery who develop serious complications with overwhelming blood loss and require stabilization/resuscitation prior to reconstruction and completion of the operation.
3. **Patients whose fascia cannot be closed.** This category includes patients who may be physiologically stable but may have extremely swollen abdominal contents from a prior resuscitation (e.g., DCS) or loss of fascial domain (e.g., giant ventral hernias) such that they cannot be primarily closed. Figure 1 depicts a patient who required TAC while waiting for bowel edema to resolve. The abdomen must be kept open until the patient is ready for a definitive fascial closure with mesh or other modalities to prevent fascial closure under tension.
4. **Patients with severe intraabdominal infections or necrotizing fasciitis of the abdominal wall.** This includes those with severe, necrotizing pancreatitis or a large amount of purulent material in the abdomen requiring repeated washouts. Patients with severe abdominal wall infections who are likely to need repeat debridement are also included in this group.
5. **Patients having a planned repeat exploration or second look surgery.** In this group are patients with intraabdominal pathology that may require another laparotomy in 48 to 72 hours. For example, a vascular surgery patient with mesenteric ischemia who undergoes a small bowel resection: 48 hours later, the patient needs to be reopened to check for additional ischemic bowel.

Once a patient is left open, a TAC is performed so that the patient can be transported to the ICU for further management. In some situations, such as with massive liver injury, the abdominal viscera may be packed with laparotomy pads to create direct pressure on bleeding surfaces prior to a TAC. As stressed before, the practice of closing the fascia under tension must be avoided to prevent IAH and ACS and to prevent wound complications such as infection and dehiscence. For hemodynamically stable patients who can withstand the prolonging of an elective operation, several options to achieve a tension-free abdominal closure do exist, some of which are discussed later in this chapter.

DISADVANTAGE AND LIMITATIONS OF TEMPORARY ABDOMINAL CLOSURE

It is important to recognize several issues and disadvantages associated with TAC. First and foremost, the open abdomen and lack of fascial reapproximation appears to create an initial inflammatory response, leading to activation of neutrophils, macrophages, and an inflammatory cascade that causes systemic inflammatory response syndrome (SIRS). Given this trajectory, it is imperative to carefully consider whether the abdomen should be left open, and one must strive to get the patient's fascia reapproximated, either primarily or with interposed mesh, as soon as feasible. Some more immediate difficulties in managing an open abdomen are fluid loss from the exposed bowel and peritoneum and the need to keep patients intubated in most cases and deeply sedated. Patients may also develop secondary peritonitis, and they have high complication rates; complications include infection, sepsis, and fistula formation. Moreover, a large number of patients with an open abdomen cannot be primarily closed. Instead, they need an intermediate mesh placement, and many require skin grafting and an eventual large ventral hernia repair.

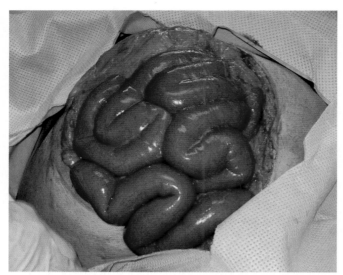

FIGURE 1 An abdomen that cannot be closed due to significant bowel edema and displacement of small intestine secondary to a massive retroperitoneal hematoma. This situation calls for a temporary abdominal closure.

TEMPORARY ABDOMINAL CLOSURE

Once the decision has been made to leave the abdomen open, the most optimal TAC technique should be used. This technique should be based on the experience of the surgeon and the practice environment. An ideal TAC should have the following attributes:

- Easily encompasses the bowel and abdominal viscera
- Allows enlargement of the abdominal cavity in situations of massive bowel, tissue, or retroperitoneal edema without inducing IAH and while preventing ACS
- Is expansible but also sturdy enough to permit the tamponade effect of packing the liver or other bleeding surfaces
- Does not damage the fascia and prevents fascial retraction
- Contains and quantifies fluid loss
- Prevents adhesion formation between viscera and abdominal fascia
- Promotes removal of infectious materials
- Is quick to apply and remove
- Has a good primary fascial closure rate

Table 1 compares the most common methods of TAC. Although the earliest forms of TAC, the towel clip closure and Bogotá bag closure, are mentioned in the table, these have been largely replaced by more improved options. Similarly, polypropylene (Prolene; Ethicon, Somerville, NJ); polytetrafluoroethylene (PTFE) (Gore-Tex; W.L. Gore & Associates, Flagstaff, Ariz.); biologic mesh, such as human acellular dermal matrix, or HADM (Alloderm; Lifecell, Branchburg, NJ); and bovine acellular collagen matrix (Surgimend; TEI Biosciences, Boston, Mass.) are rarely used anymore for TAC. These materials were abandoned for a number of reasons. Polypropylene is notorious for developing fistulas and is difficult to remove from the bowel; PTFE, although relatively inert, limits tissue granulation, is not well incorporated in the fascia, and carries a high risk of mesh infection. The biologic mesh matrix products are too expensive for temporary use and may not provide enough tensile strength, especially in heavily infected fields, where they have been known to "melt away."

Commercial and "Homemade" Vacuum Closure Devices

In the United States, most surgeons use a vacuum closure device, such as the commercially available VAC abdominal dressing (Kinetic Concepts Inc., San Antonio, Tex.) or the vacuum-pack closure device

described by Barker and colleagues. These devices create a negative-pressure silo that contains the abdominal contents, is somewhat expansible, and enables measurable fluid removal. The negative pressure is applied medially up through the open abdomen, minimizing fascial retraction and loss of abdominal domain. These dressings are also very quick and easy to apply, and they can be used in situations of massive bowel swelling. Although several variations of the negative-pressure TACs exist, most include these key features:

A fenestrated inner layer of an inert, pliable material (e.g., polyethylene) that is placed on top of the viscera to prevent it from forming adhesions to the abdominal wall, contain the abdominal viscera, and allow fluid movement.

A middle layer of foam or towels that helps generate suction, keeps the bowel moist, and provides some support to the dressing. The suction helps prevent the fascia from retracting and provides a mechanism for fluid and infectious effluent removal.

A suction mechanism with major force applied to the middle layer.

An outer layer made up of an adhesive polyurethane sheet to create an airtight seal around the entire apparatus and enable measurement of fluid loss and generation of negative pressure through the dressing. Figures 2 through 5 illustrate the ABThera VAC device (Kinetic Concepts Inc.). Figure 6 illustrates the "homemade" Barker dressing, which uses materials readily available in the operating room (OR) to create a vacuum pack.

Technical Tips for Vacuum Dressing Placement

Although it appears to be quite simple, experience in proper placement and application of the dressing does help avoid subsequent complications, the most dreadful of which is enteroatmospheric fistula formation. It is essential to place polyurethane between the bowel and the middle layer to prevent direct suction pressure on the bowel, which will cause fistula formation. One technique is to insert this innermost layer before releasing the Bookwalter, Omni, or other abdominal wall retractor. This practice ensures that the polyurethane sheet has been placed in far enough laterally. In addition, the use of ostomies or feeding tubes must be avoided in patients with an open abdomen. A nasoduodenal feeding tube can be used until the patient is ready to be closed. If an ostomy must be done, it should be placed as laterally in the flanks as possible to preserve enough normal abdominal wall for subsequent mobilization and closure.

An airtight seal of the outermost layer is essential for all vacuum dressings. It is important to keep the skin area dry prior to application of this outer adhesive layer. In cases of substantial fluid spillage, cut strips of adhesive dressing can be placed horizontally across the middle layer to stabilize the open abdomen, then the skin can be quickly dried again, and the outer adhesive layer can be applied. Special attention must be given to the suprapubic area to ensure that negative pressure is generated. This can be confirmed by ensuring that the entire abdominal dressing is "sucked in," as soon as suction is applied. If an airtight seal is not accomplished, the adhesive drape must be removed, the skin redried, and outer dressing reapplied. It is important to get an excellent, dry seal in the OR, because it is usually difficult to reinforce this dressing in the intensive care unit (ICU).

Outcomes of Vacuum-Based Temporary Abdominal Closures

In most cases both the VAC and vacuum pack have excellent outcomes, with a primary fascial closure rate reported between 70% and 80% and a mean closure time between 6 and 10 days. Both methods have a reported 15% complication rate. The most common complications are fistula formation (5% to 7%), intraabdominal abscesses (4% to 6%), and delayed small bowel obstruction (4%). Most recently, Kinetic Concepts has introduced a newer dressing, called the *KCI ABThera negative-pressure dressing*. This product has a sponge

TABLE 1: Various Methods of Temporary Abdominal Closure

Closure Technique	Description	Advantages	Disadvantages
Skin only (towel clip closure, running suture of skin)	Serial application of towel clips or suture	Rapid	Does not prevent IAH; may interfere with radiography or angiography
Bogotá bag	3 L IV bag, Steri-drape (3M; St Paul, Minn.), Silastic bag, plastic bag rapidly sutured to skin	Inexpensive, inert, nonadherent	Risk of evisceration, loss of abdominal domain, risk for IAH; fluid losses difficult to quantify
Absorbable mesh	Suturing of absorbable mesh to skin or fascial edges	Can be applied directly over bowel; allows for drainage of peritoneal fluid	Rapid loss of tensile strength (in the setting of infection), potentially large-volume late ventral hernia; risk for bowel fistula; damage to fascial edges from repeated suturing
Wittmann patch (Star Surgical, Burlington, Wis.)	Suturing of artificial burr (i.e., Velcro) to fascia, staged abdominal closure by application of controlled tension	Good tensile strength, allows for easy reexploration and eventual primary fascial closure	Poor control of third-space fluid, adherence of bowel to abdominal wall, potential for fistulas
Vacuum-pack closure	Bowel covered with plastic sheet and towel or laparotomy pads; flat drains attached to wall suction and outer adhesive layer	Inexpensive, uses available materials; moderate control of fluid; suction provides constant medial traction, preventing loss of domain; high success in fascial closure	Difficult to quantify suction; unknown whether full benefits of negative-pressure therapy are realized
Modified "sandwich" vacuum pack	3 L irrigation bag placed on bowel; three fascial sutures placed to retain "domain"; NG tubes used for suction, ostomy bag used to bring NG tube through outer adhesive dressing	Same as vacuum-pack closure but is thought to retain fascial domain and further improve primary fascial closure; inert innermost layers help prevent fistulas	Does not use innermost, perforated layer, which may make fluid removal somewhat difficult; unknown whether benefits of negative-pressure therapy are realized
Negative-pressure therapy; VAC (vacuum-assisted closure) abdominal dressing system (Kinetic Concepts, Inc., San Antonio, Tex.)	Reticulated polyurethane foam dressing over the plastic covering of the bowel; negative pressure is controlled with a computer-controlled vacuum pump that applies a constant, regulated pressure to the wound surface and a sensing device to prevent uncontrolled fluid (e.g., blood) drainage	Increase in blood flow, a reduction on abdominal wall tension, reduction in size of the abdominal wall defect, decreased bowel edema, and potential removal of inflammatory substances that accumulate in the abdomen during inflammatory states; edema and third-space losses can be controlled	Expensive; not available at all institutions, in austere environments, or in most less developed countries; mechanism of action not fully understood, but does lead to hyperossification; full relationship to fistula not studied well enough

IAH, Intrabdominal hypertension; *NG,* nasogastric

embedded in the innermost layer that reaches out to the paracolic gutters, which makes it easier to apply and improves fluid removal. Outcomes for this newer product have not been reported.

Another vacuum-based TAC that has excellent reported outcomes is the *modified sandwich vacuum pack,* described by Navasaria and Nicols from the University of Cape Town in South Africa. This technique uses an inner layer made up of an emptied 3 L irrigation bag and nasogastric tubes used to create a vacuum suction. It also uses a few large fascial sutures to keep medial traction on the wound and preserves abdominal domain. Results comparable to the VAC have been reported, with minimal complications. The technique is depicted in Figure 7, and the entire apparatus costs less than $20.

MANAGEMENT OF THE PATIENT WITH AN OPEN ABDOMEN

Initial Management

In November 2009, the Open Abdomen Advisory Panel published the first recommendations for management of patients with open abdomens. They recognized that open abdomen patients present a complex critical care problem in that the patient is between operations, and the goal of critical care is to stabilize, resuscitate, and prepare the patient for the next step toward closure of the abdomen. After the initial damage control operation, patients require immediate

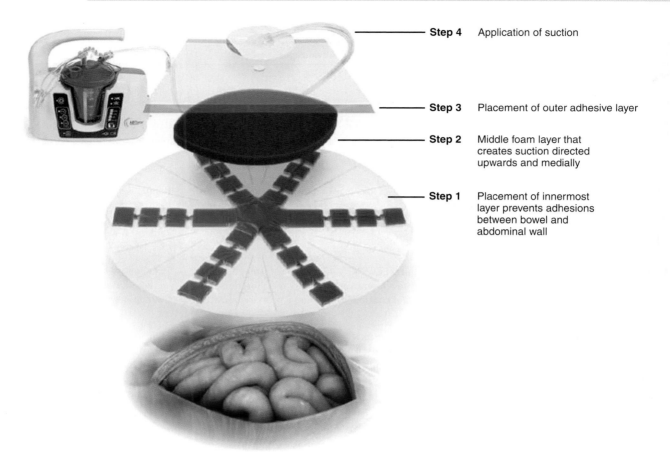

Step 4   Application of suction

Step 3   Placement of outer adhesive layer

Step 2   Middle foam layer that creates suction directed upwards and medially

Step 1   Placement of innermost layer prevents adhesions between bowel and abdominal wall

FIGURE 2   The ABThera VAC system (Kinetic Concepts, Inc.) that is currently replacing their VAC open abdomen system. Recently introduced in the United States, the ABThera features a foam that extends out laterally to assist in volume removal. *(Image courtesy Kinetic Concepts, Inc.)*

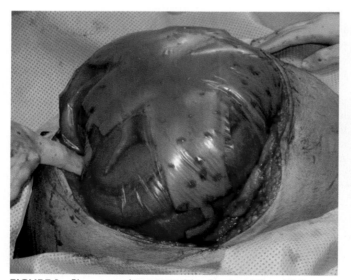

FIGURE 3   Placement of innermost layer for the ABThera VAC (Kinetic Concepts, Inc.), which uses an innermost layer with an embedded foam that fans out laterally, which makes it easier to apply and also assists in lateral paracolic fluid and effluent removal.

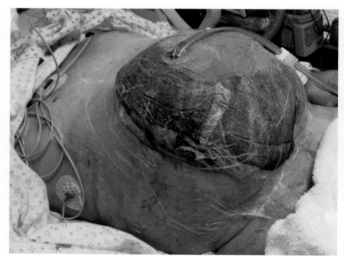

FIGURE 4   VAC dressing on patient in Surgical ICU. This dressing was easily applied despite an extremely swollen bowel and massive retroperitoneal bulging.

rewarming, correction of coagulopathy and acidosis, and most likely, massive resuscitation.

For all patients, it is important to determine the source of metabolic derangements and correct them as quickly as possible. If the patient is thought to have sepsis, broad-spectrum antibiotics should be initiated. Indicated hemodynamic monitoring should be liberally employed, including invasive modalities (e.g., Swan-Ganz catheters), especially in older trauma patients, where it is difficult to determine the end point of resuscitation. Overresuscitation in this patient population has been shown to increase complications and length of stay in the ICU.

It must also be remembered that even with the VAC dressing, it is possible to develop IAH and ACS, especially when abdominal packing is used. If ACS is suspected, intraabdominal pressure can still be measured using the conventional bladder pressure technique; if ACS is suspected, the patient should be returned to the OR for reexploration and replacement of the TAC.

Once patients are stabilized, they usually need to return to the OR within 48 to 72 hours for reexploration and possible definitive closure. However, if patients become acutely unstable or develop signs of acute hemorrhage, they may need to return immediately to the OR for reexploration. Not all patients can be closed on their first trip back

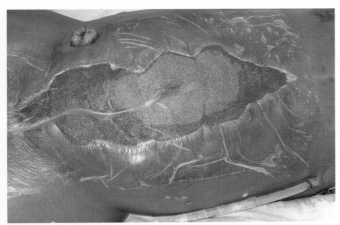

FIGURE 5   Application of a VAC dressing after two take-backs and construction of an iliostomy. Note the ostomy is placed very laterally. *(Photo courtesy Dr Elliott Haut, Johns Hopkins Acute Care Surgery, Baltimore, Md.)*

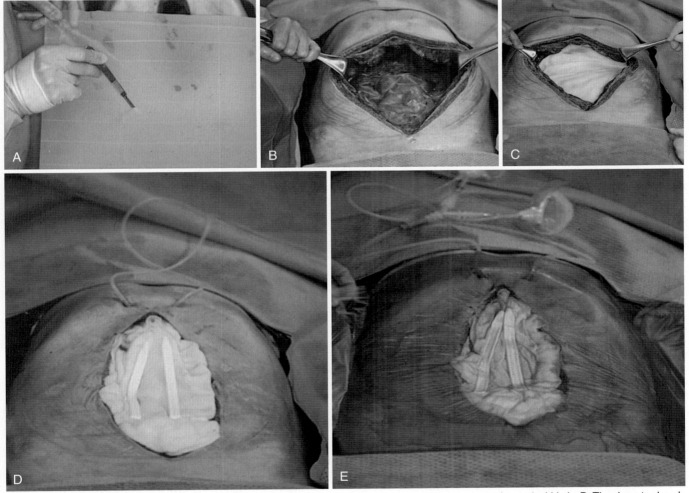

FIGURE 6   The Barker vacuum-pack technique. **A,** The polyethylene sheet is perforated multiple times with a scalpel blade. **B,** The sheet is placed over viscera and beneath the peritoneum/abdominal wall. **C,** A moist towel is placed over the polyurethane and positioned below the skin edges. **D,** Suction drains are placed. **E,** An outer adhesive dressing is applied, and the drains are hooked up to wall suction. *(Courtesy Donald H. Barker, MD, Department of Surgery, University of Tennessee, Chattanooga.)*

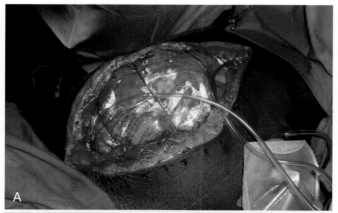

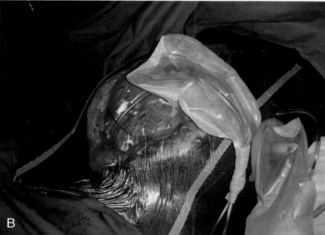

FIGURE 7   Modified sandwich vacuum-pack technique from South Africa. A sturdier inner plastic material is used, and suction is generated using nasogastric tubes. Three large fascial sutures are also placed. To ensure an airtight seal, the nasogastric tubes are brought through the outer adhesive layer through ostomy bags. *(Courtesy Dr. P. Navasaria, Department of Surgery, University of Cape Town, South Africa.)*

to the OR. In this case, the same principles that dictated leaving the patient open in the first place will apply at this juncture.

Subsequent Critical Care Management

Stabilization, resuscitation, correcting any metabolic derangements, and treatment of any infection remain the priorities in managing a patient with an open abdomen. In a critically ill patient, fluids should not be restricted to prevent bowel edema, because any organ hypoperfusion from hypovolemia will have much worse sequelae. One strategy that has been useful in such circumstances is the use of buffered hypertonic saline, which acts as an excellent volume expander that decreases or restricts edema and is also thought to retard innate inflammatory mediators. One caveat with using hypertonic saline is that development of hyperchloremic metabolic acidosis must be avoided.

Patients should begin enteral nutrition as soon as possible, and they must be deeply sedated to prevent evisceration and fully mechanically ventilated with an acute TAC. Once the patient has been resuscitated and is ready to be volume mobilized, diuresis can be considered to aid closure. Unless the patient has a known or suspected infection, antibiotics are not needed beyond the initial 24 hour surgical-site infection prophylaxis, as there is no indication for empiric antibiotics to cover an open abdomen.

Subsequent Take-Backs to the Operating Room

At 2- to 3-day intervals, the patient should be returned to the OR to irrigate the abdomen and perform the necessary therapeutic maneuvers (e.g., bowel anastomosis, drainage of purulent collections). Some centers advocate doing take-backs in the surgical ICU on hemodynamically stable patients who only require a washout. We usually perform the first take-back in the OR and any subsequent take-backs where significant surgery is required (e.g., bowel anastomosis or ostomy creation). At each surgery, fascia is brought together by tension-free sutures, and the intervening defect continues to get smaller and smaller. By the third or the fourth visit, fascial approximation is usually possible in a high percentage of patients, particularly if the patient has recovered from the acute insult and can tolerate diuresis. Data suggest that patients who remain open at day 8 are unlikely to have a primary closure and are at increased risk for serious complications, including wound infections and fistulas. Given this and the significant SIRS caused by an open abdomen, most authors recommend alternative closure techniques in patients who cannot be primarily closed by 8 days, unless there is some compelling reason, such as the continued need for fascial debridement, to keep the abdomen open. Figure 8 describes an algorithm for managing the open abdomen.

Definitive Closure of the Abdomen

Once the patient has been resuscitated and is ready for closure, the best-case scenario is primary fascial closure. We generally place interrupted, nonabsorbable nylon sutures (Ethilon; Ethicon, Somerville, NJ) or a very slow-absorbing suture like Maxon (Covidien, Mansfield, Mass.). In a setting of colonic perforation or heavy contamination, the skin should be left open. Some authors suggest the use of retention sutures, but we do not routinely place them. Retention sutures do help prevent bowel evisceration and may be used in situations where wound infection and subsequent dehiscence is suspected, as long as they are placed in a way that they do not increase intraabdominal pressures. It must be reiterated that the fascia must not be closed under tension, as this may lead to IAH and ACS. One simple technique to gauge the effect of bringing the fascia together is to use Kocher clamps to simulate reapproximation of the fascia before attempting to primarily closure. If significant force is required to reapproximate the fascia, or if the patient's airway pressures rise acutely, the risk of developing postoperative ACS is high, and the patient should not be primarily closed.

OPTIONS FOR CLOSURE WHERE FASCIA CANNOT BE PRIMARILY REAPPROXIMATED

If the fascia cannot be reapproximated, skin flaps can be raised to gain some medial length in the fascia. The fascia can also be advanced by releasing the lateral obliques; however, a full component separation is not recommended for the acute closure of an open abdomen. For patients who need mesh to bridge a gap between fascial edges, the options include biologics such as HADM, absorbable mesh such as Vicryl (Ethicon), and composite meshes. Biologics are very attractive, as they promote tissue regeneration and revascularization and can be used in a contaminated field; however, they cannot be used in heavily infected fields, because the matrix disintegrates.

Most biologics use a cross-linked structure and have a tendency to develop significant laxity over time; therefore they must be stretched and sutured in as tautly as possible. Most authors suggest that the overlying skin wound should be closed if a biologic mesh is used, to promote wound regeneration and incorporation of the mesh. HADM (Alloderm) has been on the market longest and has been used both as an interposition graft to close the fascial defect (Figure 9) and as an overlay to buttress fascia that has been primarily reapproximated. The reported hernia rate with HADM is about 17%, and few complications are reported.

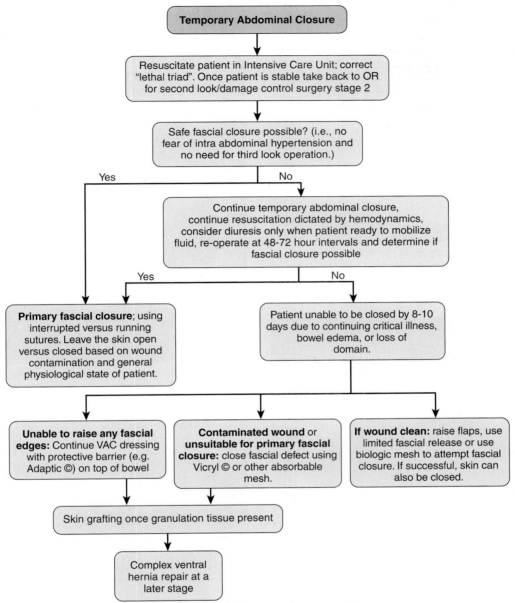

FIGURE 8   Algorithm for managing an open abdomen.

Other biologic mesh products such as Surgimend and Surgisis (porcine small intestine submucosa; Cook Medical, Bloomington, Ind.), Permacol (acellular porcine dermal collagen; Tissue Science Lab, Covington, Ga.), and Veritas (bovine pericardium, Synovis, St. Paul, Minn.) have also been used, but no long-term studies have been conducted to determine superiority of one product over the other. If the wound is infected, or if the fascial defect is extremely large, an absorbable mesh may be used (Figure 10).

Once granulation tissue grows through the mesh, a split-thickness skin graft can be placed, which will result in a large ventral hernia that will need to be repaired in the future. In difficult situations, where no fascial edges are apparent, and mesh cannot be used (Figure 11), a split-thickness skin graft can be directly placed onto the bowel, once granulation tissue has grown over it. As discussed before, permanent mesh should not be placed in direct contact with the bowel; however, it can be used as part of a composite mesh, as long as absorbable mesh is placed against the patient. Another

composite mesh, described by Wolfgang and colleagues, utilizes both HADM and Vicryl in the setting of infected wounds. If the HADM fails, the Vicryl mesh ensures that the patient's abdomen remains closed. If the HADM works well, the patient avoids a skin graft and late ventral hernia repair.

LONG-TERM MANAGEMENT AND CLOSURE

Many patients develop large ventral hernias after an open abdomen. This, of course, can be expected in patients closed with an absorbable mesh and overlying skin graft (Figure 12). Careful planning is required before attempting to repair these hernias, and the patient must be completely recovered from any complications suffered during hospitalization. The patient should also be well nourished and physiologically optimized.

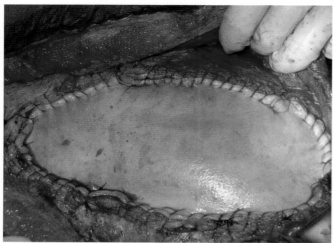

FIGURE 9 HADM (Alloderm) used as an interposition mesh where the fascia could not be primarily closed. Note that the HADM is placed, stretched, and sutured in as tautly as possible. *(Courtesy Richard Redett, MD, Johns Hopkins Plastic and Reconstructive Surgery, Baltimore, Md.)*

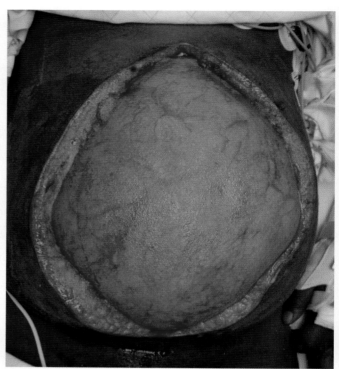

FIGURE 11 Open abdomen with fascia completely retracted. Healthy granulation tissue above the bowel allows direct placement of a split-thickness skin graft without underlying mesh. The patient will develop a large ventral hernia. *(Courtesy Dr. Elliott Haut, Johns Hopkins Acute Care Surgery, Baltimore, Md.)*

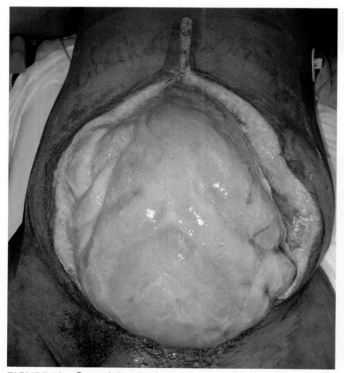

FIGURE 10 Open abdomen after several days of a temporary abdominal closure, where the fascia cannot be primarily closed and a mesh closure is required. *(Courtesy Dr. Elliott Haut, Johns Hopkins Acute Care Surgery, Baltimore, Md.)*

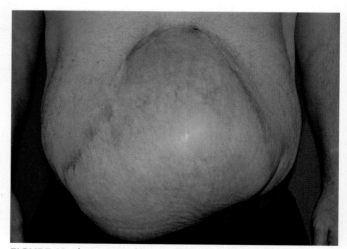

FIGURE 12 Large ventral hernia after closure of the fascia with Vicryl mesh (Ethicon) and placement of split-thickness skin graft. *(Courtesy Dr. Richard Redett, Johns Hopkins Plastic and Reconstructive Surgery, Baltimore, Md.)*

Another important aspect is to allow sufficient time for remodeling of any adhesions that may have occurred between the mesh or fascia and viscera. One key indicator of remodeling is the ability to completely pinch the skin away from the underlying mesh in the abdominal defect (Figure 13). This separation indicates that the patient is ready for repair of the ventral hernia. Many general surgeons will request assistance from plastic surgeons, especially if tissue expanders or complex tissue rearrangement is required. The steps in reconstruction are:

1. Assess overlying skin and place tissue expanders prior to surgery if necessary.

2. Excise the skin graft and completely remove previously placed mesh.

3. Perform extensive lysis of adhesions to release viscera from overlying fascia.

4. Reapproximate fascia, which may require one or all of the following:
   a. Raise large skin flaps and dissect skin and subcutaneous tissue from anterior fascia.

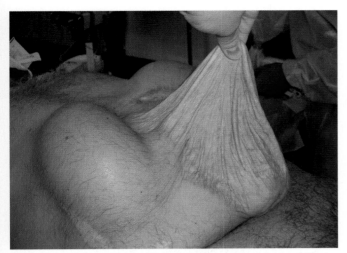

FIGURE 13   The overlying skin graft can be easily pinched and lifted off the underlying structure, suggesting that the patient is ready for a ventral hernia repair. Note placement of tissue expanders. *(Courtesy Dr. Elliott Haut, Johns Hopkins Acute Care Surgery. Baltimore, Md.)*

  b. Perform component separation, in which the aponeuroses of the abdominal oblique muscles are transected longitudinally, allowing the fascia to be pulled medially; the posterior sheath of the rectus may be similarly transected to gain further length (Figure 14).
  c. Use of mesh; if the fascia does not come together despite component separation, mesh can be placed as an underlay or as an interposition graft; most authors suggest the use of HADM or other biologics for this purpose.
5. Onlay mesh on top of the fascia for reinforcement. If a HADM underlay or interposition has been placed, we generally apply a polypropylene mesh as an overlay. If no underlay was required, HADM or polypropylene is placed as an onlay mesh to reinforce the fascia. Mesh is placed lateral enough to cover any fascial incisions made for component release or muscle relaxation (Figure 15).
6. Drains are placed to draw off accumulated fluid for closure of skin.
   Most patients are ready for hernia repair 12 to 19 months after discharge from their initial hospitalization. Recent outcome studies suggest that the most important step in reconstruction is tension-free, primary fascial closure; techniques such as component separation, which enable this, should be liberally employed. The most important patient factor predicting hernia recurrence is body mass index; the larger the patient, the higher the chance of hernia recurrence.

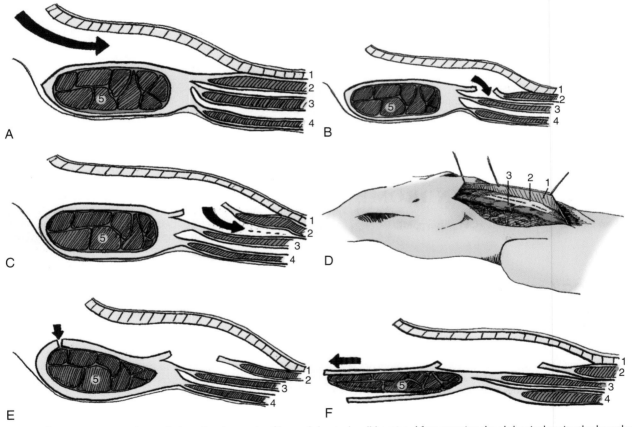

FIGURE 14   Component separation technique for the repair of large abdominal wall hernias. After entering the abdominal cavity, the bowels are dissected free from the ventral abdominal wall. **IA,** The skin and subcutaneous fat (*1*) are dissected free from the anterior sheath of the rectus abdominis muscle (*5*) and the aponeurosis of the external oblique muscle (*2*). **IB** and **IC,** The aponeurosis of the external oblique muscle (*2*) is transected longitudinally about 2 cm lateral from the rectus sheath, including the muscular part on the thoracic wall, which extends at least 5 to 7 cm cranially of the costal margin. **ID,** The external oblique muscle (*2*) is separated from the internal oblique muscle (*3*) as far laterally as possible. **IE** and **IF,** If primary closure is impossible with undue tension, a further gain of 2 to 4 cm can be reached by separation of the posterior rectal sheath from the rectus abdominis muscle (*5*). Care must be taken not to damage the blood supply and the nerves that run between the internal oblique and transverse muscles (*4*) and enter the rectus abdominis muscle at the posterior side. *(Reproduced with permission from de Vries Reilingh TS, van Goor H, Rosman C, et al, "Components separation technique" for the repair of large abdominal wall hernias, J Am Coll Surg 196[1]:32–37, 2003.)*

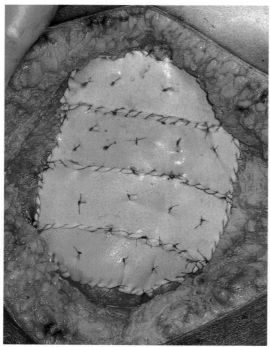

FIGURE 15   HADM (Alloderm) onlay mesh placed after component separation technique was used to primarily repair a large ventral hernia. Note that the HADM extends out laterally past all fascial incisions. *(Courtesy Dr. Richard Redett, Johns Hopkins Plastic and Reconstructive Surgery, Baltimore, Md.)*

SUMMARY

Few contemporary surgery modalities rival the open abdomen in improving mortality in the severely injured or critically ill patient. Improvements in temporary abdominal closure methods and definitive abdominal closure will continue to improve mortality and quality of life for patients who require damage control surgery or for those with ACS.

SUGGESTED READINGS

Barker DE, Green JM, Maxwell RA, et al: Experience with vacuum-pack temporary abdominal wound closure in 258 trauma and general and vascular surgical patients, *J Am Coll Surg* 204(5):784–792, 2007.

Campbell A, Chang M, Fabian T, et al and the Open Abdomen Advisory Panel: Management of the open abdomen: from initial operation to definitive closure, *Am Surg* 75(suppl 11):S1–S22, 2009.

Navsaria PH, Bunting M, Omoshoro-Jones J, et al: Temporary closure of open abdominal wounds by the modified sandwich vacuum-pack technique, *Br J Surg* 90(6):718–722, 2003.

Rodriguez ED, Bluebond-Langner R, Silverman RP, et al: Abdominal wall reconstruction following severe loss of domain: the R. Adams Cowley Shock Trauma Center algorithm, *Plast Reconstr Surg* 120(3):669–680, 2007.

Rotondo MF, Schwab CW, McGonigal MD, et al: "Damage control": an approach for improved survival in exsanguinating penetrating abdominal injury, *J Trauma* 35(3):375–382, 1993.

MANAGEMENT OF EXTREMITY COMPARTMENT SYNDROME

J. Bracken Burns, DO, and Eric R. Frykberg, MD

ETIOLOGY AND PATHOPHYSIOLOGY

A number of osteofascial compartments exist within the human body. In focusing on the extremities, there are three such compartments in the upper arm, three in the forearm, two in the thigh, and four in the lower leg. These compartments are bound by a relatively inflexible tissue envelope. This envelope commonly comprises fascia, bone, and muscle, but other structures such as skin, epimysium, and external compressive dressings may also contribute to the restrictive envelope. It is important to know the anatomic structures contained in these compartments to appreciate the consequences of their compromise.

Extremity compartment syndrome is a complex clinical condition that arises from a fairly simple concept. Basically, compartment syndrome is the result of elevated tissue pressures within a confined space that leads to tissue ischemia. On the vascular level, the pathophysiology involves decreased capillary perfusion related to the increased compartment pressure. It is the progressive venous hypertension from compression of venules that leads to the clinical manifestations of ischemia. This venous hypertension is perpetuated by transudative fluid escaping into the interstitial space, which further leads to venous collapse. Arterial inflow then opens venous channels at higher drainage pressures, which results in a decreased pressure gradient between the arterial and venous circulation. This reduces capillary blood flow and tissue perfusion. The resultant tissue ischemia stimulates vasodilatation, which then leads to further fluid transudation. A vicious cycle then develops of progressively worsening compartmental hypertension and tissue ischemia that progresses to tissue necrosis, as the arteriolar circulation is compromised. Once systemic toxicity develops from the consequent inflammatory process; infection; electrolyte abnormalities, especially hyperkalemia from cellular necrosis; acute renal failure; rhabdomyolysis; and acidosis, true compartment *syndrome* is present. *Crush syndrome* is largely synonymous with this entity (Figure 1).

The etiology of extremity compartment syndrome is often related, but not exclusive, to trauma to an extremity. Either reduction of the size of the compartment or, more commonly, volume expansion within the compartment can lead to extremity compartment syndrome (Box 1). Patients who are most at risk for this syndrome include those with major artery and venous injuries, extremity skeletal fractures, soft-tissue injuries, crush injuries, or delayed reperfusion of an injured and ischemic extremity (Box 2). Iatrogenic causes include dressings, splints, and casts that are too tight or incomplete surgical decompression.

Several factors influence the tolerance of extremity tissues to increased compartmental pressures, and these may determine the ultimate outcome of this condition in specific clinical settings. The duration and level of pressure elevation directly correlates with the extent of irreversible tissue loss and functional deficit. Peripheral nerves are more sensitive to an ischemic insult than other tissues, and chronic

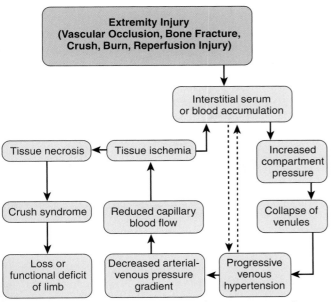

FIGURE 1   Pathophysiologic evolution of compartment syndrome.

BOX 1:   Causes of extremity compartment syndrome

Compartment size restriction	Crush injury
Limb compression	Massive soft tissue injury
Saturday night palsy	Exertion injury
Lloyd Davies positioning	Electrical burns
External compression	Insect, spider, and snakebites
Casts	Ischemic reperfusion injury
Splints	Systemic inflammatory
Military antishock trousers	response
Compartment volume	Septic shock
expansion	Extravasation of intravenous
Vascular injury	fluids
Bone fracture	Primary blast injury

atherosclerotic vascular disease reduces the ischemic threshold of extremity tissues. Shock and limb elevation both reduce the arteriovenous pressure gradient and therefore further aggravate the deleterious effects of compartment syndrome. Hypothermia and ice application also exacerbate this condition by inducing vasoconstriction, thereby inhibiting arterial perfusion.

DIAGNOSIS

In an alert and responsive patient, the diagnosis of fully developed extremity compartment syndrome may be made by physical examination. In patients with a decreased level of consciousness, in uncooperative patients, in those with spinal cord injury, and in the earliest stages of the process, an accurate physical exam may be difficult to obtain. The most common symptom of extremity compartment syndrome is the classic sign of tissue ischemia, pain out of proportion to the apparent extremity insult or injury and out of proportion to the physical findings. The most common physical sign is pain on passive stretch of the muscles in an involved compartment. Other common clinical manifestations of compartment syndrome include sensory and motor abnormalities, palpable tenseness or swelling over a compartment, and overlying skin blistering, in addition to typical laboratory indications of tissue damage such as hyperkalemia, acidosis, and myoglobinuria.

BOX 2:   Conditions associated with high risk of extremity compartment syndrome

Popliteal vessel injury
Combined arterial/venous injury
Prolonged ischemia (>4–6 hours)
Massive soft tissue injury (i.e., crush)
Prolonged or severe shock
Ligation/thrombosis of major artery or vein
Combined arterial and bone or soft tissue injury
Elevated compartment pressure

It is important to emphasize that the development of any such clinical sign represents an advanced stage of this condition, as these signs evidence tissue damage that is already established, and this reflects a high risk of long-term disability. The ideal goal of treatment is to intervene *before* these signs develop, to prevent tissue damage as much as possible by maintaining a high level of suspicion in those settings that pose a high risk of compartment hypertension (see Box 2). Any sensory abnormality suggests nerve ischemia, which must be acted on promptly, as nerve tissue is most sensitive to this insult and will progress most rapidly to nerve loss and long-term morbidity as a result.

The diagnosis of extremity compartment syndrome should never rely on the status of the peripheral pulses or other signs of vascular integrity. A palpable pulse does not exclude compartment syndrome, because major extremity vessels typically remain patent long after irreversible tissue necrosis has developed from microvascular compromise at the capillary level. Conversely, an absent distal pulse mandates evaluation for a vascular injury; this is rarely a feature of extremity compartment syndrome.

Direct measurement of intracompartmental pressures is perhaps the most accurate and specific diagnostic test for compartment hypertension, and it provides additional objective data in patients with an unreliable examination or questionable diagnosis. Compartmental pressures may be measured by a variety of techniques including a needle-catheter device connected to a syringe and manometer, wick catheters, slit catheters, and direct needle puncture with a handheld solid state transducer device (STIC catheter; Stryker Surgical, Kalamazoo, Mich.). All emergency departments should have similar pressure-measuring devices.

Normal tissue pressures are 5 to 10 mm Hg. Pressures higher than this are likely to indicate some level of tissue compromise, and many authors advocate levels of 25 to 30 mm Hg as the point at which treatment interventions should occur. The diagnosis of compartment syndrome should not rely on this value in isolation but should incorporate the entire clinical picture. The more risk factors and clinical signs and symptoms that are found, the lower the threshold for intervention should be.

TREATMENT AND SURGICAL TECHNIQUE

Although nonsurgical management with osmotic diuretics such as mannitol, ice packs, or extremity elevation have been tried, these have not proven effective, may cause more harm than benefit, and may delay proper treatment with a consequent risk of limb morbidity or loss. If the diagnosis of compartment syndrome is made, the only appropriate and effective treatment in most settings is prompt surgical decompression, or *fasciotomy*, of the involved compartments. By incising the investing fascia, the critical element of increased tissue pressure is allowed to dissipate to restore normal capillary perfusion. This must be done as early and as rapidly as possible, as delay is directly correlated with increased tissue damage and loss.

BOX 3: Below-the-knee compartments and anatomic contents

Anterior Compartment	Posterior Compartment
Extensor muscles	Soleus muscle
Tibialis anterior muscle	Gastrocnemius muscle
Extensor hallucis longus muscle	Plantaris tendon
Extensor digitorum longus muscle	**Deep Posterior Compartment**
Peroneus tertius muscle	Deep flexor muscles
Deep peroneal nerve	Flexor hallucis longus muscle
Anterior tibial artery and veins	Tibialis posterior muscle
	Flexor digitorum longus muscle
Lateral Compartment	Politeus muscle
	Tibial nerve
Peroneus longus muscle	Posterior tibial artery and veins
Peroneus brevis muscle	Peroneal artery and veins
Superficial peroneal nerve	

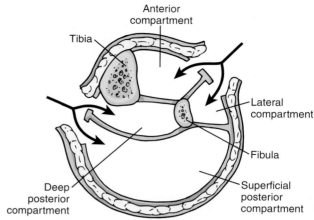

FIGURE 2 Anatomy of lower leg compartments and location of incisions for double-incision four-compartment fasciotomy.

The most important principle to follow in performing a fasciotomy is to widely open the compartments and fully incise overlying epimysium and skin along the entire length of the incisions; these can be constricting enough to prevent complete decompression, which allows the vicious cycle of progressive tissue ischemia to continue. Care must also be taken to avoid placing tight dressings, casts, or splints over these wounds for the same reason. In most clinical scenarios, all compartments of the involved extremity should be opened, as there are no reliable clinical indicators correlating with low enough risk to safely leave one or more decompressed. Exceptions may include low-energy penetrating mechanisms, such as stab wounds, in which the trajectory of injury is clearly localized. The techniques for fasciotomy depend on the anatomy of the involved extremity.

Below-the-Knee Four-Compartment Fasciotomy

The compartments below the knee include the anterior, lateral, superficial posterior, and deep posterior compartments. These are the most common locations of extremity compartment syndrome, because of the tenuous blood supply and vulnerability to injury. Knowledge of the structures contained in these compartments is essential to appreciate the consequences of their compromise (Box 3). Three techniques are described for fasciotomy below the knee. These include double-incision four-compartment fasciotomy, single-incision four-compartment fasciotomy, and fibulectomy-fasciotomy.

Fibulectomy-fasciotomy involves a single lateral incision over the fibula followed by a subperiosteal removal of the fibula, which widely opens all four compartments of the leg. Although this technique provides the widest exposure and most effective decompression, it is seldom used, as it is also the most invasive, with the highest risks of nerve and blood vessel damage and long-term disability from loss of the fibula. The anterior tibial artery is closely associated with the medial fibular surface and is quite vulnerable to disruption with this technique. Single-incision four-compartment fasciotomy also involves a single lateral incision along the length of the fibula, but the medial compartments are incised through dissection around and behind the fibula, leaving this bone in place to reduce disability. This requires much blind dissection with uncertain effectiveness at decompressing all compartments, and again, a risk of nerve and vessel damage is present.

The most commonly employed technique is the double-incision four-compartment fasciotomy (Figure 2). A lateral longitudinal incision is made in the skin midway between the tibia and fibula to expose the investing fascia deep to the subcutaneous layer, extending from the head of the fibula to the ankle. A small transverse incision is then made in the investing fascia to identify the intermuscular septum, which divides the anterior and lateral compartments, to ensure proper identification of the separate compartments. The anterior compartment is opened by longitudinally incising the fascia 2 cm posterior to the anterior edge of the tibia along the entire length of the leg. A similar, more posterior longitudinal incision is used to open the lateral compartment, and this is made 1 cm posterior to the intermuscular septum. Care must be taken to avoid the superficial peroneal nerve, which passes superficially in front of the fibula head in the lateral compartment and can lead to foot drop if injured.

The superficial posterior and deep posterior compartments are approached through a second medial longitudinal skin incision placed 2 cm posterior to the posterior border of the tibia. The superficial posterior compartment is opened by a longitudinal incision in the exposed fascia. The deep posterior compartment is opened by detaching the soleus muscle from the posterior tibial periosteum and making a longitudinal fascial incision just posterior to the tibia. Caution should be taken to avoid the posterior tibial artery, as it is superficially located in this latter compartment. Although the deep posterior compartment is the most difficult to open, it is the most important to decompress in any setting that poses a high risk of compartmental hypertension, as it contains the tibial nerve and both the posterior tibial and peroneal arteries—the most important contributors to viability and function of the foot.

Above-the-Knee Three-Compartment Fasciotomy

Compartment syndrome of the thigh is relatively uncommon. Thigh compartment syndrome may occasionally be seen following civilian trauma in patients with femur or pelvic fractures or ligation of major venous structures such as the inferior vena cava, common iliac vein, or external iliac vein. Recent reports have indicated a higher incidence in U.S. combat casualties in the Middle East following blast injuries from improvised explosive devices (IEDs).

The thigh has three compartments: *anterior, medial,* and *posterior* (Box 4). Thigh compartment fasciotomy is performed by making an anterolateral longitudinal skin incision along the iliotibial tract. The fascia over the vastus lateralis muscle is opened longitudinally, and the anterior leaf of the fascia is elevated. The vastus lateralis muscle is freed of its posterior attachments, and the intermuscular septum lateral to the posterior compartment is incised (Figure 3). This decompresses the posterior compartment. Often this is satisfactory to decompress the medial compartment, but compartment pressures should be checked in the medial compartment after decompressing the anterior and posterior compartments. If the compartment

BOX 4: Thigh compartments and anatomic structures

Anterior Compartment	Medial Compartment	Posterior Compartment
Sartorius muscle	Gracilis	Hamstrings
Quadriceps muscles	Adductors	Biceps femoris
Rectus femoris	Adductor longis	Semitendinosis
Vastus lateralis	Adductor brevis	Semimembranosis
Vastus intermedius	Adductor magnus	Inferior gluteal artery
Vastus medialis	Obturator nerve	Profunda femoris artery
Femoral artery and vein	Obturator artery	Sciatic nerve

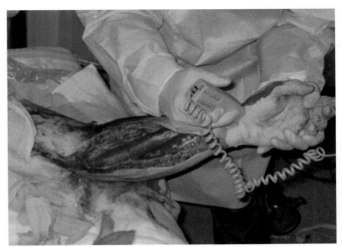

FIGURE 4   Fasciotomy of the volar compartment of the arm through a curvilinear longitudinal incision. Persistent hand ischemia required extension onto the palmar surface across the wrist.

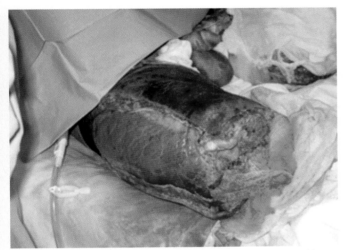

FIGURE 3   Thigh compartment syndrome from blast injury and burn after lateral fasciotomy; amputation above the knee was required. Note the bulging of the swollen vastus lateralis muscle.

pressure is still elevated in the medial compartment, an incision is made through the skin and fascia overlying the adductor muscles.

Below-the-Elbow Three-Compartment Fasciotomy

Upper extremity compartment syndrome is seen much less frequently, attributable to the more robust vascular supply with increased arterial and venous collaterals and better venous drainage. Most cases are related to major extremity trauma, particularly involving the ipsilateral major vasculature.

The volar and dorsal compartments of the forearm are both decompressed through longitudinal incisions extending from the elbow to the wrist. These may be extended onto the hand and digits if necessary. The dorsal incision should also open the mobile wad compartment at the lateral portion of the antecubital fossa. The volar incision should be S-shaped as it crosses the elbow or wrist crease to prevent disfiguring contractures, and it should then arc medially, as it progresses toward the wrist, to preserve the blood supply to the skin flap (Figure 4).

Wound Care

The fasciotomy wound should be covered with moist sterile dressings that are changed frequently. Alternatively, a vacuum-assisted closure device can be applied to the wound. It is imperative that all obviously necrotic tissue be debrided and frequent evaluation of the wound be undertaken with ongoing debridement if necessary. Range-of-motion exercises should be instituted early to inhibit contractures.

Most fasciotomy incisions may be closed after 3 to 7 days. Delayed primary skin closure may be performed if undue tension is not required, which can be confirmed by compartment pressure monitoring. The fascial incisions should not be approximated. Most full-blown cases of compartment syndrome cannot undergo primary wound closure because of extensive muscle bulging, in which case split-thickness skin grafting is required.

Another method for promoting wound closure involves securing vessel loops to the skin in a "shoelace" pattern across the skin at the time of fasciotomy. Gradual and careful tightening is then carried out daily. This technique promotes wound approximation and can avoid another operative procedure for closure.

Results

Infection is the most common complication of extremity fasciotomy, and it is documented in as many as 40% of cases; however, these cases are most likely the result of underlying tissue necrosis from treatment delay, as infection of a clean open wound should not occur with proper wound care. Long-term functional disability has also been reported in a substantial number of patients. In virtually all of them, however, limb loss or limb morbidity is directly attributable to the severity of the original insult or injury and not the fasciotomy itself.

Published reports have advocated the avoidance of fasciotomy in injured limbs in which the clinical picture reliably indicates long-standing compartment syndrome, with muscle necrosis already established, as a means of avoiding infection of these tissues and to prevent a release of toxic metabolites, which may occur if the tissues are uncovered. However, such an approach must be very cautiously applied, if it is used at all, as it is impossible to reliably assess the level of injury or recoverable tissue without direct visualization. Also, without debriding devitalized tissue, the patient could be vulnerable to life-threatening complications from rhabdomyolysis, hyperkalemia, and renal failure.

Many studies of extremity compartment syndrome have documented some correlation between early performance of fasciotomy after severe extremity injury, before the clinical manifestations develop, and lower rates of limb morbidity and amputation. This is the rationale for aggressively applying *prophylactic* fasciotomy to otherwise asymptomatic limbs in high-risk settings (see Box 2) to prevent compartment syndrome from ever developing. This may not only prevent the morbid limb-threatening and life-threatening complications, but it will also provide a better cosmetic result, as the incision would most likely be amenable to primary closure rather than skin grafting. If the decision is made to clinically observe a high-risk extremity, rather than immediately perform a fasciotomy, compartment pressure measurement must be an integral part of this management to prevent the development of major complications; fasciotomy is performed promptly once tissue pressures exceed 20 mm Hg.

The decision to perform a fasciotomy is a clinical judgment that must involve an assessment of the individual patient and the specific injury. An understanding of the pertinent anatomy, surgical techniques, and risk/benefit ratio of observation versus definitive treatment is essential. Generally, an aggressive approach of early and liberal extremity fasciotomy will provide the best results, in view of the low morbidity of this procedure and the substantial risk of limb dysfunction, loss, or rhabdomyolysis if definitive treatment is delayed.

SUGGESTED READINGS

Feliciano DV, Cruse PA, Spjut-Patrinely V, et al: Fasciotomy after trauma to the extremities, *Am J Surg* 156:533–538, 1988.

Finkelstein JA, Hunter GA, Hu RW: Lower limb compartment syndrome: course after delayed fasciotomy, *J Trauma* 40:342–346, 1996.

Matsen FA, Krugmire RB: Compartmental syndromes, *Surg Gynecol Obstet* 147:943–949, 1978.

McDermott AGP, Marble AE, Yabsley RH, et al: Monitoring acute compartment pressures with the STIC catheter, *Clinic Orthoped* 190:192–195, 1984.

Mubarak SJ, Owens CA: Double-incision fasciotomy of the leg for decompression in compartment syndromes, *J Bone Joint Surg* 59:184–187, 1977.

Vitale GC, Richardson JD, George SM, Miller FB: Fasciotomy for severe blunt and penetrating trauma of the extremity, *Surg Gynecol Obstet* 166:397–401, 1988.

Williams AB, Luchette FA, Papconstantinou HT, et al: The effect of early versus late fasciotomy in the management of extremity trauma, *Surgery* 122:861–867, 1997.

BURN WOUND MANAGEMENT

James J. Gallagher, MD

OVERVIEW

A *burn wound* is a practical term for damage and/or loss of skin resulting in a large wound that is often impractical or impossible to close without tissue flaps or grafts. Instead of a line that can be hidden in a natural crease, under hair, or in the umbilicus, the burn scar is often broad and visible. The etiology is diverse, including scald injury from a hot liquid, a chemical exposure, or the flash and conductive damage caused by an electrical current. Achieving surgical excellence requires knowledge of the goals in surgical burn care: these are *closure, function,* and *cosmesis.* These goals are not mutually exclusive, and simultaneous maximization of each is the path to the best possible result.

In the immediate days and weeks following surgery, the closed wound often changes dramatically. Scar maturation can lead to reopening of wounds, dislocation of joints with loss of function, and consequent deterioration of the result. The behavior of scar tissue during maturation is multifactorial, but it is strongly influenced by the total care provided early in treatment. Surgeon follow-up and coordination with a rehabilitation therapist is needed in nearly all significant burn injuries.

Burn treatment attempts to preserve what was not destroyed; its goals are timely wound closure and the return of the patient to the preinjury state. The degree to which the patient reintegrates into society is the measure of success in burn care. The spectrum of possible long-term problems associated with the care of the burn patient is best avoided through close and complete follow-up. This chapter focuses on the unique problems associated with the evaluation and treatment of burn wounds. An effort has been made to address and aid those surgeons whose practice is not focused on burn injury management.

EVALUATION

Assessing the Patient and the Burn

The drama of burn injury and its relative infrequency compared with other types of traumatic injuries may distract the care provider from performing a thorough and complete evaluation. The systematic

principles of modern trauma care should be applied in the care of the burn patient. Early in the evaluation and treatment of a burn patient, consider whether providing treatment locally with a surgeon who is not part of a burn center is preferable to referral to a burn center. This decision is made easier by a review of the burn center transfer criteria published by the American Burn Association. This set of transfer criteria has been developed to aid physicians in identifying patients who need the specialized care offered by a burn center (Box 1).

The estimate of the burn size forms the foundation of patient care; nearly all subsequent decisions about patient treatment will be based on this estimate. The calculation of the percent of the total body surface area (TBSA) burned is best done under the supervision of an experienced practitioner. Multiple studies have demonstrated the surprising lack of congruity between the estimates of burn size at a referring institution and the burn center estimate. It is often helpful with larger and scattered burns to write down each of the body area estimates and sum them when complete. The *rule of nines* is a commonly used way of estimating burn size (Figure 1). In children, especially toddlers, the standard rule of nines does not work well. The child's head is proportionately larger, and the lower extremities are smaller. Another helpful standard is that the patient's palm represents approximately 1% of the TBSA.

Useful Points for Estimating Burn Size

- Do not include first-degree burns in the estimate.
- Superficial second-degree burns blister and lose the epidermis.
- It is possible to estimate burn size before thorough cleaning of wounds.
- In second-degree burns, it is often difficult or impossible to assess burn depth before thorough cleaning of the wounds.
- Exposed dermis in a superficial second-degree burn is moist with blanching redness and is painful.
- Deeper burns are less sensitive; they may be red, but they will not blanch with pressure.
- Dryness and hair that is easily removed are signs of a deep wound.
- Third-degree burns are dry, leathery, and insensate.

No proven and widely accepted diagnostic tool is currently available to guide the clinician in assessing the depth of the burn and thereby evaluating the ability of the wound to heal without the need for surgery. Much work has been done and is ongoing to find a reliable, objective, and practical method for determination of burn depth. The clinical examination of burn depth by an experienced clinician remains the standard for determining the need for surgery.

BOX 1:　Burn center referral criteria

Partial thickness burn greater than 10% total body surface area

Burns involving the face, hands, feet, genitalia, perineum, or major joints

Third-degree burns

Electric burns (including lightning)

Chemical burns

Inhalation injury

Burn injury with preexisting medical conditions that could complicate patient management, prolong recovery, or affect mortality rate

Burn injury with concomitant trauma, in which the burn injury poses the greatest risk of morbidity or mortality (If the trauma poses the greatest immediate risk, the patient should first be stabilized in the trauma center before transfer to the burn facility. Decisions should be made according to regional medical control plans and triage protocols.)

Children with burns in hospitals without personnel or equipment qualified for care of children

Burn injuries in patients who will require special social, emotional, or long-term rehabilitative intervention

Data from American Burn Association ABLS Advisory Committee: Advanced burn life support course, Chicago, 2001, American Burn Association; and Johnson RM, Richard R: Partial-thickness burns: identification and management, *Adv Skin Wound Care* 16:178–187, 2003.

Do not underestimate the impact of early, accurate decision making and treatment planning by an experienced surgeon in achieving excellent results. The benefit of early wound excision and grafting is proven. Allowing a wound to declare its healing potential over weeks before operating leads to several significant problems that are best avoided. Painful daily dressing changes lead to excessive pain medications and the attendant complications with those, as well as the risk of a psychologic pain syndrome. A wound that remains incompletely closed for more than 21 days is at high risk for hypertrophy and contracture formation with loss of function over the long term. Conversely, an inexperienced surgeon who attempts surgery on a wound that would have otherwise healed removes viable tissue that would have the natural regenerative capacity to heal had it been left in place. It is therefore the challenge of the care provider to be simultaneously aggressive and conservative with the burn wound in decision making, wound care, and surgical treatment.

Burn wound evaluation should be done after light cleansing and before any topical treatment is placed. The surgical team should evaluate and determine the treatment for the wound. If burn center transfer is indicated, contact the burn center for directives about wound care for the patient in transit. Application of a topical treatment may preclude the use of dressings designed to adhere to wounds until closed. Typically, receiving burn centers will ask that smaller wounds be kept in a clean, moist dressing, and larger wounds in dry dressings, to prevent excessive loss of heat.

The need for formal burn resuscitation is not usually present with a burn of less than 10% to 15% of the body surface. Larger burns stimulate a systemic inflammatory response, which is treated with fluid to prevent hypovolemia, hypoperfusion, and the sequelae of tissue ischemia from shock. Burn fluid formulas are designed as a guide to the inception volume of resuscitation. True rates of fluid and volumes required are dictated by the condition of the patient and an assessment of the end points of resuscitation.

Large burns have an absolute need for nutritional supplementation, preferably with tube feedings. Speed of epithelialization, formation of granulation tissue, and immunocompetence are dependent on adequate nutrition. When to intervene with smaller and

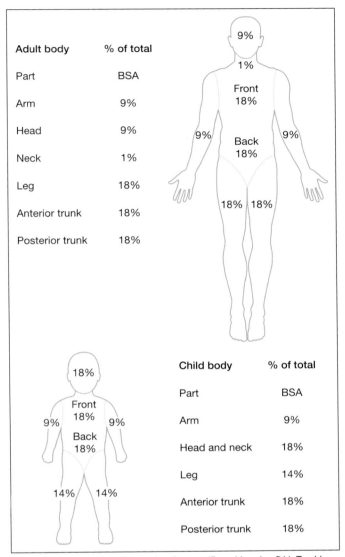

Adult body	% of total
Part	BSA
Arm	9%
Head	9%
Neck	1%
Leg	18%
Anterior trunk	18%
Posterior trunk	18%

Child body	% of total
Part	BSA
Arm	9%
Head and neck	18%
Leg	14%
Anterior trunk	18%
Posterior trunk	18%

FIGURE 1　Diagram of the rule of nines. *(From Herndon DN: Total burn care, ed 3, Philadelphia, 2007, Saunders Elsevier, p 84.)*

medium-sized burns is best guided by clear caloric goals and a good accounting of intake.

Assessing the Need for Decompression

Following burn injury, the identification and treatment of elevated tissue pressure can avoid the loss of deeper tissues and eliminate a profound cause of morbidity. Tissue that has suffered burn injury forms edema as a result of the loss of capillary integrity and the movement of fluid from the intravascular compartment to the injured tissue interstitium. The larger the burn, the greater the edema, which forms even in unburned tissues in large burns. In normal tissues, the edema formation does not cause an immediate problem. However, burned skin is less elastic than normal skin. These two factors together may result in high levels of tissue pressure that can lead to deep tissue loss similar to a classic compartment syndrome. Releasing the increased tissue pressure from a burn injury does not normally require the decompression of the deep fascial compartments as in a classic compartment syndrome. In burn injury the restriction is at the level of the burned skin. Full-thickness incision of the burned skin or eschar to an edge of normal skin usually results in resolution of the

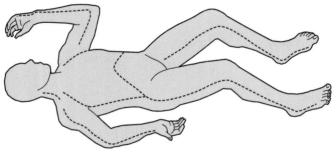

FIGURE 2 Anatomic diagram of preferred escharotomy sites, illustrating the site and orientation of decompressive escharotomy incisions for each body part.

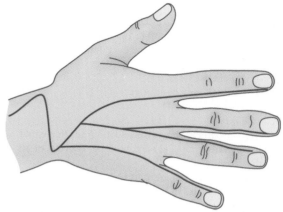

FIGURE 3 Recommended location of decompressive escharotomy of the hands. *(From Green D, Hotchkiss R, Pederson W, et al: Green's operative hand surgery, ed 5, Philadelphia, 2005, Churchill Livingstone Elsevier, p 2164.)*

increased pressure. Figures 2 and 3 give the recommended locations of decompressive escharotomies on the hands and body.

Circumferential burns are often considered for decompression; however, the presence of a circumferential burn is not an automatic indication for decompression. In patients with burns that are partial thickness, the incisions for decompression can be a significant cosmetic issue. In a cooperative patient with a small- to medium-sized burn, careful fluid administration with elevation when possible, coupled with serial exams looking for increased tissue pressure, is a safe option. In contrast, larger burns (greater than 50% TBSA) almost universally require decompression of circumferentially burned extremities, and possibly deep fascial decompression as well.

INHALATION INJURY

By nature of the mechanism of injury, many burns are associated with an inhalation injury (IHI) to the lungs. Significant morbidity and mortality can be attributed to IHI, and it has been shown to be an independent predictor of mortality. Severe injury is obvious, and often the patient is intubated at the scene. More difficult are those patients in whom there are some signs of inhalation injury without significant clinical compromise. Thoughtful decision making prior to intubation is critical to avoid the morbidity associated with an unnecessary artificial airway and mechanical ventilation.

In a stable patient the evaluation for IHI is made after a complete history of the incident is taken that focuses on assessing the amount of time spent in a closed space with the smoke. IHI is best understood as two pathologic processes: first, the chemical injury to the lung parenchyma that develops over several days, similar to acute respiratory distress syndrome (ARDS); second, a direct thermal injury to the upper airway. Early intubation can be lifesaving for the direct thermal injury to the airway to avoid its loss from edema, which will form rapidly. The parenchymal injury without damage to the upper airway is not necessarily best treated with intubation. The stable patient can be observed in a monitored setting, with intubation and mechanical ventilation reserved for those patients who deteriorate.

ELECTRICAL INJURY

Burn injury from a conductive electrical source is a particularly difficult clinical problem that requires a rapid and aggressive surgical approach. The extent of damage can be misleading on routine physical examination, as the amount of tissue damage to deep structures can be severe but is hidden by intact overlying skin. This dead tissue can create a compartment syndrome with further tissue loss. In addition, pigment from the dead and damaged muscles can rapidly produce renal failure, which increases the likelihood of mortality. Additionally, dead, undebrided muscle is an excellent medium for bacterial colonization and sepsis. The multiple possible long-term sequelae of conductive electrical injury and the complexity of the care required dictate that, once a patient

with such an injury is identified, he or she should be transferred promptly to a burn center.

CHILD ABUSE

Intentionally inflicted burn injury is a method used frequently for direct child abuse and/or to cover up other kinds of child abuse. The surgeon caring for a burned child must remain vigilant to the possibility and must obtain an absolutely clear understanding of the circumstances surrounding the burn injury. It is usual practice to have multiple practitioners interview the involved adults and the child separately and then discuss as a group the circumstances reported by the adults and the child, before the injury is attributed to an accidental cause.

Warning Signs for Child Abuse

- Lack of splash marks in scald injury
- Straight-line distribution of skin injury with immersions
- Contact burns that are evenly injured
- A halo of scaled buttocks skin around unburned area, indicating the child was held down with force during the immersion
- Unburned adults
- A previous history of burn injury

OPERATIVE CARE OF THE BURN WOUND

General Principles of Care

A meticulous preoperative plan will dictate the steps of the appropriate procedure, which will decrease operative delays and optimize results. Intraoperative positioning and patient draping are done based on the wound and any proposed graft donor site. To address the entire wound adequately, the surgeon must identify any areas that have retained the ability to heal spontaneously with good wound care, versus those that will require surgery to achieve closure. All wounds, including those not included in the operative treatment plan, are routinely cleaned and dressed as part of the procedure. This affords the opportunity for the surgeon to thoroughly clean the wounds and examine the patient under anesthesia in a way that might not be otherwise possible.

With a burn greater than 50% to 60% of the TBSA, rapid closure is the prime directive to save the patient's life. Closure of the wound is the best defense against the ongoing risk of sepsis, loss of lean body mass, and death. During the early period, when focus is on closure, consideration of the two remaining goals, normal function and good cosmesis, can greatly improve the complete result for the patient long term. The discussion that follows will focus on less extensive burns.

Preparing the Wound Bed

Approaching the Burn Wound

The basic principles of burn care involve the efficient removal of all the dead tissue, without damaging or sacrificing living tissue, while minimizing blood loss. Small wounds may be completely excised and either closed primarily or with a flap. Areas that will require grafting on an extremity can be safely and confidently excised under tourniquet; this technique minimizes blood loss associated with debridement. The determination of living versus dead tissue is best made with complete exsanguination of the extremity followed by inflation of the tourniquet. The remaining red to purple staining after complete exsanguination is a reliable marker for compromise. Healthy dermis is characterized by a pearly white appearance. Fat tissue that is compromised is a dull yellow to orange color; the yellow of healthy fat is bright. Care must be taken when using this technique in a chronic burn wound and in extremities with clinical evidence of venous stasis, as the dermal coloration may be misleading.

Tangential excision is the most common method for removal of dead tissue. Specially made tangential excision knives are used, including the dermatome, which may be used as a tool for debridement. It is important to complete the excision to the surgeon's satisfaction in one stage and then to achieve hemostasis, as this will shorten the procedure and limit blood loss. Very large areas can be done in steps. To achieve hemostasis of a large surface area after tangential excision, use clamps or cautery on vessels with pulsatile blood flow. Do not spend excessive time before application of a moist dressing with epinephrine and mild compression. The majority of bleeding points do not require direct attention, and compressive dressings may be left in place for 10 to 15 minutes before removal. Thrombogenic products can be added to the wound bed in an effort to further minimize blood loss; however, the cost must be considered.

On the trunk, tourniquet excision is not possible, and blood loss can be significant. The bleeding pattern and tissue appearance are used to determine tissue viability and completeness of excision. Tangential excision that removes dead tissue yet remains within the dermis is characterized by diffuse bleeding from the entire cut surface. When it is necessary to remove the full thickness of skin to reach a viable tissue bed, bleeding is pulsatile and moves from the perforating branches to the skin. Tumescent fluid containing epinephrine beneath the wound will limit blood loss; however, reliance of bleeding pattern as a guide to the adequacy of the excision is compromised. Reading of the wound requires attention to the color and quality of the tissue, such as in excision under tourniquet. Anecdotally, the use of tumescent fluid under the wound bed can lead to increased seromas and hematomas under the skin grafts. Burn wounds of great depth over a large area may require excision at the level of the fascia; this can greatly limit blood loss and increase efficiency, but the resulting marked functional and cosmetic impact must be considered with this approach.

SPECIAL CONSIDERATIONS

Exposed vital structures such as bone, periosteum, tendon, peritenon, and nerve require extra consideration. These structures are often poor beds for a skin graft to "take" in, which may lead to graft failure. Worse still, the resulting wound will leave the delicate structure at risk of further compromise. Consider use of a dermal template, which can bridge gaps in the robustness of the wound bed at the site of the delicate structure. This occurs by inosculation of blood vessels into the dermal template from the surrounding viable tissue, such as muscle, fat, or remaining deep dermis. The dermal template can also provide a layer between the skin graft and the structure below to allow smooth

and separate movements of each. Dermal templates are available off the shelf and can provide temporary wound closure. Disadvantages associated with the use of dermal templates include the 2 weeks or more such templates take to mature, the requirement for a second procedure for skin graft overlay after they mature, and the careful handling required to prevent infection. The benefits of decreased scarring and improved function in the long term are not well proven.

Placing the Skin

- Place the skin under some stretch, aided by attaching one edge and then pulling it toward the other edge.
- Trim the skin as it is fitted to the wound.
- The skin graft should contact the wound bed completely, which can be difficult with deep contours.
- Avoid meshing skin whenever possible; this is an absolute rule on exposed areas such as the hands and face.
- Anticipate that seams between grafts will become visible scars and areas of more intense contraction, and plan their orientation appropriately.
- Staples, sutures, glues, and other closure devices are all used depending on the need. In children, consider fixation that is absorbable or sutures that are easily removed to facilitate aftercare.

Donor Sites

The creation of a donor-site wound is necessary in burn wounds that require a skin graft. The goal of donor-site location selection is to minimize the impact of the harvest. Factors to consider in choosing a donor site are 1) cosmesis, 2) healing potential, 3) intraoperative positioning and draping, 4) pain, and 5) practical postoperative positioning. It is important to counsel the patient that the harvest site will create an additional permanent scar.

When approaching the donor site, remember never to trust the dermatome calibration: visually inspect the gap created by the chosen setting. Routinely it is set at 6/1000 to 12/1000 of an inch. It can be useful to attempt to pass a #15 knife blade tip into the gap. The knife should enter partially and glide the length of the dermatome without dropping in entirely. This technique will ensure that the breadth of the gap is less than 10 to 12/1000 of an inch. Start the dermatome before contact with the skin and continue until it is lifted off the skin. Good positioning of the patient and the surgeon will yield the best harvest. It is routine to use mineral oil on the skin to promote smooth gliding of the dermatome with advancement. Watch the skin as it comes out of the dermatome to be sure of what you are harvesting. Do not rush the skin harvest: If the skin coming out of the dermatome is not satisfactory, keep the dermatome running and communicate with your assistants to try to improve things. If there is no improvement, lift off and abort the harvest attempt and reassess. Only rarely can a donor-site harvest area be immediately reharvested. An attempt that yields poor skin will lengthen the procedure, harm the cosmetic result, and increase morbidity.

Many dressing choices are available for the donor site. In those patients with very poor healing potential—such as those on chemotherapy, the infirm, and the immunocompromised—consider grafting the donor site with meshed autograft, homograft, or xenograft to speed closure of the donor site. In these patients, minimization of open wounds is a great concern.

The scalp is a possible donor site, as the skin obtained is a good color match for face, neck, and upper chest, and it can be a reliable donor site in patients with poor healing potential as a result of other chronic disease. When done properly in an individual with hair, the donor site is invisible just weeks after the procedure. A scalp skin harvest typically yields 3% to 4% of the body surface area before meshing.

An anesthetic scalp block placed before harvest can alleviate much of the donor site pain early in the postoperative period. Late pain with the scalp donor site is usually less than with other donor sites. When the skin is carefully taken, healing is rapid and reliable but with some risk of postsurgical alopecia from excessive harvest depth. In addition, a lack of attention to hairlines during harvest will leave a visible scar; this can be avoided by marking the hairlines before harvest and staying 1 to 2 cm within them. Harvesting a graft from the scalp should never be attempted unless appropriate tumescent infiltration with lidocaine and epinephrine in a balanced salt solution has been done. Attempting harvest without having placed appropriate tumescent fluid will result in excessive blood loss from the scalp, which is difficult to control. Approximately 500 mL of tumescent fluid is routine for a complete adult scalp harvest.

To harvest a scalp graft, remove the hair from the area with clippers before entering the operating room; shave the scalp with a razor after the patient is under anesthesia, and instill the tumescent fluid with a 14 gauge spinal needle moving about the area. You will recognize the appropriate depth by the relative ease of infiltration. Tending to the burn wound debridement at this point will allow the 10 to 15 minutes required for the epinephrine to have effect without adding to the operative time.

When wound-bed preparation of the burn is complete, return to the head, and harvest the needed skin based on the open wound area. The principle of wound-bed preparation followed by skin harvest can be extended broadly, as this approach often minimizes excessive harvest and decreases operative time. Two people are required to perform the scalp harvest properly, with the one holding the head directed by the operator of the dermatome. The dressing chosen to cover the donor site is then applied, followed by a snug head wrap.

Dressings

A grafted wound bed requires a period free of shear forces during which attachment of the skin graft to the wound bed can take place. Additionally, the skin graft requires a moist environment free from significant bacterial contamination. The creation of a dressing to address these goals is as critical to success as the other aspects of burn surgical care. Postoperative position, nursing care, and patient compliance, especially in children, can be major issues.

A grafted extremity is easily dressed with oil-based fine gauze, clean dressing, and a splint; however, the task becomes more difficult with grafting that involves the anterior shoulder and lateral neck. Options include a tie-on bolster in conjunction with a neck collar and axillary splint. A negative-pressure dressing can be considered if

a good circumferential seal can be obtained with or without splinting depending on the mobility of the wound.

Special problems are encountered with small children and their ability to work their way free of a dressing, so consider this as you plan the procedure. When the grafted areas require a complex dressing, it is good practice to discuss postoperative plans with nursing and rehabilitation staff and with the patient—or in the case of a child, with the patient's parents—to increase the likelihood of success. Postoperative prone positioning, for example, may be an excellent choice for grafts placed on the back; however, such a plan is unlikely to succeed if it is not discussed with nursing, rehabilitation, and the patient before surgery. An unusual position can be tried with the patient before surgery, and bed modifications can be made to prepare for the patient after surgery. Innovative dressings are possible if the goals are understood, the options are known, and open communication takes place with everyone involved. A dressing failure may lead to massive graft loss and a return to the operating room.

SUMMARY

This chapter on burn wound management is offered with the surgeon whose practice is not burn focused in mind. An effort has been made to offer advice to avoid problems and treat burns that, in the judgment of the treating physician, do not require a burn center. For a more complete discussion of burn care, the reader is directed to the suggested readings list. Burn centers can also be contacted for advice on burns not thought to require transfer to the burn center. Utilization of the burn center as a source of education on best practices, as well as for tertiary referral, is encouraged.

SUGGESTED READINGS

Alvarado R, Chung KK, Cancio LC, et al: Burn resuscitation, *Burns* 35(1):4–14, 2009.

Greenhalgh DG, Saffle JR, Holmes JH IV, et al: *J Burn Care Res* 28(6):776–790, 2007.

Thompkins RG, Remensnyder JP, Burke JF, et al: Significant reduction in mortality for children with burn injuries through the use of prompt eschar excision, *Ann Surg* 208(5):577, 1998.

Janzekovic Z: A new concept in the early excision and immediate grafting of burns, *J Trauma* 21:827, 1981.

BURNS: FLUID, NUTRITION, AND METABOLICS

Bradley J. Phillips, MD

OVERVIEW

When an individual suffers a burn over more than 20% of his or her body surface area (10% in children), a life-threatening situation develops. This is due to direct cellular damage and the effects of cytokines that alter the properties of semipermeable cell membranes, and it results in a massive shift of fluid into extracellular spaces. Consequently, hypovolemic shock occurs, and in addition, significant effects in many endocrine systems cause changes in metabolism such as hyperglycemia, inappropriate growth hormone levels, repressed androgen levels, and increased protein catabolism. Hypovolemic shock necessitates immediate and careful fluid

resuscitation, while the induced hormone changes, which can be prolonged for weeks or months, need to be addressed through a variety of treatments aimed at stabilizing or counteracting the effects of the metabolic alterations. Speed is of the essence; in children, delays in starting fluid resuscitation of just a few hours greatly increase mortality rate.

FLUID

Moderate or extensive burn injuries induce hypovolemic shock and vascular compartment imbalances that require immediate attention. Although heat is the destructive agent in regard to burned tissue, the transfer of thermal energy induces cellular responses distal to the injury site, such as the release of histamine, bradykinin, vasoactive amines, hormones, prostaglandins, leukotrienes, other cytokines, and neutrophils. An end result of this cascading phenomenon is endothelial cell damage related to the oxidation and release of lipid peroxidation products, which vastly increases capillary permeability.

Research has shown that fluid movement under these conditions is governed by several factors that follow Starling's equation, which describes fluid movement across capillary beds. While net filtration rate increases, interstitial compliance—a measure of the pressure required to change the volume of the interstitial space between cells—also increases, allowing initial edema to expand. Because of collateral damage to the lymphatic system near injury sites and the significant increase in interstitial fluid, the lymphatic system becomes overwhelmed. In addition, extensive cell membrane depolarization as a result of shock protein factors and activation of proteases involved with programmed cell death (apoptosis) lead to widespread homeostatic disruption.

The goal is therefore to stabilize patients through the active phase of fluid resuscitation by tailoring the amount of fluids required to meet adequate tissue perfusion without exacerbating burn-associated edema. Inotropic, nutritional, and pharmacologic support is also initiated to maintain cardiovascular output, counteract anaerobic metabolism, ensure sufficient oxygen delivery, and optimize nutrient supplementation to the entire body. Although cytokine and antioxidant research is still in its infancy, it is hoped that by addressing the biochemical sources of burn-induced cellular dysfunction, adjunctive treatments can be devised that will lower the mortality rates associated with burn injury over a large surface area.

Fluid Management: First 24 Hours

Formal fluid resuscitation should commence immediately in adults between the ages of 15 and 50 years with partial- or full-thickness burns over 20% or more of the total body surface area (TBSA). In children up to age 15 years and adults older than 50 years, the threshold for active fluid resuscitation should be 10% TBSA. Crystalloid, usually isotonic Ringer's lactate solution, is the most commonly used fluid, and a wide variety of formulas are available to determine how much fluid should be given. The percentage of burned surface area should be calculated using a Lund–Browder chart or the rule of nines, in which each body area represents a specified percent of the total, including the head (9%); trunk (18%); upper, mid, and low back and buttocks (18%); each arm (9%); the groins (1%); and each leg (18%).

There is no evidence to suggest that one formula is better than another; rather, it is suggested that practitioners become familiar with one specific formula to understand the intricacies involved in acute management. The Parkland formula is the most commonly used approach in the United States (4 mL/kg per %TBSA burned; Box 1 and Table 1), with half of the total volume given in the first 8 hours after the burn injury and the remainder infused over the next 16 hours. It is important to note that for the purposes of appropriate resuscitation, time begins when the burn injury occurred, and the rate of infusion should be gradually decreased at 8 hours rather than instituting a "step" change. Although other solutions besides lactated Ringer's have been studied, there is no evidence that they provide superior results. However, if significant impairment of liver function is evident prior to resuscitation, normal saline should be used in lieu of Ringer's lactate; bicarbonate or Plasmalyte B can also be substituted.

End Points and Monitoring

Fluid resuscitation should generally be titrated to a urine output of 0.5 mL/kg/h or approximately 30 to 50 mL/h in most adults and older children (>50 kg). Despite this guideline, there has been a tendency to overresuscitate patients, prompting a debate about safety. Although it is important to ensure that patients with a large portion of the TBSA burned (>40%) are adequately resuscitated, whether driven by aggressive preload points or higher usage of opiates and other analgesics, overresuscitation can lead to abdominal compartment syndrome (ACS). If the intraabdominal pressure exceeds 25 mm Hg during the resuscitation process, swift intervention is required to ensure that ACS does not develop.

BOX 1: Parkland formula for adults

> 4 mL Ringer's lactate per kilogram per percentage of total burned surface area
>
> 4 mL RL / kg / % TBSA

TABLE 1: Parkland formula for children (first 24 hours)

Resuscitation Volume	Maintenance Volume (Weight)
4 mL Ringer's lactate/ kg/%TBSA	0–10 kg: 4 mL/kg 10–20 kg: 40 mL/h + 2 mL/kg/h > 20 kg: 60 mL/h + 1 mL/kg/h

RL, Ringer's lactate

In some instances, monitoring urine output and vital signs may not be sufficient parameters for determination of adequate resuscitation. For example, in diabetic patients, significant glycosuria can cause an osmotic diuresis that leads to an artificially high urine output. Likewise, patients on long-standing diuretics may exhibit lower than desired urine outputs despite receiving an adequate resuscitation volume. Because of such discrepancies, several studies of critically ill patients have suggested that invasive monitoring could allow more precise titration of resuscitation fluid to compensate for an apparent oxygen deficit. The enthusiasm for pulmonary artery catheters to drive aggressive hemodynamic goals has been tempered in recent years because of comprehensive cost-effectiveness analyses and other noninvasive methods allowing real-time capture of objective data.

The most promising invasive approach to date, intrathoracic blood volumes (ITBV), is based upon the transpulmonary double-indicator dilution technique (temperature and dye dilution); it employs a central venous catheter and fiberoptic thermistor catheter inserted into the femoral artery. ITBV-guided resuscitation may be useful in permitting preload restoration with improved peripheral oxygen delivery. Whatever method is chosen, it is important to reach adequate end points in an efficient and timely manner to decrease the likelihood of multiorgan dysfunction.

Other Resuscitation Fluids

Hypertonic Saline

The introduction of hypertonic saline (HTS) was built on the work of Monafo and colleagues (1973), who proposed the idea that increasing plasma osmolality might moderate the shift of intravascular water into extracellular spaces. By providing a concentrated sodium load, it was thought that less total resuscitation volume would be required than with traditional methods.

Although early work indicated promising results, a seminal study published in 1995 by Huang and colleagues found that resuscitation with HTS was associated with a twofold increase in mortality rate due to renal failure. Furthermore, after 48 hours, it was determined that patients resuscitated with HTS had the same cumulative fluid loads as those receiving conventional Ringer's lactate, and they also developed systemic hypernatremia. In addition, this study revealed that HTS did not cause the kidney to increase its output. As other reports have since elucidated, in the presence of increasing ADH levels and hyperaldosteronism, relative hypovolemia and hyperosmolarity after HTS administration could act concomitantly to stimulate further increases in ADH and thus promote frank and prolonged sodium retention. A more recent Cochrane review and meta-analysis has since lowered the relative risk of mortality to 1.49 for HTS resuscitation versus resuscitation with Ringer's lactate. However, given the risks associated with hypernatremia, there is little reason to recommend an HTS approach in routine burn resuscitation. Rather, its advantage may lie in its use on the battlefield, during mass casualty events, or in expert hands when conventional resuscitation fails.

Colloid

The concept of adding colloid to crystalloid-based resuscitation schemes lies in the theory that colloid can decrease the amount of free plasma lost to interstitial spaces by exerting an oncotic force. Following the experience of the Shriners Burn Institute in Galveston, Texas, the work of Demling and others added a more scientific rationale regarding colloid use, suggesting that it was not helpful until membrane semipermeability had begun to recover. Based on their findings, colloids are usually not considered until 8 to 12 hours after a burn.

Subsequently, research has focused on the different types of colloids and their associated risks and benefits. In 1998, a meta-analysis that examined crystalloid versus colloid and crystalloid resuscitation in burn patients found an excessive risk (risk ratio, 1.21) with colloid use. Despite wide confidence intervals (0.88 to 1.66), these conclusions had a chilling effect on colloid usage, particularly in the United Kingdom. A more recent meta-analysis, however, reduced this risk to 1.01 for use of plasma or albumin.

Although albumin has been criticized because of its small molecular size in relation to the enlarged pore sizes of the semipermeable membrane, it has been used extensively since the 1950s, when it became commercially available. Moreover, studies have consistently failed to demonstrate superior outcomes with its usage. Theoretically, high molecular weight synthetic dextran should be advantageous because of its larger molecular size; however, convincing results are absent because of a lack of human studies. Gelatin and hydroxyethyl starch are also promising alternatives, but they require additional clinical studies to demonstrate efficacy.

To date, the most recent recommendation in regard to colloid usage has been that of Pham and colleagues (2008), who suggest that if colloids are utilized, they should be given late in the first 24 hours of resuscitation. Common dosages are 2.5 g/dL crystalloid (Galveston formula) or 20% to 60% of calculated plasma volume at a rate of 0.5 mL/%TBSA/kg/h (Parkland formula). In both adults and children, my preference is to consider colloid (5% albumin, 1 mL/kg/hr) at hour 12 if objective data do not meet predesigned end points.

Fluid Management After 24 Hours

The goal of fluid management after 24 hours is to replace fluids on a maintenance basis as cellular semipermeable membranes begin to recover. Most formulas provide some latitude on how this is accomplished. For example, the Parkland formula suggests using dextrose-saline at a maintenance rate of 1.5 mL/%TBSA/kg/h, and the Galveston formula proposes Ringer's lactate at a rate of 3750 mL/m^2 plus 1500 mL/m^2 BSA for maintenance requirements, with half the total volume given during the first 8 hours and the remainder in the next 16 hours. Depending on the requirements of the patient, D5W can be added as necessary.

Even during active resuscitation with intravenous fluids, enteral feeding should begin as early as possible and should not be interrupted. Depending on serum albumin levels, protein replacement may be necessary. Aggressive monitoring and replacement of serum electrolytes should also be encouraged. In the absence of the syndrome of inappropriate ADH (SIADH), cerebral salt wasting (CSW), or HTS therapy, serum sodium levels reflect total body water and should be used as an adjunctive measure in trying to understand the status of the patient's intracellular and extracellular compartments.

Pediatric Resuscitation

Children are more sensitive to aggressive resuscitation than adults because of their lower physiological reserves and glycogen stores. The classic goal for resuscitation in children weighing less than 30 kg is a urine output of 1 mL/kg/h, although ranges of 1.0 to 1.5 mL/kg/h are acceptable, provided there are no signs of underresuscitation or over-resuscitation. Adult end points in regard to urine output are more appropriate for children approaching 50 kg in weight. For the first several hours of therapy, urine output should be monitored every 15 minutes.

If venous access is difficult to obtain in children younger than 8 years, bone marrow compartments in the anterior tibial plateau, medial malleolus, anterior iliac crest, and distal femur can be cannulated using a 16 gauge spinal needle and a gravity drip with rates up to 100 mL/h. In general, the threshold for initiating invasive monitoring in children should be more conservative; if undertaken, femoral or internal jugular triple-lumen catheters should be used in preference to pulmonary artery catheters.

In terms of burn injury, children are at higher risk for complications and also require higher maintenance volumes compared with adults because of their larger surface/volume ratios. Children under 4 years of age are at higher risk of mortality, especially in cases of high percentage TBSA burns and/or inhalation injury. Calculating fluid requirements from burned surface areas also necessitates a more precise approach using age-appropriate charts, because the rule of nines is inaccurate in growing children. The Galveston formula uses 5000 mL/m^2 BSA plus 2000 mL/m^2 BSA for the first 24 hours, with half the volume given in 8 hours. For the second 24 hours, 3750 mL/m^2 BSA plus 1500 mL/m^2 BSA for maintenance fluid is required.

Pharmacologic Support

Although the study of inotropic/hemodynamic support in the burn population has received intermittent attention, evidence-based reviews from the sepsis/shock literature support two recommendations, albeit with only C-level evidence; first, vasopressor preference for septic shock is norepinephrine or dopamine titrated to maintain a mean arterial pressure of 65 mm Hg or higher. However, unlike "pure septic" patients, many burn intensivists try to avoid use of catecholamine infusions in the setting of burn injury for fear of wound-bed impairment (dermal conversion or subsequent graft loss). The second recommendation suggests inotropic support with dobutamine, when cardiac output remains low despite adequate fluid resuscitation.

In the future, it is quite possible that the practice of supplemental colloid infusions may diminish in favor of antioxidant therapy and other pharmacologic manipulations. In particular, early results from studies of high-dose intravenous vitamin C have been promising.

Inhalation Injury

Inhalation injury is always a risk factor for mortality regardless of age or burn size, because it can directly lead to pulmonary failure and subsequent organ malperfusion. Although less common in younger children compared with older children and adults, evaluation to determine the presence of suspected smoke or chemical inhalation should always be performed. I believe in the objective assessment of bronchoscopy as an independent assessment tool to establish a proper diagnosis. The need for ventilatory support always increases fluid requirements secondary to insensible fluid losses, and clinicians should take this into account when focusing on resuscitation end points.

In the setting of a known inhalation injury, many physicians will increase the initial Parkland formula to 6 mL/kg/%TBSA burned, instead of 4 mL/kg/%TBSA burned. This guideline should be viewed as a rough estimate, and objective criteria need to continue to be followed closely.

When Resuscitation Fails: What Should Be Done?

Approximately 13% of all deaths resulting from burn injury are related to a strategic failure, and although it can be difficult to predict which patients are most at risk, three possible causes should be considered: *overresuscitation, underresuscitation,* and the *ABCs.*

Overresuscitation implies excess fluid infusion beyond the actual plasma volume required to restore the vasculature to normal. Empirically, if more than 250 mL/kg of fluid has been given in the first 24 hours, overresuscitation should be suspected regardless of the patient's status, excluding patients with very large surface area burns. Such a volume does not necessarily mean that overresuscitation has actually occurred, but rather that its presence should be ruled out. Key steps in the evaluation are to 1) determine whether an abdominal compartment syndrome is developing by measuring bladder pressure, and 2) ensure intraocular pressure is less than 30 mm Hg, as excessive pressure in the eye can cause devastating vision loss. Bladder pressure can be quickly measured by attaching a pressure monitor to the Foley catheter, which will yield an approximation of the intraabdominal pressure. If abdominal pressure exceeds 30 mm Hg, aggressive measures should be considered immediately.

Another consideration in overresuscitation is to minimize fluid replacement. This may be an instance in which HTS could prove useful provided hypernatremia is not present. In extreme cases, plasma exchange can be instituted, a process that involves a continuous blood cell separator in which platelet-poor plasma fractions are rejected, and fresh frozen plasma contributes to the addition of 1.5 times the calculated blood volume. Several studies have reported success with this technique in adults, children, and adolescents.

Even though underresuscitation is less common, it can be seen in patients who have an extensive burned surface area (>70%); in very young children, especially those resuscitated in rural facilities and then transferred to burn units; and in those with severe inhalation injury. Although no straightforward parameter is available to confirm underresuscitation, insufficient urine output (1.0 to 1.5 mL/kg/h or less in adults), very low cardiovascular indices, and known delays in resuscitation may provide clues. When such a situation is suspected, the rate of fluid infusion should be increased with the addition of small boluses as necessary. Switching to another formula that focuses on the burned surface area as the basis for fluid calculations, one that is more generous with maintenance requirements or one that uses colloid, may also be appropriate. Finally, the burned surface area should be recalculated to ensure that the resuscitation volume has not been grossly underestimated.

If strategic failure is still apparent without evidence of underresuscitation, overresuscitation, or other likely causes, then the ABCs—*a*irway, *b*reathing, and *c*irculation—should be reviewed. Failure to maintain a patent airway or the presence of depressed ventricular function (left ventricular stroke work index) are two common causes that can be quickly evaluated with pulse oximetry, end-tidal capnography, and bedside echocardiography. Transient right-sided heart failure, especially in younger children, is often seen and can lead to malperfusion. Severe lung injury remains a challenge in all burn settings and, if thought to be a major reason for inadequate resuscitation, aggressive mechanical support up to and including extracorporeal membrane oxygenation (ECMO) should be instituted.

NUTRITION

The goal of nutritional support is to meet the energy requirements of the hypermetabolic response associated with burn-induced injury, while minimizing protein catabolism. As a result of the stress involved in burn injury, metabolic rates increase significantly, and the body switches from glucose to amino acids as its major energy source to meet this demand.

Perhaps one of the most important steps in supporting burn patients is to begin enteral feeding as soon as possible, preferably within 24 hours. Although from an evidence-based medicine point of view, limited randomized controlled trial data are available to support the concept, but the weight of evidence is sufficient to show benefits. These include improved humoral and cellular immunologic responses, lower levels of inflammatory mediators, decreased cortisol and higher insulin levels, preservation of gastrin secretion and motility of the gastrointestinal tract, lower intestinal ischemia and reperfusion injury, reduced intestinal permeability, less body weight loss, shorter periods of antibiotic treatment, and lower mortality and complication rates.

Caloric Requirements

The process of nutritional support begins with an estimation of caloric requirements. In general, it takes resting energy expenditure (REE) levels approximately 100 to 150 days to reach normal values in patients with moderately sized burns (20% to 40% TBSA) and up to 250 days for patients with larger burns (>75%). Using indirect calorimetry, the gold standard for estimating REE, can be difficult in the first few days, especially if the patient requires respiratory support. Although various equations are available to estimate REE, none is truly satisfactory, even with adjustments for stress. Thus, indirect calorimetry should be conducted periodically to ensure that estimated caloric requirements are reasonable; however, this procedure is not usually feasible for children. Commonly used equations are the Harris-Benedict, Curreri, and Ireton-Jones equations for adults and the Wolfe equation for children (Table 2). Because so many formulas have been published, burn units usually choose an equation with which they have gained proficiency and to which they have made appropriate adjustment factors for burn stress. The issue of weight in these equations has led to discussions of the specific weight to be used. Because of the impracticalities in weighing patients undergoing resuscitation, the preburn weight is preferred, followed by an ideal body weight (males: 50 + {[2.3 × Height in inches] − 60}; females: 45.5 + {[2.3 × Height in inches] − 60}). In the case of obese patients, actual weight usually overestimates REE, and thus ideal or adjusted body weight (0.25 × [Actual body weight − Ideal body weight]) is often used instead.

Because indirect calorimetry provides a respiratory quotient (RQ), this parameter is often used to determine whether underfeeding or overfeeding is occurring. An RQ above 1.0 has traditionally been interpreted as overfeeding, a value of 1.0 indicates pure carbohydrate utilization, and a value less than 0.85 implies underfeeding. However, a recent study has suggested that interpretation of the RQ in isolation could be very misleading. Interestingly, the often criticized empirical target of 30 kcal/kg/day for caloric needs has been shown to be a factor in outcomes: individuals with a caloric intake greater than 30 kcal/kg/day have lower rates of mortality and complications and shorter treatment durations for their burn injuries. Because this relationship may not be directly causal, and results are preliminary, these findings should not change current practice; however, they do highlight the need for more research involving nutritional support and therapy.

Nutritional Formulas

Once caloric needs have been established, the first goal is to provide a formula with an approximate 70:30 carbohydrate-fat composition. Protein requirements should be assessed separately. In general, burn patients require 1.0 to 1.5 g/kg/day of protein to minimize loss of lean body mass; severely burned patients may require in excess of 2 g/kg/day. A simple way to estimate protein requirements is to determine the ratio of nonprotein calories (NPC) to 1 g of nitrogen (Table 3), which will vary from 150:1 for small burns to 100:1 for patients with a high percentage of total burned surface area. Once the nutritional regimen has been established, monitoring of the patient can be accomplished using a short half-life protein, such as prealbumin,

TABLE 2: Equations used to predict resting energy expenditure with adjustment factors

Equation	Calculation of Kilocalorie Requirement
Benedict-Harris (adults only; usually underestimates caloric requirements)	Males: $66.5 + (13.8 \times W) + (5 \times H) - (6.8 \times Age)$ Females: $65.5 + (9.6 \times W) + (1.7 \times H) - (4.7 \times Age)$ Adjustment factor: $\times 1.2$ (minor burns) to 2.1 (major burns)
Curreri (adults; usually overestimates caloric requirements)	16–60 y: $(25 \times W) + (40 \times \%TBSA)$ > 60 y: $(25 \times W) + (60 \times \%TBSA)$
Ireton-Jones (highly variable among patients)	$1925 + (5 \times W) - (10 \times Age) + (281 \times Sex) + (292 \times Trauma) + (851 \times Burn)$ Sex: male = 1, female = 0 Trauma: yes = 1, no = 0 Burn: yes = 1, no = 0
Wolfe (children)	$BMR^* \times 2$, with BMR calculated by age as: ≤3 y: $60.9 \times W - 54$ (males); $61.0 \times W - 51$ (females) 3 to 10 y: $22.7 \times W + 495$ (males); $22.5 \times W + 499$ (females) 10 to 18 y: $17.5 \times W + 651$ (males); $12.2 \times W + 746$ (females)

*Use actual or ideal body weight

W, Weight, measured in kilograms; *H*, height, measured in centimeters; *BMR*, basal metabolic rate

TABLE 3: Estimating protein requirements and ratios

TBSA (%)	Protein Requirement*	NPC/N Ratio†
<15	1.0–1.5	150:1
15–30	1.5	120:1
31–49	1.5–2.0	100:1
≥50	2.0–2.3	100:1

*Grams per day per kilogram of body weight

†Ratio of nonprotein calories (NPC) to 1 g nitrogen

in conjunction with nitrogen-balance studies. A prealbumin value below 20 mg/dL signifies a malnourished or catabolic state; however, it must be remembered that values for this protein can take up to 2 years to reach normal ranges.

Mounting evidence suggests that trace element supplementation, as well as the vitamin and mineral content of formulas, is important. For example, adequate copper, selenium, and zinc supplements improve wound healing and reduce pulmonary infections and skin protein catabolism. Although specific recommendations for burn patients have yet to be made, it is recommended that patients receive the minimum recommended daily intake (RDI). Studies have also shown promising results for additional supplements of glutamine and leucine, a branched-chain amino acid, but further randomized controlled trials are needed to establish whether such supplements make a difference in regard to outcomes.

In adults who experience vomiting or gastric stasis with nasogastric feeding, jejunal feeding is a reasonable alternative, as it does not seem to affect the oxygen balance of the intestine. If a patient does not tolerate enteral feeding, total parenteral nutrition (TPN) should be considered, after all efforts at enteral support have been exhausted.

Burn patients commonly undergo early excision in the first 24 to 48 hours after injury, and provision for continued enteral feeding should be made, as this is both safe and effective. Often, this requires a predesigned agreement between burn surgeons, nurses, and the anesthesia team.

Finally, in patients who were malnourished or in those who had metabolic disturbances prior to their burn injury, the possibility of refeeding syndrome exists. Although this is unlikely to appear during the resuscitation period, at-risk patients should have potassium, phosphate, and magnesium levels checked, and deficiencies should be remedied before thiamine is administered prior to feeding.

Pediatric Nutrition

Determining caloric needs in children is especially vital, as their glycogen stores are usually unequipped to meet metabolic demands during resuscitation. Children, especially very young children, can usually tolerate enteral feeding within a few hours of injury. Herndon has recommended that enteral feeding with milk is the best approach, as it is well tolerated, inexpensive, and palatable. However, the low sodium content of milk may require additional sodium supplementation. Commercially available hyperosmolar formulas will need to be diluted to half or three-quarters strength to prevent diarrhea.

For longer term enteral feeding, caloric requirements should be calculated using a suitable equation, such as the Wolfe formula (see Table 3). Protein requirements are much higher in children compared with those of adults, typically in the range of 2.5 to 4.0 g/kg/day. In young children, it is important to remember two other points: 1) the gastrointestinal tract may be functionally immature, which may exacerbate malabsorption; and 2) renal overload is possible using nutritionally dense products, and thus renal clearance tests, such as blood urea nitrogen (BUN) and creatinine, should be conducted periodically.

METABOLICS

Several changes in metabolism occur following a burn injury, the most important of which are acidosis, increased glucose levels with decreased insulin response, and changes in the adrenal glands that cause a shunting of androgen production to glucocorticoids.

Insulin, insulin-like growth factor (IGF-1), and growth hormone (GH) are all interrelated with the hypothalamus-pituitary-adrenal axis, and they are greatly perturbed by burn injury. In general, larger burns cause greater decreases in levels of IGF-1 and GH in parallel with higher concentrations of cytokines, such as IL-1β. Moreover, because IGF-1 is involved with cell growth, increasing protein anabolism, reducing the hepatic acute phase response, and assisting with dermal and epidermal regulation, acute depression of this factor causes impaired wound healing and loss of protein balance, which translates into loss of lean body mass. In addition, because the effects of GH are mediated through IGF-1, young children are especially vulnerable to protein loss. Trials of recombinant GH in children have been positive, although it is common to observe an increase in insulin requirements. As results in adults have been variable, recombinant GH is not indicated in this patient population. Studies of administration of IGF-1 and IGFBP-3, its principal binding complex, at rates of 1 to 4 mg/kg daily in burn injuries has generally met with success by improving muscle protein synthesis, particularly in children. However, the expense of such treatment, along with the availability of other less expensive agents, will likely preclude its widespread use.

Following burn injury, insulin secretion can increase, but more importantly, insulin resistance also rises. Insulin resistance occurs when the body's sensing mechanisms detect hyperglycemia and attempt to counteract the condition with increased insulin secretion. However, because cell receptors are not functioning normally, the dose-response relation between insulin and its receptors is dysfunctional, resulting in even more secretion of insulin. This imbalance can last several months, and burn intensivists have traditionally instituted insulin protocols to manage hyperglycemia. However, recent research has revealed that this may not be an optimal approach.

Following research in patients with type II diabetes, Kasper and colleagues tested the hypothesis that activation of the renin-angiotensin system (RAS) following burn injury is responsible for inhibiting insulin action. The RAS plays an important role in restoring blood pressure following hypovolemic shock, and it increases feelings of thirst as well as increasing fluid resorption by the kidneys. By administering losartan, an RAS blocker, to rats with full-thickness burns and comparing the results to those of rats given a placebo, these researchers demonstrated a dramatic difference: rats given losartan did not develop insulin resistance. Although losartan is an Food and Drug Administration–approved drug for hypertension, it is not known whether shutting down the RAS will have long-term deleterious effects. Nevertheless, it is hoped that this important conceptual breakthrough will lead to better protocols for managing hyperglycemia by manipulating mechanisms responsible for insulin resistance.

To compensate for the lack of androgen production, exogenous administration of testosterone has been studied to determine its effectiveness in increasing protein synthesis. Although most studies have reported achieving a desired target of net amino acid balance, it appears its mechanism differs between adults and children. In adults receiving testosterone, protein synthetic efficiency increases and protein catabolism is decreased, whereas testosterone stimulates protein synthesis in children. Due to the undesired side effects of testosterone, the search for an alternative led to trials with oxandrolone, a synthetic androgen. Today, the benefits of oxandrolone have been widely recognized, and it has subsequently replaced testosterone.

Metabolic Acidosis

Originally thought of as a consequence of oxygen deficit, research suggests that acidosis is a result of increased glucose flux, which in turn reflects increases in glycolysis rather than oxidative phosphorylation. In addition, full-thickness burns result in the local release of lactate, which also contributes to acidosis. Although serum lactate can be used as a guide to modify oxygen-demand goals, levels should not be used in isolation. If significant acidosis is present, 1 ampule/L of sodium bicarbonate can be added to resuscitation fluid, but base deficit alone should not be used to titrate further bicarbonate administration.

Glucose and Insulin

Hyperglycemia is a normal response to burn injury, and more severe burns induce higher glucose levels and greater resistance to insulin, particularly in muscle cells. Several studies in critical care have demonstrated considerably better outcomes in regard to mortality and morbidity rates when an insulin infusion or administration protocol is utilized to maintain normal glucose levels. Although randomized controlled trial data are lacking for burn patients, several prospective case studies suggest benefits from instituting an insulin protocol. For example, intensive insulin protocols with target glucose values of less than 120 mg/dL have been implemented that achieved mean daily blood glucose levels of 116 mg/dL with only a 5% incidence of hypoglycemic episodes (defined as serum glucose <60 mg/dL) per protocol day. Hypoglycemic episodes can be addressed by holding insulin infusions or administration of D_{50} if necessary.

Metformin has also been successfully used to manage insulin resistance, but caution is advised based on reports of associated lactic acidosis. A longer term alternative to insulin infusion in children is the use of fenofibrate, which has been found in one randomized controlled trial to improve insulin sensitivity, insulin signaling, and mitochondrial glucose oxidation.

Protein Metabolism

One of the major issues associated with burns is that, within a few days of injury, depression of androgen production occurs as glucocorticoid synthesis increases. The large increases in circulating cortisol and catecholamines significantly elevate REE, particularly in adults and older children. Although protein anabolism, primarily in muscle, is relatively unaffected, protein catabolism significantly increases. It is believed that the increase in protein catabolism is driven by the significantly higher levels of cortisol, which increase the expression of myostatin, a member of the transforming growth factor superfamily.

Two approaches are currently used to address the issue of protein catabolism. As catecholamines are a primary mediator of hypermetabolism, use of β-blockers should improve muscle metabolism, and studies involving propanolol have indeed found net increases in muscle protein balance. Other studies have also concluded that propanolol does not adversely affect inflammation and immune function as exemplified by rates of infection or sepsis. Moreover, an additional benefit of β-blockers may include reduced key cytokine levels, such as tumor necrosis factor-α and IL-1β.

Another approach has used oxandrolone, a synthetic anabolic steroid. Since the late 1990s, studies employing relatively low doses in adults (10 to 20 mg/day) and children (0.1 mg/kg twice daily) have confirmed increased protein synthesis from intracellular pools of amino acids, while not affecting inward transport of amino acids and thus leading to a zero net balance of muscle protein metabolism. Other benefits resulting from oxandrolone administration include a reduction in burn-induced proinflammatory cytokines, an anticorticosteroid action that appears to be the result of crosstalk between androgen and glucocorticoid receptors that involves multiple pathways; it results in preservation of lean body mass; increases in serum prealbumin, total protein, and testosterone; and decreases in acute-phase proteins. In addition, oxandrolone downregulates the expression of the *Adapt 78* gene, an "adaptive response" stress gene that suppresses calcineurin production. Long-term use of oxandrolone in children with severe burns is also a useful preventive measure against suppression of bone growth. Most studies show that the combination of exercise with oxandrolone administration is the best approach to the long-term rehabilitation of burn patients, leading to improved cardiopulmonary performance and muscle strength.

In terms of timing, β-blockers can be introduced 4 to 6 days after initiating resuscitation, and oxandrolone is introduced approximately 1 week following burn injury. No studies to date have addressed using both approaches simultaneously to address whether there may be any synergistic or adverse effects.

SUMMARY

Immediate resuscitation of burn patients is necessary to stabilize their critical condition and prevent further complications, such as organ dysfunction and sepsis. Although many different resuscitation formulas can be successfully utilized, the key is to ensure that underresuscitation and overresuscitation do not occur by observing the patient's response, rather than adhering to strict equations and end points. Likewise, invasive monitoring should only be undertaken when the patient's response dictates the need for more information. Although colloids may be a useful adjunct following crystalloid resuscitation, HTS should be reserved for special situations under expert care. Adjunctive measures, such as inotropic and pharmacologic support, may be helpful, but should be used with caution, especially in children. Instituting enteral feeding early and properly managing nutrition following resuscitation is central to avoiding complications. Moreover, use of insulin protocols, β-blockers, and oxandrolone are all viable options available to burn specialists in managing and treating this challenging and complex patient population.

SUGGESTED READINGS

Fluid

Demling RH: The burn edema process: current concepts, *J Burn Care Rehabil* 26:207–227, 2005.

Friedrich JB, Sullivan SR, Engrav LH, et al: Is supra-Baxter resuscitation in burn patients a new phenomenon? *Burns* 30:464–466, 2004.

Klein MB, Hayden D, Elson C, et al: The association between fluid administration and outcome following major burn: a multicenter study, *Ann Surg* 245:622–628, 2007.

Oda J, Yamashita K, Inoue T, et al: Resuscitation fluid volume and abdominal compartment syndrome in patients with major burns, *Burns* 32:151–154, 2006.

Nutrition

Chan MM, Chan GM: Nutritional therapy for burns in children and adults, *Nutrition* 25:261–269, 2009.

Flancbaum L, Choban PS, Sambucco S, et al: Comparison of indirect calorimetry, the Fick method, and prediction equations in estimating the energy requirements of critically ill patients, *Am J Clin Nutr* 69:461–466, 1999.

Schulman CI, Ivascu FA: Nutritional and metabolic consequences in the pediatric burn patient, *J Craniofac Surg* 19:891–894, 2008.

Metabolics

Gauglitz GG, Herndon DN, Jeschke MG: Insulin resistance postburn: underlying mechanisms and current therapeutic strategies, *J Burn Care Res* 29:683–694, 2008.

Herndon DN, Hart DW, Wolf SE, et al: Reversal of catabolism by beta-blockade after severe burns, *N Engl J Med* 345:1223–1239, 2001.

Jeschke MG, Finnerty CC, Suman OE, et al: The effect of oxandrolone on the endocrinologic, inflammatory, and hypermetabolic responses during the acute phase postburn, *Ann Surg* 246:351–362, 2007.

FROSTBITE AND COLD INJURIES

Paul N. Manson, MD

OVERVIEW

The several types of localized cold injuries may be classified according to the temperature that produces them, either *freezing* or *nonfreezing* temperatures. *Trench foot, immersion hand and foot,* and *chilblains* are produced by cold, but not freezing, temperatures; *frostbite* is produced by freezing temperatures. Trench foot and immersion hand and foot are principally seen in military populations, whereas chilblains and frostbite are more commonly seen in civilian populations.

Cold injuries may be further divided into *localized cold injuries,* such as frostbite, and *generalized cold injuries,* which include hypothermia. Frequently, localized cold injuries such as frostbite do *not* coexist with systemic hypothermia. Localized cold injuries have in common the fact that they are produced by exposure to cold stimuli and the fact that they occur at the extremities of circulation. Localized cold injuries may be seen in the cheeks, nose, ears, and face but are primarily seen in the hands and feet. Cold injuries in the face tend to be superficial because of the blood supply; whereas serious cold injuries are almost exclusively confined to the extremities, a small margin of difference exists between the injuries that produce superficial versus deep injury.

TRENCH FOOT

Trench foot is usually seen in military populations and occurs with exposure to above-freezing temperatures, generally over a prolonged period of time. The presence of moisture is important in its pathogenesis. Chronic symptoms produced following recovery from the acute injury are those of pain, paresthesia, and a particular susceptibility to cold.

IMMERSION FOOT AND HAND

Immersion foot and hand are seen following prolonged exposure to cold but not to freezing water. Following the recovery from the acute episode, major nerve paralysis may be seen as well as chronic vasospastic cold sensitivity and pain. Pain and parasthesias are commonly seen after all types of cold injuries.

CHILBLAINS

Chilblains represent the mildest form of cold injury and occur after prolonged exposure to cold and wet conditions. The symptoms consist of burning and itching and are associated with a mild dermatitis. Vesicles and hemorrhagic lesions may be seen in the acute period.

The chronic condition is characterized by cold sensitivity, itching, paresthesias, and skin eruptions that may be reddish lesions, vesicles, or superficial ulcers. The chronic condition may be treated by protection from cold and heat to avoid production of dermatitis symptoms and pain. The role of sympathetic denervation in the management of the chronic condition has been suggested but not established. Some feel it may be helpful in chronic, well-established symptoms requiring treatment. Chilblains do not produce tissue loss; thus they require no reconstruction.

FROSTBITE

Frostbite occurs from exposure to freezing temperatures. The period of exposure required for its production may be short or long, depending on environmental conditions, moisture, and protection. Frostbite has been classified into degrees of injury depending on the depth of damage. Often, several degrees of injury will be seen in the same extremity, with the damage increasing as it progresses from proximal to distal.

First-Degree Frostbite

First-degree frostbite is a superficial skin injury characterized by numbness, edema, and erythema. The injury is similar to first-degree burn in that it heals spontaneously, in terms of the epithelium, in 1 to 2 weeks. Superficial desquamation may occur, and regeneration is usually complete with decreased but adequate skin appendages (Figure 1).

Second-Degree Frostbite

In second-degree frostbite, partial-thickness skin injury occurs that is characterized by numbness, edema, erythema, and vesiculation. The vesicles may be filled with either clear or bloody fluid. The partial-thickness skin injury heals in 2 to 4 weeks (Figure 2). The quality of the regenerated skin depends on the depth of the injury to the dermis and parallels thermal burn injuries in that deep, second-degree injuries heal with thin atrophic skin with reduced numbers of skin appendages.

Third-Degree Frostbite

Third-degree frostbite represents full-thickness skin loss. Following the injury, a nonviable segment of full-thickness skin loss is observed that may be seen initially as a gray-blue patch, or death of the skin may follow an initial period of reactive hyperemia after 24 to 72 hours. Eventually, a black eschar forms in each case and generally separates slowly in 1 to 3 months (Figure 3).

Fourth-Degree Frostbite

Fourth-degree frostbite signifies necrosis of all deep tissue parts, down to and sometimes including bone. Black, mummified tissues are present with the initial episode. If the mummified area becomes infected, it softens and becomes swollen and macerated at the margin with viable tissue.

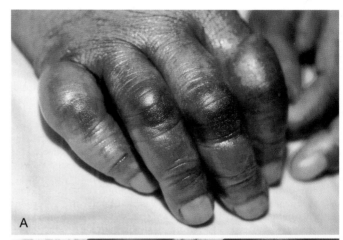

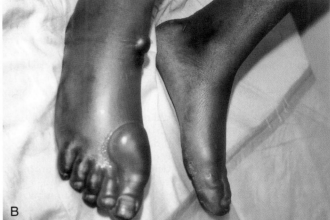

FIGURE 2   **A,** Second-degree frostbite in the fingers. Vesicles and swelling are seen. **B,** Second-degree frostbite in the feet. Vesicles and swelling are seen.

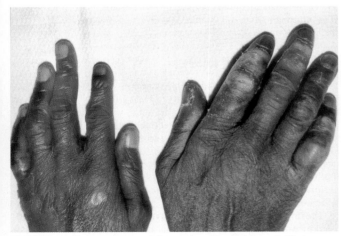

FIGURE 1   First- and second-degree frostbite. Epidermal skin loss and peeling are seen.

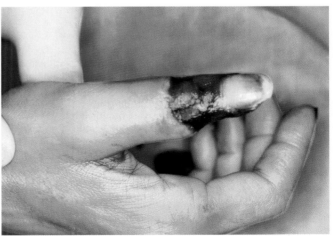

FIGURE 3   Third- and fourth-degree frostbite with tissue death; note demarcation beyond the interphalangeal joint.

Pathophysiology of Frostbite

Two pathophysiologic mechanisms are responsible for the production of frostbite: one is vasoconstriction and damage to the microcirculation in the *zone of vascular stasis,* which results in progressive vascular thrombosis. The second is direct damage to the cells or cellular toxicity. Experts disagree on the exact importance of these two mechanisms, and the importance of each mechanism varies according to the amount of tissue freezing that occurs and the local conditions, such as circulation.

Progressive Vascular Thrombosis

Capillary damage is produced by direct cold injury to vessel wall cells and by a pathologic anoxic vasculitis in the microcirculation. Cold injury may directly injure sensitive vascular epithelial cells resulting in thrombosis. The vasoconstriction may also produce anoxic damage to additional capillary epithelial cells, which is followed by a low-grade vasculitis or inflammation of the epithelium. After the circulation is reestablished, a period of hyperemia occurs, followed by circulatory stasis. If the anoxic damage has been sufficient, a vicious cycle of injury occurs that has at its basis an inflammatory response.

The cycle begins with adherence of white blood cells and platelets to the damaged endothelial cells in the vascular lumen and hyperpermeability of the capillary beds mediated by histamine and 5-hydroxytryptamine, which are released from mast cells with the production of tissue edema. This reaction is most marked in the *zone of circulatory stasis,* which is the zone that undergoes progressive vascular thrombosis. Degeneration of adrenergic nerves from anoxic damage produces an accumulation of norepinephrine at the margin of the frozen area, which aggravates vasoconstriction and produces more ischemia (Figure 4). Platelet adhesion and aggregation occur on damaged capillary endothelium, and with the sluggish circulation, the capillaries and small arteries thrombose over a 24 to 72 hour period, resulting in progressive vascular thrombosis.

Tissue injury occurs both from direct damage to cells and from the vasoconstriction anoxia, which results in vascular stasis and thrombosis. Following the state of decreased circulation, a state of *reactive hyperemia* occurs that may or may not be associated with a *no-reflow phenomenon,* in which capillary thrombosis occurs in the zone of stasis. The pathology of tissue repair is similar to that of burn injuries in that epithelium migrates to cover the wound from the surviving remnants of sweat glands, hair follicles, and margins of the living wound. The quality of the skin produced is proportional to the depth of damage. Deep injuries include necrotic nerve, muscle, and bone and are healed by scar following the shedding of dead tissue. Frequently, autoamputation occurs following ischemic necrosis and gangrene. Left untreated, the process is generally dry and progresses without infection over several months.

Environmental Influences

A number of environmental factors may influence the production of cold injuries, and one of the most significant is the ambient temperature. The effects of temperature may be modified by wearing protective clothing that provides insulation proportional to its thickness and weight. The effects of temperature are modified by the presence of wind and wet conditions, which accelerate heat loss. Wet conditions increase heat conduction to the environmental air, whereas wind accelerates the loss of heat in the air. Siple has developed a *wind child index* (WCI) to reflect the magnitude of the contribution of wind in heat loss. The heat loss would be the same at 20° F with a wind of 45 miles an hour as it would be at a temperature of −40° F with a wind of 2 miles an hour.

Clothes provide insulation proportional to their weight and thickness; one quarter of an inch equals one clothing unit. Clothing layers should be light to allow activity and to trap air in multiple layers to be effective at retaining body heat. Sweating wets the clothing, reducing

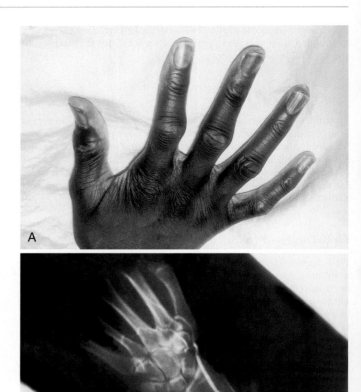

FIGURE 4   A, Second-degree frostbite. Note poor capillary perfusion of nailbed of middle finger. **B,** Arteriogram of patient in **A,** demonstrating loss of distal circulation secondary to intense vasoconstriction. The ulnar artery flow ceases in the forearm, and the palmar arch and digital vessels are not seen.

the insulation value. The importance of light clothing that permits work (heat production) is emphasized; however, the proper use of protective clothing is important. In one study, 65% of those suffering frostbite had inadequate protective clothing, whereas 20% had adequate clothing but were wearing it improperly. Only 15% of frostbite victims had adequate clothing and were wearing it properly. And as mentioned earlier, moisture accelerates heat loss.

Prevention of Cold Injury

Two ways to prevent cold injury are 1) by increasing heat production and 2) by decreasing heat loss. Heat loss may be decreased by avoiding wetness or contact with metal, which accelerates heat loss, and by wearing adequate protective clothing. The extremities have a large surface-to-mass ratio and thus represent prime sites for heat loss. Other factors may affect the circulation to extremities, such as the presence of arterial occlusive disease; some feel that the presence of a frostbite injury ought to prompt an examination for an arterial occlusive lesion or conditions such as diabetic neuropathy.

The importance of inactivity and immobility in reducing heat production, producing orthostatic edema, and decreasing circulation has been emphasized in studies on military frostbite. Malnutrition, hemorrhage, anemia, and the use of tobacco and alcohol have all been implicated in the increased susceptibility to frostbite injuries. Acclimatization and cold tolerance probably occur. African-Americans have increased susceptibility to cold injuries, probably owing to less frequent waves of cold-induced vasodilation and thus less effective skin warming. Military experience has emphasized the importance of working and keeping active so as to increase heat production, and the importance of avoiding sweating to avoid wetness and replacing wet with dry clothing are emphasized.

Superficial Versus Deep Frostbite

Frostbite in the head and neck area is generally superficial, and the face is not subject to the same vasoconstrictive phenomena as are the extremities. The drying potential of cold in the facial area is manifested in chapped lips, nose, and mucous membranes. Facial frostbite is generally superficial, whereas serious frostbite is usually confined to the extremities.

Mills believes that the differentiation of frostbite into first-, second-, third-, and fourth-degree injuries is cumbersome and not clinically useful. He believes that frostbite can only be classified as superficial (tissue remains soft) or deep (tissue is hard). It is initially difficult to tell the depth of the injury, and the differentiation can only be accomplished after rewarming and following a period of observation. In the face, a small white patch of tissue may be seen that clears up over the course of a week.

In the extremities, mild frostbite is manifested by pallor, paresthesias, and a dull yellow color of the skin. Ice crystals may be observed. The area is numb, and after rewarming, a prickly, itchy sensation or aching pain occurs. Following rewarming, reactive hyperemia is observed superficially as are deeper injuries, hypersensitivity, and paresthesias. Deep frostbite is differentiated by the absence of circulation upon rewarming or upon the progression (progressive vascular thrombosis) to full-thickness tissue loss (eschar formation). The tissue may remain insensitive following rewarming and may be seen as a blue-gray patch with absent circulation. Burning pain, paresthesias, and thick-walled blisters containing blood may follow rewarming in full-thickness tissue injury.

The history of the injury is important in predicting tissue loss. Important factors include the duration of the exposure, the temperature, the protective clothing worn, the contact with metal or moisture, and the presence of previous symptoms that would indicate reduced arterial circulation; these include claudication, Raynaud phenomenon, and superficial phlebitis. It is important to assess whether underlying vascular disease is a contributing factor in patients with frostbite.

Therapy of Frostbite

Contrary to popular belief, there is no place for vigorous rubbing of frostbitten tissue; this merely accelerates damage to skin. There is also no place for slow thawing, and especially not for the application of snow or other measures that would increase tissue damage, although a frozen part should not be allowed to thaw if refreezing is likely to occur.

Management of frostbite is carried out in accordance with the guidelines popularized by Mills. Obviously the patient's general condition should be assessed and other injuries detected and managed. Shelter should be obtained, wet garments removed, and the part wrapped in warm, dry covers or blankets, being careful to avoid trauma. The benefit of antibiotics has been difficult to establish, and although some prescribe them as they would for burn injuries, others believe they are not appropriate. Cultures should be done so that appropriate antibiotic treatment can be instituted if infection occurs. Long-term care includes physical therapy, neurologic rehabilitation, psychological support, and counseling for management of specific localized injuries.

Hospitalization

Patients with serious frostbite, such as frostbite of the extremities, should be hospitalized.

Rewarming

On admission, the frozen areas should be properly rewarmed in an agitated water bath at a precisely controlled temperature ranging from 104° to 108° F (40° to 44° C) for 15 to 30 minutes. The rewarming may be stopped when the digital flush representative of a hyperemic state of perfusion is observed. Rewarming is often painful, implying that a free-radical reaction is present upon reperfusion. Excessive rewarming results in further tissue damage, and it should be avoided. The temperature is quite critical: excessive temperatures (>44° C) cause heat damage, and lower temperatures (<38° C) are ineffective. Rewarming may be painful, and narcotic analgesics may need to be given. The pain associated with rewarming is felt to be a reperfusion injury secondary to free-radical generation.

Dressings

It has been generally recommended that open treatment or light dressings be utilized with cold injuries, keeping the blisters intact and bathing the affected area once or twice daily in an antiseptic solution (hydrotherapy). Most affected areas heal spontaneously if infection is prevented, and compression dressings are not necessary.

Hands should be splinted in a functional position as should feet. Nonadherent dressings (petrolatum or Xeroform) assist gentle treatment of the skin areas. It has been our experience that ointments macerate the areas and may contribute to increased infection. Dry treatment is preferred wherever possible. The value of prophylactic antibiotics has not been shown, and they should only be employed prophylactically for a short duration, from 48 to 72 hours.

Management of Blisters

Robson has shown that blisters contain increased amounts of thromboxane derivatives, which can accelerate production of progressive vascular thrombosis and dermal ischemia similar to that observed in thermal injury. Therefore, therapeutic advantage may be obtained from debriding the blisters. He recommends treatment of affected frostbite areas with topical aloe vera (Dermaide Aloe), aspirin, and antibiotics; however, the effectiveness of this treatment has not been clearly shown. Tetanus prophylaxis is also recommended.

Elevation and Splinting

It is important that the affected part be elevated and splinted in a position of function according to the usual principles of treatment of significant extremity injuries. Gentle exercise that includes range-of-motion exercises is important, as is physical therapy.

Surgical Intervention

Early surgical intervention is not necessary in the usual frostbite injury, but it may be necessary if acute progressive infection occurs. Full demarcation of dead tissue may take several weeks or 2 to 3 months, and the general recommendation is that the process of separation of tissue be allowed to progress spontaneously. Some feel that surgery may be appropriate at 3 weeks, if the demarcation is clear. Escharotomy may be necessary when circumferential extremity constriction occurs due to an unyielding third-degree eschar.

Therapy of Microcirculation

The damage to the microcirculation has been treated with anticoagulation, hyperbaric oxygen therapy, and free-radical scavengers. Agents such as heparin have been shown to slightly increase tissue survival in experimental frostbite tissue injury, as have free-radical scavengers. Clinical experience has not confirmed a definite advantage of these medications. It has been difficult to demonstrate the clinical effectiveness of agents such as low molecular weight dextran in preventing sludging, and although steroids have been recommended for vasculitis, the evidence for their beneficial effect has not been confirmed clinically; ultrasound treatments have been suspected of increasing tissue damage. Robson's recommendations have been employed by some to limit the progressive vascular thrombosis. Hyperbaric oxygen may be of limited value but must be begun early, although most question its effectiveness.

Sympathectomy

Regional sympathetic blockade has been used to decrease the pathologic vasoconstriction and sympathetic response. Based on the theory of the importance of progressive vascular damage in serious frostbite, several authors have advocated early surgical or chemical sympathectomy. At one time, I used intraarterial reserpine to regionally block the sympathetic nervous system (chemical sympathectomy). Arteriograms have demonstrated significant proximal vasospasm a considerable distance proximal to the demonstrated area of frostbite (see Figure 4).

Recently, Rakower attempted to define the patient populations that benefited from sympathectomy according to Doppler ultrasound and digital plethysmographic examinations done after rewarming. Patients had digital plethysmograms and Doppler ultrasound mapping of digital vessels, and three degrees of vascular response to cold were found. The most common was the *hyperdynamic response,* implying patent digital vessels; this response was clinically apparent as warm, red digital tissue. Regional sympathectomy was troublesome in these patients. Patients with a *normal* or *hypodynamic response* had evidence of vascular compromise at the digital, palmar, or pedal arch level and benefited from regional sympathectomy by chemical mechanisms. Patients with the hyperdynamic response did not have severe pain, whereas patients with a normal or decreased vascular response had ischemic pain, stiffness, and coldness in the digital areas. It thus seems possible that sympathectomy might be utilized for a group of patients who could most benefit from it.

Supporters of regional sympathectomy claim beneficial effects such as earlier cessation of pain, more rapid decrease of tissue inflammation and edema, improved tissue salvage, quicker demarcation, and earlier healing. Additionally, there is some evidence that regional sympathectomy provides significant diminution of the late sequelae of frostbite: impaired circulation, hyperhidrosis, pallor, vasospasm, and pain symptoms. It is claimed that extremities that have been subjected to a cold injury are able to perceive repeated significant cold injuries more accurately than extremities without sympathectomy.

Chronic Changes

Patients suffering the chronic sequelae of frostbite may benefit from sympathectomy in that sympathetic overactivity (hyperhidrosis and vasoconstriction) and cold sensitivity are reduced. The symptoms represent diminished circulation and reflect pallor, vasospasm, and pain symptoms. Lubrication of atrophic skin and protection from extreme temperatures are important. It is important that the parts affected be prevented from further cold exposure, as they are unusually more susceptible to cold injury. Flatt has advocated digital artery sympathectomy for patients with troublesome digital symptoms.

Radiographic and Joint Changes

Degenerative joint disease may be seen in severe cases, and stiff painful joints with fibrosis may be a sequela of moderately severe frostbite.

Intrinsic Muscle Atrophy

Flatt has described intrinsic muscle atrophy and fibrosis in severe frostbite. It may be possible to minimize the intrinsic muscle damage of contracture with proper physiotherapy, splinting, and appropriate exercise.

Injuries in Children

Injuries to epiphyseal growth centers may result from even minor cases of frostbite, with joint changes being radiographically demonstrable even 6 months after injury. These changes may result in short digits, deviation of the digits, and osteoarthritis. Parents should be advised that these sequelae are possible despite appropriate therapy of frostbite during the period of injury.

HYPOTHERMIA

Hypothermia must be excluded, and the management of frostbite should include general and specific measures that include restoration of core body temperature (Box 1). In patients with hypothermia (temperature <35° C), the hypothermic condition must be corrected prior to specific treatment of frostbite. Death may occur at a body temperature of 28° C.

Hypothermia is defined as a core body temperature below 35° C (95° F); it is principally seen in the military or secondary to outdoor recreation, homelessness, or substance abuse. Hypothermia has been classified into three general types: 1) mild (90° to 94° F); 2) moderate (80° to 89° F); and 3) severe (less than 80° F). In mild hypothermia, the patient is shivering, complaining of being cold, and displaying mental confusion, but the patient is normotensive. In moderate hypothermia, the patient becomes more confused and is often agitated, delirious, or combative, and the shivering ceases. Muscle spasticity, dilated pupils, and slow respirations are present. At this stage, mild myocardial irritability is encountered. In severe hypothermia, the patient becomes comatose, has a flaccid paralysis, and begins to develop apnea; eventually, this progresses to ventricular fibrillation and death.

BOX 1: Therapy of frostbite

Correct systemic hypothermia (<35° F)
General measures (includes detection of other injuries)
Rapid rewarming of frozen extremities (15 to 30 minutes, until a digital flush is observed in 104° to 108° F agitated water and topical antiseptic)
Tetanus immunization
Antibiotics if necessary
Aspirin 325 g q6h for 72 hours
Open or light dressings
Clear blebs: debride
Hemorrhagic blebs: keep intact
Topical aloe vera, antithromboxanes
Infected blisters: debride, antibiotics, antiseptics
Functional splinting, elevation
Cleanse twice daily in antiseptics
Avoid macerating dressings
Surgery
Await clear demarcation
Access spontaneous epithelialization
Consider regional sympathectomy in those with troublesome, persistent symptoms and normal or low vascular response after rewarming

---

The body responds physiologically to lowered temperatures by increasing cardiac output with tachycardia. Hypotension then follows with apnea, bradycardia, and an increase in total peripheral vascular resistance with decreased cardiac output and an increase in mean arterial pressure. Cardiac arrhythmias and sudden death occur in this sequence, following ventricular ectophy and atrial fibrillation. Cardiac standstill occurs with a body temperature below 21° C (70° F). The blood becomes more viscous with each drop in temperature, and hemoconcentration is seen related to cold diuresis. Sludging occurs in the peripheral vessels, respiratory depression follows, and pulmonary edema accompanies rewarming. A decrease in the ability to clear bronchial secretions is seen, along with a diminished cough reflex resulting in *cold bronchorrhea*. Metabolic acidosis follows rewarming, and *cold diuresis* results in hypovolemia.

Treatment

When the victim is identified in the prehospital setting, removal of wet clothing and replacement by dry clothing should be performed. No massage, friction rubbing, or manipulation should be performed. Patients who have sustained cardiopulmonary arrest should undergo resuscitation according to standard protocols, and patients have been salvaged followed rewarming. In the field, only passive warming is undertaken, because active rewarming can lead to myocardial arrhythmia and hypotension that can only be managed by precise, in-hospital monitoring.

In the hospital, accurate recording of temperature and vital signs is imperative. Complete examinations of the blood including CBC, electrolytes, liver function tests, coagulation, and arterial blood gas analyses are performed urgently. The workup should include toxicology screens to assess the effects of alcohol or other sedatives. A Foley catheter is inserted with a urimeter, and urine volumes are monitored. Several large-bore intravenous cannulas are inserted to combat the inevitable hypotension that occurs following rewarming. Continuous electrocardiographic (ECG) monitoring and a chest x-ray or appropriate extremity x-rays for trauma are obtained. The intensive care setting is mandatory, as is serial blood work; hypoglycemia should be excluded also, as should narcotic overdose. Passive rewarming at the rate of 0.5° to 2° C hourly results in a slow increase in body temperature, and warm, humidified oxygen should be provided.

Suggested Readings

Britt LD, Dascombe WH, Rodriguez A: New horizons in management of hypothermia and frostbite injury, *Surg Clin North Am* 71:345, 1991.

Fritz RL, Perrin DH: Cold exposure injuries; prevention and treatment, *Clin Sports Med* 8:111, 1989.

Heggers JP, Robson MD, Manavalen K, et al: Experimental and clinical observations on frostbite, *Ann Emerg Med* 16:1056–1062, 1987.

Manson PN, Jesudass R, Marzella L, et al: Evidence for an early free-radical-mediated reperfusion injury in frostbite, *Free Radic Biol Med* 10:7–11, 1991.

Marzella L, Jesdass RR, Manson PN, et al: Morphologic characterization of acute injury to vascular endothelium of skin after frostbite, *Plast Recon Surg* 83:67–75, 1989.

McCauley RI, Hing DN, Martin RD, et al: Frostbite injuries: a rational approach based on the pathophysiology, *J Trauma* 23:143, 1983.

Murphy JV, et al: Frostbite: pathogenesis and treatment, *J Trauma* 48–171, 2000.

Oumeish OY, Parish LC: Marching in the army; common cutaneous disorders of the feet, *Clin Dermatol* 20:445, 2002.

Reamy BV: Frostbite: review and current concepts, *J Am Board Fam Pract* 11:34, 1998.

Urschel JD: Frostbite: predisposing factors and predictors of poor outcome, *J Trauma* 30:340, 1990.

Vogel JE, Dellon AL: Frostbite injuries of the hand, *Clin Plast Surg* 16:565–576, 1989.

Washburn B, Frostbite, *N Engl J Med* 266:974–989, 1962.

Electrical and Lightning Injuries

Ryan D. Katz, MD, and E. Gene Deune, MD, MBA

BACKGROUND

The ability to harness the energy from electricity has been among mankind's greatest achievements, yet with the good that we derive from electricity comes an ever-present potential for injury.

Human beings are electrical beings. On both the macroscopic and microscopic level, from the intricately coordinated beating of our hearts to the resting membrane potentials across every cell wall, our bodies depend on a delicate balance of electrical homeostasis. This biologic balance can be disrupted by sudden and unexpected electrical transmission through the human body. Such transmissions are subject to the dictates of Ohm's law, which states that the current through an object is directly proportional to voltage (potential difference) and inversely proportional to the object's resistance (I = V/R). This law is helpful in categorizing electrical injury and lightning strikes.

The skin has an innate high resistance to electrical conduction and thus is not likely to allow the transmission of current through the body *except in the setting of high voltage*. Once current crosses the skin barrier, the resistance to electrical flow differs based on the different tissue types: it is highest for bone and tendon, lower for muscle and organs, and lowest for blood vessels and the central and peripheral nervous systems. This explains the variable pattern of tissue damage in electrical and lightning injury.

When voltage is applied to a tissue with low resistance, current can be generated through the tissue. Exogenous electrical current can disrupt cellular membrane potentials and result in an *electroporation phenomenon* in which cell membrane permeability increases, allowing for the unregulated diffusion of ions into and out of the cell. If membrane equilibrium is not reestablished in a timely fashion, a process that places demands on the cell's energy stores, cell death can result. This progressive energy depletion theory is one proposed mechanism for the phenomenon of delayed injury that is a hallmark of electrical injury.

When voltage is applied to a tissue with a high resistance, the flow of electrical current is resisted. The by-product of this flow across resistance is heat, which can generate burns. In victims of electrical and lightning injury, we often see small entry and exit site burns, but we rarely see extensive thermal injury to the skin, unless the injury is associated with ignited clothing, explosions, or other flash and flame burns. Although the total body surface area (TBSA) affected by electrical and lightning injuries is usually lower than that found in traditional thermal burns, these injuries all warrant transfer to a qualified burn center, because the internal derangements and soft-tissue injury may be extensive, progressive, and worse than they initially appear.

ELECTRICAL INJURIES

Electrical injuries have traditionally been divided into two categories: *high voltage* (>1000 V) and *low voltage* (<1000 V). Although high-voltage injuries are often associated with current transmission through a victim and extensive internal injury, low-voltage injuries can be just as devastating. Furthermore, a low-voltage electrical injury of 999 V likely has a destructive potential similar to that of a high-voltage injury of 1001 V. Thus this classification system may help the clinician determine the likelihood of current transmission through the patient, but it does more to establish the cause of injury than it does to direct the subsequent care. The treating physician should be cautious about downplaying the potential injury incurred with low-voltage insults.

Electrical burns account for up to 9% of admissions to burn hospitals and carry with them a mortality of up to 15%. There are approximately 1000 deaths per year attributable to electrical current, and the great preponderance of all electrical injuries occur in adult males. In low-voltage injuries, males are still in the majority, although the proportion of women and children is greater.

The economic impact of these injuries can be quite high and involves the direct cost of treatment as well as the indirect cost of lost productivity for both the patients and/or the family involved in their care. Many high-voltage injuries occur as work-related injuries that can be associated with legal claims, loss of employee manpower, and the cost of training a skilled replacement.

When treating a patient with an electrical injury, the physician must recognize the various ways in which the human body can be affected by electricity, including direct contact with an electrical current; "arc" phenomena, where current jumps from an charged object to the victim through the air; and flash burns, where an explosion or flame causes a surface burn rather than the transmission of current. The injuries caused by electrical energy can be complex and may be seen with associated orthopedic or neurologic trauma as well as a mixed picture of the above scenarios. This is highlighted by the example of a patient who contacts a poorly insulated power line and sustains a direct contact injury, a flame burn from a subsequent clothing fire, and a head injury from the associated fall.

Despite the potential for mixed injury patterns, a clear distinction can usually be made between *direct contact* injuries, in which current is transmitted to the victim, and *indirect* injuries such as arc and flash burn injuries, in which little to no current is transmitted. In arc and flash burn injuries, the skin is primarily affected, and the resultant injuries, mostly thermal in nature, manifest as first-, second-, or third-degree burns.

In a direct-contact injury, if the voltage is great enough, the body is subjected to a transmission of current, which can acutely cause entry and exit site burns, cardiac arrhythmias, cardiac ischemia, peripheral and central nervous system disturbances, central apnea, fractures secondary to tetany and fall, and muscle necrosis. Owing to the dissipation of heat, coagulation necrosis, massive cytokine release, microcirculatory derangements, progressive edema, and the electroporation phenomenon discussed earlier, injury often continues once the transmission has ceased. The physician treating a direct-contact injury is therefore often confronted with rising compartment pressures, progressive loss and destruction of what initially may appear to be viable tissue, the possibility of rhabdomyolysis, and subsequent acute renal failure.

Of the two types of electricity commonly used, alternating current (AC), in which the flow of charge alternates throughout a sinusoidal cycle, is felt to have more destructive potential than direct current (DC), in which the flow of charge is unidirectional. The cycling nature of AC that allows it to be carried long distances with relatively high fidelity is also one of its most dangerous characteristics, because it can cause muscle spasm and tetany throughout the transmission of current, sometimes freezing a person at the point of contact and prolonging exposure to the current. Although DC can also cause muscle spasms, this usually occurs only at the beginning and end of the current transmission and tends to force a victim away from the point of contact. Most countries use AC to meet the majority of their electricity needs, and most high-voltage injuries involve AC. However, DC is still commonly employed in everyday devices such as batteries, solar cells, and many subway systems' "third rail." Lightning is also DC.

LIGHTNING INJURIES

The risk of getting struck by lightning is dependent on a geographical area's *strike density*, defined as the frequency with which lightning strikes an area of ground; the population density; and any geographical factors that may expose or protect a person from lightning strikes. The strike density is quite different for different parts of the world; it is greatest in Africa, where some regions report more than 50 strikes/km^2 per year. In the United States, the Gulf Coast and Rocky Mountain states, particularly Florida and Colorado, have the highest strike densities and report the highest number of lightning-related injuries and deaths. For the average American, the lifetime risk of getting struck by lightning is 1 in 3000. Worldwide, the mortality rate associated with lightning strikes is quoted at 0.2 to 1.7 deaths per million people.

Lightning is an arc phenomenon of direct current generated when a large potential difference exists between the sky and the ground. The potential difference, which can exceed 2 million volts per meter, must be great enough to overcome the very high resistance of the interposing air. There need not be clouds for lightning to exist, and the common belief that lightning never strikes the same place twice is a fallacy easily disproven by the fact that lightning will often strike the lightning rods of tall buildings multiple times.

Those at risk for lightning strikes are those who whose occupation or recreation places them outdoors, although lightning can injure people indoors through telephones and electrical appliances. In particular, farming, roofing, and ranching appear to be the most dangerous occupations, and golfing, fishing, boating, camping, and field sports appear to be the most dangerous recreations.

Lightning injuries can be caused by multiple mechanisms including 1) a direct strike, 2) direct contact with an object that has been struck, 3) a side flash, 4) stride potential, or "step voltage," 5) thermal burns, 6) the shockwave from a thermoacoustic phenomenon (thunder), and 7) injury caused by a subsequent fall.

Of these different mechanisms, the direct strike and direct contact with an object that has been struck are the most dangerous and have the greatest lethal potential. *Side flash* is a phenomenon in which an object is struck, and the current arcs from the object to the victim. This more common type of injury, analogous to the flash burn described above, usually results in thermal burns with minimal to no transmission of electricity. The *stride potential* is a phenomenon in which lightning hits and travels radially along a surface, such as the ground. As it does, the electric current can contact one extremity before it contacts the other. If this occurs, a voltage difference is created between the extremities that allows current to flow through the body. In addition, a thermoacoustic shockwave (thunder) can cause ruptured tympanic membranes and concussive, blast-type injuries.

Treatment

Field Evaluation and Initial Response

Although the physics of the phenomena are different, treatment of electrical injuries and lightning strikes are similar. The rescuer or treating medical personnel must remember not to place themselves in harm's way. Prior to rescue and resuscitative efforts, the situation must be thoroughly assessed and the following questions must be rapidly answered:

- How many people are injured?
- Is the insult ongoing; that is, is the flow of electrical current still active? Is there ongoing lightning?

- How can I minimize risk to myself and to others?
- Do I have protective measures in place, such as a way to shut off power? Do I have protective clothing, backup personnel, and a backup plan?

Touching a person who is actively being injured by an electric current can result in passage of the current to the rescuer. The first step of the rescue is to therefore shut the power off if possible. If this is not possible, call for help and let trained professionals with appropriate protective gear disengage the victim from the power source. If the victim has been struck by lightning in an exposed area with a high likelihood of continued lightning activity, a "scoop and run" strategy, in which the victim is immediately transported to a hospital by emergency medical services, will remove the victim and the rescuers from the potentially dangerous environment. As it is safe to touch a person once the electrical insult has been terminated, resuscitative measures can begin almost immediately or during transport to a medical facility.

All resuscitation should begin with the fundamentals of basic and advanced life support (BLS and ACLS). Unlike traditional thermal injury, the causes of death in electrical injury are asystole, malignant cardiac arrhythmias, physical respiratory depression (diaphragm paralysis), or central respiratory depression caused by injury to the respiratory center of the brain. Early aggressive cardiopulmonary resuscitative efforts can therefore prove lifesaving. As the cardiac and respiratory sequelae of electrical injury can be progressive and prolonged, prompt transfer to a qualified burn center for cardiac monitoring and perhaps ventilatory support are warranted.

In-Hospital Evaluation and Treatment

Upon arrival at the hospital, any patient who has sustained an electrical injury or lightning strike should be managed the same as a trauma. BLS and ACLS should be augmented by the principles of Advanced Trauma Life Support (ATLS), confirming the presence of a definitive airway, adequate venous access for volume resuscitation, and adequate exposure for a full primary and secondary survey. Close attention should be paid to the possibility of associated injuries, as these patients may have suffered multiple catastrophic events at once: electrical transmission injury, prolonged tetany leading to fractures or respiratory collapse, blast injury with concussive blast effects including ruptured tympanic membranes, thermal injury from associated fires, inhalational injury from associated fires, and falls from a height. Often the cutaneous burns from these injuries are small, but the need to assess the victim for the possible transmission of electricity is critical. Flash burns, arc burns, and low-voltage injuries with a low likelihood of current transmission can often be managed as a purely thermal injury with supportive care that includes intravascular volume support based on the TBSA of the burn, topical antibiotics for superficial burns (first degree and superficial second degree), and debridement and skin grafting for full-thickness or deep burns with a low probability of healing in a timely fashion; it is prudent to plan a skin graft for a wound not expected to heal in 2 to 3 weeks.

When managing patients with an isolated thermal injury with greater than 20% TBSA and second- or third-degree burns, a good guide for fluid resuscitation is the Parkland formula (4 mL/kg/%TBSA delivered over 24 hours; with half the volume delivered in the first 8 hours after the burn). If arrhythmias or ECG changes are detected, the patient should be admitted for continuous cardiac monitoring, even if the size of the visible burn is small. Though permanent cardiac injury and myocardial ischemia are rare in the setting of electrical injury, prolonged arrhythmias are not, and these may require medical or electrical treatment as delineated in ACLS.

In high-voltage electrical injuries, including lightning strikes, the potential for the transmission of electrical current through the body is high. Regardless of whether the injury occurs as a result of alternating or direct current, the transmission of electrical current through the body can simultaneously affect multiple organs and

structures—skin, muscle, bone, central nervous system, heart, and kidneys—all of which should be addressed by the treating physician.

Skin

As the largest organ of the human body, the skin represents the first barrier to electrical transmission and has a high resistance to the flow of electrical current. During a direct-contact injury, a significant amount of heat is therefore generated at the skin level. This often results in full-thickness burns at the site of entry and exit, which have been described as having the appearance of a bull's-eye. When limited and superficial, the cutaneous burns associated with electrical injury can be readily treated with dressing changes and topical antibiotics. Commonly used topical antibiotics include bacitracin, mupirocin silvadene 1% cream, sulfamylon 5% solution or ointment, and silver solution or dressings. The uses, benefits, and side effects of these treatments can be found in Table 1.

All burns should be evaluated for thickness and documented on a burn diagram (e.g., Lund-Browder; Figure 1). This will help determine the involved TBSA, which will guide the volume resuscitative efforts. Particular attention should be paid to the presence of circumferential full-thickness burns and eschar, as the inelastic nature of these injuries can lead to extremity ischemia and decreased chest compliance (Figure 2). When circumferential eschar is recognized, early escharotomy, release of the skin down to the level of the fat, should be performed. This is often performed at the bedside with either a scalpel or electrocautery and should never be delayed (Figure 3).

Interestingly, after a direct lightning strike, red blood cells close to the surface of the skin can extravasate, leading to erythematous markings in a fernlike, branching pattern. This pattern, called a *keraunographic marking,* or *Lichtenberg figure,* is pathognomonic for a lightning strike and does not represent thermal injury. If present, it requires no specific treatment and is evanescent, usually disappearing within hours (Figure 4).

Muscle

One of the most devastating sequelae of electrical injury is the progressive destruction of muscle, which is likely triggered by electroporation of the myocyte and heat generated from the underlying bone. As injured muscles swell, compartmental pressures rise, and the microvascular circulation to the muscles becomes compromised. Frank compartment syndrome is a common late finding that is not to be missed. Even if soft on initial exam, compartments will become tense with aggressive fluid resuscitation and progressive muscle death. Frequent compartment checks are therefore of paramount importance. If suspicion of compartment syndrome exists, formal fasciotomy should be promptly performed.

The hallmark of compartment syndrome is *pain with passive stretch of the muscles involved.* In an intubated patient, or in one with an altered mental status secondary to sedation or injury, pain may be difficult or impossible to appreciate, and an invasive method to measure compartment pressures can be used. At pressures within 10 to 20 mm Hg of the diastolic pressure, or within 30 mm Hg of the mean arterial pressure, the ischemic threshold of muscle is approximated, and fasciotomies should be performed. Compartment syndrome should be a clinical diagnosis, and the physician should be guided by his or her overall clinical picture. Fasciotomies should *never be delayed* if the compartment pressure measurements do not correlate with the physician's level of concern.

Necrotic skin and muscle should be debrided early and initially covered with sterile dressings, allograft skin, or a biologic dressing. This decreases the overall necrotic tissue burden and potential sources of infection and sepsis. It also limits fluid loss. For smaller, localized wounds after fasciotomy or debridement, a vacuum dressing can be used. This negative-pressure dressing decreases wound bacteria counts and promotes vascularization of the wound bed. Once the

TABLE 1: Topical antibiotics

Topical Antibiotic	Uses	Notes	Side Effects
Bacitracin	Superficial burns (first degree)	Helps keep wounds moist	Anaphylaxis (rare)
	Raw wounds with injured or disrupted epithelium	Mupirocin should be used if superficial MRSA infection is confirmed	
Silvadene (silver sulfadiazine)	Superficial and intermediate-thickness burns (second- and small third-degree burns)	Broad-spectrum antimicrobial coverage	Self-limited leukopenia, usually does not mandate discontinuing the drug
		Does not penetrate eschar	May cause irritation in those with sulfa allergy
Sulfamylon (mafenide acetate)	Intermediate-thickness burns and deep burns	Broad-spectrum antimicrobial coverage	Pain on application
	Traditionally used when cartilage is exposed or with threatening exposure (e.g., ear burns)	Penetrates eschar	As a carbonic anhydrase inhibitor, it can cause metabolic acidosis
Silver solution (silver nitrate)	Superficial and intermediate-thickness burns covering a large %TBSA	Broad-spectrum antimicrobial coverage	Chronic use can lead to electrolyte abnormalities (hypnatremia and hyponatremia)
		Stains sheets and dressings black	Methemoglobinemia (rare)
		Needs to be applied to dressings repeatedly to keep them moist (every 4–6 hr)	

MRSA, Methicillin-resistant *Staphylococcus aureus; TBSA,* total body surface area

wound bed has stabilized and appears clean and without evidence of infection or ongoing muscle death, a skin graft can be placed or, if possible, the wound can be closed primarily. If the patient is lacking donor sites for a skin graft, cultured epithelial autografts (CEAs) are an option for definitive coverage. Although highly susceptible to mechanical disruption and shear, these cells can be harvested from a small donor site (1 cm² full-thickness skin or superficial shave) and expanded in the laboratory to meet the total coverage needs of the patient. These autografts are also more susceptible than traditional skin grafts to the presence of bacteria and should therefore only be applied to clean wounds.

It is more often the rule than the exception that multiple trips to the operating room for debridement are warranted. Trips to the operating room should be made frequently for debridement of nonviable structures and for testing of muscle viability. Healthy muscle should have a brick-red appearance and should twitch with manual or electrical stimulation from the electrocautery. Nonviable muscle will appear pale or gray and will not twitch with stimulation. Because an inflated tourniquet can cause a pressure or ischemic neurapraxia, the best way to assess muscle viability is with *the tourniquet down.* At the end of each debridement, the surgeon should decide on the anticipated return based on the appearance of the wound. It is common for trips to the operating room to occur as frequently as every 2 to 3 days in the acute setting. Despite aggressive surgical intervention, the amputation rate in high-voltage A/C injuries remains quite high—up to 40%, including "minor" amputations of isolated fingers or distal phalanges.

Bone

Sustained tetany or associated trauma from a blast or fall can result in fractures. The workup of victims of electrical injury should therefore be a trauma workup, once the patient is stable, that includes a radiographic examination of the cervical spine, any obviously deformed

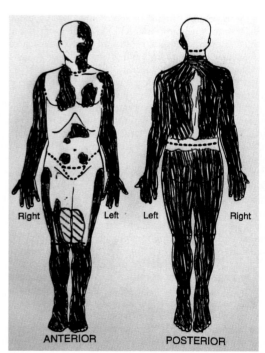

FIGURE 1 Example of a burn diagram documenting extent of the TBSA affected by the burn.

extremity, or any part in which the patient complains of significant pain. Consultation with orthopedic or plastic surgeons for fracture management is appropriate. Though definitive fracture repair may often be delayed for patient stability and an adequate wound bed, the diagnosis of fractures should not.

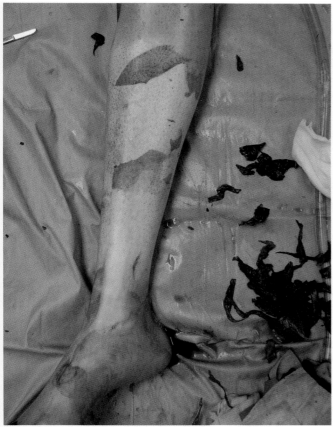

FIGURE 2 Circumferential full-thickness (third-degree) burn of the lower extremity in a burn victim. This requires an urgent escharotomy. Note the second-degree burn over the proximal portion of the leg. The second-degree burn is partial thickness and has a shiny, wet, weepy appearance.

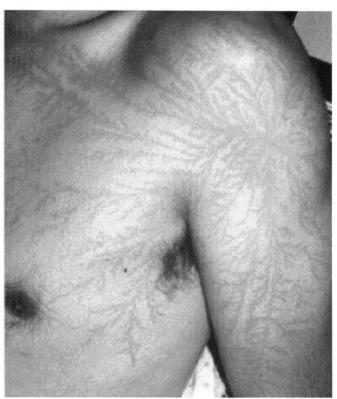

FIGURE 4 The fern-like keraunographic marking, or Lichtenberg figure, is pathognomonic for a lightning strike and does not represent thermal injury. *(From Bartholome CW, Jacoby WD, Ramchand SC: Cutaneous manifestations of lightning injury, Arch Dermatol 111[11]:1466–1468, 1975, American Medical Association. All rights reserved.)*

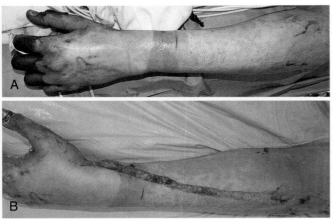

FIGURE 3 **A,** Circumferential full-thickness (third-degree) burn of the upper extremity. **B,** Postescharotomy.

Heart

Early malignant arrhythmias or asystole are often the initial cardiovascular collapse and are the primary cause of death in direct lightning strikes. Though resuscitation can be successful, prolonged rhythm disturbances are common and warrant continuous cardiac monitoring. Unstable arrhythmias should be managed medically or with cardioversion or defibrillation. These rhythm disturbances are usually transient, and late cardiac complications are rare. Myocardial ischemia is also rare but can occur, and suspicion of myocardial ischemia should prompt early cardiology consultation. Creatine kinase (CK) and CK-MB fraction levels are poor indicators of myocardial injury, which is better monitored with serial physical exams, serial electrocardiograms, and troponin levels.

Kidney

The profound muscle insult with electrical transmission injuries can cause rapid and progressive myocyte death, which can lead to release of myoglobin and result in rhabdomyolysis and acute renal failure. Rhabdomyolysis can be diagnosed by the presence of myoglobin in the urine. Though myoglobin can be detected on a urinalysis, it can often be clinically appreciated by the appearance of the urine, which will become a dark brown, like cola. Treatment of this process has traditionally focused on ensuring adequate urine output. The Parkland formula is considered by some authors to represent the minimum fluid requirement necessary in the resuscitation of an electrical injury victim; others recommend more than twice that amount. These recommendations are aimed at providing adequate intravascular volume and renal perfusion pressures, the marker of which has been a urine output in the range of 1.0 to 1.5 mL/kg, which often equates to 30 to 50 mL/hr. In the face of rhabdomyolysis, maintaining urine output around 50 to 100 mL/hr may be beneficial.

In addition to volume resuscitation, some authors recommend alkalinizing the urine with sodium bicarbonate and administering

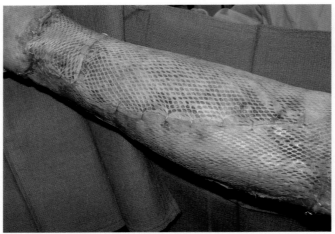

FIGURE 5   Meshed split-thickness skin graft applied to the lower extremity. Note the large surface area covered by the graft.

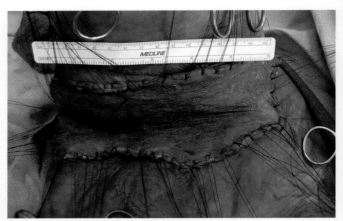

FIGURE 6   Full-thickness skin graft used to resurface an axillary scar contracture.

mannitol. Both sodium bicarbonate and mannitol are free-radical scavengers that prevent injury to the renal tubules by decreasing myoglobin precipitation. The decision to add mannitol or sodium bicarbonate to a renal protective strategy in the face of myoglobin-uria remains open for debate, as volume-replenishing strategies alone have proven effective in preventing renal failure.

Central Nervous System

Neuropathology from electrical injury can present in an acute or delayed fashion and may affect any part of the neuraxis. Centrally mediated death can occur acutely from cerebral hemorrhage, cerebral venous thrombosis, and hypoxia from respiratory depression. Transient acute injury to the nervous system occurs in up to 70% of victims of electrical injury and can include central respiratory depression, coma, seizures, blindness, deafness, aphasia, and acute autonomic insufficiency (spinal shock). Delayed and progressive neuropathology—including myelopathy, spinal muscle atrophy, ascending paralysis, and sensory loss—have also been reported. The cause of this delayed phenomenon remains largely unexplained, although MRI evidence and histopathology suggest that demyelination plays a role.

Any focal neurologic deficit or abnormal neurologic exam in the setting of electrical injury should be worked up with appropriate diagnostic imaging and serial physical exams. Timely involvement of the neurology or neurosurgery team once a lesion is recognized can be lifesaving and may limit progression of the insult.

Unique to some lightning strike injuries is the phenomenon of keraunoparalysis. This self-limiting paralysis lasts only a few hours, is accompanied by sensory loss, and typically involves the lower extremities. Patients who present with acute weakness, paralysis, or sensory deficits should, however, be presumed to have an anatomic neurologic insult, rather than keraunoparalysis, until proven otherwise with diagnostic imaging.

Technical Aspects of Surgical Management

Optimize Nutrition

Consider the early institution of protein- and calorie-rich enteral nutrition. Burn patients may require greater than 2 g/kg/day of protein—nearly twice that recommended for the postsurgical patient. If enteral nutrition is not possible, parenteral nutrition should be initiated. The metabolic demands of the burned patient in a critical care setting are enormous, and both the immune system and the process of wound healing are keenly dependent on adequate nutrition.

Nutritional goals and vitamin supplementation should be discussed daily on rounds.

Skin Grafting

Skin grafting should only be attempted once a wound bed has been adequately debrided and appears free of infectious contamination. A skin graft will not take in the presence of 10^5 organisms or more per gram of tissue. If there is a question of wound bed contamination, a quantitative culture can be sent to the lab to determine the presence and number of organisms per gram. Considering the value of donor sites in a burn victim, all attempts should be made to obtain an ideal wound bed prior to proceeding with a skin graft. Loss of a graft is an underappreciated catastrophe for the burned patient.

All skin grafts contain a portion of the dermis and thus will result in donor site scar. Split-thickness skin grafts contain only a portion of the dermis, whereas full-thickness grafts contain a majority, if not all, of the dermis. A split-thickness skin graft, often taken at 0.010 to 0.012 of an inch, can be used as a meshed graft or an unmeshed "sheet" graft. Meshed grafts have the benefit of covering a much greater surface area than their original harvested size but carry the drawback of healing with a contracted, shiny, cobblestone appearance (Figure 5). These grafts are good for concealed, low-visibility areas or for coverage of large burns. Unmeshed, split-thickness "sheet" grafts contract less than meshed grafts and heal with a smooth, unbroken appearance that is good for coverage of convex, high-visibility areas that require resurfacing but not much pliability, such as the forehead. Full-thickness grafts have the least long-term contraction and retain most of their elasticity and pliability. Full-thickness grafts are therefore a good selection for resurfacing areas that require suppleness for motion, such as the neck, elbow, and other joints. Full-thickness grafts also usually maintain their color over time and, when selected appropriately (e.g., supraclavicular skin for resurfacing the face), can provide excellent camouflage of high-visibility areas (Figure 6 and Table 2).

Donor sites can also be enhanced by tissue expansion, although this is usually performed in a delayed fashion as part of a secondary reconstructive effort, once the patient is sufficiently stable.

Biologic Dressings

If there is any question as to the adequacy of a wound bed, the wound should be covered with a biologic dressing until, after multiple debridements, it appears clean. Such biologic dressings include allograft (cadaver split-thickness skin) or xenograft (e.g., porcine skin). Both can be meshed and applied to a wound bed, and both are destined for ultimate rejection. Allograft skin will

TABLE 2: Skin grafts

Type	Benefits	Drawbacks	Technical Notes
Split thickness (meshed)	Can cover large areas	Heals with significant contraction	Grafts are usually harvested with electrical or pneumatic dermatome at 0.010 to 0.012 inch.
	Minimizes chance of fluid collection under graft	Poor cosmetic appearance	Meshed by devices set at specific ratios depending on coverage needs; a ratio of 1:2 allows for greater surface area coverage than 1:1.5.
			A vacuum dressing applied to the graft over a nonstick gauze can speed graft take, minimize shear, and help manage fluid.
Split thickness (unmeshed sheet graft)	Better cosmetic appearance compared with meshed grafts	Will not cover as much area as meshed grafts	It is useful to pierce the sheet graft at inconspicuous places to allow for fluid egress.
	Good for coverage of convex unbroken areas (e.g., forehead)	Can allow collection of fluid beneath graft, which can cause graft failure	A pressure dressing may help graft survival.
Full thickness	Maintains suppleness	Limited donor sites	A template of the defect should be designed prior to graft harvest.
	Least amount of contraction over time	Often requires bolster/pressure dressing to enhance graft take	The graft should meet the exact specifications of the template.
	May retain color	Can allow collection of fluid beneath graft, which can cause graft failure	Minimize skin waste during the reconstructive effort (e.g., leave dog ears if they appear at the closure; these can be your next graft donor sites).

revascularize if the wound bed is adequate and is thus an excellent way of determining wound-bed readiness prior to skin grafting. Xenografts are rejected *prior* to revascularization. *Allograft skin* is obtained from a cadaver and can be ordered from most hospital blood banks. It is not to be confused with *Alloderm* (LifeCell Corporation, Branchburg, NJ), which is acellular human *dermis*. Acellular dermal matrices, like Alloderm and the Integra (Plainsboro, NJ) dermal regeneration template, a bovine collagen matrix covered by a silicone sheet, can be used in select instances where reconstructing the soft tissue thickness is important—for example, with the anterior tibia, calcaneus, or posterior skull—or when coverage of structures, such as exposed tendon or bone, will likely be unsuccessful or unsightly with a skin graft alone. These soft tissue replacement options will allow vascular ingrowth but will also need skin grafting at 14 to 21 days and thus do not conserve donor sites.

Local and Regional Flaps

Small defects can often be managed with local flaps. The basic principle of reconstruction should always hold: Whenever possible, replace like with like. The power of local and regional flaps is contained within this principle, as they are similar in color, texture, and suppleness to the area undergoing reconstruction. Local flaps should be designed with attention to detail. To ensure adequate coverage, the dimensions of the defect *after debridement* should be determined prior to raising the flap. Local flaps are often good choices for nasal and hand resurfacing. Unfortunately, local and regional options are often eliminated in the setting of many burns, where skin adjacent to the wound is also typically injured. Regional flaps, when available, can provide more ample and supple tissue than local flaps; they can also include composite tissues such as bone and muscle (Figure 7).

Free Flaps

Microvascular reconstruction has now become a powerful tool in the reconstructive surgeon's armamentarium; they can provide supple, full-thickness skin, fat, and muscle or bone if needed, and free flaps allow expanded possibilities for burn reconstruction. Free flaps have high success rates at centers with dedicated microvascular teams, and they should be considered early as part of the burn reconstruction effort. In cases where there are no suitable local or regional flaps, free flaps offer the only practical and effective means to reconstruct and restore function. Free flaps have been successfully employed in such cases as severe neck contraction, extremity length preservation, limb salvage, scalp reconstruction, face reconstruction, contracture release, and resurfacing of critical areas exposed to the mechanical demands of pressure, stress, or shear (Figure 8). Although still in its infancy and highly controversial, face and hand transplantations are mentioned under the category of free flaps as ultimate examples of replacing like with like, albeit with an allograft.

Contracture Release and Z-Plasty

Burned skin and skin grafts over joints will often scar and create inelastic skin that restricts the movement of the joint. Maintenance of joint range of motion with physical therapy should be instituted as early as possible with splinting and range-of-motion exercises. Although no one therapy has been proven to prevent the progression of scar hypertrophy, silicone sheeting, pressure, taping, and massage have all shown promise. If scar contracture does form, so as to restrict range of motion, contracture release is indicated. The release usually involves "cracking" through the inelastic skin with a scalpel, extending the joint (or joints), and resurfacing them with either a full-thickness skin graft or free flap.

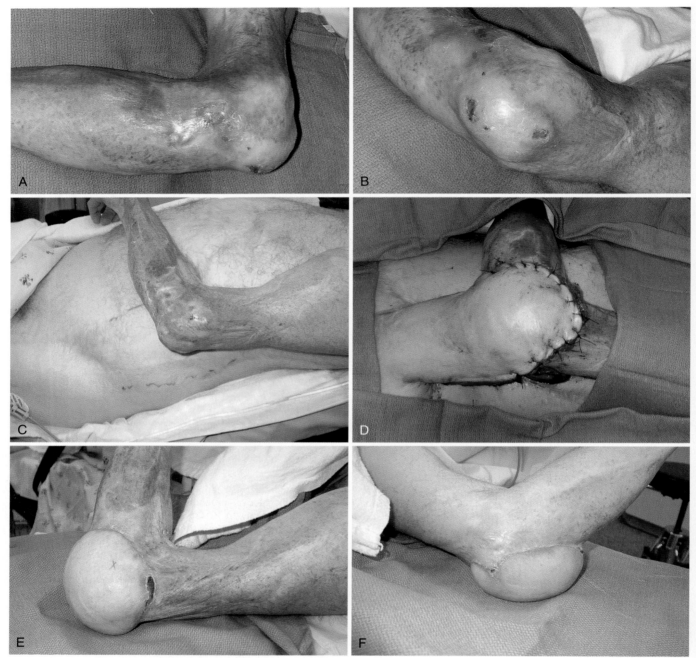

FIGURE 7   This is a 47-year-old man who sustained a high-voltage injury 25 years earlier, with a persistent unstable wound in his left elbow. Because of lack of appropriate recipient vessels in his elbow and forearm, a random chest flap was used to reconstruct the wound.

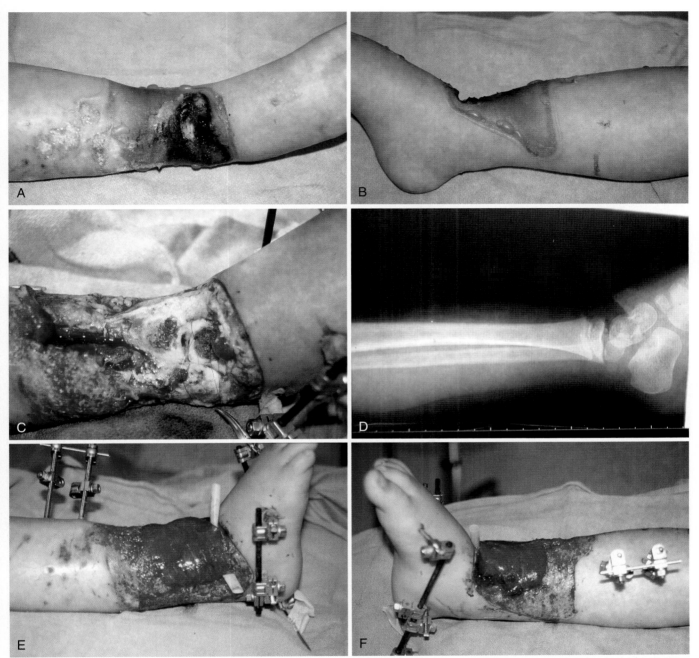

FIGURE 8   This series of pictures demonstrate the salvage and reconstruction of the lower extremity of a 4-year-old girl who tripped on a high-voltage power line. A free rectus abdominis flap covered with a split-thickness skin graft was used to resurface the soft-tissue deficit.

Continued

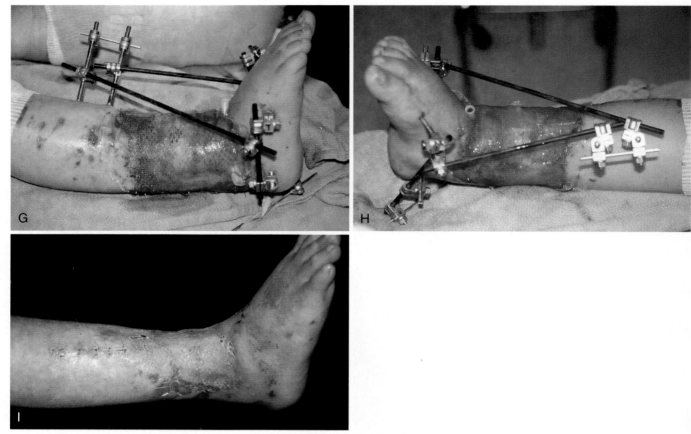

FIGURE 8 Continued.

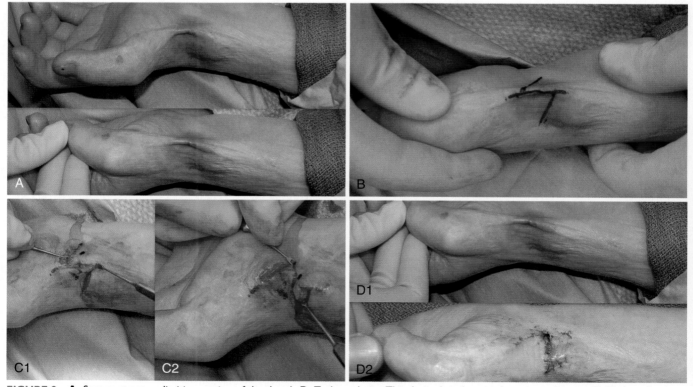

FIGURE 9 **A,** Scar contracture limiting motion of the thumb. **B,** Z-plasty design. This design lengthens and reorients the scar. **C,** Z-plasty flaps (*left*). Transposing the flaps into the original scar effectively lengthens and reorients the scar (*right*). **D,** Preoperative scar contracture (*top*). *Bottom,* A week after Z-plasty with scar effectively lengthened and reoriented.

In the scenario of a linear scar or burn that limits joint motion, a *Z-plasty* is indicated. Z-plasty comprises multiple *random* flaps, meaning they are not based on any known or named blood supply, designed in such a way as to recruit uninvolved local tissue to the involved contracture. The Z-plasty has the effect of lengthening and reorienting a scar. This effectively offloads the affected joint and redirects the line of scar tension in such a way that it can no longer restrict digit or extremity motion (Figure 9).

Suggested Readings

Arnoldo B, Purdue G, Kowalske K, et al: Electrical injuries: a 20-year review, *J Burn Care Rehabil* 25(6):479–484, 2004.

Celik A, Ergün O, Ozok G: Pediatric electrical injuries: a review of 38 consecutive patients, *J Pediatr Surg* 39(8):1233–1237, 2004.

Cherington M, Yarnell PR, London SF: Neurologic complications of lightning injuries, *West J Med* 162(5):413–417, 1995.

Haas AF, Reilly DA: Cultured epithelial autografts in the treatment of extensive recalcitrant keloids, *Arch Dermatol* 134(5):549–552, 1998.

Heckman MM, Whitesides TE, Grewe SR, et al: Histologic determination of the ischemic threshold of muscle in the canine compartment syndrome model, *J Orthop Trauma* 7(3):199–210, 1993.

Katz RD, Barbul A, et al: Nutrition and wound healing. In Horn D, Hebda P, Gosain A, editors: *Essential tissue healing of the face and neck*, Hamilton, ON, Canada, 2009, BC Decker, pp 330–337.

Lakshminarayanan S, Chokroverty S, Eshkar N, et al: The spinal cord in lightning injury: a report of two cases, *J Neurol Sci* 276(1-2):199–201, 2009.

Luce EA: Electrical burns, *Clin Plast Surg* 27:133, 2000.

Luz DP, Millan LS, Alessi MS, et al: Electrical burns: a retrospective analysis across a 5-year period, Burns (in press).

Maghsoudi H, Adyani Y, Ahmadian N: Electrical and lightning injuries, *J Burn Care Res* 28(2):255–261, 2007.

Ogilvie MP, Panthaki ZJ: Electrical burns of the upper extremity in the pediatric population, *J Craniofac Surg* 19(4):1040–1046, 2008.

Ritenour AE, Morton MJ, McManus JG, et al: Lightning injury: a review, *Burns* 34(5):585–594, 2008.

PREOPERATIVE AND POSTOPERATIVE CARE

FLUID AND ELECTROLYTE THERAPY

Timothy R. Donahue, MD, and Jonathan R. Hiatt, MD

FLUID COMPARTMENTS AND DYNAMICS

Approximately 40% to 60% of an individual's total body weight is made up of water, referred to as *total body water* (TBW). Because water content of muscle exceeds that of fat, TBW is also estimated at 60% to 70% of lean body weight. Because males, on average, have greater muscle mass than females, 60% of male body weight is water, compared with 50% to 55% of female body weight.

Body fluid compartments can be thought of as separated by selectively permeable membranes composed of endothelial or epithelial cells that are separated by intercellular junctions. "Two thirds, one third" and "three fourths, one fourth" are two simple ways to recall the approximate distribution of fluids in various compartments in a healthy subject (Figure 1). The intracellular space contains two thirds of the TBW, and the extracellular space contains one third. The extracellular space can be further divided into *interstitial* and *intravascular* or *plasma* compartments, with three fourths of the extravascular fluid in the interstitium and one fourth in the plasma.

An understanding of TBW balance includes consideration of water movement between the different compartments and of factors that determine the volume of TBW. This section examines the concepts of osmoregulation and volume regulation.

Membranes are freely permeable to water, such that the osmolalities of intracellular, interstitial, and intravascular compartments remain equal. In contrast, membranes have different permeabilities for different solutes, and solutes that cannot traverse a given membrane have the capacity to exert an osmotic force that directs water movement across that membrane; such solutes are known as *effective osmoles*. Osmotic equilibration occurs when water moves across membranes from areas of lower to higher osmolality. Such movement occurs either through intercellular junctions or via a transcellular route. Water crosses the lipid-rich cell membrane by simple diffusion or alternatively, it passes through fenestrations and water channels known as *aquaporins* that are embedded in the cell membrane.

Capillary membranes are permeable to most small solutes including sodium, potassium, glucose, and small molecular weight proteins (less than 50,000 kDa). These small solutes do not act as effective osmoles that contribute to transcapillary water movement. Rather, movement of water across capillary membranes is directed by the osmotic pressure generated by plasma proteins that are too large to cross the capillary wall, also known as *oncotic pressure,* and by the hydrostatic pressure from blood flow. Taken together, the oncotic and hydrostatic pressures are known as *Starling's forces,* and their effect on transcapillary movement can be described by *Starling's Law,* which states that net filtration is the difference between capillary and interstitial fluid hydrostatic pressures and capillary and interstitial fluid oncotic pressures. The plasma proteins are effective osmoles that hold water in the intravascular space and generate oncotic pressure, while hydrostatic pressure of the plasma opposes the oncotic pressure and forces fluid to the interstitium. At the arteriolar end of the capillary, intravascular hydrostatic pressure exceeds oncotic pressure, and fluid moves out. With the net efflux of fluid along the length of the capillary, the situation is reversed at the venous end, and fluid is drawn from the interstitium back into the intravascular space.

Although small solutes do not contribute to water movement across capillary membranes, they do act as effective osmoles that direct water movement between the intracellular and extracellular spaces across cell membranes. Sodium (Na^+) and potassium (K^+) are the principal determinants of extracellular and intracellular osmolality, respectively; they are unable to diffuse passively across the lipid-rich cell membrane. The imbalance between the intracellular and extracellular concentrations of these two solutes is

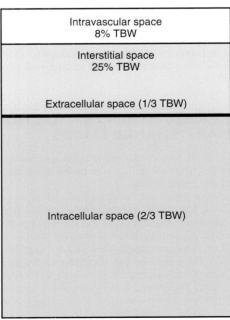

FIGURE 1 Body fluid distribution.

generated and maintained by the Na$^+$-K$^+$ adenosine triphosphatase mechanism. This transmembrane transporter exchanges three Na$^+$ molecules for two of K+ and generates a net negative cell membrane potential. Were the concentration of either of these ions to change, water would be forced to move from the compartment with lower osmolality to the compartment with higher osmolality to reestablish equilibrium. For example, if hypotonic saline (0.45% NaCl normal saline) is administered, the extracellular osmolality is lowered, and water moves from the extracellular to intracellular space causing cellular swelling. In contrast, with administration of hypertonic saline (3% NaCl normal saline), the extracellular osmolality increases, and water moves from the intracellular to the extracellular space causing cellular dehydration. Serum osmolality is maintained in a narrow range by the process of osmoregulation and is calculated using the following formula:

$$mOsm / kg = 2 \times (Na + K) + (BUN / 2.8) + (Glucose / 18),$$

where *BUN* is blood urea nitrogen and *mOsm/kg* is serum osmolality. Normal serum osmolality is 275 to 290 mOsm/kg, and variations of only 1% to 2% will stimulate mechanisms to restore the normal level, a process known as *osmoregulation.* Osmoreceptors in the hypothalamus detect plasma osmolality and stimulate the thirst mechanism and antidiuretic hormone (ADH) secretion by the posterior pituitary gland. ADH then upregulates aquaporins in the distal collecting tubules of the kidney to reabsorb free water. As a result, adult urine osmolality has a wide range that can vary from 100 to 1200 mOsm/kg depending on the serum osmolality. On average, patients with a high serum osmolality and intact renal function have a urine osmolality greater than 500 mOsm/kg. Circulatory baroreceptors also stimulate ADH secretion based on detection of plasma volume, although volume is a less potent stimulus than osmolality.

Osmoregulation can be viewed as a process distinct from but related to volume regulation. Osmoregulation describes the process by which TBW content changes to maintain normal plasma osmolality. In contrast, volume regulation is the process by which the individual components of serum osmolality, primarily sodium, change to maintain plasma osmolality.

Hormones that influence total body sodium content are the principal mediators of volume regulation. These hormones include the renin-angiotensin-aldosterone axis and atrial natriuretic peptide (ANP). Renin is secreted by the juxtaglomerular cells in response to renal hypoperfusion and/or low sodium concentration in the distal tubule as measured by the macula densa. Renin secretion leads to activation of angiotensin and release of aldosterone, both promoting sodium reabsorption. ANP released in response to atrial stretch enhances renal blood flow and inhibits sodium reabsorption in the kidney.

DAILY REQUIREMENTS AND CHOICE OF MAINTENANCE FLUIDS

Maintenance fluids replace normal sensible and insensible losses. *Replacement fluids* replace abnormal or excess losses and correct for any water or electrolyte deficits.

Sensible water losses can be quantified and occur primarily in urine and stool. Insensible losses cannot be measured and include cutaneous losses from the skin (75%) and the upper respiratory tract (25%). Normal daily sensible losses include 800 to 1500 mL in urine and 250 mL in stool, and insensible losses are approximately 8 to 12 mL/kg/day. These volumes can increase in different physiologic and pathologic conditions, including fever, hyperventilation, burns, tachycardia, and hypermetabolism. Cutaneous insensible losses increase by 10% per day for every 1° C increase in body temperature above 37.2° C. During a thoracotomy or laparotomy, insensible losses from the operative field can approach 1 L/hr.

The rate of maintenance fluid administration for both pediatric and adult patients can be calculated for a 24-hour period by the 100-50-20 rule or hourly by the 4-2-1 rule (Table 1). Patients with hypothyroidism, renal failure, and congestive heart failure will require adjustments.

The electrolyte composition of maintenance fluids is based on daily losses. Daily sodium requirement in the postoperative period is 1 to 2 mEq/kg/day, and potassium requirement is 0.5 to 1 mEq/kg/day. Postoperative maintenance fluids also include dextrose to maintain plasma osmolality and reduce short-term proteolysis. Specific electrolyte and carbohydrate requirements may vary with the clinical situation and should be monitored closely in all critically ill patients. The usual postoperative maintenance fluid for an adult is composed of dextrose 5% (D$_5$) in isotonic, half-normal saline (0.45% NaCl) with 20 mEq/L KCl. Children older than 2 years can receive the same maintenance fluids as an adult, but younger children are usually given D$_5$ hypotonic saline (0.2% NaCl) with 20 mEq KCl. Until age 2 years, the kidney has a glomerular filtration rate (GFR) that is one quarter the adult level, and the distal nephrons are unable to effectively concentrate the urine, leading to a difficulty in excreting high sodium loads.

Assessment of Fluid Status and Choice of Replacement Fluids

In the immediate postoperative period, patients may have fluid deficits resulting from preoperative or intraoperative fluid losses. During the extended postoperative period, continued excess fluid losses in the urine, skin, and gastrointestinal (GI) tract are common. Fluid management in the postoperative period requires a close assessment of fluid status and selection of an appropriate type and rate of fluid replacement.

Common signs and symptoms of low effective circulatory volume include abnormal mentation, excessive thirst, dry mucous membranes, poor skin turgor, tachycardia, hypotension, orthostatic changes in heart rate and blood pressure, oliguria, and weight loss. In the immediate postoperative period, residual anticholinergic effects of muscle relaxants may mimic some of these signs and symptoms of underresuscitation and confuse the clinical picture. In addition to clinical signs and symptoms, daily weights, serum and urine electrolytes, acid-base balance, and invasive monitoring can be used to measure volume status and assess the adequacy of resuscitation. Urine output is an excellent measure of volume status and should be at least 0.5 mL/kg/hr for adults and 1 to 2 mL/kg/hr in children. Urine output may be an inaccurate measure if the patient has renal insufficiency, is receiving diuretics, or is hyperglycemic.

Increases in either serum or urine osmolality suggest ECF depletion. Other indicators of ECF depletion include an elevated hematocrit, a BUN/creatine ratio of greater than 20:1 (prerenal azotemia), and a fractional excretion of sodium (FeNa) of less than 1%.

$$FeNa = ([Urine\ Na] \times [Plasma\ Cr] / [Plasma\ Na] \times [Urine\ Cr]) \times 100$$

TABLE I: Maintenance fluid requirements

Body Mass (kg)	Fluid Volume (mL/kg/hr)	Fluid Volume (mL/kg/day)
First 10 kg	4	100
Second 10 kg (10 to 20 kg)	2	50
Each kg > 20 kg	1	20
60 kg	100	2300

As in the case of urine output, the FeNa is altered and is not a useful indicator of volume status if the patient has underlying renal dysfunction or is receiving diuretics, most commonly furosemide.

Low serum bicarbonate and base deficit are important signs of underresuscitation. Consensus is emerging that restoration of normal acid-base status is the most reliable indicator of adequate resuscitation. Invasive monitoring of volume status and oxygen delivery, needed in cases of critical illness, include measures of central venous pressure, pulmonary artery wedge pressure, and mixed venous oxygen saturation (SvO_2).

The rate and volume of replacement fluid administration are determined by severity of the existing deficit, rate of ongoing losses, and comorbidities. Severe fluid losses that result in hemodynamic instability should be replaced with IV fluid boluses of 0.9% NaCl (normal saline, NS) or Ringer's lactate (RL) at volumes of 10 to 20 mL/kg, with boluses repeated until an adequate resuscitation is reached.

Traditional fluid strategies have encouraged the liberal use of replacement fluids and have defined *adequate resuscitation* as urine output of 0.5 to 1 mL/kg/hr. These strategies are not evidence based and are instead built on the concept that patients undergoing abdominal surgery are in a shocklike state promoted by the intravascular depletion of preoperative fasting and bowel preparation. In addition, general anesthesia decreases systemic vascular resistance, which then leads to an increased volume of distribution. A new strategy that restricts the liberal use of fluids has emerged more recently, with some evidence to show that fluid restriction improves morbidity. Potential reasons for this observation include maintenance of cardiac contractility and avoidance of 1) pulmonary edema and acute lung injury, 2) ileus and anastomotic dehiscence by decreasing fluid accumulation in the bowel wall, and 3) dilutional coagulopathy. Rather than titrating fluid output to maintain urine output, this strategy now calls for maintenance of stable daily body weights to avoid fluid overload.

The composition of various replacement fluids is shown in Table 2. NS and RL are most commonly used for replacement, because they best approach the composition of extracellular fluid. RL contains 28 mEq of HCO_3^-, whereas NS does not contain any HCO_3^- but has a greater concentration of Na^+ and Cl^- (154 mEq). Thus NS is used preferentially in patients with a metabolic alkalosis. Overuse of NS may actually worsen metabolic acidosis because of the high chloride content. Colloid solutions, such as 5% albumin, are theoretically more efficient than crystalloids in restoring intravascular volume because of the oncotic pressure afforded by the protein content. However, liberal use of colloid solutions has not been consistently shown to improve patient outcome.

The electrolyte compositions of different GI fluids are listed in Table 3. The optimal replacement for gastric losses is D_5 half NS with 20 mEq/L KCl; for pancreatic, biliary, or small intestinal losses, RL with bicarbonate; and for large intestine (diarrhea) losses, RL with 20 mEq/L KCl. If GI losses are substantial or persistent, they should be replaced on a milliliter-for-milliliter basis with the correct fluid.

DIAGNOSIS AND TREATMENT OF ELECTROLYTE DISORDERS

Sodium

Sodium is the principal determinant of serum osmolality and free-water balance. The normal range of serum sodium concentration is 135 to 145 mEq/L. Because the cell wall is sodium impermeable, sodium is an effective osmole that stimulates free-water movement across membranes.

Hyponatremia is defined as a serum sodium concentration below 135 mEq/L, and it is classified as *mild* (130 to 135 mEq/L), *moderate* (120 to 130 mEq/L), or *severe* (<120 mEq/L). Severe cases of hyponatremia or acute changes in serum sodium concentration can result in cellular edema and cerebral swelling and produce symptoms that

TABLE 2: Electrolyte composition (mEq) of parenteral fluids

Fluid	Na⁺	K⁺	Cl⁻	Ca²⁺	HCO₃⁻	Dextrose	pH
Extracellular fluid	142	4	103	5	27	0	7.4
Ringer's lactate	130	4	109	2.7	28	0	6.5
Normal saline (0.9% NaCl)	154	0	154	0	0	0	4.5
½ Normal saline (0.45% NaCl)	77	0	77	0	0	0	4.5
¼ Normal saline (0.2% NaCl)	34	0	34	0	0	0	4.5
3% Saline	513	0	513	0	0	0	4.5
5% Dextrose in water	0	0	0	0	0	50 g	4.5
5% Albumin	145	0	0	0	0	0	7.4

TABLE 3: Electrolyte composition (mEq) of gastrointestinal fluids

Source	Daily Loss (mL)	Na⁺	K⁺	Cl⁻	HCO₃⁻
Saliva	1000	30–80	20	70	30
Gastric	1000–2000	60–80	15	100	0
Pancreas	1000	140	5-10	60–90	40–100
Bile	1000	140	5-10	100	40
Small bowel	2000–5000	140	20	100	25–50
Large bowel	200–1500	75	30	30	0

include headache, lethargy, seizures, and coma (Table 4). Because of the other determinants of serum osmolality, primarily BUN and glucose, hyponatremia can occur with high, normal, or low serum osmolarities. Regardless of the serum osmolality, patients with severe or symptomatic hyponatremia should be aggressively treated with 3% NaCl hypertonic saline. Prior to treatment, it is important to calculate the sodium deficit, which is directly proportional to the TBW.

$$Na\ deficit = (140 - Serum\ Na) \times TBW$$

TBW can be estimated at 0.6 times total body weight for males and 0.55 times total body weight for females.

Rapid correction of hyponatremia with hypertonic saline can lead to central pontine myelinolysis (CPM) with potential for permanent spastic quadriparesis and pseudobulbar palsy. For this reason, the serum sodium should not be corrected more rapidly than 0.25 mEq/L/hr or 8 mEq/kg/day. Hypertonic saline (3% NaCl) should be given in 250 mL aliquots at a rate of 50 mL/hr, and serum sodium levels should be checked every 5 hours before another dose is begun. Furosemide can also be used to minimize the volume of resuscitation and aids in correcting the hyponatremia. Furosemide-induced diuresis is osmotically equivalent to administering half NS. In patients with severe head injury, central nervous system (CNS) infection, or cerebral operations, the serum sodium level should be monitored closely

TABLE 4: Signs and symptoms of electrolyte disorders

Disorder	Neurologic	Cardiovascular	Gastrointestinal	Renal	Other
Hyponatremia	Confusion, seizures, coma	Hypotension Hypertension	Salivation	Oliguria	
Hypernatremia	Confusion, seizures, coma	Fluid overload (edema)	Thirst		Tachypnea
Hypokalemia	Fatigue, weakness	Atrial arrhythmias, flat T wave, U waves	Ileus	Nephrotoxicity	
Hyperkalemia	Confusion, paralysis, areflexia	Ventricular arrhythmias, peaked T wave, prolonged PR interval, wide QRS complex	Nausea, vomiting, abdominal pain		
Hypocalcemia	Paresthesia, perioral tingling, carpopedal spasm, Chvostek sign	Ventricular arrhythmias, prolonged QT interval			Laryngospasm
Hypercalcemia	Confusion, fatigue, coma	Shortened QT interval	Abdominal pain	Renal stones, nephrogenic diabetes insipidus (long term)	
Hypomagnesemia	Weakness, cramping, hyperreflexia	Atrial ventricular arrhythmias (torsades des pointes)	Dysphagia		Refractory hypokalemia, hypocalcemia
Hypermagnesemia	Sedation, paralysis, areflexia	Atrial, ventricular arrhythmias	Diarrhea		
Hypophosphatemia	Confusion, seizures, weakness	Heart failure, respiratory failure			Bone pain
Hyperphosphatemia	Symptoms of hypocalcemia				

and replenished appropriately with 3% NaCl hypertonic saline, as outlined above, to maintain serum sodium above 140 mEq/L and minimize cerebral swelling.

Hypertonic hyponatremia occurs when BUN or glucose are elevated, thus increasing oncotic pressure and causing water to shift from the intracellular to the extracellular space. For each 100 mg/dL increase in glucose over normal, 2 mEq/L should be added to the reported sodium level. Isotonic hyponatremia, or pseudohyponatremia, occurs when elements that do not contribute to the serum osmolality are elevated, such as triglycerides and proteins. Most laboratories now correct the sodium level for these artifacts and have eliminated cases of pseudohyponatremia.

Hyponatremia most often occurs in association with low serum osmolality (hypotonic hyponatremia). Cases of hypotonic hyponatremia can be further categorized according to volume status as *hypervolemic, euvolemic,* and *hypovolemic.*

In hypervolemic hypotonic hyponatremia, the ECF and interstitium are expanded, but plasma volume is contracted, thus stimulating ADH release. Common clinical circumstances include congestive heart failure, chronic renal insufficiency, nephrotic syndrome, cirrhosis, and hypoalbuminemia. Hypervolemic hyponatremia is uncommon in the perioperative period and most often results from iatrogenic excessive administration of hypotonic fluids. It may occur in patients with advanced cirrhosis who develop hepatorenal syndrome or in renal insufficiency that occurs as a result of a low effective circulatory volume and renal blood flow. Patients with hypervolemic hypotonic hyponatremia are most effectively managed with a low-sodium diet (1500 to 2000 mg/day) and fluid restriction (1 L/day). In addition, spironolactone or amiloride can be added to promote a negative sodium balance.

Cases of euvolemic hyponatremia can result from the syndrome of inappropriate ADH secretion (SIADH), hypothyroidism, or excessive water intake (psychogenic polydipsia). Increased ADH secretion occurs transiently in the early postoperative period, after trauma, or with severe burns, but it can also occur with pulmonary malignancies, including carcinoid tumors and small-cell lung cancers, lung infections, and CNS injuries and infections. Euvolemic hyponatremia is the most common presentation of AIDS-related CNS infections. SIADH can be diagnosed by the presence of high urine osmolality (>150 mmol/kg) and high urine sodium (>20 mmol/L); it must be differentiated from adrenal insufficiency, which is accompanied by hypokalemia. SIADH is treated with fluid restriction (<1 L/day). Isotonic fluids will actually worsen the hyponatremia, because sodium is filtered in the glomerulus, and free water is reabsorbed in the distal tubule.

Hypovolemic hypotonic hyponatremia is the most common form of hyponatremia in postoperative patients. If urine sodium is greater than 20 mmol/L, the sodium loss is primarily renal in origin. If urine sodium is less than 20 mmol/L, the sodium deficit is primarily from sequestration of isotonic fluids in the extravascular (third) space or loss from the GI tract, skin, or from bleeding. Treatment of hypovolemic hypotonic hyponatremia differs from euvolemic or hypervolemic cases, because fluid restriction will only worsen the clinical picture. The sodium deficit is calculated as described above, and cases of mild or moderate hypovolemic hyponatremia are best managed by slow correction with isotonic saline.

Hypernatremia is defined as a serum sodium concentration greater than 145 mEq/L. In moderate cases, the serum sodium is 145 to 159 mmol/L; in severe cases, it is greater than 160 mEq/L. Severe hypernatremia is life threatening. Much the same as with hyponatremia, cases of severe hypernatremia or acute increases in serum sodium can result in permanent symptoms of central pontine myelinolysis (CPM). Other symptoms of severe hypernatremia include muscle weakness, restlessness, a high-pitched cry (in infants and children), insomnia, lethargy, and coma.

Hypernatremia is always associated with hypertonicity. Much like hypotonic hyponatremia, hypernatremia can occur with hypovolemia, euvolemia, or hypervolemia. Hypovolemic hypernatremia is most often seen in patients who lack free access to water and have uncontrolled fluid losses, such as infants, the elderly, and patients with mental impairments. Patients with high GI losses from nasogastric suction, vomiting, or diarrhea also are at risk for hypovolemic hypernatremia, which results from iatrogenic administration of excessive hypertonic fluids. Euvolemic hypernatremia occurs with excess loss of urinary free water in patients with neurogenic or nephrogenic diabetes insipidus. Patients with neurogenic diabetes insipidus have low ADH secretion, usually as a result of brain injury, intracerebral hemorrhage, skull base or pituitary operations, cerebral infection, or a posterior pituitary autoimmune process. Neurogenic diabetes insipidus is best diagnosed by low urine osmolality (100 mmol/kg) with hypernatremia and is treated by administration of desmopressin, an ADH analog that lacks a vasoconstrictive effect. Nephrogenic diabetes insipidus shows plasma and urine findings similar to neurogenic diabetes but results from an impaired ability of the renal tubules to respond to ADH and therefore is unresponsive to exogenous desmopressin administration.

Treatment of hypernatremia begins with calculation of the free water deficit.

$$\text{Free water deficit (L)} = [(\text{Serum Na} - 140) / 140] \times 0.6 \times \text{Weight (kg)}$$

Patients with severe (>160 mEq/L) or symptomatic hypernatremia should receive D_5 water, and patients with mild or moderate hypernatremia can be given isotonic half NS. The first half of the free-water deficit should be corrected over the first 24 hours, and the second half over the subsequent 24 hours. Serum sodium should be checked frequently; to avoid CPM, the concentration should not be reduced more than 0.5 mEq/L/hr.

Potassium

Serum potassium is maintained in a narrow range from 3.5 to 5 mmol/L, and variations in either direction from this range have potentially significant morbidity. Of total body potassium, 98% resides in the intracellular fluid compartment. Serum potassium is tightly regulated by the renin-angiotensin-aldosterone axis. Aldosterone causes secretion of potassium in the distal renal tubule.

Hypokalemia, defined as serum K^+ below 3.5 mEq/L, is encountered commonly in the postoperative period. Signs and symptoms of hypokalemia include generalized fatigue and weakness, atrial arrhythmias, ileus, and acute renal insufficiency. Flat T or U waves are seen on ECG. Causes of hypokalemia include large losses from the kidney or GI tract via nasogastric suctioning, vomiting, or diarrhea; alkalosis; catecholamine secretion; or insulin administration. Because most of the K^+ is stored intracellularly, small changes in serum K^+ reflect large changes in body stores. Low K^+ is frequently associated with hypomagnesemia and acidemia. Magnesium must first be replenished before K^+ will correct in response to exogenous administration. In patients who are both hypokalemic and acidemic, K^+ administration should precede correction of acidemia with

bicarbonate, to avoid a precipitous drop in serum K^+ as the pH increases. Potassium can be replenished orally or via IV administration. As the oral form is well absorbed, IV administration should be reserved for patients who do not tolerate the oral form or for those who have severe hypokalemia.

Hyperkalemia, defined as K^+ above 5.5 mEq/L, can lead to ventricular arrhythmias. ECG findings include, in order of progression, peaked T waves, QRS widening, shortened QT intervals, and ventricular ectopy. Chronic K^+ elevations in patients with chronic renal failure are well tolerated, but acute changes are not. Acute causes of hyperkalemia include acute renal failure, acidosis, rhabdomyolysis, cell lysis, and insulin deficiency. Pseudohyperkalemia occurs when red blood cells lyse in the collection tube; if this is suspected, the K^+ level should be rechecked.

The ischemia-reperfusion cycle poses great risk of hyperkalemia in patients who undergo reperfusion of an ischemic extremity. Severe systemic hyperkalemia may occur in response to revascularization with at least 4 to 6 hours of ischemia. We routinely administer prophylactic bicarbonate prior to reperfusion. Another cause of hyperkalemia is succinylcholine, a depolarizing paralytic agent, particularly in patients with disuse atrophy usually from prolonged bed rest, neurologic denervation syndromes, severe burns, or muscle trauma.

Hyperkalemia must be identified and treated immediately. Patients should receive at least 1 ampule of prophylactic calcium gluconate to antagonize the K^+ depolarization effect on cardiac myocytes. Treatment strategies to decrease the serum K^+ include shifting the K^+ intracellularly or eliminating it from the body altogether. Intracellular shift is promoted by administering 10 U of insulin along with 1 ampule of D_{50} to prevent hypoglycemia or giving 1 ampule of $NaHCO_3$. Potassium excretion in urine or stool is promoted by administration of a loop diuretic, such as furosemide or bumetanide, or a sodium-potassium exchange resin, such as kayexalate, either orally or as a retention enema with sorbitol. With the exchange resin, 1 mEq of K^+ is taken up in exchange for 2 mEq Na^+, and an osmotic diarrhea ensues. The retention enema should not be given to immunosuppressed patients, as it can cause rectal perforation. If these measures are unsuccessful, hemodialysis may be used as a last resort.

Calcium

Calcium is the most abundant electrolyte in the body. The normal range of serum calcium is 8.5 to 10.5 mg/dL, with 99% stored in bone. Calcium exists in bound and ionized forms. Approximately 50% of calcium circulates as the biologically active ionized form and the other 50% as the biologically inactive bound form. As most of the nonionized form is bound to albumin, the serum calcium level must be adjusted for the serum albumin level in patients who are malnourished; calcium falls 0.8 mEq/dL for every 1 g/dL reduction in serum albumin. Serum calcium concentrations are regulated by parathyroid hormone (PTH) and vitamin D. Conditions that alter PTH and vitamin D levels also indirectly alter calcium levels.

Hypocalcemia is defined as total serum concentration below 8.4 mg/dL or ionized calcium concentration below 4.5 mg/dL. Common causes of hypocalcemia include hypoparathyroidism and vitamin D deficiency. Less common causes include hyperphosphatemia, hypomagnesemia, acute pancreatitis, malnutrition, rhabdomyolysis, infusion of large volumes of fluid, and acute alkalosis secondary to hypoventilation.

Acute hypocalcemia in the postoperative period can occur in response to rapid blood transfusions and hypoparathyroidism. In the past, stored blood contained a higher concentration of citrate, which binds to and chelates serum calcium. Now that citrate has been eliminated from blood-banking techniques, this is rarely seen. Patients who undergo thyroidectomy or parathyroidectomy may become hypocalcemic after surgery.

Symptoms of hypocalcemia include perioral numbness and tingling, hyperreflexia upon stimulation of the facial nerve (Chovstek sign), and spasm of muscles of the hand and forearm with inflation of a blood pressure cuff (Trousseau sign). Prolonged QT intervals and arrhythmias also may develop.

Hypocalcemia should be treated in symptomatic patients and also in patients with total serum calcium below 7.0 mg/dL or ionized calcium below 3.0 mg/dL. Calcium may be given orally, or for severe cases intravenously, in the form of calcium gluconate or calcium chloride. Calcium gluconate has 9 mg of elemental Ca^{2+} per mL, but $CaCl_2$ has 27 mEq/mL; $CaCl_2$ must be administered by central access and in a monitored setting to avoid associated bradycardia or hypotension. Concurrent hypomagnesemia or hyperphosphatemia must be corrected first for the calcium supplementation to be effective.

Hypercalcemia is defined as serum calcium concentration greater than 10.4 mg/dL or ionized concentration greater than 5.6 mg/dL. It occurs most commonly with malignant diseases in hospitalized patients and with hyperparathyroidism in the general population. Breast cancer is the most common malignant cause. Other causes include vitamin A and D overdose, thyrotoxicosis, immobilization, excess exogenous calcium intake, granulomatous diseases, familial hypocalciuric hypercalcemia, and medications such as thiazide diuretics and lithium.

Symptoms of hypercalcemia include nausea, vomiting, altered mental status, constipation, depression, lethargy, myalgias, arthralgias, polyuria, headache, abdominal and flank pain (renal stones), and coma. Patients with symptoms or serum calcium above 14 mg/dL should be treated to avoid a hypercalcemic crisis. Goals of treatment include expansion of intravascular volume with normal saline to dilute circulating calcium and increase filtration of calcium in the kidneys. Furosemide should be administered by IV to increase renal calcium excretion and offset fluid administration.

Hypercalcemic crisis usually occurs with serum calcium levels in excess of 14 mg/dL, and it requires aggressive treatment with bisphosphonates or calcitonin in addition to fluids and diuretics. Bisphosphonates, such as pamidronate (60 to 90 mg IV), inhibit osteoclast-induced bone resorption with onset of action between 24 and 48 hours. Bisphosphonates are the best choice for long-term calcium control and for hypercalcemia due to enhanced bone resorption. Calcitonin (4 U/kg subcutaneously every 12 hours) inhibits bone resorption and decreases renal tubular resorption of calcium, with a shorter onset of action than bisphosphonates; therefore it is the better choice for short-term control of calcium.

Magnesium

Magnesium is essential for energy metabolism, protein synthesis, cell division, and calcium homeostasis. Normal serum magnesium level is 1.4 to 2.0 mEq/L. Magnesium is primarily intracellular, with less than 1% of body stores in the extracellular fluid.

Hypomagnesemia is defined as serum concentration below 1.6 mg/dL, and it often is seen postoperatively because of dilution. Alternatively, hypomagnesemia may occur as a result of poor intake or GI losses including diarrhea and biliary and enteric fistulas. Signs and symptoms rarely occur unless serum levels are below 1.0 mEq/L. Serum magnesium levels must be monitored postoperatively, because severe hypomagnesemia may cause ventricular arrhythmias such as torsades des points.

Magnesium is easily replenished with oral or IV magnesium sulfate. IV replacement is usually reserved for patients with serum magnesium levels below 1.2 mg/dL. Patients who develop ventricular arrhythmias are treated acutely with bolus doses of IV magnesium sulfate, 1 to 2 g over 3 to 5 minutes.

Hypermagnesemia is a rare disorder and usually is seen with burns, trauma, or long-term hemodialysis. *Hypermagnesemia* is defined as serum concentration above 2.8 mg/dL. Symptoms are uncommon until the serum magnesium reaches 4.0 mg/dL, at which point patients become lethargic. Treatment is similar to that for hypercalcemia. Calcium is given to stabilize cardiac myocytes, NS is given to expand the plasma volume, and loop diuretics are used to induce renal excretion.

Phosphorus

Similar to calcium, 80% of phosphorus is stored in bone, with less than 1% of total body phosphorus in the intravascular space. Normal serum phosphate ranges from 2.2 to 4.7 mg/dL.

Hypophosphatemia is defined as serum concentration below 2.5 mg/dL, and symptoms include respiratory and cardiac failure. Hypophosphatemia is frequently encountered in the postoperative period. Common causes include decreased intake and intestinal malabsorption due to vitamin D deficiency, increased renal excretion from diuretics, alkalosis, hyperparathyroidism and hungry bone syndrome, major hepatic resection, rhabdomyolysis, and refeeding syndrome. Refeeding syndrome occurs in nutritionally depleted patients who are given carbohydrates; the resultant insulin surge causes the already depleted phosphate pool to redistribute into cells. Phosphate is an essential component for the adenosine triphosphatase backbone and should be replenished when serum concentration falls below 2.0 mg/dL. Sodium or potassium phosphate can both be administered by IV or orally.

Hyperphosphatemia is defined as serum phosphate concentration greater than 5.0 mg/dL, and it rarely occurs postoperatively. Patients with renal insufficiency can become hypophosphatemic primarily because of decreased 1,25 dihydroxy-vitamin D production. These patients are also usually hypocalcemic from increased calcium precipitation, with elevated serum phosphate levels. Patients with hyperphosphatemia primarily have symptoms that result from hypocalcemia. Treatment includes expanding the plasma volume with NS and then stimulating renal excretion with acetazolamide. Acute cases of severe refractory hyperphosphatemia can be treated with hemodialysis. Patients in renal failure with chronic hyperphosphatemia are maintained on phosphate binders such as aluminum hydroxide.

Suggested Readings

Adrogue HJ, Madias NE: Hypernatremia, *N Engl J Med* 342:1943, 2002.
Adrogue HJ, Madias NE: Hyponatremia, *N Engl J Med* 342:1581, 2002.
Brandstrup B, Tonnesen H, Beier-Holgersen R: Effects of intravenous fluid restriction on postoperative complications: comparison of two perioperative fluid regimens, *Ann Surg* 238:641, 2003.
Eschempati SR, Reed RL II, Barie PS: Serum bicarbonate concentration correlates with arterial base deficit in critically ill patients, *Surg Infect* 4:193, 2003.
Jacob M, Chappell D, Rhem M: Clinical update: perioperative fluid management, *Lancet* 369:1984, 2007.
Marjanovic G, Villain C, Juettner E, et al: Impact of different crystalloid volume regimes on intestinal anastomotic stability, *Ann Surg* 249:181, 2009.
Tisherman SA, Barie PS, Bokhari F, et al: Clinical practice guideline: end points of resuscitation, *J Trauma* 57:898, 2004.

Preoperative Assessment of the Elderly Patient: Frailty

Thomas N. Robinson, MD, and Michael E. Zenilman, MD

OVERVIEW

In the previous editions of this text, this chapter focused on the preoperative workup of the elderly patient with an emphasis on well-established risk factors for adverse events. Currently, the accepted paradigm is that comorbidities in single organ systems—such as cardiac, respiratory, and renal systems—independently determine an individual's perioperative risk. Chronologic age is typically considered a minor risk factor. But, recently, chronologic age has been identified as an independent risk factor in major surgeries such as pancreaticoduodenectomy, esophagectomy, and hepatectomy. This fact is likely a result of both the stress of these major surgeries and the accumulation of physiologic compromise that occurs across multiple organ systems due to aging, creating a state defined by the term *frailty*. The older, traditional models of preoperative risk stratification do not adequately measure risk in the frail, aged patient.

The purpose of this chapter is fourfold: 1) to review the limitations of traditional preoperative assessment for geriatric patients, 2) to understand the definition of frailty, 3) to learn how to quantitatively assess for the presence of frailty, and 4) to recognize the relationship between the presence of frailty deficits measured preoperatively and adverse postoperative outcomes.

TRADITIONAL PREOPERATIVE ASSESSMENT

The purpose of preoperative assessment is to identify individuals with increased risk for poor outcomes—the so-called *vulnerable elderly*. A risk-assessment tool should affect or alter preoperative decision making. Traditional preoperative evaluation approaches risk stratify patients based on compromise in single organ systems, most notably those represented in the American Heart Association guidelines for perioperative cardiovascular evaluation (cardiac risk in noncardiac surgery). This guideline employs risk factors that include chronic renal insufficiency (creatinine >2.0), prior cerebrovascular disease, prior ischemic heart disease, and prior heart failure to stratify an individual's risk for adverse postoperative cardiac outcomes. Similar guidelines exist for preoperative risk stratification from the standpoint of other end organs, such as the lungs and liver. This traditional preoperative evaluation strategy has been accepted as comprehensive for the older adult. Although single organ system assessment cannot be ignored in the geriatric surgical patient, individual end-organ dysfunction does not capture the unique characteristics that foreshadow poor outcomes in the geriatric patient.

Geriatric patients develop a physiologic vulnerability called *frailty*, a condition that heralds a predictable perioperative course distinct from that of the older adult. Frailty distinguishes the vulnerable elderly patients from healthy, chronologically similar aged patients at less risk. With more than half of all operations in the United States being performed on patients 65 years of age and older, the knowledgeable surgeon must be able to recognize and manage the frail aged patient. Turning to the traditional preoperative assessment strategy of single end-organ assessment in the geriatric patient will miss the relevant clinical features that portend poor outcomes in the vulnerable elderly.

The clinical assessment of frailty used for preoperative risk stratification of the geriatric patient should supplement, but not replace, traditional assessment of critical end organs. For example, an older patient with unstable coronary disease or uncompensated liver disease has high operative risk irrespective of the presence of frailty. The remainder of this chapter focuses on the clinical characteristics unique to the geriatric patient that are useful in preoperative risk stratification.

FRAILTY

Frailty is defined as a state of reduced physiologic reserve associated with increased susceptibility to disability, and it results from multisystem loss of physiologic reserve (e.g., functional dependence, cognitive dysfunction, malnutrition) that culminate to create increased susceptibility to stress. Clinical characteristics common in the frail aged patient are listed in Box 1. Note that in this table, critical end organs are not factors. Clinical markers of frailty that are useful in the preoperative risk stratification of elderly surgical patients include characteristics describing function, burden of comorbidities, nutrition, and cognition.

Understanding the language used to describe frailty is necessary. Frailty traits or markers are individual clinical characteristics that characterize the frailty state. The words *trait, marker,* and *characteristic* are used interchangeably. Examples of a frailty marker or trait include functional status, burden of comorbidities, nutritional status, and cognitive function. When a frailty trait is found to be present in an elderly patient, this characteristic is referred to as a *frailty deficit*.

The concept of frailty may initially appear to be abstract and difficult to grasp. However, the experienced surgeon qualitatively recognizes frailty during the interactions commonplace to a routine preoperative clinic visit. Our goal will be to move from this qualitative, or intuitive, recognition of frailty to a scientific, quantitative approach that will reproducibly determine the presence or absence of frailty.

BOX 1: Characteristics of the frail elderly

Intrinsic Factors

Disability
Requires help with ADLs
Slow gait, impaired mobility
Functional decline
Incontinence
Falls
Multiple chronic diseases
Pressure ulcer
Failure to thrive, fatigue
Sarcopenia
Dementia
Delirium
Impaired cognition
Depression

Extrinsic Factors

Polypharmacy
Social vulnerability, living alone
Elder abuse

A Quantitative Assessment of Frailty

To move from a qualitative appreciation of frailty to a calculated, quantitative determination of frailty, the surgeon must measure individual frailty characteristics in the preoperative clinic and then sum the total number of frailty traits present in an elderly patient. Defining frailty as a composite of individual clinical traits has clinical utility. Detrimental effects on outcome are directly related to a larger number of frailty traits present in an individual, which represents increased loss of physiologic reserve. The concept of measuring frailty as a sum of deficits or problems allows the surgeon to recognize increased vulnerability to the surgical stressor by understanding that there is a relationship between a higher number of deficits present and poorer postoperative outcomes. A higher number of frailty deficits correlates with decreased physiologic reserve to withstand the operative stress. Typical community-based frailty assessment strategies define the presence of frailty when a threshold number of deficits, usually three or more, are present. A *prefrail* condition, or *relative frailty*, occurs when frailty traits are present but do not reach the threshold required for the diagnosis of frailty; for example, two frailty deficits are present, and three are required for the diagnosis. Both prefrail and frail patients are predisposed to adverse outcomes.

MEASUREMENT OF FRAILTY TRAITS

Frailty traits useful in the preoperative risk stratification of elderly surgical patients include markers of disability (function), comorbidity, nutrition, and cognition. The subsequent text describing each marker of frailty is meant to supplement Tables 1 and 2. These tables provide the practical, hands-on guide to administering and scoring the frailty assessment tools recommended for implementation in a surgeon's practice.

TABLE 1: Preoperative frailty assessment: Practical tools for the surgeon

	How to Administer the Test	Scoring
Function		
Katz ADL score	Ask about dependence in any one of six ADLs: bathing, grooming, feeding, toileting, dressing, transferring	Score 1 point for independence for each ADL (possible total of 6 points)
Timed "up and go"	Timed activity: Rise from hard chair (without use of arms), walk 10 feet, turn and return to sitting in chair	Time in seconds
Falls	Ask: "How many times have you fallen in the past 6 months?"	0 = no falls; # = number of times falls reported
Comorbidity		
Charlson index	Record conditions with assigned values: Myocardial infarction (1) Heart failure (1) Peripheral vascular disease (1) Cerebrovascular disease (1) Dementia (1) Chronic obstructive pulmonary disease (1) Connective tissue disease (1) Ulcer disease (1) Mild liver disease (1) Diabetes (1) Hemiplegia (2) Moderate to severe renal disease (2) Diabetes with end-organ damage (2) Any tumor (2) Leukemia (2) Lymphoma (2) Moderate to severe liver disease (3) Metastatic solid tumor (6) AIDS (6)	Sum values to obtain point score
Nutrition		
Recent weight loss	Review weight over time for unexplained weight loss	Calculate weight differential (6 months)
Albumin	Serum albumin	Laboratory value (g/dL)
Cognition		
Mini-Cog test	1. Ask subject to remember three words: *apple, table,* and *penny* 2. Ask subject to draw a clock, with all the numbers and hands at 11:10 3. Ask the subject to recall the three words from step 1	Three item recall: 1 point per word (3 points) Clock drawing: 2 points = accurate clock, 0 points = abnormal clock

TABLE 2: Quantifying frailty deficits

Frailty Trait Assessment	Positive Test
Function	
Katz ADL score	Dependence in any ADL (score ≤5)
Timed "up and go"	>10 seconds
Falls	One or more falls in 6 months (score ≥1)
Comorbidities	
Charlson Index	≥3 points
Nutrition	
Weight loss	>10 lb weight loss in 6 months
Albumin	<3.4 g/dL
Cognition	
Mini-Cog test	Positive test if: 1) 0 words recalled *or* 2) <3 words recalled and abnormal clock draw

Disability

Disability is defined as difficulty or dependence in one or more activities of daily living. Activities of daily living (ADLs) describe six tasks necessary for independent living: *bathing, dressing, transferring, walking, toileting,* and *feeding.* Disability has emerged as an important risk for mortality, need for postoperative institutionalization, and ultimately, higher health care costs. In a study examining 12 frailty traits measured preoperatively, logistic regression analysis found that any functional dependence was the strongest predictor of 6-month mortality. Dependence in any one of the six ADLs is considered positive for disability.

Bathing is the first ADL that requires assistance; as a result, assistance with bathing should be addressed initially to expedite the functional assessment. Excellent tools to assess functional dependence include the Katz Activity of Daily Living Score and the Barthel index. Other functional assessment tests include a recent history of falls and the timed "up and go" test, which allows the surgeon to observe an elderly patient's mobility while they perform tasks of standing, walking, and turning. This test reliably determines functional mobility and has prognostic validity for predicting falls. A recent history of unexplained falls signals frailty, because falling represents the expression of a multifactorial geriatric syndrome relating to loss of sensory input, central proprioception, and musculoskeletal function. A perioperative frailty study linked the presence of one or more unexplained falls in the 6 months prior to an operation to both postdischarge institutionalization and 6-month mortality.

Comorbidity

Comorbidity is defined as the presence of two or more disease processes. Review of Medicare databases reveals two thirds of individuals in the United States 65 years and older have two or more chronic diseases, and that one third have four or more chronic diseases. The Charlson Comorbidity Index quantifies burden of chronic disease by addressing 19 categories of comorbidity and assigning a weighted value to each comorbidity based on risk of 1-year mortality. The Charlson index has proven utility for preoperatively risk stratifying elderly patients. Other methods to define the burden of comorbidity, such as the American Society of Anesthesiologists (ASA) score and simply counting the number of outpatient medications, have not reflected poor outcomes in previous surgical frailty research.

Malnutrition

Malnutrition occurs in the oldest frail elderly because of the physiologic anorexia of aging and the associated sarcopenia. An elderly individual's unexplained weight loss therefore can be a result of a medical illness, decreased need, lack of interest, or even failure to feed. Community-based frailty indexes use weight loss of 10 lb in the previous 6 months as a measure of malnutrition, and a low preoperative albumin level is a well-recognized predictive factor of adverse postoperative outcomes in surgical patients. Results from the National Veterans Affairs Surgical Risk Study found that a low albumin level was the most important preoperative predictor for 30-day postoperative mortality.

Cognition

Cognition is a term that describes the process of thought. *Dementia* is the progressive, long-term cognitive decline that is a normal part of aging that affects areas of memory, attention, language, and problem solving. Dementia must be distinguished from delirium, an acute-onset confused state that can occur following a physiologic stress; the workup for delirium must be done in the postoperative state. Dementia screening should be performed prior to elective surgery to obtain accurate baseline assessment, but such screening cannot be performed accurately in a patient who is stressed (e.g., someone being seen for emergent surgery or a postoperative patient). Multiple screening tools exist for cognitive dysfunction, most notably the Mini-Mental Status Exam and the Mini-Cog Test. Our frailty scoring system uses the Mini-Cog Test because it is simple, brief, and can be interpreted by nonspecialists.

Other Important Frailty Markers

The frailty traits for preoperative risk described above are not comprehensive of all frailty markers previously described. For example, the Canadian Study of Health and Aging, one of the largest community-based frailty studies, used 70 clinical variables to derive their frailty index. The frailty characteristics emphasized in this chapter have proven utility in the preoperative setting. However, it is worth mentioning two other clinical characteristics of frailty that are closely related to adverse outcomes in elderly individuals: *depression* and *social vulnerability*.

Depression is common in the elderly and is not considered to be a normal part of aging. The presence of depression in the elderly increases the morbidity and mortality of common medical diseases (e.g., myocardial infarction and diabetes), and it increases 6 month mortality following cardiac surgery. Although formal diagnosis of depression requires substantial expertise, the two-question depression test is a simple tool with high sensitivity and specificity for detecting depressed mood. This test asks two simple questions about mood and anhedonia: Over the past month, have you felt down, depressed, or hopeless? Over the past month, have you felt little interest or pleasure in doing things? A positive response to either or both questions reveals the presence of a depressed mood.

Social vulnerability refers to an individual's inability to withstand a stressor from a social standpoint. Factors composing social vulnerability include social support (e.g., marital status, living alone) and social engagement (e.g., frequency of contact with family, friends, pets). Although surgeons do not commonly think of a relationship between social vulnerability and adverse outcomes, greater social vulnerability is associated with increased 5-year mortality in community-based geriatric studies. Intuitively, social vulnerability likely impacts the need for changing immediate postdischarge care plans, whether by requiring home health care or by requiring temporary institutional care.

FRAILTY AND ADVERSE SURGICAL OUTCOMES

The preoperative diagnosis of frailty predicts poor outcomes following surgery. The basic concept is that the more frailty deficits, or physiologic deficiencies, that an elderly person has or has accumulated, the more susceptible they are to having adverse outcomes to a given surgical stress in comparison with an elderly individual with fewer deficits and less baseline physiologic compromise. Gerontologists have carefully defined the relationship of frailty deficits and mortality in large community-based research on elderly individuals; the two most notable studies are the Cardiovascular Health Study and the Canadian Study of Health and Aging.

Accumulation of frailty deficits as an approach to predict the occurrence of mortality has gained wide acceptance and appears to be a concept that can be translated to global risk stratification for elderly surgical patients. In the elderly population in whom multiple chronic diseases and polypharmacy are prevalent phenomena, distinguishing operative risk simply based on the presence of chronic diseases appears inferior to summing frailty markers to stratify operative risk.

Although individual frailty markers are recognized as predictors of poor outcome in surgical patients, only recently has the entity of frailty been studied in the context of preoperative risk stratification in the elderly. Individual characteristics of frailty previously related to poor outcomes in surgical patients include cognitive dysfunction, recent weight loss, low albumin, functional dependence, and depression.

Two studies have sought to determine the relationship of frailty and adverse postoperative outcomes. Robinson and colleagues (2009) measured frailty in surgical patients 65 years and older undergoing an elective operation requiring a postoperative intensive care unit admission. Preoperative frailty markers related to both 6 month mortality and postdischarge institutionalization included impaired cognition (Mini-Cog score ≤3), recent falls (one or more in 6 months), hypoalbuminemia (albumin <3.4 g/dL), significant anemia (hematocrit <35%), any functional dependence (Katz score <6), and increased comorbidities (Charlson index ≥3). Logistic regression determined functional dependence to be the factor most closely related to the outcome of 6-month mortality. A clinical prediction rule designed to detect 6-month postoperative mortality based on frailty assessment found that the presence of four or more markers predicted 6-month mortality with high sensitivity (81%) and specificity (86%). In summary, this study found that the more frailty deficits found preoperatively, the worse the outcomes were in terms of higher 6-month mortality and postdischarge institutionalization.

In a second study, Dasgupta and colleagues (2009) recruited subjects 70 years and older prior to elective operations, mostly orthopedic, and routinely screened subjects preoperatively with the Edmonton Frailty Scale. This scale measures frailty traits that include dependence in activities of daily living, cognitive impairment, weight loss, burden of illness, and others, and it assigns points for frailty deficits. Low scores reflect a nonfrail patient, and high scores reflect an increasing burden of frailty deficits. Increasing frailty scores were directly related to increased postoperative complications, longer hospital stays, and increased need for postdischarge institutionalization.

These two studies provide powerful insight in that measurements of a higher number of preoperative frailty deficits, representing greater physiologic compromise, relate closely with increased adverse postoperative outcomes in geriatric surgical patients (Table 3). As of now, there is no validated preoperative frailty index and no absolute cutoff for the number of frailty deficits that can tell a surgeon whether or not to perform an operation. Such an algorithm will require much more patient- and operation-specific information. Factors including extent of the proposed operation, patient-centered goals, opportunity to prolong life, and potential to relieve suffering all weigh into the decision on whether to operate. Simply measuring clinical characteristics of frailty does not capture the complexities of the decision to operate.

TABLE 3: Translating frailty deficits into surgical outcomes

Lower Risk No Frailty Deficits	Higher Risk Multiple Frailty Deficits
Mild organ dysfunction	Significant organ dysfunction
Average morbidity	High morbidity
Average hospital stay	Prolonged hospital stay
Discharge to home	Discharge institutionalization
Average mortality rate	High 6-month mortality rate

An elderly individual may have a range from zero to multiple frailty deficits discovered on preoperative evaluation. The presence or accumulation of a higher number of frailty deficits, representing a higher degree of physiologic compromise, corresponds to increasing vulnerability to the adverse postoperative outcomes depicted.

TABLE 4: Risk factors for postoperative delirium

Preexisting Frailty Markers as Risk Factors for Delirium	
Dementia/cognitive dysfunction*	Low albumin
Functional dependence	Anemia
Increased comorbidities	Depression

Other Preexisting Risk Factors for Delirium	
Advanced age (>70 years)	Laboratory abnormalities (sodium)
History of alcohol abuse	
Psychotropic drug use	Sensory impairment (vision/hearing)
Narcotic use	Institutional residence

*The frailty marker of cognitive dysfunction, or dementia, has been repeatedly found to be the strongest preexisting risk factor for developing postoperative delirium.
Data from Robinson TN, Raeburn CD, Tran ZV, et al: Post-operative delirium in the elderly—risk factors and outcomes, *Ann Surg* 249:173, 2009; and Flinn DR, Diehl DM, Seyfried LS, et al: Prevention, diagnosis and management of postoperative delirium in older adults, *J Am Coll Surg* 209:261, 2009.

Delirium, a geriatric syndrome, is the quintessential postoperative inpatient geriatric complication. Given a similar surgical stress, risk factors for developing postoperative delirium are the same markers of frailty covered in this chapter (Table 4). The occurrence of delirium in the postoperative setting is associated with the occurrence of markedly worse outcomes including increased complications, longer hospital stays, increased risk of discharge institutionalization, and increased mortality rate.

The concept of a clear correlation between an increasing number of frailty deficits and poor postoperative outcomes is well established. This concept is hypothetically displayed in Figure 1. The quantitative recognition of a high number of frailty deficits measured preoperatively should alert the surgeon to prepare for adverse postoperative events, and it allows the surgeon to counsel the elderly patient accordingly. Measurement of frailty traits allows the surgeon to move from a qualitative, intuitive sense of the presence of the vulnerable aged patient to a quantitative measurement that foreshadows poor outcomes.

Implementing Frailty Assessment into a Surgical Practice

We believe that implementing a frailty scoring system in a surgeon's office to preoperatively discriminate the highly vulnerable aged patient from the elderly patient with lower risk with the objective of altering preoperative decision making will be very useful. Tables 1 and

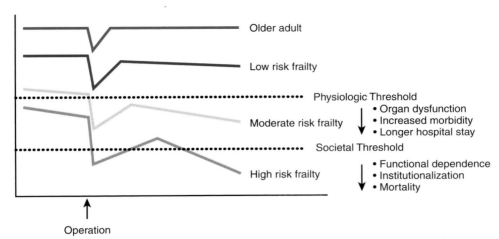

FIGURE 1   Frailty and the elderly surgical patient. This graphic depicts the hypothetical decline caused by aging and compares an older adult with elderly individuals with increasing degrees of frailty. The range of frailty from low to high risk represents a spectrum of elderly patients with no frailty deficits (low risk) to elderly patients with multiple frailty deficits (high risk). The y-axis represents reserve capacity that can be viewed from the standpoints of physiology, function, societal issues, or life expectancy. Advanced frailty, or increasing physiologic compromise represented by a higher count of frailty deficits, results in both a reduced reserve prior to an operation and an accelerated loss of reserve afterward.

2 review simple clinical tools that assess, score, and quantify the various clinical characteristics necessary to diagnose frailty. These frailty marker tests can be administered and interpreted by nonspecialists.

The practicing surgeon can implement preoperative frailty screening into their practice without excessive burden. We recommend having the person who takes vital signs perform the frailty assessment outlined in Table 1 in every preoperative patient aged 65 years and older. Completion of these seven tools that quantify the presence of individual frailty traits takes about 5 minutes. We recommend creating a scoring template that allows the assessor to rapidly mark or circle the score achieved for each test. Immediately prior to the preoperative consultation, the surgeon reviews this scoring sheet by glancing over each frailty measurement and summing the total number of frailty deficits present. A frailty deficit is determined to be present as defined by a positive test score, depicted in Table 2. The total number of frailty deficits present in an individual elderly patient is determined by the total number of positive test scores achieved. By understanding that higher numbers of positive frailty deficits correspond to increasing physiologic compromise, this process provides the surgeon prognostic information about the geriatric patient just prior to the preoperative consultation, during which the decision whether or not to operate takes place.

SUMMARY

Preoperative risk stratification of geriatric surgical patients has become increasingly important with an aging population. Utilizing frailty in the preoperative assessment provides evidence of global loss of physiologic reserve for the vulnerable elderly and therefore estimates an elderly patient's ability to withstand an operative stress. These markers may be more powerful than the traditional assessment of critical end-organ systems. The importance of frailty markers in preoperative risk stratification is gaining acceptance, as evidenced by the National Surgical Quality Improvement Project (NSQIP) adding geriatric-specific indicators into the database; for example, functional status as measured by dependence in activities of daily living and weight loss of more than 10% in the previous 6 months.

In 2008, the Institute of Medicine published "Retooling for an Aging America." Their report showed that the prevalence of chronic disease is as high as 80% in the elderly population, and that 12% of the population uses one quarter to one third of our health care resources. The report emphasized the need for multidisciplinary teams, proactive rehabilitation, and care management to address the elderly patient's unique care needs. They suggest programs to improve

the *competency* of physicians, including surgeons, in the delivery of geriatric care. Toward this end, the American Geriatrics Society has given grants to the surgical subspecialties to expand the knowledge base of surgeons in geriatrics. Multiple Internet-based geriatric educational Web portals exist with the purpose of disseminating geriatric specialty knowledge to nongeriatricians. Widely recognized sites include http://www.POGOe.org, which provides geriatric educational tools; http://champ.bsd.uchicago.edu, which offers resources and instruction for nongeriatrician educators to teach geriatric topics; http://www.eperc.mcw.edu, an end-of-life, palliative education resource center; and http://sso.efacs.org, the American College of Surgeons (ACS) Web portal with a geriatrics community.

In the future, perioperative geriatric risk will be quantified in a manner similar to the core measures that determine the quality of surgical outcomes. The ACOVE-3 (Assessing the Care of Vulnerable Elders) report from the Rand Corporation added surgical quality indicators, and Ko and colleagues (2005) included specific elderly issues such as cognition, polypharmacy, communication, and discharge planning into the optimal quality indicators for elderly patients undergoing abdominal operations. Under ACS leadership, similar elderly-specific data points have been included in the NSQIP.

As surgeons, we must embrace the aging population as a demographic inevitability and recognize the unique vulnerabilities of the aged patient to improve our surgical care of the oldest elderly.

Suggested Readings

Dasgupta M, Rolfson DB, Stolee P, et al: Frailty is associated with postoperative complications in older adults with medical problems, *Arch Gerontol Geriatr* 48:78–83, 2009.

Fried LP, Tangen CM, Walston J, et al: Frailty in older adults: evidence for a phenotype, *J Gerontol A Biol Sci Med Sci* 56:M146, 2001.

Kulminski AM, Ukraintseva SV, Kulminskaya IV, et al: Cumulative deficits better characterize susceptibility to death in elderly people than phenotypic frailty: lessons from the Cardiovascular Health Study, *J Am Ger Soc* 56:898, 2008.

McGory ML, Sekelle PG, Rubenstein LZ, et al: Developing quality indicators for elderly patients undergoing abdominal operations, *J Am Coll Surg* 201:870, 2005.

Rockwood K, Song X, MacKnight C, et al: A global clinical measure of fitness and frailty in elderly people, *CMAJ* 173:489, 2005.

Robinson TN, Eiseman B, Wallace JI, et al: Redefining geriatric pre-operative assessment using frailty, disability and co-morbidity, *Ann Surg* 250:449, 2009.

Zenilman ME, Bender JS, Magnuson TH, et al: General surgical care in the nursing home patient: results of a dedicated geriatric surgery consult service, *J Am Coll Surg* 183:361, 1996.

Preoperative Preparation of the Surgical Patient

Jerry Stonemetz, MD

OVERVIEW

From the moment the patient and surgeon decide to proceed with surgery, the preoperative time frame represents a golden opportunity to proactively manage and optimize the patient for the upcoming surgery. Unfortunately, in the vast majority of cases, this time is not managed effectively or appropriately to enhance the surgical experience or the patient's outcome. Typically, the patient receives scant instructions from the surgeon's office and may or may not be seen by the primary care provider. Ironically, this period holds the greatest opportunities to significantly improve surgical outcomes. For example, the vast majority of the Surgical Care Improvement Project (SCIP) measures require identification of at-risk patients and customized interventions to prevent common surgical complications. These include identification and prophylaxis of patients at risk for deep venous thrombosis (DVT) and pulmonary embolism (PE), preoperative administration of β-blockers, appropriate selection of antibiotics, and better glycemic control of diabetic patients.

The future of perioperative medicine will usher in advances in proactively reaching out to surgical patients during this preoperative period and delivering disease-specific management. Today's technology utilizes patient health records and online questionnaires that are tied to decision support systems to guide preoperative testing. By correctly identifying and risk stratifying surgical patients, we can tailor clinical pathways that optimize their medical conditions and better prepare them for surgery.

Today, most preoperative patients are managed using one of three methods. In the first approach, many surgical patients are given preoperative instructions by their surgeons with preoperative testing defined in preprinted letters. Frequently, these instructions inform the patient that they need to be seen by their primary medical physician for a preoperative clearance or evaluation. This system is fraught with problems that range from significant overtesting to missing key instructions that are unusual because of patient-specific conditions, such as how to manage preoperative anticoagulation.

In the second approach, some hospitals and ambulatory surgical centers (ASCs) employ specially trained nurses to call patients ahead of time to gather clinical information. If problems are identified during these calls, the nurse will typically discuss the concern with either the anesthesia team or the surgeon to determine the best solution to the problem. These systems are frequently more effective than simply relying on surgeon instructions; however, they are very dependent upon the skill and motivation of the nurse making the call. Additionally, a high percentage of patients cannot be reached by phone.

The third approach, used by a few hospitals, primarily academic centers, uses a preoperative evaluation clinic (PEC), where patients are actually seen by either trained nurses, physician assistants (PAs), or nurse practitioners (NPs) with or without the anesthesia physician's involvement. These clinics have been repeatedly demonstrated to be more effective than the previous two arrangements; however, they are significantly more expensive to implement and staff. An additional downside to these clinics is the reality that not all patients can or should be required to make a separate visit to a clinic in preparation for surgery.

I am a proponent of the preoperative clinic, based on experiences at my institution as well as on a plethora of published studies demonstrating enhanced patient safety, patient satisfaction, reduction of testing and expenses, and a significant reduction in cancellations and delays the day of surgery. However, as stipulated above, not all patients should be required to make a separate trip to the hospital for an evaluation prior to surgery.

At my institution, we have created a "preoperative road map" that is provided to our surgeons to give guidance as to which patients should be selected to come to our clinic. Additionally, this road map provides some basic algorithms that indicate what testing should be done on patients deemed appropriate to bypass the clinic. This road map was developed based on principles defined by the American Society of Anesthesiologists (ASA) Task Force on Preoperative Testing convened in 2002 and updated based on new evidence regarding specific patient conditions. Figure 1 is a diagram of the algorithm we utilize in our road map to illustrate how to triage a surgical patient. Essentially, we ask our surgeons to determine whether patients are sick or healthy. Healthy patients only need to be seen in a preoperative clinic if they are having major surgery. We define *major surgery* as specified by the American Heart Association (AHA) as involving major blood vessels, vascular or cardiac, or extensive disruption of physiology, such as an 8 hour Whipple procedure or major transplant procedure.

For a healthy patient scheduled for minor surgery, there really is no indication for much preoperative testing. Routine chest radiograph and electrocardiograph (ECG) are not warranted for most patients. We do require an ECG for all patients older than 50 years; however, that is based on local custom, and no solid evidence indicates that this should be required. Additionally, laboratory testing should also be considered only for patient conditions and surgeries that warrant the appropriate test. Minor outpatient surgery really only requires a hemoglobin on menstruating females and possibly a urine pregnancy test, unless something in the history indicates a need for further testing.

A good example of a significantly overprescribed preoperative test is coagulation studies. At most institutions, a prothrombin time/International Normalized Ratio (PT/INR) and partial thromboplastin test (PTT) are ordered on the vast majority of patients, but several problems attend ordering this test preoperatively. First, most labs have now split out the PT/INR from the PTT, and ordering a PTT adds an additional cost to the test. There are practically no preoperative patients who warrant a PTT. Exceptions are hemophiliac, and these should be identified from a basic history and physical. The PTT test represents the intrinsic coagulation pathway, and it is routinely used to monitor heparin dosing. Obviously, preoperative patients are rarely on heparin, so this test is worthless to obtain. As for the PT/INR, there are some patients for whom this test is indicated: patients with a history of liver disease or bruising and prolonged bleeding. Ironically, physicians routinely order a PT/INR on patients on anticoagulants such as warfarin, but there is little rationale for ordering this test preoperatively for these patients because they will all have abnormal values for their INR. There is a rationale for ordering the tests on the day of surgery, such as the need to document return of coagulation before any regional blocks are performed, but not a few days prior to surgery. Both of these examples illustrate how we can reduce the significant expense of unnecessary preoperative testing without affecting outcomes.

COMORBIDITIES

The road map also defines how to approach certain patient comorbidities as far as appropriate testing is concerned (Table 1). Of particular concern is the patient who is not able to achieve at least 4 mets (metabolic equivalents) of activity, which is defined as being able to climb two flights of stairs without stopping, or walking briskly for up to four city blocks. There are many reasons patients are not able to achieve this level

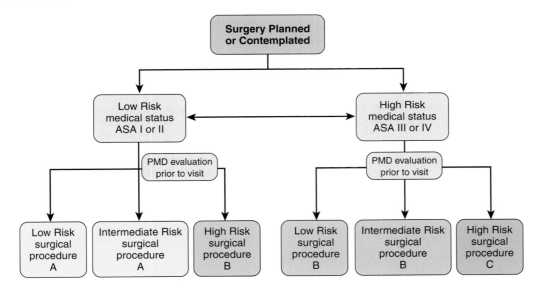

A   A – May have preanesthesia assessment done day of surgery.

B   B – Recommend preanesthesia assessment with PEC visit at least 24 hours preoperatively.
          Should have an evaluation done prior to PEC visit by PMD.

C   C – Recommend Preanesthesia consult scheduled in PEC at least 48 hours preoperatively.
          Should have an evaluation done prior to anesthesia consult by PMD.

FIGURE 1   Preoperative triage algorithm. *Low-risk medical conditions:* healthy with no medical problems (ASA I) or well-controlled chronic conditions (ASA II). *High-risk medical conditions:* multiple medical comorbidities that are not well controlled (ASA III) or extremely compromised function secondary to comorbidities (ASA IV). *Low-risk surgical procedure:* poses minimal physiologic stress (e.g., minor outpatient surgery). *Intermediate-risk surgical procedure:* medium-risk procedure with moderate physiologic stress and minimal blood loss, fluid shifts, or postoperative changes. *High-risk surgical procedure:* high-risk procedure with significant fluid shifts, possible blood loss, and anticipated perioperative stress. *PMD,* Primary medical doctor; *PEC,* Preoperative evaluation clinic *(From Johns Hopkins Preoperative Roadmap, available online at http://www.hopkinsmedicine. org/anesthesiology/Patient_Care/Preoperative_Roadmap.pdf.)*

of activity, such as arthritis or obesity, but without the patient attaining this activity level, we are not able to assess cardiac reserve. Consequently, we frequently want an echocardiogram for these patients, especially if they are scheduled for intermediate or major surgery.

The patient who represents one of our greatest challenges is the patient who is morbidly obese as defined by a body mass index (BMI) greater than 35. These patients are particularly prone to comorbidities that may seem unusual at an early age. The most concerning combination of comorbidities is the presence of morbid obesity and sleep apnea. This common combination may result in pulmonary hypertension that is undiagnosed, but it may result in perioperative death if it is not recognized and dealt with appropriately. These patients should have an echocardiogram to rule out pulmonary hypertension, but unfortunately, such patients also have a body habitus that precludes using echocardiography to assess right-heart function. In this situation, the patient may need a right-heart catheterization.

MEDICATION MANAGEMENT

Historically, implicit in our orders for nothing by mouth (NPO) after midnight, we tell patients not to take their morning medications; however, our thinking has changed dramatically based on recent evidence, and we now realize that most patients on chronic medications really should continue those medications the morning of surgery and through the perioperative period. There are exceptions, and they are listed in Table 2. Specifically, we now realize that β-blockers are important for improved surgical outcomes, and in fact they have become part of one of the SCIP measures that looks at whether a patient who is on a β-blocker as a home medication has taken this medication within 24 hours of surgery. Alternatively, a β-blocker can be administered

intraoperatively, but the preferred recommendation is to have the patient take the medicine orally before surgery. This brings into question the NPO status. We now feel that sips of water immediately prior to surgery is not a problem, and there is some evidence to suggest that clear liquids taken within 2 hours of surgery may actually reduce postoperative nausea and vomiting. Conversely, medications that are recommended to be held are described in the following sections.

Oral Hypoglycemic Agents

Oral hypoglycemic agents should be held for at least 8 hours preoperatively, which means that patients who take them in the evening should be allowed to continue these medications the night before surgery. One exception may be metformin for patients who are concomitantly going to receive contrast dye as part of their procedure. These patients should have this medication stopped at least 24 hours prior to the procedure in an attempt to reduce the risk of renal failure. The rationale for holding oral hypoglycemics comes from reports of profound lactic acidosis in patients who received the medication postoperatively and were undergoing major surgery. No studies to date have looked at the consequences of taking these medications preoperatively in minor surgery; however, I continue to recommend holding them in light of a lack of any evidence of their safety.

Insulin

We recommend that all patients hold their morning dose of insulin because they are not taking any oral glucose preoperatively. Typically, we recommend they bring their morning insulin with them to the

TABLE 1: Medical conditions that may warrant ASA III or IV status and may benefit from a preoperative assessment at a preoperative evaluation clinic

General conditions	Medical condition inhibiting ability to engage in normal daily activity; unable to climb two flights of stairs without stopping Medical condition necessitating continual assistance or monitoring at home within the previous 6 months Admission to hospital within previous 2 months for acute or exacerbated chronic condition History of previous anesthesia complication or history of malignant hyperthermia
Cardiocirculatory	History of angina, coronary artery disease, or myocardial infarction Symptomatic arrhythmias, particularly new onset atrial fibrillation Poorly controlled hypertension (systolic >160 mm Hg and/or diastolic >110 mm Hg) History of congestive heart failure History of significant valvular disease (e.g., aortic stenosis, mitral regurgitation)
Respiratory	Asthma/chronic obstructive pulmonary disease requiring chronic medication or acute exacerbation and progression within previous 6 months History of major airway surgery or unusual airway anatomy; history of difficult intubation in previous anesthetic Upper or lower airway tumor or obstruction History of chronic respiratory distress requiring home ventilatory assistance or monitoring
Endocrine	Insulin-dependent diabetes mellitus Adrenal disorders Active thyroid disease Morbid obesity
Neuromuscular	History of seizure disorder or other significant central nervous system diseases (e.g., multiple sclerosis, muscular dystrophy) History of myopathy or other muscular disorders
Hepatic/renal/heme	Any active hepatobiliary disease or compromise (e.g., hepatitis) End-stage renal disease (dialysis) Severe anemias (e.g., sickle cell, aplastic)

From Johns Hopkins Preoperative Roadmap. Available at http://www.hopkinsmedicine.org/anesthesiology/Patient_Care/Preoperative_Roadmap.pdf.

hospital, and once a blood glucose level is assessed, we can determine the appropriate dosing of the medication. We also recommend that long-acting agents, such as insulin glargine (Lantus), be reduced by half the evening before surgery, although we are not aware of any studies that demonstrate a problem with standard dosing. Finally, we also try to counsel insulin diabetic patients that if they begin to feel hypoglycemic preoperatively, they can take 8 to 10 ounces of clear apple juice—no orange juice or any juice with pulp. This should not affect their ability to proceed with surgery.

Angiotensin Converting Enzyme Inhibitors

Today many patients are started on angiotensin converting enzyme inhibitors or angiotensin receptor blockers as the preferred therapy for hypertension. Studies are adequate to illustrate that these patients have a high propensity of developing hypotension that is unresponsive to normal pressors with the induction of general anesthesia. It has been demonstrated that this hypotension is more responsive to vasopressin, presumably because this drug activates the renin-angiotensin pathway that is suppressed by these inhibitors. Exceptions to this recommendation are those patients who are prescribed these medications as therapy for congestive heart failure (CHF). These patients should take their medications in the morning on the day of surgery. Of note, some studies have indicated that continuation of these medications may have benefit as renal protection in patients undergoing major vascular or cardiac surgery; however, the current recommendations are to hold these medicines the morning of surgery except for patients with CHF.

Anticoagulants

Depending upon the specific anticoagulant prescribed and the indications, the best time to stop these drugs preoperatively will vary. Typically, we recommend stopping warfarin 5 days in advance and clopidogrel 7 days preoperatively. Some patients will require anticoagulant bridging with enoxaparin (Lovenox), which can be stopped 12 to 24 hours preoperatively. One aspect to consider is whether the patient is a reasonable candidate for regional anesthesia rather than general anesthesia. For these patients, warfarin must be stopped for at least 5 days, clopidogrel must be stopped for 7 days, and enoxaparin must be stopped for at least 24 hours. Aspirin is not a contraindication to regional anesthesia. Many surgeons want aspirin stopped 7 to 10 days preoperatively; however, mounting evidence suggests this approach should be reconsidered except in a very few select types of surgery. The rationale for this recommendation is discussed below.

Herbal Medications

In general, because there is so little control over what constitutes herbal medications, we generally recommend that these medicines be stopped at least 24 hours preoperatively. Some specific supplements may need to be held even longer: examples are fish oil and vitamin E because of reported problems with bleeding, and most importantly, any supplements that contain ephedra (Ma Huang), a major ingredient in dietary supplements such as Metabolife. This herb has been shown to cause cardiomyopathy similar to Fen-Phen, which was taken off the market years ago because of several deaths associated with its use.

Aspirin

Aspirin affects platelet function secondary to changes in the platelet that occur during platelet synthesis. Consequently, while on aspirin, a patient's platelet function is affected for the life of the platelet. Studies have demonstrated that for the vast majority of patients, essentially all antiplatelet activity will cease if aspirin is stopped for 7 days. This also means that the platelets are primarily replaced within this time frame, which explains the rationale for discontinuing aspirin 7 days prior to surgery, despite the obvious benefits to patients who need antiplatelet therapy. Unfortunately, this current practice has now been shown to have absolute detrimental effects on a specific subset of patients, specifically those who have cardiac stents in place.

The most recent recommendations from the AHA discuss patients who have had stents placed recently and patients who are past this initial critical window. To summarize these recommendations, it

TABLE 2: Guidelines for preoperative medications

As a general rule for patients scheduled for surgery with anesthesia, we recommend all medications should be continued on the day of surgery. In particular, it is *very important* for patients to take their morning dose of the following medications:
- β-Blockers and any antiarrhythmics such as digoxin or calcium channel blockers
- Asthmatic medications including inhalers, theophylline, montelukast (Singulair), and/or steroids
- GERD medication
- Statins such as atorvastatin (Lipitor), simvastatin (Zocor), and rosuvastatin (Crestor)
- Aspirin (Unless specifically told otherwise by their surgeons, patients should continue to take aspirin)
- ACE/ARB if hypertension is difficult to control without them

In addition, consider starting patients on β-blockers preoperatively if they could be considered at risk for cardiac ischemia. Exceptions to these recommendations are summarized below.

Class of Medications	Medication	Recommendations
Oral hypoglycemic agents	Metformin (Glucophage), pioglitozone (Actos), glyburide (Glynase), tolazamide (Tolinase), rosiglitazone (Avandia), glimepiride (Amaryl), all others	Hold at least 8 hours preoperatively; hold morning dose day of surgery.
Diuretics	Furosemide (Lasix), hydrochlorothiazide (HCTZ)	Hold morning dose day of surgery *unless* prescribed for CHF; patients with CHF should take their morning dose of diuretics.
ACE/ARB inhibitors	Lisinopril (Prinivil), amlodipine/benazepril (Lotrel), captopril (Capoten), benazepril (Lotensin), fisonopril (Monopril), HCTZ compounds (Prinzide, Benicar, Diovan, Avelide), candesartan (Atacand)	Hold morning of surgery *unless* prescribed for CHF; patients with CHF should take their morning dose.
Insulin	NPH, regular	Hold insulin morning of surgery; bring insulin with patient to hospital.
All herbal supplements		Stop all herbal supplements at least 24 hours prior to surgery.

ACE/ARB, Angiotensin converting enzyme/angiotensin receptor blocker; *CHF,* congestive heart failure; *GERD,* gastroesophageal reflux disease
From Johns Hopkins Preoperative Roadmap. Available at http://www.hopkinsmedicine.org/anesthesiology/Patient_Care/Preoperative_Roadmap.pdf

is important to understand that patients who have just had cardiac stents placed are at high risk of thrombosis of these stents, and consequently that is why they are maintained on antiplatelet therapy. That therapy is currently clopidogrel and aspirin. Essentially, patients who receive bare metal stents should not have surgery for 6 months after placement, unless life or limb are threatened, primarily because this dual antiplatelet therapy should not be discontinued. For patients who receive drug-eluting stents, this dual therapy should continue for at least 1 year. Obviously, any emergency surgery requires a thorough discussion of benefits and risks among the patient, the surgeon, and the cardiologist.

Our major concern now, however, is for the patient who is past this window of dual antiplatelet therapy. The AHA does recommend lifelong aspirin therapy in all of these patients. Additionally, their recommendations are that aspirin be continued up to the day of surgery except for neurosurgery and retinal surgery, where the risk of bleeding is so significant. Possibly even more important is the resumption of antiplatelet therapy. Ideally, these patients should resume their medications the day after surgery. For patients who are on dual therapy, we do recommend stopping clopidogrel 7 days prior to surgery, but we advise maintaining the 81 mg dosage of aspirin.

It is essential to understand some of the differences between clopidogrel and aspirin to understand the reasoning behind our recommendations. Clopidogrel affects platelet function in a different manner than aspirin, and it is based on the circulating platelet versus the synthesis of the platelet. As long as clopidogrel is in circulation, it will negatively affect platelet function. Consequently, we cannot reverse this antiplatelet activity by administering new platelets, as we can with aspirin. That is why we recommend stopping clopidogrel 7 days prior to surgery but continuing the low dose aspirin, which seems to be an effective dosage to prevent thrombosis of cardiac

stents. What we frequently see are cardiologists who recommend stopping both medications 5 days prior to surgery to preserve some antiplatelet therapy. Our problem with this approach is that it provides a scenario in which the antiplatelet activity cannot be reversed by administering new platelets, whereas it can if the patient is simply on aspirin. It is also important to realize that we need antiplatelet therapy, not anticoagulation, to prevent stent thrombosis. Hence, warfarin and heparin are not appropriate substitutions.

PACEMAKERS

We are seeing an increasing volume of patients with pacemakers who are coming to surgery after the pacemaker has been implanted. One of the primary reasons for this increase is the rationale that patients with extremely low cardiac function (ejection fractions <30%) benefit substantially from pacemaker insertions, and in general, these will be implantable cardioverter/defibrillators (ICDs). It is important to understand how to manage these pacemakers preoperatively. The anesthesiologist will need documentation as to the type and function of these pacemakers as well as a recent interrogation of the device. Our recommendation, based on recent studies, is that routine pacemakers need interrogations within 6 months of surgery. Exceptions to this are pacer-dependent patients and ICDs; in both of these situations, the pacemaker should have been interrogated within 3 months of surgery.

Additionally, it is important to have a discussion with the anesthesiologist as to the recommendation on how to handle the pacemaker during surgery. Their concern will be the effect of Bovie interference on the normal pacemaker function. Essentially, a pacemaker will frequently sense Bovie interference as cardiac function, and the results will depend upon what type of pacemaker is implanted. Routine pacemakers will likely sense Bovie interference as heartbeats and will suppress any discharges. This will be particularly problematic in the pacer-dependent patient, because Bovie interference may result in no pacemaker discharge, causing asystole. An alternative method of dealing with pacer-dependent patients will likely be to have the pacemaker reprogrammed into asynchronous mode, which means there will be no sensing of the pacemaker. This results in constant firing of the pacemaker at the predetermined rate. Once surgery is completed, the pacemaker can be reprogrammed back to a sensing mode.

An ICD views Bovie interference differently; it looks for signs of cardiac dysrhythmias, such as ventricular fibrillation (VFib) or ventricular tachycardia (VTach). After sensing one of these tachyarrhythmias, the ICD will attempt a cardioversion internally by emitting a shock. If it senses the Bovie instead and emits this shock, the pacemaker may in fact generate VFib or VTach. Consequently, we generally require the ICD function to be turned off prior to surgery and turned back on once the surgery has been completed.

There may be opportunities to place a magnet over the pacemaker or ICD to accomplish these goals; however, without proper documentation of what will happen with a magnet, it is not prudent to use one, because not all pacemakers function the same with a magnet. This functionality should be defined in the interrogation report. Additionally, the type of surgery may also preclude the use of a magnet and may consequently require reprogramming of the pacemaker. We advise a discussion between the anesthesiologist and surgeon prior to surgery to avoid last minute cancellations or delays.

SUMMARY

As the severity and acuity of medical problems increase in surgical patients, it will become ever more important to assess these patients prior to the day of surgery. Hospitals that cannot afford a preoperative clinic must begin to explore methods of proactively getting patient information so that rules-based logic can be applied to preoperative management.

We are quite fond of the technology that has been developed at the Cleveland Clinic, referred to as the *HealthQuest*. This computerized patient questionnaire provides a detailed profiling of the surgical patient based on yes-and-no answers to health questions, and it can be used to guide preoperative testing and analysis. The surgeon's office staff can guide patients who are not able to use the computer through the questionnaire, and this technology has significantly reduced cancellations and delays at my institution. What has not been studied, but what many believe represents an area in which the greatest opportunities exist, is in better preparing surgical patients by customizing the preoperative period to their specific surgery and comorbidities.

Finally, we strongly recommend that the anesthesia department be engaged in helping to define preoperative protocols and management, because this information is changing rapidly. We do not believe the typical surgeon should attempt to remain current on the nuances of preoperative management, rather they should come to rely on their colleagues in anesthesia to establish effective clinical guidance.

SUGGESTED READINGS

Practice advisory for perioperative management of patients with cardiac rhythm-management devices: pacemakers and implantable cardioverter-defibrillators, *Anesthesiology* 103:186–198, 2005.

Practice Advisory for Preoperative Evaluation: report by task force on preoperative evaluation, *Anesthesiology* 96(2):485–496, 2002.

Adusumilli PS, Ben-Porat L, Pereira M, et al: The prevalence and predictors of herbal medicine use in surgical patients, *J Am Coll Surg* 198(4):583–590, 2004.

Brilakis E, Banerjee S, Berger P: Perioperative management of patients with coronary stents, *J Am Coll Card* 49(22):2145–2150, 2007.

Chee YL, Crawford JC, Watson HG, et al: Guidelines on the assessment of bleeding risk prior to surgery or invasive procedures: British Committee for Standards in Haematology, *Br J Haematol* 140(5):496–504, 2008.

Comfere T, Sprung J, Kumar MM, et al: Angiotensin inhibitors in the general surgical population, *Anesth Analg* 100(3):636–644, 2005.

Di Minno MN, Prisco D, Ruocco A, et al: Perioperative handling of patients on antiplatelet therapy with need for surgery, *Intern Emerg Med* 4(4):279–288, 2009.

Fleisher L: The preoperative electrocardiogram: What is the role in 2007? *Ann Surg* 246(2):171–172, 2007.

Fleisher L, Beckman J, Brown K, et al: ACA/AHA 2007 guidelines on perioperative cardiovascular evaluation and care for noncardiac surgery, *Circulation* 116(17), 2007.

IS A NASOGASTRIC TUBE NECESSARY FOLLOWING ALIMENTARY TRACT SURGERY?

Michael J. Snyder, MD

OVERVIEW

Nasogastric (NG) tubes were an important technical advance of the early twentieth century for the treatment of intestinal obstruction and the prevention of gastric dilatation following emergency abdominal surgery. Along with other improvements in anesthesia and fluid management, NG tubes helped to significantly lower the morbidity and mortality associated with emergency surgery of the alimentary tract. As such, they were rapidly adapted by many surgeons to elective abdominal surgery. NG tubes were used so extensively that Mayo famously stated that it was more important for a surgeon to have an NG tube in his pocket than a stethoscope. Without any scientific data, NG tubes quickly became used routinely for almost all abdominal surgeries. However, over the past few decades, this blind adherence to surgical dogma has been questioned. It appears that for many patients undergoing elective abdominal surgery, the risks of the NG tube significantly outweigh the benefits.

In 1790, Hunter stretched an eel skin over whalebone to create an NG tube for enteral feeding. Although he is credited with making the first NG tube, it took almost a hundred years for Kussmaul, in 1884, to use a tube to decompress the stomach in a patient with an ileus. The modern NG tube with a blunt tip was introduced by Levin in 1921 and was widely hailed as a significant advance in the treatment of patients following abdominal surgery, and it also permitted more intense research into gastrointestinal (GI) physiology. This led to McIver revealing in 1926 that the principal source of gas in postoperative distension is swallowed air, and distension may be prevented with an NG tube. In 1932, Wangensteen published his classic studies on three patients with small bowel obstruction, demonstrating the importance of the NG tube as an adjunct to abdominal surgery. Consequently, the NG tube was rapidly adopted by almost all surgeons following any surgery on the alimentary tract. This later culminated in the American College of Surgeons (ACS) publication on preoperative and postoperative care in 1971 declaring "intestinal decompression is required after resection and anastomosis of the gastrointestinal tract."

Postoperative ileus occurs following almost every abdominal operation and is due to multiple factors. Woods and colleagues (1978) studied the physiology of intestinal function after laparotomy and found that small bowel contractile activity returns within hours. Gastric motility resumes in about a day, and colonic motor function begins in 2 to 4 days. Intestinal, biliary, and pancreatic output is diminished but not eliminated. As a result, it appears that the key step to resuming normal GI function after abdominal surgery rests with the return of colonic motility. It is not surprising, therefore, that the majority of studies concerning routine use of NG tubes involve surgery on the colon.

The rationales for using NG tubes after elective abdominal surgery are multiple. Purported benefits include preventing postoperative gastric distension and associated nausea, vomiting, and aspiration, as well as treating the bloating of postoperative ileus and diminishing aerophagia. This would potentially lead to improved patient comfort from decompression of the GI tract, a more rapid return of bowel function, fewer pulmonary complications, and a shorter hospital stay. Aerophagia is of particular concern, as it may possibly place the anastomotic suture or staple lines under tension and increase the likelihood of anastomotic leaks. Additionally, distension of the abdomen from aerophagia may predispose to wound complications and incisional hernia formation. For gastric and proximal small intestinal anastomoses, NG tubes allow for early detection of postoperative hemorrhage. Finally, in the few patients having surgery for recurrent small bowel obstructions requiring an extensive adhesiolysis, a long nasointestinal tube may plicate the bowel and diminish the possibility of recurrent obstruction.

The possible complications of NG tubes are myriad (Table 1). Problems occur with placement of the tube and with malfunction. Procedures involving intestinal tubes can be labor intensive for nursing personnel, and tubes that fail to function properly may lead to significant morbidity. Of particular concern is the development of aerophagia despite appropriate placement of the NG tube; the tube rests in the back of the throat, and this promotes air swallowing. With poorly functioning tubes, this leads to intestinal distension and ileus, precisely the symptoms the tube was supposed to prevent.

Because of the complications of NG tubes and the significant patient dissatisfaction with their use, surgeons began questioning the need for their routine placement following elective surgery of the alimentary tract. As early as 1958, Gerber wrote that NG tubes were used too often and had frequent complications. He studied 600 postoperative patients, half of whom did not receive routine NG suction. The study was nonrandomized and included patients undergoing both elective and emergency surgery. Interestingly, the average NG volume was small (75 mL). Gerber hypothesized that postoperative ileus is a natural response to the operative trauma, and because NG tubes do not improve intestinal peristalsis, it is unlikely that they would speed the return of intestinal function.

Following this article, several nonrandomized retrospective studies were published in the 1970s. Burg and colleagues (1978) presented data on 134 patients: 85 had NG tubes, and 49 did not. Only 4% of patients who did not have an NG tube initially subsequently required one to relieve postoperative distension, all following

abdominoperineal resection; 63% of patients with an NG tube placed routinely had minor complications attributed to the tube, and 22% had tubes that functioned poorly. The authors concluded that it is safe to omit routine gastric decompression after elective intestinal surgery as long as oral fluids are limited until the passage of flatus.

Several prospective randomized studies were performed to more definitely determine patients who might benefit from postoperative decompression. Reasbeck and colleagues evaluated the routine use of NG tubes in 97 patients with an intestinal suture line. This included patients with low rectal resections, colonic resections, gastric resections, gastric drainage procedures, esophageal resections, and bile duct–enteric anastomoses. They found no statistically significant differences between the two groups with regard to postoperative complications, although there was a trend to more pulmonary complications in patients with a routine NG tube.

Bauer and colleagues (1985) studied 200 patients in a prospective randomized trial to determine whether postoperative distension without an NG tube occurs after major elective abdominal surgery, and whether any wound complications can be attributed to the omission of an NG tube. In patients treated with a routine NG tube, the tube remained in place an average of 6 days. Interestingly, five patients (5%) required reinsertion of the tube sometime during their hospitalization. In patients treated without a tube initially, 6 patients (6%) required insertion of an NG tube. No pulmonary, wound, or anastomotic complications were reported in either group. The authors noted the increased comfort and mobility of the patients treated without routine NG decompression and found that 70% of their patients treated with an NG tube found the tube to be a significant source of pain.

From Denmark, Olesen and colleagues (1984) evaluated 97 patients in a prospective randomized study concerning elective colorectal surgery. They included patients receiving a colostomy, but the great majority of the patients in both the tube and nontube groups had colocolonic anastomoses. They found no statistical significant differences with regard to postoperative complications and the duration of postoperative ileus, except, interestingly, that patients in the no-tube group passed flatus significantly earlier. They hypothesized that patients in the no-tube group could be mobilized earlier with less discomfort. In addition, 11 patients in the NG-tube arm vomited despite a functioning tube, and the degree of nausea was equal between the two groups. The authors concluded that NG intubation should be performed only in those patients exhibiting postoperative gastric distension with vomiting.

Cheadle and colleagues (1985) prospectively randomized 200 patients into four study groups to assess the need for NG intubation and to evaluate any effect cimetidine might have on postoperative nausea and vomiting. They found that length of hospitalization was increased in patients treated with NG decompression, and they found a higher rate of patient discomfort with the tube. Interestingly, although cimetidine did not affect tube insertion or the incidence of vomiting, it was associated with an increased incidence of pneumonia.

MacRae and colleagues (1992) evaluated the routine need for NG tube decompression following both elective and emergent surgery involving anastomoses throughout the alimentary tract. Unlike previous studies, patients with peritonitis were included. They prospectively studied 101 consecutive laparotomies without an NG tube and compared them to 101 patients who had surgery the previous year with routine tube placement. They included patients receiving ostomies and foregut anastomoses, and colonic anastomoses were more than 30% of each group. The NG tube remained in place an average of 4.5 days, and two patients required reinsertion of the tube. In the nontube group, 9 NG tubes had to be inserted in the postoperative period; persistent nausea and vomiting was the reason for tube insertion in all but one case. The complication rate between the two groups was similar, and no differences were observed in the incidence of anastomotic leak, wound disruption, or pulmonary dysfunction. A significant improvement in the length of hospital

TABLE 1: Complications of NG tubes

Common	Uncommon	Rare
Vomiting	Esophagitis	Tracheoesophageal fistula
Atelectasis	Pneumonia	Esophageal or gastric
Sinusitis	Electrolyte	perforation
Patient discomfort	abnormalities	

stay in the no-tube group was observed, along with improvement in all phases of diet advancement. Finally, the authors concluded that 91% of patients having both routine and emergency surgery of the alimentary tract could be spared the discomfort and risk of NG intubation.

Because of the variability of the operations in other studies, Colvin (1986) and Racette (1987) and their colleagues studied purely elective colonic surgery. Colvin treated 138 patients prospectively and randomly to either an NG tube, a nasointestinal (Cantor) tube, or no tube. The no-tube group had a significantly shorter period of postoperative ileus, but hospital stay was equivalent among the three groups. The major clinical difference among the three groups was the improved patient comfort in the patients treated without any NG or nasointestinal tube. Racette and colleagues (1987) evaluated 56 patients undergoing elective colonic surgery at a community hospital. They found that atelectasis was more common in the patients treated with NG tubes and that abdominal distension occurred in 39% of the patients treated without an NG tube; 14% required insertion of a tube, and the hospital stay was prolonged in these patients.

Wolff and colleagues (1989) published one of the largest series concerning NG decompression in purely uncomplicated, elective colorectal surgery. In this series, 535 patients were prospectively randomized to either an NG tube or no tube. The authors excluded patients with peritonitis, extensive adhesions, enterotomies, previous pelvic irradiation, intraabdominal infection, pancreatitis, colonic obstruction, prolonged operating times, or a difficult endotracheal intubation, and 13% of the no-tube group required tube insertion for abdominal distension and vomiting, and 5% of the patients treated with NG tubes initially needed reinsertion of the tube sometime during their hospitalization. No difference in pulmonary or wound complications were found, and length of stay was equivalent. Importantly, repeat analysis of this same cohort of patients 5 years later did not reveal any increase in subsequent incisional hernia in those patients who had abdominal distension when no NG tube was used postoperatively. The authors concluded that routine NG decompression was unwarranted in elective colonic surgery.

To determine the effect of NG decompression in patients with bowel anastomoses, Cunningham and colleagues (1992) prospectively randomized 102 patients. Excluded were patients with peritonitis, chronic bowel obstruction, gross fecal contamination, and previous abdominal or pelvic irradiation. They found a significant improvement in the return of bowel function and diminished hospital stay in patients treated without routine NG decompression, and 8% of the patients treated without an NG tube required insertion of one for abdominal distension.

Despite all of these multiple prospective randomized studies, evaluating multiple types of patients undergoing laparotomies with or without intestinal anastomoses, NG tube use after elective surgery on the alimentary tract is still routine and unquestioned by many surgeons. As a result, two meta-analyses have tried to answer the question of whether NG decompression is necessary following elective surgery on the alimentary tract. Cheatham and colleagues published their analysis in 1995, which included 26 trials comprising 3964 patients. Not all the trials were prospectively randomized. They found that patients were started on oral intake and had fewer pulmonary complications without an NG tube. These patients, however, had greater abdominal distension and vomiting. No other complication was noted to have an increased incidence. They concluded, "For every patient requiring insertion of a nasogastric tube in the postoperative period, at least 20 patients will not require nasogastric decompression."

The second meta-analysis was performed 10 years later by Nelson and colleagues, in 2005 with an update in 2007. The update in 2007 included 33 studies involving 5240 patients, all of whom were prospectively randomized. They discovered that patients treated without an NG tube had an earlier return of bowel function and fewer pulmonary complications. The incidence of anastomotic leak was equivalent between the two groups, and length of stay was shorter without an NG tube. The authors concluded, "Routine nasogastric decompression does not accomplish any of its intended goals and should be abandoned in favor of selective use of the nasogastric tube."

Early mobilization is critical for optimal outcomes following major surgery on the alimentary tract, and an NG tube is just one more barrier to the patient ambulating. Early ambulation helps to prevent thromboembolic events and speeds the return of enteric function. Although I do not routinely use an NG tube with open or laparoscopic colon resections, some patients may benefit from NG tubes, such as those with peritonitis, severe ileus or obstruction, extensive adhesions, multiple enterotomies, or pancreatitis. I do not treat emergency patients any differently, as long as they do not have any of the above conditions. Finally, NG tubes are unnecessary for routine surgery of the alimentary tract and should be used only when indicated by the patient's condition and the pathology.

SELECTED READINGS

Baker JW: Stitchless plication for recurring obstruction of the small bowel, *Am J Surg* 116:316–324, 1968.

Bauer JJ, Gelernt IM, Salky BA, Kreel I: Is routine postoperative nasogastric decompression really necessary? *Ann Surg* 201:233–236, 1985.

Burg R, Geigle CF, Faso JM, et al: Omission of routine gastric decompression, *Dis Colon Rectum* 21:98–100, 1978.

Cheadle WG, Vitale GC, Mackie CR, et al: Prophylactic postoperative nasogastric decompression: a prospective study of its requirement and the influence of cimetidine in 200 patients, *Ann Surg* 202:361–366, 1985.

Cheatham ML, Chapman WC, Key SP, et al: A meta-analysis of selective versus routine nasogastric decompression after elective laparotomy, *Ann Surg* 221:468–478, 1995.

Colvin DB, Lee W, Eisenstat TE, et al: The role of nasointestinal intubation in elective colonic surgery, *Dis Colon Rectum* 29:295–259, 1986.

Cunningham J, Temple WJ, Langevin JM, et al: A prospective randomized trial of routine postoperative nasogastric decompression in patients with bowel anastomosis, *Can J Surg* 35:629–632, 1992.

Gerber A, Rogers FA, Smith LL, et al: The treatment of paralytic ileus without the use of gastrointestinal suction, *Surg Gynecol Obstet* 107:247–250, 1958.

McRae HM, Fischer JD, Yakimets WW: Routine omission of nasogastric intubation after gastrointestinal surgery, *Can J Surg* 35:625–628, 1992.

Nelson R, Edwards S, Tse B: Systematic review of prophylactic nasogastric decompression after abdominal operations, *Br J Surg* 92:673–680, 2005.

Nelson R, Edwards S, Tse B: Prophylactic nasogastric decompression after abdominal surgery, *Cochrane Database Syst Rev* (3) CD004929, 2007.

Olesin KL, Birch M, Bardram L, et al: Value of nasogastric tube after colorectal surgery, *Acta Chir Scand* 150:251–253, 1984.

Otchy DP, Wolff BG, Van Heerden JA, et al: Does the avoidance of nasogastric decompression following elective abdominal colorectal surgery affect the incidence of incisional hernia? *Dis Colon Rectum* 38:604–608, 1995.

Racette DL, Chang FC, Trekell ME, et al: Is nasogastric intubation necessary in colon operations? *Am J Surg* 154:640–642, 1987.

Reasbeck PG, Rice ML, Herbison GP: Nasogastric intubation after intestinal resection, *Surg Gynecol Obstet* 159:354–358, 1984.

Savassi-Rocha PR, Conceicao SA, Ferreirra JT, et al: Evaluation of the routine use of the nasogastric tube digestive operation by a prospective controlled study, *Surg Gynecol Obstet* 174:317–321, 1992.

Wangensteen OH, Paine JR: Treatment of acute intestinal obstruction by suction with the duodenal tube, *JAMA* 101:1532–1539, 1933.

Wolff BG, Pemberton JH, Van Heerden JA, et al: Elective colon and rectal surgery without nasogastric decompression: a prospective randomized trial, *Ann Surg* 209:670–675, 1989.

Woods JH, et al: Postoperative ileus: a colonic problem? *Surgery* 84:527–533, 1978.

SURGICAL SITE INFECTIONS

Lena M. Napolitano, MD

EPIDEMIOLOGY

More than 40 million inpatient and outpatient surgical procedures are performed in the United States each year, and 2% to 5% of these are complicated by surgical site infections (SSIs), the most common nosocomial infection among surgical patients and the second most common nosocomial infection overall. SSIs result in increased lengths of stay (mean, 7 days) and additional cost of about $400 to $2600 per infection—a total of $130 to $845 million per year.

Among the four health care–associated infections—pneumonia, SSI, urinary tract infection (UTI), and bloodstream infection—SSI is the second most common health care–associated infection, accounting for 17% of all health care–associated infections among hospitalized patients. A similar rate was obtained from the National Healthcare Safety Network (NHSN) from hospital data reported in 2006 through 2008, which counted 15,862 SSIs following 830,748 operative procedures, with an overall rate of nearly 2%.

DEFINITIONS

SSIs are defined in three specific categories by the Centers for Disease Control and Prevention (CDC): superficial incisional SSI, deep incisional SSI, and organ/space SSI, depending on the depth of the infection at the surgical incision site (Figure 1). In addition, the SSI must occur within 30 days after the operative procedure if no implant is left in place, or within 1 year if an implant is in place, and the infection appears to be related to the operative procedure. More specific criteria regarding these definitions are available in the CDC "Guidelines for Prevention of Surgical Site Infection."

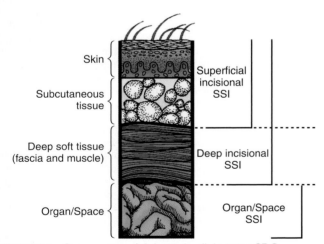

FIGURE 1 Cross-section of abdominal wall depicting CDC classifications of SSI. *Superficial incisional SSI* involves only the skin and subcutaneous tissue layer of the incision. *Deep incisional SSI* involves deep soft tissues, such as fascia and muscle layers. *Organ/space SSI* involves any part of the body opened or manipulated during the operative procedure, excluding the skin, fascia, or muscle layers (e.g., intraabdominal abscess, thoracic empyema). *(From Mangram AJ, Horan TC, Pearson ML, et al: Guideline for prevention of surgical site infection, Infect Control Hosp Epidemiol 20(4):247–278, 1999.)*

RISK FACTORS FOR SURGICAL SITE INFECTIONS

SSI risk is strongly associated with wound classification, with low risk for SSI in clean and clean-contaminated wound classes, and high risk for SSI in contaminated and dirty/infected wound classes (Table 1). In a system initially developed by the National Nosocomial Infections Surveillance System (NNIS), these three independent variables have been shown to be associated with SSI risk.

The National Healthcare Safety Network (NHSN) was established in 2005 to integrate and supersede three legacy surveillance systems at the CDC: the NNIS system, the Dialysis Surveillance Network (DSN), and the National Surveillance System for Healthcare Workers (NaSH). Similar to the NNIS system, NHSN facilities voluntarily report their health care–associated infection surveillance data for aggregation into a single national database.

The NHSN SSI Risk Index includes an American Society of Anesthesiologists (ASA) score greater than 2, classification of the wound as contaminated or dirty, and prolonged duration of operation (Table 2). Although the risk of infection increases within the wound classification, it has been shown to be also dependent within each wound class on the NNIS classification (Table 2).

Basic SSI Risk Index

The index used in NHSN assigns surgical patients into categories based on the presence of three major risk factors; the patient's SSI risk category is simply the number of these factors present at the time of the operation:

1. Operation lasting longer than the duration cut-point hours, where the duration cut point is the approximate 75th percentile of the duration of surgery in minutes for the operative procedure
2. Contaminated (class 3) or dirty-infected (class 4) wound class
3. ASA classification of 3, 4, or 5

The laparoscopic surgical approach is associated with decreased SSI incidence, and a modified risk index, adding a category of −1 for a procedure performed with a laparoscope, has been created to address this approach.

Additional patient-specific risk factors for SSI have also been identified (Box 1) that are not included in this risk index, including the presence of anemia, intraoperative blood transfusion, and colonization with resistant pathogens. This SSI risk index warrants reevaluation for the future, particularly with regard to resistant pathogens and other patient-specific risk factors that are not modifiable prior to surgical intervention. It is of paramount importance to include an SSI risk assessment in all future clinical trials in which SSI is a primary outcome measure.

TABLE 1: Wound classification and risk for SSI

Classification	Wound Class	SSI Risk
Clean	0	Low
Clean contaminated: Gastrointestinal/genitourinary tracts entered in a controlled manner	1	
Contaminated: Open, fresh, traumatic wounds; infected urine, bile or gross spillage from gastrointestinal tract	2	
Dirty/infected	3	High

TABLE 2: National Healthcare Safety Network (NHSN) Risk Index Scoring

According to the NHSN Risk Index, risk of SSI increases with degree of contamination and with more severe wound classification. Three independent variables are associated with SSI risk. Score 1 point for each:
1. American Society of Anesthesiologists (ASA) score* >2
2. Contaminated or dirty/infected wound classification
3. Length of operation above the 75th percentile for the specific operation being performed

Wound Class	All	NNIS 0	NNIS 1	NNIS 2	NNIS 3
Clean	2.1%	1.0%	2.3%	5.4%	N/A
Clean contaminated	3.3%	2.1%	4.0%	9.5%	N/A
Contaminated	6.4%	N/A	3.4%	6.8%	13.2%
Dirty/infected	7.1%	N/A	3.1%	8.1%	12.8%
All	2.8%	1.5%	2.9%	6.8%	13.0%

NHSN Risk Index Category

*ASA score ranges from 1 to 5, with 1 = normal, healthy to 5 = patient not expected to survive for 24 hours with or without operation.
NNIS, National Nosocomial Infections Surveillance System
Modified from data presented in *Am J Infect Control* 29:404-421, 2001.

Infection Prevention

Preventive measures for SSI include antimicrobial prophylaxis; diligent sterilization methods; proper ventilation of operating rooms; use of barriers; omission of shaving in favor of clipping hair, when hair removal is required; proper surgical skin preparation and surgical techniques; maintenance of normothermia; good glycemic control; and the provision of supplemental oxygen. The national Surgical Infection Prevention Project (SIP) was initiated as the first component of the Surgical Care Improvement Project (SCIP). Initiated in 2003 by the Centers for Medicaid and Medicare Services (CMMS) and the CDC, the SCIP partnership sought to substantially reduce surgical mortality and morbidity through collaborative efforts.

Despite evidence of the effectiveness of preoperative antimicrobials for SSI prevention and the publication of guidelines for antimicrobial prophylaxis, it was recognized that use of preoperative antimicrobials was often suboptimal. As part of the SIP initiative, three performance measures were developed:
- *SIP-1:* Proportion of patients in whom intravenous antimicrobial prophylaxis is initiated within 1 hour before incision
- *SIP-2:* Proportion of patients given prophylactic antimicrobials consistent with published guidelines
- *SIP-3:* Proportion of patients whose antimicrobial prophylaxis is discontinued within 24 hours after surgery

Numerous studies document that antimicrobial prophylaxis for SSI is most effective when provided 30 to 60 minutes prior to the initial surgical incision, allowing adequate blood and tissue concentrations at the time of skin incision. Risk of SSI increases when antimicrobial prophylaxis is given too early (more than 2 hours prior to skin incision) or too late (after skin incision). In a recent study of 4472 patients, SSI risk increased incrementally as the interval of time between antibiotic infusion and the surgical incision increased. These data from a large multicenter collaborative study confirmed lower SSI risk when surgical antimicrobial prophylaxis with cephalosporins and other antibiotics with short infusion times were given within 30 minutes prior to surgical incision.

BOX 1: Risk factors for the development of SSIs

Patient Factors

Ascites
Chronic inflammation
Corticosteroid therapy (controversial)
Obesity
Diabetes
Extremes of age
Hypocholesterolemia
Hypoxemia
Peripheral vascular disease (especially for lower extremity surgery)
Perioperative anemia
Prior site irradiation
Recent operation
Remote infection
Skin carriage of *Staphylococcus* species
Skin disease in the area of infection (e.g., psoriasis)
Undernutrition

Environmental Factors

Contaminated medications
Inadequate disinfection/ sterilization
Inadequate skin antisepsis
Inadequate ventilation

Treatment Factors

Drains
Emergency procedure
Hypothermia
Inadequate antibiotic prophylaxis
Oxygenation (controversial)
Prolonged preoperative hospitalization
Prolonged operative time
Intraoperative blood transfusion

Modified from National Nosocomial Infections Surveillance System (NNIS) System Report: Data summary from January 1992–June 2001 [issued August 2001], *Am J Infect Control* 29:404–421, 2001.

In addition, the correct antimicrobial must be administered to cover the potential causative pathogens, depending on the surgical procedure performed. The SCIP Pocket Card, updated in October 2010 (Table 3), provides a list of the recommended preoperative antimicrobials for specific surgical procedures.

The first report of the SIP baseline results from a systematic random sample of 34,133 Medicare inpatients undergoing surgery in U.S. hospitals in 2001 documented that only 55.7% of patients received a dose of parenteral antimicrobial prophylaxis within 1 hour before surgical incision. Antimicrobial agents consistent with published guidelines were administered to 92.6% of patients, and antimicrobial prophylaxis was discontinued within 24 hours of surgery end time for only 40.7% of patients. Interestingly, only 28% of these surgical patients had compliance with all three of these performance measures. It was concluded that "substantial opportunities exist to improve the use of prophylactic antimicrobials for patients undergoing major surgery."

We have made truly remarkable progress in the United States with appropriate perioperative antimicrobial prophylaxis since that initial published report. Compliance with SIP-1, antibiotics being given 60 minutes prior to incision, increased from 55.7% to 91.6%; compliance with SIP-2, administering guideline antibiotics, increased from 92.6% to 95.8%; and compliance with SIP-3, discontinuing antibiotics, increased from 40.7% to 87.7% (Figure 2).

Additional Strategies for Surgical Site Infection Prevention

Surgical Hand Antisepsis

Surgical hand antisepsis to destroy bacteria is routinely carried out before undertaking invasive procedures. A recent review of 10 trials confirmed that alcohol rubs used in preparation for surgery by the surgical team are as effective as aqueous scrubbing in SSI prevention.

TABLE 3: Surgical Care Improvement Project (SCIP) Pocket Card October 2009: Recommended Preoperative Antimicrobials for Specific Surgical Procedures

Surgical Procedure	Approved Antibiotics
Coronary artery bypass grafting, other cardiac or vascular intervention	Cefazolin, cefuroxime, or vancomycin* If β-lactam allergy: vancomycin[†] or clindamycin[†]
Hysterectomy	Cefotetan, cefazolin, cefoxitin, cefuroxime, or ampicillin-sulbactam If β-lactam allergy: Clindamycin + aminoglycoside Clindamycin + quinolone Clindamycin + aztreonam *or* Metronizadole + aminoglycoside Metronizadole + quinolone
Hip/Knee arthroplasty	Cefazolin, cefuroxime, or vancomycin* If β-lactam allergy: vancomycin[†] or clindamycin[†]
Colon	Cefotetan, cefoxitin, ampicillin-sulbactam, ertapenem *or* Cefazolin or cefuroxime + metronidazole If β-lactam allergy: Clindamycin + aminoglycoside Clindamycin + quinolone Clindamycin + aztreonam *or* Metronizadole + aminoglycoside Metronizadole + quinolone

*Vancomycin is acceptable with a physician, nurse practitioner, or physician assistant pharmacist-documented justification for its use. A single dose of ertapenem is recommended for colon procedures.

[†]For cardiac, orthopedic, and vascular surgery, if the patient is allergic to β-lactam antibiotics, vancomycin and clindamycin are acceptable substitutes. From Surgical Care Improvement Project Pocket Card, October 2010. Prepared by the Oklahoma Foundation of Medical Quality, the Quality Improvement Organization Support Center for Patient Safety, under contract with the Centers of Medicare & Medicaid Services (CMS), an agency of the US Department of Health and Human Services. This table does not necessarily reflect CMS policy.

There is no evidence to suggest that any particular alcohol rub is better than another. Evidence from four studies suggests that chlorhexidine gluconate–based aqueous scrubs are more effective than povidone-iodine–based aqueous scrubs in terms of the numbers of bacterial colony-forming units on the hands.

Chlorhexidine as a Surgical Site Skin Preparation

Preoperative skin antisepsis of the surgical site is performed to reduce the risk of SSI by removal of skin microorganisms. A review of six randomized controlled trials identified significant heterogeneity, and the trial results could not be pooled. In one study, infection rates were significantly lower when skin was prepared using chlorhexidine compared with iodine. No evidence of a benefit was found in four trials associated with the use of iodophor-impregnated drapes. More recent studies have documented that chlorhexidine provided superior skin decontamination and reduced SSIs compared with povidone-iodine combinations.

Appropriate Hair Removal

The preparation of the surgical site has traditionally included the routine removal of body hair; however, some studies have suggested that this is deleterious. A Cochrane systematic review of 11 randomized clinical trials, and three trials (n = 3193) that compared shaving with clipping, found that there were statistically more SSIs with shaving than with clipping (risk ratio [RR], 2.02; 95% confidence interval [CI], 1.21 to 3.36). If it is necessary to remove hair, clipping results in fewer SSIs than shaving the patient with a razor.

Normothermia Maintenance during Surgery

Perioperative hypothermia is common and adversely affects clinical outcomes. The primary beneficial effects of warming are mediated through increased blood flow and oxygen tension at the tissue level. Hypothermia may facilitate SSI in two ways. First, sufficient intraoperative hypothermia triggers thermoregulatory vasoconstriction. Second, considerable evidence indicates that mild core hypothermia directly impairs immune function, including T-cell–mediated antibody production and nonspecific oxidative bactericide by neutrophils. Randomized controlled trials have documented that perioperative warming is associated with a significant reduction in SSI and that this simple preventive strategy should be implemented in all surgical patients.

Normoglycemia Maintenance During Surgery

Perioperative hyperglycemia has been associated with increased SSIs, and previous recommendations have been to treat glucose levels above 200 mg/dL. Recent studies have questioned the optimal glycemic control regimen to prevent SSIs. A recent Cochrane systematic review included five randomized controlled clinical trials with a total of 773 patients randomized. Because of heterogeneity in patient populations, perioperative period, glycemic target, route of insulin administration, and definitions of outcome measures, combination of the results of these trials into a meta-analysis was not appropriate; however, the authors concluded that evidence was insufficient to support strict glycemic control in the intraoperative and postoperative period for the prevention of SSIs.

No randomized trials have evaluated immediate preoperative glycemic control in any setting or intraoperative and postoperative glycemic control in non-ICU patients. High-quality evidence for strict glycemic control in the intraoperative and postoperative periods among surgical ICU, cardiac, and noncardiac patients to reduce SSIs, independent of other potential benefits, is also lacking. Further large, adequately powered, well-designed randomized trials are necessary to identify the ideal target for perioperative glycemic control in patients at high risk for SSIs. Future trials should report all nosocomial infections as well as SSIs. Given the heterogeneity seen in the included trials, it would appear that trials should be targeted at very specific populations, and attempts to draw broader conclusions should not be made. At present, we should strive at least to maintain blood glucose below 200 mg/dL in the perioperative period in our surgical patients.

Supplemental Oxygen in the Perioperative Period

Several randomized controlled trials have been conducted to assess the benefit of perioperative supplemental oxygen in SSI reduction, yet meta-analyses have arrived at different conclusions. On careful review, a number of problems with the conduct of these trials has been noted: 1) SSI definition was not consistent with CDC definitions; 2) the interval for assessment of SSI was variable, ranging from 15 to 30 days; 3) SSI was captured retrospectively in some studies and was not always a primary outcome measure; 4) no assessment of the

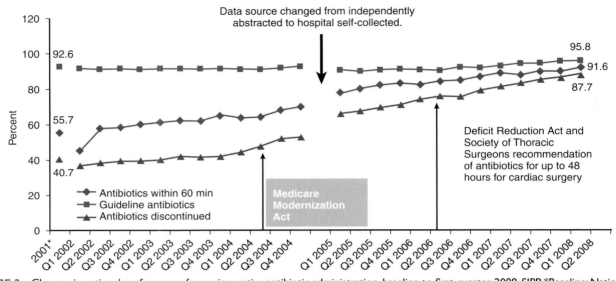

FIGURE 2   Changes in national performance for perioperative antibiotic administration, baseline to first quarter 2008, SIPP. *Baseline: National sample of 39,000 Medicare patients undergoing surgery in U.S. hospitals during 2001. (*Data from Bratzler DW, Houck PM, Richards C, et al: Use of antimicrobial prophylaxis for major surgery: baseline results from the National Surgical Infection Prevention Project, Arch Surg 140:174–182, 2005. Additional data provided by D. Bratzler, MD, 2009.*)

patient's individual risk factors for SSI was performed; 5) no control of perioperative antibiotic prophylaxis timing or selection was performed; and 6) there was variable provision of high FiO_2 supplemental oxygen in each of the studies.

Our first priority at the institutional level should be to universally implement all the evidence-based practices that reduce SSIs. The "SSI bundle" from the Institute for Healthcare Improvement includes 1) appropriate use of antibiotics, 2) appropriate hair removal, 3) perioperative glucose control, and 4) perioperative normothermia. This is one effective approach. The additional provision of increased inspired oxygen concentrations should be considered as an additional quality improvement measure, particularly in institutions with high SSI rates. A Collaborative of 44 hospitals implemented the SSI preventive strategies discussed above and documented a significant reduction in the SSI rate, from 2.3% to 1.7%, representing a 27% reduction in the first 3 months versus the last 3 months of the 1 year project. Finally, prospective SSI surveillance, including postdischarge surveillance, should be instituted to obtain accurate information regarding institutional SSI rates.

SURGICAL SITE INFECTION AND COLORECTAL SURGERY

Surgeons have held a long-standing belief that mechanical bowel preparation is an efficient strategy to reduce SSI and anastomotic leak rates following elective colorectal surgery. Recent systematic reviews have found no statistically significant evidence that patients benefit from mechanical bowel preparation, either in fewer SSIs or reduced anastomotic leak rates. In contrast, the use of nonabsorbable enteral antimicrobials to cover aerobic and anaerobic colonic bacteria, in addition to preoperative IV antibiotics, is associated with a significant reduction in SSI by at least 75%.

TREATMENT OF SURGICAL SITE INFECTION

Once superficial or deep incisional SSI is diagnosed, pathogen identification is of paramount importance. In years past, the surgical incision was opened, and dressing changes were initiated with no culture of the surgical site obtained. In today's era of multiple drug-resistant

pathogens, a Gram stain and culture of the surgical site should always be obtained to determine the optimal antimicrobial therapy required for SSI treatment.

SSI treatment includes four strategies for success: 1) early empiric antimicrobial therapy; 2) sound decision making regarding whether the surgical site should be opened; 3) pathogen identification; and 4) deescalation of antimicrobial therapy once culture results are available.

For organ/space SSI, source control and pathogen identification are both high priorities to achieve successful treatment. In the case of intraabdominal abscess, source control can be provided by either interventional radiology, percutaneous drainage, or open surgical drainage of the abscess. Abscess fluid should be sent for Gram stain and culture, and empiric antimicrobial treatment should be deescalated once culture results are available.

CURRENT CHALLENGES IN SURGICAL SITE INFECTION

There are a number of growing challenges in SSI, including resistant pathogens, an increasing elderly population, more patients with chronic diseases or immunocompromised states undergoing surgery, and more patients undergoing surgery for solid-organ transplantation and placement of prosthetic devices. We first reported that methicillin-resistant *Staphylococcus aureus* (MRSA) was the most common cause of SSI in vascular surgery patients (n = 772 over a 2-year period) in 2004. MRSA has since emerged as the leading cause of postoperative infection in vascular surgery patients, and it is associated with substantial morbidity, increased hospital lengths of stay, and higher incidences of amputation and graft removal. At that time, we advocated for empiric MRSA antimicrobial coverage in all patients with postoperative infectious complications in vascular surgery with deescalation once cultures are available, and strategies to prevent MRSA-associated SSI were recommended.

Comparison of the causative pathogens for SSI in U.S. hospitals (Figure 3) documents that *S. aureus* incidence increased from 22.5% (1986 to 2003) to 30% (2006 to 2007), with MRSA now the leading causative pathogen, comprising 49.2% of all isolates. In a study of 8302 patients readmitted to U.S. hospitals with culture-confirmed SSI from 2003 through 2007, it was noted that the proportion of

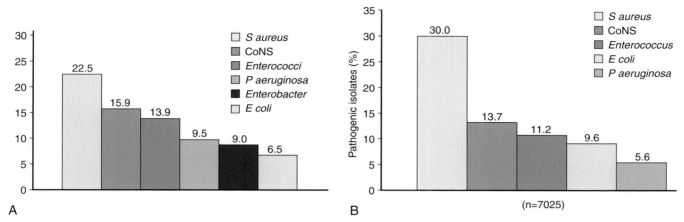

FIGURE 3   Comparison of causative pathogens for SSI in U.S. hospitals. *Staphylococcus aureus* increased from 22.5% to 30%, with MRSA now the leading causative pathogen. **A,** Pathogens associated with SSI (n = 2984) in U.S. hospitals according to the Nosocomial Infections Surveillance System (NNIS), 1986 to 2003. *S. aureus* was the most common SSI pathogen, comprising 22.5% of all isolates. The percentage of SSIs associated with gram-negative bacilli decreased from 56.5% in 1986 to 33.8% in 2003. **B,** Pathogens associated with SSI (n = 7025) in U.S. hospitals, 2006 to 2007, according to the National Healthcare Safety Network (NHSN). *S. aureus* was the most common SSI pathogen (n = 2108), with MRSA comprising 1006 (49.2%) of all isolates. CoNS, Coagulase-negative staphylococci. (**A,** *Data from Gaynes, R, Edwards JR: National Nosocomial Infections Surveillance System: overview of nosocomial infections caused by Gram-negative bacilli, Clin Infect Dis 41(6):848-854, 2005.* **B,** *Data from Hidron AI, Edwards JR, Patel J, et al: NHSN annual update: antimicrobial-resistant pathogens associated with healthcare-associated infections: annual summary of data reported to the National Healthcare Safety Network at the Centers for Disease Control and Prevention, 2006-2007, Infect Control Hosp Epidemiol 29:996–1011, 2008.*)

infections resulting from MRSA significantly increased, from 16.1% to 20.6%, and it was associated with higher mortality rates, longer hospital stays, and higher hospital costs. Based on this important finding, some have strongly advocated active screening for nasal carriage of MRSA prior to elective surgery with modification of antimicrobials for SSI prevention based on those results. Eradication of MRSA before surgery appears to lower the rates of SSI resulting from MRSA, and it is recommended.

In contrast, a prospective interventional cohort study that employed a universal, rapid MRSA admission-screening strategy among 21,754 surgical patients at a Swiss teaching hospital reported that nosocomial MRSA infection, including SSI, did not decrease; however, relatively low rates of MRSA infection (<5%) were present at the start of this study.

Most recently, a preventative "MRSA bundle" has been developed that includes five components: 1) MRSA nasal screening of patients upon admission, transfer, and discharge using polymerase chain reaction (PCR); 2) contact isolation of MRSA-positive patients; 3) standardized hand hygiene; 4) cultural transformation campaign, with staff and leadership engagement through positive deviance; and 5) ongoing monitoring of process and outcome measures.

Implementation of the MRSA bundle was associated with a significant decrease in MRSA transmission, from 5.8 to 3.0 per 1000 bed-days; a significant reduction in MRSA nosocomial infections, from 2.0 to 1.0 per 1000 bed-days; and a significant decrease in overall SSIs, with a 65% reduction in orthopedic SSIs from MRSA and a 1% decrease in cardiac SSIs from MRSA.

The proliferation of community-acquired MRSA (CA-MRSA) has also significantly impacted SSI rates. Recent studies document that CA-MRSA is replacing traditional healthcare-associated or nosocomial MRSA strains in SSIs among inpatients. A report from a large community hospital in St. Louis examined the rates of SSI resulting from *S. aureus* in a total of 122,040 surgical procedures in an earlier period (2003 to 2006) versus a later period (2006 to 2007). MRSA was identified as the SSI pathogen in 40% of all inpatients in both time periods. Interestingly, the percentage of clindamycin-susceptible MRSA, as distinguished from CA-MRSA, as a causative pathogen for SSI in inpatients rose from 9% in the early period to 19% in the later period. This increase in the rate of SSI related to CA-MRSA

was observed only among inpatients (RR, 2.2; 95% CI, 1.3 to 3.8; $P = .007$) and not among ambulatory patients. Similarly, CA-MRSA has emerged as a leading cause of healthcare-associated infections among patients with prosthetic joint SSIs.

The use of perioperative intranasal mupirocin for SSI prevention, particularly in patients with *Staphylococcus aureus* or MRSA nasal colonization, remains controversial. Reviews of multiple clinical trials documented that no reduction in SSI was seen in general surgery or cardiac surgery patients; however, in nongeneral surgery (cardiac, vascular, orthopedic) patients, the use of mupirocin was associated with a reduction in SSI. Interestingly, the surgical clinical trials did demonstrate a significant reduction in the rate of nosocomial *S. aureus* infections associated with mupirocin use (RR, 0.55; 95% CI, 0.34 to 0.89); however, this effect disappeared when the analysis only included SSIs caused by *S. aureus* (RR, 0.63; 95% CI, 0.38 to 1.04), possibly due to a lack of statistical power.

Surgical Site Infection and Financial Issues

In August of 2007, the CMS released the inpatient prospective payment system (IPPS) for fiscal year 2008 prohibiting reimbursement for eight hospital-acquired conditions. The changes were mandated by section 5001(c) of the Deficit Reduction Act of 2005. Beginning on October 1, 2008, hospitals no longer received higher payments for patients with these eight preventable conditions, or "never events." This included SSIs and mediastinitis after coronary artery bypass graft (CABG) surgery. SSI following additional surgical procedures, including certain orthopedic procedures, and SSI following bariatric surgery for obesity were subsequently added. As anticipated, CMS also confirmed the full market-basket update of 3.6% to payments for those hospitals reporting quality data, including SSI, or 1.6% for those not reporting, reflecting a 2% increase in payment as a pay-for-reporting measure (Figure 4).

SUMMARY

SSI is the leading nosocomial infection among surgical patients, and all evidence-based strategies to prevent SSI should be implemented.

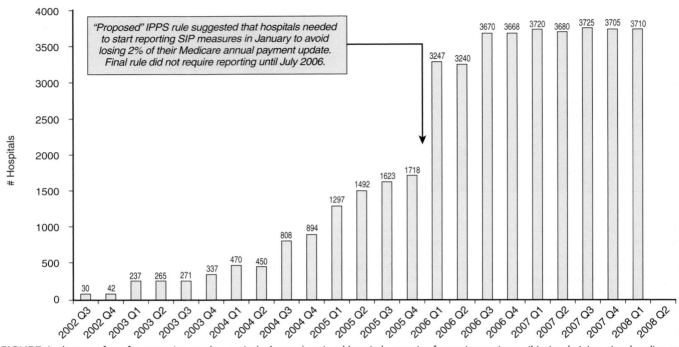

FIGURE 4   Impact of pay-for-reporting on changes in (voluntary) national hospital reporting for perioperative antibiotic administration, baseline to first quarter 2008, Surgical Infection Prevention Project (SIP). *(Data from D. Bratzler, MD, 2009.)*

SUGGESTED READINGS

Al-Niaimi A, Safdar N: Supplemental perioperative oxygen for reducing surgical site infection: a meta-analysis, *J Eval Clin Pract* 15(2):360–365, 2009.

Awad SS, Palacio CH, Subramanian A, et al: Implementation of an MRSA prevention bundle: results in decreased MRSA surgical site infections, *Am J Surg* 198:607–610, 2009.

Barie PS, Eachempati SR: Surgical site infections, *Surg Clin North Am* 85(6):1115–1135, 2005.

Bibbo C, Patel DV, Gehrmann RM, et al: Chlorhexidine provides superior skin decontamination in foot and ankle surgery: a prospective randomized study, *Clin Orthop Related Res* 438:204–208, 2005.

Brar MS, Brar SS, Dixon E: Perioperative supplemental oxygen in colorectal patients: a meta-analysis, *J Surg Res* 2009: Jul 10 (Epub ahead of print).

Bratzler DW, Houck PM, Richards C, et al: Use of antimicrobial prophylaxis for major surgery: baseline results from the National Surgical Infection Prevention Project, *Arch Surg* 140:174–182, 2005.

Campbell DA Jr, Henderson WG, Englesbe MJ, et al: Surgical site infection prevention: the importance of operative duration and blood transfusion, results of the first American College of Surgeons National Surgical Quality Improvement Program Best Practices Initiative, *J Am Coll Surg* 207:810–820, 2008.

Daroviche RO, Wall MJ, Itani K, et al: Chlorhexidine-alcohol vs. povidone-iodine for surgical site antisepsis, *N Engl J Med* 342(1):18–24, 2010.

Dellinger EP, Hausmann SM, Bratzler DW, et al: Hospitals collaborate to decrease surgical site infections, *Am J Surg* 190:9–15, 2005.

Edwards PS, Lipp A, Holmes A: Preoperative skin antiseptics for preventing surgical wound infections after clean surgery, *Cochrane Database Syst Rev* (3):CD003949, 2004.

Gaynes R, Edwards JR: National Nosocomial Infections Surveillance System: overview of nosocomial infections caused by Gram-negative bacilli, *Clin Infect Dis* 41(6):848–854, 2005.

Guenga KK, Matos D, Wille-Jorgensen P: Mechanical bowel preparation for elective colorectal surgery, *Cochrane Database Syst Rev* (1):CD001544, 2009.

Harbath S, Fankhauser C, Schrenzel J, et al: Universal screening for MRSA at hospital admission and nosocomial infection in surgical patients, *JAMA* 299(10):1149–1157, 2008.

Hidron AI, Edwards JR, Patel J, et al: antimicrobial-resistant pathogens associated with healthcare-associated infections: annual summary of data reported to the National Healthcare Safety Network at the Centers for Disease Control and Prevention, 2006-2007, *Infect Control Hosp Epidemiol* 29:996–1011, 2008.

Institute for Healthcare Improvement: Prevent surgical site infections. Available at http://www.ihi.org/IHI/Programs/Campaign/SSI.htm.

Jog S, Cunningham R, Cooper S, et al: Impact of preoperative screening for MRSA by real-time PCR in patients undergoing cardiac surgery, *J Hosp Infect* 69(2):124–130, 2008.

Kallen AJ, Wilson CT, Larson RJ: Perioperative intranasal mupirocin for the prevention of surgical site infections: systematic review of the literature and meta-analysis, *Infect Control Hosp Epidemiol* 26(12):916–922, 2005.

Kao LS, Meeks D, Moyer VA, Lally KP: Perioperative glycaemic control regimens for preventing surgical site infections in adults, *Cochrane Database Syst Rev* (3):CD006806, 2009.

Klevens RM, Edward JR Richards CL Jr, et al: Estimating health care-associated infections and deaths in U.S. hospitals, 2002, *Public Health Reports* 122:160–166, 2007.

Klevens RM, Morrison MA, Nadle J, et al: Active Bacterial Core Surveillance (ABCs) MRSA Investigators: invasive MRSA infections in the United States, *JAMA* 298(15):1763–1771, 2007.

Kourbatova EV, Halvosa JS, King MD, et al: Emergence of community-associated MRSA USA 300 clone as a cause of healthcare-associated infections among patients with prosthetic joint infections, *Am J Infect Control* 33(7):385–391, 2005.

Kurz A, Sessler DI, Lenhardt R: Perioperative normothermia to reduce the incidence of surgical-wound infection and shorten hospitalization: Study of Wound Infection and Temperature Group, *N Engl J Med* 334:1209–1215, 1996.

Malone DL, Genuit T, Tracy JK, et al: Surgical site infections: reanalysis of risk factors, *J Surg Res* 103(1):89–95, 2002.

Mangram AJ, Horan TC, Pearson ML, et al: Guideline for prevention of surgical site infection, 1999: Hospital Infection Control Practices Advisory Committee, *Infect Control Hosp Epidemiol* 20:250–278, 1999.

Manian FA, Griesnauer S: Community-associated MRSA is replacing traditional healthcare-associated strains in surgical site infections among inpatients, *Clin Infect Dis* 47(3):434–435, 2008.

Manniën J, Wille JC, Snoeren RL, et al: Impact of postdischarge surveillance on surgical site infection rates for several surgical procedures: results from the nosocomial surveillance network in The Netherlands, *Infect Control Hosp Epidemiol* 27(8):809–816, 2006.

Melling AC, Ali B, Scott EM, et al: Effects of preoperative warming on the incidence of wound infection after clean surgery: a randomized controlled trial, *Lancet* 15(358(9285)):976–980, 2001.

Morange-Saussier V, Giraudeau B, van der Mee N, et al: Nasal carriage of MRSA in vascular surgery, *Ann Vasc Surg* 20(6):767–772, 2006.

Napolitano LM: Invited critique, *Arch Surg* 144(4):366–367, 2009: for Qadan M, Akca O, Mahid SS, et al: Perioperative supplemental oxygen therapy and surgical site infection: a meta-analysis of randomized controlled trials, *Arch Surg* 144(4):359–366, 2009.

Napolitano LM: Severe soft-tissue infections, *Infect Dis Clin North Am* 23(3):571–591, 2009.

Nelson RL, Glenny AM, Song F: Antimicrobial prophylaxis for colorectal surgery, *Cochrane Database Syst Rev* (1):CD001181, 2009.

Nosocomial Infections Surveillance System: Report, data summary from January 1992-June 2001, *Am J Infect Control* 28:404–421, 2001.

Perl TM: Prevention of *Staphylococcus aureus* infections among surgical patients: beyond traditional perioperative prophylaxis, *Surgery* 134(suppl 5):S10–S17, 2003.

Popovich KF, Weinstein RA, Hota B: Are community-associated MRSA strains replacing traditional nosocomial MRSA strains? *Clin Infect Dis* 46(6):787–794, 2008.

Qadan M, Akca O, Mahid SS, et al: Perioperative supplemental oxygen therapy and surgical site infection: a meta-analysis of randomized controlled trials, *Arch Surg* 144(4):359–366, 2009.

Saltzman MD, Nuber GW, Gryzlo SM, et al: Efficacy of surgical preparation solutions in shoulder surgery, *J Bone Joint Surg Am* 91(8):1949–1953, 2009.

Schelenz S, Tucker D, Georgeu C, et al: Significant reduction of endemic MRSA acquisition and infection in cardiothoracic patients by means of an enhanced targeted infection control programme, *J Hosp Infect* 60(2):104–110, 2005.

Steinberg JP, Braun BI, Hellinger WC, et al: Trial to Reduce Antimicrobial Prophylaxis Errors (TRAPE) Study Group: timing of antimicrobial prophylaxis and the risk of surgical site infections: results from the Trial to Reduce Antimicrobial Prophylaxis Errors, *Ann Surg* 250(1):10–6, 2009.

Tanner J, Swarbrook S, Stuart J: Surgical hand antisepsis to reduce surgical site infection, *Cochrane Database Syst Rev* (1):CD004288, 2008.

Tanner J, Woodings D, Moncaster K: Preoperative hair removal to reduce surgical site infection, *Cochrane Database Syst Rev* (2):CD004122, 2006.

Taylor M, Napolitano L: Methicillin-resistant *Staphylococcus aureus* infections in vascular surgery: increasing prevalence, *Surg Infect* 5:180–187, 2004.

Trautmann M, Stecher J, Hemmer W, et al: Intranasal mupirocin prophylaxis in elective surgery: a review of published studies, *Chemotherapy* 54(1):9–16, 2008.

Van Rijen M, Bonten M, Wenzel R, et al: Mupirocin ointment for preventing *Staphylococcus aureus* infections in nasal carriers, *Cochrane Database Syst Rev* (4):CD006216, 2008.

Weigelt JA, Lipsky BA, Tabak YP, et al: Surgical site infections: causative pathogens and associated outcomes, *Am J Infect Control* 38(2):112–120, 2010.

Wilson MA: Skin and soft-tissue infections: impact of resistant Gram-positive bacteria, *Am J Surg* 186(5A):35S–41S, 2003.

Wong PF, Kumar S, Bohra A, et al: Randomized clinical trial of perioperative systemic warming in major elective abdominal surgery, *Br J Surg* 94(40):421–426, 2007.

FACT SHEETS: CENTERS FOR MEDICARE AND MEDICAID SERVICES

http://www.cms.hhs.gov/HospitalAcqCond/Downloads/HACFactsheet.pdf
http://www.cms.hhs.gov/apps/media/fact_sheets.asp

INTRAABDOMINAL INFECTIONS

Yassar Youssef, MD, and Adrian Barbul, MD

OVERVIEW

Intraabdominal infection (IAI) is a common entity encountered daily by surgeons and healthcare providers. Its most common clinical presentation, peritonitis, is the focus of this chapter. Other chapters in this textbook cover detailed descriptions of specific diseases linked to IAI.

DEFINITION

Any pathology in the abdominal cavity leading to the multiplication of microorganisms within normally sterile regions can lead to IAI. Simple contamination, such as that following the perforation of a hollow viscus, does not in itself constitute an IAI. The offending microorganisms need to overwhelm the host's defense mechanism to cause the infection.

Peritonitis is classified as *primary, secondary,* or *tertiary.* Primary peritonitis, such as spontaneous bacterial peritonitis, is a relatively rare entity that occurs in the absence of a known intraabdominal source. Adult patients with ascites and liver cirrhosis are at high risk. This monomicrobial infection is commonly caused by *Escherichia coli* or *Klebsiella* and usually is managed medically with antibiotics. Secondary peritonitis is by far the most common presentation of IAI. It results from the extension of an infection originating in an intraabdominal structure (acute appendicitis, cholecystitis) or disruption of the anatomical integrity of the gastrointestinal tract (perforated ulcer, bowel injury). It is a polymicrobial infection, usually requiring source control in addition to antimicrobial therapy. In immunocompetent patients, secondary peritonitis can evolve into an intraabdominal abscess, where the infective source is contained yet not eliminated; therefore intraabdominal abscess can be viewed as a continuum of secondary peritonitis, with which it actually shares similar microbiology. In the immunocompromised, a less well-defined entity, tertiary peritonitis, can develop. This occurs when recurrent or persistent infections fail to clear despite adequate therapy of the secondary peritonitis. Patients typically have multiple infected fluid collections with no effective sequestration of the infection. Tertiary peritonitis tends to be associated with more virulent and resistant microorganisms.

IAI may also be classified as a *community-acquired* (low risk) or *healthcare-associated* (high risk) infection, a classification useful for antimicrobial selection. Community-acquired infections are the most common and include ambulatory cases, such as acute appendicitis or cholecystitis; healthcare-associated infections occur in postoperative, hospitalized, or nursing home patients as well as in patients with recent antibiotic use.

DIAGNOSIS

History and Physical Exam

Most patients with IAI present with abdominal pain, and the diagnosis is fairly characteristic and simple (Figure 1). A careful history and physical exam may be all that is needed to determine the diagnosis and therapy in many patients with IAI. The approach

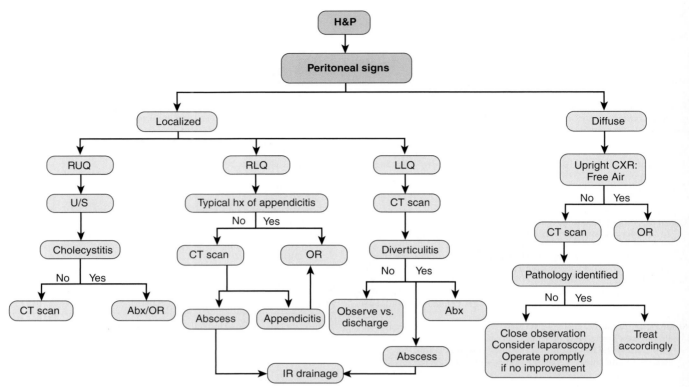

FIGURE 1 Algorithm for the diagnosis and management of patients with suspected IAI. *H&P,* History and physical exam; *RUQ,* right upper quadrant; *RLQ,* right lower quadrant; *LLQ,* left lower quadrant; *U/S,* ultrasound; *Abx,* antibiotics; *hx,* history; *IR,* interventional radiology; *CXR,* chest radiograph.

should be orderly and thorough. Onset of symptoms, type and radiation of pain, consistency and color of vomitus and stool, and associated constitutional symptoms such as weight loss, chills, fever, and anorexia should be elicited. Past medical history and recent medications may be of significance and can provide clues to the diagnosis (e.g., steroids masking the inflammatory response, β-blocker masking tachycardia, nonsteroidal antiinflammatory drugs in perforated ulcer). Alcohol abuse (pancreatitis) and drug use in addition to a menstrual history are key elements in the history. With the increased use of laparoscopy, a virgin abdomen cannot be expected based solely on the absence of scars; therefore a specific history about previous abdominal surgeries should be elicited.

The nature of the pain is helpful in arriving at a diagnosis. Biliary pain is located in the right upper quadrant with radiation to the right shoulder, and it is often associated with fatty food intake; patients with perforated ulcer remember the exact time when the pain started, and patients with pancreatitis can have severe abdominal pain with associated rigidity, mimicking a surgical abdomen. Surgery should be avoided in these patients except for complications, such as infected necrotizing pancreatitis; a history of alcohol abuse, hyperlipidemia, cholelithiasis, and certain medications (e.g. thiazides) should point to this diagnosis. Right upper quadrant pain, fever, and jaundice may be due to ascending cholangitis, requiring emergent decompression of the biliary tree. The pain of uncomplicated diverticulitis is usually localized in the left lower quadrant, except in patients with redundant sigmoid colon, where the pain can be localized to the right lower quadrant, mimicking acute appendicitis.

The initial examination should focus on signs of hemodynamic instability that include tachycardia, hypotension, pallor, dry mucous membranes, and slow capillary refill. In very ill patients, respiratory status should be assessed, along with the possible need for

mechanical ventilation and intensive care unit (ICU) admission. It is of utmost importance to rule out ruptured abdominal aortic aneurysm or ectopic pregnancy in patients seen with abdominal pain. Although the physical exam should be complete and methodical, surgeons tend to concentrate on the abdomen. The general appearance of the patient provides a relative indication of the severity of the underlying pathology. Most patients with peritonitis look unwell and distressed. They tend to lie still to prevent the occurrence of pain resulting from stimulation and movement of the parietal peritoneum. In immunocompetent patients with IAI, fever is a common finding. It is usually constant in patients with peritonitis but cyclic with intraabdominal abscess secondary to the cyclic release of bacterial toxins into the circulation; however, immunosuppressed and elderly patients may not mount a fever and may present with normothermia or even hypothermia.

Examination of the abdomen starts with inspection for evidence of distension—bowel obstruction, free air, ascites—and for abdominal wall infection and old scars; again check for small laparoscopic scars. Auscultation, thought not specific, may reveal decreased or absent bowel sounds suggestive of an ileus secondary to an infectious process. Percussion can be a sensitive way to detect peritoneal irritation, and the presence of tympany could indicate either free air or distended bowel. Rebound tenderness and involuntary guarding indicates peritonitis. Surgical scars should be assessed for incisional hernia, and the groin should be examined for inguinal hernia as well and for femoral hernia in elderly females. Check for aortic aneurysm by palpating the midline just above the umbilicus. Patients with intraabdominal abscess or a localized infective source, such as appendicitis or diverticulitis, usually have focal abdominal tenderness. Rectal exam with stool testing for blood is useful in patients with suspected bowel ischemia. Depending on the history, pelvic exam may be needed for female patients.

Diagnostic Tests

The history and physical exam will help narrow the diagnostic workup, and routine labs may reveal the presence of infection (leukocytosis) or anemia. Hydration status, renal function, and acid-base balance are assessed by electrolytes and creatinine measurement. Liver function tests and measures of amylase and lipase will help delineate biliary or pancreatic pathology. A low to moderate elevation of amylase level should be viewed with caution, however, as it could be associated with perforated ulcer or ischemic bowel. High lactate is very nonspecific but can point to possible bowel ischemia. A urinalysis should be used to test for infection as well as for pregnancy in women of childbearing age.

In a patient with a diffusely rigid abdomen, upright chest radiograph is the first, and possibly only, imaging study needed. The presence of free air is sufficient for surgical intervention, and additional diagnostic tests will add little to the clinical picture. In most instances, however, surgeons are consulted after diagnosis has been made or suggested on the basis of a computed tomography (CT) scan.

In most stable patients, the mainstay for definitive diagnosis of abdominal pathology is CT scan. It is readily available and allows good visualization of solid organs, retroperitoneum, lesser sac, pelvis, and lower lung fields; it is the best modality to diagnose acute appendicitis, diverticulitis, pancreatitis, intraabdominal abscess, and free air. It is always beneficial to use contrast enhancement, but administration may be limited by clinical factors (e.g., ileus for oral contrast, allergy or renal failure for intravenous contrast). Other modalities that are used less often in the evaluation of patients with suspected IAI include ultrasound (suspected biliary pathology), contrast radiography studies (perforated ulcer, postoperative leak), angiography (acute mesenteric ischemia), radionuclide scans (Meckel diverticulitis, HIDA for cholecystitis), paracentesis (primary peritonitis), and endoscopy (endoscopic retrograde cholangiopancreatography for cholangitis).

In high-risk patients, diagnosis of IAI is more difficult, either because of subtle and atypical presentation of the disease or inability to obtain a history. Therefore with postoperative, ICU, elderly, and immunocompromised patients who are not faring well, a high index of alertness should be maintained, and the liberal use of diagnostic tests, especially CT scans, should be encouraged. Finally, a diagnosis is not always possible or necessary in patients with suspected IAI. Surgical intervention via laparoscopy or even laparotomy should be seriously considered when there is a high index of suspicion. A negative laparotomy finding is better than a positive autopsy and should never be considered morbidity.

MANAGEMENT

Once the diagnosis of IAI is established, optimal management relies on three fundamentals: 1) patient stabilization, 2) antimicrobial therapy, and 3) source control.

Patient Stabilization

Patients with IAI are usually dehydrated and may be acidotic, and restoration of normal physiology through circulatory support is of utmost importance. The degree of dehydration depends on the cause of the infection and the severity of the peritonitis leading to third-space fluid sequestration. Patients with acute appendicitis and cholecystitis are usually mildly dehydrated and require baseline fluid maintenance, especially with anticipated early source control. Patients with diffuse peritonitis, acute pancreatitis, and postoperative infection, are usually severely dehydrated and require aggressive fluid resuscitation before source control. This resuscitation usually takes a couple of hours and should be followed by source control if needed. Monitoring of urine output and vital signs is a simple yet very effective measure to assess response to fluid resuscitation. In high-risk patients, especially in elderly patients with multiple comorbidities, resuscitation should be guided with close physiologic monitoring, including Foley catheter and central-line insertion and possible ICU admission. Analgesics should be used for pain relief, as they do not interfere with further physical examinations. A nasogastric (NG) tube can be used to decompress the stomach, preventing vomiting and aspiration as well as providing comfort for patients with bowel obstruction. An NG tube can also be used for the administration of contrast material in severely nauseated patients. When obtaining consent, especially in patients with an uncertain diagnosis, it is important to discuss all the possibilities, including temporary or permanent stoma, potential need for multiple operations, postoperative intubation for mechanical ventilation, and even death.

Antimicrobial Therapy

The aims of antimicrobial therapy in the treatment of patients with IAI are control of microorganism dissemination and elimination of pathogenic organisms remaining after source control. Therefore antimicrobial therapy should be used as an adjunct to, not a substitute for, source control. However, under some circumstances, IAI management has come to rely more heavily on conservative therapy. Acute diverticulitis is the prototype pathology in which most cases are successfully managed without surgical intervention. Small intraabdominal abscesses (less than 2 cm) and acute appendicitis with phlegmon have been managed initially by antibiotic therapy with good success. Under select circumstances, patients with a contained leak (postoperative leak or perforated ulcer) have been judiciously managed nonoperatively. With the increasing use of these conservative strategies, antimicrobial therapy plays an even more pivotal role.

Despite the guidelines outlining the use of antimicrobial therapy in the management of patients with IAI, the administration of antibiotics in patients with IAI depends largely on the preference of the treating physician. In addition, most regimens are chosen empirically without an available culture; therefore a good understanding of microbiology and knowledge of the offending microorganisms involved in IAI, as well as the trend of microbial resistance at the practiced institution, are needed for correct antimicrobial selection.

Most IAIs are caused by low-virulence enteric bacteria. The most common organisms isolated from the peritoneal fluid of these patients are the gram-negative enteric bacilli (*E. coli* followed by *Klebsiella*) and obligate anaerobes (*Bacteroides fragilis*). Anaerobe species predominate over the aerobic ones, especially in intraabdominal abscesses; and because many laboratories do not report or recover anaerobic organisms, antianaerobic coverage is always needed, even in the presence of negative cultures. In general, most microorganisms encountered in community-acquired infections are susceptible to commonly used antimicrobial regimens. Nonetheless, there is a worldwide trend of increasing bacterial resistance to a few of these agents. The problem of bacterial resistance is of even greater concern in high-risk patients with health care–associated infections, especially postoperative infection, where less *E. coli* is cultured and more antibiotic resistant and virulent strains, such as *Enterobacter* and *Pseudomonas,* are cultured. Fungal microorganism, mainly *Candida albicans,* is also more frequently encountered in nosocomial infections.

Of the isolated gram-positive cocci, *Streptococcus viridans* group organisms followed by enterococci, especially *E. faecium,* are the most frequently encountered pathogens. Although less frequently encountered in community-acquired infections, enterococci are recovered in half the patients with postoperative infections; thus some advocate adding penicillin, ampicillin, or vancomycin when treating this patient group. Although most strains are sensitive, some are resistant to this therapy, such as the vancomycin-resistant *E. faecium.*

Treatment of fungi is even more controversial. We believe that only patients at high risk for fungal infection should be treated (Box 1). Obviously, most severely ill patients will have at least two to three risk factors by the time they are admitted to the ICU. It is in this patient population that antifungal prophylaxis may be beneficial. Treatment options for high-risk patients with documented fungal infections include fluconazole for *C. albicans* and amphotericin B or caspofungin for the increasingly encountered *C. glabrata* and other *Candida* species.

Choice and *timing* of antimicrobial therapy are closely linked to treatment success, and it is thought that every hour of delay between the onset of sepsis and antimicrobial therapy increases the mortality significantly. More important is the fact that a late change in therapy, tailored to the culture, does not modify the outcomes. Thus the correct antimicrobial regimen should be started as soon as the clinical diagnosis is made, before further diagnostic tests.

Antimicrobial Regimens

Wide choices of antimicrobial therapy are available, ranging from monotherapy to combination regimens for different patient groups (Boxes 2 and 3). Monotherapy is our preference, and completing the regimen with oral forms of antimicrobial therapy is the rule and should be encouraged, once the patient is able to tolerate oral intake.

Duration of Therapy

To prevent the development of bacterial resistance and also decrease both cost and incidence of antibiotic-related infections, the duration of antimicrobial therapy should be as short as possible. Many patients have been treated with lengthy courses of such therapy despite the fact that doing so offers no advantages and may be harmful. Although there are no guidelines on the duration of therapy, antibiotics can be safely stopped in patients who improve clinically, defervesce, and normalize their white blood cell count. Antibiotics beyond one-day prophylaxis are not warranted in cases of acute appendicitis and cholecystitis in the absence of perforation at the time of source control; bowel necrosis without perforation; or gastric, duodenal, and proximal small bowel perforations repaired within 24 hours, as well as colonic and distal small bowel perforations repaired within 12 hours. Low-risk patients and most high-risk patients can have their antibiotics stopped in 3 to 5 days. Patients with severe infections and tertiary peritonitis and those with poor source control will require a prolonged antibiotic course.

Source Control

Source control is defined as the eradication of the septic source, and it aims at reducing the microorganism load to a degree that can be effectively handled by the patient's immune system and the antimicrobial therapy. Despite the fact that source control is considered the sine qua non of managing patients with IAI, as mentioned previously, a recent trend of conservative management has been adopted in many conditions.

Surgical Intervention

In most patients with IAI, such as acute appendicitis and cholecystitis, surgical intervention will involve a simple laparoscopic or open procedure for source control. Occasionally, a major resection, such as colectomy for perforated diverticulitis, is indicated. The decision to divert in these cases should be evaluated on an individual basis, taking into consideration the degree and site of infection, time to intervention, and the patient's condition and comorbidities.

A midline laparotomy is used in patients with unknown preoperative diagnosis, and peritoneal toileting should be part of the damage control. Infected fluids should be aspirated, and moist laparotomy pads should be used to swab any particulate matter. Although many surgeons still use intraoperative peritoneal lavage, there is no evidence that this technique is effective, and the use of copious irrigation in cases of localized infection or peritonitis, such as acute appendicitis, may be associated with higher rates of infected collections because of dissemination of the microorganisms in the peritoneal cavity. However, if copious irrigation is to be used, it is important to remember to suck out all the fluid at the end of the procedure.

BOX 1: Risk factors for disseminated fungal infections

Hemodialysis or placement of a central venous catheter
Neutropenia
Multiple gastrointestinal perforations or surgeries
ICU resident at time of culture
Acute renal failure
Total parenteral nutrition
Diabetes mellitus
Antibiotics use for >6 days
Cancer
Multiple trauma
Burns

BOX 2: Antimicrobial therapy for community-acquired infections in low-risk patients

Monotherapy

Cefotetan
Cefoxitin
Moxifloxacin
Ertapenem
Ticarcillin-clavulanic acid
Tigecycline

Combination Agents

Cefuroxime plus metronidazole
Cefazolin plus metronidazole
Ciprofloxacin plus metronidazole

BOX 3: Antimicrobial therapy for health care–associated infections in high-risk patients

Monotherapy

Piperacillin-tazobactam
Imipenem-cilastatin
Meropenem

Combination Agents

Ciprofloxacin plus metronidazole
Third- or fourth-generation cephalosporins (cefotaxime, ceftriaxone, cefepime, and ceftazidine) plus metronidazole
Aztreonam plus metronidazole

Excessive or radical debridement of all the fibrin on the peritoneum and bowel is not beneficial and may lead to excessive bleeding and a denuded friable intestine. Intraoperative cultures are not needed and should not lead to a change in the initial antimicrobial regimen, especially in patients who are improving clinically; however, this may be helpful in high-risk patients, in whom virulent and resistant organisms are more frequently cultured.

It is impossible to drain the entire peritoneal cavity unless six or seven drains are used. Despite relatively clear evidence that drains offer no benefits in most patients with IAI, they are still commonly used. Drains should be used only in selected cases, such as in biliary and pancreatic procedures. A soft, closed-suction drain is preferred, except in pancreatic necrosis, in which large, hard drains are required. Drains should be placed away from the bowel to prevent erosion, and they must be taken out as soon as possible.

Interventional Radiology

The recent advances in interventional radiology and percutaneous drainage techniques have shaped and undoubtedly changed the management of patients with IAI. Most intraabdominal abscesses—except pancreatic ones, which usually require open surgical drainage—can be drained with low morbidity by percutaneous techniques under ultrasound or CT guidance. It is now recognized that interventional radiology drainage related to postoperative complications, such as contained leak or perforation, is feasible and effective, especially in high-risk patients. However, not all abscesses can be drained by the less invasive technique, nor should they be. For example, two or more abscesses are better treated in an open fashion. Also, abscess in the path of bowel loops poses a risk of enterotomy and may need open drainage as well. Whatever method is chosen for drainage, it is prudent to make sure it is effective and sufficient without reliance on antimicrobial therapy. Antibiotic penetration into the abscess is minimal and often inadequate secondary to poor perfusion, mechanical barriers (fibrin), low pH, and large bacterial load.

The success rate of percutaneous drainage is more than 80% for simple abscesses but less than 50% in complex, multiloculated abscess. Cultures are usually performed on the aspirated fluid to narrow the antibiotic treatment, and satisfactory drainage is usually evidenced by clinical improvement within 48 to 72 hours; otherwise a repeat diagnostic test (CT scan) should be performed to look for any inadequate drainage, recurrence of the abscess, or complication from the primary intervention.

Laparoscopy

Minimally invasive surgery techniques have evolved to play an important role in the management of patients with suspected or confirmed IAI. Its advantages over an open technique are well established: less postoperative pain, earlier return to work, and better cosmetic results. In addition, laparoscopy is associated with fewer incisional hernias and a lower wound infection rate. Almost all pathologies leading to IAI have been managed using laparoscopic techniques with great results. However, it should be mentioned that high-risk patients may not tolerate CO_2 insufflations well, and previous surgeries and bowel distension secondary to ileus increase the risk for inadvertent enterotomy. In this population, appropriate patient selection and surgeon experience are important considerations for the use of laparoscopy.

COMPLICATIONS

Management of patients with IAI can be associated with unintended damage that occurs during the course of therapy. This "collateral damage" includes treatment failure, relaparotomies, and infectious complications.

Treatment Failure

Treatment failure can be attributed to poor source control, inadequate antimicrobial coverage, or microbial resistance. Resistant microorganisms have been linked to treatment failure, especially in health care–associated infections, and it is not uncommon to observe a prolongation or change of the antimicrobial regimen in patients with no clinical improvement. However, the most common reason for treatment failure is inadequate source control. Thus persistent clinical signs usually indicate an ongoing source of infection, and before attributing that to inadequate antimicrobial coverage or microbial resistance, a careful search for a focus of infection in the abdomen or elsewhere should be performed.

Relaparotomies

Some patients with IAI will require multiple laparotomies because of inadequate source control during the first procedure. Two strategies, *on-demand* and *planned relaparotomy,* are used in these patients. The on-demand method is used only when the patient fails to improve or deteriorates after the initial laparotomy. In the planned method, in which the fascia is usually kept open, and the abdomen is closed with a temporary method, the patient is operated on every 1 to 3 days irrespective of clinical condition.

An early use of the planned relaparotomy is in patients with mesenteric ischemia, in whom the assessment of bowel viability is not possible during the initial procedure. Other indications for planned relaparotomy include inability to obtain adequate source control during the initial procedure (e.g., infected pancreatic necrosis or multiple bowel leaks), patient instability (e.g., coagulopathy, hypothermia, or acidosis where damage control operation is needed), and patients with increased intraabdominal pressure. Except under such circumstances, we prefer the on-demand method, because it is associated with less cost, a shorter hospital stay, and fewer incisional hernias and enterocutaneous fistulas, and it has similar outcomes to planned relaparotomies. Whichever method is used, great care should be taken when reexploring the abdomen. The bowel and peritoneal surfaces are very friable and edematous; tough adhesions are formed, especially between postoperative weeks 2 and 4; and no clear anatomic planes exist, therefore the surgeon should be very gentle to prevent enterotomies, and the reexploration should be as limited as possible.

Infectious Complications

Distant and extraabdominal infections can complicate the course of patients with IAI. These include surgical site infections, urinary tract infections, pneumonia, and *Clostridium difficile* colitis among others. Lack of patient improvement should be investigated for inadequate primary source control or any of the above infectious complications.

OUTCOMES

The prognosis of patients with IAI is variable, with observed mortality in clinical trials less than 5%. However, most enrolled patients have community-acquired infection with associated low morbidity and mortality. Health care–associated infections, which are usually excluded from these trials, are associated with a demonstrated mortality of 15% to 30%. Several studies have demonstrated that preexisting conditions, such as advanced age and comorbidities, are better predictors of outcomes of IAI than the type or source of infection. Therefore, intervention for IAI should focus on treating the burden of the associated chronic disease in patients as well as the primary source of infection.

BOX 4: Important points about intraabdominal infection

- Early diagnosis is important.
- Listen to patients; they will point to the diagnosis.
- Patients with an IAI are dehydrated: take time to rehydrate and stabilize the patient before source control.
- Initiation antibiotics early: do not wait for definitive diagnosis; in septic patients, antimicrobials should be delivered in the first hour after diagnosis.
- Choose appropriate antibiotics: community-acquired IAI in low-risk patients calls for narrow spectrum agents; health care–associated IAI in high-risk patients calls for broad-spectrum agents, along with fungal and enterococcal coverage if needed.
- Be aware of the increasing antimicrobial resistance and its associated high mortality rate.
- A short course of antibiotics is best: <24 hours for simple cases, although about 3 to 5 days are needed for most patients.
- Not all patients require surgery (e.g., acute diverticulitis, contained perforation or leak), but all require fluid resuscitation and IV antibiotics.
- Effective and early source control is important.
- If no improvement is seen, make sure the source is well controlled before changing or prolonging the antibiotics course. The most common reason for treatment failure is inadequate source control, not inappropriate antibiotic selection or microbial resistance.
- Treat patient comorbidities as well as the primary disease: they will determine the final outcome.
- A paradigm shift is on the horizon for the treatment of IAI. Pathologies once considered surgical are being treated conservatively with good outcomes: be aware and up to date, and practice good judgment.

SUMMARY

Most patients with intraabdominal infections are initially seen with peritonitis. Although the clinical spectrum varies widely, most cases encountered by surgeons are community-acquired infections treated by source control and a short course of narrow-spectrum antimicrobial therapy. With improved diagnostic modalities and radiological intervention techniques, many diagnoses that previously necessitated surgical exploration—such as perforated duodenal ulcer, localized postoperative leak, and even acute appendicitis—are being treated conservatively. In the absence of good evidence, surgeons must use their experience and common sense when dealing with patients with IAIs (Box 4).

SUGGESTED READINGS

Cheadle W, Spain D: The continuing challenge of intraabdominal infection, *Am J Surg* 186(5A):15S–22S, 2003.
Mazuski J, Solomkin J: Intraabdominal infections, *Surg Clin North Am* 89(2):421–437, 2009.
Schein M: *Schein's common sense emergency abdominal surgery*, New York, 2000, Springer.
Schein M: Surgical management of intraabdominal infection: Is there any evidence? *Langenbecks Arch Surg* 387:1–7, 2002.

ABNORMAL OPERATIVE AND POSTOPERATIVE BLEEDING

Thomas H. Cogbill, MD

OVERVIEW

Abnormal perioperative bleeding may present a formidable challenge to the surgeon. Bleeding may be medication induced or the result of acquired, congenital, or technical causes. In many cases, multiple factors are responsible, and the effects are compounded. Prolonged hemodynamic instability is associated with multiple organ failure and sepsis. Furthermore, multiple blood transfusions increase the risks of bloodborne infection, transfusion reaction, and immunosuppression. For these important reasons, it is critical for the surgeon to take a systematic approach in dealing with abnormal operative and postoperative bleeding. This chapter will focus on preoperative assessment for bleeding risk, recognition of bleeding, identification of causes for bleeding, and the stepwise treatment of these conditions.

PREOPERATIVE ASSESSMENT

Cost-effective preoperative assessment of bleeding risk is essential before any surgical procedure, to identify those patients with preexisting conditions that require preoperative management to prevent bleeding and to heighten awareness of a possible bleeding diathesis. The magnitude of preoperative testing is based upon a thorough history and physical examination (Box 1). Patients without a personal or family history of bleeding disorders or abnormal bleeding associated with prior surgery, dental extractions, minor trauma, or childbirth are unlikely to have congenital coagulopathies. Patients taking no medications or dietary supplements affecting coagulation and with no history of bleeding disorders are at very low risk for perioperative bleeding. Absence of ecchymosis, petechiae, or bleeding tissues on physical examination, as well as no stigmata of liver disease, also confirms that a patient is at low risk of perioperative bleeding. Based on history and physical examination findings and the type of operation scheduled, ordering additional preoperative testing may be rational and cost effective (Table 1).

PREOPERATIVE MANAGEMENT

Herbal remedies and dietary supplements that affect coagulation should be stopped long enough before surgery to reverse their effects. Aspirin should not be routinely discontinued in the perioperative

BOX 1: Preoperative evaluation for coagulation disorders

History

- Med ications (prescription, over-the-counter, herbal supplements)
- Excessive bleeding after surgical or dental procedures
- Heavy menstrual bleeding or postpartum bleeding
- Recurrent epistaxis
- Excessive bleeding after minor trauma
- Spontaneous bruising or hematoma formation
- Chronic iron deficiency
- Liver disease
- Chronic renal disease
- Poor nutritional intake
- Family history of excessive bleeding

Physical Examination

- Petechiae
- Ecchymosis
- Mucous membrane bleeding
- Stigmata of liver disease
- Impaired wound healing
- Malnutrition

TABLE 1: Preoperative testing for coagulation abnormalities

History and Physical Examination	Planned Operation	Recommended Tests
Negative	Minor	None
Negative	Major	Platelet count, INR, aPTT
Positive	Minor or major	Platelet count, bleeding time, INR, aPTT, hematology consult, nutritional assessment

confirmed indirectly by measurement of factor VIII levels or by using assays to directly measure the amount and activity of VWF. The most common of the four VWD types, type 1, is found in 60% to 80% of patients and is the result of a quantitative defect; this is confirmed by the measurement of low levels of VWF. Type 2, which affects 20% to 30%, is the result of a qualitative defect in the *function* of VWF, but *levels* of VWF are normal; however, bleeding times are usually elevated, and the activated partial thromboplastin time (aPTT) may be slightly prolonged. Mild cases of VWD are treated with DDAVP, which causes the release of both VWF and factor VIII. More severe cases are best treated with factor VIII/VWF–specific concentrates or the administration of cryoprecipitate. Factor VIII and VWF levels can be followed sequentially to guide further administration.

Hemophilia is another congenital coagulation disorder. The two most common types are *hemophilia A* (90%) and *hemophilia B*. Both are sex-linked recessive genetic disorders. In hemophilia A, factor VIII is reduced, and in hemophilia B, factor IX is reduced. The disease is stratified as *mild* (factor level >5%), *moderate* (1% to 5%), or *severe* (<1%). Spontaneous bleeding can occur with factor levels less than 5%.

Patients with mild hemophilia A who are undergoing minor surgery can be treated effectively with IV administration of 0.3 µg/kg of DDAVP. In this situation, the increased release of endogenous factor VIII may obviate the need for recombinant factor VIII administration. For patients with moderate or severe disease undergoing major procedures, factor levels should be augmented with the administration of recombinant factor VIII and IX for hemophilia A and B, respectively. Patients undergoing minor surgery should receive enough recombinant factor VIII or IX to maintain factor levels above 30% for several days perioperatively. The levels should be maintained above 80% for several days perioperatively in patients undergoing major surgery. Neurosurgical or cardiac procedures require a factor level of 100% to be maintained for 3 to 4 days after surgery, followed by levels of 80% or greater for another week. The presence of factor-specific inhibitors should be checked and may complicate replacement therapy, which should be performed with the help of a hematology consultant.

Several other uncommon congenital factor deficiencies may be identified with specific factor assays. They may be treated with fresh frozen plasma (FFP), which contains all of the coagulation factors; cryoprecipitate, which contains factor VIII, VWF, fibrinogen, fibronectin, and factor XIII; or prothrombin complex concentrate, which contains prothrombin and factors VII, IX, and X. Recombinant activated factor VII (rF VIIa) is also available to treat patients with factor VII deficiency.

Malnutrition, hepatic failure, drugs, and malabsorption may cause vitamin K deficiency with low levels of factors VII, IX and X and prothrombin, protein C, and protein S. Warfarin also interferes with the hepatic production of the vitamin K–dependent factors. Oral or intravenous vitamin K may be administered to replenish levels.

period unless the potential risk of bleeding exceeds the thrombotic risk from withholding aspirin. Clopidogrel should be discontinued 5 days prior to elective surgery, unless it has been prescribed to prevent thrombosis after recent coronary artery stent placement. Clopidogrel should not be discontinued within 4 weeks of bare metallic coronary artery stent placement or up to 1 year after drug-eluting coronary artery stent placement. In these situations, elective surgery may need to be postponed. Emergency procedures should be performed without interrupting antiplatelet therapy. If postoperative bleeding develops, l-desamino-8-D-arginine vasopressin (DDAVP) should be administered for patients on aspirin; the antiplatelet effects of clopidogrel are reversed with platelet transfusions.

If possible, warfarin should be held for 4 days before surgery with a repeat International Normalized Ratio (INR) drawn to confirm that it is less than 1.5. Patients taking warfarin following a major venous thromboembolic event (VTE) should have elective surgery postponed for 4 to 6 weeks, until it is safe to temporarily discontinue warfarin therapy. For urgent procedures within 4 to 6 weeks of a major VTE, warfarin should be discontinued 4 days before surgery and intravenous, unfractionated heparin administered during this period as bridge therapy. Heparin can be discontinued 4 hours prior to surgery; in most cases, it is restarted within 8 to 12 hours after surgery and continued for several days, until warfarin treatment resumes and is therapeutic. A temporary inferior vena cava filter can be inserted as an alternative in this setting. Patients on warfarin to prevent arterial thromboembolism from atrial fibrillation or from mechanical heart valves have a sufficiently low risk of embolization that warfarin may be discontinued for 4 days prior to surgery and restarted as soon as the patient can tolerate liquids. Bridging therapy with heparin infusion is not usually necessary. With some mechanical heart valves, subcutaneous low molecular weight heparin (LMWH) or low-dose unfractionated heparin may be used as a bridge.

Patients with a family history of bleeding disorders must be suspected of having a hereditary coagulation abnormality. The most common inherited abnormality of coagulation is von Willebrand disease (VWD). The disorder is usually inherited in an autosomal-dominant pattern, which results in a deficiency of von Willebrand factor (VWF), a multimeric protein required for platelet adhesion. VWF also stabilizes factor VIII in the blood. The disorder can be

Drawbacks of vitamin K administration are the potential resistance to warfarin in patients anticipated to need oral anticoagulation in the near future and the potential for anaphylactic reactions in patients receiving intravenous vitamin K. FFP can also be given for vitamin K–deficient patients requiring emergent surgery.

Malnutrition and hemodialysis may cause vitamin C deficiency with troublesome bleeding due to loss of capillary integrity resulting from improper collagen formation. A preoperative serum ascorbic acid level can be measured, and if it is below 0.6 mg/dL, 500 mg of oral vitamin C replacement should be given daily.

RECOGNITION OF INTRAOPERATIVE AND POSTOPERATIVE BLEEDING

The source of intraoperative bleeding may be obvious within the operative field, but other potential sources of bleeding may be from organs remote from the operative field, organs that were injured during retraction or other operative maneuvers. Bleeding may also occur from sites within other body cavities from remote injuries or procedures, such as central venous line placement. A patient's physiologic response to blood loss may be very subtle, even in the face of a significant volume of blood loss. The systolic blood pressure may not significantly decrease until 25% to 40% of blood volume is lost. Earlier clues to ongoing bleeding may be tachycardia and decreased pulse pressure. Central venous pressure measurements are a useful adjunct, but others rely upon echocardiography for a quick assessment of cardiac volume. Changes in urine output and hematocrit usually occur late but are useful as targets for resuscitation. Measures of cardiac output and oxygen saturation can also be useful perioperatively.

Physical examination of the postoperative patient is important but may be unreliable. Drains placed near the surgical site are notoriously poor monitors of postoperative bleeding, as they can easily become plugged. It is often very difficult to detect ongoing intraabdominal hemorrhage by examination, until the abdomen is firm or distended. However, bleeding from wounds or diffuse bleeding from intravenous (IV) sites, endotracheal tubes, and bladder catheters may be early signs of coagulopathic bleeding. Often, perioperative bleeding is not readily apparent. It is incumbent on the surgeon to have a high level of suspicion for a technical cause of bleeding. Reexploration to detect occult bleeding and ligate a vessel or stop organ bleeding should be performed in a timely fashion, often in place of a time-consuming set of diagnostic tests. In the case of presumed ongoing bleeding, the risks of unchecked hemorrhage with poor organ perfusion and multiple transfusions far outweigh the risks of a potentially negative reexploration.

MANAGEMENT OF INTRAOPERATIVE AND POSTOPERATIVE BLEEDING

As mentioned above, the most likely cause of postoperative bleeding is an unligated vessel at the surgical site or an unrecognized injury near the surgical site or at a remote location. Surgically correctable technical causes should be addressed first by the surgeon. Assuming that such bleeding is due to an endogenous coagulopathic cause and blindly treating with blood-product transfusion will not be effective and has great potential for harm. Even after hemostasis has been achieved surgically, reassessment is important, as rebleeding can occur when normal blood pressure is restored and vasoconstriction subsides. Damage control techniques are advisable when obvious surgical bleeding has been controlled but generalized oozing persists. This may assist in the placement of packs for tamponade and may make reexplorations more expeditious. Only when a surgeon is confident that a missed injury or bleeding vessel is *not* the cause for ongoing hemorrhage should other potential causes be investigated.

BOX 2: Laboratory assessment for patients with ongoing bleeding after exclusion of technical causes

Complete blood count with platelet count
INR
aPTT
Bleeding time
Temperature
Arterial blood gas with pH and base deficit

After exclusion of technical causes for ongoing bleeding, the patient's temperature should be monitored, and a battery of laboratory tests should be ordered (Box 2). Coagulation cascades function optimally at 37° C. If a patient's core temperature is 35° C or less, every effort should be made to restore normothermia. Further heat loss should be prevented with elevation of room temperature. In addition, warm humidified air should be delivered endotracheally, all IV fluids and blood products should be delivered through a high-volume warming device, and external warming should be administered. In very severe cases of hypothermia, active rewarming may require arteriovenous bypass.

Similarly, the coagulation cascades function best at normal serum pH, and metabolic acidosis is frequently the consequence of hypovolemic shock. Arterial blood gas determinations are performed to sequentially measure pH and base deficit. Severe metabolic acidosis should be corrected with manipulations of ventilation settings, adequate fluid and blood resuscitation, and the IV administration of sodium bicarbonate. Parameters for adequacy of resuscitation, such as urine output and central venous pressure, should be frequently measured, until normal pH and base deficit are restored.

Coagulopathic Causes for Ongoing Bleeding

The diagnosis and treatment of coagulopathic causes for ongoing bleeding are based upon results of the laboratory assessment listed in Box 2. There are four possible categories based upon INR and aPTT results.

Normal International Normalized Ratio, Normal Activated Partial Thromboplastin Time

Platelet dysfunction, VWD, and vitamin C deficiency are most likely with this combination of findings. If the platelet count is under 20,000/mm^3, platelet transfusion should be initiated. If the platelet count is 20,000/mm^3 or greater, a measurement of bleeding time should be ordered. Medications that affect platelet adhesion should be counteracted with DDAVP, and the antiplatelet effects of clopidogrel may be reversed with platelet transfusions. If VWD is suspected, DDAVP can be administered in mild cases, and factor VIII/VWF–specific concentrates or cryoprecipitate can be given for severe cases. If the patient has chronic kidney disease, DDAVP should be administered to counteract the effects of poor platelet function. If vitamin C deficiency is suspected, a serum ascorbic acid level is ordered. If serum ascorbic acid is below 0.6 mg/dL, then 500 mg vitamin C should be administered daily. Other rare causes of coagulopathy with normal INR and aPTT may include factor VIII deficiency, hypofibrinogenemia, dysfibrinogenemia, and fibrinolytic derangements.

Normal International Normalized Ratio, Prolonged Activated Partial Thromboplastin Time

The most common cause for this scenario is a drug-induced coagulation defect, usually involving heparin or a heparin analog. For patients with an undesired unfractionated heparin effect, protamine sulfate can be administered. Rapid protamine administration can cause hypotension and anaphylaxis when given to diabetics, protamine is not effective for LMWH, and FFP will not help to reverse unfractionated heparin or LMWH effects and may exacerbate coagulopathy. To counteract direct thrombin inhibitors such as lepirudin and argatroban, FFP should be given. Additional doses of FFP are often necessary to fully reverse the anticoagulation effects of direct thrombin inhibitors.

Patients with VWD may have a slight prolongation of aPTT. These patients may require DDAVP, factor VIII/VWF–specific concentrates, or cryoprecipitate.

Although it would be unusual to make the diagnosis of hemophilia in this setting, hemophilia A should be managed with recombinant factor VIII administration, and hemophilia B should be managed with recombinant factor IX administration.

Increased International Normalized Ratio, Normal Activated Partial Thromboplastin Time

The most frequent cause for these findings is drug-induced coagulation defect involving warfarin. As above, these effects can be reversed with the administration of vitamin K or FFP. Drawbacks of vitamin K administration are warfarin resistance and the potential for anaphylactic reactions when vitamin K is given intravenously. Other causes for increased INR are poor nutrition with vitamin deficiencies and advanced liver disease. These effects are best reversed with FFP for multiple factor replacement.

Increased International Normalized Ratio, Prolonged Activated Partial Thromboplastin Time

This constellation of findings results from multiple factor deficiencies caused by disseminated intravascular coagulation (DIC), hemodilution from massive blood loss or end-stage kidney disease, or laboratory error.

The diagnosis of DIC is best confirmed by elevation of D-dimer serum levels greater than 2000 ng/mL. Additionally, thrombocytopenia, decreased fibrinogen levels, and elevated levels of fibrin degradation products are observed with DIC. The treatment of low-grade DIC is focused on identification and correction of the underlying disorder. IV heparin administration may occasionally be required. Optimal therapy for fulminant DIC is controversial and is also based upon treatment of the underlying cause. Heparin administration is added to manage endovascular thrombosis, and some have advocated using antithrombin concentrates; others have recommended the use of e-amino caproic acid to inhibit fibrinolysis.

If hemodilution is suspected as the cause of increased INR and prolonged aPTT, a multifaceted treatment approach may involve FFP, cryoprecipitate, calcium, and platelet administration. Some have recently advocated for the use of fresh whole blood in this setting. Others have recommended the use of rF VIIa.

Massive Transfusion Adjuncts

Recent civilian and military experiences with massive transfusion in trauma and surgical patients have suggested a role for several adjuncts. Some have recommended the use of fresh whole blood as opposed to component therapy in an effort to supply fresh platelets and coagulation factors with red blood cells. The early use of a high ratio of FFP to packed red blood cells (PRBCs) (>1:1.5) has been reported to be associated with both a reduced need for PRBCs and a lower risk of mortality despite an increased risk of acute respiratory distress syndrome. The lower risk of mortality has been ascribed to more timely and effective reversal of coagulopathy and hemorrhage. Finally, rF VIIa administration in the setting of significant hemorrhage in major surgical procedures has been shown to reduce the need for PRBC transfusion without an increased risk of thromboembolic complications. Mortality rates are not significantly affected. Because of the high cost of rF VIIa, the current cost/benefit ratio is only favorable in patients who require more than 40 units of PRBCs. Each of these adjuncts requires more experience in well-designed studies before parameters for their use can be better defined.

BOX 3: Principles of management of ongoing perioperative bleeding

Recognize and treat shock
Correct or exclude technical sources of bleeding
Measure temperature and treat hypothermia
Measure serum pH and treat acidosis
Measure coagulation profile and treat abnormalities appropriately
Reassess for ongoing bleeding

SUMMARY

Abnormal perioperative bleeding may result from a variety of causes, and the surgeon must be aware of all the factors involved to manage each patient appropriately. Box 3 summarizes a few of the basic principles in the management of ongoing perioperative bleeding.

SUGGESTED READINGS

American Society of Anesthesiologists Task Force on Perioperative Blood Transfusion and Adjuvant Therapies: Practice guidelines for perioperative blood transfusion and adjuvant therapies: an updated report, *Anesthesiology* 105:198, 2006.

Blee TH, Cogbill TH, Lambert PJ: Hemorrhage associated with vitamin C deficiency in surgical patients, *Surgery* 131:408, 2002.

O'Riordan JM, Margey RJ, Blake G, et al: Antiplatelet agents in the perioperative period, *Arch Surg* 144:69, 2009.

Owings JT, Letter GH, Gosselin RC: Bleeding and transfusion: approaches to the patient with ongoing bleeding. In Souba WW, editor: *ACS surgery: principles and practice*, ed 6, New York, 2007, WebMD, p 61.

Ranucci M, Isgro G, Soro G, et al: Efficacy and safety of recombinant activated factor VII in major surgical procedures: systematic review and meta-analysis of randomized clinical trials, *Arch Surg* 143:296, 2008.

Sperry JL, Ochoa JB, Gunn SR, et al: An FFP: PRBC transfusion ratio ≥1:1.5 is associated with a lower risk of mortality after massive transfusion, *J Trauma* 65:986, 2008.

Zink KA, Sambasivan CN, Holcomb JB, et al: A high ratio of plasma and platelets to packed red blood cells in the first 6 hours of massive transfusion improves outcomes in a large multicenter study, *Am J Surg* 197:565, 2009.

Exposure to Blood-Borne Pathogens in the Operating Room

Nabil N. Dagher, MD, and Andrew M. Cameron, MD, PhD

OVERVIEW

Some readers will turn to this chapter in haste after an operating room needle stick. Although more than 30 different infectious pathogens have been documented as transmissible via such exposures, by far the most concerning are the hepatitis B virus (HBV), hepatitis C virus (HCV), and the human immunodeficiency virus (HIV). What follows are current data to help gauge the risk of an exposure in terms of contracting HBV, HCV, or HIV as well as considerations in terms of initiating postexposure prophylaxis (PEP). A summary table at the end of this chapter provides current recommendations regarding management.

EPIDEMIOLOGY OF NEEDLE-STICK INJURIES

Approximately 1 million needle sticks or percutaneous exposures are reported by U.S. health care workers each year. By completion of residency, nearly 100% of surgical trainees will have reported being stuck with a needle. More than 1% of the U.S. population has chronic viral illness, and the patient population encountered in the operating room is further enriched with these diseases (Table 1).

POSTEXPOSURE PROPHYLAXIS AFTER NEEDLE-STICK INJURIES

HIV

Concern over HIV transmission has decreased somewhat in recent years, and to date there has been no case of OR transmission documented, although health care provider occupational seroconversions have occurred in other settings (n = 57 through 2001). Infection has resulted primarily through percutaneous exposures involving punctures or cuts from hollow-bore needles. Transmission can also occur via mucous membranes and nonintact skin exposures to virus in blood or body fluids. This is thought to be an inefficient event, with infection occurring after only 0.3% of exposures. Although the infected patient's viral load is likely a variable in risk of transmission, the use of viral load in assessing risk of transmission has not been established. As with HCV, HIV-contaminated blood has been almost entirely eliminated from the blood supply, and such exposures are rare today.

Diagnosis in either the patient or the exposed health care worker is first via enzyme-linked immunosorbent assay (ELISA) and then confirmed by Western blot analysis. Rapid HIV tests that give results in minutes to hours are now readily available; however, there is still no vaccine for HIV. When exposure occurs, the exposed person undergoes baseline HIV serology testing; depending on the severity of the exposure, two- or three-drug antiretroviral postexposure prophylaxis is initiated, as per Table 2. The Centers for Disease Control and Prevention (CDC) recommends that therapy be started within 72 hours of exposure, as there is a window period between exposure and the onset of systemic infection.

Hepatitis B

Of the six known hepatitis viruses, only hepatitis B and C are of concern to the surgeon. Hepatitis B is a DNA virus transmitted via contaminated blood, most commonly by sexual exposure, vertical transmission, sharing of IV drug needles, or via iatrogenic exposure to a blood product. It is highly transmissible via needle stick: an injury with a contaminated (e-antigen–positive) hollow needle results in 30% probability of transmission to a susceptible host. Most health care professionals have undergone highly effective vaccination and are at no risk if they maintain adequate titers. Therefore PEP recommendations depend on the exposed surgeon's vaccination and anti-HBV surface-antigen status (Table 3).

Those who are not protected and experience acute infection may display clinically apparent hepatitis with a jaundice episode and fever (30%). Approximately 5% of those acutely infected will remain chronically infected. Those chronically infected may simply have carrier status or may progress to cirrhosis and liver failure with elevated risk of hepatocellular carcinoma. Diagnosis of acute HBV infection is made via detection of HBSAg. HBV is preventable, and the highly effective three-dose vaccine is recommended for all health care workers as well as all newborns and children. Surgeons in high-exposure specialties—transplant surgery, orthopedics, cardiac surgery, and trauma surgery—should know their vaccination status at all times and undergo a periodic booster dose every 10 years, or when antibody titer is low. Initial treatment for exposure is shown in Table 3; treatment of chronic infection depends on HBV DNA level and alanine aminotransferase (ALT) elevation but is now usually with entecavir or tenofovir.

TABLE 1: Prevalence and risk of infectious agents in operating room

Infectious Agent	Prevalence in U.S. Population	Prevalence in an Urban Population	Risk of Transmission from Needle Stick
HIV	0.3%	25%	0.3%
Hepatitis B	0.3% (1.25 million)	3%	30%
Hepatitis C	1% (4 million)	15%	3%

TABLE 2: Recommended postexposure prophylaxis following possible HIV exposure

Exposure Type	HIV+, Class A	HIV+, Class B	Unknown HIV Status	HIV Negative
Less severe*	Two-drug basic PEP	Three-drug PEP	No PEP‡	No PEP
More severe†	Expanded three-drug PEP	Three-drug PEP	No PEP‡	No PEP

Class A: asymptomatic HIV infection or low viral load (<1500 copies/mL)
Class B: symptomatic HIV infection, high viral load
*Such as a superficial or solid-needle injury
†Such as a deep puncture with a large-bore hollow needle with visible blood
‡A two-drug PEP for source with HIV risk factors may be considered

TABLE 3: Recommended postexposure prophylaxis following possible HBV exposure

Vaccination Status of Surgeon	Anti-HBSAg Positive	Anti-HBSAg Negative
Vaccinated, known response	No treatment necessary	Give HBIg and vaccine boost
Vaccinated, no response	No tx, check for HBSAg	HBIg and revaccinate or HBIg × 3 doses
Unvaccinated	No tx, check for HBSAg	Give HBIg and vaccinate

HBSAg, Hepatitis B surface antigen; *HBIg,* hepatitis B immune globulin; *tx,* transmission

TABLE 4: Summary of PEP recommendations following needle-stick exposure

Infectious Agent	PEP Recommendation
HIV	Two- or three-drug regimen based on type of exposure
Hepatitis B	HBIg or vaccination based on immune status
Hepatitis C	None currently recommended, but some evidence supports the use of interferon

transmitted across mucous membranes, and the use of eye protection during surgery is always prudent.

Hepatitis C

In contrast to HBV, there is no vaccine for HCV, although it is inefficiently transferred by needle-stick injury, with only a 3% risk upon exposure. HCV, an RNA virus, is more commonly transmitted via sharing of needles between intravenous drug abusers, and prior to 1992, via contaminated blood products. Like HBV, acute HCV infection usually does not result in clinical hepatitis (75% are asymptomatic); however, the majority of those acutely infected will progress to chronic infection with a slow but predictable march toward cirrhosis.

Diagnosis of HCV infection is made by detection of anti-HCV antibodies in the serum, which may follow acute exposures by months, or by polymerase chain reaction identification of HCV RNA, which is detectable within 7 to 14 days. Recommended protocol following exposure is for prompt testing of the source and the surgeon. If the source of the exposure is positive for HCV, the clinician should undergo baseline and repeat testing at 3 and 6 months for anti-HCV and ALT levels. No prophylaxis or treatment with antivirals is currently recommended, though the topic is controversial: approximately 25% of those acutely infected will spontaneously clear the virus, but the antiviral treatment itself is associated with considerable morbidity. On the other hand, multiple studies have shown viral clearance rates of between 90% and 98% with initiation of a course of interferon at around 8 weeks postexposure in those who have become acutely infected, with very few necessitating discontinuation of treatment due to side effects.

Preventing Sharps Injuries in the Operating Room

Cuts or needle sticks may occur in up to 15% of operations with longer, more invasive procedures with higher blood loss showing higher rates. Surgeons and first assistants are most commonly affected, followed by scrub technicians and then anesthesiologists and circulating nurses. Most injuries (70%) involve a suture needle, 10% occur when passing a sharp instrument hand-to-hand, and 25% are inflicted by a coworker. The nondominant hand is most commonly injured, and 70% of injuries go unreported. Some data suggest that wearing two pairs of gloves may reduce the danger of infection *following* a needle-stick injury by as much as 90%, and this practice is recommended.

Use of a neutral zone to pass sharps or use of the hands-free technique (HFT) is likewise currently recommended by the American College of Surgeons (ACS), which recommends surgeons "pass sharp instruments in metal trays during operative procedures." There are limited data on the efficacy of the technique, however, and available data suggest that only a small percentage of exposures occur during instrument passages. Blunt suture needles have been studied in a prospective randomized fashion and have been shown to reduce glove perforations and sharp injuries significantly during closure of fascia and muscle, and their use is thus recommended. Finally, it is always important to remember that HIV, HCV, and HBV can all be

The Infected Surgeon

The ACS recommends that surgeons learn their HBV status and undergo vaccination if not immune. Further, if they are e-antigen positive, the recommendations state: "Surgeons should obtain expert medical advice for their own care and take appropriate measures to prevent disease transmission to patients." Regarding HCV, the college recommends that all surgeons learn their antibody status, but that "surgeons who have chronic HCV infection have no reason to alter their practice based on current information." The ACS statements on HBV and HCV and the surgeon are available at http://www.facs.org/fellows_info/statements/st-22.html.

Finally, according to the ACS: "Surgeons should know their own status for HIV infection, as they would be knowledgeable about any other disease or illness that is of concern to them personally. Treatment of HIV infection, while not curative, has been effective and is recommended. Knowledge of the HIV infection status of the individual is not to be used in the determination of suitability of the surgeon for surgical practice. The HIV status of a surgeon is personal health information and does not need to be disclosed to anyone." The ACS statement on HIV and the surgeon is available at http://www.facs.org/fellows_info/statements/st-13.html.

SUGGESTED READINGS

Berguer R, Heller PJ: Preventing sharps injuries in the operating room, *J Am Coll Surg* 199(3):462–467, 2004.

Centers for Disease Control and Prevention: *Guidelines for the management of occupational exposures to hepatitis B, hepatitis C, and HIV and recommendations for postexposure prophylaxis infection control topics.* Available online at http://www.cdc.gov/ncidod/dhqp/gl_occupational.html

Centers for Disease Control and Prevention: Updated U.S. public health service guidelines for the management of occupational exposures to HIV and recommendation for postexposure prophylaxis, *MMWR* 54(Sept), 2005. Available online at http://www.cdc.gov/mmwr/preview/mmwrhtml/rr5409a1.htm.

Chen W, Gluud C: Vaccines for preventing hepatitis B in healthcare workers, *Cochrane Database Syst Rev* (4), CD000100, 2005.

Davies CG, Kahn MN, Ghauri AS, et al: Blood and body fluid splashes during surgery: the need for eye protection and masks, *Ann R Coll Surg Engl* 89(8):770–772, 2007.

Fry DE: Occupational risks of blood exposure in the operating room, *Am Surg* 73:637–646, 2007.

Jaeckel E, Cornberg M, Wedemeyer, et al: Treatment of acute hepatitis C with interferon Alfa-2b, *N Engl J Med* 345(20):1452–1457, 2001.

Landovitz RJ: Occupational and non-occupational post-exposure prophylaxis for HIV in 2009, *Top HIV Med* 17(3):104–108, 2009.

Makary MA, Al-Attar A, Holzmueller CG, et al: Needle-stick injuries among surgeons in training, *N Engl J Med* 356(26):2693–2699, 2007.

Weiss ES, Cornwell EE, Wang T, et al: Human immunodeficiency virus and hepatitis testing and prevalence among surgical patients in an urban university hospital, *Am J Surg* 193:55–60, 2007.

ANTIFUNGAL THERAPY IN THE SURGICAL PATIENT

William H. Leukhardt, MD, and
Mark A. Malangoni, MD

OVERVIEW

More than 50% of all fungal infections occur in surgical patients. The most common and clinically relevant fungal infection in surgical patients is due to *Candida,* which is the fourth most common cause of bloodstream infections. Since noncandidal fungal infections are uncommon among most surgical patients, this chapter will emphasize infections due to *Candida* species.

Several populations of surgical patients are at risk for *Candida* infection. Included among these are patients who 1) have had solid-organ transplants, such as liver, kidney, or pancreas; 2) have undergone multiple abdominal operations; 3) are receiving parenteral nutrition; 4) have had a prolonged stay in the intensive care unit (ICU), usually defined as greater than 7 days; or 5) have been colonized with *Candida.* The mortality from systemic *Candida* infections has been reported to be between 30% and 40%, depending on the site of infection and the patient population studied. Death and complications resulting from these infections are often influenced by the high acuity of illness, significant chronic comorbid conditions, and delays in the initiation of antifungal therapy.

Although there are more than 150 species of *Candida,* only nine are pathogenic to humans. The species most commonly associated with infection are *C. albicans, C. glabrata, C. krusei, C. parapsilosis,* and *C. tropicalis.* The majority of these infections are caused by *C. albicans,* which is usually susceptible to fluconazole. However, the incidence of infection by species other than *C. albicans* is increasing, and these species are more often resistant to fluconazole. *C. glabrata* infections occur more frequently in older patients and in those who have undergone solid-organ transplantation. *C. krusei* infections are commonly associated with the prior use of antifungal therapy, hematologic malignancies, neutropenia, stem-cell transplantation, or corticosteroid use. Those infected with *C. krusei* are more commonly younger, female, and are less likely to have required parenteral nutrition or mechanical ventilation or to have a concomitant bacterial infection. Infections caused by *C. glabrata* and *C. krusei* are most commonly treated with echinocandins. *C. parapsilosis* is the least common pathogen among candidal species and is associated with the lowest mortality. Patients infected with *C. parapsilosis* are most likely to have had a recent operation and are less likely to be neutropenic or to have received corticosteroids or immunosuppressive drugs compared with those infected with other *Candida* species. *C. tropicalis* infections are less common, but infections due to this organism are the most virulent. Mucosal colonization with *C. tropicalis* is often a precursor of invasive infection.

SOURCES OF INFECTION, COLONIZATION, AND DIAGNOSIS

Candidal infections typically arise from one or more of four sites: intravascular catheters, bladder catheters, colonization of a normally sterile or uninfected location, and the gastrointestinal (GI) tract. Catheters can serve as entry points for microorganisms and, once colonized, they serve as a foreign body to which these organisms can remain attached. Indwelling central venous catheters and bladder catheters are more prone to colonization; however, even peripheral venous catheters can be sites for colonization. The presence of an indwelling device in moist areas, breakdown of the normal skin barrier, or failure to maintain appropriate aseptic catheter care can predispose to colonization.

Fungal colonization has been demonstrated to be an important risk factor for invasive infection, and that risk increases when multiple sites of colonization are present. The GI tract serves as a reservoir for candidal organisms, and overgrowth can be precipitated by changes in GI flora due to ileus, antacid use, prolonged use of antibiotics, or contamination from hospital flora. Infection can result from a breach of the GI mucosal barrier in the presence of an increased concentration of these microorganisms.

The distinction between fungal colonization and infection is not well defined. The absence of colonization makes infection unlikely. *Fungal infection* is defined as isolation of a fungal pathogen in a patient with signs and symptoms of infection. When fungal infection is suspected, cultures of the presumed site of infection should be done. Patients should also have blood cultures done whenever bloodstream infection is suspected. Neutropenic patients are sometimes treated empirically for fungal infection without confirmatory cultures, and serologic studies have not been demonstrated to improve the accuracy of diagnosis. On occasion, the presence of yeast organisms on deep tissue biopsy or on Gram stain of normally sterile sites will establish the diagnosis of infection.

INDICATIONS FOR PROPHYLAXIS

The routine use of antifungal prophylaxis has been demonstrated to reduce the incidence of candidal infections in selected high-risk patients; however, antifungal prophylaxis has not been associated with a reduction in mortality. There is concern that the widespread use of prophylactic antifungals may contribute to increased drug resistance and adverse effects; however, prophylaxis may be indicated in settings where the incidence of fungal infection is high. It is important to identify and treat sites of fungal colonization to minimize the progression to infection. This also would include treatment of mucosal sites of fungal infection.

SPECIFIC INFECTIONS

Candidemia and Invasive Candidiasis

Candidemia and invasive candidiasis (IC) represent a spectrum of disease with a high mortality. Candidemia can represent isolated bloodstream infection, hematogenous spread of an existing *Candida* infection, or it can be a manifestation of IC. Blood cultures remain the gold standard to identify candidemia and, when positive, indicate the need for treatment. However, a negative blood culture does not entirely exclude an infection due to *Candida,* because blood cultures are only 50% to 60% sensitive and can take as long as 4 days to become positive. When the diagnosis of candidemia is made or strongly suspected, all catheters should be removed and cultured, and a search for a source of invasive candidiasis should be made. All patients with candidemia or IC should be treated with a loading dose of fluconazole or caspofungin. If the patient has had recent triazole exposure, is critically ill, or has severe sepsis, an echinocandin should be given. Early appropriate treatment of candidemia is associated with improved survival, especially in patients with sepsis. These patients should have repeat blood cultures, and treatment should continue until 10 to 14 days after the last positive blood culture.

Intraabdominal Infections

The management of intraabdominal infections due to *Candida* depends in part on the isolation of these organisms on peritoneal cultures. Isolates are most frequently grown on intraoperative cultures along with various bacterial pathogens; however, in this situation, the infection is usually not caused by fungi, and antifungal therapy should not be routinely used. Intraabdominal candidal infections typically arise following the failed treatment of a previous intraabdominal infection or an anastomotic leak from an upper GI source. Patients with intraabdominal infections who have been exposed to a prolonged course of antibiotics are also at risk of developing fungal infections. Fluconazole is usually the empiric choice for treatment of these infections, unless isolates are known or suspected to be resistant to this drug. Fluconazole reaches high concentrations in peritoneal fluid and should be given in doses appropriate for systemic infection. Intraabdominal abscesses due to fungi are associated with a high failure rate when managed with percutaneous drainage, and they often require operative drainage, as well as antifungal therapy, for successful treatment.

Patients with peritoneal dialysis catheters also can develop *Candida* infections. These infections are characterized by low-grade fever, malaise, abdominal pain and tenderness, and cloudy dialysate fluid that demonstrates greater than 100 neutrophils/mm^3 on cell count. These patients should receive fluconazole and have the catheter removed, and the infection should be allowed to clear before replacing the catheter.

Urinary Tract Infections

Candida is a common pathogen found in critically ill patients with urinary tract infections (UTIs). The distinction between colonization and infection of the urinary tract is not clear. Colonization of the bladder is usually seen in patients who have had prolonged catheterization and in those who have diabetes or incomplete bladder emptying. Colonization of the urine by *Candida* in a patient who requires continued catheterization usually results in eventual growth of the organism to a concentration consistent with infection (>10^5 organisms/high power field).

Removing or replacing the catheter is the most important determinant for eradication. Antifungal therapy should be instituted if the catheter cannot be removed and in patients with immune suppression who are less likely to clear their urine of yeast after catheter removal. Oral fluconazole is effective for eradication of candiduria, especially following catheter removal. Fluconazole also can be used for *C. glabrata* UTIs, as its excretion in the urine allows for effective drug concentrations. Candiduria that persists in spite of apparent appropriate therapy can also be an indication of disseminated candidiasis with excretion of these organisms in urine.

Mucosal Infections

Oral candidiasis (thrush) appears as a whitish, patchy pseudomembrane covering the oropharynx and commonly involves the tongue, hard and soft palates, and the tonsillar pillars. Controlled trials have demonstrated the efficacy of nystatin suspensions, clotrimazole troches, oral ketoconazole, fluconazole, or itraconazole in eradicating oral candidiasis. Oropharyngeal candidiasis should be treated with fluconazole for 7 days. If symptoms do not improve within 72 hours, endoscopy should be considered, as this disease can progress to esophageal candidiasis. If no significant improvement in symptoms is observed after 1 week of treatment, therapy should be altered. Treatment should extend beyond resolution of symptoms in severely immunosuppressed patients.

Suppurative Thrombophlebitis

Suppurative thrombophlebitis is a serious intravascular infection that usually follows prolonged catheterization and candidemia. It results in persistent, high-density fungemia. Appropriate management mandates high-dose antifungal therapy, removal of the catheter, and excision of the infected vein when possible. Blood cultures may remain positive for up to 3 to 4 weeks, unless source control is obtained and the vein is excised.

Pulmonary Infection

Pneumonia due to *Candida* is rare. Growth of *Candida* on culture most often represents contamination or colonization. To establish the diagnosis of pneumonia, concentrations on quantitative culture need to reach the same threshold for a positive bronchoalveolar lavage (BAL) as bacterial pneumonia (≥10^4 to 10^5 colony-forming units/mL) and ideally should be confirmed by histopathologic evaluation.

Aspergillosis

Aspergillosis is a devastating infection that occurs primarily in surgical patients who are immunosuppressed. Transplant patients receiving corticosteroids or antirejection therapy and patients with prolonged and severe neutropenia are at particular risk for infection. Invasive pulmonary aspergillosis is the most common form of infection and usually results from airborne transmission. This disease often manifests in thrombotic and hemorrhagic events including pulmonary emboli and necrotizing bronchopneumonia. A positive sputum or BAL culture helps establish the diagnosis; however, its sensitivity is only 50%. Voriconazole is the preferred antifungal; however, the high treatment failure rate of this disease often requires a combination of one or more antifungal agents as salvage therapy.

ANTIFUNGAL THERAPY

Triazoles

There are a number of oral and intravenous triazoles available for use (Tables 1 and 2). The triazoles inhibit fungal cytochrome P450; therefore drug interactions are common. Fluconazole is the first-line empiric therapy for most fungal infections suspected to be due to *Candida*, and it can also be useful for prophylaxis. It has excellent activity against *C. albicans*, and its bioavailability when given orally is similar to intravenous administration. Fluconazole has few side effects and has good penetration into the cerebrospinal fluid. *C. krusei* is resistant to fluconazole, and approximately 20% to 25% of *C. glabrata* strains may be resistant. Recently, some strains of *C. albicans* resistant to fluconazole have been identified, and it has been postulated that resistance may have developed due to the extensive use of this drug.

Fluconazole is available in both oral and intravenous forms. Its absorption from the GI tract exceeds 90%, and absorption is not affected by foods or acidity. The recommended dose varies depending on the site of infection, but an initial loading dose that is twice the recommended daily dose should be given in all serious infections. The excellent oral bioavailability of fluconazole allows for an early switch to the oral form.

Itraconazole can be used to treat candidal esophagitis, and it is also effective against *Aspergillus* and other fungi. Voriconazole and posaconazole are triazoles approved for the treatment of candidal esophagitis and aspergillosis. They are used less frequently than fluconazole for the treatment of candidal infections because of a greater incidence of adverse effects. Voriconazole is effective against *Aspergillus* and *Candida* species, including *C. krusei*. Posaconazole is generally used for salvage therapy of invasive aspergillosis and candidiasis and is only available in oral form.

TABLE 1: Recommended treatment for fungal infections

Site	Preferred	Alternative	Duration of Therapy
Candidemia/invasive candidiasis/systemic infection	Caspofungin 70 mg loading dose, then 50 mg daily IV	Fluconazole 800 mg (12 mg/kg) loading dose, then 400 mg (6 mg/kg) daily IV or LFAmB 3–5 mg/kg daily	14 days after last positive blood culture
Peritonitis/intraabdominal abscess	Fluconazole 800 mg (12 mg/kg) loading dose, then 400 mg (6 mg/kg), daily IV caspofungin, 70 mg loading dose, then 50 mg daily IV	Caspofungin, 70 mg loading dose, then 50 mg daily IV or LFAmB 3–5 mg/kg daily	10–14 days
Urinary tract infection (invasive candidiasis not suspected)	Fluconazole 200–400 mg (3–6 mg/kg) daily IV or PO	LFAmB 3–5 mg/kg daily	4–7 days
Oropharyngeal candidiasis	Nystatin suspension 400,000 to 600,000 U four times daily	Fluconazole 200 mg once PO daily	7 days
Esophageal candidiasis	Fluconazole 200–400 mg (3–6 mg/kg) daily PO	Caspofungin 70 mg loading dose, then 50 mg daily IV	14–21 days
Suppurative thrombophlebitis	Fluconazole 400–800 mg (6–12 mg/kg) daily IV	Caspofungin 70 mg loading dose, then 50 mg daily IV or LFAmB 3–5 mg/kg daily	At least 2 weeks after last positive blood culture
Aspergillosis	Voriconazole 6 mg/kg loading dose IV, then 4 mg/kg IV twice daily	Caspofungin, 70 mg IV loading dose, then 50 mg daily IV; LFAmB 3–5 mg/kg daily	Case dependent; >2 weeks, may last months (consult indicated)

Fluconazole requires a loading dose that is twice the daily dose; begin IV then convert to oral when able; caspofungin dose in patients with liver insufficiency is a 70 mg loading dose then 35 mg/day; voriconazole should be PO after IV loading dose in patients with creatine clearance <50 mL/min.
LFAmB, Liposomal formulation of amphotericin B

TABLE 2: Antifungal agents, doses, and common adverse effects

Class	Agent	Route	Common Doses	Common Adverse Effects
Triazoles				
	Fluconazole	IV, oral	800 mg (12 mg/kg) loading dose, then 400 mg (6 mg/kg) daily	Skin rash, liver dysfunction
	Itraconazole	Oral	100–200 mg once daily up to 400 mg/day after 600 mg/day loading dose for 3 days	Nausea, vomiting, rash, liver dysfunction
	Voriconazole	IV, oral	6 mg/kg IV bid loading dose then 4 mg/kg IV twice daily; trough goal range: >1 mg/L and <5.5 mg/L	Photophobia, visual hallucinations, photosensitivity, hepatotoxicity; avoid use in patients with creatine clearance <50 mL/min
	Posaconazole	Oral	100–200 mg two to four times daily	Abdominal pain, nausea, vomiting, diarrhea, prolonged QT interval, hyperbilirubinemia, hepatotoxicity, occasional suppression of adrenal function
Azoles				
	Clotrimazole	Oral	10 mg troche five times daily	Minimal, minor local effects
	Miconazole	Topical	2% topical creams	Minor local symptoms
	Ketoconazole	Oral	200–400 mg/day as a single daily dose	Hepatotoxicity, nausea, vomiting

Continued

TABLE 2: Antifungal agents, doses, and common adverse effects—cont'd

Class	Agent	Route	Common Doses	Common Adverse Effects
Echinocandins				
	Caspofungin	IV	70 mg loading dose, then 50 mg/day	Rash, pruritus, nausea, vomiting, thrombophlebitis, headache, fever, elevated liver enzymes, leukopenia, diarrhea, hypokalemia
	Anidulafungin	IV	200 mg loading dose, then 100 mg/day; 100–200 mg/day	Diarrhea, hypokalemia, elevated liver enzymes, rash, pruritus, nausea, vomiting, thrombophlebitis, headache, fever, leukopenia
	Micafungin	IV	100 mg/day; 100–150 mg/day	Rash, pruritus, nausea, vomiting, thrombophlebitis, headache, fever, elevated liver enzymes, leukopenia
Polyenes				
	Amphotericin B	IV	Formulation dependent	Formulation-dependent anemia, headaches, chills, fever, nausea, hypotension, nephrotoxicity, tachypnea, hypokalemia, hypomagnesemia, phlebitis
	Nystatin	Oral, topical	Suspension 400,000 to 600,000 U four times daily	Nausea, vomiting, diarrhea

Echinocandins

Echinocandins are fungicidals that inhibit the synthesis of β-(1,3)-D-glucan, which results in disruption of the fungal cell wall. These drugs are available only for intravenous use, and they have few significant adverse effects. Their long half-life allows for once-daily dosing, and they are not commonly associated with drug interactions. Echinocandins are metabolized by the liver.

The echinocandins are effective against all species of *Candida* and are the drugs of choice for treatment of infections due to *Candida* strains known or suspected to be resistant to fluconazole. Caspofungin is the most commonly used of these agents, and it is also effective against aspergillosis. Caspofungin is recommended as initial empiric therapy for known or suspected candidal infections in severely immunocompromised patients, when severe sepsis or septic shock is present, and for patients who have recently received fluconazole or other triazoles. Micafungin is useful for prophylaxis against candidal infections in high-risk patients.

Polyenes

Amphotericin B was the first systemic parenteral antifungal agent, and it continues to be highly effective against *Candida* and most other fungi. Amphotericin B inhibits ergosterol, an essential component of the fungal cell wall. Its use has become limited due to the development of the triazoles and echinocandins as effective antifungal agents that have fewer and less toxic adverse effects.

Approximately 20% of patients will develop fever, hypotension, and tachycardia associated with amphotericin B infusion. To identify patients at risk for this unpredictable reaction, a test dose of 1 mg should be given intravenously, while the patient is monitored. If symptoms do not develop, the regular dose can be infused. Premedication with acetaminophen (650 mg orally or rectally) or hydrocortisone (25 to 50 mg IV) can blunt this response. Nephrotoxicity resulting from the vasoconstrictive effect of therapeutic doses of amphotericin B on afferent renal arterioles, as well as hypokalemia, are common adverse effects. Lipid formulations of amphotericin B are less nephrotoxic and have fewer side effects. Liposomal amphotericin B is preferred when amphotericin B is indicated. Nystatin is highly effective against oral and cutaneous *Candida* infections and has minimal side effects. It is not useful to treat other fungal infections.

Azoles

Clotrimazole is useful for the treatment of oropharyngeal and vulvovaginal candidal infections, miconazole is effective to treat cutaneous and vulvovaginal infections, and ketoconazole is approved for the treatment of cutaneous and mucocutaneous infections; however, ketoconazole can cause abdominal pain and GI symptoms, and the GI absorption of ketoconazole is erratic, which limits its use. None of the azoles is appropriate to use for systemic infections.

SUMMARY

All patients with serious infections should initially receive intravenous antifungal therapy followed by a transition to oral therapy when applicable. Cutaneous, mucocutaneous, vulvovaginal, and most urinary infections are usually effectively treated with topical or oral agents.

SUGGESTED READINGS

Lipsett PA: Fungal infection. In Ashley SW, editor: *ACS surgery: principles and practice,* 2007, Web MD, pp 1–16.

Patel NP, Malangoni MA: Antimicrobial agents for surgical infections, *Surg Clin North Am* 89:327–347, 2009.

Measuring Outcomes in Surgery

Justin B. Dimick, MD, MPH

OVERVIEW

Outcomes after surgery are determined in large part by where and by whom a procedure is performed. Seminal studies in pancreatic surgery, conducted nearly two decades ago, documented wide gaps in clinical outcomes between high- and low-volume hospitals. More recent studies using large, detailed clinical databases suggest similar disparities in outcomes for nearly all surgical procedures. These studies suggest substantial opportunities for improving the outcomes of surgical care.

Reducing these variations, however, has proven more difficult than finding them. Two key challenges need to be addressed before we can use outcomes measurement to reduce these disparities. First, we need to be able to accurately determine when differences in outcomes are truly due to gaps in quality. Second, we need to understand the strengths and limitations of outcomes measures as applied in the "real world." This chapter offers a brief overview of these two challenges and then closes with a discussion of emerging strategies for addressing them.

UNDERSTANDING VARIATION IN OUTCOMES

Surgeons often view variations in *outcomes* as synonymous with variations in *quality*. Traditional morbidity and mortality conferences often encourage this view by expecting surgeons to accept blame for all adverse outcomes. However, surgical outcomes may vary for other reasons. In a more complete conceptual model, the so-called calculus of quality, variation in surgical outcomes can be attributed to three contributing factors: *chance, case mix* (i.e., patient factors), and *quality of care*. Although the main themes of this chapter apply to all surgical outcomes, we will focus on surgical mortality, reflecting the predominance of this measure in the literature and ongoing quality-measurement activities.

Chance

Outcomes can vary across hospitals and surgeons simply because of good or bad luck. Provider-specific outcome measures are often based on small numbers of adverse events and surgical cases, resulting in "noisy"—that is, statistically imprecise—estimates of performance. Chance is particularly important when the event rate is low (e.g., mortality rate after cholecystectomy) or the procedure is uncommon (e.g., pancreatectomy).

Chance can cause two types of errors in quality measurement. First, extreme outcomes may be attributed to quality when they are really due to chance alone: this is a type 1 error. With many quality-measurement platforms, for example, hospitals are labeled as "outliers" if their outcomes are statistically different from those expected, such as when the 95% confidence intervals around their outcome rates fail to overlap the average. Depending on where the statistical threshold for outliers is set, some hospitals will be labeled outliers based on chance alone.

A conceptual type 1 error is often made when evaluating a provider with no deaths: the so-called *zero-mortality provider*. Although having no deaths is considered a sign of superior quality, it is also possible that such providers have no deaths simply because of chance (i.e., good luck), especially if they perform a low number of cases. In a recent study using national Medicare data for five surgical procedures, we demonstrated that *zero-mortality hospitals,* defined as no deaths during 3 years, had the same or higher mortality rates during the subsequent year. Pancreatic resection showed the most striking "zero-mortality paradox." For this operation, a history of zero mortality—that is, no deaths over a 3-year period—was associated with a 30% increased risk of death in the subsequent year; so hospitals with no deaths for this operation are more likely to be lucky than good. This paradoxic finding, that hospitals with no deaths are actually lower quality, is due to the well-known relationship between low volume and high mortality for pancreatic resection.

Type 2 errors occur when chance obscures real differences in quality. Widely recognized in clinical trials as an underpowered study, this type of error is often overlooked in quality-measurement programs. One recent study by our group examined seven surgical procedures, for which hospital mortality rates had been recommended as quality indicators by the Agency for Healthcare Quality and Research. For only one operation, coronary artery bypass graft (CABG), did the majority of U.S. hospitals perform enough cases over a 3-year period to detect with statistical confidence mortality rates at least twice the national average (Figure 1). For most procedures, few hospitals had sufficient caseloads to meet this low bar of statistical power.

Case Mix

Differences in patient characteristics such as comorbidities, functional status, indications for surgery, and so on also contribute to variation in outcomes. Some providers may have worse outcomes because they treat sicker, higher risk patients than other hospitals. When measuring provider quality, these differences in patient factors are adjusted for using statistical techniques that are now fairly standard. Although risk adjustment in comparisons of provider performance is obviously important, the evidence that differences in patient factors explain variations in surgical outcomes is mixed.

The importance of risk adjustment is a function of the population being studied. In intensive care, for example, the physiologic status of the patient—as evidenced by the Acute Physiology and Chronic Health Evaluation (APACHE) score, for example—is an important driver of outcomes, and this may vary extensively across hospitals. In contrast, with elective surgery patients tend to be very homogenous with respect to physiologic status—in other words, they all walk through the door. However, types of procedures performed at different hospitals may vary extensively. Large teaching hospitals may perform more complex, higher risk procedures than small community hospitals. Even within otherwise comparable hospitals, procedure mix varies according to the specific practices of the surgeons operating there. For this reason, adjusting for procedure mix is crucial for fair comparisons of hospitals' overall surgical morbidity and mortality rates, such as those offered by provider-driven quality improvement programs such as the American College of Surgeons National Surgical Quality Improvement Program (ACS-NSQIP).

In contrast, the importance of risk adjustment may be overstated for interpreting procedure-specific comparisons, largely because case mix usually varies little across hospitals among patients undergoing the same operation. For example, we examined publicly reported mortality rates for 35 hospitals performing isolated CABG surgery in New York state in 2000 and 2001, as derived from their state-mandated clinical registries. Observed mortality rates varied considerably, from less than 1% to more than 4%. However, risk adjustment had negligible impact in reducing apparent variation in outcomes:

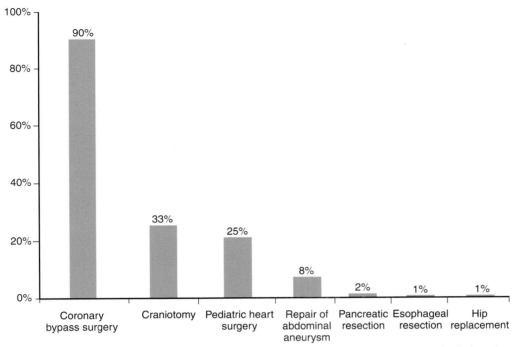

FIGURE 1   Big problems with small samples. The proportion of hospitals in the United States with sufficient caseloads (sample size) to reliably use mortality rates to measure quality.

unadjusted and adjusted hospital mortality rates were nearly identical (correlation 0.95). We conducted similar analyses of noncardiac procedures based on more recent NSQIP data and reached similar conclusions. These data are not meant to imply that patient factors are not important determinants of surgical risk. Rather, they suggest that such factors contribute little to explaining variations in procedure-specific outcomes across hospitals and surgeons.

Quality of Care

Variation in surgical outcomes that are neither a result of chance or case mix can be reasonably attributed to differences in the quality of care. For the purpose of this discussion, we consider "good quality" to comprise those details of clinical care that lead to optimal outcomes. These details are often referred to as *processes of care*. Some processes that lead to good outcomes are known and measurable, such as use of prophylactic antibiotics. However, many other processes are either unknown or unmeasurable, for example, those related to intraoperative surgical skill.

Although a list of known processes of care that potentially link to the outcomes would be extensive, payers and policy makers are currently focusing on a narrow set of perioperative care practices in their ongoing quality-measurement initiatives. These include measures aimed at reducing risks of surgical-site infection (e.g., prophylactic antibiotic administration within 60 minutes prior to surgery), venous thromboembolism, cardiac events, and ventilator-acquired pneumonia. However, recent evidence questions whether increasing compliance with this narrow set of processes will substantially reduce variation in surgical outcomes.

Based on the national Medicare population, Nicholas and colleagues (2010) noted wide variation in hospital compliance with process measures of the Surgical Care Improvement Program (SCIP), ranging from 54% in the lowest hospital tercile to 91% in the highest. However, overall process compliance was not associated with risk-adjusted mortality for any of the six procedures studied. Moreover, compliance with specific processes of care was not associated with lower rates of the adverse events each was designed to minimize;

for example, hospitals with higher rates of prophylaxis did not have lower rates of venous thromboembolism. Such data do not imply that process of care is unimportant in understanding and improving surgical mortality; they underscore the *complexity* of clinical care and the innumerable processes of care that collectively determine good outcomes after surgery. For many procedures, focusing on a limited set of individual processes will not be sufficient for understanding or reducing variation in outcomes.

In surgery, we often rely on structural measures to act as proxies for these unmeasurable and unknown processes of care. Structural variables are hospital-level resources (e.g., hospital volume) or attributes of individual providers (e.g., subspecialty training). Procedure volume is by far the most visible structural variable and has been linked to surgical outcomes for a broad range of operations. Although relatively little debate remains about the general importance of procedure volume, the strength of volume–outcome relationships varies widely by procedure. Hospital volume is most important for high-risk but relatively uncommon procedures, such as esophagectomy and pancreatectomy. For other operations—for example, CABG—hospital volume has a much weaker relationship to important outcomes. Other structural variables, such as surgeon volume and surgeon specialty, are also tightly correlated with outcomes.

Although these structural variables are useful for a narrow set of policy applications, such as selective referral, we ultimately need to understand the processes of care that explain differences in outcomes across hospitals. Once these "high-leverage" processes of care are known, they can be promoted as best practices to improve care at all hospitals. Future research should use the tools of clinical epidemiology to isolate the root causes of variation in outcomes. For example, a recent study by Ghaferi and colleagues (2009) shed light on the mechanisms underlying variations in surgical mortality rates. Using detailed, clinically rich data from the NSQIP, they ranked hospitals according to risk-adjusted mortality. When comparing the "best" to "worst" hospitals, they found no significant differences in overall (24.6% vs. 26.9%) or major (18.2% vs. 16.2%) complication rates. However, so-called failure to rescue—that is, death following major complications—was almost twice as high in hospitals with very high mortality as in those with very low mortality (21.4% vs. 12.5%,

$P < .001$). This study highlights the need to focus on processes of care related to the timely recognition and management of complications and aimed at eliminating failure to rescue and reducing variations in surgical mortality.

USING OUTCOMES TO MEASURE QUALITY

Outcome measures reflect the end result of care, from a clinical perspective or as judged by the patient. Although mortality rate is by far the most commonly used measure in surgery, other outcomes that could be used as quality indicators include complications, hospital readmission, and a variety of patient-centered measures of quality of life or satisfaction. The best example of this type of measurement is found in the NSQIP, a surgeon-led, clinical registry for feeding back risk-adjusted morbidity and mortality rates to participating hospitals. After its successful implementation in Veterans Affairs (VA) hospitals, it was introduced into the private sector with good results. Under the guidance of the ACS, hospital participation in the program continues to grow, with more than 240 hospitals currently participating.

Strengths

There are at least two key advantages of outcome measures. First, outcome measures have obvious face validity and thus are likely to get the greatest "buy in" from hospitals and surgeons. Surgeon enthusiasm for the NSQIP and the continued dissemination of the program clearly underlines this point. Second, the act of simply measuring outcomes may lead to better performance (the Hawthorne effect). For example, surgical morbidity and mortality rates in VA hospitals have fallen dramatically since implementation of the NSQIP two decades ago. No doubt many surgical leaders at individual hospitals made specific organizational or process improvements after they began receiving feedback on their hospital's performance. However, it is very unlikely that even a full inventory of these specific changes would explain the substantial improvements in morbidity and mortality rates.

Limitations

As discussed above, the Achilles heel of hospital- or surgeon-specific outcome measurement is small sample size (i.e., the role of chance). For the large majority of surgical procedures, very few hospitals or surgeons have sufficient adverse events (numerators) and cases (denominators) for meaningful, procedure-specific measures of morbidity or mortality. For example, as discussed above, a very small proportion of U.S. hospitals have adequate caseloads to reliably detect quality problems (see Figure 1). Although identifying poor quality outliers is an important function of outcomes measurement, focusing on this goal alone significantly underestimates problems with small sample sizes. Discriminating among individual hospitals with intermediate levels of performance is even more difficult.

This lack of discrimination among providers (type 2 errors) has important practical implications. When reporting outcomes in a hospital report card, we often use historic data from 2 to 3 years prior to make inferences about how a hospital is currently performing. However, some empirical data show that outcomes measures are inferior to other measures, such as hospital volume, in predicting future performance (Figure 2). Using national Medicare data, we compared the ability of historic data on hospital volume and risk-adjusted mortality (2003 to 2004) to discriminate future performance (2005 to 2006). We found that hospital volume was much better at reliably predicting future performance for less common operations, such as pancreatic resection (see Figure 2). These findings can be explained by the role of chance, as discussed above. Later in this chapter, we will discuss

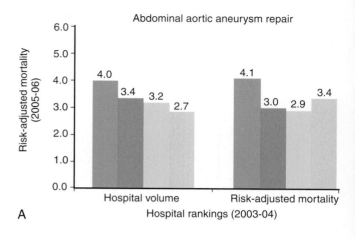

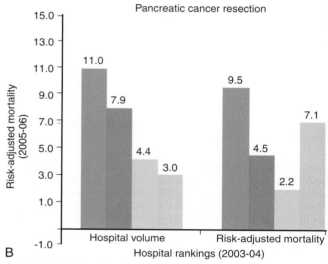

FIGURE 2   Ability of hospital rankings based on 2003–2004 mortality rates and hospital volume to predict risk-adjusted mortality in 2005–2006. **A,** Data for abdominal aortic aneurysm repair. **B,** Data for pancreatic cancer resection. *(Source: National Medicare data.)*

new tools that will help us sort out the true quality "signal" from this statistical "noise."

Another significant limitation of outcomes assessment is the expense of data collection. Reporting outcomes requires the costly collection of detailed clinical data for risk adjustment. For example, it costs over $100,000 annually for a private-sector hospital to participate in the NSQIP. Because of the expense of data collection, the program currently collects data on only a sample of patients undergoing surgery at each hospital. Although this sampling strategy decreases the cost of data collection, it exacerbates the problem of small sample size with individual procedures. As discussed later in this chapter, changes in the next iteration of the NSQIP are aimed at reducing the expense of data collection without compromising the risk adjustment.

Improving Outcomes Measurement

Although great progress has been made, the science of outcomes measurement is in its infancy. In fact, solutions are on the horizon for many of the limitations discussed above. One of the biggest limitations of surgical quality measurement is the statistical noise from the small sample sizes at most hospitals. This problem makes it difficult to isolate the quality signal from the background statistical noise. In other words, it is often hard to know whether a hospital or

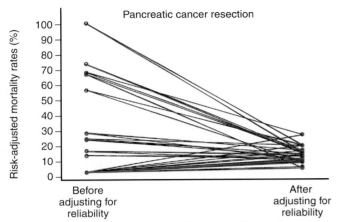

FIGURE 3   Variation in hospital mortality rates before and after adjusting for reliability. Twenty randomly sampled hospitals are shown for pancreatic cancer resection. *(Source: National Medicare data.)*

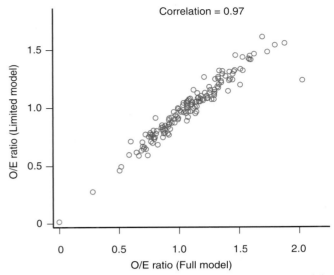

FIGURE 4   Comparison of hospital O/E ratios created using the full (up to 30 variables) versus limited model (five variables) for morbidity after five common general surgery procedures. *(Data from American College of Surgeons National Surgical Quality Improvement Program.)*

surgeon has poor performance because they provide low quality care or because they were unlucky. For obvious reasons, labeling surgeons and hospitals correctly is extremely important.

An emerging technique, *reliability adjustment,* directly addresses the problem of statistical noise. This technique, based on hierarchical modeling, quantifies and subtracts statistical noise from the measurement process. Essentially, it "shrinks" a provider's performance back toward average, unless they deviate to such an extreme that it is safe to assume they are truly different. In this way, it gives providers the benefit of the doubt. For example, Figure 3 shows the risk-adjusted mortality rates for pancreatic cancer resection in 20 hospitals before and after reliability adjustment. Prior to reliability adjustment, the mortality rates varied from 0% to 100%. After reliability adjustment, the mortality rates only varied from 2% to 22%, yielding a range of performance that is clinically more realistic. These reliability-adjusted mortality rates are much more accurate at capturing true performance, as assessed by their ability to predict future performance.

Despite increasing use in other fields, such as ambulatory care, reliability adjustment is only beginning to find applications in surgery. Perhaps the most prominent example is the Massachusetts state cardiac surgery report card, which publishes reliability-adjusted mortality rates for each hospital. This approach will also likely be applied to general and vascular surgery, as described with other changes in a recent "blueprint" for a new NSQIP. As the advantages of this technique become more widely known, there is no doubt it will become the standard technique for reporting risk-adjusted outcomes.

Another significant improvement to surgical outcomes measurement is the creation of empirically weighted composite quality measures. As payers and purchasers of health care move forward with value-based purchasing, a growing need for better measures of "global quality" becomes evident. Techniques are now emerging to create empirically weighted composite measures of surgical outcomes, and these techniques are an extension of reliability adjustment. Instead of using a single outcome, these methods combine all relevant outcomes to optimally predict a single gold standard outcome (e.g., risk-adjusted mortality). The relationships between all input measures—structure, process, and outcome—and this gold standard measure are empirically determined. A composite is then created that weights the input measures based on how reliable they are, a measure of precision, and how closely they are related to the gold-standard.

Staiger and colleagues (2009) recently published the methods for creating these measures using aortic valve replacement. They found that a composite measure of risk-adjusted mortality and hospital volume with aortic valve replacement combined with risk-adjusted mortality for other cardiac procedures explained more than two thirds of the hospital-level variation in mortality—and it was better

at predicting future performance than any individual measure. Such composite measures represent a major advance in our ability to explain variation in performance and will no doubt be widely used to profile surgeons and hospitals in the future.

Improvements in risk-adjustment are also imminent. For example, the NSQIP will be undergoing several changes that will impact risk adjustment. One major organization change will be the shift from an overall (all procedures combined) morbidity and mortality measure to procedure-specific measurement. This change will have significant impact on the risk-adjustment strategy. As discussed above, patients undergoing the same procedure tend to be a more homogenous group. As a result, it is likely that fewer variables will be necessary for risk adjustment.

To test this hypothesis, we evaluated a more limited model that used five variables, rather than the "full" model (up to 30 variables), for the five procedures targeted—colectomy, pancreatectomy, bariatric surgery, cholecystectomy, and ventral hernia repair—by the procedure-specific general surgery NSQIP module. In assessing hospital-specific outcomes, results from the limited and full-risk models were highly correlated for both mortality (range: 0.94 to 0.99 across the five operations) and morbidity (range: 0.96 to 0.99). Figure 4 shows the tight correlation (0.97) of hospital risk-adjusted morbidity (O/E ratios) for all five procedures combined. Based on these data, we believe that procedure-specific hospital quality measures can be adequately risk adjusted with a limited number of variables. In the context of the NSQIP, moving to a more limited risk-adjustment model will dramatically reduce the burden of data collection and make risk adjustment much more cost effective.

SUMMARY

Although quality is a key driver of hospital outcomes, it is also important to consider the roles of chance and patient case mix. Chance is particularly important when the number of cases per hospital is small. New techniques, such as reliability adjustment and the creation of composite measures, can be used to minimize statistical "noise" and prevent mislabeling of surgeons and hospitals. Adjustment for patient risk is obviously important, but it can be done much more efficiently. The efficiency of quality measurement platforms could be improved by focusing data collection on a smaller subset of the most important variables. Nonetheless, it is important to adjust for these differences to ensure fair comparisons and to prevent "gaming" (e.g., avoiding the sickest patients) of quality measurement systems.

Variation in outcomes that are not a result of chance and case mix can reasonably be attributed to differences in quality. Although some processes of care that lead to high-quality care are known, these explain very little of the observed variation in outcomes. Most of the processes of care that explain variations in outcomes, so-called high-leverage processes, are either unknown or unmeasurable with current methods. Using outcomes measurement to improve quality will ultimately require the use of clinical epidemiology to isolate these unknown and unmeasurable processes of care.

Suggested Readings

Birkmeyer JD, Dimick JB, Birkmeyer NJ: Measuring the quality of surgical care: structure, process, or outcomes? *J Am Coll Surg* 198:626–632, 2004.

Birkmeyer JD, Shahian DM, Dimick JB, et al: Blueprint for a new American College of Surgeons: National Surgical Quality Improvement Program, *J Am Coll Surg* 207:777–782, 2008.

Dimick JB, Birkmeyer JD: Ranking hospitals on surgical quality: does risk-adjustment always matter? *J Am Coll Surg* 207:347–351, 2008.

Dimick JB, Staiger DO, Baser O, et al: Composite measures for predicting surgical mortality in the hospital, *Health Affairs* 28:1189–1198, 2009.

Dimick JB, Welch HG: The zero-mortality paradox in surgery, *J Am Coll Surg* 206:13–16, 2008.

Dimick JB, Welch HG, Birkmeyer JD: Surgical mortality as an indicator of hospital quality: the problem with small sample size, *JAMA* 292:847–851, 2004.

Fink AS, Campbell DA Jr, Mentzer RM Jr, et al: The National Surgical Quality Improvement Program in non-Veterans Administration hospitals: initial demonstration of feasibility, *Ann Surg* 236:344–353, 2002.

Ghaferi AA, Birkmeyer JD, Dimick JB: Variation in hospital mortality associated with inpatient surgery, *N Engl J Med* 361:1368–1375, 2009.

Hofer TP, Hayward RA, Greenfield S, et al: The unreliability of individual physician "report cards" for assessing the costs and quality of care of a chronic disease, *JAMA* 281:2098–2105, 1999.

Khuri SF, Daley J, Henderson WG: The comparative assessment and improvement of quality of surgical care in the Department of Veterans Affairs, *Arch Surg* 137:20–27, 2002.

Nicholas LH, Osborne NH, Birkmeyer JD, Dimick JB: Hospital process compliance and surgical outcomes among Medicare patients, *Arch Surg* 145:999–1004, 2010.

CARDIOVASCULAR PHARMACOLOGY

Aliaksei Pustavoitau, MD, Mark Romig, MD, and Jessica Crow, PharmD

OVERVIEW

Cardiovascular pharmacology is based on manipulation of cardiac pump function and vascular function. Cardiac pump function relies on rate and rhythm, preload, contractility, and afterload. It depends on uninterrupted blood supply. Vascular function is simplistically defined by vascular tone.

CONTROL OF RATE AND RHYTHM

Problems with rate and rhythm are best described based on knowledge of ventricular myocyte action potential, or the electrical activity of the heart. Each action potential is divided into five phases characterized by distinct ionic shifts. Figure 1 shows single ventricular myocyte action potential, ionic shifts responsible for each phase, and their relationship to surface electrocardiogram (ECG). Antiarrhythmic medications modify ionic currents, thus altering electrical activity of the heart. Table 1 highlights the Vaughan-Williams classification based on the mechanism of action of each antiarrhythmic medication and the clinical indication.

TACHYARRHYTHMIAS

Supraventricular Tachyarrhythmias

Atrial fibrillation and atrial flutter are the most significant supraventricular tachyarrhythmias in the early postoperative period, affecting on average 7% of noncardiothoracic general surgery patients. Several antiarrhythmic agents are available for treatment, if the patient does not require immediate cardioversion. Amiodarone is probably the single most effective agent. A class III agent (potassium-channel blocker), it also has class I, II, and IV activity. Thus it decreases myocardial irritability, inhibits sympathetic activity, and slows atrioventricular conduction. Acutely, it functions mainly as a β-blocker. It also has a very low incidence of proarrhythmia, with a rate of *torsades des pointes* ventricular tachycardia below 1%.

β-Blockers (class II) are effective in treatment of atrial fibrillation due to attenuation of sympathetic activation in the setting of increased levels of circulating catecholamines in the perioperative period. Cardioselective β-blockers—esmolol, metoprolol, and atenolol—are particularly useful in the setting of reactive airway disorders. Esmolol has a fast onset, short half-life, and is metabolized by red blood cell esterases. Use of esmolol in high doses is limited because of the potential for ethylene glycol and methanol toxicity. Metoprolol can be given intravenously every 3 to 5 minutes, until the desired effect is achieved or further use is limited by significant hypotension. Atenolol is rarely used in the acute setting due to its long half-life, and β-blockers should be used cautiously, if at all, in the setting of hypotension, bronchospasm, and acute ventricular dysfunction. Calcium channel blockers (class IV) and digoxin (class V) are used when β-blockers are either not effective or contraindicated.

The other important arrhythmia is *paroxysmal supraventricular tachycardia*. Adenosine (class V) is effective in a majority of patients because it slows sinus rate and increases atrioventricular (AV) nodal conduction delay, thus interrupting the reentry pathways through the AV node. It can cause transient heart block or even asystole, hypotension, chest pain, dyspnea, and bronchospasm. When given intravenously, it is rapidly cleared from plasma, with duration of action of only a few seconds; it should be rapidly administered and followed by a saline flush, and it is most effective when given through the central vein. β-Blockers, calcium channel blockers, and digoxin can be used when adenosine is not effective. One exception to this rule is with Wolfe-Parkinson-White (WPW) syndrome, in which blocking the AV node will worsen arrhythmia because of the presence of accessory pathways. In this situation use of amiodarone or procainamide is the preferred treatment.

Ventricular Tachyarrhythmias

Sustained monomorphic or polymorphic ventricular tachycardia and ventricular fibrillation are associated with increased mortality. They lead to cardiac arrest, increased oxygen consumption, and exacerbation of myocardial ischemia. Prompt initiation of advanced cardiac life support (ACLS) measures is paramount to improve the outcome. Commonly this will require initiation of cardiopulmonary resuscitation (CPR), use of defibrillation or cardioversion, and administration of amiodarone or lidocaine. In addition to the above measures, injection of magnesium sulfate can be a useful adjunct when the patient presents with torsades de pointes ventricular tachycardia.

BRADYARRHYTHMIAS

Few medications are effective in treatment of bradyarrythmias. Bradycardia usually presents in the setting of myocardial ischemia. In the setting of severe bradycardia resulting from high-degree AV block (type II second-degree block or third-degree AV block) with hemodynamic compromise, an external or transvenous pacemaker

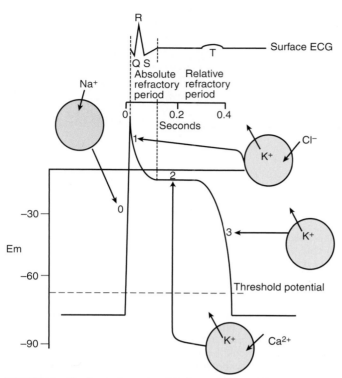

FIGURE 1 Cardiac action potential of a single ventricular myocyte. *Phase 0:* Rapid depolarization from influx of sodium through voltage-gated sodium channels. Class I antiarrhythmic agents block sodium channels and depress phase 0 depolarization, which is useful for control of both ventricular and supraventricular tachyarrhythmias. *Phase 1:* Brief repolarization caused by chloride influx and potassium efflux. *Phase 2:* Plateau phase sustained by balance of calcium influx through L-type calcium channels and efflux of potassium. Calcium channel blockers, class IV antiarrhythmic agents, inhibit slow L-type calcium channels and prolong the phase 2 plateau. β-Blockers, class II antiarrhythmic agents, also indirectly block calcium channels. Prolonging phase 2 may be useful for supraventricular tachycardias. *Phase 3:* Rapid membrane repolarization produced by potassium efflux. Class III antiarrhythmic agents block potassium channels and delay phase 2 and 3 repolarization, prolonging refraction and making the myocardium less irritable. This may be useful both in ventricular and supraventricular tachyarrhythmias. *Phase 4:* Resting membrane potential. Slow depolarization of pacemaker cells (not shown here) is governed by slow influx of sodium and calcium and reduced efflux of potassium. This phase plays a role in generation of spontaneous electrical activity. *(Modified from Meldrum DR, Cleveland JC Jr, Sheridan BC, et al: Cardiac surgical implications of calcium dyshomeostasis in the heart, Ann Thorac Surg 61:1273, 1996.)*

is a lifesaving solution. While waiting for a pacemaker, atropine is the initial treatment in this setting, although it is often ineffective for high-degree AV block. It works by inhibiting vagal cardiac influence by blocking muscarinic cholinergic receptors of sinus pacemaker cells, thus improving heart rate. Atropine dose is 0.5 mg every 3 to 5 minutes to a maximal dose of 3 mg. It crosses the blood-brain barrier, is associated with delirium, and blocks cholinergic influences in the intestines and glands. Inotropes can also be used while awaiting a pacemaker, or if pacing is ineffective.

CONTROL OF PRELOAD

A low preload state results in hypovolemic shock. Its major causes include loss of blood or body fluids via diarrhea, emesis, and so on, resulting in tissue hypoperfusion. To improve systemic oxygen

delivery, blood products are given if bleeding is the cause of hypovolemia; loss of other body fluids is corrected by replacement with balanced electrolyte solutions or colloids.

CONTROL OF MYOCARDIAL CONTRACTILITY

Myocardial dysfunction may occur as left ventricular, right ventricular, or biventricular failure. In addition, myocardial dysfunction can be related to either systolic or diastolic problems. Myocardial ischemia is the most common cause of pump failure. Finally, lack of blood ejection may be related to obstructive causes such as tamponade, tension pneumothorax, and pulmonary embolism; these require specific interventions, which are not discussed here. In general, management of cardiac failure involves treating the underlying etiologic problem while providing pharmacologic and mechanical cardiac support based on the above classification.

Myocardial Ischemia

The cornerstone in management of myocardial ischemia is to reestablish adequate coronary blood flow, ideally by percutaneous coronary intervention (PCI) within 90 minutes of presentation, and when PCI is not available, by fibrinolysis within 30 minutes. Initial management of acute coronary syndrome includes hemodynamic stabilization with inotropic and vasoactive medications and use of an intraaortic balloon pump when needed, in addition to administration of morphine, oxygen, nitroglycerin, and aspirin (MONA) while preparations are being made for revascularization. Other adjunctive medications given include β-blockers; heparin (unfractionated or low molecular weight); antiplatelet agents, such as clopidogrel; and glycoprotein IIb/IIIa inhibitors. Other medications that should be used within 24 hours of symptoms onset include angiotensin-converting enzyme inhibitors (ACEI) and 3-hydroxy-3-methylglutaryl (HMG) coenzyme A reductase inhibitor (statin) therapy.

Left Ventricular Failure

The underlying principles of managing left ventricular (LV) failure include reduction of preload with diuretics and venodilators, inotropic support, and reduction of afterload with arterial vasodilators. The most commonly used inotropes and vasopressors are summarized in Table 2. They can be divided into *adrenergic agents,* which work through activation of adrenergic receptors, and *nonadrenergic agents.* The adrenergic receptor classifications are presented in Table 3.

The apparently effective combination used to treat LV failure includes furosemide, a diuretic; nitroglycerin, especially if the patient is hypertensive and has developed coronary ischemia; and nitroprusside or nicardipine as an arterial vasodilator in a setting of hypertension. Commonly used diuretics include loop diuretics, thiazides, and potassium-sparing diuretics. The loop diuretics furosemide and bumetanide are the most potent diuretics and are used in treatment of pulmonary and systemic edema. They bind irreversibly to a chloride channel receptor site in the ascending limb of the loop of Henle, causing loss of filtered sodium and chloride. Side effects include hypovolemia, hypokalemia, hypochloremic metabolic alkalosis, hypomagnesemia, deafness, hyperuricemia (gout), and allergic skin rashes. Typical intravenous bolus doses of furosemide are 10 to 200 mg, depending on underlying renal function, and 1 to 40 mg/hr continuous infusion. Onset of diuresis begins within 15 minutes and lasts up to 6 hours. Thiazide diuretics—chlorothiazide, hydrochlorothiazide, and metolazone—inhibit sodium and chloride reabsorption in the distal nephron. Side effects are similar to loop diuretics and also include hyperlipidemia and hyperglycemia. These medications

TABLE 1: Practical Vaughan-Williams classification of antiarrhythmic medications

Class	Mechanism	Selected Medication	Doses	Indications	Side Effects
IA	Blocks sodium channels, prolongs refractory period	Procainamide	20 mg/min IV infusion until stable to a max dose 17 mg/kg, then 1–4 mg/min	Supraventricular and ventricular tachyar-rhythmias, WPW syndrome	Proarrhythmic, hypotension in setting of LV dysfunction
IB	Blocks sodium channels, shortens refractory period	Lidocaine	1–1.5mg/kg bolus, can repeat to max of 3 mg/kg, then 1–4 mg/min	Ventricular tachyar-rhythmias	Seizures
IC	Blocks sodium channels, has no effect on refrac-tory period	Propafenone	150 mg PO q8h	Supraventricular tachyarrhythmias	Proarrhythmia
II	Blocks adrenergic cardiac β_1-receptors	Esmolol Metoprolol	0.5 mg/kg bolus, 25–300 µg/kg/min 2.5–5 mg every 5 min	Supraventricular tachyarrythmias, not WPW syndrome	Bradycardia, hypotension, bronchospasm
III	Blocks potassium myocardial channels	Amiodarone Sotalol	150 mg over 10 min, then 1 mg/min for 6 hr, and 0.5 mg/kg for 18 hr 80 mg PO q12h titrated to max 640 mg/day	Supraventricular and ventricular tachyarrhythmias	Well tolerated Proarrhythmia, hypo-tension in setting of LV dysfunction
IV	Blocks AV node, slows L-type calcium channels	Verapamil Diltiazem	2.5–10 mg bolus to a max 20 mg 15–20 mg over 2 min, then 5–15 mg/hr	Supraventricular tachyarrythmias, not WPW syndrome	Hypotension in set-ting of LV dysfunc-tion
V	Works by some other mechanism	Digoxin Adenosine Magnesium	10–15 µg/kg lean body weight in three divided doses, follow levels 6 mg, then 12 mg 1 –2 g over 5–30 min	Supraventicular tachyarrhythmias *Torsades des pointes*	Interaction with amiodarone Hypotension, bron-chospasm Hypotension

LV, Left ventrtricular; *WPW*, Wolff-Parkinson-White syndrome

TABLE 2: Commonly used inotropic and vasopressor medications

Medication	Dose Range	Mechanism	Indications
Norepinephrine	1–20 µg/min	α_1, α_2, α_1	Vasoconstrictor
Epinephrine	1–20 µg/min	α_1, α_2, β_1, β_2	Inotrope and vasoconstrictor
Dopamine	1–20 µg/kg/min	α_1, α_2, β_1, β_2, dopamine	Inotrope and vasoconstrictor
Dobutamine	2–20 µg/kg/min	β_1, β_2	Inotrope and vasodilator
Phenylephrine	20–200 µg/min	α_1	Vasoconstrictor
Isoproterenol	1–20 µg/min	β_1, β_2	Inotrope and chronotrope
Milrinone	0.25–0.75 µg/kg/min	Phosphodiesterase 3 inhibitor	Inotrope and vasodilator
Vasopressin	0.01–0.04 U/min	Vasopressin V1 and V2 receptors	Vasoconstrictor in catecholamine-resistant shock

are less potent than loop diuretics, and in an acute setting, they are commonly used as cotreatment with loop diuretics. Potassium-spar-ing diuretics include aldosterone antagonists (spironolactone) and amiloride, which inhibits sodium reabsorption in the collecting duct. These are weak diuretics that exist only as oral preparations, and they can cause hyperkalemia. Spironolactone is the most useful in situa-tions with increased aldosterone production, such as with congestive heart failure and hepatic cirrhosis.

The precise use of inotropic support will depend on the clinical situ-ation. In the setting of hypertension, dobutamine, low-dose dopamine, low-dose epinephrine, or milrinone improve myocardial contractility and serve as vasodilators. They all increase myocardial oxygen con-sumption and may exacerbate infarct size. In patients with hypoten-sion, higher doses of dopamine, epinephrine, or norepinephrine are used. Isoproterenol is used for its positive chronotropic effects to main-tain heart rate after heart transplantation or in complete heart block.

Right Ventricular Failure

The right ventricle (RV) is adapted predominantly to handle volume work. Its tolerance of increased pressure load in the pulmonary vasculature is very poor. The principles of RV support are similar to LV support—lower preload, support inotropic function, and reduce afterload—but in relationship to the RV. Diuretics and nitroglycerin are effective in reducing preload, and inotropic support is provided with dobutamine, epinephrine, and dopamine. Milrinone has a particularly important role in this situation, as it also serves as a pulmonary vasodilator thus reducing RV afterload. In addition, inhaled nitric oxide (iNO) can be used for selective reduction of RV afterload (see below under Pulmonary Hypertension).

Diastolic Dysfunction

Patients with normal or near-normal ejection fraction who have signs and symptoms of heart failure are thought to have diastolic dysfunction resulting in increased diastolic ventricular pressure. It more commonly affects elderly patients, women, and those with hypertension. These patients may present with recurrent episodes of flash pulmonary edema. Treatment of patients with diastolic dysfunction includes control of systolic and diastolic hypertension; rate control of atrial fibrillation; use of diuretics to control pulmonary congestion, bearing in mind that low preload may result in significant hypotension; and coronary revascularization, if ischemia plays a significant role. Pharmacologic agents that may provide symptomatic improvement include β-blockers, ACEIs, angiotensin receptor blockers (ARBs) and calcium channel blockers.

CONTROL OF AFTERLOAD

Systemic inflammatory response syndrome (SIRS) is a universal response of the human body to an acute insult such as trauma, surgical injury, and cardiopulmonary bypass. Sepsis is a cause of SIRS in the setting of infection. It is mediated by cytokines, prostaglandins, thromboxane A2, and nitric oxide; it results in vasodilation, endothelial damage, and capillary leak. Other conditions that result in profound vasodilation include anaphylactic and neurogenic shock. The mainstay treatment of these conditions includes adequate fluid resuscitation, in the setting of relative hypovolemia; use of potent vasoconstrictors; and, when myocardial depression present, the use of inotropes (see Table 2).

In septic shock, norepinephrine is commonly used as a first-line agent. It is a potent α-agonist with minimal β-agonist effects. Dopamine is used as an alternative first-line agent in septic shock. Compared with norepinephrine, it has greater inotropic but fewer vasoconstrictive effects. This may result in more tachycardia and greater myocardial contractility and oxygen consumption, thus potentially achieving supraphysiologic hyperdynamic circulation, which has been associated with poorer outcomes in septic shock. When septic shock is associated with myocardial dysfunction, dobutamine can be added, or epinephrine can be used as a single agent. Epinephrine is associated with increased lactate concentrations, the potential to produce myocardial ischemia and arrhythmias, and reduced splanchnic blood flow. Finally, vasopressin at 0.03 U/min should be used in a setting of adequately fluid-resuscitated septic shock refractory to high doses of catecholamines. Vasopressin use is based on the rationale that septic shock is a relative vasopressin deficiency state, and the expected effect is an equivalence to norepinephrine alone; however, high doses of vasopressin are associated with coronary, splanchnic, and digital ischemia.

TREATING HYPERTENSION

Systemic Hypertension

Hypertension is prevalent in 30% of the general population and is a common problem in the perioperative period. The decision as to whether, and how aggressively, to treat systemic hypertension requires an assessment of the risk and benefit to the patient. Hypertensive emergencies are the most concerning and often require intravenous antihypertensives to attain adequate control. Although a blood pressure greater than 180/120 mm Hg is often used as a cutoff value, the true marker of hypertensive emergency is the presence of end-organ damage (Table 4).

Extra care must be taken to manage hypertension during the perioperative period, as malignant hypertension can lead to increased bleeding and vascular graft failure. In the absence of end-organ damage, severe hypertension greater than 180/120 mm Hg may also require prompt but less aggressive management. The typical goal of

TABLE 3: Effects of adrenergic and vasopressin receptor subtypes on cardiovascular system

Receptor	Location	Effect
α_1	Systemic arterioles (abdominal viscera, coronary, skin, skeletal muscle), veins, pulmonary arterioles	Vasoconstriction
α_2	Presynaptic and postsynaptic sympathetic nerve terminals, central nervous system	Vasodilation
β_1	Heart	Inotropy, chronotropy, dromotropy
β_2	Systemic arterioles (abdominal viscera, coronary, skeletal muscle), veins, pulmonary arterioles	Vasodilation
Dopamine	Systemic arterioles (abdominal viscera, renal, coronary)	Vasodilation
V_1	Vascular smooth muscle	Vasoconstriction
V_2	Renal distal convoluted tubule and collecting duct	Antidiuresis

TABLE 4: Hypertensive emergencies

Cerebrovascular	Hypertensive encephalopathy Atherothrombotic brain Infarction Intracerebral hemorrhage Subarachnoid hemorrhage
Cardiac	Acute aortic dissection Acute left ventricular failure Acute myocardial infarction
Pulmonary	Pulmonary edema
Renal	Acute glomerulonephritis
Pregnancy	Severe preeclampsia HELLP syndrome Eclampsia

HELLP, Hemolysis, elevated liver enzymes, and low platelet count therapy is to reduce the mean arterial pressure by 25% in the first hour and then reduce it to 160/100 to 110 mm Hg over 2 to 6 hours, and additional reduction may be warranted in some cases, such as with aortic dissection. However, overly aggressive reductions in blood pressure can lead to ischemic events, such as ischemic stroke and myocardial infarction, when blood pressure falls below the autoregulatory range.

Initial management of perioperative hypertension should focus on alleviating precipitating causes such as pain, hypervolemia, hypoxia, hypercarbia, and hypothermia. Rebound hypertension after withdrawal of home antihypertensive medications is another common cause of perioperative hypertension and is often adequately treated by administration of the patient's regular antihypertensives.

Both cardiac selective and non–cardiac-selective β-blockers have been successfully used in the control of hypertension. Esmolol is available only as an IV infusion, and blood pressure is reduced by reducing heart rate and contractility, thus esmolol may not be an ideal agent in patients who already have impaired cardiac output. Esmolol infusion is started with a 0.5 to 1 mg/kg loading dose administered over 1 minute, followed by a 50 µg/kg/min infusion. The infusion can be titrated up to 300 µg/kg/min. Labetalol is a non–cardiac-selective β-blocker and $α_1$-blocker. The α-blockade reduces vascular smooth muscle tone, thereby increasing vascular capacitance and directly decreasing blood pressure. The ratio of α to β effect is variable and depends on the route of administration, with a 1:3 ratio when given orally versus a 1:7 ratio when given intravenously. Labetalol can be administered orally, by intermittent IV bolus, or by IV infusion. When given orally, it is started at 100 mg twice a day, and it can be titrated up to a total combined dose of 2400 mg daily. Intravenous boluses of 20 mg of labetalol have a rapid onset of action of 2 to 5 minutes, with peak effects at 5 to 15 minutes. Repeat dosing can be given every 10 minutes up to a total dose of 300 mg. Although labetalol can be administered by intravenous infusion, the long half-life of 5.5 hours makes it difficult to titrate. β-Blockers are contraindicated in patients with bradycardia, first-degree heart block, asthma, and decompensated heart failure.

The dihydropyridine calcium channel blockers act on vascular smooth muscle tone and are potent vasodilators that reduce afterload. Unlike their nondihydropyridine counterparts, they do not act on the sinus node, which depresses cardiac contractility. Calcium channel blockers are also not associated with reflex tachycardia. Nicardipine is administered by IV infusion and has a short half-life of 2 to 4 hours. Dosing is independent of weight and starts at 5 mg/hr. The drug is titrated every 15 minutes to maximum dose of 15 mg/hr. Clevidipine has a much shorter half-life, about 1 minute, which results in much faster titration. Infusion is initiated at 1 to 2 mg/hr, and the dose is doubled every 90 seconds, up to a maximum dose of 21 mg/hr, until blood pressure control is achieved. Although sublingual nifedipine has traditionally been used to treat severe hypertension, the rapid onset and unpredictable pharmacodynamic effects have been associated with uncontrollable hypotension, stroke, myocardial infarction, and death. As such, this practice has largely been abandoned.

ACEIs act by inhibiting the production of angiotensin II, which causes renal sodium and water retention and systemic vasoconstriction. In addition, ACEIs cause vasodilation of the efferent arteriole of the kidney, which decreases perfusion pressures and glomerular filtration rate. In the volume-depleted patient, this decrease in perfusion pressure can lead to acute renal failure, which limits the usefulness of ACEIs in the surgical population. Enalaprilat is available in an intravenous formulation and is given in intermittent bolus injections every 6 hours. Dosing is started at 1.25 mg and can be titrated up to 5 mg. Peak effect is not typically seen for 1 hour, which limits its usefulness in hypertensive emergencies.

Fenoldopam is a dopamine-1 receptor agonist that acts on peripheral, renal, and mesenteric arteries to decrease peripheral vascular resistance while preserving renal blood flow. Treatment should be initiated at 0.1 to 0.3 µg/kg/min and can be titrated every 15 minutes to a maximum dose of 1.6 µg/kg/min. Fenoldopam is associated with reflex tachycardia, which can limit its clinical usefulness.

Sodium nitroprusside is a nitric oxide (NO) donor that acts directly on the arterial and venous vasculature, resulting in both preload and afterload reductions. The advantage of nitroprusside is its rapid onset of action, with blood pressure reductions seen within minutes. A starting dose of 0.3 to 0.5 µg/kg/min can be titrated to a maximum dose of 10 µg/kg/min, although effective doses normally are less than 4 µg/kg/min. Despite its clinical utility, nitroprusside use is limited by several factors: special handling is required, as exposure to light causes degradation of the drug; nitroprusside is converted to cyanide in the bloodstream with unpredictable accumulation, which can result in toxicity in as little as 6 hours; and finally, an association between increased intracranial hypertension and nitroprusside administration limits its use in patients with cerebrovascular ischemia or hypertensive encephalopathy. Its use is also associated with reflex tachycardia.

Nitroglycerin is converted to NO and acts on the vasculature primarily as a venodilator, although arterial dilation can be seen with escalating doses. The result is primarily preload reduction, which can negatively impact cardiac output. Nitroglycerin is given as an IV infusion and is started at 5 µg/min. Onset of action is rapid, and the dose can be increased by 5 µg/min every 3 to 5 minutes until a dose of 20 µg/min is reached. After that, dosing can be increased by 10 µg/min every 3 to 5 minutes until a maximum dose of 200 µg/min is achieved. As with some other direct-acting vasodilators, nitroglycerin therapy is plagued by reflex tachycardia. Nitroglycerin is not a first-line agent because of its effect on preload and cardiac output, however, this effect may be beneficial in patients with acute pulmonary edema.

Hydralazine is a potent direct-acting arteriolar vasodilator that improves cardiac afterload. It is administered intravenously in doses of 10 to 20 mg every 6 hours and can be increased to 40 mg if needed. Response is typically seen within 30 minutes. Like other bolus-dosed antihypertensives, the pharmacodynamics can be unpredictable. Reflex tachycardia also limits the clinical utility of hydralazine.

Pulmonary Hypertension

Patients with pulmonary hypertension are at increased risk of right-heart failure during the perioperative period, and they have an increased rate of morbidity and mortality. Current World Health Organization (WHO) classification divides pulmonary hypertension into five broad categories, shown in Table 5. Preoperative optimization for pulmonary hypertension should be aimed at treating the underlying cause, such as valvular lesions or chronic obstructive pulmonary disease (COPD). However, many underlying causes are not amenable to treatment in the perioperative period. General perioperative management for all classes of pulmonary hypertension should be aimed at alleviating causes of exacerbation—such as acidosis, hypoxia, hypoventilation, pain, and polycythemia—and thus should include supplemental oxygen administration and hyperventilation,

TABLE 5: Revised WHO classification of pulmonary hypertension

Class	Description
1	Pulmonary artery hypertension
2	Pulmonary hypertension with left heart disease
3	Pulmonary hypertension associated with lung disease and/or hypoxia
4	Pulmonary hypertension due to chronic thrombotic and/or embolic disease
5	Miscellaneous

bicarbonate administration for uncompensated metabolic acidosis, adequate analgesia, and avoidance of unnecessary blood transfusions. Intravascular volume should be aggressively managed to avoid increased afterload on the right heart and may require diuretic therapy. In the ICU setting, direct pulmonary artery pressure measurements using a pulmonary artery catheter can be used to guide therapy. When patients do not respond to these initial modalities, pulmonary vasodilators should be initiated.

Mainstay treatment for pulmonary hypertension involves dilating the pulmonary vasculature to reduce right ventricular afterload and improve function. Chronic treatments include calcium channel blockers, prostanoids, endothelin receptor agonists, and phosphodiesterase type 5 (PDE5) inhibitors; whenever possible these should be continued in the perioperative period.

Milrinone is a PDE3 inhibitor that prevents the breakdown of cyclic adenosine monophosphate (cAMP), which results in systemic and pulmonary vasodilation. In addition, milrinone has a positive ionotropic effect on the heart without an increase in the heart rate. The use of milrinone is often limited by its systemic hypotensive effects, which can be more pronounced if a loading dose is used. If desired, a loading dose of 50 µg/kg is given over 10 minutes, and then infusion is started at 0.375 µg/kg/min. This can be titrated up to 0.75 µg/kg/min if systemic blood pressure allows. Milrinone is also associated with atrial and ventricular arrhythmias. Because of its long half-life of 2.5 hours, which is further prolonged up to 20 hours in renal dysfunction, arrhythmias may persist even after discontinuation of infusion.

Inhaled NO (iNO) is a selective pulmonary artery dilator that acts to increase cyclic guanosine monophosphate (cGMP) to induce smooth-muscle relaxation in the precapillary arterioles. When inhaled, NO is selectively delivered to ventilated portions of the lung, thus preserving ventilation/perfusion matching. Typical dosage range of iNO is 5 to 80 parts per million (ppm), with a threshold effect on pulmonary vasculature around 10 ppm. In addition, iNO has a half-life of 15 to 30 seconds, significantly longer than endogenous NO, and it has minimal systemic effects. Abrupt discontinuation of iNO can result in return of pulmonary hypertension and subsequent ventilation/perfusion mismatching, so it should be discontinued by slow weaning. Clearance of iNO involves binding to hemoglobin and can ultimately lead to methemoglobinemia, even when dosed within an acceptable therapeutic range.

Sildenafil potentiates the effects of iNO by inhibiting PDE5 and the breakdown of cGMP. In patients who experience rebound pulmonary hypertension from iNO discontinuation, sildenafil can be instituted to facilitate iNO weaning. Sildenafil is administered orally three times per day, starting at a dose of 10 to 20 mg and titrated to a dose of 80 mg.

Prostanoids are synthetic analogues of the prostacyclin PGI_2, which acts on systemic and pulmonary vascular beds to promote vasodilation. Prostanoids are available in both inhaled and intravenous formulations. Iloprost is an inhaled prostanoid that is administered every 2 hours while the patient is awake. The starting dose is 2.5 µg, but this can be increased to 5 µg if tolerated. Epoprostenol is one of the intravenous prostanoid formulations. It is started at 1 to 2 ng/kg/min and can be titrated up by 1 to 2 ng/kg/min every 15 minutes. No maximum dose has been defined, but doses as high as 195 ng/kg/min have been described in children. Limited evidence for the use of inhaled epoprostenol also exists. Titration of both prostanoids is limited by significant systemic effects, such as pulmonary edema. Prostanoids also inhibit platelet aggregation and increase risk of bleeding.

PHARMACOLOGIC PERIOPERATIVE RISK REDUCTION

The decision to continue, discontinue, or institute new medications in the perioperative period can have a significant impact on patient outcome. The risk and benefit to the individual patient must be carefully considered when using pharmacology to modify perioperative cardiac risk.

β-Blockers are the most hotly debated medications used in the perioperative period. Patients who chronically take β-blockers have upregulation of adrenergic receptors. Withdrawal of β-blockers is associated with increased sympathetic activity; independent of surgery, it has been associated with increased cardiac morbidity and mortality. Patients are particularly at risk during the hyperadrenergic state of the perioperative period, thus β-blockade should not be discontinued. The same risk reduction has not been seen when β-blockers have been initiated during the perioperative period. Administration of β-blockers to patients without cardiovascular disease offers no cardiac benefit and has been associated with harm. Initiating β-blocker therapy during the perioperative period in patients with cardiovascular risk factors has shown reduction in cardiac morbidity and mortality. However, this benefit is outweighed by noncardiac harm, such as stroke; overall, β-blocker therapy is associated with higher mortality.

Statins act by inhibiting the HMG CoA reductase enzyme, which is the rate-limiting step in cholesterol synthesis. Traditionally thought of simply as lipid-lowering agents, mounting evidence suggests that the risk reductions seen with statins cannot be explained solely by cholesterol reduction but are likely related to modulation of inflammation, endothelial function, and coagulation. Prospective trials have shown perioperative risk reductions in patients who continue statin therapy during the perioperative period. However, there are no prospective studies addressing whether statins should be started for at-risk patients during this time.

Coronary stenting is becoming an increasingly common modality for treating cardiovascular disease. After stent placement, antiplatelet therapy with aspirin and clopidogrel is required to prevent stent thrombosis, and discontinuation during this high-risk period is associated with devastating outcomes. Bare metal stents require 1 month of dual antiplatelet therapy, and drug-eluting stents require at least 1 year of therapy. Even after completion of this period, aspirin therapy is continued for life. Careful assessment of bleeding risk versus the risk of stent thrombosis should be considered prior to discontinuing antiplatelet agents. Both aspirin and clopidogrel irreversibly inactivate platelets, and new platelet turnover is required for restoration of platelet function. As such, discontinuation of antiplatelet agents less than 5 days prior to surgery offers no benefit with regard to bleeding. Prospective studies of vascular patients who underwent surgery while continuing dual antiplatelet therapy showed increased rates of bleeding and transfusion requirements; however, no difference in long-term morbidity or mortality was found. Only the neurosurgical population has shown detriment from continuing antiplatelet agents.

SUGGESTED READINGS

American Heart Association: 2005 American Heart Association guidelines for cardiopulmonary resuscitation and emergency cardiovascular care, *Circulation* 112(suppl 24), IV1–203, 2005.

Antman EM, Hand M, Armstrong PW, et al: 2007 focused update of the ACC/AHA 2004 guidelines for the management of patients with ST-elevation myocardial infarction, *Circulation* 117(2):296–232, 2008.

Hunt SA, Abraham WT, Chin MH, et al: 2009 focused update incorporated into the ACC/AHA 2005 guidelines for the diagnosis and management of heart failure in adults, *Circulation* 119(14):391–479, 2009.

Dillinger RP, Levi MM, Carlet JM, et al: Surviving Sepsis Campaign: international guidelines for management of severe sepsis and septic shock: 2008, *Crit Care Med* 36(1):296–327, 2008.

Douketis JD, Berger PB, Dunn AS, et al: The perioperative management of antithrombotic therapy: American College of Chest Physicians evidence-based clinical practice guidelines (8th edition), *Chest* 133(suppl 6): 299S–339S, 2008.

GLUCOSE CONTROL IN THE POSTOPERATIVE PATIENT

Margarita Ramos, MD, MPH, and
Selwyn O. Rogers Jr, MD, MPH

OVERVIEW

Postoperative complications, with their attendant morbidity, cost, and mortality, remain a persistent and vexing problem in surgical care. Decreased postoperative morbidity and mortality have been targeted for quality improvement initiatives. In the pantheon of complications ranging from technical failures to communication breakdowns, postoperative infections are the most common complication; they affect an estimated 9% to 30% of all surgical patients each year, representing roughly 2 million cases per year.

Intensive glucose control in some postoperative populations has been shown to increase survival and decrease complications. Inpatient hyperglycemia has been associated with poor outcomes, prolonged length of stay, wound infection, and inpatient and outpatient mortality. This association has been demonstrated in a wide variety of patients, including critically ill surgical patients and those who have suffered myocardial infarction, stroke, pneumonia, and undiagnosed diabetes. Numerous observation studies have consistently demonstrated an almost linear relationship between blood glucose levels and adverse clinical outcomes, especially infectious ones, irrespective of diabetes status (Figure 1).

This chapter reviews the pathophysiology of stress-induced hyperglycemia, examines the association between perioperative hyperglycemia and postoperative outcomes in various settings, discusses the role for glycemic control to decrease postoperative complications, and addresses the challenges and risks in achieving glycemic control.

PERIOPERATIVE HYPERGLYCEMIA

Surgical stress, trauma, and/or critical illness can lead to the body's dysregulation of glucose homeostasis. Even surgical patients without diabetes are susceptible to stress-induced hyperglycemia. The metabolic stress response increases cortisol, glucagon, growth hormone, and epinephrine secretion, and acute hyperglycemia increases inflammatory factors. Among a host of other changes, oxidative stress decreases immune function, slows wound healing, impairs endothelial function, and promotes a procoagulant state. Poor outcomes are potentially related to cellular injury, apoptosis, tissue damage, and altered wound repair.

Diabetes is a well-known comorbidity that leads to poorer outcomes. In patients with diabetes, comorbid conditions caused by chronic hyperglycemia result in a greater need for surgical interventions, which puts those patients at a higher risk of postoperative complications compared with patients who do not have diabetes. In cardiac surgery patients who have diabetes, hyperglycemia in the perioperative period has a strong association with postoperative infection after coronary artery bypass graft (CABG). Noncardiac vascular surgical patients have a 1.7-fold and 2.1-fold increased risk of postoperative 30-day mortality with admission glucose levels in the prediabetic and diabetic range. Hyperglycemia appears to not only be an important predictor of mortality and morbidity in surgical patients without diabetes, but also a marker for surgical stress. When adjusted for severity of illness, patients with hyperglycemia are more likely to have adverse outcomes.

Perioperative Hyperglycemia and Surgical Outcomes

Cardiovascular Operations

In a study of diabetic patients undergoing cardiac surgery, lower postoperative glucose levels were demonstrated to be associated with lower postoperative infectious complications. In this observational study using historic controls, diabetic patients undergoing cardiac surgery received an intervention of intravenous insulin protocol with a goal blood glucose less than 200 mg/dL. The primary outcome was the rate of deep wound infections, including mediastinitis (Figures 2 and 3). At postoperative day 1, glucose progressively rose from 100 to 150 mg/dL to 250 to 300 mg/dL, and the deep-space infection rate rose from a nadir of 13% to a peak of 67%. As cumulative evidence mounted supporting the association of perioperative hyperglycemia and infectious outcomes following cardiac surgery, the 6 AM postoperative glucose became incorporated as a process measure for quality of cardiac surgical care in the Surgical Care Improvement Program (SCIP).

Control of hyperglycemia after CABG has been shown to not only decrease postoperative complications but also to decrease mortality. A long-term follow-up study of 970 cardiac surgery patients revealed that even after 4 years, the survival benefit was preserved in the group that had tight glycemic control during their hospital stay.

Intensive Care Unit Outcomes

In 2001, a landmark study that radically and systematically changed intensive care unit (ICU) practice, Van den Berghe and colleagues reported that intensive glycemic control with intravenous insulin protocol reduces morbidity and mortality in critically ill surgical

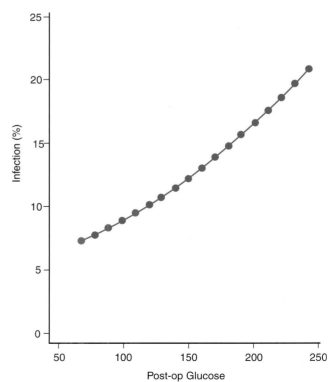

FIGURE I Adjusted probability of infection. *(From Ramos M, Khalpey Z, Lipsitz S, et al: Relationship of perioperative hyperglycemia and postoperative infections in patients who undergo general and vascular surgery, Ann Surg 248[4]:585–591, 2008.)*

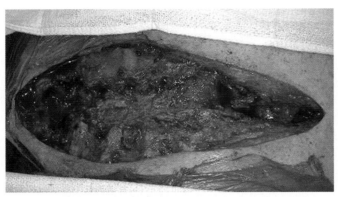

FIGURE 2 Sternal wound infection.

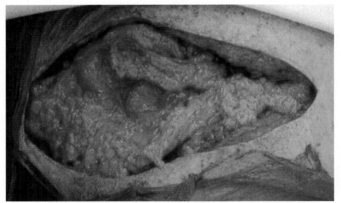

FIGURE 3 Omental flap in chest wound following sternal debridement.

patients. A large prospective trial randomized 1548 mechanically ventilated patients in the surgical ICU. The majority of these patients had undergone cardiac surgery. The intervention was an intravenous insulin infusion targeting glucose of 80 to 110 mg/dL versus conventional treatment. Mortality was significantly reduced in critically ill surgical ICU patients when intensive glycemic control was utilized, compared with conventional insulin therapy. Tight glycemic control resulted in a 34% decreased risk of mortality. For patients with ICU stays greater than 5 days, the survival benefit was even greater: 20.2% for the conventional arm compared with 10.6% for the intensive glycemic control arm. Furthermore, a 50% decrease was observed in morbidity in critically ill surgical patients with shorter ICU stays and a shorter ventilator duration in addition to lower rates of renal failure, septicemia, and polyneuropathy. The only adverse outcome was more hypoglycemia in the treatment group (5%) versus the conventional arm (0.7%).

Attempts to duplicate the findings of the Van den Berghe trials have not been successful. The Efficacy of Volume Substitution and Insulin Therapy in Severe Sepsis (VISEP) trial reported no survival benefit with intensive glucose control. Septic adults were enrolled in a factorial design paired trial of hydroxyethyl starch versus Ringer's lactate for volume resuscitation and glucose targets of 180 to 200 mg/dL versus 80 to 110 mg/dL using intravenous insulin. The trial was stopped prematurely because of a high incidence of hypoglycemia (12.1% in the intensive glucose group versus 2.1% in the conventional arm). Higher mortality rates and renal failure rates were found in the hydroxyethyl starch group compared with the Ringer's lactate group. Intensive insulin therapy was not an independent predictor of death, but hypoglycemia was. Given the early trial termination and study design, some have questioned the clinical usefulness of the results.

General and Vascular Surgery Patients

Even though the majority of the 30 million operations performed in the United States each year are for noncardiac procedures, the association between hyperglycemia and postoperative complications in noncardiac surgery patients has not been fully elucidated. Currently, serum glucose levels are routinely obtained for patients with diabetes and for those having cardiac surgery as part of their perioperative care, but this is not done for the average general surgery patient.

It is known that glucose levels are not well controlled in the perioperative period. In a retrospective case-control study of geriatric patients at risk for delirium and undergoing abdominal surgery, researchers found that 34% of patients failed to have glycemic control (<150 mg/dL of serum glucose) during the first 72 hours after surgery. Given the cumulative evidence on the positive impact of glucose control in the postoperative period in a subset of surgery patients, the need to establish the risk associated with stress hyperglycemia for a broad base of surgical patients is imperative for optimal surgical management and quality improvement.

In a recent study, we evaluated the risk of postoperative infection in patients with perioperative hyperglycemia who underwent major noncardiac surgery. Postoperative hyperglycemia was found to be strongly associated with postoperative infection rates in both general and vascular surgery patients. We analyzed data prospectively collected by trained nurse reviewers as part of the American College of Surgeons National Surveillance Quality Improvement Program (ACS-NSQIP) at our institution, supplemented by perioperative glucose levels collected over an 18-month period; in addition, 995 adult patients were studied who underwent inpatient major general and vascular surgery with 30-day follow-up. Univariate predictors of postoperative infection included postoperative hyperglycemia, age, history of diabetes, American Society of Anesthesiologists (ASA) class, operation length, and amount of blood transfused. Patients with diabetes versus those without had 15.3% and 8.8% rates of postoperative infection, respectively. Patients with diabetes who received oral agents had 9.9% infection rates, and those dependent on insulin had 21.7% rates of postoperative infection. In multivariate logistic regression analysis, risk factors associated with increased postoperative infection were ASA class, a 40-point increase in postoperative glucose level, and emergency status. Patients who are hyperglycemic in the postoperative period in the non-ICU setting have a greater risk for postoperative infection. Randomized controlled clinical trials or rigorous multiinstitutional observation studies are needed to determine the causal relationship of acute hyperglycemia and postoperative infectious complications in non-ICU postoperative settings.

The Normoglycemia in Intensive Care Evaluation and Survival Using Glucose Algorithm Regulation (NICE-SUGAR) trial provides further evidence of the role of glucose control in the critically ill postoperative patient population. This multicenter prospective randomized trial evaluated tight glycemic control compared with conventional glycemic control. Causes of mortality and length of ICU and hospital stays were similar between the two groups. However, 90-day mortality rate was higher in the intensive glucose control group, and 6.8% of patients in the group with intensive glycemic control experienced hypoglycemia as opposed to only 0.5% of patients in the conventional group. This study has swung the pendulum of tight glucose control back to advocating for moderate glucose control with a goal around 140 instead of less than 110 mg/dL. The intensive glucose control group had a 4.8% incidence of hypoglycemic events compare with 0.5% in the conventional control group. The role of hypoglycemia in adverse events and mortality remains unclear.

RISKS OF INTENSIVE GLUCOSE CONTROL

The primary risk of intensive glucose control is hypoglycemia. Of published data, this is the most common complication of intensive glycemic control (Table 1). Glucose control depends largely on the protocol

TABLE 1: Severe hypoglycemia (<40 mg/dL) with different infusion protocols

Leuven I*	Surgical	5.1%
Leuven 2†	Medical	19%
VISEP‡	Medical	17%
Yale§	Surgical	0%
Yale‖	Medical	4.3%
Glucommander¶	Surgical	2.6%
NICE-SUGAR**	Medical/Surgical	6.8%

*Van Den Berghe G, et al: *N Engl J Med* 345:1359, 2001.
†Van Den Berghe G, et al: *N Engl J Med* 354:449–461, 2006.
‡Brunkhorst FM, et al: *N Engl J Med* 358:125–139, 2008.
§Goldberg PA, et al: *Diabetes Care* 27:461, 2004.
‖Goldberg PA, et al: *J Cardiothorac Vasc Anesth* 18:690, 2004.
¶Davidson PC: *Diabetes Care* 28:2418, 2005.
**NICE-SUGAR Investigators: *N Engl J Med* 360(13):1283–1297, 2009.

and local customs. Some studies examining tight glycemic control were discontinued early because of hypoglycemia; notably, some patients are more prone to it, and some may need tighter control than others. The rates of hypoglycemia likely depend on how good the insulin infusion protocol is. Discontinuation of enteral nutrition, infrequent glucose determinations, and vasoactive agents can also contribute to hypoglycemia. Rigorous attention to the protocol and vigilance as the patient's glucose intake changes are mandatory to minimize the risk of hypoglycemia.

SUMMARY

In the past decade, convincing evidence has emerged that suggests perioperative glycemic control in certain settings, especially cardiac surgery and the surgical intensive care unit, can decrease morbidity and mortality. It remains unclear, however, whether hypoglycemia associated with intensive glycemic control is a cause of death or a marker of patient acuity. It is clear, however, that the particular intensive glycemic control protocol matters, as the rate of hypoglycemia varies across protocols and institutions. The best current evidence for intensive control rests in the population of surgical patients needing more than 5 days of critical care.

Many questions still remain: What is the optimal blood glucose level to initiate treatment? What is the best protocol to implement for glucose control, to minimize hypoglycemia? Real-time feedback loops may help to alleviate the risk of hypoglycemia, and maintaining euglycemia postoperatively is a simple and actionable step that could decrease the risk of postoperative infections and postoperative mortality.

SUGGESTED READINGS

Brunkhorst FM, Engel C, Bloss F, et al: Intensive insulin therapy and pentastarch resuscitation in severe sepsis, *N Engl J Med* 358:125–139, 2008.

Ganai S, Lee KF, Merrill A, et al: Adverse outcomes of geriatric patients undergoing abdominal surgery who are at high risk for delirium, *Arch Surg* 142:1072–1078, 2007.

Guvener M, Pasaoblu I, Demircin M, et al: Perioperative hyperglycemia is a strong correlate of postoperative infection in type II diabetic patients after coronary artery bypass grafting, *Endocr J* 49(5):531–537, 2002.

Ingels C, Debaveye Y, Milants I, et al: Strict blood glucose control with insulin during intensive care after cardiac surgery: impact on 4-year survival, dependency on medical care, and quality-of-life, *Eur Heart J* 27(22):2716–2724, 2006.

The NICE-SUGAR Study Investigators: Intensive versus conventional glucose control in critically ill patients, *N Engl J Med* 360:1283–1297, 2009.

Noordzij PG, Boersma E, Schreiner F, et al: Increased preoperative glucose levels are associated with perioperative mortality in patients undergoing noncardiac, nonvascular surgery, *Eur J Endocrinol* 156(1):137–142, 2007.

Ramos M, Khalpey Z, Lipsitz S, et al: Relationship of perioperative hyperglycemia and postoperative infections in patients who undergo general and vascular surgery, *Ann Surg* 248(4):585–591, 2008.

Van den Berghe G, Wouters P, Weekers F, et al: Intensive insulin therapy in the critically ill patient, *N Engl J Med* 345(19):1359–1367, 2001.

Zerr KJ, Furnary AP, Grunkemeier GL, et al: Glucose control lowers the risk of wound infection in diabetics after open heart operations, *Ann Thorac Surg* 63:356–361, 1997.

POSTOPERATIVE RESPIRATORY FAILURE

Sara P. Fogarty, DO, and Rhonda Fishel, MD, MBA

OVERVIEW

Postoperative pulmonary complications (PPCs) are common, and overall they increase perioperative morbidity and mortality. In fact, pulmonary complications occur more frequently than cardiac complications; they are the most costly of all postoperative complications and may increase patient length of stay dramatically. PPCs include atelectasis, infection, aspiration, bronchospasm, exacerbation of underlying lung disease, and respiratory failure requiring mechanical ventilation. The incidence of PPCs in the literature ranges from 2% to 70% depending on multiple factors, listed in Table 1.

Respiratory failure occurs with derangement of gas exchange, either oxygenation or carbon dioxide elimination. *Hypoxic respiratory failure* is defined as a PaO_2 below 60 mm Hg with a normal or low $PaCO_2$, and it is more common than hypercapnia. The most common cause is ventilation/perfusion (V/Q) mismatch. Other causes are diffusion and venous admixture. Hypercapnic respiratory failure is characterized by a $PaCO_2$ above 50 mm Hg, most commonly caused by chronic lung disease, inflammatory processes, drug overdose, neuromuscular disease, or other conditions that result in increased dead space. If these complications do occur, stabilization and further support with mechanical ventilation may be necessary.

PREOPERATIVE RISK FACTORS

Obstructive Sleep Apnea and Obesity Hypoventilation Syndrome

Over the last three decades, the obesity epidemic has resulted in acute and chronic complications, increasing patient risk of adverse events in the perioperative period. The most common of these complications

TABLE 1: Risk factors for developing postoperative pulmonary complications

Preoperative	Obesity
	COPD
	Serum albumin <3.5 g/dL
	Poor functional status, ASA class >2
	Congestive heart failure
Intraoperative	Emergency surgery
	Surgery lasting >3 hours
	Upper abdominal or thoracic surgery
	Use of pancuronium for neuromuscular blockade
Postoperative	Inadequate pain control
	Bed rest
	Poor pulmonary toilet, difficulty controlling secretions

BOX 1: Guidelines to reduce perioperative pulmonary complications in patients with OSA and obesity

- Efforts to identify OSA/COPD preoperatively
- Use of reverse Trendelenburg rather than supine positioning
- Use of CPAP/BiPAP therapy perioperatively
- Use of regional rather than general anesthesia
- Careful reversal of neuromuscular blockade
- Awake extubation following general anesthesia
- Close monitoring in the postoperative period

OSA, Obstructive sleep apnea

is obstructive sleep apnea (OSA), characterized by repeated episodes of upper airway obstruction during sleep with periods of arterial oxygen desaturation that produces a cycle of recurrent awakenings and results in daytime somnolence. OSA may contribute to a host of medical problems including depression, hypertension, and diabetes, which have all been related to hypoventilation.

The prevalence of OSA in the general surgery population has been estimated to be 1% to 9%, although as many as 77% of morbidly obese patients have OSA upon investigation using polysomnography. Obesity directly produces OSA by increasing the amount of soft tissue surrounding and narrowing the pharyngeal airway and by increasing visceral fat volume. Lung volumes and functional residual capacity (FRC) decrease, and hypoxia may result. A decreased FRC increases the propensity for atelectasis and reduced oxygen stores, resulting in rapid oxygen desaturation. Features of the obesity hypoventilation syndrome include a body mass index of 30 or higher, awake hypercapnia ($Paco_2 \geq 45$), and OSA. These patients are at increased risk for postoperative hypoxemia and/or upper airway obstruction.

Obesity is now being considered a cause of chronic respiratory failure, and it warrants a discussion of patient care between surgeon and anesthesiologist. Guidelines to help reduce perioperative pulmonary complications in patients with OSA and obesity are listed in Box 1.

Chronic Obstructive Pulmonary Disease and Smoking

Identifying and optimizing patients with chronic obstructive pulmonary disease (COPD) prior to elective surgery is one of the only modalities to reduce complications. COPD is characterized by a reduced FEV_1 (forced expiratory volume in one second) and an accelerated rate of decline of FEV_1. Although most COPD patients tolerate intubation well, hypoxemia and bronchospasm may hamper recovery. Regional anesthesia and noninvasive positive-pressure ventilation after extubation should be employed as often as possible to help reduce these complications.

A patient who currently smokes or has a recent history of smoking increases the risk of PPCs. Smoking cessation a minimum of 6 to 8 weeks prior to surgery helps decrease the need for postoperative ventilatory support and should be strongly encouraged.

Nutrition/Functional Status

Malnutrition with hypoalbuminemia is integrally linked with an increased risk of respiratory complications and subsequent failure. Wasting of the muscles of inspiration and expiration and altered immune responses in patients with chronic malnutrition lead to poor inspiratory effort and pulmonary infections. These patients are more prone to prolonged intubation, and ventilator weaning is a challenge. A fine balance between starvation and overfeeding must be reached to enable extubation. Electrolyte abnormalities such as hypophosphatemia, hypokalemia, and hypomagnesemia all contribute to muscle weakness and must be corrected. Postoperative enteral feeds high in carbohydrates can lead to increased carbon dioxide production and exacerbate pulmonary complications and must be avoided. No studies have been done to prove that preoperative total parenteral nutrition (TPN) versus oral supplementation or total enteral nutrition reduces PPCs.

Poor functional status prior to surgery is a sensitive predictor of mortality and postoperative outcomes. Patients with an American Society of Anesthesiologists (ASA) class greater than 2 have a higher overall risk of morbidity and mortality postoperatively, including respiratory complications. Congestive heart failure (CHF) is credited as the number one cause of respiratory failure in patients over the age of 65 years, and patients with CHF should be optimized with angiotensin converting enzyme (ACE) inhibitors and diuretics prior to elective surgery.

INTRAOPERATIVE MANAGEMENT: STRATEGIES AND COMPLICATIONS

Intubation, Anesthetic Management, Noninvasive Ventilation, and Positioning

Surgeons and anesthesiologists both should strive to reduce intraoperative complications and their sequelae. Intubation, especially in the obese patient, may be problematic because of anatomical constraints that include limited mouth opening and poor neck extension. Instrumentation of the airway during intubation can elicit bronchospasm, and the use of muscle relaxants decreases muscular tone and augments airway closure; both of these increase the incidence of PPCs. Aspiration may occur during intubation, resulting in devastating injury. Aspiration risk may be reduced by using cricoid pressure during intubation to occlude the upper end of the esophagus and prevent gastric contents from entering the airway. Rapid-sequence intubation (RSI) may also be used to reduce the risk of aspiration in emergency situations.

When considering the choice between regional and general anesthesia, several factors must be considered. General anesthesia with endotracheal intubation allows for improved management of ventilation, which may help reduce perioperative complications in patients with poor pulmonary function. V/Q mismatch occurs very commonly with induction of general anesthesia because of the decrease in FRC by 15% to 20%. This leads to collapse of distal small airways with resultant atelectasis. In patients with impaired capacities due to obesity or COPD, general anesthesia can markedly worsen this mismatch and result in hypoxemia.

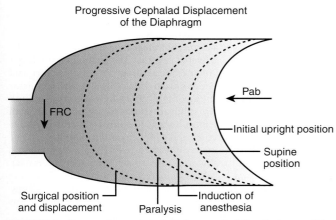

Progressive Cephalad Displacement
of the Diaphragm

FIGURE 1   Progressive cephalad displacement of the diaphragm. *Pab,* Pressure abdominal cavity. *(From Miller RD, Cucchiara RF, Miller ED Jr, et al: Anesthesia, ed 5, Philadelphia, 2000, Churchill Livingstone, p 605.)*

Regional anesthesia alone is rarely performed for major abdominal or thoracic procedures because of concerns about comfort level, analgesia, incomplete muscle paralysis, and the patients' ability to breathe. However, several case reports have been described in which abdominal surgery was completed with neuraxial anesthesia in high-risk patients, showing improved pulmonary outcomes.

Noninvasive ventilation (NIV), such as bilevel positive airway pressure (BiPAP), used intraoperatively in combination with neuraxial anesthesia may be of benefit in this patient population. BiPAP delivers a higher pressure with inspiration and a lower pressure with expiration; this differs from continuous positive airway pressure (CPAP), which delivers air at a steady pressure at all times. CPAP is employed particularly in patients with OSA, whose airways close during sleep, but whose ventilation otherwise is relatively normal.

Surgical Positioning/Factors

The position of the patient may compromise oxygenation. Supine, Trendelenburg, lithotomy, or jackknife positions, particularly in patients who are obese, further decrease FRC. Prone and reverse Trendelenburg positions help maintain FRC in all patients. Packing, abdominal insufflation, manipulation of intraabdominal organs, assistants leaning on the patient, and compression bandages can all contribute to decreased FRC and hypoxemia. Figure 1 shows the progressive displacement of the diaphragm superiorly with each insult of induction of general anesthesia, positioning, and surgery.

Upper abdominal and thoracic procedures may lead to respiratory compromise, because these incisions affect chest wall, diaphragm, and lung function. The duration of the surgical procedure (>2 hours), increases the risk of developing PPCs. Laparoscopic surgery has a decreased rate of PPCs when compared with open approaches for similar surgeries, however, insufflation of the abdominal cavity with CO_2 may lead to hypercapnia and respiratory acidosis; this should be considered in patients with impaired airflow.

Postoperative Considerations

Pain Control

Inadequate pain control can drastically affect respiratory function. Incisional pain leads to a weakened cough and poor inspiratory effort secondary to splinting or guarding, and atelectasis may follow. Poor pain control inhibits early ambulation, which may prevent deep vein thrombosis (DVT) and pneumonia. A large database search from

1966 until 2006 compared the effects of epidural analgesia with systemic analgesia when evaluating rates of postoperative pneumonia. The incidence of pneumonia following abdominal or thoracic surgery varied but was upward of 20% in patients receiving only patient-requested systemic analgesia. Only 3% to 8% of patients who received epidural analgesia developed postoperative pneumonia. The benefit of epidural analgesia decreased over the period examined because of the introduction of the patient controlled analgesia (PCA) pump and early postoperative ambulation.

Elderly or infirm patients have an increased risk for oversedation and resultant respiratory failure. Chest wall and lung compliance decrease with age, FRC is impaired, and the work of breathing is increased. Decreased cognitive abilities seen preoperatively and perhaps worsened after anesthesia makes pain assessment difficult and risks oversedation. Elderly patients usually require the same initial doses of opioids as their younger counterparts, but these requirements decrease over time and should be adjusted appropriately. Morphine has been studied extensively in the elderly, and dosing charts are available. PCA basal rates and meperidine should be avoided because of the increased risk of oversedation and delirium.

Lung-Expansion Modalities

Early ambulation, chest physical therapy, and cough should be encouraged, and incentive spirometry should be employed in the postoperative patient to prevent PPCs: all these therapies work by increasing FRC and preventing atelectasis. Patients with difficulty mobilizing secretions or those with severe atelectasis should use these modalities multiple times per day.

Complications

Atelectasis, Pneumonia, Aspiration, Bronchospasm, and Pulmonary Embolus

Atelectasis often begins in the operating room during induction of general anesthesia, and it persists postoperatively. Three mechanisms contribute to alveolar collapse: 1) compression, 2) absorption, and 3) loss of surfactant. Compression atelectasis is due to compression of lung tissue secondary to the loss of inspiratory muscle tone and cephalad displacement of the diaphragm. Absorption atelectasis can occur by complete airway occlusion, administration of 100% oxygen, or a decreased V/Q ratio. Loss-of-surfactant atelectasis implies that once alveoli have collapsed, the same region of the lung is prone to collapse again. This may be due to atelectasis impeding surfactant production. These three types of atelectasis contribute to approximately 75% of deterioration in gas exchange.

Endotracheal intubation with mechanical ventilation still prevails as the greatest risk factor for the development of nosocomial pneumonia. Other major risk factors in the nonventilated patient include major abdominal or thoracic surgery and decreased functional status. The most prevalent organisms that are of concern are *Staphylococcus aureus* and gram-negative rods including the SPACE organisms: *Serratia marcescens, Pseudomonas aeruginosa,* and *Acinetobacter, Proteus,* and *Enterobacter* species. These gram-negative organisms have a greater incidence of drug resistance and drastically increase mortality in the critically ill. Diagnosis relies heavily on clinical symptoms (tachypnea, fever, leukocytosis) and new infiltrate seen on chest radiograph. Bronchoalveolar lavage (BAL) is indicated in patients with nonresolving pneumonia; it has minimal risk of major complications and may help direct antibiotic therapy.

Aspiration is defined as the inhalation of either gastric or oropharyngeal contents into upper and lower airways, which may result in aspiration pneumonia or pneumonitis. Prior to intubation, the length of time since the patient's last meal and the presence of gastric contents must be assessed. Gastric content control is of utmost importance in the perioperative setting; minimizing intake preoperatively, increasing gastric emptying, and reducing gastric volume via naso-gastric tube decompression should be used. Acid reduction with proton pump inhibitors or H_2 blockers lessens the severity of injury if aspiration does occur. Treatment with prophylactic antibiotics is not indicated in aspiration, unless the patient presents with signs and symptoms of infection.

Bronchospasm is a sudden constriction of the muscle in the walls of the bronchioles that may occur from a variety of insults, including drug allergy, exacerbation of underlying asthma or COPD, heart failure, and instrumentation during intubation, extubation, or bronchoscopy. Treatment entails avoiding triggers and using metered-dose inhalers with bronchodilators and/or corticosteroids and ventilatory support.

Pulmonary embolus (PE) can cause acute respiratory failure in the postoperative patient. Symptoms of pulmonary embolus vary depending on the size of the clot and the status of the patient's cardiovascular system and respiratory reserves. Diagnosis is centered on multidetector computed tomographic angiography (MDCTA) to detect emboli. V/Q scan is indicated whenever MDCTA is not available or feasible, although this test is less accurate. Duplex ultrasonography is useful in demonstrating the presence of DVT but does not rule out a PE if negative. Immediate full anticoagulation is necessary in patients suspected of DVT or PE, and this reduces mortality by 20%. However, 33% of patients who receive adequate anticoagulation will develop a second PE. An inferior vena cava filter is indicated for these patients and for those who have absolute contraindications to full anticoagulation, such as severe trauma, or for those about to undergo major abdominal surgery or lower extremity surgery.

Respiratory Failure and Mechanical Ventilation

Ventilation and Oxygenation

Mechanical ventilation decreases the work of respiratory muscles. Hypoxemia and resultant acidosis is prevented by decreasing the work of breathing and therefore decreasing oxygen consumption by the body. Ventilation is a product of both respiratory rate and tidal volume, and it supplies the gas exchange needs of the body. To improve oxygenation during mechanical ventilation, applying positive end-expiratory pressure (PEEP) prevents alveolar collapse and increases FRC in a process known as *recruitment*. Understanding the basic modes of ventilation is necessary to meet patients' changing respiratory needs in the face of respiratory failure. Several basic modes are discussed.

Pressure Control Versus Volume Control

Modes of Ventilation

Volume-control ventilation—assist control (AC) and intermittent mandatory ventilation (IMV)—delivers a preset tidal volume with constant flow at a specific rate. Advantages of this mode include direct control of tidal volume and minute ventilation. Disadvantages include high airway pressures in cases of decreased lung compliance with resulting barotrauma and/or decreased venous return. Pressure-control ventilation delivers a breath with a controlled airway pressure at a set rate and time. This mode is employed in patients who have pulmonary insults with elevated risk of barotraumas, and it delivers an even distribution of ventilation in lung units with different resistances. Reduced tidal volumes secondary to increased resistance or decreased compliance may lead to hypoventilation and hypoxemia.

The most commonly employed mode is AC. Each breath given is mandatory and is delivered at a controlled volume, rate, and inspiratory time. If the patient becomes apneic, the ventilator will deliver the set minute ventilation. If there is any inspiratory effort made, the ventilator will deliver a patient-triggered breath. "Assist" accounts for the patient's inspiratory effort to trigger breathing; "control" accounts for breaths given by the machine, if the patient becomes apneic.

IMV is a partial support mode. Intermittent mandatory breaths are given at a set rate and volume, but the patient is allowed to breathe spontaneously between delivered breaths. The spontaneous breaths will have varying tidal volumes depending on patient effort and lung compliance. With synchronized IMV (SIMV), the ventilator will synchronize the beginning of inspiratory flow with the patients' own inspiratory effort. IMV is advantageous to use in patients with impaired cardiac function; intrathoracic pressure is decreased, resulting in improved venous return and a higher cardiac output.

Continuous positive airway pressure (CPAP) is a spontaneous breathing mode; all breaths are initiated by the patient, however, pressure support may be added to increase the tidal volume of these breaths. FRC is maintained by the continuous positive pressures, which improves oxygenation and decreases V/Q mismatch. This mode is commonly used as a bridge to extubation.

Acute Respiratory Distress Syndrome

Acute respiratory distress syndrome (ARDS) is a very severe form of lung injury that occurs as acute respiratory failure with hypoxemia refractory to oxygen therapy. Mortality rates from ARDS have been noted to be as high as 68%, although advances in supportive care have significantly improved since this disease process was first described in 1967. Early recognition of ARDS is paramount for treatment and reduced mortality. A high level of suspicion should be held for sepsis or pneumonia in patients who develop ARDS; these patients should be treated with broad-spectrum antibiotics, and nutrition status should be optimized with enteral or parenteral feeding. Prevention of gastrointestinal bleeding is also essential.

Much controversy surrounds the subject of mechanical ventilation for supportive care in ARDS. Multiple studies since the late 1990s have investigated the effects of mechanical ventilation in regard to patient survival. Low tidal volume, high PEEP ventilation has been shown to prevent compression atelectasis that develops secondary to severe pulmonary edema. It also decreases ventilator-induced lung injury that occurs with increased tidal volumes. Use of low tidal volume is the only modality proven to increase survival in the ARDS patient. Most deaths from ARDS are attributed to sepsis and multiorgan failure, however, overall mortality decreased over the past decade by approximately 1.1% per year, based on a recent regression meta-analysis of ARDS patients over a 12-year period. This decrease in mortality is attributed to advances in modes of ventilation and improvements in ICU care.

Modes of ventilation such as airway pressure release ventilation (APRV) and high-frequency oscillatory ventilation (HFOV) have also been used. APRV uses prolonged positive airway pressure to maintain lung volume and enhance oxygenation. Airway pressure is then released in brief, intermittent periods, aiding in CO_2 clearance. Optimal lung volume is achieved, which maximizes recruitment, limits shear forces, and improves gas exchange.

HFOV delivers small tidal volumes at a very rapid frequency, keeping alveoli open and reducing the likelihood of gas trapping. This method has been widely investigated in the pediatric and neonate population, but more recently it has been used in adult trauma patients. HFOV has been initiated in trauma patients who have high peak inspiratory pressures. It allows for constant airway pressures, which promotes oxygenation and prevents the overdistension and progressive lung injury seen with conventional ventilation settings.

Extracorporeal membrane oxygenation (ECMO) is employed in neonatal intensive care units with reported survival rates of 75%. The use of ECMO in adults with respiratory failure was first examined in the 1970s. Studies at that time showed mortality greater than 90%, and further investigation into this mode of ventilation was abandoned. Recently the Extracorporeal Life Support Organization (ELSO) registry of adult patients treated with ECMO was examined over a 20-year period. Survival rates in adults with severe respiratory failure were upward of 50%. Advanced age, diagnosis, and complications while on ECMO decreased this rate. The role and limitations of ECMO are just beginning to be understood, and further prospective studies examining its applications are underway.

Prone positioning has dated back to the 1970s as a means for countering the detrimental changes found in the lungs of ARDS patients. In the prone position, the weight of the heart and great vessels is transferred off the lung tissue. This decreases pleural pressure and promotes gas exchange and recruitment to the posterior aspects of the lungs. Additionally, blood flow goes preferentially to the anterior expanded alveoli, and V/Q matching is improved.

Criteria to Extubate

Weaning should be initiated in patients who meet criteria as dictated by several large studies produced by the American College of Chest Physicians, the Society for Critical Care Medicine, and the American Association for Respiratory Care. These criteria include 1) hemodynamic stability; 2) adequate oxygenation as measured by Pao_2/Fio_2 ratio of 150 to 200, with a PEEP range from 5 to 8 cm, H_2O, Fio_2 less than 50%, and pH greater than 7.25; 3) ability to initiate and continue to make inspiratory effort; and 4) resolution of the initial cause of acute respiratory failure. Likelihood of extubation is increased if Pao_2 is greater than 95% on Fio_2 of 40%, exhaled tidal volume is at least 5 mL/kg, and respiratory rate ranges from 10 to 30 on minimal pressure support.

Once these criteria are met, a spontaneous breathing trial (SBT) should be initiated and conducted with low levels of pressure support (5 to 7 cm H_2O) in an unsedated patient. Respiratory rate, tidal volume, hemodynamic stability, and patient comfort should be continually monitored. An SBT should last 30 to 120 minutes. The Rapid Shallow Breathing Index (RSBi) is used to determine whether an SBT is successful. RSBi is defined as the quotient of the respiratory rate in breaths per minute divided by the tidal volume. A rapid respiratory rate with small tidal volumes is indicative of respiratory muscle fatigue and correlates with an RSBi greater than 100, which is predictive of unsuccessful weaning. If a patient fails an SBT, the cause of failure should be examined. Issues with fluid balance, pain control, and bronchospasm should be corrected, and an SBT should be reattempted 24 hours after the failed trial to allow for full respiratory muscle rest.

SUGGESTED READINGS

Bapoje SR, Whitaker JF, Schulz T, et al: Preoperative evaluation of the patient with pulmonary disease, *Chest* 132(5):1637–1645, 2007.
Benditt JO: Novel uses of noninvasive ventilation, *Respir Care* 54(2):212–222, 2009.
Malhotra A, Hillman D: Obesity and the lung. Part 3: obesity, respiration, and intensive care, *Thorax* 63:925–931, 2008.
Miller RD, Cucchiara RF, Miller ED Jr, et al: *Anesthesia*, ed 5, Philadelphia, 2000, Churchill Livingstone, p 605.
Poppöng DM, Elia N, Marret E, et al: Protective effects of epidural analgesia on pulmonary complications after abdominal and thoracic surgery, *Arch Surg* 143(10):990–999, 2008.
Ware LB, Matthay MA: The acute respiratory distress syndrome, *N Engl J Med* 342(18):1334–1349, 2000.

VENTILATOR-ASSOCIATED PNEUMONIA

**Christopher M. Watson, MD, and
Robert G. Sawyer, MD**

DEFINITION

Ventilator-associated pneumonia (VAP) is defined as a new-onset pneumonia diagnosed after a minimum of 48 hours of endotracheal intubation. It is furthered divided into *early-* and *late-onset* VAP depending on whether it developed before or after 96 hours. This designation attempts to segregate patients based on the probability of infection with multidrug-resistant (MDR) pathogens, which would necessitate a more broad-spectrum regimen. Complicating this designation are the terms *health care–associated pneumonia* (HCAP) and *community-acquired pneumonia* (CAP). It is important to know these terms, however, because treatment differences do exist. HCAP occurs in individuals with specific risk factors (Box 1). CAP is assumed to occur in patients admitted 2 or fewer days prior to onset of pneumonia and have none of the risk factors for HCAP.

DIAGNOSIS

The gold-standard diagnostic modality for any pneumonia, including VAP, is lung biopsy and histology showing invasion and inflammation of involved lung tissue. Because this is obviously a high-risk, invasive procedure, alternative modes of diagnosis have been developed. Clinical suspicion for VAP may come from generalized systemic signs of inflammation, such as fever and leukocytosis, combined with new or increasing oxygen requirements, purulent sputum, and/or a persistent or new pulmonary infiltrate. The clinical pulmonary infection score (CPIS) and its modifications were developed to standardize the diagnosis of VAP, but studies to determine its validity in this regard are mixed, depending on which method of diagnosis is used: histology, quantitative broncheoalveolar lavage (qBAL), or some other method. The most accurate clinical criteria are the presence of a new or progressive radiographic infiltrate plus at least two of three clinical features: fever greater than 38° C, leukocytosis or leukopenia, and purulent secretions. Even so, these criteria are often present in the absence of pneumonia in the mechanically ventilated critically ill patient, so culture data are required for the diagnosis.

The method of culture is controversial. The most common methods used are a qBAL; blinded, protected, quantitative culturing; and a non-quantitative transbroncheal aspiration. In one randomized trial from France comparing invasive and noninvasive sampling, the use of qBAL with quantitative cultures resulted in improved survival rates, decreased days of antibiotics used, and less organ failure. These findings have been attributed to a higher false-positive culture rate in the noninvasive group.

In contradistinction to this finding, a recent Cochrane review comparing quantitative to nonquantitative cultures of respiratory secretions and invasive versus noninvasive methods found no evidence that either method reduced mortality, ICU length of stay, or antibiotic use compared with the other strategy. The recommendation of the VAP Guidelines Committee and the Canadian Critical Care Trials Group is that transbroncheal aspiration with nonquantitative culture be used as the initial diagnostic study. This only applies to patients who have not been started on empiric antibiotics prior to sampling. If prior antibiotics have been administered, the patient is immunosuppressed, or the patient has had a prolonged ICU stay or multiple previous episodes of pneumonia during the index hospitalization, qBAL may give more valid results, although no conclusive data are available to support this idea.

TREATMENT

1. Evaluate for clinical indicators of VAP (Figure 1).
2. Evaluate for risk factors for MDR pathogens.
3. Start empiric antibiotics. Select monotherapy or combined therapy for nonfermenting gram-negative bacilli (NFGNB) and obtain sputum sample (invasive or noninvasive).
4. Proceed with initial sample examination.
   a. If no bacteria are present, and the patient is not severely ill, discontinue antibiotics and look for another source of infection.
   b. If no bacteria are present, but the patient is severely ill, continue empiric therapy for VAP, and look for additional sources of infection.
   c. If bacteria are present, continue empiric therapy as recommended for VAP based on risk factors (Box 2).
5. Reevaluate finalized culture results at 48 to 72 hours.
   a. If culture results are negative or do not reveal significant growth ($<10^4$ CFU/mL), consider stopping antibiotics depending on the illness of the patient.
   b. If positive and significant growth ($\geq 10^4$ CFU/mL) is found, continue for 8 days total. Note: Some clinicians may elect to continue antibiotics for 10 to 14 days total for resistant NFGNB, but this is debated.

Once the diagnosis of VAP is considered, and after sputum and blood cultures are obtained, empiric antibiotic therapy is chosen based on risk for infection with MDR pathogens and initiated (Box 3). If VAP is suspected in a trauma patient, the physician may choose to simply categorize the patient as early or late onset (ICU length of stay ≥4 days). In trauma patients, this classification may be broadly applicable with no apparent harm. A review of a mixed ICU at our institution showed that trauma patients with VAP did better overall than nontrauma patients with VAP and that early- and late-onset VAP trauma patients behaved similarly. Although this categorization may be valid for selection in the typically younger trauma population, it should not be used for nontrauma surgical patients or transplant recipients. These patients should be categorized as either at low or high risk for VAP caused by MDR pathogens (see Boxes 1 and 2).

The clinician should also try to ascertain any history of previous infections with MDR pathogens. At most institutions, the patient's medical record will have documentation of any previous infections or surveillance cultures that were positive for MDR bacteria, including methicillin-resistant *Staphylococcus aureus* (MRSA), vancomycin-resistant enterococci (VRE), and MDR gram-negative rods. Next, consider the local prevalence of endemic pathogens and resistance patterns. In early-onset VAP patients without risk factors for MDR pathogens, monotherapy for *Streptococcus pneumoniae*, methicillin-sensitive *Staphylococcus aureus,* and *Haemophilus influenza* is

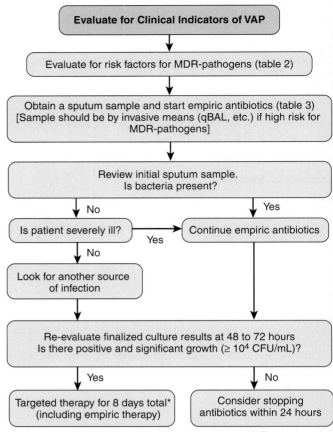

FIGURE 1   Algorithm for evaluating VAP.

recommended. Conversely, in those with late-onset VAP or with risk factors for MDR pathogens, antipseudomonal monotherapy or combination therapy for NFGNB are recommended, combined with coverage of MRSA if it is endemic. Empiric therapy should be continued until final culture results are available, at which point it is important to tailor therapy to the specific pathogens cultured in significant numbers.

Additional studies have attempted to evaluate the utility of preliminary Gram stain or initial culture results to allow early antibiotic tailoring or discontinuation. An evaluation by Fabian and colleagues of a modified treatment pathway using preliminary qBAL results (~24 hours) to discontinue antibiotic therapy was performed. If these preliminary results showed insignificant growth ($<10^4$ CFU/mL), antibiotics were discontinued. Good correlation was found between preliminary and final qBAL culture results. The false-negative rate was low and resulted in only 2.3% of patients having antibiotics

BOX 3: Empiric antibiotic selection for VAP

Early-Onset VAP and No Risk Factors for MDR Pathogens

Ceftriaxone, fluoroquinolone, ampicillin-sulbactam, or ertapenem ± macrolide

Late-Onset VAP or Risk Factors for MDR Pathogens

Antipseudomonal cephalosporin
Antipseudomonal carbapenem
β-lactam/β-lactamase inhibitor + antipseudomonal fluoroquinolone or aminoglycoside ± linezolid or vancomycin ± macrolide or fluoroquinolone

Modified from American Thoracic Society: Guidelines for the management of adults with hospital-acquired, ventilator-associated, and healthcare-associated pneumonia, *Am J Respir Crit Care Med* 171:388–416, 2005.

stopped inappropriately. In these patients, antibiotics were restarted when final culture results became available, and this interruption in treatment did not appear to affect the outcome for these patients. Importantly, patients with significant preliminary cultures had an additional pathogen cultured on final results 22% of the time; thus the preliminary results should not be used to deescalate therapy.

Multiple strategies have been evaluated to determine length of therapy. These include a predefined length of therapy, 7 or 8 days or 14 to 15 days for resistant pathogens or recurrent episodes; cessation based on clinical indicators, such as CPIS score and risk factors for MDR pathogens; or cessation based on repeat qBAL results. In a multicenter, double-blinded, randomized controlled trial, Chastre and colleagues found that 8 days of appropriate antibiotic therapy was as good as 15 days for most patients, with no difference in recurrence, superinfection, or mortality. Among patients with NFGNB, there did seem to be a higher recurrence rate but no difference in all-cause mortality. The authors appropriately caution against the rigid application of only 8 days of therapy to patients who are immunocompromised. Importantly, the length of treatment does not begin until appropriate antibiotics are selected.

More recently, a study of repeat qBAL to allow for earlier discontinuation of antibiotics has been performed. Trauma patients with VAP diagnosed by initial qBAL had repeat qBAL at day 4 of treatment. Those with less than 10^4 CFU/mL on quantitative culture had

their antibiotics stopped, and those above this threshold had antibiotics continued for 10 to 14 days. This pathway allowed for more abbreviated antibiotic usage. Because this was only an observational, case-control pilot study, the data should not be used to guide therapy until a larger trial can be performed. None of these methods have been compared in head-to-head trials.

SUMMARY

In the ICU, it is often difficult to diagnose patients with VAP. This is due to many confounding diagnoses with a similar clinical picture, such as volume overload from resuscitation and acute respiratory distress syndrome. As such, a strong index of suspicion is necessary, in conjunction with microbiologic data, to diagnose true VAP. Once suspected, appropriate broad-spectrum antimicrobials should be administered, and sputum samples should be obtained, either invasively or noninvasively, depending on patient comorbidities and length of previous antibiotic administration. Initial therapy should be based on risk factors for MDR pathogens and local antibiograms, and these should be unit specific if possible. Once final culture data are available, antibiotics should be tailored and continued for at least 8 days in most patients. Each hospital unit should develop its own criteria for more prolonged courses of antibiotics.

SUGGESTED READINGS

Canadian Critical Care Trials Group: A randomized trial of diagnostic techniques for ventilator-associated pneumonia, *N Engl J Med* 355(25):2619–2630, 2006.

Chastre J, Wolff M, Fagon JY, et al: for the PneumA Trial Group: Comparison of 8 versus 15 days of antibiotic therapy for ventilator-associated pneumonia in adults: a randomized trial, *JAMA* 290(19):2588–2598, 2003.

Hedrick TL, Smith RL, McElearney ST, et al: Differences in early- and late-onset ventilator-associated pneumonia between surgical and trauma patients in a combined surgical or trauma intensive care unit, *J Trauma* 64:714–720, 2008.

Mueller EW, Croce MA, Boucher BA, et al: Repeat bronchoalveolar lavage to guide antibiotic duration for ventilator-associated pneumonia, *J Trauma* 63(6):1329–1337, 2007.

Swanson JM, Wood GC, Croce MA, et al: Utility of preliminary bronchoalveolar lavage results in suspected ventilator-associated pneumonia, *J Trauma* 65(6):1271–1277, 2008.

EXTRACORPOREAL LIFE SUPPORT FOR RESPIRATORY FAILURE

Fizan Abdullah, MD, PhD

BACKGROUND

Extracorporeal life support (ECLS) is the term used to describe prolonged cardiopulmonary support through the use of a mechanical device. Prior to usage of this term, the term *extracorporeal membrane oxygenation* (ECMO) was used, as it is descriptive of the blood oxygenation capabilities of the technology. Both terms remain in common clinical use today. ECLS can be differentiated from standard cardiopulmonary bypass (CPB) in that it is performed using only extrathoracic cannulation, but CPB is usually instituted by transthoracic cannulation. Unlike standard CPB, which is used for short-term support measured in hours, ECLS is used for longer term support, ranging from 1 day to 4 weeks.

The first report of prolonged extracorporeal oxygenation for treatment of posttraumatic respiratory failure occurred in 1972 by Hill and associates. Bartlett, the father of ECLS technology, reported its successful use for meconium aspiration in 1976 on an abandoned baby. This was followed by Bartlett's series published in 1982, which described his use of ECMO in 45 newborns who had not responded to conventional therapy and were otherwise considered moribund by the neonatologist. Suddenly, a subset of critically ill infants—with diagnoses such as congenital diaphragmatic hernia (CDH), meconium aspiration syndrome (MAS), and persistent pulmonary hypertension (PPHN)—who would have otherwise had lethal outcomes with conventional therapies were able to be salvaged and survived.

Four prospective randomized trials of ECLS for neonatal respiratory failure demonstrated the significant positive value of the technology, but two trials of ECLS in adults with acute respiratory distress syndrome (ARDS) did not meet with nearly as much success because of variations in extracorporeal devices and technology compared with those in use today.

The successful neonatal experience and multiple subsequent single-series successes in adults with respiratory failure helped usher in an era of rapid proliferation of ECLS technology in the 1980s and 1990s, to a point that it is relatively commonplace today in most major medical centers in the United States.

CIRCUIT COMPONENTS AND MONITORS

An ECLS circuit typically contains connecting tubing, a venous reservoir, a roller pump, an artificial lung (also called an *oxygenator*), and a heat exchanger in addition to various monitoring devices. Of particular importance are the preoxygenator and postoxygenator pressure sensors, which help monitor for thrombosis or oxygenator failure, and the saturation sensors directly inserted into the circuit, which provide mixed venous and oxygen saturations. Because heparinization is required to prevent clots from forming in the circuit, whole-blood activated clotting time (ACT) is maintained at approximately 50% above normal (e.g., ACT is 180 to 200 if upper level of normal is 120).

PRINCIPLES OF EXTRACORPOREAL LIFE SUPPORT APPLICATION

The fundamental principle of ECLS is to utilize standard cardiopulmonary bypass to allow time for the intrinsic recovery of the lungs in respiratory failure. This is done by first draining venous blood, removing carbon dioxide and adding oxygen via an artificial lung, and returning the blood to the circulation either by venovenous (VV) or arteriovenous (VA) routes. A roller pump is utilized to regulate blood flow so that appropriate cardiac output and oxygen delivery can be maintained. In VA bypass, the ECLS machine provides hemodynamic support and gas exchange by removing blood from the venous cannula and returning oxygenated blood under pressure to the arterial system. In VV bypass, in which the patient does not require hemodynamic support, blood is withdrawn from the vein, oxygenated, and pumped back into the same vein. A comparison of VV and VA bypass is presented in Table 1.

After initiation, ECLS support is titrated to end points of adequate gas exchange to allow for normalization of blood gases while allowing ventilator settings to be reduced to alleviate further lung injury from barotrauma or oxygen toxicity. Typically, blood flow will be increased up to maximal flow initially, to gain full cardiopulmonary support, and then decreased incrementally until good cardiac output and gas exchange can be supported with minimal ventilator settings. Adult patients will typically receive a tracheostomy within 3 days of initiating ECLS therapy, which allows for diagnostic and therapeutic bronchoscopy and improves patient comfort. To avoid circuit thrombosis, a continuous drip of heparin is infused (to keep ACT around 180 to 200). Platelet transfusions are required to keep the platelet count above 100,000 to replenish platelets lost to consumption from contact with foreign material within the circuit. With improvements in acidosis and decreased intrathoracic pressure resulting from lower ventilator settings, cardiac output also rapidly improves, allowing for the weaning of vasoactive medications. If the patient is in renal failure, continuous hemofiltration is added by initiating diuresis using the ECLS circuit. Additionally, patient nutrition is supplied using total parenteral nutrition, which is also added to the ECLS circuit.

Over time, the degree of cardiopulmonary support is withdrawn (pump flows decrease) as the native heart and lungs recuperate and are able to restore function. Parameters such as oxygenation (pO_2), ventilation (pCO_2), and mixed venous saturation (mVO_2) are monitored during this process.

INDICATIONS

ECLS therapy can be considered for any patient suffering from any acute, reversible, high-mortality cause of pulmonary or cardiac failure. In neonates, respiratory failure requiring ECLS can be due to MAS, CDH, sepsis, PPHN, and respiratory distress syndrome (RDS). Severe respiratory failure in older children is less frequent as compared with newborns, and it is caused most commonly by viral or bacterial pneumonia. A less frequent cause of severe respiratory failure in children suited for ECLS therapy is status asthmaticus. In the most severe cases, children are unresponsive to bronchodilators, heliox, intubation, and so on, and pneumothorax can be fatal. ECLS is ideally suited in such cases, as it can provide adequate gas exchange while the lungs heal. These patients are ideal candidates for VV bypass, as they usually do not require cardiac support.

In adults, acute respiratory distress syndrome (ARDS) is by far the most common indication. ARDS patients should be identified early as candidates for ECLS, because studies have shown that patients on a ventilator for more than 5 days prior to the initiation of ECLS therapy have a lower chance of recovery. Thus, severe cases of ARDS that may require ECLS therapy include patients whose alveolar-arterial oxygen gradient is greater than 600 on the second to fourth day after intubation. Additionally, ECLS may be indicated in cases of massive pulmonary embolism, pulmonary contusions, cardiopulmonary failure with pulmonary edema, and severe hypercarbic respiratory failure (status asthmaticus or acute airway occlusion).

CONTRAINDICATIONS

Successful use of ECLS for respiratory failure is based upon the principle of reversibility of the underlying condition. Any condition in which survival would not be compatible with systemic anticoagulation

---

TABLE 1: Comparison of venovenous and venoarterial bypass approaches

ECLS Approach	Vascular Access	Advantages and Disadvantages
Venovenous bypass	*Infant and pediatric (≤4 years):* Right internal jugular vein *Older pediatric (>4 years) and adult:* Right internal jugular and femoral vein	+ Preferred gas exchange support for respiratory failure − No hemodynamic support
Venoarterial bypass	*Infant and pediatric (<4 years):* Right internal jugular vein and common carotid artery *Older pediatric (>4 years) and adult:* Right internal jugular vein and femoral artery	+ Provides gas exchange *plus* hemodynamic support − Generally requires sacrificing arterial vessels and may require distal limb perfusion catheter

is contraindicated. In neonates, evaluation before ECLS includes a head ultrasound documenting intraventricular hemorrhage (IVH) which, if present, will typically contraindicate ECLS. Concerns for IVH associated with prematurity and vessel size are also why a gestational age less than 32 to 34 weeks and weight less than 2 kg are considered relative contraindications to ECLS therapy. Lethal congenital anomalies and uncorrectable cardiac lesions are hard contraindications to ECLS. Other contraindications include major traumatic or irreversible brain injury, multiple organ failure, metastatic disease, or parental refusal. In adult patients, mechanical ventilation with a high degree of support for more than 7 days is a relative contraindication because of poor prognosis and a low chance of recovery.

CANNULATION

VV is the preferred approach in patients with respiratory failure without cardiac dysfunction. Even if the patient requires a high dose of vasoactive medications, these can be generally weaned off as the ventilator reaches rest settings. In infants, VV bypass is best performed through cannulation of the right jugular vein using a double-lumen tube. The right jugular provides the most direct access to cannula placement into the right atrium. The particular cannula selected for use is based upon the size of the vessel and desired flow rate. Patient weight can be used to assist in ensuring cannula availability preoperatively, with the final decision being made once the vessels are exposed. Guidelines for preoperative cannula selection by patient weight are presented in Table 2. It should be noted that these guidelines are appropriate to cannulas in common clinical use today. However, a new series of cannulas, including a VV cannula with bicaval venous drainage ports, has been recently approved by the FDA and is becoming available. It will be interesting to see how its differing flow characteristics and slightly different placement profile impact clinical practice.

In infants, cutdown techniques are almost universal. After placing a shoulder roll, with the infant's head turned to the left, the neck is cleansed and draped. A transverse incision is made, typically at the anterior border of the sternocleidomastoid (SCM) muscle, approximately 1 to 2 cm above the clavicle. The platysma can be divided, and the right jugular vein will typically be identified by dissecting at the anterior border of the SCM. To avoid unnecessary bleeding during the cutdown procedure, systemic intravenous heparinization (100 IU/kg) is usually given once the vessels are exposed. Once the patient is heparinized, the jugular is isolated proximally using a large tie, and the distal jugular is ligated. A venotomy is performed with a fresh knife, vessel edges are held with fine forceps, and the selected (lubricated) cannula is inserted under direct visualization.

In some instances of limited exposure or abnormal anatomy, it can be helpful to place fine Prolene stay sutures at the edges of the venotomy to hold the vessel lumen open; these also provide countertraction during cannula insertion. Commonly, a 1 cm piece of vessel loop is placed on the outside wall of the vessel under the tie to ensure that the tie can be cut free without damaging the vessel side wall at the time of cannula removal. Cannula position can be confirmed by plain radiograph or real-time echocardiogram. The portion of the VV cannula with the venous-return side holes should be sitting in the right atrium, which on plain radiograph shows the tip of the cannula, typically just above the level of the diaphragm. Ideally, blood return is aimed toward the tricuspid valve.

In VA bypass, the right carotid artery is also dissected from the surrounding structures, isolated, ligated, and an arteriotomy is made for cannula insertion. The arterial cannula is inserted into the patient so that the catheter tip is sitting in the carotid artery just before the point at which it enters the aortic arch. Generous injections of saline, via a large syringe with an angiocath, are typically used to connect the cannulas to the ECLS circuit without introducing air bubbles into the circuit. Skin is closed tightly using a Prolene suture, and the patient is fully heparinized while on ECLS support. Suturing can also be done over a piece of Gelfoam (Pfizer, New York) or Surgicel (Ethicon,

TABLE 2: Guidelines for cannula selection by patient weight

Weight (kg)	Venous Cannula (Fr)	Arterial Cannula (Fr)
2–4	8–14	8–10
5–15	12–19	12–15
16–20	19–21	15–17
21–35	21–23	17–19
35–60	23–28	17–21
>60	23–28	17–21

Somerville, NJ) to aid with hemostasis. Cannulas can then be secured to the patient by sewing them with Ethibond (Ethicon) or silk suture at the fascia posterior to the auricle. A high level of surgeon vigilance is required until the cannulas are fully secured to the crib or bed in functioning position.

In older children and adult patients, access is typically achieved by percutaneous Seldinger technique for both veins and arteries. For VV ECLS or for the venous access part of VA ECLS in an adult, a 24 to 28 Fr venous cannula is inserted into the common femoral vein and can be advanced to approximately 50 cm so that the tip sits at the junction between the inferior vena cava and the right atrium. For arterial access in VA ECLS, a 17 to 19 Fr cannula can be placed in the femoral artery. However, close attention must be paid to distal limb perfusion. If need be, limb perfusion can be reestablished by placing a catheter in the superficial femoral artery by cutdown. Alternatively, an 8 Fr arterial line can be placed into the posterior tibial artery. If blood pressure is below 50 mm Hg, the leg can be perfused using this same catheter at a rate of 100 mL/min.

DECANNULATION

Once an assessment is made that the native lungs have recovered, decannulation can be considered. This typically occurs after a period of weaning, in which the lungs demonstrate improved pulmonary compliance and improved gas exchange. Once ECLS is minimized, a trial off of ECLS is typically attempted. During such a trial in a patient on VV bypass, blood flow continues through the extracorporeal circuit, but the sweep gas through the oxygenator is discontinued. Thus, an assessment can be made of native lung function for up to a few hours.

To wean patients off of VA bypass, both arterial and venous lines must be clamped. To avoid clotting, a bridge between the two cannulas can be established and periodically flushed with heparin. Once adequate oxygenation can be demonstrated by the native lung, decannulation can occur, which typically requires that the proximal vessels be ligated in the neck. Some surgeons prefer reconstruction of neck vessels, but benefits of restoration of vessel blood flow must be weighed against the risks of distal embolization of the repaired vessel. Percutaneously placed catheters can typically be managed by application of pressure without direct repair.

OUTCOMES

Outcomes after ECLS therapy are well documented. The Extracorporeal Life Support Organization (ELSO) was founded in 1989 initially as a study group by the clinical centers using ECLS technology. One of the major functions of the organization is to maintain a registry comprising all known cases; over 35,000 cases from 170 centers in more than 14 countries are currently registered. These cases include over 24,000 newborns, 7000 children, and 2000 adults with respiratory and cardiac failure. Overall, bleeding relating to anticoagulation is the most common complication, although it is rarely life threatening.

In the neonatal population, survival to discharge ranges from 64% to 94% depending upon the underlying etiology of the respiratory failure. Patients receiving ECLS therapy for MAS, which was the most common indication, had the best survival to discharge (94%). CDH is the next most common indication in neonates, and those receiving ECLS therapy had a 52% survival to discharge. Sepsis, PPHN, and RDS complete the list of common indications in decreasing frequency with survival ranging from 64% to 84%. Long-term follow-up is also available through the registry, and 10% of survivors have some type of neurologic disability; hearing loss is the most common affliction. It is worthy of mention that with the advent of nitric oxide and new ventilator modalities, the use of ECLS for respiratory failure in the neonate has decreased substantially.

In the pediatric population, all etiology survival to discharge is approximately 55%. Viral and bacterial pneumonia are among the most common indications, with 63% and 55% survival to discharge respectively. Children placed on ECLS for treatment of ARDS survive 54% of the time. For most pediatric indications, VV access is adequate, and children have essentially normal lungs and exercise tolerance at long-term follow-up.

In the adult population, ARDS is the primary pulmonary disorder, requiring ECLS therapy in approximately half of patients; the remaining half of patients have ARDS secondary to extrapulmonary causes such as pancreatitis, trauma, or sepsis. Severe cases carry up to an 80% mortality; with ECLS this improves to 52% to 55% in the adult ARDS patient. The cause of death for those patients who do not survive is typically progressive pulmonary fibrosis from the initial insult of days of barotrauma prior to ECLS therapy or multiple organ failure from the condition that initially caused the ARDS.

SUMMARY

For the patient with a reversible underlying cause of respiratory failure, ECLS technology provides an additional supportive treatment option that allows the lung to recover up to a period of 1 month with minimal complications.

SUGGESTED READINGS

Bartlett R, Kolobow T: Extracorporeal membrane oxygenation and extracorporeal life support. In Tobin MJ, editor: *Principles and practice of mechanical ventilation*, ed 2, New York, 2006, McGraw-Hill, pp 493–500.

Duncan BW: *Mechanical support for cardiac and respiratory failure in pediatric patients*, New York, 2001, Marcel Dekker.

Van Meurs K, Lally K, Peek G, et al: *ECMO: extracorporeal cardiopulmonary support in critical care*, ed 3, Ann Arbor, 2005, Extracorporeal Life Support Organization.

TRACHEOSTOMY

Melanie W. Seybt, MD, Lana L. Jackson, MD, and David J. Terris, MD

OVERVIEW

Reports of tracheostomy date as far back as the fifteenth century; however, it was Chevalier Jackson who standardized the technique in 1909, reducing mortality rates from 25% to approximately 2%. The procedure has continued to evolve over the last century, as medical advances have improved our ability to keep critically ill patients alive, thus the most frequent indication for tracheostomy today arises with the need for long-term ventilatory support. The high incidence of complications during the transport of ICU patients combined with the increasing number of invasive procedures being performed by intensivists have in part provided the momentum to develop a safe technique for performing tracheostomy at the bedside. A traditional, open tracheostomy can be performed in the ICU, but it requires electrocautery, a surgical tracheostomy tray, and a headlight. Percutaneous dilational tracheostomy (PercTrach) was developed as an alternative to open tracheostomy and can be safely and efficiently performed in most patients.

PercTrach was first introduced in the 1950s and was associated with a high number of carotid artery and esophageal injuries from the use of sharp, unguided trocars. The procedure was essentially abandoned until 1985, when Ciaglia developed a serial dilational technique based on Seldinger principles. In 1990, bronchoscopic guidance was added and has been demonstrated to decrease the incidence of complications by nearly half. The improved visualization provided by bronchoscopy aids in ensuring appropriate placement of the guidewire, decreases the incidence of posterior tracheal wall laceration and paratracheal insertion, and confirms tracheostomy tube placement.

INDICATIONS

The most critical indication for a tracheostomy is impending airway obstruction from a bulky tumor, caustic ingestion, maxillofacial trauma, congenital anomaly, or infectious/inflammatory edema of the neck. In many of these instances, when intubation cannot safely be performed, a tracheostomy should be performed in a conscious patient under local anesthesia. The most commonly encountered indication for tracheostomy is need for long-term ventilatory support. Most otolaryngologists advocate tracheostomy after 7 to 10 days of intubation. Delays beyond 14 days can lead to increased incidence of subglottic stenosis and may lead to decreased likelihood of decannulation. In patients who have been neurologically devastated or who have a remote chance of improved respiratory status, a tracheostomy can be performed at an earlier point during the hospitalization. Excessive secretions and recurrent aspiration are also indications for tracheostomy, as it can improve pulmonary hygiene by facilitating the ability to suction bronchopulmonary secretions.

TIMING

The most appropriate timing for tracheostomy placement remains controversial. However, most would agree that when intubation is likely to extend beyond 14 days, placement of a tracheostomy is reasonable. Several studies have suggested that placing a tracheostomy in patients at 1 week or less may improve outcomes with respect to ventilator weaning, hospital stay, and nosocomial infections. By adopting the early tracheostomy model, it is likely that the procedure will be performed in patients who may have otherwise been extubated sooner (<2 weeks). Appropriate studies are still needed to indentify the ideal timing, but the trend is toward earlier surgical intervention.

For patients undergoing elective tracheostomy, every effort should be made to optimize patient status prior to surgery. Ideally, coagulopathies should be corrected to an International Normalized Ratio (INR) of less than 1.5, with more than 50,000 functioning platelets. Patients requiring positive end-expiratory pressures (PEEPs) of greater than 15 cm of water are at higher risk for complications such as subcutaneous emphysema and pneumothorax with percutaneous tracheostomy. In these patients, waiting for improved lung function may be necessary before percutaneous tracheostomy can be safely performed, or open tracheostomy can performed, as bronchoscopy is unnecessary in the open technique.

OPEN TRACHEOSTOMY TECHNIQUE

Open tracheostomy can be performed under general anesthesia in an intubated patient or under local anesthesia in a conscious patient who cannot be intubated. The first incision is made either horizontally or vertically, midway between the cricoid cartilage and the sternal notch; horizontal incisions follow relaxed skin tension lines and are substantially more cosmetic following decannulation. Electrocautery is used to continue the dissection down through the skin, subcutaneous tissue, and platysma. The sternohyoid and sternothyroid muscles are then separated in the midline (at the linea alba) with a vertical incision. These muscles are retracted laterally, and the thyroid isthmus is visualized.

Next, the cricoid cartilage is skeletonized in the midline, and a hemostat is used to undermine the isthmus of the thyroid. The thyroid is then divided with either electrocautery or suture ligatures. A cricoid hook is used to elevate the larynx so that the tracheal rings are well visualized. A horizontal incision is made between the second and third or third and fourth tracheal rings using a no. 11 blade, and the tracheal incision is enlarged using Mayo scissors. A 2-0 silk suture can be used to place stay sutures on each of the rings immediately superior and inferior to the tracheal incision. These sutures are useful for guiding the replacement of the tracheostomy tube, should the tube become dislodged in the immediate postoperative period.

Finally, a Trousseau dilator is used to dilate the tracheal incision, and the anesthesiologist slowly withdraws the endotracheal (ET) tube until the tip of the tube is visualized through the tracheal incision. Under direct vision, the tracheostomy tube is placed. The anesthesia circuit is connected to the tracheostomy tube, and CO_2 is confirmed. The tracheostomy tube flange is then secured to the skin of the anterior neck at four points using 2-0 silk sutures, and a twill tracheostomy tie is placed.

PERCUTANEOUS TRACHEOSTOMY TECHNIQUE

At our institution, a multidisciplinary team consisting of one otolaryngologist and one pulmonologist performs the procedure. Prior to the procedure, sedation and muscle relaxation are achieved through the use of intravenous agents. Bronchoscopy is used to visualize key points of the procedure, including ET tube withdrawal to the subglottis, guidewire introduction, dilation, and tracheostomy tube insertion.

A horizontal tracheostomy incision is made, and the midline anterior tracheal wall is palpated. Direct palpation of the tracheal wall through the incision causes blanching that can be visualized bronchoscopically through the ET tube (Figure 1). This facilitates identification of an appropriate location between tracheal rings two and three or rings three and four. Under bronchoscopic guidance, the ET tube is withdrawn until the tip of the tube is immediately proximal to the proposed site of percutaneous entrance into the trachea. A 14 gauge angiocatheter is then introduced into the tracheal lumen (Figure 2), a guidewire is passed through the angiocatheter, and the angiocatheter is removed (Figure 3). After a small punch is used to facilitate dilation, a single tapered dilator is introduced over the guidewire, until the stoma is dilated to an aperture of 36 Fr (Figure 4). The dilator is then withdrawn, and the tracheostomy tube is introduced over the guidewire (Figure 5). Proper intraluminal positioning is confirmed by passing the bronchoscope through the tracheostomy tube, and the flange is then secured to the skin of the anterior neck at four points

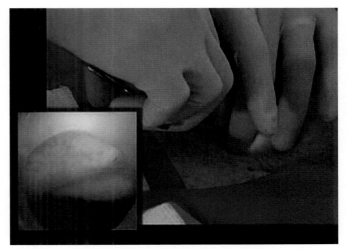

FIGURE 1 Palpation of the tracheal wall is visualized bronchoscopically to identify optimal placement.

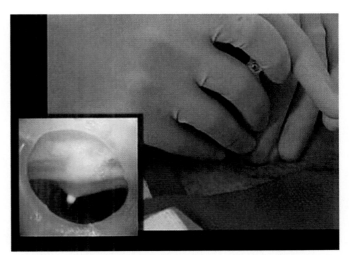

FIGURE 2 A 14 gauge angiocatheter is introduced into the tracheal lumen to place a guidewire.

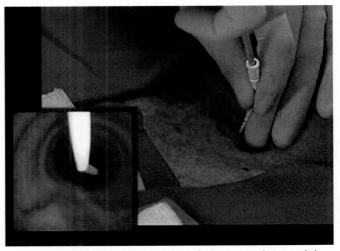

FIGURE 3 A guidewire is passed through the angiocatheter, and the angiocatheter is removed.

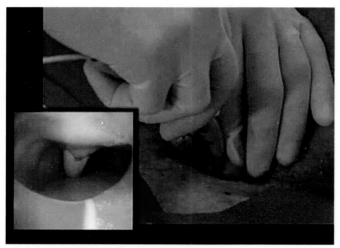

FIGURE 4   After a small punch is used to facilitate dilation, a single tapered dilator is introduced over the guidewire, until the stoma is dilated to an aperture of 36 Fr.

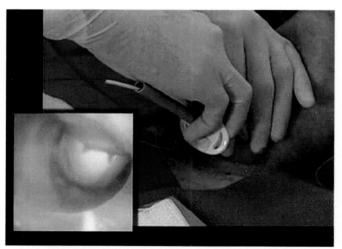

FIGURE 5   The tracheostomy tube is inserted over the guidewire.

using 2-0 silk sutures, and a twill tracheostomy tie is placed. In all cases, a surgical tracheostomy tray is available at the bedside in the event that conversion to open tracheostomy is necessary.

COMPLICATIONS

Intraoperative Complications

Pneumothorax or pneumomediastinum may occur if the cupula of the lung is violated, or if high ventilatory pressures cause dissection of air along the pretracheal fascia. Minimal tissue dissection may reduce the incidence of this complication. Additionally, the recurrent laryngeal nerve lies within the tracheoesophageal groove and is at risk for injury, if a dissection is carried laterally. A perforation of the posterior tracheal wall may result in a tracheoesophageal fistula and can lead to life-threatening mediastinitis. Careful and precise dissection when creating the tracheal incision can prevent this complication. Bleeding occurs most commonly from the anterior jugular veins, the thyroid isthmus, or the thyroid ima artery, and bleeding can be controlled with suture ligation, ultrasonic energy, or electrocautery. Hemorrhage from the carotid artery or internal jugular vein is rare.

Airway fire during tracheostomy is uncommon but can have devastating consequences. In open tracheostomy, a fire may be ignited when electrocautery is used in the presence of high oxygen concentrations by mask airway or ET tube. This risk can be minimized by decreasing oxygen concentrations to safe levels (FiO_2 <0.39) and avoiding use of electrocautery after an incision has been made in the anterior tracheal wall. Additionally, burns to the skin can occur when electrocautery is used prior to complete drying of alcohol-based skin-prep solutions.

Postoperative Complications

Bleeding that occurs within the first 48 hours after tracheostomy usually originates from the skin incision or thyroid isthmus. Packing around the tube with a hemostatic agent will often resolve any minor bleeding, and mild bleeding from a long-term tracheostomy may be from granulation tissue that can usually be cauterized using silver nitrate in an office setting. Production of copious, bright red bleeding beyond 48 hours should be evaluated for a tracheoinnominate fistula. This rare, serious complication can result from the tip of the tracheostomy tube eroding through the tracheal wall due to torsion or instability, high cuff pressure, or infection in the neck. This occurs most commonly from a low (below the third tracheal ring), suboptimally placed tracheal incision. Mortality from a tracheoinnominate fistula is around 90%. Definitive treatment requires ligation of the innominate artery.

Obstruction of the tracheostomy tube lumen is possible when thickened mucous secretions or blood clots are present. Routine care with suctioning, humidification, and frequent cleaning of the inner cannula will prevent this complication. Displacement of the tube can be fatal, particularly in the immediate postoperative period prior to maturation of the tract. Manipulation of the tube, loosening of the tracheostomy tube ties, transport of the patient, and an obese body habitus can all contribute to the tracheostomy tube becoming dislodged. Securing the tracheostomy with sutures in addition to ties will help to minimize this risk. When moving a ventilator-dependent patient with a tracheostomy, the ventilator tubing should be detached and reconnected once repositioning is completed. A second individual to attend to the tracheostomy while moving the patient can also minimize the risk of displacing the tube.

SUMMARY

Tracheostomy is a common procedure that can be safely performed in most patients. Careful attention to anatomic landmarks, precise dissection, and standardized postoperative management all contribute to minimizing complications. Including both open and percutaneous techniques in your armamentarium can be beneficial. Although exceptions do exist, most patients are candidates for percutaneous tracheostomy, which is as safe as open tracheostomy. Percutaneous tracheostomy offers the advantages of being less time consuming and less expensive than open tracheostomy in the operating room. Serious complications are rare in both percutaneous and open techniques.

SUGGESTED READINGS

Blankenship DR, Gourin CG, Davis WB, et al: Percutaneous tracheostomy: don't beat them, join them, *Laryngoscope* 114(9):1517–1521, 2004.

Kost KM: Endoscopic percutaneous dilatational tracheotomy: a prospective evaluation of 500 consecutive cases, *Laryngoscope* 115(10 pt 2):1–30, 2005.

Seybt MW, Blanchard AR, Gourin CG, et al: 100 consecutive collaborative percutaneous tracheostomies, *Otolaryngol Head Neck Surg* 136(6):934–937, 2007.

ACUTE KIDNEY INJURY

Soumitra R. Eachempati, MD, and
Philip S. Barie, MD, MBA

OVERVIEW

Acute kidney injury (AKI), or acute renal failure (ARF), as it is more commonly known, remains a common and lethal complication of critical illness. In many patients, the etiology of AKI is frequently multifactorial: hypotension and contrast agents may play a role, and AKI may exist in an individual patient, but it is generally classified as being of *prerenal, renal,* or *postrenal* origins (Table 1). The literature is replete with definitions of AKI, but the occurrence of AKI in patients is most often defined as an elevation of serum creatinine concentration of 0.5 mg/dL from baseline or the need for acute renal replacement therapy (RRT, e.g., hemodialysis). Recently, the Acute Dialysis Quality Initiative developed a consensus definition of AKI (Table 2) that incorporates *risk, injury, failure, loss,* and *end-stage renal failure* criteria for the individual patient, known as *RIFLE* criteria. These criteria assess either serum creatinine elevations, glomerular filtration rate (GFR) decrements, or urine output decrements in the determination of the different stages of AKI. These criteria also yield prognostic information regarding the status of the critically ill patient.

PREVENTION AND EARLY DETECTION OF ACUTE KIDNEY INJURY

The best management strategy for AKI entails preventing its development. Patients with sepsis, trauma, and hypovolemia and postoperative patients have been clearly identified as being at high risk for AKI. Patient groups also at risk include those receiving any nephrotoxic agents (e.g., iodinated contrast, medications), those with chronic renal insufficiency due to diabetes mellitus or hypertension, and patients with congestive heart failure, multiple myeloma, chronic infection (e.g., osteomyelitis), and myeloproliferative disorders. Whereas all hospitalized patients must have their intravascular volume status monitored to some degree, these at-risk patients require particularly close monitoring to ensure that hypovolemia is avoided and that exposure to radiocontrast media is minimized or avoided. Consequently, these high-risk patients may need frequent measurements of vital signs, central venous pressure, serum lactate concentration, urine output, or short-duration (8 to 12 hours) creatinine clearances. In the future, serum (neutrophil gelatinase-associated lipocalin [NGAL] and cystatin C) and urine (NGAL, interleukin-18 [IL-18], and kidney-injury molecule-1 [KIM-1]) biomarkers may prove useful in early detection of AKI.

Certain intravenous medications (e.g., low-dose dopamine [1.5 to 3 μg/kg/min], fenoldopam) have been suggested to prevent the occurrence of AKI. Whereas use of these agents may benefit individual patients, large studies have failed to show benefit. Low-dose dopamine may be used to promote diuresis in select patients with adequate preload; many patients do respond with increased urine output, but the course of AKI is otherwise unaffected. The indication for fenoldopam in critical care is less well defined, but it may be beneficial when hypertension must be treated while preserving renal perfusion.

Two distinct patient populations are at extremely high risk to develop AKI and warrant special consideration. The first group comprises patients with rhabdomyolysis, usually a result of crush injury but which also can occur with high fever or other clinical syndromes.

Rhabdomyolysis that needs treatment is characterized by marked elevation of creatinine phosphokinase concentration greater than 5000 U/dL or the persistent presence of urine myoglobin; treatment is by enforced alkaline diuresis, as loop diuretics result in acidified urine and are consequently not recommended for rhabdomyolysis. Patients should be monitored in an intensive care unit with central venous pressure measurement and aggressive hydration.

Myoglobin is catabolized to ferrihemate, generating reactive oxygen species (both are nephrotoxic) at a urine pH less than 5.8, so many authorities recommend maintaining urine pH above 6.0 by the continuous infusion of sodium bicarbonate. To maintain isotonicity, 150 mL of 8.4% sodium bicarbonate is added to 850 mL D5W to create the solution. Some authorities administer mannitol 25 g q6h to enforce diuresis until pigmenturia disappears, but both mannitol and sodium bicarbonate are controversial.

Another high-risk group of patients for AKI are those who have chronic kidney disease (CKD) but require iodinated intravenous contrast for a diagnostic test. Patients who have baseline creatinine concentrations above 1.5 mg/dL or baseline creatinine clearances below 30 mg/dL are at extremely high risk for superimposed AKI. These patients should receive a sodium bicarbonate infusion (50 mL of 8.4% $NaHCO_3$ added to 950 mL D5W) at 100 mL/hr for an hour prior to the contrast administration and for 6 hours thereafter. Importantly, many of these patients are also at risk for pulmonary edema and should be monitored carefully. Notably, whereas *N*-acetylcysteine infusion was previously believed to be beneficial in the prevention of AKI in certain populations with CKD, including cardiovascular patients, a recent meta-analysis has refuted this contention.

Intrinsic Acute Kidney Injury

Structural injury in the kidney is the hallmark of intrinsic AKI. The most common form is acute tubular injury (ATN), whether ischemic or cytotoxic. Although the cellular injury is observed in proximal tubules predominantly, injury to the distal nephron also occurs. The distal nephron may also become obstructed by desquamated cells and cellular debris. In contrast to necrosis, the principal site of apoptotic cell death is the distal nephron. Endogenous growth factors regulate tissue repair and recovery; administration of growth factors exogenously has been shown experimentally to ameliorate and hasten recovery from AKI. Depletion of neutrophils and blockage of neutrophil adhesion reduce AKI following ischemia, indicating that the inflammation is at least partly responsible for some features of ATN, especially in postischemic injury after transplantation.

Intrarenal vasoconstriction is the dominant mechanism for reduced glomerular filtration rate (GFR) in ATN. The mechanisms of this vasoconstriction are unknown, but tubular injury appears to play a role. Tubular obstruction causes reduced ultrafiltration, and prolonged obstruction mediates intrarenal vasoconstriction via a tubuloglomerular feedback activated when proximal tubular injury results in increased chloride load on the macula densa. The stressed renal microvasculature loses its autoregulatory capacity and becomes more sensitive to vasoconstrictive drugs and periods of systemic hypotension, which thus may provoke additional damage that can delay recovery from ATN.

A physiologic hallmark of ATN is loss of the ability to concentrate or dilute the urine (isosthenuria). The injured kidney cannot maintain a high medullary solute gradient, because solute accumulation depends on normal distal nephron function. Failure to excrete concentrated urine, even in the presence of oliguria, is a helpful diagnostic clue to distinguish prerenal from intrinsic AKI, in which urine osmolality is less than 300 mOsm/kg. In prerenal azotemia, urine osmolality is typically more than 500 mOsm/kg. Another clue to loss of concentrating ability is the development of hypernatremia in the presence of adequate urine flow.

TABLE 1: Etiologies of AKI

Prerenal Causes (Decreased Renal Blood Flow)	Intrinsic Renal Causes	Postrenal Causes
Hypovolemia	**Vascular: Large and Small Vessels**	**Ureteral Obstruction**
Renal losses (diuretics, osmotic agents, polyuria)	Trauma	Calculus
Gastrointestinal losses (vomiting, diarrhea)	Renal vein obstruction (thrombosis, ventilation with high-level PEEP, abdominal compartment syndrome)	Tumor (intrinsic or extrinsic)
Cutaneous losses (burns, exfoliative syndromes)	Microangiopathy (thrombotic thrombocytopenic purpura, hemolytic-uremic syndrome, disseminated intravascular coagulation, preeclampsia)	Fibrosis
Hemorrhage	Malignant hypertension	Ligation during pelvic surgery
Pancreatitis	Scleroderma renal crisis	
	Transplant rejection	
	Atheroembolic disease	
Decreased Cardiac Output	**Glomerular**	**Bladder Neck Obstruction**
Congestive heart failure	Antiglomerular basement membrane disease (Goodpasture syndrome)	Benign prostatic hypertrophy
Pulmonary embolism	Antineutrophil cytoplasmic antibody-associated glomerulonephritis (Wegener granulomatosis)	Prostate cancer
Acute myocardial infarction	Immune complex glomerulonephritis, systemic lupus erythematosus, postinfectious cryoglobulinemia, primary membranoproliferative glomerulonephritis	Neurogenic bladder
Severe valvular heart disease		Tricyclic antidepressants
Abdominal compartment syndrome		Ganglionic blockers
Renal artery obstruction (stenosis, embolism, thrombosis, dissection)		Bladder tumor
		Calculus
		Hemorrhage/clot
Systemic Vasodilation	**Tubular**	**Urethral Obstruction**
Sepsis	Ischemic	Strictures
Anaphylaxis	Cytotoxic	Tumor
Anesthetics	Heme pigment (rhabdomyolysis, intravascular hemolysis)	Phimosis
Drug overdose	Crystals (tumor lysis syndrome, seizures, ethylene glycol poisoning, vitamin C megadose, acyclovir, indinavir, methotrexate)	Renal calcinosis
	Drugs (aminoglycosides, lithium, amphotericin B, pentamidine, cisplatin, ifosfamide, radiocontrast agents)	Obstructed urinary catheter, ureteral stent, or ileal conduit
		Pelvic trauma, retroperitoneal hematoma
Afferent Arteriolar Vasoconstriction	**Interstitial**	
Hypercalcemia	Drugs (penicillins, cephalosporins, NSAIDs, proton-pump inhibitors, allopurinol, rifampin, indinavir, mesalamine, sulfonamides)	
Drugs (NSAIDs, amphotericin B, calcineurin inhibitors, norepinephrine, radiocontrast agents, aminoglycosides)	Infection (pyelonephritis, viral infection)	
Hepatorenal syndrome		
Efferent arteriolar vasodilation (angiotensin converting enzyme inhibitors, aldosterone receptor blockers)		
	Systemic Disease	
	Sjögren syndrome, sarcoidosis, systemic lupus erythematosus, lymphoma, leukemia, tubulonephritis, uveitis	

NSAIDs, Nonsteroidal antiinflammatory drugs; *PEEP,* positive end-expiratory pressure

BASIC PRINCIPLES OF TREATMENT OF ACUTE KIDNEY INJURY

Early intervention remains the optimal strategy in treating AKI once it has occurred. Delays in treatment of the manifestations of AKI lead to worsening dysfunction of the kidneys and other organs. Although mild AKI may develop in isolation, all patients with severe AKI also have one or more other dysfunctional organs and manifest multiple organ dysfunction syndrome (MODS). The most common pitfalls in the management of AKI are delay in diagnosis, incorrect assessment of the causes, and failure to recognize and treat not only its complications but also the other manifestations of MODS, including the underlying disorder that caused the kidney injury, which, if uncorrected, will be the most likely cause of death, not the AKI.

The most important step in diagnosing and treating AKI involves determining whether the etiology is prerenal, renal, or postrenal. However, once AKI has occurred, the clinician must treat its underlying cause while concurrently treating or possibly preventing any

TABLE 2: RIFLE criteria

	GFR Criteria	Urine Output Criteria
Risk	SCR >1.5 × baseline GFR decrease of 25%	<0.5 mL/kg for 6 hours
Injury	SCR >2.0 × baseline GFR decrease of 50%	<0.5 mL/kg for 12 hours
Failure	SCR >3.0 × baseline SCR >4.0 mg/dL GFR decrease of 75%	<0.3 mL/kg for 24 hours Anuria for 12 hours
Loss	Failure >4 weeks (either GFR or urine output criteria)	
ESRD	Failure >3 months (either GFR or urine output criteria)	

SCR, Serum creatinine; *ESRD,* end-stage renal disease; *GFR,* glomerular filtration rate; *RIFLE,* risk, injury, failure, loss, and end-stage renal failure criteria

TABLE 3: Diagnostic tests to distinguish prerenal and renal AKI

Index	Prerenal Causes	Renal Causes
FENa	<1%	>2%
Urine sodium	<10 mmol/L	>40 mmol/L
Urine/plasma osmolality	>1.5	1 to 1.5
Renal failure index	<1	>2
BUN/creatinine ratio	>20	<10

BUN, Blood urea nitrogen; *FENa,* fractional excretion of sodium
Calculation of FENa: (Urine sodium × Plasma creatinine)/(Plasma sodium × Serum creatinine) × 100
Renal failure index: (Urine sodium × Urine creatinine)/Plasma creatinine

complications of AKI that could develop. Notably, certain conditions, such as trauma and sepsis, may contribute to the development of AKI by multiple mechanisms. For example in trauma, blood loss and the concomitant proinflammatory response from massive tissue injury can lead to hypovolemia and prerenal AKI, whereas the rhabdomyolysis of trauma or the use of iodinated contrast to detect injuries can lead to intrinsic renal injury. In sepsis, the hypovolemia of sepsis can lead to prerenal AKI, but bacterial toxins or antibiotics used to treat sepsis may contribute to intrinsic causes of AKI.

Evaluation of Oliguria

The most common manifestation of the development of AKI is oliguria, which in most adults is defined as less than 0.5 mL/kg/hr based on ideal body weight. An alternative definition of oliguria is urine output below 400 mL/day. Postoperative oliguria and oliguria that occurs after injury are most likely to be due to hypovolemia or other prerenal causes. Surgical evaluation begins with a focused history and physical examination for likely causes, but if the cause is unknown or obscure, a detailed evaluation is important. Examination of the skin may reveal petechiae, purpura, ecchymosis, and livedo reticularis, which can provide clues to inflammatory and vascular causes of AKI. Ocular examination may find evidence of uveitis suggestive of interstitial nephritis or necrotizing vasculitis, whereas ocular palsy may indicate ethylene glycol poisoning or necrotizing vasculitis. Findings suggestive of severe hypertension, atheroembolic disease, or endocarditis may be observed by fundoscopy.

The most important part of the physical examination is the assessment of cardiovascular and volume status, especially for surgical patients. Vital signs taken both supine and standing (if possible) and careful examination of the heart, lungs, jugular venous pulse, skin turgor, mucous membranes, and extremities (for peripheral edema) are essential. Accurate daily records of fluid intake and urine output and daily measurements of patient weight are crucial. Medications must be reviewed, and doses should be adjusted if necessary.

Abdominal examination findings can be useful to help detect obstruction at the bladder outlet as the cause of AKI. The presence of an epigastric bruit suggests renovascular hypertension, and abdominal distension may suggest abdominal compartment syndrome (ACS). Foley catheters and other urinary conduits or stents should be inspected for patency, and intravesical pressure should be measured if ACS is suspected.

After this initial assessment, the clinician must determine whether oliguria is due to prerenal or other causes. Confirmatory tests may then be employed, such as central venous or pulmonary

artery pressure monitoring or a chest radiograph (Table 3). Notably, the detection of pulmonary edema in critically ill patients by standard anteroposterior chest radiography lacks sensitivity and specificity. Urinary electrolytes should be measured; a urine sodium concentration less than 20 mg/dL or a fractional excretion of sodium (FENa) less than 1% are consistent with a prerenal etiology: FENa above 2% suggests intrinsic disease, values between 1% to 2% are indeterminate, and the calculation is unreliable if a diuretic has been given recently. For more complex cases, a renal ultrasound should be ordered to evaluate for hydronephrosis.

Urologic and renal transplant patients pose unique diagnostic problems; the former may be leaking urine intraperitoneally and may have azotemia due to reabsorption of urea, whereas the latter may have vascular complications as well. These cases may require measurement of creatinine concentration in drain fluid or scintigraphy to assess perfusion. Eosinophils in urine sediment may suggest a drug reaction causing AKI, most frequently from β-lactam antibiotics.

In certain patients, the diagnosis of ACS needs to be excluded. In ACS, intraabdominal pressure exceeds renal capillary perfusion pressure, and the patient develops oliguria. Patients at highest risk for ACS include those with very large fluid resuscitation volumes (generally greater than 8 L), large-volume hemorrhage (generally 2 L or more), ascites, severe bowel edema, or patients with abdominal packs in place to stanch hemorrhage. Intravesical pressure is a reasonable surrogate for intraabdominal pressure; a simple method to measure intravesical pressure is to occlude the Foley catheter after the instillation of at least 50 mL, but preferably no more than 100 mL, of saline and then transducing the pressure in the hub via the sampling port proximal to the clamp. Any measurement in excess of 25 mm Hg is consistent with intraabdominal hypertension, which in the proper setting can be diagnostic for ACS.

Prompt decompression of the abdomen by laparotomy is the standard treatment for patients with high suspicion of ACS. However, bladder pressure values by this method must be interpreted cautiously in patients with CKD, neurogenic or small-volume bladders, bladder cancer, recent bladder injury, or active bacterial cystitis.

Treatment of Acute Kidney Injury of Prerenal Etiology

The management of AKI is predicated on its cause. A prerenal cause is the most common etiology of AKI in postoperative patients; it is usually the result of severe hypovolemia if not incipient or overt shock. Treating prerenal AKI entails optimizing perfusion to the kidneys and treating the cause of the hypoperfusion or shock. Importantly, in critically ill patients, a rapid consideration of all types of shock is warranted. Whereas hypovolemia is the most common etiology of shock in surgical patients, cardiogenic shock from myocardial infarction, pulmonary embolism, tension pneumothorax, or pericardial tamponade may alternatively or also be present. Other cardiac causes are manifold, including pump failure, cardiac valvular disease, or intrinsic cardiac shunts. Neurogenic shock occurs most commonly after spinal cord injury but can also occur from epidural anesthesia dosed inappropriately. Other forms of distributive shock from etiologies such as medication or transfusion reaction should also be considered. Whereas most of these causes require volume replacement and treatment of the underlying cause, in left ventricular pump failure, the patient may paradoxically have decreased renal perfusion but may require diuretics with afterload reduction for successful management.

Management of Acute Kidney Injury from Intrinsic and Postrenal Causes

Regardless of the etiology, management of AKI must avoid further insults to renal function, particularly so for intrinsic AKI, and iatrogenic complications such as fluid overload. Many patients develop secondary pulmonary organ dysfunction from hypervolemia, usually as a result of overzealous fluid management. One important goal in AKI is to maintain euvolemia so as to avoid an additional or superimposed prerenal insult. Fluid overload in the setting of AKI can be catastrophic, resulting in endotracheal intubation, prolonged mechanical ventilation, conversion of a patient with single-organ failure to MODS, and a propensity for fatal nosocomial infections. Potassium and chloride should be removed from IV solutions and minimized in enteral feedings and oral diets to preempt hyperkalemia and decrease metabolic acidosis. Frequent monitoring of serum electrolyte concentrations is crucial.

Presuming the point of obstruction has been identified in postrenal AKI, a decision must be made as to whether to relieve the obstruction or bypass it by urinary diversion. The approach is individualized depending on the site, the nature of the obstruction, the overall condition of the patient, and the degree of renal impairment. For critically ill patients, urinary diversion is often the best choice. Options include ureteral stents, suprapubic nephrostomy, and percutaneous nephrostomy.

If the patient with AKI is deemed to have adequate preload and is making some urine, the patient may be a candidate for a trial of diuretic therapy. This intervention is clearly more useful if the patient has decreased ventricular function, a history of outpatient diuretic use, or signs of hypervolemia such as hypoxemia, rales, or dyspnea. When diuretics are used, loop diuretics (e.g., furosemide, bumetanide) are generally the diuretics of choice. Lower doses of furosemide (10 to 40 mg) may be ineffective in patients with more severe AKI (serum creatinine concentration greater than 4.0 mg/dL), but patients may respond to higher doses, in the range of 80 to 200 mg, of furosemide or bumetanide (2 to 5 mg; approximate furosemide/bumetanide dosage ratio 1:40).

If an oliguric patient does not respond to a single administered high dose, there is little risk and little benefit in continuing. High doses of the loop diuretics are themselves nephrotoxic and ototoxic, and they should not be used more than once if the patient is anuric. Importantly, the diuretics do nothing to alter the natural history of the AKI but may facilitate the management of volume and nutrition to avoid the need for renal replacement therapy (RRT) if some urine output is restored. Loop diuretics can cause hypokalemia, hypomagnesemia, and metabolic alkalosis, especially after large-volume diuresis, so electrolytes should be monitored closely.

When a patient has oliguria and hypervolemia in the setting of metabolic alkalosis or a mixed picture of alkalosis and acidosis, loop diuretics should be used with caution, as they can exacerbate alkalosis. For patients with a serum sodium bicarbonate ($NaHCO_3$) concentration greater than 28 mmol/dL, acetazolamide 250 to 500 mg/dL once or twice daily is effective, provided the serum potassium and magnesium concentrations are normal, and the patient still has some renal function (creatinine clearance >30 mg/dL). For patients with severe metabolic alkalosis refractory to acetazolamide, 1% intravenous HCl is the next agent of choice prior to RRT.

COMPLICATIONS OF ACUTE KIDNEY INJURY

Deranged renal function impairs the maintenance of electrolyte homeostasis and the excretion of water-soluble toxins, thus complications of AKI are generally associated with these perturbations (Box 1). Consequently, AKI can potentially result in fluid overload, electrolyte abnormalities, and impaired clearance of toxins such as urea. These complications may manifest as hypoxemia, hyperkalemia, acidosis, or uremia—all avoidable if RRT is instituted appropriately and in a timely fashion. Left unchecked, any of these entities may be life threatening, as they may lead to arrhythmias, myocardial infarction, pericarditis, and coma. Given the potential lethality of these complications, timely RRT is especially important for critically ill patients.

Renal Replacement Therapy

The decision to institute RRT is generally made jointly by the managing inpatient service and the consulting nephrologist. In patients with immediate life-threatening complications such as severe hyperkalemia (peaked T waves by electrocardiography, serum potassium concentration >6.5 mEq/dL) or pulmonary edema causing hypoxemic respiratory failure, the decision is obvious. In other patients the timing of RRT may be subtle, depending on the clinical status of the patient. The most common indications for RRT in surgical patients are hypervolemia and metabolic acidosis, two conditions that have adverse affects on ventilated patients in particular by increasing the risk of prolonged mechanical ventilation and consequent nosocomial infection.

After the indication for RRT has been determined, the modality of the RRT must be chosen. Standardized methods of RRT include *continuous RRT* (CRRT) and *intermittent hemodialysis* (IHD); *peritoneal dialysis* is less effective, is contraindicated by recent abdominal surgery, and is falling into disuse. Both blood filtration modalities pose their own set of risks and benefits. Continuous RRT provides a creatinine clearance of 15 to 20 mL/min in addition to the patient's intrinsic clearance (usually <15 mL/min if RRT is required). The two values are summed to estimate the patient's creatinine clearance (maximum is 35 mL/min in this example) for pharmaceutical dosing purposes. By contrast, IHD provides high clearance (~300 mL/min) for brief periods (3 to 4 hours). Averaged over a 3 hour session daily, IHD might provide comparable clearance (300 mL/min × 180 min/1440 min, or ~38 mL/min). If IHD is provided on alternate days, the estimated clearance would be halved (~19 mL/min), which is less than what effective CRRT would provide over the same interval.

IHD has been the traditional first-line modality for RRT in patients with AKI or end-stage renal disease (ESRD). Maintenance outpatient IHD is often scheduled on a thrice-weekly regimen; however, in the acute setting, many patients are so catabolic that daily RRT is required, particularly at the onset. Some data indicate that

---

BOX 1: Complications of AKI requiring potentially emergent RRT

Fluid overload
Metabolic acidosis
Electrolyte abnormalities (hyperkalemia)
Uremic encephalopathy
Uremic pericarditis

early or more intensive RRT yields better outcomes, but the issue remains controversial. Because IHD only lasts 3 to 4 hours, it is more feasible for critically ill patients from a nursing perspective. IHD is superior to CRRT if rapid clearance or ultrafiltration are required, but it is more prone to cause or aggravate hypotension owing to much larger fluid shifts. Consequently, hypotensive patients may be better candidates for CRRT, which is probably safer for patients with unstable hemodynamics, particularly if vasopressors are in use. However, during CRRT the patient requires one-on-one nursing care continuously, which has implications for nurse staffing. Moreover, CRRT impedes transport for operative procedures or diagnostic tests outside the critical care setting.

Continuous RRT also poses other disadvantages compared with IHD. The extracorporeal dialysis circuit of CRRT is more prone to clotting than IHD, even if blood pressure is maintained and in the presence of concomitant anticoagulant therapy. Clotting of the CRRT circuit is detrimental, as it interrupts therapy, causes the loss of about 200 mL blood each time, and is costly. To decrease clotting, regional or systemic anticoagulation may be employed, but clotting can still occur in the presence of therapeutic anticoagulation. Newer CRRT protocols use citrate anticoagulation in the extracorporeal circuit, which may be safer for the critically ill patient than systemic anticoagulation, but this method is not widely available and can lead to hypocalcemia.

PROGNOSIS OF ACUTE KIDNEY INJURY

The prognosis of patients with AKI is directly related to the cause of renal failure and, to a great extent, to the duration of renal failure prior to therapeutic intervention. If AKI is defined by a sudden increment of serum creatinine greater than 0.5 mg/dL, but the actual increase is greater than 1.0 mg/dL, the prognosis tends to be worse. Even if renal failure is mild (peak serum creatinine <4 mg/dL), the mortality rate is about 30%. For patients who need RRT, the mortality rate is greater than 50%, but the mode of RRT (e.g., IHD vs. CRRT) does not have an impact on outcome, in that most comparative studies show equivalent results.

SUGGESTED READINGS

Barrantes F, Tian J, Vazquez R, et al: Acute kidney injury criteria predict outcomes of critically ill patients, Crit Care Med 36:1397, 2008.
Cherry RA, Eachempati SR, Hydo L, et al: Accuracy of short-duration creatinine clearance determinations in predicting 24-hour creatinine clearance in critically ill and injured patients, J Trauma 53:267, 2002.
Eachempati SR, Wang JCL, Hydo LJ, et al: Acute renal failure in surgical patients: persistent lethality despite new modes of renal replacement therapy, J Trauma 63:987, 2007.
Kellum JA, Cerda J, Kaplan LJ, et al: Fluids for prevention and management of acute kidney injury, Int J Artif Org 31:96, 2008.
Kelly AM, Dwamena B, Cronin P, et al: Meta-analysis: effectiveness of drugs for preventing contrast-induced nephropathy, Ann Intern Med 148:284, 2008.
Kindgen-Milles D, Amman J, Kleinekofort W, et al: Treatment of metabolic alkalosis during continuous renal replacement therapy with regional citrate anticoagulation, Int J Artif Org 31:363, 2008.
Palevsky P: Indications and timing of renal replacement therapy in acute kidney injury, Crit Care Med 36(suppl):S224, 2008.
Ricci Z, Cruz D, Ronco C: The RIFLE criteria and mortality in acute kidney injury: a systematic review, Kidney Int 73:538, 2008.
Schrier RW, Wang W: Acute renal failure and sepsis, N Engl J Med 351:159, 2004.
Venkataraman R: Can we prevent acute kidney injury? Crit Care Med 36(suppl):S166, 2008.

ELECTROLYTE DISORDERS

Heather L. Evans, MD, and Ronald V. Maier, MD

OVERVIEW

Electrolytes are integral to the maintenance of homeostasis within the body. Water balance, neural impulse transmission, muscle contraction, and hormone release are among the essential mechanisms mediated by electrochemical gradients. Whether inflammation is the result of trauma or infection or from excessive fluid losses or fluid administration, fluid shifts and electrolyte disorders are very common in surgical patients. Understanding the relationship between fluid and electrolytes and recognizing the consequences of imbalance are essential to avoid irreversible complications.

SODIUM

Normal Homeostasis

The distribution of total body water (TBW) between the intracellular, interstitial, and intravascular spaces is determined by the osmotic forces of each compartment (Figure 1). Because sodium and its anions account for nearly 90% of the solutes in the extracellular space, sodium is the major determinant of tonicity and osmolality. It

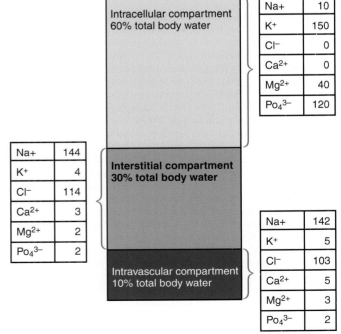

FIGURE 1 Distribution and composition (mEq/L) of total body water.

Hyponatremia

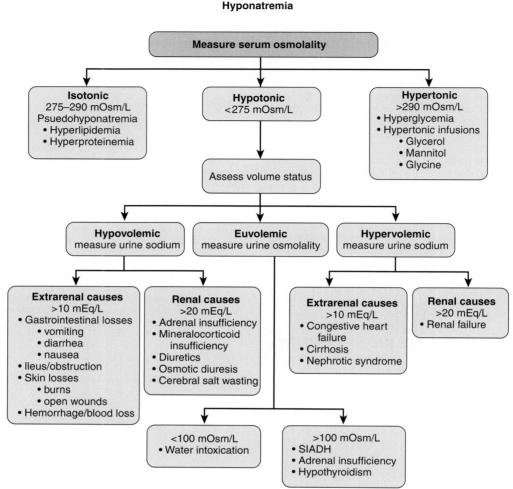

FIGURE 2   Algorithm for treatment of hyponatremia. *SIADH,* Syndrome of inappropriate antidiuretic hormone.

is important to acknowledge that although increasing total sodium content will increase the extracellular fluid volume, the plasma sodium concentration—that is, the ratio of sodium to water—is independent of the extracellular fluid (ECF) volume.

Plasma osmolality (P_{osm}) is determined by the ratio of solutes and water, whereas the extracellular volume is determined by the absolute amounts of Na^+ and water. Osmolality, normally regulated within relatively narrow limits (275 to 290 mOsm/kg), is maintained by tight control of water intake and output. The body measures serum osmolality at osmoreceptors in the supraoptic and paraventricular nuclei of the hypothalamus. When osmolality increases, the cells shrink and stimulate release of arginine vasopressin, also known as *antidiuretic hormone,* or *ADH,* from the posterior pituitary. In response to increased permeability in the renal collecting tubules, more water is retained by the kidney, and ECF volume increases. ADH release may also occur as a consequence of decreased blood volume as measured by carotid baroreceptors or atrial stretch receptors or as a result of pain, emotional stress, hypoxia, or oropharyngeal stimulation. Thirst is also stimulated with ADH release, further resulting in increased fluid intake in conscious patients. Conversely, an excess ECF will suppress the release of ADH and suppress thirst.

Serum sodium concentration, and therefore P_{osm}, is determined by changes in water balance. Total body sodium levels are regulated by the kidney via the renin-angiotensin-aldosterone axis and atrial natriuretic peptide. Changes in sodium balance are directed to maintain plasma volume and tissue perfusion, not sodium concentration.

This occurs independently of the regulation of osmolality by changes in water balance. Most disorders of sodium concentration are due to disorders of water balance; therefore, the determination of the etiology of a serum sodium imbalance begins with an assessment of the P_{osm} and an estimate of the volume status.

Hyponatremia

Hyponatremia (<135 mEq/L) is usually present as the result of an excess of body water compared with total body sodium. Identifying the underlying disorder that must be corrected to resume sodium homeostasis requires an organized approach such as that illustrated in Figure 2. Although hyponatremia is most commonly associated with hypoosmolality, low serum sodium concentrations are also possible in isotonic and hypertonic states, in which the plasma volume has been expanded by introduction of additional solutes without a change in the sodium, resulting in what has been referred to as *pseudohyponatremia.* Hyperosmolar hyponatremia results when highly osmotic aqueous solutes such as mannitol expand the plasma volume as a result of solute drag. The osmolar gap, calculated osmolality minus measured serum osmolality, can be assessed to identify the presence of undetected osmoles.

Hyperglycemia may also affect the measured sodium concentration; for every 100 mg/dL increase in serum glucose, the sodium concentration will decrease by 1.6 mEq/L. When nonaqueous solutes

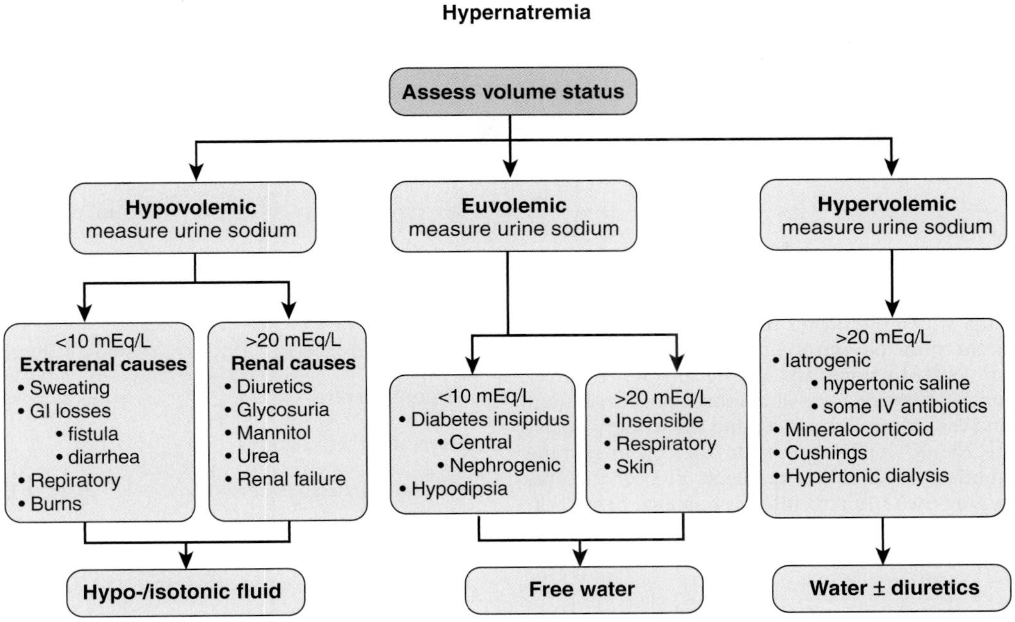

Hypernatremia

FIGURE 3   Algorithm for treatment of hypernatremia.

such as lipids and proteins are introduced into the vasculature, the relative serum sodium concentration is decreased despite a normal serum osmolality. Treatment of hyponatremia in these settings is directed at the underlying cause (e.g., glucose control).

Hypoosmolar hyponatremia occurs when free-water excretion is impaired, or the kidney's ability to produce dilute urine is exceeded. The resulting osmolar gradient shifts water into the cell, culminating in organ dysfunction. This is most clinically apparent in depression of the central nervous system due to cerebral edema. The degree of symptoms depends on both the rate and the degree of hyponatremia. As serum sodium falls below 125 mEq/L, nausea and malaise are noted. Further decrease is associated with headache, lethargy, and obtundation at levels less than 120 mEq/L; coma and seizures occur at less than 110 to 115 mEq/L.

The etiology of hypoosmolar hyponatremia may be determined by further stratifying these patients according to intravascular volume status and by urine sodium concentration. In general, patients with excessive sodium losses are hypovolemic, but those with disorders of increased total body sodium despite their low serum sodium concentration are hypervolemic. Hypovolemic hyponatremia is usually associated with excessive gastrointestinal or diuretic losses of both water and sodium, which subsequently stimulates ADH secretion that causes free-water retention and further decreases the serum sodium concentration. Hypervolemic hyponatremia is more commonly seen in edematous states of effectively reduced circulating volume such as in congestive heart failure, cirrhosis, renal failure, and nephrotic syndrome. These are thought to be mediated by progressive impairment of renal free-water excretion resulting from nonosmotic ADH release and decreased delivery of fluid to the distal diluting segment in nephrons.

Isovolemic hyponatremia occurs in a variety of clinical states involving hormonal imbalance such as glucocorticoid insufficiency, hypothyroidism, and the syndrome of inappropriate antidiuretic hormone secretion (SIADH). Polydipsia also falls into this category, although it is distinguished from the others mentioned by low urine sodium, as the kidney's ability to clear free water is exceeded by water ingestion, not an excess of ADH.

Treatment is directed at restoring Na$^+$ balance and correcting the underlying disorder. For those patients who are hypervolemic or normovolemic, water restriction is the treatment of choice. Hypovolemic hyponatremia requires restoration of circulating plasma volume with

normal saline. As the extracellular volume deficit is corrected, diuresis of free water will correct the sodium concentration. To determine the sodium deficit, the following calculation is employed:

$$Na^+ deficit = 0.6 \times Weight\ (kg) \times (140 - [Na^+])$$

Central pontine myelinolysis—a neurologic disorder characterized by pseudobulbar palsy, quadriparesis, seizures, movement disorders, and a high risk of mortality—may occur in response to rapid correction of serum sodium concentrations. It is recommended that the correction rates should not exceed 1.5 mEq/h, or 8 to 12 mEq over 24 hours, particularly among patients with chronic hyponatremia.

Hypernatremia

Hypernatremia (serum sodium >145 mEq/L) reflects a water deficit relative to sodium levels and is most commonly seen in cases of extreme dehydration. As plasma osmolality rises, ADH is released, and the urine is concentrated to a maximum of 800 to 1200 mOsm/kg. Following the osmotic gradient, water is shifted from the intracellular space, causing cells to shrink. Because of the effect on neural tissue, this disorder is characterized by irritability, weakness, and lethargy that progresses to coma and death. The etiology of hypernatremia is categorized by volume status (Figure 3). If the patient is hypovolemic, circulating plasma volume should be corrected with isotonic fluids prior to correction of the free-water deficit to maintain perfusion. Diuretics may be administered to hypervolemic patients, as sodium excretion will be achieved along with the volume of free water lost. The equation for calculating free-water deficit is as follows:

$$Water\ deficit = 0.6 \times Weight\ (kg) \times [([Na^+]_p / 140) - 1]$$

Just as in hyponatremia, acute hypernatremia may be corrected rapidly (1 to 2 mEq/hr) as compared with chronic hypernatremia (0.5 mEq/h), but to prevent cerebral edema, it should not exceed 10 to 12 mEq daily.

For central and nephrogenic diabetes insipidus (DI), pharmacologic therapy is necessary. Nasal insufflation of 1-desamino-8-D-arginine vasopressin (DDAVP) or subcutaneous injection of vasopressin corrects central DI. Agents such as chlorpropamide and carbamaze-pine may also help by potentiating ADH release. Thiazide diuretics mitigate the effects of nephrogenic DI by paradoxically decreasing urine volume. This is mediated by reduced sodium reabsorption in the distal convoluted tubule (DCT) that decreases glomerulofiltration and increases sodium and water reabsorption in the proximal tubule.

POTASSIUM

Normal Homeostasis

In contrast to sodium, which dominates the extracellular compart-ment, potassium is the principle intracellular cation, with 98% of the body's potassium located within cells. The serum $[K^+]$ is deter-mined by the relationship between potassium intake, the distribution between the cells and the extracellular fluid, and the urinary potas-sium excretion. The Na^+-K^+-ATPase pump in the cell membrane mediates the differential concentration gradients of both cations, functionally maintaining the resting membrane potential of the cell. This is described by the Nernst equation:

$$E_m = \frac{-61 \log r \, [K^+]_I + 0.01 \, [Na^+]_i}{r[K^+]_e + 0.01[Na^+]_e}$$

$$[K^+]_i = \text{Intracellular } [K^+]$$

$$[K^+]_e = \text{Extracellular } [K^+]$$

$$r = \text{Permeability constant}$$

Nerve conduction and cardiac function are among the vital pro-cesses that depend on the resting potential. Potassium also plays a role in cellular metabolism, regulating protein and glycogen synthesis.

The intracellular reservoir of potassium is a potential source of sudden, fatal hyperkalemia in certain disorders, but even slight shifts in the intracellular and extracellular balance of potassium can mark-edly disturb cellular function. Therefore it is not surprising that numerous regulatory mechanisms maintain serum K^+ within the nar-row physiologic range of 3.6 to 4.4 mEq/L. Ingested potassium is read-ily absorbed and shifted intracellularly. Insulin and catecholamines released in response to a meal promote K^+ sequestration by simulat-ing the Na^+-K^+-ATPase and the Na^+-H^+ transporter, respectively.

The kidney maintains the body's potassium balance; urinary excretion of net intake is an adaptive response mediated by the serum K^+, plasma aldosterone levels, and the delivery of sodium and water to the distal secretory site. Net renal secretion of K^+ occurs through open potassium channels in the cortical collecting duct (CCD) com-bined with a lumen-negative charge generated by the induction of Na^+ absorption by aldosterone. As the kidney is better adapted to increase than to decrease K^+ secretion, hypokalemia can occur with decreased intake. Conversely, hyperkalemia occurs primarily as a result of impairment of renal K^+ excretion.

Hyperkalemia

Hyperkalemia (K^+ > 5.0 mEq/L) is with few exceptions—thrombo-cytosis, leukocytosis, and hemolysis—indicative of either impaired excretion or impaired K^+ entry into cells (Table 1). Because the nor-mal kidney is so imminently capable of adaptive excretion, the devel-opment of hyperkalemia suggests renal dysfunction. The degree of hyperkalemia may be increased with the concomitant administration of nephrotoxic drugs or potassium supplements, two very common medical therapies. Although renal failure is the most common cause of hyperkalemia in hospitalized patients, life-threatening hyperka-lemia usually occurs in the setting of a sudden shift of intracellu-lar potassium, as seen in acute metabolic acidosis or massive tissue destruction caused by crush or ischemic injury.

TABLE 1: Etiology of potassium disorders

Hypokalemia	Hyperkalemia
Inadequate intake	Pseudohyperkalemia
Increased excretion	Thrombocytosis
Diarrhea	Leukocytosis
Renal losses	Hemolysis
Diuretic	Impaired excretion
Metabolic alkalosis	Renal failure
Osmotic dieresis	Mineralocorticoid insufficiency
Nonreabsorbable anions	Drugs
Mineralocorticoid excess	K^+-sparing diuretics
Glucocorticoids	ACE inhibitors/ARBs
Bartter and Gitelman syndromes	NSAIDs
Magnesium depletion	Heparin
Renal tubular acidosis	Cyclosporine/tacrolimus
Transcellular shift	Trimethoprim
β-Agonists	Pentamidine
Theophylline/caffeine	Transcellular shift
Insulin	β-Antagonists
Delirium tremens	Acidosis
Hyperthyroidism	Succinylcholine
Familial hypokalemic periodic paralysis	Insulin deficiency
Barium	Hypertonicity
	Familial hyperkalemic periodic paralysis
	Massive tissue destruction

ACE, Angiotensin-converting enzyme; *ARBs,* angiotensin receptor blockers; *NSAIDs,* nonsteroidal antiinflammatory drugs

Though characteristically asymptomatic, hyperkalemia can be fatal due to alteration in cellular transmembrane potential of the heart's conduction system. The first electrocardiogram (ECG) indica-tion of myocardial dysfunction is a tall, peaked T wave with a short-ened QT interval. Progressive lengthening of the PR interval and QRS duration follow, and the P wave may disappear if the hyperkale-mia continues. Ultimately, the QRS may widen into a sine wave and flatten completely, when electrical activity ceases. Any ECG changes require emergent administration of intravenous Ca^{2+} to stabilize the myocardial membrane in the hopes of preventing progression to fatal arrhythmias (Table 2). Subsequent efforts should be directed at inducing a transcellular shift in K^+ and facilitating total body losses.

After initial measures to stabilize the patient are established, the etiology of the disorder should be investigated (Figure 4). The cli-nician should first exclude excessive intake, sources of transcellular shift, and pseudohyperkalemia, which may be due to hemolysis,

TABLE 2: Treatment of hyperkalemia

Therapy	Dose	Onset	Duration
Membrane stabilization			
Calcium gluconate	1–2 g IV over 5–10 min	1–2 min	30 min
Intracellular potassium shift			
Sodium bicarbonate	50–100 mEq IV over 2–5 min	30 min	2–6 hr
Insulin and glucose	5–10 U RHI IV with 50 mL of D_{50} (25 g)	15–45 min	2–6 hr
β_2-Agonists (e.g., albuterol)	10–20 mg nebulized	20–30 min	1–2 hr
Potassium removal			
Furosemide	20–40 mg IV	5–15 min	4–6 hr
Sodium polystrene sulfonate (kayexelate)	15–60 g PO or PR	4–6 hr	4–6 hr
Hemodialysis	2–4 hr	Immediate	Duration of dialysis

RHI, Regular human insulin

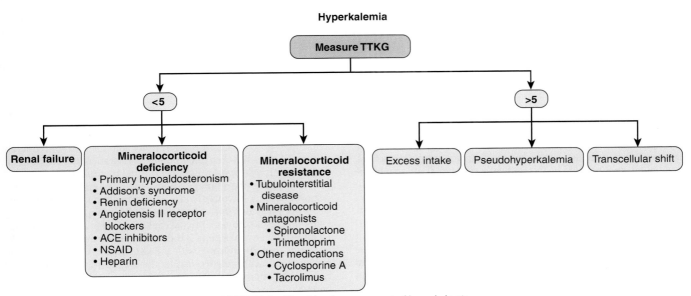

FIGURE 4 Algorithm for treatment of hyperkalemia.

thrombocytosis, fist clenching, or cachexia. If none of these is the cause, the renal response to hyperkalemia must be assessed (Figure 4). The rate of K^+ excretion is the product of urine flow and $[K^+]_u$. The transtubular K^+ gradients (TTKGs) in urine and plasma in the CCD may be estimated with the equation:

$$\text{Transtubular gradient} = \frac{[K^+]_u \times P_{osm}}{[K^+]_p \times U_{osm}}$$

The TTKG is typically less than 5 when a renal cause of hyperkalemia is present.

Hypokalemia

Hypokalemia ($K^+ < 3.6$) occurs in up to 20% of hospitalized patients. Because maintenance of the potassium concentration gradient is integral to the function of the neuromuscular junction, decreases in the serum K^+ can cause hyperpolarization that manifests as weakness, myalgias, and easy fatigability. These symptoms generally develop when K^+ goes below 2.5 mEq/L and may progress to cramps, paresthesias, ileus, and tetany. Myocardial dysfunction ranges from premature ventricular contractions and sinus bradycardia to atrioventricular block and ventricular tachycardia/fibrillation. Characteristic ECG changes include depression of the ST segment, decrease in the amplitude of the T wave, and an increase in the amplitude of U waves. Severe hypokalemia can cause rhabdomyolysis and myoglobinuria or an ascending paralysis with eventual respiratory arrest. Other pathologic sequelae include diabetes insipidus from diminished urinary concentrating ability and metabolic alkalosis from enhanced renal production of NH_3 and NH_4^+.

In the presence of ECG changes, severe myopathy, or paralysis, rapid administration of KCl should precede diagnostic intervention. Patients with severe symptoms should receive intravenous replacement to facilitate rapid correction of serum potassium levels. Administration of K^+ should not exceed 10 mEq/hr and a concentration of

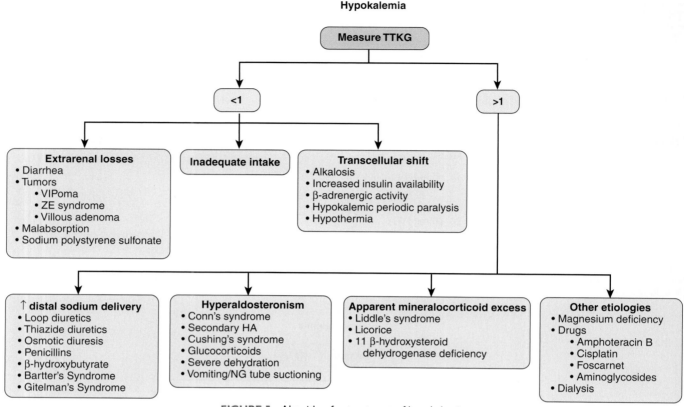

FIGURE 5 Algorithm for treatment of hypokalemia.

40 mEq/L through peripheral intravenous access or 40 mEq/hr through a central venous catheter. Because of the sequelae of possible iatrogenic hyperkalemia, continuous cardiac monitoring is essential, and the serum K^+ should be intermittently assessed. Caution must be exercised when patients are concurrently treated for a disorder with a therapy that may facilitate rapid cellular uptake of potassium (i.e., insulin infusion for diabetic ketoacidosis). In the absence of restrictions to gastrointestinal administration, particularly for the administration of chronic or subclinical hypokalemia, enteral replacement with potassium chloride or potassium phosphate preparations is the rule because gastrointestinal absorption is highly efficient. Doses range from 10 to 40 mEq and are usually administered twice daily; $[K^+]_p$ can be expected to acutely rise to 1 to 1.5 mEq/L after 40 to 60 mEq.

Hypokalemia may stem from inadequate intake, excessive losses, or transcellular shifts (Table 2). Potassium loss is mediated through the gastrointestinal tract or via renal excretion. Whether due to infection, malabsorption, tumor, or drugs, gastrointestinal losses in the form of diarrhea culminate in significant K^+ losses. By contrast, hypokalemia from gastric losses is more a consequence of excessive renal excretion; the resultant extracellular volume contraction and hypochloremia stimulate the renin-angiotensin-aldosterone axis, which induces K^+ secretion. Renal potassium losses are induced by other mean as well. Diuretic administration enhances delivery of Na^+ to the distal tubule, and hypokalemia may be exacerbated in combination with increased aldosterone because of the primary disease (e.g., cirrhosis, congestive heart failure). Mineralocorticoid excess from primary hyperaldosteronism, Cushing disease, and adrenal hyperplasia causes excessive renal K^+ losses. Presentation of Na^+ to the distal tubule in combination with a nonreabsorbable anion (e.g., beta-hydroxybutyrate in diabetic ketoacidosis) further enhances K^+ excretion.

Transcellular K^+ shifts may be caused by drugs, endogenous hormones, or acid-base disturbances. β-agonists present in decongestants and bronchodilators activate Na^+-K^+-ATPase. Similarly, the catechol response to delirium tremens may cause hypokalemia. This

physiologic response has been used in the management of hyperkalemia; high-dose nebulized β-agonists are administered to transiently decrease $[K^+]_p$. Alkalemia can promote K^+ migration into cells. In general, the $[K^+]_p$ falls by 0.4 mEq/L per 0.1 unit increase in pH.

Investigating the etiology begins with an evaluation of renal response to hypokalemia (Figure 5). Normally functioning kidneys can lower potassium excretion below 25 to 30 mEq per day. Hypokalemia that results from extrarenal causes should reveal a K^+ less than 20 mOsm/L; if hypokalemia is the result of renal dysfunction, the K^+ is greater than 20 mOsm/L with a TTKG greater than 1. Acute and chronic treatment are governed by the diagnosis. Potassium deficit can only be approximated, as serum K^+ correlates poorly with total body K^+. A useful guide is a 100 mEq decrement in total body K^+ stores for each 0.3 mEq/L fall in serum K^+. However, as intracellular K^+ repletes further losses, total body K^+ will continue to fall in the presence of relatively stable serum K^+. Furthermore, the influence of acid-base status and osmolality must be considered, as perturbations in either will induce transcellular K^+ shifts, thereby obscuring the true K^+ status.

CALCIUM AND PHOSPHATE

Normal Homeostasis

Calcium is essential for neuromuscular function, platelet adhesion, coagulation, endocrine and exocrine secretion, and bone metabolism. In addition to its role in bone structure and neuromuscular function along with calcium, phosphorus is integral in several key metabolic processes including glucose utilization, synthesis of 2,3 diphosphoglycerate, and adenosine triphosphate (ATP). Balance of calcium (Ca^{2+}) and phosphate (PO_4^{3-}) occurs via the coordinated efforts of the gastrointestinal tract, bone, and kidney functioning under the control of parathyroid hormone. Ninety-eight percent of total body

Ca^{2+} and most PO_4^{3-} are stored in bone. Plasma Ca^{2+} exists in three forms: *ionic* (50%), *protein bound* (40%), and *complexed* (10%). Fluctuations in the serum albumin level may affect the total blood calcium concentration, and normal levels of the ionized form (iCa^{2+}), the only form that is metabolically active, are preserved. Assessment of the corrected Ca^{2+} is possible with the following formula:

$$Ca^2 = \text{Measured } [Ca^{2+}] + 0.8(4 - [\text{Albumin}])$$

In response to depressed [iCa^{2+}], parathyroid hormone (PTH) is released. This induces osteoclastic bone resorption and the release of Ca^{2+} and PO_4^{3-}. Renal stimulation enhances resorption of Ca^{2+} and excretion of PO_4^{3-}. Increased calcitriol formation enhances intestinal absorption of both Ca^{2+} and PO_4^{3-}.

Hypercalcemia

Hypercalcemia (Ca^{2+} >10.4 mg/dL) is generally due to either increased bone resorption of calcium or excessive intake (Table 3). Patients commonly present with complaints of "stones, bones, moans, and psychogenic overtones" corresponding to renal (nephrolithiasis, nephrocalcinosis, DI), musculoskeletal (weakness), intestinal (nausea, vomiting, constipation), and neurologic symptoms (fatigue, depression, mental confusion) and cardiovascular manifestations (short QT, arrhythmias). Although hyperparathyroidism is the most common cause, hypercalcemia may be the earliest manifestation of malignancy, and occult cancer must be excluded. Measurement of intact PTH can distinguish between hyperparathyroidism and non–PTH-mediated hypercalcemia, most commonly because of malignancy, vitamin D intoxication, and granulomatous disease.

Asymptomatic hypercalcemia, as commonly occurs with hyperparathyroidism, infrequently needs urgent treatment. Individuals with elevated PTH should be screened for risk of progression of disease. Those patients older than 50 years with minimal calcium elevation and preserved renal function and bone mass may be carefully observed, and it is recommended that these individuals avoid drugs and practices that may aggravate hypercalcemia. Surgery is recommended for all other patients and is always an acceptable approach.

Treatment of symptomatic or acute hypercalcemia is directed at increasing calcium excretion while minimizing bone resorption. After intravenous hydration, diuretics may be administered to encourage calcium loss and may lower the calcium level by 2 to 3 mg/dL over 2 days. Bisphosphonates are employed in hypercalcemia resulting from malignancy, but they do not work rapidly. Granulomatous disease–mediated hypercalcemia may be treated with glucocorticoids (hydrocortisone 200 mg/day or prednisone 20 to 60 mg/day for 2 to 5 days). Hypercalcemic crisis (Ca^{2+} > 13 mg/dL) may require hemodialysis for acute management, particularly in patients with existing renal disease.

Hypocalcemia

Hypocalcemia (Ca^{2+} < 8.4 mg/dL) is less common than hypercalcemia and is generally due to parathyroid hormone or vitamin D disorders. Most commonly the result of chronic renal failure, hypocalcemia is also observed in critically ill patients with sepsis, burns, and acute renal failure and in surgical patients after parathyroidectomy. A careful history, physical examination, and measurement of intact PTH will assist in elucidating the cause (see Table 3). Clinical manifestations of acute hypocalcemia begin with evidence of peripheral neuromuscular excitability known as *tetany*, in which repetitive, high-frequency synaptic discharges occur after a single neural stimulus. Tetany ranges from mild signs of perioral numbness and tingling, Trousseau sign (induction of carpopedal spasm with blood pressure cuff inflation), Chvostek sign (facial muscle spasm after stimulation of facial nerve), and muscle cramps to laryngeal spasm and seizures.

TABLE 3: Etiology of calcium disorders

Hypercalcemia	Hypocalcemia
Bone resorption	PTH absent
Hyperparathyroidism	Hypoparathyroidism
Malignancy	Postparathyroidectomy
Thyrotoxicosis	Hereditary
Immobilization	Hypomagnesemia
Paget disease	PTH ineffective
Vitamin A intoxication	Chronic renal failure
Calcium absorption	Deficient active vitamin D
Increased calcium intake	Intestinal malabsorption
Chronic renal failure	Liver disease
Milk alkali syndrome	Inactive vitamin D
Vitamin D	Anticonvulsant therapy
Excessive intake	Pseudohypoparathyroidism
Granulomatous diseases	PTH overwhelmed
Drugs	Hyperphosphatemia
Thiazides	Acute pancreatitis
Lithium	Drugs
Theophylline	Protamine
Acute renal failure (rhabdomyolysis)	Heparin
Pheochromocytoma	Glucagon
Adrenal insufficiency	
Congenital diseases	
Familial hypocalciuric hypercalcemia	
Congenital lactase deficiency	
Metaphyseal chondrodysplasia	

PTH, Parathyroid hormone

Prolongation of the QT interval may progress to malignant arrhythmias such as *torsades des pointes* or heart block.

Acute, symptomatic hypocalcemia should be treated with parenteral supplementation as calcium gluconate or calcium chloride and may require continuous infusion up to 1.5 mEq/h, with frequent measuring of calcium levels and continuous cardiac monitoring. A 10% calcium chloride solution contains 273 mg calcium in a 10 mL ampule and should be administered with caution after dilution in 50 to 100 mL of D5W via central venous access only. In general, calcium gluconate is preferred, especially in peripheral infusion, because there is a risk of tissue necrosis if extravasation occurs. Because of the risk of cardiac arrest with acute increases in serum calcium, no more than 1 to 2 ampules of 10% calcium gluconate (93 mg/10 mL) should be administered in 50 to 100 mL of D5W over 5 to 10 minutes.

Because of the short duration of action, an additional continuous infusion over 4 to 6 hours may be necessary. Because PTH release also depends on adequate levels of magnesium, hypomagnesemia should be corrected prior to calcium correction. Long-term therapy depends upon the cause and includes oral calcium supplementation (1 to 2 g/day) and vitamin D administration. In concomitant renal failure, calcitriol (0.25 to 1.0 μg/day), the most active metabolite of vitamin D, should be administered.

A 10% calcium chloride solution contains 273 mg calcium in a 10 mL ampule and should be administered with caution after dilution in 50 to 100 mL of D5W via central venous access only. In general, calcium gluconate is preferred, especially in peripheral infusion, because there is a risk of tissue necrosis if extravasation occurs. Because of the risk of cardiac arrest with acute increases in serum calcium, no more than 1 to 2 ampules of 10% calcium gluconate (93 mg/10 mL) should be administered in 50 to 100 mL of D5W over 5 to 10 minutes. Because of the short duration of action, an additional continuous infusion over 4 to 6 hours may be necessary.

Hyperphosphatemia

Hyperphosphatemia (PO_4^{3-} > 5 mg/dL) is most commonly caused by diminished renal excretion (Table 4). Though often asymptomatic, its danger lies in the potential for metastatic calcification, particularly with a calcium-phosphorus product in excess of 70. In the absence of renal insufficiency, assessing urinary phosphate excretion will aid diagnosis. If increased above 1500 mg/dL, exogenous sources or cellular release from processes such as tumor lysis or rhabdomyolysis should be considered.

With preserved renal function, hydration increases the renal excretion of phosphate. In patients with renal failure, exogenous phosphates, including those from dietary protein intake, should be eliminated or reduced. Symptomatic hyperphosphatemia may require renal replacement therapy for adequate clearance. Calcium carbonate, aluminum, and magnesium can be employed to bind phosphorus in the gastrointestinal tract and diminish absorption in patients with chronic hyperphosphatemia; these agents may accumulate in patients with renal failure, and each is associated with significant side effects that include hypercalcemia, constipation, and diarrhea.

Hypophosphatemia

Hypophosphatemia (PO_4^{3-} < 2.5 mg/dL) can be the result of decreased absorption from the gastrointestinal tract, intracellular shift, or increased renal excretion (Table 4). Glucose loading, particularly in malnourished patients, can precipitate refeeding syndrome, by which rapid intracellular shifting of already diminished serum phosphate can cause extreme hypophosphatemia. Although mild hypophosphatemia is asymptomatic, severe depression of serum [PO_4^{3-}] can lead to impaired cellular energy production manifested as rhabdomyolysis, cardiomyopathy, erythrocyte dysfunction, skeletal demineralization, muscle weakness, and respiratory insufficiency. The cause should be ascertained before therapy. Dairy products are an excellent source, although phosphate salts are also available for oral use. Phosphate-binding antacids and sucralfate should be discontinued when oral phosphates are administered. In the case of symptomatic or extreme hypophosphatemia (PO_4^{3-} < 2.0 mg/dL), parenteral sources should be administered; the choice of which to use, sodium or potassium phosphate, is based on the concentration of serum potassium.

MAGNESIUM

Normal Homeostasis

Magnesium is the most common intracellular divalent cation, although two thirds is complexed to bone. Less than 1% of total body magnesium is present in the plasma. Serum Mg^{2+} circulates either

TABLE 4: Etiology of phosphate disorders

Hyperphosphatemia	Hypophosphatemia
Diminished renal excretion	Diminished intake
Renal failure	Diminished intestinal absorption
Hypoparathyroidism	Vitamin D deficiency
Hyperthyroidism	Malabsorption
Increased intestinal absorption	Diarrhea
Phosphate ingestion	Vomiting
Vitamin D excess	Cellular redistribution
Granulomatous disease	Respiratory alkalosis
Iatrogenic	Sepsis
Parenteral supplements	Ethyl alcohol withdrawal
Lipid infusion	Anxiety
Factitious	Hormone effects
Thrombocytosis	Insulin
Cellular release	Glucocorticoids
Rhabdomyolysis	Epinephrine
Tumor lysis	Cellular uptake syndromes
Lymphoma	"Hungry bone" syndrome
Sepsis	Refeeding syndrome
Malignant hyperthermia	Leukemia/lymphoma
Internal redistribution	Increased renal excretion
Acidosis	Hyperparathyroidism
	Renal tubular defects
	Hyperaldosteronism

ionized (61%), protein bound (33%) or complexed (6%). Most intracellular Mg^{2+} is bound to ATP, and because ATP is integral to all metabolic processes, Mg^{2+} is essential for life. With insufficient uptake, gastrointestinal and renal losses are restricted; in fact, renal handling of Mg^{2+} is the primary method of Mg^{2+} homeostasis, resorbed passively in the loop of Henle.

Hypermagnesemia

Hypermagnesemia ([Mg^{2+}] > 2.2 mg/dL) occurs almost exclusively in patients with renal failure, most commonly the consequence of combined excessive intake and renal insufficiency. Other causes are listed in Table 5 and include rhabdomyolysis, adrenal insufficiency, and familial benign hypocalciuric hypercalcemia. Signs and symptoms do not occur until levels exceed 5 mg/dL and are primarily neuromuscular and cardiovascular. Nausea and facial paresthesias progress to sedation, hypoventilation, decreased deep tendon reflexes, and muscle weakness. Severe sequelae of hypotension, bradycardia, and coma are

TABLE 5: Etiology of magnesium disorders

Hypermagnesemia	Hypomagnesemia
Renal failure	Diminished intake
Excess intake	Parenteral nutrition
Parenteral nutrition	Inadequate intake
Laxatives	Gastrointestinal
Enemas	Malabsorption
Antacids	Fistula
Eclampsia therapy	Diarrhea
Hypothyroidism	Pancreatitis
Adrenal insufficiency	Endocrine
Rhabdomyolysis	Hypoparathyroidism
Familial benign hypocalciuric hypercalcemia	Hyperparathyroidism
Lithium toxicity	Bartter and Gitelman syndromes
	Diabetic ketoacidosis
	Cellular redistribution
	"Hungry bone" syndrome
	Pancreatitis
	Chronic alcoholism
	Increased renal excretion
	Diuretics
	Amphotericin B
	Syndrome of inappropriate antidiuretic hormone secretion

not observed until [Mg^{2+}] exceeds 15 mg/dL. Toxicity is exaggerated with concomitant hypocalcemia, hyperkalemia, and uremia. In adults, 100 to 300 mg elemental calcium diluted in 150 mL D5W may be administered intravenously over 10 minutes to acutely antagonize the cardiovascular effects of hypermagnesemia, but the effect is temporary, and definitive treatment to lower magnesium levels is imperative. Saline hydration and loop diuretics will increase Mg^{2+} renal excretion; in the absence of preserved renal function, hemodialysis is effective.

Hypomagnesemia

Hypomagnesemia (Mg^{2+} < 1.8 mg/dL) is usually caused by insufficient intake or enhanced gastrointestinal or renal losses (see Table 5). Signs and symptoms are similar to those of other electrolyte deficiencies, which may accompany hypomagnesemia and include anorexia, nausea, vomiting, lethargy, weakness, paresthesias, mental confusion, Trousseau and Chvostek signs, tetany, seizures, and cardiac arrhythmias including ventricular fibrillation, torsades de pointes, and cardiac arrest. In addition to replenishment of all affected electrolytes, treatment should focus on correcting the cause. Serious conditions such as arrhythmias necessitate parenteral therapy, usually as magnesium sulfate (2 g intravenously over 1 to 5 minutes). Oral therapy is usually delivered in the form of magnesium oxide (250 to 500 mg orally once or twice daily).

SUMMARY

Electrolyte disorders are potentially fatal conditions. Rapid assessment and administration of lifesaving therapies should be balanced with thoughtful contemplation of the etiology of the disorder and diligent follow-up of the impact of all interventions. With all electrolyte disorders, serial measurements of serum levels to assess response to therapy are necessary, particularly in patients with renal failure.

SUGGESTED READINGS

Halperin ML, Kamel KS: Potassium, *Lancet* 352:135, 1998.
Kapoor M, Chan GZ: Fluid and electrolyte abnormalities, *Crit Care Clin* 17:503, 2001.
Kumar S, Berl T: Sodium, *Lancet* 352:220, 1998.
Rastergar A, Soleimani M: Hypokalemia and hyperkalemia, *Postgrad Med J* 77:759, 2001.
Topf JM, Murray PT: Hypomagnesemia and hypermagnesemia, *Rev Endo Met Disorders* 4:195, 2003.

ACID-BASE DISORDERS

Elizabeth Dreesen, MD, and Anthony A. Meyer, MD, PhD

NORMAL ACID-BASE METABOLISM

Normally the pH of bodily fluids is maintained between 7.35 to 7.45 and is associated with a free hydrogen concentration of approximately 40 nmol/L. This hydrogen ion concentration is approximately one millionth the concentration of Na^+, K^+, Cl^-, and HCO_3^-. Free hydrogen ions react readily with intracellular and extracellular proteins, causing alterations in their binding capacity and enzymatic efficiency, and it is for this reason that the maintenance of pH within a narrow range is critical to homeostasis.

Metabolism of carbohydrates and fats produces approximately 15,000 mmol of CO_2 daily. The production of carbonic acid (H_2CO_3) through the combination of this CO_2 with water produces a significant acid load. Additionally, the oxidation of amino acids and the hydrolysis of dietary phosphate in the typical western diet lead to the equivalent of 50 to 100 mEq of free hydrogen ion daily.

In the face of these metabolic processes, acid-base homeostasis is maintained both by changes in alveolar ventilation and by a system of extracellular and intracellular buffers. Although normal minute ventilation is approximately 5 L/min, the lungs can compensate for a nonrespiratory acidemia by hyperventilation up to 30 L/min. In addition to eliminating CO_2 through the lungs, the body regulates hydrogen ion concentration through a system of buffers that include serum bicarbonate, intracellular and extracellular proteins, and bone. In the extracellular fluid, bicarbonate is by far the most important buffer, although inorganic phosphates and plasma proteins, including albumin, also contribute. The most important intracellular buffer is hemoglobin. Controversy exists as to the contribution of bone to the buffering of acute acid loads. Clearly, however, bone buffering of chronic acidosis is associated with the loss of bone calcium in patients with end-stage renal disease. The kidneys maintain this complex buffering system by excreting the anions associated with endogenously produced acid and by regenerating the bicarbonate consumed in buffering. Renal reabsorption of virtually all filtered bicarbonate takes place in the proximal tubule, and excretion of hydrogen as ammonium ion takes place distally and can range from a normal of 30 to 40 mEq/day to over 300 mEq/day.

The complementary role of the lungs and kidneys is highlighted by the Henderson-Hasselbach equation, which demonstrates that serum pH, and thus the hydrogen ion concentration, is dependent on the ratio of serum bicarbonate to partial pressure of carbon dioxide (pCO_2):

$$pH = 6.10 + \log (HCO_3) / 0.003\ pCO_2$$

DETERMINING ACID-BASE STATUS

Commonly, acid-base status is determined through the interpretation of arterial blood gases. Mixed venous gases, however, can provide additional useful information about peripheral oxygen extraction and can contribute to a patient's peripheral perfusion and oxygen delivery. Pulmonary artery catheters are less frequently used at present; thus central venous gases are often substituted for true mixed venous gases. These venous gases can still be used to follow acid-base trends in the face of ventilator dependence and in the treatment of chronic acid-base disturbances.

By convention, *acidemia* is defined as the presence of an elevated hydrogen ion concentration or low pH in the blood. *Alkalemia* is the condition of low hydrogen ion concentration and high pH. These conditions are mutually exclusive, because the blood has only one pH at the time of any given measurement. *Acidosis* and *alkalosis*, on the other hand, refer to processes that lead to a rise or fall in hydrogen ion concentration. Because multiple metabolic derangements can coexist in the same patient, it is possible to have both an acidosis and an alkalosis, although a patient is either acidemic or alkalemic.

Like all laboratory tests, blood gas samples can be subject to contamination, which leads to erroneous results. Prolonged exposure to atmospheric conditions can result in an artificially low pCO_2 in both arterial and venous gases. When mixed venous gases are drawn through multilumen catheters, blood can be contaminated by simultaneous infusion of either basic or acidic resuscitation fluid and acidic pressors, which can alter the pH of the sample. Finally, blood gases drawn from hypothermic patients are usually "normalized" to a temperature of 37° C before being analyzed. Temperature affects the solubility of carbon dioxide, and the pCO_2 and pH of cold blood are lower than that in a warmed sample. The clinical relevance of this is unclear, but it warrants investigation as the use of therapeutic hypothermia increases.

There are three methods by which clinicians can analyze blood gases as they evaluate acid-base problems. All three evaluate the respiratory component by simply analyzing pCO_2, but they interpret the metabolic component of blood gas determination differently. The "traditional" method, popularized by Relman and Schwartz in the 1960s, is centered around the Henderson-Hasselbach equation. It uses serum bicarbonate, pH, degree of compensation, and anion gap to classify and then treat acid-base disturbances. This standard approach is often supplemented by a second method of metabolic assessment that involves measurement of *base excess*, defined as the amount of acid or base that must be added to the blood to correct the pH to 7.4, and it is often trended to follow response to therapy of acid-base abnormalities. A third approach was proposed in the 1980s by Stewart and is centered around the strong ion difference; that

is, the difference between the completely disassociated cations and anions in plasma. The Stewart approach maintains that the acid-base status is best understood through evaluation of the pCO_2, the "strong ion difference," and the plasma concentration of nonvolatile weak acids such as albumin. The critical care literature since the 1980s has contained comparative analyses of these methods but suggests that as long as the anion gap is corrected for hypoalbuminemia, the identification and treatment of acid-base disorders by the Stewart and the Relman approach are similarly effective.

Using the Relman approach to blood gas analysis, a stepwise approach can be used to determine the acid-base abnormalities present in a given situation. The first step involves examination of the pH and determining whether the patient has an acidemia or an alkalemia. The pCO_2 and bicarbonate are then evaluated to determine whether the primary disturbance is respiratory or metabolic. The next step requires assessment of the presence or absence of appropriate compensation (Figure 1). Lack of appropriate compensation indicates that a mixed respiratory and metabolic disorder is present. Finally, the anion gap should be evaluated. The presence or absence of an abnormal gap determines the differential diagnosis of a metabolic acidosis, discussed below. In a gap acidosis, protons from unmeasured acids should have been buffered by serum bicarbonate with a corresponding decrease in the measured bicarbonate. Thus, any difference between the existing gap and the normal gap (delta gap) should be approximately equal to any change from normal serum bicarbonate (delta bicarb). Difference between the delta gap and delta bicarb should suggest an additional nongap acidosis or alkalosis.

METABOLIC ACIDOSIS

The development of metabolic acidosis is the result of two processes: 1) an increase in acid production beyond the body's buffering capacity or 2) a decrease in buffering capacity itself through the loss of buffer via gastrointestinal (GI) or renal losses. These two processes can also coexist.

The differential diagnosis of metabolic acidosis is based on the presence or absence of an anion gap (AG), which is the difference between measured cations and measured anions. The gap represents the unmeasured anions, including negatively charged proteins such as albumin, phosphates, and other weak acids. Typically the gap is calculated as:

$$AG = Na^+ - (Cl^- + HCO_3)$$

with a normal AG value of 10 ± 4 mEq/L. An elevated anion gap represents the addition of unmeasured anions, including lactate and sulfates.

Although this simple method for calculating the gap is useful in most hospitalized patients, it may lead to spurious analysis and a falsely normal-appearing gap in critically ill patients. These patients often are seen with a significant decrease in serum albumin and altered phosphate metabolism. For these patients, the expected gap is lower than the usual normal range. Thus, in critically ill patients with pH lower than 7.35, the expected gap is calculated as:

$$\text{Expected AG} = 2(\text{Albumin in g}/\text{dL}) + 0.5\ (\text{Phosphate in mg}/\text{dL})$$

The *MUDPILES* mnemonic—for **m**etformin, **u**remia, **D**KA (diabetic ketoacidosis), **p**araldehyde, **i**soniazid, **l**actic acidosis, **e**thylene glycol, and **s**alicylates—is commonly used to enumerate the causes of an anion gap acidosis. However, for critically ill surgical and trauma patients, the familiar mnemonic must change (Box 1). Although the most common gap acidoses among these patients are ketoacidosis from diabetes and ethanol consumption, acidosis of renal failure, and lactic acidosis, other causes of a gap acidosis are possible that must be considered when these common causes are not present. Rhabdomyolysis, for example, is associated with release of weak organic acids from injured and dying muscle. Inhalational injury associated with

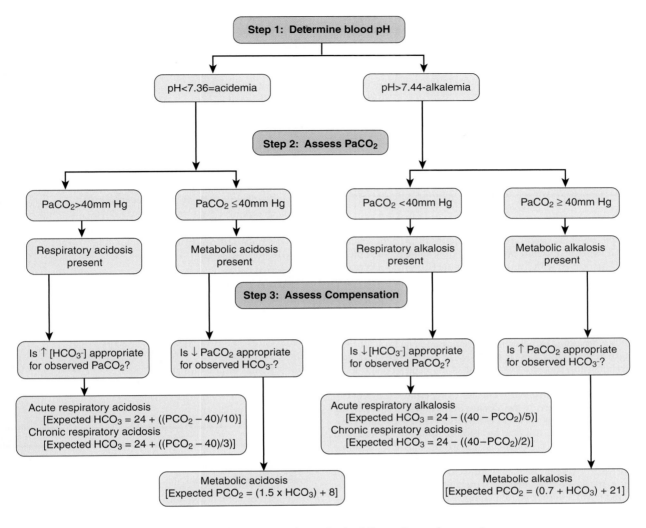

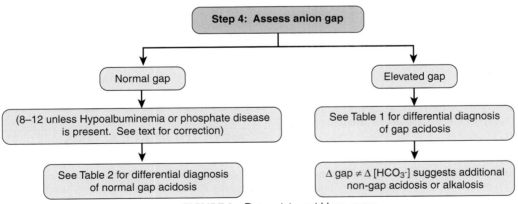

FIGURE 1   Determining acid-base status.

burns can lead to tissue hypoxia from carbon monoxide toxicity as well as the uncoupling of oxidative phosphorylation through intake of cyanide. The pressor epinephrine can drive a marked increase in the rate of glycolysis with the ensuing production of pyruvate and lactate. Use of the sedative propofol can be complicated by propofol infusion syndrome, which gives rise to profound lactic acidosis, although the mechanism is not completely understood. Propylene glycol, used as a carrier for both lorazepam and pentobarbital, is

metabolized to lactic acid at clinically significant levels when these medications are administered in high doses. Sepsis is associated with elevation in serum lactate as well, and substantial literature attests that this is not simply related to tissue hypoperfusion but also to mitochondrial dysfunction associated with inflammatory mediators and alterations in clearance of lactate. Finally, a short gut may be associated with bacterial overgrowth and the production of D-lactate as part of bacterial metabolism.

BOX 1: Causes of gap metabolic acidosis in the surgical ICU

Muscle injury: rhabodomyolysis
Uncoupling oxidative phosphorylation: cyanide
Drugs: pentobarbital and lorazepam in a carrier of propylene glycol
Propofol: infusion syndrome
Infection/sepsis: mitochondrial dysfunction
Lactic acidosis
Epinephrine
Short gut: D-lactate with bacterial overgrowth

BOX 2: Causes of nongap acidosis in the surgical ICU patient

Increased Acid Intake

Sodium chloride resuscitation
Total parenteral nutrition
Calcium chloride
Magnesium chloride

Loss of Buffer

Gastrointestinal fluid loss
Diarrhea
Drainage of pancreatic or biliary secretions
Cholestyramine
Renal loss
Renal tubular acidosis type I
Obstructive uropathy
Interstitial nephritis
Hepatorenal disease, cirrhosis
Amphotericin
Renal tubular acidosis type II
Carbonic anhydrase inhibitors
Renal tubular acidosis type IV
Diabetes mellitus
Nonsteroidal antiinflammatory drugs
Angiotensin converting enzyme inhibitors
Heparin
Adrenal insufficiency

Lactic acidosis warrants special mention. Several of the gap acidoses in the previous paragraph ultimately result in lactic acidosis through an increase in lactate production. Only some of these mechanisms are associated with frank tissue hypoperfusion, which makes lactate an imperfect indicator of tissue perfusion. Lactic acidosis may also arise from defects in lactate clearance. The majority of lactate is cleared in the liver, but up to 20% is renally cleared with both types of organ failure leading to lactic acidosis. Pyruvate dehydrogenase is a critical component of lactate clearance, and thiamine is its cofactor. Deficiency of thiamine is therefore another cause of lactic acidosis.

Nongap acidosis (Box 2) is characterized by an increase in chloride concentration with a concomitant decrease in serum bicarbonate. It can occur from an iatrogenic increase in chloride, such as that seen after resuscitation with normal saline, or infusion of hypertonic saline for elevated intracranial pressure. In the absence of the addition of acidifying substances, bicarbonate is lost in either the kidneys or the GI tract. Cholestyramine, for example, can bind bicarbonate inside the GI tract, and diversion of bicarbonate-rich duodenal, pancreatic, and biliary drainage can result in daily bicarbonate loss of several hundred milliequivalents.

Urine electrolytes may help distinguish the source of the problem, when the clinical picture is not clear. If metabolic acidosis is caused by GI loss, the normal kidney should compensate by both reabsorbing bicarbonate and excreting protons as ammonium chloride (NH_4Cl); thus pH of urine in the presence of a GI-mediated nongap acidosis should be low (<5). Additionally, because ammonium is not typically a measured electrolyte, the urine anion gap should be negative:

$$Urine\ AG = (UNa + UK) - UCl$$

By definition, bicarbonate loss from the kidneys constitutes a renal tubular acidosis. A variety of mechanisms exist for this in both the proximal and distal tubule.

Severe metabolic acidemia (pH <7.15) of any cause is characterized by alterations in many organ systems (Box 3). Treatment of metabolic acidemia should begin with identification and treatment of the underlying cause, but in the presence of cardiovascular compromise, many will treat with 2 ampules of sodium bicarbonate, followed by an infusion (3 amps $NaHco_3$ in 1 L D5W). However, the infusion of 1 ampule (50 mEq) results in the production of 1 L of CO_2 five times the usual 200 mL/min of CO_2 production. Thus the presence of lung disease significant enough to impair ventilation may result in conversion of a metabolic acidosis to a respiratory acidosis. Authors of animal research and small clinical trials challenge the efficacy of sodium bicarbonate, even in the presence of normal lung function, arguing that the decrease in ionized calcium associated with an increased pH counters the positive inotropic effects of sensitizing cells to catecholamines.

Disodium carbonate and sodium bicarbonate (carbicarb) and trishydroxymethalaminomethane (THAM) are capable of neutralizing acid without generating CO_2; however, they have shown virtually no efficacy in small clinical studies to date. Certainly, the presence of pH less than 7.15 should prompt urgent search for the cause, with the use of bicarbonate primarily as a temporizing measure.

BOX 3: Severe secondary effects of acute acidemia

Neuromuscular dysfunction

Increased cerebral blood flow
Altered mental status, stupor, coma

Cardiovascular

Decreased cardiac contractility
Arteriolar vasodilation
Cardiac dysrhythmia
Insensitivity to adrenergic stimulation

Respiratory

Impaired diaphragmatic contractility

METABOLIC ALKALOSIS

Metabolic alkalosis (Box 4) results from a primary increase in serum bicarbonate. This can occur as a consequence of loss of H+ from the GI tract or the kidney. Alternatively, excess bicarbonate reabsorption or administration of bicarbonate or a bicarbonate precursor (citrate from stored blood, acetate in total parenteral nutrition) can be responsible for metabolic alkalosis. Under normal circumstances, in the absence of hypovolemia, hypochloremia, hypokalemia, or mineralocorticoid excess, the kidney can excrete any excess bicarbonate. Each of these abnormalities diminishes the kidney's ability to excrete bicarbonate and compensate for alkalosis. The presence of hypovolemia stimulates the production of aldosterone, which activates the Na^+/H^+ exchange pumps in the collecting duct. Sodium is reabsorbed to maintain intravascular volume, but hydrogen ion is lost with the development of alkalosis.

Decrease in filtered chloride associated with hypochloremia is sensed by the macula densa and activates the renin-angiotensin-aldosterone

BOX 4: Causes of metabolic alkalosis in the surgical ICU patient

Gastrointestinal loss of chloride

Vomiting
Nasogastric suctioning
Diarrhea

Renal dysfunction

Diuretic therapy
Postcompensated hypercapnia
Penicillin
Hypokalemia

Endocrine

Hyperaldosteronism
Cushing syndrome
Exogenous steroid administration
Refeeding syndrome

Increased base intake

Sodium bicarbonate
Sodium acetate in total parenteral nutrition
Sodium citrate in massive transfusion

BOX 5: Causes of respiratory acidosis in the surgical ICU patient

Defect in central drive

Sedatives
Cerebrovascular accident
Obesity hypoventilation syndrome

Neuromuscular disease

Spinal cord injury
Myoneuropathy of critical illness

Abnormalities of the thorax

Kyphoscoliosis
Chest trauma (e.g., rib fracture, hemothorax, pneumothorax)
Pleural effusion
Restrictive effect of obesity

Abnormalities of the airway

Obstructive sleep apnea
Asthma, chronic obstructive pulmonary disease

Abnormalities of the pulmonary parenchyma

Pneumonia
Volume overload and pulmonary edema
Interstitial lung disease
Pulmonary fibrosis/acute respiratory distress syndrome

Increased CO_2 production

Fever
Seizures
Shivering
Malignant hyperthermia
Neuroleptic malignant syndrome
Overfeeding

system, with the ensuing collecting duct excretion of H^+ and creation and maintenance of alkalosis. Hypochloremia also inhibits Cl^-/HCO_3^- exchange in the collecting duct with an ensuing decrease in bicarbonate excretion. Hypokalemia results in the shift of hydrogen ions intracellularly in exchange for potassium. Intracellular acidosis enhances bicarbonate resorption in the collecting duct. Additionally, hypokalemia stimulates the H^+/K^+ pump in the collecting duct, again leading to excretion of acid and maintenance of systemic alkalosis.

The majority of alkaloses are chloride responsive and will be corrected by administration of volume, chloride, and potassium. These can be identified by the presence of urine chloride less than 20 mEq/L. Chloride-resistant alkalosis is primarily the result of mineralocorticoid excess seen in hyperaldosteronism, Cushing syndrome, and administration of exogenous steroids, including glucocorticoids, with mineralocorticoid effect. Administration of chloride will not treat these.

The sequelae of alkalemia are significant and include cerebral vasoconstriction, seizure and delirium, coronary vasoconstriction with refractory arrhythmia, and hypocalcemia with tetany. Mortality as high as 45% has been reported associated with pH of 7.55 and as high as 80% with pH higher than 7.65, and pHs in this range as a result of metabolic alkalosis call for administration of ammonium chloride or hydrogen chloride.

RESPIRATORY ACIDOSIS

Respiratory acidosis (Box 5) results from an imbalance between CO_2 production and excretion. Increased CO_2 production in surgery patients occurs most commonly as a consequence of fever, seizures, and shivering. Malignant hyperthermia can be the cause of sudden elevation of end-tidal CO_2 in an anesthetized patient. Overfeeding leads to the production of CO_2 as glucose is converted to fat, and this can also be a source of elevated CO_2. However, persistently elevated pCO_2 is more commonly associated with decreased CO_2 excretion than it is with overproduction.

Decreased CO_2 excretion arises from alterations in centrally mediated respiratory drive; the mechanical components of respiration, including airways and the musculoskeletal apparatus of respiration; or the alveolar gas exchange.

In an acute respiratory acidosis, there is little buffering capacity to compensate, because bicarbonate (HCO_3, the main extracellular buffer) cannot effectively buffer H_2CO_3. Intracellular buffers, including hemoglobin and phosphates, are the only immediate compensatory mechanism and are quite limited. Renal compensation for sustained hypercapnia begins in 6 to 12 hours, but 3 to 5 days pass before maximal compensation occurs.

The clinical manifestations of acute hypercapnia are primarily neurologic. Acute elevations to greater than 70 mm Hg produce a hypercapnic encephalopathy or CO_2 narcosis manifesting as drowsiness, depressed consciousness, or coma. The alveolar gas equation ($P_AO_2 = P_iO_2 - [P_ACO_2/\text{respiratory quotient}]$) permits calculation of the effect of hypercapnia on pO_2. In the acute setting on room air, a pCO_2 of 80 to 90 becomes life threatening because of the associated hypoxia in addition to the CO_2 narcosis. In patients breathing supplementary oxygen, however, oxygen desaturation may not occur until profound respiratory depression and CO_2 narcosis are present. Concern about airway and respiratory mechanical integrity should prompt aggressive monitoring of pCO_2 as well as oxygen saturation with blood gases or end-tidal monitoring. Ultimately, treatment of respiratory acidosis requires reversal of the underlying cause, and if this cannot be achieved promptly, mechanical ventilation must be instituted.

RESPIRATORY ALKALOSIS

Respiratory alkalosis (low pCO_2, elevated pH) arises when alveolar ventilation exceeds the ventilation needed to eliminate CO_2 (Box 6). The stimulus for this may arise centrally when the respiratory center

---

BOX 6: Causes of respiratory alkalosis in the surgical ICU patient

Primary hyperventilation

Pain
Anxiety
Closed head injury

Secondary hyperventilation

Pregnancy
Catecholamine administration
Sepsis/systemic inflammatory response syndrome
Salicylates
Fever
End-stage liver disease
Hypoxia
Severe anemia
Pneumothorax
Pulmonary embolism
Pulmonary edema
Pneumonia
Hyperventilation as a result of mechanical overventilation

---

is stimulated by medications, toxins, hormones, and inflammatory mediators associated with head injury or cerebrovascular accident. *Hyperventilation,* defined as pCO_2 less than 32 or respiratory rate greater than 20 breaths/min in a nonventilated patient, is one of the four systemic inflammatory response syndrome criteria, for example, reflecting the mediators of sepsis and their effects on respiratory drive. Centrally mediated respiratory alkalosis can also arise from pain, anxiety, and other neuropsychiatric disorders. Peripheral stimuli to hyperventilation are also common and include hypoxia as well as stimulation of pulmonary and intravascular stretch receptors in pneumonia, congestive heart failure, and pulmonary embolus.

Elevated pH is associated with increased binding of calcium to albumin, and the most common symptoms of respiratory alkalosis derive from hypocalcemia. Paresthesia and circumoral numbness are described with acute hypocalcemia. When pCO_2 drops more than 20 mm Hg, cerebral vasoconstriction occurs, and cerebral blood flow may result in alterations in consciousness. As early as 1908, the physiologist and self-experimenter Haldane actually described painful tingling in the hands and feet, numbness in the hands, and cerebral symptoms after voluntary hyperventilation. Treatment of hypocalcemia should be directed at the underlying cause.

SUGGESTED READINGS

Kellum JA, Puyana JC: Acid-base disorders. In ACS *Surgery principles and practice.* Available at http://www.acsurgery.com. Accessed September 12, 2009.

Quinn A, Sinert R: *Metabolic acidosis: treatment and medication.* Available at http://www.webmd.com. Accessed September 12, 2009.

Rose BD, Post T: *Clinical physiology of acid-base and electrolyte disorders,* New York, 2001, McGraw-Hill.

Schwartz WB, Relman AS: A critique of the parameters used in the evaluation of acid-base disorders. "Whole-blood buffer base" and "standard bicarbonate" compared with blood pH and plasma bicarbonate concentration, *N Engl J Med* 268:132, 1963.

Stewart PA: Modern quantitative acid-base chemistry, *Can J Physiol Pharmacol* 61(12):1444–1461, 1983.

CENTRAL LINE–ASSOCIATED BLOODSTREAM INFECTIONS: A NOVEL APPROACH TO PREVENTION

Raymond E. Robinson, BS, Jose M. Rodriguez-Paz, MD, and Peter J. Pronovost, MD, PhD

OVERVIEW

Intravascular catheters are used to provide beneficial medical care to patients, yet they also place patients at risk for complications that cause significant morbidity and mortality, longer hospital stays, and increased health care costs. These complications include mechanical difficulties during insertion or removal of the catheter, thrombotic events, and local and systemic infections. One of the most common and serious infectious complications, especially in the intensive care unit (ICU), is the central line–associated bloodstream infection (CLABSI), mostly attributed to the central venous catheter (CVC).

There are more than 5 million CVCs placed annually in the United States alone. An estimated 248,000 CLABSIs (82,000 ICUs), and up to 30,000 ICU deaths attributable to them, occur each year; about 90% of these infections are associated with CVC placement. Most studies of CLABSIs report attributable mortality rates between 5% and 20%, and each infection is estimated to cost about $45,000—a total cost of almost $3.7 billion annually. Substantial evidence is available to suggest that many if not most of these infections are preventable by implementing low-cost, strategic measures coupled with a change in culture.

EPIDEMIOLOGY

The National Nosocomial Infection Surveillance (NNIS) System reports CLABSI data as the number of CLABSIs per 1000 central line days ([number of CLABSIs/number of central line–days] × 1000). This allows for comparability across studies and study sites and benchmarking for hospitals involved in quality assurance and improvement efforts. An estimated 15 million central line days per year occur in the ICU alone, and hospitals reporting to the National Healthcare Safety Network (NHSN) during 2006 through 2008 reported pooled mean CLABSI rates of 1.2 per 1000 central line days in inpatient medical/surgical units and 5.5 per 1000 central line days in intensive care burn units. The 2004 NNIS report gave an overall mean of 5.2 per 1000 central line days (range, 2.8 to 12.8 per central line day). Although CVC-related CLABSI is the most common and serious infection, other vascular access device bloodstream infection rates are not insignificant and vary by device: peripheral catheters (0.5 per 1000 catheter days), arterial catheters (1.7 per 1000 catheter days), peripherally inserted dialysis catheters (2.4 per 1000 catheter days), and permanent surgically inserted vascular devices (0.1 to 1.6 per 1000 device days). Other important factors affecting CLABSI incidence include the position of the central line, severity of the patient's illness, frequency of central line manipulation, urgency of placement, hospital bed size, and unit type.

The estimated CLABSI mortality rate ranged from no impact to 35% in various studies, depending on whether they controlled for severity of illness, a potential confounder, during data analysis. Some of these studies were limited by the methods used to account for severity, which may explain the wide range of mortality rates. A newer study that adjusted for severity and matched on the basis of risk exposure found a threefold increase in mortality rates in both medical and surgical ICU patients. Another study adjusted for all confounders and found a sixfold risk of death from CLABSI among surgical ICU patients.

Finally, CLABSIs have been estimated to increase hospital length of stay by up to 22 days and ICU length of stay by 8 to 20 days, and they lengthen the duration of mechanical ventilation. This burden, coupled with the overwhelming incidence of these infections, makes them a major financial and public health challenge.

PATHOGENESIS

Several organisms are common causes of CLABSIs, and many of these organisms are antibiotic resistant. The gram-positive organisms are the most prevalent, including coagulase-negative staphylococci (37%), *Staphylococcus aureus* (12.6%, 50% oxacillin resistant), enterococci (13%, many are vancomycin resistant), gram-negative bacilli (14%), and *Candida* species (8%, many are fluconazole resistant). An increase in *Enterobacteriaceae* has also been seen, producing extended-spectrum β-lactamases and a nearly 50% increase in *Klebsiella pneumoniae* that is resistant to third-generation cephalosporins.

Several different routes are taken by organisms that colonize CVCs. These include intraluminal, extraluminal, and infusate contamination. The most common route for short-term, nontunneled, noncuffed catheters is from skin flora colonizing the insertion site and then migrating along the subcutaneous catheter tract. In cuffed, tunneled, silicone catheters and ports, the most common cause is from frequent manipulation of the device, causing colonization of the injection port, leading to intraluminal contamination. Occasionally, fluids, drugs, or total parenteral nutrition (TPN) can be the source of the infection, especially in CLABSI epidemics.

These microorganisms produce substances that not only facilitate their adherence to catheters but also interfere with antimicrobial interventions. "Biofilms" are produced by coagulase-negative staphylococci, *S. aureus*, *Enterococcus faecalis*, *K. pneumoniae*, *Pseudomonas aeruginosa*, and *C. albicans*, which contribute to lower antimicrobial effects. Adherence of coagulase-negative staphylococci, *S. aureus*, and *C. albicans* to the fibronectin and fibrin-thrombin sheath surrounding the catheter increases the potential for extraluminal infection. Some coagulase-negative staphylococci and *Candida* species produce an extracellular polysaccharide "slime" that decreases antibiotic penetration. These adherence properties and secreted films can make removal of the catheter necessary to eliminate the nidus.

PREVENTION

In 2002, the Centers for Disease Control and Prevention (CDC) published recommendations to prevent CLABSIs. These recommendations were synthesized from the available literature and evidence and mainly supported five prevention strategies: 1) appropriate hand hygiene, 2) full sterile barriers for patient and clinician/operator during central line insertion, 3) skin cleansing with 2% chlorhexidine, 4) avoidance of the femoral insertion site, and 5) removal of unnecessary lines. Even though these strategies have successfully decreased CLABSIs, they are not consistently

followed, with only 55% of patients receiving these prevention strategies. These and other effective CLABSI prevention strategies are described below.

Hand Hygiene

Substantial evidence has linked health care providers washing their hands with decreased infection rates. Even so, physician compliance remains low, ranging from 20% to 60% regardless of whether a training program is implemented to increase awareness and compliance. Washing hands with an alcohol-based product or antibacterial soap and using sterile gloves reduces infection rates.

Wearing Full Sterile Barriers During Central Line Insertion

Decreasing a patient's contact with organisms is the goal during insertion of a central line. Wearing a mask, cap, sterile gloves, and full body drape during pulmonary artery catheter insertion decreased CLABSIs twofold in one study, and another study showed an odds ratio of 6.3 in the control group (minimal barrier). Later studies also demonstrated that wearing full barriers decreased morbidity and mortality and was therefore cost effective. Data suggest the avoidance of 7 CLABSIs and 1 death for every 270 catheters placed, saving a life and a total of $68,000 (2003 dollars).

Skin Antisepsis

Sterilizing the skin for central line insertion and maintenance is pivotal in reducing CLABSIs. Povidone-iodine–based skin cleanser is still commonly used, but many studies have shown that 2% chlorhexidine solution is much better for skin antisepsis. A 2002 meta-analysis reported a 50% reduction (95% confidence interval, 0.28 to 0.88) in CLABSI rates with a chlorhexidine solution compared to a povidone-iodine solution. In a recent single-center study, ICU patients bathed with a 2% chlorhexidine washcloth instead of soap and water experienced significantly reduced primary CLABSIs (4.1 vs. 10.4 per 1000 catheter days).

Catheter Insertion Site

Skin flora is a major risk factor for CLABSIs during insertion and maintenance of a central line. Different insertion sites have been attributed with a higher density of microbes than others and are therefore attributed to higher rates of infection. Several studies have shown a two- to three-times higher risk of infection when using the jugular or femoral veins over the subclavian vein for an insertion site.

Catheter Site Dressings

Fewer changes and continuous visual inspection of the insertion site are noted benefits of transparent, semipermeable dressings. Nonetheless, data from a recent study and a meta-analysis showed that transparent dressings were comparable to gauze with respect to catheter colonization (5.7% vs. 4.6%) and CLABSIs. The dressing choice was a matter of preference that included choosing gauze dressings if blood was oozing or the patient was diaphoretic. The CDC now recommends chlorhexidine-impregnated sponges for use in patients older than 2 months of age who have short-term catheters. A large multicenter trial compared chlorhexidine-impregnated sponges to standard dressings and found reduced catheter-related infections (CRIs; 0.6 vs. 1.4 per 1000 catheter days) and CLABSIs (0.40 vs. 1.3 per 1000 catheter days).

Catheter and Central Line Removal

Daily evaluation for removal of the catheter can decrease exposure to potential complications. The longer a catheter is left in, the greater the risk of infection. Even though scheduled replacement of peripheral lines every 72 hours decreases complications like thrombophlebitis, this strategy does not lower CLABSIs from central lines, percutaneously inserted central catheters (PICCs), or hemodialysis catheters. Most studies report that more than 50% of central lines removed for a suspected bloodstream infection failed to obtain a diagnosis of CRI.

Many of these removed catheters are due to unexplained fever and mild to moderate disease. The guidelines from the Infectious Disease Society of America (IDSA) recommends that nontunneled central lines should not be routinely removed for unexplained fever and mild to moderate disease; the removal should be based on the patient's condition and appearance of the insertion site. Any patient with mild to moderate disease and without signs of insertion site infection should obtain peripheral and line cultures, insertion site cultures, exchange of the catheter over a guidewire, or a combination of these. Also, scheduled guidewire changes do not decrease CLABSI rates, but they are reportedly more comfortable and are associated with fewer mechanical complication rates than new insertions. Because the skin tract is commonly the nidus, guidewire changes are unacceptable when CLABSIs occur.

Antimicrobial- and Antiseptic-Impregnated Catheters and Cuffs

The CDC currently recommends using a chlorhexidine/silver sulfadiazine- or minocycline/rifampin-impregnated CVC in adults who require a central line for more than 5 days for CLABSI rates that stay above benchmark goals. The CDCs goals also include educating health care providers about safe insertion and maintenance practices (using 2% chlorhexidine for skin antisepsis and maximal sterile barrier precautions).

DIAGNOSIS

A CLABSI is defined as the combination of catheter colonization and at least one positive peripheral venous blood culture with the same organism (species and antibiogram) within 48 hours. There are numerous diagnostic methods for CRIs and CLABSIs, including insertion site assessment and semiquantitative and quantitative cultures of the catheter tip and subcutaneous segment. The CDC includes clinical symptoms of fever, chills, and/or hypotension and no other apparent source of bacteremia in the definition for CLABSI. Another definition, suggesting that the catheter is the nidus, includes no other apparent source of infection; isolation of a common CLABSI organism (coagulase-negative staphylococci, *S. aureus*, enterococci, *Candida*); local site infection, such as insertion site and/or tunnel-tract inflammation or purulence; or port pocket abscess with positive blood culture.

The semiquantitative roll-plate technique, which is the standard diagnosis of a CLABSI, includes culturing the external catheter surface. Given that this technique only cultures the external surface of the central line, more quantitative methods, such as vortex sonification or flushing, should be used to retrieve organisms from the internal surface of the line. The IDSA suggests one of the following methods for diagnosis: 1) positive semiquantitative or quantitative culture of the catheter, 2) simultaneous quantitative blood culture drawn through the CVC and peripheral vein with a 5:1 or greater ratio (CVC/peripheral) of culture counts, or 3) differential time to positive for both cultures (the CVC culture becomes positive 2 hours or more before the peripheral vein culture when both are drawn simultaneously). Culturing the insertion site has an 80% to 90% negative predictive value (NPV), and it can help the provider decide whether a short-term CVC can be left in place. Although the NPV is good, the positive predictive value (PPV) is not; therefore a culture of the insertion site cannot be used to diagnose a CRI.

TREATMENT

Administering the appropriate empirical antibiotics should be done after obtaining blood and catheter samples. Antibiotics must be geared toward the patient's clinical signs, severity of disease, and potential organisms. Resistance has been an increasing problem, especially in ICUs. Targeting antibiotics to the resistant or nonresistant atmosphere of the unit or hospital also needs to be considered. In antibiotic-resistant units, oxacillin-resistant *S. aureus* should be treated with vancomycin, linezolid, or quinupristin/dalfopristin; in nonresistant units, nafcillin or oxacillin can be used for empiric therapy. Additional coverage may be necessary for gram-negative rods, including *Pseudomonas,* in people who are severely immunocompromised. Empirically, cover patients suspected to have fungemia with amphotericin B or fluconazole. Target the therapy *after* the organism has been identified.

The IDSA, the American College of Critical Care Medicine, and the Society of Critical Care Medicine all suggest the removal of most nontunneled CVCs in patients with bacteremia, fungemia, unexplained sepsis, and severe disease or inflammation and/or purulence at the insertion site. If a removed catheter is significantly colonized and was replaced using a guidewire, even with a normal-appearing insertion site, the replacement must be removed and another site used.

Longer courses of antibiotic therapy are usually needed in complicated infections, such as endocarditis and osteomyelitis. No supporting data are available to suggest the duration of antibiotic treatment, but many uncomplicated bloodstream infections without permanent indwelling intravascular devices can be treated for 10 to 14 days, but persistently bacteremic patients may need 4 to 8 weeks of antibiotics. Patients who grow *S. aureus* or *Candida* from their catheter should receive 5 to 7 days of antibiotics if they have valvular heart disease or neutropenia with negative blood cultures. Indications for catheter removal include hypotension, fever for more than 48 hours after starting antibiotic treatment, septic thrombosis, and septic emboli.

One study of hemodynamically stable patients with suspected CRI found that patients could be treated without removing the catheter, allowing for three-times fewer catheter changes and similar outcomes to patients whose catheters were replaced. Critically ill patients with CLABSI are not candidates for in situ treatment. Patients with *S. aureus* or *Candida* CLABSIs must have their catheter removed and a transesophageal echocardiography performed to rule out valvular heart disease. Patients with more than 3 days of persistent positive blood cultures after catheter removal should be evaluated for endocarditis, septic thrombosis, or a metastatic infection.

Can CLABSIs Be Eliminated?

In a large collaborative prospective study (Keystone ICU Project) involving the Johns Hopkins Hospital Quality and Safety Research Group, the Michigan Health and Hospital Association Keystone Center for Patient Safety and Quality, and up to 103 ICUs predominantly in Michigan hospitals, the median CLABSI rate dropped from 2.7 per 1000 catheter days at baseline to 0 per 1000 catheter days within 3 months of implementation, using a conceptual model to increase the use of five evidence-based interventions and improve the safety culture. These reductions have been sustained for over 3 years. This model comprises the Comprehensive Unit-Based Safety Program (CUSP), the science of safety principles, and the five evidence-based recommendations from the CDC. After 18 months of implementation, bloodstream infection rates had decreased by 66% from baseline. Even though the initial funding to support hospital participation ended after the 18-month period, most of the hospitals remained committed to collecting and reporting data. In a subsequent 18-month period, 90 of 103 ICUs continued to provide data, but 13 ICUs dropped out from lack of funding. The decrease in CLABSI rates were sustained during the second 18 months, and by the end of this 36-month period, a greater than 60% reduction in infection rates and a median CLABSI rate of 0 per 1000 catheter days was seen.

What is different, and why are these interventions not widely used? The short answer: Some of these interventions are widely used and reported, and data are collected for years, but despite all the available evidence on their reduction potential, health care providers do not fully implement these interventions. A recent survey reported that maximal sterile barriers were used in 71% to 84% of CVC placements, chlorhexidine in 70% to 90%, and system-based interventions in only 40% to 60% of the 719 hospitals surveyed. Other authors found similar or worse compliance. However, hospitals that had higher safety scores, employed certified infection preventionists, and participated in a prevention collaborative had higher rates of compliance. Barriers for implementing these interventions have been described elsewhere and include fear of change, complex systems that prevent change, communication problems, patient safety not a common priority, lack of "buy in" by stakeholders, lack of feedback on the outcomes (effect on rates, level of compliance), insufficient support by leadership, and ambiguity over implementation being cost effective.

Eliminating Barriers

To start eliminating barriers, we used a model to translate research into practice to prevent CLABSI plus science of safety principles from CUSP to improve safety culture. This model involves the following:

1. **Summarize** the evidence, select interventions with the strongest evidence and lowest barriers to use, and convert them into clinical practice behaviors.
2. **Understand** the process and context of work by observing staff trying to implement the evidence-based interventions and identify barriers. In addition, talk to staff to discover firsthand what is difficult about performing the intervention.
3. **Measure** baseline performance.
4. **Ensure** that all patients reliably receive evidence-based interventions by:
   a. *Engaging* staff in the importance of the project (generally with stories and baseline data).
   b. *Educating* staff on recommended behaviors.
   c. *Executing* or redesigning the work process to make compliance easy, so patients will reliably receive evidence-based care.
   d. *Evaluating* the impact of the intervention.

SUMMARY

Most CLABSIs are preventable, and all heath care providers, especially physicians, should standardize the practices of care to ensure quality and safety. Indeed, CLABSIs are a measure of the quality of care we deliver to our patients. Moreover, the Centers for Medicare and Medicaid Services will no long pay for "preventable complications," including CLABSIs, which will impact hospital revenues. Although we have focused on the ICU, hospitals should extend these practices of standardization and safety culture to every clinical area or unit where catheters are inserted and/or managed.

SUGGESTED READINGS

National Nosocomial Infections Surveillance (NNIS) System Report, data summary from January 1992 through June 2004, issued October 2004, *Am J Infect Control* 32(8):470–485, 2004.

Edwards JR, Peterson KD, Mu Y, et al: National Healthcare Safety Network (NHSN) report: data summary for 2006 through 2008, issued December 2009, *Am J Infect Control* 37(10):783–805, 2009.

O'Grady NP, Alexander M, Dellinger EP, et al: Guidelines for the prevention of intravascular catheter-related infections, Centers for Disease Control and Prevention, *MMWR Recomm Rep* 51(RR-10):1–29, 2002.

Pronovost P, Needham D, Berenholtz S, et al: An intervention to decrease catheter-related bloodstream infections in the ICU, *N Engl J Med* 355(26):2725–2732, 2006.

Pronovost PJ, Goeschel CA, Colantuoni E, et al: Sustaining reductions in catheter-related bloodstream infections in Michigan intensive care units: observational study, *BMJ* 340:c309, 2010.

Pronovost P, Sexton B: Assessing safety culture: guidelines and recommendations, *Qual Saf Health Care* 14(4):231–233, 2005.

Pronovost P, Rosenstein B, Sexton B, et al: Implementing and validating a comprehensive unit-based safety program, *J Patient Saf* 1:33–40, 2005.

Pronovost PJ, Berenholtz SM, Needham DM: Translating evidence into practice: a model for large-scale knowledge translation, *BMJ* 337:a1714, 2008.

Rodriguez-Paz JM, Pronovost P: Prevention of catheter-related bloodstream infections, *Adv Surg* 42:229–248, 2008.

THE SEPTIC RESPONSE

Jin H. Ra, MD, José L. Pascual, MD, PhD, and
C. William Schwab, MD

OVERVIEW

Sepsis remains one of the major causes of death in both medical and surgical intensive care units (ICUs). Although its incidence continues to rise alongside an ever aging population, who are more susceptible to infection because of immunocompromise and chronic illness, the overall mortality is in slow decline. This has been mainly attributed to improvements in supportive care. Despite significant advances in technology and a better understanding of the pathophysiology of sepsis, the development of newer treatments and management strategies has failed to show consistent beneficial effects. The septic response remains a dynamic area of research for surgeons, intensivists, infectious disease specialists, and basic scientists.

DEFINITIONS

The following definitions were created by the American College of Chest Physicians and the Society of Critical Care Medicine Consensus Conference in 1992; they were revised in 2000 for the purpose of improving the collective ability to diagnose, monitor, and treat sepsis and were also developed to provide fundamental inclusion criteria for research.

- *Systemic inflammatory response syndrome* (SIRS): Systemic inflammatory response to various insults including trauma, infection, ischemia, hypersensitivity, and surgery. SIRS can be seen with a wide range of signs and symptoms, but the response is manifested by two or more of the following:
  1. Temperature greater than 38° C or less than 36° C
  2. Heart rate greater than 90 beats/min

TABLE 1: Clinical signs and symptoms of sepsis

Infection	General	Inflammatory	Hemodynamic	Tissue Perfusion
Documented or suspected	Temperature >38° C or < 36° C Heart rate >90 beats/min Respiratory rate ≥20 breaths/min Altered mental status Hyperglycemia Third spacing of fluid	WBC count <4000 or >12,000 cells/µL or ≥10% bands	Hypotension: systolic blood pressure <90 mm Hg MAP <70 mm Hg SVO_2 >70 CI >3.5 L/min/m²	Hypoxemia: (Pao_2/Fio_2 <300) Acute oliguria (urine output <0.5 mL/kg/hr) Coagulopathy Abnormal LFTs Platelet count <100,000 cells/µL Lactic acidosis Skin mottling

WBC, White blood cell; *MAP,* mean arterial pressure; *CI,* cardiac index; *LFT,* liver function tests

3. Respiratory rate greater than 20 breaths/min or pCO_2 less than 32 torr
4. WBC greater than 12,000 cells/mm³, fewer than 4000 cells/mm³, or more than 10% immature (bands) forms

- *Sepsis*: The systemic response to infection; SIRS resulting from an infectious insult
- *Severe sepsis*: Sepsis associated with organ dysfunction, hypotension, or end-organ perfusion defects
- *Septic shock*: Severe sepsis and hypotension despite adequate fluid resuscitation, along with perfusion abnormalities
- *Multiorgan dysfunction syndrome* (MODS): More than one organ with altered function, either from direct insult to the organ (primary MODS) or from altered function as a consequence of a host insult
- *Sepsis syndromes*: Used to describe the spectrum of sepsis from SIRS to MODS

EPIDEMIOLOGY

Sepsis accounts for approximately 10% to 15% of all ICU admissions, and septic shock represents about one third of these. About 25% of sepsis and over 50% of severe sepsis progress to septic shock, thus making sepsis syndromes the tenth leading cause of death in the United States. There are several risk factors for sepsis syndromes, one of which is advanced age. Patients older than 65 are about 13 times more likely to develop sepsis. African-American patients are also at increased risk, although studies cannot establish conclusively whether this is an effect of race or associated socioeconomic status. Comorbid conditions such as heart disease, diabetes, renal failure, chronic obstructive pulmonary disease, malignancy, and chronic substance abuse also substantially increase the risk of sepsis.

PATHOPHYSIOLOGY

Sepsis syndromes typically begin with a source of infection, most commonly originating from urinary, pulmonary, intestinal, or biliary systems. Spread is systemic and results in transient or nontransient bacteremia. The host's innate immunity typically reacts to the microbial antigen by triggering a systemic inflammatory response. Antigens, in particular lipopolysaccharide, an endotoxin of gram-negative bacteria, initiate a powerful host response through interactions with macrophages. These interactions result in the secretion of proinflammatory cytokines—interleukin (IL)-1β, tumor necrosis factor-α, IL-6, and IL-8—primarily by macrophages and monocytes. These cytokines then initiate a cascade of secondary mediators—leukotrienes, prostaglandins, and platelet-activating factor—that activate monocytes and result in cellular apoptosis, necrosis, nitric oxide synthetase induction, and other host-destructive processes. At the same time, antiinflammatory mediators—IL-1β receptor agonist, transforming growth factor-β, and IL-10—are released by the host in an attempt to maintain homeostasis. When homeostasis is disrupted, as in sepsis or in the case of the exaggerated proinflammatory response of SIRS, progression to end-organ dysfunction and failure may occur.

DIAGNOSIS

Characterization of the septic response should start with a thorough history and physical examination to localize the source of infection to body fluids, wounds, indwelling catheters, intravenous access lines, and other foreign bodies (Tables 1 and 2). Recent laboratory and diagnostic studies and procedures should also be scrutinized to assist in source localization.

Diagnostic testing is then performed, including blood tests such as arterial blood gas, complete blood count, serum electrolytes, liver panel, lactate, blood cultures, urinalysis and urine culture, and sputum and wound cultures. Other valuable diagnostic adjuncts include chest and abdominal radiographs, computed tomography (CT), and/or ultrasound. These diagnostic tools may also shed light on clinical evidence of organ dysfunction.

MANAGEMENT

Once the diagnosis of sepsis is made, early and aggressive interventions should be initiated (Figure 1). Multiple studies have shown that timely intervention leads to better outcomes including decreased mortality. In particular a management strategy labeled Early Goal Directed Therapy (EGDT) for Sepsis has been proposed by Rivers and colleagues emphasizing the initiation of resuscitation and treatment as early as the emergency room for community patients who arrive with sepsis. As with any critically ill patient, the general appearance and mental status of the patient should first be assessed in concert with rapid evaluation of airway and breathing for patency and adequacy. Vitals signs should be obtained, appropriate intravenous access with fluids should be started, and early transfer of the patient to the ICU is warranted. There are seven main management arms:

1. Rapid fluid resuscitation
2. Early antimicrobial therapy
3. Vasopressors and inotropes
4. Invasive and noninvasive monitoring
5. Supportive care
6. Specific treatments and adjuncts
7. Source control

TABLE 2: Signs of organ dysfunction and failure

Central nervous system	Encephalopathy Polyneuropathy/myopathy
Cardiac	Tachycardia Tachyarrhythmias Myocardial depression
Pulmonary	Acute respiratory failure Acute lung injury Acute respiratory distress syndrome
Renal	Acute renal failure
Gastrointestinal	Ileus/pseudoobstruction Gastritis Acalculous cholecystitis Pancreatitis Gut ischemia
Hepatic	Cholestasis Ischemic hepatitis
Metabolic	Hyperglycemia Hyperlipidemia
Hematologic	Disseminated intravascular coagulation Thrombocytopenia
Immunologic	Immune dysfunction
Endocrine	Pituitary, adrenal, and thyroid dysfunction

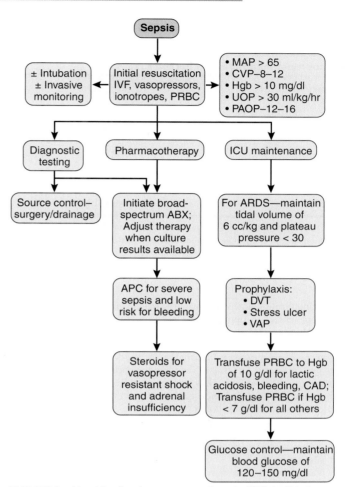

FIGURE 1   Algorithm for the treatment of sepsis. *ABX*, Antibiotics; *APC*, activated protein C; *ARDS*, acute respiratory syndrome; *CAD*, coronary artery disease; *CVP*, central venous pressure; *DVT*, deep venous thrombosis; *Hgb*, hemoglobin; *ICU*, intensive care unit; *IVF*, intravenous fluids; *MAP*, mean arterial pressure; *PRBC*, packed red blood cell; *UOP*, urine output; *VAP*, ventilator-associated pneumonia.

Initial Fluid Resuscitation

Initial isotonic fluid boluses (500 to 1000 mL) should be administered and the patient's response noted. If the patient does not respond to the fluid challenge, a second bolus is given. Hypovolemia in sepsis is mainly a result of the vasodilatory effects of nitric oxide as well as the loss of colloid oncotic pressure from leaky capillaries. Therefore isotonic fluid requirements may exceed 10 L. Although aggressive IV fluid administration is necessary for rapid intravascular volume expansion, fluid resuscitation should be titrated to clinical end points (if not using invasive monitors). These end points are mean arterial blood pressure of 65 mm Hg or greater and urine output above 0.5 mL/kg/hr. If the second bolus fails to improve the hemodynamics and tissue perfusion, then consideration for placement of invasive monitoring is warranted, such as a central line with goal central venous pressure (CVP) of 8 to 12 mm Hg and SVO_2 above 70%. Blood transfusion is also recommended during initial resuscitation for acute hemorrhage, lactic acidosis, and coronary ischemia for a goal hemoglobin of 10 g/dL. Critically ill patients who do not meet the above criteria can maintain adequate perfusion with a hemoglobin of 7 to 10 g/dL; therefore a trigger for transfusion in this population should be less than 7 g/dL. Vasopressors and inotropes can be used to reach mean arterial pressure (MAP) goals after adequate fluid and blood product resuscitation. Additional advanced monitoring using echocardiography or pulmonary artery catheters should be added if vasopressors are initiated.

Antimicrobial Therapy

Immediately after blood, urine, sputum, and wounds are cultured, empiric broad-spectrum antibiotics should be given. Although broad spectrum antibiotics should be administered early, particularly in the septic patient with shock, the type of antibiotics should subsequently be narrowed to better reflect the source of infection, the patient's immune status, and any comorbidities. Knowledge of the institution's microbial resistance patterns and the local flora is also necessary. Patients at increased risk for resistant microorganisms include those with prior exposure to antibiotics, a prolonged hospital stay, and history of colonization or infection with resistant microbes. Multiple antibiotics may be used simultaneously, although data for "double coverage" is questionable. Antifungals may also need to be considered, especially in patients hospitalized for a prolonged period of time and those who are immunocompromised: patients on chemotherapy, chronic steroids, or immunomodulators, and posttransplant patients and those with HIV/AIDS. A delay in the administration of broad-spectrum empiric antibiotic therapy in hypotensive septic patients may increase mortality by 7% to 25% for every additional hour treatment is delayed. Narrowing antibiotic coverage can be done at 48 to 72 hours from initiation, once the offending microbe is identified, or the patient clinically stabilizes.

Vasopressors and Inotropes

The use of vasopressors and inotropes is indicated when hypotension or tissue hypoperfusion persist despite adequate fluid resuscitation and anemia correction (Table 3). Current guidelines recommend

TABLE 3: Mechanism of vasopressors and inotropes used in septic shock

Vasopressor/Ionotrope	Receptor
Norepinephrine	$\alpha_1 > \beta$
Phenylephrine	α_1
Dopamine	$D > \beta_1$ and $\beta_2 > \alpha_1$ (dose dependent)
Vasopressin	V
Dobutamine	β_1 and $\beta_2 > \alpha_1$
Milrinone	Phosphodiesterase inhibitor

Action of agonists for select receptors: vasoconstrictor; α_1, β_1, ionotropic, chronotropic; β_2, ionotropic, chronotropic, vasodilator; D, vasodilator; V, vasoconstrictor, phosphodiesterase inhibitor: ionotropic, vasodilator, minimal chronotropic

norepinephrine followed by vasopressin; the goal of vasopressor and inotrope use is to optimize end-organ perfusion, and these agents should be titrated to clinical end points as in Figure 1 and Tables 4 and 5.

In the past, dopamine at dose-dependent levels was the initial inotrope of choice for septic patients. At low doses, it was thought to possess renal and mesenteric vasodilatory effects, augmenting urine output in septic patients. However, recent studies have not been able to support this theory, demonstrating instead that the increased urine output was more likely the effect of dopamine's diuretic-like properties. Furthermore, at higher doses, primarily with beta and alpha effects, dopamine may lead to tachycardia, tachydysrhythmias, and increased cardiac work. As a result, dopamine is rarely used clinically in this setting.

Vasopressin at low doses (0.01 to 0.04 U/min) has been shown to supplement norepinephrine well in resistant septic shock partly through the restoration of the relatively low levels of native vasopressin in this setting. Vasopressin will assist the reaching of clinical end points and will decrease overall pressor requirements, but it will unlikely decrease mortality. Animal studies suggest that at higher doses (>0.04 U/min), the risk of adverse cardiovascular complications may be increased. Such complications can range from arrhythmias to myocardial infarction and cardiac arrest, therefore it is recommended to use the lowest possible dose to achieve goal blood pressure.

For patients with low cardiac output after adequate fluid resuscitation and normalization of blood pressure, but with persistently reduced tissue perfusion and lactic acidosis, inotropes such as dobutamine and milrinone can be used. Both agents can increase cardiac output but may also cause significant hypotension if resuscitation is suboptimal. Phenylephrine is purely an α-agonist and can cause reflex bradycardia, therefore it is useful in patients who are hypotensive and extremely tachycardic; however, its increase in peripheral vascular resistance and lack of inotropic support can lead to decreases in cardiac output and worsening of tissue ischemia, therefore it should not be used as a first-line agent.

Noninvasive and Invasive Monitoring

Both invasive and noninvasive monitoring can be used in septic patients (see Table 5). Considerable debate about the beneficial effects of invasive monitoring remains in regard to CVP and pulmonary artery catheterization (PAC) use in septic shock in particular. These methods carry infrequent risks, such as inadvertent arterial injury, bleeding, pseudoaneurysm, pneumothorax, and pulmonary artery rupture. It remains unclear whether presumed benefits outweigh the established risks.

TABLE 4: Summary of recommendations and goals for care of the septic patient

Initial resuscitation diagnostics	MAP >65 mm Hg CVP 8–12 mm Hg UOP > 0.5 mL/kg/hr Hgb > 10g/dL History and physical examination, cultures, radiographic studies
Antibiotics	Broad-spectrum antibiotics against likely pathogens; adjust therapy when culture results are available
Source control	Surgical repair, resection or drainage of source of contamination, evacuation of infectious material
Vasopressors	MAP >65; requires fluid resuscitation and arterial catheter
Inotropes	Physiologic cardiac output; requires fluid resuscitation and PAC/echocardiography
APC	For severe sepsis with high likelihood of death; use with caution if risk of bleeding
Steroids	For septic shock unresponsive to fluid resuscitation and vasopressors; may be beneficial in relative adrenal insufficiency
Blood transfusion	Hgb of 10 g/dL for initial resuscitation for lactic acidosis, hemorrhage, and coronary ischemia; otherwise may consider goal of 7–9 g/dL
Ventilation	Tidal volume of 6 mL/kg and plateau pressure <30 cmH$_2$O for ARDS
Glucose control	Serum glucose 120–150 mg/dL; may require insulin infusion and frequent blood glucose monitoring
Renal replacement	Intermittent hemodialysis for hemodynamically stable patients; consider continuous hemodialysis for hemodynamically unstable patients;
Prophylaxis	VTE: Mechanical compression devices and heparin or low-molecular-weight heparin; use cautiously for risk of bleeding; consider inferior vena cava filter when heparin cannot be used
	Stress ulcer: histamine blocker or proton pump inhibitor
	VAP: Maintain head of bed >30 degrees in intubated patients

APC, Activated protein C; *Hgb,* hemoglobin; *MAP,* mean arterial pressure; *PAC,* pulmonary artery catheter; *UOP,* urine output; *VAP,* ventilator-associated pneumonia; *VTE,* venous thromboembolism

TABLE 5: Noninvasive and invasive monitoring devices

Noninvasive	Pulse oximetry, telemetry, blood pressure cuff measurements, TTE
Invasive	Arterial catheter, central venous catheter with continuous CVP, pulmonary artery catheter measurement, TEE, Foley catheter

Transthoracic echocardiography (TTE) has become a useful tool in assessing volume status in septic patients and is gaining wide acceptance. It provides volume as well as functional cardiac assessment. Unlike PACs, there is less error in interpreting the data, and it is not an invasive procedure. However, it is a static study, therefore serial TTEs may be needed to assess response to therapy. Its use may also be limited by availability. Transesophageal echocardiography (TEE) is also a useful tool and can provide better images than TTE, but it is invasive and not without associated risks; therefore TEE is only recommended if the TTE is indeterminate, and when accurate volume status and cardiac function evaluation is needed.

CVP may be used to assess intravascular volume in critically ill patients. CVP monitoring has been shown to be beneficial in young patients without known heart failure and with a low CVP (<6 mm Hg). However, if CVP is normal/high, or the patient is older or has heart failure, its value is not as clear. Pulmonary capillary wedge pressure (PCWP), measured through a pulmonary artery catheter, has also been used to evaluate the volume status of patients in shock. Unfortunately, several trials have shown a worse outcome with PAC use, in part attributed to improper PAC data interpretation by clinicians.

In patients requiring prolonged pressor support, the placement of an arterial line is recommended for continuous and more precise blood pressure measurements. If the patient requires more than two liters of crystalloid, a CVP should be placed to assess volume status with a goal CVP of 8 to 12 mm Hg or greater before considering pressor use. However, in the patient with impaired cardiac function, or in those in whom fluid challenges continue to fail, obtaining more advanced monitoring, such as an echocardiography or PAC, is warranted. These clinical tools may also be helpful if organ dysfunction or respiratory failure ensues. Several studies have demonstrated that noninvasive or invasive monitoring, along with critical care nursing and a closed ICU with dedicated intensivists, decreased both mortality and length of stay. Yet invasive monitoring has not been shown to clearly improve outcome when compared with noninvasive monitoring alone (Table 6).

Supportive Care

Ventilatory Support

Ventilatory support is used in septic patients for various reasons. Patients with florid sepsis may develop respiratory difficulties leading to acute lung injury (ALI) or acute respiratory distress syndrome (ARDS), which is described as development of diffuse pulmonary infiltrates, decreased pulmonary compliance, and hypoxemia ($Pao_2/Fio_2 \leq 200$) in the absence of cardiogenic failure. ALI is defined as Pao_2/Fio_2 in a range from 201 to 300. Current management guidelines recommend a "low lung stretch" protocol using low tidal volumes (6 mL/kg), positive end-expiratory pressure titrated for oxygen saturation and cardiac output, and maintained plateau pressures less than 30 cm H_2O. ARDS may also be managed with high-frequency oscillatory ventilation, prone positioning, and nitric oxide. Extracorporeal membrane oxygenation (ECMO) is used in extreme cases, and intubation should be considered in all patients in shock for whom sedation and pain control will be required to reduce anxiety and improve pulmonary compliance.

Blood Product Transfusions

Blood transfusion in ICU patients is currently withheld unless the patient is exhibiting signs of poor oxygen delivery, cardiac ischemia, or has a hemoglobin less than 7.0 g/dL. This is supported by several studies in which blood transfusion was found to have fewer benefits and more complications for patients in whom the hemoglobin goal was 10 g/dL. In particular, mortality increases were seen in younger, less ill ICU patients when packed red blood cells were transfused to maintain higher hemoglobin levels. Reasons for this include poorly deformable red blood cells in stored blood, which causes microvascular occlusion and subsequent distal tissue ischemia. Additionally, transfusions have been associated with transient immunosuppression, increased risk of infection, acute hemolytic reactions, ALI, allergic reactions, transfusion errors, and postoperative organ dysfunction.

Hemodialysis

Continuous hemodialysis in patients with sepsis and acute renal failure has shown favorable outcomes in a few studies. Hemodialysis with polymethylmethacrylate membrane filters removes a variety of proinflammatory cytokines, which are believed to drive systemic inflammation in sepsis and septic shock. Otherwise, indications for dialysis remain the same for septic as well as for nonseptic patients.

Glycemic Control

Early large randomized controlled trials have shown that tight glycemic control may reduce mortality in some critically ill populations; however, these reports have not been consistently replicated, and significant risks of hypoglycemia have been seen when goals are set too low (80 to 110 mg/dL). Current recommendations are to maintain a serum glucose level between 120 to 150 mg/dL through insulin administration.

Nutrition

Early nutrition plays a vital role in the supportive management of septic patients. Enteral feeding should begin within 24 hours of ICU admission, unless the patient has intestinal or colonic ileus, mechanical bowel obstruction, or acute peritoneal inflammation. Unlike parenteral nutrition, enteral nutrition decreases risks of infection and mortality through the promotion of local gut mucosal integrity and the reduction of bacterial translocation.

Sodium Bicarbonate

The use of sodium bicarbonate to correct acidosis continues to be controversial. It is indicated for patients with severe hyperchloremic lactic acidosis when the pH is below 7.1. Large doses of sodium bicarbonate may cause severe fluid overload, hypernatremia, postrecovery alkalosis, and a heavy CO_2 burden that must be cleared by the lungs. Therefore, treatment of the underlying disorder should be the primary goal for acidosis reversal.

Chemical Prophylaxis

The systemic inflammation that often follows sepsis can contribute to the development of deep venous thrombosis (DVT), therefore all critically ill patients should have intermittent compression boots and, if possible, subcutaneous heparin or low molecular weight heparin administered. Indications for inferior vena cava filters remain unclear but should be considered for patients in whom chemical prophylaxis is contraindicated.

TABLE 6: Timeline of implementation of recommended diagnostic and therapeutic goals

	Resuscitation	Antimicrobials	Vasopressors/ Inotropes	Monitoring	Specific Therapy	Supportive Therapy
1 hr	Initiate crystalloid fluid resuscitation (500 mL every 10 to 15 min)	Empiric, broad-spectrum, high-dose antimicrobials		Continuous ECG, arterial saturation, blood pressure and UOP		O_2; consider intubation and mechanical ventilation prior to overt respiratory distress
1–8 hr	Titrate fluid resuscitation to elimination of base deficit and normalization of serum lactate	Radiographic investigation for localization and delineation of infection source Source control if necessary	Norepinephrine if circulatory shock persists after adequate fluid resuscitation Inotropes if chloride or SVO$_2$ are persistently decreased	ICU transfer with full monitoring support Arterial catheter assessment If shock persists with >2 L resuscitation, central venous line (goal CVP ≥8 mm Hg)		Consider low-dose steroid therapy ± ACTH stimulation test
8–24 hr	Dynamic evaluation of resuscitative goals (based on clinical and invasive monitoring end points)		Consider vasopressin if shock refractory to norepinephrine	If persistently pressor dependent after 3 to 5 L crystalloid infusion, CVP ≥8 achieved, suspicion of intravascular volume depletion or limited cardiovascular reserves, echocardiography or PAC placement (initial goal PCWP 12–15 mm Hg)	Consider initiation of drotrecogin-alfa if single organ fails and APACHE II score ≥25, or two or more organ failures in absence of APACHE score	Initiate enteral feeding Consider intensive insulin therapy
>24 hr		Narrow antimicrobial regimen depending on isolation of pathogenic organisms and/or clinical improvement Reassess necessity for or efficacy of source control		Consider PAC in vasopressor-dependent patients with progressive respiratory, renal, or multiple organ dysfunction		Intensive hemodialysis therapy for renal failure Low-pressure, volume-limited ventilation for ARDS

HR, Heart rate; *MAP*, mean arterial blood pressure; *ECG*, electrocardiogram; *UOP*, urine output; *CVP*, central venous pressure; *ACTH*, adrenocorticotropin hormone; *PAC*, pulmonary artery catheter; *PCWP*, pulmonary capillary wedge pressure; *APACHE*, Acute Physiology and Chronic Health Evaluation; *ARDS*, acute respiratory distress syndrome
Modified from Kumar A, Kumar A: Sepsis and septic shock. In Gabrielli A, Layon AJ, Yu M (eds): *Critical care*, ed 4, Philadelphia, 2009, Lippincott Williams & Wilkins.

Peptic ulcer prophylaxis is also important, as sepsis is a significant risk factor for the development of acute gastritis or ulcerations. Histamine blockers and proton pump inhibitors (PPIs) are effective agents that are commonly used.

SPECIFIC TREATMENT AND ADJUNCTS

Activated Protein C

Drotrecogin alfa, or activated protein C (APC), is an inhibitor of procoagulation factors developed on the hypothesis that systemic microvascular thrombosis is the root cause of tissue ischemia and organ failure in sepsis. Although studies have shown its ability to reduce

mortality in severe sepsis with organ failure, APC carries a significant risk of bleeding. Current recommendations for its use in sepsis include the presence of two or more dysfunctional organs or an Acute Physiology and Chronic Health Evaluation (APACHE) score of 25 or higher. APC is contraindicated in patients who have intracranial bleeding, are coagulopathic, or who have had a recent (<24 hours) major operation.

Steroids

The role of cortisol supplementation in sepsis remains controversial. Large randomized studies have failed to elicit a benefit in sepsis, unless patients in shock are failing fluid and vasopressor interventions. The current regimen is 50 mg of IV hydrocortisone every 6 hours for 7 days. Benefits derived from steroid use may stem from the relative adrenal insufficiency of patients who are septic. Patients suspected of having relative adrenal insufficiency should be given supplemental hydrocortisone 50 mg every 6 hours for up to 5 days. Cortisol (cosyntropin) stimulation tests are no longer recommended in critically ill patients with sepsis.

Source Control

The main goal of source control, whether conducted by open or laparoscopic surgery or through percutaneous or endoscopic means is to drain or eliminate infected tissue or material. Prior to and concurrent with this, resuscitation and antibiotic therapy should be conducted aggressively. In patients who require a laparotomy for adequate source control, the wound may be left open in a damage-control fashion, particularly in the setting of visceral swelling. This allows for repeated washouts and the opportunity for reevaluations in subsequent explorations.

SUMMARY

The management of sepsis continues to be a challenge despite advances in medical and surgical intensive care. It is still an area of active research, and as a result, clinicians must stay abreast of the current evidence-based approaches while keeping an open mind to the novel therapies being developed.

SUGGESTED READINGS

Dellinger RP, Levy MM, Carlet JM, et al: Surviving Sepsis Campaign guidelines for management of severe sepsis and septic shock, *Crit Care Med* 34:856–870, 2004.

Kumar AN, Kumar AS: Sepsis and septic shock. In Gabrielli A, Layon AJ, Yu M, editors: *Critical care*, ed 4, Philadelphia, 2009, Lippincott, Williams & Wilkins.

Marik PE: *Handbook of evidence-based critical care*, New York, 2001, Springer.

Sena MJ, Nathens AB: Mechanical ventilation. In Souba WW, Fink MP, Jurkovic GJ, editors: *ACS surgery principle and practice*, ed 6, New York, 2007, WebMD.

MULTIPLE ORGAN DYSFUNCTION AND FAILURE

Timothy G. Buchman, MD, PhD

OVERVIEW

Multiple organ dysfunction syndrome (MODS) can be operationally defined as the functional derangement of at least two organ systems consequent to a potentially life-threatening insult. By this definition, half of all patients admitted to a surgical ICU will sustain MODS. The mortality rate of MODS is related to the number of dysfunctional organs and the degree and duration of their dysfunction. Approximately two thirds of patients with three-organ dysfunction will die. Survivors of MODS have markedly prolonged yet less complete recovery than critically ill patients who do not sustain MODS. Given the frequency, mortality, and morbidity of MODS, surgeons must know how to prevent, recognize, and treat this syndrome to mitigate its sequelae. The purpose of this chapter is to provide succinct clinical guidance.

MODS is a disease of medical progress. Prior to the Vietnam conflict, acutely ill patients with progressive organ failure simply died. Dissemination of hemodynamic monitoring, mechanical ventilation, parenteral nutrition, blood component therapies, and renal replacement therapies afforded survival to critically injured soldiers. As those supports diffused into civilian hospitals, reports began to appear describing sequential "failure" of multiple organs following rescue from previously lethal conditions. By 1975, the challenge of multiple, progressive, or sequential systems failure had become familiar to civilian surgeons. Two points are important. First, MODS describes physiology unanticipated in evolution, therefore evolved physiologic compensation mechanisms may be inappropriate. Second, whereas the original nomenclature specified *failure,* current nomenclature specifies *dysfunction;* thus the functional insufficiency is generally attributable to regulatory failure and not wholesale tissue destruction. In principle, function should be recoverable; in practice, recovery is usually incomplete and sometimes never happens.

The regulatory failures underlying MODS are linked through inflammation and immunity. Unbridled inflammation and distortions of both the innate and specific immune responses are common. In nearly every case of MODS, a trigger of widespread inflammation can be identified. In surgical units, these triggers most often include unplanned and planned injury (operations), infection, or ischemic tissues. These triggers are referred to as *sources,* thus *source control* is the foundation of both prevention and treatment of MODS. Nonviable or marginally viable tissue and inadequately controlled infection are the leading triggers of MODS, and the appearance of MODS mandates an immediate and comprehensive search for infection, ischemia, and infarction. Unless and until the source is controlled and eradicated, organ function deteriorates rapidly.

MODS may be acute, but more often it develops over several days. Early recognition and source control are essential to mitigate the severity of MODS, and tools have been developed to recognize and characterize the course of the disease. No one laboratory test has proven diagnostic or prognostic. Instead, physiologic scoring systems have been developed that aggregate functional performance of individual organs into a scale that indexes severity and predicts outcome. Three scoring systems are in current use: the MOD score, the sequential organ failure assessment (SOFA) score, and the logistic organ dysfunction (LOD) system score. Each of the scores assesses six organ systems, each has high interrater reliability, and none appears superior to the others. Given the incidence of MODS in surgical intensive care, scoring of all patients can promote timely recognition of MODS and assessment of treatment efficacy.

Over the past several decades, chemical and mechanical organ supports have become more effective so that the mortality for a given degree of derangement has declined. Unfortunately, derangements have collectively become more severe as the population has accumulated chronic illnesses that serve as a backdrop for MODS. As a consequence, the overall mortality of MODS has remained unchanged since its initial description.

SEPSIS

Sepsis describes a combination of infection and immune dysregulation and is the most common precursor of MODS among surgical patients. In addition to a rapid and comprehensive search for the source of the infection, empiric antimicrobial therapy directed against the most likely causes should be initiated without delay. In addition to consideration of the usual aerobic bacteria, some patients with specific risk factors may warrant empiric therapy with drugs directed against anaerobic bacteria (e.g., following abdominal or pelvic surgery); fungi (e.g., following certain chemotherapies); or viruses (e.g., cytomegalovirus following transplantation). Specific selection is a matter of medical judgment.

Both delay and inappropriate selection of antibiotic therapy are tightly and unambiguously linked to adverse outcomes, therefore speed of administration and accurate selection of antimicrobial therapy are essential when sepsis appears. Immediate consultation with an intensivist is recommended. Source control by excision or drainage of infected tissues should follow as soon as the patient can tolerate a procedure, and surgeons should marshal the imaging, interventional, and operative resources necessary to ensure that no time is lost controlling the source.

MECHANISMS

Neither infection nor ischemia nor injury alone appear sufficient to initiate the regulatory disruptions that culminate in MODS. Rather, multiple insults accumulate and precipitate MODS. Several theories and mechanisms have been proposed to account for this observation. The first of these was the *two-hit hypothesis,* which suggested that leukocytes were "primed" by an initial insult and "activated" by a second. The archetypal initial insult in the two-hit model is trauma-precipitated ischemia–reperfusion. In support of this theory is an extensive literature describing changes in levels of inflammatory mediators and cell numbers. Subsequent theories have pointed to organ systems that abut the environment as "motors" of organ failure. Those theories posit an initial injury that initially compromises barrier function—for example, gut or pulmonary epithelium—and leads to a leak of pathogens or mediators that are subsequently activated and disseminated as a consequence of immune disruption. In support of such theories are human and animal data demonstrating barrier failures and leaks following remote initial insults.

More recently, cytopathic hypoxia has been advanced as an explanation for widespread MODS. In this theory, sustained or repeated inflammatory stimuli lead to losses in the number and efficiency of mitochondria. Whether one or more of these mechanisms underlies a particular case of MODS is less important than their common feature of serial insults: MODS is best prevented by prevention of repeated insults to already compromised physiology.

Unfortunately, the insults include secondary effects of well-intentioned treatments such as massive fluid resuscitation, mechanical ventilation, vasopressor infusion, and blood transfusion. Although such treatments are transiently necessary to preserve life, their adverse effects dictate judicious use. More treatment is typically not better treatment in MODS, and best practices depend on clarity of physiologic objectives and on strategies to meet those objectives that minimize risk to each patient.

PHYSIOLOGIC OBJECTIVES

Brain

The physiologic objectives include freedom from pain, anxiety, and delirium. Treatment strategies include adequate perfusion and appropriate use of analgesics, anxiolytics, and antipsychotic agents. Brain dysfunction in MODS is characterized by reduced level of consciousness and also by encephalopathy, both of which are multifactorial in origin. Although no known interventions are specific to the brain and its failure modes in MODS, the brain is uniquely sensitive to accumulating organ dysfunction and therefore serves in a unique monitoring role. New or increasing encephalopathy in a critically ill patient without an alternative explanation is early MODS until proven otherwise.

Competing mechanisms have been proposed that implicate the brain (false neurotransmitters and altered blood-brain barrier permeability) as well as distant organs (altered metabolism of analgesics and anxiolytics leading to buildup of the parent compound and metabolites). Recommended supportive care includes assurance of adequate perfusion, minimization of drug treatments known to depress the sensorium, imaging to exclude structural changes, and occasionally invasive procedures to exclude a central nervous system (CNS) infection.

Lungs

The physiologic objectives for the lungs include effective gas exchange and limitation of adverse pressure-related effects on pulmonary parenchyma and circulation. The common failure modes are acute lung injury (ALI) and its more severe manifestation, acute respiratory distress syndrome (ARDS). It matters not whether the pulmonary failure is the consequence of a direct insult such as aspiration pneumonitis or a remote insult such as pancreatitis: approximately one third of patients with ARDS will die. Mechanical ventilatory support is usually required, and interventions that reduce barotrauma, volutrauma, and oxygen trauma bundled together as a lung-protective strategy appear to reduce the mortality of ARDS as much as 30%. Typical inputs include tidal volumes less than 8 mL/kg; the minimum positive end-expiratory pressure to stent the airways open (P_{flex}), and minimum oxygen concentration sufficient to maintain peripheral saturations of around 92%.

Timely intervention can truncate the course of ALI and ARDS. Use of high-frequency oscillatory ventilation (HFOV) not only achieves the lung-protective objectives but does so with minimal inflation pressures and minimal volume variation. Delays diminish effectiveness of HFOV.

Additional objectives include minimizing the risk of a ventilator-associated pneumonia (VAP), achieved by maintaining the patient in a semiupright position, and mechanical interventions that may include subglottic suctioning and antimicrobial oral care to reduce the load of bacteria that reach the injured lung. Fibrin deposition in the injured lung accompanies ALI/ARDS. Although the process is typically microscopic, accumulation of macroscopic mucus plugs is common; bronchoscopic removal of such plugs may be necessary as an adjunct or as a replacement for endogenous clearance.

Early tracheostomy appears to accelerate liberation from mechanical ventilation, minimizing pneumonia risk. However, patients with severe ARDS are vulnerable to immediate complications of tracheostomy, such as desaturation and pressure-related leaks of ventilator gases. On balance, early tracheostomy to facilitate ventilator support and liberation appears preferable to delaying tracheostomy until the later stages of recovery from lung injury.

Liver

The liver often manifests a biphasic injury pattern. Altered perfusion during an initial insult is typically reflected as a transient failure of hepatic synthetic function. International normalized ratio (INR) rises, and a brief rise in markers of liver injury (transaminases) may also be seen. The liver appears to recover, but a few days after the initial insult, multiple functions fail including synthetic, detoxification, and metabolic functions. INR rises again, patients fail to detoxify various compounds (including false neurotransmitters, discussed under "Brain"), and heme pigments begin to accumulate. Jaundice follows in severe cases. Both prevention and support involve ensuring adequate perfusion within the systemic and splanchnic circulations through careful attention to intravascular volume and also by minimizing the use of vasoconstricting drugs. Although hepatic dysfunction often causes jaundice, not all postshock jaundice is simple hepatic dysfunction. Ischemic (acalculous) cholecystitis is infrequent but should not be overlooked, especially with tenderness in the right upper quadrant or unexplained leukocytosis.

TABLE 1: Risk, injury, failure, loss, and end-stage kidney disease (RIFLE) classification

Class	Glomerular Filtration Rate Criteria	Urine Output Criteria
Risk	Serum creatinine ×1.5 over baseline	<0.5 mL/kg/hr × 6 hr
Injury	Serum creatinine ×2 over baseline	<0.5 mL/kg/hr × 12 hr
Failure	Serum creatinine ×3, or serum creatinine ≥4 mg/dL with an acute rise >0.5 mg/dL	<0.3 mL/kg/hr × 24 hr, or anuria × 12 hr
Loss	Persistent acute renal failure = complete loss of kidney function for >4 weeks	
End-stage kidney disease	End-stage kidney disease for >3 months	

For conversion of creatinine expressed in conventional units to SI units, multiply by 88.4. RIFLE class is determined based on the worst of either glomerular filtration criteria or urine output criteria. Glomerular filtration criteria are calculated as an increase of serum creatinine above the baseline serum creatinine level. Acute kidney injury should be both abrupt (within 1 to 7 days) and sustained (more than 24 hours). When the baseline serum creatinine is not known, and patients are without a history of chronic kidney insufficiency, it is recommend to calculate a baseline serum creatinine using the Modification of Diet in Renal Disease equation for assessment of kidney function, assuming a glomerular filtration rate of 75 mL/min/1.73 m². When the baseline serum creatinine is elevated, an abrupt rise of at least 0.5 mg/dL to more than 4 mg/dL is all that is required to achieve the Failure class.

Kidney

Kidney failure is currently stratified by the RIFLE classification (Table 1), which is important because acute kidney injury defined by this classification occurs in two thirds of critically ill patients, and acute kidney injury and failure defined by this classification are independently associated with in-hospital mortality. Moreover, patients who meet the mildest ("risk") criteria are at significant risk for progression to kidney injury or failure.

The kidneys have two primary failure modes. Following ischemia-reperfusion, such as with hemorrhage and transfusion, kidneys sustain an injury pattern similar to other solid organs. Vasoconstriction is predominant, tubular casts are shed, and a transient functional disturbance marked by a rise in creatinine is followed by relatively quick recovery; the entire cycle lasts 5 to 10 days. In the setting of sepsis, however, renal blood flow increases, as both afferent and efferent arterioles dilate. Efferent dilation exceeds afferent dilation and, as a consequence, a paradoxical decline in glomerular filtration rate follows, also marked by a rise in creatinine. Dysfunction tends to persist out of proportion to any perfusion compromise. In either case, ensuring adequate intravascular volume is a mainstay of therapy. Estimates of central venous volume can be made from central venous pressure (CVP) and/or from ultrasound assessment of the size and dynamics of the inferior vena cava.

Differentiating between the two failure modes may be more important when deciding whether to use fenoldopam either as a preventive or rescue agent. Although two pooled meta-analyses suggest fenoldopam has general benefit for critically ill patients at risk for or with evolving acute kidney injury, benefits and risks may be different depending on injury mechanism. From a mechanistic perspective, greater benefit would be expected in the early ischemic versus the septic setting, and no data speak to the utility of fenoldopam in established MODS.

Prevention of kidney injury is a key clinical strategy. Current practice is to minimize exposure to toxic drugs, maintain adequate intravascular volume, and initiate preemptive protective measures when risk is heightened; for example, the administration of bicarbonate or N-acetylcysteine prior to infusion of radiopacifying contrast agents.

Once MODS is established and compromises renal function, renal replacement therapy is often indicated. The classic indications include excess potassium, protons, urea nitrogen, or volume. Increasingly, excess fluid volume is used as an indication for early continuous renal replacement therapy to remove fluid that can compromise venous circulation to pressure areas. Expanded criteria include severe disturbances in sodium metabolism and a need to remove contrast agents infused for imaging. Continuous renal replacement therapies have

become a mainstay of critical care, however, no compelling data are available to suggest that intermittent dialysis is better or worse than the current practice that emphasizes continuous renal replacement therapy.

Heart

The heart is adversely affected by MODS regardless of the inciting event. If sustained or repeated ischemia-perfusion is the underlying cause, myocardial "stunning" underlies the functional impairment. Sepsis leads to a toxic myocardial dysfunction variously attributed to large (cytokine) and small (nitric oxide) inflammatory mediators. Septic dysfunction is often masked by collapse of peripheral vasomotor tone that yields high cardiac outputs in the face of an enervated heart. MODS consequent to initial hepatic failure leads to high-output cardiac dysfunction by a third mechanism involving altered splanchnic perfusion.

Emerging data suggest that whereas myocardial stunning and its immediate sequelae may be best treated with conventional sympathomimetic amines (e.g., norepinephrine for pressure and dobutamine for inotropy), patients with early cardiac dysfunction attributable to sepsis may derive added benefit from infusions of vasopressin.

Irrespective of the cause of cardiovascular dysfunction, the goal of treatment is adequate perfusion to sustain aerobic metabolism and not a particular blood pressure. Metrics of oxygen extraction (such as mixed venous oxygen saturation), of tissue oxygen content (obtained with infrared technologies) and of anaerobic metabolism (such as lactate) may be more useful than arterial pressure measurements. An indwelling bladder catheter is essential to assess renal perfusion and excretion.

Pulmonary hypertension and/or right-sided heart failure are not uncommonly observed in MODS. A search for intercurrent pulmonary embolism is often revealing. Should pulmonary hypertension become recurrent and/or severe after pulmonary embolism is excluded or addressed, treatment may be considered. The most common context is ARDS. In this setting, inhaled prostacyclin can help a marginal patient toward recovery, and it is preferred to nitric oxide owing to lower costs and a better safety profile when organ dysfunction is widespread.

Endocrine System

The effect of MODS on the endocrine system is underappreciated. Irrespective of the range selected for glucose control, nearly all patients with MODS are treated with insulin. In addition to regulating blood glucose, insulin is perhaps the most potent anabolic hormone routinely administered to critically ill patients. Yet insulin deficiency and resistance are only part of the endocrine derangement. Other endocrinopathies are more insidious and therefore are less frequently recognized or addressed.

The general feature of severe and prolonged critical illness is that the function of the hypothalamic-pituitary target axes is suppressed to nearly nil after about 10 days of critical illness; T3 and T4 measurements commonly reveal hypothyroidism, and adrenocorticotropic hormone stimulation and cortisol measurements commonly reveal adrenal failure. Supplemental thyroid hormone and corticosteroid are indicated in doses sufficient to reconstitute the normal physiologic milieu.

More controversial is the somatomedin axis. Growth hormone and insulinlike growth factor (IGF)-1 measurements will commonly reveal inadequate hormone and downstream effect. Twentieth-century prospective trials administering growth hormone (GH) to all critically ill patients without assessment of the hormone level or downstream effector status showed increased mortality. Twenty-first century replacement based on demonstrated inadequacy may be a more promising approach but currently violates a Food and Drug Administration black-box warning. Anabolic steroids such as oxandrolone may have some role in preventing or reversing the muscle wasting that accompanies MODS. Measurement of serum testosterone to demonstrate inadequate levels of the hormone should probably precede anabolic steroid prescription, so that risk-benefit-cost assessments can be made.

Nutrition Failure

Nutrition failure is common in MODS. Worse, nutrition supplementation is commonly delayed. In general, MODS patients are hypermetabolic and waste nitrogen. Even optimal supplementation does not reverse the loss and, emphatically, more is *not* better. Current treatment guidelines suggest oral feedings are at least as good and are less costly than parenteral nutrition, but either is better than starvation for more than 2 to 3 days. Enteral feeding can be performed even in the presence of adynamic ileus, with trophic effects on the mucosa and absorption of nutrients. However, enteral feeding is less beneficial and may be more risky in patients with deranged gut perfusion. High-output fistulas and massive bowel resections mandate the use of parenteral nutrition early in support.

Nutrition support should generally provide 20 (acute phase) to 30 (recovery phase) kcal/kg/day and 1.2 (acute phase) to 2 (recovery phase) protein g/kg/day. Current practice holds that glutamine is safe and should generally be provided to critically ill patients, as this amino acid is conditionally essential and a necessary fuel source for several tissues, including gut mucosa. Current practice also holds that the soy-based lipid emulsions available in the United States may deliver as much harm as benefit and are increasingly being omitted from parenteral prescriptions. In contrast, omega-3 fatty acids are generally recommended for all critically ill patients; unfortunately, no parenteral formulation is available in the United States. Finally, deficiencies of micronutrients—especially zinc, selenium, and several vitamins—are more common than previously appreciated, and the risk-benefit-cost relationship favors scheduled supplementation. Although immune-enhancing enteral feeds have been used in the past, concerns about toxic effects of these preparations in sepsis have made them less attractive in MODS patients, unless sepsis can be completely excluded.

Nutrition support will not prevent calorie-nitrogen wasting in MODS. However, given appropriate nutritional support, the wasting should be attenuated sufficient to maintain synthesis of essential proteins and immune function. Hypoalbuminemia, lymphopenia, and other signs of metabolic failure that persist or worsen in the face of adequate nutritional support should prompt a search for an uncontrolled source such as infection or necrosis, as well as screening for an undetected endocrinopathy.

TREATMENT

Early and goal-directed therapies appear important to achieve optimal recovery. Although sepsis has occupied center stage in studies of early and goal-directed therapy, there is reason to expect that early and aggressive treatment to identify and reverse other causes of MODS will produce similarly favorable outcomes. Such therapies are typically collected into bundles that specify the interventions themselves, the timing of the interventions, and physiologic targets for titration of the interventions. For example, a widely used sepsis bundle indicates targets to be achieved within 6 hours: CVP 8 to 12 mm Hg; mean arterial pressure (MAP) 65 mm Hg or greater; urine output 0.5 mL/kg/hr or more; and central venous (superior vena cava) oxygen saturation 70% or higher, or mixed venous 65% or higher. The bundle goes on to specify a method for achieving the venous oxygen target if crystalloid volume expansion is insufficient: consider further fluid; transfuse packed red blood cells (PRBCs) if required to hematocrit of 30%, and/or start dobutamine infusion, maximum 20 μg/kg/min. Follow-up studies are consistent in their confirmation of the value of timely goal-directed therapy.

TABLE 2: Sequential Organ Failure Assessment (SOFA) Score

Organ System	0	1	2	3	4
Cardiovascular* hypotension (mm Hg)	MAP >70 mm without vasopressors	MAP <70 without vasopressors	Dopamine ≤5 or dobutamine (any dose)	Dopamine >5 or epinephrine ≤0.1 or norepinephrine ≤0.1	Dopamine >15 or epinephrine >0.1 or norepinephrine >0.1
Respiratory, PaO_2/FiO_2 (mm Hg)	>400	<400	<300	<200 with respiratory support	<100 with respiratory support
Renal[†] creatinine (mg/dL)	<1.2	1.2–1.9	2.0–3.4	3.5–4.9	>5.0
Hematology, platelet count ($\times10^3/mm^3$)	>150	<150	<100	<50	<20
Hepatic, bilirubin (mg/dL)	<1.2	1.2–1.9	2.0–5.9	6.0–11.9	>12.0

MAP, Mean arterial pressure
*Adrenergic agents are administered for at least 1 hour (doses given are in μg/kg/min).
[†]Renal SOFA was modified to exclude urine output.

Two imperatives follow from this observation: First, surgeons must have a method for serially assessing their patients for the development or progression of MODS. This applies to patients in or out of the ICU. The SOFA score, derived from common measures, is the simplest to compute (Table 2). A total increment of 4 points distributed among two or more systems is a strong indicator of MODS or its progression. Second, interventions for MODS must be fast, accurate, and sustained. Surgeons who care for MODS patients only infrequently and surgeons whose clinical responsibilities preclude staying at the bedside of the ICU for extended periods are well advised to collaborate early in the patient's course with a qualified intensivist to obtain optimal outcomes.

Palliative Care

Symptom management and palliative care are frequently overlooked in treatment of the patient with MODS. An early focus on relief of pain, anxiolysis, maintenance of skin integrity, and promotion of normal intestinal function will not only mitigate subsequent complications but will also build a trust relationship among caregivers and patients and their families. Simple interventions include pressure-relief bed surfaces, prokinetic bowel regimens, conversion from shorter to longer acting analgesic medications, simplification of blood draws, and medications; these can substantially improve the experience, if not the outcome, of a prolonged stay in an ICU. Such attention ensures that the patient is treated as a whole person and not as a collection of body systems.

Perhaps more important, given the mortality of MODS, such attention to symptoms and suffering prepares patients and families for challenging decisions concerning the goals of care. Very few patients with MODS survive their critical illness and recover sufficiently to qualify for immediate discharge home. The most favorable outcome involves hospital discharge to intensive rehabilitation, where endurance and strength can be rebuilt. More often, patients cannot tolerate intensive rehabilitation at hospital discharge and become candidates to go either to a skilled nursing facility or a long-term acute care (LTAC) hospital, where mechanical support can be continued. Although discharge to a long-term care facility may be seen as a success by surgical staff, families and patients are all too often ill prepared for their likely outcomes: among older patients, multiple (two or more) ongoing organ dysfunctions acquired in and sustained through the current illness effectively precludes eventual return to a home setting and is associated with 30-day mortality rates as high as 50% following LTAC transfer. Thus persistence of organ dysfunctions requiring complex support after diligent attempts to reverse the precipitating cause, and after an interval to allow for recovery, should prompt an unblinking family meeting about the minimum quality of life acceptable to the patient in the context of the most likely outcomes of continued aggressive care.

RECOMMENDATIONS

Surgeons should be aware of several new recommendations for MODS therapies. First, intraabdominal compartment syndrome has been recognized as a reversible cause of MODS. Although many protocols now limit massive volume infusions, such infusions are occasionally lifesaving but cause complications that themselves can be life threatening. Measurement of bladder pressures should be routine after massive resuscitation, and 30 mm Hg is a reasonable point at which to perform decompressive laparotomy, if less invasive measures have failed to reverse the process. Surgeons should respond promptly to requests for decompressive laparotomy, as they can be lifesaving.

In contrast, the targets for several therapies have been revised toward less intervention. Transfusions are now appreciated to be immunosuppressive and are associated with excess mortality. In the absence of cardiac ischemia or ongoing blood loss, hemoglobin concentrations of 7 g/dL are well tolerated, and transfusion is not indicated. Recombinant erythropoietin offers no benefit and can possibly harm patients. Glucose control should be only tight enough but no tighter. Current opinion suggests that the target for blood glucose should be 150 to 180 mg/dL. More aggressive therapy increases the rate of hypoglycemia without associated benefit.

SUMMARY

MODS is a disease of medical progress that is more dysregulatory than destructive, yet it continues to have a frighteningly high mortality. Prevention of serial insults, early detection through systematic scoring, and prompt goal-directed therapy to address the underlying cause and support dysfunctional organs are mainstays of current surgical practice. Once the diagnosis of MODS has been established, management of the patient requires constant attention to the details of organ support and to the potential adverse interactions among treatments. Engagement of an integrated team of dedicated professionals, supported by expertise in intensive care medicine, is helpful to deliver, coordinate, and assess the care of the patient with MODS. Recovery is typically prolonged and incomplete.

SUGGESTED READINGS

Ziegler TR: Parenteral nutrition in the critically ill patient, *N Engl J Med* 361:1088–1097, 2010.

Mizock BA: The multiple organ dysfunction syndrome, *Dis Mon* 55:476–526, 2009.

Hotchkiss RS, Karl IE: The pathophysiology and treatment of sepsis, *N Engl J Med* 348(2):138–150, 2003.

Dematte D'Amico JE, Donnelly HK, et al: Risk assessment for inpatient survival in the long-term acute care setting after prolonged critical illness, *Chest* 124(3):1039–1045, 2003.

Broomhead LR, Brett SJ: Intensive care follow-up: what has it told us? *Crit Care* 6(5):411–417, 2002.

Baue AE: Multiple, progressive, or sequential systems failure, *Arch Surg* 110:779–781, 1975.

USE OF ANTIBIOTICS IN SURGICAL PATIENTS

Lenworth M. Jacobs, MD, MPH, and Vijay Jayaraman, MD

OVERVIEW

Surgical site infections (SSIs) are a serious problem for the patient, the practitioners managing the wound, and the environment in which the patient is being managed. Infections in surgical patients continue to be a determinant of major morbidity and mortality. One of the main objectives of successfully managing surgical patients is to avoid infection, and it is critical to understand the factors that promote and encourage infections. The three general areas are 1) the innate host defense mechanisms, 2) the causative agent, and 3) the site of the surgical infection. Antibiotic-resistant organisms are difficult to treat and require isolation practices that are an increasing challenge for hospitals. This is particularly difficult in the sick intensive care unit (ICU) patient.

SSIs are now classified and reported to organizations such as the National Hospital Safety Network (NHSN), a division of the Centers for Disease Control and Prevention (CDC), the National Institutes of Health, and the American College of Surgeons National Quality Improvement Program (ACS-NSQIP) database. NHSN data collected between 2006 and 2008 demonstrated a total of 15,862 SSIs following 830,748 operative procedures with an overall rate of 2%. One of the goals of the surgical care improvement project (SCIP) is to reduce surgical complications by 25% by 2010.

DEFINITION OF SURGICAL SITE INFECTION

The CDC adopted the term *surgical site infection* in 1992 as an improvement to using *surgical wound infection*. The new term expanded the definition of the infectious process to not only include the skin and subcutaneous tissues of surgical wounds but also the potential infection of the organ space and any implants that may have been used during the operation. The definition was created in an effort to standardize and simplify reporting practices and enable comparisons in care to be made at the global level.

The surgical site comprises the incision and the organ space. The incision is further subdivided into the superficial incision that includes the skin and subcutaneous tissues and the deep incision that includes the fascia and muscle. An SSI is defined to occur within 30 days of the operation, up to 1 year if an implant was placed, and the infection appears related to the operation.

A superficial infection involves the skin and subcutaneous tissues and is associated with purulent drainage, pain, localized swelling, and erythema (Figure 1). It is important that cellulitis not be reported as an SSI according to the CDC. The deep incisional infection involves the fascia and the muscle layers, and it requires purulence and either temperature above 38° C or localized pain and tenderness. The organ-space SSI involves any organ or space apart from the incision that was manipulated during the procedure.

PATHOPHYSIOLOGY OF SURGICAL SITE INFECTIONS

The interaction of the bacterial inoculum at the surgical site with the host defense mechanisms determines whether an infection results. These factors are also influenced by the preoperative care of the surgical site, the intraoperative techniques used by the surgeon, and the supportive therapies administered by the anesthesiologist. Widely accepted models are also available to stratify the risk of a surgical infection on a patient-to-patient basis.

Bacterial Inoculum

According to recent data from the NHSN, the most common isolates from SSIs include *Staphylococcus aureus*, coagulase-negative staphylococci, enteroccocci, and *Escherichia coli*. The surgical site needs to be contaminated with at least 10^5 colony-forming units (CFUs) per gram of tissue to markedly increase the risk of SSI. The quantity and species of bacterial inoculum will vary depending on the organ space or body cavity being operated on.

The skin has a concentration of between 10^2 CFU/cm^2 and 10^3 CFU/cm^2 depending on how dry and or exposed the particular area is. The skin is typically colonized by staphyloccocal and streptococcal species, but skin folds and regions in proximity to the anorectal area may harbor gram-negative bacilli, *Enterococcus,* and other typically gastrointestinal species (Mangram et al., 1999). The nasopharynx is home to *Streptococcus pneumoniae, Haemophilus influenza,* and *Staphylococcus aureus*. Although the nasal passages my have up to 10^3 CFU/g of organisms, the distal airway is relatively devoid of microorganisms as a result of the brisk clearance mechanisms of the bronchial tree.

A variance in the bacterial concentration is seen when samples are taken in the normal individual at different points along the alimentary tract, between the oral cavity and the rectum (Figure 2). The oral cavity typically has a concentration of up to 10^9 CFU/g in saliva. This drops to less than 10^3 CFU/g in the stomach and duodenum. The combined effect of stomach acid, bile, and pancreatic juice kills most bacteria in this region. The rapid peristalsis in this part of the alimentary tract impedes bacterial colonization, but the bacterial count continues to rise along the small intestine, and the terminal ileum has a concentration of 10^7 CFU/g in luminal content. The slow transit time within the colon allows bacteria to thrive and establish colonies in the feces-rich environment, resulting in concentrations that exceed 10^{12} CFU/g in feces.

The oropharynx is home to *Streptococci viridans* as well as *Peptostreptococcus, Fusobacterium,* and *Eikenella* species. The organisms found in the stomach and proximal small intestine are mostly gram-negative facultative aerobes such as *Escherichia coli* with some anaerobes of the *Bacteroides* species. In contrast 99% of the colonic flora consists of anaerobic organisms, predominantly *Bacteroides fragilis*. Although between 300 to 500 species of bacteria may be found on detailed examination of colonic flora, only the above mentioned strains tend to predominate as pathogens after spillage of colonic contents. The biliary tree is sterile unless it is obstructed, in which case it is most often colonized by *E. coli, Klebsiella,* and *Enterococcus* organisms.

The normal intestinal populations can be altered by therapeutics, operations, and disease states. In the stomach, acid suppression drugs or a gastric-outlet obstruction can lead to growth of bacteria found more distally in the gut. Similarly, bowel obstructions will result in bacterial overgrowth due to decreased or halted transit. An intestinal bypass procedure may result in a more favorable pH for bacteria in combination with a transit time that allows colonization. This process can sometimes be demonstrated on computed tomographic scan, when fecalization of intraluminal contents is visualized proximal to the point of a bowel obstruction.

Host Defense Mechanisms

A young, healthy, nutritionally sound patient provides the best physiologic environment to perform surgery. In the ideal situation, the operative site has an adequate blood supply to facilitate transport of

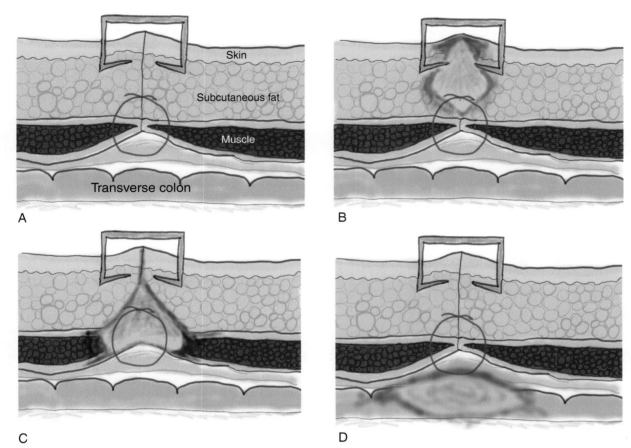

FIGURE I The definition of SSIs. **A,** Normal surgical site (midline incision above the umbilicus). Skin, subcutaneous tissue, muscle, and peritoneal layers are shown. The two layers of rectus fascia are depicted as well as a representation of the transverse colon in the deep organ space. The fascia has been closed with an appropriate suture, and the skin has been stapled. **B,** Superficial incisional SSI includes the skin and subcutaneous tissues and can extend down to level of the fascia. **C,** Deep incisional SSI also involves the muscle layers but does not enter the organ space. **D,** Organ or space SSI involves any part of the operative site other than the incised body wall layers.

oxygen, nutrients, and immune and inflammatory cells. Conversely, as the patient ages and develops underlying diseases such as diabetes, cardiovascular disease, and chronic preclinical or clinical inflammatory processes, the risk for developing infections in an elective or emergent surgical procedure increases.

In patients with diabetes an increasing hemoglobin A1c has been linked to increased SSI rates in coronary artery bypass surgery. Evidence suggests that adequate perioperative glycemic control in patients with diabetes and those without can decrease the risk of SSI. Other acquired habits such as smoking, ethanol ingestion, poor nutrition, and illicit or prescribed drug usage also has a negative influence as it relates to surgical infection. Smoking has been shown to be an independent risk factor for SSI following cardiac surgery, most likely a result of the vasoconstrictive effects of nicotine that result in delayed primary wound healing.

Obesity is a significant health issue, and severe obesity (>25% body weight) can lead to increased risk of SSI in patients undergoing many different types of procedures, from spine surgery to laparoscopic abdominal surgery to cardiac surgery. There is likely decreased perfusion to subcutaneous tissues in an obese patient, but other factors, such as length of the operation or the level of tissue trauma, may also be implicated.

The patient who is immunocompromised by either a disease process such as AIDS or preexisting cancer or a treatment regimen that includes chronic steroid medication is at an increased risk for infection. A patient who already has an underlying inflammatory

infectious process that has precipitated the need for urgent surgical intervention is also at increased risk. Appendicitis, cholecystitis, diverticulitis, and systemic sepsis will have already generated a significant bacterial challenge to the host, and the colony count of the adjacent tissues will have generated a febrile response, local peritoneal irritation, and leukocytosis.

THE SURGICAL SITE AND SURGEON TECHNIQUE

The potential for an infection is directly related to the size of the inoculum that is introduced into the surgical wound. The skin should be clean, and the inoculum of surface-derived bacteria should be minimized by a bacteriostatic or bacteriocidal fluid applied shortly before the incision. Chlorhexidene, alcohol, and iodine-based scrubs have good activity against the usual skin flora, and chlorhexidene also has excellent residual activity. Hair should not be shaved prior to the incision. The act of shaving can imbed bacteria into the skin and wound by inadvertently lacerating the dermis. Clippers remove hair but do not cause lacerations. Prior to placing an incision through a hair-bearing area, this area should be debrided with clippers, not a razor.

Meticulous operative techniques that minimize trauma to the tissues and avoid leaving necrotic tissue, seromas, or hematomas decrease the risk of infection. Minimization of tissue trauma, cautery, and blood loss all have a positive influence on the ability to minimize

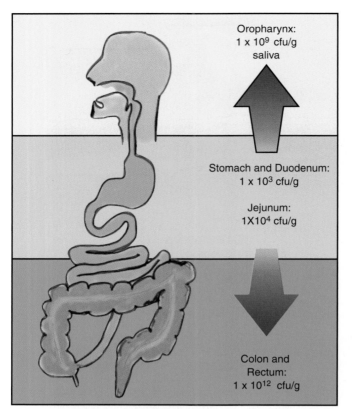

FIGURE 2   Concentration of bacteria along the gastrointestinal tract. The mouth and pharynx have a high concentration of bacteria (10^9 CFU/g). This drops to 10^3 CFU/g in the stomach because of the acidity and progressively increases along the small bowel and into the colon, where the concentration is 10^{12} CFU/g in feces.

infection. Similarly, decreasing the time spent in the operating room under anesthesia, maintaining normal tissue perfusion, and minimizing local and systemic hypotension with resultant acidosis decreases the chance of infection. The patient should have adequate tissue oxygenation, which can be enhanced by preoperative, mask-delivered hyperoxygenation. The serum glucose should be adequately controlled. Measures should also be taken to maintain an adequate core temperature during surgery. Blood and fluid losses should be anticipated and counteracted by intravenous infusion in a timely manner to maintain euvolemia.

RISK STRATIFICATION

There are several systems that have been developed to stratify the risk of SSI in a given operative procedure. One method is to evaluate the risk based on the predicted level of microbial contamination that will result in the wound. The operative procedure ranges from a clean environment—such as an elective breast procedure, which should have minimal bacterial inoculum potential—to an elective bowel procedure, in which there is a high likelihood of aerobic and anaerobic enteric organisms that are likely to be introduced into the operative field. Operations performed emergently in unprepared bowel that has already shed fecal content into the wound, such as a perforated diverticulum or a gunshot wound to the colon, have a high risk for infection.

The National Academy of Sciences National Research Council definitions of wound class were first published in 1964 and are now widely accepted. They define four wound classes: *clean* (class I), *clean-contaminated* (class II), *contaminated* (class III), and *dirty or infected*

(class IV). Although this classification was useful in stratifying the risk of infection, it did not take into account other patient-related and operation-specific factors that may affect the risk of SSI. In fact, in a class I (clean) wound, infection rates can vary from 1% to 15%.

PRINCIPLES OF ANTIBIOTIC USE

Antibiotic prophylaxis is an essential element in the armamentarium of infection prevention and management. The essential tenet is that the therapeutic goal is to obtain serum antibiotic levels greater than the minimum inhibitory concentration (MIC) for the specific bacteria that will be inoculated into the wound. The MIC refers to the concentration of antibiotic required to inhibit bacterial growth in vitro. The choice of antibiotic is dependent on the knowledge of the specific organism and its susceptibility to the antibiotic that will be selected. If this is not known, an intelligent guess based on historic evidence of bacteria associated with the injured or infected organ is appropriate.

Timing of Preoperative Antibiotics

The issue of when to give preoperative antibiotics to maximize prevention of infection is an important one. The rationale is based on principles that were elucidated by Burke and colleagues over 50 years ago. In those studies, bacteria was injected into the dermis of guinea pigs to observe the evolution of sepsis in the animal. Researchers noted a positive effect of antibiotics on the development of septic lesions, if the antibiotics were given 1 hour before staphylococci were injected. This landmark paper has influenced the way antibiotics have been administered over the years. It is important to note that administering the antibiotic more than 3 hours after staphylococci had been introduced had no effect on the size of the lesion.

Although these data have been available for over a half a century, the practice of antibiotic administration in surgery has been to administer the antibiotics at the end of the operation and continue this until the patient was discharged from the hospital. Current recommendations are to administer antibiotics at least 1 hour preoperatively in patients undergoing elective surgery. If a patient has a preexisting infection, such as cholecystitis or appendicitis, or the patient has a penetrating injury to the colon, the practice is to administer antibiotics as early as possible after the diagnosis is made.

Over the past three decades, a number of controlled trials have investigated the most efficacious method of antibiotic prophylaxis. Appropriately administered prophylactic antibiotics can decrease the risk of postoperative infection by 50%. Classen and colleagues looked at the relationship between antibiotic timing and the risk of SSI in 2847 elective clean or clean-contaminated cases in 1985 and 1986 at a large community hospital. The study showed that the lowest risk of SSI occurred when antibiotics were given between zero and 2 hours prior to making the incision. Bratzler and colleagues recommend that the first dose of antimicrobial prophylaxis be given within an hour of the incision as part of the advisory statement from the National Surgical Infection Prevention Project (2005). This recommendation forms the basis of the Surgical Care Improvement Program (SCIP) quality measures regarding perioperative antibiotics (Table 1).

The timing of delivery of prophylactic antibiotics is directly related to the pharmacodynamics of how a specific antibiotic achieves drug concentration in both the serum and the tissue. It is important to achieve a high concentration of antibiotic in the serum prior to the introduction of a bacterial inoculum. The antibiotic has to exceed the minimal inhibitory concentration of the specific bacteria in the tissues to prevent the growth and multiplication of the bacteria. This effectively allows the host's internal defense mechanisms, including white cell activation and leukocytosis, to overwhelm the bacteria in the inoculum.

In a normal host, the recommended therapeutic dose for the antibiotic used is usually sufficient to prevent SSI. In the case of a

TABLE 1: SCIP national quality measures related to antibiotic prophylaxis

SCIP 1	Prophylactic antibiotic received within 1 hour before surgical incision
SCIP 2	Prophylactic antibiotic selection for surgical patients
SCIP 3	Prophylactic antibiotics discontinued within 24 hours after surgery end time (within 48 hours after surgery end time for cardiac surgery)

Modified from the Joint Commission for Accreditation of Healthcare Organizations Specifications Manual for National Hospital Quality Measures Version 2.6b, April 2009.

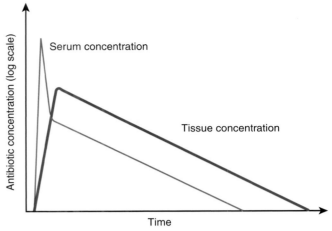

FIGURE 3 The serum and tissue concentrations of an antibiotic are shown over time from an initial intravenous dose. *(Modified from Ulualp K, Condon RE: Antibiotic prophylaxis for scheduled operative procedures, Inf Dis Clin North Am 6[3]:613–625, 1992.)*

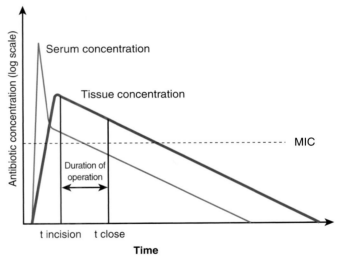

FIGURE 4 The concentrations of antibiotic in the serum and tissue during an operation. The two vertical lines represent the time of the incision (*t incision*) and the time of wound closure (*t close*). The MIC for the operation is shown with a dashed line. *(Modified from Ulualp K, Condon RE: Antibiotic prophylaxis for scheduled operative procedures, Inf Dis Clin North Am 6[3]:613–625, 1992.)*

compromised host or an overwhelming concentration of bacteria, it may be necessary to exceed the minimal bacteriocidal concentration (MBC) to prevent spreading of the infection. The type of antibiotic, as well as the specific activity of that particular antibiotic to the specific organism, enhances the body's ability to prevent an infection or to contain an infection that is already present.

Antibiotics have two main types of bactericidal activity. The first results in increasing bactericidal activity with increasing concentrations of antibiotic. Aminoglycosides, fluoroquinolones, and metronidazole all exhibit this concentration-dependent killing. The second results in increasing bactericidal activity over time of exposure to a concentration of antibiotic. The concentration is usually thought to be higher than the MIC of the antibiotic for that organism. This time-dependent killing activity is observed in vancomycin and β-lactam agents including penicillins, cephalosporins, monobactams, and carbapenems.

Ulualp and Condon described a two-compartment system comprising the central intravascular compartment and the peripheral tissue compartment to model the distribution of a preoperative antibiotic in a patient. When an antibiotic is given intravenously, it rapidly accumulates within the intravascular compartment, resulting in a peak serum concentration. The intravascular compartment equilibrates with the peripheral tissue compartment over several minutes, resulting in a peak tissue concentration. As the antibiotic is metabolized, the serum concentration falls over time. Since the intravascular compartment is in equilibrium with the tissue compartment, the tissue concentration also falls at the same rate over time.

These pharmacodynamics can be better understood in the form of an example of an antibiotic given before the start of an elective surgical procedure. A suitable example is the use of a cephalosporin in an elective clean-contaminated case, such as a scheduled sigmoid colon resection for recurrent diverticulitis. Figure 3 describes the relationship of the concentration of antibiotics with the timing of administration of antibiotic prophylaxis. The antibiotic is given intravenously and initially resides in the vascular compartment. In the initial phase, the tissue concentration rises exponentially, while the serum concentration falls as the antibiotic equilibrates between the intravascular and peripheral tissue compartments. This transient peak in serum tissue concentration of the antibiotic occurs within minutes of its administration. Once equilibrium is achieved, both the serum and tissue concentrations should fall at a similar steady rate based on the elimination half-life of the antibiotic. The tissue antibiotic concentrations lag behind the serum concentrations but remain at high levels for a longer period.

Figure 4 shows a dashed line that represents the minimum inhibitory concentration required to control the expected bacterial load in this case. The MIC should take into account the combination of residual skin flora, external contamination, and controlled contamination during the colon resection. The surgical wound is only exposed to this bacterial load between the start and finish of the case, and so the times of the incision and closure are indicated with vertical lines. In this example it is clear to see that the operative time falls within the period in which the tissue concentration of antibiotic is above

the MIC. It is important to note that the antibiotic is given prior to the incision being performed. To achieve the most effective antibiotic prophylaxis, it is essential that both serum and tissue levels are above MIC prior to the bacterial inoculum. It is also critical that the tissue levels exceed MIC prior to incision. The tissue levels must remain above the MIC for the bacteria for the duration of the operation.

The time it takes to achieve the serum concentration varies from antibiotic to antibiotic and depends on properties of protein binding, elimination route, and how quickly the antibiotic can be infused. The common cephalosporins used today achieve this well within an hour of intravenous administration, and this correlates well with data from observation studies. Vancomycin and fluoroquinolones have to be infused over a longer period of time, and so it is not appropriate to dose these antibiotics an hour before incision and expect to achieve tissue concentrations above the MIC at the time of incision. The SCIP measure asks that these antibiotics be dosed within 2 hours of the incision.

TABLE 2: Most common pathogens and recommended antibiotics based on location or type of operation

Operation	Pathogens[†]	Antibiotic Choices[‡]
Head and neck	*Staphylococcus aureus*; streptococci; oropharyngeal anaerobes (peptostreptococci)	Cefazolin (clindamycin, vancomycin*)
Gastroduodenal	Gram-negative bacilli; streptococci; oropharyngeal anaerobes (peptostreptococci)	Cefazolin, cefoxitin, cefotetan (ciprofloxacin + metronidazole)
Biliary	Gram-negative bacilli; streptococci; anaerobes	Noninfected: cefazolin Infected: cefoxitin, cefotetan, ampicillin-sulbactam (ciprofloxacin + metronidazole)
Colorectal	Gram-negative bacilli; streptococci; anaerobes	Cefoxitin, cefotetan, ampicillin- sulbactam, ertapenem, cefazolin + metronidazole (ciprofloxacin + metronidazole)
Breast	*S. aureus*; coagulase-negative staphylococci	Cefazolin (clindamycin, vancomycin*)
Cardiac	*S. aureus*; coagulase-negative staphylococci	Cefazolin, cefuroxime (clindamycin, vancomycin*)
Noncardiac thoracic	*S. aureus*; coagulase-negative staphylococci; *Streptococcus pneumoniae*; gram-negative bacilli	Cefazolin, cefuroxime (clindamycin, vancomycin*)
Vascular	*S. aureus*; coagulase-negative staphylococci	Cefazolin (clindamycin, vancomycin*)
Orthopedic	*S. aureus*; coagulase-negative staphylococci; gram-negative bacilli	Cefazolin, cefuroxime (clindamycin, vancomycin*)
Obstetric and gynecologic	Gram-negative bacilli; enterococci; group B streptococci; anaerobes	Cesearean: cefazolin (clindamycin) Other procedures, nonpregnant patient: cefazolin, cefoxitin, cefuroxime (clindamycin, vancomycin*)
Urologic	Gram-negative bacilli	Cefazolin, ciprofloxacin

Alternatives for patients with β-lactam allergy are in parentheses.
Modified from Mangram AJ, Horan TC, Pearson ML, et al: Guideline for prevention of surgical site infection, 1999, *Infect Control Hosp Epidemiol* 20(1):247–279, 1999; and Kirby JP, Mazuski JE: Prevention of surgical site infection, *Surg Clin North Am* 89:365–389, 2009.
*Vancomycin should only be used if there is a high likelihood of infection with resistant staphylococci.
†Skin flora (staphyloccocci) can cause surgical infections in all locations where a skin incision is made.
‡Clean surgical procedures do not need prophylaxis unless surgical risk is great or an implant is used.

A number of operational factors influence the effectiveness of bacterial prophylaxis. There needs to be a tight and clear coordination of the patient being sent to the operating room, arriving in the preoperative area, being given the antibiotic, and being transported to the operating suite for the incision. If the antibiotic is given, and the operative incision is delayed, the antibiotic levels in the tissue can fall below the appropriate levels during the operation. This will leave the patient unprotected and vulnerable to bacterial load during the latter portion of the operation.

Procedure-Specific Selection of Antibiotics

The second quality measure of the SCIP stipulates an appropriate selection of prophylactic antibiotic specific to the surgical procedure. At this stage the assessment for the risk of surgical infection should have already been made, based on wound class and patient factors, and the surgeon will have already decided that the patient will need prophylactic antibiotics. The antibiotic that is best suited for the space or organ being operated on is then selected. The two operation-specific factors that will determine this are 1) the species of bacteria that will be encountered during the operation and 2) the ability of the antibiotics to penetrate the tissue being operated on. Additional factors that are important in choosing the right antibiotic to use include the cost of the antibiotic and the risk of generating antibiotic resistance.

Bacterial Pathogens and Antibiotic Selection

The surgeon should be aware of the bacterial flora likely to be associated with each specific operation. Table 2 shows the bacteria associated with common general surgery operations and some recommended antibiotics. The antibiotic selected should have activity against the bacteria likely to be present in the wound. The dosage of antibiotics should be such that it has the capability to be fully effective against the bacteria.

Cefazolin is widely used for prophylaxis of SSI. It is a first-generation cephalosporin with a spectrum of activity that includes streptococcal and staphyloccal species as well as some activity against *Escherichia coli* and *Klebsiella* species. This makes it ideal for use in clean-contaminated cases of the foregut and midgut that are susceptible to skin and bowel flora as well as for clean cases that require the use of implants. It has no activity against anaerobes such as *Bacteroides* species that are encountered in colon surgery, and so it must be paired with metronidazole for those cases. Vancomycin may be substituted in patients who have penicillin or cephalosporin allergies.

Cefoxitin and cefotetan are second-generation cephalosporins that provide some coverage against staphylococcal and streptococcal species but have increased coverage against gram-negative organisms such as *E. coli*. They also provide coverage against anaerobes and are currently recommended by both the SCIP and the FDA for use in colorectal surgery prophylaxis. Unfortunately, because they have been in clinical use for over 20 years, their effectiveness against *Bacteroides* species may be diminishing.

Ampicillin-sulbactam combines ampicillin with a β-lactamase inhibitor to create a drug that has a spectrum of activity similar to that of cefoxitin that can be used for colorectal or contaminated cases. Ertapenem is a carbapenem antibiotic that has been recently approved by the FDA for colorectal prophylaxis because of its excellent activity against gram-negative bacilli and anaerobes.

The species of bacteria encountered may also vary with different hospitals. For this reason, the hospital should have an effective infection surveillance program that identifies and constantly updates the current antibiotic sensitivities for the specific hospital. This also prevents the overuse of antibiotics that may lead to the generation of multidrug-resistant organisms.

Duration of Antibiotic Therapy

The two main controversies regarding the duration of antibiotic therapy are whether to redose the prophylactic antibiotic during the case and whether to continue dosing of antibiotics postoperatively. The frequently quoted 1999 SSI guidelines set forth by the CDC committee not only recommends the intravenous dosing of an antimicrobial prophylactic agent to achieve adequate serum and tissue concentrations prior to making the incision but also to maintain these levels throughout the operation.

Redosing of Prophylactic Antibiotic During a Case

The need for redosing an antibiotic seems intuitive when considering the pathophysiology and pharmacodynamics involved. If the operation takes longer than was scheduled, if there is significant blood loss with a diminution in the antibiotic levels, or if there is an increased bacterial load during the procedure, the prophylactic effect of the antibiotic may be diluted. This can be illustrated in the example described earlier of the antibiotic use in an elective surgical case. Figure 5 shows a situation in which the tissue concentration falls below the MIC before the end of the operation. This usually happens because the duration of the case is increased because of unforeseen technical difficulties or because of a complication, but it may also occur when an antibiotic with too short a half-life is chosen. Figure 6 shows that

when the antibiotic is redosed in a timely manner, it is possible to restore the tissue concentrations above the MIC and maintain them for the duration of the operation. For effective redosing to take place, the surgeon must assess the likelihood that a procedure will take longer than expected and decide whether to administer the antibiotic.

POSTOPERATIVE ANTIBIOTIC PROPHYLAXIS

The SCIP guidelines state that antibiotics for prophylaxis should be discontinued within 24 hours of the surgery, but they make an exception for open heart surgery, in which they should be discontinued within 48 hours. After wound closure the formation of a seroma or hematoma or the presence of drains or implants may function as a nidus for a wound infection to develop. The concern is often greatest after high-risk procedures such as open heart surgery and vascular operations. Prophylactic antibiotics were often continued well into the postoperative period. Since the original recommendations from the CDC in 1999, several reviews of the literature have concluded that there is no advantage to extending the duration of antibiotic prophylaxis beyond 24 hours, and often no benefit is seen from any therapy beyond the time the wound is closed. Indeed, even in the presence of drains and tubes, the Society of Thoracic Surgeons (2006 guidelines) has made a strong statement in favor of discontinuing surgical prophylaxis after 48 hours even in the most high-risk patients.

ADVERSE EFFECTS OF ANTIBIOTIC THERAPY

When considering the duration of antibiotic prophylaxis, it is also important to consider the adverse effects of prolonged antibiotic therapy. These include the complications of antibiotic therapy, such as acute renal failure and drug hypersensitivity reactions. A complication that has significant morbidity and mortality is pseudomembranous colitis as a result of the elimination of organisms that would compete with *Clostridium difficile*. This disease is often caused by therapy with clindamycin but may also result from the use of cephalasporins and other β-lactams. The inappropriate use of antibiotics can also result in the generation of multidrug-resistant organisms. Every measure should be taken to reduce exposure of

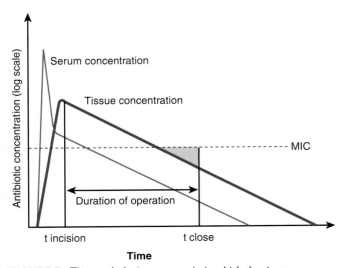

FIGURE 5 This graph depicts a scenario in which the tissue concentration falls below the MIC within the duration of the operation (*shaded triangle*). This can happen as a result of an unanticipated technical difficulty or a complication that requires additional time to manage. It can also occur when an antibiotic with a shorter half-life is used.

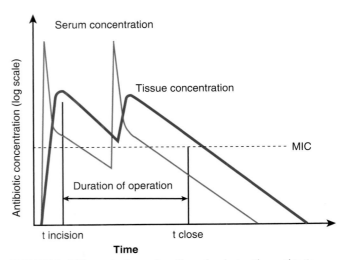

FIGURE 6 This graph shows the effect of redosing the antibiotic during an operation. When there is an indication that the operation will last longer than expected, a second antibiotic dose administered in a timely fashion (*arrow*) results in a situation in which the tissue concentration never falls below the MIC during the operation.

the patient to antibiotics beyond the period in which they are absolutely necessary.

SPECIAL CONSIDERATIONS

Colorectal Surgery

It is clear that the colon and rectum are the areas of the digestive tract most densely populated by organisms that can cause SSIs. For several years surgeons have combined oral antibiotic regimens with a mechanical bowel preparation (MBP) as part of standard antimicrobial prophylaxis. Oral antibiotics are typically neomycin and erythromycin, administered in three doses on the night before the operation. They are not well absorbed but do act to reduce the concentration of intraluminal bacteria from 10^9 to 10^7 CFU/g. The MBP generates a more significant drop in the concentration, as it removes fecal matter on which the microorganisms feed. This combination, in addition to an appropriate intravenous preoperative antibiotic, has been shown to reduce SSIs.

Over the years it has been shown that there may not be a significant benefit to MBP and oral antibiotics. A recent meta-analysis (2009) looked at 14 randomized controlled trials that compared the effect of MBP to no MBP in colorectal surgery. Surprisingly, the analysis showed that there may be an increased outcome of SSI in those patients who received MBP. There are also reports that MBP may be associated with complications such as dehydration, acute renal failure, and severe electrolyte imbalances in the elderly. It may be important to weigh the risks and benefits of this practice on a patient-to-patient basis.

Trauma

Antibiotic prophylaxis for wound infection in a trauma setting deals with wound classes in the contaminated to dirty category. A broad-spectrum antibiotic should be administered prior to exploration and may need to be redosed depending on the amount of blood loss encountered. If significant spillage has taken place, there may be a need to abandon prophylaxis and switch to a treatment course for presumed intraabdominal infection and a high likelihood of SSI.

The Eastern Association for the Surgery of Trauma (EAST) guidelines recommend a single preoperative dose of appropriate antibiotics and that therapy should not extend past 24 hours. These recommendations concur with the SCIP measures discussed earlier and are backed by level I–quality evidence. They also make a recommendation for dosing in the patient with hemorrhagic shock (level III) that is mostly based on current opinion. They suggest a twofold to threefold initial dose of appropriate antibiotic followed by a repeat dose for every 10 units of blood transfused.

SUMMARY

Infections in surgical patients continue to be a determinant of major morbidity and mortality. SSI rates are used to evaluate hospital standards and may eventually measure the individual surgeon's performance. It is important to first consider the type of operation and the patient's medical problems to use established risk stratification guidelines to decide which patients require antibiotic prophylaxis. Next the location of the operative site based on the specific surgery should determine the types of bacteria encountered. This information taken together with hospital surveillance data and the patient's allergic profile should then determine the appropriate choice of antibiotic. This antibiotic should be given at an appropriate time so that an adequate tissue concentration of antibiotic is available at the time of the incision. The correct and timely administration of prophylactic antibiotics in addition to adequate surgical site preparation and good surgical technique should result in effective prevention of surgical site infections.

SUGGESTED READINGS

Bassetti D, Akalin HE, de Lalla F: Alternatives to established surgical prophylactic practices, *J Hosp Infect* 50(suppl A):S1–S23, 2000.

Bratzler DW, Houck PM: Antimicrobial prophylaxis for surgery: an advisory statement from the National Surgical Infection Prevention Project, *Clin Infect Dis* 38:1706–1715, 2004.

Burke JF: The effective period of preventative antibiotic action in experimental incisions and dermal lesions, *Surgery* 50(1):161–168, 1961.

Classen DC, Evans RS, Pestotnik SL, et al: The timing of prophylactic administration of antibiotics and the risk of surgical-wound infection, *N Engl J Med* 326(5):281–286, 1992.

DiPiro JT, Edmiston CE, Bothren JMA: Pharmacodynamocs of antimicrobial therapy in surgery, *Am J Surg* 171:615–622, 1996.

Edwards FH, Engelman RM, Houck P, et al: The Society of Thoracic Surgeons practice guideline series: antibiotic prophylaxis in cardiac surgery. Part I: duration, *Ann Thorac Surg* 81:397–404, 2006.

Edwards JR, Peterson KD, Andrus ML, et al: National Healthcare Safety Network (NHSN) Report, data summary for 2006 through 2007, issued November 2008, *Am J Infect Control* 36:609–626, 2008.

Elsner P: Antimicrobials and the skin: physiological and pathological flora, *Curr Probl Dermatol* (33):35–41, 2006.

Falagas ME, Kompoti M: Obesity and infection, *Lancet Infect Dis* 6:438–446, 2006.

Farber MS, Abrams JH: Antibiotics for the acute abdomen, *Surg Clin North Am* 77(6):1395–1417, 1997.

Fry DE: Preventative systemic antibiotics in colorectal surgery, *Surgical Infect (Larchmont)* 9(6):547–552, 2008.

Guarner F: Enteric flora in health and disease, *Digestion* 73(suppl 1):5–12, 2006.

Hurst JR, Wilkinson TMA, Perera WR, et al: Relationships among bacteria, upper airway, lower airway and systemic inflammation in COPD, *Chest* 127:1219–1226, 2005.

Jacobs R, Wiener-Kronish J: Editorial view—endotracheal tubes: the conduit for oral and nasal microbial communities to the lungs, *Anesthesiology* 104:224–225, 2006.

The Joint Commission for Accreditation of Healthcare Organizations: *Specifications manual for national hospital quality measures*, version 2.6b. Available at http://www.jointcommission.org/performancemeasurement/ performancemeasurement/historical+NHQM+manuals.htm.

Kirby JP, Mazuski JE: Prevention of surgical site infection, *Surg Clin North Am* 89:365–389, 2009.

Levinson W, Jawetz E: *Medical microbiology and immunology examination and board review*, ed 6, 2000, McGraw-Hill.

Liesegang TJ: Prophylactic antibiotics in cataract operations, *Mayo Clin Proc* 72(2):149–159, 1997.

Luchette FA, Borzotta AP, Croce MA, et al: Practice management guidelines for prophylactic antibiotic use in penetrating abdominal trauma (EAST guidelines), *J Trauma* 48(3):508–518, 2000.

Mangram AJ, Horan TC, Pearson ML, et al: Guideline for prevention of surgical site infection. 1999 *Infection control and hospital epidemiology* 20(1):247–279, 1999.

McDonald M, Grabsch E, Marshall C, Forbes A: Single- versus multiple-dose antimicrobial prophylaxis for major surgery: a systematic review, *Aust N Z J Surg* 68:388–396, 1998.

Meakins JL, et al: Prevention of postoperative infection. In Souba WW, Fink MP, Jurkovich GJ, editors: *ACS surgery: principles and practice*, New York, 2008, BC Decker, p 17.

Nelson RL, Glenny AM, Song F: Antimicrobial prophylaxis for colorectal surgery, *Cochrane Database Syst Rev* (3):CD001181, 2009.

Novelli A: Antimicrobial prophylaxis in surgery: the role of pharmacokinetics, *J Chemother* 11(6):565–572, 1999.

Opal SM, Keusch GT: Host response to infection. *Cohen & Powdery: infectious diseases*, ed 2, St Louis, 2004, Mosby Elsevier.

Polk HC, Christmas AB: Prophylactic antibiotics in surgery and surgical wound infections, *Am Surg* 66(2):105–111, 2000.

Ulualp K, Condon RE: Antibiotic prophylaxis for scheduled operative procedures, *Inf Dis Clin N Am* 6(3):613–625, 1992.

Slim K, Vicaut E, Launay-Savary MV, et al: Updated systematic review and meta-analysis of randomized clinical trials on the role of mechanical bowel preparation before colorectal surgery, *Ann Surg* 249(2):203–209, 2009.

Song F, Glenny AM: Antimicrobial prophylaxis in colorectal surgery: a systematic review of randomized control trials, *Br J Surg* 85(9):1232–1241, 1998.

Williams REO: Benefit and mischief from commensal bacteria, *J Clin Path* 26:811–818, 1973.

Endocrine Changes in Critical Illness

John H. Adamski II, MD, MPH, Grant V. Bochicchio, MD, MPH, and Thomas M. Scalea, MD

OVERVIEW

Critical illness that includes injury, surgery, infection, and burns results in significant changes in the endocrine system. The acute phase releases hormones that shunt substrate and oxygen to the most critical organs and modulate the immune response. The prolonged response is characterized by persistent hypercatabolism. The acute phase adapts to the stress, but the prolonged phase may contribute to organ dysfunction and death (Table 1).

The hypothalamic-pituitary-adrenal (HPA) axis is essential to our stress response. Activation of the HPA axis modulates a "flight or fight" response and diverts adrenal function from mineralocorticoid to glucocorticoid production. The hypothalamus secretes corticotrophin-releasing hormone (CRH) and vasopressin, and CRH stimulates the anterior pituitary gland to release adrenal corticotrophic hormone (ACTH). Vasopressin acts with CRH to increase release of ACTH from the anterior pituitary, stimulating the release of the cortisol. Although ACTH can stimulate aldosterone and androgen secretion, these hormones are primarily regulated by the renin-angiotensin system and pituitary gonadotropins.

The adrenal cortex does not store cortisol. Normal cortisol secretion is pulsatile and has diurnal variation, with the highest levels in the morning. Hypercortisolism inhibits the HPA axis, and cortisol deficiency stimulates cortisol production. Illness can alter cortisol binding capacities, eliminate diurnal variation, and disturb the normal feedback loop. Extremely low levels of cortisol, as well as very high cortisol levels, increase mortality.

As critically ill patients enter a hypermetabolic state, they also develop distinct alterations of their carbohydrate metabolism. Increased levels of catecholamines and glucocorticoids produce hyperglycemia. Other hormones such as corticotrophin, growth hormone, and glucagons inhibit hepatic glycogenesis and peripheral glycolysis while promoting gluconeogenesis, hepatic and muscle glycogenolysis, and peripheral lipolysis. Peripheral glycolysis and the breakdown of glycogen, lipids, and (later) muscle protein provides the substrates for hepatic gluconeogenesis in the form of pyruvate, glycerol, and alanine.

The two most clinically relevant endocrine changes with critical illness are adrenal insufficiency and hyperglycemia. Rather than catalog a list of all changes, we have decided to focus on these. In this chapter, we will attempt to outline the controversies and provide the practicing clinician with guidance about these two complex issues.

ADRENAL INSUFFICIENCY

Adrenal insufficiency can be either a fundamental failure of the adrenal gland (primary adrenal insufficiency) or a failure of the hypothalamus or pituitary gland to stimulate the adrenal cortex (secondary adrenal insufficiency). The etiologies are listed in Table 2. Clinical symptoms of primary adrenal insufficiency include weakness, anorexia, weight loss, depression, fatigue, nausea, vomiting, orthostatic hypotension, and craving for salt. Physical findings may include tachycardia, hypotension, fever, mental status changes, amenorrhea, hypovolemia, and hyperpigmentation. Laboratory findings include hyponatremia, hyperkalemia, hypoglycemia, eosinophila, and normocytic normochromic anemia. These findings are similar in secondary adrenal insufficiency with a few exceptions. The lack of mineralocorticoid deficiency in secondary adrenal insufficiency limits urinary losses of water, sodium, and chloride. Hyperpigmentation as a result of ACTH elevation is only seen in primary adrenal insufficiency.

Diseases that cause outright chronic adrenal failure are rare; however, diseases that cause a disposition to adrenal failure during stress are frequent. The limitations of physical exam and the confounding effects of comorbidities or intensive care treatments make it difficult to recognize adrenal insufficiency. The absence of classic features of hypoadrenalism and the transient changes of serious illness further complicate this diagnosis. Lack of a reference standard, limitations of diagnostic testing, and an inability to develop a universal definition of adrenal insufficiency mean physicians must actively search for the diagnosis and use good common sense in developing treatment protocols.

Hemodynamic instability and hyperinflammation despite fluid resuscitation and pressor support are the hallmarks of adrenal insufficiency. Hemodynamic improvement upon cortisol administration makes the diagnosis. HPA reactivity is tested by measuring a baseline random cortisol level, followed by administration of 250 µg ACTH (cosyntropin) intravenously and assessment of cortisol levels at 30 and 60 minutes after infusion. In response to stress, the normal adrenal gland should produce cortisol levels above 18 to 20 µg/dL. This so-called *normal level* is derived from high-dose ACTH stimulation or insulin-induced hypoglycemia in patients who are not stressed or critically ill. Associated random serum cortisol levels greater than 25 µg/dL or an incremental change in baseline greater than 9 µg/dL are also considered normal responses. Using this definition, an inadequate adrenal response occurs in up to 60% of septic patients. These cutoff values have come from studies of factors associated with poor outcomes. In addition, the outcomes of treatment protocols have varied with use of high-dose (30 mg/kg) or moderate-dose (200 to 300 mg/day) glucocorticoid replacement.

A number of issues are of concern here. High-dose 250 µg ACTH is a supraphysiologic concentration that may elicit a normal cortisol response by overcoming ACTH resistance in the adrenals without adequate functional reserves. Moreover, the adrenals may already be maximally stimulated at baseline in response to illness and may be unable to show an increase of 9 µg/dL. Likewise, there are differences in sensitivity, accuracy, and reproducibility among commercially available cortisol assays. It is still unknown whether adrenal insufficiency is transient, functional, or structural during critical illness.

Alterations in protein binding, cortisol metabolism and clearance, and end-organ resistance may also influence the measurement of cortisol. A low-dose synthetic 1 µg ACTH stimulation test has been suggested to be more physiologic and sensitive for diagnosis, but data are limited. One option is testing by stimulation with low-dose 1 µg ACTH first and afterward with high-dose 250 µg ACTH in nonresponders. Regardless of what ACTH test is used, it is important to remember that test results may not reflect the adrenals' response to the stressors that accompany critical illness.

Some generalizations are outlined in Figure 1 and can be supplemented with a review of the American College of Critical Care Medicine consensus statement on the diagnosis and management of corticosteroid insufficiency in the critically ill adult patient. Classic signs and symptoms of adrenal insufficiency are not always present in the critically ill. Moreover, these findings may be masked or attributed to the disease process at hand. For instance, aggressive electrolyte protocols may mask electrolyte abnormalities. Similarly, fever and hypotension may accompany many illnesses.

Unexplained hemodynamic instability should raise suspicion of HPA dysfunction. Patients with refractory hypotension should be

TABLE 1: Overview of the endocrine system response to acute and prolonged phase of critical illness and potential interventions

Hormone	Acute Phase	Prolonged Phase	Potential Intervention
Sympathomimetic System			
Norepinephrine	++	+/=	May need vasopressor therapy if endogenous stores are inadequate
Epinephrine	++	+/=	
Somatotropic Axis			
Pulsatile GH release	+	–	Exogenous GH administration associated with increased mortality rate
GHBP	–	+	
IGF-1	–	–	
ALS	–	–	
IGFBP-3	–	–	
Hypothalamic-Pituitary-Thyroid Axis			
Pulsatile tsh release	+/=	–	No benefit of replacement and may prolong recovery to euthyroid state
T4	+/=	–	
T3	–	–	
rT3	+	+/=	
Hypothalamic-Pituitary and Lactotropic Axis			
Pulsatile LH release	+/=	–	No benefit of replacement
Testosterone	–	–	
Dehydroepiandrosterone	–	–	
Pulsatile prolactin release	+	–	
Hypothalamic-Pituitary-Adrenal Axis			
ACTH	+	–	Replace if biochemical evidence of relative insufficiency in septic shock
Cortisol	++	+/=	

ACTH, Adrenocorticotropic hormone; *ALS,* acid-labile subunit; *GH,* growth hormone; *GHBP,* growth hormone binding protein; *IGF-1,* insulinlike growth factor-1; *IGFBP-3,* insulinlike growth factor binding protein-3; *LH,* luteinizing hormone; *rT3,* reverse triiodothyronine; *T3,* triiodothyronine; *T4,* thyroxine; *TSH,* Thyroid stimulating hormone
Modified from Vanhorebeek I, Van den Berghe G: The neuroendocrine response to critical illness is a dynamic process, *Crit Care Clin* 22:1, 2006.
+, Increase from baseline; –, decrease from baseline; =, no change from baseline

given 200 to 300 mg/day of intravenous hydrocortisone in divided doses. Mineralocorticoid supplementation with 50 μg/day oral fludrocortisone is optional, as the oral route may not be available, and more than 50 mg/day hydrocortisone has sufficient mineralocorticoid activity. Hydrocortisone should be continued for 7 days and then tapered slowly, and the surgeon must have a low threshold to reinstitute steroids.

TABLE 2: Etiology of adrenal insufficiency in critical illness

Adrenal Insufficiency	Etiology
Primary	Bilateral adrenal necrosis and hemorrhage caused by sepsis, hypotension, and hemorrhage
	Unmasking of chronic known or latent primary insufficiency
	Autoimmune adrenalitis in developed countries
	Tuberculous adrenalitis in developing countries
	Infectious diseases (fungal, viral, HIV)
Secondary	Irreversible anatomic damage to the hypothalamus or the pituitary gland
	Necrosis or hemorrhage in sepsis as a result of prolonged hypotension or coagulopathy
	Unmasking of chronic known or latent secondary adrenal insufficiency caused by sepsis
	Hypothalamic or pituitary tumors
	Chronic inflammation
	Congenital adrenocorticotropic hormone deficiency
	Drug therapy
	Inhibition of early increase in adrenocorticotropic hormone caused by high-dose diazepam and fentanyl administration
	Previous treatments with glucocorticoids including topical administration
	Inhibition of steroid genesis with a single dose of etomidate
	Accelerated metabolism of cortisol by ketoconazole and cyclosporine, clarithromycin, rifampicin, and antiepileptic drugs, such as phenytoin and phenobarbital

Administration of steroid therapy in the patient with refractory hypotension is a clinical decision. Hence, ACTH stimulation tests are not always required. Adrenal testing is recommended for patients with subtle signs of adrenal insufficiency. A random cortisol level less than 25 μg/dL warrants high-dose (250 μg) ACTH testing. Failure of cortisol levels to increase greater than 9 μg/dL over baseline after ACTH stimulation suggests adrenal insufficiency, and cortisol therapy should be implemented. A random cortisol level less than 10 μg/dL is also indicative of adrenal insufficiency and justifies glucocorticoid therapy.

Hydrocortisone therapy is not warranted as an adjuvant therapy for sepsis without evidence of shock. Diagnostic testing and treatment should be started together in the unstable patient. Supplementation should be started following test results in the hemodynamically stable patient. Although dexamethasone was once advocated as a bridge to treatment pending results, it inhibits the HPA axis for a longer period and may alter test results or therapy effects. Hence, dexamethasone is no longer recommended.

HYPERGLYCEMIA

In critically ill patients, an acute sustained increase in serum glucose in response to stress is defined as *hyperglycemia*. These previously euglycemic patients typically return to their normal physiologic state once the acute process resolves. This "diabetes of injury" was once considered a compensatory response required to cope with critical stress. However, it is now known that it imposes a range of adverse

Adrenal Insufficiency in Critical Illness

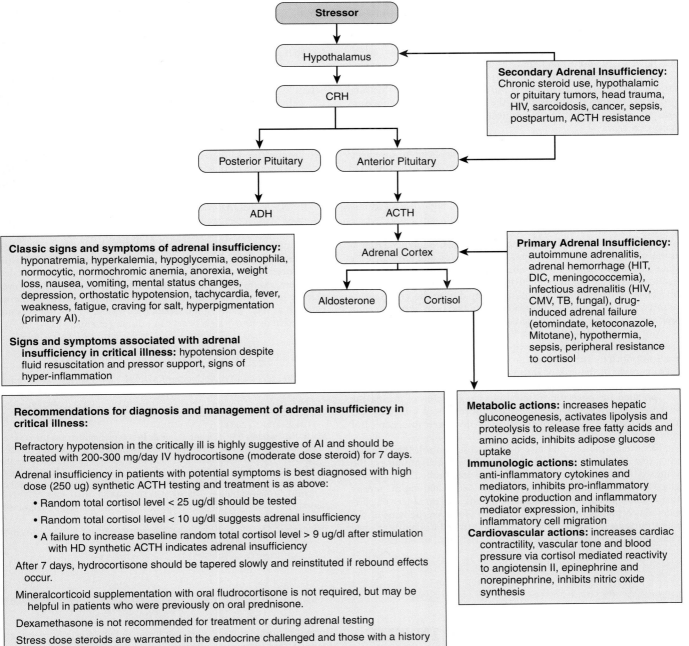

FIGURE 1   A summary of adrenal insufficiency in critical illness.

effects, including abnormal immune function, increased infection, and hemodynamic and electromyocardial disturbances. In addition, severe physical stress leads to increased insulin resistance and thus an increase in insulin requirements. Depending on the individual's capabilities to meet this increased insulin demand, hyperglycemia may occur, and a direct relationship exists between the extent of stress hyperglycemia and mortality in ICU patients.

The landmark randomized study by Van den Berghe and colleagues demonstrated the value of tight glycemic control (80 to 110 mg/dL) in surgical ICU patients. Intensive insulin therapy reduced in-hospital mortality by 34%, bloodstream infections by 46%, acute renal failure requiring dialysis or hemofiltration by 41%, and transfusion requirements by 50%. Patients receiving intensive insulin treatment were also less likely to require prolonged mechanical ventilation and intensive care. Benefits demonstrated in this study have been the stimulus for aggressive glucose control in any ICU patient who has hyperglycemia.

A review of multiple studies shows that insulin treatment decreases short-term mortality by approximately 15%. Most of these studies were performed in surgical ICU patients, thus results could not necessarily be generalized to medical ICU patients. Because medical patients tend to stay in the ICU longer, many have hypothesized that tight glucose control might even be more beneficial in the medical ICU population.

In a medical ICU, Van den Berghe and colleagues found that intensive insulin therapy (target glucose range: 80 to 110 mg/dL) significantly reduced morbidity and shortened the length of ICU and hospital stay but did not reduce mortality among the 1,200 patients included in the intention-to-treat analysis. Further post hoc analysis, however, demonstrated that the mortality of patients staying in the ICU for more than 3 days was reduced from 52.5% to 43% ($P < .01$). Clearly the issue here is the inability to identify this subgroup of patients at admission to the ICU. As with any subgroup analysis, many feel that this is a nonvalid conclusion and that this is a negative trial.

Although the majority of studies evaluating the effects of hyperglycemia have been reported in nontrauma patients, there have been increasing reports in the trauma literature on the hyperglycemic stress response and its adverse impact on outcome. Trauma patients are typically healthy prior to injury and are younger than other patients. We initially reported that elevated serum glucose on admission, defined as glucose greater than 200 mg/dL, was found to be a predictor of postoperative infection, hospital and ICU length of stay, and mortality. We then demonstrated that admission hyperglycemia is associated with significant increases in infection and mortality. We have also shown that high, worsening, and highly variable hyperglycemic patterns are highly predictive of increased ventilator days, ICU and hospital days, infection, and mortality during the first week of admission. A follow-up study demonstrated that early hyperglycemia was associated with a 17-fold increase in the odds of dying.

More significantly, the impact of glucose control after the first week persisted regardless of subsequent glucose control. Patients who were not normoglycemic in the first week of hospitalization had an 85% increase in the risk of infection and 98% increase in the risk of dying later, regardless of subsequent glucose levels. Most recently we validated the observation that tight glucose control during the first week of admission is associated with improved outcome, and the institution of a protocol significantly decreased infections and mortality.

To develop the optimal target for glucose control, the clinician must rely on clinical acumen rather than experimental findings. The improved outcomes when insulin therapy was titrated to achieve a glucose of 80 to 110 mg/dL, as opposed to 180 to 200 mg/dL, means that a blood glucose greater than 180 mg/dL can no longer be considered acceptable in critically ill patients. However, the issue of the safest range below this level is still unresolved and has not been specifically addressed in prospective clinical trials until recently.

Ideally, the optimal target for blood glucose should be defined by large prospective trials comparing two ranges. The Normoglycemia in Intensive Care Evaluation–Survival Using Glucose Algorithm Regulation (NICE-SUGAR), GluControl, and Efficacy of Volume Substitution and Insulin Therapy in Severe Sepsis (VISEP) trials compared the effects of insulin therapy titrated to 80 to 110 mg/dL versus 140 to 180 mg/dL in a prospective, randomized fashion. GluControl was stopped after the inclusion of 1109 patients. The rates of hypoglycemia and mortality in the patients who experienced at least one episode of severe hypoglycemia, defined as a blood glucose of less than 40 mg/dL, were both higher in the group randomized to the 80 to 110 mg/dL target. These data suggest that a target blood glucose between 140 and 180 mg/dL is safer than the 80 to 110 mg/dL range. Because no significant difference in overall outcome was observed between the two groups, the risk/benefit ratio was in favor of the higher glucose target. Although further confirmation of these findings is desirable, many clinicians favor this intermediate range as a target for intensive insulin therapy to prevent a higher hypoglycemia rate.

The NICE-SUGAR trial recently reported the results of their randomized prospective study, which compared tight glycemic control (80 to 108 mg/dL) versus conventional glucose control (<180 mg/dL) in ICU patients expected to be admitted for at least 3 days. The study included both medical and surgical patients admitted to 42 ICUs with the primary end point being death. Although the study concluded that there was not a benefit in mortality in patients titrated to a lower glucose level, there does appear to be a potential benefit in trauma patients, as the P value in the subanalysis was .07. The study was not powered to demonstrate a benefit in trauma patients.

SUGGESTED READINGS

Bochicchio GV, Joshi M, Bochicchio KM, et al: Early hyperglycemic control is important in critically injured trauma patients, *J Trauma* 63:1353–1358, 2007.

Cooper MS, Stewart PM: Corticoid insufficiency in acutely ill patients, *N Engl J Med* 348:727, 2003.

Marik PB, Pastores SM, Annane D, et al: Recommendations for the diagnosis and management of corticosteroid insufficiency in critically ill adult patients: consensus statements from an international task force by the American College of Critical Care Medicine, *Crit Care Med* 36:1937, 2008.

Scalea TM, Bochicchio GV, Bochicchio KM, et al: Tight glycemic control in critically injured trauma patients, *Ann Surg* 246:605–610, 2007.

Van den BG, Wouters P, Weekers F, et al: Intensive insulin therapy in the critically ill patients, *N Engl J Med* 345:1359–1367, 2001.

Zalonga GP, Marik P: Hypothalamic-pituitary-adrenal insufficiency, *Crit Care Clin* 17:25, 2001.

NUTRITION SUPPORT IN THE CRITICALLY ILL

Maria Clara Mendoza, MD, and Juan Carlos Puyana, MD

OVERVIEW

Nutrition support is usually required for critically ill patients who will not be able to return to a normal diet within 7 days of starvation. These patients require not just a replacement diet but specially tailored diets for their metabolic and therapeutic needs. Many factors, such as associated chronic illnesses and preexisting comorbidities, significantly increase morbidity and mortality when nutrition requirements are delayed, thus they constantly accumulate a caloric, proteic, and energetic debt. A significant number of critically ill patients admitted to the ICU may already have severe protein and energy malnutrition. Furthermore, once in the hospital, the risk of developing worsening malnutrition increases daily while the patient remains hospitalized. In addition, cellular function and adequate tissue healing are both completely dependent on the adequate supply of nutrients. Consequently, the incidence of postoperative complications, including nosocomial infection, increases in patients with severe malnutrition.

Even though teaching regarding the importance of early enteral nutrition (EN) and attentive attitudes toward improving nutrition intake have been more widely disseminated, it is common to see patients who have routine elective surgery submitted to unnecessary prolonged periods of starvation. Fortunately, the majority of these patients tolerate starvation well. The Society of Critical Care Medicine (SCCM) guidelines suggest that nutrition support be initiated in any critically ill patient who may go for more than 3 days without oral intake. Obviously the caveat is to simultaneously contemplate the patient's degree of metabolic burden, resulting from either trauma or postsurgical stress. Therefore the most practical approach to providing adequate nutrition support to our patients can be best simplified in a tutorial that seeks to answer the following three questions:

1. How long has it been since the patient has eaten?
2. How catabolic is the patient, and how much does the patient need to replenish his/her caloric/energy deficit?
3. How can nutrition best be provided, and what is the most appropriate route?

Prescribing Proper Nutrition

It is important to think of nutrition as an intervention that has a therapeutic effect beyond the obvious classic concept of simply supplying alimentation. This newer approach continues to solidify as more sophisticated knowledge is accrued by the increased understanding of the relationship between the inflammatory response and metabolism. Through the use of specific components, certain effects can now be targeted to ameliorate inflammation, decrease oxidative injury, and positively influence the immune response.

This chapter focuses on the indications for nutrition support, the variety of techniques available to provide it, and the results of nutrition treatment in the critically ill patient.

METABOLIC RESPONSE TO STRESS AND INJURY IN CRITICAL ILLNESS

Most critically ill patients have in common an increased metabolic rate. The initial response to stress in the severely ill patient aims at maintaining the body homeostasis; usually, the metabolic insults persist, promptly generating a catabolic state. The increase in energy requirements in critically ill patients may range between 30% to 70% above normal.

INDICATIONS

Any condition that results in the suspension of the oral intake for more than 5 to 7 days must be considered for nutrition intervention. The net negative balance of protein resulting from an increase in metabolism requires a feeding regimen to prevent deleterious effects in health state and prognosis.

NUTRITION REQUIREMENTS

Nutrition requirements differ among patients and conditions, so nutrition intervention must to be tailored for individual clinical cases.

Energy Requirements

Traditionally, caloric goals (CGs) in surgical and critically ill patients were based on an attempt to curtail the catabolic response and loss of muscle and visceral mass that invariably occur after trauma and illness. In the absence of stress, provision of small amounts of carbohydrates (400 calories/day) leads to sparing of muscle breakdown and the so called protein-sparing effect of glucose. In the presence of traumatic or septic stress, however, the provision of carbohydrates, even at CGs, fails to protect muscle mass, thus making CGs superfluous.

Several organizations—including the American College of Chest Physicians (ACCP), the American Society of Parenteral and Enteral Nutrition (ASPEN), and the Canadian Critical Care Task Force—have concluded that data are insufficient to recommend a set number of calories that should be given to critically ill patients, thus all the hospital nutrition authoritative organizations agree that CGs in surgical, trauma, and critically ill patients have never been successfully determined.

Hypermetabolism and malnourishment are common in the intensive care unit (ICU). Malnutrition is associated with increased morbidity and mortality, and most ICU patients receive specialized nutrition therapy to attenuate the effects of malnourishment. However, the optimal amount of energy that should be delivered is unknown; some studies suggest full caloric feeding may improve clinical outcomes, but other studies show that caloric intake may not be important in determining patient outcome.

The relationship between dose of nutrition and clinically important outcomes is extensively documented in the literature. Observation studies suggest that achieving targeted caloric intake might not be necessary, because provision of approximately 25% to 66% of GCs may be sufficient. Randomized controlled trials comparing early and aggressive use of EN moving intake closer to goal calories might be associated with a clinical benefit.

There is no role for supplemental parenteral nutrition to increase caloric delivery in the early phase of critical illness. Further high-quality evidence from randomized trials investigating the optimal amount of energy intake in ICU patients is needed. It would be simple to avoid overfeeding if clinicians used a reliable way of determining the caloric needs of a given patient. Most clinicians, including nutritionists, rely on population-based calculated formulas such as the Harris-Benedict formulas. These formulas were generated under conditions completely different from those faced by our critically ill patients under intensive care therapy, thus it is unclear as to whether they are applicable to that setting. More often than not, the use of such formulas leads to overfeeding in up to 30% of patients and may cause harm.

The use of indirect calorimetry could be a reliable calculator of the appropriate amount of calories needed by a given patient. Unfortunately, indirect calorimetry is labor intensive and difficult to do and is not available in many institutions. Furthermore, no significant evidence is available to suggest that performing indirect calorimetry is cost effective.

Protein Requirements

It has been suggested that a small amount of nutrients to "bathe" the gut mucosa is all that is necessary or desirable. It appears to be important to provide at least some protein, although again, how much to provide initially has not been clearly determined. In addition, the relative concentration of certain amino acids can be modified for some patients, such as those with renal or hepatic failure.

TECHNIQUES

Forms of Nutrition Intervention

There are several ways to providing nutrition and alimentation, and these vary according to the clinical practice. Different forms of nutrition intervention are frequently used in surgical and trauma patients, and each one has advantages and complications.

Controlled Starvation and Early Enteral Nutrition

Short periods of starvation have traditionally been allowed in most surgical patient populations, even in elective surgery and in critically ill patients. The suspension of oral intake is supported by the idea that it is beneficial let the bowel rest to allow complete restoration of bowel function. The benefits of early oral/enteral intake are evident, and an effort to promote individual practice changes based on this evidence would lead to better outcomes in patients. Lewis published a meta-analysis in 2001, in which he reports on 11 studies including a total of 837 patients. In six studies, patients in the intervention group were fed directly into the small bowel, and in five studies, patients were fed orally. The use of early feeding was found to reduce the risk of any type of infection (relative risk, 0.72; 95% confidence interval [CI], 0.54 to 0.98; $P = .036$). Early feeding also reduced the mean length of stay in the hospital (number of days reduced by 0.84; CI, 0.36 to 1.33; $P = .001$). Furthermore, risk reductions were also seen for anastomotic dehiscence (relative risk, 0.53; CI, 0.26 to 1.08; $P = .080$), wound infection, pneumonia, intraabdominal abscess, and mortality, but these failed to reach significance ($P > .10$). The risk of vomiting was increased among patients fed early (relative risk, 1.27; CI, 1.01 to 1.61; $P = .046$). A statistically significant increase was also observed in pulmonary complications, need for nasogastric tube decompression, and in delays in the return of bowel function. Lewis and colleagues did not report whether CGs had been met in the group of patients receiving early oral intake, and no evidence so far states definitively whether the benefits of early oral intake are independent of the amount of calories given.

Early enteral nutrition (EEN) is clearly indicated in the critically ill surgical or trauma patient. A systematic review of EEN has been published by Heyland that demonstrates a significant decrease in infection rates without an effect on mortality. Clear evidence now supports the idea that controlled short periods of starvation are not indicated in most surgical patients and that the gastrointestinal (GI) tract can be used successfully in most surgical and critically ill patients.

Permissive Underfeeding

An interesting observation about virtually all studies on EEN is the fact that in most, there is a failure to meet intake of planned caloric goals. In general, most patients on EEN meet between 50% and 70% of caloric goals. Yet there appears to be a benefit from lower caloric intake, which has raised considerable interest in the concept of "permissive underfeeding." EEN produces benefits through mechanisms independent of CGs. Starvation is associated with significant abnormalities in GI function, including mucosal atrophy and loss of GI-associated lymphoid tissue (GALT). EEN maintains normal GI function even when CGs are not met. Another possibility is that meeting CGs is associated with complications, including overfeeding. Provision of EEN is associated with an increased number of side effects, as the dietary volume delivered is increased in an attempt to meet caloric goals. In addition, calorically dense formulas with high concentrations of fat can overwhelm the digestive and absorptive capacity of the GI tract; thus investigators have noticed increased gastric residuals, bloating, and diarrhea when high volumes are delivered, or when high-fat formulas are provided to critically ill surgical and trauma patients. Furthermore, overfeeding is associated with a large number of complications and may indeed increase mortality. It negatively affects function of every organ: it could cause encephalopathy, and it increases cardiac and respiratory demands, prolongs ventilator dependency, and causes immune dysfunction. Thus the dangers of overfeeding cannot be overemphasized. Specifically, in enterally fed burn patients or highly stressed trauma patients, the onset of sepsis is commonly preceded by an inability to continue enteral feeding despite the use of a postpyloric feeding tube. The majority of these patients may also manifest hyperglycemic events. If enteral feeding is not possible, there are only two alternatives: no feeding at all or permissive parenteral underfeeding with control of glycemia. From the above discussion, parenteral underfeeding is the appropriate way of maintaining some nutrition to minimize to some degree the risk of complications.

Early Enteral Nutrition

EN has shown its greatest effectiveness when started early. Even with the significant heterogeneity among the published studies, EEN is defined as nutrition started within the first 24 to 48 hours of admission to the ICU. Across all critically ill patient populations, patients receiving EEN exhibit a clear trend toward a decrease in mortality ($P < .08$)

and infection rates. In practical terms, EEN is started as soon as the patient's hemodynamic status is stabilized. Ideally, a small-bore feeding tube is placed, and diet is started at low volumes, which are associated with decreased complications such as abdominal distension, increased gastric residuals, and vomiting. Supplementing these patients with protein to meet goals of 1.5 to 2 g/kg/day could be beneficial. Consideration to provide additional early micronutrients should also be given.

In summary, starvation is not desirable in most patients. Oral or enteral nutrition can be achieved in most surgical, trauma, and critically ill patients. EN should be started as early as possible, ideally within the first 24 hours of arrival. Meeting caloric goals is not necessary or desirable, though the degree of underfeeding that is beneficial remains undetermined.

Total Parenteral Nutrition

Compared with EN, total parenteral nutrition (TPN) offers distinct advantages and adds a number of caveats. Establishing delivery access is far simpler and more reliable when using TPN. In addition, TPN delivery does not have to be stopped for surgical procedures or trips outside of the ICU. Not surprisingly, patients on TPN consistently meet caloric goals more often than those given EN. These observations have led clinicians to advocate the use of TPN, implying that its use would be of benefit; however, this is not the case. Multiple studies have demonstrated that in surgical patients, trauma victims, and critically ill patients, TPN is inferior to EN. In the ICU, for example, 13 different studies have demonstrated that EN is associated with decreased rates of infection when compared with TPN, although there is no evidence of an effect on mortality. In critically ill trauma patients also, the use of TPN is associated with increased morbidity including more infections, a longer stay in the ICU, and prolonged ventilator dependency. A well-performed prospective randomized study demonstrated that there is no role for prophylactic TPN in surgical patients. Similarly, TPN used only as a form of achieving CGs has failed to demonstrate clear benefits in other patient populations such as trauma, surgical, and critically ill patients.

The role of TPN has therefore been progressively reduced. Nevertheless, it remains invaluable in very specific clinical circumstances, such as when 1) a nonstressed patient who has severe protein-calorie malnutrition is scheduled to undergo surgery, a perfect example is the patient scheduled to undergo esophageal surgery because of obstruction; 2) a patient is malnourished, and TPN given 7 days before surgery is associated with a significant decrease in infection rates; 3) the patient has short gut, and indefinite survival is possible thanks to the use of TPN, which can be used for long-term management or as a bridge to intestinal transplantation; or 4) patients fail oral/enteral nutrition. A frequent consult to any nutrition intervention team is the failure to achieve adequate EN support in a given patient. This is often used as an excuse to start TPN. More often, however, adequate evaluation of the patient and implementation of simple measures lead to successfully achieving adequate EN.

TPN should be implemented only after an adequate attempt at EN; however, the patient with complicated abdominal wounds that are clearly worsened by the presence of protracted fistulas that impair any healing may be candidates for TPN, at least during the early phases of wound care. It is our experience that after a brief period, which in some cases may range from several days to weeks, the combined multidisciplinary care of the wound may reach some degree of healing, allowing the re-initiation of full EN. Currently no clear guidelines define failure of EN; however, it is clear that at least early on, it is not necessary to meet CGs through the enteral route to see its benefits. There is no role for combined TPN and EN.

Doig and colleagues and the Nutrition Guidelines Investigators of the Australian and New Zealand Intensive Care Society recently published a study to determine whether evidence-based feeding guidelines could improve nutrition practices and reduce mortality in the ICU. They performed a cluster randomized trial in 36 ICUs from 27 hospitals including 1118 patients expected to remain in the ICU longer than 2 days. Despite that the introduction of the guidelines

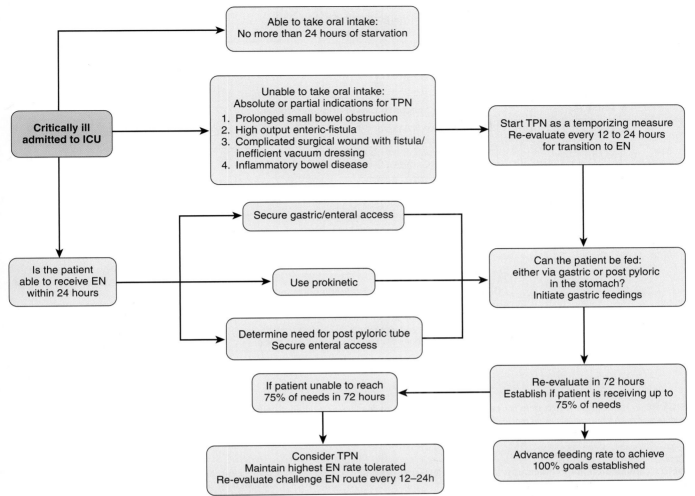

FIGURE 1   Algorithm to implement evidence-based feeding guidelines to improve nutrition practices and reduce mortality in the ICU. *(Data from Doig GS, Simpson F, Finfer S, et al: Effect of evidence-based feeding guidelines on mortality of critically ill adults: a cluster randomized controlled trial, JAMA 300[23]:2731-2741, 2008.)*

did significantly change clinical practices, promote earlier feeding, and improve nutrition adequacy, no difference was observed in clinical outcomes. Figure 1 depicts the algorithm developed to implement the guidelines in the ICU. Figure 2 depicts the management algorithm for patients who develop tube feeding–associated diarrhea.

SPECIFIC MACRONUTRIENTS AND MICRONUTRIENTS

Oral nutritional supplements (ONS) are a frequent addition to the therapy of many patients in the hospital. ONS are often concentrates of high amounts of calories with proteins and micronutrients, including vitamins, and they are heavily advertised. Little evidence, however, suggests that ONS indiscriminately administered to hospitalized patients will benefit outcome.

NUTRIENTS WITH PHARMACOLOGIC PROPERTIES

Surgery and trauma are associated with depression of adaptive T-cell function, including decreased T-cell numbers, abnormally low circulating CD4 cell counts, decreased T-cell proliferation, involution of the thymus, and depressed/delayed-type hypersensitivity (DTH).

Nevertheless, therapy to "normalize" T-cell function would be deemed necessary and desirable. Arginine supplementation is a potentially effective therapy for surgery- and trauma-induced T-cell suppression.

Independent of the arginine work, other investigators have demonstrated that several nutrients—including omega-3 fatty acids, nucleic acids, and glutamine—also affect immune function. These nutrients, along with arginine, have been incorporated and marketed as "immune-enhancing diets." At least seven of these diets exist in the market, each one with its own mix of nutrients. Interestingly, the combination and mixing of these nutrients has been done despite incomplete knowledge of their mechanisms of action, possible side effects, and unknown interactions among the various substances.

Glutamine serves as fuel for the immune cells and it increases human leukocyte antigen–DR expression on monocytes, enhances neutrophil phagocytosis, and increases heat-shock protein expression. Arginine affects the immune system by stimulating direct or indirect proliferation of immune cells. This indirect effect is possibly mediated by nitric oxide, which also enhances macrophage cytotoxicity. Furthermore, glutamine serves as a precursor for the de novo production of arginine through the citrulline-arginine pathway. Glutamine has proven beneficial in the surgical and critically ill patient, whereas arginine supplementation is still under debate. A combination of arginine, omega-3 fatty acids, and nucleotides given as a perioperative dietary supplement decreases the infection rates by about 40% in patients undergoing high-risk surgery. The benefits of this

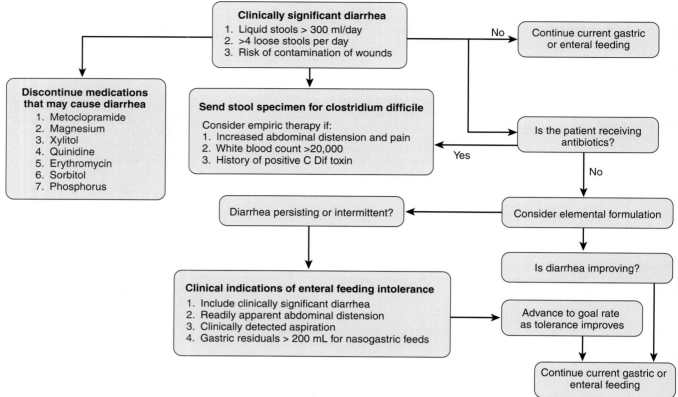

FIGURE 2   Management algorithm for patients who develop tube feeding–associated diarrhea. *(Data from Doig GS, Simpson F, Finfer S, et al: Effect of evidence-based feeding guidelines on mortality of critically ill adults: a cluster randomized controlled trial, JAMA 300[23]:2731–2741, 2008.)*

dietary combination are well demonstrated in all meta-analyses and are currently considered level I evidence of benefit.

SUMMARY

Nutrition intervention in critical care patients has changed over the years, and many questions are still unanswered. If possible, early enteral nutrition should be used in almost all cases. Specific dietary requirements differ among patients and clinical states, but specific nutrients such as glutamine and arginine could improve outcomes; many researchers are working on studies of this kind of immunonutrition.

SUGGESTED READINGS

Boelens PG, Houdijk AP, Haarman HJ, et al: Glutamine-enriched enteral nutrition increases HLA-DR expression on monocytes of trauma patients, *J Nutrition* 132:2580–2587, 2002.

Doig GS, Simpson F, Finfer S, et al: Effect of evidence-based feeding guidelines on mortality of critically ill adults: a cluster randomized controlled trial, *JAMA* 300(23):2731–2741, 2008.

Doig GS, Simpson F, Finfer S, et al: Nutrition Guidelines Investigators of the ANZICS Clinical Trials Group: effect of evidence-based feeding guidelines on mortality of critically ill adults: a cluster randomized controlled trial, *JAMA* 300(23):2731–2741, 2008.

Jones NE, Heyland DK: Implementing nutrition guidelines in the critical care setting: a worthwhile and achievable goal? *JAMA* 300(23):2798–2799, 2008.

Koretz RL, Avenell A, Lipman TO, et al: Does enteral nutrition affect clinical outcome? A systematic review of the randomized trials, *Am J Gastroenterol* 102(2):412–429, 2007.

Martindale RG, McClave SA, Vanek VW, et al: Guidelines for the provision and assessment of nutrition support therapy in the adult critically ill patient: Society of Critical Care Medicine and American Society for Parenteral and Enteral Nutrition executive summary, *Crit Care Med* 37(5):1757–1761, 2009.

Ochoa JB, Caba D: Advances in surgical nutrition, *Surg Clin North Am* 86(6):1483–1493, 2006.

COAGULOPATHY IN THE CRITICALLY ILL PATIENT

Robert F. Cuff, MD

OVERVIEW

Bleeding complications are common among critically ill patients. The focus of this chapter is to provide a working format to assess, diagnose, and treat the more common coagulation problems encountered in the critically ill patient.

INITIAL ASSESSMENT OF THE BLEEDING PATIENT

For patients who are stable but are seen with ongoing evidence of bleeding, a focused assessment that includes appropriate history, physical exam, and laboratory evaluation will guide your treatment. The most common bleeding disorders in the critical setting fall into one of three main categories: 1) anatomic vascular defects, 2) platelet disorders, and 3) coagulation cascade defects. The primary goal is to identify and categorize the etiology of the bleeding disorder so that an effective treatment regimen can be undertaken.

History

The historic evaluation includes a general personal and family history for the patient. Emphasis should be placed on any family or personal history of known inherited or acquired bleeding disorders or pre-existing systemic diseases, such as renal or hepatic failure, that may predispose the patient to a bleeding disorder. A past history of excessive bleeding following minor procedures such as dental extractions, spontaneous bleeding events such as epistaxis, or conditions such as menorrhagia may indicate an underlying platelet disorder. Previous episodes of hemarthrosis or deep-tissue bleeding are associated with a coagulation cascade defect. The majority of patients encountered in the intensive care unit (ICU) do not have an inheritable disorder but rather have an acquired or induced state of coagulopathy. Medication history should be reviewed including a history of chronic anticoagulants such as warfarin and antiplatelet agents such as aspirin, clopidogrel, or ticlidopine. Some herbal supplements also may affect hemostasis.

The second portion of the history should focus on the more immediate or event history. If this is a recent surgical patient, the intraoperative findings, medications, blood product use, and events should be reviewed with the surgeon and anesthesia team. Unexpected or greater than expected blood loss during the procedure may indicate an underlying bleeding disorder. Anticoagulants given for the procedure and the need for high-volume fluid or blood product transfusion could lead to an induced deficiency of coagulation factors and platelets. Other factors, such as hypothermia and poor tissue quality, may be causes of postsurgical bleeding.

For nonsurgical patients such as victims of trauma, the event history should be reviewed for the mechanism of trauma, potential for large-volume blood loss at the scene, and prolonged exposure prior to arrival. Often the medical history may be unavailable or unreliable in these cases, and more reliance on the physical exam and laboratory testing will therefore be needed.

Physical Examination

Assessing the location and character of the bleeding sites can provide valuable insight into the etiology of the bleeding disorder. Bleeding from a single location, such as the surgical wound or into the cavity of a recent surgery, is usually due to an anatomic vascular defect and not from a systemic bleeding disorder. Hemostatic instability resulting from rapid, large-volume blood loss is also indicative of an anatomic defect. If surgical correction is delayed, a systemic coagulopathy may develop because of consumption of coagulation factors and platelets. Slow, persistent bleeding or bleeding from multiple sites is likely to be due to a systemic coagulopathy.

Laboratory Assessment

The patient's history and findings on physical exam should help direct laboratory testing. For patients with a known inheritable coagulopathy, reassessment of their specific factor levels should be performed, in addition to general coagulation testing.

Initial testing should include a complete blood count (CBC), activated partial thromboplastin time (aPTT), international normalized ratio (INR), and fibrinogen level. This panel allows for a snapshot of the intrinsic and extrinsic coagulation arms, platelet count, and activity of the fibrinolytic system; this will often provide an answer to the type of coagulopathy and will allow for immediate treatment. Bleeding-time testing is the most useful test of platelet function but is rarely performed, as it is time consuming and user dependent. Surrogate tests such as the PFA-100 and, more recently, bedside aggregometry testing have shown more predictable, rapid results. Table 1 shows the laboratory results for some of the more common bleeding disorders.

COMMON BLEEDING DISORDERS

Platelet Disorders

Mucosal, skin, or surgical site bleeding that occurs immediately after surgery or injury and is difficult to stop characterizes bleeding as a result of platelet disorders. Once bleeding is controlled, it is rare for it to recur. Platelet disorders are due to either insufficient numbers of platelets or dysfunctional platelets despite adequate numbers.

Thrombocytopenia

Quantitative platelet disorders (thrombocytopenia) are due to either decreased production or increased destruction of circulating platelets. The more common causes of thrombocytopenia encountered in the critical care patient are listed in Table 2. For most preoperative surgical patients, platelet counts of 50,000/μL is adequate. In high-risk procedures such as cardiac or neurosurgical surgery, platelet counts over 100,000/μL are preferred.

Regardless of the etiology for thrombocytopenia, the immediate treatment is to restore adequate quantities of platelets during an acute bleeding episode. Treatment of the underlying cause should be instituted as soon as feasible to prevent further platelet loss or increased production of native platelets.

Platelet Dysfunction

Qualitative platelet disorders (platelet dysfunction) are characterized by adequate circulating platelet numbers but inability of the platelets to adhere, activate, and aggregate sufficiently to provide primary hemostasis. This inability to function normally may be inherent in the platelet at the time of production (congenital) or it may result from inactivation of a normal platelet after production (acquired).

TABLE 1: Initial laboratory results

Disorder	aPTT	PT/INR	Platelet	Fibrinogen	Bleeding Time (PFA-100)
Thrombocytopenia	Normal	Normal	Decreased	Normal	Elevated
Platelet dysfunction	Normal	Normal	Normal	Normal	Elevated
Hemophilia A and B	Elevated	Normal	Normal	Normal	Normal
von Willebrand disease	Elevated	Normal	Normal	Normal	Normal/elevated
Factor VII deficiency	Normal	Elevated	Normal	Normal	Normal
Warfarin	Normal	Elevated	Normal	Normal	Normal
Heparin/LMWH	Elevated	Normal	Normal	Normal	Normal
DIC	Elevated	Elevated	Decreased	Decreased	Elevated
Liver disease	Elevated	Elevated	Decreased	Decreased	Elevated
Lupus anticoagulant	Elevated	Elevated	Decreased	Normal	Elevated

aPTT, Activated partial thromboplastin time; *PT,* prothrombin time; *INR,* International Normalized Ratio; *LMWH,* low molecular weight heparin; *DIC,* disseminated intravascular coagulopathy

TABLE 2: Thrombocytopenia

Decreased Production	Increased Destruction
Vitamin deficiencies (vitamin B_{12}, folate)	Immune thrombocytopenic purpura
Bone marrow disease	Infection
Drugs (chemotherapy, ethanol)	DIC
Infection	Drugs (heparin, quinine, glycoprotein IIb/IIIa inhibitors)
Liver failure	Thrombotic thrombocytopenic purpura Hemolytic uremic syndrome
	Hypersplenism
	Dilutional (massive transfusion)

DIC, Disseminated intravascular coagulopathy

TABLE 3: Platelet dysfunction

Congenital	Acquired
Bernard-Soulier syndrome	Drugs (aspirin, ticlopidine, clopidogrel, NSAIDs)
Glanzmann thrombasthenia	Uremia
Storage-pool diseases	Liver disease
Platelet-type von Willebrand disease	Postcardiopulmonary bypass

NSAIDs, Nonsteroidal antiinflammatory drugs

The more common causes of platelet dysfunction encountered in the critical care patient are listed in Table 3.

Currently the most common cause of platelet dysfunction in hospitalized patients is drug therapy. Increased use of medications such as glycoprotein IIb/IIIa inhibitors, clopidogrel, and aspirin has dramatically increased the population of patients with acquired platelet dysfunction.

For patients with acute bleeding, platelet transfusion is the primary treatment for platelet dysfunction disorders. Unfortunately, if treatment is for acquired disorders, these new platelets will also become inactivated, and multiple transfusions may be required to achieve hemostasis. Bleeding in uremic patients can be improved with regular dialysis and by maintaining a hematocrit to 30% to 35%. Desmopressin (DDAVP) can also provide a transient increase in von Willebrand factor available to assist in platelet adhesion and aggregation. DDAVP may be administered at a dose of 0.3 µg/kg body weight every 12 to 24 hours for several doses.

In patients with congenital platelet disorders and postcardiopulmonary bypass, DDAVP and antifibrinolytic medications (ε-amino caproic acid or aprotinin) have been used to decrease the need for platelet transfusions. A summary of platelet disorders, their evaluation, and treatment is found in Table 4.

Coagulation Disorders

Coagulation factor disorders are a common cause of bleeding in the critically ill patient. Bleeding from a coagulation disorder is characterized by diffuse, recurrent episodes and may occur at sites unrelated to the site of operation. Coagulation factor defects are either inherited (von Willebrand disease, hemophilias) or acquired (drug induced, liver disease). Some of the more common clinically relevant coagulation disorders seen in the ICU population are listed in Table 5. Treatment for coagulation disorders consists of replacement of specific factors or broad-factor replacement with blood products (Table 6 and Box 1).

Inherited Coagulation Disorders

The diagnosis of an inherited coagulation disorder is often based on history and confirmed with abnormal coagulation panel studies (elevated aPTT and/or prothrombin time [PT]) and confirmed with specific factor studies. For patients known to have a specific inherited coagulation disorder, preoperative supplementation is recommended to prevent postoperative bleeding. The recommendations

TABLE 4: Summary of platelet disorders

Disorder	Effect	Diagnostic Test	Acute Treatment
Thrombocytopenia	Inadequate circulating platelets for primary hemostasis	Complete blood count	Platelet transfusion to greater than 50,000
Aspirin/NSAIDs	Inhibit platelet cyclooxygenase	Bleeding time (PFA-100)	Platelet transfusion
Thienopyridines (ticlopidine, clopidogrel)	Antagonist of ADP receptor, inhibits aggregation	Bleeding time (PFA-100)	Platelet transfusion
Glycoprotein IIb/IIIa antagonist (abciximab, tirofiban, eptifibatide)	Inhibit platelet aggregation	Bleeding time (PFA-100)	Discontinuation of infusion, platelet transfusion
Uremia	Inhibit platelet adhesion, aggregation, and procoagulant activity	Blood urea nitrogen, bleeding time (PFA-100)	Dialysis, DDAVP, platelet transfusion
Cardiopulmonary bypass	Thrombocytopenia, inhibit platelet aggregation	Bleeding time (PFA-100)	DDAVP, aprotinin, ε-aminocaproic acid, platelet transfusion
Antiplatelet antibodies (ITP, SLE)	Inhibit platelet aggregation	Bleeding time (PFA-100)	Platelet transfusion
Disseminated intravascular coagulation	Impaired platelet aggregation	Fibrin degradation products	Platelet transfusion
Inherited qualitative platelet disorders (Glanzmann thromboasthenia, Bernard-Soulier syndrome)	Variable platelet dysfunction	Bleeding time (PFA-100)	DDAVP, aprotinin ε-aminocaproic acid, platelet transfusion

NSAIDs, Nonsteroidal antiinflammatory drugs; *ADP,* adenosine diphosphate; *ITP,* idiopathic thrombocytopenia purpura; *SLE,* systemic lupus erythematosus; *DDAVP,* 1-deamino-8-D-arginine vasopressin

TABLE 5: Coagulation disorders

Inherited Coagulation Disorders	Acquired Coagulation Disorders
von Willebrand disease	Vitamin K deficiency
Hemophilia A (factor VIII deficiency)	Liver disease
Hemophilia B (factor IX deficiency)	Anticoagulation-associated coagulopathy (warfarin, heparin, low-molecular-weight heparin, fondaparinux, direct thrombin inhibitors)
Hemophilia C (factor XI deficiency)	Disseminated intravascular coagulation
Factor VII deficiency	Acquired factor inhibitors
Factor X deficiency	Factor V/thrombin inhibitors associated with bovine thrombin exposure
Afibrinogenemia, hypofibrinogenemia	Factor VIII inhibitors
Factor V deficiency	Cardiac bypass coagulopathy
Factor II deficiency	Dilutional coagulopathy (massive transfusions)
Factor XIII deficiency	

for the most common disorders are listed in Table 6. The most common inherited coagulation disorders are von Willebrand disease and hemophilia A and B. Other coagulation disorders are uncommon or rare and will not be discussed in detail in this chapter.

One of the more common coagulation disorders, von Willebrand disease, is caused by inherited autosomal deficiency of von Willebrand factor (vWF), a protein that plays a role in platelet adhesion and serves as a carrier protein for factor VIII, protecting it from degradation by activated protein C. As it affects both platelet function and the coagulation cascade, patients can be seen with mucosal bleeding similar to platelet defects or recurrent diffuse bleeding from failure of the intrinsic pathway. Treatment of the acutely bleeding patient includes use of DDAVP and factor VIII concentrates.

Hemophilia A (factor VIII deficiency) is an X-linked recessive trait that affects 1 in 5000 male births. The degree of severity correlates with the factor levels. Normal factor VIII levels are generally between 50% and 150% of the standard. Severe hemophilia A disease is associated with factor VIII levels less than 1%. These patients are at risk for spontaneous bleeding. Factor levels between 1% and 5% characterize moderate disease, and patients with mild disease have levels greater than 5%. Mild hemophilia patients may be undiagnosed preoperatively, as they often only have bleeding problems after a significant operation or trauma. Factor VIII inhibitors occur in up to 25% of patients with severe hemophilia A and will result in resistance to factor VIII supplementation. Treatment consists of factor VIII concentrates. Hemophilia B (factor IX deficiency) is a much less common X-linked recessive disorder. Factor levels correlate to disease severity as in hemophilia A.

Acquired Coagulation Disorders

In the critical care setting, acquired coagulation disorders are more commonly encountered than congenital disorders.

TABLE 6: Treatment of coagulation factor disorders

Bleeding Disorder	Target Factor Level	Plasma Product
Hemophilia A		
Minor surgery	>50% for 3–7 days	Recombinant (preferred) or plasma-derived monoclonal factor VIII concentrates
Major surgery	>80% to 100% for 3 days then >50% for next 7–11 days	
Cardiovascular, prostate, and neurosurgery	>100% for 3 days then 80% to 100% for days 4–7 and >50% for days 8–14	
Hemophilia B		
Minor surgery	>50% for 3–7 days	Recombinant or monoclonal plasma-derived factor IX concentrates
Major surgery	>80% to 100% for 3 days then >50% for next 7–11 days	
Cardiovascular, prostate, and neurosurgery	>100% for 3 days then 80% to 100% for days 4–7 and >50% for days 8–14	
von Willebrand Disease		
Minor surgery	>50% for 1–3 days	DDAVP or von Willebrand factor–containing factor VIII concentrates (e.g., Humate P)
Major surgery	Keep 50%–100% for 7–14 days	
Factor XI Deficiency		
Minor surgery	>30% for 3–4 days	FFP
Major surgery	>45% for 7–10 days	
Factor VII Deficiency		
Minor surgery	>15%	FFP or recombinant human factor VIIa
Major surgery	>25%	
Factor X Deficiency		
Minor surgery	>15%	FFP or prothrombin complex concentrates
Major surgery	>50% perioperatively, then >30%	
Factor V Deficiency		
Minor surgery	>25%	FFP
Major surgery	>50% perioperatively, then >25%	
Prothrombin Deficiency		
Minor surgery	20%–40%	FFP or prothrombin complex concentrates
Major surgery	20%–40%	
Afibrinogenemia or Hypofibrinogenemia		
Minor surgery	>50% to 100 mg/dL for 3 days	Cryoprecipitate
Major surgery	>50% to 100 mg/dL for 2 weeks	
Factor XIII Deficiency		
Minor surgery	>5%	FFP or cryoprecipitate
Major surgery	>5%	

DDAVP, 1-Deamino-8-D-arginine vasopressin; *FFP,* fresh frozen plasma

BOX 1: Hemostatic agents

Fresh Frozen Plasma

Contains all coagulation factors in low concentrations (1 U/mL)
Used for treatment of factor deficiency states without available factor concentrates
Used for treatment of coagulopathies associated with deficiency of multiple factors (e.g., liver disease, cardiac surgery, dilutional coagulopathy)

Cryoprecipitate

Contains factor VIII, von Willebrand factor, fibrinogen, factor XIII
Used for treatment of fibrinogen and factor XIII deficiency
Should *not* be used for treatment of factor VIII deficiency or von Willebrand disease *unless* factor VIII/von Willebrand–containing concentrates are not available

Factor VIII Concentrates (Recombinant, Plasma Derived)

Used for treatment of hemophilia A (factor VIII deficiency) and von Willebrand disease (e.g., Humate P and other von Willebrand factor–containing factor VIII concentrates)
Factor IX concentrates (recombinant, plasma derived)
Used for treatment of hemophilia B (factor IX deficiency)
Prothrombin complex concentrate
Contains vitamin K–dependent factors II, IX, and X
Used for reversal of warfarin anticoagulation in patients with serious bleeding

Activated Prothrombin Complex Concentrates

Contain activated factors II, VII, IX, and X
Used for treatment for factor VIII inhibitors

Recombinant Human Factor VIIa

Licensed for treatment of factor VIII inhibitors (e.g., used off-label for treatment of bleeding in patients with inherited platelet dysfunction, cardiac surgery coagulopathy)

Fibrin Sealants

Contain fibrinogen, thrombin, factor XIII
Used as a local hemostatic agent

Antifibrinolytic Agents (ε-Aminocaproic Acid, Aprotinin)

Inhibit the fibrinolysis by inhibiting plasmin activity or generation

Desmopressin

Induces release of von Willebrand factor and factor VIII
Used for treatment of mild von Willebrand disease and factor VIII deficiency

Coagulopathy of Liver Disease

All of the coagulation factors are synthesized by hepatocytes. Levels of the vitamin K–dependent factors and factor V decrease with progressive hepatocellular failure. Fibrinogen and factor VIII tend to be elevated in mild liver failure but decrease as liver disease progresses. Low-grade drug-induced coagulopathy occurs when the liver cannot degrade activated clotting factors, which leads to platelet dysfunction and further consumption of coagulation factors. Acute bleeding resulting from liver failure is treated with fresh frozen plasma (FFP) to replace the circulating coagulation factors and cryoprecipitate, if fibrinogen levels are less than 100 mg/dL. Platelet transfusions may also become necessary if thrombocytopenia or platelet dysfunction occurs.

Disseminated Intravascular Coagulopathy

Chronic anticoagulation therapy or perioperative anticoagulation may lead to bleeding complications for critically ill patients.

Heparin and Low Molecular Weight Heparin

Heparin potentiates the effects of antithrombin on thrombin and factors Xa and IXa. It is often used to initiate treatment for arterial and venous obstruction as well as being used intraoperatively for cardiac and vascular procedures. A history of heparin use along with an elevated aPTT is diagnostic. The anticoagulant effect of heparin disappears after a few hours but may last up to 12 hours with LMWH. For acute bleeding episodes, the effects of heparin can be reversed with intravenous protamine (1 mg protamine/100 U heparin).

Direct Thrombin Inhibitors (Bivalrudin, Lepirudin, Agatroban)

Lepirudin is a recombinant direct thrombin inhibitor approved for use in patients with heparin-induced thrombocytopenia (HIT). It is administered intravenously and monitored using aPTT (goal of 1.5 to 2.5 normal) and is excreted by the kidneys; lepirudin has a half-life of 1.3 hours, and because there is no reversal agent, it must be used cautiously in patients with renal failure.

Bivalrudin is a synthetic direct thrombin inhibitor that is administered intravenously as an alternative to heparin for patients undergoing cardiac procedures. The half-life of bivalrudin is 25 minutes in patients with normal renal function; there is no reversal agent, and dosage reductions are needed in patients with renal impairment.

Argatroban is a synthetic compound based on the structure of L-arginine, and it binds to the catalytic site of thrombin. Administered intravenously for patients with HIT, the onset of action is immediate, and the half-life is 40 to 50 minutes. It is metabolized by the cytochrome P450 enzymes in the liver and therefore is safe in renal-impaired patients, but dosage adjustments must be made for liver impairment; there is no reversal agent.

Warfarin

Warfarin is the most common orally administered vitamin K antagonist used for chronic anticoagulation. The duration of action of warfarin is 2 to 5 days, and it is monitored using the PT and INR. Many medications can alter the effects of warfarin and increase the risk of bleeding. In the critically ill patient, the most common medications include antifungals, antibiotics, amiodarone, and some loop diuretics. For patients with active bleeding, FFP and oral or subcutaneous vitamin K may be administered to restore vitamin K–dependent factors. In emergent situations, recombinant human factor VIIa (70 to 100 µg/kg body weight) is available for immediate reversal.

ANATOMIC VASCULAR DEFECTS

Bleeding from an anatomic vascular defect is usually brisk and is often fatal if not corrected. For patients without a known tissue disorder, postoperative bleeding is usually due to an arterial anastomotic leak, venous injury, or inadvertent injury to a vascular organ (liver, spleen). Minimal response to aggressive resuscitation is an indication for surgical exploration.

SUMMARY

Coagulation disorders are common in the critically ill population. It is important that the patient undergo a rapid review of history, examination, and laboratory assessment to direct an appropriate treatment plan.

Suggested Readings

Blood coagulation and anticoagulant: thrombotic, and antiplatelet drugs. In Brunton LL, Parker KL, Murri N, Blumenthal DK, editors: *Goodman & Gilman's pharmacological basis of therapeutics*, ed 11, New York, 2006, McGraw-Hill.

Marks PW: Coagulation disorders in the ICU, *Clin Chest Med* 30:123–129, 2009.

Seligsohn U, Kaushansky K, et al: Classification, clinical manifestations, and evaluation of disorders of hemostasis. In Lichtman MA, Beutler E, Kipps TJ, editors: *Williams hematology*, ed 7, New York, 2006, McGraw-Hill.

MINIMALLY INVASIVE SURGERY

LAPAROSCOPIC CHOLECYSTECTOMY

John D. Mellinger, MD, and Bruce V. MacFadyen, MD

OVERVIEW

Since its initial performance by Muhe in 1985, and subsequent description and dissemination in the late 1980s, laparoscopic cholecystectomy has not only transformed the surgical management of gallbladder disease, it has fostered a revolution in surgical practice oriented on the principle of minimally invasive access to the body's internal organs. Second only to inguinal hernia repair in terms of the number of operations done annually by general surgeons in the United States, this technique has firmly established itself as the procedure of choice for symptom-producing disease of the gallbladder. For most surgeons and surgeons in training, experience with laparoscopic cholecystectomy forms the introduction to and foundation for the development and maintenance of clinical laparoscopic skills. Review of the appropriate application of this technique, as well as a careful consideration of its conduct, is thus fundamental to the contemporary practice of surgery.

INDICATIONS

The most common indication for laparoscopic cholecystectomy is symptomatic cholelithiasis, which most frequently presents as intermittent biliary colic. Typical episodes localize to the right upper quadrant or epigastrium, may radiate to the back or right shoulder, often occur in postprandial fashion and especially after fatty food intake, and resolve spontaneously after a period of minutes to hours. Associated less specific symptoms such as bloating, nausea, and vomiting are common. Middle-aged female patients are the most likely group affected. Pregnancy, hemolytic disorders, rapid weight loss, and prior ileal resection may also be predisposing factors that heighten suspicion for the diagnosis. Patients with such a presentation should be evaluated with abdominal ultrasound, and a differential diagnosis that includes cardiac ischemia, right lower lobe pneumonia, peptic and reflux disease, malabsorptive disorders, and inflammatory or motility disturbances of the gastrointestinal tract should be considered. In patients with a negative ultrasound, microlithiasis or biliary dyskinesia may be considered. Radionuclide scanning with an iminodiacetic acid derivative and cholecystokinin-analog administration, allowing calculation of a gallbladder ejection fraction, should be considered in settings of typical symptoms and no evidence of cholelithiasis on ultrasound. An ejection fraction of less than 35% is considered abnormal and is indicative of dyskinesia, although sphincter of Oddi dysfunction or periampullary pathology unrelated to the gallbladder may cause similarly abnormal emptying function and should be considered as possible confounding issues in appropriate settings.

Fortunately, in the setting of a diminished ejection fraction, 75% or more of patients note symptomatic improvement with cholecystectomy alone. A reasonable strategy in the absence of more overt signs of a process distal to the gallbladder, such as elevated liver function studies or a dilated common bile duct (CBD) on ultrasound, would therefore be to offer cholecystectomy in such settings, deferring sphincter of Oddi manometry or other specialized evaluations for patients who do not experience relief after removal of the gallbladder. In specialized centers, endoscopic ultrasound and evaluation of bile for cholesterol crystals are available and are sometimes helpful in clarifying the diagnosis, when it remains unclear after more standard evaluations.

Acute cholecystitis may be the initial presentation of cholelithiasis in up to 20% of patients who develop symptomatic gallstone disease. These patients have lingering pain associated with persisting tenderness in the right upper quadrant, often with concomitant inflammatory signs such as leukocytosis and fever. Again, ultrasound is the most helpful diagnostic tool and may show signs of acute inflammation, such as gallbladder wall thickening or pericholecystic fluid. Nonvisualization of the gallbladder on radionuclide scanning may also be a means of inferring the diagnosis of acute cholecystitis as a harbinger of cystic duct obstruction, which is the underlying pathology of the disease entity. In less typical presentations, computed tomography (CT) may make the diagnosis while looking for other possible pathologies, again by showing inflammatory changes of the gallbladder, although the majority of gallstones are radiolucent.

Patients with acute cholecystitis are usually admitted and prepared for surgery within 24 to 48 hours. If presentation is later in the course of the illness, 72 hours or more, it may be advisable to treat the patient medically with antibiotics, and in severe cases or in highly comorbid settings, percutaneous drainage of the gallbladder should be done with surgery deferred for 4 to 6 weeks to allow the advanced inflammatory process to subside. Patients so managed have an approximately 25% relapse rate if the gallbladder is not removed within 6 to 8 weeks.

Other complicating illnesses such as gallstone pancreatitis, choledocholithiasis, and cholangitis may complicate cholelithiasis; these are typically manifested by elevations of serum enzymes, which include amylase, lipase, and liver function enzymes respectively. Elevation of these laboratory markers, clinical jaundice, and dilation of the biliary system on ultrasonography or CT should raise suspicion of the diagnosis. Magnetic resonance cholangiopancreatography (MRCP) or endoscopic retrograde cholangiopancreatography (ERCP) should be considered if the diagnosis remains unclear or nonoperative therapeutic intervention is needed.

Percutaneous transhepatic cholangiographic (PTC) approaches may also be considered, particularly if prior foregut surgery limits endoscopic access to the biliary system. In these settings, older or comorbid patients whose presenting illness was clearly related to choledocholithiasis, and who do not have lingering symptoms from residual cholelithiasis after common duct clearance by ERCP or PTC, do not necessarily need subsequent cholecystectomy, and the majority will not require a delayed cholecystectomy for symptoms over their remaining lifespan. In younger patients, cholecystectomy is appropriate after resolution of the acute common duct stone-related diathesis.

For patients with spontaneously resolving gallstone pancreatitis, it is important to remove the gallbladder after resolution of the pancreatitis, which typically will include spontaneous offending common duct stone passage, or there will be a 25% to 30% risk of recurrent pancreatitis over the next 6 to 8 weeks. Centers with facility in laparoscopic CBD exploration have reported good results with combined removal of the gallbladder and clearance of the choledocholithiasis. This approach should be considered, where local expertise allows, and offers cost and length-of-stay advantages over strategies utilizing separate ERCP and laparoscopic cholecystectomy procedures, provided the patient is stable for a general anesthetic with regard to any common duct pathology.

Other more rare indications for laparoscopic cholecystectomy may include concern for neoplastic risk in the setting of calcification of the gallbladder wall ("porcelain gallbladder"), enlarging gallbladder polyps, or very large (>3 cm) gallstones. Most gallbladder polyps are simply cholesterol depositions in the gallbladder wall, and are therefore treated based on symptoms rather than out of concern for neoplastic risk. Enlarging polyps or those greater than 1 cm in size may rarely be adenomatous and premalignant, and in such settings cholecystectomy is advised regardless of systems.

Because of the prevalence of cholelithiasis on imaging studies, a final question on indications for cholecystectomy relates to the issue of asymptomatic gallstones. Most patients with asymptomatic stones do not develop subsequent symptomatic disease, and 60% to 70% or more in some series remain asymptomatic long term. Exceptions where "prophylactic" cholecystectomy should be considered would include patients who are immunocompromised, awaiting organ transplantation, and those with sickle cell disease. Patients with diabetes do not have an increased risk of fulminant acute disease, and other than their comorbid status, they are not at risk for advanced initial presentation; accordingly, prophylactic cholecystectomy is not recommended in the setting of diabetes.

Contraindications to laparoscopic cholecystectomy are limited to patients in whom general anesthesia and pneumoperitoneum are precluded, such as with acute cardiopulmonary disease. In these settings, nonoperative strategies may serve the patient best. Advanced cirrhosis, suspicion of gallbladder carcinoma, necrotic gallbladder with extensive surrounding inflammation, Mirizzi's syndrome, concomitant acute cholangitis with sepsis unamenable to endoscopic or other nonoperative therapy, and cholecystoenteric fistulous disease are other settings in which an open approach may be advantageous. The surgeon's experience and ability to safely delineate the anatomy, determine the appropriateness of the laparoscopic approach in more complicated settings, and attend to patient safety is always the most important consideration. Pregnancy is not a contraindication to laparoscopic cholecystectomy, but the operation should be deferred until after delivery when possible. If operation during gestation is necessary, the second trimester is the most advantageous time because of the heightened risk of spontaneous abortion in the first trimester and limited peritoneal access and risk of premature labor in the third trimester.

TECHNIQUE

The patient is positioned with arms abducted on arm boards and dual monitors off the patient's shoulders, so they are respectively in a direct visual line for the surgeon standing on the patient's left and the first assistant opposite. If there is a high likelihood of cholangiographic guided intervention such as laparoscopic CBD duct exploration, it is helpful to tuck the arms to facilitate positioning of C-arm fluoroscopy and additional equipment that may be used. A foot board is useful to prevent the patient sliding on the table when in reverse Trendelenburg position.

Preparation is done from the nipples to the groins and should always include areas needed for laparotomy, should it become necessary. Antibiotic prophylaxis is controversial in elective settings but is still our routine practice: a single dose, given at the time of anesthetic induction. Bacterobilia is present in up to 25% of elderly patients and approximately 10% of the overall population, although the clinical significance is rare in uncomplicated settings. General anesthesia is required, and initial carbon dioxide pneumoperitoneum may be achieved with an open technique or with a Veress needle.

Because it facilitates safety in reoperative settings and creates a port site suitable for subsequent organ extraction, we prefer to use an open approach. A paraumbilical entry is made, as dictated by prior surgical scars and the position of the umbilicus in relation to the gallbladder fossa; stay sutures are placed, and a Hasson-type trocar is secured. Initial insufflation should be done at low-flow settings to avoid vasovagal responses and to ensure safe positioning until visually confirmed with laparoscope introduction.

A 15 mm Hg pressure limit is typically utilized, and lower pressure settings may be appropriate with pregnancy or cirrhosis. We prefer to use a 5 or 10 mm, 30-degree angled laparoscope for its visual versatility. Additional trocars are placed under laparoscopic visualization in the epigastrium, just to the patient's right of the falciform ligament (typically 10 mm) and the right subcostal area in the midclavicular and anterior axillary lines (typically 5 mm). Sizes may be decreased to 5 mm at all sites if a 5 mm laparoscope and clip applier are employed. Smaller (2 mm) and so-called needlescopic trocars have been employed but are without added significant cosmetic or recovery benefit, and these may be of limited efficacy in settings of obesity or advanced gallbladder pathology.

Various "single site" techniques have also been more recently described and typically involve placement of multiple trocars through a single paraumbilical incision and juxtaposed fascial trocar insertion sites. These techniques provide a single incision cosmetically but may limit the surgeon's retraction and exposure options compared with standard technique; their ultimate utility and efficacy remain a subject of study, especially in more complicated cases.

The patient is placed in reverse Trendelenburg position after initial trocar placement, and it is sometimes helpful, particularly if there is an enlarged left hepatic lobe or pregnancy, to rotate patients slightly to their left to facilitate exposure and venous return respectively. The gallbladder is elevated in a cephalad direction by grasping the fundus from the right lateral trocar, and the infundibulum is grasped via the midclavicular trocar and retracted laterally, toward the patient's right, to open the hepatocystic triangle. Surgeons may have assistants provide this retraction, or they may control the infundibulum themselves, which facilitates bimanual manipulation and dissection.

The visceral peritoneum is then opened over the area of the gallbladder/cystic duct junction by grasping and pulling in the opposite direction of the infundibular retraction, namely medially and inferiorly. Subsequent grasping and tearing of the investing peritoneum of the triangle itself, alternating anteriorly and posteriorly as the assistant provides opposing traction and exposure, allows the entire triangle to be divested of its peritoneal covering before any structures within it are developed. Cautery is avoided until all structures have been so exposed, and the anatomy clearly delineated, to avoid injury to biliary or vascular structures that may variably, but not uncommonly, be present and require preservation.

The cystic duct and artery are then developed by gentle dissection from the investing areolar tissues using sweeping, spreading, and gentle teasing motions of the dissecting forceps. The cystic duct

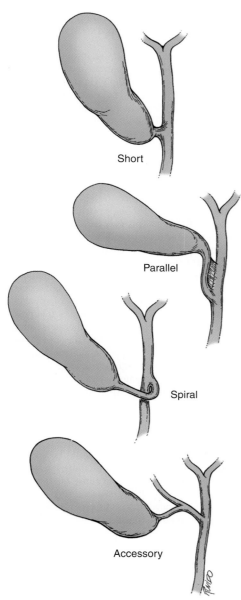

FIGURE 1 Anatomic variants of cystic duct insertion. *(From Mellinger JD: Cholecystectomy in chronic cholecystitis. In MacFadyen BV, Ponsky JL [eds]: Operative laparoscopy and thoracoscopy, Philadelphia, 1996, Lippincott-Raven, pp 203–228.)*

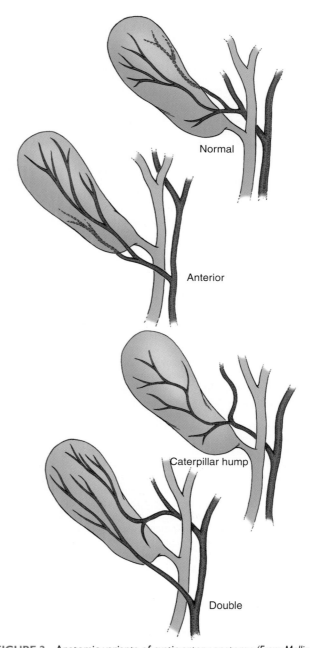

FIGURE 2 Anatomic variants of cystic artery anatomy. *(From Mellinger JD: Cholecystectomy in chronic cholecystitis. In MacFadyen BV, Ponsky JL [eds]: Operative laparoscopy and thoracoscopy, Philadelphia, 1996, Lippincott-Raven, pp 203–228.)*

and artery in particular are carefully traced to their junctions with the gallbladder proper and are developed to allow control with clips. Care should be taken to note the position of the CBD prior to clip application and to use cholangiography liberally if the anatomy is uncertain or appears atypical. It is very helpful to keep in mind the common variations of cystic duct and cystic arterial anatomy as the dissection is accomplished (Figure 1 and Figure 2). A so-called *critical view* is a useful concept at this phase, meaning that before any structures are clipped or divided, the cystic duct and artery are developed adequately to see their course to the gallbladder, with the infundibulum retracted laterally and hepatic parenchyma visible posteriorly through the window developed between those structures.

Although cholangiography has not been shown to clearly prevent bile duct injury, complete and properly interpreted cholangiograms

do help to minimize the risk of major ductal injury. The cystic duct and artery are then clipped and divided. If the cystic duct is larger or more edematous than what may be suitable for clipping, absorbable suture with intracorporeal or extracorporeal knot technique is a suitable alternative.

It is our practice to gently tease the areolar tissues that stretch between the gallbladder infundibulum and the gallbladder fossa with a dissecting forceps before using cautery, even after division of the cystic duct and artery; this is because it is not uncommon to encounter an accessory cystic artery or, more rarely, a right hepatic biliary ductal or arterial branch. If identified, such structures are carefully developed and controlled or spared as appropriate. Once this is done, the gallbladder is then mobilized off the hepatic fossa, with cautery applied with either a hook instrument or laparoscopic scissors, as the surgeon's preference dictates. The hook is useful for allowing the operator to create and direct added tension in addition to that provided by the assistant.

It is important for the surgeon to keep the dissection on the plane between the gallbladder and liver capsule to minimize the risk of bile spillage, bleeding, and postoperative bile leaks from terminal ductules in the hepatic parenchyma. Cautery application is limited during the dissection to 2 or 3 second applications to minimize the risk of establishing capacitance circuits in the abdomen that may then lead to bowel or other visceral injury. It is also important to avoid cautery application adjacent to any clips staying in the patient, as conduction of the current to these can lead to delayed thermal injuries, which can include strictures and leaks. The camera operator should carefully work during this phase, as throughout the procedure, to ensure that no instrument introduction or cautery application takes place outside the visual field, which may dynamically alter as tension and cautery are applied.

Prior to final delivery of the gallbladder, the operative area is reinspected for any evidence of bleeding, bile leakage, or insecure clips, after which the gallbladder is fully released. Reducing the insufflation pressure settings to watch for venous bleeding in the liver bed that may otherwise be offset by the pressure of the pneumoperitoneum may be wise, particularly in patients with portal hypertension. The gallbladder is then delivered via the umbilical incision after transferring the laparoscope to the epigastric port. A bag may be utilized but is not necessary if the gallbladder was not entered during dissection. If the gallbladder was entered, any spilled stones should be retrieved if possible. Scooping forceps are useful for this purpose. Although delayed sequelae of spilled stones are relatively rare compared with the number of cases in which some degree of bile spill occurs (up to 30% in some series), a variety of delayed inflammatory and infectious complications have been described, so such a spill is clearly not innocuous.

The trocars are removed under laparoscopic guidance to observe for bleeding. The fascia at the umbilical site is closed with absorbable suture, and stay sutures are placed during Hasson insertion. Fascia is typically not closed at the remaining sites, although closure of the 10 mm epigastric site may be done at the surgeon's discretion using a suture-passing device under laparoscopic guidance. Skin closure is accomplished with absorbable subcuticular suture, and dressings are applied.

In complicated settings such as acute cholecystitis, several adjunctive or alternative techniques may be useful. Perhaps the most useful technique with a tensely distended, acutely inflamed, or gangrenous gallbladder is to aspirate the organ before grasping. This can be done with a laparoscopic aspiration needle introduced through a port or a large length and caliber (14 to 18 gauge) spinal or intravenous access needle introduced directly through the abdominal wall. The gallbladder may also be opened with scissors and suctioned, although this may lead to a higher risk of stone spillage, if this entry site is not readily and persistently controlled with a grasper or suture closure through the subsequent dissection. Toothed graspers may be helpful in controlling the gallbladder once decompressed but may also increase the risk of further tearing and spill during dissection.

Adhesions are typically present in such advanced inflammatory settings but are often acute and edematous, and blunt sweeping on the plane directly on the gallbladder wall will typically allow freeing of the structure to allow subsequent grasping and retraction. As the infundibulum is exposed, continued dissection of the inflamed tissue planes is safest if it proceeds from right lateral to medial, as this achieves added retraction freedom and often allows the critical structure dissection to be commenced only after optimizing retraction and exposure.

Use of a suction/irrigation device is critical in preserving the field of view in such cases where bleeding from the inflamed surfaces can otherwise complicate visualization, and such a device often proves to be a very useful blunt dissecting instrument as well in such settings. If appropriate visualization and exposure cannot be achieved with this approach, conversion to an open procedure should be done in the interest of patient safety.

A dome or fundus-down dissection technique is also potentially useful in cases of advanced inflammation or fibrosis that obscures visualization of the hepatocystic triangle via standard techniques. In this setting, the liver may be elevated by a variety of retractors, either table or handheld, and the gallbladder is dissected off the hepatic bed so that infundibular dissection is circumferential down to the level of the cystic duct and artery. The surgeon should also remember that cholangiography can be obtained by injection into the gallbladder if needed to delineate anatomy and guide safe operative decisions, provided no impacted stone obstructs the gallbladder/cystic duct junction.

Another technique sometimes required in the setting of advanced inflammatory disease is that of leaving a portion of the posterior wall of the gallbladder on the liver. This may be done if the dissection off the liver bed is not possible in an area of advanced fibrotic change. In such settings, the surgeon should remain cognizant of the possibility of neoplasia, and if suspected, conversion to an open procedure with oncologically appropriate wide excision of the gallbladder bed and regional lymphadenectomy would be advised. If a portion of the posterior wall is left on the hepatic bed because of advanced fibrosis and nonneoplastic disease that renders removal of that portion of the gallbladder unduly hazardous, the residual mucosa is cauterized, and a temporary drain is often left in place. Drain placement is sometimes helpful in settings of advanced inflammation in general, as a means to evacuate fluid and monitor for low-grade bile leaks from the liver bed area following such difficult dissections, and this may be readily done laparoscopically by advancing a grasper from the lateral retracting port through the epigastric trocar with retrograde drain positioning (Figure 3).

According to national databases, conversion to an open procedure is required in 5% to 10% of cases, and in up to 25% of cases with severe inflammation. The surgeon should be aware that common duct injuries have been shown to be more likely very early in a surgeon's learning curve with the procedure but also later in their application of the technique, likely representing a willingness to employ it with more advanced disease as experience and confidence have grown. A paramount commitment to patient safety, steady progress of the dissection, adequate visualization and exposure, and clear delineation of all anatomy before structure division will appropriately serve the surgeon in the decision about whether to convert to an open approach. In any event, such a decision should not be seen as a failure but rather an appropriate judgment in the interest of patient safety.

As a final comment in regard to the technique of laparoscopic cholecystectomy, there is growing interest in the concept of natural orifice transluminal endoscopic surgery (NOTES) approaches to cholecystectomy. Clinical experience has been described with both transgastric and transvaginal NOTES approaches to cholecystectomy. Many of the initial reports involve hybrid techniques with laparoscopic or transabdominal access along with the transluminal approach. Meaningful benefits of this technique, as well as the risks and technical limits of such approaches, if and when they are applied on a widespread scale, remain to be determined. Expanded endoscopic and laparoscopic instrumentation capabilities will be a likely beneficial outcome of this area of endeavor, regardless of its eventual broader clinical applications or lack thereof.

COMPLICATIONS

The most common intraoperative complications encountered are bleeding and stone spillage. The latter is mentioned above and is estimated in the literature to occur in up to 30% of cases. Spillage

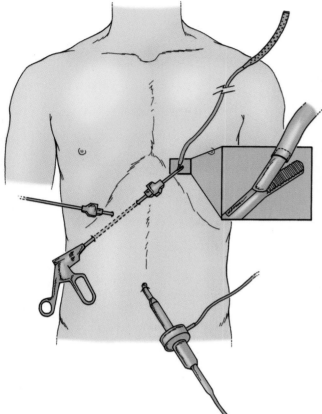

FIGURE 3 Drain placement technique. *(From Mellinger JD: Cholecystectomy in chronic cholecystitis. In MacFadyen BV, Ponsky JL [eds]: Operative laparoscopy and thoracoscopy, Philadelphia, 1996, Lippincott-Raven, pp 203–228.)*

is more likely to occur in settings of advanced or acute inflammation and should be addressed with a judicious effort to retrieve all spilled stones owing to the relatively rare, but not insignificant, well-described risk of delayed infectious and other complications of retained spilled stones. When encountered, bleeding is often seen during the dissection of the structures in the hepatocystic triangle, especially in the setting of advanced acute inflammation or chronic fibrosis. In such cases bleeding typically arises from an inadvertent trauma to a cystic artery or other communicating branch of the right hepatic artery.

The surgeon should resist the temptation to blindly use cautery or clips without first clearly delineating the anatomy. A useful technique when simple suction, irrigation, or gentle grasping and continued observation fail to allow efficient and appropriately directed control is for the assistant to use the infundibulum as a tamponade agent and push it via the grasper retracting that portion of the gallbladder into the area of bleeding (Figure 4). The surgeon may then place a fifth trocar into the abdomen, typically between the umbilicus and epigastric trocar sites, and work bimanually with suction and dissection to delineate the anatomy and allow safe control of the clearly delineated source. Inability to rapidly control bleeding should prompt conversion to an open approach. Bleeding from the hepatic bed is usually readily controlled with limited cautery application or with topical prothrombotic agents or argon plasma coagulation if necessary. Trocar-site bleeding is often seen during inspected trocar withdrawal if it does occur, and it is most efficiently dealt with by placement of transfascial sutures around the site using suture placement tools such as the Carter–Thompson device, which was designed for such placement.

Bile duct injury is the most feared complication of laparoscopic cholecystectomy, and although rare in experienced hands, it continues to be reported more frequently (0.3% to 1.0% incidence) than in series done via an open approach. Avoidance is best achieved by the measures outlined above, including avoidance of cautery early in the dissection or in proximity to major structures or clips that can act as conductors; clear visualization and demonstration of the anatomy, including liberal use of complete and properly interpreted cholangiography in unclear settings; optimization of visualization through careful clearance of any bleeding prior to control of structures during dissection; and exercising particular care in settings of advanced inflammatory disease.

Unfortunately, a high percentage of bile duct injuries are not recognized when they occur. If recognized, small tangential injuries of the common duct, such as a partial tear due to avulsion/retraction at the cystic duct insertion site, may be dealt with by T tube placement. More advanced injuries include full-thickness transections of the CBD, injuries associated with excision of a portion of the common duct or right hepatic duct mistaken for the cystic duct, or injuries associated with thermal energy; these should be dealt with via Roux-en-Y hepaticojejunostomy. Injuries recognized in the early postoperative period, manifested by jaundice or biloma formation, should be investigated with high-resolution cholangiography such as ERCP or percutaneous cholangiography. For partial-thickness injuries and low-volume leaks, sphincterotomy and/or stenting via one of these approaches may achieve control of the leak and allow healing. Endoscopic stenting in prolonged fashion may also allow successful nonoperative management of some partial-thickness injuries and partial strictures of the bile duct following operative injury. For more advanced injuries such as complete ductal division, obstruction, or excision, unless recognized very early in the course, the best option is a delayed hepaticojejunostomy reconstruction by a highly experienced biliary surgeon after thorough control of the leak and decompression of the biliary system with detailed cholangiographic delineation of the injury via percutaneous drains and catheters.

Other rare complications include trocar site hernias, which are typically at the umbilicus and most commonly occur when a preexisting umbilical hernia was not addressed at the time of surgery, or when inadequate fascial closure is accomplished at this site. If an umbilical hernia is present preoperatively, a useful strategy is to use the hernia as the initial access site and repair it at the end of the procedure. Changes in bowel habits with increased stool frequency is a relatively frequent complaint after cholecystectomy, occurring in up to 25% of patients; but in the vast majority, this resolves over a period of weeks to months after the surgery. If persistent, such complaints should be evaluated to exclude other sources of the change in bowel habits, and if none are identified, symptoms may be ameliorated with medical measures, such as fiber supplementation or cholestyramine administration.

SUMMARY

Laparoscopic cholecystectomy offers a well-attested means of control for the symptoms of gallbladder disease, by far the most common intraabdominal pathology encountered in the typical gastrointestinal surgical practice. As such, it is clearly established at this point as the procedure of choice in dealing with symptomatic disease of the gallbladder. The principles learned and repetitively applied in performing this operation form the foundation of most surgeons' skill set in minimally invasive surgical technique, both before and, by volume criteria if not otherwise, after residency training. A thorough understanding of the indications, anatomical variations, technique, and potential complications of this procedure—with attention to their prevention, recognition, and management—is thus of paramount significance in surgical education and practice.

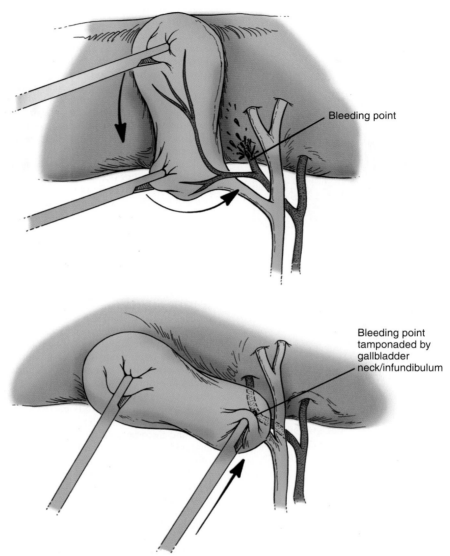

FIGURE 4   Control of bleeding in hepatocystic triangle. *(From Mellinger JD: Cholecystectomy in chronic cholecystitis. In MacFadyen BV, Ponsky JL [eds]: Operative laparoscopy and thoracoscopy, Philadelphia, 1996, Lippincott-Raven, pp 203–228.)*

Suggested Readings

MacFadyen BV, Vecchio R, Ricardo AE, et al: Bile duct injury after laparoscopic cholecystectomy: the United States experience, *Surg Endosc* 12:315, 1998.

Mellinger JD: Cholecystectomy in chronic cholecystitis. In MacFadyen BV, Ponsky JL, editors: *Operative laparosocopy and thoracoscopy*, Philadelphia, 1996, Lippincott-Raven.

Mellinger JD, Eldridge TJ, Eddelmon ED, et al: Delayed gallstone abscess following laparoscopic cholecystectomy, *Surg Endosc* 8:1332, 1994.

Olsen DO, Wolfe RS: Laparoscopic cholecystectomy: the technique. In MacFadyen BV, editor: *Laparoscopic surgery of the abdomen*, New York, 2004, Springer-Verlag.

Shamiyeh A, Wayand W: Laparoscopic cholecystectomy: early and late complications and their treatment, *Langenbecks Arch Surg* 389:164, 2004.

LAPAROSCOPIC MANAGEMENT OF COMMON BILE DUCT STONES

Joseph B. Petelin, MD, and Alejandro Arnold, MD

HISTORIC PERSPECTIVE

Choledocholithiasis is present in approximately 10% of patients seen for cholecystectomy. Definitive treatment of these patients includes cholecystectomy and clearance of the entire ductal system. In the era of open biliary tract surgery, Courvoisier answered this challenge in 1890, nearly 8 years after Langenbuch performed the first open cholecystectomy in 1882. A century later, in the late 1980s, laparoscopic cholecystectomy was introduced and soon became the standard of care for treatment of symptomatic gallbladder disease. This was followed within 2 years by the introduction of several minimally invasive techniques that have proven successful in the treatment of choledocholithiasis in the laparoscopic era of biliary tract surgery. These techniques include administration of glucagon and flushing of the ductal system; dilation and flushing of the distal common bile duct (CBD) and sphincter; balloon catheter manipulation; basket manipulation, with or without fluoroscopic guidance; and choledochoscopic manipulations.

OVERVIEW OF PATIENT MANAGEMENT

The presence of CBD stones may be determined preoperatively, intraoperatively, or postoperatively. In the first situation, the clinician must decide whether to attempt ductal treatment, such as endoscopic retrograde cholangiography and extraction, with or without sphincterotomy (ERC ± S) before operation, or to proceed directly with laparoscopic cholecystectomy (LC) and laparoscopic common duct exploration (LCDE). ERC ± S is successful in clearing the common duct in 70% to more than 90% of cases but may need to be done more than once. Similarly, LCDE is successful in clearing the duct in 70% to more than 90% of cases as well, in one setting.

In the early 1990s, however, when preoperative ERC ± S was used quite liberally for patients suspected of having CBD stones, a normal exam was documented in 40% to 60% of patients. There is no proof that this statistic has changed for the better. Moreover, these patients were exposed to the added morbidity and mortality of ERC ± S, which has been reported to be as high as 5% to 19% and 1.3%, respectively. Numerous authors have suggested that the choice of clearance method should be based on the local availability of expert endoscopists capable of a high degree of success with ERC ± S, the availability of laparoscopic and choledochoscopic equipment, the surgeon's own expertise in laparoscopic surgery, and the general condition of the patient.

When CBD stones are discovered intraoperatively, the surgeon either proceeds with LCDE, converts the case to open common duct exploration and choledocholithotomy, or leaves the stones in place for subsequent ERC ± S. Although any of these alternatives is acceptable and is associated with success rates of greater than 90%, the latter two are more costly, and open CBD exploration is associated with increased morbidity. If LCDE is unsuccessful or is not attempted, the decision regarding conversion to open common duct exploration versus postoperative ERC ± S will depend on the local availability of expert endoscopists.

The third situation, in which retained CBD stones are encountered postoperatively, is best treated initially with ERC ± S. If this is not successful, then repeat surgical intervention may be necessary. These considerations are illustrated in Figure 1.

Indications

The most common indication for laparoscopic CBD exploration is an abnormal intraoperative cholangiogram or sonogram. Preoperative studies, including unexplained elevated liver function tests; a dilated ductal system; sonographic evidence of bile duct stones; scintigraphic, endoscopic, or radiographic evidence of CBD obstruction; or a history of biliary pancreatitis, which may also warrant laparoscopic CBD exploration.

Contraindications

The first and most important contraindication to LCDE is inability of the surgeon to perform the maneuvers required for laparoscopic CBD exploration. This means lack of specialized training and expertise. Absence of any of the noted indications listed above, instability of the patient, coagulopathy, and local conditions in the porta hepatis that would make exploration hazardous, such as severe inflammation or portal hypertension, are the other potential contraindications to laparoscopic CBD exploration.

Equipment and Operating Room Setup

In addition to the basic equipment used to perform laparoscopic cholecystectomy, a number of other instruments listed in Box 1 may be required to facilitate LCDE. For maximum efficiency, these tools should be organized in a central location, preferably a mobile LCDE cart that may be moved from room to room as necessary. Operating room setup is illustrated in Figure 2.

Access to the Common Duct

Laparoscopic CBD exploration may be accomplished through the cystic duct or through a choledochotomy. Stone size; the anatomy of the triangle of Calot, including the position of the cystic duct–common duct junction; the course of the cystic duct; and the diameter of each of the ducts affect the decision as to which approach is best in a particular case. If a transcystic approach appears feasible, it is usually attempted before choledochotomy, because it is less invasive, less morbid, and is associated with better patient satisfaction. Factors that influence the route of choice are listed in Table 1. Negative influences listed in this chart have a more profound impact on selection of the access route than positive or neutral ones.

OPERATIVE TECHNIQUES

The techniques discussed below may be used with either access route, although the transcystic approach usually results in less morbidity.

Ductal Imaging

The surgeon should be skilled with his or her preferred method of intraoperative imaging of the ductal system: percutaneous cholangiography, portal cholangiography, or intraoperative ultrasonography. Although some surgeons prefer sonography, most favor fluoroscopic imaging; it has become the preferred standard for intraoperative radiologic evaluation, in contrast to static x-rays, because it is faster

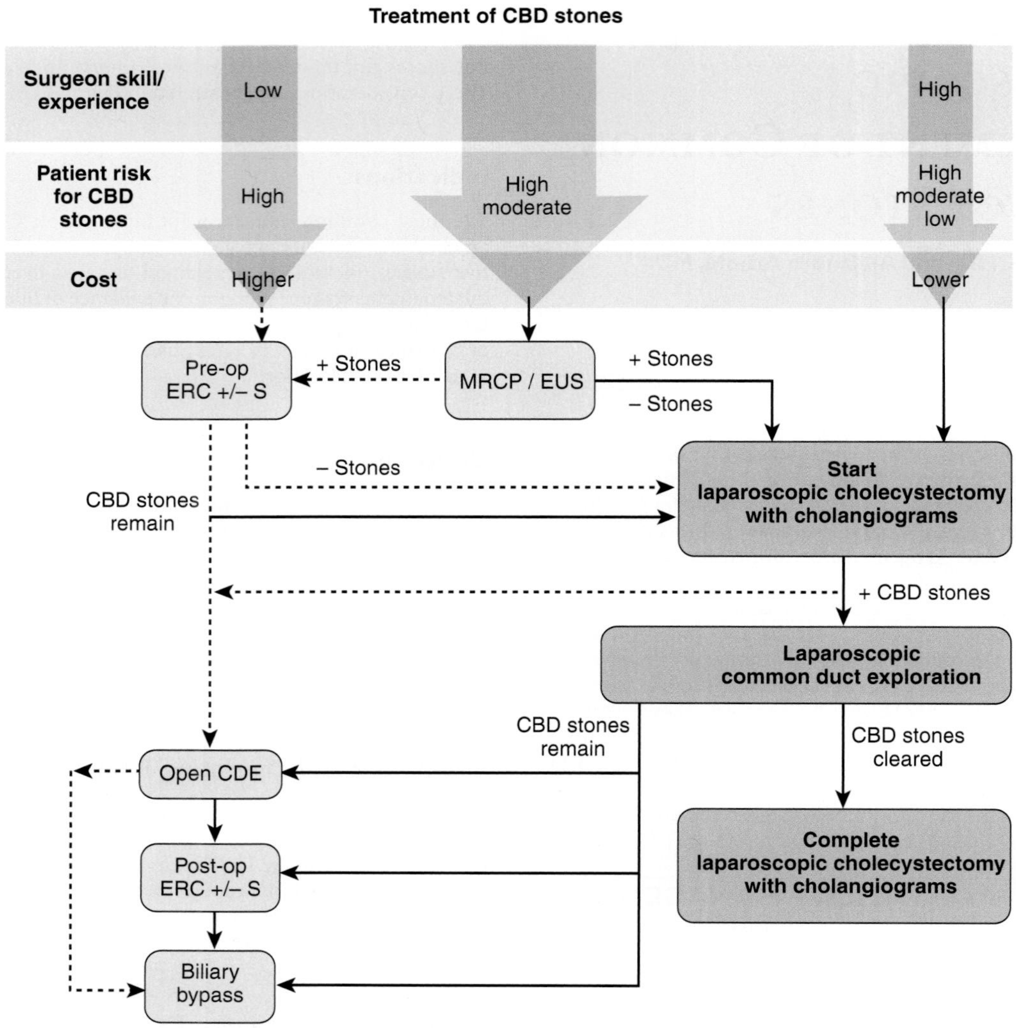

FIGURE 1   Protocol for management of common bile duct stones.

than other methods, more detailed, and allows surgeon interaction with the images in real time. The ductal system can be scanned by moving the C arm while injecting contrast material Figure 3.

Percutaneous Cholangiography

Percutaneous cholangiography employs a 14 gauge IV needle/ catheter inserted through the abdominal wall approximately 3 cm medial to the midclavicular port and directed toward the triangle of Calot. The needle is removed, and the catheter is used as a sleeve for introduction of the cholangiogram catheter; this sleeve also acts as a "miniport," which may be used for introduction of balloons and baskets during CBD exploration. The catheter is grasped with forceps, introduced through the medial epigastric port, and placed into the cystic duct. It is fixed into position with a clip loosely applied transversely across the axis of the catheter at its insertion point into the cystic duct.

Portal Cholangiography

This method requires removal of an instrument from one of the ports, usually the midclavicular port. The catheter is introduced

through this port freely or with an instrument that directs it into the cystic duct. Some instrument models also fix the catheter into the cystic duct. The major disadvantage of this technique is that it uses an existing port that would otherwise be occupied by an instrument providing exposure in the porta hepatis.

Intraoperative Sonography

With this technique, the ultrasound transducer is inserted through a 10 mm port, usually located in the epigastrium; it is placed in direct contact with the tissues to obtain real-time sonographic images. Proponents of this technology suggest that it is faster and more accurate than cholangiography, but most surgeons who advocate this base their judgment on studies comparing it to static cholangiograms. Critics have argued that fluoroscopic imaging is not only faster than sonographic imaging, but it does not require additional equipment expense, and it does not require a 10 mm port to be inserted into the epigastrium. Additionally, still images captured from fluoroscopic cholangiograms may be used as "maps" of the ductal anatomy in cases where intense inflammation obscures visual cues; this is not possible with sonography, and widespread use of laparoscopic sonography for ductal evaluation has not occurred.

BOX 1: Equipment for LCDE

Some or all of this equipment may be needed for LCDE:

- 14 gauge IV catheter, more than 2 inches long
- Fluoroscope, C-arm type
- Glucagon, 1 to 2 mg, given IV by the anesthetist
- Balloon-tipped catheters; 4 Fr is preferred over 3 and 5 Fr
- Segura-type baskets, four-wire, flat, straight, in-line configuration, <1 mm total diameter
- Guidewire 0.035 inches in diameter and >90 cm long
- Mechanical over-the-wire dilators (7 to 12 Fr), found in most urology departments
- High-pressure over-the-wire pneumatic dilator
- IV tubing for saline instillation through the choledochoscope
- Atraumatic grasping forceps for choledochoscope manipulation
- Flexible choledochoscope with light source, <3 mm diameter; a working channel >1.1 mm is preferred
- Second camera
- Second monitor or second viewing area on the primary laparoscopic monitor
- Video switcher for simultaneous same-monitor display of laparoscopic and choledochoscopic or fluoroscopic images
- Pressurized water jet (as for dental cleaning)
- Electrohydraulic or pulsed-dye lithotripter
- Absorbable polyglycolic acid suture, size 4-0 or 5-0
- T tube (transductal) or C tube (transcystic)
- Straight stent, 7 or 10 Fr
- Sphincterotome for antegrade sphincterotomy
- Side-viewing endoscope for antegrade sphincterotomy

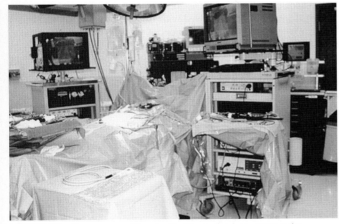

FIGURE 2   Room setup. The sterile Mayo stand containing the choledochoscope and related equipment is located next to the left-sided monitor trolley. It is moved next to the patient's left shoulder, in front of the trolley, when needed for duct exploration.

Preparation of the Access Route

Dilation of the Cystic Duct

When choledochoscopic maneuvers are attempted through the cystic duct, the duct will need to accept a 9 or 10 Fr diameter flexible scope. If the duct is not already large enough for scope insertion, it may be dilated either with over-the-wire mechanical graduated dilators or pneumatic dilators. In both situations, a guidewire (0.028 or 0.035 inches in diameter) is first inserted through the midclavicular port,

TABLE 1: Factors influencing access approach

Factor	INFLUENCE ON APPROACH	
	Transcystic	Choledochotomy
Stone Characteristics		
One stone	+	+
Multiple stones	+	+
Stones ≤6 mm diameter	+	+
Stones >6 mm diameter	–	+
Intrahepatic stones	–	+
Duct Diameters		
Diameter of cystic duct <4 mm	–	+
Diameter of cystic duct >4 mm	+	+
Diameter of common duct <6 mm	+	–
Diameter of common duct >6 mm	+	+
Cystic Duct Location		
Lateral cystic duct entrance	+	+
Medial cystic duct entrance	–	+
Posterior cystic duct entrance	–	+
Distal cystic duct entrance	–	+
Local Conditions		
Mild inflammation	+	+
Marked inflammation	+	–
Surgeon Skill Set		
Poor suturing ability	+	–
Good suturing ability	+	+

Negative factors have more influence on the approach than positive ones.
+, Positive or neutral effect; –, negative effect

through the cystic duct, and into the common duct. If graduated dilators are used, a 9 Fr size is usually the first to be advanced over the wire into the duct. Each successively larger dilator is advanced over the wire, until the duct is patulous enough to accept the scope. I have found that if a 9 Fr dilator will not initially easily enter the cystic duct, it is unlikely that dilation to a large enough diameter (11 or 12 Fr) will occur.

Pneumatic dilators may also be advanced over the wire into the cystic duct. The dilation balloon is filled using a screw-type Levine syringe, while observing changes in the duct on the video monitor and the pressure changes on the gauge attached to the dilator syringe. After dilation, the guidewire may be removed or left in place for subsequent guidance of the choledochoscope. If used to guide the scope, the wire is loaded into the distal end of the working channel of the scope and is then advanced into the ductal system over the wire.

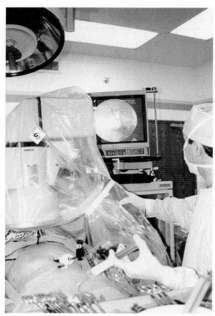

FIGURE 3 Fluoroscopic cholangiography.

Choledochotomy

Some authors prefer common duct access via a choledochotomy; others use this approach when the cystic duct cannot be dilated enough to accept passage of the scope or the largest common duct stone, or if intrahepatic pathology is suspected. Choledochotomy may be accomplished with a laparoscopic scalpel, scissors, or contact-tip laser inserted through the medial epigastric port. Avoiding the CBD blood supply, a longitudinal incision approximately 1 cm in length, or as long as the diameter of the largest stone, is usually recommended; this limits the amount time that will be spent later in closing the choledochotomy. Stay sutures, which are commonly used in open common duct exploration, are not necessary and are potentially harmful during LCDE, because they can tear out of the duct during manipulations of instruments based on an instrument fulcrum located on the abdominal wall.

Irrigation Techniques

Glucagon (1 to 2 mg IV) may be administered by the anesthetist to relieve sphincter pressure when very small stones (<3 mm diameter), sludge, or sphincter spasm are suspected to be responsible for lack of flow of contrast into the duodenum. Transcystic flushing of the duct with saline or contrast material should be attempted within 10 to 30 seconds in an attempt to gently force the debris into the duodenum; this process is monitored fluoroscopically. This technique often works well for 1 to 2 mm stones, but surgeons should not expect this method to be successful in clearing stones 4 mm and larger from the duct.

Balloon Techniques

This technique involves the use of a standard 4 Fr Fogarty balloon catheter inserted into the abdomen through the 14 gauge sleeve used to perform the percutaneous cholangiograms. The catheter is guided into the common duct through the cystic duct with forceps introduced through the medial epigastric port, and the catheter is advanced into the duodenum if possible. The balloon is inflated, and the catheter is withdrawn until resistance is met at the sphincter; the duodenum

is observed to move with the catheter at this point. The balloon is deflated, the catheter is withdrawn 1 cm, and the balloon is reinflated. This should position it in the most distal portion of the duct, just proximal to the sphincter. The catheter is then withdrawn through the cystic duct using the forceps from the medial epigastric port. Stones expressed from the cystic duct are usually removed through one of the larger ports. In the unusual event of displacement of the stone into the proximal hepatic duct, irrigation of the duct combined with operating table position changes will usually return the stone to the distal duct.

When a choledochotomy is needed, the combined use of the choledochoscope and a balloon catheter is particularly useful for stones that defy capture with a basket, even under direct vision through the choledochoscope. The balloon is inserted alongside the scope, not in the scope channel, and is advanced past the stone, inflated, and withdrawn to impact the stone against the scope. The entire scope-stone-balloon ensemble is then withdrawn through the ductal orifice. This technique is especially useful when dealing with intrahepatic stones.

Basket Techniques

Stone retrieval baskets may be inserted with or without the use of the choledochoscope. When used without the choledochoscope, the basket is inserted through the 14 gauge sleeve used for cholangiography. The basket is advanced into the common duct through the cystic duct, using forceps introduced through the medial epigastric port. The basket is opened immediately after it is advanced into the proximal CBD. The deployed wires offer not only a "soft" distal end to the catheter but also provide increased resistance when the catheter reaches the distal end of the bile duct. When the basket is located in the distal common duct, it is moved back and forth in small increments, slowly withdrawing it as the wires of the basket are being closed. Stone capture is identified when the basket fails to close completely. The device with the captured stone is removed through the cystic duct, and the stones are delivered from the abdomen as described above.

Great care must be exercised with this method so that accidental "capture" of the papilla of Vater does not occur. A fluoroscope may be used to more accurately localize the stones and basket tip. This technique, however, requires positioning of the fluoroscope in such a way as to avoid interference with movements of the forceps in the medial epigastric port. In some individuals, especially the obese, adequate fluoroscope position cannot be achieved.

Choledochoscopic Techniques

Choledochoscopic techniques are used when the conservative measures described above fail to clear the common duct (Figure 4). The choledochoscope is inserted in the most direct route to the triangle of Calot (usually via the midclavicular port) and, with or without wire guidance, into the cystic duct or the choledochotomy.

In the transcystic duct approach, if the scope will not traverse the cystic duct–common duct junction, further dissection along the lateral border of the cystic duct and CBD, or a Kocher maneuver, may allow the junction to "unwrap," thereby providing a less convoluted path into the common duct. It should be noted, however, that when a cystic duct approach is employed, access to the proximal hepatic ductal system is usually not possible, unless the cystic duct is very short or patulous and oriented at a right angle to the common duct. When a choledochotomy is used, the scope may be directed into either the proximal system or the distal bile duct.

The scope is manipulated the same way in both approaches. At the level of the skin, the surgeon initially uses an atraumatic forceps inserted through the medial epigastric port to help guide the scope into the common duct. Saline instillation through the working channel of the scope is employed at this time to expand the common duct and provide better visualization. Further manipulations require the surgeon to

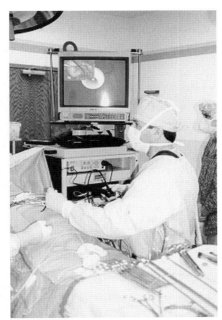

FIGURE 4   Choledochoscopic maneuvers.

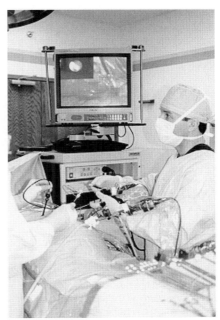

FIGURE 5   Choledochoscopic basket entrapment and extraction of bile duct stones.

use both hands on the scope in most cases. One hand controls twisting maneuvers on the body of the scope at the cannula site, while the other holds the scope head and directs the tip of the scope with the deflection lever located there. The choledochoscopic and laparoscopic images must be kept in view, either on separate monitors or preferably on the same screen with a video switcher. The surgeon manipulates the scope so that a stone is in direct view and inserts the basket into the working channel of the scope and captures the stones as described above (Figure 5).

Lithotripsy

Intraoperative electrohydraulic or laser lithotripsy techniques have seen limited use since the introduction of laparoscopic CBD exploration. The primary indications for intraoperative lithotripsy continue to be an impacted stone that defies less aggressive removal techniques or a stone that is too large to be captured and removed through the cystic duct or the choledochotomy. Electrohydraulic lithotripters (EHLs) are much less expensive than laser models and consequently have been used somewhat more frequently. EHL devices must be used with great caution, because they may cause unwanted ductal damage if the tip of the EHL probe is not accurately applied to the stone.

Occasionally, the application of a pulsatile saline jet (e.g., for dental cleaning) through the working channel of the scope may be useful in freeing stones or debris from the duct wall. The surgeon will have to configure his own adapter to connect the device to the scope, because there are no ready-made adapters for this application.

Sphincterotomy and Drainage Procedures

DePaula first described intraoperative laparoscopic antegrade sphincterotomy in Brazil in 1993. Zucker also reported success with this procedure. In this technique, a sphincterotome is passed through the working channel of the choledochoscope and through the sphincter of Oddi. The cutting action of the device is monitored by simultaneous side-viewing endoscopy of the duodenum. This technique achieves excellent results as a drainage procedure, but it is logistically quite difficult to accomplish and requires more equipment and an additional endoscopic team to be present in an already crowded operating theater. Laparoscopic antegrade sphincterotomy has not gained widespread acceptance. Others have

employed endoscopic retrograde sphincterotomy at the same time as the LCDE, but this also has not gained widespread acceptance.

Surgical biliary bypass may be indicated for patients with a dramatically dilated CBD, multiple common duct stones, nonremovable impacted distal common duct stones, retained common duct stones not amenable to ERC ± S, and obstruction secondary to tumor. Three laparoscopic operations have proven feasible: cholecystoenterostomy, choledochoduodenostomy, and choledochoenterostomy. The latter options are preferred, because cholecystoenterostomy requires patency of the cystic duct and optimal ductal configuration. In skilled hands, patency rates, morbidity, and mortality for these three options compare favorably with open techniques. These procedures require advanced technical skills, including laparoscopic suturing and knotting, therefore they should only be attempted by surgeons with proficiency in these techniques.

Completion Cholangiography

Cholangiograms are repeated after the ductal exploration is complete. If cholangiograms reveal residual stones, the surgeon must decide whether to proceed with LCDE again, convert to open CDE, perform a biliary bypass, or leave the stones in place for subsequent ERC ± S.

Completing the Cholecystectomy and Leaving the Porta Hepatis

Ligation of the Cystic Duct

The cystic duct stump is secured either during the common duct exploration, in cases in which a choledochotomy is made, or after the completion cholangiograms. If the cystic duct is dilated (> 5 mm), or if subsequent ERC ± S is planned, ligatures should be considered to secure the duct, instead of or in addition to clips, to prevent subsequent leak.

T-Tube or C-Tube Placement

A choledochotomy may be closed with or without a T tube, which is used for three reasons: 1) decompression of the duct, in the case of residual distal obstruction; 2) access for ductal imaging in the postoperative period; and 3) access for removal of residual common duct stones, should these be left after CBD exploration.

If a T tube is used, a 14 Fr T tube is prepared by removing the back wall of the T portion. The entire T tube is placed into the abdomen through a 10 mm port, and the top of the T is inserted into the common duct. The common duct closure is completed with either 4-0 or 5-0 polyglycolic acid suture or other absorbable suture in either a continuous or interrupted fashion. The magnification afforded by the laparoscope and camera allows more precise placement of the sutures than in open surgery. The suture is secured with intracorporeal ligation techniques, rather than extracorporeal techniques, because of the fragility of the duct. The security of the closure is tested by temporarily advancing the tube out of one of the 5 mm right upper quadrant ports and injecting saline through the tube. If there is a leak, the common duct closure may be resutured and tested again. During the remainder of the procedure, while the tube is completely inside the peritoneal cavity, its tip should remain occluded with a clip or ligature. The tube should ultimately exit the abdominal cavity through the port with the most direct route to the CBD.

There are many potential disadvantages to the use of T tubes. They may be associated with bacteremia, dislodgment of the tube, obstruction by the tube, or fracture of the tube. Some authors recommend broad-spectrum antibiotic coverage while the T tube is in situ. Some authors have suggested placement of a C tube through the cystic duct into the common duct for temporary postoperative biliary drainage as opposed to a T tube. Although methods of securing the C tube are not uniformly established, the technique is not unreasonable, but it is also not widely practiced.

T-tube or C-tube cholangiography should be performed before removal of the tube. Removal of T tubes postoperatively has been suggested as early as 4 days and as late as 6 weeks; the most appropriate management plan lies somewhere between these two extremes. Complications of T-tube removal include bile leaks, peritonitis, and the need for reoperation.

Primary Closure of the Choledochotomy

Despite the advantages of T-tube drainage, and because of the potential complications of T-tube placement, primary closure of the CBD without a T tube has been advocated by some in open biliary tract surgery. Shorter operative times and shorter lengths of stay have been observed with primary closure. No increase in bile leak or peritonitis has been noted with primary closure in the open-approach literature. This same technique has been employed in 33% of the one author's patients who underwent choledochotomy, and no complications were encountered in this group. Higher patient satisfaction has been associated with primary closure.

Cholecystectomy

After completion of the CBD exploration and subsequent cholangiography, the cystic duct and/or choledochotomy is secured, and the cholecystectomy is performed. The gallbladder is removed through the umbilicus, and the umbilical wound is closed at the fascial level. If a C tube or T tube has been placed, it is brought out through the most direct route through one of the existing port sites.

Drain Placement

Drains are not routinely used after transcystic laparoscopic CBD exploration but are commonly used after transductal exploration. A drain may be indicated when a choledochotomy has been performed, tissue integrity is questionable, or intense inflammation, infection, or contamination are present. If used, a closed-system suction drain is inserted in its entirety through a 10 mm port into the abdomen. The

proximal end is placed near the common duct, and the distal end is usually brought out through the abdominal wall through one of the most direct 5 mm port sites.

RESULTS

General

Thousands of successful laparoscopic CBD explorations have been reported since the introduction of laparoscopic cholecystectomy in the late 1980s. During this time, techniques have evolved that enhance the likelihood of success of the procedure. In experienced hands, successful single-stage ductal clearance rates exceed 90%. Morbidity rates have been low in these series, and mortality has occurred in less than 1% of patients.

Access Route

Most laparoscopic surgeons generally prefer the transcystic route for ductal exploration when feasible. In most series it is successful in 80% to 90% of patients. Large ductal stones are more commonly encountered by some, dictating the need for a transductal approach in approximately 90% of patients. As discussed above, there are well-defined criteria that should lead a surgeon to one or the other approach.

Operative Times

Laparoscopic choledocholithotomy takes longer than straightforward laparoscopic cholecystectomy. The mean operative time in minutes for some of the larger series varies: DePaula, 110; Petelin, 120; Phillips, 136; Franklin, 150; Millat, 140; Lezoche, 128; Gigot, 170-219; Berthou, 130; and Rhodes, 55 (basket only). Assuming that mean operative time for laparoscopic cholecystectomy in less than 1 hour, it appears that LCDE adds approximately 1 hour or more to the procedure time. Interestingly, this added time is not solely due to technical manipulations but includes equipment set-up time and often the need to perform additional surgery. It is also noted that these patients are often older, with more chronic changes in the tissues in the porta hepatis, making dissection more difficult.

Length of Stay

Whereas the length of stay (LOS) for laparoscopic cholecystectomy is generally less than 24 hours, the LOS for patients undergoing LCDE ranges from 1.3 to 7 days, depending on the severity of the disease, comorbid factors, access route, whether a T tube was placed, and whether a biliary–enteric anastomosis was created. For transcystic LCDE, the mean length of stay is 1.5 days in many large series. Length of stay for LCDE via choledochotomy is generally longer than for the transcystic approach.

Complications

Morbidity associated with LCDE occurs in approximately 8% to 10% of patients and includes those problems typically associated with general surgery and laparoscopy: nausea, diarrhea, ileus, ecchymosis, atelectasis, fever, phlebitis, urinary retention, urinary tract infection, wound infection and inflammation, biliary leak, dislodged T tube, subhepatic fluid collection, pulmonary embolus, and myocardial infarction. It is generally believed that the incidence of complications is less with a laparoscopic approach than an open approach to CBD stones.

Mortality associated with LCDE is zero to 1% in the hands of experienced laparoscopic biliary tract surgeons. This incidence is similar to that found in open surgery and relates more to the general health status of these patients than to laparoscopic CBD exploration.

Our Experience

To give a detailed overview of a typical biliary surgical practice dedicated to minimally invasive biliary tract surgery, the following data are presented. They are representative of not only our experience but also closely parallel the experience of many other advanced biliary tract surgeons.

From September 1989 through March 2010, over 5000 patients with symptomatic biliary tract disease were seen by one author. Laparoscopic cholecystectomy (LC) was attempted and completed in over 99%. Laparoscopic cholangiograms (IOCs) were performed in 97% of patients, and approximately 9.9% of IOCs were abnormal. Less than 2% underwent preoperative ERCP, and less than 1% underwent postoperative ERCP. Laparoscopic CBD exploration (LCDE) was attempted in all patients in whom CBD stones were identified, and the procedure was successfully completed in 98.5%.

Mean operating times for all patients undergoing laparoscopic cholecystectomy with or without cholangiograms or CBD exploration (LCDE) or other additional surgery was 57 minutes. Mean length of stay was 22 hours, and mean operating times for LC-only patients not undergoing LCDE or any other additional procedure was 45 minutes; mean postoperative length of stay was 17 hours for the entire series (<5 hours for cases performed in the last 10 years).

Ductal exploration was performed via the cystic duct in 85% of cases and through a choledochotomy in 15% of the cases. T tubes were used in patients in whom concern for possible retained debris or stones, distal spasm, pancreatitis, or general poor tissue quality secondary to malnutrition or infection was present. In patients who underwent choledochotomy, a T tube was placed in 67%, and primary closure without a T tube was done in 33%; no duct-related complications occurred in either group.

SUMMARY

Since 1990, surgeons throughout the world have developed a comprehensive laparoscopic solution to the problem of CBD stones. The success rate of this single-stage operation, LCDE, among accomplished laparoscopists approaches 90% or better. This compares favorably with treatment expectations in the prelaparoscopic era and addresses Perissat's challenge, that "We must move toward a management policy . . . [that] prevents patients from needing a dangerous and debilitating second operation." Biliary tract surgeons practicing in this era should have the ability to treat all benign biliary tract pathology laparoscopically in one setting, without a series of patient manipulations.

SELECTED READINGS

Arregui M, Davis CJ, Arkush AM, et al: Laparoscopic cholecystectomy combined with endoscopic sphincterotomy and stone extraction or laparoscopic choledochoscopy and electrohydraulic lithotripsy for management of cholelithiasis with choledocholithiasis, *Surg Endosc* 6:10–15, 1992.

Petelin J: Laparoscopic approach to common duct pathology, *Surg Laparosc Endosc* 1:33–41, 1991.

Petelin J: Laparoscopic approach to common duct pathology, *Am J Surg* 165:487–491, 1993.

Petelin J: Surgical management of common bile duct stones, *Gastrointest Endosc* 56(6):S183–S189, 2002.

Phillips EH: Laparoscopic transcystic duct common bile duct exploration: outcome and costs, *Surg Endosc* :1240–1242, 1995.

Rhodes M, Sussman L, Cohen L, Lewis MP: Randomised trial of laparoscopic exploration of common bile duct versus postoperative endoscopic retrograde cholangiography for common bile duct stones, *Lancet* 351:159–161, 1998.

LAPAROSCOPIC 360-DEGREE FUNDOPLICATION

Patrick R. Reardon, MD

OVERVIEW

Gastroesophageal reflux disease (GERD) affects 19 million Americans. Approximately 40% will experience heartburn more than three times per week, and 10% will suffer on a daily basis. Medical therapy, primarily with proton-pump inhibitors (PPIs), is the mainstay of treatment. Surgery has been well documented to provide effective, long-lasting control of the symptoms of GERD and provides a suitable alternative therapy in appropriate patients; currently, 360-degree fundoplication is the most widely used procedure for the surgical control of GERD.

Most procedures are now performed laparoscopically, and to achieve good results, the surgeon must first document the presence of the disease. The second necessity is to correctly perform the operation. The introduction of the laparoscopic approach to the operation significantly changed the way surgeons achieve access in performing the operation, but it did not change the principles for performance of a true and proper 360-degree fundoplication.

DEFINITION

The Montreal consensus defined GERD as "a condition [that] develops when the reflux of stomach contents causes troublesome symptoms and/or complications." Symptoms are defined as "troublesome" if they adversely affect an individual's well-being. This definition was felt to be a suitable starting point for making treatment recommendations (Table 1).

MEDICAL THERAPY

Medical therapy with PPIs remains the primary form of treatment for GERD. All patients with uncomplicated GERD should undergo a trial of medical therapy first.

DIAGNOSIS

For patients seen for first-time treatment of GERD based upon presentation with the classic symptoms of heartburn and or regurgitation, empirical therapy is appropriate. Treatment with PPIs and lifestyle modification, based on symptoms alone, is also appropriate. Relief of symptoms with initiation of medical therapy is considered confirmatory for the diagnosis. For patients who experience an extended duration of symptoms, or for those who have symptoms that suggest complicated disease—such as dysphagia, odynophagia,

TABLE 1: Symptoms used to diagnose GERD

Typical Symptoms	Extraesophageal (Atypical) Symptoms
Heartburn	Asthma
Regurgitation	Hoarseness
Chest pain	Cough
Dysphagia	Recurrent pneumonia
	Dental erosion

bleeding, weight loss, or anemia—further diagnostic testing is recommended based upon expert opinion.

TREATMENT

For patients being seen for the first time with classic symptoms of GERD, the diagnostic modality and treatment are one and the same. For long-term use, the PPI dose should be titrated down to the lowest dose that continues to control symptoms.

SURGICAL THERAPY

Diagnosis

Surgical therapy requires a higher standard for the diagnosis of GERD. Although subjective symptomatology may be adequate to initiate medical therapy, objective evidence is required to document the presence of GERD prior to considering surgical therapy. Before performing the surgical therapy, the surgeon must provide *objective* evidence of the presence of GERD.

Flexible Endoscopy

Esophagogastroduodenoscopy should be performed as the first diagnostic test in all patients being considered for the surgical therapy of GERD. Many of the diagnostic findings that constitute objective evidence for GERD may be made at the time of flexible endoscopy.

The minimum endoscopic lesion that may be considered a reliable, objective indicator of reflux esophagitis is called a *mucosal break,* defined as "an area of slough or erythema with a sharp line of demarcation from adjacent normal mucosa." These are the definitions used in the most recent version of the Los Angeles classification system. In addition, ulcers or strictures found at the time of endoscopy in patients with the appropriate clinical symptoms may be considered objective evidence of GERD. Both of these lesions require multiple biopsies to rule out malignancy.

The presence of Barrett esophagus documented by biopsy is objective evidence of GERD. *Barrett esophagus* may be defined as intestinal metaplasia arising in an endoscopically visible columnar-lined esophagus. Barrett esophagus arises when there is injury to the squamous mucosa of the esophagus, and healing occurs in the presence of an acid environment. This injury is almost always caused by GERD, although other rare causes may exist.

The diagnostic criteria proposed by Chandrasoma are also acceptable. These include the belief that an all columnar-lined esophagus is caused by, and is therefore diagnostic of, GERD. In addition, the presence of cardiac mucosa (reflux carditis) without intestinal metaplasia occurring in the esophagus is specific for and diagnostic of GERD.

The finding of one or more of these objective criteria for GERD at the time of flexible endoscopy may obviate the need for additional diagnostic testing. For this reason, strong consideration should be given to always using flexible endoscopy as the first diagnostic test in patients with suspected GERD who are being considered for surgical treatment.

Ambulatory pH Testing

24-Hour Ambulatory and Bravo Wireless pH Testing

Ambulatory esophageal pH testing, whether via a transnasal probe or a wireless Bravo capsule, is considered the gold standard for objective testing for GERD. These tests are based on the placement of a small pH sensor electrode into the distal esophagus 5 cm above the proximal border of the lower esophageal sphincter (LES). Johnson and DeMeester refined the techniques and clarified the definitions that have formed the basis for modern pH testing. DeMeester score is determined by evaluating 1) the cumulative time the esophageal pH is below 4, expressed as a percentage of the total upright and supine time; 2) the frequency of the reflux episodes, expressed as the number of episodes in 24 hours; and 3) the duration of the episodes expressed as the number of episodes lasting longer than 5 minutes per 24 hours and the time in minutes of the longest episode recorded.

Traditional 24 hour ambulatory pH testing involves the placement of a transnasal wire into the esophagus with the distal sensor located 5 cm above the upper border of the LES. The Bravo capsule is a catheter-free, radiotelemetric pH capsule that is clipped onto the distal esophageal wall 5 cm above the manometrically determined upper border of the LES. The pH data are then transmitted to a receiver worn on the patient's belt.

Impedance Manometry

More recently, multichannel intraluminal impedance recording has become available. This transnasal device combines multichannel impedance measurements with standard distal pH measurements. By measuring changes in impedance to detect the presence of liquid or gas in the esophagus, this device allows for the detection of gastric refluxate with a pH above 4. It simultaneously provides standard pH measurements. This device not only allows for the recording of non–acid reflux episodes but also facilitates the documentation of the proximal extent of the refluxate.

Barium Esophagram

For patients diagnosed with a large hiatal hernia at the time of flexible endoscopy, a barium esophagram may provide useful information for the surgeon. An esophagram performed in the upright and supine position may provide evidence of a hiatal hernia that is fixed in the mediastinum, which may indicate a shortened esophagus. This view will allow the surgeon to plan the operation and have appropriate discussions with the patient regarding the possible need for an esophageal lengthening procedure, such as a wedge Collis gastroplasty.

Indications for Antireflux Surgery

Once the diagnosis of GERD has been objectively confirmed, antireflux surgery is indicated in 1) patients who have had a good response to acid-suppressive therapy but seek an alternative therapy because of side effects or cost of medication, lifestyle considerations, and desire to avoid the lifelong need for medications; 2) those who have persistent troublesome symptoms, particularly regurgitation, despite acid-suppressive therapy with PPIs; 3) patients with complications of GERD, such as peptic strictures or Barrett esophagus; and 4) patients with extraesophageal manifestations of GERD.

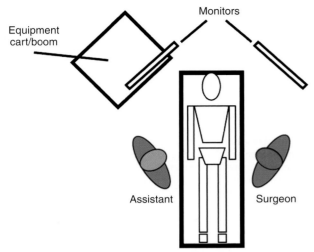

FIGURE 1   The surgeon stands on the patient's left side during dissection and on the patient's right side while suturing.

360-Degree Fundoplication

Positioning

The patient is placed in the supine position on the operating table. Where possible, both arms are tucked at the patient's sides and padded well. The table-mounted retractor holder (Mediflex, Islandia, NY) for the flexible liver retractor (Snowden-Pencer Diamond-Flex; CareFusion, San Diego, Calif.) is mounted on the patient's right side (Figure 1). For this reason, the right arm must be completely within the confines of the table to avoid pressure on the upper arm; if necessary, the left arm may be placed out on an arm board. The patient is positioned in a steep, head-up position during the operation, which necessitates that footboards be placed in the bed. Antiembolism measures should also be taken.

Port Placement

A total of five ports are used for the operation, and we initiate all of our laparoscopies with a 2 mm trocar. This technique is rapid and safe, and it allows immediate placement of a 2 mm laparoscope to confirm correct placement; angled 30-degree 5 and 10 mm laparoscopes are utilized throughout the procedure. If conditions such as an enlarged left lobe of the liver warrant moving the ports from their standard positions, abandoning a 2 mm port site results in little or no morbidity. At the conclusion of the procedure, the 2 mm trocar is utilized to close the 12 mm port site by passing a suture in a U-stitch fashion. The ports are placed as depicted in Figure 2.

The Operation

The gastrohepatic ligament is divided with a bipolar LigaSure device (Covidien, Boulder, Colo.), as bipolar devices are the safest energy source for use near the vagus nerves. Dissection is started caudally and carried cranially up to the superior aspect of the right crus. I routinely divide the hepatic vagal branch with no untoward consequences. Dissecting from right to left across the anterior hiatus, the anterior layer of peritoneum only is divided over onto the superior aspect of the left crus.

Attention is directed to the inferior aspect of the right crus, and the inferior medial margin of the right crus is almost always identifiable by a white fold of peritoneum. Blunt dissection is used to divide the peritoneum just medial to the white fold. Bluntly retracting the esophagus and vagus nerves anteriorly and to the patient's left, the right crus is gently retracted to the patient's right. The peritoneum is swept clean on its posterior aspect, utilizing a laparoscopic kitner,

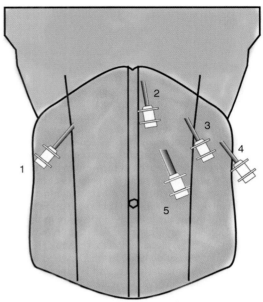

FIGURE 2   Ports 1 to 4 are 5 mm ports. Port 5 is a 12 mm port.

and then divided with the LigaSure device just medial to the right crus; this dissection is carried from posterior to anterior. Care should be taken not to dissect the peritoneum off of the right crus. When the anterior aspect of the right crus is reached, a laparoscopic kitner is used to sweep from the posterior aspect of the anterior hiatus down in a radial fashion toward the esophagus. The esophagus and vagus nerves are carefully dissected from the posterior aspect of the anterior hiatus in this manner.

Viewing from right to left posteriorly, behind the gastroesophageal junction (GEJ), blunt dissection is carried out just lateral to the inferior-most aspect of the left crus. If dissection is started inferiorly, where the left and right crura are clearly overlapping in the midline, the surgeon can avoid the mistake of dissecting just cranial to the inferior aspect of the left crus and entering the left pleural space, a particularly common mistake. Using blunt dissectors, one dissector is past-pointed beyond the esophagus and retracted anteriorly, just lateral to and parallel to the left crus. This carries the esophagus and vagus nerves anteriorly. Downward dissection with a blunt dissector just lateral and parallel to the left crus can be used to open a window in the peritoneum. Great care should be taken during this dissection, as the spleen is always just beyond the peritoneum.

Attention is then directed to the greater curve. With the LigaSure device, the short gastric arteries and veins are divided from caudal to cranial, until the left hemidiaphragm is reached. In the cranial-most portions of the dissection—where the short gastric arteries and veins are shortest, and the apposition of the stomach to the spleen is at its closest—the dissection should be carried out closer to the stomach than to the spleen. Any unintentional injury to the greater curve of the stomach may be easily oversewn; injuries to the spleen, however, tend to cause bleeding and are not so easily repaired. Once this dissection reaches the left hemidiaphragm, the peritoneum along the lateral attachments of the GEJ fat pad are divided, from posterior to anterior, until the anterior dissection is met at the anterior aspect of the left crus.

Attention is then directed to the posterior aspect of the left crus, the area where the phrenoesophageal ligament is at its thickest and is most visible. Retracting the esophagus and vagus nerves anteriorly and to the patient's right, the left crus is gently retracted to the patient's left. The posterior aspect of the phrenoesophageal ligament is swept clean with a kitner and divided just medial to the left crus. Dissection is carried from posterior to anterior, until the anterior aspect of the left crus and the anterior dissection are met. The circumferential dissection of the hiatus is now completed. During all dissection in or around the hiatus, great care should be taken to identify and preserve the anterior and posterior vagus nerves. The posterior aspect of the fundus, from the starting point of dissection of the short gastric vessels to the inferior aspect of the left crus, should be freed from all attachments.

Gentle downward traction on the GEJ fat pad makes identification of the anterior vagus nerve easy. The fat pad is then dissected away, just to the left of the anterior vagus nerve, taking care not to injure the nerve. Removal of the fat pad allows precise identification of the junction of the longitudinal muscle fibers of the distal esophagus and the serosa-lined stomach. This is the best anatomic marker for the original location of the esophageal squamocolumnar junction.

With chronic GERD, the patient may acquire a dilated end-stage esophagus. In these patients, the surgeon may mistakenly identify the distal-most portion of the tubular esophagus as the GEJ. The use of flexible endoscopy to identify the squamocolumnar junction may also lead to an incorrectly identified GEJ in patients with a columnar-lined esophagus. Finally, the inferior-most suture in the fundoplication will be placed through this area. Failure to remove the GEJ fat pad can lead to imprecise placement of this suture.

Careful circumferential dissection is then carried out around the esophagus up into the mediastinum, and a kitner and a blunt dissector are used for this purpose. Dissection is carried up to and just beyond the inferior pulmonary veins in almost all cases. The initial operation represents the surgeon's best chance for success, as failure to perform adequate mobilization may lead to the need for reoperation. When the dissection is completed, at least 3 to 4 cm of the distal esophagus should reside within the abdomen with no traction needed. A Penrose drain may be passed around the distal esophagus and secured anteriorly and may be used to manipulate the distal esophagus during this dissection. Caution should be used to avoid placing too much traction on the Penrose drain during this procedure, which may stretch the esophagus and give the surgeon a false sense of adequate mobilization.

The hiatus should be closed with at least one posterior suture in all patients. I use size 0 Surgidac for pledgeted U-stitches with Dacron felt pledgets. Suturing is performed with an Endo Stitch device (Covidien), which I believe this is the safest, most rapid way to suture for this particular laparoscopic procedure. A flexible plastic ruler is used to measure, and all patients are closed to an anteroposterior hiatal diameter of 18 to 20 mm.

Recurrent hiatal hernias and new onset postoperative hiatal hernias are the Achilles heel of laparoscopic antireflux surgery. For this reason, I bolster all hiatal closures with a saddle configuration of Dualmesh (Gore Medical, Flagstaff, Ariz.). The superior margin of the isthmus of the mesh is kept ½ cm from the inferior margin of the hiatal closure. The medial aspect of the lateral wings of the mesh are kept 3 mm away

from the hiatal edges because use of this mesh bolster appears to lower the postoperative occurrence of hiatal hernias. In my personal experience with over 300 placements of mesh in this fashion, there have been no known complications related to placement of the mesh.

Creation of an Accurate and Reproducible 360-Degree Fundoplication

A widely leveled and perhaps valid critique of antireflux surgery from our medical colleagues is the wide variability among surgeons in its technical performance and outcomes. Based on almost 20 years of training residents and fellows, I have devised a technique that should allow for the accurate reproduction of a true and concise laparoscopic 360-degree fundoplication. In a properly oriented procedure, the short gastric vessel stumps should be oriented 180 degrees opposite the completed anterior fundoplication as depicted in Figure 3.

The looseness or "floppiness" of a completed 360-degree fundoplication is determined by the distance, the additional length, between the outer circumference of the 60 Fr bougie-filled esophagus and the inner circumference of the completed fundoplication (Figure 4).

Geometry Technique for Creation of a 360-Degree Fundoplication

The circumference (c) of the 60 Fr bougie-filled esophagus was measured in 250 consecutive cases, and the esophageal diameter was calculated. Multiple linear regression analysis was then used to predict the esophageal diameter from patient characteristics. The relation can be defined by the regression equation:

$$c = [6.172 + (\text{Age} \times 0.00849) + (\text{Body surface area} \times 0.813)]$$

The diameter of the 60 Fr bougie-filled esophagus can then be calculated. The inner diameter of the completed fundoplication equals the calculated diameter of the 60 Fr bougie-filled esophagus plus additional length. The inner circumference of the completed fundoplication is calculated as c = Diameter × Π. One half of the inner circumference of the completed fundoplication is the measuring suture length (see Table 2).

A piece of 0 silk is tied to a grasper and cut to the calculated length, and a laparoscopic needle holder is used to grasp the free end of the suture, and the free end is placed at the junction of the left side of the esophagus and the greater curve of the stomach. The greater curve is gently stretched caudally, the suture is gently stretched caudally, and the grasper is rotated over and used to grasp the greater curve of the fundus. The grasper then rotates the greater curve anteriorly and to the patient's right, and the posterior fundus is gently stretched flat.

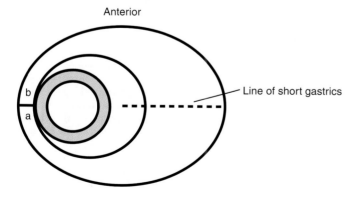

FIGURE 3 In a properly oriented 360-degree fundoplication, the short gastric vessel stumps should be oriented 180 degrees opposite the completed anterior fundoplication.

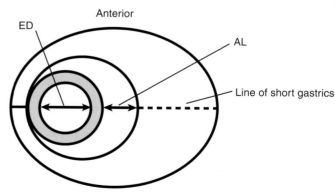

FIGURE 4 The looseness or "floppiness" of a completed 360-degree fundoplication is determined by the distance, the additional length, between the outer circumference of the 60 Fr bougie-filled esophagus and the inner circumference of the completed fundoplication.

The free end of the silk suture is then rotated posteriorly and caudally along the flattened posterior fundus, until it appears to be equidistant from the grasper on the greater curve and the junction of the greater curve in the left side of the esophagus.

Next, a traction suture is placed into the fundus, tied, and cut to a 10 cm length. The free end of the traction suture is placed against the posterior left hemidiaphragm, and the grasper on the greater curve then retracts the greater curve to the patient's left. The anterior aspect of the fundus is gently flattened by retracting gently near the lesser curve. The free end of the silk suture is then rotated onto the anterior fundus to a point that appears to be equidistant from the grasper on the greater curve and the junction of the greater curve in the left side of the esophagus. A marking suture is placed at this point, tied, and cut short (<1 cm).

Viewing from right to left behind the GEJ, the esophagus is gently retracted anteriorly. The posterior traction suture is grasped and pulled over to the right side, behind the esophagus, by pulling in a slightly cranial direction. When the insertion point on the posterior fundus is visible, it is grasped with a grasper, and the anterior traction point on the left side is grasped with a grasper. The right-sided traction point is brought over to meet the left-sided traction point at the 10 o'clock position on the superior aspect of the anterior intraabdominal esophagus. At this point, a symmetrical fundoplication should exist with the short gastric vessel stumps on the greater curve lying 180 degrees opposite the anterior fundoplication.

The fundoplication is then sutured in place, and the inferior-most suture is placed first. A pledgeted U stitch of 0 Surgidac is utilized. The suture is placed through the right side of the fundoplication 2.5 cm below the right-sided traction suture. A bite of esophagus is taken at the GEJ and just to the left of the anterior vagus nerve. The suture is passed through the left side of the fundoplication 2.5 cm below the left-sided traction suture. The superior-most suture is placed next, 2.5 cm above the first suture, which should be at or near the two previously placed traction sutures. A nonpledgeted U stitch of 0 Surgidac is utilized. A narrow, 2 to 3 mm bite of the anterior esophagus, just to the left of the anterior vagus nerve, is taken. Care should be taken not to take too large of a bite of anterior esophagus, as this will narrow the esophageal circumference when the suture is pulled tight. No pledgets should be utilized on the superior-most suture. Pledgets placed at this site will, invariably, rotate cranially and come into contact with the anterior esophagus, which may lead to erosion into the lumen over time. Immediately below the nonpledgeted suture, a pledgeted U stitch of 0 Surgidac is placed. The final suture is a pledgeted U stitch of 0 Surgidac placed halfway between the two existing platelet U stitches. When this suture is placed and tied, there should be complete apposition of the anterior length of the fundoplication.

TABLE 2: Determining additional suture length

Mean Esophageal Body Pressure on Manometry (mm Hg)	Patient Age (Years)	Additional Length	Comments
<30	Any	NA	Consider Roux-en-Y gastric bypass with 75–100 cm roux limb
30–50	Any	1.2 cm	Very loose fundoplication
>50	Any	0.9 cm	Medium tightness
>50	<30	0.6 cm	Tight fundoplication (increased risk of dysphagia is offset by need for better long-term control)

A right posterior superior gastropexy suture is then placed between the right posterior superior aspect of the fundoplication and the adjacent right crus. A right posterior inferior gastropexy suture is also placed between the right posterior inferior aspect of the fundoplication and the adjacent crura below the mesh; these sutures will help maintain a long posterior lip to the newly created flap valve within the fundoplication. This can be verified by intraoperative esophagogastroscopy with a retroflexed view. I do this routinely and recommend it to all surgeons performing this procedure.

POSTOPERATIVE CARE

Patients are started on noncarbonated full liquids within 2 hours of their arrival to the floor. If these liquids are tolerated, patients are advanced to a mechanical, soft "dysphagia diet" and are discharged home the following morning on this diet. No beef, fish, chicken, fruit, or uncooked vegetables are allowed. In addition, patients are cautioned not to lift more than 8 lb—the weight of a gallon of milk, an easy reference—or engage in vigorous activity or straining for 2 months to protect the hiatal closure.

COMPLICATIONS

Intraoperative complications are usually minor. For those surgeons who use a bougie, the esophageal perforation rate is less than 1%, and operative mortality approaches zero in experienced hands. Pleural tears are relatively common, but if no underlying injury to the lung is present, no specific therapy is required. The anesthesiologist should be notified and asked to place the patient on 10 mm Hg of positive end-expiratory pressure to avoid atelectasis from partial deflation of the lung.

OUTCOMES

For patients with typical reflux symptoms, an 80% to 90% long-term rate for relief of acid-caused symptoms can be expected. For patients with atypical reflux symptoms, the long-term cure rate ranges from 67% to 92%. Surgeons should be aware that for patients placed back on antacid medications in the postoperative period by someone other than the operating surgeon, only 25% to 30% will have documentation of recurrent acid reflux on 24-hour pH testing.

Around 6% to 9% of patients will have dysphagia that does not resolve within 60 days of the surgery. Most dysphagia is mild and is treated by modifying the diet. Complaints of gas and bloating are relatively common, but this does not keep patients from reporting an improved quality of life. Between 80% and 95% of patients queried report that they would undergo surgery again.

Surgical treatment of GERD is an equal and effective alternative to the medical therapy of this disease. For patients with documented disease who have been appropriately evaluated, laparoscopic 360-degree fundoplication provides excellent control of acid-caused symptoms, improves quality of life, and results in high levels of patient satisfaction.

SUGGESTED READINGS

Chandrasoma PT: Diagnostic atlas of gastroesophageal reflux disease: a new histology-based method, San Diego, 2007, Elsevier.

Chandrasoma PT, DeMeester TR: GERD: reflux to esophageal adenocarcinoma, San Diego, 2006, Elsevier.

Reardon PR, Scarborough T, Matthews B, et al: Laparoscopic Nissen fundoplication: a technique for the easy and precise manufacture of a true fundoplication, Surg Endosc 14:298–299, 2000.

Reardon PR, Matthews BD, Scarborough TK, et al: Geometry and reproducibility in 360 degrees fundoplication, Surg Endosc 14:750–754, 2000.

LAPAROSCOPIC APPENDECTOMY

Trevor A. Ellison, MD, and Barish H. Edil, MD

OVERVIEW

Appendectomy is the most common emergent abdominal surgery performed in the United States with approximately 250,000 appendectomies performed each year. Of the estimated 7% of the United States population diagnosed with appendicitis every year, the highest incidence is among those aged 10 to 19 years with an overall male-to-female ratio of 1.4:1.

Although open appendectomy has remained the gold standard for the treatment of acute appendicitis since McBurney first performed the operation in 1894, laparoscopic appendectomy has gained popularity since its introduction in 1980 by Semm. Even though laparoscopic appendectomy has become more popular, it has not become the gold standard but remains one more option in the surgeon's toolkit, including intervention for both uncomplicated and complicated (perforated or phlegmon associated) acute appendicitis, interval appendectomy after prior appendiceal abscess drainage, and recurrent or chronic appendicitis.

In the intervening three decades since the introduction of the laparoscopic appendectomy, many studies have looked at the outcomes of laparoscopic versus open appendectomy. The majority of studies show that the two approaches are equivalent in safety and efficacy with a few exceptions. One of the best summaries of the current literature is the 2004 Cochrane review on this subject that included 54 studies of adults and children. Results showed that laparoscopic appendectomies, as compared to open appendectomies, resulted in fewer wound infections (odds ratio [OR], 0.45; confidence interval [CI], 0.35 to 0.58); increased intraabdominal abscesses (OR, 2.48; CI, 1.45 to 4.21); longer operative time by 12 minutes (CI, 7 to 16); decreased pain on the first postoperative day (by 9 mm on a 100 mm visual analog scale; CI, 5 to 13 mm); a shorter hospital stay by 1.1 days (CI, 0.6 to 1.5); a quicker return to normal activity, including work and sports; and a higher cost of operation. The Cochrane study concluded with the recommendation that laparoscopic appendectomy should be performed unless laparoscopy is contraindicated or it is not feasible. The report also notes that females, obese individuals, and those who are employed gain the most benefit. It is also worth noting that the debate over which method is best was still not settled with the 2004 Cochrane review, and more recent randomized controlled trials suggest that the laparoscopic approach does not confer any advantages. Our institutional bias is to perform a laparoscopic appendectomy absent any contraindication to laparoscopy in the patient.

DIAGNOSIS

The classic presentation of initial periumbilical abdominal pain that migrates to the right lower quadrant followed by nausea, anorexia, and vomiting may be present in less than 50% of patients. Table 1 summarizes the sensitivity and specificity of the most common signs and symptoms of acute appendicitis.

Further workup will reveal a leukocytosis greater than 10,500 cells/mm^3 in 80% to 85% of adults with appendicitis and a neutrophilia greater than 75% in 78% of adults with appendicitis. Only 4% of those with appendicitis will have a leukocytosis less than 10,500 cells/mm^3 and a neutrophilia less than 75%. Up to a third of patients may report

urinary symptoms, and a portion of those will have pyuria, so it is important not to rule out appendicitis on the grounds of urinary tract infection symptoms and positive urinalysis.

In a young male with classic history, physical, and laboratory findings, imaging is usually not necessary and is typically reserved for questionable cases that usually involve female patients who may have gynecologic etiologies for their presenting symptoms. When considering imaging for suspected appendicitis, plain films of the abdomen, with or without contrast enema, have no role because of their low sensitivity and specificity. Instead, imaging options include ultrasound and computed tomography (CT). Acute appendicitis is diagnosed by identifying a distended, non–contrast-filled appendix, thickened appendiceal wall, and periappendiceal inflammation. CT scan is superior to ultrasound in diagnosing acute appendicitis (see Table 2), but we prefer ultrasound in women who are pregnant or potentially pregnant to avoid any radiation exposure to the fetus. If a CT scan is planned, intravenous contrast can help to define the appendiceal wall and periappendiceal inflammation, and enteric contrast can be helpful to visualize the terminal ileum and cecum to rule out terminal ileitis, but neither intravenous nor enteric contrast is absolutely necessary in straightforward cases (Figure 1).

TREATMENT

The gold standard treatment for appendicitis is appendectomy.

Equipment and Patient Positioning

To avoid delays during the operation, the surgeon should make sure all the necessary equipment is available beforehand, including the following:

- Laparoscopic tower with a full or extra gas tank
- Sterilized light cord, video cord, and gas tubing
- Entry ports (at least one 10 mm and two 5 mm)

TABLE 1: Sensitivity and specificity of clinical findings for the diagnosis of acute appendicitis

Finding	Sensitivity (%)	Specificity (%)
Signs		
Fever	67	69
Guarding	39–74	57–84
Rebound tenderness	63	69
Indirect tenderness (Rovsing sign)	68	58
Irritated iliopsoas (Psoas sign)	16	95
Symptoms		
Right lower quadrant pain	84	90
Nausea	58–68	37–40
Vomiting	49–51	45–69
Onset of pain before vomiting	100	64
Anorexia	68	36

From Paulson EK, Kalady MF, Pappas TN: Suspected appendicitis, *N Engl J Med* 348:236–242, 2003.

- A 10 mm and/or 5 mm zero degree and/or 30 degree scope
- Atraumatic graspers for bowel manipulation
- Maryland dissector and/or right-angle dissector for blunt dissection
- A stapler with vascular and bowel loads
- A containment bag

Other instruments that facilitate the operation but also add to the cost include:

- LigaSure (Covidien, Flagstaff, Ariz.)
- Harmonic scalpel (Ethicon, Somerville, NJ)
- Bipolar cautery
- Clip applier
- Laparoscopic suction irrigator

The monitor and light source should be tested to make sure they work prior to the operation, and the tower should be positioned on the patient's right, facing the left side, where the surgeons will stand. The scope tips should be placed in a container of warm water to avoid condensation when introduced into the abdomen.

Next, attention should be turned to patient positioning. First, the table should be unlocked and moved to a position in the room where the patient can be placed in Trendelenburg position without compromising the space at the head of the bed for the anesthesiologist. The patient should be placed in a supine position with the right arm out on a board to allow access to the intravenous lines and for the possible placement of more intravenous lines. The left arm should be tucked at the patient's side after egg-crate padding is placed in between the elbow and the patient. Once the patient is comfortably asleep under general endotracheal anesthesia, a nasogastric tube and Foley catheter should be placed to decompress the stomach and bladder to make more room in the abdominal cavity and to avoid any injury to these structures upon surgical entry. Both the nasogastric tube and Foley can be removed before the patient wakes up. The surgeon's assistant will stand on the patient's left side with the operating surgeon standing caudad to the assistant.

Steps of the Operation

Prior to the start of the operation, a time-out should be called, and the anesthesia, nursing, and surgical teams should introduce themselves to each other and discuss any concerns or special considerations for the case. The patient identity should be verified as well as the intended operation. At this time, the appropriate antibiotic prophylaxis should be administered; one dose within 30 minutes of incision is adequate, although we carry antibiotic coverage out for 24 hours and, in the case of perforated appendicitis, we continue coverage until the patient is afebrile and leukocytosis has normalized. Appropriate venous-thrombotic embolism prophylaxis should also be provided using compression stockings, sequential compression devices, and subcutaneous heparin as necessary.

The patient's skin is then prepped with a mixture of chlorhexidine and alcohol using short, scrubbing strokes for at least 30 seconds. The patient should be prepped from the nipples to the pubis in case an alternate diagnosis is made on the table, and the abdomen needs to be entered. The patient is then draped in the usual sterile fashion, and all the laparoscopic equipment is hooked up to the laparoscopic tower. The antifog solution pad should be placed at the edge of the drape nearest to the camera port, and the cautery scratch pad (if used) should be placed well away from this area to avoid the potential inadvertent wiping of the scope on the scratch pad.

For most of the case, the first port will accommodate the camera, the stapler, and containment bag. The decision as to whether to place the camera port above or below the umbilicus depends on the patient's size. The port can be placed in the infraumbilical ridge in the midline as long as there is at least a hand length of distance from the infraumbilical area to the appendix and at least a hand breadth distance from the infraumbilical area to the suprapubic area, where a 5 mm port will be placed. Otherwise, we prefer to place the camera port in the supraumbilical ridge in the midline. This port incision should be made so that it can be incorporated into a midline incision, should there be a change of diagnosis and operation. After local anesthetic is injected at the port site, which is done at all the port sites prior to incision, a skin incision is made to accommodate a 10 mm port, and a cutdown technique is used to expose the fascia; the needle approach to enter the abdomen is appropriate as well, depending on surgeon preference.

Once the fascia is exposed, a vertical incision is made, and a finger sweep is done on the peritoneal surface to assure that there are no adhesions that will complicate port placement. Once the port is placed, the abdomen is insufflated with carbon dioxide to 12 to 15 mm Hg. The 30 degree camera is then inserted and angled up first to assure no damage was done upon port entry. The patient is then placed in the Trendelenburg position and tilted to the left to help move the small bowel out of the right lower quadrant. To provide appropriate triangulation, we place the second port (5 mm) in the suprapubic midline, at least one hand breadth below the camera port, and the third port (5 mm) in the left lower quadrant, equidistant from the umbilical port and suprapubic port and just lateral to the rectus sheath (Figure 2). If the left lower quadrant is deemed undesirable for port entry, the alternate position for the third port is in the right upper quadrant. At this point, the surgeon operates via the two 5 mm ports, while the assistant operates the camera.

Next, attention is turned to the exploratory portion of the laparoscopy. One of the advantages of laparoscopy is the ability to do a thorough inspection of the abdomen and pelvis to exclude any other pathology associated with the patient's symptoms. Regardless of

TABLE 2: Sensitivity and specificity of imaging modalities in diagnosing acute appendicitis

Modality	Sensitivity (%)	Specificity (%)	Positive Predictive Value (%)	Overall Accuracy (%)
Ultrasound	75–90	86–100	89–93	90–94
CT scan	90–100	91–99	95–97	94–100

From Paulson EK, Kalady MF, Pappas TN: Suspected appendicitis, *N Engl J Med* 348:236–242, 2003.

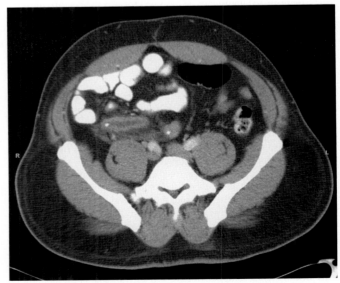

FIGURE 1 CT scan of acute appendicitis. Note the thickened appendicial wall and inflammation.

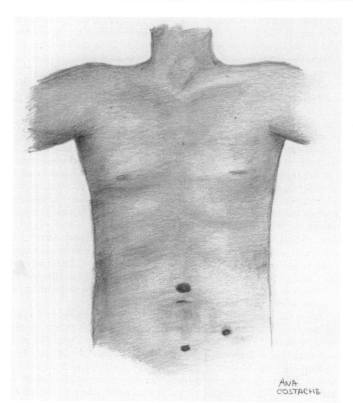

FIGURE 2   Placement of entry ports; a 10 mm supraumbilical port with 5 mm suprapubic and left lower quadrant ports. *(Courtesy Ana Costache.)*

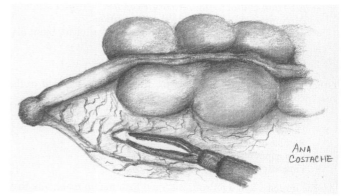

FIGURE 3   Develop a window in the mesoappendix at the base of the appendix, staying close to the appendix. *(Courtesy Ana Costache.)*

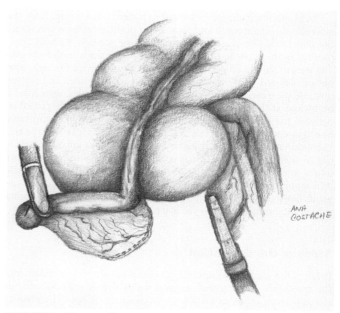

FIGURE 4   Transect the mesoappendix close to the appendix. *(Courtesy Ana Costache.)*

whether acute appendicitis is visually diagnosed, a thorough examination of the uterus, adnexa, terminal ileum, colon, gallbladder, and other viscera is carried out. Eighty-five percent of the time, the appendix is intraperitoneal, but 15% of the time, it can be retrocecal, requiring mobilization of the cecum and terminal ileum from the lateral peritoneal attachments for proper visualization. If finding the appendix is difficult, the surgeon can follow the tenia libera of the ascending colon to the cecum, where the tenia libera will converge with the other ascending colon teniae at the appendix. In addition, the terminal ileum can be followed toward the cecum, until the antimesenteric ileal fat pad is observed, which marks the termination of the ileum into the cecum. If periappendiceal fluid is present, it can be cultured at this time, if the surgeon suspects an unusual microorganism; otherwise the fluid need not be cultured, as the patient will be adequately covered by the standard, broad-spectrum antibiotic prophylaxis.

For the duration of the operation, bowel manipulation should be done with closed graspers as much as possible to avoid avulsing friable tissue, but atraumatic graspers can be used to hold the bowel when necessary. It is especially important to carefully handle the appendix, especially if it is distended and inflamed, as overhandling may cause appendiceal rupture with intraperitoneal spillage of its contents. Once the appendix is freed from the inflammation process via blunt dissection and/or exposed from its retrocecal location, the mesoappendix should be exposed. A Maryland or right-angle dissector is used to make a window at the base of the appendix to separate the base of the appendix from the mesoappendix. This maneuver must be done carefully to prevent an inadvertent puncture of the cecum at the base of the appendix or an inadvertent puncture of the cecum through the window in the mesoappendix (Figure 3). Once this window is developed, transection of the mesoappendix should be carried out close to the appendix by using a stapler with a vascular load, an energy device, or clips (Figure 4). Although some surgeons

staple the appendix first and the mesoappendix second, we favor the approach of stapling the mesoappendix first, because if the appendix is transected first and is being held by the graspers, there is the possibility of inadvertently tearing the friable mesoappendix by pulling too hard with the graspers and leaving a bleeding mesoappendix behind.

Next, the base of the appendix is exposed and transected flush with the cecum with a bowel-loaded stapler. It is important to transect the appendix completely, to avoid the complication of stump appendicitis, and at a point where there is healthy tissue, to avoid staple-line breakdown, while making sure not to narrow the cecum (Figure 5). If the endoscopic stapler is used, the tips of the stapler should always be directly visualized before firing to avoid inadvertently stapling any other structures, especially the terminal ileum.

Once the appendix is freed, the containment bag is introduced via the camera port (the 10 mm camera is switched to a 5 mm camera, placed in the left lower quadrant port), and the specimen is removed. Some surgeons will leave the containment bag with the specimen in the abdomen until they are ready to desufflate to avoid the potential necessity of reinsufflating after removing the specimen from the abdomen, but we prefer to remove the specimen so that we can finish the operation using the better quality picture of the 10 mm laparoscope.

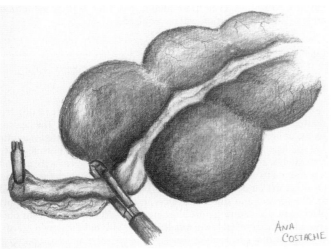

FIGURE 5 Transect the appendix flush with the cecum to avoid leaving behind any appendiceal tissue. *(Courtesy Ana Costache.)*

Next, attention is turned to the mesoappendix and appendiceal stump to ensure hemostasis and stump integrity. When necessary, the laparoscopic irrigation-suction device should be used to copiously irrigate the right lower quadrant and pelvis at this point. Special attention is given to irrigating the cul-de-sac behind the uterus in women. Once the peritoneum is clean and dry, the ports are removed under direct visualization, and the abdomen is desufflated. The patient is then put in the level supine position.

For fascial closure, only the ports that are 10 mm or greater are closed with suture. In this case, the supraumbilical camera port is closed with 2-0 absorbable suture. All port sites are then irrigated, and skin incisions are closed with 4-0 absorbable suture; alternatively, the 5 mm port skin incisions can be closed with Steri-Strips only. All incisions are then closed with Steri-Strips and a clean, dry dressing is placed on top with a clear adhesive bandage to hold everything in place.

SPECIAL CONSIDERATIONS WHILE OPERATING

Port Placement

While placing the left lower quadrant port just lateral to the rectus sheath, be careful to avoid the epigastric vessels. The vessels are usually easily seen with transillumination from the laparoscope inside the abdomen. Consider using a right upper quadrant port for retrocecal, necrotic, or ruptured appendix for added traction and in the case of pregnancy, where the uterus may be in the way of the left lower quadrant port.

Exploratory Laparoscopy

Explore the abdominal and pelvic cavity for other diagnoses that may explain the patient's symptoms. Laparoscopy is particularly beneficial with questionable diagnoses and in female patients, in whom gynecologic pathology (e.g., pelvic inflammatory disease, ectopic pregnancy, Graafian follicle rupture) may mimic appendicitis.

Tissue Handling

Use closed graspers to manipulate the bowel when possible to avoid grasping the bowel too often. Be careful when grasping an inflamed appendix, as it may rupture.

Retrocecal Appendix

When dissecting out the cecum and terminal ileum to expose a retrocecal appendix, be careful not to damage the right external iliac vessels or right ureter.

Mesoappendix

When developing the window at the base of the appendix, be aware of the appendiceal artery, a terminal branch of the ileocolic artery; it is usually at the free margin of the mesoappendix.

Stapler

Clearly identify the ileocecal junction, so it is not strictured by the staple line. Do not staple across an appendolith. Instead, milk the appendolith into the cecum before stapling. Rotate the stapler 180 degrees prior to firing to avoid catching unwanted tissue in the teeth of the stapler.

Normal Appendix

Most surgeons will face an instance in which the patient they have taken to the operating room for suspected acute appendicitis will have a normal-appearing appendix on laparoscopy; the generally held negative appendectomy rate is around 20%, although recently this has decreased somewhat as a result of the more widespread use of CT imaging prior to surgery. Upon finding a normal-looking appendix, the surgeon must decide whether to take the appendix out or leave it in. The Society of American Gastrointestinal and Endoscopic Surgeons (SAGES) reports level III, grade A evidence that if the appendix is normal, and no other pathology is appreciated in the abdomen or pelvis, the decision to remove the appendix should be based on the clinical scenario. The SAGES guidelines do note that although an appendix may appear normal macroscopically, 19% to 40% of these appendixes will have microscopic abnormalities on pathologic examination. So the decision to leave in or take out the appendix should come down to the risks of leaving in a potentially abnormal appendix versus taking out a normal appendix. Recognizing that the most common morbidity with incidental appendectomy is wound infection, which is less frequent with the laparoscopic approach, we prefer to complete the appendectomy in the face of a normal-appearing appendix, unless another pathology that explains the patient's symptoms is identified on laparoscopy.

Reasons to Proceed to an Ileocecectomy or Formal Right Hemicolectomy during Laparoscopic Appendectomy

An ileocecectomy should be performed if there is a perforation at the base of the appendix or if there is a phlegmon involving the cecum. If a carcinoid tumor over 1.5 cm or a tumor involving the base of the appendix is found, a right hemicolectomy should be performed based on the indications for those diseases.

Converting to Open Surgery

Conversion to open surgery can occur in up to 27% of laparoscopic appendectomies, so adhere to the general guidelines for converting to open surgery. Situations in which this may be called for include inadequate exposure, confounding anatomy, and failure to progress. Before opening, consider another port in the right upper quadrant for added exposure and traction, and consider a midline incision to include your port entry site, instead of placing another incision in the right lower quadrant. Besides including your previous incision, another advantage of this midline incision is that it will be away from the area of inflammation in the right lower quadrant.

COMPLICATIONS

The surgeon should be aware of the more common complications after laparoscopic appendectomy and should ensure that the signs and symptoms of these complications are relayed to the patient before discharge, so that the patient knows when to call the surgeon or go to the nearest emergency department.

Wound Infection

Wound infections after laparoscopic appendectomy occur about half as often when compared to the 5% to 10% rate after open appendectomy. The patient should call the surgeon if they experience a fever over 101.4° F or for any redness, increasing pain, increasing warmth, or drainage from the wounds. These are typically managed with antibiotics and local wound care to the port sites, and such wound infections have a much lower morbidity compared to an open appendectomy, because the incision size and subcutaneous space is less in a laparoscopic appendectomy.

Abscess

The patient should call the hospital when fever exceeds 101.4° F or for increasing or persistent abdominal pain. Management of this complication will require admission to the hospital and many times will require antibiotics and either laparoscopic or percutaneous drainage.

Bleeding

For significant bleeding, the patient may become fatigued or orthostatic, and the abdomen may become peritonitic. The patient should be told what symptoms to be aware of and should be advised to report directly to the nearest emergency department if this occurs. If symptoms are persistent, or if the patient is unstable, immediate exploration is required.

Urinary Retention

If the patient is discharged from outpatient surgery before they have voided, they must be instructed to go to their local emergency department if they have not voided within 8 to 10 hours after the operation.

Bowel Obstruction

Bowel obstruction may be caused by an ileus or by mechanical obstruction as a result of an errant staple line. The presenting symptoms may include abdominal pain, discomfort, or distension, nausea and vomiting, and dehydration. The patient should call the surgeon for readmission should any of these symptoms occur.

Recurrent/Stump Appendicitis

Recurrent appendicitis occurs when a small lumen of appendix is left behind during the operation. Patients will present with symptoms similar to their acute appendicitis and may even present many months, sometimes even more than a year, later. If these symptoms are persistent, reoperation will be required.

SPECIAL POPULATIONS

Pregnant Women

According to SAGES, laparoscopic appendectomy is safe in any trimester. This is supported with level II, grade B evidence. The laparoscopic approach offers decreased pain, leading to decreased narcotic use and its associated fetal depression; a faster return to normal activity, which will decrease the risk for venothrombotic embolisms; and less trauma to the abdominal wall, resulting in lower risk for hernias. Of note, the cutdown approach for port placement should be used for the second and third trimesters to avoid uterine injury on port placement. In planning port placement, a right upper quadrant port should replace the left lower quadrant port to avoid the gravid uterus. During the first and second trimester, preoperative and postoperative fetal heart tones should be obtained. If the operation occurs during a viable gestational age, continuous heart tones should be monitored during surgery to evaluate for fetal distress.

Extremes of Age

Laparoscopic appendectomy is safe and effective for both uncomplicated and complicated acute appendicitis in children. For elderly patients, SAGES reports that laparoscopic appendectomy may be the preferred approach, especially for those over the age of 65 because of the lower rate of complications and lower rate of death (level II, grade B evidence). Most importantly in this age group, an underlying colonic malignancy should be considered and ruled out postoperatively with a colonoscopy.

Obese Individuals

Laparoscopic appendectomy is safe and effective in obese patients, according to level II, grade B evidence. Indeed, it and may be the preferred approach (level III, grade C evidence) owing to superior exposure and decreased wound infection rates. The laparoscopic approach can also improve the ease of the operation for the surgeon in this patient population.

FUTURE DIRECTIONS

Single-incision laparoscopic surgery (SILS), also known as *single-port access* (SPA) surgery; single laparoscopic incision transabdominal (SLIT) surgery; natural orifice transumbilical surgery (NOTUS); one-port umbilical surgery (OPUS); embryonic natural orifice transumbilical endoscopic surgery (E-NOTES); and laparoscopic endoscopic single-site surgery (LESSS) are new surgical techniques that emerged in the 1990s as offshoots of natural orifice transluminal endoscopic surgery (NOTES). As such techniques are still in their infancy, there is no uniform approach. Either a single skin incision is made at the umbilicus, and a single fascial incision accommodates multiple ports, or multiple fascial incisions are made through the same skin incision after raising flaps for the multiple ports. A few of the common troubles with such approaches are the clashing of instruments, poor visualization, and sometimes the increased distance to the operative site. The impetus behind such techniques are for improved cosmesis, reduced pain, and reduced wound complications. NOTES was first trialed on uncomplicated appendicitis and cholecystitis, and we mention it here to show what may be on the horizon. Further evaluation is required to see if similar approaches are equivalent to laparoscopic or open appendectomy.

SUMMARY

Laparoscopic appendectomy has been studied extensively and is an excellent alternative to open appendectomy for appendicitis in most settings. It is particularly advantageous in clinical scenarios in which the diagnosis is in dispute; in the female population, in whom gynecologic pathologies can mimic appendicitis; and in the obese population, in whom there is better exposure and decreased wound infection.

SUGGESTED READINGS

Addiss DG, Shaffer N, Fowler BS, et al: The epidemiology of appendicitis and appendectomy in the United States, *Am J Epidemiol* 132(5):910–925, 1990.

Katkhouda N, Mason RJ, Towfigh S, et al: Laparoscopic versus open appendectomy: a prospective randomized double-blind study, *Ann Surg* 242(3):439–450, 2005.

Paulson EK, Kalady MF, Pappas TN: Suspected appendicitis, *New Engl J Med* 348(3):236–242, 2003.

Sauerland S, Lefering R, Neugebauer EAM: Laparoscopic versus open surgery for suspected appendicitis, *Cochrane Database Syst Rev* (4):CD001546, 2004.

LAPAROSCOPIC INGUINAL HERNIORRHAPHY

George S. Ferzli, MD, and Eric D. Edwards, MD

OVERVIEW

Since surgeons first began to deal with the problem of groin hernia, the search for an ideal repair has been ongoing. Tissue-based procedures were once deemed the standard of care, but they have now been largely relegated to situations involving contamination or infection. Today, the gold standard of open surgery is the anterior tension-free repair with mesh. The two most common types are the Lichtenstein technique and the "plug and patch." Novel three-dimensional mesh systems have also been tried, but data regarding the effectiveness of these methods are still unavailable. The unfortunate drawback of all these repairs is in the failure to dissect and completely reinforce the myopectineal orifice, which can lead to missed hernias and potentially higher recurrence rates. Felix (1996) demonstrated that 9% of patients undergoing laparoscopic inguinal herniorrhaphy were found to have an occult femoral hernia.

Numerous studies, with the exception of a controversial one (Neumayer, 2004), have shown that recurrence rates for primary inguinal hernias repaired laparoscopically are comparable with open tension-free repairs. There is also clear evidence that patients have less postoperative pain and return to normal activity faster after laparoscopy. The laparoscopic approach also allows recurrent hernias that were initially repaired with an open anterior approach to be corrected with a greater success rate and with less chance of injury to the cord structures. This is important, because approximately 10% of herniorrhaphies are for recurrences. Bilateral hernias can be repaired without the necessity of additional incisions. Obese patients can also benefit from the laparoscopic approach, because it avoids the wound complications that may follow extensive groin dissection.

Since the initial reports of laparoscopic extraperitoneal inguinal hernia repair by Ferzli (1992) and McKernan (1993), much has been learned regarding the technical intricacies involved in this surgery. We believe that by now, the weight of the data in favor of laparoscopy makes it the procedure of choice for most such hernias. The two most common procedures are the transabdominal preperitoneal (TAPP) repair and the totally extraperitoneal (TEP) repair. We cover the relevant anatomy, indications and contraindications, key operative steps, and potential pitfalls here. In addition, we briefly discuss our approach to patients with chronic pain after herniorrhaphy.

EVALUATING THE PATIENT

Preoperative patient evaluation should include a complete history and physical, with particular attention paid to conditions that might increase the likelihood of complications. Those with a chronic cough, constipation, or prostatism should have these problems treated prior to surgery. Risk reduction strategies, such as weight loss and smoking cessation, should be addressed when necessary.

The surgeon should note the size and reducibility of the hernia, as well as the possibility of contralateral hernia, and the umbilicus should be examined for the presence of a hernia. Peripheral nerve involvement—evidenced by anesthesia, hypesthesia, or contact dysthesia— should be documented. In men, both testicles and the cord structures should be palpated for masses, and the skin should be examined for rashes and cutaneous fungal or bacterial infection.

RELEVANT ANATOMY

A thorough understanding of preperitoneal anatomy is critical to performing a proper laparoscopy (Figure 1). The myopectineal orifice of Fruchaud is the area from which all inguinal hernias arise. This space is bound superiorly by the arch of the internal oblique and the transversus abdominis muscle, inferiorly by the Cooper ligament, medially by the rectus muscle, and laterally by the iliopsoas muscle; the inguinal ligament passes through the area obliquely. The objective of surgery is the reduction of all hernias and complete mesh coverage of the myopectineal orifice (MPO).

The space of Retzius and the space of Bogros (Figure 2) make up the working area. The space of Retzius (retropubic space) is a potential area behind the pubic symphysis, anterior to the bladder. The space of Bogros is a lateral extension of the space of Retzius and extends to the anterior superior iliac spine. To accomplish a sound repair, these spaces must be developed fully.

In the preperitoneal space, deep to the transversalis fascia, is a fascial layer analogous to the Scarpa fascia (Figure 3). The vas deferens and the gonadal vessels are enveloped by this layer. The inferior epigastric vessels, the iliac vessels, and the genitofemoral nerve are found external to this layer, in the so-called *parietal plane* of the extraperitoneal fascia. Internal to this layer, in the so-called *visceral plane*, are the bladder and its associated blood vessels. As the peritoneum is peeled off the epigastric vessels, there will still be a thin layer of tissue covering them. Similarly, when the peritoneum is peeled off the cord structures, there will still be a translucent layer covering these structures and the iliac vessels. Leaving these tissue layers intact provides a cellular barrier between important anatomic entities and the mesh, which can reduce the incidence of ischemic orchitis, fertility loss, and fibrosis around the iliac vessels caused by mesh-induced inflammation.

In laparoscopic repair, the MPO must be approached deep to this layer of extraperitoneal fascia, in the visceral plane, to avoid the risk of bleeding from the inferior epigastric vessels and the risk of nerve

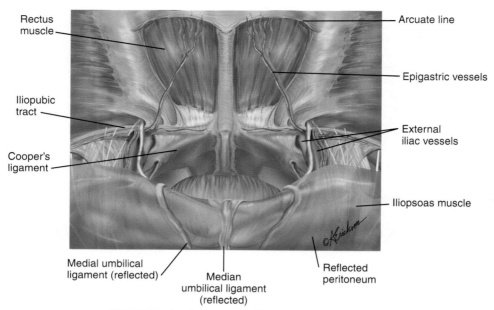

Rectus muscle

Arcuate line

Epigastric vessels

Iliopubic tract

Cooper's ligament

External iliac vessels

Iliopsoas muscle

Medial umbilical ligament (reflected)

Median umbilical ligament (reflected)

Reflected peritoneum

FIGURE 1   Inguinal anatomy. *(Courtesy Anne Erickson, CMI.)*

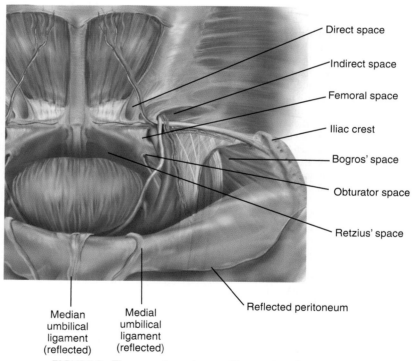

Direct space

Indirect space

Femoral space

Iliac crest

Bogros' space

Obturator space

Retzius' space

Median umbilical ligament (reflected)

Medial umbilical ligament (reflected)

Reflected peritoneum

FIGURE 2   The preperitoneal space. *(Courtesy Anne Erickson, CMI.)*

injury. Dissection lateral to the medial umbilical ligaments should occur in the visceral plane of the extraperitoneal fascia. Doing so will allow parietal nerves (genital and femoral branches of the genitofemoral nerve) and parietal vessels (inferior epigastric and external iliac) to remain in situ and undamaged. Dissection medial to the umbilical ligaments in the space of Retzius should take place in the parietal plane of the extraperitoneal fascia to avoid potential urologic complications. Identification of the correct plane is also essential for proper mesh placement (discussed below).

INDICATIONS AND CONTRAINDICATIONS

In addition to the treatment of primary inguinal hernias, the laparoscopic approach is ideally suited for the treatment of recurrent hernias initially repaired with an open anterior approach. It is equally ideal for bilateral hernias, those in athletic or obese patients, and in cases of known contralateral vas deferens injury from prior surgery.

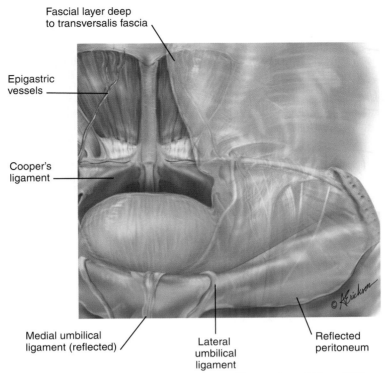

Fascial layer deep to transversalis fascia

Epigastric vessels

Cooper's ligament

Medial umbilical ligament (reflected)

Lateral umbilical ligament

Reflected peritoneum

FIGURE 3 The extraperitoneal fascial layer. *(Courtesy Anne Erickson, CMI.)*

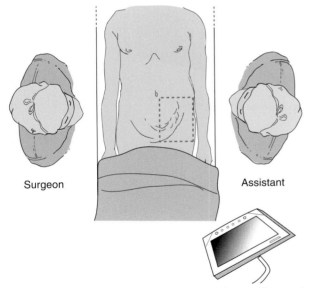

Surgeon

Assistant

FIGURE 4 Positioning of the patient and surgical team. *(Courtesy Anne Erickson, CMI.)*

Patients who are not deemed suitable for general anesthesia or who cannot tolerate pneumoperitoneum because of cardiopulmonary disease are best served with an open repair under local anesthetic. In renal transplant patients, the preperitoneal position of the transplanted organ precludes the possibility of a laparoscopic preperitoneal repair. Relative contraindications include prior surgery in the preperitoneal space, prior laparotomy, the presence of ascites, the presence of large scrotal or incarcerated or strangulated hernias, and current use of antiplatelet agents or systemic anticoagulation; however, low-dose aspirin need not be stopped preoperatively.

PREPARING THE PATIENT

Operating room setup and patient preparation are identical for the transabdominal (TAPP) and the extraperitoneal (TEP) approaches. General anesthetic with systemic paralysis is routinely used. TEP has been performed using a variety of other anesthetic techniques, including laryngeal mask airway, spinal/epidural anesthesia, and even local anesthetic. The patient is asked to void before entering the operating room, so a Foley catheter will not be necessary. The incision site is marked in the preoperative holding area.

The patient is placed supine on the operating table with the arms at the sides. Attention must be paid to proper padding of all pressure points, to avoid peripheral nerve injury. Sequential compression devices are placed on the lower extremities, and a single dose of a first-generation cephalosporin is administered prior to incision. The operating table is placed in a slight Trendelenburg position, and a single monitor is placed at the foot of the table; an irrigation setup is not routinely used. The surgeon typically stands on the side opposite the hernia (Figure 4), and an attempt should be made to reduce the hernia prior to starting the procedure.

TOTALLY EXTRAPERITONEAL INGUINAL HERNIA REPAIR

Trocar Placement

A stepwise approach is critical to performing a safe, effective, and reproducible hernia repair (Box 1). When performing a TEP, three trocars, one Hasson and two 5 mm, are placed in the midline (Figure 5). A curvilinear infraumbilical incision large enough to accommodate the Hasson is made, and dissection is carried down sharply to the level of the fascia. The anterior sheath of the rectus fascia is incised transversely on one side of the midline, and the rectus muscle is retracted laterally. An index finger is inserted into the preperitoneal space medial and parallel to the rectus muscle. Once below the line of Douglas, the finger is swept side to side (Figure 6). The peritoneum above the line of Douglas is very adherent to the overlying fascia and can be torn very easily, and this maneuver opens up the preperitoneal space sufficiently to allow placement of the trocars.

BOX 1: Steps of TEP

1. Identify the pubic symphysis in the midline.
2. Bluntly dissect the Cooper ligament bilaterally to open up the space of Retzius.
3. Identify the Hesselbach triangle and the three potential sites of herniation related to it (direct, femoral, obturator).
4. Identify and elevate the epigastric vessels.
5. Bluntly develop the space of Bogros to the level of the anterior superior ileac spine.
6. Dissect cord structures.
7. Place the mesh.

On rare occasions the finger will not cross the midline, the result of a very thick linea alba extending in the midline to the pubic symphysis. In this situation, the rectus fascia is incised transversely on the other side of the midline. S-type retractors are inserted on each side of the linea alba, lifting the right and left anterior rectus sheaths. The view will be very similar to the vocal cords (Figure 7). The linea alba is divided under direct observation, using Metzenbaum scissors. The Hasson trocar is placed in the preperitoneal space and secured to the skin with interrupted sutures in the skin. The Hasson should be placed just far enough into the preperitoneal space to allow proper insufflation, and the preperitoneal space is insufflated to 10 mm Hg; in young and muscular patients, the pressure is allowed to reach 12 mm Hg. A 10 mm 30-degree angled laparoscope is passed into the preperitoneal space and advanced tangentially to the pubic symphysis. Once this structure is encountered, the laparoscope is gently moved side to side, resulting in division of the loose areolar tissue in the parietal compartment of the extraperitoneal space (Figure 8).

Carbon dioxide (CO_2) insufflation serves as an excellent retractor of the peritoneal sac. Once this has been accomplished, the two 5

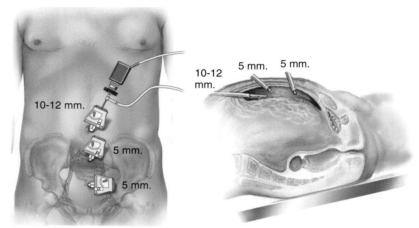

FIGURE 5   Trocar position for TEP. *(Courtesy Anne Erickson, CMI.)*

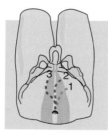

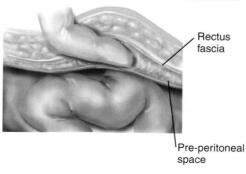

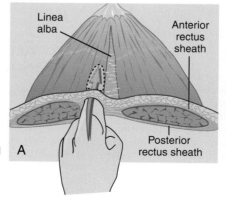

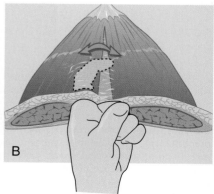

FIGURE 6   Developing the preperitoneal space in the midline. *(Courtesy Anne Erickson, CMI.)*

mm trocars are gently inserted under direct visualization in the midline of the abdomen. They should be placed as close to the umbilical trocar as possible, allowing for easier placement of the mesh. If the inferior trocar is placed too low, it can be covered by the mesh, making proper mesh placement extremely difficult. The trocars must be placed in the midline for two reasons: 1) to reduce risk of bleeding from the rectus, and 2) to increase instrument mobility in the operative space.

Some surgeons prefer to enter the extraperitoneal space using a Visiport (T2K, Redmond, Wash.) inserted through the rectus fibers. One 5 mm trocar is used in the midline, and another is inserted laterally, medial to and below the anterosuperior iliac spine through the transversus abdominis muscle. We do not find that approach desirable, because it requires an additional trocar for bilateral exploration, and insertion of the lateral trocar increases the risk of injury to the iliohypogastric and ilioinguinal nerves (Figure 9).

Dissection and Reduction of Hernias

Once the trocars have been placed in the preperitoneal space, the repair is carried out by following the steps of TEP (Figure 10). Four potential sites of hernia formation are found in the MPO: 1) the direct space, 2) the indirect space, 3) the femoral canal, and, least commonly, 4) the obturator canal. A consistent stepwise approach to the dissection of the preperitoneal space will ensure that no hernias are missed. The first step is to identify the pubic symphysis in the midline. This may be regarded as a safe harbor, a landmark by which surgeons can orient themselves, should they become confused during dissection. No dissection should be done posterior to it, as this risks injury to the bladder. Anything done should stay in the parietal plane of the extraperitoneal fascia.

Next, the Cooper ligament is bluntly swept clear in a medial to lateral direction (step 2). This should be done while staying close to the ligament and close to the pubic bone, and it should be done in a slow,

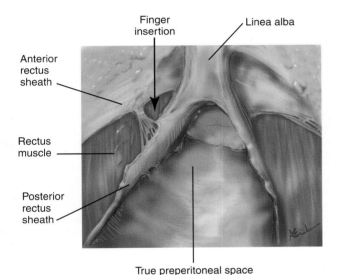

FIGURE 7 View of the developed preperitoneal space in the midline. *(Courtesy Anne Erickson, CMI.)*

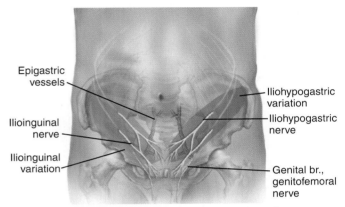

FIGURE 9 Position of the iliohypogastric and ilioinguinal nerves. *(Courtesy Anne Erickson, CMI.)*

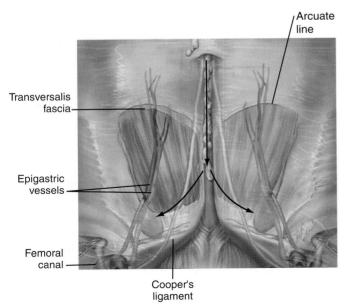

FIGURE 8 Parietal compartment of the extraperitoneal space. *(Courtesy Anne Erickson, CMI.)*

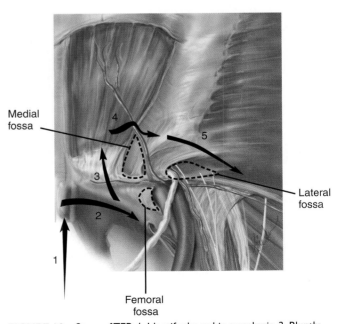

FIGURE 10 Steps of TEP: *1,* Identify the pubic symphysis. *2,* Bluntly sweep the Cooper ligament bilaterally to open up the space of Retzius. *3,* Identify the Hesselbach triangle. *4,* Elevate the epigastric vessels. *5,* Bluntly develop the space of Bogros to the level of the ASIS. *6,* Dissect cord structures. *7,* Place the mesh. *(Courtesy Anne Erickson, CMI.)*

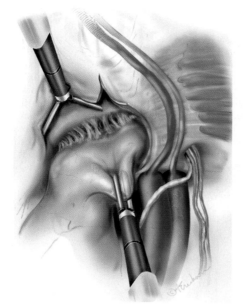

FIGURE 11   Reduction of a direct hernia sac. *(Courtesy Anne Erickson, CMI.)*

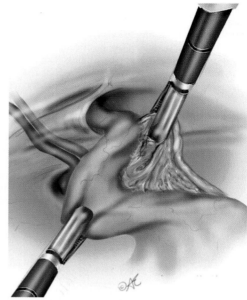

FIGURE 13   Second maneuver in dissection of an indirect hernia sac. *(Courtesy Anne Erickson, CMI.)*

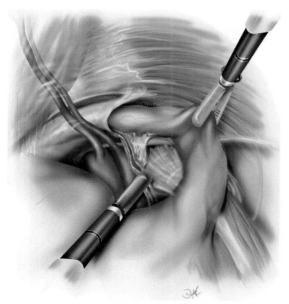

FIGURE 12   First maneuver in dissection of an indirect hernia sac. *(Courtesy Anne Erickson, CMI.)*

gentle, sweeping motion. This allows visualization of the femoral and obturator spaces and maintains the dissection in the parietal space. Any herniation in theses spaces should be reduced bluntly. Caution must be exercised when reducing a femoral hernia to avoid injury to the femoral vein and to the occasional corona mortis artery. The space of Retzius is then fully developed by dissecting the contralateral Cooper ligament in a similar fashion.

Next, the direct space located immediately superior to the femoral space is identified (step 3). The femoral and direct spaces are separated by the medial aspect of the iliopubic tract. A direct hernia will obscure the view of the Cooper ligament and is readily identifiable during the initial dissection of the preperitoneal space; convexity in the Hessel-bach triangle indicates the presence of a large, indirect hernia. A direct hernia sac is reduced by bluntly peeling it away from the attenuated transversalis fascia (Figure 11), but sharp dissection should be avoided.

Reduction of a direct hernia relies on constant, gentle traction and countertraction. When treating large, direct hernias, some surgeons suture the redundant transversalis fascia to the iliopubic tract to reduce the dead space and the potential for subsequent seroma formation.

After the inferior epigastric vessels are identified, they should be elevated so as to stay with the rectus muscle (step 4). Bleeding from the epigastric vessels or one of their branches can usually be controlled with direct pressure against the anterior abdominal wall. Occasionally, clips or judicious use of cautery are required. Dissection should remain in the visceral component of the extraperitoneal space, as dissection above the epigastric vessels will result in bleeding. When these vessels have been elevated with one grasper, blunt lateral dissection is begun with the other. This should be horizontal to the epigastric vessels. Dissection just below the level of these vessels will develop the space of Bogros (step 5); proper development of this potential space is vital to allow placement of an appropriately sized piece of mesh. The indirect space is now identifiable by finding the cord structures passing through the internal ring. The indirect hernia sac can be seen overlying the cord structures in men and the round ligament in women. It must be remembered that the vas deferens or round ligaments are always adjacent to the epigastric vessels.

If it is not possible to see the vas deferens in men or the round ligament in women, an indirect hernia is indicated. Prior to attempting reduction of that, it is important to reduce all lipomas of the cord (step 6). They are always on the upper outer quadrant of the indirect ring. Doing so makes subsequent reduction of the sac easier and lessens the chances of the patient's developing a recurrence. Reduction of the sac is accomplished by sweeping the cord structures posteromedially while holding the sac superolaterally (Figure 12).

The sac is then pivoted medially and posteriorly, while the cord structures are swept posterolaterally (Figure 13). Alternating between these two maneuvers results in separation of the cord structures from the hernia sac. The sac can then be reduced by passing it hand over hand, until it is delivered into the preperitoneal space. In female patients, the round ligament should be treated in the same manner as the vas deferens. The separation of the peritoneum from the cord structures, the nerve structures (lateral cutaneous, femoral, and femoral branches of the genitofemoral nerve), and the iliac vessels must remain within the visceral component of the extraperitoneal space. This will serve to protect these structures. Care should also be taken not to denude the psoas muscle lateral to the cord structures, and the

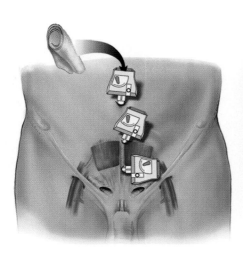
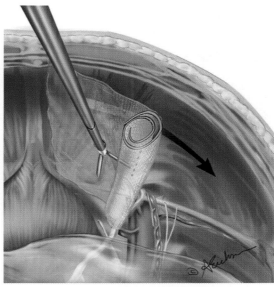

FIGURE 14   Insertion of mesh into preperitoneal space. *(Courtesy Anne Erickson, CMI.)*

membranous layer should remain intact as much as possible, even when an indirect sac is being dissected off the vas deferens. The less these cord structures are manipulated, the better.

Occult contralateral hernias can be found in 10% to 15% of patients. After reducing any hernias on the symptomatic side, it is routine to explore the contralateral side to ensure no additional hernia is present. During the dissection, any rent in the peritoneum can be problematic. If the peritoneum is violated, it is usually quite obvious. The working space may begin to collapse, the flow from the CO_2 insufflator will increase, and the patient's abdomen will become distended and tympanitic. Under spinal, epidural, or local anesthesia, pneumoperitoneum will not cause patient discomfort as long as the pressure is at 10 mm Hg. A complete dissection of the spaces of Retzius and Bogros usually allows preservation of the working room needed to complete the operation. Small tears or those distant from the site of mesh placement can be left alone as long as working room is maintained. Large tears or those close to the MPO should be closed with an Endoloop (Ethicon, Somerville, NJ). It has been our experience that decompression of the peritoneal cavity with a Veress needle in the event of a peritoneal tear is not helpful and can be dangerous. Any pneumoperitoneum present at the end of the case will resolve spontaneously.

Mesh Placement

Mesh options for hernia repair are numerous. Our preference is a 15 cm² piece of lightweight polypropylene mesh trimmed to an appropriate size, rolled tightly, and introduced tangentially through the Hasson trocar (Figure 14). It can be premoistened with saline, but there are no data to support the use of antibiotic irrigation. The Hasson trocar should be held horizontally, and the camera is withdrawn. The mesh can then be placed into the space of Retzius. The mesh should extend from the midline to the anterosuperior iliac spine minus 1 cm (minus 2 cm in patients with excessive abdominal fat) and should be diamond or kite shaped, with the "tail" extending out into the space of Bogros; lateral to the medial umbilical ligaments, the mesh should lie in the visceral plane of the extraperitoneal fascia. This placement allows parietal nerves (genital and femoral branches of the genitofemoral nerve) and parietal vessels (inferior epigastric and external iliac) to remain in situ and undamaged. Medial to the umbilical ligaments (space of Retzius), the mesh should lie more anteriorly in the parietal plane of the extraperitoneal fascia. This avoids its being in the perivesical space, directly on the bladder. The

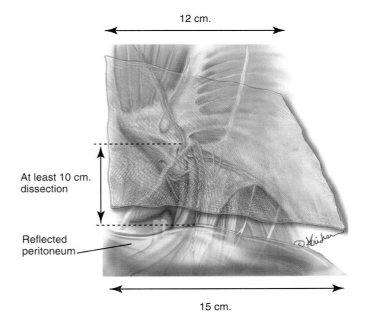

12 cm.

At least 10 cm. dissection

Reflected peritoneum

15 cm.

FIGURE 15   Mesh placement in the preperitoneal space. *(Courtesy Anne Erickson, CMI.)*

mesh is unfolded in a medial-to-lateral direction, providing coverage of the entire MPO (Figure 15).

We do not place a slit or "keyhole" in the mesh for the passage of the cord structures, as this has been shown to be a factor in the development of recurrence. Dissection to allow placement of the cord structures through the keyhole will disrupt the integrity of the membranous layer, which results in more scarring around the cord structures. For this reason we do not believe in parietalization of the cord but rather in a generous dissection of the Bogros space beyond the level of the anterior superior iliac spine. Dissection out to the anterior superior iliac spine provides at least 10 cm of distance proximal to the deep internal ring. This will diminish the likelihood of a lateral recurrence by allowing the mesh to "espouse" the lateral abdominal wall, minimizing the chance of mesh dislocation, migration, or lifting. The mesh should be slightly redundant for four reasons: 1) to allow for shrinkage of the prosthetic material, 2) to accommodate

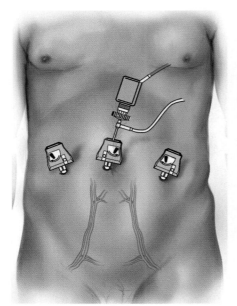

FIGURE 16   Trocar placement during TAPP. *(Courtesy Anne Erickson, CMI.)*

the protuberance of the abdominal wall, 3) to minimize the chance of groin pain resulting from taut mesh, and 4) to reduce the chance of recurrence.

It is important to understand the true purpose of mesh in the preperitoneal space. We agree with Wantz (1998), who has stated that the mesh in these cases reinforces the visceral peritoneum or sac and not the abdominal wall itself. We do not routinely tack the mesh in place, thus minimizing the risk of nerve entrapment. Some may find it helpful early in their experience to place a single tack in the Cooper ligament medially to hold the mesh in place and facilitate its lateral unfolding. However, once polypropylene comes in contact with bodily fluids, it becomes adhesive enough to stay in proper position once the preperitoneal space is desufflated.

In bilateral hernia repair, two pieces of mesh are used, and they overlap in the midline at the pubic symphysis. After placement of the mesh, it should be held in place laterally in the Bogros space and medially at the Cooper ligament. The preperitoneal space is desufflated under direct vision, and the graspers are gently removed.

Closure

The fascial defect at the umbilical trocar site is closed in an interrupted manner with an absorbable suture of appropriate size. Skin incisions are closed with staples or absorbable subcuticular sutures, and the wounds can be infiltrated with local anesthetic. We do not routinely instill lidocaine in the preperitoneal space, as some authors have advocated.

TRANSABDOMINAL PREPERITONEAL INGUINAL HERNIA REPAIR

Trocar Placement

Three trocars are used to perform a transabdominal preperitoneal (TAPP) repair, one 10 mm and two 5 mm. Pneumoperitoneum of 15 mm Hg can be established with the Veress needle through the umbilicus or with the open Hasson technique through an infraumbilical incision. The first trocar is placed in the infraumbilical position, and the other two are placed at the same level of the umbilicus, lateral to the rectus

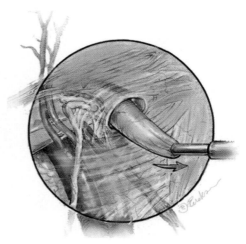

FIGURE 17   Invagination of hernia sac. *(Courtesy Anne Erickson, CMI.)*

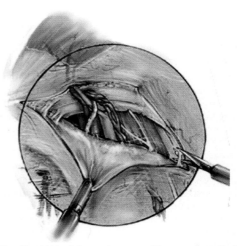

FIGURE 18   Opening of the peritoneum. *(Courtesy Anne Erickson, CMI.)*

muscles (Figure 16). Care must be taken not to injure the epigastric vessels. Use of a single incision umbilical port has recently been reported.

Dissection and Reduction of Hernias

Adhesions from prior intraabdominal surgery may need to be taken down in the standard fashion. After the hernia is identified, the contents of the sac can usually be reduced with gentle traction. A grasper is then used to invaginate the hernia sac into the abdominal cavity, with care being taken to avoid injuring the cord structures (Figure 17). Constant gentle traction will pull the sac and surrounding peritoneum from the MPO. The peritoneum is then incised 2 cm above the orifice, from the anterior superior iliac spine to the median umbilical ligament (Figure 18).

In bilateral TAPP, the median umbilical ligament should be preserved to avoid the urachus. After incision of the peritoneum, dissection in the preperitoneal space should start laterally and proceed medially. This allows development of the preperitoneal space in a safer manner. Dissecting medially without proper lateral development of the preperitoneal space increases the risk of injury to an iliac vessel or the bladder. Gentle, constant traction on the peritoneal flap combined with blunt dissection allows for the development of the preperitoneal space. Reduction of cord lipomas and hernia sacs follows the same principles outlined for a TEP repair. The use of cautery should

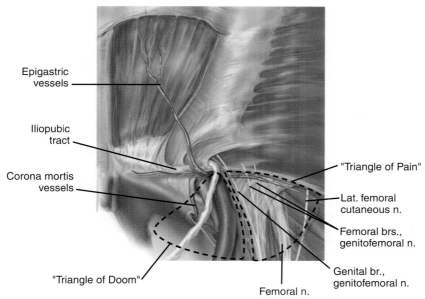

Epigastric vessels

Iliopubic tract

Corona mortis vessels

"Triangle of Doom"

Femoral n.

"Triangle of Pain"

Lat. femoral cutaneous n.

Femoral brs., genitofemoral n.

Genital br., genitofemoral n.

FIGURE 19 Triangle of pain. *(Courtesy Anne Erickson, CMI.)*

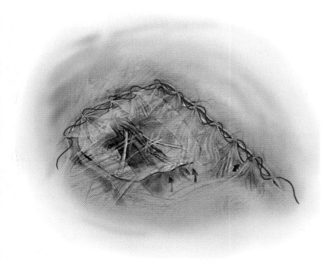

FIGURE 20 Closure of the peritoneal flap. *(Courtesy Anne Erickson, CMI.)*

be minimized to reduce risk of injury to the vas deferens and gonadal vessels. After full dissection of the MPO, attention can be turned to the mesh.

Mesh Placement

A piece of polypropylene mesh similar to that used for TEP repairs is placed in the preperitoneal space. It should be large enough to provide complete coverage of the MPO and should extend from the midline to the anterosuperior iliac spine minus 1 cm (minus 2 cm in overweight patients). As in the TEP, the mesh is not slit or keyholed; it can be fixed in place through the judicious use of sutures or any number of absorbable tacking devices, although metal tacks should be avoided. When needed, tacks can be placed in the medial aspect of the Cooper ligament and in the transversalis fascia on either side of the inferior epigastric vessels. Placement of tacks must be avoided in the "triangle of pain," an area containing many sensory nerves. It is bounded by the gonadals medially, the reflected peritoneum laterally, and the iliopubic

tract superiorly. From medial to lateral it includes the femoral nerve, the femoral branch of the genitofemoral nerve, and the lateral femoral cutaneous nerve (Figure 19). In thin patients, even properly placed tacks may cause injury to the ilioinguinal or iliohypogastric nerves.

Once the mesh is satisfactorily positioned, the peritoneal flap is used to cover it. The flap can be held in place with a tacking device or a running absorbable suture (Figure 20). To prevent the development of an internal hernia, no gaps should be left in the peritoneal closure. Lowering the pneumoperitoneum to 10 mm Hg can assist in flap closure, and trocar sites larger than 5 mm are closed with interrupted absorbable suture.

Fixing the Mesh in Place

The optimal method of mesh fixation, or whether any fixation is needed at all, are the subject of much debate. In a small study by Ferzli (2004), it was demonstrated that mesh fixation is not required when the TEP approach is used. Other small studies have shown no difference in recurrence and less postoperative pain when tacks are not used during a TEP (Ferzli, 1999; Liem, 2003). A recent retrospective study of 929 patients (1753 hernias) undergoing TEP revealed no difference in recurrence rate between the fixed and nonfixed groups. Patients in the fixed group had significantly more pain at 1 month postoperatively, more urinary retention, and a longer time to resumption of normal activity.

Biologic adhesives have been used by some, but they are costly and are also associated with an increased incidence of seroma formation (Lau, 2005). Studies of "self-gripping" mesh containing microhooks that attach to the tissue are underway (Hollinsky, 2009). Disruption of the peritoneum during TAPP seems to be the rationale for use of fixation, but the biomechanical principles of TAPP are identical to TEP. Therefore mesh fixation may not be considered mandatory (Kapiris, 2009).

TOTALLY EXTRAPERITONEAL VERSUS TRANSABDOMINAL PREPERITONEAL REPAIR

The advantages of TAPP include a larger working space and the ability to access the preperitoneal space in patients who have had prior preperitoneal violation. Contrary to what is commonly reported, TAPP does not allow the surgeon to rule out bilateral hernias by inspection alone. To exclude completely the presence of a lipoma or hernia, the MPO must be exposed. This requires incision of the peritoneum and its subsequent closure. TAPP may therefore be preferred for repairing an incarcerated hernia, as it allows for assessment of the reduced bowel. The disadvantages of TAPP when compared with TEP include a longer operative time, occasional difficulty in getting adequate peritoneal coverage of the mesh, and the need to use a tacking device. Although we favor TEP, it has not been shown to be superior to TAPP in terms of recurrence rate or the development of chronic groin pain.

MANAGEMENT OF MORE COMPLICATED HERNIAS

Treatment of Recurrences

Operations on recurrent groin hernias account for approximately 10% of herniorrhaphies, and such recurrences are fraught with risks that include testicular loss, fertility reduction, major vascular and nerve injury, and the development of chronic pain. Re-recurrence is a real concern, because each successive operation in the same groin presents an even higher risk of significant complications. Before surgery is scheduled on a recurrent hernia, a review of the operative report from any prior procedures is imperative. A discussion with the patient about the risks of serious complication should also be undertaken.

Open Recurrences

Groin hernias that recur after an open anterior approach are ideally suited to the laparoscopic approach. The chance to work in virgin tissue planes and the ability to visualize the entire MPO are two obvious advantages of laparoscopy. As previously noted, these patients also tend to experience less postoperative pain, return to normal activity faster, and have fewer complications. The surgeon can also examine the contralateral side and address any hernias discovered at that time. Numerous prospective and retrospective studies support the conclusion that both TEP and TAPP are superior to open anterior operations for recurrences. Most nonrandomized studies find equivalent rates of recurrence and complications when comparing TEP and TAPP. We prefer TEP in these situations, because with TAPP it is sometimes difficult to obtain adequate peritoneal coverage of the mesh once the repair is completed. TAPP also seems to be associated with higher rates of trocar site hernias and visceral injury. When surgery is done on an open recurrence, the previously outlined steps of the procedure and the principles behind them remain unchanged.

Special care must be taken when dealing with previously placed mesh in the preperitoneal space. The mesh is often scarred into vital structures, and aggressive attempts at removal can result in serious injury. In general it is advisable to leave old mesh in situ and place the new piece over it. On the other hand, with patients who have had prior Kugel repairs, an attempt should be made to remove the ring, as serious complications with rings have been reported.

Laparoscopic Recurrences

Laparoscopy plays a role in the repair of recurrences after an initial laparoscopic repair. But because of a significant increase in technical difficulty, extensive experience should be gained with laparoscopic repair of primary hernias before attempting this procedure. Until such experience is gained, these recurrences are probably best approached in an open manner. But when laparoscopy is employed in these particular cases, it has been our experience that TAPP is technically easier than TEP. The operative working space can be significantly reduced when attempting TEP after TEP. The contralateral space of Bogros will often fail to open up, and a full bladder will not assist in maintaining working room, should a peritoneal tear occur.

In contrast to repair of primary hernias or open recurrences, this dissection should take place in the parietal plane of the extraperitoneal fascia. It requires ligation of the inferior epigastric vessels and any associated branches. Meticulous hemostasis is essential. Postoperative hematoma may cause displacement of the mesh, and use of cautery should be minimized. The dissection should proceed as close to the rectus muscle as possible, until the MPO is visualized. There is never a hernia between the vas deferens and the epigastric vessels. If the vas deferens cannot be seen, this indicates an indirect hernia; if the Cooper ligament and femoral canal cannot be seen, a direct hernia is present; and if adhesions are present, there is no hernia. External palpation and pulling on a testicle aid in orientation. Parietalization of the cord structures is not possible because of inflammation from the prior repair.

Reduction of a recurrent hernia should be followed by placement of mesh that overlaps the defect by at least 3 cm. To gain access to the preperitoneal space when performing TAPP after TEP or TAPP after TAPP, the peritoneum is incised above the level of the mesh. The fused mesh and peritoneum are then peeled down, and the preperitoneal space is entered. As in TEP after TEP, the dissection proceeds in the parietal plane of the extraperitoneal space. Division of the inferior epigastric vessels is also required. The old mesh is difficult to cut with scissors, and cautery can be used to divide it if necessary. Reduction of any recurrences and mesh placement proceed as previously described.

Wauschkuhn (2009) reported his group's experience performing TAPP in patients who had previously undergone radical prostatectomy. When compared with those who had not had prior preperitoneal surgery, operative times were longer (59 vs. 40 minutes), morbidity was higher (5.7 % vs. 2.8%), but recurrences were similar (0.8% vs. 0.7%). Ferzli (2006) reported his experience with 21 patients undergoing TEP after TEP. Five were converted to an open repair, three for inability to open the preperitoneal space, one for bleeding, and one for tears in the peritoneum. There were no significant morbidities.

Incarcerated and Scrotal Hernias

Scrotal hernias present a challenge to the surgeon, not just because of technical issues related to the repair, but also because these patients often have significant comorbidities. When elective repair is being considered, patients should undergo cardiopulmonary evaluation to assess their fitness for surgery. Risk reduction strategies such as weight loss and smoking cessation should be attempted. Preoperative discussion should emphasize the increased risk of postoperative complications such as ischemic orchitis, testicular loss, vas deferens injury, peripheral nerve injury, and the possibility of chronic pain.

Data regarding the use of laparoscopy in repairing large scrotal hernias are limited. Both TEP (Ferzli, 1996) and TAPP (Liebl, 1999; Palanivelu, 2007; Bittner, 2008) have been successfully employed. The complication rate is higher compared with routine repairs (1.6% vs. 0.6%), mostly seromas. A Foley catheter should be placed preoperatively, both for bladder decompression and to aid in identification of bladder injury. Should the wall of the bladder be violated, the Foley bag will fill with CO_2. Confirmed or suspected preperitoneal bladder injury should be treated with a Foley catheter and a closed-suction drain placed in the preperitoneal space. A preoperative mechanical bowel preparation is performed. With use of a transabdominal approach for a scrotal hernia, the procedure is essentially unchanged from that for a typical inguinal hernia. Peritoneal closure over the mesh is easily accomplished because of the redundant nature of the hernia sac.

With use of the TEP approach, several modifications to the technique are required (Figure 21). We routinely divide the inferior epigastric vessels and open the floor of the inguinal canal at the 10 o'clock position (Figure 22). These maneuvers aid in the reduction of hernia contents. An additional trocar placed in the space of Bogros, medial to the anterior superior iliac spine on the ipsilateral side, is sometimes helpful during the dissection. If the hernia sac must be opened, it should be done at its upper outer corner. This reduces the risk of bladder or

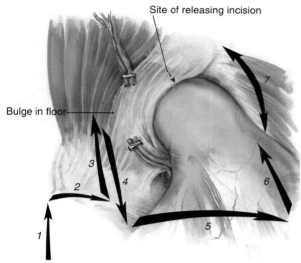

FIGURE 21   Steps of TEP for scrotal hernia: *1,* Identify the pubic symphysis. *2,* Bluntly sweep the Cooper ligament bilaterally to open up the space of Retzius. *3,* Identify the Hesselbach triangle. *4,* Move cephalad after division of inferior epigastric vessels. *5,* Cross over hernia sac to space of Bogros. *6,* Bluntly develop space of Bogros to anterior superior ileac spine. *7,* Place additional trochar in space of Bogros if needed. *8,* Reduce lipoma of the cord. *9,* Dissect indirect hernia sac. *10,* place mesh. Note the opening of the inguinal canal floor. *(Courtesy Anne Erickson, CMI.)*

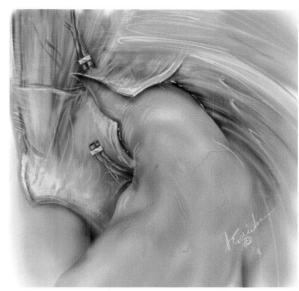

FIGURE 22   Opening the floor of the inguinal canal in a scrotal hernia. *(Courtesy Anne Erickson, CMI.)*

bowel injury, because sliding hernias composed of the bladder wall or the large intestine always develop posteromedially. The hernia sac may be sharply divided, leaving the distal end open in the scrotum. Because of the large size of the defects, the mesh should be fixed in some fashion. We prefer suturing the mesh in place to the Cooper ligament medially and to the transversalis fascia lateral to the epigastric vessels. Others have described success with suture or tack fixation medially and a biologic sealant laterally. A Jackson-Pratt drain is left in the scrotum to aid in evacuation of the seromas that will inevitably develop.

Incarcerated hernias may be repaired either by TAPP or TEP, but TAPP has the advantage of allowing the surgeon to inspect the bowel to ensure its viability. Once in the operating room, incarcerated hernias occasionally reduce spontaneously or with gentle manual pressure, once paralysis has been achieved. When the hernia remains incarcerated, the defect can be opened to aid in reduction of the sac and its contents. For direct hernias the defect can be opened with cautery at the ventromedial aspect (Figure 23). Indirect hernia defects can be opened in a similar manner by incising the abdominal wall at the ventrolateral aspect of the defect (Figure 24).

Femoral Hernias

In a large prospective study by Koch (2005), female gender was an independent risk factor for the development of inguinal hernia recurrence. Interestingly, 41% of recurrences in women were found to be femoral hernias that were not described at the original operation. Another study found the risk of developing a femoral recurrence to be 15 times higher in patients who had undergone prior inguinal hernia repair than in the general population. This fact may indicate a genetic predisposition to hernia formation. Alternatively, Chan (2008) has proposed that prior inguinal herniorrhaphy may precipitate the development of a femoral hernia.

Information regarding laparoscopic treatment of isolated femoral hernias is limited to small case series. The use of TAPP has been described for the treatment of incarcerated femoral hernias (Watson, 1993; Rebuffat, 2006; Yau, 2007). A relaxing incision in the medial border of the iliopubic tract as it recurves to form the medial border

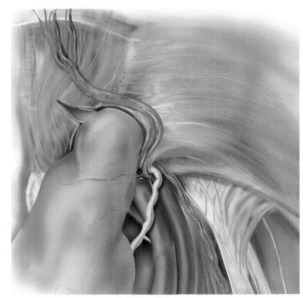

FIGURE 23   Opening the defect in an incarcerated direct hernia. *(Courtesy Anne Erickson, CMI.)*

of the femoral canal may be made to aid in reduction of the hernia sac (Figure 25). In addition, the entire MPO should be covered with a mesh patch to avoid potential complications associated with a mesh plug in the femoral space, complications that include plug migration and venous thrombosis. Rare dysfunctions such as obturator, prevascular, lateral, and medial femoral hernias should likewise be repaired with a patch rather than a plug.

Concomitant Procedures

Patients may need other surgeries performed at the same time as hernia repair. Pelvic lymph node dissections can be done then, but prostatectomy should not. Other intraabdominal procedures, such as umbilical herniorrhaphy and cholecystectomy, can be done after TEP or TAPP, once the peritoneal flap is closed.

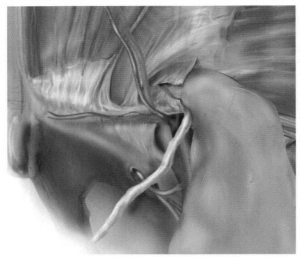

FIGURE 24   Opening the defect in an incarcerated indirect hernia. *(Courtesy Anne Erickson, CMI.)*

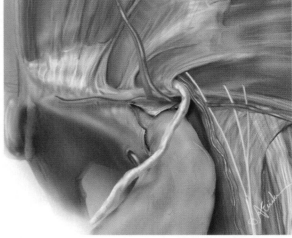

FIGURE 25   Opening the defect in an incarcerated femoral hernia. *(Courtesy Anne Erickson, CMI.)*

AFTER SURGERY

Scrotal swelling at the end of the procedure owing to CO_2 insufflation is harmless and will resolve spontaneously over the course of several hours, and patients are typically discharged home on the day of the procedure. Should urinary retention develop, a Foley catheter is placed, and the patient is sent home with a leg bag. The catheter is removed after 24 to 48 hours. Patients should be told to expect some ecchymosis, swelling, and induration. Sometimes the swelling may mimic a hernia recurrence, and they should be reassured that this is not the case.

Early recurrences are heralded by a reducible bulge, but postoperative fluid collections and induration are not reducible. If a swelling can be moved from side to side but is not reducible, it is not a recurrence and does not warrant radiologic investigation. Any fluid collections or induration will subside gradually over several weeks, and scrotum-supporting undergarments are occasionally helpful in achieving relief from postoperative swelling.

We do not advocate attempting needle evacuation of any postoperative fluid collection for several reasons: First, the bulge may in fact represent an early hernia recurrence. Second, the skin in the groin is notoriously difficult to sterilize adequately, and needle drainage may introduce bacteria into the operative site. Finally, as stated earlier, these collections will generally resolve if given enough time. Constipation should be avoided, but we do not routinely restrict patients' physical activity. Analgesia is preferably achieved with nonsteroidal antiinflammatory agents, and postprocedure antibiotics are not indicated.

MANAGING COMPLICATIONS

The risks of laparoscopic hernia repair include those inherent in any surgical procedure, such as bleeding and wound infection. Superficial infection at the trocar sites does not put the mesh at risk of infection and should be treated by opening the incision and placing the patient on a course of oral antibiotics. Care should be taken when trying to interpret CT scans in the early postoperative period; patients will always have a fluid collection in the preperitoneal space, and this does not necessarily indicate infection or active bleeding. Occasionally, the mesh itself can be mistaken for a contrast blush on CT scan. Infection in the preperitoneal space is indicated by the systemic signs and symptoms of bacterial growth and by the presence of air-fluid levels in the preperitoneal space on CT scan. These findings mandate

BOX 2: Factors associated with the development of chronic groin pain

Patient Factors

Younger age
Obesity
Presence of pain preoperatively
History of chronic pain syndromes
Being gainfully employed
Having private health insurance

Technique Factors

Use of mesh
Open versus laparoscopic approach
Inadvertent nerve injury
Intentional neurectomy
Postoperative infection or hematoma
Hernia recurrence

an open exploration with removal of the mesh if possible, copious irrigation, and the placement of wide-bore drains in the preperitoneal space.

Injuries to the bowel and the bladder are rare and should be handled according to standard surgical practice. Although it has been reported that placement of synthetic mesh is safe in the setting of a small bowel injury, we believe it is prudent to abort the hernia repair and return to the operating room at a later date. Colonic injury, even without gross spillage, is an absolute contraindication to synthetic mesh placement. Because urine is sterile, bladder injury does not necessarily prohibit the use of mesh in the initial operation. Unfortunately, the most common and most difficult complication to deal with is chronic postoperative groin pain. Grant (2004) reported that as many as 9.7% of patients experience this severely after open or laparoscopic inguinal hernia repair.

Numerous factors are associated with the development of chronic groin pain (Box 2). Some of these are quite logical, but others, like being employed and having private health insurance, are not. The best strategy for reducing the risk of chronic groin pain seems to be avoiding surgery altogether. Fitzgibbons (2006) demonstrated that watchful waiting in asymptomatic or minimally symptomatic men is a safe approach. Likewise, when a patient

BOX 3: Differential diagnosis of groin pain

Surgery

Workers' Compensation
Hernia
Recurrent hernia
Posthernia

Orthopedic

Hip disorders:
   Acetabular labral tears
   Avascular necrosis
   Chondritis dissecans
   Legge-Calvé-Perthes disease
   Osteoarthritis
   Pelvic stress fractures
   Slipped femoral capital epiphysis
   Synovitis

Urology

Cystitis
Epididymitis
Nephrolithiasis
Prostate cancer
Prostatitis
Torsion of testes
Urethral extravasation
Urinary tract infection
Vas granuloma/fibrosis

Dermatology

Lymphadenitis
Psoriasis/burn
Sebaceous cyst/hioradenitis
Thrombophlebitis/cellulitis

Neurosurgery

Disk disease
Spinal injuries, inflammation, tumors
Spondylolisthesis
Spondylolysis

Rheumatology

Connective tissue disorders
Iliopsoas bursitis
Osteitis pubis
Systemic lupus erythematosus

Neurology

Lumbosacral disorders
Neurofibromatosis

Infectious Disease

Herpes zoster
HIV/tuberculosis
Lyme disease
Psoas abscess

Sports Medicine

"Sports hernia" (adductor strains)
Gilmore's groin

Vascular

Abscess hematoma
Post–vein stripping
Pseudoaneurysm
Vascular graft

Gastroenterology

Appendicitis/adhesions
Diverticulitis
Inflammatory retroperitoneal phlegmon (pancreatitis)
Meckel diverticulum
Granulomatous colitis

Gynecology

Cesarean section
Cervical cancer
Endometriosis
Tubal/ovarian disorders

---

complains of postherniorrhaphy pain, it is important to remember that although the hernia repair is probably the culprit, a wide range of other possibilities should be considered (Box 3). Herniorrhaphy-related pain can be divided into *neuropathic, nonneuropathic,* and *visceral* pain (Box 4).

Hernia recurrence should be ruled out by physical examination and radiologic imaging such as CT or MRI. The latter has also been suggested for evaluating mesh position and inflammatory changes involving peripheral nerves in the postoperative groin. Aasvang (2009) investigated this situation and found that interobserver agreement was low in regard to postherniorrhaphy pathology. Amid (2009) observed that when educated by surgeons, radiologists were better able to identify the mesh and any peripheral nerve inflammation associated with it.

The nerves of interest in laparoscopic inguinal herniorrhaphy include the femoral nerves, the femoral branches of the genito-femoral nerves, and the lateral femoral cutaneous nerves, found in the triangle of pain. The ilioinguinal and iliohypogastric nerves are not within the dissection field but may be injured during stapling of the mesh. In neuropathic pain, physical examination may

BOX 4: Types of herniorrhaphy-related pain

Neuropathic Pain

Nerve entrapment by mesh
Nerve entrapment by suture/staples
Neuroma formation

Nonneuropathic Pain

Hernia recurrence
Excessive scar formation
Pressure from bulk of mesh
Osteitis pubis

Visceral Pain

Ischemic orchitis
Spermatic cord inflammation

elicit symptoms indicative of specific nerve involvement. Peripheral nerve blocks have also been used to elucidate the nerve or nerves involved. It is worth noting that only 20.3% of patients have a "normal" pattern of sensory distribution, as defined by modern anatomy texts (Rab, 2001). An added layer of complexity is added when consideration is given to the fact that the patterns of innervation are symmetrical in only 40.6% of patients. The initial approach in these patients is to provide reassurance that most will continue to have symptomatic improvement for as long as a year after surgery. If they desire, patients can be referred to a pain-management specialist for exploration of nonoperative alternatives such as nerve blocks, acupuncture, tricyclic antidepressants, or gabapentin.

For those who do not improve after 6 to 12 months, operative intervention should be discussed. For patients who have had open herniorrhaphies, neurectomy of the ilioinguinal, iliohypogastric, and genitofemoral nerves is currently the operation of choice. Success rates of up to 80% have been reported (Amid, 2004) with this approach. Aavsang and Kehlet (2009) used quantitative sensory testing to asses the effectiveness of mesh removal combined with neurectomy and found improvement in quantitative sensory scores and significant improvement in activities assessment scores after surgery.

In patients who have undergone laparoscopic repairs, reoperation with removal of any mesh fixation tacks may be needed if peripheral nerve entrapment is suspected. It is unknown whether open triple neurectomy would be of benefit to those who have undergone previous laparoscopic repair. Muto (2005) reported on a small series of open and laparoscopic patients who had symptomatic relief after laparoscopic ilioinguinal and genitofemoral neurectomy. Keller (2008) described a combined open and laparoscopic

approach to chronic groin pain. He examined the effectiveness of mesh removal (open or laparoscopic), neurectomy, and placement of mesh in the location opposite to the previously placed mesh. He stated that 20 of 21 patients reported improvement or resolution of their symptoms.

SUMMARY

After performing over 2,000 laparoscopic repairs, we have found that they have many advantages over open procedures. Thorough knowledge of preperitoneal anatomy, meticulous surgical technique, and a consistent, stepwise approach will result in a reproducible, highly effective treatment for inguinal hernias.

SUGGESTED READINGS

Amid PK, Hiatt JR: Surgical anatomy of the preperitoneal space, *J Am Coll Surg* 207(2):295, 2008.

Bisgaard T, Bay-Nielsen M, Kehlet H, et al: Re-recurrence after operation for recurrent inguinal hernia: a nationwide 8-year follow-up study on the role of type of repair, *Ann Surg* 247(4):707–711, 2008.

Ferzli GS, Edwards ED, Khoury GE: Chronic pain after inguinal herniorrhaphy, *J Am Coll Surg* 205(2):333–341, 2007.

Ferzli GS, Massad A, Albert P: Extraperitoneal endoscopic inguinal hernia repair, *J Laparoendosc Surg* 2(6):281–286, 1992.

Mirilas P, Mentessidou A, Skandalakis JE: Secondary internal inguinal ring and associated surgical planes: surgical anatomy, embryology, applications, *J Am Coll Surg* 206(3):561–570, 2008.

Wantz GE: Giant prosthetic reinforcement of the visceral sac: the Stoppa groin hernia repair, *Surg Clin North Am* 78(6):1075–1087, 1998.

LAPAROSCOPIC REPAIR OF RECURRENT INGUINAL HERNIAS

Jonathan Carter, MD, and Quan-Yang Duh, MD

OVERVIEW

Recurrent inguinal hernia is a commonly encountered problem in general surgical practice. Approximately 10% of patients who present with inguinal hernia have undergone a prior repair, and between 50,000 and 100,000 repairs for recurrent inguinal hernia are performed annually in the United States. Because outcomes of open repairs are worse for recurrent hernias than for primary hernias, many surgeons have turned to laparoscopy in an effort to improve results.

RATIONALE FOR LAPAROSCOPY

The best surgical approach for recurrent inguinal hernia has been evaluated in several large-scale observation studies. The largest of these was a Danish study of hernia-registry patients with recurrence after prior Lichtenstein repair. The operative re-recurrence rate was 11.3% when a second Lichtenstein repair was performed, but only

1.3% when a laparoscopic repair was performed. The laparoscopic approach was better, whether the original repair technique was a tissue-only repair (including Bassini, McVay, and Shouldice repairs), an anterior non-Lichtenstein repair with mesh, or even a primary laparoscopic repair.

Several prospective, randomized trials have also demonstrated that the laparoscopic approach is better for recurrent hernias. One study randomized 147 patients with recurrent inguinal hernia to either open Lichtenstein or laparoscopic transabdominal preperitoneal (TAPP) repair and showed less postoperative pain and shorter sick leave with the TAPP approach. Recurrence rates were similar. A second study using a similar study design in 235 patients showed fewer complications (4.4% vs. 12.2%) and fewer recurrences (2.2% vs. 5.7%) with the laparoscopic approach. A third study randomized 99 patients with recurrent inguinal hernia to either open Lichtenstein or totally extraperitoneal (TEP) laparoscopic repair and showed less chronic pain, earlier return to work, and a trend toward fewer recurrences (0 vs. 3). In the largest prospective American hernia trial to date, the Veterans Affairs Cooperative Trial randomized 1983 patients to either open Lichtenstein or laparoscopic repair. For the 9.3% enrolled with recurrent hernias, the 2 year re-recurrence rate was 10% in the laparoscopic group, which was similar to the recurrence rate for primary laparoscopic repairs. By comparison, the re-recurrence rate was 14% in the open group, more than three times the recurrence rate (4%) observed for primary open repairs.

For recurrent hernias, laparoscopy offers important advantages. First, it bypasses the need to dissect in scarred tissue planes, thereby avoiding the 3% to 5% risk of orchitis and testicular atrophy associated with redo open procedures. Second, there is less risk of chronic inguinodynia. Third, recovery time is shorter. Fourth, laparoscopy makes it possible to see the myopectineal orifice (MPO) and better identify femoral hernias, which account for 9% of recurrent hernias. It also allows for mesh to be placed easily over the entire MPO. Finally, when the diagnosis of recurrent hernia is uncertain, diagnostic laparoscopy provides a definitive diagnosis and an opportunity to repair the hernia at the same time. This avoids a groin incision and subsequent risk of wound complication.

INDICATIONS AND CONTRAINDICATIONS FOR LAPAROSCOPY

The primary indication for a laparoscopic hernia repair is recurrence after an open repair. Patients with bilateral inguinal hernias are also good candidates for the laparoscopic approach, as demonstrated by two prospective randomized trials that showed it resulted in less postoperative pain and earlier return to work with no difference in recurrence rate or complications. Some surgeons believe women should undergo laparoscopic repair for all direct and indirect inguinal hernias, because synchronous femoral hernias are found in up to 40% of patients and are frequently missed; as a result, women are known to have a higher rate of recurrence after open hernia repair. Finally, patients who engage in intense physical activity, such as professional athletes, are good candidates, because laparoscopy avoids dividing the aponeurosis of the external oblique and minimizes scar tissue between fascial layers.

Contraindications to laparscopic surgery do exist. An open approach using local anesthesia should be performed when the patient's medical condition makes general anesthesia risky. Patients with prior or planned pelvic operations (e.g., radical retropubic prostatectomy) or pelvic irradiation should undergo open repair. Patients with recurrence from a prior laparoscopic repair should undergo open repair, although good results with a TAPP approach have been reported in this circumstance. Patients at high risk for bleeding should undergo open repair, because laparoscopic repair requires blunt dissection of the peritoneum off the abdominal wall. Finally, patients with a strangulated hernia should undergo open repair, because laparoscopic repair is more dangerous for them, and a primary sutured hernia repair without mesh may be necessary if the field is contaminated. Incarcerated hernia is a relative contraindication, because traction on the intestines risks injury and contamination of an otherwise sterile field.

TECHNIQUE

Positioning

The patient is placed supine with both arms tucked, general anesthesia is induced, and the monitor is placed at the foot of the bed. If bilateral inguinal hernias are present, the more symptomatic side is repaired first. After pneumoperitoneum is established, and the trocars are inserted, the patient is placed in the Trendelenburg position.

Operative Steps for Transabdominal Preperitoneal Repair

Three trocars are used for a transabdominal preperitoneal (TAPP) repair: one 11 mm subumbilical port and two 5 mm ports placed in the same transverse plane as the subumbilical port, approximately 5 to 7 cm away. The 5 mm ports are just cephalad and medial to the anterior superior iliac spines (Figure 1). A 10 mm, 30-degree angled laparoscope should be used to inspect the groin anatomy. The inferior epigastric vessels, the spermatic vessels, and the vas deferens should be identified. These three structures form the so-called *Mercedes-Benz sign* (Figures 2 and 3). The peritoneum is incised several centimeters above the MPO, from the edge of the medial umbilical ligament laterally toward the anterior superior iliac spine. Working inferiorly, in a motion similar to opening a piece of pita bread, the surgeon should bluntly dissect the peritoneum off the transversus abdominis and transversalis fascia until the pubis, Cooper ligament, and iliopubic tract are seen.

An indirect hernia sac is usually found on the anterolateral side of the cord. When dissecting the sac, it is important to minimize trauma to the vas deferens and the spermatic vessels. If the sac is sufficiently small, it should be completely dissected free from the cord and returned to the peritoneal cavity. Occasionally, a large sac will be

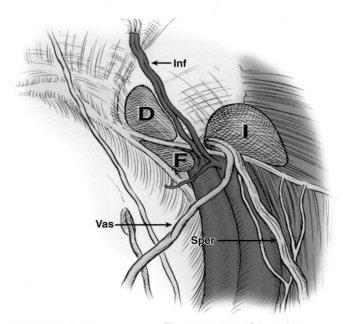

FIGURE 2   Right groin anatomy. The intersection of these three structures forms the "Mercedes-Benz" sign. *D*, Direct hernia; *F*, femoral hernia; *I*, indirect hernia; *Inf*, inferior epigastric vessels; *Sper*, spermatic vessels; *Vas*, vas deferens. *(From Takata MC, Duh Q-Y: Laparoscopic inguinal hernia repair, Surg Clin North Am 88:157–178, 2008.)*

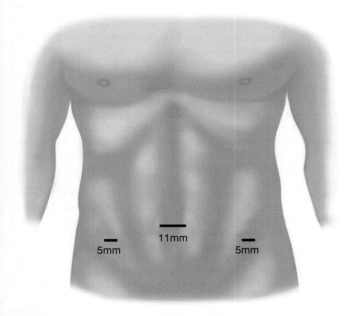

FIGURE 1   Port placement for TAPP and TEP hernia repair.

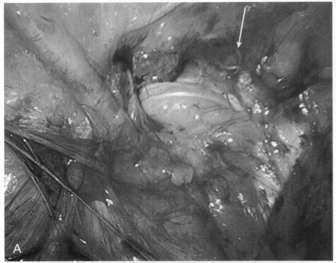

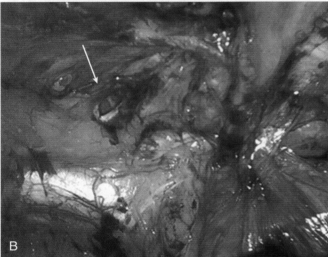

FIGURE 3   **A,** A left-sided recurrent direct inguinal hernia. **B,** An almost identical right-sided direct inguinal hernia in the same patient.

encountered, in which case it should be dissected and divided beyond the internal ring. The subsequent peritoneal defect should be closed with an Endoloop suture, because the intestine can herniate into the preperitoneal space through the peritoneal defect and become obstructed. The distal end of the transected sac should be left open to avoid formation of a hydrocele. The vas deferens and spermatic vessels are isolated and dissected free from the surrounding tissues circumferentially, creating a window inferiorly to allow for passage of the lower tail of the mesh.

For indirect hernias, we use a 12 by 16 cm flat mesh with rounded corners, slit medially so that the tails wrap around the cord structures (Figure 4). The slit in the mesh allows it to lie flat in the preperitoneal space and avoids indirect recurrence, which is the most common type of recurrence after laparoscopic repair. The tails are fixed to the Cooper ligament with two tacks, avoiding small veins that sometimes course through the region. One additional tack is placed laterally above the iliopubic tract. When fixing the mesh laterally, it is important to feel the tip of the device on the outside of the abdomen with the opposite hand to ensure that fixation occurs above the iliopubic tract; this avoids nerve injury. It is also important to completely dissect the preperitoneal space, so that the edge of the mesh does not fold. The mesh should be placed with a slight overlap of the midline to ensure adequate coverage of the MPO. Finally, the peritoneal flap is placed back in its original position to cover the mesh. We use tacks

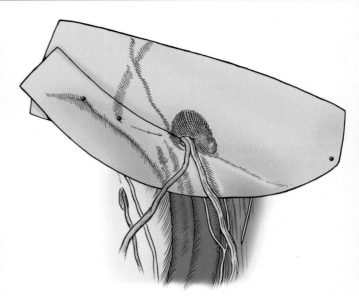

FIGURE 4   Mesh repair of right-sided indirect hernia. *(From Takata MC, Duh Q-Y: Laparoscopic inguinal hernia repair, Surg Clin North Am 88:157–178, 2008.)*

spaced closely, so that intestines cannot herniate through the peritoneum into the preperitoneal space.

Direct hernia sacs are reduced. When the peritoneum of a direct hernia sac is being reduced, a pseudosac may be present, which is actually adherent transversalis fascia that invaginates into the preperitoneal space during the dissection. This layer must be separated from the true hernia sac for the peritoneum to be released back into the peritoneal cavity. Once the pseudosac is freed, it will typically retract anteriorly into the direct hernia defect. For direct hernias, we use a preformed, contoured mesh (3DMax Mesh; C.R. Bard, Inc., Murray Hill, NJ) and anchor it with two tacks to the Cooper ligament and one tack laterally above the iliopubic tract (Figure 5). Again, peritoneum is replaced over the mesh and anchored with tacks.

Operative Steps for Totally Extraperitoneal Repair

Port placement for a TEP repair is the similar to that for a TAPP repair, except all ports are placed in the preperitoneal space. The first 11 mm port is placed using an open technique. A subumbilical transverse skin incision is made then advanced slightly off the midline, in front of the anterior rectus sheath. If the fascial incision is placed in the midline, it will enter the peritoneal cavity. The anterior sheath is opened transversely, and the rectus muscle is swept laterally and retracted anteriorly. The posterior rectus sheath is seen and left intact. The 11 mm balloon-tip port is then inserted bluntly into the preperitoneal space and the balloon is inflated. A 10 mm, 30-degree angled laparoscope is inserted and used to bluntly dissect the areolar tissue in the preperitoneal space, using a gentle sweeping motion. The preperitoneal space is dissected laterally to the anterior superior iliac spine to place the 5 mm ports. Alternatively, a balloon dissector can be used.

After the two 5 mm ports are placed, the inferior epigastric vessels, pubic bone, and Cooper ligament are identified. This dissection should be done under direct vision to avoid injury to the small veins that overlie the pubic bone and the bladder. As the Cooper ligament is exposed, a direct hernia, if present, will generally be reduced, and a pseudosac may be found. Indirect hernia sacs are managed similarly to TAPP repairs. When cord lipomas are found, they are usually located laterally along the spermatic vessels and should be reduced.

Mesh strategy is the same as for a TAPP procedure. For direct hernias, we use a preformed, contoured mesh. The contoured surface of the mesh makes it easy to manipulate, and it tends not to move

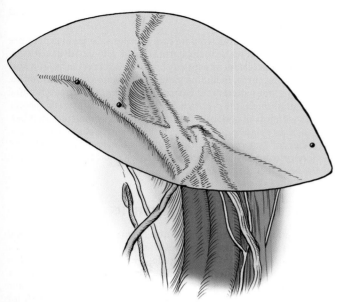

FIGURE 5   Mesh repair of right-sided direct hernia. *(From Takata MC, Duh Q-Y: Laparoscopic inguinal hernia repair, Surg Clin North Am 88:157–178, 2008.)*

within the preperitoneal space. For an indirect hernia, we use a large (16 by 12 cm) piece of flat mesh that is slit medially, passing the lower tail under the spermatic cord structures. The two tails are then overlapped and fixed to the Cooper ligament medially.

SPECIAL CONSIDERATIONS

Some open repairs—such as the Kugel mesh repair (C.R. Bard, Inc.), plug repairs, and the Prolene Hernia System (Ethicon, Somerville, NJ) repair—place mesh in the preperitoneal space. This scars the peritoneum to the mesh and increases the difficulty of laparoscopic repair for recurrent hernia. Attempts to remove the prior mesh endanger cord structures, the bladder, and the iliac vessels. If the previously placed mesh is flat, we leave it in place and place new mesh on top of it. If it protrudes, the protruding segment should be trimmed with electrocautery or shears. If a Kugel mesh is present, the ring should be inspected; if fractured, it should be removed to avoid future complications. Access to the scarred preperitoneal space via TEP repair is difficult, and a TAPP approach is safer when there is posterior mesh.

CONTROVERSIES AND FUTURE DIRECTIONS

TAPP Versus TEP

Although there are no prospective, randomized trials of TAPP versus TEP in the setting of recurrent hernia, the two approaches have been compared head-to-head in one randomized trial and several nonrandomized trials for primary hernias. The topic has also been the subject of a Cochrane review. Most studies report no difference between TAPP and TEP in length of procedure, hematomas, vascular injuries, infections, length of stay in the hospital, return to normal activity, or recurrence rate. In nonrandomized studies, more port-site hernias and visceral injuries have been associated with the TAPP approach. On the other hand, more conversions to another procedure have been reported with TEP. The major difference between the two approaches is the time it takes to learn them. When procedure length is used as

a surrogate marker for proficiency, the learning curve for TAPP is about 50 cases, whereas for TEP, it is closer to 100.

Lightweight Versus Standard Mesh

Lightweight, wide-knit polypropylene and polyester mesh have been studied in several randomized prospective studies of open hernia repairs. When compared to standard mesh, lightweight mesh is associated with a similar rate of recurrence but less pain, less sensation of a foreign body presence, faster return to work, and faster return to normal activity. Since lightweight mesh shrinks less, some surgeons believe that future trials with more statistical power will show fewer recurrences. Unfortunately, little data are available on the use of lightweight mesh in laparoscopic hernia repair. We continue to use standard mesh, because it holds its shape better in the preperitoneal space and is less apt to roll, which is a known mechanism for recurrent hernia, particularly lateral recurrences.

Mesh Fixation

Several investigators have questioned the need for mesh fixation, which has been implicated as a source of chronic inguinodynia. Two randomized trials have demonstrated no difference in recurrence rates and postoperative pain after repairs with fixation versus no fixation, suggesting fixation may not be necessary. Fibrin glue may also be used to fix mesh. In a recent comparison, less chronic inguinal pain resulted when fibrin glue was used to fix the mesh, compared to conventional stapling. No significant differences in recurrence were found, although mean follow-up was only 24 months. No published data show that absorbable tack fixation (e.g., AbsorbaTack [Covidien, Mansfield, Mass.], PermaSorb, or SorbaFix [C.R. Bard, Inc.]) reduces pain or improves outcomes.

SUMMARY

Despite improvements in open hernia repair gained over the past 30 years through the adoption of tension-free mesh techniques, recurrent inguinal hernia remains a persistent problem encountered by most general surgeons. Laparoscopic repair of recurrent inguinal hernia offers fewer re-recurrences, less acute and chronic pain, and faster return to activity when compared to redo open repairs. The major drawback is that laparoscopic hernia repair requires a significant number of cases to master, and surgeon inexperience has been shown to negate all of the benefits. For surgeons in group practice, it makes sense to have one surgeon in the group perform laparoscopic repairs, so that experience can be concentrated. For others, the best technique remains the approach the surgeon is most comfortable and experienced performing.

SELECTED READINGS

Bisgaard T, Bay-Nielsen M, Kehlet H: Re-recurrence after operation for recurrent inguinal hernia: a nationwide 8-year follow-up study on the role of type of repair, *Ann Surg* 247:707–711, 2008.

Eklund A, Rudberg C, Leijonmarck CE, et al: Recurrent inguinal hernia: randomized multicenter trial comparing laparoscopic and Lichtenstein repair, *Surg Endosc* 21:634–640, 2007.

Feliu X, Jaurrieta E, Vinas X, et al: Recurrent inguinal hernia: a ten-year review, *J Laparoendosc Adv Surg Tech A* 14:362–367, 2004.

Kouhia ST, Huttunen R, Silvasti SO, et al: Lichtenstein hernioplasty versus totally extraperitoneal laparoscopic hernioplasty in treatment of recurrent inguinal hernia: a prospective randomized trial, *Ann Surg* 249:384–387, 2009.

Neumayer L, Giobbie-Harder A, Jonasson O, et al: Open mesh versus laparoscopic mesh repair of inguinal hernia, *N Engl J Med* 350:1819–1827, 2004.

Takata MC, Duh Q-Y: Laparoscopic inguinal hernia repair, *Surg Clin North Am* 88:157–178, 2008.

Laparoscopic Ventral and Incisional Hernia Repair

Scott R. Philipp, MD, and Bruce J. Ramshaw, MD

OVERVIEW

Abdominal wall hernias are a common problem encountered by general surgeons. Despite the large volume of hernia repairs performed, there remains no single best technique. Many issues continue to influence the evolution of ventral and incisional hernia repair methods, and these create dissonance among practitioners; these include increasing laparoscopic experience, the influx of new mesh materials into the market, and a changing patient population.

Over the last decade, the laparoscopic repair of ventral and incisional hernias has been validated by several randomized trials and is one of the fastest growing minimally invasive techniques. It is based on the principles of the Rives-Stoppa repair, in which mesh is placed deep to the hernia defect and fixed with wide mesh coverage to healthy abdominal wall fascia using full-thickness permanent sutures. The laparoscopic repair differs in that mesh is placed inside the peritoneal cavity, rather than in the retrorectus position, a technique made possible by the advent of new bilayered biosynthetic materials that promote tissue ingrowth on one side and prevent adhesions on the other. This positioning of mesh against the posterior aspect of the abdominal wall with wide overlap of the hernia defect has a potential mechanical advantage over previously described inlay and onlay techniques. Intraabdominal pressure now acts to fix the mesh in place, and forces are dispersed over the entire abdominal wall. Laparoscopic ventral hernia repair allows for clear visualization of the abdominal wall, wide mesh coverage beyond the defect, and secure fixation to abdominal wall fascia.

INDICATIONS

There are three standard indications for operative repair of a ventral hernia. First, if the hernia causes pain and discomfort such that it limits a patient's ability to perform activities of daily life or significantly decreases quality of life, repair should be considered. Second, certain hernias create a bulge in the abdominal wall that negatively affects appearance, and these can be repaired for cosmetic reasons, if the risks of surgery are not prohibitive. Third, abdominal wall hernias carry a risk for incarceration and strangulation of visceral organs, the incidence of which likely varies based on several factors including defect size, location, hernia characteristics, and history of previous incarceration.

There is a fourth indication that usually occurs in combination with one of the others, and that is abdominal wall dysfunction. The abdominal wall plays an important role in balance, ambulation, lifting, and many of the activities of daily life. A ventral hernia causes a situation in which the abdominal wall musculature is displaced from its usual location, creating a discoordinated abdominal wall with the potential for loss of form and function. In the absence of pain, discomfort, negative appearance, and risk for incarceration, the presence of abdominal wall dysfunction that inhibits the performance of activities of daily life and decreases quality of life should prompt consideration for operative repair.

A laparoscopic approach may be considered in all patients with a ventral hernia. Patient selection and timing of surgery are critical for successful outcomes and avoiding complications. Surgeon experience must be accounted for, as many hernia repairs require advanced laparoscopic skills. Certain situations should be avoided early in a surgeon's learning curve, including patients with multiple comorbidities, multiple previous attempts at hernia repair, previous intraabdominal placement of mesh, the presence of enterocutaneous fistulas, chronic hernias with loss of abdominal domain, and abnormally located hernias such as epigastric, suprapubic, flank, and parastomal hernias. Regardless of surgeon experience, conversion to an open repair is not a failure or complication if performed using good surgical judgment for the benefit of the patient.

PREOPERATIVE PLANNING

In preparation for laparoscopic ventral hernia repair, patients should be counseled regarding the potential risks and benefits of surgery and must have appropriate expectations established. It is normal to have pain at incision sites and mesh suture fixation sites after surgery. In most cases this will necessitate hospital admission for adequate control of pain. In select patients, particularly those at high risk for conversion to open surgery and for large defects, preoperative placement of an epidural catheter for pain can be helpful. For larger hernia repairs, repair of incarcerated hernias, or repairs that require extensive intraabdominal adhesiolysis and bowel manipulation, prolonged hospital admission should be anticipated for adequate pain control and while awaiting resolution of postoperative paralytic ileus.

One important risk to discuss with patients is the potential for bowel injury and the management of an injury should it occur. This is particularly important for patients with large hernia defects, multiple comorbidities, multiple previous abdominal surgeries, multiple previous abdominal wall hernia repairs, and previous placement of mesh. Such patients need to be prepared for the possibility of delayed mesh placement and a second surgery with prolonged inpatient hospitalization.

All patients with morbid obesity are counseled regarding the fourfold increased risk for hernia recurrence and are sent for bariatric evaluation prior to hernia repair. Those actively using tobacco are referred for cessation therapy, and hernia repair is delayed until smoking cessation has been achieved for a minimum of 2 months.

EQUIPMENT AND MATERIALS

One important consideration in performing a laparoscopic ventral hernia repair is the choice of prosthetic material to be used in the repair. The ideal mesh would be strong and durable, resist infection, be immunologically inert, and have dual surface properties such that the abdominal wall side will facilitate tissue ingrowth and incorporation into the fascia and muscle, and the peritoneal side will minimize adherence to the visceral organs and prevent ingrowth of tissues. Any macroporous mesh placed in an intraperitoneal position should be avoided because of the long-term risk of bowel erosion, fistula formation, and small bowel obstruction. Although none are ideal, there are several mesh products available that are appropriate for intraabdominal placement (Table 1). Most mesh selection is based on personal experience and anecdotal evidence, as a paucity of human data are available comparing the long-term outcomes of different mesh use. Prospective comparative studies are needed to evaluate available mesh products for clinical outcomes.

OPERATIVE TECHNIQUE

After induction of general anesthesia, the patient is positioned supine on the operating room table with arms tucked at the sides. Prophylactic antibiotics against skin flora are routinely given, and an orogastric

TABLE 1: Available bilayer mesh products appropriate for intraabdominal placement

Mesh	Manufacturer	Fascial component	Visceral component
C-Qur	Atrium	Lightweight polypropylene	Omega-3 fatty acids
Composix	C.R. Bard	Polypropylene	ePTFE (smooth)
Composix EX	C.R. Bard	Lightweight polypropylene	ePTFE (smooth)
Dualmesh	W.L. Gore	ePTFE (rough)	ePTFE (smooth)
Duelex	C.R. Bard	ePTFE (rough)	ePTFE (smooth)
Parietex composite	Covidien	Polyester	Collagen
Proceed	Ethicon	Lightweight polypropylene	Oxidized regenerated cellulose (Interceed)
Sepramesh	C.R. Bard	Lightweight polypropylene	Hydrogel

ePTFE, Expanded polytetrafluoroethylene

tube is placed for gastric decompression, as well as a Foley catheter for decompression of the bladder. Sequential compression devices and subcutaneous heparin are utilized for deep venous thrombosis prophylaxis based on individual patient risk factors. Monitors are placed on either side of the patient with one additional monitor at the feet if necessary, depending on the location and extent of the hernia defect (Figure 1). The patient is shaved, prepped, and draped widely to allow for the lateral placement of ports, usually beyond the anterior axillary line. An Ioban drape (3M, Maplewood, Minn.) is used routinely to help avoid mesh-to-skin contact and to minimize a potential mesh infection source.

Several methods may be used to gain safe entrance into the peritoneal cavity, including the open Hasson technique, Veress needle, and direct laparoscopic guidance using a dilating optical port, among others. We routinely use blunt digital dissection through a 12 mm skin incision at either the left or right costal margin at the tip of the eleventh rib, which usually corresponds to the anterior axillary line. A 10 mm balloon-tip port is then used for secure port placement. This method, when performed well, provides a safe and effective means of gaining entrance into the peritoneal space regardless of the presence or type of intraabdominal adhesions.

We routinely place two to three additional 5 mm ports, depending on the size and position of the ventral hernia. Ports are placed in the lateral abdominal wall, far enough away from the edge of the hernia defect such that the mesh being used in the repair does not overlap them. Lateral abdominal wall adhesions must be removed prior to port placement to avoid inadvertent injuries.

All adhesions to the abdominal wall are lysed using blunt and sharp dissection (Figure 2). Electrocautery is used sparingly to avoid inadvertent thermal injury to visceral organs. Bleeding may be controlled with pressure, hemoclips, or electrocautery after all nearby visceral organs have been safely identified and cleared away. Typically, a plane is developed between the abdominal wall and the adherent abdominal contents, which allows for safe and gentle dissection. Where no discernable plane is apparent, the abdominal wall must be sacrificed to protect the bowel. This dissection must be performed with the utmost care to avoid causing, or more importantly, missing an injury to the bowel. Should an enterotomy occur, the injury needs to be repaired either laparoscopically or through an open incision. Then, the adhesiolysis may be completed, with surgeons using their best judgment to determine the appropriate timing of mesh placement. Although there are reports of placing mesh after bowel injury, we will often plan to delay mesh placement. Our practice is to admit these patients and place them on intravenous antibiotics for several days. If they do not show signs of sepsis within 3 days, it is safe to return to the operating room for delayed mesh placement. If performed within 3 to 5 days, reformation of

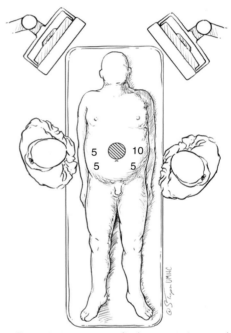

FIGURE 1 Operating room setup for laparoscopic ventral hernia repair. *(Illustration copyright University of Missouri. All rights reserved.)*

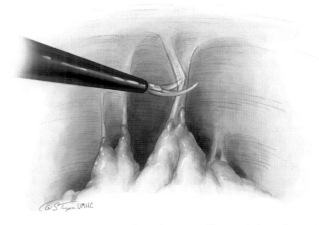

FIGURE 2 Laparoscopic adhesiolysis using blunt and sharp dissection. *(Illustration copyright University of Missouri. All rights reserved.)*

adhesions is minimal, and repeat adhesiolysis adds little time or morbidity to the operation.

After adhesiolysis the boundaries of the fascial defect are identified, and the hernia contents are reduced. This can be done with gentle traction using atraumatic laparoscopic graspers and external manual compression on the hernia (Figure 3). If omentum is incarcerated within the hernia, the major risk associated with reduction is bleeding. This can be managed with pressure, hemoclips, Endoloops, or electrocautery. If bowel is incarcerated in the hernia or densely adhered to the hernia sac, excess tension should be avoided, as this could cause a traction injury to the bowel. Sharp dissection may be necessary to dissect the bowel off of the hernia sac. In some cases it may be necessary to extend the fascial defect with sharp dissection to adequately reduce the hernia contents. The viability of incarcerated bowel must be assessed, and necrotic or nonviable bowel must be resected.

For most hernias, further dissection and exposure of the posterior abdominal wall surrounding the fascial defect is necessary prior to the placement of mesh. This may involve division of the falciform ligament and median umbilical ligament or mobilization of the bladder and exposure of the pubic symphysis and the Cooper ligaments. This is performed with electrocautery or ultrasonic dissection because of the vasculature present within these ligaments. Ultimately, this creates a flat, even surface against which the prosthetic mesh is placed.

At this point, with the hernia contents reduced, the fascial edges of the hernia defect identified circumferentially, and the posterior abdominal wall exposed to allow for wide mesh coverage, the hernia is measured. A spinal needle placed perpendicularly through the abdominal wall is used to mark the fascial edges. The pneumoperitoneum is evacuated, and the defect is measured. Alternatively, the hernia can also be measured intracorporeally using a sterile plastic ruler. If multiple hernias are present, the maximal distance between all defects is measured.

A mesh designed for intraabdominal placement is then selected to overlap all fascial defect margins by at least 5 cm. It is trimmed as necessary and then marked for orientation and placement of sutures. The four cardinal permanent sutures are then placed equidistant around the mesh, usually at the superior, inferior, and bilateral positions. Markings on the Ioban drape help to plan the site of externalization of the cardinal stay sutures. The mesh is then rolled like a scroll along its long axis with the sutures tucked in the middle.

Next, a 5 mm grasper is inserted through a port opposite the 10 mm balloon port and is brought through the abdominal wall at the balloon port site. The port is removed, the mesh is placed in the grasper, and the grasper is brought into the abdomen with the mesh. An external clamp can help push the mesh through the 10 mm incision site, and a 5 mm laparoscope may also be used to visualize mesh insertion. The balloon-tip port is then reinserted, and the mesh is unfurled and oriented inside the abdomen (Figure 4).

The cardinal sutures are then brought through the abdominal wall at predetermined positions using a transfascial suture passer (Figure 5). The Carter-Thomason suture passer has the advantages of being reusable and strong enough to easily traverse any size abdominal wall and mesh, although several other suture-passer options are available. Each individual suture is brought through the abdominal wall at a separate fascial insertion site, which results in a 1 cm wedge of abdominal wall incorporated into the suture. After each pair of sutures is brought through the abdominal wall, the next suture site is identified, and the mesh is grasped at that site. Tension is then placed on the previous sutures, as the grasper and the edge of the mesh are brought to the abdominal wall to verify appropriate placement of the next suture. In this manner, adjustments are made for a more accurate, tension-free placement of the mesh. After all four cardinal sutures are brought through the abdominal wall, tension is applied, and the mesh is evaluated for position. When the mesh is appropriately placed, the tension on the sutures should create a diamond shape on the undersurface of the mesh (Figure 6). If this does not occur, one or more sutures should be adjusted.

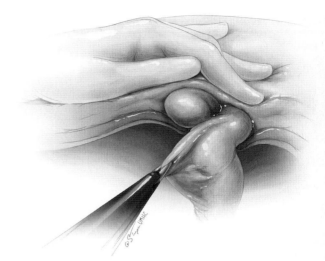

FIGURE 3   Hernia reduction using an atraumatic grasper and external manual compression. *(Illustration copyright University of Missouri. All rights reserved.)*

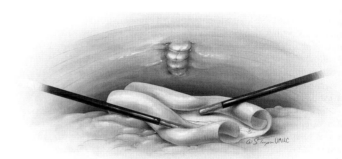

FIGURE 4   Intraabdominal positioning and orientation of the mesh. *(Illustration copyright University of Missouri. All rights reserved.)*

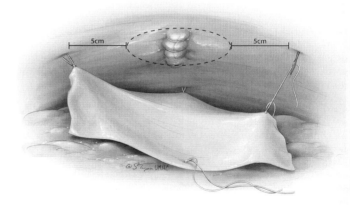

FIGURE 5   Use of the suture passer to bring the cardinal sutures through the abdominal wall. *(Illustration copyright University of Missouri. All rights reserved.)*

With the cardinal sutures holding the mesh in place, the outside of the mesh is tacked to the abdominal wall at 1 cm intervals (Figure 7). This prevents bowel or other abdominal contents from getting trapped above the mesh, while the process of mesh incorporation and neoperitonealization is occurring. We prefer to use absorbable tacks, although they are not as strong as permanent tacks and can only be

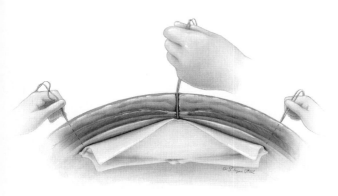

FIGURE 6 Appropriate positioning of the mesh after placement of the cardinal sutures. *(Illustration copyright University of Missouri. All rights reserved.)*

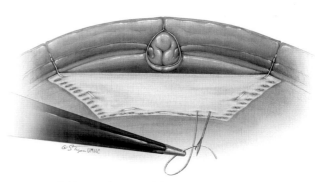

FIGURE 8 Additional fixation of the mesh with permanent sutures using a transfascial suture passer. *(Illustration copyright University of Missouri. All rights reserved.)*

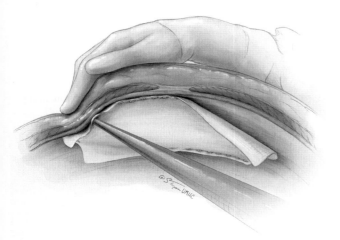

FIGURE 7 The mesh is fixed to the abdominal wall using a tacking device. *(Illustration copyright University of Missouri. All rights reserved.)*

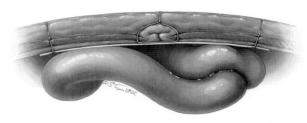

FIGURE 9 Completed positioning and fixation of the mesh. *(Illustration copyright University of Missouri. All rights reserved.)*

Postoperative care is supportive while awaiting return of bowel function. Patients with small hernias requiring minimal manipulation of bowel during surgery can be started on a clear liquid diet immediately, given oral pain medications, and potentially discharged on the day of surgery or the day after. Those patients with large, chronic hernias, those incarcerated with bowel, and those that require long and arduous adhesiolysis generally remain on NPO orders initially and are supported with intravenous fluids and patient-controlled opioid analgesia or an epidural catheter for pain control. Early ambulation and appropriate prophylaxis against deep venous thrombosis is mandatory in all patients, and all patients are encouraged to wear an abdominal binder when ambulating for the first several weeks. Follow-up in the clinic is scheduled for 3 to 4 weeks after discharge from the hospital.

A New Variation on Standard Technique

One criticism of the laparoscopic technique for ventral hernia repair is that the hernia defect is not closed, and the hernia sac is left in place. This essentially guarantees the formation of a postoperative seroma, many of which remain asymptomatic and pose no clinical problem. The published data show a postoperative seroma rate after elective laparoscopic ventral hernia repair as high as 56% based on clinical examination and 100% when evaluated radiographically by ultrasound. Up to 16% of patients will have seromas that persist for 6 weeks or longer, cause chronic pain, or become infected. Some of these patients may require therapeutic intervention.

The laparoscopic ventral hernia repair also leaves some patients with an abdominal wall bulge and persistent abdominal wall dysfunction. This is not a complication of the operation, because the hernia defect is appropriately covered, and the risk for incarceration and strangulation is eliminated. However, this is a limitation of the

used in selected cases. Patients with thick scar tissue, dense abdominal walls, and the use of expanded polytetrafluoroethylene mesh may require a permanent tacker for adequate fixation. Additional permanent transfascial sutures are then placed at 3 to 5 cm intervals around the outside of the mesh for further fixation (Figure 8). These are placed using a transfascial suture passer in a fashion similar to that previously described. At the end of the procedure, the mesh should approximate tautly and follow the curve of the abdominal wall with no wrinkles (Figure 9).

A final survey is performed to ensure that hemostasis is achieved and that no other injuries have occurred. If bowel viability was in question before, it is reevaluated now. The 10 mm balloon-tip port is removed, and the fascial defect at that site is closed laparoscopically using a 0 Vicryl suture. The remaining ports are evaluated for hemostasis, pneumoperitoneum is evacuated, and the ports are removed. Local anesthetic is injected into all port and suture sites, as these are common sources of immediate postoperative pain. Skin incisions are closed with absorbable sutures, and the skin at suture sites is inspected and released with a hemostat as needed to eliminate any permanent skin puckering. The Foley catheter and orogastric tubes are removed in the operating room for small defects. For larger defects, the Foley catheter is maintained for an additional 24 to 48 hours, should further invasive hemodynamic monitoring be indicated.

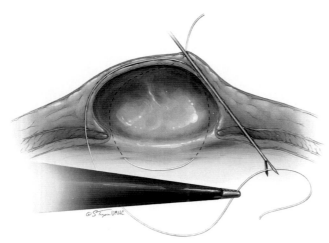

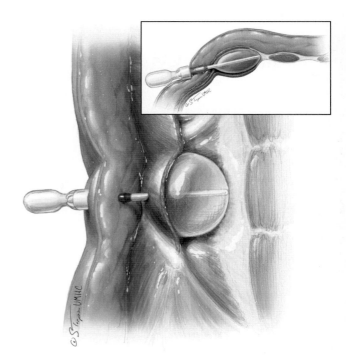

operation if the patient has a negative opinion of how they look. The lack of medialization of the rectus muscles may also have a negative impact on abdominal wall function.

In an attempt to improve cosmetic and functional outcomes and ultimately improve patient satisfaction, we have started performing a primary closure of the fascial defect using absorbable sutures prior to placement of the mesh in select patients. After complete adhesiolysis, reduction of hernia contents, and exposure of the entire fascial defect, absorbable sutures are placed in a figure-8 fashion through the abdominal wall to close the hernia defect (Figure 10). A 2 mm skin incision is made over the hernia, and a 0 polydioxanone suture is brought through the abdominal wall and healthy fascia 1 cm from the edge of the hernia and is then brought back through the other side of the hernia at a similar position using a transfascial suture passer. This is then repeated once with the same suture such that a figure-8 configuration is performed. This is repeated at 1 cm intervals until the entire defect is closed.

After all sutures have been placed, the pneumoperitoneum is evacuated, and the sutures are tied down. Pneumoperitoneum is then reestablished, and the suture line is inspected. In addition to performing primary fascial closure, we still recommend placement of a mesh with dimensions similar to what would be placed in the absence of fascial closure. In those patients whose hernia size prevents primary approximation of the fascial defect, we combine this with a bilateral laparoscopic myofascial separation of components and advancement.

Laparoscopic Myofascial Separation of Components and Advancement

Additionally, in a smaller group of select patients, a bilateral laparoscopic myofascial separation of components and advancement is performed prior to repair of the hernia. The initial port placement is performed two fingerbreadths below the costal margin at the anterior axillary line. A transverse incision is made through the skin followed by subcutaneous dissection until the external abdominal oblique musculofascial layer is exposed. This layer is incised with electocautery, and digital dissection is performed to establish a space between the two muscle layers. A 10 mm balloon-tip port is then inserted, and the dilating balloon is inflated under visualization with a 10 mm, 0-degree laparoscope (Figure 11). Appropriate position is verified by visualization of anterior and posterior muscle layers coming together medially at the edge of the rectus sheath (Figure 12).

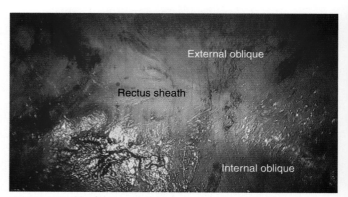

FIGURE 12   Verification of the appropriate intramuscular position by visualizing the external oblique and internal oblique musculature coming together at the edge of the rectus sheath.

Next, the balloon is deflated, and pneumatic dilation is started with carbon dioxide set at a pressure of 10. A 5 mm port in then inserted inferiorly at the lateral aspect of the intramuscular space created. Either a hook or scissors connected to electrocautery can be used to completely incise the external oblique musculofascial layer 1 to 2 cm lateral to the rectus sheath (Figure 13). This is performed superiorly to several centimeters above the costal margin and inferiorly to the pubic tubercle (Figure 14). In some cases this may require placement of an additional 5 mm medial port. To ensure maximal release and advancement, the incision is carried anteriorly through the Scarpa layer of the subcutaneous tissues. During the dissection, extra care must be taken superiorly to maintain hemostasis, as this area above the costal margin is more muscular and well vascularized. Ultrasonic dissection may be more hemostatic than electrocautery in this area.

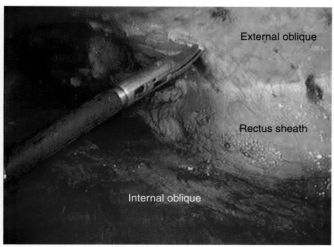

FIGURE 13   Incising the external oblique myofascial layer lateral to the rectus sheath.

External oblique

Rectus sheath

Internal oblique

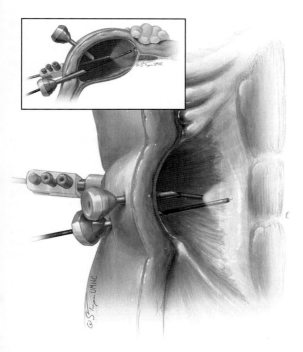

FIGURE 14   Port setup and technical depiction of laparoscopic myofascial separation of components. *(Illustration copyright University of Missouri. All rights reserved.)*

After completion of the myofascial release and advancement, this technique is repeated on the opposite side. On one side, the balloon port site is advanced through the remaining layers of the abdominal wall using digital dissection, until the peritoneal space is entered. The balloon port is then inserted through the entire abdominal wall, and pneumoperitoneum is established to 15 mm Hg with carbon dioxide. The remainder of the operation is as previously described, and at the end of the procedure, both balloon-port sites are closed with absorbable sutures using a transfascial suture passer.

There is no prospective randomized trial comparing this technique to standard laparoscopic ventral hernia repair, but this study is in progress at our institution.

ANATOMIC VARIANTS: EPIGASTRIC, SUPRAPUBIC, AND FLANK HERNIAS

Ventral hernias extending superiorly to the xiphoid process or inferiorly to the pubic tubercle pose an additional challenge for the laparoscopic surgeon. Epigastric hernias usually require high division of the falciform ligament for adequate exposure of the entire fascial defect. Anchoring transfascial sutures are not usually placed above the costal margin because of the risk for bleeding and chronic pain. In this situation, the sutures are placed lower on the mesh in position with the costal margin, and the superior aspect of the mesh is tacked to the posterior abdominal wall. It is critical that the mesh has adequate overlap of the fascial defect but not so much as to impair the normal mobility of the diaphragm or be secured in any location that would puncture the pericardium.

Complete visualization of suprapubic hernias may require mobilization of the bladder and exposure of the pubic tubercle and bilateral Cooper ligaments. Similar to transabdominal preperitoneal inguinal hernia repair, sutures and tacks must not be placed in positions that cause bleeding or chronic pain. Anchoring transfascial sutures are placed above the pubic tubercle and superior to the ileopubic tract (Figure 15). The remaining overlap of mesh can then be secured to the Cooper ligament bilaterally with tacks. Lateral fixation with sutures and tacks needs to stay superior and medial to the inguinal ligament.

Flank hernias are defined as abdominal wall defects that occur between the costal margin and the iliac crest lateral to the anterior axillary line and medial to the spine. These are challenging to diagnose by physical examination alone, as up to 50% of patients will have a persistent flank bulge after a lateral retroperitoneal incision in the absence of a hernia. Computed tomography (CT) is the procedure of choice for diagnosis and preoperative planning.

The patient is positioned in the lateral decubitus position with the hernia side up (Figure 16). Initial access and ports are placed in the midline with additional ports placed as needed. The lateral posterior peritoneum is dissected to allow access to the retroperitoneum and to expose the psoas and paraspinal muscles. This may require medial mobilization of the colon. Inferior dissection to expose the Cooper ligament and ileopubic tract and superior dissection to the costal margin may be necessary with larger hernia defects.

Once the entire hernia defect is exposed and measured, mesh appropriate for intraperitoneal placement is selected and trimmed to allow for a minimum of 5 cm hernia overlap. Mesh is secured with transfascial sutures and tacks in a fashion similar to ventral hernia repair (Figure 17). The posterior medial suture closest to the spine is the first suture placed, as this is the most critical and nonvariable suture, owing to space limitations. The same principles for epigastric and suprapubic hernia repair apply for mesh fixation in these areas during flank hernia repair as well.

RESULTS OF TREATMENT

Laparoscopic repair of ventral and incisional hernias is a well-established procedure that has been validated by several large retrospective case series and small prospective randomized trials. The majority of these studies favor the laparoscopic technique over conventional open repair with mesh because of a reduction in wound complications, mesh infections, and lower rates of hernia recurrence. A recent Veterans Administration prospective trial comparing laparoscopic versus open ventral hernia repair was terminated early by the safety review board because of a higher rate of wound complications in the open-repair group.

The largest study to effectively evaluate the safety and efficacy of laparoscopic repair of ventral hernias remains a large retrospective review of 850 consecutive patients. This series represented a complete

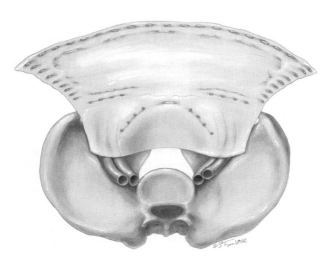

FIGURE 15 Positioning and fixation of mesh for a suprapubic hernia repair. *(Illustration copyright University of Missouri. All rights reserved.)*

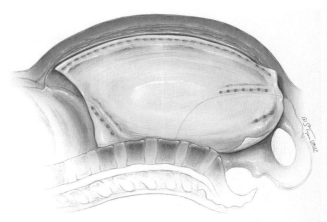

FIGURE 17 Positioning and fixation of mesh for a flank hernia repair. *(Illustration copyright University of Missouri. All rights reserved.)*

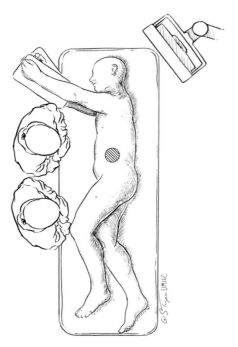

FIGURE 16 Operating room setup for laparoscopic repair of a flank hernia. *(Illustration copyright University of Missouri. All rights reserved.)*

cross-section of patients with ventral hernias, including the extremes of age, morbid obesity, various comorbidities, and previous attempts at hernia repair. The authors averaged an operative time of 120 minutes with 3.6% of patients requiring conversion to an open operation. Intraoperative complications included intestinal or bladder injury in 1.7% and one perioperative mortality due to a myocardial infarction. The most common postoperative complications included prolonged ileus in 3.0%, prolonged seroma in 2.6%, and prolonged pain in 1.6%. Over an average follow-up of 20 months, the recurrence rate was 4.7%, which compared favorably to the 12% to 52% recurrence rate seen with open ventral hernia repair.

There have been six prospective randomized trials comparing laparoscopic versus open techniques for ventral hernia repair. They consist of small study populations with short-term follow-up and use laparoscopic and open techniques that significantly vary between studies, making results difficult to interpret. Overall, these studies conclude that the laparoscopic repair of ventral hernias is a safe, feasible, and effective alternative to open ventral hernia repair, and it has the benefits of shorter operative times and hospital stays and lower incidence of postoperative complications.

Recurrence rates are thought to be lower with the laparoscopic repair, although this is not supported by these studies. A recent retrospective analysis of 331 patients found no difference in hernia recurrence at 5 years after laparoscopic versus open ventral hernia repair with mesh (29% vs. 28%). Another analysis of pooled retrospective data looked at 5,340 patients and found that laparoscopic ventral hernia repair compared with open technique was associated with significantly fewer complications (22.7% vs. 41.7%), a shorter length of stay (2.4 days vs. 4.3 days), and fewer hernia recurrences (4.3% vs. 12.1%).

Certain patient populations can expect different outcomes after laparoscopic ventral hernia repair, notably those with recurrent hernias, the morbidly obese, and current smokers. Patients with recurrent hernias are more likely to have complications and failure of hernia repair compared with patients without previous hernia repair. However, the laparoscopic repair still has fewer complications and fewer recurrences compared with the open technique. Patients with morbid obesity can expect increased recurrence rates as well—as much as four times higher. Despite the increased risk for recurrence, laparoscopic ventral hernia repair in morbidly obese patients minimizes the potential for wound and mesh complications that frequently occur for open mesh repair in this group of patients. Active tobacco smoking will also increase complications and recurrence rates, and smoking cessation has been shown to be successful in reducing perioperative complications, even when initiated as late as 4 weeks prior to surgery.

The most common complications after laparoscopic ventral hernia repair are prolonged ileus, prolonged seroma, and prolonged pain. However, the most feared complication is enterotomy, particularly a missed enterotomy. A literature review of 3,925 patients after laparoscopic ventral hernia repair showed an overall enterotomy rate of 1.78%, the majority of which were identified at the time of surgery. The only mortalities in the study were from missed enterotomies, which represented 2.8% of patients with enterotomies and 0.05% of all patients. Prompt recognition of enterotomy intraoperatively, as well as early suspicion for missed enterotomy postoperatively, is essential to limiting this complication and decreasing mortality.

SUMMARY

The laparoscopic technique for ventral and incisional hernia repair is safe and effective and can be appropriately applied to most patients. It can have the benefits of shorter operative times, decreased complications, shorter hospital stays, and lower recurrence rates. New techniques are evolving that may further decrease complications, improve abdominal wall function and cosmesis, and ultimately increase patient satisfaction.

ACKNOWLEDGEMENT

We gratefully acknowledge the assistance of Stacy Turpin for her expert and timely creation of the illustrations.

SUGGESTED READINGS

Bachman S, Ramshaw B: Prosthetic material in ventral hernia repair: How do I choose? *Surg Clin North Am* 88:101, 2008.

Cobb WS, Kercher KW, Heniford BT: Laparoscopic repair of incisional hernias, *Surg Clin North Am* 85:91, 2005.

Heniford BT, Park A, Ramshaw BJ, et al: Laparoscopic repair of ventral hernias: nine years' experience with 850 consecutive hernias, *Ann Surg* 238:391, 2003.

Jin J, Rosen MJ: Laparoscopic versus open ventral hernia repair, *Surg Clin North Am* 88:1083, 2008.

Perrone JM, Soper NJ, Eagon JC, et al: Perioperative outcomes and complications of laparoscopic ventral hernia repair, *Surgery* 138:708, 2005.

Turner PL, Park AE: Laparoscopic repair of ventral incisional hernias: pros and cons, *Surg Clin North Am* 88:85, 2008.

LAPAROSCOPIC PARASTOMAL HERNIA REPAIR

Randall O. Craft, MD, and Kristi L. Harold, MD

BACKGROUND

Between 87,000 and 135,000 enterostomies are created each year, with approximately half remaining as a permanent ostomy. Eventual formation of some degree of herniation around these stomas is so common that it is considered to be an almost inevitable consequence of ostomy formation. The artificial defect created in the abdominal wall fascia during stoma creation represents the ideal environment for hernia formation. Additional patient comorbidities that undermine the strength of the abdominal wall and may subsequently lead to an increased incidence of herniation include age, emphysema, obesity, malnutrition, steroid use, malignancy, and infection.

Most hernias occur within the first 2 years following stoma creation, but the risk of herniation can extend up to 20 years. Once established, these defects are notoriously difficult to treat. Although most parastomal hernias will be managed nonoperatively, approximately 30% to 50% will require surgical intervention secondary to complications such as obstruction, prolapse, pain, bleeding, and perhaps the most distressing for patients, a poorly fitting appliance with leakage.

OPEN REPAIR

The multitude of approaches described for addressing the parastomal hernia is a testament to the lack of a single durable repair. Traditional surgical management has consisted of stoma reversal, local tissue repair, stoma relocation, or placement of a prosthetic mesh. Stoma takedown has been universally considered the optimal treatment, but it is not always possible. Primary fascial repair has the advantages of being technically simple to perform, plus it avoids an additional laparotomy and is associated with low patient morbidity; however, recurrence rates are reported to range from 46% to 100%.

Stoma relocation is generally considered to be superior to primary fascial repair, although only a single published series has demonstrated a lower recurrence with stoma relocation compared with primary fascia repair (33% vs. 76%). Despite the lower recurrence rate, this approach effectively trades one hernia for three new potential sites for subsequent hernia formation after reoperation, including the original stoma site, the new ostomy site, and the laparotomy incision used to relocate the stoma. Open repair with mesh placed as an onlay over the defect has been attempted but is still associated with a high failure rate.

LAPAROSCOPIC REPAIR

Given the disappointing outcomes of open repair, a trend has emerged in applying the advantages of greater mesh overlap, transabdominal fixation, and avoidance of the creation of new potential hernia sites offered by a laparoscopic approach to the treatment of parastomal hernias. Two common techniques have been adapted from open intraperitoneal repairs: the Sugarbaker and keyhole approaches. Sugarbaker was the first to describe the placement of intraperitoneal mesh for the repair of parastomal hernias. His rationale for this technique was based on the premise that "the stomal bud is not disturbed so that return to normal intestinal function is rapid. In addition the colon is led out through the mesh flap valve so that further herniation out around the colon is unlikely." He described placing a circular piece of mesh around the fascial defect and securing it circumferentially, except laterally where the bowel exits into the abdominal cavity. In his series of six patients, there were no recurrences or mesh-related complications after 4 to 7 years of follow-up.

The keyhole technique uses a piece of mesh that has been cut with a "keyhole" to cover the hernia defect and surround the ostomy. However, this approach can also obstruct the enterostomy if too small a flap valve is created. We incorporated the keyhole approach early in our experience but have found the Sugarbaker technique to be technically less demanding and associated with decreased operative times and decreased recurrence rates. Reviews of current published reports of laparoscopic parastomal outcomes agree with our experience, demonstrating that use of a solid piece of mesh versus a keyhole or "slit" piece results in a lower hernia recurrence.

Early descriptions of intraperitoneal repair used polypropylene mesh. However, multiple complications of polypropylene mesh placed in direct contact with the bowel have been reported; these include erosion into the bowel, increased adhesions, and the development of enterocutaneous fistulas. These complications have been specifically noted in the setting of parastomal hernia repair. We currently prefer ePTFE for its low likelihood of forming significant intraabdominal adhesions and its relative safety for use in repairs that place it adjacent to bowel.

TECHNIQUE

After induction of general anesthesia, the patient is placed in supine position with both arms tucked at the sides. A first-generation cephalosporin is given 1 hour before the incision. A Foley catheter is placed, and a monitor is positioned on each side of the patient. The abdomen is prepped, including the ostomy, and an additional Foley balloon catheter is placed in the ostomy to assist with localization of the correct loop of intestine when dissecting adhesions (Figure 1). An Ioban drape (3M, Maplewood, Minn.) is applied to the abdomen, covering both the stoma and the inserted Foley catheter. Access to the peritoneal cavity is gained using a Veress needle placed subcostally in the left upper quadrant at the midclavicular line.

After adequate pneumoperitoneum (15 mm Hg of carbon dioxide), a 5 mm Optiview (Ethicon Japan, Tokyo) port is placed in a lateral position in the abdomen on the side opposite from the ostomy site. On the same side of the abdomen as the Optiview port, two additional 5 mm trocars are placed low and lateral in the abdomen. Lysis of any adhesions is performed using sharp dissection. At this stage, external manipulation of the Foley catheter placed in the stoma can greatly help in the identification of the loop of bowel ending in the ostomy (Figure 2). Once adhesiolysis is complete, and the entire anterior abdominal wall is visualized with the stomal loop of bowel identified, and spinal needles are used to measure the extent of the hernia defect. Any other coexisting ventral hernias are included in the measurement so that all defects are covered (Figure 3). The defect is also measured and marked on the outside of the abdomen to later center the prosthesis (Figure 4).

Next, a sheet of ePTFE, such as Gore Dualmesh (W.L. Gore, Flagstaff, Ariz.), is trimmed to a size that allows for 5 cm of overlap beyond all fascial defects. Figures are drawn on the mesh as points of reference for orienting the mesh once it has been placed intraabdominally. A single Gore-Tex suture (CV-0) is placed at the edge of the mesh on three of the four sides. Two Gore-Tex sutures are placed on the fourth side to allow the mesh to encompass the stoma, while allowing the bowel to exit through the created mesh flap valve (Figure 5). A 5 mm port is placed in the lateral abdominal wall on the opposite side of the three working ports, and a 12 mm port is placed in a position where it will later be covered by the mesh to prevent the possibility of trocar-site hernia (Figure 6).

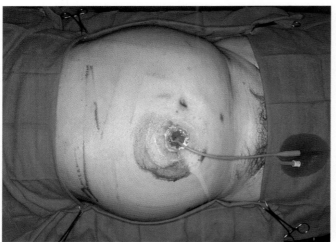

FIGURE 1 A Foley balloon catheter is in the ostomy to assist with localization of the ostomy when dissecting adhesions.

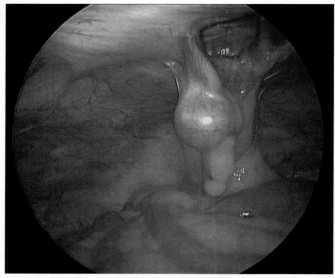

FIGURE 2 A Foley catheter in the bowel lumen assists with identifying the loop of intestine associated with an ostomy when dissecting adhesions.

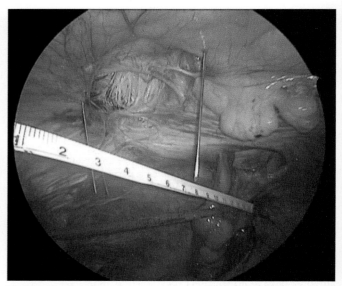

FIGURE 3 Spinal needles are used to mark the hernia defect, and a ruler is used to measure it, along with any coexisting ventral hernias.

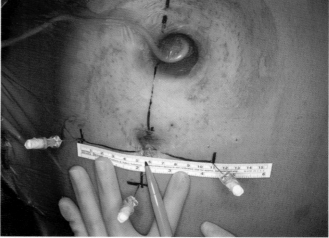

FIGURE 4 The defect is measured on the outside of the abdominal wall to later center the mesh.

The superior and inferior edges of the mesh are then simultaneously rolled toward one another to facilitate unfurling once in the abdomen. A grasper is placed in the port ipsilateral to the ostomy, and the tip of the instrument is brought out through the 12 mm port to grab the mesh and bring it into the abdomen. The mesh is unrolled and oriented based on the markings, and the open jaws of a laparoscopic atraumatic bowel grasper are used to measure a 5 cm overlap from the edge of the fascial defects. This area is marked with a spinal needle, and the transfascial sutures are passed through these sites with a suture passer (Figure 7).

It is important to orient sutures to avoid the stoma as it traverses the edge of the mesh; the mesh flap valve is created such that the stoma crosses the lateral or inferior edge. The mesh is then tacked circumferentially with spiral tacks, except at the exit site of the stoma (Figures 8 and 9). Additional size 0 Gore-Tex transabdominal sutures are placed every 4 to 5 cm circumferentially around the mesh with a suture passer. The knots are tied in the subcutaneous tissues, and the skin is released from the knot with a hemostat clamp. The 5 mm and 12 mm port sites are closed with a 4-0 monocryl suture, and the stab incisions from the transabdominal sutures are closed with skin adhesive (Figures 10 and 11).

OUTCOMES

Our institution reviewed the short-term outcomes of laparoscopic (both Sugarbaker and keyhole techniques) versus conventional open parastomal hernia repairs (primary suture repair, stoma relocation, and mesh repair). In this study, 49 patients underwent repair of symptomatic parastomal hernias that included 19 ileostomies, 13 colostomies, and 17 urostomies; 30 patients underwent 39 conventional repairs, and 19 patients underwent laparoscopic surgical repairs. Operative times were longer in the laparoscopic group (208 ± 58 vs. 162 ± 114 minutes), with a mean length of stay of 6 days equivalent for both cohorts. Mean follow-up was shorter in the laparoscopic group (20 vs. 65 months, $P \leq .001$). There were no significant differences in the incidence of surgical-site infections (11%

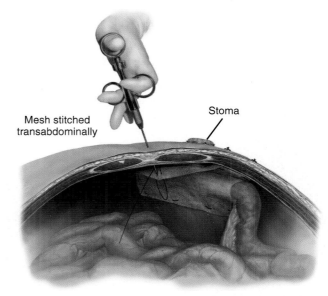

FIGURE 7 A suture passer is used to retrieve the sutures at areas marked by a spinal needle. *(From Huguet KL, Harold KL: Laparoscopic parastomal hernia repair, Op Tech Gen Surg 9[3]:113–122, 2007.)*

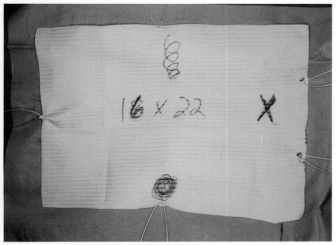

FIGURE 5 In the Sugarbaker technique, a single Gore-Tex suture is placed on three of the four sides. Two sutures are placed on the fourth side to allow the mesh to encompass the stoma in a mesh underlay fashion.

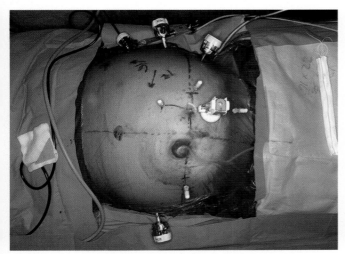

FIGURE 6 Prepped abdomen with Ioban drape showing port placement.

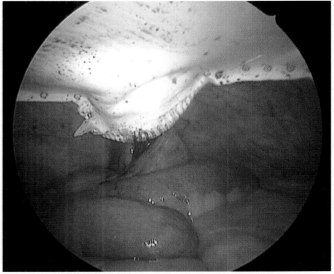

FIGURE 8 Bowel exiting over the side of the mesh with the Sugarbaker technique.

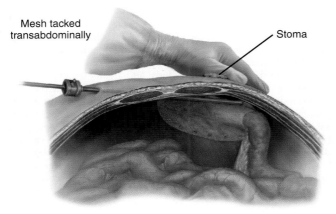

FIGURE 9 With the Sugarbaker technique, the mesh is tacked circumferentially with a spiral tacker. The surgeon uses the opposite hand for abdominal wall traction. *(From Huguet KL, Harold KL: Laparoscopic parastomal hernia repair, Op Tech Gen Surg 9[3]:113–122, 2007.)*

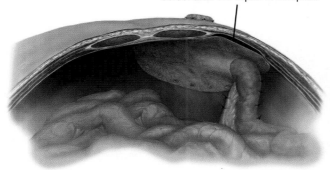

FIGURE 10 Final appearance of mesh and ostomy with the Sugarbaker technique. *(From Huguet KL, Harold KL: Laparoscopic parastomal hernia repair, Op Tech Gen Surg 9[3]:113–122, 2007.)*

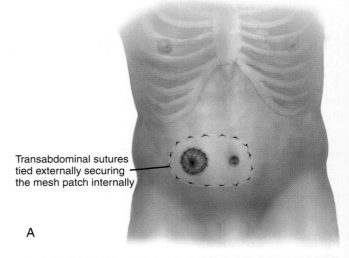

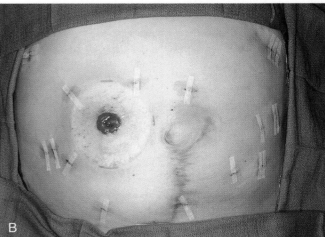

FIGURE 11 Final appearance of mesh after transabdominal sutures are placed circumferentially every 4 cm. The knots are tied in the subcutaneous tissue. *(From Huguet KL, Harold KL: Laparoscopic parastomal hernia repair, Op Tech Gen Surg 9[3]:113–122, 2007.)*

laparoscopic vs. 5% conventional, $P = .60$) or complication rates (63% laparoscopic vs. 36% conventional, $P = .67$), demonstrating that the laparoscopic approach was feasible with comparable morbidity to conventional repairs in the short term.

We subsequently evaluated our single-institution experience with 27 consecutive patients who underwent laparoscopic parastomal hernia repair with nonslit ePTFE mesh (Sugarbaker technique). All operations were completed successfully with no intraoperative complications or need for conversion to open surgery. Mean length of stay was 6 days (range, 2 to 14 days). Postoperative complications included laparoscopic reoperation for obstruction of a urinary conduit (n = 1), mesh removal for infection (n = 2), *Clostridium difficile* colitis (n = 1), pneumonia (n = 2), renal failure (n = 1), surgical-site infection (n = 1), and bowel obstruction at a site remote to the repair (n = 2). After a mean follow-up of 32 months (range, 1 to 63 months), only 1 patient (5%) had a recurrence.

The largest published multiinstitutional series consisted of 25 consecutive patients who underwent laparoscopic parastomal hernia repair with nonslit expanded polytetrafluoroethylene (ePTFE) mesh (Sugarbaker technique) followed for a median of 19 months (range, 2 to 38 months). Mean patient age was 60 years, and mean body mass index was 29 kg/m². Six of the patients had undergone previous mesh stoma repairs. The mean size of the hernia defect was 64 cm² with a mean mesh size of 365 cm². All procedures were successfully completed laparoscopically with no conversions to open surgery reported. Overall postoperative morbidity was 23% with a mean

hospital length of stay of 3.3 days. One patient death was reported because of pulmonary complications, one patient had a trocar site infection, and one patient had a mesh infection that required mesh removal. One of the 25 patients (4%) experienced a recurrence, a result similar to our own short-term outcomes.

PARASTOMAL HERNIA PREVENTION

Although the laparoscopic approach to parastomal hernia repair appears to offer comparable morbidity with a more durable repair in the short term, the ideal treatment of this entity would be primary prevention of its occurrence. It stands to reason that the effectiveness of the laparoscopic repair with nonslit mesh may be able to be accomplished by placement of a prophylactic prosthesis at the time of initial stoma creation.

Initial attempts at prophylactic mesh placement were described over 20 years ago. Abdu and colleagues prophylactically placed polypropylene mesh in 43 patients at the time of ostomy creation. Although one patient required mesh removal, there were no occurrences of parastomal hernia. Janes and colleagues conducted a randomized trial with 27 patients who received a conventional stoma and an additional 27 patients who had placement of a lightweight mesh in a sublay position at the time of ostomy creation. After 12 months of follow-up, parastomal hernia was present in 13 of 26 patients without mesh placement and in 1 of 21 in whom prophylactic mesh was placed. No incidence of wound infection, infection associated with the mesh, fistula formation, or pain was seen during the observation period.

Serra-Aracil and colleagues prospectively evaluated the use of a lightweight mesh placed prophylactically at the time of end colostomy creation, compared to standard ostomy formation alone. In this study, 27 patients were randomized to each group and were followed up clinically and radiographically with abdominal CT by an independent clinician at 1 month and every 6 months following surgery. No mesh complications were reported. In the clinical follow-up (median, 29 months; range, 13 to 49 months), 11 hernias (40.7%) were recorded in the control group compared with 4 (14.8%) in the study group ($P = .03$). Abdominal CT identified 14 hernias (44.4%) in the control group compared with 6 (22.2%) in the study group ($P = .08$).

SUMMARY

Parastomal hernia is a virtually ubiquitous complication of stoma creation. Athough the majority of hernias can be managed conservatively, nearly 50% will require surgical intervention secondary to complications. Traditional open repairs have had historically disappointing outcomes. The lessons learned from laparoscopic ventral hernia repair—namely improved mesh overlap, transbdominal prosthesis fixation, and the avoidance of an additional potential hernia site associated with a laparotomy—have recently been applied to the treatment of parastomal hernias. Although both the Sugarbaker (nonslit) and keyhole techniques have been adopted for a minimally invasive approach, the nonslit approach appears to be faster and less technically difficult, and it is associated with fewer recurrences. Although short-term outcomes are promising for this emerging technique, long-term follow-up is required to assess the ongoing durability and safety of this approach.

SUGGESTED READINGS

Craft RO, Huguet KL, McLemore EC, et al: Laparoscopic parastomal hernia repair, *Hernia* 12(2):137, 2008.

Huguet KL, Harold KL: Laparoscopic parastomal hernia repair, *Op Tech Gen Surg* 9(3):113–122, 2007.

Mancini GJ, McClusky DA 3d, Khaitan L, et al: Laparoscopic parastomal hernia repair using a nonslit mesh technique, *Surg Endosc* 21(9):1487, 2007.

Serra-Aracil X, Bombardo-Junca J, Moreno-Matias J, et al: Randomized, controlled, prospective trial of the use of a mesh to prevent parastomal hernia, *Ann Surg* 249(4):583, 2009.

Sugarbaker PH: Peritoneal approach to prosthetic mesh repair of paraostomy hernias, *Ann Surg* 201(3):344, 1985.

LAPAROSCOPIC SPLENECTOMY

Arthur Rawlings, MD, MDiv, and Brent D. Matthews, MD

OVERVIEW

The first successful splenectomy was performed in the sixteenth century, credited to Zaccarello of Palo, who removed an enlarged spleen from a woman in 1549, although later writers have suggested from his description that it was actually a large ovarian cyst. In 1893, Riegner successfully removed the spleen from a patient after a primary splenic rupture. Many of the greatest surgeons of that era went on to report successful splenectomies, even though the function of the spleen and the consequences of its removal were not yet fully understood. As these details were discovered in the twentieth century, open splenectomy remained the standard approach.

In 1991, Delaitre and Maignien reported the first laparoscopic splenectomy, and a little over 20 years later, laparoscopic splenectomy has become the operation of choice for almost all patients who are hemodynamically stable and need a splenectomy. The procedure is essentially the same, but the laparoscopic approach results in decreased abdominal wall trauma, improved cosmesis, less postoperative pain, a shorter hospital stay, and a faster return to normal activity when compared to an open splenectomy.

INDICATIONS

Laparoscopic splenectomy is limited to elective cases and stable patients in an emergent situation. The most frequent indication for a splenectomy is a hemodynamically unstable trauma patient with a splenic injury, and the most frequent indication for an elective splenectomy is idiopathic thrombocytopenic purpura (ITP). Box 1 categorizes indications for a splenectomy by various disorders.

CONTRAINDICATIONS

The two absolute contraindications to a laparoscopic splenectomy are the need for an emergent splenectomy and the inability to withstand pneumoperitoneum. Time required for setup of the laparoscopic equipment and to gain access to the abdomen, as well as the inability to adequately pack the abdomen in a trauma situation, preclude a laparoscopic approach, which effectively rules out this approach in the most common situation requiring a splenectomy.

Historically, several relative contraindications have been advocated. These include massive splenomegaly, portal hypertension, pregnancy, and obesity. As the surgical community's comfort with laparoscopic procedures has improved, reports of laparoscopic splenectomy in each of these cases have appeared in the literature. By a recent consensus statement, however, portal hypertension should still be considered a contraindication, splenectomy should be postponed during pregnancy if possible, and a hand-assisted laparoscopic splenectomy should be strongly considered for massive splenomegaly (diameter >20 cm). In addition, surgeons must make an honest assessment of their skills and comfort level before tackling these more complex cases.

PREOPERATIVE PREPARATION

Some components of patient preparation apply to all who undergo laparoscopic splenectomy, and some apply only to a specific disease state. All patients must give informed consent, or assent if the patient is a child; this should include, among other things, the possibility of conversion to an open approach, the risk of overwhelming postsplenectomy sepsis, and a portal or splenic vein thrombosis.

BOX 1: Indications for splenectomy

Red Blood Cell Disorders

Autoimmune hemolytic anemia
Hereditary spherocytosis
Elliptocytosis
Pyruvate kinase deficiency
Warm-antibody autoimmune hemolytic anemia
Sickle cell disease
Thalassemia

White Blood Cell Disorders

Hodgkin disease
Non-Hodgkin lymphoma
Chronic lymphocytic leukemia
Chronic myeloid leukemia
Hairy cell leukemia

Platelet Disorders

ITP
HIV-related ITP
Thrombotic thrombocytopenic purpura
Evans syndrome

Bone Marrow Disorders

Chronic myeloid leukemia
Acute myeloid leukemia
Chronic myelomonocytic leukemia
Essential thrombocythemia
Polycythemia vera
Agnogenic myeloid metaplasia

Storage Diseases and Infiltrative Disorders

Gaucher disease
Niemann-Pick disease
Amyloidosis
Sarcoidosis

Other Disorders/Indications

Trauma
Abscess
Cyst
Tumor
Metastases
Idiopathic splenomegaly
Portal vein thrombosis
Splenic artery aneurysm
Felty syndrome

For an elective splenectomy, all patients should receive vaccinations against meningococcal, pneumococcal, and *Haemophilus influenza* type B infections at least 2 weeks prior to the procedure. If not given before the operation, the vaccinations are generally given on the last day of admission for the splenectomy. The patients should also have some form of preoperative imaging, either computerized axial tomography or ultrasound, to assess the size of the spleen for disease states associated with splenomegaly, lymphadenopathy, or a palpable spleen on examination. The lower edge of the spleen may be palpable in a thin patient, but this becomes more difficult as the body mass index increases. Knowing the size of the spleen aids in preoperative planning for trocar placement and in assessing the difficulty of dissection and spleen retrieval.

Other preoperative preparations depend on the disease being treated. For example, ITP may require intravenous immune globulin (IVIG) or plasmapheresis to elevate the platelet count prior to the incision. Splenomegaly from chronic myeloid leukemia may respond to chemotherapy with a reduction in spleen size of 20% to 50% within a few weeks of treatment, which aids in laparoscopic splenectomy success.

Splenic artery embolization has been advocated in the past in an effort to reduce operative blood loss and to decrease the size of the spleen prior to the procedure. It has not been our practice to have patients undergo this procedure, as it can be accompanied by severe pain and ischemic complications; in addition, studies have not demonstrated a clinical benefit. If embolization is done, the surgeon must be aware of the fact that metal coils can interfere with the proper functioning of the endoscopic vascular stapler, and the coils must be avoided during the division of the splenic hilum to ensure good hemostasis.

APPROACHES

The first laparoscopic splenectomies were performed in a supine position, but after a short time, the right lateral decubitus approach became the position of choice. This "hanging spleen" technique is our preferred method, although some advocate the hand-assisted approach. This would be a reasonable choice for the surgeon who uses this as his or her primary approach to other procedures or for massive splenomegaly.

Regardless of the approach—whether open or laparoscopic, supine or hanging—a splenectomy is essentially a dividing of the vascular and avascular ligamentous attachments to the spleen. There are two major and several minor attachments: the two main ligaments are the gastrosplenic and the lienorenal ligaments. The gastrosplenic ligament contains the short gastric and the gastroepiploic vessels, and the lienorenal ligament contains the hilar vessels and the tail of the pancreas. The rest of the ligaments, such as the splenocolic and phrenosplenic ligaments, are avascular, unless the patient has portal hypertension or myeloid metaplasia.

A few other anatomical concepts must be kept in mind. First of all, no two spleens are alike. In 1942, Michaels described two types of blood supply to the spleen. The *distributive pattern* accounts for 70% of spleens (Figure 1). This consists of a short splenic trunk with several long branches (six to 12) that enter over three fourths of the splenic hilum. Generally, several transverse anastomoses will lie between the branches, which means that occluding a branch before the anastomosis with a clip or tie will not devascularize that segment of the spleen. The *magistral* or *bundled pattern* accounts for the remaining 30% of spleens (Figure 2). With this pattern, there are a few large branches (three to five) that enter the medial one fourth of the surface of the spleen. Regardless of the distribution, one key is to occlude the splenic artery distal to the pancreatic magna artery. This artery, well known to radiologists, supplies a distal portion of the pancreas. Significant pancreatitis has been reported from occlusion of the splenic artery proximal to this arterial branch. It must also be kept in mind that the tail of the pancreas is within 1 cm of the splenic hilum in approximately three fourths of all patients and that it is in direct contact with the spleen in 30% of patients, therefore careful attention to hilar dissection is needed to avoid a pancreatic injury.

Right Lateral Approach

As stated earlier, the first description of a laparoscopic splenectomy was of an anterior approach, but since then, the right lateral approach has become the position of choice for most surgeons. Prior to positioning the patient in a right lateral decubitus position on a beanbag,

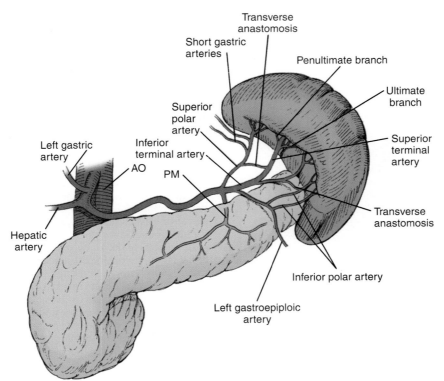

FIGURE 1 Distributed vascularization. By definition, the splenic trunk is short, and many long branches (six to twelve) enter over three fourths of the medial surface of the spleen. The branches originate between 3 to 13 cm from the hilum. Outside the spleen, the arteries also present frequent transverse anastomoses with each other, which according to Testud arise at a right angle between the involved arteries, as with most collaterals. This means that the application of hemostatic clips or the embolization of coils occluding a branch of the splenic artery before such an anastomosis may fail to devascularize the corresponding splenic segment. *AO*, Aorta, *PM*, Pancreatic magna. *(From Poulin EC, Thibault C: The anatomical basis for laparoscopic splenectomy, Can J Surg 36[5]:485–488, 1993.)*

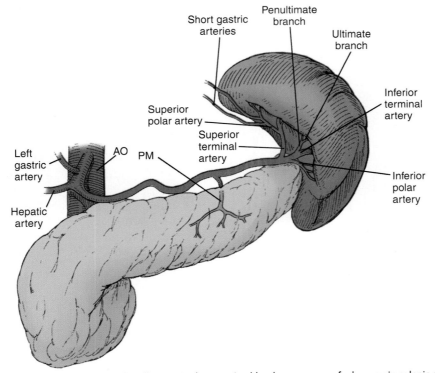

FIGURE 2 Bundled (magistral) vascularization. The bundle type is characterized by the presence of a long main splenic artery that divides into short terminal branches near the hilum. In this type, the splenic branches enter over only a fourth to a third of the medial surface of the spleen. These branches are large, few (three to four), originate 3.5 cm on average from the spleen, and reach the center of the organ as a compact bundle. *AO*, Aorta, *PM*, pancreatic magna. *(From Poulin EC, Thibault C: The anatomical basis for laparoscopic splenectomy, Can J Surg 36[5]:485–488 1993.)*

the patient undergoes endotracheal intubation. A Foley catheter and an orogastric tube are inserted, and sequential compression devices are applied to the lower extremity. A weight-appropriate first-generation cephalosporin is given within 1 hour of the incision.

After this preparation, the patient is positioned so the center between the iliac crest and the lateral costal margin is at the break of the bed. This is usually about the level of the umbilicus. The patient

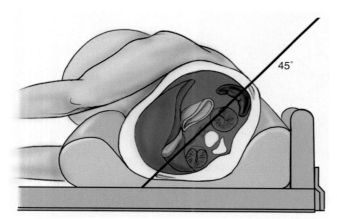

FIGURE 3 The "leaning spleen" technique requires a 45-degree tilt using a beanbag or jelly roll positioning pad. *(From Hunter JG [ed]: The atlas of minimally invasive surgical operations, New York, McGraw-Hill [in press]. Reprinted with permission.)*

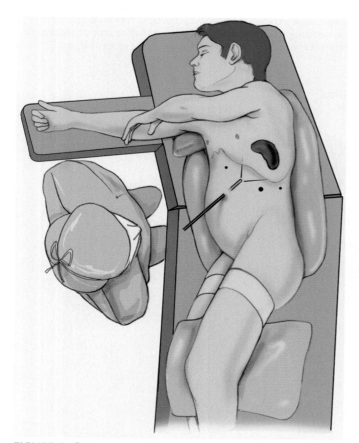

FIGURE 4 Patient, port, and laparoscope positions for the "leaning spleen" technique. *(From Hunter JG [ed]: The atlas of minimally invasive surgical operations, New York, McGraw-Hill [in press]. Reprinted with permission.)*

is rolled left side up to 45 degrees of midline with the left arm resting across the chest on an elevated arm board (Figure 3), and an axillary roll is placed. The legs are flexed, and ample padding is used to protect the knees and ankles. The table is flexed, and the beanbag is deflated. Some people use a kidney rest, but we have not found that necessary. After the patient is appropriately positioned, the hips, shoulders, and knees are padded and secured to the bed with Velcro straps or wide silk tape. Before draping, the table is fully tilted to the left, right, Trendelenburg, and reverse Trendelenburg positions to assure that the patient can tolerate it if need be during the procedure. The patient is prepped from nipples to knees and from the table anteriorly to the table posteriorly. A wide prep is necessary, as the surgeon must be prepared to introduce a hand port or convert to an open approach at a moment's notice during the case.

The surgeon stands on the patient's right side, and the assistant stands on the left. Access to the abdomen can be gained by Veress needle or via a cutdown technique; we prefer a cutdown technique. We have found S retractors and pediatric Kochers especially helpful in this regard. Initial access to the abdomen is obtained near the tip of the tenth or eleventh rib, depending on body habitus and spleen size. A 10 mm trocar is inserted, and the abdomen is insufflated to 15 mm Hg. Under direct visualization, a 5 mm trocar is placed in the epigastrium, and a 12 mm trocar is placed in the anterior axillary line. The splenic flexure is taken down with an ultrasonic dissector, and a 5 mm trocar is placed in the left flank as necessary. We use a 30-degree, 10 mm scope, thus the need for the first 10 mm port. The endoscopic stapler requires a 12 mm port, and this trocar site usually serves as our extraction site (Figure 4).

After all the trocars are placed, the first order of business is to look for accessory spleens. This should be done at the beginning of the case for two reasons: First, the tissue is most likely not stained with blood at the onset, making identification of a small accessory spleen easier than at the end of the case. If an accessory spleen is identified, it can usually be readily removed with an ultrasonic dissector. Clips should be avoided, as they can interfere with the use of a stapler later. The second reason to look for accessory spleens early is that it is easy to overlook or shortchange this step at the end of the case, especially if it has been a particularly difficult one.

For dissection we prefer the ultrasonic dissector, although bipolar vessel sealers have been used effectively by others (Figure 5). The

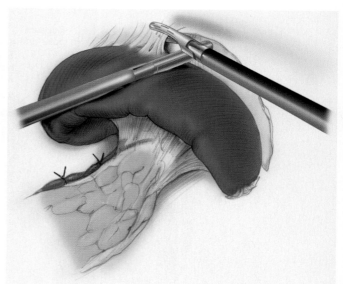

FIGURE 5 The spleen is released by dividing the peritoneal reflection with the Harmonic Scalpel (Johnson & Johnson Gateway, Piscataway, NJ). *(From Hunter JG [ed]: The atlas of minimally invasive surgical operations, New York, McGraw-Hill [in press]. Reprinted with permission.)*

ultrasonic dissector is used to divide the splenocolic ligament, which leaves a small peritoneal handle on the spleen that can be used to manipulate it. Attention is then directed to the gastrosplenic ligament and the short gastric vessels it contains. Our preference is to divide all of the short gastric vessels to allow the spleen to fall away, giving maximum exposure to the distal pancreas and splenic hilum. Generally, we would use the ultrasonic dissector to divide the short gastric arteries. If the splenectomy is for thrombocytopenia, and the patient is at a higher risk of bleeding, we will use clips to occlude the vessels. Care must be taken later to make sure that no clips are in the endovascular stapler when it is used to divide the hilar vessels. This division of the short gastric vessels is really no different from their division in a laparoscopic Nissen fundoplication.

With maxim exposure of the distal pancreas and splenic hilum, we search again for any accessory spleens, because up to 85% of them are found within the splenic hilum. Some surgeons isolate and ligate the splenic artery at this time if the case is done for thrombocytopenia, although this is not our practice. Immediately after ligation of the artery, if significant thrombocytopenia and bleeding is a concern, platelets can be given.

Next, the remainder of the splenocolic ligament and the phrenocolic ligament are divided. This should allow for elevation of the spleen to identify the hilar structures and to dissect out the hilum. As almost one third of all patients have a pancreas that abuts the spleen, care must be taken to dissect it free from the hilum. Careless dissecting or use of the stapler in this area can lead to injury to the tail of the pancreas. After the hilum has been dissected out, it is divided with an endovascular stapler (Figure 6), and multiple firings are typically required. Some surgeons prefer to dissect out the individual vessels in the hilum and divide them separately. Our practice is to take the hilum en masse with the stapler. Once divided, the spleen should be free from all of its abdominal attachments. The staple line and splenic bed are inspected for hemostasis and possible pancreatic injury. If pancreatic injury is suspected, the injury is oversewn, and a 19 Fr Blake drain is placed near the tail of the pancreas. Otherwise, we do not routinely leave a drain.

The next step is to remove the spleen. Extracting the spleen, especially a large one, can be the most difficult part of the operation. We prefer a sturdy bag for extraction and typically use the LapSac (Cook Medical, Bloomington, Ind.). Several techniques are available to place the spleen in the bag. If the spleen is normal size or smaller, it might be amenable to being picked up and dropped into a bag opened with two laparoscopic graspers (Figure 7). Others leave the spleen hanging by a small peritoneal attachment to the diaphragm and maneuver the bag over the spleen. One technique that works well for a larger spleen is to manipulate it away from the left upper quadrant, place the bag in the splenic bed against the diaphragm, and "boat" the spleen into the bag.

The opening of the bag is pulled out through the 12 mm port site. The spleen is morcellated and extracted with ring forceps being careful not to puncture the bag. If there is a concern with the diagnosis, communication with the pathologist before the case is essential to ensure that the diagnosis can be made from a morcellated specimen. Otherwise, the opening will have to be enlarged to remove the spleen in toto. If the spleen is enlarged and has to be removed in toto for the pathologist, we would elect to do a hand-assisted approach. The incisions are closed at the end of the case in standard fashion for any laparoscopic procedure.

Anterior Approach

The anterior approach was the first approach used for a laparoscopic splenectomy. Although replaced by the right lateral approach by most surgeons, it still has application in certain situations. It should be considered in patients who are undergoing concomitant procedures, such as laparoscopic splenectomy and cholecystectomy or distal pancreatectomy. It should also be considered when doing a splenectomy in the super morbidly obese.

For the anterior approach, we prefer to place the patient in lithotomy position with the surgeon positioned between the legs as in a laparoscopic Nissen fundoplication (Figure 8). A supine position with the surgeon on the patient's right side is reasonable as well. Usually, five trocars are needed rather than the four used for the right lateral position. Even though the patient is placed in a head-up and left-side-down position, more retraction is usually needed to see the critical structures. The case proceeds roughly in the same manner as the right lateral approach, except that it is usually a more caudal to cranial dissection.

Next, the splenocolic ligament is divided, and the short gastric vessels are divided in similar fashion to a laparoscopic Nissen fundoplication. This approach requires more direct manipulation of the spleen for exposure, so care must be taken to avoid tearing the

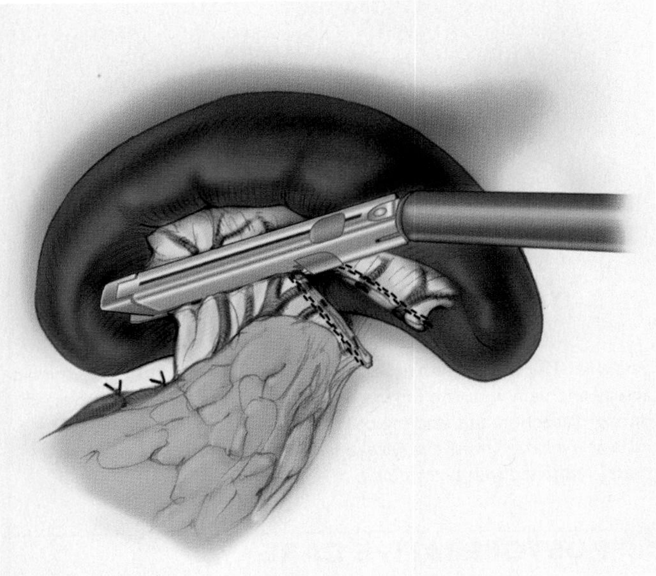

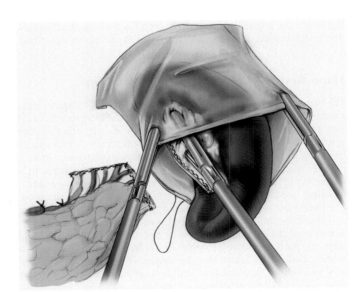

FIGURE 6 The splenic blood supply is controlled in the splenic hilum with a linear cutting stapler. *(From Hunter JG, [ed]: The atlas of minimally invasive surgical operations, New York, McGraw-Hill [in press]. Reprinted with permission.)*

FIGURE 7 The spleen is pushed into a sturdy specimen bag opened in the left upper quadrant. *(From Hunter JG [ed]: The atlas of minimally invasive surgical operations, New York, McGraw-Hill [in press]. Reprinted with permission.)*

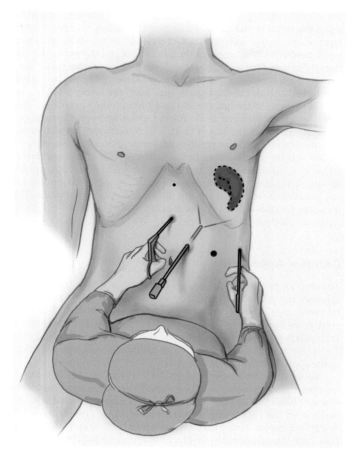

FIGURE 8   Patient and port locations for supine positioning. *(From Hunter JG [ed]: The atlas of minimally invasive surgical operations, New York, McGraw-Hill [in press]. Reprinted with permission.)*

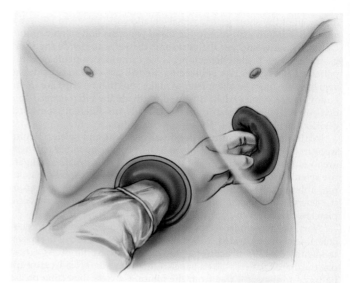

FIGURE 9   A hand port may be used if necessary to remove the spleen intact. *(From Hunter JG [ed]: The atlas of minimally invasive surgical operations, New York, McGraw-Hill [in press]. Reprinted with permission.)*

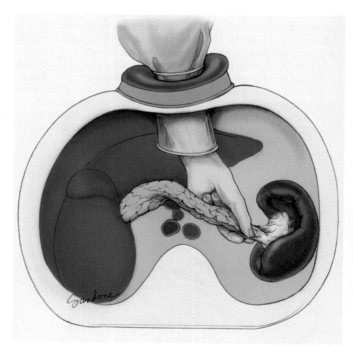

FIGURE 10   With the hand port, it is possible to control the splenic artery and vein with the fingers by encircling the tail of the pancreas during dissection and stapling of the hilum. *(From Hunter JG [ed]: The atlas of minimally invasive surgical operations, New York, McGraw-Hill [in press]. Reprinted with permission.)*

capsule. After the anterior hilum of the spleen is exposed, a blunt instrument is passed behind the spleen to elevate it. The tail of the pancreas is carefully dissected from the hilum, and the splenic vessels are taken en masse with an endovascular stapler. The remaining ligaments are divided, freeing the spleen from all its attachments. The spleen is placed in a bag and extracted as previously described.

Hand-Assisted Laparoscopic Splenectomy

The hand-assisted approach has been suggested as a bridge to laparoscopy for those less experienced in laparoscopic procedures. It also provides an extra level of comfort for manipulating a large spleen, with delicate vessels and the pancreas attached, and should be strongly considered for massive splenomegaly (diameter >20 cm).

The hand-assisted approach can be used with the patient in a supine or right lateral position. Our preference would be for a modified right lateral decubitus position with a 45-to 60-degree elevation. The hand port is placed through an upper midline incision (Figure 9). Usually two other ports are placed, a 10 mm trocar for the camera at the tip of the eleventh rib and a 12 mm trocar more laterally and inferiorly for the endoscopic stapler. The splenectomy proceeds much as described earlier, except that the surgeon's nondominant hand can now be used for manipulation and demonstration of structures for dissection and division with the ultrasonic dissector and endoscopic stapler (Figure 10). Once the spleen is free from its abdominal attachments, it is delivered out through the hand port. This can be very helpful in a patient with splenomegaly and would also be our choice if the pathologist needed an enlarged spleen removed in toto.

POSTOPERATIVE CARE

For elective splenectomy, the Foley catheter and orogastric tube can be removed in the operative room or in recovery. The patient is admitted to a general floor, started on clear fluids, and advanced to a general diet as quickly as can be tolerated. Pain is controlled mainly with oral analgesics. If the patient was receiving steroids prior to the procedure, he or she may need a quick taper of oral steroids after the splenectomy. The patient is allowed to shower after 24 hours and generally returns to normal activity over the course of the next couple of weeks.

COMPLICATIONS

The most feared complication is overwhelming postsplenectomy sepsis. Fortunately, the overall incidence of this is low (3.2%); however, the mortality rate is extremely high (40% to 50%). Patients must be counseled that their risk is the highest in the first 2 years after their splenectomy, but that they have a lifelong increase in risk, with roughly one third of infections occurring more than 5 years after splenectomy. This is why vaccinations against meningococcal, pneumococcal, and *H. influenzae* type B infections at least 2 weeks before an elective splenectomy are so important.

Portal or splenic vein thrombosis is potentially life threatening, and it can occur months after surgery. The risk is generally 0.7% to 14% after a splenectomy but can reach as high as 80% in high-risk patient populations. Those include, but are not limited to, patients with myeloproliferative disorders associated with hypercoagulopathy, hematologic malignancy, and splenomegaly. Symptoms are usually vague: diffuse abdominal pain, nausea, fever, and decreased appetite. A high index of suspicion is needed in the postoperative period, and the patient should be sent for a color Doppler sonogram or contrast-enhanced CT if portal or splenic vein thrombosis is suspected.

The tail of the pancreas abuts the spleen in almost one third of patients. Injury to it during dissection does occur from time to time. If suspected, we oversew the injury, leave a 19 Fr Blake drain in place, and check the output for amylase after the patient is back on a general diet; the drain can be removed if no pancreatic leak is evident. If the amylase is elevated, the drain remains in place, the patient is put on a low-fat diet, and the output is checked on a weekly basis. The drain is removed after the leak resolves.

RESULTS

No prospective randomized trial comparing laparoscopic splenectomy with open splenectomy has been published, however, two recent meta-analyses have been published. One looked at 135 case series for ITP with a total of 2623 patients in the analysis. This study showed that the complication rate was lower for a laparoscopic splenectomy when compared to an open splenectomy (9.6% vs. 12.9%); mortality was lower for a laparoscopic splenectomy as well (0.2% vs. 1.0%). The other study examined 51 case series with a total of 2940 patients for an elective splenectomy. The operative times were longer for a laparoscopic splenectomy when compared to an open splenectomy (180 vs. 114 minutes), and the length of stay was shorter for a laparoscopic splenectomy (3.6 vs. 7.2 days). The complication rate (15.5% vs. 26.6%) and mortality rate (0.6% vs. 1.1%) were lower for a laparoscopic splenectomy as well.

SUMMARY

The most common indication for a splenectomy is a splenic injury in a hemodynamically unstable patient. Such a patient is not a good candidate for a laparoscopic splenectomy; however, almost any elective case would be best served by a laparoscopic approach. These patients have a shorter hospital stay, fewer complications, and a quicker return to activity over an open approach.

SUGGESTED READINGS

Habermalz B, Sauerland S, Decker G, et al: Laparoscopic splenectomy: the clinical practice guidelines of the European Association for Endoscopic Surgery, *Surg Endosc* 22(4):821–848, 2008.

Heniford B, Park A, Walsh R, et al: Laparoscopic splenectomy in patients with normal sized spleens versus splenomegaly: Does size matter? *Am Surg* 67(9):854–857, 2001.

Kercher K, Matthews B, Walsh R, et al: Laparoscopic splenectomy for massive splenomegaly, *Am J Surg* 183(2):192–196, 2002.

Kojouri K, Vesely S, Terrell D, George N: Splenectomy for adult patients with idiopathic thrombocytopenia purpura, *Blood* 104(9):2623–2634, 2004.

Melman L, Matthews B: Current trends in laparoscopic solid organ surgery: spleen, adrenal, pancreas, and liver, *Surg Clin N Am* 88(5):1033–1046, 2008.

Poulin E, Thibault C: The anatomical basis for laparoscopic splenectomy, *Can J Surg* 36(5):484–488, 1993.

Tessier DJ, Pierce RA, Brunt LM, et al: Laparoscopic splenectomy for splenic masses, *Surg Endosc* 22(9):2062–2066, 2008.

Winslow ER, Brunt LM: Perioperative outcomes of laparoscopic versus open splenectomy: a meta-analysis with an emphasis on complications, *Surgery* 134(4):647–653, 2003.

LAPAROSCOPIC GASTRIC SURGERY

Jayleen Grams, MD, PhD, and Barry A. Salky, MD

OVERVIEW

Minimally invasive surgery has revolutionized many gastric operations, such as paraesophageal hernia repair, Nissen fundoplication, and gastric bypass. Progress has been slower for other benign conditions, as well as malignant ones, for various reasons. For some indications, this slow progress is a result of low incidence. Since Goh and colleagues reported the first laparoscopic gastric resection for chronic peptic ulcer in 1992, a minimally invasive approach has been described for virtually all antiulcer operations: truncal vagotomy with pyloroplasty, resection with reconstruction with or without vagotomy, highly selective vagotomy, gastroenterostomy, and modified Graham patch. However, advances in understanding of *Helicobacter pylori* pathology and medical therapy with histamine 2 (H2) blockers and proton-pump inhibitors (PPIs) have drastically reduced the overall number of operations performed.

The reasons for slow progress to minimally invasive techniques are more complex in the case of tumor resection. Although laparoscopic wedge resection of benign and gastrointestinal stromal tumors (GISTs) is now generally accepted, the minimally invasive approach has been adopted more slowly in malignant tumor resection, particularly in the West, when compared to Eastern countries such as Japan and Korea. This is partly attributable to a higher incidence of gastric adenocarcinoma in Eastern countries; aggressive screening so that gastric cancer is detected early, when it is more amenable to laparoscopic or even endoscopic resection; and a different distribution with more mid and distal stomach cancers in the East versus more proximal cancers in the United States. Furthermore, laparoscopic resection for gastric adenocarcinoma is technically challenging, especially when it requires a formal lymphadenectomy. The long-term oncologic safety has yet to be determined, but preliminary data suggest laparoscopic resection results in the short-term postoperative benefits of a laparoscopic approach with similar oncologic outcomes to open resection.

Contraindications to a laparoscopic approach consider the patient's inability to tolerate pneumoperitoneum, hemodynamic instability, and extensive prior upper abdominal surgery, as well as disease status—ability to access mass, size of tumor, invasion to adjacent organs, and metastasis—and surgeon experience and preference. Importantly, preoperative evaluation and primary operative principles remain the same regardless of approach.

OPERATIVE APPROACH

Positioning and Port Placement

The patient is typically placed in a supine split-leg position with arms abducted on arm boards, but the arms may also be tucked at one or both sides and appropriately padded (Figure 1). The patient should be securely positioned for placement into moderate to steep reverse Trendelenburg position. The monitors may be positioned above each of the patient's shoulders or, if on overhead booms, directly above the patient's head. The primary surgeon generally stands between the patient's legs but may need to move into position on the patient's right or left side, such as for distal gastrectomy; the camera assistant is usually on the left side of the patient. An endoscope should be present or readily available, as intraoperative endoscopy is invaluable both for localization of pathology and to test the integrity of any closure or anastomosis.

An example of port placement is shown in Figure 2 but will vary in number and location depending on the specific operation performed. In general, four to five ports will be necessary; this includes a camera port, working ports, and a port for liver retraction. Most of the ports can be 5 mm, but at least one 12 mm port will be necessary if performing a stapled resection, and it can also be used for specimen retrieval using a bag. The camera port is typically introduced in the midline at or just above the umbilicus. Positions of the ports may need to shift toward 1) the xiphoid if operating on the proximal stomach or in a very obese patient or toward 2) the umbilicus if operating on the distal stomach, to avoid working directly above the area of interest, or when creating a jejunojejunostomy, such as when performing Roux-en-Y reconstruction. As in all laparoscopic operations, the primary principle guiding placement of the working ports is triangulation of the target area.

For each technique described, diagnostic laparoscopy is performed and may include laparoscopic ultrasound examination of the liver with careful inspection of the peritoneal surfaces, liver, and lesser sac, if the operative indication is cancer. Prior to any resection, it is important to communicate with the anesthesia team to be certain that there are no enteric tubes present, including an esophageal stethoscope. After resection or reconstruction, the integrity of the staple line or sutured closure may be tested under saline using insufflation, by filling the stomach with methylene blue dye, or with intraoperative endoscopy. All specimens are removed using a retrieval bag.

Technique

Wedge Gastrectomy

Wedge gastrectomy is the most common method of resecting benign and gastrointestinal stromal tumors of the stomach. The goals are identical with open operative technique: complete resection of the mass with negative margins without compromising the lumen of the stomach and with no direct manipulation of the tumor to avoid rupture and peritoneal seeding. The tumor may readily be seen if it is an exophytic or subserosal lesion on the anterior stomach wall or if it was marked preoperatively during endoscopy. However, intraoperative endoscopy may be useful to localize the tumor, especially if it is endophytic or located on the posterior wall of the stomach.

For tumors on the anterior wall of the stomach, the tumor is elevated either by grasping normal stomach wall near the tumor with an atraumatic grasper or by placing traction sutures on either side of the mass (Figure 3). Most commonly, a linear stapler (blue load) is applied across a cuff of normal stomach beneath the lesion to achieve negative margins. If margin status is in question, endoscopy and intraoperative pathology should be used. Active bleeding from the staple line may be controlled with electrocautery, clips, oversewing, or bioglue.

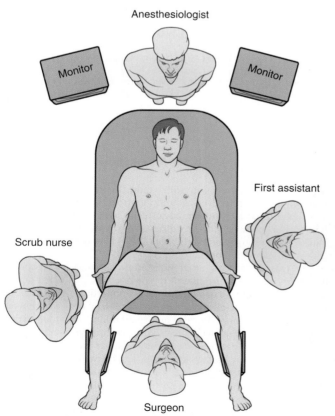

FIGURE I Operating room arrangement for laparoscopic gastric surgery.

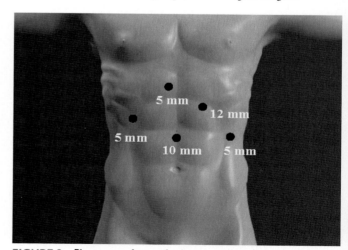

FIGURE 2 Placement of ports for laparoscopic gastric resections. *(From Novitsky YW Kercher KW, Sing RF, et al: Long-term outcomes of laparoscopic resection of gastric gastrointestinal stromal tumors, Ann Surg 243:738–747, 2006.)*

To expose lesions along the greater curvature, the greater omentum may be mobilized by dividing the gastrocolic omentum and short gastric arteries using a laparoscopic coagulating energy source such as the Harmonic Ace (Ethicon Endo-Surgery Inc., Cincinnati, Ohio) or LigaSure (Covidien, Boulder, Colo.). Wedge gastrectomy may then be performed as described above. For lesser curvature lesions, the lesser omentum is mobilized between the gastric serosa and vagus nerve to preserve innervation to the pylorus.

For exophytic or subserosal posterior wall lesions, the lesser sac is entered by mobilizing the omentum. The greater curvature or posterior stomach may then be retracted or rotated to expose the mass, and wedge resection is performed (Figure 4). An alternative approach through an anterior gastrotomy is useful for an endophytic or submucosal lesion on the posterior wall (Figure 5). Again, intraoperative endoscopy may be useful in localizing the lesion, and ultrasonic shears or electrocautery can be used to create an anterior gastrotomy overlying it. The lesion is elevated by either grasping the normal stomach near the mass or by placing traction sutures, and a linear stapler may be used for wedge resection as previously described. The anterior gastrotomy may be closed with a single layer of running intracorporeal suturing (our preference) or by placing full-thickness traction sutures along the gastrotomy and firing a linear stapler on the stomach wall below the sutures.

When more precise control of resection or closure is needed, such as when there is concern about narrowing the lumen of the stomach for antral masses or those at the gastroesophageal junction, the surgeon should consider excising the mass using the ultrasonic shears, followed by closure of the defect at a right angle to the gastric axis by intracorporeal suturing. Intraoperative endoscopy may be used to assess the lumen as well as to perform a leak test after closure of the defect. If the lesion is large, distal gastrectomy with reconstruction may be needed.

Distal Gastrectomy

If distal gastrectomy is being performed for peptic ulcer disease, truncal vagotomy may be performed with ultrasonic shears and clips applied to the proximal and distal resected ends. An energy device is used to mobilize the stomach by dividing the gastrocolic and lesser omentum, the short gastric arteries as necessary, posterior attachments, and by including distal mobilization beyond the pylorus to the proximal duodenum (Figure 6). This distal resection site is identified by visualizing the whitish rings of the pylorus or the vein of Mayo and is confirmed by identifying the Brunner glands on intraoperative frozen pathology. The right gastroepiploic and right gastrc arteries may be divided with an energy device. The duodenum is then transected using a laparoscopic linear stapler (blue or white load). The stump may be reinforced or imbricated with 3-0 silk in a running or interrupted layer, but we usually do not do this. The proximal stomach is also transected with serial firings of a linear stapler (blue loads). The

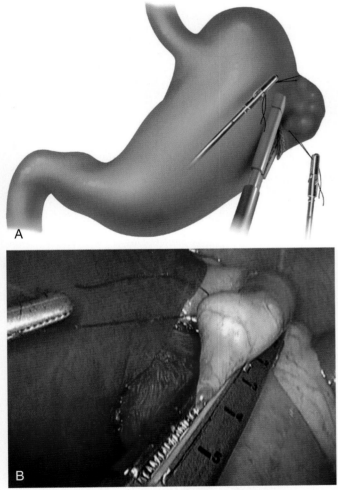

FIGURE 3   Resection of an anterior wall or greater curvature lesion. *(B from Song KY, Kim SN, Park CH: Tailored approach of laparoscopic wedge resection for treatment of submucosal tumor near the esophagogastric junction, Surg Endosc 21:2272–2276, 2007.)*

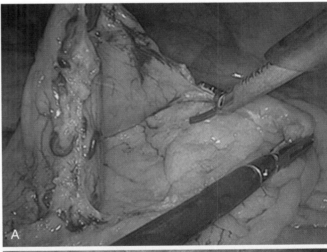
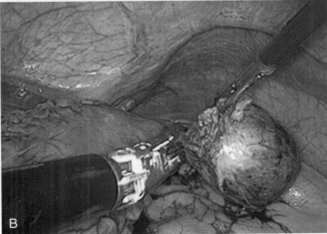

FIGURE 4   Resection of posterior wall exophytic lesion. **A,** Approach through the lesser sac. **B,** Resection with a laparoscopic linear cutting stapler.

specimen may be removed through an enlarged 12 mm port site in a retrievable bag.

A Billroth II loop gastrojejunostomy is then constructed in either a retrocolic or antecolic fashion on the posterior gastric wall, according to surgeon preference (Figure 7). We prefer an antecolic reconstruction, especially when resection is for cancer. The ligament of Treitz is exposed by retracting the transverse colon cephalad; a portion of proximal jejunum, approximately 30 cm distal to the ligament of Treitz, is chosen for a stapled or sutured anastomosis to the stomach. The common opening is closed in two layers of running 2-0 Vicryl with intracorporeal suturing and knot tying. The omentum can be bisected if the loop of jejunum does not easily reach the stomach, but the loop may need to be created in a retrocolic position. The mesenteric defect is closed with a permanent suture.

Alternatively, a laparoscopic or hand-assisted approach has been described using a 5 cm epigastric midline incision. The mobilized stomach may then be exteriorized through this incision for resection and creation of a Billroth I or Billroth II anastomosis. For gastric cancer, the greater and lesser omentum and D1 and/or D2 lymph nodes are mobilized with the stomach for resection en bloc. For resections of greater than 50% of the stomach, a Roux-en-Y gastroenterostomy may be performed.

Total Gastrectomy

Methods similar to those described above for distal gastrectomy are used to mobilize the mid and distal stomach. Proximal mobilization of the stomach will require complete division of the short gastric arteries, posterior attachments, and the phrenoesophageal ligament, and a laparoscopic energy device may be used. A linear stapler or energy device is used to divide the left gastric artery. An Endoloop or clip may then be applied for additional security. The distal esophagus must also be mobilized, which can largely be accomplished by blunt dissection in an avascular plane; however, a laparoscopic energy

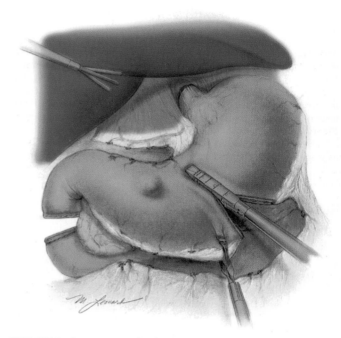

FIGURE 6   Laparoscopic distal gastrectomy. *(From Tessier DJ, Matthews BD: Resection of nonadenomatous gastric tumors. In Soper NJ, Swanström LL, Eubanks WS [eds]: Mastery of endoscopic and laparoscopic surgery, ed 3, Philadelphia, 2009, Lippincott Williams & Wilkins.)*

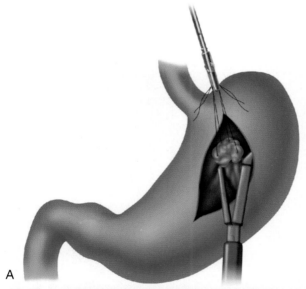

A

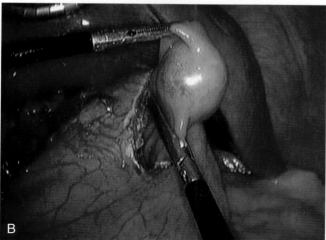

B

FIGURE 5   Transgastric resection of a posterior wall lesion. *(B from Song KY, Kim SN, Park CH: Tailored approach of laparoscopic wedge resection for treatment of submucosal tumor near the esophagogastric junction, Surg Endosc 21:2272–2276, 2007.)*

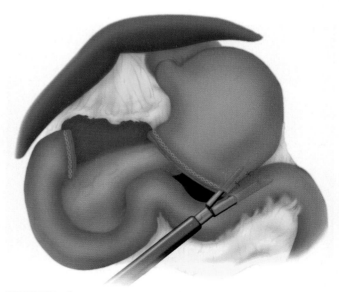

FIGURE 7   Laparoscopic creation of a Billroth II gastrojejunal anastomosis.

device may be used to divide small branches to the esophagus from the aorta. The distal esophagus is then transected using a linear stapler, and ultrasonic shears or electrocautery are used to make a small defect for the stapler anvil.

The round disc at the top of the anvil of a circular end-to-end anastomosis stapler is flipped to be in line with the anvil shaft and is secured to the cut proximal end of a nasogastric tube (Figure 8). This is then passed orally, and the tip is guided through the opening at the staple line in the distal esophagus and brought out through a port until the anvil tip appears. The nasogastric tube is then disconnected and removed from the abdomen.

Reconstruction with a Roux-en-Y gastrojejunostomy is performed next (Figure 9). The transverse colon is retracted cephalad to expose the ligament of Treitz, and a linear stapler is used to divide the proximal jejunum approximately 30 cm from the ligament of Treitz. A stapled jejunojejunostomy is made, allowing for at least a 60 cm Roux limb. The left upper quadrant port is removed, and the circular stapler is introduced through the abdominal wall into an enterotomy made at the stapled end of the Roux limb. The stapler is advanced distally, the pin is deployed on the antimesenteric border and joined to the anvil, and the stapler is fired. The open end of the Roux limb is closed with a linear stapler. Additional interrupted 3-0 silk sutures may be placed for reinforcement. Mesenteric defects are closed with a running 3-0 silk suture. Again, if the procedure is performed for cancer, proper en bloc resection of the greater and lesser omentum and proper lymphadenectomy need to be performed.

Special Considerations

It is important at all times to consider the best oncologic result and to convert to an open procedure whenever the surgeon does not think this can be achieved laparoscopically. This may include cases in which localizing or accessing the tumor, assessing margins, or resecting the tumor safely is difficult, especially in the case of a large GIST. Conversion to a hand-assisted procedure has been reported for improved tactile feedback and gentle manipulation, particularly when resecting a large or thin-walled GIST to minimize the risk of tumor rupture. If a GIST is very large, neoadjuvant therapy with imatinib may be effective in shrinking the tumor to allow organ preservation and laparoscopic resection. Most published reports of laparoscopic resection of GISTs have a mean tumor size of 4 to 5 cm, and although no long-term follow-up data are available, no significant difference in oncologic outcomes at 2 to 3 years have been observed.

An intragastric approach has been used for endophytic or submucosal lesions, especially those near the esophagogastric junction (Figure 10). Endoscopy is used to localize the mass and insufflate the stomach, and at least two or three balloon-tipped trocars are percutaneously introduced into the stomach lumen under direct endoscopic visualization. Normal saline or a dilute solution of epinephrine (1:100,000) are injected circumferentially into the submucosal plane to facilitate dissection. The lesion is enucleated from the submucosal–muscular junction using electrocautery or ultrasonic shears and is then removed using a retrieval bag, usually transorally. The remaining defect may be left open or closed with suturing.

The gastrotomy sites may be closed in routine fashion after removing the ports from their intragastric position. This approach has the added benefit of not creating a full-thickness defect and thus has a decreased risk of postoperative leaks. At the beginning, prior to insufflation, a transabdominal port for a 5 mm laparoscopic camera may also be placed for laparoscopic visualization while obtaining percutaneous intragastric access. In another recently described technique, endoscopic submucosal dissection is combined with laparoscopic seromuscular resection for transmural tumor excision.

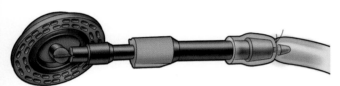

FIGURE 8 Anvil of a circular end-to-end anastomosis stapler secured to the cut end of a nasogastric tube.

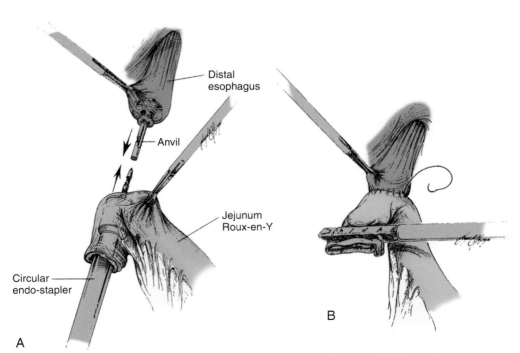

FIGURE 9 Laparoscopic Roux-en-Y gastrojejunal anastomosis after total gastrectomy. *(From Goh PMY, Cheah WK: Laparoscopic gastrectomy for cancer. In Zucker KA (ed): Surgical laparoscopy, ed 2, Philadelphia, 2001, Lippincott Williams & Wilkins.)*

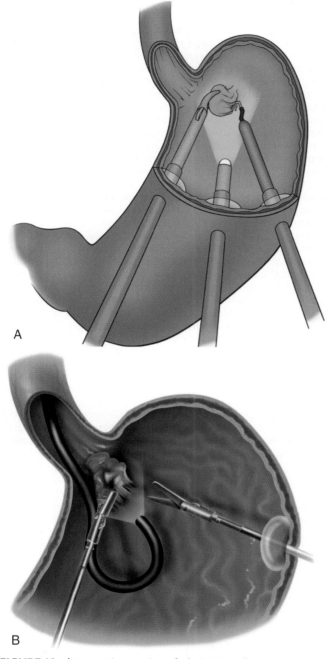

A

B

FIGURE 10   Intragastric resection of a lesion near the esophagogastric junction. **A,** Using the laparoscope for visualization. **B,** Using the endoscope.

SUMMARY

A minimally invasive approach has become the preferred method of treatment in benign diseases such as gastroesophageal reflux, para-esophageal hernia, and obesity. Although long-term data are lacking, current short-term data support improved postoperative outcomes and oncologic safety of laparoscopic resection of benign and malignant tumors by experienced surgeons. However, these laparoscopic operations can be technically difficult, and the surgeon should have the requisite laparoscopic skill set, including intracorporeal suturing, in combination with a solid open experience in these operations. Novel approaches are continually being developed, and future surgeons will need to be skilled in intraluminal approaches to therapy.

Suggested Readings

Hiki N, Yamamoto Y, Fukunaga T, et al: Laparoscopic and endoscopic cooperative surgery for gastrointestinal stromal tumor dissection, *Surg Endosc* 22:1729–1735, 2008.

Huscher CGS, Mingoli A, Sgarzini G, et al: Totally laparoscopic total and subtotal gastrectomy with extended lymph node dissection for early and advanced gastric cancer: early and long-term results of a 100-patient series, *Am J Surg* 194:839–844, 2007.

Kitano S, Shiraishi N, Uyama I, et al: A multicenter study on oncologic outcome of laparoscopic gastrectomy for early cancer in Japan, *Ann Surg* 245:68–72, 2007.

Novitsky YW, Kercher KW, Sing RF, et al: Long-term outcomes of laparoscopic resection of gastric gastrointestinal stromal tumors, *Ann Surg* 243:738–747, 2006.

Shehzad K, Mohiuddin K, Nizami S, et al: Current status of minimal access surgery for gastric cancer, *Surg Oncol* 16:85–98, 2007.

Laparoscopic Management of Crohn's Disease

Alessandro Fichera, MD, and Konstantin Umanskiy, MD

OVERVIEW

Despite significant advances in medical management of Crohn's disease (CD) with the introduction of immunomodulators and biologic agents in the late 1990s, patients with CD are still frequently referred for surgery; the lifelong need for surgery has been reported to be as high as 82%. Patients with CD have traditionally been considered poor laparoscopic candidates because of the panintestinal nature of the disease, with "skip" lesions, inflammatory complications, and the use of aggressive and often morbid medical management that increases the risk of postoperative complications. However, minimally invasive approaches have been developed for CD over the past 2 decades and in single-institution retrospective small studies have been shown to improve cosmetic results and potentially reduce postoperative ileus and hospital stay. The impact of laparoscopy on short- and long-term recurrence rates has been poorly studied, and although small, single-institution studies, including ours, recently have shown recurrence rates similar to those after open surgery, definitive large prospective studies to adequately answer this important question are lacking.

Modern principles of surgical management dictate that intestinal resections should be limited, without wide margins of normal tissue. Greater understanding of the clinical course of CD has led to a more conservative strategy, with surgery reserved for the treatment of complications of the disease and bowel-sparing approaches advocated. The indications for laparoscopic surgery for CD do not, and should not, differ from conventional open surgery (Figure 1). Relative contraindications to a laparoscopic approach include critically ill patients unable to tolerate pneumoperitoneum because of hypotension or hypercarbia, patients with dense adhesions or extensive intraabdominal sepsis (abscess, free perforation, complex fistula), and difficulty in identifying the anatomy (previous surgery, obesity, adhesions). Because CD is commonly categorized according to the affected intestinal site, we will discuss the indications for surgery, surgical technique, and results as they pertain to the specific segment of the gastrointestinal tract.

STOMACH AND DUODENUM

Gastroduodenal involvement in CD is reported in only 2% to 4% of cases and is rarely confined to only the gastroduodenal segment, and 96% of patients have disease elsewhere. About one third of patients affected by gastroduodenal CD will require surgical intervention in their lifetime, most commonly for obstruction resulting from stenotic disease. Options for surgical management of complicated gastroduodenal CD include bypass, stricturoplasty, and, less frequently, resection. Although complex stricturoplasties and resections should be approached through a laparotomy, laparoscopy is a viable alternative in patients in need of a bypass. Traditionally, the gold standard for treating obstruction of the duodenum has been to bypass the duodenum via a gastrojejunostomy. An associated highly selective vagotomy is preferred over a truncal vagotomy to reduce the incidence of vagotomy-related diarrhea.

OPERATIVE TECHNIQUE: LAPAROSCOPIC GASTROJEJUNOSTOMY

Gastrojejunostomy can be performed in either an antecolic or a retrocolic fashion with a stapled anastomosis. If the colon is not involved, most surgeons prefer a side-to-side retrocolic approach, in which a window is made in the avascular plane of the transverse mesocolon to expose the posterior wall of the stomach. Care is taken to identify the middle colic artery to avoid injuring it. The most proximal loop of jejunum that lies tension free next to the greater curvature of the stomach is selected. Two stay sutures are placed to hold the stomach and bowel together, an enterotomy and gastrotomy are made, and the linear stapler is inserted and fired. The gastrotomy and enterotomy are closed using one or two layers of interrupted 3-0 sutures or with an additional firing of a laparoscopic stapler.

Outcomes

Although the available studies are very small, a more favorable experience with duodenal stricturoplasty, compared with bypass surgery for the treatment of duodenal CD, has been reported in terms of reoperation for recurrence and complications. However, if the duodenal stricture is lengthy, multiple strictures are present, or the tissues around the stricture are too rigid or unyielding, a stricturoplasty should not be performed, and an intestinal bypass procedure should be undertaken instead.

SMALL BOWEL

The small bowel is the most frequently affected gastrointestinal site in CD. Although any portion of the small bowel may be diseased, the terminal ileum is most commonly involved. Ninety percent of patients with CD of the small bowel experience symptoms resulting from obstructive or septic complications. A complete assessment of the gastrointestinal tract is mandatory prior to surgery to evaluate the full extent of disease and any associated complications that may require management before surgical intervention. Small bowel follow through or enteroclysis can adequately assesses the entire small intestine. CD is a relative contraindication for capsule endoscopy because of the high incidence of strictures. If the patient is seen initially with a fever or an abdominal mass, a CT scan should be obtained to assess for the presence of an intraabdominal abscess amenable to percutaneous drainage.

OPERATIVE TECHNIQUE: LAPAROSCOPY-ASSISTED SMALL BOWEL RESECTION

A planned small bowel resection is preceded by exploration of all four abdominal quadrants and the entire small bowel for evidence of coexisting CD, because up to 15% of patients will present with skip lesions. If areas of stenosis are suspected on serosal inspection, these should be marked with either an intracorporeal suture or a clip for subsequent identification upon exteriorization of the specimen. Matted loops of small bowel or omentum are often found adjacent to the diseased segment, especially if the terminal ileum is involved. Care must be taken to adequately mobilize the affected areas, and often mobilization of the ascending colon is needed. The matted loops of bowel can then be separated with a combination of blunt and sharp dissection, and the area to be resected can be inspected extracorporeally.

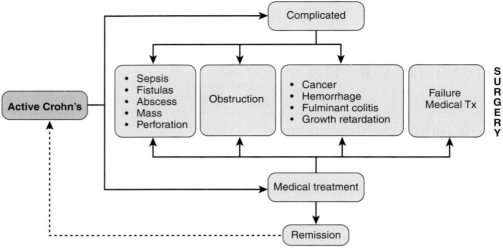

FIGURE 1   Indications for surgery in CD. *(© 2009 University of Chicago.)*

Division of the thickened mesentery of the involved small bowel is often the most challenging aspect of the procedure. The introduction of hand-activated advanced bipolar laparoscopic devices that allow for safe control of vessels up to 7 mm in diameter has dramatically improved our ability to complete these operations laparoscopically. Although the anastomosis could be completed intracorporeally, we prefer to exteriorize the specimen to construct the anastomosis extracorporeally. The bowel may be anastomosed in an end-to-end, end-to-side, or side-to-side fashion using a handsewn or a stapled technique. In our practice the bowel is anastomosed in a double-layered, handsewn, either end-to-end or side-to-side fashion. Clinical data have not demonstrated a significant clinical benefit for one configuration over another.

Nonresectional options such as stricturoplasty have gained popularity as an alternative to lengthy resections in the treatment of stricturing CD of the small intestine. Laparoscopy-assisted stricturoplasty is particularly advantageous when it is associated with a bowel resection, usually an ileocolic resection. The diseased area or areas can be marked with intracorporeal stitches or clips, exteriorized through a small abdominal incision needed for removal of the resected specimen, and the stricturoplasty is performed extracorporeally in a standard fashion.

OPERATIVE TECHNIQUE: LAPAROSCOPY-ASSISTED ILEOCOLIC RESECTION

Laparoscopy-assisted ileocolic resection is currently the most commonly performed laparoscopic procedure for CD. The patient is placed on the operating table in the modified lithotomy position. Every operation for CD, whether open or laparoscopic, should start with a complete examination of the entire gastrointestinal tract, starting from the ligament of Treitz. The patient is in the reverse Trendelenburg position and right lateral decubitus, with the assistant standing on the patient's left side, retracting the transverse colon into the upper quadrants, and the surgeon standing between the patient's legs, evaluating the intestine from the ligament of Treitz all the way to the ileocecal valve. This maneuver is facilitated by progressively rotating the patient from the reverse Trendelenburg to a full Trendelenburg position and left lateral decubitus.

In the presence of skip areas of involvement from CD, these are marked intracorporeally with sutures or clips to facilitate retrieval of the diseased segments when the specimen is exteriorized. A technique employing four 5 mm trocars is utilized (Figure 2). After the bowel has been evaluated in its entirety, the surgeon moves to the

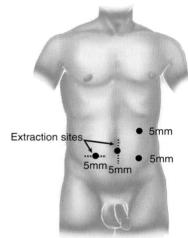

© 2007 University of Chicago

FIGURE 2   Trocar placement and specimen extraction sites for ileocolic resection. *(Reprinted from Fichera A, Peng SL, Elisseou, NM, et al: Laparoscopic vs. open surgery in patients with ileocolonic Crohn's disease: a prospective comparative study, Surgery 142[4]:566–571, 2007. © 2007 University of Chicago.)*

left side of the patient (Figure 3), and the assistant places the ileocolic pedicle under tension. The surgeon dissects the mesentery and divides the ileocolic vessels (Figure 4). The ascending colon is mobilized in a medial-to-lateral fashion in the submesenteric plane to the hepatic flexure (Figure 5), and the assistant lifts the colon to allow clear visualization of the submesenteric plane.

When the submesenteric mobilization is complete, the lateral peritoneal reflection is divided to the hepatic flexure (Figure 6). The terminal ileum is completely mobilized by dividing the peritoneum at the level of the pelvic rim to allow a tension-free anastomosis through a small incision. It is often necessary to completely mobilize the hepatic flexure to facilitate exteriorization of the specimen (Figure 7). The instruments are removed, and the umbilical port site, or occasionally the right lower quadrant port site, is enlarged for exteriorization of the specimen. In the presence of skip areas of disease marked intracorporeally, either a resection or a stricturoplasty is performed. In the presence of isolated terminal ileal disease, an ileocolic resection is performed with an extracorporeal anastomosis.

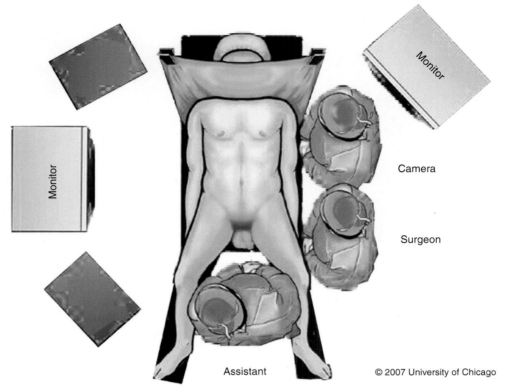

FIGURE 3   Operating room setup for ileocolic resection. *(Reprinted from Michelassi F, Hurst RD, Fichera A: Crohn's disease. In Zinner MJ, Ashley SW [eds]: Maingot's abdominal operations, ed 11, New York, 2007, McGraw-Hill, pp 521–550. © 2007 University of Chicago.)*

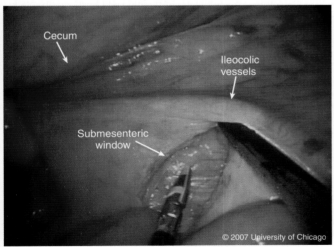

FIGURE 4   Dissection of the ileocolic vessels. *(Reprinted from Michelassi F, Hurst RD, Fichera A: Crohn's disease. In Zinner MJ, Ashley SW [eds]: Maingot's abdominal operations, ed 11, New York, 2007, McGraw-Hill, pp 521–550. © 2007 University of Chicago.)*

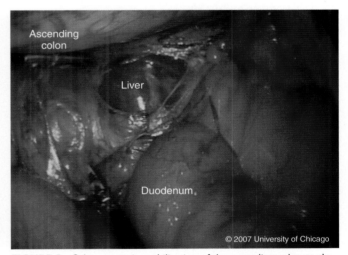

FIGURE 5   Submesenteric mobilization of the ascending colon to the hepatic flexure. *(Reprinted from Michelassi F, Hurst RD, Fichera A: Crohn's disease. In Zinner MJ, Ashley SW [eds]: Maingot's abdominal operations, ed 11, New York, 2007, McGraw-Hill, pp 521–550. © 2007 University of Chicago.)*

Outcomes

Several studies have now confirmed the short-term benefit of a minimally invasive approach in well-selected CD patients with elective, complex, and even recurrent small bowel and terminal ileal disease. The faster postoperative recovery in laparoscopic patients is due in part to the decreased use of intravenous narcotic pain medications. Resection with primary anastomosis can usually be performed with a high degree of safety, and small bowel anastomotic dehiscence rates can be kept to less than 1%. In spite of the technical challenges posed by the hyperemic and thickened mesentery, the risk of postoperative bleeding requiring surgical intervention remains very low.

COLON AND RECTUM

The indications for surgery for colonic CD should not differ between laparoscopic and conventional open surgery (see Figure 1). In the presence of multiple sites of colonic involvement, the decision to perform an ileorectal anastomosis or total proctocolectomy with an end

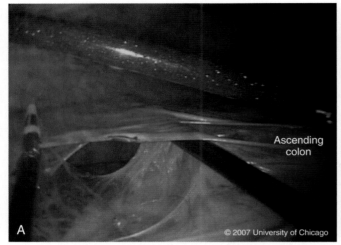

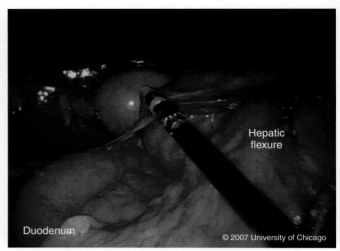

FIGURE 7   Final mobilization of the hepatic flexure. *(Reprinted from Michelassi F, Hurst RD, Fichera A: Crohn's disease. In Zinner MJ, Ashley SW [eds]: Maingot's abdominal operations, ed 11, New York, 2007, McGraw-Hill, pp 521–550. © 2007 University of Chicago.)*

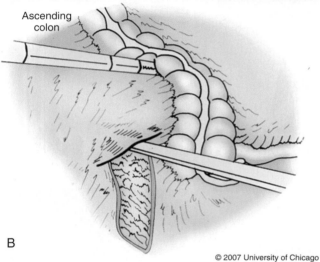

FIGURE 6   Division of the lateral attachments of the ascending colon. *(Reprinted from Michelassi F, Hurst RD, Fichera A: Crohn's disease. In Zinner MJ and Ashley SW [eds]: Maingot's abdominal operations, ed 11, New York, 2007, McGraw-Hill, pp 521–550. © 2007 University of Chicago.)*

ileostomy is determined by the degree of involvement of the distal sigmoid and rectum. Restorative procedures such as ileal pouch–anal anastomoses are typically not performed in patients with CD because of the high pouch failure rates. However, a small subset of patients, those with disease limited to the colon and rectum without any history of small bowel or perineal involvement, may be considered candidates for a restorative proctocolectomy with a J-pouch ileoanal anastomosis. In this highly selected group of patients, restorative proctocolectomy with ileal pouch–anal anastomosis has been performed with acceptable results.

OPERATIVE TECHNIQUE: LAPAROSCOPY-ASSISTED TOTAL ABDOMINAL COLECTOMY

The patient is placed in a modified lithotomy position, which is preferable to the supine position, because it allows the surgeon to access the perineum and to stand between the legs during the mobilization of the transverse colon. Both upper extremities are tucked along the side of the body with a draw sheet. We will describe the hand-assisted technique through a Pfannenstiel incision, which is our preferred

approach. The presence of the hand is particularly helpful in manipulating markedly inflamed or distended colon. The Pfannenstiel incision allows direct access to the pelvis for dissection, rectal transection, and anastomosis. If an end ileostomy is planned, we start with an incision at the ileostomy site and insert a 12 mm trocar, followed by a 5 mm camera port, at the umbilicus; a 5 mm trocar is inserted in the left lower quadrant. Otherwise we place a 5 mm camera port inferior to the umbilicus as our starting port for insufflation, followed by two additional 5 mm ports in the left lower and right lower quadrants.

Once pneumoperitoneum has been established, the feasibility of a laparoscopic approach is evaluated, and a hand-port device is placed in the suprapubic area (Figure 8). The small bowel is evaluated from the ligament of Treitz to the ileocecal valve to rule out small bowel involvement, and the right colon is mobilized as previously described. The mobilization of the transverse colon is facilitated significantly by using the hand, but care must be taken to avoid injury to the duodenum and small bowel mesentery. Placing the greater curvature of the stomach under anterior and cephalad traction facilitates exposure of the gastrocolic ligament and entry into the lesser sac. We prefer to divide the greater omentum with the specimen, 3 to 4 cm away from the greater curvature of the stomach, taking care not to injure the gastroepiploic artery.

Next, the transverse mesocolon is divided with a bipolar vessel-sealing device after division of the greater omentum and exposure of the lesser sac, proceeding from the hepatic to the splenic flexure. Chronically inflamed colon can become intimately attached to the inferior pole of the spleen, as the lienocolic ligament becomes foreshortened by inflammation. Traction on the colon or omentum could result in avulsion of the splenic capsule and result in troublesome bleeding that may require splenectomy.

It is imperative to keep the field as dry as possible with the use of a bipolar vessel-sealing device and precise and meticulous dissection. If necessary the splenic flexure can be approached, alternating the dissection between the transverse colon moving distally and the descending colon moving proximally, thus minimizing traction on the spleen and the inflamed colon. The descending colon is then mobilized by division of its lateral attachments along the white line of Toldt and the mesentery.

Once the dissection reaches the level of the pelvic brim, the colon and terminal ileum are exteriorized through the Pfannenstiel incision. When a rectal-sparing technique is used, patients with diffuse colitis are candidates for a side-to-end ileorectal anastomosis, either stapled or handsewn, provided a close endoscopic exam confirms

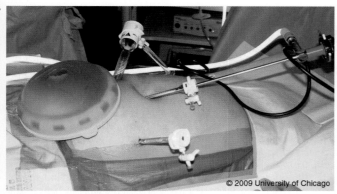

FIGURE 8 Port placement for hand-assisted total abdominal colectomy. (© 2009 University of Chicago.)

that the rectum is truly free of disease, fecal continence is satisfactory, and the patient does not have perineal complications. On the other hand, malnourished patients and those who are acutely ill should instead undergo an end ileostomy. A rectal tube is typically placed at the completion of the case for decompression of the rectal stump.

OPERATIVE TECHNIQUE: TOTALLY LAPAROSCOPIC TOTAL PROCTOCOLECTOMY

Extensive involvement of the colon and rectum or presence of dysplasia on surveillance colonoscopy requires a total proctocolectomy with permanent ileostomy. A totally laparoscopic approach virtually eliminates the risk of wound complication while providing the benefits of a minimally invasive approach.

The patient is placed in modified lithotomy position, a 12 mm trocar is inserted at the ileostomy site, and four more 5 mm trocars are placed, as shown in Figure 9. The colon is mobilized laparoscopically in a fashion similar to the hand-assisted approach described previously. The terminal ileum is intracorporeally divided and delivered through the ileostomy site. The superior hemorrhoidal pedicle is divided, after identification of the left ureter and gonadal vessels, and a totally laparoscopic proctectomy is performed in the avascular presacral space. The operating surgeon and the assistant holding the laparoscope stand on the patient's right with the second assistant on the opposite side. The rectum is mobilized to the level of the levators, and identification of the pelvic sympathetic and parasympathetic nerves is indicated to avoid postoperative urinary and sexual dysfunction. An intersphincteric dissection is completed through the perineum, the specimen is extracted (Figure 10), and the perineal wound is closed in layers with absorbable sutures.

Outcomes

Adopted rather slowly, laparoscopic colectomy in CD is nevertheless welcomed by patients who are generally young and are interested in undergoing an operation that involves minimal scarring and prompt recovery. Furthermore, patients likely require operations over a lifetime, making a minimally invasive approach more appealing, as it results in minimal intraabdominal adhesion formation. In our own series of 55 laparoscopic colectomies for colonic CD, we found potential benefits in favor of laparoscopy in regard to operative blood loss and length of stay in addition to obvious benefits of improved cosmesis and decreased risk of incisional hernia.

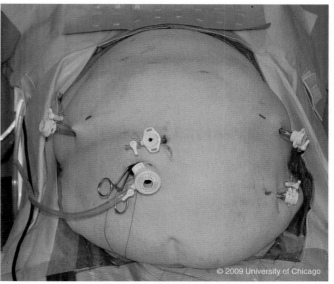

FIGURE 9 Port placement for a totally laparoscopic total proctocolectomy. This patient has had a previous laparoscopic gastric bypass for obesity. The trocar sites in the upper quadrants are from the previous operation. (© 2009 University of Chicago.)

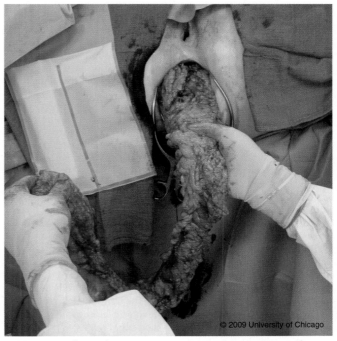

FIGURE 10 Perineal specimen extraction at the completion of a totally laparoscopic total proctocolectomy. (© 2009 University of Chicago.)

PERINEUM

The goal of surgery in anorectal CD is control of sepsis and relief of symptoms with preservation of continence. The initial approach involves a combination of drainage, seton placement, and intensive medical therapy. In selected patients, to achieve complete healing and control of sepsis, a temporary ileostomy should be considered. Another scenario for consideration of fecal diversion is the presence of active anorectal disease; although it puts the patient in need for proctectomy, it precludes definitive procedure, thus requiring creation of an end colostomy to control the sepsis prior to proctectomy.

When a temporary diversion is indicated, we prefer a diverting loop ileostomy. An end-loop ileostomy can also be constructed, if diversion is likely to be required long term. An end-loop stoma allows for better pouching, as it is similar to the end ileostomy and can be reversed without the need for laparotomy. Based on the extent of disease, a permanent stoma could be either a colostomy or an ileostomy. Laparoscopy is currently our preferred technique for fecal diversion with minimal morbidity. Moreover, laparoscopy provides useful information on the extent of disease. An initial incision at the stoma site is used to establish pneumoperitoneum and evaluate the abdomen. With the exception of emergency cases, every patient should undergo preoperative education and stoma marking by an enterostomal therapist.

OPERATIVE TECHNIQUE: LAPAROSCOPIC FECAL DIVERSION

We start similarly for both colostomy and ileostomy. The patient is placed in modified lithotomy position, and the stoma incision is made at the previously marked site. A 12 mm port is inserted, and a purse-string suture is used to cinch the anterior sheath around the port. Laparoscopic exploration is performed next to determine the feasibility of a laparoscopic operation and to determine the extent of disease. For a colostomy we place two additional 5 mm trocars in the right lower and right upper quadrants, and a 5 mm infraumbilical port is placed for the 5 mm, 30 degree camera. The lateral attachments of the sigmoid and descending colon are taken down along the white line of Toldt, and the colon is mobilized to reach the abdominal wall at the stoma opening. Evacuation of pneumoperitoneum will add additional 3 to 4 cm of bowel length sufficient to mature the stoma.

In the presence of a redundant sigmoid colon, very limited mobilization may be required. A very redundant sigmoid colon or the presence of adhesions could present a potential challenge in orienting the distal and proximal limbs. Sigmoidoscopy and insufflation with carbon dioxide, which is absorbed rapidly, can aid proper orientation. If an end stoma is planned, the colon is transected intracorporeally, and the transected proximal end is delivered through the stoma opening. Proper orientation must be maintained; when oriented correctly, the mesocolon is caudad. The abdomen is then reinsufflated, and correct orientation is confirmed with the laparoscope. The colostomy is matured in the standard fashion with slight Brooke eversion to allow better pouching.

Conversely, for an ileostomy we start at the stoma site as previously described and place two additional 5 mm trocars in the left lower and left upper quadrants, and a 5 mm infraumbilical port is placed for the 5 mm, 30 degree camera. The terminal ileum is identified by the visualization of the antimesenteric fat, the fold of Treves, and its connection to the cecum. It is essential to positively identify

the terminal ileum to assure correct orientation of the bowel. The ileum is then run proximally for at least 20 cm to ensure that an adequate length of healthy bowel is available. No mobilization of the ileum is usually required, as it almost always easily reaches the stoma site.

Once the bowel is correctly oriented, the loop of bowel is delivered through the ileostomy site. We orient the bowel so that the proximal limb is located cephalad, and the distal limb is caudad. The abdomen is then reinsufflated, and correct orientation is confirmed with the laparoscope. Some authors advocate minimizing the number of ports used for laparoscopic diverting stoma, particularly for laparoscopic ileostomy. Although this approach can be quite tempting, establishing proper orientation of the bowel can be difficult, unless adequate visualization is achieved. We find it very helpful to place two 5 mm working ports on the opposite side of the abdomen to allow precise tissue handling and improved exposure, resulting in an accurate orientation of the bowel. These benefits outweigh the minimal morbidity and cosmetic considerations of the 5 mm incisions.

Outcomes

The safety and efficacy of the laparoscopic approach for diverting ileostomy or colostomy is now well established and is our preferred method for fecal diversion.

SUMMARY

Although significant advancements have been made in the medical management of CD, surgical intervention is still required in the vast majority of patients to treat complications and palliate symptoms. Although CD presents with varying clinical manifestations requiring individualized treatment, the main goal of surgery in all individuals is to adequately relieve symptoms while avoiding excessive loss of bowel function or body disfiguration.

SUGGESTED READINGS

Fichera A, Peng SL, Elisseou NM, et al: Laparoscopy or conventional open surgery for patients with ileocolonic Crohn's disease? A prospective study, *Surgery* 142(4):566–571, 2007:discussion 571, e1.

Maartense S, Dunker MS, Slors JF, et al: Laparoscopic-assisted versus open ileocolic resection for Crohn's disease: a randomized trial, *Ann Surg* 243(2):143–149, 2006.

Milsom JW, Hammerhofer KA, Bohm B, et al: Prospective, randomized trial comparing laparoscopic vs. conventional surgery for refractory ileocolic Crohn's disease, *Dis Colon Rectum* 44(1):1–8, 2001.

Rosman AS, Melis M, Fichera A: Metaanalysis of trials comparing laparoscopic and open surgery for Crohn's disease, *Surg Endosc* 19(12):1549–1555, 2005.

da Luz Moreira A, Stocchi L, Remzi FH, et al: Laparoscopic surgery for patients with Crohn's colitis: a case-matched study, *J Gastrointest Surg* 11(11):1529–1533, 2007.

Laparoscopic Colorectal Surgery

Peter W. Marcello, MD

OVERVIEW

With the introduction of laparoscopic colectomy nearly 20 years ago, a relatively slow adoption of laparoscopic colorectal surgery into surgical practice has taken place. It is estimated that 10% to 25% of all colorectal resections are performed utilizing laparoscopy. The persistent steep learning curve, the lack of high-volume colorectal surgery by general surgeons (who perform the bulk of colonic resection in the United States), and the modest advantages reported are but a few of the reasons that the percentage of laparoscopic colorectal procedures has not dramatically risen. With the publication of several large, prospective randomized trials for colon cancer, along with the interest in single-port surgery and natural orifice surgery, there appears to be a renewed interest in minimally invasive procedures for the colon and rectum. This chapter will provide an overview of these issues and offer a current assessment of the common diseases to which minimally invasive techniques have been applied.

LEARNING CURVE

Numerous previous studies have evaluated the learning curve involved in laparoscopic colectomy. It is estimated by conventional laparoscopic techniques that the learning curve for laparoscopic colectomy is at least 20 cases but more likely 50 cases. The need to work in multiple quadrants of the abdomen, the need for a skilled laparoscopic assistant, and the lack of yearly volume has kept the learning curve relatively steep. The surgeon may also need to work in reverse angles to the camera. All of these combined add to the complexity of the procedure and result in the need to perform a number of cases before the surgeon and surgical team become proficient.

More recent publications have suggested the learning curve is more than 20 cases. In a prospective randomized study of colorectal cancer in the United Kingdom, the CLASICC trial, surgeons had to perform at least 20 laparoscopic resections before they were allowed to enter the study. The study began in July 1996 and was completed in July 2002. Despite the surgeons' prior experience, the rate of conversion dropped from 38% to 16% over the course of the study, suggesting that a minimum of 20 cases may not be enough to overcome the learning curve.

In the COLOR trial from Europe, another prospective randomized study for colon cancer that required a prerequisite experience in laparoscopic colon resection before surgeons could enter patients in the study, surgeon and hospital volume were directly related to a number of operative and postoperative outcomes. The median operative time for high-volume hospitals (>10 cases/year) was 188 minutes, compared to 241 minutes for low-volume hospitals (<5 cases/year); likewise, conversion rates were 9% versus 24% for the two groups. High-volume groups also had more lymph nodes in the resected specimens, fewer complications, and shortened hospital stays. These two relatively recent multicenter studies suggest that the learning curve is clearly greater than 20 cases and that surgeons need to perform a minimum yearly number of procedures to maintain their skills.

OUTCOMES

There may not be another area in recent surgical history that has been more heavily scrutinized than laparoscopic colorectal surgery. The plethora of accumulated data allows a careful assessment of all outcome measures for nearly every colorectal disease and procedure. In comparison to conventional colorectal surgery, the benefits of laparoscopy for colorectal procedures compared to open techniques include a reduction in postoperative ileus, postoperative pain, and a concomitant reduction in the need for analgesics; an earlier tolerance of diet; a shortened hospital stay; a quicker resumption of normal activities; improved cosmesis; and possibly preservation of immune function. This is offset by a prolongation in operative time, the cost of laparoscopic equipment, and the learning curve for these technically challenging procedures.

When reporting the outcomes of laparoscopic colectomy, a natural selection bias applies when comparing conventional and laparoscopic cases. The most complex cases are generally not suitable for a laparoscopic approach and therefore are performed via an open approach. Also, in many series the results of the successfully completed laparoscopic cases are compared to conventional cases, and the cases converted from a laparoscopic to a conventional procedure may be analyzed separately. Few studies, with the exception of the larger prospective randomized studies, leave the converted cases in the laparoscopic group as part of the "intention to treat" laparoscopic group. This clearly introduces selection bias.

Although the results of prospective randomized trials are available for almost every disease process requiring colorectal resection, the majority of studies of laparoscopic colectomy are retrospective case-control series or noncomparative reports. The conclusions regarding patient outcomes must therefore come from the repetitiveness of the results rather than the superiority of the study design. For any one study, the evidence may be weak; but collectively, because of the reproducibility of results by a large number of institutions, even with different operative techniques and postoperative management parameters, the preponderance of evidence favors a minimally invasive approach with respect to postoperative outcomes.

Operative Time

Nearly all the comparative studies provide information regarding operative times. The definition of the operative time may vary with each series, and there may be different groups of surgeons performing the laparoscopic and conventional procedures. With the exception of a few reports, nearly all studies demonstrated a prolonged operative time associated with laparoscopic procedures. In prospective randomized trials, the procedure was roughly 40 to 60 minutes longer in the laparoscopic groups. As the surgeon and team gain experience with laparoscopic colectomy, the operating times do reliably fall, but rarely do they return to the comparable time for a conventional approach.

Return of Bowel Activity and Resumption of Diet

Reduction in postoperative ileus is one of the proposed major advantages of minimally invasive surgery. Nearly all of the retrospective and prospective studies comparing open and laparoscopic colectomy have shown a statistically significant reduction in the time to passage of flatus and stool. Most series demonstrate a 1- to 2-day advantage for the laparoscopic group. Whether the reduction of ileus relates to less bowel manipulation or less intestinal exposure to air during minimally invasive surgery remains unknown.

With the reduction in postoperative ileus, the tolerance by the patient of both liquids and solid foods is quicker following laparoscopic resection. The time to resumption of diet varies from 2 days to 7 days, but in the majority of comparative studies, this is still 1 to 2 days sooner than in patients undergoing conventional surgery. Again, the physician and patient were not blinded in nearly all studies, which may have altered patient expectations. However, the overwhelming reproducible data reported in both retrospective and prospective studies of laparoscopic procedures does likely favor a reduction of postoperative ileus and tolerance of liquid and solid diets.

Postoperative Pain

To measure postoperative pain, a variety of assessments have been performed to demonstrate a significant reduction in pain following minimally invasive surgery; some studies utilize an analog pain scale, and others measure narcotic requirements. Physician bias and psychologic conditioning of patients may interfere with the evaluation of postoperative pain. There are also cultural variations in the response to pain. Three of the early prospective randomized trials have evaluated pain postoperatively, and all three have found a reduction in narcotic requirements in patients undergoing laparoscopic colectomy. In the COST study, the need both for intravenous and oral analgesics was less in patients undergoing successfully completed laparoscopic resections. Numerous other nonrandomized studies have shown a reduction in postoperative pain and narcotic usage.

Length of Stay

The quicker resolution of ileus, earlier resumption of diet, and reduced postoperative pain has resulted in a shortened length of stay for patients after laparoscopic resection when compared to traditional procedures. Recovery after conventional surgery has also been shortened, but in the absence of minimally invasive techniques, it would seem unlikely that the length of stay could be further reduced. In nearly all comparative studies, the length of hospitalization was 1 to 6 days less for the laparoscopic group. Although psychological conditioning of the patient cannot be helped and likely has a desirable effect, the benefits of minimally invasive procedures on the overall length of stay cannot be discounted. The benefit, however, is more likely a 1 to 2 day advantage only. The more recent introduction of clinical pathways, both in conventional and laparoscopic surgery, has also narrowed the gap but appears to be more reliable in patients undergoing a minimally invasive approach.

Hospital Costs

One of the disadvantages of laparoscopy is the higher cost related to longer operative times and increased expenditures in disposable equipment. Whether the total cost of the hospitalization (operative and hospital costs) is higher following laparoscopic colectomy is debatable. A case-control study from the Mayo Clinic looked at total costs following laparoscopic and open ileocolic resection for Crohn's disease (CD). In this study, 66 patients underwent laparoscopic or conventional ileocolic resection and were well matched. Patients in the laparoscopic group had less postoperative pain, tolerated a regular diet 1 to 2 days sooner, and had a shorter length of stay (4 vs. 7 days). In the cost analysis, despite higher operative costs, the overall mean cost was $3273 less in the laparoscopic group. The procedures were performed by different groups of surgeons at the institution, and although the surgeons may have introduced biases, this study was undertaken during the current era of cost containment, in which all physicians are encouraged to reduce hospital stays. The results are similar for elective sigmoid diverticular resection with a mean cost savings of $700 to $800. Clearly, if operative times and equipment expenditure are minimized, the overall cost of a laparoscopic resection should not exceed a conventional approach.

CROHN'S DISEASE

Laparoscopy in the setting of inflammatory bowel disease has its own set of unique challenges that must be overcome. For patients with CD, dissection is hampered by inflammatory changes in the mesentery, difficulty in assessing bowel involvement and identifying normal anatomic landmarks, along with the development of associated abscess and fistulous disease often seen in the patient with CD. For the patient with isolated Crohn colitis or ulcerative colitis, the challenges are more technical because of the difficulty in performing laparoscopic total colectomy.

CD of the terminal ileum seems to be the ideal application of a minimally invasive approach. The disease is usually limited to one area of the abdomen, and only mobilization with or without vascular pedicle ligation is required laparoscopically. The resection and anastomosis are generally performed extracorporeally. Patients with CD are typically young and are interested in undertaking a procedure that minimizes incisional scarring. Additionally, because many of these patients will require reoperation over their lifetime, a minimally invasive approach is appealing. More recent studies (Table 1) report a rate of conversion from 10% to 20% with the mix of complex cases (abscess, fistula, or reoperative surgery) ranging from 40% to 50%.

As expected, the outcomes following laparoscopy-assisted ileocolic resection for CD mirror those seen in other studies of laparoscopic colectomy for benign and malignant disease. In comparative studies (see Table 1), laparoscopic ileocolic resection is associated with a quicker return of bowel function and an earlier tolerance of oral diet. The quicker resolution of ileus, earlier resumption of diet, and reduced postoperative pain have resulted in a shortened length of stay for patients after laparoscopic resection compared to traditional procedures. Several prospective randomized trials compare conventional and laparoscopic ileocolic resection for refractory CD. Combined, these studies demonstrate a quicker return of bowel function and shortened length of stay with a conversion rate of 10% to 20%, but these were in elective cases in which complex abscess and fistulous disease were not present in the majority of cases.

With the loss of tactile sensation, one of the remaining concerns of performing laparoscopic surgery in the patient with terminal ileal CD is missing an isolated proximal lesion. Following ileocolic resection, many patients will develop a symptomatic recurrence proximal to the ileocolic anastomosis, but whether patients who undergo a laparoscopic procedure will be seen with unrecognized proximal disease remains unclear. However, several studies have now reported recurrence rates following laparoscopic ileocolic resection. In a recent paper, the long-term follow-up over 7 years (mean, 39 months) of 32 patients who underwent a laparoscopic ileocolic resection was compared to 29 patients who underwent open resection. The rate of CD recurrence was high but similar in both groups (48% laparoscopic, 44% conventional), as was the disease-free interval (24 months).

In another recent review of long-term outcome, the results of 39 laparoscopic and 53 conventional ileocolic resections with a 5-year follow-up were reviewed. Recurrent disease was determined by patient symptoms and was confirmed both radiographically and endoscopically in 27% of patients who underwent a laparoscopic procedure and in 29% of patients who underwent a conventional resection. Interestingly, the incidence of small bowel obstruction was significantly less in the laparoscopic group (11% vs. 35%, $P = .02$). This was thought to be due to less adhesion formation following a laparoscopic procedure.

Laparoscopic ileocolic resection for CD appears to be safe and feasible and offers the advantages seen in other reports of laparoscopic colorectal procedures. For the inexperienced laparoscopist, the initial, uncomplicated terminal ileal resection is an ideal procedure in

TABLE 1: Studies of laparoscopic resection for Crohn's disease

Author	NO. PATIENTS		OPERATIVE TIME (MIN)		LOS (DAYS)		MORBIDITY (%)		Comment
	LAP	CON	LAP	CON	LAP	CON	LAP	CON	
Alabaz (2000)	26	48	150	90	7.0	9.6	–	–	Favorable results
Bemelman (2000)	30	48	138	104	5.7	10.2	15	10	Different hospitals for each group
Young-Fadok (2001)	33	33	147	124	4.0	7.0	–	–	Laparoscopy more expensive
Schmidt (2001)	46	–	207	–	5.7	–	–	–	Safe and effective, high conversion rate
Milsom (2001)	31	29	140	85	5.0	6.0	16	28	Prospective randomized trial
Evans (2002)	84	–	145	–	5.6	–	11	–	Results improve with experience
Dupree (2002)	21	24	75	98	3.0	5.0	14	16	Laparoscopy less expensive
Shore (2003)	20	20	145	133	4.3	8.2	–	–	Laparoscopy less expensive
Benoist (2003)	24	32	179	198	7.7	8.0	20	10	Similar operative times, 17% converted
Bergamaschi (2003)	39	53	185	105	5.6	11.2	9	10	Long-term obstructio less, 11% vs. 35%

OP, Operative; *LOS*, length of stay; *LAP*, laparoscopic; *CON*, conventional

which to gain laparoscopic experience. An initial laparoscopic survey should be performed in the majority of patients with refractory ileal CD with a low threshold to alternate the approach if a complex case beyond the skill of the surgeon is encountered.

ULCERATIVE COLITIS

Few prospective randomized studies of laparoscopic total colectomy for ulcerative colitis have been done. The majority of results available for analysis are prospective and retrospective case-control studies and noncomparative reports (Table 2). Until recently there were few reports of laparoscopic proctocolectomy for patients with ulcerative colitis. However, with advances in technology and experienced gained with segmental resection, many groups have evaluated the role of laparoscopic total colectomy for inflammatory bowel disease.

The majority of reports have shown that laparoscopic total colectomy and laparoscopic proctocolectomy with and without ileoanal pouch construction is technically feasible and shares the same advantages of minimally invasive surgery as segmental colonic resection. Laparoscopic proctocolectomy has been performed in the elective setting, but it must be acknowledged that these surgeons had gained extensive experience with segmental colectomy before attempting laparoscopic proctocolectomy. There is, therefore, an underlying bias in the results, which may not be broadly applied to all surgeons.

Even though some groups perform this procedure routinely, the procedures remain technically challenging, with operative times in the 3- to 5-hour range. In an effort to reduce operative times, several groups have recently reported the use of hand-assisted techniques for restorative proctocolectomy. Several groups have performed laparoscopic total colectomy on an urgent basis for patients with unresolving acute colitis. These procedures, however, are still not recommended for the patient with toxic colitis.

The role of laparoscopic total colectomy for patients with inflammatory bowel disease is not well defined but is likely to expand as surgeons become more comfortable with segmental resection. Advantages seen in segmental resection have recently been reproduced in patients undergoing laparoscopic total colectomy. Again, although the evidence based upon study design and size for any one report is not optimal, the reproducibility of the results among many institutions provides adequate evidence to demonstrate clear

advantages of laparoscopic total colectomy for ulcerative colitis over a conventional approach. The use of hand-assisted laparoscopy for ulcerative colitis patients requiring surgery is likely another approach that may shorten operative time while maintaining the benefits of a minimally invasive approach.

DIVERTICULITIS

Laparoscopic sigmoid resection for diverticulitis remains the leading indication for minimally invasive colon resection for benign disease. The surgery is hampered by both the fibrotic changes associated with elective resection of recurrent disease and the inflammatory changes associated with acute disease. As surgeons acquire their laparoscopic skills, more complex cases involving abscess and fistulous communications have been successfully completed laparoscopically. There are now a large number of studies evaluating laparoscopic surgery for diverticulitis (Table 3). These are both large case series and nonrandomized comparative studies with open resection. Most series report an operative time of 2 to 3 hours with a conversion rate of 10% to 20%. The largest series of diverticular resection comes from a German multiinstitutional study of 1545 patients with data accumulated over 7 years at 52 institutions. The study demonstrated a low morbidity and mortality with an overall conversion rate of 6.1%. As experience increased, the percentage of complex cases increased without significantly altering the morbidity or rate of conversion. High-volume centers performed more of the complex cases with a similar conversion rate to the low-volume centers that performed less complex cases.

Nearly all comparative studies of laparoscopic to open sigmoid resection demonstrate a benefit of the laparoscopic approach, including a shorter duration of ileus and shortened length of stay, but as in other studies, with a prolonged operative time. More recent studies (Table 4) have demonstrated a cost savings with the laparoscopic approach. It should be noted that these are generally the uncomplicated elective cases with fewer patients seen with abscess or fistula formation. For more complex cases, in which the operative times are longer and the rate of conversion is higher, the cost-savings benefit of a laparoscopic approach may be lost. This highlights the importance of case selection when considering a laparoscopic approach. Less experienced surgeons should consider an early conversion of complicated diverticular resection or potentially an alteration to a hand-assisted technique, in which the difficult pelvic dissection can be guided by hand.

RECTAL PROLAPSE

As with other disease processes, the field of laparoscopy has expanded to the treatment of rectal prolapse. Full-thickness rectal prolapse repaired by an abdominal fixation procedure is potentially an ideal procedure for a laparoscopic approach, because there is no specimen to remove and no anastomosis to create. A large number of studies have evaluated not only laparoscopic fixation procedures but also the combination of sigmoid resection and rectopexy for the treatment of rectal prolapse (Table 5). The magnified view into the pelvis with the laparoscope provides unparalleled visualization into the pelvic floor, and the relative laxity of the rectal fixation to the sacrum is beneficial to performance of a laparoscopic procedure. This likely is the reason for the relatively low rate of conversion (<10%) for a laparoscopic rectopexy or resection and rectopexy in comparison to other laparoscopic colorectal procedures. The mobilization of the rectum for rectal prolapse is an ideal procedure in which to learn the laparoscopic technique of rectal mobilization, which may then be applied to other procedures, such as laparoscopic proctocolectomy or total mesorectal excision for rectal cancer.

In addition to case series results, several nonrandomized comparative studies have been done of laparoscopic versus conventional rectopexy and resection rectopexy. These studies showed a longer operative time of 45 to 60 minutes with the laparoscopic procedures but with a length of stay shortened to 2 to 3 days. Functional results following surgery were similar in laparoscopic and conventional groups, with the majority of patients reporting an improvement in incontinence and constipation. Solomon also reported a prospective randomized study of 40 patients with full-thickness rectal prolapse. This well-designed study used blinded observers and a standardized clinical pathway for both groups. As expected, the mean surgical time was 153 minutes in the laparoscopic group, compared to 102 minutes in the open group ($P < .01$). In the laparoscopic group, however, 75% of patients followed the clinical pathways, as compared to only 37% of patients in the conventional group. The mean length of stay was also less (3.9 vs. 6.6 days, $P < .01$). No differences in postoperative pain scores were observed, but total intravenous narcotic usage was less in the laparoscopic group. Functional outcomes of surgery were equivalent, and there were no recurrences of prolapse in either group, with a short mean follow-up of 24 months. Although the study is small, the outcomes mirror the results of other prospective randomized studies of laparoscopic surgery for other diseases and procedures. A later cost analysis of this study demonstrated an overall mean cost savings of $357 per patient in the laparoscopic group.

One of the major issues when discussing surgery for rectal prolapse is the rate of recurrent prolapse. For an abdominal approach, the risk of recurrence should be less than 5% to 10% over 5 years. Unfortunately, the majority of reports on laparoscopic surgery for rectal prolapse have limited follow-up (<3 years). Further long-term follow-up of these patients is needed to ensure that the rate of recurrence remains acceptable. If the rate of recurrent prolapse is confirmed to be equal to that of conventional surgery, a minimally

TABLE 2: Studies of laparoscopic colectomy for ulcerative colitis

Author	Year	No. Patients	Comment
Marcello	2000	13	Restorative proctocolectomy, favorable results
Seshadri	2001	37	25% morbidity
Hamel	2001	21	Compared to ileocolic resection, similar morbidity and length of stay
Marcello	2001	16	For acute colitis, comparative study, favorable results
Brown	2001	25	Longer operative times in laparoscopy group
Dunker	2001	35	Better cosmesis
Ky	2002	32	Single-stage procedure, good results
Bell	2002	18	Total colectomy for acute colitis, appears safe
Rivadeneira	2003	23	Hand-assisted procedure reduced operative times
Kienle	2003	59	Large study, laparoscopic colon mobilization only
Nakajima	2004	16	Hand-assisted technique, favorable results

TABLE 3: Compiled descriptive series of laparoscopic resection for diverticulitis

Study	No. Patients	Mortality (%)	Morbidity (%)	Conversion (%)	OR Time (Min)*	Resume Diet (Days)*	Flatus/BM (Days)*	LOS (Days)*
Tuech (2001)	77	0	17	14	NA	NA	NA	NA
Trebuchet (2002)	170	0	8.2	4.1	141	3.4	NA	8.5
Bouillott (2002)	179	0	15	14	223	3.3	2.5	9.3
Pugleise (2004)	103	0	8	3	190	NA	4	9.7
Schneidbach (2004)	1545	0.4	17	6.1	169	NA	NA	NA
Pessaux (2004)	582	1.2	25	NA	NA	NA	NA	NA
Schwander (2005)	363	0.6	22	6.6	192	2.8	4.0	11.8

*Median or mean values listed

OR, Operating room; BM, bowel movement; LOS, length of stay; NA, not available invasive approach to rectal prolapse appears to be an ideal operation for surgeons with laparoscopic skills.

COLORECTAL CANCER

It is estimated that more than 105,500 new cases of colon cancer and 42,000 new cases of rectal cancer were diagnosed in the United States in 2003. Prior to 2004, fewer than 5% of resections for colon and rectal cancer were being performed laparoscopically. Early in the history of laparoscopic resection of colorectal cancer, there was controversy related to the phenomenon of cancer seeding the incision sites. From 1994 to 2004, a near moratorium on laparoscopic resection for colon cancer was seen, with some national surgical societies calling for these procedures to be performed only under the auspices of randomized controlled trials or with other means of careful prospective data collection. These concerns prompted an unprecedented number of randomized controlled trials. Data from these trials, however, have banished these controversial aspects of the minimally invasive approach. The percentage of cases performed laparoscopically is

expected to increase, as more surgeons become familiar with laparoscopic techniques.

Lacy and colleagues published the first large, single-center randomized controlled trial in 2002. With median follow-up of 39 months, higher cancer-related survival for the laparoscopic arm were reported. Specifically, no difference was shown between arms for stage II cancers, but an improved survival for the laparoscopic approach in stage III cancers was observed, in which the outcome was similar to that of stage II patients. This study was followed in 2004 by the results of the large, multicenter COST study group. With almost 900 patients randomized either to the open or laparoscopic arm of the study, no differences were found in overall survival or disease-free survival. Further reassurance was provided in that only two wound recurrences were seen in the laparoscopic group and one in the open arm. Another of the large, prospective randomized studies from the United Kingdom, the CLASICC trial, has also published their results with similar findings, except a higher rate of conversions was noted. The results of these recent trials (Table 6) have demonstrated that similar oncologic resections can be achieved by experienced surgeons performing laparoscopic colorectal resections.

TABLE 4: Case-control studies pertaining to laparoscopic resection for diverticulitis

Study	N CON	LAP	MORTAL-ITY (%) CON	LAP	MORBIDITY (%) CON	LAP	CONVER-SION (%)	OR TIME (MIN)[†] CON	LAP	RESUME DIET (DAYS)[†] CON	LAP	FLATUS/BM (DAYS)[†] CON	LAP	LOS (DAYS)[†] CON	LAP	TOTAL COST ($US)[†] CON	LAP
Senagore (2002)	71	61	0	1.6	30	8[*]	7	101	107	NA	NA	NA	NA	6.8	3.1[*]	4321	3458[*]
Dwivedi (2002)	88	66	0	0	24	18	20	143	212[*]	4.9	2.9[*]	NA	NA	8.8	4.8[*]	14,863	13,953[*]
Lawrence (2003)	215	56	1.6	1	27	9[*]	7	140	170[*]	NA	NA	NA	NA	9.1	4.1[*]	25,700	17,414[*]
Gonzalez (2004)	80	95	4	1	31	19[*]	NA	156	170[*]	NA	NA	3.7	2.8	12	7[*]	NA	NA

[*]Statistically significant differences
[†]Median or mean values listed
OR, Operating room; *BM,* bowel movement; *LOS,* length of stay; *CON,* conventional surgery; *LAP,* laparoscopic surgery; *NA,* not available

TABLE 5: Recent results of laparoscopy for rectal prolapse

Study	No. Patients	Follow-up (Mo)	Procedure	Operative Time (Min) LAR/LRR	LOS (Days)	Recurrence	Comment
Heah (2000)	25	26	LR	96	7	0%	16% conversion
Kellokumpu (2000)	34	24	LR/LRR	150/255	5	7%	Constipation improved in 70%
Benoist (2001)	48	20–47	LR/LRR	—	—	MP = 8%	Suture rectopexy preferred to mesh
Solomon (2002)	20	24	LR	153	3.9	0%	Prospective randomized study
Kairiluoma (2003)	53	12	LR/LRR	127/210	5	6%	Compared with open: longer operation time, shorter LOS
D'Hoore (2004)	42	61	LR	NS	NS	FT = 4.8%	Constipation improved in 84%
Lechaux (2005)	48	36	LR/LRR	193	4–7	MP = 4.2%	Constipation worsened in 23%
Ashari (2005)	117	62	LRR	110–180	5	FT = 2.5% MP = 18%	Large study with long-term follow-up

LAR, Laparoscopic rectopexy; *LRR,* laparoscopic resection rectopexy; *FT,* full thickness; *MP,* mucosal prolapse; *NS,* not specified

TABLE 6: Prospective randomized trials comparing laparoscopic and open surgery for colorectal cancer

Baseline Characteristics	LACY 2002		COST 2004		CLASICC 2005	
	LAP	**OPEN**	**LAP**	**OPEN**	**LAP**	**OPEN**
Number assigned	111	108	435	437	526	268
Number completed	105	101	435	428	452	231
TNM Stage						
0			5%	8%		
I	27	18	35%	26%		
II	42	48	31%	34%		
III	37	36	26%	28%		
IV	5	6	4%	2%		
No. lymph nodes	11.1	11.1	12	12	12	13.5
Conversion	12 (11%)	N/A	21%	N/A	29%	N/A
OR time (min)	142	118*	150	95*	180	135
Incision length (cm)			6	18*	10	22
Short-Term Outcomes						
Hospital stay (days)	5.2	7.9*	5 vs.	6*	9	11
30-day mortality			<1%	1%	4%	5%
Postoperative complications	12%	31%*	19%	19%	33%	32%
Cancer Outcomes						
Tumor recurrence	18	28	76	84		
Distant	7	9				
Locoregional	7	14				
Peritoneal seeding	3	5				
Port site	1	0	2	1		
5-year overall survival [§]	82%	74%	79%	78%		
I	85%	94%	84%	94%		
II	75%	77%	78%	81%		
III	72%	45%	60%	63%		
5-year disease-free survival			78%	80%		
I	90%	88%	92%	96%		
II	80%	76%	82%	88%		
III	70%	45%	62%	60%		

*$P < .05$

Laparoscopic Resection for Rectal Cancer

Few randomized trials have evaluated laparoscopic resection of rectal cancer, and only one published multicenter prospective trial has compared laparoscopic to conventional proctectomy, the MRC-CLASICC trial. Compared with colonic resection, additional technical challenges are associated with operating within the confines of the pelvis. Multiple factors affect feasibility of an oncologic resection for rectal cancer: tumor factors, such as bulkiness and proximal or distal location, and patient factors, such as the width of the pelvis, obesity, presence of a bulky uterus, and potentially obscured tissue planes from prior radiation.

As would be expected, highly skilled laparoscopic surgeons who perform a large number of rectal resections on a yearly basis have reported excellent results from their institutions. However, the results of the MRC-CLASICC trial were quite different, showing a high rate of mortality (9%), morbidity (59%), and need for conversion (39%) among patients undergoing laparoscopic surgery for rectal cancer. The early oncologic outcomes from the MRC-CLASICC trial reported a higher rate of positive radial margins in the laparoscopic group (12%) compared to the open group (6%). Although this did not reach statistical significance and has not shown a higher local recurrence rate after 3 years, it is still a concerning finding, knowing that a positive radial margin can be a predictor of long-term local recurrence. Also, in a separate report from the MRC-CLASICC trial, the rate of sexual dysfunction was significantly higher in men operated on via a laparoscopic approach compared to an open technique.

A multicenter randomized trial of laparoscopic surgery for rectal cancer in Europe is currently underway, the COLOR II trial. In the United States, the American College of Surgeons Oncology Group (ACOSOG) has a multicenter randomized trial underway to compare the short-term oncologic and functional outcomes of open and laparoscopic surgery for rectal cancer. These trials must be completed to ensure the efficacy and patient safety of a laparoscopic approach for curable rectal cancer.

Technical Considerations

Following detection of a colon or rectal cancer, routine evaluation incorporates preoperative staging, assessment of resectability, and determination of the patient's operative risk. As part of this assessment, a laparoscopic approach may be contemplated. Several factors must be considered, primarily in terms of gauging the difficulty of the procedure and the likelihood of being able to perform it laparoscopically. The site of the tumor is important, as right and sigmoid colectomy are generally less technically demanding than transverse colectomy or proctectomy. Obesity, and particularly visceral obesity, may preclude laparoscopic resection, especially in the case of a rectal cancer in an obese male patient with a narrow pelvis. The patient should be informed of both laparoscopic and open alternatives and the possible need for conversion. Above all, the surgeon must have adequate experience prior to embarking on resection for a potentially curable malignancy.

Tumor Localization

A laparoscopic approach requires accurate localization of the tumor to a specific segment of the colon, as even a known cancer may not be visualized from the serosal aspect of the bowel during laparoscopy. The wrong segment of colon may be removed if accurate localization has not been performed. A variety of other options are available to localize a lesion, including preoperative colonoscopic marking with ink tattoo or metallic clips, barium enema, or intraoperative endoscopy. Preoperative endoscopic tattooing is the most common method of tumor localization. The ink is injected into the submucosa in three or four quadrants 2 cm distal to the lesion (typically 0.5 mL per site). During diagnostic laparoscopy the ink marking can be identified even at the flexures or transverse colon, and ink injection appears to be safe with few reported complications. Intraoperative endoscopy is hampered by persistent bowel distension, prolongation of operative times, and the need for equipment and an endoscopist. More recent studies have evaluated carbon dioxide colonoscopy, which allows for more rapid absorption of the intracolonic gas and may facilitate its use during laparoscopic procedures.

Operative Technique

Oncologic principles must not be compromised by a laparoscopic resection for colon cancer. Guidelines for colon cancer surgery outline recommendations for proximal and distal resection margins, based upon the area supplied by the named feeding arterial vessel; mesenteric lymphadenectomy, containing a minimum of 12 lymph nodes; and ligation of the primary feeding vessel at its base. The randomized trials of laparoscopic colectomy adhered to these standard principles and showed no significant difference in bowel margins or lymph nodes harvested. Inability to achieve these aims laparoscopically should prompt conversion to an open procedure.

The approach to colonic mesenteric mobilization and vascular pedicle ligation may vary by the surgeon's preference, patient anatomy, and cancer-related factors such as adherence of the tumor to the abdominal wall. Surgeons need to be skilled in both the lateral and medial approach to mesenteric mobilization. For right colectomy, the lateral approach begins with mobilization of the cecum and terminal ileum, a procedure most surgeons are familiar with (Figure 1). The right colon is mobilized until the duodenum and proximal ileocolic pedicle are reached. With a medial approach to the right colon, the cecum and terminal ileum are grasped and retracted laterally, tenting up the ileocolic pedicle (Figure 2). A plane is developed under the ileocolic pedicle, which will identify the sweep of the duodenum. With the laparoscope placed at the umbilicus in the majority of cases, a medial approach has become the preferred method of colonic mobilization among experienced laparoscopists.

For left colectomy, a lateral approach will begin with mobilization of the sigmoid from the pelvic inlet, until the ureter is identified (Figure 3). A medial approach to left colectomy begins with an incision at the right edge of the rectosigmoid mesentery. The inferior mesenteric pedicle is elevated, and the left ureter and left gonadal vessels are identified in the retroperitoneum (Figure 4). This approach is quite useful in cases where the cancer is adherent to the pelvic inlet or in cases of severe diverticulitis, where the sigmoid colon is densely adherent to the lateral sidewall. The medial dissection is typically uninvolved in the inflammatory process, and the left ureter can be safely freed underneath before the colon is detached laterally.

Similar guidelines exist for rectal cancer surgery, with varying levels of evidence and grades of recommendation. These include a distal margin of 1 to 2 cm, removal of the blood supply and lymphatics up to the origin of the superior rectal artery (or inferior mesenteric artery if indicated), and appropriate mesorectal excision with radial clearance. Again, the principles of adequate clearance of the primary tumor and supporting tissues should not be compromised by a laparoscopic approach.

HAND-ASSISTED LAPAROSCOPY

Hand-assisted laparoscopic colectomy has been advocated as an alternative to straight laparoscopic techniques. The reintroduction of the hand back into the abdomen during laparoscopy may overcome some of the technical challenges associated with laparoscopic colectomy. Because an extraction site is required for specimen removal, supporters of a hand-assisted approach believe the hand should be placed through that wound to facilitate dissection and mobilization of the colon. The development of sleeveless hand-assist devices provides for hand exchanges without the loss of pneumoperitoneum, allowing surgeons to perform the procedures without disruption.

Numerous randomized and nonrandomized studies have evaluated hand-assisted laparoscopic colectomy over the past 15 years. When compared to traditional laparoscopic techniques, studies suggest that operative times can be reduced, along with the need for conversion, without impacting clinical outcomes. This is true for both segmental resection with total colectomy and proctocolectomy. For segmental resection, a recent study by Chang (2005) reported on a large series of laparoscopic and hand-assisted sigmoid resections. The results of 85 straight laparoscopic sigmoid resections were compared to 66 hand-assisted procedures. Patients were well matched, with a mean body mass index of 29 kg/m^2. The rate of conversion was significantly less

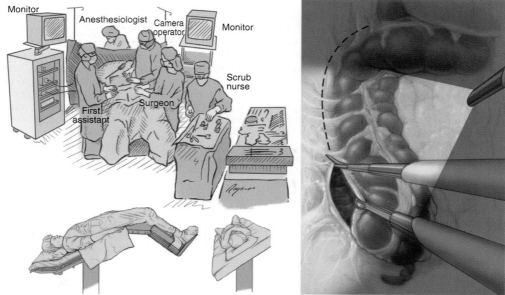

FIGURE 1   Room setup and operator positioning for laparoscopic right hemicolectomy. The patient is in the Trendelenburg position, tilted with the right side up. The peritoneum around the cecum and terminal ileum is scored to enter the correct retroperitoneal plane.

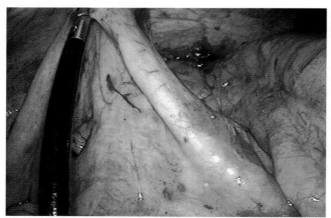

FIGURE 2   The ileocolic artery is identified by elevating the cecum at the junction of the bowel and the mesentery.

in the hand-assisted group (0% vs. 13%, $p < 0.01$) with a shortened mean operative time (189 minutes vs. 205 minutes). The mean size of the extraction was larger in the hand-assisted group (8 cm vs. 6 cm, $P < .01$), but no difference was observed in return of bowel function (mean, 2.5 days vs. 2.8 days) or the median length of stay (4 days).

More recently, we reported the results of a multicenter clinical trial, in which 95 patients with benign and malignant disease disorders were randomized to hand-assisted or straight laparoscopic colorectal surgery. This study represents the largest randomized study comparing hand-assisted techniques and traditional laparoscopy in colorectal surgery to date. Among these patients, 66 underwent left-sided segmental colonic resection. The primary outcome under study, operating time, was found to be significantly shorter among the hand-assisted group than among those who had traditional laparoscopy (175 minutes vs. 208 minutes, $P = .02$). Although not statistically significant, laparoscopy patients experienced a greater proportion of conversion than did patients in the hand-assisted group (2% vs. 12.5%, $P = .11$). In 5 of 6 cases of conversion from traditional laparoscopy, a hand-assisted technique, rather than a formal laparotomy, was successfully completed. For

both groups, other perioperative outcomes were not significantly different, including the return of bowel function, visual analog pain scores, narcotic requirements, and length of stay. The study also compared the results of total colectomy or proctocolectomy in 29 patients and found a significant decrease in skin-to-skin operative time associated with a hand-assisted technique (199 vs. 285 minutes, $P = .015$) and also the time to completion of the laparoscopic colectomy portion of the procedure (127 minutes vs. 184 minutes, $P = .015$).

For patients with inflammatory conditions associated with abscess or fistulous disease (CD and diverticular disease) and those patients requiring total colectomy, a hand-assisted approach will likely remain an invaluable tool in the armamentarium of minimally invasive techniques.

SINGLE-INCISION LAPAROSCOPIC COLORECTAL SURGERY

With the advent of single-port technology, surgeons have expanded the techniques of single-port surgery to the colon and rectum. Several series of single-incision laparoscopic colectomy and even single-incision laparoscopic restorative proctocolectomy have been published, and results so far have not demonstrated any clinical advantage to single-port colectomy, other than cosmesis, when compared to multiport laparoscopy. Whether single-incision laparoscopic colectomy will become the preferred method of laparoscopic colectomy remains to be seen. Surgeons need vast experience with multiport laparoscopy before it can even be attempted. The procedure severely limits instrument manipulations and triangulation, and it requires the surgeon to work in a confined operative field. However, this may be useful for the future application of natural orifice procedures. Single-port technique may therefore be a useful stepping stone for the future expansion of minimally invasive colorectal surgery.

SUMMARY

The field of laparoscopic colon and rectal surgery is slowly expanding. With advancement in techniques and technology, along with the further training of surgical and colorectal residents, the percentage

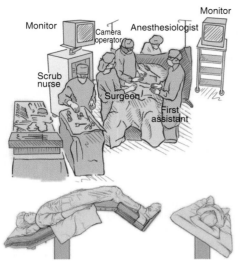

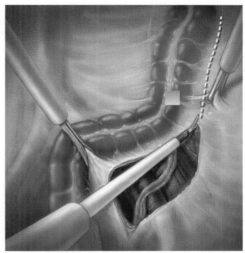

FIGURE 3   Laparoscopic left colectomy room setup. The patient is placed in the Trendelenburg position, with the left side tilted up. The left lateral peritoneal reflection is opened, and the left ureter is identified and protected. The descending and sigmoid colon are mobilized medially.

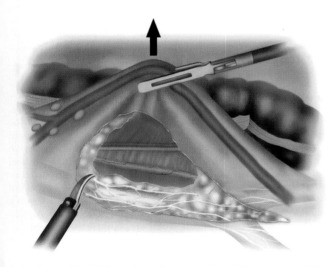

FIGURE 4   Medial dissection of the rectosigmoid mesentery with view through the mesentery of the left ureter.

of colorectal procedures performed by minimally invasive techniques will likely continue to rise. Surgeons who are more than 5 to 10 years from their residency and perform more than 20 colon resections a year should obtain advanced training and credentialing before performing laparoscopic colon resection. Hand-assisted procedures may be used to expand the field of minimally invasive colorectal surgery. The results of the large, multicenter randomized

trials for curable colon cancer have demonstrated modest short-term advantages to a laparoscopic approach, while maintaining the oncologic integrity of the operation, when performed by experienced surgeons. The laparoscopic resection of rectal cancer remains in the forefront and is likely the next area to be critically evaluated and advanced by laparoscopic surgeons. Single-incision laparoscopic colectomy may open the gates to new frontiers in minimally invasive colorectal surgery.

Suggested Readings

Lacy AM, Garcia-Valdecasas JC, Delgado S, et al: Laparoscopy-assisted colectomy versus open colectomy for treatment of non-metastatic colon cancer: a randomised trial, *Lancet* 359:2224–2229, 2002.

Nelson: H and the Clinical Outcomes of Surgical Therapy Study Group: A comparison of laparoscopically assisted and open colectomy for colon cancer, *New Engl J Med* 350:2050–2059, 2004.

Goillou PJ, Quirke P, Thrope H, et al: Short-term end points of conventional vs. laparoscopic-assisted surgery in patients with colorectal cancer (MRC-CLASICC trial): multicentre, randomised controlled trial, *Lancet* 365:1718–1726, 2005.

The COLOR Study Group: Impact of hospital case volume on short-term outcome after laparoscopic operation for colonic cancer, *Surg Endosc* 19:687–692, 2005.

Braga M, Frasson M, Vignali A, et al: Laparoscopic resection in rectal cancer patients: outcome and cost-benefit analysis, *DCR* 50:464–471, 2007.

Marcello PW, Fleshman JW, Milsom JW, et al: Hand-assisted laparoscopic vs. laparoscopic colorectal surgery: a multicenter, prospective, randomized trial, *Dis Colon Rectum* 51:818–828, 2008.

Milsom J, Bohm B, Nakajima K, editors: *Laparoscopic colorectal surgery*, ed 2, New York, 2006, Springer-Verlag.

MINIMALLY INVASIVE ESOPHAGECTOMY

Toshitaka Hoppo, MD, PhD, and Blair A. Jobe, MD

OVERVIEW

Transhiatal esophagectomy and Ivor Lewis esophagectomy are the two most commonly performed operations for esophageal pathology. Both are complex operations that can be associated with high morbidity and mortality rates. Esophagectomy is often performed in elderly patients who have many coexisting medical comorbidities, including respiratory and cardiovascular disease, therefore many surgeons have a great deal of interest in minimally invasive esophagectomy (MIE), which has the potential advantages of being a less traumatic procedure with an easier postoperative recovery and fewer wound and cardiopulmonary complications. In addition, good laparoscopic visualization may facilitate intraoperative procedures and decrease blood loss.

In 1995, DePaula and colleagues reported a small series of laparoscopic transhiatal esophagectomy. Subsequently, in 1998, Luketich and colleagues reported the combined thoracoscopic and laparoscopic approach to esophagectomy, which consisted of thoracoscopic esophageal mobilization followed by laparoscopic construction of the gastric conduit, gastric pull-up, and a neck anastomosis. A minimally invasive Ivor Lewis technique was later reported by Watson and colleagues in 1999, who described laparoscopic construction of the gastric conduit followed by thoracoscopic esophagectomy with an intrathoracic esophagogastric anastomosis.

INDICATIONS

The most common indications for MIE are resectable esophageal cancer and Barrett's esophagus with high-grade dysplasia. Rare, end-stage, benign esophageal disorders can also be ideal indications for MIE (Box 1). A laparoscopic transhiatal esophagectomy is particularly useful for patients who have lower- or middle-third early-stage tumors in conjunction with long-segment Barrett's esophagus. The anastomosis is performed in the neck and allows the surgeon to maximize the proximal margin. The limitations of this technique include a limited view of the middle and upper third of the mediastinum, leading to technical difficulty in performing the mediastinal mobilization and lymphadenectomy, limitations on the length of the gastric conduit and the potential for anastomotic tension, and the potential for recurrent laryngeal nerve injury.

In contrast, minimally invasive Ivor Lewis esophagectomy is indicated, especially for distal esophageal cancer. This procedure should not be performed for upper-third esophageal cancers because of concern over obtaining an adequate disease-free proximal margin. For upper thoracic esophageal cancers, a three-field esophagectomy or modified McKeown technique with neck anastomosis is best performed to obtain a sufficient proximal resection margin. However, this procedure is associated with high morbidity. In particular, injury to one or both recurrent laryngeal nerves has been reported in as many as 50% of patients, and the survival benefits of this approach have yet to be established in a controlled trial.

The most common type of esophageal cancer in the United States is adenocarcinoma, which usually develops in the distal esophagus associated with Barrett's esophagus, and minimally invasive Ivor Lewis and laparoscopic transhiatal esophagectomy are employed more often than the modified McKeown technique; therefore the techniques and outcomes of these two procedures are described in this chapter.

PREOPERATIVE PREPARATION

Optimal outcomes are obtained by accurate staging, risk assessment, patient selection, and choosing an appropriate approach in the surgical management; therefore it is important to assess these factors preoperatively. At our institution, computed/positron emission tomography (CT/PET) scan, endoscopic ultrasound (EUS), and minimally invasive laparoscopic staging are performed routinely prior to MIE. The possibility of conversion to an open procedure should be discussed with patients preoperatively. The surgeon should have blood products and an intensive care unit (ICU) bed available. Cardiac clearance and pulmonary function tests should be obtained to assess the risk for possible postoperative cardiopulmonary complications, such as myocardial infarction and pneumonia, which could become fatal. Maximizing pulmonary function and preventing deep vein thrombosis are critical, and all patients receive prophylactic anticoagulation in conjunction with sequential compression of the lower extremities. For thoracoscopic procedures, we use a double-lumen endotracheal tube; proper tube position is confirmed with bronchoscopy after patient positioning. If a double-lumen tube cannot be inserted, a single-lumen tube with an endobronchial blocker is used.

MINIMALLY INVASIVE IVOR LEWIS ESOPHAGECTOMY

Our current approach is to perform a minimally invasive Ivor Lewis esophagectomy, which is performed in two stages. In the first stage, laparoscopic mobilization of the stomach and construction of the gastric conduit is performed in a supine position. In the second stage, the patient is repositioned to a left lateral decubitus position for mobilization of the thoracic esophagus, removal of the esophageal surgical specimen, gastric pull-up, and construction of an intrathoracic esophagogastric anastomosis. We favor the use of a narrow (but no less than 5 cm wide) gastric tube, because it is associated with a low anastomotic leak rate and superior, long-term function. A pyloroplasty and a 7 Fr feeding jejunostomy are routinely performed.

Surgical Technique

The patient is placed supine, and the surgeon stands to the patient's right, and the assistant stands to the left. The initial step is an on-table esophagogastroduodenoscopy (EGD) to confirm the tumor's location

---

BOX 1: Indications for minimally invasive esophagectomy

Malignant disease
- Adenocarcinoma
- Squamous cell carcinoma

Premalignant disease
- Barrett's esophagus with high-grade dysplasia

Benign disease
- End-stage achalasia
- Refractory stricture
- Profound esophageal (GI) dysmotility

Multiple redo antireflux surgery

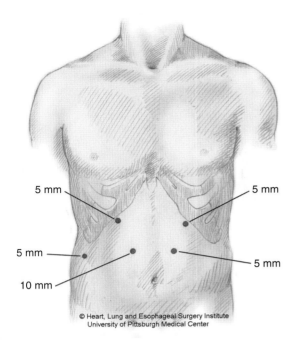

FIGURE 1 Abdominal port placement for minimally invasive Ivor Lewis esophagectomy. *(Copyright Heart, Lung, and Esophageal Surgery Institute, University of Pittsburgh Medical Center.)*

and extent and the suitability of the stomach as a conduit for reconstruction. Five abdominal trocars are placed so the entire stomach can be visualized (Figure 1). A 5 mm, 45-degree laparoscope is placed through the left paramedian port site. First, abdominal exploration is performed to rule out liver metastases and peritoneal implants. Next, the gastrohepatic ligament and the right and left crura are dissected, and the stomach is mobilized by dividing the short gastric vessels first and then the gastrocolic omentum, carefully preserving the right gastroepiploic arcade. All attachments between the posterior aspect of the stomach and anterior surface of the pancreas are divided. This dissection is carried distally, until the gastroduodenal artery is encountered. The stomach is then retracted superiorly. After dissecting the celiac and common hepatic nodal basins, and maintaining these nodes in continuity with the divided left gastric arcade, the left gastric artery is divided using a vascular stapler. Alternatively, the left gastric arcade can be divided early in the abdominal portion of the procedure from an anterior approach, if it is easily accessible.

The pyloroantral area must be mobilized until the pylorus can easily be elevated to the right crus in a tension-free manner. If this cannot be accomplished, a Kocher maneuver is required. Next, a pyloroplasty is created by opening the pylorus with the ultrasonic shears (US Surgical, Norwalk, Conn.; Figure 2, *A*) and closing the pylorus transversely in an interrupted fashion using the Endostitch device (Covidien, Mansfield, Mass.) with nonabsorbable suture (Figure 2, *B*). The gastric conduit is then created by dividing the stomach at the lesser curvature using an endoscopic stapler and preserving the right gastric vessels (Figure 2, *C*).

It is critical to remember to withdraw the nasogastric tube into the proximal esophagus prior to conduit creation. We usually begin with a 2 mm vascular stapler on the lesser omentum, a 4.8 mm stapler (green load) on the gastric antrum and body, and a 3.5 mm stapler (blue load) on the fundus, because the antrum is thicker than the other areas of the stomach. During this step, the first assistant grasps the tip of the fundus along the greater curvature and gently stretches it toward the spleen, while a second grasper is placed on the antral area, and a slight downward retraction is applied. This maneuver facilitates a straight application of the staple line, which should be

parallel to the gastroepiploic arcade. It is critical to prevent spiraling and subsequent ischemia of the conduit as the staple line is advanced proximally, and this "barber pole" deformity is prevented by ensuring consistent retraction along the line of the short gastric vessels with each staple firing. The gastric fundus of the neoesophagus (greater curvature side) is then sutured to the resection specimen (distal lesser curvature), which will ensure correct orientation of the conduit as it is delivered into the chest.

A feeding jejunostomy is placed using a needle catheter kit (Compat Biosystems, Minneapolis, Minn.). After the ligament of Treitz is identified, and insufflation pressure is reduced to 10 mm Hg, a 40 cm distal limb of jejunum is tacked to the anterior abdominal wall. An additional 10 mm port may be placed in the right lower quadrant to facilitate this step. The needle and catheter are passed into the jejunum under laparoscopic vision, and proper positioning of the catheter is confirmed by observing distension of the jejunum as air is insufflated into the catheter. The jejunum is then sutured to the anterior abdominal wall in four quadrants, and a single antitorsion suture is placed approximately 1 cm distal to the jejunostomy. After complete hemostasis is achieved, and sufficient mobilization of the gastric conduit is confirmed, the abdominal wounds are closed, and the patient is turned to the left lateral decubitus position for the thoracoscopic portion of the procedure.

The surgeon stands to the back of the patient, and the assistant stands to the front. Five thoracoscopic ports are placed (Figure 3): a 10 mm camera port for a 45-degree thoracoscope, guided by the first assistant's nondominant hand, is placed in the seventh or eighth intercostal space, just anterior to the midaxillary line. A 10 mm port for the surgeon's dominant-hand instruments is placed at the eighth or ninth intercostal space, posterior to the posterior axillary line, and is used for the ultrasonic shears. This port will be extended later as an access port to remove the surgical specimen. A 10 mm port is placed in the anterior axillary line at the fourth intercostal space and is used to insert a fan-shaped retractor to retract the lung anteriorly and expose the esophagus. Inferior to this, an additional 5 mm anterior port, for the first assistant's nondominant-hand instruments, is placed and used for suction. The last port (5 mm) is placed just anterior to the tip of the scapula and is used for retraction by the surgeon's nondominant hand. The surgeon can retract the specimen using the nondominant hand and can dissect using the ultrasonic shears with the dominant hand, while the first assistant holds the camera in his or her nondominant hand to provide exposure using the suction in his or her dominant hand.

A key initial step is to place a retracting suture through the central tendon of the diaphragm; this suture is brought out through the anterior chest wall via a 1 mm incision, and it retracts the diaphragm inferiorly and anteriorly to allow excellent visualization of the crural diaphragm and esophagogastric junction. The inferior pulmonary ligament is then divided, and the mediastinal pleura is opened anteriorly to expose the pericardium.

When performing MIE for malignancy, it is critical to resect all surrounding periesophageal lymphatic tissue en bloc with the specimen. The anterior dissection is carried superiorly, taking care to identify and protect the membranous right and left bronchi and trachea during removal of the subcarinal lymph node packet. The azygos vein arch is isolated and divided with an endoscopic vascular stapler, and all dissection proximal to the azygos arch is performed directly on the esophageal wall to prevent injury of the recurrent laryngeal nerve. The vagus nerve trunk is usually divided in this region. The posterior aspect of the esophageal mobilization is then performed by opening the mediastinal pleura within the subtle groove located anterior to the azygos vein, distal to the arch. All aortoesophageal vessels encountered during this portion of the procedure should be clipped prior to division. The thoracic duct is not included in the resected specimen, and any lymphatic branches arising from the thoracic duct are meticulously clipped and divided to prevent chylothorax. If injury of the thoracic duct is a concern, this structure can be ligated en masse at the level of the diaphragm.

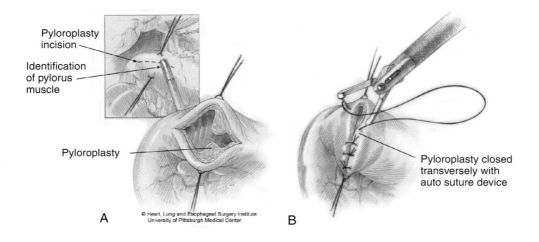

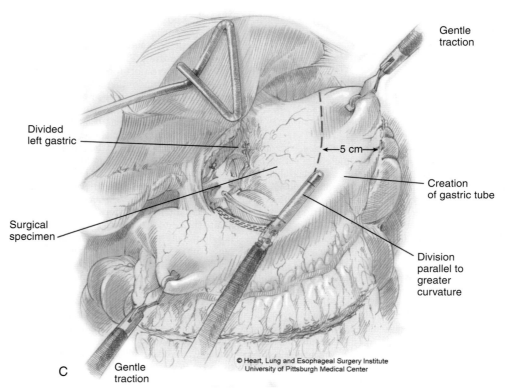

FIGURE 2 **A** and **B**, Pyloroplasty. **C**, Construction of the gastric conduit. *(Copyright Heart, Lung, and Esophageal Surgery Institute, University of Pittsburgh Medical Center.)*

After circumferential mobilization of the esophageal hiatus is performed, the esophagogastric junction with the attached conduit is pulled into the thoracic cavity, ensuring correct orientation by visualizing the staple line of the neoesophagus. Redundancy of the gastric conduit should be avoided. The neoesophagus is detached from the surgical specimen, and the remaining attachments between the specimen and contralateral pleura are divided (i.e., the medial circumferential margin). A limited thoracotomy incision (4 cm) is created at the site of the surgeon's dominant-hand port, and a wound protector is placed. The proximal esophagus is divided at the level of the azygos arch, ensuring that the site of division is proximal to the squamocolumnar junction in patients with long-segment Barrett's esophagus. The specimen is removed, and the lymph node packets are dissected and individually labeled.

The anvil of a 28 mm circular stapler is placed transthoracically through the minithoracotomy incision into the esophageal stump and secured into position with two purse-string sutures. A gastrotomy is performed along the staple line of the gastric conduit for placement of the circular stapler. The stapler is inserted through the minithoracotomy into the conduit, and the spike is deployed through the wall immediately along the greater curvature. The neoesophagus should be positioned such that there is no redundancy or tension. The anvil and stapler are engaged, and the anastomosis is created (Figure 4, *A*). After the stapler is removed, it is important to verify that the stapler contains two complete tissue rings, as this indicates that a complete circumferential anastomosis has been established. The gastrotomy is closed with a 3.5 mm linear stapler (Figure 4, *B*). A nasogastric tube is positioned through the anastomosis under direct visualization. The

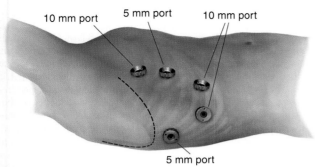

FIGURE 3 Thoracoscopic port placement. *(From Tsai WS, Levy RM, Luketich JD: Technique of minimally invasive Ivor Lewis esophagectomy, Op Tech Thorac Cardiovasc Surg 14[3]:176–192, 2009.)*

conduit is sutured to the right crus to prevent intrathoracic herniation of abdominal viscera. A closed-suction drain (Jackson-Pratt) is placed behind the anastomosis, and a 28 Fr chest tube is placed posteriorly for chest drainage; the tube exits through the camera port (Figure 4, *C*).

Results

Minimally invasive Ivor Lewis esophagectomy is technically feasible and is associated with excellent outcomes. This technique minimizes the degree of gastric mobilization, almost eliminates recurrent laryngeal nerve injury and pharyngeal dysfunction, and allows for an additional gastric resection margin in the case of cardial extension of the gastroesophageal junction tumor. Bizekis and colleagues (2006) reported that the median stay in the ICU after minimally invasive Ivor Lewis esophagectomy was 1 day. The median hospital stay was 7 days, and the mortality rate of the procedure was less than 6%. The surgical margins were negative in 98%, and anastomotic leak occurred in 6%.

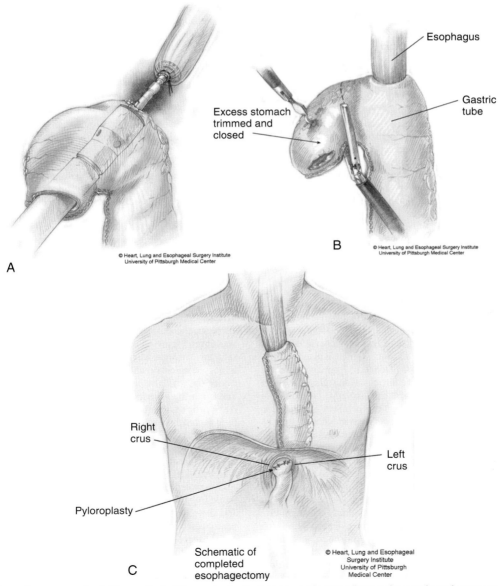

FIGURE 4 Intrathoracic anastomosis. **A,** The anvil of a 28 mm stapler is placed transthoracically into the esophageal stump, and the circular stapler is placed through the gastrotomy on the gastric conduit. **B,** The gastrotomy is closed with a linear stapler. **C,** Schema of completed esophagectomy. *(Copyright Heart, Lung, and Esophageal Surgery Institute, University of Pittsburgh Medical Center.)*

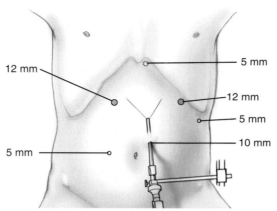

FIGURE 5 Abdominal port placement for minimally invasive transhiatal esophagectomy. *(Illustration by Corinne Sandone, Copyright Johns Hopkins University. Reprinted with permission.)*

MINIMALLY INVASIVE TRANSHIATAL (INVERSION) ESOPHAGECTOMY

Minimally invasive transhiatal (inversion) esophagectomy is a modification of the open inversion technique used for vagal preservation as described by Akiyama. Minimally invasive transhiatal esophagectomy is a totally laparoscopic approach that uses distal-to-proximal inversion of the esophagus assisted by a vein stripper introduced through a cervical esophagotomy. The advantages of this approach are inherent to the dramatic increase in mediastinal work space and improved endoscopic visualization provided as the esophagus is rolled outside-in toward the neck incision. This allows the surgeon to dissect the esophagus efficiently and safely. Additionally, patient repositioning and single-lung ventilation are not required.

Surgical Technique

The patient is placed supine and in a split-legged position, and the surgeon stands between the legs. A six-port technique is used: three 5 mm, one 10 mm, and two 12 mm ports are used (Figure 5). The primary site of access is approximately 15 cm below the left costal margin and 3 cm to the left of midline. A 45-degree laparoscope is introduced through this 10 mm port, and intraabdominal exploration is performed. The second port (12 mm), which is used for the surgeon's dominant-hand instruments, is placed 12 cm from the tip of the xiphoid process, 2 cm below the left costal margin. The third port (5 mm) is placed within the left anterior axillary line along the costal margin. This 5 mm trocar serves as the primary port site for the first assistant. The fourth port (5 mm) is created immediately to the left of the xiphoid process for placement of the Nathanson liver retractor (Cook Medical, Bloomington, Ind.) used to expose the hiatal opening and gastrohepatic omentum. The fifth port (12 mm) is placed inferior to the right costal margin immediately to the right of the falciform ligament. The trocar should enter with a slightly upward trajectory, immediately inferior to the left lateral segment of the liver. This 12 mm port provides access for the surgeon's nondominant-hand instruments and for the endoscopic stapling device. The sixth port (5 mm) is placed in the patient's right midabdomen, and this 5 mm port enables the second assistant to elevate the gastric antrum during mobilization of the greater curvature and the gastric conduit creation.

The hiatal dissection is performed by first opening the gastrohepatic omentum and then extending to the right and left crura to expose the esophagus circumferentially at the hiatus. All lymphatics

posterior to the esophagus are maintained en bloc with the esophagogastric junction. The peritoneum overlying the base of the left gastric artery is opened with the harmonic shears, and all lymphatic tissue is elevated in this region. The left gastric artery is divided at its origin. The common hepatic and celiac arcade dissection is identical to that described for the Ivor Lewis MIE. After division of the short gastric arteries, the posterior stomach is exposed, and the posterior pancreaticogastric fold and posterior gastric artery are divided. The esophagogastric junction is completely mobilized away from the left crus, continuity is established with the right-sided dissection, and the posterior esophageal window is created. The entire gastrocolic ligament is divided distally, preserving the right gastroepiploic artery, and a Kocher maneuver is performed to mobilize the duodenum and head of the pancreas.

When the stomach is completely mobilized, the gastric conduit is created with vagal preservation using the stapler inserted through the surgeon's 12 mm port, beginning approximately 6 cm proximal to the pylorus on the lesser curvature with a 45 mm stapler with a 4.5 mm staple depth (green load), proceeding cephalad along the lesser curvature with a 60 mm cartridge, ultimately resulting in a 5 cm wide gastric conduit. During conduit creation, the stomach is retracted and positioned in an identical manner to that described for the Ivor Lewis approach.

Next, a 5 cm incision is made along the anterior border of the sternocleidomastoid, and the platysma muscle is divided. The sternocleidomastoid is mobilized laterally, and the omohyoid muscle is divided. The carotid sheath should be retracted laterally, and the fascia medial to the carotid artery is opened sharply. The superior mediastinum should be easily accessed by placing a finger along the anterior spine and using blunt dissection to open this space, then the cervical esophagus is circumferentially mobilized. A vein stripper is passed distally through a cervical esophagotomy. With the nasogastric tube withdrawn, a small gastrotomy is created at the staple line. The vein stripper is passed through this opening and withdrawn through the 12 mm right upper abdominal port site (Figure 6, A). A medium anvil is attached to the vein stripper, and a 60 cm silk suture is tied to the end of the vein stripper, which is withdrawn into the peritoneal cavity. The staple line and enterotomy site are reinforced with a horizontal mattress suture. The vein stripper is withdrawn through the cervical esophagotomy, creating an outside-to-in inversion of the distal esophagus (Figure 6, B). The rolled edge of the esophagus is grasped, and mediastinal attachments are divided under direct vision (Figure 7). Lymphatics are included within the inversion, and blunt transcervical finger dissection is used to complete the inversion.

Next, the esophagus is divided at the site of the cervical esophagotomy (Figure 8), and the proximal margin of the esophagus is sent for intraoperative histologic examination. A 26 Fr chest tube is passed into the abdominal cavity through the cervical incision under the guidance of the silk suture brought up in the inversion. The tip of the gastric conduit is sutured to the end of the chest tube. After proper orientation of the gastric conduit is verified, the chest tube is gently withdrawn, and the gastric conduit is gently pulled into the cervical wound (Figure 9). It is important to push the conduit from below during this process to eliminate tension and ensure an equivalent distribution of conduit throughout the posterior mediastinum.

A stapled, end-to-side cervical anastomosis is performed. The staple line of the lesser curvature resection site is rotated posteriorly, and the gastric conduit is elevated to the skin level using a traction suture placed at the inferior aspect of the cervical incision. A vertical gastrotomy is created, and a 3.5 mm stapling device is introduced into the esophagus and gastrotomy and fired, thereby creating an end-to-side anastomosis. A nasogastric tube is then carefully passed into the conduit. The remaining enterotomy is closed in two layers, and a closed-suction drain is placed alongside the anastomosis; the surgeon must take care to ensure that the suction holes are not directly over the suture line.

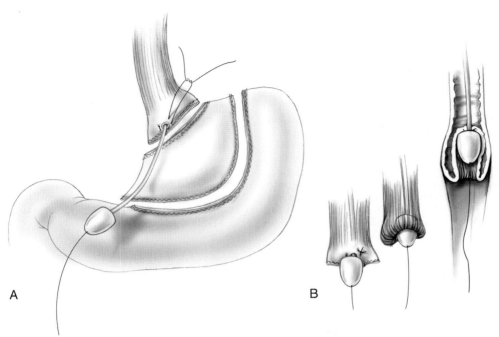

FIGURE 6   Esophageal inversion. **A,** The vein stripper exits through a small enterotomy in the gastric stump, buttressed by a horizontal mattress suture. **B,** The stripper is then pulled cephalad, inverting the esophagus. *(Illustration by Corinne Sandone, Copyright Johns Hopkins University. Reprinted with permission.)*

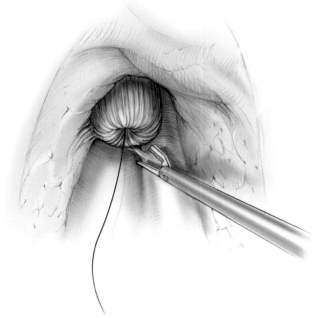

FIGURE 7   Division of the mediastinal attachment. A small posterior attachment is tented up by the inversion and can be divided under direct vision. *(Illustration by Corinne Sandone, Copyright Johns Hopkins University. Reprinted with permission.)*

Results

Recently, Perry and colleagues (2009) reported that minimally invasive transhiatal (inversion) esophagectomy is a safe and effective approach to esophageal resection with low rates of mortality and morbidity. Median ICU stay after minimally invasive transhiatal (inversion) esophagectomy was 2 days, median total hospital stay was 9 days, and the rate of recurrent nerve injury was 10%. The learning curve for this approach is approximately 10 operations in the hands of esophageal surgeons with advanced laparoscopic expertise. Perry and colleagues suggested, based on their experience, that minimally invasive transhiatal (inversion) esophagectomy is a complementary approach, best used for patients with high-grade dysplasia and early invasive cancer, while the thoracoscopic-laparoscopic approach can be reserved for more advanced esophageal cancer with or without neoadjuvant chemotherapy.

Postoperative Care

At our institution, all patients who undergo minimally invasive Ivor Lewis esophagectomy are observed overnight in the ICU, and every effort is made to extubate the patient in the operating room. Prior to extubation, therapeutic bronchoscopy is performed. Patients should be kept in reverse Trendelenburg position to minimize the possibility of aspiration with free reflux. It is crucial to correct electrolytes, especially potassium and magnesium, to prevent postoperative arrhythmia. On postoperative day (POD) 2, tube feeding through a jejunostomy tube is started at 30 mL/hour from 3 PM to 9 AM, and the rate of tube feeding is increased gradually to meet the goal rate by the time the patient is discharged. The jejunostomy tube and the nasogastric tube are flushed with small amounts of saline at each nursing shift to ensure patency, and the nasogastric tube can be removed if the output is less than 150 mL/day and the patient can make a good cough to prevent aspiration. The chest tube can be removed if the output is less than 250 mL/day and the fluid is not chylous. A Gastrografin swallow is performed on POD 4 or 5. The anastomosis is inspected for leak or stricture, and the entire conduit is inspected for leak, anatomical features, and emptying. If this swallow test is negative, patients are started on 30 to 60 mL clear fluid by mouth every 1 to 2 hours. Deep vein thrombosis prophylaxis, pulmonary toilet, and early mobilization must be considered. The patient is discharged with the ability to consume sips of liquid, tube feeding at the goal rate, and a Jackson-Pratt drain, and followed in 2 weeks at the clinic. This postoperative care protocol can be used for all types of MIE.

FUTURE PERSPECTIVE

MIE is technically feasible and can be performed as safely as conventional esophagectomy with fewer postoperative complications. However, esophagogastric anastomotic leakage is a life-threatening postoperative complication, even more so if the leakage occurs in the chest. A prospective, randomized study by Bhat and colleagues (2006) showed that pedicled omental transposition to reinforce the anastomotic suture line significantly reduced the incidence of leakage, thus decreasing the morbidity and mortality of the procedure.

Several methods have been suggested to improve perfusion, because impaired perfusion plays a significant role in the development of anastomotic leakage. It has been suggested that preoperative gastric ischemic conditioning by ligation of the left gastric vessels prior to esophagogastrectomy may decrease the rate of leakage and stricture. Experimentally, the administration of exogenous pharmacologic agents, such as vascular endothelial growth factor, has been tested as another potential strategy; however, the oncological safety of this approach has been questioned. New approaches to MIE are also under investigation. Recently, based on our experience with minimally invasive transhiatal (inversion) esophagectomy, we have attempted a transoral incisionless approach on large animal models.

SUMMARY

MIE is technically feasible and can produce therapeutic outcomes comparable to open surgery. Minimally invasive approaches can provide patients with reduced morbidity and a rapid recovery. MIE should be performed in centers with extensive experience in advanced minimally invasive esophageal surgery. Additionally, the effect on quality of life and any advantages to open surgery will need to be investigated further.

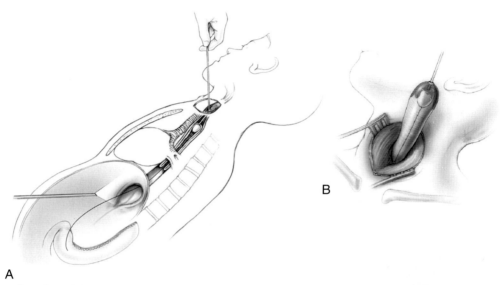

FIGURE 8   Course of esophageal inversion. **A,** Sagittal section showing the course of the esophageal inversion. **B,** Inverted esophagus as it is delivered through the cervical incision. *(Illustration by Corinne Sandone, Copyright Johns Hopkins University. Reprinted with permission.)*

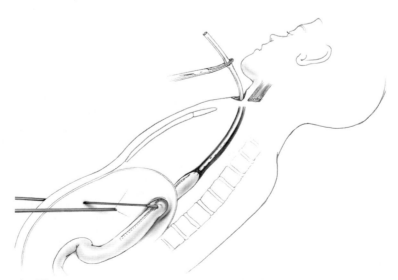

FIGURE 9   Pull-up of gastric conduit. The gastric conduit, attached to a chest tube, is guided through the mediastinum as the chest tube is gently pulled through the cervical incision. *(Illustration by Corinne Sandone, Copyright Johns Hopkins University. Reprinted with permission.)*

SUGGESTED READINGS

Luketich JD, Alvelo-Rivera M, Buenaventura PO, et al: Minimally invasive esophagectomy: outcomes in 222 patients, *Ann Surg* 238:486–495, 2003.

Kent MS, Schuchert M, Fernando H, et al: Minimally invasive esophagectomy: state of the art, *Dis Esophagus* 19:137–145, 2006.

Bizekis C, Kent MS, Luketich JD, et al: Initial experience with minimally invasive Ivor Lewis esophagectomy, *Ann Thorac Surg* 82:402–407, 2006.

Perry KA, Enestvedt CK, Diggs BS, et al: Perioperative outcomes of laparoscopic transhiatal inversion esophagectomy compare favorably with those of combined thoracoscopic-laparoscopic esophagectomy, *Surg Endosc* 23:2147–2154, 2009.

Orringer MB, Marshall B, Lannettoni MD: Eliminating the cervical esophagogastric anastomotic leak with a side-to-side stapled anastomosis, *J Thorac Cardiovasc Surg* 119:277–288, 2000.

Akiyama H, Tsurumaru M, Ono Y, et al: Esophagectomy without thoracotomy with vagal preservation, *J Am Coll Surg* 178:83–85, 1994.

Watson DI, Davies N, Jamieson GG: Totally endoscopic Ivor Lewis esophagectomy, *Surg Endosc* 13:293–297, 1999.

LAPAROSCOPIC REPAIR OF PARESOPHAGEAL HERNIAS

Steven P. Bowers, MD, and Horacio J. Asbun, MD

CLINICAL PRESENTATION

A hiatal hernia is found in up to 40% of adult Americans, however a paraesophageal hernia (PEH) is present in only 5% of patients with hiatal hernia. These hernias have been classified anatomically, with *paraesophageal hernia* defined as a hiatal hernia where the fundus of the stomach lies in the mediastinum, cephalad to the gastroesophageal junction (GEJ) (Figure 1). The natural history of hiatal hernia is that of progressive enlargement, with large sliding hiatal hernias (type I) eventually becoming mixed paraesophageal and sliding hernias over time (types III and IV). A type IV hiatal hernia denotes intrathoracic stomach with additional viscera through the hiatal defect. The type II hiatal hernia, which is classified as purely paraesophageal, is extremely rare and likely represents a variant of parahiatal hernia, which is also an uncommon occurrence.

PEH has a 3:1 female predominance, and its prevalence increases with age. PEHs are associated with obesity and kyphoscoliosis. More importantly for the surgeon, a PEH is a hiatal hernia in which the peritoneal hernia sac is not reducible with traction at operation and therefore must be surgically dissected and excised. The presence of the fixed hernia sac is also responsible for the unique presentation of patients with PEH.

Because the angle of His may be reconstituted above the diaphragm, the majority of patients with PEH do not complain of heartburn or regurgitation, although many will admit to a history of severe gastroesophageal reflux disease (GERD) symptoms in the past that improved or resolved over recent years. Because of angulation of the distal esophagus and compression by the fundus of the stomach, dysphagia is a common complaint. Relative obstruction of the stomach at the hiatus may create gas trapping or retention of particulate matter and may cause left chest pain or emesis, the most common complaints, present in 50% and 40% of patients, respectively.

The presence of a fixed mediastinal sac in PEHs creates the potential for incarceration of the stomach or other viscera in the defect. In large PEHs, more than half of the stomach herniates into the mediastinal sac. For that to happen, the stomach must twist either counterclockwise over an axis of the esophagus and pylorus (organoaxial volvulus), or alternatively, the antrum must flip either anteriorly or into the lesser sac (mesenteroaxial volvulus). Twenty percent of patients with PEH are identified as having volvulus at presentation. Early studies identified a high risk of catastrophic gastric volvulus and prompted repair of incidentally identified PEH for many years. Based on larger population studies, it has been clarified that acute gastric volvulus and strangulation are rare and generally occur in symptomatic patients. Additionally, this complication appears exclusive to patients with volvulus and is much more likely with mesenteroaxial volvulus. Urgent operation is only required in 5% of patients undergoing repair.

The Borchardt triad consists of retching without emesis, failure to pass a gastric decompression tube, and chest pain. This triad is associated with acute volvulus and requires emergent operation if the stomach cannot be promptly decompressed and the volvulus reduced. Organoaxial volvulus is surprisingly well tolerated in many patients, and if asymptomatic in elderly patients, they may be observed. The incidental finding of a retrocardiac air-fluid level on upright chest

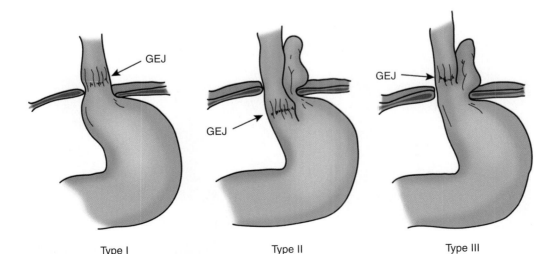

Type I   Type II   Type III

FIGURE 1   The classification of hiatal hernias is based on the position of the GEJ and the relationship of the fundus to the GEJ.

radiograph (Figure 2) is a common means of identifying an asymptomatic PEH with organoaxial volvulus.

Repetitive raking of the stomach over the crural edge with respiration can create erosion of the gastric body or fundus. These erosions are termed *Cameron ulcers*. Severe anemia from occult blood loss, or even acute upper gastrointestinal (GI) hemorrhage, is the indication for operation in 25% of patients with PEH. Although GI hemorrhage can be usually controlled via therapeutic endoscopy, the presence of either acute or chronic GI bleeding due to Cameron ulceration is an indication for surgical repair.

NONOPERATIVE MANAGEMENT

Although elective operative repair of PEH has been found to be safe and effective in numerous studies, selected minimally symptomatic patients may opt for conservative management. From a review of population studies, it has been estimated that the annual probability of developing acute symptoms is just over 1% per year, with a small reduction in quality-adjusted life-years for elderly asymptomatic patients undergoing repair. It has been calculated that if surgery for asymptomatic patients were to be performed, only one out of five patients would benefit at an age greater than 65 years, and only one

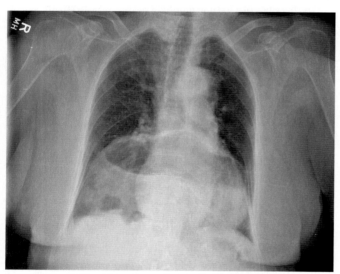

FIGURE 2   Finding of a retrocardiac air-fluid level on chest radiograph is consistent with paraesophageal hernia.

out of ten patients at an age greater than 85 years would benefit. Watchful waiting is a reasonable alternative for the initial management of patients with asymptomatic or minimally symptomatic PEH.

It is important to point out, however, that even for asymptomatic patients, watchful waiting may make a subsequent operation much more difficult if the hernia progressively enlarges over time. Therefore, when following these patients conservatively, progressive increase in size of a hernia should also be taken into consideration in the decision-making process.

PATIENT EVALUATION

The evaluation of patients suspected of having PEH should consist of upper GI contrast study, principally to confirm the diagnosis, assess the extent and type of hernia, and for preoperative planning (Figure 3). An upper endoscopy can be challenging in patients with mesenteroaxial volvulus but should be performed to exclude dysplastic Barrett esophagus. Ambulatory pH testing is not an essential part of the preoperative evaluation, as many symptoms of PEH are not related to reflux. Esophageal stationary manometry can only be performed in one quarter of PEH patients, and although an esophageal motility study can be assessed without passing the probe into the stomach, the motility study has only a limited effect on the operation, as ineffective esophageal motility is identified in fewer than 5% of patients with PEH, compared to more than 10% of patients with type I hiatal hernia and GERD. A gastric emptying study is also difficult to interpret in the setting of an intrathoracic stomach, therefore it plays little role in the physiologic evaluation of patients with PEH.

GOALS OF SURGICAL REPAIR

The goals of surgical repair of all hiatal hernias should be the same: creation of sufficient length of intraabdominal esophagus, closure of the hiatal defect, and reconstruction of the gastroesophageal antireflux barrier. The surgical repair of a PEH brings additional challenges beyond that of a type I hiatal hernia because of the more technically difficult excision of the sac, reduction of herniated contents, and closure of the larger crural defect. The authors favor a laparoscopic transabdominal approach to repair of PEH because of the decreased morbidity of the approach as well as other advantages inherent in minimal access surgery. Visualization and esophageal mobilization are facilitated by the laparoscopic approach compared to an open operation, however, population studies reveal that open and transthoracic repair techniques are still prevalent in America.

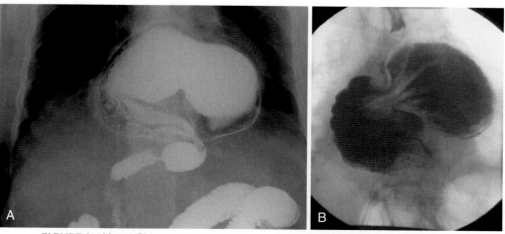

FIGURE 3   Upper GI contrast study. **A,** Organoaxial volvulus. **B,** Mesenteroaxial volvulus.

SURGICAL TECHNIQUE

Preparation and Patient Positioning

On a split-leg bed, the patient is positioned supine with the surgeon standing between the outstretched legs. Alternatively, the surgeon may stand to the patient's right side. An optically guided trocar is placed through the left rectus muscle 15 cm from the xyphoid and serves as the camera port, and additional ports are placed just inferior to the costal margins. Five trocars are utilized, with the liver retractor through the left costal margin and affixed to a table-mounted arm.

Reduction of the Sac

The short gastric vessels are first divided with ultrasonic shears to expose the base of the left crus and fully mobilize the fundus of the stomach (Figure 4). Using scissors with cautery, the leading edge of the peritoneum overlying the left pillar of the crus is divided from the base of the left crus in a counterclockwise direction around the hiatus. The hepatogastric ligament is then opened widely, dividing the hepatic branch of the vagus nerve if necessary to expose the base of the right crus. The peritoneum at the leading edge of the right pillar of the crus is similarly divided in a clockwise direction up to the apex of the hiatus. A posterior window is dissected under direct visualization in the avascular space at the six o'clock position of the hiatus, and a 6 inch Penrose drain is placed to encircle the hiatal contents, including both vagus nerves (Figure 5).

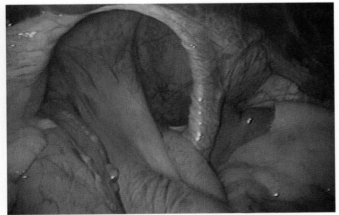

FIGURE 4 Hiatal hernia demonstrating anchoring of the fundus by the hernial sac, which prevents further reduction of the stomach into the abdomen.

Next, the sac is separated from the crural muscle and pleura and is delivered into the abdomen. Once the sac is reduced into the abdomen, the Penrose drain enables esophageal retraction and ensures the vagus nerves are kept against the esophagus to avoid injury. The sac is excised from the attachments to the fundus; the right-sided sac contains the lesser curve mesentery of the stomach and cannot be fully excised. It is not uncommon to have a posterior lipoma of the sac, which must be completely mobilized along with the sac to completely free the esophagus and fundus of the stomach from its posterior attachments.

Esophageal Mobilization

The mediastinal esophagus should be mobilized until the GEJ remains comfortably in the abdomen without tension. It is preferred to proceed from the 6 o'clock position in both clockwise and counterclockwise directions, and it is essential to identify both pleura and bluntly separate the pleura from the hernia sac. Blunt dissection aided by the ultrasonic shears enables dissection routinely to the level of the mid to upper pericardium. Adequate esophageal mobilization is ensured when, after closure of the hiatus, more than 3 cm of esophagus lies below the diaphragm without caudal traction. Endoscopy is recommended in cases of high mediastinal dissection, both to assess for esophageal injury and to definitively identify the location of the GEJ.

If the esophagus has been mobilized as high as possible into the mediastinum, and length assessment reveals inadequate esophageal length, the surgeon should consider Collis gastroplasty as an esophageal lengthening procedure. It is imperative to mobilize the esophagus such that the GEJ lies comfortably below the diaphragm, even when Collis gastroplasty is to be performed, as the fundoplication must include the GEJ. Transthoracic esophageal mobilization or even unilateral vagotomy can be used if required to reduce the GEJ below the diaphragm (Figure 6).

Crural Closure

Crural closure should be accomplished with permanent suture, until the crura approximate the empty esophagus without constriction. A combination of interrupted simple and mattress sutures with cardiovascular pledgets is preferred. The stitches are started at the base of the crura. Because the late results of the Australian randomized trial (Wijnhoven et al, 2008) revealed fewer patients with dysphagia with some component of anterior crural closure, consideration is given to place at least one anterior suture, if more than three sutures are required for closure. In this way, the anterior left crus becomes the arch of the hiatus, and the esophagus is allowed to lie in a more anatomical position. Technical tips for a successful tension-free repair include decreasing the pneumoperitoneum pressure significantly when placing and tying the crural stitches, making sure that the hernia sac has been completely dissected from

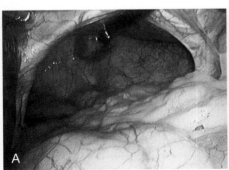 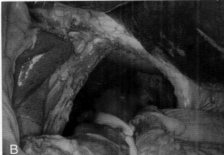 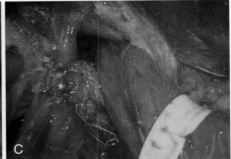

FIGURE 5 Intraoperative photos show a large hiatal defect. **A,** Prior to sac dissection. **B,** After sac dissection and excision, a Penrose drain has been passed around the gastroesophageal junction. **C,** After defect closure.

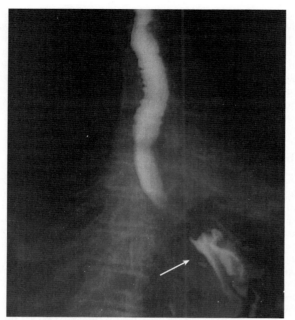

FIGURE 6 Postoperative upper GI study showing the fundoplication and gastroesophageal junction below the diaphragm.

fundoplication than preoperative evaluation. Regarding the use of a bougie, because the Portland randomized controlled trial (Patterson et al, 2000) showed a decrease in dysphagia with a bougie dilator for calibration of the Nissen fundoplication, the use of an 18 mm equivalent bougie or balloon dilator is recommended.

Gastropexy

Numerous techniques for gastropexy are available, and no data support one technique over another. Although the fundoplication serves some gastropexy function, surgeons may perform additional gastropexy to the crura, to the anterior abdominal wall, or by gastrostomy tube. Selective use of gastrostomy may be considered for patients in whom reduction of the hernia sac was more difficult or required extensive manipulation of the stomach, in those requiring urgent operation, or in those in whom adjunctive measures were needed for esophageal shortening. A laparoscopic, percutaneously placed endoscopic gastrostomy is preferred, except for patients in whom a Collis gastroplasty is needed. For those patients, a Witzel-type gastrostomy using a Foley catheter is performed.

Gastropexy is a very good option as the sole treatment for patients with acutely symptomatic mesenteroaxial volvulus, in the elderly, and in patients with multiple comorbidities. This approach has been found to be effective in diminishing the risk of recurrence of acute gastric volvulus. A laparoscopic reduction of the stomach and gastropexy via gastrostomy tubes is recommended for acute volvulus, when the surgeon is not prepared for a definitive repair or the patient would not tolerate it. In such cases, attempts at crural closure will only make subsequent operations more difficult. At least a two-point fixation is necessary in these patients, therefore two or more gastrostomy tubes are placed to avoid recurrence of the volvulus.

Short Esophagus

Several studies advocate routine Collis gastroplasty in PEH repair, and likely this would be expected to reduce the risk of recurrent hiatal hernia. Large series with objective follow-up show radiologic recurrence rates of around 10%. Most large series of selective use of Collis gastroplasty report use of the technique in only 4% to 5% of patients undergoing PEH repair. Furthermore, long-term studies in patients after Collis gastroplasty reveal that GERD-related outcomes are not as satisfactory. This is understandable, as placing the fundoplication around the neoesophagus creates at best a slipped Nissen physiology. A selective use of the Collis gastroplasty is therefore encouraged.

If the surgeon has completed the mediastinal dissection to the extent of instrument reach and laparoscopic visibility and still has insufficient intraabdominal esophageal length, esophageal lengthening is required. A stapled Collis gastroplasty is performed to excise a triangular wedge of stomach at the angle of His and can increase intraabdominal esophageal length by 2 to 3 cm. This is performed by reflecting the fundus inferiorly and using an articulated stapler through a left upper quadrant port site, with a 50 Fr bougie to prevent narrowing of the neoesophagus. A second staple firing is placed parallel to and against the bougie, directed toward the angle of His. Occasionally, in patients with esophageal foreshortening, the gastric cardia is tubularized, and stapled Gastroplasty is not required. It is essential that the subsequent fundoplication include the GEJ to prevent an aperistaltic segment of neoesophagus above the wrap and resultant severe dysphagia from late dilation of the neoesophagus above the wrap.

If the GEJ cannot be delivered to rest below the closed hiatus, and the excessively taut vagus nerves are responsible for limiting the esophageal mobilization, unilateral vagotomy can assist in delivering the GEJ below the hiatus. Otherwise, transthoracic esophageal mobilization is indicated. Fortunately, this is rarely required in initial PEH repairs.

its posterior attachments to the hiatus, preserving the serosal layer of the crura during the initial dissection.

The decision as to whether to place a permanent or biologic mesh buttress is discussed in a later section. If mesh is to be utilized, it is fixed in place as a buttress after the primary crural closure. If the crura cannot be closed, a relaxing incision in the right pillar of the crus into the mediastinal space or the right pleura is recommended. A permanent mesh is then used for interposition, covering the right crural defect. The use of a lightweight polypropylene mesh is recommended, assuring that the caudate lobe of the liver will protect the mesh from contacting the viscera.

Antireflux Operation

Although patients with PEH may not have GERD symptoms preoperatively, 30% will complain of GERD or will have endoscopic evidence of GERD following a PEH repair without an antireflux operation. It is therefore preferred to perform a fundoplication in all patients undergoing repair of PEH. Fundoplication increases the bulk of the GEJ and serves as a buttress to prevent recurrence. Furthermore, the fundoplication can also be anchored by placing a single stitch to each crus, further securing the stomach within the abdomen.

In GERD patients without PEH, esophageal motility has traditionally been used to assess whether a partial or a complete fundoplication is to be considered. It was discussed earlier, however, that in patients with PEH, there is limited value in preoperative esophageal motility testing, mainly because of the low rate of successful transnasal positioning of the motility catheter and an even lower rate of finding meaningful abnormal motility results. An intraoperative assessment of the adequacy of the fundus of the stomach to comfortably create a Nissen fundoplication is a crucial factor in helping decide what type of fundoplications is to be performed. If the fundus is thickened or fibrotic, a complete Nissen fundoplication may increase the risk of postoperative dysphagia. In this situation, a posterior hemifundoplication is to be considered. Thus, the supple or fibrotic nature of the fundus after hernia reduction and repair plays a greater role in determining the appropriateness of complete or partial

Mesh Repair of the Hiatal Defect

The reported use of hiatal mesh during PEH repair has increased, based on reports of high radiologic recurrence following primary hiatal herniorrhaphy and the reduction of this rate when using mesh. It must be stated that irrefutable high-quality evidence has shown that both permanent and biologic mesh reduce the short-term risk of radiologic recurrence. However, complete analysis of the costs and benefits of hiatal mesh can only be performed with additional considerations, including the likelihood of patients with radiologic hiatal hernia recurrence to become symptomatic and require a revision operation. In a similar manner, it is important to consider the difference in the morbidity of a revision operation when comparing reoperation for patients who had initial mesh repairs with those in whom mesh was not used.

Oelschlager and colleagues (2006) performed a multicenter, prospective, randomized trial investigating the use of a U-shaped, small intestine submucosal-based hiatal mesh as an onlay buttress, in comparison with primary suture approximation during laparoscopic PEH repair. Similar to outcomes from randomized studies investigating permanent mesh, the study authors noted that the risk of radiologic recurrence of hiatal hernia was 9%, compared to 24% in the primary repair group at 6-month follow-up. However, at 5-year follow-up, the difference seen at 6 months did not appear to have been sustained, with the two groups showing no significant difference. A similar technique is recommended when mesh is placed, with primary closure of the hiatus followed by posterior buttress of flat biologic mesh fixed to the left and right crural pillars and positioned such that it broadly covers the hiatal closure.

It appears from review of data from the highest volume American centers that 80% of recurrent hernias after nonmesh repair are of the sliding type, and that only about 10% of patients with radiologic recurrence require reoperation. Beyond this, in nonmesh patients there appears to be little correlation between recurrent hernia and recurrent symptoms. However, in a review of early series of patients after permanent and biologic mesh repair of PEH, up to 50% of patients with radiologic recurrence after mesh repair will require reoperation. It is suspected that this may be due to inflammatory adhesions of the mesh causing distortion of the fundoplication and its failure. It is speculated that the quality of the fundoplication may play a more important role in the return of symptoms than the quality of the hiatal repair. Although mesh may reduce the risk of recurrent hiatal hernia, this may be accomplished at the additional cost of GERD-related symptoms that are, at least, transiently increased.

Our reported experience with reoperation after fundoplication failure demonstrates that reoperation in the setting of prior mesh repair is associated with increased morbidity and increased rate of requiring a major esophagogastric resection even with biologic mesh, which is generally not associated with late mesh erosion. Those prior hiatal mesh patients who did not require resection were also less likely to have complete fundoplication at revision. The path to remediation after mesh repair is much more difficult than remediation in patients without mesh because of the difficulty of managing the fibrosis and adhesions caused by the mesh.

The use of biologic or absorbable, nonpermanent mesh is recommended when concern for recurrence is especially high. Such patients may include those who require an esophageal lengthening procedure or those with weak, thin crura, as well as those with large hiatal defects that pose a tense reapproximation, or for patients with prior hiatal hernia recurrences. Additionally, if the surgeon estimates that a patient would not be a candidate for reoperation if anatomic failure were to develop later, that patient would be a better candidate for mesh buttress of the hiatal repair; therefore prior to repairing a hiatal hernia with mesh, the surgeon must weigh the potential benefit of a decreased rate of recurrence against the potential risk of a subsequent major resection.

Obesity and Paraesophageal Hernia

Obesity has been clearly identified as a factor associated with anatomic failure after hiatal hernia repair. In patients with obesity (body mass index >35) and PEH, it is optimal that the patient undergo substantial weight loss prior to operation. The presence of fatty liver disease and visceral obesity significantly add to the difficulty of operation. Weight regain would be expected to increase the risk of subsequent failure after hiatal hernia repair, so consideration must be made for a bariatric operation at the time of PEH repair.

Although laparoscopic sleeve gastrectomy has been reported in a limited number of patients with PEH repair, it should be expected that the tubularized stomach would be reherniated into the mediastinum at some point postoperatively. Until longer term studies of these patients are reported, that approach may be recommended only for selected patients. The Roux-en-Y gastric bypass should be the standard operation for patients with morbid obesity and large hiatal hernia or PEH.

SUGGESTED READINGS

Allen MS, Trastek VF, Deschamps C, et al: Intrathoracic stomach: presentation and results of operation, *J Thorac Cardiovasc Surg* 105(2):253–258, 1993.

Lal DR, Pellegrini CA, Oelschlager MD: Laparoscopic repair of paraesophageal hernia, *Surg Clin North Am* 85(1):105–118, 2005.

Landreneau R, Del Pino M, Santos R: Management of paraesophageal hernias, *Surg Clin North Am* 85:411–432, 2005.

Luketich JD, Nason KS, Christie NA, et al: Outcomes after a decade of laparoscopic giant paraesophageal hernia repair, *J Thorac Cardiovasc Surg* 139(2):395–404, 2010.

Oelschlager BK, Pellegrini CA, Hunter JG, et al: Biologic prosthesis reduces recurrence after laparoscopic paraesophageal hernia repair: a multicenter, prospective, randomized trial, *Am J Surg* 244:481–490, 2006.

O'Rourke RW, Khajanchee YS, Urbach DR, et al: Extended transmediastinal dissection: an alternative to gastroplasty for short esophagus, *Arch Surg* 138(7):735–740, 2003.

Parker M, Bowers SP, Bray JM, et al: Hiatal mesh is associated with major resection at revisional operation, *Surg Endosc* , May 13, 2010:ePub.

Stylopoulos N, Gazelle GS, Rattner DW: Paraesophageal hernias: operation or observation? *Ann Surg* 236(4):492–500, 2002.

Targarona EM, Novell J, Vela S, et al: Midterm analysis of safety and quality of life after the laparoscopic repair of paraesophageal hiatal hernia, *Surg Endosc* 18(7):1045–1050, 2004.

Whitson BA, Hoang CD, Boettcher AK, et al: Wedge gastroplasty and reinforced crural repair: important components of laparoscopic giant or recurrent hiatal hernia repair, *J Thorac Cardiovasc Surg* 132(5):1196–1202, 2006.

Laparoscopic Treatment of Esophageal Motility Disorders

Arman Kilic, MD, James D. Luketich, MD, and Haiquan Chen, MD

OVERVIEW

Esophageal motility disorders can be classified as either primary motility disorders or secondary motility disorders, which are those arising from another disease process. The most common primary motility disorder of the esophagus is achalasia. Spastic or hypercontractile primary motility disorders represent a spectrum of conditions including diffuse esophageal spasm (DES), nutcracker esophagus, and hypertensive lower esophageal sphincter (LES). *Ineffective esophageal motility* is a somewhat vague term that refers to a hypocontractility of the esophagus. Another similar term is *nonspecific esophageal motility disorder;* both are used loosely in the literature and in manometry reports when a patient's esophageal dysmotility does not meet the diagnostic criteria for other, more specific diagnoses.

A multitude of disease processes can lead to secondary esophageal motility disorders. These can be stratified into malignant causes, which include both primary esophageal cancers and metastatic cancers to the esophagus, and nonmalignant causes. Nonmalignant causes include benign esophageal or gastroesophageal junction (GEJ) masses, collagen vascular diseases, neuromuscular diseases, and endocrine disorders, among others. *Pseudoachalasia* refers to conditions in which the manometric findings are indistinguishable from primary achalasia but where there is a clear, secondary cause of the motor dysfunction. For example, long-term severe dysphagia, following a tight Nissen fundoplication or as a result of other nonmalignant conditions, can obstruct the normal peristaltic process of the esophagus to some degree, leading to a "burnout" of the esophageal musculature. This mimics achalasia on manometry but generally has a very different history with a more clear antecedent problem. In this chapter, a brief overview of the current understanding of the pathogenesis, epidemiology, diagnostic approaches, and medical management of esophageal motility disorders is provided. A review of the surgical approaches to these disorders and their associated outcomes is also presented.

PATHOPHYSIOLOGY

The pathogenesis of primary esophageal motility disorders remains incompletely understood. In patients with achalasia, a consistent histologic finding is the destruction of nitric oxide–releasing neurons within the myenteric plexus of the distal esophagus. Nitric oxide release is thought to mediate esophageal peristalsis and relaxation of the lower esophageal sphincter, both of which are abnormal in achalasia. This is coupled with histologic findings of a dense inflammatory infiltrate. Whether these infiltrates represent a primary antigen-driven process or are present secondary to a primary neurodegenerative phenomenon is unclear. A viral insult in susceptible individuals that triggers an autoimmune reaction against myenteric neurons has been postulated as a potential pathophysiologic explanation.

Similar to achalasia, the hypercontractile primary motility disorders are thought to arise from a loss of endogenous nitric oxide. Given its roles in smooth muscle relaxation and peristalsis, it is clear that impaired synthesis or destruction of nitric oxide will lead to unopposed contractile stimuli and associated dysmotility patterns seen in these disorders. Ineffective esophageal motility disorders are postulated to arise from inflammation-related damage resulting from prolonged exposure to an acidic or bile-acid environment, as ineffective esophageal motility disorders are frequently associated with gastroesophageal reflux disease (GERD).

EPIDEMIOLOGY

Primary esophageal motility disorders are rare entities. Indeed, the majority of patients referred for manometry for suspected esophageal disease are found to have normal motility. The most common primary motility disorder of the esophagus is achalasia, which has an estimated incidence of 0.5 to 1 per 100,000 population. As with other chronic diseases, the prevalence of achalasia is higher than its incidence. The incidence of DES is approximately one fifth of that of achalasia. In patients referred for motility studies, approximately 25% to 33% are diagnosed with achalasia, and 4% to 10% are seen with DES. In patients experiencing noncardiac chest pain and found to have a primary esophageal motility disorder on manometry, nutcracker esophagus is the cause in 48%. Nonspecific esophageal motility disorders comprise 36%, DES 10%, hypertensive LES 4%, and achalasia 2%.

CLINICAL PRESENTATION

The classic triad of achalasia includes dysphagia to solids and liquids (present in >95% of patients), regurgitation (present in ~75% of patients), and weight loss (variable). It appears that the epidemic of obesity in the United States and other Western countries has not spared the population of achalasia patients; more and more frequently, we are seeing achalasia in patients who are significantly overweight (body mass index >30). Chest pain is seen in less than half of patients. Symptoms that mimic GERD, as well as bronchopulmonary complications, can also be seen in achalasia. This is due to the stasis of swallowed contents within the esophagus, and it may be more pronounced if the esophagus has become progressively dilated, or if there is significant candidal overgrowth.

DES is characterized by dysphagia to solids and liquids and nonexertional chest pain that is relieved by nitrates. In nutcracker esophagus, chest pain is the principal symptom in approximately 90% of patients. Hypertensive LES is also frequently associated with chest pain, although dysphagia is more commonly seen in hypertensive LES than in nutcracker esophagus. Dysphagia, chest pain, and symptoms of GERD are typically evident in patients with ineffective esophageal motor pathophysiology and, indeed, may be the underlying cause of the ineffective motility due to chronic reflux, inflammation, and damage to the esophageal musculature and innervation.

DIAGNOSIS

The diagnostic modalities used in the evaluation of esophageal motility disorders include, first and foremost, a careful history and physical examination. Once the diagnosis of a motility disorder is suspected, options for testing include esophagogastroduodenoscopy (EGD), barium esophagram, esophageal manometry, and, more recently, esophageal impedance studies. In our practice, all patients with a suspected esophageal motility disorder based on clinical presentation undergo a barium esophagram followed by EGD to rule out masses, peptic strictures, and other pathologies that may be responsible for or contributing to symptoms. In addition to providing insight into esophageal motility, a barium esophagram allows for an inexpensive assessment of associated conditions such as diverticula and hiatal hernias, which could potentially change management and in some cases may uncover abnormal anatomic findings that would increase the risk to the patient during an EGD.

The degree of esophageal body dilatation and deviation of the esophagus from the straight vertical axis can also be evaluated on barium swallow. A characteristic tapering of contrast ("bird's beak") at the GEJ is commonly seen in achalasia (Figure 1, *A*). In DES, the appearance of a "corkscrew" esophagus on barium swallow is frequently evident and aids in diagnosis (Figure 1, *B*). In the presence of a tight stricture or a very dilated esophagus, the approach to an EGD may require more careful preparation to make sure the esophagus is empty prior to sedation and attempted upper endoscopy. In addition, in experienced hands, the esophagram gives an idea of the peristaltic activity, provides a baseline anatomic assessment of the entire esophagus, and may help direct the endoscopist to a particular area of interest.

The gold standard for confirming the diagnosis of an esophageal motility disorder is manometry. The manometric criteria for the diagnosis of achalasia are 1) the absence of coordinated peristalsis and 2) incomplete relaxation of the LES. Although a hypertensive LES may be found, this is not a diagnostic criterion for achalasia; however, this is commonly and mistakenly regarded as a requirement. A subset of achalasia patients may demonstrate characteristics referred to as *vigorous achalasia,* which is essentially a DES-like picture combined with incomplete LES relaxation. DES is diagnosed when 20% or more of wet swallows demonstrate simultaneous contractions in the distal esophagus. Approximately 3% to 5% of DES patients will progress to achalasia.

Nutcracker esophagus is characterized by peristaltic contractions that exceed the 95th percentile in amplitude or are abnormally long in duration. Manometric findings in hypertensive LES include an elevated resting LES pressure with normal LES relaxation and normal peristalsis of the esophageal body. The diagnostic criterion for

ineffective esophageal motility disorder varies to some degree, but ineffective esophageal motility disorder is often diagnosed when 30% or more of wet swallows result in contractions that are either not transmitted or are of low amplitude.

TREATMENT OF ACHALASIA

Overview and Rationale for Surgery

Today, by far the most frequent first-line treatment for achalasia is laparoscopic Heller myotomy and a partial fundoplication, either Dor (anterior) or Toupet (posterior). However, two other therapies have been utilized in the past with some success: botulinum toxin injection (Botox) and endoscopic dilation. In most centers, both of these therapies have fallen into disfavor, given the low morbidity and the superior freedom from dysphagia afforded by laparoscopic Heller myotomy and a partial fundoplication.

In our practice, even in high-risk patients, we almost uniformly perform laparoscopic Heller myotomy as first-line therapy; the only caveat to this is that the most senior, experienced surgeon should be doing the high-risk cases. It should be noted, however, that such assumptions regarding the superiority of laparoscopic Heller myotomy assume the availability of a surgeon experienced in minimally invasive foregut surgery and specifically experienced with achalasia treatment. Unfortunately, this is not always the case, and few centers see enough cases to get past the learning curve inherent in the laparoscopic approach; thus it is essential that prior to surgical referral, the surgeon should be carefully queried for his training and experience in this very specialized area of surgery.

A randomized trial performed in the late 1980s showed that 95% of achalasia patients undergoing surgical myotomy had good or excellent results at 5 years, compared with 65% who had undergone endoscopic dilation. Despite this significant difference, myotomy was adopted with some hesitation as the gold standard therapy in achalasia, in part owing to the risks traditionally associated with open surgery. The emergence of minimally invasive surgery and its association with reduced perioperative morbidity reignited debate as to whether surgery should be considered the preferred treatment for this patient population. Although thoracoscopic approaches have been utilized by some surgeons, by and large this approach has fallen into disfavor by most foregut surgeons, and laparoscopic Heller myotomy has emerged as the clear procedure of choice.

A laparoscopic Heller allows for an adequate myotomy that should extend 2 to 3 cm onto the proximal stomach and 6 to 8 cm proximally onto the esophagus, thereby reducing rates of recurrent symptoms related to impaired esophageal emptying. The role of a partial fundoplication to prevent the associated reflux resulting from a long myotomy of the LES has been recently studied in a randomized trial that demonstrated significant esophageal reflux in 40% of patients without a partial fundoplication, and esophageal reflux in less than 10% if a Dor partial fundoplication was added.

A meta-analysis of six randomized trials comparing Botox to dilation demonstrated that both achieve comparable results for the first 6 months; and although both of these therapies have a higher recurrence rate than myotomy, the recurrence rate within 6 months after Botox was significantly higher (74%) than after dilation (24%). The long-term success rates of endoscopic dilation for achalasia have varied in large series, from 40% to 78% at 5 years. Several large series of laparoscopic Heller myotomy have each reported on over 200 individuals, and the outcomes have been excellent, with success in over 85% of patients. A few reports have examined the long-term (>5 years) outcomes of laparoscopic Heller myotomy for achalasia, and these have shown that it compares favorably with the dilation data. In our experience with 46 achalasia patients with extended follow-up (>5 years), 80% who underwent laparoscopic Heller myotomy experienced continued freedom from dysphagia at a mean follow-up of 6.4 years. This success rate can be improved to near

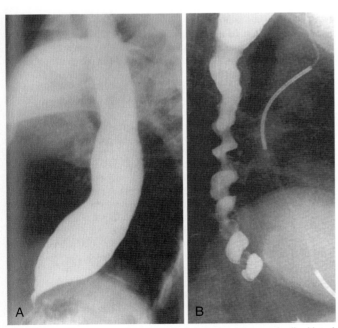

FIGURE 1 Barium esophagrams. **A,** Achalasia with a markedly dilated esophagus and "bird's beak" tapering of the distal esophagus. **B,** The corkscrew deformity that often accompanies DES. (**A,** *From Eubanks WS, Swanstrom LL, Soper NJ [eds]: Mastery of endoscopic and laparoscopic surgery, Philadelphia, 2000, Lippincott Williams & Wilkins p 175.* **B,** *From Bremner CG, DeMeester TR, Huprich JE, et al: Esophageal disease and testing, New York, 2005, Taylor & Francis, pp 27–28.*)

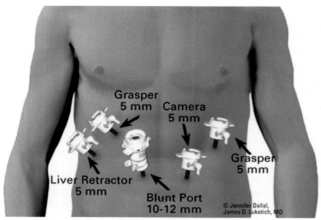

FIGURE 2 Abdominal port placement for laparoscopic Heller myotomy. *(Copyright Jennifer Dallal and James D. Luketich, MD.)*

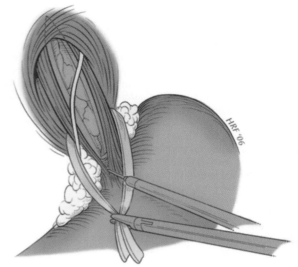

FIGURE 3 Myotomy is performed using ultrasonic shears and blunt dissection. *(From Nussbaum MS: Minimally invasive treatment of achalasia and other esophageal motility disorders. In JE Fischer, KI Bland [eds]: Mastery of surgery, vol I, ed 5, Philadelphia, 2007, Wolters Kluwer/Lippincott Williams & Wilkins. Reprinted with Permission.)*

90% when patients with a very dilated esophagus, who are much more likely to fail myotomy and ultimately require esophagectomy, were excluded.

In our experience, the outcomes of laparoscopic Heller myotomy are to some degree dependent on whether prior endoscopic therapies were utilized. Although not a universal finding of many smaller studies, in a series of 200 patients, we found that those who underwent prior dilation or Botox injections were at a slightly higher risk for myotomy failure. This may be the result of repeated trauma at the LES, causing inflammation and fibrosis and making identification of appropriate tissue planes somewhat more difficult, which increases the risk of an incomplete myotomy and perforation. Other factors that increase the failure rates of myotomy include the presence of a sigmoid esophagus, longer duration of symptoms, and lower preoperative resting LES pressure. These factors are all likely to be interrelated, because patients who are referred for repeated dilations over the course of several years have a longer duration of symptoms prior to surgery, are more prone to develop sigmoid changes as the disease process progresses, and are more likely to have lower LES pressures due to "loosening" secondary to repeated therapies. This has prompted our group, as well as some other surgeons and gastroenterologists, to advocate laparoscopic Heller myotomy as the primary therapy for achalasia in an effort to minimize the time from diagnosis to surgical intervention and optimize the chances of success.

Operative Technique, Tips, and Pitfalls

The patient is positioned supine, placed under general anesthesia, and intubated with a single-lumen endotracheal tube. An initial esophagoscopy is performed, and a "popping" sensation is often felt when passing the instrument through a tight LES; the scope is left in the esophagus for the duration of the operation. The patient is placed in the reverse Trendelenburg position, and the surgeon is positioned on the right of the operating table with the assistant on the left. We place five laparoscopic ports (5 mm) in the epigastric and subcostal areas bilaterally and in the right lateral location (Figure 2). The mediflex liver retractor is placed through the right lateral port and secured to a stationary holding device.

The gastrohepatic ligament is dissected, and the right crus is identified. We use the ultrasonic coagulating shears (US Surgical, Norwalk, Conn.) for the majority of the dissection, but other devices, such as a simple EndoShear (US Surgical) or other ultrasonic dissector, can be equally effective. The phrenoesophageal ligament is identified and divided, exposing the left crus. Following relatively modest anterior crural dissection, and taking care not to injure the vagus nerves, a limited division of the upper short gastric vessels is

performed to allow for appropriate mobilization of the gastric fundus and a tension-free anterior (Dor) fundoplication. The fat pad is then removed from the GEJ in preparation for the myotomy, and the anterior vagus nerve is swept to the patient's right.

The myotomy is initiated by carefully grasping the longitudinal fibers of the esophagus with two endoscopic graspers (Snowden Pencer, Tucker, Ga.), and the muscle is gently separated by careful spreading. This can be supplemented by a variety of maneuvers using the ultrasonic shears, hook cautery, or blunt dissection with the Endo Peanut dissector (US Surgical; Figure 3). It is important not to traumatize the mucosa, especially as the dissection extends onto the stomach. In our experience, the lower 2 to 3 cm of myotomy extension onto the stomach is the most difficult and yet the most important part of a complete myotomy.

The optimal extent of the myotomy has been debated in the literature. We extend the anterior myotomy proximally onto the esophagus for 8 to 10 cm and then extend it distally onto the stomach for 2 to 3 cm. This ensures adequate disruption of the LES barrier and facilitates esophageal emptying. Esophagoscopy is performed routinely to evaluate the completeness of the myotomy. Following the myotomy, the scope view can easily be placed into a "picture in a picture" format (Stryker Endoscopy, San Jose, Calif.), with some overlay onto the standard laparoscopic view, thereby allowing the surgical team to see the effects of the myotomy and a before-and-after assessment. This step is also useful to identify microscopic mucosal perforations. Perforations recognized during this step can be primarily repaired laparoscopically, but if any concern over the adequacy of a repair exists, an open operation should be performed to complete the repair.

Attention is then turned to the fundoplication. In our early experience, we utilized a posterior 270 degree Toupet fundoplication; however, we now prefer the Dor fundoplication for several reasons. In our opinion, the Dor more easily allows construction of a very loose fundoplication and may therefore minimize rates of recurrent dysphagia as compared to the Toupet. We have not noted a higher rate of postoperative reflux in patients receiving a Dor fundoplication compared with our historic cases using the Toupet. In addition, the Dor has the added benefit of covering the exposed mucosa from the myotomy.

The Dor fundoplication begins with a row of three 2-0 silk sutures that incorporate the medial aspect of the gastric fundus, the left edge

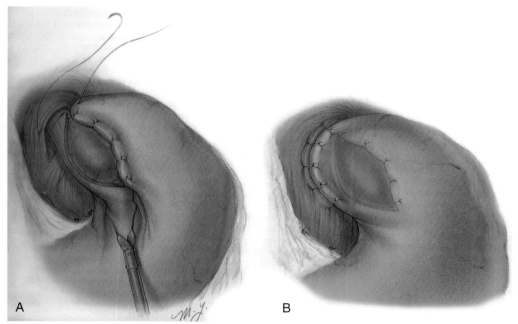

FIGURE 4   Myotomy with Dor fundoplication. **A,** First suture line. **B,** Completed Dor fundoplication. *(Reprinted with permission from Soper NJ, Swanstrom, LL, Eubanks WS [eds]: Mastery of endoscopic and laparoscopic surgery, ed 2, Philadelphia, 2005, Lippincott Williams & Wilkins, p 219.)*

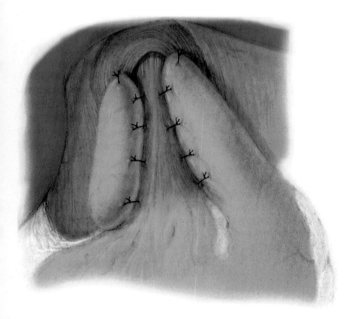

FIGURE 5   Toupet fundoplication. *(Reprinted with permission from Soper NJ, Swanstrom, LL, Eubanks WS [eds]: Mastery of endoscopic and laparoscopic surgery, ed 2, Philadelphia, 2005, Lippincott Williams & Wilkins, p 209.)*

of the myotomy, and the left crus (Figure 4). The apex of the fundus is anchored with a stitch to the anterior aspect of the right crus. The stomach is then folded over the exposed mucosa, such that the greater curvature is alongside the right crus. A second row of three 2-0 silk sutures is placed that incorporate the gastric fundus, the right edge of the myotomy, and the right crus. The patency of the partial wrap should be assessed by again passing the endoscope to ensure that the wrap is not too tight.

A Toupet fundoplication is a 270-degree posterior fundoplication performed by first passing the posterior fundus through the retroesophageal window (Figure 5). Interrupted sutures incorporating the right side of the fundus and the right edge of the myotomy are placed, followed by three to four sutures that incorporate the right side of the posterior fundus and the right crural pillar. Similarly, the left side of the fundus is secured to the left edge of the myotomy with interrupted sutures. The left side of the fundus is also secured to the left crus with interrupted sutures.

Some surgeons advocate performing this wrap over a bougie to calibrate its tightness, and the patency of the GEJ can be assessed thereafter with esophagoscopy. We have concerns about passing a bougie in the setting of a myotomy, therefore we do not recommend this. In addition, we recommend that a nasogastric tube not be placed in the perioerative period because of the risk of mucosal perforation. This fundoplication is different from the Dor in that the mucosa underlying the myotomy remains exposed. On the rare occasion that significant gastric distension develops in the first 12 to 24 hours postoperatively, we would consider performing an endoscopy instead of blind passage of a nasogastric tube.

TREATMENT OF NONACHALASIA MOTILITY DISORDERS

Medical Therapy

Because of their rare incidence, treatment algorithms for nonachalasia primary esophageal motility disorders are based on small series and expert recommendations. As with achalasia, there is no simple "cure" owing to the unknown etiology of these disorders, and treatment is aimed at improving the quality of life and improving dysphagia. Medical therapies for nonachalasia primary esophageal motility disorders include pharmacotherapy, endoscopic Botox injection, and endoscopic dilation.

Multiple pharmacotherapies similar to those used in achalasia have been employed in nonachalasia primary esophageal motility disorders with variable success. Calcium channel blockers have emerged as the principal pharmacotherapy in hypercontractile primary esophageal motility disorders, because they reduce the amplitude and duration of contractions in addition to reducing LES tone.

Because of the reduction in LES tone, aggressive antireflux therapy and monitoring via 24 hour pH studies is also frequently required in patients receiving oral calcium channel blockers. Nitrates have been used because of their ability to reduce chest pain and decrease the amplitude and duration of contractions. The effects of nitrates, however, are short lived. Antidepressants have also been shown to reduce pain in patients with hypercontractile primary esophageal motility disorders, although no effect on esophageal motility has been noted.

Similar to achalasia, Botox injections are utilized as a short-term therapy in patients with other primary esophageal motility disorders. In a study of 15 patients with hypercontractile primary esophageal motility disorders, Botox injection was associated with a good response in 11 patients. However, 120 days after injection, symptom scores returned to their pretherapy levels. Endoscopic dilation is associated with relief of dysphagia in less than 25% of patients with DES. Dilation has also been associated with symptom relief in some cases of hypertensive LES and has been noted to provide temporary subjective relief to some patients with nutcracker esophagus but is generally not effective in this patient cohort, and the preferred medical therapy is calcium channel blockers.

Surgical Therapy

Surgical therapy is typically not used in nutcracker esophagus, because myotomy is associated with symptom relief in only a small percentage of patients. However, in the minority of nutcracker esophagus patients, in whom dysphagia is the principal symptom, a Heller myotomy with partial fundoplication, performed similar to that for achalasia, has been demonstrated to be effective in reducing the symptom burden, and is, therefore, a reasonable therapeutic option in this small subset of patients.

Surgical therapy is more commonly used in DES than in nutcracker esophagus. In our experience, a significant number of patients who are referred to us with the diagnosis of DES or nutcracker esophagus are actually GERD patients who are suffering from esopagheal spasm and nonspecific esophageal motility disorders; thus we strongly recommend that any patient who carries the diagnosis of DES or nutcracker esophagus should have a 48 hour pH study (Bravo study) to assess the DeMeester score and make sure that esophageal spasm in the setting of atypical GERD symptoms is not being missed.

When a myotomy is performed for DES, the extent of the myotomy is controversial. Some surgeons will extend the proximal myotomy as high as the thoracic inlet, others extend it to the aortic arch, and others will perform the myotomy to a similar extent as in patients with achalasia. If the latter is chosen, a laparoscopic approach is reasonable, and in our practice, we would start with this, if the patient's manometry had been repeated in an experienced center, and there was a negative 24- or 48- hour pH study. However, if a long myotomy is needed—that is, if only partial relief could be obtained by doing the longest possible myotomy laparoscopically—we would consider adding a video-assisted thoracoscopic surgery (VATS) myotomy extension in rare cases. The distal extent of the myotomy should include 2 cm or more of the proximal stomach, as in achalasia. As with achalasia, this necessitates a partial fundoplication for reduction of postoperative reflux. Studies reporting on the long-term results of surgery in DES have demonstrated relief of dysphagia and/or chest pain in over 80% of patients.

The indications for and extent of myotomy in hypertensive LES patients is also debated. Again, we would repeat the manometry and perform a 24 hour pH study to rule out esophageal spasm secondary to GERD as the problem before we would consider myotomy. It is unclear whether a limited myotomy across the LES or a myotomy similar in extent to that used in achalasia is superior in this patient cohort. Either approach has been associated with symptomatic relief in small series reporting on surgery for hypertensive LES.

Ineffective esophageal motility disorders are thought to arise from damage related to GERD and may lead to more severe reflux resulting from progressively impaired esophageal emptying. As a result, the principal surgical goal is management of GERD that cannot be controlled by aggressive medical therapy. A central debate is whether to employ a partial fundoplication or a 360-degree Nissen fundoplication. As with other primary esophageal motility disorders, the balance between postoperative dysphagia resulting from a wrap that is too tight and persistent GERD resulting from a wrap that is too loose needs to be weighed. A reasonable approach is to perform a partial fundoplication in patients who have ineffective esophageal motility with dysphagia as the primary symptom or in those with complete aperistalsis of the esophageal body. In all other patients with ineffective esophageal motility, a Nissen fundoplication should be performed for optimal management of the reflux.

TREATMENT OF COMPLICATED ESOPHAGEAL MOTILITY DISORDERS

Morbid Obesity in Association with Achalasia

If a patient is seen with morbid obesity and the diagnosis of achalasia, the surgeon should consider a combined approach to include a myotomy and a small pouch with a Roux-en-Y gastric bypass. This can be a complex operation, which in some cases may be accomplished by resecting the very distal esophagus and performing an esophagojejunostomy in combination with the other steps of the gastric bypass operation. Treatment of these patients requires a multidisciplinary conference with foregut surgeons, bariatric surgeons, gastroenterologists, and bariatricians to determine the best overall care for these complex situations.

Sigmoid Esophagus

The management of sigmoid esophagus in the setting of achalasia merits special attention. The principal controversy is whether to proceed with an esophagectomy or to attempt a myotomy in this patient cohort. Essentially, the morbidity and mortality of esophagectomy need to be weighed against the likelihood that a myotomy will provide durable relief. Published studies and our own experience have demonstrated that the majority of patients (>60%) with a sigmoid esophagus derive significant symptomatic benefit from a laparoscopic Heller myotomy. The choice really boils down to sound surgical judgment and experience, age and performance status of the patient, and the patient's input. For example, in a young (40- to 65-year-old) patient with good performance status and a markedly dilated sigmoid esophagus, we would offer a minimally invasive esophagectomy (MIE), but this is in the context of our published experience of a mortality rate of near 1% for this operation. Overall, we tend to reserve MIE for patients with a markedly dilated esophagus with sigmoid loops or prior surgical failures.

Epiphrenic Diverticula

Epiphrenic diverticula are rare entities occurring in the distal 10 cm of the esophagus. They are thought to arise from esophageal motility disorders in which a pulsion force creates an outpouching of the mucosa through the muscle layer. Surgery is indicated for diverticula that produce significant symptoms. Others also advocate the use of surgery in large (>5 cm) asymptomatic diverticula as a means of preventing serious complications, such as aspiration pneumonia.

The principles of operative management include complete excision of the diverticulum, a Heller myotomy opposite the mouth of the diverticulum, extending onto the cardia of the stomach, and an antireflux procedure. A number of controversies surround this, including approach, extent of myotomy, and type of fundoplication. Several series have been published regarding the minimally invasive approach, the majority of which have been done laparoscopically. In a recent review of the literature, we found that in a cumulative experience of 85 patients, the leak rate associated with laparoscopic and/or VATS management of epiphrenic diverticula was 14%.

In our own experience, we have found that placing a drain near the myotomy site and covering the site with pleura is helpful. Any leak will most likely be small and can be managed by careful observation. The leak rate (14%) after laparoscopic management of epiphrenic diverticula is comparable to the 6% to 18% leak rate published for open Heller myotomy, although these rates are by no means ideal. This is a challenging operation that should be reserved for centers with significant experience in advanced minimally invasive esophageal surgery. We have performed these operations both laparoscopically and thoracoscopically, and in general we prefer to use a VATS approach, as it allows more certainty of complete dissection of the entire diverticulum and allows a clearer view for stapling flush with a bougie placed in the esophagus. Following the diverticulectomy, we generally perform a myotomy in a direction caudad from the diverticulum. Again, flexible endoscopy before and after the procedure will guide the degree of myotomy needed and help rule out the possibility of any leak.

In our experience, laparoscopic diverticulectomies tend to not allow a good, complete dissection of the neck of the diverticum and complete, stapled removal, although admittedly the laparoscopic view allows an easier myotomy and partial fundoplication. In some cases, we will finish the VATS, and then in the same procedure, we turn the patient supine and perform a laparoscopic extension of the myotomy onto the stomach and add a Dor fundoplication. In other cases, especially if the manometry failed to identify a clear diagnosis of a motor disorder, we have used a VATS diverticulectomy followed by a limited myotomy as far distal onto the GEJ as indicated by endoscopy. If this appears adequate from a myotomy standpoint, we may stop at this point, accepting some degree of reflux and adopting a wait-and-see approach to the absolute need for a later extension of the myotomy or addition of a partial fundoplication.

TREATMENT OF SECONDARY ESOPHAGEAL MOTILITY DISORDERS

Secondary esophageal motility disorders are associated with a wide range of disease processes, and therapy is aimed at the underlying cause. Antireflux medications, such as proton-pump inhibitors, are used when GERD symptoms are present. An important secondary esophageal motility disorder that merits discussion is pseudoachalasia, which, as the name suggests, mimics primary achalasia both radiographically and manometrically. Pseudoachalasia is often due to malignancies that infiltrate the myenteric plexus of the distal esophagus or GEJ. This underscores the importance of performing EGD in all patients suspected of having a motility disorder of the esophagus. Additionally, if we identified achalasia physiology that clearly did not exist before a Nissen fundoplication, but rather developed after construction of a tight wrap, we would perform laparoscopic redo fundoplication. This would include complete takedown of the wrap, an on-the-table EGD, a myotomy, and then a partial wrap.

SUMMARY

Esophageal motility disorders represent a spectrum of diseases that often overlap in clinical presentation, highlighting the importance of using various modalities to obtain an accurate diagnosis. Because of the unknown etiology of most esophageal motility disorders, the goal of current treatments is symptom control. Surgery has remained the most successful therapeutic intervention for these patients, and the development of minimally invasive approaches to esophageal disease has led to effective management with a minimization of morbidity. Nonetheless, advances in our understanding of these disorders are needed, and it is hoped that they will result in treatment options that aim to cure rather than palliate.

SUGGESTED READINGS

Csendes A, Braghetto I, Henriquez A, Cortes C: Late results of a prospective, randomized study comparing forceful dilatation and oesophagomyotomy in patients with achalasia, *Gut* 30:299–304, 1989.

Kilic A, Schuchert MJ, Pennathur A, et al: Long-term outcomes of laparoscopic myotomy for achalasia, *Surgery* 146: 826–831, 2009.

Patti MG, Gorodner MV, Galvani C, et al: Spectrum of esophageal motility disorders: implications for diagnosis and treatment, *Arch Surg* 140:442–448, 2005.

Schuchert MJ, Luketich JD, Landreneau RJ, et al: Minimally-invasive esophagomyotomy in 200 consecutive patients: factors influencing postoperative outcomes, *Ann Thorac Surg* 85:1729–1734, 2008.

Schuchert MJ, Luketich JD, Landreneau RJ, et al: Minimally invasive surgical treatment of sigmoidal esophagus in achalasia, *J Gastrointest Surg* 13:1029–1035, 2009.

ACHALASIA

Jeffrey Eakin, MD, and W. Scott Melvin, MD

OVERVIEW

The Greek term *achalasia* means failure to relax. Achalasia is a neurologic illness of the esophagus, which leads to progressive dysphagia, reflux, chest pain, and malnutrition. As the severity of this disease progresses, patients can develop malnutrition, dental decay, and even pulmonary complications from aspirated retained material in the distal dilated esophagus. Achalasia affects approximately 1 in 100,000 people per year, and it can occur at any age and usually has an insidious onset. The two physiologic components that constitute achalasia are an aperistaltic esophagus and a nonrelaxing lower esophageal sphincter (LES). Failure of the LES to relax creates a functional outflow obstruction of the distal esophagus. Although there is no cure for this illness, the preferred therapy to treat the symptoms and clinical sequelae associated with it, for willing and appropriate surgical candidates, is a laparoscopic modified Heller myotomy with a partial fundoplication.

PATHOPHYSIOLOGY

In the late nineteenth century, Leopold Auerbach, a German neuropathologist, discovered a layer of ganglion cells between the inner circular and outer longitudinal layer of gastrointestinal smooth muscle. This plexus of nerves is known as the *myenteric plexus* or the *Auerbach plexus*. Achalasia results from a loss of the inhibitory ganglion cells in the myenteric plexus of the esophagus, which generates an imbalance between excitatory and inhibitory input to the LES. Consequently, the LES remains in a state of excitation and fails to relax during swallowing, which leads to delayed esophageal emptying and, sometimes, trapped food in the distal esophagus. Delayed esophageal emptying generates increased esophageal pressures, which can cause pain and eventually leads to gross dilation, deformity, and elongation of the esophagus. The ensuing clinical consequences of these anatomic and functional abnormalities range from troublesome dysphagia to life-threatening pneumonia and malnutrition.

DIAGNOSIS

A clinical history of dysphagia, retrosternal pain, regurgitation of stagnant food, and weight loss should alert the surgeon to suspect achalasia as a possible diagnosis. Moreover, patients with achalasia may provide a history of pulmonary symptoms such as cough, hoarseness, frequent aspiration, and even pneumonia. Most of these patients will have been treated empirically for gastroesophageal reflux disease (GERD) with little effect. Diseases that mimic achalasia include but are not limited to malignant obstruction, GERD, benign strictures, diffuse esophageal spasm, and nutcracker esophagus. Characteristic chest radiograph findings seen in achalasia include a widened mediastinum, an air-fluid level in the esophagus, an absent gastric air bubble, and concomitant aspiration pneumonia. Any patient with dysphagia should be evaluated with a barium esophagram, which usually shows a dilated esophagus with a "bird's beak" narrowing (Figure 1) at the gastroesophageal junction (GEJ) in individuals with achalasia. A video swallow examination will demonstrate an aperistaltic esophagus, and patients who have had long-standing untreated disease may have an elongated, dilated, and tortuous esophagus known as a *sigmoid esophagus*.

All patients being evaluated for surgery should have esophagoscopy to rule out a mechanical obstruction resulting from carcinoma or other coexisting diseases. Esophagoscopy often reveals retained food in a dilated esophagus, often with significant esophagitis. The LES is tight, but usually the esophagoscope will pass through the GEJ with gentle pressure. Retained food in the esophagus is common in patients suffering from achalasia. The retained substance within the

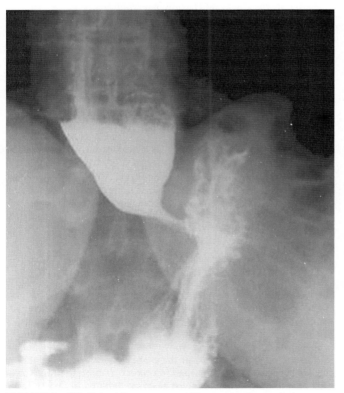

FIGURE 1 "Bird's beak" appearance of lower esophagus during an upper gastrointestinal radiographic swallow study.

esophagus should be cleared prior to an effective and safe endoscopy. Some patients will require hospitalization for 24 to 48 hours or at least a clear liquid diet prior to esophagogastroduodenoscopy to allow complete visualization.

Esophageal manometry is an essential study in the diagnosis of achalasia. Manometry is diagnostic for achalasia in most situations, because it will reveal an absence of peristalsis in the esophageal body and elevated LES pressures with failure of the LES to relax during swallowing. Pressures within the LES are often elevated from baseline and do not relax; however, many patients are seen with relatively normal baseline pressure of the LES but do not demonstrate relaxation. The technical aspects of manometry can be difficult in patients with a dilated or food-filled esophagus, so the data must be interpreted in the context of the entire clinical picture.

MANAGEMENT

Nonsurgical Management

Nonsurgical treatment options for achalasia include pharmacologic therapy, endoscopic botulinum toxin injection, and pneumatic dilation. Although each of these therapies has its own role in the management of achalasia, surgical myotomy carries the lowest rate of recurrence.

Pharmacologic Management

Medical treatment for achalasia should be reserved for individuals who are not candidates for a surgical myotomy. The primary goal of medical management is to alleviate the obstructive symptoms associated with achalasia by lowering the LES pressure via inhibition of smooth-muscle contraction. Unfortunately, pharmacologic management has many limitations, which include their moderate efficacy, inconvenience, poor side-effect profile, and their propensity for tachyphylaxis. The mainstay of medical therapy for achalasia consists of nitrates, calcium channel blockers, and endoscopic botulinum toxin injection. Anticholinergics and β-blockers have also been used for controlling symptoms. Ultimately, all of the aforementioned medications have poor long-term efficacy, because they fail to treat the underlying functional anatomic abnormality.

Nitrates

Organic nitrates have been used in cardiovascular therapy for many years, but various aspects of their pharmacology remain poorly understood. Organic nitrates generate nitric oxide production in smooth-muscle cells, which leads to smooth-muscle relaxation. Their long-term therapeutic effects are limited by the development of pharmacologic tolerance. Headaches and hypotension are common side effects that limit their usefulness in controlling this disease.

Calcium Channel Blockers

Calcium channel blockers block calcium uptake in the smooth-muscle cells of the LES. Traditionally, calcium channel blockers such as nifedipine are taken 30 minutes to 1 hour before mealtime. Rates of symptomatic relief can be up to 50%. However, similar to nitrates, patients who take these medications have a tendency to develop long-term tolerance to their effects, which results in diminished symptomatic control.

Botulinum Toxin Injection

Botulinum toxin is a bacterial neurotoxin that inhibits acetylcholine release from presynaptic cholinergic nerve terminals, which reduces neuromuscular transmission and local muscle activity. Injection of botulinum toxin into the LES reduces the LES resting pressure. Early enthusiasm regarding botulinum toxin injection as an effective long-term therapeutic option for treating achalasia has waned because of its limited period of effectiveness. Individuals undergoing endoscopic injections often require repeat injections. Although 60% to 85% of patients experience significant relief after their initial injection, half of those patients will develop recurrent symptoms within 6 months. Moreover, a major drawback of botulinum toxin injection is that it may scar the GEJ in the submucosal plane, which makes operative intervention more difficult and possibly puts the patient at increased risk for mucosal violation during a future surgical myotomy. Furthermore, gastroesophageal reflux is a substantial and common long-term side effect of treatment. In light of this, endoscopic botulinum toxin injections should be reserved for older patients, those with serious comorbidities that render them unfit for a surgical myotomy, and patients who are unwilling to undergo surgical myotomy or endoscopic pneumatic dilation.

Pneumatic Dilation

Endoscopic pneumatic balloon dilation is the oldest and most effective nonsurgical maneuver used to treat achalasia. In 1672, Sir Thomas Willis described cardiospasm and treated a patient with dilation using a sponge attached to a whalebone. Currently, pneumatic dilation offers the most reasonable remission rates for patients who are unwilling or unsuitable candidates for a surgical repair.

Many institutions use various techniques for endoscopic dilation, and many different balloon dilators are available for this procedure. In general, 30 mm diameter balloons are passed under fluoroscopic guidance through the LES and inflated. The general principle of dilatory therapy is expansion of the LES, resulting in rupture of the muscle fibers of the LES.

The results reported in the literature for endoscopic dilation are variable. Katz and colleges (1998) performed a retrospective analysis of 150 patients who underwent pneumatic dilation. They found a success rate of 91% after a median of 2.6 dilations. However, at 5 and 10 years, the calculated probability of being in remission was 67% and 50%, respectively. Pneumatic dilation is initially effective, but its utility is limited by its short-lived response and need for repeat dilations.

Perforation is the most feared complication of pneumatic dilation. Multiple studies have demonstrated that the risk of perforation is highest during the initial dilation, and risk of perforation ranges from 1% to 15% in the current international literature. Esophageal perforation can usually be treated with total parenteral nutrition and cessation of oral intake, and surgical intervention is rarely required.

Surgical Management

At the present time, surgical therapy is the most definitive treatment for symptoms related to achalasia. The first surgical myotomy was performed nearly 100 years ago by a German physician, Ernest Heller, in 1913; it consisted of two parallel myotomies on the distal esophagus. Five years later, De Brune Groenveldt modified this technique by converting it to a single anterior myotomy. Originally, a Heller myotomy was accomplished through an open approach via a thoracotomy or laparotomy.

Over the past 100 years, innumerable advances in surgical techniques and technology have allowed contemporary esophageal surgeons to approach the standard myotomy via a laproscopic or thoracoscopic approach. Nonetheless, for many reasons we will outline later, laparoscopy has become the standard approach for performing the esophageal myotomy. The advent of minimally invasive approaches to treat achalasia has led to decreased operative times, decreased incisional morbidity, reduced lengths of hospital stay, and quicker return to work in addition to greater relief from dysphagia and prevention of GERD after myotomy.

Thoracoscopic Approach

A number of retrospective analyses demonstrate the limitations of using a thoracoscopic approach to alleviate the symptoms of achalasia. The clinical disadvantages of using this approach include greater postoperative pain and morbidity. The technical drawbacks include difficulty with extending the distal myotomy onto the cardia of the stomach and decreased exposure for performing an antireflux procedure. Inability to extend the myotomy onto the cardia of the stomach leads to an increased incidence of postoperative symptomatic recurrence. Furthermore, patients undergoing thoracoscopic myotomy are more likely to develop postoperative gastroesophageal reflux because of inadequate exposure to perform an antireflux procedure.

In 2004, Abir and colleagues performed a retrospective multivariant analysis of outcomes among individuals who had thoracoscopic or laparoscopic myotomies. Abir found that dysphagia relief occurred in 76% (n = 203) and 94% (n = 499) of patients undergoing thoracoscopic and laparoscopic Heller myotomies respectively. Moreover, they also demonstrated that 35% of patients developed GERD after thoracoscopic myotomy, but only 13% of patients developed similar symptoms after a laparoscopic myotomy. These data, combined with cumulative clinical experience, have caused the laparoscopic approach to emerge as the primary exposure of choice for completing a modified Heller myotomy.

Laparoscopic Approach

Overview

A laparoscopic modified Heller myotomy with partial fundoplication is now the preferred surgical management used to treat the symptoms of achalasia. Laparoscopy has supplanted traditional approaches, such as thoracoscopy, because it offers certain clinical and technical advantages over traditional approaches to a modfied Heller myotomy. Several studies have shown that relapse rates for dysphagia after a laparoscopic modified Heller myotomy may be as low as 8% to 10% up to 9 years after surgery. Luketich and colleagues (2001) performed a retrospective analysis of 46 patients and found that 80% of patients at a mean postoperative time of 6.4 years did not have symptoms of recurrence that required reoperation, and numerous retrospective case series demonstrate similar results. Extending the esophageal myotomy onto the cardia of the stomach increases the efficacy of the myotomy and reduces the long-term risk of developing symptomatic recurrence.

A modified Heller myotomy results in the disruption of the gastrophrenic ligament and in many situations is accompanied by the dissection of the distal esophagus with the possible long-term complication of gastroesophageal reflux. The long-term consequence of this is increasingly recognized as recurrent dysphagia as a result of peptic strictures of the distal esophagus. Often the affected esophagus may not cause significant symptoms, and with a decrease in the sensation of dysphagia early, reflux symptoms are not noticed. Long-term sequelae that include esophagitis, Barrett esophagus, and stricture have been reported. Several series have demonstrated objectively that an antireflux procedure in concert with a Heller myotomy does not decrease effectiveness, and one series suggests that approximately one third of individuals may develop recurrent dysphagia as a consequense of gastroesophageal reflux strictures. Thus we currently recommend performing an antireflux procedure, either a partial posterior or anterior fundoplication, after completion of the standard myotomy (Figure 2).

Telerobotic laparoscopic surgery was introduced in the late 1990s and was quickly applied to the Heller myotomy and other foregut operations. The initial report in 2001 was followed by a multicenter series that described the benefits of the telerobotic approach. These include a stable, three-dimensional visual platform and scalable flexible arms that result in a decreased incidence of intraoperative

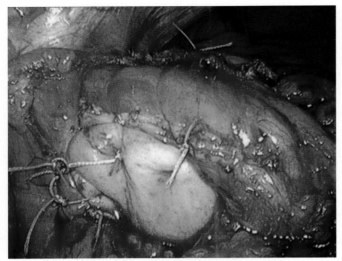

FIGURE 2 Operative completion of the Heller myotomy and posterior 270-degree Toupet fundoplication.

TABLE 1: Risk of Intraoperative Perforation

Study	Patients Treated	Perforations	Percent Perforation Rate (%)
Chapman (2004)	139	19	13.7
Bloomston (2001)	88	8	9.1
Hunter (1997)	40	6	15
Luketich (2001)	62	6	9.7
Sharp (2002)	100	8	8
Finley (2001)	98	1	1
Douard (2004)	52	3	5.8
Melvin (2005)*	100	0	0

*This study included 100 cases performed with computer-enhanced robotic telesurgery.

esophageal mucosal perforation. At centers with the available technology, robotics are regularly utilized for the surgical treatment of achalasia.

Mortality from an esophageal leak is rare following this operation. The most significant risk of surgical myotomy remains a full-thickness esophageal perforation. When identified intraoperatively, the mucosal rent can be repaired with fine absorbable sutures and buttressed with a gastric patch. It is not clear whether this changes the clinical course of the procedure, however, it usually prolongs hospitalization, as most surgeons would withhold oral feeding for a few days. The risk of intraoperative perforation is anywhere from 0% to 13% based on a review of several retrospective case studies (Table 1). Perforations of the esophagus that are not recognized intraoperatively, or that are present in the postoperative period, generally require reoperation; if not treated appropriately, these can result in a life-threatening inflammatory response. Finally, although previous pneumatic dilation and botulinum toxin injection make the surgical dissection more difficult, a myotomy can be performed safely after either of the aforementioned procedures.

Surgical Technique

After the induction of general anesthesia with neuromuscular blockade, the patient is placed in a split-leg position with the arms extended, with preventative measures taken for deep venous thrombosis. Port placement is configured such that the camera port is placed in a supraumbilical midline position. Two working ports are placed in the epigastrium in the midline for the surgeon's nondominant hand and at the midclavicular line for the dominant hand. An additional port is placed for retraction of the left lobe of the liver; this port is placed in the right upper quadrant or immediately below the xyphoid to introduce a mechanical retractor. An additional working port is placed for the surgical assistant along the left anterior axillary line, 2 cm below the subcostal margin, for manipulation of the proximal stomach. During the course of the dissection, the patient is placed in a reverse Trendelenburg position.

Anterior retraction is applied to the left lobe of the liver. The right and left crura are identified, and the dissection is carried down through the gastrohepatic ligament. An aberrant branch of the left hepatic artery can often be seen coursing through the gastrohepatic ligament. Division of an aberrant left hepatic artery is sometimes necessary to allow adequate mobilization of the distal esophagus. Our

approach includes a wide dissection of both crura and a direct visualization of the retroesophageal space. Once the left and right crura are identified, the retroesophageal space is opened, and a soft Penrose drain is placed around the distal esophagus. The remainder of the distal esophagus is mobilized using mostly blunt dissection. We limit the use of electrocautery, or energy directed toward the mediastinum, to prevent esophageal or vagal injury. Next, the dissection should continue posterior on the crura to the level of the decussation to allow complete mobilization of the distal 8 to 10 cm of the esophagus. Ligation and division of the short gastric vessels is usually unnecessary.

Once the esophagus has been fully mobilized, an anterior longitudinal myotomy should be created. Ideally, the myotomy is started approximately 2 cm proximal to the GEJ, where the esophageal muscles are easily visualized. With the hook dissector in the surgeon's nondominant hand and a curved dissector in the dominant hand, dissection can be made directly perpendicular to the esophageal wall down through the wall of the muscle to the mucosal layer. This initial dissection is the most important. Once the submucosal plane is identified, the curved dissector entering from the midaxillary line can be used to develop a plane between the mucosa and the inner muscular layer. Once this plane has been developed, the hook dissector can work superiorly to divide the muscles as far proximal as necessary. Ideally, this dissection should extend 8 cm proximal to the GEJ. At the top of the dissection, the muscle should retract circumferentially around the esophagus.

Next, the myotomy is extended distally onto the anterior stomach. Usually, the esophageal fat pad needs to be dissected free from the GEJ, and any small crossing vessels can also be divided. Clips are sometimes necessary, because some of these vessels can be quite large. It is important to carry the myotomy into the submucosal plane at least 2 cm down onto the anterior stomach. The Z line can be accurately identified by intraoperative endoscopy and by gently placing a lighted tip of the scope at the Z line. Anatomically, it can be identified by the change in the submucosal pattern of the vasculature identified at the Z line. Careful inspection should ensure that there are no perforations of the mucosa underlying the myotomy and that all muscle fibers are divided for the entire length of the myotomy.

After completing the myotomy, closure of the crura is usually necessary, even in patients without an underlying hiatal hernia. Usually a single stitch affords adequate closure of the hiatus. Finally, we perform an antireflux procedure, once the myotomy and crural repair are complete. Most commonly, a Toupet fundoplication is created by dragging a redundant portion of the anterior stomach behind the esophagus in the previously dissected retroesophageal space. The fundoplication is first created by suturing the stomach posterior to the crura, then on the right with two interrupted sutures to the cut edge of the muscle, and then directly opposite approximately 180 degrees in circumference with two sutures placed in the left lateral cut edge of the esophageal musculature.

Intraoperative flexible endoscopy is used liberally, because it allows precise identification of the Z line and thus provides clear evidence that the myotomy has been appropriately placed. Following myotomy, endoscopy can distend the esophageal mucosa and demonstrate any remaining muscle fibers that should be transected to ensure an adequate myotomy and prevent recurrence. Additionally, by air distension and intraabdominal irrigation, as well as close visual inspection, the integrity of the mucosa can be ensured, and latent esophageal perforation can be detected.

When the esophageal mucosa has been injured, it should be repaired primarily using fine absorbable sutures. If the esophageal mucosa has been compromised, an anterior Dor fundoplication should be created. This is accomplished by suturing a redundant portion of the stomach anterior to the esophagus. The fundus is fixed to the left lateral aspect of the esophageal muscle and the crura, and the more redundant portion of the stomach is mobilized to the right and anteriorly, so that the mucosal injury is covered. Two sutures should be placed on each side, incorporating the esophageal wall, crura, and the stomach. Following the completion of the myotomy and final inspection, the fascial defects for port sites larger than 5 mm are closed with suture, local anesthetic is infiltrated into the wound, and the wounds are closed in the appropriate fashion.

Robotics

Using the DaVinci robotic device (Intuitive Surgical, Sunnyvale, Calif.), an additional trocar is often needed to pass sutures; for an assistant surgeon, this trocar often can be placed in the right side of the abdomen at about the level of the umbilicus. The four-arm robotic device allows surgeons to use three working ports, placed in the midline, the left midclavicular line, and the left axillary line at the subcostal margins, so that the entire operation can be performed for the most part with the working arms of the DaVinci device. The robotic telemanipulator device is often used in this situation because of the stable, high-quality three-dimensional image and the fine dexterity afforded by the device. The myotomy and fundoplication technique using the robot or using standard laparoscopy is relatively the same.

Postoperative Care

We do not place nasogastric tubes in patients with achalasia. In general, patients are started on clear liquids immediately after surgery and are advised that a clear to full liquid diet is indicated for the first week or so as the edema clears, and we ask them to avoid carbonated beverages. The perioperative course is usually quite benign; any patient seen with fever or unanticipated complications in the immediate postoperative period should be fully evaluated for an undetected esophageal perforation. Esophageal perforations that remain undetected can be a significant source of morbidity and even mortality, especially if the diagnosis is delayed. Physical activity can resume as pain allows, although heavy activity should be avoided to prevent damage to the crura repair and injury at the larger port sites.

Recurrence

Although surgery offers great long-term results for treating achalasia, some individuals will suffer from recurrent symptoms or will have failed primary success. Few published data are available regarding the best therapeutic option for individuals with postsurgical recurrence. Failed surgical therapy could be related to an excessively tight fundoplication, an inadequate myotomy, a severely dysfunctional esophagus from long-standing disease, gastroesophageal reflux, or the interval development of a mass lesion such as a carcinoma.

Some authors suggest repeating the myotomy in individuals with recurrence, but others have shown success with postmyotomy pneumatic dilation. Little is known regarding this topic, and most of the arguments surrounding it hinge on small, nonrandomized retrospective studies. Eckardt and colleagues (2009) separated individuals with recurrence into two groups: type I and type II. Patients with type I recurrence are those with an early recurrence and persistent or recurrent hypertension of the LES; type II recurrences represent late recurrence with irreversible progression of the disease and development of megaesophagus, and the authors advocate repeat myotomy in individuals with a type I recurrence. Individuals with a type II recurrence may represent irreversible progression of disease and may require an esophagectomy to ameliorate symptoms.

SUMMARY

Achalasia is an uncommon disease, often with an insidious onset. Symptoms of progressive dysphagia can progress to malnutrition, weight loss, and even pulmonary aspiration, and flexible endoscopy should be used to rule out mechanical obstructions. Manometric and radiographic findings of an aperistaltic esophagus and nonrelaxation of the distal esophageal sphincter are indicative of the diagnosis of achalasia. Pharmacologic treatment is rarely helpful, however, endoscopic injection of botulinum toxin may provide short-term relief. Fluoroscopic or endoscopic dilation with large-caliber balloons has shown reasonable success rates but usually requires multiple procedures and comes with significant risk of perforation.

Surgical myotomy was popularized in the 1950s and modified to the standard laparoscopic approach in the 1990s. Currently, a laparoscopic approach with fundoplication should be offered as a first-line therapy in most patients, because the risk of significant perioperative complications is low, and results are excellent.

SUGGESTED READINGS

Abir F, Modlin I, Kidd M, Bell R: Surgical treatment of achalasia, *Dig Surg* 21:165–176, 2004.

Eckhardt A, Eckhardt V: Current clinical approach to achalasia, *World J Gastroenterol* 15:3969–3975, 2009.

Ferri L, Cools-Lartigue J, Cao J, et al: Clinical predictors of achalasia, *Dis Esophagus* 5:18–21, 2009.

Gockel I, Junginger T, Eckhardt V: Persistent and recurrent achalasia after Heller myotomy; analysis of different patterns and long-term results of reoperation, *Arch Surg* 142:1093–1097, 2007.

Gorodner M, Galvani C, Patti M: Heller myotomy, *Op Tech Gen Surg* 6:23–28, 2004.

Litle V: Laparoscopic Heller myotomy for achalasia: a review of the controversies, *Ann Thorac Surg* 85:743–746, 2008.

Melvin S, Dundon J, Talamini M, et al: Computer-enhanced robotic telesurgery minimizes esophageal perforation during Heller myotomy, *Surgery* 138(4):553–558, 2005.

Torquati A, Richards W, Holzman M, Sharp K: Laparoscopic myotomy, *Ann Surg* 5:587–593, 2006.

Williams V, Peters J: Achalasia of the esophagus: a surgical disease, *J Am Coll Surg* 208:151–162, 2009.

LAPAROSCOPIC ADRENALECTOMY

Alan P.B. Dackiw, MD, PhD

OVERVIEW

Laparoscopic adrenalectomy was first described in 1992 and has since become the preferred method for removal of the adrenal gland and adrenal tumors except for certain larger tumors. Several studies have compared laparoscopic adrenalectomy with open anterior or posterior adrenalectomy, documenting the enhanced recovery, shorter hospital stay, and cost effectiveness of the laparoscopic approach.

INDICATIONS AND CONTRAINDICATIONS

Adrenalectomy is indicated in any patient with a hormonally active adrenal tumor, enlarging mass, or suspected malignancy. Adrenal tumors can be generally categorized as *functional* or *nonfunctional* most functional adrenal tumors are less than 6 cm in diameter, and patients with functional tumors are excellent candidates for laparoscopic adrenalectomy. Functional tumors include aldosterone- and cortisol-producing adenomas and pheochromocytomas.

The main indication for performing an adrenalectomy with an open approach is the size of the tumor or mass in the adrenal glands. Although it may be technically feasible to remove larger tumors up to 14 cm with a laparoscopic approach, as a general rule, if a large adrenal tumor is suspected to be an adrenal cortical carcinoma preoperatively based on size and imaging characteristics, an open approach is recommended. These tumors are often soft, friable, and easily penetrable with indistinct tissue planes. An open approach to these tumors is often safer, to avoid possible tumor disruption or violation of tissue planes that may occur with a laparoscopic approach.

PREOPERATIVE PREPARATION

The importance of documenting and diagnosing function of an adrenal neoplasm preoperatively cannot be overemphasized, as the preoperative, intraoperative, and postoperative medical management of patients with hormonally active tumors is extremely important.

Pheochromocytoma

Patients with pheochromocytoma are treated preoperatively for 2 to 4 weeks with α-blockade. Phenoxybenzamine, usually at 10 mg by mouth twice daily, has been our drug of choice, as we have experienced good intraoperative blood pressure control with this regimen. The addition of β-blockade may prove necessary after institution of α-blockade, if hypertension is persistent or tachycardia ensues. Close intraoperative communication with anesthesiology colleagues cannot be overemphasized, with availability of nipride, phentolamine, and adrenergic agents following tumor removal to control blood pressure intraoperatively.

Aldosteronoma

Patients with aldosterone-producing adenomas require electrolyte monitoring and correction prior to surgery, which may require aggressive potassium replacement. This must be done with caution and closely monitored in patients who also may be receiving spironolactone or eplerenone. In some patients it may be difficult to completely normalize potassium levels preoperatively.

Cushing Cortisol-Producing Adenoma

Patients may be treated preoperatively for a brief period (5 to 7 days) with ketoconazole in an attempt to decrease and impact the significant hypercortisolemia perioperatively, which theoretically may impact blood vessel fragility and bleeding as well as wound healing. Patients are treated with 100 mg of IV hydrocortisone at induction of anesthesia and following tumor removal, followed by a dose every 8 hours until oral replacement and taper begin.

OPERATIVE TECHNIQUE

The two main techniques used today for laparoscopic adrenalectomy are the lateral transabdominal and the posterior retroperitoneal approach popularized by Gagner and Walz respectively. Interestingly, laparoscopic left adrenalectomy and laparoscopic right adrenalectomy are two anatomically and technically distinct procedures. The lateral transabdominal approach is my preferred approach for several reasons, except in certain clinical circumstances outlined below. These reasons include familiarity with laparoscopic intraabdominal anatomy and the potential to remove larger tumors and to perform laparoscopy. One of the best and most articulate early descriptions of laparoscopic adrenalectomy via a lateral transabdominal approach, which I have used in over 200 cases, was published by Smith, Weber, and Amerson.

Transabdominal Lateral Approach

By placing the patient in a lateral decubitus position, the lateral transabdominal approach allows gravity to assist in exposure of the adrenal glands, compared to a direct anterior approach, which has also been described. The day before surgery, a mild laxative is given to help decompress the colon. In the operating room, a beanbag is placed on the operating table, and the patient is secured. The iliac crest is placed directly over the table break, the bed is flexed, and the kidney rest is raised (Figure 1). Pneumatic compression boots are placed, and subcutaneous heparin and a prophylactic IV antibiotic are given.

Left Adrenalectomy

After induction of general endotracheal anesthesia, the stomach and bladder are decompressed with an orogastric tube and Foley catheter. With the patient in the right lateral decubitus position, and the iliac crest positioned over the kidney rest, the kidney rest is raised, and an axillary roll is placed. The bed is flexed, and the patient is placed in a slight reverse Trendelenburg position, which maximizes the distance between the iliac crest and the costal margin in the midaxillary line for subsequent trocar insertion. The left arm is supported on pillows on top, and the right arm is placed on an arm board, padded, and secured. The skin is then prepped and draped in the standard fashion with a wide enough skin preparation to allow open laparotomy if necessary.

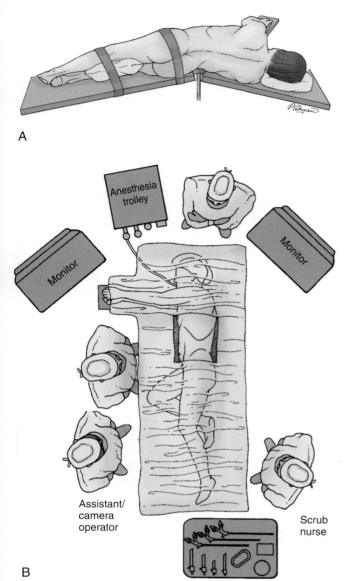

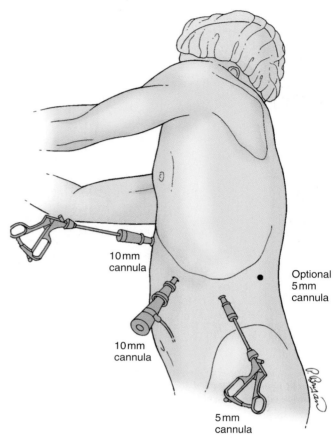

FIGURE 2   Trocar placement and instrument placement for left laparoscopic adrenalectomy. *(Modified from Smith CD, Weber CJ, Amerson JR: Laparoscopic adrenalectomy: new gold standard, World J Surg 23: 389–396, 1999.)*

FIGURE 1   A, Patient positioning for lateral approach to left laparoscopic adrenalectomy (kidney rest and table break are positioned at the iliac crest). **B,** Operating room setup and patient positioning for laparoscopic adrenalectomy. *(Modified from Smith CD, Weber CJ, Amerson JR: Laparoscopic adrenalectomy: new gold standard, World J Surg 23:389–396, 1999.)*

The procedure begins with a 12 mm skin incision in the mid-clavicular line, two fingerbreadths below the left costal margin; dissection is carried down to the level of the fascia, which is elevated between two Kocher clamps, and the peritoneal cavity is entered with a Veress needle. A leak test is performed with aspiration and irrigation of saline followed by allowing the saline to spontaneously drain into the peritoneal cavity to assure peritoneal placement of the needle. The peritoneal cavity is then insufflated to 15 mm Hg intra-peritoneal pressure, a 12 mm trocar is placed at the Veress site, and another 12 mm trocar is placed medially and laterally under direct vision. A fourth 5 mm trocar is also placed further laterally in the posterior axillary line, which facilitates lateral traction (Figure 2). A "finder" spinal needle with marcaine administered preperitoneally is often useful to guide trocar placement, especially in a patient who may have significant anterior adhesions.

The next step is to establish a plane of dissection along the anterior surface of the left kidney lateral and dorsal to the spleen and the tail of the pancreas. This is accomplished by incising the splenorenal ligament and mobilizing the spleen, allowing it to fall medially (Figure 3). The decubitus positioning facilitates this dissection and mobilization. With gravity pulling the spleen medially and away from the anterior surface of the kidney, the spleen and tail of the pancreas are dissected away from the retroperitoneum, with the superior pole of the kidney and the adrenal then exposed.

It is important to note that this dissection plane should be relatively avascular. If excessive bleeding is encountered, the wrong plane of dissection is being developed; it is relatively easy to mistake the tail of the pancreas for adrenal tissue in this area of dissection, and care must be taken not to injure the tail of the pancreas. It is also important to continue the lateral mobilization of the spleen up to the diaphragm and close to the greater curve of the stomach and short gastric vessels, until the stomach is visualized at this level; this confirms maximal mobilization of the spleen and exposure of the adrenal gland.

Dissection along the anterior surface of the kidney and adrenal continues, until the inferior pole and medial border of the adrenal are exposed. A beautiful analogy emphasized by Dr. Quan Duh is that laparoscopic left adrenalectomy is like opening a book, with the pages of the book on one side being the spleen and pancreatic tail and the pages on the other side being the anterior surface of the kidney and adrenal; the spine of the book is a line just beyond the medial edge of the adrenal gland (Figure 4).

Depending on the adrenal pathology and the amount of retroperitoneal fat, the lateral and anterior surface of the adrenal gland will become visible during this dissection. It is important to avoid

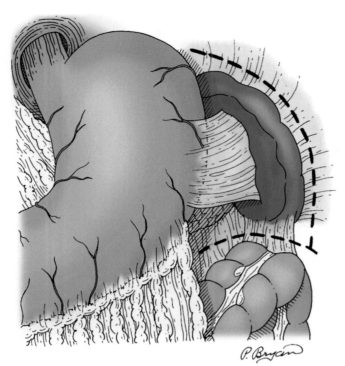

FIGURE 3   Initial planes of dissection along splenorenal and splenocolic ligaments. *(Modified from Smith CD, Weber CJ, Amerson JR: Laparoscopic adrenalectomy: new gold standard, World J Surg 23:389–396, 1999.)*

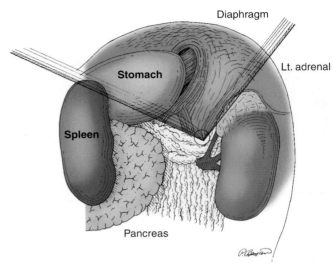

FIGURE 4   "Opening the book" as a plane of dissection with the spleen and the tail of the pancreas medially and the adrenal and kidney laterally. *(Modified from Smith CD, Weber CJ, Amerson JR: Laparoscopic adrenalectomy: new gold standard, World J Surg 23:389–396, 1999.)*

mobilizing the adrenal gland along its lateral edge too early during the exposure, because gravity allows the mobilized adrenal to fall medially and prevents visualization and access to the medial and inferior edges of the gland, and this is where the surgeon needs to expose, dissect, and clip the adrenal vein. When the retroperitoneal fat prevents clear visualization of the gland, its medial and inferior edge can be localized by palpation, as the adrenal is ballotable in the retroperitoneal tissue along the anterior surface of the kidney. In even the most obese patients, or in those with Cushing disease, this technique allows identification of the dissection plane between the anterior surface of the kidney and the inferior border of the adrenal through the Gerota fascia. Once this cleavage plane is identified, careful dissection with hook cautery eventually exposes the inferior and medial edge of the gland. In these difficult situations, intraoperative laparoscopic ultrasonography may be used to locate the gland.

The next step is isolation of the left adrenal vein. With small tumors, this is most easily accomplished by first dissecting the inferior and medial aspect of the adrenal, staying close to the gland until the vein is isolated and clipped (Figure 5). A right-angle dissector greatly facilitates this exposure and isolation. Risk of injuring the left renal vein is minimized by staying close to the adrenal gland during this dissection. The adrenal vein is then clipped with a 10 mm clip applier. Once the vein is divided, dissection continues from inferior and medial to superior and lateral, following the anterior surface of the kidney. For large tumors, early identification of the adrenal vein may be difficult. In these cases, mobilization of the gland laterally and inferiorly to find the inferior border of the gland and the adrenal vein is helpful.

Final dissection and gland excision progresses from medial to lateral and inferior to superior. The use of an ultrasonic dissector (harmonic scalpel) is especially useful to dissect posterior retroperitoneal tissues and attachments of the adrenal, but we have found monopolar electrocautery with a hook dissector to be a very effective method that allows fine and meticulous dissection in the confined

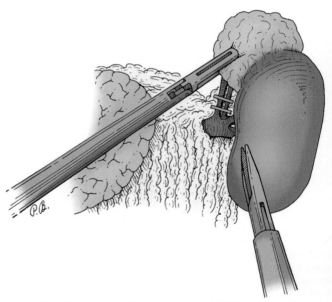

FIGURE 5   Dissection, isolation, ligation, and division of the left adrenal vein. *(Modified from Smith CD, Weber CJ, Amerson JR: Laparoscopic adrenalectomy: new gold standard, World J Surg 23:389–396, 1999.)*

space and the relatively avascular planes of dissection. The inferior phrenic artery is frequently encountered along the superior edge of the adrenal and should be sought and ligated with clips and divided. The vein may also be dissected and followed inferiorly to its junction with the left adrenal vein, which in some cases may assist in its localization.

Before specimen extraction, the operative field is carefully inspected for hemostasis, and the area is irrigated and suctioned dry. Points of bleeding from retroperitoneal fat are coagulated with electrocautery, and areas of bleeding from visible vessels are clipped. Once hemostasis is ensured, the adrenal is placed in a specimen-retrieval bag that has been inserted through the camera port. The fascia of the cannula site of extraction may need to be stretched with a Kelly clamp to facilitate removal. For large tumors, the skin or fascia incision may need to be lengthened. The operation is completed by closing the fascia of the 12 mm incisions with absorbable suture.

Right Adrenalectomy

As noted, laparoscopic right adenalectomy is an entirely different operation anatomically and technically than left adrenalectomy. For right adrenalectomy, the patient is placed in the left lateral decubitus position with the right side up; otherwise, patient positioning is identical to that described for left adrenalectomy. Pneumoperitoneum to 15 mm Hg intraperitoneal pressure is initiated with a Veress needle inserted at the midclavicular line below the right costal margin, which is the cannula site for the camera. After establishing pneumoperitoneum, the remaining cannula sites are marked four fingerbreadths away from the previously placed trocar (Figure 6). On the right, a fourth trocar in the epigastrium is always necessary for a retractor to elevate the right lobe of the liver. It is important for this trocar site to allow the angle of retractor insertion to be parallel to the undersurface of the right lobe of the liver, held by the first assistant/ camera operator. With the liver retractor positioned, the anterior surface of the right kidney and the lateral edge of the inferior vena cava can be seen clearly.

The dissection commences by creating a "hockey stick" or upside-down L-shaped incision along the retroperitoneal attachment of the right lobe of the liver and the border of the inferior vena cava (Figure 7, A). This mobilizes the right lobe of the liver and allows exposure of the anterior surface of the adrenal as the liver is pushed superiorly. The triangular ligament of the liver may also be incised to facilitate greater exposure. The medial border of the inferior vena cava is carefully exposed, looking for the right adrenal vein at the superior medial border of the adrenal, remembering that this vein is typically broad and short and enters the vena cava slightly posteriorly. We have found using a blunt-tipped right-angle dissector and laparoscopic Kittner most useful for this dissection (Figure 7, B). Rarely, an accessory hepatic vein may also be seen superiorly, and the surgeon should look for this. Once the adrenal vein has been isolated, it is ligated (Figure 7, C) with three 10 mm clips distally and two proximally. Because of the short length of this vein, the distal-most clip should be at the edge of the vena cava.

Once the right adrenal vein has been clipped and divided, dissection continues to expose and mobilize the medial edge of the adrenal. As with the left adrenal, the lateral edge should not be dissected too early, because gravity causes the laterally mobilized gland to hang over the medial edge, making visualization difficult. By dissecting from medial to lateral and inferior to superior, the superior pole of the kidney can be used as a dissection plane through the Gerota fascia, and the dissection can progress in a direction away from any anatomic danger areas (inferior vena cava and renal vein).

As with the left adrenal, monopolar electrocautery is used for most of the dissection, with the Harmonic scalpel reserved for dividing the posterior and lateral adrenal attachments. Visible vessels are clipped, and the inferior phrenic vessels are commonly encountered at the superior and lateral border of the gland. Once excised, the adrenal is placed in a specimen-retrieval bag and removed intact through the camera port.

Bilateral Adrenalectomy

Bilateral adrenalectomies are performed in the manner already described for each individual side. Because right adrenalectomy has a higher risk of conversion to open adrenalectomy because of the immediate consequences of an adrenal vein or vena cava injury, we perform left adrenalectomy first, thus the patient has the greatest likelihood of benefiting from a laparoscopic approach. Before repositioning for right adrenalectomy, the entire left adrenalectomy is completed.

Retroperitoneal Approach

This method has been popularized by Walz, and we have used it in select circumstances, including in patients with multiple prior abdominal procedures with significant adhesions or a "frozen" abdomen. The patient is positioned in the prone or semi-jackknife position with the hips flexed and the patient lying on a rectangular support that allows the ventral abdominal wall to hang through. A 12 mm transverse incision just below the tip of the twelfth rib is performed. The retroperitoneal space is reached by blunt and sharp dissection of the abdominal wall, and a small cavity is prepared digitally for insertion of one 5 mm trocar 4 to 5 cm lateral beneath the eleventh rib. This trocar is placed under finger guidance. In the same way, a 10 mm trocar is inserted 4 to 5 cm medial to the initial wound through a skin incision about 3 cm below the twelfth rib, and the trocar is directed cranially at a 45-degree angle, entering the retroperitoneum just below the twelfth rib. A blunt trocar with an inflatable balloon and an adjustable sleeve is introduced into the initial incision, and pneumoretroperitoneum is created by maintaining a carbon dioxide pressure of 20 to 28 mm Hg. Retroperitoneoscopy is performed with a 10 mm, 30-degree endoscope, which is initially introduced into the middle trocar; after the creation of the retroperitoneal space, the endoscope is placed in the trocar nearest to the spine.

After creating the retroperitoneal space beneath the diaphragm by pushing down the fatty tissue, mobilization of the upper pole of the kidney is performed; by doing so, the area of the adrenal gland

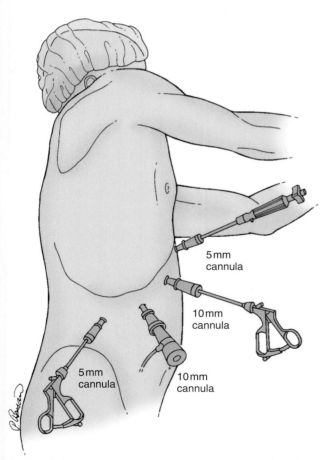

5 mm cannula

10 mm cannula

5 mm cannula

10 mm cannula

FIGURE 6 Trocar placement and instrument placement for right laparoscopic adrenalectomy. (*Modified from Smith CD, Weber CJ, Amerson JR: Laparoscopic adrenalectomy: new gold standard, World J Surg 23:389–396, 1999.*)

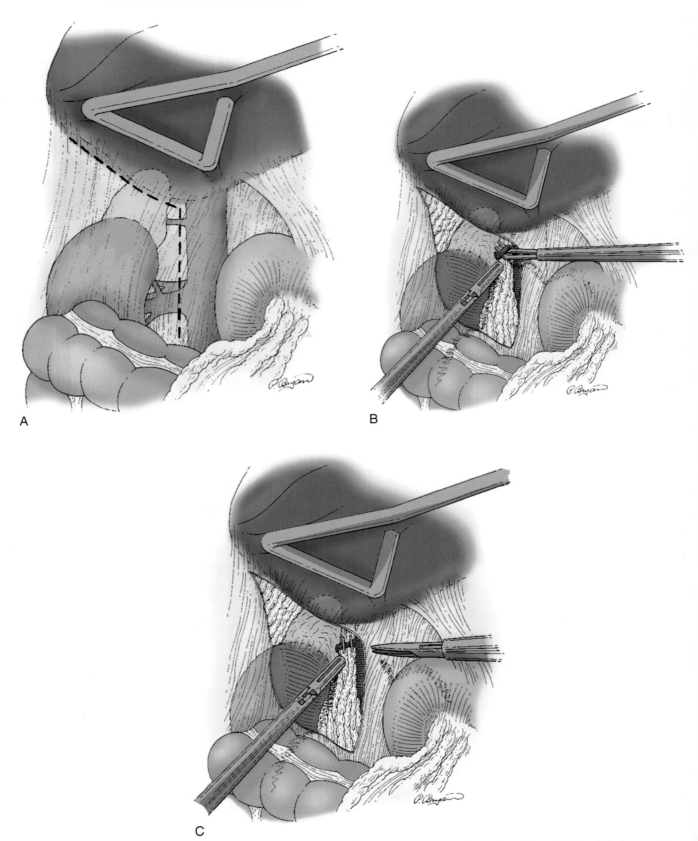

FIGURE 7   A, A "hockey stick," or L-shaped, incision is fashioned in the retroperitoenum along the border of the right lobe of the liver and the lateral border of the vena cava. **B,** The right adrenal vein is meticulously dissected using a blunt-tipped right-angle dissector and laparoscopic Kittner. **C,** Once the adrenal vein has been isolated, it is ligated. *(Modified from Smith CD, Weber CJ, Amerson JR: Laparoscopic adrenalectomy: new gold standard, World J Surg 23:389–396, 1999.)*

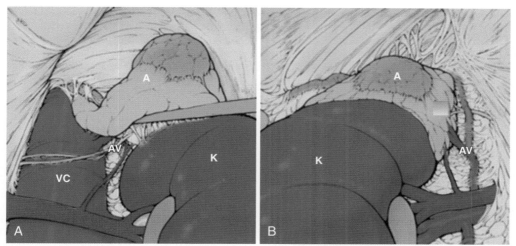

FIGURE 8   Posterior retroperitoneal endoscopic adrenalectomy. **A,** Right. **B,** Left. *AV,* Adrenal vein; *A,* adrenal; *VC,* vena cava; *K,* kidney. *(Modified from Walz MK: Minimally invasive adrenal gland surgery, [in German]. Chirurg 69:613-620, 1998.)*

is exposed. The upper pole of the kidney is then retracted by one of the instruments in the medial or lateral trocar. It may be necessary to place a fourth trocar below the first line of ports for pulling down the kidney with a retractor.

Mobilization of the adrenal gland begins medially and caudally between the inferior phrenic vein and adrenal gland. In this area on the right side, the adrenal gland arteries cross the vena cava posteriorly (Figure 8, *A*). These vessels are separated by electrocoagulation or clip application. By lifting up the adrenal gland, the inferior vena cava is visualized posteriorly in its retroperitoneal superior segment. The adrenal vein becomes visible running posterolaterally and is dissected and divided between clips.

The procedure is completed with lateral and superior dissection. For left retroperitoneoscopic adrenalectomy, the adrenal gland vein must be dissected in the space between the adrenal gland and the phrenic branch medial to the upper pole of the kidney (Figure 8, *B*) After dissection, ligation, and division of the left adrenal vein lateral to the junction with the inferior phrenic vein, dissection of the adrenal gland is continued medially, laterally, and superiorly by retracting the gland at the venous stump.

POTENTIAL COMPLICATIONS

Several complications may occur during a laparoscopic adrenalectomy. Proper padding as initially discussed for patient positioning is necessary to prevent nerve and soft-tissue compression injuries. This includes proper use of an axillary roll and avoidance of pressure to the peroneal nerve when the patient is secured to the operating table in the lateral decubitus position.

During right adrenalectomy, meticulous dissection should avoid injury to the diaphragm, liver, and gall bladder. Injury to the vena cava may require urgent conversion to laparotomy, and instruments and retraction necessary for this procedure should be available. As noted, injury to the pancreatic tail or spleen may occur during laparoscopic left adrenalectomy. As mentioned above, the plane between the adrenal and pancreatic tail should be avascular; if it is not, dissection may potentially proceed into the pancreatic tail, resulting in injury.

POSTOPERATIVE CARE

Most patients may be discharged 24 to 48 hours postoperatively, and ileus may persist for 24 to 48 hours. Patients with pheochromocytoma require postoperative hemodynamic monitoring in an intensive care unit, and those with Cushing syndrome require postoperative stress-dose steroids, followed by an oral tapering dose often over several months for up to 2 years. Patients with aldosterone-producing adenomas often experience a significant diuresis postoperatively and require close monitoring of their fluid balance and electrolytes.

LAPAROSCOPIC LIVER RESECTION

Kevin Tri Nguyen, MD, PhD, and David A. Geller, MD

OVERVIEW

Laparoscopic liver resection is expanding in the field of liver surgery. Since the introduction of laparoscopic cholecystectomy in the late 1980s, there has been a demand for minimally invasive procedures to replace the more morbid open procedures, with the hopes of minimizing incisions, reducing incisional pain, decreasing hospital stay, and providing a quicker recovery to normal function. Open operations for cancer have been slower to transition to their minimally invasive counterparts because of concerns of compromising oncologic principles and fears of port-site recurrence. Experience with laparoscopic colon resection for cancer has shown that laparoscopy does not compromise oncologic principles, nor does it potentiate carcinomatosis and port-site seeding of cancer cells. Additional concerns of liver parenchymal transection, uncontrollable hemorrhage, bile leak, and air embolism have also challenged the use of laparoscopic options for liver resection. Multiple studies have shown that these issues can be addressed laparoscopically and that liver resections are safe, feasible, and oncologically sound, with improved short-term results and comparable long-term outcomes in experienced hands. No randomized controlled trial has been performed to compare laparoscopic liver resection with open liver resection. Patient accrual in such a trial may be difficult, because multiple individual series have shown that the minimally invasive approach is safe and feasible, even with major anatomical resections.

PREOPERATIVE EVALUATION

A standard history and physical is necessary to evaluate the patient's comorbidities to determine whether the patient can undergo general anesthesia. Laboratory studies, including liver function tests and coagulation studies, can screen for liver dysfunction, nutrition status, and coagulopathy. A triphasic, contrast-enhanced computed tomography (CT) scan or magnetic resonance imaging (MRI) are essential to determine the location, multifocality, extent of the liver lesions, synchronous intrahepatic or intraabdominal pathology, proximity to major vasculature, and presence of abdominal wall varices in patients with cirrhosis and portal hypertension. Residual liver volume (future liver remnant) can be calculated from the CT scan or MRI, especially in patients with large lesions, history of cirrhosis, or history of neoadjuvant chemotherapy. For those patients with predicted insufficient residual liver mass, portal vein embolization of the planned resected lobe can trigger contralateral lobe hypertrophy and help prevent postoperative liver failure.

Appropriate patient selection is of utmost importance to a successful minimally invasive liver resection, and the first determination is whether the patient is a candidate for liver resection. It must also be discerned whether the patient will tolerate general anesthesia and pneumoperitoneum. American Society of Anesthesiologists (ASA) class 4 patients, those with severe systemic disease that is a constant threat to life, may not tolerate an operation. It must also be determined whether the tumor location is amenable to a laparoscopic approach without compromising oncologic principles. Large tumors encroaching the hilum or major vasculature, such as the IVC, may preclude a minimally invasive approach. Tumors located along the liver periphery (segments II, III, IVb, V, and VI) are most amenable to a minimally invasive approach. Tumors that are deep, superior, and posterior may require hand assistance or a hybrid approach, which we will discuss; in our opinion, resection of tumors in these locations should be attempted only by surgeons who are already advanced in laparoscopic resection of peripheral liver lesions; otherwise, an open approach is appropriate.

INDICATIONS AND CONTRAINDICATIONS

Since the first laparoscopic liver resection was described in 1992, exponential growth in laparoscopic liver resections has been reported, with almost 3000 cases reported in the English literature. The indications for laparoscopic hepatic resection include adenoma, symptomatic hemangioma, symptomatic focal nodular hyperplasia (FNH), and symptomatic giant hepatic cysts (Table 1). Although many surgeons who perform laparoscopic hepatic resection initially favored these benign lesions, minimally invasive hepatic resections for cancers—such as hepatocellular carcinoma (HCC) and colorectal carcinoma (CRC) metastasis—are now commonly reported. Indeterminate lesions, in which cancer cannot be excluded, can also be removed laparoscopically when optimally located. In addition, laparoscopic live-donor hepatectomy for liver transplantation has also been reported. Initially these were live-donor left lateral sectionectomies for adult-to-child liver transplant, with other centers expanding to live-donor hemihepatectomies for adult-to-adult liver transplant. Out of the almost 3000 laparoscopic hepatic resection cases reported in the literature, 50% of the cases were malignant tumors, and 45% were benign lesions. The majority of laparoscopic liver resection

TABLE 1: Indications and contraindications for laparoscopic liver resection

Indications	Contraindications
Benign Liver Lesions	Any contraindications to open liver resection
Symptomatic hemangioma	Patients who cannot tolerate pneumoperitoneum
Symptomatic focal nodular hyperplasia	Dense adhesions that cannot be lysed laparoscopically
Adenoma	Lesions too close to major vasculature
Symptomatic giant hepatic cyst	Lesions too large to be safely manipulated laparoscopically
Malignant Liver Lesions	Resection that requires extensive portal lymphadenectomy
Hepatocellular carcinoma	
Colorectal carcinoma metastasis	
Other	
Live donor hepatectomy for liver transplant	
Malignant lesions	
Indeterminate lesions (cannot rule out cancer)	

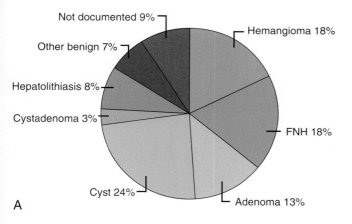

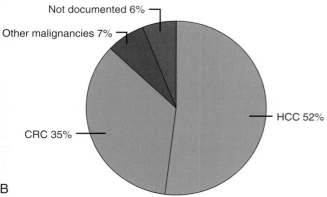

FIGURE 1 Breakdown of benign (**A**) and malignant (**B**) liver lesions resected laparoscopically. *FNH,* Focal nodular hyperplasia; *HCC,* Hepatocellular carcinoma; *CRC,* Colorectal cancer metastasis to the liver.

cases for benign lesions were performed for hepatic cysts (24%), and the remainder were for FNH (18%), hemangioma (18%), adenoma (13%), hepatolithiasis (8%), and cystadenoma (3%; Figure 1, *A*). Malignant lesions resected laparoscopically were HCC (52%) and CRC metastasis to the liver (35%; Figure 1, *B*).

Contraindications to laparoscopic liver resections include any contraindications to open liver resection, intolerance to pneumoperitoneum, dense adhesions, lesions too close to major vasculature, lesions too large to be safely manipulated laparoscopically, and resections that may require extensive dissection of the porta hepatitis (see Table 1).

EQUIPMENT

A full complement of laparoscopic equipment with 30-degree 10 mm and 5 mm scopes is recommended. A hand port (GelPort; Applied Medical, Rancho Santa Margarita, Calif.) is required for a hand-assisted approach. Ports sizes include 5 mm and 12 mm and include Hasson ports for the camera. Additional equipment includes the laparoscopic LigaSure (Covidien, Boulder, Colo.), harmonic scalpel, TissueLink (Salient Surgical Technologies, Dover, NH), clips, and Endo GIA (Covidien) 45 mm reticulating vascular (white load) staplers.

PATIENT POSITIONING AND ROOM SETUP

Patients are placed in the supine position and secured to the operating room table with thigh and shoulder straps to allow for steep rotation as needed. Sequential compression devices, a Foley catheter,

and Bovie pads are placed. Legs and arms are padded, and the arms are positioned at 60 degrees from the patient's body. Although some laparoscopic liver resection teams will use the "French position" (split-leg position), we favor having the patient supine, with the surgeon on the right side of the patient, the assistant on the left side, and two monitors placed near the head of the patient for comfortable viewing by the surgeon and assistant. The ultrasound device is placed on the left side of the patient, and the scrub nurse stands on the patient's left side near the leg.

INTRAOPERATIVE STEPS

For all minimally invasive liver resections, eight key steps are applied, irrespective of approach: 1) abdominal exploration, 2) liver ultrasonography, 3) liver mobilization, 4) inflow control, 5) parenchymal transection, 6) outflow division, 7) liver extraction, and 8) hemostasis. The use of a hand port is dependent on surgeon preference, comfort, and training.

TOTALLY LAPAROSCOPIC LEFT LATERAL SECTIONECTOMY

For a totally laparoscopic left lateral sectionectomy, a four-trocar technique is used with two 12 mm and two 5 mm ports (Figure 2, *A*). The 30-degree 5 mm or 10 mm camera is used, and the falciform ligament is divided with EndoShears or hook cautery toward the IVC and hepatic veins. The round ligament is divided with an Endo GIA stapler flush with the anterior abdominal wall and is used as a handle to retract the liver. Laparoscopic liver ultrasonography is performed to confirm tumor location, rule out synchronous lesions, evaluate proximity to major vasculature, and plan the transection plane. The bridge of the liver tissue from segment III to IVb is divided with a combination of hook cautery and LigaSure, and the left porta hepatis is dissected at the base of the round ligament with a combination of hook cautery, Maryland dissector, and right-angle clamps to clearly identify the hepatic artery and portal vein inflow to the left lateral section. Inflow control is obtained by dividing the left hepatic artery with locking hemoclips, and whenever possible, the segment IV artery branch from the left hepatic artery is preserved.

Next, the liver parenchyma is divided with the ultrasonic shears or LigaSure, just to the left of the falciform ligament, for a depth of approximately 2 to 3 cm. The segment II and III portal veins and hepatic ducts are divided inside the parenchyma with the vascular stapler (white load) after creating a tunnel in the liver parenchyma with an atraumatic Glassman dissector/grasper. The left hepatic vein is divided with a vascular stapler after thinning the parenchyma above and below it. Minimal oozing from the cut edge is cauterized with laparoscopic saline-linked cautery (TissueLink EndoSH2.0; Salient Surgical Technologies), and we do not use the argon beam coagulator because of the potential risk of air embolism from excessive intraabdominal pressure. Finally, the specimen is placed in an EndoCatch bag and is removed through an expanded umbilical incision. A Jackson-Pratt drain is placed next to the cut surface and is removed prior to discharge. For right lobe anterior lesions, a four-trocar technique is used, with port placement that mirrors the left lateral sectionectomy port sites.

HAND-ASSISTED LAPAROSCOPIC LEFT HEPATECTOMY

A hand port is used for anatomical left and right hepatic lobectomy, and it is placed as a midline 7 to 8 cm incision at the start of the operation. For left hepatic lobectomy, a periumbilical incision is made (Figure 2, *B*), and a supraumbilical incision is used for right

Totally laparoscopic
left lateral sectionectomy

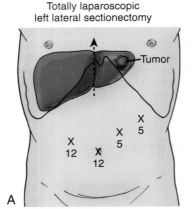

A

Hand-assisted
left hepatic lobectomy

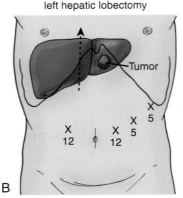

B

Hand-assisted
right hepatic lobectomy

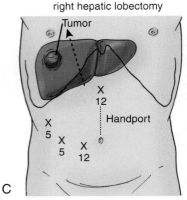

C

FIGURE 2 Port positions for laparoscopic liver surgery. **A,** Pure laparoscopic left lateral sectionectomy. **B,** Hand-assisted laparoscopic left hepatic lobectomy. **C,** Hand-assisted laparoscopic right hepatic lobectomy.

lobectomy (Figure 2, *C*), along with four trocars. For left hepatic lobectomy, the left hilar dissection is the same as with left lateral sectionectomy, except that the entire left portal vein is encircled and bulldog clamped at the base of the round ligament. The left lobe is folded to the right, exposing the ligamentum venosum, which is divided, separating the left lobe from the caudate lobe. The liver is placed back in its natural position, and the parenchyma is divided to the left of the gallbladder fossa with the harmonic scalpel and LigaSure. Large segment IV feedback veins, and the middle hepatic vein when necessary, are divided with a vascular stapler, followed by the left hepatic vein just outside the IVC. The left portal vein and left hilar plate with left hepatic duct are divided last, once the parenchyma has been divided to allow room for placement of the vascular stapler. The specimen is removed directly through the hand port.

HAND-ASSISTED LAPAROSCOPIC RIGHT HEPATECTOMY

For laparoscopic right hepatic lobectomy, the right triangular/diaphragmatic ligaments are divided, and the liver is mobilized off the IVC by dividing the short hepatic veins with LigaSure (for vessels <4 mm) or small locking hemoclips (for vessels >4 mm). We prefer to stop this dissection at the base of the right hepatic vein and proceed with right hilar dissection. After laparoscopic cholecystectomy, the right hilum is dissected with hook cautery, Maryland dissector, and right-angle and Kittner dissectors to identify the right hepatic artery, which is doubly clipped with the locking clip and divided. The right portal vein is carefully dissected free and controlled with a bulldog clamp. The liver parenchyma is then divided with a combination of harmonic scalpel, LigaSure, and Endo GIA vascular stapler. The right hepatic vein is divided inside the liver, followed by the right portal vein, and then the right hepatic ducts inside the parenchyma at the right hilar plate.

LAPAROSCOPY-ASSISTED OPEN APPROACH (HYBRID)

In the laparoscopy-assisted open approach, the right lobe is mobilized laparoscopically and delivered into the hand-port incision. The hilar dissection and liver transection are performed in open fashion through a slight extension of the hand-port incision. The hybrid approach has been described in detail by Koffron and colleagues (2007). When anticipating a right hepatectomy with this approach, we prefer to place the hand port in a right subcostal position, which gives better exposure of the liver during the parenchymal transection.

ADVANTAGES

As experience increases, it is likely that the percentage of laparoscopic liver resections will increase based on the comfort level of the surgeon. In fact, Koffron and colleagues have shifted their practice from 10% minimally invasive liver resection in 2002 to 80% of all liver resections currently, making the minimally invasive approach the preferred approach, as long as the patients meet oncologically sound safety requirements. A prospective randomized controlled trial would be best to delineate the advantages and disadvantages of laparoscopic versus open liver resection; however, such a trial may never be accomplished, as patients may resist being randomized to a more invasive procedure, when the minimally invasive option is available and has been shown to be safe. Although laparoscopic cholecystectomy is considered the standard of care for gallbladder removal, its merits were never compared to open cholecystectomy in any prospective randomized controlled trial.

Potential advantages of laparoscopic liver surgery include smaller incisions, less blood loss with decreased blood transfusion requirements, less pain, early return of oral intake, and a shorter hospital stay. Average length of stay after laparoscopic liver surgery was variable, although almost all the studies consistently showed a significant earlier discharge to home after laparoscopic liver resection. Interestingly, a cultural bias is apparent with regard to how long patients are kept in the hospital after liver resection (laparoscopic or open). Studies performed in the United States showed a length of stay of 1.9 to 2.9 days after laparoscopic liver resection. Studies from Europe showed an average length of stay of 3.5 to 8.3 days, and those from Asia reported an average of length of stay of 4 to 14.9 days after laparoscopic liver resection.

Compared with open liver resection, no differences were seen in margin-free resections, postoperative complications may have been decreased, and no differences were seen in survival outcomes with laparoscopic resection. No significant differences were seen in overall survival after laparoscopic liver resection versus open liver resection for cancer. Cherqui and colleagues (2006) showed that the overall and disease-free 3-year survival rates after resection for HCC was 93% and 64%, respectively, which was comparable to previous reports of open resections of small HCC in chronic liver disease.

Nguyen and colleagues (2009) recently reported a multiinstitutional study of the safety, feasibility, and early outcomes of laparoscopic liver resection for CRC metastasis in 109 patients performed at five major medical centers. The R0 resection rate was 94.4%, and the median tumor margin was 10 mm. The actuarial overall survivals at 1, 3, and 5 years were 88%, 69%, and 50%, respectively, and disease-free survivals at 1, 3, and 5 years were 65%, 43%, and 43%, respectively. These results are comparable to contemporaneous series of open hepatic resections for metastatic CRC. The only meta-analysis comparing laparoscopic hepatic resections (LHRs) versus open hepatic resections (OHRs) for benign and malignant tumors was conducted by Simillis and colleagues (2007), who analyzed eight studies between 1998 and 2005. At 5-year follow-up, they found comparable overall survival (61% LHR, 62% OHR) and disease-free survival (31% LHR, 29% OHR). Although initial concerns for the laparoscopic approach included possible tumor dissemination, there have been no reported cases of port site or peritoneal seeding of cancer following laparoscopic hepatic resection in more than 140 reported series.

Laparoscopy is particularly advantageous for cirrhotic patients. Several studies have shown that the laparoscopic approach leads to less blood loss and fewer postoperative complications, such as ascites and liver failure. In addition, laparoscopy improves the postoperative course by preserving the abdominal wall, improving diaphragm kinetics, maintaining collateral venous drainage, and reducing postoperative ascites.

DISADVANTAGES TO LAPAROSCOPIC LIVER RESECTION

Potential disadvantages to laparoscopic liver resection surgery include a significant learning curve. Minimally invasive liver surgery requires experience and expertise in open liver surgery, advanced minimally invasive techniques and instruments, and laparoscopic ultrasonography. At the beginning of the learning curve, the operative time may be longer than expected; however, with experience, the operative time is expected to be shorter.

Major hemorrhage is the biggest concern and the most common cause for conversion to an open procedure. Use of hand assistance during the early learning-curve period may help control potential hemorrhage, and bleeding can be decreased with appropriate planning, careful identification of the vascular structures with liberal use of ultrasonography, improved visualization and magnification, more meticulous dissection, and careful division through the liver parenchyma. Major vessels should be transected with a vascular load Endo GIA stapler. Portal control should be prepared in case the Pringle maneuver is needed, especially for major resections.

Air embolism is another potentially serious complication, particularly during laparoscopic hepatic surgery with exposed liver parenchyma and hepatic vein branches. Early manifestations can be quickly corrected by the anesthesiologist, and gas embolism during laparoscopic liver resections can be decreased by lowering the pneumoperitoneum to 10 to 12 mm Hg of CO_2. Lower central venous pressures used for open liver resections help decrease potential bleeding but may actually promote air embolism into the hepatic veins. A gasless approach with an abdominal lifting device has been advocated by some to minimize the risk of air embolism, but exposure can be compromised. If an air embolism is suspected, the patient should be placed in Trendelenburg position, and pneumoperitoneum should be released. Transesophageal echo (TEE) can be placed by the anesthesiologist to confirm the diagnosis. Use of a laparoscopic argon beam coagulator increases intraabdominal pressure and may possibly increase the risk of gas embolism.

SUMMARY

In experienced hands, laparoscopic liver resection is feasible and safe, and it provides short-term benefits. Recent studies show comparable oncologic outcomes in laparoscopic resection for HCC and CRC metastases in carefully selected patients.

SUGGESTED READINGS

Buell JF, Thomas MT, Rudich S, et al: Experience with more than 500 minimally invasive hepatic procedures, *Ann Surg* 248(3):475–486, 2008.

Cherqui D, Laurent A, Tayar C, et al: Laparoscopic liver resection for peripheral hepatocellular carcinoma in patients with chronic liver disease: midterm results and perspectives, *Ann Surg* 243(4):499–506, 2006.

Koffron AJ, Auffenberg G, Kung R, et al: Evaluation of 300 minimally invasive liver resections at a single institution: less is more, *Ann Surg* 246(3): 385–392, 2007.

Koffron AJ, Geller DA, Gamblin TC, et al: Laparoscopic liver surgery: shifting the management of liver tumors, *Hepatology* 44(6):1694–1700, 2006.

Koffron AJ, Kung RD, Auffenberg GB, Abecassis MM: Laparoscopic liver surgery for everyone: the hybrid method, *Surgery* 142(4):463–468, 2007.

Nguyen KT, Gamblin TC, Geller D: World review of laparoscopic liver resection: 2,804 patients, *Ann Surg* 250(5): 831–841, 2009.

Nguyen KT, Laurent A, Dagher I, et al: Minimally invasive liver resection for metastatic colorectal cancer: a multi-institutional, international report of safety, feasibility and early outcomes, *Ann Surg* 250(5): 842–848, 2009.

Simillis C, Constantinides VA, Tekkis PP, et al: Laparoscopic versus open hepatic resections for benign and malignant neoplasms: a meta-analysis, *Surgery* 141(2):203–211, 2007.

STAGING LAPAROSCOPY FOR GASTROINTESTINAL CANCER

B. Todd Heniford, MD, and Terri R. Martin, MD

OVERVIEW

The introduction of minimally invasive surgery or, more specifically, laparoscopy, has changed gastrointestinal surgeons' approach to most surgical disorders. This is certainly true in our staging of gastrointestinal malignancies. Laparoscopy minimizes unnecessary exploratory laparotomy, with subsequent avoidance of the associated higher morbidity for patients with metastatic disease, and it avoids the prolonged recovery of a full laparotomy in patients who often have limited survival; this way, patients can maximize their healthiest time, instead of spending up to 6 weeks recovering from an otherwise needless laparotomy. Additionally, staging laparoscopy can minimize potential delays in access to chemotherapy and/or radiation treatment for patients with unresectable disease, and it allows for appropriate selection of patients with locally advanced disease for palliative procedures. As with most procedures for benign disease, hospital length of stay is shorter, pain is minimized, and cost is reduced with staging laparoscopy when compared with staging laparotomy.

A decade or more ago, questions were raised concerning the risk of inaccurate staging using minimally invasive techniques; however, with improved technical skill and instrumentation, especially laparoscopic ultrasound, laparoscopy has proven equal to open exploration and more sensitive than computed tomography (CT) scan. The concern for the risk of port-site metastasis and peritoneal carcinomatosis as a result of laparoscopic assessment of an abdominal malignant process relative to open exploration has abated. However, controversy regarding selective versus routine use of staging laparoscopy has yet to be settled for some populations of cancer patients.

GENERAL TECHNIQUE

A proposed assessment of the indications and contraindications for staging laparoscopy for specific tumor types is listed in Table 1. Contraindications not specific to tumor type include severe adhesive disease, intolerance to pneumoperitoneum, poor cardiovascular or pulmonary status that precludes operative intervention, and uncorrectable coagulopathy.

Prior to starting a diagnostic or staging laparoscopic procedure for cancer, we make sure that adequate pathologic support is available. Most cases result in several biopsies being sent for frozen section. A phone call from the OR to the pathologist at the beginning the case frequently facilitates and speeds the care of the patient and shortens the operative time.

Using a 30- or 45-degree laparoscope, a thorough inspection of the suprahepatic and infrahepatic spaces, diaphragm, surface of the bowel, lesser sac, root of the transverse mesocolon and small bowel,

ligament of Treitz, paracolic gutters, and pelvis should be performed. In the case of pancreatic cancer, the lesser sac is opened, and the pancreas and posterior aspect of the stomach are examined. On inspection any ascites should be aspirated for cytology if suspicious or as part of a specific protocol. A biopsy of the abdominal wall, diaphragm, mesentery, or other implants should be taken and assessed using fresh frozen techniques. Peritoneal lavage is performed according to protocol or surgeon preference. Subsequently, the primary tumor—gastric, lower esophageal, or bile duct—can be assessed for possible node involvement, extraserosal invasion, and infiltration of surrounding structures.

Laparoscopic ultrasonography is often performed if gross inspection is unyielding, or if a significant chance of liver metastasis is present. Intraoperative ultrasound has an obvious and important role in surgical decision making for hepatobiliary and pancreatic malignancies. Using a multifrequency laparoscopic ultrasound probe with a flexible transducer tip, sonographic evaluation should include the deep hepatic parenchyma, portal vein and mesenteric vessels, and assessment of the organ involved with the primary tumor and associated nodes. In general, setting the probe frequency to 5 MHz, the liver parenchyma can be systematically assessed, starting from right to left anteriorly then posteriorly. Setting the probe frequency to 7 MHz, the extrahepatic bile ducts and associated nodes, as well as the

TABLE 1: Indications and contraindications for staging laparoscopy for specific tumor types

Tumor Type	Indications	Contraindications
Pancreatic adenocarcinoma	Detection of unsuspected locally advanced disease in patients with resectable disease based on preoperative imaging	Metastatic disease that is evident on CT
	Consideration of peritoneal lavage prior to definitive surgery per individual protocol	
	Selection of palliative treatment with locally advanced disease without evidence of metastatic disease	
	Assessment prior to planned neoadjuvant chemoradiation	
Gastric adenocarcinoma	T3 or T4 disease without evidence of nodal or distal metastasis	Need for palliative procedures for obstruction, hemorrhage, or perforation; proceed with surgery
	Gastroesophageal junction tumors	T1 or T2 disease can proceed with resection without diagnostic laparoscopy
	Questionable lymph nodes on imaging	
Esophageal tumors	Candidates for neoadjuvant chemotherapy Candidates for curative resection and negative preoperative imaging	
Colorectal cancer	Patients with resectable liver metastases without evidence of extrahepatic metastasis	Unresectable, nonablatable hepatic disease
Primary hepatic tumors	Candidates for curtive resection based on size and location with adequate hepatic reserve	Tumors with major vessel or organ invasion
Biliary tract tumors	Known or suspected gallbladder cancer without unresectable or metastatic disease	T1 gallbladder cancer incidentally found during cholecystectomy
	T2 or T3 hilar cholangiocarcinoma	
Lymphoma	Need for tissue diagnosis in the absence of peripheral lymphadenopathy	
	Restaging after treatment or when recurrence is suspected	

Modified from Hori Y, SAGES Guidelines Committee: Diagnostic laparoscopy guidelines. *Surg Endosc* 22(5):1353–1383, 2008.

pancreas, can be assessed. The pancreas should be imaged along the long axis in a relatively transverse plane, either directly or through the overlying omentum. For metastatic and primary liver malignancies, an ultrasound-guided core biopsy should be taken for suspicious lesions that would preclude curative resection. Color-flow Doppler imaging can be used to assess portal and hepatic vasculature and the relationship of these structures to any tumors visualized.

Because of the need for liberal adjustment of the position of the operating room table to facilitate visualizing the areas listed above, we frequently pad the patient and tape them to the operating table across the chest and the upper and lower legs. Cocooning the patient allows us the confidence to roll the patient hard one way or the other with reduced concerns that the patient will slide off of the table.

ESOPHAGEAL CANCER

Combined thoracoscopy and laparoscopy for esophageal cancer has been reported to be approximately 90% accurate in documenting nodal spread. The addition of laparoscopic sonography during staging has been reported to increase the detection rate for metastasis by 8% with little impact on the false-negative rate. Laparoscopic evaluation allows for assessment of liver and peritoneal metastasis as well as celiac nodal disease. Staging laparoscopy appears to more significantly change treatment plans for patients with lower esophageal and proximal gastric tumors when compared with those who have mid to upper esophageal lesions. At laparoscopy, enteral feeding access can be obtained if the decision to proceed with palliative or neoadjuvant therapy is anticipated. Thoracoscopic evaluation is performed in the right chest with the patient in full lateral decubitus position. Mobilization of the inferior pulmonary ligament allows for assessment of the thoracic esophagus, paraesophageal tissues, and subcarinal nodes. Major complications related to laparoscopic staging for esophageal cancer are quite uncommon.

Gastric Adenocarcinoma

Currently, routine preoperative staging in the United States for gastric adenocarcinoma includes esophagogastroduodenoscopy (EGD), CT, and staging laparoscopy. Multiple studies over the last two decades have documented the value of staging laparoscopy. Indeed, if a patient without obstructive symptoms has lymph node–positive cancer on laparoscopy and can receive chemotherapy, most never develop obstruction, bleeding, or other complaints, and they can avoid laparotomy altogether. Certainly, multimodal therapy and care at a teaching hospital have been associated with improved outcomes.

In an attempt to better define those patients who may benefit from staging laparoscopy, Sarela and colleagues reviewed 657 gastric cancer patients with minimal symptoms and no clinical evidence of metastatic disease on a previous CT scan. Multivariate analysis revealed that gastroesophageal junction lesions, diffuse tumors, or nodes greater than 1 cm in diameter were independent predictors of metastatic disease. Indeed, if one or more of these findings on CT or endoscopy were not present, diagnostic laparoscopy was always negative; therefore a preoperative CT was all that was required.

Colorectal Liver Metastases and Hepatobiliary Primary Tumors

Staging laparoscopy is seldom used in the primary treatment of colorectal cancer. Furthermore, the combination of fluorodeoxyglucose positron emission tomographic scanning (FDG-PET) and CT imaging has decreased the need for diagnostic laparoscopy for colorectal liver metastasis, but it is still occasionally used in conjunction with laparoscopic ultrasound. The overall benefit of diagnostic laparoscopy for the detection of unresectability is nearly 40% for primary liver tumors and 12% for colorectal liver metastasis. The largest study of staging laparoscopy for hepatocellular carcinoma to date was notable for avoidance of a nontherapeutic laparotomy in 16%. Routine staging laparoscopy for intrahepatic cholangiocarcinomas has resulted in avoidance of unnecessary operative intervention in 27% of patients treated at Memorial Sloan-Kettering Cancer Center. In patients with hilar cholangiocarcinomas, the addition of intraoperative ultrasound increased the yield for detecting unresectable tumors by almost 20%.

Many patients undergo percutaneous liver ablative procedures for liver cancer and metastasis in radiology suites in this country and around the world. We believe that these patients are best served by staging laparoscopy and laparoscopic, ultrasound-guided ablation if indicated. We have found that 40% of patients with unresectable disease have either extrahepatic disease or additional, often small-volume disease in the liver that was not seen on preablative imaging; therefore they are either undertreated or overtreated by ablation without staging laparoscopy with ultrasound.

Pancreatic and Periampullary Adenocarcinomas

Although the first case series of staging laparoscopy for pancreatic cancer was described by Cushchieri in 1978, minimally invasive techniques for the management of pancreatic cancer was slow to progress, compared with its use in other malignancies, for a variety of reasons. With the evolution of staging to include pancreatic helical CT imaging with fine cuts, the diagnostic yield of staging laparoscopy over the past two decades has decreased from 35% to approximately 13%, therefore some surgeons have argued for the selective use of staging laparoscopy. Evidence suggests that laparoscopy should be reserved for tumors in the body or tail of the pancreas, tumors larger than 3 cm, and with preoperative CA 19-9 levels greater than 100 U/mL. With regard to ampullary, duodenal, and distal bile duct tumors, the addition of diagnostic laparoscopy to dynamic CT scanning appears to identify an additional 10% of patients with unresectable disease.

Lymphoproliferative Diseases

Staging laparoscopy for lymphoproliferative disorders is similar to traditional staging laparotomy and can include liver biopsy, splenectomy, and lymph node sampling of iliac, celiac, portal, mesenteric, and periaortic nodes as well as excision of abnormal nodes identified preoperatively with marking of the area of excision with clips. For women, we choose to perform oophoropexy posterior to the uterus to protect the patient's fertility. The positive diagnostic yield is related to degree of tissue sampling, experience with laparoscopy, and complete mobilization of the colon, duodenum, and pancreas. We are most often called to biopsy abnormal-appearing lymph nodes in the mesentery that are seen on CT scan, either in patients with no prior history or in those with "hot" nodes on PET-CT following treatment. The entire node does not need to be removed in most cases; simply obtaining large biopsies with a cupped biopsy instrument is entirely adequate.

Prior to leaving the operating room, it is important to receive confirmation from the pathologist of the diagnosis and to ensure that the amount of tissue collected is adequate for flow cytometry or other specific tests. Morbidity is typically very limited. A core needle biopsy obtained by a radiologist is an option in some cases, especially in those with nodes that are difficult to reach surgically, such as nodes behind the renal vessels or nodes in patients who cannot tolerate anesthesia. The superior diagnostic accuracy of laparoscopic biopsy relative to percutaneous biopsy has been well documented and has been shown to be greater than 90%.

SUMMARY

Advances in preoperative helical CT, endoscopic ultrasound, and FDG-PET imaging, as well as staging laparoscopy, have given physicians more detailed information by which to tailor therapies within standard guidelines. By eliminating the need for laparotomy to assess tumor location and resectability, staging laparoscopy has gained prominence and will continue to play an important role in defining the next appropriate steps in the management of patients with gastrointestinal, hepatobiliary, pancreatic, and lymphoproliferative malignancies. Although routine use continues for esophageal and bile duct malignancies, some investigators have argued for selective employment of staging laparoscopy for gastric and pancreatic malignancies. As radiographic imaging, endoscopic ultrasound, and other assessment technologies improve, additional randomized and other prospective studies will further specify the role of laparoscopic investigation of patients with gastrointestinal malignancies.

SUGGESTED READINGS

Asoglu O, Porter L, Donohue JH, et al: Laparoscopy for the definitive diagnosis of intra-abdominal lymphoma, *Mayo Clin Proc* 80:625–631, 2005.

deCastro SMM, Tilleman EHB, Busch ORC, et al: Diagnostic laparoscopy for primary and secondary liver malignancies: impact of improved imaging and changed criteria for resection, *Ann Surg Oncol* 11:522–529, 2004.

Kooby DA, Chu CK: Laparoscopic management of pancreatic malignancies, *Surg Clin North Am* 90:427–446, 2010.

Maithel SK, Maloney S, Winston C, et al: Preoperative CA 19-9 and the yield of staging laparoscopy in patients with radiographically resectable pancreatic adenocarcinoma, *Ann Surg Oncol* 15:3512–3520, 2008.

Sarela AI, Lefkowitz R, Brennan MF, et al: Selection of patients with gastric adenocarcinoma for laparoscopic staging, *Am J Surg* 191:134–138, 2006.

Society of American Gastrointestinal and Endoscopic Surgeons: Diagnostic laparoscopy guidelines, *Surg Endosc* 22:1353–1383, 2008.

Yoon HH, Lowe VJ, Cassivi SD, et al: The role of FDG-PET and staging laparoscopy in the management of patients with cancer of the esophagus or gastroesophageal junction, *Gastroenterol Clin North Am* 38:103–120, 2009.

LAPAROSCOPIC PANCREATIC RESECTION

David A. Iannitti, MD, and Kwan N. Lau, MD

OVERVIEW

The introduction of laparoscopy to the surgical repertoire has revolutionized several procedures such as colectomy, adrenalectomy, herniorrhaphy, and cholecystectomy, among others. Increasing percentages of these types of procedures are performed on a routine basis using a minimally invasive approach. As widely reported in the literature, perioperative outcomes—such as length of stay, blood loss, and recovery—have improved significantly compared with the same indicators for open procedures. In contrast to these procedures, the adaptation of laparoscopic pancreatic surgery has been relatively slow. Initially, pancreatic procedures focused predominantly on the management of benign diseases such as pancreatitis and pseudocyst. Indeed, the proximity of the pancreas to the great vessels, coupled with the retroperitoneal location of the pancreas, were initially challenging for minimally invasive surgery. However, increased familiarity with laparoscopic techniques and with advancements in instrument technology have led many high-volume centers to routinely perform a wide range of minimally invasive pancreatic surgeries.

The first reported case of laparoscopic pancreatic resection for pancreatitis was in 1994 by Gagner and Cushieri. Several clinical series have emerged since that address management of both benign and malignant pancreatic diseases. Currently, laparoscopic enucleation, distal pancreatectomy, and Whipple procedures are performed, depending on the surgeon's level of experience and patient selection.

These procedures can be performed entirely with laparoscopy or with hand-assisted laparoscopy. More recently, the introduction of robotic operative systems has decreased the level of technical difficulty involved and has improved surgical outcomes.

LAPAROSCOPIC PANCREATICODUODENECTOMY

The Whipple procedure, or pancreaticoduodenectomy, is the only procedure for which the validity of a laparoscopic approach has not yet been verified in the literature. It is the most technically challenging laparoscopic pancreatic operation, and the proposed benefits, decreased length of stay and shortened postoperative ileus, have not been readily evident. Because of the risk of intraoperative hemorrhage and the increased potential for leakage, the safety of the procedure has also led to surgeons' hesitation to attempt it.

Gagner recently completed a review of 146 reported laparoscopic Whipple procedures and demonstrated that it can be safely performed without significant increases in the anastomotic leak rate and perioperative morbidity and mortality (Table 1). Secondary to complex upper gastrointestinal reconstruction, the length of the incision may not increase the morbidity of a Whipple procedure. Similarly, there is concern whether a laparoscopic approach can achieve adequate margins and lymphadenectomy, therefore it should only be performed in selected patients for benign conditions such as chronic pancreatitis, cystic neoplasm, intraductal pancreatic mucinous neoplasm, and neuroendocrine tumor. The role of a laparoscopic Whipple procedure remains unclear for ductal adenocarcinoma because of oncologic concerns and questionable perioperative benefits, thus it should only be performed in highly selected patients. Currently, minimally invasive pancreaticoduodenectomy should only be performed at high-volume centers and must be overseen by the institutional review board.

TABLE 1: Outcomes of laparoscopic pancreaticoduodenectomy (Whipple procedure)

Author	Approach	N	OR Time (Min)	EBL (mL)	Morbidity (%)	Mortality (%)	Fistula (%)	LOS (Days)
Gagner (2009)	Laparoscopic	146	439	142	16	1.3	7.5	18

EBL, Estimated blood loss; *LOS,* length of stay

LAPAROSCOPIC DISTAL PANCREATECTOMY

The most common indication to perform a distal pancreatectomy is for lesions located in the neck, body, and tail of the pancreas. Various approaches may be used to perform this operation, depending on whether the spleen is spared and the method used to preserve the splenic vessels. Operations include laparoscopic distal pancreatectomy with splenectomy and laparoscopic distal pancreatectomy with spleen preservation, with or without vessel preservation. The decision to perform the specific type of resection is dependent upon the size and location of the lesions relative to the pancreatic duct and vessels as well as pathology of the tumor. The body and tail of the pancreas have a more consistent duct structure and blood supply and are therefore more amendable to laparoscopic resection. In well-selected patients, benign diseases, low-grade malignancies, and adenocarcinoma are the pathologies that render patients potential candidates for a laparoscopic procedure.

Intraoperative ultrasound is useful in identifying tumors and delineating duct anatomy. It is imperative for the operating surgeon to master the technique of ultrasound and to base the operation on the information obtained. Small benign and low-grade lesions (<2 cm) located in the neck or proximal body can be managed by enucleation to preserve the tail, provided that the main pancreatic duct is not involved. The technical challenge of performing a laparoscopic pancreaticojejunostomy makes central pancreatectomy a less attractive option for midsegment lesions. The ideal resection for large tumors (>2 cm) adjacent to the duct or situated at the body and tail is a distal pancreatectomy.

Setup and Patient Position

The positioning of the patient depends on the surgeon's preference and the patient's body habitus. We utilize an operating table that can be placed low to the ground and that allows lateral rotation of up to 45 degrees and optimal split-leg positioning without stirrups. The patient usually lies supine, and both arms can be out, because the surgeon and assistant are at the level of patient's umbilicus and turned toward the patient's head. Another option is to lay the patient's left arm across the chest with the left flank elevated 45 degrees in rotation by placing a roll under the patient's left side. For the obese patient, the surgeon usually employs the "French position," with the surgeon standing between the patient's legs.

The peritoneum is usually accessed through the umbilicus. Three to four additional trocars (5 and 12 mm) are then placed, one in the epigastrium and the others in the left subcostal area, usually 15 mm apart, to allow maximum instrument flexibility. The hand-assisted device is usually placed in the left flank for an anticipated difficult procedure or distal pancreatectomy with splenectomy. High-definition video monitors are used, placed directly over the patient's head to allow a monoaxial array that allows surgeons to look in the direction of the operative field. Patients who undergo splenectomy are routinely immunized for *Streptococcus, Meningococcus,* and *Haemophilus influenzae* 2 weeks prior to the operation.

LAPAROSCOPIC DISTAL PANCREATECTOMY WITH SPLENECTOMY

Splenectomy is indicated for larger lesions, lesions that involve the vessels and hilum, or known malignancy for more thorough lymphadenectomy and oncologic staging. After establishing pneumoperitoneum, the abdominal cavity is first examined for evidence of metastatic disease. The operation commences by entering the lesser sac by dividing the gastrocolic omentum widely using an energy device, either a monopolar or bipolar cutting device or ultrasonic shears, outside the gastroepiploic arcade. The short gastric vessels are preserved if the spleen is not resected. Upon entering the lesser sac, the stomach is usually retracted by placing a suspending suture or by using an endoscopic retractor, and the anterior surface of the pancreas should be readily visible. Laparoscopic intraoperative ultrasound is used to define the pancreas and vascular anatomy as well as pinpointing the location of the lesion. Dissection is continued at the inferior border of the pancreas toward the spleen, taking care not to damage the colon. The splenocolic ligament is then divided, and the flexure is retracted caudally.

At this point, the surgeon has the option to proceed from a medial to lateral approach or vice versa; we prefer the former. The neck of the pancreas is circumferentially dissected, proceeding laterally with care to preserve the left gastric and hepatic arteries. The splenic artery should be identified, and attempts should be made to divide it outside of the pancreatic parenchyma. For patients with malignancy or chronic pancreatitis, the splenic artery may prove difficult to dissect out as a result of the underlying inflammation. In this situation, the splenic artery could be divided at a later stage along with the pancreas. Continuing the dissection at the inferior border of the pancreas toward the body and tail, the pancreas can then be lifted off the retroperitoneum with or without elevation of the splenic vein. An umbilical tape can be employed to elevate the pancreas and provide better traction to facilitate the dissection. This maneuver is called the *lasso technique.*

Next, the splenic vein is identified at the posterior border of the pancreas and divided individually or en bloc with the pancreatic parenchyma. After reconfirming the location of the lesion, the pancreas is divided. We usually prefer to divide the pancreas at its neck, just to the left of the superior mesenteric vein, as this typically represents the thinnest portion of the pancreatic substance. A laparoscopic linear stapler is routinely used, with the appropriate staple height selected depending upon the thickness of the gland. Reports support the use of bioabsorbable staple-line reinforcement to reduce pancreatic fistula formation. As such, we routinely use a 4.8 mm stapler together with bioabsorbable reinforcement. It is important not to crush the parenchyma with the stapler, while using the bioabsorbable material to evenly distribute the pressure without compromising pancreatic integrity. Another option is to transect the pancreas using a vessel-sealing device, but to date no reproducible method for dividing the pancreas to reduce the leakage rate has been reported using this approach.

Completing the mobilization of the body and tail, the posterior pancreatic dissection can be performed through a relatively avascular plane just outside Gerota's fascia, which usually includes the posterior lymph nodes. The anterior superior mesenteric lymph nodes can usually be removed along with the splenic vessel resection. As the dissection continues toward the splenic hilum at the superior border of the pancreas, an energy device or clip applier can be used to control the short gastric arteries. The specimen is ready for retrieval after the splenic attachment is divided. The specimen is removed after dividing the pancreatic tail from the spleen to allow for a smaller extraction point. The stapler line is then examined, and a drain can be selectively placed for possible seroma formation at the splenic bed, but not for anticipated leakage.

LAPAROSCOPIC DISTAL PANCREATECTOMY WITH SPLEEN PRESERVATION

The spleen can usually be preserved with benign or indeterminate lesions. The added value of splenectomy is not warranted for this type of lesion and would not improve the oncologic outcome. The spleen-preserving distal pancreatectomy can be performed in one

TABLE 2: Outcomes of laparoscopic pancreatic enucleation

	Approach	N	OR Time (Min)	EBL (mL)	Fistula (%)	LOS (Days)
Karaliotas (2009)	Laparoscopic	5	121	NA	20	11
	Open	7	92	NA	29	14
Luo (2009)	Laparoscopic	16	85	205	25	5.5

EBL, Estimated blood loss; *LOS,* length of stay; *NA,* not applicable

of two ways, depending on whether the splenic vessels are divided. Similarly, the approach to preserving the spleen relies on the condition of the splenic artery and the individual surgeon's preference. The vessel-sparing technique requires careful dissection along the superior border of the pancreas, dividing all the perforating vessels from the splenic artery into the pancreas.

Another option to preserve the spleen is to divide the splenic vessels and allow the spleen to function from the collaterals that exist from the short gastric arteries; this is known as the *Warshaw technique.* The splenic vessels are divided at the same level as the pancreas or transected just proximal to the splenic hilum. This approach requires considerable care not to divide the short gastric arteries that reside in the gastrolienal ligament and its collateral around the splenic hilum. Critics of this approach contend that the dissection involved in vessel preservation is tedious and time consuming, and many times the blood supply can become compromised as a result of secondary bleeding and/or thrombosis. Currently no definitive evidence exists to support either method as superior to the other; however, it should be noted that concern has been raised that the Warshaw technique may have the potential to increase the risk of splenic infarct and attenuate the immune response.

HAND-ASSISTED LAPAROSCOPIC PANCREATIC RESECTION

Pancreatic surgery as a whole is challenging, and performing these techniques laparoscopically adds an additional degree of technical difficulty. As such, surgeons who perform laparoscopic pancreatic resection must first master advanced laparoscopic skills and exhibit a comprehensive knowledge of hepatobiliary anatomy. The use of a hand-assisted device can provide significant advantages in terms of proprioception and retraction and dissection capability compared with a totally laparoscopic approach. It is our opinion that hand-assisted laparoscopic surgery can assist surgeons during the learning process associated with laparoscopic pancreatic resection. Additionally, this approach can enhance the confidence of the surgeon, as they teach others how to perform these operations.

Most pancreatic resections will require a sizable port (~8 cm) for specimen extraction; it is sensible to place a hand port in the beginning of the case to fully utilize the incision. Placement of the port site can be in the mid epigastrium or the left flank, but we prefer the latter, along with using a medial-to-lateral pancreatic dissection technique. Furthermore, if significant hemorrhage is encountered, the surgeon's level of confidence thus increases, because bleeding can be controlled by digital compression while other measures are attempted. Hand assistance is most useful for difficult dissections and for pancreatectomy with splenectomy.

LAPAROSCOPIC PANCREATIC ENUCLEATION

Enucleation is reasonable for small (<2 cm), benign, or low-grade tumors. To safely perform this procedure laparoscopically, the operating surgeon must master intraoperative ultrasound to locate the lesion and

BOX 1: The International Study Group of Pancreatic Fistula grading system

Grade A: Biochemical fistula without clinical sequelae
Grade B: Fistula requiring any therapeutic intervention
Grade C: Fistula with severe clinical sequelae

discern its relationship to the main pancreatic duct. The surgeon must adequately weigh the risk of increased postoperative leakage against the potential benefit of preserving pancreatic parenchyma (Table 2).

The operation begins by entering the lesser sac and thoroughly examining the pancreas using intraoperative ultrasound. Understanding the relationship of the lesion to the pancreatic duct is critical for determination of appropriateness of enucleation or resection. If the lesion is not amendable to being approached anteriorly, the inferior border of the pancreas can be mobilized, and the lesion approached posteriorly, after the pancreas is elevated. Usually, the ultrasonic shears or an energy sealing/cutting device is used to separate the lesion from the pancreatic parenchyma. Suturing the enucleation site with horizontal polypropylene sutures can be considered. Because of the higher leak rate from enucleation (see Table 2) compared with pancreatic resection, drain placement is at the surgeon's discretion.

ROBOTIC-ASSISTED LAPAROSCOPIC PANCREATIC SURGERY

In contrast to other specialties, most notably urologic and gynecologic procedures, the introduction of surgical robotic systems is still being evaluated in hepatobiliary surgery. The use of robotics in other fields has expanded exponentially in recent years, but the advantages of robotic devices in pancreatic surgery remain to be fully determined. Currently, few doubts exist that this approach provides superior optics, lighting, magnification, depth perception, range of movement, and dexterity compared with conventional laparoscopy. Hence the robotic approach provides relative ease in performing complex tasks such as intracorporeal suturing, the best example being the performance of pancreaticojejunstomy using a robotic-assisted laparoscopic device.

As with all systems, there is a learning curve for utilizing robotic systems in pancreatic surgery; however, most surgeons find that potential difficulties can be easily overcome following relatively few cases by understanding how to position the patient, dock the robot, and position the trocars. In our experience, the operative time for dissection is reduced using the robotic system as compared with its laparoscopic counterpart; in several instances, the use of a robotic device allows cases to be performed that are otherwise not possible using conventional laparoscopic approaches. Relatively few reports in the literature describe robotic pancreatic resection, however, from these initial reports, it appears that perioperative morbidity and mortality are equivalent to routine laparoscopic surgery with the exception of operative time. Further studies that compare robotic-assisted laparoscopic surgery with conventional laparoscopic surgery are needed to determine the role of these systems in pancreatic surgery.

TABLE 3: **Laparoscopic versus open distal pancreatectomy**

Authors	Approach	N	OR Time (Min)	EBL (mL)	Morbidity (%)	Mortality (%)	Fistula (%)	LOS (Day)
Matsumoto (2009)	Open	19	214	400	21	0	10.5	23.8
	Laparoscopic	14	290	247	7	0	0	12.9
Finan (2009)	Open	104	200	500	25	4.8	16.3	8.6
	Laparoscopic	44	156	100	20	0	15.9	5.8
Kooby (2008)	Open	200	216	588	57	0	18	9
	Laparoscopic	142	230	357	40	1	11	5.9

EBL, Estimated blod loss; *LOS,* length of stay

The ongoing development of instrumentation for use with the robotic arm may increase its use in pancreatic surgery.

OUTCOMES

The number of laparoscopic pancreatic surgeries has steadily increased in recent years as more surgeons master the techniques required. A growing body of literature supports the use of minimally invasive pancreatic surgery, and the characteristics of perioperative complications are becoming better classified. One example is that of pancreatic fistula, which remains a clinically challenging problem. The International Study Group of Pancreatic Fistula (ISGPF) has now provided a more consistent definition of pancreatic fistula (Box 1).

Multiple retrospective series have been published, and the perioperative profile for distal pancreatectomy is summarized in Table 3. Perioperative morbidity and mortality for laparoscopic distal pancreatectomy are comparable to open distal pancreatectomy, and clinically relevant fistula rates remain around 10% (grades B and C). The emergence of case-control series have validated the laparoscopic method, yielding a shorter length of stay, decreased estimated blood loss, and reduction of overall morbidity. Furthermore, although multiple methods of pancreatic stump management have been proposed to decrease occurrences, the incidence remains largely unchanged. Aside from conventional oversewing of the stump, common methods include using the linear stapler alone, employing staples with bioabsorbable reinforcement, application of sealant, application of tissue reinforcement such as round ligament, and the use of tissue-sealing energy devices.

Regardless of the choice of pancreatic closure, the leak rate remains comparable between open and laparoscopic approaches. In addition, risk factors reported by Weber (2009) suggest that a high body mass index (>27), estimated blood loss greater than 150 mL, and pancreatic resection greater than 8 cm may also increase the risk of pancreatic fistula formation (Box 2).

Another consideration when performing laparoscopic pancreatic operations is the potential benefit of spleen preservation. The potential of splenic infarct or bleeding from splenic artery pseudoaneurysm may increase the morbidity of performing spleen-preserving distal pancreatectomy. The morbidity profile for laparoscopic pancreatic resection may improve significantly if splenectomy is routinely performed. However, as described in the literature, overwhelming postsplenectomy sepsis (OPSS) remains a real entity, despite the relatively low incidence rate, typically well below 1%. Indeed, true incidence of OPSS may even be lower than 1%, especially after routine perioperative immunization. On the whole, the patient population susceptible to OPSS tends to be younger patients with a hematologic malignancy. Finally, the benefits of preserving the spleen must be weighed against the increases in morbidity during attempts to preserve it. With this in mind, surgeons should decide on a case-by-case basis whether to preserve the spleen.

BOX 2: Risk factors for postoperative pancreatic fistula formation

Pancreatic duct >3 mm
Body mass index >20* or >27†
Bile infection at postoperative day 1
Estimated blood loss >150 mL
Pancreatic resection >8 cm

*Per Kajiwara (2009)
†Per Weber (2009)

SUMMARY

Since its emergence as an experimental procedure 15 years ago, the outlook for the minimally invasive approach to pancreatic surgery is promising. The continuing evolution of technology for instrumentation, plus the addition of robotic surgical systems, will allow more surgeons to continue to adapt to these procedures. It is imperative that a consensus be reached as to how a curriculum should be created to educate residents and fellows in performing these complex procedures routinely.

SUGGESTED READINGS

Bassi C, Dervenis C, Butturini G, et al: Postoperative pancreatic fistula: an international study group (ISGPF) definition, *Surgery* 138(1):8–13, 2005.

Finan KR, Cannon EE, Kim EJ, et al: Laparoscopic and open distal pancreatectomy: a comparison of outcomes, *Am Surg* 75(8):671–679, discussion 679-680, 2009.

Gagner M, Palermo M: Laparoscopic Whipple procedure: review of the literature, *J Hepatobiliary Pancreat Surg* 16(6):726–730, 2009.

Iannitti DA, Coburn NG, Somberg J, et al: Use of the round ligament of the liver to decrease pancreatic fistulas: a novel technique, *J Am Coll Surg* 203(6):857–864, 2006.

Karaliotas C, Sgourakis G: Laparoscopic versus open enucleation for solitary insulinoma in the body and tail of the pancreas, *J Gastrointest Surg* 13(10):1869, 2009.

Kooby DA, Gillespie T, Bentrem D, et al: Left-sided pancreatectomy: a multicenter comparison of laparoscopic and open approaches, *Ann Surg* 248(3):438–446, 2008.

Luo Y, Liu R, Hu MG, et al: Laparoscopic surgery for pancreatic insulinomas: a single-institution experience of 29 cases, *J Gastrointest Surg* 13(5):945–950, 2009.

Matsumoto T, Shibata K, Ohta M, et al: Laparoscopic distal pancreatectomy and open distal pancreatectomy: a nonrandomized comparative study, *Surg Laparosc Endosc Percutan Tech* 18(4):340–343, 2008.

LAPAROSCOPIC BYPASS FOR PANCREATIC CANCER

R. Matthew Walsh, MD, and Sricharan Chalikonda, MD

LAPAROSCOPIC BYPASS FOR PANCREATIC CANCER

The surgical management of pancreatic cancer is typically geared toward resection. Current approaches to resection increasingly include minimally invasive techniques, including laparoscopic pancreaticoduodenectomy. Unfortunately, the majority of patients with pancreatic cancer are not candidates for resection, yet some of these patients could benefit from laparoscopic palliation of their disease.

The principle goal of palliative surgery for pancreatic malignancies is definitive palliation with minimal morbidity. Although surgical treatment is often one of several palliative options, surgery can offer durability other options lack, although this must be tempered by expected length of life and time of surgical recovery. Implementing minimally invasive surgical techniques provides the durability of surgical bypass with lower morbidity.

The surgical community is currently evaluating modeling techniques, such as the Physiological and Operative Severity Score for the Enumeration of Mortality and Morbidity (POSSUM), which uses physiologic and operative severity score to predict long-term outcome. These scoring systems have some potential to balance treatment options in patients with a limited lifespan. Incumbent in any treatment planning is accurate assessment of both disease extent and a patient's physiologic reserves. Diagnostic imaging and interventional techniques now allow for accurate preoperative staging and tissue sampling to avoid nontherapeutic laparotomies in nearly all patients. Patients with metastatic disease are typically best managed with nonsurgical palliation, because their life expectancy is limited. Expandable metallic stents are available for endoscopic treatment of biliary or gastric outlet obstructions, with surgery only necessary for treatment failures. Patients not amenable for laparoscopic palliation are those with locally advanced neoplasms that require traditional open exploration to assess resectability, and open surgical palliation and prophylactic procedures are advised for those deemed unresectable. The best patients to consider for laparoscopic surgical palliation are those with locally advanced disease that is clearly unresectable who also do not have metastatic disease on imaging. Isolated or combined palliation of biliary or gastric outlet obstruction is appropriate for laparoscopic techniques.

A minimally invasive approach to relieve malignant gastric outlet obstruction is the most straightforward procedure to perform, either as a single bypass procedure in patients with isolated symptomatic gastric outlet obstruction from pancreatic cancer; in those with symptomatic obstruction, whose biliary obstruction is already believed to be well palliated with endoscopic stenting; or in patients who have failed enteric stenting. Laparoscopic gastrojejunostomy is a reasonable option for patients with adequate nutrition status and an expected survival greater than 3 months.

The only small, comparative randomized trial of laparoscopic gastrojejunostomy versus radiologic enteric stent placement for malignant gastric outlet obstruction did show benefit in length of stay and quality of life 1 month after the stent procedure, but this study was compromised in its lack of specified disease stage and overall median survival of less than 20 weeks. Laparoscopic gastrojejunostomy does have improved outcomes when compared to open gastrojejunostomy in a similarly small, randomized trial from Italy. An antecolic laparoscopic loop gastrojejunostomy was shown to have a comparable operative time to a handsewn open technique, but it also had significantly less operative blood loss and rate of delayed gastric emptying.

Technical aspects of the operation include antibiotic and thromboembolic prophylaxis. Many surgeons prefer to place the patient in a split-leg position, although we have not found it necessary. We prefer a conventional supine position with arms tucked at the sides and a footboard for ease of placing patients in reverse Trendelenburg. It is advisable to ensure that the patient is adequately padded and secured to the table prior to prepping to avoid movement once the patient is draped.

Entry to the peritoneal cavity and establishment of pneumoperitoneum can be obtained with an open Hasson approach or via an optical trocar. We prefer to utilize an optical trocar in obese patients and in those who have had prior laparotomies, where the trocar can be placed in a remote location away from prior incisions. Once pneumoperitoneum has been established, we place the remaining trocars under direct vision.

A variety of positions and a number of trocars have been described. A lazy-U configuration is our preference (Figure 1), with trocars spaced laterally across the midline, instead of in extreme positions in the upper or lower quadrants. The midline position is centered around the umbilicus, with either a supraumbilical or infraumbilical position, depending on the distance from the xiphoid to the umbilicus and the known degree of gastric distension. Typically 2 to 3 hand widths from the xiphoid and a hand width between laparoscopic ports is preferred; a distance of 2 hand widths is necessary between the camera and any robotic port site. Generally, this is

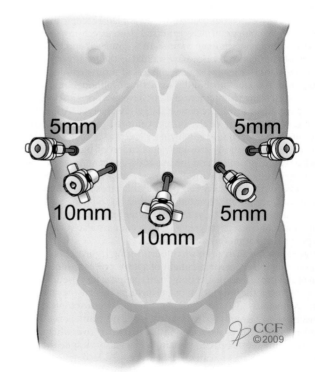

FIGURE 1 Typical port positions for surgical palliation of pancreatic cancer. This lazy-U positioning is good for double bypass; the right upper quadrant 5 mm port can usually be eliminated for an isolated laparoscopic gastrojejunostomy. *(Reprinted with permission from Cleveland Clinic Center for Medical Art & Photography, copyright 2009. All Rights Reserved.)*

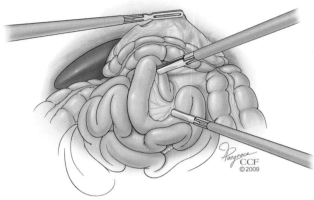

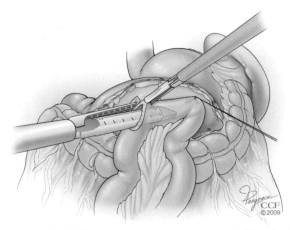

a four-port, two-person operation, where the camera port is at the umbilicus with an angled laparoscope and a 10 to 12 mm port in the right hemiabdomen for stapler insertion; the remaining two ports in the left hemiabdomen can be 5 mm.

The initial portion of the operation involves staging of the abdominal cavity with directed laparoscopic biopsy of any suspicious peritoneal or liver lesions. We also advocate surgeon-performed laparoscopic liver ultrasound and peritoneal washing for complete staging. Once the diagnostic portion of the procedure is complete, the greater omentum should be assessed for mobility. It is important to ensure that the entire omentum can be flipped superiorly over the transverse colon to visualize the ligament of Treitz. If this step cannot be performed satisfactorily, the remainder of the procedure will be very difficult to perform safely in a timely manner.

Once the omentum has been evaluated, attention is directed to the mobilization of the stomach. The preferred bypass is an isoperistaltic, antecolic, retrogastric gastrojejunostomy fashioned in the antrum. The lesser sac is entered laterally by dividing the gastrocolic portion of the greater omentum with ultrasonic shears. The omentum is widely divided, lateral to medial with division of retroperitoneal attachments, taking care to avoid injury to the middle colic vessels. The ligament of Treitz must be identified, and a loop of proximal jejunum is brought anterior to the stomach, so that it lies comfortably without tension. This maneuver is facilitated by brief Trendelenburg positioning, so that the omentum and colon can be retracted cephalad to help identify the proximal jejunum (Figure 2). A single tacking stitch is placed distally on the antrum and jejunum to ease passage of the endoscopic stapler. This can be performed using conventional sutures with laparoscopic needle drivers or with an endomechanical suturing device. Surgeons uncomfortable with intracorporeal knot tying may employ the endomechanical suturing device with extracorporeal knot tying and a knot pusher.

Once the tacking sutures are in place, we create the enterotomy and gastrotomy using hook cautery. It is helpful to create the gastrotomy and enterotomy through the 12 mm port, through which the stapler will be fired. This ensures that the stomach and jejunum will be in the correct alignment for the stapler, and it also minimizes repositioning of the assistant's instruments. We prefer a 60 mm long, 3.5 mm stapling device that enters from the right-sided trocar position (Figure 3). Depending on the patient's body habitus, a 60 mm stapler may sometimes be cumbersome, and a reticulating 45 mm stapler may be used. The enterotomy created to insert the stapler needs to be closed, and we advise handsewn laparoscopic suturing, running or interrupted, as opposed to a double-staple technique (Figure 4). If suturing is technically challenging, a double-staple technique can be

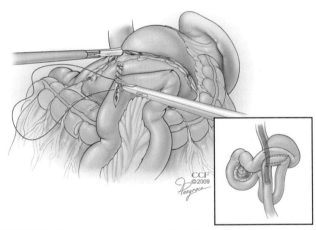

performed safely, provided that care is taken to avoid narrowing of the efferent limb. This risk can be minimized by placing an endoscope through the anastomosis into the efferent limb prior to closure. An upper endoscopy is then performed to confirm patency of the anastomosis and evaluate for leaks. A feeding tube is not typically placed in the efferent limb, although it is a feasible option for the severely malnourished, and postoperative management is aimed at early ambulation and removal of the nasogastric tube.

Surgical palliation of biliary obstruction from pancreatic cancer is advantageous for many patients and can be accomplished laparoscopically for appropriate patients. Endobiliary stenting is the palliative procedure of choice for patients with metastatic disease found on preoperative imaging or at staging laparoscopy. The laparoscopic techniques required for biliary bypass are more advanced than for an isolated gastrojejunostomy, because intracorporeal suturing and knot-tying skills are required. Acceptable candidates for laparoscopic biliary bypass include patients with locally advanced, known unresectable carcinoma without metastatic disease with satisfactory nutrition status and comorbid disease.

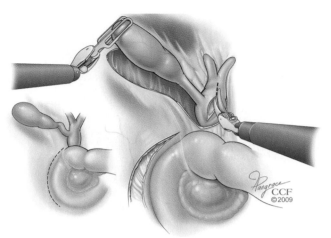

FIGURE 5   Laparoscopic robotic biliary bypass. A choledochoduodenostomy is fashioned after a wide Kocher maneuver. A Roux choledochojejunostomy can be similarly performed. *(Reprinted with permission from Cleveland Clinic Center for Medical Art & Photography, copyright 2009. All Rights Reserved.)*

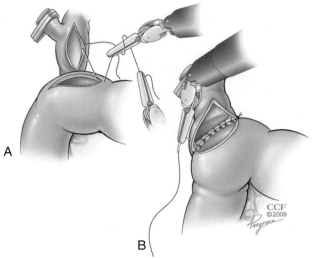

FIGURE 6   Robotic choledochoduodenostomy with interrupted absorbable sutures. **A,** Orientation of the common bile duct to bowel. **B,** Interrupted anastomosis. *(Reprinted with permission from Cleveland Clinic Center for Medical Art & Photography, copyright 2009. All Rights Reserved.)*

Types of biliary bypass include enteric bypasses to the gallbladder or bile duct. Although laparoscopic cholecystojejunostomy is the most frequently reported type of laparoscopic bypass, it should be discouraged for the same reason it is discouraged in open bypass procedures: a high rate of recurrent jaundice and biliary complications. As a general principle, an operation should not be compromised so that it can be performed laparoscopically. The operative technique may be unique to laparoscopy, but the outcomes should be equivalent (a good example is the lateral positioning for laparoscopic splenectomy), therefore we strongly advise utilizing the common hepatic or common bile duct as the biliary site for the bypass. The enteric conduit can be either a Roux limb or the duodenum, which we have long advocated; use of the duodenum spares the need for an additional anastomosis to create the Roux limb, although a good Kocher maneuver is required to mobilize the duodenum, which is not always possible laparoscopically when a bulky tumor is present.

Whenever a surgical biliary bypass is created for palliation of pancreatic cancer, a gastrojejunostomy should also be done. It is now clearly established by retrospective and prospective randomized trials that prophylactic gastrojejunostomy reduces the risk of later obstruction and can be done with a tolerable rate of delayed gastric emptying. The operative setup is similar to the one previously described. In the obese patient, the right arm may remain extended to allow for placement of a table mounted liver retractor. One additional trocar is placed laterally on the right along the arc of the lazy-U configuration, so that five trocars total are placed in the mid abdomen. An additional subxiphoid trocar is placed to retract the liver and expose the liver hilum; we prefer the Nathanson retractor for this purpose. Exposure of the bile duct is facilitated by lateral retraction of the gallbladder, leaving its removal until after the bypass is performed (Figure 5).

Should the duodenum be utilized, a wide Kocher maneuver is enhanced by rotating the patient and moving the laparoscope to one of the right lateral ports. We perform a side-to-side, fish-mouth, biliary-enteric anastomosis by longitudinally opening the bile duct and placing the longitudinal enteric opening perpendicular to it. We typically perform the anastomosis unstented, with interrupted fine absorbable sutures (Figure 6). We find this is best accomplished with robotic assistance, although standard laparoscopic suturing is also possible. The robotic-assisted biliary anastomosis is comfortable and reliable to perform, and it is easier for surgeons not as facile in intracorporeal suturing. The robot is docked into position once the enteric conduit is positioned, and the robotic instruments are used for the biliary dissection and anastomosis. The robot can then be undocked

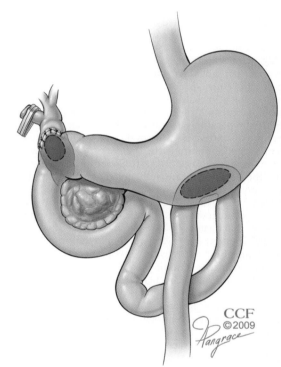

FIGURE 7   Completed laparoscopic biliary and gastric bypass for surgical palliation of pancreatic cancer. *(Reprinted with permission from Cleveland Clinic Center for Medical Art & Photography, copyright 2009. All Rights Reserved.)*

to perform the subsequent gastrojejunostomy (Figure 7). A closed-suction drain can be placed in the Morison pouch and exited through a port site. The outcome of biliary, gastric, or double bypass compares favorably to the comparable open operations when performed laparoscopically. The objective data are meager and involve highly selected patients, but it is an option whose utility will expand with time, providing adequate technical skill is available and good surgical judgment is exercised.

Suggested Readings

Artifon EL, Sakai P, Cunha JE, et al: Surgery or endoscopy for palliation of biliary obstruction due to metastatic pancreatic cancer, *Am J Gastroenterol* 101(9):2031–2037, 2006.

Cho YK, Shin JH, Oh SY: Significance of palliative gastrojejunostomy for unresectable pancreatic head carcinoma, *Hepatogastroenterology* 55:254–257, 2008.

deCastro SMM, Houwert JT, Lagard SM, et al: POSSUM predicts survival in patients with unresectable pancreatic cancer, *Dig Surg* 26:75–79, 2009.

Hamade AM, Al-Bahrani AZ, Owera AMA, et al: Therapeutic, prophylactic, and preresection applications of laparoscopic gastric and biliary bypass for patients with periampullary malignancy, *Surg Endosc* 19:1333–1340, 2005.

Kim HO, Hwang SI, Kim H, et al: Quality of survival in patients treated for malignant biliary obstruction caused by unresectable pancreatic head cancer: surgical versus nonsurgical palliation, *Hepatobiliary Pancreatic Dis Int* 7:643–648, 2008.

Mehta S, Hindmarsh A, Cheong E, et al: Prospective randomized trial of laparoscopic gastrojejunostomy versus duodenal stenting for malignant gastric outflow obstruction, *Surg Endosc* 20:239–242, 2006.

Mukherjee S, Kocher HM, Hutchins RR, et al: Palliative surgical bypass for pancreatic and peri-ampullary cancers, *J Gastrointest Cancer* 38:102–107, 2007.

Navarra G, Musolino C, Venneri A, et al: Palliative antecolic isoperistaltic gastrojejunostomy: a randomized controlled trial comparing open and laparoscopic approaches, *Surg Endosc* 20:1831–1834, 2006.

Siddiqui A, Spechler SJ, Huerta S: Surgical bypass versus endoscopic stenting for malignant gastroduodenal obstruction: a decision analysis, *Dig Dis Sci* 52:276–281, 2007.

Warner EA, Ben-David K, Cendan JC, et al: Laparoscopic pancreatic surgery: what now and what next? *Curr Gastroenterol Rep* 11:128–133, 2009.

Laparoscopic Management of Pancreatic Pseudocyst

Edward C.S. Lai, MD

OVERVIEW

Pancreatic pseudocyst represents an aftermath of pancreatic ductal disruption of both inflammatory and traumatic origin. When the main pancreatic duct or one of its radicals is disrupted, pancreatic secretions spill into the retroperitoneum or the peripancreatic tissue planes. The inflammatory response along the serosal surfaces of the adjacent organs induces the formation of a fibrous pseudocapsule after a period of 4 to 8 weeks, at which point a pseudocyst is formed. Among patients with an acute exacerbation of chronic pancreatitis, roughly 40% of them develop a pseudocyst, compared to only 5% to 15% of those with acute pancreatitis.

PREOPERATIVE INVESTIGATIONS

When therapeutic intervention is chosen, computed tomography (CT), magnetic resonance pancreatography (MRP), and in selected cases endoscopic retrograde cholangiopancreatography (ERCP) are mandatory investigations to formulate the most appropriate treatment option. When the renal function of the patient allows, thin-sliced multidetector CT supplemented by intravenous contrast injection allows a thorough evaluation of the anatomical extent of the pseudocyst, including 1) the detection of isolated collections beside the target lesion; 2) the presence of necrotic tissue; 3) isolated functional pancreatic parenchyma from the complete disruption of the main pancreatic duct to the left of the pseudocyst, or *disconnected pancreatic tail syndrome*; 4) patency of the splenic vein, and when obliterated, features suggestive of left-side portal hypertension; and last but not least, 5) details such as the presence and thickness of any interposing large blood vessels on the interface, through which the pancreatic pseudocyst would be drained surgically or endoscopically.

In recent years, endoscopic ultrasonography (EUS) has gained increasing popularity as a one-step procedure for simultaneous evaluation and treatment, especially for small pancreatic pseudocysts that do not significantly indent into the gastric or duodenal lumen. After screening the cyst cavity for any accompanying irregularity or fine septa within the cavity, fine needle aspiration (FNA) of the cystic fluid permits evaluation for cytology, carcinoembryonic antigen (CEA), mucin, and pancreatic enzymes with the aim to differentiate the pseudocyst from cystic neoplasms of the pancreas. When coupled with color Doppler examination, EUS can accurately identify the best access site into the cyst cavity for endoscopic transmural drainage. Knowing the main pancreatic duct anatomy is helpful to guide the management. Among patients with an abnormal pancreatic duct—such as those with strictures, duct-cyst communication, and duct cutoff—percutaneous drainage has a poor outcome. On the other hand, endoscopic transpapillary drainage works well only when there is a communication between the pancreatic duct and cyst.

INDICATIONS

A decision to intervene on a pancreatic pseudocyst is indicated when the cyst measures over 6 cm in diameter, persists beyond 4 to 6 weeks from diagnosis, or results in symptoms, especially infection. With the increasing armamentarium of nonsurgical options that allow effective drainage of the pseudocyst, a joint consultation with the endoscopist and the interventional radiologist is appropriate to formulate the best therapeutic measures for the patient. Treatment should be individualized, as the underlying nature of the pancreatitis, whether acute or chronic; status of the pancreatic duct; general condition of the patient; and the availability of expertise are all relevant considerations. The use of percutaneous drainage should probably be restricted as a temporizing measure when the pseudocyst becomes infected, as experience from the United States at the turn of this century showed that percutaneous drainage carried a significantly higher complication rate, prolonged hospital stay, and increased mortality rate compared to surgical drainage. On the other hand, the use of therapeutic endoscopy is gaining wider popularity despite its rates of complete resolution, reintervention, and morbidity and mortality, which are often worse than that of laparoscopy.

Among 689 patients reported in a recent literature review, close to five times as many patients were subjected to endoscopic drainage compared to laparoscopy. The increasing use of EUS coupled with color Doppler can help to overcome many of the shortcomings associated with endoscopic drainage reported previously. Overall, endoscopic drainage resulted in a 71% success rate in the treatment of pseudocysts. Most would accept that surgery is indicated when previous nonoperative drainage procedures have failed or recurrent cysts form. Consequently, complex pseudocysts—including giant pseudocysts, multiple pseudocysts, and pseudocysts accompanied by main pancreatic duct disruption—and duct abnormalities, such as strictures and stones, are left in the hands of surgeons.

SELECTION OF DRAINAGE PROCEDURE

For decades, surgical internal drainage of pseudocysts via the gastrointestinal tract were appropriate, including cystogastrostomy, cystduodenostomy, and Roux-en-Y cystojejunostomy. Under such circumstances, the surgeon must choose the best approach according to the anatomic findings. In one recent series of 108 patients, over 90% had a cystogastrostomy compared with less than 8% who had a drainage procedure via a jejunal loop. Other options include lateral pancreaticojejunostomy and duodenal-sparing pancreatic head resection with pseudocyst incorporation with or without accompanying pancreatic duct drainage. Infrequently, pancreatic resection is indicated, especially among patients with chronic pancreatitis and abnormal duct anatomy.

LAPAROSCOPIC CYSTOGASTROSTOMY

Prior to surgery, a gastroduodenoscopy should be conducted to rule out gastric pathology such as peptic ulcer or gastritis, which can cause symptoms similar to those of a pseudocyst. For patients with acute biliary pancreatitis, a laparoscopic cholecystectomy should be considered at the same sitting.

Anterior Approach

After induction of general anesthesia, the patient is placed in a semilithotomy position to allow the surgeon to stand between the patient's legs; the assistant remains at the left side of the patient. A subumbilical cutdown is made to allow the introduction of the first 10 mm trocar. Based on the visual assessment, four additional ports are placed: a 10 mm port to the left of the umbilicus, a 12 mm port below the xiphoid, and two 5 mm ports in the right upper quadrant. A 5 mm liver retractor is inserted via a 5 mm port to retract the left lobe of the liver to the patient's right to expose the entire anterior gastric wall. An anterior gastrotomy is then made with a Harmonic scalpel to expose the posterior gastric wall, where the indentation made by the pseudocyst is clearly evident. A 12 mm laparoscopic ultrasound probe is introduced to explore the posterior gastric wall.

After localizing the pseudocyst, orientation of the intended cystogastrostomy is mapped out, depending on the thickness of the interposed walls and absence of any significant intervening blood vessels. The cyst content is aspirated, and a cystogastrostomy is made with a Harmonic scalpel to accommodate the anvil of the mechanical laparoscopic, 45 mm Endo GIA stapler (Covidien, Boulder, Colo.). Depending on the size of the pseudocyst, the cystogastric anastomosis is created with one or two staple cartridges along the longitudinal axis of the stomach, as the mechanical device allows a simultaneous cutting and securing of hemostasis.

Once the cystogastrostomy is established, the interior of the cyst is then examined with the laparoscope if possible, followed by irrigation of the cyst cavity to eliminate necrotic debris. Biopsy of the cyst

is obtained, and after complete hemostasis of the anastomotic line, the anterior gastrotomy is closed using a running continuous suture. An indwelling nasogastric tube is left, and a 15 Fr drain is left in the Morison pouch.

Intragastric Approach

After administering general anesthesia and establishing pneumoperitoneum with carbon dioxide, standard ports and a laparoscope are inserted into the peritoneal cavity. Under low intraabdominal pressure, the stomach is insufflated through a nasogastric tube with CO_2. While maintaining the laparoscopic view of the anterior surface of the stomach, special intraluminal trocars are inserted under direct vision through the abdominal and anterior gastric walls. Additional ports are placed into the gastric lumen, away from the first port, to maintain principles of triangulation in a manner similar to the first port. The 12 mm trocar is positioned close to the greater curve, oriented toward the pylorus to accommodate the later use of laparoscopic ultrasound and a mechanical stapler. After all the intragastric ports are in position, the intraabdominal pressure is lowered to allow the stomach to be insufflated to its maximal size using 15 cm of water pressure. Through one of these intragastric ports, a 5 mm, 30-degree laparoscope is passed to examine the duodenum and the gastric cavity to localize the pseudocyst by identification of the prominent convexity on the bowel wall. With the aid of preoperative CT and needle aspiration of the cyst contents, the intended site for the cystogastrostomy is determined.

An incision is made and extended to the desired length and direction with electrocautery or an EndoGIA stapler as described previously. The choice of the intended site of the anastomosis should take into consideration the possibility of subsequent debridement of the cyst through a peroral flexible endoscope. The solid contents of the cyst are removed, as they might plug the anastomosis. The debrided material is left in the gastric lumen or is pushed down into the duodenum. After the cyst is drained, the gastric trocars are withdrawn, and the stomach is deflated. Under visual guidance from the subumbilical port and two other trocars, the holes in the anterior wall of the stomach are closed.

Instead of switching views between the two laparoscopes, a flexible gastroduodenoscope can be used to provide the necessary luminal view and to replace the 5 mm intragastric laparoscope. Depending on the availability of instruments and expertise, endoscopic ultrasound can also be used to evaluate and localize the pseudocyst. The rest of the procedure is otherwise similar to that performed entirely with rigid laparoscopy as described above.

Posterior Approach

When the cyst resides close to the inferior edge of the stomach, the alternative approach to drain the pseudocyst via the gastric lumen is the posterior or extraluminal approach. A 10 mm Babcock clamp via the subxiphoid port retracts the left lobe of the liver to the patient's right. The gastrocolic ligament is divided to gain access into the lesser sac, and the pseudocyst is skeletonized to the edge where the posterior gastric wall is tightly adherent to the cyst. A needle is passed to aspirate cyst fluid for analysis, and a cystotomy is made to accommodate the mechanical stapler close to the line of adhesion. Similarly, a gastrostomy about 3 cm long is created on the posterior gastric wall just above the opening made on the cyst with the Harmonic scalpel, and an Endo GIA stapler is fired to create the cystogastrostomy. The defect for the stapler introduction is then closed by either a running suture or a hernia stapler.

Data that compare the relative merits of the anterior and posterior approach are sparse and subjective. To most investigators, the posterior approach is more advantageous in that it needs only one suture line and yields a better biopsy, although this approach is more technically demanding.

TABLE I: Published series of laparoscopic management of pancreatic pseudocyst[*]

Author	N	Conversion	LOS (Days)	Operating Time (Min)	Morbidity (%)	Mortality (%)	Follow-up (Mo)	Recurrence
Hindmarsh (2005)	15	3/15 (20%)	7	82	33	0	37	0
Davila-Cervantes (2004)	10	0	7	240	20	0	22	0
Haunters (2004)	17	0	6	100	11	0	12	0
Park & Heinford (2002)	28	1/29 (3%)	4.4	162	3	0	15.8	0
Mori (2002)	18	4/18 (22%)	8.6	NA	3/18 (17)	0	NA	0
Palanivelu (2007)[†]	90	0	5.6	86	3/90 (3)	0	54	1

[*]Each series had more than 10 cases.

[†]90 of 108 patients who had laparoscopic cystogastrostomy

LAPAROSCOPIC CYSTOJEJUNOSTOMY

Occasionally, internal drainage of the pseudocyst via the jejunum is indicated, when its contact with the posterior gastric wall is limited in area, and primarily at its most cephalic aspect, making the anastomosis only possible at the least dependent position. After the initial laparoscopic exploration, two additional 5 mm trocars are inserted. Using atraumatic laparoscopic bowel clamps, the transverse mesocolon is lifted up toward the anterior abdominal wall, thus making the bulge from the pseudocyst clearly visible. The middle colic vessels may be difficult to identify because of the thickened overlying peritoneum and saponified adipose tissue from inflammation. Taking note of where the middle colic pedicle resides, the most dependent portion of the pseudocyst is chosen for the cystotomy. After aspirating the fluid content, the cyst cavity is explored with the laparoscope. Residual solid debris is removed, and part of the cyst wall is sampled for histopathology. The cystojejunostomy can be created in a Roux-en-Y manner.

The jejunum is grasped at an appropriate distance from the ligament of Treitz, where the vascular arcade is favorable for the creation of a Roux limb. Using a harmonic scalpel, the vascular arcade is divided toward the mesenteric root. The jejunum is then divided with an Endo GIA stapler, and the distal jejunal stump is brought toward the cystotomy. The cystojejunostomy can be fashioned either using another Endo GIA stapler introduced through a 12 mm trocar placed at the left lower quadrant or by running a continuous suture. Likewise, a functional end-to-side jejunojejunostomy is performed 40 cm from the cystoenteric anastomosis, and the mesenteric defect is closed with sutures.

Postoperative Care

After the laparoscopic surgery, the indwelling nasogastric tube can be removed on the first day after surgery. As leakage from the anastomosis remains as the only specific procedure-related morbidity, the drainage fluid should be essayed for its amylase content, starting on the third or fourth postoperative day. If the concentration is acceptable, the patient is allowed to resume oral feeding. Another essay on the drainage fluid is then repeated 1 or 2 days later, and the drain is removed if the amylase concentration is low.

SUGGESTED READINGS

Aljarabah M, Ammori BJ: Laparoscopic and endoscopic approaches for drainage of pancreatic pseudocysts: a systematic review of published series, *Surg Endosc* 21:1936–1944, 2007.

Behrns K, Ben-David K: Surgical therapy of pancreatic pseudocysts, *J Gastrointest Surg* 12:2231–2239, 2008.

Cannon JW, Callery MP, Vollmer CM Jr: Diagnosis and management of pancreatic pseudocysts: What is the evidence? *J Am Coll Surg* 209:385–393, 2009.

Morton JM, Brown A, Galanko JA, et al: A national comparison of surgical versus percutaneous drainage of pancreatic pseudocysts: 1997–2001, *J Gastrointest Surg* 9:15–21, 2005.

Palanivelu C, Senthilkumar K, Madhankumar M, et al: Management of pancreatic pseudocyst in the era of laparoscopic surgery: experience from a tertiary centre, *Surg Endosc* 21:2262–2267, 2007.

VIDEO-ASSISTED THORACIC SURGERY

Amgad El Sherif, MD, and Malcolm V. Brock, MD

BACKGROUND AND HISTORY OF VIDEO-ASSISTED THORACIC SURGERY

Thoracoscopy was first performed in 1910 by a Swedish internist, Hans Christian Jacobaeus. He used a primitive, rigid cystoscope to explore the pleural space, lyse adhesions, and facilitate the collapse therapy for pulmonary tuberculosis popular in that era. Large European clinical experiences described the details of the technique and the effectiveness of thoracoscopic interventions for pleural-based pathology. Despite this enthusiastic support in Europe, vocal and influential thoracic surgeons in the United States did much to forestall the adoption of thoracoscopy in North America. This criticism was led by John Alexander, a pioneer of surgical treatment for pulmonary tuberculosis and a prominent figure in American academic thoracic surgery. Alexander expressed concern about life-threatening complications of thoracoscopy occurring in the tuberculosis sanatoriums of that day and the lack of physicians who had the adequate surgical background to handle these complications. With the advent of antibiotics, thoracoscopy was nearly abandoned except for a few European investigators who continued its use, especially for selected pleural and pulmonary processes.

With the development of more sophisticated optics technology, especially over the last decade, there has been an exponential increase in the number and variety of operations now performed with video-assisted thoracic surgery (VATS). The central goal of VATS approaches is to eliminate the need to spread the rib cage and thus reduce postoperative pain and other postthoracotomy morbidities without compromising the operative principles of an open approach. If the operation requires placement of a rib spreader, the correct term for the procedure is *minithoracotomy with VATS assistance* rather than VATS alone. With new advances in video equipment, endoscopic instrumentation, and stapling devices, VATS has pervaded the practice of general thoracic surgery worldwide, just as laparoscopy now dominates many aspects of general surgery.

OPERATIVE PREPARATION

Key steps to ensure proper patient and operating room preparation include the following:

- Patients must be carefully selected to avoid relative contraindications (Box 1).
- Experienced anesthesia personnel and selective single-lung ventilation must be provided.
- Patients must be properly situated in the full lateral decubitus position (except in thymectomy and sympathectomy).
- Patients should have appropriate padding and must be safely secured, with the operating table flexed to maximize the intercostal distances on the operative side.
- The surgeon and assistant must have an unobstructed view of all monitors.
- Flexible bronchoscopy must be performed by the surgeon to confirm double-lumen endotracheal tube position.
- Specific required instruments or staples, such as an advanced thoracoscopic tray, must be reviewed intraoperatively.

- VATS procedures should be performed in an operating room where facilities for immediate conversion to thoracotomy are readily available.
- Port placement must be carefully planned based on imaging for proper triangulation.

Proper port placement is one of the most important steps for a successful operation. The surgeon should formulate a plan for port placement from the preoperative review of the chest computed tomography (CT) scan. Figure 1 shows the standard triangulation principle of port placements that can be routinely applied to most cases, no matter the pathology. The first port is placed in alignment with the inferior superior iliac spine, usually in the seventh or eighth intercostal space, through which the video thoracoscope is usually inserted. The second port is most commonly located a fingerbreadth inferior and slightly anterior to the scapular tip. The third port is placed just posterior to the lateral border of the pectoralis major muscle, usually in the third or fourth interspace. Unlike laparoscopy in general surgery, thoracic surgeons do not routinely use trocars except for camera ports; instead, they place their instruments or the examining finger directly through the incision into the chest.

VIDEO-ASSISTED THORACIC SURGERY APPROACHES TO THE HEMITHORAX

Anatomy is an important consideration when planning a VATS approach. For example, if both lungs are equally involved with diffuse interstitial disease, a right-sided approach is preferred for a VATS-directed wedge biopsy of the lung, because there is more room to work without the heart in the way. Conversely, the left-sided approach for lung biopsy is preferred in smaller patients, in whom double-lumen endotracheal intubation may not be possible, and bronchial blockers are employed. A left-sided approach is also advised for bilateral diffuse nodular disease, in which more reliable and complete collapse can be achieved on the left side. Complete lung collapse is critical in identifying discrete nodules for biopsy. A right-sided or even bilateral approach for VATS thymectomies is preferable to avoid troublesome bleeding that can arise near the superior vena cava and innominate vein, an area difficult to address from the left thorax.

BOX 1: Relative contraindications to VATS

Dense pleural adhesions
Ventilator dependency
Noncompliant lung
Severe emphysema
Severe pulmonary hypertension
Pulmonary hilar lesions
Pulmonary lesions abutting the upper mediastinum or posterior paravertebral gutter
Small (<1 cm), deeply located pulmonary nodules
Chest wall involvement by tumor
Thoracic cavity or significant anatomic restrictions (e.g., severe scoliosis)
Inability to achieve or tolerate single-lung ventilation
Inability to achieve ipsilateral pulmonary atelectasis
Hemodynamic instability
Severe thoracic trauma or intrathoracic hemorrhage
Coagulopathy
Inadequate instrumentation or inadequate visualization

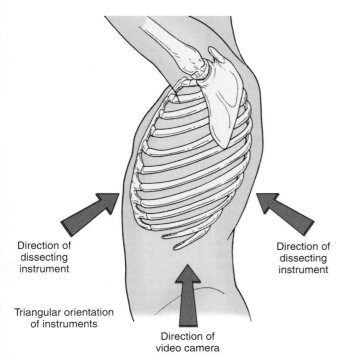

FIGURE 1 The triangulation principle of thoracoscopic port placement. The optic channel is often placed centrally and should maintain an angle of 30 to 60 degrees between it and any other instrument. Some surgeons prefer to place the optics posteriorly, both to stimulate a standard, open, posterolateral thoracotomy view and to avoid working around the assistant holding the camera. *(Modified from Hanke I, Douglas J: General approach to video-assisted thoracoscopic surgery. In Sabiston DC [ed]: Atlas of cardiothoracic surgery, Philadelphia, 1995, WB Saunders, p 544.)*

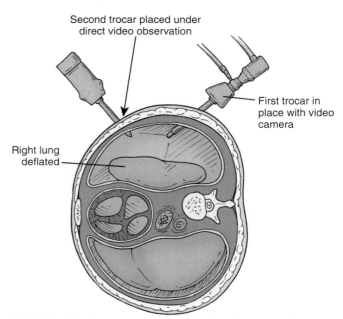

FIGURE 2 The first trocar is placed blindly with care to avoid the lung parenchyma and/or pleural adhesions. Each subsequent trocar is placed under direct vision. *(Modified from Hanke I, Douglas J: General approach to video-assisted thoracoscopic surgery. In Sabiston DC [ed]: Atlas of cardiothoracic surgery, Philadelphia, 1995, WB Saunders, p 544.)*

BASIC CONCEPTS AND CONDUCT OF VIDEO-ASSISTED THORACIC SURGERY

All VATS cases begin with an exploratory thoracoscopy. The skin incision is made directly over the intercostal space to be entered to allow increased mobility of the port and reduce postoperative intercostal neuritis. Careful introduction of a small, curved, pointed clamp (e.g., Kelly or Crile) through the intercostal muscles and pleura is made along the superior border of the lower rib of the intercostal access site chosen, to minimize injury to the intercostal vessels and nerve. The clamp is opened to widen the intercostal space.

Carbon dioxide insufflation is rarely needed to conduct VATS. Occasionally, it is used at the beginning of the procedure to facilitate a more complete and expeditious collapse of the lung. If carbon dioxide insufflation is used, the intrapleural pressure is kept below 5 mm Hg to avoid mediastinal tension and hemodynamic instability. Carbon dioxide insufflation is most often employed in surgeries when a full lateral decubitus position is not used, such as a VATS thymectomy and sympathectomy.

To avoid injury to the underlying lung and to identify the presence of local pleural adhesions, direct digital exploration of the intercostal access site, rather than blind trocar placement into the chest, is best (Figure 2). Flimsy local adhesions can be divided with blunt finger dissection. More extensive pleural symphysis in the location of the proposed initial access site may require alternative intercostal access to conduct the VATS procedure. Hemostasis of the port site should be meticulous, because even small amounts of bleeding will trickle down the trocar and onto the thoracoscope lens, interfering with the surgeon's view during the procedure.

Manipulation of the operating table is important during a VATS procedure. Typically, the table is rotated posteriorly to expose more of the anterior thorax. For cases involving an anterior lesion, a more posterior approach is achieved by rotating the table anteriorly and placing the ports more posteriorly. The use of Trendelenburg and reverse Trendelenburg positions is also helpful to allow gravity to keep the lung out of the operative field. To minimize muscular tension and fatigue in the surgeon's arms and hands, the operating table should be situated so that the handles of the instruments are at the level of the surgeon's elbow or slightly lower, thereby keeping the wrists in a neutral position and the elbows in slight extension, held slightly beyond 90 degrees. Other basic concepts include the following:

1. The thoracoscopy ports and thoracoscope are placed a distance across the chest cavity from the lesion to achieve a panoramic view of the operative field and to allow room to manipulate the instruments.
2. Place the trocar sites sufficiently apart to avoid instrument "fencing" during manipulation of the instruments.
3. After the initial port is placed, subsequent ports are inserted under thoracoscopic visualization, as are the instruments, to avoid injury to intrathoracic structures.
4. Maintain the instruments and the thoracoscope in the same 180-degree arc to maintain videoendoscopic perspective and to avoid mirror imaging.
5. The surgeon should use both hands to manipulate the instruments.
6. Manipulation and movement of the instruments should be conducted in an orderly and systematic fashion. The instruments should be manipulated serially, one by one. Random movements of multiple instruments should be avoided.
7. Avoid excessive torque on the instruments or thoracoscope.
8. Become familiar with the operation and function of the required equipment (e.g., thoracoscope, video system, stapling devices) before surgery.
9. Conversion to thoracotomy is an appropriate option when the performance of VATS is limited by availability of necessary equipment, technical assistance, or clinical condition of the patient.

10. Routinely use a retrieval device for extraction of suspected or potential neoplastic specimens. Specimen bags specifically designed for this purpose are available, but a rubber glove can also be used to prevent the unlikely complication of tumor implantation in the port site.

Instrumentation and Operating Room Setup

Most straightforward VATS procedures can be done with a 10 mm, 0 degree, rigid thoracoscope (Karl Storz Endoscopy-America, Culver City, Calif.) with a 5 mm biopsy channel. This allows a single intercostal access for the management and biopsy of many pleural-related problems. It also allows for the performance of more complex VATS interventions, such as thoracic sympathectomy cases, with one less intercostal access site. Furthermore, if used with a laser, this scope allows direct end-on viewing of the laser's effect on the target pathology. The need for the 5 mm, 30-degree and 45-degree angled thoracoscopes may arise in operations such as VATS lobectomy, minimally invasive esophagectomy (MIE), and VATS thymectomy. These smaller scopes can reduce procedure-related incisional pain.

Flexible and semiflexible thoracoscopes are available but are more difficult to use and maintain spatial orientation. Minithoracoscopes (1 to 3 mm) have been developed that offer the advantage of less patient discomfort and obviate the need for chest drainage and long hospital stays. However, these miniscopes have inferior optic definition and resolution compared with their larger counterparts.

A modern, high-resolution, charged coupled-device (CCD) video camera and high-resolution video monitors are paramount to depict the operative field accurately. At many large academic centers, high-quality three-chip CCD cameras are available from manufacturers such as Olympus, Karl Storz, Endovision, and Stryker. A photographic printer and video tape recorder complete the video endoscopic equipment setup used by most surgical teams.

Tissue Coagulation and Stapling

Monopolar electrocautery (Valleylab, Boulder, Colo.) is used during VATS for simple dissection and coagulation in a similar fashion to open surgery. Bipolar electrocautery is seldom necessary, however, it is indicated when VATS is chosen to approach paraspinous pathology (e.g., thoracic intervertebral disc disease, paraspinous neurogenic tumors) to avoid injury to central nervous system tissue.

The ultrasonic dissector–coagulator (Harmonic scalpel/Ultra-Cision LCS-Pistol Grip [5 mm]; Ethicon, Cincinnati, Ohio) works on a different principle than electrocautery. Instead of applying a current of high-frequency AC electricity, the Harmonic scalpel uses 50 kHz oscillations that result in heat and coagulation of the tissue. One important advantage of the Harmonic scalpel is that there is little threat of injury to adjacent tissue outside the grasp of the forceps's jaws or the tip of the Harmonic scalpel. Hemostasis is reliable, even when dividing blood vessels 3 or 4 mm in diameter, and the Harmonic scalpel is of particular benefit in minimally invasive esophagectomy. The recent introduction of the 5 mm Harmonic scalpel has made it the preferred instrument in VATS procedures.

Coagulation is effective in sealing blood vessels with minimal delayed bleeding. By obviating the need for individually clipping and dividing small vessels, the operation may be expedited. The primary role of electrocautery in VATS is division of simple pleural adhesions and dissection of hilar structures. Electrocautery alone is inefficient and potentially inappropriate for division of pulmonary parenchyma or larger parenchymal blood vessels. Liberal use of electrocautery to divide the fissures may result in prolonged air leaks and hospitalization.

Lung resection with the Nd:YAG laser is effective but is slow and tedious. Moreover, there is a significant learning curve for using it. With the widespread introduction of stapling devices, the use of laser during VATS procedures is limited. Adjuvant use of the Nd:YAG laser with stapled techniques may facilitate resection from difficult locations, such as the flat surface of the lower lobe, or when the nodule is deep within the substance of the lung parenchyma.

Endoscopic stapling devices are generally easy to use and reliably divide both pulmonary parenchyma and vessels, while maintaining excellent pneumostasis and hemostasis. Commonly available models include the EVC/ELC (endoscopic linear) stapler from Ethicon and the Endo GIA stapler from Covidien (Boulder, Colo.). A variety of staple sizes and stapler lengths are presently available. The Ethicon EZ-45 allows apposition of the stapler jaws and application of the staples without the need for the surgeon to change the grip. Reticulating stapler designs are of benefit in VATS lobectomies and MIE. Most pulmonary surgery can be done with the linear 30 or 45 mm stapler with white and blue loads, respectively. The 60 mm instruments are more difficult to use given the close confines of the thoracic cavity.

Buttressing staple lines is useful in pulmonary disease states, such as in chronic obstructive pulmonary disease, or during VATS lung-volume reduction surgery. Buttressing can be achieved with bovine pericardium (Peri-Strips Dry; Bio-Vascular, St. Paul, Minn.), with polytetrafluoroethylene (PTFE), and more recently with bioabsorbable products (Seamguard; R.L. Gore, Flagstaff, Ariz.). These staples can be expected to retain measurable mechanical strength for 4 to 5 weeks, and the bioabsorption process is complete after 6 months. Their main use is to decrease the duration of air leaks, chest tube drainage, and hospital stay.

Handheld Instruments

A vast array of disposable plastic instruments and trocars are available, including reusable models of thoracoscopy ports, retractors, graspers, clamps, and so on. Current instruments have limitations, such as the frequent dulling of the endoscopic scissor blades or loosening of their hinge mechanisms. This results in deterioration of the scissoring action, rendering the instrument ineffective. New technology, such as endoscopic scissors with replaceable ends, can overcome current limitations but often at an additional cost.

There is an inherent inadequacy in the design of endosurgical instruments currently used in VATS. Although the pistol-grip design works well for some applications, such as endoscopic staplers, they are awkward for detailed manipulation and dissection of tissues. Some surgeons have adapted the use of standard thoracic surgery instruments through a limited-utility thoracotomy access incision, such as in VATS lobectomy. We routinely use coaxial endosurgical instruments such as the Landreneau masher (Pilling Surgical, Horsham, Pa.) and the crocodile grasper (Snowden Pencer, Atlanta, Ga.).

SPECIFIC PATHOLOGY

Pleural Space Disease

VATS is the approach of choice for the management of pleural effusions and pleural-based masses. VATS can also be employed to manage empyemas, chest trauma with hemopneumothorax, spontaneous pneumothorax, and abdominal trauma with concerns of diaphragmatic rupture. VATS is ideal in sampling pleural fluid as well as to visualize the entire pleural space to detect disease on the visceral and parietal pleura.

VATS is especially useful in the management of the early fibro-purulent phase of empyema. Most commonly, empyema is post-pneumonic in origin (~65%), and diagnosis usually is made on clinical grounds with demonstration of infected fluid via thoracentesis. Because mortality increases rapidly as the infection remains trapped in the pleural space, VATS is employed to explore the pleural space, drain and evacuate all infected fluid and debris, and disrupt loculations. Minor loculations and adhesions are taken down, but areas of thick adhesions between the lung and the chest wall are generally left alone. Although significant risk for injury to the underlying lung is present when mobilizing adhesions in these areas with resultant bleeding or air leaks, it is unusual for these broad adhesions to be primarily responsible for limiting proper lung reexpansion. When the cause of the pleural process is in question, adequate pleural biopsies are obtained via VATS to evaluate for infectious agents or malignant etiologies. If these goals cannot be achieved via VATS, the procedure should be converted to an open thoracotomy and pleurectomy, and formal decortication is performed as needed.

VATS is also commonly performed to obliterate the pleural space (pleurodesis) to prevent reaccumulation of pleural fluid. Pleurodesis produces an inflammatory pleuritis, resulting in an obliteration of the pleural space by fusion of the parietal and visceral pleuras. The majority of malignant pleural effusions require pleurodesis, unless they have a high likelihood of clinical response to further therapy, as in lymphoma. Pleurodesis can be performed mechanically, such as with a Bovie scratch pad, or chemically, as with Talc. Talc pleurodesis is usually only employed for malignant pleural effusions but also could be considered for benign disease, if recurrent pleural effusion is a concern. Complications of mechanical pleurodesis include inadvertent injury to the thoracic duct, sympathetic ganglion, or the esophagus.

Chemoperfusion of the pleural cavity using VATS is another method of pleurodesis, if the disease is confined to one pleural cavity, with no extra thoracic metastases, and the gross removal of all local disease is achievable. The advantage of this approach is a direct exposure of any residual microscopic disease to higher drug concentrations while minimizing the toxic systemic side effects. Adding hyperthermia to chemoperfusion has been shown in some studies to increase the local tissue and cellular concentrations of the chemotherapy compared with normothermic perfusion. The drug most commonly used in intrapleural hyperthermic chemoperfusion is cisplatin. Most of the experience with this technique has been reported in patients with malignant mesothelioma and thymic malignancies, with fewer data in the treatment of stage IIIb non–small cell lung cancer. Further clinical trials will be required to determine the ideal candidates, optimal chemotherapy, as well as timing and temperature of the perfusate.

VATS is an ideal approach to diagnose pleural-based mass lesions, and the sensitivity of thoracoscopic diagnosis of pleural-based lesions approaches 100%. Benign lesions can also be completely removed by VATS. Malignant lesions usually are metastatic in origin, but VATS commonly is used for the initial diagnosis or confirmation of primary malignancy of the pleura, such as in malignant mesothelioma. Intraoperatively, a frozen section analysis should be obtained to confirm adequate tissue sampling before terminating the procedure.

VATS plays an important role in the management of clotted hemothorax after chest trauma. Early evacuation of blood from the chest cavity is critical to prevent the complications of empyema and fibrothorax. For blunt and penetrating trauma, VATS can rule out a diaphragmatic injury, particularly on the left side. Small diaphragmatic perforations may occur with few signs or symptoms and can result in bowel strangulation if not closed.

Chylothorax is an uncommon condition that arises from a broad range of etiologies, including cancer, trauma, and congenital abnormalities. A diagnosis of chylothorax is usually suspected on the basis of excess volume from the chest tube, often milky white, with chemical analysis that confirms an elevated triglyceride level. Initially, a chylothorax should be treated by complete drainage of the pleural space, reexpansion of the lung, nutrition support, and decreased oral intake. Surgical intervention should be considered within 1 week of diagnosis, if the leak does not resolve, to prevent severe protein depletion and immunosuppression. VATS can be used to drain the pleural space, identify and ligate the source of a chyle leak, and

perform a pleurodesis. Unless the exact location of the leak can be ascertained, the right side of the chest is optimal to approach and ligate the duct as closely as possible to the point at which it enters the chest through the aortic hiatus. The patient can be given a fatty enteral load (we prefer a large helping of ice cream at bedtime the day before surgery) to help identify the site of the chyle leak, as this is often difficult intraoperatively. A clip can be applied to the leaking branch of the thoracic duct if it is visible, or the duct may simply be ligated, as low in the chest as possible, by placing a ligature around all of the tissue on the vertebral column between the azygous vein and the aorta. This gross, mass ligation is performed without dissecting out the thoracic duct, and this approach is successful in 95% of cases. Postoperatively, the patient is given a fatty diet. If no additional chest drainage occurs, and the chest radiograph remains clear, the chest tube is removed.

Spontaneous pneumothoraces are due to the rupture of small blebs or bullae, usually at the lung apices. The typical patient with a primary spontaneous pneumothorax is a young, tall, asthenic male who develops acute onset of chest pain and shortness of breath, especially with exertion. A second group of patients comprising older individuals with known obstructive lung disease, usually with a bullous component, have secondary spontaneous pneumothoraces. In both patients, the general goal of treatment includes elimination of the source of the leak, full lung reexpansion, and minimization of the risk of recurrence. Surgical indications for primary spontaneous pneumothorax include recurrent pneumothorax, prolonged air leak, associated complications, and unique sociogeographic variables such as type of employment and access to medical care. VATS permits excellent visualization of the lung apex for stapling of apical blebs as definitive management of this process; apical blebs and bullae are resected with the endoscopic stapler, and a concurrent mechanical

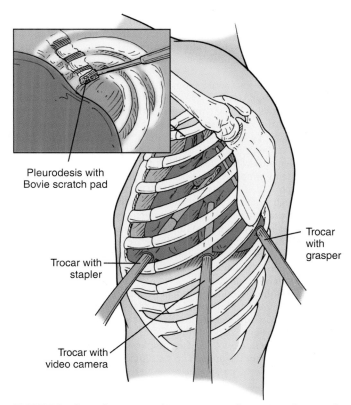

Pleurodesis with Bovie scratch pad

Trocar with grasper

Trocar with stapler

Trocar with video camera

FIGURE 3 Port placement and intraoperative illustration of an apical bullectomy and mechanical pleurodesis. *(Modified from Hanke I, Douglas J: General approach to video-assisted thoracoscopic surgery. In Sabiston DC [ed]: Atlas of cardiothoracic surgery, Philadelphia, 1995, WB Saunders, p 544.)*

pleurodesis can be performed to prevent recurrence (Figure 3). Overall this procedure has a less than 5% recurrence rate. For primary pneumothorax, a single port and a small transaxillary incision are all that is required to complete the procedure. Older patients with bullous parenchymal lung disease usually require standard triangular port placement (see Figure 1) for access to the leaking bulla and often also need a thoracotomy with muscle mobilization and transposition to obliterate a residual space.

Pulmonary Diseases

Diagnosis

VATS plays an important role in the diagnosis and therapy of many pulmonary processes, especially diffuse interstitial lung disease. Often patients with this disease are referred while on ventilator support, undergoing treatment with immunosuppressive agents such as high-dose steroids, and failing conventional therapies. Intraoperatively, at least two distinct areas should be sampled, ideally from two separate lobes. After a specimen is obtained, it should be sent for frozen section analysis to confirm that diagnostic material has been obtained. In addition, a portion of the specimen should be sent to the microbiology laboratory for cultures, including those for acid-fast bacilli, fungi, and aerobic and anaerobic bacteria. Although the operation has minimal complications, the patient's underlying pulmonary status can be the source of significant postoperative morbidity.

The malignant potential of indeterminate solitary pulmonary nodules mandates accurate diagnostic management. False-negative fine needle biopsy may unnecessarily delay the diagnosis, given the known procedure-related pneumothorax rate. The development of positron emission tomographic (PET) scanning technology has added to the management algorithm of the indeterminate solitary pulmonary nodule. Among lesions large enough to be discriminated by present-day PET, it is generally believed that a negative scan has significant predictive value. False-negative PET scans, however, may be seen among bronchioalveolar carcinomas and neuroendocrine neoplasms.

With a VATS excisional biopsy, the diagnosis of an indeterminate nodule approaches 96% sensitivity. If a malignancy is confirmed, definitive oncologic management of the malignancy can be performed at the same sitting. When a benign pathology is found, no further surgery is necessary, and the need for long-term radiographic surveillance is usually avoided. Discharge from the hospital can be anticipated within 48 hours for patients with benign pathology undergoing simple wedge resection of the peripheral pulmonary lesion. Often a VATS excisional biopsy of the indeterminate solitary pulmonary nodule can, therefore, expedite management of the patient and avoid the expense and potential complications related to percutaneous biopsy. In general, indeterminate lung nodules ideally suited for thoracoscopic excisional biopsy are less than 3 cm in diameter and are located in the outer third of the lung parenchyma, and no evidence of endobronchial extension should be seen on preoperative bronchoscopic evaluation.

It may be difficult to identify small peripheral solitary pulmonary nodules using VATS techniques. Lesions that are particularly difficult to palpate or visually localize are those of subcentimeter diameter located some distance beneath the pleural surface, and several techniques greatly facilitate VATS when employed for nodular processes of the lung. If a nodule appears to be difficult to localize by digital palpation because of its small size or deep location, radiographic localization can be performed with a guidewire or by injection with methylene blue, but we have rarely if ever used these adjuncts. Lesions can almost always be palpated by the probing index finger inserted through one of the VATS incisions, while a portion of the lung, grasped with a ring forceps, is moved to the examining finger. The surgeon developing skill with these VATS excisional biopsy

approaches will find it useful to review critically the anatomic detail of the lesion and its relationship to the lobar anatomy visualized on CT imaging.

After the lesion has been located, the nodule should not be grasped directly. Instead, the lung parenchyma just adjacent to the lesion should be grasped, and keeping in mind the location of the nodule, a wedge-type resection should be performed to encompass the lesion completely. At times, depending on the location, the lesion itself may be grasped and elevated such that the linear endoscopic stapler can be placed beneath the lesion for resection. If the nodule cannot be successfully located, or if it is in a location where wedge excision would be difficult, the procedure should be converted to an open thoracotomy, using at least one of the incisions has already been made.

Deeper lesions identified on CT imaging, such as those on the edge of an interlobar fissure, may also be candidates for VATS excisional biopsy. Attempting to resect a deep lesion may result in parenchymal injury, leading to physiologic deterioration equivalent to lobectomy. Application of endoscopic staplers through the thicker tissue of the lung can also lead to intraparenchymal hematoma, staple-line disruption, and the possibility of delayed bronchopleural fistulas. Such deep nodules may be best handled using intraoperative needle biopsy. Anatomic resection (e.g., segmentectomy or lobectomy) should usually follow when malignancy is confirmed. On some occasions, lesions can also be handled by the judicious combined application of staplers with a Nd:YAG laser resection.

VATS has proven useful not only for the removal of pulmonary nodules for diagnosis, but also for staging of lung cancer. The superior mediastinum—specifically levels II, IV, and VII—may be sampled adequately and preferentially by mediastinoscopy. For left-sided tumors, particularly left upper-lobe lesions, VATS permits excellent

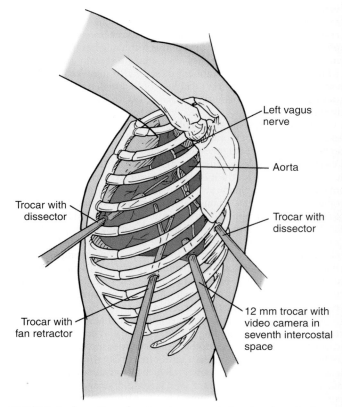

FIGURE 4 Resection of aortopulmonary window lymph nodes by VATS. *(Modified from Hanke I, Douglas J: General approach to video-assisted thoracoscopic surgery. In Sabiston DC [ed]: Atlas of cardiothoracic surgery, Philadelphia, 1995, WB Saunders, p 544.)*

exposure to the aortopulmonary window for sampling of nodal stations at level V and VI. After the chest has been entered with the videothoracoscope, the pleural cavity is explored to rule out visceral or parietal pleural involvement. With countertraction on the apical portion of the lung, the aortopulmonary window lymph nodes can be easily visualized and resected (Figure 4). Because of the proximity of the recurrent laryngeal nerve, electrocautery use should be minimized. If necessary, subcarinal lymph nodes can also be sampled to aid in planning the appropriate therapy. Thoracoscopy is also useful in ruling out unresectable T4 invasion in primary lung cancer and T3 invasion in high-risk patients.

Therapeutic Uses of VATS

VATS can be used to perform lung-volume reduction surgery for end-stage emphysema. Lung-volume reduction has been proposed to help patients with emphysema by removing hypofunctioning apical segments of the lung, thereby permitting reexpansion of the remaining lung to improve physiologic recoil. The indications for lung-volume reduction surgery have been well described in the National Emphysema Treatment Trial.

Following a thorough preoperative preparation, a bilateral VATS approach can be taken to resect the apical segments. We prefer to resect emphysematous lung tissue with staplers buttressed with either expanded PTFE or glutaraldehyde-fixed bovine pericardium. The postoperative care can be challenging, however, with the most common complications being prolonged air leak and respiratory infections. Most series report 80% of patients had significant improvement in their pulmonary status. Spirometric indices, such as forced expiratory volume at 1 second and forced vital capacity, continue to improve long after surgery.

VATS anatomic lung resection, specifically lobectomy and segmentectomy, is now widely accepted and performed by an increasing number of surgeons. VATS lobectomy was initially limited to stage I lesions or stage II lesions without extensive nodal involvement. With increasing experience with VATS lobectomy, the indications for the procedure are being extended in many groups. VATS lobectomy permits adequate visualization for a complete resection of the tumor-containing lobe, as well as allowing for a standard mediastinal lymph node dissection. It appears to be safe with low morbidity, and in experienced hands, it has equivalent short- and long-term outcomes to the open procedure. A few reports have even shown that VATS lobectomy may be an effective oncologic strategy, as patients may tolerate adjuvant chemotherapy better than with an open thoracotomy. Different groups have different preferences in port placement for VATS lobectomy of different lobes. Commonly, however, the three ports in the triangulation standard, discussed earlier, are utilized. Often, a fourth anterior utility thoracotomy, placed in the fourth space, is performed to allow for the use of standard thoracotomy instruments to complete the dissection. Few surgeons use only two incisions, one for the camera and another utility incision for dissection.

The operation follows the standard open approach, with visualization provided indirectly by the video camera and the procedure guided by the magnified appearance on the video monitor. Newly developed VATS lobectomy instruments are available; for example, the long, curved thoracoscopic right-angle retractor and the D'Amico retractor. The operating room should be ready for conversion to thoracotomy and should have a "disaster" plan in place in case the stapler misfires on the pulmonary artery or vein. Most surgeons staple the inferior pulmonary vein before the artery in lower lobe VATS lobectomies. The middle lobe can be a technical challenge in VATS lobectomy, and substantial data demonstrate that VATS lobectomy can be performed safely with results equal to those of the open approach, even after neoadjuvant chemotherapy.

Patients after VATS lobectomy procedures have reduced hospital stays, the limiting factors in discharge typically being pain control and removal of the chest tube, the timing of which should be based on cessation of air leaks and discontinuation of drainage. Overall costs may be equal for the two procedures, even though patients may be discharged a day earlier using the VATS approach, because increased intraoperative equipment costs cancel out any financial savings gained by the shorter length of stay. Most of the costs associated with a VATS lobectomy accrue during the first or second hospital day. Pain seems less with a VATS lobectomy, presumably because it obviates the need for rib spreading.

Under certain circumstances, VATS may be used for pulmonary metastasectomy. Surgical resection of all visible and palpable metastases is indicated when the primary tumor is controlled, and metastases are confined to the lung. Preoperative pulmonary function tests must confirm that a patient can tolerate the multiple wedge resections that may be required for complete resection. A common concern often voiced is that the VATS approach does not permit adequate palpation of the lung parenchyma for small lesions that cannot be seen by CT scan. Complete resection of all metastatic pulmonary lesions is the major determinant of long-term survival for patients with lung metastases. For a patient with a limited number of pulmonary nodules suspected to be metastases, a VATS resection is a reasonable option.

Mediastinal and Esophageal Diseases

Concomitant application of laparoscopic and thoracoscopic esophageal techniques is a natural fit, because they offer the patient the best chance of a cure while sparing some of the morbidity of large incisions. Totally endoscopic esophagectomy was first described by DePaula in 1995 as a laparoscopic transhiatal approach. Subsequently, the combined laparoscopic/thoracoscopic approaches, with anastomosis in either the chest or neck, became more popular, with more and more esophageal centers offering minimally invasive approaches. The three open esophagectomy techniques—transhiatal, thoracic/abdominal (Ivor-Lewis), and three-incision approaches—have been replicated with an endoscopic or endoscopy-assisted technique, both in supine and prone positions. A combination approach with thoracoscopic mobilization, laparoscopic creation of the gastric interposition, and a cervical anastomosis is currently the most popular procedure.

MINIMALLY INVASIVE ESOPHAGECTOMY

The patient is positioned on a split-leg operating table with legs spread or in regular supine position with arms out of the operating table. In prone MIE, both arms should be abducted, and care should be taken to pad and protect all extremities carefully to prevent neuropraxia or pressure ulcers during long procedures. The head is placed on a donut pad and turned to the right, to allow access to the left neck for the proximal dissection and anastomosis, and five laparoscopic ports are placed (Figure 5).

During laparoscopy, biopsies are obtained of any suspicious lesions, and these are sent for frozen section analysis. The gastroepiploic arcade is identified along the greater gastric curvature, and the gastrocolic omentum is divided, opening into the lesser sack. With a "no touch" technique, the stomach is gently elevated, and the greater curve is mobilized with the ultrasonic shears; care is taken to stay away from the vascular arcade. This dissection is taken cephalad to the left crus and inferiorly to the point at which the gastroepiploic vessels pass behind the duodenum. Retrogastric adhesions to the pancreas and retroperitoneum are divided, and the surgeon checks again for evidence of tumor invasion. Division of these adhesions exposes the left gastric pedicle, as it arises from the celiac axis. The origin of the left gastric artery is dissected free and stapled. Occasionally, a removable clip is placed across the left gastric artery to document the vascularity of the gastric replacement.

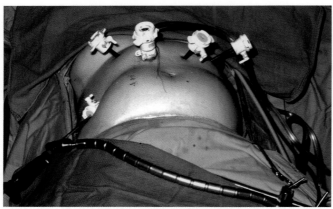

FIGURE 5 Positions of the laparoscopic ports for minimally invasive esophagectomy. (*Courtesy the University of Pittsburgh Medical Center.*)

The hepatogastric ligament is widely resected to expose the primary lymphatic basin and the celiac trunk. Attention is then directed to the greater curvature and the short gastric vessels, which are ligated with the ultrasonic shears. A narrow gastric conduit 3 cm in diameter is created with multiple firings of an endoscopic linear stapler; the first firing is immediately below the crow's foot vessels on the lesser curve in a transverse fashion. Subsequent firings follow the greater curve up to the cardia of the stomach, where the neoesophagus is then transected. Next, the mediastinum is opened by excising a rim of hiatus while pulling downward on the gastric remnant. Mediastinal dissection is performed by staying directly on the aorta, mediastinal pleura, and pericardium. This effectively leaves all lymph nodes and lymphatics with the surgical specimen.

Our preferred method for the mediastinal mobilization is simply to continue the transhiatal dissection by advancing the scope and instruments into the mediastinum, while the assistant continues to pull downward on the esophagus; this will usually allow dissection up to the carina, where the subcarinal nodes can be removed and sent separately for staging. The retrotracheal esophagus is usually mobilized by a second team from the neck incision, using a gentle finger and Kittner dissection. The remaining upper mediastinum is mobilized under laparoscopic visualization, using the long bariatric laparoscope and a long, curved sponge stick made with an aortic clamp and folded gauze. A standard laparoscopic specimen bag is placed over the nodes, and the neoplasm, together with the gastroesophageal remnant, is removed.

Another technique in removing the esophagus is the inversion method, which is useful for small cancers and benign disease. An esophagotomy is made in the cervical esophagus, and a nasogastric tube or vein stripper is passed down to the blind pouch and advanced out through a nick in the stomach and sutured. The team at the cervical incision then starts to pull on the tube or stripper, which imbricates the stomach into the esophagus. The laparoscopic team can then follow the inverting esophagus into the mediastinum and divide tissues shown to be still holding it in place. The esophagus therefore serves as its own specimen bag to prevent tumor contamination.

After dividing the cervical esophagus, a 28 Fr chest tube is then passed from the neck into the abdomen, where the gastric tube can be sewn to its end. The chest tube is withdrawn, pulling the neoesophagus along with it. Care must be taken to prevent the narrow tube from twisting and to keep the gastric mesentery from tearing as it advances into the mediastinum. The proximal tube can be resected back to freely bleeding tissue, and an anastomosis is performed using either a stapler technique or suturing in a two-layered fashion. The hiatus is loosely closed with permanent sutures, and a slight antireflux valve is created by suturing the anterior antrum

to the rim of the hiatus, creating a right-sided Dor-type repair. The narrow tube and antireflux mechanism obviate the need for a pyloroplasty. A laparoscopic feeding jejunostomy is routinely added, and a closed-suction drain is inserted through a port site and placed partly across the mediastinum, after the area is well irrigated, and hemostasis has been confirmed. A drain is likewise placed in the neck wound, with the tip directed slightly into the upper mediastinum, before the neck is closed.

Thoracoscopic/Laparoscopic Esophagectomy

We prefer a combination thoracoscopic/laparoscopic approach for MIE. This approach allows better staging with wide nodal dissections of the mediastinal esophagus. It also avoids the tedious transhiatal dissection, but it requires more complex anesthesia and the additional time needed for repositioning and reprepping the patient midway through the procedure.

There are two combined approaches to esophagectomy. The first replicates the traditional Ivor-Lewis approach with an intrathoracic anastomosis; the second involves thoracoscopic mobilization, first with subsequent laparoscopic gastric mobilization and then with a cervical anastomosis. With either choice, the gastric mobilization and tailoring are the same as described for the transhiatal approach. Choice of the laparoscopic/thoracoscopic Ivor-Lewis or three-incision procedure depends on tumor location and the surgeon's comfort with an intrathoracic anastomosis. For distal small tumors, we prefer the Ivor-Lewis approach because of the resulting larger gastric reservoir and lower stricture rates.

Laparoscopic/Thoracoscopic Ivor-Lewis

Laparoscopic/thoracoscopic Ivor-Lewis procedures begin with five laparoscopic ports placed as in a laparoscopic transhiatal resection. The abdomen is explored, the stomach is mobilized, and the gastric conduit is created. The lower mediastinum is opened by widely excising the phrenoesophageal ligament. The mediastinal esophagus is mobilized transhiatally for 5 to 10 cm, staying wide to keep the lymphatics in continuity with the esophagus. The right mediastinal pleura is then opened, and the transected stomach and neoesophagus are pushed up into the right chest. The gastric antrum is then sutured to the rim of the hiatus, or, alternatively, the hiatus can be closed with sutures around the narrow neoesophagus approximately 2 cm above the junction of the neoesophagus and antrum. This allows the surgeon to tack the anterior gastric wall to the hiatal rim to form a type of antireflux mechanism.

The patient is then repositioned on a beanbag in the left lateral decubitus position, with the usual precautions being taken to cushion any pressure points. Two 10 mm and two 5 mm ports are placed in a diamond configuration (Figure 6), the lung is swept anteriorly with a thoracoscopic lung retractor, and the mediastinum is opened from above the azygous vein to the hiatus. The azygous vein is routinely divided with a vascular stapler to allow adequate dissection. Once again, wide dissection is performed to remove all paraesophageal lymphatics, and branches of the thoracic duct should be clipped. The subcarinal nodes are removed as a packet and are sent separately for staging. The esophagus is divided at the level of the azygous vein, and the gastric conduit is brought up to it.

The anastomosis can be performed in any of several ways: hand sewn, with a circular stapler, or with a linear stapler. Use of a flexible-shaft, circular stapler is a new possibility that permits the per-oral insertion of a circular stapler; this makes intrathoracic anastomosis fairly straightforward. Next, one of the port sites is widened, and the specimen is removed and sent to the pathology laboratory to confirm clear margins. Finally, a chest tube is inserted through one of the port sites. Some groups prefer to place a removable covered esophageal stent (PolyFlex; Boston Scientific, Natick, Mass.) across

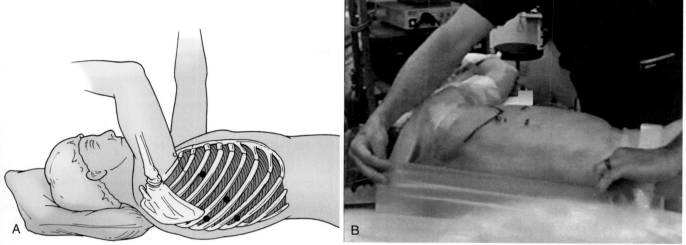

FIGURE 6 Thoracoscopic ports for a minimally invasive esophagectomy. *(Courtesy the University of Pittsburgh Medical Center.)*

the anastomosis to protect the high-risk anastomosis and prevent strictures during healing.

Three-Incision Laparoscopic/Thoracoscopic Esophagectomy

Luketich and colleagues at the University of Pittsburgh have popularized the three-incision technique, in which the same dissection, resection, and anastomosis are performed as in the techniques described previously, but the order is changed. The patient starts with a right thoracoscopy, and the esophagus is mobilized as described earlier, except that the dissection is continued to the proximal thoracic outlet. After this has been accomplished, and the node dissection has been performed, a chest tube is placed, and the patient is moved into the supine position. The abdominal portion of the procedure is performed in the standard fashion, while at the same time, a left cervical incision is made, and the cervical esophagus is mobilized. Typically, the stomach and tumor are placed in a specimen bag and withdrawn through the neck wound following transection of the cervical esophagus. A chest tube is then passed from the neck incision through the mediastinum and into the abdomen. The gastric tube is then sutured to the end of the chest tube and carefully pulled up into the neck, where an anastomosis can be performed; this can be a sutured or stapled anastomosis. A feeding jejunostomy is created by suturing a section of proximal jejunum to the anterior abdominal wall using a guidewire with an 8 Fr or 14 Fr tube. Finally, closed-suction drains are placed in the neck via one of the port sites across the hiatus.

SUMMARY

As VATS evolves, and as surgical experience with VATS increases, the demand for more sophisticated instruments, cameras, and monitors also grows. Tactile sensing, three-dimensional vision capability, and steerable instruments and cameras are all actively being developed and piloted. Close cooperation with surgeons and engineers has made this an active area of technological innovation, and the shift to minimally invasive thoracic procedures has occurred and is gaining momentum.

SUGGESTED READINGS

Anthony PC, Yim MK, Hsin Y, et al: *Video atlas of minimally invasive thoracic surgery*, Hong Kong, 2008, Chinese Press.

Krasna MJ, Mack MJ: *Atlas of thoracoscopic surgery*, London, 2002, Informa Healthcare.

McKenna RJ Jr, Houck W, Fuller CB: Video-assisted thoracic surgery lobectomy: experience with 1100 cases, *Ann Thoracic Surg* 81:421–426, 2006.

Onaitis MW, Petersen RP, Balderson SS, et al: Thoracoscopic lobectomy is a safe and versatile procedure: experience with 500 consecutive patients, *Ann Surg* 244:420–425, 2006.

Puntambekar S, Cuesta MA, editors: *Atlas of minimally invasive surgery in esophageal carcinoma*, New York, 2009, Springer.

Walker WS, editor: *Video-assisted thoracic surgery*, New York, 1999, Isis Medical Media Publications.

LAPAROSCOPIC SURGERY FOR SEVERE OBESITY

Fady Moustarah, MD, MPH, Stacy A. Brethauer, MD, and Philip R. Schauer, MD

OVERVIEW

Now considered one of the most important health issues of the twenty-first century, obesity is a complex chronic disease of mixed genetic and environmental etiology, not merely the failure of controlling caloric intake. It is associated with multiple medical comorbidities, increased health care costs, reduced quality of life, and increased risk for premature death. Although it remains primarily a problem in industrialized nations, obesity has reached pandemic proportions, affecting over 300 million people worldwide. It is estimated that two thirds of Americans are overweight or obese, and about 5% have morbid obesity (body mass index [BMI] of ≥ 40 kg/m^2). Obesity is classified as shown in Table 1.

The pathophysiology of obesity is complex and not clearly understood. In essence, obesity ultimately results from an imbalance between calorie intake and expenditure, favoring fat deposition and accumulation in the body. Bariatric procedures modify gastrointestinal (GI) anatomy and in some cases enteric hormone release to reduce caloric intake, reduce absorption, or alter metabolism to achieve weight loss. Although somewhat simplistic, these procedures have traditionally been classified as either *restrictive* or *malabsorptive* (Table 2). Restrictive operations, or restrictive components of mixed procedures, reduce the volume of the gastric reservoir or retard emptying of the upper stomach (gastric banding) to help induce a sense of fullness after eating small meals. Malabsorptive procedures divert nutrient flow and reduce the absorptive surface available for nutrients in the GI tract, but they are increasingly thought to also have a hormonal component that alters satiety and reduces caloric intake. For morbidly obese patients, the most substantial and sustained weight loss with associated improvements in comorbidities is currently best achieved with modern bariatric surgery.

Roux-en-Y gastric bypass (RYGB) remains the most commonly performed bariatric operation in North America. Other common weight-loss procedures include laparoscopic adjustable gastric banding (LAGB), biliopancreatic diversion (BPD), and BPD with a duodenal switch (BPD+DS). In the last few years, the sleeve gastrectomy (SG) has gained popularity as a primary bariatric operation, where it was initially used as a first-stage procedure in high-BMI, high-risk patients being prepared for a future BPD+DS or RYGB. Laparoscopic approaches to bariatric procedures started to emerge in the early 1990s; today, all these operations are predominantly performed laparoscopically, because of significant reduction in perioperative morbidity, mortality, recovery time, and costs.

PATIENT SELECTION

The indications for bariatric surgery established at the 1991 National Institutes of Health (NIH) consensus conference continue to be the standard for patient selection in the United States. These criteria include patients with a BMI of 40 kg/m^2 or greater or those with a BMI of 35 kg/m^2 or greater with obesity-related comorbidities. Additionally, eligible patients must be medically fit for surgery, must have failed nonsurgical methods of weight loss, and must be free of any uncontrolled psychiatric or drug dependency problems. Patients also need to demonstrate an ability and commitment to comply with the demands of surgical therapy and its aftercare. The role of a multidisciplinary team that includes a nutritionist and a mental health professional to evaluate patients preoperatively cannot be overemphasized. The team works in concert with the surgeon to assess expectations, readiness, and motivation for surgery and to confirm the absence of psychosocial factors that can jeopardize success.

Obesity-related comorbidities generally improve after surgery, but the risk of postoperative complications and death increases with the number of comorbidities present preoperatively. DeMaria and colleagues at Duke University proposed an obesity surgery mortality risk score in 2007, and five factors were identified in a multiregression analysis as predictive of mortality risk in patients undergoing RYGB. These include BMI of 50 kg/m^2 or greater, male gender, hypertension, presence of risk factors for pulmonary embolism, and age 45 years or older. The presence of two or more of these factors increases a patient's mortality risk, and this information can be used to guide patient selection and help the surgeon obtain better informed consent from patients wanting the benefits of surgery (Table 3).

Type 2 diabetes mellitus (T2DM) in particular improves remarkably after bariatric surgery. The Diabetes Surgery Summit of 2007 resulted in consensus guidelines that expand surgical indications to include patients with T2DM that is not well controlled and who have a BMI of 30 to 35 kg/m^2. Choosing the best surgical option for any one patient requires careful consideration. Each bariatric operation

TABLE 1: Classification of obesity

Category	Body Mass Index
Underweight	<18.5
Normal	18.5–24.9
Overweight	25.0–29.9
Obese	>30
Class I	30.0–34.9
Class II	35.0–39.9
Class III (morbid obesity)	>40.0

TABLE 2: Classification of common bariatric procedures

Procedure	Examples
Purely restrictive	Adjustable gastric band, sleeve gastrectomy, vertical banded gastroplasty (now offered infrequently)
Gastric restriction combined with diversion	Roux-en-Y gastric bypass
Diversionary malabsorptive procedures	Biliopancreatic diversion ± duodenal switch
Experimental metabolic operations	Duodenojejunal bypass, ileal interposition

TABLE 3: **Mortality rates of combined number of risk factors*

Class	Risk Factor†	Mortality Rate‡
A	0–1	0.31% in 957
B	2–3	1.90% in 999
C	4–5	7.56% in 119

*Data from DeMaria EJ, Portenier D, Wolf L, et al: Obesity surgery mortality risk score: proposal for a clinically useful score to predict mortality risk in patients undergoing gastric bypass, *Surg Obes Relat Dis* 3: 134-140, 2007.
†One point is assigned to each of the following mortality predictive risk factors: body mass index ≥50 kg/m², male gender, hypertension, risk of pulmonary embolism, and age ≥45 years.
‡Each rate is statistically significant from the other two by Fischer exact test.

has a risk/benefit profile that together with a patient's own risk profile and health goals should be weighed carefully by both the surgeon and patient prior to selecting a particular surgical therapy.

PATIENT PREPARATION

Weeks and sometime months before surgery, the patient should undergo medical, psychologic, and nutrition evaluation and optimization. Preoperative weight loss immediately prior to surgery is encouraged to augment medical optimization as well as to reduce liver size for improved operative exposure. However, long-term, mandatory, medically supervised diet programs often required by private insurance companies have not been proven to offer benefit and in some cases needlessly delay surgery or increase attrition. At our institution, patients are asked to adhere to an 800 to 1200 kcal/day diet for 2 weeks prior to surgery. Patients are also instructed to have only clear liquids for 2 days prior to surgery and to drink 1 L of a mechanical bowel preparation solution the day before surgery, mostly to cleanse the foregut. On the morning of surgery, a peripheral intravenous line is placed, and a first-generation cephalosporin, or an appropriate alternative in patients allergic to penicillin, is administered.

In the operating room, the patient is carefully placed in the supine position on the operating table to avoid pressure or position injury. Intermittent pneumatic compression devices are applied to the lower legs, and pharmacologic prophylaxis against thromboembolism may be given preoperatively. Under general anesthesia, a urinary catheter is placed, and the patient is safely secured on the operating table. Distribution of personnel around the operating table is variable. For all bariatric procedures at the Cleveland Clinic, the surgeon stands on the patient's right side with the first assistant across the table on the left side. Monitors are placed on both sides of the table over the patient's shoulders (Figure 1), and the camera operator directs the camera mostly to the epigastric area and left upper quadrant.

OPERATIVE PROCEDURES

Laparoscopic Roux-en-Y Gastric Bypass

We gain access to the abdominal cavity with a Veress needle inserted subcostally in the left upper quadrant along the midclavicular line, and a 5 mm optical trocar is inserted at this position after a 15 mm Hg carbon dioxide pneumoperitoneum is established. Four to five other ports are then placed, depending on the operation being performed. For the LRYGB, we use a 45-degree, 5 mm laparoscope through the initial left upper quadrant port and place five other ports under direct vision as shown in Figure 2. Steps of the operation are depicted in Figure 3.

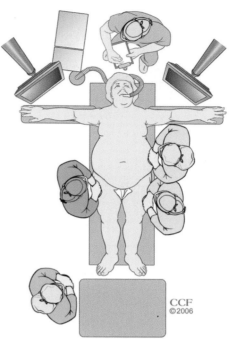

FIGURE 1   Positioning for surgery. *(Reprinted with permission from Cleveland Clinic Center for Medical Art & Photography, copyright 2005-2010. All Rights Reserved.)*

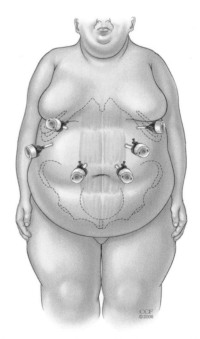

FIGURE 2   Port placement. *(Reprinted with permission from Cleveland Clinic Center for Medical Art & Photography, copyright 2005-2010. All Rights Reserved.)*

The omentum and transverse (Figure 3, *A*) colon are retracted cephalad to expose the transverse mesocolon. Anterior retraction of the mesentery here exposes the ligament of Treitz. Approximately 50 cm distal to this ligament, the jejunum is transected with an endoscopic linear cutting stapler (45 mm, 2.5 mm staple load; Figure 3, *B*). The jejunal mesentery is divided with the surgeon's choice of a stapling instrument with 2.0 mm staples, an ultrasonic scalpel, or a bipolar

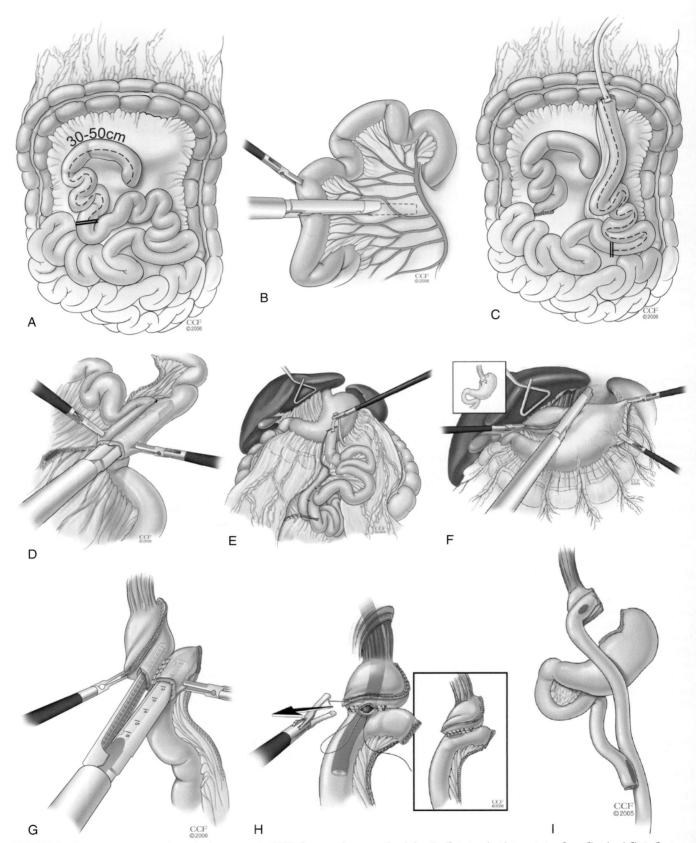

FIGURE 3 Steps in our approach to the laparoscopic RYGB. See text for procedural details. *(Reprinted with permission from Cleveland Clinic Center for Medical Art & Photography, copyright 2005-2010. All Rights Reserved.)*

energy cutting device. A short 6 cm Penrose drain is then sutured to the divided edge of the Roux limb to clearly label this intestinal segment and provide a handle for grasping and delivering the Roux limb to the pouch (Figure 3, *C*). The Roux limb is measured 150 cm distally and is sutured at that point to the end of the biliopancreatic limb. A side-to-side jejunojejunostomy (JJ) is fashioned by first making enterotomies in both small bowel limbs with the ultrasonic shears and then using a 60 mm, 2.5 mm load in the linear cutter. The common enterotomy is then closed with another 60 mm, 2.5 mm staple firing (Figure 3, *D*). The distal apex of the stapled side-to-side anastomosis is reinforced with a tension-relieving stitch, and an anti-obstruction stitch is placed at the proximal end of the anastomosis. The mesenteric defect is then closed with a running nonabsorbable stitch, and the greater omentum is split from the level of the transverse colon toward its free edge to create a path for the Roux limb and to minimize tension, as the limb is brought up to fashion a gastrojejunal (GJ) anastomosis.

Next, the patient is positioned in steep reverse Trendelenburg position, and a liver retractor is placed. The gastrohepatic ligament is opened, and the lesser omentum is divided to the edge of the stomach. The lesser sac is entered to facilitate dissection behind the posterior wall of the stomach. Before dividing the stomach, we confirm that there are no tubes or probes within the esophagus or stomach. The first gastric transection is performed horizontally just below the left gastric artery; sequential stapling is then applied in the direction of the angle of His to fashion a 15 to 20 mL pouch. It is important to exclude the fundus from the gastric pouch, and this is accomplished by directing the stapler toward the angle of His and applying lateral and downward traction on the fundus prior to closing and firing the stapler. The stomach staple lines on both sides are inspected for integrity and bleeding. Clips or suture can be applied to the staple line as necessary for hemostasis. The stomach transection point is usually determined by measuring 1 to 2 cm from the esophagogastric junction. Occasionally, pouch size may be expanded to create a well-formed tension-free gastrojejunal anastomosis.

The Roux limb is then brought up by grasping the Penrose and directing the limb through the divided omentum anterior to the transverse colon and toward the gastric pouch (antecolic, antegastric; Figure 3, *E*). Infrequently it is necessary to use the retrocolic retrogastric approach, when a short mesentery would put tension on the anastomosis. Several options are available for constructing the gastrojejunostomy; these include using a transoral circular stapler, a transgastric circular stapler, a linear stapler, or by hand sewing. All have been reported in the literature to yield similar weight-loss results with comparable safety.

At the Cleveland Clinic we use the linear stapler to create a 12 to 15 mm anastomosis. The Roux limb is sewn to the posterior aspect of the gastric pouch, leaving enough room for a posterior anastomosis. A gastrotomy at the staple line and an enterotomy at the antimesenteric border of the Roux limb are then created with the ultrasonic shears, and a 45 mm, 3.5 mm stapler is used to make a 1.5 cm stapled anastomosis (Figure 3, *G*). The common opening is then closed by running a 3-0 polyglactin (absorbable) suture from both ends, meeting in the middle over a diagnostic endoscope (Figure 3, *H*). The polyglactin sutures are tied down with the scope left in place, and an anterior row of running polyester suture is then placed as a second layer to approximate the Roux limb to the gastric pouch anteriorly, thereby oversewing the first polyglactin layer and creating a two-layer anastomosis that also incorporates the entire pouch staple line.

After placing a bowel clamp distally, the anastomosis is tested for air leaks under saline with the use of the endoscope. The GJ is then examined endoscopically for hemostasis or obstruction, and the endoscope is withdrawn. The mesenteric defect (Petersen defect) is then closed between the Roux limb and the transverse colon to minimize the risk of internal herniation at this site. A drain is placed in the left upper quadrant behind the anastomosis and over the dome of the spleen. Because of the multiple steps involved in this bypass operation, we advocate going through a checklist to ensure all steps have been completed, all specimens and sponges have been removed, and counts are correct before removing the laparoscopic ports and closing fascial incisions. Fascial defects greater than 5 mm are closed with the aid of a suture-passing device. Long-acting local anesthetic is placed in the wounds, and the skin is closed with subcuticular stitches.

Adjustable Gastric Banding

After establishing a carbon dioxide pneumoperitoneum and placing a 5 mm optical port in the left upper quadrant, a 45-degree laparoscope is inserted, and three other ports are placed under direct vision using a 15 mm, a 10 mm, and a 5 mm trocar. The left lobe of the liver is elevated with a retractor of the surgeon's choice, and the patient is placed in reverse Trendelenburg position. Attachments at the angle of His are divided, and a window in the gastrohepatic omentum (the *pars flaccida* technique) is created with a monopolar hook instrument or ultrasonic shears. The peritoneum at the base of the right crus is opened, and an articulating dissector is passed through this opening from the right crus side toward the angle of His.

Next, the gastric band is placed directly into the abdomen through the 15 mm port, and the dissector is used to pull the band behind the posterior stomach and into place around the gastric cardia, where it is then locked. Three to four nonabsorbable gastrogastric plication sutures are placed as anterior fixation sutures to reduce band slippage and stomach herniation through the band (Figure 4). The sutures should approximate stomach fundus to proximal stomach above the band but should not be too tight, to minimize the risk of band erosion. The buckle of the band should not be covered, and the tubing is brought out through the 15 mm port. The skin incision here is extended to 4 cm, and the subcutaneous fat is dissected to expose the anterior rectus sheath. The port is placed flat onto the fascia and secured, and the end of the tubing from the band is trimmed and connected to the access port at the connector. It is important to ensure that the tubing has no kinks as it enters the fascia.

Biliopancreatic Diversion with Duodenal Switch

In brief, the steps involved in the BPD+DS procedure include division of the duodenum distal to the pylorus, a pylorus-preserving vertical gastrectomy, formation of the alimentary limb via a doudeno-ileostomy, and an anastomosis of the biliopancreatic limb to the distal ileum to create a common channel 100 cm from the ileocecal valve. Figure 5, *B* shows the anatomic configuration after a BPD+DS. A 45-degree angled scope and five ports are used. A liver retractor is used to expose the greater curve of the stomach, and the duodenum is freed from its lateral attachments, taking care not to injure any hepatoduodenal ligament structures. A 45 mm, 3.5 mm linear stapler is used to divide the duodenum 2 cm distal to the pylorus.

Next, the short gastric vessels are divided all the way up to the angle of His, and a 60 Fr bougie is passed into the stomach along the lesser curve. A gastric sleeve is then resected, leaving a tubular stomach with sequential firings along the bougie to create a vertical lesser curve–based gastric pouch. The first one to two firings are usually 45 mm, 4.8 mm stapler cartridges, and then 45 mm, 3.5 mm firings can be used as the stomach is stapled and divided toward the angle of His. The remaining tubular gastric pouch usually measures about 150 to 200 mL. The resected stomach is placed into a specimen bag and extracted at the end of the case.

Next, the cecum and ileocecal valve are identified, the ileum is measured back about 100 cm, and a stitch is placed to mark the bowel at this position for the site of the enteroenteric anastomosis forming the common channel. The ileum is then measured back another 150 cm proximal to the suture and is divided at this point using a 45 mm, 2.5 mm staple. The mesentery is then divided, and a suture is placed on the distal transected bowel to mark the Roux limb, which is brought up in an antecolic fashion and connected with the duodenum. The anastomosis can then be fashioned with a linear stapler, a 2.0 cm circular stapler, or a hand-sewn technique.

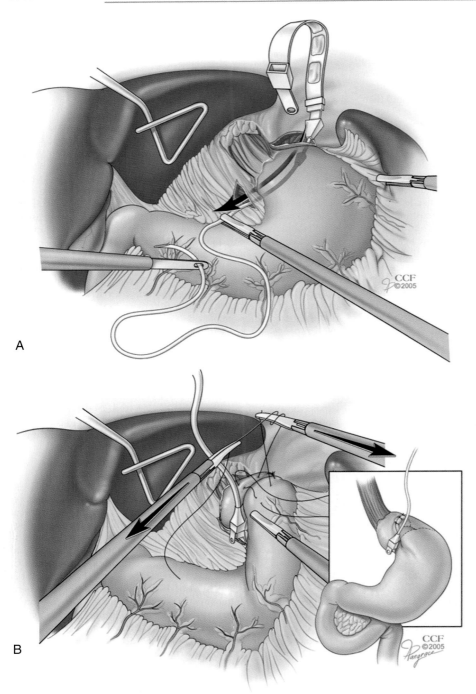

The mesenteric defect between the small bowel and transverse colon mesenteries is closed with a running suture. The Roux limb is clamped, and the endoscopist passes an upper gastrointestinal (UGI) endoscope down through the anastomosis, inspecting for bleeding and insufflating with air to perform a leak test. Next, the proximal end of the divided bowel at the aforementioned 150 cm mark, or a mark 250 cm from the ileocecal valve, forms the biliopancreatic limb; this is brought down to the 100 cm suture mark on the ileum, and a stapled enteroenterostomy is formed as described for the formation of the JJ above. The mesenteric defect between the small bowel mesentery is then closed with a running suture, and the lateral stomach specimen is removed; fascia may require widening to extract the resected stomach sleeve in a bag. Drains are placed around the

ileoduodenal anastomosis prior to removing the ports and closing fascial port sites greater than 10 mm. The standard Scopinaro biliopancreatic diversion differs from the BPD+DS in that the technique involves a horizontal distal gastrectomy to create a 250 mL stomach pouch, which is then anastomosed to a 200 cm alimentary limb joining a 50 cm common channel (Figure 5, *C*).

Sleeve Gastrectomy

Laparoscopic sleeve gastrectomy (LSG) has been employed as a primary bariatric procedure or as the first of a two-stage operation for high-risk patients, ending with a subsequent RYGB or BPD+DS

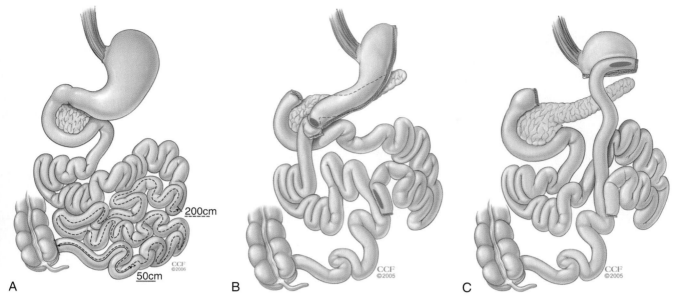

FIGURE 5 The biliopancreatic diversion. **A,** Sites of first and second small bowel transection points are marked. The 50 cm and 200 cm marks shown are for the standard (Scopinaro) BPD. For the BPD+DS these are at 100 cm and 250 cm from the ileocecal valve, respectively (250 cm alimentary limb and 100 cm common channel). **B,** BPD+DS. **C,** Standard (Scopinaro) BPD with 200 cm alimentary limb and a 50 cm common channel. *(Reprinted with permission from Cleveland Clinic Center for Medical Art & Photography, copyright 2005-2010. All Rights Reserved.)*

following a 6- to 12-month course of weight loss induced by the initial LSG. With the staged approach, weight loss from the lower risk LSG procedure is intended to reduce operative risk by improving comorbidities and reducing the technical challenges associated with high BMI patients. LSG involves a vertical resection of the stomach from the antrum up to the angle of His.

After port and liver retractor placement as described in the BPD+DS section above, the operation starts with the division of the stomach's greater curvature blood supply using a Harmonic scalpel to divide the gastrocolic and gastrosplenic ligaments close to the stomach, excluding and preserving the gastroepiploic vessels along the greater curve. Next, the narrow gastric tube is created by using a linear cutting stapler to resect the body and fundus of the stomach from the antrum, 3 to 5 cm from the pylorus, toward the angle of His alongside a calibration tube (endoscope or bougie; Figure 6).

After the first and second gastric divisions are made with the 45 mm, 4.8 mm stapler, the endoscope is inserted. The tip of the endoscope is advanced into the antrum and left in place, as the rest of the stomach is divided with sequential firings of 45 mm, 3.5 mm staple cartridges until the angle of His is reached. Care is taken not to leave fundus behind and not to apply the stapler too close to the esophagus at the last firing. We oversew the entire staple line with a running imbrication stitch, taking care not to narrow the lumen around the incisura. The resected stomach is then placed into a specimen bag and extracted through the large 15 mm port in the right upper quadrant (Figure 6, *B*).

POSTOPERATIVE MANAGEMENT

Our patients are allowed nothing by mouth immediately postoperatively. They are given supplemental oxygen to ensure O_2 saturations greater than 95%, and they are started or continued on pharmacologic prophylaxis for venous thromboembolic disease. Antibiotics are continued for the first 24 hours. Patient-controlled analgesia is administered, and patients with sleep apnea are placed on continuous positive airway pressure (CPAP) early in the postoperative period. All patients are encouraged to use incentive spirometery and to get up into the chair and ambulate within 12 to 24 hours of surgery to reduce pulmonary and thrombotic complications.

On the first postoperative day, a UGI swallow using water-soluble contrast is performed after all bariatric procedures, including gastric banding. If the swallow reveals no obstruction or leak at the gastrojejunostomy, patients are placed on a clear liquid bariatric diet formulated to include small amounts of simple sugars and calorie-reduced liquids. For gastric banding, the UGI study confirms proper band placement and patency. The diet is progressively advanced to full liquids, followed by semisoft or pureed foods in 1- to 2-week increments as tolerated. Solid food is added about 4 to 6 weeks postoperatively.

Vitamin and mineral supplementation is also started early postoperatively. Patients who undergo procedures with malabsorptive components are placed on multivitamins, iron, calcium, and vitamin B_{12} supplementation. Nausea and vomiting are treated aggressively early after surgery, especially after sleeve gastrectomy. Hospitalization is usually 2 to 4 days, and patients are discharged once clear fluids are tolerated. Drains are removed on the first postoperative visit 7 days later. If the drainage is suspicious, a repeat UGI contrast study is considered, and a sample of the drainage fluid may be sent for a salivary amylase analysis. Routine follow-up is scheduled for sleeve and bypass patients at 1, 3, 6, 9, 12, and 18 months and then yearly thereafter.

Laboratory studies for sleeve and bypass include a complete blood count, complete metabolic panel, liver function tests, iron panel, parathyroid hormone (PTH), and vitamins B_{12} and $D_{1,25}$, which are ordered at the 6-month visit and then annually. Although serious malnutrition is rare after RYGB, low levels of iron, vitamins B_{12} and $D_{1,25}$, and calcium and elevated PTH (reduced bone calcium) may occur depending on patient compliance; these should be treated with supplementation. In our practice, patients with a gallbladder but no gallstones are placed on ursodiol 300 mg twice a day for 6 months to reduce the risk of symptomatic cholelithiasis resulting from rapid weight loss. Proton-pump inhibitors or histamine-2 (H2) receptor blockers are also prescribed for bypass patients routinely for 6 months after surgery, and patients are advised to avoid NSAIDS for life to reduce marginal ulcer risk. Pregnancy is discouraged in the first year after bariatric surgery, during the period of rapid weight loss.

Patients who have had LAGB are evaluated every 2 months for the first year, then quarterly thereafter or as directed by clinical progress or weight loss response. Those who experience hunger between meals and feel minimal restriction from the band undergo band-diameter

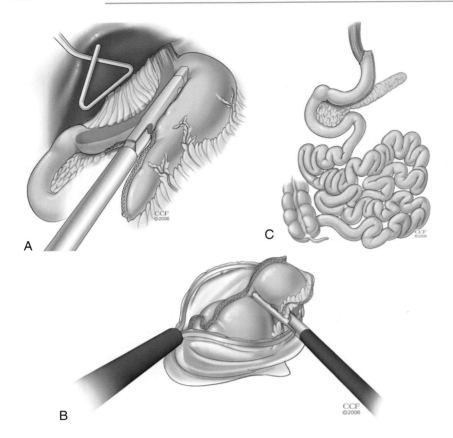

FIGURE 6 The laparoscopic sleeve gastrectomy. **A,** Creating a narrow gastric tube over a bougie or endoscope using a linear cutting stapler to excise the stomach body and fundus. **B,** Placing the resected stomach in a specimen bag before its extraction through a 15 mm port. **C,** The final anatomic arrangement after a sleeve gastric resection. (*Reprinted with permission from Cleveland Clinic Center for Medical Art & Photography, copyright 2005-2010. All Rights Reserved.*)

reduction by adding saline to the reservoir, in the clinic or under fluoroscopy, usually in 0.5 to 1.5 mL increments until the ideal fill (band "sweet spot" or "green zone") is reached, where maximum satiety is experienced without excess restriction or dysphagia. Band position and tightness can be assessed under fluoroscopy.

RESULTS

Weight Loss

Currently, bariatric surgery is the only therapeutic intervention proven to produce clinically significant and sustained weight loss (>5 years) for the majority of patients with severe obesity. On average, surgery results in 20 to 40 kg weight loss, and a 10 to 15 kg/m² reduction in BMI. In one of the earliest reports on outcomes of LRYGB, Schauer and colleagues (2000) found that the percentage of excess weight loss (%EWL) following gastric bypass was 68% at 1 year and 83% at 2 years. Other investigators have since corroborated these findings. A meta-analysis of 22,094 patients conducted in 2004 showed a mean %EWL of 61.2% in all surgical groups of patients with up to 2 years of follow-up. On further stratification by procedure, a %EWL of 48%, 62%, and 70% for AGB, RYGB, and BPD+DS respectively was observed.

In the Swedish Obese Subjects (SOS) study, the average weight loss sustained at 10 years after surgery was over 19 kg, and this was seen despite the fact that less than 5% of the patients had the RYGB (most patients had the less effective vertical banded gastroplasty). Brethauer and colleagues (2009) summarized outcomes after sleeve gastrectomy (SG) in 36 studies including a total of 2570 patients with a follow-up range of 3 to 60 months. One series with 5 year data reported a 15.7 kg/m² decrease in BMI from baseline. In 24 of the reviewed series, SG was used as a primary weight-loss procedure and resulted in an average %EWL of 60.4% over a 3- to 36-month

follow-up period, pointing to durability of the weight loss up to 3 years postoperatively.

Comorbidities

Arguably more important than weight loss are the improvements seen in medical comorbidities, overall quality of life, and longevity associated with bariatric surgery (Figure 7). The SOS study reported a significant improvement in the quality of life in the surgically treated group at 2 years, especially in the psychologic domain. Obesity-related comorbidities—such as hypertension, dyslipidemia, and especially T2DM—also improve after bariatric surgery. Schauer and colleagues demonstrated that fasting plasma glucose and hemoglobin A_{1C} levels normalized in 83% of patients in the 5 year postoperative period in a series of 1160 patients (191 with diabetes). In Buchwald's 2004 meta-analysis, T2DM completely resolved in 77% of patients and improved in an additional 9% of patients after surgery. In the same review, hyperlipidemia, hypertension, and obstructive sleep apnea improved in 70%, 79%, and 84%, respectively. Worth noting is that all bariatric operations promote weight loss and improve glucose homeostasis to some degree, but RYGB and BPD are the most effective in this regard. What is remarkable is that many patients become euglycemic well before the weight loss occurs; this observation has stimulated much interest in the metabolic role of these procedures and in how the anatomic reconfiguration and rerouting of nutrients in the GI tract affect its endocrine function.

Survival

Surgically enabled weight loss is also associated with a reduction in the risk of overall long-term mortality, as has been demonstrated by multiple studies. In 2004, the McGill Bariatric Cohort Study was the

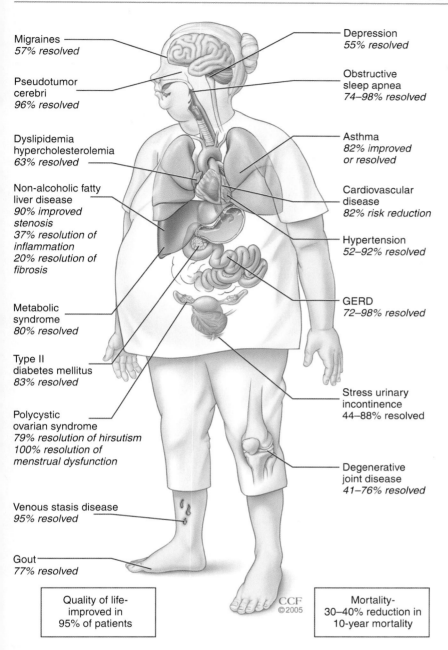

Migraines
57% resolved

Pseudotumor
cerebri
96% resolved

Dyslipidemia
hypercholesterolemia
63% resolved

Non-alcoholic fatty
liver disease
90% improved
stenosis
37% resolution of
inflammation
20% resolution of
fibrosis

Metabolic
syndrome
80% resolved

Type II
diabetes mellitus
83% resolved

Polycystic
ovarian syndrome
79% resolution of hirsutism
100% resolution of
menstrual dysfunction

Venous stasis disease
95% resolved

Gout
77% resolved

Depression
55% resolved

Obstructive
sleep apnea
74–98% resolved

Asthma
82% improved
or resolved

Cardiovascular
disease
82% risk reduction

Hypertension
52–92% resolved

GERD
72–98% resolved

Stress urinary
incontinence
44–88% resolved

Degenerative
joint disease
41–76% resolved

Quality of life-
improved in
95% of patients

CCF
©2005

Mortality-
30–40% reduction in
10-year mortality

FIGURE 7 Impact of bariatric surgery on obesity-related comorbidities. *(Reprinted with permission from Cleveland Clinic Center for Medical Art & Photography, copyright 2005-2010. All Rights Reserved.)*

first to report that a 67% excess weight loss at 5 years was associated with a relative risk reduction for mortality of 89% in a retrospective case-control analysis comparing over 1,000 surgically treated obese patients to over 5700 obese controls. The SOS study showed a survival benefit with bariatric surgery in a prospective analysis of 2,010 surgically treated patients, compared with 2037 controls with 99% follow-up at 10.9 years. The adjusted hazard ratio in the surgery group compared to the matched control group receiving conventional nonsurgical therapy was 0.71 (P = .01). A retrospective study from the University of Utah also showed a survival advantage in their surgical group with a mean follow-up of 7.1 years. The adjusted long-term mortality rate in the surgical cohort of 7925 patients decreased by 40% compared with the same size-matched control group (hazard ratio of 0.6; P < .001). Similarly, survival benefits were recently demonstrated in a higher risk Medicare population with 2 years of follow-up data. Specifically, a survival advantage was seen as

early as 6 months postoperatively in the under-65 age group and as early as 11 months in the 65-or-over age group. Studies from Europe and Australia have also confirmed survival advantages with LAGB.

POSTOPERATIVE COMPLICATIONS

Some postoperative complications are procedure specific. Clinicians caring for the bariatric surgical patient should be familiar with both early and late complications associated with different bariatric procedures to allow for early recognition and treatment of problems and prevention of long-term complications, thereby reducing morbidity and mortality in the surgically treated severely obese patient. Tables 4 and 5 outline some of the early and late postoperative complications associated with bariatric surgery and keys to recognition and management. Pulmonary embolism and

TABLE 4: Bariatric procedure-related postoperative complications

Procedure	COMPLICATIONS	
	Early Postoperative Period (<30 Days)	**Late**
LRYGB	Anastomotic leak with peritonitis Abdominal abscess Pulmonary embolism Bleeding Pulmonary complications Acute distal gastric dilation Roux limb obstruction Wound infection	Stomal stenosis Marginal ulcer Dumping syndrome Intestinal obstruction Internal hernia Incisional hernia Cholecystitis Vitamin and mineral deficiencies Weight regain Hypoglycemia
LBPD ± DS	Same as LRYGB	Same as LRYGB with the following being more common in the BPD procedure than in RYGB, if aggressive prophylactic measures are not followed postoperatively: Anemia Protein-calorie malnutrition Vitamin B_{12} deficiency Hypocalcemia Osteoporosis Fat-soluble vitamin deficiency Night blindness
LSG	Staple line leak Abscess Hemorrhage Sleeve stricture Wound infection	Intractable nausea ± vomiting Reflux symptoms Gastric dilation Weight loss failure Weight regain
LAGB	Hemorrhage Wound infection Food intolerance Reflux Nausea ± vomiting Slippage Wound infection	Reflux symptoms Erosive esophagitis Esophageal dilation Pouch enlargement Band slippage Gastric prolapse Vomiting Tubing-related problems Leakage of the reservoir Band erosion Weight loss failure Lower average weight loss

anastomotic leakage remain two important complications deserving of elaboration; we will discuss these here.

MORTALITY

Severe life-threatening complications have decreased over time, with 30 day mortality reportedly varying from 0% to 2%, depending mostly on the procedure performed, patient characteristics, and surgical volume. Buchwald's 2004 meta-analysis reported mortality rates of 0.1% for AGB, 0.5% for RYGB, and 1.1% for BPD. The SOS study reported a mortality rate of less than 0.2%. These low rates were confirmed in a 2009 report by the Longitudinal Assessment for Bariatric Surgery consortium. In a prospective multicenter cohort study evaluating the incidence of adverse outcomes in a group of patients undergoing RYGB or AGB, the overall 30-day mortality rate in 4610 evaluated patients was 0.3% with no mortality contribution from the AGB group. In addition, a total of 4.3% of patients had at least one major adverse outcome in the early postoperative period. Dreaded complications responsible for early mortality include pulmonary embolism and sepsis from a GI leakage. Both occur with a frequency of less than 1% at major centers, and they often tend to present similarly with tachycardia and respiratory distress.

Pulmonary Embolism

Postoperative pulmonary embolism (PE) remains the leading cause of death following bariatric surgery, and it can occur after discharge from hospital. The condition can be difficult to diagnose, as patients

TABLE 5: Diagnosis and management of postoperative complications after bariatric procedures

Complication	Incidence	Signs and Symptoms	Diagnosis	Management
Pulmonary embolism	<1%	Tachycardia, hypotension, hypoxia, tachypnea, chest pain, fever, extremity swelling	Helical pulmonary CT scan	Anticoagulation
			CT angiography	
			V/Q scan	
Gastrointestinal leakage	0.8%–7%	Tachycardia, hypotension, tachypnea, abdominal pain, chest pain, fever	Abdominal and Pelvic CT imaging or UGI	Surgery for irrigation, drainage, and control of abdominal sepsis to augment medical management. In stable patients, nonoperative control of sepsis with radiologic drainage and medical therapy can be considered.
			Drain fluid analysis for salivary amylase	
Bleeding	<4%	Hypotension, tachycardia, drop in hemoglobin, blood in drains	Reoperation often required	Endoscopy to treat bleeding at the GJ
			Multiple sources of bleeding to consider	Clips or suture ligation/oversewing of mesenteric or intestinal staple line bleeding
				Suture ligature for port site bleeding
Wound infection	2%–5%	Fever, swelling, erythema, discharge, pain	Clinical findings and diagnostic tests as indicated	Incision and drainage ± antibiotics
Gastric remnant dilation	≤1%	Hiccups, abdominal bloating, sepsis	Abdominal radiograph	Needle or surgical decompression
			CT of abdomen	Placement of gastrostomy tube
Dumping syndrome	Seen in up to three fourths of RYGB and BPD patients	Early satiety, nausea, cramping, and explosive diarrhea	Clinical history	Avoid foods with high simple-sugar load
		Vasomotor symptoms of flushing, sweating, palpitations, dizziness, and a feeling of needing to lie down		Consume foods high in fiber and protein
Small bowel obstruction	3% of cases	Intermittent, colicky abdominal pain occurring days to years postoperatively	CT scan of abdomen	Laparoscopic or open surgical therapy
			Small bowel series	
			Diagnostic laparoscopy	
			Referral back to bariatric surgeon for evaluation	
Marginal ulceration	<5% of cases	Nausea, vomiting, pain, bleeding	Endoscopy	Acid-suppression therapy

Continued

TABLE 5: Diagnosis and management of postoperative complications after bariatric procedures—cont'd

Complication	Incidence	Signs and Symptoms	Diagnosis	Management
			UGI contrast radiologic study	Sucralfate therapy
				Stop NSAID use and smoking
Stomal stenosis	Stenosis of GJ in 10% of cases	Occurs mostly 2 weeks to 6 months postoperatively	Endoscopy	Endoscopic balloon dilation
		Symptoms include vomiting, pain, dysphagia, and/or failure to thrive	UGI contrast radiologic study	Revisional surgery
Vitamin and mineral deficiency	Observed in malabsorptive diversional procedures	Signs and symptoms vary depending on deficiency	Blood vitamin and mineral levels	Routine follow-up with ongoing vitamin and mineral supplementation
Cholelithiasis	Up to 28% of patients require cholecystectomy within 3 yr after gastric bypass	Biliary colic or symptoms of acute cholecystitis	Ultrasound	Ursodiol for 6 months after bariatric surgery to decrease risk of gallstone formation
				Cholecystectomy for symptomatic patients
Weight regain	Can be seen in up to 25%–30% of patients at 2 to 5 years	Weight regain or leveling of weight loss	CT scan of abdomen	Medical weight management first; surgical revision then considered for failures, but at a higher risk
		Recurrence of comorbidity-related symptoms	Small bowel series	Endoscopic or endoluminal therapies
			Diagnostic laparoscopy	
			Referral back to bariatric surgeon for evaluation	

may become hypotensive and tachycardic with signs similar to those of sepsis. Nevertheless, in patients with signs of sepsis and hypoxia, the diagnosis of a PE and leak should be simultaneously considered, and appropriate imaging studies to guide diagnosis and treatment should be ordered promptly. In those whose body size precludes them from undergoing diagnostic spiral CT imaging, a pulmonary V/Q scan may be helpful; but serious consideration should be given to immediate exploration in the operating room, and if no intraabdominal pathology is found, anticoagulation can be initiated thereafter on clinical grounds.

Gastrointestinal Leak

Anastomotic and staple-line leaks have been reported to occur in 0.8% to 7% of cases. The overall mortality rate from enteric leaks after gastric bypass can be as high as 20%, and leaks remain the second leading cause of death after surgery. Leakage from the GI tract is more commonly seen with restrictive and malabsorptive procedures resulting in GI staple or anastomotic lines; early gastric leakage from a LAGB can occur but is very rare. In the case of the RYGB and BPD, leaks occur most frequently at the gastrojejunostomy but can also occur from the gastric pouch, the gastric remnant, and the jejunojejunostomy. Leakage can also occur at the gastric staple line in the case of a sleeve gastrectomy.

Again, diagnosis can be challenging in the obese patient with intraabdominal sepsis; and although fever, tachycardia, and abdominal pain are common, often the only sign is tachycardia in the absence of classic peritoneal signs, such as guarding and rebound tenderness. A heart rate greater than 120 beats/min should alert the evaluating clinician to rule out a leak, even if the patient feels and looks well. Leaks can be immediate or may present up to 1 to 2 weeks postoperatively. A negative intraoperative leak test and a UGI swallow on the first postoperative day offer reassurance regarding the integrity of the GJ anastomosis, but these tests can be falsely negative, and a leak from ischemia at any staple line may take some time to manifest. Leakage from the GJ can be contained or can result in diffuse peritonitis. If diffuse leakage is left untreated, sepsis will follow with possible multisystem organ failure. Surgical treatment involves reexploration, copious irrigation, leak containment with omental patching, and wide drainage. In select stable patients, contained leaks can be managed nonoperatively with adequate drainage, bowel rest, and antibiotics. Worth noting is that patients with leaks can also be asymptomatic at the time of diagnosis, with the only sign being a discharge or change in the color of secretion through the abdominal drain. For some patients, a drain is helpful and may avoid operative intervention, particularly in those with subclinical leaks. It is our practice to leave the abdominal drain in at least 7 to 10 days and to remove it during the first postoperative visit, if no abnormal drainage is seen.

COMPLICATIONS RELATED TO ADJUSTABLE GASTRIC BANDING

LAGB is one of the safest bariatric operations available, with a 0.05% mortality rate. Overall morbidity rates vary widely between studies, with rates as high as 20% having been reported. The most common late complication related to LAGB is gastric prolapse, or band slippage, which consists of cepahalad herniation of the stomach through the band that results in an enlarged gastric pouch and partial or complete gastric occlusion. It occurs in up to 5% of cases, but changes in the method of band placement (the *pars flaccida* technique) have reduced the incidence of this problem. Band erosion can also occur and appears to be related to surgical technique. Both of these problems usually require reoperation with removal and band replacement. Port and tubing problems include port migration, port infection, tubing disconnection, tubing kink, and port leak. They require surgical repair to maintain a functional device for weight loss. In large series, 3% to 6% of patients require removal of the band for one or more of the following conditions: failed weight loss, band erosion, esophageal dilation, or uncontrolled symptoms of reflux esophagitis or dysphagia.

SUMMARY

Bariatric surgery has evolved tremendously since the first published jejunal-ileal bypass procedure in 1954. RYGB, LAGB, SG, BPD, and BPD+DS are currently the most common procedures performed throughout the world and have been shown to have favorable risk/benefit profiles. Several randomized prospective studies have shown the laparoscopic approach to be superior to the open approach in the hands of most surgeons, as it clearly reduces perioperative morbidity. Multiple studies have highlighted the effectiveness of bariatric surgery in achieving weight loss, ameliorating comorbidities, and improving both quality of life and longevity. Better outcomes have been linked to surgeon experience and center volume. Operations tend to be more difficult in the super obese, and the use of extra ports, especially to achieve better liver retraction, may prove helpful. Revisional surgery for complications or ineffective weight loss is fraught with increased risks of morbidity and mortality. Choosing the most appropriate initial procedure for a patient remains a joint physician-patient decision that needs careful consideration. A summary of the relative advantages and disadvantages of each procedure is shown in Table 6.

TABLE 6: Comparison of commonly performed bariatric procedures

Procedure	Advantages	Disadvantages
LRYGB	Excellent proven long-term weight loss Better weight loss than restrictive-only procedures Proven improvements in medical comorbidities Mortality rate less than 1% at most centers	Malabsorption Marginal ulcer Stomal stenosis Exclusion of gastric remnant from future access Internal hernia Iron deficiency Calcium deficiency Vitamin B_{12} deficiency
LBPD ± DS	Excellent weight loss More effective for severe morbid obesity, especially BMI >70 kg/m^2 Allows for increased food intake without interfering with weight loss Preserved pylorus leads to less dumping Less risk of marginal ulcer	Increased risk of protein malabsorption Increased risk of fat-soluble vitamin malabsorption (A, D, E, K) Iron-deficiency anemia Diarrhea and flatulence more common Internal hernia Higher complication rate Higher risk of osteoporosis
LSG	Restrictive procedure with good short-term weight loss data now available Avoids risks involved with diversionary malabsorptive procedures Shorter OR time and safer in high-risk patients than bypass procedures Can be used as a stand-alone weight-loss option or as part of a staged bariatric procedure	Significant postoperative nausea and vomiting requiring pharmacotherapy Less weight loss than with diversionary procedures Long-term data on nutrition impact not yet available Has a staple line and associated risk of leakage comparable to the other common restrictive procedure, the AGB
LAGB	Lowest mortality risk Most reversible procedure Least invasive Relatively simple procedure requiring less operative time No staple line or anastomosis No malabsorption An option in the high-risk patient Band can be deflated in pregnancy	Erosion Esophageal dilation Gastroesophageal reflux disease Breakage Slippage Port site complications Frequent postoperative visits for band adjustments Failure to lose weight Lower average weight loss

In the near future, new, totally endoscopic procedures will be introduced that have great promise for further reduction of perioperative morbidity as well as cost, and they will perhaps also provide greater access for patients who may benefit from bariatric procedures. These new procedures must be subjected to the same rigorous outcome evaluation as currently accepted procedures. Stay tuned, as much lies ahead for the further development of this dynamic field of bariatric surgery.

Suggested Readings

Adams TD, Gress RE, Smith SC, et al: Long-term mortality after gastric bypass surgery, *N Engl J Med* 357(8):753–761, 2007.

Brethauer SA, Hammel JP, Schauer P: Systematic review of sleeve gastrectomy as a staging and primary bariatric procedure, *Surg Obes Relat Dis* (5):469–475, 2009.

Brolin RE: Gastric bypass, *Surg Clin North Am* 81(5):1077–1095, 2001.

Buchwald H, Avidor Y, Braunwald E, et al: Bariatric surgery: a systematic review and meta-analysis, *JAMA* 292(14):1724–1737, 2004.

Cristou N, Sampalis J, Liberman M, et al: Surgery decreases long-term mortality, morbidity, and health care use in morbidly obese patients, *Ann Surg* 240:416–423, 2004.

DeMaria EJ, Portenier D, Wolfe L: Obesity surgery mortality risk score: proposal for a clinically useful score to predict mortality risk in patients undergoing gastric bypass, *Surg Obes Relat Dis* 3:134–140, 2007.

Dixon JB, O'Brien PE, Playfair J, et al: Adjustable gastric banding and conventional therapy for type 2 diabetes: a randomized controlled trial, *JAMA* 299(3):316–323, 2008.

Favretti F, Segato G, Ashton D, et al: Laparoscopic adjustable gastric banding in 1,791 consecutive obese patients: 12-year results, *Obes Surg* 17(2):168–175, 2007.

Gagner M, Deitel M, Kalberer TL, et al: The Second International Consensus Summit for Sleeve Gastrectomy, March 19-21, 2009, *Surg Obes Relat Dis* 5(4):476–485, 2009.

Schauer P, Shirmer B, Brethauer S: *Minimally invasive bariatric surgery*, New York, 2008, Springer.

The Longitudinal Assessment of Bariatric Surgery (LABS) Consortium: Perioperative safety in the longitudinal assessment of bariatric surgery, *N Engl J Med* 361(5):445–454, 2009.

Moy J, Pomp A, Dakin G, et al: Laparoscopic sleeve gastrectomy for morbid obesity, *Am J Surg* 196(5):e56–e59, 2008.

Nguyen NT, Goldman C, Rosenquist CJ, et al: Laparoscopic versus open gastric bypass: a randomized study of outcomes, quality of life, and costs, *Ann Surg* 234(3):279–289, 2001.

Nguyen NT, Slone JA, Nguyen XM, et al: A prospective randomized trial of laparoscopic gastric bypass versus laparoscopic adjustable gastric banding for the treatment of morbid obesity: outcomes, quality of life, and costs, *Ann Surg* 250(4): 631–641, 2009.

Perry CD, Hutter MM, Smith DB, et al: Survival and changes in comorbidities after bariatric surgery, *Ann Surg* 247:21–27, 2008.

Pories WJ, Swanson MS, MacDonald KG, et al: Who would have thought it? An operation proves to be the most effective therapy for adult-onset diabetes mellitus, *Ann Surg* 222(3):339–350, 1995.

Rubino F, Kaplan LM, Schauer PR, et al: for the Diabetes Surgery Summit Delegates: The Diabetes Surgery Summit Consensus Conference: recommendations for the evaluation and use of gastrointestinal surgery to treat type 2 diabetes mellitus, *Ann Surg* 251(3):406–408, 2010.

Schauer PR, Burguera B, Ikramuddin S, et al: Effect of laparoscopic Roux-en-Y gastric bypass on type 2 diabetes mellitus, *Ann Surg* 238(4):467–484, 2003.

Schauer PR, Ikramuddin S, Gourash W, et al: Outcomes after laparoscopic roux-en-Y gastric bypass for morbid obesity, *Ann Surg* 232(4): 515–529, 2000.

Shikora SA, Kim JJ, Tarnoff ME, et al: Laparoscopic Roux-en-Y gastric bypass: results and learning curve of a high-volume academic program, *Arch Surg* 140(4):362–367, 2005.

Sjostrom L, Narbro K, Sjostrom D, et al: Effects of bariatric surgery on mortality in Swedish obese subjects, *N Engl J Med* 357(8):741–752, 2007.

Sugerman HJ, Kellum JM Jr, Engle KM, et al: Gastric bypass for treating severe obesity, *Am J Clin Nutr* 55(Suppl 2):560–566, 1992.

Thodiyil PA, Yenumula P, Rogula T, et al: Selective nonoperative management of leaks after gastric bypass: Lessons learned from 2675 consecutive patients, *Ann Surg* 248(5):782–792, 2008.

Wittgrove AC, Clark GW: Laparoscopic gastric bypass, Roux-en-Y: 500 patients—technique and results, with 3-60 month follow-up, *Obes Surg* 10(3):233–239, 2000.

Natural Orifice Transluminal Endoscopic Surgery

NOTES: What Is Currently Possible?

Erwin Rieder, MD, and Lee L. Swanstrom, MD

OVERVIEW

Despite the skepticism of some, natural orifice transluminal endoscopic surgery (NOTES) has moved beyond the vision and theory of a few free thinkers and has become clinical reality. From what was a conceptual or lab-based approach 5 years ago, multiple centers have now progressed to human NOTES procedures, including appendectomies, liver biopsies, tubal ligations, and cholecystectomies, all without major complications (Table 1). The concept is continuously expanding, as industry develops new enabling technologies for NOTES. More than 10 currently open clinical trials in humans are officially registered in the U.S. government Web-based registry (http://www.clinicaltrials.org), and it can be imagined that many more transluminal procedures are being performed by innovative surgeons worldwide.

The basic aim of scarless surgery through natural orifices such as the mouth, vagina, and anus is to dramatically reduce the surgical impact on the patient and thereby improve surgical outcomes. At minimum this concept has opened the door to a new era in minimally invasive surgery, from the avoidance of skin incisions with resulting decreases in physical and psychologic disability, offering direct patient benefits such as less pain and allowing the conversion of standard inpatient surgical interventions into outpatient clinic procedures. Eventually NOTES may even be a boon for underserved third world surgery, as it might obviate the need for a sterile operating room.

Since the first description of the feasibility and safety of peroral transgastric endoscopic access to the peritoneal cavity in a long-term survival porcine model by Kalloo in 2004, current clinical possibilities have become numerous. The first small series of successful transgastric human appendectomies, liver biopsies, and fallopian tube ligations was from Rao and Reddy in India and was presented at the annual meeting of the American Society for Gastrointestinal Endoscopy (ASGE) in 2005. Their presentation created great excitement among clinical innovators, as well as those in the medical device industry, who saw an opportunity to push the boundaries of minimally invasive surgery. To regulate this enthusiasm and prevent potential patient harm, the Natural Orifice Surgery Consortium for Assessment and Research (NOSCAR) was established under the sponsorship of the ASGE and the Society of American Gastrointestinal Endoscopic Surgeons (SAGES). Its mission is to address quality and safety issues, create guidelines, and establish training requirements. An outcomes registry of natural orifice procedures was created by NOSCAR in 2008, and many other registries worldwide have followed.

Controversy has always swirled around visionary developments in surgery. Although already a clinical reality, many surgeons still doubt the potential and clinical relevance of NOTES. Similarities to the early era of laparoscopic surgery, when the first human laparoscopic cholecystectomies were performed by Erich Mühe in 1985, can be observed. In parallel with the evolution of minimally invasive surgery, ambitious efforts have been made to transform endoscopy from serving purely diagnostic purposes to providing complex therapeutic applications. These developments have been made by both gastroenterologists and surgeons interested in interventional endoscopy. Many diseases formerly only treatable by conventional surgical interventions—such as the excision of large colon polyps, dysplastic Barrett esophagus, esophageal varyx ligation, Zenker diverticulectomy, gastrointestinal bleeding, common bile duct exploration, and others—are now more often treated by endoluminal procedures at many centers (Table 2). It can be expected that this less invasive trend is likely to continue.

The development of technologies to enable NOTES has already had an impact on current laparoscopic surgery and interventional

TABLE 1: The expanding spectrum of animal and human NOTES procedures

Procedure	Animal Studies	Human Cases
Transvaginal cholecystectomy	X	X
Transgastric cholecystectomy	X	X
Transgastric appendectomy	X	X
Transvaginal appendectomy	X	X
Transgastric gastrojejunostomy	X	
Transvaginal/transgastric liver biopsy	X	
PEG tube salvage		X
Transrectal colectomy	X	
Transesophageal Heller myotomy	X	X
Transvaginal pancreatectomy	X	

PEG, Percutaneous endoscopic gastrostomy

TABLE 2: Surgeries with endoscopic alternatives

	Open Surgery	Laparoscopy	Flexible Endoscopy
Large colon polyps	–	+	++++
Common bile duct stones	–	+	++++
Zenker diverticulum	++	–	+
Barrett esophagus ± dysplasia	+	++	+++
Pancreatic pseudocyst	–	+	+++
GI bleeding	–	+	++++
Acute colon perforation	++	+	++
Acute esophageal perforation	++	+	+++
Anastomotic leaks, foregut	+	++	+++
Anastomotic leaks, hindgut	+++	+	+
Obstructing foregut cancers	–	+	++++
Obstructing hindgut cancers	++	+	+++
Early GI cancers	–	+++	++
GI cancer staging	–	+	++++
Enteral access for feeding	–	+	++++

GI, Gastrointestinal; –, no clinical utility; +, some utility; ++, moderate utility; +++, preferred approach; ++++, gold standard approach

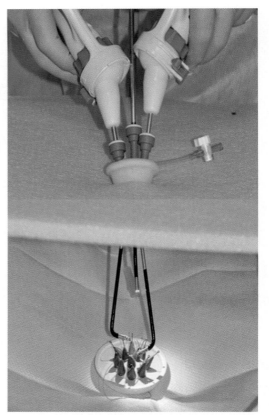

FIGURE 1 Single-port surgery is just one spin-off from NOTES.

procedures. Many such procedures and devices are approaching marketability, which leads us to question what is currently possible in natural orifice transluminal surgery.

TREATMENT AND METHODS

In NOTES, the original concept was based on a flexible endoscope entering the abdominal cavity, the retroperitoneal space, or the chest via a transesophageal, transgastric, transcolonic, or transvaginal route. It has been shown that essentially all organs can be reached by one of these approaches. Seeking to capitalize on this potential evolution in surgery, the medical device industry, as well as clinical innovators, have put a lot of effort into multiple enabling devices and novel tools for use with conventional endoscopes. In general, the adoption of NOTES into clinical practice is strongly dependent on device development. NOTES procedures using available or "standard" instrumentation are highly demanding, even for experienced laparoscopists or endoscopists. The sophisticated systems enabling pure NOTES procedures are limited in availability so far, and most remain in the prototype phase. Advanced NOTES platforms such as the Direct Drive Endoscopic System (Boston Scientific, Natick, Mass.), the EndoSamurai (Olympus, Tokyo), or the Anubiscope (Storz, Tuttlingen, Germany), all of which enable laparoscopic-like triangulation; the ability to perform intracorporeal suturing is still in the prototype phase but will prompt a huge step forward when such devices are launched (Figure 2).

The creation and closure of a viscerotomy is one of the fundamental differences between laparoscopy and NOTES. Although no adverse events such as gastric leakage have been reported in clinical cases so far, secure visceral closure is still a matter of intense debate. Several tools have been developed (e.g., the Tissue Approximation System; Ethicon, Somerville, NJ), but to date few are available for clinical use (e.g., G-Prox; USGI Medical, San Clemente, Calif.; Figure 3). Because

endoscopy. Reticulating laparoscopic instruments developed to ease requirements in minimally invasive surgery were recently adapted for single-incision surgery (SILS), in which triangulation is hampered because of a single-site approach. By adopting a crosswise approach with instruments such as graspers and scissors, it has become possible to overcome to some degree the inherent decreased traction/countertraction issues.

The umbilicus is controversially discussed as a former natural orifice by many, but SILS may be more of a bridge on the way from laparoscopic surgery to pure NOTES procedures (Figure 1). SILS and natural orifice transumbilical surgery (NOTUS) require abdominal wall incisons, which lead to somatic pain and interferes with the possibilities of pure NOTES. Even though the complexity of SILS operations is increasing, to the point that even procedures such as colonic resection have been shown to be feasible, it is yet to be determined whether single-site surgery will provide patient benefits compared to conventional laparoscopic approaches or NOTES.

An additional spin-off of the NOTES experience has been the increased interest in endoluminal natural orifice surgery (ENOS), an extension of standard interventional endoscopy in which upper abdominal procedures are performed with highly specialized surgical instruments passed through a natural orifice. Clinical trials of interventions such as endoluminal antireflux procedures, instead of laparoscopic fundoplication, and endoluminal bariatric surgeries have demonstrated the feasibility and benefits of these incisionless

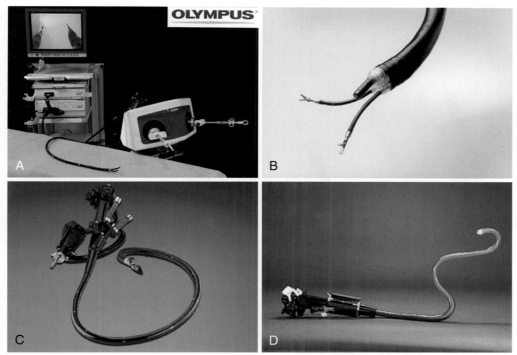

FIGURE 2 **A,** EndoSamurai (Olympus). **B,** Direct Drive Endoscopic System (Boston Scientific). **C,** Anubiscope (Storz). **D,** Transport (USGI Medical).

of this, many have opted for the transvaginal approach through the posterior fornix. Such access has long been used by gynecologists, and some surgeons have already gathered experience in colpotomy for removal of colon segments or spleens in laparoscopic surgery.

A short time after the first laparoscopy-assisted transvaginal cholecystectomy was performed in the United States, the first totally transvaginal cholecystectomy in a 30-year-old woman using a double-channel videogastroscope was reported by Marescaux and colleagues (Operation Anubis) in 2007. The procedure was done in the lithotomy position, with an additional 2 mm needle port to insufflate and monitor the pneumoperitoneum and for further retraction of the gallbladder. At no stage of the procedure was there need for additional laparoscopic assistance, and the operating time was 3 hours. In 2007, a series of four patients who had transvaginal cholecystectomy was presented by a Brazilian research group. The authors, as has become common, used a needlescopic trocar in the right upper quadrant to retract the gallbladder.

Pure NOTES, as originally conceived—that is, with the use of flexible endoscopes for transluminal procedures and no skin incisions—has proven to be time consuming and beyond the skill set of most surgeons. Because of this, more focus has been placed on transvaginal access using conventional laparoscopic instruments in addition to, or even instead of, flexible endoscopy. Many reports have followed on transvaginal cholecystectomies with the majority describing a hybrid technique with an additional 5 mm transumbilical port for insufflation, for observation of safe colpotomy, and for easier dissection enabled by increased triangulation and familiar instruments.

The hybrid approach, which uses laparoscopic techniques with NOTES, has shown to decrease the mean operative time to less than 50 minutes, which is comparable to standard laparoscopy. Other transvaginal procedures have been described worldwide, such as appendectomies, right hemicolectomies, sigmoidectomies, and even sleeve gastrectomies performed using a similar hybrid technique, and all have been shown to be safe. Even more complicated procedures, such as a pure transvaginal nephrectomy, have been shown to be feasible in humans. Of course, this is not a totally new concept; a series of laparoscopic nephrectomies with vaginal delivery via a posterior

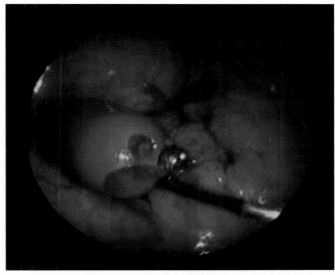

FIGURE 3 The Transport endoscope (USGI Medical) is advanced out of the stomach and into the peritoneal cavity.

colpotomy was published in 1993 by Breda and colleagues. More patients followed without any intraoperative complications, as published in 2002 by Gill and colleagues. Recently, a pure transvaginal NOTES right nephrectomy in a 58-year-old woman suffering from recurrent urinary tract infections and an atrophic right kidney was reported by Kaouk and colleagues. The transvaginal route has the potential advantage of providing easy access and closure under direct vision and at the present appears to be the only reliable technique adapted for abdominal NOTES. But it should be kept in mind that this simpler access is only available to 50% of patients at best.

Surgical endoscopists and endoscopic surgeons more familiar with flexible instrumentation have focused on the transgastric

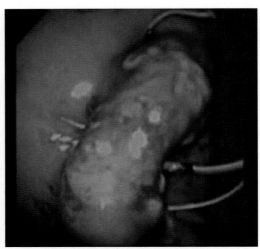

FIGURE 5   Endoluminal gastric closure after gallbladder removal.

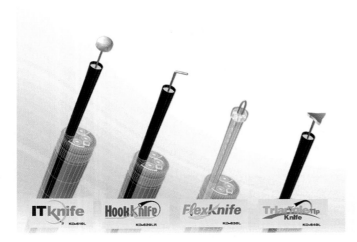

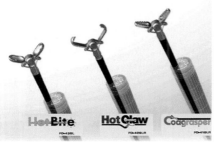

FIGURE 4   A variety of novel endoscopic instruments are useful for NOTES procedures.

approach. After transgastric endoscopic peritoneoscopies by flexible endoscopy in humans had been demonstrated, the first transgastric cholecystectomy in the United States was performed in July 2007 using an FDA-approved 18 mm four-channel shapelock-based endoscope (Transport; USGI Medical). As we perform this procedure, needle-knife cautery is used to incise the stomach at an anterior midgastric level, after routine endoscopy and gastric antibiotic lavage. A balloon dilator is used to stretch the gastrotomy to enable the scope to be advanced into the abdominal cavity (see Figure 3). The transport platform is able to lock in a retroflex position and thereby gives stable access to the gallbladder via the transgastric route. To confirm the safety of the procedure, and later the full-thickness gastric closure, a 5 mm scope is positioned transumbilically. Endoscopic dissection of the cystic duct and cystic artery is performed, adhering to principles of laparoscopic surgery. A needle port can additionally be used for retraction if needed. After clip ligation of the cystic artery and duct, further dissection proceeds with endoscopic scissors and a variety of specialized tools such as a needle knife, IT knife, or monopolar flex knife (Olympus; Figure 4). The gallbladder can then be pulled into the lumen of the stomach and removed transorally. Gastric closure is performed using the G-Prox grasper/approximation device (Figure 5).

In our first small series of patients with 1 year follow-up, we have seen fairly promising results. All patients reported satisfaction with the long-term outcomes of their procedure, and no specific gastrointestinal symptoms were observed. No evidence of esophagitis, gastritis, or erosive complications from the gastrotomy closure could be observed. However, the transgastric route currently has severe limitations. Operative times are extremely long, and the procedure requires high skill levels both for flexible endoscopy and laparoscopy. The transoral approach also requires highly flexible instruments, which restricts their size and functionality, and large specimens cannot be removed via this route.

The transrectal NOTES approach may in fact make more sense for incisionless surgery. Interestingly, more than 20 years before the

NOTES white paper was published, transanal endoscopic microsurgery (TEM), a pure natural orifice endoluminal procedure, had already been introduced. TEM has long been used for full-thickness resection of rectal tumors, followed by suture closure of the resultant defect. Although the defect was initially considered a complication, it has also been shown that transcolonic access above the peritoneal reflection during TEM does not increase short-term complications. Incisionless sigmoid and right colectomies have been described in the literature, and the advantage of the transrectal approach includes that it allows the use of rigid and flexible instruments without the need for scope retroflexion. Additionally, incorporation of the access colotomy into a subsequent anastomosis offers potential reduction in complications from leaks at the viscotomy closure site. Although not clinically applied yet, transrectal sigmoidectomy will potentially add an additional exciting approach in humans.

In the evolution of NOTES and endoluminal techniques, many traditional surgical dogmas have collapsed, such as breaching of the esophageal wall. The first clinical experience of submucosal endoscopic esophageal myotomy for esophageal achalasia without skin incision was presented in 2009. The procedure described involved a 1 cm longitudinal mucosal incision in the mid esophagus and the creation of a 3 cm submucosal tunnel with subsequent dissection of the inner circular muscle bundle for 7 cm of the distal esophagus.

RATIONALE AND JUSTIFICATION

It has been shown previously that the laparoscopic approach is as safe as conventional open surgery, and patients recover earlier and have less pain. Clinical trials have shown that the minimally invasive approach can even provide an improved outcome in oncologic parameters. The NOTES concept has already been shown to even further reduce the trauma and discomfort associated with surgery. The most recognized and discussed justifications for any effort in NOTES are patient benefits such as less pain, avoidance of unsightly wounds or incisional hernias, early recovery, and the possibility of transforming basic elective surgery into an outpatient clinic procedure.

Any developments of NOTES may also improve conventional laparoscopic surgery with subsequent benefits for the patient. SILS and devices such as needlescopic instruments can be identified as the means to an even less invasive approach. Even if surgeons were reluctant to adopt less invasive surgery, and most still are, patients will greet this effort with approval, because in the patients' view, less will always be better. It has actually been documented in several published studies that patients would prefer NOTES cholecystectomy to laparoscopic cholecystectomy for the anticipated lack of pain and visible scars. However, it must be kept in mind that the real value of pushing the boundaries in NOTES by breaching an otherwise virgin organ for transluminal access is still hypothetical and has to be evaluated within appropriate clinical trials.

NOTES: WHAT WILL BE POSSIBLE IN THE NEAR FUTURE?

We suspect that the ultimate application of NOTES is unlikely to be a standard procedure such as cholecystectomy or appendectomy, at least in the immediate future. Clinical experience to date has mostly been with hybrid procedures, using laparoscopic assistance, and mostly involves cholecystectomy or appendectomy. The focus on cholecystectomy for an initial procedure is due to its already playing a prominent role in the initial development of laparoscopic general surgery and the high number performed each year, which makes it a great candidate for meaningful pilot studies as well as randomized trials. On the other hand, cholecystectomy and appendectomy have been justifiably criticized, because both these procedures involve only a few small ports with minimal incisions and have a rapid patient recovery already.

So what should be the actual aim? It could be argued that the feasibility of large organ resection, such as colectomy done with a NOTES approach, would offer the possibility for a clear-cut patient advantage over a laparoscopic approach, avoiding as it does multiple large ports and a large hand port or specimen extraction incision. It is not even subject to the frequent NOTES criticism of violating an innocent second organ, as the colon or rectum is always breached in a colectomy. As experimental data have already shown the feasibility of transrectal sigmoidectomy in human cadavers using the transanal approach, the introduction of flexible endoscopy to the TEM platform could further ease the procedure, and the first human cases might be demonstrated soon. Additional new procedures, such as Heller myotomy and mediastinal sentinel lymph node biopsies, have been shown to be feasible in animal and cadaver studies, and previous difficulties to access structures such as mediastinal lymph nodes can be overcome.

It must be acknowledged that NOTES is not about adapting laparoscopic concepts to endoscopic surgery. Because of a change in established surgical approaches—overtubes instead of trocars, more inline instruments instead of triangulation, less need for exposure, and lower insufflation pressures—we may have to change some laparoscopic precepts and instead bring new concepts into a new surgical paradigm. Experimental data today will soon transition into the clinical setting and may thereby give access to completely new options.

NOTES is one of the most exciting current developments in minimally invasive surgery. Only a few years after its theoretical conception, many transluminal procedures without visible scars have been performed by experienced minimally invasive surgeons worldwide. Natural orifice surgery, either transluminal or endoluminal, is not simply one incision less as some argue. Procedures we would not even have thought about will become feasible because of new developments resulting from the NOTES experience in the near future, which will offer the surgeon and the patient new possibilities and alternative solutions.

SUGGESTED READINGS

ASGE/SAGES Working Group on Natural Orifice Transluminal Endoscopic Surgery: White paper, October 2005, *Gastrointest Endosc* 63:199, 2006.

Awad MM, Denk PM, Kennedy TJ, et al: NOTES transgastric cholecystectomy: outcomes at one year, *Gastrointest Endosc* 69:AB165, 2009.

Bessler M, Stevens PD, Milone L, et al: Transvaginal laparoscopically assisted endoscopic cholecystectomy: a hybrid approach to natural orifice surgery, *Gastrointest Endosc* 66:1243, 2007.

Burghardt J, Federlein M, Müller V, et al: Minimally invasive transvaginal right hemicolectomy: report of the first complex NOS (natural orifice surgery) bowel operation using a hybrid approach [in German], *Zentralbl Chir* 133:574, 2008.

Inoue H, Minami H, Satodate H, Kudo SE: First clinical experience of submucosal endoscopic esophageal myotomy for esophageal achalasia with no skin incision, *Gastrointest Endosc* 69:AB122, 2009.

Kaouka JH, Habera GP, Goela RK, et al: Pure natural orifice translumenal endoscopic surgery (NOTES) transvaginal nephrectomy, *Eur Urol* 57(4):723–726, 2010.

Zorron R, Maggioni LC, Pombo L, et al: NOTES transvaginal cholecystectomy: preliminary clinical application, *Surg Endosc* 22:542, 2008.

NOTES IN THE INTENSIVE CARE UNIT

Raymond P. Onders, MD

OVERVIEW

The ideal application for using natural orifice transluminal endoscopic surgery (NOTES) has yet to be discovered. Much of the research effort regarding application of this technique has been directed toward a variety of surgical interventions that have well-established laparoscopic approaches. To date, relatively few reports have examined the efficacy of utilizing this novel approach for its diagnostic capability outside of an operating room (OR) setting. In this chapter, two possible applications of NOTES in the intensive care unit (ICU) will be described: diagnostic abdominal exploration and therapeutic use for diaphragm pacing.

DIAGNOSTIC NOTES IN THE INTENSIVE CARE UNIT

Intraabdominal sepsis in the critically ill patient remains a challenging issue to correctly diagnose and treat in a timely manner because of poor reliability of patient exams resulting from intubation, comorbid conditions, or sedation. In autopsy series, up to 20% of those who had been ICU patients were found to have major unexpected diagnoses, and approximately half of these illnesses could have been corrected, which might have changed the patient's outcome. Computed tomography (CT) scans can be of limited use for such diagnoses and are difficult to obtain in critically ill patients who require significant support for transport. Almost 50% of patients being transported for a test will have serious complications in transit, such as hypotension, respiratory distress, central line disconnections, and dysrhythmias.

Many times, true surgical visualization of the possible pathology is needed. Taking a patient to the operating room for a laparotomy subjects them to increased risk and potential complications. Exploratory laparotomies are negative in up to 60% of patients, which greatly increases mortality rates. Bedside laparoscopy has been shown to be safe and accurate but is still rarely performed, because transporting the equipment is cumbersome. Recreating a bedside OR suite requires a significant amount of resources, including personnel and supplies, and it is extremely difficult in an urgent situation.

Flexible endoscopy at the bedside as a diagnostic tool, or for the placement of gastrostomy tubes, is a standard ICU procedure that requires minimal support from ancillary staff. Using the same equipment, NOTES can provide access to the peritoneal cavity and could decrease the number of patients with unrecognized intraabdominal catastrophic events. Several recent publications, including those for both animals and humans, have reported favorable results in the ability of a transgastric NOTES approach for evaluation of intraperitoneal structures. Not only is intraperitoneal organ assessment feasible, but basic diagnostic tasks such as tissue biopsy and aspiration of fluid collection were easily performed with currently available endoscopic devices. In my own institution's research group, a randomized animal trial comparing NOTES with laparoscopy to assess for simulated ICU pathology showed that a positive identification via NOTES was highly specific with a strong predictive value.

The peritoneal cavity is accessed by a transgastric route through a modified percutaneous endoscopic gastrostomy (PEG) technique, which is a common ICU procedure. It is a technically familiar procedure and requires instruments and materials that are widely available. This appears to be the most dependable method and involves a Seldinger technique, in which a guidewire is placed in the gastric lumen at a standard anterior site on the abdominal wall for a PEG. The endoscope and guidewire are then brought out through the mouth, and the endoscope is reinserted alongside the guidewire. A gastrotomy is performed at the site of the guidewire with needle-knife cautery to make the initial incision, followed by endoscopic balloon dilation to enlarge the gastrotomy. The endoscope is then advanced into the peritoneal cavity for visualization and systematic exploration of all four quadrants of the abdomen.

To make NOTES exploration acceptable in the ICU, the question of how best to effect gastrotomy closure remained. Numerous experimental gastrotomy closure devices have been reported, although to date none are approved for human clinical use. One aspect of NOTES in the ICU is that the gastrotomy does not have to be closed but can be managed with the use of a PEG, which negates a serious concern and barrier for the application of any NOTES procedures. Once the NOTES abdominal exploration is complete, the gastrotomy is managed by attaching a standard-pull PEG tube to the guidewire left in place during the NOTES procedure. The PEG is withdrawn back through the gastrotomy, leaving the internal mushroom bumper in the gastric lumen. When concern that the gastrotomy has become too large is an issue, additional sutures to affix the stomach to the anterior abdominal wall can be accomplished using a T-fastener technique.

The use of NOTES in the ICU began with the report of an abdominal exploration through a prematurely dislodged PEG tube, and this serves as a model for future NOTES abdominal explorations in the ICU. In this case, the peritoneal cavity was visualized, evacuation and irrigation of intraabdominal leakage was performed, and the gastric perforation was managed with the placement of another gastrostomy tube with no adverse long-term consequences. With the small but growing experience in NOTES, it is felt that abdominal exploration is feasible, although some difficulty in visualizing the right upper quadrant exists, as well as the inability to adequately view both sides of the small bowel with standard flexible endoscopes. The surgeon must also become used to the inverted and transposed orientation of the video images caused by the endoscopic retroflexion to visualize the cephalad quadrants; however, the utilization of some of the new endoscopic platforms can help with the technical limitation of the flexible endoscope.

The initial goal of NOTES in the ICU is to decide whether the patient needs to go to the OR for a more formal treatment and thus decrease the negative laparotomy rate. Small ischemic areas that may be missed with NOTES may not warrant a laparotomy, and NOTES allows for reexplorations at the bedside. It has been reported that between 60% and 90% of second-look laparotomies are negative explorations that do not require any further intervention. Many times, the disease process in this scenario is known; therefore, a specific segment

of concern or resection that would direct the endoscopist's exploration is likely. Applying a bedside evaluation may prove beneficial. A brief peritoneoscopy via NOTES could avoid the surgical complications of a negative second-look reexploration. In the small percentage of patients in whom a positive finding is identified, the patient could then be transferred to the operating room for definitive treatment.

DIAPHRAGM PACING IN THE INTENSIVE CARE UNIT

Laparoscopic implantation of a diaphragm pacing (DP) system has shown significant benefits in selected patients. The DP system is a percutaneous electrode system that overcomes patients' loss of control of the diaphragm, so that with stimulation, diaphragm negative-pressure ventilation occurs. Laparoscopically the diaphragm is mapped to identify the *motor point*, which is the area of the diaphragm where stimulation causes the greatest contraction of the diaphragm to allow ventilation. The DP then conditions the diaphragm to overcome atrophy and allows weaning of patients from ventilators. In patients with injured spinal cords, DP can completely free the patient from a ventilator, with significant improvement in quality of life, and it decreases the risk of pneumonia, which improves survival.

In patients with amyotrophic lateral sclerosis (ALS) the major cause of mortality is respiratory insufficiency, as patients lose 3% to 5% of their motor neurons monthly, leading to respiratory muscle weakness. In a recently completed multicenter trial, the use of DP decreased patients' respiratory decline and improved their ventilator-free survival. In a group of ALS patients undergoing simultaneous DP and gastrostomy, a significant improvement was seen in both 30 day mortality and 1 year survival compared with PEG alone (76% survival at 1 year with DP and PEG vs. only 23% with PEG alone). This study showed no increase in the infection rate of the implanted transperitoneal diaphragm wires when a gastrostomy was done, even though it became a contaminated case. Because of the need for PEG and DP in many patients, initial feasibility trials in animals showed that the diaphragm could be mapped with NOTES, and electrodes percutaneously implanted, leading to the possibility of ICU implantation.

TABLE 1: Physiologic effects of diaphragm pacing for intensive care unit patients

Conditioning the diaphragm	Prevents atrophy Maintains type I slow-twitch oxidative muscle fibers Avoids contraction shortening of muscle fibers Decreases weaning times
Improving posterior lobe ventilation	Decreases atelectasis Decreases ventilator-associated pneumonia Improves respiratory compliance, which decreases the work of breathing Decreases peak airway pressure, which decreases the risk of barotrauma
Maintaining negative chest pressure	Improves venous return Increases cardiac output
Overcoming acquired central sleep apnea	Decreases nighttime reintubation Improves sleep dysfunction Decreases ICU psychosis

Up to 50% of ICU patients require mechanical ventilation, and 20% are on a ventilator for over 7 days. Over 40% of this time is spent weaning a patient from mechanical ventilation after the initial event that caused intubation. Over 100,000 tracheostomies are performed in the United States yearly because of prolonged mechanical ventilation. Failure to wean from mechanical ventilation can in part be due to rapid onset of diaphragm atrophy, barotrauma, posterior lobe atelectasis, and impaired hemodynamics, which are normally improved by maintaining a more natural negative chest pressure. Ventilator-induced diaphragm dysfunction occurs very rapidly, with 50% diaphragm atrophy and conversion to the nonfunctional fast-twitch type IIb muscle fibers in less than 1 day. The growing body of literature on DP shows that use in the ICU can help overcome VIDD in several ways, as outlined in Table 1.

Patients with acute spinal cord injuries are now being implanted with the laparoscopic DP system early in their ICU course to prevent pneumonias and help with recovery. Trials are now being planned for placement of DP laparoscopically in ICU patients and during open thoracic, cardiac, and abdominal procedures to help with postoperative management. Many ICU patients presently have bedside PEGs placed to help with management, therefore NOTES may have the potential to expand the benefits of DP to this acute patient population, even in nonsurgical patients.

SUMMARY

Although in its infancy, utilization of a bedside NOTES peritoneoscopy as a diagnostic tool may play an important role for the critically ill patient in the ICU. This population inherently carries a high operative risk, and thus patients may benefit from a less invasive evaluation that can be done in a nonsterile environment at the bedside that does not require a general anesthetic. The limitations and disadvantages of NOTES exploration in the ICU are significant and include that it is invasive, and PEG alone has complications: it is limited to surface visualization, it cannot identify retroperitoneal disease, and it presents difficulties in patients with adhesions. Present trials of DP show great promise in helping to decrease mechanical ventilation in patients, and the use of NOTES to make this a bedside procedure would help to decrease the costs while increasing the benefits. Further studies are necessary and will help elucidate the roles of NOTES in these two applications.

SUGGESTED READINGS

Marks JM, Ponsky JL, Pearl JP, et al: PEG "rescue": a practical NOTES technique, *Surg Endosc* 21:816–819, 2007.

Onders RP, Elmo M, Khansarinia S, et al: Complete worldwide experience in laparoscopic diaphragm pacing: results and differences in spinal cord injured patients and amyotrophic lateral sclerosis patients, *Surg Endosc* 23(7):1433–1440, 2009.

Onders R, McGee M, Marks J, et al: Diaphragm pacing with natural orifice transluminal endoscopic surgery (NOTES): potential for difficult-to-wean intensive care unit (ICU) patients, *Surg Endosc* 21:475–479, 2007.

Onders RP, McGee MF, Marks J, et al: Natural orifice transluminal endoscopic surgery (NOTES) as a diagnostic tool in the intensive care unit, *Surg Endosc* 21:681–683, 2007.

NOTES: WHAT THE FUTURE HOLDS

Mehrdad Nikfarjam, MD, PhD, and Jeffrey M. Marks, MD

OVERVIEW

Natural orifice transluminal endoscopic surgery (NOTES) is a minimally invasive, innovative endoscopic technique in which abdominal organs are approached through natural orifices—mouth, anus, urethra, and vagina—to perform intraabdominal diagnostic and therapeutic procedures. Not since the introduction of laparoscopic cholecystectomy has the development of a new surgical technique generated so much excitement and enthusiasm. Major improvements in minimally invasive technologies have followed the NOTES revolution, in particular the advent of new instrumentation for single-site laparoscopic surgery and the growth of intraluminal surgical techniques. However, the place of NOTES in the future of surgery is uncertain and should only be speculated after an appreciation of its evolution, current achievements, and discussion of its potential benefits and limitations.

HISTORY OF NOTES

The true beginning of NOTES is controversial. Long before the current NOTES revolution, drainage procedures were being performed through various organs. The first description of a transluminal procedure probably dates to the beginnings of surgery with reports of transrectal and transvaginal drainage of collections. The modern origin of NOTES probably dates back to the first descriptions of tube-feeding gastrostomy and reports of endoscopic transgastric drainage of pancreatic pseudocysts. The first true attempt to visualize the peritoneal cavity following transvisceral puncture should, however, be attributed to Kalloo and colleagues, with the first published report in 2004 from the Johns Hopkins Hospital of an endoscopic liver biopsy in a porcine model during transgastric peritoneoscopy.

It was not until 2006, when Rao and Reddy presented the first transgastric appendectomy in a human at the Society of American Gastrointestinal and Endoscopic Surgeons (SAGES), that NOTES captured the world's imagination. The first published report of NOTES in a human occurred the following year by the team at Case Western Reserve University. In that report, the peritoneal cavity was endoscopically accessed transgastrically through the site of a prematurely dislodged percutaneous endoscopic gastrostomy (PEG), and a new gastrostomy tube was reconstituted.

The concept of NOTES has rapidly expanded from the early reports of simple transgastric peritoneoscopy and appendectomy to more complex procedures such as cholecystectomy, nephrectomy, and colectomy. Interventions performed through the rectum, vagina, and bladder have been reported, with applications predominantly in the fields of general surgery, gastroenterology, gynecology, and urology. Also evolving from NOTES is the concept of intraabdominal access through the embryonal natural orifice, the umbilicus (eNOTES). Despite the terms used, this procedure should be considered as single-site laparoscopic surgery rather than NOTES.

The number of human reports of NOTES procedures is limited given the stringent controls set in place to ensure patient safety. Most techniques described to date are hybrid techniques that combine laparoscopy and endoscopy, with very few purely NOTES procedures.

Recognizing the great excitement surrounding NOTES and possible errant development of procedures, members of SAGES and the American Society for Gastrointestinal Endoscopy (ASGE) met for the Natural Orifice Consortium for Assessment and Research (NOSCAR) in 2005 to define the principles of research in this field. They issued a white paper outlining the perceived areas for research and practice of the method, with the main principle the protection of patients by ensuring that all initial procedures would be performed under the guidance of institutional review board oversight.

TECHNIQUE

Transvaginal, transgastric, transvesical, and transcolonic approaches to the peritoneal cavity have all been described. Transvaginal access is the simplest technique in terms of closure of the access site, but it is only applicable to half the population. The transgastric approach is the most important, given that it is applicable to all patients and intuitively appears to be associated with less risk of contamination than a transcolonic approach. Transgastric NOTES is usually performed under general anesthesia, although it is applicable to conscious sedation and possibly even no sedation. Transgastric access can be achieved in a similar manner to inserting a PEG tube: A guidewire is placed in the gastric lumen and passed into the peritoneal cavity after initially incising the gastric wall with a needle knife at the chosen site. Endoscopic balloon dilation of the tract is then performed to create an adequate gastrotomy for passage of the endoscope into the peritoneal cavity (Figure 1).

Closure of the gastrostomy can be performed using several techniques with no agreement as to the most reliable technique. Full-thickness plication, clips, PEG, endoscopic suturing devices, and tunneled access have all been investigated. It is agreed that a secure, reliable, and reproducible closure is a necessity. Based on surgical principles of tissue approximation, the closure technique must avoid ischemia and tension and must provide a full-thickness closure. A major limitation of current techniques is that most achieve only superficial closure by approximation of only the gastric mucosa. This applies to techniques such endoscopic clip closure and most current commercially available suturing devices. The use of a PEG tube has had a long history of success but will invariably cause some degree of abdominal wall scarring, and it has its own associated risks and complications.

APPLICATIONS AND OUTCOMES

The clinical application of purely NOTES procedures in humans is limited, with the majority of procedures performed in conjunction with laparoscopy for safety measures. The human series of purely NOTES techniques reported to date is summarized in Table 1, although there are no actual human trials so far to compare NOTES with laparoscopy. The application of NOTES is best discussed in terms of diagnostic and therapeutic procedures.

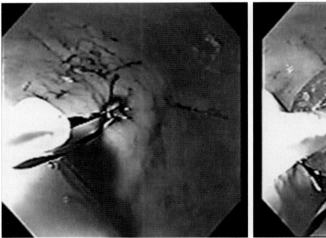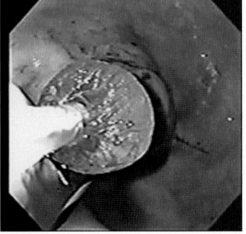

FIGURE 1   Technique of transgastric NOTES. Following gastric puncture and passage of a guidewire, the gastrotomy site is enlarged using a dilating balloon, and the peritoneal cavity is entered with the endoscope.

TABLE 1: Human studies of pure **NOTES** procedures

Author	Institution	No. Patients	Access Site	Procedure
Marks et al. (2007)	University Hospitals, Cleveland, Ohio	1	TG	PEG "rescue"
Bernhardt et al. (2008)	Medical Center Suedstadt Rostock, Rostock, Germany	1	TV	Appendectomy
Rao et al. (2008)	Asian Institute of Gastroenterology, Somajiguda, Hyderabad, India	3	TV	Cholecystectomy
Rao et al. (2008)	Asian Institute of Gastroenterology, Somajiguda, Hyderabad, India	8	TG	Appendectomy
Rao et al. (2008)	Asian Institute of Gastroenterology, Somajiguda, Hyderabad, India	3	TG	Liver biopsy
Rao et al. (2008)	Asian Institute of Gastroenterology, Somajiguda, Hyderabad, India	1	TG	Tubal ligation
Gumbs et al. (2009)	Fox Chase Cancer Center, Philadelphia, Pennsylvania	1	TV	Cholecystectomy

TG, Transgastric; *TV,* transvaginal; *PEG,* percutaneous endoscopic gastrostomy

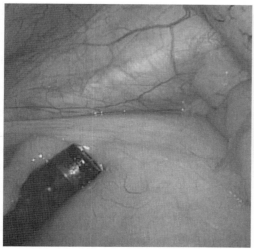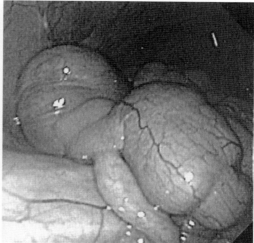

FIGURE 2 An endoscope is passed into the peritoneal cavity via transgastric puncture, demonstrating clear visualization of the cecum and appendix in the right lower quadrant.

Diagnostic

The feasibility of NOTES in terms of diagnostic procedures appears promising based on animal and human studies. Researchers at Ohio State University have published the results of transgastric peritoneoscopy in 10 patients with periampullary malignancy, in which transgastric exploration corroborated with the decision to proceed to open exploration in 9 of 10 patients. In that study, visualization of the right upper quadrant was difficult without a platform. Improved visualization has been reported by the same group with use of an endoscopic platform. A similar study investigating transgastric peritoneoscopy was performed at Case Western Reserve University in 9 patients requiring a gastrostotomy for tumor excision or retrieval of a foreign body. There was good visualization of the peritoneal cavity overall (Figure 2); however, the left upper quadrant could be clearly visualized in only one of nine cases. These human studies clearly show that with standard endoscopes, full visualization of the peritoneal cavity is limited because of the high mobility of the endoscopes. The introduction of more solid platforms in animal models has significantly improved some of the limitations of standard endoscopy and with improved stability.

Transvaginal, transcolonic, transesophageal, and transvesical NOTES procedures have been trialed in animal studies and appear to have some utility as a diagnostic tool. In studies performed in a porcine model at Case Western Reserve University, the diagnostic accuracy of transgastric NOTES was compared with laparoscopy in a randomized manner in 15 animals. Various conditions that could be encountered in an intensive care unit (ICU) setting were simulated, such as ischemic or perforated bowel and acute cholecystitis. Laparoscopy appeared to be more sensitive than NOTES overall (77.4% vs. 61.3%); however, NOTES was highly specific and had a 100% positive predictive value. To date there is no direct comparison of NOTES with other standard modalities as a diagnostic tool in humans in a randomized manner.

Therapeutic Applications

The therapeutic application of NOTES in animal studies varies and includes cholecystectomy, hysterectomy, salpingectomy, vasectomy, splenectomy, gastrojejunostomy, distal pancreatectomy, ventral and inguinal hernia repair, nephrectomy, colectomy, and diaphragm pacing. The therapeutic application of NOTES in humans to date has been limited essentially to cholecystectomy and appendectomy, with a few reports of other procedures, including tubal ligation, PEG rescue, sleeve gastrectomy, and nephrectomy. The majority of cases have been hybrid techniques. One report was done on a single series of eight patients who

underwent a pure transgastric NOTES appendectomy, and a report was also done on one patient treated by pure transvaginal NOTES appendectomy. The benefits of such procedures, compared with purely laparoscopic appendectomy, is unknown and has not been examined.

The number of reports of NOTES cholecystectomy is increasing; however, only two reports describe purely NOTES transvaginal cholecystecomy, with a total of 4 patients and only one case reported in detail. The justification of a purely NOTES procedure at this stage is uncertain, given the potential increased risk of bile duct injury during the learning phase of the procedure. Bleeding and bile leak after hybrid transgastric cholecystectomy have been reported, along with one report of a cervical esophageal tear after transgastric removal of a gallbladder containing a large stone.

BENEFITS

The true benefit of NOTES is uncertain; however, avoidance of scars and wound complications can be appreciated. Transgastric and transvaginal approaches in particular appear to be viable sites for organ retrieval. NOTES may cause less immune suppression, based on animal studies, and an overall reduction in surgical trauma may result in decreased adhesion formation, lower stress response, and quicker recovery. Proponents of NOTES emphasize the theoretical decrease in postoperative pain this technique may offer; however, in pure NOTES techniques, retained intraperitoneal gas may contribute to increased pain. What truly separates NOTES from laparoscopy is the fact that it is proposed that it can be performed in a nonsterile environment and does not necessarily require general anesthesia, which makes NOTES highly portable.

LIMITATIONS

Although few studies show a significant advantage of the NOTES approach, the technique is not clearly inferior to the conventional techniques, albeit some limitations of the current techniques are clear. The originally identified barriers to NOTES identified by NOSCAR include access to the peritoneal cavity, the technique of gastric closure, prevention of infection, development of a suturing device, maintenance of spatial orientation, development of multitasking platforms, and management of iatrogenic intraperitoneal injuries.

In terms of access to the peritoneal cavity by a transgastric route, a modified PEG technique appears to be safe. When this does not represent the ideal point of peritoneal access, endoscopic

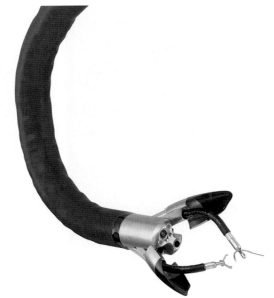

FIGURE 3   Prototype endoscope with a flexible platform and dual working channels that allow triangulation.

ultrasound-guided gastric puncture has been shown to be an effective and safe method of entry. Closure of the gastrostomy continues to be an area of research, with several endoscopic suturing devices soon to be available that are effective in achieving closure based on animal studies. In a human model, even a very low leak rate and subsequent peritonitis would not be considered acceptable.

A clear limitation of the NOTES techniques with standard scopes is an unstable platform. The inherent flexibility of the endoscope impedes achieving a stable operating field. With a transgastric approach, visualization of the upper abdomen requires retroflexion of the scope deep within the pelvis, which can be difficult to achieve. This retroflexion is also likely to lead to inversion of the image that further complicates operative procedures. The inability to manipulate tissue effectively or retract organs is also a drawback; however, more rigid and versatile platforms have now been developed that can be applied to the scope to increase maneuverability within the peritoneal cavity. In addition, the development of robotic instruments that can be passed down the working channels of the scope or built into a flexible endoscopic platform may allow greater manipulation of tissues than can be achieved by rigid instruments oriented parallel to one another (Figure 3). Some investigators have overcome the lack of maneuverability of NOTES endoscopes by addition of a second separate endoscope that is independently controlled and passed through the same or another natural orifice for performing complex procedures.

FUTURE DIRECTIONS

The NOTES revolution has made health care providers reassess the status of minimal-access technology. The true role of NOTES in surgery at present is uncertain, as no clearly defined NOTES procedure can provide a potentially improved outcome compared with laparoscopic or open surgery, and NOTES is unlikely to replace the way we successfully manage common surgical problems such as gallbladder disease. However, the interest that NOTES has generated has also resulted in increased interest in single-site surgery, with rapid development of more versatile and novel instrumentations. Many of the techniques used for NOTES will eventually be used for intraluminal surgery. The technologic improvements in visceral closure with NOTES are likely to translate to a greater number of partial- and full-thickness resections of lesions from the gastrointestinal tract. Currently, full-thickness resections of rectal lesions are performed using

rigid instruments (transanal endoscopic microsurgery) with lesions only within a certain distance from the anal verge amenable to such therapies. With improvements in NOTES technology, excision of colonic lesions might no longer be limited by such constraints, and the procedures might be applicable to other regions of the gastrointestinal tract. This concept might be termed *natural orifice intraluminal surgical endoscopy* (NOISE). The same technology used to achieve full-thickness resection of lesions may be useful for closure of defects within the gastrointestinal tract following iatrogenic perforations or as a result of varying disease processes.

In terms of diagnostic procedures, the greatest potential of NOTES appears to be in the ICU setting, in Third World regions lacking sterile facilities, and possibly in the battlefield. Essentially, NOTES appears to provide major advantages in hostile, contaminated environments, where open or laparoscopic procedures carry an extremely high morbidity. The portability of NOTES and the fact that it can be performed under minimal sedation make it a highly attractive option in these circumstances. In the ICU setting, transfer of critically ill patients for various investigations can be very hazardous, so the possibility of performing a transgastric peritoneoscopy at the bedside, similar to the performance of a PEG, may prove to be a valuable investigative tool.

As improvements continue in endoscopic technologies as a result of the NOTES revolution, some of the derivatives of NOTES instrumentation are likely to be applied to laparoscopic procedures. Flexible laparoscopes with stable platforms are in fruition and could be maneuvered into position and locked into place in performing various single-incision operations. Novel triangulating instruments are likely to be developed with multiple degrees of freedom, which could then be used for dissection, suturing, and hemostasis.

SUMMARY

The advent of NOTES signifies the beginning of a new era of minimally invasive surgical therapy. Preliminary studies demonstrate the feasibility of this technique in animal models, but further research is warranted to validate its safety in humans. NOTES is not yet ready for widespread clinical use and remains a technology without an ideal application. Ongoing fundamental research is necessary to determine the safety and benefit of these procedures, and safe and reliable access and closure techniques in particular must be established.

Whether laparoscopic procedures such as cholecystectomy and appendectomy will one day be performed routinely by NOTES techniques appears unlikely; however, the continued development of optimal instrumentation and techniques will increase its potential applicability in situations where open and laparoscopic procedures are associated with high morbidity. A major difference between NOTES and laparoscopy is that it can be performed in a nonsterile environment and possibly without general anesthesia. NOTES technology will undoubtedly improve over time and will likely occur in parallel with advancements in single-site surgery, endomucosal resection, endoscopic submucosal resection, and full-thickness endoluminal excision techniques.

Suggested Readings

Hazey JW, Narula VK, Renton DB, et al: Natural orifice transgastric endoscopic peritoneoscopy in humans: initial clinical trial, *Surg Endosc* 22(1):16–20, 2008.

Kalloo AN, Singh VK, Jagannath SB, et al: Flexible transgastric peritoneoscopy: a novel approach to diagnostic and therapeutic interventions in the peritoneal cavity, *Gastrointest Endosc* 60(1):114–117, 2004.

Marks JM, Ponsky JL, Pearl JP, et al: PEG "rescue": a practical NOTES technique, *Surg Endosc* 21(5):816–819, 2007.

McGee MF, Schomisch SJ, Marks JM, et al: Late-phase TNF-alpha depression in natural orifice translumenal endoscopic surgery (NOTES) peritoneoscopy, *Surgery* 143(3):318–328, 2008.

Voermans RP, Van Berge Henegouwen MI, Fockens P: Natural orifice transluminal endoscopic surgery (NOTES), *Endoscopy* 39(11):1013–1017, 2007.

Notes: Page numbers followed by *b* indicate boxes, *f* indicates figures, and *t* indicates tables.